INTERNATIONAL TEXTBOOK OF MEDICINE

General Editors

A. H. SAMIY, M.D.

Professor of Clinical Medicine and Chief of
Division of Medicine, New York Hospital, Cornell Medical Center
New York, New York

LLOYD H. SMITH, JR., M.D.

Professor of Medicine; Associate Dean,
University of California, San Francisco, School of Medicine,
San Francisco, California

JAMES B. WYNGAARDEN, M.D.

Director, National Institutes of Health,
Bethesda, Maryland

VOLUME I
PATHOPHYSIOLOGY
The Biological Principles of Disease

VOLUME II
MEDICAL MICROBIOLOGY AND INFECTIOUS DISEASES

Volumes I and II of the International Textbook of Medicine
have been conceived and written to follow a logical pedagogical approach
and can readily be used in conjunction with the
CECIL TEXTBOOK OF MEDICINE.

2nd edition

INFECTIOUS DISEASES AND MEDICAL MICROBIOLOGY

Edited by

ABRAHAM I. BRAUDE, M.D., Ph.D

Late Professor of Medicine and Pathology
University of California, San Diego

CHARLES E. DAVIS, M.D.

Professor of Pathology
University of California, San Diego

JOSHUA FIERER, M.D.

Associate Professor of Medicine
University of California, San Diego

1986

W. B. SAUNDERS COMPANY

Philadelphia/London/Toronto/Mexico City/Rio de Janeiro/Sydney/Tokyo/Hong Kong

W. B. Saunders Company: West Washington Square
Philadelphia, PA 19105

Library of Congress Cataloging in Publication Data

Main entry under title:

Infectious diseases and medical microbiology.

Rev. ed. of: Medical microbiology and infectious diseases / Abraham I. Braude. 1981.

1. Communicable diseases. 2. Medical microbiology. I. Braude, Abraham I. II. Braude, Abraham I. Medical microbiology and infectious diseases. [DNLM: 1. Communicable Diseases. 2. Microbiology. QW 4 I43]

RC111.I51293 1986 616.9 84–22922

ISBN 0–7216–1206–7

Infectious Diseases and Medical Microbiology ISBN 0-7216-1206-7

Last digit is the print number: 9 8 7 6 5 4 3 2 1

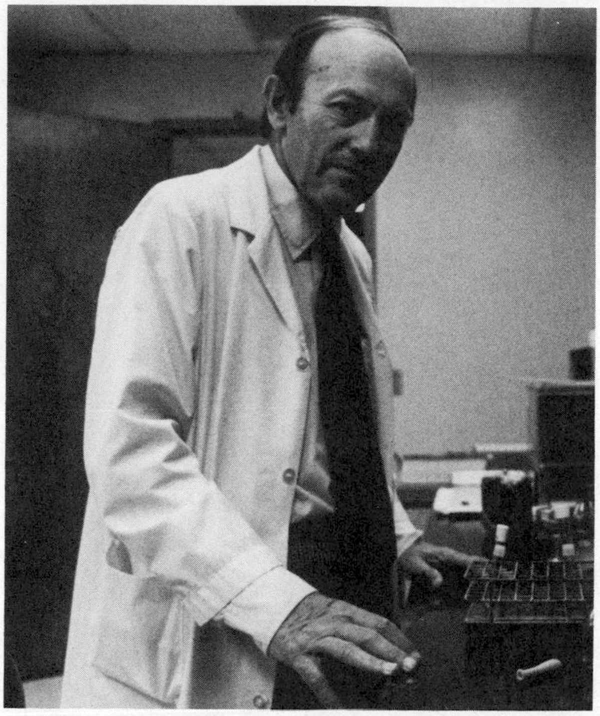

Abraham I. Braude, M.D., Ph.D.
1917–1984

IN MEMORIAM

Abraham I. Braude died suddenly and unexpectedly shortly before this edition of his textbook was completed. With his death, the scientific and medical communities have lost an important leader, and we have lost a close friend and mentor. Abe's legacy is unusually rich because he was an outstanding scientist, physician, diagnostic microbiologist, and teacher. Abe worked hard to teach all these skills to his trainees because he knew that each of these intellectual activities was enriched by the others. In his daily activities, he brought the diagnostic laboratory to the patient's bedside and used clinical observations to direct and sharpen the focus of the laboratory. He abhorred "routine work-ups" in both spheres. It is obvious from his bibliography that clinical and microbiologic problems were also the major stimuli for his own research. He approached laboratory investigation with a unique blend of intelligence, imagination, discipline, and diligence. This approach led to a number of important, original contributions that have affected the way we care for patients with infections. He taught generations of physicians to think clearly, ask intelligent questions, and apply their knowledge of microbiology to meaningful laboratory investigation and the diagnosis and treatment of patients.

This book is an appropriate tribute to Abe and his work because it places equal emphasis on the science of microbiology and the practice of clinical infectious diseases. Where it excels, the credit is due largely to a devoted partnership between Abe and his wife, Gita, our talented copy editor. We dedicate this edition to the memory of Abraham I. Braude, an extraordinary human being, and an outstanding scientist, teacher, and physician.

Charles E. Davis, M.D.

Joshua Fierer, M.D.

Contributors

YOUSEF AL-DOORY, Ph.D.
Associate Professor, Department of Pathology, The George Washington University School of Medicine, Washington D.C.; Chief, Mycology Section, Chief, Serology Section, George Washington University Hospital, Washington, D.C.
Dematiaceae: Agents of Chromomycosis

A. D. ALEXANDER, Ph.D.
Professor, Microbiology, Chicago College of Osteopathic Medicine, Chicago, Illinois
Leptospira

A. O. ANYA, Ph.D.
Professor of Zoology, University of Nigeria at Nsukka, Nsukka, Nigeria
Nemathelminthes

HOWARD ROBERT ATTEBERY, D.D.S.
Oral Microbiologist, Children's Hospital and Health Center, San Diego, California
Anaerobic Gram-Positive Cocci; Fusobacteria; Veillonella; Vincent's Infection

HERMAN BAER, M.D.
Professor of Pathology, University of Florida, College of Medicine, Gainesville, Florida; Medical Director, Autopsy Services, Shands Teaching Hopsital and Clinic, T. H. Miller Health Center, Gainesville, Florida
Classification and Identification of Bacteria; Moraxella, Kingella and Acinetobacter

ANN SULLIVAN BAKER, M.D.
Assistant Professor of Medicine, Harvard Medical School; Assistant in Medicine, Massachusetts General Hospital; Consultant in Infectious Diseases, Massachusetts Eye and Ear Infirmary, Boston, Massachusetts
Spinal Epidural Abscess; Subdural Empyema

JEFFREY D. BAND, M.D.
Clinical Associate Professor of Medicine, Wayne State University School of Medicine, Detroit, Michigan; Corporate Epidemiologist and Consultant Physician in Infectious Diseases and Geographic Medicine, William Beaumont Hospital, Royal Oak, Michigan
Legionellosis (Legionnaires' Disease and Pontiac Fever)

ALAN G. BARBOUR, M.D.
Senior Staff Fellow, Laboratory of Microbial Structure and Function, Rocky Mountain Laboratories, N.I.A.I.D., N.I.H., Hamilton, Montana
Colorado Tick Fever

LANE BARKSDALE, Ph.D.
Professor of Microbiology, New York University School of Medicine and Medical Center, New York, New York
Diphtheria Bacilli and Other Corynebacteria

ELIZABETH BARRETT-CONNOR, M.D.
Professor and Chair, Department of Community and Family Medicine, Professor, Department of Medicine, University of California at San Diego, School of Medicine, San Diego, California
Fluke Infections; Intestinal Roundworms

JOSEPH H. BATES, M.D.
Professor of Medicine and Microbiology and Immunology, University of Arkansas College of Medicine, Little Rock, Arkansas; Chief, Medical Service, John L. McClellan Veterans Administration Medical Center, Little Rock, Arkansas
Tularemia

WILLIAM R. BEISEL, M.D.
Special Assistant to the Surgeon General for Biotechnology, U.S. Army Medical Research and Development Command, Fort Detrick, Frederick, Maryland
Metabolic Effects of Infection

D. W. BELCHER, M.D.
Associate Professor of Medicine, University of Washington, Seattle, Washington; Staff Physician, MCCU, Seattle Veterans Administration Medical Center, Seattle, Washington
Dracunculiasis

FRANCISCO BIAGI, M.D.
Professor of Medical Parasitology, National University of Mexico, School of Medicine, Mexico City, Mexico; American British Cowdry Hospital, Hospital Infantil Privado, Mexico City, Mexico
Amebic Dysentery (Intestinal Amebiasis); Cutaneous Amebiasis

PERRY S. BINDER, M.D., F.A.C.S.
Associate Clinical Professor, Department of Ophthalmology, University of California, San Diego; Chief, Ophthalmic Surgery and Research, Sharp Cabrillo Hospital, San Diego, California
Ocular Fungal and Parasitic Infections; Ocular Chlamydial and Rickettsial Infections; Ocular Bacterial Infections; Ocular Inflammatory Disease

RUTH BISHOP, D.Sc.
Principal Research Fellow, Department of Gastroenterology, Royal Children's Hospital, Melbourne, Australia
Viral Gastroenteritis

ALAN L. BISNO, M.D.
Chief, Division of Infectious Diseases, and Professor of Internal Medicine, University of Tennessee Center for the Health Sciences, Memphis, Tennessee; Attending Physician, Memphis Regional Medical Center and the University of Tennessee Hospital, Memphis, Tennessee; Consulting Physician, Veterans Administration Medical Center and Baptist Memorial Hospital, Memphis, Tennessee
Rocky Mountain Spotted Fever

DONALD L. BORNSTEIN, M.D.
Associate Professor of Medicine, and Chief, Infectious Disease Section, SUNY Upstate Medical Center, Syracuse, New York; Attending Physician, State University Hospital, Crouse-Irving Memorial Hospital, Syracuse Veterans Administration Hospital; Chairman, Hospital Infection Control Committee, State University Hospital, Syracuse, New York
Bacteroides Septicemia; Clostridial Septicemia; Clostridial Myonecrosis

PAULA BRANEFORS-HELANDER, M.D.
Late Assistant Professor, University of Göteborg, Institute of Medical Microbiology, Department of Bacteriology, Göteborg, Sweden
Epiglottitis and Pseudocroup

ABRAHAM I. BRAUDE, M.D., Ph.D.
Late Professor of Medicine and Pathology, University of California, San Diego, California
Bacterial Endotoxins; Description of Antimicrobial Drugs; Mechanisms of Action of Antimicrobial Drugs; Poxviruses; Candida; The Aspergilli; The Zygomycetes; Miscellaneous Fungi; Mechanisms of Natural Resistance to Infection; Mechanisms of Acquired Resistance to Infection; Mechanisms of Immunologic Injury in Infectious Diseases; Actinomycosis; Bacterial Lung Abscess and Nocardiosis; North American Blastomycosis; Cerebral Phaeomycosis; Bancroftian and Malayan Filariasis; Dengue and Other Hemorrhagic Fevers; Lassa Fever; Sporotrichosis

RUDOLF BREZINA, M.D., Dr. Sc.
Head, Department of Rickettsiae, Institute of Virology, Slovak Academy of Sciences, Bratislava, Czechoslovakia
Epidemic (Louse-Borne) Typhus; Endemic (Murine) Typhus; Other Rickettsial Spotted Fevers

GEORGE F. BROOKS, M.D.
Professor, Laboratory Medicine, Medicine, and Microbiology and Immunology, University of California, San Francisco, California
Eikenella corrodens

S. J. D. BROOKS, M.D.
Associate Director, Family Practice Residency Program, St. Vincent's Hospital, Jacksonville, Florida; Attending Staff, St. Vincent's Hospital, Jacksonville, Florida
Bacterial Lung Abscess and Nocardiosis; Splenic Abscess

MICHAEL BROWN, M.B., F.R.C.P., F.R.C.P.E., D.T.M.&H.
Professor of Military Medicine, Royal Army Medical College, Millbank, London, England; Consultant Physician, Queen Elizabeth Military Hospital, and Honorary Associate Physician, Hospital of Tropical Diseases, London, England
Melioidosis

RICHARD E. BRYANT, M.D.
Director, Infectious Diseases Division, and Professor of Medicine, Oregon Health Sciences University, Portland, Oregon
Viral Pneumonia

ANTHONY D. M. BRYCESON, M.D., F.R.C.P.E., D.T.M.&H.
Senior Lecturer, London School of Hygiene and Tropical Medicine, London, England; Consultant Physician, Hospital for Tropical Diseases, London, England
Visceral Leishmaniasis; Cutaneous and Mucocutaneous Leishmaniasis (Oriental Sore; Espundia)

JOHN J. S. BURTON, Ph.D.
Medical Entomologist, Aramco, Saudi Arabia
Arthropods of Medical Importance

LUBOR ČERVA, R.N.Dr., D.Sc.
Senior Resident Scientist, Postgraduate Medical and Pharmaceutical Institute, Department of Tropical and Subtropical Diseases, Prague, Czechoslovakia
Amebic Meningoencephalitis

BARUN DEB CHATTERJEE, M.B.B.S., Ph.D., DIP. BACT., F.A.M.S.
Professor and Head, Department of Bacteriology and Serology, School of Tropical Medicine, Calcutta, India
Vibrios and Campylobacter

T. H. CHEN, M.D.
Research Microbiologist, Department of Biomedical and Environmental Health Sciences, School of Public Health, University of California, Berkeley, California
Yersinia, Pasteurella, and Francisella

DAVID FRANCIS CLYDE, M.D., Ph.D.
Senior Public Health Administrator, World Health Organization, Southeast Asia Region, Delhi, India
Malaria

STEPHEN N. COHEN, M.D.
Clinical Professor of Laboratory Medicine, Medicine and Microbiology, University of California San Francisco School of Medicine, San Francisco, California; Director, Clinical Laboratories, University of California Hospitals and Clinics, San Francisco, California
Infection with Pneumocystis carinii

RICHARD W. COMPANS, Ph.D.
Professor, Department of Microbiology, University of Alabama, Birmingham, Alabama
Morphology and Structure of Viruses

JAMES D. CONNOR, M.D.
Professor of Pediatrics, University of California, San Diego, La Jolla, California; Staff, University of California, San Diego, Medical Center; Consultant, Children's Hospital and Health Center; Consultant, Naval Regional Medical Center, San Diego and Camp Pendleton; and Consultant, Mercy Hospital, San Diego, California
Herpangina; Pertussis; Hand-Foot-Mouth Disease

EUGENE H. COTA-ROBLES, Ph.D.
Professor of Biology, University of California, Santa Cruz, California
The Structure of the Bacterial Cell

MANUEL CUADRA, M.D.
Professor (retired) of Infectious, Parasitic, and Tropical Diseases, Universidad Nacional Mayor de San Marcos Facultad de Medicina, Lima, Peru; Staff member, Robert Koch Institut, Associate to Virchow Krankenhaus, Berlin, Federal Republic of Germany
Bartonella bacilliformis; Bartonellosis

SCOTT F. DAVIES, M.D.
Assistant Professor, University of Minnesota Medical School, Minneapolis, Minnesota; Director, Division of Pulmonary Diseases, Hennepin County Medical Center, Minneapolis, Minnesota
Histoplasmosis; Aspergillosis

CHARLES E. DAVIS, M.D.
Professor of Pathology, University of California San Diego School of Medicine, San Diego, California; Associate Director of Microbiology, University of California, San Diego, Medical Center, San Diego, California
Classification and Identification of Bacteria; Erysipelothrix rhusiopathiae; Moraxella, Kingella, and Acinetobacter; Chromobacterium; Capnocytophaga; Cryptococcus; Paragonimiasis; Babesiosis; Cutaneous Larva Migrans (Creeping Eruption); Glanders (Farcy)

GÉRARD DE CROUSAZ, M.D.
Associate Professor, Faculty of Medicine, University of Lausanne, Lausanne, Switzerland
Tuberculous Meningitis and Tuberculoma of the Brain

GUNTHER DENNERT, Ph.D.
Associate Professor, University of Southern California; University of Southern California Comprehensive Cancer Center, Los Angeles, California
Schistosomiasis

DENNIS M. DIXON, Ph.D.
Associate Professor, Department of Biology, Loyola College, Baltimore, Maryland
Blastomyces and Paracoccidioides

A. L. DOHANY, Ph.D.
Chief, Regional Division-South, U.S. Army Environmental Hygiene Agency, Ft. McPherson, Georgia
Arthropods of Medical Importance

JEAN M. DOLBY, Ph.D.
Senior Scientific Staff, Medical Research Council, Clinical Research Centre, Harrow, Middlesex, England
Bordetella

SAM T. DONTA, M.D.
Chief, Medical Service, Veterans Administration Medical Center; Director, Infectious Disease Services, University of Connecticut, Health Center Hospitals, Newington, Connecticut
Food Poisoning

R. GORDON DOUGLAS, JR., M.D.
Professor and Chairman, Department of Medicine, Cornell University Medical College, New York, New York; Physician-in-chief, New York Hospital, New York, New York
Influenza

HERBERT L. DUPONT, M.D.
Professor and Director, Program in Infectious Diseases and Clinical Microbiology, The University of Texas Medical School, Houston, Texas; Attending Physician, Hermann Hospital, Houston, Texas
Granulomatous Hepatitis

WERNER DUTZ, M.D.
Professor and Chairman, Department of Pathology, King Saud University Medical College, Abha, Saudi Arabia
Anthrax

GEORGE A. EDWARDS, M.D.
Professor of Internal Medicine, University of Texas Southwestern Medical School, Dallas, Texas; Associate Chief of Staff for Extended Care, Veterans Administration Medical Center, Dallas, Texas
Leptospirosis

JOHN E. EDWARDS, JR., M.D.
Associate Professor of Medicine, UCLA School of Medicine, Los Angeles, California; Chief, Division of Infectious Diseases, Harbor/UCLA Medical Center, Los Angeles, California
Fungemia; Moniliasis of the Skin; Thrush of the Mouth and Esophagus

MAKOTO ENOMOTO, M.D.
Lecturer, Hamamatsu Medical College, Hamamatsu, and Lecturer, St. Marianna University, School of Medicine, Kawasaki, Japan; Consultant Pathologist, National Hospital, Shizuoka, Consultant Pathologist, Kyoritsu Kanbara Hospital, and Consultant Pathologist, Sagamihara Kyodo Hospital, Japan
Fungal Toxins

WILLIAM R. FAIR, M.D.
Chief, Urologic Surgery Service, Memorial Sloan-Kettering Cancer Center, and Professor of Surgery (Urology), Cornell University Medical College, New York, New York; Attending Surgeon, Memorial Hospital and The New York Hospital, New York, New York
Prostatitis

VLADIMIR FARKAŠ, Ph.D.
Head, Department of Biochemistry of Saccharides, Institute of Chemistry, Slovak Academy of Sciences, Bratislava, Czechoslovakia
Morphology and Structure of Fungi

JÁNOS FEHÉR, M.D., D.Sc.
Professor of Medicine and Director, 2nd Department of Medicine, Semmelweis Medical University, Budapest, Hungary
Syphilitic Hepatitis

JOSHUA FIERER, M.D.
Associate Professor of Medicine and Pathology, in Residence, University of California, San Diego, School of Medicine, San Diego, California; Director, Microbiology Laboratory, Veterans Administration Medical Center, San Diego, California
Streptobacillus moniliformis; Pseudomonas and Flavobacterium; Neurosyphilis; Herpesvirus Simiae (B Virus) Encephalitis

ROBERT H. FITZGERALD, JR., M.D.
Associate Professor of Orthopedic Surgery, Mayo Medical School, Rochester, Minnesota; Consultant, Department of Orthopedics, Mayo Clinic and Mayo Foundation, Rochester, Minnesota
Bacterial Arthritis; Bacterial Osteomyelitis

DAVID W. FLEMING, M.D.
Respiratory and Special Pathogens Epidemiology Branch, Division of Bacterial Diseases, Center for Infectious Diseases, Centers for Disease Control, Atlanta, Georgia
Legionella

ROBERTO FOCACCIA, M.D.
Assistant Professor, Infectious and Parasitic Diseases Department, Faculty of Medicine, University of São Paulo, São Paulo, Brazil; Chief of Infectious Diseases Section, Hospital das Clínicas de São Paulo, São Paulo, Brazil
Tetanus

DAVID W. FRASER, M.D.
Adjunct Professor of Medicine, University of Pennsylvania School of Medicine, Philadelphia, Pennsylvania; President, Swarthmore College, Swarthmore, Pennsylvania
Legionellosis (Legionnaires' Disease and Pontiac Fever)

LAWRENCE R. FREEDMAN, M.D.
Professor, UCLA School of Medicine, and Chair, Department of Medicine, UCLA School of Medicine, Los Angeles, California; Chief, Medical Service, Veterans Administration Medical Center, West Los Angeles, California
Infective Endocarditis and Other Intravascular Infections

STANLEY D. FREEDMAN, M.D.
Head, Division of Infectious Diseases, Scripps Clinic and Research Foundation, and Associate Clinical Professor of Medicine, University of California, San Diego, California; Director of Graduate Medical Education, Green Hospital of Scripps Clinic, La Jolla, California
Whipple's Disease; Psittacosis

CHANTAL FRELAND, Ph.D.
Former Teaching Assistant in Bacteriology at the Nantes University Medical School, Nantes, France; Chef de Service, Laboratoire de Biologie Médicale, Hôpital Léon Bellier, Nantes-Cedex, France
Erysipeloid

R. G. GARRISON, Ph.D.
Associate Professor, Department of Microbiology, University of Kansas School of Medicine, Kansas City, Kansas; Career Research Scientist, Veterans Administration Medical Center, Kansas City, Missouri
Sporothix schenckii

O. J. A. GILMORE, M.S., F.R.C.S. (Eng.), F.R.C.S. (Ed.)
Consultant Surgeon, St. Bartholomew's Hospital, London, England; Senior Lecturer, University of London, London, England
Appendicitis and Diverticulitis

ISAAC GINSBURG, M.Sc., Ph.D.
Professor of Microbiology and Chairman, Department of Oral Biology, Hebrew University–Hadassah School of Dental Medicine, Jerusalem, Israel
Streptococcus

M. P. GLAUSER, M.D.
Privat-Docent and Aggregé, Faculty of Medicine, University of Lausanne, Lausanne, Switzerland; Médecin-Chef, Division des Maladies Infectieuses, Départment de Médecine Interne, Centre Hospitalier Universitaire Vaudois, Lausanne, Switzerland
Urinary Tract Infection and Pyelonephritis

RUTH E. GORDON, Ph.D.
Professor of Microbiology (retired), Rutgers, the State University of New Jersey, Piscataway, New Jersey
Nocardia and Streptomyces

MICHAEL G. GROVES, D.V.M., M.P.H., Ph.D.
Director, Infectious Disease Research Program, U.S. Army Medical Research and Development Command, Fort Detrick, Maryland
Babesiosis

DONALD G. GUINEY, M.D.
Associate Professor of Medicine, University of California, San Diego, California; Attending Physician, University of California, San Diego Medical Center, San Diego, California
Resistance to Antimicrobial Drugs

ASHLEY T. HAASE, M.D.
Professor of Microbiology, University of Minnesota, Minneapolis, Minnesota; Head of Department of Microbiology, University of Minnesota, Minneapolis, Minnesota
Slow Infections

NANCY K. HALL, Ph.D.
Associate Professor of Pathology, University of Oklahoma College of Medicine, Oklahoma City, Oklahoma; Immunologist, Missouri State Chest Hospital, Mt. Vernon, Missouri
Histoplasma capsulatum

H. HUNTER HANDSFIELD, M.D.
Associate Professor of Medicine, University of Washington, School of Medicine, Adjunct Associate Professor of Epidemiology, University of Washington, School of Public Health and Commmunity Medicine, Seattle, Washington; Director, Sexually Transmitted Disease Control Program, Seattle–King County Department of Public Health, Seattle, Washington
Lymphogranuloma Venereum, Chancroid and Donovanosis

GARY D. HARRIS, M.D.
Associate Professor and Deputy Chairman for Education Programs, The University of Texas Health Science Center, San Antonio, Texas; Staff Physician, Audie L. Murphy Memorial Veterans Hospital, and Staff Physician, Medical Center Hospital, San Antonio, Texas
Common Pneumonias Due to Pyogenic Cocci; Common Gram-Negative Bacillary Pneumonias

HERBERT S. HEINEMAN, M.D.
Clinical Professor of Medicine, Jefferson Medical College, Thomas Jefferson University, Philadelphia, Pennsylvania; Consultant in Medicine, Mercy Catholic Medical Center, and Director, Public Health Laboratory, Philadelphia Department of Public Health, Philadelphia, Pennsylvania
Bacterial Brain Abscess; Shock in Infectious Diseases

PHILIP HIGGINBOTTOM, M.D.
Division of Infectious Diseases, Scripps Clinic and Research Foundation, La Jolla, California
Relapsing Fever

SHALOM Z. HIRSCHMAN, M.D.
Director, Division of Infectious Diseases, and Professor of Medicine, The Mount Sinai School of Medicine, City University of New York, New York, New York; Attending Physician, The Mount Sinai Hospital, New York, New York
Viral Hepatitis; Hepatitis Viruses

MONTO HO, M.D.
Professor of Medicine, Microbiology, and Pathology, University of Pittsburgh School of Medicine and Graduate School of Public Health, Pittsburgh, Pennsylvania; Chief of Infectious Diseases and Director of Clinical Microbiology, Presbyterian University Hospital, Pittsburgh, Pennsylvania
Interferon and Interference; Central Nervous System Infections Caused by Togaviridae and Related Agents

BETTY C. HOBBS, D.Sc., Ph.D., Dip. Bact., F.R.C. Path., F.R.S.H.
Director (Retired), Food Hygiene Laboratory, Central Public Health Laboratory, London, England; Consultant Microbiologist, Christian Medical and Brown Memorial Hospital, Punjab, India
The Clostridia

PATRICIA A. HOFFEE, Ph.D.
Professor of Microbiology, Department of Microbiology, School of Medicine, University of Pittsburgh, Pittsburgh, Pennsylvania
Bacterial Genetics

THOMAS ALLAN HOFFMAN, M.D.
Associate Professor of Medicine, University of Miami School of Medicine, Miami, Florida; Attending Physician and Chief, Division of Infectious Diseases, Jackson Memorial Hospital, Miami, Florida
Meningococcemia; Purulent Bacterial Meningitis

TOR HOFSTAD, M.D.
Associate Professor, Medical Faculty, University of Bergen, Bergen, Norway; Honorary Consultant, Haukeland Hospital, Bergen, Norway
Bacteroides

MARIAN C. HORZINEK, D.V.M., Ph.D.
Professor of Virology, Veterinary Faculty, and Head, Department of Virology, State University Utrecht, Utrecht, the Netherlands
Togaviruses

PETER M. HOWLEY, M.D.
Chief, Laboratory of Tumor Virus Biology, National Cancer Institute, National Institutes of Health, Bethesda, Maryland; Anatomic Pathologist, National Cancer Institute, National Institutes of Health, Bethesda, Maryland
Papovaviruses

CAROLYN COKER HUNTLEY, M.D.
Late Emeritus Professor of Pediatrics, Bowman Gray School of Medicine, Winston-Salem, North Carolina
Visceral Larva Migrans

ROBERT R. JACOBSON, M.D., Ph.D.
Chief of the Clinical Branch, National Hansen's Disease Center, Carville, Louisiana
Leprosy

W. G. JOHANSON, JR., M.D.
Professor of Medicine and Chief, Division of Pulmonary Diseases, The University of Texas Health Science Center, San Antonio, Texas; Staff Physician, Audie L. Murphy Memorial Veterans Hospital, Staff Physician, Medical Center Hospital, San Antonio, Texas
Common Pneumonias Due to Pyogenic Cocci; Common Gram-Negative Bacillary Pneumonias

ANSSI JOKIPII, M.D.
Associate Professor, Department of Medical Microbiology, University of Turku, Turku, Finland; Docent, University of Helsinki, Helsinki, Finland
Giardiasis; Cryptosporidiosis; Isosporiasis; Balantidiasis

LIISA JOKIPII, M.D.
Docent, Department of Serology and Bacteriology, University of Helsinki
Giardiasis; Cryptosporidiosis; Isosporiasis; Balantidiasis

M. COLIN JORDAN, M.D.
Professor of Medicine and Microbiology, University of Minnesota School of Medicine, Minneapolis, Minnesota; Head, Section of Infectious Diseases, University of Minnesota Hospitals, Minneapolis, Minnesota
Infectious Mononucleosis Due to Epstein-Barr Virus and Cytomegalovirus

HARVEY S. KANTOR, M.D.
Associate Professor of Medicine and Pathology, and Chief, Division of Infectious Diseases, Chicago Medical School, North Chicago, Illinois; Chief, Section of Infectious Diseases, Veterans Administration Medical Center, North Chicago, Illinois; Consultant in Infectious Diseases, Naval Regional Medical Center, Great Lakes, Illinois
Bacterial Enteritis; Antibiotic-Associated Colitis Due to Clostridium difficile

DENNIS L. KASPER, M.D.
Associate Professor of Medicine, Harvard Medical School, Boston, Massachusetts; Chief, Division of Infectious Diseases, Beth Israel Hospital; Associate Director, Channing Laboratory, Brigham and Women's Hospital, Boston, Massachusetts
Peritonitis

DAVID A. KATZENSTEIN, M.D.
Assistant Professor of Medicine, University of Minnesota, Minneapolis, Minnesota
Amebic Liver Abscess

HERBERT E. KAUFMAN, M.D.
Boyd Professor of Ophthalmology, and Pharmacology and Experimental Therapeutics, and Head, Department of Ophthalmology, Louisiana State University School of Medicine, Director, LSU Eye Center, Louisiana State University Medical Center, New Orleans, Louisiana
Viral Keratoconjunctivitis

PATRICK J. KELLY, M.D.
Professor of Orthopedic Surgery, Mayo Medical School, Rochester, Minnesota; Consultant, Department of Orthopedics, Mayo Clinic and Mayo Foundation, Rochester, Minnesota
Bacterial Arthritis; Bacterial Osteomyelitis

GERALD T. KEUSCH, M.D.
Professor of Medicine and Chief, Division of Geographic Medicine, Tufts University School of Medicine, Boston, Massachusetts; Attending Physician, New England Medical Center, Boston, Massachusetts
Typhoid Fever; Yersinia Enteritis; Malnutrition and Infection

MOGENS KILIAN, D.D.S., Ph.D.
Professor of Microbiology and Immunology, Royal Dental College, Aarhus, Denmark; Professor and Chairman of Oral Biology, Royal Dental College, Aarhus, Denmark
Haemophilus

THEO N. KIRKLAND, M.D.
Assistant Clinical Professor of Pathology and Medicine, University of California, San Diego, California; Staff Physician, Veterans Administration Medical Center, San Diego, California
Coccidioidomycosis

ALEXANDER L. KISCH, M.D.
Formerly Associate Professor of Internal Medicine, University of New Mexico, School of Medicine, Albuquerque, New Mexico
Plague

STEVE KOHL, M.D.
Professor of Pediatrics, Program of Infectious Diseases and Clinical Microbiology, University of Texas Medical School, Houston, Texas; Attending Pediatrician, Hermann Hospital, Consulting Infectious Disease Expert, Department of Pediatrics, M. D. Anderson Hospital and Tumor Institute, Houston, Texas
Granulomatous Hepatitis

REISAKU KONO, M.D., M.P.H.
Professor of Microbiology, Saitama Medical School, Saitama Prefecture, Japan
Enteroviral Infections Other Than Poliomyelitis

TERESA LAGERGÅRD, Ph.D.
Department of Medical Microbiology, Göteborg University, Göteborg, Sweden
Epiglottitis and Pseudocroup

LYNN A. LANCASTER, M.D.
Clinical Instructor of Pathology, University of California, San Diego, School of Medicine, San Diego, California; Director of Microbiology, Donald N. Sharp Memorial Hospital, San Diego, California
Anaerobic Gram-Positive Cocci; Fusobacteria; Veillonella; Fusarium; Vincent's Infection

HOWARD W. LARSH, Ph.D.
Emeritus Research Professor of Microbiology, University of Oklahoma; Norman, Oklahoma, Director of Research and Laboratories, Missouri State Chest Hospital, Mt. Vernon, Missouri
Histoplasma capsulatum

WILLIAM LAWSON, M.D., D.D.S.
Professor of Otolaryngology, Mount Sinai Medical Center, New York, New York; Chief, Otolaryngology, Bronx Veterans Administration Hospital, Attending Physician, Mount Sinai Hospital, City Hospital Center at Elmhurst, Elmhurst, New York
Otitis Media and Otitis Externa

DONALD L. LEAKE, M.A., D.M.D., M.D.
Professor of Oral and Maxillofacial Surgery, Schools of Dentistry and Medicine, and Director, The Dental Research Institute, U.C.L.A., Los Angeles, California; Chief, Oral and Maxillofacial Surgery, Harbor–UCLA Medical Center, Torrance, California
Bacterial Parotitis

D. L. LEE, B.Sc., Ph.D.
Professor of Agricultural Zoology, Department of Pure and Applied Zoology, University of Leeds, Leeds, West Yorkshire, England
Classification and Anatomy of Parasites

AMORN LEELARASAMEE, M.D.
Associate Professor, Infectious Disease Unit, Faculty of Medicine, Siriraj Hospital, Mahidol University, Bangkok, Thailand; Staff, Department of Medicine, Siriraj Hospital, Bangkok, Thailand
Dengue and Other Hemorrhagic Fevers

FRITZ LEHMANN-GRUBE, M.D.
Head, Division of Clinical Virology, Heinrich-Pette-Institut für Experimentelle Virologie und Immunologie an der Universität Hamburg, Hamburg, Federal Republic of Germany
Arenaviruses; Lymphocytic Choriomeningitis

STANLEY M. LEMON, M.D.
Associate Professor of Medicine and Microbiology and Immunology and Chief, Division of Infectious Diseases, The University of North Carolina, Chapel Hill, North Carolina; Attending Physician, North Carolina Memorial Hospital, Chapel Hill, North Carolina
The Herpesviruses

A. MARTIN LERNER, M.D.
Clinical Professor of Medicine, Wayne State University School of Medicine, Detroit, Michigan; Consultant, Microbiology Laboratory, Sinai Hospital of Detroit, Detroit, Michigan
Myocarditis and Pericarditis

WILLIAM LESTER, M.D.
Retired, Sawyer, Michigan. Formerly Professor of Medicine, University of Chicago, Pritzker School of Medicine, Chicago, Illinois.
Tuberculosis; Nontuberculous Mycobacterial Infection

ALBERTO THOMAZ LONDERO, M.D.
Professor of Medical Mycology, Department of Microbiology and Parasitology, University of Santa Maria, Santa Maria, Brazil; Attending Medical Mycologist, University Hospital, Santa Maria, Brazil
Chromoblastomycosis; Paracoccidioidomycosis (South American Blastomycosis)

W. H. R. LUMSDEN, D.Sc., M.D., F.R.C.P.E., F.R.S.E.
Emeritus Professor of Medical Protozoology, London School of Hygiene and Tropical Medicine, University of London, London, England; Senior Research Fellow, Department of Bacteriology, University of Dundee Nineweus Hospital and Medical School, Dundee, Scotland
Trypanosomiasis

WILLIAM R. McCABE, M.D.
Professor of Medicine and Microbiology, Boston University School of Medicine, Boston, Massachusetts; Director, Division of Infectious Diseases, Boston University School of Medicine, and Director, Maxwell Finland Laboratory for Infectious Diseases, Boston City Hospital, Boston, Massachusetts
Gram-Negative Bacteremia

RICHARD V. McCLOSKEY, M.S., M.D.
Professor of Medicine, Jefferson Medical School, Thomas Jefferson University, Philadelphia, Pennsylvania; Albert Einstein Medical Center, Mt. Sinai Daroff Division, Department of Medicine, Philadelphia, Pennsylvania
Diphtheria

J. ALLEN McCUTCHAN, M.D., M.Sc.(Epid.)
Associate Professor of Medicine, University of California, San Diego, California; Attending Physician, University of California, San Diego, Medical Center; Research Director, Owen Clinic, San Diego, California
Gonococcemia; Factitious and Delusional Illnesses Simulating Infections; Acquired Immunodeficiency Syndrome; Gonococcal and Chlamydial Genital Infections

ZELL A. McGEE, M.D.
Professor of Medicine and Pathology, University of Utah School of Medicine, Salt Lake City, Utah; Director, Center for Infectious Diseases, Diagnostic Microbiology, and Immunology; Chief, Division of Infectious Diseases, Department of Medicine, University of Utah School of Medicine, Salt Lake City, Utah
Mycoplasmas; Cell Wall–Defective Bacteria

RIMA McLEOD, M.D.
Assistant Professor of Medicine, Pritzker School of Medicine, University of Chicago, Chicago, Illinois; Attending Physician, Michael Reese Hospital and Medical Center, Chicago, Illinois
Toxoplasmosis

G. PHILIP MANIRE, Ph.D.
Kenan Professor of Microbiology, Vice Chancellor and Dean of the Graduate School, University of North Carolina, Chapel Hill, North Carolina
The Chlamydiae

FRANÇOIS MARIAT, D.Sc.
Institut Pasteur, University of Paris, Paris, France
Sporothrix schenckii

MELVIN I. MARKS, M.D.
Professor of Pediatrics and Director, Pediatric Infectious Disease Service; and Adjunct Professor of Microbiology/Immunology, University of Oklahoma Health Sciences Center, Oklahoma City, Oklahoma; Head, Pediatric Infectious Disease Service, Oklahoma Children's Memorial Hospital, Oklahoma City, Oklahoma
Pleurodynia; Mumps

HORACIO FIGUEROA MARROQUIN, M.D.
Emeritus Professor, University of San Carlos, San Carlos, Guatemala
Cutaneous Onchocerciasis

FRANCIS D. MARTINSON, M.B., Ch.B. (Ed.), F.R.C.S. (Eng. & Ed.)
Professor and Head, Department of Otorhinolaryngology, College of Medicine, University of Ibadan, Ibadan, Nigeria; Consultant, Department of Otorhinolaryngology, University College Hospital, Ibadan, Nigeria
Phycomycosis (Zygomycosis)

CHRISTOPHER MATHEWS, M.D.
Assistant Professor of Clinical Medicine, University of California, San Diego, California; Director, Owen Clinic, University of California, San Diego, Medical Center, San Diego, California
Acquired Immunodeficiency Syndrome

GERALD MEDOFF, M.D.
Professor of Medicine, Microbiology and Immunology, Washington University School of Medicine, St. Louis, Missouri; Physician, Barnes Hospital, Staff Physician, V.A. Hospital, Consultant, The Jewish Hospital of St. Louis, Consultant, The Children's Hospital of St. Louis, St. Louis, Missouri
Pulmonary Cryptococcosis; Cryptococcal Meningitis

MARIAN E. MELISH, M.D.
Associate Professor of Pediatrics, Tropical Medicine, and Medical Microbiology, John A. Burns School of Medicine of The University of Hawaii, Honolulu, Hawaii; Infectious Disease Consultant, Kapiolani Women's and Children's Medical Center, Honolulu, Hawaii
Staphylococci; Kawasaki Syndrome (The Mucocutaneous Lymph Node Syndrome); Impetigo; Pyogenic Skin Infections; Staphylococcal Scalded Skin Syndrome; Staphylococcal Toxic Shock Syndrome

JOSEPH L. MELNICK, Ph.D.
Distinguished Service Professor and Chairman, Department of Virology and Epidemiology, Baylor College of Medicine, Houston, Texas
Classification of Viruses

BURT R. MEYERS, M.D.
Professor of Medicine, Division of Infectious Diseases, Mount Sinai School of Medicine, New York, New York; Attending Physician, Mount Sinai Hospital, New York, New York
Ludwig's Angina; Otitis Media and Otitis Externa; Endophthalmitis; Pulmonary Mucormycosis

WAYNE M. MEYERS, M.D., Ph.D.
Chief, Division of Microbiology, and Registrar, Leprosy Registry, Armed Forces Institute of Pathology, Washington, D.C.
Mycobacterial Infections of the Skin

JOSEPH H. MILLER, M.S., Ph.D.
Professor Emeritus of Tropical Medicine and Medical Parasitology, Section of Medical Parasitology, Department of Microbiology, Immunology and Parasitology and Section of International and Tropical Medicine, Department of Medicine, LSU Medical Center, New Orleans, Louisiana; Visiting Staff, Charity Hospital of New Orleans, New Orleans, Louisiana
The Protozoa

DAVID I. MINKOFF, M.D.
Clinical Instructor, Pediatric Infectious Disease, and Nursing School Instructor of Pediatrics, University of California, San Diego, California; Staff, Children's Hospital, San Diego, California, and Infection Control Officer and Chairman, Committee on Pharmacy and Therapeutics, Palomar Hospital, Escondido, California
Herpangina; Hand-Foot-Mouth Disease

JOSÉ LISBÔA MIRANDA, M.D.
Professor of Dermatology, Director, Department of Internal Medicine, Centro de Ciências Biológicas e da Saúde, Universidade Gama Filho, Rio de Janeiro, Brazil; Chief of Dermatology, Hospital Universitário Gama Filho, Universidade Gama Filho, Rio de Janeiro, Brazil
Lobomycosis

SAROJ K. MISHRA, Ph.D.
Microbiologist, Waksman Institute of Microbiology, Rutgers University, Piscataway, New Jersey
Nocardia and Streptomyces

JOHN Z. MONTGOMERIE, M.D., F.R.A.C.P.
Professor of Medicine, University of Southern California, Los Angeles, California; Chief, Division of Infectious Diseases, Rancho Los Amigos Hospital, Downey, California
Vertebral Osteomyelitis

PETER M. MOODIE, M.D., B.S., D.T.M.&H.
Associate Professor and Head, Department of Tropical Health, Commonwealth Institute of Health, The University of Sydney, Sydney, Australia
Yaws, Pinta, and Bejel

STEPHEN A. MORSE, Ph.D.
Professor of Microbiology and Immunology, Oregon Health Sciences University, Portland, Oregon
Neisseria and Branhamella

STEPHEN I. MORSE
Late Professor and Chairman, Microbiology and Immunology, State University of New York; Downstate Medical Center, Brooklyn, New York
Staphylococci; Staphylococcal Bacteremia

MAURICE A. MUFSON, M.D.
Professor and Chairman, Department of Medicine, Marshall University School of Medicine, Huntington, West Virginia; Associate Chief of Staff for Research, Veterans Administration Medical Center, Active Medical Staff, Cabell Huntington Hospital and St. Mary's Hospital, Huntington, West Virginia
Mycoplasma Pneumonia

DANIEL M. MUSHER, M.D.
Professor of Medicine, Microbiology and Immunology, Baylor College of Medicine, Houston, Texas; Chief, Infectious Disease Section, Veterans Administration Hospital, Houston, Texas
Lyme Disease; Spirochetes: Treponema and Borrelia; Syphilis of the Genital Tract; Syphilis

HAROLD C. NEU, M.D.
Professor of Medicine and Pharmacology, College of Physicians and Surgeons, Columbia University, New York, New York; Chief of Infectious Diseases, Hospital Epidemiologist, Columbia-Presbyterian Medical Center, New York, New York
The Pharmacology and Toxicology of Antimicrobial Agents

OLLE NYLÉN, M.D.
Associate Professor, Department of ENT, University of Göteborg, Göteborg, Sweden; Sahlgrens Hospital, Göteborg, Sweden
Epiglottitis and Pseudocroup

IDA ØRSKOV, M.D.
Collaborative Centre for Reference and Research on Escherichia (WHO), Statens Seruminstitut, Copenhagen, Denmark
Enterobacteriaceae

FRITS ØRSKOV, M.D.
Collaborative Centre for Reference and Research on Escherichia (WHO), Statens Seruminstitut, Copenhagen, Denmark
Enterobacteriaceae

MICHAEL N. OXMAN, M.D.
Professor of Medicine and Pathology, University of California, San Diego School of Medicine, San Diego, California; Chief, Infectious Diseases and Clinical Virology Sections, Veterans Administration Medical Center, San Diego, California
Herpes Stomatitis; Genital Herpes; Herpes Simplex Encephalitis and Meningitis; Varicella; Herpes Zoster; Papovaviruses; Picornaviruses

JOSEPH S. PAGANO, M.D.
Professor of Medicine and Microbiology and Immunology and Director, Lineberger Cancer Research Center, The University of North Carolina, Chapel Hill, North Carolina; Attending Physician, North Carolina Memorial Hospital, Chapel Hill, North Carolina
The Herpesviruses

ZBIGNIEW S. PAWLOWSKI, M.D.
Professor of Medical Parasitology, Medical Academy, Poznan, Poland; Senior Medical Officer, Parasitic Diseases Programme, World Health Organization, Geneva, Switzerland
Trichinellosis; Cestodiasis; Platyhelminthes

LENNART PHILIPSON, M.D., Dr. Med. Sci.
Former Professor of Microbiology, University of Uppsala, Uppsala, Sweden; Director General, European Molecular Biology Laboratory (EMBL), Heidelberg, Federal Republic of Germany
Adenovirus

ALEXANDER W. PIERCE, JR., M.D.
Professor of Pediatrics and Family Practice, The University of Texas Medical School, San Antonio, Texas
Myiasis

LEO PINE, M.S., Ph.D.
Center for Infectious Diseases, Division of Bacterial Diseases, Biotechnology Branch, Centers for Disease Control, Atlanta, Georgia
Actinomyces and Microaerophilic Actinomycetes

FRANCISCO de PAULA PINHEIRO, M.D.
Regional Advisor on Viral Diseases, Pan American Health Organization, Washington, D.C.
Yellow Fever

BOSKO POSTIC, M.D.
Professor of Medicine, University of South Carolina School of Medicine, Columbia, South Carolina; Dorn Veterans' Hospital, Columbia, South Carolina
Rabies; Rhabdovirus

ROY POSTLETHWAITE, B.Sc., M.D.
Personal Professor of Virology, Medical School, University of Aberdeen, Aberdeen, Scotland; Honorary Consultant Bacteriologist, Aberdeen Royal Infirmary and Associated Hospitals, Aberdeen, Scotland
Molluscum Contagiosum

C. R. PRINGLE, B.Sc., Ph.D.
Professor of Virology, Department of Biological Sciences, University of Warwick, Coventry, England
Genetics of Viruses

SEPPO PYRHÖNEN, M.D.
Docent, Helsinki University, Helsinki, Finland; Senior Staff Member, Department of Radiotherapy and Oncology, University Central Hospital, Helsinki, Finland
Warts

T. RAMAKRISHNAN, M.Sc., Ph.D.
Emeritus Professor, Microbiology and Cell Biology Laboratory, Indian Institute of Science, Bangalore, India
Bacterial Physiology

A. RAMACHANDRA RAO, M.B., B.S., B.S.Sc.
Madras, India
Smallpox, Vaccinia, Cowpox and Orf

G. RAMANANDA RAO, M. Pharm., Ph.D.
Associate Professor, Microbiology and Cell Biology Laboratory, Indian Institute of Science, Bangalore, India
Bacterial Physiology

GARRISON RAPMUND, M.D.
Major General, Medical Corps, Assistant Surgeon General (Research and Development), Department of the Army, Washington, D.C.
Scrub Typhus; Rickettsialpox; Trench Fever; Rickettsia

ARTHUR L. REINGOLD, M.D.
Assistant Chief, Respiratory and Special Pathogens Epidemiology Branch, Division of Bacterial Diseases, Center for Infectious Diseases, Centers for Disease Control, Atlanta, Georgia
Legionella

JACK S. REMINGTON, M.D.
Professor of Medicine, Division of Infectious Diseases, Stanford University, Stanford, California; Chief Consultant in Infectious Diseases, Palo Alto Medical Foundation Clinic, Palo Alto, California
Toxoplasmosis

DOUGLAS D. RICHMAN, M.D.
Associate Professor of Pathology and Medicine, University of California, San Diego, California; Staff Physician, San Diego Veterans Administration Medical Center, San Diego, California
Tuberculous Meningitis and Tuberculoma of the Brain; Orthomyxoviruses: The Influenza Viruses; Paramyxoviruses

DAVID L. RINGO, Ph.D.
Assistant Research Biologist, University of California, Santa Cruz, California
The Structure of the Bacterial Cell

LEON ROSEN, M.D., Dr.P.H.
Head, Pacific Research Section, Laboratory of Parasitic Diseases, National Institute of Allergy and Infectious Diseases, Honolulu, Hawaii
Cerebral Angiostrongyliasis

EDWARD BROOK ROTHERAM, JR., M.D.
Clinical Associate Professor of Medicine, University of Pittsburgh, School of Medicine, Pittsburgh, Pennsylvania; Head, Division of Infectious Diseases, Allegheny General Hospital, Pittsburgh, Pennsylvania
Liver and Subphrenic Abscess; Nonvenereal Infections of the Female Genitalia

J. L. RYAN, Ph.D., M.D.
Associate Professor of Internal Medicine, Yale University School of Medicine, New Haven, Connecticut; Chief, Infectious Disease Section, Veterans Administration Medical Center, New Haven, Connecticut
Bites: P. multocida, DF-2, S. moniliformis, and S. minor

ALBERT B. SABIN, M.D.
Senior Expert Consultant, Fogarty International Center, National Institutes of Health, Bethesda, Maryland
Poliomyelitis

FRANCISCO L. SAPICO, M.D., F.A.C.P.
Associate Professor of Medicine, University of Southern California, Los Angeles, California; Associate Chief, Division of Infectious Diseases, Rancho Los Amigos Hospital, Downey, California
Vertebral Osteomyelitis

GEORGE A. SAROSI, M.D.
Professor, The University of Texas Medical School, Houston; Professor, Division Director of General Medicine, Vice Chairman of Internal Medicine, The University of Texas Health Science Center at Houston, Houston, Texas
Histoplasmosis; Aspergillosis

MARIA C. SAVOIA, M.D.
Assistant Adjunct Professor of Medicine, University of California, San Diego; Assistant Chief, Medical Service, San Diego Veterans Administration Medical Center, San Diego, California
Staphylococcal Bacteremia

HOWARD J. SAZ, Ph.D.
Professor of Biology, University of Notre Dame, Notre Dame, Indiana
Biochemistry of Parasites: Helminths

ANDREAS SCHAFFNER, M.D.
Instructor, University of Zurich, Zurich, Switzerland; Physician, Medical Clinic and Laboratory of Clinical Mycology, Department of Medicine, University Hospital, Zurich, Switzerland
Listeria monocytogenes; Listeriosis

GILBERT M. SCHIFF, M.D.
Professor of Medicine, University of Cincinnati College of Medicine; Director of Medicine, The Christ Hospital Institute of Medical Research; Attending Staff, Cincinnati General Hospital, Holmes Hospital, Cincinnati Veterans Administration Hospital, Christ Hospital; Consultant, Children's Hospital, Jewish Hospital, Cincinnati, Ohio
Measles; Rubella

BARTHOLOMEW M. SEFTON, Ph.D.
Associate Professor, Molecular Biology and Virology Laboratory, The Salk Institute, San Diego, California
Viral Replication

SMITH SHADOMY, Ph.D.
Professor of Medicine and Pathology, Affiliate Professor of Microbiology and Immunology, Medical College of Virginia, Virginia Commonwealth University, Richmond, Virginia
Blastomyces and Paracoccidioides

KAORU SHIMADA, M.D.
Professor of Medicine and Infectious Diseases, Institute of Medical Science, Tokyo University, Tokyo, Japan; Attending Staff, Tokyo Metropolitan Geriatric Hospital, Tokyo, Japan
Cholecystitis and Cholangitis

RUDOLF SIEGERT, M.D.
Professor, Philipps-Universität Marburg, Federal Republic of Germany; Center for Hygiene and Medical Microbiology, Marburg, Federal Republic of Germany
Marburg Virus and Ebola Virus; Marburg Virus Disease; Ebola Virus Disease

SAMUEL C. SILVERSTEIN, M.D.
John C. Dalton Professor and Chairman, Department of Physiology and Cellular Biophysics, College of Physicians and Surgeons, Columbia University, New York, New York
Viral Replication

IRVING J. SLOTNICK, Ph.D.
Consulting Microbiologist, Cedars-Sinai Medical Center, Los Angeles, California
Actinobacillus and Cardiobacterium

DONALD W. SMITH, Ph.D.
Professor of Medical Microbiology, University of Wisconsin, Madison, Wisconsin
Mycobacteria

B. A. SOUTHGATE, M.B., B.S., F.F.C.M.
Senior Lecturer in Tropical Hygiene, London School of Hygiene and Tropical Medicine, London, England
Loaiasis

STEPHEN A. SPECTOR, M.D.
Associate Professor of Pediatrics, and Co-Chief, Division of Pediatric Infectious Diseases, University of California, San Diego, School of Medicine; Pediatric Infectious Diseases Consultant, University of California, San Diego Medical Center, Children's Hospital and Health Center, San Diego, and Mercy Hospital and Medical Center, San Diego, California
Immunoprophylaxis and Immunotherapy

WESLEY W. SPINK, A.B., M.D., D.Sc.
Regents' Professor of Medicine and Comparative Medicine Emeritus, University of Minnesota Medical School, Minneapolis, Minnesota; Emeritus Member of Medical Staff, University Hospitals, University of Minnesota, Minneapolis, Minnesota
Brucella; Brucellosis

SPOTSWOOD L. SPRUANCE, M.D.
Associate Professor of Medicine, Division of Infectious Diseases, Department of Medicine, University of Utah School of Medicine, Salt Lake City, Utah; University of Utah Hospital, Salt Lake City, Utah
Colorado Tick Fever

NEVILLE F. STANLEY, D.Sc., F.R.C.P.A. (Hon.), F.A.N.Z.A.A.S., F.I.B.A., M.A.S.M.
Emeritus Professor and Honorary Research Fellow, Department of Microbiology, University of Western Australia, Queen Elizabeth II Medical Centre, Perth, Western Australia
Reoviridae Pathogenic for Man

DAVID A. STEVENS, M.D.
Associate Professor, Stanford University, Stanford, California; Chief, Division of Infectious Diseases, Santa Clara Valley Medical Center, San Jose, California
Coccidioidal Meningitis

H. HARLAN STONE, M.D.
Professor of Surgery, University of Maryland School of Medicine, Baltimore, Maryland; Chief of General Surgery, University of Maryland Hospital, Baltimore, Maryland
Nonclostridial Anaerobic Cellulitis

RICHARD B. STOUGHTON, M.D.
Professor of Medicine (Dermatology), University of California, San Diego, California; Attending Physician, University Hospital, University of California, San Diego, California
Dermatophytosis

WILLARD A. TABER, Ph.D.
Professor of Biology, Biology Department, Texas A & M University, College Station, Texas
Classification of Fungi

DAVID TAYLOR-ROBINSON, M.D.
Head, Division of Sexually Transmitted Diseases, M.R.C. Clinical Research Centre; Honorary Consultant, Microbiologist, Northwick Park Hospital, Harrow, Middlesex, England
Mycoplasmas

ROBERT NICOL THIN, M.D., F.R.C.P.E.
Recognised Teacher, University of London, London, England; Consultant Physician, Department of Genito-Urinary Medicine, St. Thomas' Hospital, and St. Peter's Hospitals, London, England
Melioidosis

DORIS A. TRAUNER, M.S., M.D.
Associate Professor, Department of Neurosciences, University of California, La Jolla, California; Chief, Pediatric Neurology, University of California, San Diego, Medical Center, San Diego, California
Reye's Syndrome

WALTER P. G. TURCK, M.B., F.R.C.P.
Consultant Physician, Department of Medicine, Bury General Hospital, Bury, Lancashire, England
Q Fever; Chronic Q Fever

D. A. J. TYRRELL, M.D., F.R.C.P., F.R.S.
Director, M.R.C. Common Cold Unit, Salisbury, Wiltshire, England
Coronaviridaes

HANS A. VALKENBURG, M.D., Ph.D.
Professor of Epidemiology, Erasmus University Medical School, Rotterdam, the Netherlands
Streptococcal Pharyngitis and Tonsillitis

PAUL B. VAN CAUWENBERGE, M.D.
Senior Lecturer, State University of Ghent, Ghent, Belgium; Consultant Otolaryngologist, University Hospital, Ghent, Belgium
Paranasal Sinusitis

WILLIAM EDWARD VAN HEYNINGEN, Ph.D., Sc.D., D.Sc.
Emeritus Reader in Bacterial Chemistry, Sir William Dunn School of Pathology, University of Oxford, Oxford, England
Bacterial Exotoxins

PANKAJALAKSHMI V. VENUGOPAL, M.D.
Professor and Head, Department of Microbiology, Thanjavur Medical College, Thanjavur, India; Chief Microbiologist, Thanjavur Medical College Hospital and Raja Mirasdar Hospital, Thanjavur, India
Mycetoma

TARALAKSHMI V. VENUGOPAL, M.D.
Professor and Head, Department of Pathology, Madurai Medical College, Madurai, India; Chief Pathologist, Government Erskine Hospital, Madurai, India
Mycetoma

RICARDO VERONESI, M.D.
Professor of Infectious and Parasitic Diseases, Faculty of Medicine, University of São Paulo, São Paulo, Brazil; Chairman of Infectious Diseases Department, Hospital das Clínicas de São Paulo, São Paulo, Brazil
Tetanus

GERALD E. WAGNER, Ph.D.
Assistant Professor, Department of Microbiology, The George Washington University School of Medicine, Washington, D.C.
Dematiaceae: Agents of Chromomycosis

HENRY A. WALCH, Ph.D.
Professor of Microbiology, San Diego State University, San Diego, California
Coccidioides immitis

CRAIG K. WALLACE, M.D.
Clinical Associate Professor, Department of Medicine, Uniformed Services University of the Health Sciences, Bethesda, Maryland; Director, Fogarty International Center, and Associate Director for International Research, National Institutes of Health, Bethesda, Maryland; Medical Consultant, Naval Hospital, Bethesda, Maryland
Cholera

WARREN J. WARWICK, M.D.
Professor, University of Minnesota Medical School, University of Minnesota Hospitals and Clinics, Minneapolis, Minnesota; Head, Division of Pediatric Pulmonary Disease and Cystic Fibrosis, and Director, Cystic Fibrosis Research, University of Minnesota Hospitals and Clinics, Department of Pediatrics, Minneapolis, Minnesota
Cat Scratch Disease

TADEUSZ J. WIKTOR, D.V.M.
Professor, The Wistar Institute, University of Pennsylvania, Philadelphia, Pennsylvania
Rabies; Rhabdovirus

ROBERT P. WILLIAMS, M.D.
Professor of Microbiology and Immunology, Baylor College of Medicine, Houston, Texas
Bacillus anthracis and Other Aerobic Spore-Forming Bacilli

SHELDON M. WOLFF, M.D.
Endicott Professor and Chairman, Department of Medicine, Tufts University School of Medicine, Boston, Massachusetts; Physician-in-Chief, New England Medical Center Hospital, Boston, Massachusetts
Fever

PRISCILLA B. WYRICK, Ph.D.
Associate Professor, Department of Microbiology and Immunology, University of North Carolina School of Medicine, Chapel Hill, North Carolina
The Chlamydiae

NATHANIEL A. YOUNG, M.D.
Late Head, Viral Oncology and Molecular Pathology Sections, Laboratory of Pathology, National Institutes of Health, Bethesda, Maryland; Late Senior Attending Physician in Infectious Diseases, Clinical Center, National Institutes of Health, Bethesda, Maryland
Picornavirus

JULIUS S. YOUNGNER, Sc.D.
Professor and Chairman, Department of Microbiology, University of Pittsburgh, School of Medicine, Pittsburgh, Pennsylvania
Persistent Viral Infections

ELIZABETH J. ZIEGLER, M.D.
Associate Professor of Medicine, University of California School of Medicine, San Diego, California; Attending Physician, University of California Medical Center, San Diego, California
Cerebral Mucormycosis; Cerebral Aspergillosis

Preface To The First Edition

This book tries to do two things that haven't been done before. First, it presents a full coverage of both microbiology and infectious diseases. Second, it takes advantage of the expert knowledge of authorities throughout the world by presenting contributions from nearly 30 different countries. About one-third of the authors are from outside the United States.

The reason for combining medical microbiology and infectious diseases is simply that they are inseparable. Recognizing that neither subject can be presented properly without the other, the authors of textbooks on medical microbiology have incorporated some material on infectious diseases as well, but the clinical coverage has not been enough to help the practicing physician. The reverse is true in texts dealing with clinical infectious diseases; these usually present a summary of the microbial agents causing each disease but not enough information to give the serious students of microbiology what they need. In order to avoid a superficial coverage of either subject, we have invited distinguished authorities to contribute thorough accounts of their subjects that would give even the specialist in those fields the information he is looking for. For the most part, this approach has brought together the two related disciplines so that they fully reinforce each other; each clinical problem is backed up by whatever relevant scientific data and ideas can be marshaled to help elucidate it.

The reason for an international approach is that different environments and ecologies throughout the world breed different germs, and different infections, so that the cause and nature of the diseases differ from one part of the world to another. In order to avoid the parochial approach of inviting American professors to write about infections they seldom see, we have called upon contributors who have had an unmatched experience in dealing with the disease they write about. If nothing else, we have in this way brought together an authoritative coverage of international infections by real experts with a vast first-hand encounter with their subject. In this way we can provide physicians and microbiologists throughout the world with reliable information on infections indigenous to their region, or infections carried there for the first time by international travelers, refugees, or migrants.

The picture of infectious diseases is greatly influenced by the enormous increase in such international mobility in the last 25 years. At least 4 waves of mobility to and from underdeveloped countries can be identified, and each of these is having its impact on the worldwide problem of infection. First, the rise in tourism, cultural exchange, and business travel to and from underdeveloped countries has created a remarkable growth in air travel. In 1977 alone, there were over 600 million passengers on international flights and a substantial portion of these people were visiting, coming from, or passing through underdeveloped countries. Second, the migration of laborers has accounted for another large element of movement from underdeveloped countries. Migrant workers from Mexico to the United States are increasing in number, and even greater shifts in worker populations are going on in Europe, especially from North Africa, Turkey, the middle eastern Arab countries, and India. The third mobile group of international significance is composed of pilgrims and is best illustrated by the 2 million people who go to Mecca from all over the world during the annual pilgrimage. Finally, there are the refugees from Southeast Asia who are pouring into centers in the United States and many other countries and who often pick up tropical infections in displaced persons camps in Indochina and other way stations. The movement of these 4 large population groups carries two inevitable risks: one is to the person who gets the infection, and the other is to the community through which he passes or where he settles. Both problems were anticipated in planning this text and they are dealt with in the relevant chapters.

The international approach was not limited to selecting contributors on clinical chapters. Each country has its specialists in the basic sciences, as well, and a number of important scientists, known for the originality and scope of their research, have written chapters.

We hope that all this will add up to a useful work for anyone who has an interest in microbiology and infectious diseases. The medical student, for example, should be able to learn what he needs to know about microbiology in his preclinical studies, and then have a text on infectious diseases when he moves into his clinical years. By concentrating on microbiologic principles first, he should be equipped with the scientific background needed for undertaking an intelligent study of clinical infectious diseases. But even when he is concentrating on microbiology, he will have at hand a ready reference source with those clinical examples that clarify the basic science. Physicians, on the other hand, who use the book mainly for information about problems seen in their practice, will be able to find answers to theoretical or basic microbiologic questions that have a bearing on infectious diseases.

Finally, two explanatory notes are in order. First, medical microbiology is presented here in the strict sense so that related subjects, such as immunology, are presented only as they relate to microbiology. Whereas most immunologic concepts are taken into account with this approach, they are covered more fully and as a comprehensive unit in Volume I. Second, the clinical diseases are presented by system. This is partly because the etiologic approach was needed in the first half of this volume for dealing with specific microbial agents of disease, but mainly because most infections present themselves as a disease of a specific organ or system. We feel, therefore, that physicians can find an answer to their problem more quickly if the disease is described under the appropriate system. If he needs to know more about etiology he can refer to the chapters on specific microbial agents.

If anyone finds this work useful, he or she should know that Gita Braude, Sharon McFarlin, Elizabeth Thurlow, and Pat Campbell are the unsung heroines behind its production.

ABRAHAM I. BRAUDE

Contents

MICROBIOLOGY I

G. Dermal Infections, Exanthems, and Infestations

H. Ocular Infections

Microbiology I

A. GENERAL MICROBIOLOGY
Bacteriology

1
THE STRUCTURE OF THE BACTERIAL CELL

EUGENE H. COTA-ROBLES, PH.D.
AND DAVID L. RINGO, PH.D.

The structure of bacteria can be best understood by contrasting their cellular organization to that of the higher biologic forms—animals, plants, protozoa, algae, and fungi. In these life forms the cells are divided into internal compartments by membrane systems. These compartments (cellular *organelles*) have specific activities for the maintenance of the life functions of the cell. The nuclear compartment *(nucleus)* contains the cell's hereditary material, *deoxyribonucleic acid* (DNA). The nucleus is separated by a nuclear membrane from the rest of the cell, the *cytoplasm.* The DNA of higher cells is organized in two or more chromosomes.

Bacterial cells are not compartmentalized and therefore are considered to lack organelles. The hereditary material of bacteria consists of a single chromosome. This bacterial *nucleoid* is a single, tightly bundled, long strand of DNA that lies within the cytoplasm not surrounded by a nuclear membrane. For this reason bacteria are referred to as *prokaryotic,* that is, having a primitive nuclear structure; and higher cells are designated as *eukaryotic,* literally, having a true nucleus. All bacteria (as well as the blue-green algae) possess the prokaryotic form of organization.

In a broad sense, all types of cells function in the same manner. The information stored in the DNA is transcribed as *messenger ribonucleic acid* (mRNA), which moves from the nucleus into the cytoplasm. Here the messenger RNA attaches to ribosomes, where the genetic information is translated into specific proteins by the polymerization of amino acids. The synthesis of proteins is one of the most basic of cell processes, since virtually every metabolic activity of the cell is mediated by enzymes, the proteins that catalyze specific chemical reactions.

The basic function of a bacterial cell is to assimilate chemicals from its environment in order to grow and divide. Some bacteria perform these functions by using the simplest inorganic chemicals (carbon dioxide and minerals), and are termed *autotrophs.* Certain members of this group, photosynthetic bacteria and blue-green algae, rely on light as a source of energy and thus resemble plants in their photoautotrophic metabolism. Another and larger group of bacteria, the *heterotrophs,* use simple organic molecules from their environment as a source of energy and as building blocks for cellular material. Many of this latter group have adapted to growth within the animal body. Some are harmless symbionts, such as *Escherichia coli,* which normally inhabits the mammalian gut. Others are harmful and may cause human disease. These bacteria are termed *pathogens,* and their infection of body tissues results in a characteristic illness. Many of the features of bacterial cell structure are related, in one way or another, to their role as disease organisms and to the ways in which these diseases are treated and controlled.

The generalized structure of a typical bacterial cell is shown in Figure 1. The prokaryotic cell consists of a cell wall, a cytoplasmic membrane surrounding a cytoplasm packed with ribosomes, and a more or less central nucleoid. The figure is an example of the image produced by the electron microscope of a very thin section cut through a chemically preserved (fixed) bacterium. It is possible to determine the overall shape and size of such a bacterial cell with the light microscope, but details that are smaller than about 0.2 μm cannot be resolved (Table 1). Thus, the internal structure of the bacterium can be deduced only through the use of the higher resolving power of the electron microscope, and all such detailed knowledge has been obtained only within the past 30 years.

NUCLEOID. Embedded in the ribosome-rich cytoplasm is the bacterial genetic apparatus, the nucleoid. No boundary separates it from the rest of the cytoplasm; the nucleoid's physical segregation is maintained by the very nature of the DNA that is its make-up. The DNA consists of one very long and narrow molecule—a double helix—which if stretched to its full length would measure more than 1.0 mm long and only 0.000002 mm (2 nm) wide. Genetic analysis has shown that most of the bacterial genes are linked to one another in an orderly fashion, and, moreover, that the linkage is continuous and circular. We therefore describe the bacterial nucleoid as a single, circular chromosome. Physical studies also demonstrate that the DNA strand of the chromosome is a circle that is tightly coiled into a bundle to produce the nucleoid image shown with the electron microscope. The chromosome replicates in the growing cell in preparation for cell division. Bacterial cells divide by binary fission into two daughter cells, each of which retains a copy of the chromosome. A small percentage of the cell's genetic information is present as much smaller DNA molecules, *plasmids,* which may be present in many copies and replicate independently. Bacterial plasmids often carry the genes involved in resistance to chemotherapeutic drugs. Plasmids cannot be observed within cells by the electron microscope because they are masked by the dense cytoplasm.

CYTOPLASM. Although certain autotrophic bacteria contain internal membranes associated with photosynthesis and other special metabolic functions, the cytoplasm of

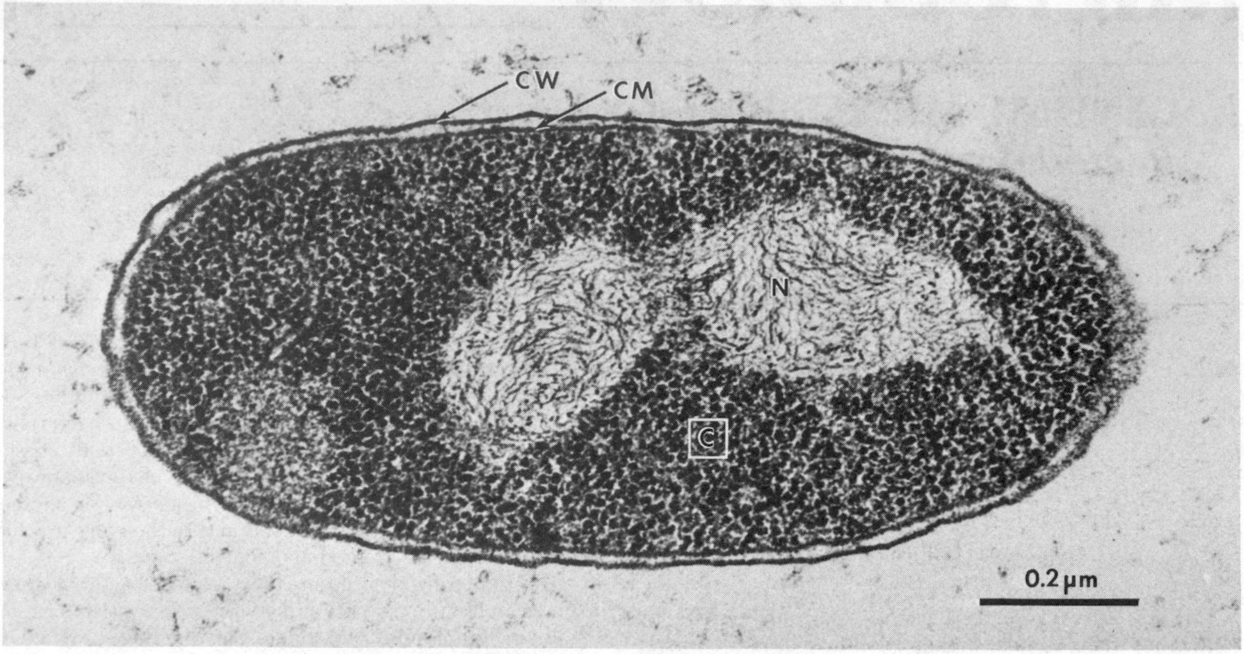

Figure 1. This electron micrograph outlines the organization that is common to all bacterial cells. The nucleoid (N) occupies the central area of the cell; the cytoplasm (C) contains many ribosomes (individual dark granules); a cytoplasmic membrane (CM) and cell wall (CW) surround the cell. This bacterium, *Alteromonas espejiana*, is a marine pseudomonad that possesses a very simple wall structure.

most heterotrophic bacteria contains only ribosomes and storage granules. Ribosomes are the site of protein synthesis, and their large numbers reflect the importance of this synthetic role in the bacterial cell. Many enzymes are present in the cytoplasm, whereas others are bound to the cell membrane. It is impossible, however, to recognize individual protein molecules with the electron microscope, except when special preparative techniques are used.

Each ribosome is a complex structure about 20 nm in diameter, and is an aggregate of several RNA molecules and many protein molecules. The ribosome consists of two major subunits, one somewhat larger than the other. Although the ribosomes of all types of cells function in a similar manner in protein synthesis, it is possible to distinguish the ribosomes of prokaryotic cells from those of eukaryotic cells by their different sedimentation velocity in the ultracentrifuge. Bacterial ribosomes have a sedimentation value of 70S (Svedberg units), whereas eukaryotic ribosomes are slightly larger and heavier with a sedimentation value of 80S. The antibiotics tetracycline, streptomycin, and chloramphenicol act by interfering with one

Table 1. UNITS USED TO DESCRIBE BACTERIA AND THEIR STRUCTURES, AND THE USEFUL LIMITS OF RESOLUTION OF THE HUMAN EYE, THE LIGHT MICROSCOPE, AND THE ELECTRON MICROSCOPE

Units:	
1 m × 10^{-3}	= 1 mm (millimeter)
1 mm × 10^{-3}	= 1 μm (micrometer or micron)
1 μm × 10^{-3}	= 1 nm (nanometer)
Limits of Resolving Power:	
Unaided human eye: 0.2 mm	
Compound light microscope: 0.2 μm	
Transmission electron microscope: 2 nm to 0.2 nm	

stage or other of protein synthesis by bacterial (70S) ribosomes.

A second class of cytoplasmic particles, which are frequently but not always found, are storage granules (Fig. 2). The presence and amount of these particles vary with the type of bacterium and its level of metabolic activity. Storage granules represent a mechanism for temporary storage of excess metabolites. Three types of such granules are common: glycogen, a glucose polymer that serves as a carbohydrate reserve; poly-β-hydroxybutyric acid, a lipid reserve; and volutin, a polyphosphate compound. These granules are often large enough to be seen with the light microscope. Volutin granules are also known as metachromatic granules because of their staining behavior; that is, they appear red when stained with methylene blue dye.

CELL MEMBRANE. The cytoplasmic membrane, a delicate structure that is only 6 nm thick, represents the true barrier between the inside and the outside of the cell. In addition to a membrane, the bacterial cell requires the presence of a cell wall to permit it to withstand the cell's osmotic pressure and other forces encountered in nature. Removal of the cell wall normally results in the rupture of the cell membrane, causing *lysis*, the dissolution and death of the cell. In an osmotically protected environment the cell may remain intact and alive even after the cell wall is removed. A cell having no wall is called a *protoplast*, if the wall is completely removed, or a *spheroplast*, if some wall fragments remain.

The selective permeability of the cell membrane determines which molecules from the cell's environment can enter the cell and which are excluded. Some molecules diffuse passively into the cell; other require active transport across the membrane by specific enzymes. Enzymes involved in cell wall synthesis and synthesis of extracellular products are lodged in the cytoplasmic membrane. The

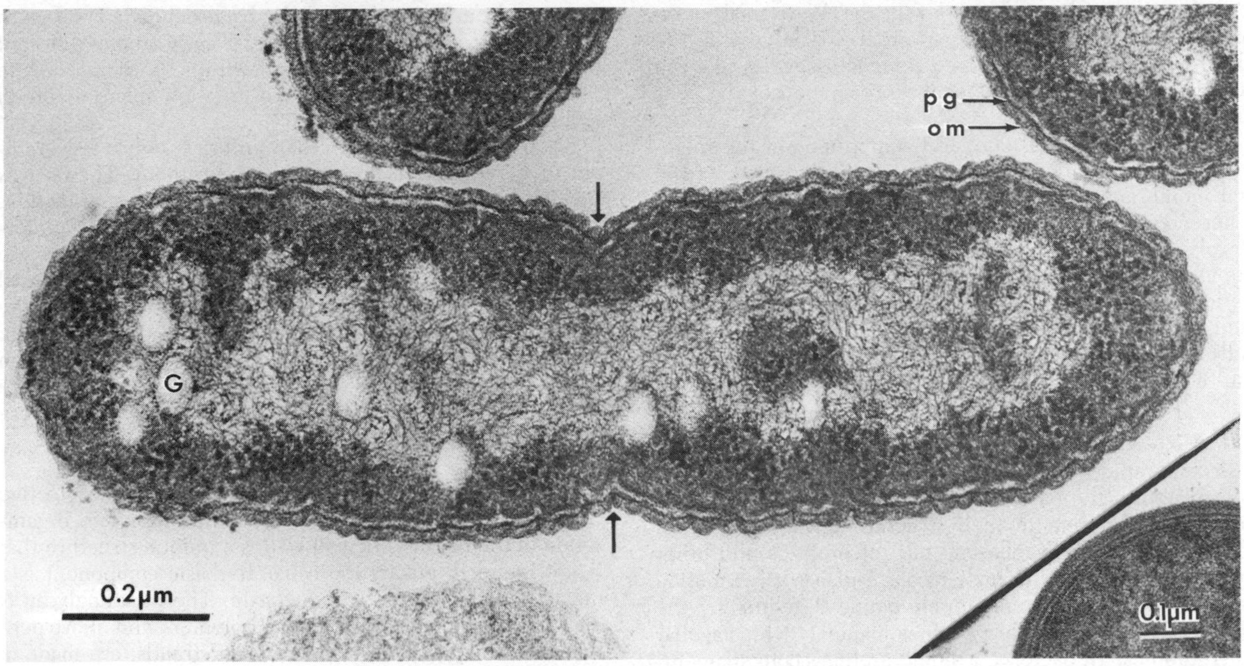

Figure 2. A typical rod-shaped gram-negative cell, *Chromobacterium violaceum,* is seen here in longitudinal and cross section. It contains several storage granules (G), probably poly-β-hydroxybutyric acid. This cell is in the process of division, as indicated by the inward constriction of the cell wall around the middle of the cell (arrows). The outer membrane and peptidoglycan layers of the cell wall may be seen. The insert at the lower right shows the wall of a gram-positive cell, *Bacillus sphaericus,* for comparison. (Insert courtesy of Drs. Stanley Holt and Donald Tipper, University of Massachusetts.)

antibiotic properties of polymyxin-B result from its interference with normal membrane permeability.

The electron transport system, the primary energy-generating system of the cell, is also located on the cell membrane. Thus, the membrane is the site where most chemical energy available through metabolism is converted into a form of energy (ATP) that can be used in the biosynthesis of cell materials or in other energy-requiring cellular reactions.

There is some evidence that the bacterial chromosome is attached to a special site on the cell membrane. This would provide a physical mechanism by which one of the two daughter chromosomes produced by DNA replication could be segregated into each of the daughter cells during cell division.

Generally, the bacterial membrane is found solely at the cell periphery. However, some bacterial cells exhibit complex infoldings or invaginations of the membrane into the cytoplasmic space (Fig. 3). These invaginations have been named *mesosomes* to distinguish them from the membrane proper and from the cytoplasm. This distinction may not be necessary, since mesosomes are not really separate bodies but rather extensions of the cell membrane. A number of efforts have been made to ascertain whether mesosomal invaginations have unique or specific functions. It has been suggested that they serve to increase the surface area of the cell membrane or that they represent specialized areas of the membrane; they are often seen in association with cell division or spore formation. However, to date no specialized functions have been conclusively

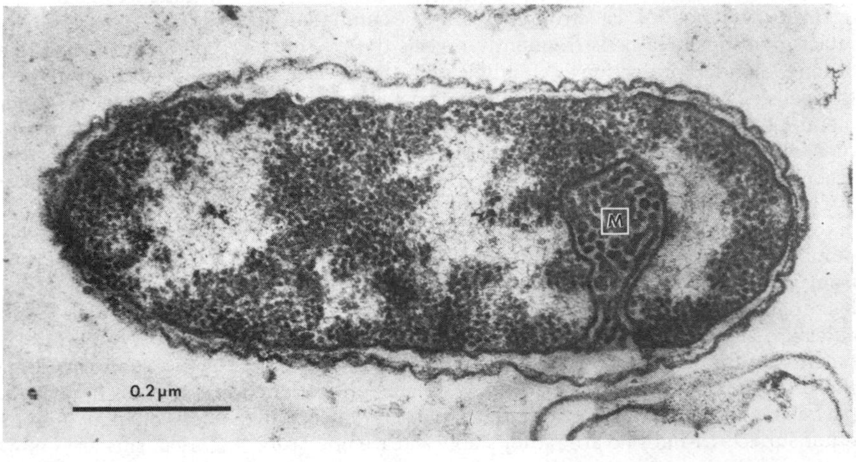

Figure 3. A *Chromobacterium violaceum* cell, showing a single large mesosome (M), a complex invagination of the cytoplasmic membrane.

demonstrated to be associated with the mesosomal membrane. Mesosomes have been observed only with the electron microscope, and some evidence suggests that the structures may be artifacts of the preparation of the cells for electron microscopy.

The appearance and chemical composition of the membrane of prokaryotic cells are quite similar to those of the cell membrane of eukaryotic cells. One notable chemical difference is that most bacterial membranes do not contain sterols (e.g., cholesterol) as do the membranes of higher life forms. In the bacterial cell, the cytoplasmic membrane performs many functions that are localized in the specialized organelles of higher cells. Thus, although the bacterial cell membrane may be simple in appearance, it is a multifunctional structure of extreme complexity.

FLAGELLA. A number of bacterial cell types demonstrate a striking rapid motility that is the product of a specialized cell structure, the bacterial *flagellum.* Bacterial flagella are completely different in their structure and mechanism of function from the flagella and cilia of protozoa and other eukaryotic cells. In the higher cells a planar wave motion is generated within a membrane-bound flagellum by the sliding action of multiple protein filaments, the flagellar microtubules. In bacteria, a single proteinaceous filament, about 15 nm in diameter, projects from the cell. At its base a complex structure, which is highly integrated with the cell wall and membrane, produces a rotary motion in the flagellar filament. The cell is driven forward by the propeller-like motion of the flagellum. The mechanism of operation of this fascinating, chemically driven rotary motor is currently under investigation.

Motility is also linked to membrane-bound receptors that identify the presence of specific molecules in the cell's environment. This phenomenon of *chemotaxis* allows bacteria to move toward higher concentrations of nutrients and away from harmful substances.

Bacterial flagella may be arranged in a diverse manner in different cell types. Some bacteria possess many flagella distributed over the entire surface of the cell (*peritrichous* flagella), whereas others possess a single flagellum or a bundle of flagella located at one pole of the cell (*polar* flagella). Special flagellar stains are used to enlarge the dimensions of the flagella artificially so that they may be observed with the light microscope. Motility versus nonmotility and the arrangement of flagella are useful diagnostic characteristics for identifying bacteria.

FIMBRIAE OR PILI. Electron microscopic examination of intact gram-negative cells frequently reveals the presence of long, slender projections extending from the surface of the cells. These projections, which originate at the cell membrane and extend through the cell wall, are of two types: the first are called *fimbriae,* or *common pili,* and the second are called *sex pili.*

The most common of these projections are the fimbriae, or common pili. Fimbriae are frequently found in large numbers (as many as several hundred per cell) projecting from the entire surface of freshly isolated gram-negative bacteria. They are made of a single protein, whose molecules are arranged in a helix to form a long filament. The function of fimbriae has not been completely clarified, but there is mounting evidence that these slender projections play a role in facilitating the adherence of bacterial cells to other surfaces. Fimbriae are rather stable and are not easily removed from the surface of the bacterial cell. The length and width of a common pilus vary greatly among different bacterial types but generally fall within the range of 3 to 15 nm in width and from 0.2 μm to a few micrometers in length.

Sex pili are less common than fimbriae; only a few gram-negative species are known to possess them. They act as specific bridges between bacterial cells during *conjugation,* a process in which unidirectional transfer of genetic information takes place between cells. The sex pilus has the form of a hollow tube, and it is believed that bacterial DNA migrates through the narrow central space of the pilus during conjugation. Sex pili are long (1 μm or more), relatively thick (about 25 nm), and very fragile. They can be broken by simple physical treatment. Very few (no more than ten) sex pili are found on bacteria that possess these fragile appendages.

CELL WALL. The wall of the bacterium confers protective rigidity to the cell. The chemical composition and organization of the prokaryotic cell wall is a unique structure that is not found in eukaryotic cells. Its basic component is a mixed polymer called *peptidoglycan.* The peptidoglycan is made of two components: linear polymers and short peptides. Linear polymers, called glycan strands, are made of two substituted hexose sugars—*N*-acetylglucosamine and *N*-acetylmuramic acid. These sugars are present in equal amounts and occupy alternate positions along the chains, which may contain dozens of sugar molecules. Short peptides—identical chains of four amino acids—attach to the glycan strand (but only to the *N*-acetylmuramic acid residues), thus forming side branches to the glycan strands. Some of these tetrapeptides are, in turn, linked to one another by other short peptides, forming cross-bridges between the glycan strands (Fig. 4). Peptidoglycan forms a single, bag-shaped macromolecule that surrounds the cytoplasmic membrane—conferring cell shape, countering the osmotic force exerted by the cell, and forming a physical barrier against the outside environment.

Besides the occurrence in peptidoglycan of the two unusual *N*-acetyl sugars, the peptide chains contain some amino acids that are found nowhere else except in bacterial cell walls. Among these are *meso*-diaminopimelic acid and the D-isomers of glutamic acid and alanine. (The amino acids found in all proteins are the L-isomers.)

Peptidoglycan is a major component in the walls of almost all bacterial cells. The composition of peptidoglycan is not absolutely uniform in different organisms; however, although considerable variation occurs in the type of amino acids in the tetrapeptide side-chain, in the type and number of amino acids that cross-link the tetrapeptides to one another, and in the extent of this cross-linking, no variation is found in the carbohydrate backbone of the glycan strand.

In a few unusual bacteria peptidoglycan is entirely lacking. The mycoplasmas (see Chapter 58) are a group of very small bacteria that have no cell wall, being only surrounded by a cytoplasmic membrane. This group of bacteria, which has several pathogenic members, is normally found in close association with eukaryotic cells. Another group, which has recently been designated the archebacteria, has a rigid wall formed of other polymers (glycoproteins and glycopeptides) instead of peptidoglycan. These organisms, such as *Halobacterium* and the methanogenic bacteria, have other unusual biochemical features and are found in extreme habitats of high temperature and salinity; no disease-causing organisms are known in this group.

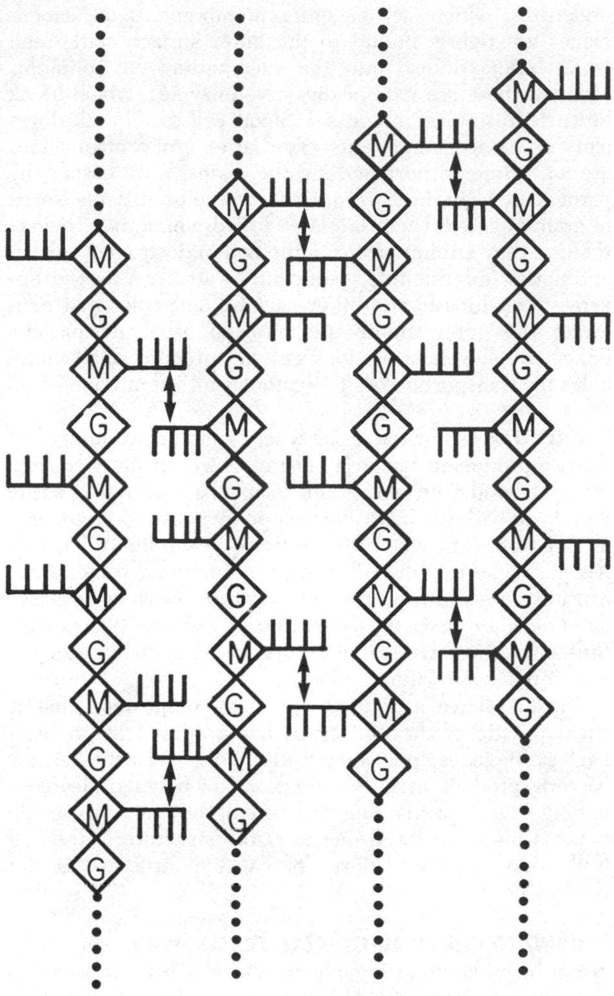

Figure 4. This diagram schematically represents the structure of peptidoglycan. The glycan strands are composed of alternating units of *N*-acetylglucosamine (G) and *N*-acetylmuramic acid (M). Tetrapeptide side chains connect to the muramic acid residues. Some of the tetrapeptides are joined by other peptides (short arrows) to form cross-bridges between the glycan strands; the degree and nature of cross-linking vary in different organisms and are generally most extensive in gram-negative bacteria.

With the exception of the archebacteria just mentioned, bacteria can be divided into two major groups on the basis of their cell wall structure. The first, *gram-negative* organisms, have a thin peptidoglycan layer adjacent to the cytoplasmic membrane, plus other major cell wall components exterior to the peptidoglycan. Examples of gram-negative bacteria are *Escherichia, Salmonella, Pseudomonas, Treponema*, and *Chlamydia*. The second, *gram-positive* organisms, have a much thicker peptidoglycan structure, consisting of many layers (although they are not visible as such with the electron microscope) of peptidoglycan, making a total cell wall thickness of 10 to 100 nm (Figs. 2 and 5). Peptidoglycan represents the major component of the gram-positive cell wall, although minor components known as teichoic acids are also present. Examples of gram-positive bacteria include *Bacillus, Streptococcus, Staphylococcus*, and *Clostridium*.

The original basis of division of bacteria into gram-negative and gram-positive forms was the staining procedure devised almost 100 years ago by the Danish physician Christian Gram. This stain, which is still in common clinical use for diagnostic purposes, involves four steps: Cells are 1) stained with crystal violet; 2) treated with iodine to form a crystal violet–iodine complex; 3) washed with an organic solvent such as alcohol; and 4) stained again with safranin. In gram-positive cells the purple dye complex is retained, whereas in gram-negative cells the dye complex is removed by the solvent. Thus gram-positive cells appear purple under the microscope; gram-negative cells are counterstained by the safranin and appear red. Although the exact mechanism of the staining reaction is not known, it appears that the staining occurs within the cell, not on the cell wall, and that the thicker peptidoglycan wall of the gram-positive cell protects the dye-iodine complex to a greater extent from the action of the solvent.

Since the cell wall of gram-positive bacteria consists of a layer of peptidoglycan that may be many times thicker than the peptidoglycan of the gram-negative cell wall, gram-positive cells tend to be sturdier and less susceptible to breakage by physical forces. In contrast, the presence in the gram-negative cell of other cell wall components in addition to peptidoglycan gives those bacteria certain advantages.

The gram-negative cell wall contains significant amounts of lipoprotein and lipopolysaccharide in association with its peptidoglycan. This layer of lipid material is seen as a membrane in electron micrographs, lying just outside the thin peptidoglycan layer (see Fig. 2); this structure is called the *outer membrane*. Although it does not have the many complex enzymatic functions of the cytoplasmic membrane, the outer membrane is known to act as an intricate molecular sieve. Permeability through the outer membrane is made possible by transmembrane channels formed by three types of outer membrane proteins. The major class of these proteins, the porins, permits passive diffusion of solutes by

Figure 5. These diagrams compare the structures of the gram-positive and the gram-negative bacterial cell walls, indicating the relative positions of the cytoplasmic membrane and the bacterial capsule.

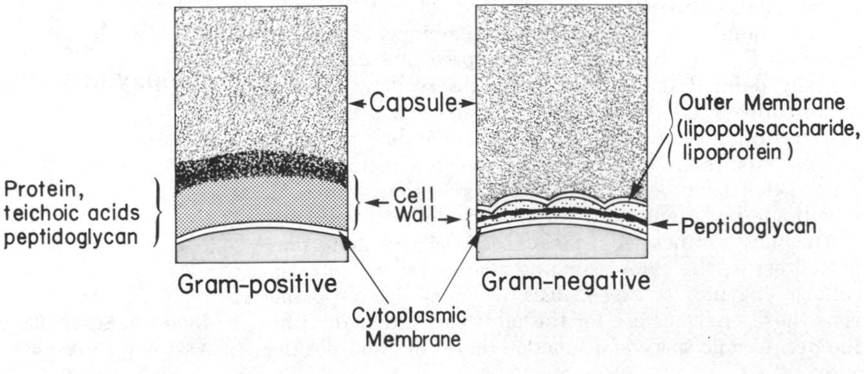

functioning as hydrophilic channels; the small size of these channels generally excludes large molecules. A second class of proteins serves as facilitators, but not as carriers, for the penetration of specific carbohydrates and nucleosides; a final group of outer membrane proteins serves as carriers for translocation of specific substrates.

An example of an advantage that gram-negative cells possess, due to the exclusion properties of the outer membrane, is a lower susceptibility to the naturally occurring hydrolytic enzyme *lysozyme*. Lysozyme is widespread in nature and specifically attacks peptidoglycan by cleaving the bonds of the glycan strand between *N*-acetylmuramic acid and *N*-acetylglucosamine. In the absence of the protective peptidoglycan layer, the bacterial cell swells excessively owing to osmotic forces. Eventually the cytoplasmic membrane ruptures from the internal pressure. The walls of gram-positive cells are generally quite sensitive to degradation by lysozyme. Gram-negative bacteria are less susceptible to such attack, since the outer membrane excludes lysozyme and prevents it from binding to its site of action on the cell wall's peptidoglycan.

The uniqueness of bacterial peptidoglycan has proved to be particularly useful in the treatment of many bacterial diseases. The biosynthesis of peptidoglycan can be disturbed by a number of antibiotics, including penicillin. The sensitive target of penicillin action is one of the final chemical reactions in peptidoglycan synthesis—the one that effects the linking of the peptide side chains. Thus, the drug prevents cross-bridges from being formed between the glycan strands. Without this bonding the integrity of the peptidoglycan is weakened, producing a fragile wall that cannot protect the cell adequately.

Since penicillin interferes with peptidoglycan synthesis, and since such synthesis does not occur in eukaryotic cells, cells of the animal body are resistant to the primary action of penicillin. Penicillin affects sensitive bacteria only when the cell wall is being synthesized, since it blocks synthesis rather than attacking existing peptidoglycan, as does lysozyme. Thus, if a penicillin-sensitive cell is not growing at the time the antibiotic is used, the cell wall will not be affected. Gram-negative bacteria are significantly less susceptible to the antibiotic action of penicillin than are gram-positive bacteria. This difference, as with lysozyme, is primarily the result of the protective effect of the outer membrane of the gram-negative cell wall, which makes it difficult for the penicillin molecule to reach its site of inhibition. However, forms of penicillin have been synthesized that can penetrate this barrier and attack gram-negative organisms.

Although we said above that bacterial cells are not compartmentalized into organelles, one important compartment does exist. This is the *periplasmic space*, defined in gram-negative bacteria as the space between the cytoplasmic membrane and the outer membrane of the cell wall (see Fig. 5). It is a functional space, not a morphologically defined space that can be observed by electron microscopy; it is occupied by small molecules that have passed through the outer membrane but not the cytoplasmic membrane and by large molecules, including enzymes, that have been transported across the cytoplasmic membrane but cannot pass through the outer membrane.

Enzymes synthesized by the bacterial cell and transported across the cytoplasmic membrane are called extracellular enzymes or *exoenzymes;* in gram-negative organisms these enzymes are for the most part retained within the periplasmic space and function there. In gram-positive organisms, which lack an outer membrane, some exoenzymes are tightly bound to the outer surface of the cell while others diffuse into the surrounding environment. Many of these are lytic or digestive enzymes, which break down large molecules, attack blood cells, or break down clots or tissue components. The latter group of enzymes are of prime importance in the damage of tissues by pathogenic bacteria. Enzymes within the periplasmic space of gram-negative bacteria play a less dramatic role; nevertheless, they are important to the cell in destroying certain antibiotics (for example, penicillin is attacked by the enzyme penicillinase) and other harmful molecules that penetrate the outer membrane. Several other periplasmic enzymes (phosphatases, for example) prepare small molecules for transport across the cytoplasmic membrane.

CAPSULE. A few bacterial types, including a number of disease-producing bacteria, manufacture an inert capsule that surrounds the entire cell. Capsular material is easily visualized with the light microscope by negative stains such as India ink. The role of the capsule in the life of bacteria has yet to be established; however, for some bacteria the capsule serves as a protective structure. Certain encapsulated cells are resistant to ingestion by animal phagocytes; thus, these bacteria cannot be destroyed by the phagocytic line of defense of animal blood.

Capsules have a defined chemical composition that is characteristic of the cell type that produces it. In most bacteria the capsule is composed of polysaccharides. A few bacteria produce capsules composed of polypeptides containing D amino acids. The structure of the bacterial capsule is not a highly ordered one as is the structure of the cell wall, thus a general form of capsule structure is not recognized.

VARIATIONS IN BACTERIAL FORM. Within the large group of prokaryotic organisms, there is a great range in the size and shape of individual cells (Fig. 6). Some are at the limit of visibility of the light microscope; others are as

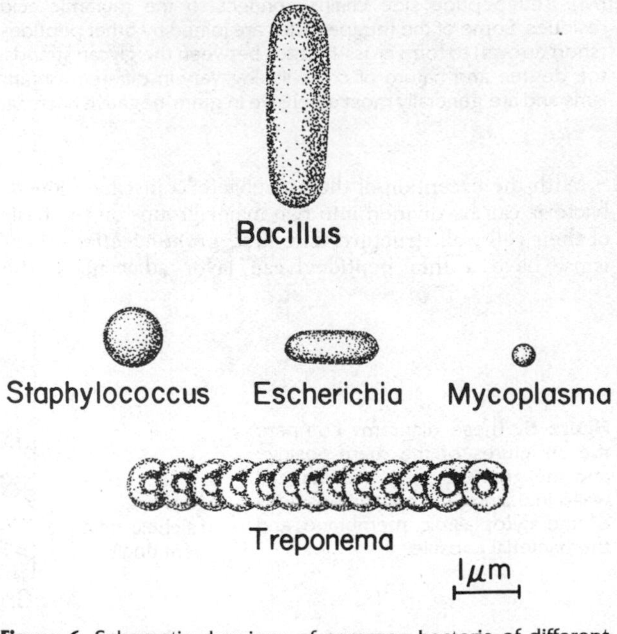

Figure 6. Schematic drawings of common bacteria of different sizes and shapes are illustrated here.

large as some eukaryotic cells. Common cell shapes include spheres (cocci), rods (bacilli), comma shapes (vibrio), and spirals (spirillum, spirochete). Cell size and shape are valuable diagnostic characteristics and are readily seen with the light microscope.

Another diagnostic characteristic of bacteria is the way in which cells do or do not remain associated during growth. They may exist as solitary individuals, or they may remain attached in random clusters, in linear chains, or in ordered sheets or packets.

Although all the cells of an individual animal originate from a single fertilized egg cell, they show many forms in the adult, meaning that they have *differentiated* to perform certain specialized functions within the organism. When a single bacterial cell divides many times to form a colony of cells, the cells in that colony may be associated in characteristic spatial arrangements, as described previously, but all individuals are usually identical in form. Differentiation of cells as found in higher organisms does not occur in bacteria; but something akin to it occurs when special cells are formed with certain reproductive functions. The myxobacteria and the actinomycetes are examples of bacteria that have elaborate growth habits and produce fruiting bodies that bear spores.

Of more practical importance are the formation of *endospores* by certain gram-positive organisms. An endospore results when part of a cell, including the nucleoid and some cytoplasm, is walled off from the rest of the mother cell. A complex multilayered wall structure then forms around it (Fig. 7). The total process is called *sporulation.* The resulting endospore demonstrates no metabolic activity and is highly resistant to radiation, chemicals, desiccation, and heat. This dormant stage represents a powerful mechanism for both dispersal and cell survival under adverse conditions. Since spores are relatively large refractile bodies, they may be seen with the light microscope. Their presence or absence and the position of the spore within the mother cell (median or terminal) are another set of useful diagnostic characteristics.

Under favorable circumstances the endospore is able to germinate rapidly. Metabolic activity resumes, and the spore swells and breaks open to release a cell identical to the one that originally produced the endospore. Such a cell, although again sensitive to heat and other adverse environmental conditions, can resume normal growth.

The organization of endospores differs substantially from that of vegetative (growing) cells. New structures are produced during sporulation as a result of the expression of specific bacterial genes. Among the new structures formed is a spore coat composed of a thin yet highly organized layer of extremely hydrophobic proteins. Also produced is the spore cortex, which lies between the spore coat and the significantly reduced cell protoplast. The cortex may be thick and is composed of a unique peptidoglycan; as such it may be analogous to the cell wall of the vegetative cell. As the spore is forming, large amounts of calcium are taken up, and corresponding quantities of dipicolinic acid are synthesized. This chemical combination appears to be responsible for the spore's heat resistance.

The production of endospores is limited to a small number of bacterial types, primarily *Bacillus, Clostridium,* and *Sporosarcina.* However, because of the extreme resistance of endospores to inactivation by physical and chemical means, endospore-forming bacteria are of major importance to human society. Most nonspore-forming bacteria are readily destroyed by boiling, but much higher temperatures are required to kill endospores (for example, autoclaving at 121° C for 20 minutes). Thus, sterilization procedures must acknowledge the high resistance of bacterial endospores even though the actual number of endospores in a given environment may be rather small.

SUMMARY. Bacteria are enormously diverse in their form, habitat, and metabolic patterns. The outline of bacterial cell structure presented here represents a series of rather broad generalizations. They are based, of necessity, on those organisms that have been the subject of the most thorough investigation because of their importance in med-

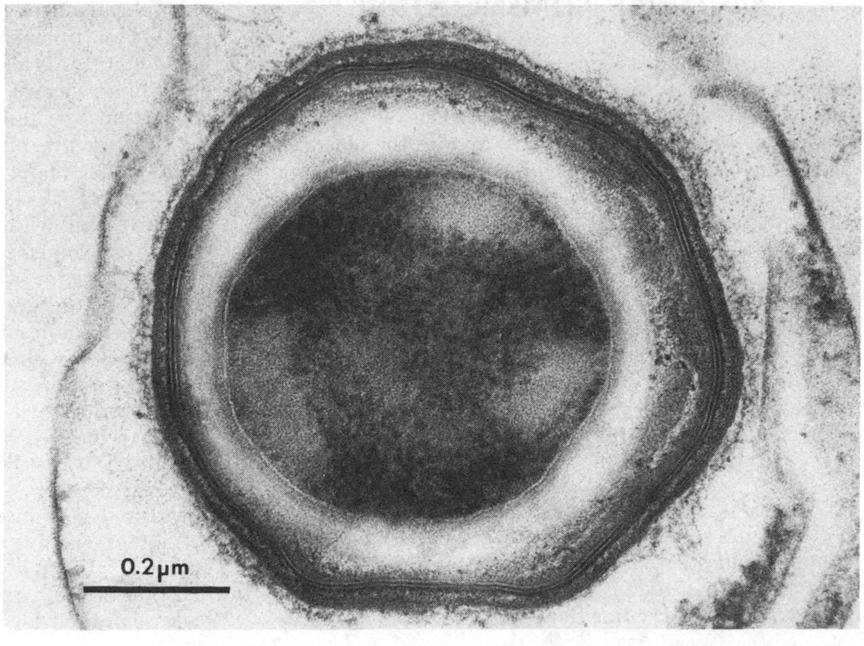

Figure 7. This electron micrograph of a bacterial endospore of *Bacillus sphaericus* illustrates the complex layer structure of the spore wall. The spore is surrounded by remnants of the mother cell. (Courtesy of Drs. Stanley Holt and Donald Tipper, University of Massachusetts.)

icine, industry, or laboratory research. Consequently, gaps in our knowledge and exceptions to our generalizations will occur, particularly among the less common and more poorly studied groups of bacteria.

We can draw an overall conclusion, however: Although bacteria are generally smaller and appear simpler in their organization than the cells of animals and plants, this simplicity is only relative. Bacteria perform a variety of cellular functions common to all living systems and other functions that are peculiar to the prokaryotic kingdom; their biochemical and physiologic machinery is quite complex.

References

Costerton, J. W., Ingram, J. M., and Cheng, K. J.: Structure and function of the cell envelope of Gram-negative bacteria. Bacteriol Rev 38:87, 1974.

Doetsch, R. N., and Sjoblad, R. D.: Flagellar structure and function in Eubacteria. Annu Rev Microbiol 34:69, 1980.

Fox, G. E., et al.: The phylogeny of procaryotes. Science 209:477, 1980.

Fuller, R., and Lovelock, D. W., (eds.): Microbial Ultrastructure, New York, Academic Press, 1976.

Greenwalt, J. W., and Whiteside, T. C.: Mesosomes: Membranous bacterial organelles. Bacteriol Rev 39:405, 1975.

Holt, S. C., Gauthier, J. J., and Tipper, D. J.: Ultrastructural studies of sporulation in *Bacillus sphaericus*. J Bacteriol 122:1322, 1975.

Kandler, O., and König, H.: Chemical composition of the peptidoglycan—free cell walls of methanogenic bacteria. Arch Microbiol 118:141, 1978.

Kleppe, K., Overbö, S, Lossius, I.: The bacterial nucleoid. J Gen Microbiol, 112:1, 1979.

Nikaido, H., and Nakae, T.: The outer membrane of Gram-negative bacteria. Adv Microb Physiol 20:163, 1979.

Osborn, M. J., and Wu, H. C. P.: Proteins of the outer membrane of Gram-negative bacteria. Annu Rev Microbiol. 34:369, 1980.

Salton, M. R. J., and Owne, P.: Bacterial membrane structure, Annu Rev Microbiol, 30:451, 1976.

Schleifer, K. H., and Kandler, O.: Peptidoglycan types of bacterial cell walls and their taxonomic implications. Bacteriol Rev 36:407, 1972.

Stanier, R. Y., Adelberg, E. A., and Ingraham, J.: The Microbial World, Englewood Cliffs, N.J., Prentice-Hall, Inc., 1976.

Stanier, R. Y., Rogers, H. J., and Ward, J. B. (eds.): Relations Between Structure and Function in the Procaryotic Cell, No. 28 of Symposia of the Society for General Microbiology, London, Cambridge University Press, 1978.

2

CLASSIFICATION AND IDENTIFICATION OF BACTERIA

CHARLES E. DAVIS, M.D.
AND HERMAN BAER, M.D.

Classification is the orderly arrangement of sets of organisms into a system; nomenclature deals with the naming or labeling of these organisms; and the recognition and allocation of an unknown organism is called identification. Classification, nomenclature, and identification are the three interdependent essentials of taxonomy.

BACTERIAL NOMENCLATURE

The naming of bacteria is subject to the rules and recommendations of the Bacteriological Code; the need to comply with the Code has been responsible for many changes in bacterial nomenclature. As with the nomenclature of higher organisms, bacterial nomenclature is binomial: The designation of the genus is given first, with the first letter capitalized; the species designation, which is given a lower case first letter, follows the designation of the genus.

The shifting of an organism into a different genus will automatically change its generic name. Since there are no rules for classification, the rearrangement of organisms is more or less left to the whim of the taxonomist. Frequent changes of the generic designations of bacteria are the unfortunate consequence.

BACTERIAL CLASSIFICATION

The classification of higher organisms is designed to reflect natural relatedness and phylogenetic relationships. It is hierarchic, proceeding from the large taxonomic groups to the species. In bacteria, studies of phylogenetic relationships are only beginning (see further on). In general, the hierarchic approach has met with limited success in bacterial classification, and its use has been sharply reduced in the 1974 edition of *Bergey's Manual of Determinative Bacteriology*, the standard work on bacterial classification. The species is the fundamental unit of bacterial classification, and taxonomic ranks higher than the genus have limited importance, with the exception of the family Enterobacteriaceae (see Chapter 31).

In the conventional approach to bacterial classification, the genera of medically important bacteria are grouped together according to certain easily observable and relatively constant properties.

Staining Reactions. The *gram reaction* is by far the most important of these properties. The gram stain, which was devised by Christian Gram in 1884, divides bacteria into two fundamentally different categories, gram-positive and gram-negative. Infected material obtained directly from patients or from small portions of bacterial colonies or liquid cultures is allowed to dry in air and is heat fixed on glass slides before treatment with gram's reagents. All conventional bacteria are stained purple by crystal violet, the primary dye of the gram stain. After treatment with gram's iodine (3 per cent I_2-KI at pH 8.0), which complexes with the crystal violet, only gram-positive bacteria resist decolorization with alcohol, ether, or acetone. Because they have retained the crystal violet, gram-positive bacteria do not color with safranin, the red counterstain used in the last step of the gram stain. Gram-negative bacteria stain red from the safranin because they lose the crystal violet when treated with decolorizing agents. The gram-positive cell wall itself does not stain. Instead, it presents a permeability barrier to elution of the crystal violet-iodine complex from the interior of the cell by the decolorizing agent. Gram-negative walls contain lipopolysaccharide and thinner, less complex peptidoglycan (see Chapter 1) that do not resist penetration of the cell by the decolorizers.

Another staining reaction used in the classification of bacteria is the *Ziehl-Neelsen (acid-fast) stain.* Mycobacteria (Chapter 44) are difficult to stain by ordinary techniques because of their high content of waxes and lipids. They are stained red, however, when they are flooded for five to seven minutes with carbol fuchsin that is kept steaming hot by placing the glass slide over a flame or on a hot plate during the staining. All bacteria are stained by this procedure, but only mycobacteria retain the carbol fuchsin when treated with 3 per cent HCl in alcohol (acid-fast). After decolorization, other bacteria are stained by a cold counterstain such as methylene blue to contrast with the red mycobacteria. Nocardia (see Chapter 45) do not stain with the conventional Ziehl-Neelsen stain but remain red (acid-fast) if they are decolorized either by 1 per cent sulfuric acid or brief exposure to 3 per cent HCl. The "firmly bound" lipids of mycobacteria, which are resistant to extraction by organic solvents, are responsible for the acid-fastness of mycobacteria (see Chapter 44).

Morphology. Microscopically, bacterial cells can be identified as either spherical (cocci) or rod-shaped (bacilli). Cocci may be arranged singly, or in pairs, clusters, or chains. Rod-shaped bacteria may be straight and regular or they may be club-shaped, curved, or spiral-shaped, or they may have pointed ends. Microscopic examination reveals the presence of spores. With the help of special staining procedures, the presence, number, and arrangement of flagella are noted. Flagella may be distributed over the entire surface of the cell (peritrichous) or they may be limited to the poles (polar).

Metabolic Reactions. The reaction to atmospheric oxygen separates bacteria into aerobic, facultative (capable of either aerobic or anaerobic growth), and strictly anaerobic organisms. The study of nutritional requirements, or the ability to grow on certain kinds of culture media, provides useful information for classification. The mode of attack on carbohydrates, usually glucose, is of taxonomic significance: Glucose is degraded anaerobically in the absence of atmospheric oxygen by the so-called fermentative organisms. Oxidative organisms require atmospheric oxygen for the degradation of glucose. Other organisms fail to metabolize glucose at all. This fermentative (F) versus oxidative (O) metabolism of carbohydrates is determined in the so-called OF test in which part of the media is exposed to air and part is anaerobic. Other characteristics thought to be of fundamental taxonomic significance include the enzyme catalase, which decomposes H_2O_2, and oxidase, which transfers hydrogen directly from its substrate to oxygen.

The properties just described and others have been used successfully by bacteriologists for many years to classify bacteria and have been accepted as fundamental and important; that is, they were weighted heavily in the classification. With the help of these properties, medically important bacteria can often be divided to the generic level, or placed into a group of genera. This is illustrated in the following list in an oversimplified fashion for the classification of some medically important gram-positive cocci:

Facultatively anaerobic, arranged in clusters, catalase-positive:
- fermentative: *Staphylococcus*
- oxidative: *Micrococcus*

Facultatively anaerobic, arranged in pairs or chains, catalase-negative: *Streptococcus*

Anaerobic, arranged in clusters, catalase-variable: *Peptococcus*

The definition of the various species within a genus is based on a set of physiologic and biochemical characteristics, including the degradation of carbohydrates, amino acids, and a variety of other substrates. Certain characteristics are quite constant and highly discriminating—they separate otherwise very similar species. For example, among all species of staphylococci, the production of coagulase is unique to *Staphylococcus aureus* and has become part of the definition of the species.

Coagulase is an enzyme that causes clotting of citrated or oxalated plasma by reacting with the coagulase-reacting factor (prothrombin) to activate thrombin. Coagulase-positive staphylococci usually also produce clumping factor ("bound coagulase") that causes macroscopic agglutination of the staphylococci when they are mixed with plasma on a glass slide. More commonly, bacterial species are defined by means of a whole pattern of biochemical properties.

Many bacterial species have been subdivided further by a variety of techniques, including antigen analysis, biochemical reactions, and susceptibility to bacteriophages—viruses that penetrate and lyse bacteria. The resulting serotypes, biotypes, and phage types have considerable clinical and epidemiologic significance.

The fact that the conventional scheme of bacterial classification is artificial and based on arbitrarily chosen criteria has not detracted from its great practical usefulness. Although it has never been possible to define the concept of the bacterial species satisfactorily, the operational value of the concept of bacterial species to medicine and epidemiology has been immense.

In recent years, new approaches to bacterial classification have evolved in an effort to supplant the conventional taxonomy by a more rational system. These include the Adansonian method of classification, or numerical classification, and the study of DNA-relatedness.

ADANSONIAN AND NUMERICAL CLASSIFICATION. Numerical classification was developed by Adanson and applied by him successfully to the taxonomy of groups of higher organisms. Instead of studying a relatively small number of properties considered to be important, a very large number of characteristics is examined, each of which is assigned equal weight. Taxonomic groups are established on the basis of the overall similarity of organisms. Similarity between two organisms can be expressed as the similarity coefficient, which is defined as the percentage of shared properties among all the properties tested. (Only those tests that give a positive result with at least one of the organisms are used for determination of the similarity coefficient.) If two organisms show a similarity coefficient of about 90, they are likely to belong to the same species.

The massive amounts of data generated by the study of a large number of properties of a great many strains is best handled by a computer. The greatest value of this so-called numerical taxonomy or numerical classification system lies in the re-evaluation of the conventional classification of groups of bacteria. Numerical classification has confirmed the appropriateness of the classification of many organisms and has suggested the reclassification of others.

CLASSIFICATION BY DNA-RELATEDNESS. The emerging field of genetic or molecular taxonomy is based on the analysis of bacterial DNA (Brenner and Falkow, 1971). In contrast to conventional taxonomy, this method can be expected to discover phylogenetic relationships among organisms and therefore provide a truly natural classification.

The degree to which organisms are related can be evaluated by the number of genes they have in common. Organisms of the same species would be expected to share most of their genes. As a consequence, the nucleotide composition and sequence of their DNA should be very similar. Techniques for determining the nucleotide sequence of nucleic acids are available, and the complete base sequence of several small viruses is known. It seems likely that this will have a major impact on the recognition of phylogenetic relationships among viruses. However, it is not practical to determine the base sequence of the much larger bacterial chromosome at the present time. Other criteria to determine the DNA-relatedness of two bacteria include the comparison of the nucleotide base composition of their DNA, the degree to which their DNA will hybridize, and the ability of their DNA to undergo recombination.

The nucleotide base composition of DNA varies widely among different groups of bacteria and is characteristic for bacteria of the same genus. Since adenine (A) pairs with thymine (T), and guanine (G) pairs with cytosine (C), the percentage of each nucleotide in double-stranded DNA can be expressed by the formula AT + GC = 100 per cent. It is customary to express the base composition of DNA in terms of its GC content, which can vary from 22 per cent to 74 per cent for bacterial DNA. Bacteria with a different GC content have few base sequences in common and therefore have different genes and cannot be closely related. Conversely, organisms with a similar GC content may or may not be closely related, since a similarity in GC content does not necessarily mean that the base sequences are similar. For example, *E. coli*, a gram-negative bacillus of the family Enterobacteriaceae, and certain species of *Bacillus*, spore-forming gram-positive bacilli, have a GC content of 50 per cent, but are clearly unrelated. Determination of the nucleotide base composition is a powerful tool in reassessing the conventional classification of bacteria, and it is widely used for that purpose. For example, the genus *Micrococcus* appeared reasonably homogeneous by the usual bacteriologic criteria; however, some micrococci were found to have a GC content of 30 to 37 per cent, which corresponds to the GC content of staphylococci, instead of 66 to 75 per cent, which is typical of the other micrococci. Hence, these micrococci have been reclassified as staphylococci.

Hybridization is used to determine the degree to which base sequences of the DNA of two organisms are shared, or "homologous." The procedure for the hybridization experiment is performed as follows: The DNA of one organism is made radioactive biosynthetically, extracted from the bacteria, sheared into small fragments, and mixed with a large excess of nonradioactive DNA from the other organism. The mixture is heated to achieve separation of the DNA into single strands. After cooling, the complementary strands of DNA reanneal into double-stranded DNA. If the two organisms are related, they have many base sequences in common, and radioactive fragments will reanneal with nonradioactive complementary DNA. The percentage of radioactive DNA bound to nonradioactive DNA can be used to estimate the degree of complementarity and therefore the genetic relatedness between the organisms. Hybridization has been used extensively to study DNA homology between members of the family Enterobacteriaceae and has great potential for supplying new information on the taxonomy of other groups of organisms.

Under certain conditions, DNA can be transferred from one organism to another by the mechanisms of transformation, transduction, and conjugation (see Chapter 4). The transferred (donor) DNA can recombine with the resident (host) DNA to produce a genetic change that may manifest itself as a newly acquired property—for example, antibiotic resistance. It is assumed that two organisms are closely related if their DNA can recombine. Recombination generally involves small pieces of DNA that are equivalent to only a few genes, and many factors other than gene similarity influence recombination rates. It must also be kept in mind that transfer of extrachromosomal genetic material (plasmids) can occur between organisms that are taxonomically unrelated.

Transformation and recombination have been used successfully for taxonomic studies of *Neisseria*, *Moraxella*, and related organisms, but recombination is less universally applicable than other methods of determining DNA-relatedness.

BACTERIAL IDENTIFICATION

Bacterial classification is a basic science; in contrast, bacterial identification is an applied discipline of microbiology with great practical significance. The identification of a bacterium suspected of being the cause of an infection is one of the major tools for the objective diagnosis of infectious diseases. The approach to the identification of bacterial isolates in the diagnostic laboratory is quite different from that taken by the bacterial taxonomist in the classification of a new or unknown organism. The taxonomist will study as many characteristics as possible; time and cost are of little concern. In contrast, in order to be clinically useful and relevant, the identification of a clinical isolate must be provided as quickly as possible. Economics and practicality dictate the use of only a minimal number of diagnostic tests (Bartlett, 1974). Thus, by necessity, identification in the clinical laboratory will always represent a compromise between accuracy on the one hand, and speed and economy on the other. Just how this compromise is made will determine the quality of a laboratory.

The practical limitation on the number of properties that can be used for identification of bacteria makes the selection of the diagnostic tests very important. The same properties of bacteria that are used in the conventional classification are employed in the identification of clinical isolates. For this reason, identification is sometimes referred to as "classification in reverse."

A hierarchic set of tables permits the identification process to proceed in a rational, stepwise fashion. A logical, practical example of a hierarchic set of diagnostic tables for medically important bacteria is presented by Cowan and Steel (1974). In the first stage of identification, the unknown organism is assigned either to a single genus or to a group of genera with the help of a small number of characteristics. The groups of organisms established by the first set of tests are differentiated to the species level by one or two additional sets of biochemical or serologic tests. The obvious advantage of this stepwise approach to identification is that it requires fewer tests than the shotgun approach, in which a very large number of tests is performed initially.

A diagnostic key is indispensable for the objective identification of clinical isolates in the modern laboratory. Nevertheless, a key is useless without consideration of the time-honored methods of the Gram stain, colonial morphology, and growth characteristics.

Examples of diagnostic keys or flow sheets based on these stable characteristics are given in Tables 1 through 7. The first-stage tables (Tables 1 and 2) classify medically important bacteria according to their gram reactions and microscopic morphology. This type of classification system reflects the thinking of the experienced microbiologist when he analyzes gram stains of primary material from patients and is often the only guide to treatment during the first 24 hours. The second-stage tables (Tables 3 through 7) illustrate the identification of medically important bacteria according to growth characteristics, ability to grow in the presence of oxygen, colonial morphology, pigment production, motility, and the presence of certain stable enzymes such as catalase, oxidase, or coagulase. These simple observations permit the rapid determination of the genera of many bacteria and both the genera and species of a surprisingly large number of bacteria. More important, attention to these major, easily established properties prevents naive errors. Laboratories that use the gram stain and pure single colony bacteriology as the cornerstones of bacterial identification will not misidentify a gram-negative bacillus as a gram-positive bacillus or a coccus just because the biochemical reactions are similar.

Third-stage tables that involve second or third subcultures into biochemical media are not included in this chapter. When a subculture into one or two simple, defined media permits identification of a bacterium to the species level, this step is included in the second-stage tables. The appendix to this chapter provides a glossary explaining some of these reactions. Additional information about the definitive identification of medically important species is provided in Part One of this book.

Gram-positive bacteria (Table 1) are easily divided into cocci and bacilli on the basis of microscopic morphology. Careful consideration of cell shape as well as the usual search for chains or tetrads virtually always separates streptococci from staphylococci. *Clostridium* and *Bacillus* cannot be differentiated from one another by gram stain and microscopic morphology, but are readily differentiated from the other gram-positive bacilli. The typical club-shaped, palisading *Corynebacterium* and the extensively branched, beaded, filamentous *Nocardia* or *Actinomyces israelii* are also distinctive, but the remainder of the gram-positive rods are more difficult to separate microscopically. *Propionibacterium*, *Listeria*, and *Erysipelothrix* are usually indistinguishable from diphtheroids (corynebacteria). In contrast, *Propionibacterium* and *Erysipelothrix* may also be filamentous and indistinguishable from other filamentous bacteria with rudimentary branching. Although extensive branching is a uniform characteristic of *A. israelii* and *Nocardia*, the other *Actinomyces* species and *Arachnia* may exhibit only rudimentary branching. *Nocardia* may be separated from *Actinomyces* and *Streptomyces* by its tendency to retain carbol fuchsin in the acid-fast stain. The

Table 1. CLASSIFICATION OF MEDICALLY IMPORTANT BACTERIA BY STAINING REACTIONS AND MICROSCOPIC MORPHOLOGY*
FIRST-STAGE TABLE

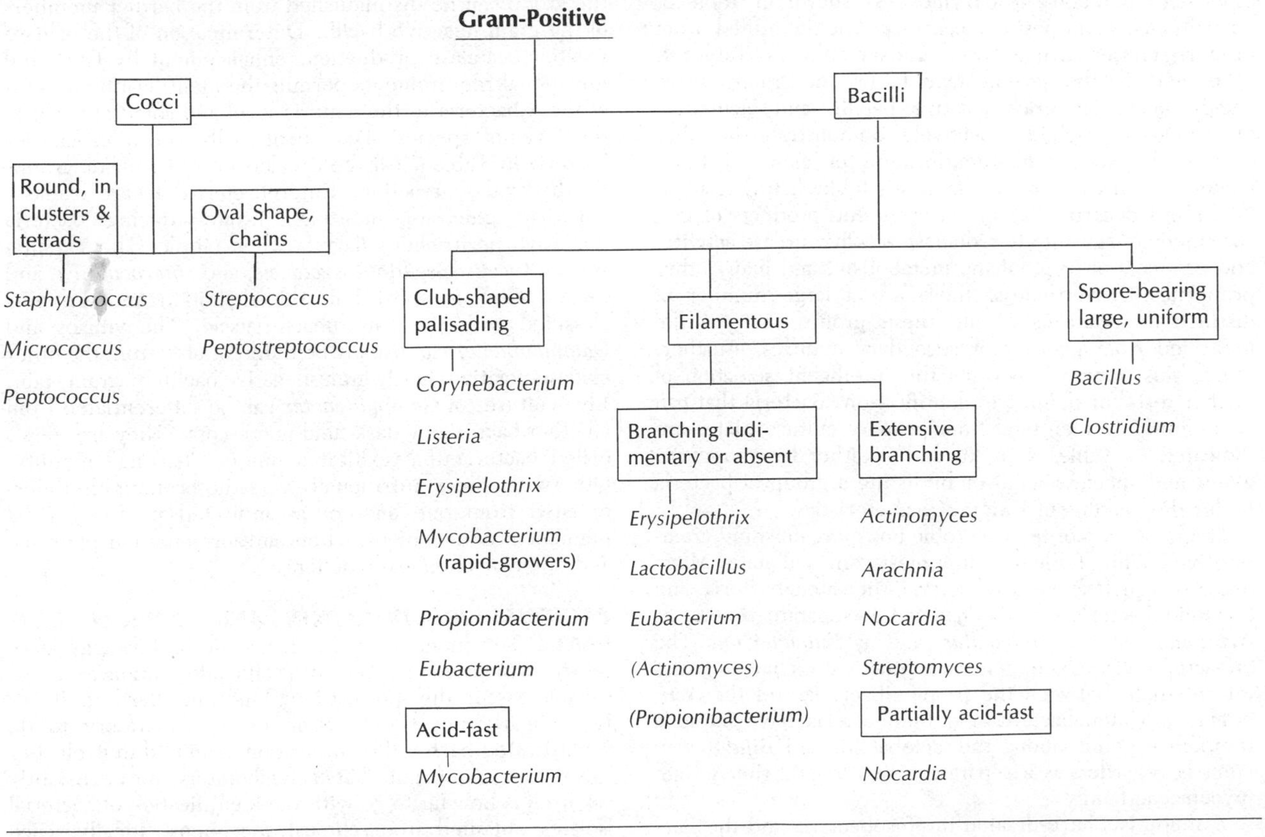

*Bacteria are listed in parenthesis when another shape or arrangement occurs more commonly.

rapid-growing, atypical mycobacteria, which take the gram stain well, may be distinguished from other club-shaped bacteria by the Ziehl-Neelsen stain.

The gram-negative bacteria shown in Table 2 are more difficult to separate by microscopic morphology, but can readily be separated into cocci, the pleomorphic group, and the uniformly shaped, larger Enterobacteriaceae-Pseudomonas group. In addition, the following bacteria can frequently be identified accurately by microscopy: *Neisseria* (kidney-shaped diplococci with flattened apposing edges), the *Acinetobacter-Moraxella* group (a mixture of *Neisseria*-like and bacillary forms), *Brucella* (tiny, faintly staining bacilli), *Bacteroides* (small, uniformly encapsulated bacilli with occasional filamentous forms), *Haemophilus* (similar to *Bacteroides* but more pleomorphic with a larger population of filamentous forms), *Fusobacterium nucleatum* (severely pointed with a rigid, crystalline appearance), *Fusobacterium necrophorum* (spheroplastic), and *Vibrio* (when markedly comma-shaped). *Campylobacter* can usually be differentiated from *Vibrio* and all other bacteria by its small, gull-shaped or spiral appearance and its poor staining with safranin. Generally, the Enterobacteriaceae cannot be separated microscopically from one another or from the other bacteria listed in the group with uniform shape. Although most of the coccobacillary, pleomorphic bacteria may be confused with one another, the source of the clinical specimen aids the microbiologist. A spinal fluid is more likely to contain *Haemophilus influenzae;* a surgical wound, *Bacteroides;* and a cat or dog bite, *Pasteurella multocida*.

The second-stage table for identification of gram-positive cocci best illustrates the usefulness of microscopic and colonial morphology, selective media, and simple techniques for detection of enzymes. As shown in Table 3, virtually all gram-positive cocci can be identified from properly chosen primary or secondary cultures. Tables 4, 5, 6, and 7—the second-stage tables for gram-positive bacilli, anaerobic gram-negative bacilli, and facultative gram-negative bacilli, respectively, demonstrate the other end of the spectrum. Identification of many of these bacteria requires complete diagnostic tables listing fermentation and decarboxylation patterns, end products of glucose metabolism, nitrate reductase activity, urease activity, end products of tryptophane metabolism, and many other properties. Nevertheless, there are a large number of distinctive organisms among these groups that can be identified from primary or secondary cultures. Furthermore, this approach permits the intelligent selection of further tests for definitive identification. Bacteria that can be definitively identified from primary culture plates are indicated in Tables 4, 5, 6, and 7 either by giving the genus and species names or by listing a group of bacteria under the heading of Unique Characteristics.

The taxonomy of the anaerobic nonspore–forming gram-positive bacilli (Table 4) is in a most confused state. Many organisms such as the ramibacteria, the catenabacteria, and the bifidobacteria have been listed as separate genera, as *Actinomyces*, as *Lactobacillus*, and as *Eubacterium*. The eubacteria are given generic status with characteristics intermediate between the propionibacteria and the *Actinomyces*. Catenabacteria and ramibacteria have found a temporary home among the lactobacilli, and *Bifidobacterium* is regarded as a separate genus among the Actinomycetaceae family.

Taxonomists have divided the fusobacteria and the *Bacteroides* (Table 5) on the basis of end products of glucose metabolism. Fusobacteria produce predominantly butyric acid from glucose metabolism, whereas *Bacteroides* produce a mixed acid pattern. This rational approach to taxonomy with a precedent among the Enterobacteriaceae (butylene glycol versus mixed acid fermentation patterns—see Chapter 31) has not greatly disturbed the older, morphologic method of characterizing fusobacteria as the anaerobic gram-negative bacilli with pointed ends. The pleomorphic, spheroplastic bacterium that was best known to microbiologists as *Bacteroides funduliformis* has now been reclassified as *F. necrophorum* because it produces primarily butyric acid from glucose fermentation. The tendency to split *Bacteroides* into multiple species on the basis of minor differences in fermentation patterns and end products of glucose metabolism has resulted in confusion, however. For example, the bile-resistant (or enhanced) *Bacteroides* that were once considered to be one species *(B. fragilis)* were first divided into five subspecies of *B. fragilis*, and then each subspecies was granted full species status. Despite this confusion, most *Bacteroides* that clearly cause disease can be assigned to a definable species.

Tables 6 and 7 are the most extensive and complicated because there are more recognized species of facultative and aerobic gram-negative bacilli than there are in the other groups. Nevertheless, this approach to identification works well. The fastidious bacteria listed in Table 6 generally produce smaller, more delicate colonies on blood agar than the Enterobacteriaceae, *Pseudomonas*, and vibrios (Table 7). Furthermore, they are inhibited or fail to grow on selective media such as eosin-methylene blue (EMB) or MacConkey agar. Although most of these bacteria cannot be differentiated from one another by gram stain, the group can be distinguished from the hardier members of the gram-negative bacilli. Determination of the oxidase reaction, catalase production, enhancement by CO_2, and nutritional requirements permits the identification of most of these bacteria to the generic level and some of them to the level of species. The nutritionally versatile, hardier bacteria in Table 7 can be divided into two major groups by the oxidase reaction. Enterobacteriaceae are oxidase-negative, glucose-fermenting, nitrate-reducing bacteria that have peritrichous flagella when motile. The *Yersinia* species *(pestis, pseudotuberculosis,* and *enterocolitica)* and certain *Erwinia* species fit this definition and are now classified with the Enterobacteriaceae. The vibrios and *Campylobacter* can usually be differentiated from the other oxidase-positive, hardy gram-negative bacilli by gram stain. Live cultures of *Campylobacter* can be differentiated from all other bacteria by dark-field microscopy. They are spiral, coiled bacteria that exhibit a unique "darting" motility. Otherwise, these nutritionally versatile bacteria are differentiated from one another as indicated in Table 7 by pigment production, oxidation and fermentation patterns, and other biochemical reactions.

BACTERIAL IDENTIFICATION AND CLINICAL RELEVANCE. The function of the diagnostic bacteriology laboratory is to provide clinically useful information at a reasonable cost in the shortest length of time (Bartlett, 1974). It is clearly not the function of the laboratory to do sophisticated bacterial identification as an end in itself. For this reason, a question that each laboratory must constantly ask itself is how far to go with the identification of bacterial isolates obtained from clinical specimens. Ideally, each

Text continued on page 18

Table 2. CLASSIFICATION OF MEDICALLY IMPORTANT BACTERIA BY GRAM STAIN AND MICROSCOPIC MORPHOLOGY
FIRST-STAGE TABLE

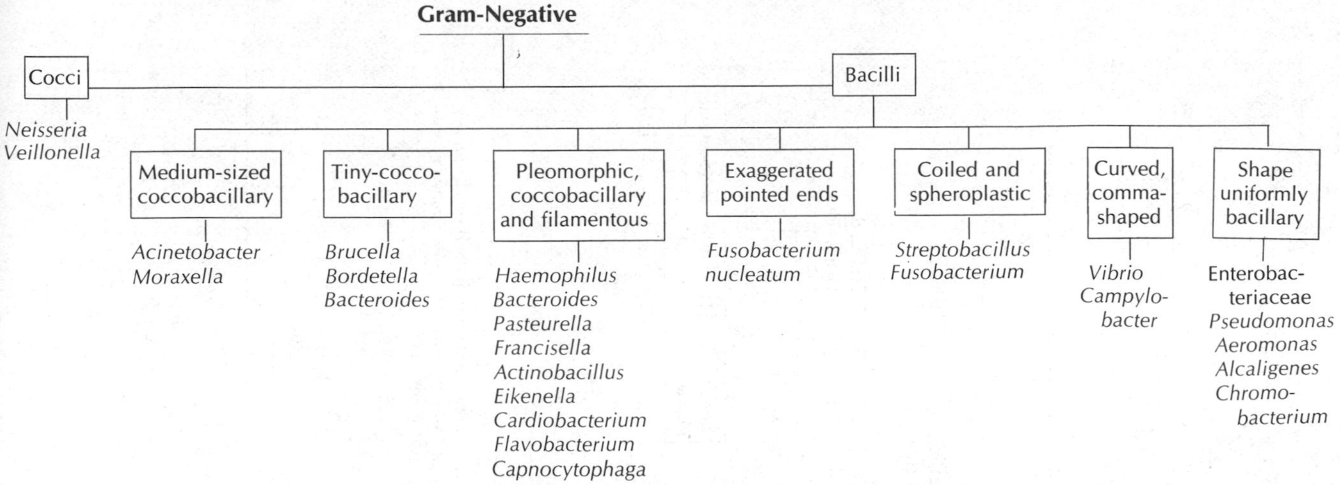

*Although the chemical composition and ultrastructure of the cell walls of *Chlamydia, Rickettsia, Legionella,* and the spirochetes suggest that they are gram-negative bacteria, they are omitted from the table because they stain poorly or not at all with Gram's reagents.

Table 3. IDENTIFICATION OF GRAM-POSITIVE COCCI
SECOND-STAGE TABLE

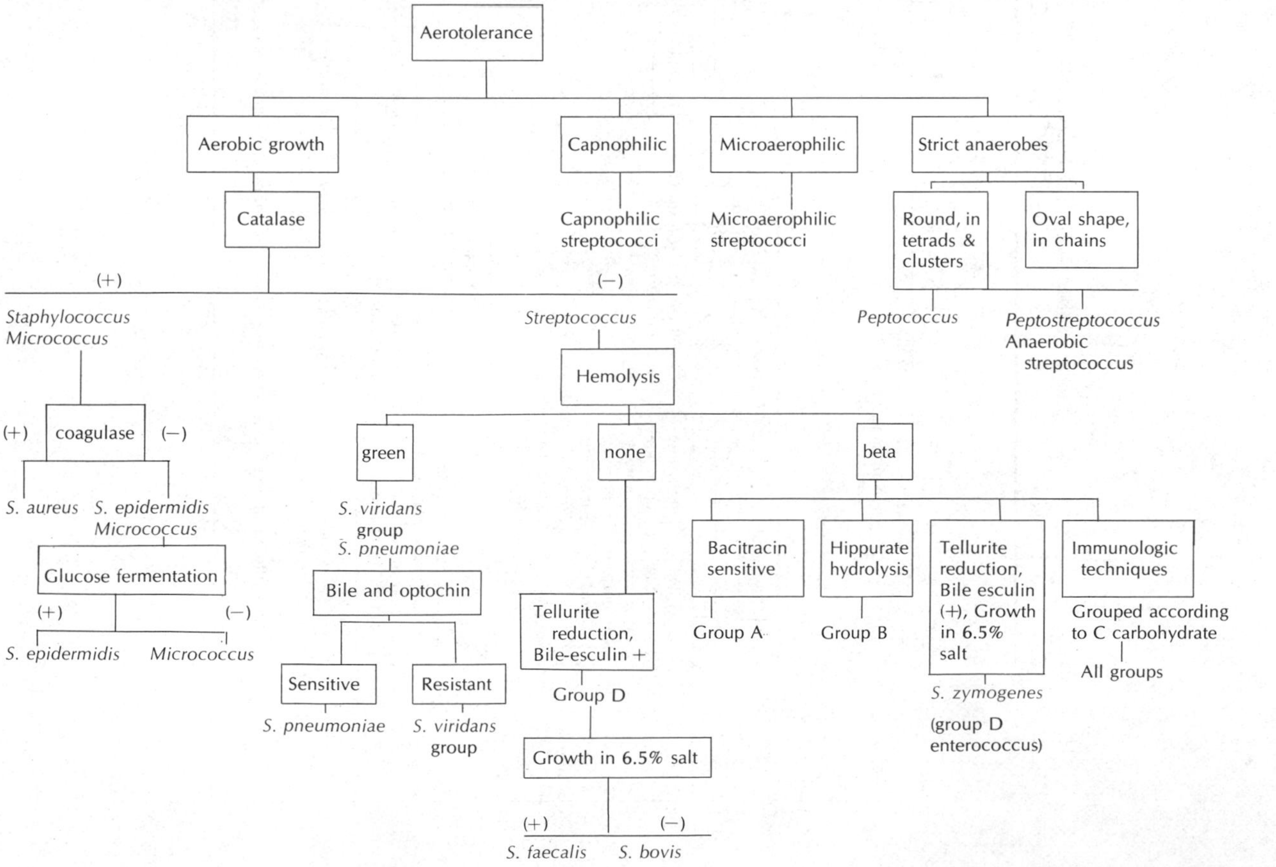

Table 4. IDENTIFICATION OF GRAM-POSITIVE BACILLI
SECOND-STAGE TABLE

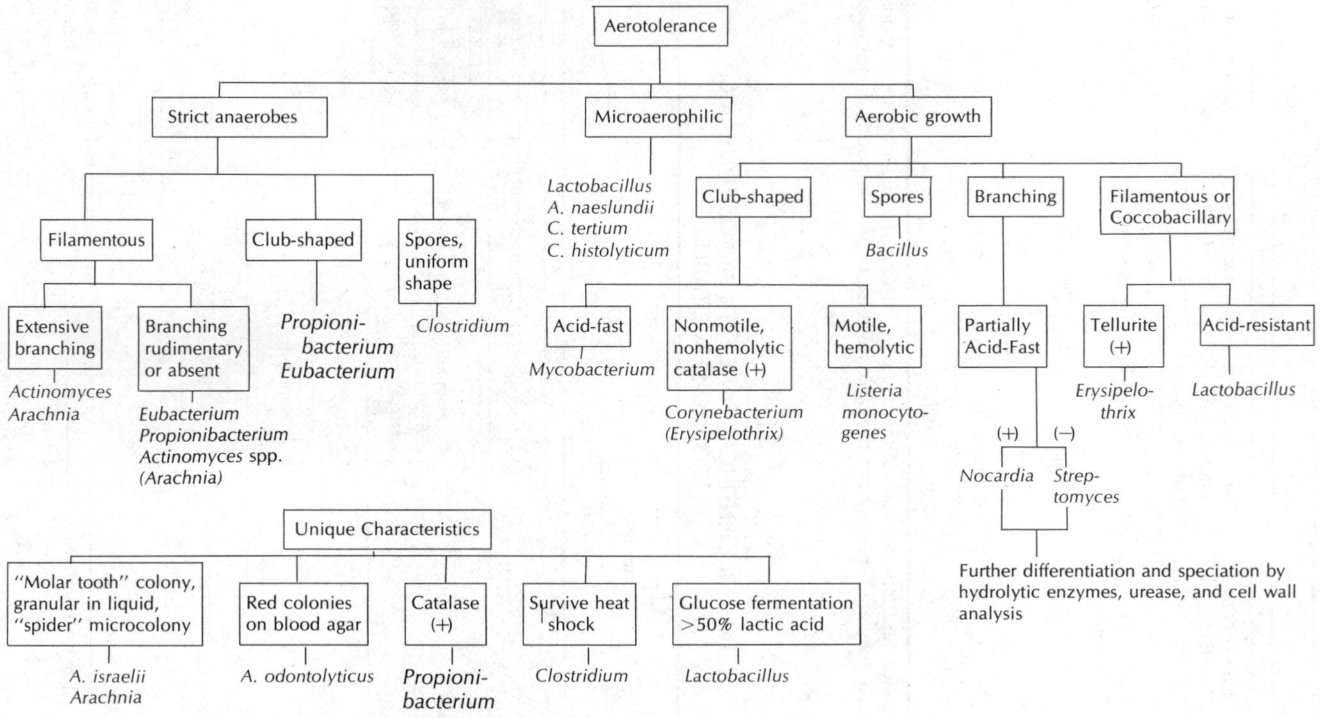

Further differentiation of anaerobic gram-positive bacilli by biochemical reactions and GLC of metabolic products

Table 5. IDENTIFICATION OF STRICTLY ANAEROBIC GRAM-NEGATIVE BACTERIA SECOND-STAGE TABLE

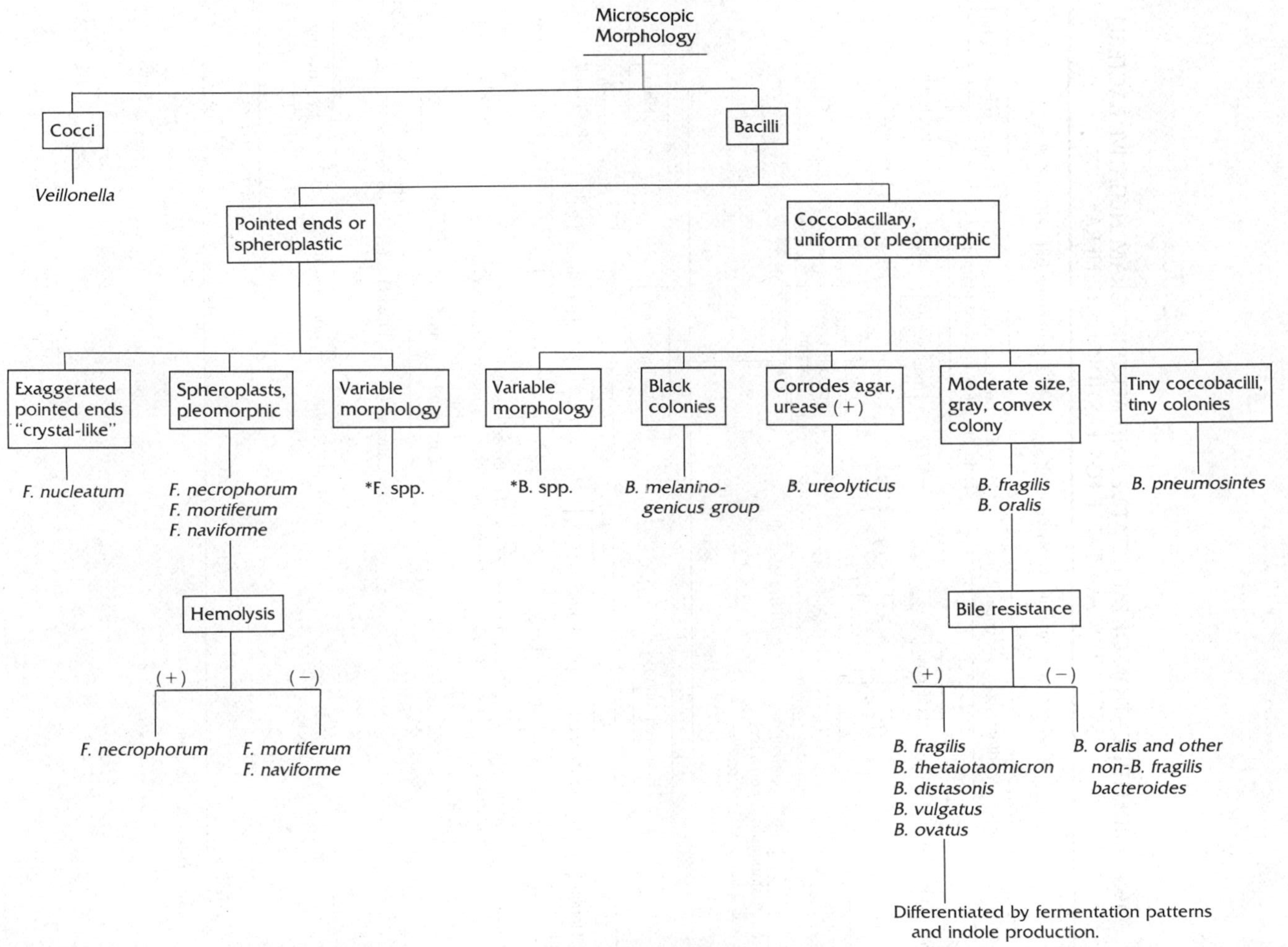

*F. species and B. species are differentiated by biochemical profiles and gas-liquid chromatography of metabolic products of spent cultures. Fusobacteria produce predominantly butyric acid from glucose fermentation. Bacteroides produce a mixed pattern of succinic, acetic, formic, and others.

Table 6. IDENTIFICATION OF FACULTATIVE AND AEROBIC GRAM-NEGATIVE BACTERIA SECOND-STAGE TABLE FOR FASTIDIOUS GENERA*

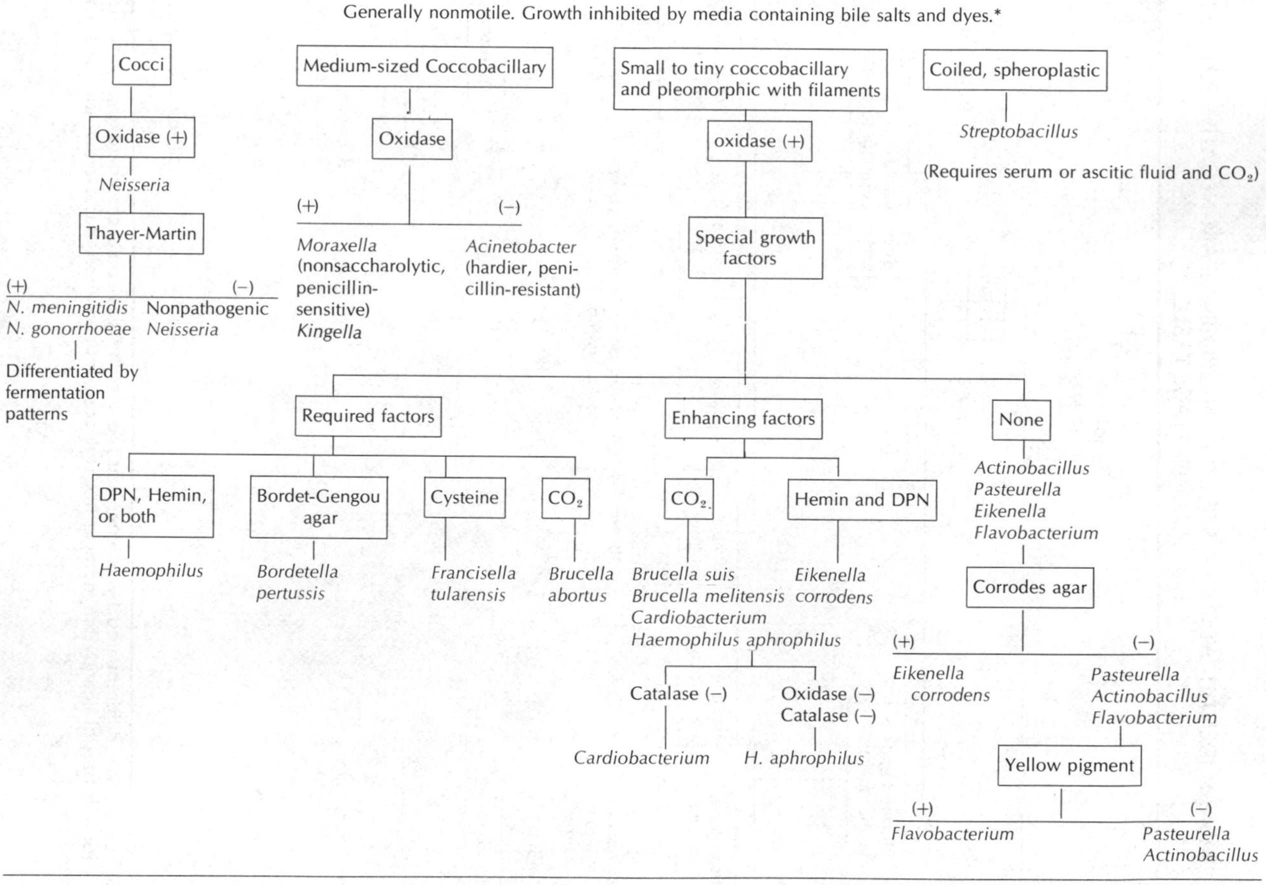

*See Table 7 for nutritionally versatile genera.

Table 7. IDENTIFICATION OF FACULTATIVE AND AEROBIC GRAM-NEGATIVE BACTERIA
SECOND-STAGE TABLE FOR NUTRITIONALLY VERSATILE GENERA*

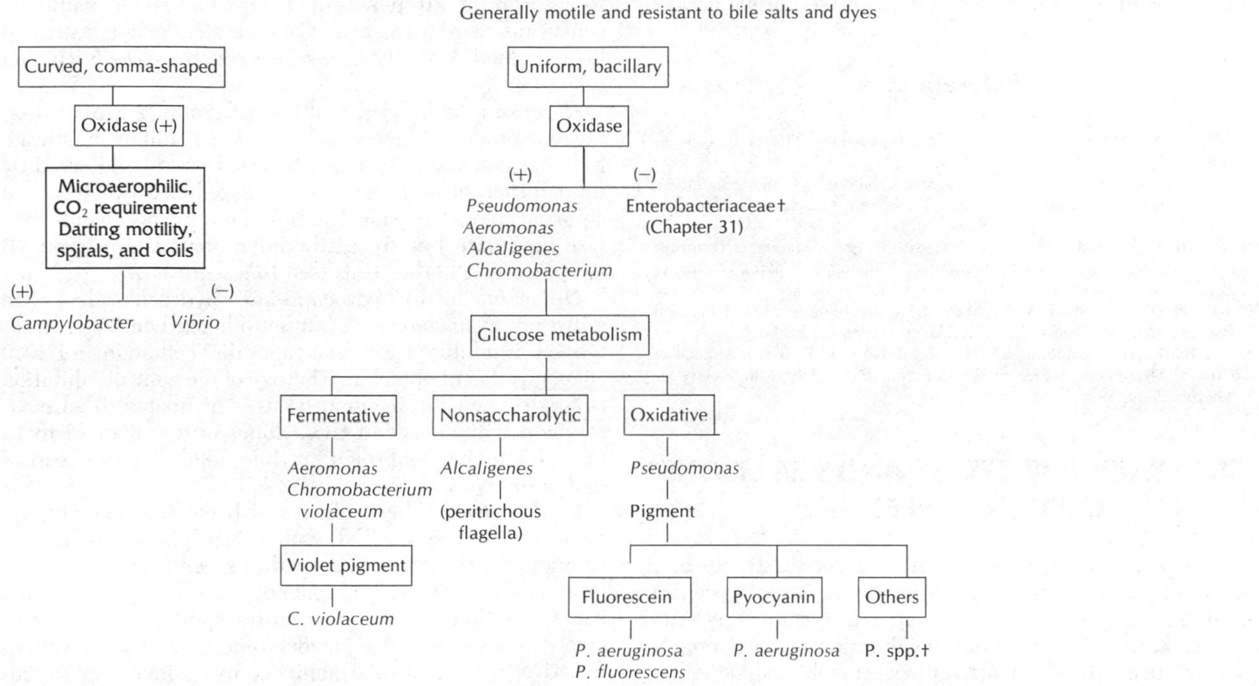

*See Table 6 for fastidious genera.
†Most organisms identified to species by fermentation patterns, oxidation patterns, production of nitrate reductase, urease, and occasionally by characteristic pigment.

organism could be identified fully to reflect the current status of bacterial classification, but this is not always feasible. The amount of work and the cost involved could be prohibitive. Furthermore, this approach would generate an enormous amount of clinically irrelevant data. Reporting the identity of all organisms regardless of potential pathogenic significance from a site normally inhabited by indigenous flora will confuse and frustrate most physicians. It is customary in most diagnostic laboratories to establish the identity of all organisms isolated from a specimen of a normally sterile anatomic site, but to identify and report only known pathogens from sites normally inhabited by indigenous flora. This approach is universally accepted for certain specimens (e.g., feces) but remains controversial for other specimens (e.g., throat and lower respiratory tract). This decision becomes especially important for specimens from immunocompromised patients who may be infected with opportunistic members of the normal flora.

References

Bartlett, R. C.: Medical Microbiology. Quality, Cost and Clinical Relevance. New York, John Wiley & Sons, 1974.

Brenner, D. J., and Falkow, S.: Molecular relationships among members of the enterobacteriaceae. In Caspari, E. W. (ed.): Advances in Genetics, Vol. 16. New York, Academic Press, 1971, pp. 81–118.

Buchanan, R. E., and Gibbons, N. E. (eds.): Bergey's Manual of Determinative Bacteriology. 8th ed. Baltimore, Williams & Wilkins Company, 1974.

Cowan, S. T., and Steel, K. J.: Manual for the Identification of Medical Bacteria. 2nd ed. Cambridge, Cambridge University Press, 1974.

Lennette, E. H., Spaulding, E. H., and Truant, J. P. (eds.): Manual of Clinical Microbiology. 2nd ed. Washington, D.C., American Society for Microbiology, 1974.

GLOSSARY FOR TERMS AND REACTIONS USED IN TABLES 1–7

Bacitracin sensitivity. Group A β-hemolytic streptococci are differentiated from other β-hemolytic streptococci by inhibition of growth around a paper disc containing 0.04 unit of bacitracin. Any zone of inhibition is considered a positive test. Many green streptococci (α-hemolytic streptococci) are sensitive to this concentration, so hemolysis must be carefully evaluated. Other β-hemolytic streptococci are inhibited only rarely by the bacitracin disc.

Bile-"positive." Capable of growth in bile. Group D streptococci grow on agar containing 40 per cent oxgall bile. *Streptococcus faecalis* and *S. zymogenes* (the penicillin-resistant enterococci) can be differentiated from other group D streptococci (such as *S. bovis*) because the enterococci will also grow in broth containing 6.5 per cent NaCl. Growth of the intestinal *Bacteroides*, especially *B. fragilis*, is enhanced in the presence of 20 per cent oxgall bile. The growth of other *Bacteroides* is inhibited.

Bile soluble. The addition of an equal volume of 10 per cent oxgall bile or deoxycholate to turbid broth cultures or saline suspensions of *S. pneumoniae* (the pneumococcus), but not to *S. viridans* or other α-hemolytic streptococci, clears the cultures within 30 minutes because the pneumococci are lysed. Bile and optochin (see further on) activate an autolytic enzyme of pneumococci, L-alanine-muramyl amidase, which acts on the peptidoglycan and actually causes the lysis.

Bile-esculin. A medium that differentiates group D streptococci from all other streptococci because only group D grows on bile *and* hydrolyzes esculin. It does not differentiate the enterococci from the other group D streptococci (see *Bile-"positive"*).

C carbohydrate (group-specific C antigens). An antigenic layer of the cell wall of streptococci that lies just outside the peptidoglycan layer. β-hemolytic streptococci may be separated into groups A through O by precipitin reactions of acid extracts of the bacteria against group-specific antisera prepared in rabbits (Lancefield grouping scheme).

Catalase. An enzyme that decomposes hydrogen peroxide to H_2O and free oxygen. In the laboratory, catalase is usually tested for by adding 3 per cent H_2O_2 directly to colonies on solid agar or by transferring a colony directly to a drop of 30 per cent H_2O_2. Immediate bubbling constitutes a positive test. Catalase should not be tested for on blood agar plates because red blood cells contain catalase.

Hippurate hydrolysis. Cultures of group B streptococci, but not other streptococci, break down sodium hippurate to benzoic acid and glycine. A positive test is detected by the addition of ninhydrin, which is reduced by glycine to a purple color. Occasional strains of enterococci will hydrolyze hippurate but are easily differentiated from group B streptococci by other tests (see *Bile sculin*).

Optochin. Ethylhydrocupreine hydrochloride. The growth of *S. pneumoniae*, but not other α-hemolytic streptococci, is inhibited around a paper disc containing a 1:4000 concentration of optochin. The size of the zone of inhibition is larger when the pneumococcus is incubated in an environment without added CO_2. Zones of less than 12 to 15 mm should be confirmed by bile solubility (see earlier definition).

Oxidase test. When colonies of bacteria containing cytochrome C are flooded with methylphenylenediamine compounds, they turn black within seconds because of the production of a colored compound, indophenol oxide. Many bacteria with functional electron transport systems contain cytochromes other than cytochrome C and are oxidase-negative in spite of their ability to use oxidative phosphorylation as a major energy source.

Pyocyanin. A bluish green, diffusible phenazine pigment produced only by *Pseudomonas aeruginosa*.

Spheroplasts (spheroplastic). Bacteria that assume bizarre, swollen shapes because of a lack of integrity of the peptidoglycan. Spheroplasts usually form because of damage to the peptidoglycan by cell wall–active antibiotics such as penicillin, but occur spontaneously in *Streptobacillus moniliformis* and *Fusobacterium necrophorum*.

Tellurite (sodium tellurite). Diphtheria bacilli, group D streptococci, *Erysipelothrix*, and a few other bacteria can reduce tellurite and form black colonies in media containing this compound.

Thayer-Martin media: Chocolate agar (laked blood agar or blood agar with enrichments) with the antibiotics colistin, vancomycin, and nystatin added to inhibit the normal bacterial flora of the mouth and vagina. Pathogenic *Neisseria* (the gonococcus and meningococcus), but not nonpathogenic *Neisseria*, grow on Thayer-Martin agar.

3

BACTERIAL PHYSIOLOGY

T. RAMAKRISHNAN, M.SC., PH.D.
AND G. RAMANANDA RAO, M. PHARM., PH.D.

The origin of all free energy reaching this planet is the nuclear fusion reactions taking place in the sun. With the exception of chemoautotrophic bacteria, all living organisms draw energy from this source—either directly or indirectly. As in all other living organisms the requirement of energy for microorganisms is fundamental and essential. This need is explained by the fact that several processes involved in the biosynthesis of proteins, nucleic acids, and polysaccharides require the input of energy (endergonic), that is, having a positive change in free engery ($\Delta F'$ value). These thermodynamically unfavorable reactions are made possible under conditions in living organisms by coupling them with energy-yielding, or exergonic, reactions (negative change in $\Delta F'$ value).

The release of energy in exergonic reactions and the manner in which energy is trapped, stored, and utilized for endergonic reactions are some of the fascinating aspects of bacterial metabolism. The central role of adenosine triphosphate (ATP) in energy exchanges in biologic systems was postulated by Fritz Lipmann and Hermann Kalckar in 1941 (Lipmann, 1941). It consists of three molecular species, adenine, D-ribose, and a triphosphate unit (Fig. 1).

The α- and β-phosphates and the β- and γ-phosphates are connected by acid anhydride linkages called energy-rich bonds and are symbolized by a wriggle bond (~). The electrostatic repulsion between the negatively charged phosphate groups, which results from their close proximity, is reduced when ATP is hydrolyzed. The high potential energy of ATP is due to the fact that adenosine diphosphate (ADP) and P_i enjoy greater resonance stabilization than ATP. The presence of this energy in ATP makes it the most functionally important compound in biologic systems.

In addition to ATP, a variety of other energy-rich compounds occur in biologic systems. They include 1) derivatives of phosphoric acid such as triphosphates of guanosine (GTP), cytidine (CTP), and uridine (UTP); and 2) derivatives of carboxylic acids, which include acyl thioesters such as acetyl coenzyme A. In fact, some of these compounds, such as phosphoenolpyruvate and creatine phosphate, have a higher potential energy than ATP.

ATP is formed by a number of reactions that are all of the general type ADP + X ~ P → ATP + X, where X ~ P is a high-energy intermediate. ATP is formed by two mechanisms in bacteria—substrate level phosphorylation and oxidative phosphorylation.

Substrate Level Phosphorylation. In this mechanism the energy required for the conversion of ADP to ATP is supplied by high-energy metabolic intermediates such as phosphoenolpyruvate, succinyl coenzyme A, or creatine phosphate—a compound regarded as a store of high-energy phosphate.

The energy is released from the high-energy phosphate bonds in the substrate by means of substrate oxidation. This can be illustrated by reactions occurring in the glycolytic cycle (Fig. 2). The oxidation of glyceraldehyde 3-phosphate to 1,3 diphosphoglyceric acid by nicotinamide-adenine dinucleotide (NAD) produces a high-energy phosphate bond through the carboxy-linkage (as indicated by ↓) in the following manner:

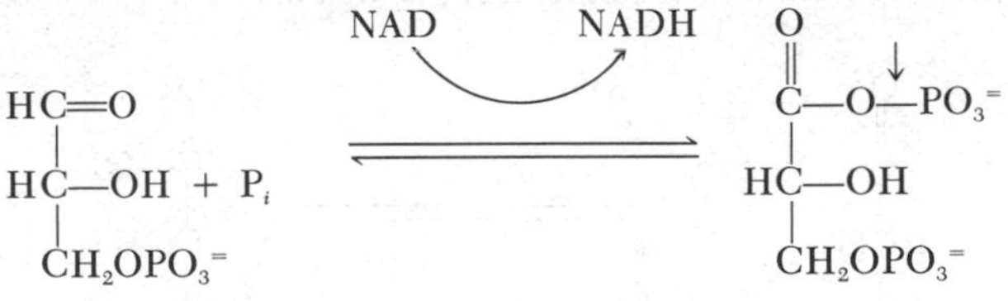

Glyceraldehyde-3-phosphate   1,3-Diphosphoglyceric acid

$$\text{Phosphoenolpyruvate} + \text{ADP} \longrightarrow \text{Pyruvate} + \text{ATP}$$

$$\text{Succinyl coenzyme A} + \text{ADP} \xrightarrow{\text{GDP}} \text{Succinate} + \text{ATP} + \text{Coenzyme A}$$

$$\text{Creatine phosphate} + \text{ADP} \longrightarrow \text{Creatine} + \text{ATP}$$

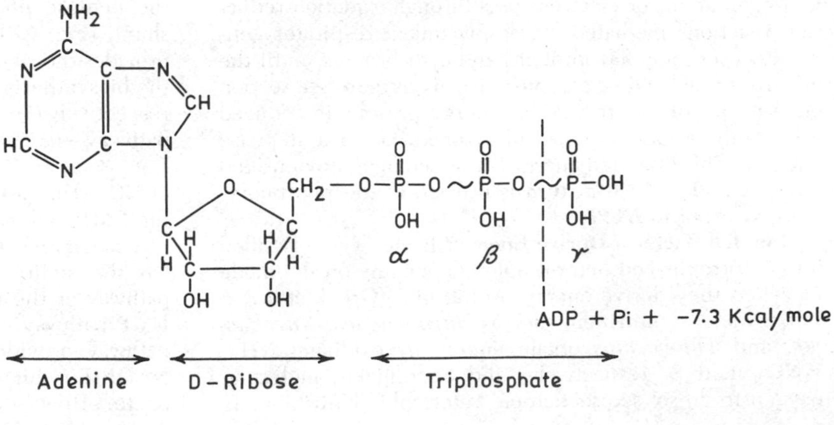

Figure 1. Structure of ATP and energy release.

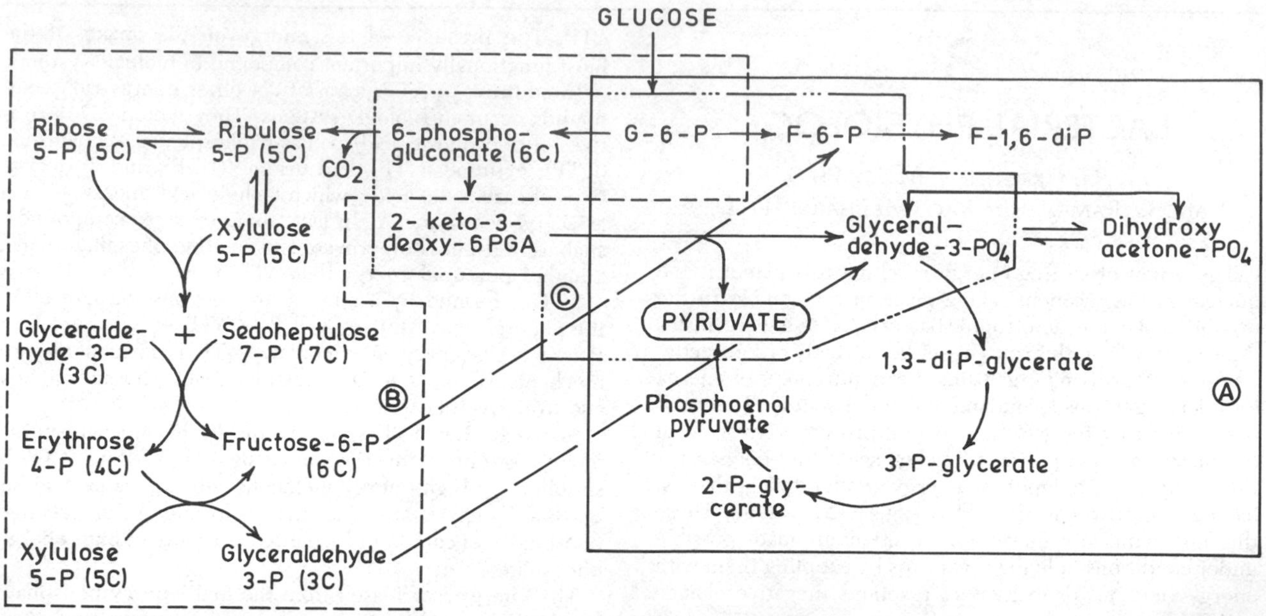

Figure 2. Pathways involved in the metabolism of glucose to pyruvate A, Embden Myerhof pathway (EMP): B, pentose-phosphate pathway; and C, Entner-Doudoroff pathway. In EMP, one molecule of fructose-1,6 diphosphate is split into two three-carbon compounds, glyceraldehyde 3-phosphate and dihydroxyacetone phosphate. Two molecules of ATP are needed to start the pathway, but four molecules of ATP are formed by the fermentation of glucose to pyruvic acid.

This high-energy phosphate bond is then transferred to ADP to form a molecule of ATP, as follows:

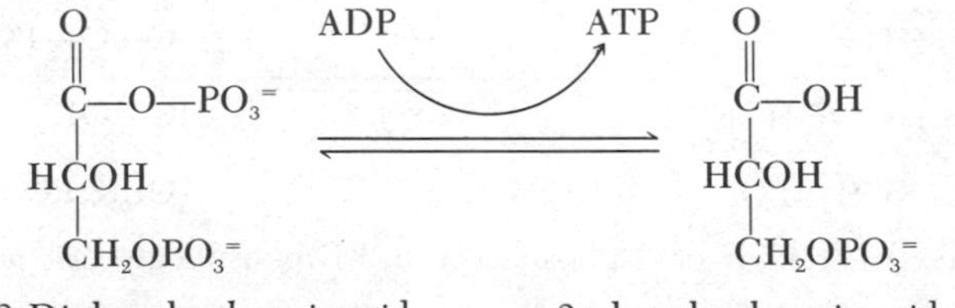

1,3-Diphosphoglyceric acid 3-phosphoglyceric acid

It should be noted that formation of the high-energy phosphate bond in 1,3-diphosphoglyceric acid is accompanied by the transfer of electrons to NAD to form NADH (reduced NAD).

Oxidative Phosphorylation. This phosphorylation is associated with electron transport. It is a coupled process wherein reduced substrates are oxidized with concomitant phosphorylation of ADP to ATP. During this process hydrogen atoms or electrons pass through oxidation-reduction reactions mediated by closely linked respiratory enzymes, especially flavoproteins and cytochromes, until the electrons reach a final acceptor, usually oxygen (see section on Aerobic Respiration). The energy present in reduced coenzymes is not released all at once but in a stepwise manner. This liberated energy is trapped in an unidentified form, X ~ P, which in turn is utilized in the phosphorylation of ADP to ATP.

How Do Bacteria Derive Energy? Bacteria are classified into autotrophs and heterotrophs, depending on the mode in which they derive energy. Autotrophs (Greek *autos* = self, *trophe* = nutrition) such as *Nitrosomonas*, *Nitrobacter*, and *Thiobacillus* obtain energy by oxidizing NH_4^+, HNO_2, and S, respectively, and by utilizing molecular oxygen to do so (see section on Autotrophic Nutrition). In heterotrophs (Greek *heteros* = another), preformed organic compounds such as polysaccharides, fats, and proteins are oxidized either aerobically (respiration) or anaerobically (fermentation), with release of energy. In respiration, molecular oxygen serves as the ultimate hydrogen acceptor, whereas in fermentation (which was defined by Pasteur as life without air) organic compounds serve as both electron donors and acceptors.

The brilliant contributions of Embden, Meyerhof, and Parnas led to the elucidation of the major pathway used by bacteria for the fermentation of glucose (Meyerhof, 1942). This pathway is termed the Embden-Meyerhof-Parnas (EMP) pathway, or glycolysis, and describes the conversion of glucose to pyruvic acid (Fig. 2*A*). This series of reactions also occurs in mammalian cells. Pyruvic acid is further metabolized to alcohol in yeast and to lactic acid in muscle. In the vast majority of bacteria, glucose is metabolized through the EMP pathway to pyruvate (Fig. 2*A*).

In obligate aerobic bacteria, which do not possess the EMP pathway, glucose is metabolized to pyruvate through the pentose phosphate pathway (hexose monophosphate shunt) (Fig. 2*B*). The reaction sequence of this pathway provides the ribose and erythrose-4-phosphate essential for the biosynthesis of nucleic acids and aromatic amino acids, respectively (Horecker, 1962). Another intermediate of this pathway—namely, ribulose-5-phosphate—is converted to ribulose-1,5-diP, the acceptor of CO_2 in autotrophic fixation of CO_2. The net yield of ATP is half that characteristic of the EMP pathway.

A facultative aerobic organism such as *Escherichia coli* has the ability to degrade glucose by either the EMP pathway or the pentose phosphate pathway. Whereas the EMP pathway gives more energy, the pentose phosphate pathway provides more reducing power in the form of NADPH (reduced nicotinamide adenine dinucleotide phosphate). However, a balance between these two pathways

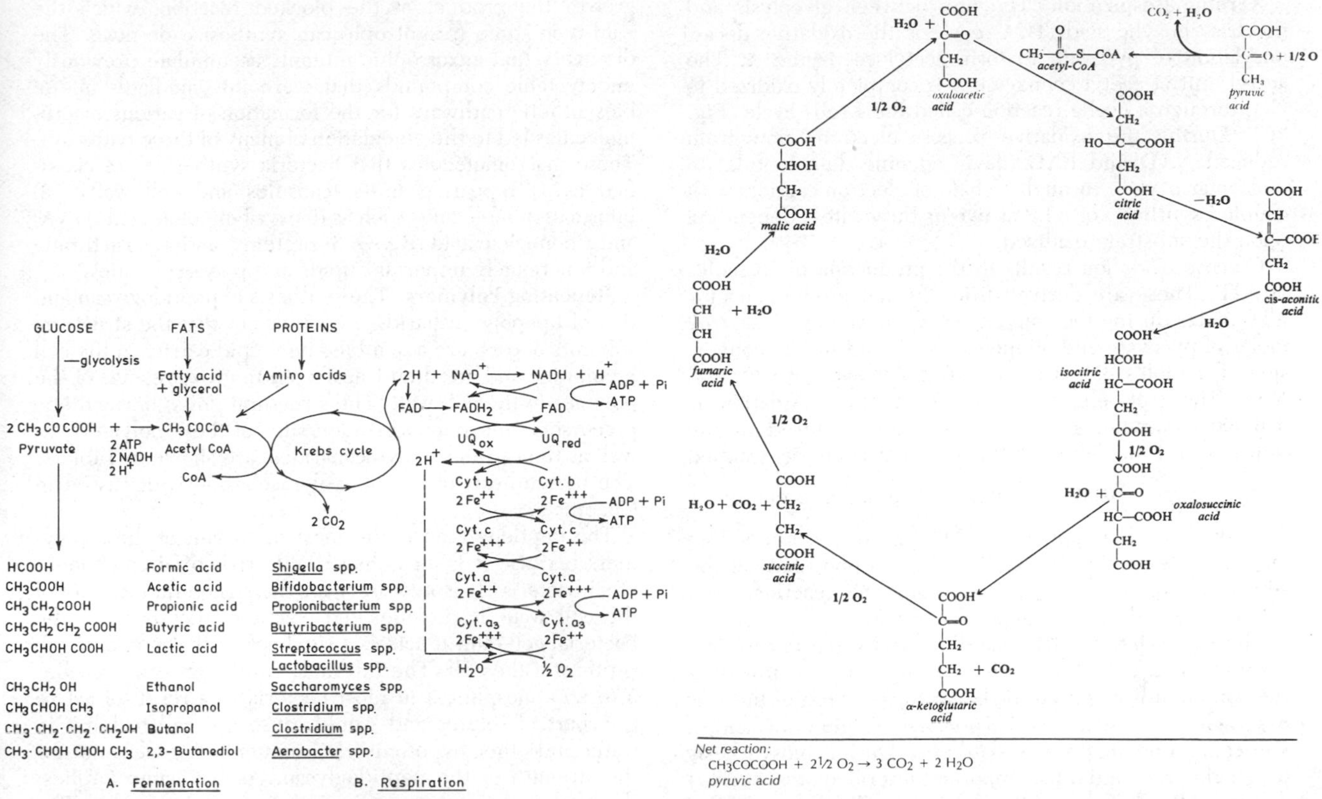

Figure 3. A, Key role of pyruvate in the formation of fermentation products and B, its oxidation through respiration, yielding ATP.

is controlled by phosphofructokinase, which phosphorylates fructose-6-P to fructose-1,6-diP. When the intracellular level of ATP increases, phosphofructokinase is strongly inhibited. As a result, phosphorylation of fructose-6-P is restricted, and the carbon flows via the pentose phosphate pathway. Increased levels of ATP similarly inhibit carbon flow through the EMP pathway under aerobic conditions and is termed the *Pasteur effect.*

In many species of aerobic bacteria glucose is metabolized by the Entner-Doudoroff pathway (Fig. 2*C*). In this pathway, 6-phosphogluconate of the pentose phosphate pathway is converted to 2-keto-3-deoxy-6-phosphogluconate (instead of ribulose 5-P as in the pentose phosphate pathway). The enzyme aldolase cleaves this into pyruvate and glyceraldehyde-3-P, intermediates in glycolysis. The latter is metabolized via the EMP pathway.

Pyruvate occupies a key position in carbohydrate fermentation. As a result of the conversion of glucose to pyruvate, NAD is reduced. Additional fermentations yield different products from pyruvate (Fig. 3*A*) and cause reoxidation of NADH, so that the oxidation-reduction balance of the cell is restored. In medical microbiology, one of the more important fermentations of pyruvate is the mixed acid fermentation by *Enterobacteriaceae*, such as *Escherichia coli* and *Shigella* spp. The reaction produces formic, lactic, and succinic acids, as well as a number of other products. The production of formate and acetate involves decarboxylation of pyruvate by the series of reactions below:

E. coli and *Salmonella* spp. have an enzyme system (formic hydrogenlyase) that produces molecular hydrogen and CO_2 from formate: $HCOOH \rightarrow H_2 + CO_2$. The production of large amounts of hydrogen ion in the mixed acid fermentation is important in the laboratory identification of *E. coli.* Similarly, the ability of *E. coli* and most *Salmonella* spp. to produce H_2 and CO_2 from formate distinguishes them from *S. typhi* and *Shigella* spp., which cannot break down formate to these gases.

$$\text{(1)}\quad \underset{\text{pyruvate}}{CH_3COCOOH} + \underset{\text{coenzyme A}}{HSCoA} \longrightarrow \underset{\text{acetyl CoA}}{CH_3\overset{\overset{\displaystyle O}{\|}}{C}SCoA} + \underset{\text{formic acid}}{HCOOH}$$

$$\text{(2)}\quad \underset{\text{acetyl CoA}}{CH_3\overset{\overset{\displaystyle O}{\|}}{C}SCoA} + \underset{\text{phosphoric acid}}{H_3PO_4} \longrightarrow \underset{\text{acetyl phosphate}}{CH_3\overset{\overset{\displaystyle O}{\|}}{C}{-}O{-}PO_3H_2} + \underset{\text{coenzyme A}}{CoA\text{-}SH}$$

$$\text{(3)}\quad \underset{\text{phosphate}}{\text{Acetyl}} + ADP \longrightarrow \underset{\text{acetic acid}}{CH_3COOH} + ATP$$

Aerobic Respiration. The link between glycolysis and the tricarboxylic acid (TCA) cycle is the oxidative decarboxylation of pyruvate to form acetyl coenzyme A. The acetyl unit of acetyl coenzyme A is completely oxidized to CO_2 through a cyclic reaction called the Krebs cycle (Fig. 3*C*). During the oxidative process electrons flow from reduced NAD and FAD (flavin adenine dinucleotide) to molecular oxygen through a chain of electron carriers with coupled synthesis of ATP at two or three sites, depending upon the substrate oxidized.

Glucose oxidation results in the production of 38 moles of ATP. These are derived from the net production of 2 ATP moles during the conversion of 1 mole of glucose to 2 moles of pyruvate and 36 moles of ATP during the conversion of 2 moles of pyruvate to 6 moles each of CO_2 and H_2O. The free energy change of glucose oxidation is 686,000 cal./mole. If 7000 calories are required in the synthesis of 1 mole of ATP, the efficiency of energy trapped is $\frac{7000 \times 38}{686,000} \times 100 = 39$ per cent. Since free energy of ATP synthesis may approach 12,000 cal./mole, depending on the concentrations of ADP, ATP, and phosphate at the actual site on the enzyme catalyzing the reactions, the efficiency could be as high as 60 per cent.

The Glyoxylate Cycle. In addition to its role in terminal respiration, the TCA cycle is also important in providing the compounds required for biosyntheses. One of these is α-ketoglutarate, which is the precursor of glutamic acid, a key compound in protein synthesis. During biosynthesis α-ketoglutarate and other important intermediates, such as 4-carbon dicarboxylic acids, are continually removed from the TCA cycle and must be resynthesized from acetate. For this resynthesis of TCA intermediates, bacteria use a modified TCA cycle in which the reaction sequence between isocitric acid and malic acid (Fig. 3*C*) is changed through the glyoxalate bypass, which short-circuits the reactions that lead to the evolution of carbon dioxide. The bypass excludes the following reactions:

$$\text{Isocitrate} \rightarrow \alpha\text{-ketoglutarate} \rightarrow \text{succinate} \rightarrow \text{fumarate} \quad (\searrow CO_2)$$

This bypass consists of two enzymatic reactions:

$$\text{1) Isocitrate} \xrightarrow{\text{isocitrate lyase}} \text{succinate} + \text{glyoxylate}$$

$$\text{2) Acetyl CoA} + \text{glyoxylate} \xrightarrow{\text{malate synthase}} \text{malate} + \text{CoA-SH}$$

Thus, acetate is not used as a source of energy, but rather as a precursor of malic and other 4-carbon dicarboxylic acids.

CH(OH)COOH
|
CH_2COOH
malic acid

BIOSYNTHESIS. Microorganisms offer several advantages for biosynthetic studies, including rapid growth, the ability to synthesize all cell components, and the homogeneity of the cell population. Beadle and Tatum (1941) isolated mutants having a block in a metabolic pathway resulting from a lack of or defective activity of key enzymes. Such mutants (auxotrophic mutants) require for their growth the product of the blocked reaction, which the wild-type strain (prototroph) can synthesize de novo. The discovery that auxotrophic mutants accumulate previously undetectable compounds that were intermediates in the biosynthetic pathways for the formation of various macromolecules led to the elucidation of many of these pathways. These macromolecules that bacteria synthesize are classified as 1) repeating units (capsules and cell walls), 2) information molecules such as deoxyribonucleic acid (DNA) and ribonucleic acid (RNA), 3) proteins, and 4) structurally and functionally important lipids and polysaccharides.

Repeating Polymers. The synthesis of peptidoglycan and that of lipopolysaccharide are similar in that the structural subunits of each are assembled on a lipid carrier in the cell membrane and are then transferred to growing ends of the polymer in the cell wall. The structural units, biosynthetic precursors, and polymerization sites of these polymers, as well as the capsular polysaccharides, are shown in Table 1. The biosynthesis of the lipopolysaccharide is discussed in Chapter 6.

The peptidoglycan is the most important of these polymers because it is an indispensable structural component of all bacteria. It is necessary for the structural integrity of the cell wall, it provides the characteristic shape of the bacterial cell, and it acts as a rigid corset that prevents the rupture of the cell. The internal osmotic pressure reaches 5 to 20 atmospheres in most bacteria as a result of active transport of solutes and would cause the cell to burst in water and other hypotonic environments if it were not for the strength of the peptidoglycan. As the name implies, the peptidoglycan is composed of sugar and peptides. The basic unit of the sugar is a disaccharide containing *N*-acetylglucosamine and *N*-acetylmuramic acid:

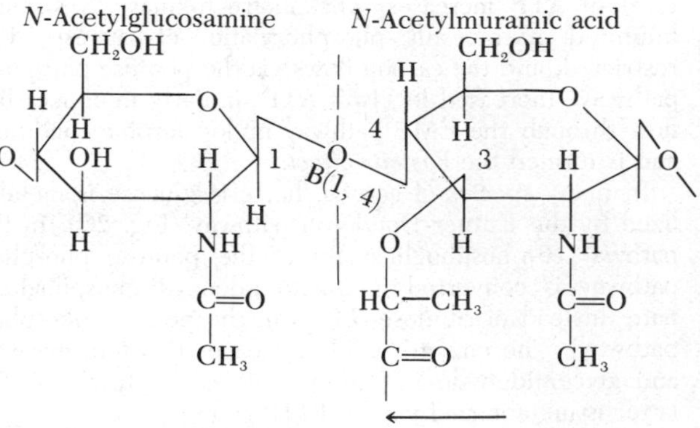

Muramic acid is a derivative of *N*-acetylglucosamine, to which lactic acid is incorporated at the 3-position. The two sugars in the disaccharide are linked at the β-1,4-position. The peptide is attached at the arrow through an amide linkage between L-alanine and the carboxyl group of muramic acid. The peptidoglycan is thus made up of polysaccharide chains linked together by peptides. The polysaccharide chains are composed of repeating units of the *N*-acetylmuramic acid *N*-acetylglucosamine disaccharide. In *E. coli* the cross-linking peptide strands consist of L-alanine, D-glutamic acid, α,ε-diaminopimelic acid (DAP), and finally D-alanine to form a tetrapeptide. The free carboxyl groups in the D-alanine residues are also attached to the NH_2 group of the diaminopimelic acid in adjacent tetrapeptides to produce a cross-linked structure. In staphylococci a

Table 1. CAPSULAR AND CELL WALL POLYSACCHARIDES IN BACTERIA

1 Polysaccharides	2 Repeating Unit	3 Linkage	4 Precursors	5 Site of Polymerization	6 Organisms
Capsular					
Dextran	Glucose	β-1,6	Sucrose	Synthesized within the cell but excreted	*Leuconostoc* spp.
Levan	Fructose	α-2,6	Sucrose	″	*Pseudomonas* spp.
Cellulose	Glucose	β-1,4	GDP-glucose	Cytoplasm	*Acetobacter xylinum*
Glycogen	Glucose	α-1,4	ADP-glucose	Cytoplasm	*Clostridium* spp.
Polyglutamic acid	D-glutamic acid	γ-glutamyl	Glutamate ATP	Cytoplasm	*Bacillus anthracis*
Pneumococcus type III polysaccharide	Glucuronic acid Glucose	β-1,4 β-1,3	UDP-glucuronic acid UDP-glucose	Cell membrane	*Streptococcus pneumoniae*
Cell wall					
Glycopeptide	GlcNAc-MurNAc-pentapeptide	β-1,4 (between sugars). Tetrapeptide side chain is attached to the -COOH of the lactic group of MurNAc	UDP-MurNAc UDP-GlcNAc Glycyl tRNA	Cell membrane murein subunit is added to the growing chains in the cell wall through the participation of bactoprenol-P-P	Gram-positive bacteria such as *Staphylococcus aureus, Micrococcus lysodeikticus* (high content)
Lipopolysaccharide	*Core:* (KDO-heptose)-glu-gal-glu-GlcNAc *Specific side chains:* (-rha-man-gal-)$_n$ abequose	Side chain sugars are attached with their reducing groups toward the core (1→ 4, 1 → 6 and so forth)	*Core:* UDP-(glu-gal-GlcNAc) *Side chain:* GDP-(gal-man)-TDP-rha	Repeating side chain subunits are constructed by attachment to bactoprenol on membrane and then transferred to the "open" end of the growing polymer of the wall	Gram-negative true bacteria. Best studied in *Salmonella* spp.
Cell wall teichoic acids	Glycerol or ribitol substituted at OH groups with sugars or amino acids	Phosphodiester	Glycerol or ribitol, D-alanine, glucose succinate, oligosaccharides	Covalently linked to peptidoglycan at C6-hydroxyl of *N*-acetylmuramic acid	Gram-positive bacteria such as staphylococci, streptococci, *Lactobacillus,* and *Bacillus*
Lipoteichoic acids	Glycerol substituents	Phosphodiester	Fatty acid substituted glycerophosphate, & glycerol teichoic acid	Membrane	All gram-positive bacteria

second chain composed of five glycine molecules—$(Gly)_5$—is used to connect neighboring peptides.

Synthesis of the peptidoglycan begins in the cytoplasm with formation of *N*-acetylglucosamine-6-phosphate (Glc NAc-6-P) from fructose-6-phosphate, glutamine, and acetyl CoA.

GlcNAc-6-P is attached to a nucleoside diphosphate (as generally occurs when sugars are polymerized) to form uridinediphospho-*N*-acetylglucosamine (UDP-GlcNAc). UDP-*N*-acetylmuramic acid (UDP-MurNAc) is then produced by the following reaction involving phosphoenolpyruvate and 2H:

$$\text{UDP-GlcNAc} + CH_2{=}\underset{\displaystyle OPO_3H_2}{\underset{|}{C}}{-}COOH \xrightarrow{2H} \text{UDP-MurNAc}$$

phosphoenol
pyruvate

The cross-linking pentapeptide is then attached, first by addition of L-alanine to the lactyl carboxyl group of UDP-MurNAc, followed by serial addition of the remaining four amino acids. The formation of each peptide bond requires ATP and a specific enzyme.

The second step in peptidoglycan synthesis is the transfer of UDP-GlcNAc-MurNAc pentapeptide to the carrier lipid, bactoprenol—a C_{55} polyisoprenoid alcohol with the formula

$$CH_3\overset{CH_3}{C}{=}CHCH_2(CH_2\overset{CH_3}{C}{=}CHCH_2)_9CH_2\overset{CH_3}{C}{=}CHCH_2OH.$$

This carrier lipid is the site of disaccharide formation, which results from the addition of acetylglucosamine (from UDP-GlcNAc) to the C_4 hydroxyl group of *N*-acetylmuramic acid. At this stage the β-1,4-linked disaccharide forms the following complex with the carrier lipid:

```
GlcNAc-MurNAc-P-P-Lipid
        |
    L-alanine
        |
    D-glu—COOH ←—— amidation
        |
Pentaglycine ——→ L-lysine
        |
    D-alanine
        |
    D-alanine
```

Note that the muramyl pentapeptide is connected to the lipid by a pyrophosphate bridge (PP). Further changes occur, depending on the species. In *S. aureus,* for example, the pentaglycine bridge is attached to L-lysine by sequential addition of glycine from glycyl-tRNA. There is also amidation of the γ-carboxyl group of D-glutamic acid.

After the disaccharide-pentapeptide unit is constructed, it is transferred from the carrier lipid to the peptidoglycan in the cell wall, where the peptidoglycan is elongated and cross-linked by transpeptidation between peptide bridges. This is achieved in *S. aureus* when D-alanine is split from D-alanyl-D-alanine, so that a peptide bond can form between the carboxyl group of the residual D-alanine and the terminal amino group of a neighboring pentaglycine chain. This reaction completes the synthesis of the cell wall peptidoglycan.

In addition to the differences in structure of the peptidoglycan of *E. coli* and *S. aureus,* there are differences in other cell wall components. Characteristic lipopolysaccharides are found in *E. coli* and all other gram-negative bacteria, but never in gram-positive bacteria. In contrast, teichoic acids are found only in gram-positive bacteria. Teichoic acids are cell wall polymers composed of long chains of either glycerol or ribitol. These chains are linked (to each other) by phosphodiester bonds and contain substitutions of both amino acids and monosaccharides. In some bacteria they are connected to the cell wall through muramic acid-6-phosphate. Glycerol teichoic acids have the general formula

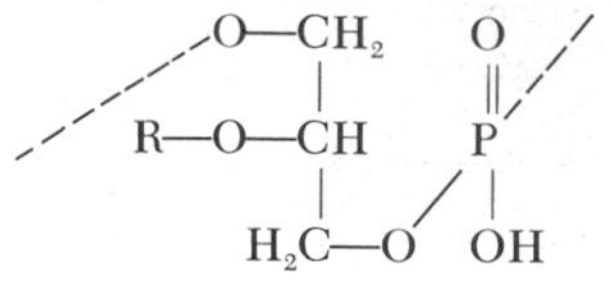

The R group is often D-alanine. The formula for ribitol teichoic acid is generally

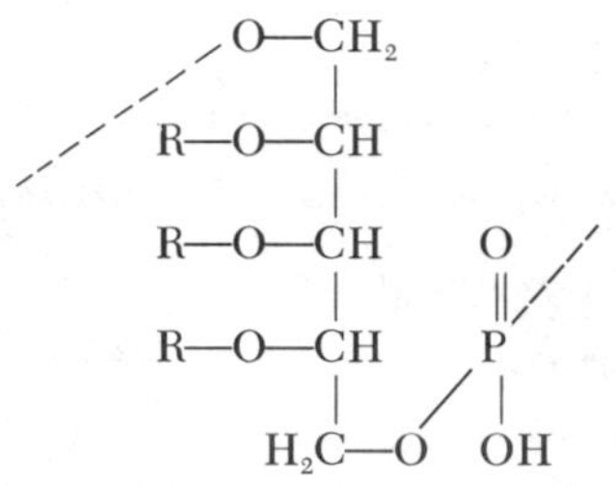

The R group substitution may also be D-alanine but is often *N*-acetylglucosamine, glucose, oligosaccharides, or succinate. Both types of teichoic acid are bound to the peptidoglycan and may be important surface antigens in streptococci, staphylococci, and other gram-positive bacteria. In addition, glycerol teichoic acid is bound to a glycolipid in the cytoplasmic membrane of all gram-positive bacteria and is known as lipoteichoic acid. In spite of their widespread occurrence, the physiologic role of lipoteichoic acids is not well understood. They may participate in the synthesis of peptidoglycan-associated teichoic acids, in binding Mg^{++} ions at the cell surface, and in regulating cell division. In the pneumococci, the lipoteichoic acid, which contains choline, inhibits autolysis of the cell wall and prevents pneumococcal cells from separating, so that they form chains. This is brought about by inhibition of the autolytic enzyme mucopeptide amidohydrolase (Höltje and Tomasz, 1975).

Information Molecules. DNA, RNA, and proteins are polymers composed of subunits (monomers). The subunits are linked to one another in a linear sequence by a phosphodiester bond (DNA and RNA) or a peptide bond (protein). The biosynthetic relationship between these macromolecules is shown in Figure 4. Three types of reactions are involved in the genetic flow from DNA→RNA→protein: replication, transcription, and translation.

In replication, free deoxyribonucleotides are assembled linearly to form an identical replica of the original DNA structure for hereditary transmission. The basis for the exact replication of a DNA strand is the base complementarity between adenine and thymine and between guanine and cytosine as proposed by the Watson and Crick model. DNA polymerase in extracts of *E. coli* has been found to catalyze the sequential addition of deoxyribonucleotides to the free 3′-OH ends using the opposite intact strand as template (Fig. 5*A*). There are three different DNA polymerases in *E. coli*, designated I, II, and III.*

DNA-dependent RNA polymerase brings about polymerization of ribonucleotide triphosphates to form a polynucleotide strand having complementarity with the DNA strand that served as a template. This process is called transcription (Fig. 5*B*). In viruses in which the genotype is RNA, its replication involves the synthesis of a complementary strand, which then serves as a template for production of new viral RNA (Fig. 5*C*). In RNA synthesis, adenine pairs with uracil and guanine pairs with cytosine. As shown in Figure 4, three classes of RNAs are formed in the cells by transcription: ribosomal RNA (rRNA), transfer RNA (tRNA), and messenger RNA (mRNA).

Proteins. The phenotype of microorganisms is determined and manifested both directly and indirectly by its structural and enzymic proteins. The mRNA specifies the sequence of amino acids in a protein. Ribosomes provide nonspecific surfaces on which the charged (aminoacyl) tRNA molecules bind, transfer their amino acids to the nascent polypeptide, and are released as uncharged tRNAs (Fig. 4). The sequence of three nucleotide bases (triplet code) in mRNA specifies which amino acid is to be added onto the growing chain. Since there are 64 possible codons from A, U, G, and C, some of the 20 amino acids are specified by multiple codons.

The sequence of molecular events that occur in the lengthening of a polypeptide chain on the surface of 70S ribosome are summarized in Chapter 20.

The amino acids required for protein synthesis are either provided in the medium or synthesized from precursors. All open chain amino acids are synthesized from four precursors: oxaloacetate, pyruvate, α-ketoglutarate, and 3-phosphoglycerate. Among the aromatic amino acids, histidine is derived from pentose and phosphate, and others (for example, tyrosine and tryptophane) from a condensation of D-erythrose-4-phosphate and phosphoenolpyruvate. When amino acids are present in the growth medium, precursor synthesis is prevented through end-product inhibition (see section on Regulation of Growth at end of chapter).

CHEMICAL COMPOSITION AND NUTRITION

Chemical Composition of Bacteria. The main chemical elements in the bacterial cell are nitrogen, carbon, oxygen,

*The function of different polymerases is not clear, except with respect to DNA repair (repair of the patch) by polymerases and ligase. Polymerases II and III can repair more extensive genetic damage than polymerase I. Polymerases II and III restore wide areas of DNA injury (1000 to 3000 nucleotides), a process known as "long patch" repair. Polymerase I carries out only "short patch" repair limited to 10 to 30 nucleotides of an injured DNA molecule. Such injury can occur from ultraviolet irradiation that causes pyrimidine dimer formation (e.g., thymine-thymine, thymine-cytosine, or cytosine-cytosine dimers). These dimers form through the linkage of 5,6 unsaturated bonds of adjacent pyrimidines to form a cyclobutane ring, which distorts the DNA helix and causes replication errors. Repair in the light involves separation of the dimers by photoligase in the presence of light (photoreactivation). Repair in the dark is more complex and requires excision of the dimer by endonucleases and re-establishment of the continuity of the DNA molecule.

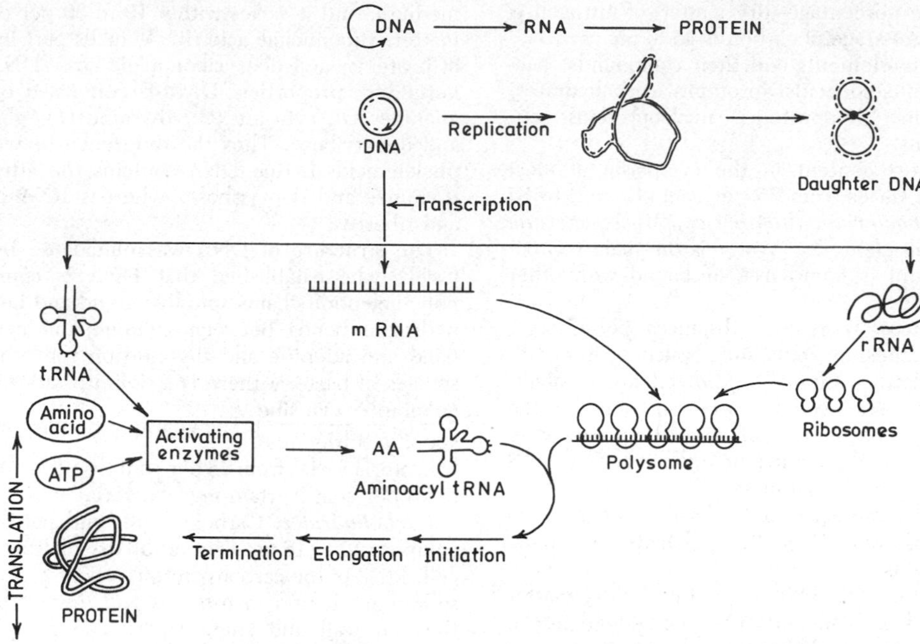

Figure 4. Biosynthetic relationship among DNA, RNA, and proteins.

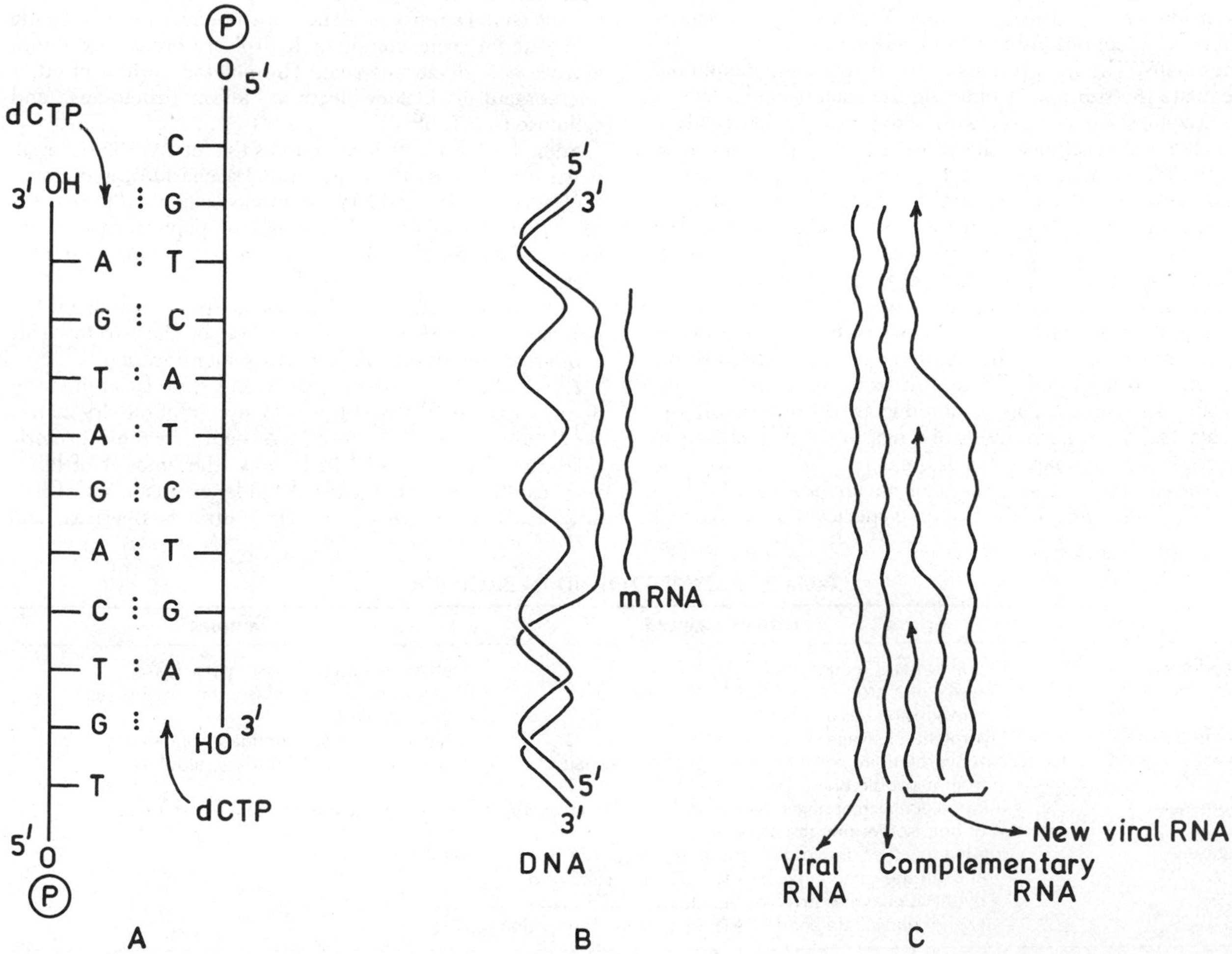

Figure 5. Diagram showing A, the action of DNA polymerase, B, RNA polymerase, and C, replication of viral RNA.

and hydrogen. The percentage (dry matter) of nitrogen is 8 to 15 and the percentage of carbon is 45 to 55.

From the various elements and their compounds, bacteria synthesize nucleic acids, proteins, carbohydrates, lipids, glycoproteins, lipoproteins, nucleoproteins, enzymes, and vitamins.

Water. The water content in the cytoplasm of most species of bacteria varies from 75 per cent *(E. coli)* to 85 per cent (*Corynebacterium diphtheriae, Mycobacterium tuberculosis, Vibrio cholerae*). Water is the main component of the cell and is found free or bound with other component substances.

Mineral Substances. Inorganic substances (phosphorus, sulfur, sodium, magnesium, potassium, calcium, iron, silicon, chlorine) and trace elements (molybdenum, cobalt, boron, manganese, zinc, copper) are also found in the bacterial cell. The total amount of mineral substances in bacteria grown on standard nutrient media varies from 2 to 14 per cent of the microbial mass.

Dry Matter. The organic part of the dry matter of bacteria consists of proteins, nucleic acids, carbohydrates, lipids, and other compounds.

Proteins. More than 50 to 80 per cent of the dry matter of the bacterial cell is made up of proteins found in the cytoplasm, nucleoid, cytoplasmic membrane, and other cell structures (see Chapter 1).

In nucleoproteins, the prosthetic group is made up of nucleic acids. Similarly in lipoproteins the prosthetic group is made up of either fats (lipids) or fat-like substances (lipoids). Lipoproteins are found within the cell as semisolid inclusions. The lipoproteins of the cytoplasmic membrane regulate the substances entering the bacterial cell.

Enzymes are proteins with active groups that catalyze biochemical reactions. The protein part of the enzyme is known as the apoenzyme and the active (prosthetic) group catalyzes the specific chemical reaction. In some cases the active, or prosthetic, groups are not bound firmly to the protein (apoenzyme) and are easily separated from it, whereas others can bind themselves to different proteins. These freely existing nonprotein catalysts involved in biochemical transformations are known as coenzymes. Another group of enzymes contain hemin compounds as the active group. Enzymes concerned with oxidation belong to this group. Enzymes act as oxidoreductases, transferases, hydrolases, lyases, isomerases, and ligases. Their functions in bacteria are summarized in Table 2.

Nucleic Acids. The amount of nucleic acids in the bacterial cell depends on the bacterial species and the nutrient medium, and it varies within 10 to 30 per cent of the dry matter. Ribonucleic acid (RNA) takes part in the synthesis of proteins, and deoxyribonucleic acid (DNA) determines hereditary properties. DNA is composed of adenine (A), guanine (G), cytosine (C), thymine (T), phosphoric acid, and deoxyribose. Thus the difference between these two nucleic acids is that DNA contains the nitrogenous base, thymine, and deoxyribose, whereas RNA contains uracil and ribose.

The structure of DNA was elucidated by Watson and Crick, who established that DNA is composed of two polynucleotide chains spirally wound and held together by hydrogen bonds between guanine and cytosine on one hand and adenine and thymine on the other. For every species of bacteria there is a definite ratio of paired bases $\frac{\text{guanine + cytosine}}{\text{adenine + thymine}}$. The guanine + cytosine (GC) content of bacteria varies from 28 per cent (some lactobacilli species) to 73 per cent (certain mycobacteria).

Carbohydrates. Carbohydrates and polyatomic alcohols compose 12 to 18 per cent of the dry matter in the bacterial cell. Most of the carbohydrate is a polysaccharide complex, sometimes bound to proteins and lipids, that is found in the cell wall and slime layer. The cytoplasm of many bacteria has a comparatively large amount of inclusions, chemically resembling glycogen or starch.

The polysaccharides of the capsules of types II, III, and VIII pneumococcus belong to the group of compounds that do not contain nitrogen. They are polymers of aldobionic acids, and during complete hydrolysis break down into glucose and glucuronic acid. The polysaccharides of other microorganisms include dextrans, levans (fructosans), and cellulose (see Table 1).

Some bacteria have hexosamines that on hydrolysis break down into monosaccharides, aminosaccharides, and amino acids (types I, IV, and XIV pneumococcus, *C. diphtheriae, M. tuberculosis*). Acid hydrolysis of polysaccharides releases galactose, glucose, fructose, and other monosaccharides.

The type specificity in *Salmonella* spp. depends on the polysaccharide side chains of their lipopolysaccharides. This is of great significance in laboratory identification.

Lipids. In those bacteria that do not store fat in the form of inclusions, lipids constitute 10 per cent of the dry matter (in *C. diphtheriae* it is only 5 per cent). In those bacteria that store fats as special inclusions, the amount of lipids reaches 40 per cent. Bacterial lipids are made up of free fatty acids (26 to 28 per cent), neutral fats, waxes, and

Table 2. ENZYMES FOUND IN BACTERIA

Type	Reaction Catalyzed	Examples
Oxidoreductase	Oxidation and reduction	Dehydrogenase, oxidase, peroxidase
Transferase	Transfer of a group containing C, N, P, or S from one substrate to another	Transaminase, transferase, transmethylase, transketolase
Hydrolase	Hydrolytic cleavage	Esterase, amidase, peptidase, phosphatase
Lyase	Nonhydrolytic removal of chemical group, usually from a double bond	Decarboxylases, deaminase, aldolase
Isomerase	Intramolecular rearrangements as in the interconversion of one isomer into the other	Isomerase, racemase, epimerase, mutase
Ligase	Joining together of two different molecules, or of two ends in the same molecule. The reaction catalyzed by these enzymes involves the cleavage of a high-energy phosphate bond in ATP or another energy donor.	Synthetases

phospholipids (see Chapters 6 and 25 for discussion of lipids in gram-negative bacteria, tubercle bacilli, and corynebacteria).

Nutrition

Transport of Nutrients. The phospholipid bilayer, which constitutes the bacterial cell membrane, is a barrier to the passage of most nutrients into the cytoplasm because nutrients are largely water soluble (polar). There are, however, proteins embedded in the membrane, with an average molecular weight of 30,000, that can actively transport into the cell a variety of molecules, including amino acids, lactose, glucose, galactose, and sulfate. This active transport allows the nutrient to reach a concentration within the cell that is thousands of times greater than on its exterior. In order to meet the work requirement for such transport against a concentration gradient, energy must be supplied by metabolic processes within the cell.

Another set of proteins, known as permeases, also facilitate transfer of nutrients into the cytoplasm, but this process requires no energy because the substrate moves from a higher concentration outside the cell to a lower concentration inside. The process is sometimes called "facilitated diffusion" and differs from simple diffusion in that the permease discriminates among substrates (Cohen and Monod, 1957). In other words, a specific permease selectively binds certain substrates, but not others, on the outside of the cell and catalyzes their movement across the cell membrane into the cell. Facilitated diffusion is much less important for transport in bacteria than is active transport. Transport of glycerol into *E. coli.* is an example of facilitated diffusion.

Specific permeases are also responsible for a third type of transport known as "group translocation." In contrast to facilitated diffusion, group translocation involves a chemical change in the substrate, and the reaction requires metabolic energy. Group translocation is typified by the phosphotransferase system that can transfer fructose, glucose, mannose, mannitol, and other sugars against a concentration gradient. The system is composed of two enzymes and a small heat stable carrier protein, HPr. Energy is provided by the energy-rich phosphate bond of phosphoenolpyruvate. The first enzyme, enzyme I, catalyzes the transfer of phosphate (P) to the carrier protein HPr in the following reaction:

$$\text{P-enolpyruvate} + \text{HPr} \rightarrow \text{pyruvate} + \text{P-HPr}$$

The activated carrier protein, P-HPr, then reacts with free hexose so as to carry hexose across the membrane into the cell as hexose-6-phosphate. A second enzyme, enzyme II, catalyzes phosphorylation of the sugar as follows:

$$\text{P-HPr} + \text{hexose} \rightarrow \text{hexose-6-P} + \text{HPr}$$

There is a specific enzyme II for each hexose.

Species of bacteria vary in the method of transport used to carry nutrients into a cell. In addition, simple diffusion allows passage into the cell of substances present in high concentration outside the cell. Water is the most important substance that passes across the cell membrane by passive diffusion.

Types of Nutrition. *Autotrophic,* chemosynthetic, and photosynthetic bacteria can produce organic substances from inorganic compounds. They do not require organic carbon compounds and synthesize the component parts of their cell by absorbing carbon dioxide, in addition to water and simple nitrogen compounds (ammonia and its salts, nitrate, and others). Nitrifying bacteria and many sulfur bacteria belong to the autotrophic microbes. They synthesize complex substances at the expense of the energy they receive from the oxidation of ammonia to nitrites *(Nitrosomonas)* and nitrates *(Nitrobacter)* and the oxidation of sulfur, sulfides, and thiosulfates to sulfuric acid and its salts *(Thiobacillus thiooxidans).*

Some species of microorganisms—anaerobic purple and green sulfur bacteria *(Thiorhodaceae, Chlorobacteriaceae)*—contain chlorophyll and use radiant energy for photosynthesis.

The autotrophic bacteria use carbon dioxide as the sole source of carbon and cannot absorb more complex carbon compounds. For this reason, such organisms cannot be pathogenic for humans and animals.

Heterotrophic bacteria require organic carbon (carbohydrates and keto, amino, and fatty acids), inorganic substances, trace elements, and vitamins. Heterotrophic bacteria can be subdivided into 1) saprophytes and 2) parasites.

1) *Saprophytes* (Greek *sapros* = decaying, phyton = plant) live at the expense of organic substances found in the surrounding environment. These include most species of bacteria inhabiting our planet.

2) *Parasites* make up a comparatively small number of species of bacteria that, in the process of evolution, have adapted themselves to a parasitic mode of life. However, this division of heterotrophic bacteria into saprophytes and parasites is not absolute. Certain species of bacteria pathogenic to man can exist in the environment as saprophytes, and, conversely, some saprophytes under unfavorable conditions can cause disease in humans and animals.

Nutrients Essential for Growth. The majority of bacteria develop only on complex media containing peptone (a product of enzymatic breakdown of meat and other protein substances), meat extract, and products of similar biologic origin, which contain all the nutrients in the form of high molecular weight compounds essential for growth.

NITROGEN. According to the character of nitrogen nutrition, bacteria have been subdivided into a number of groups including those that function by: 1) fixing atmospheric nitrogen; 2) absorbing mineral forms of nitrogen (ammonium sulfate); 3) assimilating ammonium salts, nitrates, or nitrites in the presence of amino acids or purines; 4) growing in the presence of individual amino acids or their mixtures; and 5) growing in protein nutrient media.

CARBON. The sources of carbon for bacteria may be different carbohydrates, polyhydric alcohols, or organic acids. According to their ability to synthesize complex compounds, bacteria may be divided into four groups. 1) Those that obtain carbon from carbon dioxide and nitrogen from inorganic compounds. These organisms use radiant energy (light). Autotrophs that are capable of chemosynthesis obtain energy by the simple process of oxidation of inorganic compounds (nitrifying bacteria, sulfur bacteria, some iron bacteria). 2) Those that derive carbon and obtain energy from organic carbon compounds and nitrogen from its inorganic compounds (the majority of saprophytes). 3) Those that obtain carbon and energy from organic carbon compounds and nitrogen from amino acids (majority of commensals). 4) Those that absorb carbon and obtain energy from organic compounds, obtain nitrogen from a complex of many amino acids, and require one or more vitamins (pathogenic bacteria).

VITAMINS. Besides peptones, carbohydrates, fatty acids, and inorganic elements, bacteria require special substances—vitamins or growth factors that function as coenzymes. As coenzymes, vitamins act as acceptors or donors of chemical groups or H atoms, which are transferred to or from the substrate by various enzymes. These are summarized in Table 3.

Some bacteria do not require a supplement of vitamins to the nutrient medium because they can synthesize these compounds. Others grow poorly on vitamin-free media, but their growth is enhanced upon the addition of vitamins. Bacteria such as pneumococcus and hemolytic streptococcus cannot be cultivated without vitamins. *Hemophilus influenzae* requires supplements of hemin and NAD for growth.

The amount of vitamins in the nutrient medium is expressed in micrograms, and they are required in concentrations varying from 0.001 to 10 mg/L. The concentrations of vitamins in bacterial cells (parts per million of dry weight) vary with different species but have the following ranges: nicotinic acid 210 to 250, riboflavin 44 to 67, thiamine 9 to 26, pyridoxine 6 or 7, pantothenic acid 90 to 140, and folic acid 3 to 15.

Intestinal microflora supply humans and animals directly with vitamins. Many bacteria participate in the vitamin metabolism of plants, in enriching food products with vitamins, and in producing vitamins.

INORGANIC SUBSTANCES. Potassium exerts a catalytic action and activates enzyme systems. Calcium participates in nitrification, in nitrogen fixation by soil microorganisms *(Azotobacter)*, and in the production of gelatinase. Iron is found in the respiratory enzymes and functions as a catalyst in oxidation processes. Trace elements are incorporated into the structure of the active groups of some enzymes. Sulfur is a constituent of cysteine and methionine and of the coenzymes CoA and cocarboxylase. Phosphorus is a constituent of nucleic acids, phospholipids, ATP, and NADP. Magnesium is a cofactor for enzymes, and serves to bind enzymes to substrates. Cobalt is a constituent of vitamin B_{12}. Manganese, zinc, and copper are also essential for the activity of certain enzymes.

BACTERIAL GROWTH. The growth of bacteria represents the increase in mass of bacterial cytoplasm as a result of the synthesis of cellular material.

Bacteria reproduce by simple transverse division, vegetative reproduction that occurs in different planes and produces many different cellular arrangements (clusters, chains, pairs). The transverse division of bacteria not only is a process of cell division of one mother cell into two equal daughter cells, but also represents a continuous separation of daughter cells from the mother cell so that the former in their turn become mother cells.

The rate of cell division differs among bacteria. It depends on the species of microorganism, age of culture, nutrient medium, temperature, concentration of carbon dioxide, and other factors.

The length of the generation of *E. coli*, *Clostridium perfringens*, and *Streptococcus faecalis* is 20 minutes in nutrient broth medium, whereas for the cells of a mammalian tissue culture it is 24 hours, Thus, bacteria reproduce about 100 times faster than a tissue in culture. The increase in the number of cells can be expressed in the following way:

1-2-4-8-16-32 N (number of cells)

0-1-2-3- 4 - 5 n (number of generations)

The total amount of bacteria (N) after n generations will be equal to 2^n per cell of seeded material. If we take the original amount of bacteria inoculated into the nutrient medium as a single individual, and the time for one division as 30 minutes, theoretically, the total amount of bacteria produced per 24 hours would be $N = 2^{48}$. Given a division every 20 minutes, in 36 hours the microbial mass will be equal to 400 tons. Thermophilic microbes divide even more rapidly.

However, in natural as well as in artificial conditions the reproduction of bacteria is on a considerably smaller scale. It is limited by a number of internal and external factors described in the section on regulation of growth. Figure 6

Table 3. VITAMINS AND THEIR COENZYME FUNCTION IN BACTERIA

Vitamin	Coenzyme Form	Transfer Reaction in Which Coenzyme Collaborates
Thiamine	Thiamine pyrophosphate (TPP)	Oxidative decarboxylation of α-keto acids
Nicotinamide	Nicotinamide-adenine dinucleotide (NAD)	Hydrogen transfer in fermentation and respiration
	Nicotinamide-adenine dinucleotide phosphate (NADP)	NAD reversibly transfers electrons by coupling to different enzymes
Riboflavin	Flavin mononucleotide (FMN) Flavin adenine dinucleotide (FAD)	Hydrogen transfer in respiration. FAD is an electron acceptor for the oxidizing enzymes known as flavoproteins. FAD similar in action to NAD
Pyridoxine	Pyridoxal phosphate (PALP)	Catalyzes completely different reactions varying from amino-transfer and decarboxylation to racemization. It is the coenzyme of amino acid metabolism and the active group for amino transferases, decarboxylases, lyases, and synthetases. In all cases it acts by combination of its aldehyde group with the amino group of the substrate
Pantothenic acid	Coenzyme A (CoA) adenosine 3′5′ diphosphate + panthotheine phosphate	Transfer of acyl groups—All acyltransferases transfer acyl groups to or from CoA
Folic acid	Tetrahydrofolate (THFA)	Acts as a carrier of methyl, hydroxymethyl, formyl, or formimino groups
Biotin	Biotin	Carboxyl transfer; energy is derived from ATP
Cobalamine	B_{12} coenzyme	Methyl transfer; isomerase reactions

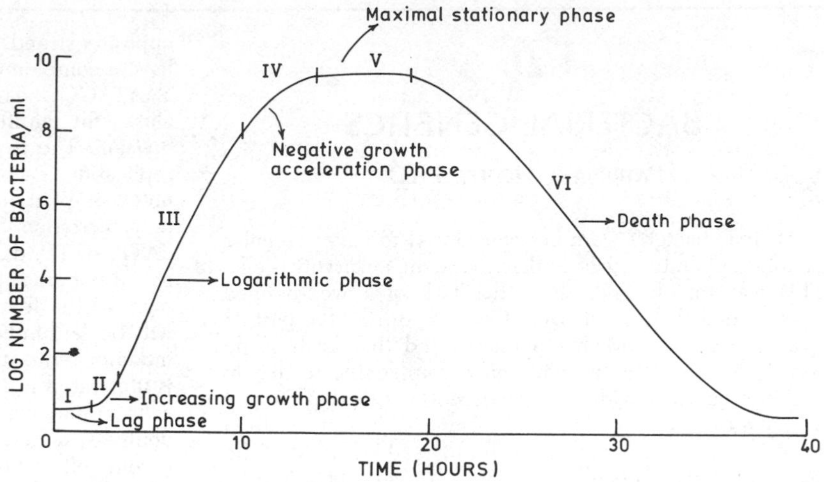

Figure 6. Bacterial growth curve.

illustrates schematically the rate of growth expressed as the number of cells per milliliter of the medium.

There are six principal phases of reproduction that are designated in Figure 6 by Roman numerals:

I. An initial *lag phase* represents a period of physiologic adjustment, during which the cells may need to synthesize new enzymes and re-establish minimal intracellular concentrations of substrates, enzymes, and inorganic ions.

II. A phase of *increasing growth* rate reflects the randomness of adjustment of individuals in the population and the increase in the rate of growth of each individual as the rates of its separate metabolic processes become maximum.

III. A phase of *logarithmic growth* is characterized by a maximal division rate and decrease in cell size. The "growth rate" of a culture is usually expressed in terms of cell doubling time, which is equated with generation time. This rate is influenced by temperature, the nature of the carbon source, the concentration of an essential nutrient if very low, the variety of nutrients available, and, for facultative anaerobes, the O_2 tension.

IV. A phase of *declining growth* rate represents the cessation of growth as a consequence of the exhaustion of the various nutrients in the medium.

V. A maximal *stationary phase* occurs when the number of newly produced bacteria is almost equal to the number of organisms that die because of the lack of essential nutrients.

VI. The *death phase* is a consequence of the loss of selective permeability and of lysis—disintegration of cells.

The length of these phases is arbitrary, for it can vary depending on the species of bacteria and the conditions of cultivation. Thus, *Escherichia coli* divide every 20 minutes, *Salmonella typhi* divide every 25 minutes, *Streptococcus pyogenes* divide every 30 minutes, and *Mycobacterium tuberculosis* divide every 18 hours under optimal growth conditions.

Regulation of Growth. The biosynthetic pathways involved in growth are controlled by *feedback regulation.* The enzyme that mediates the first reaction in the pathway is inhibited by the end product or end products of the pathway, a process designated *end product inhibition.* This process prevents an accumulation of the end product or its intermediates. It assures the balanced operation of both catabolic and biosynthetic pathways.

The mechanism of end product inhibition is not known, but it is thought that the binding of the end product distorts the enzyme and creates a conformational change in the site for substrate attachment, so that the enyzme no longer binds properly to its substrate. An important example of this phenomenon is the inhibition of pyrimidine biosynthesis by cytidine triphosphate (CTP). The synthesis of cytidine begins when the enzyme aspartic transcarbamylase (ATCase) catalyzes the condensation of carbamyl phosphate and aspartic acid with the production of carbamyl aspartic acid as follows:

$$\text{Carbamyl phosphate} + \text{aspartic acid} \xrightarrow{\text{ATCase}} \text{carbamyl aspartic acid}$$

The end product of this reaction is CTP, which inhibits aspartic transcarbamylase and prevents overproduction of the pyrimidine. This control of enzyme function is called *allosteric,* a term that refers to the fact that the enzyme inhibitor has a different shape, or structure, than the substrate, whose attachment to the enzyme is prevented (Monod et al., 1963). Another device for controlling metabolic pathways is known as *catabolite repression.* This phenomenon, described in Chapter 4, represses synthesis of the enzyme.

References

Beadle, G. W., and Tatum, E. L.: Genetic control of biochemical reactions in Neurospora. Proc Natl Acad Sci USA 27:499, 1941.

Cohen, G. N., and Monod, J.: Bacterial permeases. Bacteriol Rev 21:169, 1957.

Höltje, J.-V., and Tomasz, A.: Lipoteichoic acid: a specific inhibitor of autolysin activity in *Pneumococcus.* Proc Natl Acad Sci USA, 72:1690, 1975.

Horecker, B. L.: Pentose Metabolism in Bacteria. New York, John Wiley & Sons, 1962.

Lipmann, F.: Metabolic generation and utilization of phosphate bond energy. Adv Enzymol 1:99, 1941.

Meyerhof, O.: Intermediate carbohydrate metabolism. *In* A Symposium on Respiratory Enzymes. Vol. 3. Madison, University of Wisconsin Press, 1942.

Monod, J., Changeux, J., and Jacob, F.: Allosteric proteins and cellular control systems. J Mol Biol 6:306, 1963.

4

BACTERIAL GENETICS

PATRICIA A. HOFFEE, PH.D.

At first, bacteria were not considered to have a regular genetic apparatus such as that found in eukaryotic cells. This was mainly because of the lack of a well-defined nucleus and their small size. However, during the past 35 years extensive work has demonstrated that bacteria do have a form of genetic inheritance comparable to that in higher organisms, with the main exception that they contain a haploid genome in almost all instances. In fact, bacteria have been used as a model system to establish most of the basic concepts of molecular genetics (Hayes, 1968; Stanier et al., 1970; Watson, 1976).

MOLECULAR ASPECTS

The Bacterial Chromosome: Its Structure and Replication. In the intact bacterial cell there is a single, continuous molecule of deoxyribonucleic acid (DNA) that makes up the chromosome. This molecule has a molecular weight of about 3×10^9 and is a closed circle. The molecular structure of this chromosome was determined by the Nobel prize–winning work of Watson and Crick (Watson, 1976; Watson and Crick, 1953). It is composed of a double helix made of two complementary strands of polynucleotides that contain purine and pyrimidine bases arranged along a backbone of alternating deoxyribose and phosphate groups (Fig. 1). The two strands are held together by hydrogen bonds that occur between a purine and a pyrimidine. This bonding is formed specifically between the pyrimidine thymine and the purine adenine (A-T base pair), or between the pyrimidine cytosine and the purine guanine (G-C base pair) (Fig. 2). Thus, the sequence of bases on one strand always has a complementary sequence of bases on the opposite strand; that is, the sequence ATTATCCG will have a complementary sequence on the opposite strand of TAATAGGC. The presence of the complementary strands allows for faithful replication of the chromosome during division. The two strands separate at a particular origin of replication, each strand acting as its own template, and a new complementary strand is made by the enzymatic polymerization of the deoxyribonucleotide subunits—dATP, dTTP, dCTP, and dGTP. Because of the specificity of the bonding, the new strands will be the exact complement of the template strand, and the genetic information will be faithfully transmitted to the daughter cells. This mode of replication is referred to as *semiconservative* and is illustrated in Figure 3. By this mechanism the daughter cells in the first generation will have one strand of the double-stranded DNA molecule that originated from the parent cell and one new strand. In the second generation, two of the daughter cells will have no strand from the original parent cell. The mechanism of semiconservative replication was demonstrated by the experiment of Meselson and Stahl (1958) in which the parent cell DNA was labeled with heavy nitrogen and the pattern of distribution of the heavy label was then followed through several generations (Fig. 3).

In order for each daughter cell to receive a copy of the chromosome at cell division some control must be maintained over the replication of the chromosome. It is hypothesized that the bacterial chromosome has some attachment point on the cell membrane so that replication can be synchronized with cell division. A model proposed by Jacob and Brenner (1963), referred to as the *replicon model,* proposes that there is a specific point on the chromosome that is activated by an "initiator" protein. Replication begins at this point on the chromosome and then proceeds in a bidirectional manner until the whole chromosome has been

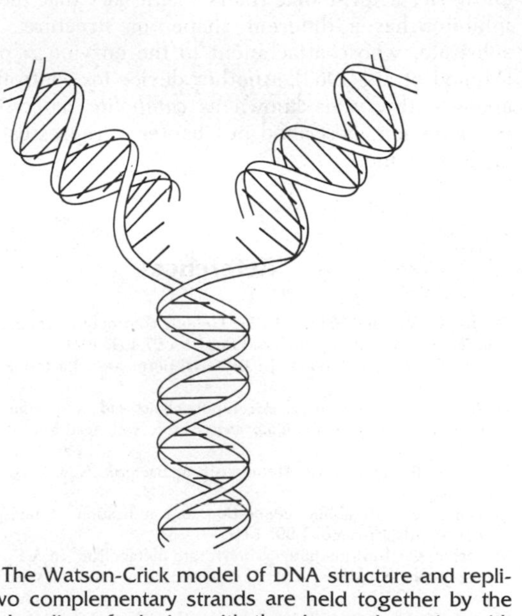

Figure 1. The Watson-Crick model of DNA structure and replication. Two complementary strands are held together by the hydrogen bonding of adenine with thymine, and guanine with cytosine. The strands unwind during replication, and each strand acts as a template for the synthesis of the new daughter strands.

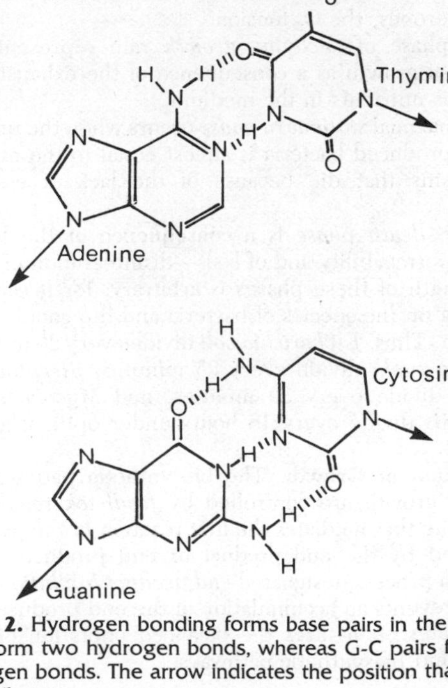

Figure 2. Hydrogen bonding forms base pairs in the DNA. A-T pairs form two hydrogen bonds, whereas G-C pairs form three hydrogen bonds. The arrow indicates the position that binds to deoxyribose.

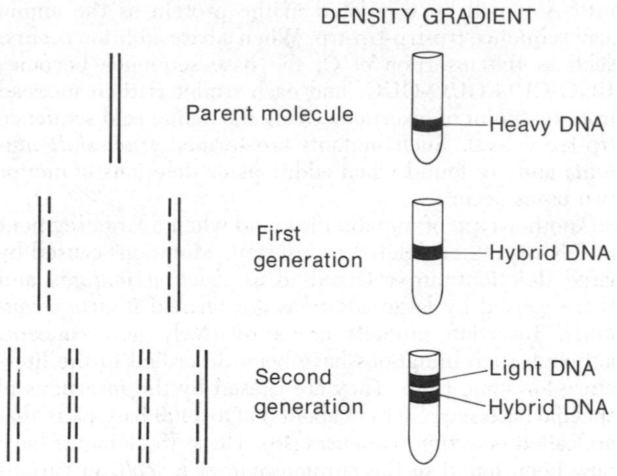

Figure 3. Semiconservative replication of DNA in *E. coli* as demonstrated by the experiment of Meselson and Stahl (1958). The DNA of the parents is labeled with ^{15}N, so that it appears heavy in a density gradient. After one generation in ^{14}N medium, the DNA from the first generation progeny is hybrid in density, since it has one strand of heavy DNA and one strand of light DNA. After the second generation, DNA of light density begins to appear along with the DNA of hybrid density. This pattern of density bands is consistent with semiconservative replication.

replicated. Numerous proteins are involved in the replication process, and a number of them have been identified by the isolation of mutants of *Escherichia coli,* which are temperature-sensitive for DNA replication (a temperature-sensitive mutant is one that can function normally at a permissive, or lower, temperature and is unable to do so at a nonpermissive, or higher, temperature; see section on Mutation). At least five specific genes have already been identified as being involved in the process of replication, and several other ones have been postulated but have yet to be identified.

The Chromosome as a Functioning Unit. All the genetic potential of the bacterial cell is contained in the base sequence of the DNA molecule. (However, many bacteria contain extrachromosomal elements also of DNA that can confer additional genetic potential on a cell; see section on Gene Transfer in Bacteria). In order for this information to be expressed in the cellular behavior of the cell a number of complex processes must occur. The first process involves the transcription of the DNA base sequence into a ribonucleic acid molecule that will serve as a message—hence the name messenger ribonucleic acid (mRNA). Segments of the DNA molecules are transcribed into mRNA by the action of an enzyme called RNA polymerase. This enzyme can polymerize ribonucleotides (ATP, GTP, CTP, and UTP) into a complementary strand of RNA, so that the presence of A in the DNA will result in U in the RNA, G in the DNA will give C in the RNA, T in the DNA will result in A in the RNA, and C in the DNA will give G in the RNA. Each discrete segment of DNA will specify an RNA message that will eventually be translated into a protein molecule. Such a segment or sequence of bases in the DNA is referred to as a *gene.* The mRNA molecule is translated into protein by the protein-synthesizing machinery of the cell, which is made up of activated amino acids, transfer RNA (tRNA), and ribosomes. The mRNA and the tRNA, which has a specific amino acid attached, come together on the surface of the ribosome. The tRNA molecule has a triplet of bases on one end that is complementary to a triplet of bases on the mRNA. Each tRNA molecule finds its complementary triplet on the mRNA, and the amino acid that it carries is put into a peptide linkage with the amino acid of the preceding tRNA molecule. As the ribosome moves along the mRNA, the peptide grows by the addition of each amino acid in a sequential manner until the complete mRNA has been translated into a sequence of amino acids. The sequence of bases in the DNA represents a code that was broken some 15 years ago. Each triplet of bases in the DNA (a *codon*), and thus in the mRNA, specifies a particular amino acid. So whenever this codon appears in the DNA, a particular amino acid will be found in a particular position in the protein coded for by that segment of DNA. This genetic code is presented in Figure 4. Any possible sequence of three bases specifies an amino acid; thus AAU will specify asparagine, whereas AAG will specify lysine. The exceptions are the three codons UAG (amber), UAA (ochre), and UGA (opal). These codons do not specify an amino acid and are involved in the termination of peptide synthesis. They are called *nonsense codons.* In order for the proper DNA sequences to be read at the appropriate times and in the right way, various mechanisms of control of transcription have evolved in bacterial cells. Some of these mechanisms will be discussed later in this chapter.

Although the detailed work on the genetic code and its translation and transcription led to a universal hypothesis of colinearity of the gene and its protein, recent work with viruses and mammalian cells suggests that other mechanisms of gene structure exist. It is now known that in some viruses there exist overlapping genes in which codons are read in different phases, so that the same sequence of bases

First	Second U	Second C	Second A	Second G	Third
U	phe	ser	tyr	cys	U
U	phe	ser	tyr	cys	C
U	leu	ser	(ochre)	(opal)	A
U	leu	ser	(amber)	trp	G
C	leu	pro	his	arg	U
C	leu	pro	his	arg	C
C	leu	pro	gln	arg	A
C	leu	pro	gln	arg	G
A	ile	thr	asn	ser	U
A	ile	thr	asn	ser	C
A	ile	thr	lys	arg	A
A	met, fmet	thr	lys	arg	G
G	val	ala	asp	gly	U
G	val	ala	asp	gly	C
G	val	ala	glu	gly	A
G	val	ala	glu	gly	G

Figure 4. The genetic code. The combinations of the four bases give 64 possible triple codons, which are listed with their amino acid assignments. Three codons, UAA (ochre), UAG (amber), and UGA (opal), do not code for any amino acid and are the nonsense codons that are used for termination signals.

in the DNA may code for more than one protein. In mammalian cells the DNA contains interdispersed base sequences referred to as "introns" and "exons." A complete RNA transcript is made from the DNA, the intron sequences are removed from the RNA, and the exons or remaining sequences are joined together to form the final mRNA molecule. In this way discontinuous sequences of bases in the DNA can code for a single polypeptide. RNA splicing has not been found in bacteria.

MUTATION

Molecular Basis of Mutation. A mutation is defined as a change in the base sequence of the DNA. In many cases such a base change will result in an altered amino acid sequence of a protein that will, in turn, alter the normal functioning of that protein. In addition, the base change will be propagated when the DNA is replicated. Thus, a mutation is characterized by its effect on cell growth or metabolism and by its stability in the progeny cells. The base change can occur in the DNA by one of two mechanisms: 1) substitution of one base pair by a different base pair, or 2) an addition or deletion of a base pair or a segment of DNA during breakage of the sugar-phosphate backbone of the DNA. Single base pair changes are referred to as point mutations. Such mutations can occur spontaneously during replication or repair of the DNA or can be increased in rate of appearance by chemicals or physical agents that can interact with the DNA molecule. Chemicals that can enhance the rate of mutation are called mutagens. The first group of mutagens includes base analogues, which are incorporated into the DNA in place of the natural base. These analogues have an increased tendency to pair with the wrong base during replication, which results in the replacement of one base pair by a different base pair. Such base analogues include compounds such as bromouracil, an analogue of thymine, and 2-aminopurine, an analogue of adenine. A second group is composed of compounds that chemically alter bases in the DNA and thus alter their pairing ability. These compounds include chemicals such as nitrous acid and alkylating reagents, of which the most powerful is *N*-methyl-*N*-nitroso-*N'*-nitroguanidine (nitrosoguanidine). The third group consists of still other chemicals, such as the acridine dyes, that cause mutation by intercalating between stacked base pairs in the DNA, which results in the insertion or deletion of base pairs during replication.

Substitution of one base pair by another may lead to a change in a codon that results in the replacement of the original amino acid in the protein by a new amino acid. For example, if there is a change from a A-T pair to a G-C pair in the DNA, one might have a change in the codon in the mRNA from UCG to CCG and thus a change in the amino acid sequence in which serine is replaced by proline. This type of change, in which one amino acid replaces another in the protein, is referred to as a *missense mutation*. If the base change results in production of one of the codons UAA, UGA, or UAG no amino acid is placed in the polypeptide chain, and termination of peptide synthesis occurs. This type of change, in which no amino acid is designated by the codon, is termed a *nonsense mutation*.

Whenever additions or deletions of single base pairs occur, such as with acridine dyes, there is a change in the reading frame of the mRNA so that all codons from the point of insertion or deletion are misread. For example, if the base sequence UGG-UGG-UGG-UGG occurs in the mRNA it will be translated in the protein as the amino acid sequence trp-trp-trp-trp. When a base addition occurs, such as the insertion of C, the base sequence becomes UGG-CUG-GUG-GUG, and each triplet is then misread from the point of insertion, giving the amino acid sequence trp-leu-val-val. Such mutants are termed *frameshift mutants* and are found when additions or deletions of one or two bases occur.

Another type of mutation is found when a large segment of DNA is either deleted or inserted. Mutations caused by large deletions are referred to as *deletion mutants* and those caused by large additions are termed *insertion mutants*. Insertion mutants are a relatively new concept, although such mutations have been described in the literature for some time. They are caused by the insertions of specific base sequences of about 800 to 1400 base pairs that are called *insertion sequences* (IS). These IS elements have now been found in the chromosome of *E. coli*, in various bacterial viruses, and in plasmids, and they act as a mechanism for joining pieces of DNA that occur in bacterial cells.

Just as mutations occur in the forward direction, as described previously, similar chemical changes occur that can result in getting back the original or a pseudooriginal phenotype. These changes, referred to as *reversions*, will be dependent in type on the kind of forward mutation that initially occurred. For example, in the case of base substitution, a reversion can simply be the change of the same base pair back to the one that was originally present. If the triplet UCG mutated to CCG, it could revert back to UCG by a change in the same base pair. Such revertants are termed *true revertants* and are genetically identical to the original parent. In addition, there are revertants that result not from changing the mutated initial base pair but from changing a base pair at another site in the DNA. Such a revertant, in which a second mutation compensates for the original mutation, is referred to as a *suppressor mutation*. They can occur within the same gene as the original mutation *(intragenic)* or they can occur in a gene outside the gene in which the initial mutation occurred *(extragenic)*. Intragenic suppression can correct both point mutations and frameshift mutations. Extragenic suppression is usually the result of a mutation occurring in a gene that codes for a product involved in translation, such as a tRNA molecule. The secondary mutation corrects the original defect by recognizing this defect as normal for translation. An important class of extragenic suppressors are those that correct a nonsense mutation. Some of these suppressors have been shown to be the result of a mutant tRNA that now recognizes the nonsense codon as one of the sense codons, and allows an amino acid to be inserted into the peptide chain and its synthesis to continue. Deletion mutants are not capable of reversion, but insertion mutants can revert to the original genotype of the parent cell by a simple loss of the inserted sequence.

The Phenotypic Expression of Mutation. The preceding discussion gives one an understanding of what mutation is at the molecular level. However, such mutations, or changes in the base sequence of DNA, can be recognized only if they have an effect on the phenotype of the bacterial cell or virus that is being studied. Early in the study of bacteriology the apparent rapidity with which mutations occurred in bacteria and the selection of such mutants by the environment made it difficult to accept that bacteria had a genetic apparatus like that found in eukaryotic systems. It was as if the bacterial cell was altered as a direct response to environmental changes. The acceptance of bacterial cells as having a genetic makeup similar to that of other living organisms came with the classic experiment of Luria and Delbrück in 1943. This experiment, called the *fluctuation test*, is diagrammed in Figure 5. To understand the fluctuation test one must remember that a culture of bacteria grows exponentially, with each cell giving rise to two daughter cells until the culture reaches stationary phase. If, during growth, mutations arise spontaneously in bacteria, the point of time during the growth cycle at which the mutation occurs will determine how many cells will carry that mutation at the end of the growth cycle. For example, if we start with a dilute culture of *E. coli* that is sensitive to the presence of streptomycin (str^s will not grow in the presence of streptomycin), and if the theory of spontaneous mutation is true, there is the probability a mutation that will make a cell resistant to the action of streptomycin (str^r) will occur at any point in the growth cycle. If this mutation occurs early during the growth of the culture, at the end of the growth phase there will be a large number of str^r cells that will have been derived from the original mutant cell. If the mutation occurs late during the growth of the culture, at the end of the growth phase there will be only a few cells that are str^r. The number of str^r cells present in the population at the end of the growth phase is determined by plating out an aliquot of the cells on a nutrient agar plate containing streptomycin. The str^s cells will be killed, and only the str^s cells will grow into colonies. If mutation in bacteria does not occur spontaneously, but instead is directed by the environment, the number of cells that become str^r at the end of the growth phase will be independent of time. The fluctuation test sets up a large number of independent cultures, each started from a few str^s cells, to test this hypothesis. The cultures are allowed to grow for a definitive amount of time in the absence of streptomycin, and a sample from each culture is then plated on a nutrient agar plate containing streptomycin. If mutation is spontaneous, the number of resistant cells present in the independent tubes at the time of plating will show a large fluctuation, the number present being dependent on the time at which the mutation occurred. If mutation is not a random event, all the cultures will have the same number of resistant colonies, since exposure to streptomycin occurs at the same time, and all cells have the same probability of becoming resistant. In all instances that were tested, a large fluctuation in the number of mutant cells occurred, providing evidence for the theory of spontaneous mutation in bacteria. This type of analysis is important today as one of the best methods for providing evidence for the occurrence of mutation, particularly in the newly developing field of somatic cell genetics.

Although the results of the fluctuation test convinced most workers that bacteria undergo spontaneous mutation, there were a few workers who objected to the statistical nature of the data. These doubters were finally convinced by the development of the replica plating or indirect selection technique of Lederberg and Lederberg in 1952. The technique of replica plating is diagrammed in Figure 6. Although it was initially used to provide evidence that one could select a mutant cell without ever having that cell come into contact with the selecting agent, replica plating is now a valuable technique for the scoring of numerous genetic markers in a large number of colonies with a minimum amount of work. The technique involves using a square of velveteen, which has a raised surface, and placing it over the flattened surface of a wood block with a diameter slightly less than the size of a petri dish. A plate containing colonies of bacterial cells is pressed against the velveteen, and the cells are transferred to the cloth. Sterile plates containing various selective media are then inverted onto the fabric and replicas of the initial plate are transferred to the selective media. By sequential plating, picking, and growing of the cells, as shown in Figure 6, one can eventually isolate a colony of bacteria, the progeny of which are all resistant to the selective agent, even though they never came into contact with the agent. Thus, bacteria are constantly undergoing mutation, and any change in the environment can select a cell that has a growth advantage over the parent cells.

Mutation Rate. The rate at which mutation occurs is expressed as a probability of the event occurring per cell generation, or each time one cell divides to form two new cells. To determine the mutation rate it is necessary to know within a specified time the increase that has occurred in the number of cells and in the number of mutations. The mutation rate (a) can be expressed as $a = \frac{M_t - M_0}{N_t - N_0}$, where M_0 is the number of mutations present at time zero

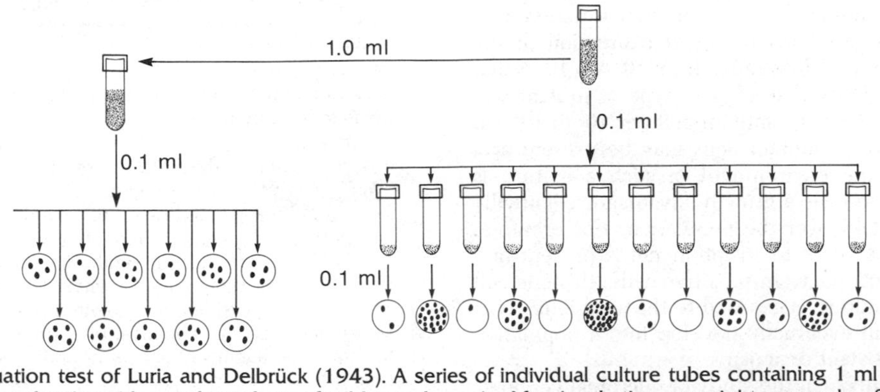

Figure 5. The fluctuation test of Luria and Delbrück (1943). A series of individual culture tubes containing 1 ml of nutrient medium are inoculated at low density with equal numbers of wild-type bacteria. After incubation overnight, a sample of each tube is plated on nutrient agar containing a selective agent such as streptomycin. Resistant cells will appear as colonies on the plates. A large fluctuation is seen in the numbers of resistant cells from different tubes, supporting the theory of spontaneous mutation. The control tube on the left is sampled multiple times to determine the fluctuation caused by random error.

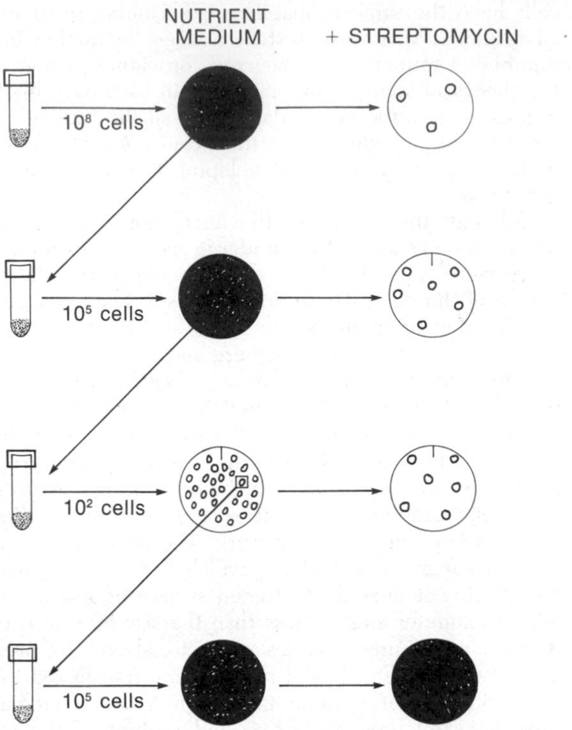

Figure 6. Replica plating or indirect selection of Lederberg and Lederberg (1952). Streptomycin-sensitive cells, 10^8, are spread on a nutrient medium and the plate is incubated to allow growth that will be confluent. The cells on the plate are then replicated using a sterile velveteen cloth to a sterile plate containing streptomycin. A few colonies develop after overnight incubation. The location on the original plate of resistant cells is determined by comparing the plates. The cells on this area are removed and transferred to fresh nutrient broth and allowed to grow. The procedure is repeated until an isolated clone is picked, the progeny of which are all streptomycin resistant.

and M_t is the number present at time t, and N_0 is the number of cells present at time zero and N_t is the number of cells present at time t. Another method for the determination of mutation rate is based on the use of the fluctuation test. If there are tubes found in the fluctuation test in which no mutations are present at the time of plating, the mutation rate can be determined from the Poisson distribution, where $\ln P_0 = -m$. Although it is difficult to get an absolute value for the mutation rate because of various problems in lag of expression of the phenotype, in general, values range from 10^{-6} to 10^{-9}; that is, there is a probability that a given type of mutant will be present to the extent of 1 mutant cell per 10^6 to 10^9 cell divisions. Even though mutant cells may be present at a low frequency, if the environment of such a culture is altered to give these cells a growth advantage, eventually this cell type will take over the population. For example, if one cell that is resistant to streptomycin is present in a population of 10^8 streptomycin-sensitive cells, this one cell will survive if the culture is exposed to the antibiotic. That one mutant cell will eventually develop into a population of streptomycin-resistant organisms.

Selection Procedures. In the study of microbial genetics, selection of specific mutant phenotypes depends on the ability to alter the environment of bacterial cells. It is from the study of mutants with altered growth properties and altered control mechanisms that one can begin to understand the normal and infectious properties of microorganisms. Thus, the basis for the study of microbial genetics is the ability to select from a large population a few cells that have the genetic characteristics one wishes to study. To this end various standard selection procedures have been developed to enable one to isolate particular types of mutant cells. Most of these studies have been done with *E. coli* or *Salmonella typhimurium,* because of the ability of these gram-negative enteric bacteria to grow on a minimal medium consisting of only salts, trace metals, and a carbon and nitrogen source. Provided with one of a variety of carbohydrates these bacteria have all the necessary enzymes and proteins to make all their necessary growth requirements, including amino acids, purines, pyrimidines, vitamins, and other metabolic intermediates. The organisms (as isolated from nature) with these genetic capabilities are referred to as *wild-type* cells. Cells isolated from the wild type that differ in one or more genes are designated as *mutants.* Mutant strains with additional growth requirements are termed *auxotrophs.* The nomenclature used to designate these strains is given in Table 1. The compound usually is listed by the first three letters of the name, hence *ara* for arabinose and *his* for histidine, followed by + or −. Resistance or sensitivity to a particular environment is designated as s or r. The following procedures have been developed to isolate various classes of mutants.

RESISTANCE. This is the easiest type of mutant to isolate. The procedure involves plating a large number of sensitive organisms in the presence of the selective agent. Surviving clones are purified and are resistant to that agent. This method can be used to isolate cells resistant to bacteriophages, antibiotics, chemicals, or physical agents such as ultraviolet light or x-rays.

AUXOTROPHS. This type of mutant is difficult to isolate because the parent cells grow as well as the mutant under all conditions. The method for the isolation of auxotrophs makes use of the fact that the parent will grow under conditions in which the mutant will not. The antibiotic penicillin, which kills only growing cells, is used. Wild-type cells are placed in a minimal glucose medium containing penicillin and are incubated for 18 to 20 hours. During this time wild-type cells grow and are killed by the action of penicillin. Any auxotrophs present are not able to grow because of the lack of a specific growth factor and so are

Table 1. NOTATION OF GENETIC MARKERS

+:	Ability to utilize a carbohydrate or synthesize an intermediate, usually wild-type
−:	Lack of ability to utilize a carbohydrate or synthesize an intermediate, usually mutant
	Examples:
ara⁺:	Ability to utilize arabinose as a carbon and energy source
ara⁻:	Inability to utilize arabinose as a carbon and energy source but will utilize other sugars
his⁺:	Ability to synthesize histidine
his⁻:	Inability to synthesize histine, requires histidine for growth, histidine auxotroph
s:	Sensitivity to agent—chemical or antibiotic
r:	Resistance to agent—chemical or antibiotic
	Examples:
str^s:	Sensitive and will not grow in the presence of streptomycin
str^r:	Resistant and will grow in the presence or absence of streptomycin

not killed by penicillin. The surviving cells are plated on a supplemented medium in the absence of penicillin. To select for a particular mutant among the survivors, the clones can be tested by replica plating on a large number of media containing different supplements; that is, a *his*$^-$ auxotroph will be selected for by looking for growth on a medium with histidine, but no growth will occur when histidine is omitted. Using the penicillin method of selecting auxotrophs, mutants in nearly all known biosynthetic pathways that are coded for by the bacterial chromosomes of *E. coli* and *S. typhimurium* are now available.

FERMENTATION-NEGATIVE MUTANTS. A fermentation-negative mutant is a strain that has lost the ability to use a particular carbohydrate as a carbon and energy source but can still use other carbohydrates for growth. These mutants generally are deficient in the specific enzymes necessary for the catabolism of the specific carbohydrate. For example, mutants unable to use the carbohydrate lactose are deficient either in a protein necessary for the transport of the sugar into the cell or in the enzyme β-galactosidase, which catalyzes the breakdown of lactose into galactose and glucose. Such mutants can be isolated by combining the penicillin selection procedure with the identification of the specific mutant on a differential medium such as eosin-methylene blue (EMB) lactose medium or McConkey's lactose medium, in which the lactose-fermenting colonies give a color reaction (due to acid production) and the lactose-negative cells (*lac*$^-$) show a lack of color. For the penicillin selection, the sugar lactose is used in place of glucose in the minimal medium with penicillin. Lactose-negative cells that are not growing survive, whereas the growing lactose-positive cells are killed.

CONDITIONAL LETHAL MUTANTS. Conditional lethal mutants have a mutation that is expressed under one set of environmental conditions but not under others. The environmental conditions in which the mutation is expressed do not permit growth and are referred to as *nonpermissive conditions*. Similarly, when the mutation is not expressed, conditions permit growth and are called *permissive conditions*. A major class of such mutants are temperature-sensitive (*ts*) mutants. Such *ts* mutants will grow at a lower temperature (25° C) but will not survive at a higher temperature (42° C), whereas the wild-type cells are capable of growing at both temperatures. These mutants usually have a missense mutation that results in the production of a protein that will function normally at a low temperature but not at the higher temperature. A second class of conditional lethal mutants result from a nonsense mutation. Such mutants can grow only in the presence of a secondary mutation or in a suppressor strain that allows for correction of the mutational defect at the translational level. Conditional lethal mutants are extremely valuable, since they allow the isolation, where no other selection procedure exists, of mutants defective in essential functions. A *ts* mutant can be isolated by plating cells at the permissive temperature and then, by replica plating, screening clones that will not grow at the nonpermissive temperature. The defective function must then be determined by biochemical analysis of the *ts* mutants.

GENE TRANSFER IN BACTERIA. Bacteria can exchange genetic material; however, the mechanisms of exchange differ strikingly from genetic exchange in eukaryotes. The three methods of gene transfer that occur in bacteria—*transformation*, *conjugation*, and *transduction*—have several features in common: 1) Only fragments of the chromosome of one parent (called the donor cell) are usually transferred to a second cell (called the recipient cell). 2) Fragments of the donor chromosome are assumed to pair with the homologous regions of the recipient chromosome. 3) After pairing, the genetic material of the donor usually replaces its allelic material on the recipient chromosome to yield haploid recombinants. This is referred to as *replacement integration*. 4) In some special instances, certain genetic elements (plasmids or bacteriophages) can recombine in total with the bacterial chromosome to form a composite molecule containing all the genetic material from both DNA molecules. This type of recombination is referred to as *additive recombination*.

Transformation. Transformation is gene transfer resulting from the uptake by a recipient cell of naked DNA released by a donor cell. For example, DNA released or purified in the laboratory from a donor strain that is *str*^{r} is mixed with cells that are *str*^{s}. An aliquot of the mixture is plated on a nutrient medium containing streptomycin, and approximately 1 in 100 cells plated are capable of growth. Thus, resistance to streptomycin has appeared with a frequency of 10^{-2}. These *str*^{r} cells do not arise from mutations, since mutation to *str*^{r} occurs with a frequency of only 1 in 10^8 cells plated, but rather must result from the transfer of the *str*^{r} DNA to the recipients. This type of gene transfer was originally described by Griffith in 1928 while working with the pneumococcus. This organism is virulent to mice only if the strains produce a polysaccharide capsule and hence have a smooth appearance during colony growth. If the capsule is absent, as in rough strains, virulence is also absent. Griffith showed that injection into a mouse of heat-killed smooth strains of pneumococci plus live rough strains killed the mouse and that live smooth pneumococci appeared in the dead mouse. He did not understand the mechanisms involved but suggested the name of "transforming factor" for the agent responsible for this phenomenon. In 1944, Avery, Macleod, and McCarty showed that the factor involved was DNA.

Transformation takes place in a large number of gram-negative and gram-positive bacteria, including *Pneumococcus, Hemophilus, Bacillus, Neisseria, Streptococcus, Xanthomonas,* and *Rhizobium*. Studies on transformation have been carried out in the laboratory, in most cases with *Pneumococcus, Hemophilus,* or *Bacillus*. More recently it has been found that *E. coli* also can undergo transformation if high concentrations of calcium ion are present.

In the interaction of transforming DNA with recipient cells, three determinants appear to be of major importance:

The size of the DNA. DNA that can transform cells has a minimum molecular weight of about 5×10^5 but may be as large as 10^8. Double-stranded DNA is many times more efficient for transformation than are single-stranded DNA structures.

The concentration of the DNA. Transformation is a function of DNA concentration. At a concentration of DNA below 100 mμg/ml, the number of transformants is proportional to the DNA concentration. This indicates that each transformant arises from the interaction of a recipient with a single molecule of transforming DNA. DNA that is foreign to the bacterial recipient DNA can also be taken up if it is double-stranded. Thus, *Pneumococcus* can take up calf thymus DNA. Such foreign DNA, however, does not integrate into the recipient DNA and thus cannot transform.

The physiologic state of the recipient cell. In order for a recipient cell to take up DNA it must be in a physiologic state called *competence*. The period in the growth cycle when competence appears can vary with each bacterial species but generally appears near the end of the growth phase, just before the stationary phase (Fig. 7). This is usually a transient state, but cells can be maintained in the competent state by freezing at −40° C in 10 to 15 per cent glycerol. Competence is genetically controlled, and a protein can be extracted from competent cells that can make noncompetent cells competent. The mechanism of action of this protein, as well as the biochemical basis for competence, is unknown.

In the process of transformation, double-stranded DNA binds to the surface of the recipient cells. This DNA is cut by a membrane-bound endonuclease, and entry of the DNA is initiated. The uptake of the DNA occurs with digestion of one of the two complementary strands and the entrance into the cell of the other strand of DNA. This single-stranded piece of DNA is then integrated into the recipient cell at the homologous region of DNA replacing the recipient allele. The initial recombinant formed has a short region of the DNA that is part donor DNA and part recipient DNA. However, during the first replication cycle each strand of DNA is replicated faithfully and a new haploid cell emerges that now carries some new genetic information derived from the donor cell.

Conjugation. Conjugation is gene transfer that occurs between sexually differentiated bacteria. It requires cell-to-cell contact between two viable cells, a donor, or male cell, and a recipient, or female cell. Conjugation was discovered in 1946 by Lederberg and Tatum and was shown to differ from transformation. The gene transfer they described was resistant to the action of DNase and needed physical contact between two cells.

In conjugation, the donor, or male strain, always transfers its genetic material to the recipient, or female strain. Genetic material does not go from the female to the male cell.

The Sex Factor. Male cells differ from female cells by possessing a factor called the fertility factor, or *F factor*. The F factor, a typical plasmid, is a small, circular DNA molecule, about 2 per cent of the size of the bacterial

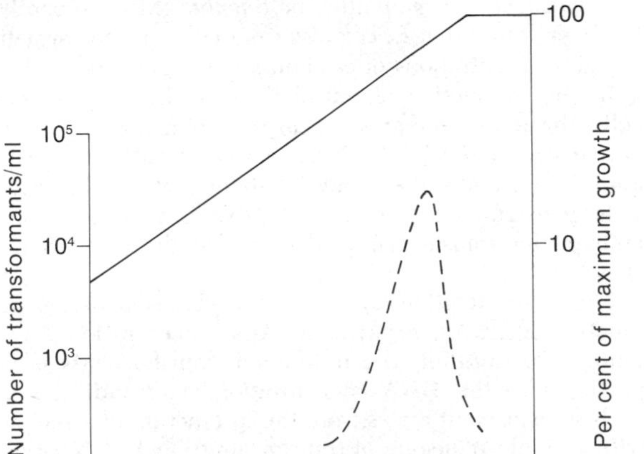

Figure 7. The appearance of competence during cell growth. During cell growth (—) samples are removed from the culture and tested for their ability to be transformed (--). Competence peaks in late log phase.

chromosome. It can exist within bacterial cells and replicate independently of the host chromosome. Male cells carrying the F factor can be recognized by the presence on the cell surface of a protein appendage referred to as an *F pilus* (see Chap. 1). The F pilus serves as a receptor site for the binding of various male-specific bacteriophages that can contain either DNA or RNA. The genetic information for the synthesis of the F pilus is contained in a series of genes located in the F factor. When the F factor is in the autonomous state, that is, not associated with the chromosome, the host cells are referred to as *F^+ cells.* F^+ cells are capable of transferring the F factor to recipient, or *F^- cells*, upon cell-to-cell contact. Within a short time as many as 70 percent of the F^- cells can become F^+ cells. However, the F^+ cells remain F^+, suggesting that the factor must be replicated sometime during or before the transfer to the F^- cells. In a cross between an F^+ and an F^- cell one can detect a few recombinants for some bacterial markers with a frequency of about 10^{-5}.

Hfr Strains. In 1950, Cavelli isolated a male strain of bacteria that was unusual in that it had a 1000-fold increase in the frequency with which recombinants appeared, and it did not transfer the F factor to the recipients except in very rare instances. Such strains, and there are many now that have been isolated, are called *Hfr strains*, or high frequency of recombination strains. These strains arise in F^+ populations and are the result of the association of the F factor with the bacterial chromosome (see later discussion).

With the finding of Hfr strains that showed such high recombination values, the kinetics of the conjugation process could be investigated. Such studies were initiated in the late 1950s by Jacob and Wollman with the development of interrupted mating experiments. An interrupted mating experiment is performed by mixing together male and female cells in a ratio of 1 Hfr to 20 female cells. The female cells contain a series of genetic defects, for example: *thr*⁻, auxotrophic for threonine; *leu*⁻, auxotrophic for leucine; *lac*⁻, unable to ferment lactose; *gal*⁻, unable to ferment galactose; *azi*ˢ, sensitive to azide; T_1^s, sensitive to the phage T1; and *str*ʳ, resistant to streptomycin. In contrast, the male strain carries the opposite markers, that is, sensitive to streptomycin, resistant to azide and T1, prototrophic for threonine and leucine, and able to ferment both lactose and galactose. The two cultures are mixed at high density for five minutes, and are then diluted to stop additional pair formation. At this point samples are removed at timed intervals. The samples are agitated violently to break up the mating pairs; then aliquots are plated on various selective media to determine what genetic information has been transferred from the Hfr strain to the recipient strain. The media are made so that neither parent strain is able to grow. For example, including streptomycin will eliminate growth of the Hfr; the absence of threonine or leucine will prevent growth of F^- cells unless they have received the respective genes from the donor. Data from a typical mating experiment are shown in Figure 8. Several things are characteristic of these experiments: 1) The curves do not go through the origin. Thus, if the mating is interrupted at zero time no recombinants are formed. However, the longer the mating time, the more genetic material is transferred, so that at 30 minutes all the tested markers have appeared in the recipient—some to a greater and some to a lesser extent. 2) The time that a curve begins to rise represents the time of entry of the marker into the recipient. Thus, 18 minutes is the time that lactose enters

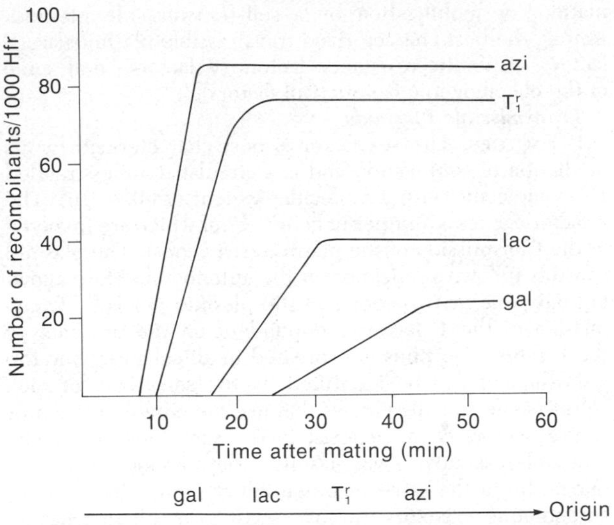

Figure 8. Interrupted mating between Hfr and F^- cells. An Hfr strain is mixed with a genetically marked F^- strain (see text). At the specified time, samples are taken, the mating is stopped by vigorous agitation, and aliquots are plated on various selective media. The data are summarized in the bottom arrow and give the order of transfer of the markers from the Hfr to the F^- cell.

the recipient. 3) The timed order of transfer reflects the order of genes on the chromosome and is characteristic of a particular Hfr strain. In the example in Figure 8, the first marker to enter the recipient is the azide gene, followed by T1, *lac*, and *gal*, in that order. Since the time of entrance is dependent on their location on the chromosome, one can construct a chromosome map by timing the genes entering the F^- cell. Such mapping is usually only accurate within one minute.

Different Hfr strains vary in the time that certain markers enter the recipient and in their point of origin (defined as the part of the chromosome that is first to enter the recipient), but the order of genetic markers with respect to each other does not change. Let us assume that we have three different Hfr strains, and the genetic markers are represented as A, B, C, D, and E, with O representing the point of origin. Interrupted mating experiments between each Hfr and the same recipient give the following pattern of gene transfer. Hfr-1 transfers the markers as O-D-C-B-A-E, Hfr-2 transfers the markers as O-A-B-C-D-E, and Hfr-3 transfers the markers as O-B-C-D-E-A. All the data, however, are consistent if we assume that the chromosome is a circular structure that can be broken at any point. The point of rupture becomes the point of origin of transfer, but the direction of transfer can be either clockwise or counterclockwise, as shown in Figure 9. Indeed, this is exactly what happens. The F factor, which exists in the cytoplasm, will sometimes associate itself with the bacterial chromosome. It does so as illustrated in Figure 10. The circular DNA structure that is the F factor will associate with specific areas on the chromosome. The two circular structures will break and recombine with one another, allowing complete integration of the F factor DNA into the chromosomal DNA. The point at which the F factor integrates will determine the point of origin of a particular Hfr strain as well as the direction of marker transfer. During the transfer, part of the F factor will be the last marker to enter the F^- cell. The entire chromosome

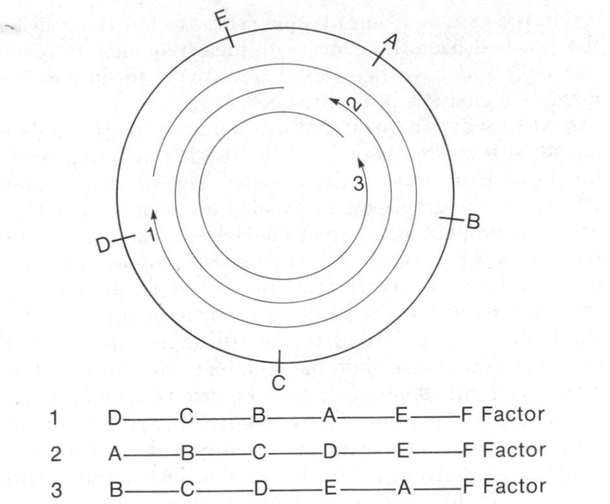

Figure 9. Genetic evidence that the bacterial chromosome is a circular structure. Data from interrupted mating experiments with Hfr 1, Hfr 2, or Hfr 3 and the same F^- strain give the order of transfer of markers as shown, with the F factor the last marker to enter. These data are consistent with a circular chromosome, which can be broken at various points.

is not usually transferred during the mating, since it is ruptured before the end is transferred explaining why the F^- recipient in a cross with an Hfr strain does not become male.

F-PRIME FACTORS. Hfr strains are not always stable, and sometimes the F factor will be lost from the chromosome, once again giving an F^+ cell. In most cases this reversal results in the original F factor as well as the complete bacterial chromosome. Occasionally, however, the F factor will bring with it part of the bacterial chromosome and is then called an F-prime (F′) factor. These F′ factors are designated by the bacterial genes they carry. For example, if an F factor carries the genes for lactose fermentation it

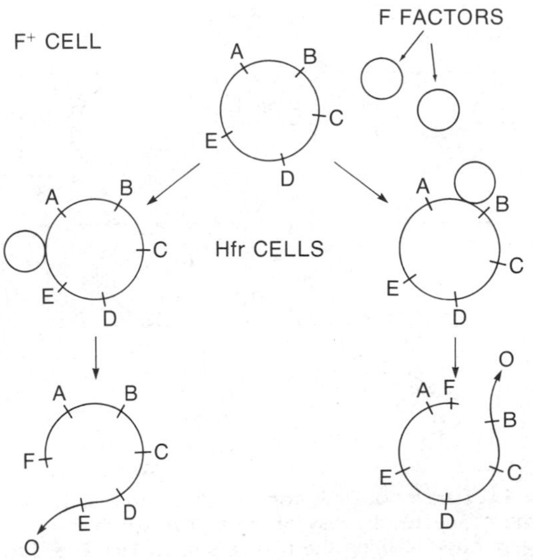

Figure 10. Association of the F factor with the bacterial chromosome. The F factor can integrate into the chromosome at various sites that have an area of base pair homology. The site of integration will determine the point of origin for the Hfr during transfer of the DNA to an F^- cell.

is referred to as an F′-*lac* plasmid. These factors can transfer the attached bacterial genes with high frequency to recipient cells and have been used extensively to do complementation analyses in bacteria cells.

KINETICS OF TRANSFER. When a culture of Hfr cells is mixed with an excess of F^- cells, the Hfr cell attaches to the F^- cell by way of the F pilus. The tip of the pilus attaches to the gram-negative wall of the recipient, and the cells are brought into direct contact—presumably by retraction of the F pilus. When pair formation occurs there is some form of signal that initiates replication of the chromosome at the site of the F factor integration. As the chromosome is replicated in the Hfr strain, one parental strand of DNA passes into the recipient cell, and the other remains in the donor cell (see Figure 11). In both the donor and the recipient cells complementary strands are synthesized during the transfer. Rarely is the entire chromosome transferred, although plasmids not associated with the chromosome are transferred in total by the same mechanisms. The piece of chromosome that is transferred to the recipient is presumed to align itself with the homologous region on the recipient chromosome, followed by replacement of the recipient allele by the donor allele. The progeny of the initial recombinant event are thus haploid. In the case in which F′ factors are transferred to the recipient cells, the progeny of the recombination event become partially diploid for the genes carried on the F factor. This is true even if the F′ factor integrates into the chromosome, because it does so by additive recombination.

Plasmids. The F factor discussed previously is a prototype of other small extrachromosomal genetic elements that exist in bacterial cells. These elements, termed *plasmids,* replicate autonomously and often confer new genetic properties on the bacterial host cell. The plasmids can be divided into two major classes: *transmissible plasmids,* which have the ability to initiate their own transfer by cell-to-cell contact; and *nontransmissible plasmids,* which lack the ability to promote their own transfer by cell-to-cell contact. Nontransmissible plasmids can be transferred from one bacterial cell to another by transduction, or transformation, or mobilization by a self-transmissible plasmid. Among the best characterized transmissible plasmids are F factors, antibiotic resistance factors (R factors), and some of the colicinogenic factors (Col factors).

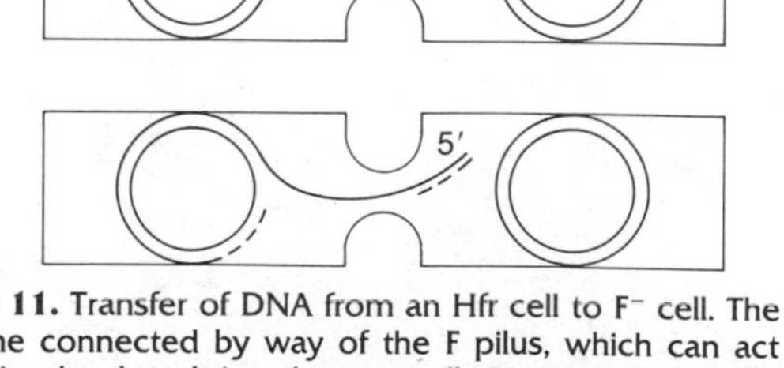

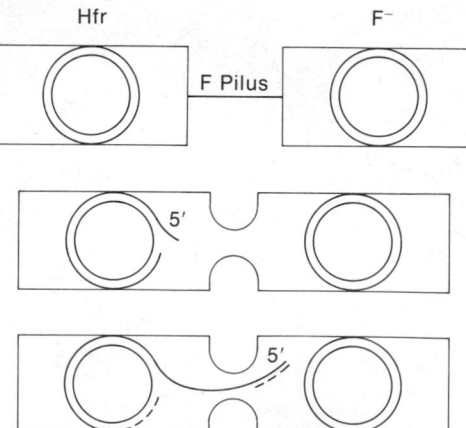

Figure 11. Transfer of DNA from an Hfr cell to F^- cell. The cells become connected by way of the F pilus, which can act as a grappling hook to bring the two cells in contact. The chromosome in the donor breaks and begins replication with the transfer of one of the original donor DNA strands into the F^- cell. The DNA enters the F^- cells with a leading 5′ end and is replicated inside the F^- cell. Simultaneous replication of the donor DNA occurs in the Hfr cell.

Transmissible Plasmids

F FACTORS. The sex factor is best characterized for its mediation of conjugation and is a circular double-stranded DNA molecule with a molecular weight of 60×10^6. The F factor carries a number of genes, 13 of which are involved in the transmission of the plasmid (*tra* genes). The plasmid controls its own replication in the autonomous state allowing only one or two copies of the plasmid per cell. Transmission of the F factor is dependent on the presence of the F pilus. The pilus is expressed in all cells carrying the F factor and can be identified by the sensitivity of such cells to male-specific viruses that use the pilus as a receptor site. F factors cannot coexist in the same cell with some types of plasmids. Two plasmids that cannot coexist are said to be in the same incompatibility group. In addition, autonomous F factors cannot coexist in a cell that has an integrated F factor (Hfr strain). All transmissible plasmids studied to date appear to have analogous *tra* systems for the transfer of the plasmid from cell to cell.

R FACTORS. The R factors are plasmids that carry genes determining resistance to antibiotics. Some R plasmids consist of two components, the RTF, or resistance transfer factor (analogous to the F factor), and the r determinants. The r determinant portion of the R factor carries one or more genes that code for proteins that abolish the effectiveness of various antibiotics. The RTF component is similar in size to the F factor, but the r determinant component varies in size, depending on the number of genes carried. In general, the composite R factors have a molecular weight of about 60 to 70 $\times 10^6$. The two components of the R factor are connected by insertion sequences (see further on) on both sides of the r determinant to give a single, closed double-stranded circular DNA molecule. Transfer of the R factor from cell to cell is dependent on a pilus structure. Unlike the F^+ cells, however, cells carrying the R factor do not usually express the pilus on the surface of the cell. Only newly infected cells express the pilus, allowing for a rapid transfer of the R factor from R^+ to R^- cells, followed by a repression of the pilus formation after several generations. The structure of the pilus of the R factor differs from that of the F pilus. One group of R factors, however, has an F-like pilus (that is, sensitive to F-specific viruses), whereas other R factors code for other types of pili (that is, I-like pili). R factors can be grouped by incompatibility or compatibility with each other and with the F factor. (See Chapter 21 for further discussion of R factors.)

Other transmissible plasmids in *E. coli* have been associated with toxins that produce diarrhea in animals and in man. Certain *E. coli* produce two enterotoxins, a low molecular weight heat-stable toxin (ST) and a heat-labile toxin (LT), that have many properties similar to cholera toxin. The *E. coli* ST and LT are both coded for by plasmid genes and are often associated with the presence of drug-resistant factors and, in some porcine strains, the production of alpha hemolysin and the K88 antigen responsible for attachment to the bowel mucosa. It appears that LT and ST may be coded for by the same plasmid.

COL FACTORS. Colicinogenic factors are plasmids that code for bactericidal substances called *colicins* or *bacteriocins.* These substances are proteins that kill closely related strains of bacteria that do not carry the same plasmid. As with the F factor and the R factor, the Col factors are closed, double-stranded circular DNA molecules. Col factors that are transmissible and classified as group II have a molecular weight of 60 to 110 $\times$ 10^6. They carry a *tra* system analogous to the F factor, allowing transfer by cell-to-cell contact. The Col factors are designated by capital letters. Group II contains the factors B, I, and V. These factors show controlled replication and have one or two copies per cell. Like the F factor they code for a pilus structure that is involved in their transmission from cell to cell. Col factors can also transfer chromosomal genes and form strains analogous to Hfr strains. The colicins produced act by binding to receptors in the outer membrane of sensitive bacterial cells. After some rearrangement, they come into contact with the cytoplasmic membrane and exert their effect. The different colicins act in killing sensitive cells by a variety of mechanisms that include degradation of DNA and RNA, interference with the energy system of the cells, and inactivation of ribosome structure with inhibition of protein synthesis. It appears that only a few cells in a Col^+ population actually produce the colicin, whereas most of the cells are in a repressed state similar to that seen in lysogenic cells. Like lysogenic cells, the repression is destroyed by exposing the cells to agents such as mitomycin C. Although most of the studies on colicins have been in gram-negative organisms, recent work has focused on similar substances produced by gram-positive organisms. For example, in the group D streptococcus there has been described a streptocin that appears to be coded for by genes on a self-transmissible plasmid.

Nontransmissible Plasmids

COL FACTORS. The nontransmissible Col factors include the factors E_1, E_3, K, and D. These plasmids are much smaller than the transmissible plasmids and have molecular weights from 3 to 6 $\times$ 10^6. This group of Col factors also differs from group II by having between 5 and 25 copies of the factor produced per chromosome-equivalent under a variety of growth conditions, suggesting a relaxed control of replication.

STAPHYLOCOCCAL PLASMIDS. The best known plasmid occurring in *Staphylococcus* carries a gene for the determination of penicillinase, rendering the bacterial cell resistant to the action of penicillin. Other plasmids also occur in this organism, giving resistance to other antimicrobial agents. Self-transmissible plasmids have not been described in the staphylococcus, but transfer of plasmids by transduction has been shown to occur both in vitro and in vivo.

Insertion Sequences and Recombination of Plasmids. Plasmids have the ability to recombine with each other as well as with the bacterial host chromosome. This ability is mainly due to the presence in the plasmids and in the bacterial chromosome of insertion sequences (IS). Insertion sequences are segments of DNA that have a specific base sequence and range in length from 800 to 1400 base pairs. They have been designated as IS1, IS2, IS3, IS4, and so on. The insertion sequences IS1, IS2, and IS3 are found at numerous points on the *E. coli* chromosome. Identical IS elements are found in various R factors, lambda phages, and F factors. The presence of these common base sequences allows for these various genomes to recombine and form new combinations of genes. Insertion sequences belong to a group of elements known as transposable elements, defined as segments of DNA that, as discrete genetic and physical entities, can move from one position in a genome to another position in the same or different genome. The IS elements are elements containing no known genes unrelated to the insertion function. More complex elements are the *Tn elements,* which contain IS segments usually as an inverted repeat on either end of the DNA fragment and additional genes unrelated to the insertion function. Many of the Tn elements are translocatable drug-resistance elements such as Tn10 (a tetracycline-resistant element) that can translocate from its position on an R factor to the bacterial chromosome and then to a bacteriophage. Other drug-resistance Tn elements have been described, such as Tn5 (kanamycin resistance) and Tn9 (chloramphenicol resistance), and are often referred to as *transposons.* More complex transposable elements are the plasmids or viruses that can contain both IS segments and Tn elements in addition to other genes needed for replication and transmission, that is, R factors. Thus, insertion sequence elements can act as sites for joining various DNA segments and allowing for new arrangements of genes in bacteria. This process results in optimal growth of the bacteria under a variety of changing environmental conditions and helps ensure survival.

Transduction. Transduction is the transfer of genetic information from a donor cell to a recipient cell by way of a virus vector. For the most part transduction is carried out by temperate DNA-containing bacteriophages. A temperate phage is a virus that can either lyse or lysogenize a host cell upon infection. In the lysogenic response, the genes of the virus that are responsible for initiating the lytic response are repressed, and the viral DNA is integrated into the host DNA by a mechanism similar to the integration of the F factor. In the integrated, or *prophage,* state the virus genes replicate with the host cell genes and all daughter cells will have a viral gene integrated into their chromosome. Bacterial cells that have a viral genome integrated into their chromosome are called *lysogenic cells.* They differ from nonlysogenic cells in two respects: 1) they are immune to superinfection by the same type virus, and 2) they usually can be induced to produce virus particles without infection from the outside. A repressor gene product produced by the virus maintains the repressed and integrated state by preventing transcription of the lytic genes of the virus. Induction of a lysogenic cell to enter the lytic cycle occurs when this repressor protein is destroyed or prevented from functioning.

There are three major types of transduction: 1) *generalized transduction,* in which any genetic marker can be transduced, and the donor DNA is integrated by replacement of the recipient allele; 2) *specialized* or *restricted transduction,* in which only markers that are adjacent to the site where the viral DNA is integrated into the host DNA are transduced, and integration is usually by additive recombination; 3) *abortive transduction,* in which any marker can be transduced, but the DNA is not integrated into the recipient chromosome.

Generalized Transduction. To carry out generalized transduction, a bacterial culture is infected with a temperate virus under conditions of low multiplicity of infection (moi) of about 0.01 to 0.1 phage particle per cell. The culture is then allowed to grow through several cycles of phage development until most of the cells have been infected and lysed. During the maturation of the viral particles an occasional mistake is made and instead of packaging viral DNA, host DNA of the same size is put into the viral protein coat. These particles, which are now the *transducing particles,* are characterized by the fact that they contain only host DNA and no phage DNA. When an appropriately marked recipient strain is then mixed with this lysate at an moi of 5 phage particles to each cell, some cells will be infected by both a normal particle and a transducing, or defective, particle. By plating aliquots of the infected culture on appropriate selective media, one selects for transductants that now have donor DNA incorporated into the recipient DNA. Such generalized transductants can be selected for any genetic marker and arise at a frequency of about 10^{-5} or one transductant for every 10^5 phage particles added. The transductants are characterized by being stable once they are formed, which is a result of the fact that the donor DNA has replaced the recipient DNA during the process. The size of the DNA that can be transduced is dependent on the size of the virus but is generally about 1 per cent of the size of the bacterial chromosome. Only closely linked genetic markers can be cotransduced on the same DNA particle, which enables transduction to be used for the genetic mapping of closely linked genes.

Abortive Transduction. During the process of generalized transduction, as described previously, there are instances when the donor DNA that is injected into the recipient cells does not integrate into the recipient DNA. These cells are referred to as *abortive transductants*. The piece of donor DNA exists in the recipient cell and is capable of functioning normally; however, it is not capable of being replicated. The result is that only one cell at any time in the population derived from the initially infected cell carries the DNA piece. The other daughter cells will receive, upon cell division, products coded for by the DNA and thus will be capable of carrying out several cell divisions until the protein product has become diluted out. As a result only minute colonies are formed by abortive transduction, although they may appear at 100 times the frequency of stable generalized transductants. Abortive transductants are seen only if two negative phenotypes happen to be defective in different genes, and thus, it is a useful method for carrying out complementation analyses.

Specialized Transduction. Specialized transduction is limited to genes that are adjacent to the site of prophage integration. This is clearly due to the mechanism by which specialized transducing particles are formed. Such particles can be generated only by starting with a bacteria culture that has been made lysogenic. Such a culture of cells when treated with short doses of ultraviolet light will lose the active viral repressor protein and begin to enter the lytic cycle. During this process the viral DNA is detached from the host DNA by a reversal of the mechanism by which it had been integrated. In the majority of cases this detachment is performed without any mistake, and a normal virus genome is released. However, in 1 in 10^6 cells this excision will result in a mistake, and a particle will be released that now carries part of the viral DNA and part of the bacterial DNA (Fig. 12). In the case of lambda phage, the host DNA carried will be either the genes for galactose fermentation or the genes for biotin synthesis. These two loci occur on either side of the integrated virus. These particles are referred to as *λdgal* or *λdbio*, which stands for lambda-defective galactose or biotin. The particles are termed defective because they are missing part of the viral genes and cannot carry out a normal productive infection of a bacterial cell without the presence of a normal viral particle. They will, however, inject their hybrid DNA into a recipient cell. The DNA will integrate at the homologous site on the recipient DNA by adding to the chromosome rather than by replacing the recipient allele. The transductants produced are therefore partially diploid for this region of

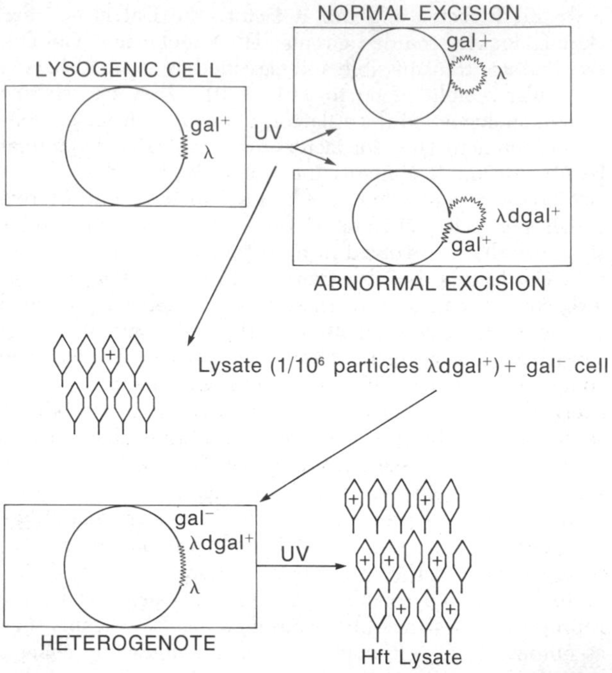

Figure 12. Specialized transduction of the galactose genes in *E. coli* by lambda phage. A lysogenic cell is treated with UV light to cause cells to undergo the lytic cycle. In nearly all cells, excision of the virus is normal, and normal virus particles result. In one in 10^6 cells, abnormal excision takes place giving a defective particle $\lambda dgal^+$. The presence of $\lambda dgal^+$ particles in the lysate can be shown by mixing the lysate with a gal^- strain and selecting for gal^+ transductants. Many of these transductants will be heterogenotes and will carry both $\lambda dgal^+$ and normal λ. Ultraviolet irradiation of these cells yields a lysate that is half normal particle and half $\lambda dgal^+$ particles or an HFT lysate. These result because the normal λ particles will provide the functions missing in $\lambda dgal^+$ and allow its replication in each cell.

the bacterial chromosome and are termed *heterogenotes*. In addition to carrying the defective particle, most of these transductants will also carry a normal phage genome and thus can be considered to be doubly lysogenic. The presence of the donor DNA is detected by infecting a *gal*⁻ recipient with the lysate produced by ultraviolet irradiation of the lysogenic cells and then plating samples onto plates containing EMB-galactose medium. Cells that have received the galactose genes will give dark clones with a green sheen on this medium. If these galactose-positive clones are picked and restreaked, it is found that they are unstable. That is, in 1 in 10^3 cell divisions, segregation of a galactose-negative clone will result. This is due to the loss of the *λdgal* particle in some cells at division. The initial number of galactose-positive transductants found is about 1 in 10^5 galactose-negative cells infected. If, however, one starts with a heterogenote clone and treats it with ultraviolet light to produce the lysate, a lysate is found that can now transduce the *gal* genes at a very high frequency. About 1 in 10 gal^- cells infected can become galactose-positive. These lysates are referred to as *IIFT*, or *high-frequency transducing*, lysates. They occur because the lysate from the heterozygote has many particles carrying the *gal* genes, approximately one half of the viral particles produced. This is a result of the presence in the heterogenote of a normal virus particle that allows for replication of the defective particle in each cell in the culture.

REGULATION OF GENE EXPRESSION. Bacteria have evolved rather intricate and elegant mechanisms to control the phenotypic expression of their genotype. In catabolic pathways, the enzymes needed for the breakdown of a substrate are expressed only if the substrate is available in the environment. In anabolic pathways, if the end-product is available in the environment the enzymes needed for the synthesis of that product are not expressed. When mutants became available that had lost their ability to control the synthesis of the enzymes involved in these pathways, an understanding of what was occurring at the molecular level began. The basic mechanism of control was elaborated by the work of Jacob and Monod in 1961 and is referred to as the *operon theory*. In this theory they describe two major classes of genes: 1) *structural genes*—genes that specify the structure of a specific protein such as an enzyme, and 2) *regulatory genes, or sites*—genes, or sites, on the chromosome that control the rate of synthesis of the structural genes. The operon is defined as a group of contiguous structural genes showing coordinate expression, together with their closely linked controlling sites. The best understood operon, that concerned with the catabolism of lactose, is diagrammed in Figure 13. This type of control is referred to as *negative control*, since the presence of a repressor protein, which is bound to a site on the DNA called the operator site, prevents the synthesis of the mRNA from the structural genes. In the presence of the substrate or inducer, the structure of the repressor product is altered so that it no longer binds to the DNA, and mRNA production begins. The site at which mRNA synthesis is initiated by RNA polymerase is called the promoter site. This is also the site for the action of another regulator molecule, the cAMP activator protein–cAMP complex.

Mutations that occur in the structural genes usually result in the loss of enzyme activity caused by the alteration of the protein structure. Mutations that occur in the regulatory gene or controlling sites result either in strains that cannot be induced to produce enzymes *(noninducible)* or in strains that always produce the enzymes, even in the absence of the inducer *(constitutive)*. To determine whether such mutations have occurred in the regulator gene or in the operator site, partial diploid studies are carried out using F′*lac* factors that carry different forms of the mutated genes (Fig. 14). In a diploid study, constitutivity is recessive to the wild-type inducible state if the regulator has been altered but is dominant to the wild-type inducible state if the alteration has occurred in the operator site. If the regulator has been altered to give a noninducible state, this is dominant to both inducibility and constitutivity (Fig. 15).

A more complex but similar control pattern is seen in the pathway for the catabolism of arabinose. This operon is under *positive control*. Positive control differs from negative control in that it requires the presence of an activator protein to initiate mRNA transcription by RNA polymerase. Diploid studies in a positive control system give a different pattern from that seen in a negative control system. In this case alteration of the regulator to give the noninducible state is recessive to the wild-type inducible state. Likewise, constitutivity is dominant to noninducibility (Fig. 15). These results are consistent with a requirement for the presence of an activator protein to get expression of the operon.

Catabolite repression is an additional control mechanism

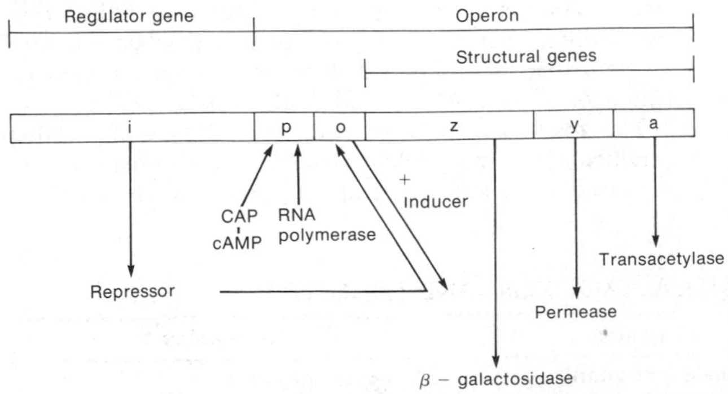

Figure 13. The operon model for regulation of lactose fermentation. The repressor, the product of the regulator gene, prevents the synthesis of mRNA for the structural genes, z, y, and a, by binding to the operator site O. Addition of the inducer prevents the repressor from binding at O, and mRNA synthesis is initiated at the promoter, or p, site by RNA polymerase. The promoter site also has a binding site for the CAP-cAMP complex.

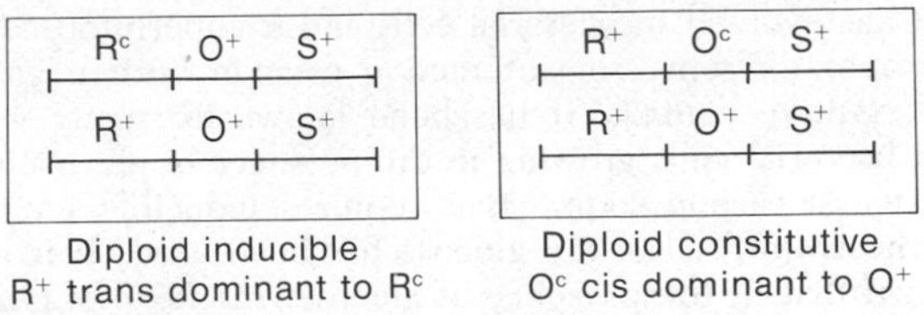

Figure 14. Differentiation of constitutive mutants as mutations in the regulator gene (R^c) or the operator site (O^c) in an operon under negative control. Partial diploids are constructed with F′-lac plasmids and then assayed for S enzyme activity after growth in the presence and absence of the inducer. Mutations in the R gene are constitutive because of the lack of repressor, and these are recessive and inducible in the presence of a wild-type repressor. Mutations in the O site are constitutive because they do not bind repressor and thus are dominant and still constitutive in the presence of the wild-type repressor.

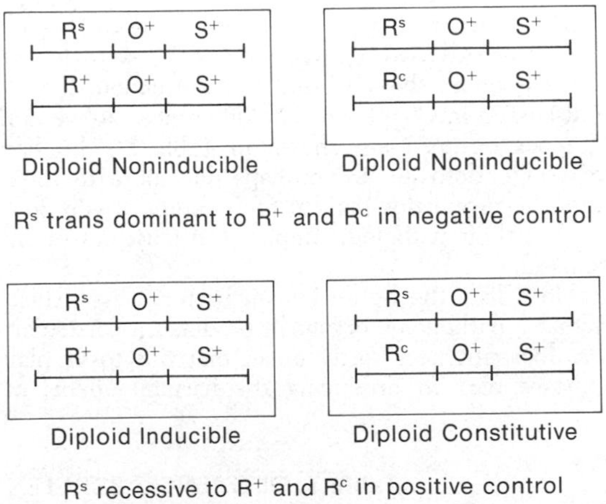

Figure 15. Differentiation of negative and positive control by partial diploid studies. R^s, or noninducible, strains in a negative control system result from the production of a mutated repressor that no longer binds the inducer and thus remains attached to the operator site. This R^s repressor will also bind to the operator site on the opposite DNA strand and thus is dominant both to wild type and constitutivity. The R^s, or noninducible, state in positive control systems results from lack of production of an activator protein. Thus, the absence of the product makes the R^s state recessive to either the presence of the wild-type activator or an altered R^c constitutive activator.

that has evolved in bacterial cells and is superimposed on the operator-repressor interaction seen in both negative and positive control. It has been known for many years that bacterial cells growing in the presence of glucose will not use a carbon source that requires inducible enzyme synthesis until all of the glucose has been used. It is now known that in the presence of glucose, the level of cAMP in bacterial cells drops from 10^{-4} M to 10^{-7} M. cAMP is essential for the initiation of mRNA transcription. This compound binds to a protein called CAP or *catabolite gene activator product*, and this complex interacts with the DNA at the promoter site to stimulate transcription. This is a general control mechanism added to the very specific controls seen within each catabolic pathway.

References

Avery, O. T., Macleod, C. M., and McCarty, M.: Studies on the chemical nature of the substance inducing transformation of pneumococcal types. J Exp Med 79:137, 1944.

Griffith, F.: The significance of pneumococcal types. J Hyg 27:113, 1928.

Hayes, W.: The Genetics of Bacteria and their Viruses. 2nd ed. New York, John Wiley & Sons, 1968.

Jacob, F., and Brenner, S.: Sur la Régulation de la synthése du DNA chez les bacteries: l'hypothèse du replicon. C R Acad Sci (Paris) 256:298, 1963.

Jacob, F., and Monod, J.: Genetic regulatory mechanisms in the synthesis of proteins. J Mol Biol 3:318, 1961.

Jacob, F., and Wollman, F.: Sur les processus de conjugaison et de recombination genetique chez *E. coli*. Ann Inst Pasteur 91:486, 1956.

Lederberg, J., and Lederberg, E. M.: Replica plating and indirect selection of bacterial mutants. J Bacteriol 63:399, 1952.

Lederberg, J., and Tatum, E. L.: Gene recombination in *E. coli*. Nature 158:582, 1946.

Luria, S. E., and Delbrück, M.: Mutations of bacteria from virus sensitivity to virus resistance. Genetics 28:491, 1943.

Meselson, M., and Stahl, F.: The replication of DNA in *Escherichia coli*. Proc Natl Acad Sci USA 44:671, 1958.

Stanier, R., Doudoroff, M., and Adelberg, E. A.: The Microbial World. 3rd ed. Englewood Cliffs, N.J., Prentice Hall, 1970.

Watson, J. D.: The Molecular Biology of the Gene. 3rd ed. New York, Benjamin Company, Inc., 1976.

Watson, J. D., and Crick, F. H. C.: Genetic implications of the structure of DNA. Nature 171:964, 1953.

5

BACTERIAL EXOTOXINS

WILLIAM EDWARD VAN HEYNINGEN, PH.D., SC.D., D.SC.

There are not more than four or five infectious diseases for which we have a reasonably clear understanding of the means by which the infecting organism brings about its harmful effects. The ability of the organism to grow in the body is not the same thing as its capacity to produce disease, for there is no intrinsic reason why the mere presence of a very small weight of infecting organisms in the body of the patient—from a few micrograms in tetanus to 100 mg at most in anthrax—should be harmful. The idea that pathogenic organisms produce poisons is an old and obvious one, and it is indeed a fact that many pathogenic bacteria do produce antigenic poisons, usually known as toxins. There are two types of toxins—the exotoxins, which are discussed in this chapter, and the endotoxins, which are discussed in Chapter 6. The differences between these two types of toxin are shown in Table 1. The harmful effects of endotoxins are perhaps due more to their immunologic properties than to their comparatively low toxicity, but their pathologic importance must not be underestimated.

Table 2 lists the better-known bacterial exotoxins. The fact that a pathogenic organism produces a particular exotoxin does not necessarily mean that this toxin plays an important part in producing the harmful effects of the infectious disease. In most cases there is no good reason for concluding whether it does or does not. The criteria that must be considered in coming to the conclusion that it does are listed in Table 3. These criteria need not all be fulfilled, and the toxins that fulfill at least some of them, or are relevant to those that do, are shown in bold type in Table 2. These are the toxins that we will discuss in this chapter, and in doing so we will be obliged to dismiss a number of well-known toxins, such as the staphylococcal and streptococcal hemolysins, that are of great scientific interest but no proven medical relevance.

Further reading (the references in this chapter should be consulted as much for their lists of references as for their texts): van Heyningen, 1970.

NEUROTOXINS

TETANUS TOXIN (TETANOSPASMIN). The harmful effects of tetanus are entirely due to this toxin, which fulfills all of the criteria in Table 3. Tetanus toxin is one of the most poisonous toxins known—purified preparations of the toxin may contain 100 million lethal doses (mouse) per milligram (i.e., 1 g kills two million tons of living matter). It is also one of the most dangerous toxins known. Reliable statistics on tetanus do not exist, but the toxin kills perhaps two million people every year, mainly newborns (*tetanus neonatorum*, or umbilical tetanus), in underdeveloped countries of Asia, Africa, and South America.

The toxin acts only on the nervous system, without producing any morphologic changes. The disease is characterized by a spastic paralysis, which nearly always in-

Table 1. DIFFERENCES BETWEEN BACTERIAL EXOTOXINS AND ENDOTOXINS

	Exotoxins	Endotoxins
Parent organisms	gram-positive and gram-negative	gram-negative
Chemical nature	simple protein	protein-lipid-polysaccharide
Stability to heating (100°C)	labile	stable
Detoxification by formaldehyde	detoxified	not detoxified
Neutralization by homologous antibody	complete	partial
Biologic activity	individual to toxin	same for all toxins
Toxicity compared with strychnine as 1	100 to 1,000,000	0.1

Table 2. EXOTOXINS OF PATHOGENIC BACTERIA

Bacterium	Disease Caused in Man	Toxins
Bacillus anthracis	anthrax	**complex lethal and edema-producing toxins?**
Bordetella pertussis	whooping cough	**lethal and dermonecrotizing toxins?**
Clostridium botulinum	botulism	**6 type-specific lethal neurotoxins**
Cl. oedematiens	gas gangrene	lethal, hemolytic, or dermonecrotizing
Cl. difficile	necrotizing enterocolitis	necrotizing enterotoxin
Cl. perfringens	enteritis necroticans and gas gangrene	**alpha, lethal, dermonecrotizing, hemolytic*** **enterotoxin**
Cl. septicum	gas gangrene	alpha, lethal, hemolytic
Cl. sordellii	gas gangrene	1. edema-producing toxin 2. hemorrhagic toxin
Cl. tetani	tetanus	1. **tetanospasmin, lethal, neurotoxic** 2. neurotoxin, nonspasmogenic 3. tetanolysin, lethal, cardiotoxic, hemolytic
Corynebacterium diphtheriae	diphtheria	**diphtheria toxin, lethal, dermonecrotizing**
Escherichia coli	diarrhea	1. **heat-labile enterotoxin** 2. heat-stable enterotoxin
Pseudomonas aeruginosa	pyogenic infections	**exotoxin A**
Staphylococcus aureus	pyogenic infections, enterotoxemia	1. alpha, lethal, demonecrotizing, hemolytic† 2. **exfoliating toxin** 3. **enterotoxin**
Streptococcus pyogenes	pyogenic infections, scarlet fever, rheumatic fever	1. Dick toxin, erythrogenic, nonlethal 2. Streptolysin O, lethal, hemolytic, cardiotoxic 3. streptolysin S, lethal, hemolytic
Vibrio cholerae *Vibrio El Tor*	cholera	**cholera toxin, lethal, enterotoxic**
Salmonella typhimurium	enteritis	**enterotoxin?**
Shigella shiga	dysentery	**enterotoxin**
Yersinia pestis	plague	murine toxin

*Plus 8 other exotoxins (beta → kappa).
†Plus 3 other lethal or hemolytic toxins (beta, gamma, delta).

volves the jaw muscles (lockjaw) and the muscles of deglutition, and by generalized convulsions (Fig. 1). The spasticity is due to the action of the toxin in blocking presynaptic inhibition in the central nervous system, particularly in the spinal cord and cerebellum, which it reaches by ascending in the nerves by retrograde axonal transport, after uptake from the anaerobically replicating organisms near the wound of entry (which is often so small as to be undetectable *post mortem*). Apart from eradication of the organisms with penicillin to prevent formation of more toxin, treatment of tetanus is aimed at controlling convulsions by curarization. However, the toxin can also block neuromuscular transmission (like botulinum toxin; see below), and it also, perhaps indirectly, causes overactivity in the sympathetic nervous system, with drastic swings in blood pressure and heart rate.

The toxin blocks both evoked and spontaneous transmitter release at the central and peripheral synapses on which it acts. The mechanism of action is not understood, and neither are the factors that determine its specificity with respect to particular synapses. Its effects are long-lasting, and it appears that, at least at peripheral synapses, restoration of function requires sprouting of new nerve terminals.

What is known about the structure of the toxin is shown in Figure 2. The toxin is a simple protein, apparently consisting of two components, a "heavy" and a "light" polypeptide chain bound together by a peptide bond that is easily "nicked" by proteolytic enzymes in the culture filtrate, and a disulfide bond that is easily cleaved by reduction. The two chains are further held together by noncovalent forces that can be broken with urea or sodium

Table 3. CRITERIA FOR JUDGING WHETHER TOXINS ARE RESPONSIBLE FOR THE HARMFUL EFFECTS OF AN INFECTIOUS DISEASE

1. The organism produces a toxin.
2. Virulent strains produce the toxin; avirulent do not.
3. The organism produces disease without multiplying profusely or spreading extensively.
4. The blood and lymph are sterile.
5. Organs and tissue at a distance from the site of infection are affected.
6. Introduction of sterile cell-free toxin into animals produces symptoms mimicking the disease.
7. The clinician sees toxic effects in the patient: peripheral vascular collapse; direct action on the heart muscle; central or peripheral nervous system affected (see Figure 1).
8. The disease can be prevented by immunization against the toxin.

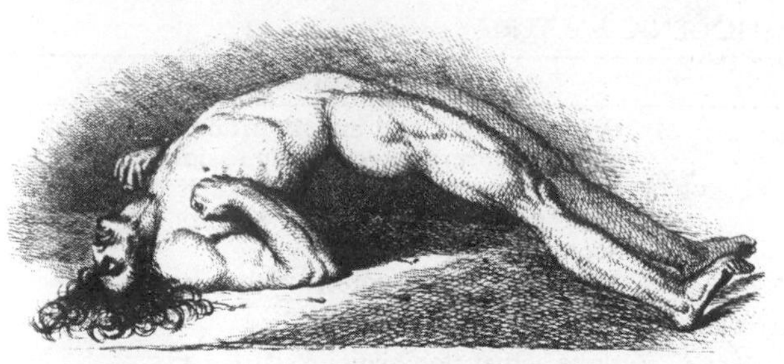

Figure 1. Sir Charles Bell's drawing (1832) of a British soldier suffering from tetanus (lockjaw) as a result of wounds received at the Battle of Corunna. Note the spastic paralysis opisthotonus resulting from opposing muscles pulling against each other, owing to tetanus toxin blocking synaptic inhibition.

dodecyl sulfate. These chains are inert and antigenically distinct when separated, but can be recombined to form the fully toxic protein.

The mode of action of the toxin at the molecular level has not been determined, but several recent experiments show direct effects of the toxin on release of neurotransmitters from synaptosomes and cultured cells. The well-known specific binding of tetanus toxin to nervous tissue (Wassermann-Takaki phenomenon, 1898) is due to the binding of the toxin to certain gangliosides. The gangliosides are components of the cell membranes of most tissues, and are particularly concentrated in nervous tissue. Since they consist of a water-insoluble ceramide moiety and a water-soluble oligosaccharide moiety (Fig. 3), they are amphipathic—i.e., they are both water-soluble and fat-soluble, and are therefore well suited to play a role in cell membranes. Tetanus toxin shows a particular affinity for the sialidase-sensitive ganglioside GGnSSLC, which contains two sialosyl residues attached to the internal galactosyl residue, and can bind with it in a ratio of 3 to 4 molecules ganglioside to 1 molecule toxin (Table 4). It is the only "heavy" component of the tetanus toxin molecule that combines with ganglioside.

Other bacterial toxins, notably cholera toxin, and certain other biologically active proteins also bind to gangliosides (Table 4). The significance of this will be discussed below.

Further reading: van Heyningen, 1963; S. van Heyningen, 1980; Mellanby and Green, 1981.

BOTULINUM TOXINS. Botulism generally assumes the form of food poisoning resulting from the ingestion of toxins preformed by *Clostridium botulinum* growing on

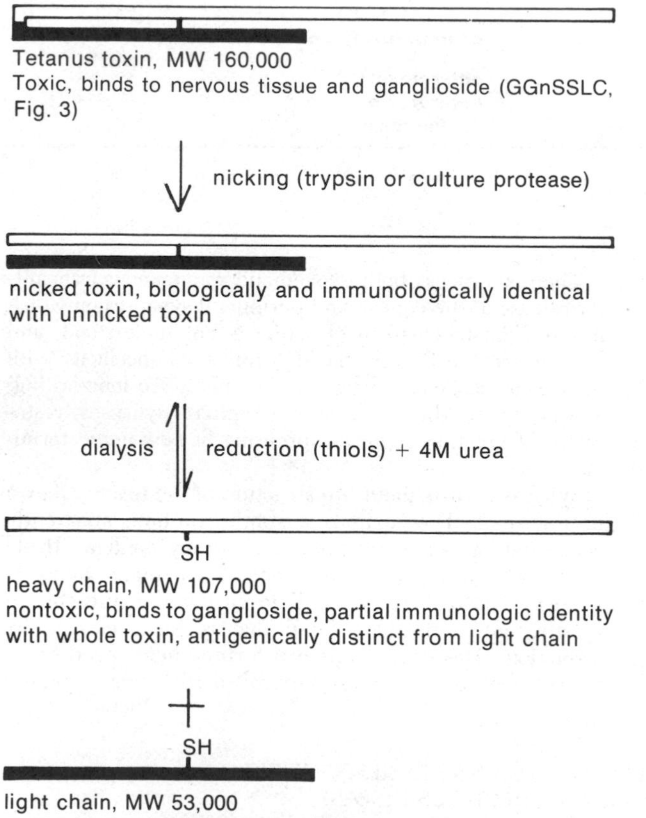

Figure 2. Diagrammatic representation of the structure of tetanus toxin. As in Figures 4, 5, and 6, the black and white bands represent polypeptide chains. In each figure the lengths of these bands are proportional to their relative molecular weights, but note the different scales. Folding of chains by noncovalent bonds is not depicted and the only folding shown is that known to be due to disulfide bonds (—S—S—) from one part of a chain to another. These disulfide bonds can be broken by reduction with thiols (to convert —S—S to —SH + SH—), and restored by dialysing away the thiols. The fact that a protein denaturing agent (urea) is also necessary to separate the light and heavy chains of tetanus toxin suggests that they are held together by noncovalent bonds in addition to the covalent disulfide and peptide bond (see cholera toxin, Fig. 6).

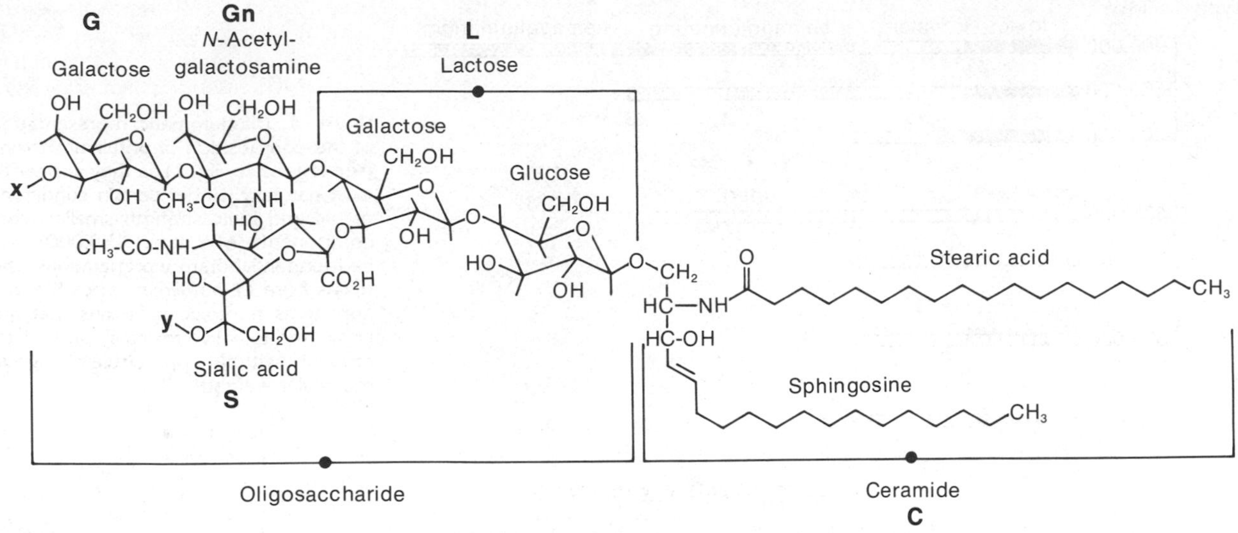

Figure 3. Structures of some of the best-known gangliosides. The bond attaching the sialosyl (S) residue to the galactose moiety of the lactose (L) residue is sialidase- (that is, neuraminidase) insensitive. When sialosyl residues substitute for X or Y they are attached by sialidase-sensitive bonds. GGn = H; y = H: Monosialosylganglioside SLC (GM3); G = H; y = H: Monosialosylganglioside GnSLC (GM2); x = H; y = H: Monosialosylganglioside GGnSLC (GM1); x = S; y = H: Disialosylganglioside SGGnSLC (GD1a); x = H; y = S: Disialosylganglioside GGnSSCL (GD1b); x = S; y = S: Trisialosylganglioside SGGnSSLC (GT1). (The shorthand names in brackets are more widely used but are not self-explanatory.)

food. There are six serologic types, A to F, of the organism, each producing an immunologically type-specific toxin. These toxins have different molecular weights, but they all have apparently the same neurotoxic activity. Only Types A, B, E, and F are known to affect man. Figure 4 shows that these toxins appear to be aggregates of two or three kinds of protein components—toxic, inert, and hemagglutinating. Only the Type A toxin contains the hemagglutinating component, and in the Types B and E toxins the toxic components are produced by the organism as inert protoxins that are converted by proteolytic enzymes into active toxins with no detectable change in molecular weight.

Botulinum toxin is as toxic as tetanus toxin; like tetanus toxin, it acts only on nervous tissue, and does not directly cause any detectable morphologic change in this tissue. It apparently has no central action, and seems to act only peripherally at the neuromuscular junctions, where (like tetanus toxin) it blocks both evoked and spontaneous release of acetylcholine from cholinergic motor nerve endings.

Nothing is known of the action of the toxin at the molecular level. The toxic component of the toxin (Fig. 4) has a molecular weight of about 150,000 (similar to that of tetanus toxin). It can be separated from the inert and hemagglutinating components without loss or change in character of the toxicity. Nothing is known of the structure of this toxic component.

Botulinum toxin is bound to synaptic membranes and to gangliosides under different physical conditions (pH, salt concentration) from those suitable for the binding of tetanus toxin. Perhaps these differences may be related to the different conditions under which these toxins block synaptic transmission in the laboratory. Thus, the in vitro effect of botulinum toxin on a phrenic nerve diaphragm preparation can be seen within 30 minutes of adding the toxin to the

Table 4. BIOLOGICALLY ACTIVE PROTEINS BINDING TO GANGLIOSIDE RECEPTORS

Protein	**Receptor**	**Target**
PROTEIN	RECEPTOR	TARGET
Tetanus toxin[1]	GGnSSLC>SGGnSSLC>SGGnSLC>GGnSLC	synaptic transmission
Botulinum toxin[2]	not identified—sialidase labile?	synaptic transmission
Cholera enterotoxin[3]	GGnSLC only	adenylate cyclase
E. coli enterotoxin[4]	GGnSLC only	adenylate cyclase
Staphylococcus alpha-toxin[5]	SGGlnLC[6]	cell membrane?
Vibrio parahaemolyticus toxin[7]	SGGnSSLC	?
Thyrotropin hormone[8]	GGnSSLC>SGGnSSLC>GGnSLC>GnSLC=SLC>SGGnSLC	adenylate cyclase
Human chorionic gonadotropin[9]	SGGnSSLC>SGGnSLC>GGnSSLC>GnSLC>GGnSLC	adenylate cyclase
Interferon[10]	GnSLC	cell reaction to virus
Sendai virus[11]	not identified—sialidase labile?	?

1. van Heyningen (1963); 2. at pH 5, Mellanby and Pope (1976); 3. van Heyningen (1973); 4. Pierce (1973); 5. Kato and Naiki (1976); 6. Gln = *N*-acetyl-glucosamine (this ganglioside so far found only in red blood cells); 7. Takeda et al. (1976); 8. Mullin et al. (1976); 9. Lee et al. (1976); 10. Besancon et al. (1976); 11. Bergelson et al. (1982). See first edition for complete references to this table.

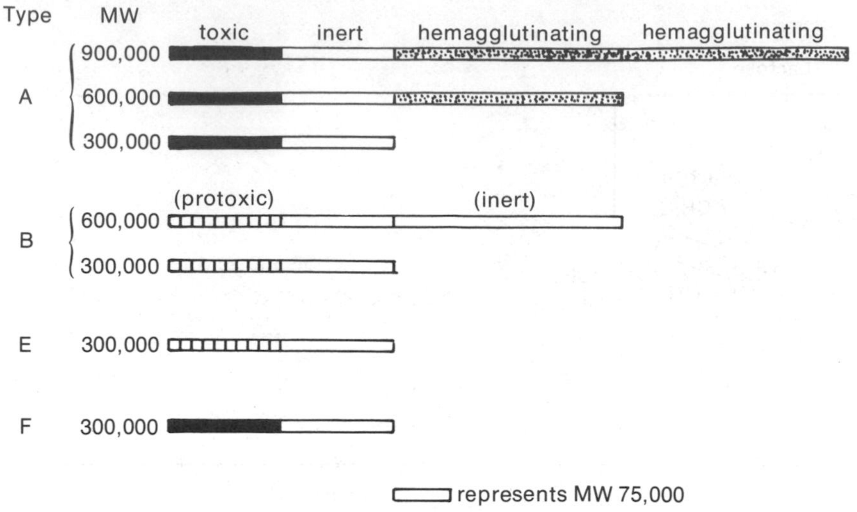

Figure 4. Diagrammatic representation of the composition of botulinum toxins (see legend to Fig. 2) as they appear to exist naturally. Under certain conditions of pH and ionic strength smaller toxic components (MW about 150,000) may be found in laboratory preparations. The toxins from *Cl. botulinum* types B and E appear as nontoxic protoxins that are converted to active toxins by proteolytic enzymes without appreciable change in molecular weight.

bathing medium, whereas the similar effect of tetanus toxin can be reproduced only by injecting the toxin into the living animal and studying a nerve-muscle preparation isolated some hours later.

Infant botulism results from ingestion of *Cl. botulinum* spores, their survival of the passage through the infant stomach, followed by their vegetation and consequent toxin production in the gut. This would mean that, contrary to previously held opinion, botulism can be an infectious disease (in infants) and an exotoxinosis.

Further reading: Arnon *et al*, 1978; Sugiyama, 1980; Cohen and van Heyningen, 1982.

TOXINS BLOCKING PROTEIN SYNTHESIS

DIPHTHERIA TOXIN. Diphtheria toxin is produced only by lysogenic strains of *Corynebacterium diphtheriae* infected with a bacteriophage carrying the *tox* gene, which carries the structural information for the synthesis of the toxin. The expression of this information is regulated, at least in part, by the bacterial host. The toxin must be considered responsible for the harmful effects of diphtheria since it fulfills all the criteria listed in Table 3. Unlike tetanus and botulinum toxins, diphtheria toxin appears to act on all tissues. It kills cells, as may be seen when it is injected intracutaneously, as in the Schick test. In the diphtheria patient or the experimentally injected animal, the effect of the toxin is best seen in the heart muscles and the adrenal glands.

It acts by blocking protein synthesis in susceptible cells by inhibiting polypeptide synthesis. The toxin inhibits the polypeptide synthesis by catalyzing the following reaction:

$$NAD^+ + \underset{\text{active}}{EF\text{-}2} \rightleftharpoons \underset{\text{inactive}}{ADPR\text{—}EF\text{-}2} + \text{nicotinamide} + H^+$$

EF-2 is the elongation factor–2, which is required for translocating polypeptide-transfer RNA from the acceptor site to the donor site on the eukaryotic ribosome. It is inactivated by being coupled with the adenosine diphosphate ribose (ADPR) resulting from the cleavage of nicotinamide adenine diphosphate (NAD).

The structure of diphtheria toxin is shown in Figure 5. It consists of two peptide chains, A and B, linked together by easily cleavable peptide and disulfide bonds. Only the A (active) part of the diphtheria toxin molecule is responsible for the reaction above, resulting in the inactivation of elongation factor–2, and this active part must therefore be considered as an enzyme. The other part (B, binding) of the toxin molecule is responsible for binding the toxin to the membranes of susceptible cells and facilitating the entry of A into the cytoplasm of the cell, where it catalyzes the reaction above. The whole toxin AB is toxic to susceptible animals or whole cells, whereas part A is not toxic to animals or whole cells, but will catalyze the reaction in cell extracts. On the other hand, the whole toxin AB is ineffective in cell extracts. Cells from species of animals that are relatively insusceptible to diphtheria toxin (e.g., mice) do not contain the receptor for the B component and therefore do not bind toxin, but protein synthesis in extracts from these cells is blocked by A. This important concept of a bipartite (AB) toxin was first revealed with diphtheria toxin, and has led to similar concepts for other toxins and biologically active proteins (see below).

Although the target of diphtheria toxin—that is, the substrate for the enzymic A component—has been identified (NAD + EF-2), the receptor for the toxin—that is, the substance in the susceptible cell membrane to which the B component binds—has not yet been identified. It may be very difficult to do so, since the affinity constant of diphtheria toxin for susceptible cells is low compared with that of other toxins and since very few molecules of toxin are bound per cell. Partial identification of a receptor has been claimed, but this needs confirmation and elaboration.

Further reading: Boquet and Pappenheimer, 1976; Collier, 1975; Collier, 1977; Murphy, 1976; and Pappenheimer and Gill, 1973; Cohen and S. van Heyningen, 1982.

***PSEUDOMONAS AERUGINOSA* EXOTOXIN A.** A lethal, necrotizing toxin (exotoxin A) is produced by most clinical isolates of *Pseudomonas aeruginosa*. The organism is an "opportunistic" pathogen that commonly infects patients who have genetic immunodeficiency, or are being treated with immunosuppressive drugs, or suffer from extensive burns. Exotoxin A is mentioned here because it is similar to diphtheria toxin insofar as it catalyzes the reaction of NAD with EF-2 to form ADPR—EF-2 and thereby blocks protein synthesis in animals, cells, and cell extracts. But there are differences. Unlike whole diphtheria toxin, the whole exotoxin A (MW about 66,000) is active

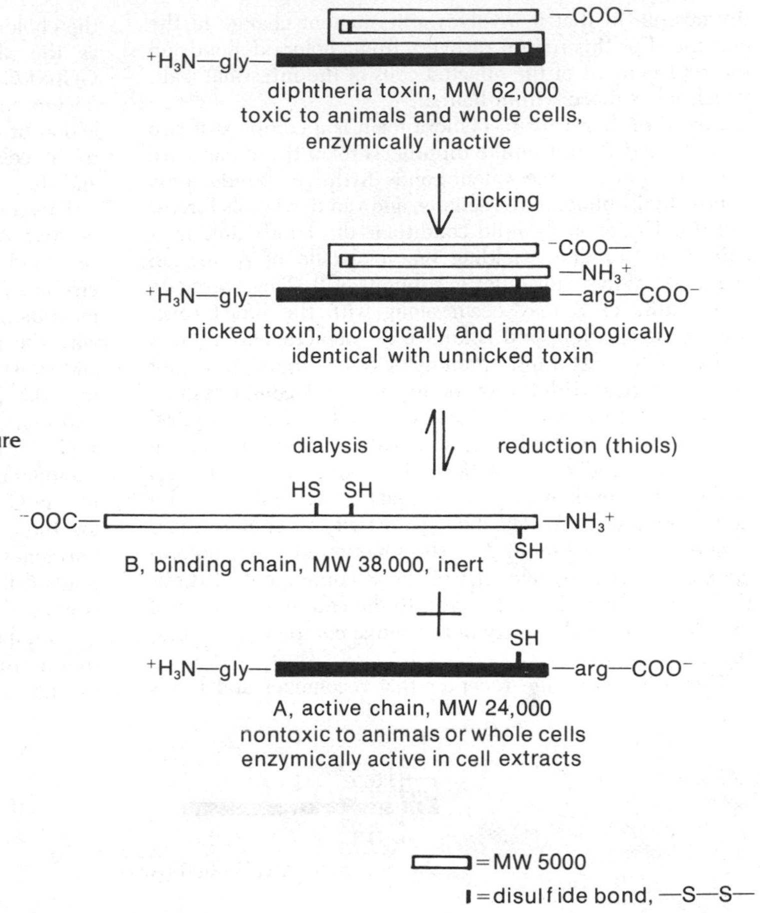

Figure 5. Diagrammatic representation of the structure of diphtheria toxin (see legend to Fig. 2).

in cell extracts as well as on whole cells; and although a smaller product of natural proteolysis (MW about 33,000) appears to be more active than the whole toxin in cell extracts, it is also active on whole cells. The toxins also differ in their relative toxicity to different species of animals and cell lines, which suggests that they bind to different receptors. There is no immunologic relationship between the two toxins.

Further reading: Collier, 1975; Cohen and S. van Heyningen, 1982.

ENTEROTOXINS

An enterotoxin is a toxin produced in the intestinal tract by an infecting organism. This toxin causes diarrhea or vomiting. This effect generally results from the direct action of the toxin on the intestinal wall (e.g., cholera), but may also follow the absorption of the toxin into the bloodstream and its action elsewhere, as is thought to be the case with the staphylococcal enterotoxins. Acute gastroenteritis is a global medical problem, particularly severe in terms of morbidity, mortality, and economic impact in the less developed countries of the world. Many of these enteropathies are enterotoxinoses.

Further reading: van Heyningen, 1983.

CHOLERA TOXIN. Cholera toxin, diphtheria toxin, and tetanus toxin are the three toxins that are quite certainly responsible for the harmful effects of the diseases caused by their parent organisms. Cholera is a disease of acute diarrhea, which may be so severe that a patient may lose up to 30 liters of watery stools in a day. Death follows the consequent dehydration. The toxic nature of cholera was recognized by John Snow in 1849, well before the germ theory of disease was established, and then reaffirmed 35 years later by Robert Koch, who postulated a cholera toxin; but the existence of such a toxin was not proved until another 75 years later, when S. N. De showed that cell-free culture filtrates of *Vibrio cholerae* promoted fluid accumulation when introduced directly into the gut. The toxin gene resides in the chromosomes of both biotypes, *V. cholerae* and *V. El Tor*, and both serotypes, Ogawa and Inaba. Cholera toxin causes diarrhea by stimulating a net output of chloride and bicarbonate ions by the immature crypt cells, and inhibiting the absorption of sodium-coupled chloride ions by the mature brush border cells of the villi of the small intestine. These actions follow an increased output of adenosine-3′:5′-cyclic monophosphate (cyclic AMP), which results from stimulation of the enzyme adenylate cyclase (AC) by the toxin. The toxin acts on all eukaryotic cells containing this enzyme (and containing a particular ganglioside in the membrane; see below), besides those of the intestinal mucosa, and brings about a great diversity of effects, including increase in capillary permeability when injected into the skin, morphologic changes in Chinese hamster ovary (CHO) cells and in adrenal tumor cells (together with increased steroidogenesis), increased glycogenolysis in liver cells, and lipolysis in fat cells. The stimulation of adenylate cyclase by cholera toxin differs from that caused by hormones such as epinephrine and thyrotropin in that it involves a permanent change in the enzyme. For this reason recovery from cholera depends on the replacement of the affected cells of the intestinal wall, which takes place within hours.

Like diphtheria toxin, cholera toxin is a complex of two parts, A and B, but unlike diphtheria toxin these parts are held together by noncovalent bonds (hydrogen bonds, ionic bonds, hydrophobic interactions, and van der Waals forces, Fig. 6). Under fairly mild conditions the bonds linking A and B are broken, yielding one molecule of A and an aggregate of five molecules of subunits of B. This aggregate of subunits of B may occur along with the intact toxin during purification, and is known as "choleragenoid"; it is biologically inert, and immunologically almost (but not quite) identical with the whole toxin. Part A comprises two parts, held together by a peptide bond and a sulfhydryl bond. The peptide bond is usually nicked by natural proteolysis, and on reduction with a thiol the sulfhydryl bond is also broken to yield a smaller fragment A2 and a larger fragment A1. The biologic activity of cholera toxin resides in the fragment A1. The function of the "choleragenoid" aggregate, like that of the B component of diphtheria toxin, is to bind the toxin to the cell membrane and thus to facilitate the entry of the active component A1 into the cell.

The cell membrane receptor that recognizes and binds the choleragenoid part of cholera toxin has been identified as the sialidase (or neuraminidase)- stable ganglioside GGnSLC, generally known as GM1 (Table 4). Cells that do not contain this ganglioside are not susceptible to the action of the toxin, but if the ganglioside is simply added to the cells it becomes incorporated into their membranes and they become susceptible to this toxin.

The A1 fragment, like diphtheria toxin fragment A, is inactive on the whole cell but active on broken or lysed cells and on extract of the cells; it appears also to be an enzyme catalyzing the cleavage of NAD into ADPR and nicotinamide. In this case the ADPR is thought to combine with the regulatory component of adenylate cyclase (AC), and so irreversibly to stimulate the catalytic component of the AC. The regulatory component binds guanidine triphosphate (GTP), and is closely associated with, or is itself, a GTP-ase. As long as GTP is bound to the regulatory component the AC is active; when the GTP is hydrolyzed by the GTP-ase, it is inactive (this appears to be the basis for the natural, reversible regulation of AC activity by hormones). When ADPR is bound to the regulatory component of AC the GTP-ase is inactivated and the AC thus is irreversibly stimulated.

An important concept with wide implications is revealed by diphtheria and cholera toxins. This concept holds that biologically active proteins can have two distinct and sep-

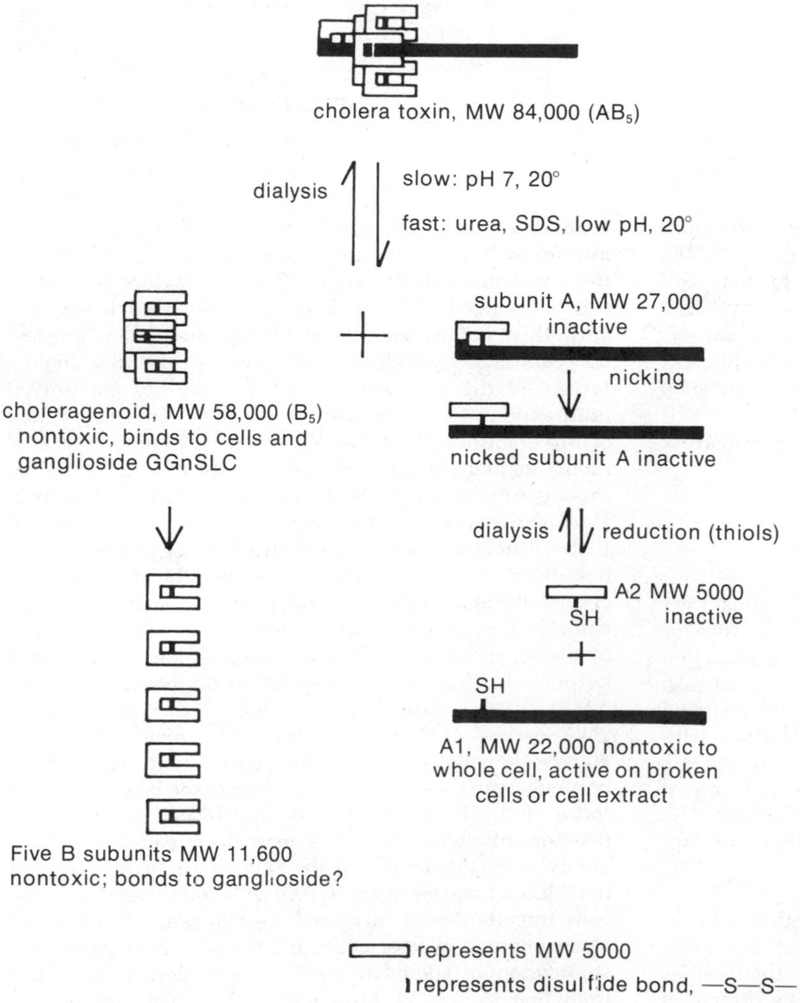

Figure 6. Diagrammatic representation of structure of cholera toxin (see legend to Fig. 2). The A component is held to the B (choleragenoid) component by noncovalent bonds (hydrogen bonds, van der Waals forces, etc.) as are the subunits of the B component. The A2 and A1 fragments of the A component are held together by a nickable peptide bond and a reducible disulfide bond.

arable parts, one part binding to the cell surface receptor and the other acting on a target within the cell. It is likely that the *Escherichia coli* enterotoxin is similarly constituted (see below); and it may be significant that tetanus toxin appears to consist of two separable components that are inactive singly but active again when rejoined, and that one of these components is responsible for the binding of tetanus toxin to the ganglioside that appears to be the receptor for the toxin in nervous tissue. The concept of a bipartite active protein is not restricted to bacterial toxins. The toxic proteins abrin and ricin from the seeds of two unrelated plant families are similarly composed. The A components both block protein synthesis by interfering with polypeptide chain elongation (as does diphtheria toxin), in this case by inactivating the 60S ribosomal subunits. The cell membrane receptors for the B chains of both toxins are similar and appear to contain lactose residues. Fully active hybrids of ricin A/abrin B and abrin A/ricin B can be constituted.

Further reading: S. van Heyningen, 1983.

***ESCHERICHIA COLI* ENTEROTOXIN.** Enteropathogenicity and the ability to produce both a heat-stable small molecular and a heat-labile protein enterotoxin is conferred on *E. coli* by an enterotoxin plasmid (Ent$^+$). It is likely that these strains of *E. coli* contribute very heavily to enterotoxic enteropathies throughout the world. We will be concerned only with the heat-labile toxin that bears many resemblances to cholera toxin: (1) it stimulates adenylate cyclase, with the same consequences; (2) it cross-reacts immunologically with cholera toxin and choleragenoid; i.e., antisera to cholera toxin and choleragenoid neutralize both toxins, antisera to coli toxin neutralizes cholera toxin poorly; (3) both toxins bind to the ganglioside GGnSLC (but see below). There are, however, some differences. Coli toxin, properly purified, is exactly like cholera toxin. This may be due to association of the toxin with other materials in the culture filtrate. It is also several orders of magnitude less toxic than cholera toxin, even taking into account the impurity of the preparations tested. Coli toxin appears to be synthesized as a protoxin, which is converted to the active form by proteolytic enzymes (thus it may be fully active in the gut, which contains trypsin-like enzymes, and inactive in the skin). Partially purified coli toxin preparations from several laboratories show faint bands in SDS gel corresponding to molecular weights of 23,000 to 30,000, and when *E. coli* is treated with the antibiotic polymyxin a protein of MW 23,000 is obtained that is very similar to cholera toxin A1 active component, but has some activity on whole cells.

Some workers have found that the ganglioside GGnSLC binds coli toxin as well as it binds cholera toxin; others find that coli toxin is far less readily bound. The results suggest that coli and cholera toxins have the same active component and bind to the same receptor but differ in their binding capacity. This might be connected with variations in the structure of coli toxin and its possible association with other components of culture filtrates that block binding capacity to varying degrees and thus affect toxicity.

Further reading: Cohen and S. van Heyningen, 1982.

OTHER ENTEROTOXINS. *Salmonella enteritidis* and *S. typhimurium* have been reported to produce enterotoxins possessing similarities to the *E. coli* enterotoxin, and *S. typhimurium* has been reported to produce a heat-labile factor inducing capillary permeability in rabbit skin, like *V. cholerae* and *E. coli* enterotoxins. These observations have not been confirmed, but might be important in future considerations of the intestinal effects of salmonella infections.

Shigella dysenteriae produces an exotoxin that appears to be as potent as botulinum toxin in producing flaccid paralysis in rabbits. The toxin is in fact not a neurotoxin but causes hemorrhages in the spinal cord of the rabbit, which leads to edema, and thus to pressure on nerves. This toxin is a cytotoxic enterotoxin capable of causing fluid accumulation in ligated ileal loops of the rabbit. The role of this toxin in the pathogenesis of shigellosis has not been determined. There has been some evidence that toxin-producing strains of *S. dysenteriae* are no more pathogenic than invasive atoxic strains, but it has been proposed that both toxinogenesis and invasiveness play a role in the disease.

Food poisoning due to contamination by *Bacillus cereus*, *Clostridium perfringens*, *Staphylococcus aureus*, and *Vibrio parahaemolyticus* is now recognized as a health hazard. *B. cereus* culture filtrate induces fluid accumulation in ligated rabbit ileal loops and an increase in capillary permeability in the skin. Apparently an enterotoxin is produced, but as yet little is known about its nature or its medical significance. Sporulating cultures of *Cl. perfringens* cause fluid accumulation in the gut, possibly owing to decreased absorption rather than increased secretion. A diarrheagenic and emetic toxin, different from the other known toxins of *Cl. perfringens*, has been isolated, with a molecular weight of 35,000. Little is known about the mode of action of the toxin, but it is likely that it is an important factor in *Cl. perfringens* food poisoning. The staphylococcus produces five enterotoxins, A to E, that can be differentiated serologically but have similar physicochemical properties (MW 26,000 to 30,000) and gastrointestinal effects, causing diarrhea and vomiting. The emetic effect is neurologically mediated. The site of the emetic action of these toxins has been shown to be in the abdominal viscera, and the sensory emetic stimulus reaches the vomiting center via the vagus and sympathetic nerves. The diarrheagenic mechanism has not yet been elucidated. The toxins seem most active on the middle segment of the small intestine where they enhance secretory activity without blocking absorption of sodium or water.

Vibrio parahaemolyticus is a major cause of seafood-borne gastroenteritis in Japan and elsewhere. The organism produces a heat-stable protein of MW 45,000 that is hemolytic, cardiotoxic, and capable of causing fluid accumulation in ligated rabbit ileal loops, causing degenerative changes at the same time (unlike cholera toxin). This toxin is blocked by a sialidase-sensitive ganglioside (Table 4).

Further reading: Takeda et al., 1976; and van Heyningen, 1971.

OTHER TOXINS

***CLOSTRIDIUM PERFRINGENS* ALPHA TOXIN.** This toxin is discussed in order to show that a fatal disease resulting from an infection by an organism producing a lethal exotoxin need not necessarily be an exotoxinosis. *Clostridium perfringens* is the main causative organism of gas gangrene, a disease resulting from the infection of deep penetrating wounds, and characterized by tissue destruction and toxemia and shock. Several toxins are produced, including a proteolytic collagenase (kappa), a cardiotoxic oxygen-labile hemolysin (theta), and a tissue-necrotizing oxygen-stable hemolysin (alpha). The alpha toxin is an enzyme, a phospholipase C, which catalyzes the cleavage of phosphoryl choline, phosphoryl ethanolamine, and other compounds from phospholipids. Gas gangrene can be prevented in experimentally infected animals by prophylactic active or passive immunization against the alpha toxin, but not against the other toxins. In view of this, and of the undoubted fact that the injection of a lethal dose of alpha toxin can produce symptoms of shock, it is not unreasonable to suggest that *Cl. perfringens* gas gangrene is an exotoxinosis, like tetanus, diphtheria, and cholera, which were discussed earlier.

However, the situation in gas gangrene is much more complicated. Although alpha antitoxin gives good protection when infection is initiated in slightly damaged muscle, it gives little or no protection when infection is initiated in severely damaged muscle, or in slightly damaged muscle when the bacteriostatic action of serum proteins (transferrin) is lowered by pretreating the experimental animals with iron compounds. It would seem that the protective role of alpha antitoxin is due not so much to its neutralizing the lethality of the toxin, but rather to its neutralizing the ability of the toxin to cause tissue necrosis and so pave the way for further growth of the organism. In effect, the role of antitoxin is bacteriostatic. But if other factors prevail that favor bacterial growth, such as severe tissue damage, or if the bacteriostatic action of serum proteins is lowered, then massive growth of the organism results in a number of effects, such as removal of oxygen from the environment; fall in redox potential; marked changes in vascular permeability; loss of plasma protein; and severe hemoconcentration. It may be that these conditions are responsible for the fatal shock of gas gangrene.

Further reading: Bullen, 1970; and Arbathnott, 1982.

ANTHRAX TOXINS. The anthrax bacillus produces three different proteins, a protective antigen (PA), a lethal factor (LF), and an edema factor (EF), which are biologically active only in certain combinations: PA + LF are lethal. EF is itself an adenylate cyclase (rather than a host cell AC stimulator), but is active only in the presence of a factor (calmodulin) that can be found in Chinese hamster ovary cells (and presumably in the affected host). PA is presumed to promote the entry of EF and LF into host cells. It seems likely that these toxins are responsible for the harmful effects of anthrax, but their role has not yet been as clearly defined as those already discussed.

Further reading: S. van Heyningen, 1982.

PERTUSSIS TOXINS. The pertussis organism also secretes an AC, stimulated by calmodulin, and a lethal toxin, which, like cholera toxin, activates AC in the host. As in the case of anthrax toxin, it seems likely that pertussis toxins are responsible for the harmful effects of (and immunity to) whooping cough, but this role has not been clearly defined.

Further reading: Pittman, 1970, and S. van Heyningen, 1982.

STAPHYLOCOCCAL EXFOLIATIVE TOXIN. Some phage group II strains of staphylococci are responsible for an exfoliative dermatitis (staphylococcal scalded skin syndrome, SSSS) in very young infants, and more rarely in older children and adults. The epidermis can be displaced at the slightest touch, like the skin of a ripe peach, and more than half the body may be denuded to give an appearance resembling severely scalded skin. It is distressing to endure, and to see, but it passes quickly and is rarely fatal, since the denuded areas dry up and the skin is rapidly replaced. The effect can be reproduced experimentally in newborn mice by infecting the skin with group II staphylococci or by injecting sterile culture filtrates. In children and adults exfoliation may also result from sensitivity to certain drugs, including sulfa compounds, phenylbutazone and barbiturates, but in these latter cases the splitting of the skin occurs at the dermoepidermal junction, whereas SSSS is characterized by intraepidermal splitting.

The exfoliative effect of group II staphylococcal skin infection is a clear case of a harmful effect of an infection being due to an exotoxin. This toxin (exfoliatin) has been freed of other active staphylococcal products and purified. It is a protein with reported molecular weights ranging from 24,000 to 33,000. Reports on its heat stability also vary, and it may be that there is more than one form of the toxin. Nothing is known about the mode of action of the toxin at the molecular level.

Further reading: Taylor, 1976.

IMMUNIZATION AGAINST EXOTOXINOSES

Since some or all of the harmful effects of some infections are entirely due to exotoxins, and since these exotoxins are antigenic, the question arises whether protection against the diseases can be obtained by passive or active immunization against the relevant exotoxins. Active immunization obviously has only prophylactic possibilities because adequate levels of antibodies can be attained only some weeks after injection of the antigen. Therapeutic passive immunization is of limited value because exotoxins are rapidly fixed to their susceptible cells, and once fixed they cannot be neutralized by antitoxin. In fact, the bound toxin may not remain on the surface of the cell, where it can be reached by antitoxin, for more than a few minutes. In the case of diphtheria and cholera toxins we know that the active components, A, of the toxins are rapidly "eclipsed," and pass into the interior of the cell where they are unavailable to antitoxin. In the case of cholera toxin we know that the cell-binding component, B, which also has most of the antitoxin-binding capacity, remains on the surface of the cell while the A component acts inside; in the case of diphtheria toxin it is not yet known what happens to the B component; in either case the cell-damaging A component is sheltered from antitoxin.

Although antitoxin probably has little therapeutic value, there may be circumstances in which it might have some prophylactic value if it is administered soon enough, especially in suspected tetanus and diphtheria, before all the toxin has reached its susceptible tissue.

Active immunization can be achieved in advance of infection by injecting toxoid, that is, toxin that has been rendered nontoxic without affecting its antigenicity, by treatment with agents such as formaldehyde or glutaraldehyde. Obviously it is feasible to consider actively immunizing only subjects that are at risk, such as children against diphtheria and tetanus, and soldiers against tetanus and gas gangrene. Pregnant women should also be immunized against tetanus to protect their babies from umbilical tetanus. It is not feasible to immunize infants against SSSS, for example, because the disease is very rare. It may be possible to immunize soldiers against gas gangrene toxin, but, as we have seen, it is likely that only those who receive wounds that do not bring about much tissue damage will be protected. This might still be worthwhile.

It might be instructive to compare the problems of active immunization against the three frank exotoxinoses we have already discussed: diphtheria, tetanus, and cholera.

People who have had diphtheria are probably immune to it, or at least to its worst effects, for the rest of their lives; they have been exposed to enough toxin to ensure this. The same state of affairs can be achieved by active immunization with purified toxoid. In developed countries where active immunization with diphtheria toxoid is carried out extensively, diphtheria has more or less disappeared. In countries where active immunization is not practiced, it is rife, and only survivors of the disease, or people who have had frequent contact with the organism without getting diseased, are immune.

People who have had tetanus and survived are no more immune to the disease than people who have not had it. The reason for this is that a sublethal (or lethal) dose of tetanus toxin is such a small amount of antigen (a few picograms or nanograms) that it is quite inadequate to elicit immunity. In Brazil and in India there is some evidence that some members of the indigenous populations may have protective levels of antitoxin in their sera, probably as a result of frequent experience of sublethal amounts of toxin. Active immunity to the disease is easily attained by immunization with the purified toxoid. In the early phase of World War I, when immunization was not practiced, the incidence of tetanus in the British Army was nearly 7 in every 1000 wounded; in World War II only 35 British soldiers died of tetanus and there are good reasons to doubt whether half of them had in fact been immunized.

How effective is antitoxic active immunization against cholera? The answer is still being sought. Although cholera is a frank exotoxinosis, it is otherwise a very different disease from either diphtheria or tetanus. For one thing, the toxin acts enterally, not parenterally as in the other two diseases, and for another, the disease is very quick, with the time interval between onset and death being measured in hours rather than days. The enteral nature of the disease suggests that for the actively produced antitoxin to be effective it must be present in the small intestine, secreted from the wall of the intestine in the form of IgA antibodies. Research is at present being conducted on the practical means of bringing about such enteral active immunity to the toxin. The rapid course of the disease means that there is not enough time for the anamnestic response of antibody production to secondary antigenic stimulus to play an important part. Protection therefore must probably depend on there being sufficient antibody present enterally at the time of infection.

If effective antitoxic immunity to cholera toxin can ever be achieved, it will have the very important added advantage that such immunity will also be effective against many *E. coli* diarrheas, since cholera antitoxin neutralizes *E. coli* toxin.

References

Arnon, S. S., Midura, T. F., Damus, D., Wood, R. M., and Chin, J.: Intestinal infection and toxin production by *Clostridium botulinum* as one cause of sudden infant death syndrome. Lancet 1:1273, 1978.

Boquet, P., and Pappenheimer, Jr., A. M.: Interaction of diphtheria toxin with mammalian cell membranes. J Biol Chem 251:5770, 1976.

Bullen, J. J.: Role of toxins in host-parasite relationships. In Ajl, S. J., Kadis, S., and Montie, T. C. (eds.): Microbial Toxins I. New York and London, Academic Press, 1970, p. 233.

Cohen, O., and van Heyningen, S. (eds.): Molecular Action of Toxins and Viruses. Amsterdam, New York, Oxford, Elsevier Biomedical Press, 1982.

Collier, R. J.: Diphtheria toxin: Mode of action and structure. Bacter Rev 39:54, 1975.

Collier, R. J.: Inhibition of protein synthesis by exotoxins from *Corynebacterium diphtheriae* and *Pseudomonas aeruginosa*. In Cuatrecasas, P. (ed.): The Specificity and Action of Animal, Bacterial and Plant Toxins. London, Chapman and Hall, 1977, p. 67.

Mellanby, J., and Green, J.: How does tetanus toxin act? Neuroscience 6:281, 1981.

Murphy, J. R.: Structure activity relationships of diphtheria toxin. In Bernheimer, A. W. (ed.): Mechanisms in Bacterial Toxinology. New York, London, Sydney, Toronto, John Wiley and Sons, 1976, p. 31.

Olsnes, S., and Pihl, A.: Abrin, ricin, and their associated agglutinins. In Cuatrecasas, P. (ed.): The Specificity and Action of Animal, Bacterial and Plant Toxins. London, Chapman and Hall, 1977, p. 129.

Pappenheimer, A. M., Jr., and Gill, D. M.: Diphtheria. Science 182:353, 1973.

Pittman, M.: Pertussis toxin: the cause of the harmful effects and prolonged immunity of whooping cough. A hypothesis. Rev. Infect. Dis. 1:401, 1979.

Sugiyama, H.: Clostridium botulinum neurotoxin. Microbiol. Rev. 44:419, 1980.

Takeda, Y., Takeda, T., Honda, T., and Miwatani, T.: Inactivation of the biological activities of the thermostable direct haemolysin of Vibrio parahaemolyticus by ganglioside GT1. Infect Immun 14:1, 1976.

Taylor, A. G.: Toxins and the genesis of specific lesions: enterotoxin and exfoliatin. In Bernheimer, A. W. (ed.): Mechanisms in Bacterial Toxinology. New York, London, Sydney, Toronto, John Wiley and Sons, 1976, p. 195.

van Heyningen, S.: Tetanus toxin. Pharmacol. Ther. 11:141 1980.

van Heyningen, S.: Diphtheria toxin: Which route into the cell? Nature 242:293, 1981.

van Heyningen, S.: Bacterial toxins and cyclic AMP. Nature 299:782, 1982.

van Heyningen, W. E.: The exotoxin of *Shigella dysenteriae*. In Kadis, S., Montie, T. C., and Ajl, S. J. (eds.): Microbial Toxins Volume IIA. New York and London, Academic Press, 1971, p. 255.

van Heyningen, W. E.: Gangliosides as membrane receptors for tetanus toxin, cholera toxin and serotonin. Nature 249:415, 1974.

van Heyningen, W. E., and Seal, J. R.: Cholera. The American scientific experience, 1947–1980. Boulder, Westview Press, 1983.

6

BACTERIAL ENDOTOXINS

Abraham I. Braude, M.D., Ph.D.

The lipopolysaccharides (LPSs) in the outer membrane of the cell wall of gram-negative bacteria can cause hypotension, shock, fever, intravascular coagulation, and death. Because of this toxicity, and because they are incorporated within the bacterial cell wall, they are called endotoxins. Exotoxins, by contrast, are not structural components of the cell, and are released from the bacteria, so that their biologic activity is far greater in the culture filtrates than in the parent cell suspension. Although endotoxin may also escape into surrounding fluids, the whole cell of gram-negative bacteria retains the major portion of the endotoxic activity.

CHEMICAL STRUCTURE OF ENDOTOXINS

The toxic LPSs or endotoxins of smooth bacteria are macromolecules composed of three main regions: lipid A, core polysaccharide, and "O" antigens (Fig. 1).

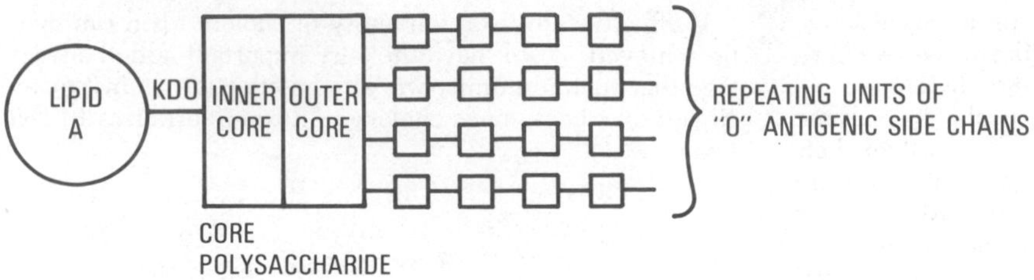

Figure 1. Diagram of lipopolysaccharide showing three main regions: lipid A, core, and "O" antigens. Note key position of KDO as a link between lipid A and polysaccharides. KDO is attached via a ketoacidic linkage to glucosamine residues of lipid A.

Each of these regions has a unique composition. The "O" antigens are made up of a series of repeating oligosaccharide units, each composed of three or four different hexoses. There may be as many as 10 such units in the smoothest gram-negative bacteria. The "O" antigens vary with each species and serologic type of organism. In rough bacteria, the "O" antigens are lost through a mutation that deprives the bacteria of enzymes required to synthesize the "O" antigen or attach them to the core. These rough bacteria thus lose hydrophilic surface properties provided by the abundant external sugars and no longer form smooth suspensions in liquid cultures (Fig. 2) or smooth colonies on solid media.

Lipid A. The key to isolation of lipid A is KDO, a unique sugar with the formula 2-keto-3-deoxyoctonate (Heath and Ghalambor, 1963). A disaccharide of KDO links lipid A to the core region, and mild acid hydrolysis will cleave the ketosidic linkage of KDO to lipid A, yielding water-insoluble preparations of lipid A with a molecular weight of approximately 2000. Another approach to the isolation of lipid A is through the use of mutants that synthesize a defective polysaccharide containing only lipid A and KDO. Mutants without lipid A have never been isolated, and therefore it appears indispensable for survival of bacteria.

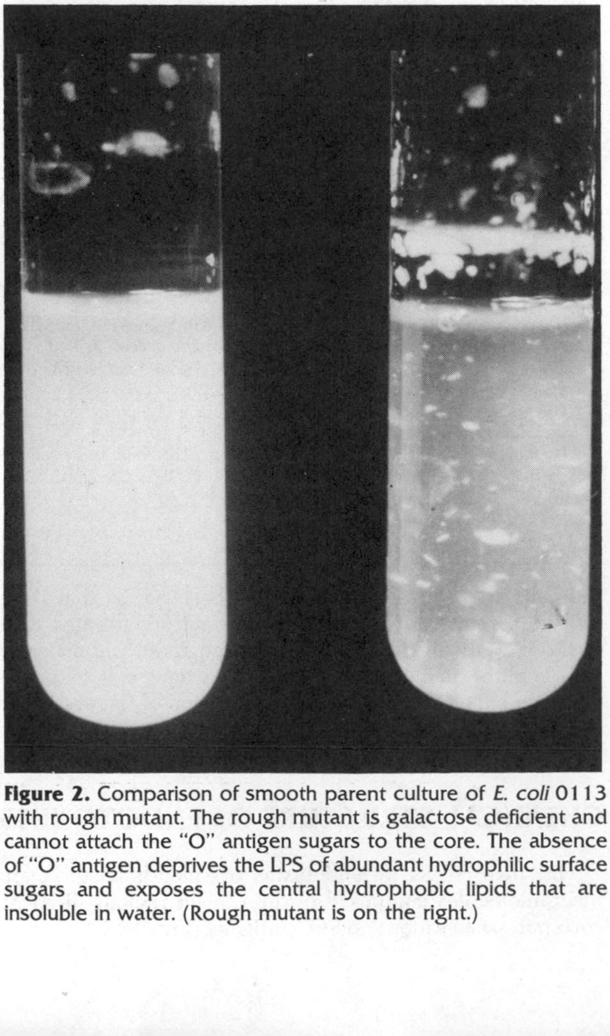

Figure 2. Comparison of smooth parent culture of *E. coli* 0113 with rough mutant. The rough mutant is galactose deficient and cannot attach the "O" antigen sugars to the core. The absence of "O" antigen deprives the LPS of abundant hydrophilic surface sugars and exposes the central hydrophobic lipids that are insoluble in water. (Rough mutant is on the right.)

Lipid A in most gram-negative bacilli of medical importance is composed of glucosamine-phosphate, long-chain fatty acids, and ethanolamine. [In certain saprophytes such as *Rhodopseudomonas*, glucosamine is absent from the lipid A (Hase and Rietschel, 1976)]. Thus, lipid A is an unusual phospholipid that uses D-glucosamine instead of glycerol as a skeleton. Disaccharides of glucosamine have β1,6 linkages in *Salmonella, Shigella, Escherichia coli, Yersinia, Fusobacterium, Pseudomonas*, and *Proteus*. The 14-carbon fatty acid β-hydroxymyristic (3-hydroxy-tetradecanoic) acid is attached to the glucosamine subunit by amide linkages (Fig. 3). In lipid A of *E. coli*, for example, β-hydroxymyristic acid is linked to each glucosamine molecule of the disaccharide by esterification of the hydroxyl group on position 3 of glucosamine and by acylation of the amino group on position 2. Other long-chain fatty acids are incorporated into lipid A by substituting the OH groups of β-hydroxymyristic acid with lauric acid, myristic acid, and 3-hydroxymyristic acid. Other β-hydroxy-fatty acids containing 10 to 17 carbon atoms are characteristic of different bacteria. In *Pseudomonas*, the lipid A contains β-hydroxymyristic acid as in the enteric bacteria. These long-chain fatty acids give lipid A its lipoidal characteristics.

The glycosidic diphosphate moiety has a high affinity for such metals as Mg^{2+}, Ca^{2+}, and Cd^{2+}, which probably stabilize the outer membrane of gram-negative bacteria by forming ionic bridges between LPS molecules (Strain et al., 1983).

Core Polysaccharide. This region contains not only KDO, the link to lipid A, but also heptose, phosphate, ethanolamine, and three hexoses. The hexoses, which consist of galactose, glucose and *N*-acetyl glucosamine, are designated the outer core, whereas the remainder is called the inner core. Much of the information on core sugars was obtained by examination of *Salmonella* mutants that were blocked in different steps in the biosynthesis of the core. These blocks resulted from defective activity of enzymes involved in transfer (transferase) or synthesis (synthetase; epimerase) of sugars. The sugars are transferred as sugar-nucleotides, usually as derivatives of uridine diphosphate (UDP) or guanosine diphosphate (GDP). The enzymes are associated with the cytoplasmic membrane where they catalyze the stepwise addition of the sugar-nucleotides to the nonreducing terminus of the growing core polymer. The inner core is constructed in the membrane by stepwise addition of KDO, heptose phosphate, and ethanolamine, followed by the hexose units of the outer core (Nikaido, 1973).

In rough mutants containing only KDO and heptose in

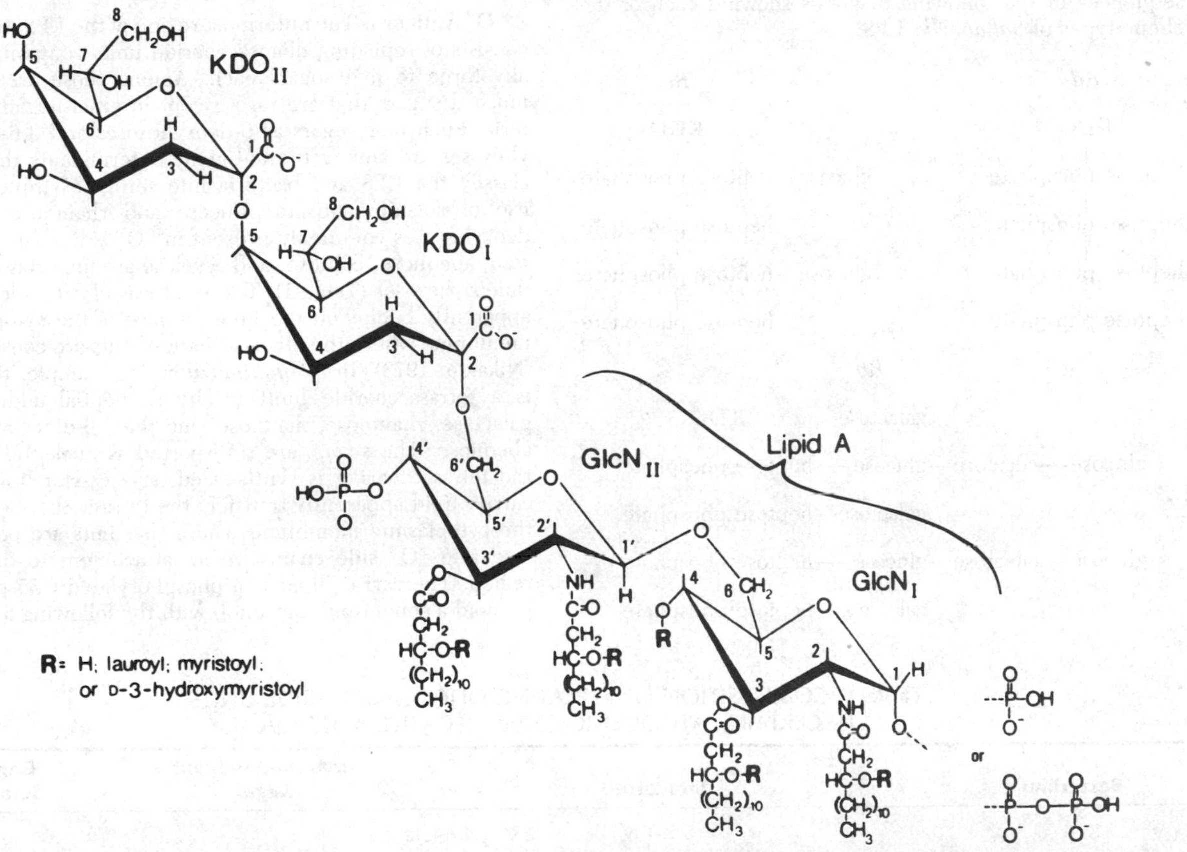

Figure 3. Diagram of proposed structure of lipid A from E. coli. Note the following key structural features. 1) The skeleton of lipid A is a disaccharide of D-glucosamine (GlcNβ1→6GlcNβ1) instead of glycerol. 2) The 14 carbon compound, β-hydroxmyristic acid, is linked to each glucosamine molecule of the disaccharide by esterification of the hydroxyl groups on position 3, or by acylation of the amino groups on position 2. 3) All of the OH groups of β-hydroxymyristic acid are substituted with the saturated long chain fatty acids indicated by R. Lauric acid (*N*-dodecanoic) has 12 carbon atoms and myristic acid (*n*-tetradecanoic) has 14. 4) The disaccharide of KDO, with the structure KDOα 2 →5KDOα 2→, is linked to the C6′ position of glucosamine ($G1cN_{II}$) (α = αanomeric configuration of KDO; 2→5 = linkage between C_2 on KDO_{II} and C5 on KDO_{I}). 5) Phosphate groups at C1 are high affinity binding sites for such metals as Ca^{2+}, Mg^{2+}, and Cd^{2+}. By forming ionic bridges between LPS molecules, these metals could stabilize the outer membrane of gram-negative bacteria. (From Strain, S., Fesik, S., and Armitage, I.: Structure and metal-binding properties of lipopolysaccharides from haptoselus mutants of *Escherichia coli* studied b ^{13}C and ^{31}P nuclear magnetic resonance. J Biol Chem 258:13466, 1983.)

the core, the LPS is designated chemotype Rd (Lüderitz et al., 1966). Such mutants lack the enzyme UDP-glucose synthetase so that synthesis of the core is not completed. In mutants with LPS designated Rc, the enzyme UDP galactose-4-epimerase is deficient so that glucose, but not galactose, is synthesized and incorporated into the core. The molecular weight of the Rc mutant is about 10,000. In chemotype Rb, the LPS contains all basal sugars except *N*-acetyl glucosamine, but the deficient enzyme has not been identified. In chemotype Ra, the core LPS is completed but the "O" side chains cannot be attached. The stepwise buildup of the core can be appreciated from its sugar sequences in the following diagrams showing each of the chemotypes of *Salmonella* LPS:

Rd

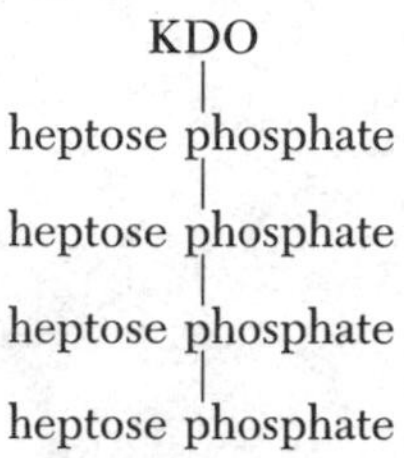

Rc

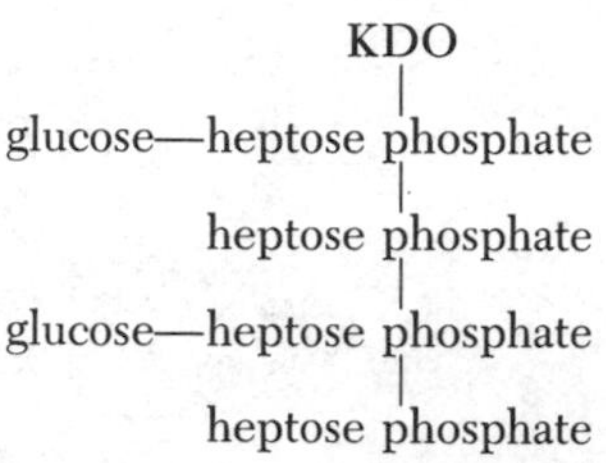

Rb

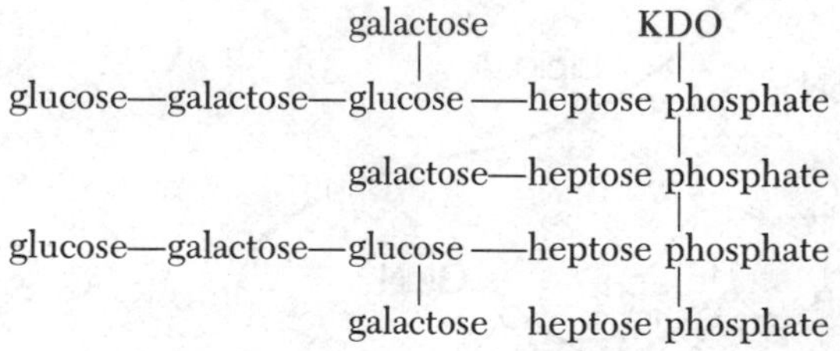

Ra

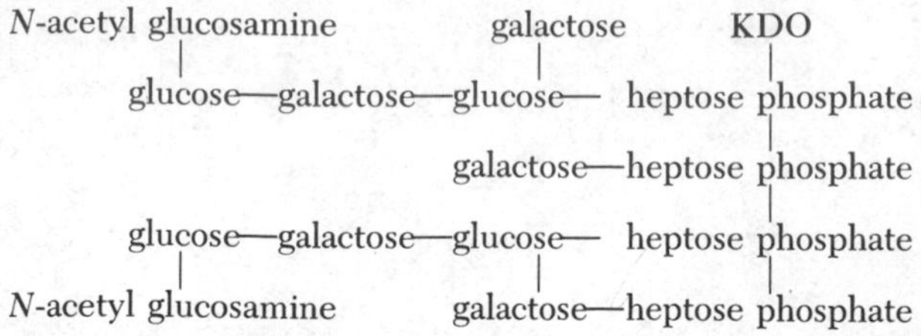

"O" Antigens. The outermost region of the LPS molecule consists of repeating oligosaccharide units containing usually three to five sugars each. Among these are certain unusual sugars that are rare except in gram-negative bacteria. Such rare sugars as 6-deoxyhexoses and 3,6-dideoxyhexoses are among the antigenic determinants that help classify the LPS and bacteria into serotypes through the use of specific antisera. Fucose and rhamnose are 6-deoxyhexoses commonly present in "O" side chains. Paratose, abequose, colitose, and tyvelose are important α-3,6-dideoxyhexoses (Table 1). The synthesis of "O" side chains apparently begins on the inner surface of the cytoplasmic membrane where the oligosaccharide units are constructed (Nikaido, 1973). In *S. typhimurium*, for example, the unit is a tetrasaccharide built up by sequential addition of galactose, rhamnose, mannose, and the 3,6-dideoxyhexose abequose. The sugars are transported as nucleotides, and the tetrasaccharide is synthesized on a carrier lipid. The carrier lipid apparently transfers the tetrasaccharide across the cytoplasmic membrane where the units are polymerized into "O" side chains before attachment to the core region. The carrier lipid is a phosphorylated C55 polyisoprenoid alcohol (undecaprenol) with the following formula:

Table 1. COMPOSITION OF REPEATING OLIGOSACCHARIDE UNITS IN CERTAIN PATHOGENIC GRAM-NEGATIVE BACTERIA

Bacterium	Structure	Immunodominant Sugar	Group or Serogroup
Salmonella typhosa	α-Tyv (on Man) α-Glc (on Gal) 2—(α)—Man—1,4—Rha—1,3 α-Gal—1	α-Tyvelose	D
Salmonella typhimurium	α-Abe (on Man) α-Glc$_{1,4}$ (on Gal) 2—d—Man—1,4—Rha → α-Gal—1	α-Abequose	B
Salmonella paratyphi	α-Par$_{1,3}$ (on Man) α-Glc$_{1,4}$ (on Gal) 2—α-Man—1,4—Rha—1,3—α-Gal—1	Paratose	A
Salmonella thompson	Glc (on third Man) Man—1,2—Man, 1,2—Man 1,2—Man—1	Glucose	C_1
Salmonella anatum	6—B Man—1,4—Rha—1,3 α-Gal—1	Mannose	E_1
Shigella flexneri	Ac 6—Glc Nac—1,2—Rha—1,4—Rha—1	Rhamnose	2a

Glc = glucose; Gal = galactose; Rha = rhamnose; Man = mannose; Par = paratose; Glc Nac = *N*-acetyl glucosamine; Ab = abequose; Tyv = tyvelose; Ac = acetyl

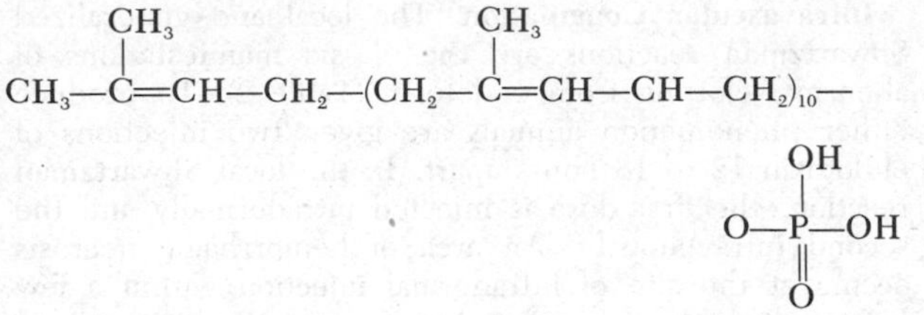

This carrier lipid is probably identical to that which functions in the biosynthesis of cell wall peptidoglycan.

The chemical structure of many O-specific side chains has been determined by biosynthetic studies. The composition of the repeating oligosaccharide units in these side chains is given for certain pathogenic gram-negative bacilli in Table 1. It should be noted that for each repeating unit there is one or more immunodominant sugar that is most responsible for the serologic specificity of antiserum against each "O" antigen (Lüderitz et al., 1966). It is the sugar with the highest affinity for the reactive site of the "O" antibody, as determined by its ability to inhibit serologic reactions. From Table 1 it can be seen that the immunodominant sugar may be a terminal nonreducing sugar in the side chain (α-tyvelose in *S. typhosa*) or main chain (rhamnose in *S. flexneri*). It may also be a nonterminal sugar in the main chain.

BIOLOGIC ACTIVITY OF ENDOTOXINS

Injections of small doses of endotoxins into experimental animals bring about dramatic changes in blood pressure, clotting, body temperature, circulating blood cells, metabolism, humoral immunity, cellular immunity, and resistance to infection. A large dose is lethal. These changes can be elicited with LPS from gram-negative bacteria or the intact organisms. There are many ways to isolate LPS but the most widely used is the phenol-water method of Westphal et al. (1952). The organisms are extracted with 45 per cent aqueous phenol at 65 to 68°C. After cooling, the LPS is recovered in the aqueous phase, and must then be separated by ultracentrifugation from RNA, which also partitions into the aqueous layer. In rough organisms, the LPS is hydrophobic and is found mainly in the phenol phase; recovery from the aqueous phase is poor. Rough LPS is best extracted by a solvent containing phenol, petroleum ether, and chloroform and recovered by ultracentrifugation (Galanos et al., 1969).

General Response to LPS. After intravenous injection of LPS the physiologic and biochemical changes depend on its dose and the animal species. In most animals (rabbits, dogs, monkeys, swine) injection of LPS in doses ranging from 0.1 to 100 μg will cause rapid onset of fever, neutropenia, and hypotension. The onset of neutropenia occurs almost immediately after injection of LPS, but fever and hypotension follow quickly, usually within 30 minutes. With large doses of LPS the hypotension may become irreversible and cause fatal shock. The pattern of fever, neutropenia, and hypotension has also been seen in patients given LPS or intravenous typhoid vaccine for fever therapy.

Fever. The most detailed studies of fever after injection of LPS have been carried out in rabbits. After intravenous injection of 0.1 μg LPS from most smooth bacteria the temperature begins to rise after a latent period of 10 to 20 minutes and reaches a peak at about 70 minutes. After the first peak the temperature declines slightly but starts to rise again at 2 hours and reaches a second higher peak at about 3 hours. The second peak alone is dose-dependent; it is absent with minimal pyogenic doses of LPS and gradually increases with rising doses until it reaches a ceiling that cannot be exceeded. According to current concepts the fever occurring after intravenous injection of endotoxin is mediated by a protein released from mononuclear phagocytes and is designated endogenous pyrogen (EP) (see Chapter 91). No latent period precedes the rise in fever after injection of EP because it stimulates the fever centers in the preoptic anterior hypothalamus directly without the intermediate reaction between pyrogen and mononuclear phagocytes that occurs with LPS. It is possible, however, that endotoxin itself can stimulate the fever centers directly because the amount of LPS needed to cause fever after injection into the cerebrospinal fluid is only one-thousandth that required by intravenous injection, and the latent period is less after intraspinal injection (Bennett et al., 1957). These findings would suggest that fever production requires EP in bacteremia but not in meningitis (e.g., meningococcemia vs meningococcal meningitis).

One of the classic features of endotoxin fever is tolerance (Fig. 4). The tolerance phenomenon occurs after repeated injections of the same dose of LPS and is characterized by a diminution in the height and duration of fever with

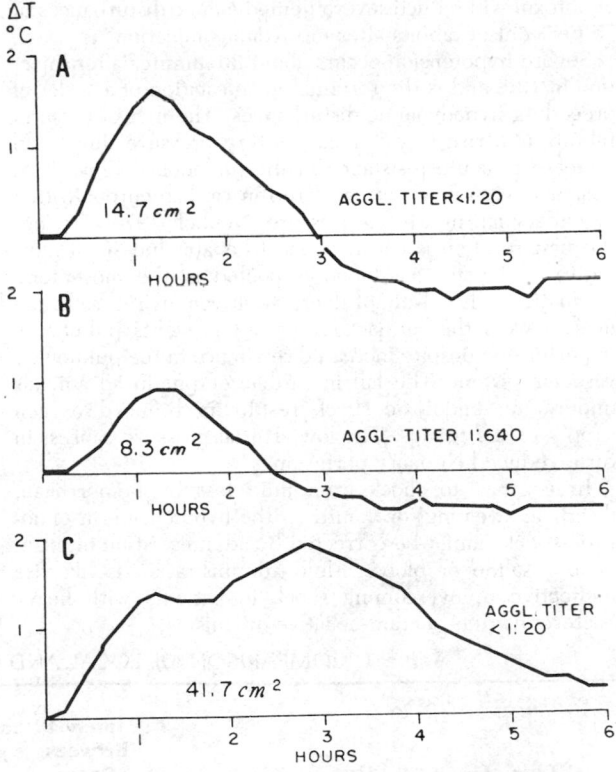

Figure 4. A comparison in rabbits of A, early tolerance, B, late tolerance, and C, no tolerance to the pyrogenic activity of lipopolysaccharides. Note biphasic fever peaks in nontolerant rabbits and disappearance of second peak after tolerance develops. Curve "A" is produced in rabbits challenged 24 hours after one I.V. injection and curve "B" after the last of seven daily I.V. injections of 1.0 μg of endotoxin. Curve "C" was obtained in control rabbits with no prior injections (Milner, 1973.)

successive injections. In rabbits this causes mainly a decline in the second peak. Two forms of tolerance are seen: (1) *early* tolerance, which is seen within 12 hours of the first injection; and (2) *late* tolerance, which appears gradually over several days. Early tolerance has been attributed to depletion of EP, or to a refractory response of the heat centers, which protects against sustained hypothermia. Late tolerance results from an immune reaction in which circulating antibody neutralizes LPS. Late tolerance can be transferred passively with serum, and causes accelerated disappearance of LPS into the reticuloendothelial system (Carey et al., 1958).

These febrile reactions are seen in nearly all mammals, including humans. In fact, man is far more sensitive to the pyrogenic action of LPS than any other animal, requiring 10 times less LPS than rabbits for the same febrile response (Wolff, 1973). Man also exhibits a longer latent period between injection of LPS and onset of fever and the fever curves are always monophasic. In tolerant human subjects the monophasic fever disappears completely, whereas tolerant rabbits maintain a monophasic response.

Rats and mice are exceptions to the rule that LPS injection causes fever in mammals. These two rodents respond to injection of LPS by a depression in body temperature.

Hypotension. The blood pressure may fall in animals given the small doses of endotoxin required to produce fever, but sustained hypotension and shock usually require larger doses of LPS. For example, 100 μg *Escherichia coli* endotoxin will induce severe hemodynamic disturbances in 75 per cent of rabbits after intravenous injection.

Severe hypotension occurs about 30 minutes after injection of LPS and is the terminal manifestation of a series of preceding hypodynamic disturbances. The first of these in rabbits is a rise in pulmonary artery pressure due to an increase in acute resistance in the pulmonary veins. This obstruction to flow causes a drop in cardiac output with a secondary fall in arterial pressure (Neuhof, 1975). In dogs the first reaction is constriction of hepatic and small mesenteric veins so that blood is pooled in the mesenteric circulation. The resultant decrease in venous return to the heart lowers the cardiac output but prevents pulmonary hypertension despite increased resistance in the pulmonary vascular system. The fall in cardiac output in all animals undergoing endotoxic shock results in reduced oxygen supply to the tissues. The low arterial pressure causes, in turn, reduced coronary perfusion.

In contrast to shock from fluid loss by hemorrhage, diarrhea, sweating, or vomiting, the hypotension in endotoxic shock cannot be corrected by administration of intravenous saline or blood. Fluid administration is likewise ineffective in overcoming shock in patients with heavy bacteremia due to gram-negative organisms.

Intravascular Coagulation. The local and generalized Shwartzman reactions are the classic manifestations of abnormal clotting from endotoxin (Table 2). To produce either phenomenon animals are given two injections of endotoxin 12 to 18 hours apart. In the local Shwartzman reaction, the first dose is injected intradermally and the second intravenously. An area of hemorrhagic necrosis occurs at the site of intradermal injection within a few hours after the second injection. In the generalized Shwartzman reaction both injections of LPS are given intravenously and the animals develop bilateral cortical necrosis of the kidneys within a few hours after the second dose.

Both reactions are the result of intravascular coagulation and the selective occlusion of small vessels by fibrin. The mechanism proposed for the local reaction involves two steps: first, the intravenous dose initiates intravascular coagulation with production of fibrin polymers; second, these polymers are trapped in the skin vessels that had been injured by the inflammatory reaction around the intradermal dose of LPS. There is no renal cortical necrosis because most of the circulating fibrin is cleared by the reticuloendothelial system (RE). In the generalized Shwartzman reaction, the first intravenous dose of LPS initiates coagulation and the second blocks RE removal of fibrin. The excess circulating fibrin is then filtered by the glomerular capillaries, which become occluded so that the renal cortex is infarcted. Small vessels in other organs may also filter fibrin. Both local and generalized reactions can be prevented by anticoagulants such as heparin.

The mechanism by which endotoxin initiates coagulation is not clear but there is good evidence that both intrinsic (plasma) and extrinsic (tissue) factors are involved (Morrison and Ulevitch, 1978). Clotting via the *intrinsic* pathway appears to be initiated when endotoxin activates Hageman factor (XII) through a reaction involving the negatively charged phosphate residues of lipid A. Hageman activation requires that a complex be formed between endotoxin and Hageman factor, probably by binding it to lipid A. Activation of Hageman factor eventuates in clotting because it initiates steps leading to the conversion of prothrombin to thrombin. The *extrinsic* pathway has been implicated because blood leukocytes are needed for both the local and generalized Shwartzman reactions, which are prevented by nitrogen mustard and other agents that cause leukopenia. Among the leukocytes, monocytes are currently regarded as the important circulating mediator cell for releasing the tissue factor (TF) that initiates clotting through the extrinsic pathway. TF is a lipoprotein in the plasma membrane of various cells, which complexes with factor VII and calcium ions to activate factor X. Activated factor X then converts prothrombin to thrombin.

The intravascular coagulation that leads to the general-

Table 2. COMPARISON OF LOCAL AND GENERALIZED SHWARTZMAN REACTIONS

Type of Reaction	First Dose	Second Dose	Interval Between Doses *(Hours)*	Dose of Endotoxin (mg), e.g., *E. coli* 0111 LPS *First*	*Second*	Manifestations of Reaction	Clinical Example
Local Shwartzman	Intradermal	Intravenous	21–24	0.25	0.03	Hemorrhagic necrosis of skin	Meningococcal purpura
Generalized Shwartzman	Intravenous	Intravenous	21–24	0.125	0.03	Bilateral renal cortical necrosis	Bilateral renal cortical necrosis in *E. coli* septicemia of pregnancy

ized Shwartzman reaction depletes clotting factors such as fibrinogen, platelets, and prothrombin. During intravascular coagulation, fibrinolysis is activated so that fibrin-degradation fragments (or fibrin split-products) accumulate in the blood. These fragments become anticoagulants since they inhibit both proteolysis of fibrinogen by thrombin and the polymerization of fibrin monomer to form a clot. In addition, the split-products inhibit platelet aggregation. This combined effect of split-products on clotting and platelet function can cause serious bleeding in patients whose clotting factors are consumed by disseminated intravascular coagulation in meningococcemia and other severe infections caused by gram-negative bacteria (Davis and Arnold, 1974).

In Vitro Coagulation. The addition of endotoxin to whole blood markedly shortens clotting time by activating Hageman factor and by stimulating leukocytes to release TF.

Endotoxin also clots the lysate prepared from the amebocytes of the horseshoe crab, *Limulus polyphemus* (Levin and Bang, 1964). This reaction has become important because clotting occurs in the presence of extremely small concentrations of endotoxin. The limulus lysate contains a clottable protein that forms a gel when exposed to as little as 0.0005 μg/ml of LPS. Endotoxin activates a high molecular weight (84,000) enzyme, which then reacts with a clottable protein to produce a gel. This reaction has been used to detect endotoxin in drugs, fluids, and other materials prepared for injection into patients. Limulus lysate has also been used to demonstrate endotoxin in the blood and spinal fluid of patients with gram-negative bacterial infections.

Disturbances in Circulating Blood Cells. Severe neutropenia occurs within minutes after injection of LPS into rabbits and other animals and persists at levels less than 10 per cent of normal for 4 hours. The neutropenia is followed by leukocytosis, with normoblasts and many other immature cells appearing in the circulation. The neutropenia results from sequestration of neutrophils in capillaries of the lung and other organs; and the leukocytosis results from the release of granulocytes from the bone marrow. Higher doses of LPS are required for neutropenia than for leukocytosis, probably because the numbers released from the marrow mask the mild sequestration of neutrophils produced by small doses. Because human beings cannot tolerate the relatively large doses given to rabbits and other animals, neutropenia has not always been observed in human studies but leukocytosis is constant and reproducible in them (Wolff, 1973).

One explanation for increased leukocyte production after injection of LPS is release of colony-stimulating factor (CSF), a glycoprotein that stimulates granulocytes and macrophages to proliferate from precursor cells. The term colony-stimulating factor refers to the ability of CSF to stimulate single cells to proliferate and grow as colonies in soft agar cultures. After an injection of endotoxin into mice, there is a striking increase in serum CSF during the period of granulocytopoiesis that precedes the release of marrow granulocytes into the peripheral blood. This is followed by a wave of proliferation and differentiation of granulocytes in the marrow (Pluznik, 1983).

The number of circulating platelets also falls rapidly after intravenous injection of LPS, and they are found in leukocyte-platelet thrombi or platelet-aggregates in small vessels of the lung and liver. As the platelets decrease, there is a simultaneous release from them of platelet constituents such as serotonin and platelet factor 8. This rapid drop in platelets requires complement. From in vitro experiments it appears that endotoxin also causes platelet lysis through a reaction that requires the alternative pathway of complement. Primates, including man, appear to be much less susceptible to thrombocytopenia after endotoxin injection than are lower mammals, and primate platelets do not seem to react to endotoxin in vitro. In contrast to rabbit platelets, which undergo massive aggregation in platelet-rich plasma, human platelets do not aggregate when exposed to endotoxin (Morrison and Ulevitch, 1978).

Lymphocytes decrease less precipitously than granulocytes and platelets and return more slowly to the circulation. They are also unaffected by tolerance. Daily injections of the same dose of endotoxin elicit a shorter period of neutrophil response. These tolerant animals develop only a brief period of neutropenia and a brisk rise in circulating neutrophils that begins between 1 and 2 hours after injection of endotoxin. Lymphocytes, on the other hand, maintain their slow decline in tolerant animals.

Immune Reactions: Cellular

Lymphocytes. Endotoxin stimulates proliferation of bone marrow-derived (B) lymphocytes (Peavy et al., 1973). This mitogenic effect of B lymphocytes results from the action of lipid A. It is demonstrated morphologically by transformation of B lymphocytes to blast cells and biochemically by increased synthesis of RNA, DNA, and protein. The phenomenon is seen in vitro with mouse lymphocytes, but not human or rabbit lymphocytes. It appears that stimulation by LPS of B cell mitosis results in division and differentiation into cells that secrete at a high rate the specific antibodies that are genetically determined for each cell. If such a reaction occurs in vivo, it could explain the increased nonspecific resistance to infection that occurs in mice shortly after an injection of endotoxin.

This idea is supported by the fact that mice (C3H/H_eJ) whose B lymphocytes do not proliferate when exposed to LPS also fail to develop increased resistance to infection when injected with LPS. The defective response of B lymphocytes to LPS is genetic and is accompanied by increased resistance of the mice to LPS toxicity (Sulzer and Goodman, 1977).

Macrophages. LPS stimulates macrophages to release interleukin 1 (IL1), an important mediator of macrophage functions. IL1 enhances the antibody response of B cells and stimulates the generation of cytotoxic T cells. LPS also activates macrophages most probably by a direct effect of lipid A on the cell membrane and without the mediation of T lymphocytes (Rosenstreich et al., 1977). Activation of macrophages by LPS causes them to increase in size, become more adherent to glass, exhibit greater random migration, and carry out increased phagocytosis. There is increased phagocytosis of certain bacteria, complement (C3b)-coated particles, and IgG antibody-coated particles. Activated macrophages are metabolically more active, showing an increased consumption of glucose via the hexosemonophosphate shunt. They also increase their production of certain enzymes such as collagenase, lactic dehydrogenase (cytoplasmic), and acid phosphatase (lysosomal). Electron microscopy reveals hypertrophy of the Golgi region and an increase in the number and size of lysosomes. As little as 1 μg/ml of LPS will stimulate increased phagocytosis in vitro, and similar concentrations in vivo will cause activation of the reticuloendothelial system so that endotoxin and various colloidal particles are cleared more rapidly from the circulation. These properties of activated macrophages might also contribute to the nonspecific resistance to infection observed in animals after injection of endotoxin. The influence of endotoxin on macrophages in vivo can be seen in exudates; after intraperitoneal injection of endotoxin, macrophages that exhibit various properties typical of activation accumulate.

One effect of LPS on macrophages is increased release of certain lysosomal enzymes, such as acid phosphatase, into the surrounding medium (Allison et al., 1973). Proteolytic enzymes, such as collagenase and plasminogen activator, are also released. Since plasmin (activated plasminogen) would cause fibrinolysis and collagenase could disrupt connective tissue, it is easy to imagine how macrophages might mediate certain toxic effects of LPS. Prostaglandins, a group of biologically active aliphatic acids, have also been implicated as mediators of LPS toxicity upon release from macrophages. Prostaglandins E and F are synthesized and released in large amounts from mouse macrophages after exposure to LPS. Since prostaglandins cause increased vascular permeability, vasodilatation, vasoconstriction (especially by prostaglandin F_2 in the pulmonary circulation), decreased cardiac output, and contraction of smooth muscle (uterus, bowel, bronchi), they could account for the cardiovascular effects, abortion, and diarrhea produced by endotoxin. This idea gains support from the finding that in C3H/H_eJ mice, which are genetically resistant to LPS toxicity, the macrophages do not secrete increased levels of prostaglandins upon exposure to endotoxin. Moreover, levels of prostaglandins are elevated in susceptible animals after injection of endotoxin, and indomethacin, which inhibits prostaglandin synthesis, also prevents certain toxic effects of endotoxin.

Endotoxin is taken up by macrophages by pinocytosis. The endotoxin is first adsorbed onto the cell membrane and then enters the cell through membrane invaginations. Peritoneal macrophages of guinea pigs are reported not to detoxify ingested endotoxin in vitro, but information on macrophages of other species in vitro and in vivo is too limited for general conclusions on cellular detoxification.

Large doses of endotoxin (e.g., 50 μg/ml *Escherichia coli* LPS) will kill macrophages in vitro.

Immune Reactions: Humoral

Antibody. Injection of endotoxin or infection with gram-negative bacteria stimulates circulating antibody to LPS. Smooth endotoxins stimulate primarily antibody to the "O" antigenic side chains and endotoxin from rough bacteria, antibody to the core. Antibody to lipid A has also been described after injection of bacterial cells of *Salmonella Minnesota* R595, which have the glycolipid KDO–lipid A on their surface. Antibody to each of these antigens ("O," core, lipid A) can be demonstrated by adsorbing LPS from smooth or rough organisms to the surface of red cells and then testing the antisera for their ability to cause hemolysis (in the presence of complement) or hemagglutination. Antibody to these antigens can also be demonstrated by precipitation reactions, precipitation-inhibition with individual sugars, enzyme-linked immunoabsorption, and bactericidal reactions in the presence of complement. Antibodies against LPS are both IgM and IgG. When lipid A is removed from the "O" polysaccharides by mild acid treatment, the "O" antigenic unit can no longer stimulate the formation of antibodies unless it is coupled to protein. The uncoupled, lipid-free O antigen is thus a nonantigenic hapten and can be identified only by in vitro reactions with specific antibody.

Antibody to "O" or "core" antigens can prevent toxicity of LPS, including the local Shwartzman and generalized Shwartzman reactions and death. The protection by "O" antibody is specific and limited to homologous LPS, whereas that from core antibody provides broad protection against LPS from a wide range of bacteria with unrelated "O" antigens (Braude et al., 1977; Ziegler et al., 1982).

The ability of LPS to stimulate antibody is independent of T lymphocytes. In this respect, LPS differs from most protein and cellular antigens that require a cooperation between T and B lymphocytes, in which the T lymphocytes activate the B lymphocytes to synthesize immunoglobulin.

Complement. Endotoxins can activate the complement system so that the various components are consumed and their activity disappears from serum (Mergenhagen et al., 1973). This activation can occur through either the classic or the alternative pathway, depending on the preparation of LPS. Activation of the classic pathway begins with activating of C1, which in turn catalyzes the assembly of C4,2 into the enzyme C3 convertase. C3 convertase activates C3 and the remaining components of complement. The first step in the reaction occurs in the presence of specific antibody against LPS, i.e., either IgG or IgM. After LPS combines with the Fab portion of the antibody, its Fc portion binds with C1 through its subunit C1q, and C1 becomes activated. There is also evidence that LPS from rough strains, as well as lipid A, can bind C1 directly and thereby activate the classic pathway without participation of antibody to LPS (Morrison and Ulevitch, 1978).

When the alternative pathway is activated by LPS, the first two steps of the classic pathway are omitted. Instead, LPS causes the enzymatic activation of a protein that can cleave C3. The activated protein, designated C3 activator, splits C3 into C3A and C3B. The C3B activates the remaining complement components.

Activation of complement by either pathway can kill gram-negative (but not gram-positive) bacteria. Complement activated by the classic pathway kills bacteria more rapidly, and rough bacteria are generally more susceptible than smooth bacteria to this bactericidal action. It has been suggested that this difference in susceptibility to killing by the complement system is due to the greater ability of LPS from rough bacteria to activate the more efficient classic pathway.

Complement can also be activated by endotoxin in vivo (Spink et al., 1964; Gilbert and Braude, 1962). Endotoxins obtained by trichloroacetic extraction (Boivin preparation) are more effective in lowering complement levels in vivo. The initial hypotensive response to endotoxin is dependent on complement activation, and in patients with shock due to gram-negative bacteremia the levels of C3 are reduced (McCabe, 1973). These findings suggest that bacteremic shock may be mediated to some extent through a reaction between endotoxin and complement.

Adjuvant Effect. When endotoxin is injected intravenously along with a protein antigen, the subsequent antibody response to the protein antigen begins earlier, increases faster, and reaches a higher level than in controls given no endotoxin (Johnson, 1983). This enhancement of antibody response by endotoxin in known as its adjuvant effect, and explains the well-known clinical observation that incorporation of typhoid vaccine with diphtheria or tetanus toxoid produces more antitoxin. Endotoxin does not need to be given by the same route as the protein antigen, but for maximal effect it should be given at the same time or within 6 hours of the antigen. Repeated injections of endotoxin, leading to tolerance to LPS toxicity, also abolish the adjuvant effect. The mechanism of the adjuvant effect of LPS is unknown. Since LPS can be detoxified by succinylation without losing its adjuvant activity, LPS toxicity does not seem essential for the adjuvant effect.

Stimulation of Interferon Activity. When endotoxin is injected intravenously into experimental animals peak levels of 1B interferon in the serum are reached within 2 to 3 hours (Youngner and Stinebring, 1966). Earlier data suggested that endotoxin caused the release of preformed interferon, but more recent evidence indicates that endotoxin and viruses stimulate synthesis of antigenically similar interferon.

Other Effects

Abortion. Injections of sublethal amounts of endotoxin can interrupt pregnancy in mice (Zahl and Bjerknes, 1943). The abortion is accompanied by placental hemorrhage and is apparently related to serotonin release. Endotoxins obtained from smooth or rough gram-negative bacteria, as well as lipid A, are abortifacient.

Tumor Necrosis. Endotoxin causes hemorrhagic necrosis of tumors in guinea pigs, rats, mice, and man. Most studies have been done with transplantable sarcomas of mice. The tumor becomes hemorrhagic 4 hours after the intravenous injection of crude or purified endotoxins and may undergo extensive necrosis and complete regression. The appearance of the necrotic tumor has suggested a similarity to the local Shwartzman reaction, but no thrombosis is observed in the hemorrhagic tumor.

Metabolic Effects. Intravenous injection of LPS causes changes in carbohydrates, lipids, iron, and sensitivity to epinephrine (Fiser et al., 1974). The level of blood glucose rises to a maximum within 2 hours after injection of LPS and then declines to severe hypoglycemic levels in shocked animals. This reaction is accompanied by rapid depletion of total body carbohydrate and impaired synthesis of glucose and glycogen (Berry, 1975). Administration of glucose or pyruvate fails to restore gluconeogenesis or glycogen synthesis to normal.

Hyperglyceridemia has been found in rabbits and rhesus monkeys after intravenous endotoxin (Lequire et al., 1959). It has also been seen in patients during septicemia due to gram-negative bacteria, but not gram-positive bacteria. It appears that endotoxin elevates serum triglyceride concentrations by interfering with the activation of lipid-clearing enzymes and with the clearance of lipids by the reticuloendothelial system.

Hypoferremia occurs in mice and rats after injection of small doses (0.1 μg) of LPS and can be used as a bioassay for endotoxin.

The increased susceptibility to epinephrine is manifested by its ability to produce skin hemorrhages after intradermal injection in rabbits given intravenous LPS simultaneously, or after intradermal injections of mixtures of LPS and epinephrine (Thomas, 1956). As little as 5 μg of intradermal epinephrine and 1 μg of intravenous LPS can produce hemorrhagic necrosis resembling the local Shwartzman reaction. In contrast to the Shwartzman reaction, the epinephrine lesion is not blocked by heparin or nitrogen mustard, but is prevented by cortisone, dibenzaline, and chlorpromazine, which do not prevent the Shwartzman. This reaction to epinephrine may reflect either an increased sensitivity of the arterioles to adrenergic stimulation or an increased release of catecholamines at the peripheral nerve endings resulting from endotoxin activation of the sympathetic nervous system. The combined effects of local catecholamines and injected epinephrine might cause sufficient vasoconstriction to infarct the skin, whereas neither could do so alone.

ALTERATION OF LPS TOXICITY

Reduced Toxicity. The toxicity of LPS can be reduced in vivo with antiserum or by inducing tolerance, as described earlier. It can also be reduced by the administration of cortisone (Chedid and Boyer, 1955) or polymyxin B sulfate. Cortisone prevents death when given before lethal doses of endotoxin are injected. When polymyxin B is injected before or together with endotoxin it can neutralize the Shwartzman reactions and prevent death of mice from endotoxin (Rifkind and Hill, 1967). Polymyxin B acts by disrupting the structure of LPS.

Although relatively resistant to heat, the toxicity of endotoxin can be abolished in vitro by dry heat at 170°C for 3 hours. It is also detoxified by acid hydrolysis at elevated temperatures (0.1 N acid), by alkaline hydrolysis, and by oxidation with periodate, H_2O_2, or permanganate. It can be reversibly inactivated by a heat-labile factor in serum that appears to depolymerize LPS. Sodium dodecyl sulfate and sodium deoxycholate are also reputed to inactivate LPS by depolymerizing it; after removal of these agents the LPS reaggregates and toxicity is restored.

Potentiation of Toxicity. A variety of procedures can potentiate LPS toxicity in experimental animals. One mechanism is reticuloendothelial blockage by thorium dioxide, which enhances the ability of endotoxin to kill animals and eliminates the increased resistance to the Shwartzman reaction and fever (tolerance) that follows repeated injections of endotoxins (Beeson, 1947). Colloidal iron saccharate, trypan blue, and lead acetate all enhance LPS toxicity when injected. A high molecular weight polygalactose, known as carrageenan, can increase the lethality of endotoxin by 100- to more than 3000-fold (Becker and Rudbach, 1978). Carrageenan is believed to function as a macrophage toxin by destabilizing the lysosomal membrane. All these agents probably enhance the toxicity of LPS by impairing macrophage function and blocking the reticuloendothelial system.

Other techniques for potentiating LPS toxicity are adrenalectomy (Parant and Chedid, 1971), mycobacterial infection, and high environmental temperatures. The mechanisms involved in lowering resistance to endotoxin by these procedures are unknown. Hypersensitivity to endotoxin, induced by repeated small intraperitoneal injections, increases the lethality of endotoxin for mice. These hypersensitivity deaths resemble anaphylaxis, occurring within 2 hours after challenge with endotoxin (Braude, 1975).

References

Allison, A., Davies, P., and Page, R.: Effect of endotoxin on macrophages and other lymphoreticular cells. J Infect Dis 128(S):204, 1973.

Atkins, E., and Bodel, P.: Fever. N Engl J Med 286:27, 1972.

Becker, L., and Rudbach, J. A.: Potentiation of endotoxicity by carrageenan. Infect Immun 19:1099, 1978.

Beeson, P.: Effect of reticuloendothelial blockage on immunity to the Shwartzman phenomenon. Proc Soc Exp Biol Med 64:146, 1947.

Bennett, I. L., Jr., Petersdorf, R. G., and Keene, W. R.: Pathogenesis of fever: evidence for direct cerebral action of bacterial endotoxins. Trans Assoc Am Physicians 70:64, 1957.

Berry, L. J.: Metabolic effects of endotoxin. In Schlesinger, D. (ed.): Microbiology 1975. Washington D.C., American Society for Microbiology, 1975, p. 315.

Braude, A.: Opposing effects of immunity to endotoxin: hypersensitivity versus protection. In Urbaschek, B., Urbaschek, R., and Neter, E. (eds.): Gram-Negative Bacterial Infections. New York, Springer-Verlag, 1975, p. 69.

Braude, A., Ziegler, E., Douglas, H., and McCutchan, J.: Antibody to cell wall glycolipid of Gram-negative bacteria: induction of immunity to bacteremia and endotoxemia. J Infect Dis 136(S):167, 1977.

Carey, F., Zalesky, M., and Braude, A.: Studies with radioactive endotoxin. III. The effect of tolerance on the distribution of radioactivity after intravenous injection of *Escherichia coli* endotoxin labeled with Cr^{51}. J Clin Invest 37:441, 1958.

Chedid, L., and Boyer, F.: Etude comparative du pouvoir antitoxique de la cortisone et de la chlorpromazine. Ann Inst Pasteur 88:336, 1955.

Davis, C., and Arnold, K.: Role of meningococcal endotoxin in meningococcal purpura. J Exp Med 140:159, 1974.

Fiser, R., Denniston, J., and Beisel, W.: Endotoxemia in the rhesus monkey; alterations in host lipid and carbohydrate metabolism. Pediatr Res 8:13, 1974.

Galanos, C., Lüderitz, O., and Westphal, O.: A new method for the extraction of R lipopolysaccharides. Eur J Biochem 9:245, 1969.

Gilbert, V., and Braude, A.: Reduction in serum complement in rabbits after injection of endotoxin. J Exp Med 116:477, 1962.

Hase, S., and Rietschel, E. T.: Isolation and analysis of the lipid A backbone, lipid A structure of lipopolysaccharides from various bacterial groups. Eur J Biochem 63:101, 1976.

Heath, E. C., and Ghalambor, M. A.: 2-keto-3-deoxyoctonate, a constituent of cell wall lipopolysaccharide preparations obtained from *E. coli*. Biochem Biophys Res Commun 10:340, 1963.

Johnson, A.: Adjuvant action of bacterial endotoxins on antibody formation: A historical perspective. In Nowotny, A. (ed.): Beneficial Effects of Endotoxins. New York, Plenum Press, 1983, p. 249.

Lequire, V., Hutcherson, J., Hamilton, R., and Gray, M.: The Effects of bacterial endotoxin on lipid metabolism. I. The responses of the serum lipids in rabbits to single and multiple injections of Shear's polysaccharide. J Exp Med 110:293, 1959.

Levin, J., and Bang, F.: The role of endotoxin in the extracellular coagulation of limulus blood. Bull Johns Hopkins Hosp 115:265, 1964.

Lüderitz, O., Staub, A. M., and Westphal, O.: Immunochemistry of O and R antigens of Salmonella and related Enterobacteriaceae. Bacteriol Rev 30:192, 1966.

McCabe, W.: Serum complement levels in bacteremia due to gram negative organisms. N Engl J Med 288:21, 1973.

Mergenhagen, S., Snyderman, R., and Phillips, K.: Activation of complement by endotoxin. J Infect Dis 128(S):78, 1973.

Milner, K.: Patterns of tolerance to endotoxin. J Infect Dis 128(S):229, 1973.

Morrison, D., and Ulevitch, R.: The effects of bacterial endotoxins on host mediation systems: A review. Am J Path 93:527, 1978.

Neuhof, H.: Changes in hemodynamics and gas metabolism after endotoxin injection. In Urbaschek, B., Urbaschek, R., and Neter, E. (eds.): Gram-Negative Bacterial Infections. New York, Springer-Verlag, 1975, p. 259.

Nikaido, H.: Biosynthesis and assembly of lipopolysaccharide and the outer membrane layer of Gram-negative cell wall. In Leive, L. (ed.): Bacterial Membranes and Walls. New York, Marcel Dekker, Inc., 1973, p. 131.

Parant, M., and Chedid, L.: Sensibilization de la souris aux endotoxines par la surrénalectomie ou par l'administration d'actinomycine D. C R Acad Sci (D) (Paris) 272:1308, 1971.

Peavy, D., Shands, J., Adler, W., and Smith, R.: Selective effects of bacterial endotoxins on various subpopulations of lymphoreticular cells. J Infect Dis 128(S):83, 1973.

Pluznik, D.: Endotoxin induced release of colony-stimulating factor. In Nowotny, A. (ed.): Beneficial Effects of Endotoxin. New York, Plenum Press, 1983, p. 397.

Rifkind, D., and Hill, R.: Neutralization of the Shwartzman reactions by polymyxin B. J Immunol 99:564, 1967.

Rosenstreich, D., Glode, L., Wahl, L., Sandberg, A., and Mergenhagen, S.: Analysis of the cellular defects of endotoxin-unresponsive mice. In Schlesinger, D. (ed.): Microbiology 1977. Washington, D.C., American Society for Microbiology, 1977, p. 314.

Spink, W., Davis, R., Potter, R., and Chartrand, S.: The initial stage of canine endotoxin shock as an expression of anaphylactic shock: studies on complement titers and plasma histamine concentrations. J Clin Invest 43:696, 1964.

Strain, S., Fesik, S., and Armitage, I.: Structure and metal-binding properties of lipopolysaccharides from heptoseless mutants of *Escherichia coli* studied by ^{13}C and ^{31}P nuclear magnetic resonance. J Biol Chem 258:13466, 1983.

Sulzer, B., and Goodman, G.: Characteristics of endotoxin. Resistant low-responder mice. In Schlesinger, D. (ed.): Microbiology 1977. Washington D.C., American Society for Microbiology, 1977, p. 304.

Thomas, L.: The role of epinephrine in the reactions produced by the endotoxins of Gram-negative bacteria. I. Hemorrhagic necrosis produced by epinephrine in the skin of endotoxin-treated rabbits. J Exp Med 104:865, 1956.

Westphal, O., Lüderitz, O., and Bister, F.: Uber die extraktion von Bakterien mit Phenol/Wasser. Z Naturforsch 7b:148, 1952.

Wolff, S. M.: Biologic effects of bacterial endotoxins in man. J Infect Dis 128(S):251, 1973.

Youngner, J. S., and Stinebring, W. R.: Comparison of interferon production in mice by bacterial endotoxin and statolon. Virology 29:310, 1966.

Zahl, P., and Bjerknes, C.: Induction of decidua-placental hemorrhage in mice by the endotoxins of certain gram-negative bacteria. Proc Soc Exp Biol Med 54:329, 1943.

Ziegler, E., McCutchan, J. A., Fierer, J., Glauser, M. M., Sadoff, J., Douglas, H., and Braude, A. I.: Treatment of gram-negative bacteremia and shock with human antiserum to a mutant *Escherichia coli*. N Engl J Med 307:1225, 1982.

Virology

7
MORPHOLOGY AND STRUCTURE OF VIRUSES

RICHARD W. COMPANS, PH.D.

Viruses were first distinguished from other microorganisms on the basis of size, as determined by filtration techniques. Most infectious virus particles, or *virions*, are smaller than any bacteria, and are below the limit of resolution of the light microscope. The smallest virions are 20 to 30 nanometers in diameter (1 nanometer, nm, = 10^{-9} meter) and are the simplest agents known to cause infectious diseases of man.

Virions may also be distinguished from other microorganisms by the fact that they contain only one type of nucleic acid, either DNA or RNA. RNA-containing viruses are unique in possessing this type of nucleic acid as their genetic material.

Virions lack metabolic activity and do not possess ribosomes or many of the enzymes necessary for their replication, although they may contain certain specialized enzymes, as discussed in Chapter 9. As a consequence, viruses depend on cellular processes for their replication and are obligate intracellular parasites. The replication process involves intracellular dissolution of the virion into its macromolecular components, followed by synthesis of viral proteins and nucleic acids, whose structures are specified by the viral genome. The individual viral macromolecules are then assembled into progeny virions in yields as high as thousands of particles per infected cell. This type of replication cycle differs markedly from division by binary fission, which is the process by which bacteria multiply.

METHODS FOR ANALYSIS OF VIRUS STRUCTURE. Filtration through membranes with graded pore sizes provided the earliest information on the size characteristics of different viruses. Ultracentrifugation studies enabled estimates of virus particle size before viruses could be visualized in the electron microscope. The ultracentrifuge is still essential for the concentration and purification of viruses, both of which are prerequisites for direct biochemical analyses. Differential centrifugation enables viruses to be concentrated and partially purified; alternatively, many viruses may be concentrated by precipitation with reagents such as ammonium sulfate or polyethylene glycol. Virus particles may be purified by density gradient centrifugation in various media, the choice of which depends on the buoyant density as well as the stability of the virion. The most common are aqueous solutions of sucrose or potassium tartrate for the less dense and more fragile viruses, and cesium chloride solutions for the more stable viruses.

The structure of viruses can be examined directly by electron microscopy. If purified or concentrated virus suspensions are available, negative staining is usually the method of choice for specimen preparation. The procedure involves drying a suspension of virions in an aqueous solution of a heavy atom salt such as uranyl acetate or sodium phosphotungstate, which forms an electron-dense background. Virions, or other biologic structures, stand out as electron-lucent particles by this staining method, and the fine structure of the particles can be seen with high resolution (see Figs. 4 and 6). Virus-infected cells may also be examined in thin section by electron microscopy after embedding in suitable polymers, and this approach has afforded much information on the intracellular aspects of virus replication.

The recent growth of *molecular virology* as an experimental science has yielded a wealth of information on the molecular structure and replication processes of viruses. Cell culture systems are available for propagation and assay of most animal viruses. Extensive use is made of radioisotopic labeling with specific precursors that are incorporated into viral macromolecules—for example, nucleosides into nucleic acids or amino acids into proteins. The sizes of viral components may be estimated by procedures such as gel electrophoresis. Advances in techniques for molecular cloning and nucleic acid sequencing have enabled the determination of the complete nucleotide sequence of viral genomes. The amino acid sequences of the encoded proteins can then be deduced as well from the genetic code.

GENERAL STRUCTURAL ORGANIZATION OF VIRUSES. The simplest virions consist solely of nucleic acid enclosed in a protein coat. Early electron microscopic observations indicated that most virions were either rodlike or roughly spherical particles, and chemical analyses of plant viruses demonstrated that they contained only a small percentage of nucleic acid—for example, 5 per cent for tobacco mosaic virus (TMV). Crick and Watson suggested that the viral coat consisted of multiple identical subunits, which would enable a limited amount of nucleic acid to direct the synthesis of a large amount of coat protein. Subsequent biochemical analyses and x-ray diffraction studies of virus crystals have demonstrated such a subunit structure. The protein subunits form a symmetric shell, termed the *capsid*. The capsid together with the nucleic acid is designated the *nucleocapsid*. Two types of capsid symmetry are observed in viruses: *helical* for the viruses that appear rodlike, and *icosahedral* for the "spherical" viruses. Although the simplest virions consist solely of the naked nucleocapsid, many are more complex and possess an outer lipid-containing membrane, termed the *viral envelope*. Schematic diagrams of the structural components of virions and their designations are shown in Figure 1.

The nucleic acid is contained within the nucleocapsid and is thus protected by the viral protein from degradation by nucleases. In addition to serving a protective function, the external proteins of the virion are important for specific interactions with receptors on host cells in the initial stages of the infection process, and are the antigens that elicit an immune response following virus infection. Lipid-containing virions are much more labile than are virions consisting of naked nucleocapsids, and are sensitive to lipid solvents or detergents.

Although there is no limit to the number of different sizes and shapes of viruses that could conceivably exist, only a few structural types have been observed. This finding forms the basis for a rational classification of animal viruses into families with common structural features, as discussed in Chapter 8. Classification is based on the size and structure of the viral nucleic acid, the size and symmetry of the capsid, and the presence or absence of an envelope. Viruses that are classified together on the basis of structure also replicate by similar processes, and frequently exhibit other similarities in their interactions with host cells. A

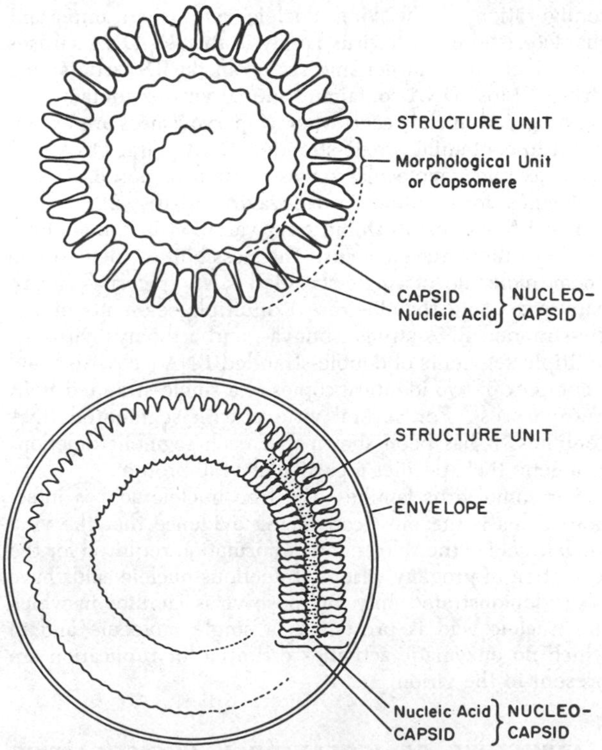

Figure 1. Schematic cross sections through virus particles, illustrating the structural components and the terms used to describe them. Above: "spherical" virus with a naked icosahedral capsid. Below: enveloped virus with a helical nucleocapsid. (Modified from D.L.D. Caspar et al., Cold Spring Harbor Symp Quant Biol 27:49, 1962.)

Table 1. STRUCTURAL PROPERTIES OF ANIMAL VIRUSES

Virus Family	Molecular Weight of Viral Nucleic Acid $\times 10^{-6}$	Capsid Symmetry	Presence of Envelope	Diameter of Virion (nm)
DNA Viruses				
Parvoviridae	1.5–2	icosahedral	−	20
Papovaviridae	3–5	icosahedral	−	45–55
Adenoviridae	20–25	icosahedral	−	75
Herpesviridae	100	icosahedral	+	150
Iridoviridae	150–250	icosahedral	+ or −	125–300
Poxviridae	160–200	complex	+	240 × 300
RNA Viruses				
Picornaviridae	2.6	icosahedral	−	25–30
Caliciviridae	2.6	icosahedral	−	35–40
Togaviridae	4	icosahedral	+	50–70
Arenaviridae	4–5	helical (?)	+	80–300
Bunyaviridae	4–5	helical (?)	+	80–100
Orthomyxoviridae	4–5	helical	+	90–120
Paramyxoviridae	6–7	helical	+	120–150
Rhabdoviridae	3.8	helical	+	70 × 170
Coronaviridae	5–6	helical	+	80–120
Retroviridae	3–4	icosahedral	+	100–120
Reoviridae	12–15	icosahedral	−	70–80

total of 17 different families of animal viruses have been identified, six containing DNA genomes, and 11 containing RNA genomes (Table 1). In addition, several additional virus families have been suggested. A more detailed description of the morphology and biologic properties of these agents is presented in Chapter 8.

VIRAL NUCLEIC ACIDS. The molecular weight and configuration of the viral nucleic acid is an important characteristic of each virus family (Table 1). DNA viruses vary much more in genome size than do RNA-containing viruses. Most DNA-containing animal viruses contain double-stranded nucleic acid, whereas parvoviruses are exceptional in containing single-stranded DNA. Viral DNA may occur as linear molecules, or as covalently closed circular molecules (for example, in papovaviruses, Fig. 2).

The RNA viruses exhibit great variation in the configuration of their nucleic acids. The possibilities include one linear molecule of single-stranded RNA (picorna-, toga-, paramyxo-, and rhabdoviruses), multiple segments of single-stranded RNA (arena-, bunya-, and orthomyxoviruses), multiple segments of double-stranded RNA (reovirus), and a complex of two identical copies of a single-stranded RNA (retroviruses). For several viruses with segmented RNA genomes, it has been shown that each segment functions as a gene that specifies a particular viral protein.

For some virus families, the free nucleic acid is infectious. This is the most convincing evidence that the viral nucleic acid is the sole genetic information required for the formation of progeny virions. Infectious nucleic acids have been demonstrated only for those virus families in which the nucleic acid is present as a single molecule and in which no enzymatic activities essential for replication are present in the virion.

STRUCTURE OF ICOSAHEDRAL NUCLEOCAPSIDS. An icosahedron consists of 20 equilateral triangular faces, and has 12 vertices at which five triangular faces meet (Fig. 3). It exhibits axes of fivefold symmetry through each vertex, threefold symmetry at the center of each triangular face, and twofold symmetry at the midpoints of the edges between two faces. The simplest icosahedral viruses possess 60 identical asymmetric protein subunits (structure units), three of which are positioned on each of the triangular faces of the particle. The icosahedral capsid is formed, and maintains its stability, by means of protein-protein bonds between adjacent subunits. Most icosahedral viruses, how-

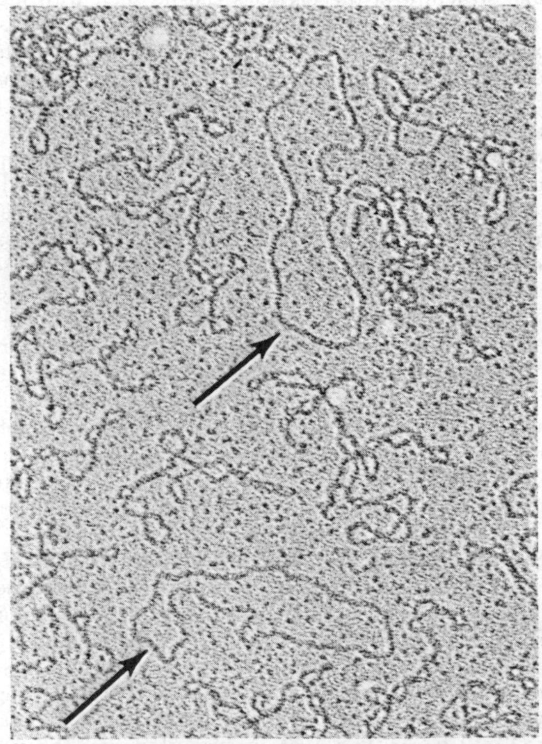

Figure 2. Electron micrograph of the DNA genome of a papovavirus (simian virus 40). Most molecules are in a circular configuration containing several superhelical twists, although some molecules (arrows) are seen as open, untwisted circles. One strand of the DNA is broken in such molecules, which enables unwinding of the twists. Courtesy of Dr. Patricia Hale. Magnification: × 70,000.

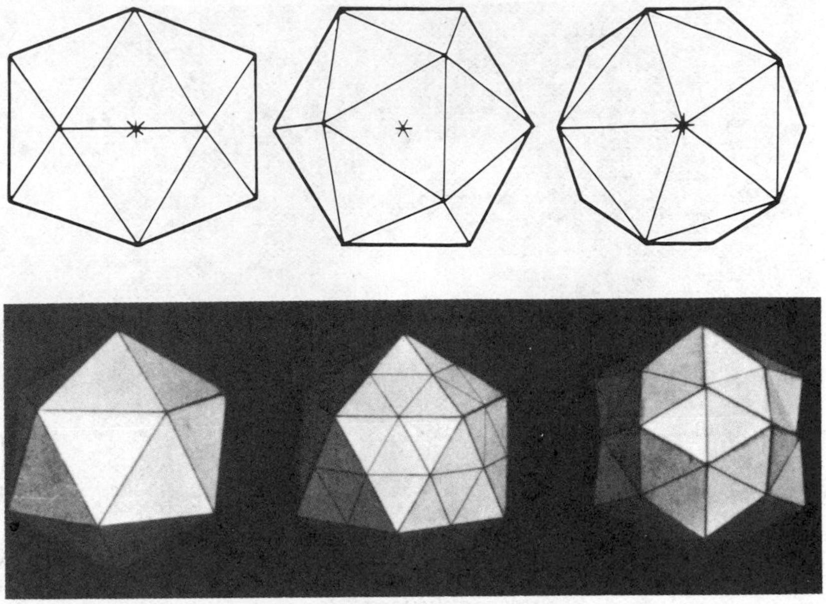

Figure 3. Structural features of an icosahedron. Above, diagrams of an icosahedron viewed along different axes of symmetry (*). From left to right, the structure is viewed along a twofold, threefold, and fivefold axis of symmetry. Below, examples of the subdivision of an icosahedron into surfaces of different triangulation numbers. From left to right, T = 1; T = 4; T= 3. (The lower portion is taken from Caspar and Klug, Cold Spring Harbor Symp Quant Biol 27:1, 1962.)

ever, are larger and possess many more protein subunits. Frequently, such subunits are arranged in clusters, which form the *morphologic units*, or *capsomers*, that are the subunits visible by electron microscopy. The most common pattern of clustering results in formation of groups of five (pentamers) found at the vertices, and groups of six (hexamers) found on faces of the particle. The adenovirus capsid (Fig. 4) is an example of a complex icosahedral structure exhibiting these types of morphological units.

The triangular facets of an icosahedron may be further subdivided into smaller equilateral triangles, and the term *triangulation number* is used to indicate the number of smaller units present on each face. Only certain triangulation numbers are possible, which are given by the relationship $T = h^2 + hk + k^2$, where h and k are any integers. Thus, some of the possible triangulation numbers are 1, 3, 4, 7, 12, and so on. An icosahedron capsid with 60 structure units corresponds to a T = 1 structure, whereas capsids with more subunits have higher triangulation numbers, with three structure units on each of the subtriangles. If these are clustered into pentamers and hexamers, the number of morphologic units in the capsid is equal to 10 T + 2. Thus, a capsid of triangulation number T will consist of 12 pentamers and 10 (T–1) hexamers.

Although simpler viruses may have only one type of structural subunit, more complex particles contain several types of protein as capsid components. Each protein is specified by a particular viral gene; thus, virions contain the same set of capsid proteins irrespective of the host cell of origin. Viruses with large genomes can direct the synthesis of more types of proteins than can viruses with more limited genetic information, and for DNA viruses there is a good correlation between genetic information content and complexity of the capsid. For adenoviruses, the *hexon* subunit found on the faces of the particle consists of a different polypeptide species from that contained in the *penton* (vertex) subunit, and another distinct protein, the *fiber*, radiates outward from each vertex of the particle. Some icosahedral particles contain internal core proteins associated with the nucleic acid that differ from those of the capsid, whereas in other virus types, the nucleic acid is directly associated with the capsid proteins. At least one icosahedral virus, reovirus, contains two distinct capsid layers. Treatment of reovirus particles with proteases removes the outer capsid layer and reveals an internal capsid that also appears to exhibit icosahedral symmetry.

For icosahedral viruses, the dimensions of each virion are uniform, as a result of identical protein-protein interactions that determine the structure of each particle. The capsid of an icosahedral virus is designed to accommodate the viral genome and size constraints would preclude the packaging of significantly larger nucleic acid molecules. However, the presence of viral nucleic acid is not essential for the assembly of the capsid, and aberrant particles are produced by infected cells, including empty icosahedral capsids devoid of any nucleic acid. The size and organization of empty capsids are very similar to those of fully infectious virions; thus it is apparent that the capsid proteins possess the shapes and bonding characteristics that cause them to form a particular structure.

HELICAL NUCLEOCAPSIDS. A helical arrangement of protein subunits has been found by crystallographic analysis of plant viruses such as TMV. As shown in Figure 5, the RNA is in a helical arrangement in the TMV particle, and lies in a groove at a radius of 4 nm from the cylindric axis. The particle has a central hollow core 4 nm in diameter and an overall particle diameter of 18 nm. Virus particles consist of a single type of structural protein arranged as repeating units, with interactions between adjacent subunits as well as between the protein and the viral RNA. Helical nucleocapsids occur in many RNA viruses but have not been observed in DNA animal viruses. The helical ribonucleoproteins in animal viruses are flexible, whereas many plant viruses are rigid rods. The flexibility of such nucleocapsids requires that there be no rigid bonds between protein subunits in adjacent turns of the helix. Animal viruses containing helical nucleocapsids all have a lipid-containing envelope; examples of some enveloped viruses with helical nucleocapsids are shown in Figure 6. In such viruses, flexibility of the helix allows folding of the nucleocapsid for enclosure within the viral membrane.

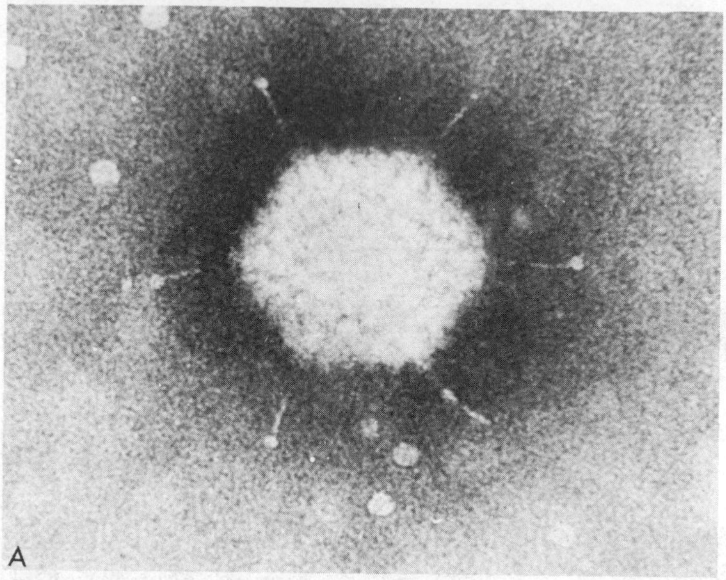

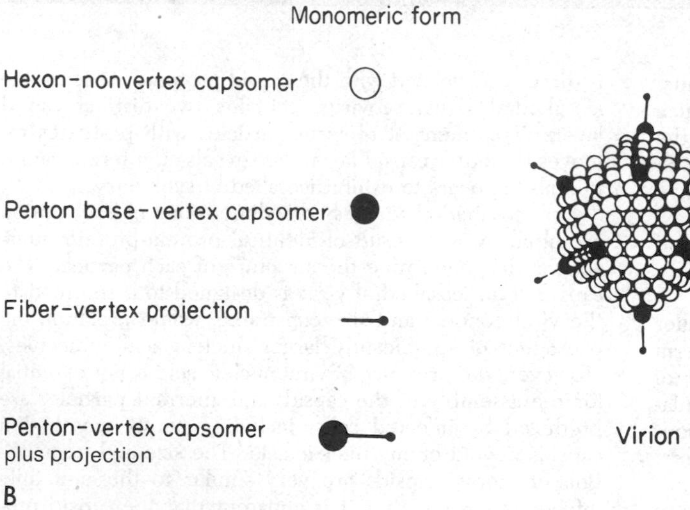

Figure 4. A, adenovirus particle negatively stained with sodium silicotungstate, illustrating the icosahedral capsid structure with fibers projecting from each of the vertices. (From Valentine and Pereira: J Mol Biol 13:13, 1965; supplied courtesy of Dr. N. G. Wrigley). B, schematic diagram of the structure of an adenovirus particle, illustrating the different capsid proteins and their arrangement, as well as the terms used to describe the individual structural components. (From E. Norrby: J Gen Virol 5:221, 1969.)

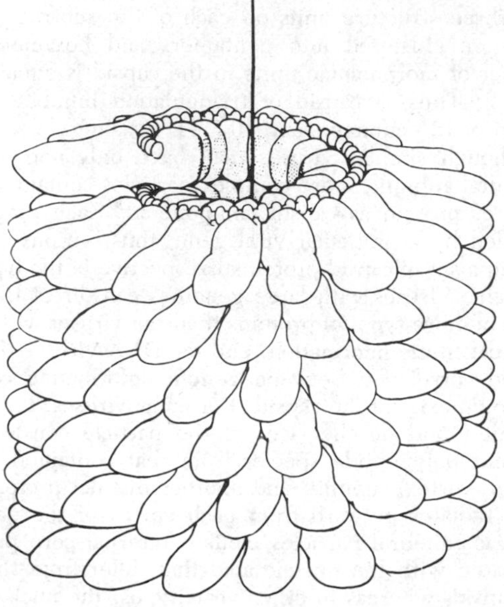

Figure 5. Schematic diagram of the structure of tobacco mosaic virus based on x-ray diffraction studies. The RNA is coiled between the turns of the protein subunits; there are 49 nucleotides and about 16 ⅓ protein subunits in each turn of the helix. The central hole is about 4 nm in diameter, and the overall diameter of the helix is 18 nm. (From Caspar and Klug: Cold Spring Harbor Symp Quant Biol 27:1, 1962.)

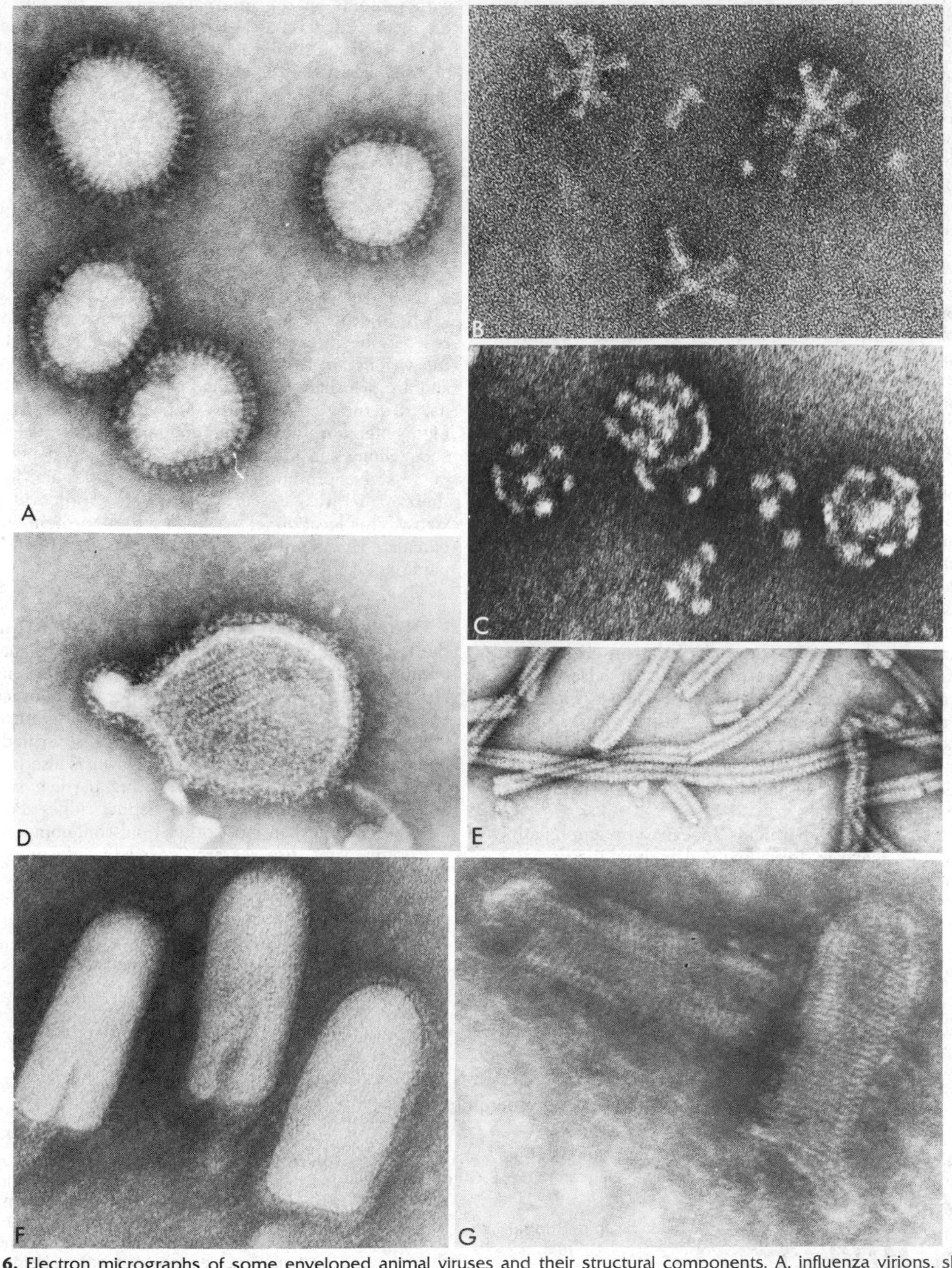

Figure 6. Electron micrographs of some enveloped animal viruses and their structural components. A, influenza virions, showing prominent surface spikes protruding from the viral membrane. The spikes consist of two types of glycoproteins, the hemagglutinin and neuraminidase. Isolated hemagglutinin spikes (B) consist of rodlike subunits that usually aggregate into rosette-like clusters because one end of the spike is hydrophobic; this end anchors the spike to the membrane. Isolated neuraminidase spikes (C) are mushroom-shaped, and also aggregate into characteristic clusters. D, Parainfluenza (SV5) particle penetrated by stain, revealing the internal helical nucleocapsid. E, Isolated SV5 nucleocapsids, some of which are broken into short fragments. The helical structure has a central hollow core, and the turns of the helix give the structure a herringbone-like appearance. F, Rhabdovirus (vesicular stomatitis) particles showing the bullet shape that is characteristic of this virus family. G, Partially disrupted vesicular stomatitis virions, in which the structure of the tightly coiled internal ribonucleoproteins can be observed. B and C are from Laver and Valentine, Virology 38:105, 1969 (Courtesy of Dr. W. G. Laver). D and E are from Compans and Nakamura, CRC Handbook Series in Clinical Laboratory Sciences, Section H, Volume 1, pp. 361–385, 1978. Magnifications: A, × 200,000; B and C, × 500,000; D, × 175,000; E, × 200,000; F and G, × 300,000.

The length of the helical nucleocapsid is determined by the length of the viral RNA molecule; for TMV, a particle length of 300 nm is observed. The TMV protein can aggregate by itself to form rods of the same diameter as the virion but of random length, due to the absence of the RNA as a length-determining factor. It is also possible for TMV protein to form helices with RNA from other sources, or with synthetic polynucleotides, indicating that the protein does not show strict specificity for a particular nucleic acid sequence for the interactions that lead to the assembly of the helical virus.

VIRAL ENVELOPES. More than half of the established families of animal viruses contain lipids as major structural components, which are present in a limiting membrane, or *envelope*. The lipids are acquired during the maturation process, which usually occurs by budding at a cellular membrane. Thus the viral lipids are acquired from a membrane of the host cell, and are similar to that membrane in composition; they are arranged in the form of a bilayer similar to that in other biologic membranes. The viral envelope is asymmetric with respect to the distribution of carbohydrate components, as are cellular membranes: glycoproteins and glycolipids are found only on the external surface. The virion glycoproteins are virus-specific (that is, the polypeptide backbone is coded by the viral genome); however, the carbohydrate portion may vary with the host cell type and is synthesized by cellular enzymes. Viral glycoproteins form projections or spikes on the external surface of the virion. These glycoproteins are essential for viral infectivity and are responsible for adsorption of viruses to receptors on cell surfaces. They are also the antigens of importance in immunity to such viruses, in that antibody directed against the viral glycoproteins will neutralize virus infectivity. Host cell membrane proteins are excluded from the viral membrane during the assembly of lipid-containing viruses.

Viral envelope glycoproteins appear to be amphipathic; that is, they have hydrophobic and hydrophilic domains. The isolated glycoproteins form rosette-like clusters (Fig. 6*B*) presumably because they aggregate by their hydrophobic ends. The hydrophobic end appears to be involved in anchoring of the glycoprotein to the viral membrane and may extend into or traverse the lipid bilayer to interact with proteins on the internal surface of the virion. Such interactions may be essential for the assembly process. The complete three dimensional structure of some viral glycoproteins has recently been determined by x-ray crystallography.

Virus-specific proteins are also components of the internal surface of the envelope. In the case of viruses with icosahedral nucleocapsids, the lipid membrane with its associated glycoproteins may be wrapped closely around the capsid itself, although intervening proteins may be present in some instances. For enveloped viruses with helical nucleocapsids, a specific membrane or matrix protein is usually found in association with the inner surface of the envelope.

The morphology of some representative enveloped viruses is shown in Figure 6. The overall shapes and sizes of the virions are features characteristic of each virus family and are primarily determined by the arrangement of internal structural components. Some enveloped viruses are highly pleomorphic and may contain multiple nucleocapsids and genomes in a single envelope. All enveloped viruses possess glycoprotein spikes, but the shapes and lengths of these structures are also a distinctive property of each virus. The location of each structural protein has been elucidated in many enveloped viruses, as depicted for the parainfluenza virion in Figure 7.

OTHER TYPES OF VIRUS STRUCTURE. Poxviruses are the largest and most complex viruses infecting man, containing about 30 or more different types of protein in the virion. They have no capsid with either helical or icosahedral symmetry (Fig. 8). The virion contains DNA encased in a core structure, with two structures termed lateral bodies adjacent to the core. A lipid layer is also present in an envelope structure. The resulting particle is oblong, and the surface is covered with distinct ridges. Poxviruses are more stable than most other lipid-containing viruses.

Certain plant diseases are caused by infectious nucleic acid molecules that lack any protein coat, and are named *viroids*. The known plant viroids are small, covalently closed, circular RNA molecules. It is possible that viroids may also cause certain diseases of animals or man in which no conventional virus has been identified.

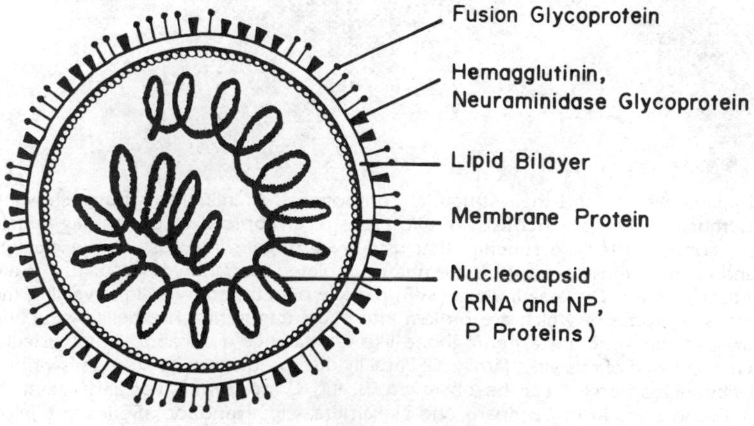

Figure 7. Schematic diagram of the arrangement of structural proteins in a parainfluenza virion. Two types of glycoproteins form projections on the external surface of the lipid bilayer, and a membrane protein lines the inner surface of the bilayer. The helical nucleocapsid is coiled inside the envelope, and consists of the viral RNA and a nucleoprotein (NP) as well as other minor proteins (P) which may possess RNA polymerase activity. (From Compans and Nakamura, CRC Handbook Series in Clinical Laboratory Sciences, Section H, Volume 1, pp. 361–385, 1978).

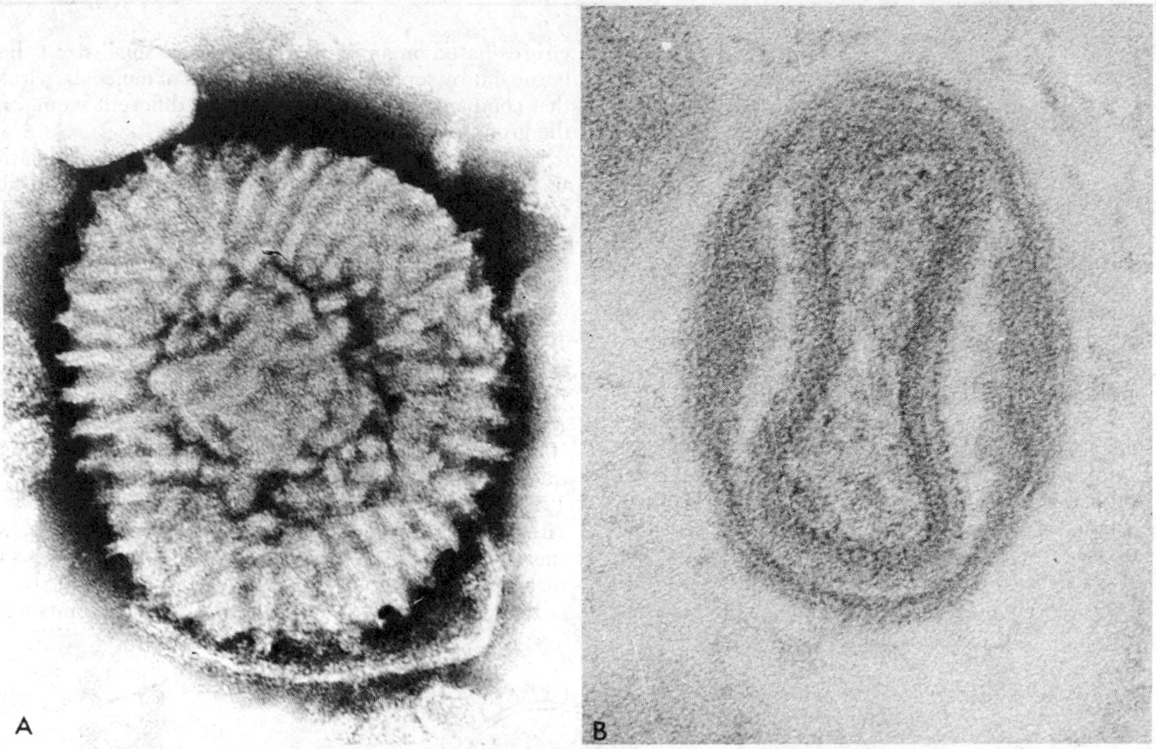

Figure 8. Electron micrographs of vaccinia (poxvirus) virions. A, Negatively stained particle showing ridges or tubular elements covering the surface. B, Thin section of vaccinia virion showing a central biconcave core, two lateral bodies, and an outer membrane. A is from Dales, S.: J Cell Biol 18:51, 1963; B is from Pogo and Dales: Proc Natl Acad Sci U.S. 63:820, 1969. (Courtesy of Dr. Samuel Dales.) Magnification: A, × 228,000; B, × 220,000.

References

General

Caspar, D. L. D., and Klug, A.: Physical principles in the construction of regular viruses. Cold Spring Harbor Symp Quant Biol 27: 1–24, 1962.

Crick, F. H. C., and Watson, J. D.: Structure of small viruses. Nature 177:473, 1956.

Methods

Brenner, S., and Horne, R. W.: A negative staining method for high resolution electron microscopy of viruses. Biochem Biophys Acta 34:103, 1959.

Brakke, M. K.: Density gradient centrifugation. In Maramorosch, R., and Koprowski, H. (eds.): Methods in Virology Vol. II. New York, Academic Press, pp. 93–117, 1967.

Elford, W. J.: The sizes of viruses and bacteriophages and methods for their determination. In Doerr, H., and Hallauer, C. (eds.): Handbuch der Virusforschung. Vienna, Springer.

Maizel, J. V.: Acrylamide gel electrophoresis of proteins and nucleic acids. *In* Fundamental Techniques in Virology. Habel, K., and Salzman N. P. (eds.): New York, Academic Press, pp. 334–362, 1969.

Viral Nucleic Acids

Air, G. M.: DNA sequencing of viral genomes. *In* Fraenkel-Conrat, H., and Wagner, R. R. (eds.): Comprehensive Virology. New York, Plenum Press, Vol. 13, pp. 205, 1979.

Shatkin, A. J.: Animal RNA viruses: genome structure and function. Ann Rev Biochem 43:643, 1974.

Icosahedral Nucleocapsids

Finch, J. T., and Klug, A.: The structure of viruses of the papillomapolyoma type. III. Structure of rabbit papilloma virus. J Mol Biol 13:1, 1965.

Valentine, R. C., and Pereira, H. G. Antigens and the structure of adenovirus. J Mol Biol 13:13, 1965.

Helical Nucleocapsids

Caspar, D. L. D.: Assembly and stability of the tobacco mosaic virus particle. Adv Prot Chem 18:37, 1963.

Compans, R. W., Mountcastle, W. E., and Choppin, P. W.: The sense of the helix of paramyxovirus nucleocapsids. J Mol Biol 65:167, 1971.

Viral Envelopes

Compans, R. W., and Klenk, H. D.: Viral membranes. *In* Fraenkel-Conrat, H., and Wagner, R. R. (eds.): Comprehensive Virology. New York, Plenum Press, Vol. 13, pp. 293–407, 1979.

Viral Glycoproteins

Varghese, J. N., Laver, W. G., and Colman, P. M.: Structure of the influenza virus glycoprotein antigen neuraminidase at 2.9 A° resolution. Nature 303:35, 1983.

Wilson, I. A., Skehel, J. J., and Wiley, D.C.: Structure of the haemagglutinin membrane glycoprotein of influenza virus at 3A° resolution. Nature 289:366, 1981.

Other Types of Virus Structure

Dales, S.: The structure and replication of poxviruses as exemplified by vaccinia. In Dalton, A. J., and Haguenau, F. (eds.): Ultrastructure of Animal Viruses and Bacteriophages. New York, Academic Press, pp. 109–129, 1973.

Diener, T. O.: Viroids: The smallest known agent of infectious disease. Ann Rev Microbiol 28:23, 1974.

8
CLASSIFICATION OF VIRUSES

JOSEPH L. MELNICK, PH.D.

Until about 1950, so little was known about viruses other than their pathogenic effect in causing diseases that they were classified according to the diseases they caused rather than the properties of the virus particle. Now, we are close to the end of an important phase of discovery and characterization of animal viruses. The knowledge thus gained concerning the viruses themselves has made it possible to establish broad groupings for these agents. It appears that most of the major groups of viruses of vertebrates—at least of man and the animals important to man—have been recognized and described. Many of these virus groupings, initially established on tentative and provisional bases, now appear to form real families and genera, in which the members are indeed related in fundamental ways. For example, the validity of the original grouping of the enteroviruses based on an enteric habitat and small size is being borne out by sophisticated techniques of molecular virology that compare the genetic makeup of different members of the group and their mode of replication.

The shift in emphasis—from sketching the broad outlines of the virus kingdom based on disease causation to filling in essential details about the viruses themselves—has been recognized by the change in the name of the International Committee on Nomenclature of Viruses (ICNV) to the International Committee on Taxonomy of Viruses (ICTV). The first report of the ICNV was published in 1971 (Wildy, 1971). Work of the Study Groups and Subcommittees of the ICTV is proceeding, and reports from these groups in their special areas of virology appear regularly in *Intervirology,* the journal of the Virology Section of the IUMS (International Union of Microbiological Societies). Subsequent reports of the ICTV have been published (Fenner, 1976; Matthews, 1979; Matthews, 1982). Other reviews on virus taxonomy and its historical development (e.g., Matthews, 1983) and on taxonomy of vertebrate viruses (Melnick, 1982a; Murphy, 1983) also are available.

Figures 1 and 2 serve as useful reference points for the

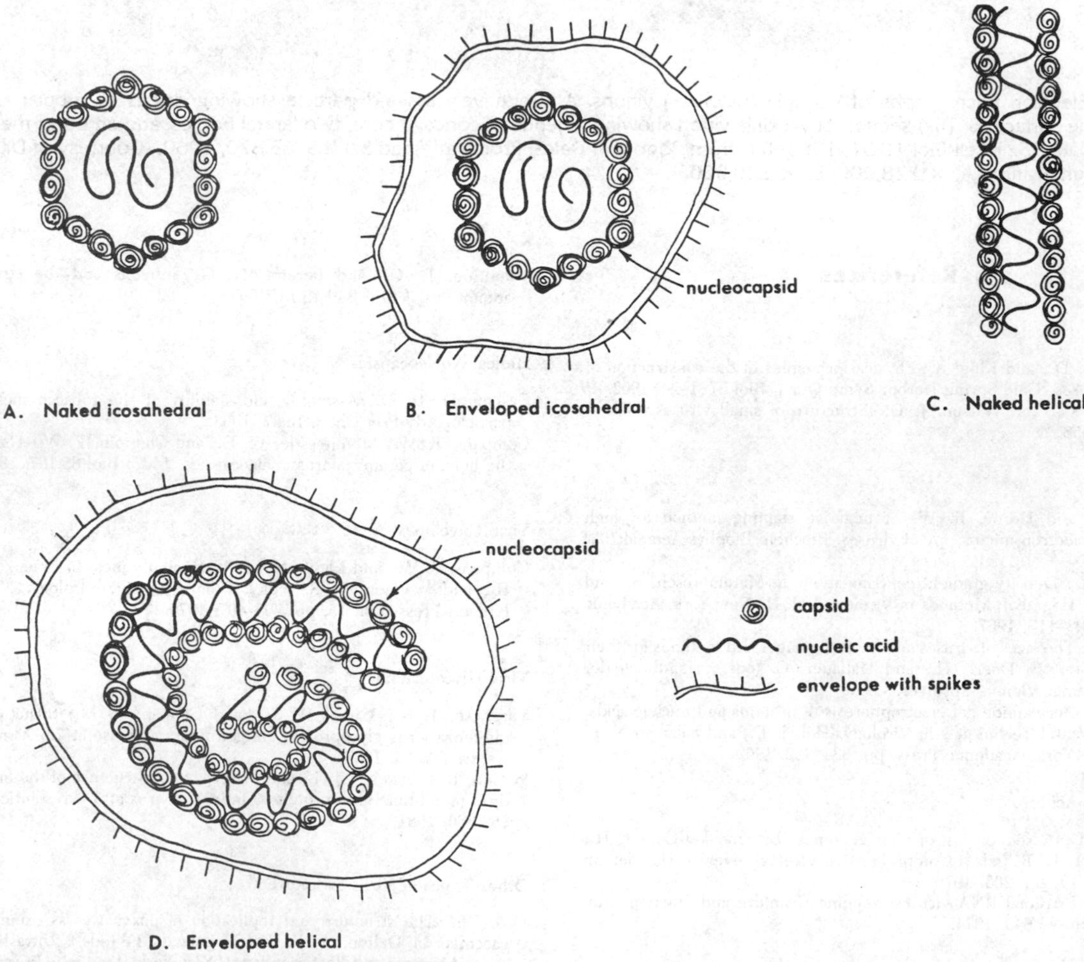

Figure 1. Schematic diagram of simple forms of virions and their components. The naked icosahedral virions resemble small crystals; the naked helical virions resemble rods with a fine regular helical pattern in their surface. The enveloped icosahedral virions are made up of icosahedral nucleocapsids surrounded by the envelope; the enveloped helical virions are helical nucleocapsids bent to form a coarse, often irregular coil, within the envelope. (From Davis, B. D., et al.: Microbiology, New York, Hoeber Medical Division, 1967.)

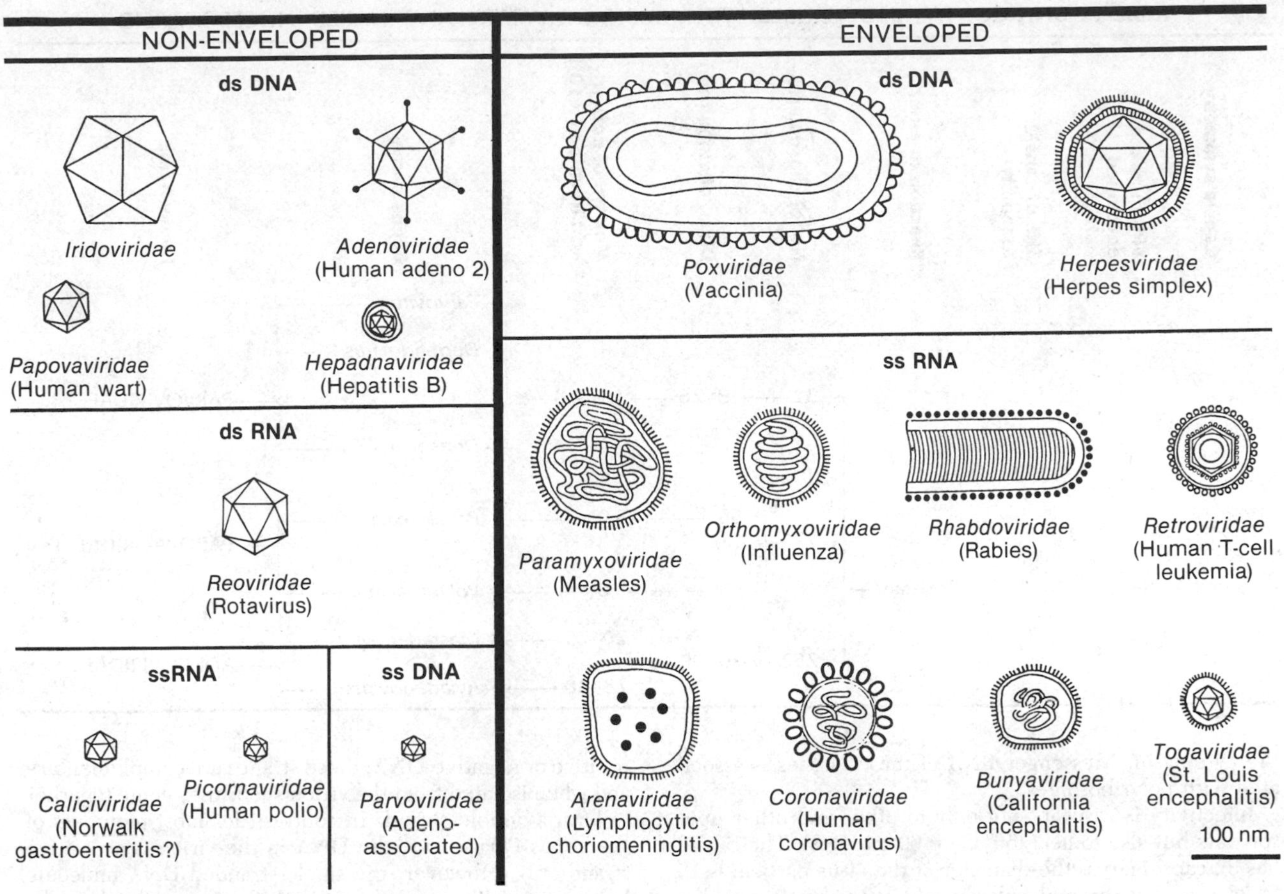

Figure 1. Schematic diagram of simple forms of virions and their components. The naked icosahedral virions resemble small crystals; the naked helical virions resemble rods with a fine regular helical pattern in their surface. The enveloped icosahedral virions are made up of icosahedral nucleocapsids surrounded by the envelope; the enveloped helical virions are helical nucleocapsids bent to form a coarse, often irregular coil, within the envelope. (From Davis, B. D., et al.: Microbiology, New York, Hoeber Medical Division, 1967.)

following discussion of classification based upon properties of the virus particles. Comparison of these figures also shows how rapidly knowledge of virus composition and structure has advanced. Figure 1 is taken from a text first published in 1967 (Davis et al., 1967); it remains fundamentally applicable in current virology. However, Figure 2, a diagram prepared about ten years later (Fenner and White, 1976) and now updated, not only draws upon additional information gained in the interim but also illustrates the wide variety of size and structure that is found among viruses of vertebrates.

Tables 1 to 5 are schematic diagrams showing separation of viruses of vertebrates into 18 families (Melnick, 1982a). Table 1 describes viruses that have a DNA genome, cubic symmetry, and a naked nucleocapsid; Table 2 describes DNA-containing viruses with envelopes or complex coats. RNA-containing viruses are presented in three tables: Table 3, those with cubic capsid symmetry; Table 4, those with helical symmetry; and Table 5, those with capsid architecture either asymmetric or unknown. Commentaries follow on the viruses that have been assigned to these groups, a few of which are still tentative.

DNA VIRUSES

PARVOVIRIDAE

(Bachmann et al., 1979; Matthews, 1982)

Originally named picodnaviruses to reflect their small size and DNA-containing genome (Mayor and Melnick, 1966), the family **Parvoviridae** now includes three named genera, *Parvovirus, Densovirus,* and *Dependovirus* (adeno-associated viruses). A typical member is adeno-associated satellite virus, several serotypes of which are indigenous to man—but as yet with no known disease association in human beings. Reading from the lefthand side of Table 1, these are DNA-containing viruses that have cubic symmetry and a naked (unenveloped) nucleocapsid; during replication, capsid assembly takes place in the nucleus of the host cell. For the DNA viruses whose capsid assembly takes place in the nucleus (not only parvoviruses, but also papovaviruses, adenoviruses, and herpesviruses), a phase of replication—that is, viral protein synthesis—occurs in

Table 1. DNA-CONTAINING VIRUSES WITH CUBIC SYMMETRY AND NAKED NUCLEOCAPSID

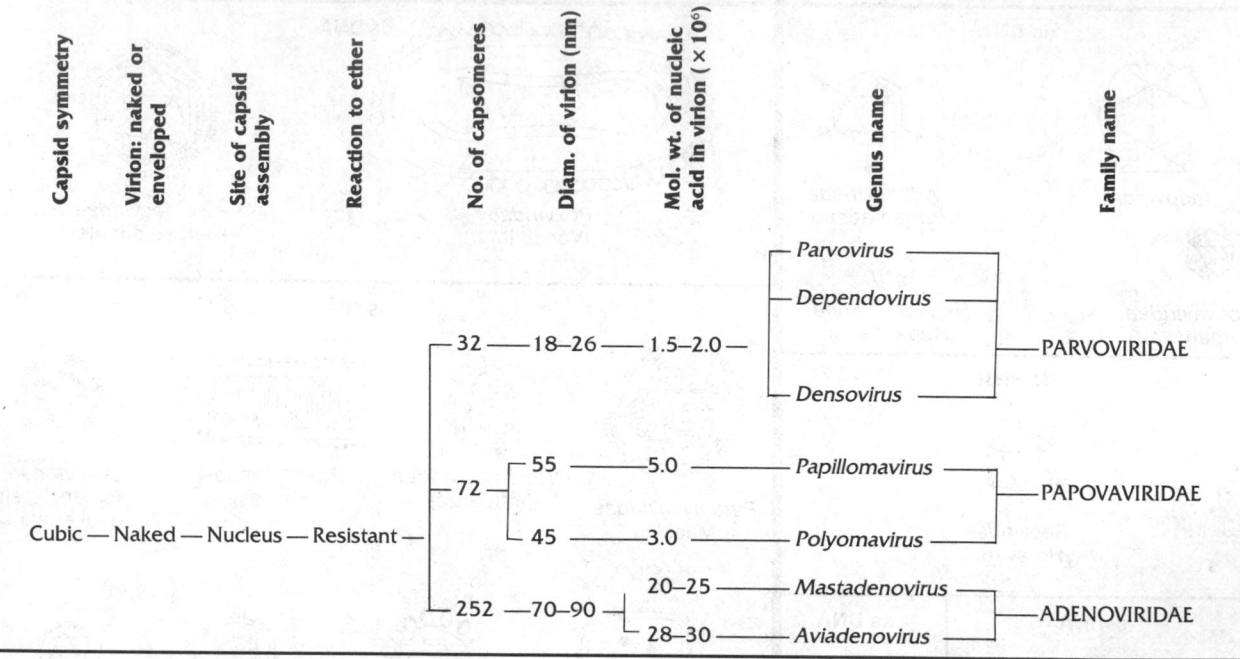

Capsid symmetry	Virion: naked or enveloped	Site of capsid assembly	Reaction to ether	No. of capsomeres	Diam. of virion (nm)	Mol. wt. of nucleic acid in virion ($\times 10^6$)	Genus name	Family name
Cubic	Naked	Nucleus	Resistant	32	18–26	1.5–2.0	*Parvovirus*	PARVOVIRIDAE
							Dependovirus	
							Densovirus	
				72	55	5.0	*Papillomavirus*	PAPOVAVIRIDAE
					45	3.0	*Polyomavirus*	
				252	70–90	20–25	*Mastadenovirus*	ADENOVIRIDAE
						28–30	*Aviadenovirus*	

the cytoplasm. Messenger RNA of these viruses is associated with polyribosomes.

Infectivity is resistant not only to ether and other lipid solvents but also to heat (56° C for 60 minutes). The capsid has 32 capsomeres, the diameter of the virus particle is 18 to 26 nm, and the molecular weight of the nucleic acid is 1.5 to 2.0 × 10^6. The genus *Parvovirus* includes autonomously replicating viruses of several animal species (cat, cow, dog, goose, mink, mouse, pig, rabbit, rat). Two members of the genus have been found to be associated with disease problems of human beings. Parvovirus B19 has been shown to cause a transient shutdown of red blood cell production by killing the late erythroid progenitor cells. This shutdown presents particular problems for individuals who are already suffering from hemolytic anemias, such as sickle cell anemia, causing aplastic crises. A virus named RA-1, which is associated with rheumatoid arthritis, is another newly identified member of the genus. A host range mutant of feline panleukopenia known as canine parvovirus induces acute enteritis with leukopenia in young and adult dogs as well as myocarditis in puppies. Infections with this virus have reached enzootic proportions around the world. Members of the *Densovirus* genus also replicate autonomously; they are viruses of insects, but also can produce cytopathic effects in cultures of certain vertebrate cells (L cells).

In contrast, adeno-satellite viruses (genus *Dependovirus)* are defective; that is, they cannot multiply in the absence of a replicating adenovirus, which serves as a "helper virus"—herpesvirus can act as a partial helper. Satellite viruses occur in cow, chicken, dog, horse, human, and monkey hosts.

Parvoviridae are the only DNA-containing viruses of vertebrates whose DNA genome is single-stranded within the virion; all the others (see Tables 1 and 2) have double-stranded DNA. In the case of adeno-satellite viruses and densoviruses, separate virions contain single strands of positive or negative DNA; these strands are complementary and when isolated from the virion shells they come together to form a double strand. In contrast, for most members of the genus *Parvovirus*, the DNA in the virion is a positive strand only. However, the single-stranded DNA molecule has a hairpin-like structure at both the 5′ and the 3′ ends. In some members of this genus, plus-strand DNA is also incorporated in variable proportions and about 1 per cent of the virions form double strands similar to the self-complementary strands of the other two genera. Members of the *Parvovirus* genus show marked preference for actively dividing cells, have been shown to be transmissible transplacentally, and are receiving attention for their special disease potential in fetuses and neonates (Kilham and Margolis, 1975). One possible member has been associated with acute viral gastroenteritis of man.

HEPADNAVIRIDAE

(Robinson et al., 1982; Melnick, 1982b)

Although hepatitis B virus has not been officially placed by the ICTV, ample evidence has accumulated for the formation of a new virus family, and the name **Hepadnaviridae** is appropriate, reflecting the DNA-containing genomes of its members, and their replication within hepatocytes (Robinson et al., 1982).

Hepatitis B virus of man and three similar viruses found in woodchucks, Beechey ground squirrels, and Pekin ducks share many basic ultrastructural, molecular, and biological features. To date, it appears that the family consists of a single genus, *Hepadnavirus;* as the longest-recognized and most-studied member, human hepatitis B virus would become type 1.

The members of the family share the following properties (Robinson et al., 1982): (i) Characteristic ultrastructure of the virion: a double-shelled particle 40 to 50 nm in diameter with a core 27 nm in diameter and incomplete forms (22-nm spheres and filaments). (ii) Circular viral DNA with length corresponding to DNA of 3,200 base pairs, and containing a single-stranded region. (iii) Virion DNA polymerase that repairs the single-stranded region in the viral DNA. (iv) Polypeptide covalently attached to the 5′ end of the long DNA strand. (v) Characteristic surface, core, and "e" antigens in the virion. (vi) Characteristic virion polypeptides. (vii) Sharing of some DNA and virion polypeptide homology. (viii) Protein kinase activity in the virion core. (ix) Liver tropism. (x) Persistent infection with large amounts of incomplete viral forms continuously in the blood. (xi) Infection associated with hepatitis, hepatocellular carcinoma, and immune-complex-mediated extrahepatic tissue injury.

As mentioned, three viruses similar to hepatitis B virus are found in woodchucks (*Marmota monax*), in Beechey ground squirrels (*Spermophilus beecheyi*), and in Pekin ducks (*Anas domesticus*). All members of the virus group share some antigens, as well as similar morphology and behavior in the infected host—formation of large amounts of excess viral coat protein in the form of small spherical and tubular particles—as well as association with chronic hepatitis and hepatocellular carcinoma.

PAPOVAVIRIDAE

(Melnick, 1962; Melnick et al., 1974a; Matthews, 1982)

These relatively small, ether-resistant viruses contain double-stranded DNA in circular form. Many are unusually heat-stable, surviving temperatures that inactivate most viruses. Other properties are shown in Table 1. The representatives that infect human beings are the papilloma or wart virus and SV40-like viruses such as JC virus, which has been isolated from the brain tissue of patients with progressive multifocal leukoencephalopathy (PML), or BK virus, which has been isolated from the urine of immunosuppressed recipients of renal transplants. Other members include papilloma viruses of several vertebrate species, polyoma and K viruses of mice, and vacuolating viruses of monkeys (SV40) and of rabbits. These viruses have relatively slow growth cycles characterized by replication within the nucleus. Papovaviruses produce latent and chronic infections in their natural hosts. Many produce tumors, particularly in experimentally infected rodents, serving as model systems to study viral carcinogenesis.

There are two genera, *Papillomavirus* and *Polyomavirus*. Each virus species contains a distinct surface antigen, but all members of a genus share a common antigen revealed by disrupting the virions. Concern has been expressed at the use of "polyomavirus" for the human viruses, since these viruses of man, such as JC and BK, have *not* been shown to be "polyoma" in character—that is, "produce many types of tumors in the host." For example, even though antibodies against BK virus are widespread in the population, human tumors and human malignant cell lines were negative when analyzed for BK virus–specific DNA sequences. Because the probes used could detect one copy of BK virus DNA if only 10 percent of the cells were tumor cells, the results are very strong evidence that the tumors analyzed did not have a BK virus etiology. The tumors tested represent about 50 per cent of all types of cancers in the United States; thus there is no evidence that this "polyomavirus" is involved in production of these tumors in the human host. The Study Group of experts recommended that the term polyomavirus should not be used as a generic name to include the human JC and BK viruses (Melnick, 1974a; and 1981 Report of the Study Group to the ICTV), but the ICTV Executive Committee overruled the Study Group recommendation.

ADENOVIRIDAE

(Wigand et al., 1982)

The adenovirus virion is a nonenveloped isometric particle with icosahedral symmetry. The particles are 70 to 90 nm in diameter, with 252 capsomeres, each 8 to 9 nm in diameter; 240 are hexons; there are 12 vertex capsomeres (or penton bases), which are antigenically distinct from the hexons and carry one or two filamentous projections. The adenovirus genome is a single linear molecule of double-stranded DNA (with molecular weight 20 to 30 $\times$ 10^6). At least 33 serotypes infect man, and there are distinct serotypes for a number of other species. Adenoviruses have a predilection for mucous membranes and may persist for years in lymphoid tissue. Some cause acute respiratory diseases, febrile catarrhs, pharyngitis, and conjunctivitis. Human adenoviruses rarely cause disease in laboratory animals, but certain serotypes do produce tumors in newborn hamsters. Common antigens are shared by all mammalian adenoviruses (*Mastadenovirus* genus); these antigens are different from the corresponding antigens of members of the genus *Aviadenovirus*.

HERPESVIRIDAE

(Roizman et al., 1981; Matthews, 1982)

The herpesvirus family is a heterogeneous group of viruses identified by their structure. As shown in Table 2, the particle consists of a DNA-containing core enclosed by an icosahedral capsid with 162 hollow cylindric capsomeres. The enveloped virion is 120 to 200 nm in diameter and consists of 4 structural components. The core consists of a fibrillar spool on which the DNA is wrapped. The ends of the fibers are anchored to the underside of the capsid shell. The capsid (100 to 110 nm in diameter) is an icosahedron with 5 capsomeres on each edge; it contains 150 hexameric and 12 pentameric capsomeres. Surrounding the capsid is a tegument consisting of globular material. The envelope, a bilayered, lipid- and protein-containing membrane, surrounds the tegument. The double-stranded DNA of various herpesviruses differs considerably in size (92 to 102 $\times$ 10^6 molecular weight), cytosine and guanine content (44 to 74 per cent), and structural complexity. The DNA of herpesviruses is sufficiently large to carry the genetic code for 80 to 100 proteins, of which about 50 have been observed.

Herpesviruses are noteworthy for their ability to establish latent and/or persistent infections, which may last for the lifetime of the host, even in the presence of circulating antibodies. Special interest has been generated by the association of EB herpesvirus with human Burkitt lymphomas and nasopharyngeal carcinomas and by the possible role of the genital herpesvirus, herpes simplex type 2, in cancer of the uterine cervix. Several simian herpesviruses have been shown to be oncogenic in experimentally infected animals. Herpesvirus infections of heterologous species are in many cases very serious; examples are the fatal

Table 2. DNA-CONTAINING VIRUSES WITH ENVELOPES OR COMPLEX COATS

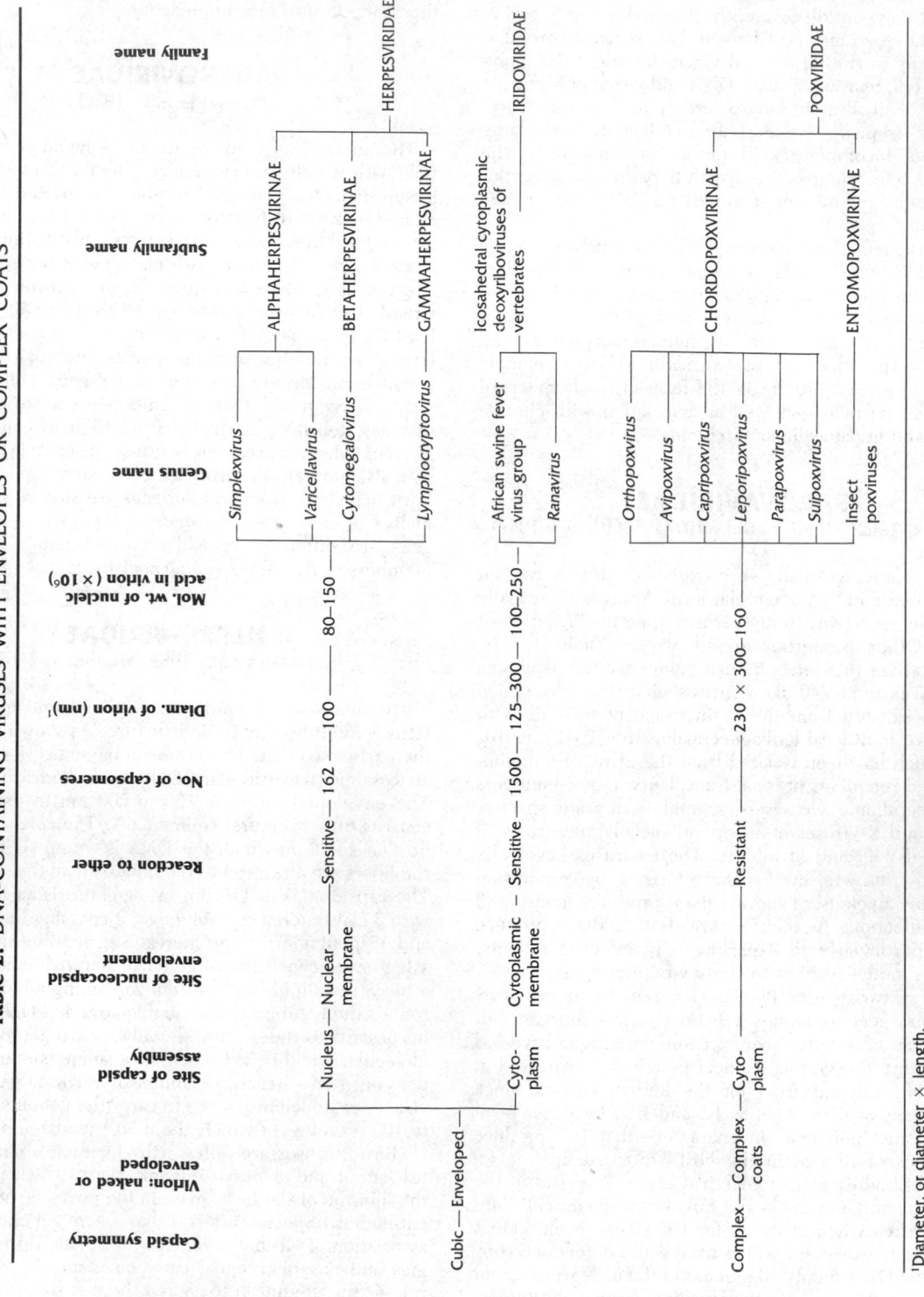

Capsid symmetry	Virion: naked or enveloped	Site of capsid assembly	Site of nucleocapsid envelopment	Reaction to ether	No. of capsomeres	Diam. of virion (nm)[1]	Mol. wt. of nucleic acid in virion ($\times 10^6$)	Genus name	Subfamily name	Family name
Cubic	Enveloped	Nucleus	Nuclear membrane	Sensitive	162	100	80–150	*Simplexvirus*	ALPHAHERPESVIRINAE	HERPESVIRIDAE
								Varicellavirus		
								Cytomegalovirus	BETAHERPESVIRINAE	
								Lymphocryptovirus	GAMMAHERPESVIRINAE	
		Cyto-plasm	Cytoplasmic membrane	Sensitive	1500	125–300	100–250	African swine fever virus group	Icosahedral cytoplasmic deoxyriboviruses of vertebrates	IRIDOVIRIDAE
								Ranavirus		
Complex	Complex coats	Cyto-plasm		Resistant		230 × 300	160	*Orthopoxvirus*	CHORDOPOXVIRINAE	POXVIRIDAE
								Avipoxvirus		
								Capripoxvirus		
								Leporipoxvirus		
								Parapoxvirus		
								Suipoxvirus		
								Insect poxviruses	ENTOMOPOXVIRINAE	

[1]Diameter, or diameter × length.

infection of man by one of the simian herpesviruses, so-called B virus, and the infection of cattle by swine pseudorabies virus. Human diseases include oral and genital herpes; chickenpox and shingles due to varicella/zoster virus; cytomegalic inclusion disease; and infectious mononucleosis. Subfamilies have now been established to include most of the members of this large virus family, and genera have been proposed (Roizman et al., 1981; Matthews, 1982). The subfamilies are as follows (see Table 2): **Alphaherpesvirinae** are viruses similar to herpes simplex virus of man. The table includes only genera for which humans are the natural host: *Simplexvirus* (herpes simplex viruses), and *Varicellavirus* (varicella/zoster virus). (The B virus of monkeys is considered to be a possible member of this genus.) **Betaherpesvirinae** are the cytomegaloviruses. **Gammaherpesvirinae** are viruses like EB virus of man; EB virus (*Lymphocryptovirus)* is the only member that infects human beings. Proposals also have been made for definition of species within the genera.

IRIDOVIRIDAE

(Bellett, 1978; Matthews, 1982)

The best-known members of this family are the members of the insect iridescent virus group (for example, *Tipula* iridescent virus), now placed in the genus *Iridovirus*. However, other members of this family include important pathogens of vertebrates: African swine fever virus and many viruses of frogs and fish. No human iridovirus is known. Vertebrate iridoviruses are enveloped; iridoviruses that infect insects contain a lipid fraction in the virion as an integral part of the icosahedral shell, but do not have envelopes as such.

POXVIRIDAE

(Fenner, 1979; Matthews, 1982)

These large viruses are brick-shaped or ovoid with a complex virion structure. The virion contains more than 30 structural proteins and several viral enzymes including a DNA-dependent RNA polymerase. This is the major DNA-containing virus family whose members replicate entirely within the cytoplasm. The genus *Orthopoxvirus* includes smallpox virus and the other poxviruses of man. Some of the animal poxviruses (for example, monkeypox) can infect humans, and with the eradication of smallpox from the world it has been speculated that human infections by these agents might be detected more frequently. Two subfamilies have now been defined: **Chordopoxvirinae,** to include the poxviruses that infect vertebrates (genera *Orthopoxvirus, Avipoxvirus, Capripoxvirus, Leporipoxvirus, Parapoxvirus,* and *Suipoxvirus)* and **Entomopoxvirinae,** the poxviruses that infect insects.

RNA VIRUSES

PICORNAVIRIDAE

(Melnick et al., 1974b; Cooper et al., 1978; Matthews, 1982)

These are shown at the top of Table 3. Members of this family—the smallest of the viruses with RNA genomes—are classed into four genera and into several hundred species. At least 70 members of the *Enterovirus* genus infect man; these include polioviruses, coxsackieviruses, echoviruses, and in recent years, new enterovirus serotypes that are assigned sequential numbers, i.e., enteroviruses 68-72 (Melnick et al., 1974). Well over 100 viruses that infect human beings belong to the genus *Rhinovirus*. Large numbers of agents from both of these genera are indigenous to other hosts. The two other genera are *Cardiovirus,* a rodent agent that may also infect man, and *Aphthovirus,* which includes the economically important foot-and-mouth disease viruses of cattle. The caliciviruses, once thought to belong to the **Picornaviridae,** have recently been shown to differ in both virus structure and method of replication, and have been placed in a separate family (see below).

The picornavirus genome is one piece of linear, single-stranded RNA of low molecular weight (about 2.5×10^6). The RNA is infectious and serves as its own messenger for protein translation. The virion is about 27 nm in diameter; there are 4 major polypeptides (of molecular weights 33,000, 27,000, 23,000, and 6,000). The enteroviruses and cardioviruses are acid-stable and have a buoyant density in CsCl of about 1.34 g/cm^3; in contrast, the rhinoviruses and aphthoviruses are acid-labile and have a higher buoyant density, about 1.4 g/cm^3.

The diseases caused by picornaviruses range from severe paralysis (paralytic poliomyelitis) to aseptic meningitis, hepatitis, pleurodynia, myocarditis, skin rashes, and common colds; inapparent infection is very common. Different viruses may produce the same syndrome; on the other hand, the same picornavirus may cause more than a single syndrome. After decades of investigation hepatitis A virus has been established as enterovirus type 72 (Matthews, 1982; Gust et al., 1983).

CALICIVIRIDAE

(Schaffer et al., 1980; Matthews, 1982)

The genome is a single molecule of infectious, single-stranded, positive-sense RNA, of molecular weight 2.6 to 2.8. The virion is 36 to 39 nm in diameter, with 32 cup-shaped surface depressions (capsomeres?) arranged in icosahedral symmetry. There is no lipid and no envelope, and there is a single major structural polypeptide rather than several as seen with the picornaviruses. Only one genus, *Calicivirus,* has been proposed; the type species is vesicular exanthema of swine virus (VESV), type A; a number of other serotypes infect cats and sea lions. Possible members include the Norwalk gastroenteritis virus of man, and also other viruses with calicivirus morphology that cause gastroenteritis in humans, calves, and swine.

REOVIRIDAE

(Matthews, 1982; Murphy, 1983)

For members of **Reoviridae,** the virion has an isometric nucleocapsid 60 to 80 nm in diameter, with icosahedral symmetry. There is no lipid envelope, but there are two

Table 3. RNA-CONTAINING VIRUSES WITH CUBIC CAPSID SYMMETRY

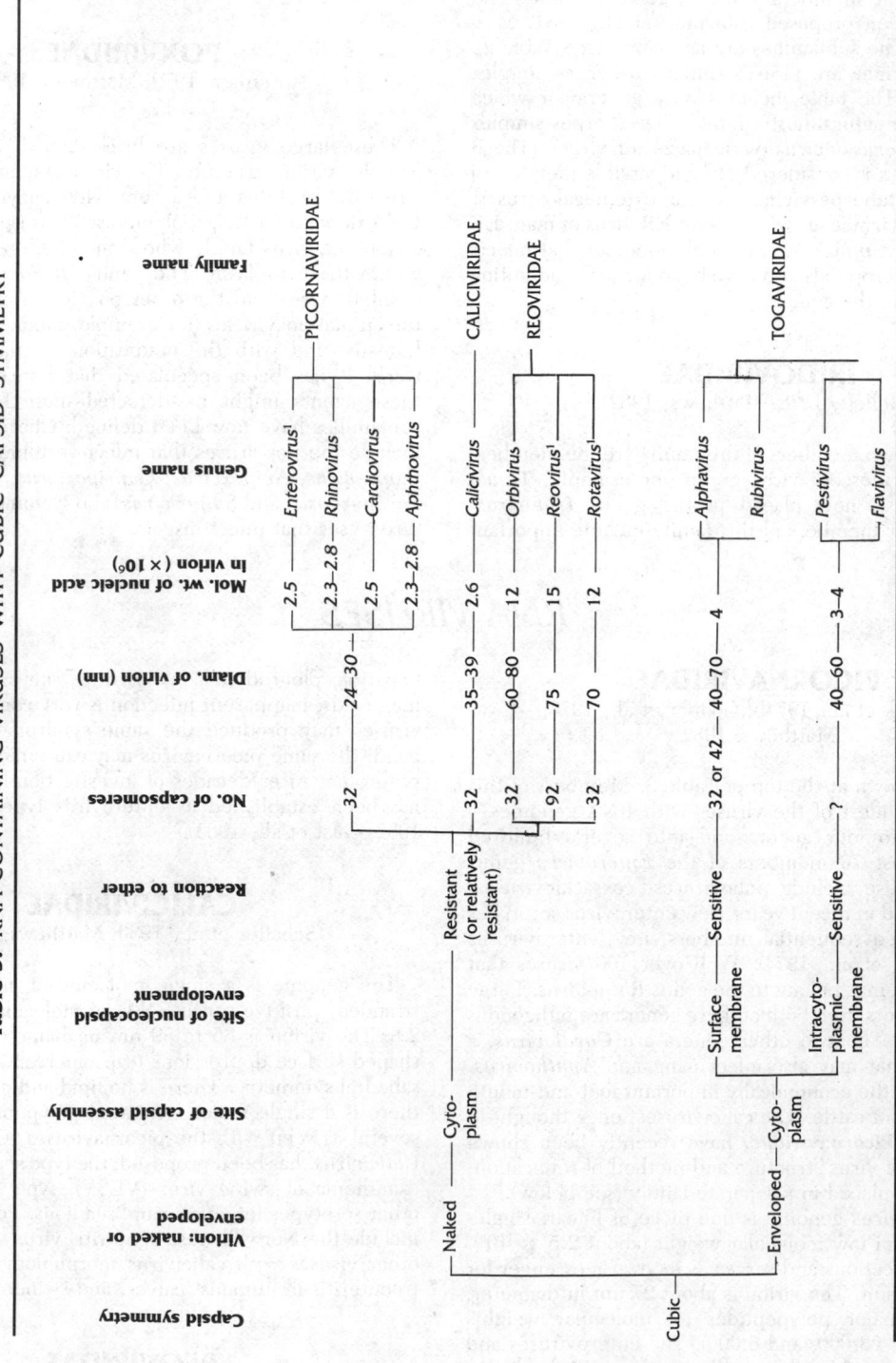

Capsid symmetry	Virion: naked or enveloped	Site of capsid assembly	Site of nucleocapsid envelopment	Reaction to ether	No. of capsomeres	Diam. of virion (nm)	Mol. wt. of nucleic acid in virion (× 10⁶)	Genus name	Family name
Cubic	Naked	Cyto-plasm		Resistant (or relatively resistant)	32	24–30	2.5	*Enterovirus*[1]	PICORNAVIRIDAE
							2.3–2.8	*Rhinovirus*	
							2.5	*Cardiovirus*	
							2.3–2.8	*Aphthovirus*	
					32	35–39	2.6	*Calicivirus*	CALICIVIRIDAE
					32	60–80	12	*Orbivirus*	REOVIRIDAE
					92	75	15	*Reovirus*[1]	
					32	70	12	*Rotavirus*[1]	
	Enveloped	Cyto-plasm	Surface membrane	Sensitive	32 or 42	40–70	4	*Alphavirus*	TOGAVIRIDAE
								Rubivirus	
			Intracyto-plasmic membrane	Sensitive	?	40–60	3–4	*Pestivirus*	
								Flavivirus	

[1]Most of the RNA-containing viruses are sensitive to pH 3 treatment; exceptions are the enteroviruses, reoviruses, and rotaviruses.

protein coats. The particle with the outer coat removed is termed the core. Cores have 12 spikes with 5-fold symmetry arranged icosahedrally. The genome consists of 10 to 12 pieces of linear double-stranded RNA with a total molecular weight of 12 to 20 × 10^6. Three of the genera in this family infect vertebrates: *Reovirus*, *Orbivirus*, and *Rotavirus*. The capsomeres of the orbiviruses are unusually large (10 to 15 nm wide) and appear ring-shaped. The human reoviruses are found in the bowel but their association with disease is not clear. Some orbiviruses have been considered to be arboviruses. The diseases caused by orbiviruses include Colorado tick fever of man, blue-tongue of sheep, African horsesickness, and epizootic hemorrhagic disease of deer.

The members of the genus *Rotavirus* that infect human beings are increasingly recognized as major pathogens, responsible for a large share of nonbacterial infantile diarrhea. The gastroenteritis syndrome they cause is clinically very severe and is one of the commonest childhood illnesses throughout the world; in developing countries it is a leading cause of death. Much of the initial study of the rotaviruses was accomplished by electron microscopy and immune microscopy, and rotaviruses that infect man have been isolated in cell cultures only recently, and with difficulty.

In addition to the members of **Reoviridae** that infect vertebrates, there are other groups within the family: the cytoplasmic polyhedrosis viruses of insects, and two genera of reoviruses of plants (Matthews, 1982; Murphy, 1983).

Reoviridae no longer stand alone as the only RNA-containing vertebrate viruses whose RNA genome is double-stranded rather than single-stranded. A newly recognized group—as yet unnamed—is characterized by a bisegmented genome; these viruses have not been classified previously but were often discussed in conjunction with **Reoviridae** because of the nature of their genome. This new group includes infectious pancreatic necrosis virus of fish, infectious bursal disease virus of chickens, and *Drosophila* X virus (Dobos et al., 1979; Murphy, 1983). The term **Birnaviridae** has been suggested informally as a family name.

TOGAVIRIDAE

(Porterfield et al., 1978)

Members of this family include most arboviruses* of antigenic groups A and B, now classed in the genus *Alphavirus* (group A) and the genus *Flavivirus* (group B), and in newly designated genera, which include nonarbo togaviruses, rubella (*Rubivirus*), and the mucosal disease virus group (*Pestivirus*). The virions are spherical and 40 to 70 nm in diameter, and have a lipoprotein envelope with lipid and virus-specified glycopeptide tightly applied to an icosahedral nucleocapsid. The genome is a single molecule of single-stranded RNA. The alphaviruses and flaviviruses include many of the major human arboviral pathogens: the viruses of Venezuelan, eastern, and western equine encephalitis are alphaviruses, and the viruses of yellow fever, dengue, Japanese encephalitis, St. Louis encephalitis, Omsk hemorrhagic fever, and Russian spring-summer encephalitis are flaviviruses. Rubella virus thus far is the only member placed in the genus *Rubivirus*. Members of the *Pestivirus* genus include the viruses of hog cholera, bovine virus diarrhea, and other animal viruses. The Subcommittee on Interrelationships Among Catalogued Arboviruses (SIRACA) of the American Committee on Arthropod-borne Viruses has published a report on the structure of the *Alphavirus* genus. Using degrees of antigenic relatedness, they have developed a hierarchical system that includes the terms group (genus), complex (subgenus), type (species), and variety or serovariant (subspecies) (Calisher et al., 1980).

*One important and well-known virus group name that does not appear in the diagrams is a category based on ecologic properties, the *arbovirus group* (Berge, 1975). The more than 350 arthropod-borne viruses survive through a complex cycle involving vertebrate hosts and arthropods that serve as vectors, transmitting the viruses by their bites. This grouping, based on transmission, remains a useful one despite the wide diversity of its members in regard to properties of the virion. The vast majority of arboviruses now have been sufficiently well-characterized to permit their taxonomic placement. Their classic serologic interrelationships previously delineated by arbovirologists are paralleled by morphologic similarities, and have provided vital clues that can speed the taxonomic location of large numbers of viruses. Once some of the members of a classic serologic group have been characterized in terms of biophysical and biochemical properties, attention of taxonomists can be focused on their antigenic relatives. Arboviruses now are included in a number of families, chiefly **Togaviridae, Bunyaviridae, Rhabdoviridae, Arenaviridae,** and **Reoviridae.**

ORTHOMYXOVIRIDAE

(Dowdle et al., 1975) (See Table 4)

All orthomyxoviruses recognized to date are influenza viruses. The virions may be spherical, elongated, or filamentous. For most members of the family, there are "spikes" projecting from the surface of the envelope; these are glycosylated protein peplomers 10 to 14 nm long and 4 nm in diameter, consisting of two types, the hemagglutinin and the neuraminidase. (In the nomenclature of variants of influenza type A, which arise frequently either as minor variants or as major new strains, the designation of these two antigens as H_1N_1, H_3H_2, and so on, supplies an important part of the information needed about new strains—their relatedness, if any, to strains that circulated previously—as a guide to the probable degree of immunity in the population.) During replication the helical nucleocapsid is first detected in the nucleus, whereas the hemagglutinin and neuraminidase are formed in the cytoplasm. The virus matures by budding at the cell surface membrane. The genus *Influenzavirus* has been established and includes viruses of type A and type B; type C is considered a "probable genus." Antigenic variation is common, particularly among members of type A. Recombination occurs with high frequency within types but not between types or genera. Type A influenza viruses include agents of human, equine, and swine influenza and of fowl plague. Only human strains are known for types B and C.

PARAMYXOVIRIDAE

(Kingsbury et al., 1978)

Usually spherical, these virions may also be pleomorphic; filamentous forms may be several micrometers long. On the lipid bilayer envelope are surface projections. Virions are formed in the cytoplasm by budding from the plasma membrane. Paramyxovirus infectivity is sensitive to ether, acid, and heat. The genera include the following: *Paramyxovirus* (parainfluenza viruses, mumps virus, Newcastle disease virus, Yucaipa and other avian paramyxoviruses); *Morbillivirus* (the viruses of measles, canine distemper,

Table 4. RNA-CONTAINING VIRUSES WITH HELICAL SYMMETRY

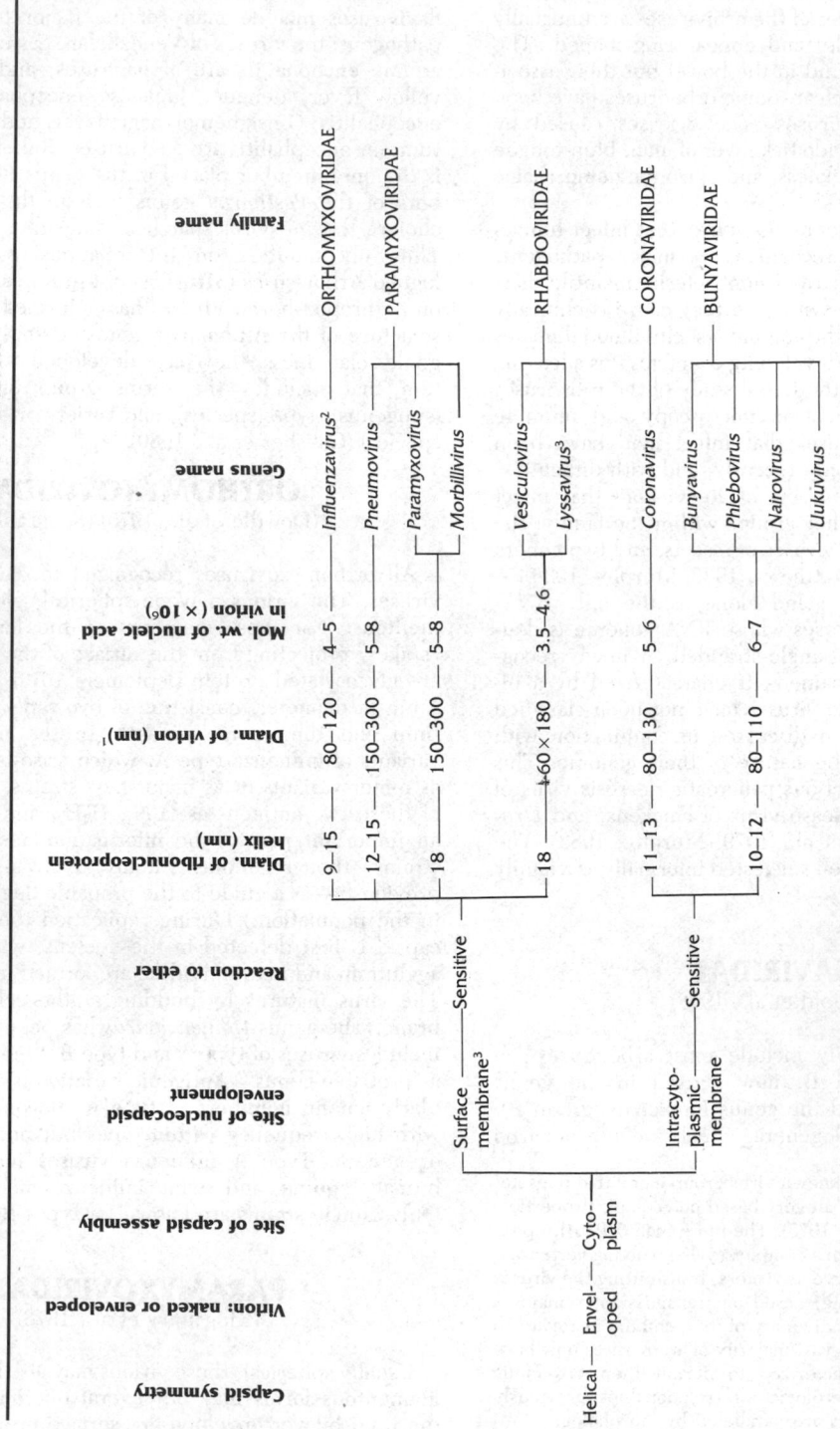

Capsid symmetry	Virion: naked or enveloped	Site of capsid assembly	Site of nucleocapsid envelopment	Reaction to ether	Diam. of ribonucleoprotein helix (nm)	Diam. of virion (nm)[1]	Mol. wt. of nucleic acid in virion ($\times 10^6$)	Genus name	Family name
Helical	Enveloped	Cytoplasm	Surface membrane[3]	Sensitive	9–15	80–120	4–5	*Influenzavirus*[2]	ORTHOMYXOVIRIDAE
					12–15	150–300	5–8	*Pneumovirus*	PARAMYXOVIRIDAE
					18	150–300	5–8	*Paramyxovirus*	
								Morbillivirus	
					18	60 × 180	3.5–4.6	*Vesiculovirus*	RHABDOVIRIDAE
								Lyssavirus[3]	
			Intracytoplasmic membrane	Sensitive	11–13	80–130	5–6	*Coronavirus*	CORONAVIRIDAE
					10–12	80–110	6–7	*Bunyavirus*	BUNYAVIRIDAE
								Phlebovirus	
								Nairovirus	
								Uukuvirus	

[1]Diameter, or diameter × length.
[2]Influenza type C probably is a separate genus, but has not yet been so designated.
[3]Rabies virus buds predominantly from intracytoplasmic membranes.

rinderpest, and peste-des-petits-ruminants); and *Pneumovirus* (respiratory syncytial viruses of man and of cattle, and pneumonia virus of mice). **Paramyxoviridae** are genetically stable and genetic recombination does not occur.

RHABDOVIRIDAE

(Brown et al., 1979; Matthews, 1982)

Members of this family have enveloped virions that are rod-shaped, resembling a bullet (with one end rounded and the other flattened) or bacilliform. Enclosed within the lipoprotein envelope and membrane protein is the long tubular nucleocapsid with helical symmetry. Members of some genera multiply in arthropods as well as in vertebrates or higher plants; others multiply only in insects. Infectivity is sensitive to ether, acid, and heat. The genera that infect vertebrates are *Lyssavirus* (including rabies virus, Duvenhage virus, and Mokola virus, all of which infect man; Lagos bat virus; and several agents isolated as yet only from insects), and *Vesiculovirus* (including vesicular stomatitis virus and a number of antigenically interrelated viruses from various animal species). Marburg virus, a simian virus highly pathogenic for man, is rhabdovirus-like in most properties but has very elongated forms. Further study of Marburg and Ebola viruses indicates that the RNA and proteins of these viruses have physicochemical properties that are distinct from those of the rhabdoviruses.

CORONAVIRIDAE

(Tyrrell et al., 1978)

The family is named for unique petal-shaped or club-shaped peplomers that project from the envelope; in negatively stained electron micrographs these projections form a fringe resembling the solar corona. The interior structure of the virion is believed to be a loosely wound, helically symmetric nucleocapsid. The genome consists of one large molecule of single-stranded RNA. Infectivity is sensitive to ether, acid, and heat. Nucleocapsids develop in the cytoplasm and mature by budding through intracytoplasmic membranes. Several serotypes of human coronaviruses have been isolated from patients with acute upper respiratory tract illnesses, primarily through the use of human embryonic tracheal and nasal organ cultures. There are distinct coronaviruses that infect a number of animal species.

BUNYAVIRIDAE

(Bishop et al., 1980; Matthews, 1982)

This family is the largest and most recently recognized taxonomic grouping assigned to an antigenically interrelated set of arboviruses. There are at least 200 members, more than 145 belonging to the Bunyamwera supergroup of serologically interrelated arboviruses. With the taxonomic placement of this large group, the vast majority of the viruses of the classic arbovirus groupings—initially based on ecological properties and subdivided by serological interrelationships—have been assigned to families on the basis of biophysical and biochemical characteristics.

The virions are spherical; they develop in the cytoplasm, mature by budding through intracytoplasmic membranes and have lipid-containing envelopes.

The nucleic acid consists of three molecules of negative-sense single-stranded RNA; the ribonucleocapsids (three) are composed of circular, long helical strands, 2.0 to 2.5 nm in diameter, sometimes supercoiled, with lengths of 0.2 to 3.0 μm. Subdivision of the family **Bunyaviridae** into genera reflects both antigenic supergroup relationships and molecular similarities and differences. The genus *Bunyavirus* includes at least 124 viruses, most of them belonging to 13 serologically cross-related groups; several ungrouped arboviruses also are included; most of these agents are mosquito-transmitted. Among the members are the virus of California encephalitis, and also the La Crosse virus, which causes human encephalitis with occasional fatal outcome, as well as other viruses that cause febrile diseases in man. Other bunyaviruses cause disease in some ruminants. The genus *Phlebovirus* includes the virus of *Phlebotomus* (sandfly) fever of man, Rift Valley fever virus, and at least 28 other viruses. The agents are predominantly sandfly-borne, but some have been recovered from mosquitoes. A wide variety of vertebrates, especially rodents, may be infected. Rift Valley fever, a serious pathogen of sheep, has caused large epidemics among humans in Africa.

The genus *Nairovirus*, named from the virus of Nairobi sheep disease, has as its prototype the more intensively studied Crimean-Congo hemorrhagic fever virus. Nairoviruses are predominantly tick-transmitted. At least 19 serotypes belong to this genus. Members of the genus *Uukuvirus* are tick-transmitted. The genus includes the type species, Uukuniemi virus, and 6 other viruses. They have been isolated in nature but have no known pathogenicity for man.

Human illness caused by Hantaan virus has been recognized in the Far East as Korean hemorrhagic fever, and a variant is known in Scandinavian and Eastern European countries as epidemic nephropathy (Lee, 1982). The illness has been collectively named "hemorrhagic fever with renal syndrome" or "muroid virus nephropathy." Recent studies show the virus to be a member of **Bunyaviridae**. It has a labile membrane and a tripartite single-stranded RNA genome. The most common natural hosts are mice (in Korea) and voles (in Europe). There have been several instances of infection of staff members handling laboratory rats infected with the virus, both in the Far East and more recently in Europe. In Belgium, there also have been sporadic cases with no apparent link to an outbreak or to each other.

RETROVIRIDAE

(Vogt, 1977; Matthews, 1982) (See Table 5)

This family includes all of the RNA tumor viruses once referred to as "oncornaviruses"; they are now assigned to a subfamily, **Oncovirinae;** other subfamilies are **Lentivirinae** (the slow viruses of the maedi/visna group) and **Spumavirinae** (the foamy virus group—agents that form syncytia in cell cultures). Members of the **Retroviridae** characteristically have a reverse transcriptase (RNA-dependent DNA polymerase) within the virion. For the most thoroughly studied members, the lipoprotein envelope encloses an inner shell with icosahedral symmetry and a central core or nucleocapsid containing a possibly helical ribonucleoprotein. The genome contains duplicate copies of high-molecular-weight single-stranded RNA of the same polarity as viral messenger RNA. The virion contains a reverse transcriptase enzyme (RNA → DNA). Infectivity is

Table 5. RNA-CONTAINING VIRUSES WITH ARCHITECTURE UNSYMMETRIC OR UNKNOWN

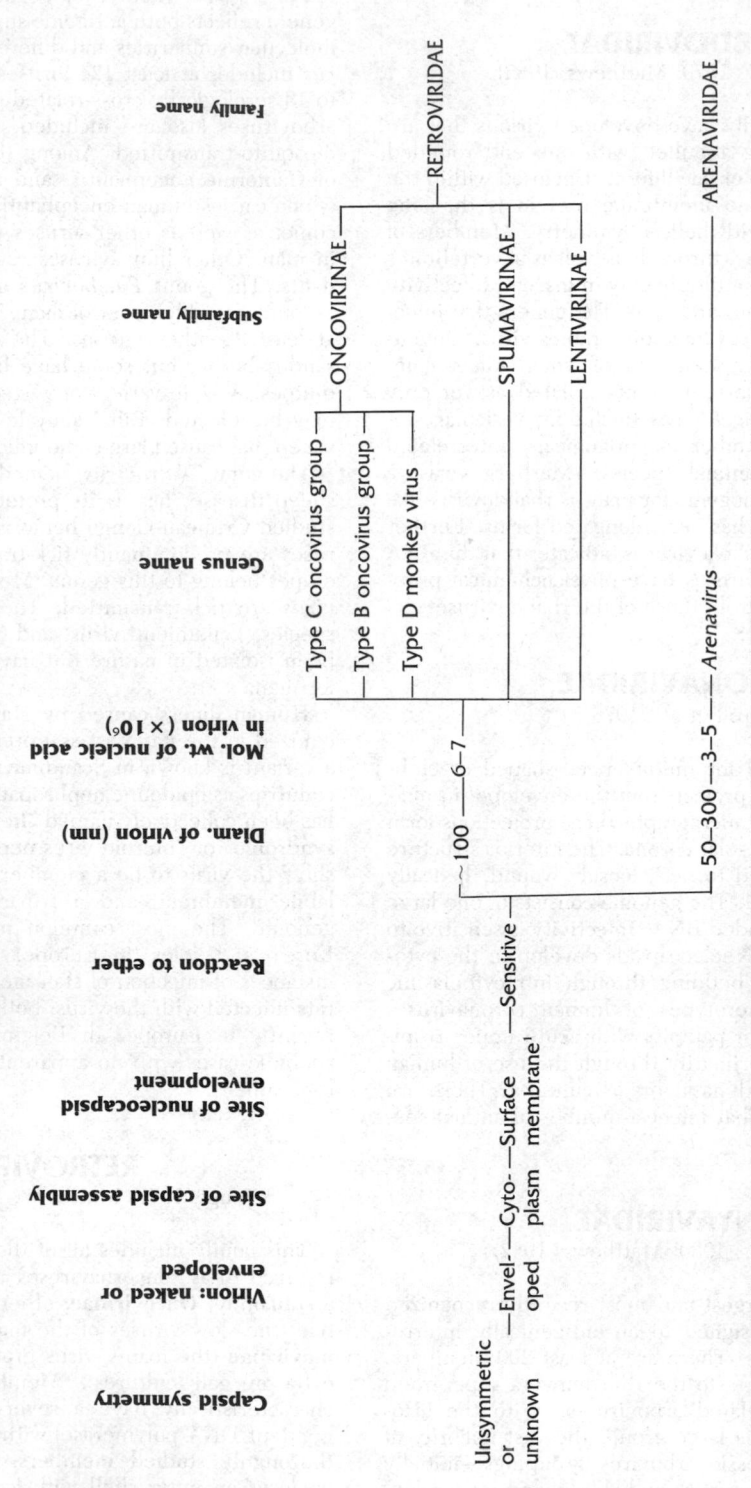

Capsid symmetry	Virion: naked or enveloped	Site of capsid assembly	Site of nucleocapsid envelopment	Reaction to ether	Diam. of virion (nm)	Mol. wt. of nucleic acid in virion ($\times 10^6$)	Genus name	Subfamily name	Family name
Unsymmetric or unknown	Enveloped	Cytoplasm	Surface membrane[1]	Sensitive	~100	6–7	Type C oncovirus group	ONCOVIRINAE	RETROVIRIDAE
							Type B oncovirus group	ONCOVIRINAE	RETROVIRIDAE
							Type D monkey virus	ONCOVIRINAE	RETROVIRIDAE
								SPUMAVIRINAE	RETROVIRIDAE
								LENTIVIRINAE	RETROVIRIDAE
					50–300	3–5	*Arenavirus*		ARENAVIRIDAE

[1]Members of Spumavirinae bud into intracytoplasmic vacuoles.

ether-, acid-, and heat-sensitive. Replication proceeds off an integrated "provirus" DNA copy in infected cells. It was through the studies of retroviruses that the cellular "oncogenes" became recognized (Bishop, 1982). In the case of the subfamily **Oncovirinae,** all normal cells of several animal species contain integrated copies of genes of the endogenous species of oncovirus. The oncovirus genes may be unexpressed but can be activated by physical and chemical agents, by superinfection with other oncoviruses, and even by herpesviruses. According to certain morphologic, antigenic, and enzymatic differences, oncoviruses also have been divided into A, B, and C (and possibly D) types of viruses. With some exceptions, oncoviruses fall into host-species-specific groups of agents inducing either leukemias or sarcomas—that is, leukemia-sarcoma complexes of avian, murine, feline, or hamster oncoviruses; other groups are murine mammary tumor virus and primate oncoviruses. One of the primate oncoviruses is the monkey mammary tumor virus (MoMTV).

Recently, members of the subfamily **Oncovirinae** have been shown to cause human disease. These include the agents generally known as the human T-cell leukemia viruses and the agent known as the lymphadenopathy-associated virus. There are at least three types of human T-cell leukemia viruses, and type 3 apparently is identical to the lymphadenopathy-associated virus; this serotype seems to be the etiological agent of AIDS (acquired immune deficiency syndrome).

ARENAVIRIDAE

(Pfau et al., 1974; Rawls and Leung, 1979)

Members of this family have spherical or pleomorphic virions with a dense lipid bilayer membrane that bears surface projections; within the virion core are electron-dense RNA-containing granules about 20 to 30 nm in diameter that resemble ribosomes. Most member viruses have a single restricted rodent host in which persistent infection occurs; spread to other mammals and to man can take place, but is unusual. Members include lymphocytic choriomeningitis virus (LCM virus), which infects mice but may spread to man; Lassa virus; and members of the Tacaribe complex (Junin and Machupo viruses of South American hemorrhagic fevers, Pichinde virus, and several other viral agents that have been isolated as yet only from arthropods). Some arenaviruses (for example, Junin and Machupo, and Lassa) are very serious pathogens when they do spread to man.

EMERGING PROBLEMS IN VIRUS CLASSIFICATION

There are other known viruses about which information is insufficient to permit their taxonomic classification. This is the status of the non-A, non-B hepatitis viruses; of agents responsible for some immune complex diseases and for some "slow" virus diseases; and of some viruses of gastroenteritis.

Some of the present and developing problems that viral taxonomists will have to meet are those posed by the recently discovered forms of life called viroids and prions, and also by viral hybrids (between unrelated viruses), pseudotypes, pseudovirions, and recombinant DNA.

VIROIDS

Viroids constitute a recently discovered class of infectious agents smaller than viruses. They are known to cause several diseases of plants (for example, potato spindle tuber disease), and may ultimately be found to cause disease in man and higher animals. (For example, the agent of scrapie disease of sheep—one of the puzzling "slow viruses" not yet placed taxonomically—may, according to recent findings, prove to be a DNA molecule similar in size to a viroid.) Viroids exhibit the characteristics of nucleic acids in crude extracts; that is, they are insensitive to heat and to organic solvents but are sensitive to nucleases. They do not appear to possess a protein coat.

Plant viroids are single-stranded, covalently closed circular RNA molecules (molecular weight 70,000 to 120,000) consisting of about 360 nucleotides and are characterized by a highly base-paired rodlike structure with unique properties. Each is arranged into 26 double-stranded regions separated by 25 regions of unpaired bases embodied in single-stranded internal loops; there is a loop at each end of the rodlike molecule. These features provide the viroid RNA molecule with structural, thermodynamic, and kinetic properties very similar to those of a double-stranded DNA molecule of the same molecular weight and G + C (guanine plus cytosine) content.

Viroids replicate by an entirely novel mechanism in which infecting viroid RNA molecules are copied by the host enzyme normally responsible for synthesis of nuclear precursors to messenger RNA. Thus, DNA-dependent RNA polymerase purified from healthy plant tissue is capable of synthesizing linear viroid RNA copies of full length from viroid RNA templates in vitro (Diener, 1984).

Comparative sequence analysis of a major group of plant viroids reveals striking similarities with the ends of transposable genetic elements. These similarities have led to speculation that viroids may have originated from transposable elements or retroviral proviruses by deletion of interior portions of the viral DNA.

PRIONS

Besides the suggestion that the agent of scrapie might be similar to viroids (see above), other hypotheses have been proposed for the structure and nature of this agent. A concept recently proposed (Prusiner, 1982) is that the agent may be a small *pro*teinaceous *in*fectious particle, the *prion*. A number of lines of evidence are set forth for consideration, including the marked resistance of the scrapie agent to procedures that attack most nucleic acids, its inactivation by procedures directed against proteins, its heterogeneity of size, and other novel properties. The evidence assembled is not claimed to rule out the possibility that a very small nucleic acid may be present, buried within a tightly packed protein shell; neither does it rule out the possible presence of a highly unusual nucleic acid whose coat or chemical structure protects it from most procedures that inactivate nucleic acids.

If prions are eventually shown to be devoid of nucleic acid, then they would indeed be unique among microorganisms, and many new questions would be raised, including that of the mode whereby an infectious protein could replicate.

VIRUS HYBRIDS

The fact that virus hybrids can exist in nature should be more widely recognized. If the simian papovavirus SV40 had not already been known as a virus before the discovery of SV40-adenovirus hybrid particles, these particles would have presented viral taxonomists with a very confusing puzzle. The hybrid particles, in which portions of SV40 genome material are covalently linked to adenovirus genetic material and encased within an adenovirus coat, would have seemed to be a new and very strange virus that reacted antigenically like an adenovirus (of the serotype from which its coat was derived) but whose progeny had many properties altogether different from other members of the adenovirus group (Rapp and Melnick, 1966).

PSEUDOTYPES AND PSEUDOVIRIONS

Pseudotypes may arise during replication in co-infected cells: the genome of one virus may become encapsulated in the heterologous protein coat encoded by the second virus.

During viral replication the capsid sometimes encloses *host* nucleic acid rather than viral nucleic acid. The resulting particles, called *pseudovirions,* look like ordinary virus particles when observed by electron microscopy, but they do not replicate. Pseudovirions theoretically might be able to transduce cellular nucleic acid from one cell to another.

RECOMBINANT DNA

Recently developed techniques allow DNA to be cleaved into specific pieces by use of restriction endonucleases from bacteria. The distinct fragments can be recombined and replicated. The genomic materials from two distinct viruses multiply together, and these new forms pose new problems for classification (Smith et al., 1983).

References

Bachmann, P. A., et al.: Parvoviridae: Second Report. Intervirology 11:248, 1979.

Bellett, A. J. D.: The iridescent virus group. Adv Virus Res 13:225, 1968.

Berge, T. O.: International Catalogue of Arboviruses Including Certain Other Viruses of Vertebrates. DHEW Publication No.(CDC) 75-8301, Washington, D.C., U.S. Government Printing Office, 1975.

Bishop, D. H. L., et al.: Bunyaviridae. Intervirology 14:125, 1980.

Bishop, J. M.: Oncogenes. Sci Am 246:80, 1982.

Brown, F., et al.: Rhabdoviridae. Intervirology 12:1, 1979.

Calisher, C. H., et al.: Proposed antigenic classification of registered arboviruses. I. Togaviridae, *Alphavirus*. Intervirology 14:229, 1980.

Cooper, P. D., et al.: Picornaviridae: Second Report. Intervirology 10:165, 1978.

Davis B. D., Dulbecco, R., Eisen, H. N., Ginsberg, H. S., and Wood, W. B., Jr.: Microbiology. New York, Hoeber Medical Division, 1967.

Diener, T. O.: Portraits of viruses: Portrait of the viroid. Intervirology, 22:1, 1984.

Dobos, P., et al.: Biophysical and biochemical characterization of five animal viruses with bisegmented double-stranded RNA genomes. J Virol 32:593, 1979.

Dowdle, W. R., et al.: Orthomyxoviridae. Intervirology 5:245, 1975.

Fenner, F., Classification and Nomenclature of Viruses: Second Report of the International Committee on Taxonomy of Viruses. Intervirology 7:1, 1976.

Fenner, F.: Portraits of viruses: The poxviruses. Intervirology 11:137, 1979.

Fenner, F., and White, D. O.: Medical Virology, 2nd ed. New York, Academic Press, 1976.

Gust, I. D., et al.: Taxonomic classification of hepatitis A virus. Intervirology 20:1, 1983.

Kingsbury, D. W., et al.: Paramyxoviridae. Intervirology 10:137, 1978.

Lee, H. W.: Korean hemorrhagic fever. Prog Med Virol 28:96, 1982.

Matthews, R. E. F.: Classification and Nomenclature of Viruses: Third and Fourth Reports of the International Committee on Taxonomy of Viruses. Intervirology 12:129, 1979, and 17:1, 1982.

Matthews, R. E. F. (ed): A Critical Appraisal of Viral Taxonomy. Boca Raton, Florida, CRC Press, 1983.

Mayor, H. D., and Melnick, J. L.: Small deoxyribonucleic acid-containing viruses (picodnavirus group). Nature 210:331, 1966.

Melnick, J. L.: Papovavirus group. Science 135:1128, 1962.

Melnick, J. L.: Taxonomy and nomenclature of viruses, 1982. Prog Med Virol 28:208, 1982a.

Melnick, J. L.: Classification of hepatitis A virus as enterovirus type 72 and of hepatitis B virus as hepadnavirus type 1. Intervirology 18:105, 1982b.

Melnick, J. L., Tagaya, I., and von Magnus, H.: Enteroviruses 69, 70, and 71. Intervirology 4:369, 1974.

Melnick, J. L., et al.: Papovaviridae. Intervirology 3:106, 1974a.

Melnick, J. L., et al.: Picornaviridae. Intervirology 4:303, 1974b.

Murphy, F. A.: Current problems in vertebrate virus taxonomy. *In:* Matthews (ed.): A Critical Appraisal of Viral Taxonomy, pp. 37-61, Boca Raton, Florida, CRC Press, 1983.

Pfau, C. J. et al.: Arenaviruses. Intervirology 4:207, 1974.

Porterfield, J. S., et al.: Togaviridae. Intervirology 9:129, 1978.

Prusiner, S. B.: Novel proteinaceous particles cause scrapie. Science 216:136, 1982.

Rapp, F., and Melnick, J. L.: Papovavirus SV40, adenovirus and their hybrids: Transformation, complementation and transcapsidation. Prog Med Virol 8:349, 1966.

Rawls, W. E., and Leung, W. C.: Arenaviruses. *In:* Fraenkel-Conrat and Wagner (eds.): Comprehensive Virology, Vol. 14, p. 157. New York, Plenum, 1979.

Robinson, W. S., et al.: The hepadna virus group: hepatitis B and related viruses. *In:* Szmuness, Alter, and Maynard (eds.): Viral Hepatitis: 1981 International Symposium, p. 57. Philadelphia, Franklin Institute Press, 1982.

Roizman, B., et al.: Herpesviridae: definition, provisional nomenclature, and taxonomy. Intervirology 16:201, 1981.

Schaffer, F. L., et al.: Caliciviridae. Intervirology 14:1, 1980.

Smith, G. L., Mackett, M., and Moss, B.: Infectious vaccinia virus recombinants that express hepatitis B virus surface antigen. Nature 302:490, 1983.

Tyrrell, D. A. J., et al.: Coronaviridae: Second report. Intervirology 10:321, 1978.

Vogt, P. K.: Genetics of RNA tumor viruses. *In:* Fraenkel-Conrat and Wagner (eds.): Comprehensive Virology, Vol. 9, p. 341. New York, Plenum, 1977.

Wigand, R., et al.: *Adenoviridae:* Second Report. Intervirology 18:169, 1982.

Wildy, P.: Classification and Nomenclature of Viruses: First Report of the International Committee on Nomenclature of Viruses. Monogr Virol, Vol. 5, Basel, S. Karger, 1971.

9
VIRAL REPLICATION

BARTHOLOMEW M. SEFTON
SAMUEL C. SILVERSTEIN, M.D.

Viruses can be thought of as packaged genes that can move from one cell to another or from one organism to another and can replicate. There is enormous diversity in the structure of viral genomes. They can be RNA or DNA, single-stranded or double-stranded, linear or circular, and can comprise either one or multiple segments. The means by which these very different molecules are propagated are dictated in large part by their structure. Mechanisms of virus replication are therefore extremely diverse and often very different from the process by which cellular genetic information is replicated and expressed.

Viruses are obligatory intracellular parasites. To propagate, they must gain access to a host organism and penetrate into the cytoplasm or nucleus of susceptible target cells. Transfer from organism to organism is passive. In most cases, infection occurs as the result of ingestion or inhalation of the virus. In specialized cases, however, virus transmission occurs by way of an insect vector or contaminated hypodermic needles or blood.

Although all viruses are dependent on cellular functions for their replication, the extent of this dependence varies greatly. Viruses with very small genomes, such as the papovaviruses and the parvoviruses, encode only one viral protein that is involved in replication and expression of the viral genome. All other functions are performed by cellular enzymes. The viruses with very much larger genomes, such as the herpesviruses and the poxviruses, can afford the genetic luxury of encoding numerous viral enzymes that play a role in replication of the virus. Nevertheless, even viruses with extensive coding capacity are very dependent on host cell organelles and biosynthetic machinery for their replication and produce progeny virions from nucleotides, amino acids, lipids, and carbohydrates that are synthesized by cellular enzymes.

The viral life-cycle consists of a fairly limited number of essential steps. The virus must bind to a susceptible cell; gain entry to either the cytoplasm or the nucleus; succeed in having the viral particle uncoated; direct the synthesis of templates for the replication of the genome and the formation of mRNA; synthesize progeny genomes, mRNAs, and the proteins that comprise the viral particle; assemble virions; and, if the infection is productive, achieve the release of the progeny particles from the host cell. In most cases, viruses also direct the synthesis of non-structural proteins that play a role in replication but are not components of the virion. The ways in which these steps are carried out vary enormously.

Virus infection usually leads to the lysis and death of the host cell, but not always. Under some circumstances persistent productive infection results. This is the typical outcome of the infection of a cell by a retrovirus. A persistent infection is possible if the release of progeny virus does not kill the host cell and the viral genome is not lost by segregation during mitosis. This is most likely to occur with viruses with DNA genomes, which can become integrated into cellular chromosomes, and with enveloped viruses, which can be released from the host cell without cell lysis. Some infections are latent rather than productive. This is often seen with herpesviruses. In a latent infection, the viral genome remains stably associated with the host cell, but progeny virus are not produced. Latently infected cells maintain the potential for virus production. Other infections may be abortive. Virus replication is initiated but there is no production of progeny nor stable association of the virus with the host cell.

INITIATION OF A VIRAL INFECTION. Virus infection is initiated by the binding of the virus to the surface of a host cell. There is often frank specificity in this process. For example, poliovirus normally can infect human cells but not mouse cells. Yet, if the necessity for the viral particle to bind to the host cell is circumvented by introduction of the RNA genome of the poliovirus directly into mouse cells, the virus replicates as well as it does in human cells. It is likely, therefore, that mouse cells are resistant to infection by poliovirus because they lack a suitable receptor. Similarly, reovirus type 3 infects mouse neurons readily, whereas reovirus type 1 does not. The basis for this restriction of replication is revealed clearly by the behavior of a virus which is a recombinant between type 1 and type 3. A virus that possesses nine genes from type 1 and only the viral hemagglutinin gene from type 3 replicates in neurons as well as a virus containing all 10 type 3 genes. Because the product of that single type 3 gene both confers the ability to infect neurons and is the protein responsible for binding the virus to host cells, it is clear that neurons are resistant to infection by reovirus type 1 because the type 1 hemagglutinin does not recognize receptors on neurons and not because type 1 virus cannot produce progeny in these cells.

The term virus receptor is somewhat of a misnomer. The normal function of the cell surface molecules to which viruses bind is certainly not as receptors for viruses. In fact, such a property could and would be selected against quickly. The proteins or lipids that function as receptors almost certainly carry out some essential function in an uninfected cell and are commandeered by infecting viruses. An attractive idea is that viruses enter cells by binding to the receptors for molecules such as hormones, which are normally taken up by the cell. To date, no molecule that functions as a virus receptor has been identified.

Not all viruses bind to receptors that have a limited distribution. The myxoviruses, for example, appear able to bind to almost any glycoprotein or glycolipid that contains sialic acid. Since this nine carbon sugar is a common component of the oligosaccharide side chains of glycoproteins and glycolipids, these viruses have, in theory, the ability to bind to nearly any cell, save those of insect origin.

THE ENTRY OF VIRUSES INTO HOST CELLS. Although some cells resist infection because the virus cannot bind to the cell, resistance to infection may also be determined at the stage of virus entry. This is most apparent in the case of the avian RNA tumor viruses, which appear to bind to both sensitive and resistant cells with equal avidity, but to penetrate only susceptible cells. Viral replication cannot be initiated until the virus gains access to either the cytoplasm or the nucleus of the host cell.

Fusion. The mechanism of virus penetration is best understood in the case of Sendai virus, a paramyxovirus also known as "hemagglutinating virus of Japan." Sendai virus is a large enveloped virus that contains two viral glycoproteins on its surface. One, termed HN, binds the virus to cell surface receptors that contain sialic acid. The other, termed F, catalyzes the fusion of the viral envelope with the plasma membrane of the cell. Membrane fusion simultaneously transfers the virus into the cytoplasm, where Sendai virus replicates, and uncoats it (Fig. 1, steps A1 and A2). This appealingly simple process could, in theory, be used by all enveloped viruses. Although there is some reason to think that the herpesviruses and the coronaviruses also enter a cell by the fusion of their envelopes with the plasma membrane of the infected cell, it is almost certain that most enveloped viruses enter a cell by endocytosis.

Endocytosis. Enveloped viruses such as the alphaviruses, the rhabdoviruses, and the orthomyxoviruses bind initially to receptors that are distributed randomly on the cell surface. Binding appears to stimulate lateral migration of the receptors and the receptor:virus complex can soon be found in specialized depressions or pits in the plasma membrane. These pits are coated on the cytoplasmic side with an electron dense layer composed largely of a single protein, clathrin (Fig. 1, step B1), and are frequently referred to as coated pits. The receptor:virus complexes are then engulfed and the resulting vesicles, called endosomes, enter the cytoplasm carrying the virus:receptor complex (Fig. 1, step B2). At this point, the virus has entered the cell, but is still separated from the cytoplasm by the membrane of the endosome. Entry to the cytoplasm is achieved by exploiting a special property of endosomes. Like the membrane of the lysosome, the membrane of the endosome contains a proton pump, and the interior of the vesicle becomes acidified rapidly. Acidic pH induces in one of the surface glycoproteins of orthomyxoviruses a conformational change that enables it to catalyze membrane fusion. Fusion of the viral membrane with that of the vesicle then releases the internal components of the virus into the cytoplasm—simultaneously uncoating the particle (Fig. 1, steps B3 and B4). Thus, the glycoproteins of most enveloped viruses appear able to stimulate membrane fusion. They differ, however, in the pH at which they have this activity. The F glycoprotein of Sendai virus is active at neutral pH, whereas the glycoproteins of the alphaviruses, the rhabdoviruses and the orthomyxoviruses acquire this activity only when exposed to acidic pH.

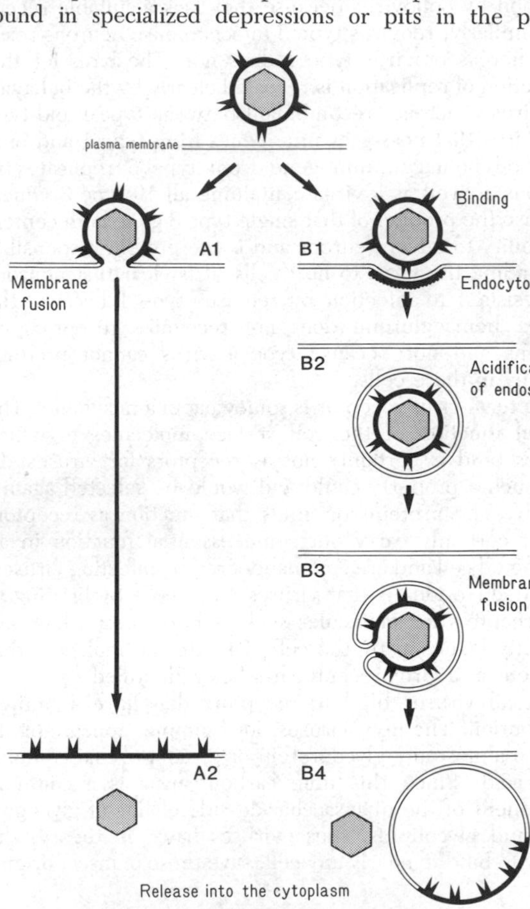

Figure 1. The entry of enveloped viruses occurs by two different mechanisms. Some viruses, such as the paramyxoviruses, undergo membrane fusion with the plasma membrane of the infected cell (step A1) and enter the cytoplasm directly (step A2). Other enveloped viruses, such as alphaviruses, rhabdoviruses, and orthomyxoviruses, enter the cell by endocytosis. Bound to their receptors, they are engulfed by coated pits (step B1). They then enter the cytoplasm in vesicles termed endosomes, which become acidified rapidly (step B2). The lowered pH renders the viral glycoproteins competent to catalyze membrane fusion and the viral cores are released into the cytoplasm (steps B3 and B4).

Little is known about how nonenveloped viruses enter a cell. They must be able to penetrate cellular membranes, but it is not clear whether this occurs at the cell surface or in an endocytic vesicle.

The method by which a virus enters into a host cell has important implications for host-parasite interactions, especially for the host's immune response. The immune system can interfere with virus replication by direct inactivation of free virus, or by the lysis of infected cells. Extracellular virus is inactivated by neutralizing antibodies and by antiviral antibody and complement. Similarly, infected cells carrying viral antigens on their surface are susceptible to lysis mediated by either antiviral antibody and complement or virus-specific cytotoxic T cells. Entry by endocytosis may have a selective advantage for an enveloped virus because it minimizes immune attack on a newly infected cell. As a necessary consequence of the fusion of the viral membrane with the plasma membrane, the surface proteins of the paramyxoviruses become integral components of the surface of the newly infected cell (Fig. 1). Such a cell, therefore, is immediately recognizable as an infected cell and is prone to immune lysis. In contrast, entry of the virus by endocytosis leaves no evidence of virus infection on the cell surface (Fig. 1). Viral antigens do not appear on the surface of the infected cell until late in infection when particles are being assembled and released.

Virus can also enter cells by inducing fusion of infected cells with their uninfected neighbors. This eliminates the need for extracellular virus and allows the virus to evade direct neutralization by antibody and complement. However, because the induction of cell fusion requires the presence of viral proteins on the surface of the infected cell, this mechanism of virus spread does not prevent immune lysis of the infected cell.

REPLICATION OF THE GENOME AND GENE EXPRESSION. Despite the fact that much of what we know about the molecular biology of cells has come from work with animal viruses, many of the mechanisms of gene expression and genome replication used by viruses bear little resemblance to the mechanism of cellular gene expression.

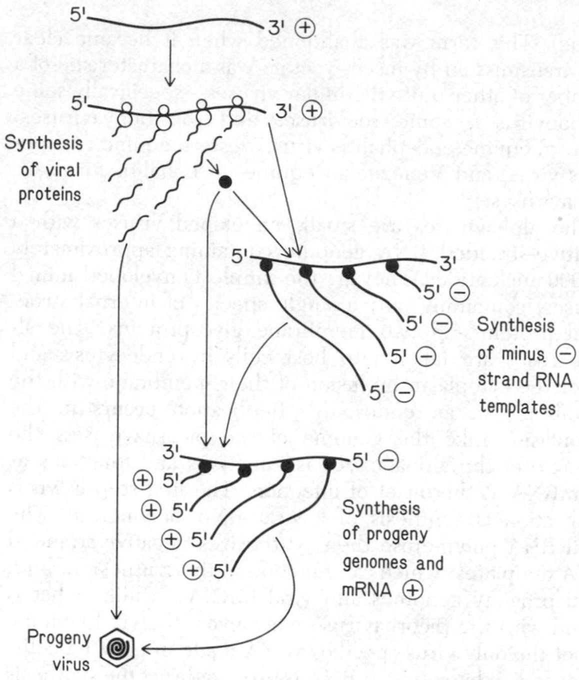

Figure 2. Replication of the picornaviruses. The plus-stranded genomic RNA of the infecting virus participates directly in the first two steps of viral replication. First, it serves as mRNA to direct the synthesis of viral proteins. Secondly, it is used by two of the newly synthesized viral polypeptides as template for the synthesis of viral minus-strand RNA. The minus-strand RNA is then used as template for the synthesis of additional plus-strand RNAs. The newly synthesized plus-strand RNA can then either function as mRNA, to direct the synthesis of more viral polypeptides, or assemble with viral structural proteins to form progeny virions.

In a fundamental sense, genome replication and mRNA synthesis are similar. In both cases, synthesis of the progeny strand or strands is initiated at the 3′ end of a template and the polymerase moves toward the 5′ end. As a consequence of the anti-parallel nature of base-pairing, the 5′ end of the progeny strand is synthesized first and the chain grows in a 5′ to 3′ direction (see Figs. 2 and 7). The synthesis of DNA differs in one important way from the synthesis of RNA. No known DNA polymerases can initiate DNA synthesis. All must be provided with a primer, which they can extend. In contrast, most RNA polymerases do not require primers and can initiate chains.

In most cases, viral mRNAs resemble cellular mRNAs in structure. They contain a methylated guanosine cap at their 5′ ends and a tail of approximately 200 adenylate residues at their 3′ ends. This imitation of cellular mRNAs is presumably the result of the fact that the synthesis of viral proteins requires that the viral mRNAs be translated efficiently by the cellular protein synthetic machinery.

One of the essential steps in virus replication is the production of templates for the synthesis of (1) progeny viral genomes and (2) viral mRNAs. For viruses with double-stranded DNA genomes, the same template can be used for both processes. For many other viruses, however, the template used for genome replication is different from that used for mRNA synthesis. Template synthesis requires an enzyme capable of copying the viral genome. In the case of viruses with double-stranded DNA genomes, both replication of the genome and synthesis of mRNA can, in theory, be carried out entirely by host enzymes. Such is not the case for viruses with RNA genomes. Animal cells have no enzymatic activity capable of transcribing RNA. This function, therefore, requires at least one viral gene product.

POSITIVE-STRANDED RNA VIRUSES

Viruses possessing single-stranded RNA genomes that are of the same sense or sequence as the viral mRNA are termed positive-stranded. Correspondingly, viruses with single-stranded RNA genomes that are complementary to viral mRNA are termed negative-stranded. There are four groups of well characterized positive-stranded RNA viruses—the picornaviruses, the alphaviruses, the coronaviruses, and the retroviruses. These viruses all replicate in the cytoplasm of the infected cell.

Picornaviruses. The enteroviruses, the rhinoviruses, and hepatitis A virus are all members of the picornavirus family. These viruses are small, nonenveloped, icosahedral, and have small, single-stranded RNA genomes. The genome of poliovirus, the best studied virus of this group, contains 7,433 nucleotides and encodes at least 8 polypeptides. The 3′ end of the genome is similar in structure to that of cellular mRNA in that it is polyadenylated. The 5′ end of the genome is unusual. Rather than containing a methylated guanosine cap like cellular RNAs, the genome has bound to it, through a phosphodiester bond, a small viral protein termed VPg. Since deproteinized poliovirus virion RNA is infectious, although much less so than the intact viral particle; neither VPg nor the other proteins present in the virion are essential for replication.

As is the case with other viruses possessing RNA genomes, the synthesis of both progeny picornavirus genomes and viral mRNA requires an enzyme capable of transcribing an RNA template into RNA. Since cells do not contain such an activity, the first step in the replication of picornaviruses must be the synthesis of a viral RNA-dependent RNA polymerase (Fig. 2). At the onset of infection, VPg is cleaved from the uncoated genomic RNA, which is then translated by cellular polyribosomes. Despite the fact that the RNA lacks a cap structure, it functions as an efficient mRNA. Two of the polypeptides produced by translation of the genomic RNA then participate in the transcription of the same viral RNA that functioned as mRNA for their synthesis. RNA replication first involves synthesis of minus-strand RNA, using the genomic RNA as template (Fig. 2). The newly synthesized minus-strand is then transcribed into progeny genomes and into mRNAs. Unlike what occurs in most viral infections, poliovirus specifies only a single species of viral mRNA. This mRNA is identical to genomic RNA, except that it lacks the terminal protein, VPg.

This single viral mRNA directs the synthesis of at least 8 different viral polypeptides. Since eukaryotic ribosomes cannot initiate protein synthesis at internal initiation codons, protein synthesis, which is initiated near the 5′ end of the genome, is terminated only after a translate of 2,207 amino acids has been synthesized. The individual viral polypeptides are produced by proteolytic processing of this enormous translation product (Fig. 3). Two types of processing occur. Two cleavages occur before completion of the synthesis of the viral polypeptide chain. Since the substrate of the protease is the nascent chain, this type of proteolytic processing is termed nascent cleavage. Later, 8 cleavages of the three primary viral polypeptide precursors produce the mature proteins that participate in replication of the viral RNA and in formation of the particle. The cleavages that occur during virion formation are termed maturational cleavages. A virus-encoded protease is responsible for

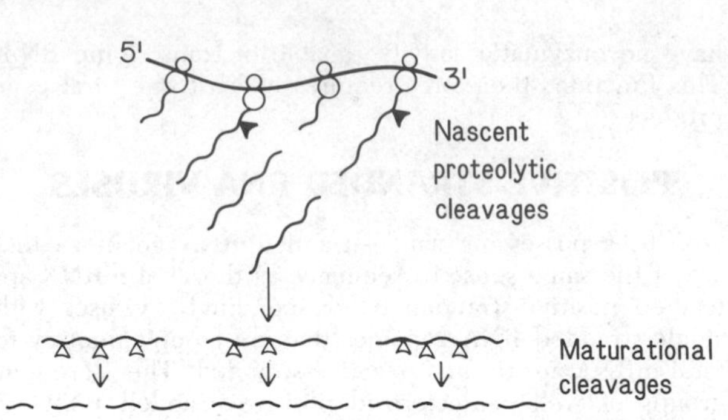

Figure 3. All of the poliovirus gene products are produced by proteolytic processing of a single precursor polypeptide. Two fundamentally different types of processing occur. Two cleavages occur before completion of the single viral translation product. These are termed nascent cleavages. Others occur only later. Some produce the viral replicase proteins. Others produce the structural proteins found in the virion.

processing most of the protein precursors. Because there is only a single picornaviral mRNA, all of the viral gene products—both those that can function catalytically and those that are purely structural—are produced in approximately equal amounts.

Virion formation occurs in the cytoplasm of the infected cell. This process appears not to be catalyzed. Rather, it is apparently driven simply by the affinity of the viral subunits for each other and begins spontaneously when the concentration of viral progeny genomes and virion structural proteins becomes sufficient. Virus is released only when the cell dies and breaks open. Lysis of the cell results in part from the inhibition of its macromolecular synthesis by the virus. Whether this is the only factor leading to cell lysis is uncertain.

Alphaviruses. The alphaviruses are members of the Togavirus family. They are transmitted in nature by arthropod vectors, most often mosquitoes. These viruses were previously called group A arboviruses (*ar*thropod-*bo*rne). This term was abandoned when it became clear that transmission by insect vectors was a characteristic of a number of other quite dissimilar viruses—specifically some rhabdoviruses, some reoviruses and the bunyaviruses. Eastern equine encephalitis virus, western equine encephalitis virus, and Venezuelan equine encephalitis virus are alphaviruses.

The alphaviruses are small, enveloped viruses with a positive-stranded RNA genome containing approximately 12,000 nucleotides. They are the simplest enveloped animal viruses, containing only a single species of internal structural protein and two membrane glycoproteins. The alphaviruses are taken into host cells by endocytosis and enter the cytoplasm by fusion of their membrane with the membrane of an endosome. Replication occurs in the cytoplasm. Like the genome of the picornaviruses, the genome of the alphaviruses is infectious and functions as an mRNA at the onset of infection. The first step in virus replication is synthesis of a viral RNA polymerase. The viral RNA polymerase then synthesizes negative-stranded RNA templates, which can function in the synthesis of both viral progeny genomes and viral mRNAs. Unlike what is found with the picornaviruses, however, the viral genome is not the only virus-specific mRNA made in infected cells. A second, subgenomic mRNA is used to direct the synthesis of the viral structural proteins. This mRNA appears to be identical in sequence to the 3′ third of the viral genome. The production of a separate mRNA for the viral structural proteins allows independent control of the abundance of the enzymatic viral proteins and the structural viral proteins.

As is the case with the picornaviruses, the number of polypeptide gene products produced during infection exceeds the number of viral mRNAs. Each mRNA encodes several proteins that are produced from large primary translates by proteolytic processing. Virus assembly occurs at the surface of the infected cell. As with all enveloped viruses, assembly involves the interaction of the nucleocapsid, in the cytoplasm, with a portion of a membrane that contains the viral glycoproteins.

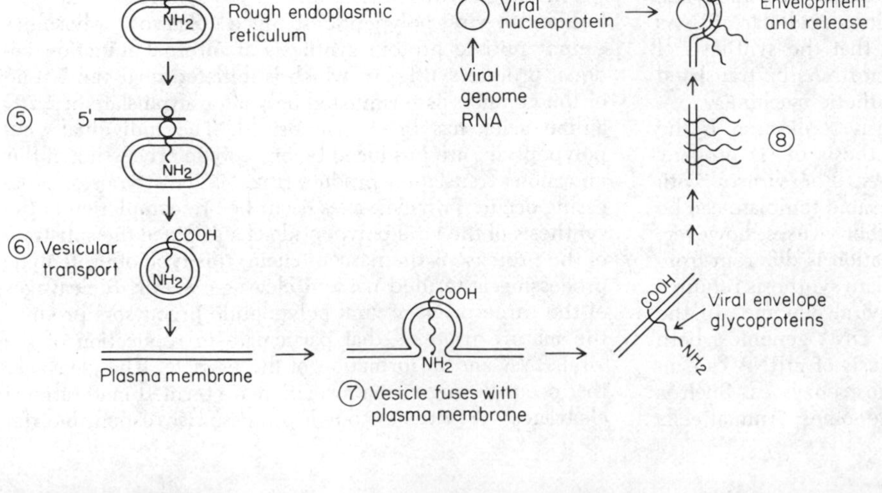

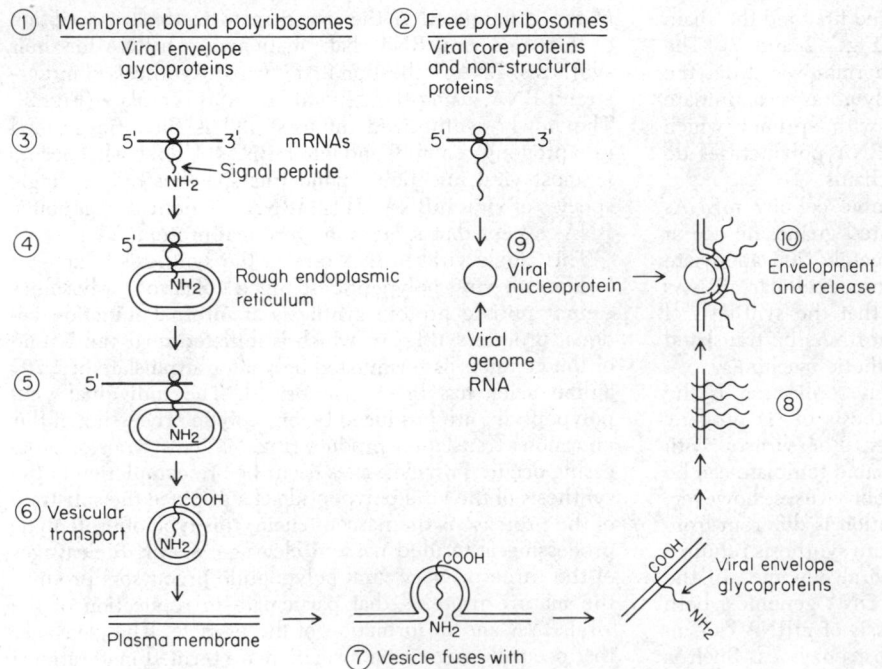

Figure 4. Formation of viral envelope glycoproteins and the assembly of enveloped viruses. See text for details.

In general, viral membrane proteins reach the site of virus maturation by a very different route from that of the internal components of the virus (Fig. 4). Viral membrane glycoproteins are synthesized with a leader or signal peptide at their amino termini, which functions as a sorting signal to direct the nascent polypeptide chain to the endoplasmic reticulum. As protein synthesis proceeds, most of the polypeptide chain is translocated across the membrane into the lumen of the endoplasmic reticulum. The viral mRNA therefore encodes both the primary sequence of the viral envelope glycoproteins and the information that initiates the transport of the protein to the cell surface.

In the membrane of the endoplasmic reticulum, the viral glycoproteins are anchored in an intracellular membrane in the same conformation that they assume at the cell surface—a portion of the polypeptide chain is exposed in the cytoplasm and most of the polypeptide chain is on the non-cytoplasmic (luminal) side of the membrane. From here they are transported, embedded in an intracellular membrane, to the site of virus assembly, which in most cases is the surface of the cell. The mechanism by which transport occurs is understood only incompletely but appears to resemble in many respects the transport of cellular plasma membrane glycoproteins, such as the histocompatibility antigens, to the surface of the cell. The mechanism of synthesis, modification, and transport of the two glycoproteins of the alphaviruses through the Golgi apparatus to the cell surface appears to be a good model for the process by which the glycoproteins of all enveloped viruses reach the site of virus assembly.

Virion assembly has two steps. First, the single internal viral structural protein assembles with the newly synthesized viral genome in the cytosol and an icosahedral nucleocapsid is formed (Fig. 4). The nucleocapsid then binds to regions of the plasma membrane that contain the viral glycoproteins. Recognition of such portions of the membrane almost certainly involves protein:protein interaction between the surface of the nucleocapsid and the tail of the viral membrane protein that is exposed on the cytoplasmic face of the membrane. The nucleocapsid then becomes enveloped in a membrane consisting of cellular lipids and viral glycoproteins (Fig. 5). Like the assembly of viruses in the cytoplasm, envelopment of viruses is most probably an example of self-assembly. The driving force is the strength of the interaction of the viral nucleocapsid with the readily deformable lipid bilayer. Virus is released by a process that resembles in certain respects the entry of the virus into the cellular cytoplasm, only here the polarity is reversed. The process must involve some form of fusion between membranes but is not understood in any detail. The result of this process is the release of mature virus into the extracellular fluid and reconstitution of an impermeable cellular plasma membrane. Lysis of the infected cell is not necessary for virus release. Production of enveloped viruses by a process of budding through the plasma membrane is a mechanism that permits persistent virus infection. Release of the virus from the host cell is not necessarily injurious and, provided inhibition of essential host cell functions does not occur, virus production and cell replication can co-exist. The process by which the alphaviruses assemble and are released from the host cell is essentially the same as the mechanism employed by all enveloped viruses except the herpesviruses and the poxviruses.

Coronaviruses. The coronaviruses are large, pleomorphic enveloped viruses with unusually large, positive-stranded genomes. Genome size is estimated to approach

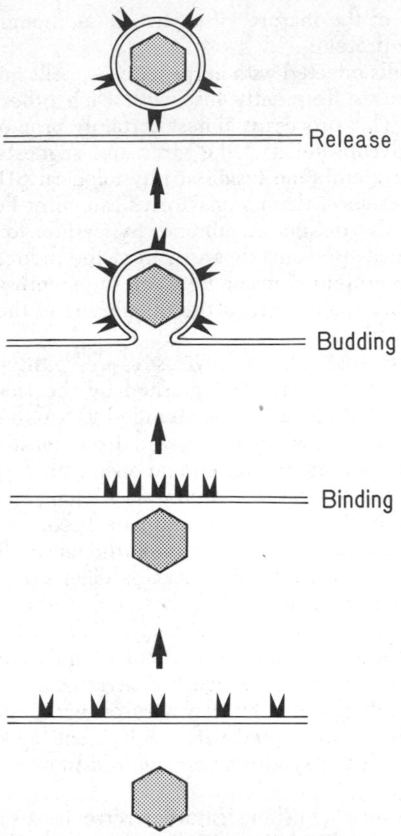

Figure 5. Enveloped viruses assemble in cellular membranes and exit from the cytoplasm in a process called budding. The envelopement of membrane-containing viruses occurs in cellular membranes. The preformed viral nucleocapsid binds tightly to regions of a membrane containing the viral glycoproteins. Additional viral glycoproteins accumulate at the site and the nucleocapsid becomes enveloped as a result of the strength of the interaction between the internal and external viral components. Virus release involves membrane fusion and leads to reconstitution of the cellular membrane. The process is essentially the reverse of the mechanism of entry employed by the same viruses (see Fig. 1). The mechanisms by which viruses that mature at the plasma membrane and viruses that mature at internal membranes are formed are fundamentally the same.

20,000 nucleotides. These viruses have been isolated from most species of vertebrates and cause diverse diseases. They are a frequent cause of colds in humans. Fundamentally, the replication of the coronaviruses resembles that of the other positive-stranded viruses. There are, however, a number of distinguishing features. First, coronaviruses use many viral mRNAs to direct the synthesis of the viral proteins. These comprise an overlapping, co-terminal family, with the sequences of any mRNA being contained entirely in all of the larger mRNAs. The use of multiple mRNAs permits precise control of the abundance of the viral gene products. Little proteolytic processing occurs in polypeptide production. Rather, most of the mRNAs direct the synthesis of a single gene product.

Virus maturation is also unusual. Unlike most enveloped viruses, which assemble at the plasma membrane of the infected cell and are released directly into the extracellular fluid, the coronaviruses assemble at intracellular membranes and the enveloped particles are therefore released into intracellular vesicles. Although this process releases the virus from the cytoplasm of the infected cell, it does not lead to escape from the cell. This appears to occur by secretion of the mature virus particle as though it were a secretory protein.

Like cells infected with herpesviruses, cells infected with coronaviruses frequently fuse with each other and form syncytia. This process is almost certainly promoted by the surface glycoproteins of the virus and suggests that they can cause membrane fusion at physiological pH. It seems likely, therefore, that coronaviruses can enter host cells by fusion at the plasma membrane. Syncytium formation by infected cells presumably arises from the induction by the viral glycoprotein of fusion between the membranes of two cells, rather than between the membrane of the virus and that of a cell.

Retroviruses. The retroviruses are positive-stranded RNA viruses that are distinguished by the fact that they replicate by using a double-stranded DNA intermediate. These viruses have been isolated from most vertebrate species. Rare examples have rapid oncogenic activity. Most isolates cause leukemia, but only after a long latent period. Occasionally, the viral DNA template becomes integrated into the chromosomes of cells of the germ line and is passed on to descendants in a mendelian manner. Retroviruses that are acquired by inheritance rather than infection are termed endogenous viruses. They are ubiquitous in many animal populations, particularly mice and domestic fowl. Recent evidence suggests that humans too are susceptible to infection by retroviruses with one virus of humans being associated with adult T cell leukemia, and another with the syndrome of acquired immunodeficiency (AIDS).

Another distinguishing feature of retroviruses is that they are biochemically diploid. They contain two identical single-stranded RNAs of approximately 9,000 nucleotides and a diverse collection of small cellular RNAs. Whether these viruses are functionally diploid is not known. Synthesis of the DNA intermediate requires an enzyme that will copy RNA into DNA. This is a reaction that does not occur in uninfected cells and is carried out during retroviral infection by a virus-coded RNA-dependent DNA polymerase called reverse transcriptase. Perhaps surprisingly, the first step in viral replication, following entry and uncoating, is not use of the positive-stranded genome as an mRNA to direct the synthesis of the reverse transcriptase. Rather, the reverse transcriptase is contained in the viral particle.

Like all DNA polymerases, reverse transcriptase requires a primer to initiate synthesis. This primer is a cellular transfer RNA that is base-paired to a site very near the 5′ end of the viral genome. It is here that DNA synthesis is initiated and synthesis continues until the end of the viral genome is encountered. Synthesis is necessarily discontinuous since the end of the genome is less than 150 nucleotides from the site of initiation of DNA synthesis. The initiated chain is then transposed to the 3′ end of one of the genomic subunits—where it anneals by virtue of the terminal redundancy of the genome—and synthesis is continued. The final product of DNA synthesis is a double stranded DNA molecule which is 300 to 1300 nucleotides longer than its RNA template (Fig. 6). The termini of this molecule are identical and the repeated structure is called the long terminal repeat (LTR) in order to distinguish it from the short terminal repeat in the genome.

With high efficiency, the DNA intermediate with two LTRs is integrated into the chromosomal DNA of the host cell. This integration is precise in that the ends of the LTRs always constitute the ends of the integrated DNA. The integrated DNA is called the provirus, in analogy with the integrated form of a bacteriophage genome, which is

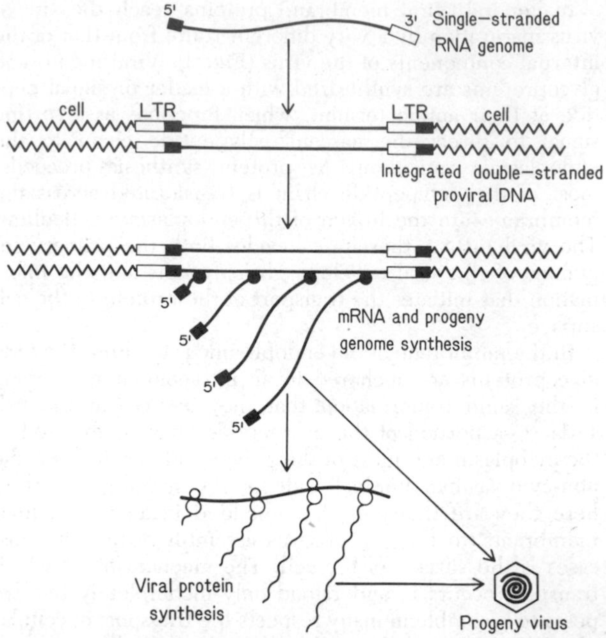

Figure 6. The retrovirus life-cycle. The single-stranded RNA genome of the retroviruses is transcribed into double-stranded DNA by the virion-associated reverse transcriptase. When integrated into chromosomal DNA, the viral DNA, or provirus, is longer than the RNA from which it is derived. The two ends of the provirus are identical and arise from duplication of sequence information present at both the 5′ and the 3′ ends of the genome. The provirus is the template for the synthesis of viral mRNA and viral genomes by a cellular RNA polymerase.

called a prophage. The site of integration of the provirus in the chromosome of the host cell is apparently random.

Progeny genomes and viral mRNAs are synthesized by a cellular RNA polymerase. The promoter for RNA synthesis is present in the LTR. Retroviruses specify 3 mRNAs. Two of these resemble cellular mRNAs in that they are encoded by non-contiguous regions of the provirus and are produced by splicing of a larger precursor. One mRNA is identical in sequence to the viral genome. All of the viral structural proteins are produced by proteolytic processing of precursor proteins. Assembly and envelopment of the virus occur at the plasma membrane and are in no way damaging to the cell. With few exceptions, retroviruses are not cytocidal and establish a persistent infection. Retrovirus production can occur for years with no obvious deleterious effects to the infected cell.

The acutely transforming retroviruses carry additional genetic information not present in the genomes of their more benign relatives. The genes responsible for transforming activity are cellular in origin and have entered the viral genome as a result of illegitimate recombination between the provirus and cellular DNA. They play no role whatsoever in viral replication.

NEGATIVE-STRANDED RNA VIRUSES

As is implied by their name, the negative-stranded RNA viruses have single-stranded RNA genomes that are complementary to the viral mRNA. The rhabdoviruses, the paramyxoviruses, the orthomyxoviruses and the bunyaviruses are the best studied of this class of virus. All of these viruses are enveloped and all package their genomes in helical nucleocapsids.

The replication of a negative-stranded virus requires a viral RNA-dependent RNA polymerase. Since the genome is the opposite sense to the viral mRNAs, it cannot direct the synthesis of such an enzyme. mRNA for a replicase can only arise by transcription of the genome. However, synthesis of mRNA for the viral transcriptase cannot occur in the absence of the viral transcriptase. This apparent predicament is avoided because the viral RNA polymerase is incorporated in the virus particle. Thus, the necessity of synthesizing a viral enzyme at the onset of infection is circumvented and RNA synthesis can commence as soon as the particle is uncoated.

Rhabdoviruses. Rhabdoviruses are rod- or bullet-shaped enveloped viruses of moderate size. Vesicular stomatitis virus and rabies virus are the best known members of this group. The rhabdovirus particle is simple in composition, consisting of only five species of polypeptide, the lipids in the viral envelope and a single piece of genomic RNA containing approximately 11,400 nucleotides. In fact, the proteins found in the virion are the only viral gene products. The first step in viral replication is the synthesis of viral mRNA by the virion-associated polymerase. Rhabdoviruses specify 5 mRNAs (Fig. 7). Each encodes one of the five proteins found in the virion. Unlike the multiple mRNAs produced in coronavirus-infected cells, the rhabdovirus mRNAs do not overlap in sequence. Both structural proteins and the two polypeptide components of the viral RNA polymerase are synthesized. Because each mRNA encodes only a single gene product, essentially no proteolytic processing of the proteins is needed.

Synthesis of progeny minus-strand genomes requires a full-length positive-strand template. The products of primary viral RNA synthesis, the viral mRNAs, cannot function as templates in this process since they each contain only a portion of the viral genetic information. Replication of the genome, therefore, requires the synthesis of another form of positive-stranded RNA—one which is a copy of the complete viral genome. Whether this process is carried out by the same enzyme that synthesizes the sub-genomic mRNAs is not known.

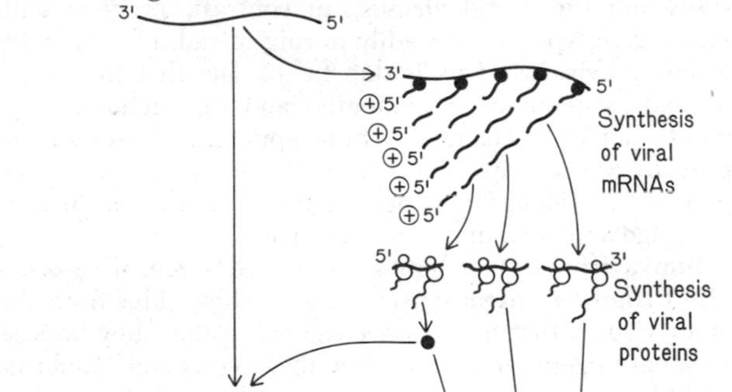

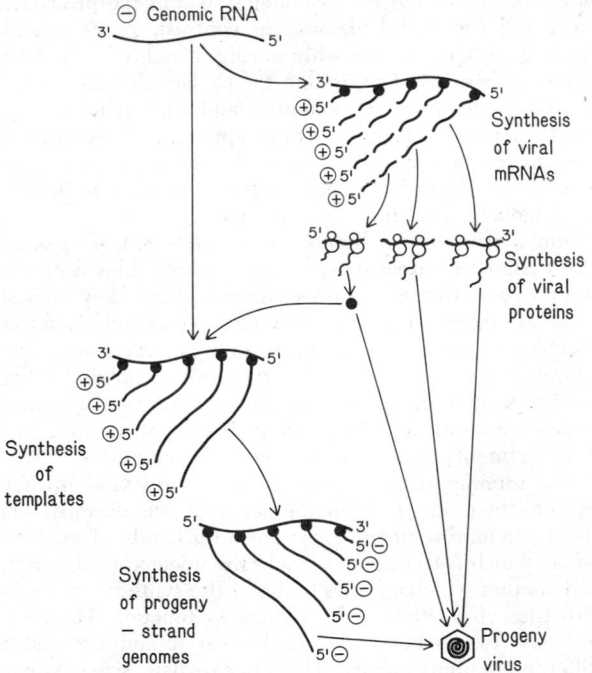

Figure 7. Rhabdovirus replication. The negative-stranded genome of the infecting rhabdovirus has two functions at the onset of infection. First, it serves as template for the synthesis of five subgenomic plus-stranded mRNAs by the virion-associated RNA polymerase. Secondly, it serves as template for the synthesis of a full-length plus-strand RNA. This full length RNA does not function as mRNA but rather is used as template for the synthesis of progeny viral genomes. The 5 subgenomic RNAs direct the synthesis of the 5 viral proteins.

The helical viral nucleocapsid is assembled in the cytoplasm of the cell. In addition to the single internal structural protein of the virus, the two polypeptide components of the viral RNA polymerase must be incorporated into the maturing particle. The nucleocapsid interacts with a portion of the plasma membrane that contains on its surface the single viral membrane glycoprotein and on its cytoplasmic face a viral matrix protein. The interaction of the nucleocapsid with such a portion of the cellular plasma membrane drives envelopment and release of progeny virions from the infected cell.

Paramyxoviruses. Measles and mumps viruses are the clinically most important members of the paramyxovirus group. These viruses, however, are difficult to study in cell culture systems. For this reason, much of our information about the biochemistry of paramyxovirus replication is derived from studies of simian and avian paramyxoviruses.

In many respects, paramyxoviruses resemble rhabdoviruses, particularly in their mode of replication. The principal difference between the paramyxoviruses and the rhabdoviruses is found in the structure and the function of their membrane glycoproteins. Whereas the rhabdoviruses possess a single surface protein that carries out both binding the virus to the host cell receptor and induction of fusion of the viral membrane with the membrane of an endosome, receptor binding and membrane fusion are carried out by separate paramyxovirus proteins. These proteins are termed HN and F. Binding is a property of the HN protein which interacts with a cell surface receptor containing sialic acid. This protein is also a neuraminidase that catalyzes the hydrolysis of *N*-acetyl neuraminic acid, otherwise known as sialic acid, from oligosaccharide chains. The role of this activity in viral replication is uncertain. It does, however, reduce the tendency of progeny virions to rebind to cells which have already been infected. The F protein catalyzes membrane fusion and hence is responsible for penetration of the virus into the host cell. It is the best example of a viral glycoprotein that can induce membrane fusion at physiological pH.

The F protein has two forms. One, termed F_o, is a single polypeptide chain that is inactive in promoting membrane fusion. Proteolytic processing of F_o activates it. The two polypeptides produced by the proteolytic activation, F_1 and F_2, remain together as a heterodimer. The protease that activates F_o is cellular in origin. Cells that lack such a protease can be infected but produce noninfectious virus particles. As a result, infection of such cells is generally limited and populations of cells lacking an appropriate protease are relatively resistant to infection.

The replication of paramyxoviruses resembles the replication of the rhabdoviruses. mRNA synthesis is initiated by a virion-associated RNA polymerase. A family of non-overlapping sub-genomic mRNAs is produced, each of which encodes a single viral polypeptide. Formation of the helical nucleocapsid occurs in the cytoplasm and assembly of the mature, enveloped particle occurs at the plasma membrane.

Orthomyxoviruses. The functions of the enveloped glycoproteins of the orthomyxoviruses and the paramyxovi-

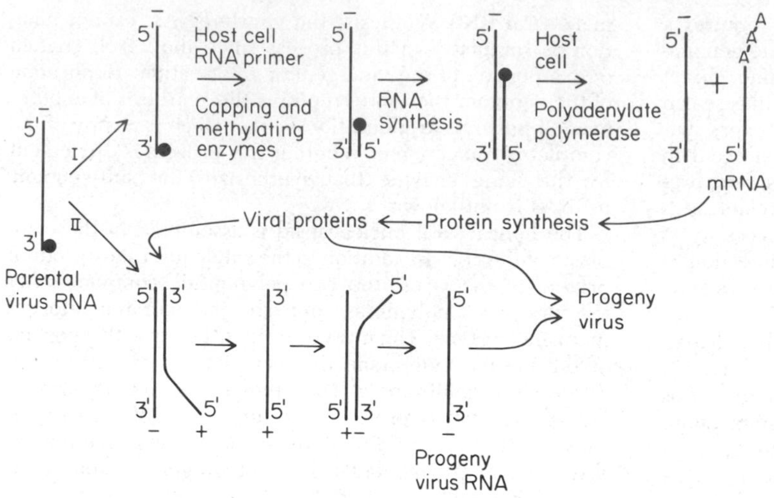

Figure 8. Replication of influenza virus RNA. Pathway I. Viral messenger RNAs are synthesized by the virion-contained RNA transcriptase (●), using the parental genome RNAs as templates. Proteins encoded by these messengers form an RNA polymerase. This enzyme synthesizes positive-stranded RNA copies of each of the segments of the parental genome (pathway II). These positive strands serve as templates for progeny negative-stranded RNAs.

ruses are very similar. It is for this reason that these viruses were both originally termed myxoviruses. In contrast, the structures of the viral genomes are profoundly different. Orthomyxoviruses are large, enveloped viruses, which contain 8 segments of negative-stranded RNA. Unlike most other RNA viruses, they appear to replicate, at least partially, in the nucleus. Like the paramyxoviruses, they bind to a receptor that contains sialic acid. This is a property of a surface glycoprotein, the hemagglutinin or HA glycoprotein. They also contain a second viral glycoprotein, termed NA, which is a neuraminidase. Uptake occurs by endocytosis and the hemagglutinin promotes entry by membrane fusion after acidification of the endosome. The influenza viruses are orthomyxoviruses.

Like all negative-stranded viruses, the orthomyxoviruses carry a virion-associated RNA polymerase that synthesizes viral mRNA at the onset of infection. Orthomyxovirus mRNA synthesis, however, is unlike that which occurs with any other virus (Fig. 8). The 10 viral mRNAs are all shorter than the genomic segment that encodes them. Moreover, these mRNAs have heterogeneous 5′ ends. The heterogeneity results from the use of fragments from the capped 5′ ends of cellular RNA as primers for the viral mRNAs. A nuclease cleaves cellular RNA to generate capped oligonucleotides approximately 10 to 15 nucleotides long. These oligonucleotides, which are not complementary to the viral template RNA, then function as primers and are extended to generate the viral mRNAs. Because transcription is terminated before the end of the template has been reached, the nucleotide sequences at the 5′ ends of the templates are not represented in the mRNAs. Except for the missing terminal nucleotides, eight of the 10 mRNAs are essentially complete transcripts of the 8 genomic segments. The two additional mRNAs arise from splicing of two of the viral mRNAs to produce smaller mRNAs, which contain only a portion of the information encoded in the template. Apparently both the production of the primers for mRNA synthesis and the splicing of the two viral RNAs must occur in the nucleus and this is the reason that nuclear function is essential during the initial stages of orthomyxovirus infection. Like the mRNAs of the rhabdoviruses and the paramyxoviruses, each orthomyxovirus mRNA encodes a single viral gene product.

Replication of the genome requires the use of plus-strand templates. The viral mRNAs cannot serve this purpose since they lack sequences complementary to the 5′ termini of the genomic segments. Consequently, plus-strand templates that are complete copies of the genomic RNAs must also be made.

The assembly of the helical nucleocapsid of the orthomyxoviruses is a potentially difficult task. An infectious particle must contain all eight genomic RNAs. How at least one copy of each segment is incorporated into the maturing particles is not understood. Maturation of the virion occurs at the plasma membrane where the nucleocapsid is enveloped by a portion of the membrane containing the two viral glycoproteins, HA and NA, and an internal viral membrane or matrix protein termed M.

Progeny carrying genetic traits derived from two parental viruses arise only very rarely during infection with viruses with non-segmented RNA genomes such as the picornaviruses and the rhabdoviruses. In contrast, progeny with mixed genotypes arise readily during mixed infection with orthomyxoviruses. This is due to the fact that the orthomyxovirus genome is segmented and that genomic segments can be exchanged. These apparently recombinant progeny are perhaps better termed re-assortants since the process by which they are produced does not involve breakage and rejoining of nucleic acid.

Bunyaviruses. The bunyaviruses are a recently recognized family of insect-borne viruses. They differ from the other viruses that have insect vectors in that they possess segmented genomes. Rift Valley fever virus and California encephalitis virus are members of this very large virus group. The virus particle is very simple, containing two species of membrane glycoprotein, one internal structural protein, a viral RNA-dependent RNA polymerase, and three segments of negative-stranded genomic RNA.

The number of viral gene products and viral mRNAs exceeds the number of genomic segments significantly. The small genomic segment gives rise to a family of mRNAs, one of which is translated to yield the nucleocapsid protein and another which appears to direct the synthesis of a nonstructural viral polypeptide of unknown function. The genes for these two proteins apparently overlap and are read in different reading frames. The intermediate size genomic segment encodes the two viral glycoproteins and, by elimination, the largest segment encodes the viral polymerase.

The structure of the genomic segments is novel. They appear circular when examined by electron microscopy. The circles are not covalently closed because denaturation renders each of the segments linear. The circular structure observed in the native segment results from the 5′ end of each segment being complementary to the 3′ end of the same segment. Annealing of these two ends leads to formation of a circular molecule held together by a double-stranded panhandle. A necessary consequence of this complementarity is that the 3′ ends of both the plus-strand and the minus-strand RNAs are identical in sequence. The nucleotide sequence recognized during initiation of transcription of both the plus and minus strands should therefore be identical and could be carried out by a single viral polymerase. Use of a single viral enzyme to synthesize all of the forms of viral RNA is clearly of advantage to a virus with limited genetic information.

As is observed with the orthomyxoviruses, mixed infection leads to frequent release of recombinant progeny. Exchange of genomic segments apparently occurs readily.

VIRUSES CONTAINING DOUBLE-STRANDED RNA GENOMES

Reoviruses, rotaviruses, and the orbiviruses comprise the reovirus family. These viruses have genomes which consist of 10 to 12 segments of double-stranded RNA. They are icosahedral in structure, containing two layers of structural protein, and are not enveloped. Like other RNA viruses, their replication requires an RNA-dependent RNA polymerase. Since their genomic segments cannot function as mRNAs, being double-stranded, reoviruses carry their own RNA polymerase in the virion. The reoviruses are taken up by endocytosis and activation of the virion-associated RNA polymerase may result from fusion of the endocytotic vesicle with lysosomes and proteolytic digestion of the outer layer of the virion by lysosomal proteases.

The virion-associated RNA polymerase synthesizes plus-stranded RNA in the partially-uncoated viral core in a manner analagous to the synthesis of RNA on a double-stranded DNA template (Fig. 9). That is, the parental double strands are conserved and the progeny strand is released from the viral core. The released plus-stranded RNA then first serves as mRNA for the synthesis of both the viral structural proteins and additional viral RNA polymerase subunits and is then packaged into nascent core particles. Here it is transcribed once by newly synthesized viral RNA polymerase to yield progeny double-stranded genomes. These can in turn serve as templates for the synthesis of more viral mRNA. Again, synthesis of plus-strand RNA is conservative, and involves no displacement of either of the strands of the template.

As with the orthomyxoviruses, it is not understood how the virion accomplishes faithful packaging of one copy each of the 10 to 12 genomic subunits in each progeny virion. It is clear, however, that this sorting of subunits occurs when the positive-stranded single strands of RNA are assembling into pre-virions. Virus assembly occurs in the cytoplasm and virus release follows lysis of the infected cell. Recombinant progeny are produced during mixed infection because of exchange of genomic segments.

VIRUSES CONTAINING DNA GENOMES

Papovaviruses. The papovaviruses are small, icosahedral, nonenveloped viruses with circular, double-stranded DNA genomes. Included in this group are SV40 virus, a monkey virus; mouse polyomavirus; JC virus and BK virus, two human viruses; and the wart or papillomaviruses. The replication of the papillomaviruses is much less well understood than is that of the other members of this group. It is clear, however, that the papillomaviruses differ fundamentally from the best studied members of this family, SV40 virus and mouse polyomavirus (see Chapter 62), and they will not be discussed in this chapter.

The genome of the polyomaviruses is very small. It contains only 5200 base-pairs of DNA. These viruses encode only a very limited number of proteins and must therefore depend greatly on host cell enzymes for replication. Mouse polyomavirus binds to a receptor containing sialic acid and probably is taken up by endocytosis. As with other viruses with DNA genomes, papovavirus gene expression is subject to temporal control. Before replication of the viral genome, only half of the genome is expressed. This phase of the replication cycle is referred to as early. After the onset of viral DNA synthesis, the other half of the genome, which encodes the viral structural proteins, is expressed. This is the so-called late phase of viral replication. The viral particle contains a single major structural protein and two minor ones. Approximately half of the genetic information in the genome is used to encode these three proteins.

Papovaviruses, and most other viruses with DNA genomes, replicate in the nucleus of the host cell. Papovaviruses depend heavily on host cell functions for both the replication of the viral genome and for the synthesis and processing of the viral mRNAs, all of which are normally carried out in the nucleus. Presumably as a means by which to facilitate viral DNA replication, the papovaviruses stimulate cellular DNA replication and induce the synthesis of all the cellular enzymes involved in DNA synthesis. How this occurs is not known.

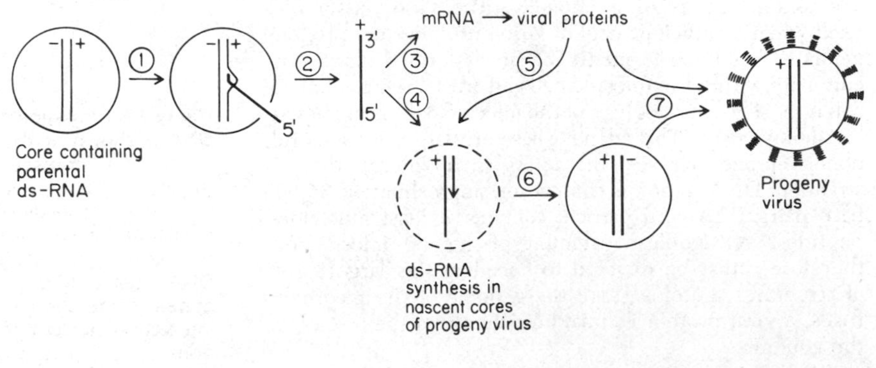

Figure 9. Replication of reovirus double-stranded RNAs. Following lysosomal uncoating, the core, containing parental double-stranded (ds) RNA, is released into the cytoplasmic matrix (*encircled 1*). Enzymes within the core synthesize and export single-stranded RNA plus strands (*encircled 2*). Progeny plus strands serve as messengers (*encircled 3*) for the synthesis of viral proteins (*encircled 5*), or as templates (*encircled 4*) for double-stranded RNA formation. Completed cores (*encircled 6*) containing all ten segments of double-stranded RNA combine with outer capsid proteins (*encircled 7*) to form progeny virions. See text for further details.

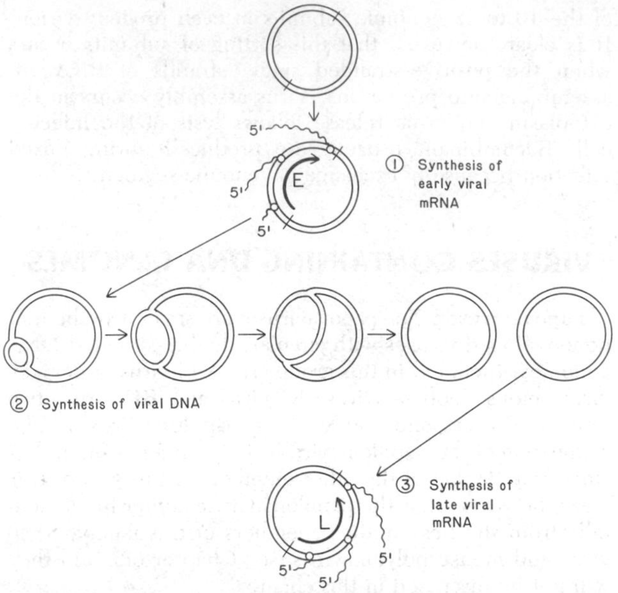

Figure 10. Papovavirus replication. In the nucleus of the infected cell, the region of the papovavirus genome encoding the early proteins, labeled E, is transcribed by cellular enzymes to yield two or three transcripts (step 1). One of these encodes the large T antigen. The large T antigen stimulates both the replication of the viral DNA genome (step 2) and the expression of the region of the genome encoding the viral structural proteins (step 3).

Early in infection, only the region of the genome encoding a protein termed the large T antigen is expressed (Fig. 10). The transcription of the early region of the genome is presumably carried out by a cellular RNA polymerase. Large T antigen initiates both viral DNA synthesis and the expression of the region of the viral genome encoding the structural proteins. With the exception of large T antigen, all the enzymes involved in the replication and expression of the viral genome appear to be cellular. The limited amount of genetic information in the viral genome is used with enormous efficiency. Some viral genes overlap. This is true of both the gene for large T antigen, which also encodes a second viral protein of unknown function termed small T antigen, and a region of the genome that encodes a short stretch of all three structural proteins. Five viral mRNAs direct the synthesis of the five SV40 virus gene products. These arise from two primary transcripts, one produced early and one produced late, which are then spliced to yield 2 and 3 mRNAs, respectively.

Replication of the circular genome is initiated at a single site and proceeds bidirectionally. The virion assembles itself when a sufficient pool of virion proteins and progeny genomes has been formed. The newly-formed viruses accumulate within the infected cell and are released following cell lysis. The cause of lysis of the infected cells is unknown.

Adenoviruses. The adenoviruses are large, icosahedral, nonenveloped viruses that possess a linear, double-stranded DNA genome comprising approximately 35,000 base pairs. The viral particle contains at least nine polypeptides. A significant amount of genetic information, therefore, must be devoted to encoding this large family of structural proteins. Like the genome of the picornaviruses, a viral protein is linked covalently to the 5′ ends of the genome.

Adenovirus gene expression occurs sequentially. Many distinct sets of early, intermediate, and late RNA transcripts are produced. The proteins encoded by some of the early genes apparently induce the expression of the late viral genes. Most of the viral structural proteins are encoded by a family of mRNAs that are all derived from a single precursor RNA (Fig. 11). This precursor RNA undergoes two fundamentally different forms of processing. For one, it undergoes splicing. A tripartite leader sequence is juxtaposed to any of the several regions of the precursor that encode the individual late gene products. For another, it is cleaved at a number of specific sites downstream from the coding regions and polyadenylated. As many as 20 different late mRNAs are produced from a single precursor RNA. All contain the same leader RNA but differ in their coding regions and their sites of polyadenylation.

Both viral mRNA synthesis and viral genome replication appear to be carried out largely by cellular enzymes in the nucleus of the infected cell. The linear adenovirus genome necessarily undergoes a different mode of replication from that of the circular papovavirus genome (Fig. 12). The terminal protein may play a role in the initiation of the synthesis of progeny strands. A single daughter strand is synthesized on the double-stranded template, displacing the parental strand that is of the same sequence. The displaced single strand then serves as a single-stranded template for the synthesis of a complementary strand and a linear, double-stranded molecule is regenerated.

Adenoviruses are released from infected cells by lysis. Infection is usually cytocidal. On rare occasions, cells transformed by adenovirus have been isolated. These invariably contain only an incomplete virus genome. Present in all adenovirus-transformed cells, however, are two specific early viral genes whose products may play a role in cellular transformation.

Parvoviruses. The parvoviruses are very small, stable, icosahedral, nonenveloped viruses with single-stranded DNA genomes. They have only recently been linked to disease in humans. Adeno-associated virus, minute virus of mice, and B19 virus are the best known members of this group.

The parvoviruses appear to encode two structural proteins and one or two nonstructural proteins. The functions of the nonstructural proteins are unknown. It is suspected

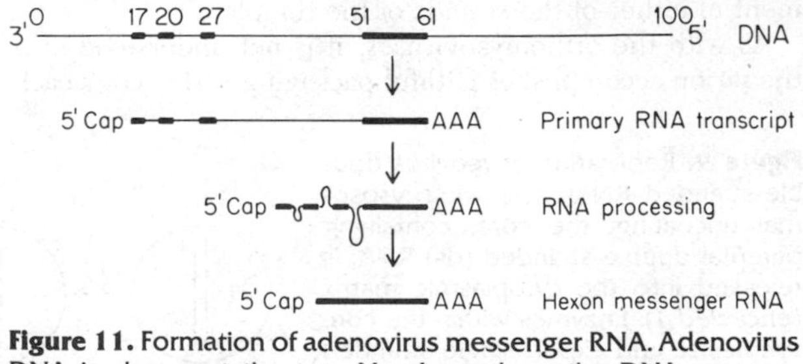

Figure 11. Formation of adenovirus messenger RNA. Adenovirus DNA is shown at the top. Numbers along the DNA are map coordinates representing the percentage of the distance from the left to the right ends of the DNA of any specific nucleotide sequence. For instance, the bulk of the hexon messenger RNA is encoded by the segment of DNA that lies between 51 and 61 per cent of the distance from the 3′ to the 5′ ends of the DNA. Heavy lines (———) = DNA or RNA sequences that appear in the completed messenger RNA. Light lines (——) = intervening nucleotide sequences. See text for further explanation.

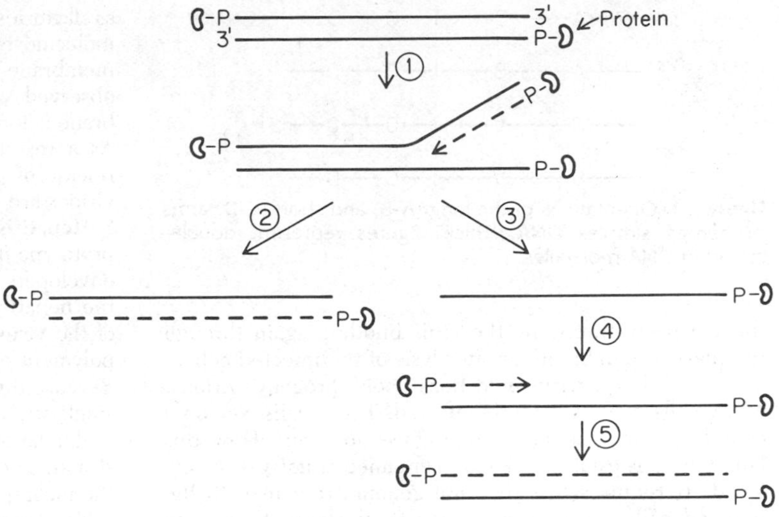

Figure 12. Replication of adenovirus DNA. Solid lines (———) signify parental DNA strands. Dotted lines (---) indicate newly synthesized DNA. DNA synthesis is initiated at the 3′ end of one strand of the double-stranded DNA molecule (*encircled 1*). An adenovirus protein-nucleotide complex may be required to initiate DNA replication. Completion of DNA elongation produces one double-stranded progeny DNA molecule (*encircled 2*) and one single-stranded parental DNA molecule (*encircled 3*). A complementary DNA strand is formed on the parental single strand (*encircled 4*), giving a second molecule of double-stranded DNA (*encircled 5*).

that they play a role in replication of the viral genome. Parvoviruses are unusually dependent on the host cell. Nondividing cells cannot be infected with parvoviruses, presumably because they do not contain enzymes essential for the replication of the parvovirus genome. Unlike the papovaviruses, the parvoviruses appear unable to induce the host cell to express the functions on which it depends.

Three viral mRNAs direct the synthesis of the three or four viral gene products. Two mRNAs are apparently produced by differential splicing of a single, full-length transcript of the viral genome. The other is produced by initiation at an internal site.

Replication of the single-stranded DNA genome necessarily proceeds by a process different from that by which double-stranded DNA genomes are replicated. The genome serves as the primer for its own replication. This is possible because the termini of the genome are novel. They each consist of two blocks of DNA which are the complements of each other. Both ends can therefore form structures called hairpins and the base-paired 3′ end can be extended by a DNA polymerase to copy the genome. This mode of replication deals efficiently with the problem of a primer for the DNA polymerase but in its simplest form is reductive and unable to yield complete progeny genomes. Complete viral genomes are produced through a complicated process involving site-specific nuclease action and strand displacement.

Herpesviruses. Herpesviruses are relatively large, spherical, enveloped viruses. They contain an icosahedral core and a very large—approximately 150,000 base pairs—double-stranded linear DNA genome. The DNA is packaged in the form of a toroid wound around a spool. Herpes simplex virus, cytomegalovirus, Epstein-Barr virus, and varicella-zoster virus are the best known members of this group.

The virus most probably enters by fusion of its envelope with the plasma membrane of the host cell. This seems likely because infection with herpesviruses frequently leads to extensive fusion of infected cells with one another. As discussed above, fusion of cells late in infection usually results from the insertion into the cellular plasma membrane of a viral glycoprotein, which can promote membrane fusion at physiological pH. Since a herpesvirus membrane protein can catalyze fusion late in infection, it is highly likely that it performs this same function at the onset of infection.

Herpesviruses replicate in the nucleus of the infected cell. Transcription appears to be carried out, at least initially, by a cellular RNA polymerase. This is suggested most strongly by the fact that herpesvirus genomic DNA is itself infectious. Subsequent viral gene expression is strictly controlled. At least three classes of viral gene products have been defined and they are expressed sequentially. The first of these, termed alpha proteins, are required for the expression of the genes encoding the beta proteins. The beta proteins are required, in turn, for the expression of the genes encoding the gamma proteins. The site of action of a number of the viral proteins, therefore, appears to be the nucleus. As a consequence, the proteins must migrate to the nucleus after their synthesis on polysomes in the cytoplasm. Because virus assembly begins in the nucleus, this is also the case for many of the viral structural proteins.

Elucidation of the mechanism of viral genome replication has been hampered by the variable structure of the genome. Four equally abundant isomers have been detected. The genome has two domains, termed L and S, which can be organized in any of four configurations (Fig. 13). Virus-coded enzymes play a prominent role in the replication of the genome. Notable among these are a viral DNA polymerase and a viral thymidine kinase. The thymidine kinase is not essential for the infection of all cells, but may facilitate viral DNA synthesis in quiescent cells. This enzyme has a noticeably broader substrate specificity than do cellular thymidine kinases and thus renders viral replication more sensitive to inhibition by nucleotide analogues such as E-5-(2-bromovinyl)-2′-deoxyuridine (BVDU) and 9-2(2-hydroxyethoxymethyl)guanine (acyclovir) than the replication of uninfected cells.

Virus assembly is a complex process. The virus assembles at least partially within the nucleus of the infected cell. Envelopment and exit from the nucleus may both occur by budding of the nascent virion through the inner lamella of nuclear membrane. The details of this process are not well understood. Budding through the nuclear membrane does not lead directly to the release of the virus from the infected cell. Release may occur by secretion of the preformed virion by way of the endoplasmic reticulum and

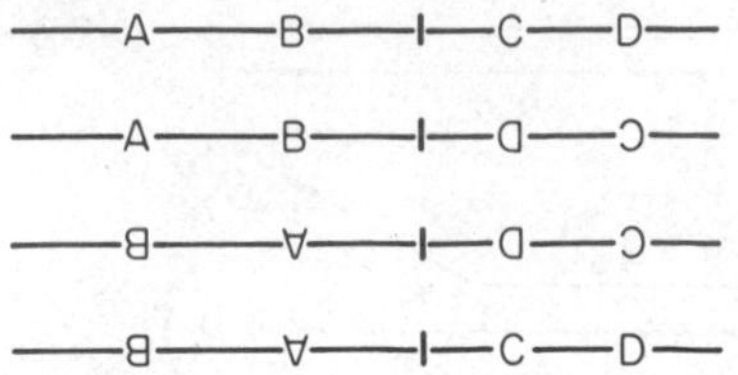

Figure 13. Orientations of the long (A-B) and short (C-D) arms of herpes simplex DNA. "Stick" figures represent double-stranded DNA molecules.

the Golgi apparatus, by the virus budding again through the plasma membrane, or after lysis of the infected cell.

Not all herpesvirus infections yield progeny virions. Many cells become latently infected. These cells contain a complete viral genome but produce no virus. How this latent state is established and maintained is not yet understood. It requires that the viral genome remain with the infected cell, either as a chromosomal element or as an episome that replicates as rapidly as the host cell, and that the expression of the viral genome be repressed.

Poxviruses. The poxviruses are by far the largest of all animal viruses. The brick-shaped viral particle is complex in structure, consisting of a viral core, lateral bodies, and an envelope. The virion contains approximately 30 structural polypeptides and a number of virus-coded enzymes. The genome of these viruses is correspondingly large, ranging in size from 120 to 200 million daltons. Although linear in structure, the two linear strands of the viral genome are cross-linked at their termini.

Poxviruses are unique among viruses with a DNA genome in that they replicate in the cytoplasm of the infected cell. Entry and uncoating occur in two steps. First, fusion of the viral envelope with the surface of the host cell or the membrane of an endosome releases the DNA-containing core of the virus into the cytoplasm. This activates the transcription of early viral genes by a virion-associated RNA polymerase. The product of one of these early mRNAs then regulates the further uncoating of the core of the virion (Fig. 14).

Viral DNA replicates and progeny virions are formed in circumscribed areas of the cytoplasm that are referred to as factories. The replication process of this enormous molecule is not well understood. Acquisition of the viral membrane occurs by a different mechanism from that observed with other enveloped viruses. The lipid membrane is formed in the cytoplasm by a process of accretion. As a result, envelopment does not lead immediately to release of the virus from the infected cell. Most progeny virions are released from the host cell only after cell lysis.

Hepatitis B Virus. Human hepatitis B virus is the prototype of a unique virus group. The virion is apparently enveloped and contains on its surface a protein carrying the hepatitis B surface antigen HBsAg. The nucleocapsid of the virus contains the hepatitis B core antigen, a DNA polymerase and a very unusual circular DNA genome. Because the genome consists of two linear, complementary single strands of DNA that are of unequal length, it contains both a large gap in the plus strand and a nick in the minus strand. The DNA-dependent DNA polymerase will extend the incomplete viral plus strand in vitro.

The means by which this novel genome is replicated seems to be as unusual as is the structure of the genome. This DNA virus appears to use a single-stranded RNA as an intermediate in DNA replication. Replication apparently involves copying of the minus strand of the DNA genome into plus-strand RNA, which can function as both mRNA and as template for the synthesis of minus-strand DNA. The minus-strand DNA produced by reverse transcription of the plus-strand RNA then serves as template for plus-strand synthesis. The initiation of DNA synthesis may involve a viral polypeptide that is found covalently linked to the terminus of the genomic DNA.

Unlike the disease induced by hepatitis A virus, a picornavirus, which is generally self-limited, infection by hepatitis B virus can progress to a chronic infection. This difference between the two diseases may derive from the fact that the genome of hepatitis B virus is DNA, and hence can be integrated into chromosomal DNA, and from the fact that the hepatitis B virus particle is enveloped, and hence can be released from the infected cell without cell death. Persistent infection with hepatitis A virus may be less likely simply because it is a nonenveloped virus with an RNA genome.

Novel Virus-Like Agents. There is considerable evidence

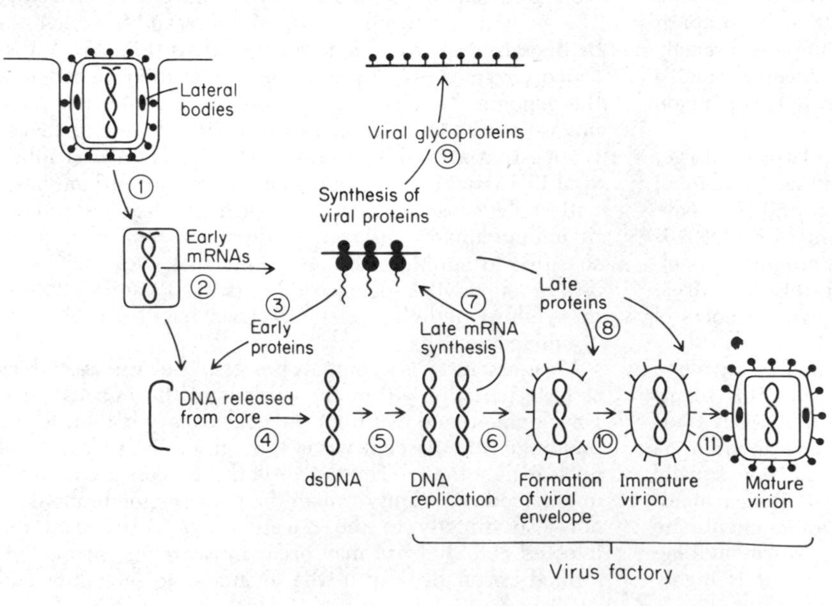

Figure 14. Poxvirus replication. Infecting virus is shown at upper left. Progeny virus at lower right. See text for an explanation of the numbered intermediate steps.

for the existence of infectious agents that are even more primitive than viruses. The degenerative neurological diseases Scrapie, Kuru, and Jakob-Creutzfeldt disease all may be caused by very small infectious agents for which the name prion has been proposed. The Scrapie agent appears to consist of protein, which is essential for infectivity, but to lack detectable nucleic acid. How such an entity might replicate is unclear at the present time. One possibility is that the agent is actually encoded by a cellular gene and, after entry into the host, is able to stimulate the synthesis of additional prion molecules. It is still possible, however, that the Scrapie agent is a very small, unusual virus.

Viroids comprise a second class of small, primitive infectious agents. Viroids are infectious molecules of RNA that have been found to cause a variety of diseases of plants. They appear to consist only of a single-stranded, circular, largely self-complementary molecule of RNA. It is unlikely that they encode a protein. As is the case with prions, it is not known how these agents replicate. Presumably they depend on host cell enzymes for their replication. This is reasonable because there is evidence that uninfected plant tissue contains enzymes that can replicate RNA. There is no evidence to date that viroids infect animals.

References

General

Fraenkel-Conrat, H., and Wagner, R. R.: Comprehensive Virology. Vols. 1–17. New York, Plenum Press, 1974–1977.

Luria, S. E., Darnell, J. E., Jr., Baltimore, D., and Campbell, A.: General Virology. New York, John Wiley and Sons, 1978.

Receptors for Viruses

Weiner, H. L., Powers, M. L., and Fields, B. N.: Absolute linkage of virulence and central nervous system cell tropism of reoviruses to viral hemagglutinin. J Infect Dis 141:609, 1980.

Virus Penetration

Helenius, A., Marsh, M., and White, J.: The entry of viruses into animal cells. Trends Biochem Sci 5:104, 1980.

Scheid, A., and Choppin, P. W.: Identification of biological activities of paramyxovirus glycoproteins. Activation of cell fusion, hemolysis, and infectivity by proteolytic cleavage of an inactive precursor protein of Sendai virus. Virology 57:475, 1974.

Picornaviruses

Kitamura, N., Semler, B. L., Tothberg, P. C., Larsen, G. R., Adler, C. J., Dorner, A. J., Emini, E. A., Hanecak, R., Lee, J. J., van der Werf, S., Anderson, C. W., and Wimmer, E.: Primary structure, gene organization and polypeptide expression of poliovirus RNA. Nature 291:547, 1981.

Alphaviruses

Strauss, E. G., Rice, C. M., and Strauss, J. H.: Complete nucleotide sequence of the genomic RNA of Sindbis virus. Virology 133:92, 1984.

Retroviruses

Bishop, J. M.: The molecular biology of RNA tumor viruses: a physician's guide. N Engl J Med 303:675, 1980.

Weiss, R., Teich, N., Varmus, H., and Coffin, J.: RNA Tumor Viruses. Cold Spring Harbor, Cold Spring Harbor Laboratory, 1982.

Rhabdoviruses

Banerjee, A. K., Abraham, G., and Colonno, R. J.: Vesicular stomatitis virus: mode of transcription. J Gen Virol 34:1, 1977.

Formation of Membranes of Enveloped Viruses

Rothman, J. E., and Lodish, H. F.: Synchronised transmembrane insertion and glycosylation of a nascent membrane protein. Nature 269:775, 1977.

Simons, K., and Garoff, H.: The budding mechanism of enveloped animal viruses. J Gen Virol 50:1, 1980.

Myxoviruses

Bouloy, M., Plotch, S. J., and Krug, R. M.: Globin mRNAs are primers for the transcription of influenza viral RNA in vitro. Proc Natl Acad Sci USA 75:4886, 1978.

Lamb, R. A., and Lai, C.-J.: Sequence of interrupted and uninterrupted mRNAs and cloned DNA coding for the two overlapping nonstructural proteins of influenza virus. Cell 21:475, 1980.

Reoviruses

Joklik, W. K.: Structure and function of the reovirus genome. Microbiol Rev 45:483, 1981.

Papovaviruses

Acheson, N. H.: Lytic cycle of SV40 and polyoma virus. In *DNA Tumor Viruses*. J. Tooze, ed. pp. 125–204. Cold Spring Harbor, Cold Spring Harbor Laboratory, 1980.

Adenoviruses

Flint, S. J., and Broker, T. R.: Lytic infection by adenoviruses. In *DNA Tumor Viruses*, J. Tooze, ed. pp. 443–546. Cold Spring Harbor, Cold Spring Harbor Laboratory, 1980.

Persson, J., and Philipson, L.: Regulation of adenovirus gene expression. Curr Topics Microbiol Immunol 97:157, 1982.

Parvoviruses

Rhode, S. L., and Paradiso, P. R.: Parvovirus genome: Nucleotide sequence of H-1 and mapping of its genes by hybrid-arrest translation. J Virol 45:173, 1983.

Herpesviruses

Roizman, B.: The organization of the herpes simplex virus genomes. Ann Rev Genet 13:25, 1979.

Poxviruses

Moss, B.: Poxviruses. In *The Molecular Biology of Animal Viruses*. Volume 2. pp. 849–890. D. P. Nayak, ed. New York. Marcel Dekker. 1978.

Hepatitis B Virus

Summers, J., and Mason, W. S.: Replication of the genome of a hepatitis B-like virus by reverse transcription of an RNA intermediate. Cell 29:403, 1982.

Prions and Viroids

Diener, T. O., McKinley, M. P., and Prusiner, S. B.: Viroids and prions. Proc Natl Acad Sci USA 79:5220, 1982.

Prusiner, S. B.: Novel proteinaceous infectious particles cause Scrapie. Science 216:136, 1982.

10

THE GENETICS OF VIRUSES

C. R. PRINGLE, B.SC., PH.D.

INTRODUCTION: THE SIGNIFICANCE OF VIRUS GENETICS. The science of virus genetics is concerned with the origin and mechanism of variation of viruses. The variability of viruses and the extent to which it is heritable have great importance for human medicine. The surface antigens of some viruses are inherently stable, and the diseases associated with these infectious agents can be controlled by vaccination (e.g., rubella, measles, rabies) or in exceptional circumstances even eradicated (e.g., smallpox). Other viruses exist as a range of antigenic types (e.g., the enteroviruses and rhinoviruses) or appear to change progressively in response to the development of immunity in their host (e.g., the antigenic drift of influenza virus). Control of these agents by vaccination is more difficult and ultimately may depend on accurate prediction of the potential evolution of the antigens of these viruses. Indeed, the design and development of appropriate influenza virus vaccines in anticipation of epidemics and even pandemics could become one of the principal applications of virus genetics in human medicine.

Viruses that cause diseases characterized by short incubation period, recurrent infection, and aviremia may be difficult to combat by vaccination and may be controllable only by chemotherapy. Suitable antiviral drugs have not been developed yet, and progress towards successful chemotherapy of virus infection depends on clear discrimination of virus-specific processes from those processes that are part of the biosynthetic apparatus of the host cell and essential for the viability of both the virus and its host. The isolation of virus mutants helps to identify these virus-specific processes, defining appropriate targets for pharmacologic attack and allowing a rational approach to antiviral chemotherapy.

Assessment of the oncogenic potential of a virus requires knowledge of the nature of its genome. To be oncogenic, the genome of the virus must exist as DNA at some stage to permit integration of viral information into the genome of the host cell and to produce a heritable change (transformation) in the growth properties of the cell. However, integration by itself does not invariably cause transformation and may not be obligatory in all cases. For example, the papillomaviruses exist in an episomal association with the genome of their host cell. Determination of what is critical for virus-induced transformation and oncogenesis requires additional analysis of the organization and function of the viral genome.

THE NATURE AND CODING CAPACITY OF VIRAL GENOMES. The viruses of man and animals exhibit great diversity of genome structure. From a genetic standpoint, viruses fall into three distinct categories: the *DNA-containing viruses*, the *RNA-containing viruses*, and the viruses endowed with reverse transcriptase (the *retroviruses*), whose genome alternates between RNA in the virion and proviral DNA in the host cell.

The DNA viruses, with the exception of the poxviruses, multiply in the nucleus of the host cell, and messenger RNA (mRNA) is transcribed by the host cell transcriptase. Hence, the naked genome of these viruses is infectious. The RNA viruses multiply predominantly in the cytoplasm, and since the host cell is unable to replicate RNA molecules, an RNA polymerase (or the information for its synthesis) must be introduced with the virus. It is an accepted convention to call a single-stranded RNA molecule the positive strand if it functions as the messenger for protein synthesis, and to call its complement the negative strand (or antimessage). The genome of RNA viruses may be represented by a positive or negative strand or both. The genome of positive-strand RNA viruses is infectious because it functions as mRNA for synthesis of the entire complement of viral proteins including the RNA replicase. The genome of negative-strand RNA viruses, on the other hand, is not infectious because it cannot replicate or be translated directly into protein. Consequently, the nucleocapsid of these viruses includes an RNA transcriptase to initiate synthesis of mRNA in the infected cell. The genome of retroviruses functions as mRNA and is therefore the positive strand; however, this RNA is not infectious, and the reverse transcriptase enzyme is a part of the structure of the virion. The proviral DNA form of these viruses is infectious, however.

The diverse nature of the viral genome can be rationalized by regarding the genome as a particular stage in the cycle of replication of nucleic acids sequestered in an extracellular particle. This concept is illustrated in Figure 1. The only stage, excluding the replicative intermediates, not represented in known viruses, is the RNA:DNA intermediate in the reverse transcription pathway.

The *information capacity* of the genome is determined by the universal coding assignment of three nucleotides per amino acid. Therefore, 1500 nucleotides (or nucleotide pairs in the case of double-stranded nucleic acid) are required for an average-sized protein of 500 amino acids. The information content of different viruses is indicated in Table 1, together with other characteristics that define the properties of the genome. The genomes of DNA viruses differ by as much as fiftyfold in coding capacity, whereas the RNA viruses vary only within a threefold range (or fourfold if the retroviruses are included). A large proportion of the genome of the large DNA viruses, e.g., herpes simplex virus, is concerned with regulation of DNA synthesis, since nearly half of all *ts* mutants (see Mutation and Mutants) have DNA-negative phenotypes. This is probably reflected in the complex biology of herpesviruses and their tendency to cause latent infection.

These estimates of the information content of the viral genome are minimum values and do not take account of proteolytic cleavage and other modifications of primary gene products. Analysis of the genome of the small single-stranded DNA bacteriophage ΦX174 has shown that polypeptides of entirely different amino acid sequence can be transcribed from the same polynucleotide by displacement of the triplet reading frame; thus gene E of ΦX174 lies entirely within gene D, and gene B within gene A. Similarly, functionally distinct gene products can be obtained by translation of mRNA from a fixed point with occasional read-through of a specific stop signal resulting in two polypeptides with overlapping sequences (e.g., the A and A′ proteins of bacteriophage Qβ). Many examples of expansion of coding capacity are now known in animal viruses: for instance, in the papovaviruses by reading of common genome sequence in different reading frames; the occurrence of overlapping genes in at least 2 of 8 subunits

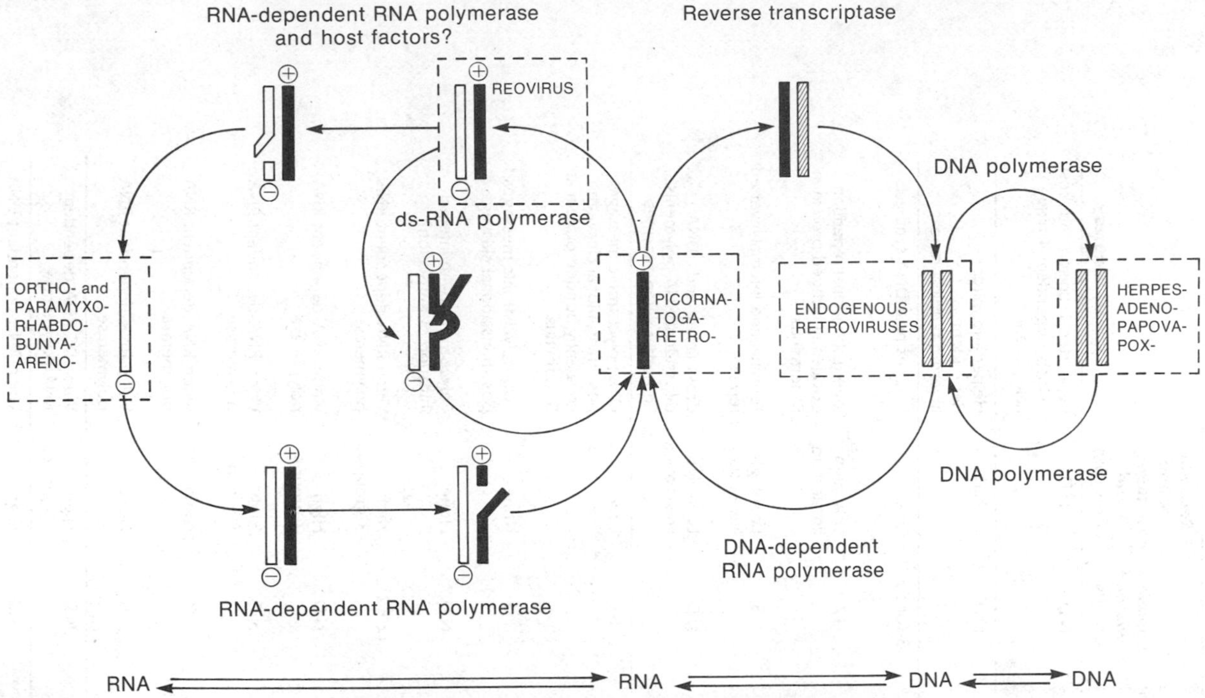

Figure 1. Replication of nucleic acid and sequestration of viral genome.

RNA replication follows the five-intermediate model proposed by Spiegelman. Reovirus replication follows a different path because there is no displacement of strands, and the parental duplex RNA is conserved. Positive strands are shown as black; negative strands are shown as white. DNA strands are indicated by cross-hatching. The stages of the nucleic acid replication cycles sequestered in extracellular virus particles are indicated by dashed lines.

The segmentation of the genome of some RNA viruses is not considered here, because subdivision of the genome is probably a form of transcriptional control. The single-stranded DNA viruses have been omitted for simplicity. The only form among known viruses not represented is the RNA:DNA intermediate in the reverse transcription cycle.

of the influenza virus genome, and the presence of polypeptide specifying information in both strands of the adenovirus genome, etc. Polyomavirus also conserves the coding potential of its genome by utilizing host proteins as structural components of the virion (Table 1).

MUTATION AND MUTANTS. Mutation can be defined as a discontinuous event that results in a change in information content. Virus mutants arise spontaneously or can be induced by chemical or physical agents (mutagens). *Mutagens* that have proved effective with human and animal viruses include base analogues (5-fluorouracil and 5-azacytidine for RNA viruses and 5-bromodeoxyuridine for DNA viruses), alkylating agents (ethyl methane sulfonate, among others), intercalating agents (proflavine and NTG), deaminating agents (nitrous acid), hydroxylamine, and ionizing and ultraviolet irradiation. The base analogues are incorporated into the genome, and mutations are produced by miscoding during replication. The other mutagens induce mutation by direct chemical change of the nucleic acid. Frameshift and nonsense (polypeptide chain-terminating) mutants of human or animal viruses are very rare and have been identified unequivocally in only a few cases. Most induced mutants appear to be missense mutants in which substitution of an amino acid modifies the functional activity of a gene product. The advent of genetic engineering and the introduction of recombinant DNA technology into animal virology has increased the scope of mutagenesis, and directed site-specific mutagenesis is now possible with most DNA viruses.

Mutants may have specific phenotypes such as resistance to heat inactivation or an inhibitory drug; for instance, mutants of poliovirus resistant to guanidine hydrochloride have played an important role in mapping the poliovirus genome. In general, however, mutants with specific phenotypes are less useful than conditional lethal mutants, in which a single common phenotype (e.g., inability to multiply at high temperature) is sufficient to provide mutants with lesions in any gene that is indispensable for normal replication. This is because a change in amino acid sequence of any polypeptide can produce a conformational change that affects the stability of a protein at high temperature. *Conditional lethal mutants* of animal viruses are almost exclusively temperature-sensitive (*ts*) mutants. Host-restricted mutants, analogous to the amber-ochre mutants of prokaryotes, are rare probably because mammalian cells with the characteristics of the suppressor strains of prokaryotes have not been identified. However, recently, a suppressor tRNA gene from *Xenopus laevis* has been introduced into mouse cells, creating an appropriate host cell for the production of suppressor-sensitive (i.e., polypeptide chain-terminating, or "nonsense") mutants of animal viruses.

Extensive changes in polynucleotide sequence of the genome can occur by rearrangement, duplication, and deletion. Spontaneous *deletion mutants* of viruses are common and occur in all virus groups. Particles with defective genomes frequently interfere specifically with the replication of the undeleted genome and are known as DI (defective interfering) particles. It has been suggested that

Table 1. THE PHYSICAL AND GENETIC CHARACTERISTICS OF THE GENOMES OF ANIMAL VIRUSES

Group[a]	Example	Site of Replication	Nucleic Acid: Type	Strand in Virion	Form	Infectivity	MW × 10^6	Genetic Properties: Relative Coding Capacity[b]	Complementation Groups	Recombination Frequency and Grouping	Special Features
Parvo	Murine minute	Nucleus	SS-DNA	—	Linear	?	1.7	3–4	N.D.	N.D.	Replicates in unison with host; mitosis-dependent. Unique hair-pin ends
	Adeno-associated	Nucleus	SS-DNA	− and +	Linear	Yes	1.8	3–4	N.D.	N.D.	Helper and mitosis-dependent. Inverted terminal repeat
Papova	SV40	Nucleus	DS-DNA	+/−	Super-coiled helix	Yes	3.0	3	3 (or 5)	Low	Induces host DNA synthesis
Adeno	Adeno 5	Nucleus	DS-DNA	+/−	Linear	Yes	23.0	23	12	Low-high linear map	Inverted terminal repetition. Covalently bonded protein at 5′ terminus
Herpes	HSV-2	Nucleus	DS-DNA	+/−	Linear	Yes	100.0	100	18	Low-high linear map	Terminal and internal inverted repeats
Pox	Vaccinia	Cytoplasm	DS-DNA	+/−	Linear	No	160.0	160	N.D.	Low-high linear map	Cross-linked ends. DNA-dependent RNA polymerase and other virion enzymes
Picorna	Polio-1	Cytoplasm	SS-RNA	+	Linear	Yes	2.6	5	Nil	Low linear map	One polycistronic message, post-translational cleavage; covalently bonded protein at 5′ terminus
Alpha	Sindbis	Cytoplasm	SS-RNA	+	Linear	Yes	4.0	8	6	None	Two polycistronic messages; post-translational cleavage
Flavi	Dengue	Cytoplasm	SS-RNA	+	Linear	N.D.	4.0	8	N.D.	None	Polycistronic (with internal initiation of translation?)
Bunya	Maguari	Cytoplasm	SS-RNA	−	3 unique subunits	No	6.4	13	(2 × 2)	High 3 groups	Virion RNA-dependent RNA polymerase
Arena	Pichinde	Cytoplasm	SS-RNA	−	2 unique subunits	No	3.2	6	N.D.	High 2 groups	Virion RNA-dependent RNA polymerase
Orthomyxo	Influenza	Cytoplasm Nucleus	SS-RNA	−	8 unique subunits	No	5.0	10	N.D.	High 8 groups	Virion RNA-dependent RNA polymerase
Paramyxo	Sendai	Cytoplasm	SS-RNA	−	Linear	No	7.0	14	7	None	Virion RNA-dependent RNA polymerase
Rhabdo	Vesicular stomatitis	Cytoplasm	SS-RNA	−	Linear	No	4.0	8	6	None	Virion RNA-dependent RNA polymerase
Diplorna	Reo	Cytoplasm	DS-RNA	+/−	10 unique subunits	No	15.0	15	N.D.	High 10 groups	Virion DS-RNA-dependent RNA polymerase
Retro	Rous sarcoma	Nucleus and cytoplasm	SS-RNA	+	2 identical subunits	RNA no DNA Yes	6.0	6	N.D.	High	Virion RNA-dependent DNA polymerase

[a]The papilloma, corona, irido, and orbi have been omitted because of lack of information.
[b]The number of possible gene products, assuming that an average sized protein contains 500 amino acids.

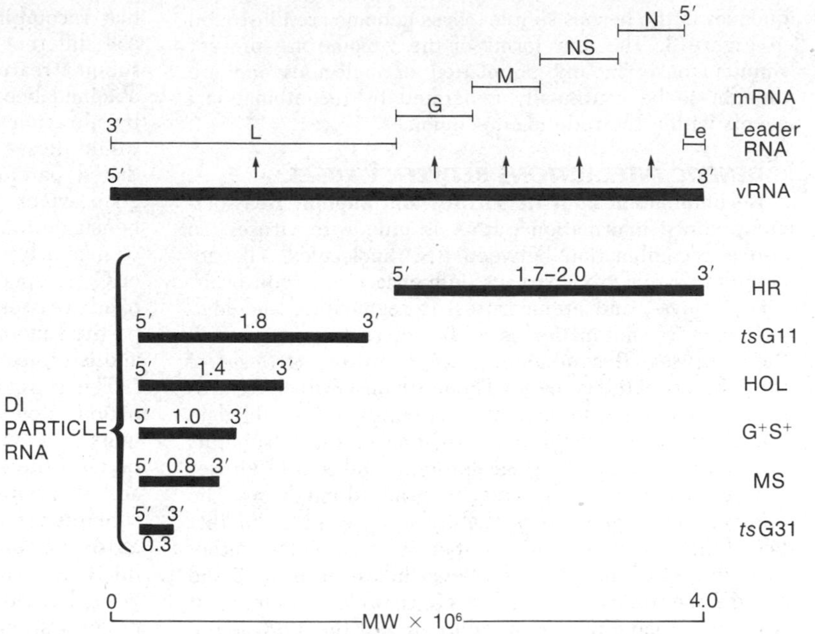

Figure 2. Physical maps of DI particle RNA of vesicular stomatitis virus (VSV).

The DI particles of VSV are deletion mutants. The physical location of the RNA from six different DI particles (HR, *ts*G11, HOL, G^+S^+, MS and *ts*G31) are illustrated. All these DI particles have interfering activity with homotypic virus. The HR DI particle is unique in its ability to interfere heterotypically. It is also the only DI particle that contains complete viral genes.

the generation of DI particles is responsible for the self-limitation of many virus diseases by moderating the course of infection until an immune response is developed. Figure 2 illustrates the extent of the deletions observed in some DI particles of the rhabdovirus vesicular stomatitis virus (VSV). Usually deletion mutants can only multiply with the assistance of a helper virus. This complex relationship is exemplified best in the leukemia-sarcoma viruses, in which the mammalian sarcoma viruses lack genetic information for envelope protein (and internal proteins according to the strain), and these viruses are entirely dependent on the "helper" leukemia virus for normal maturation.

The deletion of sequences in DI particles of papovaviruses, on the other hand, may be accompanied by rearrangements, reiteration of sequences, and substitutions of extraneous host DNA. Indeed, *duplications* and rearrangements are characteristic features of the normal genome of the herpes viruses and presumably have arisen by mutational events during the evolution of these viruses. The location and orientation of the redundant (duplicated) se-

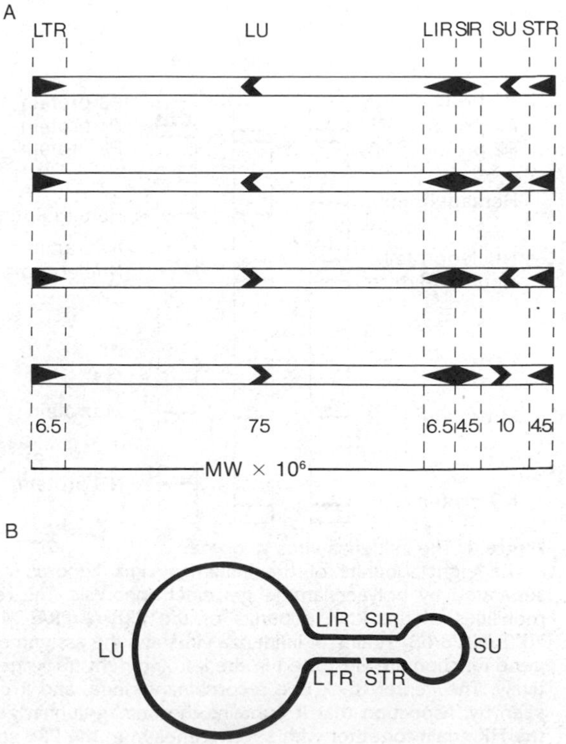

Figure 3. The herpes simplex virus genome. *A,* The four arrangements of the genome of herpes simplex virus. LTR = long terminal repeat; LU = long unique region; LIR = long internal repeat; SIR = short internal repeat; SU = short unique region; STR = short terminal repeat. Inversion of the long and short regions is indicated by arrows and could occur as a result of internal recombination within the redundant sequences. *B,* The homology of the internal and terminal repeat regions. This double ring structure is observed in electronmicrographs of single-stranded DNA following self-annealing.

This arrangement of genome is characteristic for herpes simplex viruses Type 1 and Type 2 but not for other members of the herpes group. The least complex herpesvirus genome is that of channel catfish virus, which lacks a short unique region and has no internal redundancy.

quences in the herpes simplex virus genome are illustrated in Figure 3. The four forms of the genome are present simultaneously in any population of molecules and are thought to be continually generated by recombinational events within the redundant sequences.

GENETIC INTERACTIONS BETWEEN VIRUSES

Recombination in RNA Viruses and Subunit Reassortment. Since informational RNA is unique to viruses, so also is recombination between RNA molecules. The genome of several RNA viruses (influenza virus, reo-, orbi-, rota-, bunya-, and arenaviruses) is segmented, and high frequency recombination is a characteristic feature of all these viruses. Recombination occurs by *reassortment* of the subunits of the genome. The mechanism which ensures that the correct complement of subunits is assembled in the mature virion is still unknown. Each of the 10 subunits of reovirus codes for a single protein, and hybrid viruses can be selected from the progeny of mixed infections. The influenza virus genome is slightly more complex in that two of the genome subunits contain information for synthesis of more than one protein. Nevertheless, if the PR8 and Hong Kong strains, for example, are crossed, a recombinant with the Hong Kong hemagglutinin and the PR8 neuraminidase can be selected by exposure to anti-PR8 hemagglutinin and anti–Hong Kong neuraminidase sera. The genomic subunits of different strains of influenza virus (and similarly their gene products) have different electrophoretic mobilities in polyacrylamide gel, and by analysis of the subunits present in specific recombinants, it has been possible to map completely the influenza virus genome. The coding assignment of the subunits of the genome of the PR8 and Hong Kong strains, and a recombinant with the hemagglutinin of Hong Kong (HK) and the neuraminidase of PR8 are illustrated in Figure 4. From the relative mobilities of the subunits, it is apparent that only the hemagglutinin subunit has been exchanged in this particular recombinant. In any cross of two influenza viruses, 254 different recombinants (i.e., $[2]^8-2$) are possible by subunit rearrangement. This particular recombinant was obtained because one of the parents had been irradiated by ultraviolet light, so that most viable progeny viruses would derive all their genomic segments from the unirradiated parent with the exception of the hemagglutinin gene, which was selected against by exposure to anti-PR8 hemagglutinin. Reassortment can occur freely among strains of type A influenza (but not with strains of type B or C) irrespective of time and place of origin. On the other hand, reassortment among bunyaviruses, which have tripartite genomes, is confined to serologically related viruses and is subject to a complex pattern of restrictions.

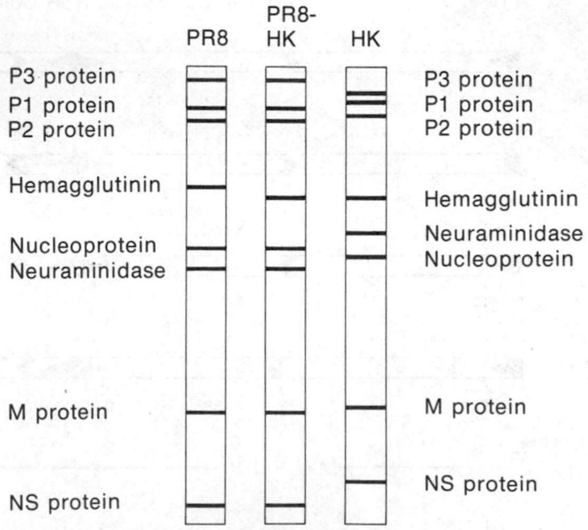

Figure 4. The influenza virus genome.
The eight subunits of the influenza virus genome can be separated by polyacrylamide gel electrophoresis. The relative mobilities of the RNA subunits of the PR8 (A/PR/8/34) and HK(A/HK/8/68) strains of influenza virus and the assignments of gene function are illustrated in the left and right tracks, respectively. The center track is a recombinant clone, and it can be seen by inspection that it contains the hemagglutinin gene of the HK strain together with seven genes from the PR8 strain.

The retroviruses also exhibit high frequency recombination. However, although the genome exists as two subunits, the mechanism is not independent reassortment because the two components of the genome are identical, and therefore the particles are genetically *diploid.* The subunits of the retrovirus genome are linked by base pairing at their 5′ end as an inverted dimer, and transcription is initiated from primers (tryptophan tRNA in Rous sarcoma virus) located close to the 5′ ends. Synthesis of a complete progeny strand necessitates a jump from the 5′ end of one strand to the 3′ end of the same or the other strand of the dimer. Hence, each round of transcription provides an opportunity for intermolecular recombination, which could account for the high frequency of recombination.

Recombination has not been detected in any negative-strand RNA virus with an unsegmented genome, but it does occur at low frequency with at least some positive-strand RNA viruses (see Table 1). *Genetic maps* of poliovirus and foot-and-mouth disease virus (FMDV) have been constructed from crosses of *ts* mutants. In both cases, the mutants were oriented relative to the locus for resistance to the inhibitor guanidine and then arranged in a linear order on the basis of the recombination frequencies observed in crosses of pairs of mutants. The reality of recombination in FMDV has been confirmed by oligonucleotide mapping of the genome of recombinants. The genetic map of poliovirus is illustrated in Figure 5. Analysis of the properties of the constituent *ts* mutants defines the different coding regions. The organization of the genome of FMDV is probably similar to that of poliovirus, but the gene order in other RNA viruses differs from the picornavirus pattern. For example, in Sindbis virus and VSV the coat protein genes are located centrally or towards but not at the 5′ end. These differences probably reflect different modes of transcription and translation. In fact, the genome of picornaviruses is polycistronic and not partitioned into genes, since the entire genome is translated directly into a single giant polypeptide, which is subsequently cleaved into smaller polypeptides, which are the functional gene products. *Post-translation cleavage* is probably a feature of all positive-strand viruses, because in eukaryotic cells, initiation of translation occurs at only a single site in all mRNA. (The flaviviruses, however, may prove exceptions to this generalization.)

The gene order of avian sarcoma virus has been established by a combination of genetic and physical methods to be the following: 5′-*gag-pol-env-src*-3′, in which *gag* is the gene for the precursor of the internal proteins, *pol* is the gene for viral polymerase, *env* is the gene for the surface glycoproteins, and *src* is the sarcomagenic sequence. In avian leukemia viruses, the *src* gene is not present.

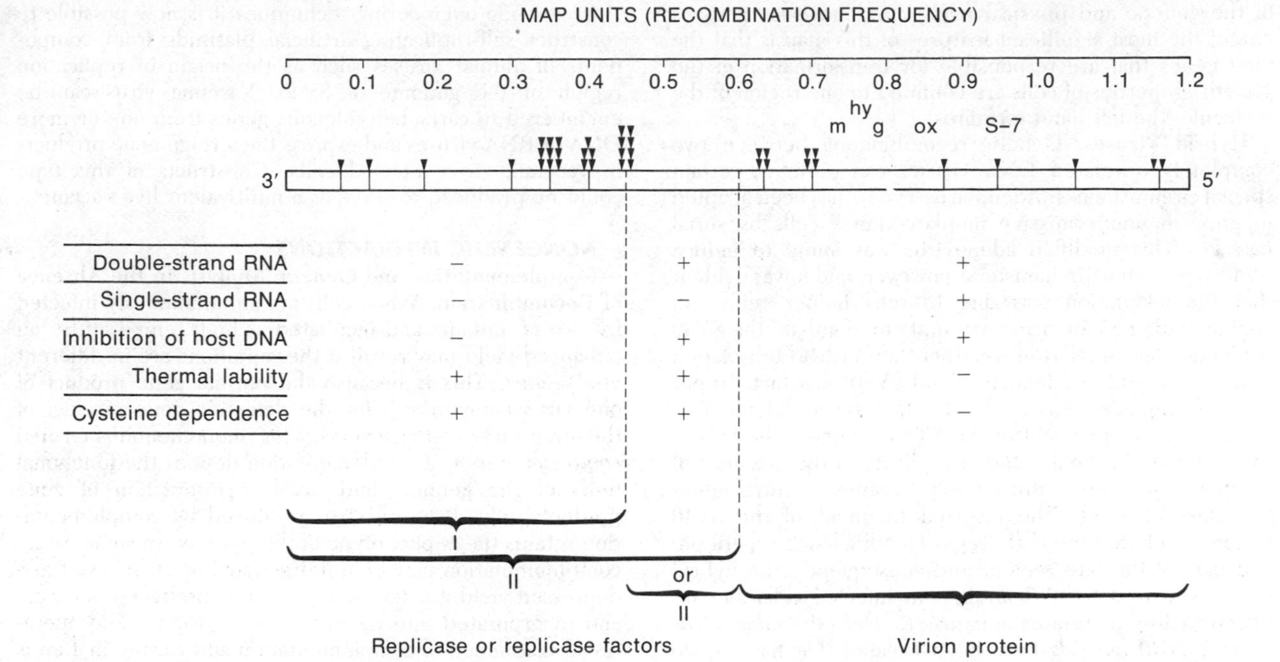

Figure 5. The picornavirus genome.

Recombination map of 39 *ts* mutants of poliovirus Type 1 and the assignment of gene function. The symbol indicates the map position of a *ts* mutant. Identification of gene function is summarized in the lower part of the figure. The loci of four inhibitors of multiplication all fall within the coat protein region. The inhibitors are guanidine (g), dextran sulfate (m), and derivatives of hydantoin (hy), oxadiazole (ox), and pyrimidine carboxylate (S-7).

The genetic map of foot-and-mouth disease virus, an unrelated picornavirus, closely resembles that of poliovirus. Thirty-five mutants have been arranged in a linear sequence extending over 0.7 map units. Again, the locus of the guanidine inhibitor falls in the presumptive coat protein region.

Recombination in DNA Viruses and Correlation of Physical and Genetic Maps. Recombination between DNA viruses does not require any exceptional mechanisms, since the enzymes capable of recombining DNA molecules preexist in the host cell. Genetic maps of the genomes of polyomavirus, SV40 virus, adenovirus, and herpes simplex virus have been derived from crosses of *ts* mutants and correlated with physical maps of the genome. In adenovirus, for example, the *physical mapping* of cross-over events was achieved by isolating recombinants between *ts* mutants of two serologically distinct strains of adenovirus, whose DNA differed in their pattern of cleavage by restriction endonucleases. (Restriction endonucleases are bacterial enzymes that recognize particular nucleotide sequences in double-stranded DNA and cleave specific phosphodiester bonds within these sites to produce unique DNA fragments that can be separated by electrophoresis in polyacrylamide gel). Since the genome of the recombinant contains sequences from each parent, the position of the cross-over event can be determined by comparison of the types of DNA fragment produced. The location of mutants to particular regions of DNA can also be determined by *marker rescue* experiments in which *ts* mutant-infected cells are coinfected with individual fragments of the DNA of wild-type virus obtained by restriction endonuclease treatment. The genetic and physical maps of the genome of adenovirus and the two papovaviruses, SV40 and polyoma, have been aligned by these methods, and mapping of the more complex herpes simplex virus is progressing rapidly. Genetic mapping is an important step towards the goal of defining the specific features of viral biosynthesis. Analysis of the properties of the different mutants locates the regions of the molecule that code for particular proteins. Figure 6 illustrates early results which first showed the alignment

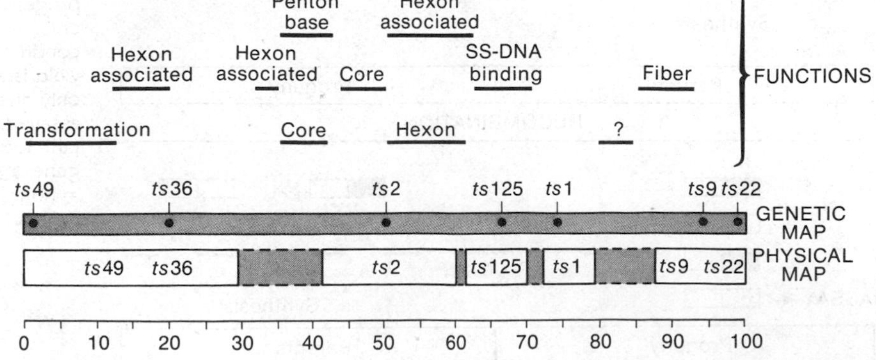

Figure 6. The adenovirus genome.

An early genetic map of *ts* mutants of adenovirus Type S obtained by crosses of seven mutants is compared with the location of the same seven mutants obtained by physical mapping where fragments of adenovirus DNA generated by restriction endonuclease treatment are used to rescue *ts* mutants. There is no discrepancy between the two maps. The presumptive gene functions of the various regions are also illustrated.

of the genetic and physical maps of adenovirus. Perhaps one of the most significant features of this map is that the viral genes that are responsible for transformation of the growth properties of cells are confined to one region of the molecule (the left hand terminus).

Hybrid Viruses. Genetic recombination between two completely unrelated DNA viruses can occur in certain special circumstances. Adenovirus Type 7 has been adapted to grow in nonpermissive monkey-kidney cells by serial passage. This modified adenovirus was found to induce SV40-type tumors in hamsters, however, and it was evident that the adaptation was due to the "helper" effect of contaminating SV40 virus. Attempts to eliminate the SV40 component by antiserum treatment led instead to isolation of a true hybrid of adenovirus and SV40, in which 10 per cent of the adenovirus genome had been deleted and replaced by 75 per cent of the SV40 genome. The hybrid was defective and only able to replicate in the presence of "helper" adenovirus, presumably because essential genes had been deleted. The inserted fragment of the SV40 genome included the early region (with a small repetition) and part of the late region, and consequently the hybrid virus expressed SV40 T-antigen in infected cells and induced SV40-type tumors in hamsters. *Defective adenovirus Type 2-SV40 hybrids* have been isolated that have up to one half of the adenovirus genome deleted and more than one genome equivalent of SV40 inserted.

Nondefective adenovirus Type 2-SV40 hybrids have also been isolated with 4.5 to 7.1 per cent of the adenovirus genome deleted and substituted by 7 to 59 per cent of the SV40 genome. Again, it is the early region of the SV40 genome that is inserted. Evidently the region of the adenovirus genome between map positions 0.79 and 0.86 (see Fig. 6), where all the deletions occur, is not essential for replication. The generation of these nondefective hybrids was a unique event, since it has not been possible to produce this hybrid again. Nevertheless, it illustrates that under rare circumstances DNA viruses at least have the potential to acquire genes from other DNA viruses, and how a nononcogenic virus might become oncogenic.

By genetic engineering techniques it is now possible to construct self-replicating artificial plasmids from components of animal viruses such as the origin of replication region of the genome of SV40. Vaccinia virus can be engineered to carry heterologous genes from one or more DNA or RNA viruses and express the foreign gene products in vaccinia virus–infected cells. Constructs of this type could be produced to serve as a multivalent live vaccine.

NONGENETIC INTERACTIONS

Complementation and Genetic Analysis in the Absence of Recombination. When cells are simultaneously infected by two *ts* mutants and incubated at high temperature, an enhanced yield may result if the mutations are in different viral genes. This is because the normal gene product of one virus compensates for the defective gene product of the other virus and vice versa. This phenomenon is termed *complementation*. Complementation defines the functional units of the genome and involves interaction of gene products only. Progeny virus produced by complementation retains the *ts* phenotype of the parents. In some cases, complementation may be unidirectional or even result in a depressed yield if a defective protein is produced in excess and incorporated into the majority of virions. The operational distinction of complementation and recombination is illustrated in Figure 7. Mutants can be grouped according to their ability to complement other mutants, and the number of complementation groups gives a minimum estimate of the number of genes in the genome of any virus (Table 1). In addition, complementation facilitates analysis of the organization of the genome of viruses (such as the unsegmented negative-strand RNA viruses) that do not undergo recombination. The example of the rhabdovirus VSV illustrates the value of this approach. Five proteins are present in the virion of VSV, and no other virus-specified proteins have been detected in infected cells. The existence of six groups of complementing mutants points to the existence of another VSV protein, as yet undetected. Further study of the properties of *ts* mutants may lead to identification of this putative VSV protein and

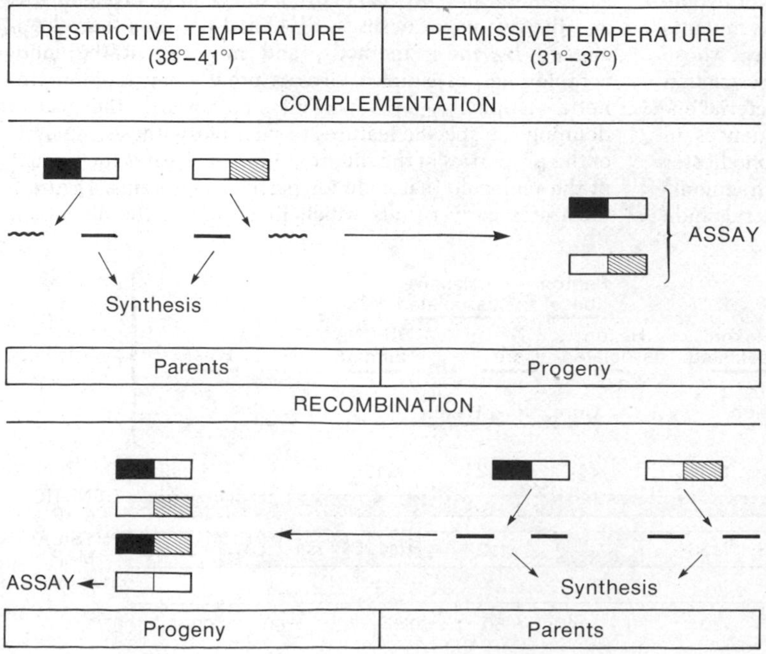

Figure 7. The operational distinction between complementation and recombination using temperature-sensitive mutants.

In complementation the mixed infection is conducted at restrictive temperature, and the yield is assayed at permissive temperature. The progeny are temperature-sensitive like the parents. In recombination the mixed infection is conducted at permissive temperature, and the yield is assayed at restrictive temperature. Thus, only one of the recombinants (the nonmutant) is assayed, since the parents and the double mutant recombinant are restricted. ▭ = normal gene; ■▨ = independent *ts* mutants; —— = normal gene product; 〰 = defective gene product.

its function. Identification of gene functions in this way provided the first confirmation that the RNA-dependent RNA polymerases of negative-strand viruses and the RNA-dependent DNA polymerase (reverse transcriptase) of retroviruses are virus-specified enzymes.

Phenotypic Mixing and Pseudotypes. Two different viruses multiplying in the same cell may produce progeny with the phenotypic characteristics of both parents. This phenomenon is particularly evident among enveloped viruses that mature by budding from membranes, but it is also prevalent among nonenveloped viruses. For instance, influenza virus can acquire antigens from serologically related strains and also from quite unrelated parainfluenza viruses and rhabdoviruses. The majority of phenotypically mixed particles contain antigens from both parents and can be neutralized by antisera to both viruses. A minority may be entirely invested by the envelope of the heterologous virus. This could have important epidemiologic consequences, since it would allow a virus to survive and persist in an apparently immune population.

The defective avian and mammalian sarcoma viruses exist only as *pseudotypes*, i.e., as phenotypically mixed particles whose envelope proteins are donated by the nondefective helper leukemia virus. Pseudotypes are also produced when cytolytic viruses (VSV is often used experimentally) multiply in cells chronically infected with oncornaviruses (the oncogenic retroviruses). Virions with the envelope antigens of avian leukosis virus and the nucleocapsid of VSV, designated VSV (ALV), and the reciprocal pseudotype ALV (VSV), have been identified among the progeny following VSV infection of chick embryo cells carrying avian leukosis virus. Pseudotype formation is also known to occur between DNA viruses (herpes simplex) and RNA viruses (VSV).

Production of pseudotypes of VSV can be used as a sensitive probe for detection of cryptic RNA tumor virus agents, as an aid in the study of membranes and host restriction, or as a rapid method of assay of such agents as mouse mammary tumor virus in which the alternative in vivo assay is lengthy and difficult. However, pseudotypes of the ALV (VSV) type constitute a potential biohazard. The leukemogenic and sarcomagenic viruses of animals are characteristically host-restricted, and envelopment in a membrane provided by an unrestricted virus like VSV could enable the oncogenic virus to reach cells that are normally inaccessible, with unpredictable consequences.

Phenotypic mixing is not confined to envelope proteins. The α mutants of Rous sarcoma virus, for example, have part of the polymerase gene deleted (as well as the entire envelope gene), and they can only be propagated in the presence of a helper virus that contributes the polymerase and envelope functions.

Host-Induced Modification. Host-induced modification, i.e., nonheritable phenotypic variation, can occur in certain circumstances. The lipid and the carbohydrate portions of the glycolipids and glycoproteins of the viral envelope are contributed by the host cell and therefore vary according to the cell of origin. For instance, the glycoproteins of arthropod-borne viruses released from insect cells lack sialic acid, while the same virus propagated in mammalian cells may possess sialic acid. However, in general this variability does not appear to have important biologic consequences.

DETERMINATION OF VIRULENCE, DISEASE POTENTIAL, AND ONCOGENICITY. The factors that determine the pathogenic potential of viruses can be defined by study of the effects of mutations in specific genes. For instance, study of temperature-sensitive mutants of reovirus revealed that mutation in a late function of the viral genome resulted in a change of disease pattern. Wild-type reovirus is lethal for newborn rats, whereas *ts* mutants exhibit greatly reduced virulence. In the case of one mutant (*ts* B1), although the majority of animals survived infection with high doses of virus, later in life progressive neurologic disease developed, which culminated in death. The assembly of the outer capsid is defective in *ts* B1-infected cells, and it was proposed that intracellular accumulation of viral nucleocapsid is responsible for the altered disease pattern.

Mutations affecting *neurovirulence* have been described frequently. One mutant of measles virus is less neurovirulent than wild-type measles virus in suckling hamsters. Hydrocephalus, a response to infection normally masked by the dominant neurologic signs, is a consequence of infection with this mutant. On the other hand, *ts* mutants of VSV often exhibit enhanced neurovirulence for newborn hamsters. However, there is no specific association of neurovirulence with a particular gene. The alteration in disease pattern is related more to the increased survival time of infected animals.

The virulence of avian influenza (fowl plague) virus appears to be influenced by many factors; so far no one gene has been implicated as a major determinant of virulence, and probably the same is true for human influenza virus. However, the virulence of the avian parainfluenza virus (Newcastle disease virus) for chickens is dependent on extracellular cleavage of an envelope glycoprotein (the F, or fusion, protein). Mutation affecting the sensitivity of this protein to proteolytic cleavage influences host range in vitro and virulence in vivo. Furthermore, there are known mutants of a murine parainfluenza virus that differ in the sensitivity of the F protein to cleavage by specific proteases and, as a consequence, their ability to infect different cells.

The role of viruses in *oncogenesis* can also be approached by study of the properties of mutants. Transformation defective (*td*) mutants of Rous sarcoma virus occur spontaneously and are predominantly deletion mutants in which part or all of the sarcoma determinant (the *src* gene) is missing. These mutants are still oncogenic, however, because they retain the ability to induce leukosis. The genome of *td* deletion mutants and the naturally occurring avian leukosis viruses are similar in size. The *src* gene sequences of different avian sarcoma viruses are homologous, indicating that they have been conserved in evolution. *Src* sequences can be detected also in the normal cells of several avian species, including Japanese quail (which has no inducible endogenous retrovirus). The prevalence of these *src*-related sequences suggests that the *src* gene of avian sarcoma viruses, which is a function not required for virus multiplication, was acquired from the cell at some time in the past. The *src* gene is one example of a class of oncogenic (*onc*) genes found only in retroviruses. More than twenty different *onc* genes are now recognized, each derived from a different cellular homologue and associated with a different retrovirus.

The origin of the *onc* gene in mammalian sarcoma viruses is more complex. The Harvey and Kirsten strains of murine sarcoma virus appear to have acquired rat genome sequences (*ras*) and transforming ability during passage in rats. The Moloney strain of murine sarcoma virus, on the other hand, acquired oncogenic sequences (*mos*) and transforming ability during passage in mice, and there is no sequence homology between the *mos* gene of the Moloney virus and the *ras* genes of the Harvey or Kirsten viruses.

Almost all *ts* mutants of avian sarcoma virus that affect transformation are late mutants. Temperature-shift experiments with *ts* mutants have shown that transformation is dependent on the continuous activity of a viral gene. The *src* gene product is a 60,000 M.W. phosphoprotein, but its precise function in transformation has still to be elucidated.

Cells transformed by SV40 virus carry viral DNA sequences integrated into their chromosomes. All or only part of the SV40 genome may be present. Study of cells transformed by *ts* mutants of SV40 virus showed that expression of an early gene function of SV40 only was necessary for initiation and maintenance of the transformed state. However, there seems to be no single chromosomal site of integration of SV40 (in rat cells at least), and the number of insertions of the SV40 genome or its early genes is variable in different cell lines.

Similarly, the isolation of *ts* mutants of adenovirus that failed to transform rodent cells at nonpermissive temperature showed that a viral gene product was required at least for initiation of transformation by adenovirus. These mutants map at one end of the adenovirus genome, and only those fragments of the adenovirus genome obtained by restriction endonuclease digestion that contain the left-hand end are able to transform cells; no more than 8 per cent of the genome is required to cause transformation.

Certain herpesviruses can also induce tumors in vivo and transform cells in vitro, and the transforming region of the genome has been located for both herpes simplex viruses type 1 and type 2. Current opinion favors the idea that herpesvirus-induced oncogenic change occurs by a hit-and-run mechanism and does not depend on persistence of herpesvirus genes.

Recent data have linked certain oncogene products (viral transforming proteins and their normal cellular homologues) to different growth factors. For example, the product of the *sis* oncogene (the transforming gene of simian sarcoma virus) is almost identical to one of the two protein chains comprising platelet-derived growth factor (PDGF), and *erbB* (an oncogene identified in avian erythroblastosis virus) closely resembles the receptor for epidermal growth factor (EGF). Consequently, transformation may be a result of constitutive expression of any of the controlling elements in the normal mitogenic pathway.

Transfection experiments in which cells are coinfected with the DNA of individual oncogenes have defined two of the stages in transformation. Normal fibroblasts can be fully transformed by two different oncogenes in conjunction, but not by either alone, and two complementing groups of oncogenes have been defined. The *myc* oncogene of avian myeloblastosis virus, the large T antigen gene of polyoma virus, or the *Ela* gene of adenovirus (left-hand terminus) are required to establish immortalization and belong to the same complementation group. The *ras* oncogene of murine sarcoma virus and the middle T antigen gene of polyoma virus constitute the other complementation group, which is responsible for morphologic change and anchorage independence. The gene products of the first complementation group bind to nuclear structures, and those of the second orientation bind at the plasma membrane. These results emphasize the multistep nature of transformation and show that the DNA viruses and the oncogenes associated with retroviruses apparently modify the same cellular functions.

EVOLUTION IN ACTION. Human influenza A virus undergoes dramatic changes in its surface antigens (*antigenic shift*) at intervals, causing severe pandemics. Between pandemics, the virus is constantly changing in a more progressive manner (*antigenic drift*). The available evidence supports the hypothesis that antigenic drift occurs by accumulation of small mutational changes, whereas antigenic shift is the result of hybridization between a human influenza virus and a virus maintained in a reservoir species. The pandemic of 1918 was caused by a strain that may have acquired an antigenically novel hemagglutinin by recombination with a swine influenza virus. Reconstruction experiments in animals have confirmed that hybridization between different influenza virus strains can occur in vivo. For example, reciprocal recombinants of swine influenza and fowl plague virus (FPV) have been obtained from pigs, despite the inability of FPV to multiply efficiently in this host animal.

The history of the introduction of *myxomatosis* into Australia illustrates that evolutionary changes may occur in both the virus and its host. Myxomavirus was extremely lethal for European rabbits when it was liberated in Australia in 1950 as a pest control measure: mortality rates were in excess of 99 per cent. However, attenuated variants soon made their appearance and within 3 to 4 years they became dominant, because reduced virulence favored survival of animals from one season to the next and allowed a susceptible population to be reestablished each year. Following appearance of the initial attenuated variants, there was a corresponding increase in the genetic resistance of the host animal, so that the mortality induced by a standard virulent strain fell from over 90 per cent to 25 per cent in 5 years. Thus, a milder disease and stable endemicity were evolved by changes in the disease potential of the virus and the genetic resistance of the host animals. It is possible that similar factors have had a similar influence in the evolution of endemic virus disease in man.

References

The Nature and Coding Capacity of Viral Genomes

Baltimore, D.: Expression of animal virus genomes. Bacteriol Rev 35:235, 1971.

Luria, S. E., Darnell, J. E., Jr., Baltimore, D., and Campbell, A.: General Virology, Third Ed., New York, John Wiley and Sons, 1978.

Watson, J. D.: Molecular Biology of the Gene, 2nd ed. New York and Amsterdam, W. A. Benjamin Inc., 1970.

Weisbeek, P. J., Borrias, W. E., Langeveld, S. A., Baas, P. D., and van Arkel, G. A.: Bacteriophage ΦX174: gene A overlaps gene B. Proc Natl Acad Sci USA 74:2504, 1977.

Mutation and Mutants

Fenner, F.: Conditional lethal mutants of animal viruses. Curr Topics Microbiol Immunol 48:1, 1969.

Fraenkel-Conrat, H., and Wagner, R. R.(eds.): Comprehensive Virology, Vol. 9: Regulation and Genetics, The Genetics of Animal Viruses. New York and London, Plenum Press, 1977.

Huang, A. S., and Baltimore, D.: Defective viral particles and viral disease processes. Nature (London) 226:325, 1973.

Pringle, C. R.: Conditional lethal mutants of vesicular stomatitis virus. Curr Topics Microbiol Immunol 68:85, 1975.

Genetic Interactions Between Viruses

Fenner, F., McAuslan, B. R., Mims, C. A., Sambrook, J., and White, D. O.: The Biology of Animal Viruses, 2nd ed. New York and London, Academic Press, 1974.

Kelly, T. J., Jr., and Nathans, D.: The genome of simian virus 40. Adv Virus Res 21:86, 1977.
Palese, P.: The genes of influenza virus. Cell 10:1, 1977.
Tooze, J. (ed.): The molecular Biology of Tumour Viruses.
Weiss, R. A., et al. (eds.): The Molecular Biology of Tumor Viruses. RNA Tumor Viruses. Cold Spring Harbor, New York, Cold Spring Harbor Laboratory, 1982.

Determination of Virulence, Disease Potential, and Oncogenicity
Fenner, F., and Ratcliffe, F. N.: Myxomatosis. London and New York, Cambridge University Press, 1965.
Klein, G.: Advances in Viral Oncology, Vol. I. Oncogene studies. New York, Raven Press, 1982.
Palese, P., and Kingsbury, D. W.: Genetics of Influenza Virus. Vienna and New York, Springer-Verlag, 1983.

11

PERSISTENT VIRAL INFECTIONS

JULIUS S. YOUNGNER, SC.D.

The attention of medical virologists has been focused primarily on acute febrile diseases. Acute infections, such as influenza, smallpox, and measles, have incubation periods of days to weeks, well-defined symptoms, and closely associated pathologic manifestations. In individuals who recover from acute viral infections, both cellular and humoral mechanisms operate during the incubation period and the virus usually disappears from the body within several weeks after the first symptoms appear. The period in which virus can be isolated from clinical specimens is very limited; in most cases virus is demonstrable only briefly before and after the onset of clinical disease. In virus infections, such as poliomyelitis and mumps, the pattern of acute disease and recovery is often more difficult to study, since the infection may be subclinical and produce no clearly recognizable or characteristic symptomatology.

Increasing attention is being devoted to persistent viral infections in which the infectious agent is present for long periods of time. Infections of this type are diverse and difficult to classify with precision. A great variety of viruses, patterns of pathogenesis, and clinical entities contribute to the complexity of this group of infections (Table 1).

CLASSIFICATION OF PERSISTENT VIRAL INFECTIONS IN HUMANS AND ANIMALS. Persistent viral infections can be classified into three general categories: (1) latent infections, (2) chronic infections, and (3) slow infections (Fenner and White, 1976).

Latent Infections. In this type of persistence, the virus disappears after acute primary disease and reappears during recurrences of disease. There may be one or more such recurrences after long intervals. The best understood diseases in this class are caused by members of the herpesvirus group, herpes simplex, and varicella-zoster viruses.

Table 1. PERSISTENT VIRAL INFECTIONS OF HUMANS

Virus Classification					
Genome	***Group***	**Agent**	**Disease**	**Virus Presence***	**Mechanism of Pathogenesis†**
DNA	Herpesvirus	Herpes simplex virus (Types 1 and 2)	Herpes	Latent	Cytolysis
		Varicella-Zoster virus	Zoster	Latent	Cytolysis
		Cytomegalovirus	Cytomegalo-inclusion disease	Latent	Cytolysis
			Mononucleosis	Latent	Transformation
		EB virus	Mononucleosis	Latent	Transformation
			Lymphoma	Latent	Transformation
DNA	Papovavirus	JC virus	Progressive multifocal leuko-encephalopathy (PML)	Minimal	Cytolysis
		BK virus	?	Latent	?
		Human papilloma virus	Warts	Overt	Transformation
DNA	Adenovirus	Adenovirus (many types)	?	Latent	?
DNA	Unclassified	Hepatitis B virus	Hepatitis	Overt	Immunopathology(?)
?		Non A/B hepatitis virus	Hepatitis	Overt	Immunopathology(?)
RNA	Paramyxovirus	Measles	Subacute sclerosing panencephalitis (SSPE)	Minimal	Cytolysis
RNA	Togavirus	Rubella	Fetal anomalies	Overt	Inhibition of cell division(?)
			Panencephalitis		Cytolysis(?)
?	?	Creutzfeldt-Jakob agent	Spongiform encephalopathy	Overt	Cytolysis
		Kuru agent	Spongiform encephalopathy	Overt	Cytolysis

*Latent = infective virus cannot be demonstrated, except during active or recrudescent symptoms of disease.
Minimal = infective virus difficult to demonstrate; may be absent or present in exceedingly small numbers.
Overt = infective virus usually demonstrable with or without presence of symptoms.
†Cytolysis = lesions result from cell destruction by virus.
Transformation = lesions due to cell proliferative response to infection in the absence of cytolysis.
Immunopathology = lesions due to specific virus antigen-antibody complex reactions in affected tissues.

The most common manifestation of herpes simplex is a recurrent vesicular eruption ("cold sores"), which appears most commonly at the mucocutaneous junctions around the lips or nostrils. These eruptions progress to pustules and crust formation and then disappear. The virus remains latent in the sensory cells of the trigeminal nerve ganglion between attacks (Stevens, 1975). The mechanism that is responsible for reactivation of virus is not fully understood. Nonspecific stimuli, such as respiratory infection, fever, or sunlight cause the virus to spread from the trigeminal ganglion via the sensory nerves to the areas of the skin supplied by the nerves. The relapses of herpes simplex occur despite the presence of circulating antibody in patients with recurring disease. The virus probably passes directly from cell to cell without release; this protects the virus from exposure to antibody in the body fluids.

A similar pattern of latency is seen in herpes zoster, a disease due to reactivation of virus latent in dorsal root or cranial nerve ganglia, many years after childhood varicella. In herpes zoster, which mainly affects adults, painful vesicles erupt in an area of skin supplied by a sensory nerve fiber from a single dorsal root. Most commonly affected are the thoracic nerves; less frequently the ophthalmic nerve of the trigeminal ganglion may be involved.

Disseminated infection with cytomegalovirus, a ubiquitous member of the herpesvirus group, is seen when immunosuppressive therapy, neoplasms, acquired immunodeficiency syndrome (AIDS), or other debilitating diseases lower resistance of the patient. Reactivation of latent cytomegalovirus is frequently seen in renal transplant recipients; these reactivations are often not associated with any overt signs or symptoms of disease. The site of latency of cytomegalovirus is not clearly established. In some cases, cytomegalovirus infection may be transmitted during the transfusion of large volumes of fresh blood, and reflects the widespread occurrence of healthy carriers of cytomegalovirus.

Chronic Infections. Persistent infections in this class have a common characteristic: virus is always demonstrable and often is shed. Disease symptoms may be absent or associated with immunopathologic manifestations. A good example of chronic human infection is hepatitis B, a disease associated with varying degrees of hepatic necrosis, and usually contracted by transmission of virus in blood from a chronic carrier (Committee on Viral Hepatitis, 1975). A large amount of a virus-associated antigen (HB-Ag) is commonly present in the serum. This antigen usually disappears rapidly after an acute clinical or subclinical infection. However, in about 5 per cent of infected individuals, HB-Ag may persist in serum in high concentration for years. Although the concentration of infective virus is lower than the HB-Ag, sera from such carriers are highly infectious for recipients of blood transfusion, staff of renal dialysis units, and drug addicts who use unsterilized syringes.

Sera from patients acutely or chronically ill with hepatitis B infection contain antigen-antibody complexes that may play a role in the pathogenesis of acute and chronic hepatic disease. In addition, there is evidence that the glomerulonephritis and polyarteritis nodosa seen in some HB-Ag carriers may be caused by antigen-antibody complexes.

Another example of a chronic infection in humans is the rubella syndrome seen in infants infected in utero with rubella virus during the first 16 weeks of pregnancy. Such infants have various disorders and defects due to generalized infection with rubella virus, and it is usually possible to isolate virus from almost any of their organs. Maternal antibody may inhibit the spread of virus but does not eliminate virus-producing cells. These cells divide at a slower rate than normal uninfected cells, probably giving rise to some of the developmental abnormalities common in infants with rubella syndrome.

Slow Infections. Diseases in this group have many of the characteristics of the chronic infections described in the previous section. However, they differ from chronic infections in several important characteristics. Slow infections have very long incubation periods ranging from months to years; the disease has a long, chronic, and progressive course, and the outcome is usually fatal (Kimberlin, 1976).

The viruses that cause slow infections are heterogeneous. Nononcogenic retroviruses cause visna, maedi, and progressive pneumonia, which are slowly progressive infections of sheep. Another group of agents is poorly defined and difficult to isolate and assay—namely, the agents that produce subacute spongiform encephalopathies in sheep (scrapie), in mink (mink encephalopathy), and in humans (kuru and Creutzfeldt-Jakob disease). The agents of these diseases resemble viruses in that they pass filters with small pore diameters and can be transmitted to experimental animals. The resistance of these agents to irradiation, chemicals, and heat, and their failure to elicit a detectable antibody response in infected hosts indicate that they are not typical viruses. A third group of agents is made up of conventional viruses that produce slow, degenerative diseases of the central nervous system in humans: subacute sclerosing panencephalitis (measles and rubella viruses) and progressive multifocal leukoencephalopathy (JC virus, a papovavirus). Table 2 summarizes the characteristics of slow virus infections of humans.

Spongiform Encephalopathies. Kuru was the first chronic degenerative disease of the central nervous system of humans proved to have a viral etiology. This disease occurred only among a group of about 50,000 highland New Guineans. The classic studies of Gajdusek (1977) revealed that the kuru agent was spread by ritualistic cannibalism and had an incubation period of from four to 20 years. The incidence of the disease has declined since the early 1960s, when the practice of cannibalism was discouraged. All attempts to cultivate the agent of kuru in cell cultures have been unsuccessful. However, transmission experiments have shown that intracerebral inoculation of brain tissue from kuru victims into chimpanzees and monkeys causes the animals to develop symptoms of kuru after an incubation period of about two years.

The importance of the studies of kuru has been illuminated by the demonstration that a rare, progressive, fatal neurologic disease of humans, Creutzfeldt-Jakob disease, is due to an agent with many of the characteristics of the kuru virus. Creutzfeldt-Jakob disease is characterized by presenile dementia with symptoms due to lesions in the cerebral cortex (status spongiosus) and lesions in the spinal cord. The disease is reproduced in chimpanzees and other monkeys by intracerebral inoculation of brain tissue from victims of the disease; the incubation period in experimental animals is about one year. The natural route of infection is not known, but the disease has been accidentally transmitted via a corneal graft (Duffy et al., 1974). Transmission has also been reported via electrodes used for electroencephalography from a patient with the disease to other patients in whom the electrodes were subsequently implanted (Bernoulli et al., 1977).

Table 2. SLOW VIRUS INFECTIONS OF HUMANS

Disease	Site	Pathology	Viruses
Kuru	Brain	Spongiform encephalopathy, especially in cerebellum	Filterable agent transmissible to chimpanzees and monkeys
Creutzfeldt-Jakob disease	Brain and spinal cord	Spongiform encephalopathy	Filterable agent transmissible to chimpanzees and monkeys
Subacute sclerosing panencephalitis (SSPE)	Brain	Neuronal degeneration	Measles and rubella viruses
Progressive multifocal leukoencephalopathy (PML)	Brain	Multiple foci of demyelination in cerebral hemispheres and cerebellum	Human papovavirus (JC virus)

Subacute Sclerosing Panencephalitis (SSPE). This severe chronic neurologic disease is seen in children and young adults several years after primary, and usually uncomplicated, measles (ter Meulen et al., 1972). Affected children have high titers of measles antibody in their serum and spinal fluid. The earliest signs of illness are personality and behavioral changes with intellectual impairment. The disease progresses to convulsions, myoclonal spasms, and increasing neurologic deterioration leading to coma and death. At postmortem there is electron microscopic evidence of measles virus infection, but measles virus cannot be recovered directly. Only by cocultivation of brain tissue with permissive indicator cells can infective measles virus be recovered. Despite the presence of high levels of specific antibody in serum and cerebrospinal fluid, the progress of the disease is not arrested. The factors involved in determining the occurrence of this slow complication of measles in rare individuals are not known. Chronic infection with rubella virus infrequently produces a progressive neurologic disease resembling SSPE (Weil et al., 1975).

Progressive Multifocal Leukoencephalopathy (PML). This is a rare disease that occurs only in patients whose immunologic responsiveness has been severely compromised by such preexisting conditions as leukemia, reticulosis, or immunosuppressive therapy. There are varied neurologic signs, such as dementia, incoordination, and impaired vision; the disease is usually fatal in three or four months. On autopsy, multiple foci of demyelination are found in the cerebral hemispheres and cerebellum; the brain stem and basal ganglia may also be affected. Most cases are due to a papovavirus (JC virus) but some are caused by a virus almost identical to SV40, another papovavirus. These viruses can be grown in human fetal glial cell cultures. Another serotype of papovavirus (BK virus) has been recovered from the urine and genitourinary tract of patients undergoing immunosuppression to prevent rejection of transplanted kidneys. BK virus has not yet been associated with any specific clinical disease (Padgett and Walker, 1976).

Infections with both JC and BK viruses appear to be widespread, since serologic surveys show that many people have antibody to these agents. However, the type of disease caused by primary infection with these viruses during childhood or early adolescence has not been identified. The site of viral latency in the body before reactivation is also not known.

In spite of the increased understanding of the etiology of the slow virus diseases described above, the causes of the most important demyelinating diseases of the central nervous system—that is, multiple sclerosis, the common presenile dementias, and Parkinson's disease—are all still obscure. In the case of multiple sclerosis, common viruses such as measles and parainfluenza type 1 have been suggested as the causative agent in the recent past. However, these associations have so far not stood up to thorough and critical investigation.

PERSISTENT VIRAL INFECTION AT THE CELLULAR LEVEL. The complexities involved in studying persistent infections in humans and the difficulties in establishing model systems in animals have led to intensive efforts to use cell culture models of persistent viral infection. Infection of permissive cells with lytic viruses in culture usually leads to productive infection, the release of large numbers of progeny viruses, and cell death. However, many animal viruses that are considered to be highly cytocidal can establish infections of cell cultures that result in long-term multiplication of the virus while at the same time the cells continue to grow and divide. These stable virus-host cell relationships can be classified into several general categories.

Cell Culture Models of Persistent Viral Infections. The classification that follows is oversimplified because, in many systems, cells may be protected by several mechanisms that may function simultaneously or sequentially. Despite these complexities, the following classification is useful in understanding the model systems that have been established in cell cultures (Walker, 1968). The salient characteristics of these model systems are summarized in Table 3.

Class I. Carrier State in Genetically Resistant Cells. In this type of infection a majority of the cells is genetically resistant. However, permissive (susceptible) cells continually appear and these cells, when infected by free virus in the medium, permit a normal cycle of virus replication and the release of progeny. Characteristically, viral specific antibody or other antiviral factors, such as interferon, are not required to maintain the stable carrier state. Only a small proportion of the cells is infected; when persistently infected cells are cloned, infected cells are destroyed and the clones obtained are free of virus. The clearest examples of this type of carrier culture are infections of a human cell line (HeLa) by poliovirus and Coxsackie virus, members of the picornavirus group.

Class II. Carrier State in Permissive Cells Protected by Antibody in the Medium. In this type of carrier culture only a small fraction of the genetically susceptible cells is infected; most cells are protected from infection by the presence of antiviral factors, usually antibody, in the medium. Removal of the antibody from the medium results in the spread of the infection and destruction of the cell culture. Infected cells do not divide and grow into colonies except in the presence of antibody in the medium. In the absence of antibody, the cell clones obtained are virus-

Table 3. CLASSIFICATION OF PERSISTENTLY INFECTED CARRIER CULTURES

Class of Carrier Culture	Antiviral Antibody Required	All or Most Cells Infected	Infected Cells Can Divide and Form Colonies	Infection Cured by Antiviral Antibody	Interfering Factors Produced in Medium
I. Genetically resistant cells	No	No	No	Yes	Yes or No
II. Permissive cells protected by antibody in medium	Yes	No	No	Yes	Yes or No
III. Permissive cells protected by interference or interferon	No	No	No	Yes	Yes
IV. Regulated infections	No	Yes	Yes	No	Yes or No
V. Virus DNA integrated into the host cell genome	No	Yes	Yes	No	No

free. The best-documented example of this type of carrier state is the persistent infection of various human cell lines by herpes simplex virus.

Class III. Carrier Cultures of Permissive Cells Protected by Interference or Interferon. The general characteristics of this class of persistently infected cells are the following: only a small fraction of the cell population is infected at any time; infected cells do not divide and cannot be cloned; cell clones, when obtained, are free of virus; endogenously produced interfering factors are always present in the culture medium; therefore, antibody or other antiviral factors do not have to be provided for establishment or maintenance of the carrier state. The relative importance of different endogenously produced interfering factors, such as defective-interfering virus particles and interferon, will be considered below.

An outstanding feature of cultures of this type is that the cells are resistant to superinfection by the carried virus or by heterologous viruses, even though only a small fraction of the cells is infected and producing virus at any given time. However, when the infections are cured by prolonged exposure to antibody, the cured cells are just as susceptible to the homologous and heterologous viruses as the original cell line, indicating that genetically resistant cells do not arise during the carrier phase. There are many examples of Class III carrier cultures involving paramyxoviruses and togaviruses.

Class IV. Carrier Cultures in Which the Infections Are "Regulated." The first three classes of persistently infected cells that were described above have important common characteristics. Only a small fraction of the cell population is infected at any given time, infected cells do not divide and grow into colonies but are killed by virus, and clones of cells that are obtained form the carrier culture are free of virus. In contrast, the "regulated" infections of Class IV have the following properties: (1) a high proportion, sometimes all, of the cells in the culture are infected; (2) infected cells can divide and grow into clones that consist of infected cells; (3) antibody or other antiviral factors are not required to establish or maintain the persistently infected state and the culture is not cured of virus by the addition of antibody to the medium; (4) although carrier cultures of this type are fully resistant to superinfection by the homologous virus, they exhibit no resistance to unrelated viruses.

Little is known about the mechanisms by which the "regulated" infections prevent the virus from going through the usual replicative events and cell destruction characteristic of cytocidal infections. The designation "regulated" infection seems appropriate because there seems to be some sort of intracellular regulation or control not yet understood. A large variety of enveloped, budding, RNA viruses can establish this type of persistence—for example, the paramyxoviruses (mumps, measles, parainfluenza viruses 1 and 3, Sendai), rubella, and rabies viruses.

Class V. Carrier State Due to Virus DNA Integration into the Host Cell Genome. Another model for persistent infections involves the integration of the viral genome into the DNA genome of the host cell, an event that would permit the long-term maintenance of viral genetic information in infected cells. There is strong evidence in cell culture systems that persistence by some members of the papovavirus, adenovirus, and herpesvirus groups is maintained by this mechanism. However, in most instances rigorous proof is lacking that genomes of these DNA viruses are integrated into the host cell chromosome in humans or animals. Even in cell culture models, the mechanisms by which the viral genomes are regulated and the phenomena associated with activation are mostly unknown.

There is convincing evidence that visna virus, an RNA C-type retrovirus, which causes a persistent inflammatory demyelinating disease of the central nervous system of sheep, replicates via a DNA intermediate that is integrated into the host cell genome (Haase, 1977). The reverse transcriptase present in the visna virion is responsible for the transcription of a DNA copy of the RNA genome, and it is this DNA intermediate that is inserted into the host DNA.

The possibility has been raised that some enveloped cytolytic RNA viruses, such as paramyxoviruses and togaviruses, which do not contain reverse transcriptase, have the choice of alternate pathways of nucleic acid synthesis and can employ an integrated DNA intermediate for maintaining long-term persistence in infected cells. This mechanism, which is yet to be proved, will be considered in more detail below.

Virus-Specific Factors That May Be Involved in the Establishment and Maintenance of Persistent Infections

Mechanisms of Persistence of DNA Viruses. Herpes simplex, varicella-zoster, and cytomegaloviruses, all members of the herpes-virus group, probably establish persistence in which the virus remains latent; the DNA genomes are present as cytoplasmic or nuclear plasmid forms in either a completely regulated or a nonreplicating state. Also likely is the possibility that in some instances a less tightly controlled, very slowly replicating state may be involved. In either case there is no a priori need to postulate integration as a means of perpetuating the infection.

In regard to the papovaviruses, the best-studied example is SV40, a virus of simian origin that is related to human papovavirus (JC virus) associated with progressive multifocal leukoencephalopathy. SV40 virus maintains a latent state in cell cultures by integration of the viral DNA into the host genome; such cells may contain up to 10 copies of SV40 DNA per cell (Doerfler, 1975). In the case of human papilloma virus, a papovavirus that causes warts, the mechanism by which the viral DNA persists is not yet known.

There is strong circumstantial evidence that persistence of adenovirus in certain cell systems is maintained by the integration of the viral genome into the host cell DNA (Doerfler, 1975). There is, however, no rigorous proof of this mechanism, and the manner in which adenoviruses persist in adenoids and tonsils of humans is unknown. Also unknown are the mechanisms of persistence of the SV40-related viruses, JC and BK, which are isolated from patients with progressive multifocal leukoencephalopathy or from immunosuppressed patients shedding these viruses in their urine.

The only definitive information concerning integration of viral DNA of herpesviruses comes from studies of the Epstein-Barr (EB) virus that is associated with infectious mononucleosis, Burkitt's lymphoma, and nasopharyngeal carcinoma (Klein, 1973). There is evidence that both in lymphoblastoid cell lines and in the tumors, the EB virus DNA is maintained in two physical states; a linear form integrated into cellular DNA, and a circular, extrachromosomal plasmid.

In summary, although there is some understanding of the state of the viral DNA in cell culture systems latently infected with some papovaviruses (except papilloma virus), adenoviruses, and EB virus, there is little definitive information concerning other herpesviruses. With the exception of EB virus, little is known about the mechanisms of DNA virus latency in man or animals. The mechanism by which the viral genomes are controlled and regulated during latent infection and, more particularly, the phenomena associated with reactivation are, at this time, poorly understood.

Mechanisms of Persistence of RNA Viruses. A number of different mechanisms, which are not necessarily mutually exclusive, have been proposed to explain the persistence of ordinarily cytolytic RNA viruses in cell cultures. Although there is some evidence that these mechanisms may operate in animal models, there is no direct support at this time for their involvement in human disease (Rima and Martin, 1976).

Role of Defective-Interfering (DI) Particles. Evidence is accumulating that defective particles capable of interfering with the replication of homologous standard virus occur spontaneously in almost every virus system that has been studied (Huang, 1973). Serial passage of viruses at high multiplicities of infection (high virus per cell ratios in the inoculum) results in the production of DI particles that have the following general characteristics: (1) they contain normal structural capsid proteins; (2) a portion of the viral genome is missing (in reality they are deletion mutants); (3) they can replicate only in cells coinfected with the homologous virus helper; and (4) they can interfere specifically with the replication of homologous standard virus.

It has been postulated that the production of DI particles may regulate the synthesis of virus in persistent infections by specifically inhibiting production of the homologous standard virus, thereby damping down infection (Huang and Baltimore, 1970). There is some evidence that this concept is plausible even for a highly cytolytic virus. When vesicular stomatitis virus (VSV), a rhabdovirus, is passaged serially at high multiplicity in susceptible Chinese hamster ovary cells, and the relative concentrations of standard VSV and DI particles are determined at each passage, there is a cyclical overlapping pattern of production of complete virus and production of DI particles. This pattern, based on serial high multiplicity passages, serves as a theoretical model for persistent infection.

Evidence concerning the possible role of DI particles in persistent infection is provided by a model system involving a line of hamster cells (BHK-21) persistently infected with VSV (Holland and Villarreal, 1974). A mixture of infective standard virus and large numbers of DI particles is required to establish the initial persistent infection. During the course of the infection, more DI particles are generated.

Synthesis of DI particles has been implicated in maintenance of measles virus persistence in human cell lines, and in cultured cells persistently infected with such diverse viruses as reovirus, rabies, several togaviruses, and lymphocytic choriomeningitis virus. The precise relationship of DI particles to autointerference and to persistence is not well understood. Although it is evident that DI particles play an important role in many carrier cell cultures, much more work is needed to prove a role for DI particles in persistent infections in animals and humans.

Role of Temperature-Sensitive (TS) Mutants. A body of information has accumulated that shows that viruses recovered from persistent infections often differ in biologic properties from the standard virus used to initiate the infection. Quite commonly, when compared to wild-type viruses, the agents recovered from persistently infected cells produce smaller plaques in cell cultures and are less able to infect experimental animals. In many model systems, there is a natural selection of ts mutants* that replace the standard virus population during the evolution of the persistently infected state (Youngner and Preble, 1980). Such ts viruses occur in a variety of host cells persistently infected with agents such as mumps, measles, rubella, Sendai, Newcastle disease, Sindbis, Western equine encephalomyelitis, and vesicular stomatitis viruses. Selection of ts mutants in persistent infections is not limited to any particular class of virus or type of cultured cell. In fact, one report (Valentine et al., 1969) describes a commonly occurring spontaneous ts mutant of bacteriophage Qβ that causes a persistent infection of its bacterial host, *Escherichia coli*.

The reasons why ts mutants are selected under conditions of persistent infection are not fully understood, but the following is known. In the cases of such viruses as VSV, Newcastle disease virus, and Sindbis, ts mutants interfere strongly with the replication of standard virus at both permissive and nonpermissive temperatures, interference occurring before or at the level of RNA transcription. Second, ts mutants of VSV are rescued by standard virus at nonpermissive temperatures; in effect, ts mutants act as conditionally defective interfering (DI) viruses at the nonpermissive temperature. As a result, the replication of ts virus tends to be dominant at the nonpermissive or partially restrictive temperature, thereby explaining why ts mutants

*Temperature-sensitive (ts) conditional lethal mutants have been described for many different viruses (Fenner, 1969). These ts viruses occur in low frequency spontaneously and in higher frequency after exposing standard virus to mutagens. Ts viruses replicate well at low temperatures (31 to 33° C) and poorly at higher temperatures (38 to 40° C); in contrast, standard wild-type viruses replicate almost equally well at both permissive and nonpermissive (restrictive) temperatures.

are selected. Also, since under these conditions ts mutants tend to be less cytocidal and the replication of standard virus is suppressed, an explanation is provided of why ts mutants tend to be selected and why this selection leads to the maintenance of persistent infections.

Despite these observations, the presence of multiple genetic alterations in viruses isolated from persistently infected cells mandates caution in attributing to any one defect a key role in the establishment and maintenance of a persistent infection. Any genetic alteration that converts a lytic virus-cell interaction to a noncytocidal one has the potential to cause a persistent infection.

There is much evidence that ts mutation plays a role in the establishment and maintenance of many persistent infections in cell cultures. However, in animals and humans the relationship of these observations to persistence is not yet established.

Role for Defects in Host Contributions to Virus Replication. It is likely that increasing evidence will appear dealing with the importance of defects or alterations in virus assembly and release in persistent infections, particularly those involving enveloped viruses. The yield of these viruses from persistently infected cells is often less than in cytocidal infections, and frequently no infective virus is produced. Several mechanisms could operate in such a system.

Specific protein cleavages, especially of viral envelope glycoproteins, are important steps in virus maturation (Scheid and Choppin, 1976). In some paramyxoviruses, cleavage is accomplished by a host enzyme and activates virus activities such as cell fusion, hemolysis, and viral penetration of host cells. The host range and tissue tropisms in large measure depend on the presence in host tissue of the appropriate activating protease. Since virus mutants have been isolated in the laboratory that require different proteases for activation, the possibility exists that infection of a tissue not normally susceptible to a given virus may result from the appearance of a mutant that can be activated by a protease present in that tissue. In addition, infection by a cytocidal virus of a cell that cannot cleave the progeny viral glycoprotein could result in persistent infection without the production infective virus. If proper cleavage reactions fail in paramyxoviruses, mature but noninfective virus is produced, whereas failure of cleavage in togaviruses prevents virus assembly. It is possible that specific proteolysis of viral proteins by host enzymes is important in many persistent infections.

Possible Role of Integrated Viral Genomes. DNA copies of RNA virus genomes are integrated into chromosomes of cells persistently infected by tumorigenic retroviruses and by visna virus, a retrovirus that causes persistent central nervous system disease in sheep. There have been several reports that DNA copies of usually cytocidal single-stranded RNA viruses have been integrated into the genome of persistently infected host cells (Simpson and Iinuma, 1975; Zhdanov, 1975). The viruses involved include respiratory syncytial virus, SV5, measles, Sindbis, and tickborne encephalitis virus. A mechanism proposing an integrated DNA intermediate of usually cytolytic RNA viruses raises questions concerning (1) the source of the RNA-dependent DNA polymerase that initially transcribes the RNA of the infecting virus into a DNA copy, (2) the nature of the integration of this DNA copy into the host cell DNA, and (3) the regulation of the expression of the integrated DNA copy of the viral RNA. Some workers have not found DNA intermediates in cells persistently infected with several cytolytic RNA viruses (Haase et al., 1977).

There is abundant evidence, however, that a DNA integration mechanism is not necessary for persistence of RNA viruses. In many instances the viral genome persists as RNA, replicates independently of the host cell genome, and passes from one daughter cell to another for generations, with viral products demonstrable at any stage.

Other Mechanisms. The intact animal probably has more mechanisms for establishing and maintaining persistent infections than cultured cells possess. Both nonspecific resistance factors (fever; interferon production) and specific immunity complicate the situation. Much more information is needed to understand how virus-infected cells are eliminated in the body. The role of antibody modulation of viral antigens from the cell surface in persistent infection in the animal must also be clarified (Joseph and Oldstone, 1975).

References

Bernoulli, C., Siegfried, J., Baumgartner, G., Regli, F., Rabinowitiz, T., Gajdusek, D. C., and Gibbs, D. J.: Danger of accidental person-to-person transmission of Creutzfeldt-Jakob disease by surgery. Lancet 1:478, 1977.

Committee on Viral Hepatitis: Symposium on Viral Hepatitis. Am J Med Sci 270:2, 1975.

Doerfler, W.: Integration of viral DNA into the host genome. Curr Top Microbiol Immunol 71:1, 1975.

Duffy, P., Wolf, J., Collins, G., De Voe, A. G., Streeten, B., and Cowen, D.: Possible person-to-person transmission of Creutzfeldt-Jakob disease. N Engl J Med 290:692, 1974.

Fenner, F.: Conditional lethal mutants of animal viruses. Curr Top Microbiol Immunol 48:1, 1969.

Gajdusek, D. C.: Unconventional viruses and the origin and disappearance of kuru. Science 197:943, 1977.

Haase, A. T., Stowring, L., Ventura, P., Traynor, B., Johnson, K., Swoveland, P., Smith, M., Britten-Darnall, M., Faras, A., and Morayan, O.: Role of DNA intermediates in persistent infections caused by RNA viruses. In Schlessinger, D. (ed.): Microbiology–1977, Washington, American Society for Microbiology, 1977, p. 478.

Holland, J. J., and Villarreal, L. P.: Persistent noncytocidal vesicular stomatitis virus infections mediated by defective T particles that suppress virion transcriptase. Proc Natl Acad Sci USA 71:2956, 1974.

Huang, A. S.: Defective interfering viruses. Ann Rev Microbiol 27:101, 1973.

Huang, A. S., and Baltimore, D.: Defective viral particles and viral disease processes. Nature 226:325, 1970.

Joseph, B. S., and Oldstone, M. B. A.: Immunologic injury in measles virus infection. II. Suppression of immune injury through antigenic modulation. J Exp Med 142:864, 1975.

Kimberlin, R. H. (ed.): Slow virus diseases of animals and man. Frontiers in Biology. Amsterdam, North-Holland Publishing Co., 1976.

Klein, G.: The Epstein-Barr virus. *In* Kaplan, A. S. (ed.): The herpesviruses. New York, Academic Press, 1973, p. 521.

Padgett, B. L., and Walker, D. L.: New human papovaviruses. Prog Med Virol 22:1, 1976.

Rima, B. K., and Martin, S. J.: Persistent infection of tissue culture cells by RNA viruses. Med Microbiol Immunol 162:89, 1976.

Scheid, A., and Choppin, P: Protease activation mutants of Sendai virus. Activation of biologic properties by specific proteases. Virology 69:265, 1976.

Simpson, R. W., and Iinuma, M.: Recovery of infectious proviral DNA from mammalian cells infected with respiration syncytial virus. Proc Natl Acad Sci USA 72:3230, 1975.

Stevens, J. G.: Latent herpes simplex virus and the nervous system. Curr Top Microbiol Immunol. 70:31, 1975.

ter Meulen, V., Katz, M., and Múller, D.: Subacute sclerosing panencephalitis: a review. Curr Top Immunol 57:1, 1972.

Valentine, R. C., Ward, R., and Strand, M.: The replication cycle of RNA bacteriophages. Adv Virus Res 15:1, 1969.

Walker, D. L.: Persistent viral infection in cell cultures. In Sanders, M., and Lennette, E. H. (eds.) Medical and Applied Virology. St. Louis, Missouri, Warren H. Green, Inc., 1968, p. 99.

Weil, M. L., Itabashi, H. H., Cremer, N. E., Oshers, L. S., Lennette, E. H., and Carnay, L.: Chronic progressive panencephalitis due to rubella virus simulating subacute sclerosing panencephalitis. N Engl J Med 19:994, 1975.

Youngner, J. S., and Preble, O. T.: Viral persistence: Evolution of virus populations. *In* H. Fraenkel-Conrat and R. R. Wagner (eds.): Comprehensive Virology, Plenum Press, New York, Vol. 16; 73, 1980.

Zhdanov, V. M.: Integration of viral genomes. Nature 256:471, 1975.

12

INTERFERON AND INTERFERENCE

MONTO HO, M.D.

The story of interferon illustrates how an obscure phenomenon originally of interest only to laboratory scientists can become important for the whole field of biomedical and clinical sciences (Stewart, 1979; Ho, 1982). In the 1930s and 1940s, virologists were already familiar with "viral interference." They found that, for example, if virus A was injected into an experimental animal at the same time or shortly before virus B, the replication of virus B would be inhibited. Virus A, the "interfering virus," frequently interfered even if it was inactivated or made non-infectious by heat or ultraviolet irradiation. No satisfactory explanation for this phenomenon was provided until 1957 when Isaacs and Lindenmann did a classic experiment, described in Figure 1.

The experiment formed the basis of a simple but important discovery. This was that viruses can induce in cells an antiviral substance, interferon, which in turn inhibits the replication of the challenge virus. In many ways, interferon is an ideal antiviral substance. It is relatively non-toxic, and it is broadly effective against a large number of RNA and DNA viruses. Further, since interferon is produced by cells under "natural" conditions of viral infections in animals, it was thought that a novel antiviral defense system was discovered.

However, we now realize that interferon is much more than a natural antiviral cytokine and lymphokine. It has broad effects on humoral and cellular immunity, phagocytosis, inflammation, and cellular proliferation. It interacts with other substances such as the interleukins and prostaglandins to modulate the immune system.

INDUCTION AND PRODUCTION. Interferon is a cellular protein. In this respect it is like hormones, enzymes, antibodies, and other cellular proteins. Such proteins are usually made by specialized cells, but as far as we know all

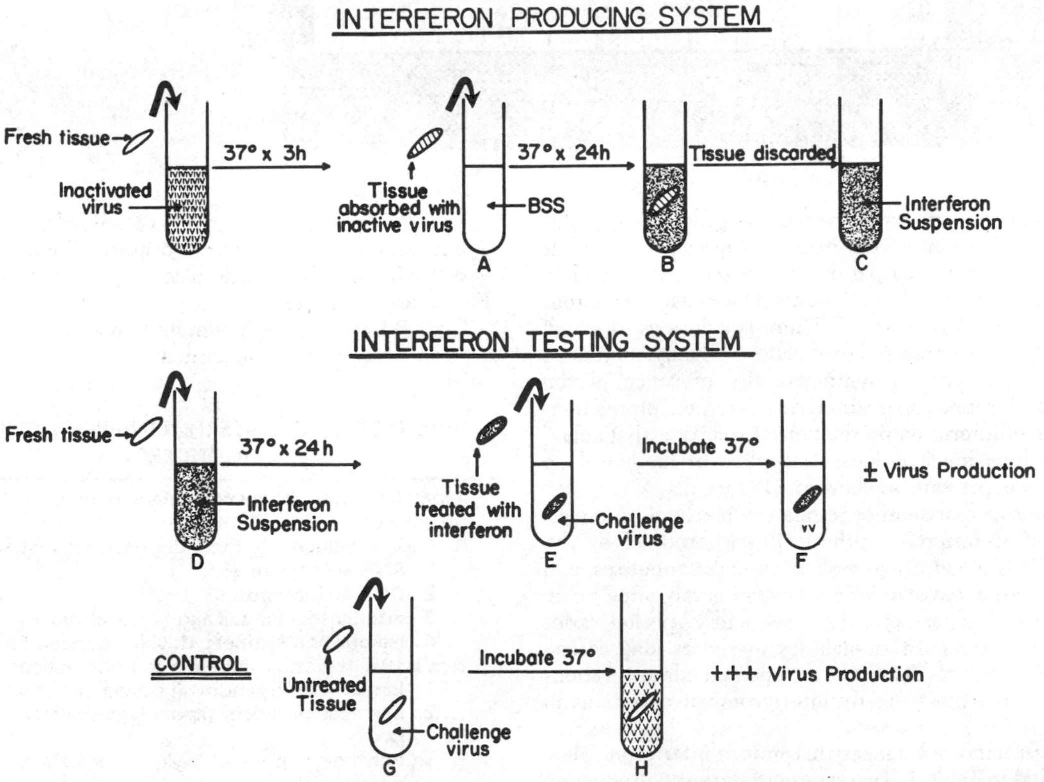

Figure 1. Scheme of a system for producing and testing interferon. (From Ho, M.: Interferons. N Engl J Med 266:1260, 1962.)

Fragments of chick chorioallantoic tissue are bathed in a suspension of inactivated Type A influenza virus (interfering virus). The tissue absorbed with the inactivated virus was incubated for 24 hours (A, B). A substance called "interferon" was released (C). Its presence was demonstrated in the "Interferon Testing System." Fresh tissue fragments are treated in the suspension containing interferon (D). The treated tissue (E) along with untreated controls (G) is inoculated with a "challenge virus." Virus production in treated and control tissue is measured. The degree of reduction in (F) as compared with (H) represents the potency of interferon. This testing system is still the conceptual basis for all methods of interferon assay.

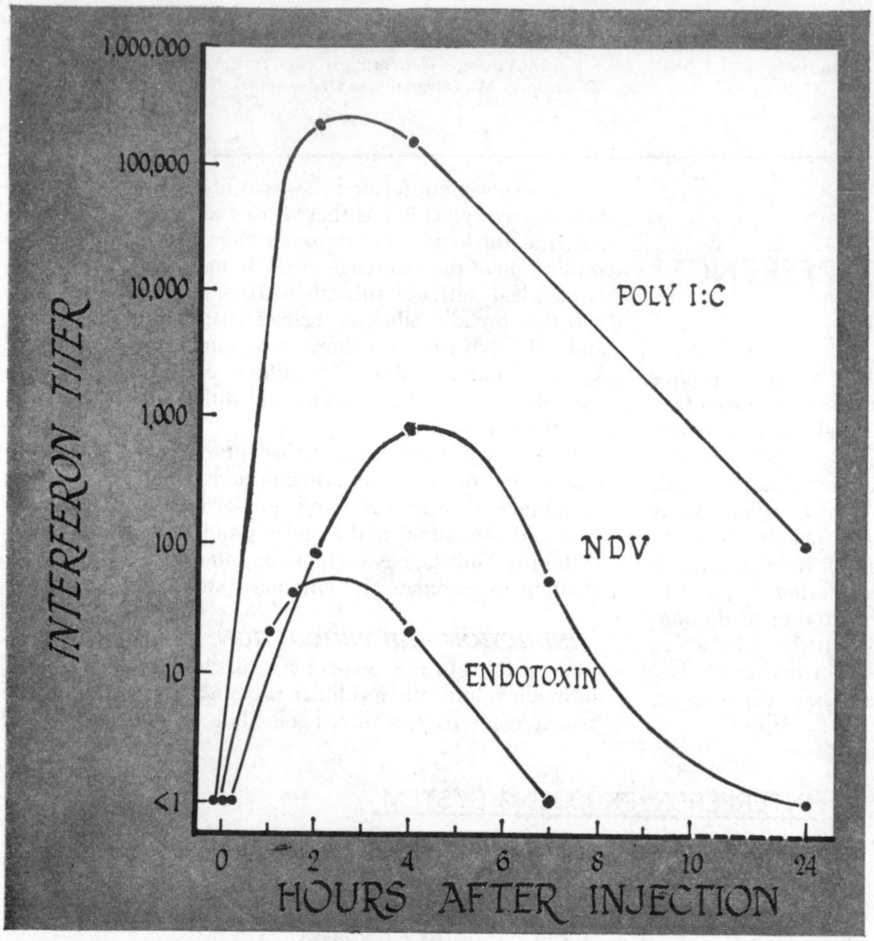

Figure 2. The appearance of interferon in the serum of a rabbit after injection of *E. coli* lipopolysaccharide (endotoxin), Newcastle disease virus (NDV), or a complexed synthetic double-stranded ribonucleic acid, polyriboinosinic-polyribocytidylic acid (poly I:C). Note the marked variation in the effectiveness of these three inducers, and that maximum interferon levels are only transiently maintained. (From Ho, M.: Factors influencing the interferon response. Arch Int Med 126:136, 1970.)

cells can make interferon if given the appropriate stimulus ("induced"). The interferon-making capacity of cells is ordinarily not expressed; it is "repressed." It is widely believed that when cells are "induced" to make interferon, this capacity is "derepressed." There is a curious aspect of "derepression" of interferon production. Usually in induced or derepressed protein synthesis, the presence of the inducer or derepressor guarantees continued production. In the case of interferon production, it is a "one-shot affair" no matter how much inducer is applied or for how long the inducer is present, as shown in Figure 2.

This suggests that another regulatory mechanism in cells that inhibits interferon synthesis is triggered off by the inducer. Cells in culture as well as animals cannot respond to an interferon inducer for varying intervals after being induced. This "hyporeactive" or "refractory" period varies from hours to days. In animals it may be as long as one week and is a serious deterrent to repeated administrations of inducers to achieve steady interferon concentrations in tissues.

There are many substances that induce interferon. They are classified in Table 1. Two types of interferon production may be distinguished. Type 1 follows stimulation with specific, known inducers. These inducers are divided into two classes, A and B. The type of interferon induced is α and β, represented in man by leukocyte and fibroblast interferon.

Class A inducers are good inducers that induce the production of 1000 units/ml or more of interferon in cell culture or in the bloodstream of animals. They contain double-stranded RNA, or may form such RNA in the course of cell infection. Newcastle disease virus and poly I:C (see Fig. 2) are examples.

Class B inducers are moderate to poor inducers that may act only when injected in animals. They are a motley group

Table 1. TYPES OF INTERFERON PRODUCTION AND INDUCERS

I. Type I Interferon Production: (α and β Interferon). Stimulated by Inducers
  A. Class A Inducers (good inducers, double-stranded RNA):
    1. RNA animal viruses
    2. DNA animal viruses
    3. Plant, insect fungus and bacterial viruses
    4. Natural and synthetic double-stranded RNA's
  B. Class B Inducers (moderate to poor inducers):
    1. Intracellular organisms (bacteria, rickettsia, protozoa)
    2. Bacterial products (lipopolysaccharides, polysaccharides)
    3. Polymers (polycarboxylic, polysulfates, polyphosphates)
    4. Low molecular weight substances (tilorone, cycloheximide, etc.)

II. Type II Interferon Production: (γ Interferon). Specific and Nonspecific Immune Induction
  A. Immune Specific Induction
  B. Nonspecific Stimulation of T Lymphocytes by Mitogens

of macromolecular substances often without effect in fibroblast or epithelial cell cultures. Some are microorganisms that infect intracellularly, usually macrophages. It is assumed that uptake by macrophages is necessary in induction by many of these substances.

Type II is the production of γ interferon by specific and nonspecific immunologic activation of lymphocytes, usually T lymphocytes. Although this important phenomenon produces only moderate amounts of interferon, it may be an effector limb of cell-mediated immunity. Interferon γ may be considered a lymphokine.

During immune specific induction, interferon is produced by sensitized lymphocytes upon exposure to specific antigen. The sensitizing antigen may be a viral antigen, or nonviral antigens such as PPD, diphtheria, or tetanus toxoid. Interferon-γ is also produced during cellular immune responses; for example, in mixed lymphocyte reactions. Immune induction may occur in vitro or in the animal.

Interferon is also produced when lymphocytes are stimulated by nonspecific mitogens such as phytohemagglutinin, pokeweed antigen, and concanavalin A. Its production during clonal expansion of lymphocytes may mediate a number of responses. For example, interferon produced by concanavalin A–activated suppressor T cells may be essential for their suppressor activity.

An important advance that has made pure α, β, and γ interferon available in abundant quantities for clinical trials has been the rapid and effective application of recombinant DNA cloning methods from research laboratories to industry. For example, interferon-α was cloned by first isolating interferon mRNA from KG-1, a human myeloblast cell line induced with Sendai virus. The interferon gene (cDNA) was prepared from the mRNA in vitro by reverse transcriptase. It was then annealed by appropriate enzymes to a plasmid, which was inserted into *E. coli.* A producer clone of this bacterium was then selected that could be used to make interferon in unlimited quantities (Goeddel et al., 1980). All three types of interferon can now be produced industrially by using recombinant methods or methods relying on conventional human cell cultures and appropriate inducers.

PROPERTIES OF INTERFERON. Interferon is a class of proteins heterogeneous at several levels. Each species or genus has its unique interferons, although there are wide stretches of amino-acid-sequence homologies between similar interferons of different species. Thus, for example, chick interferons are not effective in rabbits and humans. For each species there are, as mentioned above, three major types of interferons, α, β, and γ. Human interferon-α is a protein of about 20,000 daltons with 165 amino acids. From analysis of the amino acid sequences of cloned alpha interferons, at least 12 subtypes have been discovered to date. Natural leukocyte interferon represents a mixture of unknown composition of these subtypes plus a small amount of interferon-beta. The structures and amino acid sequences of β and γ interferons are also known.

The specific activity of interferon is comparable to the most potent hormones. There are about 2×10^8 antiviral units in 1 mg of pure interferon. Cloned materials can easily reach 50 per cent purity, whereas the best natural interferon prepared from leukocytes rarely exceeds 1 per cent purity.

Interferon is much more than a natural antiviral substance. It is now apparent that it is a pleiotropic regulatory protein and a lymphokine. It is a potent modulator of humoral and cellular immunity with a unique ability to stimulate natural killer (NK) cell activity. Interferon is thought to be the primary regulatory substance of NK activity in the body.

The paradoxical effects of interferon on immunity are illustrated by the fact that a small dose of interferon in mice enhances the production of antibody to sheep red blood cells, while a high dose (5,000 to 10,000 units) inhibits such production. The effect of interferon on delayed hypersensitivity is related to timing rather than dose (DeMaeyer and DeMaeyer-Guignard, 1980). When given 24 hours before the antigen, interferon inhibits subsequent sensitization. When given a few hours after the antigen, sensitization is enhanced.

Interferon can activate macrophages and enhance phagocytosis. It is highly reactive with cell membranes and one of its actions is to increase the surface antigens on lymphocytes. It inhibits the proliferation of many cells, including tumor cells. This action, plus its effect on the immune system, may be the basis of the anti-cancer effect of interferon. Interferon may also be a mediator of inflammation. For example, it is a potent pyrogen, the mechanism of which is still unclear. At this point, the complex biologic properties of interferon make it a candidate for eliciting many physiologic and pathologic responses in the body. In most cases, however, its precise role is unknown. Its role in therapeutics is also unclear, despite a mounting number of clinical trials.

MECHANISM OF ACTION OF INTERFERON. A great deal has been learned about the mechanism of action of interferon, particularly its antiviral aspects. Interferon has no direct antiviral action, but it inhibits the replication or release of viruses. To do this, new protein synthesis is required. Interferon is active to some extent against virtually all viruses, but some are more susceptible than others. The togaviruses, myxoviruses, and poxviruses are very susceptible. The herpesviruses and picornaviruses are less so. Adenoviruses are resistant.

Kerr and Brown (1978) discovered an enzyme in interferon-treated cells that synthesized a hitherto unknown class of adenylates, oligomers of 2′, 5′-isoadenylate. The usual adenylate in the body links ribose to adenylic acid at the 3′ to 5′ sites. This new class of molecules can activate specifically an intracellular ribonuclease F, which degrades mRNA (including viral mRNA), and hence inhibits protein synthesis and translation of viral proteins.

Another mechanism by which interferon is thought to act is by inducing protein kinases. One of these found in interferon-treated cells can phosphorylate eIF-2, one of the initiation factors of protein translation. Phosphorylation inactivates the initiation factor and thereby inhibits protein synthesis, including viral protein synthesis (Lebleu et al., 1976).

Interferon may inhibit the assembly and release of certain retroviruses. It may also inhibit the transcription of some viruses; the earliest one described was SV-40. At this time, one can say that interferon induces many proteins in cells, which may inhibit viral replication in various ways, but in terms of real understanding, the wheat has not yet been separated from the chaff.

The mechanism by which interferon mediates its many non-antiviral actions is still unclear. The first step of its action is thought to be binding to specific receptors on cells. These may be different for the three types of interferons, particularly for interferon-γ, which is a much more potent immunomodulator than the other two types. How it acts on cell membranes to produce its membrane-modulating effects, including its unique ability to increase expression of Dr antigens on macrophages and effects on the cytoskeletal system, and whether this is related to signals that initiate the synthesis of antiviral proteins are unknown.

Interferon may be important in various immunologic disorders. Circulating interferon has been found in systemic lupus erythematosus (SLE) and other autoimmune diseases. An acid labile α interferon has been found in the blood of patients with SLE or the acquired immunodeficiency syndrome (AIDS) (Preble et al., 1982). Whether these interferons merely represent a byproduct of in vivo immunologic reactions or whether they mediate an actual pathologic or defense response is unclear.

ROLE OF INTERFERON IN HOST DEFENSE. Interferon is a novel antiviral substance produced in the course of natural virus infections and after immunologic reactions, but its relative importance among specific and nonspecific antiviral defenses is uncertain. There is no "experiment in nature" in which a viral infection may be observed in an animal whose capacity to make interferon or react to it is genetically deficient. Quite possibly, a congenital absence of the interferon system is incompatible with life. Indirect evidence suggests that interferon plays an important role in host defense. Viral infections in mice run a more lethal course if interferon formed is neutralized by specific antiserum against interferon (Gresser et al., 1976).

The discovery that lymphocytes activated by mitogens and sensitized lymphocytes exposed to specific antigens produce interferon adds another dimension to the role of interferon in host defense. Interferon is one of the many lymphokines, such as migration inhibition factor, which help explain how cellular immunity works. A number of viruses, particularly the Herpetoviridae, produce more frequent and more severe infections when cellular immunity is suppressed. One method by which cellular immunity is assumed to work is by release of interferon-γ from sensitized T lymphocytes that come in contact with viral antigen. This mechanism should be particularly effective in the lesions, such as the vesicles of herpes simplex or herpes zoster, where there is an abundance of viral antigens and inflammatory lymphocytes.

THERAPEUTIC ROLE AS AN ANTIVIRAL SUBSTANCE. There are two ways to use the interferon system therapeutically. One may administer either an inducer of interferon or interferon itself. In animals the administration of "inducer" may be effective against viral infections. "Hyporeactivity" to repeated induction is an intrinsic problem of this method. It limits the efficacy of repeated administration of inducer and places a limit on the amount of interferon that can be induced, but it is not insurmountable. A more serious problem has been the toxicity of practically every inducer that has been carefully studied. Some of the best and chemically purest inducers, such as synthetic double-stranded polyribonucleotides, are prohibitively toxic. The search for nontoxic inducers, either by molecular manipulation of polyribonucleotides or by search for new types of inducers, continues, although not as vigorously as before.

Interferon has its limitations as an antiviral. It does not eradicate viral infections. While its specific antiviral activity is high, as little as 0.001 μg possesses detectable antiviral activity, but its antiviral activity at any dose is incomplete so that it cannot cure or prevent a viral infection even with relatively large amounts.

Both natural (leukocyte) and cloned α interferons have been tested clinically against a large number of viral infections and tumors. So far controlled clinical trials have been undertaken only against viral infections. It has been found efficacious in the following circumstances (Djeu and Zoon, 1983):

1. In reducing time required for healing of acute herpetic keratitis.
2. In reducing morbidity and the time required for healing of herpes zoster in patients with non-Hodgkin's lymphoma.
3. In reducing morbidity of varicella in children with hematopoietic malignancies.
4. For prevention and amelioration of the symptoms of the common cold when interferon was given intranasally after experimental inoculation of rhinoviruses.
5. For reduction of morbidity but not infection with cytomegalovirus after renal transplantation.
6. For eradicating individual lesions of verruca vulgaris (warts), caused by a papilloma virus, when interferon is given intradermally.
7. In reducing shedding of the herpesvirus in the mouth after microsurgical decompression for trigeminal neuralgia.

In uncontrolled trials, interferon has also reduced markers (DNA polymerase) for the complete virus (Dane particles) in the blood stream of patients with chronic active hepatitis (Greenberg et al., 1976). But it does not consistently affect HBsAg, and it has not been proven that the clinical course of chronic active hepatitis is improved. Interferon has not ameliorated the outcome of rabies.

It is possible that interferon will have a place in treating one or more viral diseases listed above. Its exact role has not been determined because many of the trials were very limited in design, and its toxicity may restrict its use.

Being a natural substance, interferon was originally thought to be devoid of significant toxicity. It has now been administered in large quantities (as much as 50 to 100 million units a day) after the cloned material became available. Although severe toxicity and death are rare, fever, malaise, and fatigue are common. Reversible depression of the bone marrow, particularly of the granulocytes, is almost always seen. In the case of the common cold, the toxicity of interferon and the disease it treats are about the same severity.

In uncontrolled trials, interferon has been effective against a number of papilloma virus infections. The most important is laryngeal papillomatosis, a self-limited disease of children that frequently produces dangerous airway obstruction.

In uncontrolled phase 1 and phase 2 trials, interferon also seems to have some efficacy against certain malignancies. These include osteogenic sarcoma, non-Hodgkin's lymphoma, carcinoma of the breast, renal cell carcinoma, some acute and chronic leukemias including hairy cell leukemia, Kaposi's sarcoma in AIDS, and malignant melanoma when interferon was given intralesionally. In most of these diseases, interferon was not notably superior to standard therapy. More trials are needed to determine whether interferon has a place as a primary or adjunct agent in anti-cancer therapy.

In view of its pleiotropic effects, it is not surprising that interferon has been tested as therapy for a number of chronic diseases of undetermined etiology. Foremost among these is multiple sclerosis. Many trials are in progress following one report that interferon-β given intrathecally reduces the number of relapses in this disease (Jacobs et al., 1982). Definitive results are not yet available.

OTHER TYPES OF VIRAL INTERFERENCE. There are three types of viral interference that are not mediated by interferon.

Receptor Interference. One type of interference is based on competition for specific viral receptors. Infection by a myxovirus, such as Newcastle disease virus, may be interfered with if cell receptors are occupied or blocked by a prior infection. Another example of this type of interference may be found in the avian leukoviruses. It is used to study the relatedness of these agents and their titration. For example, inapparent infection of chick cells by one leukovirus will abrogate cellular receptors for this and related agents, so that a superinfection by a related transforming or cytocidal agent will be interfered with.

Intracellular Homologous Interference. Another type of interference involves competition for limiting factor *within cells* among homologous or homotypic viruses. Examples are known among many viruses, such as influenza virus, vesicular stomatitis virus, and poliovirus. The best studied example is the ability of defective particles to interfere. These defective interfering particles (DIP) explain "autointerference" and may have a modifying role on viral infections. They are discussed in Chapter 11.

Interference by Heterologous Agents. This is also intracellular and may be based on repression of transcription or translation. One example is so-called "intrinsic interference," which depends on a protein (not interferon) specified by the interfering virus. A number of viruses, such as rubella virus or measles virus, may interfere in chick embryo fibroblast cultures with the replication of Newcastle disease virus. This type of interference may be used to titer noncytopathic or nonreplicating virus.

References

DeMaeyer, E., and DeMaeyer-Guignard, J.: Immunoregulatory action of type 1 interferon in the mouse. Ann N Y Acad Sci 350:1, 1984.

Djeu, J. Y., and Zoon, K. C.: Proceedings of Interferon Workshop. Office of Biologics, National Center for Drugs and Biologics., September 28–30 1983, Elsevier, N. Y., 1984.

Greenberg, H. B., Pollard, R. B., Lutwick, L. I., Gregory, P. B., Robinson, W. E., and Merigan, T. C.: Effect of human leukocyte interferon on hepatitis B virus infection in patients with chronic active hepatitis. N Engl J Med 295:517, 1976.

Goeddel, D. V., Yelverton, E., et al.: Human leukocyte interferon produced by *E. coli* is biologically active. Nature (Lond) 287:411, 1980.

Gresser, I., Tovey, M. G., et al.: Role of interferon in the pathogenesis of viral diseases in mice as demonstrated by the use of anti-interferon serum. I. Rapid evolution of encephalomyocarditis virus infection. J Exper Med 144:1305, 1976.

Ho, M.: Recent advances in the study of interferon. Pharmacol Rev 34:119, 1982.

Isaacs, A., and Lindenmann, J.: Virus interference. I. Interferon. Proc Roy Soc B 147:258, 1957.

Jacobs, L., O'Malley, J., Freeman, A., Murawski, J., and Ekes, R.: Intrathecal interferon in multiple sclerosis. Arch Neurol 39:609, 1982.

Kerr, I. M., and Brown, R. E.: ppA2'p5'A2'p5'A: An inhibitor of protein synthesis synthesized with an enzyme fraction from interferon-treated cells. Proc Natl Acad Sci USA 75:256, 1978.

LeBleu, B., Sen, G. C., Shaila, S., Cabrer, B., and Lengyee, P.: Interferon double-stranded RNA, and protein phosphorylation. Proc Natl Acad Sci USA 73:3107, 1976.

Preble, O. T., Black, R. J., Friedman, R. M., Klippel, J. H., and Vilcek, J.: Systemic lupus erythematosus: presence in human serum of an unusual acid-labile leukocyte interferon. Science 216:429, 1982.

Stewart, W. E., II: The Interferon System. Vienna and New York, Springer-Verlag, 1979.

MYCOLOGY

13

MORPHOLOGY AND STRUCTURE OF FUNGI

VLADIMIR FARKAŠ, PH.D.

The fungi (Latin: *fungus,* mushroom) can be defined as eukaryotic, thallus-forming organisms *(Thallobiota)* that lack both chlorophyll and chemolithotrophic machinery. Consequently, they can produce structural elements neither from carbon dioxide via photosynthesis nor from inorganic matter. For this reason they depend on external sources of organic carbon. The fungi can live as saprophytes on dead organic matter or as parasites on other organisms, mainly plants, but also animals and man. (For the taxonomic position of fungi, see Chapter 14.)

The vegetative body of the fungus, the *thallus,* is never differentiated into roots, stem, and leaves, and the fungi have no specialized vessels for transport of water and nutrients as in vascular plants. The fungi can form only a plectenchymatic type of "tissue" consisting of aggregates of cells largely retaining their individuality. In certain cases, as in sexual processes, the cells can communicate by means of hormone-like compounds.

In the vegetative phase the fungal population grows essentially as an undifferentiated group of similar cells. The differentiation occurs in the second developmental phase, known as the reproductive or fruiting phase. The hyphae that penetrate into the growth medium or spread over its surface absorbing the nutrients are called *vegetative mycelium.* The vegetative mycelium projects above the surface of the medium as *aerial mycelium* bearing reproductive structures. Some parasitic fungi produce special branches of the vegetative mycelium called *haustoria* (s. *haustorium*), which penetrate into the cytoplasm of host cells and absorb the necessary nutrients.

REPRODUCTION. The fungi usually reproduce by means of motile or nonmotile *spores;* however, in many cases even small fragments of viable mycelium are sufficient to initiate growth of a new individual. The spores can be one-celled, two-celled, or many-celled. They are derived from the parent thallus and contain all the genetic information

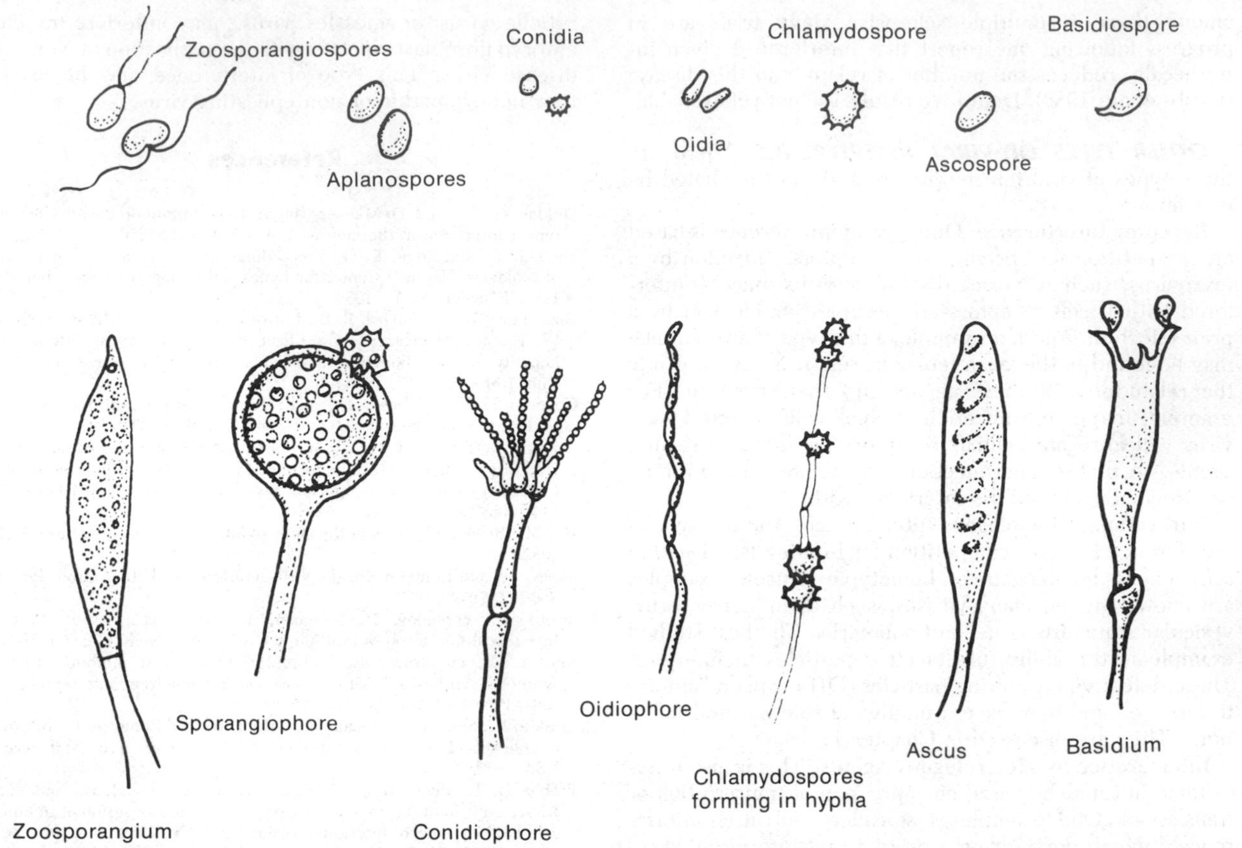

Figure 1. Different types of reproductive structures and spores in fungi. (After Encyclopedia of Science and Technology. Vol. 5. New York, McGraw-Hill Book Company, 1971, p. 117.)

necessary for the development of a new thallus. The shapes of spores and the mode of sporulation are important characteristics in classification and identification of fungi (Fig. 1).

The spores can arise either asexually by differentiation of the thallus or sexually as a result of fusion of parent haploid nuclei. This is followed by formation of a sexual zygote and by restoration of the haploid state by meiosis. The sexual process is initiated by fusion of pairs of motile or nonmotile sexual cells *(gametes)* of opposite sexes or by somatic copulation of undifferentiated vegetative hyphae (Fig. 2).

MORPHOLOGY. Morphologically, the fungi represent a very heterogeneous group of microorganisms. Some fungi grow as single cells *(yeasts)*, others as multinuclear filaments *(molds)*. Certain fungi, including many human pathogens, exhibit dimorphism—that is, they can grow as yeast or as mold (Fig. 3). Both mycelial and yeast forms of pathogenic fungi may cause superficial or deep systemic infections in humans. The biochemical nature of dimorphism is poorly understood. The yeast–mold transitions of the fungal phenotype can be influenced by temperature, nutrition, redox potential, partial pressure of carbon dioxide, and other environmental factors. The two morphologic types of the same organism are distinctly different in the chemical composition of their cell walls.

Yeasts. Yeasts are unicellular fungi that reproduce by budding or fission; the latter can be considered as a broad-base type of budding. Yeast cells are spherical or ellipsoidal, usually about 3 to 10 μm in diameter and 5 to 30 μm in length. Different species of yeast differ in their mode of budding (apical, lateral, bipolar, multipolar) and in other details. Yeast cells grow by a somewhat uniform extension of the cellular surface of the growing bud. During budding the nucleus of the mother cell divides, and one daughter nucleus passes into the bud. The two cells are then separated by a crosswall, called a *septum*, and after a certain period the bud breaks away. A birth scar is visible on the daughter cell, and a prominent bud scar remains on the mother cell's wall surface. The chemical composition of the bud scar with the septum usually differs from that of the rest of the cell wall. The bud scars remain as permanent structures on the surface of the walls, and their number indicates the age of the cells (Fig. 4).

Molds. The principal living unit of a mold is a *hypha*. Hyphae are about 3 to 12 μm diameter and can reach several centimeters in length. The hyphae grow by elongation at the tip *(apex)*. In older portions of the hypha lateral branches arise that then develop like the main hypha. The densely packed, interwoven hyphae constitute web-like *mycelia*, which are visible as macroscopic fungal *colonies* (Fig. 5).

In lower fungi the hyphae are usually not divided by septa into individual cells, but rather the whole mycelium is coenocytic—that is, it contains many nuclei in nonseparated cytoplasm. Regular septation observed in higher fungi does not change the coenocytic character of the hyphae because the septa have fine pores that ensure the continuity of the cytoplasm.

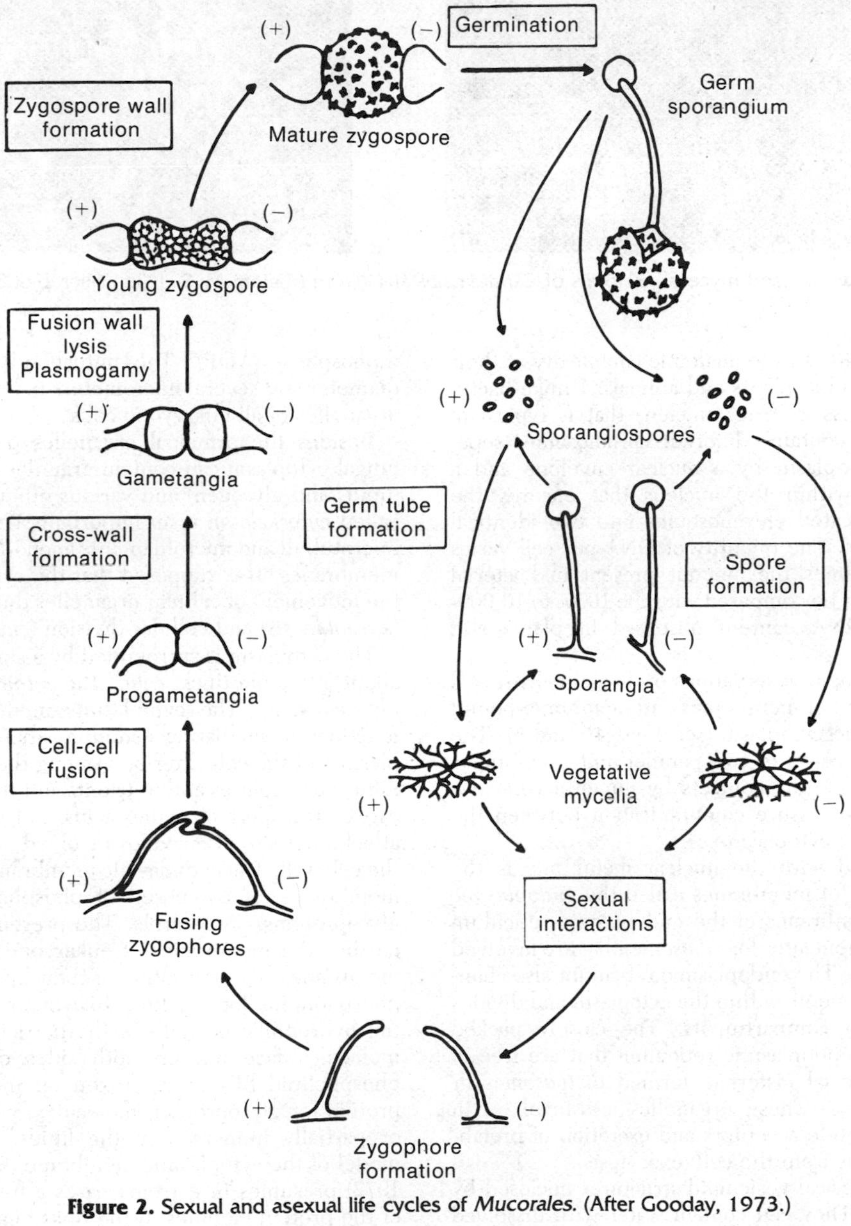

Figure 2. Sexual and asexual life cycles of *Mucorales.* (After Gooday, 1973.)

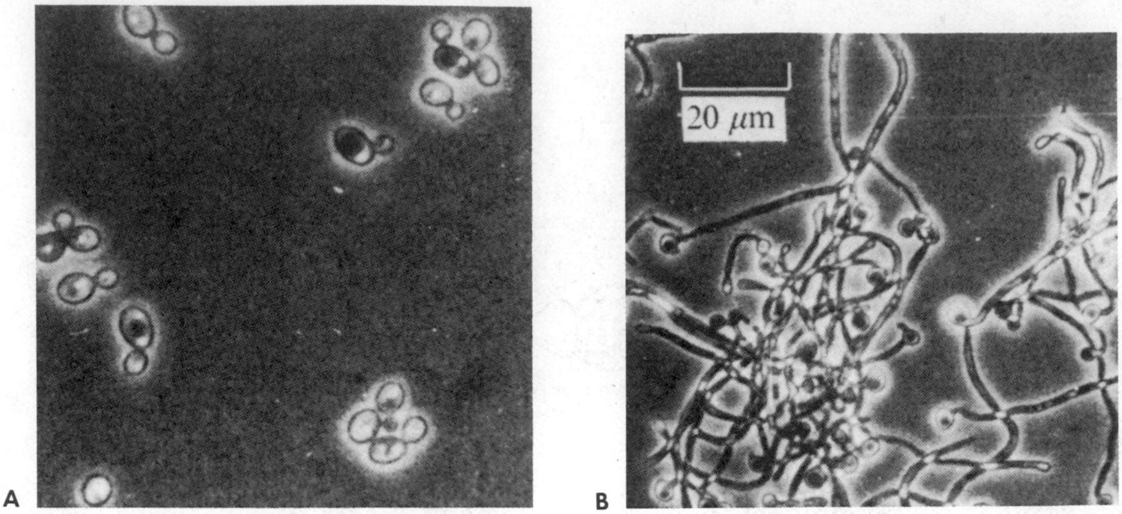

Figure 3. Yeast *(A)* and mycelial *(B)* forms of *Candida albicans.* (From Mariott, M. S.: J Gen Microbiol 86:115, 1975.)

ULTRASTRUCTURE. In the anatomic complexity of their cells the fungi resemble plants and animals. Unlike bacteria, the fungi possess a "true" nucleus that is typical of eukaryotic cells; it contains different chromosomes separated from the cytoplasm by a nuclear envelope and a mitotic apparatus within the nucleus that ensures the separation of duplicated chromosomes into two identical parts during mitosis. The quantity of DNA per cell varies from four to ten times the amount present in bacterial cells. This figure can be compared with the 1000- to 10,000-fold increase of DNA content observed in plants and animals.

Electron microscopic observations on fungal cells reveal a complicated system of membranes and membrane-bound organelles within the cytoplasm (see Figs. 4B and 6). The *nuclear envelope* consists of two parallel unit membranes perforated at their mutual contacts by numerous *nuclear pores.* Nuclear pores assure communication between the nucleoplasm and the cytoplasm.

Closely associated with the nuclear membrane is the complicated system of membranes called the *endoplasmic reticulum.* The membranes of the endoplasmic reticulum serve as the attachment sites for *ribosomes* that are involved in protein synthesis. The endoplasmic reticulum also channels different components within the cytoplasm and divides the cytoplasm into compartments. The closely packed membranes of the endoplasmic reticulum that are free of ribosomes form special cisternae termed *dictyosomes* or the *Golgi apparatus.* These organelles are involved in glycosylation of peptide acceptors and excretion of prefabricated glycoproteins from the cell (exocytosis).

Vacuoles are spherical vesiculoid structures enclosed by a unit membrane. They can contain water with dissolved solutes, gases, polymetaphosphate granules (volutine), waste products of cellular metabolism, and various hydrolytic enzymes used for breakdown of polymeric substances. Small vacuolar bodies derived from the membranes of the endoplasmic reticulum or from the cisternae of the Golgi apparatus can convey prefabricated glycoproteins to the cell exterior.

Metabolic energy is produced in *mitochondria* in the form of adenosine 5′-triphosphate (ATP) through respiration-mediated oxidative phosphorylation of adenosine 5′-diphosphate (ADP). The mitochondria, about 1 μm in diameter and several micrometers in length, are ubiquitous organelles of all eukaryotic cells.

Besides the principal organelles described above, the fungal cytoplasm can contain granules of reserve materials (lipids and glycogen) and various other inclusions. The so-called *cytoskeleton* is an important structure, consisting of microtubuli and microfilaments anchored to various cellular membranes. It is supposed that the cytoskeleton organizes the movement of cellular organelles during nuclear division (*karyokinesis*) and cellular division (*cytokinesis*).

The cytoplasm is surrounded by a single unit membrane, about 8 to 9 nm thick, called the *cytoplasmic membrane* or *plasmalemma.* The cytoplasmic membrane fulfills many functions in mediating communication between the cytoplasm and the cell exterior. Among these functions are the diffusion of solutes and nutrients and the passive and active carrier transport of amino acids and sugars. It is also an attachment site of enzymes involved in the biosynthesis of the cell wall. The cytoplasmic membrane, like other cellular membranes, is composed of phospholipids, proteins (or glycoproteins) and sterols. The presence of sterols distinguishes the membranes of eukaryotic cells from bacterial membranes. By association of their lipophilic portions, the phospholipids form a lipid bilayer or sandwich, whereby the hydrophilic portions of the participating phospholipid molecules face out on both sides of the bilayer. The phospholipid bilayer is broken up in places by globular protein (or glycoprotein) molecules, which are completely or partially immersed in the lipids. The "fluid mosaic" model of the cytoplasmic membrane (Singer and Nicolson, 1972) presumes in extreme cases a free lateral movement of the protein globules in the lipid bilayer.

The space between the cytoplasmic membrane and the cell wall, called the *periplasmic space,* contains soluble macromolecular precursors of the cell wall and various extracellular hydrolases that cleave the oligomeric substrates to monomers before their transport into the cell. A three-dimensional model of a fungal cell is shown in Figure 7.

CELL WALLS. In the great majority of fungi the outer surface of the cytoplasmic membrane is covered by a rigid

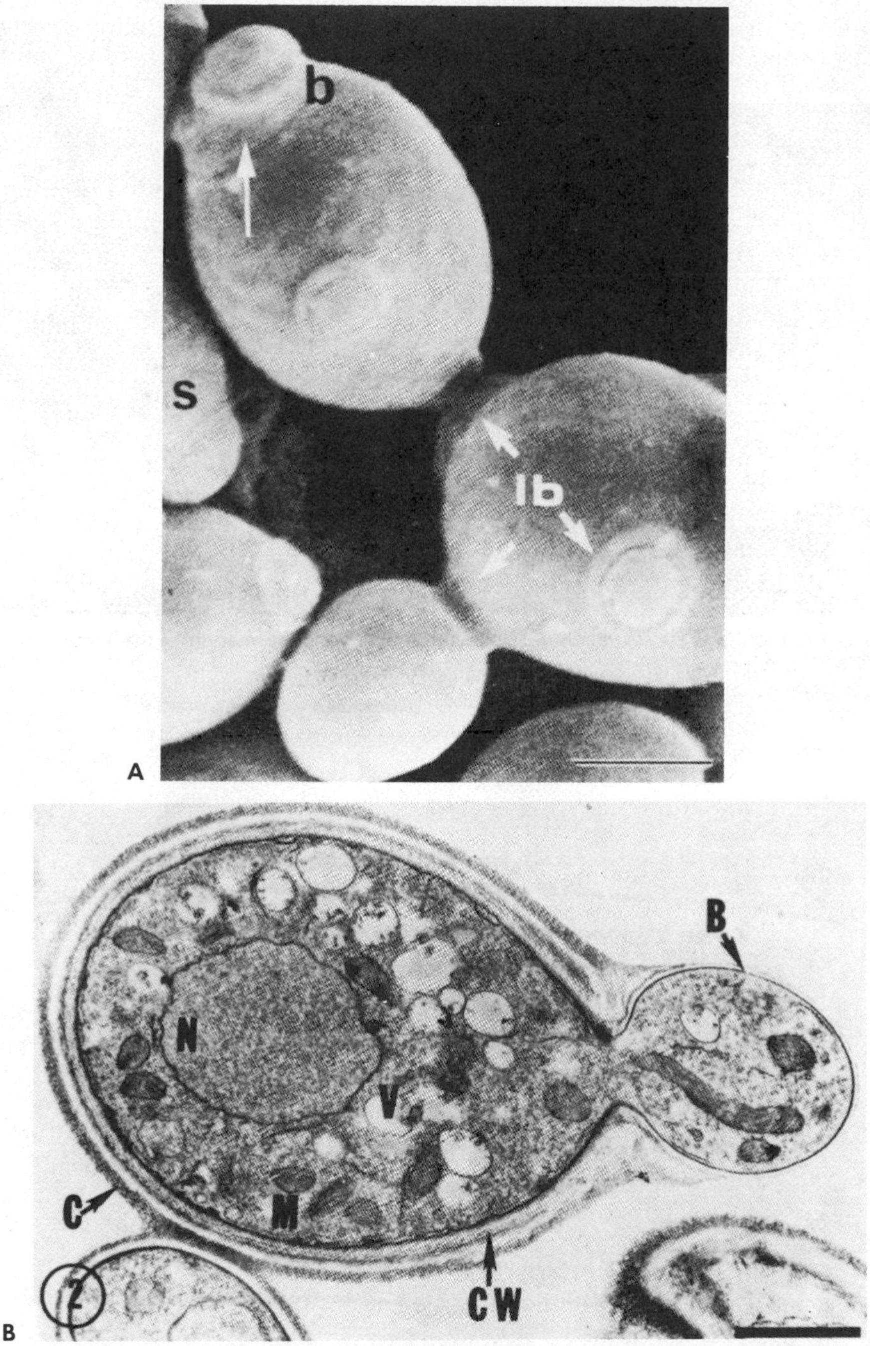

Figure 4. *A,* Scanning electronmicrograph of the cells of *Candida slooffii* showing lateral budding (1b), bud scar (b) and a birth scar (s). Bar indicates 1 μm. (From Watson, K., and Arthur, H.: J Bacteriol 130:312, 1976.)

B, Electronmicrograph of an ultrathin section through the cell of *Cryptococcus neoformans.* C, capsule; CW, cell wall; M, mitochondria; N, nucleus; V, vacuole; B, bud. Bar indicates 1 μm. (From Peterson, E. M., Hawley, R. J., and Calderone, R. A.: Can J Microbiol 22:1518, 1976.)

A

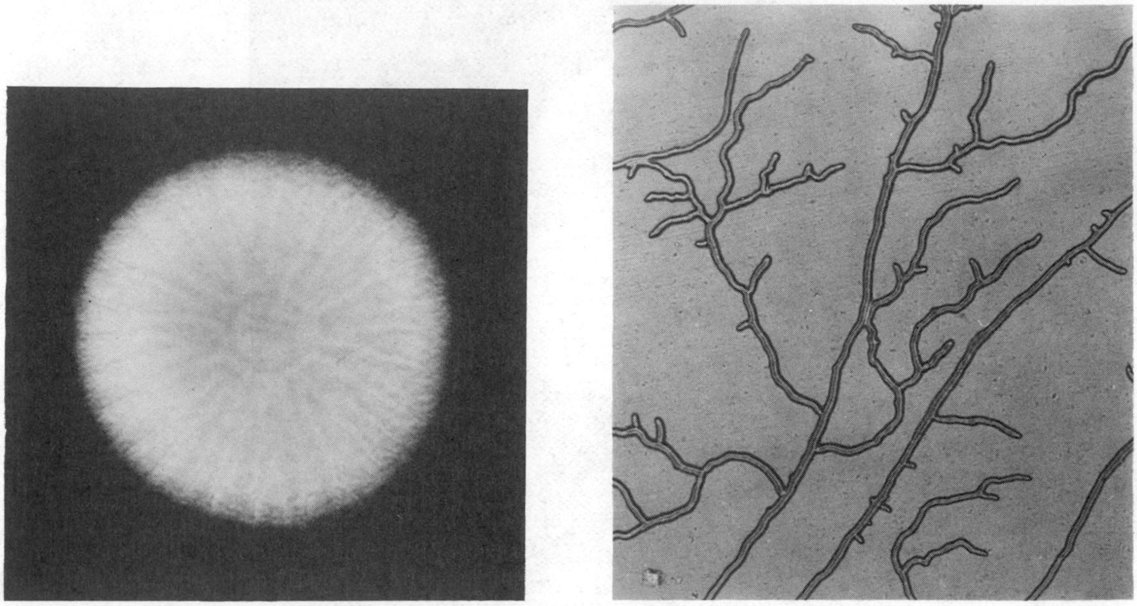

Figure 5. *A,* Colony of the mold *Aspergillus niger. B,* Microphotograph from the margin of the same colony showing individual hyphae. Bar represents 50 μm.

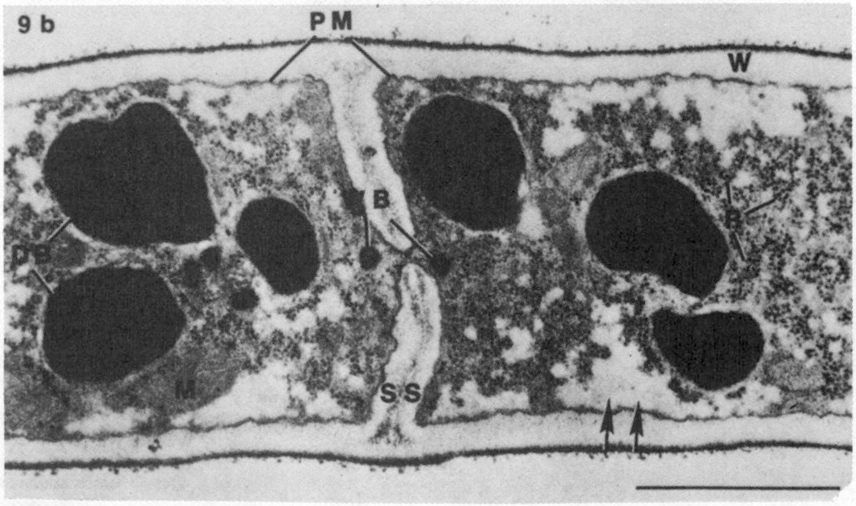

Figure 6. Electronmicrograph of sectioned hyphal cell of *Phialophora dermatitidis.* W, cell wall; R, ribosomes; DB, dense bodies; WB, Woronin bodies; M, mitochondria; SS, single septum. Double arrows indicate polysaccharide storage areas. Bar indicates 1 μm. (From Oujezdsky, K. B., Grove, S. N., and Szaniszlo, P. J.: J Bacteriol 113:468, 1973.)

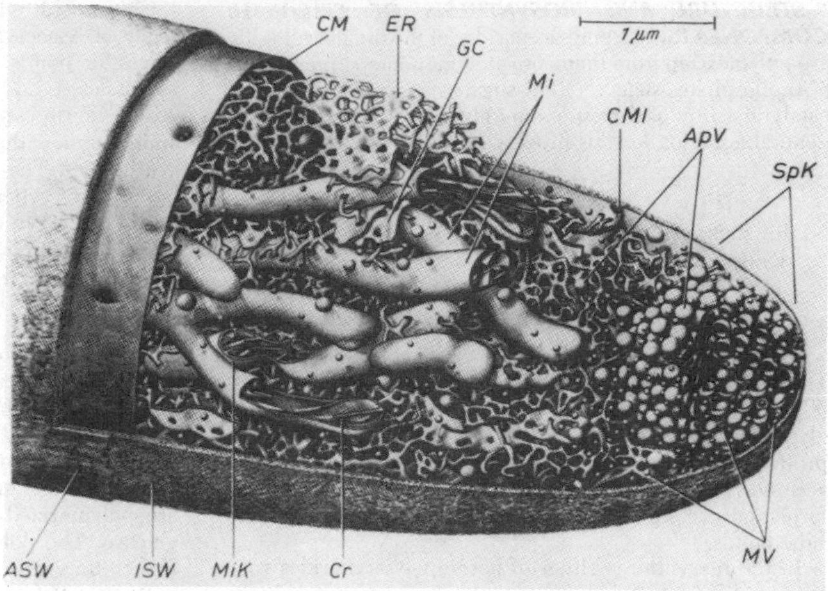

Figure 7. A three-dimensional model of the apical region of a hypha of *Polystictus versicolor.* ApV, apical vesicles; ASW, outer wall layer; CM, plasmalemma; CMI, invaginations of the plasmalemma (lomasome); Cr, mitochondrial cristae; ER, endoplasmic reticulum; GC, Golgi cisternae; ISW, inner fibrillar wall layer; Mi, mitochondria; MiK, mitochondrial membrane; MV, microvesicle; SpK, Spitzenkörper. (From Girbardt, M.: Protoplasma 67:413, 1969.)

cell wall. The primary role of the cell wall is to determine and to maintain cellular morphology. Dissolution of the cell walls by special lytic enzymes liberates osmotically fragile *protoplasts* that are shaped spherically by hydrostatic forces. Under suitable conditions (osmotic stabilizers, nutrition) the protoplasts can regenerate the cell wall on their surface. Lowering the osmolarity of the medium causes lysis of the protoplasts and kills them.

Besides their morphogenetic role, the cell walls mediate the interactions of the fungus cells with their environment, other cells, and the infected host.

Chemical Composition. The fungal walls are composed of polysaccharides, protein-polysaccharide complexes, variable amounts of lipids, and lesser quantities of other components.

Polysaccharides, which represent about 80 to 90 per cent of the dry matter of the cell walls, are composed of amino sugars, hexoses, hexuronic acids, methylpentoses, and pentoses (Bartnicki-Garcia, 1970). Owing to their distinctive physicochemical properties, the different polymers fulfill specific functions in the cell walls. The crystalline, insoluble polysaccharides, such as cellulose, chitin, and beta-glucans, form the wall skeleton that is responsible for the mechanical strength and morphology of the walls. The amorphous homo- and heteropolysaccharides, often in association with proteins, act as cementing substances, constitute the carbohydrate moieties of extracellular enzymes, and form the immunodeterminant groups of wall antigens.

Wall Architecture. The organization of individual components within the wall can be different in various genera of fungi and can vary with the age of the cells. The older parts of the walls are usually thicker, more rigid, and more resistant to hydrolytic enzymes.

Refined electron microscopic techniques coupled with cytochemical staining and selective action of purified polysaccharide-hydrolases have revealed that several layers of building material exist within the fungal cell wall. The general picture is that the outer surface of the wall is smooth or slightly granular in texture and is composed of amorphous glycoprotein material, whereas the skeletal, microcrystalline component is prominent in the layer adjacent to the cytoplasmic membrane (Fig. 8). The spaces between the fibrils of the microcrystalline layer, the *wall matrix,* are filled with an amorphous component that also penetrates the periplasmic space. Some yeasts (e.g., *Cryptococcus* spp.) produce viscous polysaccharide capsules on the outer surface of the cell wall. The chemical nature of the capsular slime closely resembles that of the protein-polysaccharides from the cell walls. A great portion of the capsular material is released into the medium during growth.

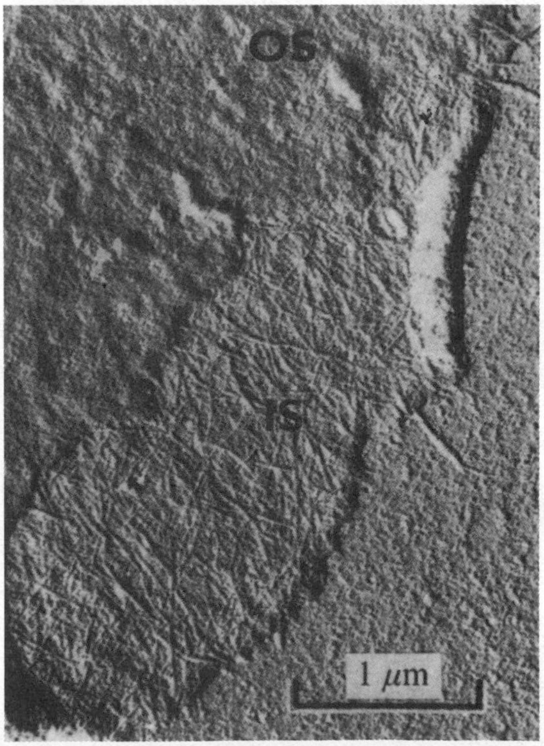

Figure 8. Electronmicrograph of an isolated empty hyphal wall of *Pythium accanthicum* showing granular outer surface (OS) and microfibrillar inner surface (IS) of the cell wall. (From Siestma, J. H., Child, J. J., Nesbitt, L. R., and Haskins, R. H.: J Gen Microbiol 86:29, 1975.)

STRUCTURE AND BIOSYNTHESIS OF CELL-WALL COMPONENTS. The polysaccharides of the fungal cell walls are polymerized from their activated monomers, nucleoside 5′-diphosphate sugars (NDP-sugars; Fig. 9) under the catalytic action of corresponding glycosyl transferases. The general equation for this process is

$$\underset{\text{donor}}{\text{NDP}-\text{sugar}} + \underset{\text{acceptor}}{(\text{sugar})_n} \xrightarrow{\text{glycosyl transferase}} \underset{\text{product}}{(\text{sugar})_{n+1}} + \text{NDP}$$

The result of the transglycosylic reaction is the lengthening of the saccharidic chain of the acceptor molecule by one glycosyl unit. A single carbohydrate unit as well as the product from the preceding reaction can serve as the acceptor. The multiple repetition of this process leads to formation of long chains of glycosyl units linked by glycosidic bonds.

In the biosynthesis either of heteropolysaccharides containing different carbohydrate units, or of polymers containing different glycosidic bonds, specialized glycosyl transferases catalyze the transfer of a specific sugar and the formation of a specific glycosidic bond. The following are examples of biosynthesis of some principal cell-wall constituents in fungi.

Chitin. Chitin is a linear polysaccharide composed exclusively of *N*-acetyl-D-glucosamine units linked by beta-1,4 glycosidic bonds. Owing to low solubility the linear chitin molecules tend to form microcrystalline aggregates in water. Chitin is polymerized from UDP-*N*-acetyl-D-glucosamine under the catalytic action of the enzyme chitin synthetase. The enzyme is located in the cytoplasmic membrane, where it can exist in two interconvertible forms, as active enzyme or as temporarily inactive zymogen. The interconversion of the two forms of chitin synthetase is supposed to play a decisive role in regulation of biosynthesis of the cell wall and, consequently, of fungal morphogenesis.

Glucans. Various polymers of glucose represent important cell-wall constituents in many fungi. The insoluble cellulose and beta-glucans (i.e., those containing only beta-glycosidic bonds) form, together with chitin, the skeletal portion of the walls, whereas the alpha-glucans are usually amorphous and are located in the wall matrix. Most glucans are polymerized by transglycosylic reactions from UDP-glucose. The polymerizing enzyme, glucan synthetase, is, like chitin synthetase, localized in the plasmalemma.

Protein-Polysaccharide Complexes. Protein-polysaccharides, or glycoproteins, are the center of much interest because they are both structural components of the cell walls and determinants of biologic specificity on cell surfaces. Structurally, the fungal wall glycoproteins exhibit many similarities with surface protein-polysaccharide com-

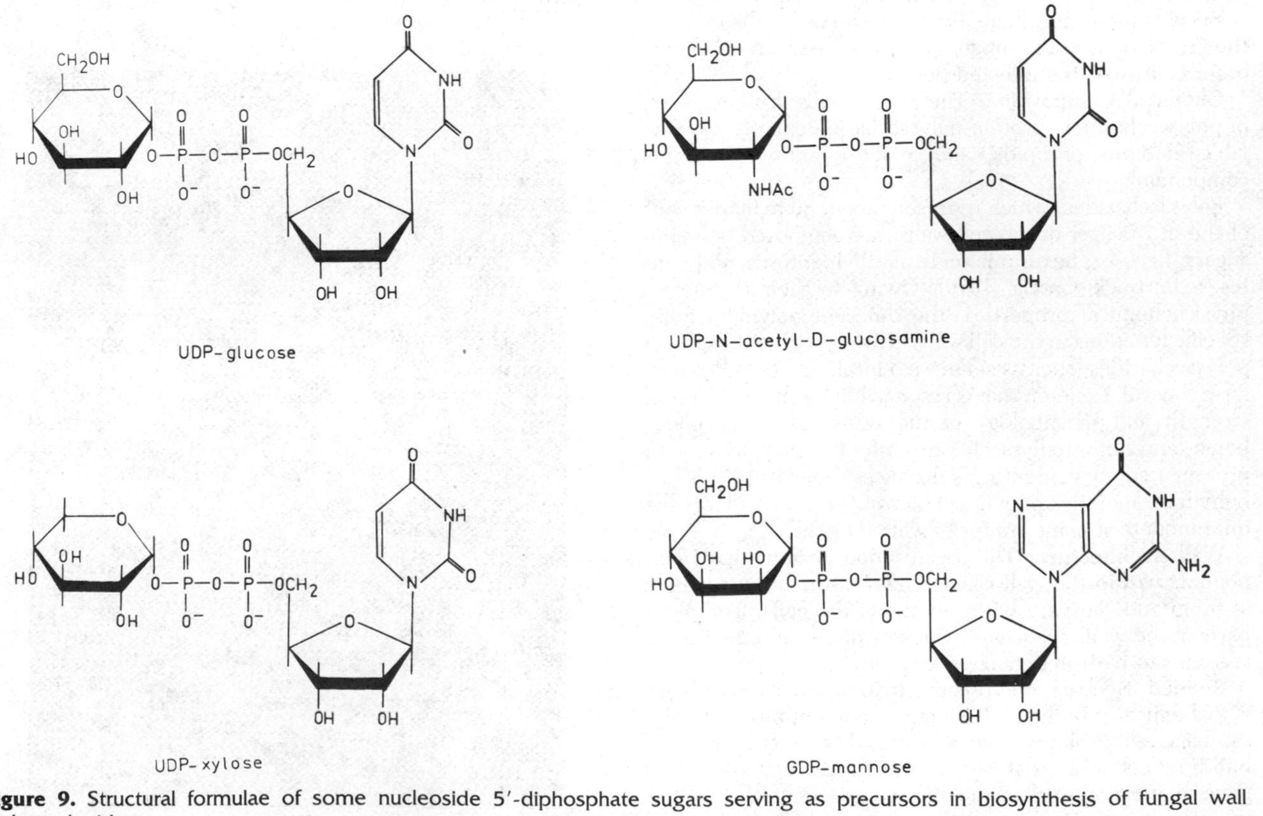

Figure 9. Structural formulae of some nucleoside 5′-diphosphate sugars serving as precursors in biosynthesis of fungal wall polysaccharides.

plexes from higher organisms. For this reason the glycoproteins of fungi are used as models to study various aspects of glycoprotein structure, function, and biosynthesis.

So far, the most systematic studies on fungal glycoproteins have been performed with yeast mannan (Cohen and Ballou, 1981). The polysaccharide moiety of yeast mannan consists of an alpha-1,6-linked polymannose backbone to which short side chains of mannosyl units linked by alpha-1,2 and alpha-1,3 glycosidic bonds are attached. The whole polysaccharide is linked via a diacetylchitobiose bridge to an asparaginyl residue in the protein part of the molecule. Besides that, short manno-oligosaccharides containing alpha-1,2 and alpha-1,3 glycosidic links are attached directly to the hydroxyaminoacids serine and threonine by O-glycosidic bonds (Fig. 10).

Biosynthesis of the relatively complex structure of yeast mannan requires participation of a whole set of mannosyltransferases, each of them catalyzing the formation of a specific linkage. The precursor of mannosyl units in the biosynthesis of yeast mannan is guanosine 5′-diphospho mannose (GDP-Man). The transfer of mannosyl units from their donor to the acceptor can proceed either in a single step or through lipophilic intermediates such as dolichol-monophosphate mannose (Fig. 11). It is assumed that the involvement of dolichols is necessary in those reactions that take place in a lipophilic environment, as for example on the surface or inside the membranes of the endoplasmic reticulum, and for the transfer of glycosyl units from their hydrophilic cytoplasmic precursors (NDP-sugars) into the lumen of cisternae of endoplasmic reticulum, where the final stages of carbohydrate polymerization take place. The biosynthesis of the great part of the "inner core" of yeast mannan proceeds while the product is attached to the dolichol carrier (Fig. 12).

The mannan of *Candida albicans* has a structure very similar to that depicted in Figure 10. The difference is that the mannan from *Candida albicans* contains a much higher proportion of unsubstituted mannosyl units in the polymannose backbone and, in addition, contains longer side branches that reach the size of a heptasaccharide. The side chains containing terminal alpha-1,3-linked mannosyl units are immunodeterminant groups in the mannan antigens, and the intensity of the precipitin reaction with antibodies induced by whole cells increases with the length of the side chains in the mannan.

Surface antigens from other fungi have usually more complex structures than the yeast mannans. The polysaccharide portions of these antigens can be chemically characterized as neutral or acidic heteropolysaccharides, composed of hexoses, pentoses, methylpentoses, and, in acidic heteropolysaccharides, uronic acids. For example, the capsular glucurono-xylo-mannan from *Cryptococcus neoformans* has a branched structure in which a linear alpha-1,3-linked polymannose chain is substituted at positions C-2 by beta-glycosidically linked glucuronic acid or xylose, with the xylose predominating (Fig. 13).

Glycosylation of nascent proteins takes place in dictyosomes and in the smooth endoplasmic reticulum. In the course of this process the formed glycoproteins are packed into vesicles derived from the original membrane systems and carried toward the cytoplasmic membrane. The carrier vesicles fuse with the membrane and discharge their contents into the cell exterior (Fig. 14). A portion of the supplied glycoproteins remains entrapped in the periplasm or anchored to the cell wall, and the other part diffuses into the surrounding medium. Some of the extracellular glycoproteins exhibit enzymatic activity; they act as hydrolases of various kinds. The hydrolytic action of these enzymes facilitates the growth and penetration of the fungus into the solid substrate or the invaded tissue.

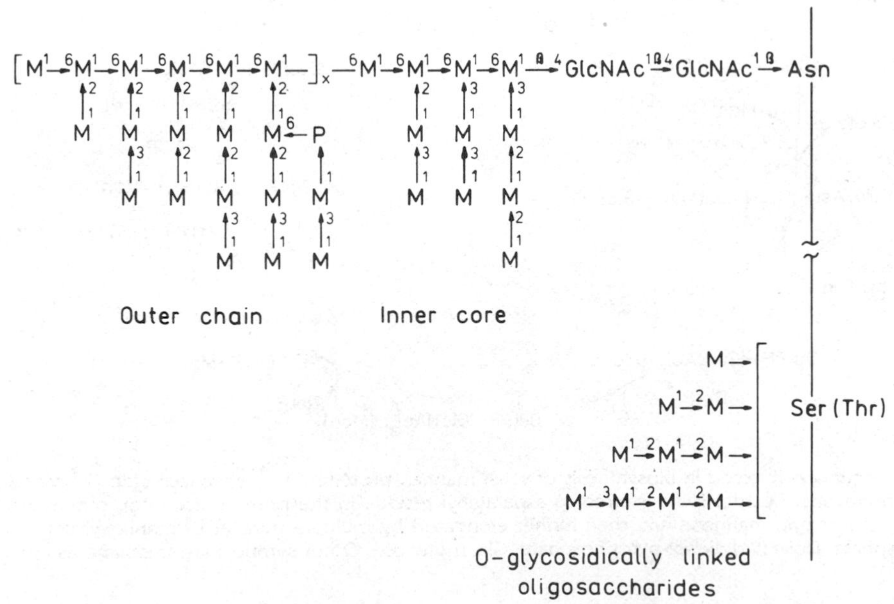

Figure 10. Structure of mannan from the cell walls of the yeast *Saccharomyces cerevisiae* (modified from Cohen and Ballou, 1981). M, mannopyranose residue; GlcNAc, *N*-acetyl-D-glucosamine; P, orthophosphate; Asn, asparagine; Ser, serine; Thr, threonine.

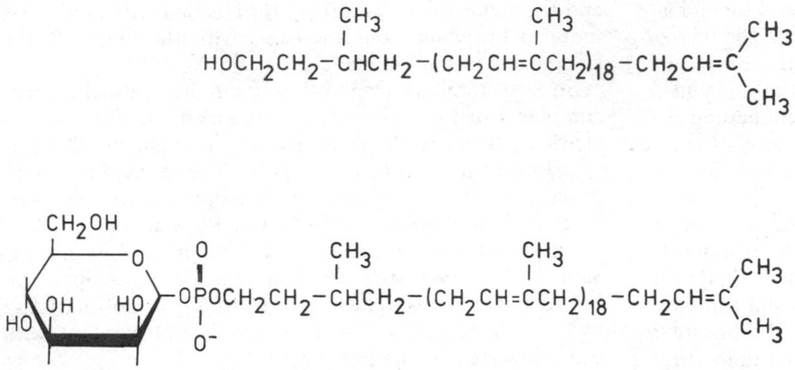

Figure 11. Structural formulae of dolichol and dolichol monophosphate-mannose.

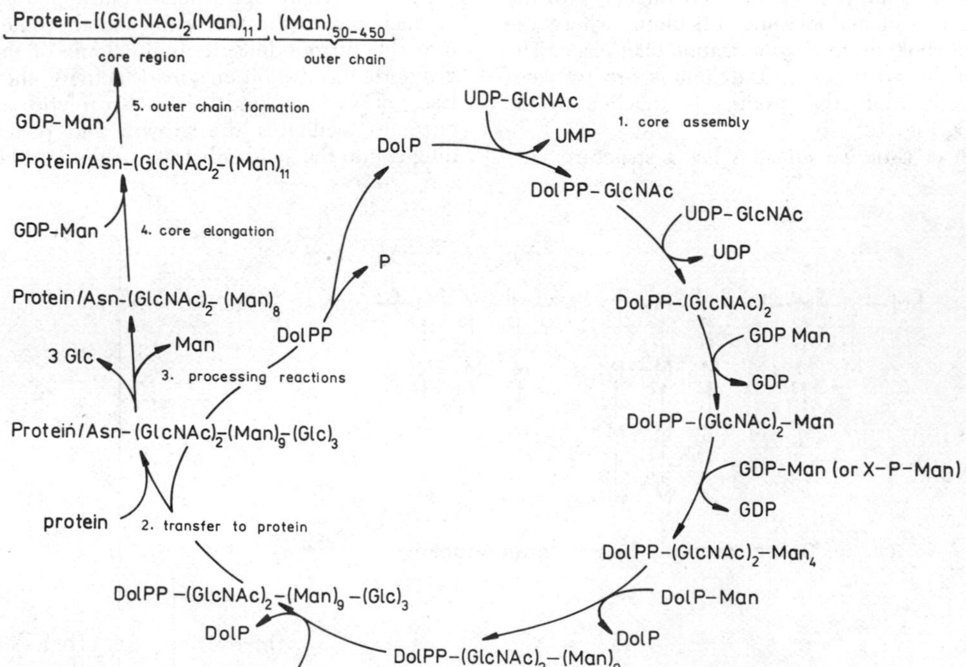

Figure 12. Reaction sequence involved in biosynthesis of yeast mannan-proteins. The oligosaccharide $Glc_3Man_9GlcNAc_2$ assembled on the dolichol-pyrophosphate carrier is transferred to asparaginyl residue in the peptide acceptor, processed by removal of the three glucosyl units and of one mannose and then further elongated by multiple transfer of mannosyl units from GDP-mannose. Dol-P, dolichol-phosphate; Dol-PP, dolichol-pyrophosphate; Glc, D-glucose. Other symbols are the same as in Figure 10.

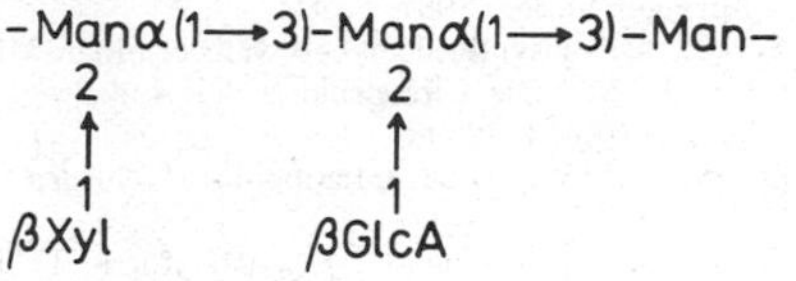

Figure 13. Structure of acidic polysaccharide from capsules of *Cryptococcus neoformans.* Man, mannopyranose residue; Xyl, xylopyranose residue; GlcA, glucuronic acid residue.

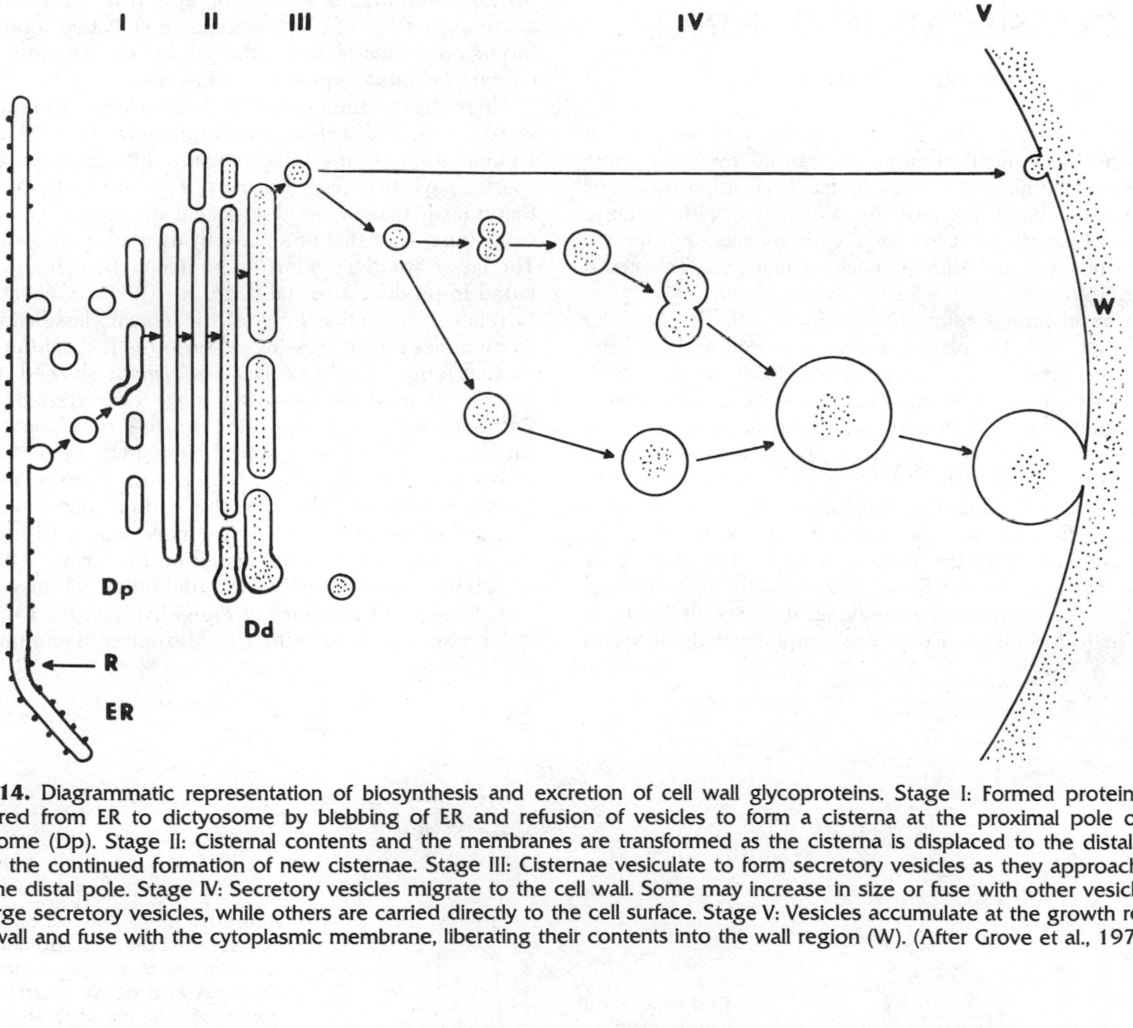

Figure 14. Diagrammatic representation of biosynthesis and excretion of cell wall glycoproteins. Stage I: Formed proteins are transferred from ER to dictyosome by blebbing of ER and refusion of vesicles to form a cisterna at the proximal pole of the dictyosome (Dp). Stage II: Cisternal contents and the membranes are transformed as the cisterna is displaced to the distal pole (Dd) by the continued formation of new cisternae. Stage III: Cisternae vesiculate to form secretory vesicles as they approach and reach the distal pole. Stage IV: Secretory vesicles migrate to the cell wall. Some may increase in size or fuse with other vesicles to form large secretory vesicles, while others are carried directly to the cell surface. Stage V: Vesicles accumulate at the growth region of the wall and fuse with the cytoplasmic membrane, liberating their contents into the wall region (W). (After Grove et al., 1970.)

References

Bartnicki-Garcia, S.: Cell wall composition and other biochemical markers in fungal phylogeny. In Hasborne, J. B. (ed.): Phytochemical Phylogeny. New York and London, Academic Press, 1970, p. 81.

Cohen, R. E., and Ballou, C. E.: Mannoprotein: structure. In Tanner, W., and Loewus, F. A. (eds.): Encyclopedia of Plant Physiology. New Series, Vol. 13B, Plant Carbohydrates II. Berlin, Heidelberg and New York, Springer Verlag, 1981, p. 441.

Farkaš, V.: Biosynthesis of cell walls of fungi. Microbiol Rev 43:117, 1979.

Girbardt, M.: Die Ultrastruktur der Apikalregion von Pilzhyphen. Protoplasma 67:413, 1969.

Gooday, G. W.: Differentiation in *Mucorales.* Symp Soc Gen Microbiol 23:269, 1973.

Grove, S. N., Bracker, C. E., and Morré, D. J.: An ultrastructural basis for hyphal tip growth in *Pythium ultimum.* Am J Botany 57:245, 1970.

Mariott, M. S.: Isolation and chemical characterization of plasma membranes from the yeast and mycelial forms of *Candida albicans.* J Gen Microbiol 86:115, 1975.

Oujezdsky, K. B., Grove, S. N., and Szaniszlo, P. J.: Morphological and structural changes during the yeast-to-mold conversion of *Phialophora dermatitis.* J Bacteriol 113:468, 1973.

Peterson, E. M., Hawley, R. J., and Calderone, R. A.: An ultrastructural analysis of protoplast-spheroplast induction in *Cryptococcus neoformans.* Can J Microbiol 22:1518, 1976.

Sietsma, J. H., Child, J. J., Nesbitt, L. R., and Haskins, R. H.: Chemistry and ultrastructure of the hyphal walls of *Pythium accanthicum.* J Gen Microbiol 86:29, 1975.

Singer, S. J., and Nicolson, G. L.: The fluid mosaic model of the structure of cell membranes. Science 175:720, 1972.

Watson, K., and Arthur, H.: Cell surface topography of *Candida* and *Leucosporidium* yeasts as revealed by scanning electron microscopy. J Bacteriol 130:312, 1976.

14

CLASSIFICATION OF FUNGI

WILLARD A. TABER, PH.D.

Fungi live in soil, on plants, in water, and occasionally on man. Most plant diseases are caused by fungi; most diseases of animals are caused by bacteria and viruses. For this reason fungi are usually associated with botany, whereas bacteria are associated with zoology. For an overview of fungi and their impact on man, see Taber and Taber, 1967.

The term fungus refers to nonphotosynthetic plant-like forms that resemble plants in possessing cell walls and the glyoxylate bypass of the Krebs cycle. Fungi resemble both plants and animals in being eukaryons—that is, they possess nuclei, mitochondria, endoplasmic reticula, more than one chromosome, protoplasmic streaming, and the capacity to synthesize steroids. They differ from bacteria, which are prokaryons, and which lack the above structures and activities. Whether microscopic or macroscopic in size (Fig. 1), fungi are united by the possession of hyphae (Fig. 2) or hypha-like structures. Fungi vary greatly in structural detail, and consequently a single all-inclusive definition is difficult to formulate. Fungi are nonphotosynthetic forms that consist of multinucleated cytoplasm within a much-branched system of tubes (the hyphae of filamentous fungi), of naked multinucleated cytoplasm (the plasmodium of Myxomycota), or of single vegetative cells that multiply by formation either of buds (the yeasts) or of motile spores (certain primitive aquatic phycomycetes).

There are a minimum of 50,000 species of fungi (Ainsworth, 1968b) distributed in approximately 4000 genera. Enumeration of fungal taxa is made difficult because some species have two generic names. This results from the fact that fungal taxa are based on sexual structures even though many fungi exist that produce only asexual spore structures. The latter are given a form-type name. If such a fungus is found to produce a sexual stage, it is given a second name to relate it to similar fungi of the sexual classification. As an example, recent crossings of various strains of the deadly asexual fungus *Cryptococcus neoformans* showed it to be capable of producing a sexual stage characteristic of the Basidiomycetes and according to the provisions of the International Code of Botanical Nomenclature was given a second name, *Filobasidiella neoformans.* The species name is usually retained although the ending may have to be changed to conform to the new generic name. Either name can be used, but the name based on the sexual state takes preference taxonomically. For definition of mycological terms, see the *Dictionary of Fungi* (Ainsworth, 1971).

All fungi are placed either in Myxomycota or Eumycota.

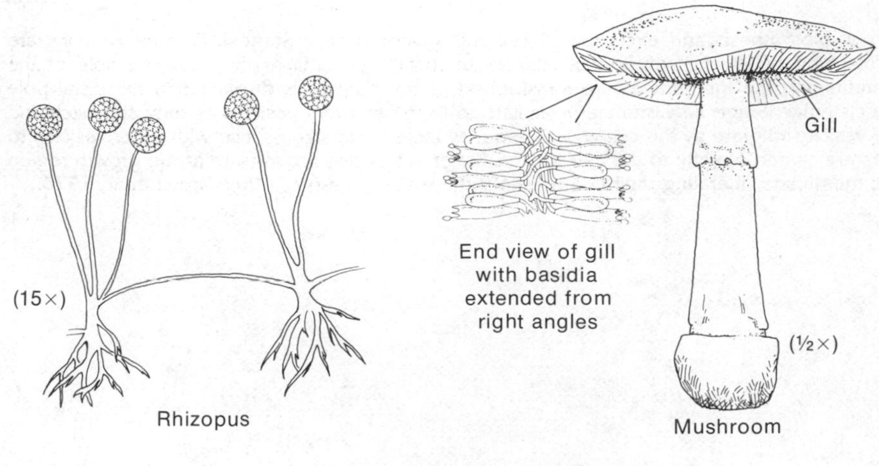

Figure 1. *(Left)* Asexual sporangiospores are borne in sporangia that are supported on sporangiophores. Rhizopus also possesses rhizoids at the base of the sporangiophore. *(Right)* Basidiocarp of Amanita sp. Basidiospores are borne on basidia.

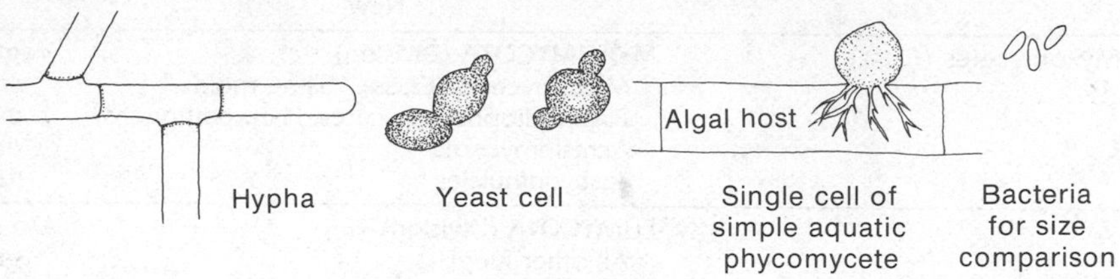

Figure 2. Vegetative or assimilative forms of growth of fungi. *(Left)* Hyphal form with branches. *(Center)* Yeast form of growth in which proliferation occurs by budding. *(Right)* Unicellular growth characteristic of certain simple phycomycetes. Approximate size of a bacterium is shown for comparison. Bacteria are always very narrow.

SOME CHARACTERISTICS OF REPRESENTATIVE FUNGI

MYXOMYCOTA. The Myxomycota as represented by the common myxomycetes, or slime molds, possess a vegetative or assimilative phase that consists of a naked mass of multinucleated cytoplasm, the plasmodium. This plasmodium increases in size as it crawls over the substrate consuming small forms of life and soluble nutrients (Fig. 3). When food or water supply becomes limited, the plasmodium is transformed into spore-bearing sporangia. Meiosis precedes either formation or germination of these spores. A spore breaks open and approximately four amoeboid or flagellated cells escape and feed on surrounding nutrients. Pairs of such cells functioning as gametes fuse (Fig. 3) and develop into the 2N plasmodium. Myxomycete plasmodia or sporangia can be found on logs, fallen leaves, or grass after rains. None is known to be pathogenic to animals although the related Plasmodiophoromycetes are pathogens of certain plants. For descriptions of species, see Martin and Alexopoulos, 1969.

EUMYCOTA

Mastigomycotina. Mastigomycotina are nonplasmodial fungi that produce motile cells. Motility is by flagella of the eukaryotic type. Many species, such as some of the Chytridiomycetes, consist of a single cell with rhizoids (Fig. 2), which becomes transformed into a sporangium containing motile spores. Chytridiomycetes possess one posterior flagellum, Hypochytridiomycetes possess one anterior flagellum, and the Oomycetes possess two flagella and in addition are usually mycelial (Table 1). Oomycetes also possess a female oogonium and a male antheridium (Table 1). The fertilized oosphere in the oogonium becomes an oospore. The oospore germinates by germ tube, which develops into mycelium or hyphae. Some species of Saprolegnia can parasitize aquatic animals, producing a woolly halo of mycelium around the host. The Oomycetes consist of four orders, Saprolegniales, Leptomitales, Lagenidiales, and Peronosporales. The Peronosporales embrace many plant pathogens, such as the downy mildews, which cause severe crop losses. The asexual spores of some can produce germ tubes as well as flagella, and this group represents a transition to nonmotile terrestrial forms of fungi.

Zygomycotina. Zygomycetes are nonmotile phycomycetes that possess coenocytic hyphae, thick-walled sexual spores called zygospores (Table 1), and sporangia containing asexual spores (Hesseltine, 1973). Most species produce woolly aerial mycelium when grown on spoiled foods or agar in a Petri plate. The aerial hyphae may fill the air space of a Petri plate culture; other fungi do not. Some species are homothallic. That is, hyphae developing from one spore can produce the sexual spore. Others are heterothallic, and hyphae of different mating types must fuse before sexual spores can be produced. Hormones are involved in hyphal attraction. Several species are pathogenic to man (Table 2) and their invasiveness is associated with diabetes. These fungi grow rapidly on sugars and are frequently referred to as sugar fungi. Members of the Entomophthorales attack insects, grow in association with amphibians, or grow in ground litter. Dead flies killed by *Entomophthora muscae* may be seen fixed to window panes and surrounded by a halo. The halo consists of sporangia shot off from the fungus growing on the fly.

Ascomycotina. There are approximately 15,000 species of ascomycetes distributed in 1950 genera. Ascomycetes

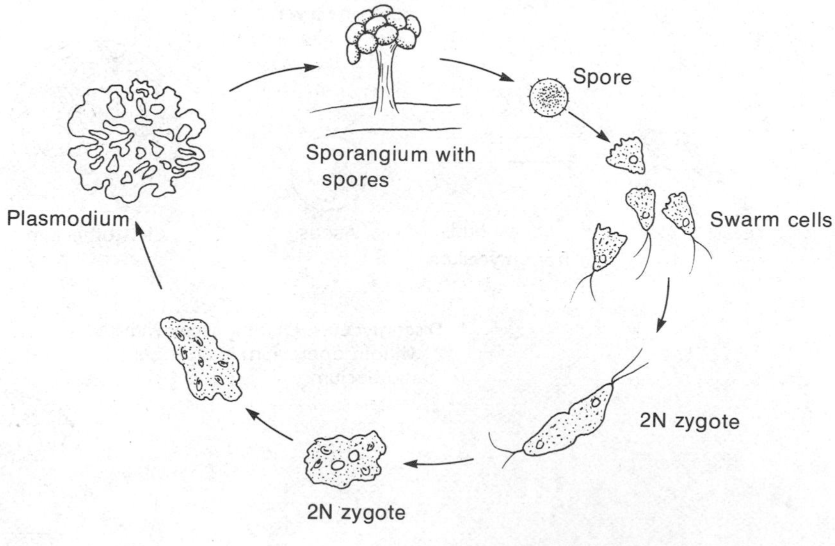

Figure 3. Life cycle of myxomycete.

Table 1. OVERVIEW OF THE FUNGI

Old	New	Characteristics
Myxomycetes (Class)	MYXOMYCOTA (Division) Myxomycetes (Class). "Slime molds." Plasmodiophoromycetes. Plant pathogens. Acrasiomycetes "Labyrinthulales"	Vegetative phase is a plasmodium that consists of fused or single amoeba. Creeps over surface of substrate. Some produce dry spore-bearing structures that resemble fungal structures.
	EUMYCOTA (Division) All other fungi.	Do not creep over substrate. Spread by growing. Vegetative phase a hypha, yeast cell, or single cell.
Phycomycetes-Oomycetes Aquatic phycomycetes, many are plant pathogens	Mastigomycotina (Subdivision) Chytridiomycetes (Class) Hyphochytridiomycetes Oomycetes	Asexual spores are motile owing to flagella. Hyphae, when present, multinucleate (coenocytic) without regular cross walls (septa).
Phycomycetes-Zygomycetes	Zygomycotina (Subdivision) Zygomycetes (Class) Sexual spore is a zygospore and asexual spore is usually a sporangiospore (borne within a sporangium). Human pathogens are found among: Rhizopus, Absidia, Mucor, and Basidiobolus. Trichomycetes (on or in arthropods)	Coenocytic hyphae without regular perforated septa but no motile spores.
Ascomycetes Ascocarp is a structure housing or supporting asci. It forms around the developing asci of the Euascomycetes. Loculoascomycetes possess a hollowed-out stroma in which asci subsequently develop.	Ascomycotina (Subdivision) 1. Euascomycetes. Unitunicate ascus (no classification). Hemiascomycetes (Class). Yeast or yeast-like. No ascocarp; no ascogenous hyphae. Yeasts usually have no hyphae. Plectomycetes. Round asci scattered throughout cleistothecium-type ascocarp; asci dissolving. (Human pathogens: dermatophytes, Histoplasma, some Aspergillus are members of this group.) Pyrenomycetes. Ascocarp usually a perithecium bearing oblong asci from one layer. Discomycetes. Oblong ascus with or without operculum in an (open) apothecium.	Coenocytic hyphae with simple perforated septa. Usually have an ascocarp. Always have ascus and ascospore.

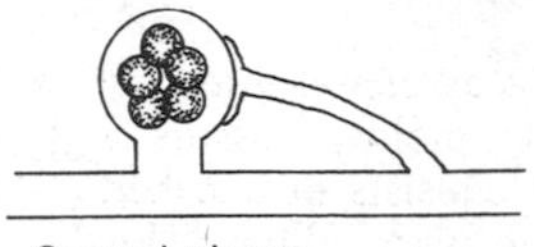
Sexual phase

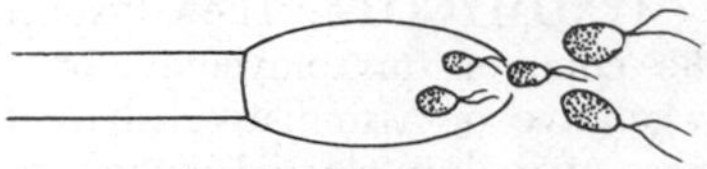
Asexual phase

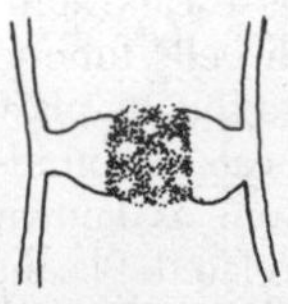
Sexual spore

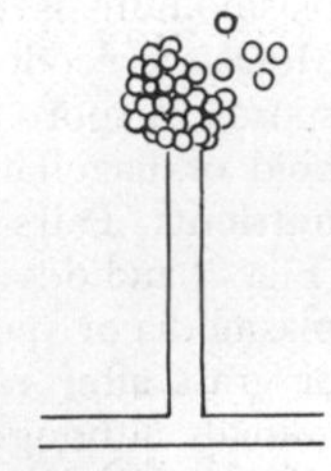
Asexual spore

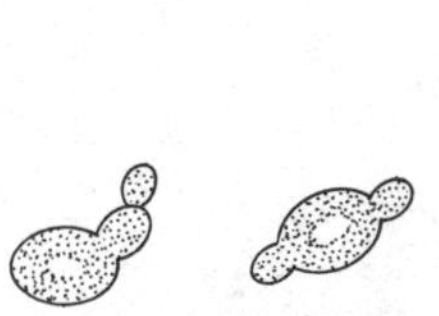
Yeast

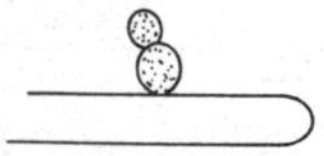
Yeast buds from mycelium

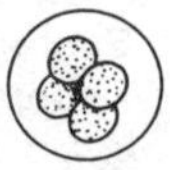
Ascus

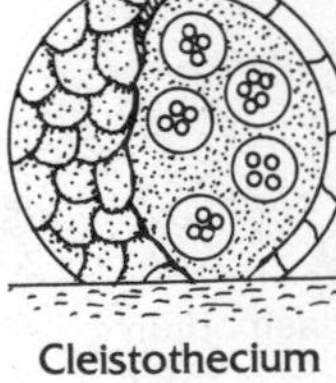
Cleistothecium ascocarp

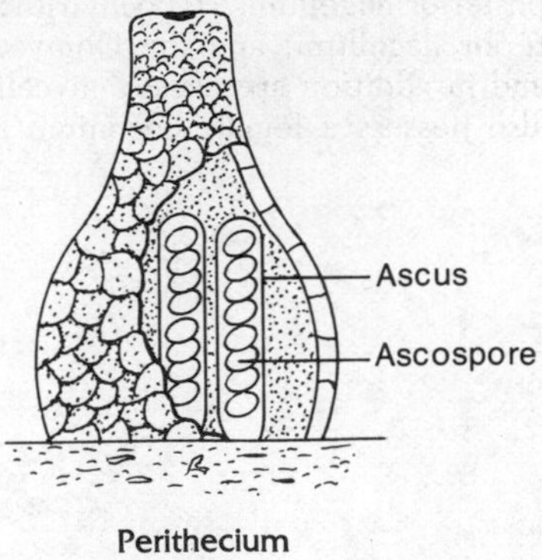

Perithecium ascocarp

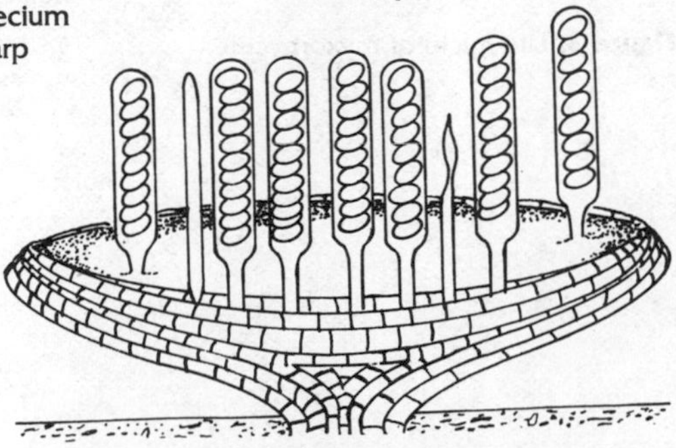
Apothecium ascocarp

Table 1. OVERVIEW OF THE FUNGI (*Continued*)

Old	New	Characteristics
	2. Loculoascomycetes (Class) Bitunicate (two-layered) ascus in a hollowed-out stroma. May resemble perithecium or black tar spots. Piedraia hortae on man. 3. Laboulbeniomycetes. Minute, on arthropod exoskeletons.	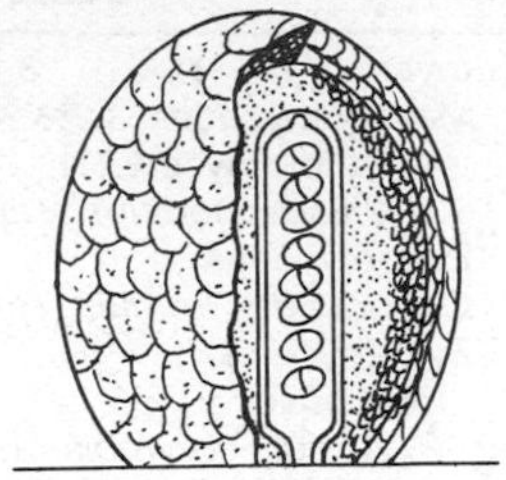

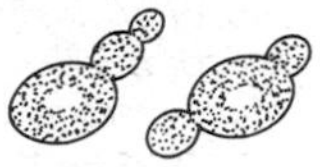

Old	New	Characteristics
Fungi Imperfecti (Most fungi growing on laboratory Petri plate cultures are Deuteromycotina or Zygomycetes.)	Deuteromycotina (Subdivision) (asexual fungi) Blastomycetes (Class). Yeasts. Hyphomycetes. Spores borne in open on hyphae. Cöelomycetes. Spores borne in (enclosed) pycnidium or on acervulus cushion breaking plant tissue epidermis.	Yeast or hyphal fungi without a sexual phase. If a sexual phase is found, both names can be used. Many are now known to be ascomycetes or to have ascomycetous affinities. Hyphae are coenocytic with perforated septa. Candida, Cryptococcus, Torulopsis, Pityrosporum.

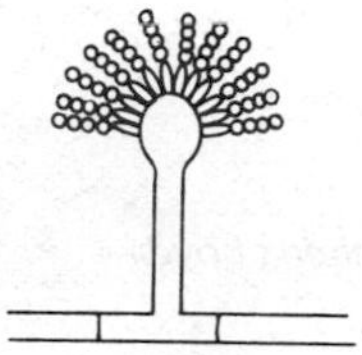
Aspergillus

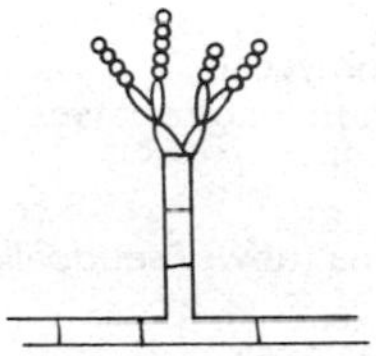
Penicillium

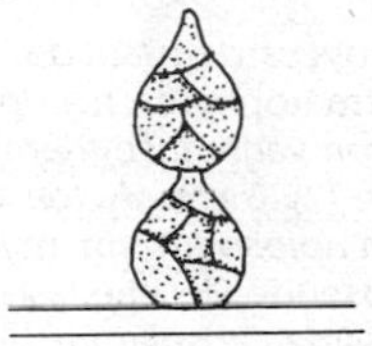
Alternaria

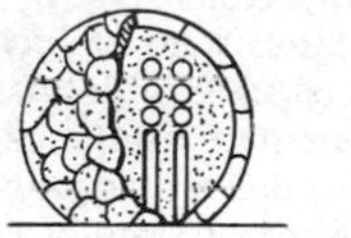
Phoma

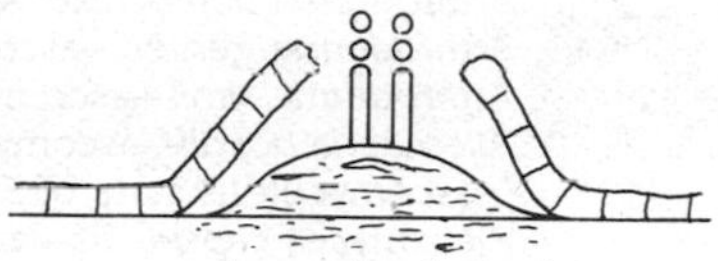
Acervulus in leaf

Old	New	Characteristics
Basidiomycetes	Basidiomycotina (Subdivision) Coenocytic hyphae with complex perforated septa and often with two nuclei per compartment. Basidium and basidiospore, and often clamp connection characterize the subdivision. The human pathogen *Cryptococcus neoformans* recently found to be asexual phase of the basidiomycete *Filobasidiella neoformans.* Teliomycetes (Class). Rusts and smuts. No basidiocarp. Hymenomycetes. Spores shot off. Mushrooms. Gasteromycetes. Spores not shot off; in an enclosed basidiocarp.	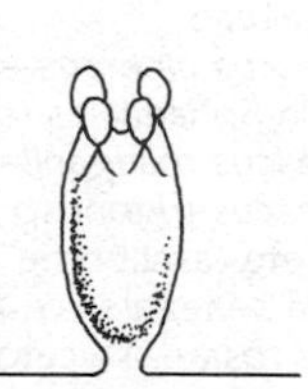 Basidium with spores

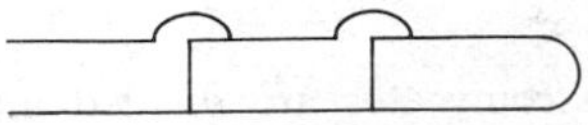
Hypha with clamp connection

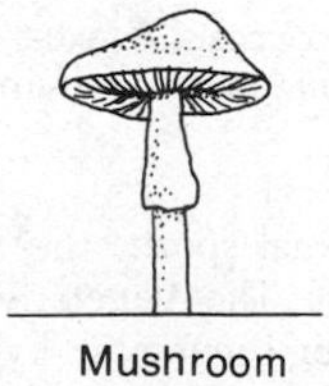
Mushroom

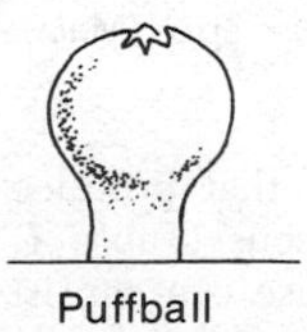
Puffball

Table 2. FUNGAL TAXA THAT CAUSE DISEASES OF MAN OR OTHER PRIMATES

- Eumycota
  - Mastigomycotina
    - Chytridiomycete (?)
      - *Rhinosporidium seeberi*
  - Zygomycotina
  - *Coccidioides immitis* (?) Coccidioidomycosis. Taxonomic location uncertain
  - Zygomycetes
    - Mucorales
      - *Absidia corymbifera*
      - *Absidia ramosa*
      - *Hyphomyces destruens* (?)
      - Mortierella spp. (questionable)
      - *Mucor circinelloides*
      - *Mucor pusillus*
      - *Mucor ramosissimus*
      - *Rhizopus arrhizus*
      - *Rhizopus oryzae*
    - Entomophthorales (usually grow on insects or in ground litter)
    - *Basidiobolus haptosporus* (tropical)
    - *Entomophthora coronata*
  - Ascomycotina
  - Euascomycete (unitunicate ascus; ascocarp wall built around developing asci)
    - Hemiascomycete (yeast or yeast-like)
      - Endomycetales
        - *Endomyces geotrichum*, ascomycetous state of *Geotrichum candidum*
        - *Pichia guilliermondii* (yeast). Sexual state of *Candida guilliermondii*
    - Plectomycete (globose asci borne at different levels in ascocarp; asci dissolving)
      - Eurotiales (cleistothecium)
        - Gymnoascaceae
          - *Ajellomyces dermatitidis*—ascomycetous state of *Blastomyces dermatitidis.* Blastomycosis
          - *Arthroderma benhamiae*—ascomycetous state of the dermatophyte *Trichophyton mentagrophytes*
          - *Arthroderma gertleri*—ascomycetous state of *Trichophyton vanbreuseghemii*
          - *Arthroderma simii*—ascomycetous state of dermatophyte (?) *Trichophyton simii*
          - *Allescheria boydii*—ascomycetous state of *Monosporium apiospermum,* mycetoma (now: *Pseudoallescheria boydii*—ascomycetous state of *Scedosporium apiospermum,* pseudoallescheriasis)
          - *Ajellomyces capsulatus*—ascomycetous state of *Histoplasma capsulatum,* histoplasmosis
          - *Nannizzia cajetani*—ascomycetous state of dermatophyte (?) *Microsporum cookei*
          - *Nannizzia fulva*—ascomycetous state of dermatophyte *Microsporum fulvum*
          - *Nannizzia grubyia*—ascomycetous state of dermatophyte *Microsporum vanbreuseghemii* (probably not pathogenic)
          - *Nannizzia gypsea*—ascomycetous state of dermatophyte *Microsporum gypseum*
          - *Nannizzia incurvata*—ascomycetous state of dermatophyte *Microsporum gypseum* (same asexual state as above)
          - *Nannizzia obtusa*—ascomycetous state of dermatophyte *Microsporum nanum* (various animals)
          - *Nannizzia persicolor*—ascomycetous state of dermatophyte *Microsporum persicolor* (various animals)
        - Eurotiacea (Trichocomataceae?)
          - *Sartorya fumigata*—ascomycetous state of *Aspergillus fumigatus* (?), aspergillosis
      - Microascales (perithecium; asci at various levels, usually spheric, asci dissolving)
        - Microascaceae
          - *Microascus cinereus*—ascomycetous state of *Scopulariopsis cinerea* (von Arix, 1974). Dermal. This genus placed by von Arx in Sphaeriales (see Muller and von Arx, 1973).
          - *Microascus manganii*—ascomycetous state of *Scopulariopsis albo-flavescens.* Dermal
          - *Microascus trigonosporus*—ascomycetous state of Scopulariopsis
  - Loculoascomycete (asci borne in locules of hollowed-out ascostroma; bitunicate ascus)
    - *Leptosphaeria senegalensis.* Mycetoma
    - *Neotestudina rosatti.* Mycetoma
    - *Piedraia hortae.* Black piedra (tropical) nodules as ascostroma on hair
- Deuteromycotina (asexual state, often, of ascomycetes; if sexual and asexual states are known, fungus will have two names with sexual name taking preference)
  - Blastomycetes (asexual yeasts)
    - Cryptococcaceae
      - *Cryptococcus neoformans.* Cryptococcosis. Asexual state of Basidiomycete *Filobasidiella neoformans*
      - *Pityrosporum* spp. *(Malassezia furfur).* In the stratum corneum; pityriasis versicolor

are those fungi that produce the sexual spore, the ascospore, in an ascus (Table 1, Fig. 4). The vegetative or assimilative phase can consist of either coenocytic hyphae compartmentalized by regularly placed simple perforated septa (crosswalls) or yeast cells. An ascus usually contains eight ascospores but certain species can produce four and others more than eight ascospores.

Ascomycetes are divided into three major categories: Euascomycetes, which possess a unitunicate ascus and usually an ascocarp (Table 1) that forms around the developing asci; Loculoascomycetes, which possess a bitunicate ascus (Fig. 4) that is formed within a cavity or locule hollowed out of a stroma that may superficially resemble an ascocarp; and Laboulbeniomycetes, which are minute

Table 2. FUNGAL TAXA THAT CAUSE DISEASES OF MAN OR OTHER PRIMATES *(Continued)*

Candida albicans. Candidiasis
Candida guilliermondii
Candida parapsilosis
Candida stellatoidea
Candida tropicalis
Trichosporon beigelii. White piedra
Trichosporon cutaneum
Geotrichum candidum (white, moist colony but not a yeast—no buds). See below
Torulopsis glabrata. Secondary invader (= *Candida glabrata*)
Hyphomycetes (filamentous, spores borne in open)
Moniliales
Moniliaceae (hyaline or light colored except for *Aspergillus niger*)
Trichophyton (see also Arthroderma in Ascomycetes) dermatophyte
T. schoenleinii; T. rubrum; T. mentagrophytes; T. concentricum; T. verrucosum; T. violaceum; T. tonsurans; T. simii (monkeys); *T. ajelloi* (?); *T. megninii*
Microsporum (see also Nannizzia in Ascomycetes). Dermatophyte
M. canis; M. gypseum; M. audouini; M. ferrugineum; M. fulvum; M. vanbreuseghemii (?); *M. cookei* (?)
Epidermophyton floccosum. Dermatophyte
Geotrichum candidum (wet, white growth with yeast-like arthrospores formed by fragmentation of hyphae)
Cephalosporium (now *Acremonium) mycetoma*
Sporothrix schenkii (white at first, becoming black with age), sporotrichosis (a yeast when growing in the body; hyphal otherwise)
Coccidioides immitis (Phycomycete?). Coccidioidomycosis (spherule in the body, hyphal otherwise)
Histoplasma capsulatum (see Ascomycetes) (yeast in the body; hyphal otherwise)
Blastomyces dermatitidis (see Ascomycetes) (yeast in the body; otherwise hyphal)
Paracoccidioides brasiliensis (Chrysosporium?) (yeast in the body; otherwise hyphal)
Chrysosporium parvum (= *Emmonsia parva)*
Pencillium commune. Pulmonary
Aspergillus fumigatus (see Ascomycetes). Pulmonary, aspergillosis
Aspergillus niger. Otomycosis, fungus balls
Paecilomyces lilacinus
Scopulariopsis brevicaulis (see Ascomycetes). In nails
Fusarium solani, F. oxysporum, F. nivale. Keratitis
Madurella mycetomi, M. grisea. Mycetoma
Monosporium apiospermum (see Ascomycetes) Mycetoma (*Scedosporium apiospermum*)
Dematiaceae (hyphae black or black-green)
Cercospora apii subcutaneous (now known as *Mycocentrospora acerina* [Rippon, 1982])
Torula bantiana. Banti's mycosis (*Cladosporium bantianum*)
Cladosporium carrionii
Cladosporium trichoides. Cladosporiosis
Cladosporium werneckii. On hands
Curvularia lunata and *C. geniculata.* Mycetoma
Phialophora (at least one species pathogenic to both man and certain trees)
P. compacta. Chromomycosis
P. dermatitidis. Chromomycosis
P. gougerotii. Phaeosporotrichosis
P. jeanselmei. Mycetoma
P. parasitica. Subcutaneous
P. pedrosoi. Chromomycosis
P. repens. Mycetoma
P. richardsiae. Phaeosporotrichosis
P. spinifera. Granulomatous lesion
P. verrucosa. Chromomycosis
Coelomycetes (asexual spores in an enclosed pycnidium or on an acervulus)
Sphaeropsidales
Macrophoma spp. Keratitis
Pyrenochaeta romeroi. Mycetoma
Loboa loboi (never cultured). Lobo's disease
Prototheca zopfii. Probably a fungus but may be an algal mutant

*For a list of rare fungal diseases, see Rippon, 1982.

nonmycelial ascomycetes living exclusively on the exoskeletons of insects and mites (Benjamin, 1973). Certain species of Euascomycetes can also possess a stroma, but if so, the ascocarp develops in or on top of it. The stroma is composed of pseudoparenchymatous tissue (see Taber and Taber 1973 for a review of structures). Unexplainably, the concept Euascomycete is not employed taxonomically.

EUASCOMYCETES

Hemiascomycetes. Yeast and yeast-like fungi that produce unitunicate asci but not in an ascocarp are placed in this class. At least one, *Pichia guilliermondii*, is pathogenic to man.

Plectomycetes. Plectomycetes are normally filamentous ascomycetes that produce a simple closed ascocarp, the cleistothecium, containing globose, dissolving asci at various heights in the ascocarp (Table 1). Many of the human pathogenic fungi are members of this class and most are in the Family Gymnoascaceae. *Histoplasma capsulatum, Blastomyces dermatitidis, Paracoccidioides brasiliensis,* and the unrelated *Sporothrix schenkii* grow as true yeasts in human tissue and as hyphae elsewhere in nature. Note that the first three names represent the asexual forms of these fungi, the forms generally observed. Names of the sexual and asexual forms are listed in Table 2. Many of the dermatophytes are members of this group. Note that dermatophytes are housed in three asexual genera: Trichophyton, Microsporum, and Epidermophyton; and note that those producing a sexual state are also members of either Arthroderma or Nannizzia (Table 2). Microascus produces a perithecium (Table 2) but here is placed in the Plectomycetes because the spheric asci are produced scattered throughout the ascocarp. Muller and von Arx (1973) place Microascus in the Sphaeriales to be considered below.

Pyrenomycetes. This class houses those ascomycetes that produce oblong unitunicate asci in a perithecium that is an ascocarp containing an ostiole, or opening, at the top. Asci originate from one layer of cells rather than being distributed throughout the ascocarp as with Plectomycetes. The spores are usually one-celled. Some cleistothecial "analogs" of perithecial forms do exist, however. The ascospores of most pyrenomycetes are shot out of the ascus, but in a very few genera, such as Chaetomium and Melanospora, the asci dissolve and spores ooze out. Virtually all live on plant tissue or in the soil and probably none is a human pathogen if Microascus is considered to be a Plectomycete.

Discomycetes. Cylindric unitunicate asci are produced on, or supported on, an open saucer-like ascocarp, the apothecium (Table 1). None is known to be a human pathogen.

LOCULOASCOMYCETES. Ascomycetes possessing bitunicate asci in the locule or cavity of a "hollowed-out" ascostroma are placed in this class (Luttrell, 1973). The asci are usually thick-walled with an apical dimple and a distinct shoulder (Fig. 4). Ascopores are usually multiseptate and dark colored. *Testudina rosatti* causes mycetoma (Table 2) and *Piedraia hortae,* which grows as ascostroma on hair, causes black piedra.

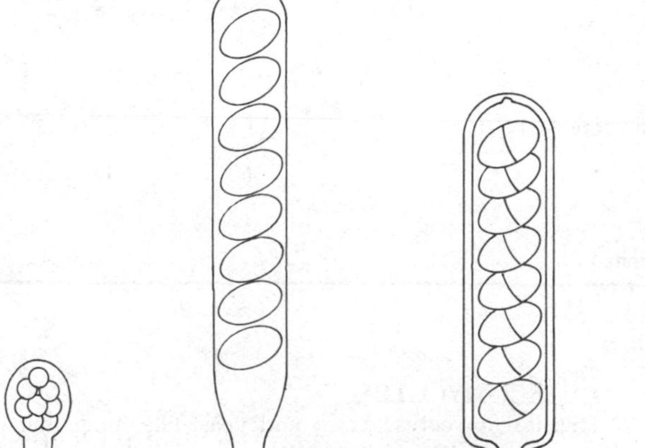

Figure 4. Asci and ascospores.

LABOULBENIOMYCETES. These are minute, nonmycelial ascomycetes that grow on the exoskeletons of insects. Benjamin (1973) reviews this unique group of fungi that may or may not be pathogens of insects and certain mites.

Basidiomycotina. Basidiomycetes are those fungi that produce sexual spores, basidiospores, on a basidium (Table 1, Fig. 1). As with the ascus, nuclear fusion and meiosis take place in this cell. Mating types occurring at one or two loci exist. These segregate as a result of meiosis, and the four basidiospores that are the direct product of meiosis contain the two or four different mating types. Germinated basidiospores are haploid and contain as a rule one nucleus per compartment. There are no sexual organs in the basidiomycetes (except rusts) and the nuclei differing in mating type are brought together as a result of fusion of hyphae derived from basidiospores of different mating types. These secondary hyphae usually contain two nuclei per compartment. The perforated septa dividing the coenocytic mycelium into compartments often possess ornamentations that distinguish them from the simple septa of the ascomycetes.

TELIOMYCETES. This class unites basidiomycetes not having basidiocarps. The plant pathogens, rusts and smuts, and the sexual stage of the human pathogen *Cryptococcus neoformans (Filobasidiella neoformans)* are members of this class.

HYMENOMYCETES. Mushroom (Fig. 1; Table 1) and other fleshy basidiomycetes bearing basidia on gills, pores, smooth surfaces, or spines are allocated to this class. In all cases, spores are shot off of the basidium.

GASTEROMYCETES. Basidiomycetes producing spores that are not shot off are placed in this class. Basidia are contained within an enclosed basidiocarp, such as that of the puffball (Table 1).

Deuteromycotina. The Class Deuteromycotina (Fungi Imperfecti) unites those fungi producing asexual spores or no spores at all. As indicated earlier, many are now known to produce sexual spores under conditions such as certain environmental conditions or presence of two mating types, and such fungi are assigned two names. Most fungi observed growing on Petri plate cultures will be Deuteromycotina or Zygomycotina. Probably the vast majority of Fungi Imperfecti are ascomycetes or were derived from comycetes. The pathogenic yeast *Cryptococcus neoformans* and the yeast *Candida scottii* along with a few others are asexual yeasts of basidiomycetes, however.

BLASTOMYCETES. Asexual yeasts are placed in this class. There are approximately 17 genera of asexual yeasts, 17 genera of ascomycete yeasts, and five genera of basidiomycete yeasts, as described by Kreger-van Rij (1973), whose work provides keys to genera of all yeasts. Identification keys are also given in the following publications: Lodder, 1970; Barnett and Pankhurst, 1974; and DeHoog, 1977.

HYPHOMYCETES. Most Fungi Imperfecti observed in the laboratory are members of this class, which embraces those asexual fungi producing spores on hyphae not contained within sporocarps (Table 1). Approximately 595 genera are recognized in the latest treatment, described by Kendrick and Carmichael (1973). They do not assign genera to families and they base their classification of genera on four properties: 1) Saccardoan spore group, which indicates shape and number of compartments of the spore, 2) arrangement of conidia, 3) color of conidia, and 4) type of conidiogenous cell.

The Hyphomycetes can be divided into five form families: Moniliaceae—mycelia and spores colorless or bright colored (except for the black *Aspergillus niger*, which otherwise conforms to the characteristics of the moniliaceous Aspergillus); Dematiaceae—mycelia and spores black, dark green or dark brown; Stilbaceae—conidiophores united into vertical fascicles called synnemata or coremia; Tuberculariaceae—sporophores borne on an acervulus-like cushion of hyphae infecting a plant; Mycelia Sterilia—spores not produced.

Aspergillus flavus and *Aspergillus fumigatus* cause pulmonary diseases and are unique in being the only non-Zygomycete fungi that grow deep in tissue in mycelial rather than yeast form. The asexual forms of the dermatophytes are also placed in the Moniliaceae or Hyphomycetes. Dark-spored Phialophora and Cladosporium are dematiaceous fungi.

COELOMYCETES. Those fungi producing asexual spores in an enclosed sporocarp, the pycnidium, or in the cushion-like structure, the acervulus, are placed in this class (Table 1). There are approximately 500 genera (Sutton, 1973). *Macrophoma* spp. and *Pyrenochaeta romeroi* cause diseases in man.

HABITAT OF HUMAN PATHOGENIC FUNGI

Fungal diseases can be divided into systemic mycoses, subcutaneous mycoses, and superficial mycoses. Of those causing systemic mycoses and subcutaneous mycoses (histoplasmosis, coccidioidomycosis, sporotrichosis, blastomycosis, aspergillosis, and candidiasis), only *Candida albicans*, the causal agent of candidiasis, normally lives in man. The rest live in soil or on plant products. Some of the dermatophytes live in soil and it is now believed (Rippon, 1982) that some of the dermatophytes have become so well adapted to man that they now normally live on him. This conclusion is based on the observation that some of the human dermatophytes have not been isolated from soil. Ainsworth (1968a) discusses the fungi parasitizing vertebrates.

References

Ainsworth, G. C.: Fungal parasites of vertebrates. In Ainsworth, G. C., and Sussman, A. S. (eds): The Fungi. Volume III. New York, Academic Press, 1968a, p. 211.

Ainsworth, G. C.: The number of fungi. In Ainsworth, G. C., and Sussman, A. S. (eds): The Fungi. Volume III. New York, Academic Press, 1968b, p. 505.

Ainsworth, G. C.: The Dictionary of Fungi. 7th ed. Kew, Surrey, England, Commonwealth Mycological Institute, 1971.

Barnett, J. A., and Pankhurst, R. J.: A new key to the yeasts. A key for identifying yeasts based on physiological tests only. Amsterdam, North Holland Publishers, 1974.

Benjamin, R. K.: Laboulbeniomycetes. In Ainsworth, G. C., Sparrow, F. K., and Sussman, A. S. (eds): The Fungi. Volume IVA. New York, Academic Press, 1973, p. 223.

DeHoog, G. S., and Hermanides-Nijhof, E. J.: The black yeasts and allied genera. Baarn, Holland, Centraalbureau voor Schimmelcultures, 1977.

Hesseltine, C. W., and Ellis, J. J.: Mucorales. In Ainsworth, G. C., Sparrow, F. K., and Sussman, A. S. (eds): The Fungi. Volume IVB. New York, Academic Press, 1973, p. 187.

Kendrick, W. B., and Carmichael, J. W.: Hyphomycetes. In Ainsworth, G. C. Sparrow, F. K., and Sussman, A. S. (eds): The Fungi. Volume IVA. New York, Academic Press, 1973, p. 323.

Kreger-van Rij, N. J. W.: Endomycetales, basidiomycetous yeasts and related fungi. In Ainsworth, G. C., Sparrow, F. K., and Sussman, A. S. (eds): The Fungi. Volume IVA. New York, Academic Press, 1973, p. 11.

Lodder, J. (ed): The Yeasts, a Taxonomic Study. Amsterdam, North Holland Press, 1970.

Luttrell, E. S.: Loculoascomycetes. In Ainsworth, G. C., Sparrow, F. K., and Sussman, A. S. (eds): The Fungi. Volume IVA. New York, Academic Press, 1973, p. 135.

Martin, G. W., and Alexopoulos, C. J.: The Myxomycetes. Iowa City, The University of Iowa Press, 1969.

Muller, E., and von Arx, J. A.: Pyrenomycetes. In Ainsworth, G. C., Sparrow, F. K., and Sussman, A. S. (eds): The Fungi. Volume IVA. New York, Academic Press, 1973.

Rippon, J. W.: Medical Mycology. Philadelphia, W. B. Saunders, 1982.

Sutton, B. C.: Coelomycetes. In Ainsworth, G. C., Sparrow, F. K., and Sussman, A. S. (eds): The Fungi. Volume IVA. New York, Academic Press, 1973, p. 513.

Taber, W. A., and Taber, R. A.: The Impact of Fungi on Man. Boulder, Col., Educational Programs Improvement Corporation, 1967.

Taber, W. A., and Taber, R. A.: Ascomycetes. In Lechevalier, H. A., and Laskin, A. I. (eds): Handbook of Microbiology. 2nd ed. West Palm Beach, Fl., CRC Press, 1978, p. 97.

von Arx, J. A.: The Genera of Fungi Sporulating in Pure Culture. Cramer, Liechtenstein, Vaduz, 1974.

15

FUNGAL TOXINS

MAKOTO ENOMOTO, M.D.

Mycotoxicosis is a disease caused by fungal toxins (mycotoxins), and should be distinguished from *mycosis* caused by opportunistic infections of fungi. Fungi include mushrooms, molds, mildews, blights, rusts, and yeasts. Generally, fungi are valued for the organic fermentation they produce and as a source of many antibiotics. In addition, edible mushrooms are used as human food.

Mycotoxicoses known to be related to human disease are shown in Table 1. Among them are ergotism and mushroom poisoning *(mycetismus)*, which are known in many countries.

MUSHROOM POISONS. The poisonous principles of mushrooms of the genus Amanita are cell-destroying cyclic peptides, such as hepatotoxic "phalloidin" and "amanitin," each representing two groups of lethal sulfur-containing cyclopeptides, the phallotoxins and amatoxins. The phallotoxins act on the endoplasmic reticulum and filamentous actin of liver cells, whereas the amatoxins act on the nucleus. After the isolation from *Amanita muscaria* of muscarine, which excites the parasympathetic nervous system, centrally active substances of isoxazole type, like "muscimol," "ibotenic acid," and "tricholomic acid," have been discovered in it and in other mushrooms (Wieland, 1968).

ERGOT. Widespread epidemics of ergotism, popularly known as St. Anthony's fire, were caused by a fungus, *Claviceps purpura*, infecting rye and other cereal grains during the Middle Ages. When ingested, the ergotized grain produced either cardiovascular effects, such as vasoconstriction and gangrenous symptoms, or neurologic changes, including convulsions and confusion. It is an interesting fact that the ravages of ergotism during the Middle Ages in Europe were largely alleviated by the introduction of new dietary staples such as potatoes and maize.

The first chemically pure alkaloid exhibiting the typical biologic properties of ergot was named ergotamine by Stoll and Hofmann (1970). Ergot alkaloid is a highly variable mixture. The ergot alkaloids have been used as therapeutic agents because of their ability to cause vasoconstriction and contraction of the uterus, and to affect the central nervous system. One of the alkaloids, lysergic acid diethylamide (LSD), is a well-known prototype of hallucinogens.

CARCINOGENIC MYCOTOXINS. Mycotoxicosis received attention in recent years upon discovery of a number of carcinogenic mycotoxins contaminating human and animal foods. The infrequent reports of human intoxication attributable to fungal toxins in foods may be explained by the absence of dramatic acute effects. Acute mycotoxicosis is common in livestock, fish, birds, and experimental animals that eat moldy feed polluted by mycotoxins. A series of outbreaks of unexplained hemorrhage and/or hepatic injury in domestic animals and "spontaneous" hepatic tumors in hatchery-raised fish and laboratory animals resulted from mycotoxin contamination of feed. Of major importance in this regard is a group of hepatocarcinogenic aflatoxins produced by *Aspergillus flavus* (Detroy et al., 1971; Butler, 1974). Luteoskyrin and cyclochloritine isolated from culture of *Penicillium islandicum* were also shown to be responsible for acute hepatic damage, cirrhosis, and tumors of the liver in mice and rats. The type of injury depended on the amount of mold metabolites produced (Uraguchi, 1971; Enomoto and Ueno, 1974). Table 2 shows the animals susceptible to both the carcinogenic and the toxic actions of several important mycotoxins.

The *aflatoxins* are a group of secondary metabolites produced by *Aspergillus flavus* and *A. parasiticus.* They are a mixture of chemically related compounds, derivatives of difuranocoumarin. Aflatoxins B_2 and G_2 are dihydro derivatives of the parent aflatoxins B_1 and G_1. Aflatoxins P_1, M_1, and Q_1 are hydroxylated derivatives of aflatoxin B_1. Aflatoxin M_1 has been recovered from milk, feces, and urine of various mammals, including humans who ingested aflatoxin B_1. In monkeys and chickens, conjugates of aflatoxin P_1 have been detected in the urine in addition to M_1. Aflatoxin B_1 is the most potent carcinogen, followed by G_1, B_2, and M_1 in order of decreasing carcinogenic potency.

Aflatoxin B_1 suppresses synthesis of DNA, RNA, and protein and inhibits the polymerase in rat liver cells. These changes are reflected in the segregation of nucleolar granules and fibrils, capping of the nucleolus, and disruption of the cytoplasmic rough endoplasmic reticulum in liver cells. Aflatoxin B_1 also causes increased activity of DNase and other lysosomal enzymes in the liver or pancreas of rats. The active metabolite is though to be an epoxide such as B_1-2,3-epoxide.

Table 1. MYCOTOXICOSIS IN MAN

Disease *(Date of outbreaks)*	**Location** *(Reported)*	**Fungal Toxins**	**Species of Fungus**	**Symptoms**
Mushroom poisoning (sporadic)	Distributed	Phallotoxin, Amatoxin	Amanita (*A. phalloides, verna, bisporigera, tenuifolia, muscaria)*	Vomiting, diarrhea, jaundice
		Muscarin		Hallucination, excites parasympathetic nervous system
Ergotism, "St. Anthony's fire" (Middle Ages)	Central Europe, U.S.A., India	Ergot alkaloids (ergotamine, ergostine, lysergic acid derivative)	*Claviceps purpurea, pasali*	Lassitude, muscular pain, gangrenous symptoms, convulsion, confusion
Alimentary toxic aleukia or specific angina (1913, 1942–1955)	USSR, Japan	Trichothecenes	Fusaria (*F. poae, sporotrichoides, tricinctum, graminearum*, etc.) Cephalosporium, Trichothecium, Stachybotrys, Myrothecium, Trichoderma	Vomiting, diarrhea, fever, hemorrhagic rash, necrotic angina, leukopenia, sepsis, etc.
Onyalai (1904–1975)	Africa	Not determined	*Phoma sorghina*	Hemorrhagic bullae in the mouth, thrombocytopenia
Aflatoxicosis	Africa, India, Thailand	Aflatoxins	*Aspergillus flavus, parasiticus*	Edema, anorexia, abdominal pain and distention (ascites), jaundice, Reye's syndrome (Thai children)
Luteoskyrin poisoning	Japan*	Luteoskyrin	*Penicillium islandicum,* Mycelia Sterilia	Anorexia, edema, jaundice

*Accidental case

Table 2. MYCOTOXINS KNOWN TO PRODUCE CANCER IN ANIMALS BY ORAL ADMINISTRATION

Carcinogenic Mycotoxin	***Animal Species Susceptible to Both the Carcinogenic and Toxic Effects*** *(target organs)*	***Regular* Dosage*** *(ppm in diet)*	***Animal Species Sensitive Only to the Toxic Effects***
Aflatoxin B_1	Rat (liver, kidney, colon); trout, duck, guppy, ferret, newborn mouse, salmon, medaka,† monkey, marmoset (liver); sheep (liver, nose)	0.5–1.5 (rat)	Turkey, mink, cattle, guinea pig, swine, dog, hamster, rabbit, pheasant, quail, chicken, cat, frog
Aflatoxin G_1	Rat (liver, kidney); duck, medaka† (liver)	1–3 (rat)	
Aflatoxin B_2	Rat, duck (liver)		
Aflatoxin M_1	Rat, trout (liver)		Duckling
Sterigmatocystin	Rat, velvet monkey, medaka† (liver); mouse (blood vessel)	10–50 (rat)	Guinea pig
Luteoskyrin	Mouse, rat (liver)	30–100 (mouse)	Rabbit, chicken, monkey, medaka†
Rugulosin	Mouse (liver)	200 (mouse)	Rat
Griseofulvin	Mouse (liver)	5000–10,000 (mouse)	Rat

*Oral carcinogenic dosage per day in the representative animal shown in parentheses.
†Medaka is a small aquarium fish (*Oryzias latipes*) (Hatanaka et al., 1982).
(From Enomoto, M.: Carcinogenicity of mycotoxin. In Uraguchi, K., and Yamayaki, M. (eds): Toxicology, Biochemistry and Pathology of Mycotoxins. Tokyo, Kodansha International, Ltd., 1977.)

Sterigmatocystin was first isolated from a culture of *Aspergillus versicolor* and was also found to be a metabolite of *A. nidulans* and Bipolaris species. Sterigmatocystin is a derivative of difurano-xanthone and has a difuranmethoxybenzene ring in its structure, just as aflatoxins have. Consequently, these two mycotoxins can be derived from a common intermediary in their biosynthesis. Sterigmatocystin is carcinogenic to the rat and mouse. A high incidence of liver cell carcinoma was observed in rats surviving a dose of 0.75 or 1.5 to 2.25 mg/rat/day (Van der Watt, 1974). Mice fed a dose of 0.1 to 0.25 mg/mouse/day in their diet for 55 or 51 weeks, respectively, developed angiosarcomas of the liver and dorsal brown-fat tissue (Enomoto et al., 1982). The relatively high carcinogenic potency of sterigmatocystin and the wider distribution of this mycotoxin in Japan and South Africa suggest that it may present a more formidable danger than aflatoxins. The metabolic fate of sterigmatocystin in mammals is unknown.

Luteoskyrin and *rugulosin* are anthraquinone pigments. Both induce acute hepatic centrilobular toxic lesions in mice and rats and liver cell adenoma or carcinoma in mice. Rugulosin has less carcinogenic activity than luteoskyrin, but rugulosin is produced by a number of common contaminants of foodstuffs, such as *Penicillium rugulosum, P. brunneum,* and *P. tardum* (Enomoto and Ueno, 1974).

MYCOTOXINS AND HUMAN LIVER CANCER. Data from Thailand, Kenya, Mozambique, and Swaziland provide strong circumstantial evidence of a causal relationship between aflatoxin ingestion and liver cancer incidence in man (Wogan, 1976). The evidence for human aflatoxicosis has also been increasing. Outbreaks of hepatitis in both man and dogs in West India were traced to consumption of spoiled maize heavily contaminated with *Aspergillus flavus*. Aflatoxins were detected in these contaminated samples and in serum samples of a few patients (Krishnamachari et al., 1975). The symptoms of high fever and rapidly progressive jaundice and ascites and the morphologic changes in the liver suggested toxic hepatitis. There was centrilobular scarring with varying degrees of occlusion of the hepatic veins, severe cholangiolar proliferation with cholestasis, and syncytial giant cells of liver-cell origin (Tandon et al., 1977). In Thai children aflatoxin presents the picture of Reye's syndrome, i.e., fatty liver and encephalopathy (Shank et al., 1971). Recent outbreak of acute hepatitis in the Machakos district of Kenya seems to be caused by eating maize that contained as much as 12 ppb of this mycotoxin (Ngindu et al., 1982). The chronic and carcinogenic effect of aflatoxins in man is potentially more important than acute toxicosis but is difficult to prove. Aflatoxin has been detected in human urine, milk, biopsy specimens of liver, and autopsied liver or other tissues by improved chemical methods of aflatoxin analysis (Pong et al., 1974) or immunoassay with antibody against aflatoxin B_1. Yet its role in neoplastic transformation of the liver is not proved by its presence in liver tissue any more than that of viruses that are frequently found in human livers with carcinomas.

In evaluating the danger from fungal toxins after long-term exposure, one must take into account the fact that experimental evidence linking cirrhosis and liver cancer has not been convincing, especially with respect to aflatoxins or sterigmatocystin. Liver cirrhosis and cancer were consistently associated with high incidence rates only in rats and mice fed moldy rice infested with *Penicillium islandicum.* The metabolites of this fungus contain both hepatocarcinogenic luteoskyrin and cirrhogenic cyclochlorotine. These facts suggest that in man liver cirrhosis itself is attributable to the combined effects of other factors, such as hepatitis virus, cirrhogenic mycotoxin, or nutritional agents. Further studies are needed to give definitive evidence of the relationship between liver cell cancer and carcinogenic mycotoxins other than aflatoxins. If prevention of mycotoxin contamination in human foodstuffs results in a decrease in human liver cancer it would be convincing evidence for the positive role of carcinogenic mycotoxins in human carcinogenesis (Fig. 1).

ALIMENTARY TOXIC ALEUKIA (ATA). Alimentary toxic aleukia has been endemic in Siberia and the Amur region of the U.S.S.R. since 1913. The causal agents are the Fusarium species, which grow on overwintered moldy cereals and other crops and produce burning sensations of the mouth, anorexia, vomiting, and diarrhea (Stage I), followed by depression of all bone marrow and thrombopoiesis (Stage II). Fever, hemorrhagic rash, bleeding from gums and nose, necrotic angina, extreme leukopenia, and agranulocytosis with general sepsis occur in the final stage (Stage III) (Joffe, 1971). Death occurs six to eight weeks after ingestion of large amounts of toxin. Skin testing is reliable for toxic assay of overwintered grains. The only prophylactic measure against ATA is the elimination of polluted grain from food.

After the isolation of diacetoxyscirpenol from *Fusarium scirpi*, a number of trichothecene compounds, including T2-toxin, trichothecolon, nivalenol, fusarenon-X, verrucarin A, roridin A, and neosolaniol, have been isolated from imperfect fungi, including Cephalosporium, Fusarium, Trichoderma, Myrothecium, and Stachybotrys species (Bamburg and Strong, 1971; Smalley and Strong, 1974). At present these trichothecenes are considered to be responsible for human ATA because of their characteristic biologic activities in animals. Mice exhibit decreased activity shortly after administration of these trichothecene samples, followed by diarrhea, loss of reaction against skin stimulation, lowered body temperature, and lethargy. The animals usually die from 12 to 72 hours after administration of toxins. Histologic examination reveals marked cytotoxic changes in tissues with actively dividing cells, such as the mucosa of the gastrointestinal tract, lymph follicles, thymus, and bone marrow (Saito et al., 1969, 1974).

ONYALAI. Onyalai is an acute purpuric disease endemic in Africa since 1904. It is attributed to the mycotoxin of *Phoma sorghina* isolated from millet and grain sorghum (Rabie et al., 1975).

CARDIAC BERIBERI. Acute cardiac beriberi was an enigmatic toxic disease prevalent in Japan until 1950. Many patients still suffer from this disease in Southeast Asia. Although the disease is considered a vitamin B_1 deficiency, Japanese investigators attribute it to a fungal toxin of rice and other staple foods. Citreoviridin isolated from *Penicillium citreo-viride* Biourage causes an acute poisoning in the cat and monkey, characterized primarily by an ascending paralysis like that in human beriberi (Uraguchi, 1971; Ueno, 1974). An antithiamine effect of citreoviridin, which inhibits thiamine diphosphate-dependent liver transketolase of the rat, probably plays a role in causing cardiac beriberi in man (Datta and Ghosh, 1981). Cardiac damage occurs in mice given xanthoascin (Takahashi et al., 1976) from *Aspergillus candidus*, a frequent contaminant of human foodstuffs in Southeast Asia. Cardiac muscle undergoes vacuolar degeneration and necrosis followed by cardiac dilatation (Ohtsubo et al., 1976).

OTHERS. Toxin-producing fungi were occasionally encountered during exploration for antibiotics, but were given little attention. Except for griseofulvin, cancer production was usually found in animals only after parenteral administration of antibiotics, including mitomycin C, streptozotocin, penicillin G, azaserine, daunomycin, elaiomycin, and actinomycin D, L, and S. The hepatocarcinogenicity of griseofulvin, the secondary metabolite of *Penicillium griseofulvin* and *patulum*, was proved in mice by the oral administration of a daily dosage of 5000 to 10,000 ppm. An

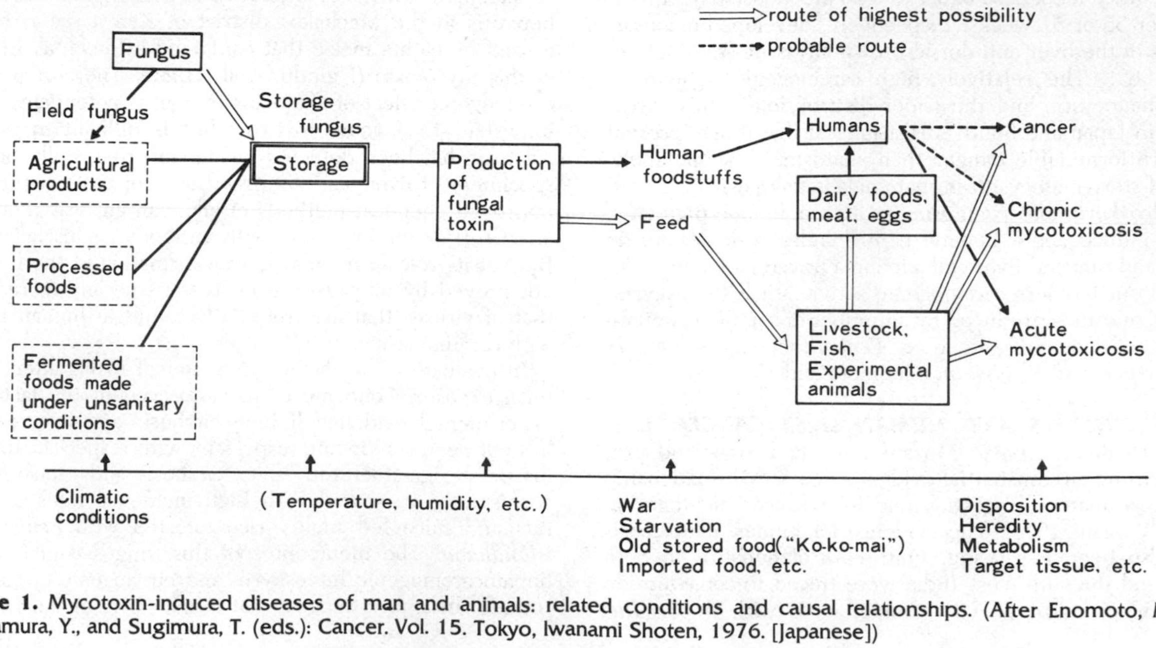

Figure 1. Mycotoxin-induced diseases of man and animals: related conditions and causal relationships. (After Enomoto, M.: *In* Yamamura, Y., and Sugimura, T. (eds.): Cancer. Vol. 15. Tokyo, Iwanami Shoten, 1976. [Japanese])

interesting finding is the production of cytoplasmic aggregates, Mallory bodies, in mouse liver cells by griseofulvin treatment, just as in alcoholic men. Formation of Mallory bodies involves cytoskeletal disorders of the liver cells, in particular, tonofilaments and possibly other forms of cytokeratin (Denk, 1981).

Cytochalasins isolated from *Chaetomium globosum* inhibit a variety of cellular activities, including cell division, motility, secretion, and phagocytosis, presumably through their interaction with the filamentous actin in cells (Yahara et al., 1982).

References

Bamburg, J. R., and Strong, F. M.: 12,13-Epoxytrichothecenes. In Kadis, S., Ciegler, A., and Ajl, S. J. (eds.): Microbial Toxins. Vol. 7. New York, Academic Press, 1971, p. 207.

Butler, W. H.: Aflatoxin. In Purchase, I. F. H. (ed.): Mycotoxins. Amsterdam, Elsevier Scientific Publishing Company, 1974, p. 1.

Datta, S. C., and Ghosh, J. J.: Production and purification of *Penicillium citreoviride* toxin and its effect of TPP-dependent liver transketolase. Folia Microbiol 26:408, 1981.

Denk, H.: Rearrangement of the hepatocyte cytoskeleton after toxic damage: involution dispersal and peripheral accumulation of Mallory body material after drug withdrawal. Eur Cell Biol 23:241, 1981.

Detroy, R. W., Lillehoj, E. B., and Ciegler, A.: Aflatoxin and related compounds. In Ciegler, A., Kadis, S., and Ajl, S. J. (eds.): Microbial Toxins. Vol. 6. New York, Academic Press, 1971, p. 4.

Enomoto, M., and Ueno, I.: *Penicillium islandicum* (toxic yellowed rice)—luteoskyrin-islanditoxin-cyclochlorotine. In Purchase, I. F. H. (ed.): Mycotoxins. Amsterdam, Elsevier Scientific Publishing Company, 1974, p. 303.

Enomoto, M., Hatanaka, J., Igarashi, S., Uwanuma, Y., Ito, H., Asaoka, S., Iyatomi, A., Kuyama, S., Harada, T., and Hamasaki, T.: High incidence of angiosarcomas in brown-fat tissue and livers of mice fed sterigmatocystin. Fd Chem Toxic 20: 547, 1982.

Hatanaka, J., Doke, N., Harada, T., Aikawa, T., and Enomoto, M.: Usefulness and rapidity of screening for the toxicity and carcinogenicity of chemicals in medaka, Oryzias latipes. Jpn J Exp Med 52:243, 1982.

Joffe, A. Z.: Alimentary toxic aleukia. In Kadis, S., Ciegler, A., and Ajl, S. J. (eds.): Microbial Toxins. Vol. 7. New York, Academic Press, 1971, p. 139.

Krishnamachari, K. A. V., Baht, R. T., Nagarajan, V., and Tilak, T. B. G.: Hepatitis due to aflatoxicosis. Lancet 1:1061, 1975.

Ngindu, A., Johnson, B. K., Kenya, P. R., Ngira, J. A., Ocheny, D. M., Nandwa, H., Omondi, T. N., Jansen, A. J., Ngare, W., Kaviti, J. N., Gatei, D. and Siongok, T. A.: Outbreak of acute hepatitis caused by aflatoxin poisoning in Kenya. Lancet 6:1346, 1982.

Ohtsubo, K., Horiuchi, T., Hatanaka, Y., and Saito, M.: Hepato- and cardiotoxicity of xanthoascin, a new metabolite of *A. candidus*. Link to mice. Jpn J Exp Med 46:277, 1976.

Pong, R. T. L., Husaini, and Karyadi, D.: Aflatoxin and primary hepatic cancer in Indonesia. Presented at the V World Congress of Gastroenterology, 1974.

Rabie, C. G., Van Rensburg, S. J., Van der Watt, J. J., and Lübben, A.: Onyalai—the possible involvement of a mycotoxin produced by *Phoma sorghina* in the aetiology. S A Med J 49:1647, 1975.

Richer, C., Paccalin, J., Larcebeau, S., Faugeres, J., Morard, J-L, and Lamant, M.: Présence d'aflatoxine B_1 dans le foie humain. Biologie Générale 223, 1975.

Saito, M., Enomoto, M., and Tatsuno, T.: Radiomimetic biologic properties of the new scirpenol metabolites of *Fusarium nivale*. Gan 60:599, 1969.

Saito, M., and Ohtsubo, K.: Trichothecene toxins of *Fusarium* species. In Purchase, I. F. H. (ed.): Mycotoxins. Amsterdam, Elsevier Scientific Publishing Company, 1974, p. 263.

Shank, R. C., Bourgeois, C. H., Keshamra, N., and Cahndavimol, P.: Aflatoxins in autopsy specimens from Thai children with an acute disease of unknown aetiology. Food Cosmet Toxicol 9:501, 1971.

Smalley, E. B., and Strong, F. M.: Toxic trichothecenes. In Purchase, I. F. H. (ed): Mycotoxins. Amsterdam, Elsevier Scientific Publishing Company, 1974, p. 199.

Stoll, A., and Hofmann, A.: The chemistry of ergot alkaloids. In Pelletier, S. W. (ed.): Chemistry of the Alkaloids. New York, Van Nostrand Reinhold, 1970, p. 267.

Takahashi, C., Yoshihira, K., Natori, S., and Umeda, M.: Xanthoascin, a new metabolite isolated from *Aspergillus candidus*. Chem Pharm Bull 24:613, 1976.

Tandon, B. N., Krishnamurthy, L., Koshy, A., Tandon, H. D., Ramalingaswami, V., Mathur, M. M., and Mathur, P. D.: Study of an epidemic of jaundice, presumably duc to toxic hcpatitis, in Northwest India. Gastroenterology 72:488, 1977.

Ueno, Y.: Citrioviridin from *Penicillium citreo-viride* Biourage. In Purchase, I. F. H. (ed.): Mycotoxins. Amsterdam, Elsevier Scientific Publishing Company, 1974, p. 283.

Uraguchi, K.: Pharmacology of mycotoxins. In Raskova, H. (ed.): International Encyclopedia of Pharmacology and Therapeutics. Section 71. Oxford, Permagon, 1971, p. 143.

Van der Watt, J. J.: Sterigmatocystin. In Purchase, I. F. H. (ed.): Mycotoxins. Amsterdam, Elsevier Scientific Publishing Company, 1974, p. 369.

Wieland, T.: Poisonous principles of mushrooms of the genus Amanita. Science 159:946, 1968.

Wogan, G. N.: The induction of liver cell cancer by chemicals. In Cameron, H. M., Linsell, D. A., and Warwick, G. P. (eds.): Liver Cell Cancer. Amsterdam, Elsevier Scientific Publishing Company, 1976, p. 121.

Yahara, I., Harada, F., Sekita, S., Yoshihira, K., and Natori, S.: Correlation between effects of 24 different cytochalasins on cellular structures and cellular events and those on actin in vitro. J Cell Biol 92:69, 1982.

Parasitology

16

CLASSIFICATION AND ANATOMY OF PARASITES

D. L. Lee, B.Sc., Ph.D.

The parasites that will be mentioned in this chapter belong to the Protozoa, Platyhelminthes, Nematoda, and Acanthocephala.

SUBKINGDOM PROTOZOA

The protozoa are now regarded as a subkingdom rather than as a phylum. They are unicellular eukaryotic cells that contain similar organelles to those found in higher eukaryotic organisms. The Society of Protozoologists has recently agreed on a major re-classification (see Levine et al., 1980; Cox, 1981) and it has been adopted for this edition. Those groups that contain parasites of man are given below.

Phylum Sarcomastigophora

Locomotor organs are flagella, pseudopodia, or both.

Subphylum Mastigophora (The Flagellates)

One or more flagella present on trophozoite; asexual reproduction by binary fission; sexual reproduction unknown in many groups. Free-living and parasitic classes.

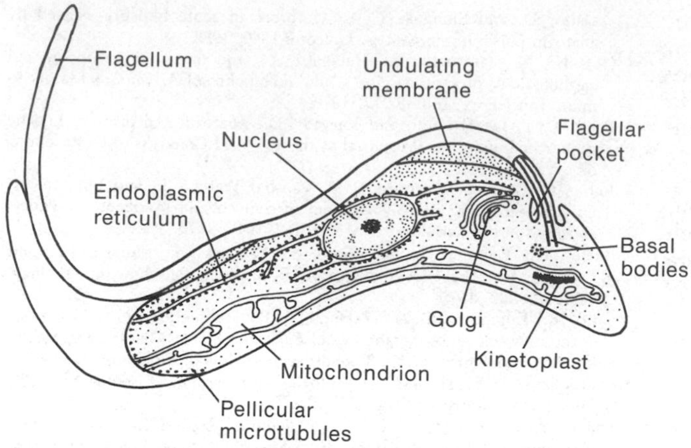

Figure 1. Diagram to show the internal structure of a *Trypanosoma* species, as revealed by electron microscopy. Note the elongate mitochondrion with tubular cristae, the undulating membrane and the kinetoplast.

CLASS ZOOMASTIGOPHOREA

Order Kinetoplastida. One to four flagella; kinetoplast.

Suborder Trypanosomatina. One flagellum, free or attached to body by undulating membrane (Fig. 1); all species parasitic *(Trypanosoma, Leishmania)*.

Order Retortamonadida. Two to four flagella, one runs posteriorly and is associated with a cytostome; harmless parasites of man *(Retortamonas, Chilomastix)*.

Order Diplomonadida. Four pairs of flagella; body bilaterally symmetric; two similar nuclei *(Giardia)* (Fig. 2).

Order Trichomonadida. Four to six flagella, one trailing and associated with undulating membrane if present; axostyle and parabasal body; no cystic stage *(Trichomonas, Pentatrichomonas, Dientamoeba)* (Fig. 3).

Subphylum Opalinata

Parasites of amphibia, fish, and snakes; numerous cilia in rows over body; two to many nuclei of one type.

Subphylum Sarcodina

The amebae; locomotion by means of pseudopodia.

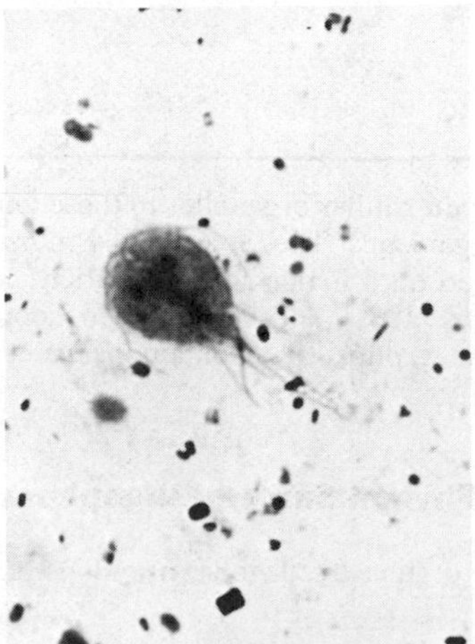

Figure 2. Photomicrograph of *Giardia.* Note the two nuclei and four pairs of flagella.

SUPERCLASS RHIZOPODA

CLASS LOBOSEA. Pseudopodia broad and blunt (lobopods), rarely long and thin (filiform).

Order Amoebida. Naked; single nucleus; multiply by binary fission; many produce resistant cysts *(Entamoeba)* (Fig. 4).

Order Schizopyrenida. Temporary flagellated stage in life cycle *(Naegleria)*.

Phylum Apicomplexa

Characteristic apical complex seen with electron microscope (Fig. 5); cilia and flagella absent except on microga-

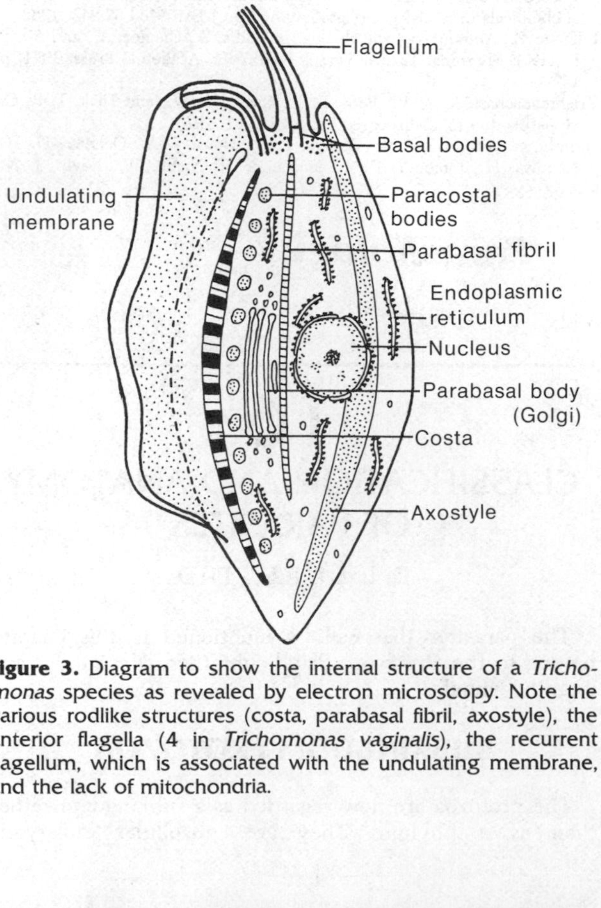

Figure 3. Diagram to show the internal structure of a *Trichomonas* species as revealed by electron microscopy. Note the various rodlike structures (costa, parabasal fibril, axostyle), the anterior flagella (4 in *Trichomonas vaginalis*), the recurrent flagellum, which is associated with the undulating membrane, and the lack of mitochondria.

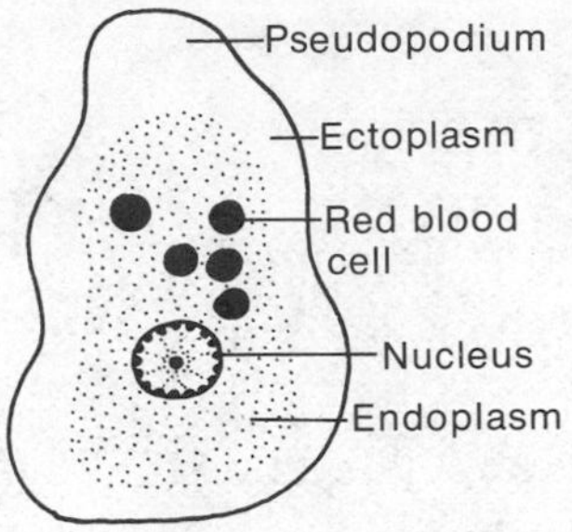

Figure 4. Diagram to show the structure of a trophozoite of *Entamoeba histolytica* as revealed by light microscopy. Note the ingested red blood cells, the characteristic appearance of the nucleus, the ectoplasm, and the endoplasm.

metes; life cycle usually has feeding stages (trophozoites), asexual multiplication (merogony), sexual stages (gametogony) and formation of spores and sporozoites (Fig. 5) (sporogony).

CLASS SPOROZOEA. Infective stages are sporozoites resulting from sporogony.

SUBCLASS COCCIDIA. Trophozoites are intracellular parasites.

Order Eucoccidiia. Merogony present; asexual and sexual phases in life cycle; parasitic in epithelial and blood cells of vertebrates and invertebrates.

Suborder Eimeriina. Micro- and macrogametes develop independently (no syzygy); zygote nonmotile; oocyst present; sporozoites (Fig. 5) enclosed in sporocyst. *(Eimeria, Isospora, Toxoplasma, Sarcocystis.)*

Suborder Haemosporina. Micro- and macrogamete develop independently (no syzygy); zygote motile; oocyst present; sporozoites naked; schizogony in vertebrate host and sporogony in invertebrate host *(Plasmodium, Haemoproteus, Hepatocystis)* (Fig. 6).

SUBCLASS PIROPLASMIA. No spores; small, nonpigmented parasites of erythrocytes of vertebrates, occasionally in other cells; transmitted by an invertebrate host, usually a tick.

Order Piroplasmida. *(Babesia, Theileria.)*

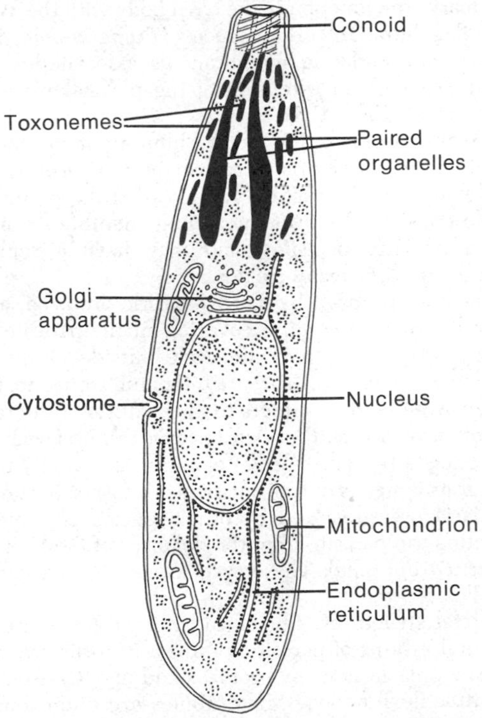

Figure 5. Diagram to show the internal structure of a sporozoite, as revealed by electron microscopy. Note the paired organelles and associated taxonemes or dense bodies (the function of these is unknown but they may be concerned with penetration of the host cell), the conoid with its reinforcing rings, the mitochondria, and the cytostome.

Phylum Ciliophora

Cilia are present in at least one stage of life cycle; two different types of nucleus (Fig. 7); sexual reproduction by conjugation.

CLASS KINETOFRAGMINOPHOREA

SUBCLASS VESTIBULIFERIA. Cilia simple, uniform over body; oral apparatus inconspicuous.

Order Trichostomatida. Cytostome at base of a vestibule; cilia normally uniform but asymmetric in some *(Balantidium)* (Fig. 7).

CLASS OLIGOHYMENOPHOREA. Oral apparatus apparent.

SUBCLASS HYMENOSTOMATIA

Order Hymenostomatida. Cilia of buccal cavity fused to form membranelles; cilia uniform over body *(Tetrahymena)*. (Most species free living but much used in study of protozoan physiology.)

For general references to the classification of protozoa see Baker, 1982; Cox, 1981; Levine, 1973; Levine et al., 1980.

Anatomy of Protozoa

The protozoan cell resembles cells of higher animals in that it may contain some, or all, of the structures (organelles) found in the metazoan cell. The protozoon consists of a mass of cytoplasm enclosed by a limiting membrane

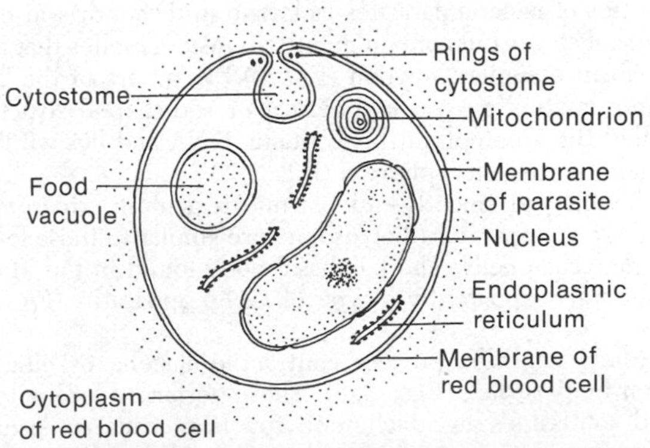

Figure 6. Diagram to show the internal structure of a trophozoite of *Plasmodium* as revealed by electron microscopy. Note the membrane of the red blood cell around the parasite, the cytostome, the food vacuole containing cytoplasm from the red blood cell, and the so-called "mitochondrion," which lacks cristae but sometimes contains whorls of membranes.

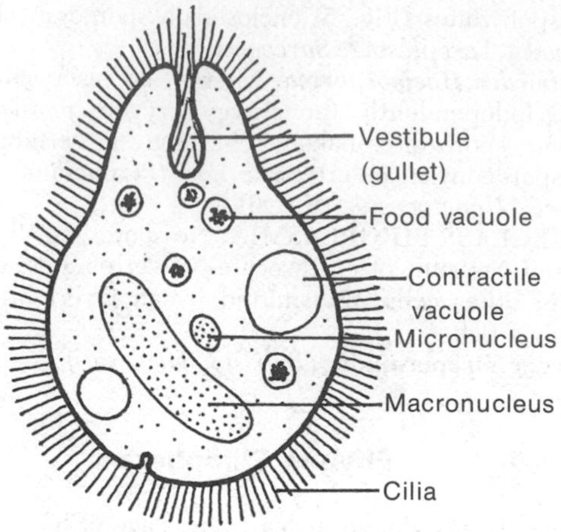

Figure 7. Diagram to show the structure of *Balantidium coli* as revealed by light microscopy. Note the uniform cilia over the surface, the micro- and the macronuclei, the two contractile vacuoles, the vestibule or gullet at the base of which lies a cytostome, and the food vacuoles.

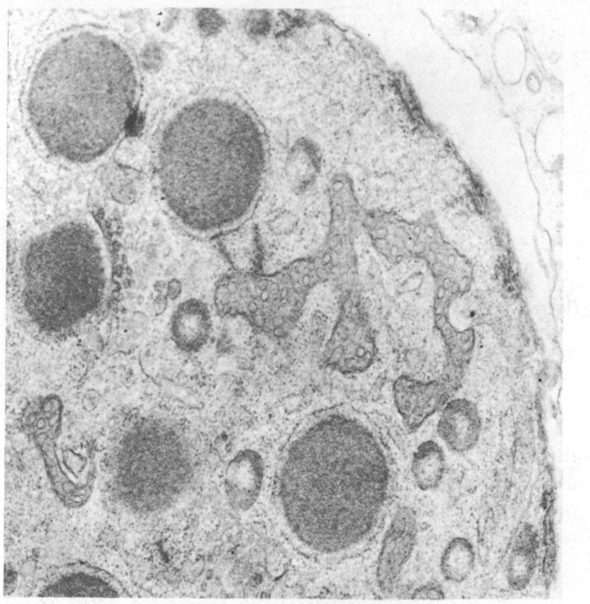

Figure 8. Electron micrograph of a section through a macrogamete of *Eimeria* to show the structure of the mitochondria. Note the tubular nature of the cristae.

(plasmalemma or pellicle) and contains one or more nuclei, mitochondria, endoplasmic reticulum, ribosomes, Golgi apparatus (dictyosome, parabasal body), centrioles, flagella, cilia, microtubules, and fibrils. Some protozoa, and specific stages in the life cycle of others, lack certain of these organelles. In some groups—for example, the Sarcodina—the cytoplasm is divided into an outer, clearer ectoplasm and an inner, denser endoplasm that contains most of the organelles (Fig. 4). Some protozoa contain contractile vacuoles (Fig. 7) and some contain skeletal rods (Fig. 3), which do not occur in metazoan cells.

The nucleus is similar to that of the metazoan cell. The ciliates have two different types of nucleus; one is the sexual nucleus (micronucleus), and the other is the asexual nucleus (macronucleus) (Fig. 7). In *Entamoeba* the nucleoprotein is arranged around the periphery of the nuclear membrane in a characteristic pattern (Fig. 4).

The mitochondria are similar to those found in the cells of higher organisms, but the cristae (infoldings of the inner membrane) are usually tubular rather than plate-like (Figs. 1, 8). Certain species are apparently anaerobic and lack mitochondria (*Trichomonas* (Fig. 3), *Entamoeba*). Some species of malaria parasites lack true mitochondria in their asexual stages but contain membranous organelles that may perform a similar function (Fig. 6). Members of the Trypanosomatina possess a spherical or rod-shaped structure called the kinetoplast; this contains DNA and lies within a single, large mitochondrion (Fig. 1).

Rough and smooth endoplasmic reticulum, ribosomes, and Golgi apparatus (dictyosome) are similar to those found in metazoan cells. The parabasal body found in the Mastigophora is apparently a type of Golgi apparatus (Figs. 1, 3).

Many protozoa possess contractile flagella or cilia on their body surface (Figs. 3, 7). These perform a locomotory, and sometimes an attachment, function. Cilia are usually shorter and more numerous than flagella, but they have a similar internal structure consisting of nine pairs of microtubules arranged around the periphery of the flagellum and two single fibrils in the center; this is called the axoneme. The whole flagellum is enclosed by an extension of the limiting membrane of the protozoan. Cilia and flagella arise from a basal body or kinetosome within the cell (Figs. 1, 3). This basal body is a hollow cylinder about 1.5 μm in diameter and is composed of nine outer double or triple microtubules that connect with the outer microtubules of the flagellum; the two central microtubules of the flagellum are not present in the basal body. A basal plate marks the junction of the basal body with the axoneme of the flagellum. In certain species (*Trypanosoma*, *Trichomonas*) an undulating membrane is associated with the flagellum and is an extension of the plasmalemma of the body surface (Figs. 1, 3).

In many protozoa the outer, limiting membrane is a typical plasma membrane, but in certain groups it is a more complicated structure and is called the pellicle. The pellicle consists of two or more unit membranes in some species (malaria parasites) and may have a sculptured appearance, as in many ciliates.

Cysts are produced by many parasitic protozoa, and the cyst wall forms a protective covering for the parasites when they spend part of their life cycle outside of their host (*Entamoeba*, *Eimeria*, *Isospora*). Granules arise inside the protozoan and are secreted to the exterior, where their contents coalesce and harden to form the cyst wall. Cysts are produced by some species of parasitic protozoa that use a vector as a means of transmission to another host (oocysts of malaria parasites) and by other species as a means of protecting the parasite from the defenses of the host (tissue cysts of *Toxoplasma*). These cysts usually have a softer and more flexible wall.

Skeletal structures, fibers, and microtubules are found in several groups of parasitic protozoa. Fibrils are present in the cytoplasm of many protozoa and may have a skeletal or contractile function. Microtubules are often found beneath the limiting membrane (Fig. 1) as well as in the flagellum (Figs. 1, 3) and may have a skeletal or locomotory function. Some may also play a role in the transport of materials within the cell. Larger skeletal structures, such as the costa and the axostyle of *Trichomonas* (Fig. 3), are also found in certain groups of protozoa.

Contractile vacuoles are unusual in parasitic protozoa but they do occur in parasitic ciliates *(Balantidium)* (Fig. 7) and in the amebae *Naegleria* and *Hartmanella,* which occasionally infect man. The contractile vacuole is a vesicle or vacuole that pulsates in a rhythmic manner and opens to the outside through a small pore in the limiting membrane.

Many parasitic protozoa possess a mouth, or cytostome, through which food particles are ingested. This cytostome may be a small depression on the surface of the body (Figs. 5, 6) or may lie at the base of a groove or cytopharynx, where it is usually associated with one or more flagella (Fig. 7).

Further reading on the structure of protozoa: Adam *et al.*, 1979; Baker, 1982; Kreier, 1977, 1978; Sleigh, 1973; Vickerman and Cox, 1967).

Phylum Platyhelminthes

The platyhelminthes are worms that are usually flattened dorsoventrally, bilaterally symmetric, and without true segmentation. The digestive tract is incomplete or absent. The excretory system is the flame cell type and there is no body cavity, circulatory system, or respiratory system. The nervous system consists of a pair of anterior ganglia from which extend longitudinal nerves connected by transverse commissures. Individuals are hermaphroditic, with a few exceptions. The body is covered by a cytoplasmic epidermis or tegument (formerly thought to be a secreted cuticle in the Trematoda and Cestoidea).

The classification given here is incomplete because particular attention was given to parasites that attack man. For details of the complete classification see the references at the end of each section.

CLASS DIGENEA (FLUKES). Adult worms are typically leaf-shaped, but cylindric forms exist. A cup-shaped sucker surrounds the mouth (oral sucker) and a second sucker (acetabulum) is situated on the ventral surface. Almost all species are endoparasitic as adults and live in the alimentary tract, bile duct, blood vessels, lungs, bladder, or other organs of the vertebrate host.

The classification of the Digenea is controversial. The system described here is based on the system proposed by La Rue (1957) and used by Erasmus (1972), Noble and Noble (1982) and Cox (1982), but reference should be made to Yamaguti (1958) and to Dawes (1956).

SUPERORDER ANEPITHELIOCYSTIDIA. Cercaria with thin excretory bladder; tails simple or forked; stylet absent.

Order Strigeatida. Miracidia with one or two pairs of flame cells; cercaria with forked tail.

Suborder Strigeata. Superfamily Schistosomatoidea (= Bilharziidae). Sexes separate; adults live in blood vessels of mammals and birds. *(Schistosoma.)*

Order Echinostomida. Cercariae with cyst-producing gland cells. Cercariae encyst on vegetation or in molluscs.

Suborder Echinostomata. Superfamily Echinostomatoidea. (*Fasciole hepatica, Fasciolopsis buski, Echinostoma ilocanum.*)

Suborder Paramphistomata. Superfamily Paramphistomatoidea. (*Gastro discoides = Gastrodiscus hominis.*)

SUPERORDER EPITHELIOCYSTIDA. Cercaria with thick-walled excretory bladder; tail of cercaria single, reduced in size, or absent; miracidium with a single pair of flame cells.

Order Plagiorchiida. Oral stylet usually present in oral sucker of cercaria.

Suborder Plagiorchita. Superfamily Plagiorchioidea. (*Dicrocoelium dendriticum; Paragonimus westermani.*)

Order Opisthorchiida. Cercaria have no oral stylet.

Suborder Opisthorchiata. Superfamily Opisthorchioidea. (*Opisthorchis = Clonorchis sinensis; Heterophyes heterophyes; Metagonimus yokogawai.*)

Anatomy of the Digenea

The life cycle of the digeneans consists of some or all of the following stages: egg, miracidium, mother sporocyst, daughter sporocyst, redia, cercaria, metacercaria, and adult.

The egg shell should correctly be referred to as an egg capsule. It is usually oval and light to dark brown, and may be operculated (Fig. 9). The egg capsule of the human blood flukes *(Schistosoma)* is nonoperculate and bears a terminal spine *(S. haematobium)*, a lateral spine *(S. mansoni)* (Fig. 10), or a lateral knob *(S. japonicum)*.

The miracidium is a ciliated, bullet-shaped, free-swimming larva in most species (Figs. 11, 12). Ciliated epidermal plates on the outer surface are separated from each other by extensions of the subepidermal layer that lie beneath the plates (Fig. 12). The anterior end of the miracidium bears an apical papilla that lacks cilia but carries the openings of the apical and penetration glands. Most miracidia possess a pair of eyespots, each of which is a pigmented cup containing a lens. The cerebral mass, which lies behind the eyespots, is connected by nerves to the eyespots, the sense organs, the apical papilla, and the posterior end of the larva. Sense organs occur on the apical papilla and also laterally on the body of the miracidium. The posterior part of the miracidium contains the germinal cells that may form clusters of cells called germ balls. The miracidium possesses one or more pairs of flame cells (Figs. 12, 20).

In most species the miracidium develops into a sporocyst (Fig. 13) after penetration of a suitable snail host. It loses its ciliated epidermal plates, the subepidermal layer de-

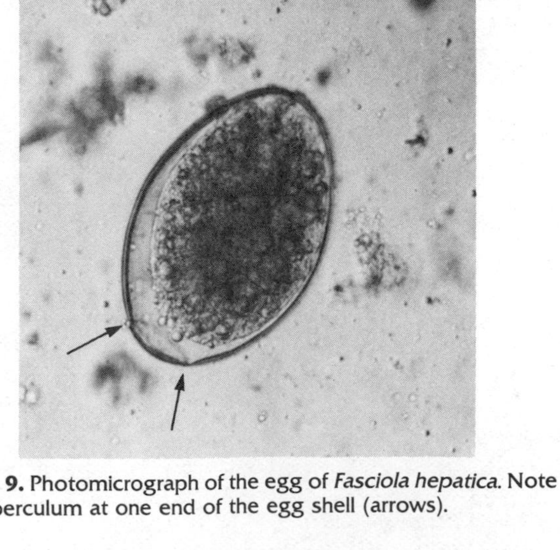

Figure 9. Photomicrograph of the egg of *Fasciola hepatica.* Note the operculum at one end of the egg shell (arrows).

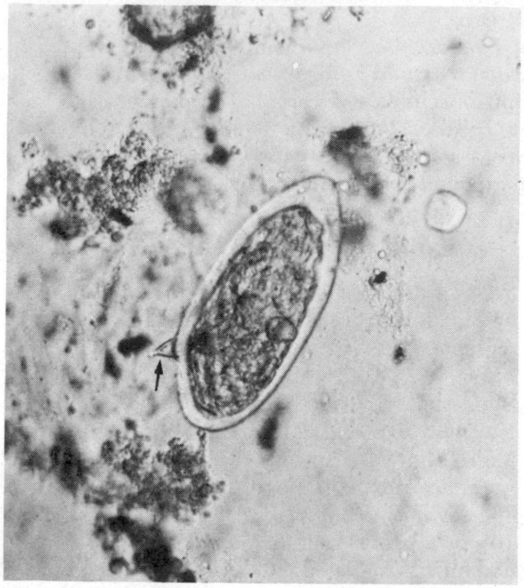

Figure 10. Photomicrograph of the egg of *Schistosoma mansoni.* Note the lack of an operculum and the characteristic spine on the egg shell (arrow).

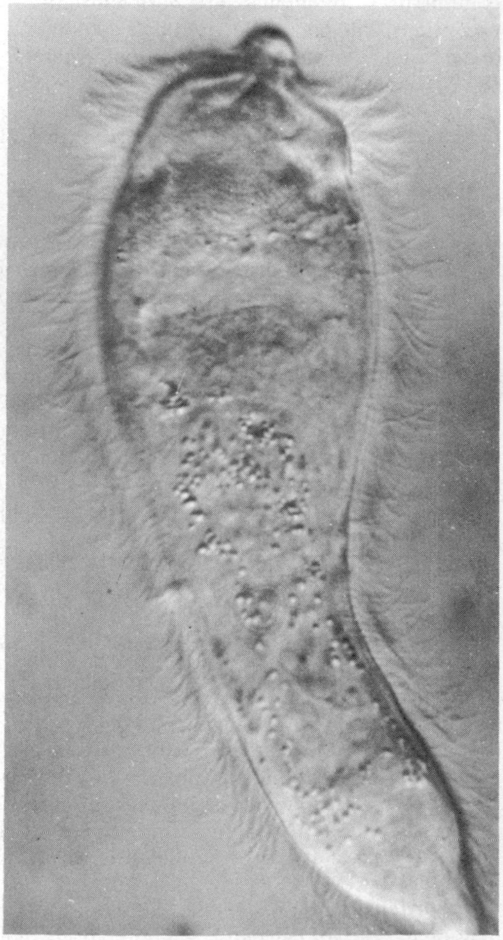

Figure 11. Photomicrograph of the miracidium of *Schistosoma mansoni* (Nomarski interference microscopy). Note the ciliated epidermis and apical papilla.

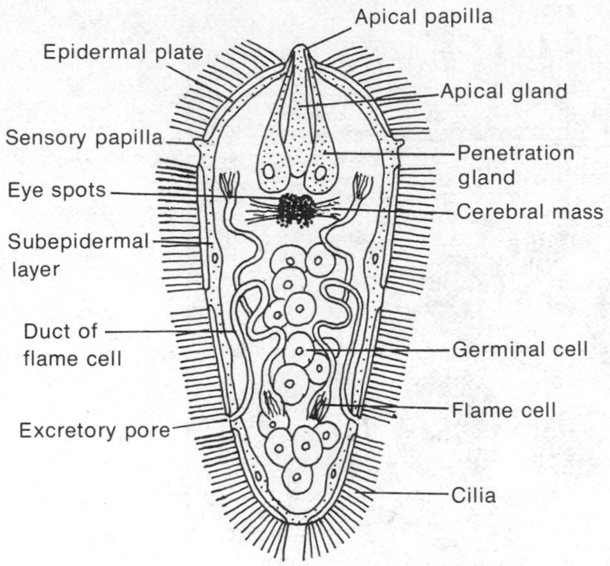

Figure 12. Diagram of a miracidium. Note the ciliated epidermal plates, the subepidermal layer, which becomes the body wall of the sporocyst, the apical papilla with its associated glands, the flame cells with their collecting ducts, and the germinal balls.

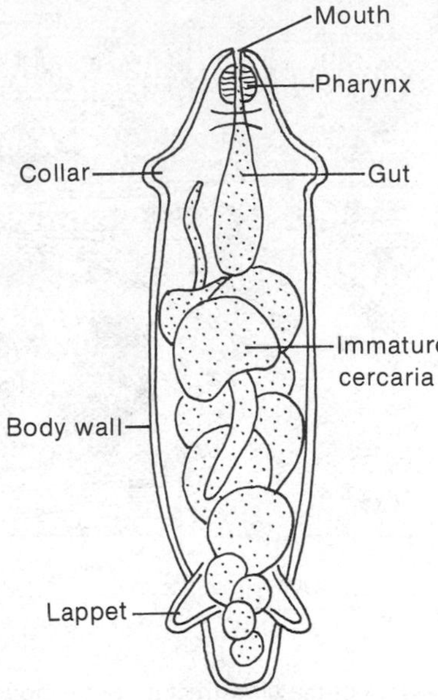

Figure 14. Diagram of a redia. Note the presence of a simple gut, the collar, lappets (2), and germinal balls, which develop into cercariae.

velops into the new outer layer or tegument, and the larva becomes an elongated sac containing germinal cells. These germinal cells subsequently give rise to daughter sporocysts (as in the schistosomes) or to rediae that escape through a birthpore.

The redia is not present in all species. It is an elongate developmental stage that possesses a mouth, muscular pharynx, and a simple sac-like gut (Fig. 14). It usually bears a ridge-like collar around its anterior end and a pair of lobe-like lappets near the posterior end. The outer covering is a thin tegument (Fig. 15) that covers circular and longitudinal muscles and a cellular layer. The body

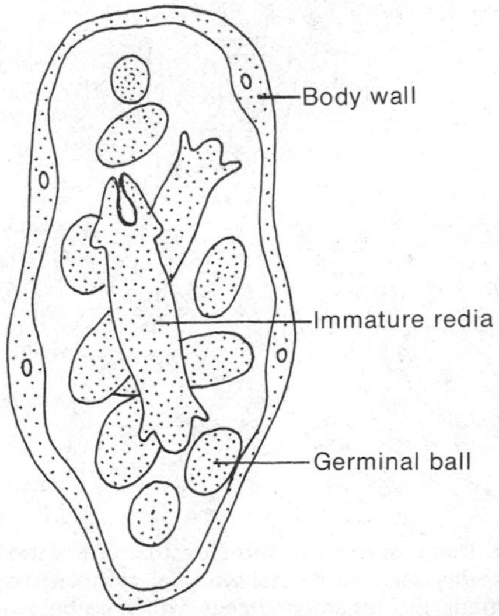

Figure 13. Diagram of a sporocyst. Note the sac-like appearance and the germinal balls, which develop into rediae (or into daughter sporocysts or cercariae in those species that lack a redia stage).

cavity contains germinal cells, germinal masses, and developing daughter rediae or cercariae (Fig. 14). The excretory system consists of flame cells that open into two lateral excretory canals.

The cercaria arises from germinal masses within the daughter sporocysts (as in the schistosomes) or within the rediae. They vary in appearance according to the species (Fig. 16 A, B) but have a cylindric or globular body and a muscular tail that is used in locomotion. The tail may be simple or forked (Fig. 16 A, B); both the body and the tail are covered by a cytoplasmic tegument. An oral sucker surrounds the mouth, and most species also have a ventral sucker. The rudimentary digestive system consists of a mouth, muscular pharynx, esophagus, and a pair of blind-ended ceca. A cerebral ganglion lies just behind the oral sucker and supplies nerves to various parts of the cercaria. Some species possess pigmented eyespots. The cercaria also possesses a well-developed excretory system of flame cells and collecting ducts.

Gland cells secrete the metacercarial cyst in those species that encyst, or secrete materials such as an adhesive substance or enzymes if the cercaria penetrates a second intermediate host or the final host. Penetration glands (Fig. 16 A) are a characteristic feature of the cercariae of schistosomes and they secrete several substances. Cystogenous gland cells, which are usually more widely scattered around the body of the cercaria, give rise to the wall of the metacercarial cyst (Fig. 16 B) in those species that form a cyst *(Fasciola hepatica)*. The tail of the cercaria, which is well-supplied with muscles and mitochondria, is shed when the cercaria penetrates another host or encysts.

The cercaria of many species *(Fasciola hepatica)* encyst upon vegetation, whereas others penetrate a second intermediate host *(Opisthorchis sinensis)* and encyst inside the tissue; these stages are called the metacercaria. The cercaria of schistosomes penetrates the skin of the final host and becomes an active schistosomule; the schistosomule lacks the tail of the cercaria and has discharged its penetration glands.

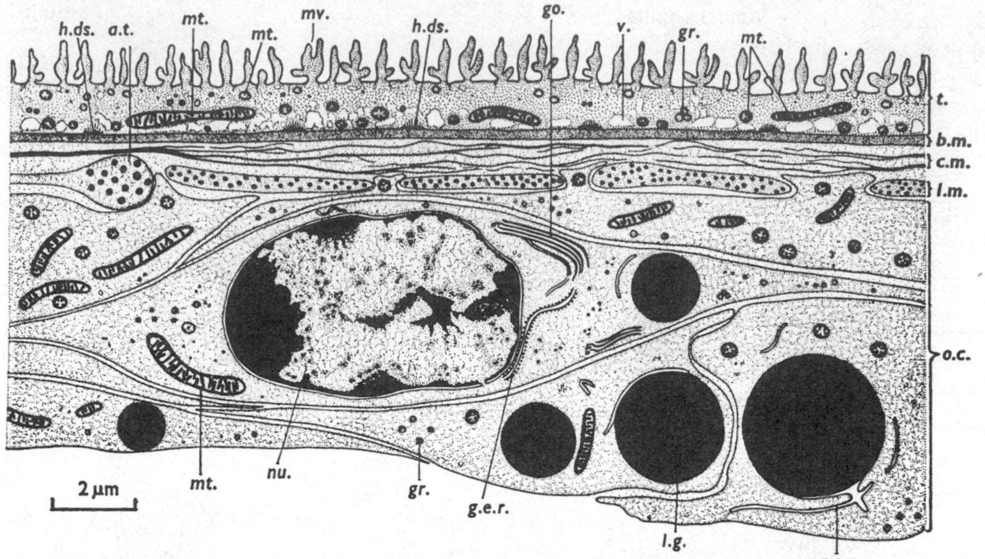

Figure 15. Diagram of the ultrastructure of the body wall of a redia. Note the extension of the surface into branched microvilli. a.e.r., agranular endoplasmic reticulum; a.t., axon terminal; b.m., basement membrane; c.m., circular muscle; g.e.r., granular endoplasmic reticulum; go., Golgi complex; gr., granule; h.ds., half-desmosome; l.g., lipid globule; l.m., longitudinal muscle; mt., mitochondrion; mv., microvillus; nu., nucleus; o.c., overlapping cell; t., tegument; v., vacuole. (Reproduced with permission from G. Rees: *Parasitology* 56, 1966.)

The adult digenean is covered with a syncytial cytoplasmic epidermis called the tegument, the nucleated portions of which lie below the main outer layer (Fig. 17). The tegument contains mitochondria, dense rod-shaped bodies of unknown function, endoplasmic reticulum, vacuoles, and, in some species, spines that extend from the surface of the tegument (Fig. 17). Nuclei and lateral cell walls are not present in the outer covering. Nucleated cells make contact with the main tegument by means of cytoplasmic tubes (Fig. 17). These cells contain endoplasmic reticulum, mitochondria, Golgi apparatus, and ribosomes. The tegument of adult schistosomes is covered by a series of membranes that may be important in evasion of the immune response of the host.

The terminal mouth of the adult leads to a muscular pharynx, esophagus, and a pair of blind-ending intestinal ceca in most species (Fig. 18). The wall of the ceca consists of a single layer of epithelial cells lying upon a basement

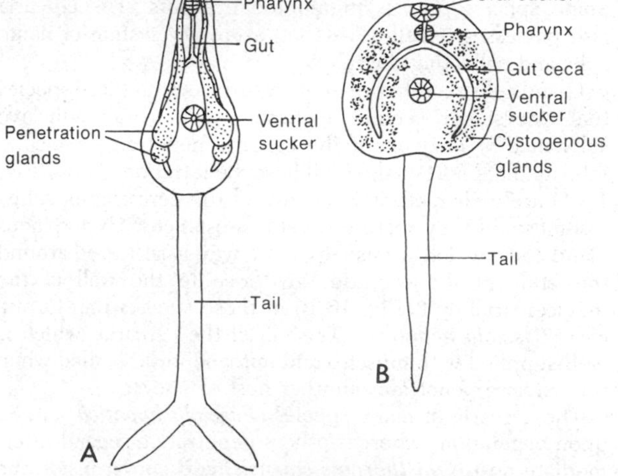

Figure 16. A, Diagram of a schistosome-type cercaria. Note the bifurcate tail, the penetration glands, and the sucker. B, Diagram of a *Fasciola*-type cercaria. Note the unbranched tail, the lack of penetration glands, the cystogenous glands, which produce the wall of the metacercaria, and the suckers.

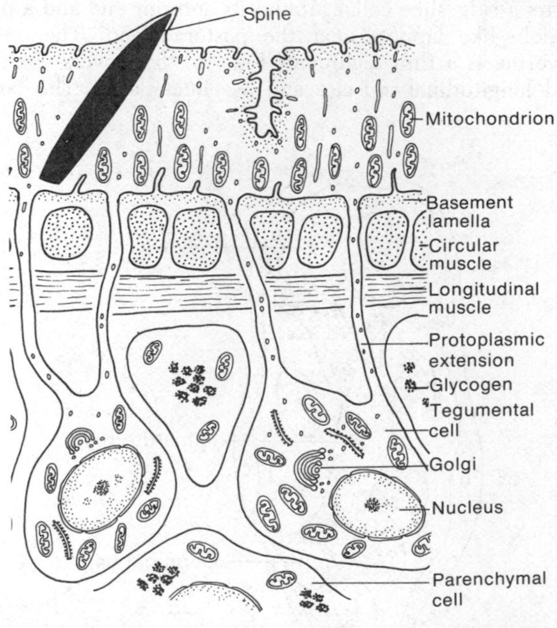

Figure 17. Diagram to show the ultrastructure of the body wall of *Fasciola hepatica*. Note the syncytial cytoplasmic nature of the tegument, the tegumental cells, which lie below the tegument but connect with it by processes, the muscle layers, and the spine. The nuclei of the tegument lie in the tegumental cells and not in the tegument itself. (Based on Threadgold; Quart J Microscopical Sci. 104, 1963.)

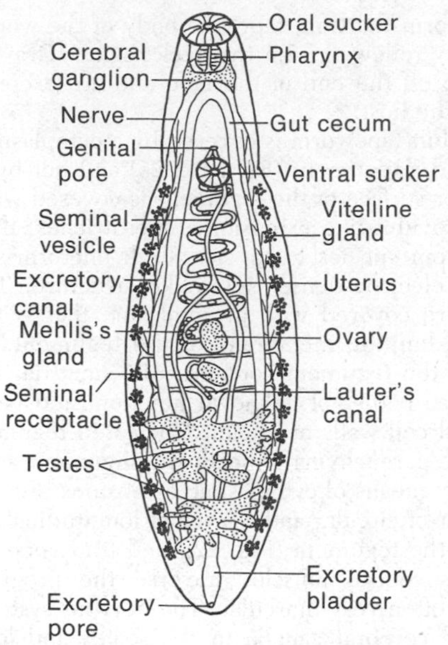

Figure 18. Diagram to show the morphology of a digenetic trematode *(Opisthorchis-Clonorchis sinensis).*

lamella; a thin layer of muscle surrounds the cecal wall. The surface of the cells that line the cecal lumen is covered with long microvilli (Fig. 19). These intestinal cells are capable of secretion and absorption.

The excretory system consists of flame cells (Fig. 20) and collecting ducts, which open either directly to the outside from two large lateral excretory tubules or into a bladder that opens to the exterior (Fig. 18). A system of lymph channels occurs in some species but little is known about them.

The nervous system consists of a pair of cerebral ganglia from which longitudinal nerves arise (Fig. 18). Transverse commissures connect these longitudinal nerves. Nerves extend from the ganglia and from the longitudinal nerves to supply the sense organs, suckers, muscles, and other organs of the body.

A layer of circular and a layer of longitudinal muscles lie beneath the tegument (Fig. 17). The muscle fibers contain thick and thin myofilaments, and an extension of the sarcoplasm contains the nucleus, mitochondria, and endo-

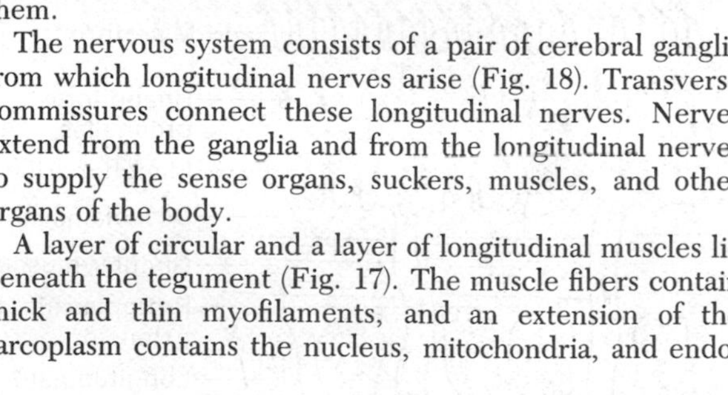

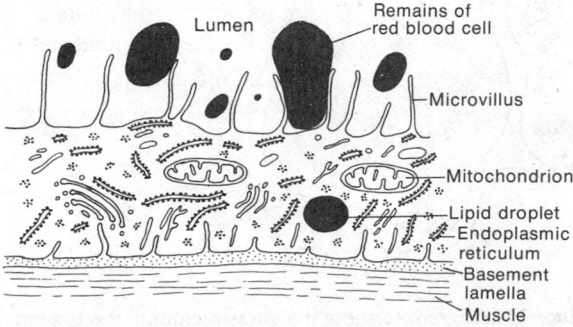

Figure 19. Diagram to show the ultrastructure of part of the gut ceca of *Schistosoma mansoni.* Note the long, widely spaced microvilli and the partly broken-down red blood cells. (Drawn from an electron micrograph in Morris, A.P. *Experientia,* 24, 1968.)

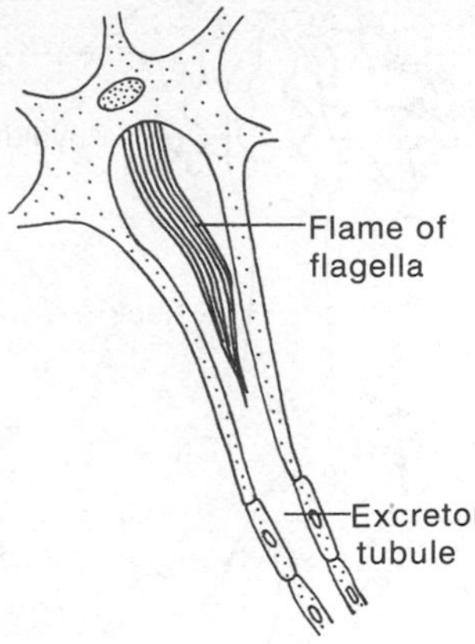

Figure 20. Diagram of a flame cell (highly magnified).

plasmic reticulum of the muscle cell. The muscle fibers appear nonstriated in the adult worm, but the muscles in the tail of the cercaria are striated.

The parenchyma consists of large cells that lie in contact with the various tissues and organs of the body; there is no body cavity in the adult worm.

Most digeneans are hermaphroditic but the sexes are separate in the schistosomes. Figure 18 shows a diagram of the reproductive system of a typical digenean. There is usually a single ovary and one or more testes, which may be either compact or branched organs. Yolk for the eggs is produced by paired vitelline glands that may be branched or compact. A characteristic chamber called the ootype lies between the oviduct and the uterus. A series of small cells that form the Mehlis' gland are associated with the ootype. This combined structure is important in the formation of the egg capsule. The uterus, which is usually long and full of eggs, opens to the exterior at the genital atrium. Spermatozoa pass from the testes along the vas deferens to a seminal vesicle and an eversible cirrus.

For further reading on the structure and anatomy of trematodes see Hyman, 1951a; Grassé, 1961; Erasmus, 1972; Smyth and Halton, 1983; Dawes, 1956; Yamaguti, 1958; and Noble and Noble, 1982.

CLASS CESTODA. The class Cestoda consists of hermaphroditic worms, which, as adults, are parasitic in the alimentary tract of vertebrates. They are commonly called cestodes or tapeworms.

SUBCLASS EUCESTODA. The long, ribbon-like body consists of 4 to 4000 proglottids and a scolex with adhesive organs at the anterior end of the worm.

Order Pseudophyllidea. Scolex with two bothria (Fig. 21B), length varies from a few millimeters to 25 meters. Mainly parasites of fish except for *Dibothriocephalus latus* (= *Diphyllobothrium latum*), which is parasitic in man.

Order Cyclophyllidea (= Taenoidea). Scolex with four muscular suckers (acetabula) and often with one or more rows of hooks on the tip (rostellum) of the scolex (Fig. 21C); proglottids well defined. Includes most tapeworms of higher animals and man *(Taenia, Echinococcus, Hymenolepis).*

For further reading on the classification of tapeworms see Wardle and McLeod, 1952; Wardle et al., 1974; Smyth, 1969; Voge, 1969; Hyman, 1951a; Joyeux and Baer, 1961; and Yamaguti, 1959.

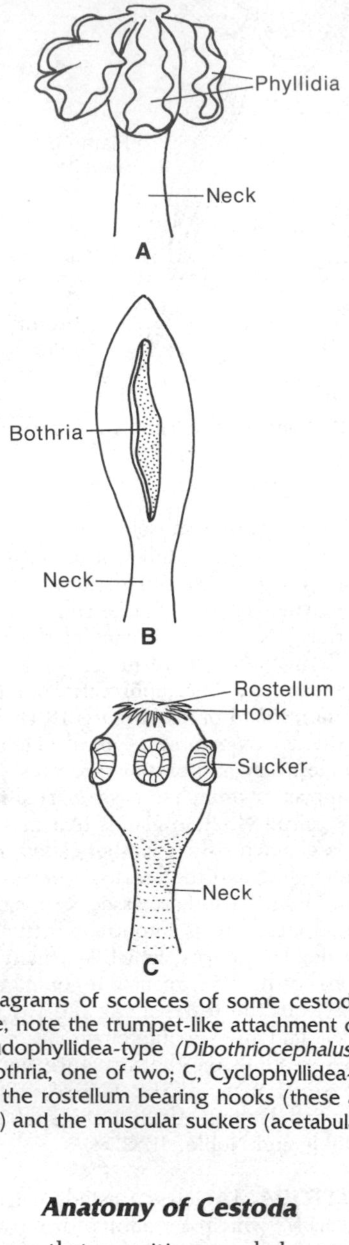

Figure 21. Diagrams of scoleces of some cestodes. A, Tetraphyllidea-type, note the trumpet-like attachment organs (phyllidia); B, Pseudophyllidea-type *(Dibothriocephalus latus),* note the slit-like bothria, one of two; C, Cyclophyllidea-type *(Taenia solium),* note the rostellum bearing hooks (these are absent in some species) and the muscular suckers (acetabula).

Anatomy of Cestoda

All tapeworms that parasitize man belong to the Eucestoda. They are mostly slender, elongate, white or cream-colored worms with a body consisting of few to many segments (proglottids). Each proglottid contains a complete set of male and female reproductive organs at some stage in development. There are no circulatory, respiratory, or skeletal organs and there is no alimentary system. Larval stages develop in one or more intermediate hosts.

The head is an attachment organ (scolex) that is armed with suckers of various sorts (bothria are slit-like grooves, Fig. 21B; phyllidia are trumpet-like or leaf-like structures, Fig. 21A; acetabula are muscular suction cups, Figs. 21C, 23) and may or may not also possess hooks. The anterior end of the scolex may be formed into a rostellum (Figs. 21C, 23). The neck lies behind the scolex and is a zone of proliferation from which immature proglottids are formed. These proglottids pass through a phase when they increase in size, develop gonads (mature proglottids), and fill the uterus with eggs (gravid proglottids) (Fig. 23). These proglottids form the thin, tape-like body of the worm and are constantly renewed from the neck region. Gravid proglottids drop off the end of the tape and are excreted in the feces of the host.

The adult tapeworm is covered by a cytoplasmic epidermis called a tegument (Figs. 22, 25) and not by a cuticle. The outer surface of the tegument is covered with numerous microvillus-like extensions (microtriches) that vary in length from species to species; each microthrix is tipped with an electron-dense, spine-like structure. The microtriches are covered with a membrane that is continuous with the limiting membrane of the tegument. The cytoplasm of the tegument contains mitochondria, small electron-dense bodies of unknown function, and vesicles, but no lateral cell walls or nuclei. Nucleated tegumental cells lie in the parenchyma beneath the tegument and connect with it by means of cytoplasmic extensions (Fig. 22).

A layer of circular and a layer of longitudinal muscle lie beneath the tegument (Fig. 22), and transverse, diagonal, and dorsoventral muscles traverse the proglottid. The scolex is often very muscular. The nervous system consists of paired cerebral ganglia in the scolex and longitudinal nerves that run along the lateral margins of the worm. Sensory receptors are present on the scolex and on the proglottids. The excretory system consists of flame cells (Fig. 20), collecting vessels, and longitudinal excretory canals (dorsal and ventral) located along the lateral margins of the worm (Figs. 23, 25). Transverse canals link the longitudinal canals in each proglottid (Fig. 23).

All of the organs and tissues of the body are embedded in a cellular parenchyma (Fig. 25); there is no body cavity.

The worms are usually hermaphrodites (Figs. 24, 25), but in many species the male organs ripen before the

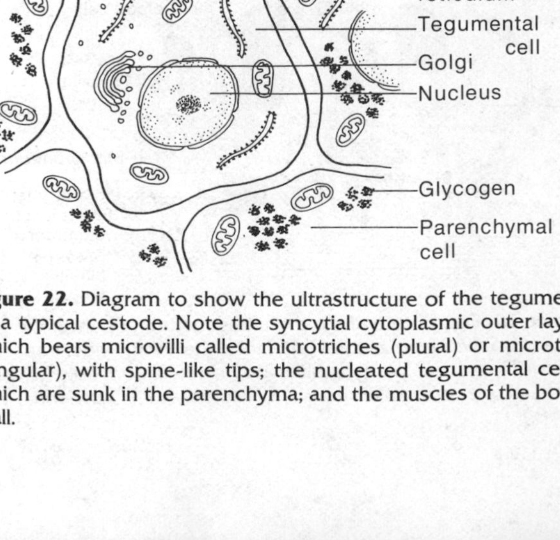

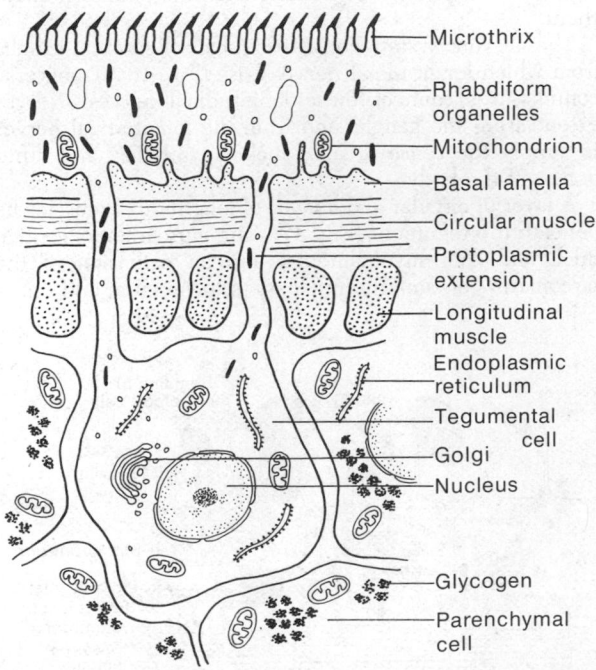

Figure 22. Diagram to show the ultrastructure of the tegument of a typical cestode. Note the syncytial cytoplasmic outer layer which bears microvilli called microtriches (plural) or microtrix (singular), with spine-like tips; the nucleated tegumental cells, which are sunk in the parenchyma; and the muscles of the body wall.

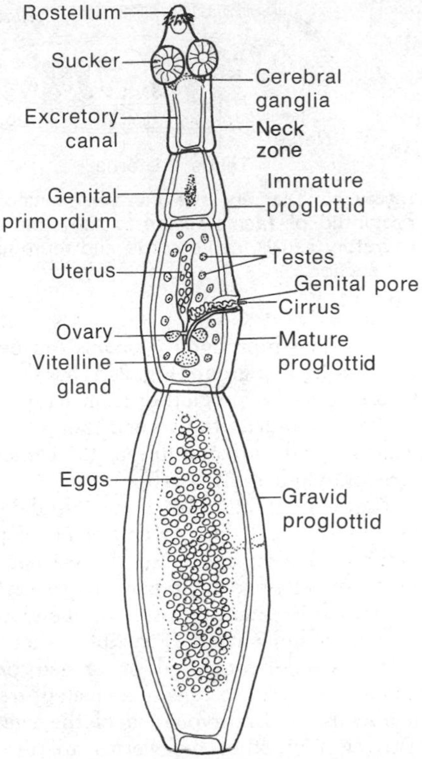

Figure 23. Diagram of adult *Echinococcus* granulosus to show various anatomic features of a cyclophyllidean cestode.

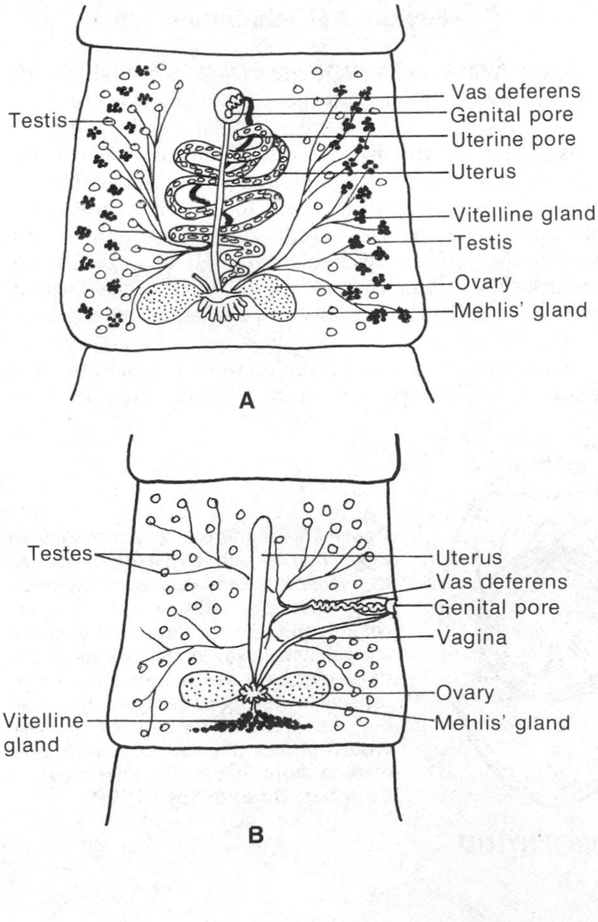

Figure 24. A, Diagram of a mature proglottid of *Dibothriocephalus latus* to show the reproductive system. Note the scattered nature of the vitelline glands. Excretory canals and nerves omitted from the diagram. B, Diagram of a mature proglottid of *Taenia saginata* to show the reproductive system. Note the compact vitelline gland. Excretory canals and nerves omitted from the diagram.

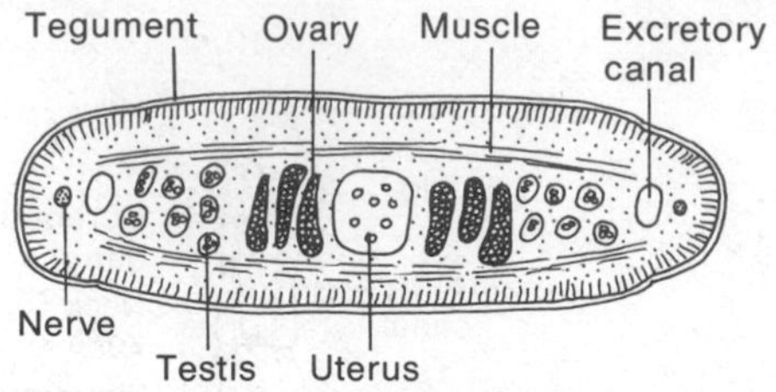

Figure 25. Diagram of a transverse section through a mature proglottid of *Taenia solium* to show the arrangement of the excretory canals, nerve cords, and reproductive organs within the section.

female. The reproductive organs can be divided into two groups: the first group (Fig. 24A) has the vitellaria scattered throughout the proglottid or in laterally situated masses (Pseudophyllidea); the second group has compact vitelline glands usually situated toward the center of the proglottid (Cyclophyllidea) (Fig. 24B).

The egg of cestodes varies in different groups, but essentially it has four layers, or envelopes, enclosing the embryo. These layers are the capsule, outer envelope, inner envelope (which may be subdivided to form the embryophore), and oncospheral membrane (Fig. 26). The pseudophyllidean egg (Fig. 26) has an operculum, and a thick capsule composed of tanned protein. It usually hatches in water to release a ciliated, free-swimming larva (coracidium). Embryonation of the egg occurs in water. The eggs of other tapeworms are usually embryonated when laid and do not have a free-living aquatic stage in the life cycle. They fall into three types: type 1 has a thin capsule and a thin embryophore (*Hymenolepis*); type 2 has an outer tanned protein capsule and a thick, striated embryophore (Fig. 26) (*Taenia, Echinococcus*); and type 3 has a shell formed by the egg and not by the vitellaria (*Stilesia*).

In the Pseudophyllidea, of which *Dibothriocephalus latus* is the most important species to man, the egg hatches in water to release a ciliated larva (coracidium). This coracidium contains an oncosphere or hexacanth embryo (Fig. 26) that carries three pairs of hooks. The cilia are shed when the coracidium is eaten by a copepod and the oncosphere migrates to the body cavity, where it develops into a procercoid larva. This larval stage is a small worm-like creature that possesses a tail-like appendage containing the oncospheral hooks. When the infected copepod is eaten by a suitable fish, the larva migrates to the muscles of the fish and develops into a plerocercoid larva. The plerocercoid of *Dibothriocephalus latus* is an undifferentiated worm with a poorly developed scolex at the anterior end. When ingested by the final host, this larva differentiates into the adult worm.

In the order Cyclophyllidea, which includes most of the tapeworms parasitic in man, there are three types of larvae. The oncosphere (Fig. 26) hatches from the egg and is a six-hooked embryo that penetrates the tissues of the intermediate host. The oncosphere then develops into a cysticercoid larva or into a cysticercus, depending upon the species. The cysticercoid larva develops as a small cyst or bladder in which the scolex of the future adult is retracted (Fig. 27A) as in *Hymenolepis nana*. The cysticercus (often called the bladderworm) consists of a rounded, fluid-filled cyst or bladder within which the scolex of the future adult is invaginated (Fig. 27B) as in *Taenia solium*. A coenurus larva is a large cysticercus in which several inverted scoleces (protoscoleces) develop from the inner (germinal) layer of the bladder wall (Fig. 27C) as in *Multiceps*. A hydatid cyst is a form of coenurus and is a large bladder that buds off numerous daughter cysts (brood capsules) from the germinal layer of the bladder wall. Each of these brood capsules contains several inverted scoleces (protoscoleces) (Figs. 27, 28).

For further reading on the structure and anatomy of cestodes see Wardle and McLeod, 1952; Wardle et al., 1974; Smyth, 1969; Voge, 1969; Hyman, 1951a; Grassé, 1961; Yamaguti, 1959; Noble and Noble, 1982.

Phylum Aschelminthes

CLASS NEMATODA (ROUNDWORMS). Nematodes are found in most habitats and there are many species. They are important parasites of man, animals, and plants, but many species are free living. This classification will concentrate on those groups that are important in human disease. Some authorities regard the nematodes as a separate phylum (Maggenti, 1976), whereas others regard them as a class in the phylum Aschelminthes (Hyman, 1951b; De Coninck, 1965; Anderson et al., 1974). The classification given here is incomplete as particular attention has been given to parasites that attack man.

Nematodes are slender, cylindric worms, usually tapered at both ends (Fig. 29), that range in length from less than

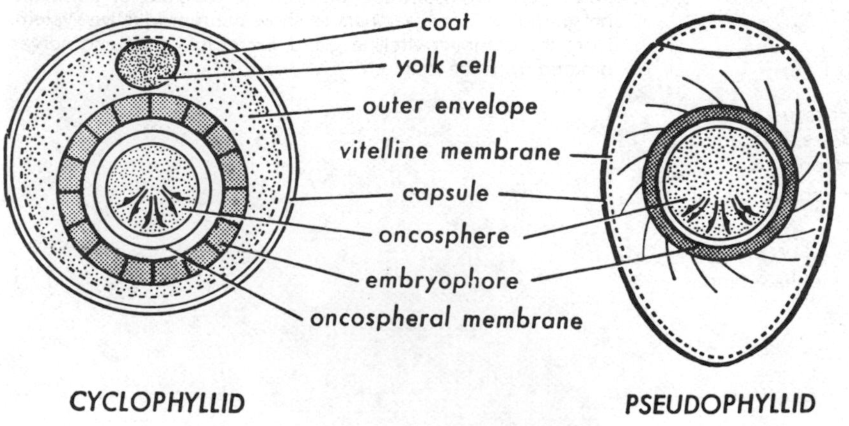

Figure 26. Diagrams of a cyclophyllidean egg *(Taenia)* and a pseudophyllidean egg *(Dibothriocephalus)*. Note the thick, toughened egg capsule with its operculum, and the ciliated embryophore (coracidium larva) in the pseudophyllidean egg, and the lack of a thick egg capsule in the egg of the cyclophyllidean but the presence of a thick, striated embryophore. (Reproduced, with permission, from Smyth: The Physiology of Cestodes, Oliver & Boyd 1969.)

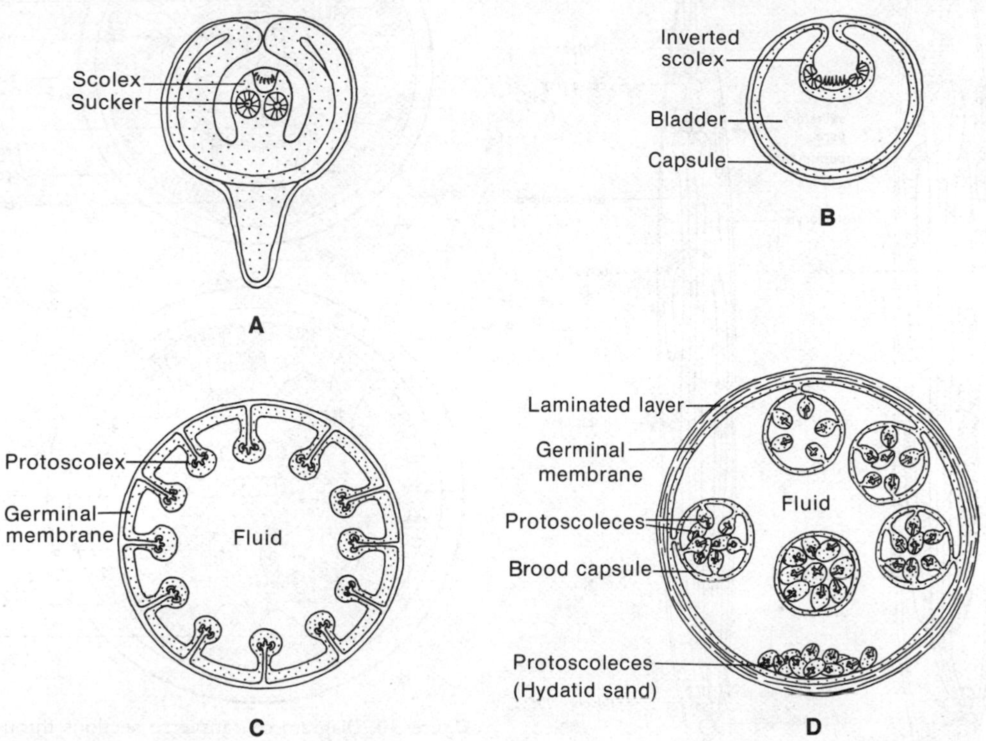

Figure 27. Diagrams of A, cysticercoid larva; B, cysticercus larva; C, coenurus larva; and D, hydatid cyst.

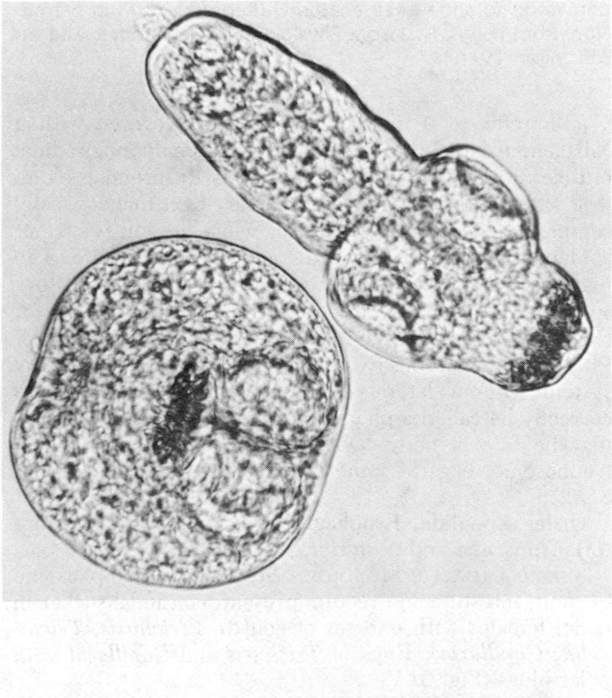

Figure 28. Photomicrograph of protoscoleces of *Echinococcus* granulosus, one is evaginated and the other invaginated.

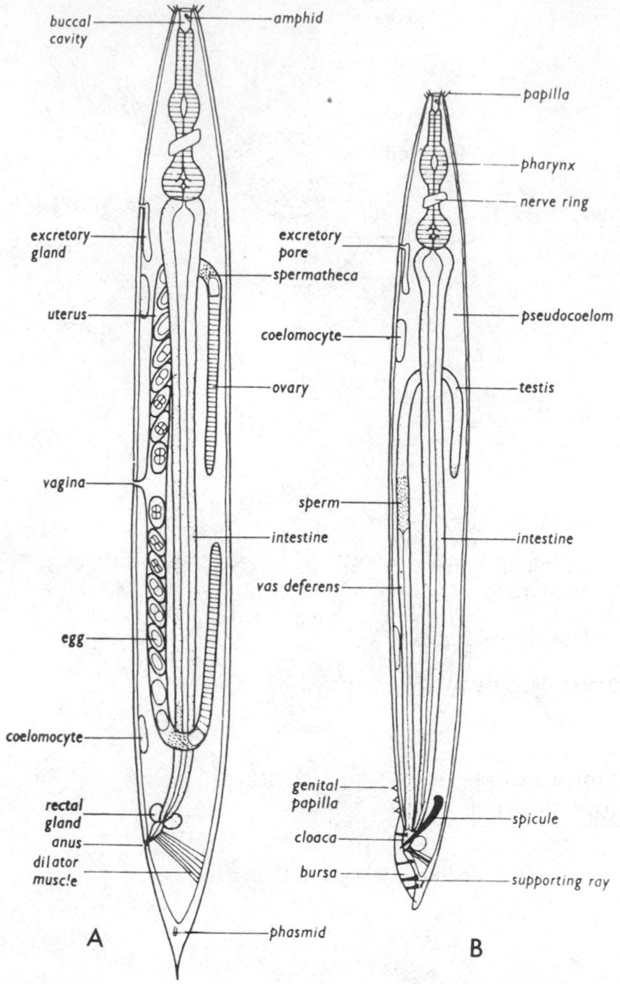

Figure 29. Diagram of a generalized female (A) and male (B) nematode to show their anatomy. (Reproduced, with permission, from Lee & Atkinson: Physiology of Nematodes, 2nd ed. Macmillan 1976.)

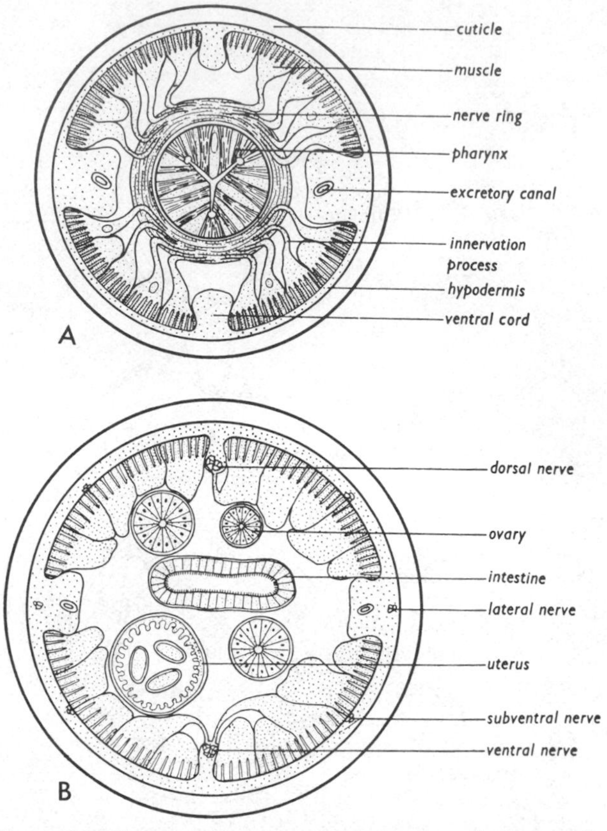

Figure 30. Diagram of transverse sections through the esophageal (A) (should more correctly be called pharynx) and middle (B) regions of a female nematode to show the arrangement of the tissues and organs. (Reproduced with permission from Lee & Atkinson: Physiology of Nematodes, 2nd ed. Macmillan 1976.)

a millimeter to 9 meters. The body is covered with a collagenous cuticle, is unsegmented, has only longitudinal muscles in the body wall, has a body cavity (pseudocoelom) (Fig. 30), and has a straight alimentary tract that is usually complete. The excretory system, when present, does not contain flame cells. The sexes are usually separate. The male has a cloaca that usually contains one or two copulatory spicules.

SUBCLASS ADENOPHOREA (= APHASMIDIA). Phasmids (caudal sensory organs) (Fig. 29) absent; excretory system without lateral canals; esophagus (should more correctly be called a pharynx) cylindric, esophageal glands may be free in body cavity and form a stichosome or a trophosome; eggs of some species have polar plugs (Fig. 31A).

Order Enoplida. Esophagus cylindric, usually with anterior muscular and posterior glandular parts.

SUPERFAMILY TRICHUROIDEA. Stichosome or trophosome present; intestine and rectum present; no caudal sucker in male; females with one set of gonads. *(Trichuris, Trichinella, Capillaria).* Eggs of *Trichuris* and *Capillaria* with polar plugs (Fig. 31A).

SUBCLASS SERCENENTEA (= PHASMIDIA). Phasmids present (Fig. 29); excretory system usually with paired lateral canals (Fig. 33); stichosome or trophosome absent; eggs without polar plug.

Order Rhabditida. Parasitic generation (females only) alternating with free-living generations (males and females); parasitic in lungs of amphibia or small intestine of vertebrates. *(Strongyloides stercoralis.)*

Order Tylenchida. Stylet present in buccal cavity. Feed on plants or fungi; some species parasitic in body cavity of insects.

Order Strongylida. Male has copulatory bursa with

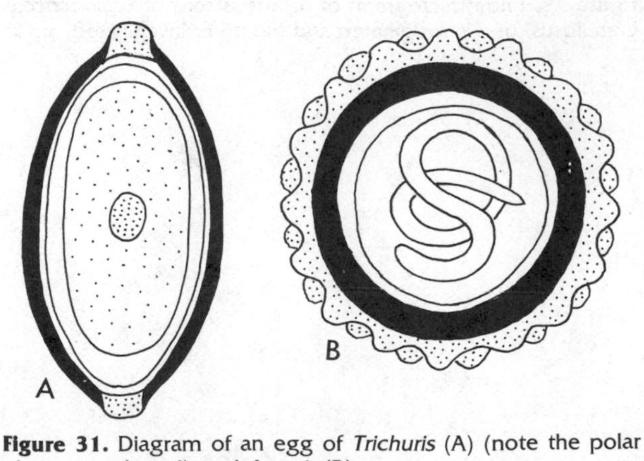

Figure 31. Diagram of an egg of *Trichuris* (A) (note the polar plugs at each end), and *Ascaris* (B).

supporting rays (Fig. 32); usually two spicules; ovejector of female with well-developed sphincter muscles. Mouth and buccal cavity variable in size and shape. Excretory system H-shaped and with two large glands (Fig. 33 , B). Parasitic in vertebrates.

SUPERFAMILY ANCYLOSTOMATOIDEA. Buccal capsule large, strongly cuticularized; lips absent; mouth with teeth and cutting plates (Fig. 34) or unarmed. Parasitic in intestine of mammals. *(Necator americanus, Ancylostoma duodenale.)*

SUPERFAMILY STRONGYLOIDEA. Buccal cavity variable, sometimes surrounded by ring of projections (corona radiata); no teeth or cutting plates. Parasites of intestine, respiratory tract, or urinary tract of mammals and birds. *(Strongylus, Oesophagostomum.)*

SUPERFAMILY TRICHOSTRONGYLOIDEA. Buccal cavity small (Fig. 35), cuticle around head often inflated; longitudinal cuticular ridges often present. Parasites of alimentary tract or respiratory tract of mammals. *(Trichostrongylus colubriformis.)*

SUPERFAMILY METASTRONGYLOIDEA. Buccal cavity small; copulatory bursa often reduced; vulva near anus; longitudinal cuticular ridges absent. Mainly parasites of respiratory tract of mammals. Intermediate host usually a gastropod, oligochaete, crustacean, or occasionally a vertebrate. *(Metastrongylus* spp., *Angiostrongylus cantonensis.)*

Order Oxyurida. Male without copulatory bursa, one or two spicules; excretory system H-shaped (Fig. 33D); esophageal bulb present; body usually short and stout. Parasitic in lower intestine, colon, or rectum of vertebrates or hindgut of insects. *(Enterobius vermicularis.)*

Order Ascaridida. Usually three or six lips; esophagus variable in form but not divided into short muscular and long glandular parts; excretory system a modified "H" system (Fig. 33E). Usually parasitic in intestine of vertebrates.

SUPERFAMILY ASCARIDOIDEA. Mouth surrounded by three lips (Fig. 36); buccal cavity and esophagus simple.

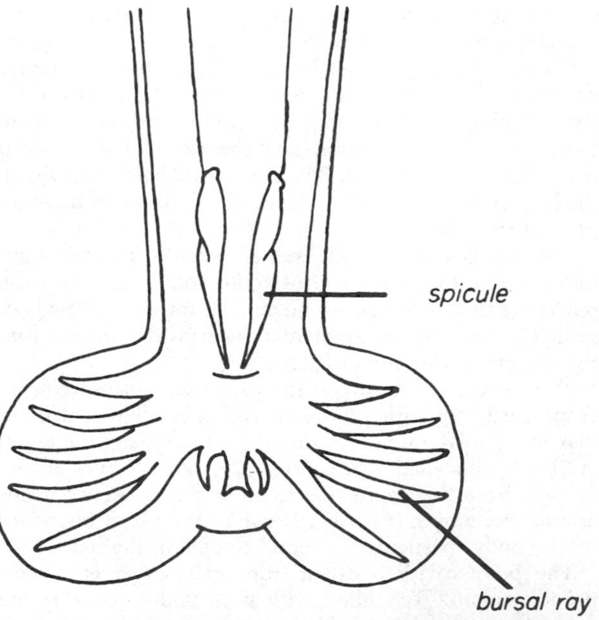

Figure 32. Diagram of tail of a male trichostrongyle to show the copulatory bursa and spicules. (Reproduced with permission from Lee & Atkinson: Physiology of Nematodes, 2nd ed. Macmillan 1976.)

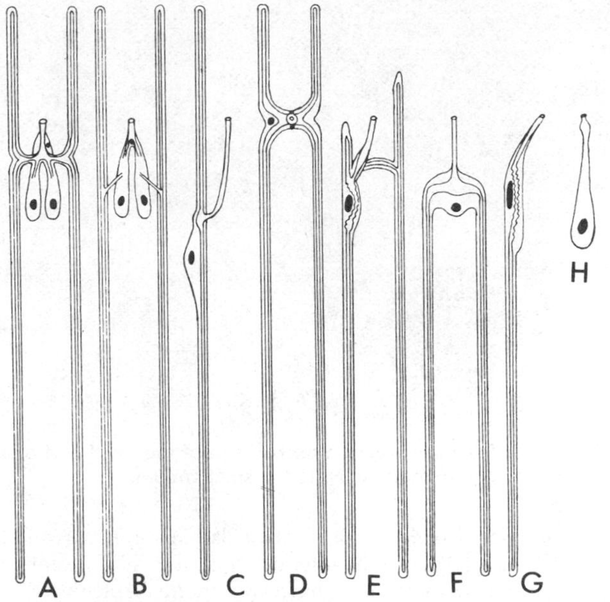

Figure 33. Representative types of excretory system found in nematodes. A, Rhabditoid-type, an H-shaped system with two subventral glands, the lateral canals are embedded in the lateral cords (see Fig. 30); found in the Strongylida. B is a variant of A found in *Oesophagastomum.* C, Tylenchoid type. D, Oxyuroid type, an H-shaped system lacking subventral gland cells. E, Ascaroid type. F, Cephaloboid type. G, Anisakid type, a reduced form of E. H, Single ventral cell type present in Chromadorina, Manhysterina, and Enoploidea. (Reproduced with permission from Lee & Atkinson: Physiology of Nematodes, 2nd ed. Macmillan 1976. Based on originals by Chitwood and Chitwood, 1950.)

Tail of male usually curved or coiled. *(Ascaris lumbricoides, Toxocara canis.)*

SUPERFAMILY HETEROCHEILOIDEA (= ANISAKOIDEA). Esophageal ventriculus (glandular modification of esophagus, which extends posteriorly beside the intestine) present; intestinal cecum often present. Parasitic in stomach of mammals *(Anisakis).*

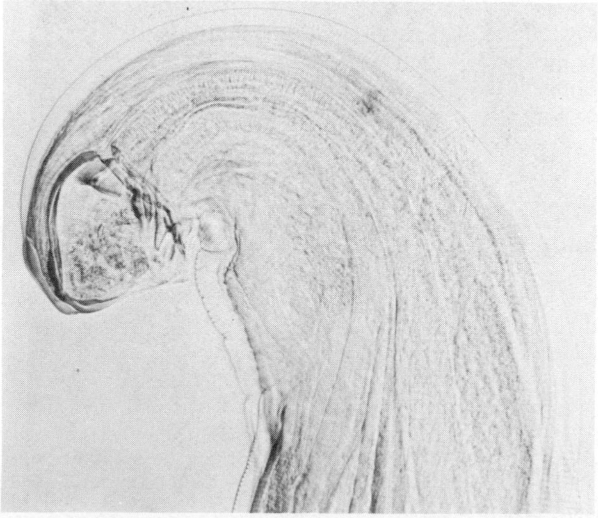

Figure 34. Photomicrograph of the head end of *Ancylostoma duodenale.* Note the cutting plates at the opening of the mouth and the teeth at the base of the buccal cavity.

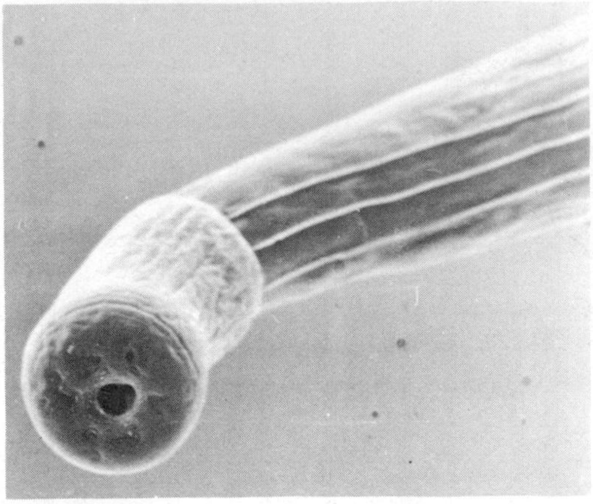

Figure 35. Scanning electron micrograph of the head end of a trichostrongyle nematode. Note the small mouth.

Order Spirurida. Usually two lateral lips surround mouth; esophagus with anterior muscular and posterior glandular part; most males have two unequal spicules.

Suborder Camallanina. Larvae without cephalic hooks; esophageal glands usually uninucleate.

SUPERFAMILY CAMALLINOIDEA. Buccal cavity well developed. Parasites of gut.

SUPERFAMILY DRACUNCULOIDEA. Buccal cavity weakly developed; six conspicuous labial papillae present. Usually parasitic in tissues of host. *(Dracunculus medinensis.)*

Suborder Spirurina. Larvae with cephalic hooks; esophageal glands multinucleate.

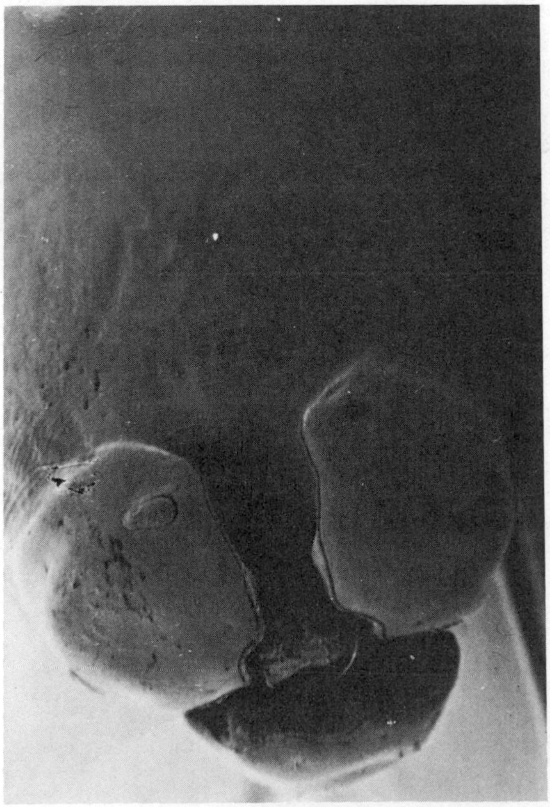

Figure 36. Scanning electron micrograph of the head end of *Ascaris.* Note the three lips.

SUPERFAMILY GNATHOSTOMATOIDEA. Cuticular outgrowths (pseudolabia) overlie and replace lips; cuticle on inner face folded to form projections that interdigitate with projections on adjacent pseudolabium. Head sometimes bulbous. Parasites of gut and tissues. *(Gnathostoma spinigerum.)*

SUPERFAMILY THELAZIOIDEA. Buccal cavity variable, sometimes long and thin; mouth usually without definite lips. Parasites of eye cavity of mammals and birds, lungs of mammals, or intestine of fishes. *(Thelazia.)*

SUPERFAMILY SPIRUROIDEA. Buccal cavity never long and cylindric, but well cuticularized; two lateral lips surround mouth. Vulva near middle of body; males usually have two unequal spicules. Parasites of alimentary tract, respiratory tract, eye cavity, nasal cavity, or sinuses of vertebrates. *(Gongylonema pulchrum.)*

SUPERFAMILY FILARIOIDEA. Lips absent; ovoviviparous; first larva a microfilaria. Parasites of tissues and tissue spaces of vertebrates; transmitted by arthropod vectors. *(Wuchereria bancrofti, Onchocerca volvulus, Loa loa.)*

For further information on the classification of nematodes see Hyman, 1951b; de Coninck, 1965; Chitwood, 1969; Maggenti, 1976; Anderson, Chabaud, and Willmott, 1974; Yamaguti, 1961; Noble and Noble, 1982.

Anatomy of Nematoda

The typical nematode is a spindle-shaped, unsegmented, and bilaterally symmetric worm (Fig. 29) that is round in cross-section (Fig. 30). The internal organs of the male and of the female are shown in Figures 29 and 30.

The body wall has an outer collagenous cuticle, a cellular or syncytial hypodermis, and a layer of longitudinal muscle (Fig. 30). The cuticle lines the buccal cavity, esophagus (more correctly called the pharynx), excretory pore, rectum, cloaca, and vulva. Teeth, cutting plates, stylets, and spicules are formed from toughened and hardened cuticle. The cuticle is basically three layered, but further subdivisions often occur. The outer surface of the cuticle is superficially annulated and may also be formed into finlike structures (alae) or ridges that run along the length of the body. The hypodermis lies between the cuticle and the longitudinal muscles of the body wall. It is normally a thin layer of cytoplasm but it projects into the body cavity along the middorsal, midventral, and the lateral lines to form four ridges or cords (Fig. 30). The lateral cords are usually the largest and contain the excretory canals when these are present (Fig. 30).

The muscles of the body wall are spindle shaped, longitudinal cells that have a contractile and a noncontractile portion (Fig. 37). There are no circular muscles in the body wall. The muscles are innervated by arms that extend from the muscle to the nerves (Fig. 30).

The nervous system consists of a ganglionated circumesophageal ring with a large ventral, a smaller dorsal, and two or more lateral nerves running from it along the length of the hypodermal cords (Figs. 29, 30). Nerves extend forward from the nerve ring to innervate the sense organs around the mouth (Fig. 38). Sense organs occur elsewhere on the body, particularly around the tail of the male.

The body cavity is not a true coelom and is called a pseudocoelom. It is filled with fluid under pressure and forms the hydrostatic skeleton of the nematode.

The alimentary system is usually complete. There is a mouth surrounded by lips (Fig. 38) (these may be reduced

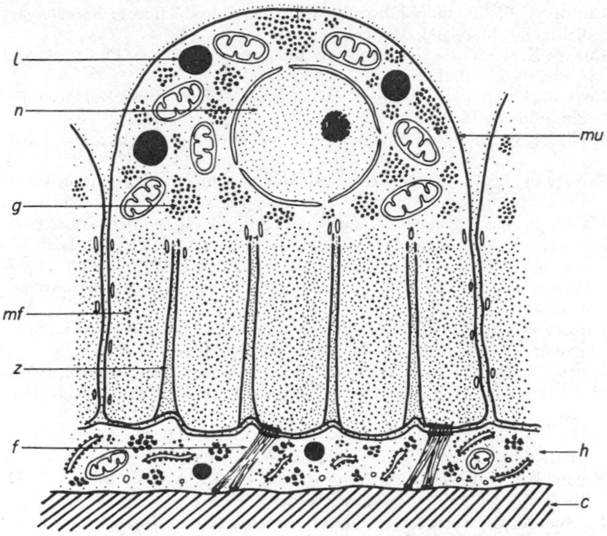

Figure 37. Diagram of a section through a longitudinal muscle of the body wall of a nematode to show the internal structure of the muscle and the association with the hypodermis and the cuticle. c, cuticle; f, fibres connecting muscle to cuticle; g, glycogen; h, hypodermis; l, lipid; mf, myofilaments; mu, muscle; n, nucleus; z, z-band region of muscle. (Reproduced with permission from Lee & Atkinson: Physiology of Nematodes. 2nd ed. Macmillan 1976.)

in number from the normal six, or may be absent), a buccal cavity of varying shape and size, a muscular and glandular esophagus (pharynx), which usually has a triradiate lumen, a straight intestine, a rectum (cloaca in the male), and anus (Figs. 29, 30). The intestine consists of a single layer of epithelial cells that carry microvilli on the lumen side (Fig. 30B).

The excretory system varies in structure from group to group and is absent in some species. There are two basic types—a glandular system and a tubular system (Fig. 33). The glandular system is found in many free-living nematodes and consists of a ventral gland cell situated in the body cavity near the base of the esophagus. It usually has a terminal ampulla that opens to the exterior on the ventral surface. The tubular system varies in structure but is basically an H-shaped system with a lateral canal in each lateral cord. It is united by a transverse canal in the anterior end of the nematode (Fig. 33 D, E). This opens

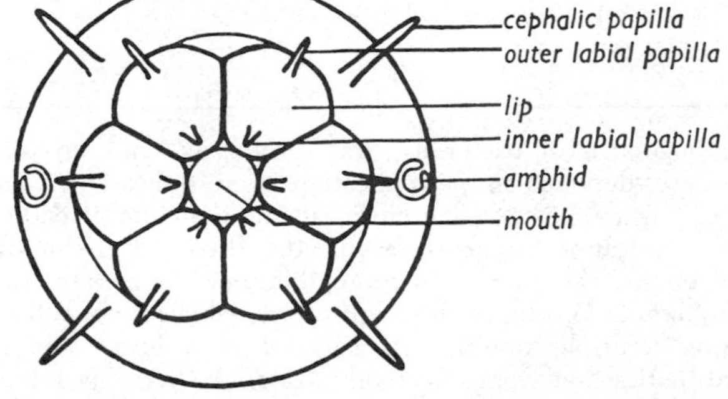

Figure 38. En face view of a nematode head showing the position of the mouth, lips, amphids, labial sensillae, and cephalic sensilla (usually called papilla). (Redrawn from Jones: Plant Nematology. H.M.S.O. 1959.)

to the exterior through a common excretory duct and pore on the ventral surface. The Strongylida also contain a pair of glands in the pseudocoelom and these open into the transverse excretory canal just behind the excretory pore (Fig. 33A, B); although these are called excretory glands they appear to have a secretory rather than an excretory function. The excretory system contains no flagella or cilia.

The sexes are usually separate, and males are frequently smaller than females. The males have one or two testes, each opening into a seminal vesicle and then into a common vas deferens. The vas deferens opens into a cloaca (Fig. 29). Many males possess one or two copulatory spicules that lie in pouches connected to the cloaca (Fig. 32). In some groups of nematodes (Strongylida) the area around the cloaca is expanded to form a copulatory bursa (Fig. 32). Females have one or two ovaries that open into an oviduct(s) and a uterus or uteri (Fig. 29). The uterus often ends in a ovejector that is usually very muscular and opens to the exterior via the vagina and vulva. The eggs of nematodes are essentially ovoid and have three main layers (Fig. 31), the middle layer containing a chitin-protein complex. The sperm of nematodes are ameboid.

Nematodes have no circulatory or respiratory organs and lack true flagella.

The larval stages are really juveniles, since they are similar in structure to the adults but without sex organs. All nematodes moult four times, and any structural changes that occur during the life cycle, such as modifications to the buccal cavity or to the cuticle, occur during the moult.

For further reading on the structure and anatomy of nematodes see Bird, 1971; Chitwood and Chitwood, 1950; Hyman, 1951b; Croll, 1976; and Lee and Atkinson, 1976.

Phylum Acanthocephala

These worm-like parasites live as adults in the intestine of vertebrates and as larvae in arthropods. They are distinguished by their spined anterior proboscis, which may be retracted into the main body of the worm. A digestive system is completely absent and there are no circulatory or respiratory structures. The sexes are separate; the males possess a posterior bell-like bursa.

Order Archiacanthocephala. Proboscis spines are concentric; contain protonephridia, eight cement glands in male. Parasitic in terrestrial hosts *(Moniliformis, Macracanthorhynchus)*.

Order Palaeacanthocephala. Proboscis spine in alternate radial rows; no protonephridia; usually six cement glands in males. Parasitic mainly in aquatic hosts.

Order Eoacanthocephala. Proboscis spines arranged radially; no protonephridia; cement gland syncytial. Parasitic in aquatic hosts.

Anatomy of Acanthocephala

Adult acanthocephala are unsegmented worms in which the sexes are separate (Fig. 39 A, B). Most species are 1 to 2 cm long, but a few, notably *Macracanthorhynchus hirudinaceus* from pigs, are longer and can reach 45 cm. The body is divided into an anterior praesoma that contains the retractable spiny proboscis together with its associated structures, and a larger posterior portion called the metasoma that includes the other organs and tissues of the body. The body wall consists of about five layers. There is

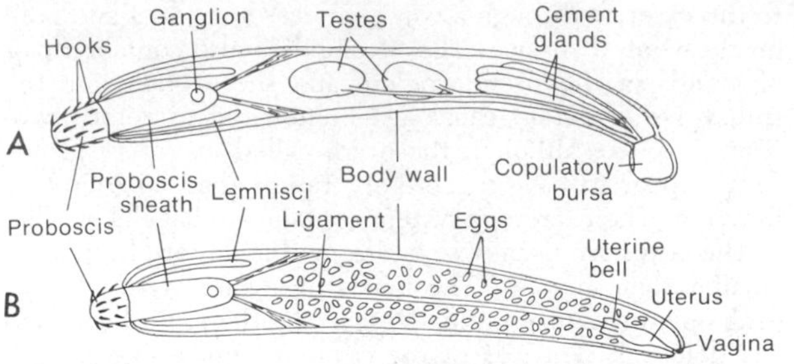

Figure 39. Diagram of a male (A) and female (B) acanthocephalan to show their internal anatomy. Note the spiny proboscis and the lack of an alimentary system.

a thin outer epicuticle, a tough cuticle penetrated by numerous pores that lead into canals of the striped layer. This striped layer merges into the fibrous felt layer. The innermost layer of the body wall is the thickest layer and is called the radial layer. It contains nuclei, mitochondria, ribosomes, and other cellular constituents, but has no lateral cell walls. The radial layer is separated from the circular and longitudinal muscles of the body wall by a basement lamella. There is a body cavity but it is not a true coelom. There is no alimentary tract in this group of worms. Food is taken up across the body wall. There are no circulatory or respiratory structures; nephridia are present in some groups but not in others. A nerve ganglion associated with the proboscis sheath sends nerves to various regions of the body. The male reproduction system consists of a copulatory bursa, a number of cement glands (usually six to eight), a pair of testes, and a sperm duct that leads to the genital pore. The female system has no persistent ovary; ova develop on a ligament in the body cavity and are set free in the body cavity, where they are fertilized. The eggs are sorted in a uterine bell and pass through a uterus to the genital pore.

For further reading on the Acanthocephala see Hyman, 1951b; Crompton, 1970; and Noble and Noble, 1982.

References

Adam, K. M. G., Paul, J., and Zaman, V.: Medical and Veterinary Protozoology, 2nd ed. Edinburgh, Churchill Livingstone, 1979.

Anderson, R. C., Chabaud, A. G., and Willmott, S: CIH keys to the nematode parasites of vertebrates. No. 1. Commonwealth Agricultural Bureaux, Farnham Royal, Slough, U. K. 1974.

Baker, J. R.: The Biology of Parasitic Protozoa. London, Edward Arnold, 1982.

Bird, A. F.: The Structure of Nematodes. New York, Academic Press, 1971.

Chitwood, B. G., and Chitwood, M. B.: An Introduction to Nematology. Baltimore, Maryland, Monumental Printing Co., 1950.

Cox, F. E. G.: A new classification of the parasitic protozoa. Protozoological Abstracts 5:9, 1981.

Cox, F. E. G. (ed.): Modern Parasitology. Oxford, Blackwell Scientific Publications, 1982.

Croll, N. A.: The Organization of Nematodes. New York, Academic Press, 1976.

Crompton, D. W. T.: An Ecological Approach to Acanthocephalan Physiology. Cambridge, Cambridge University Press, 1970.

Dawes, B.: The Trematoda. Cambridge, Cambridge University Press, 1956.

de Coninck, L.: Classe des nématodes. In Grassé, P-P (ed.): Traité de Zoologie. IV Némathelminthes (Nématodes). Paris, Masson et Cie, 1965.

Erasmus, D. A.: The Biology of Trematodes. London, Edward Arnold, 1972.

Grassé, P-P. (ed.): Platyhelminthes, Mesozoaires, Acanthocephales, Nemertiens. Traité de Zoologie IV. Paris, Masson, 1961.

Hyman, L. H.: The Invertebrates. Vol. II. New York, McGraw-Hill, 1951a.

Hyman, L. H.: The Invertebrates. Vol. III. New York, McGraw-Hill, 1951b.

Joyeux, C., and Baer, J. G.: Classe des Cestodaires. In Grassé, P-P. (ed.): Traité de Zoologie, IV. Paris, Masson et Cie, 1961.

Kreier, J. P. (ed.): Parasitic Protozoa, Vol. I, 1977; Vol. II, 1978; Vol. III, 1977; Vol. IV, 1977. New York, Academic Press.

La Rue, G. A.: The classification of digenetic trematodes: a review and a new system. Exp Parasitol 6:306, 1957.

Lee, D. L., and Atkinson, H. J.: Physiology of Nematodes. London, Macmillan Press, 1976.

Levine, N. D.: Protozoan Parasites of Domestic Animals and of Man. Minneapolis, Burgess Publishing Co., 19 .

Levine, N. D., Corliss, J. O., Cox, F. E. G., Deroux, G, Grain, J., Honigberg, B. M., Leedale, G. F., Loeblich, A. R., Lom, J., Lynn, D., Meringeld, E. G., Page, F. C., Pojansky, G., Sprague, V., Varra, J. and Wallace, F. G.: A newly revised classification of the protozoa. J Protozool 27:37, 1980.

Llewellyn, J.: The evolution of parasitic platyhelminths. Symposia of the British Society for Parasitology 3:47, 1965.

Maggenti, A. R.: Taxonomic position of Nematoda among the Pseudocoelomate Bilateria. In Croll, N. A. (ed.): The Organization of Nematodes. New York, Academic Press, 1976.

Noble, E. R., and Noble, G. A.: Parasitology. The Biology of Animal Parasites. Philadelphia, Lea and Febiger, 1982.

Sleigh, M.: The Biology of Protozoa. London, Edward Arnold, 1973.

Smyth, J. D.: The Physiology of Cestodes. Edinburgh, Oliver & Boyd, 1969.

Smyth, J. D. and Halton, D. W.: The Physiology of Trematodes. Cambridge, Cambridge University Press, 1983.

Vickerman, K., and Cox, F. E. G.: The Protozoa. London, John Murray, 1967.

Voge, M.: Systematics of cestodes—present and future. In Schmidt, G. D. (ed.): Problems in Systematics of Parasites. Baltimore, University Park Press, 1969.

Wardle, R. A., and McLeod, J. A.: The Zoology of Tapeworms. Minneapolis, University of Minnesota Press, 1952.

Wardle, R. A., McLeod, J. A., and Radinovsky, S.: Advances in the Zoology of Tapeworms 1950–1970. Minneapolis, University of Minnesota Press, 1974.

Yamaguti, S.: Systema Helminthum. I. The Digenetic Trematodes of Vertebrates. New York, Interscience Publishers Inc., 1958.

Yamaguti, S.: Systema Helminthum II. Cestodes of Vertebrates. New York, Interscience Publishers Inc., 1959.

Yamaguti, S.: Systema Helminthum III. The Nematodes of Vertebrates. New York, Interscience Publishers Inc., 1961.

17

BIOCHEMISTRY OF PARASITES: HELMINTHS

HOWARD J. SAZ, PH.D.

In order to understand the mode of action of anthelmintic agents, it must be realized that the metazoan parasites differ from other disease-causing organisms in several important pharmacologic as well as biochemical respects. Pathogenesis of bacterial, viral, protozoan, and mycotic diseases depends on the replication or multiplication of the invading pathogens. Therefore, agents that inhibit pathogen replication will arrest or cure the disease. In helminth infections, the picture is quite different. Generally, the problem is to remove the adult worm, which is not reliant upon multiplication for its survival in a host. Hence, antibiotics that work effectively against bacteria by inhibiting macromolecular synthesis have little or no value in the chemotherapy of helminth infections.

What are the vulnerable sites for drug action in helminths? Anthelmintics are inhibitory primarily at one of two sites. Many, but not all, anthelmintics inhibit either muscle contraction or energy-generating processes within the parasites. The effect on energy generation may be direct or indirect. For example, some anthelmintics inhibit cellular transport, decreasing the availability of substrates within the cell, thereby lowering ATP levels. Table 1 lists some anthelmintic compounds and their reported sites of inhibition. Although the inhibitions noted may account for the chemotherapeutic effect of each of these compounds, it is not established that these inhibitions represent their primary modes of chemotherapeutic action. At any rate, the importance of studying the biochemistry of the metazoan parasites now becomes more obvious. A better understanding of parasite biochemistry would help to explain how anthelmintics act. It would also aid in pointing out possible sites of inhibition that are unique to the parasite metabolism and therefore suggest the design of drugs that are more toxic for the parasite than for the host. In the remainder of this chapter we will discuss the biochemistry of the metazoan parasites with emphasis on their energy metabolisms, since this area is susceptible to drug action.

Before 1950, most biochemists were concerned primarily with elucidating the concept of unity in biochemistry. They were struck by the biochemical similarities of all living tissues. However, small groups of scientists, particularly the pharmacologists and the immunologists, began to stress the fact that tissues even from related species were biochemically distinct in some respects. These considerations gave rise to studies of comparative biochemistry. It is now readily accepted that differences exist both at the subtle level of protein or enzyme structure and kinetics and at the more obvious metabolic level.

Krebs and Najjar (1948) were the first to report that enzymes carrying out the same reaction in different animal species could be antigenically different. Antisera to purified yeast glyceraldehyde-3-phosphate dehydrogenase inhibited the yeast enzyme, but not the corresponding enzyme isolated from rabbit muscle. Similarly, certain enzymes of *Schistosoma mansoni* were immunologically distinct from the corresponding enzymes of rabbit muscle. Thus, the protein structures of the host and parasite enzymes are different.

Such structural differences between corresponding host and parasite enzymes may account for the specificity of some anthelmintics. For example, the trivalent organic antimonials, such as stibophen and potassium antimony tartrate, have been used to treat both schistosomiasis and filariasis. As with numerous other anthelmintics, the antimonials destroy the parasites by inhibiting energy metabolism, in this case by inhibiting glycolysis. Specifically, in schistosomes, filariids, *Ascaris*, and the rat tapeworm *Hymenolepis diminuta*, the antimonials are potent inhibitors of the glycolytic enzyme phosphofructokinase. Most important, and presumably because of differing protein structures, the mammalian phosphofructokinase is not affected by therapeutic concentrations of antimonials. Only slight inhibition of the mammalian enzyme occurs even at levels of drug 80- to 100-fold higher than those that inhibit the parasite enzyme almost completely (Mansour and Bueding, 1953; Saz and Dunbar, 1975).

Striking differences also exist between the metabolic pathways of the parasites and their hosts. This first became obvious at the level of overall metabolism. Although all helminths examined can consume oxygen, none can catalyze the complete oxidation of substrates to carbon dioxide and water. All helminths examined accumulate end products of metabolism other than, or in addition to, carbon dioxide and water. The same is true of the parasitic protozoans. Thus, in contrast to their mammalian hosts, terminal aerobic respiration in parasites is either absent or rate limiting. Similarly, it appears that many helminths surprisingly have lost their ability to synthesize long chain fatty acids de novo and must rely on their host to supply these important nutritional components (Meyer et al., 1966). Such an abbreviated lipid metabolism occurs in the cestodes *Spirometra mansonoides* and *Hymenolepis diminuta;* the nematode *Ascaris lumbricoides;* and the trematode *Schistosoma mansoni.*

Although the oxidative capacity of all helminths is limited, some are obligate aerobes and are destroyed rapidly by anaerobiosis. In contrast, others require no oxygen for energy metabolisms and survive equally well in the presence or absence of oxygen. Relatively few parasites have

Table 1. REACTIONS INHIBITED BY ANTHELMINTIC COMPOUNDS

Anthelmintic Agent	Site of Inhibition
Trivalent antimonials	Phosphofructokinase
Niridazole	Phosphorylase phosphatase
p-Rosaniline	Glycogen accumulation
	Acetylcholine esterase
Praziquantel	Ca^{2+} transport
Cyanine dyes (Dithiazanine)	Respiration
	Glucose uptake
Chlorsalicylamide (Yomesan)	Electron transport phosphorylation
Dichlorophen	
Desaspidin	
2,4-Dihexanoyl-6-methyl phloroglucinol	
Closantel	
Tetramisole	Neurotransmission
	Fumarate reductase
Thiabendazole	Fumarate reductase
Cambendazole	Tubulin assembly
Mebendazole	Glucose and amino acid uptake
Dibenzylamines	Glucose transport

been cultured through their life cycles in vitro, making it difficult to assess their oxygen requirements for growth. Investigators have determined oxygen requirements mainly from survival time in air of a given stage of the parasite. Among worms that have been completely or partially cultured, a gradation of oxygen requirements exists ranging from highly aerobic to anaerobic. It has been suggested that oxygen may even inhibit the normal development of some parasites. In all helminths and in all stages of their development, however, oxygen can be consumed even though it may be deleterious to survival. In many instances, when the energy metabolism appears to be anaerobic, neither the physiologic significance nor the mechanism of this oxygen consumption is understood. It must be borne in mind that we are dealing with complex developmental stages in the life cycles of the helminths. In a given parasite, some of these stages may be aerobic while others are not. Shifts or changes in the metabolism of the parasites occur upon development from one stage to another. Almost nothing is known of the mechanisms by which these "switches" in metabolism occur. Examples of this "switching" phenomenon will be discussed below.

In many respects, the helminths resemble the facultative and obligate anaerobic bacteria. A wide range of fermentation products is formed, indicating the utilization of terminal electron acceptors other than oxygen. More simply stated, rather than oxygen being reduced to H_2O, other organic compounds take the place of oxygen and accept electrons, resulting in an accumulation of fermentation products. Some of the helminths are homolactate fermenters, accumulating lactate as the sole fermentation product. This also occurs in rapidly contracting muscle and mammalian red blood cells, and in certain bacteria and numerous other organisms. Most helminths accumulate an array of fermentation products that might include volatile fatty acids, succinate, lactate, and neutral volatile compounds such as ethanol and acetylmethylcarbinol (acetoin). In general, all of these products arise from either pyruvate or succinate, or from both of these acids. Therefore, the carbohydrate metabolisms of most helminths studied might be divided into two categories. The first group would comprise those parasites, such as the schistosomes and filarial worms, that rely entirely on glycolysis and a few adjunct reactions for their energy metabolisms. Products of these fermentations would include lactate or ethanol and possibly acetate and acetylmethylcarbinol (acetoin). The second group of parasites, as exemplified by *Ascaris* and *Hymenolepis diminuta*, rely on a similar series of reactions, but can also fix carbon dioxide into phosphoenolpyruvate, leading to the formation of a C_4 dicarboxylic acid, which in turn could give rise to succinate, propionate, and other volatile fatty acids. A representative sampling of a few parasites and their type of metabolism are listed in Table 2 together with the products formed by each worm. In the remainder of this chapter, examples of the "primarily glycolytic helminths" and the "CO_2-fixing helminths" will be discussed. A limited number of examples of each type of parasite will be examined.

PRIMARILY GLYCOLYTIC HELMINTHS

Schistosomes. The schistosomes constitute one of the most prevalent of the parasitic helminths that infect man. It is not surprising, therefore, that *Schistosoma mansoni* was one of the first helminths whose pathway of carbohydrate metabolism was elucidated (Bueding, 1950). This blood fluke was found to utilize glucose very rapidly. In one hour an amount of glucose equivalent to approximately one fifth of its dry weight was dissimilated by a schistosome. Essentially all of the glucose carbon that disappeared from the medium was recoverable as lactate carbon, indicating

Table 2. GLYCOLYTIC AND CO_2-FIXING HELMINTHS AND PRODUCTS FORMED

Parasite	Fermentation Products
Glycolytic	
Schistosoma mansoni	Lactate
Schistosoma haematobium	Lactate
Schistosoma japonicum	Lactate
Brugia pahangi	Lactate
Dipetalonema viteae	Lactate
Litomosoides carinii	Lactate, acetate, CO_2
Dirofilaria uniformis	Lactate
Dracunculus insignis	Lactate
Angiostrongylus cantonensis	Lactate
CO_2-fixing	
Ascaris lumbricoides	Succinate, volatile fatty acids
Heterakis gallinae	Succinate, propionate
Trichuris vulpis	Succinate, volatile fatty acids
Trichinella spiralis (larvae)	Acetate, propionate, volatile fatty acids
Oesophagostomum radiatum	Acetate, propionate, lactate, 2-methylbutyrate, 3-methylbutyrate, isobutyrate
Hymenolepis diminuta	Succinate, acetate, lactate
Moniezia expansa	Succinate, lactate
Echinococcus granulosus (cysts)	Succinate, lactate, acetate, ethanol
Taenia taeniaformis (adults and larvae)	Succinate, lactate, pyruvate, acetate, ethanol, glycerol
Spirometra mansonoides (spargana and adults)	Propionate, acetate, succinate, lactate
Echinostoma liei	*n*-Valerate, propionate, acetate, *n*-hexanoate
Fasciola hepatica	Acetate, propionate, lactate
Paragonimus westermani	Acetate, formate, propionate, *n*-valerate, 2-methylbutyrate, *n*-caproate
Moniliformis dubius	Succinate, lactate, acetate, ethanol

that these organisms were homolactate fermenters, almost quantitatively converting the glucose utilized to lactate by the reactions of glycolysis (Fig. 1).

It is of particular interest that these blood flukes, living free in the aerobic environment of the bloodstream, should still employ the anaerobic reactions of glycolysis as their sole source of carbohydrate energy metabolism. Presumably, glucose concentrations in the blood are always sufficiently high to allow the parasite the extravagance of such a wasteful metabolism. Further evidence in support of the anaerobic nature of this energy metabolism comes from several sources. First, the rates of glucose utilization, as well as the rates of lactate formation, by the schistosomes are the same under either aerobic or anaerobic conditions of incubation. Second, a group of compounds referred to as the cyanine dyes (of which the anthelmintics dithiazanine and pyrivinium chloride are members) inhibits oxygen uptake almost completely in the schistosomes, but has no effect upon their rate of glycolysis or their survival. Third, during in vitro incubation of adult schistosomes for 12 days, their gross morphology, motor activity, frequency of sex pairings, rates of glucose utilization, and lactate formation were the same in the presence or absence of oxygen. However, egg production was essentially stopped when oxygen was omitted. It is not known if oxidative metabolism is required for energy to produce eggs, or whether another

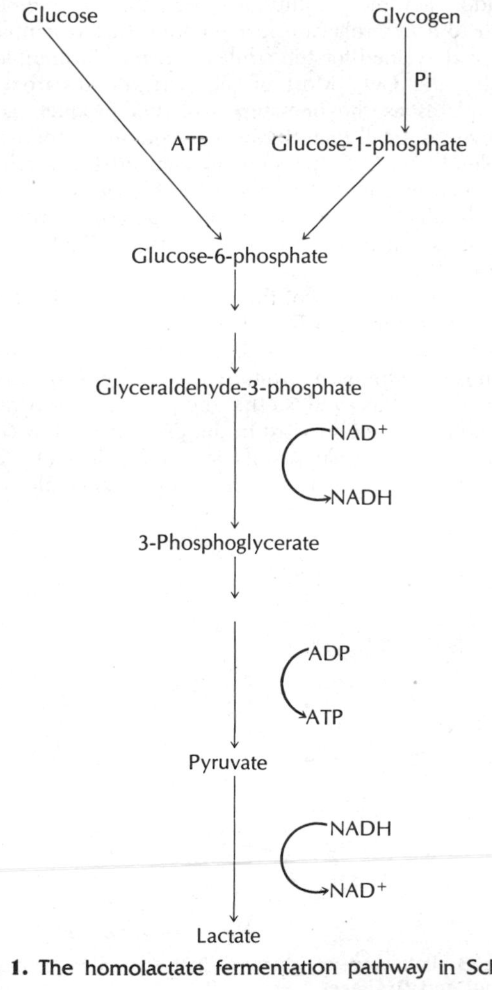

Figure 1. The homolactate fermentation pathway in Schistosomes.

non-energy-yielding reaction is essential for the developmental processes within the egg. Reports indicate that one non-energy-yielding reaction, tanning of the egg shell, is needed for maturation. Tanning requires the oxidation of some phenolic compounds with oxygen. There is little question, however, that for survival the adult parasite requires little or no oxygen.

The importance of carbohydrate metabolism to the schistosomes is indicated by evidence other than their rapid utilization of exogenous glucose and endogenous glycogen. As mentioned, the trivalent antimonials impair carbohydrate utilization by inhibiting phosphofructokinase, which, in turn, destroys the parasite. Glycolysis, therefore, is vital for schistosomes. Another example concerns the antischistosomal drug niridazole. Its first detectable effect is to lower glycogen levels of the male *S. mansoni*. Glycogen is depleted through accelerated utilization. Glycogen phosphorylase catalyzes this degradation of glycogen in tissues, including those of the schistosomes. This enzyme has two rapidly interconvertible forms, the "inactive" b form and the "active" a form (Fig. 2). Phosphorylase a is formed by the phosphorylation of phosphorylase b. Normally, when glycogen utilization is no longer necessary, glycogen phosphorylase a is converted back to the "inactive" phosphorylase b by the removal of phosphate as catalyzed by phosphorylase phosphatase. Niridazole inhibits phosphorylase phosphatase, thereby preventing the removal of the "active" glycogen phosphorylase a. As a consequence, in the presence of niridazole the phosphorylase continues to break down glycogen, depletes the parasite of stored glycogen, and kills it. Unfortunately, niridazole also lowers muscle glycogen in patients and causes muscular weakness. These findings further indicate the importance of carbohydrate metabolism to schistosomes.

Relatively little is known of the metabolism of other developmental stages of the schistosomes. The cercariae appear to differ from the schistosomules and adults. Cercariae oxidize all three carbons of pyruvate to CO_2, indicating (but not proving) the operation of a tricarboxylic acid cycle. In support of this possibility, some of the intermediates of the tricarboxylic acid cycle also are utilized by cercariae. Schistosomules, on the other hand, show a much reduced pyruvate catabolism and appear to resemble more closely the adults. The factors that regulate this shift from an apparent aerobic metabolism of the cercariae to the more nearly anaerobic metabolism of the adults (and presumably the schistosomules) are obscure.

Filarial Worms. Most filarial parasites that infect man are not amenable to biochemical studies, since they have not been reared in sufficient quantities in laboratory animals. This difficulty has been overcome partially by utilizing other filarial systems as models. Of these models, the three that have received most attention from the biochemical point of view are these: *Litomosoides carinii,* the adult form of which invades the pleural cavity of cotton rats or jirds; *Dipetalonema viteae,* which matures in the subcutaneous tissues of jirds or hamsters; and *Brugia pahangi,* which normally invades lymphatics but for experimental purposes is much more readily recovered from the peritoneal cavity of jirds when they are infected intraperitoneally. Of these three species, only *B. pahangi* can infect man.

L. carinii was the first of this group of parasites to be reared in small animals, studied biochemically, and employed routinely for the screening of antifilarial compounds. Diethylcarbamazine (Hetrazan) was discovered by using

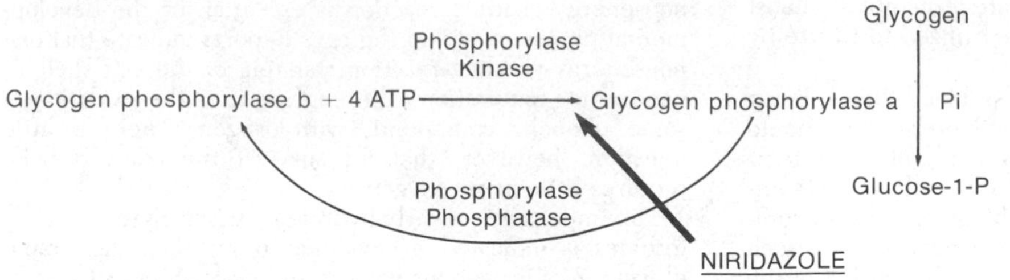

Figure 2. The mechanism of the stimulation of glycogen breakdown by niridazole.

this screen. Subsequently, another series of compounds, the cyanine dyes (for example, dithiazanine) was found to eliminate *L. carinii* infections in cotton rats. Cyanines strongly inhibit oxygen uptake of the parasite, which requires this gas for survival. Unfortunately, dithiazanine was without effect on those filariids that infect man. This disparity between the effectiveness of the cyanine dyes on these closely related species was disappointing and raised the question of the ways *L. carinii* differed from the other filariids.

A probable answer to this question has been arrived at by comparing the energy metabolisms of *L. carinii, B. pahangi,* and *D. viteae.* The motility of *L. carinii* adults ceases almost completely within one hour of anaerobic incubation, whereas aerobically, the parasites maintain good motility for several days. Therefore, *L. carinii* is an obligate aerobe. In contrast to this, both the motility and survival of *B. pahangi* and *D. viteae* is the same aerobically or anaerobically. Thus, oxygen does not appear to be required for motility or maintenance in either of these two parasites.

In accord with the apparent lack of an oxygen requirement for the motility of *B. pahangi* and *D. viteae,* subsequent studies have demonstrated that, in vitro, both of these parasites are homolactate fermenters, as was found with the schistosomes. All of the glucose carbons utilized could be accounted for as lactate. No other products were detected. If the filarial worms that infect man are similar in their energy metabolism to *B. pahangi* and *D. viteae,* then they too would need no oxygen for survival, and depression of oxygen consumption by the cyanine dyes would be expected to have little or no effect upon them. On the other hand, the trivalent antimonials that inhibit the anaerobic reactions of glycolysis at the level of phosphofructokinase were once used for treating filarial infections but later abandoned because of their toxicity.

In contrast with *B. pahangi* and *D. viteae,* adult *L. carinii* are obligate aerobes. This pleural cavity-invading parasite is a heterolactate fermenter. That is, it accumulates other fermentation products in addition to lactate. Approximately 50 per cent of the glucose carbon it dissimilates aerobically is recovered as lactate. Acetate, CO_2, acetylmethylcarbinol (acetoin), and one or more unidentified products also accumulate. Presumably energy is derived from this further metabolism, since under anaerobic incubation the fermentation shifts toward a homolactate fermentation but the parasite dies. Studies employing various species of ^{14}C-glucose as substrates indicate that essentially all of the respiratory CO_2 formed arises from the 3 and 4 carbons of glucose with very little arising from the other carbon atoms of glucose (Wang and Saz, 1974). According to the glycolytic sequence of reactions, the 3 and 4 carbons of glucose give rise to the carboxyl carbons of pyruvate, which, in turn, would be lost as CO_2 in the oxidative decarboxylation to acetate. Since almost no CO_2 arises from the 1,2 or 5,6 carbons of glucose, presumably acetate is not further oxidized and the tricarboxylic acid cycle is not a quantitatively significant energy-yielding pathway in *L. carinii.* The findings suggest that the aerobic requirement of *L. carinii* may reside completely in one system, the oxidative decarboxylation of pyruvate to acetate and CO_2. A summary of the metabolic energy pathways of the three filariids is outlined in Figure 3.

As might be expected, the metabolisms of the adult and microfilarial stages differ from each other. The microfilariae lose their motility in the absence of oxygen, but even after seven days of anaerobic incubation the reintroduction of air results in full restoration of motility. Therefore, although oxygen is required for motility, it does not appear to be required for survival of the microfilariids.

Under aerobic conditions, *B. pahangi* microfilariae switch to a heterolactate fermentation that resembles the process described for the adult *L. carinii,* forming lactate, acetate, and CO_2. Most of the pyruvate decarboxylated accumulates as the one-step oxidation product, acetate. However, a small quantity of the acetate may be oxidized completely to CO_2, presumably via a tricarboxylic acid cycle mechanism. When the microfilariae are incubated anaerobically they become nonmotile and concurrently shift their metabolism toward total lactate accumulation (Rew and Saz, 1977).

A further indication of the coupling of motility with the aerobic metabolism of *B. pahangi* microfilariae is obtained when they are incubated with the anthelmintic levamisole. Levamisole inhibits neuromuscular transmission (possibly by ganglionic blockade) so that the parasites are paralyzed. Aerobic incubation in vitro in the presence of low concentrations of levamisole results in a rapid loss of motility. After this loss of motility, the energy metabolism shifts

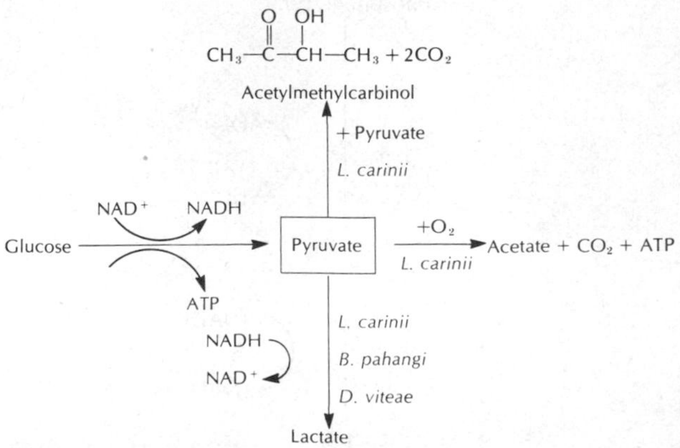

Figure 3. Pathways of glucose dissimilation in *L. carinii, B. pahangi,* and *D. viteae.*

toward lactate production, mirroring an anaerobic metabolism. The effects of levamisole on the metabolism of the microfilariid appear to be secondary to the paralysis because loss of motility from levamisole blockade reduces the energy requirement. The lowered energy requirement may cause a secondary shift toward an anaerobic lactate-forming metabolism. These findings indicate a tight coupling between motility and aerobiosis in these microfilariae.

CO_2-FIXING HELMINTHS

Ascaris lumbricoides. Although all helminths examined dissimilate carbohydrates to triose via the glycolytic pathway, many of them have evolved another sequence of reactions leading to the accumulation of succinate or products derived from succinate. This succinate-forming pathway requires the fixation of carbon dioxide and has the potential of yielding additional energy (ATP) for the worm. *A. lumbricoides*, the parasitic intestinal roundworm, has served as the model system in elucidating this pathway. Increasing numbers of species of organisms that accumulate succinate under reduced oxygen tension and appear to obtain energy for survival by employing this "*Ascaris* pathway" are being reported. In addition to many of the parasitic helminths and protozoans, numerous free-living metazoans, such as the intertidal molluscs, which spend part of their life cycle under anoxic conditions burrowing in the sand, bottom and deep dwelling fish, and diving mammals such as seals and porpoises, as well as ischemic or anoxic rat hearts, are all reported to use this pathway of succinate formation. Therefore, the pathway reported initially for *Ascaris* represents an important sequence in many organisms, including some mammals, in which it is a means of obtaining additional energy during oxygen deprivation to the tissues.

It has long been known that *Ascaris* survives equally well under aerobic or anaerobic conditions. The presence of CO_2 in the environment enhances survival. Adult *Ascaris*, therefore, can obtain energy for survival via anaerobic pathways. Accordingly, the organism is not sensitive to cyanide and levels of cytochrome c oxidase are so low as to be of doubtful physiologic significance. Accumulation of hydrogen peroxide in the presence of air indicates the existence of a flavin terminal oxidase rather than the usual cytochrome system, although it has been postulated that cytochrome o, which can react directly with oxygen to give hydrogen peroxide, may be involved in terminal respiration. Due to a deficiency of catalase, hydrogen peroxide accumulates and is toxic to the tissues of the worm.

Succinate and a mixture of volatile fatty acids comprise the major fermentation products of *Ascaris* metabolism. Volatile acids formed include acetate, propionate, traces of butyrate, pentanoate (valerate), tiglate (2-methylcrotonate), 2-methylbutyrate, and 2-methylvalerate. Lactate is not a fermentation product of intact *Ascaris* adults. The current concept of the carbohydrate fermentation pathway in *Ascaris* muscle is illustrated in Figure 4 (Saz, 1971, 1981). According to this pathway, the glycolytic enzymes of *Ascaris* muscle, which are present in the cytosol portion of the cell, function similarly to those of the host tissues up to the point of phosphoenolpyruvate (PEP) accumulation. At this point the metabolism of the parasite diverges from that of the host. In *Ascaris*, cytoplasmic pyruvate is not formed from PEP, since pyruvate kinase activity is barely detectable and of doubtful physiologic significance. Instead,

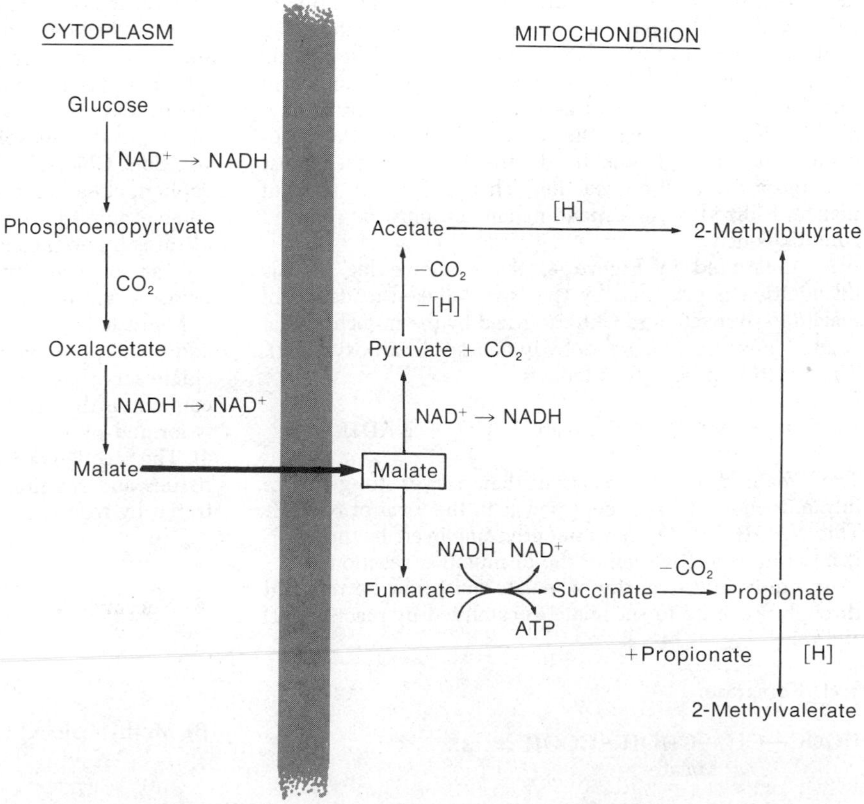

Figure 4. Pathway for the dissimilation of glucose and the formation of succinate and volatile acids in *Ascaris lumbricoides* muscle.

the cytoplasmic PEP carboxykinase catalyzes the fixation of carbon dioxide into PEP to form oxalacetate according to the following reaction:

$$\text{PEP} + CO_2 + \text{IDP(GDP)} \rightleftharpoons \text{Oxalacetate} + \text{ITP(GTP)}$$

In this reaction a substrate level phosphorylation of inosine diphosphate or of guanosine diphosphate takes place to form the corresponding energy-rich triphosphate. This conserves the energy of the phosphate bond of PEP as is accomplished by the pyruvate kinase reaction of the host tissues. Therefore, up to this point, identical amounts of energy are recovered from both pathways.

In order for glycolysis to continue, the NADH formed at the glyceraldehyde dehydrogenase level of glycolysis must be reoxidized back to NAD^+ so that another molecule of glyceraldehyde may be oxidized. In mammalian tissues this would be accomplished by the lactate dehydrogenase reaction, wherein pyruvate is reduced to lactate with NADH as the electron donor, thus reforming NAD^+. In *Ascaris*, however, cytoplasmic pyruvate is not formed and lactate is not an end product. Instead of employing lactate dehydrogenase, the parasite uses its cytoplasmic malate dehydrogenase for this function. Oxalacetate formed from the PEP carboxykinase reaction as illustrated above is reduced with NADH to form malate and regenerate NAD^+ as follows:

$$\underset{\text{(Oxalacetate)}}{HOOC{-}CH_2{-}CO{-}COOH} + NADH + H^+ \rightleftharpoons \underset{\text{(Malate)}}{HOOC{-}CH_2{-}CHOH{-}COOH} + NAD^+$$

Malate then permeates through the mitochondrial membrane and serves as the substrate for the mitochondrion of the nematode. In contrast with mammalian mitochondria, evidence indicates that a functional tricarboxylic acid cycle is absent from the *Ascaris* organelles. The roundworm mitochondria function and generate energy anaerobically. Under these conditions, the malate that enters the mitochondrion cannot be oxidized directly, but rather must undergo a dismutation reaction. That is, for each mole of malate oxidized, a corresponding amount must be reduced simultaneously.

As illustrated in Figure 4, the oxidative leg of this dismutation is provided by the NAD^+-linked oxidation of malate to pyruvate and CO_2 catalyzed by the mitochondrial "malic" enzyme (malate dehydrogenase decarboxylating). This reaction proceeds as follows:

$$\text{l-Malate} + NAD^+ \rightleftharpoons \text{Pyruvate} + CO_2 + NADH + H^+$$

The "malic" enzyme reaction then serves to generate intramitochondrial reducing power in the form of NADH. This NADH will be subsequently employed in the ATP-generating reductive leg of the dismutation reaction.

An equivalent quantity of malate must now be reduced through fumarate to succinate as catalyzed by reactions (1) and (2):

(1) Fumarase:

$$\underset{\text{Malate}}{HOOC{-}CH_2{-}CHOH{-}COOH} \rightleftharpoons \underset{\text{Fumarate}}{HOOC{-}CH{=}CH{-}COOH} + H_2O$$

(2) Fumarate Reductase:

$$\underset{\text{Fumarate}}{HOOC{-}CH{=}CH{-}COOH} + NADH + H^+ \xrightarrow{\nearrow ATP} \underset{\text{Succinate}}{HOOC{-}CH_2{-}CH_2{-}COOH} + NAD^+$$

NADH formed from the "malic" enzyme reaction donates electrons to fumarate, thereby accumulating succinate. The fumarate reductase reaction differs dramatically from the corresponding mammalian enzyme, succinate dehydrogenase. It does not catalyze a simple reversal of the succinate dehydrogenase system found in host tissues. The mammalian succinate dehydrogenase passes electrons directly to flavins, bypassing NAD^+. In contrast, the fumarate reductase of *Ascaris* couples with NADH, which, in turn, passes the electrons to a presumed flavin. This transfer of electrons from NADH to flavin would be analogous to a Site I phosphorylation of mammalian electron transport and, as would be expected, electron-transport-associated ATP is generated by the *Ascaris* fumarate reductase reaction. Therefore, this reaction provides energy for the cell in excess of that which would be obtained by the homolactate fermentation, providing an advantage to the succinate-forming organisms. For each glucose molecule fermented, two malates would enter the mitochondrion, but one half of the malate would be oxidized and one half would be reduced to succinate. Thus, 1 mole of ATP would be formed in the fumarate-reductase reaction for each mole of glucose dissimilated over this pathway.

The fumarate reductase and its associated reactions of electron transport are of great importance for chemotherapeutic and other reasons. A number of anthelmintic agents such as thiabendazole, cambendazole, and tetramisole inhibit the reduction of fumarate, although it is not clear whether this inhibition would constitute or contribute to the primary site of action. A number of other anthelmintics uncouple the phosphorylation system associated with this reaction. Chlorsalicylamide (Yomesan), desaspidin, dichlorophen, closantel, and phloroglucinol derivatives constitute some examples. The fumarate reductase pathway of metabolism is by no means limited to *Ascaris*, but appears to be a means of anaerobic energy generation in numerous other parasitic and free-living forms (Table 2).

Many helminths, including *Ascaris* adults, accumulate additional products that arise from succinate; that is, succinate serves as the precursor for these products. The most common is the three-carbon volatile acid propionate, which is formed by an overall decarboxylation of succinate (Fig. 4). The reaction occurs in two steps as it does in mammalian tissues and requires the coenzyme A derivatives as illustrated by reactions (A) and (B) below:

$$\text{(A) Succinyl-CoA} \underset{}{\overset{\text{Mutase (Coenzyme } B_{12})}{\rightleftharpoons}} \text{Methylmalonyl-CoA}$$

$$\text{(B) Methylmalonyl-CoA} \overset{\text{Propionyl-CoA Carboxylase (Biotin)}}{\rightleftharpoons} \text{Propionyl-CoA} + CO_2$$

Mammalian tissues generally employ these reactions in a direction opposite to that shown. Propionate is utilized by means of CO_2 fixation to form succinate. As a consequence, propionate is a glycogenic fatty acid in mammals. That is, it can give rise to succinate that, in turn, can go on to form glycogen. In *Ascaris*, however, the reaction operates primarily in the reverse direction, toward propionate accumulation. What controls the direction of this sequence in *Ascaris* is not understood completely. However, the fact that propionyl-CoA is further metabolized by the nematode, as will be discussed below, may pull the reaction in the indicated direction. It also may be significant that the apparent K_m values of the purified *Ascaris* propionyl CoA carboxylase for Mg^{2+}–ATP and propionyl CoA are similar to those reported previously for the corresponding human and pig liver enzymes. However, the K_m of the *Ascaris* muscle enzyme for bicarbonate is approximately 10-fold higher than those of the mammalian enzymes, indicating why the nematode enzyme might function physiologically in the direction of the decarboxylation of succinyl CoA. Since the methylmalonyl-CoA mutase requires vitamin B_{12}, those parasites that form propionate contain high levels of this vitamin (Tkachuck et al., 1977). In contrast, those helminths that form primarily succinate, lactate, or products unrelated to propionate do not contain appreciable amounts of vitamin B_{12}.

Pyruvate, formed as a product of the "malic" enzyme reaction (Fig. 4), is a precursor of acetate that arises within the mitochondrion. In mammalian tissues the oxidative decarboxylation of pyruvate to acetate and CO_2 results in the generation of ATP, since the reaction is linked to the electron transport system with oxygen acting as the terminal electron acceptor. Pyruvate utilization by *Ascaris* is particularly interesting in that acetate is formed anaerobically. What substitutes for oxygen as the electron acceptor is still not known, but it is possible that the oxidation of pyruvate may be coupled to the formation of the volatile fatty acids 2-methylbutyrate and 2-methylvalerate. Whether or not ATP is generated in the nematode by this anaerobic oxidative decarboxylation is unknown.

The mechanism by which *Ascaris* muscle forms its major fermentation products, 2-methylbutyrate and 2-methylvalerate, is not completely understood. However, acetyl CoA and propionyl-CoA are precursors to these volatile fatty acids. Incubating various radioactive substrates with *Ascaris* muscle preparations, then isolating the fermentation products formed and chemically degrading these products to determine the distribution of isotope in the carbon atoms of each have led to a postulation of the pathways for the formation of the two branched-chain volatile acids (Fig. 5). Observations are consistent with the hypothesis that 2-methylbutyrate is formed after a condensation of the carboxyl carbon of acetyl-CoA with the number-two carbon of propionyl-CoA. The condensation product would be the coenzyme A derivative of methylacetoacetate, which possesses the appropriate carbon skeleton and could be reduced to 2-methylbutyrate. A similar series of reactions appears to account for the formation of the six carbon branched chain volatile acid, 2-methylvalerate. In this case, two molecules of propionyl-CoA condense to form the corresponding C_6 keto acid, which would then be reduced to 2-methylvalerate. Preliminary evidence indicates that the NADH-linked reduction of the double bond in tiglyl-CoA to form 2-methylbutyryl-CoA in *Ascaris* mitochondria is associated with electron-transport-generated ATP. Rotenone, a specific inhibitor of the Site I (NADH→flavin) electron-transport-associated phosphorylation in mammalian tissues, also inhibits this *Ascaris* system. Although it was thought that these reactions were unique to *Ascaris*, it was reported recently that the clinically important lung

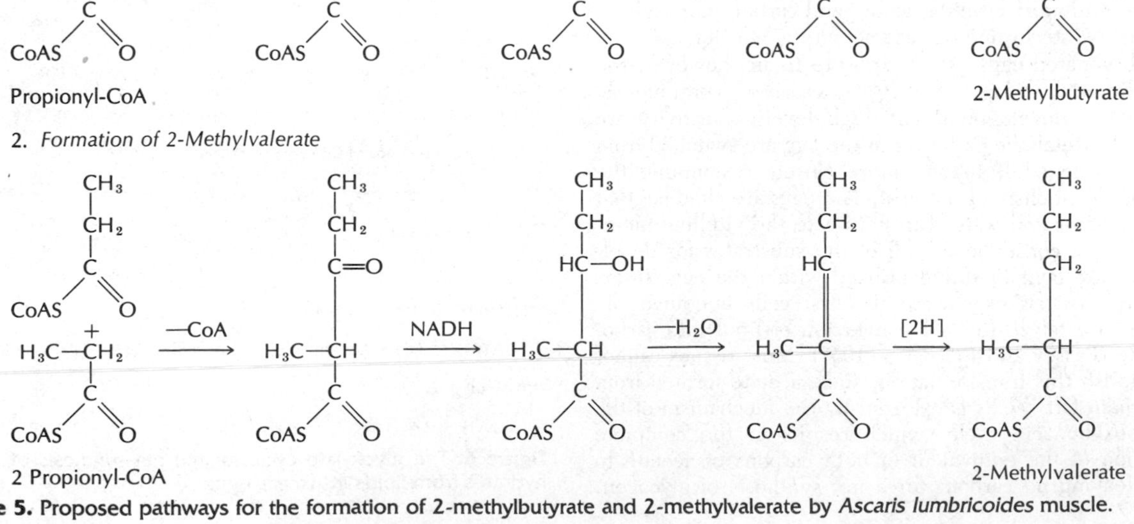

Figure 5. Proposed pathways for the formation of 2-methylbutyrate and 2-methylvalerate by *Ascaris lumbricoides* muscle.

fluke *Paragonimus westermani* also accumulates 2-methylbutyrate as a fermentation product. In addition, the stomach worm *Oesophagostomum radiatum*, *Echinostoma liei*, and the saprophytic swamp worm *Alma emini* have been reported to accumulate 2-methylbutyrate.

Normally, human tissues do not accumulate significant levels of propionate or propionyl-CoA. However, some of the intermediates of this pathway (Fig. 5) accumulate diagnostically in the serum and urine of children affected with the rare, but usually fatal genetic disease propionic acidemia (Truscott et al., 1979). This disease results from a failure to convert propionyl-CoA to succinate. Possibly, the high propionate levels that develop in the blood drive the reactions depicted in Figure 5, thereby accumulating the observed intermediates.

Although many of the reactions in the energy pathways of *Ascaris* and its host are similar or almost identical, others are distinct and therefore vulnerable to chemotherapeutic attack. The fumarate reductase system is vital to the adult ascarids, but of minor, if any, physiologic importance to the mammalian host. Thus, interference with the fumarate reductase reaction should be detrimental to the parasite, but not to the host. As stated above, many anthelmintics inhibit some component of the fumarate reductase electron transport system. Accordingly, succinate formation and the fumarate reductase pathway are common among other parasites and invertebrates (Table 2). On the other hand, the formation of the branched-chain volatile acids seems to be of great importance in the overall economy of *Ascaris* and *Paragonimus*, but may be of lesser importance to other parasites. Therefore, each parasite may have unique as well as common features in its biochemical arsenal of reactions. Each parasite is in some ways similar to and in some ways different from other parasites and from the host tissues, indicating that each worm should be examined independently.

In contrast to the adult *Ascaris*, fertilized eggs laid by the female in the intestines cannot develop past the single-cell stage until they are passed out and gain access to oxygen. The eggs require oxygen to initiate and maintain development. At any stage, growth and differentiation may be arrested by removing oxygen. Yet the potential for continued development remains even after extended periods of anaerobiosis, and normal maturation may be resumed merely by the introduction of air. Unlike adults, respiration of the eggs is highly sensitive to the cytochrome oxidase inhibitors cyanide, azide, and carbon monoxide in the dark. Cytochrome oxidase activity is not detectable in unembryonated eggs. After exposure to air, however, the cytochrome oxidase activity increases continuously throughout development and high levels of activity are attained. Metabolic pathways in the egg are switched from those of the adult to one more closely resembling the aerobic metabolism of the host. The eggs are cleidoic; that is, only gases and water can permeate the vitelline membrane. As a consequence, all of the substrates for development are contained and utilized within the egg. Interestingly, *Ascaris* eggs were the first cells unequivocally shown to catalyze the net conversion of lipid into carbohydrate (Passey and Fairbairn, 1957). Most tissues cannot accomplish this transformation, since acetate formed from long-chain fatty acids is oxidized by the mechanism of the tricarboxylic acid cycle, which results in the complete oxidation of the equivalent of both carbons of acetate to CO_2, leaving no carbons for a net synthesis of glycogen. Hence, no *net* synthesis of carbohydrate can take place from lipid. However, the glyoxylate cycle pathway in certain bacteria, plant cells, and *Ascaris* eggs allows for this conversion of lipid into carbohydrate (Fig. 6), thereby allowing the egg to utilize its stored lipids to replenish depleted carbohydrate stores for subsequent use.

The first molt in the *Ascaris* life cycle occurs within the eggs, resulting in formation of the second stage larvae that are released from the eggs on hatching in the upper intestine. The second molt occurs in the lungs of the host and the third stage larvae make their way up the bronchial tree to the esophagus to be swallowed back down to the intestine. Before or shortly after entering the intestine the third molt to the fourth stage occurs. Cytochrome c oxidase activity is present in each stage from the developing egg through the third (lung) stage larvae. When the larvae molt to the fourth stage, the cytochrome c oxidase activity is lost, indicating a shift from aerobic to an anaerobic metabolism. Factors that control the "switchovers" from anaerobic to aerobic metabolism in the developing egg and from aerobic to anaerobic in going from the third to the fourth larval stages are unknown.

Hymenolepis diminuta. The large intestinal tapeworm of the rat, *Hymenolepis diminuta*, also has served as a biochemical model for studying parasitic helminths. There is little doubt that this cestode is an anaerobe, since it has been cultivated from larva through adult in a CO_2-containing anaerobic environment. Oxygen may be detrimental to normal development. Another cestode, *Hymenolepis nana*, which infects humans, has also been cultivated. This cultivation also requires a CO_2-containing anaerobic gas phase. It is noteworthy that both the adult and larval stages were cultivated anaerobically. This is different from the larval stages of *Ascaris*, most of which require oxygen.

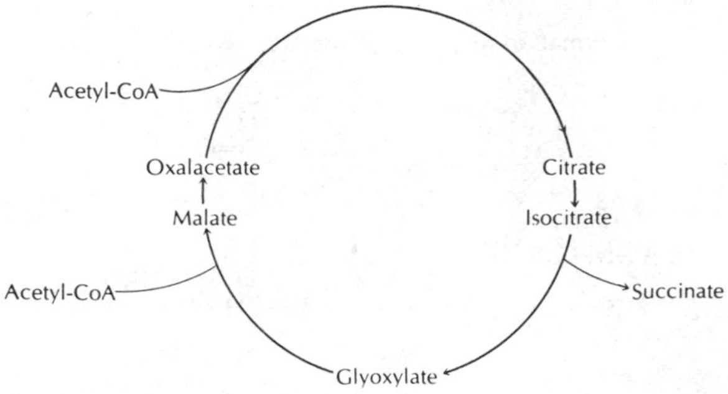

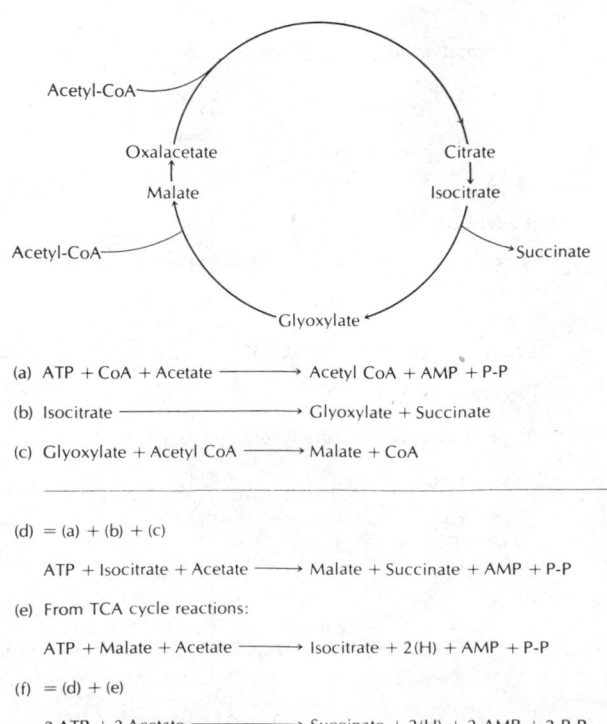

(a) ATP + CoA + Acetate ⟶ Acetyl CoA + AMP + P-P

(b) Isocitrate ⟶ Glyoxylate + Succinate

(c) Glyoxylate + Acetyl CoA ⟶ Malate + CoA

(d) = (a) + (b) + (c)

ATP + Isocitrate + Acetate ⟶ Malate + Succinate + AMP + P-P

(e) From TCA cycle reactions:

ATP + Malate + Acetate ⟶ Isocitrate + 2(H) + AMP + P-P

(f) = (d) + (e)

2 ATP + 2 Acetate ⟶ Succinate + 2(H) + 2 AMP + 2 P-P

Figure 6. The glyoxylate cycle for the net synthesis of carbohydrates from lipids in *Ascaris* eggs.

Hymenolepis diminuta adults accumulate succinate as the major fermentation product. Smaller quantities of acetate and lactate also are produced. Succinate is formed by a pathway involving CO_2 fixation, a "malic" enzyme, and fumarate reductase, as was described in *Ascaris*. The tapeworm also is similar to *Ascaris* in other respects. The tricarboxylic acid cycle does not appear to be of physiologic significance as an energy-yielding pathway in *H. diminuta*. Mitochondrial ATP generation from the fumarate reductase reaction is inhibited by chlorosalicylamide (Yomesan), desaspidin, dichlorophen, and some of the phloroglucinol derivatives, and the cestode has lost its ability to synthesize long-chain fatty acids de novo.

Unlike *Ascaris* metabolism, succinate is a terminal fermentation product in *H. diminuta* in that it is not further utilized. The adult cestode does not form propionate from succinate, and in accordance with this does not contain appreciable levels of vitamin B_{12}. Another interesting difference between *Ascaris* and *H. diminuta* was uncovered upon comparing their respective "malic" enzymes. In the case of the former, the oxidative decarboxylation of malate is coupled with NAD^+ (see text above for reaction). In the cestode, the reaction is coupled specifically with $NADP^+$. This is important because the reducing power generated by these mitochondrial reactions must be further employed in the specific NADH-requiring fumarate reductase reaction, which presumably will not accept directly from NADPH. To overcome this discrepancy, *H. diminuta* adults contain an active $NADP^+$:NAD^+ transhydrogenase as a constituent of their inner mitochondrial membranes. This activity is not detectable in *Ascaris*. The $NADP^+$:NAD^+ transhydrogenase provides the *H. diminuta* fumarate reductase with NADH by reaction with the NADPH formed in the "malic" enzyme reaction as follows:

1. $\text{l-Malate} + NADP^+ \rightleftharpoons \text{Pyruvate} + CO_2 + NADPH + H^+$

2. $NADPH + NAD^+ \xrightleftharpoons{\text{Transhydrogenase}} NADH + NADP^+$

3. $\text{Fumarate} + NADH + H^+ \xrightarrow{ADP \curvearrowright ATP} \text{Succinate} + NAD^+$

Fasciola hepatica. Although it seems clear that some of the helminths possess primarily, if not solely, an anaerobic energy metabolism as in the cases of the homolactate fermenters and the cestodes that have been cultured anaerobically, it is difficult to assess the physiologic significance of oxygen in the energy metabolisms of many other worms. One of the indications that oxygen plays a role in the metabolism of an organism is when the presence of oxygen alters the rate or type of metabolic products formed (for example, Pasteur effect). It has been known for many years that the liver fluke *Fasciola hepatica* exhibits such an effect of oxygen, but it has only recently been indicated that oxygen may serve as a terminal electron acceptor in the energy metabolism of the parasite.

During the adult phase of its life cycle, *F. hepatica* resides in the bile duct, a habitat of low oxygen tension. Therefore, the major part of the trematode's energy metabolism may be expected to be anaerobic. The major end products of either aerobic or anaerobic incubation are acetate and propionate, with considerably smaller quantities of lactate. Incubation of the fluke in air, however, decreases the amount of propionate formed but does not alter acetate formation. Therefore, oxygen may play a role in the energy metabolism of this parasite even though it appears to be predominantly anaerobic in this respect. Recent evidence indicates that either fumarate or oxygen may serve as the terminal respiratory acceptor of electrons. In both cases, phosphorylation of ADP to ATP is associated with the transport of electrons. If oxygen competes with fumarate as terminal acceptor, then aerobically less fumarate and hence less propionate would accumulate. Therefore, although the liver fluke is similar to *Ascaris* in most of its energy-forming pathway, aerobic oxidations may be of considerably greater physiologic significance to this trematode than they are to the nematode.

SUMMARY. Of those anthelmintics whose mode of action has been examined, most appear to act by inhibiting either neurotransmission or interrupting the energy-yielding reactions of the parasites. These inhibitions are possible because many of the components of the parasite tissues differ from those of the host.

No two helminths will have completely identical biochemical reactions. Differences exist not only between parasite and host, but also between any two parasites. These differences may be at the subtle level of enzyme or protein structure and kinetics or at a more obvious level of pathways, reactions, and products. The key, in examining the energy metabolism of the parasites, is that each organism is different and is a separate biochemical entity. Some helminths, such as *Hymenolepis diminuta* and *Hymenolepis nana*, appear to be anaerobic in all stages of development. Others are capable of a complete or major anaerobic energy metabolism in one or more developmental stages, but require aerobiosis during other parts of the life cycle. Still other parasites are obligate aerobes in one or more of their developmental forms.

Most parasitic worms possess one of two types of energy metabolism; either they are primarily glycolytic, or they are glycolytic but also depend, for part of their energy supply, on the fixation of CO_2 and the formation of succinate or products arising from succinate. Many worms employ both pathways and accumulate lactate as well as succinate. Generally, where this is found, the succinate pathway is dominant. Schistosomes and the filarial worms *Brugia pahangi* and *Dipetalonema viteae* are the best examples of glycolyzing helminths, since in vitro they are all homolactate fermenters and do not appear to require oxygen for energy generation. *Litomosoides carinii*, another filarial worm, is an example of a primarily glycolyzing parasite that forms mostly lactate but also requires oxygen for survival, presumably for the single-step energy-yielding oxidative decarboxylation of pyruvate to acetate and CO_2. Many other parasites accumulate acetate; some require air for this reaction, others accomplish this oxidative decarboxylation anaerobically. Little is known about the mechanism or energetics of the anaerobic oxidative decarboxylation of pyruvate to acetate in the helminths.

Ascaris and to some extent *Hymenolepis diminuta* have served as models for parasites that require CO_2 fixation and succinate formation for their energy needs. Many anthelmintics inhibit either the fumarate reductase reaction or the ATP-generating electron transport system associated with it. The role of oxygen in the parasites that form succinate is still not clear. In some—for example, *F. hepatica*—oxygen appears capable of partially competing with fumarate as the terminal electron acceptor. Other parasites, such as *Ascaris* and *Hymenolepis*, will take up oxygen, but the parasites survive equally well without air.

Progress has been slow in the field of parasite biochemistry for many reasons, but some of the biochemical relationships that exist between the host and parasite systems are emerging. Pathways and reactions of greater physiologic significance to the parasite than to the host are being recognized, thereby designating areas that may be amenable to chemotherapeutic attack. However, the giant void between recognizing vulnerable pathways and designing specific inhibitors of these pathways must still be bridged.

References

Bueding, E.: Carbohydrate metabolism of *Schistosoma mansoni*. J Gen Physiol 33:475, 1950.

Krebs, E. G., and Najjar, V. A.: The inhibition of d-glyceraldehyde 3-phosphate dehydrogenase by specific antiserum. J Exp Med 88:569, 1948.

Mansour, T. E. and Bueding, E.: The actions of antimonials on glycolytic enzymes of *Schistosoma mansoni*. Br J Pharmacol 9:459, 1954.

Meyer, F., Kimura, S., and Mueller, J. F.: Lipid metabolism in the larval and adult forms of the tapeworm *Spirometra mansonoides*. J Biol Chem 241:4224, 1966.

Passey, R. F., and Fairbairn, D.: The conversion of fat to carbohydrate during embryonation of *Ascaris* eggs. Can J Biochem Physiol 35:511, 1957.

Rew, R. S., and Saz, H. J.: The carbohydrate metabolism of *Brugia pahangi* microfilariae. J Parasitol 63:123, 1977.

Saz, H. J.: Facultative anaerobiosis in the invertebrates: Pathways and control systems. Am Zoologist 11:125, 1971.

Saz, H. J.: Energy metabolisms of parasitic helminths: Adaptations to parasitism. Ann Rev Physiol 43:323, 1981.

Saz, H. J., and Dunbar, G. A.: The effects of stibophen on phosphofructokinases and aldolases of adult filariids. J Parasitol 61:794, 1975.

Tkachuck, R. D., Saz, H. J., Weinstein, P. P., Finnegan, K., and Muller, J. F.: The presence and possible function of methylmalonyl CoA mutase and propionyl CoA carboxylase in *Spirometra mansonoides*. J Parasitol 63:769, 1977.

Truscott, R. J. W., Pullin, C. J., Halpern, B., Hammond, J., Haan, E., and Danks, D. M.: The identification of 3-keto-2-methylvaleric acid and 3-hydroxy-2-methylvaleric acid in a patient with propionic acidemia. Biomed Mass Spectrom 6:294, 1979.

Wang, E. J., and Saz, H. J.: Comparative biochemical studies of *Litomosoides carinii*, *Dipetalonema viteae*, and *Brugia pahangi* microfilariae. J Parasitol 60:361, 1974.

18

ARTHROPODS OF MEDICAL IMPORTANCE

A. L. DOHANY, PH.D.
JOHN J. S. BURTON, PH.D

The animals within the phylum Arthropoda are characterized by bilateral symmetry, a chitinous exoskeleton, and paired jointed appendages (Borror et al., 1981). This phylum, the largest of all animal phyla, contains species that transmit some of the most important diseases known to man, including malaria, yellow fever, plague, dengue, typhus, and the encephalitides. The majority of the arthropods of medical importance are contained within two large classes: Insecta (insects) and Arachnida (mites, ticks, spiders, and scorpions) (Furman and Catts, 1982).

The purpose of this chapter is to provide an overview of the arthropods of medical importance. Specific relationships between the arthropods and their animal hosts will be covered in chapters pertaining to the diseases they cause or transmit.

CLASS: INSECTA

Order: Diptera

FLIES AND MOSQUITOES. Adult Diptera or true flies have only a single pair of wings. The hind wings are modified into a pair of small stalked knobs called halteres (balancing organs). The mouth parts of adult biting Diptera are broadly classed as piercing-sucking, and those of filth flies as sponging-lapping.

The Diptera are the most important arthropods medically, and Culicidae (mosquitoes) is the most important family within the group. The activities of Diptera in relation to man can be placed in three categories. (1) As *disease vectors*, they are capable of rapid dissemination of infection either by biologic transmission (e.g., malaria, filariasis) or by mechanical transmission (e.g., typhoid, anthrax) (Chamberlain and Sudia, 1961). (2) As *pests*, the persistence of flies can interrupt and interfere with human activity over broad geographic areas. (3) As *allergens*, biting Diptera sometimes produce rather severe reactions in man, depending on the immune system of the individual (Feingold, 1973). Scratching the site of the reaction can lead to secondary infection.

Family: Culicidae

MOSQUITOES. Mosquitoes can be recognized by their relatively long and slender wings, with scales along the wing veins and posterior margin, and by their long, forward-projecting sucking proboscis. Only the females suck blood. The males can be distinguished by the much greater plumosity of the antennae.

There are a number of medically important genera. Living specimens of *Anopheles* (subfamily Anophelinae) are readily distinguishable by their resting and biting posture (Fig. 1). Their body plane is generally at a considerable angle to the substrate, giving the impression that they are standing on their heads. The palpi of both sexes are long like the proboscis. The eggs float singly on the water surface, and the larvae lie parallel to and just below the surface. Certain species in this genus are exclusively responsible for the biologic transmission of the four species of human malaria *(Plasmodium)* as well as simian malaria. They are also known to transmit filariasis (both *Wuchereria* and *Brugia*), as well as some viruses of man, notably that producing O'nyong-nyong fever in Africa.

The genera *Aedes* and *Culex* (subfamily Culicinae) hold their thoracic-abdominal plane essentially parallel to the substrate during resting and biting (Figs. 2 and 3). Palpi of the male are long like the proboscis; those of the female are short. The eggs of *Aedes* are laid singly, most commonly on moist substrate above the water line; those of *Culex* are laid in groups (rafts) on the water. The larvae of this subfamily hang head down into the water and contact the surface film only with an elongated respiratory siphon.

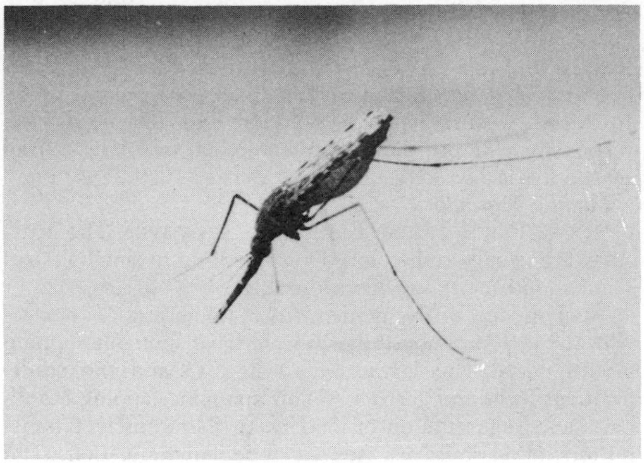

Figure 1

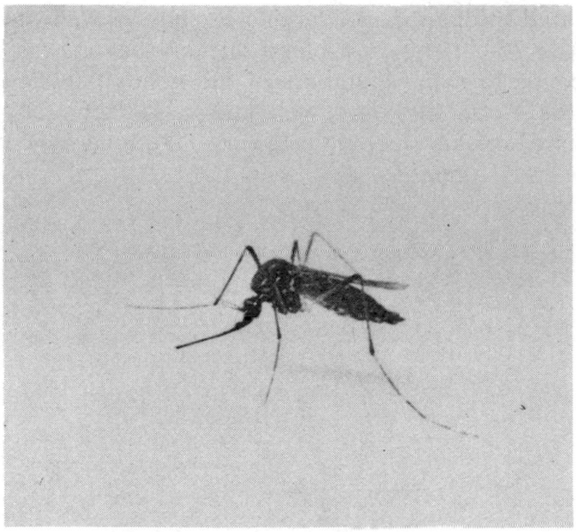

Figure 2

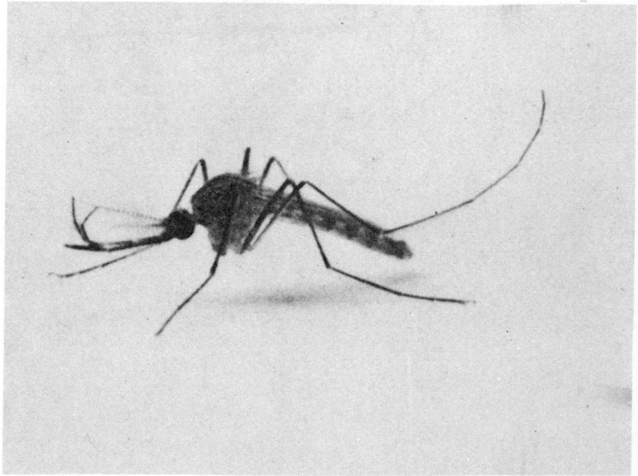

Figure 3

Figures 1–3. *Anopheles, Aedes* and *Culex* mosquitoes in typical resting positions.

Aedes mosquitoes are best known for transmitting viral diseases, and *A. aegypti* is clearly the most important disease vector in this genus. Yellow fever and dengue are the major viral diseases transmitted by *Aedes*, but they are also known to transmit chikungunya and encephalitis viruses. Several species also transmit filariasis. *Culex* mosquitoes may be most important as vectors of filariasis (*Wuchereria*), but they also have significant roles in the transmission of viral encephalitis, including Japanese encephalitis, western and eastern equine encephalitides, and St. Louis encephalitis.

Some other genera are important vectors of *specific* diseases; e.g., *Mansonia* mosquitoes are the principal vectors of *Brugia*. Larvae of this genus obtain oxygen peculiarly by attaching to the submerged parts of aquatic plants rather than at the water surface, a characteristic that complicates control measures.

Toxorhynchites mosquitoes (subfamily Toxorhynchitinae) are beneficial. The adults do not suck blood; instead they live on plant juices. The larvae are predaceous and may partially control the larvae of other mosquito genera locally.

Family: Simuliidae.

Black Flies. Black flies are small (1 to 5 mm) and have stout bodies that are usually dark in color (Fig. 4). Their antennae contain 9 to 12 segments (usually 11) and are without arista (long sensory hairs). The wings are broad and are folded over the body when at rest. The anterior wing veins are strong and the legs are relatively short and stout.

The genus *Simulium* transmits the filarial worm *Onchocerca volvulus* in Africa and in Central and South America (Smith, 1973). *Onchocerca* typically causes subcutaneous swellings and may cause blindness when the organism migrates into the eyes. Black fly attacks may also be serious. Irritation, allergic reactions, toxemia, and secondary infections may complicate the bites of simulia (Smith, 1973).

Family: Ceratopogonidae

Biting midges. Biting midges are very small (0.6 to over 4 mm), have piercing-sucking mouth parts, and usually

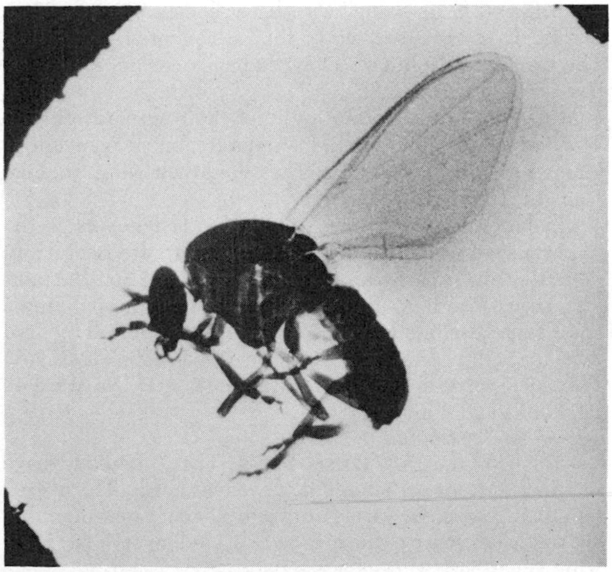

Figure 4. A slide-mounted specimen of the family *Simuliidae*, black flies.

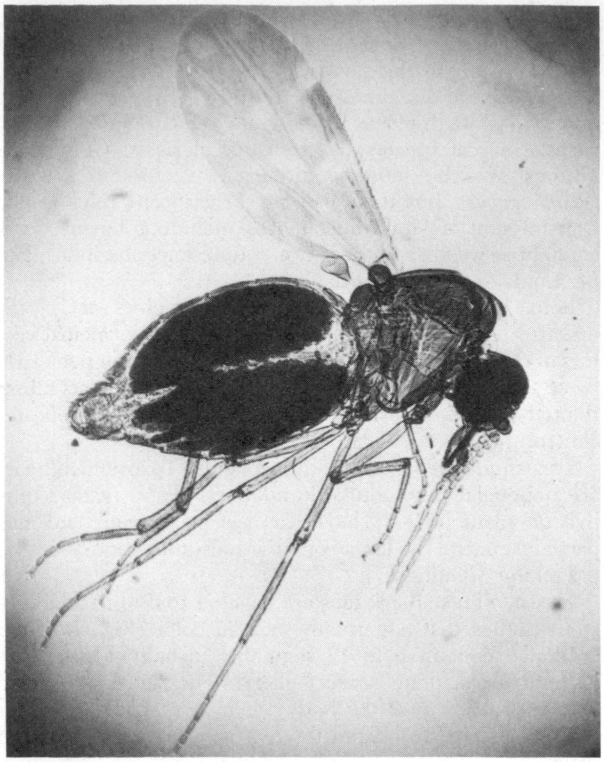

Figure 5. A slide-mounted specimen of a biting midge, *Culicoides.*

have 14 apparent antennal segments (Fig. 5). Their wings are sometimes speckled, have reduced venation, and are folded over the body when at rest. The most important genera are *Culicoides, Lasiohelea,* and *Leptoconops.*

These flies can be a major nuisance to man. Bites may become irritated and secondarily infected. Several species of filaria are transmitted by *Culicoides.*

Family: Psychodidae

SAND FLIES AND MOTH FLIES. The *Psychodidae* are small flies (1.5 to 4 mm) with hairy bodies (Fig. 6). They usually have rounded wings that are pointed at the tip. The wings have numerous longitudinal veins but few if any basal cross veins.

Moth flies are important only for their nuisance effects. They are often found around sewage treatment plants or in kitchen or bathroom drains. They hold their wings rooflike over the body when at rest.

Phlebotomine sand flies, of which *Phlebotomus* is the important genus, are best known as vectors of visceral and dermal leishmaniasis throughout Central and South America, Africa, southern Europe, and eastward through India and China. Bartonellosis (*Bartonella*) is transmitted by sand flies in South America. Sand fly fever, a nonfatal viral disease, occurs from the Mediterranean area eastward to Sri Lanka and China.

Family: Tabanidae

HORSE FLIES AND DEER FLIES. The *Tabanidae* have medium to stout bodies and large convex heads. The overall length of *Tabanidae* varies from 5 to 30 mm. Their piercing-sucking mouth parts have broad, blade-like stylets. Their wing venation is very characteristic (Figs. 7 and 8).

Horse flies and deer flies are vicious biters of man and animals, producing a large wound that can become secondarily infected. They can be efficient mechanical vectors of disease when their mouth parts have been recently contaminated with pathogenic organisms. Anthrax (*Bacillus anthracis*) and tularemia (*Pasteurella tularensis*) are diseases known to be transmitted in that manner (Krinsky, 1976). In Africa, several species of deer flies (*Chrysops*) are responsible for the biologic transmission of loiasis caused by the filaria *Loa loa.*

Family: Muscidae

HOUSE FLIES, TSETSE FLIES, AND RELATIVES. The Muscidae are usually dull-colored and medium to small in size. Their mouth parts vary considerably.

Most species of the genus *Musca,* including *M. domestica,* the common house fly (Fig. 9), have sponging-lapping mouth parts. The larvae breed in filth and the adults frequent feces and garbage. Their sponging-lapping mouth parts and regurgitation of food make them efficient transmitters of various diseases by food contamination. The diseases that house flies are known to transmit include: many bacterial diseases such as dysenteries, typhoid, and paratyphoid; protozoan diseases including amebic dysentery; helminthic diseases; and viral infection such as poliomyelitis.

Piercing-sucking mouth parts suitable for blood sucking are found throughout the family. *Stomoxys calcitrans* (Fig. 10), the stable fly, is a blood sucker that may transmit pathogens to man. Members of the genus *Glossina* (Fig. 11), the tsetse flies, are well known for their ability to transmit African sleeping sickness (*Trypanosoma rhodesiense* and *T. gambiense*).

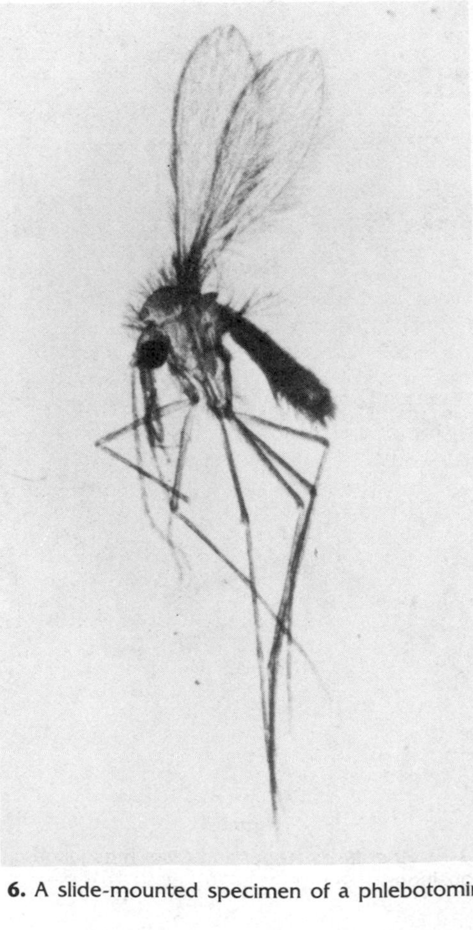

Figure 6. A slide-mounted specimen of a phlebotomine sand fly.

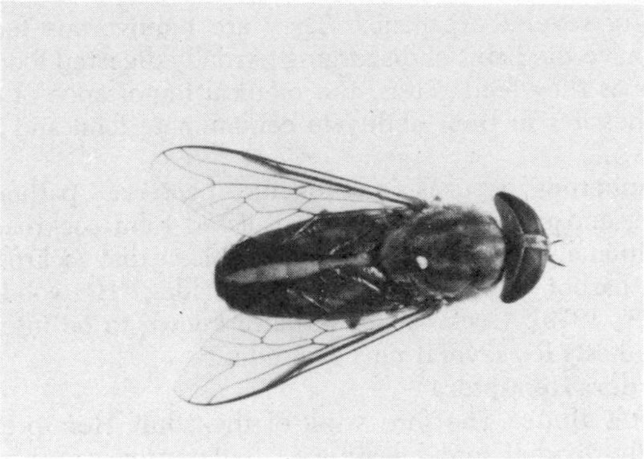

Figure 7

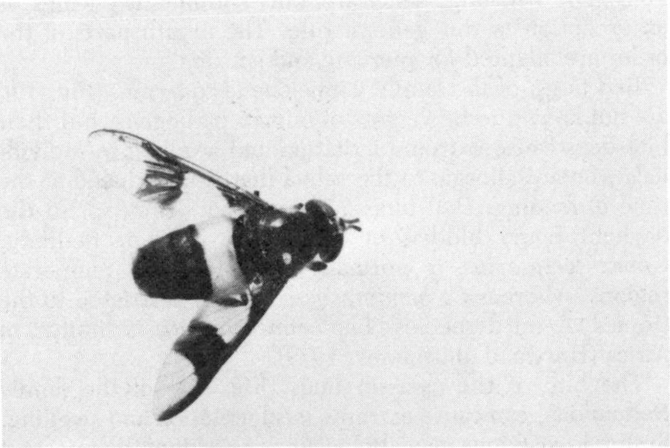

Figure 8

Figures 7–8. Pinned specimens of a horsefly, *Tabanus*, and of a deer fly, *Chrysops*, showing their stout bodies and large convex heads.

Various members of this family and the following two families are known to cause myiasis, with the fly larvae living, at least temporarily, in man. Larvae may enter the body by several routes. For example, they may be ingested in contaminated food, or the adult fly may deposit eggs at body orifices or in wounds.

Families: Calliphoridae and Sarcophagidae

BLOW FLIES AND FLESH FLIES. Many of the blow flies (Calliphoridae) are metallically green or blue (Fig. 12) and have an antennal arista that is plumose nearly to the tip. The flesh flies (Sarcophagidae) (Fig. 13) have a black and gray variegated pattern (not metallic). If the antennal arista is plumose, the plumosity does not extend to the tip of the antenna.

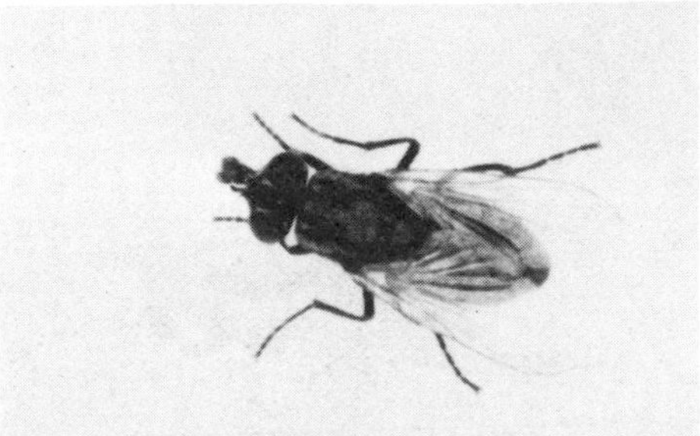

Figure 9. A specimen of the common house fly, *Musca domestica*.

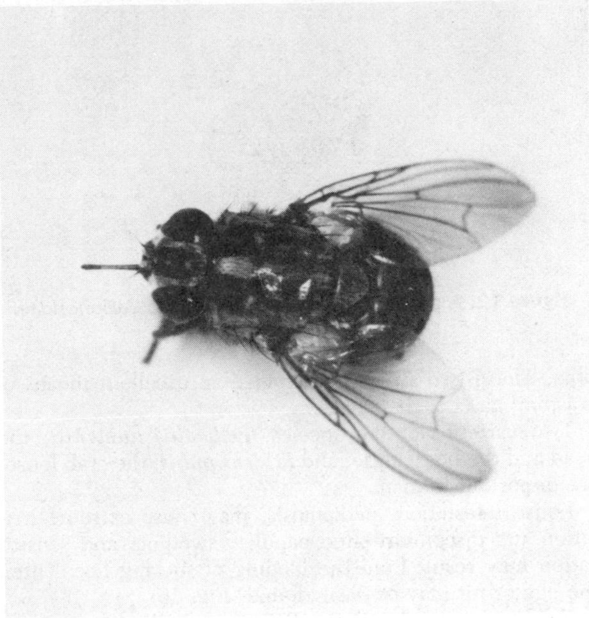

Figure 10. A pinned specimen of *Stomoxys calcitrans*, the stable fly.

In both families, the larvae generally feed on carrion and excrement. Some are known to cause myiasis. The larvae of some species are able to pierce the skin. Adult flies are able to transmit dysentery by contaminating food.

Order: Anoplura

SUCKING LICE. The sucking lice are small (1.5 to 3 mm) wingless insects (Figs. 14 and 15) with piercing-sucking mouth parts. The tarsi of the legs are usually reduced. The single tarsal claw is opposed by a toothed projection on the

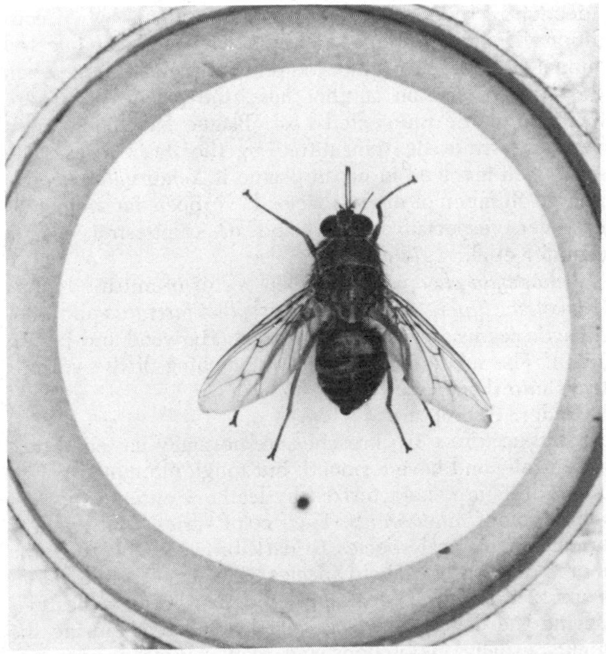

Figure 11. A pinned specimen of *Glossina*, a tsetse fly, showing a distinct hatchet-shaped wing cell.

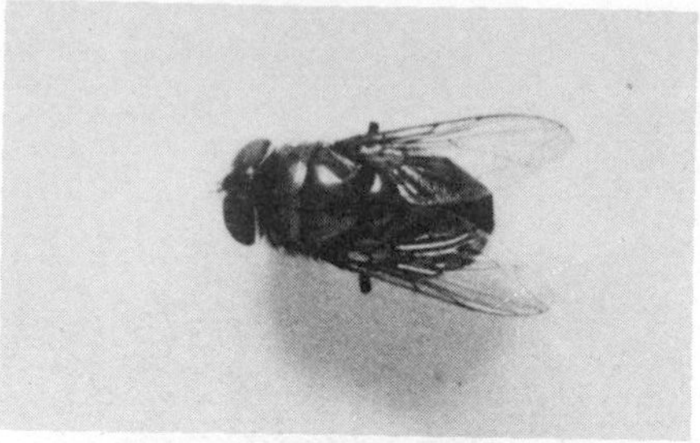

Figure 12. A pinned specimen of a blow fly, *Calliphoridae.*

tibia. These two structures provide an excellent means of grasping hairs of their hosts.

Two varieties of the species, *Pediculus humanus*, the head and the body louse, and *Pthirus pubis*, the crab louse, are important to man.

Louse infestation, pediculosis, may cause extreme irritation and discomfort. Red papules, swelling, and sensitization may result from the feeding of sucking lice. Often the egg or nit may be easily found (Fig. 16).

Epidemic relapsing fever (*Borrelia recurrentis*) is transmitted by crushing an infected body louse on the skin. Epidemic typhus or louse-borne typhus (*Rickettsia prowazekii*) and trench fever (*R. quintana*) may be transmitted to humans either by the feces of the louse or by crushing the body of the louse (Hunter et al., 1976). Transmission from the salivary glands of the louse is not involved in any of these diseases.

Order: Siphonaptera

FLEAS. Fleas, which are well known for their jumping ability, are wingless insects (Fig. 17) with laterally compressed bodies. The usual size varies from 1.5 to 4 mm. Their mouth parts are adapted for piercing-sucking. Only adult fleas feed on mammals. The larvae and pupae are normally found in soil or bedding. Fleas are the vector of bacterium *Yersinia pestis*, which causes plague. Plague, an infection of rodents, is transmitted to humans when conditions become favorable. Fleas that have fed on an infected animal often develop a blocked proventriculus. Then, when they try to feed on another host, the plague bacilli are forced into the uninfected host. Plague bacilli have also been shown to be transmitted by the flea's feces. The major flea involved in urban plague is *Xenopsylla cheopis*; a large number of other species have been incriminated, however, especially in sylvatic or campestral plague (Hunter et al., 1976).

Xenopsylla cheopis is the main vector of murine typhus (*Rickettsia typhi*), although *Nosopsyllus fasciatus* and *Leptopsylla segnis* are suspected vectors (Harwood and James, 1979). The mode of infection is scratching of the vector's feces into the skin.

Order: Orthoptera

COCKROACHES. Cockroaches are normally flattened dorsoventrally and have a smooth but tough integument (Fig. 18). Adults are characterized by leathery outer wings and membranous inner wings. Their color varies from green to orange in tropical species to dark brown to black in the more common household species. The size of adults varies from 12 to 40 mm. Most species remain in dark locations during the day and can be seen feeding only during the night, usually in kitchens and food storage areas when lights are suddenly turned on.

Circumstantial and experimental evidence indicates that cockroaches could be involved in the mechanical transmission of several organisms. They are omnivorous feeders and have the habit of disgorging partially digested food and feces as they feed. Thus, the medical importance of cockroaches lies in their ability to contaminate food and foodstuffs.

Numerous viruses, pathogenic bacteria, pathogenic fungi, and protozoa have been isolated from cockroaches. Additionally, the list of different organisms that cockroaches may harbor experimentally is quite long (Harwood and James, 1979). Cockroaches are also known to be intermediate hosts for several rat nematodes.

Order: Hemiptera

TRUE BUGS. The fore wing of the adult Hemiptera is usually divided into a leathery basal portion and a membranous apical portion. The hind wing is totally membranous. The bed bug, which has only rudimentary wings, is an exception to this general rule. The mouth parts of the order are adapted for piercing and sucking.

Bed bugs, of the family Cimicidae (4 to 5 mm) (Fig. 19), are not known to be vectors of human pathogens, but their bite does cause extreme irritation and swelling in individuals who are allergic to the saliva that is introduced at the time of feeding. Bed bugs are nocturnal. They spend the daylight hours hidden in cracks, crevices, or bedding. *Cimex lectularius* is normally found in the temperate regions, whereas *C. hemipterus* is usually restricted to the tropics. A third species, *Leptocimex boueti*, is limited to Africa (Harwood and James, 1979).

The bite of the assassin bugs (Fig. 20), of the family Reduviidae, can cause extreme local irritation and swelling. Systemic reactions may also occur as a result of the injection of foreign protein.

Chagas' disease (*Trypanosoma cruzi*), normally found in South and Central America, is transmitted by several genera of reduviids. This disease is transmitted when the reduviid defecates while feeding (Faust et al., 1968). The feces are then transported by the fingers to the conjunctiva of the eye or the mucosa of the mouth or nose. Although these bugs are large (up to 25 mm) and formidable in appearance, they are seldom disturbed during feeding because their bite is painless and they usually feed at night.

Order: Coleoptera

BEETLES. The adults of the order Coleoptera have two pairs of wings. The outer pair is thickened to form wing covers called elytra, while the inner pair is membranous (Fig. 21). The mouth parts are formed for chewing.

Some families of beetles are known for their ability to

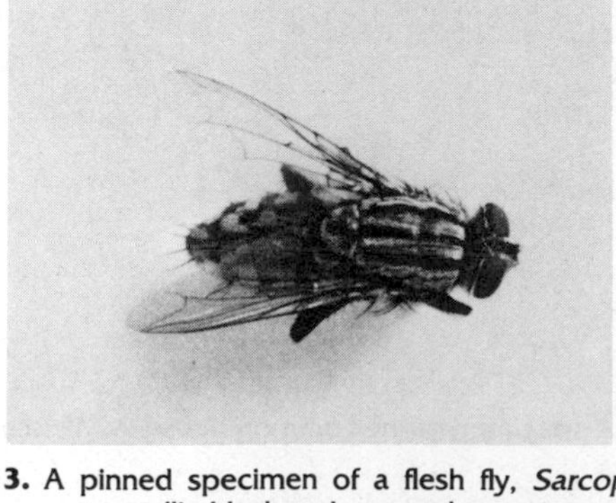

Figure 13. A pinned specimen of a flesh fly, *Sarcophagidae*, showing a non-metallic black and gray color-pattern.

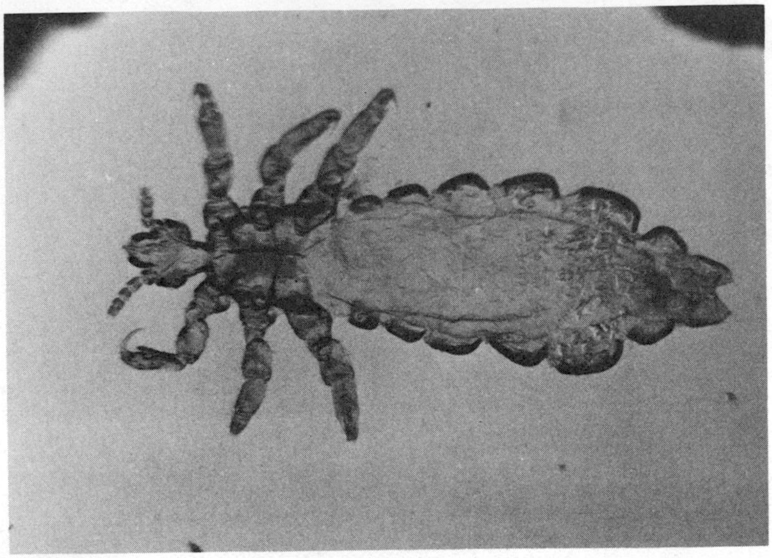

Figure 14. A slide-mounted specimen of the human body louse, *Pediculus humanus*.

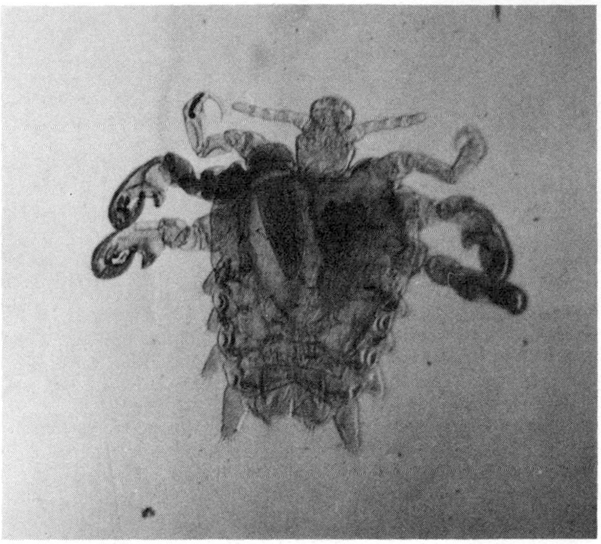

Figure 15. A slide-mounted specimen of the pubic louse, *Pthirus pubis*, showing the distinctive tarsal claws used for grasping hairs.

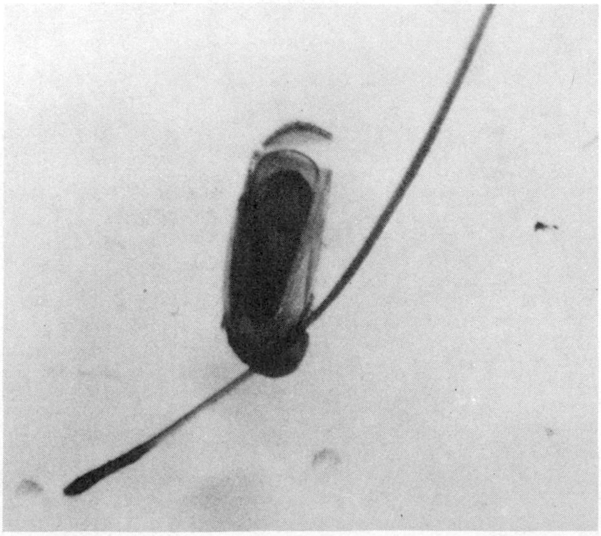

Figure 16. Egg of a sucking louse cemented to a hair.

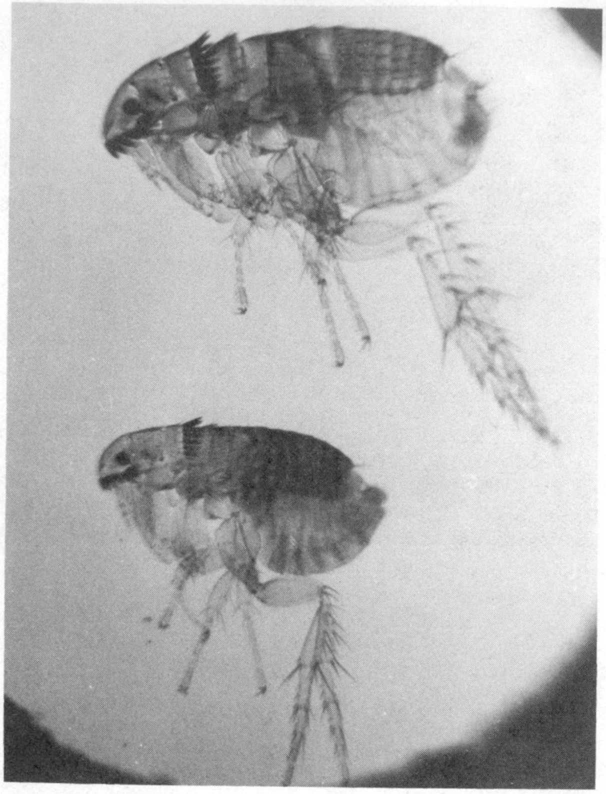

Figure 17. Male (top) and female (bottom) adult *Siphonoptera*, showing their lack of wings and their strong hind legs.

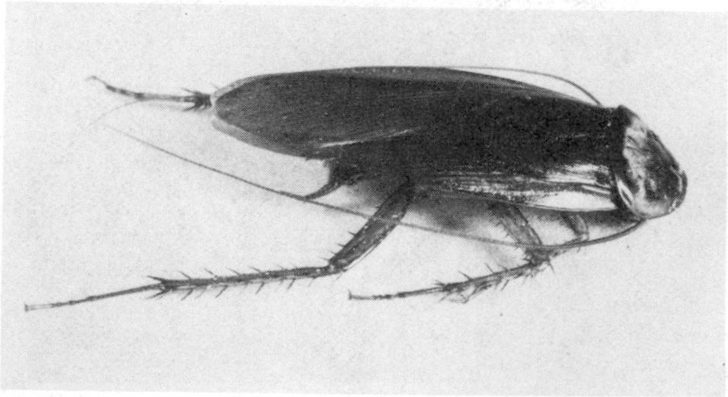

Figure 18. Specimen of the cockroach, *Periplaneta americana.*

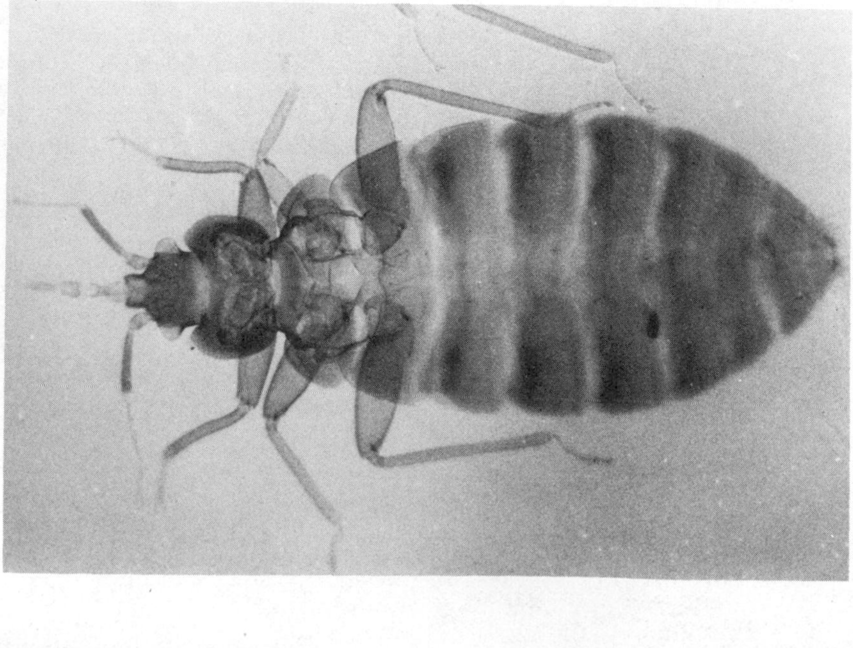

Figure 19. A slide-mounted specimen of *Cimex*, showing rudimentary wings.

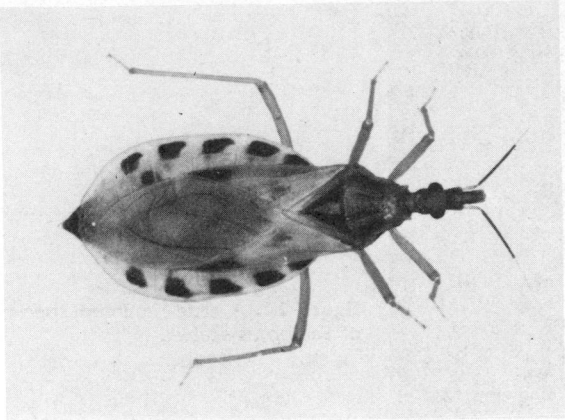

Figure 20. A specimen of a reduviid, *Triatoma*.

produce blisters by discharging their body fluids onto the skin. The "Spanish fly" (*Lytta vesicatoria*) (10 to 15 mm) is perhaps the best known vesicating beetle. Blisters are formed when this beetle is crushed on the skin.

Order: Lepidoptera

BUTTERFLIES AND MOTHS (CATERPILLARS). The adults of the Lepidoptera (butterflies and moths) may be separated from other insects by their two pairs of membranous wings that are covered with overlapping scales. Their mouth parts are adapted for siphoning. Larvae (caterpillars) are usually cylindrical in shape and have three pairs of thoracic legs and two to five pairs of abdominal legs or prolegs (Fig. 22).

Contact with poison hairs on the external surface of some caterpillars causes a stinging dermatitis. The urticating fluid is released when the tips of the hairs are broken upon contact.

Order: Hymenoptera

BEES, WASPS, HORNETS, AND ANTS. The Hymenoptera usually have two pairs of membranous wings with hind wings that are smaller than the fore wings (Fig. 23), but some members of the order, notably most of the ants, are wingless. The abdomens of the females are usually provided with a stinging apparatus.

The effects of a Hymenoptera sting may range from moderate, temporary pain and slight local swelling to shock and death.

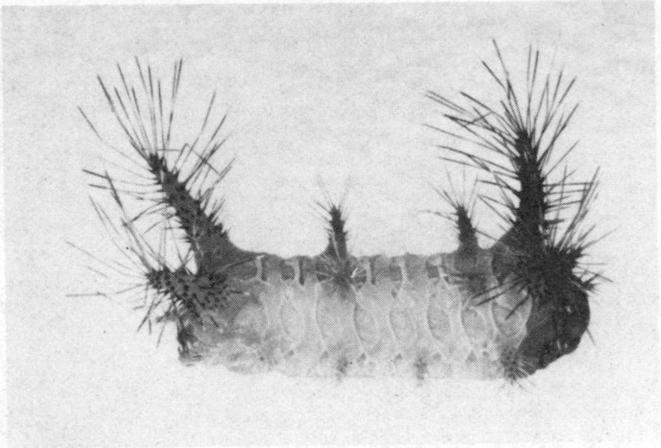

Figure 22. A specimen of a lepidopterous larva, showing its urticating hairs.

CLASS: ARACHNIDA

SUBCLASS: ACARI

MITES AND TICKS. The subclass Acari is composed of the arthropods that are commonly referred to as ticks and mites. These arthropods are distinctive in that they have two body regions, an idiosoma (fused abdomen and cephalothorax) and a gnathosoma (mouth parts) (Krantz, 1978). Adult Acari usually have four pairs of legs, but larvae have only three pairs.

Only two species of mites are fully adapted parasites of man: the skin mite, *Sarcoptes scabiei* (0.3 to 0.5 mm) (Fig. 24), and the follicle mite, *Demodex folliculorum* (0.4 mm) (Fig. 25). *Demodex folliculorum* may not cause any disease in man; it may only be a commensal. However, *Sarcoptes scabiei* can cause extreme itching and keratotic crusts covering large numbers of mites. *Demodex* and *Sarcoptes* cause the condition commonly known as mange in animals.

A large number of mites and ticks can parasitize man if their normal host is not available. Additionally, another large group of mites may affect man by biting and causing dermatitis (Krantz, 1978). This group includes many mites that feed on plants and organic matter and that come into contact with man only accidentally.

Scrub typhus or chigger-borne rickettsiosis (*Rickettsia tsutsugamushi*) is transmitted by the larvae of the trombiculid mite or chigger (Fig. 26). The disease occurs throughout Asia in a triangle roughly bound by India, northern Australia, and northern Japan. All known vectors are in the genus and subgenus *Leptotrombidium* (Traub and Wisseman, 1974). The small (0.2 to 0.4 mm), six-legged larvae

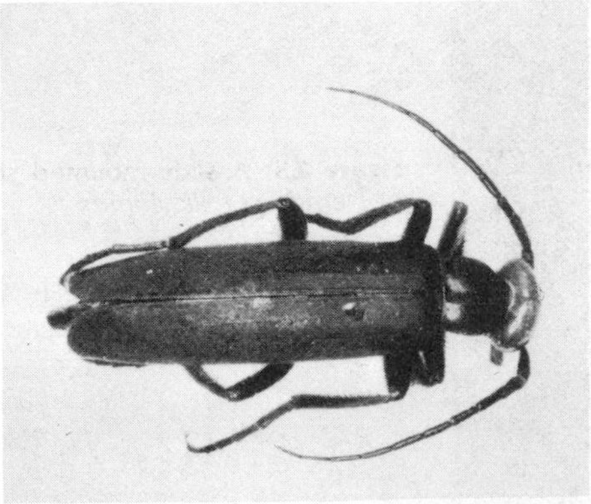

Figure 21. A pinned specimen of a blister beetle, showing its thick wing covers or elytra.

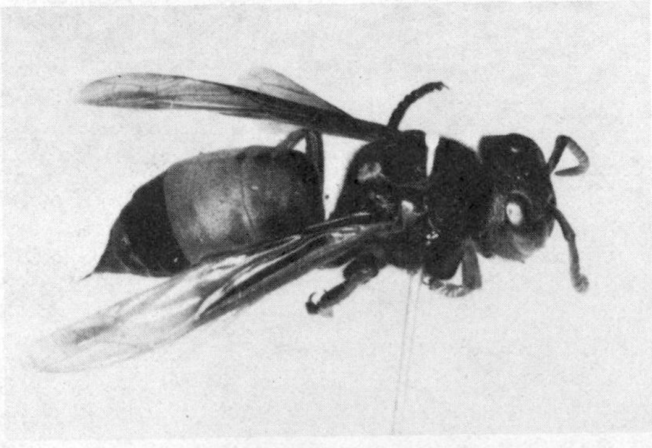

Figure 23. A pinned specimen of an adult hymenopteran, showing a stinger on the terminal abdominal segment.

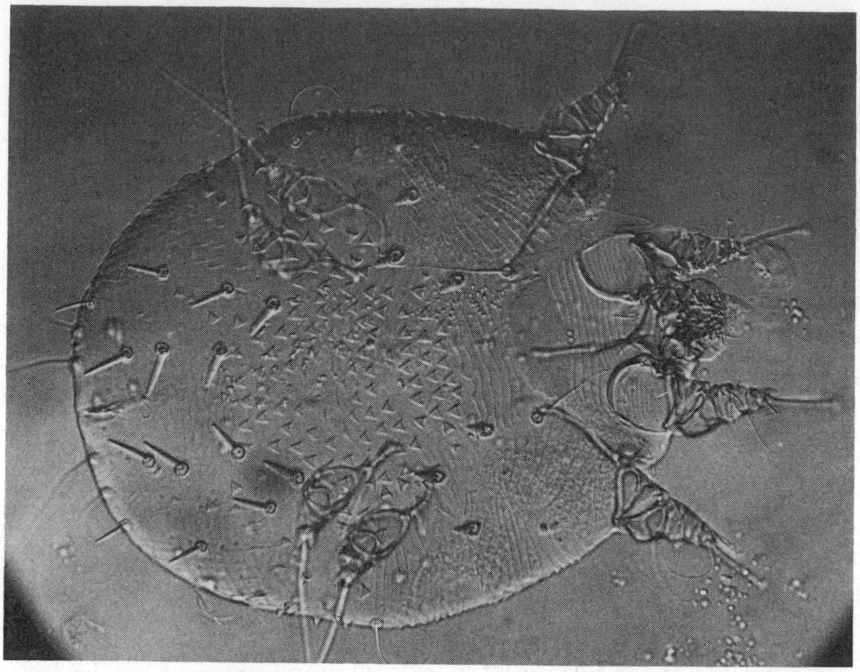

Figure 24. A slide-mounted specimen of *Sarcoptes scabiei.*

normally feed on small rodents but will attack man if he is in the chiggers' habitat. Feeding by these mites is often inapparent until the onset of the disease.

Rickettsialpox (*Rickettsia akari*) reported from the United States and the Soviet Union is transmitted by nymphs and adults of the house mouse mite, *Liponyssoides sanguineus.* Although this disease is apparently uncommon, it may be more widely spread than has been reported, since a similar disease has been described from Africa and the causative organism has been isolated from wild rodents in Korea.

A number of mites commonly referred to as house dust mites have been associated with the production of allergens that cause bronchial asthma and rhinitis (Wharton, 1976). Although a large number of different genera may occur in dust samples, species of the genus *Dermatophagoides* (0.2 to 0.4 mm) have proved to be the most important in relation to allergies. Dust mites are normally found in beds and furniture and under beds, feeding on human dander.

Ticks (superfamily Ixodoidea) can be differentiated from the other acari by the presence of a sensory structure known as Haller's organ on the first pair of tarsi. Also, many species have a toothed hypostome (Fig. 27). Generally, adult ticks are relatively large (0.3 to 5 mm) in comparison to other acari and have a leathery appearance (Fig. 28). Ixodoidea is composed of three families: Ixodidae, or hard ticks; Argasidae, or soft ticks; and Nuttalliellidae,

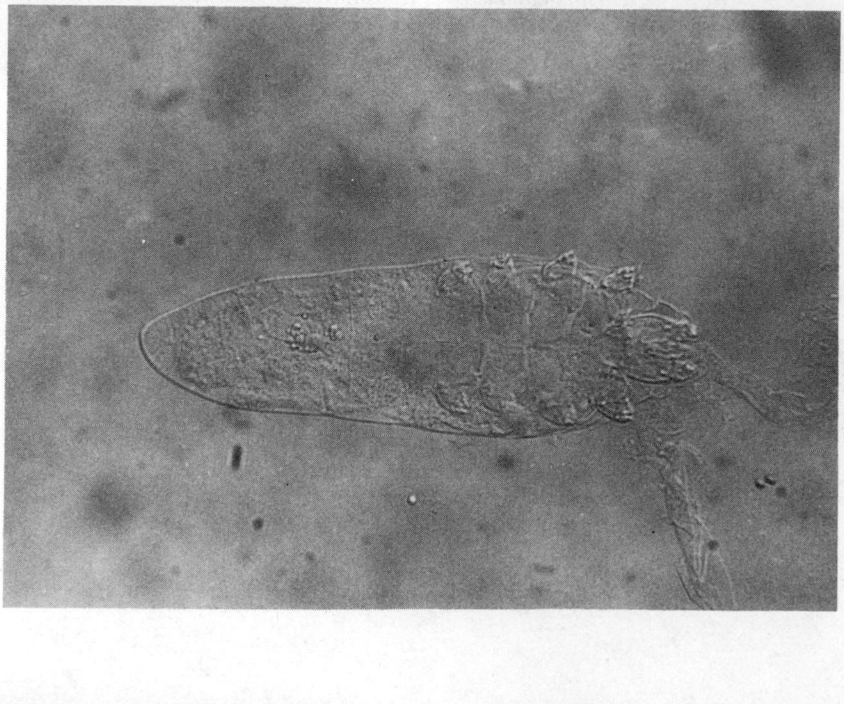

Figure 25. A slide-mounted specimen of *Demodex folliculorum.*

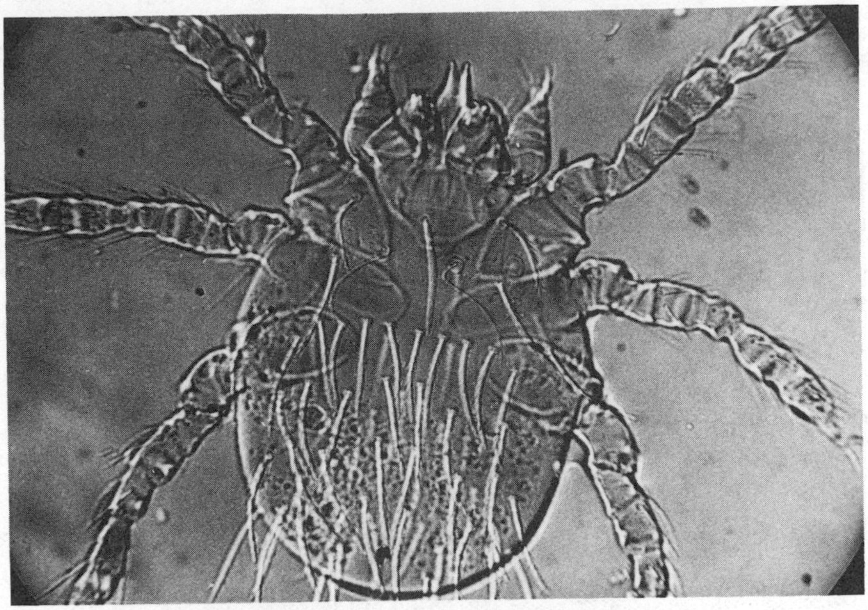

Figure 26. A slide-mounted specimen of a *Leptotrombidium* chigger.

an intermediate represented by a single species. Of the vast number of tick-borne diseases, by far the largest number are transmitted to man by the Ixodidae (Balashov, 1972).

Harwood and James (1979) list eight factors that make ticks such good vectors of mammalian diseases. Ticks are persistent bloodsuckers, slow feeders, highly sclerotized, and relatively free of natural enemies. They also have a wide host range, a long life span, ability to transmit the disease agents transovarially, and a great reproductive potential. Ticks are known to transmit arboviruses, rickettsiae, bacteria, spirochetes, and piroplasms to man. Additionally, ticks may cause paralysis in man.

By far the largest number of diseases transmitted to man by ticks are caused by arboviruses. The majority fall into the category known as the Russian spring-summer complex (flavivirus or antigenic group B).

SUBCLASS: SCORPIONES

SCORPIONS. Scorpions are easily recognizable by their long, five-segmented, tail-like post-abdomen that terminates in a bulbous sac with a prominent stinger. Anteriorly, the pedipalps are enlarged and resemble an additional pair of legs, and the last two segments are modified to form pincers (Fig. 29).

Scorpions are nocturnal by nature, remaining hidden in the daytime under stones, litter, and lumber. The sting usually results from accidental contact with a scorpion, such as accidentally stepping on it, placing one's foot in its

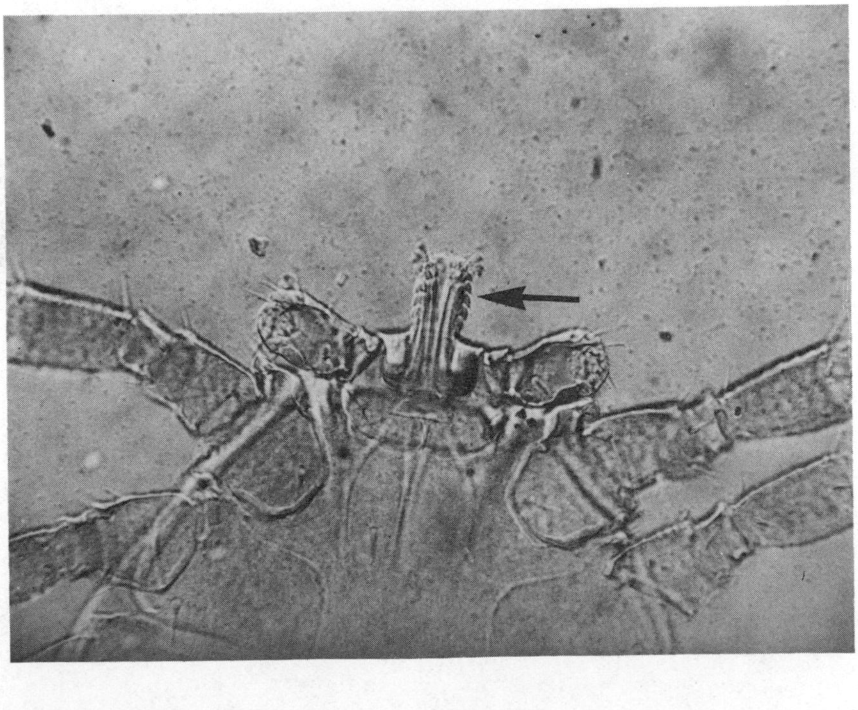

Figure 27. A slide-mounted specimen showing the hypostome (arrow) of a tick.

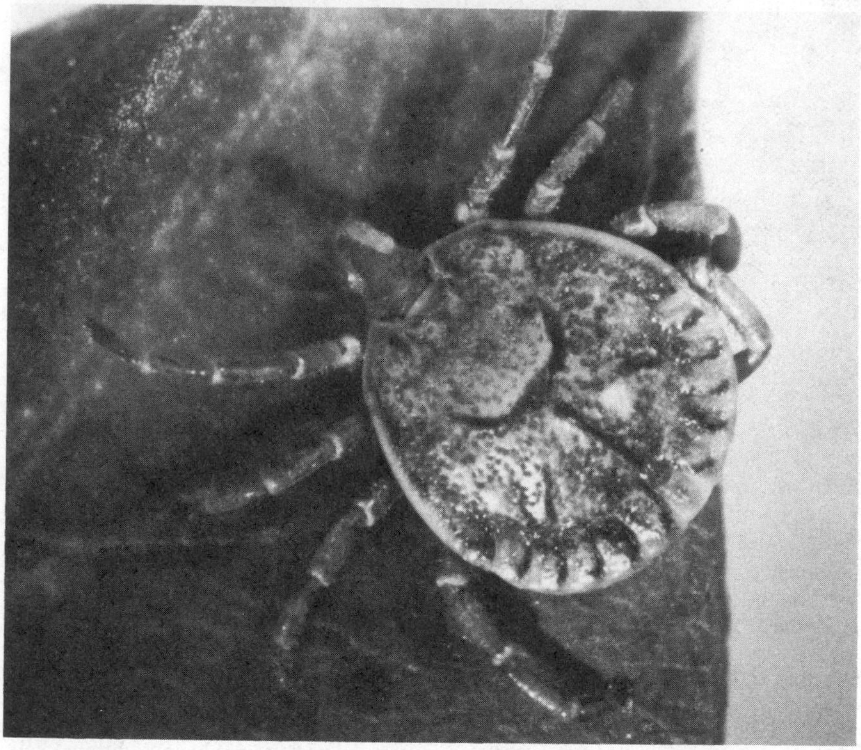

Figure 28. A specimen of an adult tick, Ixodidae.

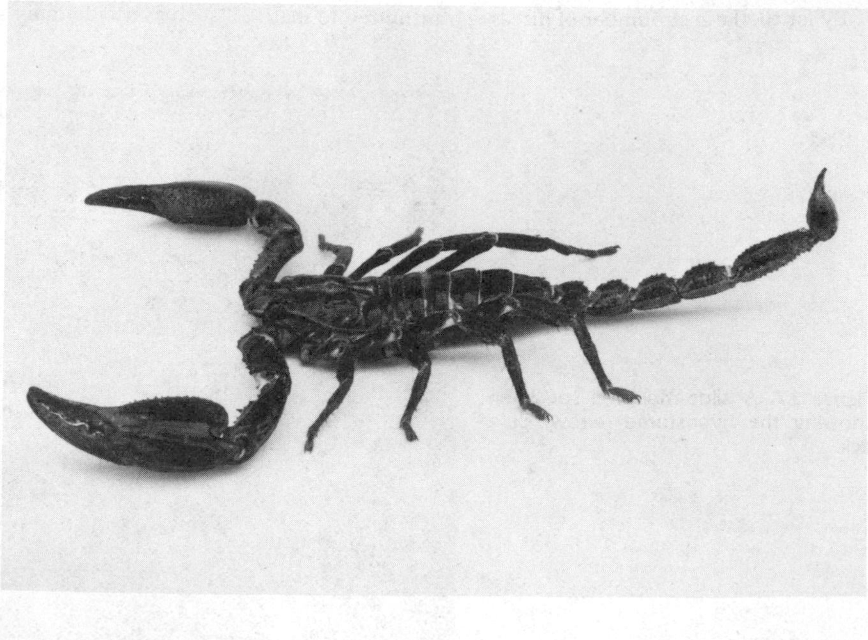

Figure 29. Scorpion, showing the bulbous sac and prominent stinger.

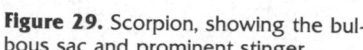

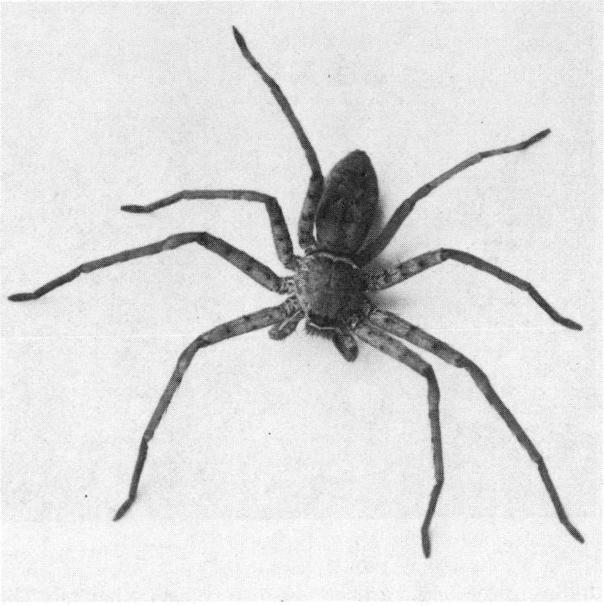

Figure 30. Spider, characterized by the prominent body division of the cephalothorax and abdomen.

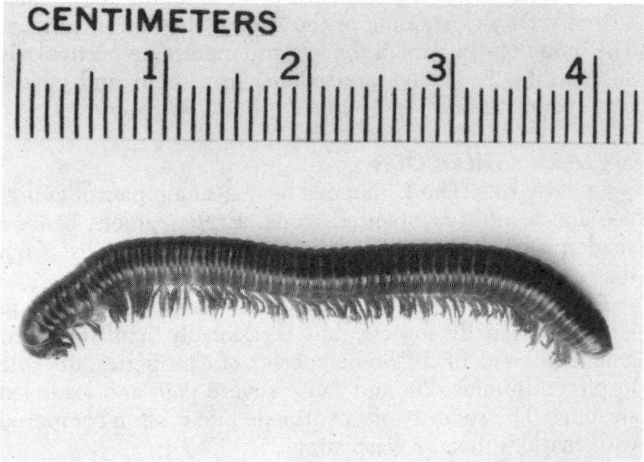

Figure 31. Millipede, bearing 2 pairs of legs per body segment.

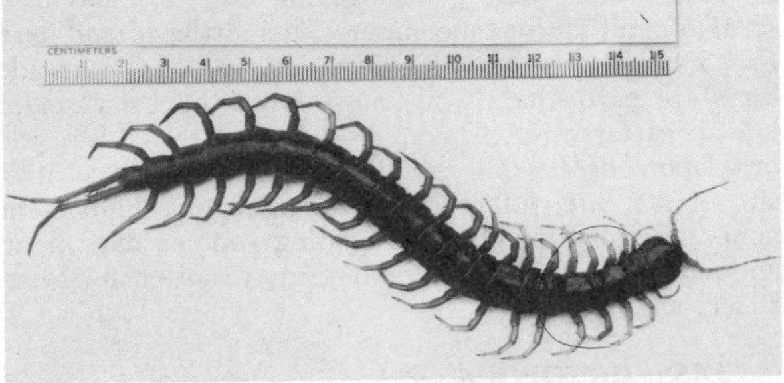

Figure 32. Centipede, bearing a single pair of legs per segment.

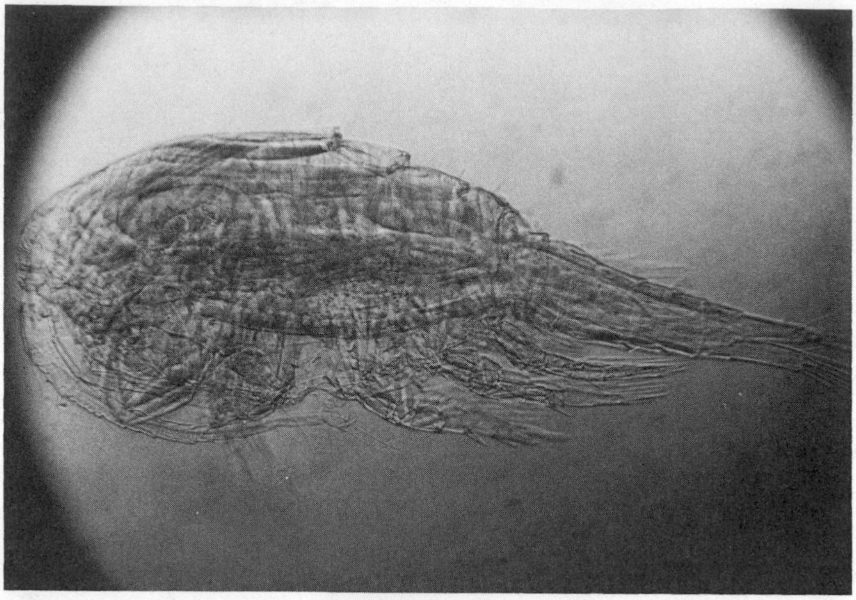

Figure 33. A slide-mounted specimen of a copepod, *Cyclops.*

hiding place (e.g., a boot), or disturbing its habitat. The sting of the scorpion can be very dangerous, depending upon the species. Areas such as Mexico, southwestern United States, parts of South America, and North Africa west of Egypt are known to have particularly dangerous species. The severity of the sting is not necessarily related to the size of the scorpion; the smaller species are often more dangerous. Children are more seriously affected. Pain is usually associated with the sting, but swelling and discoloration at the site may or may not occur, depending upon the species of scorpion. The sting of dangerous species can be fatal, particularly to children.

SUBCLASS: ARANEAE

SPIDERS. The spiders have two body parts, cephalothorax and abdomen, and four pairs of legs (Fig. 30). The cephalothorax is separated from the abdomen by a narrow constriction, the pedicel. The eyes are simple and antennae are absent. All spiders have silk glands that produce silk through spinnerets located near the rear of the abdomen. The legs are borne on the cephalothorax.

All spiders feed by injecting venom into their prey, but relatively few species are of medical importance. Two types of effects are commonly noted from spider bites: the formation of a necrotizing ulcer and systemic symptoms. The bite of *Loxosceles* spp., brown recluse or fiddle-back spiders, causes necrotic ulcers on the skin, a condition termed loxoscelism. In mild cases the necrotic ulcer may be slow to heal, leaving a disfiguring scar. In severe cases erosion of all mucous membranes, hemorrhage, and death may occur (Southcott, 1976). Systemic reactions from spider bites are particularly well known from the hairy spiders known as tarantula, Theraphosidae, and the "black widows," *Latrodectus* spp. Swelling and pain may occur at the site of the bite, followed by burning and aching in the general area of the bite. Circulating venoms may induce abdominal cramps. Untreated bites may cause convulsions, shock, and death.

CLASS: DIPLOPODA

MILLIPEDES. Members of the class Diplopoda are multi-segmented and multi-legged arthropods. Each body segment bears two pairs of legs (Fig. 31). Most species of millipedes feed on decaying organic matter and many species are equipped with offensive stink glands.

The stink glands of the millipede may have the capability of forcefully ejecting secretions. This liquid may cause severe pain and staining of the skin at the site of contact. The lining epithelium of the eye and mouth are particularly susceptible. Erythema and edema may occur and persist for several weeks.

CLASS: CHILOPODA

CENTIPEDES. The Chilopoda have a single pair of antennae and a multi-segmented trunk. Each segment bears a single pair of legs (Fig. 32). Paired poison claws arise from the first trunk segment.

The venom of the poison claws of centipedes is used to kill prey, usually insects, but occasionally small reptiles, mammals, and birds. Some species of centipedes are able to pierce human skin and cause severe pain and localized swelling. The severity of a centipede bite is often compared with that of a bee or wasp sting.

CLASS: CRUSTACEA

CRAYFISH, SHRIMP, CRABS, LOBSTERS, AND COPEPODS. Crustaceans typically have two pairs of antennae and five or more pairs of legs.

Crustaceans play an important part in the life cycle of a number of helminths by acting as intermediate hosts. Species of copepods, especially *Cyclops* (Fig. 33), are intermediate hosts for the broad tapeworm, *Diphyllobothrium latum,* and for the guinea worm of Africa, *Dracunculus medinensis.*

References

Balashow, Y. S.: Bloodsucking ticks (Ixodoidea)—vector of diseases of man and animals (1968). Misc Pub Entomol Soc Am 8:161, 1972.

Borror, D. J., DeLong, D. M., and Triplehorn, C. A.: An Introduction to the Study of Insects. 5th ed. Philadelphia, W.B. Saunders Co, 1981.

Chamberlain, R. W., and Sudia, W. D.: Mechanism of transmission of viruses by mosquitoes. Ann Rev Entomol 6:371, 1961.

Feingold, B. F.: Introduction to Clinical Allergy. Springfield, Ill., Charles C. Thomas, 1973.
Furman, D. P., and Catts, E. P.: Manual of Medical Entomology. 4th ed. Palo Alto, Calif., National Press Books, 1982.
Harwood, R. F., and James, M. T.: Entomology in Human and Animal Health. 7th ed. New York, Macmillan, 1979.
Hunter, G. W., III, Swartzwelder, J. C., and Clyde, D. F.: Tropical Medicine, 5th ed. Philadelphia, W. B. Saunders Co., 1976.
Krantz, G. W.: A Manual of Acarology. 2nd ed. Corvallis, Ore., State University Book Stores, Inc., 1978.
Krinsky, W. L.: Animal disease agents transmitted by horse flies and deer flies (Diptera: Tabanidae). J Med Entomol 13:225, 1976.
Smith, K. G. V. (Ed.): Insects and Other Arthropods of Medical Importance. London, Trustees of the British Museum (Natural History), 1973.
Southcott, R. V.: Arachnidism and allied syndromes in the Australian Region. Records Adelaide Children's Hosp 1:97, 1976.
Traub, R., and Wisseman, C. L., Jr.: The ecology of chigger-borne rickettsiosis (scrub typhus). J Med Entomol 11:237, 1974.
Wharton, G. W.: House dust mites. J Med Entomol 12:577, 1976.

PRINCIPLES OF ANTIMICROBIAL CHEMOTHERAPY OF INFECTIONS

19
DESCRIPTION OF ANTIMICROBIAL DRUGS

Abraham I. Braude, M.D., Ph.D.

CLASSIFICATION

Antimicrobial drugs may no longer be classified according to the organisms they inhibit because their spectra can be broadened by minor adjustments in structure or dosage. Classification of antibiotics and synthetic antimicrobial drugs is based instead on chemical structure or biochemical effects. Since the biochemical effects are considered in the next chapter, "Mechanisms of Action of Antimicrobial Drugs," a chemical classification will be presented here. All antimicrobial drugs are ring compounds; otherwise, the various groups have little structural similarity.

THE PEPTIDES. The penicillins, cephalosporins, bacitracin, and polymyxins are the most important peptide antibiotics. Their molecular weight seldom exceeds 3000. For this reason they are too small to be antigenic and stimulate neutralizing antibodies that would cause them to lose activity with continued administration. Small nonantigenic peptide antibiotics are a lucky evolutionary by-product in the molds and bacteria that produce these antimicrobial agents. They are small because they are synthesized by a pathway that does not depend on the elaborate system for coding amino acids and their sequences required for protein synthesis. It is likely that microbial peptides, including peptide antibiotics, evolved before the process of protein synthesis via nucleic-acid coding on ribosomes. Since the functions performed by peptides were later taken over by microbial proteins, the peptides can be regarded as "fossils" (Bodanszky and Perlman, 1969). The fact that the majority of these antibiotics have a cyclic structure is also consistent with the idea that they once performed a functional role in microbial metabolism because cyclic structures are found in enzymes and other functional proteins.

The Penicillins. The common nucleus of the penicillins is 6-aminopenicillanic acid, a cyclic dipeptide of L-cysteine and D-valine (Fig. 1). These are arranged in a basic structure consisting of a thiazolidine ring joined to a β-lactam ring. Individual penicillins differ with respect to the side chains attached to the common nucleus. The most important of the naturally occurring penicillins is penicillin G, containing a benzyl side chain (Fig. 1). Penicillin V is obtained when phenoxyacetic acid is added as a precursor to the fermentation medium so that a phenoxymethyl side chain becomes attached to the pencillin nucleus. This compound is well suited for oral use because of its resistance to gastric acid. Other penicillins are prepared by the synthetic addition of various groups as side chains to 6-aminopenicillanic acid after it has been isolated from *Penicillium* fermentation media. Depending on their chemical structure, these side chains can broaden the antimicrobial spectrum, protect the penicillin nucleus from acid hydrolysis, or protect it against penicillinase. In ampicillin, for example, the presence of an amino group in the phenyl radical of benzylpenicillin produces a compound both resistant to acid and more active against gram-negative bacteria than penicillin G. If a carboxyl group is introduced instead, as in carbenicillin, the spectrum is altered so that the compound becomes the only penicillin derivative with activity against *Pseudomonas aeruginosa*. None of these modifications, however, confers resistance to staphylococcal penicillinase. This was first accomplished in the synthesis of methicillin by the introduction of methoxy groups at positions 2 and 6 on the benzyl ring so that affinity of the substrate site for penicillinase is reduced 10,000 times (Novick, 1962). This modification did not achieve acid resistance, but the synthesis of isoxazolyl penicillin introduced a series of products with combined resistance to penicillinase and gastric acid. Oxacillin and dicloxacillin are the most widely used of these doubly resistant penicillins.

These and other penicillin derivatives have been modified further to improve their blood levels, broaden their antimicrobial spectrum and reduce side effects. The conversion of ampicillin to amoxicillin, by the introduction of a hydroxyl radical at the para position in the benzyl side chain, improves absorption. Absorption is also improved by conversion of amoxicillin to pivampicillin, the pivaloyloxymethyl ester of ampicillin. After absorption, pivampicillin is hydrolyzed first to pivalic acid and the hydroxymethyl ester of ampicillin; these are then hydrolyzed within 15 minutes to ampicillin and formaldehyde. Either modification provides blood levels after oral administration that are approximately twice that obtained with ampicillin (Neu, 1974).

The acid lability of carbenicillin in the stomach has been

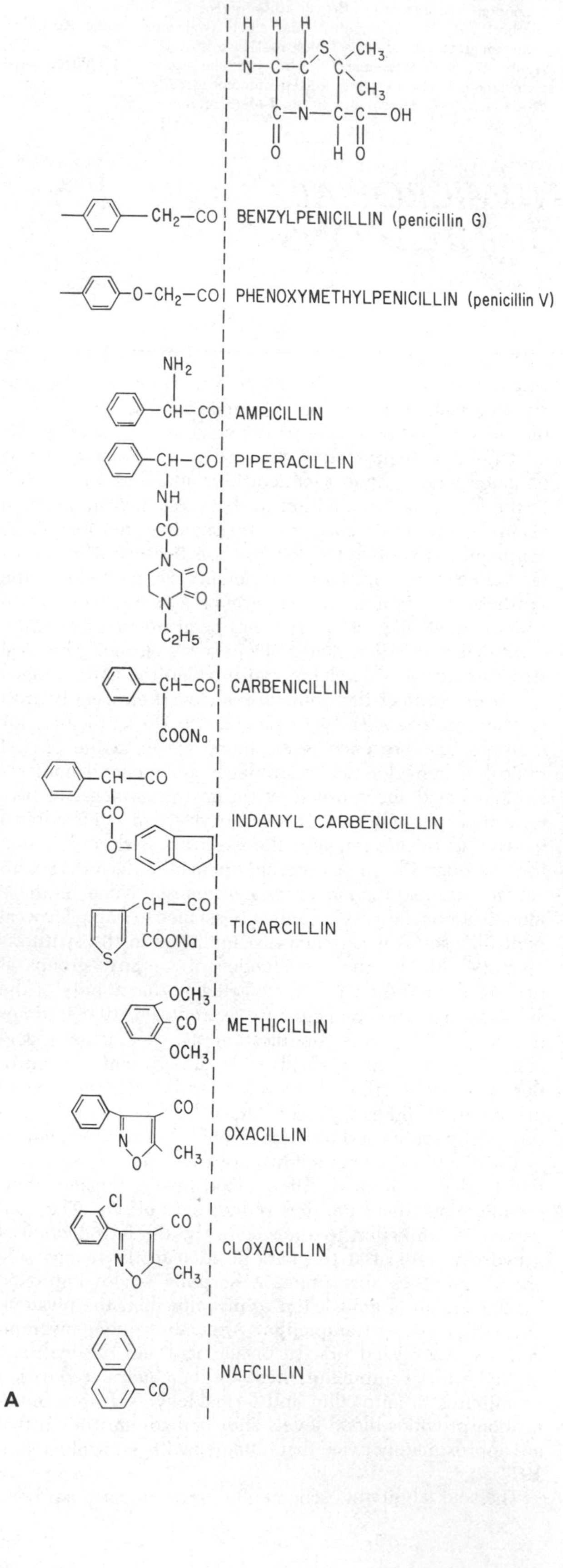

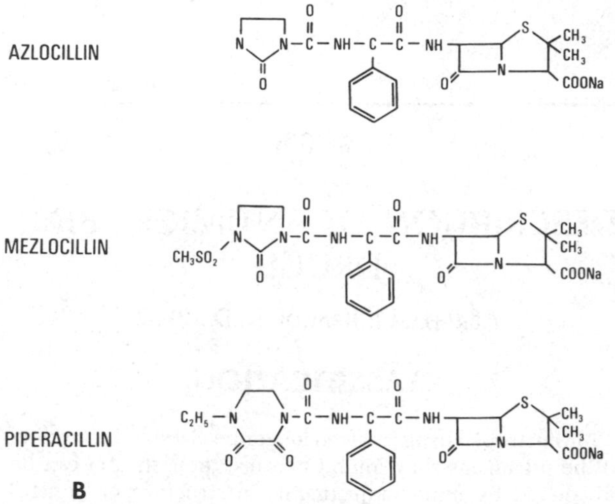

Figure 1. *A,* The side chains responsible for the biologic differences in each of the penicillins are shown to the left of the dotted line, and 6-aminopenicillanic acid is on the right. The last four side chains protect the β-lactam ring from the action of penicillinase. *B,* Substitutions on the free aminogroup of ampicillin are used to synthesize azlocillin, mezlocillin, and piperacillin, and thereby increase the range and potency of antibacterial action of the substituted compound.

overcome by converting it to the 5-indanyl ester, as indanyl-carbenicillin. In this compound the α-carboxylic acid moiety of carbenicillin is bound through ester linkage to 5-indanol and hydrolyzed after ingestion to active carbenicillin. The carbenicillin is then well absorbed. If the benzyl group in carbenicillin is replaced with the 5-carbon thienyl ring, the resulting compound, ticarcillin, is two to four times more active against *Pseudomonas aeruginosa*, but remains acid labile and must be given parenterally. Somewhat greater activity against *P. aeruginosa* is obtained with piperacillin. In this antibiotic, ampicillin is bound through its amino group to a derivative of piperazine. Similar substitutions on the free amino group of ampicillin were used to synthesize mezlocillin and azlocillin, which also show improved activity against *P. aeruginosa* (Fig. 1a). This substitution converts the amino group to a ureido group and the 2 drugs are, therefore, known as ureidopenicillins (Neu, 1983).

The Cephalosporins. The common nucleus of the cephalosporins resembles 6-aminopenicillanic acid but differs by having a dihydrothiazine ring, instead of a thiazolidine ring, attached to the β-lactam ring (Fig. 2). The active nucleus, known as 7-aminocephalosporanic acid, can also be manipulated chemically to yield more active and useful derivatives (Hewitt, 1973). The basic advantages of the cephalosporin nucleus are its innate resistance to staphylococcal penicillinase and its safety in patients with allergy to penicillin. These properties are retained in cephalothin (Fig. 3), in which the side chain at the 7-position increases its potency and range of activity. Another derivative, cephalexin (Fig. 3), has a different side chain at the 7-position that confers resistance to gastric acid and allows good absorption from the alimentary tract. Cefazolin (Fig. 3), with substitutions at both the 7- and 3-positions, can be injected intramuscularly without pain and possesses greater activity than cephalothin against certain bacteria.

Cefoxitin is derived from cephamycin C, which has a methoxy group at position 7 in 7-aminocephalosporanic acid. The methoxy group is responsible for the total resistance of this group to all β-lactamases, including that of all *Bacteroides fragilis*. At the same time, however, the 7α-methoxy group reduces antibacterial activity (Fig. 3). On other cephalosporins, such as cefotaxime, ceftizoxime, and cefuroxime, the β-lactamase resistance is increased by the α-methoxyimino group at the 7-acyl site; in cefotaxime and ceftizoxime the antibacterial activity is increased through the 5-aminothiazol group, which is joined to the methoxyimino group (Fig. 3a).

In addition to enhancing β-lactam resistance in cephalosporins, the 7α-methoxy group increases the β-lactamase resistance of the oxa-β-lactam drugs, of which moxalactam is the most important. Oxa-β-lactams have the same structure (Fig. 3a) as the cephalosporins except that oxygen is present in the place of sulfur in the dihydrothiazine ring. This difference accounts for greater antibacterial action in moxalactam. Moxalactam also differs from the cephalosporins in its ability to inactivate most of the chromosomally mediated cephalosporinases of gram-negative bacteria (Labia, 1982).

Bacitracin. This antibiotic is produced by a strain of *Bacillus subtilis*, which was isolated from the dirty compound fracture of a girl named Tracy and called "bacitracin" out of joint deference to the bacillus and patient (Johnson et al., 1945). The antibiotic consists of a mixture of polypeptides, the most important of which is bacitracin A. Like the penicillins, it contains a thiazolidine ring but does not have their β-lactam ring. In bacitracin A the thiazolidine ring is a condensation product of isoleucine and a cysteine residue and is attached through L-leucine to a peptide composed of D- and L amino acids (Fig. 4).

The Polymyxins. These cyclic polypeptides are also produced by a spore-forming aerobic bacillus, *Bacillus polymyxa*. Their detergent activity on bacteria can be attributed to two unique components: an amino acid, α,γ-diaminobutyric acid (DAB), and a C9 fatty acid, 6-methyloctanoic acid (Fig. 5). The cationic α-amino groups of DAB and the hydrophobic side chain of the fatty acid give the polymyxins the surface-active properties of a cationic de-

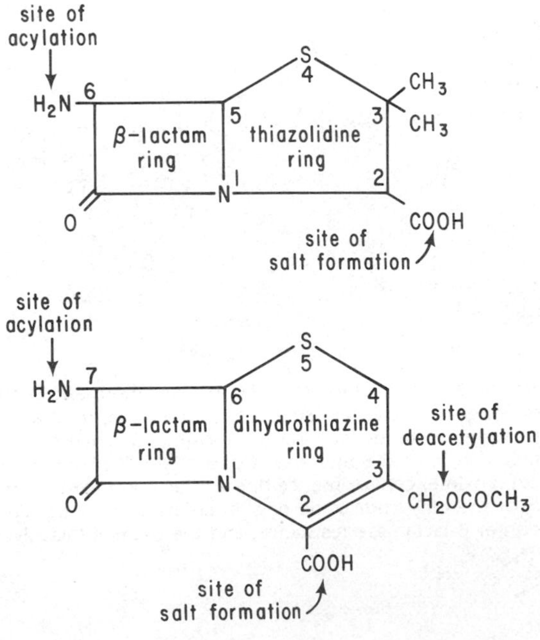

Figure 2. Comparison of penicillin nucleus, 6-aminopenicillanic acid (upper figure), with cephalosporin nucleus, 7-amino-cephalosporanic acid (lower diagram). The main difference in the two compounds is the thiazolidine ring in penicillin and the dihydrothiazine ring in the cephalosporins. Most penicillin derivatives are produced by addition of side chains at the acylation site. Cephalosporin derivatives vary in the chemical groups at the acylation site, and at the deacetylation site as well. For this reason, much greater variation in derivative antibiotics is possible with the cephalosporins than the penicillins.

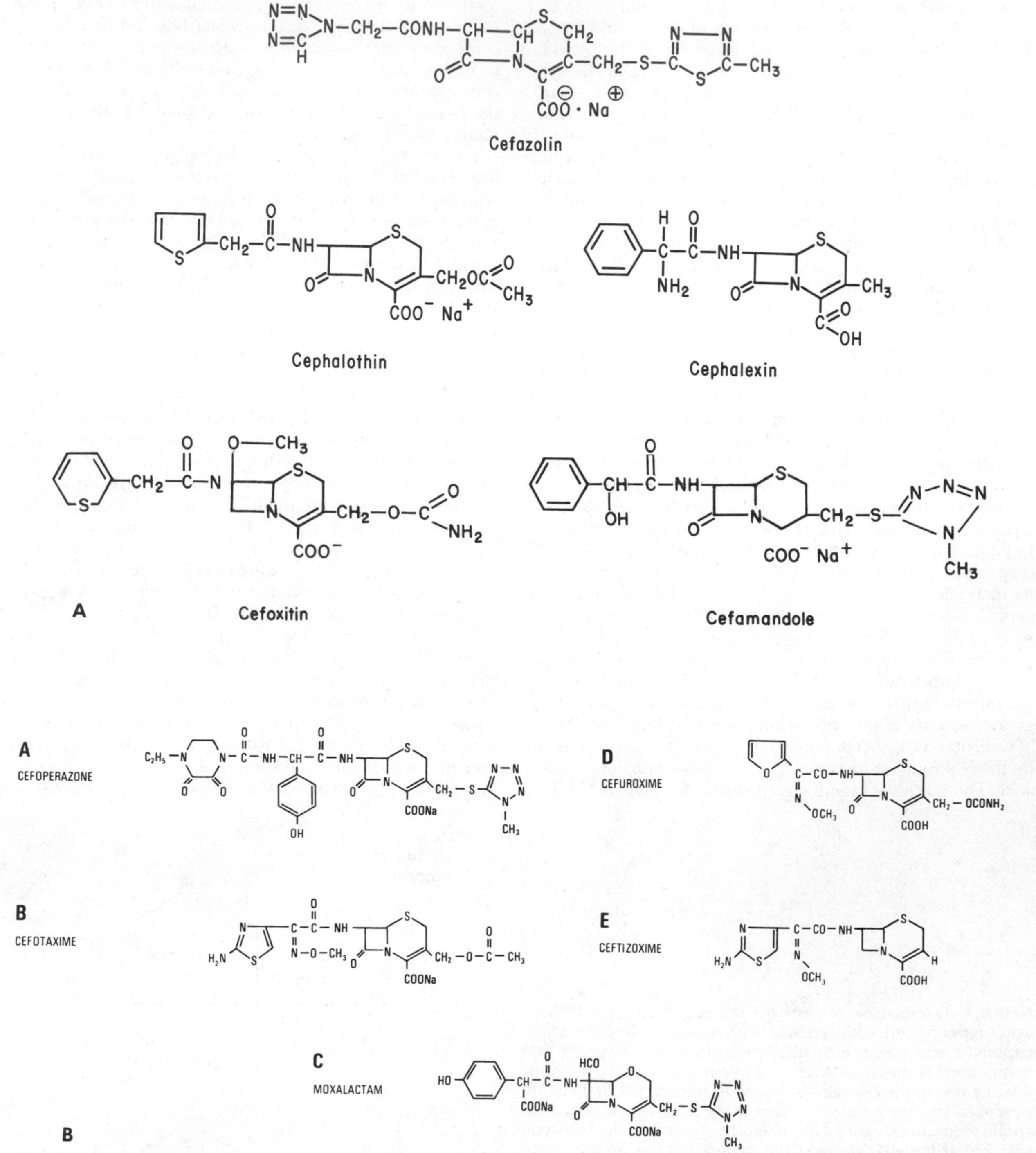

Figure 3. *A*, Structural formulas of five important cephalosporin derivatives illustrate differences in side chains at acylation and deacetylation sites. In general, substitutions at the 7-acyl site determine β-lactamase resistance and spectrum of antibacterial activity. Changes at the deacylation site (position 3) govern mainly the half-life in the circulation and absorption from the alimentary tract. In cefoxitin, e.g., the methoxy group at the 7-position results in total β-lactamase resistance. *B*, Structural formulas of cefotaxime, ceftizoxime, cefuroxime, cefoperazone, and moxalactam. Note that in moxalactam, oxygen is present in place of sulfur in position 5 of the dihydrothiazone ring. In cefotaxime, ceftizoxime, and cefuroxime, the α-methoxyimino group (A) at the 7-acyl site helps confer β-lactamase resistance, and the 5-aminothiazolyl group (B) to which it is attached improves the antibacterial activity.

BACITRACIN A

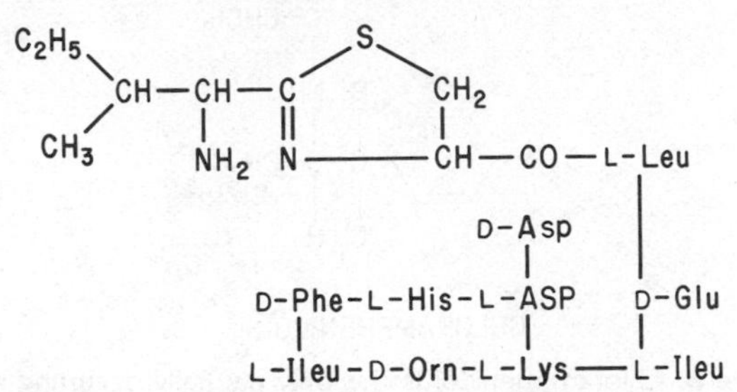

Figure 4. Like penicillin, bacitracin A contains a thiazolidine ring. It is a condensation product of isoleucine and cysteine, in contrast to that of penicillin which contains D-valine and L-cysteine. Bacitracin lacks the β-lactam ring of penicillin.

tergent. Only two of the polymyxins, B and E, are used in clinical medicine. Polymyxin E is generally known as colistin.

THE AMINOGLYCOSIDES. The aminoglycosides are derived from different species of *Streptomyces* and are composed of amino sugars. In contrast to penicillin, they are organic bases rather than acids. Streptomycin, neomycin, kanamycin, and paromomycin—listed in order of discovery—are all members of this group. They resemble each other because of the inositol residue and the prominent basic groups, ranging from three in streptomycin to six in neomycin. They differ in the sugars attached to inositol and in the guanidine groups of streptomycin (Fig. 6). This similarity in structure accounts for common toxic effects on patients and bacteria.

POLYMYXIN B

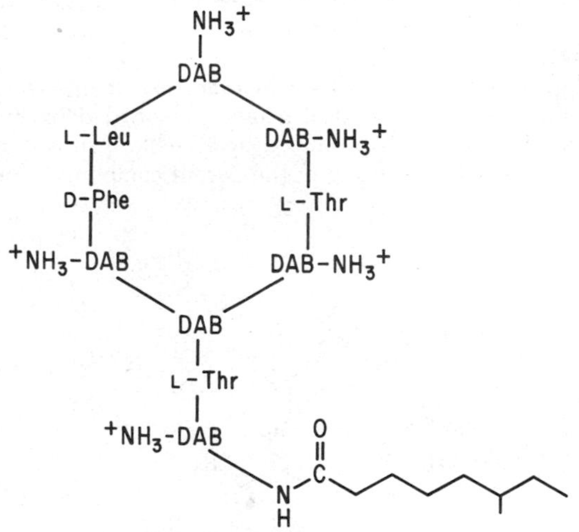

Figure 5. Diaminobutyric acid (DAB) is present in all polymyxins, including colistin (polymyxin E). The terminal residue of DAB is acetylated by 6-methyloctanoic acid, the C9 fatty acid at the bottom of the structural formula. The cationic α-amino group of DAB and the hydrophobic fatty acid are responsible for the surface-active properties of the cationic detergent.

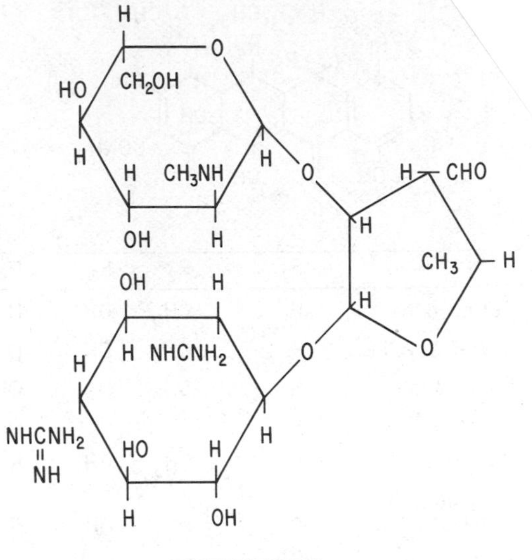

STREPTOMYCIN

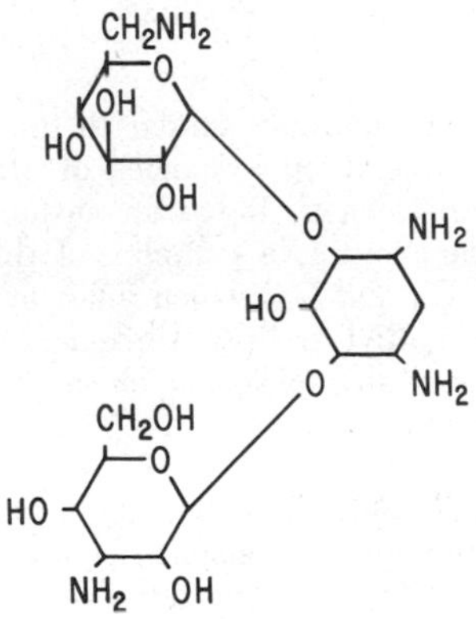

KANAMYCIN

Figure 6. The basic structure of the aminoglycosides, illustrated by kanamycin and streptomycin, is that of a polycationic compound composed of amino sugars and connected by glycosidic linkages. In streptomycin, the inositol residue common to both compounds is in the form of streptidine (the bottom sugar with two guanido groups), and in kanamycin it is deoxystreptamine (the central sugar with two amino groups). Amikacin and tobramycin are related structurally to kanamycin. In amikacin the lower amino group in the diagram of the deoxystreptamine nucleus (position 1) is replaced with a side chain consisting of:

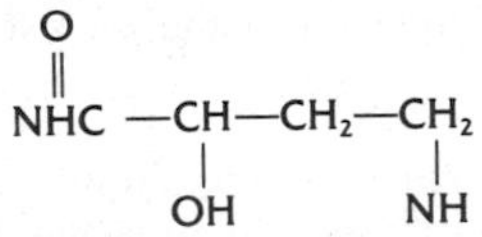

in order to increase its resistance to bacterial inactivating enzymes. In tobramycin the main differences from kanamycin are the absence of the first two hydroxyl groups in the upper ring and the presence of an amino group at position 1.

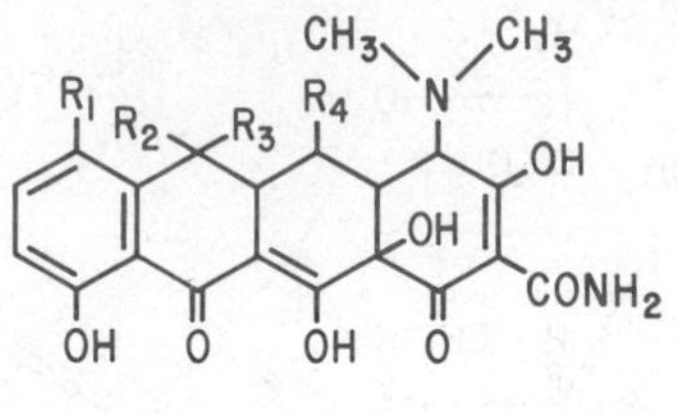

	R_1	R_2	R_3	R_4
Tetracycline	H	CH_3	OH	H
Oxytetracycline	H	CH_3	OH	OH
Doxycycline	H	CH_3	H	OH
Methacycline	H	CH_2		OH
Chlortetracycline	Cl	CH_3	OH	H
Demethylchlor-tetracycline	Cl	H	OH	H
Minocycline	$N(CH_3)_2$	H	H	H

Figure 7. The compounds of this group are named in relation to the basic structure of tetracycline and on the basis of substituted chemical groups at one or more of the four R positions.

Gentamicin is structurally similar to these aminoglycosides but is produced by a species of *Micromonospora* rather than *Streptomyces.* It has an inositol residue with two amino sugars and is a complex of three antibiotics (designated C_1, C_2, and C_{1A}) which differ in structure only by one or two methyl groups. Amikacin and tobramycin are related structurally to kanamycin as indicated in the legend to Figure 6.

THE TETRACYCLINES. The tetracyclines are so named because their common hydronaphthacene nucleus contains four fused rings (Fig. 7). Chlortetracycline (Aureomycin) was the first tetracycline compound described, and oxytetracycline (Terramycin) was discovered 2 years later, in 1950. Both compounds were produced by strains of *Streptomyces.* Although tetracycline was made by the catalytic reduction of chlortetracycline, all other compounds in this group are named in relation to the basic structure of tetracycline. In chlortetracycline a hydrogen is replaced by chlorine, and in oxytetracycline it is replaced by a hydroxyl ion. Demeclocycline (Declomycin) is chlortetracycline without the 6-methyl group, and doxycycline is oxytetracycline without the 6-hydroxyl group. These minor structural differences have less effect on their antimicrobial spectra than on stability in solution and pharmacologic properties. Chlortetracycline not only is less stable than the other tetracyclines but is the least stable of any important antibiotic.

CHLORAMPHENICOL. Chloramphenicol is the only naturally occurring antibiotic with nitrobenzene in its structure (Fig. 8). This chemical grouping probably accounts for its toxicity to both bacteria and patients. Its tendency to cause aplastic anemia is explained by its benzene ring, a component of most organic substances involved in that disorder. Its ability to compete with messenger RNA for ribosomal binding is explained by its spatial similarity to uridine-5-phosphate.

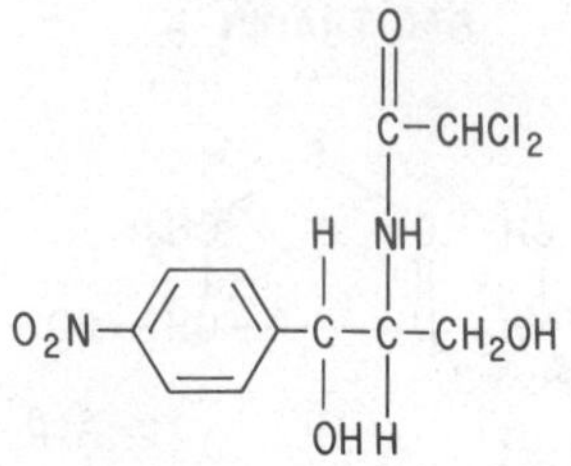

CHLORAMPHENICOL

Figure 8. Chloramphenicol is the only naturally occurring antibiotic with nitrobenzene in its structure, a property that may account for its tendency to cause aplastic anemia.

THE MACROLIDES. Erythromycin, isolated from *Streptomyces erythreus,* is the only important member of the macrolides. The basic structure is a large lactone ring to which unusual sugars are attached (Fig. 9). The term "macrolide" refers to the large ring, formed from a chain of 14 to 20 carbon atoms by lactone condensation of a carboxyl and hydroxyl group. The other 37 macrolides, such as oleandomycin, spiramycin, kitasamycin, and carbomycin, differ from erythromycin both in the structure of the lactone ring and in the attached sugars. Since the other macrolides have the same spectrum but are less potent than erythromycin, they are not widely used.

The avermectins, a group of macrolide-like compounds, possess an unusually broad spectrum of activity against certain nematodes, including the human filarial parasite *Onchocerca volvulus* (Aziz et al., 1982).

CLINDAMYCIN AND LINCOMYCIN. Despite some similarity in the biologic effects of clindamycin and erythromycin, their chemical structures are totally dissimilar. In contrast to the macrolides, clindamycin and lincomycin consist of an amino acid joined to a sulfur-containing amino sugar. The amino acid is trans-L-4-*n*-propyl hygric acid, and the amino sugar in lincomycin is methyl-α-thiol lincosaminide (Fig. 10).

Clindamycin is a synthetic modification of lincomycin. As indicated by its chemical name, 7-chloro-7-deoxylincomycin, clindamycin is produced by a 7-chloro substitution of the 7(R)-hydroxyl group of the parent compound, linco-

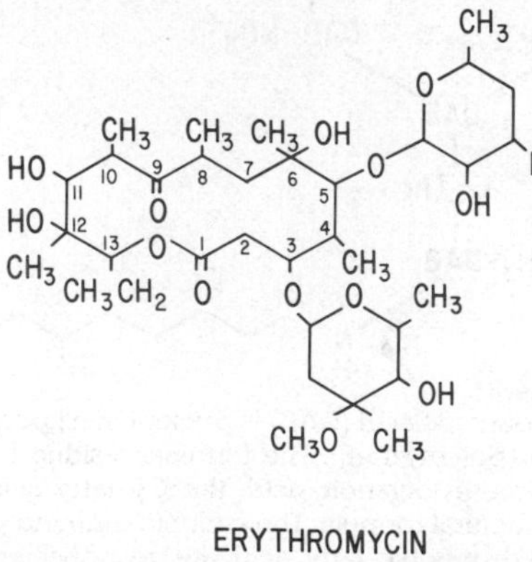

ERYTHROMYCIN

Figure 9. Erythromycin is the only important member of a group of 37 different compounds known as macrolides. The term "macrolide" refers to the large lactone ring formed from a chain of 14 to 20 carbon atoms by lactone condensation.

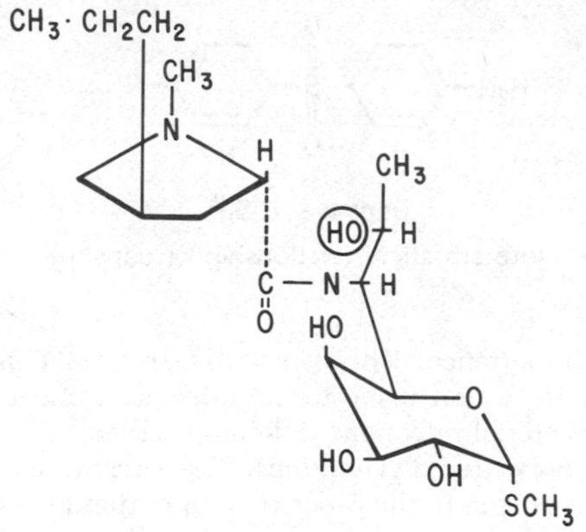

LINCOMYCIN

Figure 10. The sulfur-containing amino acid, methyl-α-thiol lincosamide, is named for the parent compound which was obtained from a mold growing in Lincoln, Nebraska. The circle indicates the 7-hydroxyl group where a chloro group is substituted in clindamycin.

mycin. These modifications in structure appear to increase absorption, blood levels, and antibacterial activity.

THE RIFAMYCINS. The rifamycin antibiotics are fermentation products of *Streptomyces mediterranei*. Their basic structure is an aromatic ring compound spanned by an aliphatic bridge. The most active of the original compounds, rifamycin B, was not well absorbed after ingestion. After the chemical structure of various rifamycins was determined in 1963, it was possible to synthesize a great many semisynthetic derivatives (Wehrli and Staehelin, 1971). Rifampin is the most important of these because it is orally effective in tuberculosis and leprosy, and in infections by various gram-negative and gram-positive bacteria. The special features of rifampin, shown in Figure 11, are the double ring compound, the long aliphatic bridge, and the side chain: CH = N — N ⬡ N — CH_3. The ring is a naphthohydroquinone and is the chemical grouping responsible for the red color of the antibiotic. The importance of the rifamycins lies not only in their currently important derivative, rifampin, but also in the great potential for new derivatives with activity against many different microorganisms, including viruses and fungi.

RIFAMPIN

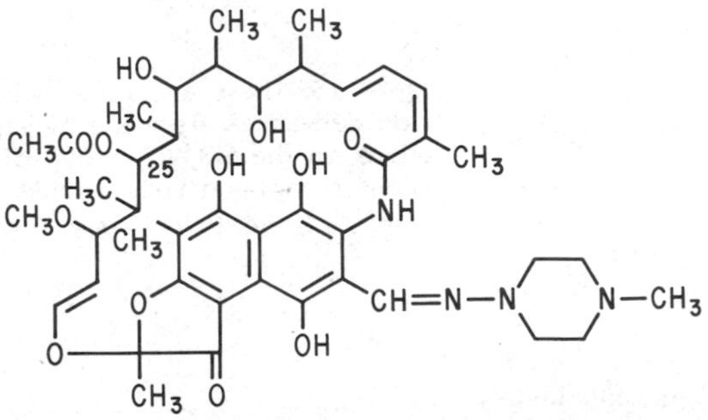

Figure 11. The basic structure of rifampin is the double ring compound spanned by a long aliphatic bridge, and the side chain.

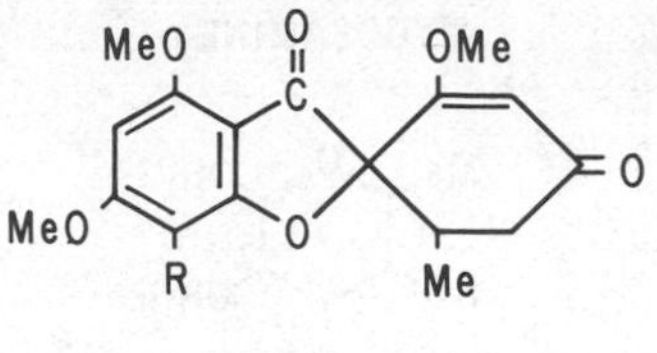

GRISEOFULVIN

Figure 12. Griseofulvin is a spirocyclic compound formed from acetate units. The condensed ring system of griseofulvin resembles that of the tetracyclines (Fig. 7).

VANCOMYCIN. Vancomycin is a bactericidal antibiotic produced by *Streptomyces orientalis*. The structure of vancomycin has been determined by x-ray analysis (Sheldrick et al., 1978). The principal units in the structure are a disaccharide linked to three aromatic rings: N-methylleucine, aspartic acid, and a biphenyl system. These units are connected by secondary amide bonds to form a tricyclic molecule containing N-terminal N-methylleucine and two free carboxyl groups.

GRISEOFULVIN. Although derived from *Penicillium* molds, griseofulvin is active against fungi rather than bacteria. Discovered in 1939 in London, by A. E. Oxford, griseofulvin was used against plant fungi before its value against human dermatophytes was demonstrated (Oxford et al., 1939). It has a spirocyclic structure formed from acetate units (Fig. 12).

THE POLYENES. Amphotericin B, nystatin, and pimaricin are polyenes. These antifungal antibiotics are classified as polyenes because the molecules contain a series of carbon atoms with four or five conjugated double bonds. Nystatin and amphotericin also possess the aminodeoxyhexose, mycosamine (Fig. 13), which is not present in many of the polyenes that are unsuitable for medical use (Dutcher et al., 1956). Their extensive unsaturation makes them unstable compounds, especially in acid or alkaline solutions. They are also unstable in light and air. Although the exact formula has not been worked out for either one, amphotericin B is known to be a conjugated heptaene lactone linked with mycosamine and has the tentative formula $C_{46}H_{73}O_{20}N$ (Fig. 14). It was first isolated in 1956 from *Streptomyces nodosus* and remains the most important antifungal drug in clinical medicine.

SYNTHETIC ANTIMICROBIAL DRUGS

The Sulfonamides. The term "sulfonamide" refers to derivatives of sulfanilamide, or π-aminobenzenesulfona-

PARTIAL STRUCTURE FOR AMPHOTERICIN B

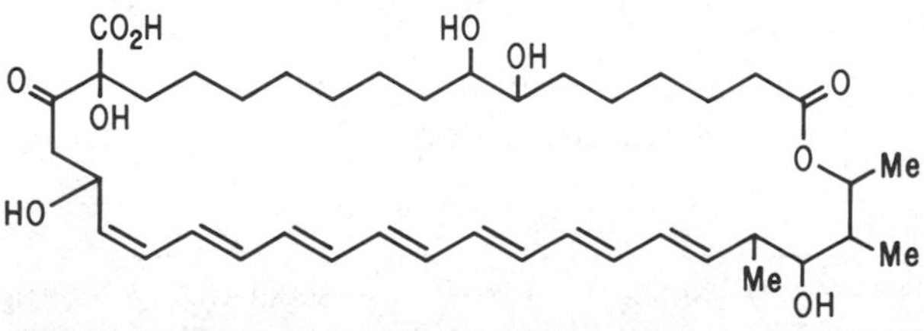

Figure 13. Amphotericin B is called a polyene because it contains a series of carbon atoms with multiple conjugated double bonds.

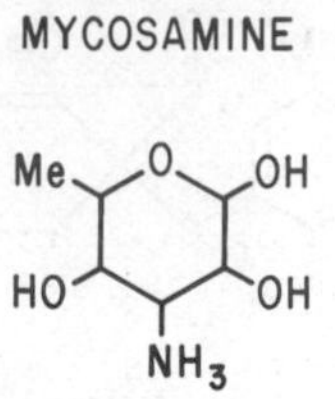

Figure 14. This amino sugar, mycosamine, is linked to a polyene in both amphotericin B and nystatin.

mide (Fig. 15), the first antimicrobial shown to be effective systemically for the treatment of human bacterial infection (Long and Bliss, 1937). Thousands of sulfonamides have been synthesized, but only a dozen are of value for patients.

Most derivatives are made by substitutions on the sulfonamide group (SO_2NH_2), since these increase the antimicrobial activity. The para-NH_2 group, on the other hand, must remain free, or become free, after hydrolysis. Succinylsulfathiazole (Sulfasuxidine) is a good example of how the para-NH_2 group becomes free after slow hydrolysis from its inactive form to the active sulfathiazole. The substitutions on the SO_2NH_2 group of other sulfonamides are shown in Fig. 15.

The Sulfones. As is evident from the structural formula of dapsone in Figure 16, sulfones are related to sulfonamides but lack the sulfonamide group and its broad antibacterial spectrum. Instead, the sulfones are limited in antibacterial activity to the leprosy bacillus.

Clofazamine. This lipid-soluble phenazone dye is used for sulfone-resistant leprosy (Fig. 17). It is superior to dapsone because it is both anti-inflammatory and antibacterial, and controls lepra reactions.

Isoniazid and Ethionamide. Isoniazid was the first modern chemotherapeutic agent synthesized (1912), but its value in tuberculosis was not appreciated until 1952 (Fox 1953). It is the hydrazide of isonicotinic acid (Fig. 18). Ethionamide is also a derivative of isonicotinic acid.

The Diaminopyrimidines. The diaminopyrimidine compounds were first synthesized as analogs of the nitrogenous bases found in DNA. Pyrimethamine, for example, was prepared as a thymine analog. This drug and trimethoprim are the only two members of this group that are of practical

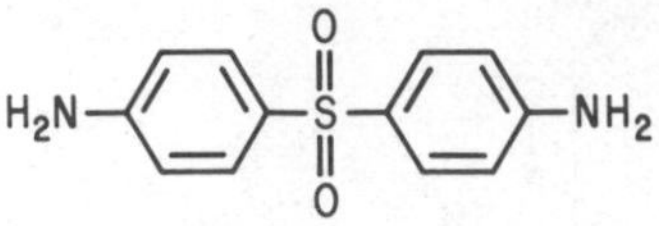

Dapsone, U.S.P.

Figure 16. Note structural relationship of dapsone to sulfonamides.

medical importance. Their formulas are given in Figure 19. Both are useful in protozoal infections, and trimethoprim in bacterial infections (Hitchings, 1969).

The Fluorinated Pyrimidines. The substitution of fluorine for hydrogen in the 5-position on pyrimidines was first made in order to produce the pyrimidine analog 5-fluorouracil, a potent antimetabolite for mammalian cells and useful in cancer chemotherapy. Another fluorinated pyrimidine, 5-fluorocytosine (5FC), does not seem to be metabolized in mammalian cells and has no activity against cancer cells. The activity of 5FC against microorganisms seems to be related to its conversion to 5-fluorouracil by deamination (Lacroute, 1969) (Fig. 20).

The Nitrofurans. The nitrofurans are derivatives of the 5-membered ring sugars known as furans and possess a nitro group in the 5-position. The chief nitrofuran available for clinical application is shown in Figure 21 and is the only sugar derivative with clinically important antibacterial properties.

Quinine and the Quinolines. Quinine shares the quinoline ring with the aminoquinolines (Fig. 22). For many centuries quinine was the standard treatment for malaria. Although displaced as the drug of choice after World War II by various synthetic antimalarials, it has become important again for treating chloroquine-resistant falciparium infections. Quinidine is the dextrorotatory isomer of quinine and also has antimalarial properties but is not used in malaria because its absorption is less than that of quinine. Quinine is manufactured by extraction from cinchona bark because synthesis is too expensive.

The most important member of the aminoquinolines is chloroquine, a 4-aminoquinoline with the structure shown in Figure 23. The main parts of the molecule are the quinoline nucleus composed of a double ring and the alkyl

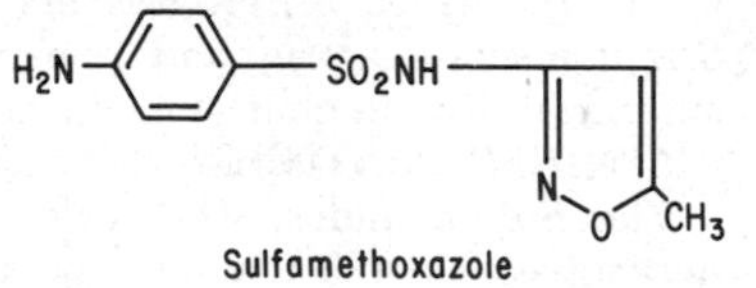

Sulfamethoxazole

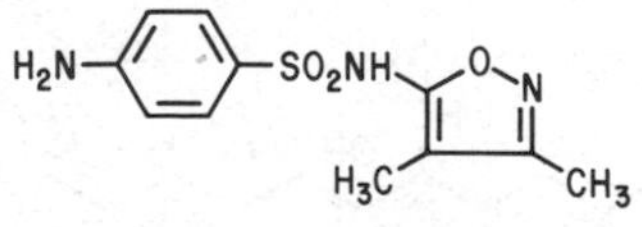

Sulfisoxazole, U.S.P.

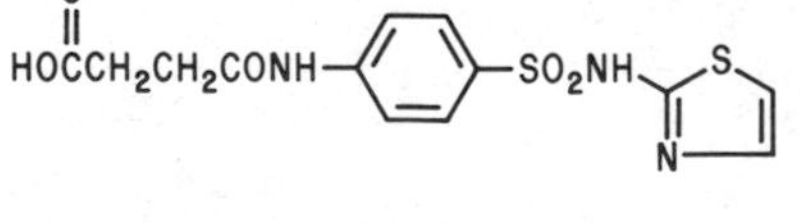

Succinylsulfathiazole, U.S.P.

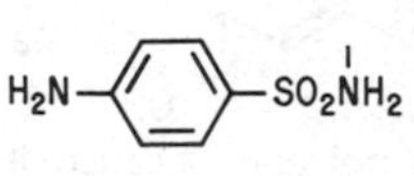

Sulfanilamide

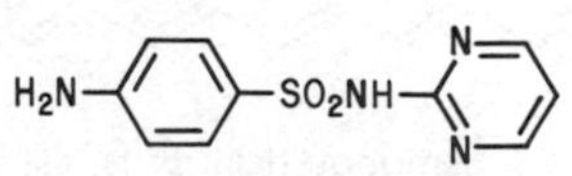

Sulfadiazine, U.S.P.

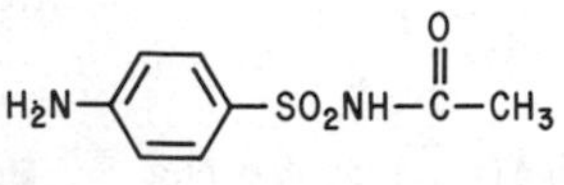

Sulfacetamide, N.F.

Figure 15. These and other sulfonamide derivatives are made by substitutions on the SO_2NH_2 group of the parent compound sulfanilamide. The para-NH_2 group must remain free.

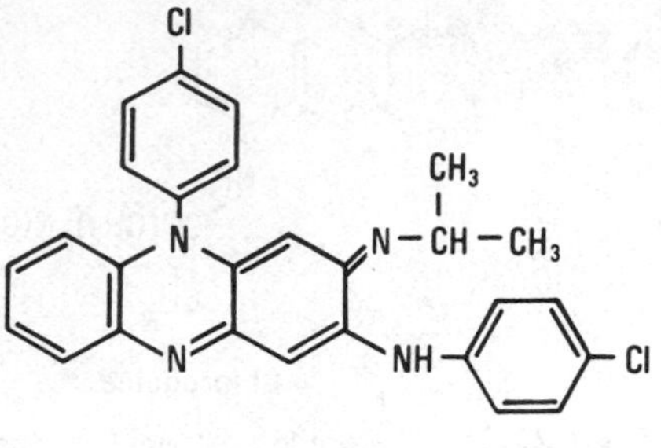

CLOFAZIMINE

Figure 17. This lipid soluble phenazine dye is useful in leprosy and other mycobacterial infections. It is unique among antimicrobials because it suppresses both the inflammation and the infecting organism.

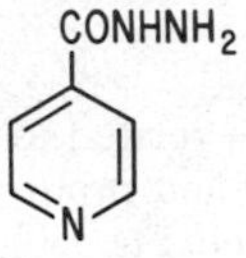

ISONIAZID

Figure 18. The drug isoniazid is a derivative of isonicotinic acid.

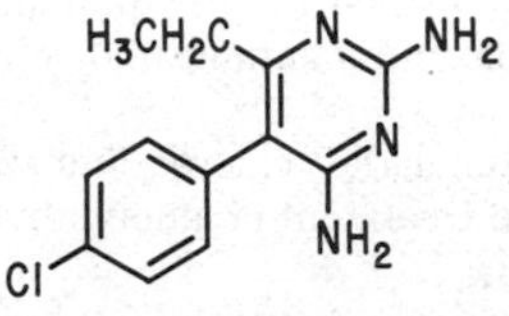

Pyrimethamine

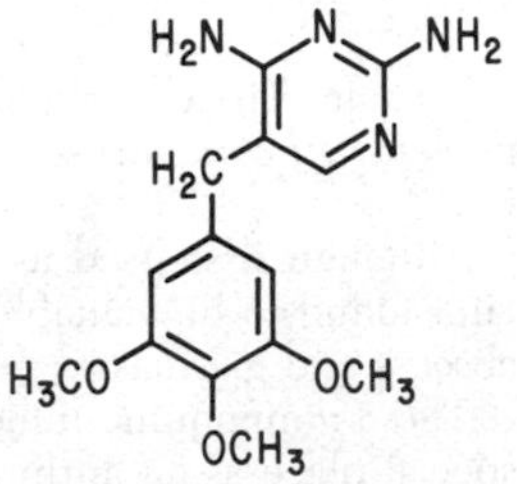

Trimethoprim

Figure 19. These diaminopyrimidines were first synthesized as analogs of the nitrogenous bases found in DNA.

DEAMINATION OF
5-FLUOROCYTOSINE TO 5-FLUOROURACIL

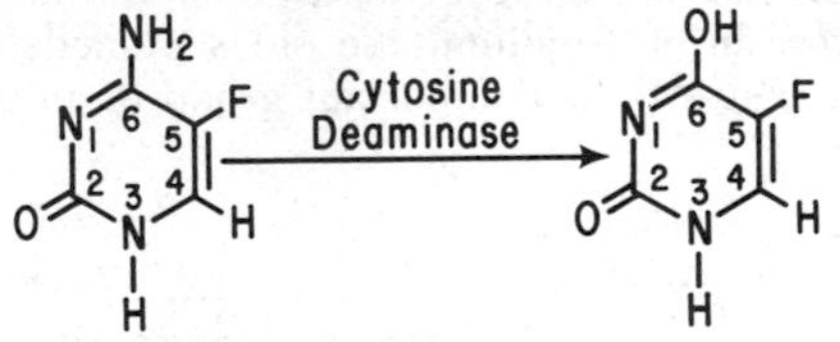

5-Fluorocytosine

5-Fluorouracil

Figure 20. The activity of 5-fluorocytosine against microorganisms seems to be related to its conversion to 5-fluorouracil.

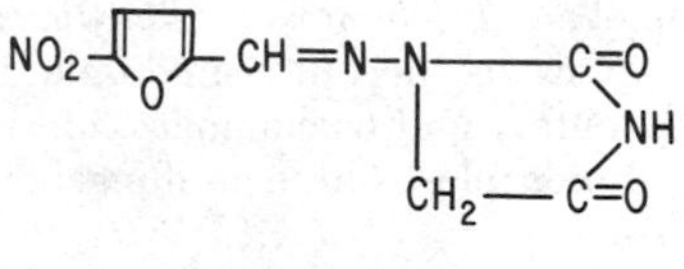

FURADANTIN

Figure 21. The nitrofurans are the only synthetic sugar derivatives with clinically useful antibacterial properties.

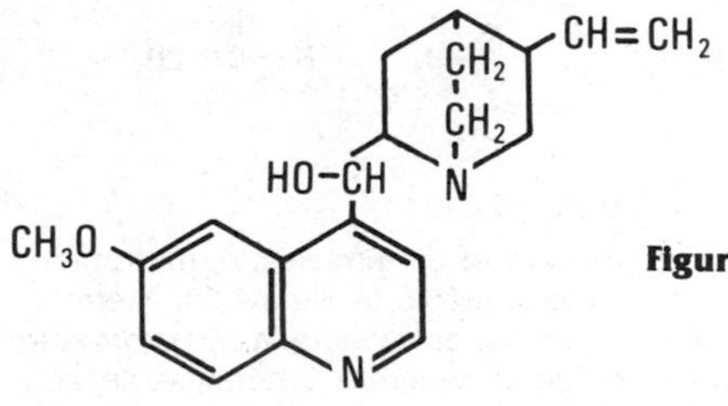

QUININE

Figure 22. Quinine.

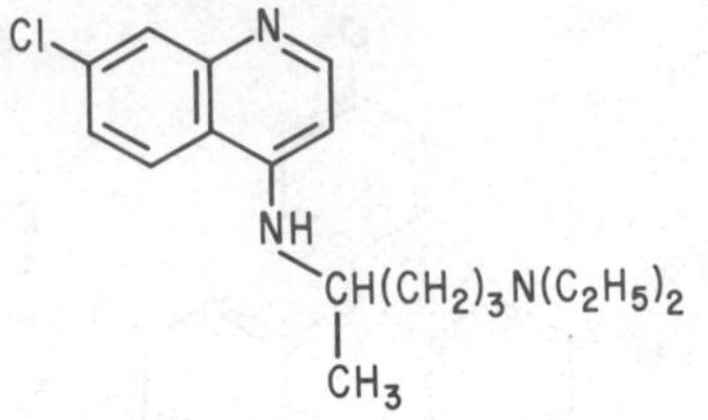

Chloroquine

Figure 23. The Cl atom in position 7 is necessary for maximum antimalarial activity of chloroquine. The length of the side-chain is also critical in allowing the drug to intercalate between the stacked base pairs of the DNA double helix. Thus, the two positively charged nitrogens are separated by 7.5 Å, which is the distance required to bridge the narrow groove of the helix and thereby link to the phosphodiester group in the complementary strands (Hahn, F. E.: in Antibiotics III. Mechanism of Action of Antimicrobial and Antitumor Agents (eds. J. W. Corcoran and F. E. Hahn), Springer-Verlag, Heidelberg, pp. 58–78, 1975).

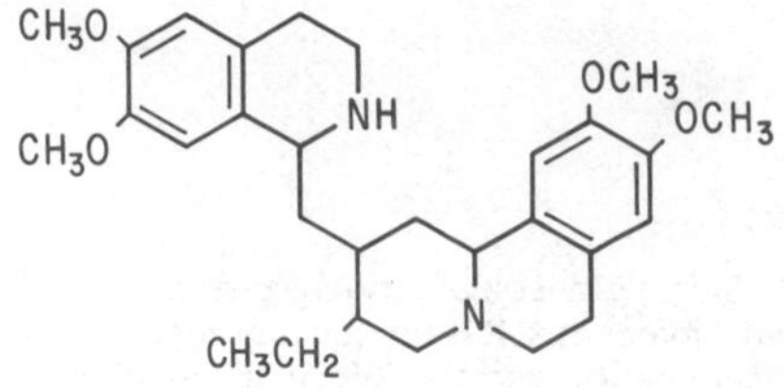

EMETINE

Figure 25. Emetine. This is the structure of the active principle of ipecac.

side chain. The chlorine atom in position 7 of the quinoline nucleus appears necessary for maximum antimalarial activity.

Although first used as an antimalarial, chloroquine was later found to be valuable in the treatment of amebic liver abscess and giardiasis.

The 8-aminoquinoquinoline, primaquine, (Fig. 24) has a special place as an antimalarial drug because it is the only compound that eradicates the exoerythrocytic stage of the parasite in the liver and thus achieves a radical cure of malaria. Before killing the schizonts in the hepatic tissue, primaquine is converted to quinoline-quinone derivatives by demethylation and oxidation. It is also the best gametocidal drug and prevents spread of malaria.

Emetine. Emetine is the oldest amebicidal drug and the active principle chiefly responsible for the clinical efficacy of ipecac in amebic infections. Emetine hydrochloride is obtained from ipecac as a hydrated hydrochloride (Grollman, 1966) (Fig. 25).

Nitroimidazoles. Metronidazole (Fig. 26) is the most widely used amebicidal drug. It is a nitroimidazole derivative active against two groups of anaerobic organisms, the anaerobic bacteria and the pathogenic protozoa, including amebae, *Trichomonas*, *Giardia*, and *Balantidium*. Tinidazole is another nitroimidazole drug effective in amebic dysentery and trichomonas infections.

Imidazoles. Three antifungal drugs, clotrimazole, miconazole, and ketoconazole, are imidazoles that are related to the nitroimidazoles used for anaerobic bacteria and protozoa (Figs. 26 and 26a). The benzimidazoles (see Fig. 30) are potent anthelmintics. Clotrimazole is limited to topical use for ringworm and moniliasis of the skin, but miconazole can be given intravenously for generalized fungus infections. Ketoconazole, the newest imidazole, is well absorbed orally and is effective against dermatophytoses, mucocutaneous candidiasis, and several deep seated mycoses.

The Anthelmintics (Bueding, 1969). The simplest structure of the anthelmintics, a group of nitro ring compounds, is that of piperazine, a drug used unsuccessfully at first for the treatment of gout but later found to be highly effective against *Ascaris* and *Enterobius* worms. Modification of piperazine (Fig. 27) by substituting a diethylcarbamyl group at the 1-position and a methyl group at the 4-position created diethylcarbamazine, a drug that can kill adult filaria and microfilaria. Bephenium is a quaternary amine and resembles acetylcholine in both structure and function (Fig. 28). The anticestodal drug, niclosamide (chlorsalicylamide), resembles closely the structure of desaspidin, the active principle of oleoresin of aspidium, the oldest remedy for tapeworms (Fig. 29). Another important group of anthel-

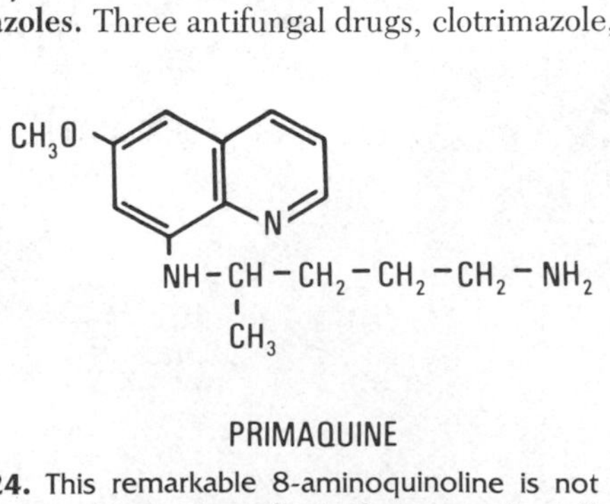

PRIMAQUINE

Figure 24. This remarkable 8-aminoquinoline is not only the sole compound that can eradicate the exoerythrocytic stage of malaria from the liver, but is also the best gametocidal drug. In other words, it achieves radical cure and prevents spread of malaria.

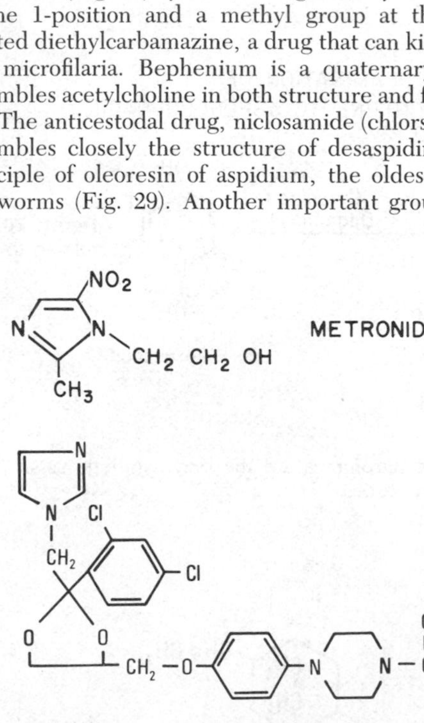

A METRONIDAZOLE

B KETOCONAZOLE

Figure 26. *A* and *B*. Comparison of nitroimidazole, metronidazole, with the imidazole, ketoconazole in Figure 6a. Metronidazole attacks anaerobic organisms only (bacteria and protozoa) after the nitro group is reduced, whereas ketoconazole acts against fungi, which are aerobic. Compare also the benzimidazoles (Fig. 30), which are also active against anaerobes—the intestinal worms.

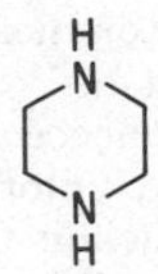

PIPERAZINE

Figure 27. Piperazine has the simplest structure of the anthelmintics.

mintics are the substituted benzimidazole compounds. One of these, thiabendazole, is effective against various round worms, while mebendazole in the only anthelmintic effective against both tapeworms and round worms. The formula of thiabendazole is shown in Figure 30. The only compound with a close structural resemblance to antibacterial drugs is niridazole, which is derived from a nitrothiazole nucleus (Fig. 31). Its structure is related to that of nitrofurantoin and metronidazole, two agents with antibacterial activity.

One of the most important new anthelmintics is praziquantel (Fig. 32) a synthetic isoquinoline that is remarkably effective in cysticercosis, the larval form of *Taenia solium*, the pork tapeworm. It is also valuable in schistosomiasis chlonorchiasis, paragonimiasis, and various tapeworm infections.

MICROBIAL SUSCEPTIBILITY TO DRUGS

The antimicrobial activity of a drug is generally expressed as its minimum inhibitory concentration in nutrient broth or agar. The test conditions would seem far removed from those in infected tissues or body fluids, but there is a remarkable correlation between successful treatment of the patient and inhibitory concentrations in the laboratory.

Microbial inhibition is measured either by serial dilution or by diffusion of antibiotics. In the dilution tests the antibiotic is diluted serially in broth or agar, and results are expressed as the lowest concentration that inhibits growth of a standard bacterial inoculum at 37° C. Three

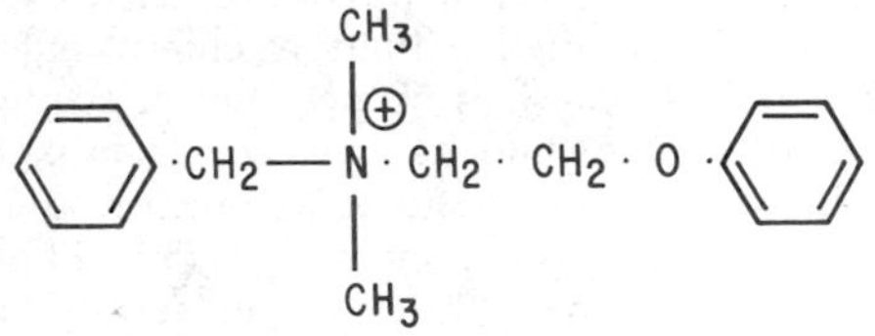

BEPHENIUM

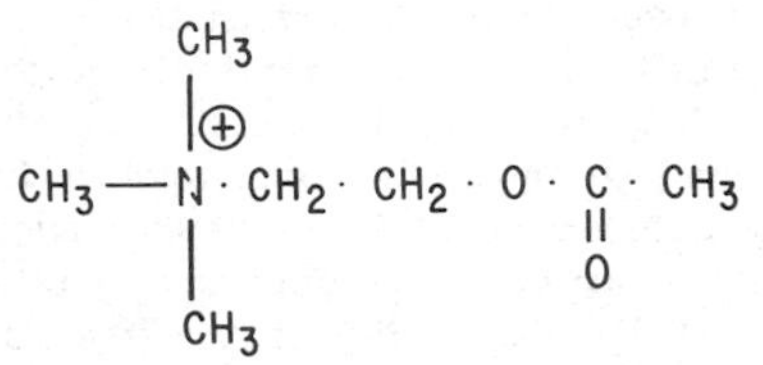

ACETYLCHOLINE

Figure 28. The anthelmintic bephenium resembles acetylcholine in structure and action. Bephenium paralyzes nematodes by causing membrane depolarization of muscle in the worms.

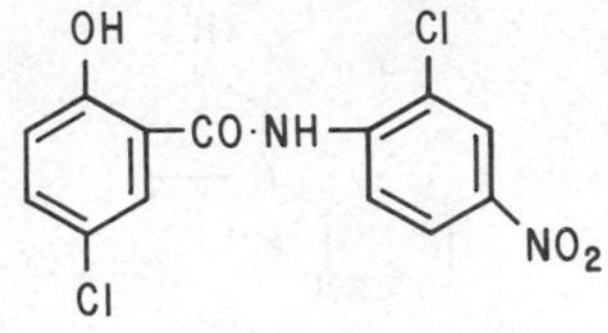

NICLOSAMIDE

Figure 29. Niclosamide resembles in structure desaspidin, the active principle of oleoresin of aspidium, an old remedy for tapeworms.

diffusion tests are used: the disk test, the filter strip, and the gradient plate. In the disk test, antibiotics are incorporated into filter paper disks, and the minimum inhibitory concentration is calculated indirectly from the diameter of the inhibitory zone (Bauer et al., 1966; Ericsson et al., 1954) (Fig. 33). Long filter paper strips can be used instead of disks. The strips have the advantage of measuring inhibitory concentrations against multiple strains of bacteria that are streaked perpendicularly to the strip.

The gradient plate is prepared by pouring agar with a given concentration of antibiotic in square Petri dishes that are tilted so that the agar solidifies on a slant. The plate is then placed on a flat surface and an equal volume of agar without antibiotic is poured over the slanted agar to provide a horizontal layer, as shown in Figure 34. The antibiotic diffuses into the upper layer to give a perfect linear gradient ranging from zero to the concentration present in the original layer. Multiple strains can be streaked on the agar surface along the gradient. The minimum inhibitory concentration is directly related to the distance bacterial growth extends from the zero end of the gradient.

The gradient plate method is the best quantitative method for laboratories that need to perform sensitivity on many strains because multiple organisms can be examined on one plate and there is little room for error (Braude et al., 1954). The disk test is the most widely used (despite a number of disadvantages) because it lends itself to commercial distribution and has been publicized. It is not quantitative, however, and can only indicate in a general way whether an organism is very, moderately, or not susceptible to an antibiotic. It has been standardized for use mainly with rapidly growing bacteria, such as *Enterobacteriaceae*, but is not suitable for testing sensitivity of many slow-growing organisms. It is not reliable for testing susceptibility to drugs that diffuse slowly, such as the polymyxins. Another limitation with the disk method is the occasional failure to detect strains of staphylococci that are resistant to penicillin (Sherris and Washington, 1980). These resistant staphylococci are easily recognized by tests for penicillinase. The simplest is a rapid capillary tube assay that should be carried out routinely in all laboratories

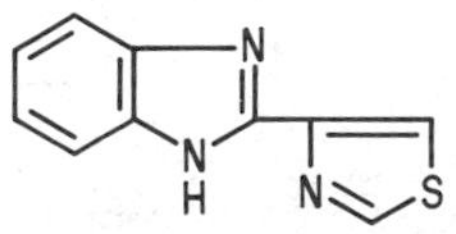

Thiabendazole

Figure 30. Thiabendazole is the best anthelmintic among several hundred substituted benzimidazole compounds.

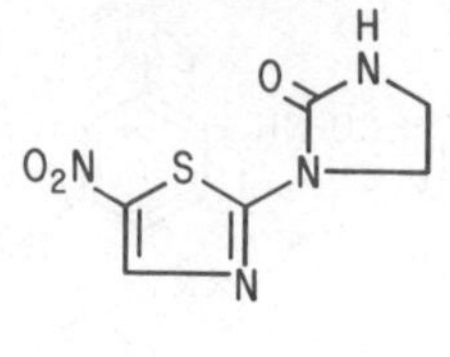

NIRIDAZOLE

Figure 31. Niridazole. Note structural similarity of this anthelmintic to the antibacterial drug nitrofurantoin.

(Rosen et al., 1972). It is based on the change in pH that occurs when staphylococcal penicillinase hydrolyzes penicillin to penicilloic acid.

The values given below for antibiotic sensitivity are derived from either dilution methods or the gradient plate and are a composite of results from our laboratory and several other representative laboratories.

THE COCCI. With the exception of certain staphylococci, gonococci, and enterococci, cocci remain exquisitely sensitive to penicillin G (benzylpenicillin). Pneumococci, hemolytic streptococci, meningococci, anaerobic streptococci, and *Streptococcus viridans* are usually inhibited by less than 0.1 μg/ml and frequently by as little as 0.01 μg/ml (Table 1), although a few strains of each of these bacteria display some resistance to penicillin. This resistance is a special problem when resistant pneumococci occasionally cause meningitis (Chapters 21 and 165). Although such resistance amounts only to 0.5 to 1 μg/ml, this is high enough to exceed levels of penicillin in the spinal fluid that can be reached by parenteral therapy. This degree of resistance is not enough to block the effectiveness of penicillin in the lung, joints, blood, or paranasal sinuses where high levels of penicillin are achieved. Staphylococci are seldom sensitive to penicillin. Staphylococci that produce penicillinase cannot be treated with benzylpenicillin at any dosage. The number of staphylococci that produce penicillinase varies among hospitals. At the University Hospital in San Diego 90 per cent do so. Before 1960, 95 per cent of gonococci were sensitive to 0.1 μg/ml benzylpenicillin, but now less than half are inhibited by this concentration, and 1.0 μg/ml is necessary to inhibit 95 per cent of gonococcal strains in many communities. Complete resistance to penicillin is produced by penicillinase-producing gonococci, which appeared in 1976. This plasmid-determined resistance is common in the Phillipines, but quite rare in the United States.

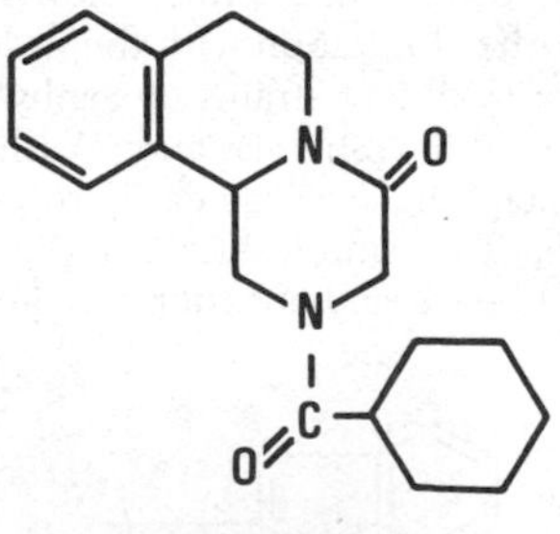

PRAZIQUANTEL

Figure 32. This synthetic isoquinoline is the first medical cure for cerebral cysticercosis, the larval stage of *Taenia solium* infection. It is also valuable against schistosomiasis and other helminth infections.

In contrast to those gonococci and staphylococci that have lost initial sensitivity, enterococci have always been relatively resistant to penicillin G. Enterococci generally grow readily in 1.0 μg/ml and usually require 3 to 6 μg/ml for inhibition.

Modification of penicillin G to acid-resistant or penicillinase-resistant compounds causes loss in antibacterial power. In penicillin V and ampicillin the loss of activity against most cocci is usually slight; in fact, ampicillin is more active than penicillin G against the enterococci. *Neisseria* show the biggest differences in sensitivity between penicillin V and G, with the meningococcus and penicillin-sensitive gonococci requiring concentrations of penicillin V four times greater than those of penicillin G for inhibition.

The penicillinase-resistant penicillins show greater loss of activity against penicillin-sensitive cocci. Methicillin is 35 to 40 times less active than penicillin G against streptococci and penicillinase-negative staphylococci. Cloxacillin, oxacillin, and dicloxacillin are approximately 8 to 12 times less active than penicillin G against pneumococci, various streptococci, and penicillinase-negative staphylococci (Hammerstrom et al., 1966; Sutherland et al., 1970). The same, except for a little more activity against the pneumococcus, is true for nafcillin. All four inhibit penicillinase-producing staphylococci in a range of 0.15 to 1 μg/ml.

The related group of penicillinase-resistant antibiotics, the cephalosporins, are also less active than penicillin against all cocci (Table 2). The new cephalosporin, cefotaxime, approaches benzylpenicillin in potency in vitro against the group A streptococcus and the *Neisseriaceae* but otherwise the cephalosporins are considerably less active against cocci than is benzylpenicillin (Kayser, 1971). The cephalosporins are so inactive against the enterococcus that they are useless in infections with that organism (Benner, 1968; Sabath et al., 1973).

Tetracyclines have lost some of their potency against cocci. In all species of cocci, strains have appeared that are too resistant for treatment with this group of antibiotics. Resistance to tetracyclines has been most marked among the enterococci, but many staphylococci have also developed resistance beyond the limits of clinical efficacy. In certain hospitals as many as 50 per cent of staphylococci show such resistance while staphylococci from patients in outpatient clinics remain sensitive. So much resistance has developed among strains of pneumococci (5 to 23 per cent) and group A streptococci (20 to 40 per cent) (Matsen et al., 1969) that tetracyclines cannot be relied on for the treatment of pneumonia or sore throat unless sensitivity tests establish their susceptibility. Among anaerobic gram-positive cocci, tetracycline resistance is a lesser problem. In contrast to the aerobic gram-positive cocci, over 90 per cent of *Neisseria* remain sensitive to the tetracyclines, which can cure most cases of gonorrhea. One tetracycline, minocycline, has also been somewhat effective in treating pharyngeal carriers of meningococci (Guttler et al., 1971). The in vitro susceptibility of sensitive strains of cocci to the tetracyclines is shown in Table 3.

Certain tetracycline analogs seem to be more active in vitro against cocci that are resistant to other tetracyclines (Steigbigel et al., 1968). Minocycline is the best example of this phenomenon since it inhibits in low concentrations

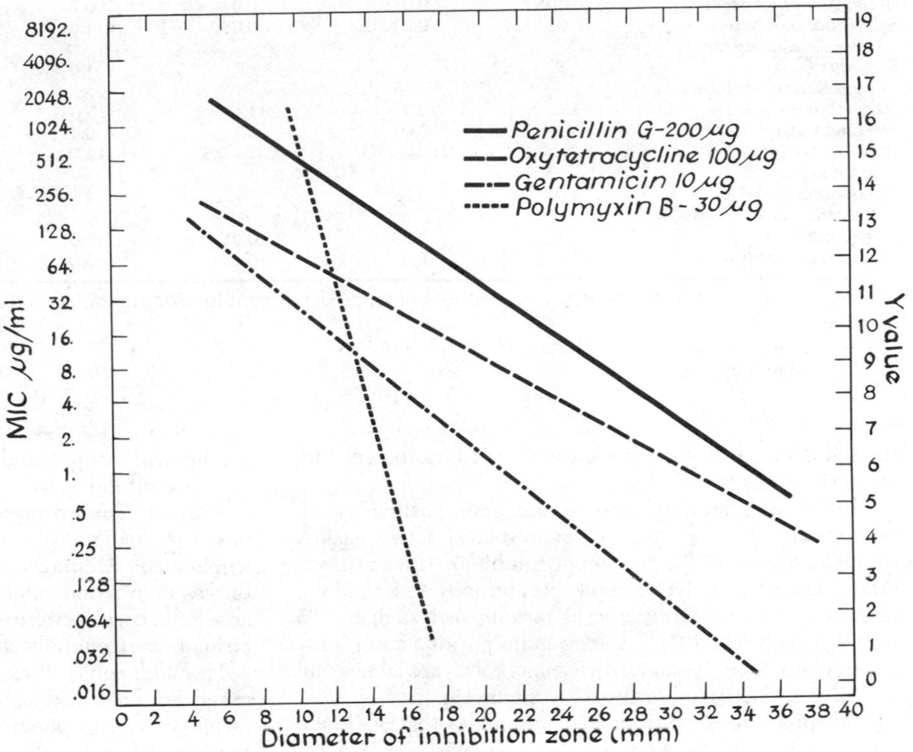

Figure 33. Determination of antibiotic sensitivity by disk method is based on correlation between zone diameter and minimum inhibitory concentration. Regression lines for minimum inhibitory concentrations and inhibitory zone diameter are shown for penicillin G (200 µg), oxytetracycline (100 µg), gentamicin (10 µg), and polymyxin B sulfate (30 µg). (From Stamey, T. A.: Urinary Infections. © 1972, The Williams and Wilkins Co., Baltimore, p. 45.)

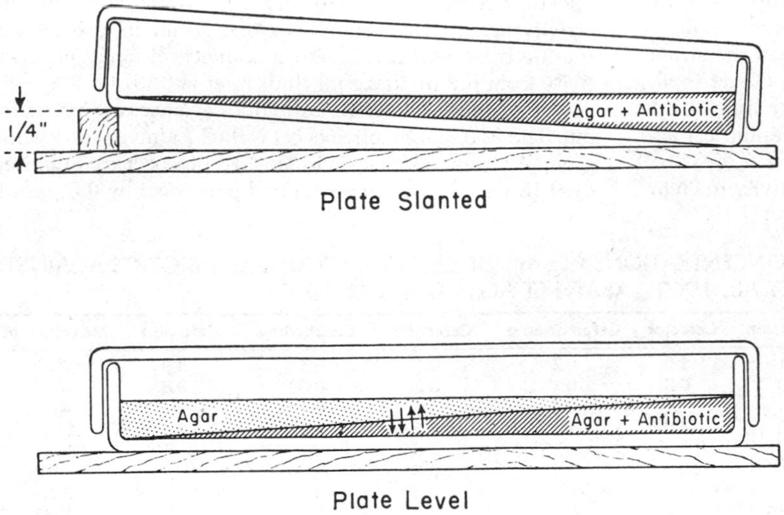

Figure 34. Diagram of procedures used for preparing gradient plates. The extreme right end of the completed plate (bottom) is where the gradient begins; there is initially no dilution of antibiotic at this point. Halfway across the plate (arrows) there is a twofold dilution of antibiotic. At the extreme left there is virtually no antibiotic and its concentration is zero. Thus a uniform linear gradient is formed by the vertical diffusion of antibiotic. (From Braude, A. I., Banister, J., and Wright, N.: Use of the gradient plate for routine clinical determinations of bacterial sensitivities to antibiotics. Antibiot Annu p. 1134, 1954–1955.)

Table 1. USUAL MINIMUM INHIBITORY CONCENTRATIONS (μg/ml) OF PENICILLIN DERIVATIVES AGAINST COCCI

	Benzyl-penicillin	Phenoxymethyl-Penicillin	Ampicillin*	Methicillin	Oxacillin	Dicloxacillin	Nafcillin
Pneumococcus	0.01	0.03	0.02	0.1	0.5	0.15	0.04
Group A streptococcus	0.005	0.015	0.02	0.2	0.02	0.05	0.02
Staphylococcus aureus (penicillinase-negative)	0.03	0.03	0.05	1.0	0.30	0.15	0.40
S. aureus (penicillinase producer)	R	R	R	1.0	0.40	0.10	0.50
Streptococcus faecalis	3.6	3.2	1.6	> 25.0	> 25.0	—	25.0
Streptococcus viridans	0.01	0.01	0.1	0.1	—	—	0.06
Gonococcus (penicillin susceptible)	0.01–0.5	0.03–> 3.0	0.03–0.5	12.0	12.0	0.06–4.0	—
Gonococcus (penicllin resistant; penase negative)	4.0	4.0					
Meningococcus	0.03	0.25	0.05	6.0	—	6.0	6.0
Peptostreptococcus	0.2	0.5	0.2	2.0	0.6	2.0	< 25.0

*The activity of amoxicillin is very similar to that of ampicillin, except for *Streptococcus faecalis.* Amoxicillin inhibits most strains of *S. faecalis* at 0.6 μg/ml.
R = Resistant to all concentrations.
– = Inadequate data.

staphylococci, group A streptococci, and enterococci that are resistant to tetracycline.

Clindamycin inhibits most of the gram-positive cocci, but not the *Neisseriaceae.* Clindamycin is active against staphylococci, and the minimum inhibitory concentration (MIC) against hemolytic streptococci (groups A, B, and C), pneumococci, and *Streptococcus viridans* is less than 0.05 μg/ml (Chadwick, 1971). Among gram-positive cocci, only enterococci are resistant. Anaerobic cocci are almost all sensitive to 1.0 μg/ml or less of clindamycin.

The spectrum of erythromycin resembles that of clindamycin except for the *Neisseriaceae* (Chadwick, 1971; Griffith and Black, 1970). Most strains of gonococci and meningococci are inhibited by 1.0 μg/ml of erythromycin. The pyogenic streptococci and pneumococci are inhibited by 0.04 μg/ml, and sensitive staphylococci by 0.4 μg/ml. Staphylococci sometimes become resistant to erythromycin, especially in the hospital. Strains of group A streptococci (Sanders et al., 1968) and pneumococci are rarely resistant, but in some large hospitals over half the strains of enterococci are resistant to erythromycin (Toala et al., 1969). Other enterococci range in sensitivity from 0.1 to 1.5 μg/ml erythromycin. Most anaerobic streptococci also fall in this range of sensitivity (Martin et al., 1972).

The cocci do not show the exquisite sensitivity to chloramphenicol often found with other antibiotics, but most cocci are inhibited by 1 to 4 μg/ml and acquired resistance is unusual. The average pneumococcus or group A streptococcus, for example, is inhibited by 3.0 μg/ml of chloramphenicol. Meningococci tend to be more sensitive, with the average strain inhibited by 1.0 μg/ml. Staphylococci, anaerobic cocci, enterococci, gonococci, and *Streptococcus viridans* are generally sensitive to 4 μg/ml or less.

The aminoglycosides are less active against cocci than other antibiotics that interfere with protein synthesis. Streptococci and pneumococci are naturally resistant, and the *Neisseria* generally show only marginal sensitivity. The staphylococci are an exception, because kanamycin and gentamicin are both highly active against them, and some strains are sensitive to streptomycin (Simon, 1968).

Staphylococci range in sensitivity to gentamicin from 0.1 to 1.0 μg/ml, and to kanamycin from 0.4 to 4.0 μg/ml. Spectinomycin is the only aminoglycoside with enough activity against the gonococcus to warrant its use for the routine treatment of gonorrhea. Gonococci range in sensitivity from 6.2 to 25 μg/ml (Judson et al., 1974).

One of the most active antibiotics against cocci is rifampin. The MIC for staphylococci is 0.02 μg/ml or less, while group A streptococci and viridans streptococci are inhibited by 0.12 μg/ml, meningococci and gonococci by 0.5 μg/ml,

Table 2. USUAL MINIMUM INHIBITORY CONCENTRATIONS (μg/ml) OF CEPHALOSPORIN ANTIBIOTICS AGAINST COCCI (LEVISON ET AL., 1969, SABATH ET AL., 1973, NEU, 1983)

	Cephalothin	Cephalexin	Cefaclor	Cefamandole	Cefazolin	Cefotaxime	Cefoxitin	Moxalactam
Pneumococcus	0.6	3.1	1.0	0.2	0.1	0.3	3.0	2
Group A streptococcus	0.1	1.0	0.8	0.1	0.2	0.03	0.8	4
Group B streptococcus	0.4			0.4		0.1		4
Staphylococcus aureus	1.6	6.0	4.0	1.6	0.6	3.1	6	4–16
Staphylococcus epidermidis	0.6–25	12.0		1–25	1.0	8	6.3–50	8–32
Streptococcus faecalis	50.0	50.0	60.0		50.0	> 128	> 50.0	> 128
Streptococcus bovis	0.4					0.8		3.1
Streptococcus viridans	0.4	6.25		0.4	0.3	0.4	12.0	8–32
Gonococcus (B-lactam sensitive)	4.0	4.0	0.02–2.0	3.1	4.0	0.05	0.5–4.0	0.06
Gonococcus (penicillin resistant; B-lactamase negative)		2.0–> 50					1.0–8.0	
Gonococcus (B-lactamase +)		2.0–25.0					1.0–4.0	
Meningococcus	1.6	100.0				0.02	0.5–1.5	0.05

Table 3. USUAL MINIMUM INHIBITORY CONCENTRATIONS (μg/ml) OF TETRACYCLINES AGAINST SENSITIVE STRAINS OF COCCI

	Tetra-cycline	Doxy-cycline	Mino-cycline
Staphylococcus aureus	0.3	0.8	0.8
Group A streptococcus	0.3	0.2	0.2
Pneumococcus	0.3	0.1	0.1
Peptostreptococcus	1.6	0.8	0.8
Gonococcus	0.8	0.8	0.8
Gonococcus (penicillin resist; penase neg)	8.0	—	—
Gonococcus (penase pos)	8.0	—	—
Meningococcus	0.8	0.8	0.8

group B streptococci by 1.0 μg/ml and anaerobic streptococci by 1.6 μg/ml (Lester, 1972). Many pneumococci are inhibited by less than 1.0 μg/ml but 4.0 μg/ml are needed to inhibit 90 per cent of strains. Only enterococci have too much innate resistance for clinical effectiveness of the drug. Acquired resistance to rifampin among staphylococci and other cocci occurs readily and limits its usefulness.

Only one other antibiotic, vancomycin, deserves brief mention for its use against cocci. Its main value is for enterococcal or staphylococcal endocarditis in patients with severe penicillin allergy (Friedberg et al., 1968). The MIC for vancomycin against enterococci is 0.3 to 3.0 μg/ml and for staphylococci, it is 5.0 μg/ml or less.

Most other antimicrobials have little place in the treatment of coccal infections. The polymyxins are inactive against cocci, and antimicrobials other than antibiotics are of such limited value that they need not be discussed here. An exception is trimethoprim, whose antimicrobial spectrum is described later.

THE BACILLI. Penicillin G is highly effective against all gram-positive bacilli and many gram-negative bacilli. Most enteric bacilli are relatively resistant but the penicillin derivatives, ampicillin, carbenicillin, pipericillin, ticarcillin, azlocillin, and mezlocillin usually inhibit these gram-negative rods in concentrations that can be reached in infected body fluids. The gram-positive rods, *Listeria monocytogenes, Actinomyces israelii,* the clostridia, *Erysipelothrix rhusiopathiae, Bacillus anthracis,* and *Corynebacterium diphtheriae,* are all very sensitive to penicillin, and most are inhibited by less than 0.1 μg/ml. Certain important gram-negative rods such as *Haemophilus influenzae, Pasteurella multocida, Streptobacillus moniliformis,* and most *Bacteroides* other than *Bacteroides fragilis* are also sensitive to penicillin in a range of 0.5 to 2.0 μg/ml (Table 4). Despite impressions to the contrary, ampicillin is not superior to penicillin G against *H. influenzae*. Most careful studies in the United States have shown that the MIC of both antibiotics against *H. influenzae* ranges from 0.2 to 1.6 μg/ml, with a median near 0.8 μg/ml (McLinn et al., 1970). A few strains have developed resistance, but since this is mediated by a β-lactamase, both drugs are ineffective against them.

Enteric bacilli are considerably less sensitive to penicillin G than the rods listed in Table 4 (Sabath et al., 1973; Steigbigel et al., 1967). Table 5 shows the greater susceptibility of these organisms to ampicillin, carbenicillin and various later penicillin derivatives. These penicillin derivatives inhibit sensitive strains of *Proteus mirabilis* and *E. coli* at a concentration of 3.0 μg/ml or less, and are active in a range achieved clinically against all gram-negative bacilli listed except for a few strains of each species that has developed resistance.

The older cephalosporins differ from the penicillins and the newer cephalosporins in the poor activity of the former against *H. influenzae* (Table 6). Another notable difference is the greater activity of most cephalosporins against *Klebsiella pneumoniae* than that shown by ampicillin and penicillin G. *Enterobacter aerogenes, Serratia,* indole + *Proteus,* and *Pseudomonas* are resistant to the older cephalosporins (Edmondson and Sanford, 1967) but not to most of the newer ones (Table 6a). *E. aerogenes* is especially sensitive to cefotaxime, ceftizoxime, and moxalactam; *S. marcescens* to cefoperozone, cefotaxime, ceftizoxime, and moxalactam; and *P. aeruginosa* to cefoperozone, ceftizoxime, and moxalactam.

Erythromycin and clindamycin are effective in vitro against *Bacteroides* (Martin et al., 1972) and the gram-positive rods, but not against enteric gram-negative bacilli. Erythromycin also shows activity against *H. influenzae* and *B. pertussis.* Table 7 compares the activities of these two antibiotics against bacilli. The activity of clindamycin against *Campylobacter fetus* subsp. *jejuni* is noteworthy.

All the rods, both gram-positive and gram-negative, were initially sensitive to the tetracyclines and chloramphenicol, but some resistance has developed among the enteric bacilli. Table 8 shows that *Pseudomonas aeruginosa,* indole + *Proteus,* and most *Serratia* are beyond the reach clinically of chloramphenicol and tetracycline.

The aminoglycosides differ from other antibiotics in the weakness of their inhibitory action against anaerobes (Martin et al., 1972) but show potent in vitro activity against nearly all other bacilli. The usual MIC of streptomycin, kanamycin, and gentamicin against aerobic gram-negative bacilli is given in Table 9. Two MIC values are given for a number of enteric bacteria because of differences in sus-

Table 4. USUAL MINIMUM INHIBITORY CONCENTRATIONS (μg/ml) OF BENZYLPENICILLIN AGAINST SENSITIVE BACILLI

Gram-positive rods	
Listeria monocytogenes	0.2
Actinomyces israelii	0.06
Clostridium perfringens	0.16
Bacillus anthracis	0.02
Corynebacterium diphtheriae	0.08
Erysipelothrix rhusiopathiae	0.03
Gram-negative rods	
Hemophilus influenzae	0.8
Hemophilus ducreyi	1.0
Pasteurella multocida	0.4
Streptobacillus moniliformis	0.01
Bacteroides oralis	1.6
Bacteroides melaninogenicus	1.0
Fusobacterium nucleatum	0.8
B. actinomycetems comitans	6.25
Eikenella corrodens	2.0
Campylobacter jejuni	20.0
Legionella pneumophila	3.2
Bordetella pertussis	0.5

Table 5. COMPARISON OF USUAL MINIMUM INHIBITORY CONCENTRATIONS (μg/ml) OF SEVEN PENICILLIN DERIVATIVES FOR ENTERIC GRAM-NEGATIVE RODS

	Benzyl-penicillin	Ampicillin*	Ticarcillin	Carbenicillin	Azlocillin	Piperacillin	Mezlocillin
E. coli	100.0	1.6–500	16–>128	12.0	8–>128	3.1–500	8–>128
P. mirabilis	50.0	1.0–32.0	0.5–16	1.6	0.5–16	0.8	0.5–16
K. pneumoniae	> 100.0	25.0–400.0	> 128	> 200.0	32–>128	> 200.0	8–>128
Enterobacter aerogenes	> 500.0	20.0–250.0	2–>128	6.0	2–>128	50.0	4–>128
S. marcescens	> 500.0	40.0–100.0	32–>128	12.0–400.0	32–>128	3.1–500	64
P. aeruginosa	> 500.0	> 200.0	32–128	50.0–100.0	3–128	12.0	16–>128
Proteus vulgaris	> 100.0	3.0–100.0	16–64	2.0–25.0	16	2	16
Other indole + Proteus	> 100.0	3.0–50.0	16–64	1.0–12.0	16	1.6–500	16
Salmonella species	12.0	6.0		12.0	4–>128	1.6–500	4–>128
Pseudomonas pseudomallei	25.0	10.0		> 100.0			

*Amoxicillin activity against gram-negative rods is very similar to that of ampicillin except that amoxicillin is approximately four times as active against Salmonella strains (Neu, 1974).

Table 6. USUAL MINIMUM INHIBITORY CONCENTRATIONS (μg/ml) OF CEPHALOSPORINS FOR PATHOGENIC BACILLI

	Cefazolin	Cephalothin	Cefaclor	Cephalexin	Cefoxitin
Gram-positive rods					
Listeria monocytogenes	—	2.0	—	64.0	—
Actinomyces israelii	—	2.0–> 100		—	0.5–32.0
Clostridium perfrigens	—	0.6	12.0	1.2	1.2
Bacillus anthracis	—	0.6	—	2.0	—
Gram-negative rods					
Haemophilus influenzae	40.0	6.0–10.0	1.0	6.0–20.0	2.0
Pasteurella multocida	—	0.6	—	2.0	—
Bacteroides fragilis	> 200.0	25.0	> 100	25.0	10.0
Bacteroides oralis	—	0.1	—	—	—
Bacteroides melaninogenicus	—	0.2–6.0	—	—	1.0
Fusobacterium nucleatum	2.0	1.0	—	—	2.5
E. coli	0.4	6.0	3	12.0	3.0
P. mirabilis	8.0	6.0	6	20.0	1.0
K. Pneumoniae	5.0	6.0	12	20.0	4.0
E. aerogenes	6.0–400.0	50.0–> 400.0	> 100	> 100.0	> 75.0
S. marcescens	> 400.0	> 100.0	—	> 100.0	> 200.0
P. aeruginosa	> 400.0	> 400.0	—	> 100.0	> 100.0
Indole + *Proteus*	200.0	100.0–400.0	> 100	> 100.0	125.0
Salmonella spp.	6.0	2.0	0.8	4.0	3.0
Shigella spp.	1.0	8.0	0.8	12.0	—
Pseudomonas pseudomallei	—	> 1000.0	—	—	—

— = Inadequate data. The antibacterial activity of cephradine is nearly identical to that of cephalexin.

Table 6A. USUAL MINIMAL INHIBITORY CONCENTRATIONS (μg/ml) OF β-LACTAMASE RESISTANT CEPHALOSPORINS AGAINST PATHOGENIC BACILLI (JORGENSEN ET AL., 1980; KAYE ET AL., 1980; JONES AND BARRY, 1983)

	Cefoxitin	**Cefoperozone**	**Cefotaxime**	**Ceftizoxime**	**Cefuroxime**	**Moxalactam**
Gram positive rods						
Listeria monocytogenes	100	50	8	2	0.12	> 64
Actinomyces israelii	0.06		0.12			0.5
Clostridium perfringens	1	3.1–> 100	2–4		4	0.5
Clostridium difficile	64		128		> 128	100
Gram negative rods						
Haemophilus influenzae	3.1	0.1	0.06	0.05–1.6		0.8
Pasteurella multocida	0.5		0.06		0.06	0.06
Bacteroides fragilis	6.3–5.0	50–100	25–100	3.1–25	16	6
Bacteroides melaninogenicus	0.2–50	0.4–100	0.06–2		1	10
Fusobacterium nucleatum	3–50	0.8–12	0.5	0.5–128	0.5	0.6
E. coli	1.6–6.3	2	0.06–0.12	.06	2–4	0.06–12
S. marcescens	16–64	3–12	0.25–4	8	> 128	0.5–10
K. pneumoniae	3.1	5	0.1	0.1	2–4	0.125
E. aerogenes	> 128	32–> 128	0.06–4	8	4–64	0.12–0.5
P. aeruginosa	> 200	5–20	20–60	2–12	> 128	8–32
P. mirabilis	3.1	1.5	0.12	0.06	1.6–25	0.3
M. morganii	12.5	1.3–25	0.06	0.026	16–32	0.125
P. rettgeri	8–128	1.3–25	0.06–1	0.02–6	8–32	0.06–0.5
Yersinia enterocolitica	16	2	0.03–0.5		4	0.25
B. actinomycetem comitans	6.2		0.4		0.8	
Salmonella spp	2–7	0.4–25	0.08–25	0.04	1.6–6.3	0.1
Providencia spp	4	4	1	0.04		
Citrobacter freundii	2–128	0.4–12	0.06–1	0.1	4–16	0.25
Acinetobacter anitratus	64–128	70	16–32	6.3–25	32–64	32–64
Aeromonas hydrophila	4–64	2	0.06		2	0.06
Campylobacter jejuni			3–6		160	12.5–50
Shigella spp	25	0.4–6	0.025	0.025	12.5	0.2
Legionella pneumophila	1.0	32			3	32

Table 7. USUAL MINIMUM INHIBITORY CONCENTRATIONS (μg/ml) OF ERYTHROMYCIN, LINCOMYCIN, AND CLINDAMYCIN AGAINST SUSCEPTIBLE BACILLI

	Erythromycin	Cindamycin
A. israelii	0.12	—
L. monocytogenes	2.0	—
C. diphtheriae	1.6	—
C. perfringens	1.5	0.8
B. anthracis	0.6	—
H. influenzae	3.0	6.0
P. multocida	3.1	—
B. fragilis	2.0	0.2
B. oralis	0.1	0.1
B. melaninogenicus	0.4	0.01
F. nucleatum	1.6	0.4
C. jejuni	0.5	0.8
B. actinomycetems comitans	6.25	12.5
Eikenella corrodens		64.0
Legionella pneumophila	< 0.5	

— = Inadequate data.

ceptibility between "street" and "hospital" strains and because of variations from one community or hospital to another. The in vitro sensitivities of *Salmonella* and *Brucella* are misleading because streptomycin and kanamycin are not effective in treating brucellosis or *Salmonella* infections.

The polymyxins—polymyxin B and colistin methane sulfonate—are also impotent against the anaerobes, as well as the gram-negative bacilli, *Proteus, Serratia, Brucella,* and *P. pseudomallei.* Most strains of *E. coli, K. pneumoniae,* and *P. aeruginosa* are inhibited by 2.5 μg/ml or less of either drug. *Salmonella, Shigella,* and *H. influenzae* are even more sensitive (0.2 to 0.4 μg/ml), but the polymyxins are seldom used to treat infections by these three groups of organisms.

Rifampin is effective against *H. influenzae* (Atlas and Turck, 1968; Kunin et al., 1969), *H. ducreyi, Legionella* spp and actinobacilli. It also inhibits *Listeria monocytogenes* in therapeutically achievable concentrations (< 0.25 μg/ml). The enteric gram-negative bacilli, on the other hand, generally have too much innate resistance for rifampin therapy in most infections by these bacteria (Table 10).

Among the sulfonamides, sulfadiazine and sulfisoxazole will inhibit most enteric bacilli in concentrations of 8 to 64 μg/ml in the absence of acquired resistance. Of the gram-negative rods, *P. aeruginosa* is most likely to be innately resistant to these concentrations. Acquired resistance to sulfonamides is so common among all bacteria, however, that sensitivity tests are usually needed to predict results.

Many gram-negative bacilli are also susceptible to nalidixic acid in concentrations of 20 to 50 μg/ml. *Klebsiella, E. coli, P. mirabilis,* and indole + *Proteus* organisms are often sensitive, while *P. aeruginosa* is uniformly resistant. Resistance tends to develop so rapidly, however, that it can appear overnight during treatment with nalidixic acid (Ronald et al., 1966; Stamey et al., 1969).

Metronidazole, a drug with potent activity in anaerobic infections, can inhibit *B. fragilis* and other species of the family *Bacteroidaceae.* Concentrations of 3.1 μg/ml inhibit most *B. fragilis* (Tally et al., 1972).

OTHER PATHOGENIC MICROORGANISMS

Mycobacteria and Nocardia. Mycobacteria show a different pattern of drug suceptibility than that of most bacteria (Table 11). Among antibiotics in general use in various bacterial infections, only the aminoglycosides and rifampin are active enough to warrant extensive use in tuberculosis and other mycobacterial infections (Lester, 1972; Raleigh, 1972). In fact, the most important antituberculosis drug, isoniazid, has no sigificant inhibitory effect on any other group of bacteria. The same is true of ethambutol and pyrazinamide. Despite its spectacular activity against human and bovine tubercle bacilli, isoniazid is inactive against most mycobacteria. Some other mycobacteria, especially *Mycobacterium kansasii,* are very sensitive to rifampin (but not rifamycin) and are moderately sensitive to streptomycin (Lorian and Finland, 1969). This organism is also sensitive in vitro to erythromycin. The major difference in susceptibility between the human and bovine tubercle bacillus is that *M. tuberculosis* var. *bovis* is resistant to pyrazinamide while *M. tuberculosis* var. *hominis* is sensitive. The slight sensitivity of the human tubercle bacillus to tetracycline has had some practical implications in combined drug therapy for preventing

Table 8. USUAL MINIMUM INHIBITORY CONCENTRATIONS (μg/ml) OF CHLORAMPHENICOL AND TETRACYCLINE AGAINST GRAM-POSITIVE AND GRAM-NEGATIVE RODS

	Chlor-amphenicol	Tetracycline
A. israelii	3.0	3.0
L. monocytogenes	5.0	1.0
C. diphtheriae	0.5	0.3–1.0
C. perfringens	3.0	3.0
B. anthracis	1.5	4.0
H. influenzae	2.0	2.0
H. ducreyi	< 1.0	< 1.0
B. pertussis	2.0	2.0
P. multocida	1.5	3.0
B. fragilis	6.0	1.0–25.0
B. oralis	1.5	0.5
B. melaninogenicus	1.5	1.0
F. nucleatum	3.1	6.2
E. coli	6.0–12.0	6.0–50.0
E. aerogenes	20.0	50.0–> 100.0
K. pneumoniae	10.0	50.0–> 100.0
S. marcescens	25.0	100.0
P. mirabilis	6.0–12.0	50.0–100.0
Indole + *Proteus*	50.0	25.0
P. aeruginosa	> 100.0	> 100.0
Y. enterocolitica	3.0	6.0
B. abortus	3.0	1.0
P. pseudomallei	6.4	1.6
Salmonella spp.	2.0	1.0
Shilgella spp.	2.0	8.0
Vibrio cholerae	1.25	1.05
Vibrio parahaemolyticus	3.1	3.1
B. actinomycetem comitans	0.8	1.6
Campylobacter jejuni	12.5	3.1
Legionella pneumophila	0.8	

Table 9. SENSITIVITY IN VITRO OF GRAM-NEGATIVE BACILLI TO AMINOGLYCOSIDES

	Usual Minimum Inhibitory Concentrations (μg/ml)			
	Streptomycin	***Kanamycin***	***Gentamicin****	***Amikacin***
H. influenzae	8.0	4.0	2.0	—
B. pertussis	4.0	2.0	1.0	—
P. multocida	25.0	—	—	—
E. coli	4.0–25.0	3.0	2.0	2.0–4.0
E. aerogenes	4.0–25.0	2.0–10.0	0.5–2.0	1.4–2.0
K. pneumoniae	6.0–100.0	2.0–10.0	1.0–4.0	1.8
S. marcescens	>100.0	10.0	4.0	3.2
P. mirabilis	6.0–>100.0	2.0–>100.0	0.3–5.0	1.2–2.0
Indole + *Proteus*	6.0–>100.0	2.0–>100.0	2.0	—
P. aeruginosa	50.0	>100.0	1.0–4.0	3.0–6.0
P. pseudomallei	>200.0	25.6	50.0	—
Y. enterocolitica	6.0–>100.0	6.0	—	—
B. abortus	2.0	1.5	0.3	—
Salmonella spp.	4.0–16.0	3.0	0.8	—
Shigella spp.	3.0–10.0	5.0	2.0	—
Francisella tularensis	0.4	—	—	—
Vibrio cholerae	20.0	—	—	—
B. actinomycetem comitans	—	—	6.25	12.5
H. ducreyi	32.0	8.0		
Legionella pneumophila			0.8	1.6

*Tobramycin activity against gram-negative bacilli is similar to that of gentamicin except that tobramycin is twice as active against *P. aeruginosa* and less active against some *Serratia.*

— = *Inadequate data.*

resistance to another antituberculous drug, but not for primary treatment.

Nocardia asteroides, the only important acidfast bacillus other than the mycobacteria, is resistant to most antimycobacterial drugs. In general, strains of *Nocardia* show considerable variation in susceptibility to a given drug but are usually sensitive in vitro to the sulfonamides, tetracyclines, and cycloserine. The most consistently active antibiotic in vitro is minocycline, which inhibits 90 per cent of nocardial strains at a concentration of 3.1 μg/ml (Bach et al., 1973). Erythromycin inhibits 40 per cent of strains at 0.8 μg/ml, but the others are resistant to > 100 μg/ml. These in vitro results, based on standard testing methods, are probably not applicable to clinical therapy because the sulfonamides have been the most consistently successful drug for treating human nocardiosis even though *Nocardia* strains are highly resistant (> 1600 μg/ml) to sulfonamides in vitro unless tiny inocula (< 100 organisms) are used. Likewise, a number of patients have not responded to antibiotics that inhibited the infecting strain of *Nocardia* in low concentrations in vitro.

Mycoplasma. *Mycoplasma pneumoniae*, the cause of primary atypical pneumonia, is the only mycoplasma that has been proved to cause human infection, although *Ureaplasma* has been implicated in nongonococcal urethritis. Both organisms are resistant to drugs that affect the mucopeptide of bacteria because this structure is not present in mycoplasma. Their in vitro sensitivities are given in Table 12 (Braun et al., 1970; Niitu et al., 1970). Erythromycin and tetracycline are active against them, while clindamycin is ineffective.

Yeasts and Fungi. Amphotericin B, 5-fluorocytosine, nystatin, miconazole, ketoconazole, and griseofulvin are the major drugs given for treating fungus infections. Amphotericin B, 5-fluorocytosine, ketoconazole, and miconazole are active against the fungi causing deep mycoses, and griseofulvin against dermatophytes. Nystatin is used only topically. The sulfonamides, clotrimazole, and hydroxystilbamidine have some antifungal properties, but toxicity (clotrimazole, hydroxystilbamidine) or narrow spectrum (sulfonamides) greatly limit their use. Their activity against sensitive strains in vitro (Artis and Baum, 1961; Drouget, 1970; Drutz et al., 1968; Hildick-Smith, 1968; Larsh et al., 1957; Shadomy, 1970; Shadomy et al., 1973; Sterr et al., 1972; Watson and Neame, 1960) is summarized in Table 13.

Table 10. SENSITIVITY OF GRAM-NEGATIVE BACILLI TO RIFAMPIN (THORNSBERRY ET AL., 1983)

Organism	**Usual Minimum Inhibitory Concentrations (*μg/ml*)**
E. coli	2.5–6.0
P. mirabilis	4–8
Indole + *Proteus*	32
P. aeruginosa	64
S. marcescens	64
Acinetobacter spp.	8
Citrobacter freundii	32
K. pneumoniae	32
E. aerogenes	64
B. acetinomycetem comitans	0.8
Legionella pneumophila	0.03
Legionella micdadei	0.03
Salmonella spp.	7.5
Shigella spp.	2.5
P. pseudomallei	50.0
H. influenzae	0.2–0.8
H. ducreyi	0.02

Table 11. DRUG SENSITIVITY OF MYCOBACTERIA

	Usual Minimum Inhibitory Concentrations (μg/ml)				
	M. tuberculosis* var. *hominis	***M. kansasii***	***M. marinum***	***M. intracellulare***	***M. fortuitum***
Isoniazid	0.2	>25.0	>25.0	>25.0	>25.0
Rifampin	0.1	0.1–0.5	0.6	10.0	>20.0
Ethambutol	1.0	5.0	—	—	>20.0
Streptomycin	0.3–6.0	12.0–25.0	2.0–10.0	12.0–25.0	>100.0
Kanamycin	8.0	>5.0	5.0	—	—
Erythromycin	>32.0	1.0–2.0	—	32.0	>32.0
Tetracycline	10.0	—	—	—	16.0
PAS	1.0	>10.0	>2.0	—	>10.0
Pyrazinamide	18.0–20.0	>100.0	50.0	>100.0	—
Cycloserine	5.0–20.0	>50.0	50.0	—	>100.0
Gentamicin	3.6–6.0	3.0	—	3.0	25.0

— = Inadequate data.

Griseofulvin inhibits virtually all dermatophytes at a concentration of less than 0.5 μg/ml. *Microsporum canis, M. gypseum, M. audouinii, Epidermophyton floccosum, Trichophyton mentagrophytes, T. rubrum, T. tonsurans, T. versicolor,* and all other clinically significant dermatophytes are susceptible in tube dilution tests to this concentration, or less, of griseofulvin (Roth et al., 1959). Miconazole is less active against dermatophytes than griseofulvin, inhibiting most of these skin fungi at 32 μg/ml or less; it is especially active against *E. floccosum* (< 0.125 μg/ml). Miconazole is useful when applied topically in ringworm.

SYNERGISM. A few important drugs are more active in the presence of another. The second drug can potentiate by increasing permeability. Thus, the aminoglycosides are more active with penicillin, while rifampicin, 5-fluorocytosine, and tetracycline are potentiated against fungi by amphotericin B. By injuring the mucopeptide of the cell wall, penicillin facilitates entry so that more of the aminoglycoside can reach the ribosomes (Moellering et al., 1971; Zimmermann et al., 1971). Amphotericin B alters permeability by binding with sterols so that more 5-fluorocytosine can enter the cells and inhibit nucleic acid synthesis through its action on pyrimidine biosynthesis (Medoff et al., 1971). This idea is the basis for the combined treatment of cryptococcosis with amphotericin B plus 5-fluorocytosine, and of enterococcal endocarditis with streptomycin and penicillin. More than 50 μg/ml streptomycin and more than 100 μg/ml penicillin are required to kill most enterococci, but many of these are killed by 6.25 μg of streptomycin in the presence of 6.25 μg penicillin or less (Wilkowske et al., 1970). In other words, one-fourth or less of the minimum bactericidal concentration of each drug alone killed enterococci in combination. Similar synergism against enterococci occurs with penicillin plus kanamycin and with penicillin plus gentamicin.

A second drug can also potentiate by reinforcing the metabolic disturbance of the first. This approach is used for synergism between trimethoprim and sulfonamides, two drugs that block two sequential steps in folinic acid synthesis (Bushby, 1969). Maximum potentiation occurs

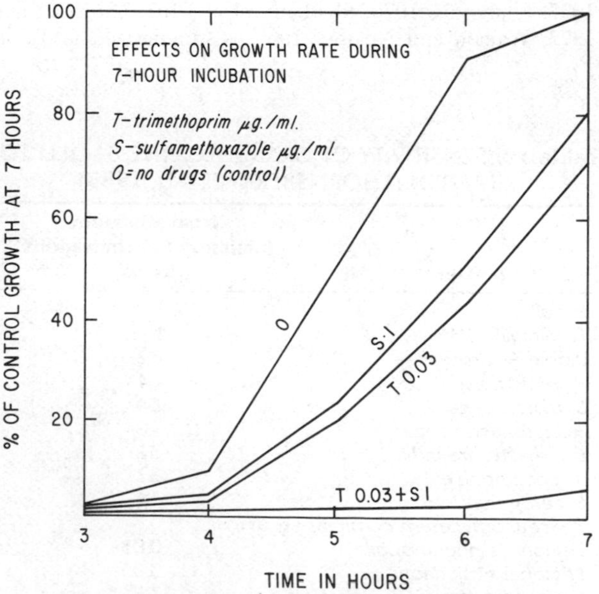

Figure 35. Synergism between trimethoprim and sulfamethoxazole on growth inhibition of *E. coli.* (Modified from Bushby, S. R. M.: Combined antibacterial action *in vitro* of trimethoprim and sulphonamides. Postgrad Med J 4:17, Nov. 1969.)

Table 12. IN VITRO SENSITIVITY OF MYCOPLASMAS TO ANTIBIOTICS

	Usual Minimum Inhibitory Concentrations (μg/ml)	
	M. pneumoniae	***Ureaplasma***
Tetracycline	1.6	0.4
Erythromycin	0.025	1.6
Lincomycin	20.0	200.0
Chloramphenicol	12.0	1.6
Streptomycin	1.0	1.6
Polymyxin	—	500.0
Kanamycin	—	3.1
Gentamicin	—	6.2
Clindamycin	—	6.2–50.0

— = Inadequate data.

Table 13. USUAL MINIMUM INHIBITORY CONCENTRATIONS (μg/ml)

	Amphotericin	5-Fluorocytosine	Clotrimazole	Ketoconazole	Miconazole
Cryptococcus neoformans	0.4–1.0	0.5–4.0	1.6	0.125	0.5
Coccidioides immitis	0.5	>100.0	0.4	1.0	3.0
Aspergillus fumigatus	>40.0	50.0–>100.0	1.6	—	8.0–16.0
Blastomyces dermatitidis	0.4–0.8	25.0	0.2	—	1.0
Candida albicans	2.0–4.0	0.5–500.0	4.0–16.0	0.5	1.0
Candida glabrata	0.5–2.0	0.5–5.0	2.0–8.0	—	16.0–64.0
Histoplasma capsulatum	0.1–0.8	>100.0	3.0	0.2–0.4	0.5
Sporothrix schenckii	0.1–0.6	>100.0	0.5–10	—	2.0
Zygomycetes	0.03–>2.5	>100.0	0.8	—	1000.0
Pseudallescheria boydii	3–>100	>100.0	0.6–4	0.8–5	0.05
Phialaphora spp.	0.1–>100	—	0.6>100	—	0.08–64.0
Basidiobolus spp.	0.1–12.5	>200.0	—	0.1–1.5	0.1–12.5
Conidiobolus spp.	0.1–0.4	200.0	—	0.2–1.6	0.1–3.1

— = Inadequate data.

when the two drugs are present in proportions corresponding to their respective MIC when acting singly. Trimethoprim is usually about 20 times more active than sulfamethoxazole, the sulfonamide with which it is usually combined. When the two drugs are mixed according to this ratio (20 sulf:1 trimethoprim), they potentiate each other against many organisms, including streptococci, pneumococci, *S. aureus*, *H. influenzae*, *B. pertussis*, *K. pneumoniae*, *E. coli*, *Salmonella*, *Shigella*, *Proteus*, and gonococci. Examples are given in Table 14 and Figure 35 which give the minimum inhibitory concentrations of each drug when they are combined in a ratio of 1 part trimethoprim and 20 parts sulfamethoxazole (Bushby, 1969). The results show a potentiation of at least 20-fold for each drug against most organisms when used in combination.

SERUM CONCENTRATIONS OF ANTIMICROBIAL DRUGS. The aim of chemotherapy is to get enough drug into the infected tissues to inhibit or kill the pathogenic organism. In other words, the drug level must exceed the minimum inhibitory concentration. The levels of drug that can be anticipated in serum after different routes of administration are listed in Tables 1 and 2 in Chapter 22. By comparing these levels to the minimum inhibitory concentrations given in the preceding tables, an estimate can then be made of appropriate drugs and dosage for a given infection. These estimates will be modified, in turn, by the pharmacologic considerations discussed in Chapter 22. Renal failure, diffusion barriers, and the type of inflammatory reaction, if any, must be taken into account in selecting a drug and determining its dose.

Table 14. SYNERGISM BETWEEN TRIMETHOPRIM AND SULFAMETHOXAZOLE (BUSBY, 1969; CARLSON ET AL. 1983)

	Usual Minimum Inhibitory Concentrations (μg/ml)*			
	Sulfamethoxazole Alone	***Trimethoprim Alone***	***Sulfamethoxazole in Combination***	***Trimethoprim in Combination***
Streptococcus pyogenes	100.0	1.0	1.0	0.05
Pneumococcus	30.0	2.0	2.0	0.1
S. aureus	3.0	1.0	0.3	0.015
H. influenzae	10.0	1.0	0.3	0.015
K. pneumoniae	100.0	3.0	4.0	0.2
E. coli	3.0	0.3	1.0	0.05
Salmonella typhimurium	10.0	1.0	0.3	0.05
Shigella sonnei	>10.0	1.0	0.3	0.05
N. gonorrhoeae	5.0	18.3	4.0	2.3
B. fragilis	6.0	25.0	4.0	0.2
Fusobacterium spp.	40.0	100.0	15.0	1.0
Peptostreptococcus spp.	>100.0	>100.0	30.0	2.0
B. actinomycetem comitans	50.0	0.8	—	—
Yersinia enterocolitica		2.0	32.0	
Campylobacter jejuni	40.0	128.0	128.0	
Aeromonas hydrophila		2.0	2.0	
Vibrio parahaemolyticus		2.0	1.0	

*The levels of sulfamethoxazole usually reached in serum are 16 to 32 μg/ml and those of trimethoprim are 0.8 to 1.6 μg/ml.

References

Classification

Aziz, M., Drop, I., Diallo, S., Lariviere, M., and Porta, M.: Efficacy and tolerance of invermectin in human onchocerciasis. Lancet 2:8291:171, 1982.

Bodanszky, M., and Perlman, D.: Peptide antibiotics. Science 163:352, 1969.

Bueding, E.: Some biochemical effects of anthelmintic drugs. Biochem Pharmacol 18:1541, 1969.

Dutcher, J. D., Young, M. B., Sherman, J. H., et al.: Chemical studies on amphotericin B. I. Preparation of the hydrogenation product and isolation of mycosamine, an acetolysis product. Antibiot Annu 866, 1956–1957.

Fox, H.: The chemical attack on tuberculosis. Trans NY Acad Sci 15:234, 1953.

Grollman, P.: Structural basis for inhibition of protein synthesis by emetine and cycloheximide based on an analogy between ipecac alkaloids and glutarimide antibiotics. Proc Nat Acad Sci USA 56:1867, 1966.

Hewitt, L.: The cephalosporins—1973. J Infect Dis 128:Suppl:S312, 1973.

Hitchings, H.: Species differences among dihydrofolate reductases as a basis for chemotherapy. Postgrad Med J 45(Suppl):7, 1969.

Johnson, A., Anker, H., and Meleney, L.: Bacitracin; new antibiotic produced by member of *B. subtilis* group. Science 102:376, 1945.

Labia, R.: Moxalactam: an oxa-β-lactam antibiotic that inactivates B-lactamases. Rev Inf Dis 4:5529, 1982.

Lacroute, F.: Regulation of pyrimidine biosynthesis in Saccharomyces cerevisiae. J Bacteriol 95:824, 1968.

Long, H., and Bliss, A.: Para-amino-benzene-sulfonamide and its derivatives; experimental and clinical observations on their use in treatment of beta-hemolytic streptococci infection: preliminary report. JAMA 108:32, 1937.

Nair, S., and Cherubin, C.: Use of cefoxitin, new cephalosporin-like antibiotic, in the treatment of aerobic and anaerobic infections. Antimicrob Agents Chemother 14:866, 1978.

Neu, H. D.: Antimicrobial activity and human pharmacology of amoxicillin. J Infect Dis 129(Suppl):123, 1974.

Neu, H.: Structure-activity relations of the new β-lactam compounds and in vitro activity against common bacteria. Inf Dis Rev 5:5319, 1983.

Novick, P.: Staphylococcal penicillinase and the new penicillins. Biochem J 83:229, 1962.

Oxford, E., Raistrick, H., and Simonart, P.: XXIX. Studies in the biochemistry of microorganisms: LX: Griseofulvin, $C_{17}H_{17}O_6Cl$, a metabolic product of *Penicillium griseofulvum* Dierckx. Biochem J 33:240, 1939.

Sheldrick, G, Jones, P., Kennard, O., Williams, D., and Smith, G.: Structure of vancomycin and its complex with acetyl-D-alanyl-D-alanine. Nature 271:223, 1978.

Wehrli, W., and Staehelin, M.: Actions of the rifamycins. Bacteriol Rev 35:290, 1971.

Microbial Susceptibility to Drugs

Artis, D., and Baum, G. L.: In vitro susceptibility of 24 strains of *Histoplasma capsulatum* to amphotericin B. Antibiot Chemother 11:373, 1961.

Atlas, E., and Turck, M.: Laboratory and clinical evaluation of rifampicin. Am J Med Sci 256:47, 1968.

Bach, M. C., Sabath, L. D., and Finland, M.: Susceptibility of *Nocardia asteroides* to 45 antimicrobial agents in vitro. Antimicrob Agents Chemother 3:1, 1973.

Bauer, A. W., Kirby, W. M., Sherris, J. C., et al.: Antibiotic susceptibility testing by a standardized single disk method. Am J Clin Pathol 45:493, 1966.

Benner, E. J.: The cephalosporin antibiotics. Pediatr Clin North Am 15:31, 1968.

Braude, A. I., Banister, J., and Wright, N.: Use of the gradient plate for routine clinical determinations of bacterial sensitivities to antibiotics. Antibiot Annu 1133, 1954–1955.

Braun, P., Klein, J. O., and Kass, E. H.: Susceptibility of genital mycoplasmas to antimicrobial agents. Appl Microbiol 19:62, 1970.

Bushby, R. S.: Combined antibacterial action in vitro of trimethoprim and sulphonamides. The in vitro nature of synergy. Postgrad Med J 45 (Suppl):10, 1969.

Butler, K., English, A. R., Ray, V. A., et al.: Carbenicillin: chemistry and mode of action. J Infect Dis 122:(Suppl):51, 1970.

Carlson, J., Thornton, S., Du Pont, H., West, A., and Mattewson, J.: Comparative in vitro activities of ten antimicrobial agents againt enterobacterial pathogens. Antimicrob Agents Chemother 24:509, 1983.

Chadwick, P.: Bacteriological assessment of clindamycin, a new lincomycin derivative. J Med Microbiol 4:529, 1971.

Dixon, D., Shadomy, S., Shadomy, H., Espinel-Ingroff, A., and Kerkering, T.: Cmparison of the *in vitro* antifungal activities of miconazole and a new imidazole, R 41,400. J Infect Dis 138:245, 1978.

Drouhet, E.: Basic mechanisms of antifungal chemotherapy. Mod Treat 7:539, 1970.

Drutz, D. J., Spickard, A., Rogers, D. E., et al.: Treatment of disseminated mycotic infections. A new approach to amphotericin B therapy. Am J Med 45:405, 1968.

Edmondson, E. B., and Sanford, J. P.: The Klebsiella-Enterobacter (Aerobacter)-Serratia group. A clinical and bacteriological evaluation. Medicine (Balt) 46:323, 1967.

Eickhoff, T. C., Bennett, J. V., Hayes, P. S., et al.: *Pseudomonas pseudomallei:* susceptibility to chemotherapeutic agents. J Infect Dis 121:95, 1970.

Ericsson, H., Hogman, C., and Wickman, K.: Paper disc method for determination of bacterial sensitivity to chemotherapeutic and antibiotic agents. Scand J Clin Lab Invest 6 (Suppl):21, 1954.

Friedberg, C. K., Rosen, K. M., and Bienstock, P. A.: Vancomycin therapy for enterococcal and *Streptococcus viridans* endocarditis. Successful treatment of six patients. Arch Intern Med (Chicago) 122:134, 1968.

Griffith, R. S., and Black, H. R.: Erythromycin. Med Clin North Am 54:1199, 1970.

Guttler, R. B., Counts, G. W., Avent, C. K., et al.: Effect of rifampin and minocycline on meningococcal carrier rates. J Infect Dis 24:199, 1971.

Hammerstrom, C. F., Cox, F., McHenry, M. C., et al.; Clinical laboratory, and pharmacological studies of dicloxacillin. Antimicrob Agents Chemother 69, 1966.

Hildick-Smith, G.: Antifungal antibiotics. Pediatr Clin North Am 15:107, 1968.

Jones, R., and Barry, A.: Cefoperozone: a review of its antimicrobial spectrum, β-lactamase stability, enzyme inhibition, and other in vitro characteristics. Rev Inf Dis 5:5108, 1983.

Jorgensen, J., Crawford, S., and Alexander, O.: In vitro activities of moxalactam and cefotaxime against aerobic gram-negative bacilli. Antimicrob Agents Chemother 17:937, 1980.

Judson, F. N., Allaman, J., and Dans, P. E.: Treatment of gonorrhea—Comparison of penicillin G procaine, doxycycline, spectinomycin, and ampicillin. JAMA 230:705, 1974.

Kaye, O., Kobasa, W., and Kaye, K.: Susceptibility of anaerobic bacteria to cefoperozone and other antibiotics. Antimicrob Agents Chemother 17:957, 1980.

Kayser, F. H.: In vitro activity of cephalosporin antibiotics against gram-positive bacteria. Postgrad Med J 47 (Suppl):14, 1971.

Kunin, C. M., Brandt, D., and Wood, H.: Bacteriologic studies of rifampin, a new semisynthetic antibiotic. J Infect Dis 119:132, 1969.

Larsh, H. W., Hinton, A., and Silberg, S. L.: The use of the tissue culture method in evaluating antifungal agents against systemic fungi. Antibiot Annu 988, 1957–1958.

Lester, W.: Rifampin: a semisynthetic derivative of rifamycin—a prototype for the future. Am Rev Microbiol 26:85, 1972.

Levison, M. E., Johnson, W. D., Thorhill, T. S., et al.: Clinical and in vitro evaluation of cephalexin. A new orally administered cephalosporin antibiotic. JAMA 209:1331, 1969.

Lorian, V., and Finland, M.: In vitro effect of rifampin on mycobacteria. Appl Microbiol 17:202, 1969.

Martin, W. J., Gardner, M., and Washington, J. A., II: In vitro antimicrobial susceptibility of anaerobic bacteria isolated from clinical specimens. Antimicrob Agents Chemother 1:148, 1972.

McLinn, S. E., Nelson, J. D., and Haltalin, K. C.: Antimicrobial susceptibility of *Hemophilus influenzae.* Pediatrics 48:827, 1970.

Medoff, G., Comfort, M., and Kobayashi, G. S.: Synergistic action of amphotericin B and 5-fluorocytosine against yeast-like organisms. Proc Soc Exp Biol Med 138:571, 1971.

Moellering, R. C., Jr., Wennersten, C., and Weinberg, A. N.: Studies on antibiotic synergism against enterococci. I. Bacteriologic studies. J Lab Clin Med 77:821, 1971.

Neu, H.: Antimicrobial activity and human pharmacology of amoxicillin. J Infect Dis 129 (Suppl):S123, 1974.

Neu, H.: Structure activity relations of new β-lactam compounds and in vitro activity against common bacteria. Rev Inf Dis 5:5319, 1983.

Niitu, Y., Hasegawa, S., Suetake, T., et al.: Resistance of *Mycoplasma pneumoniae* to erythromycin and other antibiotics. J Pediatr 76:438, 1970.

Raleigh, J. W.: Rifampin in treatment of advanced pulmonary tuberculosis. Report of a VA cooperative pilot study. Ann Rev Respir Dis 105:397, 1972.

Ronald, A. R., Turck, M., and Petersdorf, R. G.: A critical evaluation of nalidixic acid in urinary-tract infections. N Engl J Med 275:1081, 1966.

Rosen, I. G., Jacobsen, J., and Rudderman, R.: Rapid capillary tube method for detecting penicillin resistance in *Staphylococcus aureus.* Appl Microbiol 23:649, 1972.

Roth, F. J., Sallman, B., and Blank, H.: In vitro studies of the antifungal antibiotic griseofulvin. J Invest Dermatol 33:403, 1959.

Sabath, L. D., Wilcox, C., Garner, C., et al.: In vitro activity of cefazolin against recent clinical bacterial isolates. J Infect Dis 128 (Suppl):S320, 1973.
Sanders, E., Foster, M. T., and Scott, D.: Group A beta-hemolytic streptococci resistant to erythromycin and lincomycin. N Engl J Med 278:538, 1968.
Shadomy, S.: Further in vitro studies with 5-fluorocytosine. Infect Immun 2:484, 1970.
Shadomy, S., Kirchoff, C. B., and Ingroff, A. E.: In vitro activity of 5-fluorocytosine against *Candida* and *Torulopsis* species. Antimicrob Agents Chemother 3:9, 1973.
Sherris, J., and Washington, J.: Laboratory tests in chemotherapy. In Lennette, E. H. (ed.) Manual Clin Microbiol, Washington, D.C., American Society of Microbiology, 1980.
Simon, H. J.: Streptomycin, kanamycin, neomycin, and paromomycin. Pediatr Clin North Am 15:73, 1968.
Smith, C. B., Wilfert, J. N., Dans, P. E., et al.: In-vitro activity of carbenicillin and results of treatment of infections due to *Pseudomonas* with carbenicillin singly and in combination with gentamicin. J Infect Dis 122 (Suppl):S14, 1970.
Stamey, T. A., Nemoy, N. J., and Higgins, M.: The clinical use of nalidixic acid. A review and some observations. Invest Urol 6:582, 1969.
Sterr, P. L., Marks, M. I., Klite, P. D., et al.: 5-Fluorocytosine: an oral antifungal compound. A report on clinical and laboratory experience. Ann Intern Med 76:15, 1972.
Steigbigel, N. H., McCall, C. E., Reed, C. W., et al.: Antibacterial action of "broad spectrum" penicillins, cephalosporins and other antibiotics against gram-negative bacilli isolated from bacteremic patients. Ann NY Acad Sci 145:224, 1967.
Sutherland, R., Croydon, E. A., and Rolinson, G. N.: Flucloxacilin, a new isoxazolyl penicillin, compared with oxacillin, cloxacillin, and dicloxacillin. Br Med J 4:455, 1970.
Tally, F. P., Sutter, V. L., and Finegold, S. M.: Metronidazole versus anaerobes. In vitro data and initial clinical observations. Calif Med 117:22, 1972.
Thornsberry, C., Hill, B., Swenson, J., and McDougal, L.: Rifampin: spectrum of antibacterial activity. Rev Inf Dis 5:5412, 1983.
Toala, P., McDonald, A., Wilcox, C., et al.: Comparison of antibiotic susceptibility of group D streptococcus strains isolated at Boston City Hospital in 1953–54 and 1968–69. Antimicrob Agents Chemother 479, 1969.
Watson, D. C., and Neame, P. B.: In vitro activity of amphotericin B on strains of *Mucoraceae* pathogenic to man. J Lab Clin Med 56:251, 1960.
Wilkowske, C. J., Facklam, R. R., Washington, J. A., II, and Geraci, J.: Antibiotic synergism: enhanced susceptibility of group D streptococci to certain antibiotic combinations. Antimicrob Agents Chemother 195, 1970.
Zimmermann, R. A., Moellering, R. C., Jr., and Weinberg, A. N.: Mechanism of resistance to antibiotic synergism in enterococci. J Bacteriol 105:873, 1971.

20

MECHANISMS OF ACTION OF ANTIMICROBIAL DRUGS

ABRAHAM I. BRAUDE, M.D., PH.D.

The key to antibiotic action is a selective toxicity for the infecting organism but not for the patient. Antibiotics can hit at least four targets in bacteria and other organisms that are either missing or less vulnerable in human cells: the cell wall, the cytoplasmic membrane, the ribosomes, and the enzymes involved in transcription of genetic information (Table 1).

CELL WALL

The cell wall is where the penicillins and cephalosporins do their damage. It is the most important target for antibiotics because it is absent in human cells. The cell wall of bacteria is a thick rigid envelope that surrounds the cell membrane, maintaining the shape of the bacteria and keeping them from osmotic damage in water and body fluids. The internal pressures of pathogenic bacteria are somewhat higher than serum and other extraceullar fluids so that the organisms would imbibe water, swell, and burst if the cell wall became defective. The rigid portion of the cell wall, known as the sacculus, is reminiscent of grape hulls in cocci and balloons in bacilli. The rigid material in the sacculus is a material composed of sugar and peptides and called mucopeptide or murein. The mucopeptide is at least four times thicker in gram-positive cells than in gram-negative cells. In *E. coli* the layer of mucopeptide is made up of polysaccharide chains linked together by peptides. The polysaccharide chains are composed of repeating units of two sugars, muramic acid and N-acetylglucosamine, as indicated in Figure 1. The cross-linking peptide strands are attached to the polysaccharide chains by a peptide bond between the carboxyl group in each muramic acid unit and the amino group of L-alanine. Another peptide bond connects L-alanine to D-glutamic acid, followed in turn by α, ε-diaminopimelic acid, and finally D-alanine to form a tetrapeptide. The free carboxyl groups on the D-alanine residues are also attached to the NH_2 group of the α, ε-diaminopimelic acid in adjacent tetrapeptides to produce a cross-linked structure (Fig. 2). In staphylococci a second chain composed of five glycine molecules is used to connect neighboring peptides so that the structure is more like that in Figure 3. The peptide group in staphylococci is also different from that in *E. coli*, as shown in Figure 4. The staphylococcal peptide lacks diaminopimelic acid and, instead, has L-lysine as the third amino acid. This is followed by D-alanyl-D-alanine at the end of the chain. The murein network in the *Staphylococcus* is completed when D-alanine is split from D-alanyl-D-alanine so that a peptide

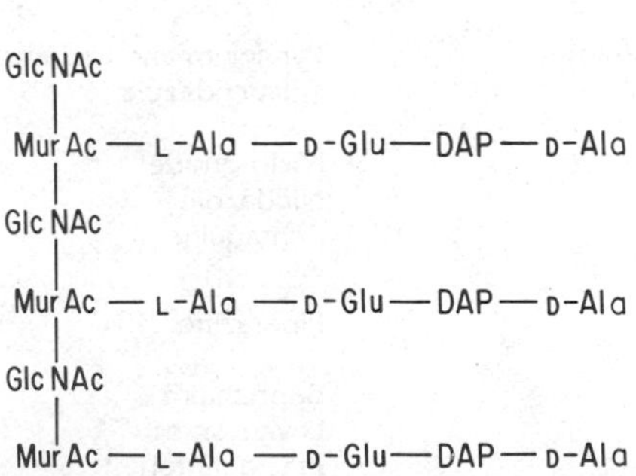

Figure 1. The rigid structure in bacterial cell walls is a sugar peptide called mucopeptide or murein. The sugar is a polysaccharide of muramic acid (MurAc) and glucosamine (GlcNAc). The peptides are composed of four amino acids: L-alanine (L-Ala), D-glutamic acid (D-Glu), α, ε-diaminopimelic acid (DAP), and D-alanine (D-Ala).

Table 1. MECHANISMS OF ACTION OF ANTIMICROBIAL DRUGS

Nature of Injury	Antimicrobial Drug	Mode of Action
Defective cell wall mucopeptide	Penicillins and cephalosporins	Prevent final peptide bond between D-alanine and glycine
	Cycloserine	As structural analogue of D-alanine, it inhibits enzymes responsible for synthesis of D-alanyl-D-alanine, an essential component of mucopeptide
	Bacitracin	Blocks transfer to cell membrane of peptidoglycan precursors from site of synthesis in cytoplasm
	Vancomycin	Complexes with D-alanyl-D-alanine of nascent peptidoglycan
Damaged cytoplasmic membrane	Polymyxins	Disorganize lipoproteins by inserting lipophobic moiety into bacterial membrane lipid
	Polyenes	React with sterols in fungal membranes so that permeability is altered
	Imidazoles	Impair structure and function of membranes by depriving them of ergosterol
Impaired function of ribosomes	Aminoglycosides	Bind to 30S ribosomal unit and inactivate initiation complexes; also interfere with attachment of tRNA and distort triplet codons so that message is misread
	Tetracyclines	Bind to 30S unit and block binding of tRNA so that new amino acids cannot be introduced into peptide chain
	Chloramphenicol	Attaches to 50S subunit or ribosomes and prevents peptide-bond formation by inhibiting enzyme peptidyltransferase
	Lincomycin	Same as chloramphenicol
	Emetine	Inhibits translocation reaction on 40S ribosome of eukaryotic cells
	Thiosemicarbazones	Disrupt polyribosomes
Impaired nucleic acid function	Rifampicin	Blocks bacterial RNA formation by inhibiting DNA-dependent RNA polymerase
	Chloroquine	Inserted between stacked base pairs in double helix and thus interferes with ability of DNA to act as a template for nucleic acid synthesis
	Quinine	Forms hydrogen-bonds with double stranded DNA so that DNA replication is stopped
	Antiviral nucleosides (5-iodo-2′-deoxyuridine, trifluorothymidine, adenine arabinoside, and ribavirin)	Compete with normal nucleic acid
	Acycloguanosine	Inhibits viral DNA synthesis by the herpes-encoded DNA polymerase. Only herpes-virus infected cells are attacked because acycloguanosine needs a virus specific thymidinekinase to phosphorulate it to acycloguanosine triphosphate
	Nalidixic acid	Inhibits DNA synthesis by attacking DNA gyrase
	5-Fluorocytosine	Converted to 5-fluorouracil which blocks thymidylate synthetase so that lethal thymine deficiency results
	Sulfonamides and diaminopyrimidines	By preventing synthesis of folic acid, they block formation of thymidine and purines needed for nucleic acid synthesis
	Metronidazole	After partial reduction of the nitro group, the activated drug inhibits DNA synthesis
Impaired energy metabolism	Pyrvinium and mebendazole	Blocks glucose uptake
	Thiabendazole	Inhibits fumaric reductase so that glucose fermentation is impaired
	Niclosamide	Blocks phosphorylation of ATP
	Niridazole	Depletes glycogen reserves
	Primaquine	Disrupts respiratory chain after conversion to quinoline diquinone, an analogue of ubiquinone
Paralysis	Piperazine	Stabilizes membrane potential of *Ascaris* muscle by hyperpolarization
	Bephenium	Depolarizes membranes (i.e., reverse of piperazine)
	Levamisole	Inhibits neuromuscular transmission by ganglionic blockade
	Praziquantel	Causes loss of intracellular calcium and hypercontractility of muscle cells in flukes and tapeworms
	Metrifonate	Inhibits cholinesterase
	Ivermectin	Blocks post synaptic transmission in nematodes by modifying release of the neurotransmitter gamma amino butyric acid

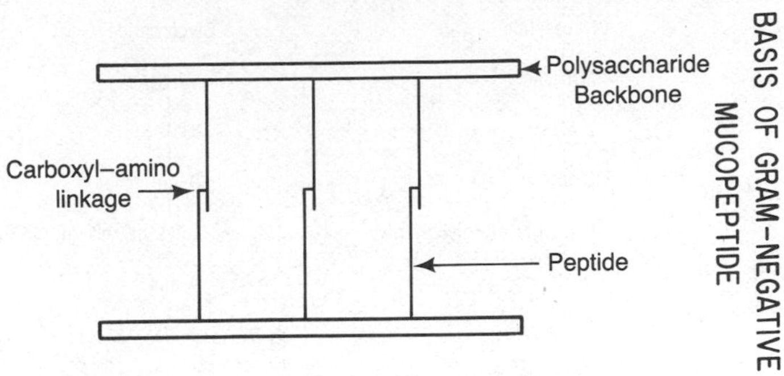

Figure 2. Cross-linking of peptide chains in gram-negative bacilli by bonds between the free carboxyl groups of D-alanine and NH_2 groups of α,ε-diaminopimelic acid. (Modified from Rogers, H. J.: The mode of action of antibiotics. In Bittar, E. E. (ed.): The Biological Basis of Medicine. Vol. 2. New York, Academic Press, 1968, p. 427.)

bond can form between the carboxyl group of the residual D-alanine and the terminal amino group of the pentaglycine chain (Fig. 4).

Penicillin is thought to prevent the final peptide bond between D-alanine and glycine (Tipper and Strominger, 1965). It has been suggested that penicillin combines with the transpeptidase responsible for this final cross linkage (the cross-linking enzyme). Since the stearic configuration of penicillin is like that of D-alanyl-D-alanine, penicillin might react with the cross-linking enzyme and inactivate it so that it could not complete the transpeptidation reaction (Fig. 5). By preventing this final step in murein synthesis, penicillin seems to have at least two deleterious effects on bacteria: (1) it inhibits multiplication; and (2) it creates weak points in the cell wall through which the growing cytoplasm can bulge (Fig. 6).

The transpeptidase enzyme is attached to the cytoplasmic membrane where it reacts with penicillin. This has been demonstrated with radioactive (^{14}C) penicillin, which combines covalently with the transpeptidase and other enzymes involved in peptidase reactions with the peptidoglycan. Because of their ability to bind penicillin and other β-lactam antibiotics these enzymes are also known as penicillin-binding proteins or PBPs (Waxman and Strominger, 1983). PBPs are identified by numbers in order of decreasing molecular weight, with PBPs 1, -2, and -3 representing those of high molecular weight (M_r 60,000 to 40,000), and -4, -5, and -6 those of low molecular weight (M_r between 49,000 and 40,000). Since binding inactivates PBPs, their function can be identified by the disturbances induced in bacterial cells exposed to β-lactam drugs that bind to specific PBPs. In *E. coli,* for example, PBP 1A and 1B are involved in cell elongation, so that their inhibition blocks elongation. PBP-2 maintains the characteristic rod-shape of *E. coli* and inhibition of this protein (by mecillinam, e. g.) causes transformation of the rods to large osmotically *stable* round cells that lyse after several hours of active growth. Although PBP-2 is not a transpeptidase, it apparently incorporates new glycan strands for cell elongation in a way that ensures rod formation. Without PBP-2, new glycan strands can be appropriated by the enzymes that synthesize septa so that the cell becomes rounded by growing in width instead of length. The reverse occurs when *E. coli* PBP-3 is inhibited by β-lactams such as cephalexin and piperacillin. By inhibiting PBP-3, they impair murein synthesis in the septum that separates dividing cells, but do not reduce linear growth. The result of blocking PBP-3 is thus to induce formation of long filaments.

PBP-4 functions as a D-alanine carboxypeptidase, which is thought to act as a secondary transpeptidase of peptidoglycan biosynthesis. In contrast to primary transpeptidases, which insert new peptidoglycan strands into the existing cell wall, the secondary transpeptidases catalyze cross-linkage of the newly incorporated strands. The two enzymes are inhibited by different β-lactam drugs: those that inhibit primary transpeptidases block growth and those that inhibit carboxypeptidase (such as cefoxitin) cause a reduction in cross-linking without affecting growth.

These observations on penicillin-binding proteins, as well as studies with bacterial mutants deficient in certain enzymes, have emphasized that the mechanism of action of a β-lactam drug depends on the type(s) of enzyme it attacks, the species of bacteria involved, the structure of the drug, and the stage in cell wall synthesis or cell division. Thus no simple explanation involving any one enzyme or covering all β-lactam drugs can account for their mechanism of action.

It should also be noted that most of the effects of β-lactam drugs on PBPs are inhibitory, producing deformity of the bacterial cell but not necessarily lysis or death. Lysis does not seem to occur unless autolysin activity is triggered by β-lactams. Such activation of autolysis is seen in *E. coli,* e. g., when cephalothin or cephaloridine bind to PBP1. Benzylpenicillin and ampicillin, which bind to PBP1 less effectively than these cephalosporins, are less effective in activating autolysis, and correspondingly less effective in producing spheroplasts. Mecillinam or 6-aminopenicillanoic acid binds strongly to PBP2 without triggering autolysin activity or killing cells; thus PBP1, not PBP2, must be suppressed to trigger autolysins. The autolysins are

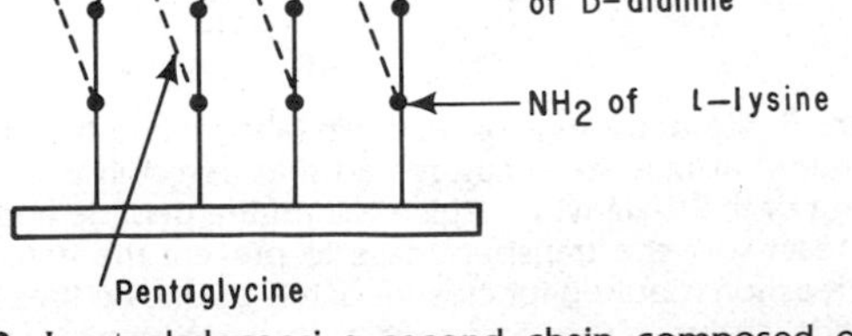

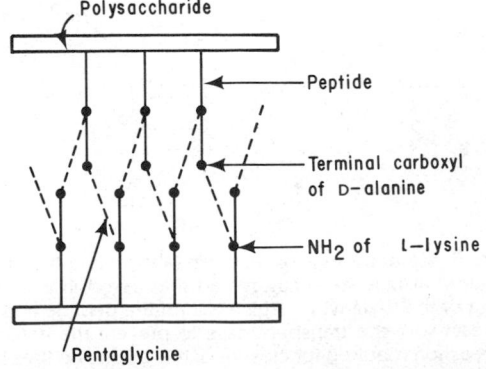

Figure 3. In staphylococci a second chain composed of 5-glycine (pentaglycine) molecules connects the neighboring peptides. (Modified from Rogers, H. J.: The mode of action of antibiotics. In Bittar, E. E. (ed.): The Biological Basis of Medicine. Vol. 2. New York, Academic Press, 1968, p. 428.)

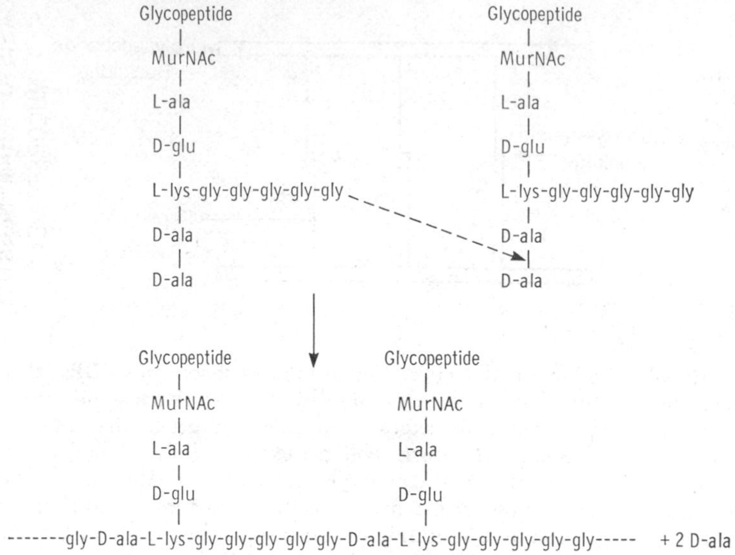

Figure 4. Mucopeptide from staphylococci. The peptide chain differs from that in *E. coli* (Fig. 1) in that staphylococcal peptide lacks diaminopimelic acid and instead has L-lysine as the third amino acid. The murein network is completed when D-alanine is split from D-alanyl-D-alanine so that a peptide bond can form between the carboxyl group of the residual D-alanine and the terminal group of the pentaglycine chain. Penicillin is thought to act by inhibiting the enzyme (transpeptidase) responsible for this cross linkage. (From Strominger, J. L.: Enzymatic reactions in bacterial cell wall synthesis sensitive to penicillins and other antibacterial substances. In Guze, L. B. (ed.): Microbial Protoplasts, Spheroplasts and L-Forms. © 1968, The Williams & Wilkins Co., Baltimore, p. 57.)

murine hydrolases and their activity is measured by release of radio-labeled amino acids (e.g., ^{3}H diaminopimelic acid) from the peptidoglycan.

Binding of the β-lactam to PBPs seems to trigger autolysin activity by different mechanisms. In the pneumococcus and some other gram-positive organisms, autolysis is suppressed by lipoteichoic acid, and autolysis is activated when β-lactams induce the release of the lipoteichoic acid from the bacterial cell so that the pneumococcal autolysin, an amidase, is free to disrupt the peptidoglycan (Thomas, 1979). In *E. coli,* the mechanism for triggering autolysins is different but not clear. Inhibition of cell wall formation by inactivation of certain PBPs activates the autolysin, possibly by creating poor cross-linkages or by causing cell wall precursors to accumulate. Even more obscure is the mechanism of killing *Streptococcus pyogenes* by penicillin *without* lysis.

The term "antibiotic tolerance" has been used to describe the dissociation between inhibition and killing of bacteria by an antibiotic that inhibits peptidoglycan synthesis. These bacteria, which have lost their autolytic activity through mutation, remain as sensitive as the wild-type organisms to growth inhibition but are resistant to lysis and killing by the antibiotic.

In comparing the action of antibiotics on gram-negative and gram-positive bacteria, it is important to take into account penetration of the outer membrane of gram negatives by β-lactam compounds. In general, gram-negative bacteria are less sensitive for several reasons, including the barrier imposed by the outer membrane. (Low efficiency β-lactamases in the periplasmic space of gram negatives also reduce susceptibility to these drugs as noted in the next chapter). Molecules of antibiotics enter through the porins (Chapter 1), which provide hydrophilic entry pores for small water-soluble substances but not hydrophobic drugs like nafcillin. Cationic antibiotics can pass through certain porins and anionic compounds are accepted for passage by others.

While β-lactam compounds block the action of enzymes that incorporate new glycan strands into the mucopeptide, it is also possible for antibiotics to prevent the synthesis or transfer of mucopeptide precursors. Such action against

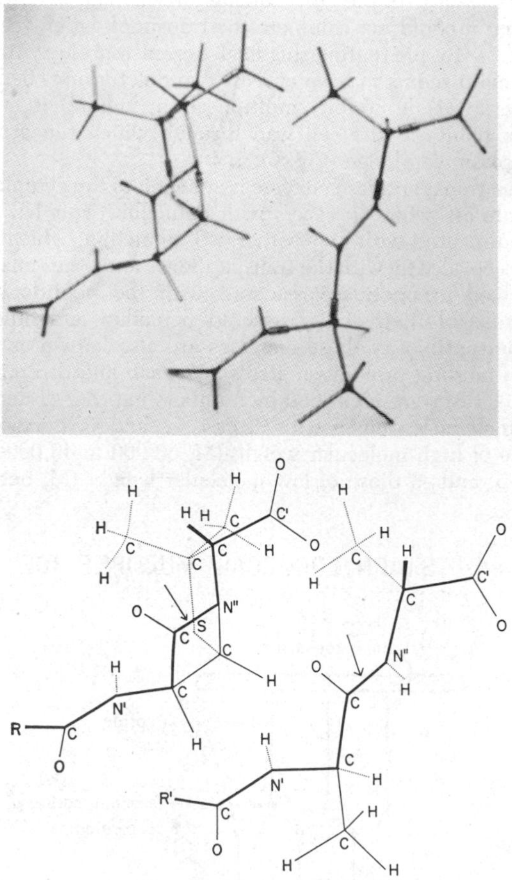

Figure 5. Stereomodels of penicillin (above) and the end of the peptide D-alanine have suggested that penicillin is a structural analog of the D-alanyl-D-alanine end of the peptide and thereby can react with the transpeptidase to prevent the transpeptidation reaction required for closure of the glycine bridges between peptide chains. (From Strominger, J. L.: Enzymatic reactions in bacterial cell wall synthesis sensitive to penicillins and other antibacterial substances. In Guze, L. B. (ed.): Microbial Protoplasts, Spheroplasts and L-Forms. © 1968, The Williams & Wilkins Co., Baltimore, p. 58.)

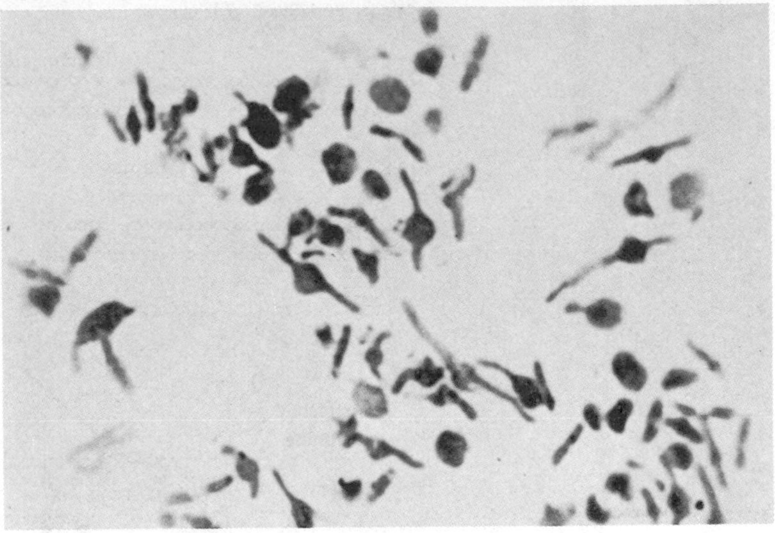

Figure 6. Effect of penicillin on cell wall of *Klebsiella pneumoniae.* Defective portions of the mucopeptide allow the high internal osmotic pressure to cause swellings in both the central and terminal portions of the rods. (From Braude, A. I., Siemienski, J., and Jacobs, I.: Protoplast formation in human urine. Trans Assoc Am Physicians 74:238, 1961.)

precursors by certain antibiotics does, in fact, take place but these are usually less important in clinical medicine. Cycloserine is a structural analog of D-alanine and competitively inhibits the enzyme responsible for synthesis of D-alanyl-D-alanine, an essential component of the pentapeptide (Neuhaus and Lynch, 1964). Bacitracin (Siewert and Strominger, 1967) blocks stages of cell wall construction that involve transfer of the sugar pentapeptide from the site of synthesis in the cytoplasm to its attachment to a lipid in the cell membrane. Bacitracin combines with the lipid soluble carrier in the membrane, undecaprenyl alcohol. Normally the lipid carrier provides a site in the membrane where the precursors can attach and be synthesized into a complete subunit of the peptidoglycan before transfer into the cytoplasm. Bacitracin blocks this reaction when it combines with the pyrophosphate derivative of undecaprenyl alcohol.

In addition to combining with enzymes or carriers involved in peptidoglycan synthesis, antibiotics can inhibit cell wall synthesis by reacting with the substrate of the enzyme. This is the mode of action of vancomycin, which complexes with the D-alanyl-D-alanine end of the newly synthesized peptidoglycan and thus inhibits the transglycosidase enzyme that polymerizes the peptidoglycan subunits brought in by the lipid carrier.

The target of vancomycin is such an integral part of the cell wall that development of resistance to the drug is virtually impossible. Resistance would require such a drastic change in cell wall structure and biosynthetic enzymes that the multiple mutations required are not a realistic consideration.

Only gram-positive bacteria are susceptible to the action of vancomycin because its molecule is too large to pass through porins in the outer membrane of gram-negative bacteria.

CYTOPLASMIC MEMBRANE

Beneath the rigid cell wall is a membrane that totally encloses the cytoplasm (Fig. 7A). This cytoplasmic membrane resembles that of human cells in possessing lipid and protein structural elements. Bacterial lipids are mainly phospholipids. Fungi contain sterols in their membranes that are not present in bacteria.

The lipoproteins in the cytoplasmic membrane of all cells account for selective permeability to water, ions, and nutrients. The polymyxins are cationic detergents that react with the phosphate groups of cell envelope phospholipids and disorganize the lipoproteins in the bacterial cytoplasmic membrane by inserting the lipophilic portion of their molecule into the membrane lipid. This causes leakage of amino acids, purines, pyrimidines, and other small molecules from inside the cell so that nucleic acids and proteins break down and the cell dies (Few, 1955, Newton, 1956). These effects can be prevented by the divalent cations Mg^{2+} and Ca^{2+}, which stabilize the membrane. It has been proposed, therefore, that polymyxins also act by competitively displacing Mg^{2+} and Ca^{2+} from negatively charged phosphate groups on the membrane lipids. The polymyxins have no effect on gram-positive bacteria, anaerobes, and certain gram negatives (*Proteus, Serratia, Brucella,* and *P. pseudomallei*). This selectivity for certain gram negatives, such as *P. aeruginosa, E. coli, K. pneumoniae,* the salmonellas, the shigellas, and *H. influenzae* may be related to their outer membrane. The outer membranes of these bacteria contain lipopolysaccharides that combine with the polymyxins, probably through phosphate groups on lipid A. It is possible that this initial complex with outer membrane lipopolysaccharides is a necessary step in bringing the antibiotic to the cytoplasmic membrane.

Amphotericin B and other polyene antibiotics also alter the permeability of sensitive cells, but only in organisms whose membranes contain sterols. For this reason they do not affect bacteria and are limited in their action against pathogenic organisms to yeasts, fungi (Fig. 7B), and certain amebae. After reacting with polyenes, sterols probably become reoriented within the membranes so that permeability is altered and leakage of small molecules (K^+, Na^+, NH_4^+, amino acids, ribose, phosphate esters) ensues. Amphotericin B is more toxic to yeast and fungal cells than to human cells because of the type of sterol in their membranes, cholesterol being the main sterol in human cells and ergosterol in fungal membranes (Kinsky, 1962). If sterol synthesis is blocked in fungi, the polyenes lose their target and are no longer effective. This occurs in fungi

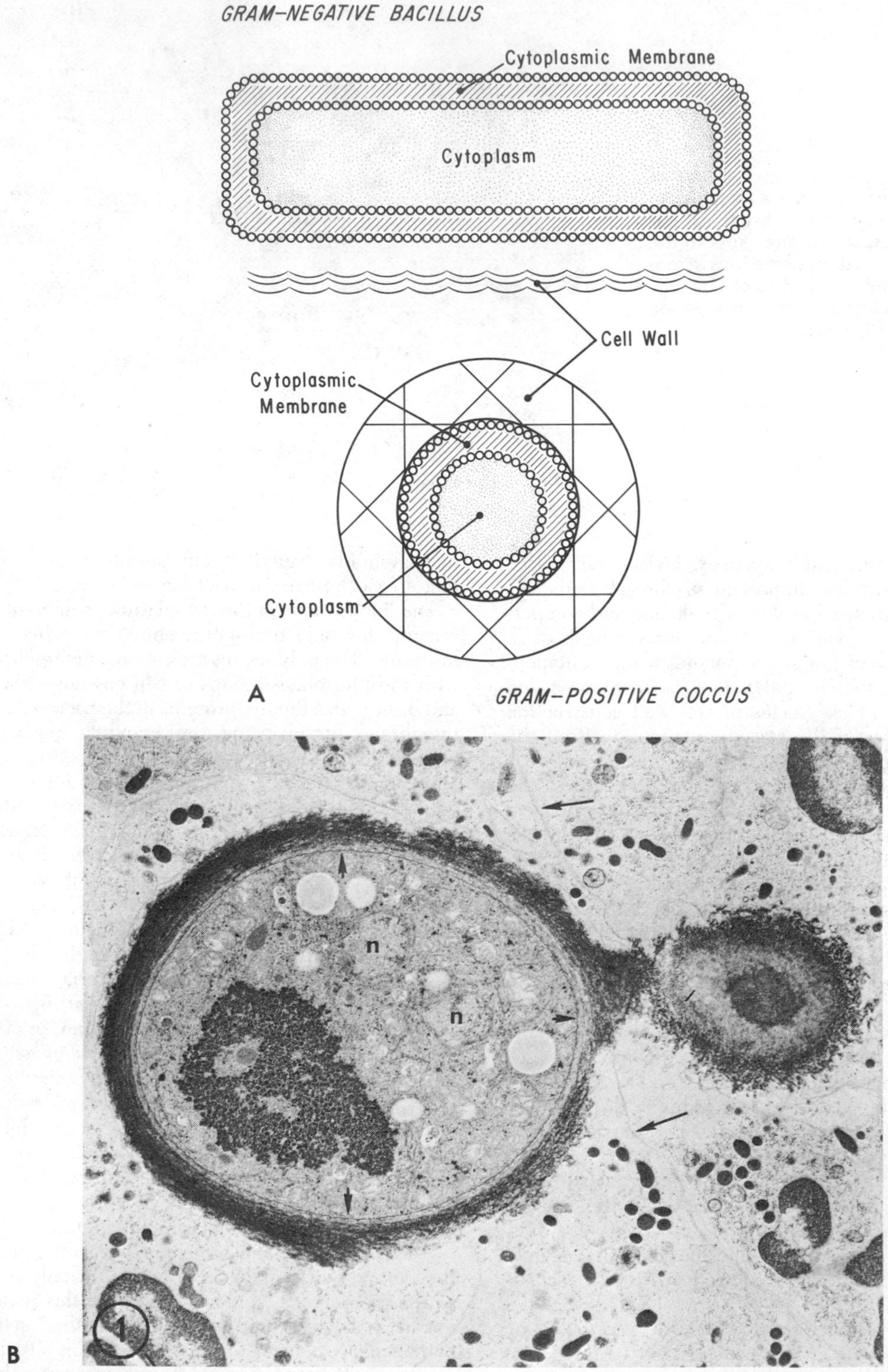

Figure 7. *A,* Bacterial cell wall and underlying cytoplasmic membrane. The circles indicate the protein, and the adjacent diagonal lines represent the lipid in the lipoprotein cytoplasmic membrane. The cytoplasmic membane is drawn out of proportion to its true relationship to the rest of the cell for purposes of illustration. In gram-negative bacilli the cytoplasmic membrane is the site of action of the polymyxins, but in gram-positive cocci it is not damaged by those drugs in usual doses. Differences in accessibility to the membrane, related to differences in cell wall, may account for these differences in susceptibility between gram-positive and gram-negative organisms.

B, Effect of amphotericin B on cytoplasmic membrane of fungi 1, 2, 3, and 4 show in vivo effect of amphotericin during treatment of human North American blastomycosis. (Courtesy Dr. Henry C. Powell.)

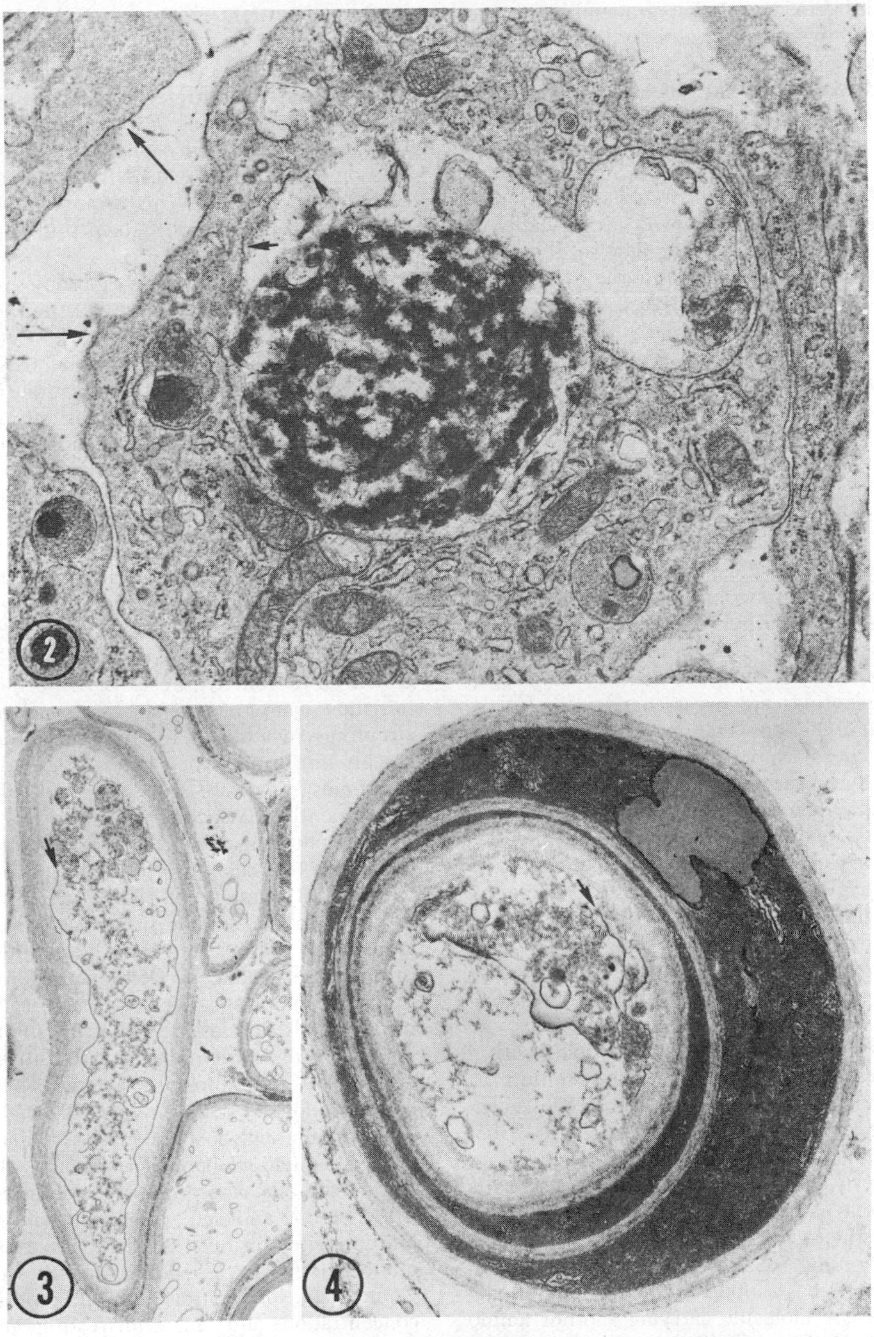

Figure 7 Continued.
1. Skin biopsy, North American blastomycosis. Budding organism: the parent cell shows two nuclei (n), numerous mitochondria, and aggregates of electron-dense material (probably glycogen) enclosed by cell membrane (arrowheads) and the rough outer coat. The surfaces of surrounding macrophages are closely opposed (arrows). ×20,000. 2. Skin biopsy, North American blastomycosis, after amphotericin treatment. Rupture of the cell membrane (arrowhead) and cytolysis. × 20,000. 3. North American blastomycosis. Fungal cells in vitro after incubation with amphotericin and 5-fluorocytosine. Note lysis of the cell membranes (arrow) and cytoplasmic degeneration. ×7000. 4. Degenerating fungal cell with electron-dense deposits in the cell wall. ×20,000.

exposed to miconazole, which inhibits ergosterol synthesis and thus interferes with the antifungal action of amphotericin B. For this reason amphotericin is of no value in patients under treatment with miconazole. By itself, however, miconazole and ketoconazole impair membrane structure and function of fungal membranes by depriving them of ergosterol. Electron microscopy in vitro and in vivo discloses that the first effect of an imidazole on fungi is a disturbance in the cell membrane structure. This is accompanied by leakage of cations and other small molecules (Voigt, 1978).

Studies with ketoconazole demonstrated that inhibition or ergosterol biosynthesis coincided with accumulation of sterols with a methyl group at C-14, and is, therefore, attributed to interference with removal of the 14 α-methyl group of lanosterol. Since it cannot replace ergosterol as a functional unit in membranes, the accumulation of lanosterol at the expense of ergosterol is harmful to the fungal cell (Van den Bossche et al., 1980).

RIBOSOMES

Ribosomes act as an assembly line where amino acids are strung together in peptide chains and proteins. The process is directed by messenger RNA (mRNA), which carries the code for protein synthesis from nuclear DNA. The message in the code is *transcribed* from DNA to RNA (Fig. 8A) and translated into the appropriate amino acid sequence by the four types of ribonucleotides in mRNA. These four ribonucleotides are prearranged in 4^3 (or 64) different triplet combinations that can specify different amino acids. Since there are 64 triplets and only 20 amino acids used in protein synthesis, many amino acids are selected by more than one triplet (or codon). Three of the codons (UAA, UAG, and UGA) code for chain termination only and do not select amino acids. Each amino acid specified by the triplet is carried to the ribosome for incorporation into the growing peptide chain by a second type of RNA, transfer RNA (tRNA). The triplet AUG (adenylyl-uridylyl-guanylyl) or GUG initiates peptide chain formation by directing tRNA carrying methionine (as N-formylmethionine) to attach to the ribosome.

The bacterial ribosomes are spherical particles with a molecular weight of nearly 3 million. They sediment in the Svedberg ultracentrifuge at a rate expressed as 70S (Svedberg units). Before protein synthesis is started, the ribosome dissociates into a 30S subunit and a 50S subunit (Fig. 8B). Protein synthesis starts when mRNA attaches to the 30S subunit and tRNA carrying methionine is bound (Fig. 8C). This is followed by recombination with the 50S subunit to form the functioning 70S ribosome (Fig. 8D). The complete 70S ribosome has another binding site for tRNA, so that a second tRNA molecule carrying another amino acid becomes attached (Fig. 8E, step 1). The first amino acid (methionine) is linked to the second amino acid by the enzyme peptidyltransferase, the two being joined by a peptide bond between the carboxyl group of formylmethionine and the amino group of the second amino acid (Fig. 8E, step 2). This beginning chain with its tRNA is translocated to the first site (donor site) after it has been vacated by the release of tRNA that had formerly carried formylmethionine (Fig. 8E, steps 3 and 4). The ribosome then moves along the chain of mRNA to the next triplet codon for further instruction. Here directions are given for the attachment of the unoccupied acceptor site of a third tRNA with its amino acid. The dipeptide on the donor site is transferred to the third amino acid, and the process of chain elongation is continued until a termination code triplet in mRNA announces that the protein chain is complete.

Since the mRNA strand is "read" by several ribosomes simultaneously, multiple proteins are synthesized simultaneously. A connecting mRNA fiber between adjacent ribosomes, which forms an assembly of as many as 100 ribosomes on a single mRNA strand, can be seen in the electron microscope. This arrangement of multiple ribosomes, each producing its own protein, is called a polyribosome.

Antibiotics that bind to ribosomes cure infections by interfering at certain points with peptide chain formation in bacteria. Thus, they may interfere with initiation of the peptide chain, the attachment of tRNA after initiation, peptide-bond formation, translocation, and the movement of ribosomes along mRNA. Among antimicrobials important in clinical medicine, the mechanism of such interference has been worked out best for five groups: the aminoglycosides, the tetracyclines, chloramphenicol, erythromycin, and emetine.

The Aminoglycosides. The mode of action of streptomycin has been examined far more than that of other aminoglycosides. Streptomycin binds to the 30S subunit of the ribosome by irreversibly combining with a specific ribosomal protein, designated P10. At this site it has three effects on protein synthesis: (1) It permits formation of the initiation complex but blocks its normal activity. When streptomycin attaches to ribosomes, they fall off the "assembly line"; i. e., they leave mRNA prematurely. These ribosomes dissociate into 30S and 50S subunits which subsequently reassociate at the normal initiation sites on mRNA, but they remain irreversibly inactivated initiation complexes that cannot form peptide bonds. (2) It interferes with the attachment of tRNA. (3) It distorts the triplet codons of mRNA so that the message is misread, the wrong amino acids are inserted into the peptide chain, and faulty proteins are produced. Of these three effects, the first is the most important cause of bacterial killing by streptomycin. Cells are killed by the accumulation of aberrant inactive initiation complexes (Luzzato et al., 1968; Ozaki et al., 1969). The third occurs only at borderline inhibitory concentrations of streptomycin (Davis, 1970).

Other aminoglycosides such as kanamycin, neomycin, and gentamicin probably act similarly, but not at the same site on the 30S ribosome as streptomycin. There is some evidence that amikacin, neomycin, and gentamicin bind to multiple sites on both 30S and 50S ribosomes, and show different effects, depending on the drug concentration. Gentamicin, for example, inhibits protein synthesis at low concentrations and causes misreading at higher concentrations.

The Tetracyclines. These drugs also bind to the 30S subunit of bacterial ribosomes and block the binding of tRNA to the acceptor site (Fig. 8E, step 1) of the bacterial ribosome as directed by mRNA (Graven et al., (1969). Spectinomycin, an aminocyclitol, inhibits translocation but does not cause misreading. In other words, tetracyclines prevent the introduction of new amino acids into the peptide chain so that protein synthesis cannot proceed.

Chloramphenicol. In contrast to the aminoglycosides and tetracyclines, chloramphenicol attaches to the larger

(50S) moiety of the ribosome. The drug prevents peptide-bond formation by inhibiting the enzyme peptidyltransferase. This enzyme is located in the 50S subunit, so that it is blocked when chloramphenicol binds to that portion of the ribosome (Pongs et al., 1973). Chloramphenicol also binds to the 30S subunit but its effects there are unknown.

Erythromycin. Like chloramphenicol, erythromycin binds to 50S ribosomal subunits and can compete with chloramphenicol for binding sites on 50S ribosomes. Like chloramphenicol, it interferes with peptidyltransferase activity. Erythromycin probably inhibits translocation (Fig. 8E, step 4).

Lincomycin. This antibiotic resembles erythromycin in its antibacterial spectrum and also acts like chloramphenicol in inhibiting protein synthesis. Thus, lincomycin binds to 50S ribosomes (but not ribosomes of *E. coli*, organisms whose growth is not inhibited by lincomycin) and also appears to block the peptidyltransferase reaction necessary for peptide-bond formation.

Emetine. This ancient amebicidal drug is an inhibitor of protein synthesis but only in eukaryotic cells such as *Entamoeba histolytica*. It inhibits the translocation reaction on the 40S ribosome. Emetine also inhibits protein synthesis in mammalian cells. This lack of selectivity may explain

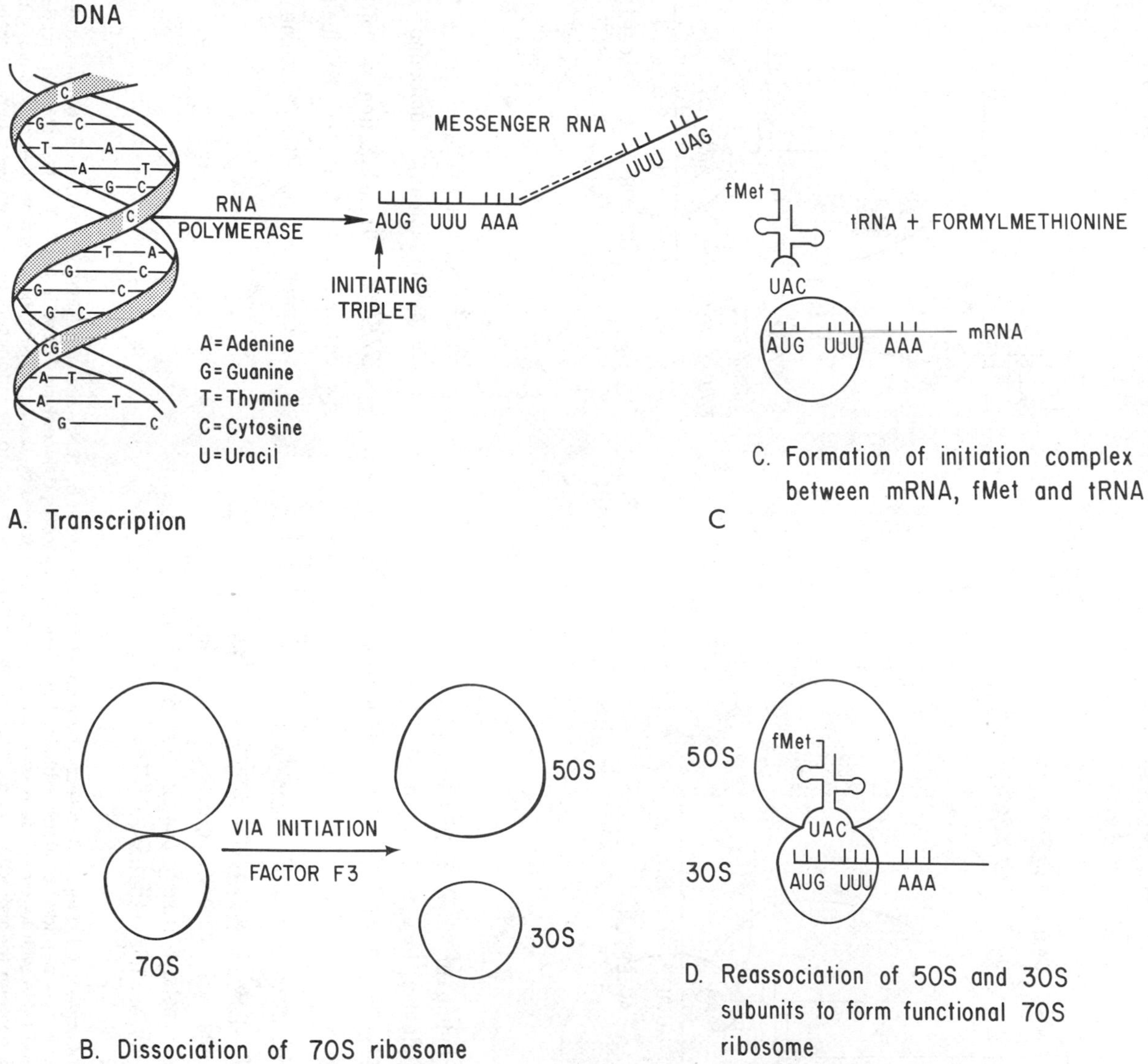

Figure 8. *A,* Messenger RNA receives the code for amino acid sequence (and thus protein synthesis) from DNA in a process known as transcription. The message is carried to the ribosomes in the form of nucleotide triplets. Since there are four nucleotides in mRNA, they can be arranged in 4^3, or 64 different triplet combinations, and each can specify one of the 20 amino acids. As each triplet reaches the ribosome it directs the attachment of a specific amino acid. Rifampin, chloroquine, 5-iodo-2′-deoxyuridine, 5-fluorocytosine, sulfonamides, pyrimethamine, and trimethoprim all interfere with transcription by one or more mechanisms as described in the text. *B,* Dissociation of the 70S ribosome is the first step in protein synthesis on ribosomes. *C,* Protein synthesis starts when mRNA attaches to the 30S subunit and then tRNA + formylmethionine are bound. The 50S subunit then reassociates and the initiation complex is completed. Streptomycin binds the 30S subunit and inactivates the initiation complex so that it cannot form peptide bonds. The tetracyclines also bind to the 30S subunit and prevent binding of tRNA. *D,* Reassociation of 50S and 30S subunits to form functional 70S ribosome.

Figure continued on following page

ELONGATION (GROWTH) OF PEPTIDE

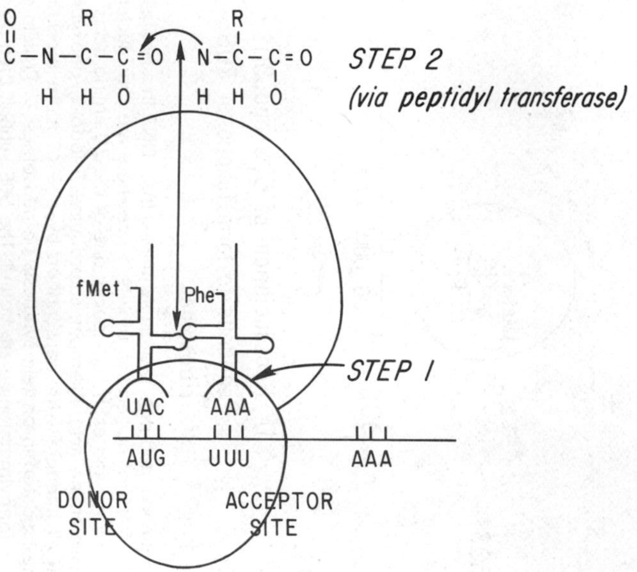

STEP I: Binding of tRNA + 2nd amino acid (e.g. phenylalanine) to acceptor site of 70S ribosome, as directed by 2nd triplet on mRNA (e.g. UUU).

STEP 2: Formation of peptide bond by reaction of amino group of newly bound amino acid (e.g. phenylalanine) with carboxyl group of methionine. The enzyme peptidyl transferase in the 50S subunit catalyzes this reaction.

E

ELONGATION OF PEPTIDE

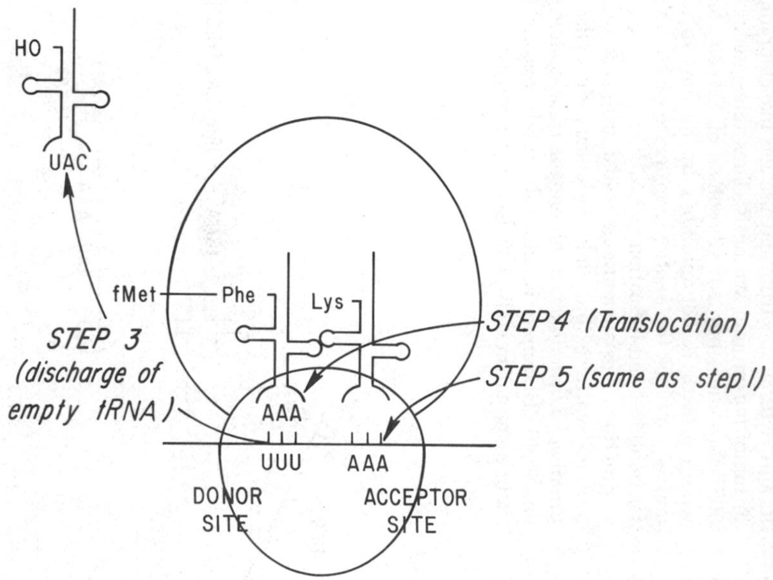

STEP 3: Discharge of empty tRNA (formerly carrying formylmethionine) from donor site on 70S ribosome.

STEP 4: Translocation of mRNA and tRNA with new peptide bond (between methionine and e.g. phenylalanine) to donor site on 70S ribosome.

E

Figure 8 Continued. *E,* Step 1: The second amino acid is brought in by tRNA after the initiation complex is completed. Step 2: This binds the two amino acids by a peptide bond and is blocked by chloramphenicol and lincomycin. Steps 3 and 4: The first tRNA is ejected from the ribosome and the second tRNA with its dipeptide is translocated to the site vacated by the first tRNA. The ribosome then moves along the chain of mRNA to the next triplet codon for instruction on the identity of the third amino acid to be introduced into the growing peptide chain. Erythromycin blocks the translocation step.

the toxicity of emetine for patients during treatment of amebic dysentery or liver abscess (Grollman, 1966).

The Thiosemicarbazones (Methisazone). If polyribosomes are disrupted, protein synthesis stops. At least one group of antimicrobials, the thiosemicarbazones, seem to interfere with protein synthesis of smallpox virus by breaking up the mRNA into smaller fragments and disrupting the ribosomes (Appleyard, 1967).

TRANSCRIPTION MECHANISMS

The information that determines the sequence of amino acids in a given protein is coded in the DNA and *transcribed* into messenger RNA (see Fig. 8A). Messenger RNA then becomes attached to ribosomes, where the code is translated into protein synthesis. Antibiotics interfering with translation act on the ribosomes, as described in the preceding section. Drugs acting on transcription may interfere either with separation of DNA strands or with the synthesis of RNA. DNA consists of two polynucleotide chains twisted about each other in the form of a double helix. During transcription these strands of the double helix separate, and one of them serves as a specific surface or *template* upon which a complementary strand of RNA is synthesized through the action of RNA polymerase. The complementary RNA strand and its template DNA differ in only two respects: the presence of deoxyribose in DNA in place of ribose, and of thymine, in place of uracil, as one of the four major bases.

A drug can interfere with the transcription process by preventing strand separation of DNA, by breaking a strand, by introducing an improper component into the replicating RNA strand, or by blocking access of RNA polymerase to the template strand. Only one clinically valuable antibiotic, rifampicin, interferes with transcription. Other antimicrobial drugs, however, active against protozoa, fungi, and viruses act by interfering with transcription.

Rifampicin. This antibiotic is the most potent inhibitor of DNA-dependent RNA polymerase in bacteria. Human DNA-dependent RNA polymerase, on the other hand, is resistant to rifampicin, so that the drug is selectively toxic for bacterial but not human cells. By binding to RNA polymerase, rifampicin inhibits the formation of all forms of RNA in bacteria and kills them (i. e., it is bactericidal) (Wehrli and Staehelin, 1971).

Nalidixic Acid. By attacking the enzyme DNA gyrase, which generates supercoiling in circular DNA, nalidixic acid selectively inhibits DNA synthesis in bacteria. The drug causes degradation of DNA and is bactericidal, but its use in clinical medicine is limited to infections of the urinary tract by gram-negative bacteria (Cozzarelli, 1980). Although supercoiling allows the extremely long strand of DNA to fit into the limited room available in the bacterial cell, the coil must be relaxed before DNA synthesis can begin. This relaxation is triggered by DNA gyrase when it nicks the linkage in a strand of the double helix. The strands of the uncoiled DNA separate at the nick and new strands are synthesized with the original strands serving as template. Naladixic acid blocks the nicking-reunion action of the gyrase that would allow DNA to uncoil and DNA synthesis to begin.

Chloroquine, Primaquine, and Quinine. The important antiprotozoal drug chloroquine inhibits nucleic acid synthesis by interfering with the ability of DNA to act as a template (Hahn et al., 1966). Chloroquine is inserted (intercalated) between the stacked base pairs of the double helix (See Fig. 23, Chapter 19). This drug inhibits nucleic acid synthesis in mammalian cells as well, but protozoa concentrate chloroquine so that their intracellular level is much higher than that in the body fluids of the patient.

The action of the γ-aminoquinoline, primaquine, is apparently different from that of quinine and chloroquine. Primaquine is probably converted to quinoline diquinone before it kills schizonts in the liver, or gametocytes in the blood. It has been proposed that it disrupts the respiratory chain of the parasite by acting as an analog of ubiquinone.

Although used in malaria for over 300 years, the exact mechanism of action of quinine is still uncertain. The drug can prevent strand separation by forming hydrogen bonds with double stranded DNA. This prevents DNA replication, transcription, and protein synthesis.

Nitroimidazoles. The selective toxicity of metronidazole and other 5-nitroimidazoles against anaerobic bacteria and protozoa probably involves reduction of the nitro group to a nitrosohydroxyl amino group. This is carried out by a reduced electron transport protein similar to ferredottin, which is important in the terminal energy metabolism of susceptible organisms. The intracellular concentration of the unreduced nitroimidazole is kept low by its metabolism so that the drug is taken up by simple diffusion to reach intracellular concentrations 50 to 100 times that in the environment (Gutteridge and Coombs, 1979). The reduced drug is lethal to anaerobic organisms because it inhibits DNA synthesis (Sigeti et al., 1983). Because the reduction of the nitro group requires a reduction-potential more negative than the 350 mV attainable during growth of aerobic bacteria, metronidazole acts selectively against anaerobes. Mammalian cells are unharmed because they lack the enzymes required for reduction of the nitro group.

5-Fluorocytosine. Like 5-iodo-2′ deoxyuridine (IUDR), this halogenated (fluorinated) pyrimidine probably acts by eventually inhibiting the action of the enzyme thymidilic acid synthetase. Cytosine is first deaminated to uracil by cytosine deaminase. 5-Fluorouracil is then converted to 5-fluorodeoxyuridylate. This fluorinated compound causes a lethal thymine deficiency by blocking the conversion of the normal deoxyribonucleotides to deoxythymidylate by thymidylate synthetase. 5-Fluorouracil is also incorporated into mRNA so that errors are produced in translation of information from DNA into protein (De Kloet, 1968).

The Sulfonamides. This group of drugs is placed here among transcription inhibitors because sulfonamides block the synthesis of thymidine and all purines. Thymidine is necessary for DNA synthesis, and the purines for nucleic acid synthesis. This action of sulfonamides is accomplished by preventing the synthesis of folic acid (pteroylglutamic acid) by microbial cells. Sulfonamides are structural analogs of para-aminobenzoic acid (PABA), an essential ingredient of folic acid (Fig. 9). Competitive inhibition of PABA utilization by sulfonamides interferes with folic acid synthesis. Folic acid functions as a coenzyme for transporting 1-carbon units from one molecule to another, reactions that are necessary for the synthesis of thymidine, purines, methionine, and serine. Folic acid metabolism in patients is not affected by sulfonamides because human cells cannot synthesize folic acid. Instead, patients must obtain folic acid in their diets. Since bacteria cannot transport exogenous folic acid into their cells, dietary folate does not interfere with the action of sulfonamide drugs. In pus,

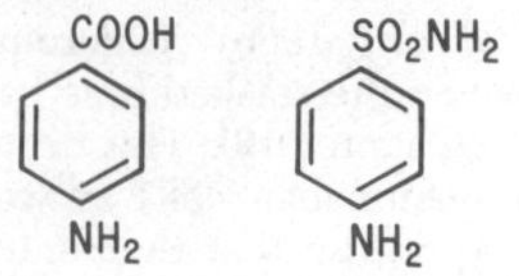

Structural relationship between
p-aminobenzoic acid (left) and
sulfanilamide (right)

Figure 9. The close structural relationship of sulfonamides to para-aminobenzoic acid (PABA) is used to explain their antibacterial effect. The competitive inhibition of PABA utilization by sulfonamides interferes with folic acid synthesis in bacteria but not in man.

however, the breakdown of cells may cause a considerable accumulation of thymidine, purines, methionine, and serine which reverse the inhibitory effect of sulfonamides on bacteria by replenishing the end products of folic acid metabolism. In this way, the sulfonamides may lose therapeutic effectiveness (Feingold, 1963).

In addition to the sulfonamides, para-aminosalicylic acid (PAS) and the sulfones (both active against certain mycobacteria) are PABA analogs and block folic acid synthesis by competitive inhibition.

The Diaminopyrimidines. Both pyrimethamine and trimethoprim, the two important members of this group, are folic acid antagonists ("antifols"). Their site of action is different from that of the sulfonamides, however. The diaminopyrimidines are structurally similar to the pteridine portion of dihydrofolate; therefore, instead of blocking PABA utilization, they prevent the conversion of folic acid to tetrahydrofolic acid by depression of the enzyme dihydrofolic reductase, as indicated in the following reactions:

$$\text{PABA} \rightarrow \text{folic acid} \xrightarrow[\text{reductase}]{\text{folic}} \text{dihydrofolic acid}$$

$$\xrightarrow[\text{reductase}]{\text{dihydrofolic}} \text{tetrahydrofolic acid } (H_4FA)$$

$$\text{Precursors} \xrightarrow{H_4FA} \text{components of nucleic acids}$$

The dihydrofolic acid reductase of protozoa and certain other pathogenic organisms is far more sensitive to trimethoprim than that of man, so that folic acid deficiency in patients given trimethoprim is not a serious problem (Hitchings, 1969).

In order to take advantage of the two vulnerable metabolic sites in protozoa and bacteria, the diaminopyrimidines are usually given in conjunction with sulfonamides. This combination has a much greater antifol action than a simple summation of the two, and, since the two sequential depression steps are present only in the parasite, the combination has markedly increased activity against infection without an increased toxicity for patients.

Antiviral Nucleosides. Four of the important antiviral compounds are synthetic nucleosides composed of nucleic acid bases or their derivatives and linked to ribose or analogs of ribose. These compete with normal nucleic acid precursors and thus inhibit synthesis of viral nucleic acids (Richman and Oxman, 1978).

The first of these to be used effectively for treatment of virus infections is 5-iodo-2′ deoxyuridine (IUDR), which is widely used topically for treatment of herpes simplex infection of the cornea. Because of its resemblance to thymidine, it is phosphorylated by thymidine kinase and incorporated as a triphosphate into viral and cellular DNA instead of thymidine. This results in mismatching during the replication and transcription of the substituted DNA. Although IUDR is toxic to multiplying mammalian cells, it spares corneal cells because their very slow rate of division makes their DNA less vulnerable to IUDR than the more rapidly replicating viral DNA.

5-Trifluoromethyl-2′-deoxyuridine, (trifluorothymidine), which is also used for topical therapy of herpes keratitis, seems to be more effective than IUDR. As a halogenated analogue of thymidine, it is also incorporated into cellular and viral DNA so that the mode of action of IUDR and trifluorothymide are the same. The greater effectiveness of trifluorothymidine would be best explained by its much greater solubility.

The third important synthetic nucleoside of clinical value is adenine arabinoside. This analogue of adenine deoxyriboside inhibits herpesviruses and poxviruses and can be used systemically without serious toxic reactions. Adenine arabinoside is phosphorylated by the cell to the triphosphate, which selectively inhibits the viral DNA polymerase more than it does the cellular enzyme. This selective inhibition, unfortunately, does not apply to viruses like adenoviruses and papovaviruses, which have no DNA polymerase and must use the cell enzymes. Adenosine arabinoside is incorporated into viral DNA and inhibits replication of herpes viruses in a concentration of less than 3 μg/ml, and vaccina viruses at 0.5 μg/ml or less.

The fourth compound belonging to this group of antiviral agents is ribavirin 1-β-D-ribofuranosyl1*H*-1,2,4-triazole-3-carboxamide). It is phosphorylated in cells to the mono-di- and triphosphate and inhibits competitively inosine-5′-phosphate dehydrogenase. In this way it interferes with the biosynthesis of guanine nucleotides and nucleic acids. Its spectrum is broader than that of the 3 other synthetic nucleosides because it inhibits a variety of DNA and RNA viruses, including herpesviruses, influenza viruses, coxsackie B viruses, lassa fever virus, poliovirus measles, and respiratory syncytial virus.

Acycloguanosine (9-(2-hydroxyethoxymethyl guanine)) is unique among clinically useful antivirals because of its highly selective action on herpes virus-infected cells. This selectivity is explained by the need for a virus-specific thymidine kinase to phosphorylate it to acycloguanosine triphosphate, which preferentially inhibits viral DNA synthesis by the herpes-encoded DNA polymerase. Since uninfected cells cannot convert acycloguanosine to the triphosphate, the drug is specific for the virus and nontoxic to healthy tissues. Its minimum 50 per cent inhibitory concentration for viruses of the herpes group varies from 0.10 μm for herpes simplex type 1, to 1.62 μm for herpes simplex type 2, 4-5 μm for varicella zoster, and 50 to 300 for cytomegalovirus (Biron and Elion, 1980).

MECHANISM OF ACTION OF ANTHELMINTIC DRUGS

Chemotherapy for worms is based on physiologic damage rather than protein inhibition. This is because pathogenic worms are fully grown when treatment is needed. Drugs that interfere with growth through inhibition of protein synthesis can stop egg production, but egg production is not needed for worm survival.

Anthelmintics kill worms by blocking energy metabolism or by paralysis (Bueding, 1970). Pyrvinium and mebendazole, for example, interfere with energy metabolism by blocking uptake of glucose, while thiabendazole inhibits fumaric reductase, a key enzyme in fermentation of glucose (Van den Bossche, 1972). Like other intestinal microflora, worms are anaerobic and do not have the enzymes that mammalian cells use for terminal oxidation of glucose (Saz, 1970). In the generation of energy-rich phosphate during glucose metabolism in worms, electron transfer is characterized by the reduction of fumarate to succinate through the action of fumarate reductase, which serves as an electron carrier from flavoproteins to fumarate. In other words, fumarate, instead of O_2, becomes the ultimate electron acceptor in worms as in the following schema of electron transfer in worms and man:

Worms: Flavoprotein→fumaric reductase→fumarate
Man: Flavoprotein→cytochrome oxidase→O_2

This selective inhibition of fumaric reductase explains the toxicity of thiabendazole for worms, but not man.

Niclosamide, an important drug against tapeworms, interferes with energy metabolism by blocking the phosphorylation of adenosine diphosphate (ADP) and thus the formation of adenosine triphosphate (ATP) during electron transport. In other words, the high-energy phosphate required for energy by the worm is not generated in the presence of niclosamide. Niclosamide would, no doubt, show the same effect on human ATP formation, but fortunately the drug is not absorbed from the intestine. Niridazole, an effective remedy for schistosomiasis, affects energy metabolism by depleting glycogen reserves. It blocks the inhibitor of glycogen phosphorylase so that glycogenolysis becomes excessive (Bueding and Fisher, 1970).

The important paralyzing anthelmintics are piperazine, bephenium hydroxynaphthoate, levamisole, praziquantel, and metrifonate (Saz and Bueding, 1966). Piperazine produces flaccid paralysis of *Ascaris* so that the worm can be expelled from the patient by intestinal peristalsis (Del Castillo et al., 1964). It stabilizes the membrane potential of *Ascaris* muscle by hyperpolarization, but has no effect on human muscle. Hence its toxicity is fully selective for the parasite. Bephenium, which resembles acetylcholine in structure and function, has the reverse effect on nematodes. Instead of hyperpolarization and flaccid paralysis, it causes depolarization and contraction. Since the cuticle of many worms is impervious to bephenium, the drug is effective against only a few nematodes of clinical importance, including *Necator americanus, Ancylostoma duodenale*, and *Ascaris lumbricoides*. The mucosa of the human gastrointestinal tract is also impervious to bephenium, as it is to acetylcholine, presumably because these two compounds possess a quarternary nitrogen, i. e., a central nitrogen attached to four methyl groups. The poor absorption explains the low toxicity of this anthelmintic. Levamisole inhibits neuromuscular transmission, possibly by ganglionic blockade. The macrolide-like drug, ivermectin, which has potent activity against nematodes, appears to modify the release of the neurotransmitter gamma-aminobutyric acid so that postsynaptic transmission is blocked (Kass et al., 1980).

Praziquantel, the exciting new pyrazino-isoquinoline derivative, appears to cause paralysis of flukes and tapeworms by increasing the permeability of the cytoplasmic membrane so that intracellular calcium ions are lost and hypercontraction of muscle cells occurs. This effect would explain expulsion of paralyzed worms from the bowel, but not cure of cerebral cysticercosis. The drug also damages the tegument of the neck of the adult tapeworm so that blebs develop and burst. Similar damage would need to occur in order to explain the remarkable therapeutic success of the drug in cerebral cysticercosis. In schistosomes praziquantel produces severe vacuolization over multiple areas on the surface (Melhorn et al., 1981; Thomas et al., 1982).

Metrifonate, an important drug since 1960 for *Schistosoma haematobium* infection, is an organophosphorous compound that inhibits cholinesterase. The action is indirect because it seems that metrifonate must first be converted to 2,2-dichlorovinyl dimethyl phosphate to inhibit cholinesterase. In spite of the fact that metrifonate causes marked inhibition of cholinesterase in patients given the drug for bladder schistosomiasis, it is well tolerated and side effects are unusual. The paralyzed shistosomes lose their hold in bladder veins and are swept into the lung where they die.

References

Anderson J. S., Meadows, P. M., Haskin, M. A., et al.: Biosynthesis of the peptidoglycan of bacterial cell walls. I. Utilization of uridine diphosphate acetylmuramyl pentapeptide and uridine diphosphate acetylgucosamine for peptidoglycan synthesis by particulate enzymes from *Staphylococcus aureus* and *Micrococcus lysodeikiticus*.. Arch Biochem 116:487, 1966.

Appleyard, G.: Chemotherapy of viral infections. Br Med Bull 23:114, 1967.

Biron, K., and Elion, G.: In vitro susceptibility of varicella-zoster virus to acyclovir. Antimicrob Agents Chemother 18:443, 1980.

Bueding, E.: Some biochemical effects of anthelmintic drugs. Biochem Pharmacol 18:1541, 1969.

Bueding, E., and Fisher, J.: Biochemical effects of niridazole on *Schistosoma mansoni*. Molec Pharmacol 6:532, 1970.

Cozzarelli, N. R.: DNA gyrase and the supercoiling of DNA. Science 207:953, 1980.

Craven, G. R., Gavin, R., and Fanning, T.: The transfer RNA binding site of the 30S ribosome and the site of tetracycline inhibition. Sympos Quant Biol 34:129, 1969.

Davis, B. D.: Streptomycin resistance and the study of ribosomal structure and function. N Engl J Med 83:1405, 1970.

De Kloet, S. R.: Effects of 5-fluorouracil and 6-azauracil on the synthesis of ribonucleic acid and protein in *Saccharomyces carlsbergensis*. Biochem J 106:167, 1968.

Del Castillo, J., De Mello, W. C., and Morales, T.: Mechanism of the paralysing action of piperazine on ascaris muscle. Br J Pharmacol 22:463, 1964.

Edwards, D. I.: The action of metronidazole on DNA. J Antimicrob Therap 30:43, 1977.

Feingold D. D.: Antimicrobial chemotherapeutic agents: the nature of their action and selective toxicity. N Engl J Med 269:957, 1963.

Few, A. V.: Interaction of polymyxin E with bacterial and other lipids. Biochim Biophys Acta 16:137, 1955.

Greenwood, D.: Mucopeptide hydrolases and bacterial "persisters." Lancet 2:465, 1972.

Grollman, A. P.: Structural basis for inhibition of protein synthesis by emetine and cycloheximide based on an analogy between ipecac alkaloids and glutarimide antibiotics. Proc Nat Acad Sci USA 56:1867, 1966.

Gutteridge, W., and Coombs, G.: Biochemistry of Parasitic Protozoa. Baltimore, University Park Press, 1977.

Hahn, F. E., O'Brien, R. L., Ciak, J., et al.: Studies on modes of action of chloroquine, quinacrine, and quinine and on chloroquine resistance. Milit Med 131(Suppl):1071, 1966.

Hitchings, G. H.: Species differences among dihydrofolate reductases as a basis for chemotherapy. Postgrad Med J 45(Suppl):7, 1969.

Kaplan, A. S., and Ben-Porat, T.: Differential incorporation of iododeoxyuridine into the DNA of pseudorabies virus-infected and noninfected cells. Virology 31:734, 1967.

Kass, I., Wang, C. Walrond, J., and Stretton, A.: Avermectin, B_{1a}, a paralyzing anthelmentic that affects interneurons and inhibitory motoneurons in ascaris. Proc Natl Acad Sci USA 77:6211, 1980.

Kinsky, S. C.: Nystatin binding by protoplasts and a particulate fraction of *Neurospora crassa*, and a basis for the selective toxicity of polyene antifungal antibiotics. Proc Nat Acad Sci USA 48:1049, 1962.

Luzzato, L., Apirion, D., and Schlessinger, D.: Mechanism of action of streptomycin in *E. coli:* interruption of the ribosome cycle at the initiation of protein synthesis. Proc Nat Acad Sci USA 60:873, 1968.

Mao, J. C., and Robishaw, E. E.: Erythromycin, a peptidyltransferase effector. Biochemistry 11:4864, 1972.

Mansour, T. E.: Chemotherapy of parasitic worms: New Biochemical Strategies 205:462, 1979.

Melhorn, H., Becker, B., Andrews, P., Thomas, H., and Frenkel, J.: In vivo and in vitro experiments on the effects of praziquantel on *Schistosoma mansoni*. Arneimettleforsch 31:544, 1981.

Neuhaus, F. C., and Lynch, J. L.: The enzymatic synthesis of D-alanyl-D-alanine. 3. On the inhibition of D-alanyl-D-alanine synthetase by the antibiotic D-cycloserine. Biochemisty (Wash) 3:471, 1964.

Newton, B. A.: The properties and mode of action of the polymyxins. Bacteriol Rev 20:14, 1956.

Ozaki, M., Mizushima, S., and Nomura, M.: Identification and functional characterization of the protein controlled by the streptomycin-resistant locus in *E. coli*. Nature (London) 222:333, 1969.

Pongs, O., Bald, R., and Erdmann, V. A.: Identification of chloramphenicol-binding protein in *Escherichia coli* ribosomes by affinity labeling. Proc Nat Acad Sci USA 70:2229, 1973.

Richman, D., and Oxman, M.: Antiviral agents. Seminars in Infectious Dis 1:200, 1978.

Saz, H. J.: Comparative energy metabolisms of some parasitic helminths. J Parasitol 56:634, 1970.

Saz, H. J., and Bueding, E.: Relationships between anthelmintic effects and biochemical and physiological mechanisms. Pharmacol Rev 18:871, 1966.

Siewert, G., and Strominger, J. L.: Bacitracin: an inhibitor of the dephosphorylation of lipid pyrophosphate, an intermediate in biosynthesis of the peptidoglycan of bacterial cell walls. Proc Nat Acad Sci USA 57:767, 1967.

Sigeti, J., Guiney, D., and Davis, C.: Mechanism of action of metronidazole on *Bacteroides fragilis*. J Inf Dis 148:1083, 1983.

Thomas, H., Andrews, P., and Melhorn, H.: New results on the effect of praziquantel in experimental cysticercosis. Am J Trop Med Hyg 31:803, 1982.

Thomasz, A.: The mechanism of the irreversible antimicrobial effects of penicillins. How the beta-lactam antibiotics kill and lyse bacteria. Ann Rev Microbiol 33:113, 1979.

Tipper, D. J., and Strominger, J. L.: Mechanism of action of penicillins: a proposal based on their structural similarity to acyl-D-alanyl-D-alanine. Proc Nat Acad Sci USA 54:1133, 1965.

Van den Bossche, H.: Biochemical effects of the anthelmintic drug mebendazole. In Van den Bossche, H. (ed.): Comparative Biochemistry of Parasites. New York, Academic Press, 1972, pp. 139-157.

Van den Bossche, H., Willemsens, G., Cools, W., Cornellissen, F., Lauwers, W., and Van Cutsem, J.: In vitro and in vivo effects of the antimycotic drug ketoconazole on sterol synthesis. Antimicrob Agents Chemother 16:287, 1980.

Van den Bossche, H., Willemsens, G., Cools, W., Lauwers, W., and Le June, L.: Inhibition of ergosterol biosynthesis in *Candida albicans* by miconazole. Curr Chemother 3:228, 1978.

Voight, W.: On the mode of action of antimycotics, especially of clotrimazole (canesten) on the ultrastructural level of human pathogenic fungi. Scand J Infect Dis Suppl 16:51, 1978.

Waxman, D., and Strominger, J.: Penicillin-binding proteins and the mechanism of action of β-lactam antibiotics. Ann Rev Biochem 52:825, 1983.

Wehrli, W., and Staehelin, M.: Actions of the rifamycins. Bacteriol Rev 35:290, 1971.

21

RESISTANCE TO ANTIMICROBIAL DRUGS

DONALD G. GUINEY, M.D.

The ability of bacteria to resist the action of antimicrobial agents is a major problem in medical microbiology. For practical purposes, resistance to an antimicrobial means that the bacteria are not inhibited by concentrations of the drug that can be achieved in patients. Bacterial resistance can be classified into two types: *intrinsic* and *acquired*. *Intrinsic* resistance refers to the natural insusceptibility of the bacteria to a given drug and is an innate characteristic shared by most or all members of a species. *Acquired* resistance means that certain strains of a bacterial species have developed the ability to resist an antimicrobial drug to which the species as a whole is naturally susceptible. This classification of resistance has important therapeutic implications. The intrinsic resistance of an organism governs which classes of drugs can be used to treat infections due to that organism. A knowledge of the prevalence and mechanisms of acquired resistance dictates which organisms need sensitivity testing (as described in Chapter 19) and profoundly influences the choice of the particular antimicrobial agent to be used for the initial therapy of an infection.

THE GENETIC BASIS OF ANTIMICROBIAL RESISTANCE

There are fundamentally different genetic mechanisms underlying intrinsic and acquired resistance. The intrinsic resistance of an organism is a stable genetic property encoded in the chromosome and shared by members of the species. Acquired resistance implies a change in the DNA of the bacteria so that a new phenotypic trait is expressed. There are two ways in which resistance can be *acquired:* (1) by mutation in the chromosome of the bacteria, or (2) by acquisition of new DNA sequences that encode a resistance function.

Mutation

Bacteria can develop resistance to some antibiotics by mutation. Like most organisms, bacteria possess a complex enzymatic machinery to replicate DNA accurately, correct errors, and repair damage to the chromosome. Therefore, the frequency of mutation in any given gene is low, about 10^{-6} to 10^{-9} per generation. Furthermore, most mutations are either silent or detrimental to the cell, and only changes at specific genetic loci result in resistance to an antibiotic. Since antibiotics inhibit essential biochemical processes in the cell, resistance mutations are usually limited to those that result in an altered protein that is less susceptible to the antibiotic but can still carry out its vital cellular function. This is why one-step mutations to antibiotic resistance are usually rare events and only occur with certain antibiotics, common examples being nalidixic acid, rifampin, and streptomycin. In each of these cases, a single base-pair change in the DNA results in an altered protein with much lower affinity for the antibiotic, but with normal enzymatic activity. Some resistance mutations affect the cell envelope and decrease the uptake of an antibiotic. However, for many antibiotics, simple mutational changes are not possible for the bacteria. With these antibiotics, resistance can be acquired by mutation only in a step-wise fashion, as a successive series of single mutations. The frequency of these multiple mutations, which essentially represent an evolutionary process, is very low, and the emergence of resistant strains by this mechanism occurs only rarely.

Acquisition Of New DNA

Most acquired resistance in medically important bacteria results from the acquisition of new DNA sequences that encode the resistance function. The obvious advantage of this mechanism to the bacterial cell is that no changes in its essential components are necessary, and it acquires the resistance genes in a "pre-formed" state. This mechanism requires genetic transfer between different bacterial cells. The new resistance genes can be integrated into the bacterial chromosome and stably inherited from generation to generation, or they can be maintained in an extra-chromosomal state on a bacterial plasmid. Drug resistance plasmids, or R plasmids, are of particular importance because they can carry resistance to many different antibiotics and often can be transferred to other bacteria.

Drug Resistance Plasmids. Bacterial plasmids are circular double-stranded DNA molecules that usually exist physically separated from the bacterial chromosome (Fig. 1). In the cell, the DNA strands are covalently-closed, without nicks or gaps, and the plasmid is "supercoiled," or twisted on itself (Fig. 1A). A single nick or break in one of the phosphodiester bonds of the DNA strand relaxes the superhelix and the plasmid is seen in its "open-circular" configuration (Figure 1B). Plasmids encode many properties of medical significance, including virulence traits, toxin production, and resistance to antibiotics. Because of heavy use of antibiotics since the early 1950's, drug resistance plasmids have become widespread in many different species of bacteria. In addition to genes coding for antibiotic resistance, plasmids also carry genetic information for DNA replication, incompatibility, and conjugal transfer. Replication refers to the duplication of the plasmid during the growth cycle of the bacterial cell, so that each daughter cell after division inherits a copy of the plasmid. DNA replication generally starts from a specific site on the plasmid molecule, the origin of replication or *ori*V. Plasmids, like phages, rely heavily on the host cell metabolism for most DNA biosynthesis enzymes, but the plasmid often contributes at least one specific protein required to initiate its own replication. Plasmids differ in their copy number (the number of plasmid molecules per cell). Larger plasmids, more than 50 kilobases in size, often are present in only one to six copies per cell, while small plasmids, usually less than 20 kilobases, may have 25–50 copies per cell. Plasmids also differ in their stability, the rate at which they are lost from a bacterial population due to deficiencies in replication or segregation so that some of the daughter cells do not get a copy of the plasmid. Plasmid stability has an important medical implication since it governs how rapidly a drug resistance plasmid is lost from bacteria when the selective pressure of antibiotic use is stopped.

Incompatibility (*Inc*) means the inability of two plasmids to co-exist stably in the same bacterial cell. It has provided a useful method of classifying plasmids into groups: all members of an *Inc* group are mutually incompatible with each other. Although the detailed mechanism of incompatibility for most plasmids is not well understood, it seems intimately connected with replication functions. Generally, plasmids of an *Inc* group share extensive DNA homology, especially in the replication regions, while plasmids of different groups have little DNA homology (Guerry and Falkow, 1971; Sharp et al., 1973; Villarroel et al., 1983). Thus incompatibility groups usually represent genetically related plasmids that may have had a common evolutionary origin. *Inc* groups have been best defined for plasmids found in *Escherichia coli* and *Pseudomonas*. There are at least 20 *Inc* groups for *E. coli* and 11 for *Pseudomonas* (Jacob et al., 1977; Jacoby and Shapiro, 1977).

Another important plasmid property is "host range," which refers to the kinds of bacteria in which a drug resistance plasmid can be maintained. Many resistance plasmids have a narrow host range and can exist only in the organism in which they are naturally found or in closely related bacteria (Datta and Hedges, 1972). Some plasmids have a broad host range, such as the *Inc*P plasmids, and can replicate in almost any gram-negative bacterium (Olsen and Shipley, 1973). Host range correlates well with incompatibility grouping, so that most plasmids in a given group have the same host range. For practical purposes, the host range of drug resistance plasmids in gram-negative bacteria has been well defined only for *Enterobacteriaceae* and *Pseudomonas*. Broad host range plasmids can exist in both *Enterobacteriaceae* and *Pseudomonas*, while narrow host range plasmids are maintained in one group of organisms but not the other. Much less is known about drug resistance plasmids in gram-positive bacteria, but incompatibility groups with different host ranges probably exist in these organisms as well.

Conjugation functions allow plasmids to be transferred between different bacterial cells during the process of mating. This transfer greatly facilitates the spread of antibiotic resistance genes in the bacterial population. Mating is a complex process in bacteria and requires a number of different structural proteins and enzymes. Plasmids that encode all the gene products required for their own transfer are called self-transmissible, or conjugative, plasmids. These plasmids are large, 35 kilobases or greater, since the transfer genes occupy a considerable amount of DNA. Smaller plasmids are nonconjugative, since they lack the self-transfer genes. However, many small plasmids can be "mobilized" or transferred by a conjugative plasmid when the two are present in the same cell.

By use of a combination of genetic and recombinant DNA technology, the various plasmids functions of drug resistance, replication, and conjugal transfer can be localized to specific regions of the circular plasmid DNA molecule. Such a functional map for one of the best studied drug resistance plasmids, the *Inc*P plasmid RK2, is shown in Figure 2.

EXCHANGE OF RESISTANCE GENES IN BACTERIA. Drug resistance genes are transferred from one cell to

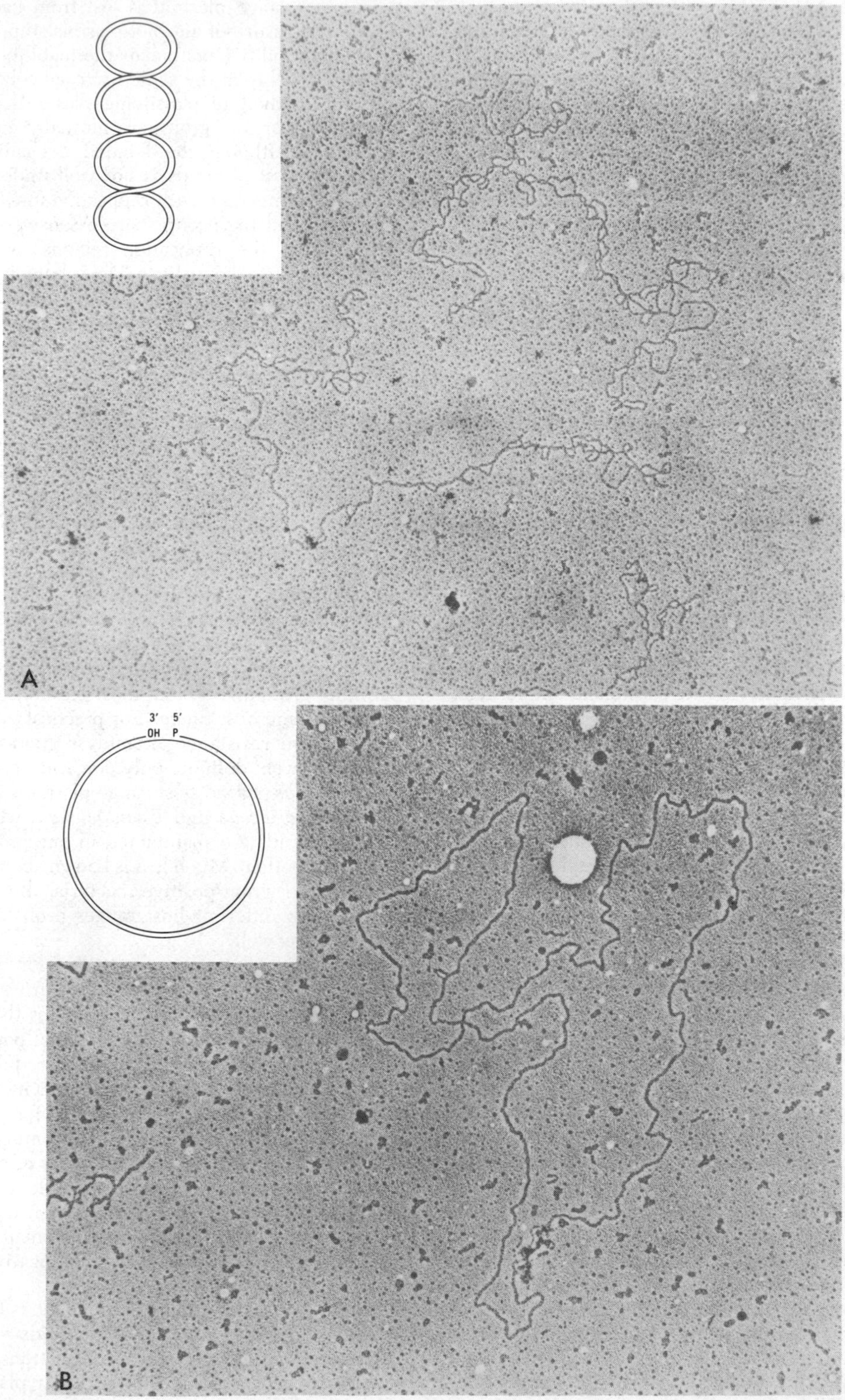

Figure 1. Physical structure of plasmid DNA. Panel A shows an electron micrograph of the supercoiled form of the plasmid, in which the DNA winds around itself like a twisted rope. Panel B shows the same plasmid after a single nick has been introduced in one of the strands; the plasmid is now in the open circular form.

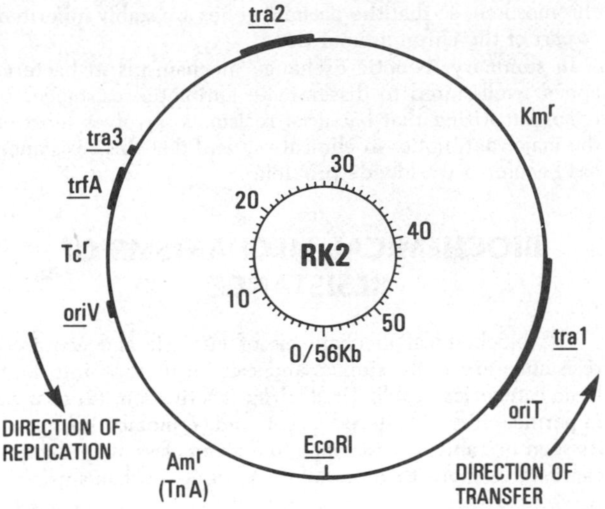

Figure 2. Map of the plasmid RK2. This plasmid has a very broad host range and can transfer to almost any gram-negative bacteria. The map is oriented with respect to the single cleavage site for the *Eco*RI restriction enzyme. The plasmid encodes tetracycline (Tc), kanamycin (Km), and transposable ampicillin (Am, TnA) resistance. The gene product of the *trf*A region interacts with the origin of replication (*oriV*) to initiate DNA synthesis. The *tra*l, 2, and 3 regions encode the conjugation system of RK2. Single-stranded DNA transfer during mating begins at the transfer origin (*oriT*). Adapted from Thomas, 1981 and Guiney and Yakobson, 1983.

another by means of the three major systems of genetic exchange in bacteria: conjugation, transduction, and transformation (see Chapter 4). Both chromosomal and plasmid resistance genes can be transferred by each mechanism, but often one system predominates in a given species of bacteria.

Conjugation. The transfer of DNA between bacteria by cell-to-cell contact is known as conjugation and is also called bacterial mating. Most conjugal transfer systems are encoded by plasmids. The process of conjugation has been studied most extensively in gram-negative bacteria, particularly *E. coli* (Clark and Warren 1979; Willetts and Skurray, 1980). The plasmid-containing donor cells have filamentous appendages on their surface called sex pili, which are required for mating (see Fig. 3). After the sex pili make contact with a recipient bacterium, the donor and recipient come into close contact and a mating bridge is formed. Only one strand of the plasmid DNA is transferred to the recipient, with the single strand in both cells serving as a template for synthesis of the complementary strand. Thus after mating, both donor and recipient contain a copy of the plasmid. In this manner, highly transmissible plasmids carrying multiple resistance genes can spread rapidly through a bacterial population. Furthermore, transfer of resistance is not limited to exchange within a particular species of bacteria. The broad host range conjugative plasmids can transfer drug resistance between most medically important gram-negative bacteria. Conjugation also occurs in gram-positive bacteria, particularly in streptococci but also in staphylococci as well (Engel et al., 1980; McDonnell et al., 1983; Forbes and Schaberg, 1983). A unique mating system has been described in enterococci: certain plasmid-free recipient strains produce "sex pheromones" that facilitate the adherence of donor and recipient cells and greatly enhance the mating process (Clewell, 1981).

Transduction. Certain bacteriophage can transfer antibiotic resistance by transduction, in which resistance genes on a plasmid or in the chromosome are incorporated into phage particles and introduced into another bacterial cell during phage infection. Some phages can transduce entire drug resistance plasmids, provided the plasmid DNA does not exceed the size limit of the phage head. Transduction is an important mechanism for the spread of nonconjugative plasmids, particularly in staphylococci (Novick and Morse, 1967). Since the host range of most phages is limited to a particular genus or species, transduction usually results in the transfer of drug resistance between closely related bacteria.

Transformation. Certain bacteria can take up free DNA molecules from outside the cell and incorporate these DNA sequences into their chromosome in the process called transformation. The naturally transformable bacteria of medical importance are *Hemophilus*, *Neisseria*, and *Streptococcus pneumoniae*. Most other organisms of clinical significance are not easily transformed, and gene exchange by this mechanism probably does not occur under natural conditions. Transformable bacteria undergo spontaneous lysis during growth, and antibiotic resistance genes on the chromosome can be taken up by drug-sensitive members of the population. Plasmids can also be transformed experimentally but it is not known if this is a significant mechanism for plasmid transfer in the natural environment. Like transduction, transformation only occurs between closely related bacteria, since foreign DNA from other species is either not taken up or rapidly degraded in the cell (Sisco and Smith, 1979).

Transposition. In addition to genetic exchange between bacteria, many drug resistance genes can move between different plasmids and the chromosome by the process of transposition shown in Figure 4 (Kleckner, 1981). A drug resistance transposon consists of one or more antibiotic resistance genes flanked on both sides by direct or inverted DNA repeats containing insertion sequences (IS). The IS

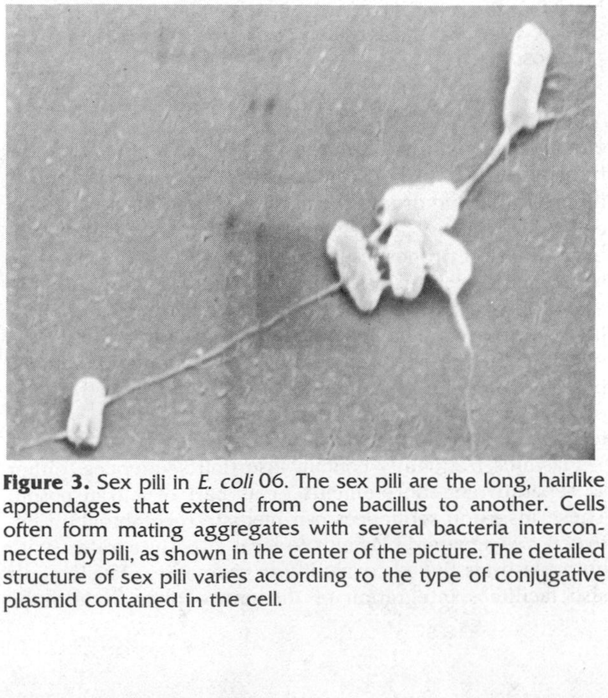

Figure 3. Sex pili in *E. coli* 06. The sex pili are the long, hairlike appendages that extend from one bacillus to another. Cells often form mating aggregates with several bacteria interconnected by pili, as shown in the center of the picture. The detailed structure of sex pili varies according to the type of conjugative plasmid contained in the cell.

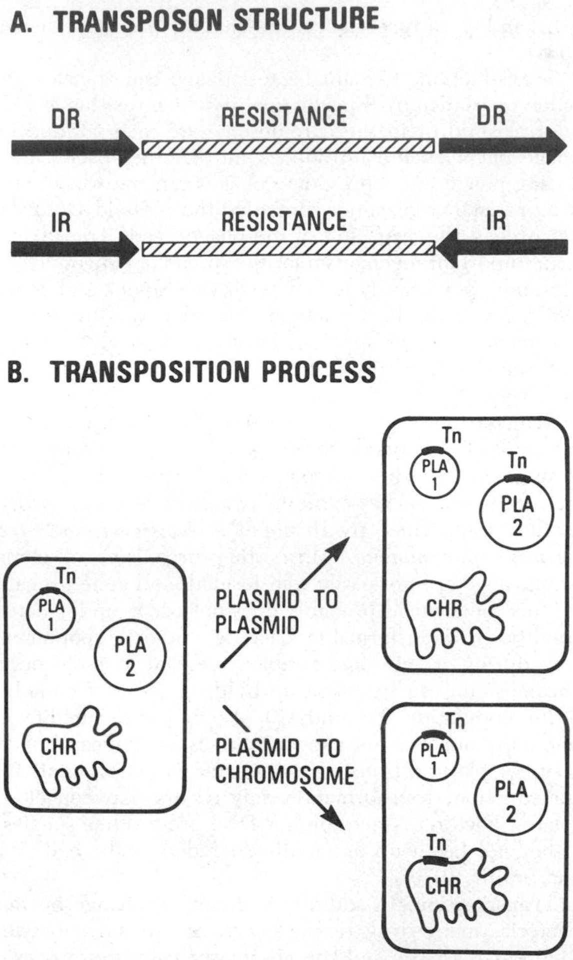

Figure 4. Transposition of antibiotic resistance in bacteria. The general structure of transposons is shown in section A. The antibiotic resistance genes are generally flanked by DNA sequences that are either direct (DR) or inverted (IR) repeats, as shown by the heavy bars with arrows. As seen in section B, the transposon (Tn) present on one plasmid (PLA-1) can transpose to another plasmid (PLA-2) or onto the chromosome (CHR). Note that the original copy of the Tn element is often retained on PLA-1, so that transposition can result in duplication of the transposon.

elements mediate the transposition process, in which the transposon is duplicated and a new copy is inserted into a different plasmid or into the chromosome. This mechanism enables drug resistance genes to spread to plasmids that have different properties or to the chromosome if the drug resistance plasmid is unstable in a particular host cell. For example, transposition of a resistance gene from a nonconjugative to a conjugative plasmid can greatly facilitate the spread of this resistance in the bacterial population. Transposons are common in nature, being found in both gram-positive and gram-negative bacteria, and encode resistance to most of the important groups of antibiotics.

Plasmids frequently contain insertion sequences, either as separate genetic elements or as part of a transposon. These insertion sequences can mediate recombination between two separate plasmids to form a "co-integrate," with both plasmids linked covalently to each other. IS elements also facilitate integration of the entire plasmid into the chromosome, so that the plasmid genes are stably inherited as part of the chromosomal DNA.

In summary, genetic exchange mechanisms in bacteria appear well-suited to disseminate antibiotic resistance. It is not surprising that bacterial resistance involves most of the major antibiotics in clinical use and that this resistance has become a worldwide problem.

BIOCHEMICAL MECHANISMS OF RESISTANCE

The biochemical mechanisms of intrinsic and acquired resistance are quite similar and can be divided into four basic categories (Table 1): (1) drug inactivation, (2) change in permeability, (3) altered target, and (4) metabolic bypass. As seen in Table 1, resistance to a given class of antibiotics can involve more than one of these basic mechanisms.

Drug Inactivation

Drugs are inactivated by enzymes that chemically modify the antibiotic so that it no longer inhibits the bacteria. Inactivation is an important mechanism of resistance for three groups of antibiotics: β-lactams, aminoglycosides, and chloramphenicol.

β-lactams. Most clinically important resistance to the β-lactams is due to β-lactamases. These enzymes hydrolyze the β-lactam ring of penicillins and cephalosporins, and the resulting acid compounds are inactive as antibiotics (Fig. 5). β-lactamases are widespread in bacteria and can be found in both gram-positive and gram-negative organisms. However, the staphylococci are the only clinically significant gram-positive organisms that can produce β-lactamase, and this gene is usually encoded by a plasmid. In contrast, many medically important gram-negative organisms have β-lactamases, and these enzymes can be either encoded by plasmids or the chromosome. β-lactamases differ in their substrate specificity, and numerous classification systems have been proposed based on the β-lactam compounds that are hydrolyzed by a given enzyme (Richman and Sykes, 1973; Sykes, 1982). For medical purposes, β-lactamases can be divided into three categories: penicillinases, cephalosporinases, and mixed enzymes. The β-lactamase of *S. aureus* is a penicillinase with very poor activity against cephalosporins. A number of gram-negative rods that cause nosocomial infections, such as *Enterobacter*, *Serratia*, and *Pseudomonas*, are intrinsically resistant to many cephalosporins due to a chromosomally encoded cephalosporinase, but are sensitive to certain penicillin derivatives such as ticarcillin and piperacillin. The most frequently encountered plasmid-encoded β-lactamases in gram-negative bacteria, the TEM enzymes, have a broad substrate profile and are active against both penicillins and cephalosporins.

Aminoglycosides. The aminoglycosides are inactivated by chemical substitution reactions involving transfer of an acetyl, phosphoryl, or adenyl group to a reactive site on the antibiotic (Benveniste and Davies, 1973; Davies and Smith, 1978). The enzymes that catalyze these reactions are therefore called acetylases, phosphorylases, and adenylases, and are further named by the specific site on the aminoglycoside molecule that is modified (see Fig. 6). Modification of the antibiotic lowers its affinity for the ribosome and produces a dual effect: less inhibition of

Table 1. MECHANISMS OF RESISTANCE TO ANTIMICROBIAL DRUGS

Category of Resistance	Antimicrobial Involved	Specific Mechanism	Genetics: *Plasmid*	Genetics: *Chromosome*
I. Drug inactivation	β-lactams	β-lactamases	+	+
	Aminoglycosides	Phosphorylases, adenylases, acetylases	+	+
	Chloramphenicol	Acetyltransferases	+	+
II. Decreased permeability	Tetracyclines	Decreased uptake, increased egress	+	+
	Aminoglycosides	Decreased uptake due to defect in respiration	−	+
	β-lactams	Change in outer membrane proteins	−	+
III. Altered target	Nalidixic acid	Mutant DNA gyrase	−	+
	Rifampin	Mutant RNA polymerase	−	+
	Streptomycin	Mutant 30S ribosome	−	+
	Erythromycin/clindamycin	Methylated 23S ribosomal RNA	+	+
	β-lactams	Change in penicillin-binding proteins	−	+
IV. Metabolic bypass	Trimethoprim	New dihydrofolate reductase	+	+
		Thymine-requiring mutation	−	+
	Sulfonamides	New dihydropteroate synthetase	+	+

protein synthesis and decreased concentration in the cell. Aminoglycoside modifying enzymes are also widespread and are found in staphylococci, streptococci, and a variety of gram-negative bacteria. They are frequently plasmid-encoded and often are present on transposons. These enzymes can also be found on the bacterial chromosome, probably as the result of transposition events. The aminoglycoside-modifying enzymes differ in their substrate specificity, so that enzymes that inactivate kanamycin, for instance, may not work on gentamicin or tobramycin. Amikacin (Fig. 6) has only two sites for modification and therefore is resistant to most inactivating enzymes.

Chloramphenicol. This antibiotic is inactivated by acetyltransferases (Fig. 7), which are a family of enzymes (usually plasmid encoded) found in both gram-positive and gram-negative bacteria. Analogs of chloramphenicol have been developed that are less susceptible to acetylation, but these are not available for clinical use.

Decreased Permeability

Blocks in permeability reduce the amount of drug that reaches its target site in the cell. The porin proteins in the outer membrane of gram-negative bacteria can act as a molecular sieve and exclude certain antibiotics from the periplasmic space. The permeability of the outer membrane for an antibiotic varies greatly in different gram-negative bacteria. In the *Enterobacteriaceae* and *Pseudomonas aeruginosa*, the outher membrane forms a significant barrier to several antibiotics (Leive, 1974; Scudamore et al., 1979; Zimmermann, 1980), while in *Neisseria* the outer membrane is quite permeable. Therefore, the properties of the outer membrane are an important determinant of the intrinsic resistance of gram-negative bacteria. In contrast, gram-positive bacteria lack an outer membrane and antibiotics have free access to the cell wall and cell membrane. Table 1 lists the antibiotics for which decreased permeability is an important resistance mechanism.

Tetracycline. Resistance to tetracycline is common and is usually mediated by plasmids in both gram-positive and gram-negative bacteria (Chopra and Howe, 1978). Several tetracycline transposons have been described. Plasmid-encoded resistance is usually inducible by low concentrations of tetracycline, but the mechanisms of resistance are not completely understood. The resistance genes specify proteins that are associated with the cyloplasmic membrane, and appear to decrease the influx of tetracycline and to pump the drug out of the cell (McMurry et al., 1980). The end result is a lower intracellular concentration of tetracycline in resistant bacteria.

Aminoglycosides. The aminoglycosides are actively trans-

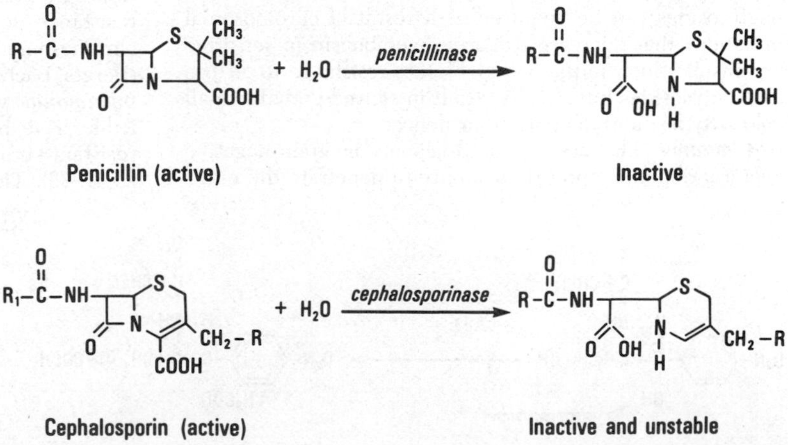

Figure 5. The β-lactamase reaction.

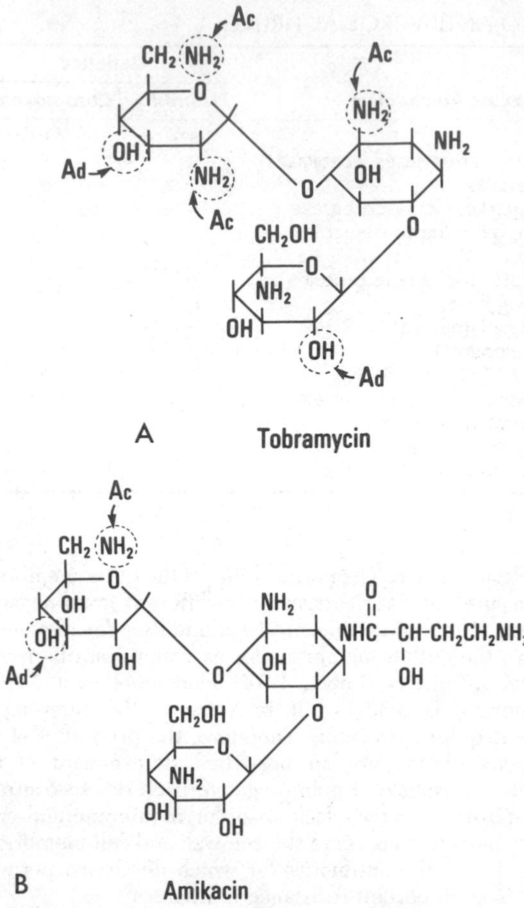

Figure 6. Chemical structure and sites available for modification of the aminoglycosides tobramycin and amikacin. Ac and Ad represent acetylases and adenylases respectively. Note that tobramycin has several sites for inactivation, but amikacin has only two.

ported across the cell membrane in sensitive bacteria by an energy-dependent process that is coupled to electron transport and oxidative phosphorylation (Bryan and Van Den Elzen, 1977). Anaerobic bacteria do not carry out oxygen-dependent electron transport and therefore are intrinsically resistant to the aminoglycosides (Bryan et al., 1979). Streptococci are also poorly susceptible to the aminoglycosides because they lack cytochromes and therefore are deficient in electron transport. Resistance to the aminoglycosides can be acquired as a result of chromosomal mutations that decrease oxidative metabolism in sensitive organisms. Such mutations give cross-resistance to all the aminoglycosides but usually result in slowed growth, small colony types, and decreased virulence.

β-lactams. The activity of β-lactams in gram-negative bacteria depends upon their ability to penetrate the outer membrane and interact with the penicillin binding proteins in the periplasmic space. The poor permeability of the outer membrane for β-lactams is an important factor in the intrinsic resistance of several gram-negative bacteria, especially *Pseudomonas aeruginosa*. Gram-negative bacteria can also acquire increased resistance to β-lactams by chromosomal mutations that change the permeability of the outer membrane proteins. The low-level resistance to penicillin in some strains of *Neisseria gonorrhoeae* is due in part to chromosomal mutations at two loci that result in changes in the outer membrane proteins (Guymon et al., 1978). In contrast, high level penicillin resistance in gonococci is due to plasmid-mediated β-lactamase production.

Altered Target

Much of the intrinsic resistance of bacteria is simply due to poor affinity of the antibiotic for its target, usually a protein but sometimes RNA or a membrane structure. Bacteria can acquire resistance by changing the target so that it no longer binds or is affected by the antibiotic.

Nalidixic acid, rifampin, and streptomycin. Bacteria become resistant to each of these agents by single-step mutations in the target proteins: DNA gyrase for nalidixic acid; RNA polymerase for rifampin; and the P10 protein of the 30S ribosomal subunit for streptomycin. Since these chromosomal mutations have no effect on virulence, resistance to these drugs is particularly likely to emerge during treatment. Plasmid-determined resistance to nalidixic acid and rifampin has not been found.

Erythromycin, lincomycin, clindamycin. These antibiotics all apparently bind to the same site on the 50S ribosomal subunit. Resistance plasmids in gram-positive bacteria encode an enzyme that methylates the 23S ribosomal RNA and blocks the action of these drugs (Lai and Weisblum, 1971). There is complete cross-resistance to all three agents. Plasmids that mediate clindamycin resistance have also been described in *Bacteroides*, but the mechanism of resistance is not known.

β-lactams. The targets for the β-lactams are the penicillin-binding proteins involved in cell wall synthesis (Wayman and Strominger, 1983). Chromosomal mutations that change the penicillin binding proteins appear to be an important mechanism of resistance in several bacteria. Resistance of staphylococci to the semi-synthetic penicillins (such as methicillin) and cephalosporins is due to decreased affinity of the penicillin-binding proteins for β-lactam antibiotics (Hartman and Tomasz, 1981). The methicillin resistance determinant in staphylococci is located on the chromosome and may be part of an insertion sequence (Berger-Bachi, 1983). Recently, isolates of *Streptococcus pneumoniae* with markedly decreased susceptibility to penicillin have been isolated, and an outbreak of a multiply resistant strain occurred in South Africa in 1977 (Jacobs et al., 1978). The South African strain has several changes in

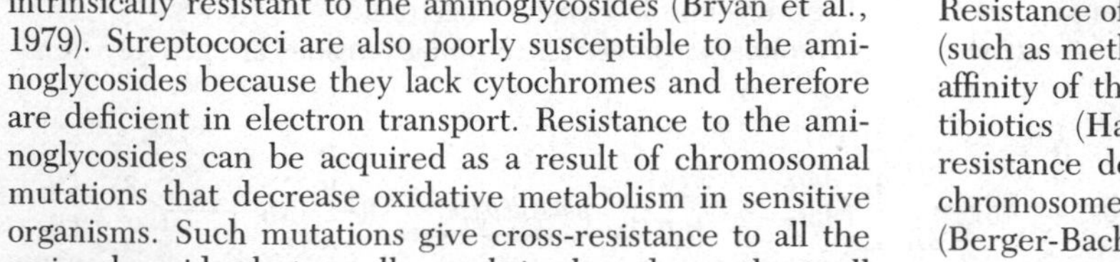

Figure 7. Inactivation of chloramphenicol by acetyltransferase.

its penicillin-binding proteins. A genetic analysis by transformation indicates that penicillin resistance in pneumococci is acquired stepwise as a series of chromosomal mutations in different genes (Zighelbåoim and Tomasz, 1981). A similar mechanism accounts for low-level penicillin resistance in gonococci. A combination of mutations affecting the penicillin-binding proteins and outer membrane proteins resulted in the stepwise acquisition of penicillin resistance (Dougherty et al., 1980). In both pneumococci and gonococci, these mutations have affected the virulence of the bacteria. The South African pneumococcal infections occurred primarily in debilitated patients, and *Neisseria gonorrhoeae* strains with chromosomally mediated penicillin resistance are not able to cause disseminated gonococcal disease.

Metabolic Bypass

Bacterial resistance to trimethoprim and the sulfonamides involves changes in folate metabolism so that the reaction inhibited by the antibiotic is bypassed. Plasmid-mediated trimethoprim resistance is due to the production of a new dihydrofolate reductase that is highly resistant to inhibition by trimethoprim (Skold and Widh, 1974). These resistance genes are often located on transposons and thus may be found in the chromosome of some isolates. Trimethoprim blocks the synthesis of thymine, and resistant bacteria can also arise as a result of thymine-requiring chromosomal mutations. Such bacteria are dependent on exogenous thymine for growth. Sulfonamide resistance is usually due to the acquisition of a plasmid encoding a new dihydropteroate synthetase that is insusceptible to inhibition by the sulfonamides (Wise and Abou-Donia, 1975). These sulfonamide resistance genes are also frequently located on transposons and are widespread in bacteria.

REGULATION OF RESISTANCE GENE EXPRESSION

The expression of antibiotic resistance in bacteria may be either constitutive or inducible (see Chapter 4). Cells that express constitutive resistance synthesize the proteins responsible for resistance whether or not the bacteria are exposed to the antibiotic. In contrast, organisms with inducible resistance do not express the resistance phenotype unless they encounter the antimicrobial agent. Exposure to low concentrations of the drug then induces synthesis of the resistance enzymes. Resistance mechanisms that are typically inducible include the *Staphylococcus* plasmid-mediated penicillinase, certain chromosomal cephalosporinases of gram-negative bacteria, and plasmid-mediated resistance to tetracycline and erythromycin. The mechanism of induction of β-lactamase and tetracycline resistance appears to fit the classic operon model, with the resistance gene under the control of a repressor protein. The antibiotic binds to the repressor and inactivates it, releasing the resistance gene for transcription and expression. Induction of erythromycin resistance conforms to a translational attenuation model in which the drug binds to ribosomes, which change the secondary structure of the mRNA for the methylase protein. The altered mRNA is more efficiently translated, synthesis of methylase increases, and the cell expresses erythromycin resistance (for a review, see Foster, 1983).

Inducible resistance has several clinical implications. Uninduced organisms may express only low-level resistance. However, antibiotic treatment of the patient will induce high-level resistance that cannot be overcome even with enormous doses of the drug. This phenomenon is particularly important in the therapy of staphylococcal infections in which penicillinase-producing isolates may initially appear relatively sensitive to penicillin but quickly become very resistant. For this reason, all *Staphylococci* should be tested for penicillinase production, and positive strains should be treated with a penicillinase-resistant drug such as oxacillin or cefazolin. Induction of the chromosomal cephalosporinases of certain gram-negative bacteria, such as *Enterobacter*, *Serratia*, and *Pseudomonas*, has been implicated in the development of resistance during therapy with the new, broad spectrum cephalosporins, which are strong inducers of β-lactamase (Sanders, 1983).

EVOLUTION OF DRUG RESISTANCE

Antibiotic resistance genes and plasmids were clearly present before the widespread use of antibiotics began in the 1950's. Davis and Anandan (1970) found transferable, multiple drug resistance plasmids in the fecal flora of villagers in a remote region of North Borneo. This community had not been exposed to antibiotics except for a few injections of penicillin given ten years previously. This study demonstrates that R plasmids were relatively common in the normal intestinal flora even without the selective pressure of antibiotic use. There is increasing evidence that R plasmids have evolved by transposition of drug resistance genes onto the plasmids that normally reside in bacteria. "Cryptic" plasmids, with no known phenotypic trait, are common in bacteria and are often self-transmissible (Hughes and Datta, 1983). The widespread nature of drug resistance plasmids in *Enterobacteriaceae* and *Pseudomonas* is mainly due to the selection of R plasmid-containing strains by the heavy use of antibiotics. However, in some bacteria, such as *Hemophilus* and *Neisseria gonorrhoeae*, the emergence of R plasmids is clearly a new phenomenon. Antibiotic resistance plasmids in *Hemophilus* arose in 1976 by transposition of resistance genes from enteric bacteria onto resident *Hemophilus* plasmids (Elwell et al., 1977; Laufs et al., 1981). The penicillinase plasmids of *Neisseria gonorrhoeae*, discovered later in 1976, are closely related to certain *Hemophilus* plasmids and were probably introduced into gonococci by conjugation or transformation (Roberts et al., 1977; Brunton et al., 1982). This spread of resistance to previously susceptible bacteria demonstrates how drug resistance plasmids can evolve under the selective pressure of antibiotic use. Due to the genetic exchange mechanisms of transposition and conjugation, the gene pools of many bacteria are interconnected, and a vast reservoir of drug resistance genes exists.

The origin of the resistance genes themselves is less clear. Since most antibiotics are natural products of soil bacteria and fungi, other soil bacteria may have evolved resistance genes as a defense mechanism. Benveniste and Davies (1972) proposed that some resistance genes have come from the very bacteria that produce the antibiotics. Those producing bacteria must have a method of protection from their own antibiotics, and many have evolved detoxifying enzymes. In support of this hypothesis, an aminoglycoside phosphotransferase (Aph) from a *Streptomyces* strain producing neomycin was shown to be closely related by sequence homology to the Aph enzyme encoded by two bacterial transposons specifying neomycin resistance (Thompson and Gray, 1983).

CLINICAL IMPLICATIONS OF ANTIBIOTIC RESISTANCE

The intrinsic resistance of a bacterial species dictates which types of antibiotics can generally be used to treat infections due to this organism. Acquired resistance has three important therapeutic consequences: 1) the patient may get a drug to which the infecting organism is resistant, resulting in a treatment failure; 2) sensitivity testing of individual isolates is required whenever the incidence of acquired resistance is significant, and 3) the development of widespread resistance may render a previously effective agent useless in treating a given infection.

In most cases, resistant organisms are present at the outset of the infection and are detected by routine sensitivity testing. The development of resistance during the treatment of an individual infection is a rare event except for a few special situations, including the therapy of cavitary tuberculosis, the use of 5-fluorocytosine for fungal infections, and the treatment of urinary tract infections with naladixic acid or streptomycin. In each of these cases, chromosomal mutations arise at a high enough frequency to result in clinically significant numbers of resistant organisms, which are selected by continued use of the antimicrobial agent and often result in relapse of the infection during treatment. Recently, emergence of resistance has been reported during therapy of serious *Enterobacter*, *Serratia*, and *Pseudomonas* infections in compromised patients using the newer cephalosporins, such as cefotaxime and moxalactam. Fortunately, the acquisition of resistance plasmids by a sensitive organism during treatment is quite unusual, so that the initial sensitivity testing is generally a reliable guide to the choice of antibiotic therapy. Nevertheless, the selective pressure of antibiotic use can lead to the acquisition and spread of drug resistance on a larger, epidemiologic scale. The patterns of acquired resistance in the hospital, the community, the nation, and even the world, are profoundly influenced by antibiotic usage.

Control of Antibiotic Resistance

Strategies to limit antibiotic resistance fall into three categories: 1) the use of more than one drug to treat an infection, 2) the development of new antibiotics that are not inactivated by bacterial resistance mechanisms, and 3) the control of antibiotic use in order to reduce the selective pressure for the emergence of resistant strains.

Combination antibiotic therapy is most useful in the prevention of chromosomal resistance. For example, if the frequency of resistance mutations for each drug is one in 10^6, then only one in 10^{12} organisms will be resistant to the two drugs in combination. This latter number is well above the usual load of organisms in an individual patient. This strategy underlies the treatment of cavitary tuberculosis with INH, ethambutol, and rifampin, and also the therapy of cryptococcal meningitis with amphotericin B and 5-fluorocytosine. Combination therapy is less useful in preventing plasmid-mediated resistance, since an R plasmid can encode resistance to several antibiotics and a bacterial cell can contain more than one R plasmid.

Considerable progress has been made in developing β-lactam and aminoglycoside antibiotics that are resistant to inactivation by bacterial enzymes. The semi-synthetic penicillins such as methicillin and oxacillin are not degraded by staphylococcal penicillinase. Similarly, newer cephalosporins, such as cefoxitin and moxalactam, are quite resistant to both the plasmid and chromosomal β-lactamases of gram-negative bacteria. Amikacin (Fig. 6) is resistant to inactivation by most of the aminoglycoside-modifying enzymes in bacteria. Nevertheless, bacteria are still capable of developing resistance to all of these agents. This problem underscores the need for stricter control in the use of antibiotics on a worldwide scale. Huge quantities of antibiotics are used each year as growth stimulants in the livestock industry. These agents select for resistant bacteria that can spread to the human population (Levy et al., 1976). In addition, antibiotics are available in many countries without a physician's prescription. The use of these agents for inappropriate indications and at suboptimal doses has undoubtedly contributed to the emergence of resistant strains. The ease and rapidity with which penicillinase-producing *Neisseria gonorrhoeae* spread from the Far East around the globe emphasizes the fact that antibiotic resistance is a worldwide public health problem.

REFERENCES

Benveniste, R., and Davies, J.: Mechanisms of antibiotic resistance in bacteria. Ann Rev Biochem 42:471, 1973.

Berger-Bachi, B.: Insertional inactivation of staphylococcal methicillin resistance by Tn551. J Bacteriol 154:479, 1983.

Brunton, J., Meier, M., Ehrman, N., Maclean, I., Slaney, L., and Albritton, W.: Molecular epidemiology of beta-lactamase-specifying plasmids of *Hemophilus ducreyi*. Antimicrob Ag Chemother 21:857, 1982.

Bryan, L. E., Kowand, S. K., and Van Den Elzen, H. M.: Mechanism of aminoglycoside antibiotic resistance in anaerobic bacteria: *Clostridium perfringens* and *Bacteroides fragilis*. Antimicrob Ag Chemother 15:7, 1979.

Bryan, L. E., and Van Den Elzen, H. M.: Effects of membrane energy mutations and cations on streptomycin and gentamicin accumulation by bacteria: a model for entry of streptomycin and gentamicin in susceptible and resistant bacteria. Antimicrob Ag Chemother 12:163, 1977.

Chopra, I., and Howe, T. G.: Bacterial resistance to the tetracyclines. Microbiol Rev 42:707, 1978.

Clark, A. J., and Warren, G. J.: Conjugal transmission of plasmids. Ann Rev Genet 13:99, 1979.

Clewell, D. B.: Plasmids, drug resistance, and gene transfer in the genus *Streptococcus*. Microbiol Rev 45:409, 1981.

Datta, N., and Hedges, R. W.: Host range of R factors. J Gen Microbiol 70:453, 1972.

Davies, J., and Smith, D. I.: Plasmid-determined resistance to antimicrobial agents. Ann Rev Microbiol 32:469, 1978.

Davis, C. E., and Anandan, J.: The evolution of R factor. A study of "preantibiotic" community in Borneo. N Engl J Med 282:117, 1970.

Dougherty, T. J., Koller, A. E., and Tomasz, A.: Penicillin-binding proteins of penicillin-susceptible and intrinsically resistant *Neisseria gonorrhoeae*. Antimicrob Ag Chemother 18:730, 1980.

Elwell, L. P., Saunders, J. R., Richmond, M. H., and Falkow, S.: Relationships between some R-plasmids found in *Hemophilus influenzae*. J Bacteriol 131:356, 1977.

Engel, H. W., Soedirman, N., Rost, J. A., van Leeuwen, W., and van Embden, J. D.: Transferability of macrolide, lincosamide, and streptogramin resistances between group A, B, and D streptococci, *Streptococcus pneumoniae*, and *Staphylococcus aureus*. J Bacteriol 142:407, 1980.

Forbes, B. A., and Schaberg, D. R.: Transfer of resistance plasmids from *Staphylococcus epidermidis* to *Staphylococcus aureus*: Evidence for conjugative exchange of resistance. J Bacteriol 153:627, 1983.

Foster, T. J.: Plasmid-determined resistance to antimicrobial drugs and toxic metal ions in bacteria. Microbiol Rev 47:361, 1983.

Guerry, P., and Falkow, S.: Polynucleotide sequence relationships among some bacterial plasmids. J Bacteriol 107:372, 1971.

Guiney, D. G., and Yakobson, E. Y.: Location and nucleotide sequence of the transfer origin of the broad host range plasmid RK2. Proc Natl Acad Sci USA 80:3595, 1983.

Guymon, L. F., Walstad, D. L., and Sparling, P. F.: Cell envelope alterations in antibiotic-sensitive and resistant strains of *Neisseria gonorrhoeae*. J Bacteriol 136:391, 1978.

Hartman, B., and Tomasz, A.: Altered penicillin-binding proteins in methicillin-resistant strains of *Staphylococcus aureus*. Antimicrob Ag Chemother 19:726, 1981.

Jacob, A. E., Shapiro, J. A., Yamamoto, L., Smith, D. I., Cohen, S. N., and Berg, D.: Plasmids studied in *Escherichia coli* and other enteric bacteria. In Bulchari, A. I., Shapiro, J. A., and Adhya, S. L. (eds.): DNA Insertion Elements, Plasmids, and Episomes. New York, Cold Spring Harbor Laboratory, 1977, p. 607.

Jacobs, M. R., Koornhof, H. J., Robins-Browne, R. M., Stevenson, C. M., Vermaak, Z. A., Freiman, I., Miller, G. B., Witcomb, M. A., Isaacson, M., Ward, J. I., and Austrian, R.: Emergence of multiply resistant pneumococci. N Engl J Med 299:735, 1978.

Jacoby, G. A., and Shapiro, J. A.: Plasmids studied in *Pseudomonas aeruginosa* and other pseudomonads. In Bukhari, A. I., Shapiro, J. A., and Adhya, S. L. (eds.): DNA Insertion Elements, Plasmids, and Episomes. New York, Cold Spring Harbor Laboratory, 1977, p. 639.

Kleckner, N.: Transposable elements in prokaryotes. Ann Rev Genet 15:341, 1981.

Lai, C. J., and Weisblum, B.: Altered methylation of ribosomal RNA in an erythromycin-resistant strain of *Staphylococcus aureus*. Proc Natl Acad Sci USA 68:856, 1971.

Laufs, R., Riess, F., Jahn, G., Fock, R., and Kaulfers, P.: Origin of *Hemophilus influenzae* R factors. J Bacteriol 147:563, 1981.

Leive, L.: The barrier function of the gram-negative envelope. Ann N Y Acad Sci 235:109, 1974.

Levy, S. B., Fitzgerald, G., and Macone, A. B.: Changes in intestinal flora of farm personnel after introduction of a tetracycline-supplemented feed on a farm. N Engl J Med 295:583, 1976.

McDonnell, R. W., Sweeney, H., and Cohen, S.: Conjugal transfer of gentamicin resistance plasmids intra- and interspecifically in *Staphylococcus aureus* and *Staphylococcus epidermidis*. Antimicrob Ag and Chemother 23:151, 1983.

McMurry, L., Petrucci, R. E., and Levy, S. B.: Active efflux of tetracycline encoded by four genetically different tetracycline resistance determinants in *Escherichia coli*. Proc Natl Acad Sci USA 77:3974, 1980.

Novick, R. P., and Morse, S. I.: *In vivo* transmission of drug resistance factors between strains of *Staphylococcus aureus*. J Exp Med 125:45, 1967.

Olsen, R. H., and Shipley, P.: Host range and properties of the *Pseudomonas aeruginosa* R factor R1822. J Bacteriol 113:772, 1973.

Richman, M. H., and Sykes, R. B.: The β-lactamases of gram-negative bacteria and their possible physiological role. Adv Microbiol Physiol 9:31, 1973.

Roberts, M., Elwell, L. P., and Falkow, S.: Molecular characterization of two beta-lactamase-specifying plasmids isolated from *Neisseria gonorrhoeae*. J Bacteriol 131:557, 1977.

Sanders, C. C.: Novel resistance selected by the new expanded-spectrum cephalosporins: A concern. J Infect Dis 147:585, 1983.

Scudamore, R. A., Beveridge, T. J., and Goldner, M.: Outer membrane penetration barriers as components of intrinsic resistance to beta-lactam and other antibiotics in *E. coli* K12. Antimicrob Ag Chemother 15:182, 1979.

Sharp, P. A., Cohen, S. N., and Davidson, N.: Electron microscope heteroduplex studies of sequence relations among plasmids of *E. coli*. J Mol Biol 75:235, 1973.

Sisco, K. L., and Smith, H. O.: Sequence specific DNA uptake in *Hemophilus* transformation. Proc Natl Acad Sci USA 76:972, 1979.

Skold, O., and Widh, A.: A new dihydrofolate reductase with low trimethoprim sensitivity induced by an R factor mediating high resistance to trimethoprim. J Biol Chem 249:4324, 1974.

Sykes, R. B.: The classification and terminology of enzymes that hydrolyze β-lactam antibiotics. J Infect Dis 145:762, 1982.

Thomas, C. M.: Molecular genetics of the broad host range plasmid RK2. Plasmid 5:10, 1981.

Thompson, C. J., and Gray, G. S.: Nucleotide sequence of a streptomycete aminoglycoside phosphatransferase gene and its relationship to phosphotransferases encoded by resistance plasmids. Proc Natl Acad Sci USA 80:5190, 1983.

Villarroel, R., Hedges, R. W., Maenhaut, R., Leemans, J., Engler, G., Van Montagu, M., and Schell, J.: Heteroduplex analysis of P-plasmid evolution: The role of insertion and deletion of transposable elements. Molec Gen Genet 189:390, 1983.

Waman, D. J., and Strominger, J. L.: Penicillin-binding proteins and the mechanism of antibiotics. Ann Rev Biochem 52:825, 1983.

Willetts, N., and Skurray, R.: The conjugation system of F-like plasmids. Ann Rev Genet 14:41, 1980.

Wise, E. M., and Abou-Donia, M. M.: Sulfonamide resistance mechanisms in *E. coli*: R plasmids can determine sulfonamide-resistant dihydropteroate synthetases. Proc Natl Acad Sci USA 72:2621, 1975.

Zighelboim, S., and Tomasz, A.: Multiple antibiotic resistance in South African strains of *Streptococcus pneumoniae:* mechanism of resistance to β-lactam antibiotics. Rev Infect Dis 3:267, 1981.

Zimmermann, W.: Penetration of β-lactam antibiotics into their target enzymes in *Pseudomonas aeruginosa:* comparison of a highly sensitive mutant with its parent strain. Antimicrob Ag Chemother 18:94, 1980.

22

THE PHARMACOLOGY AND TOXICOLOGY OF ANTIMICROBIAL AGENTS

HAROLD C. NEU, M.D.

There has been great progress in understanding the pharmacology of antibiotics. Unfortunately, it is not always possible to apply data about the biologic half-life, plasma and renal clearance, and bioavailability to clinical practice in a way that improves on the results of empirical antimicrobial therapy. Unlike the situation with anesthetics and anticonvulsants, in which serum concentrations of an agent correlate well with therapeutic effect, there has been little substantiation that serum or tissue concentrations of antibiotics correlate well with successful therapy. The reason for this is that response to therapy with antimicrobials is the result of many disparate factors in addition to the antimicrobial effect of the drugs, including the infectious and pathogenic abilities of the particular microorganism and the resistance of the patient.

Knowledge of the pharmacology of antimicrobials can, however, be used to minimize drug toxicity. Close attention to certain pharmacokinetic properties of antibiotics results in fewer adverse side effects, since many of the toxic reactions of antimicrobials are due to the accumulation of drugs in patients who have renal or hepatic dysfunction, which can be avoided by adjustments in dosage programs.

GENERAL CONSIDERATIONS. Antibiotics can be administered by oral, intramuscular, intravenous, or topical routes. After absorption, they dissolve in the plasma water. They are bound to plasma proteins and occasionally are absorbed onto erythrocytes. In the plasma, they are distributed to various extravascular tissues and fluids in which they may be free or bound. As the antibiotic is distributed into extravascular compartments, there is an initial rapid fall in plasma concentration. This initial fall in the plasma level occurs at the end of an I.V. infusion. After intramus-

Table 1. SERUM AND BODY FLUID LEVELS AFTER ORAL ADMINISTRATION OF VARIOUS ANTIBIOTICS

Drug	Unit Dose[1] (Oral)	Average Peak Level (μg/ml) Blood[2]	Urine[3]	Bile[4]	CSF[5]
Amoxicillin	0.5 g	10	1,000	10	N.A.
Ampicillin	0.25 g	1.5	50	5	N.A.
Cephalexin	0.25 g	8	500	3	N.A.
Cephradine	0.25 g	8	500	85	N.A.
Chloramphenicol	1 g	13	100	3	6
Clindamycin	0.15 g	2	30	20	N.A.
Cloxacillin	0.5 g	8	200	**	N.A.
Dicloxacillin	0.5 g	15	200	**	N.A.
Doxycycline	100 mg	2.5	100	15	N.A.
Erythromycin estolate	0.25 g	1.4	200	800	N.A.
Indanylcarbenicillin	1 g	15	600	N.A.	N.A.
Metronidazole	0.25 g	5	50	5	2
Minocycline	100 mg	25	100	15	N.A.
Norfloxacin	500 mg	4	400		N.A.
Penicillin V	0.25 g	2	300	4	N.A.
Rifampin	8 mg/kg	10	50	100	0.5
Sulfadiazine	1.0 g	25	100	25	15
Tetracycline	0.25 g	2.2	100	15	N.A.
TMP/SMX	0.16 g TMP + 0.8 g SMX	1 + 30	10 + 100	3 + 30	0.5 + 15

[1]Doses listed are the lowest doses that would normally be employed for adults or children over 32 kg. with normal renal function in the treatment of systemic infections.

[2]Blood levels are at 1–2 hours after I.M. or at the end of 20–30 minutes I.V. infusion. In most instances considerably higher serum levels are attainable with higher dosages. For example, 2 g of ampicillin would yield a peak blood level of 70–90 μg/ml, cefoxitin 2 g a peak blood level of 120–140 μg/ml.

[3]Drug concentrations may be significantly lower if the patient is producing a very dilute urine or if creatinine clearance is below 10 ml/min. Concentration based on mean levels for the first 4 hours after drug is administered.

[4]Assuming normal liver function.

[5]Meningeal inflammation; in meningitis higher doses than those listed would normally be employed resulting in higher CSF levels.

N.A. = not appropriate therapy for meningitis

** = data not available

cular injection and after oral ingestion, the initial distribution phase is obscured by the combination of slow absorption and simultaneous excretion. The continued decrease in serum levels of antibiotics is related to renal and biliary excretion and to biotransformation of some drugs. The amount of drug that reaches extravascular tissue depends not only upon the concentration gradient from serum to tissue fluid, but also on the degree of protein binding in serum and in tissues, and on the diffusibility of the agent. Diffusibility of a drug is a function of its molecular size, dissociation constant, and lipid solubility.

Although blood and tissue levels both decline after each dose, the decline in the two compartments is not usually parallel. Some tissues may avidly bind the drug, although the amount of drug bound in relation to the total dose is usually small, and the rate of decline of drug concentration is not usually affected. Locally bound drug may be extremely important from a toxicologic viewpoint, however.

The pharmacokinetics of most antibiotics are first or second order. Thus, a plot of antibiotic concentration in serum on a logarithmic scale versus time on a linear scale yields a straight line after the initial phase of absorption and distribution. The slope of the linear phase is a measure of biologic life of the antibiotic. The most commonly used measure is the time required for a 50 per cent decrease from the peak value; this is the half-life of the antibiotic. For most antibiotics, the half-life is independent of the dose, initial concentration, or route of administration.

ABSORPTION

Penicillins. There has not been any demonstration of an active transport of penicillins across the lipid protein barrier of the intestinal mucosal cell. Penicillin G is not stable in gastric acid at pH 1-2, and 50 per cent of the drug is destroyed in 20 minutes. In contrast, at pH 4-5, penicillin G is stable for four hours. Other forms of penicillin are more acid-stable, such as penicillin V, and they are well absorbed by mouth (McCarthy and Finland, 1960). Oral absorption of the semi-synthetic penicillinase-resistant penicillins (cloxacillin, dicloxacillin, and flucloxacillin) is excellent (Table 1). Oral absorption of nafcillin is erratic, and the oral absorption of oxacillin is so much less than the other penicillins that it probably should not be used orally. Methicillin is not absorbed orally owing to its acid liability. Wide variations in oral absorption exist among the aminopenicillins. Amoxicillin is well absorbed, approximately twice as well as ampicillin (Neu, 1979). The acetone derivative of ampicillin, hetacillin, is no better absorbed orally than is the parent compound. Pivampicillin, talampicillin, and bacampicillin are esters of ampicillin that are converted in the intestinal mucosa and in serum to ampicillin. These compounds produce blood levels twice those achievable with ampicillin. Cyclacillin, azidocillin, and epicillin are adequately absorbed after oral ingestion. Pivamdinocillin, a pivolyl ester of amdinocillin, formerly called mecillinam, is absorbed and converted immediately to the parent compound. None of the extended spectrum or anti-*Pseu-*

domonas penicillins (carbenicillin, ticarcillin, azlocillin, mezlocillin, and piperacillin) are absorbed orally. An indanyl ester of carbenicillin, indanylcarbenicillin, is well absorbed (Neu, 1982), as is carfecillin, another phenolic ester, but the serum and tissue levels are too low to treat systemic *Pseudomonas* infections. They both achieve adequate urinary levels. Ingestion of food at the same time as the penicillin decreases the absorption of ampicillin but not of amoxicillin, pivampicillin, or pivmecillinam; and it may increase the absorption of indanylcarbenicillin.

Cephalosporins. The orally absorbed cephalosporins are cephalexin, cephradine, cephaloglycin, cefaclor, cefatrizine, and cefadroxil. Cephalexin is extremely well absorbed even in the presence of food (Kirby and Regamy, 1973). Cephaloglycin is poorly absorbed, which results in inadequate serum levels, although urinary concentrations are adequate for the treatment of infections with susceptible bacteria. Cephradine appears to behave almost identically to cephalexin. Cefaclor is well absorbed. Esters of cefuroxime and ceftizoxime are moderately well absorbed.

Tetracyclines. With the exception of chlortetracycline, the tetracyclines are well absorbed when taken by mouth (Neu, 1978). Food, divalent cations (such as those found in antacids and milk), and iron interfere with absorption of the tetracyclines. If a patient ingests a tetracycline on an empty stomach, about 75 per cent of tetracycline hydrochloride, 55 per cent of oxytetracycline, 30 per cent of chlortetracycline, 65 per cent of demeclocycline, and 95 per cent of minocycline and doxycycline are absorbed. The absorption of both of the latter compounds is less affected by food, but iron and calcium decrease their absorption.

Macrolides and Lincinoids. Because erythromycin base is destroyed by acid it must be coated with an acid-resistant coating if it is taken by mouth. Since the coated antibiotic is absorbed in the duodenum and ileum, peak levels occur later than with erythromycin estolate or stearate, which are absorbed in the stomach (Gribble and Chow, 1981). Food does not appreciably alter the absorption of erythromycin estolate, but absorption of erythromycin stearate is decreased if it is given with food. Spiramycin, oleandomycin, and triacetyloleandomycin (all macrolides) are all absorbed orally, as are rosamicin and kitasamycin. Lincomycin is absorbed after oral ingestion but not as well as clindamycin, which produces blood levels five-fold greater. Furthermore, although food markedly impairs lincomycin absorption, food does not decrease clindamycin absorption.

Other Agents. Chloramphenicol and thiamphenicol are well absorbed orally, yielding levels equal or superior to those after intravenous injection (Bartlett, 1981). However, in the form of palmitate ester, unless particle size is well controlled, absorption may be erratic.

Fusidic acid is usually administered orally, but the amount absorbed varies considerably from one individual to another. Phosphomycin is moderately absorbed orally. Metronidazole and ornidazole are both well absorbed orally.

None of the aminocyclitol-aminoglycoside antibiotics yield levels adequate for therapeutic purposes after oral ingestion, although ototoxic serum levels of neomycin can be reached after chronic oral ingestion or after rectal dosing in patients with decreased renal function. Some aminoglycosides are, in fact, now used primarily to suppress microflora, e.g., neomycin and paromomycin. Vancomycin, which is not an aminoglycoside is not absorbed orally.

All the sulfonamides (except sulfaguanidine, succinylsulfathiazole, and phthalylsulfathiazole) are well absorbed after oral administration. Trimethoprim and pyrimethamine are also well absorbed orally (Wormser and Keusch, 1979). All of the urinary "antiseptics" (such as methenamine, furadantoin, nalidixic acid, oxolinic acid, and cinoxacin) are absorbed when taken orally but yield inadequate serum levels to treat infections outside the urinary tract. Urinary levels are, however, adequate to treat urinary tract infections. Newer carboxy quinolines such as pipemidic acid, enoxacin, ciprofloxacin, and norfloxacin are moderately well absorbed orally.

Among the antituberculosis drugs (isoniazid, para-aminosalicylic acid, ethambutol, pyrazinamide, ethionamide, thiacetazone, and rifampin), all are absorbed orally.

Antifungal agents that can be given orally are 5-fluorocytosine, clotrimazole, griseofulvin, and ketoconazole. However, the orally absorbed clotrimazole is rapidly converted to an inactive form. Antiviral agents that are taken orally are amantadine, methisazone, and acylovir.

Parenterally Administered Agents. In general, intramuscular (I.M.) administration of antibiotics is safe and effective. However, a number of the antibiotics cannot be given frequently by intramuscular administration because of pain on injection, and others probably should not be used this way since oral administration yields levels greater than those achieved by I.M. injection. Intramuscular routes should not be relied on in patients in shock, in obese individuals, or in diabetics because poor perfusion from the injection sites may reduce absorption.

Among the penicillins, crystalline penicillin G, given I.M., is so rapidly cleared from the body that it yields inadequate serum levels unless given frequently. Indeed, when used in prophylaxis for dental procedures to prevent endocarditis in people with valvular heart disease, it should be given no more than 30 minutes before dental work is begun. Penicillin combined with procaine produces low levels for 12 hours and is satisfactory to treat hemolytic streptococcal or pneumococcal infections. Doubling the dose of procaine penicillin does not double the serum level unless the dose is given at two sites. Benzathine penicillin G is a repository salt of penicillin that provides tissue and serum levels for 15 to 30 days (depending upon the size of the dose used) that will treat syphilis or streptococcal pharyngitis and will prevent recurrences of rheumatic fever. In general, in adults the levels of penicillinase-resistant penicillins produced by I.M. injection are below those needed for serious systemic staphylococcal illness. Ampicillin, carbenicillin, ticarcillin, and the newer broad spectrum penicillins yield serum levels after I.M. injection that are adequate to treat gram-positive infections or urinary infections but not to treat systemic infections with gram-negative bacteria such as *E. coli*, *Pseudomonas*, *Klebsiella*, and *Enterobacter*. Indeed, relatively high serum levels are needed to treat most gram-negative infections with agents such as carbenicillin, so they should be administered every four hours by intravenous infusion.

Cephalothin, cephapirin, cephacetrile, and cefoxitin are too painful to be given by the I.M. route. Cefamandole can be given by I.M. injection, but cephaloridine and cefuroxime yield slightly higher serum levels. Cefazolin yields the highest serum levels of all the cephalosporins after either intravenous or intramuscular administration (Kirby and Regamey, 1973). Cefotaxime, ceftizoxime, and moxalactam all can be given by the I.M. route but it is preferable to administer cefoperazone intravenously. Cef-

Table 2. SERUM AND BODY FLUID LEVELS AFTER PARENTERAL ADMINISTRATION OF VARIOUS ANTIBIOTICS

Drug	Unit Dose[1] (Parenteral)	Average Peak Level (μ/ml)			
		Blood[2]	Urine[3]	Bile[4]	CSF[5]
Amdinocillin	1.0 g I.V.	70	> 1000	5–30	1–5*
Amikacin	7.5 mg/kg I.M. or I.V.	25	200	5	5
Ampicillin	1.0 g I.V.	35	500	10	3*
Azlocillin	3.0 g I.V.	190	> 2000	100	20
Aztreonam	1.0 g I.V.	160	> 1000	5–10	1–5*
Carbenicillin	4.0 g I.V.	250	> 1000	50	20
Cefamandole	1.0 g I.V.	70	1000	100	N.A.
Cefazolin	1.0 g I.V.	110	> 1000	50	N.A.
Cefmenoxime	1.0 g I.V.	70	> 1000	30	1–10*
Cefoperazone	2.0 g I.V.	250	> 1000	> 100	N.A.
Cefotaxime	1.0 g I.V.	80	> 1000	15	1–30*
Cefoxitin	1.0 g I.V.	70	1000	25	1–5
Cefsulodin	1.0 g I.V.	70	> 1000	5–10	1–10*
Ceftazidime	1.0 g I.V.	80	> 1000	5–10	1–20*
Ceftizoxime	1.0 g I.V.	80	> 1000	10–20	1–30
Ceftriaxone	1.0 g I.V.	150	> 1000	200	1–20*
Cephalothin	1.0 g I.V.	70	500	10	0.7
Cephapirin	1.0 g I.V.	70	500	10	N.A.
Chloramphenicol	1.0 g I.V.	15	100	3	10
Clindamycin	0.6 g I.V.	15	30	40	N.A.
Gentamicin	1.5 mg/kg I.M. or I.V.	6	50	2	1
Kanamycin	5.0 mg/kg I.M. or I.V.	20	200	5	5
Methicillin	2.0 g I.V.	80	1000	30	1
Metronidazole	8.0 mg/kg I.M.	25	100	20	10
Mezlocillin	3.0 g I.V.	190	> 2000	100	1–20
Moxalactam	1.0 g I.V.	100	> 1000	60	1–30*
Nafcillin	1.0 g I.V.	70	150	40	2
Oxacillin	1.0 g I.V.	70	500	2.5	1
Penicillin G	3 million units I.V.	115	300	15	6
Piperacillin	3.0 g I.V.	190	> 2000	50	20
Ticarcillin	3.0 g I.V.	190	> 2000	50	20
Tobramycin	1.5 mg/kg I.M. or I.V.	6	50	2	1
Vancomycin	0.5 g I.V.	10	100	3	3

[1]Doses listed are the lowest doses that would normally be employed for adults or children over 70 lbs with normal renal function in the treatment of sytemic infections.
[2]Blood levels are at 1–2 hours after I.M. or at the end of 20–30 minutes I.V. infusion. In most instances considerably higher serum levels are attainable with higher dosages. For example, 2 g of ampicillin would yield a peak blood level of 70–90 μg/ml, cefoxitin 2 g a peak blood level of 120–140 μg/ml.
[3]Drug concentrations may be significantly lower if the patient is producing a very dilute urine or if creatinine clearance is below 10 ml/min. Concentration based on mean levels for the first 4 hours after drug is administered.
[4]Assuming normal liver function.
[5]Meningeal inflammation; in meningitis higher doses than those listed would normally be employed resulting in higher CSF levels.
N.A. = not appropriate therapy for meningitis
* = at higher dose

tazidime and aztreonam can be administered intramuscularly (Neu, 1982c).

Most of the tetracyclines can be given by either intramuscular or intravenous routes, although the acid pH of tetracycline solutions causes phlebitis. Chloramphenicol as an ester with succinate can be used intravenously, but, given intramuscularly, the ester is not hydrolyzed, and blood levels are inadequate. Lincomycin and clindamycin can be given by either the I.M. or the I.V. route, but rapid infusions should be avoided. Erythromycin is usually too painful to use by the I.M. route, but, as lactobionate or gluceptate, it can be given intravenously. Vancomycin can be given only intravenously since I.M. injection produces sterile abscesses.

All of the aminoglycosides (amikacin, dibekacin, gentamicin, kanamycin, netilmicin, sisomicin, and tobramycin) yield effective serum levels after I.M. injection or I.V. infusion (Neu, 1982a). Streptomycin and spectinomycin are given only by the I.M. route. Rifamide is administered by I.M. injection. It is also possible to give isoniazid by I.M. injection. Amphotericin is given only by I.V. infusion. Pentamidine isethionate is given I.M. since there is an increased risk of hypotension when it is given intravenously. Adenosine arabinoside is given by intravenous infusion, as is acylovir.

Nearly all antibiotics that can be administered I.M. can be given intravenously (some exceptions are mentioned above). In general, higher peak blood levels are produced by equal doses of intravenously administered antibiotics (Table 2). If a drug can be safely administered by either route, intravenous administration is preferred when: (1) absorption from I.M. sites cannot be relied upon; (2) the volume of the required dose precludes I.M. injection; or (3) there is a risk of hemorrhage from the trauma of the injection.

Topical Absorption of Antibiotics. Antibiotics can exert their antibacterial effect when used as topical agents. The degree of absorption of antibiotics from the skin varies widely, but in the presence of denuded or burned skin, even poorly absorbed agents may be absorbed sufficiently to accumulate and produce toxic reactions (Breen et al., 1972). Topical administration of penicillins and cephalosporins is probably unwise, since not only does it promote the selection of resistant bacterial species, but it is also a means of sensitization of the patient by coupling the beta-lactam to body proteins. Aminoglycosides can be absorbed through burned skin to a degree sufficient to produce renal toxicity and ototoxicity if combined with parenteral use of the agents. In contrast, topical use of silver sulfadiazine, mafenide, and silver nitrate has been effective and safe as a therapeutic maneuver in reducing bacterial colonization of the wound eschar and thereby preventing wound sepsis. Compounds such as bacitracin, vancomycin, and aminoglycosides, which can be incorporated into fibrin material but are not bound to the protein, can inhibit entrapped bacteria. In general, however, the topical use of antibiotics should be avoided.

ELIMINATION OF ANTIBIOTICS. Antibiotics may be removed from the body by renal mechanisms (glomerular filtration, tubular secretion, or both), by secretion into the bile, by enzymatic inactivation in the liver, or inactivation rarely by renal dipeptidoses (Kropp et al., 1982).

Renal Excretion. Most antimicrobials are excreted by the kidney as active compounds (Table 3). The renal clearance of compounds within the same class of drug may vary widely. All penicillins, which are weak anions, are cleared from the body by proximal tubular secretion, but the rate of clearance of the penicillins varies somewhat. Thus the half lives of the penicillins vary from 40 minutes for penicillin G to 66 minutes for carbenicillin. Renal clearance of oxacillin is half that of dicloxacillin, accounting to some extent for differences in serum levels. Amoxicillin and ampicillin are cleared equally by the kidney, and the clearances of carbenicillin, ticarcillin, azlocillin, mezlocillin, and piperacillin are similar. Some of the difference in the half-lives of penicillins is due not only to differences in renal clearance but to differences in metabolism. For example, only 5 per cent of carbenicillin is metabolized to penicilloic acid versus 17 per cent of penicillin G.

The renal clearance of cephalosporins is by tubular secretion for some agents whereas others are cleared by glomerular filtration and some are also metabolized. Cephaloridine differs from the other cephalosporins because it is both excreted by glomerular filtration and actively transported into the proximal tubule cell, where it can accumulate to toxic levels. Cephalosporins, such as cefamandole, cefuroxime, cefoxitin, cefotaxime, cefmenoxime, and ceftizoxime all are rapidly secreted by renal tubular cells. Moxalactam, ceftazidime, cefsulodin, and aztreonam are cleared by glomerular filtration. Only 25 per cent of cefoperazone is excreted by the kidney. Ceftriaxone is excreted by the kidney since 60 per cent is recovered in the urine over a 24-hour period (Neu, 1982c).

The excretion of many beta-lactam compounds, both penicillins and cephalosporins, can be blocked by probenecid, which seems to bind to the transport protein in the renal tubule and thereby competitively interferes with the tubular transport of the antibiotics (Table 3).

All the aminoglycosides are excreted by glomerular filtration. There may be a minor role for tubular secretion. In the presence of decreased renal function, the aminoglycosides accumulate. Even in normal individuals, part of a dose is not excreted, and variable amounts, depending on the particular aminoglycoside, bind to renal cortical tissue. Vancomycin is also excreted by the kidney via glomerular filtration. Polymyxins, polymyxin B and colistimethate, are excreted by the kidney, but the mechanism is unclear. Polymyxins also bind to renal tissue.

That amount of tetracycline not eliminated in the feces is excreted by the kidney with the exception of chlortetracycline, which is metabolized, and doxycycline, which is excreted into the intestine.

Renal excretion accounts for only a small fraction of the elimination of erythromycin, other macrolides, chloramphenicol, lincomycin, and clindamycin.

Sulfonamides are partly filtered and partly reabsorbed and secreted, depending on the nature of the individual drug. The solubility of sulfonamides in the urine depends on the drug concentration, which is a function of the plasma concentration and state of hydration, the urinary pH, and the temperature and inherent solubility of the drugs and their acetylated derivatives. Trimethoprim appears to be handled by both glomerular filtration and tubular secretion, and renal clearance increases with acidity. Quinolines are excreted by glomerular filtration.

If the hepatic clearance of rifampin is exceeded, the excess drug, as well as the desacetyl derivative, is cleared by the kidney. Isoniazid, both the free form and the acetylated derivative, and ethambutol are cleared by the kidney.

Hepatic Elimination. Although the liver can secrete weak anions such as the beta-lactam compounds, hepatic clearance of penicillins (except for nafcillin and dicloxacillin) is not significant. In the presence of combined hepatic and renal insufficiency, however, carbenicillin and ticarcillin do accumulate.

Many antibiotics are converted in the liver to compounds that are either less active or inactive. Cephalothin, cephapirin, and cephacetrile are all converted by hepatic esterases to desacetyl derivatives, which are much less active than the parent compounds. Isoniazid is also modified in the liver by acetylation, as are sulfonamides (Hughes, 1953). Chloramphenicol is converted by glucuronyltransferase to the inactive glucuronide, which is then excreted by renal tubular secretion. Although rifampin is converted in the liver to a desacetyl derivative, this metabolite retains significant activity against bacteria and mycobacteria. The desacetyl rifampin is excreted in bile but is reabsorbed in the intestine to reenter the enterohepatic circulation and thereby maintain prolonged serum levels (Cohn, 1969). Rifampin induces the microsomal liver enzymes responsible for its excretion, thereby resulting in a shorter half-life and lower peak blood levels after chronic therapy. Cefotaxime is converted to a desacetyl derivative that is only slightly less active than the parent compound except against *Morganella* and *Pseudomonas*. Cefoporazone is excreted to a major degree by the liver. Ceftriaxone is partially excreted by the liver (Neu, 1982c).

Although erythromycin, lincomycin, clindamycin, fusidic acid, and doxycycline are excreted in bile, this route does not account for all of the drug excreted, and it seems probable that there are other mechanisms of inactivation.

Table 3. PHARMACOKINETIC PROPERTIES OF ANTIBIOTICS

Antibiotic	Oral Absorption	Major Excretion Route	Protein Binding (%)	Serum Half-Life: *Normal (h)*	Serum Half-Life: $C_{cr} < 10$ [1] *(h)*	Hepatic Metabolism Excretion	Dose Adjustment in Renal Failure	Effect of Probenecid	Serum Level Affected by: *Hemodialysis*	Serum Level Affected by: *Peritoneal Dialysis*
Amdinocillin	No	R–T	20	1	4	No	Minor	Yes	Yes	Yes
Amikacin	No	R–G	0	2	35–50	No	Major		Yes	Yes
Amoxicillin	Yes	R–T	17	1	6–18	No	Yes	Yes	Yes	Yes
Amphotericin	No	Nonrenal	90	24	24	No	Minor		No	No
Ampicillin	Yes	R–T	17	1	6–18	No	Yes	Yes	Yes	Yes
Azlocillin	No	R–T	50	1	4	Yes	Minor	Yes	Yes	Yes
Aztreonam	No	R–G	50	2	6	No	Major	No	Yes	No
Carbenicillin	No	R–T	50	1	10–15	Yes	Major	Yes	Yes	Yes
Cefaclor	Yes	R–T	15	1	2	No	No	Yes	Yes	Yes
Cefamandole	No	R–T	70	0.5	9	No	Yes	Yes	Yes	Yes
Cefazolin	No	R–T	85	1.9	20–30	No	Major	Yes	Yes	Yes
Cefmenoxime	No	R–T	50	1	15–20	No	Minor	Yes	Yes	No
Cefonicid	No	R–G, T	70	3–4	—	No	Major	Yes	Yes	Yes
Cefoperazone	No	R, L	90	2	3–6	Yes	Minor		Yes	No
Cefotaxime	No	R–T	50	1	2–4	Yes	Minor	Yes	Yes	Yes
Cefotetan	No	R–G	80	4–6	—	No	Major	Yes	Yes	?
Cefoxitin	No	R–T	70	0.5	9	No	Yes	Yes	Yes	Yes
Cefsulodin	No	R–G	60	1.8	10	No	Major	Yes	Yes	No
Ceftazidime	No	R–G	27	1.8	14	No	Major	No	Yes	No
Ceftizoxime	No	R–T	50	1.5	20	No	Minor	Yes	Yes	Yes
Ceftriaxone	No	R–T Liver	90	6–8	9–15	Yes	Minor	No	Yes	No
Cefuroxime	No	R–T	50	1	20	No	Yes	Yes	Yes	Yes
Cephacetrile	No	R–T	70	0.5	3–8	Yes	Yes	Yes	Yes	Yes
Cephalexin	Yes	R–T	15	1	8–20	No	Yes	Yes	Yes	Yes
Cephaloridine	No	R–G, T	50	1.5	25	No	Avoid		Yes	Yes
Cephalothin	No	R–T	70	0.5	3–8	Yes	Yes	Yes	Yes	Yes
Cephapirin	No	R–T	70	0.5	3–8	Yes	Yes	Yes	Yes	Yes
Cephradine	Yes	R–T	15	1	8–20	No	Yes	Yes	Yes	Yes
Chloramphenicol	Yes	L	25	1–2	3–5	Yes	Minor		Yes	Yes
Chlortetracyline	Yes	L	55	6	7–11	Yes	Avoid		No	No
Ciprofloxacin	Yes	R	28	4–6	?	No	?	No	?	?
Clindamycin	Yes	L	94	2–2.5	6–10	Yes	Minor		No	No
Cloxacillin	Yes	R–T	94	0.5	1–2	Yes	Minor	Yes	Yes	No
Colistimethate	No	R	< 10	5	50–70	No	Avoid		No	No
Demethylchlortetracycline	Yes	R	50	10	50	Yes	Avoid		Yes	Yes
Dibecacin	No	R–G	0	2	35–50	No	Major		Yes	Yes
Dicloxacillin	Yes	R–T	97	0.5	1–2	Yes	Minor	Yes	No	No
Doxycycline	Yes	L	90	15–20	15–20	Yes	No		No	No
Erythromycin	Yes	L	18	1.5	4–6	Yes	No		No	No
Ethambutol	Yes	R–G	< 10	4	7–10	No	Major		Yes	Yes
Flucloxacillin	Yes	R–T	96	0.5	1–2	Yes	No		No	No
5-Fluorocytosine	Yes	R–G	< 10	3–6	70	No	Yes		Yes	Yes

Fosfomycin	Yes	R–T	0	2		No	?	?	?	?
Fusidic acid	Yes	R	28	4–6	?	No	?	?	?	?
Gentamicin	No	R–G	0	2	35–50	No	Major		Yes	Yes
Imipenem	No	R–T		1	4	Yes	Major	No	No	No
Isoniazid	Yes	L, R	< 10	1–4	1–4	Yes	Minor		Yes	Yes
Kanamycin	No	R–G	0	2	35–50	No	Major		Yes	Yes
Lincomycin	Yes	L	70	4	10–15	Yes	No		No	No
Methenamine	Yes	R		4		No	Avoid		—	—
Methicillin	No	R–T	35	0.5	4	No	Minor	Yes	No	No
Metronidazole	Yes	R, L	20	6–14	14–20	No	Major		Yes	
Mezlocillin	No	R–T	50	1	4	Yes	Minor	Yes	Yes	Yes
Minocycline	Yes	R, L	90	15	35	Yes	Major		No	No
Moxalactam	No	R–T	60	2	19	No	Major		Yes	
Nafcillin	Yes	R–T	90	0.5	1–2	Yes	Minor		No	No
Nalidixic acid	Yes	R	93	1–2	6	No	Avoid	Yes		
Neomycin	No	R–G	0	2	50	No	Avoid		Yes	Yes
Netilmicin	No	R–G	0	2	35–50	No	Major		Yes	Yes
Nitrofurantoin	Yes	R		0.3	1	No	Avoid			
Norfloxacin	Yes	R–G	30	4–6	?	No	Avoid	Yes	Yes	Yes
Oxacillin	Yes	R–T	94	0.5	1–2	No	Minor	Yes	Yes	
Oxytetracycline	Yes	R	35	10	50	Yes	Avoid		No	No
Para-aminosalicyclic acid	Yes	R	70	1	25	Yes	Avoid		No	No
Paromomycin	No	R–G	0	2	50	No	Avoid		Yes	
Penicillin G	Yes	R–T	60	0.5	2–6	No	Minor	Yes	Yes	Yes
Penicillin V	Yes	R–T	80	1	1–2	No	Minor	Yes	No	No
Pentamidine	No	R		—	—	No	—			
Piperacillin	No	R–T	50	1	4	Yes	Minor	Yes	Yes	Yes
Pivamdinocillinam	Yes	R–T	20	1	4	No	Minor	Yes	Yes	Yes
Polymyxin B	No	R	< 10	5	40–70	No	Avoid		No	No
Pyrimethamine	Yes	Nonrenal		2–5	20	No	Major			
Quinine	Yes	Nonrenal	70	4	—	Yes	Major		Yes	No
Rifampin	Yes	L	70	1.5–5	1.5–5	Yes	Minor		No	No
Sisomicin	No	R–G	0	2	35–50	No	Major		Yes	Yes
Spectinomycin	No	R–G	0	2	35	No	Avoid		—	—
Streptomycin	No	R–G	0	2	25	No	Major		Yes	Yes
Sulfadiazine	Yes	R	50	2–5	12–25	Yes	Major		Yes	Yes
Sulfamethoxazole	Yes	R	70	5–11	25	Yes	Major		Yes	Yes
Sulfisoxazole	Yes	R	50	5–7	12	Yes	Major		Yes	Yes
Temocillin	No	R–G	90	4	15	No	Major	No	Yes	No
Tetracycline-HCl	Yes	R	55	6–8	50	Yes	Avoid		No	No
Thiamphenicol	Yes	R–G	30	3	5	Yes	Minor		Yes	Yes
Ticarcillin	No	R–T	50	1	12–17	Yes	Major	Yes	Yes	Yes
Tobramycin	Yes	R	60	10	25	No	Major		Yes	Yes
Trimethoprim	No	R–G	40	11	20–60	No	Major		Yes	Yes
Vancomycin	No	R	0	2	30–50	No	Major		Yes	Yes

[1]Creatinine clearance less than 10.
R = renal, T = tubular, G = glomerular,
L = liver

Some drugs may be bound to tissues, as appears to be the case with amphotericin, aminoglycosides, and certain quinolones that disappear from serum but can be detected in urine for months after the last dose has been administered (Craig and Kunin, 1976).

The metabolism of antibiotics can be altered by other drugs that diminish the microsomal degradation system of the liver or by intrinsic liver disease. Thus, toxic concentrations of free drug may develop in patients with liver failure. There is no way to predict the blood level of hepatically excreted or metabolized antibiotics in patients with liver disease.

DISTRIBUTION. The tissue distribution of antibiotics can be considered as consisting of three major areas: (1) highly perfused lean tissues, such as the heart, lung, and hepatoportal system; (2) less well perfused tissues, such as muscle and skin, representing lean tissue mass; and (3) tissues of negligible perfusion, such as ligaments, cartilage, and some areas of bone. Concentrations of antibiotics in the heart, lung, and liver are equivalent to the levels in serum. However, the level of antibiotic found in normal tissues may not represent the amount in infected tissue since inflammation alters blood flow. Certain "barriers" in the body markedly alter the concentration of antibiotic in a compartment such as the brain and CSF (blood-brain and blood-cerebrospinal fluid barriers) and the aqueous and vitreous barriers in the eye between the ocular fluid and plasma water). Some agents cannot cross tissue barriers such as the prostatic acini because of ionization of the drug.

Many antibiotics are bound to serum proteins, principally to albumin (Craig and Welling, 1977). The amount of an antibiotic bound to protein usually represents only a small fraction of the antibiotic in the body. If a drug is 50 per cent bound to albumin, only 10 per cent of the total drug is bound. The precise effect that protein binding of antibiotics has on biologic activities is poorly understood. Only the free antibiotic has antibacterial action. Most antibiotic receptor sites lie below the outer membrane of the bacterial cell wall and, if an antibiotic is bound to a protein the size of albumin, it cannot reach its receptor, e.g., penicillin receptors of the inner wall or aminoglycoside receptors on ribosomes in the cytoplasm of the bacterium. On the other hand, protein binding of some antibiotics acts as a temporary store of the agents and thereby prevents large fluctuations in the concentrations of free drug in the body fluids. Indeed, some penicillins have never been used clinically since, as a result of low protein binding, there is rapid tubular secretion, and they are cleared from the body too rapidly to be effective.

Antibiotics differ greatly in protein binding from one class to another and markedly within a class, as illustrated in Table 3. For example, aminoglycosides are not protein-bound, while penicillins range in protein binding from 17 per cent for ampicillin and amoxicillin to 97 per cent for dicloxacillin. The values given in the literature for the protein binding of antibiotics show a marked variation from one study to another, depending upon the technique used to measure protein binding. Protein concentration, pH and presence of other substances alter the binding and probably do so in vivo since the serum binding of antibiotics in uremic patients is markedly less for certain agents, and uremic patients have higher levels of free drug. If other competing compounds are present in the serum, the amount of each substance bound to protein depends on the relative affinity of each agent for the particular protein receptor site.

Florey and associates studied the distribution of penicillin into tissues in 1946 and showed that there was penicillin in wound exudates eight hours after an intramuscular injection of penicillin. This observation has been confirmed and extended by recent studies utilizing a variety of model systems that have shown that antibiotics that are not highly protein-bound reach peak levels in tissue one to two hours after administration, but highly protein-bound antibiotics reach peak levels later and remain in the tissue for longer periods. Using a fibrin clot model, Barza and colleagues (1974) found that there was an inverse correlation between penetration of beta-lactam antibiotics into the clot and the degree of protein binding. With a chamber implanted in an animal, it has been shown that highly protein-bound agents penetrate the chambers best and remain for the longest period.

Although protein-bound drug is also carried to tissue sites, the amount of free drug in serum governs the level of free drug in tissues. This is important since it might be thought that leakage of serum into an area of inflammation would provide a higher concentration of drug than one could achieve on the basis of diffusion of unbound drug. However, it is unlikely that inhibitory levels of an antibiotic will be achieved at sites of infection if the concentration of free drug in serum never reaches inhibitory levels.

Highly protein-bound agents tend to be excluded from areas of the body in which a complex carrier system across a lipid-protein barrier is needed to transport antibiotics. Protein binding also delays the removal of drugs handled by glomerular filtration, but, in the case of tubular secretion, even a highly protein-bound antibiotic can be eliminated rapidly without eliminating a volume of plasma fluid that contains the drug.

TISSUE BINDING. Many body tissues can inactivate antibiotics by binding them and releasing small amounts so slowly that the agent is ineffective. This is particularly true of the polymyxin class and the antifungal polyene antibiotics. Polymyxin B and E bind to acid phospholipids present in mammalian tissues. Polyene antibiotics are taken up in the reticuloendothelial system. Intracellular ligands in liver tissue bind penicillins, cephalosporins, tetracyclines, and chloramphenicol. Nucleic acid debris, acid proteins, and high concentrations of divalent cations, such as calcium and magnesium, decrease the activity of aminoglycosides. Inert materials, such as fecal material, can inactivate aminoglycosides; and calcium, iron, or magnesium salts in the intestine chelate tetracyclines, rendering them inert.

DISTRIBUTION OF ANTIBIOTICS TO SPECIFIC BODY AREAS

Pulmonary. Concentrations of most antibiotics within the lung are satisfactory, provided there is some blood flow (Neu, 1980). There is a wide variation in the concentrations of penicillins and tetracyclines in sputum. Peak sputum levels occur about two hours after the drugs are administered and are dose-dependent, although disproportionately higher sputum concentrations are achieved at higher doses (Pennington, 1981). Levels of carbenicillin and ticarcillin are only 5 per cent of simultaneous serum levels. Appreciable levels of the cephalosporin antibiotics, cefoxitin and cefuroxime, are reached in bronchial secretions within one hour after an intravenous dose. Cephalothin concentrations in sputum are approximately 25 per cent of the serum level. Tetracycline concentrations in sputum are generally low and do not seem to vary with the degree of purulence. Although sputum concentrations of tetracyclines are low, levels in bronchial epithelium and lung are close to serum levels. Aminoglycoside levels in bronchial secretions are appreciable, but, because of charge properties, they may be less effective in sputum than other agents. Chloramphenicol, because of its lipid solubility and small size, achieves high concentrations in sputum and bronchial secretions. Trimethoprim also achieves effective levels in sputum and bronchial secretions. All of the antituberculosis agents (isoniazid, ethambutol, rifampin, and others) reach appreciable levels in pulmonary tissue.

It has not been established that either sputum or bronchial concentrations of antibiotics influence therapy of pneumonia.

Pleural, Pericardial, and Ascitic Fluid. Most of the penicillins, cephalosporins, sulfonamides, macrolides, clindamycin, chloramphenicol, fusidic acid, and antituberculosis drugs diffuse into serous cavities. Aminoglycosides, such as tobramycin and gentamicin, diffuse slowly into the peritoneal cavity, but, once equilibrium with extracellular fluid is achieved, the serum levels are lower than predicted because of the increased volume of distribution. Peritonitis increases the rate at which aminoglycosides enter ascites. In most cases, it is unnecessary to inject antibiotics into the peritoneum, but penicillins, cephalosporins, and aminoglycosides can be added safely to peritoneal dialysis fluids.

Bone. Penicillins, tetracyclines, cephalosporins, and the lincomycin-clindamycin antibiotics penetrate bone and bone marrow (Pancoast and Neu, 1980). Levels of these antibiotics in infected bone are greater than in normal bone. Administration of semisynthetic penicillinase-resistant penicillins or cephalosporins at the time of surgery yields bone hematoma levels adequate to inhibit most staphylococci. Further injection over the next 24 to 48 hours causes continued incorporation of antibiotic into the wound site hematoma, which, during this period, continues to develop. Tetracycline binds to bone in areas in which bone is being laid down. Tetracyclines temporarily depress normal skeletal growth, but permanent effects on the skeleton have not been seen. New cephalosporins all achieve concentrations in bone adequate to inhibit most *Enterobacteriaceae* and *Haemophilus*. Ceftazidime and aztreonam achieve concentrations in bone adequate to treat *Pseudomonas*. It is not established whether the high calcium environment of bone depresses aminoglycoside activity, but these drugs have been used successfully to treat osteomyelitis due to *Pseudomonas* and *Serratia*. Antituberculosis drugs (isoniazid, rifampin, and ethambutol) all achieve therapeutic concentrations in bone.

Synovial Fluid. Most antibiotics used in the treatment of joint infections enter inflamed joints adequately so that intra-articular instillation of antibiotic is unnecessary (Pancoast and Neu, 1980). The penicillins, cephalosporins, chloramphenicol, tetracycline, lincomycin, and clindamycin reach peak levels in joint fluid about one to two hours after administration and are present in the synovial fluid at levels equal to or in excess of those in serum for the next four to six hours. Aminoglycosides (kanamycin, gentamicin, tobramycin, and amikacin) all reach therapeutic levels in synovial fluid in the presence of inflammation. Measurement of antibiotic activity in joint fluid should be done and the drugs instilled only if patients do not respond to treatment. Polymyxins are not transported into synovial fluid in adequate concentrations and must be injected into the joint.

Ear, Sinuses, and Tears. Most of the penicillins, including penicillin G, penicillin V, ampicillin, and amoxicillin, reach levels in middle ear fluid in acute otitis adequate to eradicate the major organisms involved in this infection (Neu, 1981). Amoxicillin and bacampicillin yield higher middle ear fluid levels than ampicillin. Cephalosporins reach the middle ear but, with the exception of cefaclor, their concentrations are too low to inhibit most strains of *Haemophilus influenzae*. Erythromycin, sulfonamides, and trimethoprim achieve adequate middle ear fluid levels. In chronic otitis in which there is a great deal of scarring, middle ear fluid levels of penicillins are often inadequate, and perhaps in these situations large doses of the drugs are needed. In such situations benzathine penicillin does not yield adequate levels.

Concentrations of antibiotics in sinuses have been shown to be adequate for ampicillin, amoxillin (and the other aminopenicillin esters), tetracyclines, erythromycin, sulfonamides, and trimethoprim. High concentrations of sulfonamides, minocycline, and rifampin are present in the lacrimal secretions, which bathe the posterior pharynx where meningococci are harbored, explaining the value of these agents for the prophylaxis of meningococcal disease.

Eye. Very few antibiotics penetrate the eye well. Measurements in patients undergoing cataract extraction or in rabbit models to determine tissue levels in the eye have been disparate. In general, the levels of penicillins and cephalosporins in the aqueous are less than 10 per cent of the peak serum level and so inhibit only highly sensitive bacteria such as pneumococci or streptococci (Barza, 1980). The penicillinase-resistant penicillins (methicillin, oxacillin, and others) do not penetrate the aqueous of noninflamed eyes, but, in the presence of infection, achieve levels adequate to inhibit staphylococci, provided large doses are given intravenously. Cefamandole can reach levels in the aqueous high enough to inhibit streptococci and staphylococci. Aminoglycosides do not achieve adequate aqueous levels when given by I.M. or I.V. injection. Chloramphenicol given orally or I.V. yields measurable levels in the aqueous, but not if injected subconjunctivally as the succinate salt (McPherson et al., 1968). Amphotericin concentrations are not measurable when the drug is administered parenterally.

Subconjunctival instillation of aminoglycosides, gentamicin, or tobramycin has produced levels adequate to treat experimental *Pseudomonas* infection in the rabbit eye. Amphotericin has also been administered by this technique. No significant penetration of any antibiotic into the vitreous has been demonstrated, and aminoglycosides have been injected intracamerally on rare occasions.

Skin. Highly protein-bound penicillins and cephalosporins have not achieved high concentrations in skin windows. Tetracyclines and clindamycin concentrate in skin tissue, accounting for their effectiveness in the treatment of acne. Minocycline, because of its high lipid solubility, has the greatest concentration in skin among the tetracyclines. Chloramphenicol also achieves excellent levels in skin tissues but obviously should not be used for skin infections unless other agents are not available. In second and third degree burns, antibiotics do not penetrate the subeschar level, and even sensitive bacteria can proliferate in this area although serum levels are very high.

Kidney. Renal parenchymal concentrations of antibiotics differ in relation not only to renal blood flow but also to the state of hydration and the presence of other drugs within the kidney that compete for transport mechanisms (Whelton and Walker, 1982). In general, it has been stated that cure of urinary tract infection is related to urinary levels rather than to serum levels (Stamey, 1972). This is well substantiated by compounds such as nalidixic acid or the nitrofurantoins that are effective in the treatment of urinary tract infections in spite of inadequate serum levels. In the treatment of pyelonephritis, high concentrations within medullary, cortical, and papillary interstitial fluid may be important. Penicillin G and ampicillin levels are two to eight times the serum level. Similar findings have been made for cephalosporins. Aminoglycosides concentrate in the renal cortical tissue, which undoubtedly contributes to the development of proximal tubular cell damage. Bound gentamicin may also function as an antibiotic, however. The renal cortical concentrations of tobramycin and netilmicin are considerably less than those of gentamicin.

In the presence of markedly decreased renal function, oral ampicillin, cephalexin, and trimethoprim-sulfamethoxazole still give urinary concentrations adequate to treat infections by most urinary bacteria. In contrast, nitrofurantoins (Sachs et al., 1968), methenamine, and nalidixic acid do not yield urine levels in renal failure necessary to treat urinary infection unless toxic serum levels are achieved. The parenterally administered penicillins (carbenicillin and ticarcillin) and parenteral cephalosporins (such as cephalothin, cefazolin, cefamandole, and cefoxitin) yield adequate intrarenal and urinary concentrations even in the presence of markedly decreased renal function. Cefotaxime, moxalactam, ceftizoxime, and cefoperazone all yield therapeutic concentrations in urine until creatinine clearances fall below 5 ml/min. (Neu, 1982a).

Prostate. The high degree of ionization and protein binding of most antibiotics excludes most antibiotics from the prostate (Stamey, 1972). In acute inflammatory prostatic infections, this is not a consideration since the acute inflammatory process allows the antibiotics to enter the infected gland. Although some sulfonamides, erythromycin, and rifampin enter the normal gland, they are usually not effective against the bacteria that cause chronic prostatitis (Fair et al., 1979). Trimethoprim achieves prostatic fluid levels eight-fold greater than serum levels, and doxycycline (Garnes, 1973) and minocycline also achieve high prostate levels.

Placenta. Penicillin G, ampicillin, amoxicillin, tetracyclines, clindamycin, lincomycin, erythromycin, cephalothin, and cephaloridine reach effective levels in fetal blood within a short time after administration to the mother. Penicillins cross the placental barrier poorly if they are very highly bound to proteins. Aminoglycosides, trimethoprim, and metronidazole cross the placenta, as do the antimalarial quinolines. Penicillin G, ampicillin, erythromycin, and clindamycin reach therapeutic concentrations in amniotic fluid readily, but only negligible amounts of streptomycin, tetracycline, and chloramphenicol are found there (Philipson, 1979).

Central Nervous System. Only lipid-soluble compounds reach the brain readily because of the blood-brain barrier created by tight intracellular junctions and specialized cells surrounding the brain capillaries (Rall, 1971; Norby, 1978). Chloramphenicol achieves high brain tissue levels. In the presence of inflammation, such as a brain abscess, penicillin G, ampicillin, methicillin, oxacillin, and nafcillin achieve levels of antibiotic high enough to be measured. Lincomycin and clindamycin do not produce adequate brain tissue levels nor do the aminoglycosides. Vancomycin does achieve levels in the brain in the presence of inflammation. Trimethoprim and many of the sulfonamides achieve adequate levels in brain tissue. Metronidazole produces adequate levels in brain tissue–brain pus to eradicate anaerobic bacteria. Unfortunately, with most of the antibiotics, the kinetics of entry into the brain and the rate of decline of brain levels are unknown.

The level of antibiotics in the cerebrospinal fluid (CSF) is a function of lipid permeability, protein binding, and the secretion and removal of weak anions by the transport systems of the choroid plexus and other sites in which CSF is formed. CSF levels of most agents except chloramphenicol, trimethoprim, some sulfonamides, isoniazid, and 5-fluorocytosine are low in the absence of inflammation. Penicillins not only have difficulty passing through the blood-brain barrier into the CSF but are removed from the CSF by active transport. Penicillin G and ampicillin can achieve adequate CSF levels in the presence of inflammation (Barrett et al., 1966). Oxacillin, nafcillin, and methicillin administered at high doses (12 g/day) yield CSF levels adequate for the treatment of staphylococcal meningitis. Vancomycin also achieves adequate CSF levels, but older cephalosporins do not. Relapses of meningitis due to pneumococcus and meningococcus have occurred in patients being treated with cephalothin. Cefamandole and cefoxitin do not yield CSF levels adequate to treat most organisms. Cefotaxime, moxalactam, ceftizoxime, and ceftriaxone enter the CSF in the presence of inflammation in concentrations adequate to inhibit *S. pneumoniae, H. influenzae, N. meningitidis,* and most *E. coli* and *K. pneumoniae* but not *Pseudomonas.* Moxalactam does not yield adequate levels to treat *S. pneumoniae* or group B streptococci. Table 4 lists the CSF levels of the newer cephalosporins and the CSF bactericidal indices for important bacteria. The tetracyclines enter CSF but to a lesser extent than does chloramphenicol. The concentration of a tetracycline is about 10 per cent of the serum level. Minocycline penetrates normal CSF more readily than the other tetracyclines. Erythromycin does not enter the CSF in the absence of inflammation. Although chloramphenicol produces CSF levels adequate to treat pneumococci, meningococci, and *Haemophilus*, the levels needed to eradicate some gram-negative bacteria may be higher than those that are usually achieved. Aminoglycosides do not penetrate the CSF adequately, and intrathecal administration or intraventricular injection via an Omaya reservoir is necessary to treat *Pseudomonas* or multi-resistant Enterobacteriaceae. Polymyxins do not enter the CSF and must be given intrathecally for the treatment of central nervous system infections.

Amphotericin B achieves concentrations in CSF that are sufficient to treat cryptococcal meningitis but not meningitis due to *Coccidioides immitis* or amebas (Atkinson and Bennett, 1978). Rifampin and ethambutol enter the CSF with inflammation to give levels adequate to treat most mycobacteria. Quinine and pyrimethamine enter CSF and brain tissue in concentrations that inhibit Plasmodia. Adenosine arabinoside and acylovir enter both brain tissue and CSF in concentrations adequate to inhibit growth of herpes simplex virus.

Intracellular. Many antibiotics do not enter phagocytic

Table 4. PARENTERAL CSF BACTERICIDAL LEVELS BASED ON MBCS OF INFECTING ORGANISMS AND CONCENTRATIONS OF DRUGS ACHIEVED IN THE CSF

	CSF Bacterial Index					
	Cefotaxime	***Ceftixoxime***	***Ceftriaxone***	***Cefoperazone***	***Ceftazidime***	***Moxalactam***
Group B streptococci	10–60	10–60	10–60	5–20	(2–10)[1]	(2–5)[1]
Escherichia coli	10–100	10–50	10–100	(2–25)[2]	10–100	10–100
Streptococcus pneumoniae	10–60	10–50	10–100	5–50	(2–20)[1]	(2–5)[1]
Haemophilus influenzae	10–200	10–200	10–300	5–40	10–100	10–300
Neisseria meningitidis	10–200	10–200	10–300	10–20	10–100	10–300
Klebsiella pneumoniae	10–200	10–100	10–100	(2–50)[1]	10–100	10–200
Pseudomonas aeruginosa	(< 10)[1]	(< 10)[1]	(< 10)[1]	(< 10)[1]	(2–10)[1]	(< 10)[1]
Serratia marcescens	(2–5)[1]	(2–10)[1]	(2–5)[1]	(10)[1]	(2–10)[1]	(2–10)[1]
Listeria monocytogenes	0	0	0	0	0	0

[1]( ) not uniformly adequate.
[2]( ) not adequate if strain TEM β-lactamase type.

cells, such as polymorphonuclear cells and macrophages. Chloramphenicol, tetracycline, trimethoprim, rifampin, and isoniazid all enter these cells, and this property may be important in the eradication of intracellular bacteria. The uptake of amphotericin by the reticuloendothelial system may contribute to its destruction of fungi within these cells.

MODIFICATION OF ANTIBIOTIC PROGRAMS IN THE PRESENCE OF RENAL FAILURE. For some antibiotics, little or no dosage adjustment is required in the presence of renal failure, either because they are eliminated by extrarenal mechanisms or because the margin of safety is so great that accumulation does not result in toxicity, (Appel and Neu, 1983). With the aminoglycosides, vancomycin, anti-*Pseudomonas* penicillins, sulfonamides, and trimethoprim, major adjustments in dosage are necessary. There are a number of methods available to adjust dosage in the presence of renal failure. These are based on the assumption that the drugs are eliminated in an exponential fashion and that the rate of elimination is proportional to the glomerular filtration rate. In order to reach a therapeutic level in critically ill patients with a decreased renal function, it is necessary to administer a loading dose of antibiotics. Dosage adjustments may be made by giving an initial dose and then subsequent doses at prolonged intervals, which are calculated from the serum creatinine or creatinine clearance. The alternative method is to give the loading dose and then a fraction of the usual dose at the usual interval for the drug. This method avoids the high peak and low trough concentrations that result from the former, but, in some animal studies, aminoglycosides administered this way are more nephrotoxic.

Aminoglycosides require dose adjustment most commonly even when there is only moderate renal insufficiency because their toxic to therapeutic ratio is so narrow. Since, in hospitalized patients, medications are conveniently administered at certain regular intervals, Table 5 shows a method for estimating the dose to be given at fixed intervals to provide effective but safe peak blood levels for all degrees of renal insufficiency. The creatinine clearance can be estimated from the serum creatinine as follows:

$$C_{cr} = \frac{(140 - \text{Age})\ \text{Wt}^*}{72\ \text{Cr}}$$

*Weight in kilograms.

Table 5. AMINOGLYCOSIDE DOSING CHART

1. Select loading dose in mg/kg (ideal weight) to provide peak serum levels in range listed below for desired aminoglycoside.

Aminoglycoside	**Usual Loading Doses**	**Expected Peak Serum Levels**
Tobramycin Gentamicin Netilmicin	1.5 to 2.0 mg/kg	4 to 10 μg/ml
Amikacin Kanamycin	5.0 to 7.5 mg/kg	15 to 30 μg/ml

2. Select maintenance dose (as percentage of chosen loading dose) to continue peak serum levels indicated above according to desired dosing interval and the patient's corrected creatinine clearance.

Percentage of Loading Dose Required for Dosage Interval Selected

C(c)cr (ml/min)	***Half Life[1] (hr)***	***8 hr***	***12 hr***	***24 hr***
90	3.1	84%	—	—
80	3.4	80	91%	—
70	3.9	76	88	—
60	4.5	71	84	—
50	5.3	65	79	—
40	6.5	57	72	92%
30	8.4	48	63	86
25	9.9	43	57	81
20	11.9	37	50	75
17	13.6	33	46	70
15	15.1	31	42	67
12	17.9	27	37	61
10	20.4	24	34	56
7	25.9	19	28	47
5	31.5	16	23	41
2	46.8	11	16	30
0	69.3	8	11	21

[1]Alternatively, one half of the chosen loading dose may be given at an interval approximately equal to the estimated half life.

Modified from Sarubii, F.A., and Hull, J.H.: Amikacin serum concentrations: prediction of levels and dosage guidelines. Ann Intern Med 89:612, 1978.

This method provides only an estimate of the serum levels that will be obtained, and these levels should be measured. If this method is followed, the blood levels may fall below the minimal inhibitory concentration toward the end of the interval between doses, but there is no evidence that sustained levels above the MIC are necessary.

All techniques for dosage adjustment are guides to therapy and should be confirmed by measuring serum levels. Checking the serum level at the time of anticipated peak concentrations (just after an I.V. dose or 30 to 60 minutes after an I.M. dose) and just before the next dose establishes both whether the levels are adequate and if the agents are accumulating unduly.

Effects of Peritoneal Dialysis and Hemodialysis. Because patients who are treated by dialysis have minimal or no renal function, no antibiotic is eliminated in the urine. However, many antibiotics are removed by dialysis, and during that procedure they are eliminated at a constant rate. The exact rate of elimination depends both on the characteristics of the drug (i.e., protein binding, charge, and molecular weight) and on the conditions of dialysis (such as the machine that is used, the flow-pressure relationships, and the duration of dialysis). Table 3 provides data on which antibiotics can be removed by dialysis. If a drug is removed, it is necessary to administer an additional dose after dialysis. It is possible to add the antibiotic to the peritoneal dialysate at the same concentration that is desired in the blood. If that is done, it is not necessary to administer additional doses of the antibiotic. If the toxic to therapeutic ratio is narrow, drug concentration should be measured just before and just after dialysis to determine whether safe but effective concentrations have been attained. If that is not possible, then drugs with a wider margin of safety should be used.

TOXICOLOGY OF ANTIMICROBIAL AGENTS. Antimicrobial agents cause direct toxicity, can interact with other drugs to influence the toxicity of the other agent, or can by alteration of microbial flora result in infection with organisms that are normally saprophytic (Table 6). Table 7 lists the frequency of side effects.

Hypersensitivity Reactions. Almost any antimicrobial agent has the potential of being an antigenic stimulus and provoking an immunologic reaction due either to immunoglobulins or to sensitized lymphocytes, but in fact the most common agent to do this has been penicillin G or one of the other penicillins. Penicillins are widely dispersed in nature and contaminate milk products and other foods so that individuals who have never received penicillin for medical reasons have been otherwise exposed to them.

The incidence of true hypersensitivity reactions to penicillins is thought to be between 0.1 and 5 per cent. Four immune mechanisms invoked to explain allergic reactions to penicillins are listed in Table 8. Patients are not allergic to penicillin itself but to breakdown or metabolic products of the penicillin. These products function as haptens to form antigens after forming covalent bonds with proteins. The components consist of a major antigenic component benzylpenicilloyl (BPO) which is about 95 per cent of breakdown products. Minor determinants are the important cause of immediate IgE-mediated reactions. Major determinants are only occasionally related to immediate reactions, but they do cause accelerated IgE-mediated reactions. IgG responses to the major determinant are responsible for hemolytic anemia and immune complex-mediated diseases.

Table 6. MAJOR TOXICITIES OF SELECTED ANTIMICROBIAL AGENTS

Agent	Mechanism	Signs
Hematologic		
Chloramphenicol	Inhibits protein synthesis	Reversible anemia, leukopenia
Chloramphenicol	Damages stem cell	Aplastic anemia
Sulfonamides	G-6-PD deficiency	Hemolytic anemia
Carbenicillin and ticarcillin	Platelet aggregation inhibited	Bleeding
Moxalactam	Platelet aggregation inhibited	Bleeding
Cefamandole Moxalactam Cefoperazone	Prothrombin deficiency	PT, increased bleeding
Nervous System		
Aminoglycosides	Binds hair cells of organ of Corti	Deafness
Aminogylcosides	Binds vestibular cells	Vertigo
Aminoglycosides	Competitive neuromuscular blockade	Respiratory paralysis
Polmyxins	Noncompetitive neuromuscular blockade	Respiratory paralysis
Penicillins and cephalosporins	Cortical stimulation	Myoclonic seizures
Gastrointestinal Rifampin, isoniazid and tetracyclines Nitrofurantoin	Liver cell damage	Hepatitis
Neomycin	Villous damage	Malabsorption
Clindamycin, lincomycin	Clostridium difficile	Diarrhea
All agents	Altered bowel flora C. difficile	Diarrhea

Late reactions to penicillins account for 80–90 per cent of all reactions. They begin days to weeks after the initiation of penicillin therapy. No definite allergic mechanism has been established for the morbilliform eruptions. Overall only 0.02 per cent of courses of penicillin treatment are associated with serious IgE-mediated allergic response. Furthermore, there is no evidence that individuals with a history of atopic allergic reactions are more prone to an allergic reaction when given a penicillin (Greene and Roseblum, 1971).

Positive skin tests with benzylpenicilloyl polylysine and with penicillin G, benzylpenicilloic acid, and benzylpenicilloate predict who will have immediate reactions to penicillins (Voss et al., 1966). An immediate wheal and flare reaction to the major and minor determinants after skin pricks or intradermal injection indicates a high probability of immediate (2 to 30 minutes) anaphylactic or accelerated (1 to 72 hours) urticarial reactions (with wheezing, pharyngeal edema, or local inflammation) to penicillins. Negative skin tests virtually rule out an anaphylactic reaction, although they do not exclude late cutaneous reactions.

Ampicillin produces rashes twice as frequently as do other penicillins (7 per cent versus 3 per cent). The mechanism of this reaction is not understood. The rash occurs in almost all individuals with Epstein-Barr virus infection (infectious mononucleosis) and cytomegalovirus infections. Rechallenge of these individuals with penicillin does not elicit a reaction. Allergic cross-reactions with cephalosporins in patients allergic to penicillins are uncommon, probably less than 2 per cent. Recent studies have demonstrated that patients with positive penicillin skin

Table 7. EXAMPLES OF SIDE EFFECTS OF VARIOUS ANTIMICROBIAL AGENTS

	Side Effects				
Antibiotic or Chemotherapeutic Agent	***Allergic***	***Hematologic***	***Nephrotoxic***	***Hepatotoxic***	***Neurotoxic***
Penicillin G	++	+/−	+/−		+
Cloxacillin, dicloxacin, oxacillin, nafcillin	++				+/−
Amoxicillin, ampicillin	++				+/−
Azlocillin, mezlocillin, piperacillin	++				+/−
Carbenicillin, ticarcillin	++	+			+/−
Cephaloridine	+	+/−	++		
Cephalosporins (except cephaloridine)	+	+/−			
Cefoperazone, moxalactam	+	++	−	−	−
Tetracyclines	+/−	+/−		+/−	
Chloramphenicol	+/−	+			+/−
Thiamphenicol	+/−	+			
Streptomycin	++	+/−	+/−		++
Amikacin	+/−		+		++
Gentamicin, tobramycin	+/−		+		++
Polymyxin B, colistin	+/−		+		++
Erythromycin	+/−				
Clindamycin	+/−			+/−	
Fusidic acid	+/−				
Vancomycin	+/−		+/−		+
Rifampin	+	+	+	++	+
Isoniazid	+/−	+/−		+	++
Ethambutol	+/−			+/−	++
Amphotericin B	+/−	+/−	++	+/−	+/−
Flucytosine		+		+	
Ketoconazole	+				
Griseofulvin	+	+/−	+/−	+	+
Nitrofurantoin	++	+/−		+/−	++
Nalidixic acid	+/−	+/−			+
Sulfonamides	++	+/−	+/−	+/−	
Trimethoprim	+/−	+/−			

++ = frequent
\+ = rare
+/− = very rare

tests can receive the cephalosporin drugs without anaphylaxis or accelerated reactions (Saxon, 1983).

Anaphylaxis and serum sickness have been associated with most of the other antimicrobial agents but are uncommon for erythromycin, clindamycin, and chloramphenicol. Serum sickness due to antigen-antibody complexes has complicated treatment with sulfadiazine and sulfathiazole. Hypersensitivity reactions including urticaria, periorbital edema, wheezing, and even anaphylaxis have occurred following use of tetracyclines.

Drug fever mediated via sensitized lymphocytes has been associated with all antimicrobials. Indeed, allergy to cephalosporins is manifest more often as fever than as a rash. Isoniazid can produce a syndrome indistinguishable from systemic lupus erythematosus that is presumably on an allergic basis. Both penicillins and sulfonamides have produced a nonspecific vasculitis similar to Henoch-Schönlein purpura.

Skin Reactions. Cutaneous reactions ranging from urticaria, fixed drug eruptions, and photodermatitis to exfoliative dermatitis, toxic epidermal necrolysis, and erythema nodosum have been reported with antimicrobial agents of every class. Sulfonamides and penicillins are the most common offenders. Tetracyclines and antituberculosis medications (such as isoniazid, ethambutol, rifampin, and particularly para-aminosalicylic acid) have produced dermatologic reactions. Antimalarials have produced alopecia. Nalidixic acid, griseofulvin, chlortetracycline, and demethylchlortetracycline cause photosensitivity. This reaction is probably phototoxic rather than photoallergic and apparently results from conversion of the drug by light to a noxious agent. It can range from intense sunburn and

Table 8. CLASSIFICATION OF REACTIONS TO PENICILLINS

Type of Reaction and Immune Mechanism	**Penicillin Determinant**	**Clinical Syndrome**
I. IgE antibody	Minor components	Anaphylaxis Laryngeal edema Early onset of urticaria (< 72 hours)
II. Cytotoxic antibody	Major components	Hemolytic anemia
III. Antigen-antibody complexes	Major components	Serum sickness
IV. Delayed hypersensitivity	Cytotoxic antibody	Contact dermatitis
Idiopathic	Unknown	Maculopapular drug eruptions Nephritis Late onset of urticaria Fever

loosening of the nails with tetracyclines to bullous skin eruptions with nalidixic acid. For unknown reasons, chlorination makes the tetracyclines phototoxic.

Hematologic Reactions. Pancytopenia and aplastic anemia have been produced by chloramphenicol. The incidence of aplastic anemia is estimated at one in 60,000. There are two types of marrow reaction to chloramphenicol. In one type, which occurs in nearly everyone after prolonged serum levels over 25 μg/ml, there is gradual development of anemia and mild thrombocytopenia. Serum iron increases, and the reticulocyte count falls. Bone marrow cells show maturation arrest with vacuolization of the cytoplasm of erythroid cells. These changes reverse if chloramphenicol is discontinued. The second type of marrow depression is not reversible or dose-related. It has occurred in individuals who have had multiple exposures to the drug and is characterized by fatal aplastic anemia. Its occurrence in identical twins raises the question of genetic predisposition (Nagao and Mauer, 1969).

Hemolytic anemia occurs in individuals with glucose-6-phosphate dehydrogenase deficiency who take eight aminoquinolines, such as quinacrine, sulfonamides, nitrofurans, sulfones, nalidixic acid, and chloramphenicol. Immune hemolysis has developed during treatment with PAS, penicillins, and cephalosporins. With cephalosporins, most positive Coombs' tests are false-positives, and hemolysis is very rare (Borg and Kammer, 1983). Hemolysis due to membrane damage occurs with amphotericin, but most of the anemia seen with amphotericin results instead from marrow suppression (Brandiss et al., 1964).

Leukopenia and agranulocytosis have followed use of chloramphenicol, penicillins, cephalosporins, sulfonamides, dapsone, trimethoprim, and 5-fluorocytosine. In most instances, the reaction is reversible. In some cases leukopenia due to penicillins and cephalosporins is dose-related, and reduction in dose causes the white count to become normal (Parry and Neu, 1982). Sulfisoxazole has produced a pseudo Pelger-Huët anomaly of white cells.

Thrombocytopenia can result from an immunologic reaction with penicillins, sulfonamides, cephalosporins, and rifampin. Direct damage to platelets has occurred with other antibiotics. Trimethoprim produces thrombocytopenia, leukopenia, and megaloblastic anemia by interference with the dihydrofolate reductase enzyme (Kahn et al., 1968). When penicillins, particularly carbenicillin, are given in high doses, most recipients develop defective platelet function within 24 hours. Carbenicillin and ticarcillin, and, to a lesser degree, piperacillin, azlocillin, and mezlocillin impair the function of platelets by decreasing their sensitivity to aggregation by adenosine diphosphate (ADP). Moxalactam, which contains a carboxyl group on its acyl side chain, also causes this abnormality. Since ADP is the physiologic agent responsible for aggregation of platelets into plugs that repair blood vessels, prolonged bleeding can develop. Platelet function remains abnormal for several days after the drugs have been discontinued (Somani et al., 1983).

Cephalosporins, which contain a methylthiotetrazole group at the 3 position of the dihydrothiazine ring, appear to produce some alteration in prothrombin synthesis with resultant prolongation of prothrombin times. Bleeding caused by prothrombin increase has followed use of cefamandole, cefoperazone, and moxalactam. It may also occur with cefmetazole, cefpyramide, and cefotetan, which also contain this chemical moeity. The prolongation of PT can be corrected by administration of oral or parenteral vitamin K (Neu, 1982b).

Cardiovascular Toxicity. Most cardiovascular toxicity occurs with antiparasitic drugs. Emetine and pentamidine can cause hypotension and electrocardiographic changes. Quinine depresses conduction velocity. Rapid injection of large doses of a potassium salt of penicillin can produce cardiac arrest. Miconazole has produced hypotension and arrhythmias. Pentamidine administered intravenously produces hypotension and cardiac arrhythmias.

Gastrointestinal Toxicity. Many antibiotics produce gastrointestinal complaints that vary from hairy tongue to enterocolitis. Severe diarrhea progressing to pseudomembranous enterocolitis has occurred with all antibiotics, but particularly with ampicillin, indanylcarbenicillin, tetracyclines, chloramphenicol, lincomycin, and clindamycin. The mechanism for this toxicity appears to be alteration of intestinal flora. Proliferation of *Clostridium difficile* and accumulation of toxin within the colon has been established as the cause of this syndrome (Bartlett, 1981). Administration of vancomycin orally at 125 mg every 6 hours will treat this problem. Nonabsorbable aminoglycosides, such as neomycin, produce malabsorption of fat, protein, carbohydrates, and digoxin (Neu, 1982a). Oral neomycin causes striking villous shortening, round cell infiltration of the upper small bowel, and crypt-cell damage. This mucosal injury, plus an interaction of neomycin with bile salts, are responsible for malabsorption.

HEPATIC TOXICITY. Cholestatic jaundice has followed use of tetracyclines, erythromycin estolate, oxacillin, nitrofurans, and sulfonamides. Tetracyclines, taken in doses above 2 g/day during the third trimester of pregnancy or postpartum, have produced hepatic damage with extensive fatty changes in the liver and a fatality rate of 80 per cent (Schultz et al., 1963).

Antituberculosis agents are the antimicrobials most often associated with hepatocellular toxicity. Isoniazid produces hepatitis, but the incidence of this side effect varies with the age of the patient. The risk of individuals below 20 years of age developing hepatitis due to isoniazid is 0.03 per cent, while those above 35 years, the risk is over 1 per cent. Approximately 10 per cent of children receiving isoniazid develop abnormal liver chemistry values, but clinical signs of hepatitis are extremely rare in children. Toxicity due to isoniazid is not related to previous hepatic disease but is more common in rapid acetylators of isoniazid, suggesting that the toxic component is the acetyl derivative. Para-aminosalicylic acid, ethionamide, and pyrazinamide have produced fulminant hepatic necrosis. Rifampin is infrequently associated with liver toxicity but seems to increase the likelihood of isoniazid toxicity.

Sulfonamides may produce both hepatocellular and cholestatic liver damage. Nitrofurantoin produces serious hepatocellular damage in some people. Penicillins (penicillin G, ampicillin, oxacillin, and carbenicillin) rarely produce hepatitis and usually in association with a general allergic reaction. Erythromycin, many of the penicillins, and cephalosporins produce elevations in serum glutamic-oxaloacetic transaminase by mechanisms that are unexplained.

Respiratory Toxicity. Nitrofurantoin produces two forms of pulmonary reaction (Hailey et al., 1969). In the acute form, chills, fever, cough, and dyspnea begin 2 to 10 days after the antibiotic is started. X-rays reveal diffuse alveolar infiltrates, and there usually is an eosinophilia. This reaction resolves when the drug is stopped. The second reaction to nitrofurans is a chronic one that occurs after the patient has taken the drug for a prolonged period, usually months. Dyspnea, cough, and cyanosis develop gradually. The x-ray shows diffuse basilar interstitial infiltrates, and pulmonary function studies show restrictive lung disease. Partial recovery occurs if the drug is stopped.

Metabolic Toxicity. Hypoglycemia can follow pentamidine administration. Use of large doses of penicillins, particularly the anti-*Pseudomonas* agents like carbenicillin, present such a large load of nonreabsorbable anion to the distal tubule that hypokalemia results. Carbenicillin also can produce sodium overload since it contains 4.7 mEq/g and is given in doses of 24 to 40 g/day. Demethylchlortetracycline produces nephrogenic diabetes insipidus (Singer and Rotenberg, 1973). Amphotericin B and outdated tetracyclines produce renal tubular acidosis and hypokalemia.

Renal Toxicity. Many factors intrinsic to the kidney make it particularly vulnerable to nephrotoxic reactions to antimicrobial agents (Fig. 1) (Appel and Neu, 1977). The most common form of renal damage due to penicillins is an acute interstitial nephritis that has been associated with methicillin therapy but can occur with any penicillin. Fever, eosinophilia, and rash commonly antedate or accompany the renal lesion. Urinalysis may reveal white cells, casts, and proteinuria, but microscopic hematuria is most common. Urinary output is normal at first, although the serum creatinine and urea nitrogen increase. With discontinuation of the drug, the renal function of most patients returns to normal. Renal biopsy shows patchy tubular damage with interstitial edema, accumulation of lymphocytes, monocytes, eosinophils, and plasma cells. Glomeruli are normal. Most of the evidence suggests that this is a hypersensitivity reaction. Antitubular basement membrane antigens have been demonstrated in the serum in methicillin nephritis; and IgG, C_3, and a methicillin antigen were present in a linear pattern along the tubular basement membrane (Border et al., 1974).

Nephrotoxicity due to cephaloridine is dose-related (Silverblatt et al., 1973). There is proximal tubular damage due to accumulation of high intracellular concentrations of the drug in cortical tubular cells. The other cephalosporins have not been convincingly shown to be nephrotoxic.

Polymyxins bind to proximal tubular cells and damage cellular membranes. The aminoglycosides vary in their nephrotoxic potential ranging from neomycin, the most toxic agent, to streptomycin, the least toxic. Gentamicin and amikacin appear to be more nephrotoxic in animals than tobramycin, but clinical differences among the agents are difficult to establish. Gentamicin damages proximal tubules with loss of renal tubular enzymes, concentrating ability, and the development of intracytoplasmic bodies that seem to be injured cellular organelles. Aminoglycoside nephrotoxicity is dose-related and seems to be increased by simultaneous administration of cephalosporins. The overall incidence of nephrotoxicity due to aminoglycosides is about 5 to 10 per cent.

Crystallization-producing obstructive nephropathy, allergic and hypersensitivity reactions, precipitation of hemoglobin casts secondary to drug-induced hemolysis, and an intrinsic toxic effect have all been reported as secondary to sulfonamide therapy. Whether trimethoprim produces nephrotoxicity is unclear, but it does seem to alter handling of creatinine by the kidney.

Amphotericin can cause renal vasoconstriction and damage to proximal and distal tubular cells with intratubular calcium deposits. Renal abnormalities occur in about 25 per cent of patients who receive the drug. Most of the toxicity due to amphotericin is reversible, provided less than 5 g have been given. The primary disturbance is distal tubular acidosis (Burgess and Birchall, 1972). The drug seems to produce a permeability defect that allows the

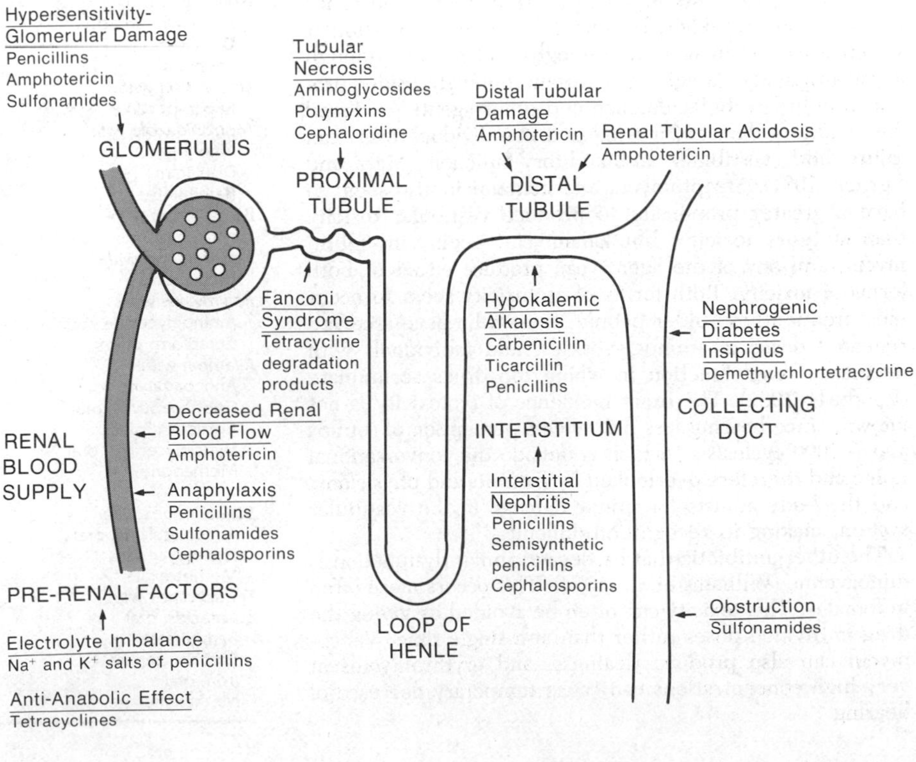

Figure 1. Nephrotoxic sites of antimicrobial agents.

tubular cells to leak potassium and become permeable to hydrogen ions. Hydrogen ions then pass from tubular urine into the cells. The overall picture of amphotericin toxicity to the kidney is one of azotemia, acidosis, hypokalemia, and polyuria. Daily supplements of 100 mg of potassium are often needed after even small doses of amphotericin.

Neurologic Toxicity. Peripheral neuropathy has been produced by isoniazid most often in patients who acetylate the drug slowly. It is dose-related and can be reversed by pyridoxine (La Du, 1972). Ethionamide also produces peripheral neuropathy. High concentrations in the blood of nitrofurans, polymyxins, and emetine cause peripheral neuropathy in patients with decreased renal function. Metronidazole also produces peripheral neuropathy. Polymyxins and aminoglycosides produce a reversible neuromuscular blockade resembling myasthenia gravis (Warner and Sanders, 1971). This toxicity is dose-related and has followed use of the agents as a peritoneal lavage. The drug produces a competitive blockade at the myoneural end-plate. Aminoglycosides probably compete with acetylcholine for receptor sites so that the end-plate is not depolarized. Neostigmine reverses this paralysis (Ream, 1963). Polymyxins also produce a noncompetitive prolonged depolarization due to calcium depletion, which can be reversed by calcium (Zauder et al., 1966).

Central nervous system excitation and seizures can be induced by isoniazid, amantadine, and penicillin. Penicillin-induced seizures are myoclonic and more frequent in elderly patients and following cardiopulmonary by-pass (Seamans et al., 1968). Direct instillation of methicillin, oxacillin, or cephalosporins into the ventricles when CSF shunts are installed usually does not produce seizures. Cycloserine also causes seizures.

Ototoxicity. Aminoglycosides vary in their potential to produce deafness. Neomycin is the most ototoxic, followed by kanamycin, gentamicin, and amikacin. Tobramycin and netilmicin are less ototoxic. Deafness is the result of damage to the hair cells of the organ of Corti. The mechanism for this reaction is unknown. Sensory cells of the vestibular system are also damaged by aminoglycosides, and, although it was originally thought that certain aminoglycosides produced only vestibular damage and other agents produced only auditory damage, it is clear that individual drugs can injure both vestibular and auditory function (Matz and Lerner, 1981). Streptomycin and gentamicin also seem to have a greater propensity to produce vestibular toxicity than auditory toxicity, but kanamycin, neomycin, tobramycin, and any of the agents can produce either or both forms of toxicity. Both forms of ototoxicity seem to occur most frequently in older people, those who have received repeated doses of aminoglycosides, and individuals with decreased renal function in whom the drugs accumulate (Bendush, 1982). The exact incidence of ototoxicity is not known, since hearing loss first affects perception of sounds above 2000 cycles/sec, which is outside the conversational range and therefore overlooked by patients and physicians, and the body adjusts for minor damage to the vestibular system, making its recognition difficult.

The other antibiotic that causes vestibular dysfunction is minocycline (Williams et al., 1974). This occurs more often in females. This toxicity can often be avoided by giving the drug in divided doses rather than at a single time. Vancomycin can also produce deafness, and erythromycins at very high concentrations can cause temporary decrease of hearing.

ALTERATION OF MICROBIAL FLORA. Alteration of intestinal flora by use of antibiotics allows overgrowth of *Candida*, which often results in thrush or vaginitis and may cause disseminated candidiasis in patients with depressed resistance (Kirck and Remington, 1976). Prolonged use of oral penicillins as prophylaxis against recurrent rheumatic fever has been complicated by colonization of the oropharynx with streptococci that are relatively resist-

Table 9. DRUG INTERACTIONS OF ANTIMICROBIAL AGENTS WITH OTHER COMPOUNDS

Interacting Drugs	Adverse Effect
Aminoglycoside antibiotics with:	
Cephaloridine	Nephrotoxicity
Cephalothin and other cephalosporins	Nephrotoxicity
Curariform drugs	Neuromuscular blockade
Digoxin	Possible decreased digoxin effect
Ethacrynic acid	Ototoxicity
Furosemide	Ototoxicity
Methoxyflurare	Nephrotoxicity
Polymyxins	Nephrotoxicity
Aminosalicylic acid (PAS) with:	
Probenecid	Aminosalicylic acid toxicity
Amphotericin B with:	
Curariform drugs	Curare effect
Digitalis	Digitalis toxicity
Cephaloridine with:	
Aminoglycoside antibiotics	Nephrotoxicity
Ethacrynic acid	Nephrotoxicity
Furosemide	Nephrotoxicity
Cephalosporins with:	
Aminoglycoside antibiotics	Nephrotoxicity
Chloramphenicol with:	
Dicoumarol	Excessive anticoagulation
Phenytoin	Phenytoin toxicity
Hypoglycemics, oral	Hypoglycemia
Erythromycin with theophylline carbamazepine	Excess theophylline
Griseofulvin with:	
Anticoagulants, oral	Decreased anticoagulant effect
Isoniazid with:	
Aluminum antacids	Decreased isoniazid effect
Disulfiram	Psychotic episodes, ataxia
Phenytoin	Phenytoin toxicity
Lincomycin with:	
Kaolin-pectin	Decreased lincomycin effect
Metronidazole with:	
Alcohol	Antabuse-like reaction
Disulfiram	Psychosis
Barbiturates	Decreased metronidazole
Moxalactam with:	
anticoagulants	Increased anticoagulant effect
Nalidixic acid with:	
Dicoumarol	Prolonged prothrombin time
Polymyxins with:	
Aminoglycoside antibiotics	Nephrotoxicity
Curariform drugs	Neuromuscular blockade
Rifampin with:	
Anticoagulants, oral	Decreased anticoagulant effect
Contraceptives, oral	Decreased contraceptive effect
Corticosteroids	Decreased corticosteroid effect
Hypoglycemics, oral	Possible decreased effect
Methadone	Methadone withdrawal symptoms
Sulfonamides with:	
Anticoagulants, oral	Anticoagulant effect
Hypoglycemics	Sulfonylurea hypoglycemia
Methotrexate	Leukopenia
Tetracyclines with:	
Antacids, oral	Decreased effect of tetracyclines
Barbiturates	Decreased doxycycline effect
Carbamazepine	Decreased tetracycline effect
Iron, oral	Decreased effect of tetracyclines
Methoxyflurane	Nephrotoxicity

ant to penicillin. Superinfection due to enterococci and *Pseudomonas* has followed use of the new broad-spectrum cephalosporins, particularly moxalactam.

A serious problem that has resulted from the use of newer antimicrobial agents has been the development of resistant bacteria, particularly of *Enterobacter* (John et al., 1982) and *Citrobacter* to broad spectrum β-lactamase stable cephalosporins. It is clear that development of infection in hospitalized patients frequently is due to the acquisition of a particular flora that is resistant to common antimicrobial agents. Excessive use of antimicrobial agents results in the selection of such a flora. Serious fungal, enterococcal, and *Pseudomonas* infections have followed use of some of the newer cephalosporins. Alteration of intestinal flora is most likely to occur with antimicrobial agents, which are highly excreted into the intestine via the bile. An extremely broad-spectrum agent imipenem does not alter intestinal flora since it doesn't undergo biliary excretion. A drug such as aztreonam does not alter intestinal flora since it has neither gram-positive nor anti-anaerobic activity. Pseudomembranous colitis due to overgrowth of *C. difficile* has been discussed.

DRUG INTERACTIONS. Penicillins can inactivate aminoglycosides when the two are mixed in the same solution. Drug interactions within the patient are numerous and may result in increased toxicity of an agent or a decreased effect of a drug (Table 9). These antibiotic reactions with other agents in vivo involve a change in the metabolism of a compound. Microsomal enzymes that destroy more drug may be induced or there may be competition for enzymes involved in inactivation of both drugs. Binding to receptor sites on proteins or tissues, so that the second drug is blocked, may make more drug available. Competition for excretory pathways in the kidney or liver may result in accumulation of a drug.

REFERENCES

Appel, G. B., and Neu, H. C.: The nephrotoxicity of antimicrobial agents. N Engl J Med 296:663,722,784, 1977.

Appel, G. B., and Neu, H. C.: Infection and antibiotic usage in patients with renal diseases. In Martinez-Maldonado, M. Handbook of Renal Therapeutics. New York, Plenum Press, 1983, p. 227.

Atkinson, A. J., and Bennett, J. E.: Amphotericin B pharmacokinetics in humans. Antimicrob Agents Chemother 13:271, 1978.

Bang, N., and Kammer, R. B.: Hematologic complications associated with β-lactam antibiotics. Rev Infect Dis 5(Suppl): 20:380, 1983.

Barrett, F. F., Eardley, W. A., Yow, M. D., et al: Ampicillin in the treatment of acute suppurative meningitis. J Pediatr 69:343, 1966.

Bartlett, J. C.: Antibiotic-associated pseudomembranous colitis. Hosp Pract 16:85, 1981.

Bartlett, J. C.: Chloramphenicol. Med Clin N Am 66:91, 1982.

Barza, M.: Treatment of bacterial infections of the eye. In Remington, J. S., and Swartz, M. N. (eds.): Current Clinical Topics in Infectious Diseases. New York, McGraw Hill, 1980, p. 158.

Barza, M., Brusch, J., Bergeron, M., et al: Penetration of antibiotics into fibrin loci in vivo. III. Intermittent vs. continuous infusion and the effect of probenecid. J Infect Dis 129:73, 1974.

Bendush, C. L.: Ototoxicity: clinical considerations and comparative information in The Aminoglycosides. A. Whelton and H. C. Neu (eds) New York, Marcel Dekker, 1982, p. 453.

Border, W. A., Lehman, D. H., Egan, J. D., et al: Antitubular basement-membrane antibodies in methicillin-associated interstitial nephritis. N Engl J Med 291:381, 1974.

Brandiss, M. U., Wolff, S. M., Moores, R., et al: Anemia induced by amphotericin B. JAMA 189:663, 1964.

Breen, K. J., Bryant, R. E., and Levinson, S. D.: Neomycin absorption in man. Ann Intern Med 76:211, 1972.

Brummett, R. E., and Fox, K. E.: Studies of aminoglycoside ototoxicity in animal models. In Whelton, A., and Neu H. C., (eds.): The Aminoglycosides. New York, Marcel Dekker, 1982, p. 4191.

Burgess, J. L., and Birchall, R.: Nephrotoxicity of amphotericin B, with emphasis on changes in tubular function. Am J Med 53:77, 1972.

Cohn, H. D.: Clinical studies with a new rifamycin derivative. J Clin Pharmacol 9:118, 1969.

Craig, W. A., and Kunin, C. M.: Significance of serum protein and tissue binding of antimicrobial agents. Ann Rev Med 27:287, 1976.

Craig, W. A., and Welling, P. C.: Protein binding of antimicrobials: clinical pharmacokinetics and therapeutic implications. Clin Pharmacokin 2:252, 1977.

Fair, W. R., Crane, D. B., Schiller, N., et al: A re-appraisal of treatment in chronic bacterial prostatitis. J Urol 121:437, 1979.

Finland, M., and Neu, H. C.: Tobramycin. J Infect Dis 134(Suppl): 1-234, 1976.

Florey, T. E., Turton, E. C., and Duthe, E. S.: Penicillin in wound exudates. Lancet 2:405, 1946.

Garnes, H. A.: Doxycycline levels in serum and prostatic tissue in man. Urology 1:205, 1973.

Green, G. R., and Rosenblum, A.: Report of the Penicillin Study Group: American Academy of Allergy. J Aller Clin Immunol 48:331, 1971.

Gribble, M. J., and Chow, A. W.: Erythromycin. Med Clin N Am 66:79, 1982.

Hailey, F. J., Glascock, H. W., Jr., and Hewitt, W. F.: Pleuropneumonic reactions to nitrofurantoin. N Engl J Med 281:1087, 1969.

Hughes, H. B.: On the metabolic fate of isoniazid. J Pharmacol Exp Ther 109:444, 1953.

John, J. F., Jr., Sharbaugh, R. J., and Bannister, E. R.: *Enterobacter cloacae:* bacteremia, epidemiology, and antibiotic resistance. Rev Infect Dis 4:13, 1982.

Kahn, S. B., Fein, S. A., and Brodsky, I.: Effects of trimethoprim on folate metabolism in man. Clin Pharmacol Ther 9:550, 1968.

Kirby, W. M., and Regamey, C.: Pharmacokinetics of cefazolin compared with four other cephalosporins. J Infect Dis 128(Suppl):341, 1973.

Kirck, J. A., and Remington, J. S.: Opportunistic invasive fungal infections in patients with leukaemia and lymphoma. Clin Haemotol 5:249, 1976.

Kropp, H., Sundelof, J. G., Hajdu, R., et al: Metabolism of thienamycin and related carbapenem antibiotics by the renal dipeptidase, dihydropeptidase-1. Antimicrob Agents Chemother 22:62, 1982.

La Du, B. N.: Pharmacogenetics: defective enzymes in relation to reaction to drugs. Ann Rev Med 23:453, 1972.

LeFrock, J. L., Molavi, A., and Prince, R. A.: Clindamycin. Med Clin N Am 66:103, 1982.

Levine, B. B., Redmond, A. P., Fellner, M. J., et al: Penicillin allergy and the heterogeneous immune responses of man to benzylpenicillin. J Clin Invest 45:1895, 1966.

McCarthy, C. G., and Finland, M.: Absorption and excretion of four penicillins: penicillin G, penicillin V, phenethicillin and phenylmercaptomethyl penicillin. N Engl J Med 263:315, 1960.

McPherson, S. D., Jr., Presley, G. D., and Crawford, J. R.: Aqueous humor assays of subconjunctival antibiotics. Am J Opthalmol 66:430, 1968.

Matz, G. J., and Lerner, S. A.: Prospective studies of aminoglycoside ototoxicity in adults. In Lerner, S. A., Matz, G. J., and Hawkins, J. E., Jr. Aminoglycoside Ototoxicity. Boston, Little Brown and Co., 1981, p. 327.

Mitchell, J. R., Zimmerman, H. J., Ishak, K. G., et al: Isoniazid liver injury: clinical spectrum, pathology and probable pathogenesis. Ann Intern Med 84:181, 1976.

Nagao, T., and Mauer, A. M.: Concordance of drug-induced aplastic anemia in identical twins. N Engl J Med 281:7, 1969.

Neu, H. C.: A symposium on the tetracyclines. A major appraisal. Bull NY Acad Med 54:141, 1978.

Neu, H. C.: Drugs five years later - amoxicillin. Ann Intern Med 90:356, 1979.

Neu, H. C.: Optimal antibiotic therapy in bronchopulmonary infection. Infection 8(Suppl 1):62, 1980.

Neu, H. C.: Clinical pharmacology of the antimicrobial agents for infections in the ear, nose and throat. Ann Otol Rhinol Laryngol 90:2, 1981.

Neu, H. C.: Antistaphylococcal penicillins. Med Clin N Am 66:51, 1982.

Neu, H. C.: Pharmacology of aminoglycosides. In Whelton, A., and Neu, H. C. (eds.): The Aminoglycosides. New York, Marcel Dekker, 1982a, p. 125.

Neu, H. C.: The new beta-lactamase-stable cephalosporins. Ann Intern Med 97:408, 1982b.

Neu, H. C.: The in vitro activity, human pharmacology and clinical effectiveness of new β-lactam antibiotics. Ann Rev Pharmacol Toxicol 22:599, 1982c.

Neu, H. C.: Carbenicillin and ticarcillin. Med Clin N Am 66:61, 1982d.

Neu, H. C.: The use of cephalosporins in the treatment of bacterial meningitis. In Sande, M., and Root, R. (eds.): Contemporary Issues in Infectious Diseases. New York, Churchill Livingstone, 1983.

Norby, R.: A review of penetration of antibiotics into CSF and its clinical significance. Scand J Infect Dis 14(Suppl):296, 1978.
Pancoast, S. J., and Neu, H. C.: Antibiotic levels in human bone and synovial fluid. Ortho Rev 9:49, 1980.
Parry, M. F., and Neu, H. C.: The safety and tolerance of mezlocillin. J Antimicrob Chemother 9(Suppl A):273, 1982.
Pennington, J. E.: Penetration of antibiotics into respiratory secretions. Rev Infect Dis 3:67, 1981.
Philipson, A.: Pharmacokinetics of antibiotics in pregnancy and labour. Clin Pharmacokin 4:297, 1979.
Rall, D. P.: Drug entry into brain and cerebrospinal fluid. In Brodie, B., and Gillette, J. R. (eds.): Handbook of Experimental Pharmacology: Concepts in Biochemical Pharmacology, Part 1. New York, Springer-Verlag, 1971, p. 240.
Ream, C. R.: Respiratory and cardiac arrest after intravenous administration of kanamycin with reversal of toxic effects by neostigmine. Ann Intern Med 59:384, 1963.
Sachs, J., Geer, T., Noell, P., et al: Effect of renal function on urinary recovery of orally administered nitrofurantoin. N Engl J Med 278:1032, 1968.
Saxon, A.: Immediate hypersensitivity reactions to β-lactam antibiotics. Rev Infect Dis 5(Suppl 2):368, 1983.
Schultz, J. C., Adamson, J. S., Jr., Workman, W. W., et al: Fatal liver disease after intravenous administration of tetracycline in high dosage. N Engl J Med 269:999, 1963.
Seamans, K. B., Gloor, P., Dobell, R. A. R., et al: Penicillin-induced seizures during cardiopulmonary by-pass. A clinical and electroencephalographic study. N Engl J Med 278:861, 1968.
Silverblatt, F., Harrison, W. O., and Turck, M.: Nephrotoxicity of cephalosporin antibiotics in experimental animals. J Infect Dis 128(Suppl):367, 1973.
Singer, I., and Rotenberg, D.: Demeclocycline-induced nephrogenic diabetes insipidus. In vivo and in vitro studies. Ann Intern Med 79:679, 1973.
Somani, P., Smith, M. R., Gohara, A., et al: The effect of mezlocillin, ticarcillin and placebo on blood coagulation and bleeding time in normal volunteers. J Antimicrob Chemother 11(Suppl C):33, 1983.
Stamey, T.: Urinary infections. Baltimore, The Williams & Wilkins Co., 1982, p. 161.
Voss, H. E., Redmond, A. P. and Levine, B. B.: Clinical detection of the potential allergic reactor to penicillin by immunologic tests. JAMA 196:679, 1966.
Warner, W. A., and Sanders, E.: Neuromuscular blockade associated with gentamicin therapy. JAMA 215:1153, 1971.
Whelton, A., and Walker, W. G.: Intrarenal antibiotic distribution in health and disease. Kidney Internatl 6:131, 1974.
Williams, D. N., Laughlin, W., and Lee, Y.: Minocycline: possible vestibular side effects. Lancet 2:744, 1974.
Wormser, G. P., and Keusch, G. T.: Trimethoprim-sulfamethoxazole in the United States. Ann Intern Med 91:420, 1979.
Zauder, H. L., Barton, N., Bennett, E. J., et al: Colistimethate as a cause of postoperative apnoea. Canad Anaesthiol Soc J 13:607, 1966.

B. SPECIFIC MICROBIAL AGENTS OF DISEASE

1. Aerobic Bacteria Or Facultatively Anaerobic Bacteria

GRAM-POSITIVE COCCI

23 STAPHYLOCOCCI

STEPHEN I. MORSE, M.D.*
REVISED AND UPDATED BY MARIAN E. MELISH, M.D.

The staphylococci make up the medically most important genus in the family *Micrococcaceae*. There are three species: *Staphylococcus aureus* is responsible for most cases of staphylococcal disease in man; *S. epidermidis* usually causes minor skin lesions; and the newly recognized species *S. saprophyticus* may produce bladder infection.

MORPHOLOGY. Staphylococci are nonmotile, nonspore forming, gram-positive cocci; in old cultures, or after ingestion by phagocytes, they may appear gram negative. Individual cells have a diameter of 0.7 to 1.2 μm and are characteristically grouped in irregular aggregates that resemble clusters of grapes, hence the name *staphylo* from the Greek *staphylē*—bunch of grapes. Cell division takes place in successive perpendicular planes, but there is incomplete separation of the daughter cells and, instead of residual attachment along the division plane, the attachment point is usually eccentric to the division plane, resulting in irregular aggregates (Tzagaloff and Novick, 1977). Moreover, daughter cells may shift from their original site of attachment. Although clusters are usually seen in pathologic material and in growth on solid media, staphylococci often form short chains in liquid culture.

Some *S. aureus* strains possess distinct capsules, as demonstrated by the India ink method, electron microscopic techniques, or the Quellung reaction with specific capsular antiserum (Morse, 1978). Encapsulation may be more frequent in vivo than after cultivation in vitro.

The peptidoglycan of staphylococcal cell walls is characterized by unique pentaglycine bridges that link the tetrapeptides attached to the muramic acid residues (see Chapter 20). The pentaglycine bridges are specifically susceptible to the action of the enzyme lysostaphin, thereby providing a useful means of identifying the genus.

Osmotically unstable L forms, deficient in cell wall material, can be induced by agents that affect cell wall synthesis or structure—for example, penicillin or lysostaphin—and can be propagated in vitro in hypertonic medium. Small colony variants of *S. aureus* (G forms) occur when microbial growth is inhibited by a variety of agents, including antimicrobials, but also may appear spontaneously. Both L and G forms are resistant to many drugs, especially those affecting the cell wall, and it has been postulated that recrudescent *S. aureus* disease is sometimes due to reversion of persisting dormant L or G forms to invasive parental organisms.

This attractive hypothesis has been extensively investigated with negative results. At this time there is no evidence that L and G forms are important causes of bacterial persistence in clinical infections.

*Deceased.

On solid media, most strains of S. *aureus* produce a characteristic golden-yellow *(aureus)* carotenoid pigment; however, colonial coloration may vary from white to orange. S. *epidermidis* colonies usually are white and those of S. *saprophyticus* are white to greyish-white. Colonies of staphylococci are sharply defined, round, convex, and measure 4 mm in diameter. On blood agar, S. *aureus* is usually surrounded by a zone of clear (β) hemolysis. Strains of S. *aureus* may produce one or more of four distinct hemolysins with different hemolytic specificities; therefore, the occurrence and extent of hemolysis depends upon both the strain and the source of blood. Some S. *epidermidis* strains are also hemolytic, whereas S. *saprophyticus* is nonhemolytic.

ANTIGENIC COMPOSITION

Species Antigens. The species-specific antigens of staphylococci are cell wall teichoic acids. In S. *aureus*, the antigen is a ribitol teichoic acid composed of a linear backbone of ribitol linked by phosphodiester bridges. *N*-acetylglucosamine is attached to the C4 position of the ribitol residues, and ester-linked *D*-alanine is attached to approximately 50 per cent of the C2 residues. The antigenic determinant is the glucosamine moiety, which may be in either α or β glycosidic linkage to ribitol. In most strains both types of glycosidic linkage are found, but in some only one is present. Therefore, antisera that will react with both anomers must be used for immunochemical determination of the species. Similarly, teichoic acids with both specificities must be used when testing for the presence of serum antibodies.

The S. *epidermidis* species-antigen is a glycerol teichoic acid in which glucose residues, in either α or β glycosidic linkage, are attached to a glycerol phosphate backbone and constitute the antigenic determinant. Cell walls of S. *saprophyticus* contain ribitol teichoic acid of two types. One has *N*-acetylglucosamine residues, whereas the other has glucose residues. Both may be present in the same strain.

Cellular Antigens of S. Aureus

Capsules. The few strains of S. *aureus* that are encapsulated in vitro tend to be more virulent in animals, and anticapsular antibodies protect against experimental disease. The capsule of one group of strains is a polymer of glucosaminuronic acid; that of another contains mannosaminuronic acid; and components characteristic of the peptidoglycan, e.g., glycine, alanine, and glucosamine, are found in the capsules of other strains.

Protein. Protein A (agglutinogen A) is a surface component of most strains of S. *aureus*. Depending upon the method of isolation, the molecular weight of protein A ranges between 13,000 and 42,000. Although the bulk of protein A is covalently linked to the peptidoglycan, approximately one third is released extracellularly. The most striking property of protein A is its nonspecific interaction with the Fc portion of the IgG of a wide range of mammalian species. The result of the interaction may be either precipitation or the formation of soluble complexes. In the case of human IgG, protein A reacts with subclasses IgG1, IgG2, and IgG4, but not IgG3. Protein A also binds to some samples of human IgM and IgA2. The interaction with the Fc portion of IgG produces a variety of biologic effects, including: activation of complement by both the classical and the alternative pathways; local wheal and flare reaction; the Arthus phenomenon; local and systemic anaphylaxis; inhibition of phagocytosis of opsonized particles through competition with the Fc receptors of phagocytes for the Fc portion of opsonic antibody (Peterson et al., 1977); and in vitro induction of proliferation of both human T lymphocytes and B lymphocytes (Sakane and Green, 1978). Protein A is also a true antigen and reacts with the Fab portion of specific antibody.

Clumping Factor (Bound Coagulase). Unencapsulated strains of S. *aureus* clump when suspended in fibrinogen-containing solutions. There are apparently specific receptors on the bacterial surface for fibrinogen and the clumping is due to cross-linkage of the cells by fibrinogen. The receptors have not been characterized.

Extracellular Antigens and Products of S. Aureus

Coagulase. S. *aureus* has the unique ability to clot a variety of mammalian plasmas. Clotting is caused by an extracellular product, coagulase (or free coagulase), which exists in several antigenically different forms, all having the same mechanisms of action. Virtually all naturally occurring strains of S. *aureus* produce coagulase, and since tests for coagulase are simple to perform, the *aureus* species is usually identified by coagulase production rather than by serologic, physiologic, or biochemical tests. Coagulase-positive staphylococci are by definition S. *aureus*.

Coagulase does not clot fibrinogen directly but first reacts with a plasma constituent, coagulase-reacting factor (CRF), which is most probably prothrombin, to form a thrombin-like substance. The fibrinopeptides formed during clotting are identical to those produced by the action of thrombin on fibrinogen and, as in the case of thrombin-mediated clotting, diisopropyl-fluorophosphate (DFP) blocks the reaction.

Hemolysins. Four distinct hemolytic exoproteins are produced by coagulase positive staphylococci. The purified forms of three of these, α, γ, and δ toxins, are "membrane damaging toxins" that have other potent biologic effects that may be more important than their ability to lyse red blood cells. These three toxins may affect the course of infection because they activate T and non-T lymphocytes. Each hemolysin exhibits a characteristic lytic and cytotoxic spectrum against erythrocytes and other cells of different species. All cause clear (β) hemolysis of susceptible erythrocytes. The hemolytic toxins are all antigenic proteins whose action can be neutralized by specific antisera.

α-Toxin (α-hemolysin) is the most common hemolysin in clinical isolates of coagulase-positive staphylococci. Alpha toxin is extremely potent and causes lysis of many other cells. Injected intravenously in mammals, it seriously affects the central nervous system so that respiratory paralysis and death follow rapidly. It causes dermonecrosis at the site of subcutaneous infection. Rabbit erythrocytes and granulocytes are particularly susceptible to lysis while human erythrocytes are 100-fold less sensitive and human granulocytes are not lysed. Binding to surface receptors on susceptible cells is the first step in its action. Alpha toxin has complex interactions with polymorphonuclear leukocytes. At low doses (< 10 hemolytic units) it inhibits chemotaxis but enhances phagocytosis and intracellular killing. Cell lysis occurs at higher doses. The overall effect of α toxin at the site of infection is not clearly understood.

β-Hemolysin is found in many strains of animal origin but is produced by less than 20 per cent of human strains. It is a "hot-cold" hemolysin; lysis is maximal only after blood agar plates or toxin-erythrocyte mixtures are held at low temperatures after incubation at 37°C. β-Hemolysin is a sphingomyelinase, which, in the presence of magnesium ions, catalyzes the breakdown of sphingomyelin to *N*-acylsphingosine and phosphorylcholine. Erythrocyte susceptibility is directly correlated with sphingomyelin content. Sheep, human, and guinea pig erythrocytes contain decreasing amounts of sphingomyelin and are decreasingly susceptible to β-hemolysin. β-Hemolysin is toxic for experimental animals only in high doses.

γ-Toxin consists of two components that act in concert to induce hemolysis. γ-Toxin is inhibited by sulfonated polymers, including agar, and hence its activity is not readily seen on blood agar plates. Rabbit, human, and sheep erythrocytes are susceptible to lysis.

δ-Toxin consists of aggregates of low molecular weight subunits and has a broad range of lytic and cytotoxic activity.

Leucocidin. In addition to the leukocytotoxic effects of some of the hemolysins, *S. aureus* also produces a distinct nonhemolytic leukocytotoxic substance, Panton-Valentine (P-V) leucocidin. P-V leucocidin contains two components, F (electrophoretically fast moving) and S (slow moving). Both are required for activity, and antibody to either component neutralizes toxicity. Human and rabbit polymorphonuclear leukocytes and macrophages are susceptible.

As with the α, γ, and δ toxins, the exact role of leucocidin on host defenses and the establishment of infection is unknown. When these cytotoxic exoproteins are purified they have such potent biologic effects that it is tempting to speculate that they may be important in invasiveness and virulence of coagulase-positive staphylococci. Coagulase-negative staphylococci do not produce these exoproteins and are much less invasive. Nevertheless, the precise biologic role of these exoproteins must still be worked out. In contrast, staphylococcal enterotoxins and epidermolytic toxins have clearly demonstrable specific effects in human disease.

Enterotoxins. Five chemically and immunologically related enterotoxins (designated a-e) are produced by *S. aureus*. These proteins have a molecular weight of 3.5×10^4, are relatively heat stable, and only moderately susceptible to trypsin digestion (Bergdoll et al., 1974). They cause vomiting that is thought to be mediated by effects on the central nervous system. Preformed enterotoxin in food contaminated by *S. aureus* causes the most common form of food poisoning. Intravenous administration of enterotoxins to laboratory animals causes hypotension, cardiovascular collapse, and death. The significance of these properties in naturally occurring human disease is unknown.

Epidermolytic Toxins. Certain *S. aureus*, primarily nontypable strains that are lysed by Group II phages, produce one or both of the epidermolytic toxins. Both are proteins (also known as epidermolysins and exfoliatins) with similar low molecular weights and isoelectric points (M.S. ~ 26,000 daltons, pI 7.1). They have different amino acid compositions and do not cross-react immunologically. Epidermolytic toxin A is chromosomally determined while epidermolytic toxin B is plasmid mediated. These toxins separate the cells of the stratum granulosum of the epidermis and lyse their intercellular contact without destroying the cells. The site of action is limited to the upper epidermis of certain susceptible species: man, other primates, mice, and hamsters. The epidermolytic toxins cause the dermatologic manifestations of the Staphylococcal Scalded Skin Syndrome.

Toxic Shock Syndrome Toxin 1. This exoprotein with a molecular weight of 24,500 daltons and an isoelectric point of 7.1 was isolated independently by Bergdoll (1981) and Schlievert (1981). It is called Staphylococcal Enterotoxin F (SEF) by Bergdoll and Pyrogenic Exotoxin C (PEC) by Schlievert. Since these two preparations are immunologically and chemically identical, agreement has been reached on a new name, Toxic Shock Syndrome Toxin 1. It is the most reliable marker for identifying staphylococci associated with Toxic Shock Syndrome. In its purified state, it is pyrogenic for rabbits and activates lymphocytes. Intravenous infusions cause hypotension and azotemia in rabbits and baboons. It is not yet proven to be the mediator of the shock and multisystem damage characteristic of the syndrome.

A number of other extracellular substances with biologic activity are also produced by *S. aureus*. These include staphylokinase (fibrinolysin), hyaluronidase, and phospholipase.

The wide variety of antigenic components and extracellular products found in *S. aureus* is not seen in either *S. epidermidis* or *S. saprophyticus*. Some strains of *S. epidermidis* cause β-hemolysis owing to a hemolysin termed ε-hemolysin, which is similar to the *S. aureus* δ-hemolysin. *S. saprophyticus* is not hemolytic.

METABOLISM. *S. aureus* and *S. epidermidis* are facultative anaerobes that ferment sugars with the formation of large amounts of lactic acid, as occurs in lactic acid bacteria (Baird-Parker, 1974). They also resemble the spherical lactic acid bacteria in the low G + C content (30 to 35 moles per cent) of their DNA, but staphylococci possess heme-containing enzymes that allow normal respiratory metabolism, which is absent in lactic acid bacteria. The most important of these respiratory enzymes in staphylococci are cytochromes a, b, and o, which contain firmly bound prosthetic groups capable of donating or accepting electrons as they undergo oxidation or reduction. They are bound to the cell membrane of the staphylococcus and, with a group of quinones (menaquinones), form the membrane-bound electron transport system. The quinones are nonprotein carriers of relatively low molecular weight. Catalase, another heme enzyme possessed by staphylococci, is important for splitting hydrogen peroxide and preventing accumulation of this highly toxic compound. In the diagnostic laboratory, catalase activity helps distinguish staphylococci from streptococci, which are catalase deficient. Of particular usefulness in species differentiation is the capacity of *S. aureus* to ferment mannitol and to grow in concentrations of sodium chloride that are inhibitory for other microorganisms—for example 7.5 per cent NaCl. *S. aureus* also produces a heat-stable nuclease, not found in the other species. In contrast to *S. aureus* and *S. epidermidis*, *S. saprophyticus* grows very poorly under anaerobic conditions.

Although capable of anaerobic growth, *S. aureus* and *S. epidermidis* grow better aerobically. Moreover, they exhibit different metabolic activities under aerobic and anaerobic conditions. For example, oxygen is necessary for pigment production, and nonpigmented colonies of *S. aureus* grown anaerobically will develop their characteristic yellow color upon exposure to air (aerochromogens; compare with photochromogens among mycobacteria, Chapter 44). Glucose, lactose, maltose, and mannitol are energy sources for staphylococci anaerobically. These sugars are also metabolized in air, and so are other hexoses, pentoses, disaccharides, and sugar alcohols. The products of glucose metabolism change from lactic acid during fermentation to acetate and CO_2 in air. S. *epidermidis* produces nitrite from nitrate when grown in air but may not do so under anaerobic conditions because nitrate reductase does not function in the absence of air. For reduction of nitrate, oxygen is required not as a terminal electron acceptor but for the biosynthesis of a cytochrome, which mediates electron transfer to nitrate.

GENETICS. Many of the properties and products of S. *aureus* are genetically controlled by plasmids. Plasmid regulation of antibiotic resistance, especially through the production of penicillinase (β-lactamase), is of profound clinical importance (Lacey, 1975).

In contrast to R-factors in gram-negative bacteria, penicillinase plasmids do not tend to carry other antibiotic resistance markers, with the exception of erythromycin. Hence, multiple drug resistance mediated by plasmids is unusual in S. *aureus*. There appear to be two molecular classes of staphylococcal resistance plasmids. The larger of these has a molecular weight of 20×10^6, may be isolated as a covalently closed ring molecule, and its replication appears to depend on cell division so that only one (or at most a few) copy occurs in each cell. The other type is much smaller and has a molecular weight in the range of 3×10^6. The smaller type may carry resistance determinants for tetracycline or chloramphenicol and multiply independently of cell division so that multiple copies are produced in each cell. As with gram-negative bacteria, chloramphenicol resistance is mediated by staphylococcal plasmids through the enzyme chloramphenicol acetyltransferase. In contrast, however, to the constituent enzymes of gram-negative R-factors, the penicillinase and acetyltransferase of resistant staphylococci are inducible (see Chapter 4). Transfer of genetic material between strains of S. *aureus* occurs by transduction. Most strains of S. *aureus* are lysogenic, and lysogenic bacteriophages belonging to serologic group B are capable of generalized transduction, in which bacterial DNA (rather than phage DNA) is incorporated with the phage particle. Spontaneous prophage induction and subsequent transduction occurs in mixed cultures in vitro and more importantly transduction occurs in vivo in animals and humans carrying an appropriate lysogenic donor and a suitable recipient strain of S. *aureus* (Novick and Morse, 1968). In addition to transduction, bacteriophages also exert genetic control by the process of phage conversion as in the production of staphylokinase and β-hemolysin. Under highly specialized circumstances, transformation reactions can occur, but conjugation as a means of genetic transfer in staphylococci is not seen.

PATHOGENIC PROPERTIES. Staphylococci produce two types of disease, invasive and toxigenic. The hallmark of invasive staphylococcal infection is abscess formation. Tissue destruction at the site of inoculation is followed rapidly by hyperemia and vigorous accumulation of many polymorphonuclear leukocytes. The center of the lesion soon becomes necrotic and a fibrin wall is formed at the site of intensive hyperemia surrounding the lesions. The mature lesion consists of a fibrin wall surrounded by inflamed tissues and enclosing a central liquified core of pus containing staphylococci and leukocytes. Live bacteria may persist within these lesions. As pus accumulates, it may drain towards the skin surface or into adjacent tissues, where it forms sinus tracts and secondary abscesses. This type of reaction may be seen in staphylococcal infections of the skin and subcutaneous tissues, lymph nodes, joints, renal tissues, liver, parotid glands, muscles, lung, and long bones.

In addition to local extension, coagulase-positive staphylococci may spread hematogenously from the focus of infection—even from small or trivial abscesses. Bones, joints, and heart valves may become infected by hematogenous dissemination. Skin and wounds, which are the usual ports of entry, are remarkably resistant to infection, but this natural resistance is lowered dramatically by the presence within the wound of foreign bodies such as sutures and bits of soil or gravel. Natural resistance is also affected by ecchymosis, hemorrhage, and vascular insufficiency. Poor personal hygiene also predisposes to staphylococcal skin infection. Moist, macerated skin is invaded more easily, as shown by the higher frequency of staphylococcal skin infections in intertriginous areas and tropical climates.

Infections of hair follicles (folliculitis) and sweat glands (hiradenitis) are extremely common. Furuncles and carbuncles result from local extension and amalgamation of multiple smaller lesions. Less well-localized infections like cellulitis of the subcutaneous tissues also occur. Surgical and traumatic wounds are more frequently infected by staphylococci than any other organism.

Deep tissue infections of multiple organs generally result from hematogenous dissemination. Severe disseminated staphylococcal infection is not infrequent in healthy individuals; malnourished people are even more susceptible and S. *aureus* is second only to *Pseudomonas aeruginosa* as a cause of bacteremia in cancer patients. Osteomyelitis, septic arthritis, septic thrombophlebitis, and acute bacterial endocarditis are relatively common. Liver, spleen, and pancreatic abscesses are less common results of bacteremia. Liver abscess may also complicate biliary disease, ascending cholangitis, or biliary surgery. Muscle abscesses are rare in temperate climates and developed countries but are common in tropical areas. Staphylococci may reach the lungs either by aspiration or hematogenously. Inhalation pneumonitis occurs most commonly in infants under 1 year and as a secondary invader after aspiration or influenza pneumonia in any age group. It begins as a localized unilateral, peribronchial infiltrate but spreads rapidly. Effusions, abscesses, pneumatoceles and bronchopleural fistulas with pneumothorax are common complications. Hematogenous staphylococcal pneumonia is characterized by multiple metastatic foci in both lungs, and is encountered regularly in patients with endocarditis, focal infections of other organs, and in intravenous drug abusers,

Coagulase negative staphylococci are a ubiquitous part of the normal flora of the skin and respiratory tracts and are so non-invasive that infection of normal people is very rare. Bacteremia and focal infection occur in neonates and immunocompromised persons. Serious infections with coagulase negative staphylococci are frequently associated with colonization of prosthetic heart valves, cerebrospinal fluid shunts and intravenous catheters. S. *saphrophyticus* is a frequent cause of urinary tract infection in young, sexually active women.

There are now three clinical syndromes in which the major manifestations are mediated by exotoxins instead of tissue invasion or bacteremia. These are staphylococcal food poisoning, the various forms of skin disease due to epidermolytic toxin (Scalded Skin Syndrome), and the recently described Toxic Shock Syndrome.

The most common form of food poisoning is due to ingestion of preformed staphylococcal enterotoxin. Contamination of foods by enterotoxin-producing staphylococci is followed by a period of incubation at warm or room temperatures during which bacteria multiply and enterotoxin is produced. Cooking will not destroy these heat stable toxins. Nausea, vomiting, and occasionally diarrhea occur abruptly one to six hours after eating contaminated food. In most cases recovery occurs promptly without therapy although fluid and electrolyte replacement is required occasionally.

The various skin changes of the Staphylococcal Scalded Skin Syndrome (SSSS) are caused by epidermolytic toxin. Two generalized forms of SSSS occur. The first is characterized by painful, total body erythroderma, followed by widespread bullae formation and superficial skin separation. In the second generalized form of SSSS, which is milder than the first, tender scarlatiniform erythroderma occurs without significant skin loss. The two generalized forms are the result of hematogenous dissemination of toxin from a distant focus of infection. The infection itself may be serious but is more often a trivial focus such as bacterial conjunctivitis. The generalized forms of SSSS are seen most often in children under 5 years; less than 20 cases have been reported in adults, all of whom either have had severe staphylococcal infections or have been immunocompromised. The presence of specific antitoxic antibody, nearly universal over the age of 10 years, protects against disseminated disease. Bullous impetigo represents a localized form of SSSS in which the toxin is produced at the site of skin infection and causes only local bullae. Organisms, toxin, and inflammatory cells can all be found within the skin lesion, while other areas of the skin remain normal. Bullous impetigo can develop and progress despite antitoxic immunity.

Toxic Shock Syndrome was first described in 1978 but not recognized widely until 1980 when approximately 1000 cases from different locations were reported to the U.S. Centers for Disease Control. Occurring primarily in young women during their menstrual periods but occasionally in men and children with focal staphylococcal infection, the illness is hyperacute with abrupt onset of fever, followed by vomiting, diarrhea, and abdominal pain and myalgias. Within 2 to 3 days, patients develop a fine faint erythroderma resembling but milder than the exanthema of scarlet fever. Generalized mucous membrane hyperemia is manifested by conjunctival injection, pharyngitis, and strawberry tongue. There is also renal involvement with elevated BUN and creatinine, hepatocellular disease with elevated transaminase values, decreased serum calcium and phosphorus concentrations, abnormal hematologic values with thrombocytopenia and lymphocytopenia. Since most patients have had negative blood cultures, the shock and multiorgan dysfunction is thought to be mediated by a toxin or toxins disseminated hematogenously from a focal infection. The most common focal infection has been vaginal colonization with *S. aureus* in menstruating women who were using vaginal tampons. Focal infections in men and children have included abscesses, surgical and traumatic wound infections, and pneumonia with effusion. Staphylococci isolated from patients with Toxic Shock Syndrome have been universally penicillin resistant and likely to belong to phage group 1. The most reliable marker of these staphylococci is that they produce an intracellular protein toxin, Toxic Shock Syndrome Toxin 1. This exotoxin causes fever, hypotension, renal, hepatic, and muscle damage in experimental animals and is likely to be the major pathogenic mediator of the syndrome.

IMMUNITY. Staphylococcal infections are frequent and recurrent throughout life. All but the youngest infants have had considerable antigenic exposure. Invasive *S. aureus* disease often occurs despite humoral antibodies to multiple cellular components. In experimental animals and in human studies only anticapsular antibodies appear to confer any protection. Since encapsulated organisms seldom cause infections, this protective effect is of little significance. Overall, there is little evidence that humoral immunity either prevents or modifies staphylococcal infection, except in the case of the staphylococcal scalded skin syndrome, in which specific antitoxin to the epidermolytic toxins prevents the generalized forms of the disease.

The effects of cell mediated immunity are more complex and controversial. Although cell-mediated immunity does not prevent infection, it may modify its course. In experimental animals, cell-mediated immunity may restrict the spread of organisms from the inoculation site but, as in the case of tuberculosis, local reactions are often more severe. Thus, the characteristic morphology and confinement of the staphylococcal abscess may be related to the effects of cell-mediated immunity.

Man has a high innate resistance to *S. aureus* disease, but resistance can be readily decreased by local factors. For example, intradermal injection of as many as 10^8 to 10^9 organisms usually causes no abscess, but if a suture containing as few as 10^2 organisms is passed through the skin and tied, marked abscess formation occurs, often requiring surgical and antimicrobial therapy. Other local factors, particularly those that impede circulation, enhance susceptibility to staphylococcal disease.

There is considerable evidence that colonization of normal human skin or mucosa with one strain of *S. aureus* inhibits colonization with another strain, a phenomenon known as bacterial interference. This has been used therapeutically in the case of epidemics in newborn nurseries. The neonate is purposefully colonized in the nares with an avirulent strain of *S. aureus*, and suprainfection with an epidemic virulent strain is thereby prevented. The nature of the inhibition is unknown but may be based upon competition for nutrients, or, more likely, the production of bacteriocins.

The prime defense against staphylococcal infection is an intact phagocytic system. Staphylococcal infections are most severe in those with granulocytopenia or defective phagocytosis or intracellular killing by leukocytes. Patients with Chronic Granulomatous Disease frequently develop persistent and multifocal staphylococcal infections because phagocytosed staphylococci are not killed but transported to distant sites. A unique susceptibility to severe recurrent and persistent *S. aureus* infections is also a major feature of Job's syndrome (Hyper-IgE syndrome). In this condition patients develop multiple and recurrent staphylococcal infections frequently characterized by a decreased inflammatory response. Immunoglobulin E levels are massively increased (over 1000 IU/ml) and chemotaxis sometimes declines. The IgE is predominantly directed at the staphylococcus. An attractive hypothesis is that IgE that is bound to mast cells and basophils may react with staphylococcal antigens at the site of infection and thereby liberate bioactive substances, including histamine and slow reacting substance. These, in turn, may impair neutrophil function.

LABORATORY DIAGNOSIS. The diagnosis of staphylococcal disease is suggested by the finding of gram-positive cocci in clumps in pathologic material, but final diagnosis is achieved only by culture and appropriate tests. The characteristic β-hemolysis and yellow pigmentation strongly point to S. *aureus*, and selective media are useful, but a positive coagulase test is required for definitive identification. The test is performed by adding an aliquot of a broth culture or an inoculum from agar to 0.5 ml of rabbit plasma (either undiluted or diluted 1:10). Most strains produce clotting within three hours of incubation at 37°C, but cultures should be held overnight before a negative result is reported.

Identification of individual strains of S. *aureus* is often epidemiologically useful. Serologic tests are complex and typing sera are not readily available for routine use. Determining the spectrum of antibiotic resistance (resistogram) is simple but imprecise. Phage typing is the most useful technique and is based upon the susceptibility of S. *aureus* to lytic phages. The phages used for typing are divided into groups that have similar, but not identical, host range.

Typing phages for S. *epidermidis* strains are at present not available for general use and strains are usually distinguished by their patterns of resistance to antimicrobials, or their metabolic and biochemical properties (biotypes).

Strains of coagulase-negative staphylococci, isolated from urine, can be identified as S. *saprophyticus* by their poor growth anaerobically and their resistance to novobiocin (M.I.C. > 2.0 μg/ml, Baird-Parker, 1974).

DRUG SUSCEPTIBILITY. When penicillin was first introduced, the vast majority of strains of S. *aureus* were susceptible. Depending upon the geographic area, 80 per cent or more of strains occurring in the population-at-large are now penicillin-resistant. Because the prevalence of penicillin-resistant strains in the general community is now as high as it is in the hospital, penicillin resistance must now be presumed for all staphylococcal infections until sensitivity testing is performed. Resistance is due to the plasmid-mediated enzyme penicillinase, which is a β lactamase that splits the β lactam ring of the penicillin nucleus (Lacey, 1975). In severe staphylococcal disease, unless the strain is sensitive to penicillin, penicillinase-resistant penicillins such as oxacillin and methicillin are the drugs of choice. In patients allergic to penicillin, cephalosporin derivatives may be used. Combined therapy with an aminoglycoside such as gentamicin is often employed, but there is no clear evidence that such combinations are more effective than the use of the bactericidal penicillins or cephalosporins alone. Vancomycin is used in patients who are allergic to the penicillins and cephalosporins.

Methicillin-resistant staphylococci have assumed increasing importance as a cause of both nosocomial and community acquired infection, first in the British Isles and Europe and more recently in North America. Methicillin-resistant staphylococci are resistant to all anti-staphylococcal penicillins and frequently to multiple drugs, with varying susceptibilities to cephalosporins and aminoglycosides. Vancomycin is the treatment of choice for serious infections with methicillin-resistant staphylococci.

Tolerance is the term used to describe strains of staphylococci with a marked discrepancy between the concentration of an antibiotic necessary to inhibit their growth and the concentration necessary to kill them. Mean inhibitory concentrations for tolerant strains are similar to those for sensitive strains but the mean bactericidal concentrations are 8- to 100-fold higher. These strains of staphylococci are usually tolerant to all anti-staphylococcal penicillins and cephalosporins. The mechanism of tolerance seems to be a deficiency of the autolytic enzymes necessary to complete the destruction of the bacterial cell. Most tolerant strains are eventually killed by the usual concentrations of antibiotics after 48 hours of incubation. The frequency of tolerance among staphylococci varies geographically. The clinical significance of tolerance is unknown but some authorities recommend that staphylococci from patients with poor clinical responses or serious infections (endocarditis, bacteremia, multifocal abscesses) be tested for tolerance. Addition of an aminoglycoside such as gentamicin and/or rifampin to the anti-staphylococcal penicillin or cephalosporin may produce a more rapid clinical response. A randomized controlled trial is needed to assess the need for amplified therapy in serious infections with antibiotic tolerant strains.

Infections due to S. *epidermidis* are often caused by strains resistant to a variety of antimicrobial agents, and therapy of deep-seated disease may be very difficult. Strains of S. *saprophyticus* are generally sensitive to penicillin.

Superficial staphylococcal abscesses generally do not require antimicrobial therapy. Local application of moist heat, immobilization, and incision and drainage usually suffice. In both serious and minor staphylococcal disease, infected foci such as foreign bodies or necrotic bone or tissue must be removed.

EPIDEMIOLOGY. S. *aureus* is ubiquitous. Approximately 40 per cent of adults are asymptomatic carriers. Colonization begins in the neonatal period. The nares and the conjunctivae are the usual carrier site, but organisms can be found on skin and mucous membranes, and occasionally in the gut. S. *aureus* is extremely hardy and survives in the air and on inanimate objects and surfaces for long periods of time. It is likely that person-to-person transmission is more important than environmental contamination. Persons with minor staphylococcal infections frequently transmit infection to others, especially in the home or hospital, through close contact and sharing of towels and other personal items. Intravenous abuse of "street drugs" has become a major cause of staphylococcal endocarditis in urban areas of North America and Europe. Nosocomial transmission of S. *aureus* among neonates, surgical patients and recipients of intravenous therapy has been a major problem, but patient segregation, strict routines for hand washing between patients, and frequent changes of intravenous cannulas and needles have reduced its frequency. The transmission of S. *epidermidis* in neurosurgery, cardiac surgery and neonatal nurseries is now a major problem that demands equally effective control measures.

Because of the widespread occurrence of S. *aureus*, it is inappropriate to consider methods to prevent acquisition of strains in a normal population. However, in "at risk" patients, such as newborns and patients in hospitals with serious underlying disorders, it is imperative that individuals with open lesions be isolated.

References

Baird-Parker, A. C.: *Micrococcaceae.* In Buchanan, R. E. and Gibbons, N. W. (eds.): Bergey's Manual of Determinative Bacteriology. 8th ed. Baltimore, Williams and Wilkins, 1974, p. 483.

Bergdoll, M. S., Crass, B. B., Reiser, R. F., Robbins, R. N., and Davis, J. P.: A new staphylococcal enterotoxin, enterotoxin F, associated with toxic shock syndrome *Staphylococcus aureus* isolates. Lancet 1:1017, 1981.

Bergdoll, M. S., Huang, I. Y., and Schantz, E. J.: Chemistry of the staphylococcal enterotoxins. J Agr Food Chem 22:9, 1974.

Bernheimer, A. W.: Interactions between membranes and cytolytic bacterial toxins. Biochim et Biophysica Acta 344:27, 1974.

Cohen, J. O.: The Staphylococci. New York, John Wiley and Sons Incorporated, 1972.

Forsgren, A.: Immunological aspects of protein A. In Schlessinger, D., (ed.): Microbiology-1977. Washington, D.C., American Society for Microbiology, 1977, p. 353.

Jeljaszewiez, J. (ed.): Staphylococci and Staphylococcal Diseases. New York, Gustav Fischer Verlag, 1976.

Lacey, R. W.: Antibiotic resistance plasmids of *Staphylococcus aureus* and their clinical importance. Bacteriol Rev 39:1, 1975.

Melish, M. E., and Glasgow, L. A.: The staphylococcal scalded-skin syndrome: development of an experimental model. N Engl J Med 282:1114, 1970.

Morse, S. I.: Staphylococci. In Davis, B. D., Dulbecco, R., Eisen, H. N., and Ginsberg, H. S. (eds.): Microbiology. 3rd ed. Hagerstown, Harper and Row, 1978.

Novick, R. P., and Morse, S. I.: In vivo transmission of drug resistance factors between strains of *Staphylococcus aureus.* J Exp Med 125:45, 1968.

Peterson, P. K., Verholf, J., Sabbath, L. D., and Quie, P. G.: Effect of protein A on staphylococcal opsonization. Infect Immun 15:760, 1977.

Sakane, T., and Green, I.: Protein A from *Staphylococcus aureus*—a mitogen for human T lymphocytes and B lymphocytes but not L lymphocytes. J Immun 120:302, 1978.

Shlievert, P. M., Shands, K. N., Dan, B. B., Schmid, G. P., and Nishimura, R. D.: Identification and characterization of an exotoxin from *Staphylococcus aureus* associated with toxic shock syndrome. J Infect Dis 143:509, 1981.

Tzagaloff, H., and Novick, R. P.: Geometry of cell division in *Staphylococcus aureus.* J Bact 129:343, 1977.

Wiseman, G. M.: The hemolysins of *Staphylococcus aureus.* Bacteriol Rev 39:317, 1975.

24

STREPTOCOCCUS

ISAAC GINSBURG, M. SC., PH.D.

Since the discovery of the streptococcus by Billroth and Ehrlich in 1877, it has received special attention because it is involved in numerous diseases of humans and lower animals. Few other microorganisms of medical importance can elaborate as many exotoxins and enzymes and also produce serious infections in virtually any tissue. Certain streptococci also are notorious for inducing nonsuppurative sequelae that affect the heart, kidney, joints, and brain, and take the form of rheumatic fever, acute glomerulonephritis (AGN), and chorea (Wannamaker, 1981; Holm and Christensen, 1982).

Although some streptococci are human pathogens, others are integral parts of the normal flora of the mouth and bowel. The normal streptococcal flora may, however, invade the bloodstream and cause septicemia, usually associated with endocarditis. Streptococci in the mouth are involved in the pathogenesis of dental caries. Certain streptococci are also important in the dairy industry.

The genus *Streptococcus* belongs to the family Streptococcaceae. The most important species of streptococci with pathogenic properties for man are *Streptococcus pyogenes* (group A streptococci), *Streptococcus pneumoniae* (pneumococci), *Streptococcus agalactiae* (group B), *Streptococcus faecalis* (enterococci—group D) and viridans streptococci (a heterogenous group of different species (Tables 1 and 2). The guanine + cytosine content of streptococcal DNA ranges from 33 to 44 moles per cent. Analysis of DNA-RNA homology among streptococci (including pneumococci) discloses a close relationship except for *S. faecalis* (Weissman et al., 1966). Numerical taxonomic analyses are the basis for recent taxonomic revisions (Bridge and Sneath, 1983).

MORPHOLOGY. Streptococci are gram-positive, usually nonmotile cocci that are arranged in chains. Growth occurs by elongation on the axis parallel to the chain and division is at right angles in the equatorial plane. Whereas certain streptococci—that is, pneumococci and the oral streptococci—grow in pairs or relatively short chains in liquid medium, the hemolytic streptococci grow in longer chains. These do not elongate indefinitely, since in some cases the streptococci produce a "dechaining factor."

The most typical colonies of *S. pyogenes* are disk-like, matt (dull), and 0.5 to 2.0 mm in diameter. The matt colonies are derived from younger mucoid colonies whose hyaluronic acid capsules become dehydrated. If plate cultures are sealed to prevent dehydration, the colonies of group A streptococci remain mucoid. With loss of virulence the matt form reverts to small, smooth colonies with a dry, glistening surface or to typical rough colonies.

When grown on blood agar, various streptococcal groups can modify hemoglobin. Most oral streptococci and *Streptococcus pneumoniae* modify hemoglobin to green pigments (biliverdin and other heme compounds) and are designated α-hemolytic, whereas most Lancefield groups A, B, C, and G streptococci (see below) produce a discrete clear zone of true hemolysis around the colonies; this is known as β-hemolysis. Most *S. faecalis* species do not modify hemoglobin. These characteristics aid in rapid preliminary screening of different streptococcal groups, but final classification depends on detailed biochemical, serologic, and genetic analysis of streptococci (Facklam and Wilkinson, 1981) (See Table 1).

METABOLISM. Streptococci are facultatively anaerobic, acidogenic, and acidophilic. Growth in media that lack body fluids is usually poor but it may be greatly enhanced by the addition of serum proteins and reducing agents in the form of sulfhydryl compounds. Most streptococci virulent for humans show an absolute demand for at least 12 amino acids, 3 purines and pyrimidines, 4 vitamins, certain divalent metals, and an energy source like glucose. Growth is sometimes enhanced by certain peptides (streptogenin).

Luxurious growth in fluid media always forms aggregates (floccules) that fall to the bottom, leaving a relatively clear supernatant fluid. Growth of bacteria in the submerged floccules is inhibited by lactic acid, which is formed from glucose by glycolysis. Excellent growth is usually obtained on brain heart infusion media, in Todd-Hewitt broth, or on complete synthetic media. Growth is facilitated by constant neutralization of the lactic acid and rich growth is

Table 1. DIFFERENTIATION OF COMMON GROUPABLE STREPTOCOCCACEAE

Category	β-Hemolysis	Group Antigen	Fermentation of: *Trehalose*	*Sorbitol*	Hydrolysis of: *Hippurate*	*Esculin*	Growth in: *6.5% NaCl*	*40% Bile*	Inhibition by: *Bacitracin*	*SXT*	*Penicillin (0.5) units)*	*CAMP Factor*
S. pyogenes	+	A	−	−	−	−	−	−	+	−	+	−
S. agalactiae	+	B	−	−	+	−	V	−	(−)	−	+	+
S. equisimilis	+	C	+	−	−	−	−	(−)	(−)	+	+	−
S. faecalis	V	D	+	+	(−)	+	+	+	−	−	−	−
S. bovis	−	D	V	−	−	+	−	+	−	(+)	(+)	−

+ = positive
− = negative
(−) (+) = occasional exception
V = variable
SXT = sulfamethoxazole-trimethoprim

achieved in a chemostat (steady-state culture) in a complete synthetic medium.

All streptococci ferment glucose, maltose, and most of them ferment lactose and sucrose. They all give a negative catalase reaction. They all lack cytochrome systems and are thus resistant to azide, which facilitates their isolation. The major end product of fermentation is lactic acid. A most important characteristic of certain viridan streptococci (normal flora of the oral cavity) is the synthesis of polysaccharides from sucrose (dextrans) and fructose (levans). The mucoid appearance of streptococcal colonies grown on 5 per cent sucrose is used to classify these streptococci (Table 2). Certain streptococci liquefy gelatin and about half of the *S. pyogenes* strains hydrolyze casein.

Cell Wall Structure. The rigid cell of streptococci has several layers of a linear polymer that is composed of *N*-acetylglucosamine-*N*-acetylmuramic acid (the peptidoglycan, PPG) held together by peptide bridges (Wannamaker and Matsen, 1972) and forming a three-dimensional lattice. The PPG accounts for about 40 to 80 per cent of the wall. In most β-hemolytic strains the PPG is attached covalently to a surface polysaccharide, the C carbohydrate. The streptococcus cell wall is extremely resistant to degradation by lysosomal enzymes of mammalian leukocytes (Ginsburg, 1979). The peptidoglycan is an attachment site for bacteriocins and bacteriophages, which may change genetic and biochemical properties of streptococci (see section on streptococcal bacteriocins).

Many strains of hemolytic streptococci produce a prominent capsule in young cultures that is composed of hyaluronic acid in Group A streptococci. It is not immunogenic and is susceptible to streptococcal hyaluronidase.

Streptococci also possess characteristic surface polymers known as teichoic (TA) and teichuronic acids. These acids contain polyglycerol phosphate and alanine and are covalently linked to the PPG. Certain strains belonging to Lancefield's groups A, B, C, D, and G possess receptors for serum proteins, i.e., albumin, fibrinogen, IgG, IgA, and beta-2 microglobulin. The streptococcus receptor that binds IgG is a protein rich in aspartic acid, glutamic acid, lysine, and alanine. The receptor for IgG interacts via the Fc portion, possibly with the CH2 domain. It is heat labile and trypsin sensitive and can be visualized by immunoelectron microscopic analysis. It is probably responsible for agglutination of streptococci by nonimmune sera and may be a virulence factor. IgG attached to streptococcal Fc

Table 2. DISTINGUISHING FEATURE AMONG MEMBERS OF VIRIDANS GROUP OF STREPTOCOCCI

Species	Lancefield Group Antigens	Levan (L) or Dextran (D) from Sucrose	Fermentation of: *Inulin*	*Raffinose*	*Salicin*	*Lactose*	*Trehalose*	*Mannitol*	Hydrolysis of: Hippurate	Esculin	Arginine
S. sanguis	H	(+) (D)	+	±	+	(+)	(+)	0	0	±	±
S. salivarius	K (?)	(+) (L)	+	+	+	±	±	0	0	(+)	0
S. mitis	O (?), M (?)	∓ (D)	0	0	±	+	∓	0	0	0	∓
*S. milleri**	A, C, F, G,	0	0	∓	+	+	(+)	0	0	(+)	(+)
S. anginosus-constellatus	F, G, L.	0	0	∓	+	0	+	0	0	±	∓
S. mutans	none	+ (D)	+	±	+	+	+	+	0	(+)	0

*Includes S. MG-intermedius and minute strains of A, C, and G.
+ = always
± = usually +
∓ = rarely +
0 = never
? = questionable
(+) = occasional exception

receptors may induce anti-IgG antibodies, which may then interact with tissues via their IgG content (Holm and Christensen, 1982).

The triple layered cytoplasmic membrane (75 to 90 Å) is composed of lipoprotein that differs in structure and content from that of L-forms and has at least 29 different antigens, of which eight are exposed on the outer surface of the membrane and 11 are on the inner membrane or unexposed. The cell membrane is attached by hydrophobic interaction with the glycolipid moiety of lipoteichoic acid (LTA). LTA consists of chains of polyglycerol phosphate units that may contain sugar or amino sugar substituents covalently linked to a glycolipid. The LTA extends through the width of the wall and is intertwined with the M-protein in surface fimbria, held together by ionic interaction. The LTA is haptenic when extracted from the streptococci by phenol, but is highly immunogenic when bound to the streptococcal cells. Although only a fraction of the LTA is spontaneously released into the medium during growth, the bulk of LTA may be released by phenol, lysozyme, extracts of human leukocytes, a variety of cationic polyelectrolytes, and by penicillin treatment. Although LTA's function is not fully known, it is possible that it is involved in the attachment of the streptococci to cell surfaces. LTA may serve as a carrier of various streptococcal antigens and bind them to the membranes of host cells. LTA may also regulate the autolytic wall enzymes thought to function in cell division and cell wall lysis. Penicillin causes lysis of streptococcal cells by removing LTA. LTA of all streptococci cross-react immunologically among themselves and with LTA of other gram-positive bacteria.

The cytoplasm of streptococci contains proteins (including enzymes) and nucleic acids. A high degree of antigenic heterogeneity is a particular characteristic of the nucleoprotein fraction.

ANTIGENIC COMPOSITION

Group-Specific Carbohydrate. Rebecca Lancefield laid the ground for the serologic classification of streptococci into at least 18 groups (A-R) on the basis of the group-specific carbohydrate, the "C carbohydrate." Groups A, B, and C "C carbohydrates" are composed of branched polymers. The carbohydrate is covalently linked to the PPG. They can be extracted with either hot formamide, hot TCA, autoclaving, or enzymatic digestion with lysozyme and *Streptomyces albus* enzymes. The carbohydrate probably protects the peptidoglycan against lysozyme. It accounts for approximately 30 to 50 per cent of the dry weight of the cell wall and about 10 per cent of the intact cell, and may be found on both sides of the PPG. The polysaccharide of group A streptococci, which is composed of a terminal *N*-acetyl glucosamine (NAGA) and rhamnose, may be cleaved by *N*-acetylglucosaminidase of human macrophages. Upon cleavage of the terminal NAGA, a structure known as the A-variant antigen is left; rhamnose is the antigenic determinant. Certain rabbits develop antibodies of restricted heterogeneity after immunization with C polysaccharide. Like myeloma proteins, these antibodies also show selectivity of expression of allotypic specificity on both the heavy and light chains. The discovery of this response, which may be genetically determined, has opened new horizons in immunogenetics and approaches to host genetics of streptococcal infections and their sequelae (see below) (Eichman et al., 1971).

The group-specific antigen of Group D streptococci is a teichoic acid, not a carbohydrate, and it is a component of the cytoplasmic membrane, not of the cell wall.

Type-Specific M-Proteins. These are almost exclusively found in group A streptococci. M-proteins are surface antigens (Fox, 1974). They are responsible for the virulence of group A streptococci by virtue of their unique antiphagocytic characteristic; when lost, virulence is lost. The large M-protein complex contains hair-like structures (fimbria or pili) on the cell wall that are probably attached to it by covalent bonds. As protein antigens, they confer type specificity upon Group A streptococci; about 80 types are known. M-protein has been released from the streptococci by extraction with HCl, sonic oscillation, pepsin digestion, phage lysis, extraction with guanidine, and by nonionic detergents. The M-protein molecule has been purified. It is a heat- and acid-stable protein, soluble in alcohol, has a molecular weight of 40,000, and an isoelectric point of 5.3. It possesses multiple subunits, all having identical serologic activity. M-protein is susceptible to proteases, including streptococcal proteinase, which can prevent typing by digesting this antigen. The conformation and molecular dimensions of the M protein show close structural relationship to tropomyosin. It exists as a stable dimer and contains about 70 per cent alpha helix. Each fiber on the cell wall consists of a single M protein molecule made of two chains in a coiled structure (see also section on Vaccination).

Until recently, all preparations of M-protein were contaminated with non-type-specific polypeptides. These strongly associated proteins give rise to non-type-specific antibodies and also elicit local and systemic hypersensitivity reactions. Beachey and his colleagues have separated M-protein from these contaminants and their preparation is both immunogenic and nontoxic.

T Antigen. In addition to the type-specific M-protein, group A streptococci possess another set of protein antigens known as the T-system. The T-protein can be isolated by peptic, tryptic, or pancreatic digestion of heat-killed streptococci. It is protease-resistant, insoluble in alcohol, antigenic in the cell, and antigenic when cell free. It is not related to virulence, and antibodies against it are not protective. Some T-antigens are restricted to a single M-type whereas others may be shared by several M-types. The T-system is employed for typing those group A strains that either fail to synthesize M-protein or to which no anti-M-type serum is available (see *Laboratory Diagnosis*).

R Antigen. Certain types of group A streptococci possess R antigens that can also be found among groups B, C, G, and L streptococci. The antigen is a nonprotective protein that cross-reacts with grouping and typing antisera that contain antibodies to the R protein. This antigen is not commonly employed for classification and its biologic significance is still not known.

Group A Streptococci

PATHOGENETIC PROPERTIES. The most prominent pathogen for humans is *Streptococcus pyogenes* belonging to Lancefield's groups A and C (see also *Infections by Other Streptococci*). Pyogenic streptococci (Groups A and C) produce large amounts of extracellular products during growth in vitro in defined media or in human tissues. At least 25 different antigens are detected in concentrated culture supernatants by immunoelectrophoresis with pooled human γ-globulin or rabbit sera hyperimmune to streptococcal extracellular products (Ginsburg, 1972). Only a few of these products have been identified, and a small number purified. Of the numerous factors elaborated by the group A streptococcus, few have been implicated in the pathogenesis of tissue damage in animal models.

The major virulence factor of group A streptococci is the type-specific M-protein that deters phagocytosis. M-proteins, along with LTA, are a prominent component of fimbriae, the structures responsible for adherence of streptococci to pharyngeal and tonsillar epithelium. LTA adheres to cellular attachment sites composed of a lipid-binding region on fibronectin. Whether the hyaluronic acid capsule also has significant antiphagocytic activity in natural infections is less certain. (See below.)

Extracellular Toxins. Streptococcal infection is probably facilitated by extracellular products, some of which are cytopathic (Ginsburg, 1972; Alouf, 1980).

Streptolysins. The majority of group A, C, and G streptococci elaborate two distinct hemolysins called streptolysins O and S. The hemolytic zones around streptococcal colonies on blood agar, under aerobic conditions, are primarily due to streptolysin S (SLS). Both hemolysins are cytopathic for mammalian cells and block phagocytosis, presumably by impairing both chemotaxis and ingestion by leukocytes and disrupting their lysosomes. (Ginsburg, 1972; Alouf, 1980).

Streptolysin O (SLO). This oxygen-labile protein antigen has a molecular weight of approximately 70,000. It is synthesized only by growing streptococci. It possesses a labile SH-group and is hemolytic or cytolytic only under reducing conditions. Its activity is strongly inhibited by cholesterol and other sterols. SLO is also cardiotoxic. The observation that rheumatic fever is not associated with infection of the skin due to group A streptococci suggests that cholesterol in the epidermis may inhibit a toxic effect of SLO that is involved in the development of rheumatic fever. It may cause interstitial myocarditis in experimental animals and systolic arrest of perfused mammalian hearts, probably caused by inducing the release from atria of acetylcholine and irreversibly damaging the A-V conducting system (Alouf, 1980).

Streptolysin S (SLS). This oxygen-stable nonantigenic peptide with a molecular weight of approximately 2800 is synthesized by both growing and resting cells and is found on the surface of washed streptococcal cells as a cell-bound hemolysin. The extracellular SLS is a loosely bound peptide formed from a precursor that is tightly bound to the streptococcus membrane and can be activated by sonication. The loosely bound peptide can be released into the surrounding medium by a variety of carrier molecules such as serum albumin, α-lipoproteins, yeast RNA, nonionic detergents (tweens and tritons) and especially LTA, which may be the physiological carrier of SLS. Upon release by the carriers, the hemolysin becomes recognized as SLS. Extracellular SLS is thus a complex between a carrier molecule and a hemolytic peptide. The peptide can be transferred among the various carriers and finally to the surface of mammalian cells. Studies with liposomes composed of various phospholipids showed that the fluidity of the phospholipid hydrocarbon chain in the membrane is important for SLS to function as a lytic agent. After the interaction with membrane phospholipids the hemolytic peptide is inactivated. SLS activity is strongly inhibited by lecithin and β-lipoproteins but not by cholesterol. RBCs treated with SLO show distinct "lesions" similar to those caused by complement; no such lesions have been shown to be induced by SLS. Upon intravenous injection, SLS causes necrosis of liver and kidney tubules and massive intravascular hemolysis. It can induce a chronic arthritis when injected intra-articularly (Ginsburg 1972).

Erythrogenic Toxin. Most group A streptococci produce one (or more) of three immunologically distinct erythrogenic toxins known today as Streptococcal Pyrogenic Exotoxins, which were first described by the Dicks. In addition to causing fever and rash, SPE enhances susceptibility to lethal endotoxin shock, injures macrophages, alters antibody response to red blood cells, is mitogenic for lymphocytes, and alters the blood-brain barrier permeability. SPEs also enhance skin reactivity to themselves or other antigens in a sensitized host. SPE has been purified and crystallized from culture supernatant fluid of certain streptococcal strains. It has 1×10^7 rabbit skin doses per mg N and a molecular weight of approximately 29,000. It contains 80 per cent protein and hyaluronic acid; the latter probably acts as a carrier and is not associated with toxicity. The symptoms of scarlet fever are believed due to both the primary toxicity of SPE and the secondary effects of hypersensitivity; the typical scarlatinal rash is due to the latter. The role, if any, played by SPE in the pathogenesis of streptococcal infections and their sequelae is not established. SPE is probably produced under the direction of a temperate phage (Wannamaker, 1981; Bloomster and Watson, 1982).

Proteinase. Most group A streptococci elaborate an SH-dependent proteinase precursor (M.W. = 44,000), which can be converted to an active proteinase by reducing agents and by proteases. Proteinase paradoxically destroys M-protein. This protease acts on several naturally-occurring proteins as well as on some synthetic substrates. The intravenous injection of reduced proteinase causes massive myocardial and skeletal muscle necrosis in rabbits and release of chondroitin 4,6 sulfate-protein complexes into the circulation resulting from proteolysis of cartilage and ground substance. It is immunogenic and the specific antibodies that develop neutralize the proteolytic activity of this enzyme. Its role in the pathogenesis of streptococcal infections is not known.

Streptokinase (SK). Most group A and C strains produce SK, an activator of the fibrinolytic system of human blood. SK is a protein with a molecular weight of approximately 47,000. It converts a proactivator present in plasma to an activator, which converts plasminogen to the proteolytic enzyme, plasmin. Plasmin splits fibrinogen, fibrin, and other proteins. SK may be a virulence factor of streptococci by lysing blood clots and fibrin precipitates which facilitates bacterial spreading. Preparations of SK derived from group C streptococci have been widely employed for debriding surface infections, for enhancement of wound healing, for treatment of fibrinous exudates, and for the lysis of intravascular thrombi.

The Spreading Factors. Several extracellular products of streptococci are regarded as "spreading factors" because they promote spread of streptococci in tissues by liquefying and reducing the viscosity of inflammatory exudates. Group A strains elaborate hyaluronidase, four serologic varieties of deoxyribonucleases (A, B, C, and D), and a ribonuclease. All these enzymes are immunogenic (see *Laboratory Diagnosis*).

Nicotinamide Adenine Dinucleotide Glycohydrolase (NADG). Some strains belonging to groups A, C, and G elaborate NADG. At one time this enzyme was thought to be associated with leukotoxicity of streptococci, presumably because of its ability to affect leukocyte metabolism. Now it is believed that leukotoxicity is due to cell-bound SLS. The role of NADG in pathogenicity of streptococci is not known. Production of NADG by streptococci is sometimes used in serologic differentiation of certain strains (see *Laboratory Diagnosis*).

Opacity Factor (OF). Certain group A strains opacify horse serum through the action of a highly immunogenic lipoproteinase. Conflicting reports have been made on whether OF and M protein are physicochemically linked or genetically related. There is also circumstantial evidence that the OF and M protein antigen are plasmid borne. The role played by OF in the pathogenesis of streptococcal infections is not known.

Cardiohepatic Toxin (CHT). Supernatant fluids of group A streptococci grown in a chemostat contain an undefined low molecular weight toxin(s) that cause extensive myocardial, diaphragmatic, and hepatic lesions in rabbits. The role, if any, of this toxic agent in the pathogenesis of streptococcal infections is not known.

Cell-Associated Toxic Agents

M Protein. Purified M protein precipitates fibrinogen and interacts with fibrin lysates and fibrinomonomer complexes. It clumps platelets and leukocytes, lyses PMN leukocytes, and inhibits the migration of leukocytes in capillary tubes. It is highly immunogenic and complexes of M protein and immunoglobulins localize in the glomeruli in glomerulonephritis (see below). M protein impairs complement activation via the alternative pathway and the concomitant binding of C3b to the bacterial walls. Streptococci that lose their M protein can still attach to PMN leukocytes by fibronectin, which serves as an adhesin and may thus function as a nonspecific opsonin.

Peptidoglycan-Polysaccharide Complexes (PPGPS). Although streptococci are readily killed after phagocytosis by PMNs and macrophages, intracellular digestion of their cell walls is extremely slow, either because C polysaccharride and teichoic acid shield them from lysozyme or cross-linking and *O*-acetylation of the peptidoglycan prevents its degradation (Ginsburg, 1979). Cell wall components of streptococci persist within macrophages in inflammatory sites in experimental animal models for very long periods. Such laden macrophages secrete large amounts of lysosomal enzymes capable of destroying connective tissue (Davies et al., 1974; Ginsburg, 1979). Macrophages laden with undegraded streptococcal cell walls are translocated from one tissue site to another, which may explain the dissemination of granulomatous lesions (Ginsburg, 1979). It has been proposed that post streptococcal sequelae (rheumatic fever) are associated with localization and persistence of undegraded wall components (Ginsburg, 1979).

Biologic Properties of Peptidoglycans (PPG). Isolated and partially purified PPG can cause the following: fever, the localized Shwartzman reaction, nonspecific resistance to infections, enhancement of lesions induced by pyogenic bacteria, enhanced immunologic response to other antigens (adjuvant effect), inhibition of macrophage migration, tumor inhibition, impaired phagocytosis by PMN, activation of complement, and lysis of platelets. Undegraded complexes of PPG and other polysaccharide moieties have induced granulomatous inflammation in the skin, heart, joints, and liver of laboratory animals. It appears that the size of the PPG molecule and its association with the naturally occurring polysaccharide moiety of the cell wall is of utmost importance for the expression of toxicity, immunogenicity, and persistence in tissues. The probability that different individuals may degrade streptococcal cell walls to different entities may explain the enigma that poststreptococcal sequelae affect only certain patients (see below).

Lipoteichoic Acid (LTA). This membrane-associated haptene is probably the major surface component of streptococci responsible for surface hydrophobicity. It may be responsible for the attachment of streptococci to mammalian cells. It sensitizes a variety of mammalian cells to agglutination and lysis by antibodies and complement (passive immune lysis). LTA can cause arthritis after intra-articular injection in preimmunized rabbits. It can cause resorption of bone (via cyclic AMP and prostaglandins) in culture and nephrocalcinosis in laboratory animals. It releases lysosomal enzymes from macrophages and may also regulate the autolytic wall enzymes in a bacteria. The binding sites for LTA on mammalian cells may be associated with fibronectin (Ginsburg, 1979; Beachey, 1981).

Streptococcal Plasmids and Bacteriophages. Plasmids may be important in genetic changes of streptococci that affect their ecological, taxonomic, and pathogenetic status. Plasmids have been isolated from nearly every species of streptococci examined and those that mediate resistance to macrolide antibiotics have been the most thoroughly investigated extrachromosomal elements found in streptococci. A plasmid originating in one streptococcus species can be transferred to and maintained by a heterologous species. Resistance to macrolides can be transferred with high efficiency by temperate phages obtained by UV light induction of a naturally resistant strain. Multiple antibiotic resistance in *S. faecalis* is also plasmid borne. Streptococcal bacteriophages have been examined for their role in toxigenicity (production of SPE), resistance to phagocytosis (Wannamaker, 1981), and production of M-protein. Both M-protein and the closely linked serum opacity factor (OF) have been transduced.

The recent findings that group A and C streptococci possess a potent phage-associated cell wall lysin may shed light on the autolysis of group A streptococci. This phage-associated lysin may function as a muramidase to cleave streptococcal peptidoglycans that are extremely resistant to lysozyme. Peptidoglycan may be the main streptococcal component to persist in macrophages and to induce chronic inflammatory lesions (see above).

Streptocins. These bacteriocins are low molecular weight antibiotics produced by almost all species of streptococci. Streptococcal bacteriocins kill other species of streptococci and other gram-positive bacteria but not gram negatives. They inhibit DNA, RNA, and protein synthesis and block uptake and incorporation of glucose. The determinant of streptocin A can be transduced to group A strains of different types. The role played by bacteriocins in the ecology and pathogenicity of streptococci is not clear but some evidence indicates that they help regulate the normal streptococcal flora of the oropharynx and exclude pathogens such as *S. pneumoniae* (Johanson et al., 1970).

SEQUELAE OF ACUTE STREPTOCOCCAL INFECTIONS.

A unique characteristic of group A streptococci is their ability to induce nonsuppurative sequelae in susceptible individuals. These are rheumatic fever (RF), chorea, and acute glomerulonephritis (AGN). They may follow overt or inapparent infections. The onset of these complications may be two to three weeks after infection. The common denominator among these diverse late complications of group A streptococcal infections is the failure to isolate living streptococci or their products from the affected tissue. The failure to duplicate these sequelae in lower animals has hampered research into the pathogenesis of these syndromes. Our present concepts are based on circumstantial evidence and no mechanism can be considered proved or accepted by most investigators in this field.

There are several absolute requirements for the development of rheumatic carditis and arthritis. First, group A streptococci must have been present; second, the infection must have been localized in the upper respiratory tract; third, a streptococcal antibody response, often exaggerated, must occur.

The importance of the site of infection for the development of RF has been stressed; many observations suggest that RF does not develop after streptococcal infection of the skin. The factors that localize streptococci to the throat are not fully understood, but LTA is implicated in anchoring streptococci to the surface of epithelial cells.

Current Theories of Pathogenesis. The numerous theories proposed to explain how group A streptococci initiate sequelae fall under several headings: (a) the "rheumatic" toxin; (b) autoimmunity and immunopathology; (c) genetic and anatomic aberrations; (d) a combination of these theories.

Is There a "Rheumatic Toxin"? Several extracellular substances elaborated by group A streptococci can induce myocardial, endocardial, hepatic, articular, and renal lesions in laboratory animals (see above). As a rule, none of the lesions fully resemble the human lesions of RF, and no clinical manifestations similar to those seen in humans have been duplicated in the animals. Undegraded peptidoglycan-polysaccharide complexes (PPGPS) of the cell wall have produced rheumatic-like granulomatous lesions in mice and rabbits. Another approach suggests that in early streptococcal pharyngitis certain susceptible patients develop acute myocardial and articular injuries explainable by diffusible "toxins." None of the "toxic" theories have been based on firm ground and all data have been obtained from experimental models (Ginsburg, 1972; Glynn, 1975; Ginsburg, 1979; Wannamaker, 1981; Unny and Middlebrooks, 1983).

Immunopathology, Autoimmunity. Several investigations have proposed that complexes formed between streptococcal products and autologous antibodies (for example, SLO–anti-SLO complexes) may localize in tissues and damage them by activating complement (serum sickness type), or through cell-mediated immunity (CMI). Sensitized T lymphocytes may then interact with streptococcal antigens to cause the release of lymphokines.

The theory of autoimmunity gained favor because substances in mammalian cardiac tissue can act as autoantigens and because certain streptococcal toxins can release such antigens. However, the theories implicating autoimmunity in RF have been stated only in general terms, with no focus on precise mechanisms, and have been overshadowed by theories implicating immunologic cross-reaction between streptocococcal antigens and components of mammalian tissues.

The phenomenon of crossed immunity between mammalian and bacterial constituents (the concept of molecular mimicry) is well established (Kaplan, 1976; Zabriskie, 1976; Wannamaker, 1981; Unny and Middlebrooks, 1983). Several antigens in group A streptococcal cell walls and protoplast membranes have been isolated. These cross-react with glycoproteins of the heart valves, sarcolemma of cardiac and skeletal muscle, bundle of His, synovial fluids, glycoprotein of glomerular basement membrane, human fibroblasts, endothelial cells, astrocytes, cytoplasm of subthalamic and caudate nuclei, and histocompatibility antigens (Kaplan, 1976; Zabriskie, 1976). Despite the presence in human sera of cross-reactive antibodies and their elution from myocardium of patients with RF, there is no evidence that such antibodies have any relationship to the lesions of rheumatic fever. It is interesting that no bound cross-reactive globulin is found in Aschoff bodies. There is no evidence that the cross-reactive antibodies are cytotoxic to mammalian cells. The heart-reactive antibodies that are adsorbable with streptococcal membranes do appear to be useful diagnostically, however, because such antibodies tend to persist in rheumatic patients (Wannamaker, 1981).

Genetic and Anatomic Aberrations. Despite speculations about genetic factors in rheumatic fever, no clear-cut genetic patterns have been detected. Also, no consistent association with specific HLA antigen has been found. Many observations, however, have shown that rheumatic fever patients tend to develop exaggerated humoral and cellular responses to various streptococcal antigens but not to non-streptococcal antigens. On the other hand, rheumatic patients may have fewer histocompatibility antigens than normal controls. A possible linkage to Ir genes could bring on less response to certain streptococcal antigens so that streptococci survive longer and elaborate more toxins. None of these observations have explained the pathogenesis of rheumatic fever (see Wannamaker, 1981). Another line of thought would suggest that the "rheumatic patient" may possess direct anatomical routes (probably lymphatic channels) that connect the tonsils with the heart through which streptococci and some of their extracellular toxins and undegraded cell wall components migrate and damage the heart (Wannamaker, 1973; Wannamaker, 1981; Unny and Middlebrooks, 1983).

Migratory arthritis is part of the rheumatic syndrome. The similarity of the tissue alterations in the joints of rheumatic patients to those induced experimentally by anaphylactic and delayed hypersensitivity reactions suggest that the human joint disease may be caused by such mechanisms. As a rule, neither viable streptococci nor their extracellular or cellular constituents are found within the inflamed joints. A decrease in both early and late components of complement within the synovial fluid of RF patients suggests local activation by immune complexes. Although the streptococcus antigen that could be present in these complexes has not been identified, this phenomenon may point to the mechanism of arthritis in rheumatic fever. Arthritic lesions can be induced in laboratory animals by the intra-articular injection of Streptolysin S, by a pool of extracellular products, by soluble cell wall components, by L-forms, and by lipoteichoic acid (LTA) (Ginsburg et al., 1977; Ginsburg, 1979).

Acute Glomerulonephritis (AGN). One of the most common complications of upper respiratory and skin infections with group A streptococci is AGN. It is an old observation that acute RF and AGN rarely, if ever, occur in the same person at the same time (Stollerman, 1975). AGN is probably caused by special nephritogenic strains. The pharyngeal M-types 12, 14, and 49 and a family of "impetigo" streptococcal strains belonging to the following serologic complexes: T-3/13/B3264/12 (related to the M serotypes (22, 33, 39, 41, 43, 52, 56); T8/25/Imp19(M-types 2, 8, 25, 55, 57, 58); and T5/11/12/27/44 (M-types 11, 59, 61) are all associated with AGN. The latter pyoderma strains were previously unrecognized owing to lack of specific antisera for typing them. The factors elaborated by these skin strains, which endow them with nephritogenicity, is not understood. Furthermore, in spite of the detailed serologic, epidemiologic, and renal morphologic studies, the pathogenesis of nephritis remains unknown. The theories regarding pathogenesis of AGN can be summarized under four main headings and are based primarily on experimental models (Ginsburg, 1972; Wannamaker, 1981; Holm and Christensen, 1982).

The Nephrotoxin. Streptolysin S, M-protein, autolysates of nephritogenic streptococci, extracts of streptococcal cell walls, solubilized protoplast membranes, and undefined diffusible agents released by certain nephritogenic streptococci (nephrotoxin) can cause renal disease in laboratory animals but not the full spectrum of clinical and pathologic changes seen in humans.

Immunologic Cross-Reactivity. Cross-reactive antigens between soluble components of glomerular basement membranes are chemically and immunologically similar to antigens of protoplast membranes of nephritogenic streptococci. Antibodies to protoplast membranes can cause glomerular lesions.

Autoantibody. Extracts of kidneys that had been mixed with streptococci were claimed to give rise to nephrotoxic antibodies. Although this theory was favored by several investigators, the results were controversial and could not be duplicated in several other laboratories.

Immune Complex Disease. Immunofluorescent and electron microscopic analysis of kidneys obtained from patients with AGN showed localized immune complexes and complement in the glomeruli. The nature of the antigenic substance in these complexes and its possible relationship to streptococci is still controversial. Recently, a new antigen called endostreptosin was isolated from the plasma membrane of nephritogenic streptococci and implicated as the antigen involved in the pathogenesis of AGN. Antibodies to this antigen react with renal biopsies of patients with glomerulonephritis but only within the first days of the disease (Holm and Christensen, 1982). It has also been suggested that immune complexes can be obtained when streptococcal enzymes modify the chemical composition of IgG; the altered IgG then interacts with autoantibodies that recognize both native and altered globulin. Such complexes can cause glomerular lesions.

Despite the numerous models established, none are satisfactory analogs to the human disease (Wannamaker and Matsen, 1972; Wannamaker, 1981).

IMMUNITY. Infections with group A streptococci that possess M-antigen are usually followed by a type-specific humoral immunity. If the anti-M antibodies disappear, they can be recalled by small booster doses of homologous M antigen. The anti-M antibodies are mainly IgG. They appear slowly (over 30 to 60 days) and are opsonins (Stollerman, 1975). None of the antibodies that are regularly produced against C-polysaccharide, T antigen, teichoic acid, or the numerous extracellular enzymes and other factors can prevent infection. Type-specific antibody can be detected by opsonization, mouse protection, or chain elongation in vitro. These tests are difficult to perform in a routine bacteriologic laboratory.

LABORATORY DIAGNOSIS

Tests for Streptococcal Antibodies. Antibodies against streptolysin O, streptokinase, hyaluronidase, DNase-B, proteinase, and NADG are measured to diagnose recent streptococcal infections. Proof of a streptococcal infection is based, in part, upon an increase in one or more of these antibodies. Although antistreptolysin O (ASO) titration in patients' sera is the most common test, it is often advantageous to measure other antistreptococcal antibodies. The streptozyme test is a two-minute slide hemagglutination procedure that quantitatively measures multiple antibody (A-STZ) to streptococcal extracellular products. The reagents are sheep RBC sensitized simultaneously with streptolysin-O, deoxyribonuclease-B, hyaluronidase, streptokinase, and NADG. A-STZ correlates well with ASO in the sera of rheumatic fever patients. Moreover, the A-STZ test detects a higher incidence of elevated antistreptococcal antibodies than does one ASO test. The specificity of the test (no antibodies to cellular elements of streptococci are detected with this reagent), its high reproducibility, the ease of performance, and the minimal quantities of patient serum required indicate that the test helps estimate antibody response to streptococcal infection whenever the performance of a battery of tests for individual antibodies is impractical and expensive (Fernandez et al., 1983).

Culture of Group A Streptococci. Specimens must be transported to the laboratory without delay, because cotton swabs may contain substances that inhibit group A streptococci. Viability is well maintained in swabs transported in a silica-gel. Use of enrichment media (for example, Pike's broth) increases the isolation rate of group A streptococci compared with direct plating on blood agar. The growth on blood agar is screened for complete (β) hemolysis. Sheep blood is preferred because it inhibits the growth of *Hemophilus hemolyticus*, a β-hemolytic saprophyte commonly found in the throat. Overgrowth of other microorganisms can be prevented by various selective agents in the media. Group A streptococci can be tentatively identified, rapidly and easily, with bacitracin disks. About 90 per cent of group A streptococci are inhibited by disks containing 0.04 unit of bacitracin, whereas most group B, C, and G streptococci are resistant. Definitive identification is made by demonstrating the C carbohydrate of group A by immunofluorescence with group-specific antiserum, or by precipitin tests with C carbohydrate extracted from the bacteria, or by agglutination of latex beads or fixed *S. aureus* that are coated with specific antibody (co-agglutination).

Rapid Methods. Several rapid (<1 hour) tests have been developed for detection of Group A streptococci in pharyngeal exudates. These tests are based either on immunologic detection of the C carbohydrate from material extracted directly from swabs or on the detection of the enzyme pyrrolidonylaminopeptidase in the exudate. This enzyme is specific for *S. pyogenes*. These rapid methods are 80 to 95 per cent sensitive when compared with throat cultures and are 100 per cent specific. If culture facilities are not available, these rapid assays are an expensive but acceptable alternative.

DRUG SUSCEPTIBILITY. No group A streptococcus strain has been shown to be resistant to penicillin. This makes penicillin the drug of choice in the treatment of streptococcal infections and in prevention of rheumatic fever. The MIC for penicillin G is usually 0.01 μg/ml, and even lower concentrations are effective in the presence of phagocytes. About 40 per cent of strains are resistant to tetracycline and sulfadiazine. Resistance to erythromycin is uncommon and is mediated by a plasmid. Streptococci are resistant to polymyxins, kanamycin, and streptomycin. All strains are susceptible to cephalosporins and vancomycin.

EPIDEMIOLOGY

Upper Respiratory Infections. Understanding of the pathogenesis of streptococcal infections, their nonsuppurative sequelae, and their epidemiology depends on the distinction between a "carrier" state and acute streptococcal upper respiratory infection. Group A streptococci cultured from acute sore throats contain large amounts of M-protein. Pharyngitis and tonsillitis occur most frequently in children from 5 to 15 years of age. A child is not likely to reach the age of ten without having encountered group A streptococci. However, group A streptococci can be cultured from up to 20 per cent of asymptomatic schoolchildren's throats. Organisms isolated from many carriers do not contain M-protein and probably are not epidemiologically significant.

Transmission occurs via droplets from respiratory secretion of patients or from healthy carriers. Both food and milk may be sources for occasional outbreaks. Organisms recovered from clothing, bed, or house dust are usually noninfective. Control of hemolytic streptococcal disease is difficult because many infections are either exceedingly mild or inapparent, and persons with subclinical infections can disseminate streptococci. Overcrowding allows the explosive spread of single serotypes, especially among civilians.

Peak incidence occurs between December and May in temperate zones.

Pyoderma. Occurrence is usually confined to the summer and early fall in hot and tropical climates. It mostly affects preschool children and infants. Transmission may be aided by insects. Poverty, filth, and overcrowding are major predisposing factors. The same streptococcus type is often found in throats and in pyoderma lesions.

PREVENTION. Infections with group A streptococci may be prevented by therapeutic intervention during epidemics or by prophylactic drugs given to those at high risk, in boarding schools, orphanages, and military camps in which infections are endemic. Impetigo may be prevented by improved skin hygiene. Epidemics are best halted by antibiotic treatment of all cases.

Streptococcal Vaccine. Since the immunity to group A streptococci is type-specific, and since about 80 types are known to be present in different populations, the rationale for preparing an adequate vaccine depends on the distribution of the major M-types in a particular population. Immunization, if available, should aim to prevent both suppurative and nonsuppurative complications. The preparation of a vaccine should also take into consideration the risk of inducing delayed hypersensitivity reactions, the elimination from the M-protein of antigens cross-reactive with heart, and the elimination from M-protein of covalently bound lipoteichoic acid (LTA). Preliminary field trials have used M-protein in alum given either subcutaneously or intrapharyngeally. Seventy-five per cent of the subjects immunized revealed a primary opsonic response to the vaccine with no reactions. Immunization did not prevent colonization of the throat, but protected against clinical illness. Since protective immune responses can be evoked by native and synthetic fragments that present only limited regions of M protein devoid of the regions that cross-react with heart, such fragments can perhaps be employed for vaccination. Furthermore, hybridoma antibodies raised against the homologous type streptococci acted as opsonins and protected mice against challenge infections with the homologous strain (Hasty et al., 1982). The main question is how many serological types warrant inclusion in the safer new vaccine.

OTHER β-HEMOLYTIC STREPTOCOCCI PATHOGENIC FOR HUMANS

Group B Streptococci (*Streptococcus agalactiae*)

Although *S. agalactiae* (group B streptococci) (GBS) has been long recognized as an important bovine pathogen that is transmitted to humans, during the 1970s GBS were clearly identified as an important neonatal pathogen. There are two well recognized forms of the disease: early-onset and late-onset. Early-onset disease occurs within the first few days of life, develops rapidly, and has a high mortality, most often from sepsis and pneumonia. In contrast, late-onset disease occurs in the first month of life, is often insidious, and is commonly associated with meningitis (Patterson et al., 1976; Anthony et al., 1977; Anthony, 1981). Unlike group A streptococci, the GBS grow as gray, flat, relatively large colonies usually surrounded by a zone of β-hemolysis caused by a streptolysin S–like hemolysin. Nonhemolytic variants occur.

ANTIGENIC STRUCTURE. The cell wall of group B streptococci contains as a major constituent, a group-specific carbohydrate composed of rhamnose, *N*-acetylglucosamine and galactose. *L*-rhamnose is the significant component of the antigenic determinant. External to the group substance, the capsular antigens form the major type-specific antigens Ia, Ib, II, and III, which are composed of galactose, glucose, glucosamine, and sialic acid. Type Ic contains the Ia carbohydrate antigen plus a protein antigen. Both human and bovine strains are found in all types, at different frequencies.

Products. In addition to the SLS-like hemolysin, GBS produce a CAMP factor. The CAMP phenomenon is complete hemolysis of sheep RBC resulting from the interaction of a protein exoproduct of GBS with the α-hemolysin of *S. aureus*. It is demonstrated in both hemolytic and nonhemolytic strains. GBS hydrolyze hippuric acid and elaborate a potent extracellular neuraminidase, which may function as a virulence factor.

IMMUNITY. Type-specific antibody confers protection. Studies of sera from postpartum women and infants with type III GBS disease indicate a correlation between inadequate levels of type III-specific antibody and susceptibility to GBS infection. Human immunoglobulins suitable for I.V. administration are opsonic for multiple strains of GBS in vitro and protect animals against experimental infections. Such passively administered IgG could offer protection against GBS to premature infants who are either at high risk of infection or already ill.

Prophylactic Antibiotics. Although treatment of all neonates with penicillin has been recommended, intrapartum penicillin therapy of colonized women appears to reduce vertical transmission of GBS and to prevent both maternal and neonatal disease. There is concern, however, that exposure of all neonates to penicillin might increase neonatal infections with penicillin-resistant pathogens, and possibly increase the incidence of penicillin allergy. Hence, only institutions having a high incidence of early onset of GBS disease might use penicillin (Fischer et al., 1983).

Concentrations of penicillin required to inhibit GBS are very low, but higher than for group A streptococci. Most GBS are also sensitive to erythromycin, clindamycin, and chloramphenicol, but often resistant to tetracyclines.

Group C Streptococci

These comprise three streptococcal species, all of which cause human infections. Of the three, *S. equisimilis* (Table 1) is found most often, frequently in cultures from the pharynx and occasionally in cultures from impetiginous lesions. Whether *S. equisimilis* causes pharyngitis is debatable. Group C streptococci have never been proved to cause acute glomerulonephritis or rheumatic fever. The natural habitat of *S. equi* and *S. zooepidemicus*, which are found primarily in animals, is unknown. Several isolates of each of the strains have been obtained from the sputum, pus, and blood of patients with abscesses and pneumonia. Group C streptococci elaborate numerous extracellular products many of which are similar to those produced by group A strains. The major virulence factor of the group C strains is their hyaluronic acid capsule. Streptokinase-streptodornase (deoxyribonuclease) preparations produced from Group C streptococci are used to dissolve thrombi and to debride fibrinous exudates on skin lesions.

Group G Streptococci

Group G strains may be part of the vaginal flora and may occur normally in the pharynx, in the gastrointestinal tract or on the skin. Serious infections due to group G strains include puerperal and neonatal septicemia, otitis media, pharyngitis, pneumonia and empyema, meningitis, peritonitis, arthritis, and cellulitis. A recent report documented 38 patients suffering from bacteremia with this streptococcus group (Auckenthaler et al., 1983). The most frequently documented portal of entry of group G streptococci is the skin. In addition to the upper respiratory infection, there have been reports of subacute bacterial endocarditis caused by these streptococci. Group G strains also produce extracellular products similar to these elaborated by groups A and C strains.

Group D Streptococci (S. faecalis, S. faecium, S. durans, S. bovis, S. equinus)

The group D antigen is unique among the streptococci in that it is a glycerol teichoic acid containing D-alanine and glucose, is probably located in the region of the wall, and may not be linked through a primary bond with the wall components. The type-specific antigen is a cell-wall carbohydrate that is composed of D-glucose and NAGA, and also contains rhamnose. In order to preserve the type-specific antigens of Group D streptococci, they must be released from the cells not by the routine hot HCl method but by lysozyme or by lytic or autolytic enzymes.

METABOLISM. Carbohydrate metabolism is chiefly homofermentative in all these groups. Glucose is fermented to lactic acid. An oxidative pathway also can be utilized by *S. agalactiae*, which yields lactic acid, acetic acid, acetylmethylcarbenol, and carbon dioxide. A noncytochrome iron-containing chromophore appears to be utilized, and oxygen is the terminal electron receptor in this reaction.

LABORATORY IDENTIFICATION. Non-Group A hemolytic streptococci are usually distinguished from Group A by their resistance to an 0.04 unit bacitracin disk. However, because up to 5 per cent of Group A streptococci are also resistant and a like percentage of other Groups are sensitive, this is not a definitive test. β-Hemolytic streptococci are identified with specific antibody against the C carbohydrate. It is often difficult to identify the Group D strains serologically and they are identified by their hydrolysis of esculin in the presence of 40 per cent bile (Table 1). Group D streptococci are divided into enterococci (including *S. faecalis, S. faecium, S. zymogenes*) and nonenterococcal species (*S. bovis, S. equinis*). This distinction, which is based on the ability of enterococci to grow in hypertonic salt media, has therapeutic implications. Thus, *S. bovis*, which cannot grow in 6.5 per cent NaCl, is sensitive to penicillin and *S. bovis* endocarditis can be cured with penicillin. On the other hand, *S. faecalis* grows in 6.5 per cent NaCl, is resistant to penicillin and *S. faecalis* endocarditis requires an aminoglycoside plus penicillin for cure. Group B strains hydrolyze hippurate and produce a soluble hemolysin that acts synergistically with the α-hemolysin of *Staphylococcus aureus* (CAMP phenomenon).

DRUG SUSCEPTIBILITY. β-Hemolytic streptococci, other than Group D, are uniformly susceptible to less than 1.0 unit/ml of penicillin G. Ninety per cent are also susceptible to erythromycin and clindamycin, but up to 50 per cent of recently isolated strains of Group B are resistant to tetracycline. Nonenterococcal Group D streptococci are also susceptible to penicillin, but enterococci are much less so. Enterococci are somewhat more susceptible to ampicillin than to penicillin G and show variable susceptibilities to chloramphenicol, tetracycline, and erythromycin. They are susceptible to vancomycin. Synergism between penicillin and aminoglycoside antibiotics is important in the treatment of enterococcal endocarditis. The combination is bactericidal in concentrations of each drug that are only one tenth that required to kill the enterococcus when either acts alone. An exception is *S. faecium*, which is resistant to killing by the combination of penicillin and aminoglycosides.

EPIDEMIOLOGY. Groups B, C, and G streptococci are often isolated from the nasopharynx. Group D predominates in the gastrointestinal tract, but as many as 30 per cent of normal people have Group B streptococci in their feces. Group B streptococci can also be isolated from the genital tract of 30 per cent of normal women. Neonatal colonization with Group B streptococci is common, but the risk of disease is probably less than 5 per cent. Serotype III Group B streptococci are often acquired by infants in the nursery as well as in utero or at delivery. These bacteria may spread from infant to infant or from nurses to infants, because many nurses may be colonized.

The Viridans Group

The most important and numerous streptococci in the human mouth belong to the viridans group. They are subdivided into the species *S. salivarius*, *S. mitis*, *(S. mitior)*, *S. sanguis*, *S. mutans*, and *S. milleri* (Table 2). Each of these species is serologically heterogeneous and has characteristic physiological properties that make its identification and classification possible. When grown on blood agar most strains are α-hemolytic, i.e., cause partial destruction of red cells about the colony with a green discoloration. Most oral streptococci establish themselves in the human mouth within the first few months of life (Gehring, 1981). About 50 per cent of bacterial endocarditis is caused by these bacteria.

Viridans streptococci usually form a narrow zone of α-hemolysis around their pinhead colonies. No exotoxins or hydrolytic enzymes similar to those produced by pyogenic streptococci are found in culture supernatants. Several of the streptococci elaborate a constitutive extracellular glycosyltransferase and a fructosyltransferase responsible for the synthesis from sucrose of large capsules of dextran and levan respectively. Certain of the streptococci also accumulate intracellular polysaccharides of the amylopectin type, which may play an important role in the initiation of dental caries (Tanzer, 1976).

Their cell wall structure is essentially that of the pyogenic streptococci. They possess peptidoglycan, wall teichoic acid, and membrane-associated lipoteichoic acid.

METABOLISM. Viridans streptococci resemble pneumococci both culturally and in Gram stains, but unlike pneumococci they have no well-developed autolytic systems and are not lysed by bile salts. The viridans streptococci are fastidious and grow luxuriantly only in heart infusion broth or in media rich in protein. They are microaerophilic and acidophilic, and the major product of fermentation is lactic acid. This heterogenous group can, however, be subdivided by its ability to ferment inulin, raffinose, salicin, lactose, and trehalose, and to release ammonia from arginine (Table 2).

PATHOGENIC PROPERTIES

Dental Caries. Four recognized species, *S. sanguis*, *S. mitis*, *S. salivarius*, and *S. mutans*, are associated with dental caries in humans, rats, and in monkeys. *S. mutans* appears to be the most virulent and is the only species recognized that consistently initiates decay affecting smooth enamel surfaces. This pathogenic potential is probably related to its ability to adhere and accumulate on the surface of the teeth and to form large bacterial plaque deposits. It can synthesize high molecular weight dextrans and other glucans from sucrose but not from other sugars. The extracellular polysaccharides enable them to adhere to surfaces. It has the unique property of aggregating in the presence of very small amounts of high molecular weight dextran, indicating the presence on its surface of specific receptors. Small fragments of dextran prevent plaque formation and tooth decay in laboratory animals presumably by functioning as glycosyl acceptors for dextransucrase, thereby inhibiting synthesis of high molecular weight polymers.

Dental caries may be looked upon as an infectious disease and studies with monoinfected gnotobiotic animals show that *S. mutans* can spread among members of hamster or rat colonies, colonize the mouth, and induce carious lesions in animals fed high sucrose diets. Thus, the unique combination of streptococci, sucrose, and tooth surface are prerequisite for the initiation of caries.

Bacterial Endocarditis. Most strains of viridans streptococci can adhere to and produce infection of previously damaged human heart valves. The chemical nature of the receptors has not been identified.

Brain and Liver Abscesses. One species, *S. milleri*, is being increasingly recognized as a virulent pyogenic organism responsible for many cases of frontal lobe brain abscess (de Louvois, 1978) and liver abscess. It is more readily isolated in the presence of increased CO_2 (capnophilic) and has been erroneously regarded in the past as microaerophilic because of this special gas requirement.

VACCINATION AGAINST DENTAL CARIES. Experiments with a vaccine against dental caries showed that monkeys injected with *S. mutans* developed antibodies that could be detected in gingival fluid. Such antibodies (mostly IgG) seem to be responsible for a substantial decrease in the incidence of fissure caries but had no effect on the incidence of carious lesions on smooth surfaces (Lehner et al., 1976). More recently, three protein antigens have been isolated from *S. mutans* that can replace the whole *S. mutans* vaccine in conferring immunity against dental caries. Protection is associated predominantly with serum and crevicular fluid IgG antibodies. Effective immunization of monkeys with the new protein antigens requires induction of very active T helper cells, which help B cells to produce IgG antibodies (Lehner et al., 1976).

STREPTOCOCCUS PNEUMONIAE (Pneumococcus)

The pneumococcus is a *Streptococcus* that forms α-hemolytic zones on blood agar and readily undergoes spontaneous autolysis. It causes pneumococcal pneumonia, septicemia, otitis media, and meningitis.

MORPHOLOGY. The cell is characteristically ovoid or lanceolate. They are usually arranged in pairs, but chains are also present in infected secretions and in cultures.

Pneumococci grow well on meat infusions supplemented with serum or blood under reducing conditions. Pneumococcal colonies are 1 mm in diameter, raised, smooth, and circular. Type 3 strains grow as larger mucoid colonies. When autolysis occurs, the center of the pneumococcal colony becomes depressed. Growth in the presence of antiserum may yield chains of unencapsulated variants that produce small, granular, rough colonies.

ANTIGENIC STRUCTURE. About 82 pneumococcal types are recognized. Typing is based on variation of the chemical composition of the capsular polysaccharide. Eighty-seven per cent of strains isolated from cases of lobar pneumonia in adults fall into types 12, 14, 15, 17–20, 22, 23, and 33.

The different types of capsular polysaccharides differ serologically and chemically. Thus, the polysaccharide antigen of Type 1 pneumococci contains galacturonic acid, galactose, fucose, and glucosamine; that of type 2 contains rhamnose, glucose, and glucuronic acid; type 3 is a polymer of cellobiuronic acid that consists of alternate residues of glucose and glucuronic acid. The isolated capsular polysaccharides are immunogenic in man and mice, but not in horses or in rabbits unless they are injected with a protein carrier. Human beings injected with 30 to 60 μg of pneumococcal polysaccharide produce antibodies that protect them against pneumonia.

Some capsular surface polysaccharides crossreact immunologically with other α-hemolytic streptococci, with capsular polysaccharides of *Klebsiella* or *Salmonella*, and with blood group substances. The capsule swells when treated with specific antibodies (the Quellung reaction). The cell wall of pneumococci is composed of a peptidoglycan similar in structure to the group A streptococci. In addition, a C-substance reacts with C-reactive protein. The binding site is probably choline, which forms part of the wall teichoic acid. The key role of choline in susceptibility to lysis by bile salts and penicillin is evident when pneumococci are grown in the presence of ethanolamine instead of choline. With ethanolamine they form chains and are no longer solubilized by bile salts nor lysed by penicillin. The choline-containing lipoteichoic acid is a powerful inhibitor of the homologous autolytic enzyme *N*-acetylmuramyl-L-alanine amidase, which is lost from the cell in the presence of penicillin so that autolysis is no longer inhibited. Pneumococci also possess protein antigens similar to the streptococcal M-proteins, but unlike the streptococcus this pneumococcal protein antigen is not associated with virulence.

LABORATORY DIAGNOSIS. *Streptococcus pneumoniae* is bile soluble and inhibited by optochin (ethylhydrocupreine). The nutritional requirements are complex, but they can be grown readily on infusion agars supplemented with 5 per cent blood. About 8 per cent of strains require increased CO_2 for growth during primary isolations. The white mouse is exquisitely sensitive to many pneumococcal types (type 14 is a notable exception) and pneumococci can be isolated from sputum by injecting it intraperitoneally into a mouse. The mouse will eliminate other bacteria but die from pneumococcal septicemia; its heart blood will contain only pneumococci. This is the most sensitive way of isolating the pneumococcus from sputums, but it is rarely necessary if blood agar is inoculated and the growth examined with a dissecting microscope.

Pure cultures are identified as *S. pneumoniae* by capsular swelling. A diagnostic reagent, "Omni-serum," which contains antibodies to all 82 capsular polysaccharides, has been employed for rapid identification (obtained from Statens Serum Institut, Copenhagen, Denmark). This serum can also be used to identify by counterimmunoelectrophoresis (CIE) capsular polysaccharide in the blood and urine of patients with pneumonia and the cerebrospinal fluid (CSF) of patients with meningitis. The CIE technique gives rapid diagnosis and can identify pneumococcal infection even in patients whose CSF has been sterilized by antibiotics.

PATHOGENICITY. The capsular polysaccharide makes the pneumococcus virulent. Like the M-protein of group A streptococci, this surface polysaccharide deters phagocytosis by both polymorphonuclear leukocytes and macrophages. On the other hand, decapsulated pneumococci or encapsulated organisms opsonized with specific antibodies are readily taken up by phagocytes. Complement may also be opsonic for some types, even in the absence of specific antibody. Solubilized polysaccharide, which may persist in the circulation, may overcome host resistance by binding with circulating antibodies. The polysaccharide, being resistant to degradation by host enzymes, may also contribute to immune paralysis by overwhelming the mononuclear phagocytic system. The polysaccharide may thus remain within phagocytic cells for the life of the animal without inciting an inflammatory response.

No pneumococcal toxin is known to be definitely related to pathogenicity. Upon washing and autolysis, pneumococci release a cell-bound lysin that is antigenically related to streptolysin O. A neuraminidase, which cleaves terminal *N*-acetyl-neuraminic acid from glycoprotein substrates on cell membranes, may be involved in the neurotoxicity of meningeal infections. In the presence of immunoglobulin, platelets are aggregated by heat-killed bacteria; this may play a role in the pathogenesis of disseminated intravascular coagulation seen in severe infections. It is believed that lethality depends entirely on the ability of the organism to grow extracellularly and that toxins are not significant lethal factors. Strains of pneumococci elaborate an extracellular protease that can cleave IgA into Fab and Fc fragments, so that the immunoglobulin cannot block their adherence to mucosal surfaces. As a result, colonization and infection by the pneumococcus is facilitated. Increased susceptibility to pneumococcal infections has been observed: (1) in infants under six months, who usually do not develop adequate amounts of opsonins and who are deficient in naturally occurring antibodies and serum complement; (2) in immunoglobulin disorders, especially hypogammaglobulinemia, Wiskott-Aldrich syndrome, and multiple myeloma; (3) in pulmonary disease where mechanisms for clearance of pneumococci from the lung are disturbed; (4) in alcoholics, whose tendency to aspiration and neutropenia (from folate deficiency) interferes with natural resistance in the lung; and (5) after splenectomy.

DRUG SUSCEPTIBILITY. Although most pneumococci are susceptible to less than 0.03 μg/ml penicillin G, acquired resistance to this antibiotic has been described in South Africa, New Guinea, and elsewhere. South African strains are resistant to 2 to 10 μg/ml of penicillin, a level 100 times greater than that of the MIC for the susceptible strains. Resistant strains have penicillin-binding protein patterns that differ from those of sensitive strains. Tetracycline, erythromycin, and vancomycin resistance have also been reported. Multiple drug resistance, not associated with β-lactamase production, has also been described (see Chapter 21).

PROPHYLAXIS. A polyvalent pneumococcal vaccine has been made for prophylaxis of pneumococcal infection. The vaccine consists of highly purified capsular polysaccharides from the 23 most prevalent or invasive pneumococcal types accounting for at least 80 per cent of pneumococcal disease isolates. The vaccine has lowered the attack rate of pneumococcal pneumonia and bacteremia but the results in infants are discouraging because the antibody titers after vaccination were not higher than those in unvaccinated infants (Quie et al., 1981).

EPIDEMIOLOGY. Infection with pneumococci occurs through droplets released from infected patients. Whether or not soiled clothing and blankets can serve as infective material has not been established. There is no animal reservoir. Intrafamily spread and asymptomatic infection occurs frequently, especially in association with viral upper respiratory infections.

REFERENCES

Alouf, J. E.: Streptococcal toxins (Streptolysin O, Streptolysin S, Erythrogenic toxin). Pharmac Ther 11:661, 1980.

Anthony, B. F.: Group B streptococcal infections. In Textbook of Pediatric Infectious Diseases. Feigin, R. D. and Cherry, J. D. (eds.). W. B. Saunders Co., Philadelphia, p. 995, 1981.

Anthony, B. G. and Okada, D. M.: The emergence of Group B streptococci in infections in newborn infants. Ann Rev Med 28:353, 1977.

Auckenthaler, R., Hermans, P. E., and Washington, J. A.: Group G Streptococcal Bacteremia: Clinical study and review of the literature. Rev Infect Dis 5:196, 1983.

Beachey, E. H.: Bacterial adherence: adhesion-receptor interactions mediating the attachment of bacteria to mucosal surfaces. J Infect Dis 143:325, 1981.

Bloomster, T. G., and Watson D. W.: Recent trends in streptococcal pyrogenic toxin production by Group A streptococci. In Basic Concepts of Streptococci and Streptococcal Diseases. S. E. Holm and P. Christensen, (eds.). Reed Books, Ltd., Fox Lane North Chertsey, Surrey, England, 1982.

Bridge, P. D., and Sneath, P. H. S.: Numerical taxonomy of Streptococcus. J Gen Mic 129:587, 1983.

Davies, P., Page, R. C., and Allison, A. C.: Changes in cellular enzyme levels and extracellular release of lysosomal acid hydrolases in macrophages exposed to group A streptococcal cell wall substance. J Exp Med 139:1962, 1974.

de Louvois, J.: The bacteriology and chemotherapy of brain abscess. J Antimicrob Chemother 4:395, 1978.

Eichman, K., Brown, D. G., and Krause, R. M.: Influence of genetic factors on the magnitude and the heterogeneity of the immune response in the rabbit. J Exp Med 134:48, 1971.

Facklam, R., and Wilkinson, H. W.: The family Streptococcaceae (Medical Aspects). In The Prokaryotes Handbook on Habitat, Isolation and Identification of Bacteria. Starr, M. P., Stolp, H., Trouper, H. G., Balows, A., and Schlegel, H. G. (eds.). Volume II, Springer Verlag, Berlin, Heidelberg, New York, p. 1573, 1981.

Ferenandez, C., Daasch, V. N., and Folds, J. D.: Streptococcal serology. Clin Mic Newsletter 5:73, 1983.

Fischer, G., Horton, R. E., and Edelman, R.: 1983 summary of the National Institute's of·Health Workshop on group B Streptococcal infections. J Inf Dis 148:163, 1983.

Fox, E. N.: M Proteins of group A streptococci. Bact Rev 38:57, 1974.

Gehring, F. J.: The genus Streptococcus and dental diseases. In The Prokaryotes Handbook on Habitat, Isolation and Identification of Bacteria, Starr, M. P., Stolp, H., Trouper, H. G., Balows, A., and Schlegel, H. G. (eds.). Volume II, Springer Verlag, Berlin, Heidelberg, New York, p. 1598, 1981.

Ginsburg, I.: Mechanism of cell and tissue injury induced by group A Streptococci: Relation to poststreptococcal sequelae. J Infect Dis 126:294, 1972.

Ginsburg, I.: The role of lysosomal factors of leukocytes in the biodegradation and storage of microbial constituents in infectious granulomas. In Lysosomes in Applied Biology and Therapeutics. Dingle, J. T., Jacques, P. J., and Shaw, I. H. (eds.): North Holland Publishing Company, Amsterdam, New York, Oxford, p. 327, 1979.

Ginsburg, I., Zor, U., and Floman, Y.: Experimental models of streptococcal arthritis: Pathogenetic role of streptococcal products and prostaglandins and their modification by anti-inflammatory agents. In Glynn, L. E., and Schlumberger, H. D. (eds.): Experimental Models in Chronic Inflammatory Diseases. Berlin, Springer Verlag, 1977, 256.

Glynn, L. E.: Rheumatic fever. In Gell, P. G. H., Coombs, R. R. A., and Lachmann, P. J. (eds.): Clinical Aspects of Immunology. 3rd ed. Oxford, London, Blackwell Scientific Publications, 1975, p. 1079.

Hasty, D. L., Beachey, E. H., Simpson, W. A., and Dale, J. B.: Hybridoma antibodies against protective and nonprotective antigenic determinants of a structurally defined polypeptide fragment of Streptococcal M protein. J Exp Med, 155:1010, 1982.

Holm, S., and Christensen, P. (eds.): Basic Concepts of Streptococci and Streptococcal Diseases. Reedbooks Ltd., Fox Lane North Chertsey, Surrey, England, 1982.

Kaplan, M. H.: Antoimmunity in rheumatic fever: Relationship to Streptococcal antigens cross-reactive with valve fibroblasts, myofibers and smooth muscle. In Dumonde, D. C. (ed.): Infection and Immunity in the Rheumatic Disease. Oxford, Blackwell, Scientific Publication, 1976, p. 113.

Lehner, T., Challacombe, S. J., and Caldwell, J.: Immunologic basis for vaccination against dental caries in rhesus monkeys. J Dent Res 55:c166, 1976.

Patterson, M. J., and Hafeez, A. El.B.: Group B streptococci. Bact Rev 774:40, 1976.

Stollerman, G. H.: Rheumatic fever and streptococcal infection. New York, Grune and Stratton, 1975.

Tanzer, J. M., Freedman, M. L., Woodid, F. N., et al.: Association of *Streptococcus mutans* virulence with synthesis of intracellular polysaccharide. Special Supplement to Microbiology Abstracts, 3:597, 1976.

The Pneumococcus, A Symposium. Edited by Quie, P. G., Giebink, S., and Winkelstein, J. A.: Rev Infec Dis Vol. 3(2), 1981, pp. 183-395.

Unny, S. K., and Middlebrooks, R. L.: Streptococcal rheumatic carditis. Microbiol Rev 47(1):97, 1983.

Wannamaker, L. W., and Matsen, J. M.: Streptococci and Streptococcal Diseases. Recognition, Understanding and Management. New York, Academic Press, 1972.

Wannamaker, L. W.: The chain that links the heart and the throat. Circulation 48:9, 1973.

Wannamaker, L. W.: Immunology of Streptococci. In Nahmias, A. J., and O'Reily, R. J. (eds.): Immunology of Human Infections Part I. Bacteria, Mycoplasm, Chlamydia and Fungi. New York and London, Plenum Medical Book Company, 1981, p. 47.

Weissman, S. M., Reich, P. R., Somerson, N., and Cole, R.: Genetic differentiation by nucleic acid homology. IV. Relationships among Lancefield groups and serotypes of Streptococci. J Bacteriol 92:1372, 1966.

Zabriskie, J. B.: Rheumatic fever: A streptococcal-induced autoimmune disease? In Dumonde, D. C. (ed.): Infection and Immunology in the Rheumatic Diseases. Oxford, Blackwell Scientific Publications, 1976, p. 97.

25

DIPHTHERIA BACILLI AND OTHER CORYNEBACTERIA

LANE BARKSDALE, PH.D.

Diphtheria is a contagious disease of man in which *Corynebacterium diphtheriae* colonizes the mucous membranes of the fauces and pharynx (sometimes extending to the larynx and the trachea). This is *faucial (laryngeal,* etc.) *diphtheria.* When colonization occurs on the subcutaneous tissue (of the skin) *cutaneous diphtheria* may result.

THE DISCOVERY OF DIPHTHERIA, CORYNEBACTERIUM DIPHTHERIAE, DIPHTHERIAL TOXIN, AND ANTITOXIN

Just one century ago, in most countries of the world, diphtheria was a dreaded disease with a case fatality rate of about 8 per cent (see Table 1).

The history of our coming to understand diphtheria and to devise a means of combating *diphtheritic death* stands as a model investigation of the etiology of an infectious disease and as a lasting tribute to the clinicians and microbiologists concerned (Andrewes et al., 1923). It was the astute French physician Pierre Fidèle Bretonneau who (from 1821 to 1826) conceived the clinical entity diphtheria to be characterized by the formation of a tightly adhering membranous growth (the pseudomembrane) on the mucous membranes of the throat, sometimes extending into the trachea. At that time, before bacterial agents of disease were known, Bretonneau's clear delineation of the specific clinical condition of diphtheria was the beginning of separation of one throat infection from another, for example, diphtheria from streptococcal pharyngitis. The question "can diphtheria be transmitted from one human subject to another?" was asked by Bretonneau and answered by Trendelenburg (1879), who showed that injection of pseudomembranous material from human cases of diphtheria into pigeons and rabbits gave rise to pseudomembranes. Thus the pseudomembrane of diphtheria was transmissible. With these important facts to go on, Friedrich Loeffler began a painstaking investigation into the cause(s) of diphtheria. Being a student in the laboratory of Robert Koch (see *Mycobacterium tuberculosis*), he was disposed to think that diphtheria might have a bacterial etiology. He also accepted the idea of Bretonneau that diphtheria was a singular disease, in the sense that physicians of Bretonneau's day considered smallpox to be singular.

Loeffler's approach to the microscopic examination of material from diphtheritic lesions was essentially that employed today. The staining of smears from some pseudomembranes with alkaline methylene blue revealed to him club-shaped bacilli containing reddish, spheroidal inclusions (metachromatic granules), as shown in Figure 1. Loeffler also knew that diphtheria bacilli growing in vitro often assumed a unique shape (Fig. 2). In smears from 22 cases of clinical diphtheria *he was able to demonstrate bacilli in only 13.* From 6 of these he isolated diphtheria bacilli in culture (on inspissated serum slants). Thus, it was not possible for Loeffler to isolate the causal agent in every case of diphtheria. To the present day, such has been a common experience of bacteriologists. He also isolated diphtheria bacilli from one normal child. Thus, he realized that *the isolation of diphtheria bacilli from the human throat does not necessarily mean that that throat is a diphtheritic one.* He observed that diphtheria and streptococcal pharyngitis *could occur together.* To this day *streptococcal infections sometimes occur simultaneously with diphtheria.* Thus, a diagnosis of diphtheria may require sophisticated clinical judgment backed up with careful bacteriology.

Loeffler's experimental infections in animals led to the discovery that diphtheria bacilli tended to remain at the site where they had been injected, although autopsy of those animals revealed damage to organs far from that site. The *connection* between diphtheria bacilli at a superficial location (in experimentally infected animals) and damage to distant organs with subsequent death was shown by Roux and Yersin (1888) to be the filterable poison diphtherial toxin. It remained for Behring and Kitasato (1890) to discover that antibodies prepared against diphtherial toxin could neutralize its toxicity, thus providing a means of rescuing patients from diphtheritic death by *passively* immunizing them against diphtherial toxin.

Table 1. DECLINE IN THE CASE FATALITY RATE FOR DIPHTHERIA IN ENGLAND ACCORDING TO RETURNS FROM THE HOSPITALS OF THE METROPOLITAN ASYLUMS BOARD*

Year	Case Mortality Per Cent	Year	Case Mortality Per Cent
1889	40.7	1909	9.4
1890	33.5	1910	7.8
1891	30.6	1911	8.4
1892	29.3	1912	6.2
1893	30.4	1913	6.2
1894	29.3	1914	7.9
1895	22.8	1915	8.4
1896	21.2	1916	6.8
1897	17.7	1917	6.7
1898	15.4	1918	7.7
1899	13.9	1919	9.3
1900	12.3	1920	8.6
1901	11.1	1921	8.8
1902	11.0	1922	8.7
1903	9.7	1923	6.8
1904	10.0	1924	7.0
1905	8.3	1925	5.0
1906	8.8	1926	4.9
1907	9.6	1927	4.0
1908	9.7		

*Antitoxin came into general use in the treatment of diphtheria in 1895. During the same period the diagnosis of diphtheria began to pick up mild cases that previously may have fallen into some other clinical category. There was probably a slow but general improvement in living standards including personal hygiene. General immunization with toxoid was not begun until more than 20 years after the gathering of the data in this table. (Data from Wilson, G. S., and Miles, A. A.: Topley and Wilson's Principles of Bacteriology and Immunity. 4th ed. Baltimore, The Williams and Wilkins Company, 1955).

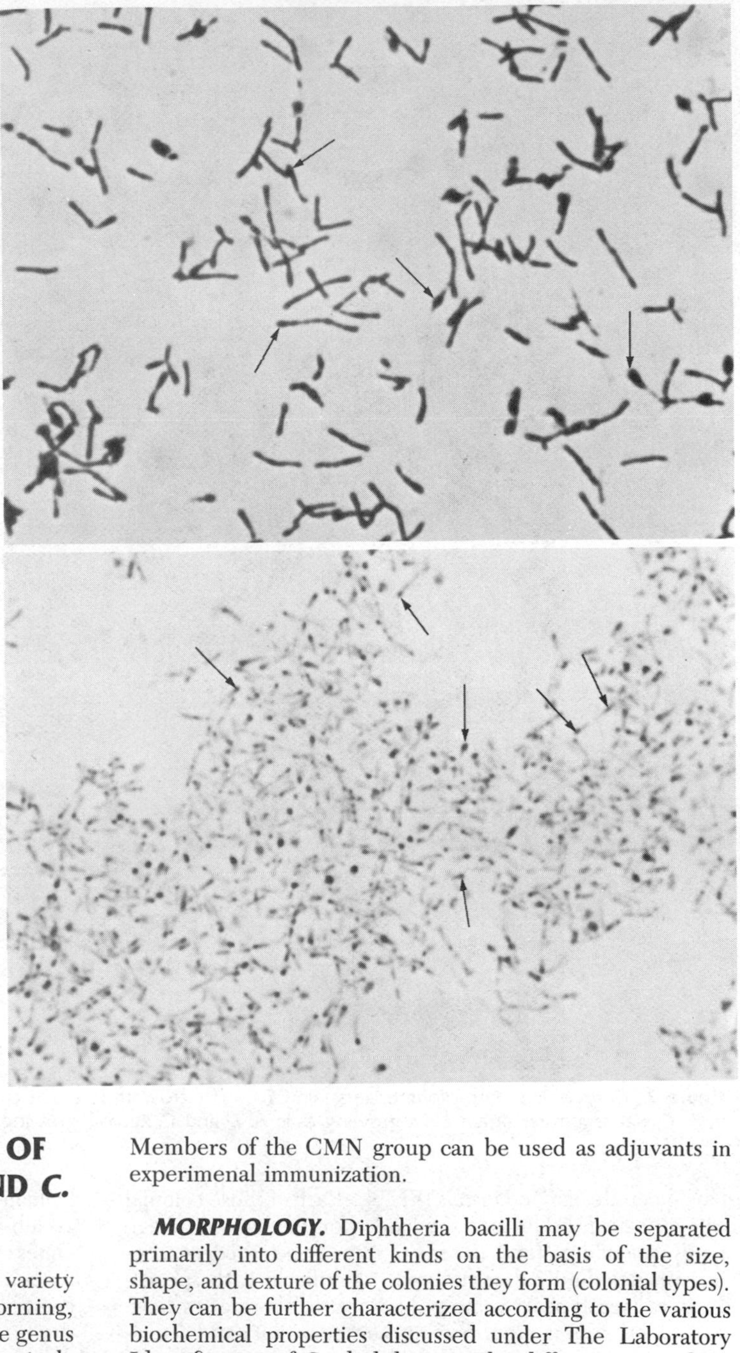

Figure 1. *Corynebacterium diphtheriae,* strain $C7_S(^-)^{tox-}$ grown on Loeffler's Medium with added phosphate. *Upper,* Cells stained by the method of Gram. Arrows indicate swollen areas, "club shapes." See text. *Lower,* Cells stained with alkaline methylene blue. Arrows indicate metachromatic granules. Compare these shapes with those found in tissue culture (Fig. 2) and those found under conditions ideal for maximal growth (Fig. 3, upper). ×2000. Courtesy K.-S. Kim.

CHEMICAL BASIS OF TAXONOMY OF THE GENUS *CORYNEBACTERIUM* AND *C. DIPHTHERIAE*

Corynebacterium is the Latin name applied to a variety of tapered, gram-positive, nonmotile, nonspore-forming, rod-shaped bacteria. Their closest relatives are in the genus *Nocardia* and the genus *Mycobacterium,* collectively known as the CMN group (Barksdale, 1970). This group of organisms share a basic cell wall peptidoglycan of cross-linked subunits containing *meso*diaminopimelic acid, L-alanine, and D-alanine to which are covalently bonded polysaccharides consisting of arabinose and galactose (arabinogalactan) and some mannose as arabinomannan. In addition, the cell walls of organisms of each of the three genera contain ester-linked, β-hydroxylated, α-branched, long-chain fatty acids of characteristic carbon lengths ranging from about C_{28} to C_{90} (corynomycolic, C_{28} to C_{40}, nocardomycolic, C_{40} to C_{56} and mycolic (mycobacterial), C_{60} to C_{90}, acids). These mycolic acids are important constituents of the outer cell walls and such cell-surface-associated conjugates as trehalose dimycolates (cord factors) (Fig. 3). Members of the CMN group can be used as adjuvants in experimenal immunization.

MORPHOLOGY. Diphtheria bacilli may be separated primarily into different kinds on the basis of the size, shape, and texture of the colonies they form (colonial types). They can be further characterized according to the various biochemical properties discussed under The Laboratory Identification of *C. diphtheriae.* The difference in colony morphology reflects certain essential differences in the cell surfaces of individual diphtheria bacilli. These surface peculiarities affect the manner in which individual bacilli pile up to form a colony. To identify diphtheria bacilli, knowledge of the colonial type is useful. The three most common types of colony are (1) smooth, (2) dwarf-smooth, and (3) semirough (rough strains of *C. diphtheriae* lack characteristic surface antigens present in semirough organisms).

When the strains that are smooth also produce diphtherial toxin, they are called *mitis* (Fig. 4) (McLeod, 1943; Robinson, 1934). Similarly, toxin-producing strains of the dwarf-smooth variety have been termed *intermedius* and certain starch-fermenting, toxin-producing rough strains

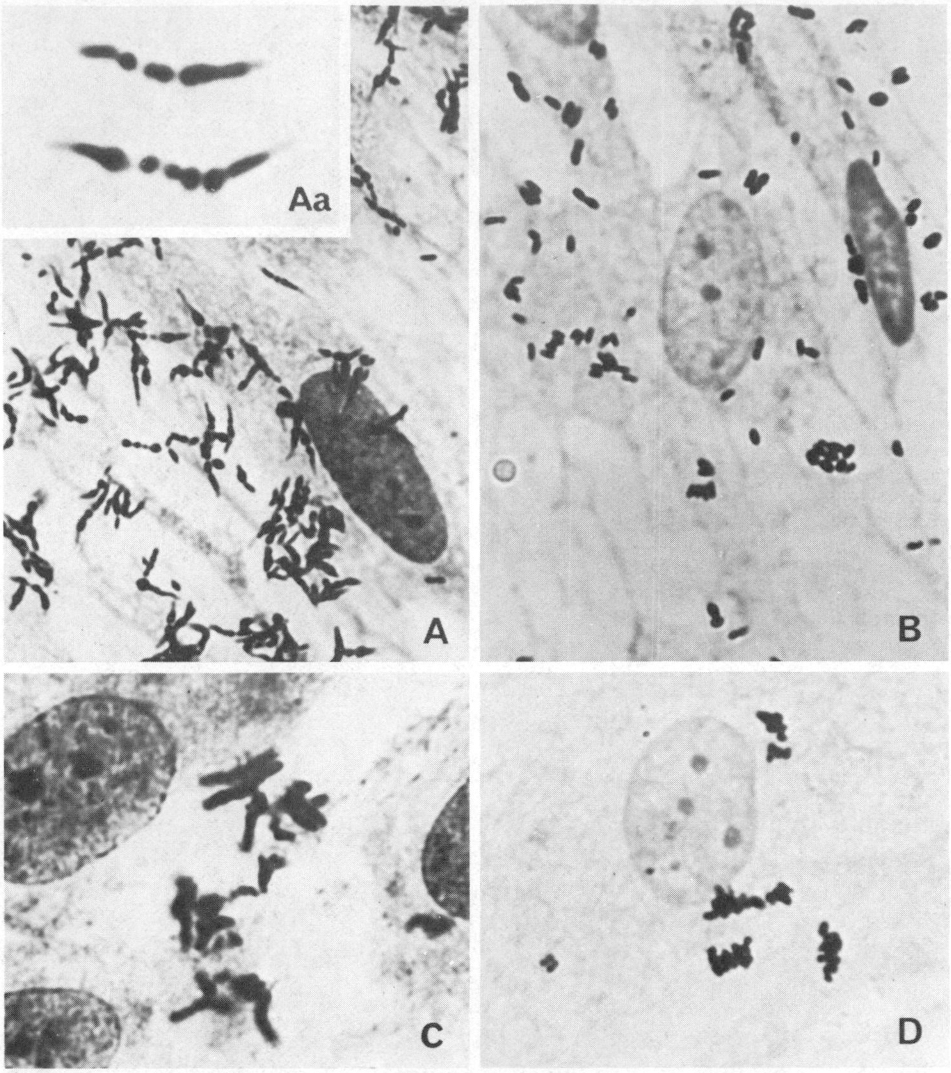

Figure 2. *Corynebacterium diphtheriae* strain $C7_s(-)^{tox-}$ growing in tissue culture, *A* and *Aa. B* and *C, diphtheriae gravis* growing as in *A. C, Bacterium sp.* strain 22M growing as in *A. D* and *C,* xerosis growing as in A. × 3,000. Courtesy K.-S. Kim.

have been designated *gravis* (Fig. 4). Each of these colonial categories can be further subdivided on the basis of phage types (specific patterns of sensitivity to selected corynebacteriophages) and antigenic types identifiable with specific antisera (serotypes). Some public health laboratories have also typed strains according to their sensitivity to bacteriocins (see Chapter 4). Individual cells of semirough strains of *C. diphtheriae* tend to be short and stubby. Cells of smooth strains are much longer, whereas the cells of dwarf-smooth strains are intermediate in length.

Common to cells of diphtheria bacilli and most other corynebacteria are certain properties which can be observed with the light microscope: (1) When growing in tissue their cell walls have in them thin spots that are leaky to the Gram stain; they are gram-variable. (2) Old cells store phosphate as polymetaphosphate, localized as phosphate glass and known as metachromatic granules. When bacilli containing such granules are stained with a metachromatic dye, e.g., alkaline methylene blue, the granules stand out as reddish refractile bodies against a blue background (see Fig. 1). (3) Bacilli with thin spots tend to balloon out at one end of the cell and assume a shape like a club (coryne-, coryneform, corynebacterium). Misshapenness of this sort is called pleomorphism. In smears from tissue, the pleomorphism of smooth strains is more exaggerated than that of dwarf-smooth and rough strains. Thus, the bizarre morphology of diphtheria bacilli from a pseudomembrane associated with infection by a *mitis* strain could be more readily recognized than that from a membrane associated with a *gravis* infection.

Since in each of the colonial categories (*gravis, mitis,* and *intermedius*) there are a number of serologic and phage types, the species *C. diphtheriae* has the potentiality for accommodating to the defenses of the human host much as do Group A *streptococci* and *pneumococci.* Thus, persons who have experienced infection with one type of *C. diphtheriae* may later be infected with another type. When this happens in young adults or older individuals having adequate levels of circulating antitoxin, the second infection is apt to be of little consequence to the individual though it may be of some importance in the epidemiology of the disease (see Chapter 96).

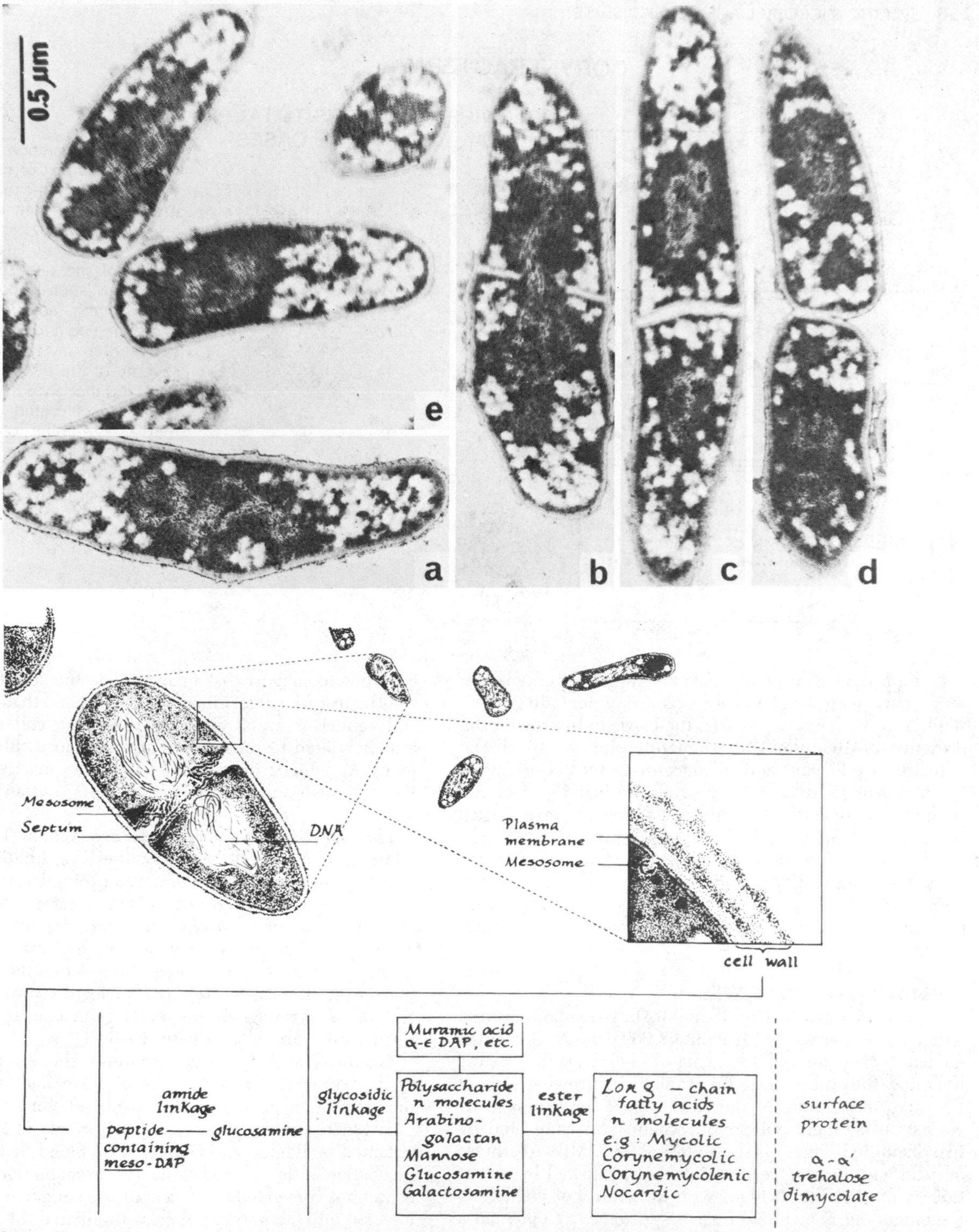

Figure 3. *Upper,* An electron micrographic record of cell division as it occurs in logarithmically growing *C. diphtheriae,* $C7_s(-)^{tox-}$. Division time = 60 minutes. *A,* Initiation of septum formation by ingrowth of membrane. *B,* Well-developed septal initials showing "layers" of the components of the cell envelope. *C,* Two cells still connected showing that the septum consists of two full complements of membrane and envelope components. *D,* Beginning of separation of cell doublets. *E,* The "snapping" involved in the pulling apart of two corynebacterial cells, showing the characteristic taper from septal to distal end. Electronopaque areas, peculiar to actively growing cells, seem not to be glycogen but may represent lipid associated with loci of intense biosynthetic activity. ×51,000. Bar = 0.5 µm. From data of Sheila Heitner.

Lower, Diagrammatic sketch of an actively growing bacterial cell representing a composite of the CMN group. A "resting" cell with metachromatic granule is shown. A portion of the envelope of an actively growing cell has been expanded to show the relation of the complex envelope to the cytoplasmic membrane. A portion of the wall is shown to consist of murein, arabinogalactan-mannan linked to species of long-chain, α-branched. β-hydroxylated fatty acids, the mycolic acids, and to dimycolates of trehalose and to a surface protein antigen. The mureins and arabinogalactans are distinctive from genus to genus as are the mycolic acids—for example, mycolic *(Mycobacterium),* corynemycolic and corynemycolenic *(Corynebacterium),* and nocardomycolic *(Norcardia).* In general terms, the murein-arabinogalactan is a heat-stable O antigen; the heat-labile surface protein antigen is the K antigen. Drawing by James E. Ziegler. Rearrangement by Kwang-Shin Kim. Reproduced with permission of Bacteriological Reviews.

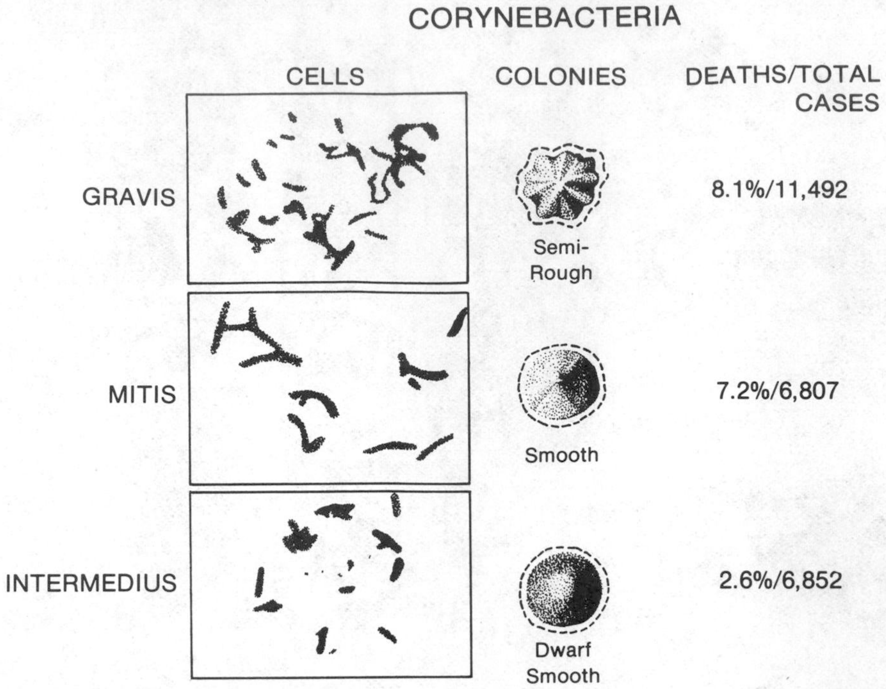

Figure 4. Separation of toxinogenic strains of *Corynebacterium diphtheriae* on the basis of the morphology of their colonies. In a series of 25,000 cases of diphtheria studied in England, outbreaks of the disease could be related to specific colony types (*gravis, mitis,* and *intermedius*), and there was a rough correlation between colony type and clinical severity of the disease. It should be noted that once these colonial types are cultivated in complex media, a number of nutritional and colonial mutants grow out. Thus, in order to keep a stock culture of a model of any one of the colony types, repeated reisolation of that type is necessary.

C. diphtheriae and Salts of Tellurium. Most corynebacteria share with certain other organisms, including some staphylococci and some yeasts, the capacity to grow in the presence of 100μg/ml potassium tellurite, to reduce the tellurite to tellurium and to concentrate the tellurium (as the metal or its sulfide) in the cells, so that the bacterial colonies that develop on tellurite agar appear grayish black to jet black. The growth of most streptococci, some staphylococci, and other members of the throat flora is inhibited on tellurite agar. For over 60 years a variety of tellurite media have been used for the selective cultivation of *C. diphtheriae* (see The Laboratory Identification of *C. diphtheriae*).

PATHOGENIC PROPERTIES

Diphtherial Toxin. Diphtherial toxin is a simple protein with a molecular weight of about 62,000 daltons. It is lethal for man in amounts of 130 ng/kg of body weight. Toxin is liberated into the extracellular milieu by growing cells of *C. diphtheriae* and is therefore called an exotoxin. It consists of a single polypeptide chain cross-connected by two disulfide bridges, as shown in Figure 5. Mild treatment of toxin with trypsin (termed "nicking") followed by reduction of its disulfide bridges with dithiothreitol yields two fragments: an N-terminal fragment A (m.w. 21,000) and a C-terminal fragment B (m.w. 39,000); see Pappenheimer (1977).

Although the only biologic activity directly associated with the intact toxin molecule is the ability to inactivate a variety of animal cells, fragment A behaves as a diphosphopyridine nucleotidase (NADase) as well as an adenosine diphosphoribosyl transferase. This latter function of fragment A stops protein synthesis in the test tube by covalently linking the adenosine diphosphoribose moiety of nicotinamide adenine dinucleotide to eukaryotic elongation factor 2 (EF2) (Collier, 1975). This *enzymatic activity of fragment A* (liberated from diphtherial toxin) operationally places toxin in the category of a proenzyme. There is good evidence to suggest that toxin fixes to the sensitive animal cells by its carboxy terminal end (Fig. 5) and that proteolytic and reductive steps occurring near the cell surface (or infolds related to the process of endocytosis) liberate fragment A, which, once inside the cell, inactivates EF2. Enough such inactivation would stop protein synthesis, leading to cell death.

The Genetic Control of Toxin Production. The genetic information required for the synthesis of diphtherial toxin is carried in the genomes of certain temperate corynebacteriophages as the gene *tox*. This information gains expression in strains of *C. diphtheriae* undergoing lysis by the phage as well as in lysogenic strains that carry tox^{+} in the prophage state (Fig. 6). Integration of *tox*-containing prophages into the corynebacterial nucleoid assures perpetuation of the toxinogenic character from one generation of toxinogenic corynebacteria to the next.

Toxoid. The early efforts at immunizing against diphtherial toxin with graded doses of toxin and, later, with mixtures of toxin and antitoxin (horse) sometimes led to unfortunate accidents. A satisfactory nontoxic antigen was obtained by Ramon and Glenny, who found that prolonged incubation of diphtherial toxin with formalin under alkaline conditions converted it into a nontoxic antigen which, when injected into laboratory animals, stimulated the production of antitoxin. Formalin interacts with the tyrosine residues of toxin, effecting their cross-linkage with the ε-amino groups of constituent molecules of lysine. Toxoid is unable to fix to animal cells and it cannot be split into A and B fragments. It lacks, therefore, all of the properties of toxin except antigenicity and the capacity to interact with antitoxic antibody. This remarkably stable antigen has served for more than 50 years as satisfactory prophylactic agent against death from diphtheritic intoxication (see also Schick Test).

In the early days of production of toxoid for immunization, it was necessary to find an exceptional strain of *C. diphtheriae* that produced large amounts of toxin. Park and

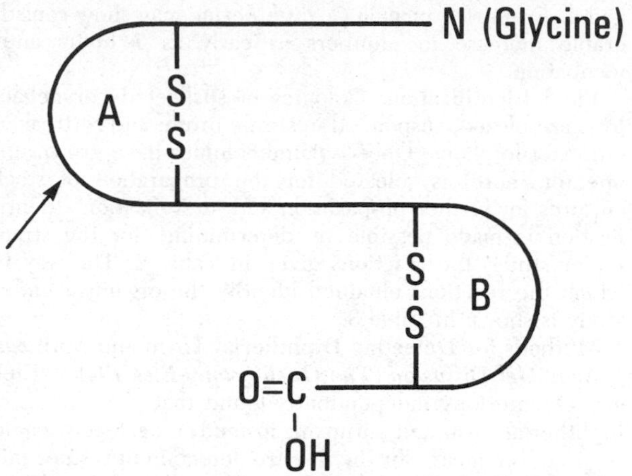

Figure 5. A molecule of diphtherial toxin schematically represented as a single polypeptide chain. At one terminus is the amino group of glycine; the amino acid functioning as the carboxy ($-\overset{\overset{O}{\|}}{C}-OH$) terminal is not known. The molecule is interconnected by disulfide bridges between cystine residues. At the bend shown by the arrow is a sequence of three arginines. Trypsin acts to nick toxin at the arrow point. When such nicking action is followed by exposure of the molecule to dithiothreitol, the disulfide bridges are broken and two fragments of toxin result. The smaller piece (from the arrow point back to the terminal glycine residue) has been designated fragment A. The larger piece (from the arrow point to the carboxy terminus) has been designated fragment B. Fragment A is the enzymically active fragment responsible for the following group transfer reactions:

1. NAD^+ + EF2 ⇋ ADP-ribosyl EF2 + nicotinamide + H^+
2. NAD^+ + HOH ⇋ ADP-ribose + nicotinamide + H^+
3. NAD^+ + toxin ⇋ ADP-ribosyl-toxin + nicotinamide + H^+

EF-2 = elongation factor 2. See text. Fragment B is thought to be important for the fixing of diphtherial toxin to receptors on toxin-sensitive cells.

Williams discovered an *avirulent* diphtheria bacillus, the Park-Williams Number 8 strain (PW8), which is used throughout the world in the "manufacture" of diphtherial toxoid. In suitable media the PW8 strain can produce 300 μg toxin protein/10^9 bacilli/ml, or around 300 mg per liter.

Invasiveness or Virulence of *C. diphtheriae*. In Figure 6 are listed the properties of a smooth strain of *C. diphtheriae*, $C7_S(-)^{tox-}$, carrying no tox^+ prophage and the properties of $C7_S(\beta)^{tox+}$, a lysogenic strain carrying prophage β^{tox+}. Antigenically, these two strains are identical except for the synthesis of diphtherial toxin by the toxinogenic strain. Each of the strains can colonize the pharyngeal mucous membranes of susceptible people and produce a pseudomembrane. Invasiveness in *C. diphtheriae* is associated with production of a dimycolate of trehalose, a so-called cord factor (see Chapter 44), which can inactivate the mitochondria of mammalian cells. *C. diphtheriae* can survive in pharyngeal mucus by producing a neuraminidase (sialidase) capable of cleaving residues of *N*-acetylneuraminic acid, NANA (sialic acid), from parent molecules such as mucins, the glycoproteins of cell surfaces, and gangliosides. In addition, these corynebacteria liberate an *N*-acetylneuraminic acid lyase which can split NANA into its constituents, *N*-acetyl mannosamine and pyruvate. Pyruvate markedly stimulates growth of corynebacteria and other members of the CMN group.

***THE LABORATORY IDENTIFICATION OF* C. DIPHTHERIAE.** At present, *C. diphtheriae* is not sought in the average diagnostic laboratory *unless* a death from diphtheria has occurred. In many countries there are few if any laboratory technicians who have had first-hand experience with *C. diphtheriae*. Yet diphtheria occurs in at least one major city of the world each year. The problem of diagnostic inadequacy of laboratories is compounded by deficiencies in contemporary textbooks regarding the characterization of diphtheria bacilli. The deficiencies include (1) inadequate

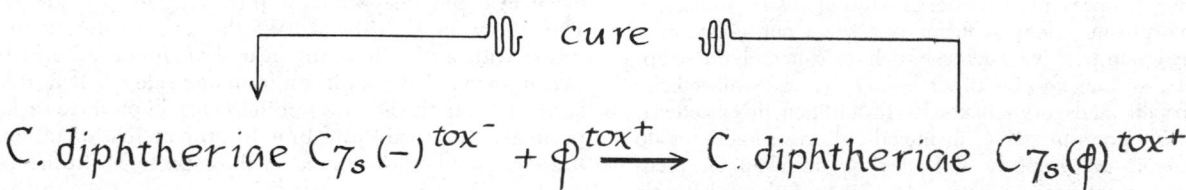

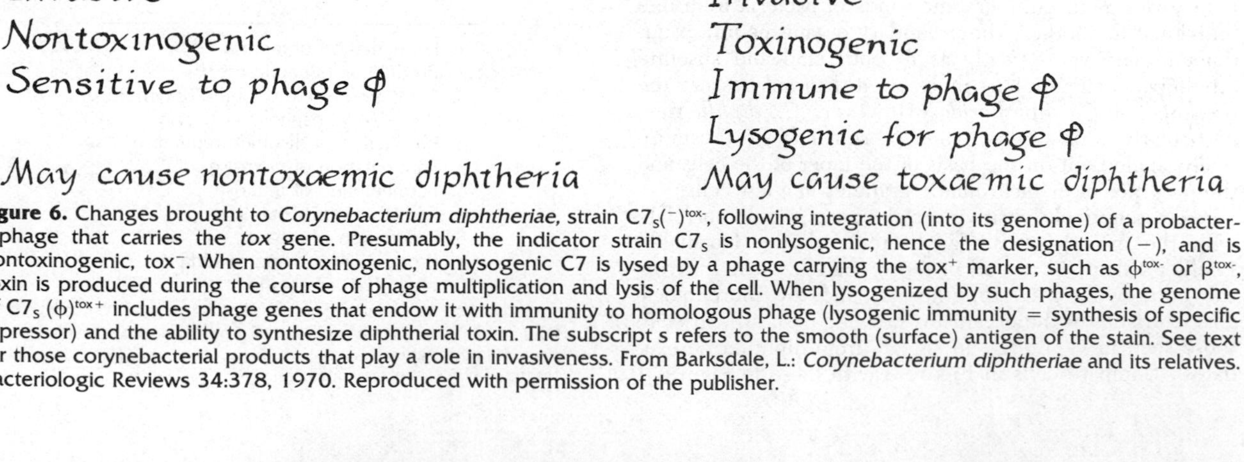

Figure 6. Changes brought to *Corynebacterium diphtheriae*, strain $C7_S(^-)^{tox-}$, following integration (into its genome) of a probacteriophage that carries the *tox* gene. Presumably, the indicator strain $C7_S$ is nonlysogenic, hence the designation (−), and is nontoxinogenic, tox^-. When nontoxinogenic, nonlysogenic C7 is lysed by a phage carrying the tox^+ marker, such as ϕ^{tox-} or β^{tox-}, toxin is produced during the course of phage multiplication and lysis of the cell. When lysogenized by such phages, the genome of $C7_S\ (\phi)^{tox+}$ includes phage genes that endow it with immunity to homologous phage (lysogenic immunity = synthesis of specific repressor) and the ability to synthesize diphtherial toxin. The subscript s refers to the smooth (surface) antigen of the stain. See text for those corynebacterial products that play a role in invasiveness. From Barksdale, L.: *Corynebacterium diphtheriae* and its relatives. Bacteriologic Reviews 34:378, 1970. Reproduced with permission of the publisher.

definitions of "pleomorphism" in general and with regard to *C. diphtheriae* in particular; (2) absence of a clear statement of the relationship existing between nontoxinogenic and toxinogenic *C. diphtheriae* (see Fig. 6); and (3) erroneous fermentation patterns (repeated from earlier textbooks) by which various corynebacteria are identified.

Procedures. Smears are prepared from diphtheritic membrane, and media are inoculated for enrichment of numbers of diphtheria bacilli and for primary isolation. *Note*: Corynebacteria thrive in a CO_2-rich environment, e.g., 10 per cent in air. A candle jar provides satisfactory levels of CO_2.

The diphtheritic membrane (pseudomembrane, see Figs. 1 and 2 in Chapter 96) is usually so tenacious that rubbing it with a cotton swab will remove only some of its outermost material. More of the fibrinous exudate may be obtained by using a bacteriologic loop (steel) that has been opened into a hook. Pulling away bits of pseudomembrane with such a device often results in slight bleeding. This behavior is in contrast to that of the easily removable exudate found in uncomplicated streptococcal pharyngitis. Some of the pseudomembrane so obtained is used for inoculating (1) a slant of Loeffler's medium supplemented with 2.5 gm K_2HPO_4/liter, (2) a blood agar plate, and (3) a Mueller-Miller tellurite or Tinsdale tellurite agar plate. From the remainder, smears should be prepared for future reference and for (1) the Gram stain and (2) staining with alkaline methylene blue. The former should provide an assessment of the different kinds of bacteria present in the exudate; the latter indicates whether or not any of the tapered, pleomorphic rods present contain polyphosphate (metachromatic) granules. Corynebacteria growing in a low phosphate environment produce very few metachromatic granules. This probably explains the limited numbers of granules found in *C. diphtheriae* in smears from tissues. The tapered ends of *C. diphtheriae* (see Figs. 1 and 2) will appear more exaggerated with the methylene blue stain than with the Gram stain. The exaggeration of the taper is most striking with *mitis* strains and less so with *intermedius* and *gravis* strains. Tapering of these rods is stressed here because it represents a particular kind of misshapenness or pleomorphism. Pleomorphism per se is not uncommon among gram-positive bacteria such as α-hemolytic streptococci, certain species of *Actinomyces*, propionibacteria, lactobacilli, and corynebacteria. In addition, fusobacteria, ordinarily gram-negative, in mixed cultures sometimes do not decolorize properly and may be mistaken for pleomorphic gram-positive rods. Any one of these bacteria might grow well in and about a streptococcal sore throat or a diphtheritic membrane. Since the normal pharyngeal flora varies as to numbers and kinds of bacteria from one individual to another, the secondary organisms in a pseudomembrane vary greatly as to both kind and absolute numbers. Their numbers more often than not obscure the presence of *C. diphtheriae*. However, *C. diphtheriae*, particularly *mitis* strains, when present may be presumptively singled out on the basis of the taper of the cells and the presence of metachromatic granules in a few cells.

A presumptively positive set of smears should correlate with the growth of similar bacteria on the inoculated Loeffler's slant, in use all of these years because it favors the outgrowth of *C. diphtheriae*, and the morphologic characteristics of the organisms growing on it are closer to those seen in vivo (e.g., in smears from diphtheritic exudates). Compare cells in Figure 3 with those in Figures 1 and 2. From rich inocula *C. diphtheriae* may show considerable increase in numbers as early as 7 hours after incubation.

Final Identification. Colonies of suspected corynebacteria are picked, suspended in sterile broth, and restreaked onto sterile plates. Once isolated colonies have grown up, one (or more) is selected for the preparation of stock cultures for further propagation and identification. Identification is made possible by determining, for the strain under study, the reactions given in Table 2. The way in which the reactions obtained identify the organism under study is shown in Table 3.

Methods for Detecting Diphtherial Toxin and Antitoxin

Agar Gel Diffusion (The Ouchterlony-Elek Plate). Elek and Ouchterlony independently found that precipitates of diphtherial toxin and antitoxin, formed in agar gels, could be used as a means for the in vitro detection of toxinogenic strains of *C. diphtheriae*. A horse serum agar plate (Petri dish) is poured and, before the agar has hardened, a strip of filter paper (1.6 × 8 cm), previously dipped into horse antitoxin (500 au/ml) and drained of excess liquid, is placed across the center of the agar surface. The Petri dish, its lid ajar, is kept in a 37° C incubator until dry. Onto the dry surface of the plate in well separated parallel lines (Fig. 7) are streaked known toxinogenic and nontoxinogenic strains of *C. diphtheriae* and the unknown organisms being tested. Cotton swabs, soaked in heavy bacterial cultures and then freed of excess liquid by expression against the sides of the culture tubes, are useful for introducing each of the bacterial cultures onto the plate. A satisfactory positive control is the toxinogenic avirulent PW8 strain, and a suitable negative control is the nontoxinogenic mutant of *C. diphtheriae gravis*, HF. Consider as unknown organisms to be tested strains $C7_S(-)^{tox-}$ and $C7_S(\beta)^{tox+}$. Each is streaked so that it is growing next to the known toxinogenic strain, PW8. If, during growth on the antitoxin-containing agar plate, toxin is produced, then a line of toxin-antitoxin precipitate will become visible in the agar, as can be seen to the left of the PW8 strain. When gradients of identical precipitates of antigen-antibody are formed from different loci in agar gels, they will fuse, producing an arc of identity. Thus, between C7 (β) and PW8 the diffusing toxins interacting with antitoxin in the agar have produced arcs between toxin (C7 (β)) antitoxin from one side to toxin (PW8) antitoxin from the other. Diphtheria bacilli produce various proteins other than toxin. In most preparations of antitoxin there are antibodies to some of these proteins. In the case

Table 2. TEN PROPERTIES USEFUL FOR SEPARATING MEMBERS OF THE GENUS *CORYNEBACTERIUM**

1. Fermentation of lactose
2. Production of catalase†
3. Formation of iodinophilic polymer from glucose-1-phosphate
4. Production of disulfide reductase
5. Fermentation of dextrose
6. Fermentation of maltose
7. Fermentation of starch
8. Production of urease
9. Production of pyrazinamidase
10. Hydrolysis of gelatin

*The author is much indebted to M. C. Pollice and Ioan T. Sulea for data supporting this Table.
†In the absence of exogenous hemin.

of C7(−)$^{tox-}$(Fig. 7) an anomalous protein has formed a precipitate with its antibody. Between strain PW8 and strain HF anomalous antigen-antibody precipitates have formed showing no arc of identity.

Intradermal Skin Tests. Necrosis by diphtherial toxin can readily be seen following the introduction of minute amounts of toxin into the skin of shaved rabbits or guinea pigs. Neutralization of toxicity by antitoxin specifically identifies the toxin. Bacterial cultures may similarly be tested intradermally for their capacity to produce toxin. For example, at numbered multiple sites on the back of a rabbit, *known* and *test cultures* are injected at time zero, antitoxin is given intravenously at time *t* (usually 3½ hours later), and at time *t* + 30 minutes *the same cultures* are injected at new (prime) sites. The reactions are read daily up to 96 hours. When diphtherial toxin is present, necrosis will occur at the sites inoculated at time *t* but not at the sites inoculated 30 minutes after the administration of antitoxin. Necrosis at both sites indicates the production of a toxin not neutralized by diphtherial antitoxin, i.e., a toxin immunologically distinct from diphtherial toxin.

IMMUNITY: THE SCHICK TEST. In 1913 Bela Schick described a skin test for the detection of circulating antitoxin in human subjects. Once in use, it became clear that a modified Schick test would also detect delayed hypersensitivity to other products of *C. diphtheriae*. In the modified Schick test used at New York University Medical School for over 30 years, minute amounts of toxin are injected at one site (on the forearm) and toxoid at a second site. There are five pairs of reactions possible. (1) If at 48 to 96 hours there is no reaction at either site, the subject has sufficient circulating antitoxin to neutralize the dose of toxin and shows no allergy to corynebacterial products. This rather positive capacity has been designated as *the Schick-negative reaction*. (2) If there is *necrosis* at the toxin site and no

Table 3. FORMULATION OF SPECIES OF *CORYNEBACTERIUM* ACCORDING TO THE 10 PROPERTIES LISTED IN TABLE 2*

Species	Above the line	Below the line
C. diphtheriae mitis:	2 3 4 5 6	1 7 8 9 10
C. diphtheriae gravis:	2 3 4 5 6 7	1 8 9 10
C. diphtheriae intermedius:	2 3 4 5 6	1 7 8 9 10
C. diphtheriae variety *ulcerans:*	2 3 4 5 6 7 8 10	1 9
C. kutscheri:	2 3 4 5 6 8 9	1 7 10
C. minutissimum:	2 3 4 5 6 9	1 7 8 10
C. pseudotuberculosis (ovis):	2 3 4 5 6 8	1 7 9 10
C. pseudodiphtheriticum: (hofmanni)	2 3 4 8 9	1 5 6 7 10
C. renale:	2 3 4 5 ⑨	1 6 7 8 10
C. xerosis:	2 3 4 5 9	1 ⑥ 7 8 10

*Numbers above the line indicate positive traits. Numbers below the line indicate negative traits. Circled numbers below the line indicate that a very occasional strain may be positive; circled numbers above the line indicate that a very occasional strain may be negative. Sucrose has not been included. Most *C. xerosis* are sucrose positive; some *C. diphtheriae mitis* are sucrose positive, as are some strains of *C. minutissimum* and *C. kutscheri.* Note that the pattern $\frac{2\ 3\ 4}{1}$ is common to each of the 10 species. The three types of *C. diphtheriae* differ only with regard to starch fermentation. However, when this pattern is supplemented with colonial morphology on tellurite agar and cellular morphology (under the microscope), as shown in Figure 4, precise identification can readily be accomplished. Those laboratories using sheep's blood agar plates with a concentration of erythrocytes low enough to reveal feeble hemolysis will be able to separate hemolytic *mitis* strains from nonhemolytic *gravis* and *intermedius* strains. *Note:* To obtain the most prompt and reliable test reactions, actively growing corynebacteria should be washed with saline, resuspended as a thick slurry and inoculated into test media so that each tube receives 100 million or more bacteria.

Note: Among gram-positive bacillary organisms that might conceivably be isolated from the human throat are *Actinomyces viscosus, A. propionica, A. pyogenes, Bacterionema matruchotii, Corynebacterium diphtheriae,* (as well as *C. ulcerans* and *C. pseudotuberculosis*) *C. pseudodiphtheriticum, C. xerosis, Nocardia asteroides* and *Rothia dentocariosa*. All, except *C. diphtheriae, C. ulcerans* and *C. pseudotuberculosis*, produce pyrazinamidase.

The author is much indebted to M. C. Pollice and Joan T. Sulea for data supporting this table.

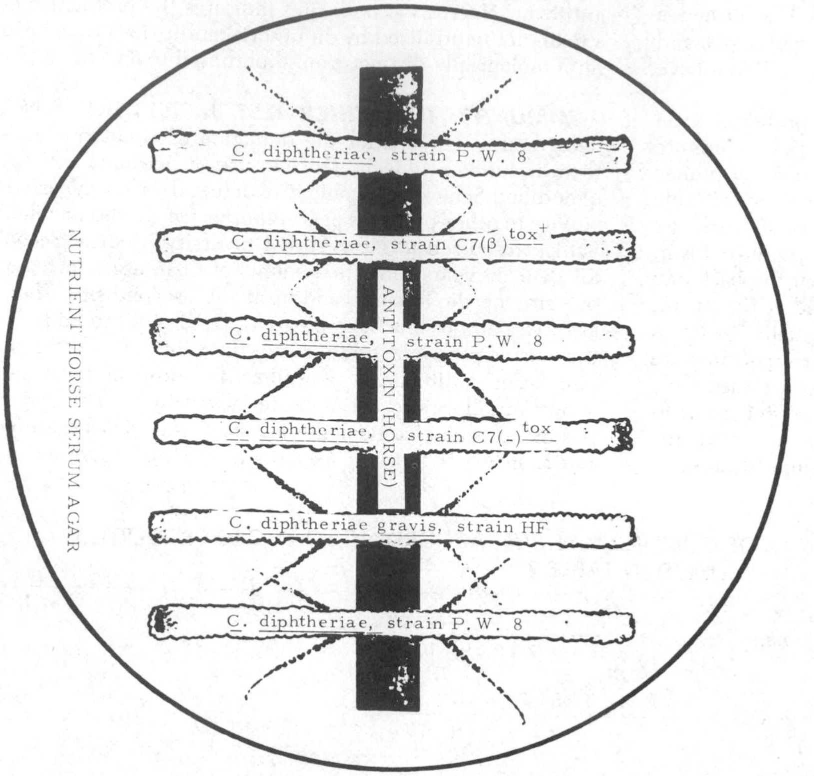

Figure 7. Diagram of an Elek/Ouchterlony plate (see text for details) for the in vitro detection of diphtherial toxin. Cultures of strains of *C. diphtheriae* have been streaked at right angles to the central strip of filter paper soaked in antitoxin. See text for information concerning each of the different strains of diphtheria bacilli and the antigen-antibody precipitates formed in their vicinities.

reaction at the toxoid site, the subject has insufficient circulating antitoxin to neutralize the toxin. This relatively negative condition is designated as *the Schick-positive reaction.* (3) An *immediate wheal* and *erythematous reaction* at both sites at about 35 minutes post injection indicates circulating IgE specific for the injected products. (4) An *erythematous reaction* at *48* to *96 hours* at both sites indicates that there has been enough circulating antitoxin to neutralize the toxin administered and that in addition the subject shows delayed allergy to corynebacterial products. This has been called *the pseudoreaction.* (5) *Necrosis* at the test site and *delayed allergy* at both sites indicate insufficient circulating antitoxin to neutralize the toxin and an allergy to corynebacterial products. This has been called *the combined reaction.*

Over the years the examination of human populations with the Schick test has given various insights into immunobiology (Barksdale, 1980). It has revealed that carriers of *C. diphtheriae* do not necessarily have detectable levels of circulating antitoxin. It has revealed that circulating antitoxin per se does not prevent the onset of a diphtheritic infection. And, most recently, it has led to the discovery that about 1.5 to 2 per cent of the human population cannot respond to immunizing doses of toxoid with the production of detectable levels of circulating antitoxin. As long as these people are around and as long as diphtheria bacilli continue to be carried in populations, there will probably be occasional deaths from diphtheria.

SENSITIVITY OF DIPHTHERIA BACILLI TO ANTIBIOTICS. Although *C. diphtheriae* is sensitive to a variety of antibiotics active on gram-positive organisms, including chloramphenicol, erythromycin, kanamycin, methicillin, penicillin G, rifampin, streptomycin, and tetracycline, the antibiotics that have been most thoroughly examined in relation to cases of diphtheria and carriers of diphtheria bacilli are penicillin G and erythromycin. Of 337 strains of *C. diphtheriae* isolated from cases of diphtheria, 90 per cent were sensitive to the aforementioned antibiotics, and all to gentamicin. The minimal inhibitory concentrations of antibiotics for *C. diphtheriae* are as follows (μg/ml): penicillin G, 0.08; erythromycin, 1.6; chloramphenicol, 0.5; and tetracycline, 1.0.

OTHER CORYNEBACTERIA. Listed in Table 3 are most of the species of *Corynebacterium* encountered in material from human and animal sources. Those that are of significance in diphtheritic infections are *C. diphtheriae* and sometimes *C. ulcerans.* Rare infections with *C. pseudotuberculosis (ovis)* have been reported in human subjects whose occupation put them into intimate contact with animals. *C. pseudotuberculosis (ovis)* causes infections in sheep and horses. *C. xerosis,* originally isolated from the conjunctiva, is one of those "background" corynebacteria from which *C. diphtheriae* must be differentiated. Aside from its distinguishing properties given in Table 3, *C. xerosis* tenaciously retains crystal violet, in contrast to the leaky, gram-variable reaction given by *C. diphtheriae* to the Gram stain. *C. pseudodiphtheriticum (C. hofmanni)* (Table 3) is another species of *Corynebacterium* that was originally isolated from normal throats and sometimes is encountered in routine bacteriologic study of the throat and upper respiratory tract. Among corynebacteria associated with genitourinary infections is a group designated *C. genitalium. C. kutscheri* is found in overt and latent infections of mice. *C. renale* is the cause of pyelonephritis in cattle.

Organisms that have been wrongly listed as belonging

to the genus *Corynebacterium* include *C. pyogenes*, now known as *Actinomyces pyogenes*, and *Propionibacterium acnes*, formerly *C. acnes*. *A. Pyogenes* under natural conditions produces suppurative lesions in cattle, sheep, pigs, and goats and has been associated with pharyngitis and ulcers of the skin in humans. Although the bacillary shape assumed by *A. pyogenes* has led to its confusion with *Corynebacterium*, unlike the latter its cells show no taper and contain no metachromatic granules.

A group of metabolically inert gram-positive rods are tentatively assigned to this genus and called the JK Group. They grow slowly on blood agar, producing small, nonhemolytic colonies. Gram stain reveals small, somewhat beaded coccobacillary forms that are often in a cuneiform pattern. They are catalase-positive, nonmobile, oxidase-negative, urease-negative, and do not reduce nitrates. Glucose and maltose are fermented slowly in serum-supplemented broth. The JK Group is uniformly resistant to the antibiotics used to treat infections caused by gram-positive bacteria with the exceptions of vancomycin (100 per cent sensitive) and erythromycin (about 50 per cent sensitive).

References

Andrewes, F. W., Bulloch, W., Douglas, S. R., Dreyer, G., Gardner, A. D., Fildes, P., Ledingham, J. C. G., and Wolf, C. G. L.: Diphtheria, Its Bacteriology, Pathology and Immunology. London, Medical Research Council, His Majesty's Stationery Office, 1923.

Barksdale, L.: *Corynebacterium diphtheriae* and its relatives. Bacteriol Rev 34:378, 1970.

Barksdale, L.: The immunobiology of diphtheria. In Nahmias, A. J., and O'Reilly, R. J. (eds.): Immunology of Human Infection. Part I in Comprehensive Immunology, Vol. 8. R. A. Good and S. B. Day (eds.) New York, Plenum Medical Book Company, 1980.

Collier, R. J.: Diphtheria toxin: mode of action and structure. Bacteriol Rev 39:54, 1975.

McLeod, J. W.: The types mitis, intermedius and gravis of *Corynebacterium diphtheriae*, a review of observations during the past ten years. Bacteriol Rev 7:1, 1943.

Pappenheimer, A. M., Jr.: Diphtheria toxin. Ann Rev Biochem 46:69, 1977.

Robinson, D. T.: Further investigations on the *gravis, mitis* and "intermediate" types of *C. diphtheriae: type stability. J Path Bact 39:551, 1934.*

26

LISTERIA MONOCYTOGENES

ANDREAS SCHAFFNER, M.D.

DEFINITION AND MORPHOLOGY. *Listeria monocytogenes* (Hulphers, 1911; Murray et al., 1926) is a facultatively anaerobic, nonsporulating, beta-hemolytic, gram-positive bacillus with variable microscopic morphology. In direct smears from infected sites the cells usually appear as cocci, diplococci, or short rods. They may be found singly, in short chains or in palisades that resemble corynebacteria (Chapter 25). On solid media coccobacillary forms and short rods predominate. In broth cultures longer bacillary forms prevail. After 2 to 5 days in culture, the cells tend to become gram-negative although the cell walls retain the typical structure of gram-positive bacteria. At room temperature the cells produce flagella (usually 1 to 4) and display tumbling motility, a unique characteristic of this genus. *L. monocytogenes* is usually non-motile at 37° C because of loss of flagella at this temperature.

L. monocytogenes grows on most ordinary media at atmospheric gas tensions over a broad range of temperatures (+3 to +42° C). Growth is optimal between 30 and 37° C and is stimulated by increased carbon dioxide tensions. Within 18 to 24 hours on colorless media, *L. monocytogenes* forms small, round, slightly elevated colonies that are bluish-gray in color when visualized by obliquely transmitted light. Colonies on blood agar are surrounded by a narrow zone of beta-hemolysis which is typically opaque. On solid media colonies dissociate into rough, smooth, and intermediate types. Rough colonies consist of filamentous organisms and bacilli, the smooth of coccal forms. Under special conditions (low temperature and media either rich in sugars or supplemented with serum) the organism forms a mucopolysaccharide capsule (Smith and Metzger, 1962).

L. monocytogenes is distinct from the non-hemolytic, non-pathogenic and antigenically distinct bacilli which have variously been assigned either to the genus *Listeria* or a new genus called *Murrayi*.

ANTIGENIC COMPOSITION. Several serogroups and serovarieties (12 to 15) can be differentiated by agglutination tests based on various somatic (0) and flagellar (H) antigens. Serotyping is performed by specialized reference laboratories and can be used as an epidemiologic tool or an auxiliary method of identification. Although two serotypes (4b and 1/2a, corresponding to Paterson's type 1) are most frequently isolated from infections, there is no direct evidence that certain serotypes are more virulent than others. It should be noted that the former serovariants 4f and 4g with numerous subvarieties do not belong to *L. monocytogenes* proper, but to a related nonpathogenic species of *Listeria* that has been named *L. innocua* (Seeliger and Schoofs, 1978).

L. monocytogenes shares several antigens such as the Rantz antigen (of unknown chemical composition) with other gram-positive bacteria. Difficulties in serodiagnosis of listeriosis have been attributed to such cross-reactive antigens (Gray and Killinger, 1966).

METABOLISM. Many of the metabolic and growth characteristics of *L. monocytogenes* reflect its capacities to live freely in soil and sewage and to colonize the mammalian intestine. Like the enterococci, it grows well in high concentrations of bile and salt. Since it also hydrolyzes esculin, it can be misidentified as an enterococcus (see Diagnosis, below). It is sensitive to hydrogen ions, however, and cultures die rapidly when the pH falls below 5.0. *Listeria* ferments a broad range of carbohydrates to lactic acid without the production of gas. Although the metabolism is said to be essentially homofermentative, acetoin is also produced because *Listeria* is Voges-Proskauer positive (See Enterobacteriaceae, Chapter 31). Glucose, levulose, mannose, maltose, lactose, trehalose, salicin, and glycerol are regularly fermented and esculin is hydrolyzed. Mannitol, arabinose, and glycogen are not metabolized. The ability to ferment most other carbohydrates is variable.

Except for the fermentation of carbohydrates, *Listeria* is not very active metabolically. It reduces hydrogen peroxide but does not form indole, hydrogen sulfide, or urease. It is oxidase negative. Nitrate is not reduced. The organism is non-proteolytic and does not liquefy gelatin. Strains of *Listeria* isolated from infections invariably produce a soluble, filterable, beta-hemolytic protein.

PATHOGENIC PROPERTIES. *L. monocytogenes* is a natural pathogen for humans, many other mammals, wild and domestic birds, and fish (Gray and Killinger, 1966). Strains of human and animal origin do not differ in serotype, virulence or pathogenic properties, but the course of infection varies with the affected animal species. The three most important forms of listeriosis are: 1) septicemia, 2) meningoencephalitis, and 3) infection of the contents of the pregnant uterus. All three forms occur in humans. Intrauterine infection late in pregnancy causes neonatal listeriosis. In ruminants, in which listeriosis can cause economically important losses, meningoencephalitis is the most common manifestation of listeriosis. In monogastric experimental animals, like rabbits and mice, the septicemic form is most common (Gray and Killinger, 1966). During septicemia, the organisms lodge preferentially in the liver and spleen where they multiply and usually cause focal necrosis and mononuclear infiltration (Mackaness, 1961). In other cases there is marked polymorphonuclear leukocyte infiltration and abscess formation. Infection of pregnant animals regularly leads to infection of the uterus, placenta, and fetus resulting in either abortion or neonatal listeriosis, depending on the gestational stage. After transplacental infection, newborn rabbits usually die of septicemia with hepatic necrosis or, if they survive for several days, with signs suggestive or meningoencephalitis, a spectrum of disease that resembles human neonatal listeriosis (Gray and Killinger, 1966).

L. monocytogenes can penetrate the intact conjunctiva and cornea and probably the abraded skin. The potential of the organism to penetrate the intact occular surface and provoke local infection in laboratory animals can be used diagnostically. Hemolysin production differentiates pathogenic from nonpathogenic *Listeria*, but no direct link between virulence and hemolysin production has been made. Furthermore, isolates of serogroup 5 are more hemolytic than other *L. monocytogenes* but not more virulent for mice (Seeliger et al., 1982). The hemolysin is also cytotoxic to several lines in culture. The pathogenic relevance of the monocytogenic factor of *Listeria*, an extractable lipid which provokes monocytosis in rodents, has no other recognized effect. This phenomenon, from which the species name *monocytogenes* was derived, is a characteristic feature of listeriosis in rodents but not in humans.

L. monocytogenes is considered a facultative intracellular pathogen (Mackaness, 1961) because it locates preferentially in the liver and spleen of laboratory animals with a propensity to multiply intracellularly.

NATURAL AND ACQUIRED IMMUNITY. *Listeria monocytogenes* is frequently isolated from the environment and the human gastro-intestinal tract. Relative to the abundance of *Listeria* in the environment, overt clinical disease is rare and commonly takes a benign, self-limited course in immunocompetent people.

Our understanding of the resistance factors responsible for this impressive immunity stems primarily from studies of experimental infection in laboratory animals. Extrapolation of these findings to human immunity is speculative, since the manifestations of listeriosis and resistance to disease differ greatly among different animal species and strains.

Mucosal resistance to *Listeria* is limited. Instillation of a saline suspension into the conjunctival sac of mice, rabbits or guinea pigs, even without scarification leads to local invasion followed within 24 to 72 hours by marked purulent keratoconjunctivitis. A similar phenomenon has been observed after accidental inoculation of the human eye (Anton, 1934). In guinea pigs gastro-enteric mucosal resistance to an oral challenge of *Listeria* can be overcome by neutralizing the gastric acid with bicarbonate and paralyzing the intestine with opium (Racz et al., 1972). Keratoconjunctivitis or gastroenteritis is a self limited localized disease in normal (but not immunosuppressed) animals. Hematogenous infection of the contents of the pregnant uterus after conjunctival or oral challenge indicate however that the local lesions are regularly accompanied by transient bacteremia (Gray and Killinger, 1966). The benign course of listeremia points to important host defense mechanisms that protect the immunocompetent animal from overwhelming infection after *Listeria* has breached mucosal resistance.

Like other gram-positive bacteria *L. monocytogenes* is resistant to complement even in the presence of specific antibody. Rabbits and rats produce alternative, humoral listericidal factors, probably cationic proteins, similar to or identical with beta-lysin (Czuprynski and Balish, 1981). This factor is released, at least in part, from platelets during the process of coagulation. Because heparin increased the susceptibility of rats to *Listeria*, it was proposed that this factor contributes to the relatively strong resistance of rats compared to mice which lack it (Davies et al., 1981). Early non-specific resistance of mice to *Listeria* appears to depend on the phagocytes of the RES. Macrophages, mainly in the spleen and liver, phagocytose circulating *Listeria*, restrict intracellular multiplication, and prevent overwhelming, rapidly fatal disease (Newborg and North, 1980). T lymphocyte dependent activation of macrophages is required, however, for control of high challenge doses and the ultimate elimination of *L. monocytogenes*. This important contribution of cell mediated immunity has been well documented by studies of nude mice, selective suppression of cell mediated immunity by Cyclosporin A, and transfer of protective immunity by lymphocytes from convalescent mice (Lane and Unanue, 1972; Schaffner et al., 1983). Judged by attempts to transfer protective immunity with anti-listeria sera, acquired humoral immunity is of little importance in resistance to listeriosis (Mackaness, 1961). Immunization with live, but not with heat-killed organisms, stimulates protective immunity in mice (Wirsing von Koenig et al., 1982).

DIAGNOSIS. Diagnosis of listeriosis depends on culture. In the past the use of special enrichment methods (Gray's cold enrichment technique) or the use of selective media was advocated. These procedures are valuable for the isolation of *Listeria* from heavily contaminated material such as feces but are not required for the isolation of the organism from most clinical specimens. Recognition of *Listeria* may, however, be hampered by the failure to

Table 1. DIFFERENTIATION OF *L. MONOCYTOGENES* FROM MORPHOLOGICALLY SIMILAR AND RELATED ORGANISMS

Species	Morphology	Motility 22c	Catalase	Hemolysis	Anton-Test*	Salicin
L. monocytogenes	coccoid, rods	+**	+	beta	+	+
Non-pathogenic *Listeria*#	coccoid, rods	+**	+$	–	–	+
Corynebacterium spp.	coccoid, rods	–	+/–	–/+	–	–
Erysipelothrix rhusiopathiae	slender rods	–	–	alpha	–	–
Lactobacillus spp.	rods	–	–	alpha	–	+/–
Streptococci$$	cocci	–	–	+/–	–	+

*Kerato-conjunctivitis in rabbits after inoculation of bacteria into the conjunctival sac.

**Characteristic tumbling, pinwheel type of motility in dark field. In stabbed semi-solid agar at room temperature an "umbrella" pattern of motility radiates from the inoculation channel.

$Rarely negative.

#*L. grayi, L. grayi,* biovar *murrayi, L. innocua.*

$$*Streptococcus faecalis* (variety zymogenes) may be hemolytic and motile. Since *L. monocytogenes* is also bile-esculin positive, coccoid forms can easily be confused with enterococci unless careful attention is given to the catalase test and the type of motility.

differentiate *Listeria* from other bacteria, such as "diptheroids" or streptococci. The most important criteria for differentiation of *L. monocytogenes* from similar organisms are given in Table 1.

Serodiagnosis is of little help in the diagnosis of listeriosis because of cross-reactive and/or natural antibodies (Gray and Killinger, 1966). The diagnostic use of more specific antigens has not been exploited.

DRUG SUSCEPTIBILITY. *L. monocytogenes* is susceptible to a broad range of antimicrobial agents. Ampicillin (<2 μg/ml), penicillin G (< 2 μg/ml), erythromycin (<1 μg/ml), trimethoprim (< 0.5 μg/ml), gentamicin (< 5 μg/ml), clindamycin (< 2 μg/ml), chloramphenicol (< 5 μg/ml), and vancomycin (< 5 μg/ml) inhibit the growth of *L. monocytogenes* in vitro. While inhibition is obtained at these concentrations, which are readily attained in vivo, in vitro killing often requires much higher concentrations, for example, 5 to 250 μg/ml for ampicillin and penicillin (Tuazon et al., 1982). The combination of gentamicin and ampicillin is synergistic in vitro and in a rabbit model of meningitis (Scheld et al., 1979).

EPIDEMIOLOGY. *L. monocytogenes* is ubiquitous, being found all over the world. It is found in a high percentage of environmental samples including surface water, soil, and vegetation. It is also isolated frequently from the feces of normal people and cattle. Animal contact appears to have only a minor influence on the carrier rate (Table 2). Several older studies found lower carrier rates (1 to 5%) but the results are difficult to compare because of differences in isolation techniques (Bojsen-Moller, 1972). Only pathogenic isolates of *Listeria monocytogenes* (established by hemolysis, serotyping, or pathogenicity in laboratory animals) should be evaluated in epidemiological surveys.

People usually become colonized and infected from environmental sources. Direct transmission of listeriosis from animals to man has been documented only rarely, for

Table 2. EPIDEMIOLOGY OF *L. MONOCYTOGENES**

Prevalence in Environment		Incidence of Human Disease†	
Population	***Rate (%)****	***Population***	***Rate***
Human feces			
random, NL 1972	11.9		
abattoir workers, NL 1972	13.3	U.S. 1971	0.51/10⁶
random, EU 1978	10.7	Northern EU, 1958–67	0.8–2.7/10⁶
Animal feces			
cattle, NL 1969	15.0		
Environment			
surface water, NL 1958–77,	11.9		
NL 1981	21.0		
sewage, NL 1976	93.0		
soil, vegetation, GB 1975	7.2		

*% of individuals or sample positive for pathogenic strains of *L. monocytogenes.* NL—Netherlands; EU—Europe; GB—Great Britain; U.S.—United States.

†Listeriosis is a reportable disease in Europe but not in the U.S., so figures for the latter may be underrated.

example, in veterinarians with listeric skin pustules (Gray and Killinger, 1966). A few instances of transmission by milk from cows with mastitis have been noted. Case clusters of human listeriosis have been attributed to contamination of vegetables by sheep manure from flocks with known cases of "circling disease" (Schlech et al., 1983). On the other hand, a large scale survey in the Netherlands showed that contamination of surface water stemmed largely from sewage draining from cities (Dijkstra, 1982). Raw sludge from sewage plants used as fertilizer contaminates the soil and *Listeria* persists for many months in such an environment (Watkins and Sleath, 1981). Listeriosis is more common in urban than rural populations and seasonal or yearly variations in the incidence of listeriosis in humans and animals do not correlate (Larsson, 1979). These are strong arguments that the epidemiology of listeriosis in humans and animals is largely independent. The capacity of *Listeria* to grow at low temperatures permits the organism to grow in refrigerated food and might be of epidemiologic importance.

Except for transplacental transmission, and possible infection during birth, human-to-human transmission has not been documented. There is circumstantial evidence of rare instances of nosocomial transmission of listeriosis in nurseries (Larsson, 1979).

References

Anton, W.: Kritisch experimenteller Beitrag zur Biologie des *Bakterium monocytogenes*. Zentr Bakteriol Parasitol Abt I Org 131:89, 1934.

Bojsen-Moller, J.: Human listeriosis. Diagnostic, epidemiological and clinical studies. Acta Pathol Microbiol Scand B 229 (suppl.):13, 1972.

Czuprinski, C. J., and Balisk, E.: Killing of *Listeria monocytogenes* by conventional and germfree rat sera. Infect Immun 33:348, 1981.

Davies, W. A., Ackerman, V. P., and Nelson, D. S.: Mechanism for nonspecific immunity to *Listeria monocytogenes* in rats mediated by platelets and the clotting system. Infect Immun 33:477, 1981.

Dijkstra, R. G.: The occurrence of Listeria monocytogenes in surface water of canals and lakes, in ditches of one big polder and in the effluents and canals of a sewage treatment plant. Zbl Bakt Hyg I Abt Org B 176:202, 1982.

Gray, M. L., and Killinger, A. H.: *Listeria monocytogenes* and listeric infections. Bacteriol Rev 30:309, 1966.

Hülphers, G.: Lefvernekros kanin orsakad af en ej förnt beskrifven bakterie. Sven Vet Tidskr 16:265, 1911.

Lane, F. C., and Unanue, E. R.: Requirement of thymus (T) lymphocytes for resistance to listeriosis. J Exp Med 135:1104, 1972.

Larsson, S.: Epidemiology of listeriosis in Sweden 1958–74. Scand J Infect Dis 11:47, 1979.

Mackaness, G. B.: Cellular resistance to infection. J Exp Med 116:381, 1961.

Murray, E. G. D., Webb, R. A., Swann, M. B. R.: A disease of rabbits characterized by large mononuclear leukocytosis, caused by a hitherto undescribed bacillus *Bacillus monocytogenes* (n. sp.). J Pathol Bacteriol 29:407, 1926.

Newborg, M. F., and North, R. J.: On the mechanism of T cell-independent anti-*Listeria* resistance in nude mice. J Immunol 124:571, 1980.

Paterson, J. St.: The antigenic structure of organisms of the genus Listerella. J Path Bact 48:25, 1940.

Racz, P., Tenner, K., and Mero, E.: Experimental listeric enteritis. 1. An electron microscopic study of the epithelial phase in experimental *Listeria* infection. Lab Invest 26:694, 1972.

Schaffner, A., Douglas, H., and Davis, C. E.: Models of T cell deficiency in listeriosis: The effects of cortisone and cyclosporin A on normal and nude BALB/c mice. J Immunol 131:450, 1983.

Scheld, W. M., Fletcher, D. D., Fink, F. N., and Sande, M. A.: Response to therapy in an experimental rabbit model of meningitis due to *Listeria monocytogenes*. J Infect Dis 140:287, 1979.

Schlech, W. F., Lavigne, P. M., Bortolini, R. A., et al.: Epidemic listeriosis—evidence for transmission by food. New Engl J Med 308:203, 1983.

Seeliger, H. P. R., and Finger, H.: Analytical serology of *Listeria*. In Kwapinski, J. B. G. (Ed.): Analytical serology of microorganisms. J. S. Wiley and Sons, Inc., vol. 2, 1969.

Seeliger, H. P. R., Schweitenbrunner, A., Pongrek, G., and Hof, H.: Special position of strongly haemolytic strains of the genus *Listeria*. Zbl Bakt Hyg I Abt Orig A 252:176, 1982.

Smith, C. W., and Meztger, J. W.: Demonstration of a capsular structure on *Listeria monocytogenes*. Pathol Microbiol 25:499, 1962.

Tuazon, C. U., Shamsuddin, D., and Miller, H.: Antibiotic susceptibility and synergy of clinical isolates of *Listeria monocytogenes*. Antimicrob Agents Chemother 21:525, 1982.

Watking J., and Sleath, K. P.: Isolation and enumeration of *Listeria monocytogenes* from sewage, sewage sludge and river water. J Appl Bacteriol 50:1, 1981.

Wirsing von Koenig, C. H., Finger, H., and Hof, H.: Failure of killed *Listeria monocytogenes* vaccine to produce protective immunity. Nature 297:233, 1982.

27

ERYSIPELOTHRIX RHUSIOPATHIAE

CHARLES E. DAVIS, M.D.

Erysipelothrix rhusiopathiae is a facultatively anaerobic, gram-positive bacillus that shares many characteristics with *Listeria monocytogenes* (Chapter 26), corynebacteria, lactobacilli, and certain streptococci. The technique of numerical taxonomy, and the guanine plus cytosine content of its DNA indicate a closer relationship to *Listeria*, lactobacilli, and some streptococci than to coryneform bacteria but no definite relationship to any family of bacteria. In the eighth edition of Bergey's Manual of Determinative Bacteriology (1974), *Erysipelothrix* and *Listeria* have been removed from the chapter on coryneform bacteria and placed in the *Lactobacillus* chapter as genera of uncertain affiliation. *Erysipelothrix* may be more closely related to lactobacilli than *Listeria*. *Listeria*, but neither *Erysipelothrix* nor lactobacilli, synthesizes catalase, cytochromes, and isoprenoid quinones (Collins et al., 1978).

Erysipelothrix was first recovered from mice in 1880 by Koch. In 1882, Löffler and Pasteur and Thuillier independently isolated *Erysipelothrix* from pigs with erysipelas. Only two years later, Rosenbach isolated the same organism from an erysipeloid lesion of a patient and established it as the cause of erysipeloid by inoculating himself with the isolate. Although *Erysipelothrix* is still isolated from zoonotic skin infections of patients and from rare cases of septicemia and endocarditis, its major importance is the economic loss associated with outbreaks of swine erysipelas.

MORPHOLOGY. *Erysipelothrix rhusiopathiae* is a gram-positive, nonmotile, nonsporulating bacillus that may form either smooth or rough colonies on primary isolation. Smooth colonies are entire, convex, transparent, and about 1.0 mm in diameter. There may be a blue sheen by reflected light. Broth cultures are uniformly turbid. Rough colonies are larger and granular with a matte appearance on agar and flocculent with hair-like projections in broth.

Cells from smooth colonies are small, slender, straight or slightly curved bacilli that measure from 0.2 to 0.4 μm in width by 0.5 to 2.5 μm in length. Cells from rough colonies vary from short forms to long chains of bacilli. Some are filamentous and beaded like the actinomycetes. Others may have large, fundus-like swellings.

Fully developed colonies on blood agar are surrounded by a zone of greening that may clear on further incubation. Colonies on tellurite agar are pinpoint and gray at 24 hours, but they become larger and jet black by 48 to 72 hours.

ANTIGENIC COMPOSITION. *Erysipelothrix* has been divided into at least 22 serotypes according to cross-agglutination studies against heat-resistant, acid-soluble antigens (Kucsera, 1973; Norrung, 1979). These antigens are thought to be peptidoglycans of the cell wall. Most isolates from swine fall into serotypes 1 and 2.

Although Pasteur and Thuillier successfully immunized swine against *Erysipelothrix* in 1883 with live organisms attenuated by passage through rabbits, little was known about the protective antigen until recently. White and Verway (1970 and 1970a) found that soluble protective antigens in culture supernatants contained a glycolipoprotein that was probably derived from the cell wall, since 75 per cent of the protective activity was destroyed by pretreatment of the antigen with muramidase. Trypsin and heat also destroyed part of the protective activity of this antigen, which was soluble in butanol but unaffected by lipase or ribonuclease.

Animals immunized with either the vaccine of Pasteur and Thuillier or cell-free culture supernatants develop agglutinins to whole bacteria.

METABOLISM. *Erysipelothrix rhusiopathiae* is microaerophilic. It will grow when exposed to atmospheric concentrations of oxygen but grows best in reduced oxygen tension with 5 to 10 per cent carbon dioxide. *E. rhusiopathiae* multiplies at temperatures of 16 to 41° C. Optimum growth occurs at 33 to 37° C. It obtains the energy for growth by glycolysis and does not produce catalase, cytochromes, or isoprenoid quinones even when grown aerobically. All strains produce acid but no gas from glucose, galactose, fructose, and lactose.

Riboflavin and oleic acid are required for growth. Acid production from carbohydrates is poor in 1 per cent peptone water. Five per cent rabbit serum or yeast autolysate should be added to the sugar in 1 per cent peptone water.

One of the unique metabolic properties of *Erysipelothrix* is the production of hydrogen sulfide. Among gram-positive organisms, only a few species of streptococci and *Bacillus* show this characteristic. *Erysipelothrix* acidifies the butt of Kligler's iron agar by producing organic acids from glucose by the process of anaerobic respiration with thiosulfate as the electron acceptor. In this acid environment, thiosulfate is broken down to sulfite and H_2S gas by the enzyme thiosulfate reductase, which is produced in most bacteria that generate H_2S.

PATHOGENIC PROPERTIES. *Erysipelothrix* is a natural pathogen primarily of mice, fish, swine, and man. Sheep, turkeys, other wild and domestic fowl, dolphins, and other cetaceans are also susceptible to natural infections. In swine, *Erysipelothrix* produces three clinical types of disease: acute fatal septicemia, red rhomboid-shaped skin lesions ("diamond skin disease"), and chronic disease with endocarditis of the mitral valves. Arthritis is a frequent complication of all forms of swine erysipelas and may also occur independently of the other manifestations. Laboratory mice die of overwhelming septicemia after intraperitoneal inoculation.

Erysipelothrix causes skin infections in man that are called erysipeloid because they resemble streptococcal erysipelas. These lesions usually occur on the hand after contact with infected animals or animal products. Arthritis of nearby joints is common (see Chapter 259).

The virulence of different strains of *Erysipelothrix* for mice varies, but most strains kill mice. Variations in virulence are independent of serotype, biochemical properties, and protein composition as determined by patterns on electrophoresis and electrofocusing (White and Mirikitani, 1976) but serotypes 1 and 2 are the most common causes of swine erysipelas. The virulence factors have not been determined, but virulence is related to rapid growth and the production of neuraminidase (Krasemann and Muller, 1975). Inoculation of a partially purified glycoprotein from culture filtrates into the skin of rabbits causes necrosis. Intravenous inoculation of this product also causes high fevers in rabbits (Leimbeck et al., 1975).

The pathogenesis of *Erysipelothrix* arthritis has been extensively studied because it is a prominent feature of swine erysipelas and erysipeloid in man (Chapter 259). It has been used as a laboratory model of relapsing, erosive arthritis because its histopathology and course are similar to rheumatoid arthritis (Hadler, 1976). Intravenous inoculations of whole live organisms causes polyarthritis in swine, dogs, and rabbits. Rabbits develop heterologous rheumatoid factor (Astorga, 1969) and polyarthritis after injection of dead organisms and cell-free culture extracts (White et al., 1971). This cell-free extract contains murein and many proteins. Some of these products bind rapidly to the synovium, persist for as long as six months, and cause cytopathic changes in synovial cell cultures after a single brief exposure (White et al., 1976). The exact antigen or antigens responsible for this effect have not been isolated, but it is clear that the pathogenic factors do not require the continuing presence of the organism.

IMMUNITY. Active immunization with the live attenuated vaccine of Pasteur and Thuillier protects against swine erysipelas, although experimental mice are not protected against some of the unusual serotypes of *Erysipelothrix* (Wood, 1979). This protection is probably mediated by antibody because passive protection with antiserum provides effective prophylaxis for at least two weeks. The protective antigen in this preparation is a glycolipoprotein that is destroyed by lysozyme (White and Verway, 1970 and 1970a). The immune response after vaccination with either whole cells or cell-free culture extracts may be monitored by the titer of agglutinins to *Erysipelothrix*. Immunization is effective after a single inoculation. Swine do not develop clinical arthritis after immunization. Polyarthritis from culture extracts develops only after multiple intravenous inoculations. This arthritis does not seem to be primarily an antibody-mediated autoimmune phenomenon, since persistence of bacterial antigens in the synovium has been demonstrated (White et al., 1976).

Natural human infection with *E. rhusiopathiae* also stimulates the production of agglutinins, but patients undergo relapses and reinfections. Immunization of swine probably does not prevent colonization of the tonsils and gastroin-

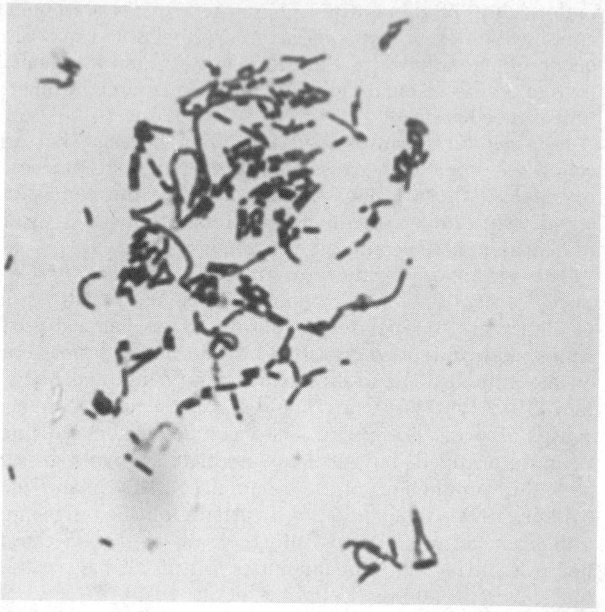

Figure 1. Gram stain appearance of rough colony of *E. rhusiopathiae.* Note predominance of filamentous beaded bacilli.

testinal tract. It is possible that swine are more effectively immunized by vaccination than man is by natural infection because swine are reimmunized by colonization with *Erysipelothrix* (see Epidemiology, below).

Crude culture extracts are cytopathic for synovial cells and probably mitogenic for lymphocytes (White and Mirikitani, 1976), but the role of cellular immunity against this bacterium has not been determined.

LABORATORY DIAGNOSIS. Gram stains of aspirates or biopsies from erysipeloid or blood cultures from patients with septicemia and endocarditis may reveal coccobacillary, coryneform, or filamentous gram-positive bacilli. Forms that are almost indistinguishable from streptococci are not uncommon either from infected material or from primary isolation plates. Growth is enhanced by carbon dioxide, reduced oxygen tension, and 5 per cent serum. Both smooth and rough colonies (see Morphology, above) usually produce a zone of greening on blood agar. This zone may clear on further incubation. Gram stains of smooth colonies usually reveal coccobacillary or coryneform bacilli, while smears of the larger rough colonies often show a predominance of filamentous, beaded bacilli that may resemble actinomycetes or lactobacilli (Fig. 1).

Two unique cultural features of *Erysipelothrix* should prevent confusion with any other gram-positive rod. Except for a few species of *Bacillus* and a few streptococci, *E. rhusiopathiae* is the only gram-positive bacterium that will produce H_2S in Kligler's iron agar incubated in air. It also produces a unique appearance in gelatin stab cultures if the tube is incubated at temperatures low enough to keep the gelatin in a solid state. Bead-like colonies with lateral filamentous growth develop and resemble a test-tube brush.

Erysipelothrix is nonmotile, and is negative for catalase, oxidase, and indole production; it does not reduce nitrate to nitrite. It makes acid but not gas from glucose, lactose, galactose, and fructose. Some strains make acid from mannose (10/14) and xylose (4/14) (White and Mirikitani, 1976). It makes an acid slant and butt in Kligler's iron agar and triple sugar iron agar with enough H_2S formation to blacken the butt. Key biochemical reactions are shown in Table 1.

Erysipelothrix can be easily differentiated from *Listeria* (Chapter 26) because *Listeria* is motile and beta-hemolytic and does not produce H_2S (Table 1). *Erysipelothrix* is resistant to neomycin and kanamycin, but *Listeria* is not. Intraperitoneal inoculation of mice with a 24- to 48-hour culture of *Erysipelothrix* kills mice within two to three days but will not cause keratoconjunctivitis when dropped into the eye of a rabbit. *Listeria* causes keratoconjunctivitis in rabbits. *Erysipelothrix* can be differentiated from all lactobacilli and corynebacteria by the production of H_2S in KIA or TSI slants. Corynebacteria also produce catalase except for *C. pyogenes* and *C. haemolyticum*, which are beta-hemolytic.

DRUG SUSCEPTIBILITY. *E. rhusiopathiae* is exquisitely sensitive to penicillin (0.0025 to 0.02 μg/ml), ampicillin, the semisynthetic penicillins, the cephalosporins, erythro-

Table 1. CHARACTERISTICS OF *ERYSIPELOTHRIX RHUSIOPATHIAE*

Test or Compound	Reaction	Comment
Alpha-hemolysis	+	
Beta-hemolysis	−	*Listeria, C. pyogenes,* and *C. haemolyticum* are +
Motility	−	*Listeria* is +
H_2S in KIA or TSI	+	*Listeria,* corynebacteria and lactobacilli are −
Nitrate reduction	−	
Catalase	−	*Listeria* and most corynebacteria are +
Esculin hydrolysis	−	*Listeria* is +
Glucose	A[a]	*Erysipelothrix* produces acid without gas from carbohydrates
Lactose	A	
Fructose	A	
Galactose	A	
Mannose	A(10/14)	
Xylose	−(10/14)	
Resistance to neomycin and kanamycin	+	*Listeria* is sensitive
Pathogenic for mice	+	
Keratoconjunctivitis in rabbits	−	*Listeria* is +
Per cent G + C	36.5%	*Listeria* is 38%

[a]A few drops of rabbit serum or yeast autolysate should be added to carbohydrate tests if the base is 1 per cent peptone water.

mycin, and clindamycin. It is also susceptible to readily achievable levels of tetracycline. Some strains are only moderately sensitive to chloramphenicol. It is resistant to the aminoglycosides, vancomycin, sulfonamides, and polymyxin.

EPIDEMIOLOGY. *Erysipelothrix* lives on dead and dying organic matter in the environment. It can be isolated in large numbers from the slime covering the bodies of fish and has been isolated from the soil of pig pens as long as five years after an outbreak of swine erysipelas. The organism tolerates high salt concentrations and develops as well in sea water as it does in fresh water.

Erysipelothrix also colonizes many animals including fish, cetaceans, wild and domestic birds, and rodents, especially mice and rats. Its primary economic importance is in agriculture, in which significant losses of poultry and swine are common. *Erysipelothrix* colonizes a high percentage of apparently normal swine. In one recent study (Stephenson and Berman, 1978), the tonsils of 62 out of 63 normal pigs were colonized by *Erysipelothrix* at slaughter. The organism is widely distributed throughout Europe and the United States. Tissue (primarily spleens) of hogs from 2633 herds in 46 states of the United States were contaminated with *E. rhusiopathiae* in another recent study (Harrington and Ellis, 1975). In this study, the swine came from herds in which hog cholera was suspected, and 21.1 per cent were infected with *Erysipelothrix*.

Hogs and other wild and domestic animals can probably be infected either through the skin or through the alimentary canal. The tonsils may be one of the major foci of infection in hogs. Hogs and poultry probably acquire Erysipelothrix primarily from the soil of their pens, but uncooked garbage and rodents may also be a major source of swine infection. The peak incidence of swine erysipelas occurs in the summer. The peak incidence of human disease occurs in the fall and winter shortly after outbreaks of swine erysipelas.

E. rhusiopathiae infection is primarily an occupational disease in humans. Farmers, abbatoir workers, poultry workers, fishermen, and housewives acquire the infection through skin abrasions while handling infected meat. Occasionally, cases of septicemia and endocarditis have no apparent preceding skin infection. Some investigators believe that these infections may be acquired through the gastrointestinal tract after ingestion of improperly prepared infected meat or fish. Human-to-human transmission has never been proved.

Disease in domestic animals and humans can be prevented by immunization of animals with the vaccine of Pasteur and Thuillier and by improved practices of animal husbandry. Housewives and those at occupational risk should handle meat and fish cautiously and wear gloves when possible.

References

Astorga, G.P.: Immunologic studies of an experimental chronic arthritis resembling rheumatoid arthritis. Arthritis Rheum. 12:589–596, 1969.

Collins, M. D., Jones, D., Goodfellow, M., and Minnikin, D. E.: Isoprenoid quinone composition as a guide to the classification of *Listeria*, Brochothrix, *Erysipelothrix*, and Caryophanon. J Gen Microbiol 111:453, 1979.

Hadler, Nortin H.: A pathogenetic model for erosive synovitis. Lessons from animal arthritidies. Arthritis and Rheumatism 19:256–266, 1976.

Harrington, R., and Ellis, E. M.: Salmonella and Erysipelothrix infection in swine: A laboratory survey. Am. J. Vet. Res. 36:1379–80, 1975.

Jones, D.: The taxonomic position of *Listeria*. *In* M. Woodbine (ed.): *Problems of Listeriosis*. Leicester University Press, Leicester, 1975, pp. 4–17.

Krasemann, C., and H. E. Muller: The virulence of *Erysipelothrix rhusiopathiae* strains and their virulence production. Zentrabl. Bakteriol. [ORIG A] 231 (1–3), 206–213, 1975.

Kucsera, G.: Proposal for standardization of the designations used for serotypes of *Erysipelothrix rhusiopathiae* (Migula) Buchanan. Int. J. Syst. Bacteriol. 23:184–188, 1973.

Leimbeck, R., K. H. Bohm, H. Ehard, and L.-Cl Schulz: Studies of the toxic components of *Erysipelothrix rhusiopathiae:* Detailed characterization of an extracted endotoxin. Zentrabl. Bakteriol. [ORIG A] 232 (2–3), 266–286, 1975.

Nørrung, V.: Two new senotypes of *Erysipelothrix rhusiopathiae*. Nord Vet Med 31:462, 1979.

Stephenson, E. H., and D. T. Berman: Isolation of *Erysipelothrix rhusiopathiae* from tonsils of apparently normal swine by 2 methods. Am. J. Vet. Res. 39:187–188, 1978.

White, R. R., and W. F. Verway: Isolation and characterization of a protective antigen-containing particle from culture supernatant fluids of *Erysipelothrix rhusiopathiae*. Infect. Immun. 1:380–386, 1970.

White, R. R., and W. F. Verway: Solubilization and characterization of a protective antigen of *Erysipelothrix rhusiopathiae*. Infect. Immun. 1:387–393, 1970(a).

White, T. G., J. L. Puls, and F. K. Mirikitani: Rabbit arthritis induced by cell-free extracts of *Erysipelothrix*. Infect. Immun. 3:715–722, 1971.

White, T. G., F. K. Mirikitani, and P. Hargrove: The effect of bacterial extracts on synovial cells in tissue culture. *In Vitro* 12:702–707, 1976.

White, T. G., and F. R. Mirikitani: Some biological and physical-chemical properties of *Erysipelothrix rhusiopathiae*. Cornell Vet. 66:152–163, 1976.

Wood, R. L., and R. A. Packer: Isolation of *Erysipelothrix rhusiopathiae* from soil and manure of swine-raising premises. Am. J. Vet. Res. 33:1610–1620, 1972.

Wood, R. L.: Specificity in response of vaccinated swine and mice to challenge exposure with strains of *Erysipelothrix rhusiopathiae* of various serotypes. Am J Vet Res 40:795, 1979.

28

BACILLUS ANTHRACIS AND OTHER AEROBIC SPORE-FORMING BACILLI

ROBERT P. WILLIAMS, PH.D.

MORPHOLOGY. The genus *Bacillus* is a member of the family Bacillaceae. The bacteria are rod-shaped, and the majority are motile by means of lateral flagella. An important exception is *Bacillus anthracis,* which lacks flagella and is not motile. Formation of a single endospore in the vegetative bacterium is a dominant feature of the genus. Spores may be oval or spherical, and may be located centrally, subterminally, or terminally. The presence of spores causes the vegetative cell to swell in some species. Capsules are present in a few species, particularly *Bacillus anthracis,* whose virulent strains synthesize a polypeptide capsular material composed of repeating units of D-glutamic acid.

The bacteria can be divided into two groups depending on the size of the vegetative cell (Table 1). In small cell species the bacterium has a width of 0.6 to 0.8 μm and a length of 1.5 to 3 μm; in large cell species, the width is 1.0 to 1.5 μm and the length 2 to 5 μm. Although usually gram positive, some species show a variable reaction, particularly if the stain is made from samples taken in the later stages of growth. Sometimes globules of a reserve metabolic material, poly-beta-hydroxybutyrate, are seen in vegetative bacteria of *B. anthracis, B. cereus,* and related species.

The structure of the endospore and its location within the vegetative cell are characteristics useful for taxonomy (Table 1). In morphological Group I, which includes *B. anthracis, B. cereus,* and *B. subtilis,* the spore is oval, has a central location, and does not distend the vegetative cell. Vegetative cells of *B. subtilis* do not contain globules of poly-beta-hydroxybutyrate. Spores of Group II, including *B. macerans* and *B. polymyxa,* cause the vegetative cell to swell. These spores usually are located centrally but also may be found subterminally or terminally. Under the electron microscope, thin sections of these spores show a thick spore coat with several prominent longitudinal, parallel ridges on the surface. The ridges are not seen on spores of other species. *B. sphaericus* is included in Group III, in which the spores are round, are located terminally, and cause the vegetative cell to swell. The endospores of *B. cereus, B. anthracis,* and *B. thuringiensis* are enclosed within a loose outer coat, the exosporium.

The different species have an enormous range of colonial morphology that can vary according to the composition of the medium. Isolated colonies may be quite rough and may spread over the surface, particularly if the agar is moist. Pigments sometimes color colonies yellow, pink, red, or even black.

B. anthracis grows in vitro in long chains that look like a jointed bamboo rod. In vivo, the chains are shorter, and single bacilli or pairs of rods may be seen (Fig. 1). When grown in culture, no capsule can be seen around anthrax bacteria unless they are grown under an increased tension of carbon dioxide. Capsules are readily apparent around the bacteria when smears from infected animals are examined, particularly if a polychrome stain is used (Fig. 1). When grown on conventional media in air, encapsulated anthrax bacteria, the virulent form, grow as rough colonies. But when the same bacteria are incubated on media containing bicarbonate in an atmosphere of increased carbon dioxide, the colonies are mucoid and smooth (Fig. 2), and capsules are readily seen around the rods (Fig. 3). No other species of *Bacillus* grows in this fashion under these conditions. *B. anthracis* forms spores only under aerobic conditions; thus, spores are not seen in the circulating blood of infected animals.

ANTIGENIC COMPOSITION. The genus *Bacillus* forms an antigenically heterogeneous group. However, data about the definitive antigenic composition of the various species are scant. Vegetative cells and spores contain different antigens. Since the bacteria usually are motile, flagellar or H antigens are also present. Unfortunately, except for *B. cereus* and *B. thuringiensis,* in which serotyping schemes have been developed based upon agglutinins formed against the H antigens, the antigenic composition of the genus has been of little help in distinguishing species or strains from one another.

Spores and vegetative cells are antigenically distinct, although some investigators claim that vegetative antigens can be found in spores. Spore antigens can distinguish among the small cell species of the genus, but differentiation among large cell species is less successful. Injection of autoclaved spores into animals produces agglutinins and precipitins to the spores. If live spores are injected, antibodies against both the spore and the vegetative cell develop. The precipitinogens seem to be mainly species-specific, while the agglutinogens show subspecies distribution.

Vegetative cell, spore, and flagellar antigens show different levels of specificity. Considerable cross-reaction occurs among species with respect to vegetative cell antigen. Spore antigens seem to provide the highest species specificity, whereas flagellar antigens show the greatest strain specificity within species. Spores of *B. anthracis* and *B. cereus* can be differentiated by quantitative immunofluorescence.

A serotyping scheme has been developed based on agglutination with the H antigen of *B. cereus* and has been used in epidemiologic studies of outbreaks of food poisoning caused by the bacteria. Strains of *B. cereus* were classified into 23 serotypes by the scheme and about 90 per cent of the strains isolated from the vomiting type of food poisoning could be typed. Of strains isolated from other types of food poisoning and infections, only about 50 per cent are typable.

The capsular polypeptide of *B. anthracis* is antigenic, although antibodies against it are not protective against infection. Only one capsular type of *B. anthracis* is known. An antigenic polysaccharide is a component of the cell wall of *B. anthracis.* Antibodies to the polysaccharide cross-react with sera prepared from vegetative cells of *B. cereus.* Whereas *B. anthracis* seems to possess only one type of cell-wall antigen, several types are present in *B. cereus* and *B. megaterium.* However, little success has been achieved in the serologic identification of strains of *B. cereus* on the basis of cell-wall antigens. The complex protein toxin produced by *B. anthracis* also is antigenic (Table 2).

Table 1. CHARACTERISTICS USEFUL TO DIFFERENTIATE BETWEEN SOME SPECIES OF *BACILLUS*[a]

Characteristic	**Morphological Group and Species of *Bacillus*[b]**														
	Group I								***Group II***						***Group III***
	anthracis	*cereus*[c]	*coagulans*	*firmus*	*licheniformis*	*megaterium*	*pumilus*	*subtilis*	*alvei*	*brevis*	*circulans*	*laterosporus*	*macerans*	*polymyxa*	*sphaericus*
Morphologic															
Gram stain	+	+	+	+	+	+	+	+	v	v	v	v	v	v	v
Size[d]	l	l	s	s	s	l	s	s	s	s	s	s	s	s	s
Motility	−	v	+	v	+	v	+	+	+	+	v	+	+	+	+
Spore shape[e]	o	o	o	o	o	o	o	o	o	o	o	o	o	o	r
Spore location[f]	c	c	cts	c	c	c	c	c	cts	cts	cts	c	t	cts	t
Swelling of vegetative cell	−	−	v	−	−	−	−	−	+	+	+	+	+	+	+
Capsule	+[g]	−	−	−	+	v	−	−	−	−	−	−	−	+	−
Biochemical															
Casein hydrolysis	+	+	v	+	+	+	+	+	+	+	v	+	−	+	v
Catalase	+	+	+	+	+	+	+	+	+	+	+	+	+	+	+
Fermentations (acid)[h]															
Arabinose	−	−	v	v	+	v	+	+	−	−	+	−	+	+	−
Glucose	+	+	+	d	+	+	+	+	+	+	+	+	+[i]	+[i]	−
Mannitol	−	−	v	+	+	v	+	+	−	v	+	+	+	+	−
Xylose	−	−	v	v	+	v	+	+	−	−	+	−	+	+	−
Citrate utilization	v	+	v	−	+	+	+	+	−	v	v	−	v	−	v
Gelatin liquefaction	+	+	−	+	+	+	+	+	+	+	+	+	+	+	v
Hemolysis on sheep blood agar[j]	−	+	n	n	n	n	n	±	n	n	n	n	n	n	n
Lecithinase activity	+	+	−	−	−	−	−	−	−	−	−	+	−	−	v
Nitrate reduction	+	+	v	v	+	v	−	+	−	v	v	+	+	+	−
Starch hydrolysis	+	+	+	+	+	+	−	+	+	−	+	−	+	+	−
Voges-Proskauer reaction	+	+	v	−	+	−	+	+	+	−	−	−	−	+	−
Anaerobic growth[k]	+	+	+	−	+	−	−	−	+	−	v	+	+	+	−
Growth in 0.001% lysozyme	+	+	−	−	−	−	v	v	+	v	v	+	−	v	v
Growth at pH <6	+	+	+	−	+	+	+	+	−	v	v	−	+	+	v
Growth in 7% NaCl	+	v	−	+	+	+	+	+	−	−	v	−	−	−	v
Growth at 50°C	−	−	+	−	+	−	+	+	−	+	+	v	v	−	−

[a]Data obtained principally from Bergey's Manual of Determinative Bacteriology, 8th ed., Cowan and Steel, Manual for the Identification of medical Bacteria, 2nd ed., and Parry, Turnbull, and Gibson, A Colour Atlas of *Bacillus* Species.

[b]Variable reactions indicated by v; d indicates delayed reaction; n indicates reaction not reported in the manuals.

[c]*B. cereus* var. *mycoides* is not listed as a legitimate species in Bergey's Manual but is often mentioned in the literature and seen in the laboratory. This variant grows as large, rhizoid colonies whose outgrowths may cover the agar surface. The variant usually is not motile, in contrast to *B. cereus.* The insect pathogen *B. thuringiensis* also has identical reactions to *B. cereus* but can be differentiated by the presence of a parasporal crystal in cultures that have sporulated. The crystals can be stained or seen by phase contrast microscopy (see Parry et al.).

[d]l represents large (width 1.0 to 1.5 μm and length 2 to 5 μm); s represents small (width 0.6 to 0.8 μm and length 1.7 to 3 μm).

[e]o represents oval; r, round.

[f]c represents central; t, terminal; and s, subterminal.

[g]Demonstration of capsule requires special growth conditions (see text).

[h]In media containing $(NH_4)_2HPO_4$ and the appropriate sugar.

[i]Gas also is produced.

[j]Presence of hemolysis eliminates possibility of *B. anthracis* but lack of hemolysis may be characteristic of other species also.

[k]In broth containing glucose.

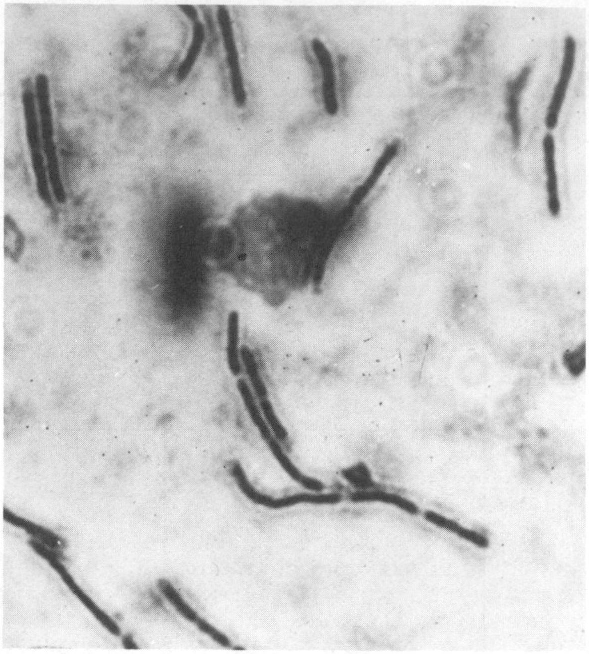

Figure 1. Blood smear from a moribund guinea pig infected with *B. anthracis*. Smear was stained with polychrome methylene blue.

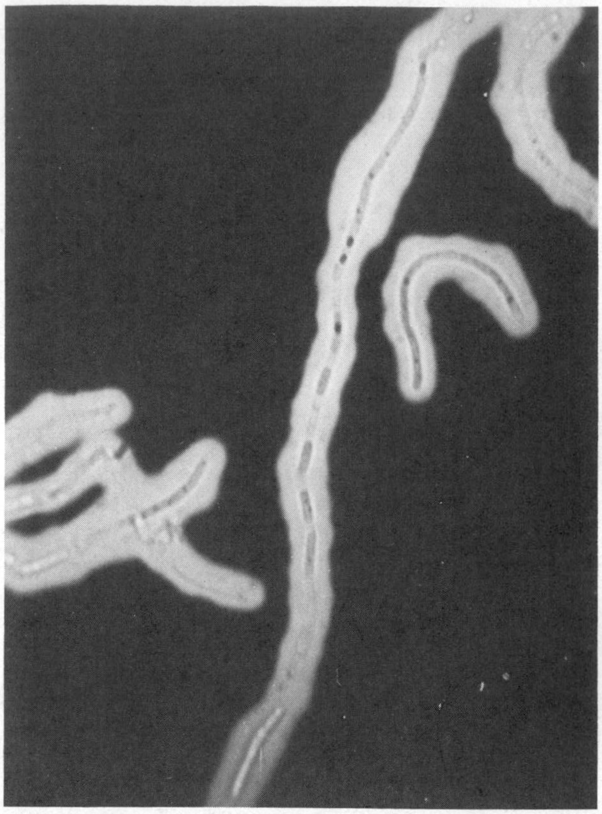

Figure 3. Smear of bacteria stained with India ink from colonies of *B. anthracis* grown in a candle jar on bicarbonate medium. Note the abundant capsule around the bacteria.

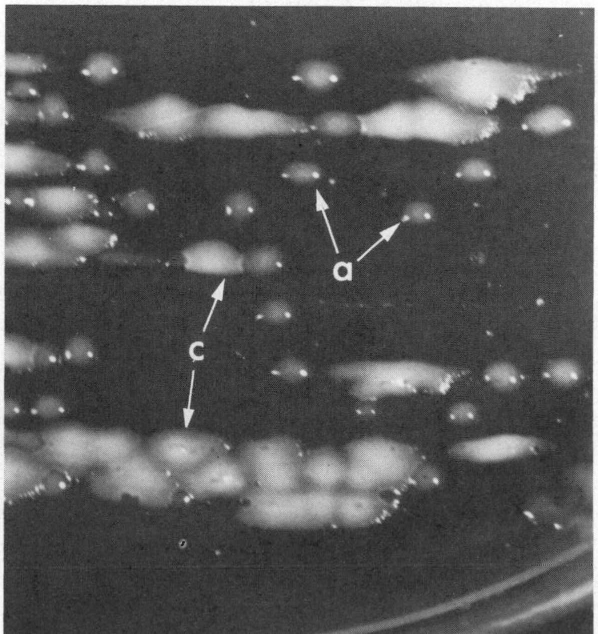

Figure 2. Colonial morphology of virulent *B. anthracis* (smooth colonies, a) and *B. cereus* (rough colonies, c) when grown on nutrient agar containing 0.7 per cent of sodium bicarbonate and incubated at 35°C in a candle jar.

METABOLISM. The great diversity among species of *Bacillus* is exemplified by their metabolism. The bacteria are classified as aerobes, but most species are facultative anaerobes, although growth occurs best aerobically. All are chemoheterotrophs and can dissimilate a variety of organic substrates such as amino acids, organic acids, and sugars to obtain carbon and energy by aerobic respiration, anaerobic respiration, or fermentation. Adenosine triphosphate (ATP) usually is generated from an aerobic electron transport chain.

Growth requirements range from simple to complex. Most species grow readily on nutrient agar or peptone media. *B. subtilis* grows on a minimal medium containing glucose, citrate, ammonium phosphate, and the usual mineral salts. *B. cereus* requires the addition of certain amino acids, whereas *B. anthracis* needs in addition thiamine, and its growth is stimulated by adenine, guanine, and uracil. Some of the insect pathogens have a more fastidious nutrition and require factors for growth that have not been identified.

Most species grow optimally at pH 7, but some species can grow under alkaline conditions at pH 9, while a few tolerate acidic conditions as low as pH 2. The optimal temperature for growth of the majority of species is 30 to 45° C. *B. stearothermophilus* is thermophilic and grows vigorously at 65° C. Other extreme thermophiles occur in the genus, but these species have not been well characterized. They grow in hot, moist environments such as hay stacks, where they decompose plant material. A few species are psychrophiles and grow at temperatures below 25° C.

Fermentation of glucose can yield a mixture of end products depending upon the species. Initial dissimilation of the sugar is through the Embden-Meyerhof pathway. *B. cereus* and other large cell species of Group I produce 2,3-butanediol, glycerol, and carbon dioxide and small amounts of lactate and ethanol. *B. anthracis* can grow anaerobically on sugars, but *B. megaterium* cannot. A small cell variety of Group I, *B. subtilis*, also cannot grow anaerobically on glucose, perhaps because the enzyme for reduction of triose phosphate to glycerol is missing, but in air this bacterium does produce large quantities of 2,3-butanediol. *B. licheniformis* is unique in the genus because it can carry out denitrification. Another unique member of Group I, *B. fastidiosus* utilizes uric acid as the only source of energy, carbon, and nitrogen, producing ammonia, carbon dioxide, and cell material.

Good growth of species in Group II occurs only on utilizable carbohydrates. *B. polymyxa* produces 2,3-butanediol from glucose but not glycerol. *B. macerans* ferments glucose with the formation of ethanol, acetone, acetate, formate, carbon dioxide, and H_2. Both species can dissimilate starch and pectins, and they participate in the retting of flax. When grown anaerobically, both species can fix atmospheric nitrogen.

Species of Group III such as *B. sphaericus* do not use carbohydrates effectively as sources of energy because they lack fermentative ability. They utilize amino and organic acids as oxidizable substrates. Many strains produce urease, which hydrolyzes urea to form ammonia, and during growth of these bacteria the pH of the medium rapidly becomes alkaline.

The different species produce an abundance of extracellular products including antimicrobial substances, enzymes, pigments, and in some cases toxins. With few exceptions, primarily among the insect pathogens and thermophiles, catalase is formed. Amylase, collagenase, hemolysin, lecithinase, phospholipase, protease, and urease are some of the other enzymes that can be found in cultures. *B. anthracis* does not synthesize hemolysin, and this deficiency is used to separate this pathogen from other members of the genus. The enzyme activities, fermentation reactions, and other characteristics of metabolism form the basis for the differentiation of the several species of *Bacillus* (Table 1).

Several species produce pigments, two of which have been identified. Pulcherrimin, the ferric salt of the pyrazine compound pulcherriminic acid, is synthesized by strains of *B. cereus*, *B. licheniformis*, and *B. subtilis*. An aromatic compound, protocatechuic acid, is formed by *B. anthracis*, probably as a derivative of shikimic acid. When complexed with iron in various proportions, protocatechuic acid causes liquid cultures to vary in color from brown to pink to red. Virulent strains of *B. anthracis* reportedly produce more protocatechuic acid than avirulent strains. Unidentified pigments formed by some species are black, tan, or yellow.

B. cereus and *B. anthracis* synthesize toxins that cause disease in humans (Tables 2 and 3). Cultural conditions, particularly the tension of carbon dioxide, are critical for synthesis of anthrax toxin. If cultures of *B. cereus* are rapidly transferred in broth, they produce an uncharacterized toxin that is extremely lethal for guinea pigs and mice. A toxin from *B. thuringiensis* also is lethal for mice. Toxins from *B. lentimorbus*, *B. popilliae*, and *B. thuringiensis* are lethal for insects.

Production of antimicrobial substances prior to the onset of sporulation is characteristic of the genus. These compounds are linear or cyclic polypeptides with a molecular weight of about 1400. Many of the amino acids in the peptides are of the D configuration. Biosynthesis of the peptides does not involve transfer ribonucleic acid (tRNA) and ribosomes; their assembly instead is directed by a protein enzyme. Examples of these antimicrobial compounds are bacitracin, gramicidin, polymyxin, and tyrocidine.

The peptidoglycan of the vegetative cell wall usually is similar to the type found in gram-negative bacteria. The diamino acid, *meso*-diaminopimelic acid, is present but in some species is replaced with lysine. The cortex of spores contains a unique peptidoglycan that contains three repeating subunits: a muramic acid unit without attached amino acids; a muramic acid unit attached to an alanine residue; and a muramic acid unit attached to L-alanine, D-glutamic acid, *meso*-diaminopimelic acid, and D-alanine.

The guanine plus cytosine content of the DNA of species ranges from 32 to 53 moles per cent. The DNA base composition of *B. cereus* and *B. anthracis* is similar but not the same, indicating that these two species are related but not identical. Relationships between some species have been studied by use of genetic recombination mediated by transformation or by transduction, or by use of DNA-to-DNA hybridization. Because the DNA of *B. subtilis* is readily transferred, and the bacteria grow well on a minimal medium, this species has been used extensively for studies of bacterial physiology and genetics. Mutants, both natural and induced, of various species can differ in nutritional requirements, sensitivity to drugs and bacteriophage, heat resistance, and, in the case of *B. anthracis*, virulence and production of capsule and toxin.

Table 2. ANTHRAX TOXIN: COMPOSITION AND BIOLOGICAL EFFECTS

Factor[a]	Chemical Nature	Toxic Effect[b] Edema	Toxic Effect[b] Lethal	Antigenic Activity	Immunogenic Activity
Edema factor (EF); I	Protein, carbohydrate	−	−	+	−
Protective antigen (PA); II	Protein	−	−	+	+
Lethal factor (LF); III	protein	−	−	+	−
EF + PA		+	+	+	+
EF + LF		−	−	+	+
PA + LF		−	+	+	+
EF + PA + LF[c]		+	+	+	+

[a]The descriptive terms and acronyms are the American terminology. The Roman numerals are the British terms.
[b]Edema tested in guinea pig skin; lethal effect in mice.
[c]Complete toxin that would simulate the substances present in infected animals.

Table 3. COMPARISON OF TWO ENTEROTOXINS PRODUCED BY *BACILLUS CEREUS*[a]

Characteristic	Type of Enterotoxin: *Diarrheal*	*Emetic*
Clinical syndrome		
Incubation period	8 to 16 hr	1 to 5 hr
Diarrhea	Very common	Fairly common
Vomiting	Occasional	Very common
Duration of illness	12 to 24 hr	6 to 24 hr
Foods implicated	Meat products, soups, vegetables, puddings, sauces	Fried or boiled rice
Serotypes of *B. cereus* involved	1, 2, 6, 8, 9, 10, 12, 19	1 (majority) 3, 4, 5, 8, 12, 19
Enterotoxin[b]		
Molecular weight	*ca.* 50,000	<5,000
Stability to heat	−	+
Fluid accumulation in ligated rabbit ileal segment	+	−
Increased vascular permeability in guinea pig or rabbit skin	+	−
Lethal for mice after intravenous injection	+	−
Stimulation of adenylate cyclase-cAMP system in intestinal epithelial cells	+	−
Response when fed to rhesus monkeys	Diarrhea	Vomiting

[a]From Gilbert, et al., 1981.
[b]Except for molecular weight, data obtained from cell-free culture filtrates.

Formation of endospores is one of the most salient characteristics of *Bacillus*. The process is complex. Essentially, the phenomenon involves cell differentiation in which morphologic, biochemical, genetic, and physical changes occur in the bacteria. Endospores are a normal stage in the life history of *Bacillus*, but their biologic function is unknown. Their high resistance to inimical environments has survival value, and the mode of life of these bacteria depends upon the accumulation of spores in nature. Asporogenous mutants have little capacity to survive.

The initiation of endospore formation begins as the exponential growth of vegetative cells ends and the cultures approach the stationary phase as a result of limitation of nutrients, particularly sources of nitrogen and carbon. Synthesis of polypeptide antimicrobial substances commences, and cytologic changes begin in the vegetative cell. Morphologically, the mature endospore consists of a core, the spore protoplast, which contains the nucleus and the enzymes needed for subsequent germination. A complex envelope surrounds and protects the core. The innermost layer is the spore membrane, the original cytoplasmic membrane of the forespore, which contains normal peptidoglycan. External to this membrane is the cortex, the thickest layer of the envelope. The relatively impermeable spore coat is the most superficial layer of most spores, although it may be enclosed by an exosporium in some species.

Mature endospores are less easily stained than vegetative cells and are highly refractile. They have no detectable metabolism, are highly dehydrated, and can survive for decades in a state of dormancy. Spores are highly resistant to deleterious treatment by chemical agents, enzymes, heat, ionizing radiation, and ultraviolet light. Boiling for 10 minutes, dry heat at 140° C for three hours, or autoclaving for 20 to 30 minutes at 15 pounds of steam pressure kills most spores. Alcohols, phenols, heavy metal ions, and detergents are poor agents for killing spores. When an endospore is placed in an environment with favorable nutritional conditions, it germinates to produce a single vegetative cell.

PATHOGENIC PROPERTIES. Susceptible animals injected with *B. anthracis* develop a massive septicemia. Even in the natural infection, the number of bacilli in the blood is so great that they can be seen in stained smears. These observations led to the early conjecture that death from anthrax was caused by blockade of capillaries that prevented oxygenation of tissues. In 1955, British investigators demonstrated that sterile plasma obtained from guinea pigs dying of anthrax was lethal when injected into guinea pigs or mice. The presence of masses of bacteria in the blood was not required, because termination of bacteremia by administration of streptomycin did not prevent death of guinea pigs once the critical number of *B. anthracis* was reached. This number was about 1/300 of the number of bacteria present at death in untreated animals. The investigators concluded that a toxin caused death.

Anthrax toxin is a complex substance that contains three factors (Table 2): edema factor (EF), protective antigen (PA), and lethal factor (LF), or factors I, II, and III respectively. Various combinations cause edema or are lethal. The most lethal is a combination of the three. Problems arise in precise interpretations of the effects of mixtures because of the difficulty of recombining three relatively unstable proteins in the appropriate proportions. Purified protective antigen is immunogenic and has been used as a vaccine for humans. The toxin complex is produced by virulent, encapsulated and avirulent, nonencapsulated *B. anthracis* and production is mediated by a plasmid. Structural genes from the plasmid for synthesis of protective antigen recently have been cloned in *Escherichia coli*. For manufacture of protective antigen, cultures of avirulent, nonencapsulated *B. anthracis* are used.

The purified toxin complex interferes with phagocytosis and the bactericidal activity of serum. The toxin also increases vascular permeability. The decrease in circulating blood volume plus capillary thrombosis produced by the toxin may account for death from anthrax by secondary shock. The virulence of *B. anthracis* apparently depends upon both the ability to produce the toxin complex and the possession of a capsule. The presence of bicarbonate or serum is required in the medium for production of both the capsule and the toxin. Although the capsule is antigenic, it is not immunogenic. However, the capsule does interfere with phagocytosis and probably plays a role in the pathogenicity of anthrax.

The complex nature of anthrax toxin has left unresolved the precise nature of its pathogenic effects. Paradoxically, some animals such as mice are very susceptible when challenged with spores but relatively resistant when toxin is given intravenously. In contrast, dogs and rats are resistant when injected parenterally with spores but succumb to small doses of toxin. In addition, various animal species show different pathophysiologic responses to injection of the substance. Edema factor is an adenylate cyclase synthesized in an inactive form by *B. anthracis*. A heat-stable compound, probably calmodulin, activates the enzyme within the cytoplasm of eukaryotic cells to increase markedly the intracellular concentration of cAMP. Protective antigen may bind to cell receptors to permit binding and entrance of edema, and perhaps, lethal factors. What part these events play in pathogenesis of anthrax is still unknown. Other factors with pharmacologic activity are produced by *B. anthracis*, such as a material with epinephrine-like activity and a cardioactive substance. The bacteria also produce protocatechuic acid that combines with iron to form pigment in liquid cultures of *B. anthracis*. The role, if any, of these substances in the pathophysiology of anthrax is unknown. Other species of *Bacillus* produce a variety of extracellular metabolites with antibiotic, hemolytic, lethal, lipolytic, or proteolytic activity, but their association with the occasional pathogenicity of the bacteria is unknown.

Two enterotoxins are produced by *B. cereus* during exponential growth (Table 3), one that causes diarrhea and the other vomiting. The diarrheal toxin is produced readily on media such as brain-heart infusion broth containing added glucose. Detection of emetic toxin was difficult at first because ordinary media do not support its production, but growth on a medium prepared from rice permitted its isolation. The diarrheal enterotoxin causes increased vascular permeability and necrosis of rabbit skin, fluid accumulation in rabbit ileal loops, and is lethal for mice when injected intravenously. A significant relationship is found between the signs and symptoms of infections caused by *B. cereus* and the ability of the isolated strains to induce necrosis of rabbit skin and hemolysis in blood agar. Phospholipolytic activities are not associated with pathogenicity of *B. cereus* or with the enterotoxins. Strains of *B. cereus* produce amounts of the diarrheal toxin that vary from undetectable to considerable. Loss of the capacity to produce toxin after transfer in the laboratory led to the speculation that elaboration of the toxin might be under the control of plasmids or bacteriophages. This speculation has not been confirmed.

Some species of *Bacillus* are pathogenic for insects but not for vertebrates. *B. lentimorbus* and *B. popilliae*, which grow readily and produce large numbers of spores in the hemolymph of Japanese beetles, cause milky disease that is lethal for the insects. During sporulation, *B. thuringiensis* forms a crystalline protein that lies adjacent to the spore. After ingestion by larvae of *Lepidoptera*, this parasporal protein dissolves in the gut and effects paralysis of the caterpillar. A specific strain of *B. thuringiensis* also is lethal for larvae of *Diptera*, and its use as a bacterial pesticide may provide means to control mosquitoes and flies.

IMMUNITY. Louis Pasteur in 1881 dramatically established that herbivorous animals developed immunity to anthrax. He immunized a group of sheep with a vaccine made from an attenuated strain of *B. anthracis*. When later challenged with virulent *B. anthracis*, all 25 vaccinated animals survived, while an equal number of unvaccinated controls did not. Because the attenuated Pasteur vaccine sometimes caused severe disease in vaccinated animals, its use has been supplanted by a suspension of viable spores prepared from a nonencapsulated, avirulent strain of *B. anthracis*. This vaccine is not approved for human use, and occasional cases of disease still occur in vaccinated animals. Both of these vaccines probably produce immunity by release of toxin by growing bacteria.

Second attacks of anthrax in man are rare, and humans probably are relatively resistant to the disease. Manufacturing plants that process wool have large numbers of spores in the air and dust that is inhaled by workers, yet few cases of inhalation anthrax occur in spite of the fact that some of the particles in the dust are of a size that could reach the alveoli. Nor is cutaneous anthrax common in such plants. Antibodies to protective antigen were found in workers who were not immunized and who had no history of anthrax. This serologic evidence suggests that inapparent or mild forms of anthrax occur in humans to provide an antibody response and immunity.

Vaccines of killed bacilli evoke no significant immunity probably because they cannot grow and produce anthrax toxin. Antibody against the polypeptide capsule is not protective except in mice. The complex, purified anthrax toxin is both antigenic and immunogenic, but isolated edema and lethal factors are only antigenic (Table 2). Protective antigen is immunogenic. A vaccine prepared by precipitation and concentration of protective antigen by addition of aluminum potassium sulfate to sterile culture filtrates was calculated to be 92 per cent effective in an exposed, susceptible population of humans. Antibody can be measured by complement fixation, agar gel precipitation, or indirect microhemagglutination tests. The latter procedure is the most sensitive.

Acquired immunity to anthrax apparently involves primarily antibody to the toxin, although the antiphagocytic nature of the capsule suggests that it also may be important. Some animals have a high natural immunity to anthrax. Rats and dogs are only slightly susceptible to infection, but the nature of their immunity is unknown. Guinea pigs, mice, and rabbits are very susceptible, and reportedly one virulent *B. anthracis* is lethal after injection into a mouse. The natural disease occurs primarily in herbivorous animals such as cattle, sheep, and horses, who possess little immunity.

Whether other species of *Bacillus* evoke an immune response is unknown. Except for food poisoning, primarily by *B. cereus*, other species cause no well-defined infection. Apparently there is little or no immunity to the enterotoxins produced by *B. cereus* (Table 3).

LABORATORY DIAGNOSIS. An isolated, hemolytic colony of an aerobic, spore-forming, gram-positive, motile bacillus often is dismissed by the microbiology laboratory as an unimportant contaminant. But the increasing frequency with which severe infections caused by *Bacillus* is being reported mandates that the laboratory consult with the clinician before discarding such cultures. If the specimen originated from a seriously ill patient or from an unusual source or was isolated in large numbers in repeated specimens, the physician should be notified so that the results can be interpreted in terms of the clinical findings.

Identification of the species of *Bacillus* usually can be made by evaluation of several morphologic and biochemical characteristics and speciation confirmed by additional tests (Table 1), although speciation may not be made quickly because of the number of species and the fact that variant strains are common. The bacteria most often encountered in humans grow readily on common nutrient media. Specimens should be obtained from patients prior to administration of antimicrobial therapy and inoculated onto 5 per cent horse or sheep blood agar. The cultures are incubated at 35 to 37° C in air for 24 to 48 hours. Hemolytic, catalase-positive colonies of gram-positive bacilli that contain spores can then be identified by a series of commonly used biochemical tests that include lecithinase production, the Voges-Proskauer reaction, starch hydrolysis, glucose fermentation, and anaerobic growth (Table 1). Experienced technicians may make a preliminary identification from the morphologic appearance of the colonies. Recently, differential agglutination of vegetative bacteria by various lectins was reported as a procedure to distinguish species of *Bacillus*. In particular, *B. anthracis* could be rapidly differentiated from other species.

When *B. cereus* is suspected as a cause of food poisoning, the food can be cultured to isolate the bacteria, or isolation of *B. cereus* from the stool or vomit of patients can be attempted. If more than 10^5 bacteria per gram of food are identified as *B. cereus*, and other pathogens are absent, the diagnosis is confirmed. Serologic typing of isolated strains can be done for epidemiologic purposes, but the antisera developed by the Food Hygiene Laboratory in London are available only in a few centers. *B. licheniformis* and *B. subtilis* also may be isolated from foods and incriminated as causes of food poisoning.

Although *B. anthracis* is seldom encountered in an average hospital or public health laboratory, it can be confused with the more common *B. cereus* or encapsulated *B. megaterium*. The three species can be differentiated easily (Table 4). The "string of pearls" phenomenon is observed when *B. anthracis* is inoculated onto agar containing penicillin (0.05 to 0.5 units per ml). After incubation for about three to six hours, the areas where growth might occur are examined microscopically for the presence of large spherical bacilli in chains, the "string of pearls." Animals injected subcutaneously with *B. anthracis* develop an overwhelming infection within 36 to 48 hours, and smears from the blood or spleen show numerous encapsulated bacteria. Suspensions should be diluted and made in saline to avoid nonspecific deaths.

Samples from cutaneous anthrax lesions should be obtained carefully. Fluid can be taken from the vesicles with a Pasteur pipette, or less preferably, with a syringe and needle or swab, and used for smear and culture. Tentative identification can be made if a smear shows short chains of large gram-positive rods, perhaps with a few spores. Pulmonary anthrax cannot be diagnosed by culture because the sputum rarely contains bacteria; a blood culture usually is positive. Blood cultures also should be obtained to diagnose intestinal anthrax. Specimens for diagnosis in animals are best taken from the jugular vein.

The fluorescent antibody stain for *B. anthracis* is presumptive because *B. megaterium* and *B. cereus* also fluoresce with the antiserum. Cultures for fluorescent staining must be grown in carbon dioxide to permit capsule production. This test and the test for susceptibility to gamma bacteriophage are obtainable only in certain laboratories such as the Center for Disease Control in the United States. Serologic diagnosis for anthrax is not valuable because the disease is of short duration, although procedures such as an agar gel precipitation test, complement fixation, and indirect microhemagglutination have been used to detect antibody. Selective media for isolation have been unsatisfactory because they inhibit growth of *B. anthracis*.

B. anthracis can be isolated from contaminated wool and hair. The material should be soaked in detergent or dilute potassium hydroxide. After thorough soaking, the sample is teased, heated to 65° C for five minutes, and centrifuged. The sediment is cultured, and suspicious colonies are identified.

Any competent microbiology laboratory can handle *B. anthracis* safely. Aerosols should be avoided, and use of a biological safety hood is advisable, particularly if contaminated materials are examined. Animals should be inocu-

Table 4. CHARACTERISTICS USEFUL FOR DISTINGUISHING *B. ANTHRACIS, B. CEREUS,* AND *B. MEGATERIUM*

Characteristic	*B. anthracis*	*B. cereus*	*B. megaterium*
Hemolysis on sheep's blood agar	−	+	−
Motility	−	+	+
Lecithinase production	+	+	−
Peptonization of litmus milk	−	+	±
Fermentation of salicin	−	±	−
Specific fluorescent antibody stain	+	−	−
Appearance of colonies grown on bicarbonate (0.7%) nutrient agar[a]			
In air	(Rough)[b]	Rough	No growth
In 5% CO_2 or candle jar	Smooth	Rough	Rough
Growth in penicillin (10 U/ml) agar	−	+	−
String of pearls reaction	+	−	−
Pathogenicity for mice by intraperitoneal or subcutaneous injection	+	−	−
Positive capsular stain for bacteria from spleen[c]	+	−	−
Susceptibility to specific gamma bacteriophage	+	−	−

All cultures incubated at 36 to 37°C.
[a]Bicarbonate must be sterilized separately by filtration and added to agar.
[b]*B. anthracis* may not grow under these conditions.
[c]Stained by Loeffler's methylene blue stain (polychrome methylene blue stain).

lated only when adequate facilities are available for isolation, but reasonable identification of *B. anthracis* can be made without use of animals. Benches should be washed with 5 per cent carbolic acid (phenol) or 5 per cent hypochlorite, and instruments should be autoclaved to reduce the possibility of contamination.

DRUG SUSCEPTIBILITY. With one exception, broad spectrum antimicrobial agents are usually effective against species of *Bacillus*. The exception is penicillin. *B. cereus* in particular produces a beta-lactamase that renders penicillin ineffective for treatment. Chloramphenicol, erythromycin, penicillin, tetracyclines, and sulfonamides have been used to treat anthrax. About 24 to 48 hours after treatment with penicillin, *B. anthracis* disappears from cutaneous lesions, although signs of the disease may persist. The bacteria are reported to persist longer after treatment with chloramphenicol or tetracycline. However, some patients with cutaneous anthrax recover without treatment, another indication that humans are relatively resistant to the disease. *B. anthracis* is resistant to neomycin and polymyxin. Other species of *Bacillus* usually are sensitive to chloramphenicol, gentamicin, kanamycin, and tetracyclines. Treatment of infections caused by these organisms usually involves initial treatment with a broad spectrum antibiotic, followed by laboratory tests on the isolated organism to determine sensitivities. *B. subtilis* is susceptible, *B. pumilus* less so, to ampicillin, cephalothin, methicillin, and penicillin G. *B. cereus* is resistant to these drugs as well as to sulfonamides and trimethoprim. Infections of the eye caused by *B. cereus* have been treated with some success by a combination of clindamycin and gentamicin.

EPIDEMIOLOGY. Gram-positive, aerobic, spore-forming bacilli are ubiquitous in the environment. They are found in decaying organic matter, dust, soil, vegetables, and water, and some species are part of the normal flora. From these sources, the bacteria can readily cause infections in debilitated, immunosuppressed, or traumatized patients. However, except for *B. anthracis*, members of the genus unfortunately are not considered pathogenic. But the opportunity for infection with other species is increasing with the prolonged survival of patients with severe illnesses. When the bacteria are isolated from blood, body fluids, or infections of closed spaces, they should not be dismissed as contaminants, particularly if patients are receiving immunosuppressive or myelosuppressive drugs, are undergoing hemodialysis, or are drug addicts. *Bacillus* species are common contaminants of heroin samples and associated injection paraphernalia. Although the true prevalence is unknown, infection caused by the bacteria occurs more frequently than is appreciated. They have been documented as causes of bronchopneumonia, meningitis, ocular infections, septicemia, osteomyelitis, endocarditis, abscesses, and several other types of infections. *B. cereus* is one of the most destructive bacterial pathogens of the eye.

The diarrheal type of gastroenteritis caused by *B. cereus* is associated with a wide range of foods, whereas boiled and fried rice is primarily implicated in the emetic disease (Table 3). Several serotypes are found in outbreaks of diarrhea, but Serotype 1 predominates in cases of vomiting, perhaps because the spores of this type are more resistant to heat, and they survive in cooked rice. Outbreaks of food poisoning caused by *B. cereus* have been reported from Asia, Australia, Europe, and North America. The diseases may be more common than reported because they are easily confused with the more frequent outbreaks of food poisoning caused by staphylococci and *C. perfringens*. Thorough cooking and refrigeration of foods help control gastroenteritis effected by *B. cereus*.

B. anthracis is a saprophytic bacterium that can become a facultative parasite. The bacteria probably survive in soil in a dynamic state in which they undergo cycles of germination and sporulation depending upon conditions in the microenvironment. Contamination of the soil originally occurs when infected animals soil the ground with blood and excreta that contain vegetative bacteria. Sporulation ensues in the aerobic environment outside of the body. In an alkaline, calcareous soil that is poorly drained, the spores germinate in decayed vegetation. When the weather becomes dry, spores form, and, if grazing animals inadvertently ingest them, an outbreak of anthrax can occur. Such focal areas may remain contaminated indefinitely, with *B. anthracis* undergoing cycles of germination and sporulation. The dependency of the cycle upon the environment may account for the seasonal occurrence of anthrax in the late summer and early fall subsequent to previous rain, as well as for the sporadic outbreaks of the disease.

Anthrax primarily afflicts herbivorous animals. It is one of the major livestock diseases in the world and affects thousands of cattle, goats, horses, and sheep annually. Carnivorous animals can be infected secondarily if they feed on infected carcasses, but the disease is not spread from animal to animal. About a third of the cases in animals occur in Europe, with the major portion of infections occurring in Asia and Africa. The disease is enzootic in Asia Minor, Central and South America, Africa, and Southeast Asia, where epizootics periodically are reported in wild and domestic animals. Anthrax today is the most important cause of wildlife mortality in Southern Africa. In the United States, sporadic cases occur in the Gulf coast and midwest states and in California. The disease may be more prevalent than reported because many sudden deaths in animals, the typical outcome of an infection, may not be recognized as anthrax.

As many as 20,000 to 100,000 cases of anthrax in humans are estimated to occur worldwide per year, but such figures are unreliable because many countries do not report the disease. Anthrax was a formidable scourge in England in the mid-19th century, when fatal outbreaks of "woolsorter's disease" (inhalation anthrax) among textile workers led to legislation to control the disease. Today in industrial countries anthrax still is predominantly an occupational disease in the textile and tanning industries. Wool, hair, hides, and bone meal imported from countries where the disease is prevalent in animals contain large numbers of spores. Workers are exposed to the spores in the air and dust of plants and while handling the contaminated materials. However, although the bacteria are widespread, the number of cases of disease is few. Cutaneous infections (malignant pustule) are most common when spores invade the skin of the head, neck, or arms through cuts or abrasions. If properly treated, the mortality is nil. Inhalation anthrax is rare but almost uniformly fatal. Although industrial anthrax is the most commonly reported form of the disease, agricultural anthrax may be widespread among farmers in countries where the disease is epizootic. Several thousand cases in humans reportedly have occurred recently in Zimbabwe, probably as a result of disruption of control measures in animals. Intestinal anthrax that has a high mortality occurs when meat from diseased animals is eaten. Veterinarians occasionally develop anthrax from contact with infected animals or carcasses. Cases of disease now occur in amateur craftsmen who use raw wool contaminated with anthrax spores. There are no age or sex differences in cases. Industrial anthrax has no seasonal incidence, but agricultural cases are most common in the late summer and early fall. No human anthrax was reported in the United States in 1979, one case in 1980, and none in 1981 and 1982.

Control of anthrax requires elimination or reduction of contact with infected animals. Carcasses of animals that died from anthrax must be incinerated or buried with lime deep in the soil. Autopsies should not be done if anthrax is suspected to avoid recontamination of the soil. Potential focal areas for growth of *B. anthracis* can be eliminated by proper drainage or tillage. If anthrax does occur, infected animals must be treated, and the exposed herd quarantined and vaccinated with the viable spore vaccine. This vaccine protects for about one year. Immunization and improved working conditions in industry seem to be responsible for the progressive decline of human cases of anthrax, so that the disease now is rare in the United States and Europe. Vaccine prepared from protective antigen can be used to immunize exposed individuals who handle materials contaminated with anthrax spores. Antibody titer declines rapidly; booster doses of the vaccine are suggested at six months or one year to maintain immunity.

References

Cole, H. B., Ezzell, J. W., Jr., Keller, K. F., and Doyle, R. J.: Differentiation of *Bacillus anthracis* and other *Bacillus* species by lectins. J Clin Microbiol 19:48, 1984.

Gilbert, R. J., Turnbull, P. C. B., Parry, J. M.: *Bacillus cereus*: Their part in food poisoning and other clinical infections. *In* Berkeley, R. C. W. and Goodfellow, M. (eds.): The Aerobic Endospore-forming Bacteria: Classification and Identification. New York, Academic Press, 1981.

Leppla, S. H.: Anthrax toxin edema factor: A bacterial adenylate cyclase that increases cyclic AMP concentrations in eukaryotic cells. Proc Nat Acad Sci USA 79:3162, 1982.

Mikesell, P., Ivins, B. E., Ristroph, J. D., Vodkin, M. H., Dreier, T. M., and Leppla, S.: Plasmids, Pasteur, and anthrax. ASM News 49:320, 1983.

Parry, J. M., Turnbull, P. C. B., and Gibson, J. R.: A Colour Atlas of *Bacillus* Species. London, Wolfe Medical Publications Ltd., 1983.

Siegman-Igra, Y., Lavochkin, J., Schwartz, D., and Konforti, N.: Meningitis and bacteremia due to *Bacillus cereus*. A case report and a review of *Bacillus* infections. Isr J Med Sci 19:546, 1983.

Stephen, J.: Anthrax toxin. Pharmacology and Therapeutics 12:501, 1981.

Turnbull, P. C. B.: *Bacillus cereus* toxins. Pharmacol Ther 13:453, 1981.

Turnbull, P. C. B., Jorgensen, K., Kramer, J. M., Gilbert, R. J., and Parry, J. M.: Severe clinical conditions associated with *Bacillus cereus* and the apparent involvement of exotoxins. J Clin Pathol 32:289, 1979.

Van Ness, G. B.: Ecology of anthrax: Anthrax undergoes a propagation phase in soil before it infects livestock. Science 172:1303, 1971.

Vodkin, M. H., and Leppla, S. H.: Cloning of the protective antigen gene of *Bacillus anthracis*. Cell 34:693, 1983.

GRAM-NEGATIVE COCCI AND COCCOBACILLI

29

NEISSERIA AND BRANHAMELLA

STEPHEN A. MORSE, PH.D.

NEISSERIA

The genus *Neisseria* is one of four genera included in the family *Neisseriaceae*. The other genera in the family are *Branhamella*, *Moraxella*, and *Acinetobacter* (see Table 1). Members of the genus *Neisseria* inhabit the mucosal surfaces of warm-blooded animals. The genus includes two species that are pathogenic for man: *Neisseria gonorrhoeae* (the gonococcus) and *Neisseria meningitidis* (the meningococcus). It also includes several species (*N. flavescens, N. cinerea, N. mucosa, N. perflava, N. sicca*, and *N. lactamica*) that rarely cause disease and that may be part of the normal flora and therefore can be confused with gonococci and meningococci.

Descriptions of a condition resembling gonococcal urethritis can be found in the earliest recorded histories of man. The disease, gonorrhea, was named by Galen in about A.D. 130 (*gonos*, seed; *rhoia*, flow). Galen had the mistaken impression that the disease was due to a morbid loss of semen. Gonorrhea was known to be of venereal origin in the 13th century, but was thought to be an early symptom of syphilis. It was not until the middle of the 19th century that gonorrhea and syphilis were clearly differentiated. *N. gonorrhoeae*, the causative agent of gonorrhea, was first described by Neisser in 1879 in smears of purulent exudates from patients with acute gonorrhea and from newborn infants with conjunctivitis. The gonococcus was first cultivated by Leistikow and Loeffler in 1882. Bumm showed that the gonococcus fulfilled Koch's postulates in 1885.

Table 1. TAXONOMY AND NOMENCLATURE OF THE NEISSERIACEAE

Genus I.	Neisseria
Species:	*N. gonorrhoeae*
	N. meningitidis
	N. lactamica
	N. sicca
	N. flavescens
	N. subflava (includes *N. flava, N. perflava*)
	N. mucosa
	N. cinerea
Genus II.	Branhamella
Species:	*B. catarrhalis* (formerly *N. catarrhalis*)
	B. ovis (formerly *N. ovis*)
	B. caviae (formerly N. caviae)
Genus III.	Moraxella
Species:	*M. lacunata*
	M. nonliquifaciens
	M. bovis
	M. osloensis
	M. phenylpyruvica
	*M. urethralis** (formerly *Mima polymorpha* var *oxidans*)
Genus IV.	Acinetobacter
Species:	*A. calcoaceticus* (formerly *Bacillus anitratus, Herrelea vaginicola,* or *M. lwoffi*)

*Tentatively placed in this genus.

N. meningitidis is the causative agent of meningococcal meningitis (formerly called epidemic cerebrospinal meningitis). The disease can occur in epidemic form. It was first recognized as a contagious disease early in the 19th century. Outbreaks were eventually described on all continents, and the prevalence of the disease, particularly among military personnel, became apparent. The causative organism was first described by Marchiafava and Celli (1884) in meningeal exudate. In 1887, Weichselbaum isolated the organism in pure culture and described it in detail as the characteristic bacterium found in six cases of acute cerebrospinal meningitis.

MORPHOLOGY. *Neisseriae* are gram-negative cocci, 0.6 to 1.0 μm in diameter. The organisms are usually seen in pairs with their adjacent sides flattened. Tetrads or clusters are occasionally seen. Negatively stained cells display a rugose outer cell surface that is characteristic of many gram-negative bacteria. The presence of a capsule on *N. gonorrhoeae* has not been irrefutably demonstrated. *Neisseria* do not possess flagella; however, twitching motility may sometimes be observed with piliated organisms. Spores are not produced.

Thin sections of gonococci or meningococci grown in vitro exhibit cell structures in electron micrographs similar

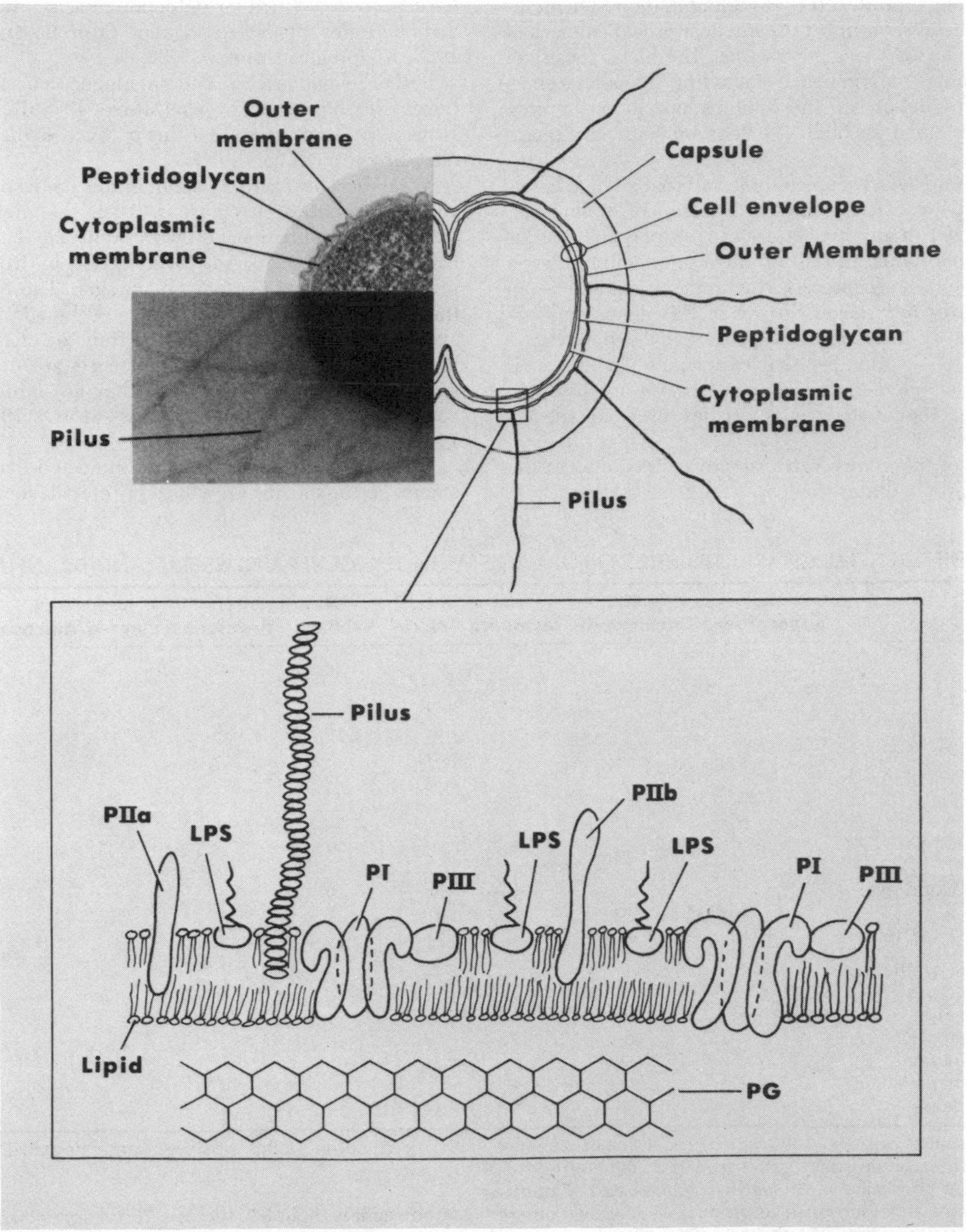

Figure 1. Structures and characteristics of the gonococcal cell envelope. Abbreviations: PI, protein I; PIIa, PIIb, protein IIs; PIII, protein III; LPS, lipopolysaccharide; PG, peptidoglycan. From Brooks and Donegan, 1984. (Used with permission of Edward Arnold (Publishers) Ltd.)

to those of other gram-negative bacteria (Fig. 1). An undulating outer membrane, approximately 7.5 to 8.5 nm in thickness, appears as a bilayered structure. The periplasmic space, between the cytoplasmic membrane and the outer membrane, contains a thin, electron-dense layer, approximately 6.0 nm in diameter, which corresponds to the peptidoglycan layer of the bacterial cell envelope. The chemical composition of the purified peptidoglycan from *N. gonorrhoeae* consists of muramic acid, glutamic acid, alanine, *meso*-diaminopimelic acid, and glucosamine in approximate molar ratios of 1:1:2:1:1 respectively (Morse, 1978; Roberts, 1977). The peptidoglycan layer and the outer membrane adhere to each other at regular intervals around the periphery of the cell.

Cell wall blebs produced by budding of the outer membrane have been seen in broth- and agar-grown cultures of *N. meningitidis* and *N. gonorrhoeae*. The blebs consist of outer membrane components, including lipopolysaccharide. The production of these blebs occurs on rapidly growing cells since no blebs are seen on stationary phase cells.

Metabolism. *Neisseria* are aerobic and contain high levels of cytochrome *c* oxidase activity (Morse, 1978; Roberts, 1977). However, many species are capable of growth under anaerobic conditions by using nitrite (or nitrate) as a terminal electron acceptor. Cytochrome *c* oxidase is an important taxonomic characteristic of this genus and can be measured by reduction of *N,N*-dimethyl-*p*-phenylenediamine (or tetramethyl-*p*-phenylenediamine). The principal species included in the genus *Neisseria* are listed in Table 2, together with characteristics used in species differentiation.

Members of the genus *Neisseria* are restricted as to the number of carbohydrates that can be utilized (Morse, 1978; Roberts, 1977). Carbohydrates are utilized by oxidative pathways, resulting in the accumulation of acetic acid. Under some conditions, lactic acid and acetylmethylcarbinol are produced. *N. gonorrhoeae* and *N. meningitidis* dissimilate glucose by a combination of the Entner-Doudoroff and pentose phosphate pathways. Each species of *Neisseria* exhibits a characteristic pattern of acid production from specific carbohydrates (see Table 2) that can be used for speciation. Oxidative organisms such as the *Neisseria* spp. produce less acid than do fermentative organisms. In addition, *Neisseria* spp. produce ammonia from amino acids, so that any acid produced from carbohydrate may be partially or completely neutralized if the concentration of amino acids is high. Both rapid and growth-dependent tests have been developed for detection of acid production from carbohydrates by *Neisseria* spp. (Morella and Bohnhoff, 1980; Knapp and Holmes, 1983).

Both the gonococcus and meningococcus have a functional tricarboxylic acid cycle (Morse, 1978; Roberts, 1977). However, the utilization of this pathway is markedly influenced by growth conditions.

N. gonorrhoeae and *N. meningitidis* are fastidious organisms (the gonococcus more so than the meningococcus) with complex nutritional growth requirements. Both organisms are sensitive to growth inhibition by free fatty acids present in various peptones or in agar. The toxic effect of the free fatty acids can be eliminated by adding a binding agent, such as soluble starch, serum, or charcoal, to the medium. Gonococci and meningococci are unique among gram-negative bacteria because they are inhibited by low concentrations of gonadal steroids (Morse, 1978; Roberts, 1977).

A survey of gonococcal isolates indicated that there were stable, strain-specific growth requirements for amino acids,

Table 2. DIFFERENTIAL CHARACTERISTICS OF ORGANISMS IN THE GENERA NEISSERIA AND BRANHAMELLA*

	N. gonorrhoeae	N. meningitidis	N. lactamica	N. sicca	N. subflava†	N. flavescens	N. cinerea	N. mucosa	B. catarrhalis
Acid from:									
Glucose	+	+	+	+	+	−	−	+	−
Maltose	−	+	+	+	+	−	−	+	−
Lactose	−	−	+	−	−	−	−	−	−
Fructose	−	−	−	+	v	−	−	+	−
Sucrose	−	−	−	+	v	−	−	+	−
Growth on:									
TM, or MTM, or NYC medium§	+	+	+	−	−	−	−	−	d
Chocolate or blood agar at 22°C	−	−	v	v	v	+	−	+	+
Nutrient agar at 35°C	−	−	+	+	v	+	+	+	−
Polysaccharide synthesis from 5% sucrose	ø	ø	?	+‡	d	+	−	+	−
Production of H_2S	−	−	−	+	+	+	?	+	−
Presence of capsule	v	d	?	v	+	−	?	+	+
Reduction of nitrate	−	−	−	−	−	−	−	+	+
Reduction of nitrite¶	+	d	+	+	+	+	+	+	+
Deoxyribonuclease	−	−	−	−	−	−	−	−	+

*+, most strains positive (≥90%); −, most strains negative (≥90%); d, some strains positive, some negative; v, character inconsistent within single strain; ø, no growth on medium with 5% sucrose

†New species consisting of *N. subflava, N. flava,* and *N. perflava*

‡*N. sicca* forms an iodine-positive product when grown on trypticase soy agar without 5% sucrose. This reaction, which does not occur with *N. subflava,* may be used as a differentiating characteristic

§T.M., Thayer-Martin medium, MTM, modified Thayer-Martin medium; NYC, New York City medium.

¶0.001% (w/v) nitrite. Higher concentrations of nitrite (≥0.1%) are toxic for many species.

pyrimidines, purines, and vitamins. These requirements differ among certain strains that have a block in metabolic pathway as a result of a deficient or defective enzyme. These differences in growth requirements are determined by attenuated culture in a minimal medium with defined constituents adequate to permit growth of normal (wild) strains of gonococci. Auxotrophs are detected by their need for a specific nutrient not present in the defined medium, i.e., for the product of the blocked enzymatic reaction or other metabolites that are not required by wild-type organisms. Auxotyping is based on the particular nutrient or nutrients required. Isolates from different geographic areas frequently differ in auxotype. Auxotyping has also been useful in epidemiologic studies.

Many strains of *N. gonorrhoeae* require increased atmospheric carbon dioxide concentrations (ca. 4 to 8 per cent) for initial isolation. This requirement is often lost after repeated subculture. An exogenous source of carbon dioxide is required during the lag phase. This requirement may be met by either the addition of bicarbonate ions or gaseous carbon dioxide. During exponential growth, the exogenous source is replaced by metabolically generated carbon dioxide. Meningococci are less stringent in their requirement for carbon dioxide.

Gonococci and meningococci typically undergo autolysis in older cultures or when suspended in appropriate buffers. In *N. gonorrhoeae*, autolysis results from a combination of peptidoglycan hydrolysis and destabilization of the cell membranes (Morse, 1978; Roberts, 1977). The presence of divalent cations (Mg^{2+} or Ca^{2+}) will prevent cellular lysis but will not inhibit peptidoglycan hydrolysis.

The pathogenic *Neisseria* have an optimum growth temperature that ranges from 36 to 39°C. The maximum growth temperature is ca 41°C and the minimum growth temperature is ca 24°C. The inability of *N. gonorrhoeae* and *N. meningitidis* to grow at 22°C distinguishes these species from most of the nonpathogenic species of *Neisseria*. The pH range for growth varies from strain to strain. Many strains will grow in media buffered over a pH range of 6.0 to 8.0.

NEISSERIA GONORRHOEAE

Colony Phenotypes. Variation in the colony characteristics of *N. gonorrhoeae* were noted as early as 1904. However, it was not until the 1960's that gonococcal colony morphology was correlated with infectivity (Kellogg et al. 1963, 1968). These studies by Kellogg and his colleagues provided the basis for investigations that have continued to the present time. Four morphologically distinct colony types were initially described and designated 1,2,3, and 4 (T1, T2, T3, T4). The colony types 1 and 2 were small, usually about 0.5 mm in diameter, and had different color and convexity characteristics.

Freshly isolated strains consist of type 1 and type 2 colonies. When gonococci are nonselectively subcultured there is a shift in colony type such that types 3 and 4 predominate after only a few subcultures. The four colony types can be readily maintained in vitro by selective subculture during colony visualization with a dissecting microscope.

Organisms from type 1 and type 2 colonies are piliated and retain virulence when they are inoculated experimentally into the urethra of the human or chimpanzee male, or intravenously into chicken embryos. Organisms from colonial types T3 and T4 lack pili and are considerably less virulent.

Colony types 1 and 2 have opaque and transparent colony variants when observed with light transmitted from a polished substage mirror. Colony type 3 is opaque while colony type 4 is transparent. In reality, the opacity/transparency variants exist as a continuous spectrum from very opaque colonies to very transparent colonies. The opacity/transparency of the colonies has been correlated with the presence or absence of one or more of a group of outer membrane proteins termed protein II's. Photographs showing the spectrum of opaque and transparent colonies have been published (Swanson, 1982).

The terminology of gonococcal colony morphology has evolved so that multiple colony phenotypes are described for the original four colony types described by Kellogg and co-workers. Nomenclature systems and their relationship to one another are presented in Table 3. Recent studies (James and Swanson, 1978) indicated that there were opacity/transparency differences in isolates from different anatomic sites and different types of clinical infections. Gonococci from men with symptomatic urethritis tend to form small opaque colonies. Similar colony phenotypes are isolated from the cervix at mid-cycle. However, small transparent colony phenotypes predominate in cervical isolates at or near the time of menstruation. Transparent colony phenotypes also predominate among isolates from salpingitis patients obtained by laparoscopy and culture of fallopian tubes, in urethral isolates from asymptomatic men, and in genital, blood and joint fluid isolates from disseminated gonococcal infections. Nasopharyngeal isolates usually form opaque colonies; rectal isolates may form either opaque or transparent colonies.

Gonococci from any given strain appear to have the ability to undergo reversible transitions in colony phenotype from piliated to nonpiliated, and from opaque to transparent types. Rearrangement of the gonococcal genome may be involved in these transitions. However, environmental factors may also be of importance.

Pili. Metal-shadowed electronmicrographs of *N. gonorrhoeae* reveal hairlike filaments, known as pili, extending from the surface. Pili have a diameter of ca 6 nm and are found on the surface of gonococci from colony types 1 and

Table 3. CLASSIFICATION SCHEMES FOR GONOCOCCAL COLONY PHENOTYPES

Scheme 1*	Scheme 2†	Scheme 3‡
T1	P^+Op	P^+O^-
	P^+Tr	P^+O^+
		P^+O^{++}
T2	$P^{++}Op$	P^+O^{+++}
	$P^{++}Tr$	P^+O^{++++}
T3	P^-Op	P^-O^-
		P^-O^+
		P^-O^{++}
T4	P^-Tr	P^-O^{+++}
		P^-O^{++++}

*Kellogg et al., 1963.

†Draper et al., 1980. P^-, non-piliated; P^+, piliated; P^{++}, heavily piliated; Op, opaque; Tr, transparent

‡Swanson, 1982. P^-, non-piliated; P^+, piliated; O^-, transparent; O^+ to O^{++++}, increasing colony opacity.

2; gonococci from colony types 3 and 4 are devoid of visible pili. The presence of pili on *N. gonorrhoeae* is not unique. Nonpathogenic *Neisseria* spp. and *N. meningitidis* also possess pili. Short pili (175 to 210 nm in length) are seen only on nonpathogenic species, whereas long pili (up to 4300 nm) are seen on organisms of both nonpathogenic and pathogenic species. There is no consistent relationship between colonial morphology and pili among the nonpathogenic *Neisseria* spp. and *N. meningitidis*.

Gonococcal pili have been purified and are primarily protein in nature. Pili purified from different gonococcal strains possess subunit molecular weights between 17,500 and 21,000 as estimated by sodium dodecyl sulfate polyacrylamide gel electrophoresis. Each pilus consists of up to 10,000 of these subunits, termed pilin, that aggregate to form filamentous structures 1000 to 4000 nm in length. More than 50 serotypes of pili are known to exist. However, structural domaines are shared between serologically unrelated strains. The amino-terminal amino acid sequence is identical for the first 49 residues in pili purified from two serologically unrelated strains and for the first 24 residues in pili purified from three other serologically unrelated strains. Gonococci apparently have the ability to alter their pili. Four types of pili showing little antigenic cross-reactivity and different adhesive properties are produced by variants of a single gonococcal strain.

A potential antiphagocytic role for pili has been proposed to explain the decreased association of piliated gonococci with human polymorphonuclear leukocytes as compared with nonpiliated gonococci. This role has been challenged, and the association of the gonococcus with polymorphonuclear leukocytes has been ascribed to another protein surface factor (leukocyte association (LA) factor). On the other hand, there is considerable evidence that gonococcal pili play an important role in the attachment of the gonococcus to host cells. Pili appear to recognize specific binding sites on host cell surfaces. It is noteworthy that the greatest attachment of purified pili is to cells that are histologically the most similar to the actual sites of gonococcal infection. It has been postulated that pili overcome the long-range electrostatic repulsion between the negatively charged gonococcal and host cell surfaces.

Outer Membrane Proteins. The gonococcal outer membrane differs from that of the *Enterobacteriaceae* in that it does not function as an effective barrier to hydrophobic molecules due to the presence of phospholipid bilayer regions. The gonococcal outer membrane contains relatively few proteins, with one to several proteins predominating. The major outer membrane is called protein I. The orientation of protein I within the outer membrane resembles a hairpin with both ends inserted in the membrane. Cross-linking analysis indicated that protein I exists as a trimer. This protein forms channels in bilayers and probably functions as a porin. The diameter of the pore is larger than those of other gram-negative bacteria, providing a partial explanation for the extreme sensitivity of gonococci to various hydrophilic antibiotics that penetrate the outer membrane through these water-filled protein channels. Protein I is the principal protein involved in serological systems based on outer membrane antigens. Peptide mapping indicates two groups of protein I molecules. Monoclonal antibodies have been used to subdivide further each group and has led to a better understanding of the epidemiology of gonococcal infections. Antibodies against protein I are bactericidal and opsonic.

Another major outer membrane protein is called protein III. Protein III is surface-exposed and exists as a complex with protein I within the outer membrane. Protein III possesses antigenic determinants common to diverse strains of *N. gonorrhoeae*.

An interesting group of outer membrane proteins have been called protein II. These proteins may be variably present depending upon the colony phenotype (opaque). Protein IIs may have an attachment function. More than one molecular weight species of this protein can be present in a single strain. Protein IIs exhibit heat-modifiable behavior in SDS-polyacrylamide gels. As a group, they are sensitive to *in situ* proteolysis, share considerable apparent structural homology, and exhibit common antigens. All protein IIs influence colony phenotype (degree of opaqueness). Rearrangement of the genome may be involved in the expression of protein IIs.

Lipopolysaccharides. Gonococcal lipopolysaccharide has not been as extensively characterized as that from *Escherichia coli* or *Salmonella typhimurium*. SDS-polyacrylamide gel electrophoresis of gonococcal lipopolysaccharide indicates that it is a relatively small molecule devoid of O-antigen repeat units. Serological analysis indicates that there are three distinct antigenic determinants. These have been designated the common, variable, and serotype antigens. The common antigen is found on all gonococcal lipopolysaccharides, whereas the variable antigen may or may not be present. There are at least six different serotype antigens that are serologically analogous to the O-*antigen* of enterobacterial lipopolysaccharide. The role of gonococcal lipopolysaccharide in the pathogenesis of natural infection and in promoting virulence is unclear. Gonococcal lipopolysaccharide contains a site(s) that is important in killing by normal human serum, and may be the toxin associated with ciliary loss in the fallopian-tube tissue culture model.

GENETICS. The chromosome of the gonococcus has approximately 1.5×10^6 nucleotide pairs and a molecular weight of 9.8×10^8. Approximately 95 per cent of the strains isolated in the United States contain a 2.4×10^6 dalton plasmid. It is lacking in ca. 50 per cent of Canadian isolates, particularly those with a Pro^- Cit^- Ura^- auxotype. There has been no function ascribed to the presence of this plasmid and it remains phenotypically cryptic. A smaller percentage of gonococcal strains contains a 24.5×10^6 dalton plasmid. This plasmid is a sex factor capable of promoting the transfer of chromosomal genes and R-plasmids via conjugation.

Genetic transformation readily occurs with *N. gonorrhoeae*. Unlike most bacteria, the gonococcus is competent for transformation throughout the growth cycle. All strains of *N. gonorrhoeae* examined have been found competent for genetic transformation. Transformation frequencies are significantly higher ($>10^3$-fold higher) with piliated cells than with nonpiliated cells.

Conjugation has recently been described in *N. gonorrhoeae*. Only strains harboring the 24.5×10^6 dalton plasmid serve as donors. There is no relationship between colony type (and presumably the presence of pili) and the ability to serve as donor.

No bacteriophage has been described for *N. gonorrhoeae*, and transduction has not been reported in the gonococcus.

EPIDEMIOLOGY. The only natural host for *N. gonorrhoeae* is the human. An estimated 2 million cases of gonorrhea were treated in the United States during 1982. The annual incidence of reported gonorrhea in the United States tripled between 1963 and 1975. This increase in incidence has leveled off in the last few years and has begun to decline. Nevertheless, gonorrhea is still a significant worldwide problem.

The gonococcus is susceptible to drying and will die within one to two hours. Because it cannot survive for long away from its host, and because it can produce primary infection only on certain specific epithelial surfaces, the gonococcus is almost always venereally transmitted.

The highest attack rate for gonorrhea occurs between the ages of 20 and 24 years in men, and 18 and 24 years in women. Because of numerous biases in case detection and reporting, the true male-female ratio for new cases of gonorrhea is unknown but is probably close to 1:1 in large populations.

There are several factors that contribute to the incidence of uncomplicated gonorrhea. Some host-related factors are as follows: the number of sexual partners; patterns of contraceptive use; population mobility; homosexuality; and recidivism. An increase in the resistance of the gonococcus to therapeutic antibiotics may also be an important factor.

Behavioral factors predisposing to gonococcal infection also increase the risk of acquiring other sexually transmitted diseases. Such diseases are prevalent in groups with a high incidence of gonorrhea, and populations or individuals with any sexually transmitted disease should be screened for gonorrhea.

PATHOGENIC PROPERTIES. Not everyone exposed to gonorrhea acquires the disease. It is uncertain whether this is due to variations in virulence or in the size of the inoculum, to nonspecific resistance, or to specific immunity. Several potential virulence factors (pili, outer membrane proteins, lipopolysaccharide) have been discussed in a preceding section. All strains of *N. gonorrhoeae* can remove iron from transferrin; fewer strains have the ability to remove iron from lactoferrin. The gonococcus elaborates a cytotoxic factor that damages ciliated epithelial cells in fallopian tube cultures. In addition, gonococci and meningococci produce an extracellular protease that cleaves a pro-thr bond on the heavy chain of the IgA_1 subclass of IgA. Cleavage of this bond results in a loss of antimicrobial activity. Only human, gorilla, and chimpanzee IgA are cleaved by this protease. Because IgA is the antibody subclass that predominates in secretions, this enzyme may be important in pathogenesis of infection. Recently, gonococcal IgA protease has been cloned in *E. coli* and mutants of gonococci have been constructed that lack enzyme activity (Koomey et al., 1982). Analysis of these mutants in appropriate model systems will provide insight into the biological significance of this protease as it pertains to the relationship of the gonococcus with its host.

It is not yet known whether gonococci produce chemotaxin in the absence of serum antibody and complement, but a polymorphonuclear (PMN) leukocyte inflammatory response is often apparent within 2 to 3 days after infection. Many gonococci stimulate formation of the chemotactic factor C5a when incubated with normal human serum plus complement. However, strains associated with both asymptomatic infections in men and disseminated infections (Arg^- Hyx^- Ura^-) are less reactive than other strains in this respect. Gonococci are present both on and within PMN leukocytes. Piliated cells tend to remain extracellular, often in clumps, whereas nonpiliated cells are readily ingested and killed. Normal human serum contains opsonic IgG, which cross-reacts with gonococcal protein I. Acquired IgA and IgG serum antibodies enhance the association of gonococci with PMN leukocytes in vitro. Pilus-specific antibody is known to be opsonic and to prevent attachment of gonococci to epithelial cells.

Resistance to the complement-mediated bactericidal action of serum has been associated with the ability of gonococci to cause disseminated disease in individuals with a functionally intact complement pathway. The bactericidal activity of NHS is mediated, in part, by IgM antibodies that recognize determinants on the gonococcal lipopolysaccharide. The molecular basis of serum resistance of *N. gonorrhoeae* has not been fully defined. A number of reports have suggested that changes in the lipopolysaccharide, protein I, and colony opacity-related protein II species contribute to the sensitivity of gonococci to NHS. Recently, three genetic loci (*sac*-1, *sac*-2, *sac*-3) have been described, which govern the level of serum resistance of *N. gonorrhoeae*. The gene products of these loci have not been identified. However, it has been postulated that the expression of these loci modifies the cell envelope structure in some fashion enabling the gonococcus to evade the bactericidal activity of NHS. Environmental factors can affect the phenotypic expression of serum resistance by *N. gonorrhoeae*.

Gonococci can activate either the classical or alternative complement pathways. Both serum-sensitive and -resistant strains activate complement. Recent studies indicate that there is a difference between the molecular configuration of the C5b-9 complex bound to serum-sensitive and serum-resistant organisms. Apparently, bactericidal antibody causes killing of serum-resistant gonococci by changing the molecular configuration of C5b-9 bound to the bacterial membrane.

DRUG SUSCEPTIBILITY. Sulfonamides were used extensively to treat gonorrhea until the end of World War II, when sulfonamide resistance of gonococci became extensive. Fortunately, penicillin was introduced at about the same time as the sulfa drugs were losing effectiveness. Initially, gonococci were extremely sensitive to penicillin with minimum inhibitory concentrations (MIC) ranging from 0.003 to ca 0.03 units/ml. Treatment with a single injection of 150,000 units of penicillin produced cure rates of 90 per cent or more.

By the mid-1950s, gonococci with reduced sensitivity to penicillin were isolated from various parts of the world. This low-level resistance was not due to a β-lactamase but necessitated higher doses of penicillin. At the same time, gonococci developed low-level resistance to several other antibiotics, including tetracycline, chloramphenicol, and erythromycin. The use of streptomycin for therapy has resulted in resistance to levels of streptomycin far in excess of achievable serum levels of this drug.

β-Lactamase-producing strains of *N. gonorrhoeae* were first reported in 1976. The β-lactamase was active against penicillin G, ampicillin, and cephalosporins. The β-lactamase-producing strains possess either a 3.2×10^6 or 4.4×10^6 dalton plasmid. Loss of this plasmid results in loss of β-lactamase production. Some strains which possess the 4.4×10^6 dalton plasmid also possess a 24.5×10^6 dalton sex factor capable of mediating the conjugal transfer of the resistance factor. It is generally believed that the 4.4×10^6 and 3.2×10^6 dalton plasmid are genetically related and originated in an enteric bacterium. β-Lactamase-producing strains now account for as many as 60 per cent of all gonococcal isolates in certain areas of the Philippines, and these strains are increasingly common elsewhere in Asia. In the United States, infections caused by β-lactamase-producing strains remained at a low level from 1976 through 1980. Recently, microepidemics of such infections have occurred in many areas of the United States. Penicillin-resistant strains of *N. gonorrhoeae* may be successfully treated with other drugs, including spectinomycin. However, spectinomycin resistance has also been reported. Prompt screening of all isolates for β-lactamase and active contact tracing are important in controlling the spread of these strains.

IMMUNITY. The natural route of infection by *N. gonorrhoeae* brings the organism into direct contact with mucosal surfaces. However, it is still not clear to what extent gonococcal infection stimulates local immunity and whether any subsequent secretory immune response will protect against subsequent infection (Griffiss, 1976).

Repeated infections with *N. gonorrhoeae* are common. The development of serologic and biochemical typing schemes will allow differentiation between reinfection and infection with a new strain. It is also not clear whether disseminated infection elicits protective antibody. At present there is no vaccine. However, candidate vaccines consisting of pilus protein or protein I are under evaluation.

LABORATORY DIAGNOSIS. A gram stain of urethral or endocervical exudate is considered diagnostic for gonorrhea when typical gram-negative diplococci are seen within leukocytes. The results are considered equivocal if only extracellular gram-negative diplococci are observed, and negative if no gram-negative diplococci are observed. The sensitivity and specificity of the gram stain of urethral exudate approaches 100 per cent. The specificity of the gram stain of endocervical exudate obtained after the cervix is wiped clean to remove vaginal secretions also is high, but the sensitivity is less than 60 per cent.

In men with uncomplicated gonorrhea, culture specimens should be obtained from the anterior urethra and inoculated onto a selective medium such as Modified Thayer-Martin (MTM) medium, Martin-Lewis (ML) medium, or Modified New York City (MNYC) medium. Cultures should be incubated in a candle jar or CO_2 incubator for 24 to 48 hours, in an environment of at least 70 per cent humidity. Oxidase-positive colonies composed of gram-negative diplococci are presumed to be *N. gonorrhoeae*. Fluorescent antibody staining, coagglutination, or the production of acid from glucose, but not maltose, sucrose, or fructose, may be used for confirmation. An additional specimen should be obtained from the anal canal and pharynx of homosexual men and processed as above.

For women with uncomplicated gonorrhea, culture specimens should be obtained from the endocervix and anal canal and processed as described above. An additional pharyngeal culture may increase the diagnostic yield.

Some stains of *N. gonorrhoeae* are inhibited by the concentration of vancomycin in the selective medium (>3 μg/ml). Arg^- Hyx^- Ura^- strains are particularly susceptible to vancomycin. These stains are often associated with both disseminated infections and asymptomatic urethral infections. To avoid failure of confirmation of disseminated infection by culture of the blood, joint fluid, or skin lesions, both selective and nonselective mediums should be used. Many gonococcal isolates are inhibited by the sodium polyanethol sulfonate present in standard liquid blood culture medium. The inhibitory effect can be reversed by the addition of 1 per cent gelatin to the medium.

NEISSERIA MENINGITIDIS

ANTIGENIC COMPOSITION

Capsule. The capsular polysaccharides of *N. meningitidis* provide the basis for grouping these organisms. The serogroups and the chemical composition of their capsular polysaccharide, where known, are listed in Table 4. Capsular polysaccharides of groups A and C meningococci are effective vaccines against meningococcal disease in children and adults. Protection is provided through complement-mediated bactericidal antibodies that persist for at least five years after a single parenteral injection of vaccine. Antibodies against group A and C polysaccharides are responsible for most of the opsonic activity against meningococci. The group B capsular polysaccharide is not immunogenic for humans.

Outer Membrane Proteins. Serogroups B and C meningococci have been subdivided into serotypes based upon the presence of outer membrane proteins. The majority of both group B and group C disease is caused by one serotype, type 2. The type 2 antigens from groups B and C meningococci are chemically and serologically identical. Antibodies against the serotype antigens are bactericidal in the presence of complement.

Lipopolysaccharide. Meningococci can be classified serologically into lipopolysaccharide immunotypes. There are at least 11 lipopolysaccharide immunotypes of *N. meningitidis*. There is no apparent correlation between the occurrence of a lipopolysaccharide immunotype and a polysaccharide serogroup or protein serotype in *N. meningitidis* except that immunotypes 10 and 11 have been observed only in serogroup A organisms. Tsai et al. (1983) reported that meningococcal lipopolysaccharides lacked repeating 0 side chains and had molecular weights similar to those of rough enteric lipopolysaccharide that were estimated to be in the range of 4,200 to 5,000.

Purified meningococcal lipopolysaccharide is highly toxic, and is as lethal for mice as is the lipopolysaccharide from *E. coli* or *S. typhimurium*. However, meningococcal lipopolysaccharide is five-to ten-fold more effective than enteric lipopolysaccharide in eliciting a dermal Shwartzman reactions in rabbits (Davis and Arnold, 1974). Salari et al. (1982) found that meningococcal lipopolysaccharide suppressed leukotriene B_4 synthesis in human polymorphonuclear leukocytes. The loss of leukotriene B_4 deprives the leukocytes of a strong chemokinetic and chemotactic factor.

Normal human sera contain bactericidal antibodies directed at some meningococcal lipopolysaccharide determinants (Griffiss, 1982). Humans develop antibodies against meningococcal lipopolysaccharide during systemic disease. However, a role for these antibodies in immunity to meningococcal infection has yet to be demonstrated.

Table 4. CHEMICAL COMPOSITION OF THE CAPSULAR POLYSACCHARIDES OF *N. MENINGITIDIS* (FROM DEVOE, 1982. USED WITH PERMISSION OF THE AMERICAN SOCIETY FOR MICROBIOLOGY).

Serogroup	Components*	Structural repeating unit
A† (homopolymer)	ManNAc, phosphate, NAc and OAc	ManNAc-(1-P$\xrightarrow{\alpha}$6)--- 3 ⋮ OAc
B (homopolymer)	NeuNAc	NeuNAc-(2$\xrightarrow{\alpha}$8)---
C‡ (homopolymer)	NeuNAc, OAc	NeuNAc-(2$\xrightarrow{\alpha}$9)--- 7 8 ⋮ ⋱ OAc OAc
W-135 (disaccharide repeating unit)	Gal, NeuNAc	6-*D*-Gal (1$\xrightarrow{\alpha}$4)-NeuNAc (2$\xrightarrow{\alpha}$6)---
X	GlcNAc, phosphate	DOGlcNAc(1-P$\xrightarrow{\alpha}$4)---
Y (BO)§ (disaccharide repeating unit)	Glc, NeuNAc, OAc	6-*D*-Glc(1$\xrightarrow{\alpha}$4)-NeuNAc(2$\xrightarrow{\alpha}$6) ⋮ O-Ac
Z (monosaccharide-glycerol repeating unit)	GalNAc, glycerol phosphate	*D*-GalNAc, (1$\xrightarrow{\alpha}$1′)-glycerol-(3′-P$\xrightarrow{\alpha}$4)---
29-e (disaccharide repeating unit)	GalNAc, KDO, OAc	*D*-GalNAc(1$\xrightarrow{\beta}$7)-KDO(2$\xrightarrow{\alpha}$3)--- 4,5 ⋮ O-Ac
L (trisaccharide repeating unit)	GlcNAc, phosphate	3-*D*-GlcNAc(1→3)-*D*-GlcNAc(1-3)-*D*-GlcNAc (1-P-

*The abbreviations used are: Gal, galactose; Glc, glucose; GlcNAc, *N*-acetylglucosamine (2-acetamido-2-deoxy-*D*-glucose); KDO, 3-deoxy-*D*-manno-octulosonic acid; ManNAc, *N*-acetylmannosamine (2-acetamido-2-deoxy-*D*-mannose); NeuNAc, *N*-acetyl neuraminic acid (sialic acid); OAc, *O*-acetylated; NAc, *N*-acetylated; phosphate, phosphodiester linkage.

†Group A is substituted with *O*-acetyl at C_3 on ca. 70% of the ManNAc-P residues.

‡Group C is substituted on C7 or C8 with 1 mol of *O*-acetyl per mol of sialic acid. One-quarter of the sialyl residues are not acetylated. Some di-*O*-acetylated (C7 and C8) may exist.

§The Y polysaccharide contains 1.3 mol of *O*-acetyl per NeuNAc residue. The most probable site for acetylation is C3, C4, or C7. ^{13}C nuclear magnetic resonance studies have shown that the serogroup BO polysaccharide is identical to serogroup Y although BO contains 1.8 mol of *o*-acetyl per mol of NeuNAc.

PATHOGENIC PROPERTIES. The fatality rate in meningococcal disease before the use of antibiotic or sulfonamide therapy was sufficiently high (75 to 90 per cent) to suggest that the meningococcus possesses the necessary mechanisms to overcome or evade all host defenses. The virulence of *N. meningitidis* depends in part upon the antiphagocytic properties of its capsule. Antibodies directed against the capsular polysaccharide are opsonic and bactericidal. In the host, meningococci behave as extracellular parasites. Although they are often visible within polymorphonuclear leukocytes, there is no evidence that they can multiply intracellularly. The lipopolysaccharide is responsible for much of the pathophysiology. Meningococci can remove iron from transferrin and lactoferrin. *N. meningitidis* strains are piliated on initial isolation. Piliation is rapidly lost upon subsequent subculture. There is little or no correlation between colonial morphology and piliation of *N. meningitidis*. Meningococci produce IgA proteases, which may contribute to the survival of the organism in some host environments.

EPIDEMIOLOGY. The meningococcus usually inhabits the human nasopharyngeal area without causing disease (Griffiss, 1976). This carrier state may last for days or months and is important because it provides a reservoir for meningococcal infections and enhances the immunity of the host. From 3 to 30 per cent of normal individuals are carriers at any given time, yet few develop meningococcal disease. Even during epidemics of meningococcal meningitis in military recruits, when the carrier rate may reach 95 per cent, the incidence of systemic disease is less than 1 per cent (Goldschneider et al., 1969, 1969a). Carriers of meningococci are usually over 21 years of age, but the attack rates of disease are highest in children: with group B, under 5 years of age; with group C, 4 to 14 years of age. The low incidence of disseminated disease after colonization suggests that host rather than bacterial factors play an important determining role.

Meningococci can establish systemic infections only in individuals that lack serum bactericidal antibodies directed against capsular or noncapsular antigens of the invading strain, or in patients deficient in the late acting complement components (C_5 thru C_9). In addition, those deficient in IgM are at greater risk from meningococcal infections than normal hosts.

The bactericidal activity of IgM and IgG is blocked by IgA (Griffiss, 1982). IgA synthesis is thought to be stimulated by gut organisms with surface antigens that cross-react with those of *N. meningitidis*. The IgA induces susceptibility by blocking immune lysis.

Meningococcal meningitis occurs sporadically and in epidemics, with highest incidence during the late winter and early spring. Most epidemics are caused by group A strains, but small outbreaks have occurred with both group B and group C strains. Sporadic cases are generally caused by group B, group C, and group Y strains, with groups B and C alternating in predominance. Whenever group A strains become prevalent, the incidence of meningitis increases markedly.

DRUG SUSCEPTIBILITY. The usual minimal inhibitory concentrations of antibiotics against the meningococcus are as follows (μg/ml): benzylpenicillin 0.03, ampicillin 0.05, methicillin 6.0, dicloxacillin 6.0, cephalothin 1.6, cephalexin 10.0, tetracycline 0.8, minocycline 0.8, rifampin 0.2, chloramphenicol 1.0, and erythromycin 1.0. Penicillin is the most potent and is the drug of choice in treatment, although useless in prophylaxis (see Chapter 16). Chloramphenicol has less in vitro activity than penicillin but penetrates the cerebrospinal fluid so well that it is an acceptable alternative in meningococcal meningitis for patients who cannot take penicillin. Rifampin, minocycline, and sulfonamides are sometimes used for eliminating meningococci from pharyngeal carriers. During World War II sulfonamides were remarkably effective in eliminating the carrier state but many strains of meningococci are now resistant to that drug.

Meningococci and gonococci can exchange genetic information. These species can be isolated together from infected individuals. A strain of *N. meningitidis* was recently identified that harbored the 4.5 megadalton β-lactamase plasmid and the 24.5 megadalton transfer plasmid common to penicillinase-producing strains of *N. gonorrhoeae* (Dillon et al., 1983).

IMMUNITY. Group A and group C capsular polysaccharide vaccines are available (Gotschlich et al., 1969, 1969a). These vaccines are highly protective against strains of these serogroups. Protection is provided through complement-mediated bactericidal antibodies that persist for at least five years after a single parenteral injection of vaccine. The capsular polysaccharide from serogroup B organisms is not immunogenic for humans.

LABORATORY DIAGNOSIS. Specimens of blood, spinal fluid, and nasopharyngeal secretions should be examined for the presence of *N. meningitidis* in cases of suspected meningococcal disease. Specimens should be collected before treatment with antimicrobial agents because they reduce cultural isolation. However, smears may still show gram-negative diplococci, and counter-immunoelectrophoresis will detect meningococcal capsular polysaccharide. The CSF should be cultured on chocolate or blood agar in either a candle jar or a CO_2 incubator. The presence of oxidase-positive colonies consisting of gram-negative diplococci provides a presumptive identification of *N. meningitidis*. Production of acid from glucose and maltose, but not from sucrose, lactose, or fructose, may be used for confirmation. The serologic group may be determined by a slide agglutination test, using first polyvalent then monovalent antisera.

Nasopharyngeal specimens must be obtained from the posterior nasopharyngeal wall behind the soft palate. Specimens should be inoculated onto selective medium (modified Thayer-Martin) and processed as above.

Gram-stained smears of CSF may be diagnostic. However, organisms in CSF smears are often more difficult to find than in pneumococcal meningitis. Quellung tests may be of value.

Branhamella. *B. catarrhalis* (formerly *N. catarrhalis*) are gram-negative cocci that morphologically resemble *Neisseria*. Other relevant characteristics are presented in Table 2. This organism was formerly placed in the genus *Neisseria*; however, studies of DNA base content, fatty acid composition, and genetic transformation showed that it did not belong in that genus. *B. catarrhalis* should be considered more than a harmless commensal of the mucous membranes of humans. It is an infrequent, yet significant, cause of severe systemic infections such as meningitis and endocarditis (Doern et al., 1981). It has also been implicated as a pathogen in otitis media (Bluestone and Shurin, 1974) and acute maxillary sinusitis in children (Wald et al., 1981), and in acute pulmonary infections in coal miners (Ninane et al., 1978). *B. catarrhalis* may be isolated from clinical syndromes indistinguishable from gonococcal urethritis (Doern and Gantz, 1982) and gonococcal opthalmia neonatorum (Spark et al., 1979). Thus, a false diagnosis of a gonococcal infection is possible when that diagnosis is based solely on clinical presentation and on the finding of intracellular gram-negative diplococci in gram-stained smears of exudates. Many strains of *B. catarrhalis* produce a β-lactamase of chromosomal origin. This enzyme is apparently more active against penicillin congeners than against cephalosporin congeners (Doern et al., 1980).

References

Bluestone, C. D. and Shurin, P. A.: Middle ear disease in children. Pediatr Clin North Am 21:379, 1974.

Brooks, G. F. and Donegan, E. (eds.): Gonococcal Infections. Baltimore and London, Edward Arnold Ltd, 1984.

Davis, C. E., and Arnold, K.: Role of meningococcal endotoxin in meningococcal purpura. J Exp Med 140:159, 1974.

DeVoe, I. W.: The meningococcus and mechanisms of pathogenicity. Microbiol Rev 46:162, 1982.

Dillon, J. R., Pauze, M., and Yeung, K-H.: Spread of penicillinase-producing and transfer plasmids from the gonococcus to *Neisseria meningitidis*. Lancet i:779, 1983.

Doern, G. V. and Gantz, N. M.: Isolation of *Branhamella (Neisseria) catarrhalis* from men with urethritis. Sex Trans Dis 9:202, 1982.

Doern, G. V., Miller, M. J., and Winn, R. E.: *Branhamella (Neisseria) catarrhalis* systemic disease in humans. Arch Int Med 141:1690, 1981.

Doern, G. V., Siebers, K. G., Hallick, L. M., and Morse, S. A.: Antibiotic susceptibility of beta-lactamase-producing strains of *Branhamella (Neisseria) catarrhalis*. Antimicrob Agents Chemother 17:24, 1980.

Draper, D. L., James, J. F., Brooks, G. F., and Sweet, R. L.: Comparison of virulence markers of peritoneal and fallopian tube isolates with endocervical *Neisseria gonorrhoeae* isolates from women with acute salpingitis. Infect Immunity 27:882, 1980.
Goldschneider, I., Gotschlich, E. C., and Artenstein, M. S.: Human immunity to the meningococcus. I. The role of humoral antibodies. J Exp Med 129:1307, 1969.
Goldschneider, I., Gotschlich, E. C., and Artenstein, M. S.: Human immunity to the meningococcus. II. Development of natural immunity. J Exp Med 129:1327, 1969a.
Griffiss, J. M., and Artenstein, M. S.: The ecology of the genus *Neisseria*. Mt Sinai J Med 43:746, 1976.
Griffiss, J. M.: Epidemic meningococcal disease: synthesis of a hypothetical immunoepidemiologic model. Rev Infect Dis 4:159, 1982.
James, J. F. and Swanson, J.: Studies on gonococcus infection. XIII. Occurrence of color/opacity colonial variants in clinical cultures. Infect Immunity 19:332, 1978.
Kellogg, D. S. Jr., Cohen, I. R., Norins, L. O., Schroeter, A. L., and Reising, G.: *Neisseria gonorrhoeae* II. Colonial variation and pathogenicity during 35 months in vitro. J Bacteriol 96:596, 1968.
Kellogg, D. S. Jr., Peacock, W. L. Jr., Deacon, W. E., Brown, L., and Pirkle, C. I.: *Neisseria gonorrhoeae* I. Virulence genetically linked to clonal variation. J Bacteriol 85:1274, 1963.
Knapp, J. S. and Holmes, K. K.: Modified oxidation-fermentation for detection of acid production from carbohydrates by *Neisseria* spp. and *Branhamella catarrhalis*. J Clin Microbiol 18:56, 1983.
Koomey, J. M., Gill, R. E., and Falkow, S.: Genetic and biochemical analysis of gonococcal IgA_1 protease: cloning in *Escherichia coli* and constructing of mutants of gonococci that fail to produce the activity. Proc Natl Acad Sci USA 72:7881, 1982.
Morello, J. A. and Bohnhoff, M.: *Neisseria* and *Branhamella*, p. 111. In Lennette, E. H. et al. (eds.): Manual of Clinical Microbiology, third ed. American Society for Microbiology, Washington, D. C., 1980.
Morse, S. A.: The biology of the gonococcus. Crit Rev Microbiol 7:93, 1978.
Ninane, G., Joly, J., and Kraytman, M.: Bronchopulmonary infection due to *Branhamella catarrhalis*. 11 cases assessed by transtracheal puncture. Br Med J 1:276, 1978.
Roberts, R. B. (ed.): The Gonococcus. New York, John Wiley and Sons, 1977.
Salari, S. H., DeVoe, I. W., and Powell, W. S.: Inhibition of leukotriene B_4 synthesis in human polymorphonuclear leukocytes after exposure to meningococcal lipoplysaccharide. Biochem Biophys Res Commun 104:1517, 1982.
Spark, R. P., Dahlberg, P. W., and LaBelle, J. W.: Pseudogonococcal opthalmia neonatorum. *Branhamella (Neisseria) catarrhalis* conjunctivitis. Am J Clin Pathol 72:471, 1979.
Swanson, J.: Colony opacity and protein II compositions of gonococci. Infect Immunity 37:359, 1982.
Tsai, C-M., Boykins, R., and Frasch, C. E.: Heterogeneity and variation among *Neisseria meningitidis* lipopolysaccharides. J Bacteriol 155:498, 1983.
Wald, E. R., Milmoe, G. J., Bowen, A., Ledesma-Medina, J., Salamon, N., and Bluestone, C. D.: Acute maxillary sinusitis in children. N Engl J Med 304:749, 1981.

30

MORAXELLA, KINGELLA AND ACINETOBACTER

CHARLES E. DAVIS, M.D.
HERMAN BAER, M.D.

Moraxella, *Kingella* and *Acinetobacter* are gram-negative, strictly aerobic, coccobacillary rods that do not produce flagella or spores. Their classification has changed repeatedly and there are numerous synonyms for some of the species. Seven species are currently included in the *Moraxella* genus: *M. lacunata* (the diplobacillus of Morax and Axenfeld), *M. bovis, M. nonliquefaciens, M. phenylpyruvica, M. osloensis, M. urethralis* (formerly Mima polymorpha and CDC group M4), and *M. atlantae* (formerly CDC group M3). The validity of the first 5 species has been confirmed genetically by transformation studies. *Kingella* consists of 3 species: *K. kingae, K. indologenes*, and *K. denitrificans* (formerly TM-1). *K. kingae* was previously classified as CDC group M-1 and more recently as *M. kingii*. It was reclassified because it differs biochemically and genetically from the *Moraxella*. *Acinetobacter* is considered in Bergey's Manual to consist of one species, *A. calcoaceticus*. This species includes both saccarolytic (formerly *Herellea vaginicola*) and nonsaccharolytic strains (formerly *Mima polymorpha*, variety nonoxidans).

All 3 genera are currently included in the family Neisseriaceae (see Chapter 29, Table 1). *Moraxella* is genetically and phenotypically related to the other members of this family, especially *Branhamella*, but *Acinetobacter* is a hardier, nutritionally versatile organism that shows no significant genetic homology with the other *Neisseriaceae*. Although the G + C content of both *Moraxella* and *Acinetobacter* is in the range of 40 to 47 per cent, DNA hybridization studies show very limited homology (Henriksen, 1976). *Kingella* is genetically unrelated to *Neisseria*, *Moraxella*, or *Acinetobacter* but is included in the family Neisseriaceae because of a number of phenotypic similarities. The G + C content of *K. kingae* is about 47%, *K. indologenes* 49%, and *K. denitrificans* 54% (Snell and LaPage, 1976).

MORAXELLA AND KINGELLA

MORPHOLOGY. The chief reason for regarding *Moraxella, Acinetobacter*, and *Kingella* as closely related bacteria is their microscopic morphology. In stained smears of wild organisms obtained directly from patients or the environment, they are short, plump bacteria that tend to occur in pairs and to be so coccoid that they may be confused with *Neisseria*. Careful examination almost always reveals some bacillary forms that increase in number with repeated passages in culture. *Moraxella* and *Kingella* are usually fastidious and produce small colonies. Colonies from freshly isolated strains of *M. nonliquefaciens, M. bovis, K. kingae*, and *K. indologenes* spread and corrode agar surfaces after incubation for several days in a humid environment. This type of growth is associated with polar fimbriae of about 5 nm diameter. Fimbriae are often lost during passage, and only fimbriated cells show the twitching motility that appears to cause the spreading phenomenon. Nonfimbriated bacteria neither corrode agar surfaces nor exhibit twitching motility (Henriksen, 1976). Because the twitching motility and corrosion are difficult to demonstrate by routine procedures, *Moraxella* and *Kingella* are still considered nonmotile for purposes of differentiation from flagellated bacteria in the diagnostic laboratory. The polar fimbriae appear to determine competence in transformation.

Capsules may or may not be present. Cell walls have not been extensively studied.

M. bovis and *K. kingae* produce beta-hemolytic colonies on sheep and rabbit blood agar plates. The other species of both genera are nonhemolytic.

ANTIGENIC COMPOSITION. Because *Moraxella* and *Kingella* are not important pathogens, few studies of antigenic composition have been undertaken. Instead, the purpose of serologic studies has been to confirm taxonomic relationships. Studies of a collection of *Moraxella* species and a few *Acinetobacter* strains show serologic relationships between *M. lacunata, M. bovis,* and *M. nonliquefaciens.* There was no cross-reactivity with the other *Moraxella* species or *Acinetobacter.*

METABOLISM. *Moraxella* and *Kingella* are relatively fastidious and grow best on rich media such as blood agar. In the case of *M. lacunata,* this fastidiousness is due in part to inhibition by fatty acids and other media components that can be neutralized by the addition of binding agents such as starch, charcoal, or serum.

Moraxella are mesophilic and obligately aerobic. They grow poorly at room temperature and not at all at 5°C. They do not attack sugars. All *Moraxella* are oxidase positive when tested by *N,N*-dimethyl-*p*-phenylenediamine, a characteristic demonstrated by Baumann et al. (1968) to be associated with the presence of cytochrome C in the electron transport system. *Moraxella* species are chemoorganotrophs that use only a limited number of organic acids, alcohols, and amino acids as carbon and energy sources. Little is known about specific growth requirements. *M. osloensis,* but not the other species, will grow in mineral medium with acetate and ammonium salts. Only *M. bovis* fails to produce detectable catalase activity. Nitrogen can be obtained from reduction of nitrate by *M. lacunata, M. nonliquefaciens,* most strains of *M. phenylpyruvica,* and occasional strains of *M. osloensis. M. bovis* and *M. lacunata* are proteolytic and digest blood serum in Loeffler's medium. The other species are nonproteolytic. Only *M. phenylpyruvica* degrades urea. *M. osloensis* can utilize ammonium as the sole nitrogen source.

Kingella are also oxidase positive, nonproteolytic, chemoorganotrophs but can ferment carbohydrates weakly. Growth is independent of hemoglobin derivatives, NAD, and CO_2. Few amino acids, organic acids, or alcohols are attacked. All species are catalase, gelatinase, and urease negative. Only *K. denitrificans* synthesizes nitrate reductase and only *K. indologenes* produces indole from tryptophan.

PATHOGENIC PROPERTIES. *Moraxella* and *Kingella* inhabit the mucous membranes of animals. They rarely cause systemic disease even when defense mechanisms are impaired. In the last century, *M. lacunata* was described by Morax and Axenfeld as a cause of keratoconjunctivitis in man, but this infection has essentially disappeared. *M. bovis* causes epizootic keratoconjunctivitis of cattle, a condition that causes severe economic losses in the livestock industry. *M. caprae* and *M. equi,* which are indistinguishable bacteriologically from *M. lacunata,* are isolated from keratoconjunctivitis of goats and horses, respectively. *M. phenylpyruvica, M. osloensis,* and *M. nonliquefaciens* are part of the indigenous flora of mammals and are virtually nonpathogenic, except for occasional isolation of *M. nonliquefaciens* from corneal ulcers and keratitis in debilitated patients (Cobo et al., 1981). *M. urethralis* and *M. atlantae* are rare causes of local and systemic infections in compromised patients. Although *Kingella species* are equally rare causes of infection, there have been several reports of endocarditis, osteomyelitis, and septic arthritis (Rabin et al., 1983; Davis and Peel, 1982, and Redfield et al., 1980).

Because they rarely cause disease, there have been few studies of possible pathogenic properties. *M. bovis* needs fimbriae to colonize mucous membranes and cause bovine disease. Fimbriae are probably also responsible for the adhesiveness of *M. nonliquefaciens* and *K. kingae,* but nonfimbriated *Moraxella* and *Kingella* also adhere readily to mucosal surfaces. Because both genera have a typical gram-negative wall, they presumably contain LPS, but its toxicity has not been studied.

LABORATORY DIAGNOSIS. *Moraxella* and *Kingella* should be considered when the gram stain reveals deep-staining, gram-negative diplococci accompanied by definite bacillary forms. Colonies are small and delicate, and some strains may grow only on agar enriched with blood or serum (*M. lacunata* and *M. bovis*). *M. bovis* and *K. kingae* are beta-hemolytic.

All species of *Moraxella* are oxidase positive, nonmotile by standard tests, indole negative, nonsaccharolytic, and penicillin sensitive. They are differentiated from *Acinetobacter* with 100 per cent accuracy by their oxidase positivity and penicillin sensitivity and from *Kingella* by their catalase positivity and inability to ferment glucose. Although *M. bovis* is catalase negative, it is never isolated from people. *Moraxella* are more difficult to differentiate from several unnamed bacteria that resemble *Moraxella* phenotypically (M-5, and M-6). M-5 is usually isolated from infections of dog bites, but M-6 colonizes the mucosa of the respiratory tract. Careful attention to yellow pigment production (M-5, and M-6), inability to utilize acetate (M-5 and M-6), and catalase negativity (M-6) will usually separate these unusual isolates. *Moraxella* are differentiated from one another by the diagnostic characteristics shown in Table 1. *M. lacunata* is recognized by its requirement for enrichment with blood or serum and enhancement of growth by CO_2; *M. bovis* by its beta-hemolysis and catalase negativity; and *M. phenylpyruvica* by production of urease and phenylalanine deaminase. *M. nonliquefaciens* can usually be separated from *M. osloensis* by failure to grow on MacConkey agar and by production of nitrate reductase. *M. osloensis* is hardier than other *Moraxella* and produces colonies that approach those of *Acinetobacter* in size and character. *M. phenylpyruvica* is a very fastidious organism that deaminates phenylalanine and grows poorly even in complex media.

The 3 species of *Kingella* are usually easy to differentiate from one another and from other fastidious bacteria that pit or corrode agar surfaces. Major identifying characteristics are listed in Table 2. Catalase negativity and the ability to ferment carbohydrates distinguish *Kingella* from most other bacteria. *Kingella* do not grow well in peptone-based carbohydrate media, and fermentation reactions should be tested in agar or broth supplemented with ascitic fluid or serum. *K. kingae* is beta-hemolytic, *K. indologenes* produces indole, and *K. denitrificans* reduces nitrate to nitrite and nitrogen gas. *K. denitrificans* was originally called TM-1 because it grows on Thayer-Martin agar, an otherwise selective medium for pathogenic *Neisseria.* It can be differentiated from pathogenic *Neisseria* by its catalase negativity and nitrate reductase.

DRUG SUSCEPTIBILITY. *Moraxella* and *Kingella* are uniformly sensitive to penicillin and most other antibiotics. *K. denitrificans* is resistant to vancomycin and the polymyxins. *M. bovis* is resistant to 2.5 μ/ml of cloxacillin, which is sometimes incorporated into blood agar as a selective medium for cultures of bovine keratoconjunctivitis.

Table 1. DIAGNOSTIC CHARACTERISTICS OF MORAXELLA

Test or Substrate	*lacunata*	*bovis*	*nonliquefaciens*	*osloensis*	*phenylpyruvica*	*atlantae*	*urethralis*
Enrichment[1]	[required]	±	0	0	0	0	0
β-Hemolysis	0	[+]	0	0	0	0	0
Oxidase	+	+	+	+	+	+	+
Catalase	+(w)	[0]	+(w)	+(w)	+(w)	+	+
CO_2 enhancement	+	0	0	0	0	0	0
MacConkey agar	NG	NG	NG	+(w) or NG	+(w) or NG	+	+
Citrate	0	0	0	0	0	0	[+]
Nitrate reduction	+	0	+	−or+ (28%)	+ (64%) or−	0	0
Phenylalanine deaminase	0	0	0	0	[+]	0	[+]
Urease (Christensen's)	0	0	0	0	[+ (95%)]	0	0
Acid from carbohydrates	0	0	0	0	0	0	0
Acetate	0	0	0	[+]	0	0	[+]
Penicillin sensitivity	S	S	S	S	S	S	S

[1]With blood or 3% rabbit serum; (w) = weak; NG = no growth; 0 = negative; S = sensitive; [ ] = reaction of major importance in identification.

ACINETOBACTER

Acinetobacter calcoaceticus is the only species recognized in *Bergey's Manual*, but it is customary to divide the species into strains that oxidize carbohydrates and strains that fail to attack carbohydrates. Some diagnostic schemes subdivide both of these groups into hemolytic and nonhemolytic biotypes. The oxidative strains have been known by a variety of names, including *Herellea vaginicola, Moraxella glucidolytica, Bacterium anitratum,* and *Acinetobacter anitratus*. Synonyms for the nonoxidizing strains include *Moraxella lwoffi, Mima polymorpha* var. nonoxidans, B5W-organism, and *Acinetobacter lwoffi*.

MORPHOLOGY. The microscopic morphology of *Acinetobacter* is indistinguishable from that of *Moraxella* and *Kingella*. The nonsaccharolytic strains of *A. calcoaceticus* were presumably named *Mima* because they mimicked *Neisseria*. Larger cells, typical bacilli, and filamentous forms can be found in most cultures. *Acinetobacter* strains generally grow more vigorously than *Moraxella* and *Kingella* and produce butyrous colonies resembling those of the Enterobacteriaceae.

Electron microscopy of thin sections of *Acinetobacter* has revealed a multilayer cell envelope typical of gram-negative bacilli. Chemical studies of the LPS and peptidoglycan confirm their similarity to the equivalent cell wall

Table 2. DIAGNOSTIC CHARACTERISTICS OF MORAXELLA AND OTHER CORRODING BACILLI

Test or Substrate	Kingella *kingae*	Kingella *indologenes*	Kingella *denitrificans*	Eikenella	A. actinomycetemcomitans	Moraxella	Hemophilus, aphrophilus	Cardiobacterium hominis	Capnocytophaga
Oxidase	+	+	+	+	[0orW)	+	0	+	[0]
Catalase	0	0	0	0	[+]	[+[1]]	[0]	0	0
β-hemolysis	[+]	0	0	0	0	0[1]	0	0	0
Indole	0	[+]	0	0	0	0	0	[+]	0
Urease	0	0	0	0	0	0[2]	0	0	0
Nitrate reduction	0	0	[+]	+	+	V	+	0	OorV
Nitrite reduction	0	0	[+]	0	0	0[3]	N.D.	0	0
Acid from CHO[4]	+	+	+	[0]	+	[0]	+	+	+
glucose	+	+	+	0	+	0	+	+	+
maltose	+	+	+	0	+	0	+	+	+
sucrose	0	[+]	0	0	[0]	0	[+]	+	+
fructose	0	[+]	0	0	N.D.	0	N.D.	N.D.	V
mannose	0	[+]	0	0	N.D.	0	N.D.	N.D.	+
Penicillin sensitivity	+	+	+	+	0	+	+	+	+
CO_2	I	I	I	E	EorR	I	R	EorR	R
Pigment (Pale yellow)	0	0	0	[+]	0	0	0	0	[+]
Growth on Thayer-Martin media	0	0	[+]	0	0	0	0	0	[+]

Key: A = Actinobacillus; W = weak; 0 = negative; + = positive; [ ] = reaction of major importance in identification; E = enhanced; R = required; I = indifferent; v = variable; N.D. = not done. Reactions partly taken from Henriksen and Bovre, 1976; Snell and La Page, 1976; and Lennette et al., *Manual of Clinical Microbiology,* 3rd ed., Am. Soc. Microbiol., Wash., D.C., 1980.

[1]except *M. bovis*; [2]except *M. phenylpyruvica*; [3]except *M. urethralis*; [4]in ascitic or serum supplemented media.

structures of Enterobacteriaceae. Capsules have been seen in electron micrographs and characterized chemically and serologically. Some strains of *Acinetobacter* display twitching or gliding motility that depends on polar fimbriae. The relationship of genetic competence to fimbriae has not been studied.

ANTIGENIC COMPOSITION. Fluorescein-labeled antisera to capsular antigens have identified 28 serotypes of saccharolytic acinetobacters and suggested that there are different serotypes of nonsaccharolytic acinetobacters (Marcus et al., 1969). Juni (1978) studied the capsules of two strains of *Acinetobacter* and found that one was composed of L-rhamnose and D-glucose and the other of glucose and galactose. The capsule that was composed of rhamnose and glucose cross-reacted in precipitin studies with antisera to groups B and G streptococci and type XIII pneumococci.

The peptidoglycan of saccharolytic and nonsaccharolytic strains is similar and contains muramic acid, glucosamine, alanine, D-glutamic acid, and m,-diaminopimelic acid, a composition characteristic of peptidoglycans of chemotype I (Horisberger, 1977). Neither the LPS nor the polar fimbriae of *Acinetobacter* have been characterized antigenically, but the LPS is a polyclonal activator. Cross-reactions between chlamydial antibody and *A. calcoaceticus* are directed at a heat stable, nondialyzable, water-soluble antigen (Brade and Brunner, 1979).

METABOLISM. Acinetobacters are strictly aerobic chemoorganotrophs that are versatile in the utilization of organic compounds for carbon and energy sources. None has specific growth requirements and most can grow in a mineral medium containing a single organic carbon and energy source. Nitrate is not reduced to nitrite or other reduced compounds but ammonium and nitrate salts can be used as nitrogen sources. Urease-producing strains can substitute urea for these compounds.

Acinetobacters capable of using glucose as a source of carbon and energy degrade this compound exclusively via the Entner-Doudoroff pathway. Acinetobacters lack enzymes for the direct phosphorylation of hexoses, and the first step for entry into the Entner-Doudoroff pathway is the oxidation of glucose to gluconic acid (Juni, 1978).

Acinetobacters that produce acid from glucose, lactose, mannose, arabinose, and xylose produce a glucose dehydrogenase that oxidizes D-glucose to D-gluconolactone. Oxygen is the ultimate electron acceptor for the particulate form of this enzyme, which is tightly complexed to cytochrome b (Hauge, 1960). Nonsaccharolytic acinetobacters lack glucose dehydrogenase (Juni, 1978).

All the enzymes of the tricarboxylic and glyoxylate cycles have been demonstrated in either cell-free extracts or ethanol-grown cells of *Acinetobacter*. Acinetobacters contain functional electron transport pathways consisting of cytochrome a_1, a_2, o, d and b as well as flavin. All can be reduced with NADH or succinate and re-oxidized by oxygen. As expected for an oxidase-negative organism, *Acinetobacter* does not contain cytochrome C.

Pathways used by this versatile organism for biosynthesis and for the degradation of aromatic and alicyclic compounds, hydrocarbons, and 2,3-butanediol are similar to those of the pseudomonads and have been extensively reviewed by Juni (1978). *Acinetobacter* strains produce a polyanionic emulsifier (emulsan) and utilize chlorinated biphenyl compounds, characteristics that may be useful in control of pollutants. *Acinetobacter* also synthesizes antineoplastic enzymes. A succinylated *Acinetobacter* glutaminase-asparaginase has been used to treat patients with carcinoma and leukemia.

Most strains grow well at mesophilic temperature ranges of 35 to 37°C. Some strains grow well at 5°C. The optimal pH for growth is about 7.

PATHOGENIC PROPERTIES. *Acinetobacter* is common in the environment and has been isolated from a nearly unlimited variety of clinical specimens. In most cases *Acinetobacter* can be dismissed as a contaminating or colonizing strain, but it is occasionally isolated from patients in whom its pathogenic role is indisputable. When *Acinetobacter* is isolated in mixed culture, the clinical situation and the culture results must be carefully evaluated before the diagnosis of *Acinetobacter* infection is accepted.

Acinetobacter behaves essentially like any other gram-negative, aerobic, opportunistic pathogen. Because of its low pathogenicity, the organism rarely, if ever, causes infection in otherwise healthy individuals. The number of nosocomial infections by *Acinetobacter* has increased in recent years. Several outbreaks of nosocomial *Acinetobacter* septicemia have been reported, and indwelling intravenous catheters were suspected as the portal of entry of the organisms. Nosocomial *Acinetobacter* pneumonia most often affects patients who are severely debilitated and have undergone major surgery or trauma. The pneumonia may be necrotizing. Abscesses, pleural effusions, and septicemia are occasional complications. Acinetobacter urinary tract infection is usually associated with an indwelling bladder catheter. Postoperative surgical infections by *Acinetobacter* usually involve complicated procedures in severely ill patients or implantation of a prosthetic orthopedic device.

Some strains of *Acinetobacter* produce fimbriae. The role of these structures in the usual habitat of this free-living bacterium is unknown. The adherence of *Acinetobacter* to epithelial cells is related to its ability to adhere to hydrocarbons and is associated with hydrophobic interactions (Rosenberg et al., 1981).

Since *Acinetobacter* seldom causes disease, there have been few studies of possible pathogenic properties. The heteropolysaccharide capsules may prevent phagocytosis by severely ill patients who may be deficient in opsonins or phagocytes.

Acinetobacter contains a typical trilaminar, gram-negative cell wall, and its LPS has been isolated and partly characterized chemically. Its biologic activity for people has been proven by typical endotoxin reactions in 23 patients who were hemodialyzed with contaminated fluid (Kantor et al., 1983).

IMMUNITY. Healthy people resist colonization and infection by *Acinetobacter*. Since severely ill, immunocompromised patients are frequently colonized and occasionally infected, it is likely that normal resistance mechanisms play a role in preventing *Acinetobacter* infection. The relative importance of natural versus acquired immunity is unknown. The heteropolysaccharide capsule is antigenic in animals and it is likely that both the *Acinetobacter* capsule and LPS stimulate antibody production in human beings. It is possible that natural resistance to infection is partly related to the known cross-reactions between *Acinetobacter* capsules and those of Streptococcus B and G and *S. pneumoniae* type XIII.

Table 3. DIAGNOSTIC CHARACTERISTICS OF *ACINETOBACTER CALCOACETICUS**

Test or Substrate	Anitratus Biotypes *anitratus*	Anitratus Biotypes *hemolyticus*	Lwoffii Biotypes *lwoffii*	Lwoffii Biotypes *alcaligenes*
Oxidase	0	0	0	0
Catalase	100	100	100	100
Hemolysis	[0]	[100]	[0]	[100]
Growth on MacConkey agar	100	99	99	100
SS agar	[1]	[90]	[1]	[93]
Nitrate reduction	0	0	0	0
Motility	0	0	0	0
Oxidation-Fermentation	[Ox]	[Ox]	[I]	[I]
glucose	100	100	0	0
galactose	100	100	0	0
mannose	99	96	0	0
xylose	100	100	0	0
10% lactose	100	98	0	0
sucrose	0	0	0	0
fructose	0	0	0	0
Urease	72	22	25	6
Hydrolysis of:				
gelatin	[0]	[99]	[0]	[100]
lecithin	[0]	[98]	[8]	[94]
tween 80	100	100	100	100
starch	0	0	0	0

*Modified from Gilardi, 1978. Results are given as per cent positive. I = inactive; Ox = oxidative attack on carbohydrates; [ ] indicates key reactions for distinguishing biotypes.

LABORATORY DIAGNOSIS. Although the microscopic morphology of *Acinetobacter* is indistinguishable from that of *Moraxella* and *Kingella*, the colonial morphology is usually quite different. Acinetobacters produce larger, butyrous colonies on most standard laboratory media; *Moraxella* and *Kingella* produce smaller, more fragile colonies and some strains of *Moraxella* require media enriched with blood or serum. Unlike *Moraxella* and *Kingella*, Acinetobacters are strongly catalase positive, oxidase negative, and resistant to penicillin. They are easily differentiated from *Pseudomonas* by the oxidase reaction and from Enterobacteriaceae by their failure to reduce nitrate and their lack of reactivity in triple sugar iron agar or Kligler's iron agar. Acinetobacters also give uniformly negative results in the following tests: indole, H_2S, decarboxylation of lysine, ornithine, and arginine, and deamination of phenylalanine. The remainder of the laboratory characteristics of the saccharolytic (var. anitratus) and the nonsaccharolytic (var. lwoffi) strains are given in Table 3. Although only one species is recognized by bacterial taxonomists, the variation in diagnostic characteristics makes it more convenient in the diagnostic laboratory to divide both the saccharolytic and the nonsaccharolytic strains into hemolytic and nonhemolytic biotypes.

ANTIBIOTIC SUSCEPTIBILITY. *Acinetobacter* is resistant to penicillin, ampicillin, the cephalosporins, and chloramphenicol. The susceptibility to tetracycline varies but many strains are susceptible to doxycycline and minocycline. Most strains are sensitive to the aminoglycosides and the acylampicillins.

EPIDEMIOLOGY. *Acinetobacter* is not part of the indigenous flora of man or animals, but it is commonly found in soil and water. The organism is occasionally recovered in specimens obtained from non-hospitalized patients, but it is much more prevalent in hospitalized patients. *Acinetobacter*, like many other aerobic gram-negative organisms, frequently contaminates moist environments in the hospital, e.g., respirators, humidifiers, and sinks. Patients acquire the organism either by direct contact with an environmental reservoir of the organism, or indirectly from members of the hospital staff who carry the organism on their hands. Nosocomial colonization by *Acinetobacter* may involve the respiratory tract, intestinal tract, urogenital tract, and the moist intertriginous areas of the skin. The severity of illness seems to be the most important risk factor for nonsocomial colonization.

Fluorescein-labeled antisera to capsular antigens can be used as an epidemiologic marker for tracing the source of nosocomial infections.

References

Baumann, P., Doudoroff, M. and Stanier, R. Y.: Study of the Moraxella group. I. Genus *Moraxella* and the *Neisseria catarrhalis* group. J Bacteriol 95:58, 1968.

Brade, H., and Brunner, H.: Serological cross-reactions between *Acinetobacter calcoaceticus* and chlamydiae. J Clin Microbiol 10:819, 1979.

Buchanan, R. E., and Gibbons, N. E. (eds.): Bergey's Manual of Determinative Bacteriology. 8th ed. Baltimore, The Williams and Wilkins Company, 1974, pp. 426–438.

Cobo, L. M., Coster, D. J., and Peacock, J.: *Moraxella* keratitis in a nonalcoholic population. Br J Ophthalmol 65:683, 1981.

Davis, J. M. and Peel, M. M.: Osteomyelitis and septic arthritis caused by *Kingella kingae*. J Clin Path 35:219, 1982.

Gilardi, G. L.: Identification of miscellaneous glucose non-fermenting gram-negative bacteria. *In* G. L. Gilardi, (ed.): *Glucose Non-fermenting Gram-negative Bacteria in Clinical Microbiology*. CRC Press, West Palm Beach, 1978, p 45.

Hauge, J. G.: Purification and properties of glucose dehydrogenase and cytochrome b from *Bacterium anitratum*. Biochim Biophys Acta 45:250, 1960.

Henriksen, S. D.: *Moraxella, Neisseria, Branhamella*, and *Acinetobacter*. Annu Rev Microbiol 30:63, 1976.

Henriksen, S. D. and Bovre, K.: Transfer of *Moraxella kingae* Henriksen and Bovre to the genus *Kingella* gen. nov. in the family Neisseriaceae. Int J Syst Bacteriol 26:447, 1976.

Horisberger, M.: Structure of the peptidoglycans of *Moraxella glucidolytica* and *Moraxella lwoffi* grown on hydrocarbons. Arch Microbiol 112:297, 1977.

Juni, E.: Genetics and physiology of *Acinetobacter.* Annu Rev Microbiol 32:349, 1978.
Kantor, R. J., Carson, L. A., Graham, D. R., Petersen, N. J., and Favero, N. S.: Outbreak of pyrogenic reactions at a dialysis center. Association with infusion of heparinized saline solution. Am J Med 74:449, 1983.
Lennette, E. H., Spaulding, E. H., and Truant, J. P.: *Manual of Clinical Microbiology*, 3rd ed., Am. Soc. Microbiol., Wash, D.C., 1980.
Marcus, B. B., Samuels, S. B., Pittman, B., and Cherry, W. B.: A serologic study of *Herellea vaginicola* and its identification by immunofluorescent staining. Am J Clin Pathol 52:309, 1969.
Rabin, R. L., Wong, P., Noonan, J. A., and Plumley, D. D.: *Kingella kingae* endocarditis in a child with a prosthetic aortic valve and bifurcation graft. Am J Dis Child 137:403, 1983.
Redfield, D. C., Overturf, G. D., Ewing, H., and Powars, D.: Bacteremia, arthritis, and skin lesions due to *Kingella kingae*. Arch Dis Child 55:411, 1980.
Rosenberg, M., Perry, A., Bayer, E. A., Gutnick, D. L., and Rosenberg, E.: Adherence of *Acinetobacter calcoaceticus* RAG-1 to human epithelial cells and to hexadecane. Infect Immun 33:29, 1981.
Snell, J. J. S. and La Page, S. P.: Transfer of some saccharolytic *Moraxella* species to *Kingella* Henriksen and Bovre 1976 with descriptions of *Kingella indologenes* sp. nov. and *Kingella denitrificans* sp. nov. Int J Syst Bacteriol 26:451, 1976.

GRAM-NEGATIVE RODS

31
ENTEROBACTERIACEAE

Frits Ørskov, M.D.
Ida Ørskov, M.D.

Enterobacteriaceae are a family of five tribes (Table 1) of closely related, nonspore-forming gram-negative bacilli that ferment glucose and, except for some strains of *Erwinia*, reduce nitrates to nitrites. They are found widespread in nature, and many genera are important normal inhabitants of the intestinal flora of mammals. Others, like the typhoid bacillus, the Shiga bacillus, and the plague bacillus, are historically and medically among the most important bacterial pathogens encountered by man. The plague bacillus, *Yersinia pestis*, and the other *Yersinia* species are discussed more extensively in Chapter 37 for historical reasons and because they cause clinical syndromes similar to those caused by *Francisella* and *Pasteurella*. Most members of the family can be opportunistic pathogens.

The taxonomy and nomenclature used in this chapter are in accordance with the eighth edition of Bergey's Manual of Determinative Bacteriology. It is, however, anticipated that a coming edition of that manual will contain proposals for certain changes in nomenclatural and taxonomic praxis, most of them based on DNA homology studies.

Table 1. FAMILY ENTEROBACTERIACEAE

Tribes	Genera
I Escherichieae	Escherichia Edwardsiella Citrobacter Salmonella Shigella
II Klebsielleae	Klebsiella Enterobacter Hafnia Serratia
III Proteeae	Proteus Providence (*Proteus inconstans*)
IV Yersinieae[a]	Yersinia
V Erwinieae	Erwinia

[a]This tribe is discussed in depth in Chapter 37.

MORPHOLOGY. Enterobacteriaceae are relatively short, 2 to 3 μ by 0.4 to 0.6 μ, rod-shaped, gram-negative bacteria. Most genera are so similar microscopically and colonially that they cannot be differentiated from one another reliably without the use of differential media or a battery of biochemical tests. Most Enterobacteriaceae are motile, and motility is always dependent upon the production of peritrichous flagella. Many strains produce pili or fimbriae. Fimbriae are proteinaceous adhesive structures that are found on many strains from all species of Enterobacteriaceae. Some special fimbriae play a role as necessary adhesive organelles during the first phases of the pathologic process. Strains that can serve as donors of plasmid DNA during conjugation also produce sex pili. Several members of the family produce capsules or microcapsules that are composed of acidic polysaccharides. The capsules of *Klebsiella* and the microcapsules that are more typical of *Escherichia coli* and some other Enterobacteriaceae can be recognized by capsular swelling and by immunoelectron microscopy. The capsules and microcapsules of Enterbacteriaceae are referred to as K antigens except for the microcapsule of *Salmonella typhi*, which is called the Vi (virulence) antigen.

Enterobacteriaceae contain the typical, lipid-rich multilayered cell wall of gram-negative bacteria. The outer layer contains the lipopolysaccharide (LPS) that is responsible for many of the toxic and biologic properties of these organisms. LPS contains complex oligosaccharide side chains that determine O antigen specificity. The peptidoglycan forms a distinct layer of the cell wall between the LPS and the cytoplasmic membrane but is neither as thick nor as complex as that of gram-positive bacteria. Enterobacteriaceae contain 5 to 10 per cent lipoprotein in the cell wall. This substance is intermixed with the LPS and covalently linked to the peptidoglycan. It does not form a distinct layer. Unlike gram-positive bacteria, Enterobacteriaceae do not produce teichoic acid.

Enterobacteriaceae grow on most common media and on media with concentrations of bile salts and aniline dyes that inhibit most gram-positive bacteria. Colonies are circular, convex, entire, and more or less glistening and mucoid, depending partly on the production of polysaccharide surface structures. Unencapsulated mutants, which have also lost the O antigenic polysaccharide side chains of the LPS, produce flat, granular, irregular colonies that are referred to as "rough." The highly motile *Proteus* spp. may move away from the original point of inoculum on solid media and produce the swarming phenomenon. Some strains produce hemolysins on blood agar. Some strains of *Serratia* produce a nondiffusible red pigment called prodigiosin. *Enterobacter agglomerans* (classified by some taxonomists as the Herbicola group of *Erwinia*) produces yellow colonies. Other *Erwinia* strains that are infrequently isolated from man produce blue or pink pigments. The rest of the Enterobacteriaceae are unpigmented.

ANTIGENIC COMPOSITION

General. Most genera of Enterobacteriaceae can be subdivided into serotypes by antibody raised against their antigenic surface components. The O, K, and H antigens are the fundamental serotyping antigens because of the great variety of their chemical composition and their antigenic stability. The properties of these antigens are relatively stable because they are chromosomally determined. Serotyping is used to establish the precise identification of strains isolated during outbreaks and epidemics. As certain serotypes are closely associated with special pathogenic properties, antigenic analysis may also be important diagnostically.

O Antigens. The O antigens are the polysaccharide side chains of the LPS and the backbone of analytic antigenic systems. LPS is a highly complex molecule (see Chapter 6), which consists of three regions (Luderitz et al., 1971): (1) Lipid A, which is buried in the outer membrane of the cell wall, is responsible for many of the biologic properties of LPS. (2) The LPS core, which is linked to lipid A and expresses R (rough) specificity, is partly hidden in S (smooth) forms by the attachment to the core of O antigens. (3) The O-specific polysaccharides of the bacterial S forms are the chemical basis for the serologic classification of Enterobacteriaceae into hundreds of complex O antigen groups, e.g., *Salmonella* into 65 and *E. coli* into more than 170 such groups.

O antigenic analysis is carried out by bacterial agglutination.

K Antigens. K antigens are polysaccharides that usually contain acidic groups. When well developed, they form microscopically distinct capsules. K antigens are determined either by the capsular swelling technique, in which the capsule is made visible by the addition of specific antiserum, or by countercurrent immunoelectrophoresis. Bacterial agglutination can also be used, but the results may be difficult to interpret because of the many other surface antigens (Ørskov and Ørskov, 1978). Capsules can interfere with phagocytosis and serum bactericidal activity.

H Antigens. Flagella are protein organelles that determine the H antigen specificity of motile members of the family. Many *Salmonella* strains show phase variation, i.e., the H antigens of a single strain may occur in either one or both of two serologically different phases called Phase 1 and Phase 2. Serologic determination is performed by agglutination techniques.

Fimbrial or Pili Antigens. Most Enterobacteriaceae may develop fimbriae (or pili). These will usually be the so-called type 1 fimbriae. General serologic analysis of fimbrial antigens is not yet available.

The K88 and K99 antigens of *E. coli* are fimbrial, proteinaceous antigens that are important colonization factors of strains associated with diarrhea in young pigs and calves. They received the K label at a time when their true nature was not recognized and may, therefore, soon receive the new designation of F antigens. Special fimbrial adhesive antigens are now recognized in many pathogenic Enterobacteriaceae, e.g. the colonization factor antigens of human enterotoxigenic *E. coli* strains and the F antigens (P fimbriae) found in strains associated with urinary tract infections.

Serotypes. Serotyping schemes, such as the Kauffmann-White scheme (Kauffmann, 1966), are based on the systematic examination of the antigenic specificities and cross-reactions between the surface antigens. Complete analysis may require numerous cross-absorption and cross-reaction tests.

The table below shows the basic agglutination-absorption experiment used in Enterobacteriaceae serology. Two strains, A and B, react mutually in antisera A and B. By reciprocal absorption followed by agglutination, it is shown that both strains contain a common and a specific antigenic factor. The two absorbed sera are called factor sera. Strain A might be given the antigenic designation of 1,2 and Strain B the designation of 1,3, where 1 represents the common factor and 2 and 3 the specific factors.

	Antiserum A		***Antiserum B***	
	Unabsorbed	***Absorbed by B***	***Unabsorbed***	***Absorbed by A***
Antigen A	+	+	+	0
Antigen B	+	0	+	+

Some typical examples of serotypes are:

Salmonella 1,4,5,12:b:1,2 (*S. paratyphi* B), where 1,4,5,12 represents the O antigen and b:1,2 the two phases of the H antigen.

Klebsiella 01:K1, or just K1, because the 0 antigens of *Klebsiella* are not usually determined.

Escherichia coli O1:K1:H5 or 1:1:5.

Shigella II:1,3,4 (*Shigella flexneri* 2a), where both II and 1,3,4 stand for O antigen determinants, II for the so called type-specific O factor and 1,3,4 for the group factors.

Simplified serologic labels can be found in the literature, e.g., when *E. coli* O111 and O75 are described as serotypes, even though they are O groups. The serotype of strains belonging to these O groups could be O111:H2 or O75:K100:H5.

Specific

Escherichia coli. The *E. coli* antigenic scheme now comprises 170 O antigens, 103 K antigens, and 56 H antigens. Most of the K antigens are polysaccharides, but a few proteinaceous, fimbrial antigens, which confer adhesiveness on enterotoxigenic *E. coli*, are presently listed as K antigens. They have, however, recently been established as a special group of antigens (F antigens). Since many O, K, and H antigens can be combined in different ways, the number of possible serotypes is very high. Fortunately, some are more common than others, both among the special serotypes associated with disease and among the flora of the normal colon. Consequently, most routine laboratories use only a limited number of antisera that correspond to certain "pathogenic" serotypes. More detailed serologic analysis should be carried out in specialized national or international centers.

Salmonella. *Salmonella* strains are serotyped by the Kauffmann-White scheme, which has divided this genus into more than 1500 serotypes (Kauffmann, 1966). The O and H antigens in this highly complex scheme were defined only after extensive cross-absorption and cross-agglutination tests. More than 65 O-antigenic groups have been described. Several strains contain more than one O antigen factor. This means that more than one determinant has been found on the O-specific side chain of the LPS molecule, e.g., O factors 1,2,12 in *Salmonella paratyphi* A. Lysogenization by converting bacteriophages can bring about modification of certain O antigens.

Only one K antigen, the Vi antigen, is important for *Salmonella* serotyping, and it is usually associated only with *S. typhi*.

H antigens, the flagellar antigens, can be found in two alternative phases in many *Salmonella* cultures. One is called "specific phase," or Phase 1, and the other "nonspecific phase," or Phase 2. During subculture of the two types, the population of each gives rise to cells of the alternative phase. The Kauffmann-White scheme first divides *Salmonella* into O groups. Strains of the same O group are then subdivided according to their H antigen.

Fimbriae can interfere with serotyping by blocking antigenic sites of the other surface antigens.

Shigella. *Shigella* is closely related to *E. coli* phenotypically and genetically. When these groups were given taxonomic status, *Shigella* strains had been isolated primarily from patients with severe dysentery, while *E. coli* was considered to be a harmless, normal inhabitant of the mammalian intestinal tract. The fact that otherwise typical *Escherichia* strains may cause dysentery has underscored the similarities between the two groups. By differences in O antigens and minor biochemical differences *Shigella* is subdivided into four subgroups: *S. dysenteriae*, *S. flexneri*, *S. boydii*, and *S. sonnei*. The first three of these can be subdivided into several serotypes based on further analysis of O antigens. Capsular polysaccharide antigens have not been demonstrated in *Shigella*. Fimbrial antigens have been described but are not used for serotyping.

Edwardsiella and *Citrobacter*, are usually not serotyped.

Klebsiella. This genus is characterized by a rich variety of K antigens but a small number of different O antigens. Thus, antigenic analysis of *Klebsiella* strains is based on testing the organism against about 80 antisera to different K types.

Enterobacter, *Hafnia*, *Serratia*, and *Proteus* are usually not serotyped, although typing schemes have been described.

Yersinia. The frequent association between *Yersinia enterocolitica* and diarrhea has been established only recently. Serotyping is based on O and H antigens.

METABOLISM. Enterobacteriaceae are facultative anaerobes. They possess a respiratory electron transport system that enables them to grow aerobically at the expense of a rich variety of oxidizable organic compounds. Organic acids, amino acids, and carbohydrates are utilized by all members of the family, and some can use aromatic compounds. They are oxidase negative because their electron transport system does not include cytochrome C. All except one species of *Shigella* produce catalase. Under anaerobic conditions, growth becomes strictly dependent upon carbohydrate fermentation. Many monosaccharides, disaccharides, and polyalcohols can be fermented by members of this group. Polysaccharides are utilized less commonly, but some plant pathogens (*Erwinia*) do attack pectin. All, except some species of *Erwinia*, reduce nitrates to nitrites.

Enterobacteriaceae ferment sugars by the Embden-Meyerhof pathway (Chapter 3). The pyruvic acid produced by this fermentation can be catabolized through several different pathways. All Enterobacteriaceae cleave pyruvate to formic acid. This unique cleavage is not encountered in any other bacterial fermentation. Formic acid does not always accumulate because many Enterobacteriaceae synthesize formic hydrogenlyase, which converts formic acid to hydrogen and carbon dioxide. The remainder of the pyruvic acid is broken down either by mixed-acid fermentation or by butylene glycol (butanediol) fermentation. Enterobacteriaceae that metabolize glucose by the mixed-acid fermentation produce succinic acid by one pathway, lactic acid by another, and acetic acid and ethanol by the third. Enterobacteriaceae that use the butylene glycol fermentation convert a major portion of the pyruvate to a different end product, 2,3-butanediol, which is formed by an additional independent pathway. Although bacteria that use the butylene glycol pathway also produce succinic, lactic, and acetic acids, the neutral end products (butanediol and ethanol) predominate, and the total amount of acid formed per mole of glucose is much less than in the mixed-acid fermentation. Two simple tests on cultures in glucose-peptone broth divide the Enterobacteriaceae into two groups according to which fermentation pathway they use. The methyl red test detects those that use the mixed-acid fermentation because they produce enough acid from glucose to convert this indicator to its red, acidic form. The Voges-Proskauer test detects the butylene-glycol fermentation because acetoin, an intermediate in this pathway, is oxidized to a diacetyl form at an alkaline pH and complexes with creatine in the media to form a pink compound. The mixed-acid pattern is typical of the Escherichieae and Yersinieae tribes, and the butylene glycol pattern is typical of the Klebsielleae tribe.

All Enterobacteriaceae produce formic acid, but only those that synthesize formic hydrogenlyase produce gas. The production of butanediol also results in a net production of CO_2, but the CO_2 is very soluble in water and does not cause observable gas in the medium. Gas formation is a property of differential value in identification of Enterobacteriaceae, since it differentiates the gas formers of the genus *Escherichia* from *Salmonella typhi* and *Shigella* spp. and the gas forming *Enterobacter* from *Serratia*.

The ability to ferment lactose, a disaccharide, depends on the possession of β-galactosidase and is a characteristic of considerable diagnostic importance in this family. Utilization of lactose also depends upon a specific galactoside permease, which facilitates the entry of lactose into the cell. Lactose fermentation is characteristic of *E. coli*, *Klebsiella*, *Citrobacter*, and *Enterobacter* and is absent from *Shigella*, *Salmonella*, and *Proteus*. Some *Shigella* species produce β-galactosidase but cannot ferment lactose because they lack a permease.

PATHOGENIC PROPERTIES

General. The natural habitat of many Enterobacteriaceae is the mammalian intestine. Some, like *E. coli*, are found in the normal healthy intestine; others, like *Salmonella*, *Shigella*, *Yersinia*, and enteropathogenic *E. coli*, can be considered to be pathogenic.

Although many Enterobacteriaceae are part of the normal intestinal flora, they are also "opportunistic" pathogens that may cause fatal infections when the normal host defenses are insufficient, e.g., in newborns, in patients in terminal stages of disease or in patients receiving immunosuppressive therapy. Enterobacteriaceae are the most common causes of infection of the obstructed biliary and urinary tracts and, along with the intestinal anaerobes, the major cause of infection of the soiled peritoneum. Enterobacteriaceae, especially *E. coli* and *Klebsiella*, are now the most common causes of septicemia in hospitalized patients.

Endotoxin. All Enterobacteriaceae synthesize endotoxin. Lipid A seems to be responsible for most of the potent biologic activities of endotoxin. Endotoxin is extensively discussed in Chapter 6, but it is important to point out in this chapter that many of the symptoms of invasive disease caused by Enterobacteriaceae can be ascribed to endotoxin.

Among these effects are: (1) pyrogenicity: microgram doses of LPS given intravenously cause a diphasic rise of the temperature of humans and many experimental animals; (2) consumption of complement: the survival rate of patients with enterobacterial septicemia is inversely related to the complement level; (3) consumption of coagulation factors: hemorrhage and fibrin deposition occur in patients and are equivalent to the Shwartzman phenomenon in experimental animals; and (4) shock: injection of larger doses of LPS causes hypotension, irreversible shock, and death. Similar symptoms can be caused by the presence of large numbers of Enterobacteriaceae in the blood.

Enterotoxins. Enterotoxin-producing *E. coli* strains have been the subject of intensive investigation in recent years. These protein exotoxins, which are genetically determined by transferable plasmids, play a prominent role in the pathogenesis of diarrhea in animals and man. Enterotoxin-positive strains colonize but do not invade the small intestine. There are at least two types of enterotoxins; one is called ST (thermostable toxin) and the other LT (thermolabile toxin). Diarrhea occurs as a result of water and electrolyte loss caused by enterotoxin-induced adenyl or guanyl cyclase activity of the epithelial cells. LT (the thermolabile toxin) is immunogenic but ST is not. Enterotoxigenic *E. coli* also affects infant pigs and calves, causing great economic loss to farmers. Enterotoxins have now been detected in other species of Enterobacteriaceae, notably in *Yersinia enterocolitica*.

Exotoxin. Some human isolates of *E. coli* produce a hemolysin that is encoded for by a chromosomal gene. By genetic manipulation (transposon mutagenesis), it has been shown that the hemolysin enhances the virulence of these strains in animal models of peritonitis and pyelonephritis. Hemolytic *E. coli* are more common in clinical isolates than in fecal specimens, indirect evidence that the hemolysin is a virulence factor. The important toxic effect of the hemolysin is probably damage to leukocyte membranes. It inhibits WBC chemotaxis and phagocytosis and kills PMN's in higher concentrations.

Colonization Factors. Many enterotoxigenic strains produce special, plasmid-determined fimbriae (or pili) that play an important pathogenic role as adhesive structures. Experimental evidence suggests that these structures make it possible for enterotoxin-producing *E. coli* to deliver their toxin close to the intestinal epithelial cells.

The best known colonization factor is the K88 antigen of the *E. coli* strains that causes diarrhea in piglets. Enterotoxin-producing strains are not virulent for piglets if they have lost the K88 antigen or if the pigs have been immunized with K88. The K99 antigen plays a similar role in diarrhea of calves. Other colonization factors, CFAI and CFAII, have been identified in human enterotoxigenic strains. These fimbrial antigens are mediated by transferable plasmids. It has been proposed that all fimbrial antigens be designated F antigens.

A Pap pilus that binds to digalactoside residues promotes adherence to uroepithelial cells and to RBC (the mannose-resistant hemagglutinin). *E. coli* that cause pyelonephritis in children have this pilus (90%). It binds to the P^k antigen on erythrocytes and a globoside or a trihexosyl ceramide on epithelial cells.

K Antigens. K antigens are acidic polysaccharides that probably promote pathogenicity primarily by interfering with phagocytosis.

E. coli K1 strains cause a very high percentage of neonatal meningitis without an equivalent increase in either gastrointestinal colonization or septicemia. The sialic acid-containing K1 capsule cross-reacts immunologically with the capsule of serogroup B meningococci. The reasons for this unique predilection for the meninges are not known. K1, K2, K5, K12, and K13 are the most common K types associated with infections of the urinary tract. Certain O types—O1, O2, O4, O6, O7, O8, O9, O11, O18, O22, O25, and O75—are also more commonly associated with urinary tract and other extraintestinal infections. Strains with these O and K antigens are commonly found in the intestine, and it is uncertain whether they are especially virulent or are just more prevalent.

Specific

E. COLI DIARRHEA. Three groups of special *Escherichia* strains are associated with three types of intestinal disease (Table 2). The enterotoxigenic *E. coli* species (ETEC), which were discussed above, cause diarrhea in piglets and calves, traveler's diarrhea in man, and a cholera-like disease in the people living under poor hygienic conditions in developing countries.

Another group of special *Escherichia* serotypes (EIEC), which are related to certain serotypes of *Shigella*, is invasive into the epithelial cells of the human colon and can cause dysentery-like disease. These serotypes have also been associated with food poisoning.

A third group of special serotypes is associated with diarrhea in institutionalized infants in developed countries and are also common causes of infantile diarrhea in developing countries. These special serotypes, which are not

Table 2. *ESCHERICHIA COLI* AND ACUTE DIARRHEA

	Enteropathogenic EPEC	Enterotoxigenic ETEC	Enteroinvasive EIEC
Pathogenic mechanism	Unknown*	Enterotoxin (LT, ST)	Epithelial cell invasion
Age groups affected	Infants	Infants and adults	Adults and infants
Epidemiology	Sporadic cases and outbreaks	Sporadic cases and outbreaks	Sporadic cases and outbreaks
O groups associated	2, 55, 86, 111, 114, 119, 125, 126, 127, 128, 142, 158	6, 8, 15, 25, 27, 78, 148, 159	28ac, 29, 112ac, 124, 136, 143, 144, 152, 164, 167

From Rowe, B.: *Escherichia coli* in acute diarrhoea. Lab-Lore 7:449, 1977, modified.

*Toxins and adhesive factors have been described recently in some EPEC strains.

commonly found in the normal intestine, have been called the enteropathogenic *E. coli* (EPEC). They do not invade the epithelial cells of the small intestine, and for many years it was thought that they did not produce enterotoxins. Recently, toxins have been detected in some EPEC strains. The pathogenic mechanism of these strains has not yet been completely elucidated; however, the close association of these highly specialized serotypes with severe outbreaks of diarrhea cannot be disputed.

Extraintestinal Infections. A limited number of highly defined O:K:H:F serotypes play a role as invasive pathogens in extraintestinal diseases.

The Col V plasmid appears to be highly associated with isolates of *E. coli* that cause extraintestinal infections. These plasmids, in addition to encoding the bacteriocin, encode the synthesis of aerobactin and the aerobactin receptor protein in the outer membrane of *E. coli*. This iron-scavenging system confers a selective advantage on bacteria that must multiply in the iron-poor environment within the infected host.

Salmonella. More than 1500 different serotypes have been described, all of which should be considered as potentially pathogenic to man. Several cause generalized infection in specific animals, such as *S. typhimurium* in mice and *S. typhi* in man. Most serotypes can cause enteritis in many different animals when large numbers of organisms are ingested.

ENTERIC FEVER. In humans, enteric fever is caused by *S. typhi* or *S. paratyphi* A, B, and C, depending on the geographic location. Other *Salmonella* serotypes are occasionally isolated from cases of enteric fever. A relatively small oral inoculum of the strains of *Salmonella* that cause enteric fever can initiate disease. The organisms invade the mucosa and the mucosal macrophages of the small intestine, multiply in local lymph nodes, spread through the lymphatics to the bloodstream, and disseminate to many organs. *S. typhi* and *S. paratyphi C (S. hirschfeldii)* frequently produce the Vi antigen, which is composed of a simple polymer of *N*-acetyl galactosaminuronic acid. This substance is elaborated as a thin, outermost layer and is equivalent to K antigen.

Salmonella septicemia may be caused by some other serotypes, notably *S. choleraesuis*. This infection is characterized by high remittent fever and bacteremia usually without involvement of the intestinal tract. Focal suppuration, meningitis, osteomyelitis, pneumonia, and endocarditis may occur.

ENTERITIS (FOOD POISONING). Most other *Salmonella* serotypes can cause enteritis in man when ingested in large numbers. Typically, these strains cause disease after ingestion of food in which the *Salmonella* strain has had the opportunity to multiply. The disease is often labeled food poisoning, but invasion and multiplication are probably a necessary part of the pathogenesis. The incubation period ranges from 8 hours to 3 days. The disease is usually limited to the local intestinal lymph nodes. Some serotypes, e.g., *S. typhimurium, S. enteritidis, S. heidelberg,* and *S. adelaide*, are more frequently associated with this disease, but almost all strains have caused enteritis. Some *Salmonella* strains also produce enterotoxins.

Shigella. *Shigella* causes bacillary dysentery in man and higher apes. This enteritis is localized to the mucosa of the terminal ileum and colon. The bacteria invade the colonic epithelial cells, where they multiply and cause mucosal ulcerations. One of the serotypes, *Shigella dysenteriae* Type 1 (the Shiga bacillus), also produces a special exotoxin that was earlier described as a neurotoxin. Recent reports have shown that a similar toxin is produced by many strains of *Shigella* and *E. coli*. Virulent *Shigella sonnei* strains contain a 120-megadalton plasmid that is absent in avirulent strains (Sansonatti et al., 1981).

Yersinia. *Yersinia pestis*, the cause of plague, is discussed in Chapter 37. *Y. pseudotuberculosis* and *Y. enterocolitica* may cause mesenteric lymphadenitis and acute and chronic arthritis. *Yersinia enterocolitica* is now recognized as one of the common causes of diarrhea in humans. Adhesive properties, enterotoxin production, and local invasiveness are characteristic of pathogenic strains.

Other Enterobacteriaceae. The other members of the family are primarily causes of opportunistic infections. Several reports have suggested an association of the *Klebsiella* group with enterotoxic diarrhea, but there is no current evidence to suggest that there is a regular association of the enterotoxin plasmid with any serotype of *Klebsiella*.

Proteus species are found regularly in the mammalian intestine. These urease-producing bacteria, which break down urea to ammonium, are so frequently associated with stones of the urinary tract that the isolation of *Proteus* from the urine alerts clinicians to this possibility.

Table 3. DISTINGUISHING CHARACTERISTICS OF THE FIVE PRIMARY GROUPS (TRIBES)

	Tribe I Escherichieae	Tribe II Klebsielleae	Tribe III Proteeae	Tribe IV Yersinieae	Tribe V Erwinieae
Fermentation pattern	Mixed acid	2,3-Butanediol		Mixed acid	Mixed acid and 2,3-butanediol
M.R.	+	D	+	+	
V.P.	—	D	D	—	D
Phenylalanine deamination	—	—	+	—	D
Nitrate reduction	+	+	+	+	D
Urease	—	D	D	D	—
KCN, growth in	D	+	+	—	D
Optimal temp. for growth	37 C	37 C	37 C	30–37 C	27–30 C
G + C, %	50–53	52–59	39–42	45–47	50–58

From Buchanan, C. E., and Gibbons, N. E. (eds.): Bergey's Manual of Determinative Bacteriology, 8th ed. Baltimore, The Williams & Wilkins Company, 1974.
G + C = Guanine + cytosine
D = different reactions from different genera or species

Table 4. MAIN BIOCHEMICAL CHARACTERS OF PRIMARY GROUPS I TO IV

	GROUP I					GROUP II				GROUP III PROTEUS	GROUP IV YERSINIA
	Escherichia	Edwardsiella	Citrobacter	Salmonella	Shigella	Klebsiella	Enterobacter	Hafnia	Serratia		
Catalase	+	+	+	+	D[a]	+	+	+	+	+	+
Oxidase	−	−	−	−	−	−	−	−	−	−	−
β-Galactosidase	+	−	+	D	d	+	+	+	+	−	+
Gas from glucose at 37 C	+	+	−	+	−	d	+	+	d	D	−
KCN (growth on)	−	−	−	D	−	+	+	+	+	+	−
Mucate (acid)	+	−	+	D	−	d	d	−	−		
Nitrate reduced	+	+	+	(+)	+	+	+	+	+	+	+
G + C, moles %	50–51			50–53		52–56	52–59	52–57	53–59	39–42 (*morganella* = 50)	45–47
Carbohydrates (acid from)											
Adonitol	−	−	−	−	−	d	+	−	d	D	D
Arabinose	+	−	+	+		+	+	+	−	−	+
Dulcitol	d	−	d	D	d	d	−	−	−	−	−
Esculin	d	−	d	−			D	−	−	d	D
Inositol	−	−	−	d	−	+	D	−	d	D	−
Lactose	+ or ×	−	+ or ×	D	D	D	+	−	−	−	−
Maltose	+	+	+	+		+	+	+	+	D	+
Mannitol	+	−	+	+	D	+	+	+	+	D	+
Salicin	d	−	d	−	−	+	+	−	+	d	D
Sorbitol	+	−	+	+		+	+	−		−	D
Sucrose	d	−	d	−	D	+	+	− or ×	+	D	D
Trehalose	+	−	+	+		+	+	+	+	d	+
Xylose	d	−	+	+	D	+	+	+	d	D	D
Related C sources											
Citrate	−	−	+	+	−	d	+	+	+		−
Gluconate		−		−	−	+	+	+	+		
Malonate	−	−	d	D	−	D	+		−		−
d-Tartrate	d	−	+	D		d	−	−			D
M.R.	+	+	+	+	+	D	−	−	−	+	+
V.P.	−	−	−	−	−	D	+	+	D	d	−
Protein reactions											
Arginine	d	−	d	+	−	−	D	−	−	−	−
Gelatin hydrolysis	−	−	−	D	−	(d)	(+)	−	+	D	−
H_2S from TSI	−	+	D	+	−	−	−	−	−	D	D
Indole	+	+	D	−	D	d	−	−	−	D	D
Lysine decarboxylated	+	+	−	+	−	d	D	+	+	d	−
Ornithine	d	+	d	+	d	−	+	+	+	D	D
Urea hydrolyzed	−	−	(+)	−	−	d	(d)	−	−	D	D
Glutamic acid	−	−	−	−	−	−				+	
Phenylalanine	−	−	−	−	−	−	−	−	−	+	−

[a]D = different reactions given by different species of a genus; d = different reactions given by different strains of a species or serotype; × = late and irregularly positive (mutative).

From Buchanan, C. E., and Gibbons, N. E. (eds.): Bergey's Manual of Determinative Bacteriology, 8th ed. Baltimore, The Williams & Wilkins Company, 1974.

IMMUNITY. The intestinal tract of the newborn mammal is colonized shortly after birth by several different groups of bacteria including the Enterobacteriaceae. Of the many bioserotypes or clones of *E. coli*, only a limited number are highly prevalent. Immune reactions take place, and low titers of anti-Escherichia antibodies develop against the more common serogroups. The *E. coli* flora undergoes changes with time, age, and diet and is also dependent on the bacteria that are continuously taken in by mouth. Thus, some of the so-called natural antibodies are determined by immune reactions to the gram-negative intestinal bacteria. Antigenic cross-reactions that occur between different species of Enterobacteriaceae may be of importance for protection against intestinal diseases, and similar cross-reactions also exist between Enterobacteriaceae and pathogenic organisms from quite different bacterial groups. Thus, immune reactions to normal intestinal *E. coli* may protect against the invasion of many different bacteria; for example, *Haemophilus influenzae* Type b, which has a capsule that is serologically similar to the capsular antigen K100 of *E. coli*.

Escherichia coli. People living in an area in which enterotoxigenic *E. coli* strains are widely distributed are more resistant to disease from this type of organism than visitors coming from areas with few enterotoxigenic strains. Experimental evidence suggests that this immunity may be mediated by antibody production either to the heat-labile toxin or to colonization factors such as pili or K antigens. Vaccines against enterotoxigenic *E. coli* are widely used in animals and may soon be available for human diarrhea.

Salmonella. Enteric fever provides some protection against the infecting serotype. Vaccination with TAB vaccine against *S. typhi* and *S. paratyphi* A and B has been given for more than 50 years to travelers going to parts of the world in which these diseases are endemic. The vaccine provides some protection against exposure to smaller doses of *S. typhi*. An attenuated live vaccine against *S. typhi* has been shown to be highly protective in trials in developing countries.

Shigella. People living in geographic areas in which *Shigella* species are endemic acquire some immunity to the disease. There are no effective vaccines, probably because most *Shigella* vaccines have not been able to increase the local intestinal defenses.

LABORATORY DIAGNOSIS. Enterobacteriaceae are easy to cultivate either directly from feces, urine, or blood or from swabs of feces held in Stuart's medium. In addition to blood agar or nutrient agar, specimens that may contain Enterobacteriaceae are plated onto media that are both selective and differential. These media incorporate bile salts (MacConkey's agar, deoxycholate agar) or dyes (eosin-methylene blue or bromthymol blue) to inhibit gram-positive bacteria, lactose as the sole fermentable substrate, and a pH indicator (e.g., methylene blue), so that colonies that make acid from lactose are colored. Strains that do not ferment lactose are able to grow on the peptone provided in the media but are colorless because they do not produce acid.

Salmonella and *Shigella* are very resistant to bile salts and certain dyes and can be selected by plating directly on media (e.g., Salmonella-Shigella agar, Hektoen agar) that partly inhibit *E. coli* and the other Enterobacteriaceae. Further selection is accomplished by culturing feces into selenite or tetrathionate broth for 18 to 24 hours before subculturing onto the selective solid media.

Final identification of Enterobacteriaceae is established by a battery of biochemical tests, agglutination with appropriate O, K (Vi), and H antisera, and occasionally by phage typing. A limited number of biochemical tests (Table 3) separates the five tribes. In practice, identification to the species level is usually accomplished easily in one step by selecting certain differential tests from the major biochemical characteristics of Enterobacteriaceae listed in Table 4. A typical battery of these tests, which will differentiate between the major species of the *Escherichia* and *Klebsiella* groups, is given in Table 5. Tables 6 and 7 highlight the limited number of tests necessary to separate the species of *Klebsiella* and *Enterobacter*, respectively. Most *Klebsi-*

Table 5. DIFFERENTIATION OF MAJOR GENERA OF ESCHERICHIEAE AND KLEBSIELLEAE

	E. coli	**Edwardsiella**	**Shigella**	**Salmonella**	**Citrobacter**	**Klebsiella pneumoniae**	**Enterobacter aerogens**	**Hafnia**	**Serratia marcescens**
KIA	A/AG	K/AG	K/A	K/AG	K or A/AG	A/AG	A/AG	K/AG	K/A or AG
H_2S (KIA)	−	+	−	+	+ or −	−	−	−	−
Indole	+	+	− or +	−	−	− or +	−	−	−
Methyl red	+	+	+	+	+	−	−	+ or −	− or +
Voges-Proskauer	−	−	−	−	−	+	+	+ or −	+
Citrate (Simmons)	−	−	−	d	+	+	+	(+) or −	+
Motility	+	+	−	+	+	−	+	+	+
Urease	−	−	−	−	−	+	−	−	−
KCN	−	−	−	−	+ or −	+	+	+	+
Lysine decarboxylase	d	+	−	+	−	+	+	+	+
Ornithine decarboxylase	d	+	d	+	d	−	+	+	+
Gas from glucose	+	+	−	+	+	+	+	+	− or +
Lactose	+	−	−	−	d	+	+	− or (+)	− or (+)
Salicin	d	−	−	−	d	+	+	d	+
Sorbitol	+	−	d	+	+	+	+	−	+
Raffinose	d	−	d	−	d	+	+	−	−
Rhamnose	d	−	d	+	+	+	+	+	−
Gelatin liquefaction (22°C)	−	−	−	−	−	−	− or (+)	−	+

+ = 90% or more positive in 1 to 2 days; − = 90% or more negative; d = different biochemical types; (+) delayed positive; − or + = majority of cultures negative; + or − = majority positive; KIA = Kligler's iron agar; K = alkaline or no change; A = acid; G = gas.
Modified from Edwards, P. R., and Ewing, W. H.: Identification of Enterobacteriaceae, 3rd ed. Minneapolis, Burgess Publishing Co., 1972.

Table 6. DIFFERENTIATION OF KLEBSIELLA SPECIES

	K. pneumoniae	K. ozaenae	K. rhinoscleromatis
Urease	+	− or +	−
Methyl red	− or +	+	+
Voges-Proskauer	+	−	−
Citrate (Simmons)	+	− or +	−
Malonate	+	−	+ or −
Lysine decarbosylase	+	− or +	−
Gas from glucose	+	+ or −	−
Lactose	+	(+) or −	(+) or −

+ = 90% or more positive in 1 to 2 days; − = 90% or more negative; − or + = majority of cultures negative; + or − = majority positive; (+) = delayed positive.

Modified from 8th ed., Bergey's Manual of Determinative Bacteriology, 1974; and Lannette et al., Manual of Clinical Microbiology, 2nd ed., Am Soc Microbiol, Wash., D.C. 1974. In the ninth edition of Bergey's Manual 4 species are described in the genus *Klebsiella: K. pneumoniae, K. oxytoca* (produces indole and liquefies gelatin), *K. terrigena,* and *K. planticola.* The last two species are mainly of soil and plant origin. *K. ozaenae* and *K. rhinoscleromatis* are subspecies of *K. pneumoniae.*

ella isolates are typical strains of *K. pneumoniae; K. ozaenae* and *K. rhinoscleromatis* are unusual isolates. *K. oxytoca,* which differs from *K. pneumoniae* by indole production and gelatin liquefaction, is isolated more frequently. *Enterobacter aerogenes* is the most commonly isolated *Enterobacter* species, but *E. cloacae* and *E. agglomerans* are isolated fairly frequently. *E. agglomerans (Erwinia herbicola)* is still classified with the *Erwinia* in the 8th edition of Bergey's Manual (1974), but many medical diagnostic laboratories have followed the suggestion of Ewing and Fife (1972) and classified it with *Enterobacter.*

There are three species or biotypes of *Citrobacter* that can be separated from one another by a limited number of biochemical tests (Table 8). *Citrobacter freundii* is by far the most common isolate. Most laboratories do not recognize *Citrobacter intermedius* (not listed in Table 8—see 8th ed. Bergey's Manual of Determinative Bacteriology) and regard strains that are either H_2S negative, indole positive, or ornithine-positive as variants of *C. freundii. C. diversus* is the biotype of Citrobacter that combines these 3 divergent characteristics with the inability to grow in KCN and inability to decarboxylate lysine.

Table 7. DIFFERENTIATION OF ENTEROBACTER SPECIES

	E. aerogenes	E. cloacae	E. agglomerans
Urease	−	+ or −	− or +
Lysine decarboxylase	+	−	−
Ornithine decarboxylase	+	+	−
Adonitol	+	− or +	−
Inositol (acid)	+	− or +	− or +
Inositol (gas)	+	−	
Esculin	+	− or +	d
Yellow pigment	−	−	+ or −

+ = 90% or more positive in 1 to 2 days; − = 90% or more negative; − or + = majority of cultures negative; + or − = majority positive; d = different biochemical types.

Modified from Edwards, P. R., and Ewing, W. H.: Identification of Enterobacteriaceae. 3rd ed., Minneapolis, Burgess Publishing Co., and Ewing, W. H., and Fife, M. A.: *Enterobacter agglomerans* (Beijerinck) Comb. Nov. (The Herbicola-lathyri Bacteria.) Int J Syst Bacteriol *22*(1):4–11, 1972.

Table 8. DIFFERENTIATION OF CITROBACTER SPECIES

	C. freundii	C. diversus
Citrate (Simmon's)	+	+
Indole	−	+
H_2S (KIA)	+	−
Ornithine decarboxylase	− or +	+
Lysine decarboxylase	−	−
KCN	+	−

+ = 90% or more positive in 1 to 2 days; − = 90% or more negative; d = different biochemical types; − or + = majority negative; KIA = Kligler's iron agar.

Modified from 8th ed. Bergey's Manual of Determinative Bacteriology, 1974; and Ewing, W. H.: Differentiation of Enterobacteriaceae by Biochemical Reactions, Revised. DHEW Publication No. (CDC) 74-8270, May, 1974.

The biochemical reactions used to differentiate between *Salmonella* and *Shigella* species are listed in Tables 9 and 10. *Shigella* can be differentiated to the species level by a combination of the indicated biochemical tests and simple agglutination tests with four O antisera. Speciation of *Salmonella* is an entirely different matter. The Salmonella species *S. typhi, S. paratyphi* A, *S. arizona* (formerly Arizona), and *S. choleraesuis* can be identified biochemically and have distinct serotypes. More than 1500 other bioserotypes are now grouped together as *S. enteritidis* and differentiated mainly by serologic methods (see below).

Biochemical differentiation of the *Proteus* tribe is usually easily accomplished by the tests listed in Table 11.

Table 12 lists the major differential characteristics of the *Yersinia* species, which are discussed more extensively in Chapter 37. Although *Yersinia* has recently been reclassified in the family Enterobacteriaceae, it is discussed separately for historic reasons and because it causes clinical syndromes similar to those of *Francisella* and *Pasteurella.*

Erwinia, another recent addition to the family of Enterobacteriaceae, also cause classification problems. These organisms are plant pathogens or commensals and are isolated infrequently from human sources except for the Herbicola group (*Enterobacter agglomerans*). *Erwinia* are usually divided into three groups: the Amylovora group (sometimes referred to as "true *Erwinia*"), the Herbicola group (*E. agglomerans*), and the Carotovora group (pectobacteria). The Amylovora group is frequently nitrate-negative, attacks glucose primarily oxidatively, fails to grow at 37°C, and is isolated very infrequently from humans. Since this group fits the definition of Enterobacteriaceae poorly and is rarely isolated from humans, we will not deal with it further in this chapter. *E. agglomerans* (Herbicola group) is characterized in Table 7. The Carotovora group (pectobacteria) is occasionally isolated from man and is biochemically similar to the *Klebsiella* tribe but also grows better at room temperature than at 37°C; reactions are given at both temperatures.

As indicated in the tables, most Enterobacteriaceae can be differentiated to the species level by biochemical tests. Serologic methods are used most frequently for the identification of *Shigella, Salmonella,* and certain serotypes of *E. coli.* Although *Shigella* can frequently be speciated by the tests shown in Table 10, the identification is always confirmed by agglutination with O antisera. Shigellae have no special capsular antigens and no H antigens since they

Table 9. DIFFERENTIATION OF MAJOR SPECIES OF SALMONELLA

	S. typhi	**S. choleraesuis**[a]	**S. enteritidis**	**S. paratyphi A**	**S. arizonae**
H_2S (KIA or TSI)	$+^w$	d	+	− or +	+
Citrate (Simmons)	−	(+)	+	− or (+)	+
Lysine decarboxylase	+	+	+	+	+
Ornithine decarboxylase	−	+	+	+	+
Gas from glucose	−	+	+	+	+
Dulcitol	− or(+)	− or +	+	+	−
Trehalose	+	−	+	+	
Arabinose	−	−	+	+	+
Rhamnose	−	+	+		+
Malonate	−	−	−	−	+
O group	D	C_1	All groups	A	Arizona[b]

[a]H_2S positive strains are referred to as *S. choleraesuis* var. *Kunzendorf.*

Salmonella are now named either *S. typhi, S. choleraesuis,* or *S. enteritidis,* serogroup—. *S. paratyphi* A and *S. arizonae* are included in this table because they can be identified biochemically and because *S. arizonae* was considered a separate species until recently.

Precise identification is made in reference centers by extensive cross agglutination tests and occasionally by phage typing.

+ = 90% or more positive in 1 to 2 days; − = 90% or more negative; d = different biochemical types; (+) = delayed positive; − or + = majority of cultures negative; + or − = majority positive; A = acid, KIA = Kligler's iron agar; TSI = triple sugar iron agar.

[b]S. arizona is agglutinated by commercial Arizona antisera and by some specific salmonella antisera.

Modified from 8th ed. Bergey's Manual of Determinative Bacteriology, 1974; and Edwards, P. R., and Ewing, W. H.: Identification of Enterobacteriaceae, 3rd ed., Minneapolis, Burgess Publishing Co., 1972.

are nonmotile. Salmonellae are speciated by the Kauffmann White scheme described previously under Antigenic Composition. Most laboratories use only O and Vi antisera for preliminary identification of salmonellae and send their isolates to reference laboratories for final identification. If *S. typhi* is suspected in the clinical laboratory, it is important to attempt agglutination with Vi antisera, because the Vi antigen may block access to the O antigenic sites by O antisera. Blocking of O agglutination by either Vi or H antigens may be removed by boiling. *S. typhi* should be suspected when a *Salmonella*-like organism (Table 10) fails to utilize citrate as the sole carbon source, produces no gas from glucose, produces little or no H_2S, and fails to decarboxylate ornithine. A *Salmonella* with these biochemical reactions that agglutinates with Vi antisera before boiling and with O antisera after boiling should be identified as *S. typhi.* A *Salmonella* that agglutinates with C_1 antisera and has typical *Salmonella* reactions, except for failure to produce H_2S, is identified as *S. choleraesuis.* All other salmonellae are customarily identified as *S. enteritidis,* Group—, according to the group of O antisera with which they agglutinate, and are sent to reference laboratories for final identification.

Enteropathogenic E. coli. The *E. coli* bioserotypes associated with diarrhea constitute a special problem because they cannot be differentiated from other *E. coli* on existing media.

Enterotoxigenic *E. coli* (ETEC) isolated from diseases of pigs are usually hemolytic, so that only hemolytic colonies are tested with agglutinating antisera against the serotypes that cause piglet diarrhea. No similar characteristic trait is known for strains that are enteropathogenic to human beings. However, some serotypes harbor enterotoxin plasmids more frequently than others. This finding may simplify the screening for enterotoxigenic strains, but it will not represent a definitive test.

The laboratory identification of enterotoxigenic strains is very time-consuming and is ordinarily a research procedure. Single colonies of each specimen are tested for LT (heat-labile) enterotoxin by determining their influence on the morphology of adrenal (Y1) or Chinese hamster ovary cells (CHO) in tissue culture. ST (heat-stable) enterotoxin is detected in infant mice by peroral or intragastric injections of suspected colonies followed by measurement of fluid accumulation (weight gain) of the total intestinal tract. Both toxins can be detected by fluid accumulation in the

Table 10. DIFFERENTIATION OF SHIGELLA SPECIES

	S. dysenteriae	**S. flexneri**	**S. boydii**	**S. sonnei**
Indole	d	d	d	−
Lactose (acid)	−	−	−	(+)
Mannitol	−	d	+	+
Sucrose	−	−	−	(+)
Dulcitol	d	d	d	−
Xylose	d	d	d	−
Ornithine decarboxylase	−	−	−	+
Rhamnose	d	d	d	+
Raffinose	−	d	−	d
O groups	A	B	C	D

+ = 90% or more positive in 1 to 2 days; − = 90% or more negative; d = different biochemical types; (+) = delayed positive.

Modified from 8th ed. Bergey's Manual of Determinative Bacteriology, 1974; and Edwards, P. R., and Ewing, W. H.: Identification of Enterobacteriaceae, 3rd ed., Minneapolis, Burgess Publishing Co., 1972.

Table 11. DIFFERENTIATION OF PROTEUS TRIBES[a]

	P. vulgaris	P. mirabilis	Morganella[a]	P. rettgeri	P. inconstans[a] A	P. inconstans[a] B
Phenylalanine deaminase	+	+	+	+	+	+
Urease	+	+ or (+)	+	+	–	–
Indole	+	–	+	+	+	+
H_2S (KIA or TSI)	+	+	–	–	–	–
Lysine decarboxylase	–	–	–	–	–	–
Ornithine decarboxylase	–	+	+	–	–	–
Moles % G + C	39	39	50	39	41	41
Gas from glucose	+	+	+ or –	– or +	+ or –	–
Esculin	d	–	–	+	–	–
Inositol	–	–	–	+	–	+
Maltose	+	–	–	–	–	–
Mannitol	–	–	–	+ or –	–	– or +
Mannose	–	–	+	+	+	+
Rhamnose	–	–	–	+ or –	–	–
Adonitol	–	–	–	+ or –	+	–
Spontaneous swarming	+	+	–	–	–	–
Penicillin sensitivity	–	+	–	–	–	–

[a]*P. inconstans* subgroups A and B (8th ed., Bergey's Manual of Determinative Bacteriology) were formerly known as *Providencia alcalifaciens* and *Providencia stuartii*. *Morganella* was previously known as *P. morganii*.

+ = 90% or more positive in 1 to 2 days; – = 90% or more negative; d = different biochemical types; (+) = delayed positive; – or + = majority of cultures negative; + or – = majority positive.

Modified from Edwards, P. R., and Ewing, W. H.: Identification of Enterobacteriaceae. 3rd ed. Minneapolis, Burgess Publishing Company, 1972, and 8th ed., Bergey's Manual of Determinative Bacteriology, 1974.

"rabbit ileal loop," which is even more forbidding as a routine test. The isolation of pure LT and ST has been followed by the introduction of several serological tests. The simplest one is probably the Biken test. Recently developed DNA probes for LT and ST may become important diagnostic tools in the future.

Invasive *E. coli* can be detected by the capacity of a few drops of an overnight culture to cause keratoconjunctivitis in guinea pigs or rabbits; these strains are also invasive in tissue cultures.

The so-called enteropathogenic serotypes (EPEC) from infantile diarrhea can be detected by screening colonies with appropriate antisera. Because not all of the strains identified by serologic methods will be pathogenic, it is important that several EPEC serotypes have recently been shown to produce enterotoxin and adhesive factors.

Table 12. DIFFERENTIATION OF YERSINIA SPECIES

	Y. pestis	Y. pseudotuberculosis	Y. enterocolitica
Motility			
22°C	–	+	+
37°C	–	–	–
Urease	–	+	+
Esculin	+	+	– or +
Rhamnose	– or +	+	–
Salicin	+ or –	+	–
Sucrose	–	–	+
Ornithine decarboxylase	–	–	+
Indole	–	–	+ or –

+ = 90% or more positive in 1 to 2 days; – = 90% or more negative; – or + = majority negative; + or – = majority positive.

Modified from 8th ed., Bergey's Manual of Determinative Bacteriology; and Lennette et al., Manual of Clinical Microbiology, 2nd ed., Am Soc Microbiol, Wash., D.C., 1974.

DRUG SENSITIVITY. Except for benzyl penicillin, Enterobacteriaceae are intrinsically sensitive to achievable serum and tissue concentrations of most antimicrobials when they are first introduced, including the new broad-spectrum penicillins and cephalosporins. Resistant strains are selected quickly, however, because the Enterobacteriaceae in the normal intestinal tract are frequently exposed to antibiotics directed at other, more invasive bacteria. Furthermore, some genera of Enterobacteriaceae are intrinsically resistant to certain antimicrobials. Some examples of this property include the resistance of *Proteus* spp. and *Serratia* to polymyxins, the resistance of *Proteus* spp. to tetracycline, and the resistance of *Enterobacter* to cephalothin. *Klebsiella* is usually resistant to aminobenzyl-penicillin (ampicillin) but sensitive to the cephalosporins. *Proteus mirabilis* is unique among the Enterobacteriaceae species for its sensitivity to benzylpenicillin. Rapid selection of resistant mutants may occur when Enterobacteriaceae are exposed to nalidixic acid, rifampin, or the aminoglycosides as single antimicrobial therapy. All Enterobacteriaceae are intrinsically resistant to achievable levels of erythromycin and the other macrolides.

Most of the genetic determinants of resistance, however, are carried on transferable plasmids that have been responsible for the appearance of an increasing number of multiresistant Enterobacteriaceae. The use of antibiotics for treatment of disease and as food additives in animal breeding has exerted a powerful selection pressure for antibiotic-resistant strains. When the use of antibiotics is restricted, the number of resistant strains in that area decreases (Falkow, 1975).

Thus, the antimicrobial sensitivities of individual species of this important family of bacteria are unpredictable. They vary from broad sensitivity to complete resistance to the tetracyclines, aminoglycosides, the sulfonamides, cephalosporins, polymyxins, chloramphenicol, ampicillin, and carbenicillin. For this reason, antimicrobial sensitivity tests must be conducted quickly and accurately to ensure effective therapy against enterobacterial infections.

EPIDEMIOLOGY

Escherichia coli. The source of infection with the three types of *E. coli* diarrhea described above is human. Few cases exist that point to direct transfer of pathogenic strains from domestic animals to human beings. The enteropathogenic types (EPEC), are transferred nosocomially in nurseries and wards directly or indirectly from one child to another. The ultimate source of human enterotoxigenic strains (ETEC) is probably the infected patient, but transmission is indirect, possibly through contaminated food. The finding of the same highly defined serotypes among enterotoxigenic strains isolated all over the world indicates that the same clones of bacteria have spread around the world. Enterotoxigenic piglet diarrhea strains spread from country to country within a short period of time and demonstrated how easily special pathogenic strains could be globally disseminated.

The epidemiologic characteristics of *E. coli* strains from dysentery-like disease (EIEC) are the same as those of *Shigella* (see below).

Salmonella. Typhoid and paratyphoid bacteria are primarily human parasites, and the corresponding diseases originate from human sources, i.e., either sick patients or carriers. Some geographic differences occur, e.g., *S. paratyphi* C is found primarily in Eastern Europe and Asia, while *S. paratyphi* A is found in the Americas and India.

Typhoid fever in developing countries is often waterborne in contrast to paratyphoid fevers. Shellfish, especially oysters, are an important source of typhoid fever but are rarely the source of paratyphoid fever. Milk and other dairy products are often vehicles for typhoid and paratyphoid infections. A small percentage of clinical cases of typhoid fever become chronic carriers and excrete the organism indefinitely. In developed countries, it is often possible to trace nonimported cases of typhoid fever to such carriers.

Salmonella enteritis, associated with many different serotypes, such as *S. typhimurium, S. newport, S. adelaide,* and others, is often described under the heading of food poisoning. It is true that large infectious doses are generally necessary to cause disease, but the pathogenesis includes inflammation of the mucosal tissues and often involves the local lymph nodes. Human *Salmonella* enteritis is associated with consumption of food contaminated either directly or indirectly by an infected animal, e.g., pig, fowl (eggs), cattle, and others. *S. typhimurium* is the most widespread of the serotypes causing enteritis, but the predominant *Salmonella* serotype varies in different geographic areas. Patterns of prevalence change with time as new serotypes are introduced and spread within certain geographic locations. The present close contact between countries and the extensive exchange of travelers and food products have also increased the exchange of pathogenic *Salmonella* serotypes. The same applies, of course, to other pathogenic (and nonpathogenic) Enterobacteriaceae.

Shigella. Human cases are always the source of infection, so the prevalence of bacterial dysentery is highly dependent on sanitary conditions. Bacillary dysentery is endemic in many developing countries. In countries with better conditions of public health, this disease is often confined to institutions or to outbreaks caused by contamination of dairy products. In the highest developed countries, shigellosis is rare and often imported. Chronic carriers are uncommon. *Shigella dysenteriae* Type 1 (the Shiga bacillus) causes the most severe disease.

PREVENTIVE MEASURES. Sanitary measures are all important to control enteric diseases caused by *Salmonella, Shigella,* pathogenic *E. coli,* and other Enterobacteriaceae, e.g., control of water, food, milk, and sewage disposal. Carriers (of *Salmonella*) must not be allowed to work as food handlers.

References

Buchanan, C. E., and Gibbons, N. E. (eds.): Bergey's Manual of Determinative Bacteriology. 8th ed. Baltimore, The Williams & Wilkins Company, 1974, pp. 290–340.

Edwards, P. R., and Ewing, W. H.: Identification of *Enterobacteriaceae.* 3rd ed. Minneapolis, Burgess Publishing Company, 1972.

Ewing, W. H.: Differentiation of Enterobacteriaceae by Biochemical Reactions, Revised. DHEW Publication No. (CDC) 74–8270, May, 1974.

Ewing, W. H., and Fife, M. A.: Enterobacter agglomerans (Beijernick) Comb. Nov. (the Herbicola-Lathyri bacteria). Int J System Bacteriol 22(1):4, 1972.

Falkow, S.: Infectious Multiple Drug Resistance, London, Pion Limited, 1975.

Kauffmann, F.: The Bacteriology of *Enterobacteriaceae.* Copenhagen, E. Munksgaard, 1966.

Lennette, E. H., Spaulding, E. H., and Truant, J. P.: Manual of Clinical Microbiology, 2nd ed. American Society of Microbiology. Washington, D.C. 1974.

Lüderitz, O., Westphal, O., Staub, A. M., and Nikaido, H.: Isolation and chemical and immunological characterization of bacterial lipopolysaccharides. In Weinbaum, G., Kadis, S., and Ajl, S. J. (eds.): Microbial Toxins. Vol. 4. New York and London, Academic Press, 1971, pp.145–233.

Ørskov, F., and Ørskov, I.: Serotyping of *Enterobacteriaceae* with special emphasis on K determination. In Norris, J. R., and Bergan, T.(eds.): Methods in Microbiology. Vol. 11. London and New York, Academic Press, 1978.

Ørskov, I., Ørskov, F., Jann, B., and Jann, K.: Serology, genetics and chemistry of O and K antigens of *Escherichia coli.* Bacterial Rev 41:667, 1977.

Rowe, B.: *Escherichia coli* in acute diarrhoea. Lab-Lore 7:499, 1977.

Sack, R. B.: Human diarrhea disease caused by enterotoxigenic *Escherichia coli.* Ann Rev Microbiol 29:333, 1975.

Sansonnetti, P. J., Kopecko, D. J., and Formal, S. B.: *Shigella sonnei* plasmids: Evidence that a large plasmid is necessary for virulence. Infect Immun 34:75, 1981.

32

VIBRIOS AND CAMPYLOBACTERS

BARUN DEB CHATTERJEE, M.B.B.S., PH.D., DIP. BACT., F.A.M.S.

Vibrios

Facultatively anaerobic comma shaped gram-negative bacilli with polar flagellation are called *vibrios*. These chemorganotropic bacteria having respiratory and fermentative metabolism are grouped under the family *Vibrionaceae* as (a) *Vibrio cholerae,* (b) Noncholera vibrios (NCV) or Nonagglutinating (NAG) vibrios, (c) *Aeromonas hydrophila,* and (d) *Plesiomonas shigelloides.* The earliest designation, *Vibrio gindha,* Pfeiffer 1896 (Chalmers and Waterfield, 1916) is preferred to NCV or NAG vibrios, since these organisms produce cholera-like disease and agglutinate in homologous antisera. They do not possess the O1 antigen of *V. cholerae* but share the same H antigen. As such, these bacteria have been currently described as Non-O1 *V. cholerae,* although according to the priority of nomenclature they should be named *V. cholerae* biotype *gindha.* The taxonomic position of *Vibrio parahaemolyticus* is unsettled: being peritrichous it is not a vibrio. Although related to other genera as shown in Table 1, *V. parahaemolyticus* is provisionally described here until its status is clarified. Likewise, *Vibrio vulnificus* and *Vibrio metchnikovii* are considered here for the time being.

In the tropics, cholera vibrios are the principal but not the sole agents of acute dehydrating rice water diarrhea. Cholera syndrome may be related to a range of pathogens of widely different taxons—for example, Non-O1 *V. cholerae, v. parahaemolyticus, A. hydrophila, P. shigelloides,* and enterotoxigenic *E. coli* (Chatterjee and Neogy, 1972).

VIBRIO CHOLERAE

(*vibrio*, which vibrates; *cholerae*, an intestinal disease, first seen by Pacini (1854); Robert Koch (1883) rediscovered it, cultured it, and, attributed its pathogenic rôle)

MORPHOLOGY. Cells are slightly curved, gram negative, 0.5 by 1.5 to 3.0 μm, and occur singly (Fig. 1). Bacilli rarely appear straight, spherical, and, if joined, S- or C-shaped and as spirilla. The cholera vibrios are fimbriated and show fast linear motility by a long wavy polar flagellum (Fig. 2). They are essentially noncapsulated, but occasionally a cell may look encapsulated. In smears from mucus flakes of rice water stool, bacilli lie parallel to each other like "fish in a stream," presumably because of the degenerating spirilla forms. Cells are vividly stained by dilute carbol fuchsin.

On nutrient agar, the organism produces semitransparent, low convex, 2 to 3 mm round colonies that suspend uniformly in saline. In one week, the growth is overlaid by minute secondary colonies and develops needle-shaped crystals underneath. Colonies may undergo variation to (1) dwarf, (2) entirely opaque, (3) centrally opaque with smooth periphery, and (4) reversible rugose varieties.

After primary isolation in bile salt agar (BSA) and lactose teepol agar (LTA), the conspicuously transparent, flat colonies of cholera vibrios are readily differentiated from the opaque raised ones of coliforms. Under stereo-plate microscopy, the cholera vibrios on BSA exhibit greenish to red-bronze iridescence with fine granular transparency.

Colonies appear opaque-yellow on thiosulfate citrate bile salts-sucrose (TCBS) agar, translucent-yellow on sucrose teepol tellurite (STT) agar (Chatterjee et al., 1977), translucent bluish gray on thiosulfate citrate bile salts–sucrose lauryl sulfate agar (Vibrio agar), grayish translucent on lauryl sulfate tellurite agar (Cholera medium), and gelatin taurocholate tellurite (GTT) agar. While BSA and LTA inhibit gram-positive bacilli, others suppress coliforms as well, thus permitting vibrios to grow in pure form. The slide agglutination with antisera can be done from isolates of all media except TCBS and Vibrio agar, for which, because of the stickiness, subculture on nutrient agar is necessary.

ANTIGENIC COMPOSITION. Cholera vibrios possess heat labile flagellar (H) and heat stable somatic (O) antigens. The former is a protein, the latter a lipopolysaccharide. Three fractions of the O antigen: A, B, and C determine Ogawa (AB), Inaba (AC), Hikojima (ABC), and one unusual (A) serotype. In vivo conversion from Ogawa to Inaba and the reverse is a rare possibility. The isolates from chronic carriers even if appearing smooth may lack O antigen because of S-R variation. Detection of such a variant is facilitated by the "rough" antiserum, made against the O antigen-deficient strain. A common O antigenic factor shared by cholera vibrios, brucella species, *Y. enterocolitica* serotype IX, and *C. terrigena* may confuse serologic diagnosis.

The outer membrane protein has a molecular weight of 48,000; this is common for all bioserotypes of *V. cholerae.* Because it is immunogenic in man, it has prospects in vaccination. Unlike *Enterobacteriaceae,* the lipopolysaccharide of *V. cholerae* does not possess 2-keto-3-desoxyoctonate and galactose; instead it contains a large amount of glycine and ammoniacal radicals.

METABOLISM. Cholera vibrios are facultative anaerobes and can multiply at 16° to 42°C and pH 6.4 to 9.6. Optimum growth occurs aerobically, at 37°C, pH 8.0 to 8.2, in ordinary media and even on minimal synthetic medium containing sources of carbon, nitrogen, and salts. Higher pH (8.5 to 9.5) is beneficial but a lower one (pH 4.0) is lethal, so that strains grown in media containing glucose do not survive. In Table 2, the various distinctive characters of *V. cholerae* are presented.

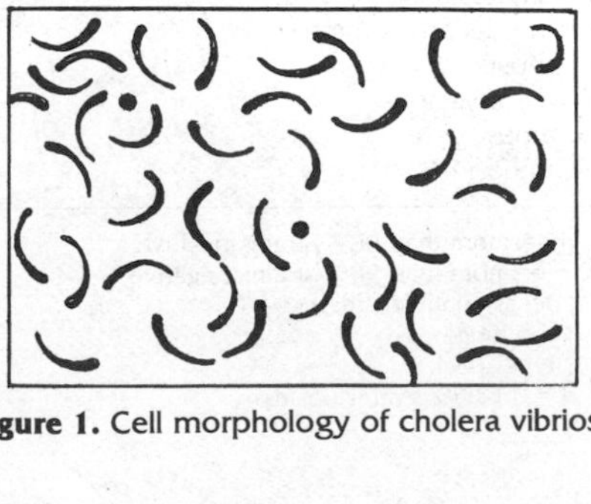

Figure 1. Cell morphology of cholera vibrios.

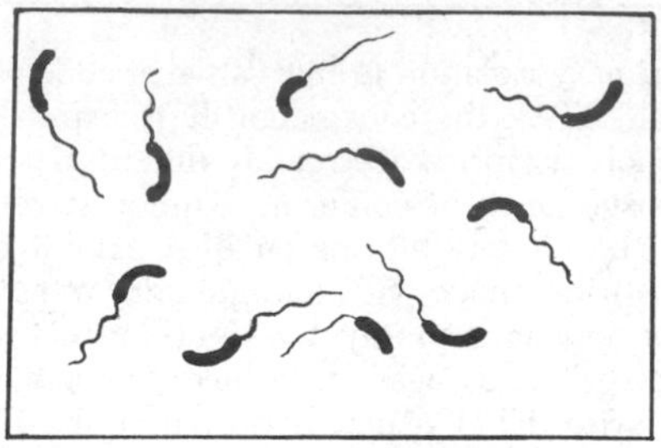

Figure 2. Long, wavy polar flagella of cholera vibrios.

V. cholerae differs from *V. cholerae* biotype El Tor (El Tor vibrio, named for its discovery in El Tor lazeret of Sinai Peninsula). The *V. cholerae* (classic vibrio) is sensitive to 50 IU polymyxin B disk (or 15 μg/ml in nutrient agar) and 1 RTD group IV cholera phage, whereas the El Tor is resistant to these. Only El Tor produces acetoin and agglutinates with chicken, sheep, and human erythrocytes. Further, El Tor causes distinct opacity and a pellicle in nutrient broth, whereas the *V. cholerae* creates minimum turbidity and no pellicle. Until 1962, El Tor strains were hemolytic, but subsequent isolates have not been.

With four lytic phages and standard laboratory strains, classic vibrios exhibit five lytic patterns and El Tor is distributed into six types by five phages. However, phage typing provides limited information in tracing the source of infection, because in actual practice, wild strains of the classic and El Tor strains comprise only two phage types, and the El Tor phages are unstable. Strains of El Tor vibrio isolated from clinical cases from the year 1961 onward, almost invariably show lysogenization by a specific temperate phage called the "kappa" phage. Such strains are identified by their capacity to elicit turbid plaques on *V. cholerae* H 218. By detecting "kappa" phage lytic mutants in their feces, bacteriologically negative cases of El Tor cholera and their contacts can be identified. The *V. cholerae* is resistant to "kappa" phage; El Tor acquires susceptibility after eliminating the temperate phage.

PATHOGENIC PROPERTIES. Evidence suggests that low gastric acid predisposes to attacks of cholera, a finding in keeping with the in vitro susceptibility of *V. cholerae* to low pH. The infective dose in natural infections is probably less than that causing disease in volunteers (10^6).

After bypassing the acid gastric barrier, the organisms reach the favorable alkaline medium in the small bowel, where they penetrate the mucus barrier of the small gut by elaborating mucinase, anchor to the gut mucosa and colonize, and liberate enterotoxin to cause acute rice water diarrhea. The toxin, irreversibly fixed to the intestinal mucosa, stimulates adenyl cyclase, which in its turn builds up cAMP to trigger outpouring of isotonic fluid. Cholera toxin is a protein of molecular weight 84,000 and comprises synergistically acting toxin and toxoid moieties. Experimentally, the toxin produces diarrhea in nine day old rabbits and mongrel dogs. It causes dilatation and fluid accumulation in the ligated loops of adult rabbits, induces rounding of cells and steroidogenesis in clonal cell lines of Y-1 and OS-3 adrenal tumor cells in tissue culture, and elongation of Chinese hamster ovarian (CHO) cell line. The ELISA test is the most sensitive tool in toxin detection.

The toxin moiety consists of six light subunits (L) and one heavy subunit (H). While the former helps adherence to the receptor (GM_1 ganglioside) of the cell membrane, the latter performs the toxic activity.

However, other metabolites of cholera vibrios, like vascular permeability factor, cytolysin and hemolysin do not appear to be related to the pathogenesis of cholera.

IMMUNITY. An attack of cholera confers short-lived immunity to reinfection. Within a few weeks after onset of the disease, there is rise of both serum antibodies (agglutinins [IgM], vibriocidal antibody [IgM], antitoxin [IgG]) and coproantibody (IgA), which persists for three months, but shortly afterwards falls to low titer. It is well known that the IgM and IgG lose their normal functions within the gut lumen because of enzymatic inactivation, and because complement-mediated bactericidal activity as well as complement-dependent phagocytosis are not operative in the anticomplementary intestinal contents. However, it

Table 1. ALLIANCE OF *V. PARAHAEMOLYTICUS* TO DIFFERENT FERMENTATIVE, GRAM-NEGATIVE BACTERIA

Characters	*V. parahaemolyticus*	*Pasteurella*	*Yersinia*	*Lucibacterium*	*Aeromonas*	*Vibrio*‡
Cells : coccoid	+	+	+	−	−*	−
Capsule	+	+	−	−	+	−
Flagella : polar and peritrichous	+	−	−	+	−	−
Swarming	+	−	+	+	−	−
Growth in 0% NaCl conc.	−	+	+	−	+	+
Oxidase	+	+	−	+	+	+
β-galactosidase	−	−	+	?	+	+
Lysine decarboxylase	+	d	−	+	−	+
Zoonosis	+	+	+	−	+	−
Tissue invasion	+	+	+	?	+	−
Luminescence	−	−	−	+	−	−
GC ratio : 46	+	+†	+	+	−	−

+ = more than 90% strains positive
− = more than 90% strains negative
*occasionally positive
† top range
‡ type species
d = 11-89% strains positive

Table 2. DISTINGUISHING FEATURES OF VIBRIO AND ALLIED PATHOGENS
(ALL SINGLE POLAR FLAGELLATED, RAPIDLY MOTILE, POSITIVE TO CATALASE, AND OXIDASE TESTS)

Characters	*V. cholerae*	*Non-01 V. cholerae*	*A. hydrophila*	*P. shigelloides*	*V. parahaemolyticus*	*V. vulnificus*	*C. jejuni*
Cells:							
curved	+	+	−	−	−	−	+
coccoid	−	−*	−*	−	+	+	−
Flagella							
lophotrichous	−	−	+	+	+	+	−
peritrichous	−	−	−	−	+	?	−
Capsule	−	+	+	+	+	+	−
Motility: corkscrew-like	−	−	−	−	−	−	+
Facultative anaerobic	+	+	+	+	+	+	−
Microaerophilic	−	−	−	−	−	+	+
Growth:							
TCBS agar	+	+	−	−	+	+	NT
SS agar	−	−	+	+	−	−	−
Skirrow's medium	d	+	−	−	?	?	+
0% NaCl in gelatin agar	+	+	+	+	−	−	NT
7% NaCl in gelatin agar	−	−	−	−	+	+	NT
KCN broth	d	d	+	−	−	?	NT
O-F test: fermentative	+	+	+	+	+	+	−
Gas from: glucose	−	−	d	−	−	−	−
Acid from							
glucose	+	+	+	+	+	+	−
mannitol	+	+	+	−	+	+	−
inositol	−	−	−	+	−	−	−
Current Heiberg groups	I	(I II V)	(I III IV V)	VI	VII	V	−
Acid from							
mannose	+	+ − +	+ + − +	−	+	+	−
sucrose	+	+ + −	+ + + −	−	−	−	−
arabinose	−	− − −	− + + −	−	+	−	−
β-galactosidase	+	+	+	+	−	+	−
Arginine dihydrolase	−	−	+	+	−	−	−
Lysine decarboxylase	+	+	−	+	+	+	−
Ornithine decarboxylase	+	+	−	+	+	d	−
Nitrate reduction	+	+	+	+	+	+	−
Methyl red	d	d	+	+	−	+	−
Voges-Proskauer	−	d	d	−	−	−	?
Indole	+	+	+	+	d(weak)	+	?
Citrate utilization	d	+	d	−	−	+	?
Hydrolysis							
gelatin	+	+	+	−	+	+	?
casein	+	+	+	−	+	+	−
Tween 80	+	+	?	−	+	+	?
starch	+	+	+	−	+	+	−
esculin	−	−	d	−	+	?	?
Hemolysis							
sheep cell suspension	−	d	d	−	−	?	−
0/129 sensitivity	+	+	−	+	+	+	−
Moles per cent GC	47	46–48	57–63	51	46	46–48	32–35
Mice: s.c. injection bacteremia	−	+	+	+	+	+	NT
Saprophytic existence	−**	+	+	−	+	+	−

+ = more than 90% strains positive
d = 11–89% strains positive
− = more than 90% strains negative
NT = not tested
*occasionally positive
**toxigenic strains
S.C. = subcutaneous

is believed that the antibacterial antibody prevents attachment of the organism to the gut mucosa, whereas the antitoxic immunity inhibits fixation of the toxin.

Likewise, the cholera vaccines, inactivated parenteral (preferably inactivated by formalin than by phenol—with or without adjuvant) and live or killed oral varieties, without exception, impart protection for three to nine months only. The efficacy of vaccines is further limited by their failure to prevent epidemics, death, and inapparent cases and carriers. Although cholera is a toxin-mediated disease, current studies on human volunteers indicate that antibacterial immunity is more protective than antitoxic immunity.

LABORATORY DIAGNOSIS. Prompt diagnosis of cholera caused by *V. cholerae* alone is made by immobilizing the organism in feces with the O-1 antiserum. This phenomenon is observed under the dark field or phase contrast microscope. The indirect immunofluorescence technic is an effective alternative. On the other hand, the following procedure gives the precise diagnosis of the cholera syndrome.

Collection. Fecal samples are collected asceptically in sterile containers with soft rubber catheters (No. 22 or 24), previously lubricated in sterile liquid paraffin. Rectal swabs are not recommended because they often become dry if sampling is inadequate or if the interval between collection and inoculation is too long. If cotton swabs are used they should be soaked in Sorensen's buffer, pH 7.4, before autoclaving. A sample that cannot be inoculated soon after collection should be kept in Cary-Blair's transport medium, which is ideal for vibrios, shigella, salmonella, and *E. coli.*

Culture. Since a range of pathogens is expected in rice water stool, a semiquantitative approach sheds light on the role of organisms, especially in mixed infections (Chatterjee and Neogy, 1972). Usually one of these agents is found in high numbers (10^6 to 10^9/ml), whereas others constitute a minor proportion (10^1 to 10^4/ml). A calibrated loop (0.01 ml; 4 mm internal diameter) is filled with neat, 1/10 and 1/100 dilutions of feces in sterile saline containing 0.1 per cent peptone, and streaked on selective media as for a urine culture.

Six hours of enrichment in alkaline peptone water (with 3 per cent NaCl), pH 9.2 enhances isolation of cholera vibrios, Non-O1 *V. cholerae*, and *V. parahaemolyticus.* For the salmonella, aeromonas, and plesiomonas species, 18 hour enrichment in selenite F broth is recommended. Subculture on selective media after preliminary enrichment allows identification of pathogens.

Media. Colony counts of cholera vibrios, Non-O1 *V. cholerae*, and *V. parahaemolyticus* are done from TCBS or STT agar. The SS agar provides similar information on salmonella, aeromonas, plesiomonas, and pseudomonas; the desoxycholate citrate agar (DCA) is primarily used for salmonella and shigella species, and the MacConkey agar is used for *E. coli.*

Identification. Oxidase-positive isolates on TCBS or STT agar that ferment sucrose are tested in cholera polyvalent and (if necessary) "rough" antisera. Cholera vibrios showing agglutination are divided into Inaba, Ogawa, or (rarely) Hikojima serotypes by specific sera and classic or El Tor biotypes after noting sensitivity to phage IV and polymyxin B (and/or hemagglutination of sheep cells). Contrarily, the sucrose fermenters not reacting with cholera sera are identified as Non-O1 *V. cholerae* on the basis of decarboxylase-dihydrolase tests. Of the sucrose nonfermenting colonies, the Heiberg group VII strains, showing growth at 7 per cent but not in 0 per cent NaCl concentrations and a negative β-galactosidase reaction are identified as *V. parahaemolyticus* biotype 1; whereas those of Heiberg group V, lacking the halophilic property with a positive β-galactosidase test are regarded as Non-O1 *V. cholerae* (Table 2). *V. parahaemolyticus* is subjected to serotyping and the Kanagawa test (see below). The oxidase-positive colonies off MacConkey agar and DCA are treated in a similar manner.

The nonlactose-fermenting, oxidase-positive colonies from SS agar are tested for their oxidation-fermentation (O-F) reaction: *C. terrigena* is negative, whereas *P. aeruginosa* is oxidative. The fermentative breakdown of glucose suggests aeromonas and plesiomonas species. They are identified from the results of mannitol and inositol fermentation and decarboxylase tests (Table 2, Fig. 3).

DRUG SUSCEPTIBILITY. The mean inhibitory concentrations (MIC) in μg/ml for cholera vibrios are as follows: tetracycline 2.5, chloramphenicol 1.5, streptomycin 25, paromomycin 25, viomycin 200, and neomycin 20 to 30. The cholera vibrios are also sensitive to disks of ampicillin (2 μg), sulfisoxazole (4 μg), and polymyxin B (100 IU). Only 2.5 per cent of the global strains are not susceptible to one of these agents. The resistance is chromosomal in origin and seldom, if ever, mediated by plasmids. Strains of El Tor vibrio with plasmid-borne multiple drug resistance have been found in Tanzania and Bangladesh.

EPIDEMIOLOGY. From remote times, *V. cholerae*, the pathogen of Asiatic cholera has been endemic in the vicinity of the Ganges and Brahmaputra rivers in Eastern India and Bangladesh. Over the 19th and early part of the present century, a series of six pandemics originated from the endemic focus in which areas of Asia, Europe, Africa, and America were devastated. During 1923 to 1960, it produced seasonal epidemics within India and Bangladesh with occasional extension to the neighboring countries.

In 1961, the biotype El Tor was implicated in the seventh pandemic, which, since 1937 had been causing bouts of mild cholera in the Sulawesi island of Indonesia. It spread to all states of Southeast Asia in 1961 to 1962, states of mainland Asia within 1963 to 1969, and, gradually replaced the classic vibrio. Later on, it also invaded Africa, Europe, and South USSR, and, to a minor extent, Canada and Australia. However, very recently the classic vibrio has started reappearing in Bangladesh. There have been cases of imported cholera in nonendemic areas owing to rapid air travel.

Under natural conditions, cholera vibrios produce attacks of diarrhea, inapparent cases, and carrier states in no other animals than man. The ratio of overt to asymptomatic infection is 1:24. The former group is twenty times more infective than the latter. Incubation period ranges from one to five days, and, the infectivity 5 to 14 days. The bacterium is transmitted from man to man by the fecal oral route through food and drink. It is particularly prevalent in overcrowded and unsanitary conditions with sharing of common water sources and latrines.

In endemic areas, such as India, Philippines, and Bangladesh, the outbreak occurs before, during, and after the monsoon. In the interepidemic periods, the endemicity continues through a sort of "silent epidemic," moving from the carriers to inapparent cases or vice versa.

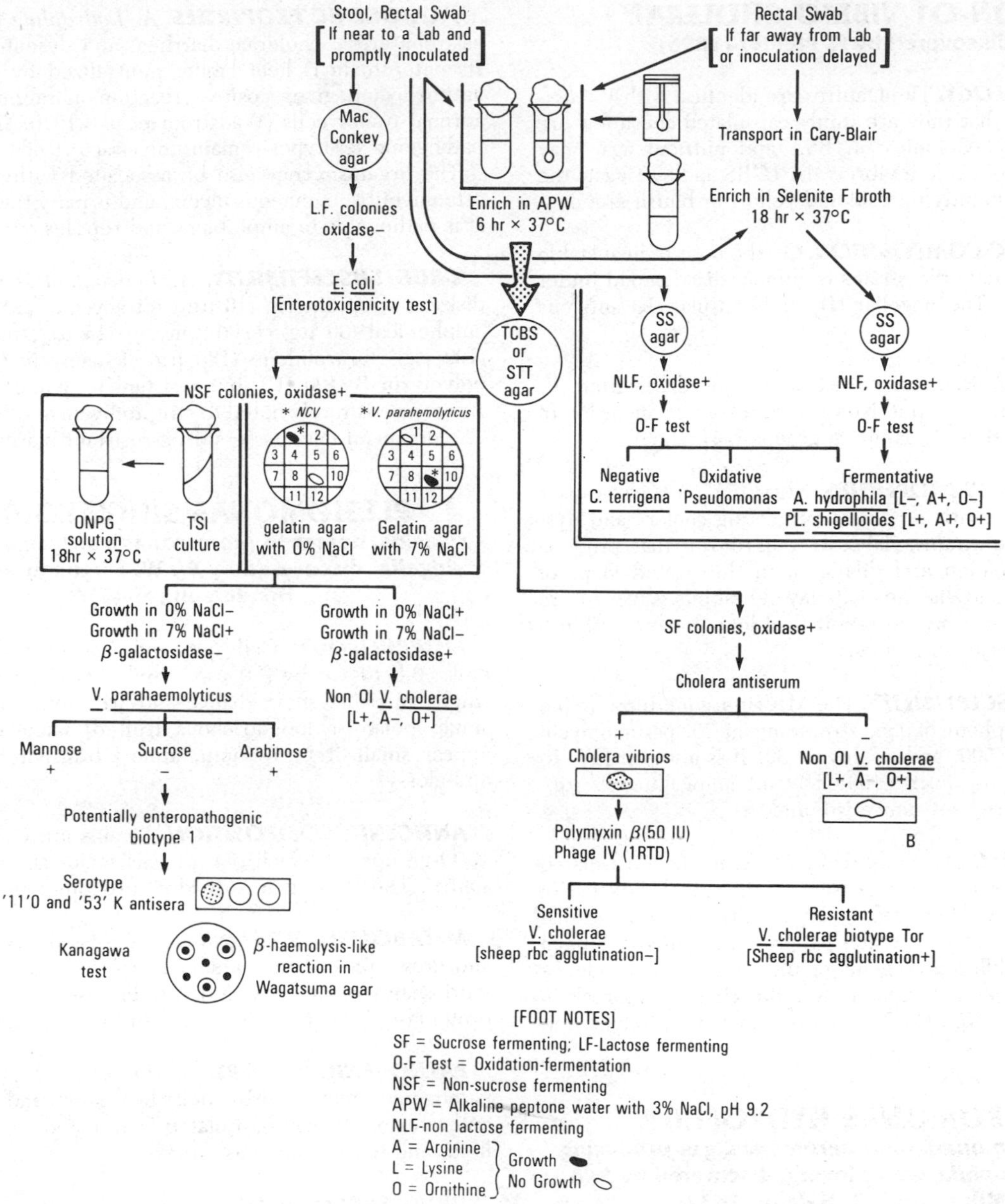

Figure 3.

In comparison to the classic biotype, El Tor proliferates faster, is more resistant to environmental conditions, and produces many more cases, carriers, and newer foci of infections. An El Tor epidemic runs a protracted course rather than the explosive pattern of the Asiatic cholera. The Inaba and Ogawa serotypes, respectively, predominate among the isolates of *V. cholerae* and *V. cholerae* biotype El Tor.

Age old convictions on the epidemiology of cholera are undergoing a thorough shakeup. Contrary to the popular belief that cholera vibrios are short lived in nature, they survive well in water, soaked garments, and sweets. Furthermore, the organism has a natural habitat in coastal and inland waters, so that the environment is not necessarily contaminated by human excreta. The infective dose of *V. cholerae* is significantly lower in an alkaline medium. Strangely enough, the marine strains are non-toxigenic and their role in human diarrhea is unknown.

Cost benefit analyses point to the superiority of hygiene and improved sanitation over cholera vaccines. Water borne epidemics are most effectively controlled by water chlorination and least so by vaccination. Vaccination is economically justified only when the case incidence exceeds 8 per 1000 population, which is hardly seen in practice. Although the immunity is serotype specific, one biotype induces nearly equal protection against the other. However, vaccination is indicated in persons moving from a cholera-free area to the endemic zone.

NON-O1 VIBRIO CHOLERAE
(discovered by R. Pfeiffer (1896))

MORPHOLOGY. The features are identical with *V. cholerae*, except that they are thinly capsulated and a few are coccobacillary. Colonies on BSA and nutrient agar may mimic those of cholera vibrios. In TCBS and STT agar, the colonies are slightly mucoid and yellow or bluish green.

ANTIGENIC COMPOSITION. On the basis of heat stable somatic antigens, the strains of human diarrhea fall under 60 O-groups. The flagellar (H) and capsular (K) antigens are heat labile.

METABOLISM. Characteristics do not differ from *V. cholerae* (Table 2), but Non-O1 *V. cholerae* in order of prevalence belong to Heiberg groups I, II, and V.

PATHOGENIC PROPERTIES. Non-O1 *V. cholerae* causes mild gastroenteritis or illness simulating cholera and dysentery. Some strains elaborate enterotoxin that produce fluid accumulation and dilatation in the ligated loops of adult rabbits and diarrhea in 9 day old rabbits. Live culture of certain strains invade rabbit ileal loop mucosa within 6 hours (Chatterjee et al., 1979).

DRUG SUSCEPTIBILITY. The MIC in μg/ml: tetracycline 1.5, chloramphenicol 1.5, streptomycin 75, paromomycin 50, viomycin 500, and neomycin 30. It is also sensitive to disks of polymyxin B (100 IU) and ampicillin (25 μg). Sometimes drug resistance is found.

EPIDEMIOLOGY. Non-O1 *V. cholerae* can be isolated usually from natural waters, sewage, flies, and the feces of cold-blooded and hot-blooded animals, but not from normal human stool. These organisms produce sporadic human diarrhea in different regions of the world. The incidence commonly rises before and after the cholera outbreak in eastern India. Non-O1 *V. cholerae* does not produce epidemics.

AEROMONAS HYDROPHILA
(*aer*, gas; *monad*, unit; *aeromonas*, gas-producing one; *hydrophila*, water loving, discovered by A. A. Miles and E. T. Halnan (1937))

MORPHOLOGY. Cells are gram-negative, thinly capsulated, straight rods, or coccobacilli, 1.0 to 4.4 μm, arranged singly, in pairs and short chains, and rapidly motile by one or more terminal flagella.

On nutrient agar, the colonies are 2 to 3 mm, translucent, smooth, round, and convex after 18 hrs at 30° to 37° C. Broth culture shows diffuse turbidity with or without pellicle.

METABOLISM. *A. hydrophila* is a facultative anaerobe and is nonfastidious. Its generation time is short. Growth occurs at 21° to 40°C, pH 5.5 to 9.0, but some biochemical characters (Table 2) are better elicited at 22°C than 37°C—for example, gas from carbohydrates, production of acetoin, and utilization of citrate. Whereas the aerogenic biotype produces acetoin and H_2S from cysteine, the anaerogenic one is negative to these tests.

PATHOGENIC PROPERTIES. *A. hydrophila* causes mild gastroenteritis, choleraic diarrhea, and dysentery in man. Its enterotoxin is heat labile, neutralized by the cholera antitoxin and gives positive reaction in rabbit loops and adrenal tumor cells (Wadström et al., 1976). The enteropathogenic serotypes remain uncharacterized.

The organism may also be associated with bacteremia, osteomyelitis, cutaneous ulcers, and urinary tract infection. It is pathogenic to amphibians and reptiles.

DRUG SUSCEPTIBILITY. *A. hydrophila* is sensitive to disks of streptomycin (10 μg), tetracycline (30 μg), chloramphenicol (30 μg), erythromycin (15 μg), nalidixic acid (100 μg), furazolidone (100 μg), kanamycin (5 μg), and polymyxin B (100 IU), but resistant to ampicillin (25 μg). Resistance is rarely noted to streptomycin and tetracycline. The organism may possess drug-resistant plasmids.

PLESIOMONAS SHIGELLOIDES
(*Plesios*, nearer to *(aeromonas)*; *shigelloides*, like *shigella*; discovered by W. W. Ferguson and N. D. Henderson (1947))

MORPHOLOGY. Cells are rod shaped with rounded ends, 0.8 to 1.0 by 3.0 μm, thinly capsulated, arranged singly, in pairs, short chains, and are rapidly motile with single polar or lophotrichous (tufted) flagella. Colonies appear small, 1 to 1.5 mm, almost transparent, convex, and glossy.

ANTIGENIC COMPOSITION. Strains are classified into 16 O-groups, of which one reveals major sharing with *S. sonnei*. The H antigen is divided into four types.

METABOLISM. *P. shigelloides* is a facultative anaerobe and grows on ordinary media at 18° to 37°C. Unlike the vibrios and aeromonas, it lacks diastase, lipase, DNase, proteinase, hemolysin (Table 2), and has no biotypes.

PATHOGENIC PROPERTIES. The organism is an enteropathogenic agent by virtue of its heat labile and heat stable enterotoxins. It may be isolated from blood, cerebrospinal fluid, and feces of animals.

DRUG SUSCEPTIBILITY. It is usually sensitive to disks of streptomycin (10 μg), tetracycline (10 μg), chloramphenicol (25 μg), kanamycin (30 μg), gentamicin (10 μg), paromomycin (30 μg), furazolidone (100 μg), but resistant to ampicillin (25 μg).

VIBRIO PARAHAEMOLYTICUS
(*para*, like; *haema*, blood; *parahaemolyticus*, like *haemolytica*; discovered by T. Fujino (1951))

MORPHOLOGY. Cells are ellipsoidal, gram-negative, capsulated rods, 0.5 to 1.4 μm by 0.4 to 0.6 μm, slightly pleomorphic, arranged singly, in pairs, short chains and small clusters; filaments are rare but consistent (Fig. 4). Adverse conditions or aging produces marked pleomorphism. Strains grown on nutrient agar containing 3 per cent NaCl after two or three days show involution forms—for example, bipolar staining, spheroplasts, slender rods with

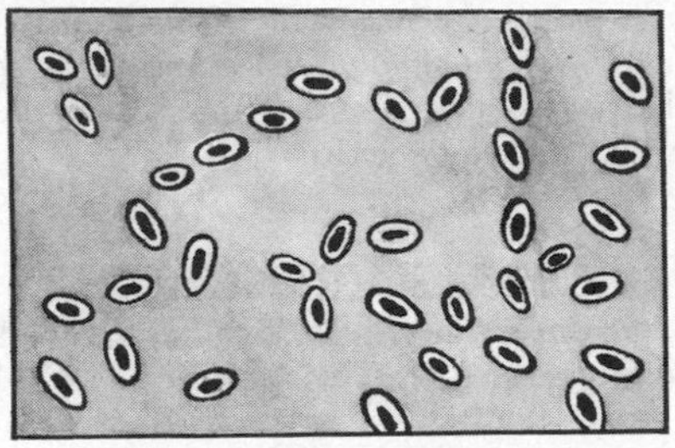

Figure 4. Well formed capsule of *V. parahaemolyticus.*

tapering ends, and clubs. Broth culture at 37°C reveals polar flagellated cells with rapid linear motility. Contrarily, 18-hr growth at 22° to 28°C on semisolid agar and 5-hr nutrient agar culture at 37°C disclose feebly motile peritrichous and polar flagellated cells (Fig. 5). The polar flagella are thick and wavy but the lateral ones are thin, fragile, and curly (Chatterjee, 1974).

The organism produces dome-shaped, off-white, sticky colonies in meat extract agar that measure 2 to 3 mm in diameter. With time, the culture is slowly covered by minute daughter colonies. Colonies of the enteropathogenic variety are bluish green on TCBS and STT agar but others are yellow and a little bigger. Somctimes a smooth colony exhibits wrinkled opaque transformation at the center with unaltered periphery; this is reversed on subculture at 22°C. An old culture in agar slant may show brown coloration of the medium and a bunch of needle shaped crystals underneath. Growth on semisolid agar at 22°C may show swarming.

ANTIGENIC COMPOSITION. *V. parahaemolyticus* possesses flagellar (H), capsular (K), and somatic (O) antigens, having 2, 53, and 11 types respectively. Flagellar antigenicity and agglutinability are better developed at 22° to 28°C than 37°C. Since these H antigens are shared by all strains, they do not help in classification. Serotyping is based on O and K antigens. The enteropathogenic serotypes are: 01:K38, 01:K56, 02:K3, 03:K4, 03:K33, 04:K8, 04:K9, 04:K11, 04:K12, 04:K13, 04:K55, 05:K12, 05:K15, 05:K17, 05:K30, 05:Cal/Ka, 05:K47, 08:K20, 08:K21, 08:K22, 09:K23, 010:K19, and 010:K24. They are rarely distributed in the fish and water.

METABOLISM. *V. parahaemolyticus* differs sharply from the other members in that it gives a negative test for β-galactosidase and fails to grow in NaCl-deficient media. In order to cultivate the organism in gelatin agar, at least 0.1 per cent NaCl is needed. Table 2 shows characteristics of enteropathogenic strains grouped under the biotype 1. It differs from the biotype 2 (*V. parahaemolyticus* biotype *alginolyticus*), which ferments sucrose, produces acetoin, and grows in 10 per cent NaCl. There are intermediate forms between the biotypes 1 and 2. *V. parahaemolyticus* is proteolytic and saccharolytic but essentially nonhemolytic for suspended red cells of different species. Yet, most (> 90 per cent) of strains from cases of human diarrhea and their contacts show the Kanagawa phenomenon—that is, a reaction resembling β-hemolysis in Wagatsuma agar during overnight incubation at 37°C. On the other hand, the isolates of fish, food, and water are Kanagawa-negative after overnight incubation and positive only after 48 hours. Growth on Wagatsuma agar, with its high pH, excess NaCl and fermentable carbohydrate like mannitol is a test for hemodigestion rather than for true hemolysis.

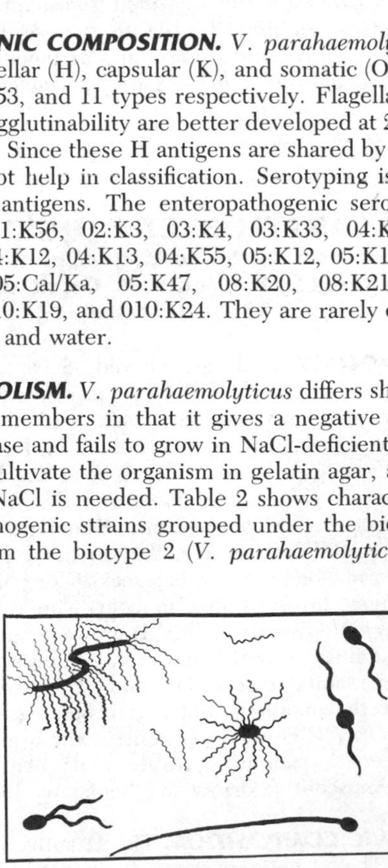

Figure 5. Polar and peritrichous flagella of *V. parahaemolyticus.*

The media for methyl red (MR), V-P, and decarboxylase-dihydrolase tests being salt free are supplemented with 0.5 per cent NaCl. Results of the MR test, KCN tolerance, and citrate utilization are negative in media having 0.5 per cent NaCl (Table 2), but can be reversed if the same media are modified with 3 per cent NaCl (Chatterjee, 1974).

An "aberrant biotype" of *V. parahaemolyticus* (Group F, EF-6, *Vibrio fluvialis*) usually grows in 7 per cent NaCl, ferments sucrose and arabinose, but reacts negatively in lysine and ornithine decarboxylase tests, and in indole and V-P tests. Like *A. hydrophila* it reveals arginine dihydrolase activity. It is Kanagawa positive whether isolated from the environment or diarrhea stools. The organism can be isolated from cold blooded animals and water (Chatterjee, 1974; Lee et al., 1981).

PATHOGENIC PROPERTIES. *V. parahaemolyticus* is enteropathogenic even though it is nonenterotoxic and Sereny negative. For want of a better substitute, the Kanagawa phenomenon continued to be the yardstick of pathogenicity. But whereas the strains recovered from human gastroenteritis are almost invariably Kanagawa positive, those of incriminated foodstuffs and the environment are Kanagawa negative. The Kanagawa positive strains are characterized by a more rapid adherence to the monolayer culture of human fetal intestinal cells, stronger cytotoxic effects on the HeLa cell line, and greater accumulation of fluid in ligated rabbit ileal loops. Microscopy shows that *V. parahaemolyticus* and its "aberrant biotype" invade and colonize within the mucosal epithelial cells and lamina propria of these loops. This is accompanied by acute inflammation, degeneration and erosion of the villi, the process at times spreading into the deeper layers. Recent diarrheal isolates irrespective of their Kanagawa reactions are almost always invasive but those from the environment are rarely so (Chatterjee et al., 1979).

LABORATORY DIAGNOSIS. The steps of investigating *V. parahaemolyticus* food poisoning are shown below in addition to those already indicated in connection with the cholera syndrome.

Food Bacteriology. Demonstration of numerous organisms in the food strongly supports the diagnosis. Accordingly, 50 g of food are homogenized and diluted 1/10 and 1/100 in sterile saline with 0.1 per cent peptone. The neat and diluted samples are streaked on TCBS or STT agar with a calibrated loop for quantitation. A similar quantity of homogenized food is also put up for enrichment in alkaline peptone water (pH 9.2) containing 3 per cent NaCl.

Isolation and identification of *V. parahaemolyticus* from

feces are already discussed under *V. cholerae*. The isolates of food and feces are compared by serotyping and the Kanagawa test; they may reveal multiple serotypes, of which one remains dominant.

DRUG SUSCEPTIBILITY. MIC in μg/ml are as follows: streptomycin 15 to 25, tetracycline 2.5 to 6, and chloramphenicol 0.5 to 2.5. It is also sensitive to disks of kanamycin (5 μg), polymyxin B (50 IU), colistin (10 μg), cephalothin (30 μg), furazolidone (100 μg), but resistant to ampicillin (25 μg). The organism produces β-lactamase.

EPIDEMIOLOGY. *V. parahaemolyticus* is a free-living bacterium. It is distributed all over the world in offshore sea water and marine animals. In eastern India where the inland water is slightly brackish it is found in pond water and its fish; it is also recovered from flies and sewage.

The organism produces sporadic diarrhea and food poisoning in Japan, Southeast Asia, Australia and the United States. The food poisoning may break out suddenly in a community after eating from a common source. It is occasionally lethal in Japan. The "aberrant biotype" is associated with sporadic and epidemic forms of gastroenteritis in Bangladesh. It is rarely isolated from human diarrhea in Calcutta.

Fish is most often responsible for infection. In Japan more than 70 per cent of summer food poisoning cases are produced by *V. parahaemolyticus* after eating uncooked or undercooked fish. Since adequate cooking reduces the risk of infection, the incidence of food poisoning is much lower in other countries. However, the food may be recontaminated by the pathogen after cooking owing to poor kitchen hygiene. Its short generation time (ten minutes) allows it to attain infective numbers (10^5 to 10^7 viable cells in human volunteers) rapidly at ambient temperature. The housefly and the blue-bottle fly may act as mechanical vectors by transporting *V. parahaemolyticus* from human feces or fish to food (Chatterjee et al., 1978). This explains the incidence of diarrhea in strict vegetarians.

VIBRIO VULNIFICUS

(*vulnus*, wound; *ficus*, relation; discovered by R. E. Weaver and N. J. Enrenkranz (1975))

Vibrio vulnificus is a gram negative, halophilic, lactose-positive bacterium sharing features with *V. parahaemolyticus* (Table 2). It is divided into biotypes 1 and 2, which are pathogenic to man and eels, respectively. The biotype 1 produces indole and ornithine decarboxylase, it usually grows at 42°C, and ferments mannitol and sorbitol. The biotype 2 is negative to these tests.

The organism is found in the marine environment, i.e., in coastal water, sediment, and oysters. It infects middle aged persons during summer months in Japan, Belgium, and USA. Attacks of septicemia follow 18 hours after ingestion of contaminated raw oysters. The cases of wound sepsis, but not usually of septicemia, are evident 12 hours after contact with sea water.

VIBRIO METCHNIKOVII

(*metchnikov*, a scientist; discovered by M. N. Gamaleia (1888))

The organism is widely distributed in natural water. Although it may rarely be identified from human stool, its pathogenicity is doubtful. It is lactose, sucrose, and arginine dihydrolase positive and oxidase and arabinose fermentation negative and thus differs from *V. parahaemolyticus*.

Campylobacters

Microaerophilic, gram negative, curved spiral bacilli with polar flagellation are called *campylobacters*. Because of their morphology and darting motility they were previously regarded as *vibrios*. However, they are microaerophilic, capnophilic, not facultatively anaerobic, and have longer spirals (8 μm), corkscrew movement, long generation time, negative oxidation fermentation test, and lower GC content of DNA (30 to 35 moles % Tm). Unlike obligate anaerobes, they possess superoxide dismutase and catalase. Campylobacteriosis is a zoonosis having venereal and fecoral routes of transmission. It causes abortion, in animals but not in man. Other diseases are presented in Table 3.

These chemorganotropic bacteria with respiratory metabolism are grouped under family *Spirillaceae* as I. genus *Campylobacter: Campylobacter jejuni, Campylobacter intestinalis, Campylobacter sputorum*, and others (Table 3), and II. genus *Spirillum*, which includes *Spirillum minor* (Smibert, 1978). Since the innovation of selective coproculture by Dekeyser et al. (1972) there has been tremendous advancement in the understanding of *C. jejuni*. *Campylobacter coli* is a variant of *C. jejuni* rather than a different species. The overall features of campylobacters are given in Table 3.

CAMPYLOBACTER JEJUNI

(*campylo*, curved; *bacter*, rod; *jejuni*, portion of small gut. Discovered by F. S. Jones, M. Orcutt and R. Little (1931) from cattle)

MORPHOLOGY. Cells are curved, S- or gull-shaped gram-negative, slender rods 1.5 to 5 μm by 0.2 to 0.5 μm and occur singly, in pairs and chains with three to five spirals. They transform to spheroplasts in 4 to 5-day-old cultures. The organism bears a long polar flagellum at one or both ends. It shows rapid linear or corkscrew motility.

The colonies are small 1 to 2-mm diameter and look flat, watery, or turbid with an irregular spreading margin, and tend to swarm along the line of streak. Older plates reveal round, convex, brownish gray mucoid colonies with entire edges. *C. jejuni* is nonhemolytic. It grows in nutrient broth producing diffuse turbidity and scanty deposit. Stock cultures can be maintained only in liquid nitrogen or at −20°C in FBP broth containing nutrient broth, agar (0.12 per cent), $FeSO_4$, 7 H_2O (0.05 per cent), sodium metabisulfite (0.05 per cent), sodium pyruvate (0.05 per cent), and glycerol (1 per cent) (Skirrow and Benjamin, 1980).

ANTIGENIC COMPOSITION. The H antigen is uncharacterized. The O antigen shows type-specific and cross-

Table 3. DIFFERENTIAL FEATURES OF CAMPYLOBACTERS (ALL GRAM-NEGATIVE, POLAR FLAGELLATED RODS, OXIDASE-POSITIVE AND OXIDATION FERMENTATION TEST NEGATIVE)

	Growth Potentiality								
Species Characteristics	**Glycine 1%**	**NaCl 3.5%**	**Bile 1%**	**Sodium Selenite 0.1%**	**Temp 25°C**	**Temp 42°C**	**Reservoirs**	**Mode of Transmission**	**Pathogenicity**
Catalase +, H_2S- (on TSI), Nitrate Reduction −									
C. fetus	−	−	+	−	+	−	Bull:genital tract	Venereal	Abortion and infertility in cattle
C. intestinalis	+	−	+	+(R)	+	−	?	Oral (?)	Systemic infection and rarely diarrhea in human. Abortion in sheep and cattle.
C. jejuni	+	−	+	+(R)	−	+	Cattle, sheep, goats, birds, pigs: gut lumen	Oral	Diarrhea and rarely septicemia in man. Abortion in sheep. Bluecomb disease and enteritis in turkeys. Dysentery in pigs.
Catalase-, H_2S + (on TSI), Nitrate Reduction +									
C. sputorum	+	−	+	?	+	−	Man: oral cavity	?	?
C. bubulus	+	+	−	+(R^d)	d	d	Cattle, sheep: genital tract	?	?
C. mucosalis	−	−	−	?	?	?	Pigs: oral cavity	Oral	Intestinal adenomatosis, necrotic enteritis, regional ileitis and proliferative enteropathy in pigs.
Catalase +, H_2S + (on TSI), Nitrate Reduction ?									
C. fecalis	+	d	d	+(R)	−	+	Sheep: gut	?	?

+ = more than 90% strains positive; − = more than 90% strains negative; d = 11–89% strains positive; R = reduction.

reactive fractions. The bacterium is classified into 21 serotypes of which seven: O1, O2, O4, O5, O7, O9, and O11 are commonly associated with human diarrhea. These types are also frequently isolated from chicken, swine, and cattle.

METABOLISM. *C. jejuni* is microaerophilic and capnophilic. It cannot grow under aerobic and strict anaerobic conditions. Growth occurs optimally at 5 per cent oxygen with 8 per cent carbon dioxide and 87 per cent hydrogen or nitrogen concentrations, 37°C and pH 7.2. Other attributes are presented in Table 3. Table 4 shows the characteristics of the three biotypes isolated from human diarrhea (Skirrow and Benjamin, 1980). *C. jejuni* produces H_2S in cysteine-containing media but not in TSI. Slants having 0.1 per cent sodium selenite support growth with evidence of reduction. Sixty per cent of the strains reveal alkaline phosphatase activity, hydrolysis of casein, ribonucleic, and deoxyribonucleic acids.

PATHOGENIC PROPERTIES. *C. jejuni* diarrhea is more common in children (5.8 per cent) than adults (2.3 per cent). The infection often mimics acute dysentery. Asymptomatic carriers are unusual: it has been recorded in 1.3 per cent Belgian and 13 per cent South African children. *C. jejuni* diarrhea is due to acute enterocolitis. The mucosa of jejunum looks hemorrhagic and necrotic, while that of colon shows inflammatory changes with or without crypt abscesses. Septicemia and meningitis are rare complications.

It shows heat labile enterotoxin but reacts negatively to the Sereny test. HeLa cells show surface adhesion and penetration by the organism. Three-day-old chicks fed orally with 9 × 10^7 cells of *C. jejuni* manifest diarrhea within 24 to 48 hours. Histological study shows invasion of the lamina propria of the ileum and cecum with cellular infiltration but no ulceration. Diarrhea is induced in gnotobiotic puppies with or without microinvasiveness of the colon.

IMMUNITY. In developing countries, the incidence of diarrhea caused by *C. jejuni* is high (30 per cent) during the first 8 months of life. Thereafter it declines, presumably because of gut immunity resulting from intense transmission as in the case of enteropathogenic *E. coli*. The bactericidal antibody is type specific, whereas, the agglutinating and complement-fixing antibodies are cross absorbed by other campylobacters. Mere presence of bactericidal antibody is not the *sine qua non* of active infection, since it is demonstrable in 20 to 25 per cent of normal controls in endemic areas.

Table 4. CHARACTERISTICS OF THE BIOTYPES OF *C. JEJUNI*

Tests	*C. jejuni*	*C. jejuni* Biotype *coli*	*C. jejuni* Biotype NART
Temperature (°C)			
25	–	–	–
30.5	–	+	+
37	+	+	+
43	+	+	+
45.5	d	d	+
Hippurate	+	–	–
Triphenyl tetrazolium chloride (40g/l)	S	R	S
NaCl 1.5%	–	–	+
H_2S in iron medium	d	–	+
Nalidixic acid (30 μg/disk)	S	S	R
Metronidazole (5 μg/disk)	d	d	R

S sensitive, R resistant, d variable, + growth, – no growth. NART nalidixic acid resistant thermophilic campylobacter.

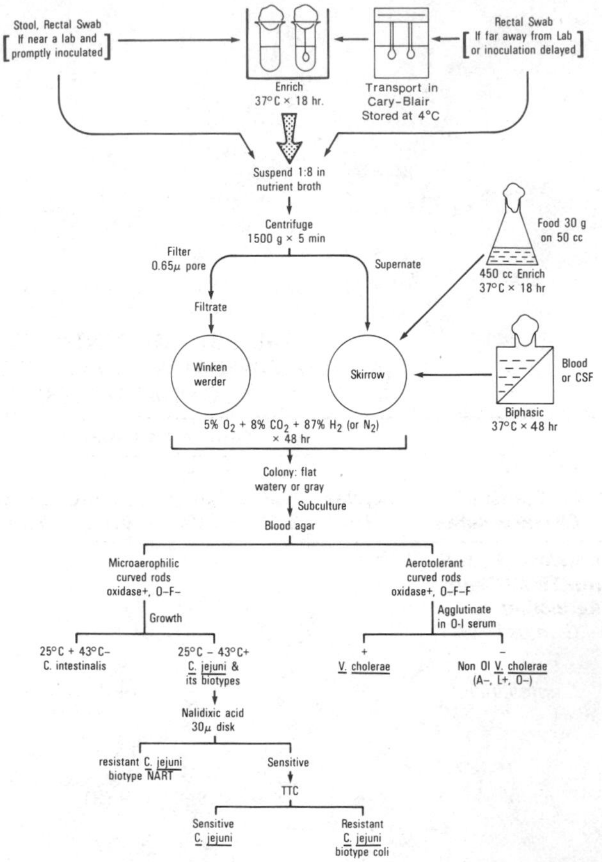

Figure 6. Laboratory diagnosis of *C. jejuni* diarrhea.

LABORATORY DIAGNOSIS

Acute Diarrhea. Fecal samples are collected similarly to *V. cholerae* as outlined in Figure 6, diluted 1:8 in nutrient broth and centrifuged at 1500 × g for 5 minutes. Isolation of *C. jejuni* is facilititated by the procedure of twofold selection. At first, the fecal supernate is passed through a 0.65 μ filter and then the filtrate is cultured on the Winkenwerder's thioglycolate blood agar with bacitracin (25 IU/ml), novobiocin (5 μg/ml), and actidione (50 μg/ml) (Butzler, 1978). The filter permits passage of *C. jejuni* and a few other small microbes but eliminates a large bulk of the gut flora.

More conveniently, the supernate of the stool suspension is directly streaked on Skirrow's (1977) medium, containing 5 per cent laked horse blood agar with vancomycin (10 μg/ml), polymyxin B (2.5 IU/ml), and trimethoprim (5 μg/ml). Better selection is achieved by using rifampicin (10 μg/ml) and cyclohexamide (100 μg/ml) instead of vancomycin and by doubling the concentration of polymyxin B and trimethoprim (Preston medium). Without agar, this medium is suitable for enrichment culture.

The suspected colonies are screened under 10× lens and subcultured on blood agar for microaerophilism and aerotolerance. Microaerophilic growth is stained by 1:10 dilution of carbol fuchsin for 30 seconds to demonstrate cell morphology. The strains showing oxidase reaction but no sugar fermentation or H_2S production on TSI are accepted as *C. jejuni*. Other tests are detailed in Table 4. Skirrow's medium permits profuse growth of other gram-negative curved rods like *V. cholerae* and non-O1 *V. cholerae*. Their dwarf colonies are particularly confused with *C. jejuni* but may be differentiated by aerotolerance and biochemical tests (Chatterjee et al. 1982).

The isolates are serotyped with 21 antisera by slide agglutination.

Food Bacteriology. Since *C. jejuni* is relatively short-lived at the ambient temperature, proper storage of food samples is necessary if culture is delayed. Refrigeration (at 4°C) in an atmosphere of 100 per cent nitrogen is ideal for all sorts of specimens. Alternatively, milk is preserved at 4°C in an oxygen-free medium after addition of 0.01 per cent sodium bisulfite. Solid food is refrigerated in an equal volume of Cary-Blair medium. Quantitition and enrichment culture follow as usual.

Pathogenicity Test. Diarrhea is demonstrated by feeding three-day-old chicks with live culture of *C. jejuni*.

Serodiagnosis. This is done by showing fourfold rise of bactericidal antibodies in the paired sera of patients. The increase of specific IgG titers can be demonstrated by the fluorescent antibody technique in which the autologous isolate is used as an antigen (Blaser et al., 1979).

Meningitis or Septicemia. CSF or blood is cultured in biphasic medium containing brucella broth and brucella agar under microaerophilic condition for 48 hours. Identification of *C. jejuni* is established by the above procedure.

DRUG SUSCEPTIBILITY. The minimal inhibitory concentrations in μg/ml for *C. jejuni* are: streptomycin 2 to 4; neomycin 8; kanamycin 0.01 to 3.12; gentamicin 0.19 to 1.56; tetracycline 0.8; ampicillin 1.56; erythromycin 2 to 8; chloramphenicol 4; cephalothin 50; carbenicillin 200. It is resistant to penicillin (5 units), polymyxin B (1024 units), and bacitracin (120 units). Tetracycline resistance is sometimes encountered.

EPIDEMIOLOGY. *C. jejuni* is one of the commonest agents of diarrhea. It poses a global problem and infects all age groups. A wide range of wild and domestic animals act as reservoirs of infection by harboring the organism in the gut. The carrier rates (per cent) in healthy animals are: ducks 88.3, pigs 54.2, chicken 23.8, sheep 13.6, rabbits 11.3, goats 2.7, cattle 2.5, and dogs 0.5. Human gastroenteritis is a zoonosis in which man does not act as an end host. The transmission of *C. jejuni* follows fecal contamination of raw cow's milk, water, poultry, pork, and ham. Handling of sick pets carries similar risk. Milk is a common vehicle of infection in the UK and USA. Only 500 cells of *C. jejuni* in milk can precipitate an attack of diarrhea. The infection usually gives rise to sporadic cases at times with family clusters. Single source outbreak may be recorded in which contaminated milk or water is implicated. Attacks are more common in summer than winter and more frequent in rural than urban settings.

Foodstuffs other than milk do not apparently support multiplication or survival of *C. jejuni* (unlike *Salmonella*); they are cooked before consumption. Salting of meat prevents infection. The red meat carcasses have a small potential to allow growth of *C. jejuni* at pH 6.4 but not at its normal pH of 5.8. The contamination is detected in the flanks but is of the low order (ca 1 to 10 cm^2). However, 54 to 62 per cent of fresh chicken may disclose contamination. The organism survives in meat for one week if refrigerated, and keeps longer under deep freezing (−20°C). The preventive measures include breast feeding of infants, pasteurization of milk, chlorination of water, irradiation or lactic acid treatment of meat, proper kitchen hygiene, and isolation of sick pets.

CAMPYLOBACTER INTESTINALIS

(*intestinalis*, relating to gut. Discovered by A. Florent (1959) from bovine genitalia)

On primary isolation the colonies are small, 1-mm diameter, flat, and opalescent with irregular margins. The color varies from gray to dirty brown. They are nonhemolytic. Colonies tend to spread along the line of streaking. They become mucoid after one week. After subculture, cut glass colonies showing reflecting facets may develop. Rough colonies are small, finely granular, and opaque. The organism grows in nutrient broth and produces H_2S in cysteine-containing media. Growth on 0.1 per cent sodium selenite slants is associated with signs of reduction. It does not elaborate alkaline phosphatase. Other features are shown in Table 3. The drug sensitivity pattern is like that of *C. jejuni*.

Debilitated subjects are prone to infection with *C. intestinalis*, revealing septicemia without splenomegaly. There may be meningitis, meningoencephalitis, abortion, enteritis, thrombophlebitis, septic arthritis, and jaundice with splenomegaly.

UNCLASSIFIED CAMPYLOBACTERS. Fennel and coworkers (1984) described slow-growing, catalase-positive campylobacterlike microorganisms from the feces of homosexual men with diarrhea. These isolates were divided into three types based on phenotypic differences. All three grew on Skirrow's medium at 37°C but not at 25°C. Type 3 grew at 45°C. All types utilized glycine, grew on 0.04 per cent TTC but not 2 per cent NaCl, and did not make H_2S or hydrolyze hippurate. All were inhibited by nalidixic acid and types 1 and 2 were inhibited by cephalothin. The DNA of all three types was related but did not hybridize with DNA from other catalase-positive campylobacters.

SPIRILLUM MINOR

(*spirillum*, small spiral; *minor*, little. Discovered by H. V. Carter (1888) from rats)

Cells are spiral, 3 to 5 μm by 0.2 to 0.5 μm with tapering ends. The organism is amphi-lophotrichous and actively motile. It is demonstrated by the Leishman, Wright, or Giemsa stains. *S. minor* produces rat bite fever in Japan and Far East, which is characterized by relapsing fever, macular rash, and regional lymphadenopathy adjacent to the site of bite. It is not cultivable.

The bacterium can be identified from the stained smear of bite wound, aspirate of lymph node, and blood. Dark ground microscopy of the heparinized blood is worthwhile. The disease is reproduced in mice or rats after inoculation but more typically in guinea pigs. The infection responds to penicillin and tetracycline.

References

Blaser, M. J., Berkowitz, I. D., Laforce, F. M., Cravens, J., Reller, B., and Wang, W. L. L. : Campylobacter enteritis: Clinical and epidemiological features. Ann Intern Med 91:179, 1979.

Butzler, J. P., J. D. Williams (ed:) Infection with Campylobacters. In: Modern Topics in Infection. London. William Heinemann Medical Books Ltd. p. 214. 1978.

Chalmers, A. J., and Waterfield, N. E. : Paracholera caused by *Vibrio gindha*. Pfeiffer 1896. J Trop Med Hyg 19:165, 1916.
Chatterjee, B. D. : Epidemiologic and taxonomic status of *Vibrio parahaemolyticus*. In: Fujino T., Sakaguchi, G., Sakazaki, R. and Takeda, Y. (eds.) : International Symposium on *Vibrio parahaemolyticus*. Tokyo, Saikon Publ. Co., 1974, p. 177.
Chatterjee, B. D., and Neogy, K. N. : On the etiology of choleraic diarrhoea. Indian J Med Res 60:531, 1972.
Chatterjee, B. D., De, P. K., and Sen, T. : Sucrose teepol tellurite agar : A new selective indicator medium for isolation of *Vibrio* species. J Infect Dis 135:654; 136:716, 1977.
Chatterjee, B. D., Mukherjee, A., and Sanyal, S. N. : A test for invasive *Vibrio parahaemolyticus* in rabbit small bowel. Bull Calcutta Sch Trop Med 27:4, 1979.
Chatterjee, B. D., De, P. K, Hati, A. K., and Tandon, N. : Fly borne *Vibrio parahaemolyticus*. Trop Geogr Med 30:499, 1978.
Chatterjee, B. D., Pan, G., and Khatua, S. P. : Acute infantile diarrhoea : Selectivity of Skirrow's medium for *Campylobacter fetus* ssp. *jejuni*. Proceedings V National Congress, Indian Association of Medical Microbiologists. p. 127, 1982.
Dekeyser, P., Gossuin-Detrain, M., Butzler, J. P., and Sternon, J. : Acute enteritis due to related vibrio : First positive stool cultures. J Infect Dis 125:390, 1972.
Fennell, C. L., Totten, P. A., Quinn, T. C., *et al.*: Characterization of *Campylobacter*-like organisms isolated from homosexual men. J Infect Dis 149:58, 1984.
Lee, J. V., Shread, P., Furniss, A. L., and Bryant, T. N. : Taxonomy and description of *Vibrio fluvialis* sp.nov. (Synonym Group F vibrios, Group EF-6). J Appl Bacteriol 50:73, 1981.
Skirrow, M. B. : Campylobacter enteritis : A new disease. Brit Med J 2:9, 1977.
Skirrow, M. B., and Benjamin, J.: '1001' Campylobacters: Cultural characteristics of intestinal campylobacters from man and animals. J Hyg Camb 85:427, 1980.
Smibert, R. M. : The genus Campylobacter. Ann Rev Microbiol 32:673, 1978.
Wardström, T., Ljungh, A., and Wretlind, B. : Enterotoxin, haemolysin and cytotoxic protein in *Aeromonas hydrophila* from human infections. Acta Path Microbiol Scand Sec B 84:112, 1976.

33 PSEUDOMONAS AND FLAVOBACTERIUM

JOSHUA FIERER, M.D.

PSEUDOMONAS

In clinical microbiology laboratories, most of the nonfermentative gram-negative rods that are isolated from patients belong to the genus *Pseudomonas* and of these, *P. aeruginosa* accounts for about two-thirds of the isolates. Species other than *P. aeruginosa* that are primarily environmental organisms are sometimes called pseudomonads. This term has no toxonomic validity. This chapter will concentrate on *P. aeruginosa* because it is the only commonly isolated pathogen in this genus. The characteristics that define this genus are shown on Table 1. For a more complete review of the microbiology of this genus, see Clarke and Richmond, 1975, and Hugh and Gilardi, 1980.

MORPHOLOGY. The *Pseudomonaceae* are short, unicellular, straight or slightly curved, gram-negative rods that measure 0.5 to 1 μm by 1.5 to 4 μm. They do not form spores. When motile, they have one or more polar flagella that are visible with the light microscope only when special stains are used; the flagella are unsheathed in most species. Fimbria are also made by some species; they are polar in most species but peritrichous in *P. cepacia* (Palleroni, 1975). On light microscopy, the cells do not show any unusual features except for those species that accumulate poly-β hydroxybutyrate in granules. These granules can be seen with a phase microscope or by staining with sudan black. With electron microscopy, it is evident that the bacteria have a typical multilayered cell wall of gram-negative bacteria, similar in appearance to the cell wall of *Enterobacteriaceae*. In addition, with proper fixation, an outer slime layer can be detected surrounding individual cells and sometimes encasing multiple cells, creating a microcolony.

Colonial morphology varies so widely from species to species, and even within a single species, that it is impossible to generalize about the appearance of *Pseudomonas* colonies on agar. All species of *Pseudomonas* grow well on simple nutrient agars and on common selective media such as EMB and McConkey's agars. The colonial morphology of *P. aeruginosa* is quite diverse. Phillips (1969) described six colony types on nutrient agar: 1) Flat, with irregular edges, a grey-green metal sheen, with or without a pocked surface; 2) Raised, smooth, with entire edges resembling *Enterobacteriaceae* colonies; 3) Raised, rough; 4) Rugous; 5) Dwarf; and 6) Mucoid. Types 1 and 2 account for about 90 per cent of isolates. Mucoid strains do not usually maintain this form when passaged in vitro and turn into type 1 colonies when passed on standard media (Chan et al., 1984). Colonies of *P. stutzeri* are rugous. Young colonies of *P. pseudomallei* are usually smooth but turn rugous with prolonged incubation. Many strains of *P. aeruginosa* secrete a hemolysin that completely lyses red cells in blood agar.

The fluorescent group of *Pseudomonas (P. aeruginosa, P. fluorescens,* and *P. putida),* under suitable conditions, produces water or chloroform soluble fluorescent and nonfluorescent pigments that diffuse into the agar. Pyocyanin is a distinctive blue pigment produced by most strains of *P. aeruginosa*. It is not fluorescent. Pyoverdin (fluorscein) is a yellow, fluorescent pigment made by most strains of *P. aeruginosa* and *P. fluorescens*. Strains of *P. aeruginosa* that make both pyoverdin and pyocyanin are common, and they stain the agar green. About 5 per cent of strains of *P. aeruginosa* make rust-red pigments (pyrubins). Other species of *Pseudomonas* may produce other diffusible nonfluorescent pigments. Pigment production is influenced by temperature of incubation and cation content of the agar. Some uncommonly isolated species, e.g., a *P. vesicularis*, can produce cell-associated carotenoid pigments that impart a yellow color to their colonies. *P. cepacia* may secrete a yellow pigment when grown on a Kligler's iron agar slant.

Table 1. CHARACTERISTICS OF THE GENUS *PSEUDOMONAS*

Glucose Oxidized	+
Glucose Fermented	−
Catalase	+
Cytochrome C Oxidase	+*
Gram-negative Rods	+
Polar Flagella	+**
Spores	−
Photosynthetic	−

*Strains of *P. maltophilia* are negative
**P. mallei* is non-motile

METABOLISM. *Pseudomonas* organisms are aerobes. They derive their energy from oxidation and do not ferment sugars. Denitrifying species, which includes *P. aeruginosa*, can grow anaerobically utilizing nitrate as the terminal electron receptor in the presence of certain carbon compounds. To carry out nitrate respiration, nitrate and nitrite reductases are induced in the presence of nitrate and the absence of oxygen (Clarke and Ornsten, 1975). Nitrate respiration differs from nitrate assimilation, a process that converts nitrates to ammonia for assimilation into organic compounds.

The growth requirements for most species of *Pseudomonas* are extremely simple. They will grow in aqueous solutions of mineral salts with ammonium ions as the only nitrogen source and can use a variety of simple organic compounds as energy sources. They will utilize carbohydrates, alcohols, saturated and unsaturated fatty acids, amino acids, amines and amides (Clarke and Ornsten, 1975). Not all species can utilize all these different substrates. Differences in ability to utilize these organic compounds are useful taxonomic features. The ability to metabolize such a wide variety of substrates implies many specialized catabolic pathways that are regulated in response to environmental demand.

P. aeruginosa utilizes the Entner-Douderoff pathway to metabolize hexoses to intermediates that enter the tricarboxylic acid cyle (TCA). The TCA cycle is central to both catabolism and biosynthesis by *Pseudomonas*. Acetate is utilized by most *Pseudomonas* and in the process, cells regenerate C4 dicarboxylic acids for the TCA cycle (Clarke and Ornsten, 1975). The ability to use certain amides for growth, especially acetamide, is characteristic of *P. aeruginosa;* it is converted to acetate and NH_{4+}.

Most species of *Pseudomonas* produce extracellular enzymes that degrade macromolecules, a process that is important for nutrition. *P. aeruginosa* secretes several proteinases and phospholipase C (the hemolysin). *P. maltophilia* and *P. putrefaciens* secrete a DNAase.

PATHOGENIC PROPERTIES. *P. aeruginosa* is not a successful parasite, but it is a virulent opportunistic pathogen. Pseudomonas infections occur almost exclusively in hospitalized patients with severely lowered host resistance. *P. aeruginosa* produces infections by virtue of its ability to invade damaged natural barriers, e.g., burned skin, or intact mucous membranes left unguarded by the absence of functional polymorphonuclear leukocytes. Once having gained entrance to tissue, the organism exhibits a peculiar tropism for blood vessels which it invades from the adventitial side, producing medial necrosis and thrombosis (Ziegler et al., 1975). This tropism has not been explained.

P. aeruginosa infections are characterized by fever and *Pseudomonas* bacteremia may be complicated by septic shock. It is likely that the organisms' LPS is responsible for these manifestations. The importance of LPS in the pathogenesis of *Pseudomonas* infections is shown by the ability of antibody to the homologous immunotype of LPS to protect granulocytopenic mice from death after intravenous infection. Antibody in this system both neutralizes LPS and is opsonic. Antibody to the core component of LPS, which is not opsonic, also reduces mortality in experimentally infected granulocytopenic animals and in bacteremic humans (Ziegler et al., 1975 and 1982). This is strong evidence that the toxic properties of LPS contribute greatly to the lethality of *Pseudomonas* infections.

In addition to its potent endotoxin, *P. aeruginosa* synthesizes a variety of exotoxins that also contribute to virulence. Exotoxin A is the best characterized of these toxins (Liu et al., 1973). It is a prototoxin with two important subunits; one subunit is responsible for binding to the host cell membrane, the other enzymatically catalyzes the transfer of ADP-ribosyl (ADPR) from NAD to elongation factor 2 (EF2):

$$\text{NAD} + \text{EF2} \xrightarrow{\text{Exotoxin A}} \text{ADPR–EF2} + \text{nicotinamide.}$$

As a result, EF2 is inactivated and cannot promote ribosomal translocation along mRNA (Iglewski et al., 1975). This brings protein synthesis to a halt. Exotoxin A has the same mechanism of action as diptheria toxin even though the two toxins are not structurally or antigenically similar. Although the exact role of exotoxin A in natural infection is not established, there is suggestive evidence that it does contribute to virulence in experimental *Pseudomonas* infections. Toxin is found in the serum of infected mice and antitoxin enhances their survival, if the infecting strain is toxigenic (Saelinger et al., 1977). The same antiserum has no effect on outcome if the infecting strain is non-toxigenic (Pavolovskis et al. 1977). In humans, pre-existing antibody to exotoxin A correlates with survival from *P. aeruginosa* bacteremia (Pollack and Young, 1976).

Although exotoxin A and diphtheria toxin both produce the same metabolic defect, there are major differences between the infections. Unlike diphtheria, antibody to exotoxin A does not completely prevent disease. Furthermore, *P. aeruginosa* is locally and systemically invasive and infection with *C. diptheria* but not *P. aeruginosa* results in neuritis or myocarditis. In *Pseudomonas* infections, exotoxin A may exert its primary effect by producing local necrosis and by inhibiting phagocyte function, allowing the organism to penetrate through important physical barriers.

Other exo-enzymes that may function as exotoxins are made by *P. aeruginosa*. These include phospholipase C (the hemolysin), elastase, and two other broad spectrum proteases. These enzymes may contribute to vascular necrosis, and local tissue destruction, especially ocular and pulmonary damage. When tested in a model of naturally occurring *P. aeruginosa* infections in minks, immunization with a vaccine, made from toxoids of the elastase and a protease, increased the survival of the immunized minks during an enzootic of pneumonia (Homma et al., 1983).

Mucoid strains of *P. aeruginosa* produce an extracellular alginic acid matrix that encases the bacteria in vivo (Lamm et al., 1980). The alginate interferes with the opsonic activity of antibody directed to the LPS but not with the bactericidal activity of complement (Baltimore and Mitchell, 1980). With the exception of the mucoid strains isolated from patients with cystic fibrosis (Thomassan and Demko, 1981) nearly all pathogenic strains of *P. aeruginosa* are resistant to killing by complement (Young and Armstrong, 1972).

The virulence factors of *P. pseudomallei* are very poorly characterized. The organism contains an LPS that probably is responsible for the manifestations of the acute septicemic forms of infection including the renal lesions that resemble Shwartzman reactions.

ANTIGENIC STRUCTURE. Several sets of antisera have been developed for serotyping *P. aeruginosa*. The Fisher scheme (Fisher et al., 1969) is probably based on antibody to LPS and distinguishes 7 serotypes. The Homma scheme (Homma, 1974) distinguishes 18 sterotypes. There is no correspondence between the two schema and neither set

Table 2. DIFFERENTIAL CHARACTERISTICS OF NONFERMENTING GRAM-NEGATIVE BACILLI ISOLATED FROM HUMANS

Characteristic	Pseudomonas	Eikenella	Acinetobacter	Alcaligenes	Flavobacterium	Moraxella	Kingella
MacConkey Agar	+	−	+	+	+ or −	+ or −	−
Oxidase	+	+	−	+	+	+	+
Catalase	+	−	+	+	+	+	−
Motility	+**	−	−	+	−	−	−
Pigment	+ or −	+*	−	−	+*	−	−
Nitrate Reduction	+ or −	+	−	+ or −	−	+ or −	−
Urease	+ or −	−	+ or −	−	+ or −	−**	−
Susceptible to Pencillin	−	+	−	−	−	+	+

*Pale yellow colonies.
**Except for one species; non-motile mutants are rare.
+This genus is weakly fermentative if broth is supplemented with ascites or serum.

of sera reacts with all clinical isolates. In addition to LPS, the glycoprotein is antigenic as are several outer membrane proteins. Pyocins (bacteriocins) produced by *P. aeruginosa* are also antigenic and immune serum neutralizes the bactericidal effect of the pyocin. Convalescent sera from people infected with *P. aeruginosa* also inhibit some bacteriocins, indicating that antibodies are formed during natural infection (Allen and Kelly, 1975).

For epidemiological purposes, combinations of serotyping, pyocin typing (production of or sensitivity to pyocins), and phage typing have been used to identify and distinguish epidemic strains. No one system is completely satisfactory and combinations of two or three typing schemes are often used.

IMMUNITY. Normal adults have a high degree of natural immunity to all species of *Pseudomonas*, other than *pseudomallei.* Immunity depends primarily on the ability of normal serum to opsonize bacteria that are then engulfed and killed by polymorphonuclear leukocytes (Young and Armstrong, 1972). The principal opsonin in normal serum is activated C3 but antibody to the oligosaccharide side chain of LPS and to surface glycolipid potentiate the effectiveness of complement (Bartell and Kriskszens, 1980). Pre-existing antibody to the core of LPS strongly correlates with survival from *P. aeruginosa* sepsis (Pollack et al., 1983). There is also evidence that antibody to exotoxin A increases survival in humans and experimental animals infected with exotoxin A producing strains of *P. aeruginosa* (Pavolovski et al., 1977).

Patients with abnormal PMN, as in chronic granulomatous disease, or acute myelogenous leukemia, are susceptible to *P. aeruginosa* infections because their PMN are not bactericidal. It is not understood why patients with third degree burns and cystic fibrosis are so susceptible to *P. aeruginosa* infections although the former have defects in PMN function (McManus, 1983) and have lost an important physical barrier that normally resists colonization and invasion by *Pseudomonas.*

Compared to immunity to *P. aeruginosa*, natural immunity to *P. pseudomallei* is much less effective since healthy people can be infected. In endemic areas most infections are asymptomatic, but even in those who have asymptomatic infection, viable organisms can persist in tissue for years. This implies that even acquired immunity cannot always eradicate infection. In experimental animals, immunization with heat-killed bacteria stimulates an antibody response but is not protective. Immunization with live, attenuated mutants stimulates partial immunity; on subsequent challenge with a virulent strain, it requires a larger inoculum to cause disease (Dannenberg et al., 1960). It is not known what accounts for the protection induced by live infection.

LABORATORY DIAGNOSIS. Members of the genus *Pseudomonas* usually can be distinguished easily from other non-fermentative gram-negative bacilli by using simple characteristics such as ability to grow on McConkey's agar, pigmentation, oxidase and catalase reactions, and motility. The clinically important non-fermenting bacteria that may be confused with *Pseudomonas* include *Acinetobacter, Alcaligenes, Flavobacterium, Moraxella, Kingella,* and those strains of *Eikenella* that do not pit the agar (Table 2).

Pseudomonas grow well on all commonly used nonselective media and on EMB and McConkey's agar. Isolation of any species of *Pseudomonas* from a blood culture indicates serious infection except for "pseudobacteremia" due to contaminated blood drawing equipment. Isolates from sputum or wounds may or may not be significant. Since these are common environmental bacteria that can colonize open wounds or mucosal surfaces, their mere presence is not synonymous with infection. However, serious attention should be paid to the isolation of *P. aeruginosa* from any specimen from a patient whose numbers of functional PMN are below normal.

P. Aeruginosa. This is usually easily identified (Table 3). Colonies have a characteristic "fruity" odor (reminiscent of corn tortillas), colonial morphology, and extracellular pigment. Motile, non-fermentative, oxidase-positive bacteria that grow at 42°C and have a characteristic antibiotic susceptibility pattern can usually be identified as *P. aeruginosa* if they produce an extracellular pigment. Nonpigmented, polymyxin-resistant strains may be harder to identify. They should be tested for gluconate and maltose oxidation, arginine dihydrolase and DNAase activity (Table

Table 3. CRITERIA FOR IDENTIFICATION OF *P. AERUGINOSA*

Monotrichous Polar Flagella	+ (97)
Oxidize Glucose	+ (100)
Oxidize Maltose	− (4)
Cytochrome C Oxidase	+ (100)
Arginine Dihydrolase	+ (100)
Oxidize Gluconate	+ (60)
Growth at 42°C	+ (100)
Susceptible to Polymyxin	+ (95)
Pigment Production	+ (95)

Uniformly negative reactions: Lactose, H_2S, LDC, ODC, indole, VP (acetoin). Per cent of strains having a positive result shown in parenthesis.

Table 4. BIOCHEMICAL CHARACTERISTICS OF *P. PSEUDOMALLEI*

Cytochrome C Oxidase	+
Oxidize Glucose	+
Oxidize Maltose	+
Utilize Citrate	+
Lysine Decarboxylase	−
Arginine Dihydrolase	+
Nitrate to Gas	+
Accumulate β-hydroxybutyrate	+
Fluorescent Pigment	−
Growth at 42°C	+

3). *P. aeruginosa* can be differentiated from *P. fluorescence* by growth at 42°C, utilization of acetamide, and inability to utilize lactose, sucrose, or maltose. *P. putida*, which is sometimes isolated from wounds but rarely causes disease in people, is the third "fluorescent" *Pseudomonas*. It does not grow at 42°C, does not utilize acetamide or gluconate, and can be differentiated from *P. fluorescens* by hippurate hydrolysis and inability to oxidize lactose or sucrose.

P. Pseudomallei. Isolation of *P. pseudomallei* from clinical material is always of diagnostic significance. Although this species grows well on all common media, it is often not isolated from patients with the subacute or chronic forms of melioidosis (see Chapter 113). For that reason, serological tests have been used to diagnose infection. Both CF and hemaggutination assays give positive reactions in infected patients. However, neither test differentiates between active and inactive (subclinical) infection. A new indirect-immunofluorescent assay for IgM antibody appears to be able to identify active infections (Ashdown, 1981).

Colonies of *P. pseudomallei* may resemble *P. cepacia* or *P. stutzeri*. Many strains of *P. pseudomallei* are pigmented and have a yeasty odor. Colonies vary from rugous to mucoid. The important biochemical characteristics of this species are shown in Table 4. These organisms are resistant to polymyxin and sensitive to sulfa in vitro. They have three or more polar flagella (Redfearn et al., 1966). All identifications should be confirmed with specific antiserum.

Antibiotic Sensitivity. *P. aeruginosa* is one of the most inherently antibiotic-resistant organisms encountered in the clinical laboratory. Resistance is due both to permeability barriers and to enzymatic inactivation. The latter can be coded for either by chromosomal or episomal genes. Strains that are resistant to all aminoglyosides may have mutations that affect transport of these antibiotics (Bryan et al., 1980). Such strains grow slowly and form dwarf colonies.

The usual sensitivities of each of the important species of *Pseudomonas* are shown in Table 5. Inherent resistance to certain species of *Pseudomonas* polymyxins (colistin) is a useful taxonomic feature. In practice, the in vitro susceptibility of each isolate should be determined since many species can acquire resistance to antibiotics that are usually effective.

EPIDEMIOLOGY. *P. aeruginosa* infections occur primarily in hospitalized patients. These organisms are found naturally in water and soil and their metabolic versatility allows them to grow in ecological niches that could not support the growth of many other genera. Bacteria can be introduced into the hospital on apparently innocuous items such as flowers and fresh vegetables. They are often in potable water and can proliferate in water faucets from which they can be transferred to medical equipment (Fierer et al., 1967) and to the hands of staff or patients. Strains introduced into intensive care units can spread from patient to patient via colonized staff (Lowbury and Fox, 1954). Their relative resistance to disinfectants makes it difficult to eliminate *Pseudomonas* from the hospital environment (Lowbury and Fox, 1954). In leukemic patients, most infections are from their endogenous microflora, occurring after *P. aeruginosa* has colonized the patient's nasopharynx or gut (Schimipf et al., 1972). It is not known why *P. aeruginosa* has such an affinity for patients with hematologic malignancies, but *P. aeruginosa* has a selective advantage over other bacteria in these hosts because of their natural resistance to most antibiotics and to the chemotherapeutic drugs used to treat the malignancies.

The incidence of infections due to *P. maltophilia* and *P. cepacia* is much lower than the incidence of *P. aeruginosa*. However, the epidemiology of these infections seems to be similar. Most infections are nosocomial and occur after massive numbers of bacteria are inadvertently introduced into patients, usually because of the failure of a disinfectant or a sterilizing procedure (Ederer and Matsen, 1972; Zuravleff and Yu, 1982). Infection due to other species of *Pseudomonas* occur too infrequently to generalize about their epidemiology (Gilardi, 1972). They are all environmental bacteria, however.

The epidemiology of *P. pseudomallei* infection sets it apart from other members of this genus. In contrast to the worldwide distribution of most *Pseudomonas* organisms, this species appears to have a geographic distribution limited only to those countries that lie between 20°N and 20°S latitude. It has been reported from all large land masses within these tropical latitudes except Africa (Howe et al., 1971). However, there is indirect evidence that the organism is also natural in Africa (Bremmelgaard et al., 1982). The bacteria live in the clay layer of soil and during the rainy season appear in stagnant, muddy surface water

Table 5. ANTIBIOTIC SUSCEPTIBILITY OF COMMONLY ISOLATED PATHOGENIC *PSEUDOMONAS* ORGANISMS

	Piperaceillin*	Cefaperzone*	Cefoxitin	Cephalothin*	Tetracycline	Chloramphenicol	Trimethoprim-Sulfamethoxazole	Gentamicin*	Thienamycin
P. aeruginosa	±	±	−	−	−	−	−	+	±
P. fluorescens	+	+	−	−	+	−	−	+	+
P. pseudomallei	−	−	−	±	+	+	−	−	−
P. maltophilia	−	−	−	−	±	±	+	+	±
P. cepecia	+	+	−	−	−	±	+	−	−
P. stutzeri	+	+	−	−	+	±	+	+	+

\+ = >80% susceptible
± = 50%–80% susceptible
− = <50% susceptible
*Representative of a class of similar antibiotics

(Thomas et al., 1979). It infects rodents and grazing animals as well as people but it is not a zoonosis. Human-to-human transmission is extremely rare. People appear to be infected by direct inoculation or inhalation of contaminated soil. Subclinical infection is extremely widespread in endemic areas as judged by serological surveys of healthy residents (Howe et al., 1971). *P. pseudomallei* infections occur outside the endemic areas when latently infected people move to temperate climates. A latent infection can reactivate years later, usually following some stressful situation.

FLAVOBACTERIUM

Flavobacteria are a heterogeneous group of organisms that were originally assigned to that genus on the basis of yellow pigmentation. The genus is currently restricted to oxidase-positive, nonmotile, gram-negative bacilli. Motility distinguishes it from the genus *Cytophaga*, which consists of thin, delicate, rodlike bacteria that glide along the surface of solid media and show "flexing" motility in suspension. Less than a dozen species, all of which have DNA with a G+C content of 30 to 42 per cent, belong to the genus *Flavobacterium* (Holmes et al., 1982; Shewan and McMeekins, 1983).

MORPHOLOGY. In gram stains, it is a slender rod that is sometimes curved and may appear encapsulated in clinical specimens. Colonies of *F. meningosepticum* are smooth, entire, grayish white, and small (1 to 1.5 mm) after 24 hours incubation on blood agar, which is often discolored blue-green due to proteolysis. Some, but not all, strains of *F. meningsepticum* turn pale yellow with prolonged incubation at room temperature. The other species of *Flavobacterium* produce brighter yellow pigments after only 24 hours and *F. odoratum* (M-4f Group) has a characteristic pleasant, fruity odor. The yellow pigment is associated with the outer membrane of these organisms. It is an incompletely characterized alcohol-soluble compound termed "flexirubin," which is also found in many strains of *Cytophaga* and *Flexibactium*.

ANTIGENIC COMPOSITION. There are six serotypes of *F. meningosepticum* (A–F). Most cases of meningitis are due to Type C, but all types have been associated with meningitis.

METABOLISM. *F. meningosepticum* is an obligate aerobe. It is proteolytic and saccharolytic. About a third of the isolates are temperature sensitive and will not grow at 42°C.

PATHOGENIC PROPERTIES AND IMMUNITY. *F. meningosepticum* is the only species that has an unambiguous claim to pathogenicity, and even this species at best is considered to have low virulence. This organism infects neonates primarily, especially premature infants, in whom it causes sepsis and meningitis (Dooley et al., 1980). Nothing is known that explains the neurotropism of this species. There have been a few reported cases of septicemia in adults, all of whom had serious underlying diseases such as leukemia, renal failure, and cancer. A few cases of iatrogenic but self-limited septicemia were associated with a temperature-sensitive strain.

LABORATORY DIAGNOSIS. Nonpigmented strains of *F. meningosepticum* may be difficult to identify. It is nonmotile, oxidase-positive, and catalase-positive, and it grows slowly, if at all, on MacConkey agar. It does not grow on SS agar. A small amount of indole is produced by some strains and can be detected using a sensitive method such as Ehrlich's reagent. If a peptone-based oxidation-fermentation medium is used, glucose and maltose are slowly converted to acid in the tube that is not overlayed with mineral oil. Glucose is more rapidly oxidized in media without peptone. All strains digest casein and hydrolyse DNA, gelatin, and esculin. Nearly all strains produce beta-D-galactosidase.

The differential characteristic of *Flavobacterium* and other oxidase-positive, nonmotile, nonfermentative gram-negative bacilli are given in Table 6.

DRUG SUSCEPTIBILITY. Characteristically, *F. meningosepticum* is resistant to penicillins, first-generation and second-generation cephalosporins, tetracycline, and polymyxin (Harrington and Perlino, 1981). Many strains are sensitive to erythromycin and rifampin. There is variable sensitivity to vancomycin, novobiocin, clindamycin, and chloramphenicol. Both erythromycin and rifampin have been used successfully to treat meningitis. With the Kirby-Bauer method, some resistant strains may appear sensitive to amikacin.

EPIDEMIOLOGY. *Flavobacterium* spp. have been isolated from many fresh-water and ocean-water samples as well as from marine plants and animals. They are also widely distributed in soil. Many species have been recovered from water samples taken in hospitals. *F. meningosepticum* infections occur sporadically and in nursery epidemics. In the latter, contaminated sink water has frequently been implicated as the source of the organisms. *F. meningosepticum* are relatively resistant to chlorine and

Table 6. CHARACTERISTICS OF *FLAVOBACTERIUM* AND OTHER OXIDASE-POSITIVE, NONMOTILE, NONFERMENTATIVE GRAM-NEGATIVE BACILLI

	Yellow or Tan Pigment	Reduces Nitrate	Urease	Penicillin	Polymyxin B
Flavobacterium meningosepticum	+[1]	0	3%	R	R
Flavobacterium odoratum	+	0	+	S(20%)	R
Moraxella lacunata	0	+	0	S	S
Pseudomonas paucimobilis	+	0	0	S(49%)	S(70%)
II B	+	80%	8%	R	R
II J	+	0	+	S	S
II F	+	0	0	S	S

R = Resistant S = Sensitive

[1]Often nonpigmented unless held at room temperature for up to five days.

chlorhexidine disinfectant. Sporadic cases of meningitis may result from colonization of the infant during delivery. It has been postulated that vaginal colonization can result from douching with contaminated water.

References

Pseudomonas

Allen, J. C. and Kelly, P. C.: Antigenic heterogeneity among pyocins of *Pseudomonas aeruginosa*. Inf Immun 12:318, 1975.

Ashdown, L. R.: Relationship and significance of specific immunoglobulin M antibody response in clinical and subclinical melioidoses. J Clin Micro 14:361, 1981.

Baltimore, R. S. and Mitchell, M.: Immunological investigations of *Pseudomonas aeruginosa*: Comparison of susceptibility to opsonic antibody in mucoid and nonmucoid strains. J Inf Dis 141:238, 1980.

Bartell, P. F. and Kriskszens, A.: Influence of anti-slime glycoprotein serum on the interaction between *Pseudomonas aeruginosa* and macrophages. Infect and Immunity 27:777, 1980.

Bremmelgaard, A., Bygbjery, I. B., and Hocby, N.: Microbiological and Immunological Studies in a case of human melioidoses diagnosed in Denmark. Scand. J Inf Dis 14:271, 1982.

Bryan, L. E., Nicas, T., Holloway, B. W. and Crowther, C.: Aminoglycoside-resistant mutation of *Pseudomonas aeruginosa* defective in cytochrome C_{522} and nitrate reductase. Antimicrob Agents Chemother 17:71, 1980.

Chan, R., Lam, J. S., Lam, K., and Cesterson, J. W.: Influence of culture conditions on expression of the mucoid mode of growth of *Pseudomonas aeruginosa*. J Clin Micro 8, 1984.

Clarke, P. H., and Ornsten, L. N.: Metabolic Pathways and Regulation–Part I and II. In Clarke, P. H. and Richmond, M. H. Genetics and Biochemistry of *Pseudomonas*. John Wiley and Sons, London, 1975.

Dannenberg, A. M. and Scott, E. M.: Melioidosis: Pathogenesis and immunity in mice and hamsters. III. Effect of vaccination with avirulent strain of *Pseudomonas pseudomallei* on the resistance to the progress of respiratory melioidesis caused by virulent strains; all-or-none aspects of this disease. J Immunol 84:233, 1960.

Ederer, G. M. and Matsen, J. M.: Colonization and Infection with *Pseudomonas cepacia*. J Infect Dis 125:613, 1972.

Fierer, J., Taylor, P. M. and Gezon, H.: *Pseudomonas aeruginosa* epidemic traced to delivery-room resuscitators. N Engl J Med 276:991, 1967.

Fisher, M. W., Devlin, H. B. and Gnabasik, F. J.: New immunotype schema for *Pseudomonas aeruginosa* based on protective antigens. J Bacteriol 98:835, 1969.

Gilardi, G. L.: Infrequently encountered *Pseudomonas* species causing infection in humans. Annals Int Med 77:211, 1972.

Homma, J. Y.: Serological typing of *Pseudomonas aeruginosa* and several points to be considered. Jpn J Exp Med 44:1, 1974.

Homma, J. Y., Abe, C., Yanagawa, R., and Noda, H.: Effectiveness of immunization with multicomponent vaccines in protection against hemorrhagic pneumonia due to *Pseudomonas aeruginosa* infection in mink. Rev Inf Dis V. 5, Suppl 5:S858, 1983.

Howe, C., Saupath, A. and Spotnity, M.: The *Pseudomallei* Group: A Review. J Inf Dis 124:598, 1971.

Hugh, R., and Gilardi, G. L.: Pseudomonas. In Lennette, E. H., Balows, A., Hausler, W. J., Jr., and Truant, J. P. (eds.) Manual of Clinical Microbiology, Third Edition. American Society for Microbiology, 1980.

Iglewski, B. H. and Kabat, D.: NAD-dependent inhibition of protein synthesis by *Pseudomonas aeruginosa* toxin. Proc Natl Acad Sci USA 72:2284, 1975.

Lam, J. B., Chan R., Lam, K. and Costersen, J. W.: Production of mucoid microcolonies by *Pseudomonas aeruginosa* within infected lungs in cystic fibrosis. Infect Immun 28:546, 1980.

Lowbury, E. J. L. and Fox J. E.: The epidemiology of infection with *Pseudomonas* pyocyanea in a burns unit. J Hyg (Cambridge) 52:403, 1954.

Lui, P. V., Yoshii, S., and Hsieb, H.: Exotoxins of *Pseudomonas aeruginosa*. II Concentration, purification and characterization of exotoxin A. J Infect Dis 128:514, 1973.

McManus, A. T.: Examination of neutrophil function in a rat model of decreased resistance following brain trauma. Rev Inf Dis 5, Suppl 5: S989, 1983.

Palleroni, N. J.: General Properties and Taxonomy of the Genus *Pseudomonas*. In Clarke, P. H. and Richmond, M. H. Genetics and Biochemistry of *Pseudomonas*. John Wiley & Sons, London, 1975.

Pavolovskis, O. R., Pollack, M., Callahan, L. T., III, and Iglewski, B. H.: Passive protection by antitoxin in experimental *Pseudomonas aeruginosa* burn infections. Infect Immun 18:596, 1977.

Phillips, I.: Identification of *Pseudomonas aeruginosa* in the clinical laboratory. J. Med Microbiol 2:9, 1969.

Pollack, M. and Young, L. S.: Protective activity of antibodies to exotoxin A and lipopolysacchride at the onset of *Pseudomonas aeruginosa* septicemia in man. J Clin Invest 63:276, 1976.

Pollack, M., Huang, A. I., Prescott, R. K., Young, L. S., Hunter, K. W., Cruess, D. F. and Tsai, C-M.: Enhanced survival in *Pseudomonas aeruginosa* septicemia associated with high levels of circulating antibody to *Escherichia coli* endotoxin core. J Clin Invest 72:1874, 1983.

Redfearn, M. S., Palleroni, V. J. and Stanier, R. X.: A comparative study of *Pseudomonas pseudomallei* and Bacillus mallei. J Gen Microbiol 43:293, 1966.

Rudolph, H. and Gilardi, G. L.: *Pseudomonas*. In Lennett, E. H. Manual of Clinical Microbiology, 3rd Ed. Amer Soc Microbiology, Washington, D. C., 1980.

Schimpff, F. S. C., Young, V. M., Greene, W. H., Vermeulen, G. D., Moody, M. R. and Wurnick, P. H.: Origin of infection in acute nonlymphocytic leukemia. Annals Int Med 77:707, 1972.

Saelinger, C. B., Snell, K., and Holder, I. A.: Experimental studies on the pathogenesis of infections during *Pseudomonas* infection of burned skin tissues. J Infect Dis 136:555, 1977.

Thomas, A. D., Forbes-Faulkner, J. and Parker, M.: Isolation of *Pseudomonas pseudomallei* from clay layers at defined depths. Amer J Epi 110:515, 1979.

Thomassan, M. J. and Demko, C. A.: Serum bactericidal effect on *Pseudomonas aeruginosa* isolates from cystic fibrosis patients. Infect Immun 33:512, 1981.

Wilkinson, S. G.: Composition and structure of lipopolysaccharides from *Pseudomonas aeruginosa*. Review of Inf Dis 5, Suppl 5:S941, 1983.

Young, S. L. and Armstrong, D.: Human immunity to *Pseudomonas aeruginosa* I and II. J Infect Dis 126:257, 1972.

Ziegler, E. J., McCutchan, J. A., Douglas, H. and Braude, A. I.: Prevention of lethal *Pseudomonas* bacteremia with epimerase-deficient *E. coli* antiserum. Trans Assoc Am Physicians 88:101, 1975.

Ziegler, E. J., McCutchan, J. A., Fierer, J., Glauser, M. P., Sadoff, J. C., Douglas, H. and Braude, A. I.: Treatment of gram-negative bacteremia and shock with human antiserum to a mutant *Escherichia coli*. N Engl J Med 307:1225, 1982.

Zuravleff, J. J. and Yu, V. L.: Infections caused by *Pseudomonas maltophilia* with emphasis on bacteremia. Rev Infect Dis 4:1236, 1982.

Flavobacterium

Dooley, J. R., Nims, L. J., Lipp, V. H., et al.: Meningitis of infants caused by *Flavobacterium meningosepticum*. Report of a patient and analysis of 63 infections. J Trop Pediatr, 26:24, 1980.

Harrington, S. P., and Perlino, C. A.: *Flavobacterium meningosepticum* sepsis: disease due to bacteria with unusual antibiotic susceptibility. South Med J, 74:764, 1981.

Holmes, B., Owen, R. J., and Hollis, D. G.: *Flavobacterium spiritvorum*, a new species isolated from human clinical specimens. Int J Syst Bacteriol, 32:157, 1982.

Shewan, J. M., and McMeekin, T. A.: Taxonomy (and ecology) of *Flavobacterium* and related genera. Annu Rev Microbiol, 37:233, 1983.

34

BRUCELLA

WESLEY W. SPINK, A.B., M.D., D.SC.

MORPHOLOGY. Members of the genus *Brucella* occur as small, nonmotile, noncapsular, gram-negative bacilli or coccobacilli that do not form spores and are not acid-fast. They vary from 0.4 to 1.5 μm in length and 0.4 to 0.8 μm in width. Young colonies are pinpoint in size, moist, translucent, and glistening. Six species of *Brucella* are recognized, some with several biotypes. The most significant species in human disease are *Brucella melitensis*, *Brucella abortus*, and *Brucella suis*, which cause contagious abortion in goats (melitensis), cattle (abortus), and swine (suis), and are shed in their milk. *Brucella neotomae* has been identified in the desert wood rat *(Neotoma lepida)* in the western United States. *Brucella ovis* is an important pathogen in sheep, causing chiefly ram epididymitis. *Brucella canis* is found in dogs, especially in the beagle family, and causes epidemic abortions in kennels. Neither *B. neotomae* nor *B. ovis* has been known to cause human illness, and *B. canis* has resulted in only a few recognized human cases. *Brucella neotomae* grows as smooth colonies on solid media and is probably a derivative of *B. abortus*. *Brucella ovis* and *B. canis* reproduce as rough colonies, and both are probably variants of *B. suis*. Several brucellaphages have been recognized for all three species, but their use is of limited value in differentiation. Further discussion centers on the three classic species: *melitensis*, *abortus*, and *suis*, and some of their biotypes. These and other members of the genus are closely related as determined by DNA hybridization. The G & C content of their DNA ranges from 56 to 58 moles per cent (Brinley-Morgan and McCullough, 1974).

Brucella cells contain nucleoprotein, protein, lipopolysaccharide, and polysaccharide antigens. A soluble polysaccharide fraction elicits an immediate localized reaction when injected intradermally into an infected subject, whereas the nucleoprotein material produces a delayed response.

METABOLISM. Although *Brucella* may sometimes be cultivated on chemically-defined media containing amino acids, glucose, and B vitamins (nicotinic acid, thiamine, and biotin), the fastidious nutritional requirements of *Brucella* are ordinarily met by tryptose or trypticase broth and agar. Brucella organisms are obligate aerobes. Growth at 37° C requires several days, and for some strains (*abortus*) added carbon dioxide is essential. Neither acid nor gas is produced from carbohydrates in peptone media, catalase activity is variable, and urease is present in *B. suis* and *B. melitensis*. Hydrogen sulfide is produced by all three species, but in variable amounts. All species except *B. neotomae* and *B. ovis* are usually oxidase-positive (Brinley-Morgan and McCullough, 1974). The differential metabolic requirements of the three species and their subtypes are discussed later under Laboratory Diagnosis.

Brucella organisms are killed in 3 minutes at 143° to 145° F, that is, at temperatures used for pasteurization. They are also killed by gastric juice so that persons who ingest the organism are infected by *Brucella* less easily than those who are exposed through skin abrasions (Garrod, 1939; Morales-Otero, 1929).

PATHOGENIC PROPERTIES. The three classic species of *Brucella* are highly invasive, gaining entrance into the body through the oral or ocular mucosae or through abrasions of the skin. The organisms can invade the respiratory tract. A state of bacterial hypersensitivity much like that in tuberculosis is induced. Strains having attenuated virulence such as those used in immunization programs in cattle (*B. abortus* strain 19) can cause human illness when accidentally injected through the skin during the procedure of vaccination. When this occurs in veterinarians having a previous history of brucellosis, an immediate localized reaction takes place at the site of entry of the organisms, which is accompanied by a systemic response with chills and fever. This is due to the acquired *Brucella* hypersensitivity caused by the previous infection (Spink, 1956).

ANTIGENIC COMPOSITION. The basic antigenic components of *Brucella* as defined by Wilson and Miles (1932) with quantitative agglutinin-absorption tests distinguish *B. melitensis* from *B. abortus* and *B. suis*. These species all possess A and M antigen in different proportions; in *B. melitensis* the ratio of A and M is 1:20 and in *B. abortus* it is 20:1. This permits the production of specific monovalent sera for agglutination tests with *melitensis* or *abortus*. From a practical point of view a standardized *Brucella* antigen for diagnostic agglutination tests can be prepared from cultures of any one of the three species.

Brucella organisms produce no exotoxins but, as in all gram-negative bacteria, the lipopolysaccharide (LPS) in their cell wall is an endotoxin. *Brucella* endotoxins have the same chemical and biologic properties as the endotoxins of enteric bacilli (see Chapter 6). The O-specific side chains of *Brucella* LPS are lost when smooth (S) strains undergo dissociation to rough (R) strains. This S→R transformation occurs more readily than in enteric bacteria and is accompanied by loss in virulence and serologic specificity. The loss in virulence implies that the complete LPS is a virulence factor. This implication is supported by the fact that patients with brucellosis uniformly develop hypersensitivity to *Brucella* LPS, and that certain important clinical manifestations can be reproduced in these patients with LPS (Spink, 1956).

A prominent feature of *Brucella* infection is intracellular parasitism of the macrophages and histiocytes of the reticuloendothelial system. Focal aggregates of the parasitized cells produce granulomas of the liver, spleen, and bone marrow. In experimental animals the pathologic response varies with the species (Braude, 1951). In infections of guinea pigs caused by *B. abortus*, there is marked splenomegaly, little if any suppuration, and no discernible ill health. Guinea pigs infected with *B. suis*, on the other hand, develop extensive suppurating granulomas of the liver, bones, and testicles. *B. melitensis* infections are intermediate in their tissue damage, but more disabling than the other two.

IMMUNITY. Recovery from brucellosis is accompanied by an effective, but not total, acquired immunity to subsequent attacks of the disease. The humoral immune response can be evaluated by measuring bacteriolysins, precipitins, and agglutinins in the serum. Cellular immunity is associated with acquired hypersensitivity, as it is in tuberculosis, and can be detected with the use of *Brucella* antigens for skin tests.

Evidence for immunity against brucellosis has been demonstrated by the remarkable protection afforded cattle, sheep, and goats through the use of vaccines containing living organisms with attenuated virulence.

LABORATORY DIAGNOSIS

Bacteriologic. A definitive diagnosis of brucellosis is made through the isolation of *Brucella* from body fluids or tissues (Alton et al., 1975). For this purpose the culture media of tryptose or trypticase broth and agar is recommended. Liquid media are employed for primary isolation and subcultures on agar slants and plates are used for identification. For the majority of specimens such as blood, cerebrospinal fluid, urine, and minced tissue suspensions, the double medium of Castaneda is recommended. The medium is prepared under sterile conditions and stored in 4 oz rubber-stoppered glass bottles until ready for use. Twenty ml of broth are added to each bottle and then 10 ml of melted agar are layered on one of the wide flat sides. Ten per cent of the bottled air should be displaced with CO_2. After the bottle is inoculated with suspected material, it is incubated at 37° C for a minimum of 2 to 3 weeks. After 48 to 72 hours minute colonies of *Brucella* may be detected on the agar surface. Subcultures should be made on agar plates by withdrawing material through the rubber stopper with a needle and syringe every 4th, 7th, 15th, and 21st day. The agar plates should be placed in a jar containing 10 per cent CO_2. Usually organisms can be detected for identification within a week after the primary culture is made.

The isolation of *Brucella* from heavily contaminated substances is possible by the intraperitoneal injection of the material into guinea pigs.

Colonies appearing on the agar surface should be transferred to agar plates and to broth suspensions. A suspected culture of *Brucella* reveals small gram-negative bacilli or coccobacilli. Discrete colonies appearing within 48 to 72 hours should be examined by indirect light. Freshly isolated smooth colonies are gray, translucent, sharply edged, and about 0.5 mm in size. *Brucella* organisms tend to dissociate, especially in broth cultures, from smooth to rough forms, revealing morphologic changes and a decrease in virulence. Rough colonies are flat, dull, opaque, and granular. Mucoid colonies are slimy in consistency.

The observations made by direct examination of the colonial morphology can be supplemented quickly by exposing the organisms to acriflavine and to crystal violet. After a drop of fresh acriflavine solution in a concentration of 1:1000 is added to a loopful of suspended smooth colonies on a slide, examination under low-power magnification shows that the colonies remain in suspension, but rough colonies are immediately agglutinated, and mucoid variants form threads. When a fresh culture of *Brucella* on a plate is flooded with a fresh 1:40 dilution of crystal violet, the smooth colonies are not stained, whereas dissociated rough forms appear red and purple with radial cracks on the surface. Only smooth forms should be used for identification with *Brucella* antiserum because rough variants not only lose their antigenic specificity but also become autoagglutinable owing to loss of their O side chains.

A presumptive identification of *Brucella* can be readily made by mixing a drop of high titer human or rabbit anti-*Brucella* serum with a suspended drop of smooth organisms on a slide when agglutination of *Brucella* occurs. Further substantiation is obtained with the tube-agglutination test and by using appropriate controls of a known *Brucella* culture, anti-*Brucella* serum, and a serum without *Brucella* antibody.

Having identified a culture as belonging to the genus *Brucella*, it is necessary to determine the species of *Brucella*. For practical purposes the aim is to distinguish between the three principal species: *melitensis*, *abortus*, and *suis*. Methods that are used are indicated in Table 1.

CO_2 Requirement. The vast majority of the initial isolates of *B. abortus* strains require the addition of 10 per cent CO_2 for optimal growth. After many subsequent subcultures, particularly in broth, this requirement is reduced or lost. Strain 19 *B. abortus*, used widely in the United States for vaccinating cattle, does not require added CO_2.

Inhibitory Action of Fuchsin and Thionin. Freshly prepared agar plates with either of these dyes from a stocked solution should be used. The test is performed by dividing a plate into four segments and streaking suspensions of each of the known three species on three segments, and the unknown on the fourth. One set of two plates, one with fuchsin and one with thionin, is placed in a jar with 10 per cent CO_2 added and incubated at 37° C. A second set of plates is incubated without added CO_2. Growth is checked at 48 and 72 hours. The results listed in Table 2 distinguish among the three species.

H_2S Production. The three species can be differentiated by the amount of S liberated from agar slants by reproducing organisms. This is determined by suspending in tubes dried filter strips that have been soaked in a 10 per cent solution of lead acetate and then noting the intensity of the black precipitated sulfide on the paper. Each of three tubes contain one of the known species of *Brucella* and the fourth has the unknown culture. The tubes are incubated at 37° C for 4 days with 10 per cent CO_2 added to each tube. Every 24 hours the strips are examined and replaced by fresh ones. The degree of blackening is measured from 0 to 4+. A typical series of observations is as follows:

Day	Abortus	Melitensis	Suis	Unknown
1	+	0	++	+
2	++	0	+++	+
3	±	0	++++	±
4	0	0	+++	0

The "unknown" is *B. abortus*. H_2S production is most intense with *B. suis* and is not observed with *B. melitensis*.

Urease Activity. Most *Brucella* strains split urea to form ammonia. This activity can be measured by adding urea to

Table 1. TESTS FOR DISTINGUISHING AMONG THE SPECIES OF BRUCELLA

1. Requirement of added CO_2 for growth
2. Inhibitory action of basic fuchsin and thionin on growth
3. Production of H_2S
4. Urease activity
5. Inhibitory action of bacteriophage on growth
6. Agglutination with monospecific serum
7. Oxidative-metabolic tests

Table 2. INHIBITING ACTION OF FUCHSIN AND THIONIN ON BRUCELLA

B. melitensis	Growth on all six plates
B. abortus	Growth only in CO_2 and with fuchsin
B. suis	Growth with and without CO_2 but only with thionin

the media along with phenol red as an indicator. A loopful of known *Brucella* organisms and an unknown culture is added to the surface of an agar slant and observed at room temperature. *Brucella suis* produces a pink color of the medium almost immediately, reaching a maximum intensity within 15 to 30 minutes, whereas the color change with *B. abortus* takes several hours. The color change with *B. melitensis* occurs more slowly than with *B. abortus* and the overall results are variable.

Thus, the H_2S and urease tests are most specific in identifying strains of *B. suis*.

Inhibitory Action of Brucella Bacteriophage. Tb (Tbsili) phage, originally isolated in the U.S.S.R., is specific for most *abortus* strains. This test is rarely necessary in a routine diagnostic laboratory. If it is necessary, assistance should be sought from one of the FAO/WHO Research Centers for Brucellosis.

Agglutination with Monospecific Serum. For practical purposes the foregoing procedures for the differentiation of *Brucella* species can be adapted to a diagnostic laboratory. Thus, *B. suis* can be readily distinguished from *abortus* and *melitensis* cultures. The vast majority of fresh isolates of *B. abortus* can be differentiated from *melitensis* and *suis* cultures because of the requirement of added CO_2 for optimal growth of *abortus*. However, on rare occasions some difficulty may be encountered in differentiating *abortus* cultures from those of *melitensis*, especially if the CO_2 requirement for the former is not definite. For this reason the use of monospecific absorbed agglutinating serum can be helpful. An example from our laboratory using monospecific anti-*abortus* and anti-*melitensis* sera is shown in Table 3.

The "unknown" in Table 3 is not *B. melitensis*, but it still could be *B. suis* on the basis of this single procedure. The H_2S and urease tests will make the final distinction.

Although many *Brucella* isolates have been studied intensively on a world-wide basis, the taxonomy of the *Brucella* species is focused on three basic species. Nevertheless, on the basis of biologic and metabolic studies, some strains cannot be strictly assigned to *abortus, suis,* or *melitensis*. These strains have not been classified as new species but rather as biotypes of one of the three. Three biotypes of *B. melitensis* are recognized, two of which have antigenic properties of *abortus* strains as determined with monospecific agglutination sera. Some isolates of *abortus* strains do not require additional CO_2 for growth; in others agglutinins for *melitensis* predominate. Nine types of *abortus* are known. There are four biotypes of *suis*. Although the classic strain forms H_2S readily, three do not, including type 4, which is found in reindeer, and type 2, found in the Danish hare and swine.

Serologic. If *Brucella* organisms are not isolated, the diagnosis can sometimes be made by testing the serum of patients for antibody. The most reliable serologic test is the tube-dilution, saline-agglutination test using a standardized *B. abortus* antigen. The test has minor limitations as far as specificity is concerned. Cross-agglutination with *Vibrio cholera*, *Yersinia enterocolitica*, and *Francisella tularensis* occurs in the sera of patients who have either had these diseases or have been vaccinated for them. The antigen-serum mixtures should be incubated for 48 hours at 37° C and then examined. Titers of 1:100 and above are significant, though on occasion healthy individuals who have had the disease months and years previously may have titers of 1:100 or below, rarely higher. "Blocking antibodies" may interfere with a clear-cut reading so that the lower dilutions reveal little or no agglutination, and the higher dilutions show incomplete agglutination. When such blocking is present, centrifuging the mixtures at 3000 rpm may reveal further clumping. The presence of blocking antibody can also be detected by incubating the suspect serum with a known serum of high antibody content. The known serum is then diluted with antigen and incubated, and if blocking is occurring the titer will be lower than in the untreated serum.

Agglutination tests on the sera of patients suspected of *B. canis* infections must be done with antigens prepared from *B. canis* (Alton, et al., 1975). The specificity of the test with canine sera is improved by adding 2-mercaptoethanol to the test diluent, but the importance of this reagent for tests with human sera has not been determined.

Although agglutinins are rarely absent in patients with active disease, especially in those with blood cultures that reveal *Brucella* organisms, the interpretation of agglutinin titers of 1:100 or less is often difficult when the cultures remain sterile. The *Brucella* agglutinin in active disease is IgG antibody, whereas in those who have recovered from the disease it is IgM. The type of antibody present in the serum may be differentiated by adding 2-mercaptoethanol to the antigen-antibody mixtures. Under these circumstances IgM dissociates and no agglutination occurs.

Other serologic tests carried out in some laboratories include the complement-fixation, the Coombs'-antiglobulin, and the fluorescent antibody tests. Additional serological tests are described in the WHO guide (Elberg, Ed. 1981).

Drug Susceptibility. It is not necessary to carry out routinely in vitro drug sensitivity tests on isolated strains of *Brucella* for the purposes of human therapy. Extensive clinical experience in several areas of the world has shown that tetracycline is the drug of choice for the treatment of

Table 3. DIFFERENTIATION OF ABORTUS AND MELITENSIS CULTURES USING MONOSPECIFIC SERUM

	Monospecific Anti-Abortus Serum				**Monospecific Anti-Melitensis Serum**			
	1:20	***1:40***	***1:80***	***1:160***	***1:20***	***1:40***	***1:80***	***1:160***
B. abortus	+++[a]	+++	+++	+++	0	0	0	0
B. melitensis	0	0	0	0	++++	+++	+++	+++
Unknown	+++	+++	+++	+++	0	0	0	0

[a]Degree of agglutination ranges from 0 to ++++.

brucellosis. In severe illness tetracycline can be supplemented with streptomycin. An alternate drug for tetracycline is chloramphenicol.

Tests in vitro also show that the tetracycline antibiotics are the most effective. Tetracycline, for example, inhibits 95 per cent of strains in a concentration of 0.02 μg/ml, and is more bactericidal for *Brucella* than is generally appreciated (Hall and Manion, 1970). Chloramphenicol is approximately 100 times less active against *Brucella* than tetracycline. Streptomycin is as active in vitro as chloramphenicol but the aminoglycoside is not effective in clinical therapy, presumably because it does not effectively enter the cells in which *Brucella* organisms are living.

EPIDEMIOLOGY. Brucellosis is one of the zoonoses—that is, a disease transmitted directly or indirectly from animals to man. The disease is very rarely transmitted from one person to another. The most common animal reservoirs are sheep, goats, cattle, hogs, and caribou, although other domestic animals can harbor the organisms. The prevalence of human disease will depend on the concentration of the animal populations just mentioned, the incidence of animal disease, and the efficiency of disease eradication programs in animals.

Where disease is prevalent in sheep and goats (*B. melitensis*) there will be a high incidence of human infection transmitted through the milk and cheese of these animals. Likewise, brucellosis in cattle (*B. abortus*) results in human disease by ingestion of unpasteurized dairy products. Hogs and caribou infected with *Brucella* (*B. suis*) transmit disease to veterinarians, farmers, and packing-house workers who handle infected tissues and vaginal discharges of aborting animals. The frequent association of *B. abortus* with fistulous withers in horses provides another source of potential infection. *Brucellae* will survive in dry soil for 40 to 60 days after it is soiled by animal discharges or tissues, and in milk for 10 days at 10° C. Unpasteurized cheese preserves the vitality of these organisms for up to 2 months, but they do not survive in ripened, aged cheeses. Viable Brucellae can be recovered for long periods in refrigerated meat and material in the pickling process (Elberg, 1981).

Eradication programs in domestic animals include testing and slaughtering infected animals. Vaccination has been successful in sheep and goats, and in cattle. Prophylactic vaccines in humans are not feasible. The successful eradication program of bovine brucellosis in the United States has markedly reduced the incidence of human brucellosis from 3500 cases reported in 1950 to only 185 cases in 1981. In other parts of the world, however, animal and human brucellosis is still widespread. The disease is still prevalent in Mexico, Central and South America, much of Africa, France, Italy, Spain, the Middle East, India, Australia, Polynesia, and New Zealand. For a comprehensive review of the problem throughout the world up to 1980 consult the WHO Guide (Elberg, 1981).

References

Alton, G. G., Jones, L. M., and Pietz, D. E.: Laboratory Techniques in Brucellosis. 2nd ed. Geneva, World Health Organization, 1975.

Braude, A. I.: Studies on the pathology and pathogenesis of experimental brucellosis. I. A comparison of the pathogenicity of *Brucella abortus*, *Brucella melitensis*, and *Brucella suis* for guinea pigs. J Inf Dis 89:76, 1951.

Brinley-Morgan, W. J., and McCullough, N. B.: *Brucella*. *In* Bergey's Manual of Determinative Bacteriology. 8th ed. Baltimore, The Williams & Wilkins Company, 1974, p. 278.

Elberg, S. S. (ed.): A Guide to the Diagnosis, Treatment, and Prevention of Human Brucellosis, Document VPH/ 81.31 (1981).

Garrod, L. P.: A study of the bactericidal power of hydrochloric acid and of gastric juice. St. Barth Hosp Rep 72:145, 1939.

Hall, W., and Manion, R.: In vitro susceptibility of *Brucella* to various antibiotics. Appl Microbiol 20:600, 1970.

Meyer, M. E.: Advances in research on brucellosis, 1957–1972. In Bradley, C. A., and Cornelius, C. E. (eds.): Advances in Veterinary Science and Comparative Medicine. Vol. 18, New York, Academic Press, 1974, p. 231.

Morales-Otero, P.: Experimental infection of *Brucella abortus* in man: Preliminary report. Puerto Rico J Public Health and Trop Med 5:144, 1929.

Spink, W. W.: The Nature of Brucellosis. Minneapolis, University of Minnesota Press, 1956.

Wilson, G., and Miles, A. A.: The serologic differentiation of smooth strains of the *Brucella* group. Br J Exp Pathol 13:1, 1932.

35

BORDETELLA

JEAN M. DOLBY, PH.D.

Bordetella pertussis is virulent for man and is the cause of whooping cough. *B. parapertussis* also causes whooping cough in children, and *B. bronchiseptica* is an animal pathogen of the upper respiratory tract rarely transmissible to man.

MORPHOLOGY. All three species are minute, gram-negative, nonacidfast coccobacilli 1 × 0.3 to 0.5 μm; *B. pertussis* is shown in Figure 1. *B. bronchiseptica* is the only motile species, and *B. pertussis* is the only one that is capsulated. Pili have been demonstrated on *B. pertussis* (Morse and Morse, 1976).

ANTIGENIC COMPOSITION. The three members of the species are more closely related antigenically to each other than to *Haemophilus* and *Brucella*, with which one or the other has been classified. Some of the antigens are common to the genus *Bordetella*, some are shared by only two of the three species, and some are species- or even strain-specific. Most antigens are protein or lipopolysaccharide components of the bacterial cell wall.

When freshly isolated, *B. pertussis* organisms are nutritionally exacting (phase I). They can be slowly adapted to grow on less complex media (phase IV) and have lost most of the Phase I antigens (Leslie and Gardner, 1931; Standfast, 1951). Phase IV organisms can still be identified, however, because the lipopolysaccharide of their cell walls retains the ability to elicit "bactericidal antigen" as do Phase I cells (Dolby and Ackers, 1975).

More rapid loss of Phase I properties occurs in cells grown in a medium containing (a) magnesium sulfate, to give C-mode cells (Lacey, 1960; Idigbe et al., 1981) or (b) 500 μg/ml nicotinic acid (Pusztai and Joo, 1967). Phase IV cells and C-mode cells may be similar; Phase IV cells and cells grown in high concentrations of nicotinic acid are not (Table 1). Initially at least, the loss of antigens is reversible, and cultivation on complex media causes reversion to typical Phase I cells.

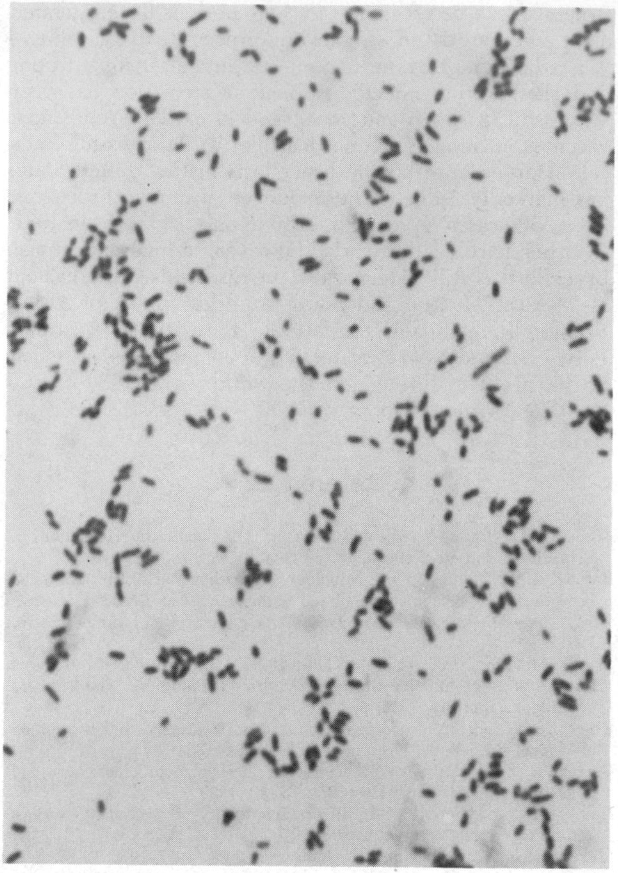

Figure 1. *B. pertussis*, phase 1, grown 18 hours on Bordet-Gengou agar medium at 36°C and stained with carbol-fuchsin (× 3000).

By simple immunodiffusion techniques, about 20 precipitin lines denoting antigen-antibody systems of Phase I antigens can be demonstrated. By chemical methods, 35 proteins can be demonstrated in the cell walls of Phase I *B. pertussis;* Phase IV cells have only two less protein bands which cannot account for all the antigens lost (Parton and Wardlaw, 1975; Wardlaw et al., 1975). Electronmicroscope photographs show more differences between Phases I and IV than are apparent from protein analysis.

B. parapertussis and *B. bronchiseptica* grow on simple media upon isolation, and cultivation on complex media does not alter their antigenic make-up.

Table 1 lists some of the defined antigens of *B. pertussis*, and Table 2 shows those shared by other *Bordetella* organisms. A few are discussed below.

(1) The agglutinogens are a heterogeneous group of antigens that stimulate antibodies including the relatively heat-labile K antigens, protein components of the wall, and the less specific heat-stable lipopolysaccharide components. The K antigens are demonstrable in cells heated at 56° C and in vaccine but are destroyed at 100° C; they are numbered 1 through 14, of which 1 through 7 and 13 are found in *B. pertussis*, 1 through 6 being specific (Andersen, 1953; Eldering et al., 1957). Agglutinogen 1 is found in all *B. pertussis* organisms together with one or more of all of the others, usually in the combinations 3 and 6, 2 and 4. Serotypes are distinguished on the basis of agglutinogens (K antigens), which are stable characteristics with the exception of variable strains of serotypes 1,2,3 (Bronne-Shanbury and Dolby, 1976).

(2) The histamine-sensitizing factor for mice (HSF), the lymphocyte-promoting-factor (LPF) responsible for the leukocytosis-inducing property of *B. pertussis* and islet-activating protein (IAP) that stimulates insulin and can cause fasting hypoglycemia may all be one antigenic protein moiety of the cell wall, called "pertussigen" (see Munoz et al., 1981a). The protein may also promote the formation of IgE (reaginic antibody) by eliminating the suppressor activity of T-lymphocytes (Morse, 1976) and be responsible for experimental allergic encephalomyelitis in rats (Munoz et al., 1981a).

(3) Hemagglutinating activity has now been attributed to two antigens, the pili (fimbrial hemagglutinin, F-HA) and the lymphocyte-promoting factor, part of "pertussigen" (LPF-HA). References to the earlier work, realization of the dual nature and purification are given by Munoz et al. (1981b) and Ashworth et al. (1982).

(4) The protective antigen (PA), which confers protection in mice against an intracerebral challenge and is equated with protection in children (see below), is the most important antigen(s). It has been difficult to determine if it is a separate entity from the antigens described above. Earlier protection tests in mice have suggested that it is, but Munoz et al. (1981b) have shown that pertussigen detoxified with glutaraldehyde is protective in mice. This activity is associated with LPF-HA but not F-HA.

Protection experiments are now being carried out in animal models directed against intranasal challenges and should be assessed cautiously (see below); Stanbridge and Preston (1974) have implicated agglutinogen in marmosets; F-HA and LPF-HA both appear to be involved in mice (Sato et al., 1981) and in rabbits (Ashworth et al., 1982).

Some antigens of *B. parapertussis* and *B. bronchiseptica* that are shared with *B. pertussis* and the species-specific ones are shown in Table 2. *B. bronchiseptica* is antigenically heterogeneous.

METABOLISM. Phase I *B. pertussis* requires a complex medium; the original solid one of Bordet and Gengou (1906) and still used in a modified form contains starch, peptone glycerol, and 33 per cent blood. Increasingly

Table 1. ANTIGENIC RELATIONSHIP OF *B. PERTUSSIS* AND DERIVATIVES

Antigen	Phase I	Phase IV	Nicotinic-Acid-Grown	C-Mode
K agglutinogens 1–6	+	–	–	–
HSF, LPF-HA, IAP[a]	+	–?	–	–
"Bactericidal antigen"	+ or ±	as ph I	as ph I	
"Protective antigen"	+	–	–	–
Heat labile toxin	+	–		–
Antigen stimulating opsonin	+	+	–	
Fimbrial hemagglutinin	+	–	–	

[a]HSF = histamine-sensitizing factor; LPF = lymphocytosis-promoting factor; HA = hemagglutinin; IAP = islet activating protein

Table 2. ANTIGENIC RELATIONSHIPS IN THE GENUS *BORDETELLA*

Antigen		B. Pertussis	B. Parapertussis	B. Bronchiseptica
K agglutinogens 7–14		7,13	7–11, *14*	7–11, *12*, 13
Toxin		+	+	+
Pertussis "bactericidal antigen"		+ or ±	−	−
Fimbrial hemagglutinin		+	+	+
HSF, LPF-HA etc (see Table 1)		+	−	−
Precipitinogen	Pertussis LPS[a]	+	−	variable
	Parapertussis LPS	−	+	variable
	Bronchiseptica LPS	variable	variable	+
Protection by Vaccine against	Pertussis	+	−	variable
	Parapertussis	−	+	variable
	Bronchiseptica	variable		+

[a]LPS = lipopolysaccharide; other abbreviations see Table 1

defined liquid ones have been suggested (Cohen and Wheeler, 1946; Lacey, 1954; Stainer and Scholte, 1970) on which *B. pertussis* may be grown for a vaccine. *B. parapertussis* and *B. bronchiseptica* present no problems and can be grown on nutrient agar, broth, and citrate agar. None of them ferment carbohydrates or reduce nitrates to nitrites. *B. pertussis* does not possess a urease, but the other two do.

All three species derive energy from oxidative deamination so that suitable buffering is necessary to retain the optimum pH at about 7.6. Amino acids essential to the metabolism of *B. pertussis* are cysteine and glutamic acid or proline, without which the others cannot be utilized. Growth factors nicotinic acid, glutathione, and ferrous salt are necessary (Rowatt, 1955).

The blood in the agar medium absorbs inhibiting substances and allows growth from small inocula of *B. pertussis*. Albumin or charcoal can be used instead. The subject has been reviewed by Rowatt (1957) and Parker (1976).

B. pertussis produces extracytoplasmic adenylate cyclase during growth which may control growth; the enzyme is lost on degradation to phase IV (Hewlett et al., 1978; Idigbe et al., 1981). *B. bronchiseptica* and *B. parapertussis* produce less enzyme than *B. pertussis*.

PATHOGENIC PROPERTIES. *B. pertussis* is virulent for humans (Bordet and Gengou, 1906) and so is *B. parapertussis* (Bradford and Slavin, 1937; Eldering and Kendrick, 1938). The organisms are not invasive but attach themselves to the ciliated epithelium of the upper respiratory tract (Rich, 1932) causing catarrh, lasting about 2 weeks, and then paroxysmal coughing and "whooping," which may last 4 to 6 weeks (Miller et al., 1982). *B. bronchiseptica*, mainly a disease of animals, attaches to ciliated epithelium in the same way (Bemis et al., 1977). In exposed humans, it causes chronic catarrh and spasmodic cough (McGowan, 1911; Brown, 1926). In experimental situations, ciliated epithelium elsewhere can become the target of *B. pertussis*, as shown in Figure 2. The surface component of the bacterial cell upon which this attachment depends is obviously of great importance in pathogenicity. The adherence antigen of Holt (1972), may be F-HA (Sato et al., 1981). Toxin, common to all three species is dermonecrotic and paralyzes the cilia. It is intracellular (Cowell et al., 1979). Another toxin with anti-ciliary activity has been demonstrated (Goldman et al., 1982). Little is known of the contribution to pathogenesis of these and other biologically active components.

IMMUNITY. Successful immunization has been achieved with parenteral vaccination of children with a whole cell *B. pertussis* vaccine (Medical Research Council, 1951; 1956), and the incidence of whooping cough has been reduced to a very low level in communities with a high acceptance of vaccine (Kendrick, 1975). A cell-free but not purified absorbed bacterial extract has also been effective (Medical Research Council, 1959). The effect of vaccination on pertussis in the United Kingdom is shown in Figure 3. *B. parapertussis* vaccine is similarly used with success in areas in which parapertussis is prevalent. An experimental study on vaccination in dogs with *B. bronchiseptica* has

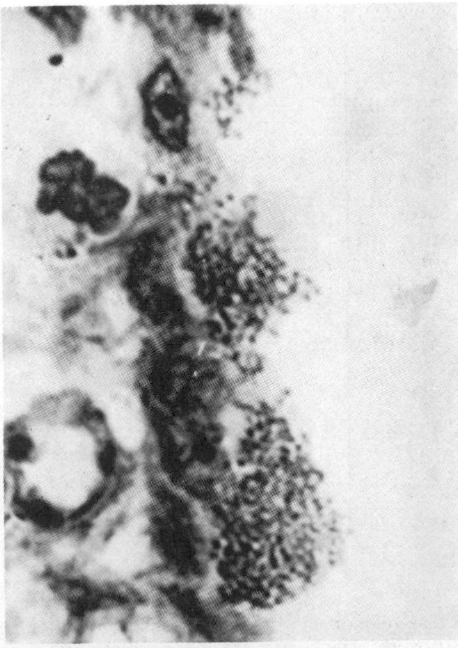

Figure 2. *B. pertussis* on the ependymal cells of mouse brain 24 hours after infection, Giemsa stain (× 1500). (From Iida, T., et al.: Jap J Exp Med 32:490, 1962.)

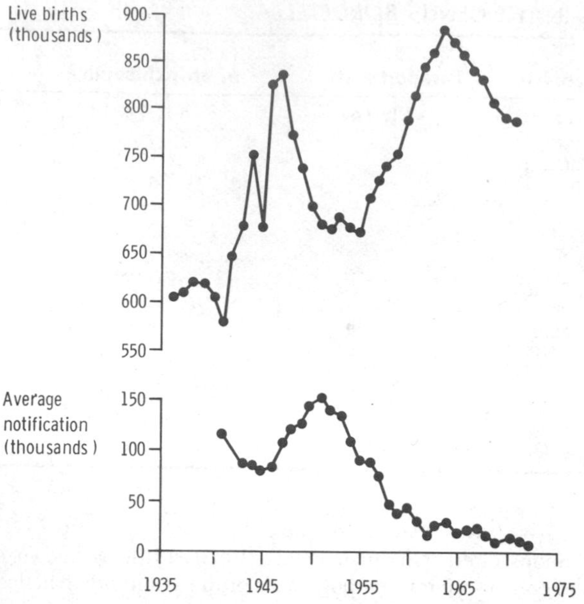

Figure 3. Annual live births and average whooping cough notifications in the United Kingdom from 1940 to 1975. Widespread vaccination was introduced in 1957 at the time that the number of births increased—whooping cough notifications continued to decrease. (From Miller, C. L., et al.: Lancet 2:510, 1974.)

been reported (Bemis et al., 1977) and in pigs with a novel vaccine (Shimizu, 1978).

The ability of vaccine to protect mice against an intracerebral but not an intranasal challenge was correlated with the success of the vaccine in children (Standfast, 1958), as shown in Figure 4. This correlation is the basis of the international assay of vaccine in mice (World Health Organization, 1964). Protection of the mouse against an intranasal challenge follows vaccination by all *B. pertussis* organisms, including Phase IV (Logan et al., 1959) and is due to antibody against lipopolysaccharide, which reduces the infection to sublethal levels from which mice recover. Such vaccine is not effective in children (Standfast, 1958). These animal models must be examined with care to determine exactly what is being measured and to understand the pathology (Pittman et al., 1980).

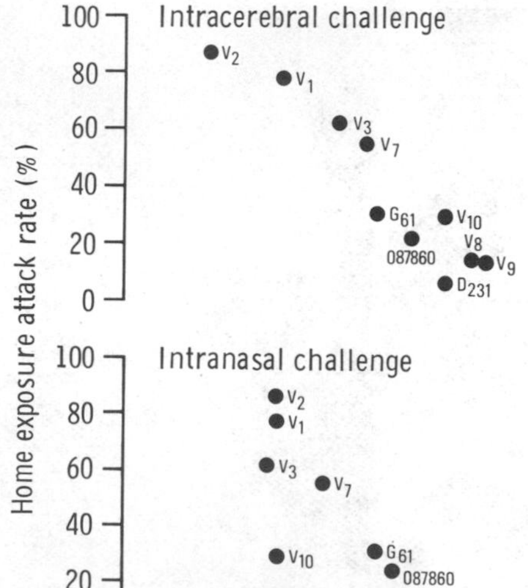

Figure 4. The relationship between mouse protection tests and home exposure attack rate for ten pertussis vaccines: (*top*), close relationship by intracerebral mouse challenge (*bottom*), no relationship by intranasal mouse challenge. (From Standfast, A. F. B.: Immunology 1:135, 1958.)

The vaccine is a suspension of detoxified, inactivated cells of *B. pertussis* in Phase I. A course consisting of a minimum of 12 units in three doses is recommended and without the addition of alum in areas in which poliomyelitis is prevalent. Both 7S and 11S immunoglobulins protect mice against intracerebral infection (Dolby et al., 1975); secretory IgA is probably effective in nasopharyngeal clearance in rabbits (Ashworth et al., 1982). Passive transfer of lymph node cells from immune animals is also protective, but the responsible cell type is unknown (Adams and Hopewell, 1970; Dolby et al., 1975). Mice can be immunized by repeated oral vaccine (Hof et al., 1976). This route may offer a new approach to human immunization (Maurer et al., 1979, quoted by Ashworth et al., 1982).

LABORATORY DIAGNOSIS. Organisms can be cultured in the 1st or 2nd week of the disease from the posterior nasopharynx by using swabs made from 16-cm lengths of thin wire wrapped with cotton wool. Unless plated immediately, the swabs should be held in a tube containing 0.2 ml of 1 per cent casamino acids and plated within 4 to 6 hours onto solid media (Bordet-Gengou or blood-charcoal medium) containing 0.25 to 0.3 unit of benzyl penicillin per ml and, if possible, 2 μg/ml of M&B 938 (4:4 diamidino phenylamine dihydrochloride) (Lacey, 1954). The identity of the isolated *Bordetella* can be checked by agglutination and growth characteristics: *B. parapertussis* grows on nutrient agar with brown pigment formation; *B. bronchiseptica* grows on nutrient agar without forming pigment.

Fluorescent-labeled antipertussis serum to a strain of 1,2,3,4 serotype has given good diagnostic results on smears from nasopharyngeal swabs (Kendrick et al., 1961). A greater success rate has been obtained by using a combination of culture and labeled antibody than by either method alone (Chalvardjian, 1966). Serological diagnosis has also been attempted (Macaulay, 1981; Viljanen et al., 1982) but is difficult.

DRUG SUSCEPTIBILITY. *B. pertussis* is sensitive *in vitro* to several antibiotics; erythromycin is best, but chloramphenicol, kanamycin, and oxytetracycline are moderately effective (Bass et al., 1969a). None of these has any effect on the course of the disease, but they reduce the infectivity of the patients (Bass et al., 1969b; Altemeir and Ayoub, 1977).

EPIDEMIOLOGY. Pertussis and parapertussis are spread by droplet infection, particularly during the catarrhal stage. *B. parapertussis* may account for 0.5 to 5 per cent of all whooping cough (Linneman, 1977). *B. bronchiseptica* is very rare in man.

B. pertussis infection occurs sporadically the world over (Raska, 1970), mainly in children up to 8 to 10 years old, and an attack probably confers immunity of 15 to 20 years, or the same duration as vaccination. The disease incidence undulates (Fig. 5). Newborns are particularly susceptible,

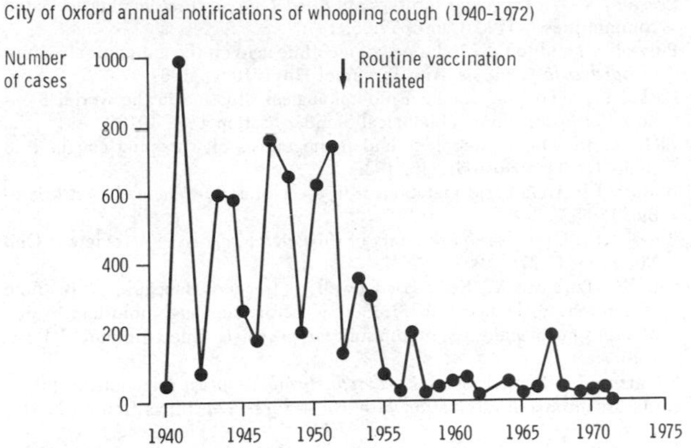

Figure 5. The seasonal fluctuation of *B. pertussis* in Oxfordshire, England. (From Warin, J. F.: Proc Roy Soc Med 67:374, 1974.)

but it is still not known whether transfer of immunity from the mother to her baby is impossible, or whether transmissible immunity at child-bearing age is low (Kendrick et al., 1945). Adult vaccination is not recommended, even though the adult population may be susceptible in countries with successful vaccination campaigns (Linneman et al., 1975). Partial immunity decreases the severity of the disease (Miller and Fletcher, 1976), which may pass undiagnosed and may be a source of subsequent infection (Kurt et al., 1972).

A high vaccination rate (greater than 80 per cent) can protect a community. At the beginning of a vaccination campaign, babies should be inoculated at 1, 2, and 3 months of age, but, as these grow up to be immune siblings, the vaccination of the newborn can be postponed to begin at 3 months. Later vaccination produces less general reaction to the vaccine and enables pertussis to be combined with diphtheria and tetanus toxoids (Dudgeon, 1976).

There has been concern in Northern Europe about the rare (1:100,000) brain damage to vaccinated children similar to that occasionally found after infection (Byers and Moll, 1948). This concern has led to a decline in vaccine acceptance and subsequent increase in incidence of whooping cough. The debate and its consequences have been summarized for the United Kingdom by D. L. Miller and colleagues (1982).

Over the last 30 years, there has been a change in the infecting serotype of *B. pertussis* in some countries, from predominantly 1,2,4 to 1,3,6 (Blaskett et al., 1971; Bronne-Shanbury et al., 1976). It has been suggested that this may be influenced by vaccination (Preston, 1976), particularly by vaccine from which one serotype is missing. Vaccine containing the main serotypes is now made, and the consequences are awaited with interest.

References

Adams, G. J., and Hopewell, J. W.: Enhancement of intracerebral infection of mice with *Bordetella pertussis*. J Med Microbiol 3:15, 1970.

Altemeir, W. A., and Ayoub, E. M.: Erythromycin prophylaxis for pertussis. Pediatrics 59:623, 1977.

Andersen, E. K.: Serological studies on *H. pertussis, H. parapertussis* and *H. bronchisepticus*. Acta Pathol Microbiol Scand 33:202, 1953.

Ashworth, L. A. E., Fitzgeorge, R. B., Irons, L. I., Morgan, C. P., and Robinson, A.: Rabbit nasopharyngeal colonization by *Bordetella pertussis*: the effects of immunization on clearance and on serum and nasal antibody levels. J Hyg (Camb) 88:475, 1982.

Bass, J. W., Crast, F. W., Kotheimer, J. B., and Mitchell, I. A.: Susceptibility of *Bordetella pertussis* to 9 antimicrobial agents. Am J Dis Child 117:276, 1969a.

Bass, J. W., Klenk, E. L., Kotheimer, J. B., Linneman, C. C., Smith, M. H. D.: Antimicrobial treatment of pertussis. J Pediatr 75:768, 1969b.

Bemis, D. A., Greisen, H. A., and Appel, M. J. G.: Pathogenesis of canine Bordetellosis. J Infect Dis 135:753, 1977.

Blaskett, A. C., Gulasekharam, L. M. S., and Fulton, L. C.: The occurrence of *Bordetella pertussis* serotypes in Australia, 1950–70. Med J Aust 1:781, 1971.

Bordet, J., and Gengou, O.: Le microbe de la coquelucheuse. Ann Inst Pasteur 23:415, 1906.

Bradford, W. C., and Slavin, B.: An organism resembling *Hemophilus pertussis*. Am J Public Health 27:1277, 1937.

Bronne-Shanbury, C. J., and Dolby, J. M.: The stability of serotypes of *Bordetella pertussis* with particular reference to serotypes 1,2,3,4. J Hyg (Camb) 76:277, 1976.

Bronne-Shanbury, C. J., Miller, D., and Standfast, A. F. B.: The serotypes of *Bordetella pertussis* isolated in Great Britain between 1941 and 1968 and a comparison with serotypes observed in other countries over this period. J Hyg (Camb) 76:265, 1976.

Brown, J. H.: *Bacillus bronchisepticus* infections in a child with symptoms of pertussis. Bull Johns Hopkins Hosp 38:147, 1926.

Byers, R. K., and Moll, F. C.: Encephalopathies following prophylactic pertussis vaccine. Pediatrics 1:437, 1948.

Chalvardjian, N.: The laboratory diagnosis of whooping-cough by fluorescent antibody and by culture methods. Can Med Assoc J 95:263, 1966.

Cohen, S. M., and Wheeler, M. W.: Pertussis vaccine prepared with Phase-I cultures grown in fluid medium. Am J Public Health 36:371, 1946.

Cowell, J. L., Hewlett, E. L., and Manclark, C. R.: Intracellular Localization of the dermonecrotic toxin of *Bordetella pertussis*. Infect Immun 25:896, 1979.

Dolby, J. M., and Ackers, J. P.: Taxonomic distribution of the antigen eliciting bactericidal antibody for *Bordetella pertussis*. J Gen Microbiol 87:239, 1975.

Dolby, J. M., Dolby, D. E., and Bronne-Shanbury, C. J.: The effects of humoral, cellular and non-specific immunity on intracerebral *Bordetella pertussis* infections in mice. J Hyg (Camb) 74:85, 1975.

Dudgeon, J. A.: Immunising procedures in childhood. In Hull, D. (ed): Recent Advances in Paediatrics. London, Churchill-Livingstone, 1976, p. 169.

Eldering, G., Hornbeck, C., and Baker, J.: Serological study of *Bordetella pertussis* and related species. J Bacteriol 74:133, 1957.

Eldering, G., and Kendrick, P. L.: Bacillus para-pertussis: A species resembling both *Bacillus pertussis* and *Bacillus bronchisepticus* but identical with neither. J Bacteriol 35:561, 1938.

Goldman, W. E., Klapper, D. G., and Baseman, J. B.: Detection, isolation, and analysis of a released *Bordetella pertussis* product toxic to cultured tracheal cells. Infect Immun 36:782, 1982.

Hewlett, E. L., Underhill, L. H., Vargo, S. A., Wolff, J., and Manclark, C. R.: *Bordetella pertussis* adenylate cyclase: regulation of activity and its loss in degraded strains. In Manclark, C. R., and Hill, J. C. (ed)., International Symposium on Pertussis. National Institutes of Health, Bethesda, p. 81, 1978.

Hof, H., Finger, H., Korner, L., and Milke, L.: Effectiveness of orally administered *Bordetella pertussis* vaccine in mice. Dev Biol Stand 33:47, 1976.

Holt, L. B.: The pathology and immunology of *B. pertussis* infections. J Med Microbiol 5:407, 1972.

Idigbe, E. O., Parton, R., and Wardlaw, A. C.: Rapidity of antigenic modulation of *Bordetella pertussis* in modified Hornibrook medium. J Med Microbiol 14:409, 1981.

Iida, T., Kusano, N., Yamamoto, A., and Shiga, H.: Studies on experimental infection with *Bordetella pertussis*. Bacteriological and pathological studies on the mode of infection in the mouse brain. Jpn J Exp Med 32:471, 1962.

Kendrick, P. L.: Can whooping cough be eradicated? J Infect Dis 132:707, 1975.

Kendrick, P. L., Eldering, G., and Eveland, W. C.: Fluorescent antibody techniques. Am J Dis Child 101:149, 1961.

Kendrick, P. L., Thompson, M., and Eldering, G.: Immunity response of mothers and babies to injections of pertussis vaccine during pregnancy. Am J Dis Child 70:25, 1945.

Kurt, T. L., Yeager, A. S., Guenette, S., and Dunlop, S.: Spread of pertussis by hospital staff. J Am Med Assoc 221:264, 1972.

Lacey, B. W.: A new selective medium for *Haemophilus pertussis* containing a diamidine, sodium fluoride and penicillin J. Hyg (Camb) 52:273, 1954.

Lacey, B. W.: Antigenic modulation of *Bordetella pertussis*. J Hyg (Camb) 58:57, 1960.

Leslie, P. H., and Gardner, A. D.: The phases of *Haemophilus pertussis*. J Hyg (Camb) 31:423, 1931.

Linneman, C. C.: *Bordetella parapertussis*. Recent experience and review of literature. Am J Dis Child 131:560, 1977.
Linneman, C. C., Ramundo, N., Perlstein, P. H., Minton, S. D., Englender, G. S., McCormick, J. B., and Hayes, P. S.: Use of pertussis vaccine in an epidemic involving hospital staff. Lancet 2:540, 1975.
Logan, J. E., Griffiths, B. W., and Mason, M. A.: Specificity of the clearance phenomenon in the lungs of pertussis-immunised mice following intratracheal administration of radio-iodinated pertussis vaccine. Can J Microbiol 5:405, 1959.
Macaulay, M. E.: The IgM and IgG response to *Bordetella pertussis* vaccination and infection. J Med Microbiol 14:1, 1981.
McGowan, J. P.: Some observations on a laboratory epidemic principally among dogs and cats in which animals affected presented the symptoms of the disease called 'distemper.' J Pathol Bact 15:372, 1911.
Medical Research Council: Vaccination against whooping cough. Investigation. Br Med J 1:1464, 1951; Relation between protection of children and laboratory tests. Ibid 2:454, 1956; Final report. Ibid 1:994, 1959.
Miller, C. L., and Fletcher, W. B.: Severity of notified whooping cough. Br Med J 1:117, 1976.
Miller, C. L., Pollock, T. M., and Clewer, A. D. E.: Whooping cough vaccine, an assessment. Lancet 2:510, 1974.
Miller, D. L., Alderslade, R., and Ross, E. M.: Whooping cough and whooping cough vaccine: The risks and benefits debate. Epidemiol Rev 4:1, 1982.
Morse, S. I.: Biologically active components and properties of *Bordetella pertussis*. Adv Appl Microbiol 20:9, 1976.
Morse, S. I., and Morse, J. H.: Isolation and properties of the leukocytosis- and lymphocytosis-promoting factor of *Bordetella pertussis*. J Exp Med 143:1483, 1976.
Munoz, J. J., Arai, H., Bergman, R. K., and Sadowski, P. L.: Biological activities of crystalline pertussigen from *Bordetella pertussis*. Infect Immun 33:820, 1981(a).
Munoz, J. J., Arai, H., and Cole, R. L.: Mouse-protecting and histamine-sensitizing activities of pertussigen and fimbrial haemagglutinin from *Bordetella pertussis*. Infect Immun 32:243, 1981(b).
Parker, C.: Role of the genetics and physiology of *Bordetella pertussis* in the production of vaccine and the study of host-parasite relationships in pertussis. Adv Appl Microbiol 20:27, 1976.
Parton, R., and Wardlaw, A. C.: Cell envelope proteins of *Bordetella pertussis*. J Med Microbiol 8:47, 1975.
Pittman, M., Furman, B. L., and Wardlaw, A. C.: *Bordetella pertussis* respiratory tract infection in the mouse: pathophysiological responses. J Infect Dis 142:56, 1980.
Preston, N. W.: Prevalent serotypes of *Bordetella pertussis* in nonvaccinated communities. J Hyg (Camb) 77:85, 1976.
Pusztai, S., and Joo, I.: Influence of nicotinic acid on the antigenic structure of *Bordetella pertussis*. Ann Immunol Hung 10:63, 1967.
Raska, K.: Whooping cough: Epidemiological situation in the world. Symposia Series in Immunobiological Standardisation 13:4, 1970.
Rich, A. R.: On the aetiology and pathogenesis of whooping cough. Bull Johns Hopkins Hosp 51:346, 1932.
Rowatt, E.: Amino-acid metabolism in the genus *Bordetella*. J Gen Microbiol 13:552, 1955.
Rowatt, E.: Growth requirements of *Bordetella pertussis*: A review. J Gen Microbiol 17:279, 1957.
Sato, Y., Izumiya, K., Sato, H., Cowell, J. L., and Manclark, C. R.: Role of antibody to leukocytosis-promoting factor haemagglutinin and to filamentous haemagglutinin in immunity to pertussis. Infect Immun 31:1223, 1981.
Shimizu, T.: Prophylaxis of *Bordetella bronchiseptica* infection in guinea pigs by intranasal vaccination with live strain ts-S34. Infect Immun 22:318, 1978.
Stainer, D. W., and Scholte, M. J.: A simple, chemically defined medium for the production of phase I *Bordetella pertussis*. J Gen Microbiol 63:211, 1970.
Stanbridge, T. N., and Preston, N. W.: Experimental pertussis infection in the marmoset: Type specificity of active immunity. J Hyg (Camb) 72:213, 1974.
Standfast, A. F. B.: The phase I of *Haemophilus pertussis*. J Gen Microbiol 5:531, 1951.
Standfast, A. F. B.: Comparison between field trials and mouse protection tests against intranasal and intracerebral challenges with *Bordetella pertussis*. Immunology 1:135, 1958.
Viljanen, M. K., Ruuskanen, O., Granberg, C., and Salmi, T. T.: Serological diagnosis of pertussis: IgM, IgA and IgG antibodies against *Bordetella pertussis* measured by enzyme-linked immunosorbent assay (ELISA). Scand J Inf Dis 14:117, 1982.
Wardlaw, A. C., Parton, R., and Hooker, M. J.: Loss of protective antigen, histamine sensitising factor and envelope polypeptides in cultural variants of *Bordetella pertussis*. J Med Microbiol 9:89, 1975.
Warin, J. F.: Immunisation: Balancing the risks. Proc R Soc Med 67:374, 1974.
World Health Organisation: Requirements for pertussis vaccine. Technical Reports Series No. 274, 25-40, 1964.

36

HAEMOPHILUS

MOGENS KILIAN, D.D.S., PH.D.

The organisms of the genus *Haemophilus* are small, gram-negative, nonmotile, and nonspore-forming, facultatively anaerobic rods, which require accessory factors for in vitro growth. The name *Haemophilus* refers to the fact that these growth factors are contained in blood cells and may be supplied to ordinary growth media by the addition of blood or its derivatives. Robert Koch was the first to observe bacteria of the genus *Haemophilus* in conjunctivitis exudates in Egypt (Koch, 1883). However, the isolation and description of another Haemophilus organism in 1892 by Koch's colleague Richard Pfeiffer caused more sensation (Pfeiffer, 1892). Pfeiffer's bacillus was isolated from purulent sputum and postmorten lung cultures of patients succumbing to influenza during the pandemic of 1889 through 1892. The discovery was published as "the exciting cause of influenza," and the organism was accordingly designated *Haemophilus influenzae* by a committee of the American Society of Bacteriologists. Following the discovery in 1933 of the influenza virus, the actual etiologic agent of epidemic influenza, interest in *H. influenzae* vanished for several years.

The precise role played by *H. influenzae* in the pandemic of 1890 and again in that of 1918 through 1919 is still not clear. The view was held by a number of investigators of the 1918 pandemic that the unprecedented severity of the disease reflected the concurrent interplay of a virus and Pfeiffer's bacillus. This thesis was strengthened by the subsequent demonstration by Shope (1931) that the synergistic effect of a Haemophilus organism (*H. suis*) and swine influenza virus is essential for both natural and experimental swine influenza. Because *H. influenzae* has clearly not played a similar part in more recent pandemics, the importance of viral and bacterial synergism in the pathogenesis of the human disease needs further study (Michaels et al., 1977).

MORPHOLOGY. Bacteria of the genus *Haemophilus* tend to be pleomorphic (Fig. 1). In samples of pathologic material such as cerebrospinal fluid, the bacteria are predominantly coccobacillary, sometimes simulating diplococci and erroneously suspected of being meningococci or pneumococci. In older cultures, or when grown under unfavorable conditions, the rods become elongated and frequently appear filamentous. The pleomorphic appearance is most prominent among the X-factor independent species.

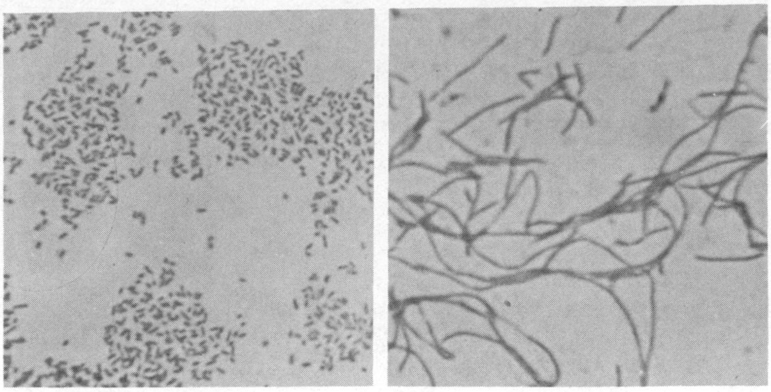

Figure 1. Variations in microscopic appearance of Haemophilus organisms (Gram-stained smears × 800).

Colonies formed on solid media are 1 to 3 mm in diameter after incubation for 24 hours. Young cultures (8 to 18 hours) of encapsulated strains on translucent solid media are characteristically iridescent (produce a rainbow effect) when examined in obliquely transmitted light. Strains of some species are β-hemolytic (Table 1).

ANTIGENIC COMPOSITION. Virtually all strains of *H. influenzae* isolated from serious infections have capsules that are antiphagocytic. Six distinct capsular serotypes, designated a through f, have been described by Pittman (1931); these are identified by agglutination, precipitation, or quellung tests performed with specific antisera.

The capsules of all six types are negatively charged, high-molecular weight polysaccharides with a disaccharide repeat unit. All except types d and e contain phosphate (for review see Sutton et al., 1982).

Strains causing meningitis and other invasive infections virtually all belong to serotype b. The type b capsule is a phosphodiester-linked ribose-ribitol copolymer. It is structurally and serologically closely related to the cell-wall teichoic acid of gram-positive bacteria and the capsular polysaccharides of certain serotypes of pneumococci and enterobacteria (Table 2).

A number of subtypes of *H. influenzae* have been defined on the basis of differences in outer membrane protein profiles (Loeb and Smith, 1980; Barenkamp et al., 1982).

The lipopolysaccharide of *H. influenzae* is similar to the endotoxin of enteric bacilli with regard to composition and biological properties (see Chapter 6).

METABOLISM. Haemophilus organisms grow very poorly on ordinary laboratory media. The hemophilic nature of these bacteria is due to their inability to carry out the biosynthesis of either one or two substances present in blood cells (as well as in most other cells). The two growth factors were first recognized as a heat-stable substance referred to as the *X-factor* and a heat-labile substance referred to as the *V-factor*. The requirement for these factors has been used for the definition of the genus as well as for its internal subdivision into species. *H. influenzae* thus requires both X- and V-factors for growth, whereas most other species require only one (Table 1).

Both X- and V-factors are vital in the metabolism and growth of living cells. The X-factor is used in the biosynthesis of respiratory cytochromes and has been identified as hematin or certain precursors. The V-factor, which is involved in oxidation-reduction processes, can be replaced by one of the two co-dehydrogenases, NAD or NADP.

Optimal growth occurs in rich media to which the two growth factors have been added. The growth on ordinary blood agar is very poor, since only the X-factor is directly available to the bacteria in satisfactory quantities. Both growth factors may be liberated into the medium either by peptic digestion of the blood (Fildes medium) or by briefly

Table 1. PRINCIPAL DIFFERENTIAL CHARACTERISTICS AND PRIMARY HABITAT OF THE COMMON SPECIES OF THE GENUS *HAEMOPHILUS*[a]

	X-Factor Required	V-Factor Required	Hemolysis	Indole	Glucose, Acid	Sucrose, Acid	Lactose, Acid	Xylose, Acid	Nitrate Reduction	CO_2 Required	Primary Habitat
H. influenzae	+	+	−	d[b]	+	−	−	+	+	−	pharynx
H. haemolyticus	+	+	+	d	+	−	−	+	+	−	pharynx
H. ducreyi	+	−	−	−	−	−	−	−	+	−	(genital organs)
H. parainfluenzae	−	+	−	−	+	+	−	−	+	−	oral cavity and pharynx
H. parahaemolyticus	−	+	+	−	+	+	−	−	+	−	oral cavity and pharynx
H. aphrophilus	d	−	−	−	+	+	+	−	+	+	oral cavity
H. paraphrophilus	−	+	−	−	+	+	+	−	+	+	oral cavity

[a]Ref.: Kilian, 1976.
[b]d = differences observed

Table 2. BACTERIAL SPECIES POSSESSING ANTIGENS CROSS-REACTIVE WITH THE CAPSULAR/POLYSACCHARIDE OF *H. INFLUENZAE* TYPE bb

Baccillus alvei
Bacillus pumilus
Escherichia coli K 100
Lactobacillus plantarum
Staphylococcus aureus
Staphylococcus epidermidis
Streptococcus faecalis
Streptococcus pneumoniae types 6, 15a, 29, 35a
Streptococcus pyogenes (group A)

Refs.: Alexander, 1965; Argaman et al., 1974; Bradshaw et al., 1971.

heating the medium (chocolate agar and Levinthal's medium).

Various microorganisms (e.g., staphylococci) excrete the V-factor and may support the growth of haemophili on media deficient in this growth factor. This satellite phenomenon, which is illustrated in Figure 2, is widely used for the demonstration of this growth requirement.

All *Haemophilus* species reduce nitrate, and all, except for *H. ducreyi*, are heterofermentative. In addition to the requirement for growth factors, fermentation reactions and other biochemical characteristics are useful for the identification of the *Haemophilus* species (Table 1).

PATHOGENIC PROPERTIES

H. influenzae. *H. influenzae* is the most important *Haemophilus* species in human medicine. From a clinical point of view the species may be divided into two groups: 1) capsulated strains of serotype b, which cause several serious infectious diseases, usually associated with bacteremia; and 2) noncapsulated strains and capsulated strains of other serotypes than type b, which are implicated in various surface infections of mucous membranes.

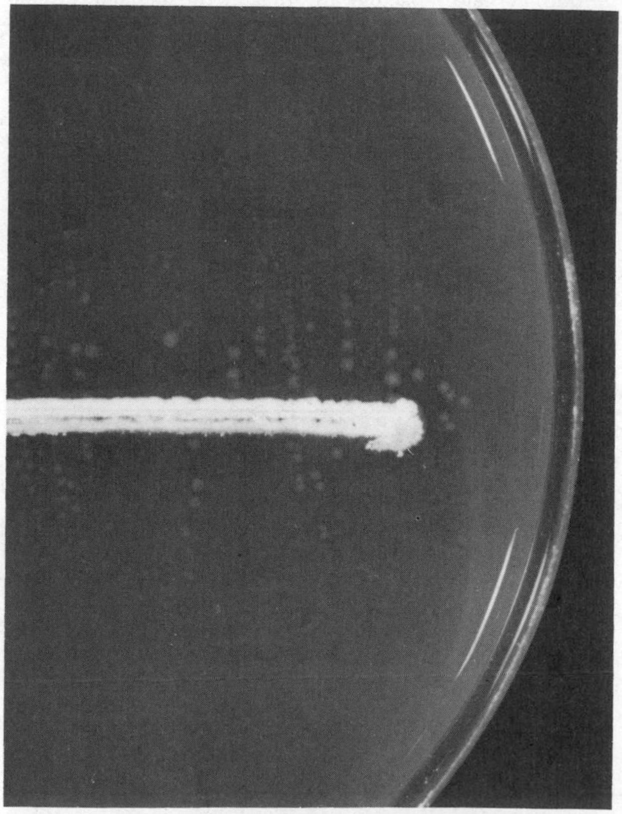

Figure 2. Satellite phenomenon: Colonies of *H. influenzae* growing on an agar plate cross-inoculated with a staphylococcus. The agar medium is autoclaved blood agar that lacks the V-factor.

H. influenzae serotype b is among the three leading causes of bacterial meningitis, the others being meningococci and the pneumococci. *H. influenzae* meningitis is more strictly a disease of early childhood than the two other forms. About 80 per cent of all cases occur between the age of 2 months and the end of the 3rd year (Fig. 3). Adults are rarely affected.

Epiglottitis is another serious disease caused by *H. influenzae* serotype b. It is associated with bacteremia and results in an acute obstruction of the air passages due to swelling of the epiglottitis. It is less common than *Haemophilus* meningitis and the children affected are usually somewhat older.

Invasion of the bloodstream by *H. influenzae* (mainly serotype b) may result in suppurative arthritis, osteomyelitis, and pericarditis. Primary *H. influenzae* pneumonia occurs in all age groups but is uncommon (for review see Turk and May, 1967).

Noncapsulated strains of *H. influenzae* are frequently involved in surface infections of the mucous membranes of the respiratory tract and attached sinuses. In healthy individuals such organisms constitute a minor proportion of the bacteria inhabiting the upper respiratory tract mucosa. However, helped by preceding virus infections, allergic reactions, or dysfunctions, noncapsulated *H. influenzae* may become predominant and enter normally sterile locations. Typical results of such disturbances are otitis media, sinusitis, bronchitis, bronchiectasis, and acute exacerbations of cystic fibrosis.

With a similar pathogenesis noncapsulated *H. influenzae* may become implicated in conjunctivitis. The predisposing conditions are trachomatous or viral infections, or obstruction of the lacrimal duct. A closely related organism, *H. aegyptius* ("Koch-Weeks bacillus") is associated with a more acute, purulent, and contagious form of conjunctivitis. This disease occurs as seasonal endemics, especially in hot climates.

The known virulence factors of *H. influenzae* include the capsule, the endotoxin, a ciliostatic factor, and an IgAl protease.

The polysaccharide capsule protects the organism against phagocytosis in the absence of specific antibody. Serotype b strains appear to be the most invasive of the *H. influenzae* because their capsular polysaccharide is most effective in resisting the action of serum complement (Sutton et al., 1982).

An extracellular toxin-like factor with the ability to arrest the mobility of cilia of the respiratory mucosa has been detected in *H. influenzae*.

Strains of *H. influenzae* and *H. aegyptius* produce an extracellular protease capable of cleaving a specific peptide bond in the hinge region of subclass 1 of IgA, the principal mediator of specific immunity on mucous membranes. A similar IgAl protease is excreted by meningococci, pneumococci, and gonococci, and is likely to facilitate the colonization and penetration of these bacteria (for review see Kornfeld and Plaut, 1981; Kilian et al., 1983).

H. ducreyi. This organism was first described by Ducrey (1889) in purulent discharge from the venereal "soft chancre" or "chancroid." The organism is recognized as the etiologic agent of the disease. However, it is often isolated

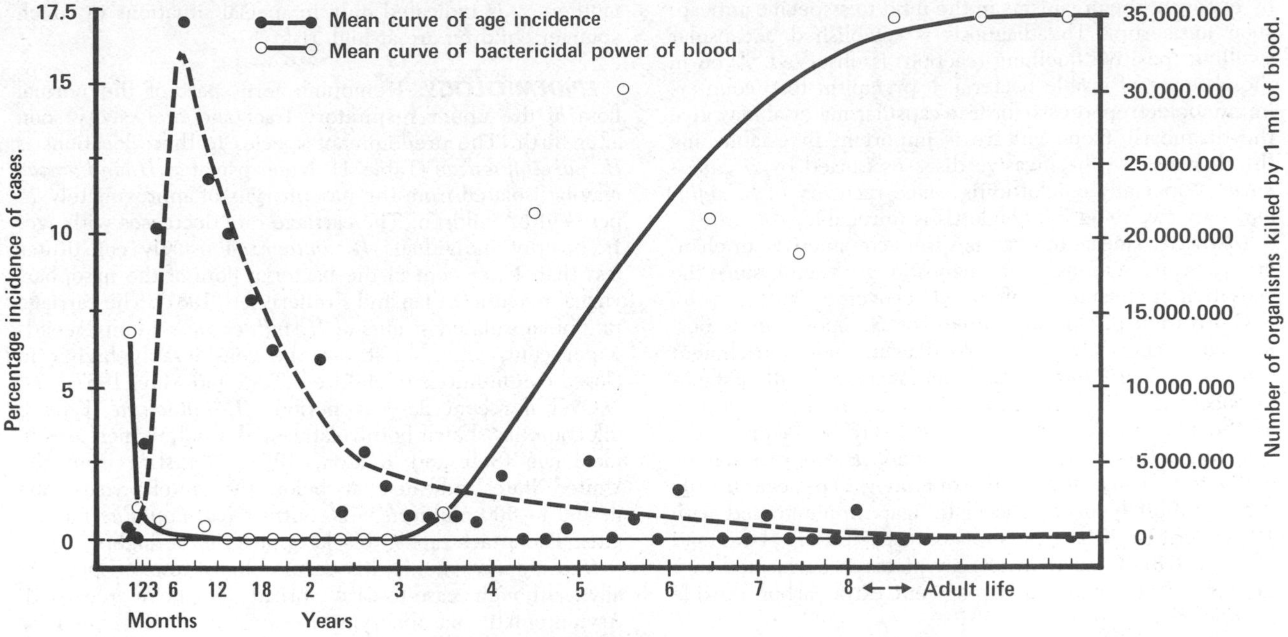

Figure 3. Relation of the age incidence of *H. influenzae* meningitis to bactericidal activity in the blood. (From Fothergill, L. D., and Wright, J.: J Immunol 24:281, 1933. © (1933) The Williams & Wilkins Co., Baltimore.)

together with poorly staining, gram-positive rods, which have been misidentified as *H. ducreyi*. In purulent material collected from ulcerative lesions or bubonic lymph nodes, the organism appears as chains of small gram-negative coccobacilli often located intracellularly.

Other Haemophilus Species. The species found indigenously in the oral cavity, *H. parainfluenzae*, *H. parahaemolyticus*, *H. aphrophilus*, and *H. paraphrophilus*, like other oral bacteria, occasionally cause subacute endocarditis and brain abscesses in predisposed patients (for review see Albritton, 1982). *H. haemolyticus* occurs in the healthy upper respiratory tract and is nonpathogenic. Colonies of β-hemolytic hemophili may be mistaken for those of hemolytic streptococci on blood agar.

IMMUNITY. The characteristic age distribution of *H. influenzae* meningitis was found to be inversely related to that of a serum bactericidal factor to that organism (Fig. 3). This finding suggests that immunity in the newborn is acquired from the mother transplacentally (IgG antibodies), is lost within the first months of life and then gradually restored by natural immunization during childhood. The age-related distribution of serum bactericidal activity depicted in Fig. 3 conforms closely to concentrations of antibodies against the serotype b capsule (polyribosylribitolphosphate, PRP) (Anderson et al., 1972, 1977).

Anti-PRP antibodies enhance phagocytosis of the organism, and protect against experimental *H. influenzae* serotype b meningitis in an infant rat model (Moxon, 1981; Gigliotti and Insel, 1982).

Surveys of the prevalence of *H. influenzae* serotype b carriage among infants and children suggest that exposure to this bacterium alone is insufficient to explain the acquisition of anti-PRP antibodies in most individuals aged more than 3 to 4 years (Sell et al., 1973). However, there is growing evidence that "natural" antibody, and hence protective immunity to *H. influenzae* serotype b infection, is acquired, in part, as a result of cross-reactive antigenic stimulation by members of the normal bacterial flora (Table 2).

Children with *H. influenzae* meningitis develop surprisingly low levels of anti-PRP antibodies (Norden et al., 1976). In patients under 2 years of age, an antibody response is even undetectable (Anderson et al., 1972; Sell and Karzon, 1973). This apparent failure of infants below the age of 2 years to respond to the serotype b capsular polysaccharide has also been observed in clinical trials with PRP vaccines (Peltola et al., 1977; Robbins et al., 1982).

In contrast to meningitis patients, children with epiglottitis react with high levels of antibody to the capsular antigen of *H. influenzae* Type b. The magnitude of the antibody response correlates with increasing age of the patients. Although the pathogenesis of the disease is largely unknown, the dramatic changes taking place in the epiglottis are likely to be a result of a local allergic reaction.

Acute sinusitis, otitis media, or bronchial infection due to noncapsulated *H. influenzae* strains results in significantly raised serum levels of complement-fixing antibodies against somatic antigens. This antibody response may be used as a diagnostic indicator (Turk and May, 1967).

Although the natural route of infection by *H. influenzae* starts at mucosal surfaces, the protective role of the secretory immune system is unknown. Systemic *H. influenzae* serotype b infection does induce detectable nasopharyngeal anticapsular antibody of the S-IgA class. However, the fact that *H. influenzae* can cleave IgAl antibodies may render this antibody response functionally insufficient.

LABORATORY DIAGNOSIS. Haemophili do not survive well in clinical specimens. Whenever possible a suitable transport medium should be used for transportation of swabs for throat or nose cultures or scrapings from the conjunctivae or chancroid lesions.

If gram-negative rods resembling *H. influenzae* are found in normally sterile material, such as cerebrospinal fluid or pleural fluid, an immediate diagnosis can be made by exposing the organisms in the fluid to a specific anticapsular antiserum. The diagnosis is established if capsular swelling (positive quellung-reaction) is observed. Even in the absence of visible bacteria, a precipitin test (counterimmunoelectrophoresis) for free capsular material may give the diagnosis. Blood culture is important in establishing the diagnosis of the invasive diseases caused by *H. influenzae*, especially epiglottiditis, since recovery of *H. influenzae* by swabbing the epiglottis is unreliable.

Likewise, smears of scrapings from conjunctivae or chancroid lesions, although not diagnostic, are useful, since the causative organisms are often not recovered.

Cultivation of clinical samples for *H. influenzae* is performed on chocolate (heated blood) agar, Fildes enrichment agar, or ordinary blood agar cross-inoculated with a staphylococcus (Fig. 2). For primary isolation from sources such as the respiratory tract, advantage may be taken of the selective action of bacitracin (300 mg/l). *H. ducreyi* may be cultivated on an agar medium containing 30 per cent freshly drawn rabbit blood or chocolate agar supplemented with 10 per cent Iso-Vitalex plus vancomycin 5 μg/ml (Hammond et al., 1978). Incubation of agar plates is performed in a mixture of air plus 5 to 10 per cent extra carbon dioxide (candle jar).

Identification of isolated strains is done by determining the growth factor requirements and by performing selected biochemical tests (Table 1). The V-factor requirement can be demonstrated by observing the satellite phenomenon, preferably on autoclaved blood agar. The X-factor requirement is difficult to determine on agar media, since most media contain small quantities of hematin. It is most clearly established by a biochemical detection of the in vitro ability of strains to carry out some of the steps involved in the biosynthesis of hematin (porphyrin test).

DRUG SUSCEPTIBILITY. Most Haemophilus strains are susceptible to penicillin and its derivatives, chloramphenicol, sulfonamides, trimethoprim, and the tetracycline group. These antibiotics have been extensively used to treat infections caused by these organisms. For the treatment of *Haemophilus* meningitis, chloramphenicol and ampicillin are particularly effective. However, since 1974 an increasing number of *Haemophilus* isolates have been found to be resistant to ampicillin due to plasmid-mediated β-lactamase production (Katz, 1975; Sykes et al., 1975). In some areas of the world with extensive use of antibacterial drugs, the prevalence of ampicillin resistance among *Haemophilus* strains is approaching 50 per cent. More recently, plasmid-mediated resistance against chloramphenicol and tetracycline have likewise been recorded. Some of the resistance plasmids in *H. influenzae* are closely related to R-plasmids in gonococci and enterobacteria (Laufs et al., 1979). Large plasmids coding for resistance to one to three antibiotics are transferable between strains of *H. influenzae* and between strains of *H. influenzae* and *Escherichia coli* by a conjugation-like mechanism (Thorne and Farrar, 1975; van Klingeren et al., 1977). The same transfer mechanism has been demonstrated in *H. ducreyi* (Brunton et al., 1979).

The choice of initial therapy in acute *Haemophilus* infections should depend on the prevalence of resistance to ampicillin and chloramphenicol in the particular area. Subsequent revision of the chemotherapy is done according to the results of the bacteriologic examination. Rifampin is sometimes used for eliminating *H. influenzae* serotype b from nasopharyngeal carriers. However, prophylactic chemotherapy is indicated only in special situations in which younger children are at high risk.

EPIDEMIOLOGY. Hemophili form part of the normal flora of the upper respiratory tract and oral cavity soon after birth. The predominant species in these locations is *H. parainfluenzae* (Table 1). Noncapsulated *H. influenzae* may be isolated from the nasopharynx of approximately 75 per cent of children. The carriage rate decreases with age. In healthy individuals *H. influenzae* usually constitutes less than 1 per cent of the bacterial flora of the nasopharyngeal mucosa (Kilian and Frederiksen, 1981). The carriage rate of capsulated strains of *H. influenzae* seldom exceeds 5 per cent, although it may be considerably higher in closed communities of children (Turk and May, 1967).

Over a recent 25-year period, *H. influenzae* Type b infection has shown both relative and absolute increases in incidence (Sell and Karzon, 1973). Statistics from the United States indicate that, before the age of 5 years, one in 400 to 500 children will contract *Haemophilus* meningitis. The attack rate in blacks appears to be higher.

Haemophilus meningitis occurs almost always sporadically, although case-to-case spread has been recorded. Asymptomatic nasopharyngeal carriage of *H. influenzae* Type b is common in homes in which *Haemophilus* meningitis occurs. It seems that the organism must pass through one or two partially immune contacts before it can cross the meningeal barrier.

The mortality rate of untreated *H. influenzae* meningitis is close to 90 per cent. Antimicrobial therapy reduced mortality dramatically, but deaths from meningitis remain a problem. In surviving patients, disabling and permanent central nervous system residua occur with high frequency.

Attempts to develop a vaccine against *H. influenzae* serotype b infections have been hampered by the low immunogenicity of PRP in infants. Current studies are testing the possibility of improving the immunogenicity of PRP through combinations with outer-membrane proteins or lipopolysaccharide of *H. influenzae*. PRP complexes with T-dependent carriers, such as the pertussis vaccine or a conjugate with diphtheria toxoid, are being investigated (Sell and Wright, 1982).

References

Albritton, W. L.: Infections due to *Haemophilus* species other than *H. influenzae*. Annu Rev Microbiol 36:199, 1982.

Alexander, H. E.: The Hemophilus group. In Dubos, R. J. (ed.): Bacterial and Mycotic Infections in Man. 3rd ed. Philadelphia, J. B. Lippincott Company, 1958, p. 470.

Anderson, P., Peter, G., Johnston, R., Jr., Wetterlow, L. H., and Smith, D. H.: Immunization of humans with polyribophosphate, the capsular antigen of *Hemophilus influenzae*, type b. J Clin Invest 51:39, 1972.

Anderson, P., Smith, D. H., Ingram, D. L., Wilkins, J., Wehrle, P. F. and Howie, V. M.: Antibody to polyribophosphate of *Haemophilus influenzae* type b in infants and children: Effect of immunization with polyribophosphate. J Infect Dis 136:57, 1977.

Argaman, M., Lui, T-Y., and Robbins, J. B.: Polyribitolphosphate: An antigen of four gram-positive bacteria cross-reactive with the capsular polysaccharide of *Haemophilus influenzae* type b. J Immunol 112:649, 1974.

Barenkamp, S. J., Munson, Jr., R. S., and Granoff, D. M.: Outer membrane protein and biotype analysis of pathogenic nontypeable *Haemophilus influenzae*. Infect Immun 36:535, 1982.

Bradshaw, M. W., Schneerson, R., Parke, F. C., and Robbins, B.: Bacterial antigens cross-reactive with the capsular polysaccharide of *Haemophilus influenzae* type b. Lancet 1:1095, 1971.

Brunton, J. L., MacLean, I., Ronald, A. R., and Albritton, W. L.: Plasmid mediated ampicillin resistance in *H. ducreyi*. Antimicrob Agents Chemother 15:294, 1979.

Fothergill, L. D., and Wright, J.: Influenzal meningitis: The relation of age-incidence to the bactericidal power of blood against the causal organism. J. Immunol 24:273, 1933.

Gigliotti, F. and Insel, R. A.: Protection from infection with *Haemophilus influenzae* type b by monoclonal antibody to the capsule. J Infect Dis 146:249, 1982.

Hammond, G. W., Lean, C. J., Wilt, S. C., and Ronald, A. R.: Comparision of specimen collection and laboratory techniques for the isolation of *Haemophilus ducreyi*. J Clin Microbiol 7:39, 1978.

Katz, S. L.: Ampicillin-resistant *Haemophilus influenzae* type b: A status report. Pediatrics 55:6, 1975.

Kilian, M.: A taxonomic study of the genus *Haemophilus*, with the proposal of new species. J Gen Microbiol 93:9, 1976.

Kilian, M. and Frederiksen, W.: Ecology of *Haemophilus*, *Pasteurella* and *Actinobacillus*. In: Kilian, M., Frederiksen, W. and Biberstein, E. L. (eds.): *Haemophilus*, *Pasteurella* and *Actinobacillus*. p. 11. London, Academic Press, 1981.

Kilian, M., Thomsen, B., Petersen, T. E. and Bleeg, H. S.: Occurrence and nature of bacterial IgA proteases. Ann NY Acad Sci 409:612, 1983.

Kornfeld, S. J. and Plaut, A. G.: Secretory immunity and the bacterial IgA proteases. Rev Infect Dis 3:521, 1981.

Laufs, R., Kaulfers, P.-M., Jahn, G. and Teschner, U.: Molecular characterization of a small *Haemophilus influenzae* plasmid specifying β-lactamase and its relationship to R factors from *Neisseria gonorrhoeae*. J Gen Microbiol 111:223, 1979.

Loeb, M. R. and Smith, D. H.: Outer membrane protein composition in disease isolates of *Haemophilus influenzae*: pathogenic and epidemiological implications. Infect Immun 30:709, 1980.

Michaels, R. H., Myerowitz, R. L., and Klaw, R.: Potentiation of experimental meningitis due to *Haemophilus influenzae* by influenza A virus. J Infect Dis 135:641, 1977.

Moxon, E. R.: Immunology of *Haemophilus influenzae* infections. In: Nahmias, A. J. and O'Reilly, R. J. (eds.): Immunology of human infections. Part I: Bacteria, mycoplasmae, chlamydiae, and fungi. p. 113, New York, Plenum Press, 1981.

Norden, C. W., Michaels, R. H., and Melish, M.: Serologic responses of children with meningitis due to *Haemophilus influenzae* type b. J Infect Dis 134:495, 1976.

Peltona, H., Kayhty, H., Sivonen, A. and Mäkela, H.: *Haemophilus influenzae* type b capsular polysaccharide vaccine in children: a double-blind field study of 100,000 vaccinees 3 months to 5 years of age in Finland. Pediatrics 60:730, 1977.

Pittman, M.: Variation and type specificity in the bacterial species *Haemophilus influenzae*. J Exp Med 53:471, 1931.

Robbins, J. B., Schneerson, R. and Parke, Jr. J. C.: A review of the efficacy trials with *Haemophilus influenzae* type b polysaccharide vaccines. In: Sell, S. H. and Wright, P. F. (eds.): Epidemiology, immunology and prevention of disease. p. 255, New York, Elsevier Biomedical, 1982.

Sell, S. H. W., and Karzon, D. T. (eds.): *Hemophilus influenzae*. Nashville, Vanderbilt University Press, 1973.

Sell, S. H. and Wright, P. F. (eds.): *Haemophilus influenzae*. Epidemiology, immunology and prevention of disease. New York, Elsevier Biomedical, 1982.

Shope, R. E.: Swine influenza: Experimental transmission and pathology, J. Exp Med 54:349, 1931.

Sutton, A., Schneerson, R., Kendall-Morris, S. and Robbins, J. B.: Differential complement resistance mediates virulence of *Haemophilus influenzae* type b. Infect Immun 35:95, 1982.

Sykes, R. B., Matthew, M., and O'Callaghan, C. H.: R-factor mediated β-lactamase production by *Haemophilus influenzae*. J Med Microbiol 8:437, 1975.

Thorne, G. M. and Farrar, Jr. W. E.: Transfer of ampicillin resistance between strains of *Haemophilus influenzae* type b. J Infect Dis 132:276, 1975.

Turk, D. C., and May, J. R.: *Hemophilus influenzae*. Its clinical importance. London, The English Universities Press Ltd., 1967.

Van Klingeren, B., van Embden, J. D. A. and Dessons-Kroon, M.: Plasmid-mediated chloramphenicol resistance in *Haemophilus influenzae*. Antimicrob Agents Chemother 11:383, 1977.

37

YERSINIA, PASTEURELLA, AND FRANCISELLA

T. H. Chen, M.D.

The new genus *Yersinia*, of the family Enterobacteriaceae, comprises the species Y. *pestis*, Y. *pseudotuberculosis*, and Y. *enterocolitica* (Bergey's Manual of Determinative Bacteriology, 1974). *Pasteurella* is now restricted to the type species *P. multocida* and a number of other closely related animal pathogens. *Francisella tularensis* is a species of another new genus, *Francisella*. These microorganisms are the causes of plague (*Y. pestis*), yersiniosis (*Y. pseudotuberculosis* and *Y. enterocolitica*), pasteurellosis (*P. multocida, P. haemolytica* et al.), and tularemia (*F. tularensis*). Although they are primarily rodent, other mammalian, and fowl parasites, they are also responsible for severe human infections.

Yersinia Pestis and Plague

MORPHOLOGY. *Yersinia pestis*, the causative agent of plague, was independently discovered by Kitasato and Yersin during the great epidemic in Hong Kong in 1894 (Bibel and Chen, 1976). The bacilli (small, oval, pleomorphic rods with rounded ends) are nonmotile and form no spores. They vary considerably in size (average 1.5 × 0.7 μm), stain readily with the basic aniline dyes, and are gram-negative. With the use of such stains as Wayson's, Giemsa's, and Gram's, the central part of the bacillus is often left colorless, yielding the so-called bipolar staining. Thus, the overall morphology of plague bacilli in a smear resembles a scattering of various sized "safety pins" (Fig. 1). In cultures grown at 37° C, envelopes can be demon-

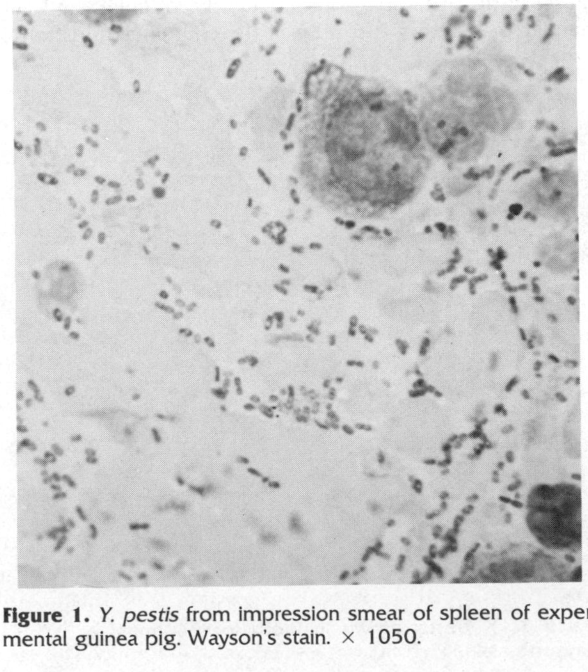

Figure 1. *Y. pestis* from impression smear of spleen of experimental guinea pig. Wayson's stain. × 1050.

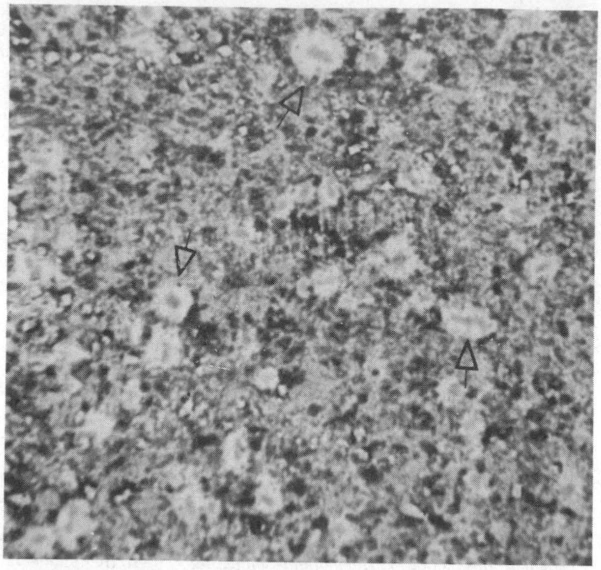

Figure 2. *Y. pestis* grown on blood agar at 37° C for 72 hours. India ink preparation. Note the envelope antigen around the organisms (arrows). × 1050.

strated by negative staining with India ink (Fig. 2). When the organisms are cultivated under suboptimal conditions (with media containing 2 to 4 per cent sodium chloride, i.e., "salt agar"), these involuted forms become very large and take on a striking diversity of shapes, becoming large globular, oval, or pyriform yeastlike bodies.

On blood agar plates *Y. pestis* grows well but slowly. The pinpoint, transparent colonies become gray and grossly visible after 48 hours and, following 72 hours of incubation, enlarge up to 3 to 4 mm in diameter. If growth is prolonged, particularly at lower temperatures, the colonies have a "fried egg" appearance. Those grown at 37° C for 72 hours, because of the gelatinous surface antigen (envelope) of this organism, are more abundant and have a stringy consistency when tested with a wire loop. In broth *Y. pestis* causes little turbidity, appears slightly granular, and collects at the bottom and sides of the container, illustrating

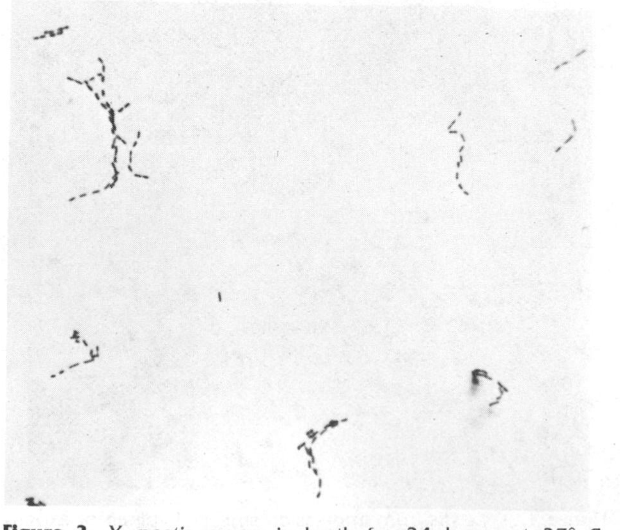

Figure 3. *Y. pestis* grown in broth for 24 hours at 37° C. Wayson's stain. × 1050.

its stalactiform growth property. A feathery vortex can be seen when the culture is gently shaken. In smears from young broth cultures, the bacilli generally emerge in chains, sometimes of considerable length, exhibiting a streptobacillary configuration (Fig. 3).

METABOLISM. Although biochemical tests are not used extensively to identify this microorganism, they may help to distinguish it from other species of *Yersinia* (Buchanan and Gibbons, 1974) (Table 1). The two most important distinctive characteristics of *Y. pestis* are (1) slower alkali production from nitrogenous constituents than other species of *Yersinia* and (2) no hydrolysis of urea. Thus this strain, cultivated on deoxycholate citrate agar plates for 48 hours at 37° C, grows scantily in reddish, pinpoint colonies while the medium retains its original pink hue. *Yersinia pseudotuberculosis* bacilli, in contrast, grow plentifully within this period of time in large opaque colonies that (like the medium in general) become yellow. *Yersinia pestis* grows in urea medium without hydrolyzing it. The urease of *Y. pseudotuberculosis* strains reddens the urea medium within 24 hours (Thal and Chen, 1955).

ANTIGENIC COMPOSITION. *Yersinia pestis* contains at least 19 different antigenic components recognizable by gel diffusion and/or biochemical methods (Albizo and Surgalla, 1970; Chen, 1965; Chen, 1972), 15 of which are shared by the closely related *Y. pseudotuberculosis*. Some of these 19 antigenic constituents of *Y. pestis* have been isolated in pure form, and five components (Fraction 1, the V and W antigens, exotoxin, and endotoxin) correlate well or at least somewhat with immunogenic activity and virulence (see Pathogenic Properties later in this chapter), whereas the remainder bear little or no relationship to plague immunity and infection.

Fraction 1. Fraction 1 or "envelope antigen," which was first isolated in a highly purified state by Baker et al., 1974, is a principal antigen involved with both virulence and immunity. Envelope antigen consists of two serologically identical components, 1A and 1B, which appear to differ chemically only in respect to a carbohydrate moiety in the former and its absence in the latter. Bennett and Tornabene (1974) reported that the soluble Fraction 1 antigen of *Y. pestis* exists as aggregates more than 300,000 in molecular weight, and that each aggregate can be further separated into a single antigenic subunit of 15,000 to 17,000 MW by dissociation with 0.1 per cent mercaptoethanol in 0.25 per cent sodium dodecyl sulfate (SDS) at 95° C for 5 minutes. These subunits reaggregate into a variety of large structures upon removal of the SDS. Chen and Elberg (1977) have confirmed these physicochemical observations by scanning electron microscopy.

V and W. In 1956, Burrows and Bacon demonstrated that the virulent *Y. pestis* strain contains two additional antigens, designated V and W, which are not produced by most avirulent strains of *Y. pestis* (Burrows and Bacon, 1956). They believed that these components were responsible for the virulence of a strain. V antigen is a protein with a molecular weight of 90,000, and the W antigen is a lipoprotein of 145,000 MW. The titers of both antigens fall upon prolonged storage at 5° C or after lyophilization, but not upon storage at −20° C. Thus, V and W are unstable antigens.

PATHOGENIC PROPERTIES. Plague is a highly fatal disease with fever and enlarged suppurative lymph nodes

Table 1. COMPARISON OF THE PHYSICAL AND METABOLIC CHARACTERISTICS OF *YERSINIA* AND *P. MULTOCIDA*[a]

	Yersinia			
	Pestis	***Enterocolitica***	***Pseudo-tuberculosis***	**Pasteurella multocida**
Growth in MacConkey's	+	+	+	−
Growth at 5°C	−	⊕	−	−
Motile	⊖	+ (22°)	+ (22°)	−
Nitrate	+	+	+	+
Citrate	−	−	−	−
Oxidase	−	−	−	v
Indole	−	d	−	+
Urease	−	⊕	⊕	−
β-Galactosidase	+	+	+	−
Ornithine decarboxylase	−	⊕	−	+
Phenylalanine deaminase	·	−	−	·
Fermentations				
lactose	−	−	−	−
glucose	·	·	·	+
galactose	(+)	+	+	+
sucrose	−	⊕	−	+
rhamnose	v	−	+	−
salicin	v	−	+	−
inositol	·	·	·	−
sorbose	−	−	+	−
adenitol	−	−	+	−
esculin	+	⊖	+	−

[a] v, variable reaction; >50% of stains are +; circled reactions are most helpful in differentiating between species.

(buboes); occasionally septicemia and pneumonia also occur. In experimental plague, the term "virulence" defines the comparative lethality of different strains as measured in LD_{50}. Virulent strains have lower LD_{50} levels than avirulent strains. Low virulence resulting from repeated cultivation in artificial media will be restored to full virulence by passage through susceptible animals (guinea pigs), in which selection occurs and the nonvirulent organisms are killed by phagocytes.

The virulence determinants of a strain are complex and are associated with its specific antigens (see Antigenic Composition) and nutritional factors. In *Y. pestis*, the determinants of virulence consist of the capacity to (1) develop an elaborate envelope of Fraction 1 antigen, (2) produce V and W antigens, (3) synthesize a surface structure that permits absorption of hemin from the medium and pigments, (4) synthesize purines, (5) generate toxins, and (6) link the production of pesticin, coagulase, and fibrinolytic factors. The major functions of the six virulence determinants are as follows:

Fraction 1, V, and W. Fraction 1, a surface envelope antigen, protects organisms grown in vivo against phagocytosis (Chen and Meyer, 1954) so that they can multiply and induce fatal infection. However, certain non-enveloped strains that still produce V and W antigens retain considerable virulence. Indeed, it has been contended that these components are also responsible for virulence (Burrows and Bacon, 1956).

In an effort to clarify the relationship of Fraction 1 and V and W antigens to the virulence of *Y. pestis*, Donovan et al. (1961) studied the infectivity and lethality of two antigenically different strains, enveloped MP6 (wild strain, F+, V and W+), and nonenveloped M23 (mutant strain, F−, V and W+). They found that a single bacterium of the enveloped strain, intradermally injected, could cause fatal infection in the guinea pig. Nonenveloped strains, able to produce V and W antigens, lose their lethality but can maintain the capacity to establish infection (skin lesions, buboes, and fever); death does not ensue if the organism is injected in nontoxic dosages. Thus the strain possessing the envelope antigen would appear to be more virulent.

Further studies of the Fraction 1 and V and W antigens by Cavanaugh and Randall (1959) have elucidated the process of plague infection. Following the injection of bacilli in the phagocytosis-susceptible state from the blocked flea into a host (plague-blocked fleas contain nonenveloped [F−, V and W+] virulent *Y. pestis* because the organisms are grown at a temperature lower than 37° C), most organisms were ingested by polymorphonuclear leukocytes (PMN) and destroyed, while the minority, engulfed by monocytes, survived and multiplied. Later the pathogens were released in a well-enveloped form (F+, V and W+) that was resistant to phagocytosis by both PMN and monocytes. These phagocytosis-resistant, enveloped organisms establish fatal infection.

Janssen et al. (1963) found no strict correlation between virulence and the envelope antigen's ability to resist phagocytosis. The well-enveloped avirulent strains (F+, V and W−) were more resistant to ingestion by nonsessile phagocytes than nonenveloped strains that produced V and W antigens. Hence these authors concluded that the primary factors in determining the virulence of *Y. pestis* were, rather, the V and W antigens, which permit survival and multiplication of the organisms within the phagocytic cells (monocytes). Apparently the factors determining virulence are Fraction 1, associated with resistance to phagocytosis, and the V and W antigens, associated with the capacity for intracellular multiplication. In contrast, an avirulent (F+, V and W−) strain of *Y. pestis* cannot multiply extensively and is destroyed by phagocytic activity.

Pigmentation. Virulent strains grown on a defined medium ("pigmentation medium" containing hemin) (Jackson and Burrows, 1956) form dark brown (P+) colonies; others produce whitish or straw-colored (P−) colonies in the same medium. To demonstrate high virulence, both for guinea pigs and mice, it is insufficient for a strain to produce only Fraction 1 and V and W antigens (F+, V and W+); it must also be able to absorb hemin (P+) from the medium. Nonpigmented colonies consist of avirulent organisms. Loss of pigmentation will result in the loss of virulence. For example, the avirulent, living vaccine strain EV76 is F+, V and W+ but P−.

Purine. Many nutritional factors can differentiate virulent from avirulent *Y. pestis*. As noted above, fully virulent strains possessing the properties of F+, V and W+, and P+ must also synthesize purine (Pu+) to grow in the host. If a mutant strain derived from a fully virulent one loses the ability to synthesize purine (Pu−), a considerable loss of virulence and failure to produce disease result. However, if purine is injected into mice simultaneously with the bacilli, disease develops (Burrows, 1955).

Toxins. All of the fully virulent strains have produced toxins (Ts+), which are doubtless responsible for death from plague, suggesting that toxigenicity is a significant virulence determinant.

Two classes of toxins have been isolated and characterized from the plague bacillus. One, a soluble, heat-labile, formalin-sensitive exotoxin, is composed of two active proteins of toxin A (associated with the cytoplasmic membrane) and toxin B (within the cytoplasm) with molecular weights of 240,000 and 120,000, respectively (Montie et al., 1966). These two proteins are highly toxic for rats and mice: the LD_{50} is less than 1 μg in the mouse, as determined via the intravenous route (Ajl et al., 1958). The other, an insoluble, heat-stable lipopolysaccharide endotoxin contained in the cell wall (Albizo and Surgalla, 1970), has an intraperitoneal LD_{50} of about 500 μg in guinea pigs and mice and an intravenous LD_{50} of 32 μg in rabbits. Both the exotoxin and the endotoxin contribute to or account for death in plague, acting respectively on the peripheral vascular system to produce hemoconcentration and shock and on the spleen and liver to produce gross damage and endotoxic shock.

Yet many avirulent strains produce about the same amount or more toxin than the virulent strains (Englesberg et al., 1954); none are fatal, however, if the number of injected bacilli is below the toxic death level. Toxicity alone, then, is inadequate to render an organism virulent.

PCF Complex. Pesticin, a bacteriocin with *N*-acetylglucosaminidase activity, along with factors with coagulase and fibrinolytic activity, is correlated with virulence and apparently is linked on a plasmid (Ben-Gurion and Hertman, 1958; Beesley et al., 1967; Ferber and Brubaker, 1979).

In summary, the pathogenic properties of *Y. pestis* are complex. To cause fatal infection, a strain should possess all virulent features, i.e., F+, V and W+, P+, Ts+, Pu+, and PCF+. Absence of one or more factors will cause loss of virulence. Still, there are some strains with all of the known determinants of virulence that, surprisingly, remain not fully virulent. Perhaps the final determinant of virulence is the *quantity* in which these substances are present.

IMMUNITY. Those who recover from plague appear to be protected from a second attack or at least incur a milder form on reinfection. Antibodies to three of nineteen recognized antigens correlate well with immunity, and the remainder have no bearing on plague immunity. The three most important immunogens are Fraction 1, exotoxin, and endotoxin.

Antibodies in immunized animals cannot eradicate *Y. pestis* in the absence of phagocytic cells. In the blood of immune hosts, plague bacilli are more readily phagocytized than in the blood of the nonimmune because Fraction 1 antibodies act as opsonins. Antibody to Fraction 1 is the principal protective factor against plague in animals as well as in man, as concluded from the positive correlation found between Fraction 1 antibody (CF and PHA titers), the opsonocytophagic index, and resistance to virulent infection following immunization by Fraction 1. Phagocytosis by neutrophils and macrophages of virulent *Y. pestis* directly parallels the development of Fraction 1 antibodies. Immunity to *Y. pestis* infection ultimately depends upon the ability of the macrophage to inactivate and to resist cytotoxic effects of the intracellular organism. Factors other than antibody that are produced by a subpopulation of lymphocytes from spleens of specifically immunized animals are essential for this macrophage function (Wong and Elberg, 1977).

Albizo and Surgalla (1970) isolated and purified the endotoxin and showed that endotoxin can contribute significantly to death in plague. Rabbits can be immunized and develop monospecific antibody that reacts with *Y. pestis* endotoxin. This antitoxin has a curative value, despite the fact that the antitoxic antibodies of exotoxin and endotoxin are not considered essential for serotherapy. Only in near-terminal cases, or when excessive antibiotic therapy may have caused the lysis of numerous bacilli, is antitoxin needed to neutralize the toxin.

Prevention of plague by vaccination has been practiced since the advent of the Haffkine vaccine in 1897. Thereafter, many investigators developed various vaccines, which were prepared as (1) killed broth cultures of *Y. pestis*, (2) chemically inactivated, agar-grown cultures of *Y. pestis*, (3) certain antigenic fractions of *Y. pestis*, or (4) live, attenuated plague strains. At present, the recommended regimen of immunization consists of administering two intramuscular injections, one month apart, of 1×10^9 formalin-killed plague bacilli preserved with phenol in physiologic saline (0.5 ml), followed by a booster dose of 4×10^8 bacilli (0.2 ml) 4 to 12 weeks after the second dose. Measurable levels of antibody can be maintained by booster inoculations given at intervals of not less than six months apart. When administered parenterally, attenuated live *Y. pestis* in repeated revaccinations has been effective during interepidemic periods (Payne et al., 1956). Severe local and systemic reactions have occurred, however, and there is no proof of the efficacy of this vaccine in preventing pneumonic plague. Oral administration of live attenuated EV76 (Paris) F vaccine is efficacious against both bubonic and pneumonic plague in the very susceptible vervet (*Cercopithecus aethiops*) (Chen et al., 1976, 1977). Thus the prospect that an oral, live, avirulent vaccine will be effective for human immunization is promising.

LABORATORY DIAGNOSIS. The clinical diagnosis of plague must be confirmed by conventional bacteriologic procedures. Smears from bubo aspirates, sputum, and blood should be stained with Gram's stain and also with Wayson's reagent. The direct smear should show gram-negative bipolar staining bacilli. A pure culture may be obtained after 48 to 72 hours from such material, with the use of the blood agar plate and infusion broth tube. *Yersinia pestis* grows slowly on blood agar, requiring 48 hours for macroscopic visibility, especially at 37° C. Touched with a wire loop, the 72-hour-growth colonies exhibit some stickiness. *Yersinia pestis* is nonmotile and never displays turbidity in standing broth culture tubes. A feathery vortex can be seen when the tube is gently shaken. Confirmation can also be achieved by specific bacteriophage lysis at 20° C. At a temperature of 37° C, but not 20° C, this phage can also lyse *Y. pseudotuberculosis*. Passive hemagglutination (PHA) is the most specific and sensitive serologic procedure (Chen and Meyer, 1954, 1966). Positive results can usually be obtained after about five to seven days of illness. Enzyme-linked immunosorbent assay (ELISA) and radioimmunoassay (RID) techniques with Fraction I antigen for serodiagnosis do not surpass conventional PHA in reliability, simplicity and economy. Although ELISA and RID attain higher titers and detect class-specific antibody for determining the time-frame of infection, they are more useful for research than clinical diagnosis (Hill and Matsen, 1983).

Inoculation of the plague specimens into mice and guinea pigs produces bacteremia and death within two to seven days. The appearance of the bacilli in these animals, combined with the pathologic changes induced by the infection, helps identify *Y. pestis*. Direct fluorescent antibody techniques allow screening of the cultures and detection of the organisms in infected material (Moody and Winter, 1959) (Fig. 4). Assay for isocitrate lyase gives uniformly positive results for *Y. pestis* but consistently negative findings for other *Yersinia* species and rarely all *Enterobacteriaceae* and pseudomonads (Hillier and Charnetzky, 1981).

DRUG SUSCEPTIBILITY. *Yersinia pestis* is susceptible to sulfonamides and antibiotics, including streptomycin, tetracycline, kanamycin (Cantey, 1974), and chloramphenicol. Trimethoprim-sulfamethoxazole is at least as active in vivo and in vitro as streptomycin and chloramphenicol (Nguyen Van Ai et al., 1972a, b).

EPIDEMIOLOGY. Plague, primarily a naturally occuring disease of rodents and mammals, infects over 200 species of wild rodents, which are frequently incriminated hosts for *Y. pestis* (Pollitzer and Meyer, 1961). Humans may become victims of the disease through an aberrant interruption of the rodent-flea-rodent sequence or through the handling of infected animals. Usually bubonic plague in humans is transmitted by a bite from fleas (*Xenopsylla cheopis*, rat flea; *Diamanus montanus*, squirrel flea; *Pulex irritans*, human flea) that have previously sucked blood from a plague-infected animal or human. Plague bacilli (as many as 10^7/ml) are present in rat blood during the acute stage, and the flea becomes infected by feeding on the diseased rat (Douglas and Wheeler, 1943). As ingested bacilli multiply in the midgut of the flea, massive infection eventually blocks the proventriculus to the extent that little or no blood can pass. During feeding, some bacilli mix with the blood of the new host and are regurgitated into the wound of the bite, transmitting about 25,000 to 100,000 bacilli. Thus, under natural conditions, transmission from rodent to rodent or human is always mediated by infected fleas. Generally the bubonic form proceeds to the secondary pneumonic form and may lead to person-to-person "droplet" transmission of primary pneumonic plague without the insect vector.

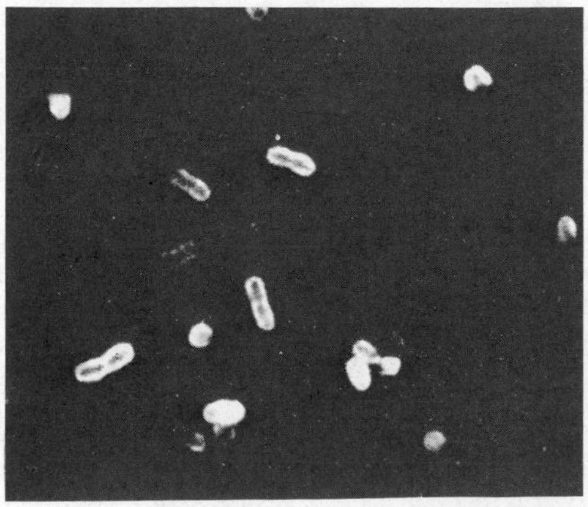

Figure 4. Smear of *Y. pestis* strain 195/P stained with fluorescent Fraction I specific antibody. × 1000. (From Quan, S. F., et al., Am J Trop Med Hyg14:424, 1965.)

The most prevalent vector species for transmitting plague is *Xenopsylla cheopis*, the rat flea, because of its longevity as a reservoir of plague bacilli and the more frequent impediment of its proventriculus than in other types of fleas. Infected fleas can sometimes survive for 396 days (Pollitzer and Meyer, 1961), suggesting that possibly fleas carry infection from one epizootic season to another, even in the absence of definitive hosts. The human flea, *Pulex irritans*, is a relatively ineffective vector but can transmit plague from person to person under certain circumstances. *Diamanus montanus*, the common squirrel flea, is also an important vector and is a far more serious threat in introducing plague into rat populations in rural and perhaps urban areas (Meyer and Holdenride, 1949). The danger of human plague in an area can be measured by the "flea index" (the average number of fleas per rat). An *X. cheopis* index of at least 3 appears to prevail during epidemics.

Plague now occurs in Central and South Africa, South America, and Asia. In the United States, rural plague has been discovered in ground squirrels, prairie dogs, jack rabbits, voles, pack rats, and other animals in 15 states. A minimum of 50 rodent species is involved in enzootic and epizootic plague (Meyer, 1965). Under natural conditions, camels, sheep, coyotes, deer, dogs, and cats can contract plague infection, either by feeding on infected carcasses or, as in the case of dogs and cats, by acting as mechanical conveyances transporting the infected fleas to their owners (Christie et al., 1980; Rollag et al., 1981). One hundred thirty-nine cases were recognized in the United States from 1973 to 1982, all acquired from areas of wilderness in the enzootic western states (Center for Disease Control, 1983).

The incidence of plague continues to decline only because the epidemics are under control, rather than because the disease has been eradicated. It is now, in fact, firmly established in endemic foci. Plague is still a potential danger, due to the vast areas of wilderness in which infection persists and the increasing use of wilderness areas for recreational purposes.

Yersinia Pseudotuberculosis and Yersiniosis

MORPHOLOGY. *Yersinia pseudotuberculosis*, a pleomorphic, coccoid-appearing, oval or rod shaped microorganism, is gram-negative and measures 0.8 to 6.0 × 0.8

μm. Some strains disclose bipolar staining with Wayson's stain. Neither spores nor definite capsules are detectable, but at 22° C a viscous layer may be visible in India ink preparations. When cultured between 20 and 30° C, the organism is motile, and examination by scanning electron microscopy reveals peritrichous flagella (Fig. 5) (Chen and Elberg, 1977).

METABOLISM. A facultative anaerobe, *Yersinia pseudotuberculosis* ferments the sugars in Table 1 to acid (but no gas). It has both a urease and a β-galactosidase. It can be distinguished from *Y. enterocolitica* and *Y. pestis* by its fermentation of adonitol (Table 1).

ANTIGENIC COMPOSITION. The multiplicity of antigens in *Y. pseudotuberculosis* is exemplified by the variety of somatic (O) antigens present in different strains. Fifteen somatic and five flagellar (H) antigens have been defined by Thal and Knapp (1971), and a diagnostic antigenic scheme of 6 serotypes (I to VI) based on type-specific thermostable somatic O antigens has been proposed. In diagnostic work it is sufficient to identify the O group.

Many of the antigenic components of *Y. pseudotuberculosis* are shared with those of *Y. pestis*. Indeed, extensive investigation of the antigenic structure of both *Yersinia* species has revealed 17 antigenic components, 15 of which are common to both (Burrows and Bacon, 1956, 1960; Lawton et al., 1960; Larrabee et al., 1965). A protein-lipopolysaccharide complex, protective factor (PF), has been isolated from avirulent *Y. pseudotuberculosis* type IV and *Y. pestis* strains (Lawton and Surgalla, 1963). Burrows and Bacon (1960) demonstrated that only newly isolated *Y. pseudotuberculosis* strains also produce V and W antigens identical to those of *Y. pestis*. (The importance of these two antigens is discussed in the preceding section on the antigenic composition of *Y. pestis*.)

Exotoxins have been isolated mainly in group III strains of *Y. pseudotuberculosis*, although they may also be found in some other groups. Despite the fact that each of these exotoxins is unique, they are immunologically identical (Thal, 1954, 1966).

Certain O antigens of *Y. pseudotuberculosis* are related to *Salmonella* antigens, and group II and IV strains can be agglutinated by sera from patients infected with *Salmonella*.

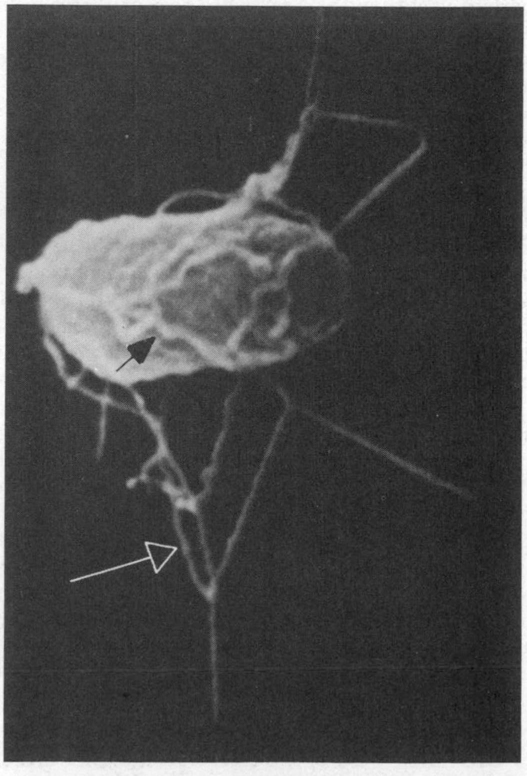

Figure 5. *Y. pseudotuberculosis* Type I bacillus cultured at 22° C for 48 hours. Note the prominent flagella (arrows). Scanning Electron Micrograph. × 43,000. (From Chen, T. H., and Elberg, Sanford S.: Infect Immun 15:972, 1977.)

PATHOGENIC PROPERTIES. In man, *Y. pseudotuberculosis* causes diarrhea, lymphadenopathy with necrosis, and septicemia, and may be severe and even fatal. Generally, however, the human disease is localized to the mesenteric lymph nodes and commonly has a benign course. Intracellular survival and reproduction contributes to its virulence (Besednova et al., 1975). A plasmid has been associated with the formation of V and W antigens and pathogenicity (Gemski et al., 1980).

IMMUNITY. Immunization against yersiniosis caused by *Y. pseudotuberculosis* has been of wide interest because this pathogen is intimately related antigenically to *Y. pestis* (see Antigenic Composition). Guinea pigs recovered from yersiniosis become immune to reinfection, and active immunity in these animals can be induced by inoculation with suspensions of avirulent, live Type IV strain 32 *Y. pseudotuberculosis* (Thal, 1962). Such immunization will also protect them from infection with *Y. pestis*. Yet guinea pigs so immunized or recovered from *Y. pestis* remain susceptible to yersiniosis. The relationship of the PF antigen to plague and yersiniosis immunity is still unclear. Injection of PF antigen protects guinea pigs as early as the first day by increasing nonspecific resistance to infection. Anti-*Y. pestis* serum usually agglutinates a variety of strains of *Y. pseudotuberculosis*, and anti-*Y. pseudotuberculosis* R serum also reacts with nonenveloped *Y. pestis* strains.

LABORATORY DIAGNOSIS. The diagnosis of yersiniosis is confirmed by isolating *Y. pseudotuberculosis* from the affected blood, liver, spleen, lymph nodes, or feces, or by demonstrating the presence of specific antibodies in the serum. *Y. pseudotuberculosis* is easily cultured in ordinary media. Specimens should be processed by direct culture on plate and by the cold enrichment method using phosphate buffered saline. The cold enrichment cultures are held for at least 4 weeks at 4° C and should be subcultured once weekly on solid media (e.g., MacConkey's agar, Salmonella-Shigella agar) at 35° C for isolation (Oberhofer and Podgore, 1980). The smooth phase produces a uniform turbidity in broth and a sediment after 24 hours. The rough phase strains grow without generating turbidity. On solid media, transparent colonies reach diameters of 0.5 to 1.0 mm in 24 hours. The pathogen grows abundantly in large opaque colonies on deoxycholate citrate agar, whereas *Y. pestis* grows scantily in reddish pinpoint colonies (Thal and Chen, 1955).

Biochemical and growth characteristics also should be assayed (Table 1). The commercial specific typing sera containing agglutinins for types of *Y. pseudotuberculosis* will not agglutinate *Y. pestis*. Likewise, *Y. pseudotuber-*

culosis bacteriophage will lyse all strains of this organism but will not lyse *Y. pestis*. Further, *Y. pestis* phage will lyse *Y. pseudotuberculosis* at 37° C but not at 22° C. For these reasons, two sets of cultures should be prepared for incubation at two different temperatures (Gunnison et al., 1951). The two simple media that are used to differentiate plague and *Y. pseudotuberculosis* bacilli, namely urea and deoxycholate citrate agar, are extremely useful (Thal and Chen, 1955). *Yersinia pseudotuberculosis* grown below 30° C, but not at 37° C, is motile.

DRUG SUSCEPTIBILITY. *Yersinia pseudotuberculosis* is sensitive to chloramphenicol, kanamycin, tetracycline, and streptomycin, and some strains are sensitive to penicillin or ampicillin.

EPIDEMIOLOGY. Rodents and birds constitute the primary reservoirs of yersiniosis. Mice and rats, although apparently resistant to natural infection, shed the organisms for weeks in their urine and feces. Thus the resistant rodents may be the carriers and would seem to play an important epidemiologic role in spreading the disease (Mair, 1973).

Yersinia pseudotuberculosis inhabits a diversity of mammals, which are probably the main sources of most human infections. Evidence indicates that the strains isolated from man and animals possess the same cultural, biochemical, and pathologic characteristics. Most human cases can be attributed to contact with or ingestion of contaminated food and drinking water, and the consistent involvement of the abdominal organs in this disease also suggests that transmission may be oral.

Yersinia Enterocolitica and Yersiniosis

MORPHOLOGY. *Yersinia enterocolitica* was originally isolated at autopsy from abscesses in two cases of human septicemia (Hässing et al., 1949). The microorganism is a gram-negative, facultative anaerobe of oval or coccoid shape with dimensions of 0.5 to 1.0 × 1.0 to 3.0 μm. Capsules (envelope) may be present in some strains and/or clinical specimens. The bacterium is easily grown on both blood agar and selective media. Its temperature relationships are characteristic: Peritrichous flagella are demonstrated when it is cultivated at 25° C. Although the optimal temperature for growth is 30° to 37° C, *Y. enterocolitica* multiplies less rapidly at this range than other enteric pathogens. The outstanding temperature feature of the organism useful for differentiation is its ability to replicate readily at low temperatures (4° C). Refrigeration in 2 per cent peptone water of the specimen (from feces or lymph nodes) results in selective enrichment. Upon primary isolation, this bacterium produces smooth colonies, 0.5 to 2.0 mm in diameter, that in subculture often exhibit R forms. When cultivated in broth, either turbidity or a pellicle with clear supernatant and sediment is visible.

METABOLISM. *Yersinia enterocolitica* can be distinguished from *Y. pestis* and *Y. pseudotuberculosis* by its fermentation of sucrose, cellobiose, and sorbose and its production of ornithine decarboxylase. Also fermented are arbutin, galactose, and sorbitol, forming acid without gas. β-galactosidase (o-nitrophenol-B-D-galactoside) and, in some biotypes, indole is synthesized. Acetoin is produced at 25° C, especially in fresh isolates, but absent at 37° C and often after numerous subcultures. Urease is not evident at 25° C but is clearly found in cultures grown at 37° C; subculturing promotes expression. Certain atypical rhamnose-fermenting or sucrose-negative strains have been isolated, and may constitute new species (Brenner et al., 1976).

ANTIGENIC COMPOSITION. Thirty-four different O antigens have been established in *Y. enterocolitica* (Wauters et al., 1972). In 1973 Knapp and Thal proposed a revision of the serologic scheme on the basis of only six O-antigen groups. Serotype O:9 cross-reacts with *Brucella abortus* (Ahvonen, 1969). The cross-reacting antigens were isolated by hot phenol-water extraction of the respective bacteria and identified as lipopolysaccharides. Presently, six K antigens of the envelope have been described, some of which are related to fimbriae. H antigens, associated with motility, number at least 19. However, as motility is dependent on temperature and biotype, this serology still needs improvement (Wauters, 1981). V and W antigens of *Y. enterocolitica* are immunologically identical to those of *Y. pestis* and *Y. pseudotuberculosis* (Carter et al., 1980).

PATHOGENIC PROPERTIES. Pathogenicity in *Y. enterocolitica* is complex with major strain variation in virulence factors; no current single assay correlates with virulence. Invasiveness has been demonstrated in HeLa cell culture (Lee et al., 1977; Une, 1977). Other tests include conjunctivitis in the guinea pig (Sereny reaction) and mucosal penetration of the rabbit or mouse ileum (Carter, 1975; Une and Zen-Yoji, 1979; Robbins-Browne et al., 1979; Feeley et al., 1979). Enterotoxin, a heat-stable, mercaptoethanol-inactivated substance of 10,000 daltons, is produced in vitro only at temperatures below 30° C (Pai and Mors, 1978; Pai et al., 1978; Okamoto et al., 1982). Its minimal effective dose in suckling mice is 25 ng. The enterotoxin resembles that of *Escherichia coli*, but although common in nearly all isolates, its role in pathogenicity, indeed its synthesis in vivo, is yet unknown (Schiemann, 1981). Plasmids mediate dependence on calcium, survival in serum, conjunctivitis, and pathogenicity in white mice (Heesemann et al., 1983). The production of V and W antigens has been linked with plasmids of 40 to 48 megadaltons (Gemski et al., 1980; Bolin et al., 1982). Iron enhances virulence in certain serotypes. In vitro, iron neutralizes the bactericidal property of serum (Robins-Browne et al., 1979); an accidental overdose of iron in two children preceded septicemia of *Y. enterocolitica* type O:3 (Melby et al., 1982). Laird and Cavanaugh (1980) found that only virulent strains of *Yersiniae* autoagglutinate in tissue culture media at 36° C (but not at 26° C). The mechanism and correlative principle are yet undetermined.

IMMUNITY. Maximal antibody titers are demonstrable in patients by the agglutination test within one or two weeks, declining within two months. Carter et al. (1979) protected mice against intravenously inoculated *Yersinia* by vaccination with heat-killed cells of the same strain. Serum, but not splenic cells, could transfer this immunity to normal mice. Delayed hypersensitivity was not manifested after recovering from infection. Immune serum produced enhanced phagocytosis in vitro. Contrary to that observed in human infection with *Y. enterocolitica* O:3 (Robins-Browne et al., 1979), serotype O:8 is resistant to killing by mouse antibody and complement (Carter et al., 1979).

LABORATORY DIAGNOSIS. *Yersinia enterocolitica* has been confirmed as the causative infection by isolation of organisms from the affected blood, urine, feces, mesenteric lymph nodes, appendices (Pai et al., 1982), wounds, abscesses, or demonstrating the presence of specific antibodies in the serum, the latest method being enzyme-linked immunosorbent assay (ELISA) (Granfors, 1979). The cold enrichment technique by which specimens are held in phosphate-buffered saline or broth at 4° C for 3 weeks improves cultural isolation of *Y. enterocolitica* in convalescent and asymptomatic subjects (van Pee and Stragier, 1979; Pai et al., 1979). The *Yersinia* species, *enterocolitica* and *pseudotuberculosis*, can be differentiated by their biochemical reactivity, bacteriophage susceptibility, but apparently no longer by pathogenicity for laboratory animals. Whereas *Y. enterocolitica* was once considered nonpathogenic for mice, guinea pigs, and rabbits by subcutaneous, intraperitoneal, or intravenous injection (Knapp and Thal, 1963) and *Y. pseudotuberculosis* pathogenic for all these animals, some North American strains of *Y. enterocolitica* have now been found to be lethal for mice and gerbils (Carter et al., 1973; Quan et al., 1974; Carter, 1975). Both species are motile at 22° C, but not at 37° C.

Because of cross-reacting antibodies, yersiniosis and brucellosis are indistinguishable by the agglutination and complement fixation tests, a situation that has caused great confusion in brucellosis eradication work in cattle. The two diseases can now be differentiated, however, by electroimmunoassay (Huewell, 1975); an H agglutination test, since *Brucella* is not motile (Mittal and Tizard, 1979); and an ELISA procedure (Lindberg et al., 1982).

DRUG SUSCEPTIBILITY. Most strains of *Y. enterocolitica* are sensitive to polymyxin, gentamicin, kanamycin, chloramphenicol, streptomycin, and cefotaxime (Goldstein et al., 1982).

EPIDEMIOLOGY. Apparently *Y. enterocolitica* is distributed worldwide. Reservoirs of this organism are extensive, and it has been isolated from sick and healthy animals, both wild and domestic. Common sources include livestock, especially swine (Asakawa et al., 1979; Schiemann and Fleming, 1981), dogs and cats, cage birds and pigeons, deer, rodents, mink, and chinchilla. Isolates have been obtained also from fruit and vegetables and from fresh water and drinking water (Harvey et al., 1976; Eden et al., 1977); fish may harbor the bacterium. The peak infectious periods of autumn and winter have been linked to a waterborne route, the cold water temperature being conducive to growth and selection. However, strong evidence implicates contaminated food as the major source of human infections. Milk products were incriminated in two recent epidemics in New York State (Black et al., 1978; Shayegani et al., 1983).

Serotype O:8 is common in the United States, O:3 and O:5 in Japan, O:9 in northern Europe, and O:3 in Canada. The last group has been rare in the United States despite the common border and high frequency of population and trade movement. This situation may be changing; serogroup O:3 apparently is becoming established in New York City (Bottone, 1983). Serotypes from wild animals tend to differ from those in human infections, but O:8 strains have been detected recently in the United States in a natural reservoir, pigs (Doyle et al., 1981). One study has associated flies in the mechanical spread of the bacterium from farm yard to kitchen (Fukushima et al., 1979).

Pasteurella Multocida and Pasteurellosis

MORPHOLOGY. *Pasteurella multocida* is an ellipsoid gram-negative rod or a coccobacillus, ranging from 1.0 to 1.8 × 0.3 to 0.5 μm in size with bipolar-staining capsules (when present), which are best demonstrated by negative staining, as with India ink or Giemsa's stain. *Pasteurella multocida* is nonsporogenous and nonmotile at both 22 and 37° C. Its optimal growth temperature is 37° C. Small, nonhemolytic, gray colonies form on blood agar, but most nonhemolytic strains create a brownish discoloration in the blood medium. Broth cultures of smooth or mucoid strains are evenly turbid, while the rough strain produces floccular or granular deposits.

METABOLISM. *Pasteurella multocida* is an aerobe (or facultative anaerobe) that will not grow on MacConkey's agar. It produces acid from galactose, mannose, and sucrose, and most strains ferment mannitol, sorbitol, and xylose (lactose is not fermented). Indole and H_2S are also usually produced, as well as ornithine decarboxylase. The organism is urease-negative and catalase-positive.

Pasteurella haemolytica is quite similar to *Pasteurella multocida* but can be differentiated by its ability to grow in media with bile salts (MacConkey's agar), its hemolysin, and its failure to produce indole.

ANTIGENIC COMPOSITION. *Pasteurella multocida* has both capsular polysaccharide and somatic lipopolysaccharide antigens, which can be used to serotype the pathogen. The antigenic structure correlates with strain virulence and host susceptibility (Collins, 1977). Bain (1955) and Dhanda (1960) both isolated a mouse-protective protein antigen from some of their strains of *P. multocida*. On the basis of the capsular antigen, Carter (Carter and Annau, 1953; Carter, 1972a), using the indirect hemagglutination (IHA) test, separated *P. multocida* into four serotypes (A to D). Later, a new type (E) was added (Carter, 1961, 1963) and type C was discarded, narrowing the serotypes to A, B, D, and E.

Pasteurella multocida also contains a number of smooth, somatic, lipopolysaccharide antigens. The rapid agglutination test (Carter, 1972b) has been used for subtyping strains classified in the same capsular serotype category. The arabic numeral is utilized for the specific somatic antigen, followed by a capital letter designating the capsular antigen. So far, 12 specific O antigens have been identified, e.g., 1:A, 3:A, 11:B (Namioka and Bruner, 1963; Chengappa et al., 1982).

Endotoxins and their component lipopolysaccharides have been isolated from whole cells and cell walls. They are toxic for mice and pyrogenic in rabbits (Bain and Knox, 1961). Type E lipopolysaccharide is antigenic for rabbits, and mice can be passively immunized with this antiserum (Perreau and Petit, 1963).

PATHOGENIC PROPERTIES AND IMMUNITY. *Pasteurella multocida* represents an animal parasite of considerable economic and veterinary importance, especially to cattlemen and fowl ranchers (Collins, 1977). It is so highly pathogenic for mice and rabbits that only one to ten cells of a smooth or mucoid variant usually kill a mouse. Infrequently, it may be found in the throats of healthy people (Smith, 1959), and under conditions of stress or debilitation of the host, the parasite, previously benign, may penetrate beneath the mucous membrane and cause disease. Most infections take one of three clinical patterns: local infection by cat scratch or animal bite, respiratory tract infection, or systemic infections such as meningitis and bacteremia. Serotype A strains may be correlated with respiratory infections by their 10-fold higher ability to adhere to the mucosa of the nasopharynx by fimbriae (Glorioso et al., 1982).

Agglutinins in the sera of patients with generalized infection can be detected by hemagglutination. (Normally, no antibodies are present in the patient with a localized wound infection.) It is not known if these antibodies are bactericidal or antitoxic, although evidence indicates that the immunity is humorally mediated (Collins, 1973). Domestic animals (cattle) and birds (poultry) are often immunized with a killed vaccine conveying protection against pasteurellosis. Viable, attenuated, oral vaccines have also proved effective in turkeys and chickens. No vaccine exists for humans.

LABORATORY DIAGNOSIS. Specimens from infected wounds, nasal secretions, sputum, pleural or spinal fluid, blood and post-mortem tissues should be placed on 5 per cent blood agar. Pure cultures can be further identified as *P. multocida* by their inability to grow on MacConkey's agar, biochemical reactions, lack of motility at both 22 and 37° C, sensitivity to penicillin, and high pathogenicity for mice. Bacteriophage can also be used for identification of *P. multocida* (Gadberry and Miller, 1977).

DRUG SUSCEPTIBILITY. *Pasteurella multocida* is inhibited by drugs at the following average concentrations (μg/ml): chloramphenicol (1.5), tetracycline (3.0), penicillin (0.4), and erythromycin (3.1). Chang and Carter (1976), studying the multiple drug resistance of *P. multocida* and *P. hemolytica*, observed that penicillin and tetracycline are not consistently effective. Chloramphenicol proved most efficacious; only 4 of 403 isolates were resistant to this drug.

EPIDEMIOLOGY. *Pasteurella* species can survive for only a short time outside the host; thus, the reservoir of infection is probably a healthy carrier. Mammals, birds, and people can be reservoirs for *P. multocida*. Human infections are acquired from animal bites, and 15 per cent of cat bites and dog bites treated in United States and Russian hospitals have yielded positive cultures of *P. multocida* (Francis et al., 1975). Most respiratory and septicemic infections occur in farmers. Most human isolates are Serotype A or D (Carter, 1962, 1984). On occasion, the organism is discovered in the throats of healthy individuals exposed to infected animals (Smith, 1959), so the possibility of interhuman spreading by nasopharyngeal excretions, urine, and feces must be considered (Hubbert and Rosen, 1970). *Pasteurella multocida* may remain in the host for a long time, later asserting its pathogenic properties when resistance to the infection diminishes. In animals, pasteurellosis has been characterized as a disease of debility. In fact, stress in livestock during transportation is responsible for the illness known as "shipping fever."

Francisella Tularensis and Tularemia

In 1911, McCoy, exploring plague in California ground squirrels, discovered a disease characterized by lesions similar to those of plague. The following year, he and Chapin isolated the causative organism of this plaguelike disease by means of coagulated egg yolk medium and named it *Bacterium tularense*, after Tulare County, California. After previous assignment to several genera, this organism is now known by its own genus name, *Francisella*, in honor of Francis, a pioneer investigator of the disease in humans (Francis, 1921a, b), who infelicitously termed it "tularemia" to indicate its ability to cause septicemia.

MORPHOLOGY. *Francisella tularensis* is small and aerobic, measuring 0.2 × 0.2 to 0.7 μm. A gram-negative, nonmotile, noncapsular, nonspore-forming bacillus, it is highly pleomorphic, often appearing as a rod or coccus and always singly. The bacterium forms minute, transparent droplike colonies on blood-glucose-cystine agar. Colonies may reach a diameter of 4 mm after two to five days of incubation and are readily emulsified. They require more cystine than is present in the ordinary nutrient medium.

METABOLISM. The optimal growth temperature of *F. tularensis* is 37° C. Most strains ferment glucose, maltose, mannose, fructose, and dextrose, creating acid without gas. The organism is grown in medium containing cystine or cysteine and produces H_2S.

ANTIGENIC COMPOSITION. Several strains of *F. tularensis* have been studied by serologic methods, but no immunologic types have emerged. Agglutinins appear during the 2nd and 3rd weeks of illness and reach a peak two or three months after infection. Cross-reactions with *Brucella melitensis* and *B. abortus* do occur, but rising titers for *F. tularensis* in the convalescent phase will confirm this infection.

Treatment of aqueous suspensions of *F. tularensis* with ethyl ether yields an ether-soluble, immunogenic antigen that protects mice from death following challenge with more virulent strains of *F. tularensis* (Larson, 1945; Bell et al., 1952). Up to 23 antigenic factors have been determined by comparative immunoelectrophoresis of combined ether, ethanol, and water extracts (Holm et al., 1980). Ether-water extracts of strain SCHU S4 from stationary-phase, liquid-grown, saline suspensions have been demonstrated to stimulate better antibody formation in rabbits than antigens obtained by other chemical procedures. Thus they provide a good crude antigenic mixture for further purification and the production of related monospecific antisera (Nutter, 1971).

PATHOGENIC PROPERTIES. *Francisella tularensis* is a facultative, intracellular parasite that may persist for many years in the organs (Carr and Kadull, 1957). Direct human contact with infected vertebrates and the discharges or bites of arthropods (deerflies and ticks) generally evoke tularemia. The persistent immune response and the occasional tendency of the disease toward relapse and chronicity are probably attributable to prolonged intracellular survival.

Jellison (1970) and Russian scientists have observed two types of *F. tularensis* that differ in virulence and biochemical reactions but not antigenically. The highly virulent strains, mainly isolated in North America, can kill mice, guinea pigs, and rabbits (Bell et al., 1955). They are usually isolated from tick-borne tularemia in rabbits. They utilize glycerol and produce citrulline ureidase. One to 100 of these highly virulent bacilli produce necrotic nodules of the lung, spleen, and liver. The low-virulence strains kill rabbits only when the dose is at least 5×10^9 organisms; they do not utilize glycerol or generate citrulline ureidase. This type is primarily associated with rodents; it may also be transmitted by ticks but is frequently associated with water and occurs in both the western and eastern hemispheres. It has been reported that *F. tularensis* yields both a heat-labile toxin and an endotoxin (Landay et al., 1968).

IMMUNITY. An attack of tularemia confers solid lifelong immunity. Agglutinins appear during the 2nd or 3rd week of illness and persist for years. A live, attenuated strain of *F. tularensis* has been used to immunize both animals and people and has afforded significant protection against the pathogen (Eigelsbach and Downs, 1961). In the United States, live vaccine in volunteers protected 10 of 14, whereas the cell wall antigen and the killed vaccine protected few or none against intracutaneous or respiratory-route challenge infection (McCrumb, 1961; Saslaw et al., 1961a, b). Burke (1977), in an effort to determine the incidence of tularemia in laboratory workers, compared the number of individuals vaccinated with the phenol-killed Foshay vaccine and those given the live, avirulent vaccine and demonstrated that the live vaccine was more protective; the incidence of typhoidal tularemia fell from 5.70 to 0.27 cases per 1000, whereas the incidence of ulceroglandular tularemia remained constant, although the clinical signs and symptoms were much milder than in those vaccinated with the killed vaccine. At present, vaccination with the live, attenuated vaccine is indicated only for persons at high risk, such as laboratory workers.

Francisella tularensis induces both humoral and cell-mediated immune responses. With membranes or whole bacteria as antigen, T lymphocytes from vaccinated individuals were stimulated to transform to blast cells. The reaction was macrophage dependent (Tarnvik and Hom, 1978; Koskela and Herva, 1982).

LABORATORY DIAGNOSIS. A definitive diagnosis of tularemia is usually achieved by a combination of bacteriologic, serologic, and animal inoculation methods. *F. tularensis* cannot be grown in ordinary media but thrives on coagulated egg yolk, enriched blood glucose-cystine agar, and thioglycollate broth. It can be isolated from sputum, pharyngeal exudate, scrapings, and biopsy material from local lesions or gastric washings when it is cultured on specific media, such as blood-glucose-cystine agar, or when guinea pigs are inoculated. Enriched media with incorporated antibiotics (penicillin, 100,000 U/ml; polymyxin B sulfate, 100,000 U/ml; and cycloheximide, 0.1 mg/ml) may be of value when clinical specimens harboring normal flora are cultured for *F. tularensis*. Colonies may appear in two to four days and should be identified by the rapid slide agglutination test with specific antiserum. For fast screening of cultures and detection of the organism in infected material, it is possible to use the Dieterle spirochete stain (Gallivan et al., 1980) or preferably fluorescent antibody techniques (Yager et al., 1960). Cultures should be incubated for two weeks before being discarded as negative, and culture plates should be enclosed in polyethylene bags to reduce desiccation during the prolonged incubation period. It is also of value to determine the dependence of the organism upon special media (the possible requirement for extra cystine or sulfhydryl compound) for growth.

Guinea pigs, mice, and hamsters die with characteristic lesions two to seven days after subcutaneous or intraperitoneal inoculation of *F. tularensis*. Animal inoculation is particularly valuable when the specimen is contaminated with other organisms that tend to overgrow *F. tularensis* in culture. At autopsy there is hemorrhagic edema at the site of inoculation and whitish necrotic lesions of the liver, spleen, lung, and bone marrow, yielding positive cultures.

Berdal and Søderlund (1977) observed that specimens grown on selective chocolate agar (containing 7.7 μg/ml colistin, 12.5 μg/ml nystatin, 0.5 μg/ml lincomycin, and 5 μg/ml trimethoprim lactate) at 37° C in 5 per cent CO_2 for two to three days gave rise to smooth colonies of *F. tularensis*, 0.1 to 1.0 mm in diameter, in cultures that were either pure or only slightly contaminated. Thus, the selective chocolate agar medium might be a practical supplement to non-selective media.

Agglutinins appear during the 2nd or 3rd week of illness and reach peak titer at two to three months. Only rising titers are indicative of recent infection, since previous infections with the same or other organisms can cause detectable antibody titers which may persist for years. Cross-reactions with *Brucella* immune sera may occur, but they can be distinguished by comparative agglutination tests performed with antigens of both species, since the homologous titers are much higher than the heterologous ones. The enzyme-linked immunosorbent assay, which can be more than 10-fold as sensitive as the tube agglutination procedures, can be of diagnostic use by detecting rising titers after the first week of illness (Carlsson et al., 1980).

Delayed hypersensitivity reactions to the tularemia skin test may be an early diagnostic aid because the positive reaction may be obtained during the first week of illness (Buchanan et al., 1971).

DRUG SUSCEPTIBILITY. *Francisella tularensis* is susceptible to streptomycin, kanamycin, tetracycline, chloramphenicol, and gentamicin (Mason et al., 1980).

EPIDEMIOLOGY. Tularemia is a sporadic disease, largely limited to lagomorphs (rabbits, hares) and rodents in certain areas of enzootic infection. Humans are an accidental end host. Human infections have been traced to a broad variety of sources, including ectoparasites, vertebrates, aerosols and contaminated water. *Francisella tularensis*, originally isolated from California ground squirrels in 1912, has since been found in innumerable species of wild animals (muskrats, beavers, woodchucks, water rats, voles, skunks, deer, dogs, cats, and rabbits) throughout North America and primarily in Europe, Russia, Turkey, and Japan. The insects that are most significant in the transmission of tularemia and that keep the infection active in vertebrates are lice, mites, and ticks (Meyer, 1965).* The propagation

**Haemaphysalis leporispalustris*, rabbit tick; *Amblyomma americanum*, Lone Star tick; *Dermacentor andersoni*, common wood tick; *D. variabilis*, dog tick; *Chrysops discalis*, bloodsucking deerfly.

of *F. tularensis* in nature depends upon the wood tick and dog tick, feeding on cottontail and jack rabbits and many other rodents. Animals naturally infected with *F. tularensis* can therefore serve as reservoirs.

In the United States, there are two distinct types of tularemia, the highly virulent and the low-virulent forms. The former is tick-borne from the rabbit; the low-virulent, rodent form is contracted from water contaminated by water rats. Low-virulent strains growing in water and mud can infect muskrats and then trappers. Tularemia in humans, however, is largely transmitted by direct contact with the blood or other tissue fluids of infected rodents. Vector-borne tularemia in the United States, mainly conveyed by ticks and deerflies (Boyce, 1975), has a mortality rate of 7.5 per cent in untreated cases.

References

Yersinia pestis

Ajl, J., Jr., Rust, J., Jr., Hunter, D., Woebke, J., and Bent, D. F.: Preparation of serologically homogeneous plague murine toxin and its reactions with physical, chemical and enzymatic agents. J Immun 80:435, 1958.

Albizo, J. M., and Surgalla, M. J.: Isolation and biological characterization of *Pasteurella pestis* endotoxin. Infect Immun 2:229, 1970.

Baker, E. E., Somer, H., Foster, L. E., Meyer, E., and Meyer, K. F.: Antigenic structure of *Pasteurella pestis* and the isolation of a crystalline antigen. Proc Soc Exp Biol Med 64:139, 1947.

Ben-Gurion, R., and Hertman, I.: Bacteriocin-like material produced by *Pasteurella pestis*. J Gen Microbiol 19:289, 1958.

Bennett, L. G., and Tornabene, T. G.: Characterization of the antigenic subunits of the envelope protein of *Yersinia pestis*. J Bacteriol 117:48, 1974.

Beesley, E. D., Brubaker, R. R., Janssen, W. A., and Surgalla, M. J.: Pesticins III. Expression of coagulase and mechanism of fibrinolysis. J Bacteriol 94:19, 1967.

Bibel, D. J., and Chen, T. H.: Diagnosis of plague: An analysis of the Yersin-Kitasato controversy. Bacteriol Rev 40:633, 1976.

Buchanan, R. E., and Gibbons, N. E. (eds.): Bergey's Manual of Determinative Bacteriology. 8th ed. Baltimore, The Williams & Wilkins Company, 1974.

Burrows, T. W.: The basis of virulence for mice of *Pasteurella pestis*. *In* Mechanisms of Microbial Pathogenicity. Fifth Symposium of the Society for General Microbiology. Cambridge, Cambridge University Press, 1955, p. 152.

Burrows, T. W., and Bacon, G. A.: The basis of virulence in *Pasteurella pestis*. An antigen determining virulence. Br J Exp Pathol 37:481, 1956.

Burrows, T. W., and Bacon. G. A.: V and W antigen in strains of *Pasteurella pseudotuberculosis*. Br J Exp Pathol 41:38, 1960.

Cantey, J. R.: Plague in Vietnam. Clinical observation and treatment with kanamycin. Arch Intern Med 133:280, 1974.

Cavanaugh, D. C., and Randall, R.: The role of multiplication of *Pasteurella pestis* in mononuclear phagocytes in the pathogenesis of fleaborne plague. J Immunol 83:348, 1959.

Christie, A. B., Chen, T. H., and Elberg, S. S.: Plague in camels and goats: Their role in human epidemics. J Infect Dis 141:724, 1980.

Center for Disease Control: Annual Summary 1982. Morbid Mortal Weekly Rep 3:142, 1983.

Chen, T. H.: The antigenic structure of *Pasteurella pestis* and its relationship to virulence and immunity. Acta Trop (Basel) 22:97, 1965.

Chen, T. H.: The immunoserology of plague. In Kwapinski, J. B. (eds.): Research in Immunochemistry and Immunobiology. Vol. 1. Baltimore, University Park Press, 1972, p. 223.

Chen. T. H., and Elberg, S. S.: Scanning electron microscopic study of virulent *Yersinia pestis* and *Yersinia pseudotuberculosis* Type I. Infect Immun 15:972, 1977.

Chen, T. H., Elberg, S. S., and Eisler, D. M.: Immunity in plague: Protection induced in *Cercopithecus aethiops* by oral administration of live, attenuated *Yersinia pestis*. J Infect Dis 133:302, 1976.

Chen, T. H., Elberg, S. S., and Eisler, D. M.: Immunity in plague: Protection of the vervet (*Cercopithecus aethiops*) against pneumonic plague by the oral administration of live attenuated *Yersinia pestis*. J Infect Dis 135:289, 1977.

Chen, T. H., and Meyer, K. F.: Studies on immunization against plague. VII. A hemagglutinin test with the protein fraction of *Pasteurella pestis*: A serologic comparison of virulent and avirulent strains with observations on the structure of the bacterial cells and its relationship to infection and immunity. J Immunol 72:282, 1954.

Chen, T. H., and Meyer, K. F.: An evaluation of *Pasteurella pestis* Fraction-I-specific antibody for the confirmation of plague infections. Bull WHO 34:911, 1966.

Donovan, J. E., Han, D., Fukui, G. M., and Surgalla, M. J.: Role of the capsule of *Pasteurella pestis* in bubonic plague in the guinea pig. J Infect Dis 169:154, 1961.

Douglas, J. R., and Wheeler, C. M.: Sylvatic plague studies. II. The fate of *Pasteurella pestis* in the flea. J Infect Dis 72:18, 1943.

Englesberg, E., Chen, T. H., Levy, J. B., Foster, L. E., and Meyer, K. F.: Virulence in *Pasteurella pestis*. Science 119:413, 1954.

Ferber, D. M., and Brubaker, R. R.: Mode of action of pesticin: N-acetylglucosaminidase activity. J Bacteriol 139:495, 1979.

Hill, H. R., and Matsen, J. M.: Enzyme-linked immunosorbent assay and radioimmunoassay in the serologic diagnosis of infectious diseases. J Infect Dis 147:258, 1983.

Hillier, S. L., and Charnetzky, W. T.: Rapid diagnostic test uses isocitrate lyase activity for identification of *Yersinia pestis*. J Clin Microbiol 13:661, 1981.

Jackson, S., and Burrows, T. W.: The pigmentation of *Pasteurella pestis* on a defined medium containing hemin. Br J Exp Pathol 37:570, 1956.

Janssen, W. A., Lawton, W. D., Fukui, G. M., and Surgalla, M. J.: The pathogenesis of plague: A study of the correlation between virulence and relative phagocytosis resistance of some strains of *Pasteurella pestis*. J Infect Dis 113:139, 1963.

Meyer, K. F.: *Pasteurella* and *Francisella*. In Dubos, R. J., and Hirsch, J. G. (eds.): Bacterial and Mycotic Infections. 4th ed. Philadelphia, J. B. Lippincott Company, 1965, p. 659.

Meyer, K. F., and Holdenride, R.: Rodents and fleas in a plague epizootic in a rural area of California. Puerto Rico J Public Health Trop Med 24:201, 1949.

Montie, T. C., Montie, D. B., and Ajl, S. J.: A comparison of the characteristics of two murine-toxic proteins from *Pasteurella pestis*. Biochim Biophys Acta 130:406, 1966.

Moody, M. D., and Winter, C. C.: Rapid identification of *Pasteurella pestis* with fluorescent antibody. III. Staining *Pasteurella pestis* in tissue impression smears. J Infect Dis 104:288, 1959.

Nguyen Van Ai, Nguyen Duc Hanh, Pham Van Dien, and Nguyen Van Le: Action *in vitro* and *in vivo* of trimethoprim-sulfamethoxazole on *Yersinia pestis*. Bull Soc Pathol Exot 65:759,1972a.

Nguyen Van Ai, Nguyen Duc Hanh, Pham Van Dien, and Nguyen Van Le: Successful treatment of bubonic and septicaemic plague by trimethoprim-sulfamethoxazole. Preliminary note. Bull Soc Pathol Exot 65:770, 1972b.

Payne, F. E., Smadel, J. E., and Courdurier, J.: Immunologic studies on persons residing in a plague epidemic area. J Immunol 77:24, 1956.

Pollitzer, R., and Meyer, K. F.: The ecology of plague. In May, J. M. (ed.): Studies in Disease Ecology. New York, Hafner Publishing Company, 1961, p. 433.

Rollag, O. J., Skeels, M. R., Nims, L. J., Thilsted, J. P., and Mann, J. M.: Feline plague in New Mexico: Report of five cases. J Am Vet Med Assoc 179:1381, 1981.

Thal, E., and Chen, T. H.: Two simple tests for the differentiation of plague and pseudotuberculosis bacilli. J Bacteriol 69:103, 1955.

Wong, J. F., and Elberg, S. S.: Cellular immune response to *Yersinia pestis* modulated by product(s) from thymus-derived lymphocytes. J Infect Dis 135:67, 1977.

Yersinia pseudotuberculosis

Besednova, N. N., Timchenko, N. F., Gorshknova, R. P., and Somov, G. P.: An interaction of the causative agent of pseudotuberculosis with the peritoneal macrophages of the immune and nonimmune organism. Zh Mikrobiol Epidemiol i Immunobiol (10):39, 1975.

Burrows, T. W., and Bacon, G. A.: The basis of virulence in *Pasteurella pestis*. An antigen determining virulence. Br J Exp Pathol 37:481, 1956.

Burrows, T. W., and Bacon, G. A.: V and W antigens in strains of *Pasteurella pseudotuberculosis*. Br J Exp Pathol 41:38, 1960.

Chen, T. H., and Elberg, S. S.: Scanning electron microscopic study of virulent *Yersinia pestis* and *Yersinia pseudotuberculosis* Type I. Infect Immun 15:972, 1977.

Gemski, P., Lazere, J. R., Casey, T., and Wohlhieter, J. A.: Presence of a virulence-associated plasmid in *Yersinia pseudotuberculosis*. Infect Immun 28:1044, 1980.

Gunnison, J. B., Larson, A., and Lazarus, A. S.: Rapid differentiation between *Pasteurella pestis* and *Pasteurella pseudotuberculosis* by action of bacteriophage. J Infect Dis 88:254, 1951.

Larrabee, A. R., Marshall, J. D., and Crozier, D.: Isolation of antigens of *Pasteurella pestis*. I. Lipopolysaccharide-protein complex and R and S antigens. J Bacteriol 90:116, 1965.

Lawton, W. D., Fukui, G. W., and Surgalla, M. J.: Studies on the antigens of *Pasteurella pestis* and *Pasteurella pseudotuberculosis*. J Immunol 84:476, 1960.

Lawton, W. D., and Surgalla, M. J.: Immunization against plague by a specific fraction of *Pasteurella pseudotuberculosis*. J Infect Dis 113:39, 1963.

Mair, N. S.: Yersiniosis in wildlife and its public health implications. J Wildlife Dis 9:64, 1973.

Oberhofer, T. R., and Podgore, J. K.: *Yersinia pseudotuberculosis*: Use of cold-temperature enrichment for isolation. J Clin Microbiol 11:106, 1980.

Thal, E.: Untersuchungen über *Pasteurella pseudotuberculosis* und besonderer Berücksichtigung ihres immunologischen Verhaltens. Nord Vet Med 6:829, 1954.

Thal, E.: Oral immunization of guinea pigs with avirulent *"Pasteurella pseudotuberculosis."* Nature 194:490, 1962.

Thal, E.: Immunobiologische Studien an *Yersinia pseudotuberculosis* (Syn. *Pasteurella pseudotuberculosis*). Schweiz Arch Tierheilkd 108:372, 1966.

Thal, E., and Chen, T. H.: Two simple tests for the differentiation of plague and pseudotuberculosis bacilli. J Bacteriol 69:103, 1955.

Thal, E., and Knapp, W.: A revised antigenic scheme of *Yersinia pseudotuberculosis*. Symp Ser Immunobiol Stand 15:219, 1971.

Yersinia enterocolitica

Ahvonen, P., Janssen, E., and Aho, K.: Marked cross-agglutination between *Brucellae* and a subtype of *Yersinia enterocolitica*. Acta Pathol Microbiol Scand 75:291, 1969.

Asakawa, Y., Akahane, S., Shiozawa, K., And Honma, T.: Investigations of source and route of *Yersinia enterocolitica* infection. (Karger, Basel). Contrib Microbiol Immunol 5:115, 1979.

Black, R. E., Jackson, R. J., Tsai, T., Medvesky, M., Shayegani, M., Feeley, J. C., Macleod, K., and Wakelee, A. M.: Epidemic *Yersinia enterocolitica* infection due to contaminated chocolate milk. N Engl J Med 298:76, 1978.

Bolin, I., Norlander, L., and Wolf-Watz, H.: Temperature-inducible outer membrane protein of *Yersinia pseudotuberculosis* and *Yersinia enterocolitica* is associated with the virulence plasmid. Infect Immun 37:506, 1982.

Bottone, E. J.: Current trends of *Yersinia enterocolitica* isolated in the New York city area. J Clin Microbiol 17:63, 1983.

Brenner, D. J., Steigerwalt, A. G., Falcao, D. P., Weaver, R. E., and Fannin, G. R.: Characterization of *Yersinia enterocolitica* and *Yersinia pseudotuberculosis* by deoxyribonucleic acid hybridization and by biochemical reaction. Int J Syst Bacteriol 26:180, 1976.

Carter, P. B., Varga, C. F., and Keet, E. E.: New strain of *Yersinia enterocolitica* pathogenic for rodents. Appl Microbiol 26:1016, 1973.

Carter, P. B.: Pathogenicity of *Yersinia enterocolitica* for mice. Infect Immun 11:164, 1975.

Carter, P. B., MacDonald, T. T., and Collins, F. M.: Host responses to infection with *Yersinia enterocolitica*. (Karger, Basel). Contrib Microbiol Immunol 5:346, 1979.

Carter, P. B., Zahorchak, R. J., and Brubaker, R. R.: Plague virulence antigen from *Yersinia enterocolitica*. Infect Immun 28:638, 1980.

Doyle, M. P., Hugdahl, M. B., and Taylor, S. L.: Isolation of virulent *Yersinia enterocolitica* from porcine tongues. Appl Environ Microbiol 42:661, 1981.

Eden, K. V., Rosenberg, M. L., Stoopler, M., Wood, B. T., Highsmith, A. K., Skaliy, P., and Wells, J. G.: Waterborne gastrointestinal illness at a ski resort. Isolation of *Yersinia enterocolitica* from drinking water. Public Health Rep 92:245, 1977.

Feeley, J. C., Wells, J. G., Tsai, T. F., and Puhr, N. D.: Detection of enterotoxigenic and invasive strains of *Yersinia enterocolitica*. (Karger, Basel). Contrib Microbiol Immunol 5:329, 1979.

Fukushima, H., Ito, Y., Saito, K., Tsubokura, M., and Otsubki, K.: Role of the fly in the transport of *Yersinia enterocolitica*. Appl Environ Microbiol 38:1009, 1979.

Gemski, P., Lazere, J. R., and Casey, T.: A plasmid associated with pathogenicity and calcium dependency of *Yersinia enterocolitica*. Infect Immun 27: 682, 1980.

Goldstein, E. J., Cherubin, C. E., Corrado, M. L., and Sierra, M. F.: Comparative susceptibility of *Yersinia enterocolitica, Eikenella corrodents*, and penicillin-resistant and penicillin-susceptible *streptococcus pneumoniae* to beta-lactam and alternative antimicrobial agents. Rev Infect Dis 4 Suppl Sept-Oct 1982.

Granfors, K.: Measurement of immunoglobulin M (IgM), IgG, and IgA antibodies against *Yersinia enterocolitica* by enzyme-linked immunosorbent assay: persistence of serum antibodies during disease. Clin Microbiol 9:336, 1979.

Harvey, S., Greenwood, J. R., Pickett, M. J., and Mah, R. A.: Recovery of *Yersinia enterocolitica* from streams and lakes of California. Appl Environ Microbiol 32:352, 1976.

Hässig, A., Karrer, J., and Pusterla, F.: Über Pseudotuberkulose beim Menschen. Schweiz Med Wohenschr 79:971, 1949.

Heesemann, J., Keller, C., Morawa, R., Schmidt, N., Siemens, H. J., and Laufs, R.: Plasmids of human strains of *Yersinia enterocolitica*: molecular relatedness and possible importance for pathogenesis. J Infect Dis 147: 107, 1983.

Hurwell, B.: Differentiation of cross-reacting antibodies against *Brucella abortus* and *Yersinia enterocolitica* by electroimmunoassay. Acta Vet Scan 16:318, 1975.

Knapp, W., and Thal, E.: Untersuchungen Über die Kulturell-biochemischen, serologischen, tierexperimentellen und immunologischen Eigenschaften einervorläufig *"Pasteurella* X" benannten Bakterienart. Zbl Bakt (Abt I. orid.) 190:472, 1963.

Knapp, W., and Thal, E.: Die biochemische Charakterisierung von *Yersinia enterocolitica* (Syn. *"Pasteurella* X") als Grumdlage eines vereinfachten O-Antigenschemas. Zol Bakt (Abt I, org.) 223:88, 1973.

Laird, W. J., and Cavanaugh, D. C.: Correlation of autoagglutination and virulence of *Yersiniae*. J Clin Microbiol 11:430, 1980.

Lee, W. H., McGrath, P. P., Carter, P. H., and Edie, E. L.: The ability of some *Yersinia enterocolitica* strains to invade HeLa cells. Can J Microbiol 32:1714, 1977.

Lindberg, A. A., Haeggman, S., Karlson, K., Carlsson, H. E., and Mair, N. S.: Enzyme immunoassay of the antibody response to *Brucella* and *Yersinia enterocolitica* 09 infections in humans. J Hyg 88:295, 1982.

Melby, K., Slordahl, S., Gutteberg, T. J., and Nordbo, S. A.: Septicaemia due to *Yersinia enterocolitica* after oral overdoses of iron. Br Med J 285:467, 1982.

Mittal, K. R., and Tizard, I. R.: A simple technique to differentiate between animals infected with *Yersinia enterocolitica* IX and those infected with *Brucella abortus*. Res Vet Sci 26:248, 1979.

Okamoto, K., Inoue, T., Shimizu, K., Hara, S., and Miyama, A.: Further purification and characterization of heat-stable enterotoxin production by *Yersinia enterocolitica*. Infect Immun 35:958, 1982.

Pai, C. H., and Mors, V.: Production of enterotoxin by *Yersinia enterocolitica*. Infect Immun 19:908, 1978.

Pai, C. H., Mors, V., and Toma, S.: Prevalence of enterotoxigenicity in human and nonhuman isolates of *Yersinia enterocolitica*. Infect Immun 22:334, 1978.

Pai, C. H., Sorger, S., Lafleur, L., Lackman, L., and Marks, M. L.: Efficacy of cold enrichment techniques for recovery of *Yersinia enterocolitica* from human stools. J Clin Microbiol 9:712, 1979.

Pai. C. H., Gillis, F., and Marks, M. I.: Infection due to *Yersinia enterocolitica* in children with abdominal pain. J Infect Dis 146:705, 1982.

Quan, T. J., Meek, J. L., Tsuchiya, K. R., Hudson, B. W., and Barnes, A. M.: Experimental pathogenicity of recent North American isolates of *Yersinia enterocolitica*. J Infect Dis 129:341, 1974.

Robins-Browne, R. M., van Vuuren, C. J. J., Still, C. S., Miliotis, M. D., and Koornhof, H. J.: The pathogenesis of *Yersinia enterocolitica* gastroenteritis. (Karger, Basel). Contrib Microbiol Immunol 5:324, 1979.

Robins-Browne, R. M., Rabson, A. R., and Koornhof, H. J.: Generalized infection with *Yersinia enterocolitica* and the role of iron. Contrib Microbiol Immunol 5:277, 1979.

Schiemann, D. A., and Fleming, C. A.: *Yersinia enterocolitica* isolated from throats of swine in eastern and western Canada. Can J Microbiol 27:1326, 1981.

Shayegani, M., Morse, D., DeForge, I., Root, T., Parsons, L. M., and Maupin, P. S.: Microbiology of a major foodborne outbreak of gastroenteritis caused by *Yersinia enterocolitica* serogroup 0:8. J Clin Microbiol 17:35, 1983.

Une, T.: Studies on the pathogenicity of *Yersinia enterocolitica*. II. Interaction with cultured cells *in vitro*. Microbiol Immunol 21:365, 1977.

Une, T., and Zen-Yoji, H.: Investigations on the pathogenicity of *Yersinia enterocolitica* by experimental infections in rabbits and cultured cells. (Karger, Basel). Contrib Microbiol Immunol 5:304, 1979.

van Pee, W., and Stragier, J.: Evaluation of some cold enrichment and isolation media for the recovery of *Yersinia enterocolitica*. Antonie Van Leeuwenhoek 45:465, 1979.

Wauters, G., Le Minor, L., Chalon, A. M., and Lassen, J.: Supplement au schema antigenique de *"Yersinia enterocolitica."* Ann Inst Pasteur Lille 122:951, 1972.

Wauters, G.: Antigens of *Yersinia enterocolitica*. In Bottone, E. J. (Ed.) *Yersinia enterocolitica*. Boca Raton, Florida, CRC Press, 1981, p. 48.

Pasteurella multocida

Bain, R. V. S.: Studies on hemorrhagic septicemia of cattle. IV. A preliminary examination of antigens of *Pasteurella multocida* Type I. Br Vet J 111:492, 1955.

Bain, R. V. S., and Knox, K. W.: The antigens of *Pasteurella multocida* Type I. II. Lipopolysaccharides. Immunology 4:122, 1961.

Carter, G. R.: A new serological type of *Pasteurella multocida* from central Africa. Vet Rec 73:1052, 1961.

Carter, G. R.: Animal serotypes of *Pasteurella multocida* from human infections. Can J Public Health 53:158, 1962.

Carter, G. R.: Immunological differentiation of Type B and E strains of *Pasteurella multocida*. Can Vet J 4:61, 1963.

Carter, G. R.: Improved hemagglutination test for identifying Type A strains of *Pasteurella multocida*. Appl Microbiol 24:162, 1972a.

Carter, G. R.: Agglutinability of *Pasteurella multocida* after treatment with hyaluronidase. Vet Rec 91:150, 1972b.

Carter, G. R., and Annau, E.: Isolation of capsular polysaccharides from colonial variants of *Pasteurella multocida*. Am J Vet Res 14:474, 1953.

Carter, G. R.: The epidemiology and pathogenesis of pasteurellosis in man. Vet Med Sm An Clin 79:629, 1984.

Chang, W. H., and Carter, G. R.: Multiple drug resistance in *Pasteurella multocida* and *Pasteurella hemolytica* from cattle and swine. J Am Vet Med Assoc 169:710, 1976.

Chengappa, M. M., Meyers, R. C., and Carter, G. R.: Capsular and somatic types of *Pasteurella multocida* from rabbits. Can J Comp Med 46:437, 1982.

Collins, F. M.: Growth of *Pasteurella multocida* in vaccinated and normal mice. Infect Immun 8:868, 1973.

Collins, F. M.: Mechanisms of acquired resistance to *Pasteurella multocida* infections: A review. Cornell Vet 67:103, 1977.

Dhanda, M. R.: Purification and properties of the soluble antigen of *Pasteurella septica*, Type I. Indian J Pathol Bacteriol 2:59, 1960.

Francis, D. P., Holmes, M. A., and Brandon, G.: *Pasteurella multocida*. Infections after domestic animal bites and scratches. JAMA 233:42, 1975.

Gadberry, J. L., and Miller, N. G.: Use of bacteriophages as an adjunct in the identification of *Pasteurella multocida*. Am J Vet Res 38:129, 1977.

Glorioso, J. C., Jones, G. W., Rush, H. G., Pentler, L. J., Darif, C. A., and Coward, J. E.: Adhesion of type A *Pasteurella multocida* to rabbit pharyngeal cells and its possible role in rabbit respiratory tract infections. Infect Immun 35:1103, 1982.

Hubbert, W. T., and Rosen, M. N.: II. *Pasteurella multocida* infection in man unrelated to animal bite. Am J Public Health 60:1109, 1970.

Namioka, S., and Bruner, D. W.: Serological studies on *Pasteurella multocida*. IV. Type distribution of organisms on the basis of their capsular and O groups. Cornell Vet 53:41, 1963.

Perreau, P., and Petit, J. P.: Lipopolysaccharide antigens of *Pasteurella* Type E. Rev Élèvage Med Vet Pays Trop 16:5, 1963.

Smith, J. E.: Studies on Pasteurella septica. III. Strains from human beings. J Comp Pathol 69:231, 1959.

Francisella tularensis

Bell, J. F., Larson, C. L., Wight, W. C., and Ritter, S. S.: Studies on the immunization of white mice against infections of *Bacterium tularense*. J Immunol 69:515, 1952.

Bell, J. F., Owen, C. R., and Larson, C. L.: Virulence of *Bacterium tularense*. I. A study of the virulence of *Bacterium tularense* in mice, guinea pigs, and rabbits. J Infect Dis 97:162, 1955.

Berdal, B. P., and Søderlund, E.: Cultivation and isolation of *Francisella tularensis* on selective chocolate agar as used routinely for the isolation of gonococci. Acta Pathol Microbiol Scand (B) 85:108, 1977.

Boyce, J. M.: Recent trends in the epidemiology of tularemia in the United States. J Infect Dis 131:197, 1975.

Buchanan, T. M., Brooks, G. F., and Branchman, P. S.: The tularemia skin test. 325 skin tests in 210 persons: Serologic correlation and review of the literature. Ann Intern Med 74:336, 1971.

Burke, D. S.: Immunization against tularemia: Analysis of the effectiveness of live *Francisella tularensis* vaccine in prevention of laboratory acquired tularemia. J Infect Dis 135:55, 1977.

Carlsson, H. E., Lindberg, A. A., Lindberg, G., Hederstedt, B., Karlsson, K. A., and Agell, B. O.: Enzyme-linked immunosorbent assay for immunological diagnosis of human tularemia. J Clin Microbiol 10:615, 1979.

Carr, E. A., Jr., and Kadull, P. J.: Persistence of *Bacterium tularense* in man in the absence of serious clinical illness. Arch Pathol 64:382, 1957.

Eigelsbach, H. T., and Downs, C. M.: Prophylactic effectiveness of live and killed tularemia vaccines. I. Production of vaccine and evaluation in the white mouse and guinea pigs. J Immunol 87:415, 1961.

Francis, E.: Tularemia Francis 1921. I. The occurrence of tularemia in nature as a disease of man. Public Health Rep 36:1731, 1921a.

Francis, E.: Tularemia Francis 1921. A new disease of man. JAMA 78:1015, 1921b.

Gallivan, M. V., Davis, W. A., Garagusi, V. F., Paris, A. L., and Lack, E. E.: Fatal-cat transmitted tularemia: Demonstration of the organism in tissue. South Med J 73:240, 1980.

Holm, S. E., Tarnvik, A., and Sandstrom, G.: Antigenic composition of a vaccine strain of *Francisella tularensis*. Int Arch Allergy Appl Immunol 61:136, 1980.

Jellison, W. L.: Tularemia in Montana. *In* Montana Wildlife, Series 2 of Montana Animals, Montana Fish and Game Commission. Butte, McKee Printing Company, 1970.

Koskela, P., and Herva, E.: Cell-mediated and humoral immunity induced by a live *Francisella tularensis* vaccine. Infect Immun 36:983, 1982.

Landay, M. E., Wright, G. G., Pullian, J. D., and Finegold, M. J.: Toxicity of *Pasteurella tularensis* killed by ionizing radiation. J Bacteriol 96:804, 1968.

Larson, C. L.: Immunization of white rats against infections with *Pasteurella tularensis*. Public Health Rep 60:725, 1945.

McCoy, G. W.: A plague-like disease of rodents. Public Health Bull 43:53, 1911.

McCoy, G. W., and Chapin, G. W.: Further observations on a plague-like disease of rodents with a preliminary note on the causative agent, *Bacterium tularense*. J Infect Dis 10:61, 1912.

McCrumb, F. R.: Aerosol infection of man with *Pasteurella tularensis*. Bacteriol Rev 25:262, 1961.

Mason, W. L., Eigelsbach, H. T., Little, S. F., and Bates, J. H.: Treatment of tularemia including pulmonary tularemia, with gentamicin. Am Rev Respir Dis 121:39, 1980.

Nutter, J. E.: Antigens of *Pasteurella tularensis:* Preparative procedures. Appl Microbiol 22:44, 1971.

Saslaw, S., Eigelsbach, H. T., Wilson, H. E., Prior, J. A., and Carhart, S.: Tularemia vaccine study. I. Intracutaneous challenge. Arch Intern Med 107:689, 1961a.

Saslaw, S., Eigelsbach, H. T., Prior, J. A., Wilson, H. E., and Carhart, S.: Tularemia vaccine study. II. Respiratory challenge. Arch Intern Med 107:702, 1961b.

Tarnvik, A., and Holm, S. E.: Stimulation of subpopulations of human lymphocytes by a vaccine strain of *Francisella tularensis*. Infect Immun 20:698, 1978.

Yager, R. H., Spertzel, O. R., Yaeger, R. F., and Tigertt, W. D.: Domestic fowl: Source of high titer *P. tularensis* serum for the fluorescent antibody technique. Proc Soc Exp Biol Med 105:651, 1960.

38
STREPTOBACILLUS MONILIFORMIS

JOSHUA FIERER, M.D.

Streptobacillus (Actinobacillus) moniliformis is a pleomorphic gram-negative bacterium. It is nonmotile, unencapsulated, and nonacid-fast. Gram-stained smears of exudate show small rods or short filaments. When grown in serum-enriched broth, they are branching filaments that form interwoven masses. There usually is marked pleomorphism. Many filaments contain cells with rounded or fusiform swellings. After prolonged culture, tiny curved and ring forms appear.

Much of the pleomorphism of this bacterium is due to the spontaneous appearance of variants with defective cell walls, called L-phase variants (after the Lister Institute where this observation was first made). These are stable variant bacteria that lack a rigid cell wall. As a consequence, in broth they grow as small round cells, and on agar the colonies are flat and grow into the agar like *Mycoplasma* colonies. For many years this similarity in colonial morphology and in osmotic fragility between L-forms and Mycoplasmatales obscured the large and fundamental differences between these disparate microorganisms (see Chapters 54 and 58). Stable L-forms lack the mucopeptide that confers on the parent bacteria their rigidity and rod-like shape. The L-forms divide and propagate by binary fission as cell-deficient forms. Unstable L-forms revert back to parental bacteria. Protoplasts, in contrast to L-forms, are cell wall-deficient forms that are created artifically by exposing gram-positive bacteria to enzymes (e.g., lysozyme) or antibiotics such as penicillin that directly interfere with cell wall synthesis. Sometimes a stable protoplast is produced by these manipulations that can multiply without synthesizing a cell wall in the absence of the inducing agent.

ANTIGENIC COMPOSITION. The L-phase variant and the bacillus share a common antigen, but the L-phase lacks antigens present in the latter. There appears to be only one serotype of the bacillus, but the chemical nature of the antigen has not been established.

METABOLISM. Growth can occur aerobically but is equally good or better under anaerobic conditions (Wittler, 1974). A 10 per cent CO_2 atmosphere probably enhances growth. Optimum temperature for growth is 37° C. The metabolic characteristics of the organism have not been studied in detail. It is both catalase and oxidase negative and does not reduce nitrate to nitrite, nor produce indole. Urea is not hydrolyzed nor is phenylalanine deaminated. Acid but not gas is produced from dextrin, fructose, galactose, glucose, maltose, mannose, starch, and glycogen if a 1 per cent carbohydrate broth is supplemented with serum or ascites. No acid is produced from lactose, glycerol, inositol, inulin, sorbitol, rhamnose, or mannitol. Tetrazolium salt and tellurite are reduced aerobically and anaerobically though the tellurite reduction test may be only weakly positive.

IMMUNITY. The pathogenic properties of this organism have not been studied in detail. The stable L-forms do not produce disease in mice whereas bacilli do. If injected into mice, unstable L-forms revert to the bacterial form and cause disease. Vaccination with the L-form does not protect mice against challenge with the bacterial form, but a killed bacterial vaccine is protective.

LABORATORY DIAGNOSIS. Diagnosis of infection is made by isolating the bacteria from a lymph node, pus, joint fluid, or blood. Bacteria grow in ordinary blood culture media (Rogosa, 1974). This organism does not grow on nutrient agar, but on sheep blood agar it produces very small, gray, translucent, nonhemolytic colonies with entire edges after 48 to 72 hours of incubation. In serum or ascitic fluid broth, it grows as white granules or flocculent balls that sediment rapidly or stick to the side of the glass tube. Nutrient broth supplemented with 20 per cent horse serum is useful for primary isolation. Injection of pus into mice can also be used to isolate the bacterium, but care must be taken not to use naturally infected animals for such isolation.

The tube-agglutination test with whole bacterial antigen can be used for serologic diagnosis. Demonstration of a rising titer is significant. A negative test does not exclude the diagnosis.

DRUG SUSCEPTIBILITY. The organism is susceptible to penicillin (0.05 unit/ml), streptomycin, and tetracycline. The L-phase variant is resistant to penicillin, and persistent symptoms and signs may be associated with the presence of L-phase organisms in the blood during penicillin therapy. Tetracycline or streptomycin can be used in that circumstance.

EPIDEMIOLOGY. The distribution of this organism is worldwide, although human infections are rare in Europe and North America. The reservoir is infected rats or, rarely, other rodents. It may cause an epizootic disease in mice characterized by arthritis and lymphadenitis. Most human infections are acquired as the result of a rat bite (Cole et al., 1969). Consequently, it is an occupational hazard of research laboratory workers. After a bite, the incubation period is 3 to 10 days. Infection can occur as a consequence of ingesting contaminated milk (Haverhill fever or erythema arthriticum epidemicum). Some patients who live in rat-infested environments have had no history of a bite, and infection may have been food-borne.

References

Cole, J. S., Stoll, R. W., and Bulger, R. J.: Rat bite fever, report of three cases. Ann Intern Med 71:979, 1969.

Rogosa, M.: Streptobacillus moniliformis and Spirillum minus. In Manual of Clinical Microbiology, 2nd ed. American Society for Microbiology, Washington, 1974.

Wittler, R. G.: In Bergey's Manual of Determinative Bacteriology, 8th ed. Baltimore, The Williams & Wilkins Company, 1974.

39

EIKENELLA CORRODENS

GEO. F. BROOKS, M.D.

Eikenella corrodens is so named because it was characterized by Eiken (1958) and because it often produces colonies that appear to pit or corrode the agar surface. Jackson and Goodman (1972) established that Eiken's corroding bacillus would grow aerobically on appropriate media and that it also differed genetically from *Bacteroides corrodens*, an obligate anaerobe that is now referred to as *B. ureolyticus* (Chapter 50). *Eikenella corrodens* was also called HB-1 by E. O. King in her classic observations on the identification of unusual pathogenic gram-negative bacteria. It is now known that *E. corrodens* and HB-1 are the same organism (Riley et al., 1973).

MORPHOLOGY. *E. corrodens* is a small (0.5 μm wide and 1–3 μm long) gram-negative, pleomorphic, often coccobacillary rod. On Gram stain, *E. corrodens* cannot be distinguished morphologically from many organisms in the genera *Brucella, Haemophilus, Pasteurella,* and *Actinobacillus.*

E. corrodens is nonspore-forming, unencapsulated, nonmotile, and microaerophilic or capnophilic. Aerobic, but not anaerobic, growth requires media that contain hemin, such as blood or chocolate agars. Growth is also very clearly enhanced by incubation in the presence of 5 to 10 per cent carbon dioxide (Goldstein et al., 1981).

The colonial characteristics of *E. corrodens* are distinctive. After 18 to 24 hours of incubation on blood agar, tiny ("pinpoint") colonies can be seen. After 48 to 72 hours, the distinctive colonial morphology becomes apparent. Colonies reach 2 to 3 mm in diameter and are dry and flat. They spread radially, usually with an irregular periphery. The center of the colony appears moist. On close examination, particularly with a magnifying lens or a dissecting microscope, the colonies appear to pit the agar, hence the term "corroding." Actually, only about one-half of the strains pit the agar. Nonpitting colonies are often dome-shaped. In some cultures, both colonial forms appear. Corroding strains exhibit a type of movement called "twitching motility." This movement is not due to flagella, but appears to be associated with the presence of polar fimbria. Corroding strains of *E. corrodens* must be differentiated from other organisms that pit or corrode the agar surface, including the obligate anaerobe *B. ureolyticus*, *Hemophilus aphrophilus*, and some of the *Moraxella* species (see Chapter 30).

On prolonged incubation, a heavy growth of *E. corrodens* may produce very slight discoloration of blood agar that differs in appearance from alpha hemolysis of streptococci.

E. corrodens yields a characteristic musty odor, variously described as similar to hypochlorite bleach, crackers, or musty mouse cages. It cannot be differentiated from the odor of *Hemophilus* spp. Since *Eikenella* grows slowly and is most often found in mixed cultures, prolonged incubation combined with careful selection and subcultures of pinpoint colonies may be necessary to prevent overgrowth by other bacteria that grow more rapidly. Alternatively, if *Eikenella* is the probable cause of an infection, its resistance to clindamycin can be used for selection. A standard clindamycin disc can be placed on the plate to inhibit the growth of some gram-positive bacteria and anaerobes. Alternatively, clindamycin at 5 μ/ml incorporated into agar or into a modified Todd-Hewitt broth provides an effective selective medium. Selective media are particularly useful when culturing specimens from the upper respiratory tract or from infections contaminated with oral flora (Brooks et al., 1974; Slee and Tanzer, 1978).

E. corrodens will grow in complex, highly supplemented, liquid media, but do so slowly. Routine culture of specimens in liquid media is a less than optimal method for its isolation.

ANTIGENIC COMPOSITION. The cell envelope of *E. corrodens* is characteristic of gram-negative bacteria. Electron microscopic studies of *E. corrodens* have demonstrated an organized fibrous slime layer associated with the outer surface of the outer membrane and an interwoven network of fibrils (Progulske and Holt, 1980). Several antigenic components of *E. corrodens* have been described (Maliszewski et al., 1983), but all strains appear to be closely related antigenically. Antisera suitable for typing the organisms are not available.

METABOLISM AND LABORATORY IDENTIFICATION. *E. corrodens* requires hemin or blood when grown aerobically but grows without these supplements under anaerobic conditions. On subculture, it is possible to isolate variants that will grow on media without supplementary hemin or hemin-containing blood products. The failure of *E. corrodens* to grow on MacConkey agar is a useful test for its laboratory identification.

Metabolically, *Eikenella* is relatively inert. It lacks both oxidative and fermentative capabilities for carbohydrates and does not produce catalase, urease, or indole. Hydrogen sulfide production can be demonstrated for some isolates by the lead acetate paper method after prolonged incubation. The key tests for identification of *Eikenella* are a positive oxidase reaction, reduction of nitrate, and inability to attack carbohydrates. Many strains produce ornithine decarboxylase. None produces arginine dihydrolase. *Eikenella* grows well at 35 to 37° C. Some strains grow at 25° C; about one-half will grow at 42° C (Weaver et al., 1983).

The guanine plus cytosine content of *E. corrodens* is 54 to 56 per cent. In general, it shows very little DNA homology with other gram-negative bacteria.

PATHOGENIC PROPERTIES AND IMMUNITY. *Eikenella corrodens* is a common member of the gingival and dental plaque flora. On selective media, it has been recovered from 59 per cent of dental plaque samples and 33 per cent of gingival cultures, but less than 1 per cent of saliva samples (Goldstein et al., 1983a). The prevalence of *Eikenella* in samples of dental plaque from children aged 7 to 14 years was 90 per cent. Thus, *E. corrodens* is most commonly isolated from infections with contamination by the oral flora.

E. corrodens will not cause subcutaneous abscesses in rabbits unless it is injected in high inoculum mixed with streptococci, and foreign materials such as methylphenidate tablets (Brooks et al., 1974). *E. corrodens* causes endocarditis in the rabbit model (Badger et al., 1979).

Although *E. corrodens* is occasionally isolated in pure culture from human infections, it is usually isolated in association with alpha or nonhemolytic streptococci. When beta-hemolytic streptococci are associated with *Eikenella* in infections, the streptococci are usually not group A (Brooks et al., 1974). *E. corrodens* is also one of the gram-negative bacteria that are frequently isolated in association with *Actinomyces* species in the classic presentation of actinomycosis. Thus, *E. corrodens* is a common human commensal, but it appears to have relatively low pathogenicity by itself. On the other hand, it can cause necrotizing synergistic infections in association with other bacteria. It synthesizes a biologically active lipopolysaccharide (Behling et al., 1979), but endotoxic shock is not characteristic of *Eikenella* infection.

Although *E. corrodens* is most commonly isolated from purulent infections or abscesses that have been contaminated with gingival flora, it also appears in mixed intraabdominal infections. The most common sites of infection are perioral tissues, the hands and other sites with oral contamination, the lung and pleura, and intraabdominal abscesses (Johnson and Pankey, 1976; Dorff et al., 1974; Zinner et al., 1973). Occasionally, *E. corrodens* is the sole cause of infection in endocarditis (Geraci et al., 1974) or osteomyelitis, but these infections are uncommon enough that the culture results are frequently a surprise to both the clinician and the laboratory worker.

Very few patients develop precipitin antibodies against *E. corrodens* as measured in agar immunodiffusion tests. The role of host defense mechanisms in the prevention of human infections with *E. corrodens* has not been extensively studied. Some strains produce an extracellular slime that is immunosuppressive in experimental animals (Behling et al., 1979).

DRUG SUSCEPTIBILITY. Because *E. corrodens* grows slowly and poorly in liquid media, agar dilution is the only acceptable method for testing sensitivity to drugs (Goldstein et al., 1983a).

E. corrodens is sensitive to most beta-lactam antibiotics. Penicillin G, ampicillin, carbenicillin, ticarcillin, cefoxitin, cefotaxime, moxalactam, cefoperazone, piperacillin, and mezlocillin show marked or good activity against *E. corrodens*. Cefadroxil and cefamandole are relatively inactive (Goldstein et al., 1978, 1980).

E. corrodens is resistant to clindamycin and inhibited little by metronidazole and vancomycin. The aminoglycosides are also relatively inactive. Erythromycin and tetracycline are of intermediate activity against *E. corrodens*.

EPIDEMIOLOGY. Because *Eikenella* is an oral bacterium, it is found in infections associated with contamination by the oral or gingival flora. An interesting sidelight of this epidemiologic observation is the relatively frequent occurrence of *E. corrodens* in subcutaneous abscesses of drug abusers who inject methylphenidate (Brooks et al., 1974). Methylphenidate tablets contain lactose, sucrose, polyethyleneglycol, magnesium stearate, corn starch, native hydrous magnesium silicate (talc), and tragacanth, an insoluble gum. People who inject methylphenidate commonly crush the tablets in their teeth or otherwise contaminate the injection material, apparatus, or injection wound with oral secretions. The presence of the foreign materials in the methylphenidate tablet along with other oral flora such as streptococci appear to provide optimal conditions for enhancing the pathogenicity of *Eikenella corrodens*.

References

Badger, S. J., Butler, T., Kim, C. K., and Johnston, K. H.: Experimental *Eikenella corrodens* in endocarditis in rabbits. Infect Immun 23:751, 1979.

Behling, U. H., Ham, P. H., and Nowotny, A.: Biological activity of the slime and endotoxin of the periodontopathic organism *Eikenella corrodens*. Infect Immun 26:580, 1979.

Brooks, G. F., O'Donoghue, J. M., Rissing, J. P., et al: *Eikenella corrodens*, a recently recognized pathogen: Infections in medical-surgical patients and in association with methylphenidate abuse. Medicine 53:325, 1974.

Dorff, G. J., Jackson, L. J., and Rytel, M. W.: Infections with *Eikenella corrodens*. Ann Intern Med 80:305, 1974.

Eiken, M.: Studies on an anaerobic, rod-shaped, Gram-negative microorganism: *Bacteroides corrodens* n. sp.: Acta Path Microbiol Scand 43:404, 1958.

Geraci, J.E., Hermans, P.E., and Washington, J.A.: *Eikenella corrodens* endocarditis: Report of cure in two cases. Mayo Clin Proc 49:950, 1974.

Goldstein, E. J. C., Sutter, V. L., Finegold, S. M.: Susceptibility of *Eikenella corrodens* to ten cephalosporins. Antimicrob. Agents Chemother. 14:639, 1978.

Goldstein, E. J. C., Gombert, M. E., and Agyare, E. O.: Susceptibility of *Eikenella corrodens* to newer beta-lactam antibiotics. Antimicrob Agents Chemother 18:832, 1980.

Goldstein, E. J. C., Agyare, E. O., and Silletti, R.: Comparative growth of *Eikenella corrodens* on 15 media in three atmospheres of incubation. J Clin Microbiol 13:951, 1981.

Goldstein, E. J. C., Cherubin, C. E., and Shulman, M.: Comparison of microtiter broth dilution and agar dilution methods for susceptibility testing of *Eikenella corrodens*. Antimicrob Agents Chemother 23:42, 1983a.

Goldstein, E. J. C., Tarenzi, L. A., Agyan, E. D., and Berger, J. R.: Prevalence of *Eikenella corrodens* in dental plaque. J Clin Microbiol 17:636, 1983b.

Jackson, F. L. and Goodman, Y. E.: Transfer of the facultatively anaerobic organism *Bacteroides corrodens* Eiken to a new genus, *Eikenella*. Int J Syst Bacteriol 22:73, 1972.

Johnson, S. M. and Pankey, G. A.: *Eikenella corrodens* osteomyelitis, arthritis, and cellulitis of the hand. Southern Medical Journal 69:535, 1976.

Maliszewski, C. R., Shuster, C. W., and Badger, S. J.: A type-specific antigen of *Eikenella corrodens* is the major outer membrane protein. Infect Immun 42:208, 1983.

Progulske, A. and Holt, S. C.: Transmission-scanning electron microscopic observations of selected *Eikenella corrodens* strains. J Bacteriol 143:1003, 1980.

Riley, P. S., Tatum, H. W., and Weaver, R. E.: Identity of HB-1 of King and *Eikenella corrodens* (Eiken) Jackson and Goodman. Int J Syst Bacteriol 23:75, 1973.

Slee, A. M. and Tanzer, J. M.: Selective medium for isolation of *Eikenella corrodens* from periodontal lesions. J Clin Microbiol 8:459, 1978.

Weaver, R. E., Hollis, D. G., Clark, W. A., and Riley, P.: Revised tables from the identification of unusual pathogenic gram negative bacteria, Elizabeth O. King. U.S. Department of Health and Human Services, Public Health Service, Centers for Disease Control, Atlanta, Georgia, 1983.

Zinner, S. H., Daly, A. K., and McCormack, W. M.: Isolation of *Eikenella corrodens* in a general hospital. Appl Microbiol 25:705, 1973.

40

ACTINOBACILLUS AND CARDIOBACTERIUM

IRVING J. SLOTNICK, PH.D.

Actinobacillus

Cardiobacterium and *Actinobacillus* are fastidious, opportunistic gram-negative bacilli that are increasingly recognized as causes of human disease. Only one species in the genus *Actinobacillus*, *Actinobacillus actinomycetemcomitans*, has been consistently associated with human infection. The other species are pathogenic in cattle, horses, and pigs, but only rarely in man.

MORPHOLOGY. Members of the genus *Actinobacillus* are gram-negative rods, coccoid to coccobacillary in shape, 0.3 to 0.5 μm wide and 0.5 to 1.5 μm long, nonspore-forming and nonacid-fast. They often present pleomorphic coccal and long bacillary and filamentous forms. They are not distinguishable morphologically from *Brucella*, *Haemophilus*, and *Pasteurella* (Fig. 1).

In infections of animals, grayish white granules may appear in pus that are similar to but smaller (0.4 mm diameter) than the "sulfur" granules of actinomycosis. The granules contain clublike bodies emanating radially from the center, which is made up of the gram-negative bacilli and cell deposits. Care must be taken to differentiate these from granules caused by *Actinomyces* spp, *Nocardia* spp, staphylococci, Monosporium spp, fragments of caseous material, and clumps of pus cells and fibrin. A Ziehl-Neelsen stain colors the granule interior blue whereas the clubs are weakly acid-fast.

Growth is improved in increased carbon dioxide and by adding blood (5 per cent) or serum (10 per cent) to any of the common agar media. No growth occurs on *Salmonella-Shigella* (SS) or eosin-methylene blue (EMB) agar. *A. lignieresii* and *A. equuli* grow on MacConkey agar, whereas *A. actinomycetemcomitans* grows only slightly at best. Both rough and smooth types of colonies occur in primary

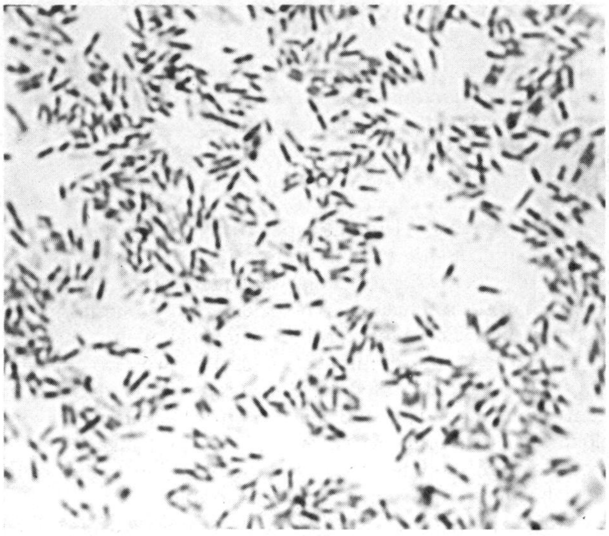

Figure 1. *Actinobacillus actinomycetemcomitans* #CS-G. Gram stain. Blood agar. 48-hours' growth. 1800×.

cultures. Rough colonies are tiny at 24 hours, ranging up to 1.0 mm in diameter and are raised, grayish, opaque, convex, tenacious, and firmly adherent to the medium. The surface appears dry and dull. In 72 hours the colony increases to 3–4 mm in diameter.

Smooth and rough colonies are the same size. They are small, discrete, convex, and semi-opaque, with entire edges and glistening surfaces. The colonies appear gray but may have a blue to yellowish hue in transmitted light. After four to five days of incubation, the colony has a domed appearance when examined microscopically. The formation of smooth colony variants is favored on continued subculture.

The center of the colonies may, after three to five days of incubation, contain a four- to six-pointed star formation, which grows into the agar, and remains when the colony is scraped away. This is more readily observed on clear media than on blood agar.

The consistency of bacterial growth on agar is strain-dependent. On blood agar growth may be butyrous and scraped up easily, or it may be adherent and difficult to remove with a loop.

Serum enriched thioglycollate, soy broths, cooked meat, and other infusion media show growth after 24 hours in air. Granular growth may follow uniform turbidity. The granules adhere to the walls of the tubes, leaving the broth fairly clear. A surface film and a heavy tenacious sediment also occur in old broth cultures. A new selective medium, TSBV (tryptic soy-serum-bacitracin-vancomycin) agar, offers promise in isolating *A. actinomycetemcomitans* from mixed flora sites (Slots, 1982).

ANTIGENIC COMPOSITION. Heat-stable polysaccharide agglutinating antigens associated with extracellular slime and several agglutinogens are formed by the actinobacilli. Antigenic relationships exist between *A. lignieresii* and *A. equuli*. Cross-reactions between *Pseudomonas mallei, Pseudomonas pseudomallei,* and *A. equuli* are well known. Common antigens occur between *A. actinomycetemcomitans* and various other *Actinobacillus* and *Haemophilus* species (Slots et al., 1982). Phillips (1967) defined six types (1 through 6) and two subtypes (1a and 4c) of *A. lignieresii* on the basis of heat-stable somatic antigens. Some host specificity in the distribution of serotypes seems to be involved, because most cattle strains belong to Type 1 and most sheep strains belong to Types 2, 3, and 4. Heat-labile antigens common to different antigenic types also occur.

Pulverer and Ko (1972) examined 100 strains of *A. actinomycetemcomitans* and delineated 6 heat-stable agglutinating antigens and 24 agglutinating patterns. Agar-gel diffusion was inferior to agglutination for typing.

METABOLISM. The actinobacilli are representative chemoorganotrophs, using only organic compounds as their source of energy. Growth is aerobic and facultatively anaerobic. Carbohydrates are fermented with production of acid and usually no gas. Fermentation reactions are weak, variable, and often delayed. The OF medium of Hugh and Leifson is not recommended for fermentation reactions because it does not support the growth of most strains of actinobacilli. Carbohydrate broths used to test reactions should be supplemented with 5 to 10 per cent sterile horse serum and not incubated more than 14 days to minimize nonspecific reactions.

Pulverer and Ko (1970) classified eight fermentative biotypes of *A. actinomycetemcomitans* on the basis of galactose, mannitol, and xylose reaction patterns. Biotypes I through IV make up most strains isolated from cases in the United States reported to the Center for Disease Control.

Optimal growth is at 37° C, with a range of 20 to 42° C. Optimal pH is 7.6, and no growth occurs at pH below 6.5. The guanine plus cytosine (G+C) content of the DNA ranges from 40.6 to 42.0 moles per cent. Capsules are not produced, but some strains produce extracellular slime. They have no flagella and are nonmotile.

PATHOGENIC PROPERTIES. Localized purulent granulomatous lesions, abscess formation in soft tissues, septicemia, endocarditis, and occasionally meningitis characterize the disease spectrum of the actinobacilli. Toxic substances identified from *A. actinomycetemcomitans* include a potent endotoxin (Kiley and Holt, 1980) and leukotoxin (Taichman et al., 1980). Subcutaneous inoculation of a pure culture of *A. lignieresii* or *A. equuli* into cattle causes an abscess like that in the natural disease, but not all strains are virulent. Experimental studies have been limited due to lack of pathogenicity for rabbits, mice, or guinea pigs.

IMMUNITY. Definitive data concerning the immune state following an overt case of actinobacillosis are meager. Repeated attacks have been singularly rare, although chronic cases can occur. Serum antibodies are formed in animals and humans, but it is not known if they are protective. Horse antiserum has been employed in the treatment of animals without conspicuous success.

Nonspecific agglutination reactions with normal sera and seronegative reactions in proven cases make serodiagnostic testing unsatisfactory (Phillips, 1967). Agglutination tests with known organisms or known antisera can be used to identify antibody or species, but commercial sources for either are not available. Antibody develops in infected patients against their own isolate (Pathak and Ristic, 1962). The sera of animals suffering from actinobacillosis frequently agglutinate the causative agent to a titer of 1:160

or higher. We observed a transitory rise to a titer of 1:320 in a patient with *A. actinomycetemcomitans* endocarditis and no rise in a second case.

LABORATORY DIAGNOSIS. Identification of culture isolates is based on biochemical reactions in Table 1.

DRUG SUSCEPTIBILITY. Streptomycin, tetracycline, and chloramphenicol inhibit all strains tested in reasonably low concentrations (Page and King, 1966). Less than 50 per cent of *A. actinomycetemcomitans* organisms are inhibited by 12.5 μg/ml of penicillin, only 35 per cent are inhibited by 3.12 μg/ml of ampicillin, and all are resistant to methicillin.

Potassium iodide is the drug of choice in the treatment of spontaneous actinobacillosis. The response is dramatic and permanent. It has been used with some success in more chronic human infections. The iodides have little bactericidal effect against *A. lignieresii*. The sulfonamides, penicillin, streptomycin, and broad-spectrum antibiotics are used to treat *A. lignieresii* and *A. equuli* infection.

EPIDEMIOLOGY. Actinobacilli are recovered with ease from the normal mouth, tonsillar area, and intestinal tract of all hosts. The genital tract may also be colonized. The oral cavity and upper respiratory tract are primary portals of entry and serve as a focal endogenous habitat.

In patients *A. actinomycetemcomitans* causes endocarditis in rheumatic or congential heart disease or opportunistic infections in malignant lymphoma and acute leukemia. Infections have followed dental manipulations, but *A. actinomycetemcomitans* causes abscesses without evidence of trauma to the area of infection (Burgher et al., 1973). A human urinary tract infection has been reported (Townsend and Gillenwater, 1969).

A. lignieresii and *A. equuli* are chiefly the cause of actinobacillosis in animals and can cause epidemics. The disease can spread rapidly in a herd, attacking up to 50 per cent of the animals within weeks. Human infections by *A. lignieresii* or *A. equuli* have occurred in farmers, animal husbandmen, veterinarians, and abbatoir personnel (Custus et al., 1944).

Cardiobacterium

The slow growing and fastidious gram-negative rod *Cardiobacterium hominis* causes a form of endocarditis with a markedly prolonged clinical course before clinical recognition. Unlike similar gram-negative bacteria it produces indole.

MORPHOLOGY. The only species in this genus is *Cardiobacterium hominis*. It is a gram-negative rod, 0.5 μm wide and 1.0 to 2.2 μm long, arranged singly, in pairs, short chains, or clusters. The rods may be uniform or pleomorphic. The pleomorphic forms have one or both ends enlarged, and resembles tear-drops or rosette clusters (Figs. 2, 3, and 4). Pleomorphism is less and organisms stain homogeneously and have *uniform dimensions* on blood agar containing yeast extract. The organism is nonspore-forming and nonacid-fast. Sudanophilic bodies and metachromatic inclusions are demonstrable.

Thin sections of *C. hominis* show a cell wall of gram-negative type with a cytoplasm containing numerous intrusive membranes disposed around the periphery of the cells, especially at the poles (Reyn et al., 1971). The cell wall consists of a unit membrane sandwiched between dense outer and inner layers. Polar caps are seen on the ends of cells. The substructure of the surface layer is unusual for a gram-negative bacterium.

C. hominis colonies on blood agar are punctiform after 24 hours, and attain a maximum size of one to two mm in 48 to 72 hours. Colonies are circular, convex, smooth, entire, glistening, opaque, and butyrous. In older colonies their center appears more opaque and grayish white than the edges. A slight greening of blood, which develops around dense growth in two to three days, becomes brownish later. Clear hemolysis is not observed.

C. hominis grows well in humidors containing filter paper strips saturated with water and in atmospheres of 3 to 5 per cent carbon dioxide.

C. hominis grows well on trypticase soy agar, tryptose blood agar with or without 5 per cent blood enrichment, chocolate agar, PPLO medium, cystine-heart agar, Casman's medium, and heart infusion agar. Moderate growth

Table 1. DIFFERENTIATION OF ACTINOBACILLUS, CARDIOBACTERIUM AND SIMILAR GENERA AND SPECIES

	Actinobacillus actinomycetem-comitans	Actinobacillus lignieresii	Actinobacillus equuli	Cardiobacterium hominis	Hemophilus aphrophilus[1]	Kingella species[2]	(HB-1) Eikenella corrodens[3]
Oxidase	−/weak	+	+	+	−/weak +	+	+
Growth on MacConkey's agar	−/slight	+	+	−	−/v[6]	−/v	−
Catalase activity	+	−/weak	−/weak	−	−	−	−
Indole production	−	−	−	+/weak	−[4]	−	−
Nitrate reductase	+	+	+	−	+[5]	+	+
LDC/ODC	−	−	−	−	−	−	+/+
Fermentative capability	+	+	+	+	+	+	−
Mol % G + C of DNA	39			58.7–60.2	40	47.3–54.8	56.2–58.2

Data adapted from Weaver et al., CDC (1983). An excellent reference for sets of key reactions to differentiate other fastidious gram-negative fermentative bacteria.

[1] *Hemophilus paraphrophilus* does not require V factor.

[2] The three known species in this relatively new genus are *Kingella kingae* (formerly *Moraxella kingae*), *K. indologenes*, and *K. denitrificans.*

[3] *Eikenella corrodens* and *Kingella* have a tendency to pit or corrode blood agar plates.

[4] Produced only by *K. indologenes.*

[5] Not reduced by *K. indologenes.*

LDC: Lysine decarboxylase; ODC: Ornithine decarboxylase.

[6] v = variable

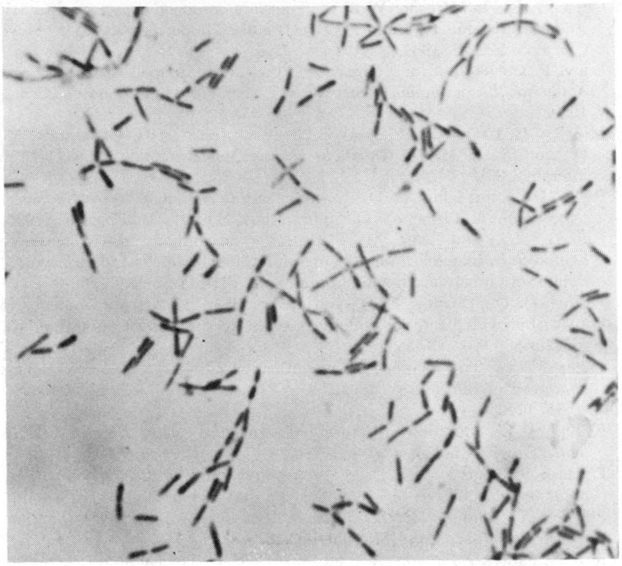

Figure 2. *Cardiobacterium hominis.* Strain #6518. Blood agar culture illustrative of a culture with singular lack of pleomorphic cell-types. Rod shape cells predominate. 1800×.

occurs on nutrient agar and Lowenstein-Jensen's medium. The organism does not grow on MacConkey's agar, Simmon's citrate, SS agar, tellurite medium, potato medium, Sabouraud's dextrose agar, phenylethylalcohol medium, EMB medium, or endo agar medium.

ANTIGENIC COMPOSITION. Antigenically, *C. hominis* is relatively homogeneous. The organisms cross-agglutinate to high titer in unabsorbed immune antisera. Antiserum absorption with heterologous strains gives residual titers indicative of varied as well as common antigenic groupings. Fluorescent-isothiocyanate-labeled antibody detects the same antigenic relationships (Slotnick and Dougherty, 1964).

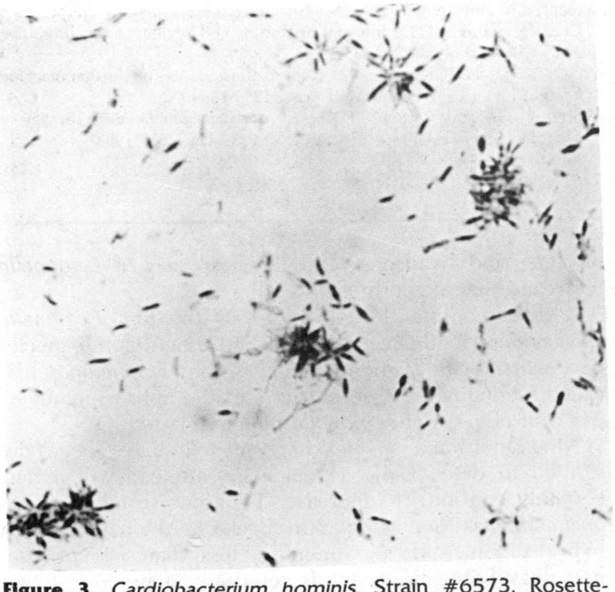

Figure 3. *Cardiobacterium hominis.* Strain #6573. Rosette-clusters in a Gram stain preparation of a blood agar culture. 1800×.

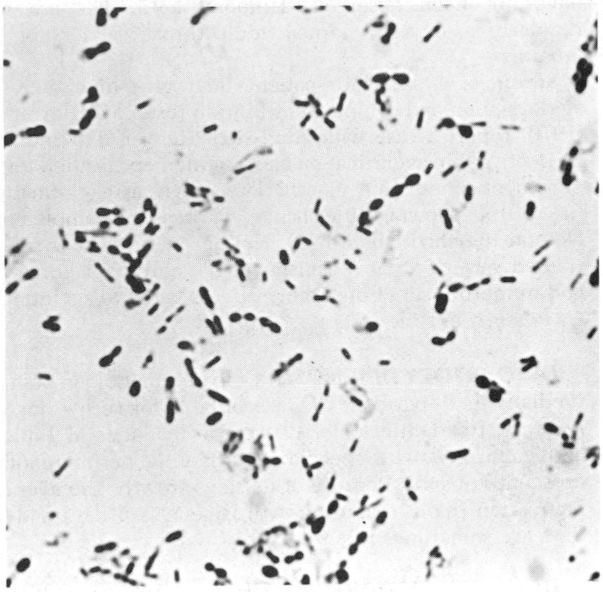

Figure 4. *Cardiobacterium hominis.* Strain #6573. Gram stain of blood agar culture illustrating tear-drop morphology and chaining tendency. 1800×.

METABOLISM. *C. hominis,* like the actinobacilli, is an aerobic, facultative anaerobic, chemoorganotroph with a fermentative, albeit weak, type of metabolism. Indole production is an important feature for distinguishing it from similar bacteria (Table 1).

C. hominis ferments carbohydrates without gas production. Fermentable substrates include glucose, sucrose, levulose, mannose, and sorbitol. Maltose and mannitol breakdown varies with individual strains. Fermentation is late and irregular in raffinose, dextrin, glycogen, and starch. Xylose, lactose, glycerol, salicin, inulin, arabinose, adonitol, dulcitol, galactose, rhamnose, trehalose, inositol, cellobiose, erythritol, melibiose, and melezitose are not attacked. Glucose is converted primarily to lactate and smaller amounts of pyruvate, formate, and propionate.

Optimal temperature for growth is 37° C. No growth occurs at 42° C or above, and only sporadic light growth occurs at 25° C. Optimal pH range is 7.0 to 7.2. Neither capsules nor flagella are produced.

PATHOGENIC PROPERTIES. Infections with *C. hominis* have been primarily associated with human endocarditis (Tucker et al., 1969; Midgley et al., 1970; Snyder and Ellner, 1969; Weiner and Werthamer, 1975; Savage et al., 1977; Perdue et al., 1974). Their low virulence is in keeping with the subacute course of the endocarditis. Infection occurs most frequently in patients with pre-existing cardiovascular defects. (Geraci and Wilson, 1982; Colebunders et al., 1982). Clinical presentation is not always typical (Wong and Chan, 1982). Isolates from other diseased sites are increasing, including the cervix, vagina, cheek, mandible, empyema fluid, and spinal fluid, as well as sputum, nose, and throat. Exotoxins are not produced. Other virulence factors are not known. *C. hominis* is not pathogenic for laboratory animals.

IMMUNITY. Immune mechanisms against *C. hominis* infection are unknown. Second attacks or chronic cases have not been observed. Humoral antibodies are not regularly formed in normal adult throat carriers of *C. hominis*.

Serum of endocarditis patients may give high titers in agglutination and complement fixation tests. Midgley et al. (1970) report a case with admission titers of 320 and 640 respectively in agglutination and complement fixation tests. Serum obtained nine months later gave an agglutination titer of 160, showing little change, whereas the complement fixation titer had fallen to 20. Neither of these sera agglutinated various other organisms in the authors' laboratory, and numerous sera from other patients failed to agglutinate *C. hominis* in slide tests.

LABORATORY DIAGNOSIS. Conventional blood culture media with 10 per cent CO_2 are suitable for recovering *C. hominis*. Its identification is based on reactions in Table 1 and confirmed with specific agglutinating or immunofluorescent antisera. Because of its slow growth, the average incubation period before growth is seen is 5 days and 14 days are sometimes required.

DRUG SUSCEPTIBILITY. *C. hominis* is susceptible to many antibiotics. Penicillin and streptomycin, either singly or in combination, are the drugs of choice. Drug resistance has not been a problem.

EPIDEMIOLOGY. *C. hominis* is part of the indigenous commensal human respiratory flora in many normal persons of all ages and both sexes. They are easily detectable with direct fluorescent antibody in the stool. They have extremely low incidence in cervical and vaginal cultures and are absent from urine.

In contrast to actinobacillosis, *C. hominis* infection does not occur in epidemics. It is primarily an infection of compromised persons. No animal host or reservoir is known, and extensive sampling of several soil and hospital environments has failed to detect these organisms.

References

Burgher, L. W., Loomis, G. W., and Ware, F.: Systemic infection due to *Actinobacillus actinomycetemcomitans*. Am J Clin Pathol 60:412, 1973.

Colebunders, R., Mertens, A., Mahler, Ch., and Parizel, G.: *Cardiobacterium hominis* endocarditis. Acta Clin Belg 37:3, 1982.

Custus, D. L., Halley, H., and Bacon, C. M.: *Actinobacillus lignieresii* endocarditis. Arch Pathol 38:332, 1944.

Geraci, J. E., and Wilson, W. R.: Symposium on infective endocarditis III. Endocarditis due to gram-negative bacteria. Report of 56 cases. Mayo Clin Proc 57:145, 1982.

Kiley, P. and Holt, S. C.: Characterization of the lipopolysaccharide from *Actinobacillus actinomycetemcomitans* Y4 and N27. Infect Immun 30:862, 1980.

Midgley, J., LaPage, S. P., Jenkins, B. A. G., Barrow, G. I., Roberts, M. E., and Buck, A. G.: *Cardiobacterium hominis* endocarditis. J Med Microbiol 3:91, 1970.

Page, M. I., and King, E. O.: Infection due to *Actinobacillus actinomycetemcomitans* and *Haemophilus aphrophilus*. N Engl J Med 275:181, 1966.

Pathak, R. C., and Ristic, M.: Detection of an antibody to *Actinobacillus lignieresii* in infected human beings and the antigenic characterization of isolates of human and bovine origin. Am J Vet Res 23:310, 1962.

Perdue, C. D., Dorney, E. R., and Ferrier, F.: Embolomycotic aneurysm associated with bacterial endocarditis due to *Cardiobacterium hominis*. Am Surg 34:901, 1974.

Phillips, J. E.: The incidence of agglutinating antibodies to *Actinobacillus lignieresii* in the sera of normal and infected cattle. J Pathol Bacteriol 90:557, 1965.

Phillips, J. E.: Antigenic structure and serological typing of *Actinobacillus lignieresii*. J Pathol Bact 93:463, 1967.

Pulverer, G., and Ko, H. L.: *Actinobacillus actinomycetemcomitans*: Fermentative capabilities of 140 strains. Appl Microbiol 20:693, 1970.

Pulverer, G., and Ko, H. L.: Serological studies on *Actinobacillus actinomycetemcomitans*. Appl Microbiol 23:207, 1972.

Reyn, A., Birch-Anderson, A., and Murray, R. G. E.: The fine structure of *Cardiobacterium hominis*. Acta Pathol Microbiol Scand [B]72:51, 1971.

Savage, D. D., Kagan, R. L., Young, A. N., and Horvath, A. E.: *Cardiobacterium hominis* endocarditis: Description of two patients and characterization of the organism. J Clin Microbiol 5:75, 1977.

Slotnick, I. J., and Dougherty, M.: Further characterization of an unclassified group of bacteria causing endocarditis in man: *Cardiobacterium hominis* gen. et sp.n. Antonie van Leeuwenhoek 30:261, 1964.

Slots, J.: Selective medium for isolation of *Actinobacillus actinomycetemcomitans*. J Clin Microbiol 15:606, 1982.

Slots, J., Zambon, J. J., Rosling, B. G., Reynolds, H. S., Christerson, L. A., and Genco, R. J.: *Actinobacillus actinomycetemcomitans* in human peridontal disease association, serology, leukotoxicity, and treatment. J Peridont Res 17:447, 1982.

Snyder, A. I., and Ellner, P. D.: *Cardiobacterium hominis* endocarditis. NY State J Med 69:704, 1969.

Taichman, N. S., Dean, R. T., and Sanderson, C. J.: Biochemical and morphological characterization of the killing of human monocytes by a leukotoxin derived from *Actinobacillus actinomycetemcomitans*. Infect Immunol 28:258, 1980.

Townsend, T. R., and Gillenwater, J. Y.: Urinary tract infection due to *Actinobacillus actinomycetemcomitans*. JAMA 210:558, 1969.

Tucker, D. N., Slotnick, I. J., King, E. O., Tynes, B., Nicholson, J., and Crevasse, L.: Endocarditis caused by *Pasteurella*-like organism: Report of four cases. N Engl J Med 267:913, 1962.

Weiner, M., and Werthamer, S.: *Cardiobacterium hominis* endocarditis: Characterization of the unusual organisms and review of the literature. Am J Clin Pathol 63:131, 1975.

Wong, M. J., and Chan, R. M.: Atypical presentation of *Cardiobacterium hominis* endocarditis. Can Med Assoc 127:511, 1982.

Wormser, G., and Bottone, E. J.: *Cardiobacterium hominis*: Review of Microbiologic and Clinical Features. Rev Inf Dis 5:680,1983.

41
LEGIONELLA

DAVID W. FLEMING, M.D.
ARTHUR L. REINGOLD, M.D.

The genus *Legionella* comprises a group of newly recognized bacterial species that are unrelated, at the family level, to other described human pathogens. Illness caused by legionellae, called legionellosis, occurs in two distinct clinical forms: *Legionella* pneumonia, a severe, acute pneumonia with multisystem involvement, and Pontiac fever, a self-limited influenza-like syndrome consisting of fever, myalgia, and headache. Individual species of *Legionella* may cause one or both of these illnesses.

L. pneumophila (lung-loving) was the first *Legionella* species described (Brenner et al., 1979) and is the species best characterized. Pneumonia caused by *L. pneumophila*, called Legionnaires' disease, accounts for approximately 85 per cent of cases of *Legionella* pneumonia.

Nine additional species of *Legionella* have been described to date (Table 1), and this number will almost certainly continue to increase. Different strains of *Legionella* are classified as separate species on the basis of DNA hybridization studies. Generally, less than 70 per cent homology between strains is required; in practice, DNA homology between currently accepted species ranges from 1 to 30 per cent.

Table 1. TAXONOMIC CLASSIFICATION OF *LEGIONELLA*

Species	Clinical Presentation
Family—Legionellaceae	
Genus—*Legionella*	
1) *L. pneumophila* (OLDA)	Legionnaires' disease or Pontiac fever
2) *L. bozemanii* (WIGA, MI-15)	Legionella pneumonia
3) *L. dumoffii* (NY-23, TEX-KL)	Legionella pneumonia
4) *L. micdadei* (Tatlock, HEBA, PPA)	Legionella pneumonia
5) *L. gormanii* (LS-13)	Legionella pneumonia
6) *L. longbeachae*	Legionella pneumonia
7) *L. jordanis*	Serologic evidence for human infection
8) *L. wadsworthii*	Legionella pneumonia
9) *L. oakridgensis*	Environmental isolates only
10) *L. feeleii*	Pontiac fever

The results of these hybridization experiments, as well as the similar morphologic and metabolic characteristics of these bacteria, have led to the creation of a new bacterial family, Legionellaceae, under which all these species are grouped. At the generic level, most authorities feel that currently recognized species should be classified on the basis of phenotypic similarities rather than genotypic differences, and that a single genus, *Legionella*, is represented.

MORPHOLOGY. Legionellae are nonspore-forming, pleomorphic, gram-negative bacilli. Colonies, which appear after 2 to 4 days of growth on BCYE agar, are 1 to 2 mm in diameter when young, flat to convex, and circular with complete edges. To the unaided eye they appear dull grey to white. Under oblique lighting, colonies have a characteristic cut glass appearance with a refractile ring of variable color depending on the species. In ultraviolet light, colonies of *L. dumoffii*, *L. gormanii*, and *L. bozemanii* fluoresce blue-white; other species appear dull yellow. Dye-containing media have been reported to be of use in species differentiation (Vickers et al., 1981).

Individual bacteria range from .3 to .9 μ in width and 2 to 3 μ in length. Filamentous forms 20 to 40 μ or longer may be observed, most commonly after prolonged growth on artificial media. Most strains have flagella, which usually are single and polar in location, although multiple flagella in a variety of positions have been described (Chandler et al., 1980). Division occurs by a pinching, non-septate process.

Electron microscopy reveals a double, 75A tripartite outer membrane typical of gram-negative bacteria (Chandler et al., 1979). An intervening peptidoglycan layer has been difficult to visualize, but diaminopimelic acid, a substance characteristic of this layer, has been identified by mass spectrometry. The bacterial cytoplasm is rich in ribosomes and may contain vacuoles that stain readily with Sudan Black B.

The cellular fatty acid composition of the legionellae as revealed by gas liquid chromatography is distinctive. Fourteen- to 17-carbon branched chain fatty acids make up greater than 60 per cent of the total profile, while other types of fatty acids, generally present in other bacteria, are absent (Moss et al., 1979). These branched-chain molecules are distinctly uncommon in other gram-negative bacteria and are present in major amounts in only a few bacterial genera.

METABOLISM. Legionellae are obligate aerobes with fastidious nutritional requirements. Optimal growth occurs at a pH of 6.9 (range 6.3 to 7.9), at 35°C (range 25 to 40°). Legionellae do not reduce nitrates, degrade urea, or ferment carbohydrates. They produce multiple aminopeptidases, which enable them to utilize L-amino acids as their primary source of energy and carbon. Arginine, leucine, isoleucine, methionine, threonine, valine, serine, and cysteine are generally considered to be essential amino acids, although amino acid requirements may vary depending on media employed (Tesh and Miller, 1981). Legionellae produce esterases that enable them to split short-chain fatty acids, and they have phosphatase activity.

Biochemical testing has not been found to be useful in species differentiation. Most species are catalase and gelatinase positive, and most, except *L. micdadei* and *L. feeleii*, elaborate a β-lactamase. *L. pneumophila*, *L. micdadei*, *L. longbeachae*, and *L. jordanis* are oxidase positive, and *L. pneumophila* and *L. feeleii* hydrolyze hippurate.

Because of their fastidious nutritional requirements, legionellae do not grow on commonly used bacteriologic media. Originally, they were cultured in embryonated hens' eggs after intraperitoneal inoculation in guinea pigs, a rickettsiologic technique (McDade et al., 1977). The first artificial medium that was found to support the growth of *L. pneumophila* was Mueller-Hinton agar supplemented with 1 per cent hemoglobin and 1 per cent IsovitaleX. Subsequently, it was determined that soluble ferric pyrophosphate and L-cysteine hydrochloride could replace these two supplements, and a new medium incorporating these two chemicals, Feeley-Gorman (F-G) agar, proved to be superior for isolating *L. pneumophila* (Feeley et al, 1978).

Legionellae are most commonly cultured on a charcoal yeast-extract medium supplemented with L-cysteine, ferric pyrophosphate, and ACES buffer (BCYE media). This medium is more sensitive than F-G agar, does not require incubation in 2.5 per cent CO_2, and results in the appearance of colonies in 2 to 4 rather than 5 to 7 days (Feeley et al.,1979). Addition of a-ketoglutarate (BCYEa), glycine, or selective antibiotics may further improve the rate of recovery of *Legionella*.

ANTIGENIC PROPERTIES. A variety of antigens have been identified in legionellae, including antigens common to gram-negative bacteria in general, to *Legionellaceae*, and to individual *Legionella* species. Additionally, serogroup-specific antigens have been identified in *L. pneumophila*, *L. longbeachae*, and *L. bozemanii*. Within *L. pneumophila*, the species that most frequently causes human illness, 8 serogroups are recognized currently. Serogroup 1 is the most commonly encountered, and accounts for approximately 80 per cent of clinical isolates.

The serogroup and species-specific antigens have been the subject of investigation, both because of their relative antigenicity, and because of their specificity and consequent use in diagnosis. The *L. pneumophila* serogroup 1 antigen has been characterized as a high molecular weight lipid-protein-polysaccharide complex. Evidence suggests that it is most likely located on the cell surface (Elliot et al., 1981), and that antibody directed against it may facilitate phagocytosis by leukocytes (Johnson et al., 1979).

Monoclonal antibodies specific for strains within *L. pneumophila* serogroup 1 have been produced recently. These antibodies permit specific subtype identification and thus are potentially useful epidemiologic tools for demonstrating the relationship between environmental and patient isolates (McKinney et al., 1983).

PATHOGENIC PROPERTIES. The ways by which *Legionella* cause illnesses are not well understood. More is known about the pathogenesis of *Legionella* pneumonia than about Pontiac fever, and about the pathogenicity of *L. pneumophila* than the other *Legionella* species.

Pneumonia caused by the *Legionella* may be patchy or confluent and involve one or more lobes. Generally, the infection is alveolar, with relative sparing of the underlying lung tissue. Abscess formation and cavitation occur infrequently. Microscopically, the intraalveolar infiltrates are composed of fibrin, desquamated alveolar lining cells, neutrophils, and macrophages, occasionally containing clusters of *Legionella* (Winn and Myerowitz, 1981). An associated leukocytoclastic vasculitis and focal septal disruption may be demonstrated on histologic section.

Legionella may spread to extrapulmonary sites during the course of illness, including the hilar and thoracic lymph nodes, kidney, spleen, liver, brain, pericardium, and myocardium (Weisenburger et al., 1981). The bloodstream is the presumed route of dissemination, and blood cultures occasionally may be positive. Whether disseminated infection is the cause of the hepatic, renal, and neurologic abnormalities frequently associated with this disease remains unclear.

The pathogenicity of *Legionella* is probably due, at least in part, to its ability to survive and multiply intracellularly, a property shared with only a few other bacterial genera including *Listeria*, *Brucella*, *Mycobacteria*, *Salmonella*, and *Staphylococcus*. The human monocyte seems particularly susceptible; phagocytized *Legionella* in cytoplasmic vacuoles appears to multiply as efficiently as in any in vitro system yet described (Winn and Chandler, 1982). This ability to survive and replicate within alveolar macrophages provides a means of increasing bacterial infectivity while avoiding the host immune system (Fig. 1).

A number of enzymes and toxins that may play a role in the virulence of *Legionella* have been described. These include extracellular proteases, phosphatases, lipases, deoxyribonucleases, and β-lactamases, as well as a cytotoxin (Thorpe and Miller, 1981). Protease activity and type appear to vary by species. *Legionella* also possesses an endotoxin as measured by gelation of Limulus amebocyte lysate by cell suspensions and by induction of pyrogenicity in rabbits (Highsmith et al., 1978). This endotoxin is probably related to, but distinct from, the heat stable lipopolysaccharide endotoxin of other gram-negative bacilli. For *L. pneumophila*, this endotoxin is associated, or perhaps synonymous with, the serogroup-specific antigen (Wong and Feeley, 1983). Besides endotoxin, *Legionella* species share a common, acid extractable, protein toxin that has been shown to suppress phagocytosis by interfering with the oxidative metabolism of the host cell. This protein has properties similar to the cytotoxin that has been isolated, and the two may be the same protein.

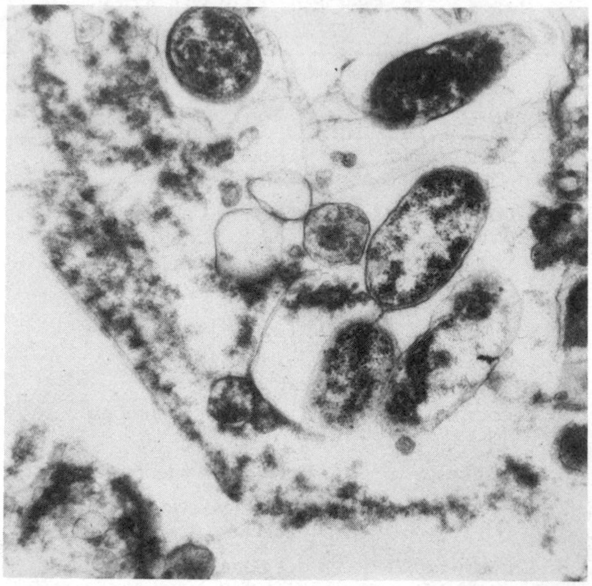

Figure 1. Electron micrograph of lung from a patient who died of Legionnaires' disease during the 1976 Philadelphia outbreak. Intracellular *L. pneumophila*, including one in the process of dividing, can be seen within a phagocytic vacuole of an alveolar macrophage. Magnification 36,450 X. Photograph courtesy of Francis W. Chandler, CDC, Atlanta, Ga.

Other unknown factors may relate to the pathogenicity of *Legionella*. For example, serial passage of *L. pneumophila* on Mueller-Hinton media results in loss of virulence, which subsequent passage of the attenuated culture through embryonated hens' eggs restores (McDade and Sheperd, 1979). Pathogenic mechanisms that account for the differences between the two forms of legionellosis have not yet been discovered.

IMMUNITY. The host response to *Legionella* infection is complex and involves both the humoral and cell-mediated components of the immune system. The relative importance of each, however, and the interactions between the two, are not well understood. *Legionella*'s ability to survive and grow within monocytes, protected from humoral immune mechanisms, further complicates understanding. Attack rates of *Legionella* pneumonia are highest in immunocompromised individuals, and most individuals with normal host defenses seem to be able to prevent serious disease.

The humoral system responds to infection by legionellae with synthesis of a variety of antibodies including IgG, IgM, and IgA, either singly or in various combinations. Antibodies are produced against serogroup-specific antigens, species-specific antigens, Legionellaceae antigens, and antigens common to other gram-negative bacteria. IgG and IgM levels can remain elevated for months to years after infection. IgA, however, is not synthesized in detectable quantities as often, nor is its production sustained as long (Wilkinson et al., 1981).

Virulent *L. pneumophila* remains highly resistant to killing by leukocytes, even in the presence of antibody. Although antibodies to *L. pneumophila*, in conjunction with complement, promote binding of the organism to polymorphonuclear cells and monocytes, only 70 per cent of an inoculum is killed (Horwitz and Silverstein, 1981). The survivors reproduce intracellularly, and the presence of antibody has no effect on this multiplication.

In contrast, stimulation of the cell-mediated immune system seems to play an important role in combating infection. Mononuclear cells respond to *Legionella* antigen with proliferation and production of cytokines, which, in turn, activate other monocytes that have not been exposed to antigen. Monocytes activated in this fashion, in contrast to those exposed to humoral antibodies, have the capability to inhibit intracellular multiplication of *Legionella* (Horwitz, 1983). Once intracellular replication has been inhibited, progression of infection is slowed, and antibody, complement, and polymorphonuclear neutrophils may become effective. Circulating sensitized monocytes that inhibit intracellular growth of legionellae persist in patients who have recovered from *Legionella* pneumonia.

Cell-mediated immunity, therefore, seems to be more important than humoral immunity in the host's response to *Legionella* infection. It is not surprising that experimental *L. pneumophila* vaccines, which stimulate primarily the humoral immune system, have been of limited success in preventing infection in animals.

LABORATORY DIAGNOSIS. Illnesses caused by *Legionella* are clinically indistinguishable from illnesses caused by a variety of other pathogens. Pontiac fever mimics many self-limited viral infections, and *Legionella* pneumonia can resemble infection caused by *Mycoplasma pneumoniae*, *Chlamydia psittaci*, *Coxiella burnetti*, and *Francisella tularensis*, as well as viral respiratory infections such as influenza. Thus, the clinical presentation only suggests the etiology, and diagnosis of legionellosis must be made by appropriate laboratory evaluation.

Commonly used stains, including H&E, gram, and Giemsa, are not effective for visualizing legionellae. The Kinyoun tissue acid-fast stain has been used to demonstrate *L. micdadei* (Myerowitz et al., 1979); other species may occasionally stain weakly with this method. The Gimenez technique has been found to be the most dependable stain for *Legionella* on smears or imprints from fresh tissue, while a modified Dieterle silver impregnation method is recommended for parafinized sections (Blackmon et al., 1979). All of these stains are nonspecific, however, and therefore are not diagnostic.

Currently, laboratory diagnosis of *Legionella* infection can be made in three ways: 1) culture of the organism from appropriate specimens; 2) detection of *Legionella* antigen; and 3) measurement of anti-*Legionella* antibody. All of these methods have been standardized primarily for *Legionella* infections caused by *L. pneumophila*. None are both 100 per cent sensitive and specific.

Legionella can be cultured from otherwise sterile clinical specimens by direct plating onto a suitable medium, such as BCYEa. If other bacterial contaminants are present, as in expectorated sputum, overgrowth is a problem. The yield from specimens from such nonsterile sites may be increased by using a semiselective medium, such as BCYEa supplemented with cefamandole, anisomicin, and polymyxin B (Edelstein, 1983). Heat or low pH treatment of this type of specimen also has been reported to increase the rate of recovery of *Legionella* (Bopp et al., 1981; Groothuis and Veenendall, 1983).

Since asymptomatic carriage of *Legionella*, if it occurs at all, is rare, recovery of the organism from a clinical specimen provides the most specific means of diagnosis. Sensitivity, however, has been reported to be as low as 65 per cent (Edelstein, 1980) when a combination of other diagnostic tests is used as a reference. Recently, advances in medium composition have increased the ease of isolating *Legionella* from clinical specimens, and this means of diagnosis, once thought to be both insensitive and technically difficult, is becoming more widely accepted today (Zarauleff et al., 1983).

Detection of *Legionella* antigen provides the best currently available method for rapid diagnosis of *Legionella* pneumonia. The direct fluorescent antibody test (DFA) is the most commonly used technique (Cherry and McKinney, 1979). Rabbit antiserum, which is *Legionella* serogroup or species specific, is labeled with fluorescein isothiocyanate and used as a stain. *Legionella* of the corresponding serogroup or species stain as fluorescent green bacilli. Appropriate specimens include sputa, trans-tracheal aspirates, bronchial washings or brushings, pleural fluids, and lung tissues. A slide is considered positive if ≥ 25 fluorescing bacteria per smear are seen in lung tissue, or ≥ 5 bacteria in other specimens. Both monovalent and polyvalent conjugates are available for most of the described *Legionella* species and serogroups (Wilkinson, 1983).

The reported sensitivity of the DFA has ranged, in different studies, from 24 to 86 per cent (Wilkinson, 1982). Factors that may affect sensitivity include specimen type, speed of processing, duration of previous antibotic exposure, and number of specimens tested per patient. False-positive interpretation has been a problem when inexperienced personnel read smears. In experienced hands, the specificity of the DFA is approximately 95 per cent. While a few *Pseudomonas* and *Bacteroides* strains have been reported to cross-react with the *Legionella* DFA stain (Cherry et al., 1978), this rarely poses a problem. With earlier reagents, *Staphylococcus* and Streptococcus occasionally fluoresced because of nonspecific antibody binding; however, this is not the case with currently available reagents.

Detection of soluble *L. pneumophila* antigen may prove to be a method of rapid diagnosis in the future. Detection of *L. pneumophila* serogroup 1 antigen excreted in urine during the course of infection by either radioimmune assay (RIA), or enzyme-linked immnosorbent assay (ELISA), appears particularly promising (Kohler and Sathapatavongs, 1983). A variety of other methods for detection of antigen, including slide agglutination and co-agglutination, indirect hemagglutination, glucose oxidase immunoenzymatic assay, and counterimmunoelectrophoresis, have been reported, but have not yet been standardized and validated.

The last method that is used to diagnose *Legionella* pneumonia, and the only method that is used to diagnose Pontiac fever, is measurement of anti-*Legionella* antibody. The indirect immunofluorescence assay (IFA) is the most commonly used technique (Wilkinson et al., 1979). The IFA has not been standardized for *Legionella* pneumonia caused by species other than *L. pneumophila*, or for Pontiac fever. In this test, *Legionella* organisms of a specific serogroup or species are heat or formalin killed, and fixed to a slide. Serial dilutions of acute and convalescent sera are added, followed by conjugated rabbit antihuman globulin. An IFA is positive if a fourfold rise in titer to ≥ 128 (for the heat-killed method) is demonstrated. A single convalescent titer ≥ 256 is considered presumptive evidence of infection, but must be interpreted with caution. Most patients seroconvert within 3 to 6 weeks after onset of symptoms; however, lags of up to several months have been reported (Kirby et al., 1979), and some patients with culture-documented infections never seroconvert. After infection, titers drop slowly and variably, averaging two dilutions in the first 18 months.

The sensitivity of the IFA test has been reported to be 78 to 91 per cent and the specificity 75 to 99 per cent (Wilkinson, 1982). Infrequent cross-reactions with other pathogens causing atypical pneumonia have been reported. Like DFA testing, IFA testing is usually performed with a polyvalent antigen preparation. The clinical usefulness of the IFA is limited because infection can be confirmed only weeks to months after the onset of illness.

As with antigen detection, other methods for measuring anti-*Legionella* antibody have been reported. These include indirect hemagglutination, microagglutination, a solid phase immunofluorescence assay, and an enzyme-linked immunosorbent assay.

DRUG SUSCEPTIBILITY. In vitro studies of drug susceptibilities suggest that legionellae are sensitive to a wide variety of antimicrobials, including rifampin, erythromycin, tetracyclines, trimethoprim-sulfamethoxazole, aminoglycosides, chloramphenicol and β-lactamase-resistant penicillins (Edelstein and Meyer, 1980). Legionellae appear resistant to β-lactamase-sensitive penicillins and cephalosporins, presumably due to the production of β-lactamase by most species. This β-lactamase is species or serotype specific, is more active against cephalosporins than penicillins, and probably is not plasmid mediated (Marre et al., 1982).

In vivo studies, however, strongly suggest that legionellae are resistant to a number of antimicrobials to which they appear to be sensitive in vitro. Only rifampin and erythromycin prevent death of infected embryonated eggs or guinea pigs (Fraser et al., 1978); aminoglycosides, penicillin, chloramphenicol, and tetracycline do not. Retrospective analysis of case fatality rates during the early outbreaks of Legionnaires' disease showed that the highest mortality occurred in patients receiving cephalosporins. Rates were lower in patients receiving aminoglycosides, chloramphenicol, ampicillin, or penicillin, and lowest in those receiving tetracycline, rifampin, or erythromycin (Thornsberry and Kirven, 1979).

This discrepancy between in vivo and in vitro studies may, to a large degree, be the result of differential penetration into macrophages by various antibiotics, and resultant differences in the antibiotic concentrations to which intracellular legionellae are exposed. In general, the greater the lipid solubility of an antibiotic, the better the penetration. Erythromycin has been demonstrated to have much better penetration into cells than tetracyclines, aminoglycosides, or chloramphenicol, which in turn have better penetration than the β-lactams (Johnson et al., 1980).

The current recommendation for treatment of *Legionella* penumonia is erythromycin at a dose of 2 to 4 g/day (15mg/kg in children) for 2 to 3 weeks. Routine drug susceptibility testing is not recommended. Rifampin may be added if the clinical response is poor, but should not be used alone because of the potential for development of drug resistance.

Because Pontiac fever is self-limited and the diagnosis is made retrospectively, drug therapy for this disease has not been evaluated and is not currently recommended.

EPIDEMIOLOGY. Legionnaires' disease was first described following the investigation of an explosive outbreak of a febrile respiratory illness among attendees of an American Legion convention in Philadelphia in 1976 (Fraser et al., 1977). In retrospect, legionellosis has been occurring for at least several decades (McDade et al., 1979) and, most likely before that time as well.

Since 1976, legionellosis has been reported from many areas of the world including Europe, Africa, Asia, North America, and Australia. Sporadic cases of *Legionella* pneumonia are recognized frequently, and can be either community acquired or nosocomial in origin. The incidence of sporadic cases in the United States is estimated at 1.2 cases per 10,000 people per year (Foy et al., 1979), and *Legionella* may be responsible for up to 4 per cent of nosocomially acquired pneumonia (Cohen et al., 1979). Serosurveys of normal populations demonstrate that the prevalence of antibody titers $\geq$ 128 to *L. pneumophila* serogroup 1 is generally 1 to 4 per cent, although much higher prevalences have been reported in presumed hyperendemic areas.

Legionella pneumonia occurs most commonly in the summer and fall. Approximately two-thirds of the patients who acquire this disease are male, and most are over 50 years old (England et al., 1981). Other factors that put individuals at risk for *Legionella* pneumonia are primarily those that cause immune system suppression. Diabetes, underlying malignancy, renal transplantation, immunosuppressive medication, and radiation therapy have all been shown to increase risk, as do smoking, heavy alcohol consumption, and chronic obstructive lung disease (Storch et al., 1979). In contrast, acquisition of Pontiac fever is much less dependent on host factors, and the attack rate among exposed individuals approaches 100 per cent.

The ecology of the *Legionella* is important in understanding the epidemiology of legionellosis. Contrary to what might be expected considering their fastidious nutrient requirements on artificial media, legionellae have been found to be an integral part of the natural aquatic environment and are commonly isolated from streams and lakes, as well as from potable water supplies (Fliermans, 1983). *Legionella*, although not thermophilic, can tolerate temperatures as high as 67° C (Skaliy and McEachern, 1979) and can survive for up to one year in tap water. *Legionella* growth has been observed in association with blue-green algae (Tilson et al., 1980) and both fresh water and soil ameba species (Rowbotham, 1980). Whether these associations are important in the growth and survival of *Legionella* in the environment, or in its pathogenicity in humans is uncertain.

The ways in which *Legionella* in the environment are transmitted to humans are not well understood. Person-to-person transmission has not been shown to occur, and direct spread from environmental sources is the presumed route of infection. As it has become clear that legionellae are common aquatic organisms, attention has focused on aerosolized contaminated water as a means of spread. Heat rejection systems (cooling towers and evaporative condensers), industrial aerosols, and recreational whirlpools that have become contaminated with legionellae have all been implicated as the sources of infection in outbreaks of both *Legionella* pneumonia and Pontiac fever (Broome, 1983).

The presence of the organism in potable water has been associated with disease in several outbreaks as well, although information is still incomplete on exactly how transmission occurs. Administration of respiratory therapy, use of room humidifers, and aerosolization via showering have all been implicated (Lancet, 1983). Since *Legionella* is common in aquatic environments and the significance of a positive environmental culture is unclear, routine environmental sampling in the absence of human illness is not recommended. When there is evidence of human disease, environmental culturing should be undertaken only as a part of an epidemiologic evaluation. Control measures, such as decontamination of water systems and cooling towers, can be difficult, expensive, and have attendant risks. Generally, they should be undertaken only after a source of infection has been implicated epidemiologically, and should be monitored for efficacy and adverse effects.

References

Anonymous. Waterborne *Legionella* [Editorial]. Lancet 2:381, 1983.

Blackmon, J. A., Chandler, F. W., Hicklin, M.D.: Pathologic features of Legionnaires' disease. In: Jones, G. L., Hebert, G. A., (eds.): Laboratory Manual "Legionnaires'" the disease, the bacterium and methodology. Atlanta, Georgia: Centers for Disease Control, 1979; HEW publication no. (CDC) 79-8375.10-12.

Bopp, C. A., Sumner, J. W., Morris, G. K., Wells, J. G.: Isolation of *Legionella* spp. from environmental water samples by low pH treatment and use of a selective medium. J Clin Microbiol 13:714, 1981.

Brenner, D. J., Steigerwalt, A. G., McDade, J. E.: Classification of the Legionnaires' disease bacterium: *Legionella pneumophila*, genus novum, species nova, of the family Legionellaceae, Familia nova. Ann Intern Med 90:656, 1979.

Broome, C. V.: Epidemiologic assessment of methods of transmission of legionellosis. Zbl Bakt Hyg 255:52, 1983.

Chandler, F. W., Cole, R. M., Hicklin, M. D., Blackmon, J. A., Callaway, C. S.: Ultrastructure of the Legionnaires' disease bacterium: a study using transmission electron microscopy. Ann Intern Med 90:642, 1979.

Chandler, F. W., Roth, I. L., Callaway, C. S., Bump, J. L., Thomason, B. M., Weaver, R. E.: Flagella on Legionnaires' disease bacteria: ultrastructural observations. Ann Intern Med 93:711, 1980.

Cherry, W. B., Pittman, B., Harris, P. P., et al.: Detection of Legionnaires' disease bacteria by direct immunofluorescent staining. J Clin Microbiol 8:329, 1978.

Cherry, W. B., McKinney, R. M.: Detection of Legionnaires' disease bacteria in clinical specimens by direct immunofluorescence. In: Jones, G. L., Hebert, G. A. (eds.): Laboratory Manual "Legionnaires'" the disease, the bacterium and methodology. Atlanta, Georgia: Centers for Disease Control, 1979; HEW publication no. (CDC) 79-8375 p91-103.

Cohen, M. L., Broome, C. V., Paris, A. L., et al.: Fatal nosocomial Legionnaires' disease: Clinical and epidemiologic characteristics. Ann Int Med 90:611, 1979.

Edelstein, P. H., Meyer, R. D., Finegold, S. M.: Laboratory diagnosis of Legionnaires' disease. Am Rev Respir Dis 121:317, 1980.

Edelstein, P. H., Meyer, R. D.: Susceptibility of *Legionella pneumophila* to twenty antimicrobial agents. Antimicrob Agents Chemother 18:403, 1980.

Edelstein, P. H.: Culture diagnosis of *Legionella* infections. Zbl Bakt Hyg 255:96, 1983.

Elliott, J. A., Johnson, W., Helms, C. M.: Ultrastructural localization and protective activity of a high-molecular-weight antigen isolated from *Legionella pneumophila*. Infect Immun 31:822, 1981.

England, A. C., Fraser, D. W., Plikaytis, B. D., Tsai, T. F., Storch, G., Broome, C. V.: Sporadic legionellosis in the United States: the first thousand cases. Ann Intern Med 94:164, 1981.

Feeley, J. C., Gorman, G. W., Weaver, R. E., et al.: Primary isolation medium for the Legionnaires' disease bacterium. J Clin Microbiol 8:320, 1978.

Feeley, J. C., Gibson, R. J., Gorman, G. W., et al.: Charcoal-yeast extract agar: primary isolation medium for *Legionella pneumophila*. J Clin Microbiol 10:437, 1979.

Fliermans, C. B.: Autecology of *Legionella pneumophila*. Zbl Bakt Hyg A255:58, 1983.

Foy, H. M., Broome, C. V., Hayes, P. S., et al.: Legionnaires' disease in a prepaid medical care group in Seattle 1963-1975. Lancet 1:767, 1979.

Fraser, D. W., Tsai, T. R., Orenstein, W., et al.: Legionnaires' disease: description of an epidemic of pneumonia. N Eng J Med 297:1189, 1977.

Fraser, D. W., Wachsmuth, K. I., Bopp, C., et al.: Antibiotic treatment of guinea-pigs infected with agent of Legionnaires' disease. Lancet 1:175, 1978.

Groothuis, D. G., Veenendaal, H. R.: Heat treatment as an aid for the isolation of *Legionella pneumophila* from clinical and environmental samples. Zbl Bakt Hyg A255:39, 1983.

Highsmith, A. K., Mackel, D. C., Baine, W. B., Anderson, R. L., Fraser, D. W.: Observations of endotoxin-like activity associated with the Legionnaires' disease bacterium. Curr Microbiol 1:315, 1978.

Horwitz, M. A., Silverstein, S. C.: Interaction of the Legionnaires' disease bacterium (*Legionella pneumophila*) with human phagocytes: I. *L. pneumophila* resists killing by polymorphonuclear leukocytes, antibody, and complement. J Exp Med 153:386, 1981.

Horwitz, M. A.: Cell-mediated immunity in Legionnaires' disease. J Clin Invest 71:1186, 1983.

Johnson, J. D., Hand, W. L., Francis, J. B., King-Thompson, N., Corwin, R. W.: Antibiotic uptake by alveolar macrophages. J Lab Clin Med 95:429, 1980.

Johnson, W., Pesanti, E., Elliott, J.: Serospecificity and opsonic activity of antisera to *Legionella pneumophila*. Infect Immun 26:698, 1979.

Kirby, B. D., Snyder, K. M., Meyer, R. D., et al.: Legionnaires' disease: clinical features of 24 cases. Ann Int Med 89:297, 1978.

Kohler, R. B., Sathapatayavongs, B.: Recent advances in the diagnosis of serogroup 1 *L. pneumophila* pneumonia by detection of urinary antigen. Zbl Bakt Hyg A255:102, 1983.

Marre, R., Medeiros, A. A., Pasculle, A. W.: Characterization of the Beta-lactamases of six species of *Legionella*. J Bacteriol 151:216, 1982.

McDade, J. E., Shepard, C. C., Fraser, D. W., et al.: Legionnaires' disease: isolation of a bacterium and demonstration of its role in other respiratory disease. N Engl J Med 297:1197, 1977.

McDade, J. E., Brenner, D. J., Bozeman, F. M.: Legionnaires' disease bacterium isolated in 1947. Ann Intern Med 90:659, 1979.

McDade, J. E., Shepard, C. C.: Virulent to avirulent conversion of Legionnaires' disease bacterium (*Legionella pneumophila*)—its effect on isolation techniques. J Infect Dis 139:707, 1979.

McKinney, R. M., Thacker, L., Wells, D. E., Wong, M. C., Jones, W. J., Bibb, W. F.: Monoclonal antibodies to *Legionella pneumophila* serogroup 1: possible applications in diagnostic tests and epidemiologic studies. Zbl Bakt Hyg A255:91, 1983.

Moss, C. W., Weaver, R. E., Dees, S. B., Cherry, W. B.: Cellular fatty acid composition of the Legionnaires' disease bacterium. In: Jones, G. L., and Hebert, G. A. (eds.): Laboratory Manual "Legionnaires'" the disease, the bacterium and methodology. Atlanta, Georgia: Centers for Disease Control, 1979; HEW publication no. (CDC) 79-8375, p 48.

Myerowitz, R. L., Pasculle, A. W., Dowling, J. W., et al: Opportunistic lung infection due to "Pittsburgh pneumonia agent." N Engl J Med 301:953, 1979.

Rowbotham, T. J.: Preliminary report on the pathogenicity of *Legionella pneumophila* for fresh water and soil amoebae. J Clin Pathol 33:1179, 1980.

Skaliy, P., McEachern, H. V.,: Survival of the Legionnaires' disease bacterium in water. Ann Intern Med 90:662, 1979.

Storch, G., Baine, W. B., Fraser, D. W., et al.: Sporadic community-acquired Legionnaires' disease in the United States: A case-control study. Ann Intern Med 90:596, 1979.

Tesh, M. J., Miller, R. D.: Amino acid requirements for *Legionella pneumophila* growth. J Clin Microbiol 13:865, 1981.

Thornsberry, C., Irven, L. A.: Antimicrobial susceptibility of the Legionnaires' disease bacterium. In: Jones, G. L., Hebert, G. A., (eds.): Laboratory Manual "Legionnaires'" the disease, the bacterium and methodology. Atlanta, Georgia: Centers for Disease Control, 1979; HEW publication no. (CDC) 79-8375, p 56-7.

Thorpe, T. C., Miller, R. D.: Extracellular enzymes of *Legionella pneumophila*. Infect Immun 33:632, 1981.

Tilson, D. L., Pope, D. H., Cherry, W. B., Fliermans, C. B.: Growth of *Legionella pneumophila* in association with blue-green algae (Cyanobacteria). App Env Micro 39:456, 1980.

Vickers, R. M., Brown, A., Garrity, G. M.: Dye-containing buffered charcoal-yeast extract medium for differentiation of members of the family *Legionnaceae*. J Clin Microbiol 13:380, 1981.

Weisenburger, D. D., Helms, C. M., Renner, E. D.: Sporadic Legionnaires' disease: a pathologic study of 23 fatal cases. Arch Pathol Lab Med 105:130, 1981.

Wilkinson, H. W., Cruce, D. D., Fikes, B. J., Yealy, L. P., Farshy, C. E.: Indirect immunofluorescence test for Legionnaires' disease. In: Jones, G. L., Hebert, G. A. (eds.): Laboratory Manual "Legionnaires'" the disease, the bacterium and methodology. Atlanta, Georgia: Centers for Disease Control, 1979; HEW publication no. (CDC) 79-8375, p 112-116.

Wilkinson, H. W., Cruce, D. D., Broome, C. V.: Validation of *Legionella* pneumophila indirect immunofluorescence assay with epidemic sera. J Clin Microbiol 13:139, 1981.

Wilkinson, H. W.: Serologic Diagnosis of legionellosis. Lab Med 13:151, 1982.

Wilkinson, H. W.: Status of serologic tests for *Legionella* antigen and antibody at the Centers for Disease Control. Zbl Bakt Hyg 255:3, 1983.

Winn, W. C., Myerowitz, R. L.: The Pathology of the *Legionella* pneumonias. Human Pathology 12:401, 1981.

Winn, W. C., Chandler, F. W.: Role of virulence factors in *Legionella* infections. Arch Pathol Lab Med 106:105, 1982.

Wong, K. H., Feeley, J. C.: Antigens and toxic components of *Legionella* in pathogenesis and immunity. Zbl Bakt Hyg 255:132, 1983.

Zuravleff, J. J., Yu, V. L., Shonnard, J. W., Davis, B. K., Rihs, J. D.: Diagnosis of Legionnaires' disease: an update of laboratory methods with new emphasis on isolation by culture. JAMA 250:1981, 1983.

Bibliography

General Reviews

1. Jones, G. L., Hebert, G. A.: Laboratory Manual "Legionnaires' " the disease, the bacterium and methodology. Atlanta, Georgia: Centers for Disease Control, 1979; HEW publication no. (CDC) 79-8375.
2. Herwaldt, L. A., Fraser, D. W.: Legionellosis: Legionnaires' disease and related diseases. In: Fishman, A. P. (ed.): Updates of pulmonary diseases and disorders. New York: McGraw Hill, 1982, p. 45.
3. Meyer, R. D.: *Legionella* infections: a review of five years of research. Rev Infect Dis 5:258, 1983.
4. Reingold, A. L., Band, J. D.: Legionellosis. In: Easmon, C. S. F., Jeljaszewicz, J. (eds.): Medical microbiology. London: Academic Press, 1982(I), p. 217.

42

CHROMOBACTERIUM

Charles E. Davis, M.D.

Chromobacterium violaceum is an oxidase positive, fermentative gram-negative bacillus that produces violet colonies on ordinary media. It is the only violet-colored pathogenic bacterium. *C. violaceum* is motile by means of either polar or polar and peritrichous flagella, depending on the medium and age of the culture. In 1956, Sneath clarified the confusion about the *Chromobacterium* genus. He was able to divide 38 strains of chromobacteria into only two groups. One grew at 37°C, but not at 4°C; the other grew at 4°C but not at 37°C. The biochemical characteristics of each group were uniform enough to propose only one species of mesophilic chromobacteria (*C. violaceum*) and another of psychrophilic bacteria (*C. lividum*). Until this study many other pigmented bacteria were referred to by some authors as species of chromobacteria. For example, pigmented *Serratia marcescens*, now a well-documented member of the family of enterobacteriaceae, was called *Chromobacterium prodigiosum* because it produced a red pigment.

C. lividum will not grow at 37°C and has never been proven to infect animals or man. Although *C. violaceum* is a common soil and water bacterium in subtropical areas, it only rarely causes infections of man and other mammals. In susceptible individuals it causes septicemia and metastatic abscesses with a clinical course similar to meliodosis (Chapter 113). Recent studies suggest that people with chronic granulomatous disease, and perhaps other neutrophil disorders, are uniquely predisposed to infection with this bacterium (Macher et al., 1982).

MORPHOLOGY. The most distinctive colonial feature of chromobacteria is the production of violacein, a violet pigment that is insoluble in water and chloroform but soluble in ethanol. It is synthesized by the bacteria from the metabolism of l-tryptophan and is chemically related to indigo. In many cultures only part of a colony is pigmented, and nonpigmented colonies develop among the more numerous ones with striking violet pigmentation. Nonpigmented variants can be selected *in vitro* on tryptophan-deficient media, and 10 nonpigmented strains were isolated from a pond in Malaysia (Silvendra and Tan, 1977). Nonpigmented strains have never been isolated from infected people or animals. Pigment is not produced anaerobically.

Round, convex, entire colonies of 1 to 2 mm in diameter are produced within 24 hours on most media. Most strains are beta-hemolytic on ox and horse blood agar, but only 50 per cent produced clear hemolysis on rabbit blood within 24 hours (Weaver and Hollis, 1980). Occasional isolates produce rough colonies that are low and conical with an undulate or erose edge. They are dull and granular in appearance and autoagglutinate in suspension. Smooth colonies produce diffuse growth in broth cultures; rough colonies sediment to the bottom of the tube.

Microscopically, *C. violaceum* is a gram-negative bacillus with rounded ends. The average size is about 0.75 by 2 microns. All are motile by means of flagella that can be identified by light microscopy after standard flagellar stains. With respect to flagella, two types of bacteria occur, those that produce only a polar flagellum regardless of growth conditions, and those that produce both lateral and polar flagella (Sneath, 1956a). It is unusual to find an organism without a polar flagellum or to see two polar flagella, unless the bacteria are dividing and the polar flagella are then always at opposite ends. Lateral flagella, usually four to six, occur in young cultures on agar and are of greater length with very short wave lengths. The shorter polar flagella persist and are usually the only flagellum present after 48 hours in culture.

Unlike most gram-negative bacteria, *C. violaceum* contains mesosomal invaginations of the cytoplasmic membrane (Rucinsky and Cota-Robles, 1974). Other cytoplasmic inclusions include fat granules, which are numerous in some strains, and polar polymetaphosphate granules that cause metachromatic staining (Sneath, 1956). Occasional strains produce a small amount of extracellular slime but definite capsules have not been demonstrated. Defective tail-like bacteriophage particles that do not cause plaques on agar overlays of any known bacterial host have been observed (Rucinsky and Cota-Robles, 1973).

ANTIGENIC COMPOSITION. Experimental animals produce agglutinating antibody to whole cells of *C. violaceum*. Sneath (1956a), however, noted that agglutination was only partial over a wide range of dilutions and suspected that there were two antigenic types within a single culture. By careful selection of strains followed by cross-absorption, he showed that the lateral and polar flagella were antigenically different and that both blocked agglutination by antibody to the "O" antigen of *C. violaceum* lipopolysaccharide.

C. violaceum synthesizes a biologically active lipopolysaccharide that is also antigenic. The structure of its lipid A is similar to that of *Salmonella* and other enterobacteriaceae, but some of the fatty acid and amino sugar substituents of the central glucosamine disaccharide differ (Hase and Rietschel, 1977). Despite these structural differences, the lipid A of *Salmonella* and *C. violaceum* are cross-protective in rabbit pyrogenicity studies. Cross-protection is lost when rabbits are challenged with the whole LPS, indicating that the oligosaccharide side chains are antigenically distinct.

METABOLISM. *C. violaceum* is a facultative bacterium that grows well either aerobically or anaerobically. It is markedly proteolytic and hemolytic for most mammalian erythrocytes. It ferments glucose and several other sugars without producing gas. It is a true mesophilic bacterium that grows optimally at temperatures of 20 to 37°C and dies rapidly at 4°C.

Two of the most interesting metabolic reactions of *C. violaceum* are produced by its active respiratory activity; namely, the production of hydrogen cyanide and the violet pigment, violacein. The bacterium has two respiratory pathways. One produces small amounts of cyanide and is azide and cyanide sensitive. The other is resistant to these poisons and evolves high concentrations of cyanide. This high cyanide pathway utilizes cytochromes a_1, d, c, and o; the low cyanide pathway utilizes only cytochromes o and c (Niven *et al.*, 1975).

C. violaceum metabolizes *L*-tryptophan by a number of enzymatic pathways that produce indole but break it down further to violacein and other indole metabolites. Among the more interesting enzymes are two mixed action oxidases, tryptophan hydroxylase and phenylalanine hydroxylase. Tryptophan hydroxylase is usually thought of as a mammalian enzyme because it is the first and rate-limiting step in serotonin synthesis. Its function in chromobacteria is to provide a precursor for violacein.

C. violaceum also produces an active lipase that binds to long chain fatty acids by hydrophobic bonds. This hydrophobic site is distinct from the catalytic site because binding increases the lipolytic activity of the enzyme (Horiuti and Imamura, 1978).

Like many other bacteria, *C. violaceum* synthesizes an *L*-asparaginase with anti-tumor activity. Since patients become sensitized to bacterial asparaginases, the *Chromobacterium* enzyme is interesting because it does not cross-react with the enzymes of *Citrobacter*, *E. coli* or *Erwinia* (Bascomb and Bettelheim, 1976).

In contrast to *C. violaceum, C. lividum* grows at 4°C, but not at 37°C. It is a strict aerobe, nonlipolytic, and only weakly proteolytic and hemolytic.

PATHOGENIC PROPERTIES. *C. violaceum* is a low grade pathogen that seems to require special circumstances to infect mammals. Although the bacterium is widely distributed in subtropical soil and water, only about 30 human infections have been reported in the literature. The portal of entry is most often the broken skin that is exposed to the water or soil of endemic areas. Human and animal infections have been reported from Malaysia, Thailand, India, Australia, New Guinea, Africa, and the Southeastern United States.

Most susceptible individuals develop fulminating septicemia that resembles meliodosis (Chapter 113). Of the 14 cases in the United States (Macher et al., 1982 and 1983) nine have died. Patients typically present with fever, infected skin lesions, and lymphadenitis. Abdominal pain is common and may be the only symptom other than fever. Pulmonary involvement may consist only of a patchy pneumonia, nodular pneumonia, or full-blown miliary disease. Several patients have been thought to have tuberculosis. At autopsy, abscesses of the lungs, liver, and spleen are the most common findings. Endocarditis has not been reported.

The characteristics of the organism that are responsible for the severe disease are not known. The endotoxin is biologically active and the clinical features of DIC have been reported, but most endotoxin-bearing bacteria cause neither such widespread metastatic abscesses nor miliary and cavitary lung disease. Some strains of *C. violaceum* produce an extracellular slime that has not been assayed for biological activity.

IMMUNITY. The skin and mucous membranes are clearly the most important barriers to chromobacteria. Many of the human and subhuman primate infections have followed skin injuries that were exposed to chromobacteria in the water or soil (Macher et al., 1982 and 1982; Groves et al., 1969), Nevertheless, only a few heavily exposed people become infected. Macher et al. (1982 and 1983) have reviewed the cases acquired in the U.S. and obtained data suggesting that defective intracellular killing is an important predisposing condition. Of the 14 cases, four have had proven chronic granulomatous disease of childhood. If one 49-year-old man who inhaled large amounts of infected water when he nearly drowned in a Florida pond is excluded, the rest of the patients are between 4 and 28 years of age. Most are 15 years or less, and Macher suggests that several of the others may have had chronic granulomatous disease or more subtle, clinically unrecognized leukocyte defects that are variants of this disease. These defects would permit the organism to multiply intracellularly and explain some of the manifestations of this disease.

Groves et al. (1969) studied 10 gibbons that died of chromobacteriosis at the National Zoo in Kuala Lumpur, Malaysia and concluded that these tree-dwelling primates were uniquely susceptible to infection. During a 3 year period all gibbons that died were autopsied and all had chromobacteriosis with widespread abscesses of the lungs, liver, and spleen. Gibbons are strictly arboreal animals who even obtain their water supply from vegetation. Only when placed in an unnatural environment such as a zoo are these animals observed to descend to the ground where chromobacteria are found. Groves postulated that their unique susceptibility might be due to complete lack of exposure to this organism or cross-reactive soil organisms. Studies of phagocytosis and killing were inconclusive (unpublished).

The roles of humoral antibody and cell-mediated immunity have not been studied but it seems likely that the first line of defense against this low-grade pathogen is the mechanical barrier of the skin. The polymorphonuclear leukocyte is probably the second.

LABORATORY DIAGNOSIS. *C. violaceum* is the only violet-pigmented pathogenic bacterium. *C. lividum*, the nonpathogenic species, will not be isolated in most diagnostic laboratories because it will not grow at 35 to 37°C. The characteristics that differentiate *C. violaceum* from *C. lividum* and *Aeromonas hydrophila* are listed in Table 1.

Table 1. CHARACTERISTICS OF *C. VIOLACEUM*[1]

Characteristic	Reaction	Comment
Violet pigment	+	*A. hydrophila* is −
Growth at 37°C	+	*C. lividum* is −
Growth at 4°C	−	*C. lividum* is +
Beta-hemolysis	+	*C. lividum* − or weak
Motility	+	both lateral and polar flagella
Oxidase[2]	+	
HCN production	+	*C. lividum* and *A. hydrophila* are −
Methyl red	−	*Aeromonas hydrophila* + (95%)
Indol[3]	−	*A. hydrophila* + (87%)
Voges-Proskauer	−	*A. hydrophila* may be + (33%)
Nitrate reduction	+	
Nitrite reduction	43%	*A. hydrophila* is −
Citrate	+ (slow)	
Lysine decarboxylase	0	
Ornithine decarboxylase	0	
Acid from:[4]		
glucose	+	*C. lividum* (95%) and *A. hydrophila*
sucrose	+	produce gas from the fermentation
fructose	+	of glucose and other sugars. *C.*
mannose	±	*violaceum* does not produce gas.
trehalose	+	*C. lividum* is −
lactose	−	
mannitol	−	*A. hydrophila* is + (99%)
maltose	−	*A. hydrophila* is + (99%)
rhamnose	−	
glycerol	−	*A. hydrophila* is + (89%)
Hydrolysis or liquefaction		
gelatin	+	*C. lividum* − or feeble
egg yolk	+	*C. lividum* −
esculin	−	*C. lividum* is +

[1]Reactions for *C. violaceum* are virtually 100 per cent except where noted. Tests that differentiate *C. lividum* or *Aeromonas hydrophila* from *C. violaceum* are noted in the COMMENT column. *A. hydrophila* is considered because it could be confused with nonpigmented mutants of *C. violaceum* (see text). Reactions are from Sneath (1956), Sivendra (1976), Groves et al., (1969), and Weaver and Hollis (1980).

[2]Some laboratories have noted variable oxidase reactions (Weaver and Hollis, 1980). Our strains from gibbons and soil and water in Malaysia (Groves et al., 1969) and all of Sneath's original 38 strains (Sneath, 1956) were positive.

[3]Nonpigmented strains do not metabolize indol further to violacein and may be indole positive.

[4]Almost all *C. violaceum* strains ferment carbohydrates *without* the production of gas, but Sivendra (1976) reported 3 aerogenic strains.

A. hydrophila is included because it would be possible to confuse it with nonpigmented mutants of *C. violaceum*. Nonpigmented *C. violaceum* has not been recognized as a cause of human or animal infections, but Sivendra and Tan (1977) isolated 10 strains from pond water in Malaysia.

DRUG SUSCEPTIBILITY. *C. violaceum* is uniformly susceptible to readily achievable levels of chloramphenicol, the aminoglycosides, and tetracycline. Patients have been successfully treated with the combination of chloramphenicol and gentamicin and gentamicin alone (Macher, 1982 and 1983). *C. violaceum* synthesizes a chromosomally mediated beta-lactamase that is related to the cephalosporinases of *Pseudomonas aeruginosa* (Farrar and O'Dell, 1976). This enzyme inactivates penicillins and all but the most cephalosporinase-resistant cephalosporins. Chloramphenicol and gentamicin appear to be the antibiotics of choice.

EPIDEMIOLOGY. *C. violaceum* has been isolated either from infections or the soil and ground water of Southeast Asia, the Philippines, India, Australia, New Guinea, the Southeastern United States (Florida, Louisiana, South Carolina, Georgia), Trinidad, French Guiana, and Senegal. All these areas are between the latitudes of 35°N and 35°S. It is clear that this mesophilic bacterium that prefers temperatures of 20 to 37°C and dies at 4°C is limited to subtropical areas where freezing either does not occur or is unusual. Furthermore, all infections in the United States have been acquired during June to September, when water and soil temperatures are optimal for *C. violaceum* (Macher et al., 1982). Infections are acquired from these environmental sources, often through open wounds. The water supplies of the gibbons in Malaysia (Groves et al., 1969) and a village in Vietnam were found to be contaminated with *C. violaceum* (Ognibene and Thomas, 1970). It is more likely that the portal of entry was broken skin than the alimentary tract, but *C. violaceum* has been isolated from the feces of people (Groves et al., 1969).

In a careful study of food, water, and soil in Florida, Koburger and May (1982) found large numbers of *C. violaceum* in the soil and water of the Gainesville area. *C. lividum*, but not *C. violaceum*, was isolated from food. This result was not unexpected since most of the food samples had been refrigerated before study. The use of two types of selective media probably contributed to the success of this study.

References

Bascomb, S. and Bettelheim, K. A.: Immunological relationships of bacterial L-asparaginases. J Gen Microbiol 92:173, 1976.

Farrar, W. E. Jr. and O'Dell, N. M.: Beta-lactamase activity in *Chromobacterium violaceum.* J Infect Dis 134:290, 1976.

Groves, M. C., Strauss, J. M., Abbas, J., and Davis, C. E.: Natural infections of gibbons with a bacterium producing violet pigment (*Chromobacterium violaceum*). J Infect Dis 120:605, 1969.

Hase, S. and Rietschel, Th.: The chemical structure of the lipid A component of lipopolysaccharide from *C. violaceum* NCTC 9694. Eur J Biochem 75:23, 1977.

Horiuti, Y. and Imamura, S.: Stimulation of Chromobacterium lipase activity and prevention of its absorption to palmitoyl cellulose by hydrophobic binding of fatty acids. J Biochem (Tokyo) 83:1381-1385, 1978.

Koburger, J. A. and May, S. O.: Isolation of *Chromobacterium* spp. from foods, soil, and water. Appl Environ Microbiol 44:1463, 1982.

Macher, A. M., Casale, T. B., and Fauci, A. S.: Chronic granulomatous disease of childhood and *Chromobacterium violaceum* infections in the Southeastern United States. Ann Int Med 97:51, 1982.

Macher, A. M., Casale, T. B., Gallin, J. I., Boltansky, H., and Fauci, A. S.: *Chromobacterium violaceum* infections and chronic granulomatous disease (Letter). Ann Int Med 98:258, 1983.

Niven, D. F., Collins, P. A., and Knowles, C. J.: The respiratory system of *Chromobacterium violaceum* under conditions of high and low cyanide evolution. J Gen Microbiol 90:271, 1975.

Ognibene, A. J. and Thomas, E.: Fatal infection due to *Chromobacterium violaceum* in Vietnam. Am J Clin Pathol 54:607, 1970.

Rucinsky, T. E. and Cota-Robles, E. H.: The intracellular organization of bacteriophage tail-like particles in cells of *Chromobacterium violaceum* following mitomycin C treatment. J. Ultrastruct. Res. 73:260, 1973.

Rucinsky, T. E. and Cota-Robles, E. H.: Mesosome structure in *Chromobacterium violaceum.* J Bacteriol 118:717, 1974.

Sivendra, R.: Unusual *Chromobacterium violaceum*: Aerogenic strains. J Clin Microbiol 3:70, 1976.

Sivendra, R. and Tan, S. W.: Pathogenicity of non-pigmented cultures of *Chromobacterium violaceum.* J Clin Microbiol 5:514, 1977.

Sneath, P. H. A.: Cultural and biochemical characteristics of the genus Chromobacterium. J Gen Microbiol 15:70, 1956.

Sneath, P. H. A.: The change from polar to peritrichous flagellation in *Chromobacterium* spp. J Gen Microbiol 15:99, 1956a.

Weaver, R. E. and Hollis, D. G.: Gram-negative fermentative bacteria and *Francisella tularensis. In* Manual of Clinical Microbiology 3rd edition. Lennette, E. H., Balows, A., Hausler, W. J. and Truant, J. P. (eds.). American Society for Microbiology, Washington, D.C., 1980, p 249.

43

CAPNOCYTOPHAGA

CHARLES E. DAVIS, M.D.

Capnocytophaga are fascinating oral bacteria that have been implicated in gingival destruction and bone resorption in patients with defective neutrophil function. They also cause septicemia in patients with hematologic malignancies and neutropenia. In 1979, the genus name of *Capnocytophaga* was proposed for the gliding, anaerobic to microaerophilic, fusiform gram-negative bacilli that produced acetate and succinate as major metabolic end products and required carbon dioxide for both aerobic and anaerobic growth (Leadbetter et al., 1979; Williams and Hammond, 1979). These catalase-negative and oxidase-negative bacteria are active fermenters, even when grown in the presence of oxygen. Three species were proposed: *C. ochracea, C. sputigena,* and *C. gingivalis.*

The name *Capnocytophaga* was chosen to emphasize the CO_2 dependence (Capno-) and the relationship to other gliding bacteria (-cytophaga). *Capnocytophaga* differs from other gliding bacteria in two important ways, however. Typical gliding bacteria (cytophaga-flexibacter-myxobacter groups) are not associated with disease, and all undergo nonfermentative, strictly respiratory metabolism in the presence of air. Most are strict aerobes.

C. ochracea, the best known species of *Capnocytophaga,* has had a short but active history. It was thought to be a variant of *Fusobacterium nucleatum* by Prevot et al. (1955), a variety of *Bacteroides oralis* (*Bacteroides oralis* var. *elongatus*) by Loesche et al. (1964), and a new capnophilic bacterium, Dysgonic-Fermenter-1 (DF-1) by Elizabeth King of the Communicable Disease Center of the U.S.A. In 1972 Holdeman and Moore recognized the identity of Prevot's (1953) and Loesche's (1964) strains. Although they found that these bacteria were capnophilic instead of obligately anaerobic, they proposed the name *Bacteroides ochraceus.*

At the same time that the new genus was proposed, other laboratories demonstrated the identity of *Capnocytophaga* with DF-1 and *Bacteroides ochraceus* (Williams et al., 1979 and Newman et al., 1979). All three were similar in colonial and microscopic morphology, biochemical reactions, metabolic end products, and DNA homologies. Guanine-cytosine ratios varied from 33 to 41 per cent. Further studies of genetic divergence in DNA homology studies supported the inclusion of all strains into one genus with three species (Williams and Hammond, 1979).

Capnocytophaga spp. colonize normal and diseased human gingiva, are associated with periodontitis, and cause septicemia in patients with hematologic malignancies and granulocytopenia.

MORPHOLOGY. Two types of colonies are produced. The more common is more typical of the gliding bacteria than ordinary eubacteria. These colonies are thin and flat with serrated edges and fingerlike projections that may extend several centimeters from the point of inoculation (Leadbetter et al., 1979). This gliding or spreading colony is more easily appreciated under oblique lighting or a dissecting microscope and can be accentuated by inoculation onto media with agar concentrations of about 3 per cent (wt/vol). These colonies may appear to pit the agar. Other colonies of the same or different strains may be round with smooth edges, especially in media with lower concentrations of agar. *Capnocytophaga* grow slowly and require 2 to 4 days to form colonies of 2 to 3 mm. Aerobic and anaerobic growth is equal in 5 to 10 per cent CO_2.

Colonies may appear to be greyish-white, pink, or yellow, but the cell mass is always yellow when scraped from the medium. The nondiffusible, cell-bound pigment is not carotenoid because its production is not inhibited by diphenylamine (Leadbetter et al., 1979).

Growth in liquid media may be either clumped or dispersed. Clumping is associated with the presence of glucose or other sugars in the medium and may be caused by the production of surface polymers that promote cell-to-cell and cell-to-glass adhesion.

Microscopically, the cells are gram-negative and fusiform. One end is tapered, and the other round or square. A single colony may contain small (2.4 to 4.2 μm by 0.38

to 0.5 μm) and large (4.8 to 5.8 μm by 0.42 to 0.6 μm) cells (Holt et al., 1979).

The typical three-layered gram-negative cell wall contains a definite periplasmic space. Mesosomes and extracellular vesicles resembling extruded lipopolysaccharide are common (Holt et al., 1979). Several extracellular appendages were noted by Holt et al. (1979). Almost half the bacteria are bounded by electron-dense, hairlike "fuzz," and fibrous material appears to join many cells. Some bacteria also seem to produce a stalklike projection at one end of the cell that may function as an attachment or holdfast element, similar to that of Caulobacter (Poindexter, 1964). This stalk and the extracellular polymers represented by the fuzz and fibrous material may promote gliding (surface translocation) and attachment to surfaces.

The major components of the peptidoglycan of *C. ochracea* are diaminopimelic acid, glucosamine, muramic acid, alanine, and glutamic acid (Murayama et al., 1982b). Structural studies have not been reported. The lipopolysaccharides of *Capnocytophaga* contain C15 fatty acids and typical LPS sugars including ketodeoxyoctulosonic acid (KDO). They are biologically active (Murayama et al., 1982b and Stevens et al., 1980a), but the LPS of *C. sputigena* is less potent in many biological assays than the endotoxins of other gram-negative bacteria (Stevens et al., 1980a).

ANTIGENIC COMPOSITION. Very little work has been done on the antigenic composition of *Capnocytophaga*. A lipid-associated protein that is common to the genus stimulates the production of precipitating antibody in rabbits that differentiates *Capnocytophaga* from other bacteria. A periodate-sensitive, carbohydrate antigen isolated from *C. ochracea* stimulated antibody specific for this species (Murayama et al., 1982a). The LPS and peptidoglycan are potent immunomodulators, and the LPS induces good antibody production in rabbits. The antigenic specificities of the LPS have not been studied.

METABOLISM. *Capnocytophaga* spp. are microaerophilic, capnophilic bacteria that will not grow in ambient air without the addition of 5 to 10 per cent CO_2. They attack carbohydrates fermentatively and do not synthesize catalase, even in the presence of oxygen. They apparently lack a complete electron transport chain.

Menaquinone (vitamin K2) is the only respiratory quinone found in a careful study of 12 strains (Collins et al., 1982). *Capnocytophaga* spp. do not synthesize cytochrome C. No strains produce hydrogen sulfide, indole, or acetylmethylcarbinol, but all ferment glucose, sucrose, maltose, and mannose (Socransky et al., 1979).

Capnocytophaga are not thought of as proteolytic organisms, but trypsinlike activity has been reported (Laughon et al., 1982), and some strains hydrolyze gelatin; all decarboxylate arginine (Socransky et al., 1979). Aminopeptidase activity has been reported (Nakamura and Slots, 1982).

Growth requirements have not been carefully studied but *Capnocytophaga* will grow on most complex media. Bile salts are inhibitory.

All species of *Capnocytophaga* synthesize on identical group of 15 carbon, saturated isobranched fatty acids that are unique to this genus (Dees et al., 1982; Collins et al., 1982).

PATHOGENIC PROPERTIES. *Capnocytophaga* has been implicated as an important factor in human periodontal disease and causes severe experimental periodontitis in gnotobiotic rats (Socransky et al., 1979). The evidence is even stronger for its participation in special types of gingival destruction and bone resorption in patients with juvenile periodontitis (Slots, 1976), diabetes mellitus, and the Papillon-Lefevre syndrome, all conditions with defective neutrophil function (Van Dyke et al., 1982). Furthermore, culture filtrates of *C. ochracea* contain a dialyzable substance that distorts the morphology of neutrophils and inhibits their migration. This neutrophil lesion, which was also present in 2 people with severe *Capnocytophaga* infections (one with severe juvenile periodontitis and one with septicemia), was corrected by eradication of the infection (Shurin et al., 1979). Whole cells of *Capnocytophaga* also cause neutrophils to release lysosomal enzymes that could be destructive to infected tissue (Tsai et al., 1978).

Extracts and whole cells of *Capnocytophaga* have many effects on other human cells. They are polyclonal activators of B cells, stimulate proliferation of splenic lymphocytes and peritoneal macrophages, and inhibit fibroblast proliferation (Bick et al., 1981; Stevens et al., 1980a; Murayama et al,. 1982b.) Since B cells and plasma cells are plentiful in periodontal lesions and the T and B cells of patients with severe periodontitis proliferate and produce lymphokines in response to oral microbes, these activities of *Capnocytophaga* may contribute to periodontitis (See Bick et al., 1981). Purified extracellular polysaccharide, on the other hand, may inhibit the responses of lymphocytes to LPS and concanavalin A (Bolton and Dyer, 1983).

All *Capnocytophaga* spp. also have a direct effect on humoral immunity. Among the oral bacteria, only *B. melaninogenicus*, an occasional strain of streptococcus, and *Capnocytophaga* synthesize an IgA protease (Kilian, 1981). IgA1 is cleaved into intact Fab and Fc fragments. Polyclonal IgG, but not IgA_2, is also broken down. This difference between *Capnocytophaga* and most other oral bacteria is analogous to the contrast between pathogenic and nonpathogenic *Neisseria* and suggests that the IgA protease is an important virulence factor.

Unlike most other oral bacteria, *Capnocytophaga* produce trypsin (Laughon et al., 1982). The proteolytic activity of trypsin could disrupt the junctional epithelium of the gingival pocket, activate latent gingival collagenases by destroying the serum collagenase inhibitor, and release chemotactic components of complement by activating the alternative complement pathway.

Finally, the morphology of *Capnocytophaga* should add to its virulence. The hold-fast stalk and the extracellular polysaccharide represented by the "fuzz" and fibrous material between cells (Holt et al., 1979) are ideal structures for adherence to the epithelium of the gingiva. The combination of gliding motility and the lubricating effect of the extracellular slime probably permit *Capnocytophaga* to translocate over the gingival surface into the gingival pocket.

IMMUNITY. Whole cells and extracts of *Capnocytophaga* stimulate antibody production and delayed hypersensitivity reactions (Murayama et al., 1982a and 1982b), but the roles of humoral and cellular immunity in resistance to infection are unknown. The LPS and peptidoglycan are strong immunomodulators that may either promote or interfere with the immune response to *Capnocytophaga* and other bacteria. The exopolysaccharide slime layer of *C. ochracea* inhibits lymphocyte proliferation (Bolton and Dyer, 1983).

The prominence of *Capnocytophaga* in periodontitis of

Table 1. BIOCHEMICAL CHARACTERISTICS OF CAPNOCYTOPHAGA[1].

Characteristic[2]	Per cent Positive		
	C. ochracea	*C. sputigena*	*C. gingivalis*
Acid from:			
glucose[3]	100	100	100
sucrose	100	100	100
maltose	100	100	100
mannose	100	100	100
fructose	89	50	12
galactose	83	0	0
amygdalin	90	25	0
cellobiose	45	0	0
glycogen	71	0	0
Reduction of:			
nitrate	8	83	4
nitrite	57	40	60
Urease	14	0	12
Lysine decarboxylase	5	0	9
Benzidine reaction	100	100	100
Hydrolysis of:			
starch	77	0	0
gelatin	14	60	17
dextran	96	17	4

[1]Modified from Socransky et al., 1979.
[2]Ribose, xylose, mannitol, and sorbitol are not attacked. Indole, H_2S, and Voges-Proskauer reactions are negative. Less than 10 per cent of *C. ochracea* ferment trehalose, salicin, and arabinose, but positive reactions are useful because the other species do not attack these sugars.
[3]By fermentation.

people with defective neutrophil function (Van Dyke et al., 1982) and the occurrence of *Capnocytophaga* septicemia primarily in patients with hematologic malignancies or granulocytopenia (Forblenza et al., 1980) suggest that the polymorphonuclear leukocyte is the major natural barrier to infection with these bacteria.

LABORATORY DIAGNOSIS. Laboratories that do not supplement aerobic cultures with 5 to 10 per cent CO_2 may confuse *Capnocytophaga* with fusobacteria or *Bacteroides* species. This error can be avoided by subculturing all anaerobic gram-negative bacilli at least once in an extinction candle jar. Within two to four days *Capnocytophaga* species will form gray, pink, or yellow colonies of 2 to 3 mm in diameter. Spreading, lightly pigmented, slow-growing colonies of fusiform bacteria should raise the possibility of *Capnocytophaga* even under anaerobic conditions. If the organism fails to grow either aerobically or anaerobically on subculture without CO_2, the isolate is probably a *Capnocytophaga* species. If the isolate forms white, entire colonies, it will be misidentified unless subcultures are made to establish the need for CO_2.

All species are active fermenters of glucose, sucrose, maltose, and mannose. Unlike fusobacteria, most are sensitive to actinomycin D and give a positive benzidine reaction. H_2S, indole, and acetylmethylcarbinol are not produced. Identification to species level is dependent on fermentation of certain sugars, hydrolysis of polymers, and reduction of nitrate (Table 1). Some isolates of *C. ochracea* cannot be differentiated from *C. sputigena*. Gliding motility is difficult to detect but can sometimes be recognized by dark field examination of log phase cultures.

ANTIBIOTIC SUSCEPTIBILITY. Strains without plasmid-mediated antibiotic resistance are sensitive to penicillin (MIC range 0.5 to 2 μg/ml), clindamycin (0.062 to 4 μg/ml), erythromycin (0.125 to 4 μg/ml), cefaclor (0.5 to 8 μg/ml), tetracycline (0.25 to 2 μg/ml), and chloramphenicol (2 to 8 μg/ml) (Sutter et al., 1981). Most strains are sensitive to the third-generation cephalosporins and newer penicillins, but they are usually more sensitive to penicillin G. All strains are resistant to colistin, nalidixic acid, and the aminoglycosides.

It is necessary to test the sensitivities of *Capnocytophaga*, however, because we have isolated a strain of *C. ochracea* that was resistant to penicillin, tetracycline, chloramphenicol, erythromycin, clindamycin, rifampin, and the aminoglycosides (Guiney and Davis, 1978 and 1982). Resistance to tetracycline, chloramphenicol, and the aminoglycosides was mediated by a large conjugative plasmid that was transferable to *E. coli* and closely related to other well-characterized *E. coli* plasmids.

EPIDEMIOLOGY. *Capnocytophaga* spp. have been isolated only from people (Williams et al., 1979) and may be obligate human commensals and pathogens, although they can cause experimental periodontitis in gnotobiotic rats. They can reach levels of 10^8 in gingival pockets and may make up to 10 to 15 per cent of the total cultivable flora (Mashumo et al., 1983). A selective medium (TBBP) made up of 4 per cent trypticase soy agar, 5 per cent sheep blood, 0.1 per cent yeast extract, 50 μg/ml of bacitracin, and 100 μg/ml of polymyxin B enhances recovery and recognition.

References

Bick, P. H., Carpenter, A. B., Holdeman, L. V., Miller, G. A., Ranney, R. A., Polcanis, K. G., and Tew, J. G.: Polyclonal B cell activation induced by extracts of gram negative bacteria isolated from periodontally diseased sites. Infect Immun 34:43, 1981.

Bolton, R. W., and Dyer, J. K.: Suppression of murine lymphocyte mitogen responses by exopolysaccharide from *Capnocytophaga ochracea*. Infect Immun 39:476, 1983.

Collins, M. D., Shah, H. N., McKee, A. S., and Knoppenstedt, R. M.: Chemotaxonomy of the genus *Capnocytophaga* (Leadbetter, Holt, and Socransky). J Appl Bacteriol 52:409, 1982.

Dees, S. B., Karr, D. E., Hollis, D., and Moss, C. W.: Cellular fatty acids of *Capnocytophaga* species. J Clin Microbiol 16:779, 1982.

Forblenza, S. W., Newman, M. G., Lipsey, A. L., Siegel, S. E., and Blackman, U.: Capnocytophaga sepsis: A newly recognized clinical entity in granulocytopenic patients. The Lancet 1 No. 8168:567, 1980.

Guiney, D. G., and Davis, C. E.: Identification of a conjugative R plasmid in *Bacteroides ochraceus* capable of transfer to *Escherichia coli*. Nature 274:181, 1978.

Guiney, D. G., and Davis, C. E.: Incompatibility and host range of pGD10 from *Capnocytophaga ochraceus*, formerly *Bacteroides ochraceus*. Plasmid 7:196, 1982.

Holdeman, L. V., and Moore, W. E. C.: *Bacteroides*. In Holdeman, L. V., and Moore, W. E. C. (eds.): Anaerobe Laboratory Manual. Blacksburg, VA, Virginia Polytechnic Institute Anaerobe Laboratory, 1972, p. 27.

Holt, S. C., Leadbetter, E. R., and Socransky, S. S.: *Capnocytophaga*: new genus of gram negative gliding bacteria. II. Morphology and ultrastructure. Arch Microbiol 122:17, 1979.

Kilian, M.: Degradation of immunoglobulins A1, A2, and G by suspected principal periodontal pathogens. Infect Immun 34:757, 1981.

Laughon, B. E., Syed, S. A., and Loesche, W. J.: API ZYM system for identification of *Bacteroides* spp., *Capnocytophaga* spp. and spirochetes of oral origin. J Clin Microbiol 15:97, 1982.

Leadbetter, E. R., Holt, S. C., and Socransky, S. S.: *Capnocytophaga*: new genus of gram negative, gliding bacteria. I. General characteristics, taxonomic considerations, and significance. Arch Microbiol 122:9, 1979.

Loesche, W. J., Socransky, S. S., and Gibbons, R. J.: *Bacteroides oralis*, proposed new species isolated from the oral cavity of man. J Bacteriol 88:1329, 1964.

Mashumo, P. A., Yamamoto, Y., Masakazu, N., and Slots, J.: Selective recovery of oral *Capnocytophaga* spp. with sheep blood agar containing bacitracin and polymyxin B. J Clin Microbiol 17:187, 1983.

Murayama, Y., Mashimo, P. A., Tabak, L. A., Levine, M. J., and Ellison, S. A.: Isolation and partial characterization of a genus common antigen and species specific antigen of *Capnocytophaga*. Jap J Med Sci Biol 35:153, 1982a.
Murayama, Y., Muranishi, K., Okada, H., Kato, K., Kotani, S., Takada, H., Tsujimoto, M., Kawasaki, A., and Ogawa, T.: Immunological activities of *Capnocytophaga* components. Infect Immun 36:876, 1982b.
Nakamura, M., and Slots, J.: Aminopeptidase activity of *Capnocytophaga*. J Periodont Res 17:597, 1982.
Newman, M. G., Sutter, V. L., Pickett, M. J., Blachman, U., Greenwood, J. R., Grinenko, V., and Citron, D.: Detection, identification, and comparison of *Capnocytophaga, Bacteroides ochraceus*, and DF-1. J Clin Microbiol 10:557, 1979.
Poindexter, J. S.: Biological properties and classification of the Caulobacter group. Bacteriol Rev 28:231, 1964.
Prevot, A. R., Tardieux, P., Joubert, L., and deCadore, F.: Researches sur *Fusiformis nucleatus* (Knorr) et son pouvoir pathogen pour l'homme et les animoux. Ann Inst Pasteur (Paris) 91:788, 1955.
Shurin, S. B., Socransky, S. S., Sweeney, E., and Stossel, T. P.: A neutrophil disorder induced by *Capnocytophaga*, a dental micro-organism. N Engl J Med 301:849, 1979.
Slots, J.: The predominant cultivable organism in juvenile periodontitis. Scand J Dent Res 84:1, 1976.
Socransky, S. S., Holt, S. C., Leadbetter, E. R., Tanner, A. C. R., Savitt, E. D., and Hammond, B. F.: *Capnocytophaga*: new genus of gram negative gliding bacteria. III. Physiological characterization. Arch Microbiol 122:29, 1979.
Stevens, R. H., Sela, M. N., Shapira, J., and Hammond, B. F.: Detection of a fibroblast proliferation inhibitory factor from *Capnocytophaga sputigena*. Infect Immun 27:271, 1980a.
Stevens, R. H., Sela, M. N., Shapira, J., McArthur, W. P., Nowotny, A., and Hammond, B. F.: Biological and chemical characterization of endotoxin from *Capnocytophaga sputigena*. Infect Immun 27:246, 1980b.
Sutter, V. L., Pyeatt, D., and Kwok, Y. Y.: *In vitro* susceptibility of *Capnocytophaga* strains to 18 antimicrobial agents. Antimicrob Agents Chemother 20:270, 1981.
Tsai, C.-C., Hammond, B. F., Baehni, P., McArthur, W. P., and Taichman, N. S. Interaction of inflammatory cells and oral micro-organisms. VI. Exocytosis of PMN lysosomes in response to gram-negative plaque bacteria. J Periodontal Res 13:504, 1978.
Van Dyke, T. E., Levine, M. J., and Genco, R. J.: Periodontal diseases and neutrophil abnormalities. In Genco, R. J. and Mengenhagen, S. E. (eds.): Host-Parasite Interactions in Periodontal Diseases. Washington, D.C., American Society for Microbiology, 1982, pp. 235–245.
Williams, B. L. and Hammond, B. F.: *Capnocytophaga*: new genus of gram-negative gliding bacteria. IV. DNA base composition and sequence homology. Arch Microbiol 122:35, 1979.
Williams, B. L., Hollis, D., and Holdeman, L. V.: Synonymy of strains of Center for Disease Control group DF-1 with species of *Capnocytophaga*. J Clin Microbiol 10:550, 1979.

ACID-FAST RODS

44
MYCOBACTERIA

DONALD W. SMITH, PH.D.

The genus *Mycobacterium* includes the causative agents of tuberculosis and leprosy, two diseases that, according to the World Health Organization, are among the main public health priorities of many of the developing countries of the world. For example, the global tuberculosis problem is estimated to be the following: 1500 million persons infected with tubercle bacilli; 20 million sputum-positive persons capable of disseminating the disease; 3 to 5 million new cases each year; and 600,000 deaths per year.

The principal species of mycobacteria that cause disease in man and other animals are listed in Table 1, along with the most common saprophytic (free living) mycobacteria.

MYCOBACTERIUM TUBERCULOSIS AND ATYPICAL MYCOBACTERIA

Morphology. Mycobacteria are slender, rod-shaped organisms that cannot be distinguished from each other by their morphology. Tubercle bacilli in tissue and in sputum smears frequently have an irregularly staining, beaded appearance. The unstained regions of the cell are presumably areas containing inclusion bodies such as glycogen and polymetaphosphate. Electron microscopic examination of mycobacteria shows a thick cell wall, mesosomes, and inclusions of lipid (Fig. 1). Mycobacteria do not form spores. They have an unusually high lipid content, greater than 25 per cent in contrast to 0.5 per cent lipid in gram-positive and 3 per cent lipid in gram-negative bacteria. The high lipid content is presumed to be responsible for their characteristic resistance to drying, alcohol, acids, alkali, and certain germicides. The high lipid content also renders the Gram stain invalid for mycobacteria. On the other hand, mycobacteria are acid-fast; this property is shared with certain species of only one other genus of bacteria, *Nocardia*. Once stained with basic fuchsin dyes, acid-fast organisms resist decolorization even with alcohol containing 3 per cent mineral acid. Acid-fastness is an

Table 1. PATHOGENIC AND SAPROPHYTIC MYCOBACTERIA

Pathogenic Mycobacteria	
Microorganism	***Disease Produced***
M. tuberculosis	Tuberculosis in man and subhuman primates
M. bovis	Tuberculosis in cattle, man and subhuman primates
*M. avium intracellulare**	Tuberculosis in birds and swine; tuberculosis-like disease in man
*M. kansasii**	Tuberculosis-like disease in man
*M. fortuitum complex** (including *M. chelonei*)	Wound infection in man
*M. marinum**	Tuberculosis in fish and cutaneous disease in man
*M. ulcerans**	Ulcerative lesions in man
M. leprae	Leprosy in man
Saprophytic Mycobacteria	
Microorganism	***Source in Nature***
M. gordonae	Soil, water Not responsible for human disease but may be isolated from sputum, gastric washings, etc.
M. terrae complex (includes *M. terrae, M. triviale, M. novum,* and *M. nonchromogenicum*)	Soil, water
M. flavescens	Soil, water
M. gastri	Soil, water

*Atypical mycobacteria.

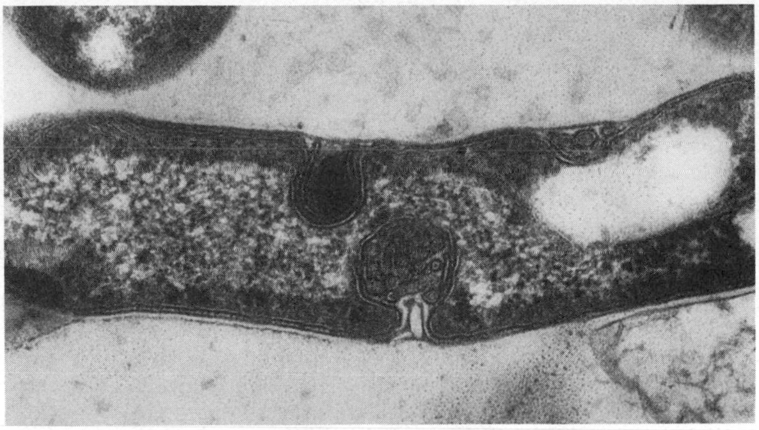

Figure 1. Section of actively growing cell of *M. tuberculosis* strain H37Rv. Note the presence of mesosomes at the initiation of cross-wall formation and the presence of vacuole-like fatty inclusion bodies. ×78,000. (From Barksdale, L., and Kim, K. S.: Mycobacterium. Bacteriol. Rev. 41:217, 1977.)

important characteristic useful in the laboratory diagnosis of all mycobacterial diseases. Although the lipids extracted from mycobacteria are weakly acid-fast and the lipid-free cell residue is not acid-fast, tubercle bacilli also become non-acid-fast after such damage as crushing the cells between glass slides or exposure to ultrasound. According to Barksdale and Kim (1977), the acid-fastness of intact mycobacterial cells depends on trapping of intracellular fuchsin. A barrier results from mycolate-fuchsin complexes that form in the cell wall.

Growth. Most pathogenic mycobacteria grow unusually slowly. The doubling time for *M. tuberculosis* is 12 to 18 hours, in contrast to 15 minutes for the Enterobacteriaceae. Although tubercle bacilli can grow on simple synthetic media, their isolation from clinical specimens requires complex media. The organism is a strict aerobe, an attribute that appears to be important in the pathogenesis of tuberculosis.

Virulent (but not avirulent) strains of *M. tuberculosis* grown on the surface of liquid or solid media characteristically form strands or cords, and this is reflected in a difference in the appearance of the colonies on solid media (Fig. 2).

Drug Susceptibility. Tubercle bacilli are inhibited in vitro and in vivo by isonicotinic acid hydrazide (INH), streptomycin (ST), para-aminosalicylic acid (PAS), thiacetazone (TH), ethambutol (EMB), and rifampin (RIF), as well as by several other more toxic drugs (e.g., ethionamide, kanamycin, cycloserine) that are used primarily in patients whose organisms are resistant to the first-line drugs (INH, ST, PAS, TH, EMB, RIF). Although antituberculosis drugs administered singly to experimentally infected animals are bacteriostatic, the combination of RIF and INH has bactericidal activity in vivo. Tubercle bacilli isolated from the sputum of inadequately treated patients may be resistant to one or more of the drugs used. This resistance is not associated with plasmids (no R factor) and is due to the selection and the eventual predominance of naturally occurring resistant mutants present in small numbers among the high populations of bacilli that develop in cavitary tuberculosis.

Lipids. Mycobacteria contain a number of unusual high molecular weight complex lipids, for example, mycosides, waxes D, trehalose-6,6'-dimycolate, and sulfolipid. A number of the complex lipids of mycobacteria contain mycolic acid, which has the general formula $C_{88}H_{176}O_4 \pm 5CH_2$. The general structure of mycolic acid from *M. tuberculosis* is:

```
      OH
      |
R—CH—CH—COOH
          |
          C24H49
```

The R group in the formula contains about 60 carbon atoms and an undetermined oxygen function and occurs in the molecule in three chains.

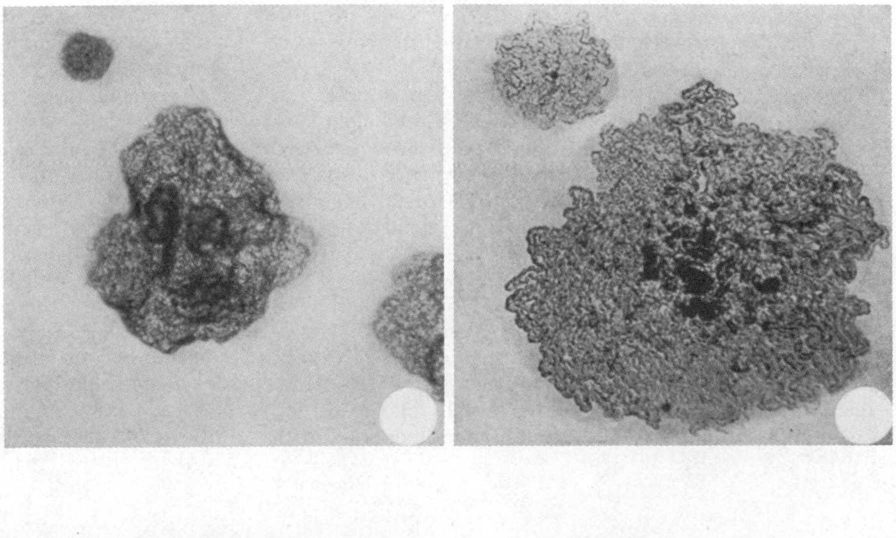

Figure 2. Colonies of virulent (H37Rv) and attenuated (H37Ra) *M. tuberculosis* grown on the surface of agar medium. *A*, H37Ra: 12-day-old culture illustrating the nonoriented heaped-up structure of the colony. *B*, H37Rv: the colonies are flat with a serpentine structure. Cording is visible at the edge of the colony as thin strands and loops. (From Middlebrook, G., Dubos, R. J., and Pierce, C.: Virulence and morphological characteristics of mammalian tubercle bacilli. J. Exp. Med. 86:175, 1947.)

The mycosides, a series of mycolic acid–containing glycolipids or glycolipid peptides, are uniquely distributed among the different species of mycobacteria, a chemically distinct mycoside associated with each species (Randall and Smith, 1964). Some of the mycosides occur on the outer surface of the cell and act as mycobacteriophage receptors. Although determination of the specific mycoside in an isolate could contribute to its identification, the steps involved are too complex for routine application.

Waxes D are a family of closely related substances composed of mycolic acid, peptides, and polysaccharides. When extracted from *M. tuberculosis*, these substances have unique adjuvant properties in that they not only enhance antibody production against a protein antigen incorporated in a wax D oil emulsion, but also induce a cell-mediated immune (CMI) response against the protein (White et al., 1958). Because of this attribute, waxes D may contribute to the pathogenesis of tuberculosis through enhancement of the CMI response (specifically, delayed-type hypersensitivity) against mycobacterial proteins. Research from several laboratories indicates that the adjuvant-active component of waxes D (and the mycobacterial cell wall) is an N-acetylmuramyl dipeptide (see Saiki et al., 1983).

Cord factor, so named because it was thought to be responsible for the cord-forming tendency of virulent tubercle bacilli grown on the surface of liquid or solid media, can be extracted from the cells with hexane. The purified material has been reported by various investigators to have the following properties: lethality for mice; inhibition of migration of polymorphonuclear leukocytes; induction of protection against virulent infection; and induction of granuloma formation. Despite this impressive array of potential contributions to virulence, the role played by cord factor in the pathogenesis of tuberculosis is unknown.

Binding of the dye neutral red, another property reported to distinguish between virulent and avirulent mycobacteria, has been shown to be due to the presence of a sulfonated glycolipid characterized as a tetraester of trehalose; again, the role of this substance in the disease process has not been elucidated.

Antigenic Structure. As is true of all other microbes, mycobacteria contain many antigens and antigenic determinants. Antibody-mediated immunity (AMI) and cell-mediated immunity (CMI) develop against many of these determinants during the course of infection; however, no association between a particular antigenic structure and virulence has been established. Various species of mycobacteria share antigenic determinants, and this is responsible for the cross-reactions observed in tuberculin skin test responses.

Pathogenic Properties. Tuberculosis epitomizes the pathogenesis of chronic infectious diseases. Virulent mycobacteria produce no potent toxins or tissue-destructive enzymes. The principal basis for their virulence lies in the fact that, though readily phagocytosed, the organisms resist the destructive properties of normal macrophages and are capable of multiplying intracellularly. This process damages tissue once CMI is activated.

The principal features in the initiation of tuberculous infection and its evolution to tuberculous disease, as revealed by studies of the disease in man and in an experimental model of tuberculosis in guinea pigs, can be summarized as follows. The organism (usually one to three), airborne as droplet nuclei coming from an individual with cavitary tuberculosis (or in the case of the guinea pig model, from an aerosol-generating device) is inhaled by a susceptible individual. Droplet nuclei less than 5μm in diameter escape the defense mechanisms of the upper respiratory tract, and usually one such particle is carried into a terminal alveolar space in the well-ventilated mid to lower lung. The small number of organisms present in the particle is readily ingested by an alveolar macrophage.

After a lag period of about three days, the organism begins to multiply slowly, with one generation occurring each 12 to 18 hours. The bacilli, accumulating intracellularly, kill the initial alveolar phagocyte, and the organisms released are readily ingested by macrophages (transformed from blood monocytes) carried to the site and replicating in response to the developing inflammatory process. This slowly evolving local lesion continues to enlarge, and about two weeks after initiation of the infection, bacilli are transported via the lymphatics to the lymph node draining that region of the lung. The fixed macrophages in the lymph node ingest the organisms, but again they continue to multiply intracellularly.

A few days later, organisms leave the lymph node and are carried via the efferent lymphatics and thoracic duct to the bloodstream. This bacillemic phase of the infection leads to the dissemination of organisms throughout the body, where they are again trapped by macrophages already present, or they are ingested by macrophages carried to the sites of deposition. Again, evidence suggests that the bacilli likely multiply inside cells at each of these sites.

About three to four weeks after infection, the CMI response has been initiated, and immune (sensitized) lymphocytes coming from lymph nodes and spleen are carried by the bloodstream to the sites of the developing microscopic lesions. The interaction between lymphocytes sensitive to mycobacterial antigens and the corresponding specific antigen presumably leads to the release of mediators (lymphokines) and in turn to the activation of macrophages and to the initiation of caseation necrosis. The joint action of the activated macrophages and the unfavorable oxygen tension at most of the sites of hematogenous dissemination are presumably responsible for the death of the mycobacteria. In contrast, the organisms that by chance lodge in the apex or the subapical area of the lungs, the kidney, or the growing ends of long bones (in children) are favored by the high pO_2 in these sites (the high pO_2 in the apical and subapical areas of the lungs results from a high ventilation-perfusion ratio). The tubercle bacillus, a strict aerobe, may survive in small numbers in these sites of high pO_2 in a slowly metabolizing, relatively dormant state.

These events can all occur without the development of symptoms; that is to say, this is tuberculous infection, but not tuberculous disease. The host-parasite interaction terminates at this stage in about 90 per cent of infected persons. The only evidence that infection has taken place is conversion of the tuberculin reaction from negative to positive (tuberculin conversion) and perhaps the later development of a calcified focus at the site of the primary respiratory implantation and perhaps at the site of the draining lymph node in the hilus of the lung. These calcified sites are called the primary complex or Ghon complex. There may also be radiologic abnormalities and even calcification in the apical and subapical areas of the lung. These are sometimes referred to as Simon's foci.

Paradoxically, if tuberculous infection is to progress to tuberculous disease, the subsequent critical events usually

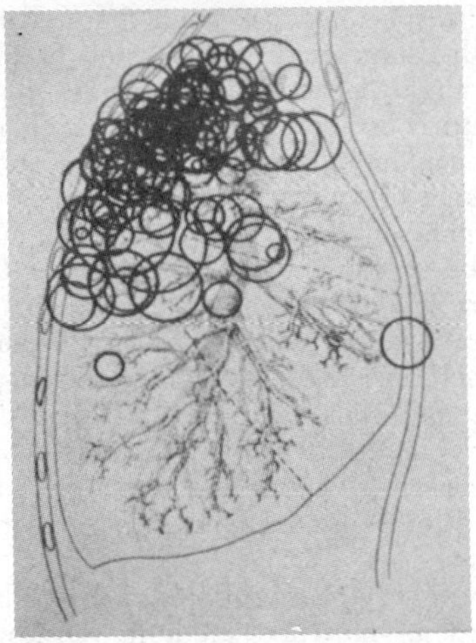

Figure 3. Location of 268 cavities in the lungs of 204 tuberculosis patients as revealed by stereoscopic radiographs. Note the tendency for cavities to occur in the apical and subapical areas of the lungs. (From Sweaney, H. C., Cook, C. E., and Kegerreis, R.: A study of the position of primary cavities in pulmonary tuberculosis. Am. Rev. Tuberc. 24:558, 1931.)

take place at the apical or subapical site seeded during the bacillemia (Fig. 3), rather than at the site of the primary respiratory implantation (primary complex). This progression occurs during the first two years of infection in about 5 per cent (recent experience in India suggests a lower percentage) of those infected and much later in life in another 5 per cent. One can postulate the following events.

There is an antecedent temporary suppression of the CMI response, perhaps due to another infection or therapy for another disease. Activated macrophages are no longer produced, and the organisms that had been dormant in the apical focus begin to multiply and within several weeks are present in relatively high numbers. Later, when the CMI response is restored, sensitive lymphocytes reappear at the site of the developing lesion, lymphokines are released, and macrophages are activated. However, because of the high level of bacillary antigen, the entire process is exaggerated, and although the population of bacilli is temporarily reduced, caseation necrosis is extensive. Some change in the lesion, which is not yet fully understood, causes the caseous mass to undergo liquefaction. This creates a favorable environment for the bacillus, and massive growth ensues, more lymphocytes infiltrate, more lymphokines are released, and the lesion enlarges. As the developing lesion erodes through a bronchus, the liquid caseum is released into the bronchial tree, coughed up, and expectorated or swallowed. This leaves a cavity in the lung, and bacilli continue to multiply in the lining of the cavity. This process is usually accompanied by low-grade fever, cough, and malaise—that is, the symptoms of tuberculous disease.

IMMUNITY TO TUBERCULOSIS. Substantial evidence from work with animal models of tuberculosis, as well as work with other diseases caused by facultative intracellular pathogens, indicates that immunity to these microbial agents is most likely due to the CMI response. Macrophages, activated as a result of the lymphokines released from the interaction of immune lymphocytes and specific mycobacterial antigen, are apparently altered so that they become competent to control the intracellular organism. The process of macrophage activation results in increases in the following: metabolic activity; membrane activity; phagocytic activity; and granule (lysosomal) enzymes (Dannenberg, 1968). It has not been established, however, which if any of these changes is responsible for the ability of the activated macrophage to limit the intracellular multiplication of tubercle bacilli. The role of CMI in the tissue-destructive aspects of the disease and in acquired resistance to tuberculosis is a clear example of the immune response as a "double-edged sword."

Human field trials reveal that injection of bacille Calmette-Guérin (BCG) vaccine, a viable attenuated strain of *M. bovis*, induces a protective response. Prospective double-blind trials of BCG vaccine in human populations have revealed discordant results. For example, in the British Medical Research Council trial (Hart, Sutherland, and Thomas, 1967), BCG showed a protective efficacy of 70 to 80 per cent. On the other hand, in the more recent trial in the Chingleput District of South India, the data seven and one-half years after intake revealed no evidence of a protective effect of BCG (Indian Council of Medical Research, 1980). It has been suggested (Clemens, Chuong, and Feinstein, 1983) that the conflicting reports on efficacy of BCG may be due in part to differences in bias in detection of cases of tuberculosis and to differences in the adequacy of statistical power. Many reports indicate that killed mycobacterial vaccines or bacillary fractions induced protective immunity in experimental animals (Smith, Wiegeshaus, and Grover, 1968); however, none of these substances has been shown yet to have application for the prevention of human disease.

EPIDEMIOLOGY OF TUBERCULOSIS (PREVALENCE, MODE OF SPREAD, PREVENTION). The *prevalence* of tuberculous infection is estimated by tuberculin test surveys of sample populations. The *incidence* of tuberculous disease is obtained from data giving the number of new cases of tuberculosis, as revealed by laboratory studies and clinical findings. The incidence of tuberculosis varies greatly from one country to another. In several of the developing countries, tuberculous infection rates are as high as 85 to 90 per cent of the general population. In these same areas the prevalence of tuberculous disease may be as high as one to two per hundred. In contrast, in some of the developed countries, rates of tuberculous infection have fallen to as low as 10 to 15 per cent, and of tuberculous disease as low as 10 to 15 per 100,000.

Transmission of tuberculosis occurs when an individual with tubercle bacilli present in his or her sputum (sputum-positive tuberculosis) coughs, sings, or otherwise creates an aerosol and a few organisms are inhaled by a nearby susceptible individual. This aerosol, referred to as a primary aerosol, is one in which droplet nuclei containing bacilli are transmitted via the air directly from the diseased person to a susceptible person. It is this primary aerosol that is most likely to be associated with transmission of the infection. In contrast, droplets of sputum that fall to the floor, bedding, or furniture are less likely to result in transmission even if they become airborne once again. This is referred to as a secondary aerosol, and successful transmission is less likely for several reasons. The most important is that the bacilli in the secondary aerosol are almost always associated (by electrostatic forces) with particles of dust or lint, and the particle size is thereby increased. Because the defense mechanisms of the upper respiratory tract are very effective in trapping and eliminating particles greater than 5μm in diameter, the organisms in the secondary aerosol are removed before they reach susceptible tissues deep in the lung. Moreover, bacilli in the secondary aerosol usually have had longer exposure to the inactivating influence of ultraviolet light. It has been shown experimentally that tubercle bacilli in an aerosol are rapidly killed upon exposure to ultraviolet light. The significance of the contrast between primary and secondary aerosol is that it focuses attention on the most important source of transmission, namely, the infectious person. It is possible to reduce transmission of tuberculosis to direct contacts of patients with positive sputum by lowering the concentration of infectious particles in the air. This can be done by means of an adequate number of air changes and by ultraviolet irradiation of the upper air in the patient's room. The concept of primary aerosol indicates that less attention need be given to the handling of bedding and objects used by the patient.

The most effective means of preventing tuberculosis is to block the transmission of the organism. This is best accomplished by early detection and treatment of patients with tubercle bacilli in their sputum. Treatment for only several weeks with isoniazid alone (despite the need for two or more drugs to prevent drug resistance) will greatly reduce the number of secondary cases among close contacts of a patient under treatment, even though organisms may still be recovered from his sputum.

LABORATORY DIAGNOSIS

Direct Microscopy. Sputum collected from the diseased person should be examined after the preparation of an acid-fast stain. A loopful of material from the sediment in the sputum container (the maximal chance of finding bacilli is realized from a study of the solid particles) is smeared on a glass slide, air-dried, and heat-fixed. Some modification of the Ziehl-Neelsen acid-fast stain is usually employed. The smear is flooded with carbol-fuchsin and then heat is applied to cause the stain to steam. After five minutes of steaming, the carbol-fuchsin is washed off with water and the smear is decolorized for up to two minutes with a reagent consisting of 3 ml of hydrochloric acid in 97 ml of 95 per cent ethanol or with 25 per cent sulfuric acid. The preparation is then washed with water and counterstained for one minute with methylene blue. After a final water wash, the slide is air-dried and examined under the oil-immersion lens of a microscope. Tubercle bacilli appear as deep-red–staining, thin-beaded, often curved rods in a blue background. The number of tubercle bacilli in a positive sputum smear could vary from a few in 20 to 30 oil-immersion fields to many in each oil-immersion field. *Fluorochrome staining* may be superior to Ziehl-Neelsen staining for the detection of tubercle bacilli in sputum. The staining reagent is tetramethyldiaminodiphenyl ketoimine (auramine O), and although most laboratories examine auramine-stained smears under ultraviolet light with a special microscope, techniques have been developed that permit use of a standard microscope and an illuminator with a special filter (Runyon et al., 1974). The fluorochrome staining procedure has the advantage of permitting the survey of a sputum smear at a lower magnification, and this speeds up the examination and increases the sensitivity of the detection of acid-fast organisms.

Digestion and Concentration. Acid-fast stains are also made after the specimen has been digested and concentrated. The digestion-concentration step breaks up tissue debris, kills nonmycobacterial organisms present as contaminants, and concentrates tubercle bacilli in a smaller volume of specimen. Digestion can be accomplished by vigorous shaking of a mixture of equal parts of specimen and 3 per cent sodium hydroxide for 30 minutes. The process can be accelerated by incorporating 0.5 per cent acetyl cysteine in 2 to 4 per cent sodium hydroxide, mixing, and allowing the suspension to stand for 15 minutes. The shorter contact time increases the number of surviving mycobacteria and thus increases the sensitivity of the technique for detection of a positive specimen. After digestion, the specimen is centrifuged, the supernatant fluid is decanted, and the sediment is used for smears and stains and for culture.

Culture. Recovery of mycobacteria from clinical specimens requires an enriched medium. Ordinarily this is some modification of Löwenstein-Jensen's (L-J) medium containing egg, potato extract, glycerine, and an inhibitory dye (often malachite green) added to retard the growth of contaminants that have survived the decontamination step. Slants of L-J medium are inoculated with the concentrated sediment. The cultures are incubated at 37° C for up to eight weeks and examined weekly for the appearance of colonies. If viable *M. tuberculosis* organisms were present in the specimen, small buff-colored, rough colonies could appear in about three weeks but may take as long as six to eight weeks to appear. Acid-fast stains made from these colonies will reveal a morphology like that described above. If growth appears within one week, the organism could be *M. fortuitum* or one of the saprophytic mycobacteria. Although a slow-growing, nonpigmented, acid-fast organism may be *M. tuberculosis*, it could also be one of the atypical mycobacteria.

ATYPICAL MYCOBACTERIA. Depending on the region of the world, mycobacteria other than *M. tuberculosis* are recovered from less than 0.1 per cent to as many as 50 per cent of individuals with tuberculosis-like diseases.* These organisms, collectively called "atypical mycobacteria," are indicated by an asterisk in the list of mycobacteria given in Table 1. Recent reports suggest that atypical mycobacteria more frequently cause disease in patients whose lung or immune response is already damaged by another disease. Atypical mycobacteria and the disease they produce differ in several important respects from classic tuberculosis. Of primary significance is that examination of close contacts of patients with disease due to an atypical mycobacterium reveals *no evidence of human to human transmission* (atypical mycobacteria have been recovered from the soil and from water). Atypical mycobacteria are more likely to be *resistant to the first-line antituberculous drugs* than is *M. tuberculosis*. Patients infected with atypical mycobacteria usually give a *negative tuberculin test* to the 5-TU test dose of tuberculin prepared from *M. tuberculosis*. Finally, atypical mycobacteria can be distinguished from *M. tuberculosis* by a series of laboratory tests, primarily biochemical tests.

*The high levels are based on recent reports from the low-prevalence areas of developed countries. In contrast, in a recent report from Madras, only one case of disease due to atypical mycobacteria was found among many thousands of cases of tuberculosis.

Identification of the Species of Mycobacteria (Speciation). Of these tests, the secretion of niacin by *M. tuberculosis* is the most important because it distinguishes this species from nearly all clinical isolates of other mycobacteria. Pigmentation is another differential feature. The production of a yellowish or orange pigment (carotene) helps delineate the relatively nonpathogenic scotochromogens (which produce pigment in the dark or light) from the more pathogenic photochromogens (especially *M. kanasii*) in which carotene is characteristically produced only in the light (photoinducible). Speed of growth is a third key property: most pathogenic mycobacteria require three weeks of incubation before they appear in primary cultures of clinical material. By contrast, colonies of the rapid growers, such as *M. fortuitum* and *M. chelonei* are usually seen in a week or less after inoculation of specimens into culture media. In addition to these biochemical tests, *M. tuberculosis* and *M. bovis* produce fatal disease in guinea pigs and the atypical mycobacteria do not. Although complete speciation requires a comprehensive series of tests, the 12 characteristic tests shown in Table 2 permit a satisfactory identification of most species. (Note, for example, that *M. avium* and *M. intracellulare* differ primarily in the proportion of strains showing photo-inducible pigmentation and the proportion that grow on MacConkey agar. This is the reason why these species were listed in Table 1 as the *M. avium intracellulare* complex.)

Drug Susceptibility Tests. Five to 10 per cent or more of cultures isolated from human specimens may contain bacilli resistant to one or more first-line antituberculous drugs. Therefore, pathogenic mycobacteria cultured from patients should be examined for susceptibility to the first-

Table 2. CHARACTERIZATION OF CLINICALLY SIGNIFICANT MYCOBACTERIA ACCORDING TO TWELVE KEY PROPERTIES*

Twelve Properties[a]

(1) Rate of growth (S = slow; F = fast)
(2) Secretion of niacin
(3) Reduction of nitrate ($NaNO_3$)
(4) Semiquantitative test for hyperproduction of catalase (column of gas bubbles, >45 mm)
(5) Stability of catalase to 68°C, 20 min
(6) Carotenogenesis constitutive (scotochromogenic)
(7) Carotenogenesis photoinducible (photochromogenic)
(8) Hydrolysis of Tween 80 after 10 days
(9) Reduction of tellurite ($KTeO_2$), 3 days
(10) Growth on media containing 5% (wt/vol) NaCl
(11) Hydrolysis of tripotassium phenolphthalein disulfate by arylsulfatase, 3 days
(12) Growth on MacConkey agar

Formulae for 17 Mycobacterial Taxa and 1 Species Complex[a]

Taxon	Above the line	Below the line
M. avium:	S ⑤ [7] [9]	3 4 6 8 10 12
M. bovis:	S	2 3 4
M. chelonei:	F ④⑤[8][9]⑩[b] 11 ⑫	2
M. flavescens:	S 3 ④ 5 ⑥ 8 [9] ⑩	
M. fortuitum[c]*:*	F ③④ 5 [8][9] 10 ⑪ ⑫	2
M. gastri:	S [12]	
M. gordonae:	S ④⑤ 6 ⑧	3 9 12
M. intracellulare:	S ⑤ ⑨ [12]	3 4 6 7 8 10 11
M. kansasii:	S ③④ 5 ⑦ 8	2 6 12
M. marinum:	S [2] [4][5]⑦⑧	3 10 11
M. phlei:	F ③ 4 5 6 8 [9] 10	
M. scrofulaceum:	S [3]④ 5 6	9
M. smegmatis:	F 3 ④⑤ 8 ⑨ 10	11
M. terrae complex[d]:	S ③ 4[c] ⑤ ⑧	6 7 10 12
M. triviale:	S 3 ④ 5 8 10 [11]	
M. tuberculosis:	S ②③ [8]	5 6 9 10
M. vaccae:	F ③ 4 5 [6] 7 8 ⑨ [10] [11]	
M. xenopi:	S ⑤ 6 [11]	9

*From Barksdale, L., and Kim, K. S.: Mycobacterium. Bacteriol Rev *41*:217, 1977.

[a]Key for reading formulae. When number N is unboxed, *N* (number above the line) = 100% strains tested was positive (e.g., *11* in *M. chelonei*); Ⓝ = 70 to 99% strains tested, positive (e.g., ⑤ in *M. avium*); [N] = 15 to 60% strains tested, positive (e.g., [7] in *M. avium*); N (number below the line) = 0.4 to 14% strains tested, positive (e.g., 3 in *M. avium*). Absence if N = 100% strains tested, negative (e.g., 11 absent in *M. avium*).

[b]*M. chelonei* subsp. chelonei fails to grow in 5% NaCl.

[c]*M. fortuitum* includes strains designated as *M. peregrinum*.

[d]*M. terrae* complex includes *M. terrae, M. nonchromogenicum* and *M. novum*.

line antituberculous drugs. If acid-fast organisms are still grown from sputum six months after the start of treatment, susceptibility tests should be done to look for drug resistance.

MYCOBACTERIUM LEPRAE

Mycobacterium leprae, the causative agent of leprosy, was discovered by Hansen in 1874. In honor of his discovery and in part to circumvent the stigma associated with leprosy, the affliction is sometimes referred to as Hansen's disease and the organism as Hansen's bacillus.

Morphology. *M. leprae* is morphologically indistinguishable from the other mycobacteria; they are rod-shaped organisms approximately 0.3 to 0.5 μm wide and 2 to 5 μm in length. *M. leprae* is acid-fast and can be stained by the Ziehl-Neelsen method.

Metabolism and Drug Susceptibility. Of paramount importance is that *M. leprae* is an obligate intracellular parasite. The microbe has not been cultured in the absence of living tissues. The generation time of the organism is exceptionally long. Estimates based on experimental infection of mouse foot pads (Shepard, 1971) indicate a generation time of 13 days. *M. leprae* is susceptible to diaminodiphenylsulfone (dapsone) and to rifampin. Inoculation tests in the mouse foot pad indicate that *M. leprae* present in the circulation of lepromatous patients is killed faster after rifampin therapy than dapsone therapy.

Antigenic Composition. *M. leprae* contains no unusual antigens. Patients infected with *M. leprae* may undergo both an antibody-mediated immune (AMI) response and a cell-mediated immune (CMI) response. Because the organism is noncultivable, the skin test reagent, called lepromin, is prepared from organisms concentrated from diseased tissue.

Pathogenic Properties. Like the tubercle bacillus, *M. leprae* produces no potent toxins or extracellular factors contributing to the disease process. The pathogenesis of leprosy appears to derive from the ability of the microbe to survive and replicate in macrophages and other host cells, especially nerve cells, and the consequent immune response to the invader. In one polar form of leprosy, lepromatous leprosy, the CMI response appears to be suppressed, and consequently the organisms accumulate in the tissues in large numbers. On the other hand, the AMI response in the lepromatous patient is not suppressed (and perhaps not even controlled), and excessive quantities of antibody are produced. The sera of lepromatous patients often contain circulating immune complexes composed of antibacillary antibody and anti-immunoglobulin. These immune complexes, which precipitate in the cold (+4° C) and therefore are called cryoglobulins, contribute to the pathogenesis of the disease. In patients with the other polar form of leprosy, tuberculoid leprosy, the CMI response appears to be intact and the bacillary population in the tissues is very low or even nondemonstrable.

Experimental infections have been produced in the foot pads of mice and in the nine-banded armadillo. Mice that have been thymectomized and x-irradiated develop a more rapidly progressive infection upon inoculation with *M. leprae*. A naturally occurring infection in armadillos in the United States is caused by an organism indistinguishable from *M. leprae* (Walsh et al., 1977).

IMMUNITY TO LEPROSY. The patient with tuberculoid leprosy appears to be making an effective immune response against *M. leprae*, and bacillary populations are reduced to a very low level. On the other hand, the patient with lepromatous leprosy appears to have either a specific or a general defect in CMI responsiveness, and bacillary populations in the tissues reach very high levels. The increased frequency of leprosy in certain families in endemic areas and the studies of Jamison and Vollum (1968) suggest that the CMI defect in lepromatous leprosy has a genetically determined component. They compared tuberculin-negative children with a family history of leprosy and tuberculin-negative children with no family history of leprosy for their response to a vole bacillus vaccine (a live attenuated antituberculosis vaccine about equal in potency to BCG). Whereas 90 per cent of the children with no family history of leprosy responded to the vaccine by converting to a positive tuberculin test, tuberculin conversion was observed in less than 20 per cent of children with a family history of leprosy.

Considering all lines of evidence, it appears that the protective host response in leprosy is the CMI response. No vaccine has been developed from *M. leprae*. Field trials with BCG vaccine have yielded discouraging results in reducing the extent of leprosy (only 20 per cent over a nine year follow-up—Bechelli et al., 1974).

LABORATORY DIAGNOSIS OF LEPROSY. The bacteriological diagnosis of leprosy is based on finding acid-fast organisms in scrapings from nasal mucosa and skin lesions or in biopsy specimens. Leprosy is differentiated from other mycobacterial diseases by demonstrating the lack of cultivability and by showing nerve involvement in histologic examination of tissue biopsies.

EPIDEMIOLOGY OF LEPROSY. Leprosy appears to be transmitted by direct contact. The disease is not highly contagious, and prolonged contact with infected persons may be required before transmission occurs. It is estimated that approximately 35 million persons have leprosy, most of them living in states in central Africa and certain regions in Asia. Prevention of leprosy in endemic areas is based on diagnosis, isolation, and treatment of infected persons.

References

Barksdale, L., and Kim, K. S.: Mycobacterium. Bacteriol Rev 41:217, 1977.
Bechelli, L. M., Lwin, K., Garbajosa, P. G., Gyi, M. M., Uemura, K., Sundaresan, T., Tamondong, C., Matejka, M., Sansarricq, H., and Walter, J.: BCG vaccination of children against leprosy: Nine-year findings of the controlled WHO trial in Burma. Bull WHO 51:93, 1974.
Clemens, J. D., Chuong, J. J. H. and Feinstein, A. R.: The BCG controversy, a methodological and statistical reappraisal. J Am Med Assoc 249:2362, 1983.
Dannenberg, A. M., Jr.: Cellular hypersensitivity and cellular immunity in the pathogenesis of tuberculosis: Specificity, systemic and local nature, and associated macrophage enzymes. Bacteriol Rev 32:85, 1968.
Hart, P. D., Sutherland, I., and Thomas, J.: The immunity conferred by effective BCG and vole bacillus vaccines, in relation to individual variations in induced tuberculin sensitivity and to technical variations in the vaccines. J Brit Tuberc Assoc 48:201, 1967.
Indian Council of Medical Research. Trial of BCG vaccines in south India for tuberculosis prevention. Indian J Med Res 72 (Suppl):1, 1980.
Jamison, D. G., and Vollum, R. L.: Tuberculin conversion in leprous families in northern Nigeria. Lancet 11(no. 7581): 1271, 1968.
Middlebrook, G., Dubos, R. J., and Pierce, C.: Virulence and morphological characteristics of mammalian tubercle bacilli. J Exp Med 86:175, 1947.

Randall, H. M., and Smith, D. W.: Characterization of mycobacteria by infrared spectroscopic examination of their lipid fractions. Zentralbl Bakteriol 194:686, 1964.

Runyon, E. H., Karlson, A. G., Kubica, G. P., and Wayne, L. G.: Mycobacterium. In Lennette, E. H., Spaulding, E. H, and Truant, J. P. (eds.): Manual of Clinical Microbiology, 2nd ed. Washington, D.C., American Society for Microbiology, 1974, pp. 148–174 (pertinent section, p. 155).

Saiki, I., Tokushima, Y., Mishimura, K., Yammamura, Y., and Azuma, I.: Activation of macrophages by quinonyl-*n*-acetyl muramyl dipeptide. Infect Immunol 40:622, 1983.

Shepard, C. C.: The first decade in experimental leprosy. Bull WHO 44:821, 1971.

Smith, D. W., Grover, A. A., and Wiegeshaus, E.: Nonliving immunogenic substances of mycobacteria. Adv Tuberc Res 16:191, 1968.

Sweany, H. C., Cook, C. E., and Kegerreis, R.: A study of the position of primary cavities in pulmonary tuberculosis. Am Rev Tuberc 24:558, 1931.

Walsh, G. P., Storrs, E. E., Meyers, W., and Binford, C. H.: Naturally acquired leprosy-like disease in the nine-banded armadillo (Dasypus novemcinctus): Recent epizootologic findings. J Reticuloendothel Soc 22:363, 1977.

White, R. G., Bernstock, L., Johns, R. G. S., and Lederer, E.: The influence of components of *M. tuberculosis* and other mycobacteria upon antibody production to ovalbumin. Immunology 1:54, 1958.

45

NOCARDIA AND STREPTOMYCES

SAROJ K. MISHRA
RUTH E. GORDON

Nocardia and *Streptomyces* are important aerobic actinomycetes known mainly for causing serious diseases of man and animals, producing potent antibiotics as well as toxic metabolites, and decomposing organic matter in the soil (Waksman, 1959). The infections caused by members of the two genera are broadly classified into two categories: 1) Nocardiosis, a generalized or systemic disease due to members of the genus *Nocardia*, principally *N. asteroides*, and occasionally to *N. caviae* (Causey, 1974) and *N. brasiliensis* (Berd, 1973, see Chapter 118). The disease is usually characterized by primary pulmonary involvement that may be pneumonic or subclinical, chronic or transitory (Emmons et al., 1977). A hematogenous dissemination may occur from the lungs to other parts of the body. 2) Actinomycetoma, a localized swollen lesion, usually on the foot, hand, or back, and involving the skin, subcutaneous tissues, fascia, and bone (Mariat et al., 1977, see Chapter 252). The pus draining through the sinuses contains granules (compact colonies of the causative microorganism surrounded by reactive cells), the size, shape, and color of which may suggest specific etiology. The chief etiologic agents are strains of *N. madurae*,* *N. pelletieri*, *N. brasiliensis*, *N. caviae*, *N. asteroides*, and *Streptomyces somaliensis*. In addition, strains belonging to other species (Table 1), namely *N. dassonvillei*, *N. autotrophica*, *S. griseus*, *S. albus*, etc., are isolated from clinical specimens. But their actual role in the etiology of disease is uncertain owing to the lack of supporting clinical, experimental, and histologic evidence. With increasing use of immunosuppressants in modern medicine, their role as "possible opportunistic invaders" should be judiciously considered.

MORPHOLOGY. Cultures of nocardiae and streptomycetes are composed of branching filaments (hyphae) approximately 1 μ in width. In stained smears the growth appears as gram-positive filaments (Fig. 1) or as fragmented forms (rods and/or coccoid bodies). Motile forms have not been reported.

In infections caused by some species of *Nocardia* (mainly *N. asteroides*, *N. caviae*, and *N. brasiliensis*), the microorganisms observed in clinical specimens are generally acidfast. Acidfastness (See Appendix in this chapter) of cultures of the same species grown in vitro is, however, a variable characteristic. In some cultures of these few species of *Nocardia*, usually those recently isolated, a high percentage (85 to 100 per cent) of the filaments and fragments retain the carbol fuchsin. Smears of other cultures reveal a decreasing range of acidfastness with only portions of the filaments resisting decolorization (Fig. 1), and many nonacidfast cultures have been observed.

Routinely, the best observation of morphologic characteristics of the nocardiae and streptomycetes is by microscopic examination (100, 200, and 400 ×) of individual, mechanically undisturbed colonies. After three to five days of incubation at 28° C, individual colonies of cultures streaked on plates of tap water agar (see Appendix) display a network of branching filaments (vegetative or substrate hyphae) that spread over the surface of the agar. (Caution: The microorganisms must be killed by formalin fumigation before opening the plate.) The vegetative hyphae normally give rise to aerial hyphae that project into the air and, therefore, appear wider and darker than the substrate hyphae (Fig. 2). Junctures of a substrate hypha and an aerial hypha can usually be clearly seen at the periphery of the colony. At the center of the colony, longer and more abundant aerial hyphae hide the substrate hyphae. After longer incubation (7 to 14 days), the aerial hyphae generally are more extensive and branching. Some are straight; some flexuous; and some form loose spirals or a variety of other forms. Under these conditions of growth, the aerial hyphae of cultures of nocardiae and streptomycetes may or may not segment into bead-like conidia (spores).

In the routine diagnostic laboratory, the microscopic appearance of the individual colonies of nocardiae and streptomycetes offers the best means of their separation from cultures of mycobacteria and corynebacteria, which do not, as a rule, produce aerial hyphae. (For other means of identifying strains of *Streptomyces*, *Nocardia*, *Mycobacterium*, and *Corynebacterium* see Species Identification.)

On the whole, the gross appearance of cultures of strains of *Nocardia* and *Streptomyces* belonging to the same species varies considerably. Figures 3 and 4 are presented to illustrate not only the diversity in appearance among cultures of the same species but also the similarity among strains of different species, for example, the likeness of certain cultures of *N. dassonvillei* to cultures of *S. griseus* (Fig. 3). The growth of some strains of *N. asteroides* (Fig.

*The authors prefer the retention of *N. madurae*, *N. pelletieri*, and *N. dassonvillei* in the genus *Nocardia* to their assignment to *Actinomadura*.

Table 1. SOME PROPERTIES OF TYPICAL STRAINS OF SPECIES OF NOCARDIA AND STREPTOMYCES OF MEDICAL IMPORTANCE

Property	*N. asteroides*	*N. carnea*	*N. caviae*	*N. brasiliensis*	*N. transvalensis*	*N. autotrophica*	*N. orientalis*	*N. aerocolonigenes*	*N. dassonvillei*	*N. madurae*	*N. pelletieri*	*S. somaliensis*	*S. lavendulae*	*S. albus*	*S. rimosus*	*S. griseus*
Acidfastness	v*	v	v	v	v	−	−	−	−	−	−	−	−	−	−	−
Decomposition of																
Adenine	−	−	−	−	v	+	−	−	+	−	−	−	−	−	+	+
Casein	−	−	−	+	−	−	+	+	+	+	+	+	+	+	+	+
Hypoxanthine	−	−	+	+	+	+	+	+	+	+	v	−	+	+	+	+
Tyrosine	−	−	−	+	+	+	+	+	+	+	+	+	+	+	+	+
Urea	+	−	+	+	+	+	+	+	v	−	−	−	v	+	v	+
Xanthine	−	−	+	−	v	v	v	−	+	−	−	−	v	v	+	+
Resistance to																
Lysozyme	+	+	+	+	+	−	−	+	−	−	−	−	+	v	+	−
Rifampin	+	+	+	+	+	−	v	−	−	v	v	−	−	+	+	−
Hydrolysis of																
Hippurate	v	−	v	−	−	v	v	v	+	−	−	−	−	v	v	v
Starch	v	v	v	v	+	+	+	+	+	+	−	v	+	−	+	+
Nitrite from nitrate	+	+	+	+	+	v	v	v	+	+	+	−	v	v	v	v
Survival at 50°C, 8 hr	+	+	+	−	+	v	v	v	+	+	+	v	−	+	+	+
Acid from																
Adonitol	−	−	−	−	+	+	+	v	−	+	−	−	−	+	+	v
1(+)Arabinose	−	−	v	−	−	v	+	+	v	+	−	−	v	−	v	v
Cellobiose	−	−	−	−	−	v	+	+	+	+	−	−	v	+	+	+
1-Erythritol	−	−	−	−	+	+	+	−	−	−	−	−	−	+	+	−
Glucose	+	+	+	+	+	+	+	+	+	+	+	v	+	+	+	+
Glycerol	+	+	+	+	+	+	+	+	+	+	−	−	+	+	+	+
i-Inositol	−	v	+	+	v	v	+	+	−	v	−	−	v	v	+	v
d(+)Lactose	−	−	−	−	−	−	+	+	−	v	−	−	v	+	+	+
d(+)Maltose	−	−	−	−	−	+	v	+	+	v	−	v	+	+	+	+
d(−)Mannitol	−	+	v	+	v	+	+	+	+	+	−	−	−	+	+	+
d(+)Melezitose	−	−	−	−	−	+	v	−	−	−	−	−	−	v	−	−
α-Methyl-D-glucoside	−	−	−	−	−	v	+	−	v	−	−	−	−	+	−	+
d(+)Raffinose	−	−	−	−	−	−	v	v	−	−	−	−	−	−	+	v
1(+)Rhamnose	v	−	−	−	−	−	v	v	v	+	−	−	−	−	−	v
d-Sorbitol	−	+	−	−	v	+	v	−	−	−	−	−	−	−	v	−
d(+)Trehalose	v	+	v	+	v	+	v	+	v	+	+	−	v	+	+	+
d(+)Xylose	−	−	−	−	−	+	+	+	v	+	−	−	v	+	v	+

*v, variable property; +, positive property; −, negative property of typical strains.

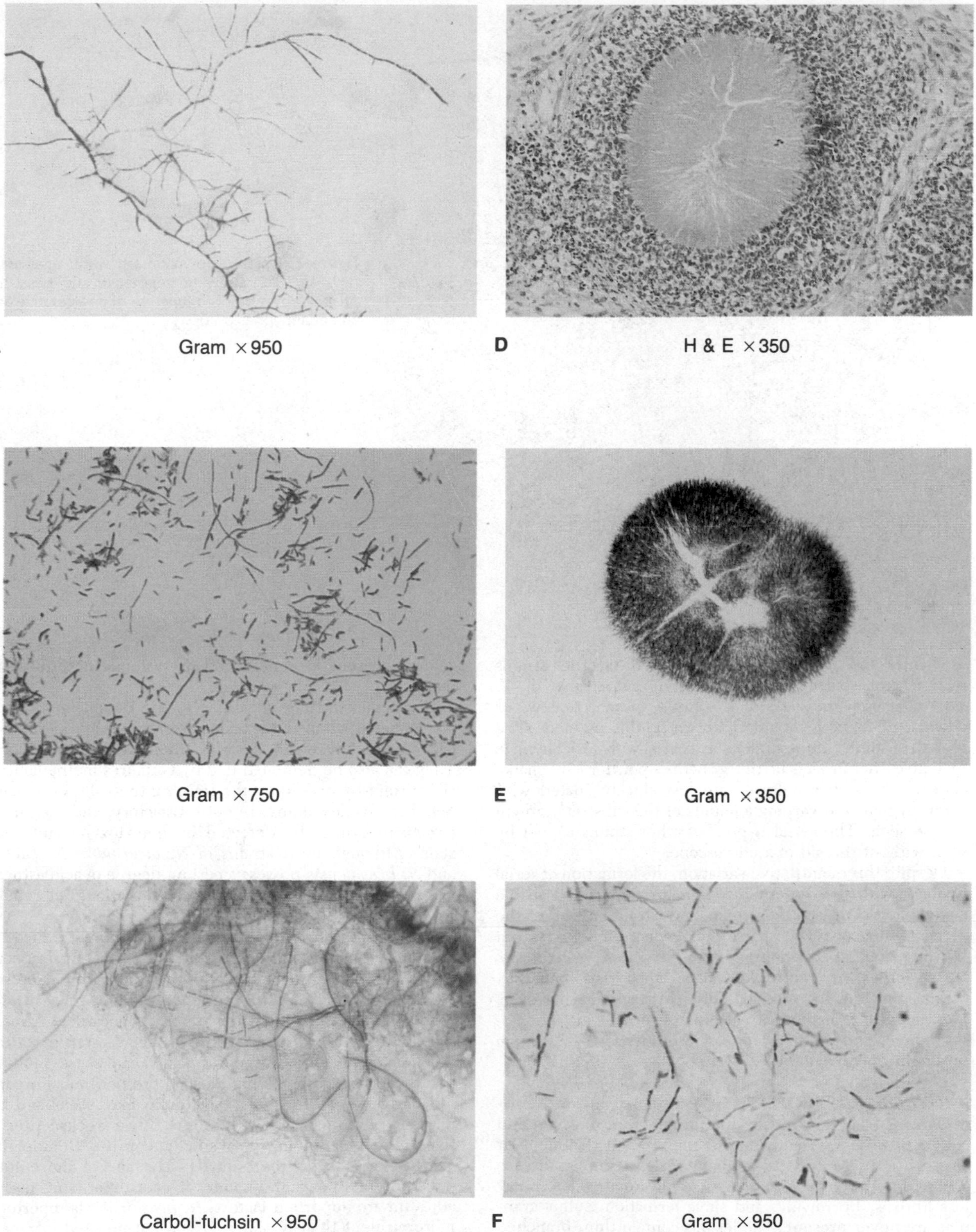

Figure 1. Microscopic morphology of some Nocardiae in culture *(A-C)* and in tissue *(D-F)*.

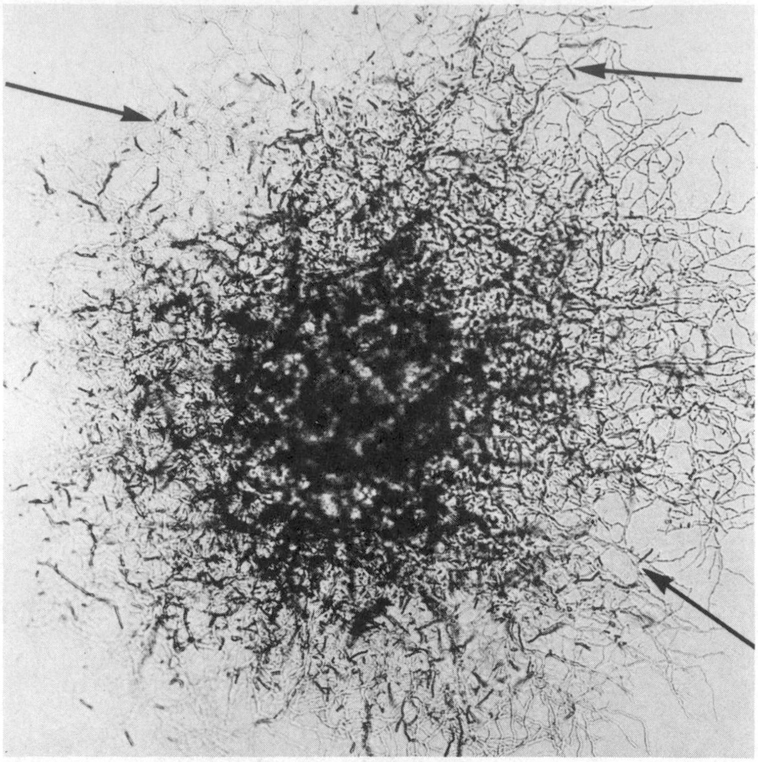

Figure 2. Colony grown on tap water agar for 4 days at 28°C, showing vegetative and aerial hyphae. Arrows point to juncture of a vegetative and an aerial hypha. ×700.

4) is thick and abundant, whereas growth of other strains is thin and sparse. Cultures of different strains of *N. asteroides* may be red, pink, purple, peach, yellow, or cream, and some form a dark brown soluble pigment. The growth of some cultures is heavily coated with aerial hyphae that give the surface of the growth a powdery or chalky appearance. Other cultures are less thickly coated with aerial hyphae and varying amounts of the substrate growth can be seen. The aerial hyphae of other strains cannot be seen without the aid of a microscope.

Despite this quantitative variation, the formation of aerial hyphae, with few exceptions, is a taxonomically reliable characteristic of the nocardiae and streptomycetes; the aerial hyphae may be sparse and even rudimentary, but they are there. Exceptions are some strains of *N. madurae*, *N. pelletieri*, *N. aerocolonigenes*, and *S. somaliensis*. Strains that do not produce aerial hyphae are, however, identifiable by distinctive patterns of physiologic, chemotaxonomic, and other morphologic properties (see section on *Laboratory Diagnosis*).

PATHOGENIC PROPERTIES. Nocardiosis due to *N. asteroides* is characterized by the formation of multiple and confluent abscesses and intense suppuration (Emmons et al., 1977). In contrast to actinomycosis, a similar disease caused by *Actinomyces israelii*, the nocardial lesions show less fibrosis, burrowing, and sinus formation; sulfur granules are never present. The lesions contain thin, branched filaments, as well as bacillary bodies, which can be demonstrated only when the sections are properly stained. Loose conglomeratory growth may sometimes be observed in the tissues, but granules and the giant cell granulomatous tissue reaction, as seen in actinomycetoma or in organs of mice experimentally infected with nocardiae (Fig. 1), are seldom present in generalized or systemic nocardiosis in man.

For demonstrating nocardiae in the tissue, best results are obtained when the sections are stained by the method of Brown and Brenn or McCallum-Goodpasture-Gram. They can also be demonstrated by Gomori's methenamine-silver stain by extending the staining time. Periodic acid–Schiff or Gridley stains are not satisfactory, and the microorganisms cannot be detected by hematoxylin and eosin stain. Although most strains of *N. asteroides*, *N. caviae*, and *N. brasiliensis* possess a certain degree of acidfastness, this property is hard to demonstrate in sections of formalin-fixed tissue.

Generalized nocardiosis can be successfully produced in laboratory animals, although suitability of animal species varies and the degree of virulence may differ from microbial strain to strain. In our experience, albino mice are the most suitable for testing pathogenicity of nocardiae. Usually a heavy inoculum prepared in 5 per cent, sterile, gastrin mucin and injected intraperitoneally can cause multiple abscess formation involving most of the peritoneal organs. Dissemination to the lungs and brain may occur and the majority of animals die within one to two weeks. Alternatively, the infection may heal spontaneously with indefinite survival of most of the animals. The age of the culture (three to five days), amount of inoculum, and use of adjuvant are important factors. *N. brasiliensis* is reportedly more virulent than *N. asteroides* when injected intraperitoneally (Kurup et al., 1970A) or in the footpads of mice (Gonzalez Ochoa, 1973). When injected intravenously, however, *N. asteroides* and *N. caviae* cause much higher mortality and morbidity than *N. brasiliensis* (Mishra et al., 1973B). Mishra and coworkers also demonstrated that cortisone administration can significantly lower host resis-

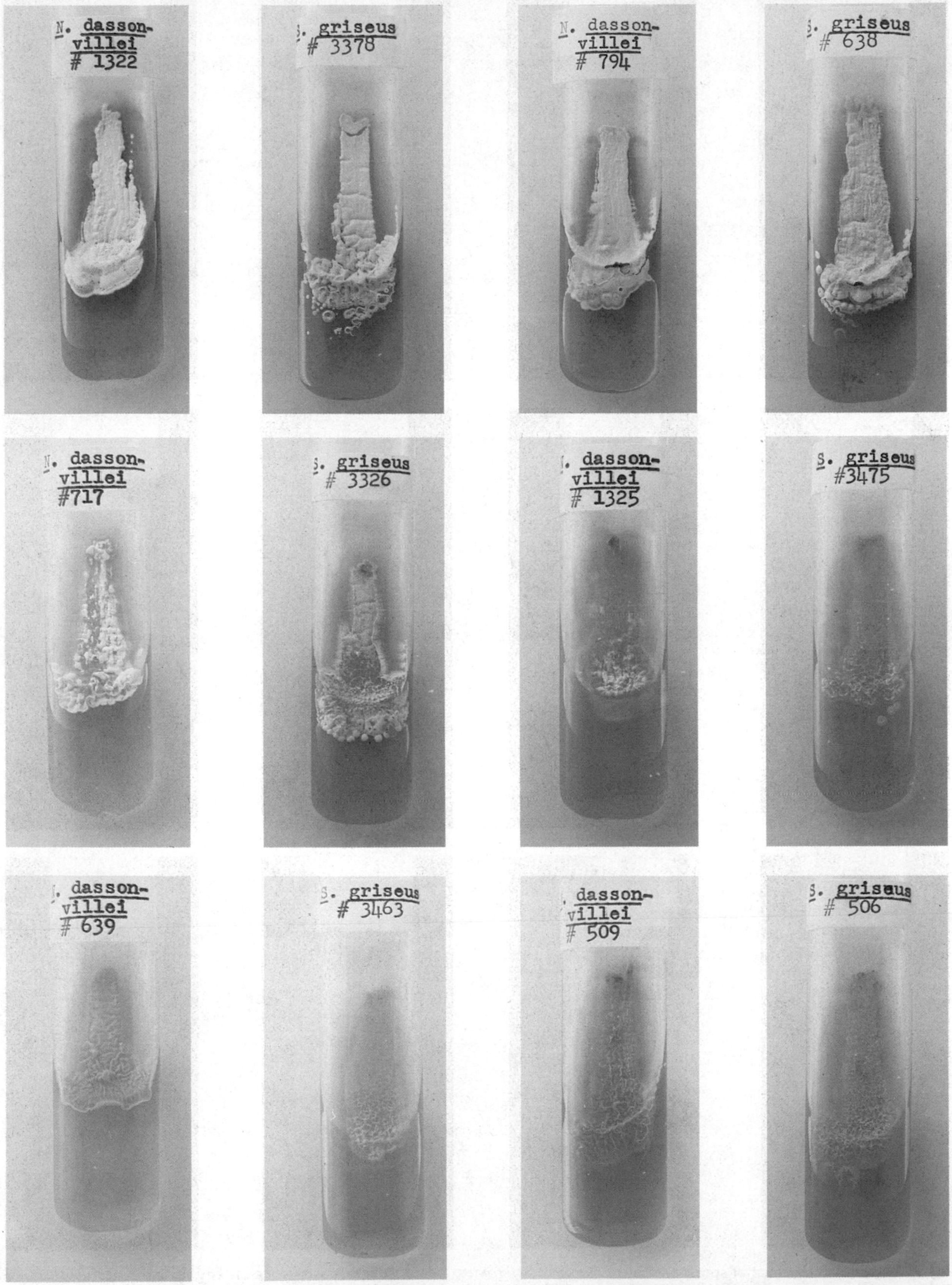

Figure 3. Gross appearance of cultures of *Nocardia dassonvillei* and of *Streptomyces griseus.* Cultures of *N. dassonvillei* and *S. griseus* grown on yeast dextrose agar for 2 weeks at 28°C and forming varying amounts of aerial hyphae. (Reproduced from J Gen Microbiol 50:235–240, 1968, with the kind permission of the editors.)

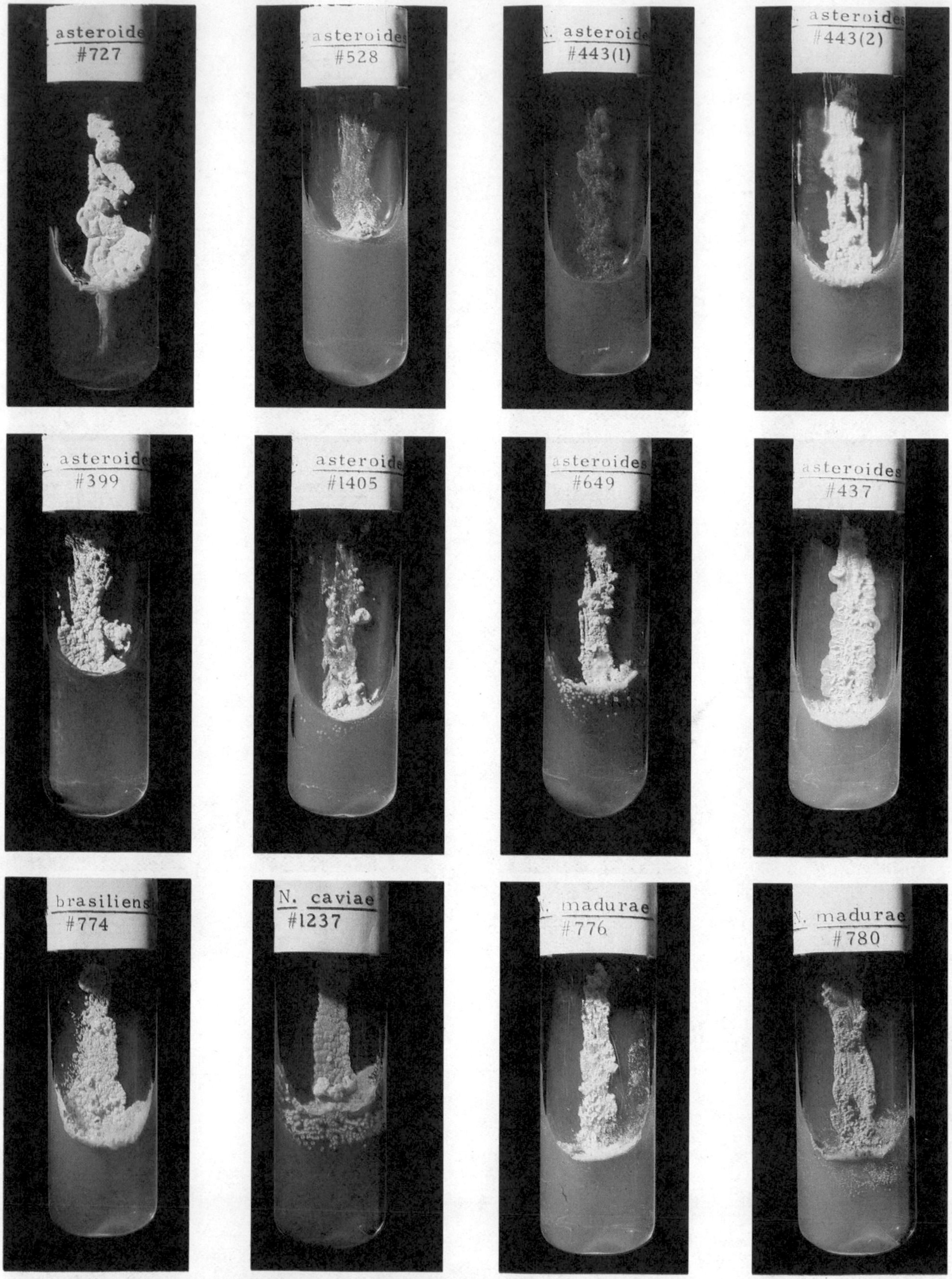

Figure 4. Gross appearance of some cultures of *Nocardia asteroides, Nocardia brasiliensis, Nocardia caviae,* and *Nocardia madurae.* Cultures grown on yeast dextrose agar for 1 week at 28° C. *N. asteroides:* no. 727, heavy growth thickly covered with aerial hyphae; no. 528, thin growth covered with aerial hyphae; no. 443(1), red-pigmented growth without macroscopically visible aerial hyphae; no. 443(2), variant of red strain with abundant aerial hyphae; nos. 399, 1405, 649, and 437, cultures forming decreasing amounts of aerial hyphae; nos. 399 and 649, cultures producing dark brown soluble pigment. *N. brasiliensis:* no. 774. *N. caviae:* no. 1237. *N. madurae:* nos. 776 and 780, cultures with different pigments.

tance to infection by the three species. The histopathologic picture of experimental nocardiosis is similar to that observed in generalized nocardiosis of man and animals. Attempts to infect mice or other laboratory animals with *N. madurae, N. pelletieri, N. dassonvillei*, and *S. somaliensis* have been, so far, unsuccessful.

LABORATORY DIAGNOSIS. Owing to the lack of a characteristic clinical syndrome and specific immunologic tests, the laboratory diagnosis of nocardiosis demands greater attention and effort than most of the other common bacterial and fungal infections. The problem is also aggravated by the in vitro sensitivity of cultures of *Nocardia* and *Streptomyces* to most of the commonly used antibiotics that are incorporated into culture media to suppress the fast-growing saprophytic or commensal bacteria and fungi. On the other hand, filaments of *N. asteroides* may occasionally survive the concentration procedure commonly used for the isolation of *Mycobacterium tuberculosis* and grow on Lowenstein-Jensen medium. Because the filaments may be very fragile and may show strong acidfastness, nocardiae may easily be mistaken for *M. tuberculosis*.

Collection of Clinical Specimens. Samples of sputum, bronchial aspirates, gastric lavage (in the case of young children who tend to swallow their sputum), surgically removed tissues (biopsies and resected lungs), cerebrospinal fluid, and midstream urine are collected under aseptic conditions. A fresh morning sample of sputum, collected in a wide mouthed, glass stoppered bottle, after the patient has thoroughly cleaned his teeth and mouth, is more productive than a 24-hour specimen. The specimen is promptly brought to the laboratory and processed immediately. Sputum is homogenized by vigorous shaking with sterile glass beads. The biopsied tissues may be homogenized with the help of glass tissue grinders. Samples of cerebrospinal fluid and urine must be concentrated by centrifugation.

Direct Examination. Smears prepared from the homogenized or concentrated specimen are stained and examined microscopically. Several fields should be searched for the presence of filaments and coccobacillary bodies. The filaments are gram positive but often take the stain irregularly, look beaded, and may sometimes be 50 μ in length. Branching is usually at right angles and tends to be at long intervals. Acidfastness, if demonstrable, is particularly helpful in differentiating *N. asteroides, N. caviae*, and *N. brasiliensis* from *N. madurae, N. pelletieri*, and *S. somaliensis*.

Direct Culture. After the initial processing, the specimens are streaked upon neutral Sabouraud's dextrose agar and yeast dextrose agar plates (see *Appendix*) and incubated at 37° C (anaerobic or microaerophilic conditions are not required for growth). These media are useful for isolating nocardiae and streptomycetes from relatively less contaminated clinical specimens such as biopsied tissues, washed grains from actinomycetoma, and cerebrospinal fluid. If the specimens are suspected of harboring a wide spectrum of contaminating microbial flora, for example, gastric lavage and sputa of patients with chronic pulmonary diseases, the chances of isolating some nocardiae are enhanced by the use of the paraffin bait technique (see *Appendix*) as described by Mishra and Randhawa (1969) and Mishra et al. (1973A). It depends on the ability of nocardiae to use as energy sources certain organic compounds, such as paraffin, which are not attacked by other aerobic bacteria.

N. asteroides and other pathogenic nocardiae and streptomycetes, although widespread in nature, are surprisingly seldom encountered as laboratory contaminants or as constituents of normal microbial flora of the human body. Isolation of *N. asteroides* from a clinical specimen, therefore, has diagnostic value. An unequivocal diagnosis of systemic nocardiosis depends upon repeated demonstration of gram-positive and partially acidfast branching filaments in the direct smear and isolation of the pathogen in culture.

Laboratory diagnosis of actinomycetoma is relatively easier. Biopsied tissue or the pus collected from the draining sinuses should be examined carefully for the presence of granules. If present, the granules should be separated from the pus and washed carefully in sterile physiologic saline. In the case of *N. brasiliensis, N. caviae*, and *N. asteroides*, the granules are soft, white to cream colored, and range from 0.5 to 1 mm in size. The grains produced by *N. pelletieri* in tissue are hard, red, pink, or occasionally yellowish in color and measure about 1 mm. The granules produced by *N. madurae* are soft, big in size, mostly white or cream, rarely pink. *S. somaliensis* produces yellowish to brown, hard granules, 0.5 to 2 mm in diameter. After gross examination, the granules are crushed, examined microscopically, and inoculated on Sabouraud's dextrose agar and yeast dextrose agar. (The paraffin bait technique is not suitable for the isolation of *N. madurae, N. pelletieri*, and *S. somaliensis* because they do not utilize paraffin as the sole source of carbon.) Although morphology of the granules and staining characteristics of the filaments present therein are fairly distinctive of some of the etiologic species, the organism must be grown in culture for its specific identification.

Single colonies, morphologically compatible with the cultures of *Nocardia* and *Streptomyces*, should be picked from the plates or tubes directly inoculated with the clinical specimens or isolated from the growth on paraffin-coated rods. After purifying the culture by serial dilution or by repeated streaking on yeast dextrose agar plates, the growth, microscopic morphology, and physiologic characteristics are studied.

Species Identification. In the absence of a reliable morphologic feature, or features, for the separation of the genera *Nocardia* and *Streptomyces*, the form of diaminopimelic acid (DAP) in the cell wall or in whole-cell hydrolysates is used to divide the genera (Lechevalier, 1977). Strains of *Nocardia* species have the *meso*-form of DAP and strains of *Streptomyces* species, the L-form.

Other properties—pigment formation, fragmentation of substrate hyphae, development of conidia, and production of an earthy odor—are possessed by some strains of nocardiae and by some strains of streptomycetes. We found no physiologic test that differentiates strains of the two genera. The key (Fig. 5) presented here for the tentative identification of strains of nocardiae and streptomycetes includes the species represented by the strains received here as isolations from patients (Mishra et al., 1980). It is designed to permit the user, in whose laboratory chromatographic determination of DAP is not feasible, to arrive at species identifications of unknown isolations with the morphologic characteristics of nocardiae and streptomycetes as though the species belonged to one genus (Gordon, 1976). If the 13 tests employed in the key (see *Appendix*) are applied to an unknown isolate and the strain is found to be, for example, cellobiose negative, glycerol positive, hypoxanthine negative, and urease positive, the strain may be

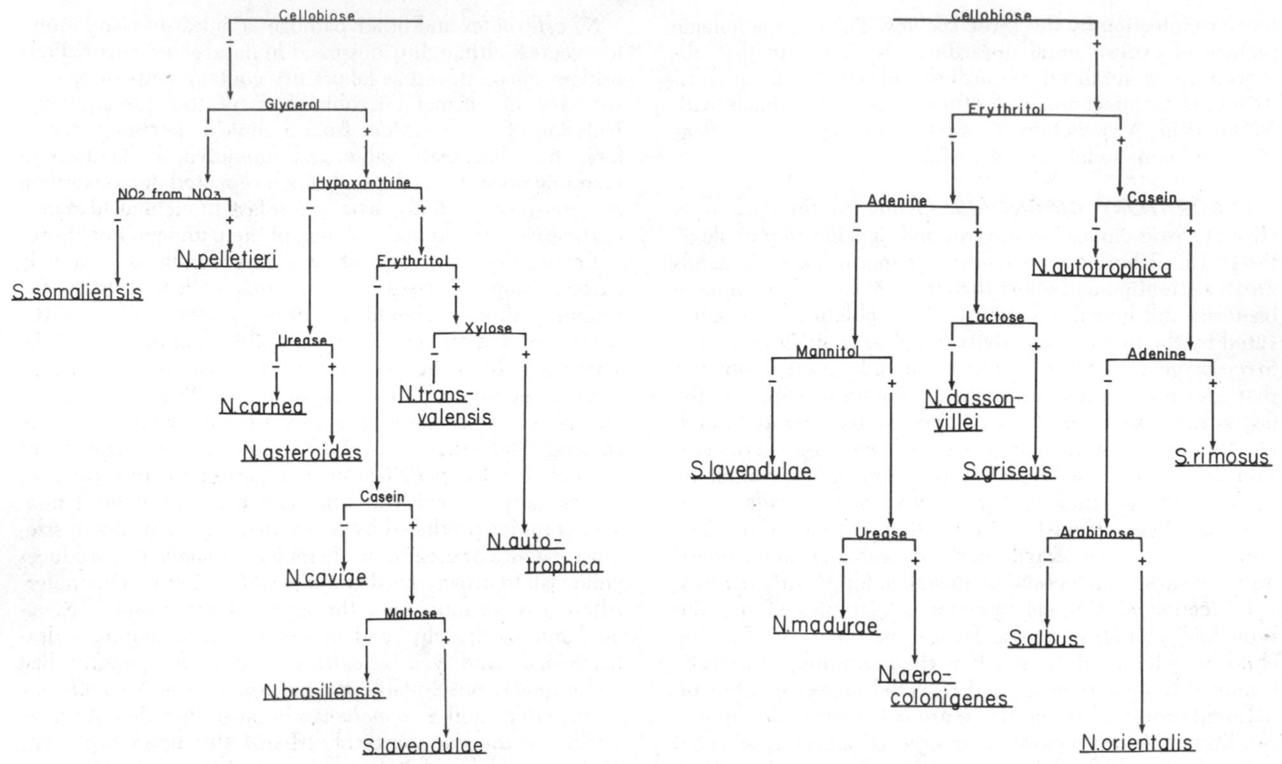

Figure 5.

tentatively identified as one of *N. asteroides*. If the remaining properties of the strain are as follows: acid formation negative from arabinose, erythritol, lactose, maltose, mannitol, and xylose; inability to decompose adenine and casein; and positive reduction of nitrate to nitrite, the tentative identification of the strain as one of *N. asteroides* is partially confirmed.

Further confirmation may be obtained by studying additional physiologic characteristics listed in Table 1 and described in detail by Gordon et al. (1974, 1977, 1978).

If chemotaxonomic examinations are feasible in the laboratory, the presence of *meso*-DAP, arabinose, and galactose in the cell walls or in hydrolysates of whole cells will provide further evidence of the strain's identity as one of *N. asteroides*. The lipids (mycolic acids) of strains of mycobacteria and of some nocardiae offer another valuable chemotaxonomic property (Lechevalier, 1976). Species lacking mycolic acids are usually nonacidfast. Among the species described in Table 1, cultures of *N. asteroides, N. carnea, N. caviae, N. brasiliensis*, and *N. transvalensis* contain LCN-A (lipid characteristic of *Nocardia* species-asteroides type) that distinguishes them from the other species in Table 1 and from strains of mycobacteria and corynebacteria. Mycolic acids apparently have no significant role in the pathogenicity of nocardiae and streptomycetes. Certain nonpathogenic species, e.g., *N. amarae*, are known to have LCN-A, whereas some of the well known pathogenic species, such as *N. madurae, N. pelletieri*, and *S. somaliensis*, do not have LCN-A or any other mycolic acids.

The importance of comparing unknown isolates with as many named strains of the various species as possible cannot be overstressed to anyone attempting to identify strains of nocardiae and streptomycetes for the first time. By applying the tests to known strains, the investigator soon learns whether each test as applied in his laboratory yields results comparable with those given here or elsewhere in the literature (Ajello et al., 1963; Goodfellow, 1971). If only a tentative identification of an isolate can be made or if the strain cannot be identified by the information provided, it should be sent to a reference laboratory (American Type Culture Collection, Rockville, Maryland; the Centers for Disease Control, Atlanta, Georgia; or any other laboratory actively engaged in the identification of aerobic actinomycetes).

The name *N. farcinica*, once considered the type species of the genus *Nocardia*, is not used here because its status is uncertain. Diversity of interpretations of Nocard's description (1888) of his strain isolated from a case of bovine farcy in Guadeloupe, the different species identity of strains purported to be Nocard's original isolate, and the assignment of causal agents of African cases of bovine farcy to the genus *Mycobacterium* (Asselineau et al., 1969) confuse present-day significance of the name. *N. asteroides* is now recognized as the type species of the genus (Skerman et al., 1980; Gordon, 1981).

ANTIGENIC COMPOSITION, SEROLOGY AND IMMUNITY. The immunology of *Nocardia* and *Streptomyces* is still poorly understood. Cross-reaction with mycobacteria and members of related genera is frequently observed. Strains of *Nocardia, Mycobacterium*, and *Corynebacterium*, which have identical cell wall sugars, seem to have some common antigenic components. Crude and purified polysaccharides, and protein derivatives, are immunologically active but both homologous and heterologous reactions may occur. Pier and Fichtner (1971), using a gel diffusion precipitin test and soluble extracellular antigens, distinguished four serotypes of nocardiae. Type I, II, and III antigens were confined to *N. asteroides;* the type IV antigen occurred in strains of *N. caviae* and *N. brasiliensis* as well as in several strains of *N. asteroides*. By comparative reciprocal intradermal sensitin tests in guinea pigs, some success has been reported in delineating *Nocardia* at the species level but not at the generic level (Magnusson, 1976). Despite the promising value of immunologic methods in demonstrating homologous antigenicity in experimental models, the diagnostic worth of sensitin tests in demonstrating immediate or delayed hypersensitivity is limited. A skin test with purified protein derivatives (nocardin-PPD) derived from *N. brasiliensis* is reported to elicit a positive reaction in patients with actinomycetoma caused by *N. brasiliensis* and to be negative in healthy individuals and patients with tuberculosis and various other diseases (Bojalil and Zamora, 1963). Similar convincing results, however, are lacking in cases of actinomycetoma caused by other species, and in cases of systemic or generalized nocardiosis.

The relationship of antibodies to immunity against infection by nocardiae and streptomycetes is not clear. Since members of the two genera are widely distributed in nature, it is logical to assume that more people are frequently exposed to these microorganisms than acquire clinical disease. The immunity may develop after a very mild or subclinical infection that diminishes spontaneously if host-defense mechanisms are not impaired. Studies by Beamann (1979) suggest that the host-defenses against nocardial infections are multifaceted and that cell-mediated immunity plays an important role.

DRUG SUSCEPTIBILITY. Strains of *Nocardia* and *Streptomyces* are sensitive to a number of antibiotics in vitro, but there is considerable strain variation and lack of correlation between the in vitro and in vivo effects. Since the first successful use of sulfadiazine in the treatment of subcutaneous nocardiosis (Lyons et al., 1943) and the demonstration of its in vitro inhibitory effect on aerobic actinomycetes (Cutting and Gebhardt, 1941), sulfonamides have remained the drug of choice in the treatment of nocardial infections. *N. asteroides* is demonstrably more sensitive to chlortetracycline, oxytetracycline, and chloramphenicol than to sulfadiazine in vitro, but sulfadiazine is more effective in vivo (Strauss et al., 1951). Sensitivity to penicillin is poor, whereas ampicillin, streptomycin, erythromycin, neomycin, gentamycin, minocycline, and many other antibiotics and chemotherapeutics are quite active against nocardiae and streptomycetes in vitro (Bach et al., 1973; Pridham and Tresner, 1974). Some of these, alone or in combination with sulfonamides, have been used in the treatment of nocardiosis and actinomycetoma. A combination of trimethoprim and sulfamethoxazole has in vitro inhibitory effect on strains of *N. asteroides* and *N. brasiliensis* at a relatively low concentration and appears to be very useful in the management of diseases caused by this group of microorganisms. Antifungal antibiotics, such as nystatin, cycloheximide, griseofulvin, and amphotericin B, are by and large not effective against *Nocardia* and *Streptomyces* infections, although occasional clinical success and in vitro inhibitory action have been reported.

EPIDEMIOLOGY. *Nocardia* and *Streptomyces* are soil-inhabiting, ubiquitous microorganisms, commonly present in the human environment. After the first report on the isolation of *N. asteroides* from soil by Gordon and Hagan (1936), several investigators have demonstrated the occurrence of *N. asteroides, N. caviae, N. brasiliensis,* and other medically important aerobic actinomycetes in the soil in many different parts of the world (Cross et al., 1976). Since their filaments are delicate and highly fragile, they are easily airborne. Systemic or primary pulmonary infection is usually acquired by inhalation of the airborne mycelial fragments or spores. Occasionally, primary lesions may develop in the gastrointestinal tract through ingestion of food contaminated with dust or water harboring nocardiae. In the case of actinomycetoma or subcutaneous manifestations, traumatic implantation of the pathogen directly into the skin is the commonest mode of infection. These microorganisms have no special affinity for any particular race, sex, age, or geographic region. Cases of systemic nocardiosis are reported from all over the world (Kurup et al., 1970B) although more frequently from America and Europe than from Asia and Africa. The differences are mainly due to the greater availability of highly specialized laboratory diagnostic facilities and an increased awareness among the investigators in those countries. Occupational relationship is not established, but farmers and laborers heavily exposed to the soil and dust are more likely to contract the infection, especially in the presence of debilitating metabolic diseases and poor nutritional and working conditions.

The etiologic agents of actinomycetoma also have a worldwide distribution, although the disease is more frequently observed in Sudan, Mexico, and certain other arid regions lying between the equator and the Tropic of Cancer. Incidentally, *N. pelletieri* and *S. somaliensis* are more commonly incriminated in the etiology of actinomycetoma in Sudan and other African countries, whereas *N. brasiliensis* and *N. madurae* are more frequently reported in Mexico. Strains of almost all the species have been isolated from cases in other countries but no etiologic or regional significance could be attached to any particular species.

APPENDIX

Acidfastness. Slides with air-dried smears of the cultures are immersed in carbolfuchsin (saturated ethanol solution of basic fuchsin, 10 ml; 5 per cent aqueous solution of phenol, 90 ml). Heat is applied and the fuchsin boiled for five minutes. The slides are washed in water, quickly dipped once in acid alcohol (concentrated HCl, 3 ml; 95 per cent ethanol, 97 ml), immediately washed again in water, and counterstained with methylene blue (saturated solution of methylene blue in 95 per cent ethanol, 30 ml; 0.01 per cent aqueous solution of KOH, 100 ml). Use of 0.5 per cent H_2SO_4 instead of acid alcohol was abandoned in this laboratory because filaments of some strains of *S. griseus* were not decolorized.

Tap Water Agar. This medium contains only 1.5 g of agar in 100 ml of tap water.

Neutral Sabouraud's Dextrose Agar. The ingredients of this agar are: glucose, 20 g; neopeptone, 10 g; agar, 20 g; distilled water, 1000 ml; pH 7.0.

Yeast Dextrose Agar. This agar comprises 10 g of yeast extract, 10 g of glucose, 15 g of agar, 1000 ml of tap water, and the pH is adjusted to 7.0.

Paraffin Bait Technique. Mix 2 ml of the homogenized specimen with 5 ml of carbon-free broth ($NaNO_3$, 2 g; K_2HPO_4, 0.8 g; $MgSO_4{\cdot}7H_2O$, 0.5g; $FeCl_3$, 10 mg; $MnCl_2{\cdot}4H_2O$, 8 mg; $ZnSO_4$, 2 mg; distilled water, 1000 ml;

pH 7.0). Introduce into the tube a paraffin-coated glass rod (sterilized by storing overnight in 95 per cent alcohol), after the alcohol has drained off. Incubate the tubes at 37° C and observe regularly up to four weeks before discarding as negative. Cream to orange growth on the paraffin rod, just above the surface of the medium, is removed and streaked on Sabouraud's dextrose agar (pH 7.0). Single colonies morphologically compatible with those of nocardiae are picked and processed further for specific identification. Better results can be obtained if, after 1 week, the paraffin rod is carefully removed from the inoculated tube and transferred to another tube containing only 6 ml of carbon-free broth.

Acid from Carbohydrates. The basal inorganic nitrogen medium contains $(NH_4)_2HPO_4$, 1 g; KCl, 0.2 g; $MgSO_4 \cdot 7H_2O$, 0.2 g; agar, 15 g; distilled water, 1000 ml. The pH value of the medium is adjusted to 7.0 before the addition of 15 ml of a 0.04 per cent solution (w/v) of bromcresol purple. After this agar is tubed and sterilized by autoclaving, 0.5 ml of a 10 per cent solution (w/v) of each carbohydrate (autoclaved separately) is added aseptically to the tubes. Cultures on slants of these carbohydrate agars are observed for acid color of the indicator after 7 and 28 days of incubation at 28° C. Tubes showing a negative reaction at 28 days are retained 4 more weeks and observed again.

Decomposition of Adenine and Hypoxanthine. Adenine (0.5 g), suspended in 10 ml of distilled water, is autoclaved, mixed carefully with 100 ml of sterile nutrient agar (peptone, 5 g; beef extract, 3 g; agar, 15 g; distilled water, 1000 ml; adjusted to pH 7.0), cooled to 45° C, mixed again, and poured onto sterile plates (60 mm diameter). Care must be taken to obtain an even distribution of the crystals of adenine throughout the solidified agar. Each culture is streaked once across a plate, incubated at 28° C, and observed at 14 and 21 days for the disappearance of the crystals underneath and around the growth. Plates of hypoxanthine are prepared, inoculated, incubated, and observed in the same way.

Decomposition of Casein. A suspension of 5 g skim milk powder in 50 ml of distilled water and a suspension of 1 g of agar in 50 ml of distilled water are autoclaved separately and cooled to 45° C. The two suspensions are then mixed and poured onto plates. Each culture is streaked once across a plate and incubated at 28° C. At 7 and 14 days the plates are examined for clearing of the casein underneath and around the growth.

A heavy inoculum is necessary in testing for the decomposition of casein, adenine, and hypoxanthine. Some cultures grow well but do not dissolve the casein or the crystals of adenine and hypoxanthine except around the larger clumps of inoculum.

Decomposition of Urea. A 10 ml amount of 15 per cent solution of urea (w/v), sterilized by filtration, is added to 75 ml of sterile urease broth (KH_2PO_4, 10 g; Na_2HPO_4, 9.5 g; yeast extract, 1 g; 0.04 per cent solution of phenol red (w/v), 20 ml; distilled water, 1000 ml; adjusted to pH 7.0). The mixture is pipetted aseptically in 2.5 ml amounts into sterile, capped tubes and inoculated with actively growing cultures. An alkaline reaction after 28 days of incubation at 28° C demonstrates the presence of urease.

Reduction of Nitrate to Nitrite. Cultures in nitrate broth (peptone, 5 g; beef extract, 3 g; KNO_3, 1 g; distilled water, 1000 ml; pH 7.0) are tested for nitrite at 5, 10, and 14 days by mixing 1 ml of culture with three drops of each of the following solutions: 1) sulfanilic acid, 8 g; 5 N acetic acid (glacial acetic acid and water 1:2.5), 1000 ml; and 2) dimethyl-α-naphthylamine, 6 ml; 5 N acetic acid, 1000 ml. (Caution: Dimethyl-α-napthylamine is carcinogenic and should be used with care.) Development of a red or yellow color (high concentration of nitrite) is proof of the presence of nitrite. In the absence of a positive reaction for 14 days, 4 to 5 mg of zinc dust are added to the tube previously tested for nitrite. The presence of nitrate (absence of reduction) is demonstrated by the development of a red color.

We thank the Foundation for Microbiology for providing color Figures 1 and 4, and Dr. A. H. McIntosh and Mrs. R. Shamy for Figures 2 and 5. Permission of the *Journal of General Microbiology* to reproduce Figure 3 is gratefully acknowledged.

References

Ajello, L., Georg, L. K., Kaplan, W., and Kaufman, L.: Laboratory Manual for Medical Mycology. Public Health Service Publication No. 994. Washington, D.C., U. S. Government Printing Office, 1963, p. G65.

Asselineau, J., Lanéele, M. A., and Chamoiseau, G.: De l'étiologie du farcin de zébus tchadiens: nocardiose ou mycobactériose? II. Composition lipidique. Rev. Élev Méd Vét Pays Trop 22:205, 1969.

Bach, M. C., Sabath, L. D., and Finland, M.: Susceptibility of *Nocardia asteroides* to 45 antimicrobial agents *in vitro*. Antimicrob Agents Chemother 3:1, 1973.

Beaman, B. L.: Interaction of *Nocardia asteroides* at different phases of growth with in vitro-maintained macrophages obtained from the lungs of normal and immunized rabbits. Infect Immun 26:355, 1979.

Berd, D.: *Nocardia brasiliensis* infection in the United States; A report on nine cases and a review of the literature. Am J Clin Path 60:254. 1973.

Bojalil, L. F., and Zamora, A.: Precipitin and skin tests in the diagnosis of mycetoma due to *Nocardia brasiliensis*. Proc Soc Exp Biol Med 113:40, 1963.

Causey, W. A.: *Nocardia caviae:* a report of 13 new isolations with clinical correlation. Appl Microbiol 28:193, 1974.

Cross, T., Rowbotham, T. J., Mishustin, E. N., Tepper, E. Z., Antoine-Portaels, F., Schaal, K. P., and Bickenbach, H.: The ecology of nocardioform actinomycetes. In Goodfellow, M., Brownell, G. H., and Serrano, J. A. (eds): The Biology of the Nocardiae. London, Academic Press, 1976, p. 337.

Cutting, W. C., and Gebhardt, L. P.: Inhibitory effect of sulphonamides on cultures of *Actinomyces hominis*. Science 94:568, 1941.

Emmons, C. W., Binford, C. H., Utz, J. P., and Kwon-Chung, K. J.: Medical Mycology, 3rd ed. Philadelphia, Lea and Febiger, 1977.

Gonzalez Ochoa, A.: Virulence of nocardiae. Canad J Microbiol 19:901, 1973.

Goodfellow, M.: Numerical taxonomy of some nocardioform bacteria. J. Gen Microbiol 69:33, 1971.

Gordon, R. E.: A taxonomist's obligation. In Goodfellow, M., Brownell, G. H., and Serrano, J. A. (eds.): The Biology of the Nocardiae. London, Academic Press, 1976, p. 66.

Gordon, R. E.: A proposed new status for *Nocardia asteroides*. In Schaal, K. P. (ed.): Actinomycetes. Stuttgart, Gustav Fischer Verlag, 1981, p. 3.

Gordon, R. E., and Barnett, D. A.: Resistance to rifampin and lysozyme of strains of some species of *Mycobacterium* and *Nocardia* as a taxonomic tool. Int J Syst Bacteriol 27:176, 1977.

Gordon, R. E., Barnett, D. A., Handerhan, J. E., and Pang, C. H-N.: *Norcardia coeliaca, Nocardia autotrophica*, and the nocardin strain. Int J Syst Bacteriol 24:54, 1974.

Gordon, R. E., and Hagan, W. A.: A study of some acid-fast actinomycetes from soil with special reference to pathogenicity for animals. J Infect Dis 59:200, 1936.

Gordon, R. E., Mishra, S. K., and Barnett, D. A.: Some bits and pieces of the genus *Nocardia: N. carnea, N. vaccinii, N. transvalensis, N. orientalis,* and *N. aerocolonigenes*. J Gen Microbiol 109:69, 1978.

Kurup, P. V., Randhawa, H. S., Sandhu, R. S., and Abraham, S.: Pathogenicity of *Nocardia caviae, N. asteroides,* and *N. brasiliensis*. Mycopathologia 40:133, 1970A.

Kurup, P. V., Randhawa, H. S., and Gupta, N. P.: Nocardiosis: a review. Mycopathologia 40:193, 1970B.

Lechevalier, H. A.: The actinomycetales: Soil or oxidative actinomycetes. In Laskin, A. I., and Lechevalier, H. A. (eds.): Handbook of Microbiology, 2nd ed. Cleveland, CRC Press, 1977, p. 363.

Lechevalier, M. P.: The taxonomy of the genus *Nocardia:* Some light at the end of the tunnel? In Goodfellow, M. Brownell, G. H., and Serrano, J. A. (eds.): The Biology of the Nocardiae. London, Academic Press, 1976, p. 1.

Lyons, C., Owen, C. R., and Ayers, W. B.: Sulphonamide therapy in actinomycotic infections. Surgery 14:99, 1943.

Magnusson, M.: Sensitin tests as an aid in the taxonomy of *Nocardia* and its pathogenicity. In Goodfellow, M., Brownell, G. H., and Serrano, J. A. (eds.): The Biology of the Nocardiae. London, Academic Press, 1976, p. 236.

Mariat, F., Destombes, P., and Segretain, G.: The mycetomas: clinical features, pathology, etiology and epidemiology. Contr Microbiol Immunol 4:1, 1977.

Mishra, S. K., Gordon, R. E., and Barnett, D. A.: Identification of nocardiae and streptomycetes of medical importance. J Clin Microbiol 11:728, 1980.

Mishra, S. K., and Randhawa, H. S.: Application of paraffin bait technique to the isolation of *Nocardia asteroides* from clinical specimens. Appl Microbiol 18:686, 1969.

Mishra, S. K., Randhawa, H. S., and Sandhu, R. S.: Observations on paraffin baiting as a laboratory diagnostic procedure in nocardiosis. Mycopathologia 51:147, 1973A.

Mishra, S. K., Sandhu, R. S., Randhawa, H. S., Damodaran, V. N., and Abraham, S.: Effect of cortisone administration on experimental nocardiosis. Infect Immun 7:123, 1973B.

Nocard, E.: Note sur la maladie des boeufs de la Guadeloupe connue sous le nom de farcin. Ann Inst Pasteur 2:293, 1888.

Pier, A. C., and Fichtner, R. E.: Serologic typing of *Nocardia asteroides* by immunodiffusion. Am Rev Resp Dis 103:698, 1971.

Pridham, T. G., and Tresner, H. D.: Family VII. *Streptomycetaceae* Waksman and Henrici. In Buchanan, R. E., and Gibbons, N. E. (eds.): Bergey's Manual of Determinative Bacteriology. 8th ed. Baltimore, Williams and Wilkins Company, 1974, p. 747.

Skerman, V. B. D., McGowan, V., and Sneath, P. H. A. (eds.): Approved lists of bacterial names. Int J Syst Bacteriol 30:225, 1980.

Strauss, R. E., Kligman, A. M., and Pillsbury, D. M.: Chemotherapy of actinomycosis and nocardiosis. Am Rev Tuberc 63:441, 1951.

Waksman, S. A.: The Actinomycetes. Vol. 1. Baltimore, Williams and Wilkins Company, 1959.

SPIROCHETES

46

LEPTOSPIRA

A. D. Alexander, Ph.D.

GENERAL CHARACTERISTICS AND MORPHOLOGY. The genus *Leptospira* consists of a large number of serologically heterogeneous strains that are distributed into two species: *L. interrogans*, which includes the parasitic members, and *L. biflexa*, which comprises the so-called saprophytic leptospires. *L. biflexa* leptospires are omnipresent in natural waters and wet soils, where apparently they are free-living. They are not known to produce infections in man or other mammalian hosts except for a few rare reports. The parasitic leptospires include the pathogenic strains known to infect man and other mammals. (Faine and Stallman, 1982).

Biflexa strains are distinguishable from pathogenic strains in the following respects: inability to infect laboratory animals; relative resistance to growth-inhibitory effects of bivalent copper ions, 8-azaguanine and aniline dyes; less fastidious nutritional growth requirements; ability to grow at low temperatures; and serologic and genetic characteristics (Turner, 1976). Members of the two complexes share no nucleotide sequences as determined by DNA-DNA annealing tests. However, leptospires within each complex can be further separated into three groups that have partial DNA homology. Leptospira-like organisms have been isolated, which generally resemble *L. biflexa* phenotypically but are genetically unrelated to any of the known genetic types. They may represent new species or genera (Brendle et al., 1974; Hovind-Hougen, et al., 1981).

Morphologically the saprophytic and parasitic leptospires are indistinguishable. Leptospires are helicoidal, flexuous organisms with semicircular hooked ends (Fig. 1). Occasional strains are straight-ended or have only one hook. The organisms usually measure 6 to 20 μm in length (range 3 to 40 μm) and approximately 0.1 μm in diameter. The coils are tightly wound with an overall diameter of 0.2 to 0.3 μm and a wavelength of approximately 0.5 μm. When examined by electron microscopy the structure of leptospires consists of a helicoidal protoplasmic cylinder that is wound about two independent axial filaments (Fig. 2). The filaments are inserted subterminally at each end with their free ends positioned toward the middle, where they usually do not overlap. The axial filaments resemble bacterial flagella structurally, in chemical composition, and in method of attachment. The helicoidal body is delineated by a cytoplasmic membrane–cell wall complex similar to that of gram-negative bacteria. The flagella and protoplasmic cylinder are enclosed by a common outer envelope or sheath (Alexander, 1980a).

In fluid media, leptospires appear to rotate alternately along their longitudinal axis, moving forward or backward without polar differentiation. The movement is characteristic because of the spinning hooked ends. In semisolid media, serpentine, boring, and flexing movements are seen. Leptospires can be seen by dark-field or phase contrast but not by bright-field microscopy. They are not readily visualized when stained with aniline dyes but can be demonstrated by the use of silver deposition techniques. Leptospires are capable of penetrating bacterial retaining filters. These attributes coupled with the fact that they do not grow on conventional media have frequently led to the mistaken identification of leptospirosis as a viral disease.

ANTIGENIC COMPOSITION. The pathogenic leptospires have distinct agglutinogenic properties that provide the basis for their differentiation. Otherwise they are indistinguishable by morphologic, cultural, and physiologic properties. The basic taxonomic group is the serovar (syn., serotype), which is included within a species. Currently, approximately 180 different serovars have been recognized on the basis of cross-agglutination and agglutinin-adsorption tests with serovar-specific rabbit antiserum (Turner, 1976). The serovars have been assembled into 20 serogroups on the basis of shared major agglutinogens. The serogroup has no taxonomic status but is used as an expedient for selection of antisera or antigens to identify isolates and to test sera. The agglutinogenic relationships do not necessarily correlate with genetic groupings. Each genetic group contains serologically diverse serovars. However, strains with major antigenic affinities appear to be genetically homologous (Brendle et al., 1974).

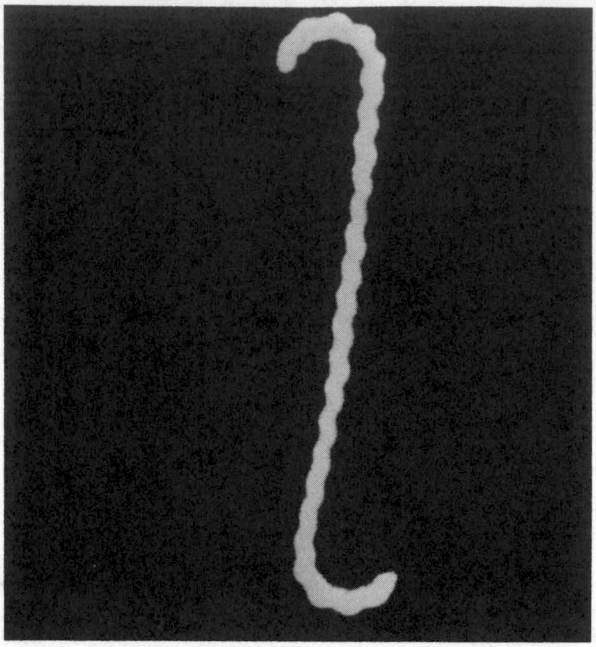

Figure 1. Leptospira. Dark-ground illumination. (Courtesy C. D. Cox, University of Massachusetts, Amherst.)

The agglutinogen, not surprisingly, has been associated with the enveloping sheath, which is composed of lipids, carbohydrates, and proteins (Johnson, 1977). Flagellar antigens have been isolated and shown to fall into eight antigenic groups by immunodiffusion techniques. They appeared to correlate best with genetic groupings (Chang et al., 1974). A variety of other antigenic substances have been extracted from leptospires by various chemical or physical treatments and have been shown to have specific or generic activity by the use of various serologic techniques. Their exact location and role in immunity and virulence needs additional study. An extract from biflexa serovars that is soluble in 50 per cent but insoluble in 95 per cent ethanol has proved to be particularly useful as a genus-specific, erythrocyte-sensitizing antigen in indirect hemagglutination and hemolytic tests (Cox et al., 1957; Sulzer et al., 1975).

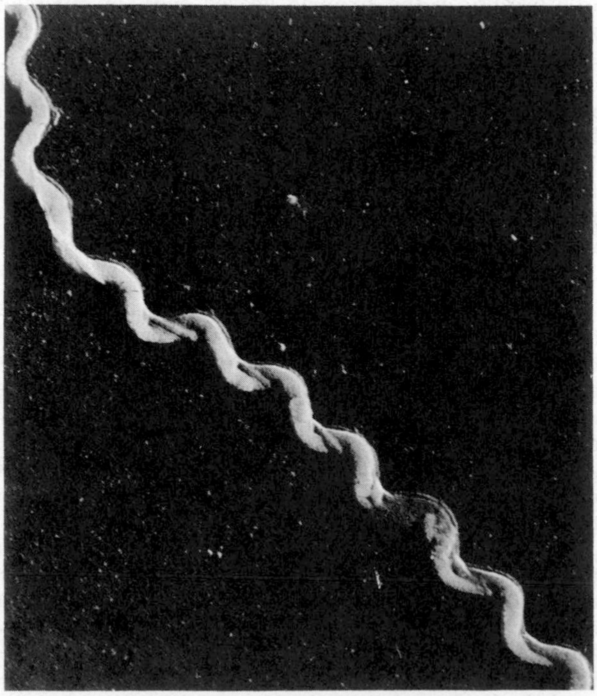

Figure 2. Electron micrograph of a portion of a leptospire. (Courtesy Armed Forces Institute of Pathology, Washington, D.C.)

METABOLISM. The pathogenic leptospires are aerobic organisms that can be grown in media containing serum, or serum components and fatty acids, at pH 6.8 to 7.8 (optimally at pH 7.2 to 7.4). Long-chain fatty acids (not carbohydrates or amino acids) are used as a source of carbon and energy. Leptospires can utilize ammonium salts or urea but not amino acids for their nitrogen requirements. Exogenous purines but not pyrimidines can be incorporated. Leptospires require thiamin and vitamin B_{12} in media. Cultures are usually incubated at 30° C. Incubation time for optimal growth ranges from a few days to 4 weeks or longer but is usually 6 to 14 days. At time of optimal growth the concentration of organism ranges from 1 to 4 $\times 10^8$/ml. Cytochrome enzymes, catalase, and enzymes of the citric acid cycle, glycolytic, and pentose pathways, and an acyl-coenzyme A dehydrogenase for β-oxididation of fatty acids have been demonstrated (Smibert, 1973).

PATHOGENIC PROPERTIES. The clinical and histopathologic findings in leptospirosis are consistent with the action of a toxin. However, attempts to isolate and identify a toxic component or product of leptospires has been elusive. Endotoxic properties of leptospires have been reported but not confirmed, nor were findings of toxic substances in lysed cultures or culture filtrates consistent (Johnson, 1976). Toxic substances have been demonstrated in extracts of infected tissues of experimental animals (Arean et al., 1964; Hanson, 1976). The nature of these toxins has not been defined. A hot-cold heat-labile, oxygen-stable hemolysin with specific activity for ruminant red blood cells is produced by some pathogenic leptospires and may be a significant factor for the hemolytic manifestations in bovine and other ruminant species (Alexander, 1976). Association of virulence with the outer envelope is suggested by findings that it is the site of the cidal action of antibody and complement and that virulent leptospires are more resistant to the antibody complement system than avirulent cells (Johnson and Harris, 1967). Pathogenicity has also been associated with production of catalase (Baseman and Cox, 1969). Pathogenic leptospires produce hyaluronidase (Yanagihara et al., 1973), which may contribute to the high invasiveness of these organisms.

IMMUNITY. Immunity in leptospirosis is best correlated with specific agglutinogenic characteristics of serovars (Alexander, 1976). Individuals who recover from infection with a specific serovar develop immunity against the same serovar but are susceptible to frank infection with antigenically different serovars. Where cross-protection was observed, it was related to common major agglutinogenic components. In accordance with this observation, the outer sheath has been found to be highly immunogenic and to have the same serologic specificity as agglutinogens (Auran et al., 1978). Intertype immunity against disease but not against infection has been demonstrated for certain serologically heterologous strains in experimental infections in hamsters and guinea pigs, and appeared to occur only between genetically homologous serovars (Alexander, 1976).

The protection afforded by specific immunoglobulins reflects their agglutinating and opsonizing properties, which enhance destruction of the organisms by phagocytosis. Cell-mediated immunity does not appear to be important in combating acute disease but its role in the development or prevention of the renal carrier state and other persistent forms of infection cannot be ruled out (Adler and Faine, 1977). Immunologic factors may be important in some of the pathogenetic features of leptospirosis. Antigen-antibody complex reactions have been suggested to explain neurologic, renal, and ocular complications that occur after the first week of disease. Autoimmune reactions have been postulated to explain lesions in the kidney and eye. Various immediate and delayed-type hypersensitivity reactions have been elicited in experimental animals (Alexander, 1976).

Vaccines are usually prepared from fixed cells. In man, vaccines have been extensively used in Japan, Italy, the USSR, and other Eastern European countries. Vaccine prophylaxis for livestock and pets is carried out in the United States and in many other countries throughout the world. Vaccines are serovar specific and usually incorporate two or more serovars, depending on the types of prevailing leptospiral infections.

LABORATORY DIAGNOSIS. Various microscopic, cultural, and serologic procedures are available for the laboratory diagnosis of leptospirosis. The selection and use of a suitable test depend on knowledge of the course of infection. After an incubation period, usually of 10 to 12 days, the disease appears abruptly, ushering in a septicemic stage persisting approximately 1 week. During this period the organisms may be found in the cerebrospinal fluid as well as in blood. The septicemic period usually ends with the appearance of detectable antibodies. Maximal antibody levels occur the third or fourth week of disease. Thereafter antibody levels gradually decline but may be detectable for years. Leptospires may be found in the urine after the first week of disease. Shedding is more pronounced during the first few weeks of convalescence; thereafter it may persist intermittently for two to three months in many cases and longer in some.

Culture. Leptospires are best demonstrated during the acute stage by culture of blood on such media as Stuart's liquid or Fletcher's semisolid, which contain rabbit serum, or EMJH medium, which contains albumin and fatty acid in lieu of serum (Vera and Power, 1980). Media are usually dispensed in test tubes in 5 ml amounts and inoculated with one or two drops of blood. At least four tubes of media, preferably from two different lots, should be used for each sample. Repeated blood cultures during the acute phase of disease are recommended. If culture medium is not immediately available at time of collection, blood may be defibrinated or mixed with anticoagulants, and subsequently cultured. Triturated clotted blood can also be used as inoculum. Spinal fluid, if available, may be cultured during the acute stage.

After the first week of disease, cultural recovery of leptospires from urine is possible in many cases. A midstream urine sample is carefully collected from cleansed genitalia and diluted 1:10 and 1:100 with media. Undiluted and diluted samples are cultured by using one or two drops of inoculum. In fatal cases leptospires may be isolated from suspensions of triturated liver and kidney. Minimal inocula of blood, urine, and tissue samples are recommended to dilute out growth-inhibitory substances. To inhibit the growth of contaminating organisms that may be present in urine or other samples, media may be supplemented with 5-fluorouracil, or with various antibiotics such as neomycin, furazolidone, cyclohexamide, or sulfathiazole, used singly or in combination (Alexander, 1980a; Sulzer and Jones, 1976).

Cultures are incubated at 30° C or in the dark at room temperature, examined at five- to seven-day intervals, and discarded if negative after six weeks of incubation.

In semisolid media a linear disk of growth is usually seen 1 to 3 cm below the surface. Fluid media become slightly turbid. On plating media containing 1 per cent agar, many strains form subsurface colonies. Plating media are useful for purifying cultures but are less satisfactory than tubed media for primary isolation. To examine cultures, a drop is placed on a slide, covered with a coverslip, and examined by dark-ground microscopy at high dry magnification (450 times). Leptospires are recognized by their characteristic morphology and motility. Cultures can be stored in screw-capped or other airtight tubes. Transfers are made at two- or three-month intervals from semisolid media, and at three to six weeks if kept in fluid media. Cultures are typed by the use of microscopic agglutination techniques. Initially the isolate employed as antigen is tested against a battery of different serovar antisera to determine serogroup affinities. It is then tested with additional antisera to elucidate further relationships. For definitive identification, agglutinin-adsorption tests are carried out. Culture typing is usually carried out in state or national laboratories, or in special WHO Leptospirosis Reference Laboratories (Faine, 1982; Sulzer and Jones, 1976).

Microscopic Examination. The concentration of leptospires in the blood of human patients is low and may not be demonstrated by dark-ground microscopic examination. In a small proportion of cases the chance of demonstrating leptospires may be increased by differential centrifugation of whole unclotted blood, first to remove cellular elements, and then to concentrate organisms in plasma (Wolff, 1954). Although the method may be valuable in establishing a rapid diagnosis, it is not recommended as a routine diagnostic procedure because artifacts such as cellular extrusions and fibrils are frequently mistaken for spirochetes. Direct microscopic methods are of value in examination of specimens in which a profuse number of leptospires may be present, such as blood and liver suspensions of hamsters or guinea pigs infected with clinical material or urine or kidney suspensions of natural animal hosts. Fluorescent-antibody staining techniques and silver deposition techniques have been used to demonstrate organisms in postmortem tissues and are especially useful if cultural and serologic tests are not possible (Alexander, 1980a; Sulzer and Jones, 1976).

Animal Inoculation. The use of laboratory animals offers no greater chance than direct culture for recovery of leptospires from blood or from other materials that can be obtained aseptically. Weanling hamsters and young guinea pigs are most commonly preferred because of their greater susceptibility to frank infection with a broad range of serovars (Wolff, 1954). The course of disease in laboratory animals varies with different serovars and also with different strains of the same serovar, and range from inapparent to lethal. Material is inoculated intraperitoneally. Heart blood for culture is taken on the fourth and sixth day after inoculation or whenever disease signs appear, and if necessary, at periodic intervals up to the twentieth day. On the twentieth day kidneys should also be cultured.

Serologic Diagnosis. The microscopic agglutination test has been most widely used. It is highly sensitive for diagnosis of recent as well as past infections and can be applied to animal as well as human sera. However, it has high specificity. Consequently, to ensure detection of antibodies that may be provoked by any of the large number of different serovars, it is necessary to use multiple serovar antigens that would cross-react with most of the known serovars that may be present. The number of test serovars may range from a few to 15 or more, depending on the number of serovars and their relative occurrence in specific geographic regions (Alexander, 1980b). Young cultures of leptospires in fluid media are used as antigen. These may be used live or be treated with formalin. Test sera are serially diluted two- to four-fold with physiologic salt solution to provide serum dilutions from 1:50 to 1:3200. Two-tenths-milliliter amounts of serum in each dilution are distributed in a series of agglutination tubes, to which is added an equal volume of antigen. The reaction mixtures are shaken, incubated at room temperature for two to three hours, shaken again, and examined for agglutination by dark-ground microscopic examination. The test has been adapted for use with microtitration techniques (Sulzer and Jones, 1976). Titers of 1:100 are considered to be significant, and may range as high as 1:25,600 or greater.

The laboriousness of the microscopic agglutination test limits its usefulness by the small laboratory. To circumvent this drawback, macroscopic-agglutination slide tests incorporating single or pooled antigens were developed and are commercially available (Alexander, 1980b). These tests are simple to perform and have good sensitivity for detecting recently or previously formed antibodies. "Genus-specific" tests have been proposed, which entail the use of specific biflexa strains known to cross-react frequently with leptospiral antibodies elicited by a large variety of pathogenic serovars (Alexander, 1980b; Faine, 1982; Turner, 1968). A hemolytic test with a "genus-specific" biflexa erythrocyte-sensitizing antigen has been used advantageously in areas of multiple leptospirosis (Cox et al., 1957; Tan, 1974). The test has been simplified by use of glutaraldehyde-fixed sensitized erythrocytes (Sulzer et al., 1975). Complement-fixation, slide agglutination, and latex particle agglutination tests with *L.* biflexa antigens are in use in some countries (Turner, 1968; Faine, 1982). Counterimmunoelectrophoresis and enzyme-linked-immunosorbent-assay (ELISA) tests have also been found to be useful for detecting leptospiral antibodies (Terpstra et al., 1980). Various fluorescent-antibody techniques have been reported for diagnosing leptospirosis but have not been widely adopted.

DRUG SUSCEPTIBILITY. Penicillin, streptomycin, tetracycline, and macrolide antibiotics are all active against leptospires in experimental animals and in vitro. Leptospires are resistant to chloramphenicol, sulfa drugs, neomycin, actidione, and isoniazid (Stahlheim, 1973).

EPIDEMIOLOGY. Leptospiroses are zoonoses that are globally distributed in a large variety of rodents and other feral and domestic mammals. Approximately 160 different mammalian species have been found to harbor leptospires (Leptospire Serotype Distributions Lists, 1966; 1975). Pathogenic leptospires have occasionally been isolated from birds, amphibians, reptiles, and ticks. The epidemiologic importance of nonmammalian hosts for leptospirosis has not been demonstrated. The distribution of the various serovars in mammalian hosts varies according to geographic region. The host range of selected serovars that are frequent causes of human disease in many parts of the world is shown in Table 1. Many serovars appear to be preferentially adapted to select mammalian hosts. For example, serovar *icterohaemorrhagiae* is primarily associated with the Norway rat, *canicola* with dogs, and *pomona* with swine and cattle. The occurrence of a specific serovar in a select host is not exclusive. The same mammalian species may be the

Table 1. HOST RANGE* FOR SOME WIDELY DISTRIBUTED, COMMONLY OCCURRING SEROVARS CAUSING HUMAN LEPTOSPIROSIS†

Serovar	Hosts: *Domestic*	Hosts: *Wild*
Icterohaemorrhagiae	dog, pig, horse, cattle	rats,‡ mice, mongoose, raccoon, muskrat, foxes, opossum, skunk, woodchuck, nutria, cavy, hedgehog, civet, apes
canicola	dog,‡ pig, cattle, cat, horse	skunk, raccoon, armadillo, mongoose, hedgehog, jackal, bandicoot, nutria, rats, vole
pomona	pig,‡ cattle,‡ goat, dog, cat, horse, sheep, water buffalo	skunk, opossum, foxes, raccoon, deer, hedgehog, mice, civet, cavy, woodchuck, vole, souslik, wolf, rabbit, sea lion
grippotyphosa	cattle, goat, sheep, swine, dog, cat	vole,‡ mice, rats, shrew, hedgehog, raccoon, skunk, fox, opossum, cavy, muskrat, weasel, mole, bobcat, leopard cat, bandicoot, rabbit, gerbil, squirrel, polecat
bataviae	dog,‡ cat, cattle	rats,‡ mice,‡ bandicoot, leopard cat, armadillo, vole, hedgehog, shrew
autumnalis	cattle, dog	mice,‡ rat, bandicoot, raccoon, opossum
australis	cattle, dog, horse	rats,‡ hedgehogs, mice, skunk, nutria, raccoon, vole, opossum, weasel, fox, bandicoot

*Based on cultural isolation.
†Source: Leptospiral Serotype Distribution Lists, 1966, 1975.
‡Known major maintenance host.

primary reservoir for several serovars. In addition, this species may be infected and serve as a carrier of serovars that occur predominantly in other hosts. Infections in natural hosts are usually inapparent, but may be morbid. Naturally occurring disease in animals has been principally observed in dogs, swine, cattle, and other livestock. Cats appear to be relatively resistant to disease. In many countries leptospirosis is an important veterinary medical problem.

In natural hosts, leptospires nest in the lumen of convoluted tubules within the kidneys, whence they are shed in the urine. The degree and duration of leptospiruria vary with the host and infecting serovar. The Norway rat infected with *icterohaemorrhagiae* sheds profuse numbers of organisms, apparently for the remainder of its natural life. Strains of *canicola* are less efficient in colonizing rat kidneys. On the other hand, in the dog *canicola* is better able to establish leptospiruria than is *icterohaemorrhagiae* (Babudieri, 1958). Shedding by infected dogs, swine, cattle, and other domestic animals may be heavy for several months after infection but is usually sparse or absent after six months. The prevalence of infection in natural hosts can be remarkably high. Carrier rates of 50 per cent or greater in Norway rats and other feral mammals, and of 10 to 50 per cent in domestic animals, are common findings in many parts of the world.

Leptospires are transmitted through contact with urine of animal carriers, either directly or by contact with damp soil or natural waters soiled by carriers. Pathogenic leptospires can survive for three months or more in neutral or slightly alkaline waters. They do not persist in brackish or acid waters. Organisms enter hosts through abrasions of the skin or through mucosal surfaces of the mouth, nasopharynx, eye, or esophagus. Individuals of all ages and both sexes are susceptible. Infection in man is accidental and is related to occupational or avocational exposure, or to contact with infected pets. Man is usually a dead-end host. Sewer workers, butchers, fish and poultry processors, miners, ditch diggers, and other individuals who work or live in rat-infested areas are at risk. Cases in dairymen, swineherds, and in abattoir workers are usually epidemiologically related to infection in livestock. Sporadic cases or epidemics have occurred in various parts of the world in agricultural workers engaged in raising flax, rice, vegetables, or sugar cane, in rubber plantation workers, and in soldiers exposed to natural waters contaminated by carriers. Common-source epidemics have occurred repeatedly in children and young adults who bathe or swim in ponds or streams located in pasturelands (Faine, 1982; van der Hoeden, 1958).

References

Adler, B., and Faine, S.: Host immunological mechanisms in the resistance of mice to leptospiral infections. Infect Immun 17:67, 1977.

Alexander, A. D.: *Leptospira*. In Lennette, E. H., Balows, A., Hausler, W. J. Jr., and Truant, J. P. (eds.): Manual of Clinical Microbiology. 3rd ed. Washington, D. C., American Society for Microbiology, 1980a, p. 376.

Alexander, A. D.: Serological diagnosis of leptospirosis. In Rose, N. R., and Friedman, H. (eds.): Manual of Clinical Immunology. 2nd ed., Washington, D. C., American Society for Microbiology, 1980b, p. 542.

Alexander, A. D.: Immunity in leptospirosis. In Johnson, R. C. (ed.): The Biology of Parasitic Spirochetes. New York, Academic Press, 1976, p. 339.

Arean, V. M., Sarasin, G., and Green, J. H.: The pathogenesis of leptospirosis: Toxin production by *Leptospira icterohaemorrhagiae*. Am J Vet Res 25:836, 1964.

Auran, N. E., Johnson, R. C., and Alexander, A. D.: Chemical composition and serological activity of leptospiral outer envelope. In Proceedings of the National Symposium on Leptospirosis, *Leptospira*, and other *Spirochaeta*, 25-27 September, 1975. Cantacuzino Institute, Bucharest. Ilexum Editure Medicala, 1978, p. 277.

Babudieri, B.: Animal reservoirs of leptospires. Ann NY Acad Sci 70:393, 1958.

Baseman, J. B., and Cox, C. D.: Terminal electron transport in Leptospira. J Bacteriol 97:1001, 1969.

Brendle, J. J., Rogul, M., and Alexander, A. D.: Deoxyribonucleic acid hybridization among selected leptospiral serotypes. Int J Systematic Bacteriol 24:205, 1974.

Chang, A., Faine, S., and Williams, W. T.: Cross-reactivity of the axial filament antigen as a criterion for classification of *Leptospira*. Aust J Exp Biol Med Sci 52:549, 1974.

Cox, C. D., Alexander, A. D., and Murphy, L. C.: Evaluation of the hemolytic test in the serodiagnosis of human leptospirosis. J Infect Dis 101:203, 1957.

Faine, S. (ed.): Guidelines for the Control of Leptospirosis. WHO Offset Publ. No. 67. Geneva, World Health Org, 1982.

Faine, S., and Stallman, N. D.: Amended descriptions of the genus *Leptospira* Noguchi 1917 and the species *L. interrogans* (Stimson, 1907), Wenyon 1926 and *L. biflexa* (Wolbach and Binger 1914) Noguchi 1918. Int J Systematic Bacteriol 32:461, 1982.

Hanson, H. E.: Pathogenesis of leptospirosis. In Johnson, R. C. (ed.): The Biology of Parasitic Spriochetes. New York, Academic Press, 1976, p. 295.

van der Hoeden, J.: Epizootiology of leptospirosis. Adv. Vet Sci 4:277, 1958.

Hovind-Hougen, K., Ellis, W. A., and Birch-Andersen, A.: *Leptospira parva* sp. nov: Some morphological and biological characters. Zentralbl Bakt Hyg Abt. 1 Orig. A 250:343, 1981.

Johnson, R. C.: Comparative spirochete physiology and cellular composition. In Johnson, R. C. (ed.): The Biology of Parasitic Spirochetes. New York, Academic Press, 1976, p. 39.

Johnson, R. C.: The spirochetes. Annu Rev Microbiol 31:89, 1977.

Johnson, R. C., and Harris, V. G.: Antileptospiral activity of serum. II. Leptospiral virulence factor. J. Bacteriol 93:513, 1967.

Leptospiral Serotype Distribution Lists According to Host and Geographic Area. Atlanta, Georgia, U.S. Dept. Health, Education and Welfare, Centers For Disease Control, 1966 (Supplement 1975).

Smibert, R. M.: *Spirochaetales*, a review. CRC Critical Reviews in Microbiol 2:491, 1973.

Stahlheim, O. H. V.: Chemical aspects of leptospirosis, CRC Critical Reviews in Microbiol 2:423, 1973.

Sulzer, C. R., Glosser, J. W., Roger, F., Jones, W. L., and Frix, M.: Evaluation of an indirect hemagglutination test for the diagnosis of human leptospirosis. J Clin Microbiol 2:218, 1975.

Sulzer, C. R., and Jones, W. L.: Leptospirosis. Methods in Laboratory Diagnosis. Revised ed. U.S. Dept. Health, Education, and Welfare, Public Health Service, Centers for Disease Control, HEW Publ. No. (CDC) 76–8275, 1976.

Tan, D. S. K., and Welch, Q. B.: Evaluation of *Leptospira biflexa* antigens for screening human sera by the microscopic agglutination (MA) test in comparison with the sensitized-erythrocyte-lysis (SEL) test. Southeast Asian J Trop Med Publ Hlth 5:12, 1974.

Terpstra, W. J., Ligthart, G. S., and Schoone, G. J.: Serodiagnosis of leptospirosis by enzyme-linked-immunosorbent-assay (ELISA). Zentralbl Bakt Hyg Abt. 1 Orig 247:400, 1980.

Turner, L. H.: Leptospirosis. II. Serology. Trans R Soc Trop Med Hyg 62:880, 1968.

Turner, L. H.: Classification of spirochaetes in general and of the Genus *Leptospira* in particular. In Johnson, R. C. (ed.): The Biology of Parasitic Spirochetes. New York, Academic Press, 1976, p. 95.

Vera, H. D., and Power, D. A.: Culture media. In Lennette, E. H., Balows, A., Hausler, W. J. Jr., and Truant, J. P. (eds.): Manual of Clinical Microbiology. 3rd ed. Washington, D.C., American Society for Microbiology, 1980, p. 965.

Wolff, J. W.: The Laboratory Diagnosis of Leptospirosis. Springfield, Ill., Charles C Thomas, 1954.

Yanagihara, Y., Taniyama, T., and Mifuchi, I.: Separation and purification of hyaluronidase of Leptospira (in Japanese). Medicine and Biology 86:83, 1973.

2. Anaerobic Bacteria

47

GRAM-POSITIVE COCCI; PEPTOCOCCUS, PEPTOSTREPTOCOCCUS, STREPTOCOCCUS (ANAEROBIC), AND SARCINA

LYNN A. LANCASTER, M.D.
HOWARD ROBERT ATTEBERY, D.D.S.

The anaerobic gram-positive cocci are a controversial and difficult group of organisms. Their pathogenicity is doubted by some (Facklam and Smith, 1976) and respected by others (Finegold, 1977; Lambe et al., 1973; Pien et al., 1972). Their classification has also been controversial, but most clinical laboratories identify anaerobic gram-positive cocci on the basis of gas-liquid chromatographic analysis of end-products of metabolism and by growth requirements for fermentable carbohydrates (Holdeman et al., 1977).

Peptococcus, Peptostreptoccus, Sarcina, and *Streptococcus* do not require fermentable carbohydrates for growth and are the most important genera of anaerobic gram-positive cocci. Streptococci produce lactic acid as the major metabolic end-product and on this basis are distinct from *Peptococci* and *Peptostreptococci*.

Gemminger, *Coprococcus*, and *Ruminococcus* require carbohydrate and, therefore, grow poorly if at all in media such as peptone yeast broth. *Gemminger* and *Coprococcus* are distinguished from *Ruminococcus* by their production of butyric acid. Members of these genera are seldom encountered in clinical infections but may be cultured from feces. See Smith (1975) for further information on alternate schemes of classification.

Gram-positive cocci that grow both in a mixture of 10 per cent carbon dioxide and air and in an anaerobic environment are microaerophilic (also called capnophilic or CO_2 dependent) cocci and are not usually classified with anaerobic cocci. However, some strains of anaerobic cocci become tolerant of air upon subculturing and confuse classification efforts. Many other strains of anaerobic cocci, on the other hand, are fastidious anaerobes and good transport and anaerobic methods are necessary for their recovery.

MORPHOLOGY. It is not possible to classify anaerobic cocci to genera by cellular morphology alone. Although peptococci are usually clumped, they also occur singly and in pairs or short chains. Peptostreptococci and anaerobic streptococci cannot be differentiated by gram stain. Peptostreptococci may cluster like peptococci and form only short chains, but chaining is usually accentuated by growth in liquid medium.

Many strains of anaerobic gram-positive cocci destain easily and appear gram-negative. This seldom presents an identification problem, however, because *Veillonella*, the only anaerobic gram-negative coccus, is much smaller than the anaerobic gram-positive cocci, with the exception of *Peptostreptococcus micros*. Anaerobic gram-positive cocci may elongate and resemble short rods. This is more common with *Peptostreptococcus productus*. Cells may be of unequal size in culture. This size differential may be so great that it gives the appearance of budding.

The cellular morphology of *Sarcina ventriculi* is distinctive from that of other anaerobic gram-positive cocci. Cells are usually about 2.0 μ in diameter, nearly spherical with flattened adjacent sides, and arranged in packets of eight or more.

The colonial morphology of *Peptococcus (Pc.)*, *Peptostreptococcus (Ps.)* and the anaerobic members of the genus *Streptococcus (S.)* is not distinctive. On blood agar plates, colonies are small (0.5 mm after 48 hours of incubation), convex, opaque, entire, and either shiny or dull. Most colonies are gray to white. *Peptococcus niger* forms small black colonies on blood agar plates. The colonies fade to gray after exposure to oxygen and may not be pigmented after repeated subculture (Wilkins et al., 1975). Some strains of *Ps. micros* and *Ps. anaerobius* also produce black colonies.

S. constellatus and *S. morbillorum* are usually alpha hemolytic; *S. intermedius* is usually not. *Ps. productus* may be nonhemolytic or give alpha or beta reactions. The other peptococci and peptostreptococci are not hemolytic except for some strains of *Ps. micros* and *Pc. prevotii* that produce a beta hemolysin.

Surface colonies of *S. ventriculi* are 1 to 3 mm after 24 hours of incubation, colorless, circular, and opaque with an irregular edge. Most strains are nonhemolytic; a few are alpha hemolytic. Subsurface colonies are frequently star-shaped or irregular.

ANTIGENIC AND BIOCHEMICAL COMPOSITION. Most studies of the antigenic composition of anaerobic gram-positive cocci have attempted to clarify their taxonomy. No antigen common to the genera *Peptococcus*, *Streptococcus*, and *Peptostreptococcus* can be produced in rabbits by immunization with whole cells or soluble proteins obtained by sonification (Graham and Falkler, 1978 and 1979). Wong et al. (1980) have prepared species-specific *Staphylococcus* protein A coagglutination reagents that can be used for species identification of bacterial saline suspensions. The technique is simple, rapid, and more sensitive than previous immunologic procedures. Antigens recognized by these antibodies have not been characterized.

Indirect fluorescent antibody techniques have been used to recognize and separate the majority of strains of *Peptococcus magnus* from *Peptostreptococcus* and other *Peptococcus* species (Porschen and Spaulding, 1974). Counterimmunoelectrophoresis of antisera to three strains of *Pc. magnus* and one strain of *Ps. anaerobius* showed that each strain was distinct (Markowitz and Lerner, 1977).

Antisera to anaerobic and microaerophilic members of the genus *Streptococcus* have been analyzed by counterimmunoelectrophoresis, tandem-crossed counterimmunoelectrophoresis and other immunologic techniques. *S. intermedius* and *S. constellatus* contain at least six common antigens and are therefore closely related. Two *S. morbillorum* strains are antigenically distinct from one another;

one has few and the other no antigens in common with *S. intermedius* and *S. constellatus*. *S. intermedius*, *S. constellatus*, and *S. morbillorum* share some antigens with *S. sanguis* and *S. mitis*. There are no common antigens between these three species and *S. mutans*. and *S. bovis* (Coleman and Lambe, 1979).

Wells and Field (1976) analyzed the long-chain fatty acids of 82 strains of anaerobic gram-positive cocci and divided them into four groups. *Ps. anaerobius* and *Pc. saccharolyticus* could be identified by unique patterns and constituted groups I and IV, respectively. Other strains that were not as distinct constituted groups II and III. Further studies have resulted in more complete characterization of the compounds separated by gas liquid chromatography (GLC) (Moss et al., 1977). Analysis of acidic and basic components of spent-growth media combined with GLC analysis of cellular fatty acids separates most species of anaerobic gram positive cocci. The occurrence of lactobacillic acid in the profiles of anaerobic streptococci and facultative streptococci supports their combination into one genus (Lambert and Armfield, 1979).

Peptococcus saccharolyticus isolates have been subjected to a wide variety of nucleic acid studies that reveal a closer relationship to staphylococci than peptococci (Ludwig et al., 1981). Studies of peptidoglycan also suggest a relationship to the staphylococci (Schleifer and Nimmerman, 1973).

Polyacrylamide gel electrophoresis of soluble cellular proteins permits clear separation of the biochemically similar species *Ps. micros* and *Pc. magnus*, which are ordinarily differentiated on the basis of size. Despite some heterogeneity, the protein components of *Pc. magnus* strains are basically similar. Analysis of reference *Pc. variabilis* strains, which some have considered synonymous with *Pc. magnus*, reveals two patterns. One strain is similar to *Pc. magnus*, while the other is distinct. Since the soluble proteins of *Pc. glycinophilus* are identical to reference strains of *Ps. micros*, they are probably identical species (Cato et al., 1983).

METABOLISM. The clinically important species of the anaerobic gram-positive cocci are listed in Table 1, together with their major end-products of amino acid and glucose metabolism.

Peptococci and peptostreptococci metabolize glucose heterofermentatively and utilize amino acids as their main sources of nitrogen and energy. The anaerobic streptococci are homofermentative, producing lactic acid as the major end product of carbohydrate fermentation. In media supplemented with Tween 80, *Ps. parvulus* shows increased fermentative ability and produces primarily lactic acid (homofermentative). Cato (1983) recommends that *Ps. parvulus* be placed in the *Streptococcus* genus.

Table 2 lists some of the metabolic activities of the anaerobic gram-positive cocci. Peptococci are not very active biochemically. *Pc. asaccharolyticus* and *Pc. indolicus* are the only clinically important anaerobic gram-positive cocci that produce indole.

Sarcina ventriculi is a fermentative bacterium; its principal products from glucose metabolism are carbon dioxide, hydrogen, ethyl alcohol, and acetic acid. It uses two pathways for conversion of pyruvate to ethyl alcohol. One is the same as that used by yeast and the other is similar to that of *Escherichia coli* (Canale-Parola, 1970).

Peptostreptococci are very sensitive to oxygen. The toxic effect of oxygen on *Ps. anaerobius* appears to be mediated in large part by H_2O_2 or a related compound. Catalase, which decomposes H_2O_2, and manganese dioxide protect organisms exposed to aerated broth (Frolander and Carlsson, 1977). Organisms are most sensitive during the exponential growth phase, but inhibitors of protein and nucleic acid synthesis fail to diminish toxicity. Certain metal ion chelators and ionophores greatly diminish killing. The precise molecular events are unknown (Nyberg and Carlsson, 1981).

Table 1. CLINICALLY IMPORTANT ANAEROBIC GRAM-POSITIVE COCCI AND THEIR MAJOR METABOLIC END-PRODUCTS FROM AMINO ACID AND GLUCOSE METABOLISM[a]

Name	Major End Products		Minor End Products
Pc. asaccharolyticus	A	H	B(SLF)
Pc. magnus	A	H	(LSF)
Pc. prevotii	A	H	B(L)
Pc. saccharolyticus	FA2		
Ps. anaerobius	A	H	(2BL, et al.)
Ps. micros	A		(LSF)
Ps. parvulus	LA		(S)
Ps. productus	A	(H)	S(LP)
St. constellatus	L		
St. intermedius	L		
St. morbillorum	L		
S. ventriculi	A2	H,CO_2	

[a]*Pc., Peptococcus; Ps., Peptostreptococcus; St., Streptococcus; S., Sarcina*; A, acetic acid; B, butyric acid; F, formic acid; L, lactic acid; P, propionic acid; S, succinic acid; H, hydrogen gas; CO_2, carbon dioxide gas; ( ), variable; 2, ethyl alcohol.

PATHOGENICITY. Isolation of the anaerobic gram-positive cocci in pure culture from some infections is the most compelling evidence for their pathogenicity. Because speciation of the anaerobic gram-positive cocci has been difficult and controversial, the older literature is of only limited value in ranking the relative frequency of isolation and pathogenicity of a given species. For example, *Peptococcus magnus* is currently the most frequently isolated anaerobic gram-positive coccus, but it was commonly identified as *Peptostreptococcus magnus* until 1972 (Pien et al., 1972). Separation of *S. intermedius* from the peptostreptococci and of *S. morbillorum* and *S. constellatus* from the peptococci is a recent change. Also, capnophilic and microaerophilic streptococci have undoubtedly been considered anaerobic and regarded as peptostreptococci by some workers.

Despite confusion over the precise identity of the species involved, it is clear that anaerobic gram-positive cocci are isolated in pure culture from a variety of processes ranging from brain abscess, meningitis, extradural and subdural empyema, liver abscess, pleuopulmonary infection, breast abscess, osteomyelitis, and other infections. Bourgalt et al. (1980), isolated *Pc. magnus* in pure culture from 32 patients. Bone and joint, soft tissue, and vascular infections were most common and were usually associated with surgery or prosthetic devices indicating a low potential for breaching normal defense mechanisms.

The anaerobic gram-positive cocci are more commonly found in mixed infections with other anerobes or facultative bacteria. The pathogenic role of the anaerobic gram-positive cocci in such conditions is unproven. About one-third

Table 2. METABOLIC REACTIONS OF GRAM-POSITIVE ANAEROBIC COCCI[a]

	Fermentation								
	Glucose	***Lactose***	***Maltose***	***Sucrose***	**Indole**	**Nitrate Reduction**	**Gelatin Hydrolysis**	**Esculin Hydrolysis**	**Catalase**
Pc. asaccharolyticus	–	–	–	–	+	–	–	–	–
Pc. magnus	$-^{w}$	–	–	–	–	–	V	–	–
Pc. prevotii	$-^{w}$	–	–	–	–	$-^{+}$	–	–	$-^{+}$
Pc. saccharolyticus	A^{w}	–	–	–	–	$+^{-}$	–	–	+
Ps. anaerobius	W^{a-}	–	$-^{w}$	–	–	$-^{+}$	$-^{w}$	–	–
Ps. micros	$-^{w}$	–	–	–	–	–	–	–	–
Ps. parvulus	A	A	A	–	–	–	–	+	–
Ps. productus	A	A	A	A	–	–	–	+	–
St. constellatus	A	–	A	A	–	–	–	+	–
St. intermedius	A	A	A	A	–	–	–	+	–
St. morbillorum	A	–	A^{w}	A	–	–	–	–	–
S. ventriculi	A	A	A^{w}	A	–	$+^{-}$	–	+	–

[a] –negative reaction; +, positive reaction; A, acid; W, weak acid; V, variable.
From Holdeman, L. V., Cato, E. P., and Moore, W. E.: Anaerobe Laboratory Manual. Blacksburg, Va., Virginia Polytechnic Institute and State University, 1977.

of intraabdominal infections contain a mixed flora of anaerobic cocci with either *Bacteroides fragilis*, clostridia, or both.

Certain bacteria act synergistically to produce infections. For example, synergistic gangrene is produced by a microaerophilic *Streptococcus* and a hemolytic *Staphylococcus aureus*. If animals are monoinoculated with individual cultures, no disease is produced, but if the organisms are combined before inoculation, typical necrotic ulcers are formed (Meleney, 1949). The basis of the synergy is production by the *Staphylococcus* of hyaluronidase and a growth factor that make the microaerophilic *Streptococcus* invasive.

The mechanisms of pathogenicity of the anaerobic cocci are unknown. Most produce ammonia that causes inflammation. Production of extracellular enzymes is limited to certain species and, with the exception of *Pc. indolicus*, is variable from strain to strain (Marshall and Kaufman, 1981). Peptocoagulase is cell-bound and secreted into the media by over 90 per cent of *Pc. indolicus* isolates. It interacts stochiometrically in an unknown fashion with prothrombin, which then catalyzes the conversion of fibrinogen to fibrin. *Pc. indolicus* is seldom a human pathogen, and the role of peptocoagulase in its pathogenicity for cattle is unknown (Switalski et al., 1978).

S. ventriculi is occasionally found in infections, especially of the gall bladder and bile ducts but never in pure culture. It is a free-living bacterium that often enters the stomach and becomes a minor member of the normal flora of humans. Prolonged gastric retention allows *Sarcina* to grow rapidly and produce so much gas from fermentable substrates that abdominal discomfort results.

IMMUNITY. Intact epithelium and the high oxidation-reduction potential of the tissues provide a high degree of resistance to the anaerobic gram-positive cocci. Leukocytes can ingest and kill *Pc. magnus* and *Ps. anaerobius* even in the absence of oxygen. The roles of humoral and cellular immunity are unknown.

LABORATORY DIAGNOSIS. Differentiation between the genera *Peptococcus* and *Peptostreptococcus* is difficult because the species are variable in morphologic, cultural, and metabolic properties and are relatively inert biochemically. Criteria established by the Anaerobe Laboratory of the Virginia Polytechnic Institute (Holdeman et al., 1977) are used by most laboratories for identification. This method requires determination of the end-products of metabolism of glucose and amino acids by gas-liquid chromatography.

Peptococci can be differentiated from peptostreptococci on the basis of the guanine plus cytosine content of their DNA. Peptostreptococci contain 33.5 moles per cent; peptococci, 35.7 to 36.7 moles per cent. Anaerobic streptococci, however, range from 33 to 44 moles per cent and analysis of end-products of fermentation is necessary for their differentiation.

Anaerobic streptococci and peptostreptococci do not synthesize catalase. Because peptococci may give weak and variable catalase reactions, a negative catalase test does not reliably separate this genus. A positive test does suggest the genus *Peptococcus*.

Peptococci usually do not form long chains. Because peptostreptococci and anaerobic streptococci both have a strong chaining tendency, absence of chaining suggests peptococci. If long chains are present, end-product analysis of glucose fermentation is necessary to differentiate peptostreptococci from anaerobic streptococci. This technique is also used to confirm the identity of peptococci.

It is seldom difficult to assign a gram-positive coccus to the genus *Streptococcus* when GLC analysis of end-products of metabolism reveals primarily lactic acid (homofermentative). No scheme for subsequent speciation is widely followed. Holdeman and Moore (1974) recognize both anaerobic and microaerophilic strains among the species *S. intermedius*, *S. constellatus*, and *S. morbillorum*. Some strains are microaerophilic on primary isolation or become microaerophilic after subculture. Others remain strictly anaerobic despite repeated subculture. The classification outlined in Tables 2 and 3 assigns both microaerophilic and strictly anaerobic isolates to species level. Alternatively, microaerophilic species may be assigned to classification schemes for the viridans streptococci. Using Facklam's (1977) criteria for speciation, Rosenblatt (1980) reclassified 30 strains of *Peptostreptococcus intermedius* as *Streptococcus* MG (20), *S. anginosus* (6), and *S. sanguis* (4). European workers have favored the classification scheme of viridans streptococci, popularized by Coleman and Williams (1972). Certain microaerophilic strains of *S. constellatus* and *S. intermedius* would be classified as *S. milleri* in their scheme (see Chapter 24). *Streptococcus milleri* refers to a hetero-

Table 3. IDENTIFICATION KEY TO THE CLINICALLY IMPORTANT ANAEROBIC GRAM-POSITIVE COCCI

Lactic acid the sole major end-product	
Esculin hydrolysis +	
Lactose +	Streptococcus intermedius
Lactose −	Streptococcus constellatus
Esculin hydrolysis −	Streptococcus morbillorum
Lactic acid not the sole major end-product	
Indole +	Peptococcus asaccharolyticus[b]
Indole −	
Sensitive to SPS[a]	Peptostreptococcus anaerobius
Resistance to SPS	
Lactose +	
Sucrose +	Peptostreptococcus productus
Sucrose −	Peptostreptococcus parvulus
Lactose −	
Glucose +	Peptostreptococcus micros
Glucose −	
Butyric acid produced	Peptococcus prevotii
Butyric acid not produced	Peptococcus magnus

[a]Sodium polyanethol sulfonate.

[b]*Peptococcus indolicus* also produces indole and is distinguished from *Pe. asaccharolyticus* by its ability to reduce nitrate to nitrite.

geneous collection of organisms with variable serologic, hemolytic, and biochemical characteristics. *S. milleri* is frequently capnophilic and closely related biochemically to *S. MG-intermedius* and *S. constellatus*. Its role in purulent abscesses of soft tissue and major viscera is well established. Characteristics of *S. milleri* are reviewed by Ball and Parker (1979) and by Poole and Wilson (1979).

Two species common in clinical specimens may be identified by simple tests. *Pc. asaccharolyticus* and *Pc. indolicus* are the gram-positive anaerobic cocci that produce indole. *Pc. indolicus* reduces nitrate but *Pc. assachrolyticus* does not. *Ps. anaerobius* is the only anaerobic gram-positive coccus highly sensitive to sodium polyanetholsulfonate (SPS) in disk susceptibility tests. Fresh isolates give larger zone sizes than stock cultures. Most other species are not inhibited but a few may show small or intermediate zone sizes. The test has an overall accuracy of 98% (Wideman et al., 1976). Hydrolysis of tyrosine in a medium containing tyrosine crystals is a simple, sensitive, and specific way of identifying *Ps. anaerobius* (Babcock, 1979).

Sarcina ventriculi can be easily distinguished by microscopic morphology. Large round cells with flattened adjacent sides in packets of eight or more are characteristic of this species, the only anaerobic *Sarcina* found in man.

A key for identification of the clinically important anaerobic gram-positive cocci is given in Table 3. This is one of several schemes that have been proposed for the identification of these bacteria.

Anaerobic and microaerophilic gram-positive cocci frequently grow slowly and may require 48 hours of incubation before becoming visible. Ultimate recovery is greatly enhanced by a full 48 hours of anaerobic incubation. Exposure to oxygen after 24 hours (despite subsequent reincubation) results in a significant reduction in frequency of isolation from clinical specimens (Wren, 1980).

Not all anaerobic gram-positive cocci can be identified. On occasion, facultative gram-positive cocci grow only anaerobically upon isolation and initial subculture (Yatabe et al., 1977). Facultative cocci may also mutate to obligate anaerobes that retain all their other original characteristics.

DRUG SUSCEPTIBILITY. All β-lactam antibiotics inhibit over 90 per cent of anaerobic gram-positive cocci at levels attainable with parenteral therapy. Penicillin G remains the drug of choice for treatment of infections with these organisms. Most peptococci, peptostreptococci, and anaerobic streptococci are inhibited by 0.1 μg/ml and 90 per cent by 0.5 μg/ml. Unusual strains of peptostreptococci and streptococci require up to 32 μg/ml for inhibition. Two μg/ml of cephalothin inhibits over 90 per cent of anaerobic gram-positive cocci (Sutter and Finegold, 1976).

Clindamycin at a concentration of 2 μg/ml inhibits most anaerobic streptococci and peptostreptococci, but over 10 per cent of peptococci are resistant to as much as 64 μg/ml. Two μg/ml of chloramphenicol inhibits approximately 90 per cent of peptococci and peptostreptococci but only 40 per cent of streptococci. Nearly all isolates of peptococci, peptostreptococci, and streptococci are inhibited by 8 μg/ml. Tetracycline resistance among anaerobic gram-positive cocci is common. Four μg/ml inhibits 36, 52, and 90 per cent of peptococci, peptostreptococci, and streptococci, respectively (Sutter and Finegold, 1976).

Metronidazole and related imidazoles are active against nearly all peptococci and peptostreptococci. Some anaerobic and all microaerophilic streptococci, however, are resistant. Goldstein (1978) found that 88 per cent of peptococci were inhibited by 0.5 μg/ml of metronidazole and 97 per cent by 2 μg/ml. All 20 peptostreptococci tested were inhibited by 0.5 μg/ml. Microaerophilic streptococci are resistant. Caution must be exercised in the use of metronidazole as sole therapy for infections thought to be caused by anaerobic gram-positive cocci because it may take repeated subcultures and several days to differentiate a microaerophilic streptococcus from a peptostreptococcus.

EPIDEMIOLOGY. Peptococci, peptostreptococci, and anaerobic streptococci are part of the indigenous microbiota of the human oral cavity, gastrointestinal tract, genitourinary system, and skin (see Table 1). *Pc. saccharolyticus* is the dominant skin organism in some individuals (Evans and Strom, 1982). These opportunistic bacteria are commonly found in infections that are closely associated with these organs.

Sarcina ventriculi is commonly found in soil and mud, and on grain, but only infrequently and in low numbers in the normal human fecal flora.

A 14-year study of clinical specimens showed that 58.5 per cent yielded anaerobes (Holland et al., 1977). Anaerobic gram-positive cocci were present in 66 per cent of these specimens. This is a major clinical concern, especially since 15 per cent of the specimens contained anaerobic cocci as the only anaerobe.

Pc. asaccharolyticus is found in about 10 per cent of human infections, *Ps. anaerobius* in 9 per cent, and *S. intermedius* in 5 per cent. *Pc. prevotti* and *Pc. magnus* are each found in about 4 per cent.

In a study of 100 anaerobic pleuropulmonary infections, peptostreptococci were recovered 19 times, 3 times in pure culture. Peptococci were recovered 15 times, always in mixed culture.

Anaerobic cocci are isolated from 1 per cent of blood cultures and make up approximately 7 per cent of anaerobic isolates. The foci of infection in anaerobic gram-positive cocci bacteremias are usually infections of the soft tissue, gastrointestinal tract, liver, female genital tract, and oropharynx.

Anaerobes have been isolated from about 3 per cent of patients with bacterial endocarditis. Anaerobic and microaerophilic streptococci make up over 90 per cent of these isolates.

Anaerobic cocci are isolated from about one-third of all abdominal infections, usually in association with *Bacteroides fragilis* and clostridia. Although anaerobic cocci and clostridia are the dominant anaerobes in biliary tract infections, they are isolated from only a small proportion of these infections.

The anaerobic gram-positive cocci are frequently found in liver abscesses and brain abscesses, and 40 per cent of abscesses of the female pelvis contain anaerobic streptococci. *B. fragilis, B. melaninogenicus*, and anaerobic streptococci are the most common isolates from septic abortions. Bacteremias from septic abortions most frequently yield anaerobic streptococci and *Bacteroides*. These two groups are also the most frequent isolates from postpartum endometritis.

One study of brain abscess reported recovery of anaerobes in 89 per cent of the cases. Peptostreptococci were the predominant organisms (Heineman and Braude, 1963). The most common isolates from chronic sinusitis are peptostreptococci (Frederick and Braude, 1974).

References

Babcock, J. B.: Tyrosine degradation in presumptive identification of *Peptostreptococcus anaerobius*. J Clin Microbiol 9:358, 1979.

Ball, L. C., and Parker, M. T.: The cultural and biochemical characteristics of *Streptococcus milleri* strains isolated from human sources. J Hyg (London) 82:63, 1979.

Canale-Parola, E.: Biology of the sugar-fermenting sarcinae. Bacteriol Rev 34:82, 1970.

Bourgault, A., Rosenblatt, J. E., and Fitzgerald, R. H.: *Peptococcus magnus*: A significant human pathogen. Ann Int Med. 93:244, 1980.

Cato, E. P.: Transfer of *Peptostreptococcus parvulus* (Weinberg, Nativelle, and Prévot, 1937) Smith 1957 to the genus *Streptococcus: Striptococcus parvulus* (Weinberg, Nativelle, and Prévot, 1937) Comb. Nov., nom. rev., emend. Int J Syst Bacteriol 33:82, 1983.

Cato, E. P., Johnson, J. L., Hash, D. E., and Holdeman, L. V.: Synonomy of *Peptococcus glycinophilus* (Cardon and Barker 1946) Douglas 1957 with *Peptostreptococcus micros* (Prevot 1933) Smith 1957 and electrophoretic differentiation of *Peptostreptococcus micros* from *Peptococcus magnus* (Prevot 1933) Holdeman and Moore 1972. Int J Syst Bacteriol 33:207, 1983.

Coleman, G., and Williams, R. E. D.: Taxonomy of some human viridans streptococci. In Wannamaker, L. W., and Matsen, J. M. (eds.): Streptococci and Streptococcal Diseases. Recognition, Understanding and Management. New York, Academic Press, 1972.

Coleman, R. M., and Lambe, D. W., Jr.: Serologic studies of *Streptococcus intermedius, Streptococcus constellatus,* and *Streptococcus morbillorum* by crossed immunoelectrophoresis. A J Clin Path 72:12, 1979.

Evans, C. A., and Strom, M. S.: Eight year persistence of individual differences in the bacterial flora of the forehead. J Invest Dermatol 79:51, 1982.

Facklam, R. R., and Smith, P. B.: The gram positive cocci. Human Pathol 7:187, 1976.

Facklam, R. R.: Physiological differentiation of viridans streptococci. J Clin Microbiol 5:184, 1977.

Finegold, S. M.: Anaerobic Bacteria in Human Disease. New York, Academic Press, 1977.

Frederick, J. and Braude, A. I.: Anaerobic infection of the paranasal sinuses. N Engl J Med 290:135, 1974.

Frolander, F., and Carlsson, J.: Bactericidal effect of anaerobic broth exposed to atmospheric oxygen tested on *Peptostreptococcus anaerobius*. J Clin Microbiol 6:117, 1977.

Goldstein, E. J., Sutter, V. L., Finegold, S. M.: Comparative susceptibilities of anaerobic bacteria to metronidazole, ornidazole, and SC-28538. Antimicrob Agents Chemother 14:609, 1978.

Graham, M. B., and Falkler, W. A., Jr.: Serological reactions of the genus *Peptostreptococcus*. J Clin Microbiol 7:385, 1978.

Graham, M. B., and Falkler, W. A., Jr.: Extractable antigen shared by *Peptostreptococcus anaerobius* strains. J Clin Microbiol 9:507, 1979.

Heineman, H. S., and Braude, A. I.: Anaerobic infection of the brain: Observations on eighteen consecutive cases of brain abscess. Am J Med 35:682, 1963.

Holdeman, L. V., Cato, E. P., and Moore, W. E.: Anaerobe Laboratory Manual. Blackburg, Va., Virginia Polytechnic Institute and State University, 1977.

Holdeman, L. V., and Moore, W. E. C.: New genus *Coprococcus*, twelve new species, and emended descriptions of four previously described species of bacteria from human feces. Int J Syst Bacteriol 24:260, 1974.

Holland, J. W., Hill, E. O., and Altemeier, W. A.: Numbers and types of anaerobic bacteria isolated from clinical specimens since 1960. J Clin Microbiol 5:20, 1977.

Lambe, D. W., Vroon, D. H., and Rietz, C. W.: Infections due to anaerobic cocci. In Ballows, A., et al. (eds.): Anaerobic Bacteria: Role in Disease. Springfield, Ill., Charles C Thomas, 1973.

Lambert, M. A. S., and Armfield, A. Y.: Differentiation of *Peptococcus* and *Peptostreptococcus* by gas liquid chromatography of cellular fatty acids and metabolic products. J Clin Microbiol 10:464, 1979.

Ludwig, W., Schleifer, K. H., Fox, G. E., et al: A phylogenetic analysis of staphlococci, *Peptococcus saccharolyticus* and *Micrococcus mucilaginosus*. J Gen Microbiol 125:357, 1981.

Markowitz, A., and Lerner, A. M.: Differentiation of several isolates of *Peptococcus magnus* by counterimmunoelectrophoresis. Infect Immun 16:152, 1977.

Marshall, R., and Kaufman, A. K.: Production of deoxyribonuclease, ribonuclease, coagulase, and hemolysins by anaerobic gram-positive cocci. J Clin Microbiol 13:787, 1981.

Meleney, F. L.: Clinical Aspects and Treatment of Surgical Infections. Philadelphia, W. B. Saunders Company, 1949.

Moss, C. W., Lambert, M. A., and Lombard, G. L.: Cellular fatty acids of *Peptococcus variabilis* and *Peptostreptococcus anaerobius*. J Clin Microbiol 5:665, 1977.

Nyberg, G. K., and Carlsson, J.: Metabolic inhibition of *Peptostreptococcus anaerobius* decreases the bactericidal effect of hydrogen peroxide. Antimicrob Agents Chemother 20:726, 1981.

Pien, F. D., Thompson, R. L., and Martin, W. J.: Clinical and bacteriologic studies of anaerobic gram-positive cocci. Mayo Clin Proc 47:251, 1972.

Poole, P. M., and Wilson, G.: Occurrence and cultural features of *Streptococcus milleri* in various body sites. J Clin Path 32:764, 1979.

Porschen, R. K., and Spaulding, E. H.: Fluorescent antibody study of the gram-positive anaerobic cocci. Appl Microbiol 28:851, 1974.

Rosenblatt, J. E.: Anaerobic cocci. In Lennette, E. H. (ed.): Manual of Clinical Microbiology, 3rd ed. Washington, D.C., American Society for Microbiology, 1980, p. 426.

Schleifer, K. H., and Nimmerman, E.: Peptidoglycan types of strains of the genus *Peptococcus*. Arch Microbiol 93:245, 1973.

Smith, L. D.: The pathogenic anaerobic bacteria, 2nd ed. Springfield, Il., Charles C Thomas, 1975.

Sutter, V. L., and Finegold, S. M.: Susceptibility of anerobic bacteria to 23 antimicrobial agents. Antimicrob Agents Chemother 10:736, 1976.

Switalski, L. M., Schwan, D., Smyth, C. J., et al.: Peptocoagulase: Clotting factor produced by bovine strains of *Peptococcus indolicus*. J Clin Microbiol 7:361, 1978.

Wells, C. L., and Field, C. R.: Long chain fatty acids of peptococci and peptostreptococci. J Clin Microbiol 4:515, 1976.

Wideman, P. A., Vargo, V. L., and Finegold, S. M.: Evaluation of the sodium polyanethol sulfonate disk test for the identification of *Peptostreptococcus anaerobius*. J Clin Microbiol 4:330, 1976.

Wilkins, T. D., Moore, W. E. C., et al.: *Peptococcus niger* (Hall) Kluyver and Van Niel 1936: Emendation of description and designation of neotype strain. Int J Syst Bacteriology 25:47, 1975.

Wong, M., Catena, A., Hadley, W. K.: Antigenic relationships and rapid identification of *Peptostreptococcus* species. J Clin Microbiol 11:515, 1980.

Wren, M. W. D.: Prolonged primary incubation in the isolation of anaerobic bacteria from clinical specimens. J Med Microbiol 13:257, 1980.

Yatabe, J. H., Baldwin, K. L., and Martin, W. J.: Isolation of an obligately anaerobic *Streptococcus pneumoniae* from blood culture. J Clin Microbiol 6:181, 1977.

48

ACTINOMYCES AND MICROAEROPHILIC ACTINOMYCETES

LEO PINE, PH.D.

Perhaps the earliest description of the actinomycotic organism was made by von Graefe (1854), who described fungal masses in granules taken from infections of the lacrimal canal. Cohn (1875) also observed a fine branching fungus in lacrimal concretions, which he named *Streptothrix foersteri*. In 1877, Bollinger published the first description of actinomycosis in cattle. This organism, resembling *Streptothrix*, was described in the tissues by Hartz (1879), who named it *Actinomyces bovis*. Israel described actinomycosis in man in 1878, and Ponfick (1880) compared human and bovine actinomycosis. Although Bujwid (1889) first isolated *Actinomyces* from human actinomycosis, it was the classic description of its morphology and physiology by Wolff and Israel (1891) that allowed later workers to identify and establish this organism as the cause of actinomycosis in man.

Silberschmidt first cultured the anaerobic actinomycete from lacrimal concretions; he compared the organisms isolated from maxillary actinomycosis of a cow, from human lacrimal concretions, and from maxillary and thoracic infections in man (Silberschmidt, 1901). Because all strains appeared identical, Silberschmidt concluded that *Streptothrix* was the correct name on the basis of taxonomic priority. Thus *Streptothrix* and names such as *Leptothrix*, *Cladothrix*, and *Leptotrichia* were used in early literature to refer to long filamentous or branching organisms. These names were used so commonly that some investigators no longer associated the *Streptothrix* or *Leptothrix* of lacrimal canaliculitis or of dental plaque with the *Actinomyces* of thoracic infections. To add to the confusion, Bostroem (1891) had earlier isolated aerobic forms of filamentous bacteria not only from human and bovine cases of actinomycosis but also from plant materials and soil. Although years later these aerobic forms were given the name *Streptomyces*, the generic name *Actinomyces* is still used today in certain countries to describe the aerobic nonpathogenic streptomycetes.

The source of the infections became apparent when Naeslund (1925) identified the bacterium as part of the normal flora of the mouth; Emmons (1935) later found *Actinomyces* in granules in tonsillar crypts. Although Erikson (1940) believed that human and bovine strains were sufficiently different to warrant separation as *Actinomyces israelii* and *Actinomyces bovis*, respectively, these species were not accepted by other workers until after World War II (Thompson, 1950; Pine et al., 1960). *A. naeslundii*, originally isolated from the mouth by Thompson and Lovestedt (1951) and Howell et al. (1959), was later found to be pathogenic for animals and man (Colemen et al., 1969).

Of great importance for taxonomy and for laboratory diagnosis was the observation that the pathogenic *Actinomyces* had no catalase, whereas coryneforms were catalase positive (Sutter, 1956). Analysis of fermentation products and cell wall composition helped delineate those actinomycetes that showed true branching or mycelial microcolonies (Cummins, 1962).

The 8th edition of *Bergey's Manual of Determinative Bacteriology* (1974) describes five genera in the family. Five species of *Actinomyces* are accepted and three others are described, but are of uncertain taxonomic status (Table 1). All species of *Actinomyces* were originally isolated from patients with actinomycosis, actinomycosis-like disease, periodontal plaque, or dental caries. The exception is *Actinomyces humiferus*, which was isolated from the soil and is nonpathogenic. Similarly, *Bacterionema matruchotii*, an oral commensal of animals, has not been associated with disease. A definitive discussion of these organisms appears in *Actinomyces, Filamentous Bacteria: Biology and Pathogenicity* (Slack and Gerencser, 1975). On the basis of a wide spectrum of characteristics, Holmberg and Nord (1975) and Schofield and Schaal (1981) have more completely defined the actinomycete species and separated them from related bacteria by using numerical taxonomy.

MORPHOLOGY. The species of bacteria in the families Actinomycetaceae and Propionibacteriaceae have gram-positive, straight or curved, branching, pleomorphic rod-like cells that are nonacid-fast, nonmotile, and nonspore-forming (Fig. 1). They are 0.2 to 0.3 μm in diameter and may vary from 0.4 to many μm in length. Cells are more branched and mycelial in early stages of growth and become fragmented, forming coccoidal and short tapered bacillary forms (diphtheroids) in the stationary phase of growth. Important differences in morphology occur (1) in infected tissues (2) in young liquid cultures, and (3) on agar plates within 24 to 72 hours (microcolonies) and after 3 to 14 days (macrocolonies).

All species that cause deep infections (except *Bifidobacterium adolescentis*) are seen in pus or infected tissues as long, nonbranching filaments or as complexes of loosely or tightly interwoven branching mycelial elements (Fig. 2). Masses of *B. adolescentis* with a morphology similar to that seen in culture have been found in human tissues. The Gram stain is the primary method for detecting actinomycetes in clinical material and for observing their morphology; however, actinomycetes may stain gram positively or negatively depending on their age and condition. Often the long hyphal elements stain gram positively only at intervals, so that they appear as masses of cocci or long chains of coccoidal elements that have been identified as streptococci (Fig. 2).

The various *Actinomyces* or *Arachnia* species form structures, called drusen, or sulfur granules or mycelial granules in tissues. Only traces of sulfur are present in sulfur granules, so the term probably derived from their yellow color in pus. *A. odontolyticus* does not invade the tissues and does not make granules. *B. adolescentis* does not form granules, although it does form compact masses of bacterial cells in human infections (Georg et al., 1965). Sulfur granules in pus or tissue are discrete yellow grains of hard consistency (Fig. 3). They are 40 to 400 μm in diameter and can be seen by naked eye, in surgical dressings.

When placed in a water or 5 per cent postassium hydroxide mounts and crushed between the coverslip and the glass slide, the mycelial and cellular elements can be seen with phase optics or Gram, methylene blue, periodic acid–Schiff, or silver methenamine stains. The sulfur granules have peripheral clubs that contain an internal mycelial

Table 1. TAXONOMIC RELATIONSHIPS OF FERMENTATIVE ACTINOMYCETES AND SIMILAR-FORM ORGANISMS ASSOCIATED WITH HUMAN OR ANINMAL DISEASE

Family[a]	Genus (Species)	Synonym	Disease	Habitat	Morphology in Disease Tissue	Cellular Morphology[c]	Pathogenicity in Laboratory Animals
Actinomycetaceae (microaerophilic, fermentative)	*Actinomyces*[b] *bovis, A. israelii, A. naeslundii, A. suis, A. viscosus, A. odontolyticus*	*Streptothrix, Cladothrix, Leptothrix, Actinobacterium*	Actinomycosis, lacrimal canaliculitis	Oral cavity, tonsillar crypts, dental plaque, calculus	Long branching mycelium or filamentous cells, sulfur granules, mycelial masses, streptococcal-like chains	Filaments, long rods, branching rods, clubs, small rods, diphtheroids	Pathogenic for mice and hamsters; forming limited or progressive abscesses in most animals when injected intraperitoneally
	Arachnia propionica	*Actinomyces propionicus*	Actinomycosis, lacrimal canaliculitis	Oral cavity, dental plaque, tonsillar crypts	Long threadlike filaments, sulfur granules; branching mycelial masses	Long branching rods, nonbranching filaments, coccoid bodies (spheroplasts)	Same as *Actinomyces*
	Bifidobacterium adolescentis[d]	*Actinomyces eriksonii*	Lung abscess, pleural fluid	Oral cavity, tonsils, intestinal tract	Small bifid rods; club-shapes; curved rods	Small singly branched rods, clubs, unbranched rods	Nonpathogenic; forms limited abscesses
	Bacterionema matruchotii	*Leptotrichia dentium, L. buccalis*	None	Dental plaque, calculus	None	Branching filaments, long filaments with terminal bacillary head	Nonpathogenic
	Rothia dentocariosa	*Nocardia salivae*	None	Dental plaque, calculus	Beaded filaments, short branching rods	Short or long branching rods, cocci, filaments	Nonpathogenic; forms limited abscesses
Propionibacteriaceae (microaerophilic, fermentative)	*Propionibacterium acnes*	*Corynebacterium acnes*	Skin abscess	Gingival plaque, skin abscesses, intestinal contents, lacrimal canal	"Diphtheroid" rods, curved rods, branched rods, irregular shapes	Diphtheroid rod-like cells	Forms limited abscesses when inoculated into mice subcutaneously or intraperitoneally
Nocardiaceae (aerobic, oxidative)	*Nocardia asteroides, N. brasiliensis, Actinomadura madurae, Actinomadura pelletiera*	*Streptothrix, Proactinomyces, Actinomyces, Streptomyces, Nocardia*	Maduromycosis	Soil	Long branching mycelial elements, granules	Nonsporulating fragmenting mycelium gives rise to rod-shaped and coccoidal elements	Pathogenic for laboratory animals depending on route of inoculation and species
Streptomycetaceae (aerobic, oxidative)	*Streptomyces somaliensis, S. paraguayensis*	*Actinomyces*	Maduromycosis	Soil	Long branching mycelial elements, granules	Nonfragmenting surface mycelium; may form chains of spores	May cause limited progressive abscesses with intraperitoneal inoculation

[a]Based primarily on the data in Bergey's Manual of Determinative Bacteriology (Buchanan and Gibbons, 1974) and Slack and Gerencser (1975). *Actinomyces humiferus*, not listed above, is isolated from the soil and is not pathogenic.
[b]*A. odontolyticus* is nonpathogenic.
[c]Grown for 24 to 72 hours in semisolid thioglycolate or Trypticase Soy Broth.
[d]Mitsuoka et al. (1974).

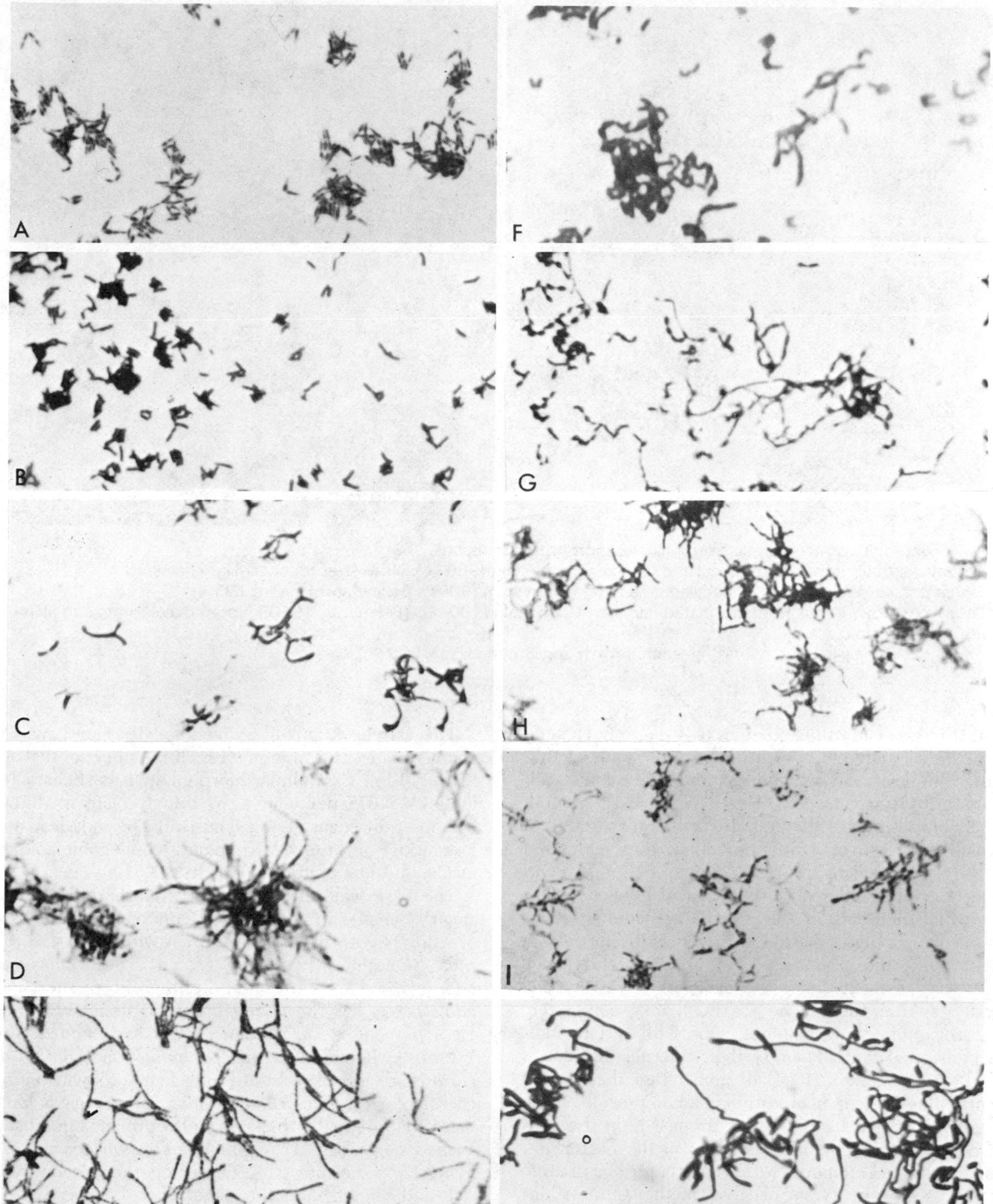

Figure 1. Cellular morphology of *Actinomyces* species grown in thioglycollate broth, Gram stain, (1200 ×) (Mycology Division, Centers for Disease Control, Atlanta, Georgia). (A) *Actinomyces bovis,* (B) *A. odontolyticus,* (C) *Bifidobacterium adolescentis (A. eriksonii),* (D) *A. naeslundii,* (E) *A. israelii,* (F) *A. israelii,* (G) *Arachnia propionica,* (H) *Propionibacterium acnes,* (I) *Rothia dentocariosa,* (J) *Bacterionema matruchotii.* Most species exhibit the range of cellular morphologies seen in Figure 2. However, the long filamentous form terminating in a bacillary head is characteristic only of *Bacterionema matruchotti* (J), whereas the bifid branching of *B. adolescentis* (C) is characteristic of the genus *Bifidobacterium.* Within the remaining species, short cells, often in pairs as V forms (A, F, and G) to long filamentous branching cells are often seen (E and F). The morphology of *P. acnes* cannot be distinguished from that of the *Actinomyces* species.

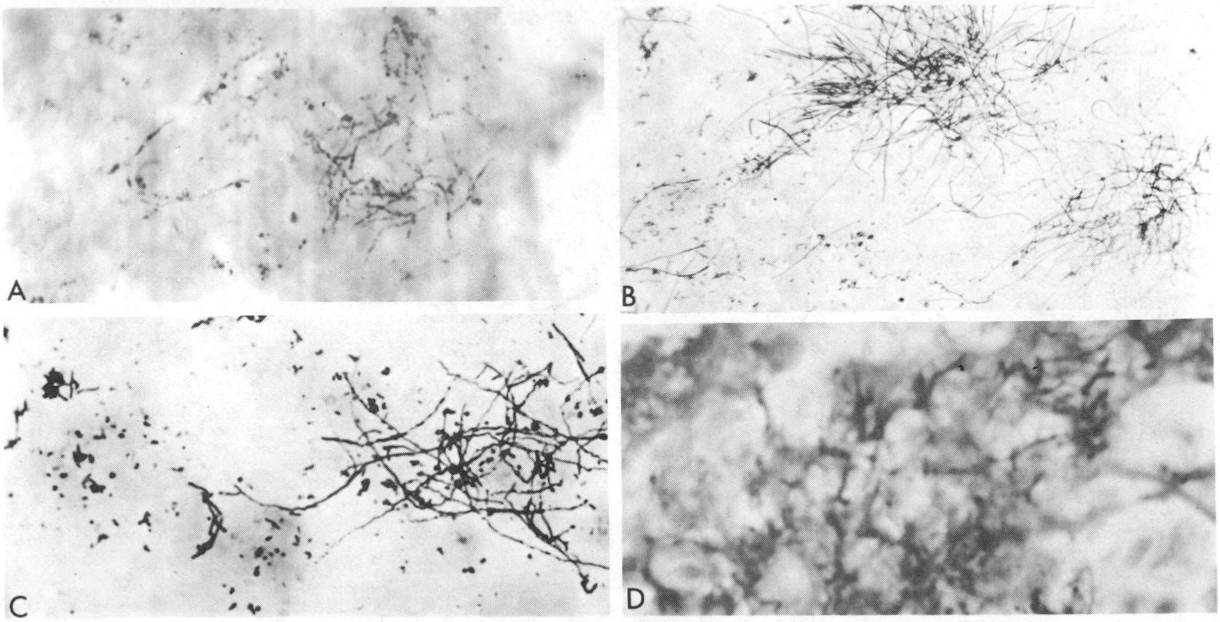

Figure 2. Morphologic aspects of microaerophilic actinomycetes in tissues.
A. *Actinomyces bovis* in pus from inoculated hamster. Gram stain (900 ×). Note streptococcal-like chains.
B. *Arachnia propionica* in pus from inoculated hamster. Gram stain (900 ×). (Pine and Hardin, 1959.)
C. Actinomyces *bovis* in pus from inoculated hamster. Gram stain (900 ×). (Pine et al., 1960.) Note coccal forms and filamentous forms without branching.
D. *Actinomyces israelii* in lung, human infection. Brown and Brenn stain (1000 ×).

filament (Fig. 4). The sulfur granules of *A. bovis* have been analyzed by a combination of histochemical stains of thin sections, chemical analyses, and electron microscope studies (Pine and Overman, 1963, 1966). Whereas the overall chemical composition of the granules was similar to that of the organism grown on culture medium, they contained some 40 to 60 per cent $Ca_3(PO_4)_2$. Some of the $Ca_3(PO_4)_2$ was poorly crystallized apatite (Frazier and Fowler, 1967). The mycelial elements of the granule are cemented together by mucopolysaccharide with the clubs forming a rosette around the periphery (Fig. 3). The clubs may measure from 3 to 20 times the diameter of the hyphae embedded within them. The $Ca_3(PO_4)_2$ may completely saturate the embedding material, simply fill certain individual cells, or form a layer at their internal periphery. Coupled with Wright's (1905) demonstration that typical sulfur granules develop in cultures containing serum, these findings suggest that $Ca_3(PO_4)_2$ deposition within the cells is caused by the biochemical activities of the bacterium. The normal hyphal elements within the center of a granule are readily seen with Gram or silver methenamine stains (Fig. 4). However, heavily calcified granules or clubs do not stain intensely, and clear observation of the cellular elements that are either within the club or embedded in the granule requires extraction of the granule with trichloracetic acid or other chemical treatment (Fig. 4).

Although sulfur granules strongly suggest *Actinomyces* infection, *Staphylococcus*, *Nocardia*, *Streptomyces*, and *Actinobacillus lignieresii* may also form "granules."

Morphology of strains even within the same species may vary greatly. In one medium a strain may be rod-shaped, and in another it may be longer, branched, or even a coccus. Similarly, morphology may change radically with various phases of growth and depleted medium.

The various strains of a given species may have cellular characteristics in common with all members of that species (Fig. 1; Table 2). Cellular morphology is best characterized in fluid (0.075 per cent agar) thioglycolate medium with 0.1 per cent sugar. Long incubation periods lead to fragmentation of branched hyphae, conversion to atypical forms, and loss of gram-positivity.

The basic cell shapes are: (1) diphtheroids, which are small branched or unbranched comma-shaped cells or V- or Y-forms with two or three cells connected, and (2) long rods, sometimes branching (Table 2). *A. bovis* and *A. odontolyticus* are most often diphtheroids or short rods. *B. adolescentis* has the characteristic Y-branched form (Fig. 1). *A. israelii*, *A. naeslundii*, *A. viscosus*, and *A. suis* are V-forms, whereas *Arachnia propionica* and *Rothia dentocariosa* are mixed rods and long filaments with numerous coccoid forms. *Bacterionema matruchotii* has a long filament that gradually thickens and terminates in a bacillary-shaped body (Fig. 1). *Propionibacterium acnes* and *Actinomyces* species are often found together in clinical materials and cannot be distinguished morphologically.

Colonial morphology is best seen on agar plates at 24 to 48 hours by transmitted light. Young colonies have two forms (Fig. 5): (1) small mycelial colonies, and (2) smooth streptococcal-like colonies without true filaments. In general, microcolonies of *A. bovis* are small, circular, translucent or opaque, and have an entire edge with a smooth or granular surface. They cannot be distinguished from similar colonies of *Streptococcus pyogenes* (Fig. 5D). Although colonies of *A. odontolyticus* and *B. adolescentis* closely resemble those of *A. bovis* described above, some isolates of *A. bovis* are petite mycelial microcolonies (Fig. 5). No mycelial colonies have been reported for *A. odontolyticus* or *B. adolescentis*. Mycelial-like colonies may be formed

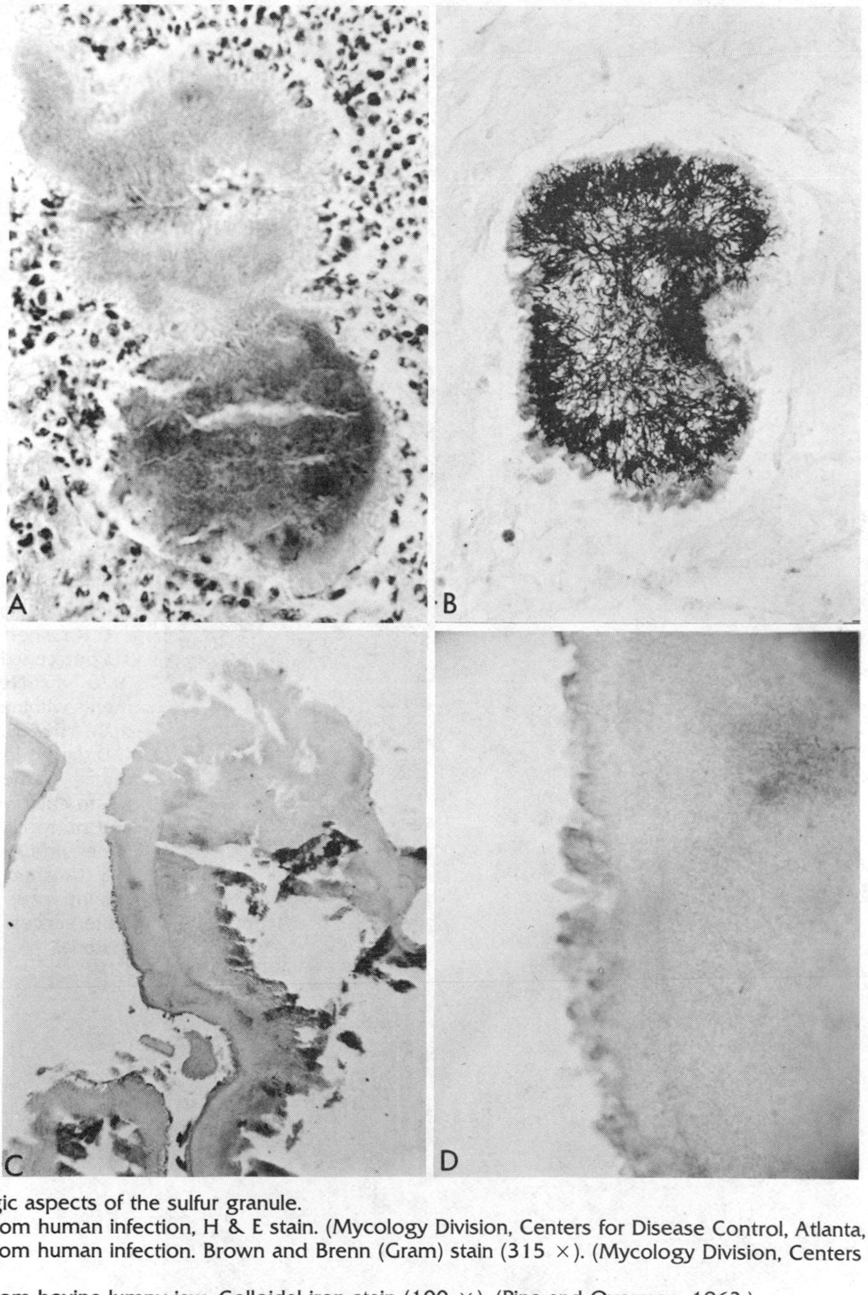

Figure 3. Morphologic aspects of the sulfur granule.

A. Sulfur granule from human infection, H & E stain. (Mycology Division, Centers for Disease Control, Atlanta, Ga.)

B. Sulfur granule from human infection. Brown and Brenn (Gram) stain (315 ×). (Mycology Division, Centers for Disease Control, Atlanta, Ga.)

C. Sulfur granule from bovine lumpy jaw. Colloidal iron stain (100 ×). (Pine and Overman, 1963.)

D. As C above (800 ×) showing peripheral arrangement of clubs.

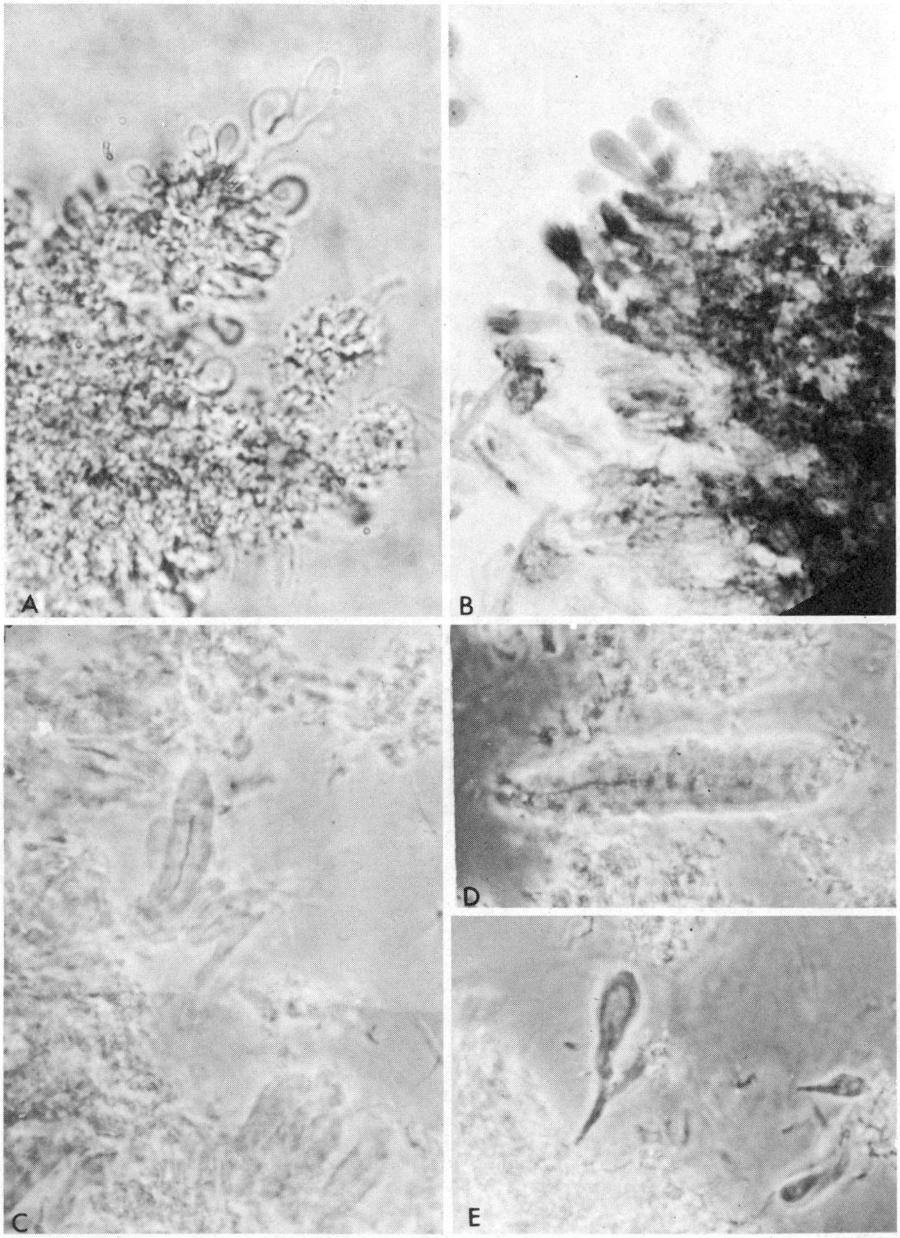

Figure 4. Sulfur granule—structure of clubs.

A. Crushed granule mounted in 10 per cent KOH showing multibranched hyaline clubs (970 ×).

B. Periodic acid-Schiff stain of sectioned granule (970 ×). Note hyaline nature of clubs and absence of clearly defined mycelium.

C. Crushed granule, digested in 10 per cent KOH; phase contrast, (970 ×). Note presence of filaments within clubs. (Pine and Overman, 1966.)

D. Large intact club showing internal filament after successive treatments with trichloracetic acid and proteolytic enzymes (970 ×). (Pine and Overman, 1963.)

E. Crushed granule, lactophenol mount; phase contrast (970 ×). Note successive layers of capsular material.

Table 2. MORPHOLOGIC ASPECTS OF THE MICROAEROPHILIC ACTINOMYCETES

Species	Morphology in Pus or Infected Tissue	Sulfur Granules	Cellular and Colony Morphology in Culture: Liquid Medium[a]	Solid Medium[b]: Microcolony	Solid Medium[b]: Macrocolony
Bifidobacterium adolescentis	Short filaments	None	Short rods, branched V and Y shape	Smooth glistening entire edge, no mycelium	Large, shiny convex colonies; circular or irregular; surface smooth or granular
Actinomyces odontolyticus	None	None	Diphtheroid, very short, pleomorphic	Smooth circular granular colonies, no mycelium	Large, circular, glistening, white, opaque colonies; red colonies on blood
A. bovis	Long filaments, branching mycelium	Typical sulfur granules, clubs calcified	Short (rarely long) branching rods	Round steptococcal-like, smooth glistening colony, no mycelium or small compact mycelium	Colonies of a wide range of morphology (see Figs. 6 and 7); white to yellow; generally adherent to agar; roughly circular with smooth, granular, raspberry or molar tooth morphology
A. suis	Long filaments, branching mycelium	Typical sulfur granules, clubs	Short branching rods	Like *A. bovis*	As above
A. israelii	Long filaments, branching mycelium	Typical sulfur granules, clubs calcified	Long branching rods	Large mycelial colonies, spider colonies	As above
A. naeslundii	Long filaments, branching mycelium	Granules, no clubs reported	Short to long branching rods	Mycelial colonies with dense centers	As above
A. viscosus	Filamentous, coccoidal	Granules, no clubs reported	Short branching rods	Like *A. bovis*	As above
Arachnia propionica	Long filaments, branching mycelium, short rods, coccoidal	Typical sulfur granules, clubs	Short branching rods, coccoidal cells, long unbranched filaments	Mycelial colonies, spider colonies	As above
Rothia dentocariosa	None	None	Short to long branched filaments, coccoidal forms	Diffuse mycelial colonies, branching filaments	As above
Bacterionema matruchotii	None	None	Long filaments with bacillary or club-shaped terminal ends, short rods	Small diffuse clumps of branching filamentous cells	As above
Propionibacterium acnes	None	None	Short pleomorphic rods, resembles *Actinomyces*	Smooth on entire edges, glistening colony, streptococcal or micrococcal-like	Small, circular, white to pink colonies

[a]Thioglycolate medium, 10 ml per tube.
[b]Brain Heart Infusion agar, incubated anaerobically or under microaerophilic conditions.

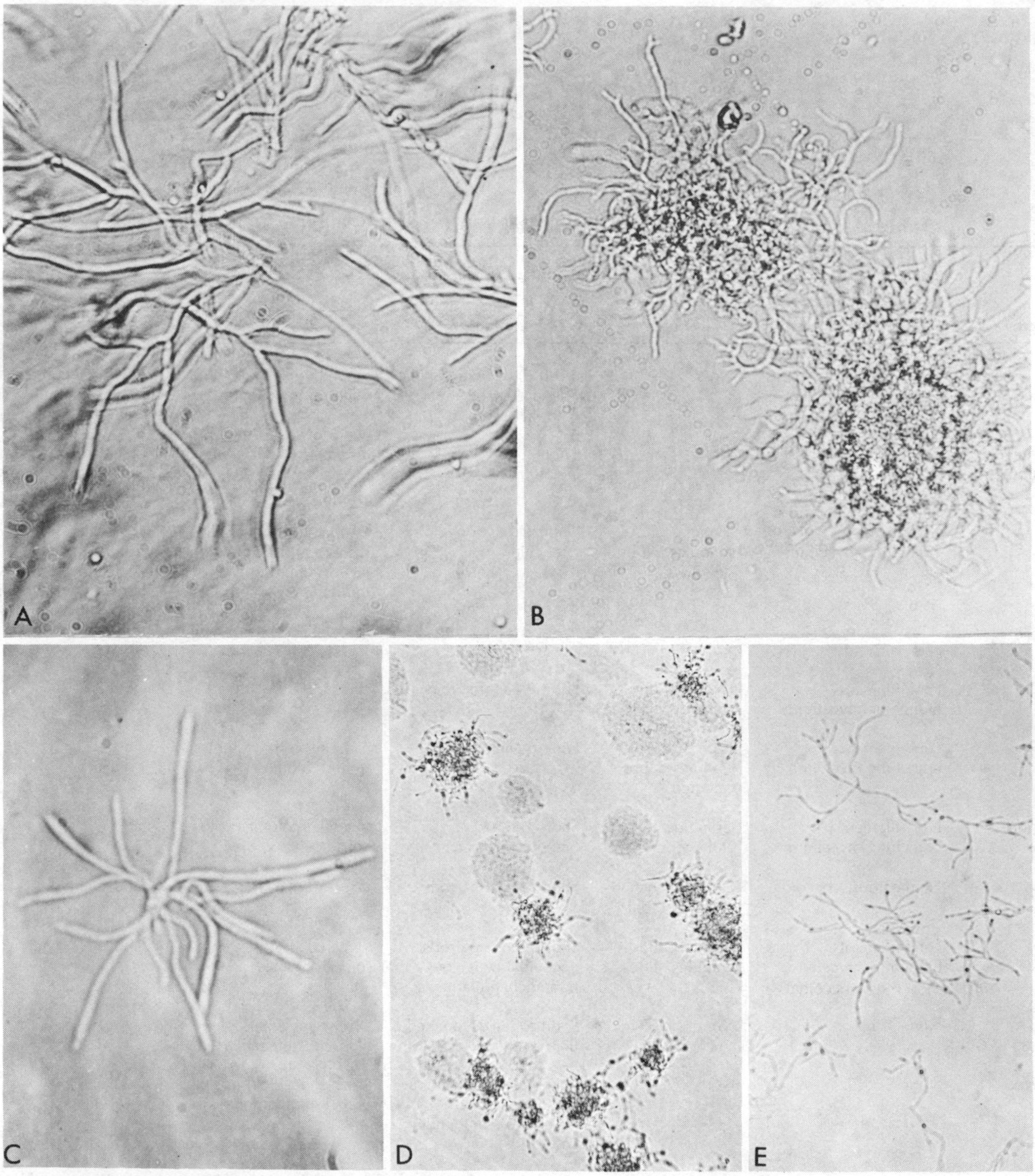

Figure 5. Microcolonies of the microaerophilic actinomycetes.

A. *Actinomyces israelii* (Howell et al., 1959). The diffuse branching colony is characteristic of the species.

B. *A. naeslundii* (Howell et al., 1959). The tightly interwoven compact mycelium of the central portion of the colony is characteristic of this species.

C. *A. viscosis* (Howell, 1963).

D. *A. bovis* (Pine et al., 1960). Spider-like and smooth circular colonies isolated from the same case of bovine lumpy jaw. Transmitted light (290 ×).

E. *Arachnia propionica* (Buchanan and Pine, 1962). Web-like mycelial colonies (430 ×).

by *Propionibacterium* species, although *P. acnes* forms only a smooth circular colony like that of *A. bovis*.

After incubation for three to seven days the microcolonies of the Actinomycetaceae develop into 1- to 3-mm diameter macrocolonies, which are described as raspberry, molar tooth, or rough colonies. The forms vary considerably (Figs. 6 and 7) with no one morphologic pattern specific for a given species. Furthermore, the smooth and matt strains of *Streptococcus pyogenes* may be confused with the macrocolonies formed by *Actinomyces* and *Arachnia* species (Fig. 6). Thus features of cellular or colonial morphology in tissues or in media that suggest *Actinomyces* or *Arachnia* may instead indicate the genera *Streptococcus, Propionibacterium, Nocardia,* and *Streptomyces* (Table 2).

ANTIGENIC STRUCTURE. *Actinomyces* antigens prepared from formalized whole cells, cell walls, soluble semipurified cell walls, or culture supernate precipitates have been used for taxonomy and serotyping (Bowden and Hardie, 1973). Also, formalized whole cells have been used to prepare hyperimmune fluorescein-tagged rabbit serum which effectively demonstrates actinomyces in infected tissue, human saliva, and dental plaque. Because of cross-reactions with sera from streptococcal infections, nocardiosis, and tuberculosis (Holm and Kwapinski, 1959; Georg et al., 1968), no satisfactory complement fixation, immunodiffusion, or hemagglutination test has been developed.

Species have been differentiated mainly by immunodiffusion, whole cell or cell wall agglutination, and fluorescent antibody staining of whole cells. Agar gel immunodiffusion has used soluble antigens either precipitated from the culture supernate by acetone or extracted from whole cells with formamide and trichloracetic acid. The protein associated with carbohydrate seems to be the serologically reactive component. Identification of species by agar gel immunodiffusion has not been entirely successful. Brock and Georg (1969) clearly separated *A. naeslundii* and *A. israelii* by agar gel diffusion, and Cummins (1968) distinguished the two serotypes of *A. israelii* using trichloracetic acid–acetone precipitated antigens from strains of *A. israelii*. These serotypes were confirmed with fluorescent antibody (Brock and Georg, 1969).

Chemical differentiation of purified cell walls (Cummins and Harris, 1958) combined with the use of whole cells for cell wall agglutination studies (Cummins, 1962) provided a definitive basis for species identification. What was once an extremely complex heterogeneous mixture of overlapping morphologic and physiologic groups was now organized primarily on the basis of a definitive chemical cell wall composition (Table 3). After delineation of these groups, their serologic relationships became clear.

The fluorescent antibody technique, which became the most fruitful and least complex serologic procedure for identifying species and serotypes, was first used by Slack (1966) to identify *A. israelii* from two patients with actinomycosis. The technique, tested with pure cultures and specific sera, has led to separations and identifications of species that correlate with those determined by other means. Nevertheless, cross-reactions occur like those between sera specific for the species *A. israelii, A. naeslundii,* and *A. viscosus* (Slack and Gerencser, 1975). All *Actinomyces* species and *Ar. propionica* have had two serotypes described; the exceptions are *A. naeslundii*, which has one, and *R. dentocariosa*, which has four or more.

Based upon the use of soluble HCl, TCA, urea, or sonic extracts, Holmberg, Nord, and Wadstrom (1975) developed a crossed immunoelectrophoresis test that they applied to the sera of nine actinomycosis patients. All sera formed precipitin lines with one or more of 10 protein or glycoprotein antigens from *A. israelii*, whereas sera from cases of tuberculosis, nocardiosis, *Candida* infection, and aspergillosis, or from normal humans did not react.

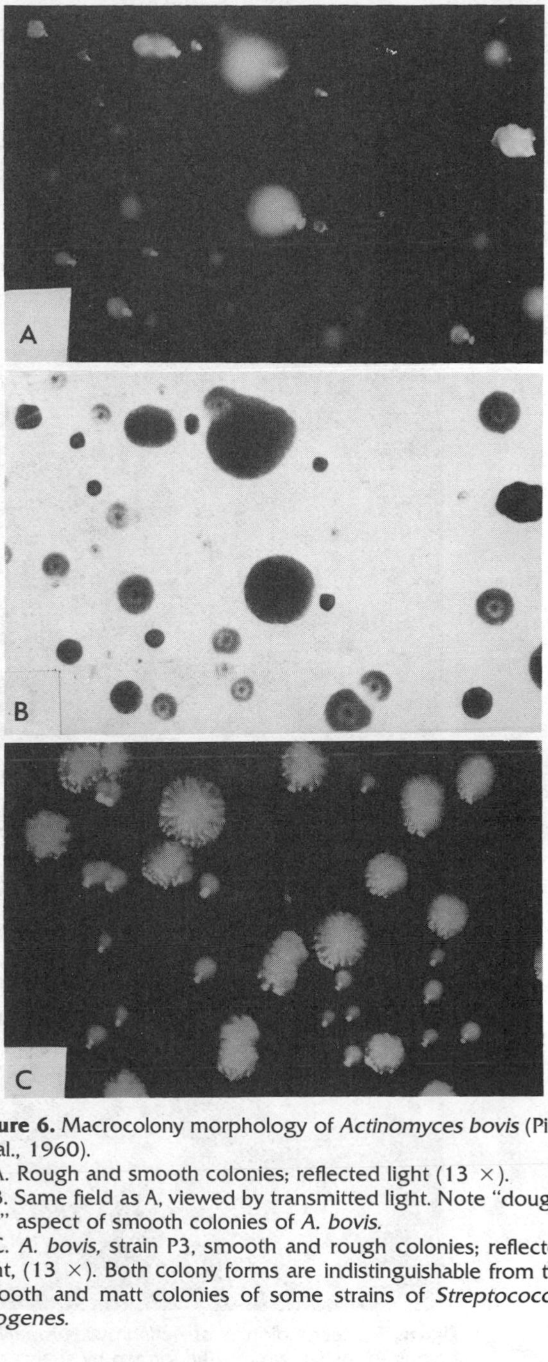

Figure 6. Macrocolony morphology of *Actinomyces bovis* (Pine et al., 1960).

A. Rough and smooth colonies; reflected light (13 ×).

B. Same field as A, viewed by transmitted light. Note "doughnut" aspect of smooth colonies of *A. bovis*.

C. *A. bovis*, strain P3, smooth and rough colonies; reflected light, (13 ×). Both colony forms are indistinguishable from the smooth and matt colonies of some strains of *Streptococcus pyogenes*.

METABOLISM. All of the Actinomycetaceae are fermentative, and their substrates are largely converted to volatile and nonvolatile acids in anaerobic, microaerophilic, or strongly aerobic conditions. Alcohols are not formed. The fermentative actinomycetes do not contain a sequence of cytochromes to oxidize the substrate for utilizable energy. A carbohydrate energy source such as sugar, alcohol,

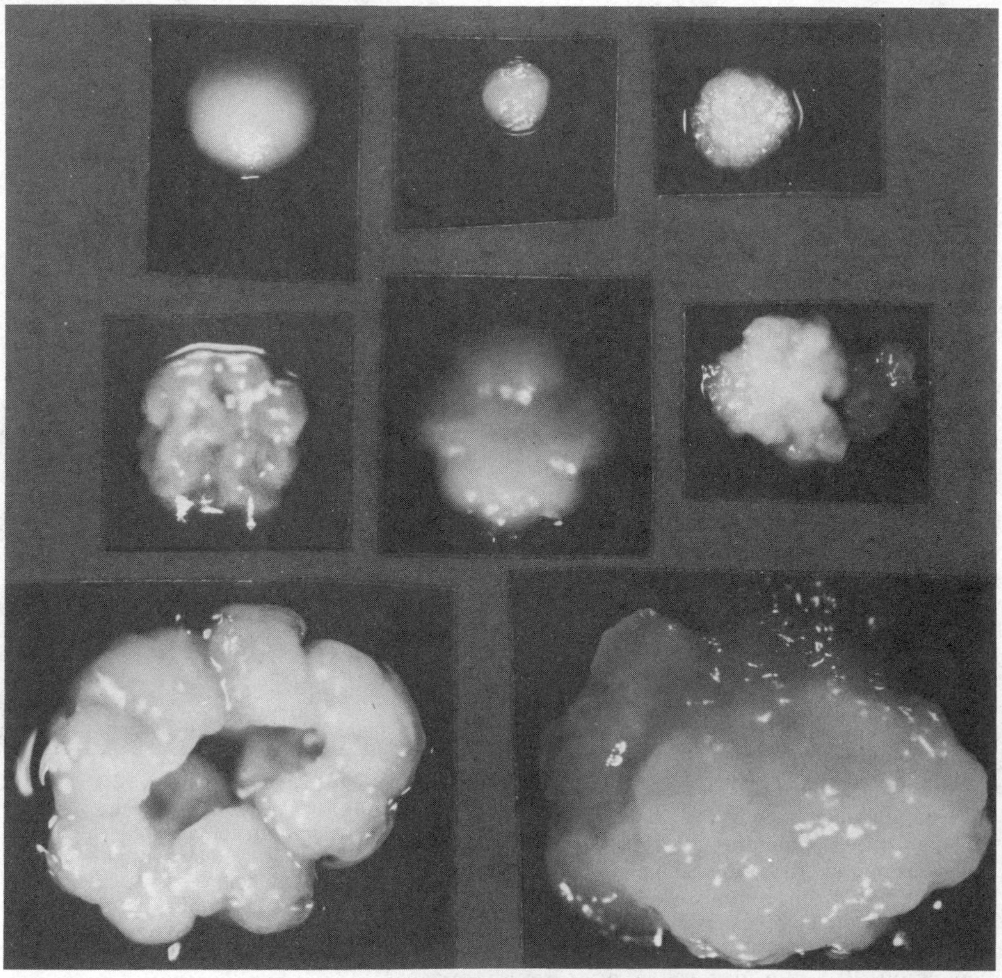

Figure 7. Macrocolonies of *Actinomyces israelii*; reflected light (23 ×) (Howell et al., 1959). The diverse colony forms shown may be formed by strains of all the species of *Actinomyces* and *Arachnia*.

Table 3. CELL-WALL COMPOSITION OF THE PATHOGENIC *ACTINOMYCES* AND RELATED SPECIES[a]

	Amino Acids[b]															
	Aspartic Acid	Lysine	Ornithine	Glycine	LL Diaminopimelic Acid	DL Diaminopimelic Acid	Galactose	Glucose	Mannose	Rhamnose	Deoxyhexose	Deoxytalose	Fucose	Arabinose
Actinomyces														
A. bovis ATCC13683	+	+	−	−	−	−	−	+	+	+	+	+	+	−
A. bovis P2R	−	+	−	−	−	−	−	+	+	+	+	+	+	−
A. humiferus	+	+	+	−	−	−	−	−	−	+	−	−	−	−
A. odontolyticus	−	+	+	−	−	−	+	+	+	−	−	−	−	−
A. suis	−	+	+	−	−	−	−	−	−	+	−	−	−	−
A. israelii/1	−	+	+	−	−	−	+	−	−	−	−	−	−	−
A. israelii/2	−	+	+	−	−	−	+	−	−	+	−	−	−	−
A. naeslundii	−	+	+	−	−	−	−	+	+	+	+	+	−	−
A. viscosus/1	−	+	+	−	−	−	+	+	−	+	+	+	−	−
A. viscosus/2	−	+	+	−	−	−	+	+	−	+	+	+	−	−
Bifidobacterium adolescentis	+	+	+	−	−	−	+	+	−	−	−	−	−	−
Rothia dentocariosa	−	+	−	−	−	−	+	−	−	−	−	−	−	−
Bacterionema matruchotii	−	−	−	+	−	+	+	+	−	−	−	−	−	+
Arachnia														
A. propionica/1	−	−	−	+	+	−	−	+	−	−	−	−	−	−
A. propionica/2	−	−	−	+	+	−	+	+	−	−	−	−	−	−
Propionibacterium														
P. acnes/1	−	−	−	+	+	−	+	+	±	−	−	−	−	−
P. acnes/2	−	−	−	+	+	−	−	+	±	−	−	−	−	−

[a]Based on data and references in Cummins (1968), Johnson and Cummins (1972), Schleifer and Kandler (1972), Pine (1973), and Cummins (personal communication).
[b]All strains have alanine and glutamic acid.

pentose, hexose, di- or trisaccharide, or starch is required for growth, but amino acids or proteins are not used. In contrast with this family, which accumulates acids in the medium, strictly aerobic genera such as *Mycobacterium*, *Nocardia*, *Actinomadura*, and *Streptomyces* oxidize their substrates mainly to carbon dioxide and water; in addition, these genera may also use amino acids and proteins for growth once the carbohydrate is completely metabolized.

Within the family Actinomycetaceae, the fermentations of glucose are best described as homolactic, heterolactic, or propionic acid (Pine, 1970). All species of *Actinomyces* are homolactic acid organisms because, given the correct conditions of growth and medium, they will ferment glucose primarily to lactic acid. Therefore, they have fructose diphosphate aldolase and use primarily the Embden-Meyerhof glycolytic scheme for catabolizing sugar. However, under anaerobic conditions when CO_2 is present, all species form acetic, lactic, and succinic acids, and traces of formic acid (Table 4). Some species use large amounts of CO_2 to synthesize succinic acid and form aspartic acid internally. Since these carbon dioxide–fixing strains lack a permease for the uptake of aspartic acid (Buchanan and Pine, 1965), CO_2 is a factor required for growth. But once growth is initiated, some members of the genus can grow aerobically, converting glucose primarily to acetic acid and CO_2.

The genus *Bifidobacterium*, however, has no fructose diphosphate aldolase or glucose-6-phosphate dehydrogenase, and glucose is degraded by the fructose-6-phosphate shunt to acetic and lactic acids. Since two moles of lactic acid cannot be formed from one mole of glucose, this fermentation is heterolactic. Acetate and lactate are formed in molar ratios approximating 3:2; only traces of other products such as formic or succinic acid are formed.

Although they contain fructose diphosphate aldolase, the species of the third group (*Ar. propionica* and *B. matruchotii*) ferment glucose to form propionic and acetic acids as the major products. Small amounts of lactic and succinic acids with considerable amounts of CO_2 are also formed in the anaerobic fermentation within the family in which CO_2 is a major product. Although the fermentations resemble those of the propionobacteria, they can differ in the quantities of products formed.

There is an excellent correlation of the cell wall mucopeptide components to the fermentation. All *Actinomyces* species except *A. bovis* have lysine, ornithine, and glutamic acid in their cell walls in a ratio of 1:1:2, and all ferment glucose homolactically. However, in *B. adolescentis* (*A. eriksonii*) ornithine or lysine occurs in a ratio of 1:1 with glutamic acid replacing one or the other within the peptide subunit (Schleifer and Kandler, 1972). The propionic acid–forming species, however, have diaminopimelic acid instead of lysine or ornithine as the dibasic component of the cell wall. These relationships of fermentation to cell wall composition are summarized in Table 4.

The identifying physiologic characteristics of the species of Actinomycetaceae are listed in Table 5. All organisms are anaerobic or facultatively anaerobic; the latter can grow in oxygen when growth is initiated with larger inocula. Carbon dioxide stimulates growth and increases the fermentation products of glucose from only lactic acid to volatile and nonvolatile acids that are more characteristic of the species. Under strongly aerobic conditions, certain species ferment glucose to acetate and the cell yields under these conditions are doubled, indicating that the use of oxygen is energy yielding and linked to growth. *Ar. propionica*, *B. matruchotii*, *A. viscosus*, and *R. dentocariosa* are aerobic or facultatively aerobic and may not require CO_2 to initiate growth. In general, CO_2 improves primary

Table 4. FERMENTATIVE CHARACTERISTICS DIFFERENTIATING GENERA OF *ACTINOMYCETACEAE* AND *PROPIONIBACTERIUM*

Genus	Oxygen Relationship	Cell-Wall Mucopeptide[a]	Fermen-tation	Major Acids Formed from Glucose	
				Anaerobic	*Aerobic*
Actinomyces	Anaerobe, facultative anaerobe	Lysine, ornithine, glutamic acid (1:1:2)	Homolactic	(Formic), acetic, lactic, succinic	CO_2, acetic
Rothia	Aerobe	Lysine	Homolactic	Lactic	Acetic, lactic
Bifidobacterium	Anaerobe	Alanine, lysine (ornithine): glutamic acid (1:1)	Heterolactic	Acetic, lactic	No growth
Arachnia	Facultative anaerobe	Glycine, alanine, glutamic acid (2:1:1) plus LL diaminopimelic acid	Propionic	CO_2, acetic, propionic, lactic, succinic	CO_2, acetic
Propionibacterium	Anaerobe	Glycine, alanine, glutamic acid (1:2:1) plus LL diaminopimelic acid	Propionic	CO_2 acetic, propionic (lactic, succinic)	CO_2, acetic
Bacterionemia	Aerobic, facultative anaerobe	Glycine, DL diaminopimelic acid	Propionic	CO_2, propionic, lactic	CO_2, acetic, propionic

[a]Data based on Schleifer and Kandler (1972).

isolation from small numbers of cells whether incubation is anaerobic or aerobic.

Although numerous primary colonies of species defined as aerobic may grow on isolation plates incubated anaerobically, they cannot be transferred under anaerobic conditions. Conversely, particularly when the inoculum is heavy, anaerobic species may sometimes grow under aerobic conditions. On occasion microcolonies of even the aerobic *Nocardia asteroides* may grow on primary isolation plates incubated anaerobically. These results suggest that for primary isolation of an actinomycete, both aerobic and anaerobic isolations should be made in CO_2.

The definition of a species as aerobic is strongly supported by the presence of catalase or of cytochromes, as shown by the benzidine test. *R. dentocariosa* is aerobic and catalase-positive. *P. acnes* and *A. viscosus* are anaerobic and facultatively anaerobic respectively, but both have catalase. This distinguishes them from all other facultative or anaerobic species within the family Actinomycetaceae.

The growth requirements of this family of organisms are complex and resemble those of lactobacilli and streptococci. A few strains of *A. israelii* require cysteine, glutamic acid, lysine, leucine, isoleucine, and tryptophan.

Of the characteristics in Table 5, acid is formed by certain strains, listed as acid-negative, only after incubation of 14 days or more. The results in Table 5 should be apparent within seven or eight days. Thus, hydrolysis of starch by *A. bovis* and *B. adolescentis* is rapidly apparent. Although a few strains of *Ar. propionica* may ferment glycerol or lactic acid after prolonged incubation, they do so less readily than *P. acnes* or other propionibacteria. Gelatin liquefaction or casein hydrolysis differentiates *P. acnes* and *A. humiferus* from all other species. Catalase production may require a short period of aerobic induction. A major source of confusion in diagnosis of actinomycosis is *P. acnes*, because it is often a contaminant. However, *P. acnes* can be differentiated from other species by its catalase and gelatin liquefaction.

PATHOGENIC PROPERTIES. *A. humiferus*, which was isolated from soil, is the only *Actinomyces* species that is not resident in the animal body. *A. bovis* has been isolated only from cows and *A. suis* only from pigs, primarily as a cause of mammary actinomycosis. In bovine and swine actinomycosis, both species appear to inhabit the oral cavity of their host as do the other species in this genus. *A. israelii* is the major cause of actinomycosis in man; although actinomycosis has been reported in dogs, deer, and other animals, species identification has been minimal. *A. israelii* causes lacrimal canaliculitis, which is not true actinomycosis because deep tissues are not penetrated. In this infection, large mycelial masses of the organism block the lacrimal canal and may erode the surface membrane without invading the underlying tissues. *Ar. propionica* also shares these characteristics with *A. israelii*. Typical actinomycosis, i.e., progressive chronic inflammatory disease, suppuration, and sinus and sulfur granule formation, is rarely caused by the other species of the family (Table 6).

Transmission of these diseases from man to man or animal to animal is unknown except after a human or animal bite; this mode of transmission is suspected in cases of swine actinomycosis. Bovine actinomycosis is attributed to injury of tissues surrounding the mandible during the chewing of roughage by the cow. In lacrimal canaliculitis the organisms are assumed to spread from the mouth or nasopharynx to the lacrimal duct by a stifled sneeze or by transfer of saliva to the eye from which it drains into the lacrimal canal. There is no evidence that *Actinomyces* normally inhabits the lacrimal canal. All other cases of actinomycosis are attributed to the direct introduction of the organism from its normal habitat in the mouth into the deeper tissues or bloodstream by physical injury. Thus, tooth extraction or dental surgery may be followed by actinomycosis of the jaw. Appendectomy, cholecystectomy, or other operations were the major factors preceding actinomycosis in most patients reported by Brown (1973). Disseminated infections are best explained by spread of the organism from the mouth or bowel into the bloodstream.

Table 5. PHYSIOLOGIC CHARACTERISTICS OF SPECIES OF *ACTINOMYCETACEAE* AND *PROPIONIBACTERIUM ACNES*[a]

Organism	Catalase	Nitrate Reduced	Nitrite Reduced	Casein and Gelatin Hydrolysis	Starch Hydrolysis	Glucose	Starch	Mannitol	Xylose	Arabinose	Glycerol	Oxygen Required	CO_2 Required	%G + C Composition of DNA
Actinomyces														
A. humiferus	−	−	−	+	+	A	A	A	A	A	A(−)	Ae	−	73 −
A. bovis	−	−	nr	−	+	A	A	−	−(A)	−	−	An	+	57–63
A. suis	−	nr	nr	−	+	A	A	A(−)	nr	A(−)	−(A)	An	+	nr
A. odontolyticus	−	+(−)	−	−	−	A	−	−	A	−(A)	(A)	Fac An	+	62
A. israelii	−	+(−)	−	−	−	A	−	A	A	A−	−	An	+	57–60
A. naeslundii	−	+	−	−	−	A	−	−	−	−	A,−	FacAn	+	63–64
A. viscosus	+	+	+−	−	+	A	A−	−	−	A−	A,−	FacAn	+	63–70
Rothia dentocariosa	+	+	+	−	−	A	−	−	−	−	A,−	FacAn	+	63–70
Bifidobacterium adolescentis	−	−	−	−	+	A	A	A	A	A	−	An	−	62
Arachnia propionica	−	+	nr	−	−	A	−	A	−	−	−(A)	FacAn	−	63–65
Bacterionema matruchotii	+−	+	+	−	+(−)	A	nr	−	−	−	−	Ae	−	50–56
Propionibacterium acnes	+	+	nr	+	−	A	−	A(−)	−	−	A(−)	An	−	57–60

[a]+, positive reaction; −, negative reaction; +−, positive and negative reactions among strains; A, acid formed but no gas; nr, not reported; Ae, aerobic; An, anaerobic; FacAn, facultative anaerobe; ( ), occurs in a few strains.

Data compiled from Pine (1973), and Slack and Gerencser (1975).

Table 6. PATHOGENICITY OF MICROAEROPHILIC ACTINOMYCETES IN MAN AND EXPERIMENTAL ANIMALS

Organism	Natural Infection: Number of Cases and Characteristics in Man	Experimental Infection: Animal	Lesions	Abscesses Formed with Mycelium, Sulfur Granules[h]
Actinomyces				
A. bovis	None	Hamster, mouse	Progressive	6/10
A. israelii	Numerous cases[a] (true actinomycosis)	Hamster, mouse	Progressive	52/66 341/397
A. naeslundii	Three cases[b] (atypical actinomycosis)	Mouse	Progressive	111/129
A. odontolyticus	One case[a] (atypical actinomycosis)	Mouse	Regressive	6/68
A. viscosus	One case[d] (atypical)	Mouse	Progressive	23/24
Arachnia propionica	Numerous cases[e] (true actinomycosis)	Mouse	Progressive	28/28
Bifidobacterium adolescentis	Several cases[f] (abscess formation)	Mouse	Regressive	34/49
Rothia dentocariosa	One case[g]	Mouse	Regressive	0/32
Bacterionema matruchoti	None	Hamster	Regressive	0/6

[a]Brown, J. R. (1973); Bowden and Hardie (1973).
[b]Coleman et al. (1969).
[c]Morris and Kilbourn (1974).
[d]Adeniyi-Jones et al. (1973).
[e]Slack and Gerencser (1975).
[f]Georg et al. (1965).
[g]Sharfen, J.: Zentralbl Bakterial [Orig A] 233:80, 1975.
[h]Data taken in part from Slack and Gerencser (1975); Animals positive/animals inoculated.

Data partially compiled from Table 11–3 in Slack and Gerencser (1975).

Of the species examined for pathogenicity (Table 6), *A. israelii*, *A. naeslundii*, *A. viscosus*, and *Ar. propionica* were equally effective in causing actinomycotic lesions in mice. These usually produced progressive lesions with mycelial filaments, mycelial clumps, and occasionally sulfur granules, unlike the abscesses formed by other species. From Table 6 and studies of dental calculus it is evident that *A. israelii* and *Ar. propionica* are the most pathogenic species for man regardless of their relative population in the mouth or on calculus. In mice and other animals these four species appear to be equally infectious and pathogenic.

The mechanisms by which species of *Actinomyces* establish a progressive infection in humans are unknown. In humans the disease is degenerative and may destroy tissue and dissolve bone. In cattle, lumpy jaw may destroy bone, but usually stimulates bone growth in the upper or lower jaw. No toxin has been implicated in actinomycosis, nor is there evidence that sulfur granules protect the bacterium from the defensive mechanisms of the host. There are sufficient reports of successful vaccine therapy to support the contention that high levels of antibody may limit the progress of the disease (Buchs, 1963). It is often stated but not proved that other bacteria contribute to the pathogenesis of *A. israelii* infections.

The oral actinomycetes are strongly associated with the formation of cavities and periodontal disease. *A. naeslundii* and *A. viscosus* are implicated in gingivitis in man and cause extensive periodontal disease in hamsters and germ-free rats (Jordan et al., 1972).

Studies with *Streptococcus mutans* indicate that dental plaque forms as a result of bacterial adherence to the tooth surface, where the bacteria colonize the salivary glycoproteins coating the enamel. The bacterium has both a soluble and a cell-associated glycosyltransferase that converts sucrose to insoluble glucans and oligosaccharides of low molecular weight. The insoluble polysaccharide precipitates on the tooth surface and, because of the affinity of the cell-bound enzyme with its substrate, the streptoccocus adheres to the polysaccharide. Other bacteria also adhere to the insoluble polysaccharides, which may be used for further bacterial growth and colonization. Plaque is the final result.

Within the plaque the fermenting bacteria form their characteristic volatile and nonvolatile acids that cause localized areas of low pH and thereby the dissolution of enamel that initiates dental caries. When the plaque becomes calcified, it is converted to calculus, and both are colonized by all the *Actinomyces* species, which become the predominant populations. Intimate contact or abrasion of the periodontal tissue by the calculus then exposes the tissue to the organism and its products, without being invaded by them.

Baker et al. (1976) summarized the immunologic events leading to the pathogenesis of gingivitis or periodontosis of 11 common oral bacteria. They strongly implicated *A. israelii*, *A. naeslundii*, *A. viscosus*, *Ar. propionica*, *P. acnes*, and a gram-negative rod as the primary causes of lymphocyte transformation. The organisms or their products sensitize lymphocytes and release lymphokines that enhance antibody production, attract phagocytic cells, and initiate processes that resorb bone and damaged tissue. Ivanyi and Lehner (1970) showed a direct correlation between the severity of periodontal disease and the degree of blastogenesis of the host's lymphocytes when the host is exposed to oral bacteria. Baker et al. (1976) showed that the lymphocytic transformations caused by the above species were the result of antigenic sensitivity and not of the bacterial walls acting as mitogens. Thus, leukocyte transformation induced by *Actinomyces* requires the sensitized leukocyte of the diseased host or immune serum. Leukocytes of patients with periodontal disease respond to sonicated dental plaque, whole *Actinomyces* cells and cell walls, and soluble cytoplasmic components. These components contain protein and neutral sugars and are specific antigens for the immune cellular response (Reed et al., 1976). These data implicate the four species above as major causes of periodontal disease by mechanisms linked with bacterial hypersensitivity. This mechanism may also explain pathogenesis of actinomycosis when the actinomycete enters into the tissues.

IMMUNITY. In the early 1920s, opsonins and agglutinins were observed in actinomycosis; more recently agar gel precipitins, hemagglutinins, and complement-fixing antibodies have been described. In a few cases, the serum precipitin response corresponded with the course of actinomycosis. Thus recovery after treatment was accompanied by a fall in precipitins.

There is a suggestion that vaccine therapy can control the disease when used alone or with surgery or antibiotics. Colebrook (1921) found that vaccine therapy was particularly successful in cervico-facial actinomycosis. There are no reports of immunity to reinfection.

DRUG SUSCEPTIBILITY. The susceptibilities of pathogenic *Actinomyces* and *Arachnia* species to drugs is shown in Table 7. Their correlation with treatment of actinomycosis is summarized by Lerner (1974). The effectiveness of penicillin is well-established in human actinomycosis (Brown, 1973; Weese and Smith, 1975). The antifungal agents amphotericin B, nystatin, and griseofulvin are not effective.

Clinical failures with penicillin and other drugs active in vitro against *A. israelii* are attributed to secondary infections with Gram-negative organisms. Weese and Smith (1975) reported that 65 per cent of 57 cases over a 36-year period had *Actinomyces* in association with other bacteria, the majority of which were Gram-positive. There have been no extensive reports of antibiotic resistance of *Actinomyces* developing during therapy. Garrod (1952) found eightfold and twentyfold increases respectively in the resistance of two strains during treatment.

LABORATORY DIAGNOSIS

Media. For primary isolation of *Actinomyces* and related organisms, Brain Heart infusion agar plates both without blood and with 5 per cent whole defibrinated animal blood should be used. Rabbit, sheep, or horse blood is recommended; human blood is not. However, *Actinomyces* broth (BBL Division of BioQuest, Becton, Dickinson and Company) with 1.5 per cent agar can be used for isolation plates or with 0.7 per cent agar for dilution tubes and for maintenance. The recommended formula for the *Actinomyces* broth is: potassium dihydrogen phosphate, 15.0 g/L; ammonium sulfate, 1.0 g/L; magnesium sulfate, 0.2 g/L; calcium chloride (anhydrous), 0.01 g/L; heart infusion broth, 25.0 g/L; dextrose, 5.0 g/L; cysteine hydrochloride, 1.0 g/L; casitone, 4.0 g/L; yeast extract, 5.0 g/L; insoluble potato starch (preferred) or soluble starch, 1.0 g/L; final pH adjusted to 6.5 to 6.8 with potassium hydroxide.

Table 7. IN VITRO SENSITIVITY OF PATHOGENIC SPECIES IN THE FAMILY ACTINOMYCETACEAE

	A. israelii	*A. naeslundii*	*A. odontolyticus*	*A. viscosus*	*A. bovis*	*A. eriksonii*[a]	*Arachnia propionica*
No strains tested	32	5	5	15	4	6	7
			μg/ml for total inhibition of colony growth				
Penicillin G	0.5	1.0	0.15	0.5	1.0	0.5	0.5
Ampicillin	2.0	2.0	2.0	1.0	2.0	2.0	1.0
Cephaloridine	0.5	0.5	0.5	1.0	2.0	0.5	1.0
Cephalothin	2.0	2.0	0.25	0.5	1.0	2.0	1.0
Cephalexin	8.0	16.0	4.0	8.0	8.0	16.0	4.0
Minocycline	1.0	1.0	0.5	1.0	0.5	0.5	0.5
Doxycycline	2.0	4.0	0.5	2.0	1.0	4.0	4.0
Tetracycline	2.0	8.0	8.0	2.0	2.0	4.0	2.0
Clindamycin	0.5	8.0	0.5	2.0	0.5	0.25	4.0
Lincomycin	1.0	4.0	0.5	2.0	2.0	0.5	2.0
Oxacillin	8.0	4.0	4.0	4.0	16.0	8.0	8.0
Dicloxacillin	3.2	16.0	8.0	16.0	32.0	16.0	16.0
Erythromycin	0.25	0.12	0.06	0.12	0.06	0.06	0.12
Chloramphenicol	8.0	8.0	4.0	8.0	32.0	4.0	8.0
Vancomycin	20.0	10.0	10.0	20.0	10.0	20.0	10.0
Rifampin	>0.5	>0.5	0.03	>0.5	0.6	>0.5	>0.5
Fusidic acid	20.0	>20.0	5.0	>20.0	>20.0	>20.0	>20.0
Novobiocin	8.0	>25.0	16.0	>25.0	16.0	>25.0	16.0

[a]*A. eriksonii* — *Bifidobacterium adolescentis*.

Data from Lerner (1974).

Fluid thioglycolate broth may also be used for dilution tubes. However different commercial products vary in sugar concentrations and in the presence or absence of cysteine or phosphate as buffer, and also in their basic complex protein extracts. Media with cysteine and phosphate are preferred. For best results the commercial fluid thiglycolate medium should be fortified with 0.2 per cent sterile rabbit serum just before use.

The Brain Heart infusion media are excellent for isolation; they are not satisfactory for maintenance. For maintenance, deep cultures are made in *Actinomyces* broth with 0.7 per cent agar. Tubes of the medium are sealed with the pyrogallol–sodium carbonate seal described below. For the maintenance of the aerobic species *R. dentocariosa*, 1.5 per cent agar slants of Brain Heart Infusion agar or Trypticase Soy Agar (BBL, BioQuest) are used.

The medium used for fermentation tests is Thioglycolate Fermentation Medium without added dextrose (BBL, BioQuest) or indicator to which 2.0 g of yeast extract (glucose free) and 2.0 ml of 1.0 per cent Brom cresol purple have been added (Slack and Gerencser, 1975). This medium is used for all species except *R. dentocariosa*, for which meat-extract peptone base is used. The formula for this medium is: meat extract, 3.0 g/L; bactopeptone, 10.0 g/L; sodium chloride, 5.0 g/L; Andrade's indicator, 10 ml/L; pH adjusted to 7.4.

All media may be prepared and stored; before use, however, they should be freshly melted or heated to eliminate absorbed oxygen. For isolation or stock cultures, the *Actinomyces* maintenance medium with 0.7 per cent agar can be tubed in 10 ml quantities and stored in anaerobic containers or with pyrogallol–sodium carbonate seals at 5°C for one year.

Steps in Laboratory Diagnosis

1. Clinical Materials. All materials should be examined under wet mounts in dilute KOH, and by Gram and acid-fast stains of thinly prepared smears. Acid-fast cells should be regarded as potential *Nocardia* or *Mycobacteria*.

Pus is examined for mycelium or sulfur granules by adding a few drops of it to 5 ml of sterile distilled water and shaking the mixture well to make a fine suspension and to lyse tissue cells. The sediment is examined in KOH mounts and by Gram stains. Granules are washed several times by passage through 4 or 5 ml of sterile distilled water and then crushed in 0.5 ml of liquid. This suspension is used to streak plates or make dilution tubes. Sulfur granules or mycelial colonies are characteristic of *Actinomyces* and *Arachnia*.

2. Preparation and Examination of Primary Isolation Cultures. Two plates each of Brain Heart Infusion agar with and without blood should be made; a series of dilution tubes in the 0.7 per cent agar–*Actinomyces* medium or in thioglycolate broth are also made. One plate each, with and without blood, should be incubated anaerobically with CO_2, and one set should be incubated aerobically with CO_2. A candle jar or Gaspak (BBL, BioQuest) is adequate for the anaerobic CO_2 systems. However, anaerobic chambers that can be evacuated and flushed with nitrogen-5 per cent CO_2 are preferred. A desiccator to which a few pea-sized granules of dry ice are added can be used for aerobic incubation with carbon dioxide. Dilution tubes made with *Actinomyces* medium are extremely effective for primary isolation, particularly if the tubes are sealed with pyrogallol-sodium carbonate. Once the tubes are inoculated, the top half of the cotton plug is cut off, and the plug is pushed into the tube, care being taken to keep the plug several inches above the agar. A second snug fitting stopper of absorbent cotton is inserted; five drops of a saturated pyrogallol solution and five drops of a 10 per cent sodium carbonate solution are added in that sequence, and the tube is rapidly sealed with a tight rubber stopper. Dilution tubes made in fluid thioglycolate may be used without the anaerobic seals. All cultures are incubated at 37° C.

All plates should be examined after 24 to 48 hours by transmitted or reflected light to observe the spider-like microcolonies of *A. israelii*, or the round entire microcolonies characteristic of *A. bovis*, *A. odontolyticus*, and *B. adolescentis*. Beta hemolysis or strong alpha hemolysis is not produced by the actinomycetes. After four to five days the macrocolonies are examined by Gram stain and for catalase.

To test for catalase a drop of a cell suspension is added to a drop of 1.5 per cent H_2O_2 on a microscope slide and covered at once with a coverslip. Catalase causes bubbles to form beneath the coverslip within 30 seconds and stream continuously to the edges. Blood agar must not be transferred with the colony, since red cells contain catalase. Also, metallic ions such as iron can catalyze the breakdown of H_2O_2. In a positive test gas formation continues for at least 20 to 30 seconds after bubbling begins. A positive catalase test suggests *A. viscosus*, *R. dentocariosa*, or contaminating bacteria.

Primary cultures should be restreaked before a stock culture is made. Cultures that appear pink and are catalase-positive may contain *P. acnes*. After moderate growth in *Actinomyces* agar deeps, the cultures may be stored at 5° C for 6 to 12 months.

*3. **Differential Physiologic Characteristics.*** Identification rests on the characteristics summarized in Tables 3, 4, and 5. The tests of Table 5 are the minimum required for generic if not species identification. Species may also be identified with the fluorescent antibody (Slack and Gerencser, 1975). Volatile and nonvolatile acids are identified by chromatography; cell wall sugars and amino acids are identified by paper chromatography after enzymatic digestion or sodium hydroxide extraction of cell walls followed by acid hydrolysis (Cummins, 1962; Boone and Pine, 1968).

EPIDEMIOLOGY. There have been no recorded epidemics of *Actinomyces* infections. The human disease occurs throughout the world and shows no propensity for any race. One clinic reported an average incidence of from one to three cases per year over 36 years, with one three-year period averaging five cases per year (Weese and Smith, 1975). Another reported about five cases per year over a 10-year period (Buchs, 1963). Distribution does not seem to be age-related, although about 80 per cent were over 20. Among 181 cases, two thirds were between 30 and 60 years old (Brown, 1973). More cases are reported in males, with only 20 to 40 per cent in females.

Thirty-five to 55 per cent of human infections occur in the head and neck, 14 to 33 per cent in the thorax, and 23 to 28 per cent in the pelvis and abdomen, of which 10 per cent may occur in the pelvic organs alone (Brown, 1973). In cattle, where 0.03 to 0.5 per cent of the herds may have actinomycosis, the disease is mainly lumpy jaw or infection of the soft tissues of the head.

Because the organisms are commensals in the mouth of the adult, it is assumed that the young are colonized by direct oral contact or through some other physical vector. Infection most often follows some physical trauma by which the organism gains entrance to the tissues. Supporting the effect of physical trauma are the reports of Henderson (1973), and Schiffer et al. (1975) relating the presence of *Actinomyces* and pelvic actinomycosis to the use of intrauterine devices. These reports represent only a few of those published recently in America, England, and Canada on this subject. In recent observations, the description of abscesses with pus containing sulfur granules, the typical aspect of the sulfur granule stained with hematoxylin and eosin, and the typical gram-positive mycelium in sections stained by the Brown and Brenn stain all support the conclusion that *Actinomyces* is associated with infections that occur during the use of intrauterine devices. Even more significant, Spence et al. (1977) have observed organisms consistent with actinomycetes in 350 pancervicovaginal (Fast) smears of patients who used intrauterine devices. In 35 of these, *A. israelii* was identified by specific fluorescent antibody. Similar stains for *A. naeslundii* were negative. These reports of IUD-associated infections have been supported by isolations of *A. israelii* from three cases by Luff and Gupta (1977) and by one fatality associated with *A. israelii* (Serotype 1) infection (Hager and Majmudar, 1979). *A. israelii* and *A. propionica* are common in the vaginas of women whether they have or have not worn an IUD (Pine et al., 1981) but the presence of the IUD increases the actinomycete population (Traynor et al., 1981) (Valicenti et al. 1982). Furthermore an association of pelvic inflammatory disease with associated tubovarian abscesses and the presence of actinomycetes has been made (Burkman et al. 1982). The overall results show *A. israelii* is a causal organism in infections resulting from the use of intrauterine devices and show that women who use IUDs or pessaries have an increased risk of infection by this organism (Christ and Haja, 1978).

References

Baker, J. J., Chan, S. P., Socransky, S. S., Oppenheim, J. J., and Mergenhagen, S. E.: Importance of *Actinomyces* and certain gram-negative anaerobic organisms in the transformation of lymphocytes from patients with periodontal disease. Infect Immun 13:1363, 1976.

Bollinger, O.: Ueber eine ne Pilzkrankheit beim Rinde. Zentralbl Med Weiss. 15:481, 1877.

Boone, C. J., and Pine, L.: Rapid method for characterization of actinomycetes by cell wall composition. Appl Microbiol 16:279, 1968.

Bostroem, E.: Untersuchungen über die Aktinomykose des Menschen. Beitr Pathol 9:1, 1891.

Brock, D. W., and Georg, L. K.: Determination and analysis of *Actinomyces israelii* serotypes by fluorescent-antibody procedures. J Bacteriol 79:581, 1969.

Brown, J. R.: Human actinomycosis. A study of 181 subjects. Hum Pathol 4:319, 1973.

Buchanan, B. B., and Pine, L.: Relationship of carbon dioxide to aspartic acid and glutamic acid in *Actinomyces naeslundii*. J Bacteriol 89:729, 1965.

Buchs, H.: Zur Klinik und Therapei der Cervicofaciaten Aktinomykose. Dtsch. Zahnaerztl Z 18:1069, 1963.

Bujwid, O.: Ueber die Reinkulter des *Actinomyces*. Zentralbl Bakteriol [Orig. B] 6:630, 1889.

Burkman, R., Schlesselman, S., McCaffrey, L., Gupta, P. K., and Spence, M.: The relationship of genital tract actinomycetes and the development of pelvic inflamatory disease. Am J Obstet Gynecol 143:585, 1982.

Cohn, F.: Untersuchungen über Bacterien. Beitr. Biol Pflanzen 1:141, 1875.

Colebrook, L.: A report on 25 cases of actinomycosis with special reference to vaccine therapy. Lancet 1:893, 1921.

Coleman, R. M., George, L. K., and Rozzell, A. R.: *Actinomyces naeslundii* as an agent of human actinomycosis. Appl Microbiol 18:420, 1969.

Christ, M. L., and Haja, J.: Cytologic changes associated with vaginal pessary use with special reference to the presence of *Actinomyces*. Acta Cytol 22:146, 1978.

Cummins, C. S.: Chemical composition and antigenic structure of cell walls of *Corynebacterium*, *Mycobacterium*, *Nocardia*, *Actinomyces* and *Arthrobacter*. J Gen Microbiol 28:35, 1962.

Cummins, C. S.: *Actinomyces israelii* type 2. In Prouser, H. (ed.): The Actinomycetales. Jena, Gustav Fischer Verlag, 1968.

Cummins, C. S., and Harris, H.: Studies on the cell wall composition and taxonomy of Actinomycetales and related groups. J. Gen. Microbiol 18:173, 1958.
Emmons, C. W.: *Actinomyces* and actinomycosis. Puerto Rico J Public Health Trop Med 11:63, 1935.
Erikson, D.: Pathogenic anaerobic organisms of the *Actinomyces* group. Med Res Council Spec Rep Ser 240:1, 1940.
Frazier, P. D., and Fowler, B. O.: X-ray diffraction and infrared study of the "sulphur granules" of *Actinomyces bovis*. J. Gen Microbiol 46:445, 1967.
Garrod, L. P.: The sensitivity of *Actinomyces israelii* to antibiotics. Br Med J 1:1263, 1952.
Georg, L. K., Coleman, R. M., and Brown, J. M.: Evaluation of an agar gel precipitin test for the serodiagnosis of actinomycosis. J Immunol 100:1288, 1968.
Georg, L. K., Robertstad, G. W., Brinkman, S. A., and Hicklin, M. D.: A new pathogenic anaerobic *Actinomyces* species. J Infect Dis 115:88, 1965.
von Graefe, A.: Koncretionen in unteren Thränenröhrchen durch Pilzbildung. Arch Ophthalmol 1:284, 1854.
Hager, W. D., and Majmudar, B.: Pelvic actinomycosis in women using intrauterine devices. Am J Obstet Gynecol 156:60, 1979.
Hartz, C. O.: *Actinomyces bovis*: ein neuer Schimmel in dem Geweben des Rindes. Dtsche Z Tier-Med 5:125 (Suppl.) 1879.
Henderson, S. R.: Pelvic actinomycosis associated with an intrauterine device. Obstet Gynecol 41:726, 1973.
Holm, P., and Kwapinski, J. B.: Studies on the detection of *Actinomyces* antibodies in human sera by use of pure antigenic fractions of *Actinomyces israelii*. Acta Pathol Microbiol Scand [B] 45:107, 1959.
Holmberg, K., and Nord, C-E.: Numerical taxonomy and laboratory identification of *Actinomyces* and *Arachnia* and some related bacteria. J Gen Microbiol 91:17, 1975.
Holmberg, K., Nord, C-E., Wastrom, T.: Serological studies of *Actinomyces israelii* by crossed immunoelectrophoresis: Taxonomic and diagnostic applications. Infect Immun 12:398, 1975.
Howell, A., Jr., Murphy, W. C., Paul, F., and Stephan, R. M.: Oral strains of *Actinomyces*. J Bacteriol 78:82, 1959.
Israel, J.: Neue Beobachtungen auf dem Gebiete der Mykosen des Menschen. Arch Pathol Anat 74:15, 1878.
Ivanyi, L., and Lehner, T.: Stimulation of lymphocyte transformation by bacterial antigens in patients with peridontal disease. Arch Oral Biol 15:1089, 1970.
Jordan, H. V., Keyes, P. H., and Bellack, S.: Periodontal lesions in hamsters and gnotobiotic rats infected with *Actinomyces* of human origin. J Periodont Res 7:21, 1972.
Lerner, P. I.: Susceptibility of pathogenic actinomycetes to antimicrobial compounds. Antimicrob Agents Chemother 5:302, 1974.
Luff R. D., and Gupta, P. K.: Actinomycetes-like organisms in wearers of intrauterine contraceptive devices. Am J Obstet Gynecol 129:477, 1977.
Morris, J. F., and Kilbourn, P.: Systemic actinomycosis caused by *Actinomyces odontolyticus*. Ann Int Med 81:700, 1974.
Naeslund, C.: Studies of *Actinomyces* from the oral cavity. Acta Pathol Microbiol Scand 2:110, 1925.
Pine, L.: Classification and phylogenetic relationship of microaerophilic actinomycetes. Int J System Bacteriol 20:445, 1970.
Pine, L.: Parasitic or fermentative actinomycetes. In Laskin, A. I., and Lechevalier, H. A. (eds.): Handbook of Microbiology. Cleveland, CRC Press, 1973, p. 212.
Pine, L., Howell, A., Jr., Watson, S. J.: Studies of the morphological physiological and biochemical characters of *Actinomyces bovis*. J Gen Microbiol 23:403, 1960.
Pine, L., and Overman, J. R.: Determination of the structure and composition of the "sulphur granules" of *Actinomyces bovis*. J Gen Microbiol 32:209, 1963.
Pine, L., and Overman, J. R.: Differentiation of capsules and hyphae in clubs of bovine sulphur granules. Sabouraudia 5:141, 1966.
Pine, L., Malcolm, G.B., Curtis, E.M., and Brown, J.M.: Demonstration of *Actinomyces* and *Arachnia* species in cervicovaginal smears by direct staining with species-specific fluorescent-antibody conjugate. J Clin Microbiol 13:15, 1981.
Ponfick, E.: Ueber Actinomykose. Berl Klin Wchnehr 17:660, 1880.
Reed, M.J., Potters, M.R., Mashimo, P.A., Genco, R.J., and Levine, M. J.: Blastogenic response of human lymphocytes to oral bacterial antigens: Characterization of bacterial sonicates. Infect Immun 14:1202, 1976.
Schiffer, M. A., Elguezabal, A., Sultana, M., and Allen, A. C.: Actinomycosis infections associated with intrauterine contraceptive devices. Obstet Gynecol 45:67, 1975.
Schleifer, K. H., and Kandler, O.: Peptidoglycan types of bacterial cell walls and their taxonomic implications. Bacteriol Rev 36:407, 1972.
Schofield, G. M. and Schaal, K. P.: A numerical taxonomic study of members of the *Actinomycetaceae* and related taxa. J Gen Microbiol 127:237, 1981.
Silberschmidt, W.: Über Actinomykose. Z Hyg 37:345, 1901.
Slack, J. M., and Gerencser, M. A.: *Actinomyces*, Filamentous Bacteria: Biology and Pathogenicity. Minneapolis, Burgess Publishing Company, 1975.
Slack, J. M., Moore, D. W., and Gerencser, M. A.: Use of the fluorescent antibody technique in the diagnosis of actinomycosis. W Va Med J 62:228, 1966.
Spence, M. R., Gupta, P. K., Frost, J. K., and King, T. M.: Cytological detection and clinical significance of *Actinomyces israelii* in women employing intrauterine contraceptive devices. Am J Obstet Gynecol 131(3):295, 1978.
Sutter, V. L.: Evaluation of criteria used in the identification of *Actinomyces bovis* with particular reference to the catalase reaction. Mycopathologica 6:220, 1956.
Thompson, L.: Isolation and comparison of *Actinomyces* from human and bovine infections. Proc Staff Meet Mayo Clin 25:81, 1950.
Thompson, L., and Lovestedt, S. A.: An *Actinomyces*-like organism obtained from the human mouth. Proc Staff Meet Mayo Clin 26:169, 1951.
Traynor, R. M., Parrott, D., Duguid, H. L. D., and Duncan, I. D.: Isolation of actinomycetes from cervical specimens. J Clin Path 34:914, 1981.
Valicenti, J. F., Pappas, A. A., Graber, C. D., Williamson, H. O., and Willis, N. F.: Detection and prevalence of IUD-associated *Actinomyces* colonization and related morbidity. J Am Med Assoc 247:1149, 1982.
Weese, W. C., and Smith, L. M.: A study of 57 cases of actinomycosis over a 36-year period. Arch Intern Med 135:1562, 1975.
Wolff, M., and Israel, J.: Ueber Reincultur des *Actinomyces* and seine Uebertragbarkeit auf Theire. Virchow's Arch [Path Anat] 126:11, 1891.
Wright, J. J.: The biology of the microorganism of actinomycosis. J Med Res 13:349, 1905.

49
THE CLOSTRIDIA

BETTY C. HOBBS, PH. D., D. SC., F.R.C.PATH., DIP. BACT.

GENERAL CHARACTERISTICS. The *Clostridium* species are gram-positive, spore-forming bacilli, motile except for *C. perfringens*, and obligate anaerobes. They vary in their requirements for reduced oxygen, and some species tolerate concentrations of oxygen not far below those found in the atmosphere.

The clostridia are biochemically active and may be saccharolytic, fermenting carbohydrate, such as *C. perfringens*, *C. septicum*, *C. oedematiens*, and *C. fallax*, and proteolytic, decomposing protein, such as *C. sporogenes*, *C. histolyticum*, and *C. botulinum*.

Most species are saprophytic, others exist as commensals in the human and animal intestine, and many are pathogenic. The pathogenic clostridia cause serious diseases such as tetanus *(C. tetani)*, gas gangrene *(C. perfringens, C. oedematiens*, and *C. septicum)*, and botulism *(C. botulinum)*. *C. perfringens* also causes gastroenteritis, usually mild but sometimes fatal in elderly and debilitated persons, and also enteritis necroticans, which is a more serious disease with high mortality. In veterinary medicine clostridia are important intestinal pathogens. They cause enterotoxemia in sheep, calves, lambs, goats, and piglets. Dysentery in lambs (*C. perfringens* Type B) and piglets (*C. perfringens* Type C) may necessitate extensive vaccination programs. Toxemias in adult animals may follow a change of diet. High carbohydrate levels may encourage the growth of clostridia and toxin formation, as in the production of epsilon toxin by *C. perfringens* Type D in pulpy kidney disease. Similarly, it is suggested by Lawrence and Walker (1976) that in Papua, New Guinea, the sudden intake of pork during feasting encourages the growth of *C. perfringens* Type C and the production of beta toxin, which cannot be destroyed because of the low level of digestive proteases in the intestine; the staple diet is sweet potato possessing a heat-stable trypsin inhibitor. The use of a *C. perfringens* Type C toxoid has given encouraging results in preventing necrotizing enteritis (Pigbel) in children (Leader, 1977).

The artificial feeding of 12 hospital-born neonates was followed by necrotizing enteritis of varying severity within ten days to six weeks. Evidence of the presence of *C. butyricum* was found in the blood of nine to ten babies examined; this organism was thought to be the invader responsible (Howard et al., 1977). Rifkin et al. (1977) described *C. sordellii* infection in adults with antibiotic-induced colitis. From 1978 onward, *C. difficile* has been suspected as the agent responsible for pseudomembranous colitis (PMC) following extensive antimicrobial treatment (Leader, 1980). Thus it seems that clostridia can grow and produce toxin under favorable conditions and in the absence of the usual flora or mechanisms that control them (Leader, 1977). It is suggested also that clostridia may be involved in the breakdown of bile salts to steroids during digestion and thus indirectly may produce conditions that predispose toward cancer (Drasar, 1982).

Aside from the medical and veterinary significance of the clostridia, many species are used commercially in the production of acids and alcohols in fermentative or digestive processes; some have been and could be used in the chemical industry when fossil fuels expire. Many species break down nitrogen and cellulose (denitrifying and degrading cellulose in the soil) and many fix nitrogen in the soil. They are prominent in decomposition processes such as silage maturation. Table 1 lists the names of some clostridia and their uses.

In food technology, the presence of mesophilic clostridia in canned nonacid foods indicates that heating has been insufficient to destroy spores of *C. botulinum*, which are the greatest hazard in canned food. In chilled or dried foods, an unusually large number of viable clostridia might indicate a hazard from *C. perfringens* or *C. botulinum*, either in the food as preserved or in its future use. Spores of the most heat-resistant clostridia are used to test the sterility of medical equipment.

Table 1. INDUSTRIAL USES OF THE CLOSTRIDIUM GROUP

C. pasteurianum	Nitrogen fixation in the soil
C. beijerinckii	Anaerobic digestion
C. cellobiofavum	Cellulose degradation
C. butyricum	Butyric acid production in butter and cheese
C. tyrobutyricum	Butyric acid production in cheese
C. butylicum	Acetic and butyric acid production from glucose; also ethyl, butyl and propyl alcohols and acetone
C. iodophilum	Acetic and butyric acid production from glucose; also ethyl and butyl alcohols and acetone
C. toanum	Butyric acid; also ethyl, butyl and isopropyl alcohols and acetone
C. acetobutylicum	Acetic and butyric acids; also ethyl and butyl alcohols and acetone. Anaerobic digestion
C. amylosaccharobutylpropylicum	Butyl and propyl alcohols from starch and sugar

CLOSTRIDIUM PERFRINGENS

MORPHOLOGY. The organism is a strongly gram-positive, nonmotile rod with blunt or square ends; it is not a strict anaerobe. On some media the bacilli may be long and slender. Human Type C strains may be large with filaments and swollen forms. Sometimes they are short and almost coccoid. Spores are rarely seen in laboratory media or in cooked foods. Sporulation may be encouraged in special media described by Ellner (1956), Duncan and Strong (1968), and Clifford and Annellis (1971); sporulating mutants have been induced. The spores are large, oval, and central and distend the organism. Capsules are mostly seen in the animal body.

The colonies are low, convex, semiopaque, and shiny; they may be round and entire, or somewhat irregular with a vine leaf appearance. Hemolysis is variable according to the strain and the animal source of the blood. It may be clear beta or partially clear alpha, sometimes with a double zone.

ANTIGENIC COMPOSITION. *C. perfringens* is divisible into five serologic types, A to E, according to the kinds and proportions of exotoxins (soluble antigens) produced. Antitoxic sera are used in the routine typing of strains. The α-toxin or lecithinase is produced by all types; it is antigenically related to the lecithinase of *C. bifermentans* and *C. sordellii.* Although agglutination is of little value in subdividing the species because of its heterogeneity, Type A strains nevertheless are further divided into a large number of serotypes by simple agglutination. This is of value for the epidemiologic study of food poisoning and gas gangrene. Bacteriocin typing is also described (Watson et al., 1982).

METABOLISM. Glucose, lactose, maltose, and sucrose are fermented, and gelatinase is produced. H_2S is formed, but not indole. *C. perfringens* may be differentiated from most other species of *Clostridium* by lactose fermentation, nitrate reduction, tests for motility and sporulation, and lecithinase activity; the Nagler reaction is a simple in vitro test for this substance.

PATHOGENIC PROPERTIES. Types A, C, and D are pathogenic for man, Type A is responsible for gas gangrene and food poisoning, and Type C for enteritis necroticans; Type A has also been incriminated in necrotizing colitis. Types B, C, D, E, and possibly A affect animals. More than 80 per cent of environmental isolates have been shown to be Type A. Infection of experimental animals and patients causes extensive blood-stained edema fluid, often with gas in the tissues, and invasion of the bloodstream. A number of exotoxins are involved.

TOXICOLOGY. There are at least 12 different soluble antigens described for *C. perfringens*. Alpha, beta, epsilon, and iota are the major lethal toxins in mice.

α-toxin is common to all types of *C. perfringens*, but it is produced in largest amount by strains of Type A. It is lethal for mice 6 to 12 hours after intravenous inoculation. It also causes necrosis after intradermal injection in guinea pigs. The lecithinase activity of alpha toxin splits lecithin to phosphorylcholine and a diglyceride and can be demonstrated by production of opalescence on egg yolk agar (Nagler reaction) and by lysis of sheep or mouse erythrocytes.

β-toxin is produced by Types B and C. It is necrotizing and lethal, but not hemolytic; it is heat-labile. It is identified by the intradermal inoculation of depilated albino guinea pigs, in which it produces a purplish necrotic area.

δ-toxin is lethal and hemolytic. It lyses sheep erythrocytes but not those of the horse or rabbit. It is produced by Types B and C.

θ-toxin is produced in greatest amount by Type C strains but can be found also in culture filtrates of Types A, B, D, and E. It is an oxygen-labile hemolysin, active against sheep and horse red cells but not very active against those of the mouse.

ϵ-toxin is produced by Types B and D, ι-toxin by Type E strains. Both toxins are lethal and necrotizing. They are detected in culture filtrates by intradermal tests in guinea pigs. Trypsinization must be used to ensure activation of the prototoxins. They are both absorbed from the intestinal tract.

κ-toxin is produced by Types A, C, E, and some strains of Type D. It is a collagenase and gelatinase and is also lethal and necrotizing.

λ-toxin is produced by Types B and E and some strains of Type D. It is a proteolytic enzyme that attacks gelatin and azocoll (commercial hide powder coupled to a dye) and also casein and hemoglobin (unlike κ-toxin).

γ- and η-toxins are lethal toxins without other demonstrable activity.

μ- and ν-antigens are a hyaluronidase and deoxyribonuclease; they may be estimated by the ACRA (acid-congo red-alcohol) test using horse synovial fluid (hyaluronic acid) (μ) and sodium deoxyribonuclease (ν) as the substrates (Oakley and Warrack, 1951).

Other soluble substances found in filtrates have included neuraminidase and fibrinolysis. The toxin patterns in relation to pathogenicity in man and animals are shown in Table 2 (Oakley and Warrack, 1953).

Enterotoxin. This component of the sporulating cells of Types A and C is responsible for food poisoning and is produced and released in the large intestine during sporulation (Skjelkvåle and Duncan, 1975). Sporulation in cooked food as in laboratory media is poor, so that the toxin is unlikely to be detected. By means of ligated loop experiments, the association between a large intake of *C. perfringens*, sporulation, and enterotoxin production in the intestine was confirmed (Duncan and Strong, 1971).

Hauschild (1973, 1975) described the purified toxin extracted from sporulated cells as a protein of approximately 36,000 MW and isoelectric point 4.3, containing 19 amino acids with a predominance of aspartic and glutamic acids, serine, and leucine. The toxicity for mice was 2000 MLD/mg N. The enterotoxin is heat-labile with a decimal reduction time of 4 minutes at 60° C. The toxin has lethal and emetic properties and causes cutaneous erythema in the guinea pig and rabbit. Antiserum against the enterotoxin was prepared by Stark and Duncan (1972).

Antienterotoxin antibodies have been found in the blood of a high proportion of persons who yet remain sensitive to the enterotoxin (Torres-Anjel and Riemann, 1975).

Biologic assays are carried out with suckling mice and the ileal loop technique; the fluorescent antibody technique may be used also. Torres-Anjel et al. (1975) described a fluorescent antibody technique for the detection of enter-

Table 2. THE SOLUBLE ANTIGENS OF CLOSTRIDIUM PERFRINGENS[a]

		α	β	γ	δ	ϵ	θ	ι	κ	λ	μ	ν
A	Gas gangrene, puerperal infection, septicemia, food poisoning:											
	Classical	++++	–	–	–	–	++–	–	++	–	–	+
	Atypical	+–	–	–	–	–	–	–	+–	–	–	–
B	Lamb dysentery, foal enterotoxemia, goats and sheep: hemorrhagic enteritis	+	+++	+	++	++	+	–	–	+++	+	+
C	Sheep toxemia, calves and lambs: hemorrhagic enteritis,	+	+++	+	++	–	+	–	+	–	–	+
	Man: enteritis necroticans	+	+	+	–	–	–	–	–	–	–	+
D	Sheep, lambs, goats, cattle: enterotoxemia	+++	–	–	++	+++	++	–	++	++	++–	++–
E	Sheep, cattle (? pathogenic)	+++	–	–	–	–	++	+++	++	++	(+)	+–

[a]+++, produced by all strains; +, ++, produced in increasing quantities; ++–, +–, present in some strains only; –, not produced. Adapted from Willis (1977).

otoxin-producing cells of *C. perfringens* Type A. Enterotoxin appeared at the end of the cell after four hours of growth and gradually spread throughout the cell (Niilo, 1977). Enterotoxin was demonstrated in the stools of patients by reversed-passive hemagglutination (RPHA) (Dowell et al., 1975). RPHA is described as the most sensitive method for measurement of enterotoxin (Niilo, 1978). A comparison of the various biological and serological methods including gel diffusion and electrophoresis is given by Stringer et al. (1982).

LABORATORY DIAGNOSIS. Pathologic material may be inoculated directly onto plates of blood agar and egg yolk agar and incubated anaerobically. Neomycin sulfate may be incorporated into the medium or spread over the surface to suppress facultative organisms. Cooked meat broth cultures may be subcultured onto the same two agar media after eight to ten hours of growth. Since the organism does not form spores in the tissue or in cooked foodstuffs, heat treatment is not required. The organism produces spores readily in feces, and heat treatment of fecal suspensions is an advantage for isolation of heat-resistant strains. Direct inoculation from a fecal sample onto blood agar (with neomycin sulfate) and subculture from cooked meat broth without heat treatment should also be carried out (Sutton et al., 1971).

C. perfringens is a minor component of the fecal flora in most, if not all, persons. The median count of *C. perfringens* in fecal samples from 50 healthy adults was 7.5×10^3 per g. The ratio of the spore count to the count of unheated material was generally of the order of 1/10 to 1/100 (Sutton, 1969). In outbreaks of *C. perfringens* food poisoning, counts of the organism in feces from patients are higher, usually 10^6 to 10^7, and the heat-resistant spore/vegetative cell count was found to be 1/2000 to greater than 1/60,000 in one outbreak reported by Sutton (1966). Thus quantitation is useful in the assessment of the significance of *C. perfringens* in the stool. The Miles and Misra (1938) technique may be used on blood agar spread with neomycin sulfate; an approximately 1/10 suspension of the fecal sample may be used as the first dilution (Sutton et al., 1971). Heavily contaminated foods responsible for outbreaks may be cultured onto blood agar with and without neomycin sulfate and incubated anaerobically. For the enumeration of small numbers of *C. perfringens* for speciation purposes, black colonies in pour plates of sulfite cycloserine agar may be preferred. A selective liquid enrichment medium for the detection of low numbers of *C. perfringens* was described by Beerens et al. (1982). The isolation of small numbers of *C. perfringens* through cooked meat or liver enrichment media may be of value in epidemiologic studies and when serological typing is carried out, but care must be taken in the interpretation of the results.

The simplest means of identification is by the reaction described by Nagler in 1939 and developed as a diagnostic test by McClung and Toabe (1947). Cultures growing on media incorporating lecithin, egg yolk agar with or without mannitol, and an indicator show an opalescent precipitate around colonies. The opalescence is due to the interaction between the lecithin in the medium and lecithinase (α-toxin) produced by the organism. It is inhibited by antiserum to the α-toxin. The antitoxin is usually spread over half the plate (half antitoxin egg yolk agar), so that single streaks of cultures across the plate show the precipitate on one half only. Several strains can be tested on one plate. Lecithinase-negative strains occur from time to time. Stringer et al. (1978) described five outbreaks due to lecithinase-negative strains, and found that in four, the serotype of the strains isolated was identical.

Other tests for identification include motility, proteolysis, nitrate reduction, and biochemical reactions; the action on litmus milk (stormy clot) is not always typical. Laboratory reactions used in differentiating *C. perfringens* from other pathogenic clostridia are summarized in Table 3.

EPIDEMIOLOGY. The organism is widely distributed in nature in soil, sewage, water, and the intestinal tract of man and animals. Wounds may be infected from spores or cells in the environment or from contaminants on the skin surrounding the lesion. Serologic studies have indicated that *C. perfringens* in postoperative gangrene frequently originates from the intestine of the patient (Parker, 1967; Ayliffe and Lowbury, 1969).

C. perfringens is an important agent of food poisoning in the United States and the United Kingdom and perhaps (unrecognized) in many other countries also. It was reported as a cause of intestinal disturbances in hospital patients as early as 1895 (Klein, 1895). Knox and MacDonald (1943), McClung (1945), Zeissler and Rassfeld-Sternberg (1949), Hobbs et al. (1953), and many subsequent workers described the role of *C. perfringens* Type A in food poisoning. *C. perfringens* Type C was described by German investigators in a more serious and often fatal food-borne disease known as enteritis necroticans. Murrell et al. (1966) described the same disease in Papua, New Guinea. The β-toxin was thought to be responsible for the more severe intestinal lesions. The enterotoxin, which is distinct from the other toxins of *C. perfringens*, was later proved to be responsible for the milder type of food poisoning due to the Type A strains.

In humans symptoms of food poisoning from Type A strains develop 8 to 24 hours after eating food heavily contaminated with the organism. Symptoms include abdominal pain, nausea, and acute diarrhea lasting 12 to 24 hours; fever is rare. Occasionally there are fatalities among elderly debilitated patients. Deaths of some malnourished children with diarrhea may be due to terminal septicemia with *C. perfringens*. There were approximately 6500 cases of *C. perfringens* food poisoning in England and Wales during the years 1973 to 1975 (Vernon, 1977), representing between 15 and 32 per cent of the annual numbers reported from all bacterial causes. In the two years 1981 and 1982 there were 2373 cases and 115 outbreaks of *C. perfringens* food poisoning. The cases represented 20 per cent of the annual numbers from all cases. The outbreaks occurred mostly in hospitals, schools, and institutions and tended to be larger (50 persons average) than outbreaks due to other organisms. Outbreaks resulting from faults in the cooling and storage of foods cooked in bulk occurred repeatedly in hospitals and schools. Means for rapid cooling and adequate cold storage of meat and poultry, and other foods cooked ahead of requirements, should be incorporated into the design of canteen kitchens and other establishments preparing food on a large scale. The importance of this measure needs emphasis in teaching.

Statistics for enteritis necroticans due to the Type C strains are not available. The disease has been reported from Germany and Papua, New Guinea ("Pigbel"), but it is rarely noted in other countries. The factors leading to

Table 3. DIFFERENTIAL LABORATORY REACTIONS OF CLOSTRIDIA PATHOGENIC FOR MAN

	Nagler Reaction (Lecithinase)	Spores[a]	Motility	β-Hemolysis	Lactose Fermentation	Glucose Fermentation	H_2S	Indole	Urease	Nitrate Reduction
C. perfringens	+	C	0	+	+	+	+	0	0	+
C. tetani	0	T	+	+	0	0	0	+	0	0
C. botulinum										
Types A, B, E, F,	0	ST	+	+	0	+	+	0	0	0
Types C, D	0	ST	+	+	0	+	+	0	0	0
Type G	0	ST	+	+	0	0	+	0	0	0
C. novyi										
Type A	+	ST	+	+	0	+	+	0	0	+
Type B	+	ST	+	+	0	+	+	0	0	+
C. histolyticum	0	ST	+	+	0	0	+	0	0	0
C. septicum	0	ST	+	+	+	+	+	0	0	+
C. sporogenes	+	ST	+	0	0	+	+	0	0	+
C. sordellii	+	C	+	+	0	+	+	+	+	+
C. difficile	0	ST	+	0	0	+	0	0	0	0

[a]T, terminal; C, central; ST, subterminal.

illness are similar to those for the Type A strains: the survival of spores resistant to heat and the multiplication of vegetative cells in the slow cooking and cooling of masses of meat. In New Guinea the spit roasting of pig carcasses eaten at feasts and the "cairn" cooking of meat by the heat of the sun encourage multiplication of the organism to large numbers. Lawrence and Walker (1976) suggest that the low protein diet of the people of the Highland of Papua, New Guinea, and the presence of heat-stable trypsin-inhibitor from sweet potatoes results in low levels of digestive proteases in the intestinal lumen. Thus there is no proteolytic activity, and the β-toxin from *C. perfringens* Type C that is normally susceptible to proteolysis is not destroyed and causes necrosis.

The heat resistance of the spores of *C. perfringens* Type A varies from strain to strain and also within strains. Some spores can survive for an hour or more in boiled meats, in which they may be protected by the meat or fat; others live for a few minutes only. Cooking stimulates (heat shock) most spores of *C. perfringens* to germinate; the activation of germination is detected at about 75 to 80° C. The optimum temperatures for growth in cooked meat are 43 to 47° C (Collee et al., 1961).

The rate of division or generation time at optimum temperatures is 10 to 12 minutes (Mead, 1969) in food favorable for growth, principally a meat medium. Cooking drives off dissolved oxygen and leaves an anaerobic environment suitable for the growth of *C. perfringens*. The resistance to heat and activation by heat of the spores during cooking, and the fast multiplication of the vegetative cells during cooling result in the food becoming a medium for an almost pure culture of *C. perfringens*. When many (millions per g) vegetative cells in cooked foods are swallowed, they survive passage through the gastric acid and become established in the intestine. In the United Kingdom and United States, outbreaks of *C. perfringens* food poisoning occur throughout the year with no seasonal prevalence. The fault lies in the prolonged storage at 30 to 50° C between cooking and eating. Without proper cooling and adequate cold storage facilities, the preparation of food in large catering establishments often leads to this type of food poisoning. In addition to outbreaks associated with hospitals, schools, and factories, there are many that follow banquets and meals prepared for touring groups. Kitchens designed to prepare a few meals are often expected to cater for many travelers, despite inadequate space and facilities.

Vegetative cells and spores of *C. perfringens* are common on raw meat and on and within poultry and fish. Their origin is assumed to be feces from man and animals. Because the spores are resistant to dehydration, they can survive for long periods in soil and dust. The ubiquitous nature of the organism makes epidemiologic investigation difficult without finer methods of typing the strains isolated. The serologic differentiation of Type A strains was originally described by Henderson (1940) and Hobbs et al. (1953). It has now been expanded widely into an international typing scheme (Hughes et al., 1976; Stringer et al., 1975; Stringer et al., 1978; Stringer et al., 1982). Approximately 82 per cent of strains may be typed by a simple slide agglutination method using a battery of 43 or more sera made up into polyvalent groups, each containing about five sera of different types. The antigenic specificity is thought to originate from the capsular material.

Serotyping is useful also for tracing the origin of infection in gas gangrene cases (Parker, 1967; Ayliffe and Lowbury, 1969).

CLOSTRIDIUM TETANI

MORPHOLOGY. The characteristic bacilli are slender, gram-positive, motile, and strictly anaerobic. The mature spores are terminal and spherical so that the bacillus has a "drumstick" appearance; immature spores are oval and terminal. Sporefree forms occur, and older cultures may be gram-negative. The organism grows as a fine rhizoidal film with a finely filamentous edge of growth; the extremely fine growth may be missed. Nonmotile variants form discrete colonies with no swarming. Antitoxin will prevent swarming. There is alpha-to-beta hemolysis on horse blood agar.

ANTIGENIC COMPOSITION. There are at least ten types of flagellar antigens. Antigenically identical neurotoxin is formed by all types. Nontoxigenic variants may be isolated from wounds of patients.

METABOLISM. No sugars are fermented except glucose rarely. *C. tetani* is nonproteolytic but produces gelatinase. H_2S is not formed, but most strains produce indole. A rennin-like enzyme gives zones of opacity around colonies on milk agar. Some strains produce deoxyribonuclease. Metabolic products include acetic, propionic, and butyric acids and ethanol and butanol.

PATHOGENIC PROPERTIES. The pathogenicity of *C. tetani* for man arises from its neurotoxic exotoxin. The neurotoxin first causes local peripheral nerve and muscle spasms. The toxin (tetanospasmin) then spreads to the anterior horn cells via the bloodstream and causes generalized convulsions. A hemolysin (tetanolysin) is also produced but is less important; it is not related to the neurotoxin and may be produced by nontoxigenic strains. Tetanospasmin and *C. botulinum* neurotoxin are the most potent poisons known. In culture, tetanospasmin is produced after the phase of active growth; it is heat-labile and is destroyed at 65° C in five minutes.

IMMUNITY. The disease may be prevented by active immunization with tetanus toxoid or passive immunization with antitetanus hyperimmune human gamma globulin. Recovered patients must be immunized because the disease is produced by amounts of toxin that are too small for immunization. Toxoid given to pregnant women prevents tetanus of the newborn.

LABORATORY DIAGNOSIS. Pathologic material should be placed directly onto culture media and incubated in cooked meat broth for two to four days under anaerobic conditions. Fresh or heated blood agar is used for subculture, and the inoculum is placed near the edge of the plate so that the spreading or swarming growth may leave the contaminants behind. For purity, subcultures may be made from the edge of the growth. Neomycin sulfate and cautious heat treatment may be used to inhibit contaminants in material containing nonmotile variants of *C. tetani.*

DRUG SUSCEPTIBILITY. The organism is sensitive to penicillin and its derivatives and to tetracycline.

EPIDEMIOLOGY. *C. tetani* is widely distributed in soil, especially cultivated soil, and in the intestinal tract of man and animals. Infection of wounds and umbilical stumps of the newborn occurs after contamination with soil and human and animal feces. Military wounds, trauma among farm workers, and injuries from auto accidents are especially subject to soil contamination and thus to tetanus intoxication.

CLOSTRIDIUM BOTULINUM

MORPHOLOGY. The bacilli are large stout rods, motile and gram-positive, especially in young cultures. Sporulation may be sparse; the spores are oval and central or subterminal.

The colonies are irregular or circular and translucent with a granular surface; they may be lobular with an indefinite spreading edge. Growth may spread over the plate. There is hemolysis on horse blood agar.

ANTIGENIC COMPOSITION. There are eight known toxicologic types, A to G, which produce antigenically distinct neurotoxins. There are minor antigenic relationships between the neurotoxins of Types C and D and between Types E and F. Walker and Batty (1964) found that the toxicologic types fell into three distinct serologic groups. Types A, B, and F are serologically related and are distinct from Types C, D, and F. Types C and D are related and are distinguishable from Type E. Walker and Batty also noted limited cross-reactions between strains of *C. botulinum* and *C. sporogenes.*

METABOLISM. Types A, B, E, and F ferment glucose, maltose, and sucrose; Types C and D ferment glucose and maltose; Type G is nonsaccharolytic. All types produce gelatinase and H_2S; indole is not produced.

PATHOGENIC PROPERTIES. *C. botulinum* Types A, B, E, and F cause botulism in man. Types C and D and more rarely A and B are pathogenic for mammals and birds. Type G has not been reported from outbreaks in man or animals. The exotoxin is responsible for the disease; the organisms do not multiply easily in the body. *C. botulinum* in wounds can give rise to botulism in a few cases (Mersam and Dowell, 1973). Toxin elaborated by *C. botulinum* in the bowel of infants can cause illness and in some instances sudden death (Midura and Arnon, 1976). It has been suggested that *C. botulinum* may be one cause of sudden infant death syndrome (Lewis, 1981).

The potent neurotoxins, although antigenically distinct, are pharmacologically similar; they are absorbed from the alimentary tract through the gastric and upper intestinal mucosa. They can be demonstrated in the blood, and they reach the peripheral nervous system. The toxin acts at the tips of the motor nerve endings at the neuromuscular junction and interferes with the release of acetylcholine. To be effective, antitoxin should be administered before the toxin becomes fixed to the tissues. The incubation period is usually less than 24 hours. Vomiting, thirst, and pharyngeal and ocular paresis occur. Voluntary muscles weaken, and death may occur within 24 hours from paralysis of the respiratory muscles. In poultry and wildfowl the condition known as limberneck gives rise to paralysis of the neck and leg muscles.

A fatal dose of toxin for man has been estimated to be between 0.1 and 1.0 μg (Schantz and Sugyama, 1974). The toxicity of the neurotoxin is about 10^3 that of *C. perfringens* α-toxin, 10^5 that of crotactin (rattlesnake venom), and 10^6 that of strychnine (van Heyningen, 1968, 1970). The toxin is described as a simple protein consisting of 19 amino acids, molecular weight about 150,000, and isoelectric point 5.6. The toxin is rapidly destroyed by boiling. Toxigenic strains may lose their toxigenicity, while naturally occurring nontoxigenic strains can revert to a toxigenic state after infection with certain phages.

IMMUNITY. Natural immunity is unlikely to occur because the lethal dose of toxin is less than that required to elicit an antibody response. Laboratory workers may be immunized with polyvalent antitoxin (A, B, and E).

LABORATORY DIAGNOSIS. The toxin in supernatants of food and gastrointestinal contents and also in serum can be detected and identified by the mouse challenge test. Mice are injected with extracts and protected with specific antitoxin. Other reliable *in vitro* serological tests are described by Stringer et al. (1982). The clinical diagnosis can be confirmed by demonstrating the toxin in blood and stool specimens. Reverse passive hemagglutination, immunofluorescence and agar plates containing specific antitoxins are also used for identification. The organism may be isolated from cooked meat cultured onto blood agar plates incubated anaerobically. Shaking the cooked meat culture with a little alcohol or benzol before subculture inhibits contaminants. Neomycin sulfate in culture media helps to repress facultative aerobic organisms. However, low concentrations of neomycin sulfate may be inhibitory to *C. botulinum* Type E. Likewise, heat treatment should be used with caution. The selection of colonies is aided by the use of egg yolk agar; with the exception of type G, *C. botulinum* produces opalescence and a pearly layer. Culture on lactose egg yolk milk agar distinguishes proteolytic and nonproteolytic variants. Types C, D, and E produce nonlactose, nonproteolytic fermenting lipolytic colonies. Also there are nonproteolytic variants of Types B and F.

EPIDEMIOLOGY. *C. botulinum* is unevenly but widely distributed throughout the world. The natural habitat is the soil. Types A and B are the most common around the world. Type E has been found in Japan, Alaska, Canada, Russia, and also near the Baltic Sea. Type G was first isolated by Gimenez and Cicarrelli (1966, 1970) from Argentinian soil. Type E occurs in fish and in mud and shore waters; toxin production may increase to levels that affect fish. Intensive growth of *C. botulinum* may occur in overstocked fish farms in which the fish are overfed. The infection is more difficult to control when the floor of the pond is earth rather than concrete.

Drought appears to encourage proliferation of the organism in mud and wildlife, such as fish, ducks, and seagulls. In foods, the germination of spores and the growth of vegetative cells are necessary for toxin production. The spores survive cooking, smoking, and salting; nitrite is required in the curing of salted meats to prevent the outgrowth of spores. Potassium sorbate inhibits the vegetative cells (Blocher and Busta, 1983). Home-preserved foods are most frequently responsible for botulism. Examples are home-canned or salted low-acid vegetables, smoked or pickled fish, and pork products cured with salt without the addition of nitrite. Cheese can become toxigenic when acid production is deficient. Processes for commercially canned foods are usually calculated to destroy the spores of *C. botulinum* that are particularly resistant to heat. Outbreaks of botulism attributable to commercially canned foods have involved both underprocessing and postprocessing contamination. Micro-leaks in cans are significant even when chlorinated water is used for cooling, because although vegetative cells may be destroyed by chlorine, spores are not. Thus, adequate methods of food preservation are important in the prevention of botulism in both commercial and home processing of foods. Nonacid foods may be particularly dangerous.

CLOSTRIDIUM NOVYI (C. OEDEMATIENS)

Type D is sometimes called *C. hemolyticum.*

MORPHOLOGY. The organism is a fairly large gram-positive bacillus that is motile and strictly anaerobic. It sporulates freely, and the spores are large, subterminal and expand the rod. In young cultures it resembles *C. perfringens.* Colonies are irregular or circular and semi-translucent with a finely lobulated or crenelated edge. The surface is finely granular. Growth may spread.

ANTIGENIC COMPOSITION. There are four types: A, B, C, and D. All strains of *C. novyi* Types A, B, and C share two somatic antigens in varying proportions. Fluorescent-labeled antiserum prepared against Type B organisms stains strains of all types.

METABOLISM. Glucose and maltose are fermented by Types A and B, but only glucose is fermented by Types C and D. All types produce gelatinase but do not attack more complex proteins. Type D produces large amounts of indole; and H_2S is formed by all strains and especially by Type D. Products of metabolism include propionic and butyric acids and small amounts of acetic and valeric acids.

PATHOGENIC PROPERTIES. Types A and B cause gas gangrene in man and animals; Types B and D are responsible for other diseases in animals. Type A is the most common clinical pathogen.

TOXICOLOGY. Eight different soluble toxic antigens have been demonstrated in culture filtrates. Types A and B produce necrotizing lethal α-toxin, which increases capillary permeability and causes the characteristic gelatinous edema of muscle seen in *C. novyi* gas gangrene. Production of α-toxin is apparently bacteriophage-dependent. Types A and B also produce lecithinase C enzymes that are hemolytic, necrotizing, and lethal (Type B).

LABORATORY DIAGNOSIS. Isolation is often difficult and slow, particularly for Type D. Media should be freshly poured or prereduced. The cysteine dithiothreitol medium of Moore (1968) is recommended for Types B, C, and D. Before culture, the material may be heated at 80° to 100° C for 10 to 15 minutes. Preliminary enrichment in cooked meat broth is of value. Reactions on half-antitoxin lactose egg yolk milk agar are species specific and type specific for Type A strains; there is a diffuse lecithinase C opalescence and a restricted pearly layer due to lipolysis. Strains of Types B and D produce opalescence only, while Type C strains are egg yolk–negative. Animal inoculation and protection tests may be used. Neomycin sulfate can be used in culture media to suppress facultative organisms.

EPIDEMIOLOGY. The organism is widely distributed in soil and (Types A and B) in the livers of healthy animals. Approximately 42 per cent of the cases of gas gangrene in World War II were due to *C. novyi.*

CLOSTRIDIUM HISTOLYTICUM

MORPHOLOGY. The bacillus is gram-positive and motile. It is not an exacting anaerobe. Spores are formed readily except under aerobic conditions. They are large, oval, subterminal, and distend the organism.

The colonies are small, circular, opaque, shiny, and grayish white with an entire edge. There is a narrow zone of hemolysis on horse blood agar.

ANTIGENIC COMPOSITION AND TOXICOLOGY. There is no division into types. Oakley and Warrack (1950) demonstrated three separated soluble antigens in culture filtrates as follows:

α-toxin, lethal and necrotizing.

β-antigen, collagenase, attacking azocoll and gelatin.

γ-antigen, proteinase, attacking azocoll, gelatin, and casein.

δ-antigen, an elastase (Oakley and Banerjee, 1963).

METABOLISM. The organism ferments no sugars. It is strongly proteolytic and attacks gelatin and more complex proteins. H_2S is formed but not indole. Acetic acid is the only volatile product.

PATHOGENIC PROPERTIES. The organism is pathogenic for man and animals. In man it is associated, together with other anaerobes, with gas gangrene infections.

LABORATORY DIAGNOSIS. The organism grows slowly aerobically but is atypical and pleomorphic without spores; growth is improved under anaerobic conditions. Colonies are easily recognized on lactose egg yolk milk agar. There is partial clearing, lactose is not attacked, and there is no typical egg yolk reaction. Neomycin sulfate may be used to eliminate facultative organisms, and differential heating may be used for the same purpose. In cooked meat broth, there is vigorous proteolysis of the meat particles.

EPIDEMIOLOGY. The organism is widely but sparsely distributed in soil and probably also in the intestinal tract of man and animals.

CLOSTRIDIUM SEPTICUM AND CLOSTRIDIUM CHAUVOEI

The characteristics of these two organisms are similar and sometimes they are considered as a single species, *C. septicum* Types A and B (*C. chauvoei*).

MORPHOLOGY. They are gram-positive bacilli, particularly in young cultures. Spores are oval and subterminal, distending the organism. They are strict anaerobes. Colonies of *C. septicum* are small with a coarse rhizoidal edge and they may spread. There is beta hemolysis on horse blood agar. *C. chauvoei* colonies are small, umbonate, irregular or circular, shiny, and semitranslucent.

ANTIGENIC COMPOSITION. *C. septicum* is divisible into two groups on the basis of the O antigen; neither group cross-reacts with *C. chauvoei*, which possesses a common O antigen (Moussa, 1959). Batty and Walker (1963) found that both organisms could be differentiated by the fluorescent antibody technique. The swarming growth of *C. septicum* can be prevented by treating plates with a polyvalent *C. septicum* O antiserum before inoculation.

METABOLISM. Both organisms ferment glucose, maltose, and lactose; in addition, *C. septicum* ferments salicin and *C. chauvoei* ferments sucrose. Both produce H_2S but not indole, both produce gelatinase and deoxyribonuclease. Acetic, butyric, and formic acids are formed.

PATHOGENIC PROPERTIES. *C. septicum* is pathogenic for man and animals and is associated with gas gangrene in man. *C. chauvoei* is pathogenic only for animals, especially ruminants.

TOXICOLOGY. *C. septicum* produces three exotoxins. The α-toxin is lethal, necrotizing, and hemolytic; the β-toxin is deoxyribonuclease; and the γ-toxin is hyaluronidase. A neuraminidase and hemagglutinin are also formed. *C. chauvoei* also produces α- β- and γ-toxins and an oxygen-labile hemolysin; all appear to be related to the corresponding antigens produced by *C. septicum*.

IMMUNITY. *C. septicum* antitoxin provides homologous protection and also protection against *C. chauvoei*. *C. chauvoei* antitoxin does not protect against *C. septicum* toxemia, because *C. septicum* produces additional toxins, in particular, the α-toxin, which is unrelated to the α-toxin of *C. chauvoei*.

LABORATORY DIAGNOSIS. Both organisms are easy to grow; *C. chauvoei* is encouraged by the presence of liver in the medium. Preliminary enrichment is helpful and neomycin sulfate may be used to discourage growth of facultative aerobic contaminants; initial heating is also useful. The organisms are egg yolk–negative. In clinical medicine, it is important to distinguish *C. septicum* from *C. chauvoei*. Animal protection tests should be used. In cooked meat medium, both organisms produce small amounts of gas, and the meat particles may become pink.

EPIDEMIOLOGY. Both organisms are found chiefly in soil and also in the intestinal tract of herbivorous animals.

CLOSTRIDIUM SPOROGENES

MORPHOLOGY. The bacillus is strongly gram-positive. Sporulation is profuse, and the spores are oval, subterminal, and distend the cell. Free spores are common. The colonies are umbonate, opaque with a grayish white center, flat, irregular or circular with a rhizoidal edge, and they may spread. There is no hemolysis.

ANTIGENIC COMPOSITION. Soluble antigens of clinical significance are not produced.

METABOLISM. Glucose and mannitol are fermented but not lactose or sucrose. Gelatin and more complex proteins are broken down. H_2S is formed but not indole. A wide range of acids and alcohols are produced, particularly acetic, propionic, isobutyric, isovaleric, and isocaproic acids.

PATHOGENIC PROPERTIES. In mixed clostridial infections *C. sporogenes* increases the virulence of pathogenic species such as *C. perfringens* and *C. septicum*. There are local putrefactive changes in inoculated muscles, especially after damage has occurred; occasionally guinea pigs may die after inoculation.

LABORATORY DIAGNOSIS. Heat treatment and neomycin sulfate may be used to suppress facultative aerobic organisms. On lactose milk yolk agar, there is restricted opalescence, and a pearly layer develops from lipase activity. Growth is surrounded by wide zones of clearing due to proteolysis of the milk. In cooked meat broth, meat particles are attacked and partly digested. A scum of fatty acids may develop on the surface. Cultures have the odor of skatole.

EPIDEMIOLOGY. *C. sporogenes* is widely distributed in nature, both in soil and in the intestinal tract of man and animals. It is not easily distinguishable from nontoxic sporulating strains of *C. botulinum.*

CLOSTRIDIUM BIFERMENTANS AND CLOSTRIDIUM SORDELLII

MORPHOLOGY. The organisms are strongly gram-positive bacilli, motile, and not exacting in their requirements. They spore readily, and the spores are large and cylindrical, usually central and slightly distending the cell. Chains of sporulating organisms are formed, and free spores are common.

The colonies of both organisms are low, convex with an entire but irregular edge, and grayish white; they may swarm. There is a narrow zone of hemolysis on horse blood agar.

ANTIGENIC COMPOSITION. Walker (1963) differentiated the two species on the basis of spore agglutinogens but not spore precipitinogens. There was no cross-agglutination or precipitation between the spores of the *C. sporogenes, C. histolyticum, C. sphenoides,* and *C. perfringens* Types A to D.

METABOLISM. Glucose and maltose are attacked but not lactose or sucrose. In addition, *C. bifermentans* ferments mannose, sorbitol, and salicin; and *C. sordellii* is urease positive. Gelatin and more complex proteins are broken down by both organisms, and H_2S and indole are produced.

Large amounts of acetic, isobutyric, and isovaleric and small amounts of propionic and isocaproic acids are formed.

PATHOGENIC PROPERTIES. Intramuscular inoculation of a pathogenic strain of *C. sordellii* kills guinea pigs in one to two days. Proteolysis of tissues may progress in the same way as that of *C. histolyticum* infections; there is hemorrhage and gas production. Rifkin et al. (1977) describe infection by *C. sordellii* in colitis induced by antibiotics.

TOXICOLOGY. Pathogenic strains of *C. sordellii* produce a lethal toxin for which antitoxic sera are available. All strains of *C. sordellii* and *C. bifermentans* produce a lecithinase C that is antigenically related to, but not identical with, the lecithinase C (α-toxin) of *C. perfringens.* There are indications that at least one other soluble antigen is produced by these organisms.

LABORATORY DIAGNOSIS. Heat treatment and neomycin sulfate in or on solid media help to inhibit facultative aerobic organisms. On lactose egg yolk milk agar there is extensive opalescence that is inhibited by *C. perfringens* Type A antitoxin, but the inhibition is seldom complete. There is no pearly layer; lactose is not fermented; zones of partial clearing indicate that milk is attacked. In cooked meat broth, the meat particles are partly digested, and a viscous mucoid deposit is produced that is peculiar to these organisms.

EPIDEMIOLOGY. Both organisms are widely distributed in the soil and in the large bowel of man and animals.

CLOSTRIDIUM DIFFICILE

MORPHOLOGY. The bacilli are long, slender, motile, gram-positive, and strictly anaerobic. The spores are large, oval, subterminal, and distend the organism. Colonies are 2 to 3 mm in diameter, white, opaque, circular with an entire margin, and nonhemolytic on horse blood agar.

ANTIGENIC COMPOSITION AND BEHAVIOR OF TOXINS. Two immunologically distinct toxins are described, a cytotoxin and an enterotoxin (Taylor et al., 1981; Libby and Wilkens, 1982). They caused similar morphological changes in tissue-culture cells but there were differences in toxin potency and cell sensitivity (Donta et al., 1982). Not all strains produce the cytotoxin (Muldrow et al., 1982). The cytotoxicity is neutralized by commercially available *C. sordellii* antitoxin (Leader, 1980). Taylor et al. (1981) describe mucosal destruction in the ileal loop of the hamster by the enterotoxin. Cholestyramine binds the toxin in the bowel lumen and is used for treatment of *C. difficile*–induced colitis.

METABOLISM. The organism is nonproteolytic and egg yolk–negative. It ferments glucose and mannitol, but not maltose, lactose, or sucrose. Indole and H_2S are not formed. There are many products of fermentation including small amounts of acetic, propionic, isobutyric, butyric, isovaleric, valeric, and isocaproic acids.

PATHOGENIC PROPERTIES. The diseases associated with *C. difficile* follow prolonged antimicrobial therapy, especially with clindamycin, but also with ampicillin, cephalosporins, trimethoprim plus sulfamethoxazole, tetracycline and chloramphenicol. These diseases include: pseudomembranous colitis (PMC), antibiotic-associated diarrhea, chronic inflammatory bowel disease, postoperative diarrhea, and neonatal diarrhea. George et al. (1982) examined fecal specimens from 223 patients and concluded that, although *C. difficile* appeared to be a major cause of PMC, it was not responsible for at least two-thirds of cases of antimicrobial agent-associated diarrhea in which PMC was not documented. The isolation of *C. difficile* or the detection of cytotoxin should not be considered diagnostic of *C. difficile*–induced disease. Falson et al. (1980) examined 2390 fecal samples for intestinal pathogens and concluded that the causative significance of *C. difficile* might be doubtful in most cases of diarrhea.

LABORATORY DIAGNOSIS. Direct and enrichment techniques should be used with base media containing antibiotic supplement including cycloserine and cefoxitin. *C. difficile* is tolerant to cresol, and paracresol (0.2 per cent) may be added to enrichment broth (cooked meat). The presence of cytotoxin in fecal supernatant can be demonstrated by means of tissue culture cells; the effect is inhibited by *C. sordellii* antitoxin.

EPIDEMIOLOGY. Walters et al. (1982) traced an outbreak of PMC in an intensive care unit to a patient who had received several antibiotics in the previous three months. After treatment with vancomycin the diarrhea stopped, but excretion of *C. difficile* continued. The organism was isolated from various sites in four cubicles for 3 to 7 weeks. Patients in two cubicles developed diarrhea and *C. difficile* and toxin were found in stools; in the previous two years

C. difficile was not found in stools from patients with diarrhea following antibiotic treatment.

ANTIBIOTIC SUSCEPTIBILITY. *C. difficile* is almost uniformly sensitive to vancomycin and it is used to treat colitis attributed to this organism.

Acknowledgements

All those whose work and research have enabled this information to be assembled are acknowledged with gratitude. The author and editors are particularly grateful to Dr. A. T. Willis for his clear exposition of the facts in his book *Anaerobic Bacteriology: Clinical and Laboratory Practice*, third edition, and for his willingness to allow some of his material to be abstracted. We are grateful also to Butterworth and Co. (Publishers) Ltd. for their permission.

References

Ayliffe, G. A. J., and Lowbury, E. J. L.: Sources of gas gangrene in hospital. Br Med J 2:333, 1969.

Batty, I., and Walker, P. D.: Differentiation of *Clostridium septicum* and *Clostridium chauvoei* by the use of fluorescent labelled antibodies. J Pathol Bacteriol 85:517, 1963.

Beerens, H., Romond Ch., Lepage, C., and Criquelion, J.: A Liquid Medium for the Enumeration of *Clostridium perfringens* in Food and Faeces. In Isolation and Identification Methods for Food Poisoning Organisms. Corry, J. E. L., Roberts, D., and Skinner, F. A. (eds.). Society for Applied Bacteriology Tech Series 17. Academic Press, 1982.

Blocher, J. C., and Busta, F. F.: Influence of potassium sorbate and reduced pH on the growth of vegetative cells of four strains of type A and B *Clostridium botulinum*. J. Food Sc., 48: 574–575, 5808, 1983.

Clifford, W. J., and Annellis, A.: *Clostridium perfringens*. I. Sporulation in a biphasic glucose-ion-exchange resin medium. Appl Microbiol 22:856, 1971.

Collee, J. G., Knowlden, J. A., and Hobbs, B. C.: Studies on the growth, sporulation, and carriage of *Clostridium welchii* with special reference to food poisoning strains. J Appl Bacteriol 24:326, 1961.

Donta, S. T., Sullivan N., and Wilkins, T. D.: Differential effects of *Clostridium difficile* toxins on tissue-cultured cells. J Clin Microbiol 15:1157–1158, 1982

Dowell, B. R., Jr., Torres-Angel, M. J., Reimann, H. P., Merson, M., Whaley, D., and Darland, G.: A new criterion for implicating *Clostridium perfringens* as the cause of food poisoning. Rev Lat-Am Microbiol 17:137, 1975.

Drasar, B. S.: Anaerobic bacteria and cancer. In Usha Gupta (ed.): Anaerobic Infections in Man. Everyman's Press, Delhi, 1982.

Duncan, C. E., and Strong, D. H.: Improved medium for the sporulation of *Clostridium perfringens*. Appl Microbiol 16:82, 1968.

Duncan, C. E., and Strong, D. H.: *Clostridium perfringens* type A food poisoning. Response of the rabbit ileum as an indication of enteropathogenicity of strains of *Clostridium perfringens* in monkeys. Infec Immun 3:167, 1971.

Ellner, P. D.: A medium promoting rapid sporulation in *Clostridium perfringens*. J Bacteriol 71:495, 1956.

Falson, E., Kaiiser, B., Nehls, L., Niygten, B., and Svodhem, H.: *Clostridium difficile* in relation to enteric bacterial pathogens. J Clin Microbiol 12:397, 1980.

George, W. L., Rolfe, R. D., and Finegold, S. M.: *Clostridium difficile* and its cytotoxin in feces of patients with antimicrobial agent-associated diarrhea and miscellaneous conditions. J Clin Microbiol 15:1049–1053, 1982.

Gimenez, D. G., and Ciccarelli, A. S.: A new type of *Clostridium botulinum*. In Ingram, M., and Roberts, T. A. (eds.): Botulism. Proceedings of the 5th International Symposium on Food Microbiology, July 1966. London. Chapman and Hall, 1966, p. 455.

Gimenez, D. F., and Ciccarelli, A. S.: Another type of *Clostridium botulinum*. Zentralbl Bakteriol Parasitol Infektionskrankh Hyg Abt I [Orig] 215:221, 1970.

Hauschild, A. H. W.: Criteria and procedures for implicating *Clostridium perfringens* in food-borne outbreaks. Can J Public Health 66:388, 1975.

Hauschild, A. H. W.: Food poisoning by *Clostridium perfringens*. Can Inst Food Sci Technol J 6:106, 1973.

Henderson, D. W.: The somatic antigens of the *Cl. welchii* group of organisms. J Hyg Camb 40:501, 1940.

Hobbs, B. C., Smith, M. E., Oakley, C. L., Warrack, G. H., and Cruickshank, J. C.: *Clostridium welchii* food poisoning. J Hyg Camb 51:75, 1953.

Hobbs, G., Crowther, J. S., Weaver, P., Gibbs, P. A., and Jarvis, B.: Detection and Isolation of *Clostridium botulinum*. In Corry, J. E. L., Roberts, D., and Skinner, F. A. (eds.): Isolation and Identification Methods for Food Poisoning Organisms. Society for Applied Bacteriology Tech Series 17. Academic Press, 1982.

Howard, F. M., Bradley, J. M., Flynn, D. M., Noone, P., and Szawatkowski, M.: Outbreak of necrotizing enterocolitis caused by *Clostridium butyricum*. Lancet 11:1099, 1977.

Hughes, J. A., Turnbull, P. C. B., and Stringer, M. E.: A serotyping system for *Clostridium welchii (Clostridium perfringens)* type A, and studies on the type-specific antigens. J Med Microbiol 9:475, 1976.

Klein, E.: On a pathogenic anaerobic intestinal bacillus, Bacillus enteritidis sporogenes. Zantralbl Bakteriol 1 Abt 18:737, 1895.

Knox, R., and MacDonald, E. J.: Outbreaks of food poisoning in certain Leicester institutions. Med Off 69:21, 1943.

Lawrence, G., and Walker, P. D.: Pathogenesis of enteritis necroticans in Papua New Guinea. Lancet 1:125, 1976.

Leader.: Clostridia as intestinal pathogens. Lancet ii:1113, 1977.

Leader.: *Clostridium difficile* and chronic bowel disease. Lancet i, 402–403. 1980.

Lewis, G. E., Jr. (ed.): Biomedical aspects of botulism. Proceedings of an International Conference, Fort Detrick, Maryland. Academic Press Inc., 1981.

McClung, L. S.: Human food poisoning due to growth of *Clostridium perfringens (Cl. welchii)* in freshly cooked chickens: Preliminary note. J Bacteriol 50:229, 1945.

McClung, L. S., and Toabe, R.: Egg-yolk plate reaction for presumptive diagnosis of *Clostridium sporogenes* and certain species of gangrene and botulinum groups. J Bacteriol 53:139, 1947.

Mead, C. C.: Growth and sporulation of *Clostridium welchii* in breast and leg muscle of poultry. J Appl Bacteriol 32:86, 1969.

Mersom, M. H., and Dowell, V. R.: Epidemiologic clinical and laboratory aspects of wound botulism. N Engl J Med 289:1005, 1973.

Midura, T. F., and Arnon, S. S.: Infant botulism. Identification of *Clostridium botulinum* and its toxins in feces. Lancet 11:934, 1976.

Miles, A. A., and Misra, S. S.: The estimation of the bactericidal power of blood. J Hyg Camb 38:732, 1938.

Moore, W. G.: Solidified media suitable for the cultivation of *Clostridium novyi* type B. J Gen Microbiol 53:415, 1968.

Moussa, R. S.: Antigenic formulae for *Clostridium septicum* and *Clostridium chauvoei*. J Pathol Bacteriol 77:341, 1959.

Muldrow, L. L., Archibold, E. R., Ninez-Montiel, O. L., and Sheehy, R. J.: Survey of the extrachromosomal gene pool of *Clostridium difficile*. J Clin Microbiol 16:637–640, 1982.

Murrell, T. G. C., Egerton, J. R., Rampling, A., Samuels, J., and Walker, P. D.: The ecology and epidemiology of the pig-bel syndrome in man in New Guinea. J Hyg Camb 64:375, 1966.

Nagler, F. P. O.: Observations on a reaction between the lethal toxin of *Cl. welchii* (Type A) and human serum. Br J Exp Pathol 20:473, 1939.

Niilo, L.: Enterotoxigenic *Clostridium perfringens* type A isolated from intestinal contents of cattle, sheep and chickens. Canad J Comp Med Vet Sci 42:357–363, 1978.

Niilo, L.: Enterotoxin formation by *Clostridium perfringens* type A studied by the use of fluorescent antibody. Can J Microbiol 23:908, 1977.

Oakley, C. L., and Banerjee, N. G.: Bacterial elastases. J Pathol Bacteriol 85:489, 1963.

Oakley, C. L., and Warrack, G. H.: The ACRA test as a means of estimating hyaluronidase deoxyribonuclease and their antibodies. J Path Bact 63:45, 1951.

Oakley, C. L., and Warrack, G. H.: Routine typing of *Clostridium welchii*. J Hyg Camb 51:102, 1953.

Parker, M. T.: Clostridial sepsis. Br Med J 2:698, 1967.

Rifkin, G. D., Fekety, F. R., Silva, J., and Sack, R. B.: Antibiotic-induced colitis: Implications of a toxin neutralized by *Clostridium sordellii* antitoxin. Lancet ii:1103, 1977.

Schantz, E. J., and Sugyama, H.: Toxic proteins produced by *Clostridium botulinum*. Agric Food Chem 22:26, 1974.

Skjelkvåle, R., and Duncan, C. L.: Enterotoxin formation by different toxigenic types of *Clostridium perfringens*. Infect Immun 11:563, 1975.

Stark, R. L., and Duncan, C. L.: Transient increase in capillary permeability induced by *Clostridium perfringens* type A enterotoxin. Infect Immun 5:147–150, 1972.

Stringer, M. F., Watson, G. N., and Gilbert, R. J.: *Clostridium perfringens* type A. Serological typing methods for the detection of enterotoxin. In Corry, J. E. L., Roberts, D., and Skinner, F. A. (eds.): Isolation and Identification Methods for Food Poisoning Organisms. Society for Applied Bacteriology Tech Series 17. Academic Press, 1982.

Stringer, M. F., Shah, N., and Gilbert, R. J.: Serological typing of *Clostridium perfringens* and its epidemiological significance in the investigation of food poisoning outbreaks. Proceedings of IAMS meeting in Szczecin, Poland, 1978.

Sutton, R. G. A.: The pathogenesis and epidemiology of *Clostridium welchii* food poisoning. Thesis (Ph.D), University of London, 1969.

Sutton, R. G. A., Ghosh, A. C., and Hobbs, B. C.: Isolation and enumeration of *Clostridium perfringens*. In Shapton, D. A., and Board, R. G. (eds.): Isolation of Anaerobes. Soc Appl Bact Tech Ser No 5 London, Academic Press, 1971, p. 39.

Taylor, N. S., Thorne, G. M., and Bartlett, J. G.: Comparison of two toxins produced by *Clostridium difficile*. Infect Immun 34:1036–1043, 1981.

Torres-Anjel, M. J., Reimann, H. P., and Tsai, Che C.: A fluorescent-antibody technique for the detection of enterotoxin-producing cells of *Clostridium perfringens* type A. Scientific Publication No. 305. New York, Pan American Health Organization (World Health Organization), 1975.

Torres-Anjel, M. J., and Reimann, H. P.: Enterotoxic *Clostridium perfringens* in selected humans. II. A cohort study. Rev Lat Am Microbiol 17:199, 1975.

Tsai, C. C., Torres-Anjel, M. J., and Reimann, H. P.: Improved culture techniques and sporulation medium for enterotoxin production by *Clostridium perfringens* type C. J Formosan Med Assoc 73:404–409, 1974.

van Heyningen, W. E.: The pathogenic actions of exotoxins. Zentralbl Bacteriol Parasitol Infect Hyg Abt I [Orig] 212:191, 1970.

van Heyningen, W. E.: Tetanus. Sci Am 218:69, 1968.

Vernon, E.: Food poisoning and salmonella infections in England and Wales 1973–1975. An analysis of reports to the Public Health Laboratory Service. Public Health 91:225, 1977.

Walker, P. D.: The spore antigens of *Clostridium sporogenes, Cl. bifermentans* and *Cl. sordellii,* J Pathol Bacteriol 85:41, 1963.

Walker, P. D., and Batty, I.: Fluorescent studies in the genus *Clostridium*. II. A rapid method for differentiating *Clostridium botulinum* types A, B, and F, types C and D, and type E. J Appl Bacteriol 27:140, 1964.

Watson, G. N., Stringer, M., Gilbert, R. J., and Mahony, D. E.: The potential of bacteriocin typing in the study of *Clostridium perfringens* food poisoning. J Clin Pathol 35:1361–1365, 1982.

Willis, A. T.: Anaerobic Bacteriology: Clinical and Laboratory Practice. Third edition. Butterworth & Co. (Publishers) Ltd. 1977.

Willis, A. T., and Williams, K.: Prevention of swarming of *Clostridium septicum*. J Med Microbiol 5:493, 1972.

Zeissler, J., and Rassfeld-Sternberg, L.: Enteritis necroticans due to *Clostridium welchii* type F. Br Med J 1:267, 1949.

50

BACTEROIDES

TOR HOFSTAD, M.D.

The genus *Bacteroides* comprises a heterogeneous group of nonspore-forming, obligately anaerobic rods that often are very pleomorphic. Their habitat is the mucous membranes of man and animals. They can be differentiated from *Fusobacterium* by their inability to produce substantial amounts of butyric acid from glucose.

The *Bacteroides* species most frequently encountered in clinical specimens are those of the *B. fragilis* group (*B. fragilis, B. distasonis, B. ovatus, B. thetaiotaomicron, B. uniformis, B. vulgatus*) followed by the black-pigmented bacteroides (*B. asaccharolyticus, B. melaninogenicus*). Other species pathogenic for man are *B. bivius, B. disiens, B. ureolyticus* and organisms of the *B. oralis-ruminicola* group.

They are an important cause of abscesses in the abdomen, pelvis, lung, and brain, usually in the company of peptostreptococci and other intestinal or oralpharyngeal aerobic or anaerobic bacteria that join with them in invading dead or dying tissues.

MORPHOLOGY. Cells of the *B. fragilis* group are nonmotile, pale-staining, gram-negative straight or slightly curved rods with rounded ends, 0.5 to 1.0 μm in diameter and 0.5 to 5.0 μm long, occurring singly and in pairs. Irregular staining, which is often bipolar, may be seen. Cells grown in fluid media containing a fermentable carbohydrate tend to be more pleomorphic than cells grown in solid media. Short filaments and, in particular, vacuolated cells may be seen in such cultures. Ovoid forms are common in some strains. *B. melaninogenicus* and *B. asacharolyticus* are nonmotile, evenly-staining, gram-negative coccobacilli, 0.3 to 0.4 μm wide and 0.6 to 2.0 μm long. Fluid cultures of some strains show larger, pale, and highly vacuolated cells, with some densely stained areas. Cells of *B. ureolyticus* are nonmotile, pale-staining, gram-negative rods, 0.5 to 0.7 μm in width and 1.0 to 3.0 μm long, occurring singly or in pairs. Filaments are occasionally seen. Other *Bacteroides* species are characterized by short to medium-sized rods, which may be pleomorphic.

The ultrastructure of *Bacteroides,* as seen in the electron microscope, is that of a gram-negative bacterium. The cell wall has an electron-dense, solid layer containing the peptidoglycan and an outer, trilaminar membrane made up of protein, lipid, and polysaccharide. A capsular polysaccharide is present in *B. fragilis* (Kasper, 1976). Encapsulation has been observed also in some isolates of other species within the *B. fragilis* group and among black-pigmented *Bacteroides*.

ANTIGENIC COMPOSITION. The best studied *Bacteroides* antigens are the cell wall lipopolysaccharides and the capsular polysaccharide of *B. fragilis.* Both are type-specific antigens. The lipopolysaccharides consist of a heteropolysaccharide portion and a covalently bound lipid component (lipid A). The structure of the heteropolysaccharide is largely unknown. Heptose, which is an essential constituent of most other bacterial lipopolysaccharides, is not present. The lipid A of the species of the *B. fragilis* group contains only trace amounts or no 3-hydroxytetradecanoic acid, another constituent typical of bacterial lipopolysaccharides. The capsular polysaccharide of *B. fragilis* has a complex and unusual chemical structure.

The outer membrane of the *B. fragilis* group contains a protein antigen that may be species specific.

GROWTH AND METABOLISM. The clinically important *Bacteroides* species grow well anaerobically on blood agar and in enriched media containing peptone and yeast extract. After two days of incubation, surface colonies of species of the *B. fragilis* group on sheep or horse blood agar become 1 to 3 mm in diameter, circular, entire, convex, semiopaque, grayish to whitish, and nonhemolytic. Colonies of some strains may be soft and shiny. The black-pigmented bacteroides grow on blood agar with entire, circular, convex to pulvinate colonies, which after incubation for two days measure 0.5 to 2 mm in diameter. Old colonies are often surrounded by flattened margins. Colonies of some strains are shiny or slightly mucoid. Colonies are whitish or slightly gray in color when young, but after two or three days of incubation they take on a slightly tan to brownish pigment, and soon become jet black. The pigment is formed earlier on agar that contains laked blood rather than intact erythrocytes. The tan and light brown colonies fluoresce pink or orange, and the darker colonies show red under ultraviolet light (365 nm). Entirely black colonies do not fluoresce. The colonies are β-hemolytic or nonhemolytic. Surface colonies of *B. ureolyticus* range from barely visible to 0.5 mm in diameter after two days of incubation. Upon continued incubation they grow to about 1 mm in diameter and are gray-white, convex or umbonate circular colonies with slightly undulating or entire margins that seem to disappear into the agar. Their ability to corrode, or pit, the agar may be lost after continued cultivation in fluid media. Colonies of most other *Bacteroides* species resemble those of the *B. fragilis* group but are usually smaller and may be β-hemolytic.

In fluid media (prereduced and anaerobically sterilized) growth of *Bacteroides* causes turbidity and, frequently, a sediment that may be smooth, ropy or stringy. A small amount of gas is produced by most strains of the *B. fragilis* group. Organisms of the *B. fragilis* group grow well in semifluid media incubated in air at 37°C. Under the same cultural conditions, other *Bacteroides* species grow slowly or not at all.

The *Bacteroides* grow best at 37° C and at a pH of about 7.0. With some exceptions they are moderate anaerobes that grow maximally in oxygen tensions of up to 3 per cent. The members of the *B. fragilis* group are the most oxygen-tolerant *Bacteroides*.

The energy metabolism of *Bacteroides* is virtually unknown. There is evidence that *B. fragilis* has a primitive type of electron transport system with cytochrome B that is linked to the reduction of fumarate. The asaccharolytic *B. ureolyticus* seems to gain energy by the transfer of electrons from hydrogen or formate to fumarate.

The organisms of the *B. fragilis* group have simple nutritional requirements. They have an obligate need of vitamin B_{12}, and the growth of most strains is stimulated by hemin and bile. Ammonium is the preferred nitrogen source rather than amino acids. A fermentable carbohydrate is essential for good growth. The other *Bacteroides* species are more fastidious anaerobes. The black-pigmented *Bacteroides* have an obligate requirement for hemin and for peptides, and many strains need vitamin K. The organisms grow well in media based on tryptone and tryptose. Serum or L-asparagine often stimulates growth. Bile is growth-inhibitory. Fumaric acid has been found to stimulate growth of *B. ureolyticus*. This organism grows best in a liver digest medium with added yeast extract and blood. Strains of several *Bacteroides* species require carbon dioxide.

Most bacteroides metabolize carbohydrates. The fermentation products include combinations of acetic, lactic, succinic, propionic, isobutyric, isovaleric, and formic acids. Butyric acid is formed by a few species but not as a major product. The organisms of the *B. fragilis* group are highly saccharolytic, giving a final pH in glucose broth of about 5.0 to 5.4. *B. ureolyticus* does not ferment carbohydrates. *B. asaccharolyticus* is highly proteolytic. The organism can hydrolyze casein, gelatin, plasma proteins, and collagen. Indole is produced by some *Bacteroides* species. Catalase, lecithinase, and lipase are usually not produced. *B. fragilis* and some other bacteroides hydrolyze aesculin. Dehydrogenases specific for different amino acids and other organic acids are present in *Bacteroides* and have been used for differentiation between members of the species.

PATHOGENIC PROPERTIES. The pathogenic *Bacteroides* species are part of the normal microflora of mucous membranes, particularly those of the gastrointestinal and upper respiratory tracts. They are harmless inhabitants unless the mucous membrane barrier is broken. The *Bacteroides*, like other microorganisms on the mucosa, may then invade the adjacent tissue and cause localized infection or spread hematogenously to the liver, lung, or brain. Following aspiration they may be carried from the mouth into the lung. These endogenous infections are not communicable from one person to another.

A requisite for *Bacteroides* infection is lowering of the redox potential by tissue necrosis, impaired blood supply, and growth of facultative microorganisms in an infected area. The importance of underlying disease was illustrated in a study of 112 patients with Bacteroidaceae bacteremia, caused mainly by *B. fragilis* (Chow and Guze, 1974). Forty-three per cent of the patients had either malignancy, arteriosclerosis, alcoholic liver disease, diabetes mellitus, or end-stage renal disease. Underlying disease was the overriding determinant of mortality. The most significant factors in nonfatal infections were old age and a history of trauma or surgery.

The most common serious anaerobic infections encountered are caused by members of the family Bacteroidaceae, especially *B. fragilis* (Finegold, 1977). This organism may be implicated in suppurative lesions of almost every part of the human body, and is the anaerobic microorganism isolated most often from microbial infections. It is also the anaerobic gram-negative rod found most frequently in pure culture. Usually, however, *B. fragilis* and other *Bacteroides* are accompanied by facultative or other anaerobic bacteria such as peptostreptococci. Other bacteria are almost universally present in infections with *B. melaninogenicus* and *B. asaccharolyticus*, probably because they satisfy the need for vitamin K.

Members of the *B. fragilis* group are isolated from two-thirds or more of intra-abdominal infections. *B. fragilis* accounts for more than half of these isolates. The isolation of *B. ovatus* and *B. vulgatus* indicates contamination with normal fecal flora. Other *Bacteroides* species are isolated less often. Black-pigmented *Bacteroides*, organisms of the *B. oralis-ruminicola* group and *B. ureolyticus* are, together with *Fusobacterium nucleatum*, the most commonly encountered anaerobic rods in anaerobic pleuropulmonary disease (empyema, lung abscess, pneumonitis). *B. bivius*, *B. disiens*, black-pigmented *Bacteroides* and *B. fragilis* are often isolated from anaerobic infections of the female genital tract. *B. fragilis* is the anaerobic organism isolated most often from soft tissue infections. In septicemic patients *B. fragilis* is isolated in 5 to 10 per cent of all positive blood cultures. The common portals of entry are the gastrointestinal and female genital tract. *Bacteroides* species are often isolated from abscesses of the liver and brain, and may be implicated in decubital ulcers (Rissing et al., 1974) and gangrene, in dental infections, and in chronic infections of the paranasal sinuses and the middle ear. Occasionally *Bacteroides* species are isolated from osteomyelitis, purulent arthritis, infective endocarditis, and urinary tract infections.

Little is known about the pathogenesis of *Bacteroides* infections (Hofstad, 1983). Synergistic mechanisms are thought to play a role in mixed infections. Two such mechanisms are known: production of a low oxidation-reduction potential by facultative organisms, and supply of an essential growth factor. The capsular polysaccharide of *B. fragilis* may protect the organism against phagocytosis and produces abscess formation in rats (Onderdonk et al., 1977). The cell wall lipopolysaccharides of *Bacteroides* species have low toxicity compared to endotoxins of the facultative enteric bacilli (Sveen et al., 1977). Certain enzymes, like neuraminidase, deoxyribonuclease, IgA protease, and heparinase, may contribute to pathogenicity. *B. asaccharolyticus* is one of the few microorganisms that produces collagenase.

IMMUNITY. Low titers of IgM antibodies against antigens from *B. fragilis* and *B. melaninogenicus* are present in normal human serum, but their protective function is not known. Normal human serum kills *B. fragilis* group strains isolated from stools, and polymorphonuclear leukocytes can phagocytose them with the help of heat-labile opsonins (Bjornson and Bjornson, 1978). A rise in IgM and IgG antibodies in patients has been observed after *B. fragilis* septicemia and local suppurative lesions. The significance of these humoral antibodies in recovery from infection is unknown.

LABORATORY DIAGNOSIS. Pus, tissue from biopsies of normally sterile sites, transtracheal aspirates, pleural and ascitic fluids, aspirates from the nasal sinuses, carefully collected materials from the root canals and periapical tissues of teeth, cervical material collected by direct visualization, and specimens of blood should be cultured routinely for *Bacteroides* and other anaerobes. It is imperative to avoid contamination with normal flora. Whenever possible specimens should be taken by aspiration in large volumes. Purulent exudate is in itself a good transport medium.

Processing of Specimens. A Gram-stained smear should always be examined for characteristic gram-negative rods that do not appear in aerobic culture. The specimen is streaked on a nonselective solid medium, preferably Brucella blood agar (tryptose agar with glucose added), and on laked blood agar containing 75 μg/ml of kanamycin and 7.5 μg/ml of vancomycin, which is selective for *Bacteroides*. The plates are incubated for two days in GasPak jars or in ordinary anaerobic jars in an atmosphere of nitrogen and hydrogen with 5 to 10 per cent carbon dioxide. An enriched liquid medium, for instance chopped-meat glucose, is also inoculated. If prereduced anaerobically sterilized (PRAS) media are not available, semifluid media can be used.

Identification. A definite identification of the members of the *B. fragilis* group, and a presumptive identification of the other frequently encountered *Bacteroides* species, can be made on the basis of cellular morphology, colonial growth, ability to grow in a medium containing 20 per cent ox bile, and a few biochemical tests (Table 1). Fermentation of carbohydrates and hydrolysis of esculin should be performed in media containing peptone and yeast extract. The indole reaction can be carried out as a spot test or in a medium containing tryptone or tryptose, which are peptones rich in tryptophan. *B. ureolyticus* produces urease, reduces nitrate to nitrite, and pits the agar. The pitting may take days to develop or may not occur.

Micromethod multitest systems for identification of *Bacteroides* species and other anaerobic bacteria pathogenic in man are sold commercially. Fluorescent antibody techniques can be used for a rapid identification of black-pigmented *Bacteroides* and *B. fragilis* group in clinical materials and in pure cultures. The commercial kits available are not yet specific enough for species identification.

DRUG SUSCEPTIBILITY. All members of the *B. fragilis* group have a similar susceptibility pattern to antibacterial drugs. Of particular importance is the fact that the *B. fragilis* group is resistant to the aminoglycoside antibiotics, and is resistant to penicillins and first generation cephalosporins. Clindamycin usually inhibits *B. fragilis* group strains in a concentration of 0.2 μg/ml. The antibiotic is active also against most other anaerobes and has produced good results in the treatment of anaerobic infections. It does not penetrate well into the central nervous system. Serious colitis is seen sometimes in patients treated with clindamycin. Metronidazole, which inhibits *B. fragilis* group strains at 3 μg/ml or less, is bactericidal in the same concentration against anaerobic bacteria including the *B. fragilis* group but inactive against aerobic bacteria. The drug has a low toxicity and crosses the blood-brain barrier, but prolonged administration in large doses has caused tumors in an animal model. Tinidazol and other imidazol derivatives have similar antibacterial activity. *B. fragilis* is regularly inhibited by chloramphenicol at a level of 5 to 8 μg/ml and by erythromycin in concentrations of 2.0 μg/ml. The β-lactamase resistant cephalosporin, cefoxitin, is active against the *B. fragilis* group. A relatively small percentage of *B. fragilis* group isolates, varying from one geographic area to another, is susceptible to tetracycline in concentrations as low as 1.0 μg/ml.

Production of β-lactamase occurs in *B. fragilis*, frequently also in *B. bivius* and *B. disiens*, and has been observed in a growing number of isolates of the black-pigmented *Bacteroides* and the *B. oralis-ruminicola* group.

EPIDEMIOLOGY AND ECOLOGY. In human subjects on a Western diet, *Bacteroides* species are the predominant organisms of the lower intestinal tract, amounting to 10^{11} or more bacterial cells per gram of dry feces. The great majority is made up of *B. vulgatus* and *B. thetaiotaomicron*. *B. fragilis* is present in a comparatively low number. *Bacteroides* is normally found in small numbers in the terminal ileum. In patients with a continent ileostomy or with intestinal blind loops, there is bacterial overgrowth, a substantial part of which is caused by members of the *B. fragilis* group. The overgrowth is regularly associated with vitamin B_{12} malabsorption and steatorrhea (stagnant loop syndrome) (Farrar et al., 1975).

Black-pigmented *Bacteroides* constitute 4 to 8 per cent of the cultivable microflora of the gingival crevices and are the predominant *Bacteroides* species of the mouth. They become established in the mouth upon eruption of the permanent teeth. Black-pigmented *Bacteroides* are members of the normal flora of the upper respiratory tract,

Table 1. DISTINGUISHING CHARACTERISTICS OF THE MOST COMMON *BACTEROIDES* SPECIES

	Morphology			Biochemical Tests							
						Fermentation of					
Species	***Cellular***	***Colony***	**Growth Inhibition 20% Bile**	***Indole Production***	***Esculin Hydrolysis***	***Glucose***	***Lactose***	***Rhamnose***	***Mannitol***	***Trehalose***
B. fragilis	Short rods with rounded ends, may be ovoid or vacuolated, may show irregular staining	Convex, white to gray, glistening, nonhemolytic.	−	−	+	+	+	−	−	−
B. distasonis			−	−	+	+	+	V	−	+
B. vulgatus			−	−	+	+	+	+	−	−
B. ovatus			−	+	+	+	+	+	+	+
B. thetaiotaomicron			−	+	+	+	+	+	−	+
B. uniformis			−	+	+	+	+	V	−	−
B. asaccharolyticus	Coccobacilli or short rods with rounded ends	Tan to black, hemolytic	+	+	−	−	−			
B. melaninogenicus			+	V	−	+	V			
B. oralis-ruminicola group	Short rods with rounded ends	Convex, white to gray, often glistening. Mostly nonhemolytic	+	−	+	+	+			
B. bivius	Short rods with rounded ends	Convex, white to gray, may be glistening and hemolytic	+	−	−	+	+			
B. disiens	Medium or short rods with rounded ends	Convex, white to gray, shiny. Mostly nonhemolytic	+	−	−	+	−			
*B. ureolyticus**	Slender rods with rounded ends	Pin-point, may be corroding, nonhemolytic	+	−	−	−	−			

+, positive; −, negative; V, variable.
*urease-positive

vagina, external male and female genitalia, and skin between the toes.

B. bivius is the predominant *Bacteroides* species of the female genital tract. *B. disiens* is part of the normal microflora of female genitalia and the upper respiratory tract. The members of the *B. oralis-ruminicola* group and *B. ureolyticus* inhabit the mouth and the upper respiratory tract. The principal habitat of other *Bacteroides* species occasionally isolated from anaerobic infections seems to be the lower intestinal tract.

Bacteroides is frequently involved in hospital infections. Infection may be facilitated by radiation and surgery, and treatment with cytotoxic drugs. A substantial number of *Bacteroides* infections is associated with surgery. The use of antibiotics that select resistant anaerobes such as *B. fragilis* is thought to predispose to infection.

A significant morbidity and mortality attend infections with *Bacteroides*. Prophylaxis would require avoidance of any condition that reduces the normal redox potential of the tissues and the introduction of the normal mucosal microflora into wounds, closed cavities, or other sites that are normally sterile. Preoperative antimicrobial therapy is of value in surgery involving the colon and the female genitalia.

References

Bjornson, A., and Bjornson, H.: Participation of immunoglobulin and the alternative complement pathway in opsonization of *Bacteroides fragilis* and *Bacteroides thetaiotaomicron*. J Infect Dis 138:351, 1978.

Chow, A., and Guze, L.: Bacteroidaceae bacteremia: Clinical experiences with 112 patients. Medicine 53:93, 1974.

Farrar, W., O'Dell, N., Achord, J., and Greer, H.: Intestinal microflora and absorption in patients with stagnation-inducing lesions of the small intestine. Am J Dig Dis 17:1065, 1975.

Finegold, S. M.: Anaerobic Bacteria in Human Disease. Academic Press, New York, San Francisco, London 1977.

Hofstad, T.: Pathogenicity of anaerobic Gram-negative rods: possible mechanisms. Rev Infect Dis 6:189, 1984.

Kasper, D. L.: The polysaccharide capsule of *Bacteroides fragilis* subspecies *fragilis:* Immunochemical and morphologic definition. J Infect Dis 133:79, 1976.

Onderdonk, A. B., Kasper, D. L., Cisneros, R. L., and Bartlett, J. G.: The capsular polysaccharide of *Bacteroides fragilis* as a virulence factor: Comparison of the pathogenic potential of encapsulated and unencapsulated strains. J Infect Dis 136:82, 1977.

Rissing, J., Crowder, J., Dunfee, T., and White, A.: Bacteroides bacteremia from decubitus ulcers. S Med J 67:1179, 1974.

Sveen, K., Hofstad, T., and Milner, K. C.: Lethality for mice and chick embryos, pyrogenicity in rabbits and ability to gelate lysate from amoebocytes of *Limulus polyphemus* by lipopolysaccharides from *Bacteroides, Fusobacterium* and *Veillonella*. Acta Pathol Microbiol Scand (B) 85:388, 1977.

51

FUSOBACTERIA

LYNN A. LANCASTER, M.D.

HOWARD ROBERT ATTEBERY, D.D.S.

Fusobacteria are anaerobic non–spore-forming gram-negative rods. The genus *Fusobacterium* belongs to the family *Bacteroidaceae* and is distinguished from other genera by production of large amounts of butyric acid with little or no isobutyric or isovaleric acids (see Laboratory Diagnosis). Members of the genus have been known by many different genus and species designations, including *Sphaerophorus, Bacteroides*, and *Fusiformis*.

Species of the genus *Fusobacterium* have been associated with humans (Moore, Holdeman, and Kelley, 1984). *F. nucleatum* and *F. necrophorum* are most commonly isolated. *F. naviforme, F. gonidiaformans, F. mortiferum, F. russi*, and *F. varium* are isolated occasionally. The other members of the genus are isolated less frequently and will not be discussed individually. For more information, refer to Moore and Holdeman, 1974; Holdeman et al., 1977: Finegold et al., 1977.

MORPHOLOGY. Fusiform is the term used to describe thin, gram-negative anaerobic rods with pointed ends. Fusiforms are not all members of the genus *Fusobacterium*, and all fusobacteria are not fusiform shaped. *Fusobacterium nucleatum* is a slender, spindle-shaped, rigid-appearing rod with tapered ends and an average length of 5 to 10 μ (Fig. 1). Central swellings and pleomorphism occur occasionally. *F. varium* is coccobacillary to bacillary with rounded ends. The variability of size and shape may make one suspect a mixed culture. The variable microscopic appearances of *F. necrophorum* correlate to some degree with cultural and physiologic properties. Type A strains are pleomorphic rods averaging 0.6 μ in width and at least 5 μ in length. Curved rods and cells with irregular pleomorphic swellings are common. Type B strains tend to be longer with pale staining areas that give the cells a beaded appearance. They are less frequently irregular or swollen. *F. mortiferum* is a markedly pleomorphic rod with tapered ends ranging from 0.5 to 2 μ in diameter and 2 to 10 μ in length. Terminal or central swellings are common and large coccoid bodies may occur (Smith, 1975). Pleomorphic cells may be short or elongated.

The colonial and microscopic morphologies of *F. nucleatum* present a unique combination that assures recognition of this species. Colonies are circular, convex, and translucent with a "flecked" appearance. Mature colonies on blood agar produce a greenish discoloration of the surrounding agar when exposed to air for 15 minutes.

Colonies of *F. varium* are minute to 1 mm in diameter, circular with entire edges, flat to low convex, and translucent with gray-white centers and colorless edges.

Colonies of *F. necrophorum* vary in appearance. Those from type A strains are low, convex, and circular; they

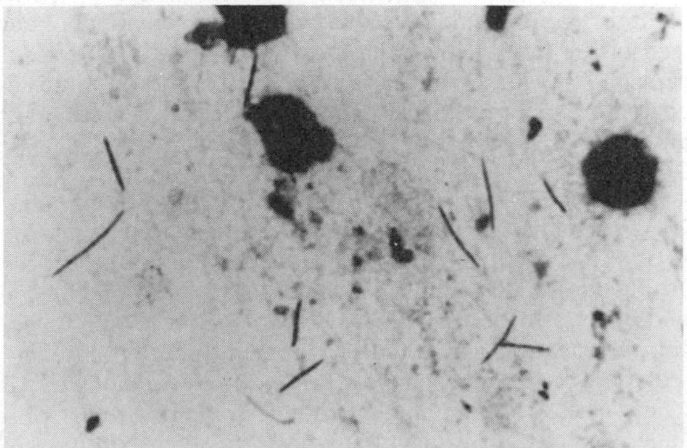

Figure 1. *F. nucleatum* in crystal violet stained smear of amniotic fluid (× 1000).

measure 2 to 3 mm in diameter. They have a smooth consistency. Type B strains often form peaked or conical colonies that are yellowish and opaque with entire margins. They are adherent and may be picked up intact or slid across the agar surface. In broth, type B strains settle out quickly, whereas type A strains form a smooth suspension.

Colonies of *F. mortiferum* are 1 to 2 mm in diameter, circular with entire to irregular edges, convex to umbonate, translucent, and smooth.

ANTIGENIC AND BIOCHEMICAL COMPOSITION. With a few exceptions, fusobacteria possess a typical endotoxic lipopolysaccharide (LPS). The LPS of *F. nucleatum* is composed of lipid A and a heteropolysaccharide. Frederiksen and Hofstad (1978) analyzed the polysaccharide component from 20 *F. nucleatum* strains and found glucosamine, glucose, L-glycero-D-manno-heptose, and a small and variable component of 2-keto-3-deoxy-octonate in each. They divided the strains into six chemotypes, according to the presence of galactose, rhamnose, and D-glycero-D-manno-heptose. At least eight O-antigen specificities are present among strains of chemotypes II and V. Antibodies to these O antigens are slightly cross-reactive. (Hofstad et al., 1979; Adnegard and Hofstad, 1983). The strains apparently share common or closely related core polysaccharides with the variable O antigen specificity determined by either chemically or structurally distinct side chains. Protein containing antigens that may be associated with the outer membrane are also responsible for broad cross-reactivity among strains of fusobacteria. The sera of a majority of normal people contain antibody to this antigen (Kristoffersen and Hofstad, 1970).

The lipid A component of *F. nucleatum* LPS is similar in chemical composition to that of *Enterobacteriaceae* (Hase et al., 1977). The fatty acids in lipid A of *F. nucleatum, F. necrophorum, F. mortiferum, F. gonidiaformans*, and *F. varium* are similar and include 3-hydroxy-tetradecanoate, *n*-tetradecanoate, hexadecanoate, n-hexadecanoate, octadecanoate, n-octadecanoate, and a compound with the properties of octadecadienoate. A 3-hydroxylated fatty acid component is characteristic of these species. *F. nucleatum* strains can be identified by the presence of 3-hydroxyhexadecanoate. Most strains of *F. russi, F. naviforme, F. plauti*, and *F. prausnitzii* form a second group characterized by the absence of 3-hydroxy fatty acids (Jantzen and Hofstad, 1981, Hofstad and Skaug, 1980). Hofstad and colleagues postulate that this second group constitutes a phylogenetically distant cluster in the genus.

Peptidoglycan of *F. nucleatum* is generally similar to that of other gram-negative bacteria, but the diaminopimelic acid in the peptidoglycan of most gram-negative species is replaced by meso-lanthionine. It is not known if this is characteristic of other members of the genus (Vasstrand et al., 1979).

METABOLISM. Fusobacteria obtain energy by metabolizing carbohydrates or peptones. Large amounts of butyric acids with small amounts of acetic and lactic acids are produced. Small amounts of propionic, succinic, and formic acids may also be produced as well as short-chained alcohols. Pyruvate is converted predominantly to butyrate and acetate. Some strains convert threonine to propionate. All strains are strong ammonia producers. Some strains produce indole. Catalase is usually not produced. Nitrates are rarely reduced. The production of hydrogen sulfide gas, volatile amines, aldehydes, and large amounts of butyric acid gives cultures a malodorous character and infections a putrid odor.

Fusobacteria are obligate anaerobes. Although they do not require an extremely low oxidation-reduction (redox) potential, some strains are very sensitive to peroxides and cannot survive exposure to air for even a few minutes. Carbon dioxide gas or bicarbonate stimulates growth. Some strains require purines, pantothenic acid, or tryptophan.

Some fusobacteria synthesize and store intracellular polysaccharides.

PATHOGENIC PROPERTIES. Because fusobacteria are part of the normal mammalian flora, they are often isolated from mixed infections with facultative bacteria or other anaerobes such as *Bacteroides melaninogenicus, B. fragilis*, or anaerobic cocci. Although it is difficult to assess the pathogenic role of normal flora in mixed infections, it is clear that fusobacteria can cause disease. Fusobacteria have been isolated many times in pure culture from the blood as well as from infections of the skin and mucous membranes. *F. nucleatum* was isolated from 18 per cent of anaerobic pleuropulmonary infections in one hospital series and was recovered four times in pure culture (Bartlett and Finegold, 1972). Fusobacteria are also one component of the fusospirochetal synergistic infections that have been demonstrated in experimental animals (Lewis and Barenberg, 1928; Smith, 1930), and *F. nucleatum* is one of the components of acute necrotizing ulcerative gingivitis (see Chapter 97, Vincent's infection). Another indicator of the pathogenicity of fusobacteria is the occurrence of metastatic lesions at sites distant from the primary lesion.

F. nucleatum and *F. necrophorum* are the species implicated most often in human and animal disease. Several studies of the LPS from both species indicate toxicity equal to that of *Salmonella* endotoxins. *F. nucleatum* LPS is similar in lethality for mice and chick embryos, rabbit pyrogenicity, and gelation of Limulus lysates to the LPS from *Salmonella enteriditis* (Sveen et al., 1977). Rabbit polymorphonuclear leukocyte migration in response to *F. nucleatum* LPS is nearly equal to that of *S. enteriditis*, but there is some strain-to-strain variability (Sveen, 1977). The endotoxins of fusobacteria have been implicated in human periodontal disease and in fatal cases of septic shock.

Cell walls of *F. nucleatum* generate complement activity by activation of the alternate pathway in guinea pig sera (Hawley and Falkler, 1977). Other workers have demonstrated that LPS activates C3 primarily by the classical pathway.

F. nucleatum synthesizes a cell wall protein that agglutinates red cells of a variety of species. The hemagglutination is calcium-dependent and does not involve pili. Antisera inhibit hemagglutination (Falkler and Hawley, 1977). Oral isolates of *F. nucleatum* also exhibit hemolytic activity following hemagglutination of human erythrocytes (Falkler et al., 1983). Falkler et al. (1979) have shown inhibition of hemagglutination by galactose but not glucose, suggesting that the protein recognizes some galactose-containing moiety. Dehazya and Coles (1980 and 1982) have isolated and purified an acidic cell wall protein with different hemagglutinating properties. Hemagglutination was not inhibited by galactose, but under certain conditions was inhibited by compounds with guanido groups. Attachment of *F. nucleatum* cell wall fragments to oral bacteria (Falkler and Burger, 1981), human oral epithelial cells, gingival fibroblasts, and white cells occurs in the same manner as hemagglutination. The role of this phenomenon in adherence to epithelial cells, bacteria, and plaque is not clear. Some workers speculate that it positively influences colonization and pathogenicity (Falkler et al., 1982).

F. necrophorum is a major pathogen of many animal species. It causes or contributes to liver abscesses of cattle, necrotizing oral infections of calves, foot rot in ungulates, and other infections. Certain strains produce a soluble protein which is toxic to leukocytes of experimental animals both *in vitro* and *in vivo*. Workers have used various *in vitro* systems to demonstrate and characterize the *F. necrophorum* leukotoxin(s) and report somewhat different properties (Fales et al., 1977; Coyle-Dennis and Lauerman, 1978, 1979; and Scanlan et al., 1982). Pathogenicity for mice correlates well with leukotoxin in limited studies.

As noted previously, *F. necrophorum* can be separated into biotypes (See Laboratory Diagnosis). Types A, B, and an uncommon intermediate type, AB, have been described. Biotypes show a significant but imperfect correlation between leukotoxin production and mouse pathogenicity. Type A strains produce the most leukotoxin and are the most pathogenic. Type B strains produce little or no leukotoxin and are least pathogenic for mice. Type B strains are isolated from abscesses less frequently and almost always in mixed culture. In addition, B types are the dominant biotype in the rumen (Berg and Scalan, 1982). The role, if any, of leukotoxins in the greater virulence of A strains for cattle is not known. Both A and B strains are isolated from human infections. There is no evidence for a role of leukotoxin in human disease.

Hemolytic strains of *F. necrophorum* are isolated more frequently from serious infections than nonhemolytic strains and are more pathogenic in experimental infections of mice. It is not known whether hemolysin is directly responsible for the increased virulence. Partially purified hemolysin has phospholipase A and lysophospholipase activity. The hemolysin is active against the red cells of a wide variety of species. Leukotoxin and hemolysin do not appear to be identical (Abe et al., 1979).

The mechanism of symbiosis between fusobacteria and spirochetes in mixed infections is unknown, but these synergistic infections usually induce necrotic lesions. Purulent tissue reactions are more common when fusobacteria are isolated in pure culture or in association with other bacteria from infections such as periapical dental abscess, brain abscess, or mastoiditis.

IMMUNITY. The sera of most adults and newborns contain IgG antibodies to protein-containing antigens of fusobacteria (Kristoffersen and Hofstad, 1970). Serum IgM specific for the LPS of strains of *F. nucleatum* appears after the first year of life and is present in most adults (Hofstad, 1974). The capacity of these antibodies to protect against invasion of the tissues by fusobacteria is unknown, and is probably not essential for defense. The cell walls of *F. nucleatum* contain a protein moiety that strongly stimulates polymorphonuclear leukocyte phagocytosis and generation of oxygen-derived free radicals (Passo et al., 1982). Serum is not required for phagocytosis. *F. mortiferum* is killed *in vitro* under aerobic and anaerobic conditions by serum alone, white cells and serum, or white cells alone (Bjornson et al., 1976).

The most important defense against invasion of the tissues by all anaerobes is the redox potential of well-oxygenated tissue (about 150 microvolts). Obligate anaerobes like the fusobacteria cannot propagate at this redox potential. Consequently, death of tissue after trauma, surgery, arterial insufficiency and infection by aerotolerant bacteria are important predisposing factors to fusobacterial infection.

The growth of facultative bacteria in the tissues may promote fusobacterial infection by lowering the redox potential, whereas other members of the normal flora may limit the growth of fusobacteria. The production of hydrogen peroxide and the superoxide ion during aerobic growth of competing microflora inhibits fusobacteria, since they synthesize little or no catalase or superoxide dismutase.

Normal human sera and saliva contain a mucinous glycoprotein that aggregates *F. nucleatum* and inhibits binding to red cells (hemagglutination). The glycoprotein-bacterium interaction is calcium ion dependent and inhibited by galactose but not glucose. These glycoproteins thus appear to bind to the hemagglutinin of the *F. nucleatum* cell wall. The influence of these proteins on oral colonization is unknown. If the glycoproteins themselves are bound to other bacteria, plaque, or cells, they might positively influence colonization by aggregating *F. nucleatum*. On the other hand, if the glycoproteins are solubilized in saliva or the gingival crevice they might cause aggregation, block binding to stationary surfaces, and inhibit colonization (Falkler et al., 1979; Smoot and Falkler, 1981).

Responses to immunization of experimental animals with *F. necrophorum* preparations have been explored. Protection of sheep and mice to subsequent challenge by lethal doses of intraperitoneally administered *F. necrophorum* can be achieved by immunization with sonicated cells. The livers of immunized mice clear the organisms in 24 hours, while the fusobacteria proliferate in mononuclear cells and cause abscesses in nonimmune mice. Since passive transfer of sera from immunized mice does not protect recipients, cellular immunity may be important (Garcia and McKay, 1978). Sonicates of *F. nucleatum* activate macrophages and helper T cells *in vitro* (Yoshie et al., 1981).

F. nucleatum is a potent inducer of polyclonal B–lymphocyte activation in vitro. Peripheral lymphocytes activated by *F. nucleatum* sonicates produce antibodies specific for *F. nucleatum* and IgM antibodies to a variety of oral bacteria. Polyclonal B–lymphocyte activation may play some role in periodontal disease (Mangan et al., 1983).

LABORATORY DIAGNOSIS. Fusobacteria are gram-negative obligate anaerobes that produce large amounts of butyric acid from fermentable carbohydrates or metabolized peptones (with little or no isobutyric or isovaleric acids). The differential reactions of the four major species are listed in Table 1.

Some strains of *F. necrophorum* are the only fusobacteria that produce lipase. A lipase-negative fusobacterium that is indole-positive and produces propionic acid from lactate is *F. necrophorum*. Most strains of *F. necrophorum* are hemolytic on horse and rabbit blood agar. Sheep red blood cells are less susceptible to this hemolysin.

F. nucleatum is the only *Fusobacterium* species with fusiform cells from colonies that show internal flecking. This species is indole-positive and does not produce propionic acid from lactate. Mannose is not fermented. Propionic acid is not produced from threonine.

F. varium is indole-variable. No propionic acid is produced from lactate. Mannose is fermented to a weak acid.

Table 1. DIFFERENTIAL CULTURE REACTIONS OF THE MAJOR FUSOBACTERIA[a]

Culture Reaction	F. Necrophorum	F. Nucleatum	F. Mortiferum	F. Varium
Microscopic morphology	L-form like	spindle-shaped	L-form like	small, variable
Beta-hemolysis	+	−	−	−
Indole	+	+	−	$+^{-}$
Esculin hydrolysis	−	−	+	−
Nitrate	−	−	−	−
Growth in 20% bile	$-^{2+}$	$-^{2+}$	4+	4+
Gas in glucose agar deeps	4+	$-^{2+}$	4+	4+
Threonine → propionate	+	+	+	+
Lactate → propionate	+	−	−	−
Lipase	+	−	−	−
Fermentation				
glucose	$-^{w}$	$-^{w}$	$+^{w}$	w^{+}
lactose	−	−	w^{+}	−
fructose	$-^{w}$	w^{-}	w^{+}	w
maltose	−	−	w^{-}	−

[a]Numbers refer to intensity of reaction. Superscripts refer to reactions of 10 to 40% of strains. +, 90% or more of strains positive; −, 90% or more of strains negative; w, weak reaction.

Esculin is not hydrolyzed. Fructose is fermented. Propionic acid is produced from threonine.

F. mortiferum is indole-negative. Esculin is hydrolyzed. Acid is produced from lactose.

A selective medium for isolation of *F. nucleatum* from subgingival plaque contains erythromycin and crystal violet as inhibitory agents. *F. nucleatum* has distinctive colony characteristics on crystal violet erythromycin (CVE) agar that permits easy separation from the few other oral organisms that can also grow on it (Walker et al., 1979). Fusobacterium egg yolk agar is a selective medium for isolation of fusobacteria. It permits rapid recognition of *F. necrophorum* by the lipase reaction (Morgenstein et al., 1981).

DRUG SUSCEPTIBILITY. Fusobacteria are highly sensitive to penicillin G, metronidazole, chloramphenicol, clindamycin, and thienamycin. They are usually sensitive to clinically achievable levels of nearly all beta-lactam antibiotics, including third generation cephalosporins and newer penicillins. Erythromycin is only moderately active *in vitro*. In the past decade many strains have become tetracycline resistant.

Strains resistant to nearly all major antibiotics including penicillin G and other beta-lactam antibiotics have been reported. Resistance to clindamycin, chloramphenicol, and metronidazole is still very uncommon.

Certain species are typically more resistant. *F. varium* is commonly resistant to penicillin G and other beta-lactams. Clindamycin and erythromycin resistance is typical. Metronidazole is highly active and inhibits all strains of *F. varium* at 1 μg/ml. Approximately one-quarter of *F. mortiferum* strains are resistant to beta-lactam antibiotics. They are sensitive to chloramphenicol, clindamycin, and metronidazole (George et al., 1981).

EPIDEMIOLOGY. Fusobacteria live in the normal mucous membranes of the mouth, bowel, and urogenital tract, and often invade underlying tissue that has been damaged by biting, other accidental trauma, surgery, tumors, or another infection. They make up about 3 per cent of the anaerobes recovered from clinical infections (Finegold et al., 1977).

Fusobacteria in the mouth and throat may contribute to periodontal disease and can cause pharyngitis. Fusobacteria may also infect any adjacent area such as the head, eyes, ears, mastoids, and sinuses. They may be aspirated into the terminal bronchioles and cause lung abscess, or spread by local or systemic circulation to cause brain abscess, meningitis, or pleuropulmonary disease. A recent literature survey showed that fusobacteria were second only to anaerobic (and microaerophilic) gram-positive cocci in their frequency of isolation from brain abscesses, anaerobic meningitis, and pleuropulmonary disease (Finegold et al., 1977).

In the preantibiotic era, *F. necrophorum* was isolated far more frequently than *F. nucleatum* from clinical infections, but *F. nucleatum* is now isolated more commonly from infections with oropharyngeal flora (Finegold et al., 1977). *F. necrophorum* pharyngeal infections, although uncommon, may result in serious septicemia accompanied by metastatic abscesses in a wide variety of organs. This syndrome, well described by Lemierre (1936), is seen most frequently in adolescents or young adults and is typically accompanied by septic jugular vein thrombophlebitis.

Fusobacteria from the gastrointestinal tract, especially *F. necrophorum* and *F. varium*, may cause intra-abdominal and perineal infections and septicemia. After *Bacteroides* and peptostreptococci, these two fusobacteria are the third most common isolates from these sites. Fusobacteria are among the most common bacteria isolated from the 70 per cent of normal postpartum uterine cavities that are culturally positive for anaerobes. They frequently colonize the genital tract of women and account for up to 20 per cent of serious pelvic infections (Gorbach and Bartlett, 1974). *F. necrophorum* has been isolated from fatal salpingitis and peritonitis associated with intrauterine devices (Maloy et al., 1981).

There is evidence that the gastrointestinal tract is colonized with fusobacteria that are ingested in the diet. Japanese ingesting a Japanese diet have fusobacteria in their stools in concentrations of 10^8 to 10^{10} (Ueno et al., 1974). *F. necrophorum* was present in ten out of ten studied, *F. varium* in two out of ten, and other fusobacteria in about five out of ten. Of 11 Americans (two black and nine Caucasian), only six had fusobacteria isolated from stool cultures. *F. varium* was present in three of six and *F. nucleatum* in three of six. None of the Americans had *F. necrophorum* in their stools. Two of the patients with

F. varium ate rice regularly. Furthermore, the number of fusobacteria steadily declined in those Japanese who switched to American diets. Thus, the numbers and species of fusobacteria in the stool are at least partly determined by diet.

References

Abe, P. M., Kendall, C. J., Stauffer, L. R., and Holland, J. W.: Hemolytic activity of *Fusobacterium necrophorum* culture supernatants due to presence of phospholipase A and lysophospholipase. Am J Vet Res 40:92, 1979.

Adnegard, B., and Hofstad, T.: O-antigenic cross reactivity in *Fusobacterium nucleatum*: chemotype V lipopolysaccharides. Acta Pathol Microbiol Immunol Scand [B] 91:93, 1983.

Bartlett, J. G., and Finegold, S. M.: Anaerobic pleuropulmonary infections, Medicine 51:413, 1972.

Berg, J. N., and Scanlan, C. M.: Studies of *Fusobacterium necrophorum* from bovine hepatic abscesses: biotypes, quantitation, virulence, and antibiotic susceptibility. Am J Vet Res 43:1580, 1982.

Bjornson, A. B., Altemeier, W. A., and Bjornson, H. S.: Comparison of the *in vitro* bactericidal activity of human serum and leukocytes against *Bacteroides fragilis* and *Fusobacterium mortiferum* in aerobic and anaerobic environments. Infect Immun 14:843, 1976.

Coyle-Dennis, J. E., and Lauerman, L. H.: Biological and biochemical characteristics of *Fusobacterium necrophorum* leukocidin. Am J Vet Res 39:1790, 1978.

Coyle-Dennis, J. E., and Lauerman, L. H.: Correlations between leukocidin production and virulence of two isolates of *Fusobacterium necrophorum*. Am J Vet Res 40:274, 1979.

Dehazya, P., and Coles, R. S., Jr.: Agglutination of human erythrocytes by *Fusobacterium nucleatum*: Factors influencing hemagglutination and some characteristics of the agglutinin. J Bacteriol 143:205, 1980.

Dehazya, P., and Coles, R. S., Jr.: Extraction and properties of hemagglutinin from cell wall fragments of *Fusobacterium nucleatum*. J Bacteriol 152:298, 1982.

Fales, W. H., Warner, J. F., and Teresa, G. W.: Effects of *Fusobacterium necrophorum* leukotoxin on rabbit peritoneal macrophages *in vitro*. Am J Vet Res 38:491, 1977.

Falkler, W. A., Jr., and Hawley, C. A.: Hemagglutinating activity of *Fusobacterium nucleatum*. Infect Immun 15:230, 1977.

Falkler, W. A., Jr., Mongiello, J. R., and Burger, B. W.: Hemagglutination inhibition and aggregation of *Fusobacterium nucleatum* by human salivary mucinous glycoproteins. Arch Oral Biol 24:483, 1979.

Falkler, W. A., Jr., and Burger, B. W.: Microbial surface interactions: Reduction of the hemagglutination activity of the oral bacterium *Fusobacterium nucleatum* by absorption with *Streptococcus* and *Bacteroides*. Arch Oral Biol 26:1015, 1981.

Falkler, W. A., Jr., Smoot, C. N., and Mongiello, J. R.: Attachment of cell fragments of *Fusobacterium nucleatum* to oral epithelial cells, gingival fibroblasts, and white blood cells. Arch Oral Biol 24:553, 1982.

Falkler, W. A., Jr., Clayman, E. B., and Shaefer, D. F.: Hemolysis of human erythrocytes by the *Fusobacterium nucleatum* associated with periodontal disease. Arch Oral Biol 28:735, 1983.

Finegold, S. M.: Anerobic Bacteria in Human Disease. New York, Academic Press, 1977.

Fredriksen, G., and Hofstad, T.: Chemotypes of *Fusobacterium nucleatum* lipopolysaccharides. Acta Pathol Microbiol Immunol Scand [B] 86:41, 1978.

Garcia, M. M., and McKay, K. A.: Intraperitoneal immunization against necrobacillosis in experimental animals. Can J Comp Med 42:121, 1978.

Gorbach, S. L., and Bartlett, J. G.: Anaerobic infections. N Engl J Med 290:1177, 1974.

George, W. L., Kirby, B. D., Sutter, V. L., et al.: Gram-negative anaerobic bacilli: Their role in infection and patterns of susceptibility to antimicrobial agents. II. Little known *Fusobacterium* species and miscellaneous genera. Rev Infect Dis 3:599, 1981.

Hase, S., Hofstad, T., and Rietschel, E. T.: Chemical structure of the lipid A component of lipopolysaccharides from *Fusobacterium nucleatum*. J Bacteriol 129:9, 1977.

Hawley, C. E., and Falkler, W. A., Jr.: Anticomplementary activity of *Fusobacterium polymorphium* in normal and C4-deficient sources of guinea pig complement. Infect Immun 18:124, 1977.

Hofstad, T.: Antibodies reacting with lipopolysaccharides from *Bacteroides melaninogenicus*, *Bacteroides fragilis*, and *Fusobacterium nucleatum* in serum from normal human subjects. J Infect Dis 129:349, 1974.

Hofstad, T., Skaug, N., and Bjornland, T.: O-antigenic cross reactivity in *Fusobacterium nucleatum*. Acta Pathol Microbiol Immunol Scand (B) 87:341, 1979.

Hofstad, T., and Skaug, N.: Fatty acids and neutral sugars present in lipopolysaccharides isolated from fusobacterium species. Acta Pathol Microbiol Immunol Scand (B) 88:115, 1980.

Holdeman, L. V., Cato, E. P., and Moore, W. E.: Anaerobe Laboratory Manual. Blacksburg, Va., Virginia Polytechnic Institute and State University, 1977.

Jantzen, E., and Hofstad, T.: Fatty acids of *Fusobacterium* species: Taxonomic implications. J Gen Microbiol 123:163, 1981.

Kristoffersen, T., and Hofstad, T.: Antibodies in humans to an isolated antigen from oral fusobacteria. J Periodontol Res 5:110, 1970.

Lemierre, A.: On certain septicemias due to anaerobic organisms. Lancet 1:701, 1936.

Lewis, J. M., and Barenberg, L. H.: Pulmonary gangrene due to spirochetes and fusiform bacilli. Am J Dis Child 37:351, 1928.

Maloy, A. L., Meier, F. A., and Karl, R. C.: Fatal peritonitis following IUD-associated salpingitis. Obstet Gynecol 58:397, 1981.

Mangan, D. F., Won, T., and Lopatir, D. E.: Nonspecific induction of immunoglobulin M antibodies to periodontal disease associated microorganisms after polyclonal human B–lymphocyte activation by *Fusobacterium nucleatum*. Infect Immunol 41:1038, 1983.

Moore, W. E. C., Holdeman, L. V., and Kelley, R. W.: Fusobacterium. In Krieg, N. R., and Holt, J. G. (eds.): Bergey's Manual of Systematic Bacteriology, vol. I. Baltimore, Williams & Wilkins, 1984, p. 631.

Morgenstein, A. A., Citron, D. M., and Finegold, S. M.: New medium selective for *Fusobacterium* species and differential for *Fusobacterium necrophorum*. J Clin Microbiol 13:666, 1981.

Nygren, H., Gunnar, D., and Nilsson, L.: Human complement activation by lipopolysaccharides from *Bacteroides oralis*, *Fusobacterium nucleatum*, and *Veillonella parvula*. Infect Immun 26:391, 1979.

Passo, S. A., Syed, S. A., and Silva, J., Jr.: Neutrophil chemiluminescence in response to *Fusobacterium nucleatum*. J Peridont Res 17:604, 1982.

Scanlan, C. M., Berg, J. N., and Fales, W. H.: Comparative *in vitro* leukotoxin production of three bovine strains of Fusobacterium necrophorum. Am J Vet Res 43:1329, 1982.

Smith, D. T.: Fuso-spirochetal disease of the lungs produced with cultures from Vincent's angina. J Infect Dis 46:303, 1930.

Smith, L. D.: The Pathogenic Anaerobic Bacteria. Springfield, Ill., Charles C Thomas, 1975.

Smoot, C. N., and Falkler, W. A., Jr.: Attachment of serum non-antibody glycoproteins to the *Fusobacterium nucleatum* found in periodontal disease. Arch Oral Biol 26:859, 1981.

Sveen, K.: Rabbit polymorphonuclear leukocyte migration *in vivo* in response to lipopolysaccharides from *Bacteroides*, *Fusobacterium* and *Veillonella*. Acta Pathol Microbiol Immunol Scand [B] 85:374, 1977.

Sveen, K., Hofstad, T., and Milner, K. C.: Lethality for mice and chick embryos, pyrogenicity in rabbits, and ability to gelate lysate from amoebocytes of *Limulus polyphenus* by lipopolysaccharides from *Bacteroides*, *Fusobacterium*, and *Veillonella*. Acta Pathol Microbiol Immunol Scand (B) 85:388, 1977.

Ueno, K., Sugihara, P. T., Bricknell, K. S., Attebery, H. R., Sutter V. L., and Finegold, S. M.: Comparison of characteristics of gram-negative anaerobic bacilli isolated from feces of individuals in Japan and the United States. In Balows, A. (ed.): Anaerobic Bacteria, Role in Disease. Springfield, Ill., Charles C Thomas, 1974.

Vasstrand, E. N., Hofstad, T., Endresen, C., and Jensen, H. B.: Demonstration of lanthionine as a natural constituent of the peptidoglycan of *Fusobacterium nucleatum*. Infect Immun 25:775, 1979.

Walker, C. B., Ratliff, D., Muller, D., et al.: Medium for selective isolation of *Fusobacterium nucleatum* from human periodontal pockets. J Clin Microbiol 10:844, 1979.

Yoshie, H., Mitsuma, T., Kozima, K., and Hara, K.: Effects of Actinomyces and Fusobacterium on humoral immune response *in vitro*. J Peridont Res 16:556, 1981.

52
VEILLONELLA

LYNN A. LANCASTER, M.D.
HOWARD ROBERT ATTEBERY, D.D.S.

Veillonella are gram-negative, obligately anaerobic cocci. They are a universal part of the indigenous oral microbiota of humans and are commonly found in the respiratory tract, intestine, and vagina. Because they occur in high numbers as parasites on the mucous membranes of man, they can be found in infected sites when the indigenous flora are transported from the protective mucous membrane barrier into deeper tissues that can also support their growth.

Veillonella are not regarded as overt pathogens, although they do exhibit some pathogenic properties. They are not found in pure culture in any infections but are always mixed with facultative bacteria or other anaerobes or both. Veillonella are spoken of as "opportunists" because they share an infected site with more aggressive and more pathogenic microorganisms, and their role in the infectious process is considered minor.

Two species of *Veillonella* are commonly seen in the literature, *Veillonella parvula* and *Veillonella alcalescens*. These species are now known to be genetically homologous, and have been combined into a single species, *Veillonella parvula*. Additional species have been proposed on the basis of DNA homology studies. (See Antigenic and Biochemical Composition.) (Holdeman et al., 1977).

MORPHOLOGY. Veillonella are small cocci that measure 0.3 to 0.5 μm in diameter. They usually appear in masses or as diplococci but occasionally as single organisms in short chains.

On blood agar plates, colonies are small, convex, translucent, and glistening with an entire edge. They are small unless pyruvate or lactate and carbon dioxide gas are added to the growth system.

ANTIGENIC AND BIOCHEMICAL COMPOSITION. Rogosa found seven major serologic groups on the basis of whole cell agglutination by rabbit antisera (Rogosa, 1965). He could clearly distinguish 21 oral strains from hamsters that possessed a distinctive antigen and were assigned to Group I. He placed 28 strains in group II, all oral isolates from hamsters, rats, and rabbits. Group III consisted of two oral strains isolated from rats. Group IV, *Veillonella alcalescens*, comprised 15 members, which included 3 from the rat, 1 from a rabbit, 4 from human bacteremias that followed dental operations, and 5 from the human mouth. Group V consisted of only two strains, one each from man and the rat. Group VI, *Veillonella parvula*, consisted of 28 strains. Most were oral strains from humans, but four were isolated from the intestinal tract of man. Group VII consisted of only three strains, two from the human mouth and one from the human respiratory tract.

Veillonella possess a typical endotoxic lipopolysaccharide that is structurally associated with an outer three-layered cell membrane (Bladen and Mergenhagen, 1964). Hofstad (1978) has extracted and analyzed the chemical components of LPS from 34 strains. All contained glucosamine, galactosamine, L-glycero-D-manno-heptose, glucose, and 2-keto-3-deoxy octonate. They could be divided into four chemotypes (I-IV), however, depending on the presence of the additional components: galactose, rhamnose, and D-glycero-D-manno heptose. The LPS possesses O-antigen specificity that resides in the side chain components of the polysaccharide moiety of the molecule (Hofstad et al., 1971).

Mays et al. (1982) have studied DNA homology of 116 strains of *Veillonella*. They included representatives of the two species and seven subspecies recognized by Rogosa and found eight genetically distinct groups with low intergroup homology. In most cases, the DNA homology groups corresponded to the type strains of the subspecies given in the eighth edition of *Bergey's Manual of Determinative Bacteriology*. The type strains of *V. parvula* ssp. *parvula* and *V. alcalescens* ssp. *alcalescens* were highly homologous and the authors proposed their combination into one species, *V. parvula*. They proposed elevation of the other subspecies, *V. dispar*, *V. atypica*, *V. rodentium*, *V. ratti*, and *V. criceti*, to species status.

Mays et al. also proposed creation of a new species, *V. caviae*, for a previously unrecognized homology group of seven strains from guinea pigs. A homology group consisting only of two human isolates was not proposed for species status. DNA from three other human isolates showed no homology with any group or each other and may represent additional species. Most human isolates belong to the species *V. atypica*, *V. parvula*, or *V. dispar*.

METABOLISM. *Veillonella* has complex nutritional requirements. Carbohydrates are not fermented (with the exception of *V. criceti*). D-ribose is, however, utilized biosynthetically and incorporated into nucleic acid (Kafkewitz and Delwiche, 1967).

For energy requirements, *Veillonella* utilizes pyruvate best but also lactate, oxaloacetate, malate, and fumarate. Veillonella also obtains energy by reducing nitrates to nitrites.

Lactate is metabolized to acetic and propionic acids and to carbon dioxide and hydrogen.

Hydrogen sulfide is produced from a number of sulfur-containing compounds such as thioglycolate, thiocyanate, thiosulfate, cysteine, cystine, and glutathione. Carbon dioxide is required for growth.

PATHOGENICITY. *Veillonella* can produce disease in experimental animals. Its lipopolysaccharide is an endotoxin that produces fever and Shwartzman reactions in rabbits.

The role of *Veillonella* in human clinical infections is not clear. It appears that *Veillonella*, the parasite of mucous membranes, is an opportunist in human infection and does not play a major role in any infection. This view has evolved because of the relative infrequency of involvement of *Veillonella* in clinical infections and the fact that it is rarely present in pure culture.

LABORATORY DIAGNOSIS. Three genera of anaerobic, gram-negative cocci that belong to the family Veillonellocae may be found in infected material. These genera are easily differentiated. *Megasphaera* is fermentative and produces abundant acid from glucose, fructose, and maltose. *Veillonella* and *Acidaminococcus* are nonfermentative (with the exception of *V. criceti*). In addition, *Megasphaera* produces butyric acid from carbohydrate growth media, while the others do not. *Megasphaera* is large, between 1.7 and 2.5 μm, which also distinguishes this genus from *Veillonella* and *Acidaminococcus*. *Veillonella* reduces nitrates, whereas *Acidaminococcus* and *Megasphaera* do not.

The criteria separating *Veillonella* from the other anaerobes are as follows: small, gram-negative cocci, 0.3 to 0.5 μm, that reduce nitrate but do not ferment. Growth is stimulated by pyruvate and lactate, and carbon dioxide is required for growth.

Separation of *Veillonella* into the seven or more species described by Mays et al. (1982) is currently not practical, or even possible, for the clinical laboratory. Distinctive phenotypic traits are not known for the proposed species. Kelley (1982) described the use of a commercially prepared panel of substrates for assay of 19 different metabolic enzymes for partial characterization of the strains. Differences in phosphoamidase, acid phosphatase, and C4 (butyrate) esterase activity made it possible to identify *V. rodentium*, *V. criceti*, *V. ratti*, and one unnamed homology group. The other proposed species were not identifiable by this technique. Until stable traits are described, the clinical laboratory should identify these isolates as *Veillonella* sp.

DRUG SUSCEPTIBILITY. *Veillonella* are usually very sensitive to penicillin, clindamycin, and N-F-thienamycin. Virtually all β-lactam antibiotics inhibit 90 per cent of strains at clinically achievable levels. The approximate concentrations necessary to inhibit 50 and 90 per cent of strains ($MIC_{50,90}$) are for metronidazole (<1 μg/ml), tetracycline (0.5 μg/ml, 32 μg/ml) and erythromycin (<2 μg/ml, 8 μg/ml) (Sutter and Finegold, 1976). Aminoglycosides and vancomycin have poor activity in vitro.

EPIDEMIOLOGY. *Veillonella* is part of the indigenous microbiota of the mouth, respiratory system, intestinal tract, and vagina of humans. The organisms are universally present in high numbers in the human mouth and might be expected in infections in which the oral flora is the primary infecting agent. *Veillonella* can on occasion be found in infections associated with the microbiota of the intestinal tract and vagina.

Veillonella can be found in transient bacteremias following dental extraction, in sinusitis, tonsillar and peritonsillar abscesses, otitis media, mastoiditis, and brain abscesses. The organisms are occasionally found in intra-abdominal infections and genitourinary infections. They are commonly found in the mixed flora of lung abscess, aspiration pneumonia, empyema, and pleuropulmonary infections. They can be seen in female genital tract infections, intrauterine infections, tubo-ovarian abscesses, and postoperative genitourinary infections. Osteomyelitis has been reported (Barnhart et al., 1983).

Veillonella has been reported in bile. Some strains can dehydroxylate bile acids, and *Veillonella* organisms have the potential to be involved in the chain of microorganisms producing chemical carcinogens from bile acids. Veillonella was found in 5 of 25 subjects with colonic polyps but not in 25 matched control subjects without polyps (Finegold et al., 1975).

Certain *Veillonella* strains are aggregated and tightly bound by oral streptococci, through a variety of mechanisms. Such interbacterial adherence probably plays a role in colonization of the mouth and dental plaque (McBride and van der Hoeven, 1981). This phenomenon is interesting because of the possible role of *Veillonella* in ameliorating the strong cariogenic effect of lactate produced by streptococci. *Veillonella* can metabolize lactate to weaker acids such as acetate and propionate (Mikx and van der Hoeven, 1975). A similar food chain probably occurs between *Actinomyces* and *Veillonella* (Distler and Kroncke, 1981).

References

Bladen, H. A., and Mergenhagen, S. E.: Ultrastructure of *Veillonella* and morphological correlation of an outer membrane with particles associated with endotoxic activity. J Bacteriol. 88:1482, 1964.

Finegold, S. M., Flora, D. J., Attebery, H. R., and Sutter, V. L.: Fecal bacteriology of colonic polyp patients and control patients. Cancer Res 35:3407, 1975.

Distler, W., and Kroncke, A.: Acid formation by mixed cultures of dental plaque bacteria *Actinomyces* and *Veillonella*. Arch Oral Biol 26:123, 1981.

Hofstad, T., Kristoffersen, T., and Macland, J. A.: Serological properties of lipopolysaccharides from strains of oral *Veillonella*. Acta Pathol Microbiol Immunol Scand [B] 79:615, 1971.

Hofstad, T.: Chemotypes of *Veillonella* lipopolysaccharides. Acta Pathol Microbiol Immunol Scand [B] 86:47, 1978.

Holdeman, L. V., Cato, E. P., and Moore, W. E.: Anaerobe Laboratory Manual. Blacksburg, Va., Virginia Polytechnic Institute and State University, 1977.

Kafkewitz, D., and Delwiche, E. A.: Utilization of D-ribose by *Veillonella*. J Bacteriol 98:903, 1967.

Kelley, R. W.: Phenotypic differentiation of some of the *Veillonella* species with the API Zym system. Can J Microbiol 28:703, 1982.

Martin, W. J.: Anaerobic cocci. In Lennette, E. H., Spaulding, E. H., and Truant, J. P. (eds.): Manual of Clinical Microbiology. Washington, D.C., American Society for Microbiology, 1974, p. 970.

Mays, T. D., Holdeman, L. V., Moore, N. E. C., Rogosa, M., and Johnson, J. L.: Int J Syst Bacteriol 32:28, 1982.

McBride, B. C., and van der Hoeven, J. S.: Role of interbacterial adherence in colonization of the oral cavities of gnotobiotic rats infected with *Streptococcus mutans* and *Veillonella alkalescens*. Infect Immun 33:467, 1981.

Mikx, F. H. M., and van der Hoeven, J. S.: Symbiosis of *Streptococcus mutans* and *Veillonella alkalescens* in mixed continuous culture. Arch Oral Biol 20:407, 1975.

Rogosa, M.: The genus *Veillonella*. IV. Serological groupings, and genus and species emendations. J Bacteriol 90:704, 1965.

Sutter, V. L., and Finegold, S. M.: Susceptibility of anaerobic bacteria to 23 antimicrobial agents. Antimicrob Agts Chemother 10:736, 1976.

53

SPIROCHETES: TREPONEMA AND BORRELIA

DANIEL M. MUSHER, M.D.

The order Spirochaetales includes the following five genera: *Treponema*, *Borrelia*, *Spirochaeta*, *Leptospira*, and *Cristispira*. This chapter will deal with the first two. Within the genus *Treponema*, organisms pathogenic for man include *T. pallidum*, *T. pertenue*, and *T. carateum*, the etiologic agents of syphilis, yaws, and pinta, respectively. These three virulent organisms have not been cultivated successfully in vitro, although in recent years *T. pallidum* has been maintained for days to weeks with limited replication in artificial media containing mammalian cells (Jenkin and Sandok, 1983). No differences among *T. pallidum*, *T. pertenue*, and *T. carateum* have been detected by microscopic, electron microscopic, or immunologic techniques, although the infections they produce in animals or humans are readily distinguishable (Turner and Hollander, 1957) and biologic differences among *T. pallidum* strains have been documented. *T. cuniculi* and *T. hyodysenteriae* cause dermal and systemic disease in rabbits and diarrheal disease in swine, respectively; *T. cuniculi* also produces experimental infection in primates. Neither of these organisms has been shown to infect people. *T. macrodentium* and *T. vincentii* may contribute to infections of the mouth and gums. Except for *T. cuniculi*, these other treponemes can all be cultivated in artificial media. Only the treponemes that are pathogenic for man will be discussed in this chapter. Much of this material is covered in depth elsewhere (Schell and Musher, 1983).

The genus *Borrelia* comprises about 18 species or strains that are pathogenic for humans, in whom they cause relapsing fever. Some of these may be distinguished serologically, although formal classification is usually based on their arthropod vectors. Their classification is imprecise also, in part, because most strains have not been cultivated in vitro. In the past few years another spirochete has been newly recognized and shown to be the etiologic agent of Lyme disease. Based on analysis of DNA base ratios and DNA homology, this organism has just (September, 1984) been designated *Borrelia burgdorferi* (see Chapter 270 on Lyme disease).

MORPHOLOGY. The pathogenic treponemes are too narrow ($\leq$0.15 μm) to be resolved by the light microscope and, therefore, are considered gram-indeterminate. Electron microscopy shows them to be wavelike organisms with tapered ends (Fig. 1). They have tight, regular spirals with a wavelength of 1.1 μm and an amplitude of 0.2 to 0.3 μm; their length ranges from 6 to 15 μm, and is usually 10 to 13 μm. Whereas some electron microscopic studies have suggested that *T. pallidum* has an amorphous external layer that stains with ruthenium red, others disagree (Hovind-Hougen, 1983); the relation of these findings to a long-hypothesized slime layer that prevents phagocytosis and inhibits early antigen processing is not known. The virulent treponemes have three to eight periplasmic flagella (formerly called axial filaments or axial fibrils) that emerge from an electron-dense area near each end of the organism. The flagella, consisting of a sheathed filament, a hook, and a basal body, are contained between the three-layered outer membrane and an electron-dense layer (peptidoglycan) that is thought to give the treponemes their wavelike configuration. The cytoplasmic membrane is within, and is adherent to the electron-dense layer. Motility of treponemes appears to depend upon flagella, with the repertoire of various kinds of motion resulting both from the presence of flagella at the ends of the organism and the ability of each set of flagella to stimulate clockwise or counterclockwise motion. Cytoplasmic tubules are present, but their function is unknown.

Borreliae are pointed, helical organisms, usually 10 to 20 μm in length. They have coarse irregular coils with variable amplitude. Because their width at the center is 0.4 to 0.5 μm, they are easily detectable in stained preparations as gram-negative, wavelike organisms. Wright's and Giemsa's stains also delineate them nicely, especially after prolonged staining. Borreliae have an outermost amorphous surface layer surrounding an outer membrane that has three distinct layers. Between the outer and the cytoplasmic membrane may be found 15 to 20 flagella that lack sheaths; they are inserted at each end of the organism by means of basal knobs.

ANTIGENIC COMPOSITION. Antibody to several outer membrane proteins of *T. pallidum* is present in serum from patients with primary syphilis; additional antibody appears as the infection progresses into secondary and early latent stages although this antibody may not persist in late stages of infection (Hanff et al., 1982). Some antigens are shared by nonpathogenic treponemes (Hanff et al., 1982; Lukehart et al., 1982; Baughn et al., 1983) and may be detected in immune complexes of patients or rabbits with secondary (disseminated) infection (Baughn et al., 1983). The relation between any of these antigens and those to which antibody is directed in standard treponemal serologic tests is not known; it seems unlikely that a common antigen would be involved since adsorption with nonpathogenic treponemes is an essential part of the FTA-ABS or MTPHA tests (see below). It should also be noted that differences among *T. pallidum*, *T. pertenue*, and *T. carateum* cannot be detected serologically. The antigenic properties of other treponemal components, e.g., mucopolysaccharides or lipopolysaccharides, have not been described.

It is not known with certainty whether cardiolipin, the antigen that stimulates production of Wassermann (VDRL, Veneral Disease Research Laboratory) antibody (see below), is a component of the treponeme or whether it is released from mammalian tissues during active treponemal infection. Favoring a treponemal origin is the observation that VDRL antibody follows clinically inapparent infection of primates with *T. cuniculi*. Favoring release from tissues is the association in experimental animals and humans between active lesions and the detection of this antibody, as well as the appearance of antibody to cardiolipin in autoimmune disease states such as systemic lupus erythematosus. Cardiolipin represents 13 per cent of the total lipid composition of *T. pallidum* (Matthews et al., 1979). However, since treponemes cannot synthesize some fatty acids, their lipid composition may simply reflect that of the tissue in which they have grown.

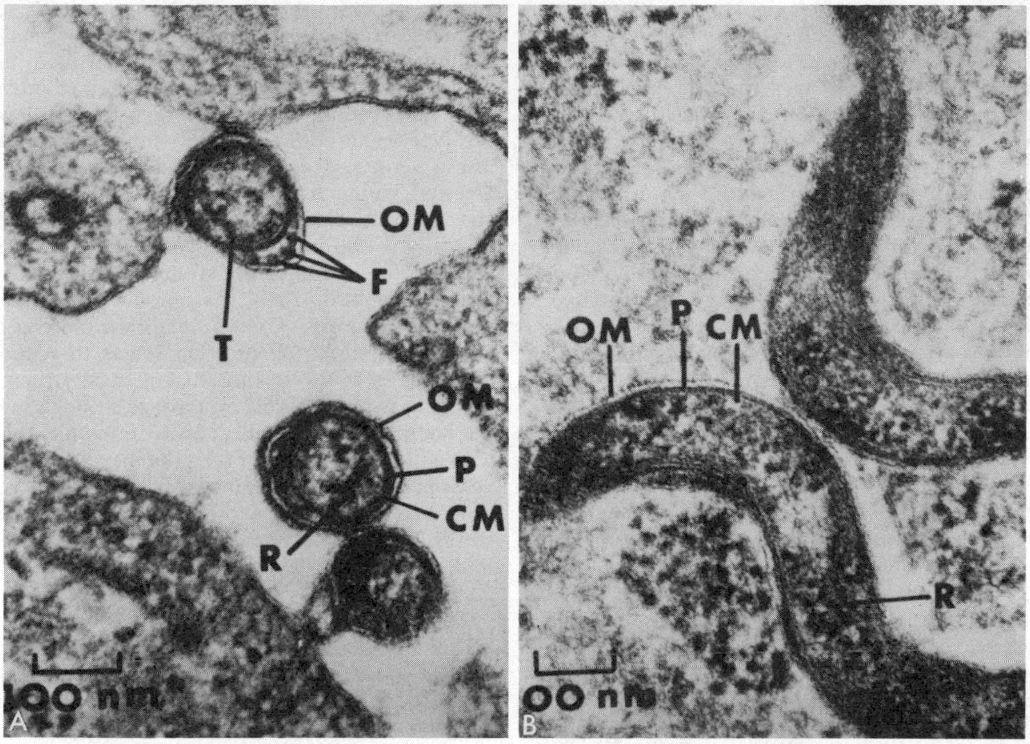

Figure 1. Ultrastructure of *Treponema pallidum.* OM—outer membrane; F—flagella; P—peptidoglycan layer; CM—cell membrane; R—ribosome; T—tubule.

Antigenic properties of borreliae have not been studied thoroughly. Antiserum to one strain of Borrelia agglutinates other borreliae as well as *T. pallidum.* Typhus-immune serum may also contain complement-fixing antibodies that react with borreliae. However, infection with one strain of *Borrelia* does not necessarily protect against others. A further problem results from the fact that relapse strains differ antigenically from the original infecting organism. In fact, whatever the serotype of an infecting *B. hermsii,* relapses are caused by other serotypes, with a distinct hierarchy in their likelihood of appearance. More recently, polyacrylamide gel electrophoresis has been used to show changes in the major protein components of borreliae as a result of passage in vitro or in vivo (Barbour et al., 1982). Antibody to cardiolipin appears in a small percentage of cases of borreliosis. Both treponemes and borreliae have ornithine and lack muramic and diaminopimelic acid in their cell walls, in contrast to *Leptospira.*

METABOLISM. *T. pallidum* has traditionally been regarded as an obligate anaerobe because it best retains motility in vitro under anaerobic conditions. Recent studies, however, have shown that *T. pallidum* takes up oxygen and degrades glucose aerobically to carbon dioxide and acetate, as well as anaerobically to pyruvate and lactate, although of 22 carbon sources studied, only glucose and pyruvate were metabolized aerobically (Baseman et al., 1976). *T. pallidum* is, in fact, better able to incorporate amino acids into proteins in the presence of 10 per cent oxygen than anaerobically, and growth of *T. pallidum* in vitro is best maintained at 3 to 5 per cent oxygen. The failure to demonstrate a functioning Krebs cycle in vitro does not exclude the possibility that *T. pallidum* has this capacity in vivo (Cox, 1983). The electrical energy needed for motility of treponemes appears to come from movement of protons and is dependent upon exchange of hydrogen, sodium, and potassium ions via conducting channels.

The metabolic characteristics of most borreliae are unknown. *Borrelia duttoni* metabolizes glucose anaerobically via the Embden-Meyerhof pathway, with pyruvate acting as the terminal electron acceptor and reducing to lactate; aerobic respiration does not appear to play a role, and the borreliae are generally considered to be anaerobic or microaerophilic. Borreliae metabolize lysolecithin (but not lecithin) to fatty acids and glycerol, and incorporate cholesterol from culture medium in vitro.

PATHOGENIC PROPERTIES. Treponemes have receptors at both ends by means of which they can adhere to a variety of mammalian cells. This adherence is blocked by antibody to *T. pallidum* and is thought to play a role in pathogenesis of infection although ultrastructural examination of infected tissues does not reveal attachment of treponemes to cells (Penn, 1981). This attachment is associated with deterioration of cultured tissues and loss of physiologic responses of cultured nerve or cardiac muscle responses in vitro (Fitzgerald, 1983). Treatment of both syphilis and relapsing fever is accompanied by an acute febrile reaction called, in the case of syphilis, a Jarisch-Herxheimer reaction. This is thought to be due to release of pyrogenic substances. Nevertheless, neither *T. pallidum* (Young et al., 1982) nor *B. hermsii* (Butler et al., 1982) has been found to contain endotoxin that reacts in the limulus assay.

IMMUNITY. Polymorphonuclear leukocytes (PMN) accumulate at a site of treponemal infection, can ingest *T. pallidum* in vitro and in vivo, and can incorporate ingested treponemes into phagocytic vacuoles (Musher et al., 1983). Nevertheless, this slowly replicating organism still manages to escape destruction by PMN.

By the time primary syphilis is diagnosed most patients have immunofluorescent and hemagglutinating antibodies to *T. pallidum*. Also present are antibodies that, together with complement, inhibit motility and eliminate infectivity of the organism (*T. pallidum* immobilizing [TPI] antibodies). Despite the antibodies, syphilis progresses and secondary lesions develop in virtually all patients unless specific therapy is given. Passive immunization with serum from rabbits that have recovered from experimental infection and are immune to rechallenge with *T. pallidum* delays and attenuates but does not prevent syphilitic lesions (Bishop and Miller, 1976). Antibody to cardiolipin does not appear to contribute to immunity.

A number of findings suggests a role for cell-mediated immune mechanisms, although the complete picture is far from clear. Infection with *T. pallidum* stimulates cellular immune mechanisms, as demonstrated by enhanced ability of macrophages from syphilitic rabbits to suppress the growth of *Listeria monocytogenes*; this reaction is mediated by thymus-dependent lymphocytes (Schell et al., 1975). However, stimulation of acquired cellular resistance by systemic injection of unrelated organisms such as *Mycobacterium bovis* (BCG) or *Propionibacterium acnes* does not protect animals against challenge with *T. pallidum*. Adoptive transfer of spleen cells from syphilis-immune rabbits failed to protect recipients against syphilitic infection, although studies using hamsters and *T. pallidum* strain *bosniae* found opposite results. Thymus-dependent lymphocytes and macrophages accumulate 7 to 10 days after intratesticular injection of rabbits coinciding with a marked decline in the number of treponemes present and the possible appearance of treponemal forms within macrophages (Lukehart et al., 1980). Ultrastructural examination supports a role for macrophages in ingesting and destroying *T. pallidum* (Sell et al., 1982).

Several findings suggest that thymus-dependent immune responses may be impaired in early syphilis: (1) in vitro blastogenic transformation of lymphocytes after stimulation with a variety of antigens is depressed; (2) delayed-type hypersensitivity to several antigens may be depressed, and (3) ability to produce IgG antibody to sheep red blood cells (a thymus-dependent humoral response) is markedly inhibited (Baughn and Musher, 1978). It is entirely possible that there is no complete immunity to *T. pallidum*. Active lesions may be brought under control and animals may be resistant to rechallenge with *T. pallidum*, but the host cannot rid itself of the infecting organism, which persists in lymph nodes. Human subjects have also been resistant to rechallenge with *T. pallidum* during latency, even though it is known that they are unable to eradicate the infecting organism (Magnuson et al., 1956).

Humoral immunity is held responsible for arresting borreliosis. Three to five days after the onset of symptoms, circulating antibodies appear that agglutinate, immobilize, and/or lyse borreliae; their appearance corresponds with clinical improvement and disappearance of these organisms from the bloodstream. Antibody also enhances uptake of borreliae by human polymorphonuclear leukocytes in vitro (Spagnuolo et al., 1982). Although these antibodies can cross-react with other borreliae, immunity is species- and strain-specific. After the initial humoral response, and as a result of mechanisms that are not understood, the infecting organism is thought to undergo a series of antigenic shifts, each one leading to the emergence of a new "relapse" serotype that is not immediately subject to humoral control. These serotypes cause a clinical relapse, which is then arrested within a few days by a newly emerging set of specific antibodies. The shorter duration and the reduced intensity of the relapses suggest antigenic cross-reactivity with the original infecting strain (Felsenfeld, 1965; Southern and Sanford, 1969). As noted above, polyacrylamide gel electrophoresis of outer membrane proteins of borreliae at different stages of infection seems to support this hypothesis. It is interesting that relapse strains appear to revert to parental forms on passage through insect vectors but not through mammalian hosts. Immunity to rechallenge with a particular strain of *Borrelia* may persist up to several years in experimental animals. In clinical reports that have described reinfection within a few months, the infecting strains have not been specifically identified. Cell-mediated immunity has not been shown to play a role in borreliosis.

LABORATORY DIAGNOSIS. Three kinds of laboratory tests are important for diagnosis of syphilis, yaws, or pinta: (1) Treponemes in exudates from suspicious lesions can be detected by darkfield microscopy. This method is sensitive if a good specimen has been obtained, especially in primary chancres, and is highly specific if care has been used to prevent contamination from oral or fecal sources. (2) Antibody to cardiolipin can be detected by a variety of flocculation tests. The most widely used is the VDRL reaction. The rapid plasma reagin (RPR) test or a modification thereof is particularly useful for screening large numbers of specimens. It is still considered best to verify and quantify positive RPR reactions by measuring VDRL antibodies. The VDRL test is reactive in about 80 per cent of patients at the time primary syphilis is diagnosed and in all patients with secondary syphilis. VDRL reactivity is closely associated with active infection, including tertiary disease of soft tissues, bones, and viscera, but the reaction may be negative in patients with cardiovascular syphilis or neurosyphilis. (3) Antibody to virulent treponemes can be detected by using an immunofluorescent technique (FTA-ABS, an abbreviation for fluorescent treponemal antibody, after absorbing the serum to be tested with nonvirulent treponemes to remove nonspecific reactivity) or a hemagglutination assay (TPHA, *T. pallidum* hemagglutination assay). These tests are positive in more than 90 per cent of patients with primary syphilis and in all patients with secondary, latent, and late infections. The same antibodies are also detectable in yaws and pinta. These tests are highly specific for treponemal infection; serum from patients with autoimmune diseases is rarely reactive. Despite the advantages of sensitivity and specificity, detection of antitreponemal antibody may not be useful in diagnosing active infection in an individual case because, once present, the antibody persists indefinitely and its presence may indicate prior rather than active infection. The greatest reliability is in obtaining a negative result and thus *excluding* a treponemal cause for a chronic lesion. It should be stressed that the recent change from a system of health care in which only central reference laboratories carried out these serologic tests to one in which most individual hospitals do them themselves has resulted in many erroneous results.

Falsely positive TPHA and falsely negative VDRL (reflecting failure to dilute serum with a prozone phenomenon) are responsible for many, but by no means all of the problems.

Borreliosis is usually diagnosed by finding loosely coiled spirochetes during microscopic examination of Wright- or Giemsa-stained peripheral blood, or during darkfield microscopic examination of the whole fresh blood. This is specific but relatively insensitive, being positive in one-quarter to one-half of patients who have relapsing fever. Injecting mice with blood from infected patients can be helpful diagnostically because it produces an obvious spirochetemia, often within two to three days, but is not practical. Results in a recent outbreak suggested that agglutination of the Proteus OX-K antigen is useful diagnostically because it is positive in at least two-thirds of cases. Antibodies that agglutinate or kill *Borrelia* have been identified but have not been shown to be of clinical value. The VDRL test is negative in borreliosis.

ANTIMICROBIAL SUSCEPTIBILITY. The virulent treponemes are highly susceptible to penicillins, cephalosporins, and tetracyclines and somewhat less so to erythromycin, clindamycin, and chloramphenicol. They are resistant to sulfonamides and aminoglycosides. Borreliae are susceptible to penicillin, aminoglycosides, tetracycline, and chloramphenicol; penicillin-binding proteins have recently been demonstrated (Barbour et al., 1982).

EPIDEMIOLOGY. *T. pallidum, T. pertenue,* and *T. carateum* infect only humans under natural conditions, although experimental infection has been produced in a variety of animals. *T. pallidum* infections have a worldwide distribution; infection is spread primarily by venereal contact but may be acquired in utero. Yaws (*T. pertenue*) is limited to tropical areas and has largely been eradicated in recent years thanks to efforts of the World Health Organization. Infection appears to spread by direct contact, although flies may possibly act as vectors. Pinta (*T. carateum*) is prevalent in areas of Central and South America and the Caribbean. It also appears to spread by contact from person to person. There is no known animal reservoir. Infection occurs sporadically in all age groups, although yaws generally begins in childhood.

In the United States relapsing fever has almost always been acquired in areas high above sea level where pine and fir trees predominate. The north rim of the Grand Canyon is recognized as a highly endemic area with tick-infested log cabins playing the predominant role (Boyer et al., 1977). Natural hosts for the infecting organism include rodents and small mammals, infection is transmitted to humans by *Ornithodorus* ticks. The reservoir of *B. recurrentis*, the classic cause of louse-borne relapsing fever, is unknown. This disease does not occur in the United States. Only human beings are clinically infected, and there is no transovarian transmission by the insect vector (*Pediculus humanus var humanus*). Elimination of rodent nests adjacent to human habitations and use of insecticide and insect repellents appear to control the spread of infection.

References

Baseman, J. B., Nichols, J. C., and Hayes, N. S.: Virulent *Treponema pallidum*: Aerobe or anaerobe. Infect Immun 13:704, 1976.

Barbour, A. G., Tessier, S. L., and Stoenner, H. G.: Variable major proteins of *Borrelia hermsii*. J Exper Med 156:1312, 1982.

Barbour, A. G., Todd, W. J., Stoenner, H. G.: Action of penicillin on *Borrelia hermsii*. Antimicrob Agents Chemother 21:823, 1982.

Baughn, R. E., and Musher, D. M.: Altered immune responsiveness associated with experimental syphilis in the rabbit: elevated IgM and depressed IgG response to sheep erythrocytes. J Immunol 120:1691, 1978.

Baughn, R. E., Adams, C. B., Musher, D. M.: Circulating immune complexes in experimental syphilis: identification of treponemal antigens and specific antibodies to treponemal antigens in isolate complexes. Infect Immun, In press.

Butler, T., Spagnuolo, P. J., Goldsmith, G. H., Aikawa, M.: Interaction of Borrelia spirochetes with human mononuclear leukocytes causes production of leukocytic pyrogen and thromboplastin. J Lab Clin Med 99:709, 1982.

Bishop, N. H., and Miller, J. N.: Humoral immunity in experimental syphilis. I. The demonstration of resistance conferred by passive immunization. J Immunol 117:191, 1976.

Boyer, K. M., Munford, R. S., Maupin, G. O., Pattison, C. P., Fox, M. D., Barnes, A. M., Jones, W. L., and Maynard, J. E.: Tick-borne relapsing fever: an interstate outbreak originating at Grand Canyon National Park. Am J Epidemiol 105:469, 1977.

Canale-Parola, E.: Physiology and evolution of spirochetes. Bacteriol Rev 41:181, 1977.

Cox, C. D.: Metabolic activities. In: R. F. Schell and D. M. Musher, eds., Pathogenesis and immunology of infection. Marcel Dekker, New York, 1983, p 57.

Felsenfeld, O.: Borreliae, human relapsing fever, and parasite-vector-host relationship. Bacteriol Rev 29:46, 1965.

Fitzgerald, T. J.: Toxic activities of *Treponema pallidum*. In: Schell, R. F. and Musher, D. M. (eds.); Pathogenesis and Immunology of Treponemal infection, Marcel Dekker, New York, 1983, p 173.

Hanff, P. A., Miller, J. N., and Lovett, M. A.: Molecular characterization of common treponemal antigens. Infect Immun 40:825, 1983.

Hovind Hougen, K.: Morphology. In: Schell, R. F. and Musher, D. M. (eds.): Pathogenesis and Immunology of Treponemal Infection. Marcel Dekker, New York, 1983, p 3-28.

Jenkin, H. M. and Sandok, P. L.: In vitro cultivation of *Treponema pallidum*. In: Schell, R. F. and Musher, D. M. (eds.): Pathogenesis and Immunology of Treponemal Infection. Marcel Dekker, New York, 1983, p 71-98.

Lukehart, S. A., Baker-Zander, S. A., Lloyd, R. M. C.: Characterization of lymphocyte responsiveness in early experimental syphilis. II. Nature of cellular infiltration and *Treponema pallidum* distribution in testicular lesions. J Immunol 124:461, 1980.

Lukehart, S. A., Baker-Zander, S. A., and Gubish, E. R., Jr.: Identification of *Treponema pallidum* antigens: comparison with a nonpathogenic treponeme. J Immunol 129:833, 1982.

Lysko, P. G., and Cox, C. D.: Terminal electron transport in *Treponema pallidum*. Infect Immun 16:885, 1977.

Magnuson, H. J., Thomas, E. W., Olansky, S., Kaplan, B. I., deMello, L., and Cutler, J. C.: Inoculation syphilis in human volunteers. Medicine 35:33, 1956.

Matthews, H. M., Yang, T-K., and Jenkin, H. M.: Unique lipid composition of *Treponema pallidum* (Nichols virulent strain). Infect Immun 24:713, 1979.

Musher, D. M., Hague-Park, M., Gyorkey, F., Anderson, D. C., and Baughn, R. E.: The interaction between *Treponema pallidum* and human polymorphonuclear leukocytes. J Infect Dis 147:77, 1983.

Penn, C. W.: Avoidance of host defences by *Treponema pallidum* in situ and on extraction from infected rabbit testes. J Gen Microbiol 126:69, 1981.

Schell, R. F., Musher, D. M., Jacobson, K., and Schwethelm, P.: Induction of acquired cellular resistance following transfer of thymus-dependent lymphocytes from syphilitic rabbits. J Immunol 114:550, 1975.

Schell, R. F., and Musher D. M.: Pathogenesis and Immunology of Treponemal Infection (multiauthored textbook). Marcel Dekker, New York, 1983.

Sell, S., Baker-Zander, S. A., and Powell, H. C.: Experimental syphilitic activities in rabbits: ultrastructural appearance of *T. pallidum* during phagocytosis and dissolution by macrophages in vivo. Lab Investig 46:355, 1982.

Spagnuolo, P. J., Butler, T., Bloch, E. H., Santoro, C., Tracy, J. W., and Johnson, R. C.: Opsonic requirements for phagocytosis of *Borrelia hermsii* by human polymorphonuclear leukocytes. J Infect Dis 145:358, 1982.

Southern, P. N., Jr., and Sanford, J. P.: Relapsing fever: A clinical and microbiological review. Medicine 48:129, 1969.

Turner, T. B., and Hollander, D. H.: Biology of the Treponematoses. Geneva, World Health Organization, Geneva, Monograph Series No. 35, 1957.

Young, E. J., Weingarten, N., Baughn, R. E., and Duncan, W. C.: Studies on the pathogenesis of the Jarisch-Herxheimer reaction: development of an animal model and evidence against a role for classical endotoxin. J Infect Dis 146:606, 1982.

3. Unique Intracellular Gram-Negative Bacteria

54
RICKETTSIA

GARRISON RAPMUND, M.D.

Rickettsiae are small bacteria that are natural parasites of certain arthropods. Some of these arthropods can transmit rickettsiae to animals, including man. Most of our knowledge of rickettsiae come from studies of the few species that are pathogenic for man.

Rickettsiae are named after the American physician, H. T. Ricketts, who first recognized rickettsiae as the cause of typhus and spotted fever and who died of typhus in 1910 while investigating the disease in Mexico.

Rickettsiae are distinct from other bacteria because of their small size, their transmission by arthropods, and their obligate intracellular parasitism. Four groups of rickettsiae are pathogenic for man: the typhus group, of which the type species is *Rickettsia prowazekii;* the spotted fever group, of which the type species is *Rickettsia rickettsii;* the scrub typhus group, composed of one species complex, *Rickettsia tsutsugamushi;* and the Q fever group, *Coxiella burnetii.* The first three groups are similar in their growth and metabolism, fine structure, and pathogenic properties in man. They differ significantly, however, in size, intracellular location, extracellular behavior, and antigenic composition. These differences distinguish the species of rickettsiae and separate the organism that causes Q fever into a different genus, *Coxiella.* Several organisms that cause disease in man have been called rickettsiae in the past but have now been reclassified. *Rickettsia quintana,* the cause of louse-borne trench fever in man, is now placed in a separate genus, *Rochalimaea,* because of its ability to grow on artificial media. *Rickettsia sennetsu,* the cause of an infectious mononucleosis-like syndrome in southern Japan and perhaps elsewhere, is now known to be related serologically to organisms of the genus *Ehrlichia,* which are pathogens of dogs and domestic ruminants. For reasons to be discussed later, *R. sennetsu* has been reclassified with the *Ehrlichia.*

MORPHOLOGY. Rickettsiae are typically short rods 0.3 to 0.7 μm by 1.0 to 2.0 μm, a size just visible by light microscopy. Pleomorphism is common. Coccobacilli, diplobacilli, and individual rods are seen in infected tissue. A developmental cycle has never been identified in rickettsiae. Some investigators have postulated that morphologic variation represents a developmental cycle, but this view is not generally accepted. It is true that rickettsiae in the logarithmic growth phase are typically rod-shaped, while those in the stationary phase are often coccoid, filamentous, or swollen, but there is no evidence that this pleomorphism reflects a developmental cycle. *C. burnetii* is smaller than pathogenic rickettsiae and is filterable through certain pore filters that trap other bacteria.

Rickettsiae are gram-negative but stain poorly by the Gram technique. Rickettsiae stain red by the Macchiavello (Fig. 1) and Giminez techniques (Giminez, 1964) and purple by the Giemsa stain. Only specific immunofluorescent antisera can differentiate rickettsiae definitely from other microorganisms by means of a staining reaction.

The ultrastructure of rickettsiae is typical of gram-negative bacteria (Anacker et al., 1967). A five-layered cell wall-plasma membrane complex (Fig. 2) surrounds the cytoplasm, which contains a large array of ribosomes and fibrouslike strands indicative of deoxyribonucleic acid. Intracytoplasmic vacuoles and invaginations of the plasma membrane are common (Figs. 2 and 3). Discrete, sharply defined nuclear structures have not been observed. *C. burnetii* contains a central fibrous body with radiating fibrils that are susceptible to treatment with ribonuclease. This suggests an organized DNA center that may be physically connected with RNA-containing ribosomes in the cytoplasm.

Several workers have demonstrated a zone on the outer surface of rickettsiae (Fig. 4). Silverman and Wisseman (1978) called this a slime layer rather than a capsule because of its tendency to slough away. This extracellular layer corresponds to an electron-lucent zone surrounding *R. prowazekii* and *R. rickettsii* in infected host cells and appears to be a complex of three distinct zones: an inner layer at the cell surface of small projections with a periodicity of 13 nm radiating outward, an intermediate clear zone, and an outer fibrous slime layer that varies in width from 25 to 130 nm. The morphologic similarities to gram-negative bacteria are striking, but there seem to be significant functional differences. The presence of a capsule in other bacteria is associated with virulence, but the avirulent

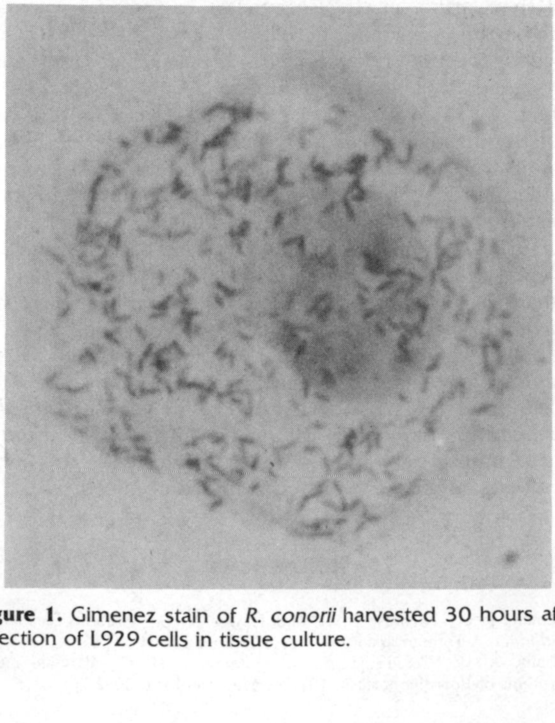

Figure 1. Gimenez stain of *R. conorii* harvested 30 hours after infection of L929 cells in tissue culture.

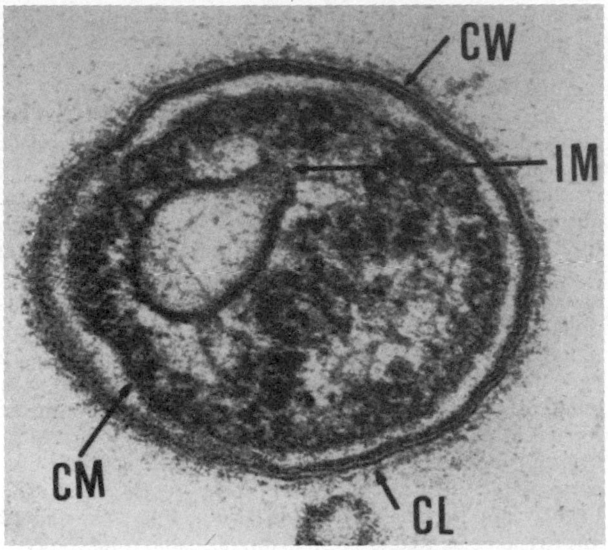

Figure 2. Thin section of *R. prowazekii.* Note capsule-like layer (CL), five-layered cell wall (CW), and intracytoplasmic membrane (IM). × 185,000 (From Anacker, R. L., et al.: J Bacteriol 94:260, 1967.)

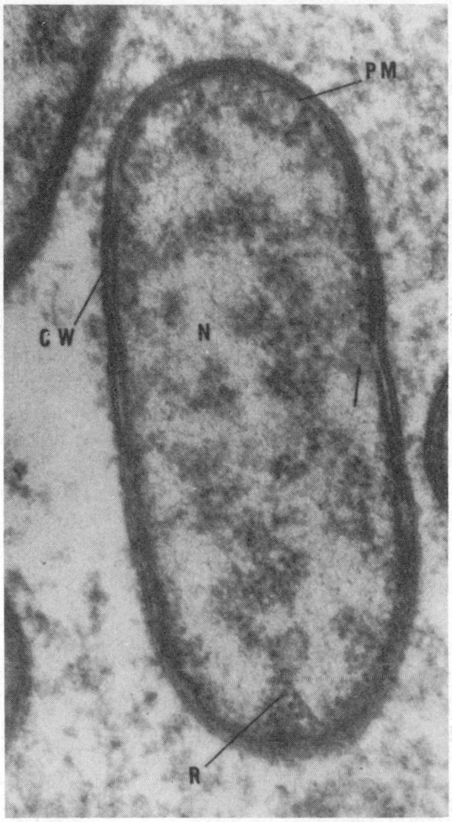

Figure 3. Thin section through several *R. quintana* cells from the intestine of an infected louse. Cell wall (CW) and plasma membrane (PM) both appear trilaminar. Arrow indicates an invagination of the plasma membrane. R indicates granules that are presumed to represent ribosomes. The "nuclear" component (N) is composed of fine filaments between the granules. × 125,000. (From Ito, S., and Vinson, J. W.: J Bacteriol 89:481, 1965.)

(Madrid E) strain of *R. prowazekii* contains the same extracellular structures as the fully virulent Breinl strain. Furthermore, the ultrastructure of rickettsiae in arthropod tissue is identical to that in mammalian tissue, and the ultrastructure of viable extracellular *R. prowazekii* in dried louse feces is identical to its intracellular morphology in the louse gut epithelium (Silverman et al., 1974). Thus, the ultrastructure of rickettsiae has not yet provided clues to the important functional properties of virulence and intracellular or extracellular survival.

The chemical composition of the rickettsial cell wall is similar to other gram-negative bacteria. It contains muramic acid, diaminopimelic acid, other amino acids, sugars, and amino sugars. Teichoic acid, a characteristic component of gram-positive bacteria, has not been found. Some years

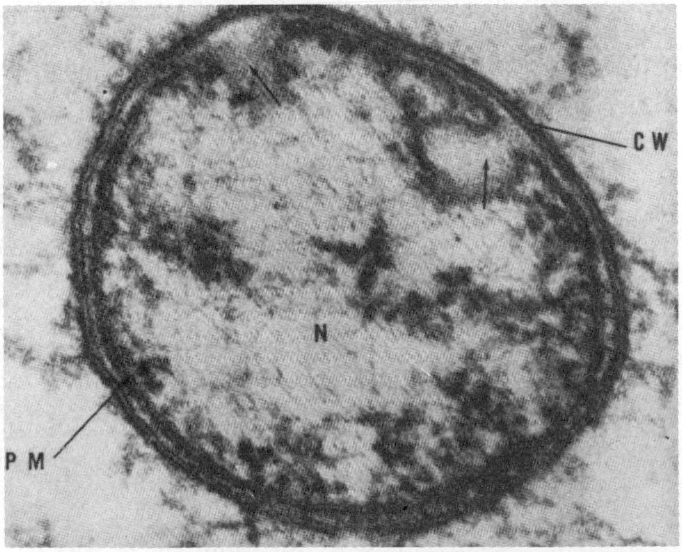

Figure 4. Transverse section of *R. quintana.* Arrows designate multiple invaginations of the plasma membrane. Symbols are the same as those in Figure 3. × 190,000. (From Ito, S., and Vinson, J. W.: J Bacteriol 89:481, 1965.)

ago, Wood and Wisseman (1967) reported that *R. typhi* had endotoxic activity that suggested the possibility that it contained a lipopolysaccharide layer. More recently, Schramek and co-workers (1976) isolated lipopolysaccharide from the typhus group, the spotted fever group, and purified cells and soluble antigen preparations of the scrub typhus group. These workers have not yet reported a full chemical analysis of this rickettsial lipopolysaccharide, but they have analyzed similar preparations of lipopolysaccharide from purified phase 1 cells of *C. burnetii* (Schramek and Brezina, 1976). The lipopolysaccharide contains 17 fatty acids, including hydroxymyristic acid, which is a common constituent of most gram-negative bacterial lipopolysaccharides. The sugar moiety of *C. burnetii* lipopolysaccharide contains mannose, glucose, galactose, xylose, heptose, and 2-keto-3-deoxyoctonate (KDO). The presence of the amino sugars, glucosamine, galactosamine, and possibly fucosamine is further evidence of the similarity of this lipopolysaccharide to that of other gram-negative bacteria. Serologic cross-reactivity between lipid A of *C. burnetii* and *Salmonella minnesota* R595 lipopolysaccharide has also been reported (Schramek and Galanos, 1981).

Rickettsiae contain both RNA and DNA. The RNA species include transfer RNA and ribosomal RNA. The size of the DNA genome is about one third that of *E. coli* and the same as or slightly smaller than that of pathogenic *Neisseria*. Myers and Wisseman (1980) reported the genome size to be about 1×10^9 daltons. Tyeryar et al. (1973) analyzed the base composition of rickettsial DNA and found a small but distinct difference in the molar percentage of guanine plus cytosine (G + C) between the typhus group (30 per cent) and the spotted fever group (32.5 per cent). Strains within each group show remarkable homogeneity of G + C content, even when isolated from widely separated geographic areas. *Rickettsia canada*, an organism that cross-reacts immunologically with members of both the typhus and the spotted fever groups, has a G + C content of 30 moles per cent, which suggests that it evolved from the typhus group. *C. burnetii* has a G + C content of 43 to 45 per cent (Schramek, 1968), distinctly different from other rickettsiae. *R. quintana's* G + C content of 38.6 moles per cent is also quite distinct. DNA-base composition can be identical in quite different organisms, however. The DNA-base ratio of typhus rickettsiae is identical to that of *Wolbachia persica*, a rickettsia-like symbiont of ticks, with significantly different metabolism from typhus rickettsiae (Weiss, 1982).

ANTIGENIC COMPOSITION. The typhus group of rickettsiae includes *R. prowazekii*, the cause of louse-borne epidemic typhus; *R. typhi*, also referred to as *R. mooseri*, the cause of flea-borne murine typhus; and *R. canada*, isolated from ticks in Ontario, Canada, and California (Philip et al., 1982). Members of this group possess common soluble antigens that are released into the aqueous phase during ether extraction of infected yolk sacs. These antigens cross-react in the complement fixation (CF) test. Members of the group can be distinguished from each other in the CF test by using washed whole rickettsial cells as the CF antigen.

The spotted fever group of rickettsiae includes representatives from all continents and Australia. Members of this group also possess common soluble antigens that are released into the aqueous phase by ether treatment of infected yolk sacs. The type species for the group, *R. rickettsii*, causes spotted fever in man in North America. Other members of this group that are pathogenic for man include Siberian tick typhus *(Dermacentroxenus sibericus)*, North Queensland tick typhus *(R. australis)*, fievre boutonneuse in the Mediterranean region *(R. conorii)*, and the cause of rickettsialpox *(R. akari)*. Washed rickettsial cells of each species are species-specific in the CF test. All spotted fever rickettsiae except *R. akari* cause acute toxic death of mice when inoculated live intravenously in high titer. In the so-called toxin neutralization test, rickettsiae and immune guinea pig sera are incubated together before inoculation. Neutralization of the toxic death is species-specific and distinguishes between members of the group. A number of strains of spotted fever rickettsiae that are generally avirulent for guinea pigs have been isolated from different tick species in the West, Southwest, and Southeast regions of the United States. Some, like *R. parkeri* and *R. rhipicephalus*, have been given species designation (Burgdorfer et al., 1975). Other workers (Tarasevich et al., 1976; Urvolgyi and Brezina, 1978) have isolated from ticks spotted fever rickettsiae that are also distinguishable from the type species of their respective regions. A number of the tick and human strains of North American origin have been examined by Philip et al. (1978) by immunofluorescence with mouse antisera. They reported that all human isolates were identical to *R. rickettsii* and that the isolates from ticks can be sorted into one of eight other serotypes. None cross-reacted with *R. akari*. Rickettsiae of one serotype were not limited to one geographic locality. The serotypes may be grouped epidemiologically according to association with either one or more than one species of arthropod. Some serotypes were recovered from only one tick species and are apparently host-specific. They include *R. parkeri* from the Gulf Coast tick *Amblyomma maculatum;* an unclassified rickettsia from the rabbit tick, *Dermacentor parumapertus;* an unclassified rickettsia isolated many times from the Pacific Coast tick, *Ixodes pacificus;* and an unclassified rickettsia from another Pacific Coast tick, *Dermacentor occidentalis*. Rickettsiae of the five other serotypes were recovered from more than one species of ticks that were widely distributed in the United States. The tick species involved were *Haemaphysalis leporispalustris, Dermacentor andersoni, Dermacentor variabilis*, and *Rhipicephalus sanguineus*. The serotype to which all human isolates belonged was also recovered from the first three of the foregoing tick species. The stability of these antigenic characteristics is not known yet, but, if they prove to be genetically stable, they offer an interesting opportunity to search for antigenic markers of virulence for man among the spotted fever rickettsiae.

The scrub typhus group of rickettsiae is antigenically much more heterogeneous than the typhus and spotted fever groups. Yet, only one species, *R. tsutsugamushi*, is recognized. Soluble antigens extracted by ether treatment of infected yolk sacs are not group-reactive in the CF test. Therefore, members of the group are identified by a mouse vaccination-challenge procedure. A laboratory mouse that survives infection with one strain is immune to all other strains. Such broad heterologous immunity is unfortunately not seen in man. Three strains (Karp, Gilliam, and Kato), all isolated from human infections, have evolved into reference strains to which all other strains are compared. The full number of immuno-types of *R. tsutsugamushi* is still not known. Using the immunofluorescence procedure, Elisberg and co-workers (1968) identified six additional serotypes (as well as Karp, Gilliam, and Kato) from an array of human, larval mite, and wild small mammal isolates from Thailand. An immunofluorescence study of 74 isolates from Pakistan (Shirai and Wisseman, 1975) found almost all to be related to Karp. The remainder cross-reacted with Gilliam and/or Kato. Antigenic heterogeneity was also found by Russian workers in the Soviet Far East and in Tadjikistan and by Japanese workers throughout Japan. A single immunologic strain does not appear to be restricted to one species of mite vector. Implications of this strain diversity for the ecology of scrub typhus have been considered in a comprehensive review by Traub and Wisseman (1974).

METABOLISM. Although rickettsiae produce some energy from independent metabolic activity, they are obligate intracellular parasites because their essential substrates must come from the host cell. Rickettsial respiration is stimulated most by glutamate, but less so by glutamine, which the rickettsia must deaminate to glutamate. Pyruvate and the dicarboxylic acid intermediates of the citric acid cycle support respiration to a much lesser extent. Glucose, glucose-6-phosphate, lactate, sucrose, and naturally occurring amino acids other than glutamate do not stimulate respiration. End products of glutamate metabolism include ammonia and carbon dioxide, but most of the amino group of glutamate is transaminated to form aspartate by glutamate-oxaloacetate transaminase. Rickettsiae have a tricarboxylic acid cycle but not a complete glycolytic sequence and pentose shunt (Coolbaugh et al., 1976). In comparison with *Chlamydia*, *R. typhi* can generate appreciable amounts of energy. It has also been shown that typhus rickettsiae synthesize levels of monophosphate and diphosphate kinases comparable to those of *Salmonella typhimurium.* The fact that *C. burnetii* does catabolize glucose is further evidence of the great difference between this organism and other rickettsiae. All metabolic studies are hindered by the difficulties of harvesting viable undamaged whole cells or extracts free of host-cell material. The development of renografin density gradient centrifugation provides highly purified viable rickettsiae. Like other bacteria, rickettsiae have an electron-transport system, including nicotinamide adenine dinucleotide (NADPH) and NADPH-dependent enzymes. Rickettsiae can synthesize small amounts of protein as measured by incorporation of radiolabeled amino acids and the inhibition of this incorporation by chloramphenicol. The phosphorylation and stimulation of endogenous levels of adenine nucleotides by glutamate metabolism indicates that rickettsiae have the potential for sustained biosynthetic capabilities. However, the paucity of other nucleotides places severe restrictions on nucleic acid synthesis. Rickettsiae also synthesize lipids, but on a minute scale, similar to their synthesis of protein. These synthetic activities require the donation from the host cell of complex energy-yielding substrates, including ATP, but rickettsiae can produce small amounts of ATP (Phibbs and Winkler, 1982).

One of the chief objectives of the studies of the metabolic pathways of rickettsiae is the definition and synthesis of an artificial medium that supports extracellular rickettsial growth. To date, this has not been achieved. Given the chemical composition and structural similarity between rickettsiae and other gram-negative bacteria, there is obviously some fundamental difference between the two that precludes extracellular growth of rickettsiae. Much attention has focused on the integrity and function of the rickettsial cell wall as a possible explanation for this difference. Moulder (1966) propounded the concept of "leakiness" of the cell wall. He suggested that rickettsial cell walls were nonspecifically porous and allowed passage of host-cell nutrients into intracellular rickettsiae, but allowed loss of essential nutrients from extracellular rickettsiae. Winkler (1976) disproved this thesis in a series of elegant experiments showing that rickettsial cell membranes are highly specialized and active rather than passive with respect to nutrient transport. He defined a carrier-mediated transport system that is very specific for ATP and ADP and the analog β, γ-methylene-ATP. The system is an obligatory exchange system in that a molecule can enter a cell only if another molecule can exit. The pool of ATP and ADP remains the same, but ATP can be acquired in exchange for ADP. Smith and Winkler (1977) defined and Zahorchak and Winkler (1983) further characterized a second highly specific system that actively transports lysine against a gradient.

Rapid death of extracellular rickettsiae can be retarded by suspension in a medium composed of sucrose and glutamate in potassium phosphate buffered to pH 7.0 (SPG). This medium, devised years ago by Bovarnick and co-workers, has been widely used to sustain rickettsiae during purification, metabolic studies, and titrations. Its performance was improved by the addition of serum albumin. Rickettsiae can be preserved for long periods frozen at minus 60° C, in whole yolk sac membranes or membranes triturated in SPG. In an effort to improve plaquing of rickettsiae, Wike et al. (1972) showed that extracellular infectivity and stability could be maintained more satisfactorily for short periods if rickettsiae were suspended in brain-heart infusion broth.

Rickettsiae multiply by transverse binary fission. Wisseman and Waddell (1975) have studied the kinetics of growth in irradiated chick embryo cells. Growth of *R. prowazekii* proceeded immediately if the inoculum was derived from rickettsiae harvested in the logarithmic phase of growth. There was a lag period of about 7.5 hours if rickettsiae were harvested in the stationary phase. The generation time of rickettsiae was slightly less than 9 hours at 34° C, and this rate continued for about 36 to 48 hours. After this period, heavily infected cells released their rickettsiae, and the cycle of growth became irregular.

Well-adapted strains of rickettsiae grow luxuriously in cell cytoplasm, often pushing the nucleus to one side, but they do not aggregate in the cytoplasm to form inclusion bodies like *Ehrlichia.* Spotted fever rickettsiae are distinguished by their ability to grow in the cell nucleus as well as the cytoplasm. *R. canada*, a member of the typhus group, also grows in the nucleus occasionally. Rickettsiae form plaques in monolayer cultures, and it is possible to clone strains. *R. rickettsii* forms plaques larger and faster than other rickettsiae. This is consistent with the independent observation that *R. rickettsii* is released from the cell and infects other cells at a much earlier stage of the growth cycle than either *R. prowazekii* or *R. tsutsugamushi.*

Rickettsiae require well-nourished host cells for growth, but the host cells do not need to multiply. It is possible, therefore, to stop host-cell metabolism with irradiation or colchicine and use these stationary cells as temporary microenvironments for the culture and study of rickettsiae. In such cells, rickettsiae may grow until the host cell bursts, but release of rickettsiae from actively metabolizing cells appears to occur also by extrusion. Schaechter and co-workers (1957) observed rickettsiae trapped in microfibrillar structures protruding from the edge of the cell. When the microfibrillae retracted, they either carried the rickettsiae back into the cytoplasm or released them to the outside. Stork and Wisseman (1976) have observed that *R. prowazekii* can infect and multiply in enucleated L and chicken embryo cells, but the rickettsiae do not achieve true exponential growth. This finding is consistent with the earlier observations of Weiss that *R. typhi* continued to grow in cells that could not synthesize protein because of treatment with cycloheximide.

PATHOGENIC PROPERTIES. Rickettsiae enter most mammalian cells by first attaching to the cell membrane and then being phagocytized. Attachment is not a casual process. Close contact is required; centrifugation of mixtures of entodermal cell cultures and rickettsiae increases attachment and penetration. Active participation of rickettsiae is also required. Rickettsial red blood cell interactions have been studied as a model of cell attachment (Ramm and Winkler, 1973). The erythrocyte was found to have a receptor for rickettsiae, a neutral lipid complex of cholesterol and palmitic acid. Energy poisons, such as potassium cyanide, inhibited both adsorption and lysis, and addition of ATP reactivated this rickettsial activity (Winkler, 1974). Scanning electronmicrographs revealed that rickettsiae adsorb end-on almost exclusively. Winkler and Ramm (1975) have also observed that rickettsiae harvested after lysing red blood cells can adsorb to other red blood cells. Lysis of human and sheep red blood cells required live rickettsiae and was associated with phospholipase A activity (Winkler and Miller, 1980). Recently, a phospholipase-associated penetration mechanism has been described for *R. rickettsii* in mouse L cells (Walker et al., 1983). Hyperimmune serum enhances phagocytosis of rickettsiae by professional phagocytes, but it does not improve phagocytosis by such nonprofessional cells as endothelial cells and fibroblasts.

Once inside the cell, virulent rickettsiae can escape from the phagosome before it fuses with the lysosome and thus survive to multiply freely in the cell cytoplasm. By contrast, the avirulent Madrid E strain of *R. prowazekii* remains in the phagosome and is destroyed when the phagosome forms and the rickettsiae are exposed to lysosomal enzymes. Phagocytosed rickettsiae coated with immune serum are destroyed in professional phagocytes but survive in nonprofessional phagocytes. In contrast, *C. burnetii* remains in the phagosome and multiplies, protected by unknown means from the lysosomal hydrolases.

For experimental work, rickettsiae are usually cultivated in fertile hen eggs, tissue cultures, and small laboratory animals. The minimum infectious dose for eggs has been estimated to be one infectious rickettsia for the Madrid E strain of *R. prowazekii*. Ley et al. (1952) also estimated that only one *R. tsutsugamushi* organism could cause human disease. The optimum growth temperature for *R. rickettsii* is about 33.5° C and for other rickettsiae about 35° C. Large numbers of rickettsiae can be harvested from infected yolk sacs of chicken embryos, and this is usually the source of rickettsiae for a wide variety of investigations and for preparation of diagnostic antigens. Many host cell-parasite relationships have been worked out in explant and continuous-cell-line tissue cultures. Small laboratory animals are used chiefly for isolation of rickettsiae from patients. Guinea pigs are the animal of choice for typhus and the spotted fever group, and the laboratory mouse for scrub typhus (see *Laboratory Diagnosis*).

The basic lesion caused by rickettsiae is a vasculitis, localized to the endothelium and smooth muscle of the vessel wall. The lesion contains rickettsiae. There is endothelial swelling, thrombosis, and vascular and perivascular necrosis. Vascular permeability is increased. The infected host displays varying degrees of hemorrhage, tissue edema, and peripheral circulatory failure. Depending on the distribution of the vasculitis, the patient develops a petechial rash, frank hemorrhage into the skin, gangrene of appendages, interstitial inflammation of major viscera, lymph node hyperplasia, and meningoencephalitis. The circulatory failure of severe rickettsial disease has been studied by Harrell and Aikawa (1949). Plasma volume is decreased, and the extravascular fluid spaces are increased. The pathophysiology has been studied in experimental hosts including the guinea pig, rabbit, and monkey. Different species of rickettsiae have typical pathophysiologic manifestations, as shown by variations in the diseases they cause in man. Each pathogenic species causes some infections in man and experimental animals, however, that are entirely inapparent and others that are so severe as to be lethal. In some geographic regions, inapparent infection is the rule. As yet, there are no defined markers that distinguish virulent from avirulent rickettsiae in terms of host response to infection, nor is there clear evidence for any mechanism of rickettsiae-induced pathophysiology other than direct cell invasion and injury by live rickettsiae. De Brito and co-workers (1968) found gamma globulin and complement in late vascular lesions of guinea pigs infected with *R. rickettsii*, which suggests that immune complex vasculitis occurs in spotted fever. More recently, Walker and Henderson (1978) studied *R. rickettsii* infection in the immunosuppressed guinea pig. They found as severe a vasculitis in the immunosuppressed as in control animals and argued that rickettsiae damage cells without the participation of immune mechanisms.

Schramek, Brezina, and Tarasevich (1976) have reported isolation of lipopolysaccharide antigens from *R. prowazekii*, *R. typhi*, *R. canada*, *R. conorii*, and *R. tsutsugamushi*. From hypothermic reactions in intraperitoneally inoculated white rats and chemical analysis, they concluded that these antigens had endotoxic properties. Other investigators have shown that rickettsial lipopolysaccharide gels *limulus* lysate and possesses platelet aggregative and leukocyte procoagulant activity (Miragliotta et al., 1981). The endotoxin hypothesis is attractive as an explanation of some aspects of rickettsial pathophysiology.

Yamada and co-workers (1978) reported activation of the kallikrein-kinin system in five patients with American spotted fever. Four had petechial rashes characteristic of vasculitis and then developed disseminated intravascular coagulation. They concluded that even if kinins do not initiate the early vascular changes, they may promote progression of the lesions.

Despite these studies of the basic pathology and pathogenic properties of rickettsiae, the virulence factors are still largely unknown. The attenuated Madrid E strain of *R. prowazekii*, in contrast to fully virulent strains, disappears quickly from the tissues of guinea pigs, so that serial passage is usually unsuccessful. It does not differ substantially from virulent strains, however, in a variety of other properties, including toxicity for mice, hemolytic activity, infectivity for body lice, antigenic characteristics, and quantity of slime layer. There is no difference in its ability to infect and grow in chicken embryo cells and a variety of other cell lines. It does differ in one important respect: in human macrophages, the Madrid E strain cannot escape from the phagosome and is killed by lysosomal hydrolases. This may be the mechanism of its attenuation.

The stability of the E strain has been questioned by Russian (Balayeva and Nikolskaja, 1972) and Slovak (Kaźar et al., 1973) workers who noted reversion to full virulence for guinea pigs after prolonged serial passage in the mouse lung and the guinea pig peritoneum. It is unclear whether this phenomenon represents selection of a virulent strain from a mixture that is predominantly avirulent or is a true back-mutation.

There have been many studies of the virulence of spotted fever rickettsiae. Long ago it was observed that inoculation of rickettsiae into guinea pigs from unfed adult ticks *(Dermacentor andersoni)* would produce immunity but no disease. If the ticks were given a blood meal before harvest and inoculation of rickettsiae, the guinea pigs became sick. Later, Spencer and Parker reexamined this phenomenon by inoculating a virulent strain of *R. rickettsii* into adult ticks and storing them for several months at refrigerator temperature. Inoculation at this point produced, as before, immunity but no disease in guinea pigs. If the ticks were warmed first or fed a blood meal, virulence for guinea pigs was restored. Close examination of this phenomenon showed that it was not caused by an increase in the number of rickettsiae. Addition of para-aminobenzoic acid (PABA), parahydroxybenzoic acid, or PABA plus coenzyme A to rickettsiae held for 60 hours at 25° C restored virulence to the stored rickettsiae. Virulence could also be restored by incubating the rickettsiae with recently fed and ground-up ticks. A recent ultrastructural analysis has validated these observations (Hayes and Burgdorfer, 1982).

Generally, the virulence of rickettsiae for laboratory animals does not parallel virulence for man. However, there does appear to be a consistent geographic difference in the virulence of scrub typhus rickettsiae for man. A strain from the Pescadores Islands, where disease is characteristically mild, was used as a live vaccine in Japan. Disease contracted during the winter months in Japan is said to be much milder than disease contracted in the warmer months. It is interesting that different mite vectors are involved in the Pescadores and during different seasons in Japan. Certainly, scrub typhus is commonly very mild in Southeast Asia, where the predominant vector mite is still another species. Because a good marker for virulence is lacking, it is not possible to examine the stability of rickettsial virulence during passage through different species of mites.

IMMUNOLOGY. Natural host resistance to infection must be considered in assessments of rickettsial virulence. Groves and co-workers examined genetic resistance to lethal infections with *R. tsutsugamushi* in over 30 inbred strains of mice. They found some strains fully resistant, some fully susceptible, and a few selectively resistant to lethal infection with the Gilliam strain of scrub typhus rickettsiae. Resistance was not due to an inability of host cells to support rickettsial growth. It was genetically dominant and controlled by a single gene or a closely linked cluster of autosomal genes (Groves et al., 1980). Susceptibility, on the other hand, was not due to inability to mount an immune response. Russian workers (Kokorin et al., 1976) analyzed the same phenomenon and noted a marked difference in the reaction of the macrophages of resistant and susceptible mice. Fatal infection was accompanied by death of macrophages and peritoneal necrosis. The resistant mice showed no clinical signs of infection but mounted an intensive macrophage reaction at the inoculation site. Most of the inoculated rickettsiae died at the inoculation site, and the macrophages remained viable. Some rickettsiae survive and persist in resistant mice for a long time without producing overt clinical disease. Anderson and Osterman (1980) have also observed a genetic basis for natural resistance to lethal infection with *R. akari* (rickettsialpox).

Rickettsiae stimulate both humoral and cellular immunity. The role of each in response to infection of man and animals is not completely understood. Humoral antibody appears in response to rickettsial infections between the seventh and fourteenth days of disease. Production of humoral antibody to *R. tsutsugamushi* requires the presence of mature T lymphocytes, and athymic nude mice did not make antibody to *R. akari*, *R. conorii*, and *R. typhi* (Jerrells and Eisemann, 1983). Passive transfer of immune serum provides protection against clinical disease in animals challenged with the same strain. Cellular immune processes also occur, as shown by the development of dermal hypersensitivity, lymphocyte transformation, and elaboration of migration-inhibiting factor.

Recent studies of *R. tsutsugamushi* and *C. burnetii* revealed some details of the immune process. Shirai and co-workers (1976) have shown that passive transfer of spleen cells from infected mice protects the recipient against challenge with homologous and heterologous strains of *R. tsutsugamushi*. The protective spleen cells were thymus-dependent lymphocytes. Subsequently, these investigators (Catanzaro et al., 1977) demonstrated that peritoneal exudate lymphocytes (PEL) were the mediators of this cellular protection. It was not possible to determine from their experiments whether PELs were the primary mediators, as they are in other bacterial infections. Subsequently, Nacy and Osterman (1979) determined that protective splenic lymphocytes elaborate lymphokines that activate macrophages. However, lymphokine activation is not restricted to professional macrophages. Mouse and human fibroblasts infected with *R. prowazekii* clear rickettsiae and suppress growth of the organism when they are treated with appropriate lymphokines (Turco and Winkler, 1983).

LABORATORY DIAGNOSIS. Isolation of rickettsiae should ordinarily be attempted only in a research laboratory. Isolation is accomplished preferably by immediate (within one hour of collection) intraperitoneal inoculation of the specimen into a suitable experimental animal. The isolation host of choice for the typhus and spotted fever groups of rickettsiae is the guinea pig and for scrub typhus the laboratory mouse. The most appropriate isolation specimen for human diagnosis is blood clot prepared as a 10 per cent suspension in skim milk or brain-heart infusion broth. Other diluents adversely affect rickettsiae. Several passages of tissue from inoculated animals at approximately 14-day intervals may be necessary before symptomatic infection develops. In guinea pigs, the only indication may be an increase in rectal temperature, which must be recorded daily from the time of inoculation. On the first passage of typhus group rickettsiae, fever does not appear until the third week after inoculation. Either brain or spleen should be harvested from the febrile animal and inoculated intraperitoneally into other guinea pigs. If no fever or other evidence of infection occurs, animals in the second or third passage are bled on day 28 for antibody studies. Antibody may be the only evidence that rickettsiae have been isolated. The only gross evidence of *R. prowazekii* infection in the guinea pig is a fibrous exudate on the spleen surface. Examination of smears taken from scrapings of the spleen surface may show rickettsiae in serosal cells. If the inoculum of rickettsiae is large, the scrotum may enlarge, and the testes may adhere to the scrotal sac. This lesion is called the Neill-Mooser reaction after the investigators who discovered it. The lesion is much more often found in *R. typhi* infections and occurs at the time of fever. In other respects, *R. typhi* infections are like those of *R. prowazekii*, except that the incubation period of established infections is shorter (three to seven days), and the Neill-Mooser reaction is more severe. The isolated rickettsiae are identified by using the rickettsiae as antigen in the CF or other serologic test against various antisera and by cross-vaccination and challenge against known rickettsiae.

The response of guinea pigs to virulent spotted fever group rickettsiae is more severe. After several passages to establish the isolate, the incubation period is shortened to two to five days, the fever course is often prolonged, and the animals may die on the sixth to eighth day. A severe scrotal reaction usually begins on the third or fourth day of fever and first consists of edema and erythema. The scrotum becomes necrotic with eventual tissue sloughing. Gangrene of the ears and footpads may also occur. As in infections with the typhus group, necropsy findings consist chiefly of a fibrinous exudate on the spleen surface and the scrotal reaction.

Scrub typhus rickettsiae are isolated by intraperitoneal inoculation of the white laboratory mouse. Several passages of infected liver, spleen, or brain may be required to establish the agent. Gross signs of infection include ruffled fur and a swollen abdomen. Necropsy reveals an enlarged spleen and mucoid peritoneal fluid. Scrapings of the peritoneal lining yield mesothelial cells containing rickettsiae in the cytoplasm.

Rickettsiae can be isolated by inoculation either into the yolk sac of the hen eggs or into tissue cultures. Adaptation to these substrates is often slow, and small inocula may be lost. Laboratory acquired infection is a constant hazard, even in the most sophisticated laboratory (Oster et al., 1977), so isolation of rickettsiae should be attempted only by experienced personnel in well-equipped facilities. Identification of rickettsiae or rickettsial antigen in the first week of disease would greatly assist clinicians to diagnose atypical cases. DeShazo and co-workers (1976) diagnosed Rocky Mountain spotted fever by the fourth day of disease in rhesus monkeys upon identification of *R. rickettsii* by immunofluorescence in primary monocyte culture. Shirai and colleagues (1978) achieved similar results in *R. tsutsugamushi* infections of monkeys and dogs. Coolbaugh and colleagues (1978) have used this procedure for the early diagnosis of a human case of scrub typhus. For pathologic specimens, Walker and Cain (1978) have described a method allowing retrospective analysis of fixed, paraffin-embedded tissue by *R. rickettsii*-specific immunofluorescence. The diagnosis of *R. rickettsii* infection may also be suggested by examination of ticks taken from patients. Burgdorfer identified *R. rickettsii* by immunofluorescent examination of the hemolymph of live ticks, and in desiccated ticks rickettsial antigen may be detected by immunofluorescence for several weeks (Kurz and Burgdorfer, 1978).

Human rickettsial antibodies are detectable by many serologic procedures. Complement fixation has been the most widely used specific test because antigens for the typhus and spotted fever groups have been available commercially or from central reference laboratories. Group-specific soluble antigen is prepared by ether extraction of infected yolk sacs of embryonated hen eggs. The antigen is inactivated. Typhus group antigen is prepared from *R. typhi*, while spotted fever is usually prepared from *R. akari*. The CF test can be made species-specific by using washed rickettsial cell suspensions as antigen. For diagnosis of spotted fever infections in various parts of the world, it is best to use the prevalent rickettsial species as antigen since *R. akari*, while broadly group-reactive, does not detect CF antibody to all the spotted fevers. Scrub typhus-soluble CF antigens are principally strain-specific, and the CF test is unsuitable for group diagnosis.

The indirect microimmunofluorescence procedure (Bozeman and Elisberg, 1963) is now widely employed for serologic diagnosis. Concentrated suspensions of rickettsiae from infected yolk sacs or cell culture are used as antigen. In the micro-technique, many antigen spots can be applied to one slide. After air drying and fixation in acetone, the slides may be stored at −70° C for later use. Philip and co-workers (1977) have compared this procedure with others for the diagnosis of both typhus and spotted fever group infections. In their hands, it was superior to the CF test for identifying disease. Herbert and co-workers (1980) have developed high-titered rickettsial species-specific fluorescent antibody to identify rickettsiae in clinical specimens, and Hechemy and co-workers (1981) have devised a reliable latex agglutination procedure for detecting serum antibody.

Rickettsial agglutination has been used for many years for the diagnosis of a variety of rickettsial infections by French workers and has been widely used by others for the diagnosis of Q fever. A microagglutination procedure (Fiset et al., 1969) conserves antigen (washed rickettsial suspensions).

Chang and colleagues (1954) performed hemagglutination with an erythrocyte-sensitizing substance (ESS) from typhus and spotted fever group rickettsiae. This antigen, which depends for its activity on a carbohydrate moiety (Osterman and Eiseman, 1978), has not been isolated from *R. tsutsugamushi*. The hemagglutination and microagglutination procedures compare favorably with the microimmunofluorescence procedure for the diagnosis of North American spotted fever (Philip et al., 1977).

Because CF antibodies are not found until the third week of disease, much effort has been expended to develop procedures for early diagnosis. The indirect immunofluorescence procedure, the indirect hemagglutination test, and the ELISA (enzyme-linked immunosorbent assay) all detect antibodies as early as the sixth to seventh day of disease. Woodward and co-workers (1976) demonstrated *R. rickettsii* in skin biopsy specimens from two patients on days 4 and 8 of illness by direct immunofluorescence. While confirming this experience in some patients, other workers have failed to identify rickettsiae in skin biopsies from patients already treated with tetracycline or chloramphenicol. Years ago, Fleck and co-workers (1960) found murine typhus antigen in the urine by indirect hemagglutination, but this early diagnostic technique has not been evaluated by others.

Specific rickettsial antibody appears by the end of the first week of disease in human and animal infections and persists in some cases for years. Rickettsemia and circulating specific antibody are detectable in the same blood specimens during disease and convalescence. Humans respond early to primary typhus infection with IgM antibodies, but this class of antibody is not recalled in recrudescent typhus. Philip and co-workers (1976) found IgM antibodies by microimmunofluorescence early in American spotted fever patients but noted its absence in 15 per cent of them. IgM antibody usually disappears within three to four months. IgG antibody usually appears by the third week of disease and persists for one or more years.

The antibody response can be suppressed by antibiotics early in the disease. Patients with American spotted fever who were treated early, especially during the first two days of illness, were less likely to be seropositive and had lower titers of antibody by the CF test during convalescence (Philip et al., 1977). Smadel (1954) also observed delayed or diminished antibody production by patients who were treated for scrub typhus by the third day of disease but there was no effect when therapy was started on the sixth day or later. It is assumed that early treatment suppresses antibody production by reducing the antigenic mass.

Antigenic cross-reactions occur between the typhus and spotted fever groups. The degree of cross-reactivity reflects not only the extent of shared antigens but also the species of host involved. Ormsbee and co-workers (1978) found that most patients who were acutely ill with epidemic typhus produced IgG and IgM antibodies to purified antigens of *R. prowazekii*, *R. typhi*, and *R. canada*. They also produced IgG, but seldom IgM, antibodies to spotted fever rickettsiae. Similarly, patients acutely ill with spotted fever produced IgG and IgM antibodies to *R. rickettsii*, *R. conorii*, and *R. akari*, as well as both classes of antibody to the typhus group. By contrast, the mouse produces species-specific rickettsial antibody. Ormsbee and co-workers (1978) have speculated that the more specific rodent antibody response reflects the greater antiquity of this host-parasite relationship. Scrub typhus and Q fever rickettsiae do not share antigens with other rickettsiae. The degree of heterologous antibody response in spotted fever and typhus infections is usually less than the homologous response, which helps clarify the serologic diagnosis of these infections. Prior immunization with epidemic typhus or spotted fever vaccine can cause confusion in the serologic findings because the anamnestic response of vaccine-induced antibody may exceed that stimulated by infection.

Rickettsiae share antigens with other bacteria. The antigens shared with *Proteus* organisms form the basis of the Weil-Felix agglutination test. For many years, this test was the only serologic test widely available for the diagnosis of rickettsial disease. The shared antigens have never been fully characterized, but years ago Castaneda described a carbohydrate antigen shared by *Proteus vulgaris* OX-19 and *R. prowazekii*. In human typhus, agglutinins occur chiefly against OX-19 and, to a much lesser extent, to the OX-2 strain. These agglutinins are rarely found in recrudescent typhus (Brill-Zinsser disease), although Ormsbee and co-workers (1977) found a brisk agglutinin response in two of five cases in Ethiopia. The cross-reactive antibody response stimulated by the spotted fever groups varies widely. Some patients produce chiefly OX-19 antibody, some chiefly OX-2, and some both. Therefore, the Weil-Felix agglutinins do not distinguish spotted fever from typhus group infections. Scrub typhus may stimulate production of agglutinins to *Proteus mirabilis* strain OXK. A titer of 1:200 or greater suggests infection. Because these antigens are commercially available, and the procedures are simple, physicians have relied on the Weil-Felix agglutination tests for rickettsial diagnosis. With the development of other procedures that use strain-specific antigens that are also noninfectious, the Weil-Felix test should be discarded. It is unreliable because agglutinins are often absent in proven rickettsial disease, especially scrub typhus. Furthermore, the presence of agglutinins may only indicate infection with *Proteus* or other bacteria. Infections with *R. akari* and *C. burnetii* do not produce Weil-Felix agglutinins.

DRUG SUSCEPTIBILITY. The growth of rickettsiae is inhibited by chloramphenicol and the tetracyclines that are given for treatment of rickettsial diseases. Penicillin and streptomycin are of no clinical value but are slightly inhibitory to rickettsiae. Sulfonamides have no effect on rickettsiae. On the other hand, para-aminobenzoic acid, an antagonist of sulfonamides, inhibits most rickettsiae, but *R. tsutsugamushi* is affected only slightly and *C. burnetii* not at all. Ormsbee and colleagues (1955) studied the relative inhibitory effect of various antibiotics in infected chicken embryos and found that the inhibitory dose of oxytetracycline for typhus and spotted fever rickettsiae was about one-eighth that of chlortetracycline, which was one third as active as chloramphenicol. Erythromycin was highly inhibitory for *R. prowazekii*, less so for spotted fever rickettsiae, and almost not at all for *C. burnetii*. Chloramphenicol is also relatively inactive against *C. burnetii*. *R. tsutsugamushi* is as sensitive to chloramphenicol and the tetracyclines in laboratory culture as the spotted fever rickettsiae. Doxycycline is highly effective clinically against the typhus group and *R. tsutsugamushi*. The MIC for *R. prowazekii* and *R. rickettsii* is about 0.1 μg/ml in vitro (Wisseman and Waddell, 1982).

Growth-inhibiting antibiotics do not eliminate viable rickettsiae from infected people. *R. tsutsugamushi* can persist in lymph nodes for years after recovery from infection. Persistence of *R. prowazekii* in patients who had survived an attack of epidemic typhus in the preantibiotic era was dramatically illustrated by recrudescent disease long after they had emigrated from endemic areas of Europe to America. Recrudescent typhus is called Brill-Zinsser disease. In laboratory animals that survive a rickettsial infection, recrudescent disease can be provoked by administration of cortisone. It is assumed that cortisone in animals mimics stress in man, which seems to modify the steady-state host-parasite relationship and permit rickettsiae to proliferate. Clinical recrudescence of other rickettsial diseases long after recovery has not been observed, but persistence of viable rickettsiae after treatment indicates that these drugs are rickettsiostatic. Continuous exposure of *R. tsutsugamushi* in cultured L-cells to high concentrations of chloramphenicol eventually sterilized the culture, but only after three weeks.

Antibiotic-resistant strains of rickettsiae have not been isolated from nature. Weiss and Dressler (1962) found that many serial passages of the Madrid E strain of *R. prowazekii* in the presence of increasing amounts of chloramphenicol did yield a substrain resistant to chloramphenicol. Resistance was not lost during 10 drugless egg passages. These workers isolated an erythromycin-resistant strain by the same procedure but could not induce resistance to tetracycline.

HOST RANGE. The human pathogens among the rickettsiae are distributed widely in many arthropods and mammals. Among the typhus group, *R. prowazekii* parasitizes both the head and body varieties of the human louse, *Pediculus humanis*. The human body louse is the major vector of classic epidemic typhus. *R. prowazekii* infects only the gut epithelium of the louse, which acquires the rickettsiae by feeding on the blood of a rickettsemic human. After a few days, proliferating rickettsiae burst the epithelial cells of the gut and appear in the louse feces. The louse usually dies from the infection within 7 to 10 days. Its salivary glands are not infected. Man acquires the infection from the louse by scratching the skin that has become contaminated with rickettsiae-containing louse feces (autoinoculation). Until recently, it was believed that the only cycle of *R. prowazekii* in nature was man-louse-man. Man was thought to be the reservoir because the louse does not pass the rickettsiae from generation to generation transovarially like other rickettsiae of ticks and mites. Bozeman and co-workers, in a remarkable series of studies, demonstrated the first nonhuman mammalian host of *R. prowazekii*, the American flying squirrel *(Glaucomys volans)*. They found enzootic foci in flying squirrels from Florida, North Carolina, Virginia, and Maryland and also recovered rickettsiae from the squirrel lice and fleas. The squirrel flea is known to feed on man. Bozeman and colleagues (1981) subsequently demonstrated that flying squirrel lice, but not other ectoparasites, could transmit the infection from squirrel to squirrel, thus maintaining rickettsiae in nature. *R. prowazekii* infection in the squirrel louse duplicates infection in the human body louse, with rickettsiae excreted in the feces. Therefore, transmission of disease to man may occur by aerosol of infected squirrel louse feces as well as by the bite of infected squirrel fleas. The strains of rickettsiae isolated from flying squirrels have been identified as *R. prowazekii* (Dasch et al., 1978). McDade and co-workers (1980) reported that sera of 7 of 1575 persons had rickettsial antibodies suggesting recent infection with *R. prowazekii*. Two of the seven patients had had contact with flying squirrels. Duma et al. (1981) described seven patients in Virginia, West Virginia, and North Carolina with *R. prowazekii* infection and Kaplan et al. (1981) suggested that patients with suspected Rocky Mountain spotted fever in winter months may have *R. prowazekii* infection. Reiss-Gutfreund reported infection with *R. prowazekii* in domestic animals and their ticks in Ethiopia that seemed to confirm earlier reports of epidemic typhus antibodies in domestic animals as well as man in the Upper Volta, Ruwanda-Burundi, and the Central African Republic. But other workers are skeptical (Burgdorfer et al., 1972).

R. typhi is found naturally in rats and mice. It is transmitted from rat to rat by the rat louse and the rat flea, *Xenopsylla cheopis*, which is usually the vector to man. Many other animals are also susceptible to *R. typhi*. The host range of *R. canada* is not well defined. It has been isolated in nature only from *Haemophysalis leporispalustris* ticks in Ontario, Canada (McKiel et al., 1967) and California.

The host ranges of the spotted fever group and scrub typhus group are discussed in the chapters on each disease.

Q FEVER RICKETTSIAE

Coxiella burnetii has been placed in a separate genus because it differs in many ways from other rickettsiae (Table 1). The differences have been summarized well by Ormsbee (1969). *C. burnetii* stains gram-positive when alcoholic iodine is used as mordant instead of aqueous iodine. Under these conditions, rickettsiae stain gram-negative. Rickettsiae release a soluble antigen when aqueous suspensions of cells are shaken in ether. *C. burnetii*, like other gram-negative bacteria, does not. Immunizing antigens of *C. burnetii* are very resistant to heat, whereas those of rickettsiae are heat-sensitive. The guanine plus cytosine molar per cent content of *C. burnetii* DNA is about 43 per cent, whereas rickettsiae have a G + C content in the range of 30 to 32.5 per cent. *C. burnetii* is remarkably resistant to physical and chemical agents. It survives in wool for seven to nine months at 20° C, at least two years in skim milk and tap water at 15 to 20° C, and for about six months in dried blood at room temperature. Disinfection of *C. burnetii* requires exposure to 5 per cent H_2O_2 or 2 per cent formaldehyde. Because of the extraordinary survival of *C. burnetii* in the extracellular environment, it probably infects man more often by the aerosol route than by tick transmission. Rickettsiae are generally transmitted to man by arthropods. The energy-producing metabolism of *C. burnetii* is quite different from that of rickettsiae. *C. burnetii* metabolizes pyruvate, synthesizes enzymes of the Embden-Meyerhof pathway, and contains many enzymes generally associated with the catabolism of glucose. Rickettsiae synthesize none of these enzymes.

The extraordinary extracellular resistance of *C. burnetii* may simply reflect its intracellular behavior, which is quite distinct from that of rickettsiae. *C. burnetii* enters the cell in phagosomes and remains there even as the phagosomes fuse with lysosomes. Not only can the organism protect itself from the harsh action of lysosomal hydrolases but the acidic environment of the phagolysosome is favorable to *C. burnetii* metabolism and replication (Hackstadt and Williams, 1981). Rickettsiae quickly escape from the phagosome and exist free in the cell cytoplasm. McCaul and Williams (1981) have proposed a developmental cycle for *C. burnetii*, based on electronmicroscopy of purified organisms grown in yolk sacs, which could explain the pleomorphism and viability in extreme environmental condi-

Table 1. DIFFERENCES BETWEEN *COXIELLA BURNETII* AND THE RICKETTSIAE

	C. Burnetii	**Rickettsiae**
Gram stain (alcohol mordant)	Gram-positive	Gram-negative
Soluble antigen released with ether	No	Yes
Immunizing antigens	Heat-resistant	Heat-sensitive
Guanine plus cytosine molar per cent	43	30 to 32.5
Usual route of infection	Aerosol	Arthropods
Embden-Meyerhof pathway	Yes	No
Persistence in phagosomes	Yes	No
Susceptibility to chloramphenicol and erythromycin	±	++++
Acute toxicity for mice	No	Yes
Phase variation	Yes	No

tions. They observed large and small cell variants. The former appeared to be similar to gram-negative bacteria, with outer and cytoplasmic membranes separated by a periplasmic space, and did not survive extreme environmental conditions. The latter had an extremely electron-dense area between the cytoplasmic and outer membranes and were viable in harsh environments. The small variant seemed to be derived by unequal cell division from an electron-dense body formed at one pole of the large variant, like an endospore. However, dipicolinic acid commonly found in bacterial spores was not found in these cells. Growth of *C. burnetii* in experimental yolk sac infections is only slightly affected by chloramphenicol and erythromycin, which are highly rickettsiostatic. *C. burnetii* is sensitive to the tetracyclines, however. Unlike certain rickettsiae, live *C. burnetii* do not cause acute toxic death of mice when inoculated intravenously in high titer. Finally, *C. burnetii* exhibits a unique phase variation, which is host-influenced. *C. burnetii* exists in nature only in Phase I. When cultivated in chick embryos, the organism shifts to Phase II but reverts to Phase I upon passage through laboratory animals. The significance of phase variation has been a topic of intense study since it was originally recognized by Stoker et al. (1955). Shift in phase is accompanied by changes in major antigenic components, pathogenicity, immunogenicity, buoyant density, agglutinability, staining properties, resistance to phagocytosis, and pyrogenicity. Phase variation appears to represent a phenotypic rather than a genotypic change. There is no discernible morphologic difference between phases of *C. burnetii*. Conversion of Phase I to Phase II resembles the smooth-to-rough variation in gram-negative bacteria, as discussed by Schramek and Mayer (1982) who showed phase variation in lipopolysaccharide constituents.

ROCHALIMAEA QUINTANA

This organism causes trench fever in man. It was originally recognized as a natural inhabitant of the gut lumen of the human body louse in the course of studies undertaken to elucidate the etiology of louse-borne epidemic typhus during World War I. Although it was called a rickettsia for many years, this organism has been reclassified into its own genus because it is usually located extracellularly and can be cultivated on cell-free media. The organism is named for the Brazilian scientist H. da Rocha-Lima, who was one of the early investigators of rickettsial diseases, and for the form of the disease, in which febrile episodes recur after every fifth (quintana) day without fever.

The organisms resemble rickettsiae in size and cell structure. The cell wall is similar to that of rickettsiae in chemical composition (Osterman et al., 1974) and in structure by electron microscopy (Ito and Vinson, 1965). It multiplies by binary fission and, like rickettsiae, metabolizes glutamine and succinate but not glucose. It is gram-negative and stains like rickettsiae in the Giminez and Macchiavello stains. It is susceptible to inactivation by standard disinfectants, but it survives for months in dried louse feces, like *R. prowazekii*.

R. quintana is distinct from all other rickettsiae in its G + C content of 38.5 moles per cent. This characteristic contributed to the recent identification of Baker's vole agent as related to *R. quintana* (see Chapter 206). This was the first isolation of a *R. quintana*-like organism in nature from a nonhuman mammalian source (Weiss et al., 1978). Weiss and Dasch (1982) have proposed the name *Rochalimaea vinsonii* for Baker's vole agent.

The second major difference between *R. quintana* and rickettsiae is its capacity to grow on cell-free media. It was first cultivated by Vinson (1966) on a blood agar base enriched with 6 per cent horse serum inactivated at 56° C for 30 minutes and 4 per cent washed, hemolyzed horse erythrocytes incubated at 37° C in a moist atmosphere of 5 per cent CO_2 in air. After 12 to 14 days incubation, colonies are round, lenticular, translucent, mucoid, and 65 to 200 μ in diameter. Colonies develop only on the surface of the agar. Organisms do not multiply without added carbon dioxide nor under anaerobic conditions. Mason (1970) developed a liquid culture medium for study of the growth cycle of *R. quintana* and noted that fetal calf serum could be substituted for the erythrocyte lysate. The growth cycle was characterized by a lag phase of approximately 24 hours, an exponential growth phase of 72 hours, and a doubling time of approximately 4.5 hours. Myers and co-workers (1972) demonstrated a growth requirement for hematin and concluded that the hematin was required as a precursor in the synthesis of various heme-proteins. *R. quintana* would not grow on hematin substitutes that satisfied other hematin-requiring bacteria. Apparently, it absolutely requires hematin for the synthesis of heme-proteins. *R. quintana* does not appear to produce H_2O_2 and is catalase-negative (Myers et al., 1972).

The only experimental host for *R. quintana* is the rhesus monkey (Mooser and Weyer, 1953), but specific antibody can be produced in rabbits and guinea pigs immunized with soluble or whole cell antigens in Freund's adjuvant (Herrmann et al., 1977). A number of serologic procedures detect *R. quintana* antibody in man, including complement fixation, passive hemagglutination; enzyme immunoassay; and radioimmunoprecipitation tests. Hollingdale and co-workers (1978) examined sera by the enzyme immunoassay method from patients with various rickettsial infections. Nine of 15 sera from patients with typhus group infections, 2 of 7 sera from *R. rickettsii* infections, and 3 of 6 sera from scrub typhus infections produced antibody to *R. quintana* antigen. Cross-reactions also occurred in guinea pigs infected with scrub typhus. These findings suggest that *R. quintana* shares antigens with rickettsiae. Seroepidemiologic studies, which have not yet been undertaken on a broad scale, must take these cross-reactions into account.

RICKETTSIA (EHRLICHIA) SENNETSU

In 1954, two Japanese groups (Fukuda, 1954; Misao and Kobayashi, 1954) reported the isolation of a rickettsia-like agent from patients with an infectious mononucleosis-like syndrome on the island of Kyushu. Subsequent studies established *R. sennetsu* to be immunologically distinct from *R. tsutsugamushi;* from *Neorickettsia helminthoeca*, the cause of salmon poisoning in dogs; and from Elokomin fluke fever agent, the cause of a similar lymphadenopathy in bears and raccoons in the Pacific Northwest of the United States (Kitao et al., 1973). Korb and co-workers (1966) in Czechoslovakia examined sera from 17 patients with clinical infectious mononucleosis. They, and other European workers, concluded that there was no good evidence to associate *R. sennetsu* with infectious mononu-

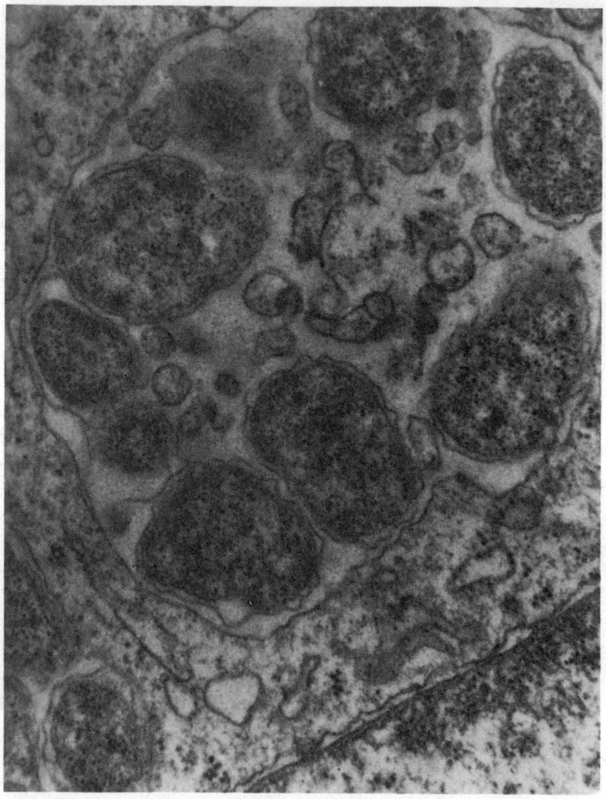

Figure 5. *R. sennetsui* in a distended vacuole. Several organisms are enclosed in a membrane-lined vacuole. Note that each organism is enclosed by a cell wall and a plasma membrane. × 30,000. (From Anderson, D. R., et al.: J Bacteriol 90:1387, 1965.)

cleosis in central Europe. Electronmicrographs show that *R. sennetsu* resides within an intracytoplasmic vesicle (Fig. 5) in contrast to other rickettsiae, which lie free in the cytoplasm (Anderson et al., 1965). Huxsoll recognized that this property was similar to that of organisms of the genus *Ehrlichia*, which is taxonomically close to *Rickettsia* but pathogenic for animals. Recent studies by Huxsoll, Ristic, and colleagues suggest an immunologic relationship between *R. sennetsu* and *Ehrlichia canis*, a tick-borne disease agent of dogs found in many parts of the world (Hoilien et al., 1982). Because of these immunologic and intracellular similarities *R. sennetsu* was removed from the Rickettsia genus and classified with the *Ehrlichia* in the 9th edition of *Bergey's Manual of Systematic Bacteriology* (1984). It is not yet known whether *E. sennetsu* is tick-transmitted to man, like *Ehrlichia*, or is transmitted by eating raw fish, like salmon poisoning in dogs. Recently, Ristic and Lewis (personal communication) have isolated a *E. sennetsu*-like agent from the blood of two febrile patients in Malaysia and have found anti-*E. sennetsu* antibodies in human sera collected in Malaysia and the Philippines, the first evidence of *E. sennetsu*-related infection outside of southern Japan. The discovery of this interesting disease agent and its relationship to *Ehrlichia* underscores the importance of considering agents of animal disease when searching for the specific etiology of obscure human febrile diseases. These studies will not always be as rewarding as those on *E. sennetsu* mononucleosis. An example of one of these febrile diseases that still remains obscure is Kawasaki disease (or mucocutaneous lymph node syndrome of infants and children), first reported by Kawasaki on the basis of 50 cases in Tokyo (see Chapter 215). Hamashima et al. (1973) reported rickettsia-like bodies by electron microscopy of skin and lymph node biopsies, but others cannot confirm these results. The unresponsiveness of the disease to antibiotics suggests an alternate etiology.

References

Anacker, R. L., Pickens, E. G., and Lackman, D. B.: Details of the ultrastructure of *Rickettsia prowazekii* grown in the chick yolk sac. J Bacteriol 94:260, 1967.

Anderson, D. R., Hopps, H. E., Barile, M. F., and Bernheim, B. C.: Comparison of the ultrastructure of several rickettsiae, ornithosis virus, and mycoplasma in tissue culture. J Bacteriol 90:1387, 1965.

Anderson, G. W., and Osterman, J. V.: Host defenses in experimental rickettsialpox: Genetics of natural resistance to infection. Infect Immun 28:132, 1980.

Balayeva, N. M., and Nikolskaya, V. N.: Enhanced virulence of the vaccine strain E of *Rickettsia prowazekii* on passaging in white mice and guinea pigs. Acta Virol 16:80, 1972.

Bozeman, F. M., and Elisberg, B. L.: Serological diagnosis of scrub typhus by indirect immunofluorescence. Proc Soc Exp Biol Med 112:568, 1963.

Bozeman, F. M., Sonenshine, D. E., Williams, M. E., Chadwick, D. P., Lauer, D. M., and Elisberg, B. L.: Experimental infection of ectoparasitic arthropods with *Rickettsia prowazekii* (GvF-16 strain) and transmission to flying squirrels. Am J Trop Med Hyg 30:253, 1981.

Burgdorfer, W., Ormsbee, R. A., and Hoogstraal, H.: Ticks as vectors of *Rickettsia prowazekii*—a controversial issue. Am J Trop Med Hyg 21:989, 1972.

Burgdorfer, W., Sexton, D. J., Gerloff, R. K., Anacker, R. L., Philip, R. N., and Thomas, L. A.: *Rhipicephalus sanguineus*: Vector of a new spotted fever group rickettsia in the United States. Infect Immun 12:205, 1975.

Catanzaro, P. J., Shirai, A., Agniel, L. D., and Osterman, J. V.: Host defenses in experimental scrub typhus: Role of spleen and peritoneal exudate lymphocytes in cellular immunity. Infect Immun 18:118, 1977.

Chang, R. S. M., Murray, E. S., and Synder, J. C.: Erythrocyte-sensitizing substances from rickettsiae of the Rocky Mountain spotted fever group. J Immunol 73:8, 1954.

Coolbaugh, J. C., Progar, J. J., and Weiss, E.: Enzymatic activities of cell-free extracts of *Rickettsia typhi*. Infect Immun 14:298, 1976.

Coolbaugh, J. C., Ho, C-M., and Fang, R. C. Y.: Diagnosis of scrub typhus by culture of blood monocytes. In Tan, D. S. K. (ed.): Proceedings of the 18th South East Asia Ministers of Education Organization Tropical Medicine Seminar. Bangkok, SEAMEO Regional Tropical Medicine Publishing Health Project, 1978.

Dasch, G. A., Samms, J. R., and Weiss, E.: Biochemical characteristics of typhus group rickettsiae with special attention to the *Rickettsia prowazekii* strains isolated from flying squirrels. Infect Immun 19:676, 1978.

deBrito, T., Tiriba, A., Godoy, C. V. F., Penna, D. O., and Jordao, F. M.: Glomerular response in human and experimental rickettsial disease (Rocky Mountain spotted fever group). A light and electron microscopy study. Pathol Microbiol (Basel) 31:365, 1968.

DeShazo, R. D., Boyce, J. R., Osterman, J. V., and Stephenson, E. M.: Early diagnosis of Rocky Mountain spotted fever. Use of primary monocyte culture technique. JAMA 235:1353, 1976.

Duma, R. J., Sonenshine, D. E., Bozeman, F. M., Veazey, J. M. Jr., Elisberg, B. L., Chadwick, D. P., Stocks, N. I., McGill, T. M., Miller, G. B. Jr., and MacCormack, J. N.: Epidemic typhus in the United States associated with flying squirrels. JAMA 245:2318, 1981.

Elisberg, B. L., Campbell, J. M., and Bozeman, F. M.: Antigenic diversity of *Rickettsia tsutsugamushi*: Epidemiologic and ecologic significance. J Hyg Epidemiol Microbiol Immunol 12:18, 1968.

Fiset, P., Ormsbee, R. A., Silberman, R., Peacock, M., and Spielman, S. H.: A microagglutination technique for detection and measurement of rickettsial antibodies. Acta Virol 13:60, 1969.

Fleck, L., Porat, S., Evenchik, Z., Klingberg, M. A.: The renal excretion of specific microbial substances during the course of infection with murine typhus rickettsiae. Am J Hyg 72:351, 1960.

Fukuda, T., Kitao, T., and Keida, Y.: Study on the causative agent of "Hyuga netsu" disease (infectious mononucleosis). Med Biol 32:200, 1954.

Giminez, D. F.: Staining rickettsiae in yolk-sac cultures. Staining Technol 39:135, 1964.

Groves, M. G., Rosenstreich, D. L., Taylor, B. A., and Osterman, J. V.: Host defenses in experimental scrub typhus: mapping the gene that controls natural resistance in mice. J Immunol 125:1396, 1980.

Hackstadt, T. and Williams, J. C.: Biochemical stratagem for obligate parasitism of eukaryotic cells by *Coxiella burnetii*. Proc Nat Acad Sci 78:3240, 1981.

Hamashima, Y., Kishi, K., and Tasaka, K.: Rickettsia-like bodies in infantile acute febrile mucocutaneous lymph-node syndrome. Lancet 2:42, 1973.

Harrell, G., and Aikawa, J.: Pathogenesis of circulatory failure in Rocky Mountain spotted fever. Medicine 28:333, 1949.

Hayes, S. F. and Burgdorfer, W.: Reactivation of *Rickettsia rickettsii* in *Dermacentor andersoni* ticks: an ultrastructural analysis. Infect Immun 37:779, 1982.

Hébert, G. A., Tzianabos, T., Gamble, W. C. and Chappell, W. A.: Development and characterization of high-titered, group-specific fluorescent-antibody reagents for direct identification of Rickettsiae in clinical specimens. J Clin Microbiol 11:503, 1980.

Hechemy, K. E., Osterman, J. V., Eisemann, C. S., Elliott, L. B., and Sasowski, S. J.: Detection of typhus antibodies by latex agglutination. J Clin Microbiol 13:214, 1981.

Hoilien, C. A., Ristic, M., Huxsoll, D. L., and Rapmund, G.: *Rickettsia sennetsu* in human blood monocyte cultures: similarities to the growth cycle of *Ehrlichia canis*. Infect Immun 35:314, 1982.

Hollingdale, M. R., Herrmann, J. E., and Vinson, J. W.: Enzyme immunoassay of antibody to *Rochalimaea quintana*: Diagnosis of trench fever and serologic cross-reactions among other rickettsiae. J Inf Dis 137:578, 1978.

Ito, S., and Vinson, J. W.: Fine structure of *Rickettsia quintana* cultivated in vitro and in the louse. J Bacteriol 89:481, 1965.

Jerrells, T. R., and Eisemann, C. S.: Role of T-lymphocytes in production of antibody to antigens of *Rickettsia tsutsugamushi* and other *Rickettsia* species. Infect Immun 41:666, 1983.

Kaplan, J. E., McDade, J. E., and Newhouse, V. F.: Suspected Rocky Mountain spotted fever in the winter—epidemic typhus? N Eng J Med 305:1648, 1981.

Kazar, J., Brezina, R., and Urvolgyi, J.: Studies on the E strain of *Rickettsia prowazekii*. Bull WHO 49:257, 1973.

Kitao, T., Farrell, R. K., and Fukuda, T.: Differentiation of salmon poisoning disease and Elokomin fluke fever: Fluorescent antibody studies with *Rickettsia sennetsu*. Am J Vet Res 34:927, 1973.

Kokorin, I. N., Chyong, D. K., Kekcheeva, N. G., and Miskarova, E. D.: Cytological investigation on *Rickettsia tsutsugamushi* infection of mice with different allotypic susceptibility to the agent. Acta Virol 20:147, 1976.

Korb, J., Kouba, K., and Kulková, H.: *Rickettsia sennetsu* and the etiology of infectious mononucleosis. Čas lék Čes 105:975, 1966.

Kurz, J., and Burgdorfer, W.: Detection of the Rocky Mountain spotted fever agent, *Rickettsia rickettsii*, in dead ticks, *Dermacentor andersoni*. Infect Immun 20:584, 1978.

Ley, H. L., Smadel, J. E., Diercks, F. H., and Paterson, P. Y.: Immunization against scrub typhus. V. The infective dose of *Rickettsia tsutsugamushi* for men and mice. Am J Hyg 56:313, 1952.

Mason, R. A.: Propagation and growth cycle of *Rickettsia quintana* in a new liquid medium. J Bacteriol 103:184, 1970.

McCaul, T. F., and Williams, J. C.: Developmental cycle of *Coxiella burnetii*: structure and morphogenesis of vegetative and sporogenic differentiations. J Bacteriol 147:1063, 1981.

McDade, J. E., Shephard, C. C., Redus, M. A., Newhouse, V. F., and Smith, J. D.: Evidence of *Rickettsia prowazekii* infections in the United States. Am J Trop Med Hyg 29:277, 1980.

McKiel, J. A., Bell, E. J., and Lackman, D. B.: *Rickettsia canada*: A new member of the typhus group of rickettsiae isolated from *Haemophysalis leporispalustris* ticks in Canada. Can J Microbiol 13:503, 1967.

Miragliotta, G., Fumarolo, D., Colucci, M. and Semerano, N.: Platelet aggregation and stimulation of leucocyte procoagulant activity by Rickettsial lipopolysaccharides in rabbits and in man. Experientia 37:47, 1981.

Misao, T., and Kobayashi, Y.: Studies on infectious mononucleosis: On the isolation of causative agents from blood, bone marrow fluid, and lymph gland with mice. Tokyo Med J 71:683, 1954.

Mooser, H., and Weyer, F.: Experimental infection of *Macacus rhesus* with *Rickettsia quintana*. Proc Soc Exp Biol Med 83:699, 1953.

Moulder, J. W.: The relation of the psittacosis group (chlamydiae) to bacteria and viruses. Ann Rev Microbiol 20:107, 1966.

Myers, W. F., and Wisseman, C. L., Jr.: Genetic relatedness among the typhus group of rickettsiae. Int J Syst Bacteriol 30:143, 1980.

Myers, W. F., Osterman, J. V., and Wisseman, C. L., Jr.: Nutritional studies of *Rickettsia quintana*: Nature of the hematin requirement. J Bacteriol 109:89, 1972.

Nacy, C. A., and Osterman, J. V.: Host defenses in experimental scrub typhus: Role of normal and activated macrophages. Infect Immun 26:744, 1979.

Ormsbee, R. A., Parker, H., and Pickens, E. G.: The comparative effectiveness of aureomycin, terramycin, chloramphenicol, erythromycin, and thiocymetin in suppressing experimental rickettsial infections in chick embryos. J Inf Dis 96:162, 1955.

Ormsbee, R. A.: Rickettsiae (as organisms). Ann Rev Microbiol 23:275, 1969.

Ormsbee, R., Peacock, M., Philip, R., Casper, E., Plorde, J., Gabre Kidan, T., and Wright, L.: Serologic diagnosis of epidemic typhus fever. Am J Epidemiol 105:261, 1977.

Ormsbee, R., Peacock, M., Philip, R., Casper, E., Plorde, J., Gabre Kidan, T., and Wright, L.: Antigenic relationships between the typhus and spotted fever groups of rickettsiae. Am J Epidemiol 108:53, 1978.

Oster, C. N., Burke, D. S., Kenyon, R. H., Ascher, M. S., Harber, P., and Pedersen, C. E., Jr.: Laboratory-acquired Rocky Mountain spotted fever. The hazard of aerosol transmission. N Engl J Med 297:859, 1977.

Osterman, J. V., Myers, W. F., and Wisseman, C. L., Jr.: Chemical composition of the cell envelope of *Rickettsia quintana*. Acta Virol 18:151, 1974.

Osterman, J. V., and Eisemann, C. S.: Rickettsial indirect hemagglutination test: Isolation of erythrocyte-sensitizing substance. J Clin Microbiol 8:189, 1978.

Phibbs, P. V. Jr. and Winkler, H. H.: Regulatory properties of citrate synthase from *Rickettsia prowazekii*. J Bacteriol 149:718, 1982.

Philip, R. N., Casper, E. A., Ormsbee, R. A., Peacock, M. G., and Burgdorfer, W.: Microimmunofluorescence test for the serological study of Rocky Mountain spotted fever and typhus. J Clin Microbiol 3:51, 1976.

Philip, R. N., Casper, E. A., MacCormack, J. N., Sexton, D. J., Thomas, L. A., Anacker, R. L., Burgdorfer, W., and Vick, S.: A comparison of serologic methods for diagnosis of Rocky Mountain spotted fever. Am J Epidemiol 105:56, 1977.

Philip, R. N., Casper, E. A., Burgdorfer, W., Gerloff, R. K., Hughes, L. E., and Bell, E. J.: Serologic typing of rickettsiae of the spotted fever group by microimmunofluorescence. J Immunol 121:1961, 1978.

Philip, R. N., Casper, E. A., Anacker, R. L., Peacock, M. G., Hayes, S. F. and Lane, R. S.: Identification of an isolate of *Rickettsia canada* from California. Am J Trop Med Hyg 31:1216, 1982.

Ramm, L. E., and Winkler, H. H.: Rickettsial hemolysis: Adsorption of rickettsiae to erythrocytes; effect of metabolic inhibitors upon hemolysis and adsorption. Infect Immun 7:93, 550, 1973.

Ristic, M., and Huxsall, D. L.: Ehrlichia. In Krieg, H. R., and Holt, J. G. (eds.): Bergey's Manual of Systematic Bacteriology. Vol. 1, Baltimore, Williams & Wilkins, 1984, p. 704.

Schaechter, M., Bozeman, F. M., and Smadel, J. E.: Study on the growth of rickettsiae. II. Morphologic observations on living rickettsiae in tissue culture cells. Virology 3:160, 1957.

Schramek, S.: Isolation and characterization of deoxyribonucleic acid from *Coxiella burnetii*. Acta Virol 12:1822, 1968.

Schramek, S., Brezina, R., and Tarasevich, I. V.: Isolation of a lipopolysaccharide antigen from *Rickettsia* species. Acta Virol 20:270, 1976.

Schramek, S. and Galanos, C.: Lipid A component of lipopolysaccharides from *Coxiella burnetii*. Acta Virol 25:230, 1981.

Schramek, S. and Mayer, H.: Different sugar compositions of lipopolysaccharides isolated from Phase I and Pure Phase II cells of *Coxiella burnetii*. Infec Immun 38:53, 1982.

Shirai, A. and Wisseman, C. L.: Serologic classification of scrub typhus isolates from Pakistan. Am J Trop Med Hyg 24:145, 1975.

Shirai, A., Catanzaro, P. J., Phillips, S. M., and Osterman, J. V.: Host defenses in experimental scrub typhus: Role of cellular immunity in heterologous protection. Infect Immun 14:39, 1976.

Shirai, A., Sankaran, V., Gan, E., and Huxsoll, D. L.: Early detection of *Rickettsia tsutsugamushi* in peripheral monocyte cultures derived from experimentally infected monkeys and dogs. Southeast Asian J Trop Med Public Health 9:11, 1978.

Silverman, D. J., and Wisseman, C. L., Jr.: Comparative ultrastructural study on the cell envelopes of *Rickettsia prowazekii*, *Rickettsia rickettsii*, and *Rickettsia tsutsugamushi*. Infect Immun 21:1020, 1978.

Smadel, J. E.: Influence of antibiotics on immunologic response in scrub typhus. Am J Med 17:246, 1954.

Smith, D. K., and Winkler, H. H.: Characterization of a lysine-specific active transport system in *Rickettsia prowazekii*. J Bacteriol 129:1349, 1977.

Stoker, M. G. P., and Fiset, P.: Phase variation of the Nine Mile and other strains of *Rickettsia burneti*. Can J Microbiol 2:310, 1956.

Stork, E., and Wisseman, C. L., Jr.: Growth of *Rickettsia prowazekii* in enucleated cells. Infect Immun 13:1743, 1976.

Tarasevich, I. V., Plotnikova, L. F., Fetisova, N. F., Makarova, V. A., Jablonskaja, V. A., Rehacek, J., Zupacico, M., Kovacova, E., Urvolgyi, J., Brezina, R., Zakarjan, A. V., and Kocinjan, M. E.: Rickettsioses studies. I. Natural foci of rickettsioses in the Armenian Soviet Socialist Republic. Bull WHO 53:25, 1976.

Traub, R., and Wisseman, C. L., Jr.: The ecology of chigger-borne rickettsioses (scrub typhus). J Med Entomol 11:237, 1974.

Turco, J. and Winkler, H. H.: Inhibition of the growth of *Rickettsia prowazekii* in cultured fibroblasts by lymphokines. J Exp Med 157:974, 1983.

Tyeryar, F. J., Jr., Weiss, E., Millar, D. B., Bozeman, F. M., and Ormsbee, R. A.: DNA base composition of rickettsiae. Science 180:415, 1973.

Urvolgyi, J., and Brezina, R.: *Rickettsia slovaca*: A new member of the spotted fever group rickettsiae. In Kazar, J., Ormsbee, R. A., and

Tarasevich, I. V. (eds.): Rickettsiae and Rickettsial Diseases. Bratislava, VEDA, 1978, pp. 299-306.
Vinson, J. W.: *In vitro* cultivation of the rickettsial agent of trench fever. Bull WHO 35:155, 1966.
Walker, D. H., and Cain, B. G.: A method for specific diagnosis of Rocky Mountain spotted fever on fixed paraffin-embedded tissue by immunofluorescence, J Inf Dis 137:206, 1978.
Walker, D. H., and Henderson, F. W.: Effect of immunosuppression on *Rickettsia rickettsii* infection in guinea pigs. Infect Immun 20:221, 1978.
Walker, D. H., Firth, W. T., Ballard, J. G. and Hegarty, B. C.: Role of phospholipase-associated penetration mechanism in cell injury by *Rickettsia rickettsii*. Infect Immun 40:840, 1983.
Weiss, E., and Dressler, H. R.: Increased resistance to chloramphenicol in *Rickettsia prowazekii* with a note on failure to demonstrate genetic interaction among strains. J Bacteriol 83:409, 1962.
Weiss, E., Dasch, G. A., Woodman, D. R., and Williams, J. C.: Vole agent identified as a strain of the trench fever rickettsia, *Rochalimaea quintana*. Infect Immun 19:1013, 1978.
Weiss, E.: The biology of Rickettsiae. Ann Rev Microbiol 36:345, 1982.
Weiss, E. and Dasch, G. A.: *Rochalimaea vinsonii.* Differential characteristics of strains of SP–nov.,the Canadian vole agent. Int J Syst Bacteriol 32:305, 1982.
Wike, D. A., Ormsbee, R. A., Tallent, G., and Peacock, M. G.: Effects of various suspending media on plaque formation by rickettsiae in tissue culture. Infect Immun 6:550, 1972.
Winkler, H. H.: Inhibitory and restorative effects of adenine nucleotides on rickettsial adsorption and hemolysis. Infect Immun 9:119, 1974.
Winkler, H. H., and Ramm, L. E.: Adsorption of typhus rickettsiae to ghosts of sheep erythrocytes. Infect Immun 11:1244, 1975.
Winkler, H. H.: Rickettsial permeability. An ADP-ATP transport system. J Biol Chem 251:389, 1976.
Winkler, H. H., and Miller, E. T.: Phospholipase A activity in the hemolysis of sheep and human erythrocytes by *Rickettsia prowazekii*. Infect Immun 29:316, 1980.
Wisseman, C. L., Jr., and Waddell, A. D.: In vitro studies on rickettsia-host cell interactions: Intracellular growth cycle of virulent and attenuated *Rickettsia prowazekii* in chicken embryo cells in slide chamber cultures. Infect Immun 11:1391, 1975.
Wisseman, C. L. Jr., and Waddell, A. D.: In vitro sensitivity of *Rickettsia rickettsii* to doxycycline. J Infect Dis 145:584, 1980.
Wood, W. H., Jr., and Wisseman, C. L., Jr.: Studies of *Rickettsia mooseri* cell walls. II. Immunologic properties. J Immunol 98:1224, 1967.
Woodward, T. E., Pedersen, C. E., Oster, C. N., Bagley, L. R., Romberger, J., and Synder, M. J.: Prompt confirmation of Rocky Mountain spotted fever: Identification of rickettsiae in skin tissues. J Inf Dis 134:297, 1976.
Yamada, T., Harber, P., Pettit, G. W., Wing, D. A., and Oster, C. N.: Activation of the kallikrein-kinin system in Rocky Mountain spotted fever. Ann Int Med 88:764, 1978.
Zahorchak, R. J. and Winkler, H. H.: Transmembrane electrical potential in *Rickettsia prowazekii* and its relationship to lysine transport. J Bacteriol 153:665, 1983.

55

BARTONELLA BACILLIFORMIS

MANUEL CUADRA, M.D.

MORPHOLOGY. *Bartonella bacilliformis* is a gram-negative intracellular bacterial parasite of red cells that causes an acute febrile anemia (Oroya fever) in Colombia, Ecuador, and Peru in persons bitten by certain species of Phlebotomus flies. The acute stage may be followed after a variable asymptomatic period by a secondary stage (verruga peruana) in which a verrucous eruption occurs.

The morphology of *Bartonella bacilliformis* varies greatly with environmental conditions. In the red cells of blood smears from patients with Oroya fever, it appears as a pleomorphic organism (Fig. 1), varying from slender bacilli to coccoid forms. Although the bacillary forms usually have a smooth surface, there are also rosary-like forms that are considered to be produced by multisegmentation of the smooth forms; later the beaded forms disintegrate into coccoid forms. During the 1st week in typical cases of Oroya fever, when the rate of red cell parasitism increases geometrically, the bacillary (vegetative) forms predominate greatly over the coccoid forms (Fig. 1, top). In the 2nd week, both forms are found in approximately equal numbers. When the fever subsides in the 3rd week (usually by lysis), the coccoid forms greatly predominate over the bacillary forms. During convalescence (an afebrile stage with profound anemia), only coccoid forms are seen (Fig. 1, bottom). Electron microscopy shows that *B. bacilliformis* lies within the red cells (Fig. 2) and that its internal structure, showing a defined cell wall, resembles that of bacteria (Cuadra and Takano, 1969). Compact masses of organisms filling the cytoplasm of capillary endothelial cells have been found in the stage of Oroya fever (Strong, 1945; Aldana, 1929; Pinkerton and Weinman, 1937–38; Alzamora Castro, 1940; Urteaga, 1948).

B. bacilliformis has been demonstrated within verruga nodules and experimental monkey nodules by light microscopy (Mackehenie and Weiss, 1926; Noguchi, 1926a, b; Noguchi, 1927a; Marquez da Cunha and Muniz, 1928;

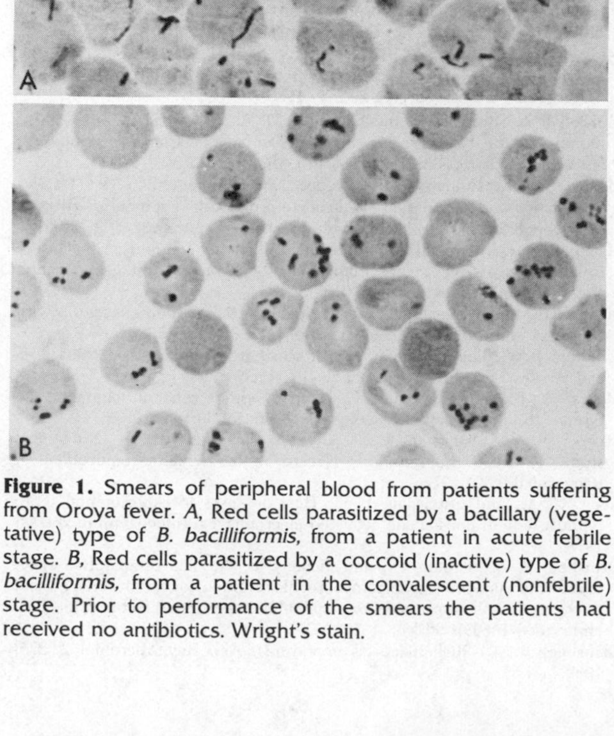

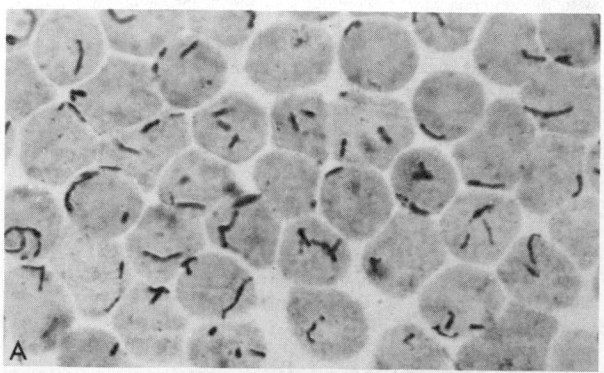

Figure 1. Smears of peripheral blood from patients suffering from Oroya fever. *A*, Red cells parasitized by a bacillary (vegetative) type of *B. bacilliformis,* from a patient in acute febrile stage. *B*, Red cells parasitized by a coccoid (inactive) type of *B. bacilliformis,* from a patient in the convalescent (nonfebrile) stage. Prior to performance of the smears the patients had received no antibiotics. Wright's stain.

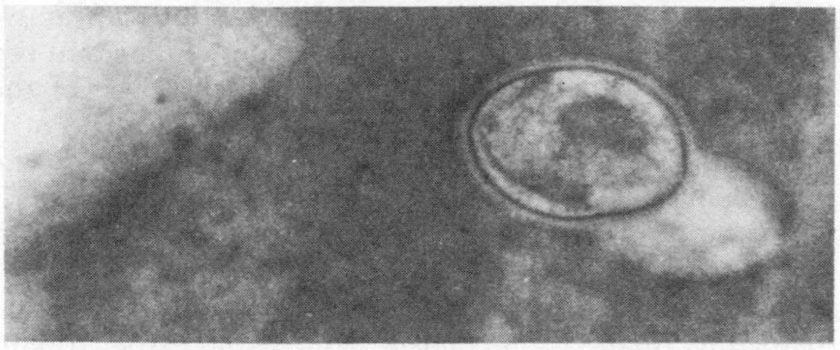

Figure 2. Thin section of a red cell parasitized by *B. bacilliformis*. The organism lies within a cavity in the red cell and shows a dense cell wall. Lead hydroxide stain. ×50,000.

Weiss, 1932; Weinman and Pinkerton, 1937a; Alzamora Castro, 1945; Ureteaga and Calderón, 1965) and electron microscopy (Recavarren and Lumbreras, 1972; Takano, 1970). Both extracellular (Recavarren and Lumbreras, 1972) and intracellular (Takano, 1970) organisms occur; they resemble those forms parasitizing red blood cells.

Inclusion-like bodies, consisting of aggregated organisms that are presumably in a stage of intracellular digestion, have also been found in the cytoplasm of the verruga cells (angioblasts) (Mayer et al., 1913; Marquez da Cunha and Muniz, 1928; Weiss, 1932; Pinkerton and Weinman, 1937–38; Noguchi, 1927b; Kikuth, 1931). Both extracellular and intracellular bacterial forms and the inclusion-like bodies develop in cultured cells (Pinkerton and Weinman, 1937). The assumption that the inclusions are composed of a viral form of *B. bacilliformis* (Aldana, 1947) is speculative.

The morphology of *B. bacilliformis* in blood agar cultures is shown in Figure 3. During active growth (3rd to 6th day at 28° C), the organisms appear in Giemsa-stained touch preparations as small rods with parallel sides, straight or slightly curved axis, slightly rounded ends, moderate variation in length (monomorphism), and arranged as single elements or in palisades. Later, pleomorphism becomes marked and increases with time of incubation. Long and short bacilli, coccobacilli, coccoid forms, short chains, diplococcoid forms, diplobacilli, and bacilli with bipolar staining closely resembling *Pasteurella* are seen. In cultures more than seven days old, coccoid forms predominate over bacillary forms, and by the 9th day, ring-shaped organisms are predominant. The coccoid forms are derived either by segmentation of the rods or by dissolution of the midportion of bipolar rods, so that the poles become freestanding. Under electron microscopy, many organisms show an envelope secondary to retraction of the cytoplasm (Fig. 4), and a defined cell wall is shown by thin sections (Cuadra and Takano, 1969) (Fig. 2). Most bacilli have single or multiple (up to 30 μm long and up to 10 in number) flagella (Fig. 4) at one pole (cephalotrica) (Peters and Wigand, 1951–1952; Perez Alva and Giustini, 1957). If transverse septation occurs centrally, two identical daughter cells result; if septation occurs eccentrically, the daughter cells are pleomorphic.

Growth of *B. bacilliformis* in liquid media produces no morphologic differences from the forms grown on solid media. Flagellated and nonflagellated forms appear in solid, semisolid, and liquid media.

MOTILITY. Free forms in plasma (wet preparations) of patients suffering from Oroya fever have not been reported, but free forms lying in the spaces between the red cells of stained blood smears are occasionally seen. Most, however,

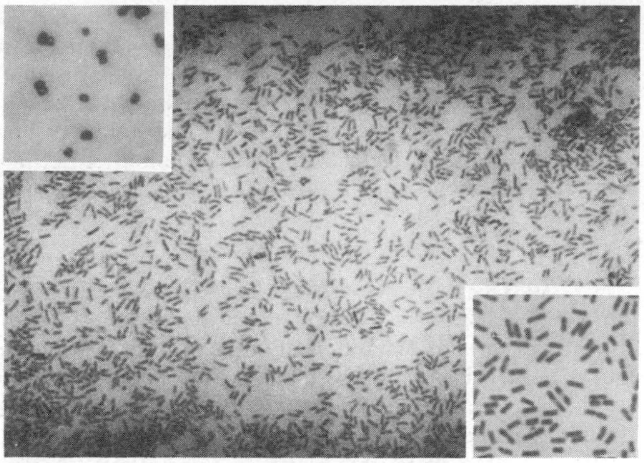

Figure 3. Touch preparation from a blood agar culture of *B. bacilliformis* (4th day of incubation at 28° C) showing monomorphic rods. For comparison see insets; touch preparations of *Staphylococcus epidermidis* (top) and *Escherichia coli* (bottom). Giemsa stain. The three organisms are shown at the same magnification (×840).

lie in ghosts of erythrocytes (Cuadra, 1957). Old reports (Barton, 1909) that the organisms move inside the red cells have not been confirmed. In cultures nonmotile forms predominate markedly over motile ones, and paradoxically, flagellated forms predominate over nonflagellated ones. Hence, the flagellated organisms are not necessarily motile. Moreover, *Bartonella* organisms growing in the semisolid medium of Noguchi may not be motile (Peters and Wigand, 1951–1952; Noguchi and Battistini, 1926) but are flagellated. Moreover, the yield of flagella increases with the time of incubation (Peters and Wigand, 1951–1952) as motility decreases.

Bartonellae can attach to red blood cells in cultures. The "parasitized" erythrocytes appear to rotate (dance) in a characteristic fashion (Cuadra, 1978). Dance is prevented, specifically, by antisera.

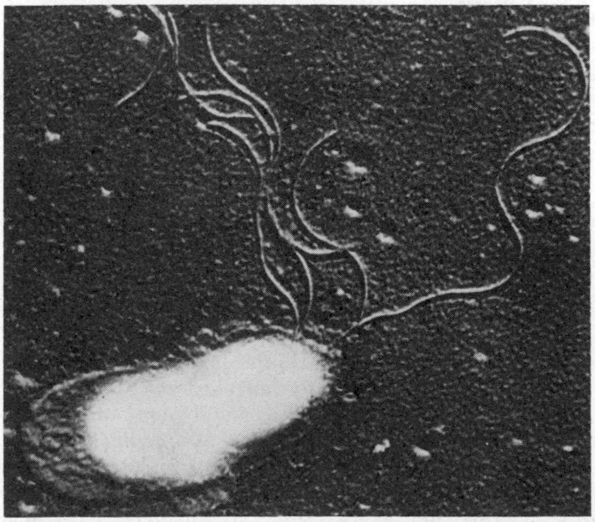

Figure 4. *B. bacilliformis* as seen by electron microscope. The organism shows a pronounced retraction of the cytoplasm and flagella emerging from a pole. Coated with palladium. × 19,000. (From Peters, D., and Wigand, R.: Z. Tropenmed Parasitol 3:313, 1951.)

B. bacilliformis is gram-negative and readily takes the Romanowsky stains (Giemsa, Wright, Leishman) in smears from patients' blood or cultures and in histologic sections of organs and verruga nodules after fixation with Ragoud's fixative (Noguchi and Battistini, 1926; Pinkerton and Weinman, 1937–1938). Flagella stain by the method of Zettnow-Fontana (Noguchi and Battistini, 1926; Pinkerton and Weinman, 1937–1938).

ANTIGENIC COMPOSITION. There have been no reports of flagellar or somatic antigens of *Bartonella*. Different clinical patterns in two different areas of Peru (Callejon de Huaylas and Rimac Valley) suggest that there are two antigenic variants of *Bartonella*. Morphologically, the strains isolated from both areas are indistinguishable. Strains isolated from the blood of Oroya fever patients cross-react in complement-fixation reactions with strains from verruga nodules (Noguchi, 1927c), and there is cross-immunity between Oroya fever and verruga (Noguchi, 1927d). No cross-reaction occurs with *Hemobartonella* or related organisms (Wigand, 1956, 1958).

CULTURAL CHARACTERISTICS. *B. bacilliformis*, a nonsporing organism, grows slowly in different bacteriologic media. In the blood broth of Hercelles (1927), the first medium devised for cultivation of *B. bacilliformis*, the organism does not produce turbidity; the change in color of the medium from red to dark reddish violet is the only indicator of growth. Both single elements and clusters of organisms can be seen under the microscope from the 3rd to the 4th day of incubation. The organisms have a marked tendency to attach to red blood cells (Cuadra, 1978). Attachment is evidenced by the "dance" of "parasitized erythrocytes" and by clumped red cells containing clusters of organisms arranged in a framework. We use both signs as indicators of growth. On blood agar, the colonies are too small for study by the naked eye. Under the stereoscopic microscope, the colonies appear from the 3rd to the 4th day of incubation to be variable in size, circular, transparent, and smooth. The colonies can also be studied microscopically on stained touch preparations (Fig. 3). A square piece of blood agar culture is removed from a Petri dish culture and placed, surface-to-surface, on a slide; when the piece is suddenly removed, a layer of organisms, arranged in colonies or singly, remains on the slide. On the leptospira-semisolid medium of Noguchi (Noguchi and Battistini, 1926), which also contains blood factors essential for growth, *Bartonella* forms clusters; the organism, predominantly coccobacillary in form, is less motile than on blood agar slants (Peters and Wigand, 1951–1952; Noguchi and Battistini, 1926). In liquid, semisolid, or on the solid media of Geiman (1941), which contain ascorbic acid and glutathione as key substances with animal serum, *Bartonella* grows well; in the liquid medium, it causes a fine dustlike deposit but neither turbidity nor clusters. The individual organisms are dispersed and are mainly nonmotile.

All media that support growth of *Bartonella* contain either whole blood or serum. Attempts to determine if the *Haemophilus influenzae* growth promoting factors V and X(I) (Thjötta and Avery, 1921) are involved have given confusing results (Jimenes, 1940; Colichón and Bedón, 1973). In comparison with *H. influenzae* or any other known bacterium, *Bartonella* slowly reaches a moderate amount of growth.

Metabolism. *B. bacilliformis* is an obligate aerobe (Noguchi and Battistini, 1926), but in blood broth the organism grows partly at the bottom on the mass of sedimented red cells and partly as a thin pellicle on the surface of the medium (Aldana, 1929, 1946). A difference in oxygen or carbon dioxide requirements therefore exists between the two populations. Growth occurs between about 20° and 37° C, but the optimal temperature is 28° C, and no growth occurs at 40° C. The pH range for growth is between 6.8 and 8.4, with an optimum level of 7.8 (Noguchi and Battistini, 1926). The organism ferments no carbohydrates (Noguchi and Battistini, 1926). No hemolysis occurs on blood agar, but in blood broth the erythrocytes attached to clusters of organisms become hemolyzed, and red cell ghosts can be seen by phase-contrast microscopy (Cuadra, 1978).

Resistance and Viability. *B. bacilliformis*, a nonsporing organism, dies within seven minutes at 56° C. Formalin, phenol, mercurochrome, neosalvarsan, and neutroflavine inhibit growth in cultures. The inhibitory concentration varies. Thus, formalin is inhibitory at 1:100,000 and phenol at 1:100 concentrations (Aldana, 1929; Noguchi, 1928a).

Viability varies with the specimen, the cultural conditions, and the strain. Thus, in citrated blood from patients with Oroya fever, the organism remains viable for four months (Aldana, 1929), and in blood clots, for nine months (Herrer, 1948) at room temperature. In the excised verruga nodule from monkeys, *B. bacilliformis* survives for about 56 days at 4° C and 28 days at room temperature; on blood agar slants or leptospira semisolid medium, it remains viable for about 50 days at 37° C and four months at 4° C or room temperature (Noguchi, 1926c). In blood broth or on blood agar slants, it survives for nine months at room temperature (Aldana, 1929). Protection of the cultures from drying by adequate stoppers, without impairing the oxygen supply (since *Bartonella* is an obligate aerobe) is essential to maintain viability. Under storage at −20° to −70° C, after freezing the cultures in the period of optimal growth (abundance of motile forms), *B. bacilliformis* remains viable for years and resists the process of lyophilization (Perez Alva et al., 1957).

PATHOGENIC PROPERTIES. *B. bacilliformis* is pathogenic only for man and causes Oroya fever and verruga peruana, which represent two successive stages of the same disease (Carrión's disease).

Inoculations of *Bartonella* into human beings have given variable results. Carrión, a medical student, was inoculated intracutaneously with juice from a verruga nodule. After 21 days of incubation, he developed Oroya fever with severe anemia and died on the 16th day of disease (Rebagliati, 1940). Strong and co-workers (1945) inoculated a man intracutaneously with verruga material, and a local verruga nodule developed but no Oroya fever. Garcia Rosell, a physician, inoculated himself accidentally with the blood of an Oroya fever patient while giving a blood transfusion (Rebagliati, 1940). A febrile illness without anemia lasted for two weeks, and then a florid verruga eruption appeared. Another physician, Kuchinsky-Godard (Mackehenie, 1937), who inoculated himself voluntarily with a culture of bartonellae, developed verruga nodules locally and at distant sites but no Oroya fever. Urteaga (1950) could induce Oroya fever in splenectomized individuals, but not in normal ones, by inoculation of parasitized blood from Oroya fever patients.

Inoculations carried out in monkeys (*Macacus rhesus* is the animal of choice) have also given variable results

(Jadassohn and Seiffert, 1910; Mayer et al., 1913; Arce et al., 1913; Noguchi and Battistini, 1926; Noguchi, 1926a, b; Marquez da Cunha and Muniz, 1928; Aldana, 1929; Weinman and Pinkerton, 1937a; Wigand and Weyer, 1952). In an effort to reproduce human bartonellosis with its two stages, infected blood from Oroya fever patients, juice from verruga nodules, infected wild sandflies, and cultures have been inoculated intravenously, cutaneously by scarification, and intra- or subdermally. Local verruga nodules occur with relative ease after cutaneous inoculation of these materials. A mild Oroya fever characterized by fever, anemia, and parasitism of the red blood cells occurs in a limited number of cases after intravenous inoculation with cultures. With parasitized blood from Oroya fever patients as the inoculum, negative results are obtained as a rule. The high degree of parasitism that usually occurs in Oroya fever patients, involving nearly 100 per cent of red cells (Fig. 1) with associated severe anemia (one million erythrocytes/mm^3), has never been obtained in monkeys (Weinman and Pinkerton, 1937a). The discrete Oroya fever induced in monkeys is very exceptionally followed by a generalized (endogenous) eruption (Noguchi, 1926a). However, it seems that anemia is produced more easily in splenectomized monkeys (Weinman and Pinkerton, 1937a).

According to older reports from Peruvian doctors, verruga peruana but not Oroya fever can be induced by inoculation of various animal species (Tamayo, 1899; Arce et al., 1913; Aldana, 1929). Noguchi confirmed the results in dogs and donkeys (Noguchi et al., 1929).

IMMUNITY. Oroya fever is an acute disease. In most nonfatal cases, recovery occurs spontaneously within two to three weeks. It is followed first by an asymptomatic "intercalary period" of variable duration (one or more weeks) and then by the verruga peruana stage, which lasts about one to three months. Chronic Oroya fever with persistent anemia and *B. bacilliformis* in peripheral red blood cells has never been reported. After spontaneous remission of the verrucous eruption, a solid lifelong immunity is established. A second attack of Oroya fever has never been reported in patients who returned to endemic areas. However, two, three, or more episodes of verruga peruana, usually accompanied by rheumatoid manifestations (verrucous rheumatism) and mild fever may occur in some individuals (chronic verruga peruana). The fact that some subjects with or without a past history of Oroya fever or verruga peruana give positive blood cultures (Howe, 1943; Weinman and Pinkerton, 1937b; Herrer, 1959) supports the existence of a state of infection-immunity (i.e., immunity depending on existing but not prior infection).

LABORATORY DIAGNOSIS. Blood smears stained with Giemsa, Wright, or Leishman stain reveal the organisms in the red cells of patients suffering from Oroya fever throughout the course of the fever and convalescent period (Fig. 1). The percentage of parasitized erythrocytes and the relative proportions of bacillary and coccoid forms should be estimated because bacillary forms, whatever the number of associated coccoid forms, are always related to the presence of fever. For this reason, the bacillary form is considered to be the active form. In contrast, in the convalescent period, when fever is absent, only coccoid forms may be encountered, although they may be parasitizing 100 per cent of red cells (Fig. 1). Thus, the coccoid form, originating from the bacillary form, is considered to be an inactive (stationary) form. Parasitized erythrocytes disappear gradually during convalescence, which, in cases with a high rate of parasitism, may last up to three weeks. By this time, the residual red cells harboring coccoid forms are spherocyte-like microcytes. The finding of pure coccoid forms in febrile patients indicates that the fever is not caused by *Bartonella* but by an associated infection, usually caused by *Salmonella* (Cuadra, 1956).

In an atypical form of the disease characterized by little or no anemia, the organisms are found with difficulty. In these cases, the thick-blood technique is of great aid. Blood cultured (28° C) in broth always produces growth of *B. bacilliformis*. The incubation time is usually three to five days and depends on the degree of parasitism of red blood cells. Blood cultures are frequently positive for *Salmonella* after a shorter incubation time. *S. typhimurium* is encountered most frequently (Cuadra, 1956).

No bartonellae are found in blood films of patients suffering from verruga peruana, although the blood cultures, and especially the cultures of excised verruga nodules, may be positive. The nodules have a characteristic histologic appearance (Rocha-Lima, 1913; Mackehenie, 1938).

The agglutination reaction was thoroughly studied by Howe (1942, 1943) in a group of 203 individuals. The titer of agglutinins appeared to be low but was of diagnostic significance. Practically all patients with Oroya fever had measurable agglutinins; in contrast, agglutinins were found in only 28 per cent of 54 patients in the verruga stage. In both Oroya fever and verruga peruana, the titer showed a tendency to decline and to disappear within a relatively short time after remission of the symptoms. In many individuals, blood cultures were positive (with or without symptoms), and agglutination tests were negative; the reverse was uncommon. In a group of 21 apparently healthy residents of endemic areas, both blood cultures and agglutination tests were negative.

The complement fixation reaction (Strong et al., 1915; Noguchi, 1928b; Aldana, 1929; Reese et al., 1950) has not been evaluated by extensive clinical trials.

DRUG SUSCEPTIBILITY. Penicillin, streptomycin, chloramphenicol, tetracycline, and erythromycin are highly effective against Oroya fever (Larrea, 1958). They produce defervescence within 24 hours, in parallel with morphologic changes of bartonellae and their disappearance from the peripheral blood cells. In vitro, *Bartonella* is highly susceptible to antibiotics and relatively resistant to sulfonamides (Wigand, 1952). Penicillin induces extraordinarily large coccoid forms in the cultures (Aldana and Tisnado Munoz, 1945; Wigand, 1952). Such forms correspond to L forms of *Bartonella* (Sharp, 1968). Resistance develops to streptomycin during treatment, whereupon the fever returns and the bacillary forms of bartonellae coincidentally reappear in the peripheral erythrocytes (Aldana et al., 1948; Cuadra, 1957).

The effectiveness of antibiotics on verruga peruana is doubtful. A comparative in vitro assay on drug susceptibility of strains isolated from Oroya fever patients with those isolated from verruga peruana patients is needed.

EPIDEMIOLOGY. Bartonellosis occurs in certain Andean valleys of Colombia, Ecuador, and Peru between 2 degrees north and 13 degrees south latitude. In Peru, the most afflicted country, the endemic foci lie between 800 and 3500 meters above sea level. The most important foci lie in valleys watered by rivers that flow into the Pacific Ocean at about 30 km. distance from the sea. Foci of minor importance are scattered in valleys with rivers that flow into the Amazon River (Rebagliati, 1940).

The inhabitants of the endemic areas constitute the reservoir. A high proportion of blood cultures of healthy individuals in those areas, with or without a past history of bartonellosis, is positive (Weinman and Pinkerton, 1937b; Howe, 1943; Herrer, 1959). Among animals, field mice have occasionally been found to harbor *Bartonella* in their blood (Hertig, 1948). The fact that some persons have contracted Oroya fever after spending the night in the forest supports the concept of an animal reservoir. Infection is transmitted by certain species of *Phlebotomus: Ph. verrucarum, Ph. pescei,* and *Ph. bicornutus* (Noguchi et al., 1929; Hertig, 1942; Herrer et al., 1959–1960). The bite of wild sandflies in the endemic areas can cause infection in monkeys (Battistini, 1931). However, the crucial experiment of transmission to man by *Phlebotomus* fed on Oroya fever patients failed. The cycle of bartonellae within *Phlebotomus* is unknown. In an epidemic area, Guaytara (Colombia), no *Phlebotomus* species were found, and only lice were present as a possible vector (Patino Camargo, 1939). *Bartonella* can multiply within the celomic cavity of lice (Wigand and Weyer, 1952). Experimentally, the infection could be transmitted from infected to normal rhesus monkeys by the bite of the tick *Dermacentor andersoni* (Noguchi, 1926d).

References

Aldana L. D.: Bacteriologia de la enfermedad de Carrión. Cron Med Lima 46:237, 1929.

Aldana, L.: Estado actual del tratamiento de la enfermedad de Carrión por la penicilina. Rev Med Per Lima 19:617, 1946.

Aldana, L.: Estados biológicos de la Bartonella en la enfermedad de Carrión. Rev Sanid Polic Lima 7:391, 1947.

Aldana, L., and Tisnodo Munoz, S.: Penicilina y enfermedad de Carrión. Rev Med Per Lima 18:343, 1945.

Aldana, L., Zubiate, P., and Contreras, F.: Un caso de verruga peruana resistente a la estreptomicina. Arch Per Pat Clin Lima 2:553, 1948.

Alzamora Castro, V.: Contribución al estudio de la bartonellosis humana o enfermedad de Carrión. Garc Med Lima 2:78, 1945.

Alzamora Castro, V.: Enfermedad de Carrión: Ensayo de etiopatogenia. Anales Fac Cien Med 23:1, 1940.

Arce, J., Mackehenie, D., and Ribeyro, R.: Estudio experimental de la enfermedad de Carrión. I. Inoculabilidad de la verruga peruana a los animales. Cron Med Line 30:394, 1913.

Barton, A.: Descripción de elementos endoglobulares en los enfermos de fiebre de verruga. Cron Med Lima 26:7, 1909.

Battistini, T.: La verrue péruvienne. (Sa transmission par le phlébotome.) Rev Sud Amér Med Chirug 2:719, 1931.

Colichón, H., and Bedón, C.: Factores que la *Bartonella bacilliformis* requiere para su crecimiento. Rev Lat Am Microbiol 15:11, 1973.

Cuadra, M.: The ability of *Bartonella bacilliformis* growing in culture to attach to red blood cells. Abstracts of the Twelfth International Congress of Microbiology. Sept 3-8, 1978, Munich, p. 178.

Cuadra, M.: Mecanismo de destrucción de los eritrocitos. La hemolisis intravascular. Anal Fac Med Lima 40:872, 1957.

Cuadra, M.: Salmonellosis complication in human bartonellosis. Texas Rep Biol Med 14:97, 1956.

Cuadra, M.: Tratamiento con cloranfenicol de casos de bartonellosis aguda (enfermedad de Carrión) en periodo de inicio. Anal Fac Med Lima 40:147, 1957.

Cuadra, M., and Takano, J.: The relationship of *Bartonella bacilliformis* to the red blood cell as revealed by electron microscopy. Blood 33:708, 1969.

Geiman, Q. M.: New media for the growth of *Bartonella bacilliformis*. Proc Soc Exp Biol Med 47:329, 1941.

Hercelles, O.: El germen de la verruga peruana. Anal Fac Med Lima 10:231, 1927.

Herrer, A.: Estudios sobre la enfermedad de Carrión en el valle interandino del Mantaro. II. Incidencia de la infección bartonellósica en la población humana. Rev Med Exper Lima 23:47, 1959.

Herrer, A.: Supervivencia de la *Bartonella bacilliformis* en la sangre coagulada de los enfermos de verruga. Rev Med Exp Lima 7:70, 1948.

Herrer, A., Blancas, F., Cornejo Ubilús, J., Lung, J. Espejo, L., and Flores, M.: Estudios sobre la enfermedad de Carrión en el valle interandino del Mantaro. I. Observaciones entomólógicas. Rev Med Exper Lima 13:27, 1959.

Hertig, M.: Phlebotomus and Carrión's disease. Am J Trop Med (suppl) 22:1942.

Hertig, M.: Sandflies of the genus *Phlebotomus*. A review of their habits, disease relationships, and control. Proceedings of the 4th International Congress of Tropical Medicine and Malaria, 1948, Washington, DC, USDA, p. 1609.

Howe, C.: Carrión's disease. Immunologic studies. Arch Int Med 72:147, 1943.

Howe, C.: Demonstration of agglutinins for *Bartonella bacilliformis*. J Exp Med 75:65, 1942.

Jadassohn, W. E., and Seiffert, G.: Ein Fall von Verruga peruviana: Gelungene Übertragung auf Affen. Z Hyg Infec Krankh, 6:247, 1910.

Jimenes, J. F.: Carrión's disease. I. Some growth factors necessary for cultivation of *Bartonella bacilliformis*. Proc Soc Exp Biol Med 45:402, 1940.

Kikuth W.: Experimentelle Untersuchungen über Oroyafieber und Verruga peruana. Z Immunforschg 73:1, 1931.

Larrea, P.: Los antibioticos en la bartonellemia humana. Arch Per Pat Clin 12:1, 1958.

Mackehenie, D.: Un caso de verruga humana por autoinoculación experimental. Rev Med Lima 23:741, 1937.

Mackekenie, D.: Estudio del noduloma verrucoso. Rev Med Lima 24:50, 1938.

Mackehenie, D., and Weiss, P.: Contribución al estudio de la verruga peruana. Gac Med Per Lima 4:51, 1926.

Marquez de Cunha, A., and Muniz, J.: Perquisas sobre la verruga peruana. Med Inst Oswaldo Cruz 21:161, 1928.

Mayer, M., Rocha-Lima, H., and Werner, H.: Untersuchungen über verruga peruviana. Münch Med Wochenschr 60:739, 1913.

Noguchi, H.: Comparative studies of different strains of *Bartonella bacilliformis* with special reference to the relation between the clinical types of Carrion's disease and the virulence of the infecting organism. J Exp Med 47:219, 1928b.

Noguchi, H.: Etiology of Oroya fever. II. Viability of *Bartonella bacilliformis* in cultures and in the preserved blood and an excised nodule of Macacus rhesus. J Exp Med 44:533, 1926c.

Noguchi, H.: Etiology of Oroya fever. III. The behavior of *Bartonella bacilliformis* in Macacus rhesus. J Exp Med 44:697, 1926a.

Noguchi, H.: Etiology of Oroya fever. IV. The effect of inoculation of anthropoid apes with *Bartonella bacilliformis*. J Exp Med 44:715, 1926b.

Noguchi, H.: Etiology of Oroya fever. VI. Pathological changes observed in animals experimentally infected with *Bartonella bacilliformis*. The distribution of the parasites in the tissues. J Exp Med 45:437, 1927a.

Noguchi, H.: Etiology of Oroya fever. VII. The response of the skin of Macacus rhesus and anthropoid apes to inoculation with *Bartonella bacilliformis*. J Exp Med 45:455, 1927b.

Noguchi, H.: Etiology of Oroya fever. VIII. Experiments on cross-immunity between Oroya fever and verruga peruana. J Exp Med 45:781, 1927d.

Noguchi, H.: Etiology of Oroya fever. XIII. Chemotherapy in experimental *Bartonella bacilliformis* infection. J Exp Med 48:619, 1928a.

Noguchi, H.: The etiology of verruga peruana. J Exp Med 45:175, 1927c.

Noguchi, H.: The experimental transmission of *Bartonella bacilliformis* by ticks (*Dermacentor andersoni*). J Exp Med 44:729, 1926d.

Noguchi, H., Shannon, R. C., Tilden, E. B., and Tyler, J. R.: Etiology of Oroya fever. XIV. The insect vectors of Carrión's disease. J Exp Med 49:993, 1929.

Noguchi, H., Muller, H. R., Tilden, E. B., and Tyler, J. R.: Etiology of Oroya fever. XVI. Verruga in the dog and the donkey. J Exp Med 50:455, 1929.

Noguchi, H., and Battistini, T.: Etiology of Oroya fever. I. Cultivation of *Bartonella bacilliformis*. J Exp Med 43:851, 1926.

Patinto Camargo, L.: Bartonellosis del Guaytara o fiebre verrucosa del Guaytara. Rev Med Lima 24:649, 689, 1939.

Perez Alva, S., and Giustini, J.: La maladie de Carrión. Étude morphologique de *Bartonella bacilliformis* au microscope électronique. Bull Soc Path Exot 50:188, 1957.

Perez Alva, S., Roger, F., and Roger, A.: La maladie de Carrión. Resistance de *Bartonella bacilliformis* au processus de lyophilisation. Bull Soc Path Exot 50:243, 1957.

Peters, D., and Wigand, R.: Neue Untersuchungen über *Bartonella bacilliformis*. I. Morphologie der Kulturform. Z Tropenmed Parasitol 3:313, 1951.

Pinkerton, H., and Weinman, D.: Carrión's disease. I. Behavior of the

etiological agent within cells growing or surviving in vitro. Proc Soc Exp Biol Med 37:587, 1937.
Pinkerton, H., and Weinman, D.: Carrión's disease. II. Comparative morphology of the etiological agent in Oroya fever and verruga peruana. Proc Soc Exp Biol Med 37:591, 1937.
Rebagliati, R.: Verruga Peruana (Enfermedad de Carrión). Imprenta Lima, Torres Aguirre, 1940.
Recavarren, S., and Lumbreras, H.: Pathogenesis of the verruga of Carrión's disease. Am J Pathol 66:461, 1972.
Reese, J. D., Morrison, M. E., and Fowler, E. M.: Complement fixation and Weil-Felix reactions in rabbits inoculated with *Bartonella bacilliformis*. J Immunol 65:355, 1950.
Rocha-Lima, H.: Zur Histologie der Verruga peruviana. Verh Dtsch Path Ges 16:409, 1913.
Sharp, J. T.: Isolation of "L" forms of *Bartonella bacilliformis*. Proc Soc Exp Biol Med 128:1072, 1968.
Strong, R. P.: Verruga peruana and Oroya fever. In Stitt's Diagnosis, Prevention and Treatment of Tropical Disease, 7th ed. vol 2. Philadelphia, The Blakiston Company, 1945, pp. 997–1014b.
Strong, R. P., Tyzzer, E. E., and Sellards, A. W.: Differential diagnosis of verruga peruana. Fifth report. J Trop Med 18:122, 1915.
Takano, J.: Enfermedad de Carrión (Bartonellosis humana). Estudio morfológico de la fase hemática y del periodo eruptivo con el microscopio electrónico. Doctoral thesis. Faculty of Medicine of the National University of San Marcos, 1970.
Tamyo, M. O.: Inoculabilidad de la verruga. Cron Med Lima 16:81, 1899.
Thjötta, T., and Avery, O. T.: Studies on bacterial nutrition. II. Growth accessory substances in the cultivation of hemophilic bacilli. J Exp Med 34:97, 1921.
Urteaga, O.: Histopatogenia de la anemia en la verruga peruana. Arch Per Pat Clin 2:355, 1948.
Urteaga, O.: Lecture at the Cathedra of Infectious, Parasitic and Tropical Diseases of the Faculty of Medicine, Lima, 1950.
Urteaga, O., and Calderón, J.: Ciclo biológico de reproducción de la *Bartonella bacilliformis* en los tejidos de pacientes de verruga peruana o enfermedad de Carrión. Arch Per Pat Clin Lima 19:1, 1965.
Weinman, D., and Pinkerton, H.: Carrión's disease. III. Experimental production in animals. Proc Soc Exp Biol Med 37:594, 1937a.
Weinman, D., and Pinkerton, H.: Carrión's disease. IV. Natural source of *Bartonella* in the endemic zone. Proc Soc Exp Biol Med 37:596, 1937b.
Weiss, P.: Contribución al estudio de la verruga peruana o enfermedad de Carrión. Rev Med Per Lima 4:5, 1932.
Wigand, R.: Morphologische, biologische und serologische Eigenschaften der Bartonellen. Stuttgart. Georg Thieme Verlag, 1958.
Wigand, R.: Neue Untersuchungen über *Bartonella bacilliformis*. 2. Verhalten gegenüber Sulfonamide und Antibiotica in vitro. Z Tropenmed Parasitol 3:453, 1952.
Wigand, R.: Serologische Reaktionen an Haemobartonella muris und Eperythrozoon coccoides. A Tropenmed 7:322, 1956.
Wigand, R., und Weyer, F.: Neue Untersuchungen über *Bartonella bacilliformis*. 3. Ubertragungsversuche auf rhesus Affen und auf Kleiderläuse. Z Tropenmed Parasitol 4:243, 1952.

56
THE CHLAMYDIAE

G. PHILIP MANIRE, PH.D.
PRISCILLA B. WYRICK, PH.D.

No other pathogenic microorganisms are better adapted for persistence and survival than the chlamydiae and no others are more widespread. Epidemiologic surveys suggest that some members of almost every species of birds and mammals may be infected with these organisms. Their ability to produce inapparent infections in these hosts is unexcelled, and individuals may be infected for extremely long periods of time without apparent harm. Estimates have been made that 10 to 20 per cent of the human population of the world is infected with chlamydiae. These organisms are ubiquitous, rarely kill their hosts, are generally highly infectious and easily transferred to new hosts, and have a remarkable ability to escape normal host immune mechanisms.

CLASSIFICATION. The genus *Chlamydia* is composed of two species, *C. trachomatis* and *C. psittaci* (Page, 1974). Although trachoma has been recognized as a specific disease for many centuries, and the first microscopic evidence of a specific causative agent was obtained early in the twentieth century, laboratory studies on these organisms began only in 1930 following the first successful isolation of *C. psittaci* from infected humans and birds. Isolation of *C. trachomatis* was not achieved until 1957. The new edition of Bergey's Manual (Moulder et al.) lists three biovars of *C. trachomatis*: mouse, lymphogranuloma venereum (LGV) and trachoma (comprising human strains other than LGV). *C. psittaci* is such a heterogeneous group that differentiation into strains or other species has not yet been accomplished on a rational basis.

It was shown very quickly that chlamydiae are strict intracellular parasites and as evidence regarding their growth and biochemical characteristics accumulated, it became obvious that these organisms are bacteria with unique characteristics. Like other bacteria they (1) contain both DNA and RNA, (2) possess a continuous cell envelope similar to that of gram-negative bacteria, (3) possess procaryotic ribosomes and synthesize their own proteins and nucleic acids, (4) possess limited but definite numbers of metabolic systems, and (5) are susceptible to a wide range of antibiotics.

The characteristics separating the two species are shown in Table 1. This classification was further justified by the finding that there is a significant DNA homology within each species but very little homology between the two, suggesting a long-standing evolutionary separation.

MORPHOLOGY. All members of the genus *Chlamydia* share a unique developmental cycle in which two distinct forms occur. These two forms are especially adapted for extracellular survival and transfer from cell to cell, and for intracellular growth. The extracellular form, generally referred to as an elementary body (EB), is a spherical bacterium 0.25 to 0.3 μm in diameter (Fig. 1). It is surrounded by a rigid trilaminar cell envelope similar in composition to those of other gram-negative bacteria. Even though it is not certain that endotoxin is present or plays a role in the pathogenesis of chlamydial infections, extraction of *C. psittaci* EB envelopes with a hot phenol-H_2O mixture produces a small quantity of a protein-free product with an electrophoretic mobility identical to R-type LPS on silver stained gels. The extracted material also gels the

Table 1. DIFFERENTIATION OF *C. TRACHOMATIS* AND *C. PSITTACI*

C. Trachomatis	C. Psittaci
Sensitive to sulfonamide	Resistant to sulfonamide
Rigid micro colonies	Diffuse micro colonies
Glycogen in inclusion	No glycogen in inclusion
Guanine + cytosine content of DNA ~ 44%	Guanine + cytosine content of DNA ~ 41%

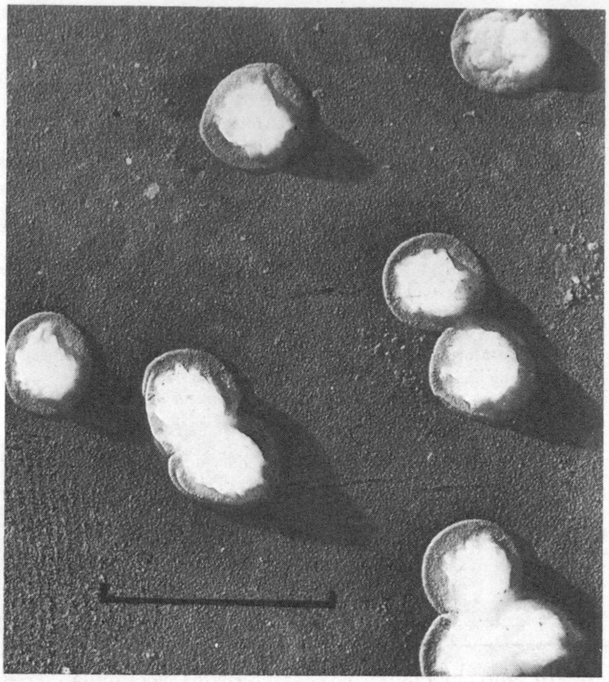

Figure 1. Shadowcast preparation of purified elementary bodies showing typical central condensation of cytoplasmic contents.

limulus lysate, and contains hydroxy fatty acids and a ketodeoxyoctanoic acid. The inner side of the envelope is composed of a continuous layer of small subunit structures in a hexagonal array (Fig. 2A). The predominant component of the outer membrane is a single surface protein (MOMP), whose characteristic subunit molecular weight varies (42.5K–45K) among strains. Recent studies suggest that the major outer membrane component is probably a glycoprotein. Both the hexagonal subunit and MOMP may serve to maintain envelope rigidity and stability. The most striking feature of the EB surface is the patch of cylindrical projections, average 18 in number, arranged in a hexagonal array (Fig. 2B). The projections appear to be anchored in the cytoplasmic membrane and protrude through a hole in the cell wall.

The cytoplasm of the elementary body is surrounded by a typical plasma membrane. The DNA and ribosomes are condensed in the center of the organisms, and in electron micrographs of shadow-cast preparations these assume a "derby hat" appearance (Fig. 1). Thin-section electron microscopy shows a similar central condensation.

The intracellular form of chlamydia, referred to here as the reticulate body (RB), is much larger than the extracellular form and differs from it in many respects (Fig. 3). It is surrounded by a trilaminar envelope that is very fragile and flexible so that pleomorphism results. The subunit layer found on the inside of the elementary body envelope is missing, and no sulfur-containing amino acids have been detected in the outer cell wall but the surface projections are retained in the RB form. Ribosomes and other cytoplasmic constituents are distributed homogeneously throughout the cytoplasm.

The genome of the organism has a molecular weight of 660×10^6 as estimated by electronmicroscopic measurements. Both *C. psittaci* and the biovars of *C. trachomatis* contain a 4.4 megadalton cryptic plasmid. As in other bacteria, the chlamydiae contain numerous proteins, which comprise 60 per cent of dry weight of the organisms, and lipids, about 30 per cent of dry weight. A summary of the differing characteristics of elementary bodies and reticulate bodies is shown in Table 2.

In a typical growth cycle, the elementary body attaches

A

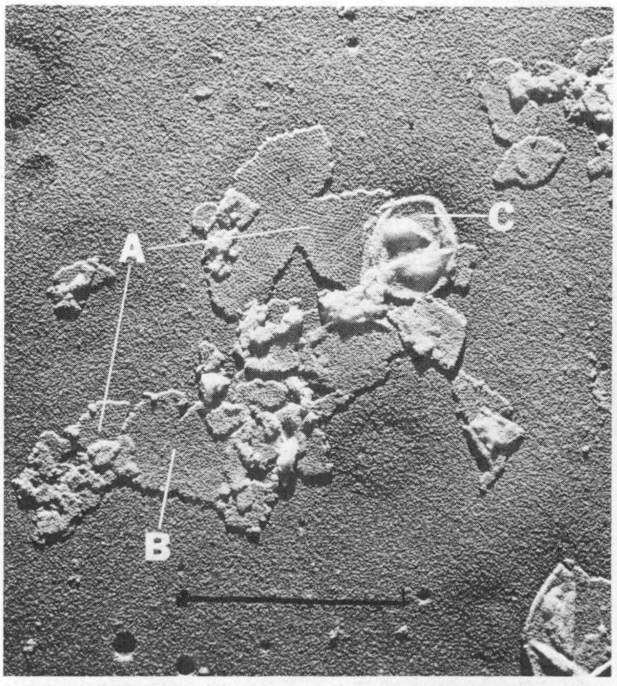

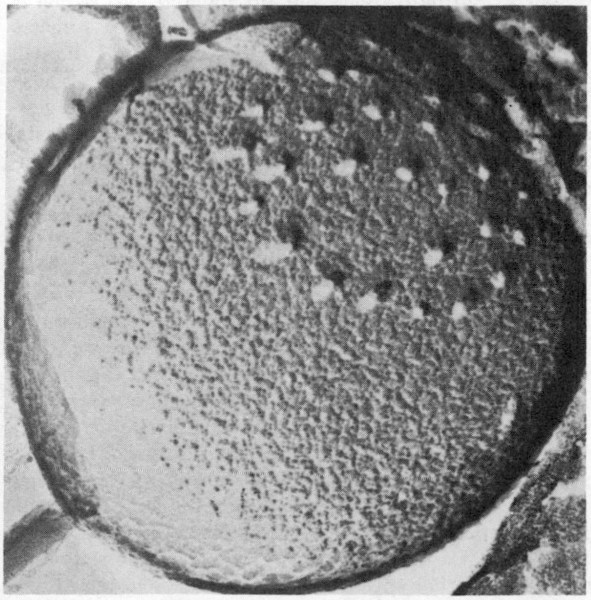

B

Figure 2. *A*, Cell envelope fragments prepared from disrupted suspensions of *C. psittaci.* Fragment A illustrates the hexagonal array of subunit structure found on the inner side of the cell envelope. Fragment B illustrates the outer granular side of the envelope. The structure C is an intact envelope. *B*, Freeze-fracture of a cell envelope of *C. psittaci* elementary body illustrating the cylindrical surface projections.

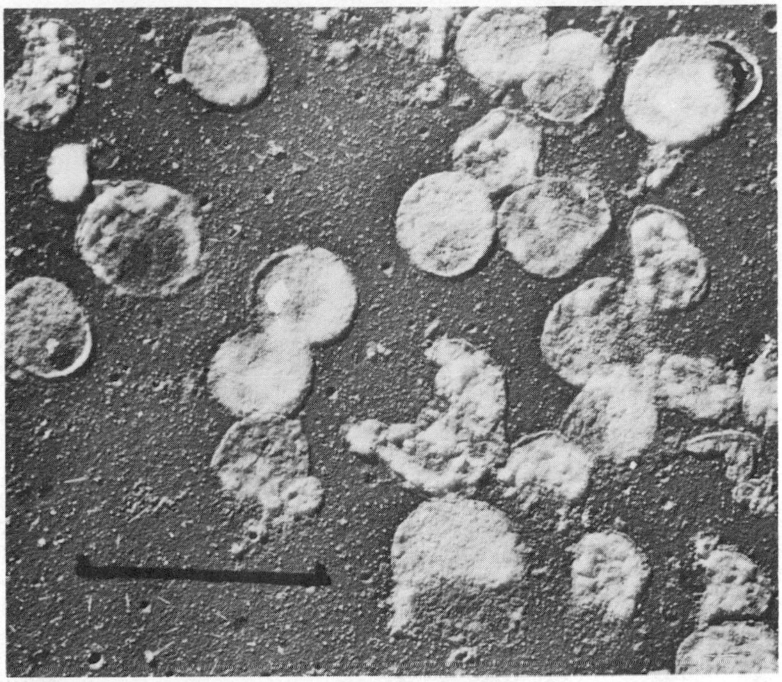

Figure 3. Shadowcast preparation of purified reticulate bodies.

to a susceptible cell by a process that involves a heat-sensitive adhesin on the surface of the organism and a trypsin-sensitive receptor on the host cell (Byrne, 1976). Since epithelial cells are not very active phagocytically but the EB are internalized quite efficiently, Byrne and Moulder (1978) have termed the uptake process "parasite-specified phagocytosis". It is insensitive to microfilament inhibitors such as cytochalasin B. The resulting phagosome membrane separates the developing colony of chlamydiae from the host cell cytoplasm throughout the active growth cycle.

There is no early fusion of lysosomes with phagosomes containing elementary bodies. However, if the elementary bodies are opsonized, there is rapid fusion of lysosomes and phagosomes, and the noninfectious chlamydiae are rapidly digested (Eissenberg, 1981).

Within 6 to 8 hours after phagosome formation, *C. psittaci* elementary bodies undergo a conversion to form reticulate bodies, and by 12 hours binary fission begins (Fig. 4). In 20 to 24 hours some of the reticulate bodies have begun to show central condensation and conversion to elementary bodies, but most continue to undergo binary fission until about 40 hours, when large numbers of elementary bodies begin to appear (Fig. 5). Following this the host cells begin to die and chlamydiae are released by lysis. It has been suggested that host cell lysosomes release into the cytoplasm hydrolytic enzymes that digest host cell constituents with consequent membrane lysis and release of chlamydiae (Todd and Storz, 1975). The developmental cycle of *C. trachomatis* organisms is the same except that it extends for 72 to 96 hours as opposed to 48 hours.

ANTIGENIC COMPOSITION. As with all bacteria, the chlamydiae have a complex antigenic structure. The major antigens under study demonstrate genus, species, and subspecies or serotype specificity. The first of these, the genus (group) antigen, is found in all chlamydiae and is a lipid-carbohydrate complex, stable when heated at 100°C for 30 minutes. Its antigenic determinant appears to be an acidic polysaccharide, similar, but not identical, to salmonella 2 keto-3 deoxy octanoic acid, and is glycosidically bound to serologically inactive neutral carbohydrates.

There are a variety of species-specific antigens on or near the surface of the envelope of chlamydiae. These protein antigens are shared by all members of a chlamydial species and appear to be highly immunogenic.

Table 2. CHARACTERISTICS OF ELEMENTARY BODIES (EB) AND RETICULATE BODIES (RB)

Characteristics	EB	RB
Morphology	Small, dense centered	Large, homogeneous
RNA:DNA	1:1	3:1
Sonication	Resistant	Sensitive
Effect of trypsin	Resistant	Sensitive, lysis
Infectivity	+	−
Toxicity	+	−
Hemagglutinin	Present	Absent
Permeability	Slight	Marked
Envelope subunit	Present	Absent
Location	Extracellular	Intracellular

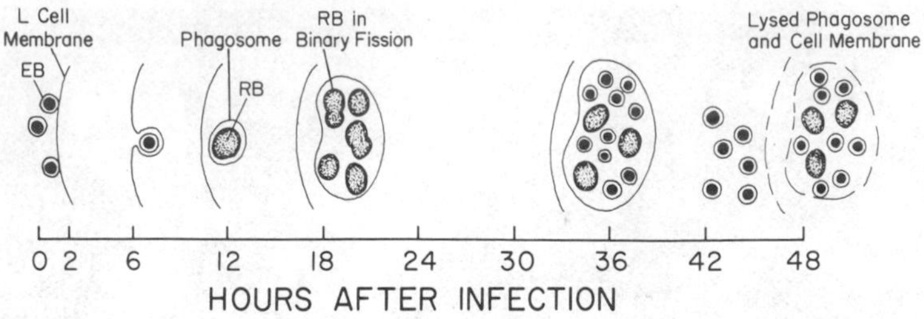

Figure 4. Schematic representation of the reproductive cycle of *C. psittaci* in L cells. (EB = elementary body, RB = reticulate body).

Serotype determinants are common only to certain isolates within a species. In *C. psittaci*, a large number of these have been demonstrated by toxin neutralization and plaque reduction tests. Among *C. trachomatis* strains, there are three serologically distinct types of lymphogranuloma venereum (LGV) agents, and 12 serotypes of the trachoma-inclusion conjunctivitis-urethritis group. The serotypes of *C. trachomatis* have been determined mostly by use of the microimmunofluorescence test (Wang and Grayston, 1970). Conflicting data have been reported concerning the chemical nature of the serotype antigens but they are probably surface exposed, are part of the MOMP, and they seem to play a major role in the development of protective immunity.

METABOLISM. The adaptation of chlamydiae for intracellular parasitism is well illustrated by their apparent total dependency on host cells for energy. They do synthesize their own macromolecules including DNA, RNA, and proteins, and they inhibit to varying degrees macromolecular synthesis in host cells, although the mechanism of this inhibition is not known. The chlamydiae contain numerous enzymes and can complete some metabolic processes, but they cannot complete the pentose cycle and do not utilize pyruvate by way of the tricarboxylic acid cycle. There is no evidence that they can generate high energy phosphate bonds, and they are completely dependent on the host cell for ATP. Mitochondrial ATP is taken up by growing RBs via a chlamydial ATP-ADP translocase. The ATP is broken down to ADP by a specific RB ATPase and the resultant proton-motive force helps to drive the transport of nutrients (Hatch, 1982). This dependence on host mitochondria gives added significance to the microscopic evidence that mitochondria accumulate around the phagosome membrane of developing inclusions (Matsumoto, 1981) and are among the last cell organelles to disintegrate in the dying infected cell.

Essentially all of the previous in vitro studies done on metabolism of chlamydiae have been conducted with partially purified organisms prepared by methods that tend to destroy the reticulate bodies. Since the reticulate bodies are the metabolically active form of chlamydiae, further studies need to be done with purified and stabilized suspensions of reticulate forms.

PATHOGENIC PROPERTIES. Chlamydia do have several properties of significance in pathogenesis, one of which is toxicity of live elementary body preparations for young

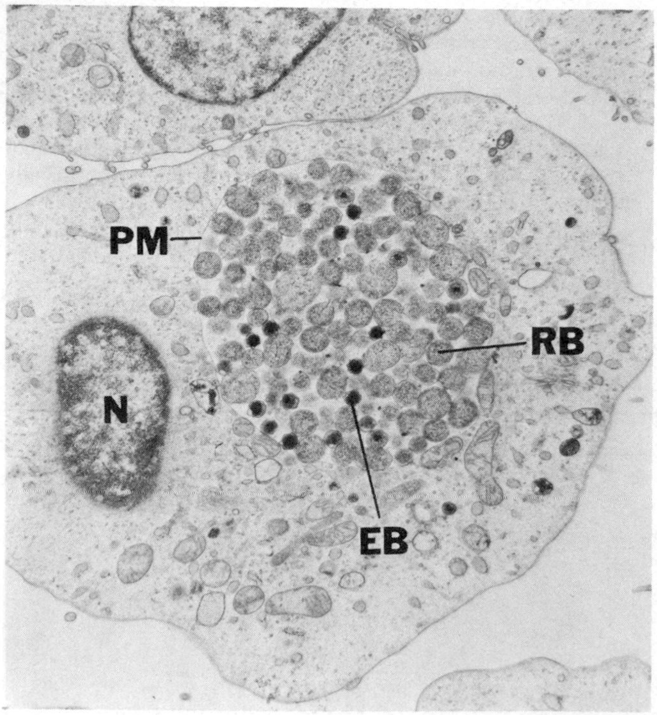

Figure 5. Thin section of L cell 30 hours after infection with *C. psittaci.* Typical reticulate bodies (RB), newly formed elementary bodies (EB) and the continuous phagosome membrane (PM) are labeled.

mice. The component responsible for toxicity cannot be separated from the elementary body, and only live infectious elementary bodies exhibit this phenomenon. Toxicity can be neutralized by specific antisera, although the organisms may remain infectious. However, both live elementary bodies and their cell envelopes will absorb antitoxin, indicating that the antigen responsible for toxin neutralization lies on the surface of the envelope.

In contrast, the reticulate body is nontoxic, and antitoxin is not absorbed by suspensions of reticulate bodies, indicating the absence of this specific antigen during the growth of chlamydiae (Christoffersen and Manire, 1969).

The relatively harmless or nontoxic nature of the developing form may well contribute to another property of chlamydiae—the ease with which these organisms establish chronic inapparent carrier states in man and animal. This lack of specific antigenicity may allow reticulate bodies to reside intracellularly for long periods of time protected from host antibody.

Hypersensitivity may also play a role in *C. trachomatis* infection in that prior vaccination or infections often produce increasingly severe clinical symptoms.

In general, *C. trachomatis* tends to produce localized infections in mucous membranes with some extension in the case of genital infections. It may also produce pneumonitis in newborn infants. *C. psittaci*, in contrast, almost always produces generalized infections involving many organs in different animal hosts.

Little information is available to explain these differences or to answer other questions about the ability of chlamydiae to damage cells, establish latent or inapparent infections, or overcome immune mechanisms.

IMMUNITY. Diseases produced by chlamydiae in animals and man tend to be chronic, and carrier states frequently develop after recovery from clinical disease. Neutralization of these organisms by specific antisera can be demonstrated in vitro, but the intracellular site of their growth probably protects the organisms from specific antibody. Humoral antibody does serve to (i) prevent attachment of the infectious elementary bodies to target host cells of the mucous membranes or (ii) cause destruction in phagolysosomes of opsonized chlamydiae ingested by macrophages. Humoral immunity is also essential for the recovery of experimental animals from genital infection (Rank, 1979).

IgM, IgG, and IgA against chlamydiae are all detectable in infected animals and man. A high IgM titer is usually seen during acute, recently acquired infections. Recent studies indicate that the quantity of *C. trachomatis* isolated from genital secretions is inversely correlated with sIgA. The speculation is that sIgA is related to shedding of organisms at mucosal surfaces (Brunham, 1983).

It is well recognized that the cell-mediated immune response plays a major role in the resistance of the host to infection with intracellular bacteria and parasitic microorganisms. The same is probably true of *Chlamydia* (Rank, 1983).

Macrophages activated by lymphokines, obtained from splenocytes from *C. psittaci* infected, immune mice, markedly suppress the intracellular development of a lymphogranuloma venereum biovar of *C. trachomatis*. The lymphokine may be a type of interferon, which has been shown to reduce the rate of *C. trachomatis* RB replication. The factor in lymphokine that activates human macrophages to inhibit *C. psittaci* replication is gamma interferon (Rothermel et al., 1983). In addition, spleen cells from *C. psittaci* infected mice lyse *C. psittaci* infected target and cell monolayers (Lammert, 1982). The induction by the host of cytotoxic cells may help to control chlamydial multiplication and the spread of infection.

Severe infection often occurs in healthy avian, and probably mammalian, carriers when they are subjected to stress, nutritional deprivation, and other traumatic events, indicating a delicate balance between host defense and chlamydial pathogenicity.

Since 1960 many trachoma vaccines produced by a variety of techniques have been tested in primates and humans. Short-term protection has been achieved in numerous instances, but subsequent susceptibility and development of hypersensitivity have been consistent long-term consequences.

LABORATORY DIAGNOSIS. In *C. psittaci* infections, the complement fixation test using the heat-resistant genus antigen has been the most commonly used serologic procedure. The organisms can be isolated without difficulty but with considerable hazard by injection of specimens into mice by various routes and into the chick embryo yolk sac, and many laboratory infections have occurred.

In *C. trachomatis* infections, recovery of the organisms from tissue culture or chicken embryo yolk sacs is a well established technique. *C. trachomatis* produces glycogen during a certain stage of its growth, which stains with iodine and results in easily recognizable inclusions. Two other common methods for recognizing inclusions in chlamydiae-infected cells are by Giemsa stain or flourescent antibody. Tissue culture is, however, time-consuming and expensive and often is not available in small diagnostic laboratories.

Two new techniques have just been reported that eliminate tissue culture, are essentially as sensitive and specific as tissue culture, and can be performed rapidly. One is a direct slide assay that detects extracellular chlamydiae in urethral or cervical smears via fluorescein-labeled monoclonal antibody and can be performed in 20 minutes (Nowinski et al., 1983). The second method is an immunoassay involving the reaction of commercially prepared "treated beads" and the patient sample for 1 hour, followed by the addition of polyclonal or monoclonal antibody to *C. trachomatis* and peroxidase labeled immunoglobulin.

The microimmunofluorescence test revolutionized the serological identification of oculogenital infection and trachoma. It served both as a method for serotyping unknown *C. trachomatis* isolates and for measuring type-specific antibodies in serum and tears. The sensitivity of these tests is compared in Table 3.

DRUG SUSCEPTIBILITY. The first specific therapy for chlamydial infections followed the discovery that these organisms are sensitive to sulfonamides and penicillin. In general, *C. trachomatis* strains are sensitive to sulfonamides and these drugs have long been used in treatment of trachoma and LGV. *C. psittaci* strains are generally resistant to sulfonamides. Therapeutic cures have been claimed with penicillin, however, treatment failures and/or relapses are common following this therapy. Its antimicrobial effect is to prevent RB binary fission and conversion of reticulate forms to elementary bodies; it does not inhibit cell infection, conversion of elementary bodies to reticulate bodies, or growth of reticulate bodies. Thus it is bacterio-

Table 3. COMPARATIVE SENSITIVITIES OF DIAGNOSTIC LABORATORY TESTS FOR *C. TRACHOMATIS* INFECTIONS

	Anatomic Site		
Test	***Conjunctiva* (*130*)[a]**	***Male Urethra* (*200*)[a]**	***Female Cervix* (*300*)[a]**
Isolation			
Tissue culture	95%[b]	100	95
Yolk sac	38	26	40
Stain of cell scrapings			
Giemsa	45	15	41
Fluorescent antibody	85	60	66
Serum antibody			
Complement fixation	50	15	40
Microimmunofluorescence	100	90	99

[a]Number tested
[b]% positive
From Schachter, J.: N Engl J Med 298:545, 1978.

static and, in vitro when penicillin is removed from the tissue culture system, the chlamydiae resume division and maturation.

Both of these drugs have been largely replaced by tetracycline. The action of these drugs on chlamydiae is the same as with other bacteria and sufficiently high levels accumulate inside cells to be effective against these intracellular parasites. The recommended course of tetracycline for psittacosis infections is 250 mg four times a day for 21 days. A major drawback is compliance. In general patients have a tendency to abbreviate the course of therapy when symptoms abate or gastrointestinal disturbances occur or candida vaginitis appears.

Double sexually transmitted infections involving both *C. trachomatis* and *N. gonorrheae* are now quite common. The frequency in men is reported to range from 15 to 35 per cent while the incidence in women approaches 65 per cent. Tetracycline alone is highly effective against *N. gonorrheae* and thus can be used in these circumstances. Some clinicians prefer a combined regimen using ampicillin with probenocid, followed by a 5 to 7 day course of tetracycline.

EPIDEMIOLOGY. In 1967 Meyer presented a comprehensive review on the distribution of chlamydiae in humans and in wild and domestic mammals and birds. More than 130 species of birds had been found to be infected then and it is probable that almost all bird species are carriers of *C. psittaci*. There is a wide range of mammals that are naturally infected. These include mice, cats, dogs, cattle, sheep, seals, and many other species. Various arthropods associated with infected animals also carry chlamydiae, but there is no evidence that arthropods play a role in disease transmission. The extent of infection in laboratory animals is illustrated by Meyer's finding that none of the colonies of mice and hamsters tested between 1940 and 1944 were free from chlamydiae.

Although clinical trachoma appears to have been diminishing since World War II, there are hundreds of millions of infected humans, primarily in Africa and Asia. Recent evidence that *C. trachomatis* is an important cause of nongonococcal urethritis and of cervicitis, and the finding of chlamydiae in 5 to 10 per cent of cervical specimens from asymptomatic women undergoing routine examinations, further confirm the extraordinarily widespread occurrence of these organisms and their role as a cause of infectious disease.

C. psittaci organisms spread from birds to man only sporadically, and outbreaks of human psittacosis occur mostly in persons processing carcasses of domestic turkeys, ducks, and other birds. There are several recorded instances of direct person-to-person transmission primarily involving hospital personnel.

Humans have been frequently infected after contact with apparently healthy birds. The organisms may be introduced from dust in birds cages and in other material contaminated with fecal materials from domestic or wild birds. Infection in humans most commonly results from inhalation of contaminated droplets or dust.

C. trachomatis is spread principally by three methods. The most common is direct contact by uninfected persons with eye secretions from infected carriers. In populations where hygiene is little practiced and where the carrier rate is very high, essentially every child is infected by contact with older carriers. The second method of transmission is sexual intercourse, resulting in acute, subacute, or inapparent infections of the genital tract of females and the genitourinary tract of males. The third method of transmission occurs during birth when the infant becomes infected during passage through the birth canal, with resulting conjunctivitis and/or pneumonitis.

References

Brunham, R. C., Kuo, C. C., Cles, L. and Holmes, K. K.: Correlation of host immune response with quantitative recovery of *Chlamydia trachomatis* from the human endocervix. Infect Immun 39:1491, 1983.

Byrne, G. I.: Requirements for ingestion of *C. psittaci* by mouse fibroblasts. Infect Immun 14:645, 1976.

Byrne, G. I. and Moulder, J. W.: Parasite-specified phagocytosis of *Chlamydia psittaci* and *Chlamydia trachomatis* by L and Hela cells. Infect Immun 19:588, 1978.

Christoffersen, G. and Manire, G. P.: The toxicity of meningopneumonitis organism (*C. psittaci*) at different stages of development. J Immunol 103:1085, 1969.

Eissenberg, R., Groppe, L., and Wyrick, P. B.: Inhibition of phagolysosomes fusion is localized to *Chlamydia psittaci*-laden vacuoles. Infect Immun 32:889, 1981.

Hatch, T. P., Al-Hossainy, E., and Silverman, J. A.: Adenine nucleotide and lysine transport in *Chlamydia psittaci*. J Bacteriol 150:662, 1982.

Lammert, Joyce K.: Cytotoxic cells induced after *Chlamydia psittaci* infection in mice. Infect Immun 35:1011, 1982.

Matsumoto, Akira.: Isolation and electron microscopic observations of intracytoplasmic inclusions containing *Chlamydia psittaci*. J Bacteriol 145:605, 1981.

Meyer, K. F.: The host spectrum of psittacosis-lymphogranuloma venereum agents. Am J Ophthalmol 63:1225, 1967.

Moulder, J. W., Hatch, T. P., Kuo, C. C., Schachter, J., and Storz, J.: In Krieg, N. R. (ed.), Bergey's Manual of Systematic Bacteriology, Ninth Edition, Volume 1, Baltimore, The Williams and Wilkins Company, 1982.

Nowinski, R. C., Tam, M. R., Goldstein, L. C., Strong, L., Kuo, C. C., Corey, L., Stamm, W. E., Handsfield, H. H., Knapp, J. J. and Holmes, K. K.: Monoclonal antibodies for diagnosis of infectious diseases in humans. Science 219:637, 1983.

Page, L. A.: Chlamydiales. In Buchanan, R. E. and Gibbons, N. E. (eds.): Bergey's Manual of Determinative Bacteriology, 8th ed. Baltimore, The Williams and Wilkins Company, 1974.

Rank, R. G., White, J. H. and Barron, A. L.: Humoral immunity in the resolution of genital infection in female guinea pigs infected with the agent of guinea pig inclusion conjunctivitis. Infect Immun 26:573–579, 1979.

Rank, R. G. and Barron, A. L.: Effect of antithymocyte serum on the course of chlamydial genital infection in female guinea pigs. Infect Immun 41:876, 1983.

Rothermel, C. D., Rubin, B. Y., and Murray, H. W.: Gamma interferon is the factor in lymphokine that activates human macrophages to inhibit intracellular *Chlamydia psittaci* replication. J Immunol 131, 1983.

Schachter, J.: Chlamydial infections. N Engl J Med 298:428, 490, 540, 1978.

Stokes, G. V.: Cycloheximide-resistant glycosylation in L-cells infected with *C. psittaci*. Infect Immun 9:497, 1974.

Storz, J. and Spears, P.: Chlamydiales: Properties, cycle of development and effect on eukaryote host cells. Curr Topics Microbiol Immunol 76:167, 1977.

Todd, W. and Storz, J.: Ultrastructural cytochemical evidence for the activation of lysosomes in the cytocidal effect of *C. psittaci*. Infect Immun 12:638, 1975.

Wang, S. P. and Grayston, J. T.: Immunological relationship between genital TRIC lymphogranuloma venereum and related organisms in a new microtiter indirect immunofluorescence test. Am J Ophthalmol 70:367, 1970.

4. Mycoplasmas and L-Forms

57 MYCOPLASMAS

ZELL A. MCGEE, M.D.
DAVID TAYLOR-ROBINSON, M.D.

Mycoplasmas, originally called pleuropneumonia-like organisms (PPLO), are the smallest of free-living organisms. In addition to their characteristic small size (smaller than some viruses), they all lack a cell wall and therefore are resistant to penicillin and other cell-wall active antimicrobials. The individual organisms are bounded by a pliable unit membrane that encloses the cytoplasm, DNA, RNA, and other metabolic components necessary for propagation on cell-free media. Mycoplasmas have a number of other characteristics that distinguish them from bacteria and viruses (Table 1). They are not related to L-phase variants of bacteria (see Chapter 58) (Hayflick, 1969; McGee et al., 1967).

Despite the superficial similarities among mycoplasmas, they comprise a heterogeneous assemblage of microorganisms that differ from one another in DNA composition, nutritional requirements, metabolic reactions, antigenic composition, and host species specificity. Taxonomically, the mycoplasmas are divided into three families: the Mycoplasmataceae and Spiroplasmataceae, which require cholesterol for growth, and the Acholeplasmataceae, which do not. All the mycoplasmas commonly isolated from humans belong to the Mycoplasmataceae. This family comprises the genus *Mycoplasma*, which contains organisms that do not hydrolyze urea, and the genus *Ureaplasma*, the organisms of which do hydrolyze urea. The latter were originally termed T strains or T mycoplasmas because of the tiny colonies they form.

Although the small size of their genome restricts the metabolic capabilities of mycoplasmas, certain species nonetheless have complex molecular mechanisms of pathogenicity by which they cause pneumonia, arthritis, keratoconjunctivitis, and mastitis in humans or other animals. Twelve species constitute the normal flora or are pathogens of humans (Table 2). Many mycoplasma species are a laboratory nuisance as occult contaminants of hybridoma cell lines and tissue cultures used for diagnostic and research purposes. Those mycoplasmas which infect plants and insects (spiroplasmas) have a helical structure. Others

Table 1. CHARACTERISTICS OF MYCOPLASMAS COMPARED TO THOSE OF BACTERIA AND VIRUSES

Characteristic	Mycoplasmas	Bacteria	Viruses
Size (diameter)	0.3 μm[a]	1–2 μm	<0.5 μm
Lack a cell wall	Yes	No	Yes
Propagate on cell-free media	Yes	Yes	No
Usually require sterol and native protein for growth	Yes	No	No
Intrinsic energy metabolism	Yes	Yes	No
Usually narrow range of host specificity	Yes	No	Yes
Growth inhibited by specific antibody	Yes	No	Yes
Resistant to cell wall-active antibotics (e.g., penicillins)	Yes	No	Yes
Resistant to antibiotics that inhibit metabolism (e.g., tetracycline)	No	No	Yes

[a]Smallest organism capable of propagation.

Table 2. MYCOPLASMAS OF HUMANS

	Species	Frequency of Isolation	Usual Site of Isolation	Nature of Disease
Nonpathogenic				
	M. orale	frequent	oropharynx	none
	M. salivarium	frequent	oropharynx	none
	M. buccale	rare	oropharynx	none
	M. faucium	rare	oropharynx	none
	M. lipophilum	rare	oropharynx	none
	A. laidlawii	very rare	oropharynx	none
	M. fermentans	infrequent	genitourinary tract	none[a]
	M. primatum	rare	genitourinary tract	none
Unknown pathogenicity	*M. genitalium*	unknown	genitourinary tract	Nongonococcal urethritis
Occasionally pathogenic				
	M. hominis	frequent[b]	genitourinary tract	Septicemia, abcess, endometritis-salpingitis, reproductive disorders (sterility, abortion, prematurity)?
	U. urealyticum	frequent[b]	genitourinary tract	Nongonococcal urethritis, septicemia? endometritis-salpingitis? reproductive disorders
Frequently pathogenic				
	M. pneumoniae	frequent[c]	oropharynx, respiratory tract	Tracheobronchitis, pneumonia, hemorrhagic bullous myringitis

[a]Reports of isolation from joint fluids in rheumatoid arthritis remain unconfirmed.
[b]Colonization frequent, disease infrequent.
[c]During disease but otherwise infrequent.

have been isolated from cattle and sheep rumen only under strict anaerobic conditions (anaeroplasmas).

MORPHOLOGY. The morphology of individual organisms varies from one mycoplasma species to another, from time to time during the growth cycle, and from one environmental condition to another. Most mycoplasmas are spherical (0.3 to 0.8 μm in diameter) and divide by binary fission. Some mycoplasmas develop branching filaments 0.3 to 0.4 μm in diameter and up to 150 μm long. These divide to produce new spherical bodies.

The morphology of four species of mycoplasmas, *Mycoplasma genitalium* (Tully et al., 1981), *M. pneumoniae. M. pulmonis* and *M. gallisepticum*, the last three of which are pathogens of the human, murine, and avian respiratory tracts respectively, is characterized by specialized structures at one or both ends of the organisms. *M. pneumoniae* and *M. genitalium* each have a tapered, filamentous tip that contains a dense, central rodlike core (Fig. 1). A specialized structure also has been observed in *M. pulmonis. M. gallisepticum* has a pear-shaped bleb at one or both ends of the organism. These structures may help

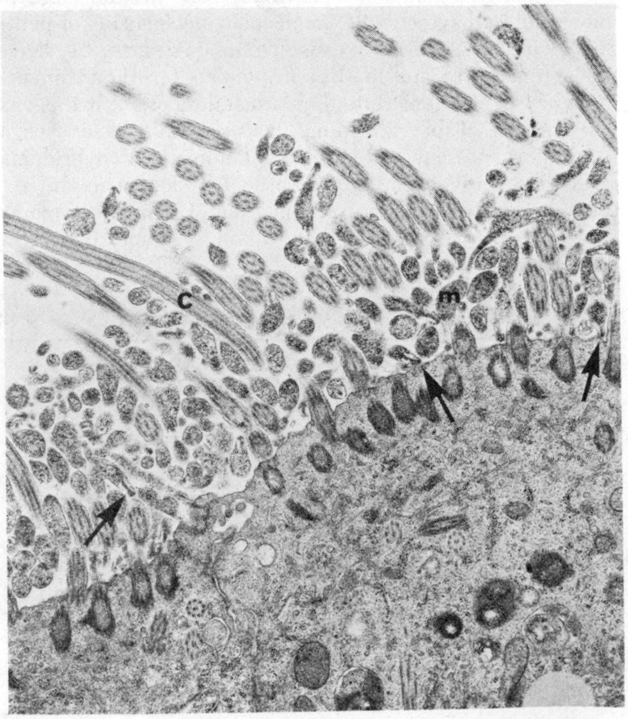

Figure 1. Electron micrograph of ciliated epithelial cells in tracheal mucosa infected with *Mycoplasma pneumoniae.* Note cilia (c) and individual organisms of *M. pneumoniae* (m) with specialized terminal structure oriented toward the membrane of the host cell (arrows). (× 13,000).

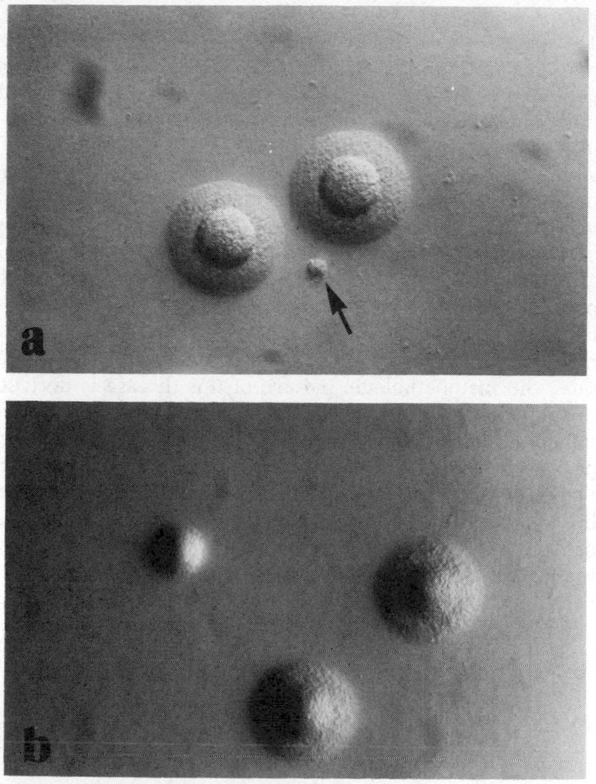

Figure 2. Colonial morphology of mycoplasmas. (*a*) Two colonies (90 μm diameter) of *Mycoplasma hominis* and one colony (15 μm diameter) of *Ureaplasma urealyticum* or T-strain (tiny colony) mycoplasmas (arrow) from urethral exudate. (*b*) Three colonies of *Mycoplasma pneumoniae* from the sputum of a patient with pneumonia. Two colonies (80 μm diameter) have a poorly defined periphery and the third, more typical of *M. pneumoniae*, lacks a periphery.

attach the organism to the respiratory or genital tract mucosa, since they usually are the point of intimate contact of the mycoplasmas with the host cell membrane (Fig. 1). They also may be involved in motion, since these four mycoplasmas exhibit gliding motility in which the organisms move tip first.

Colonies of most mycoplasma species vary in size from 50 to 600 μm and are therefore most easily viewed through clear media with a dissecting microscope. The characteristic "fried egg" morphologic appearance of mycoplasma colonies on agar medium (Fig. 2a, large colonies) is caused by an opaque central zone of growth in the agar and a translucent peripheral zone on the surface. Such typical colonies do not always develop, since development depends on the species of mycoplasma, the constituents and degree of hydration of the medium, and atmospheric conditions. Ureaplasmas generally produce small colonies (15 to 30 μm in diameter—Fig. 2a, small colony); however, on medium buffered to pH 6, typical colonies up to 300 μm may develop. On primary isolation, *M. pneumoniae* usually produces mulberry-like colonies with no translucent peripheral zone, but larger colonies with a periphery sometimes develop (Fig. 2b).

ANTIGENIC COMPOSITION. The major antigenic determinants of mycoplasmas are membrane proteins and glycolipids. The glucose- and galactose-containing glycolipids of *M. pneumoniae* are haptens, which are antigenic only when bound to membrane protein. They induce antibodies that react in tests of complement fixation, metabolism inhibition, and growth inhibition. Glycolipids of similar structure and activity are found in some other mycoplasmas, in most plants, and in human brains. The cross-reactivity of human brain tissue antigens with *M. pneumoniae* antibodies could account for the neurologic manifestations of *M. pneumoniae* infection. In contrast, a glycoprotein fraction of *M. pneumoniae*, rather than the glycolipid moiety, is involved in the development of a cell-mediated immune response to this mycoplasma species.

Several mycoplasma species, such as *M. mycoides* (bovine), *Acholeplasma laidlawii*, and *M. meleagridis* (avian), possess extracellular carbohydrates or capsule-like material. Although the function of these substances is not clear, the galactan of *M. mycoides*, which is similar to a substance found in bovine lung, may play an immunologic role in the production of pneumonia.

Antigenic relationships among mycoplasmas infecting humans have been defined by relatively specific serologic procedures (such as metabolism inhibition, growth inhibition, and immunofluorescence) that measure antibodies directed against mycoplasma membrane antigens. By means of these tests, mycoplasma "species" have been established. Species isolated from humans are distinct from each other and from those isolated from other animals. In contrast, tests employing mycoplasma cell extracts are less specific and show group relationships; thus, by immunodiffusion, common antigens are demonstrable among all the human mycoplasma species that have been tested except *M. pneumoniae*. Ureaplasmas of human origin comprise a single species, *U. urealyticum*, which has been subdivided into fourteen serotypes by such tests as metabolism and growth inhibition.

NUTRITION AND METABOLISM. Mycoplasmas require lipids and lipid precursors for synthesis of the plasma membrane (Hayflick, 1969; Razin, 1978). Animal sera provide a complex of lipoprotein and cholesterol, the latter being incorporated into the lipid bilayer membrane of sterol-requiring mycoplasmas and functioning as a regulator of the bilayer fluidity. Acholeplasmas do not need exogenous cholesterol because they synthesize saturated long-chain fatty acids and carotenoids that substitute for cholesterol in the membrane.

Mycoplasmas generally multiply at a slower rate than bacteria. The mean generation time for many mycoplasmas, including ureaplasmas, is one to three hours, and for some, six to nine hours. Most mycoplasmas are facultative anaerobes, but they will grow aerobically, some preferring this atmosphere. They utilize either glucose or arginine as a major source of energy. The carbohydrate-fermenting species catabolize glucose by glycolytic pathways, mainly to lactic acid. In most but not all mycoplasmas the respiratory pathways are flavin-terminated so that the heme compounds, cytochromes, and catalase are absent. Mycoplasmas that metabolize arginine use a three-enzyme system that converts it via ornithine to ammonia, and in so doing, supplies the organisms with ATP. A few species utilize both glucose and arginine, but ureaplasmas metabolize neither substrate. They convert urea to ammonia by means of a urease, although the need for urea as an energy source has not been established. Some metabolic properties of common human mycoplasmas are summarized in Table 3.

PATHOPHYSIOLOGY. Although *M. hominis* and *U. urealyticum* have been associated with perinatal sepsis, endometritis-salpingitis, and other genitourinary infections,

Table 3. METABOLIC PROPERTIES OF COMMON HUMAN MYCOPLASMAS

	Arginine Hydrolyzed	Glucose Fermented to Acid	Urea Hydrolyzed
M. orale	+	−	−
M. salivarium	+	−	−
M. hominis	+	−	−
M. pneumoniae	−	+	−
U. urealyticum	−	−	+

their pathogenic role in many cases is unclear. Both organisms attach to the surface of mammalian cells and replicate there, but little else is known of their pathogenic mechanisms (Cassell and Cole, 1981; Taylor-Robinson and McCormack, 1980). The pathogenicity of *M. pneumoniae*, which has been studied in humans, hamsters, guinea pigs and tracheal organ cultures, seems to depend on attachment of the specific terminal structure to neuraminic acid receptor sites on the surface of mucosal cells in the trachea and bronchi (Fig. 1). Proteins on the membrane of *M. pneumoniae* play a role in the attachment (Hu et al., 1977). The organisms do not invade the mucosal cells but appear to damage them by a toxic factor. *M. neurolyticum*, a pathogen of mice, produces a soluble protein exotoxin, but the only toxic factors definitively identified in *M. pneumoniae* so far are superoxide (O_2^-) (Lynch and Cole, 1980) and hydrogen peroxide (H_2O_2). Attachment is important in pathogenesis; disease is produced by strains of *M. pneumoniae* that produce peroxide and attach, but no disease is caused by strains that produce peroxide but do not attach. *M. pneumoniae* can also activate the classic and alternative pathways of complement and inhibit phagocytosis by alveolar macrophages.

Because fatal cases of *M. pneumoniae* pneumonia are rare, the histopathologic picture of this disease is derived mainly from infection of experimental animals. The pneumonic infiltrate is predominantly a peribronchiolar and perivascular cuffing by lymphocytes (Fig. 3a). This tissue response is followed by a change of the exudate in the bronchioles from a predominance of lymphocytes to a predominance of polymorphonuclear leukocytes and macrophages. These latter cells may, in association with antibody, help clear mycoplasmas by immune phagocytosis.

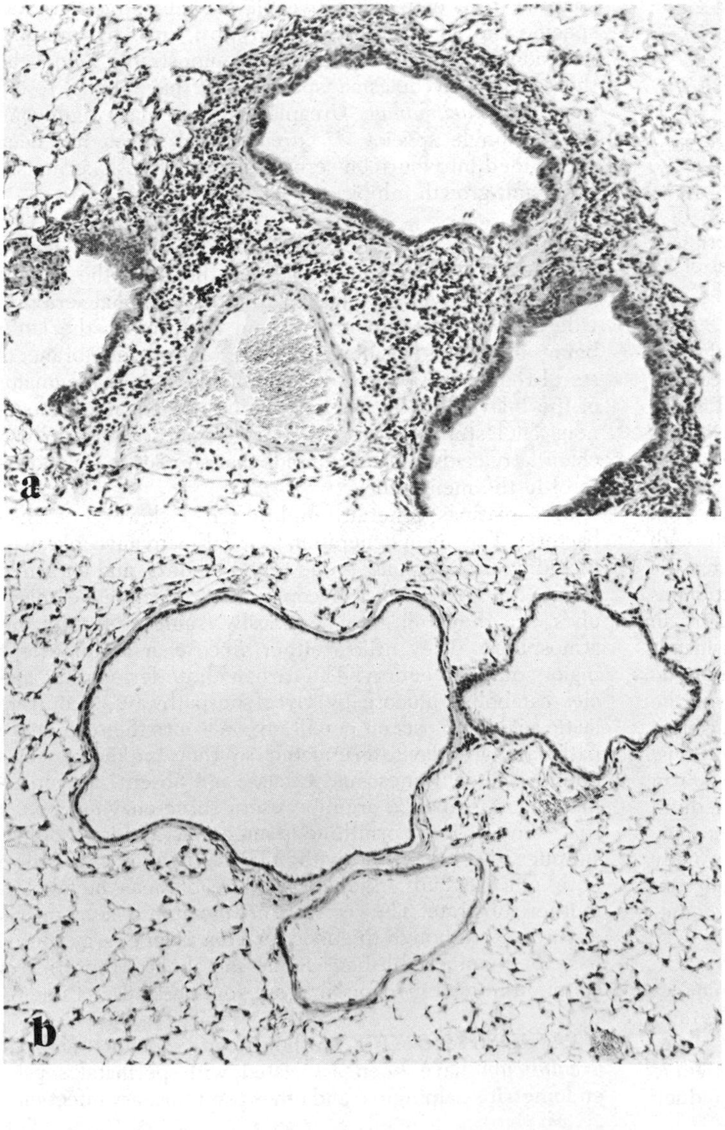

Figure 3. Pathology of pneumonia caused by *Mycoplasma pneumoniae.* Pneumonia 2 weeks after intranasal inoculation with *M. pneumoniae* of (*a*) immunologically normal hamsters (note peribronchiolar and perivascular infiltrate of mononuclear cells, predominantly lymphocytes) and (*b*) hamsters previously depleted of T-lymphocytes (note virtual absence of infiltrates). (Hematoxylin and eosin, × 176).

The rather slow development of these events in a primary infection contrasts with the markedly accelerated and often more intense response that occurs with reinfection. Some of the lymphocytes in the peribronchial infiltrate contain immunoglobulin, but most of these cells appear to be thymus-dependent. Ablation of the thymus in hamsters by various procedures prevents the development of peribronchial cuffing when these animals are challenged with *M. pneumoniae* (Fig. 3b). Many mycoplasmas serve as specific or nonspecific B cell and T cell mitogens and induce a variety of potential immunopathologic changes in infected hosts (Cassell and Cole, 1981; Fernald, 1982). At least to some extent, therefore, the pneumonia caused by *M. pneumoniae* is an immunopathologic process (Taylor and Taylor-Robinson, 1975; Fernald, 1982). Since many young children possess *M. pneumoniae* antibody, it is possible that the pneumonia that occurs in older age groups is an immunologic overresponse to reinfection, the lung being infiltrated by previously sensitized lymphocytes.

The pathophysiology of the Stevens-Johnson syndrome (erythema multiforme), meningoencephalitis, and other conditions that sometimes complicate *M. pneumoniae* infections is not understood. No firm evidence supports a pathogenic role for the antiheart and antilung antibodies that are observed in some patients with *M. pneumoniae* pneumonia.

The localization of specific receptor sites for *M. pneumoniae*, and thus the organisms of *M. pneumoniae*, in the trachea and bronchi with subsequent peribronchial infiltrates, contrasts with the localization of pneumococci in fluid-filled alveoli that are adjacent to the pleura. This may explain why pneumonia caused by *M. pneumoniae* is characterized by substernal burning and scanty production of sputum on coughing, whereas pneumococcal pneumonia is characterized by lateral pleuritic chest pain and generous production of sputum on coughing.

IMMUNITY. Antibodies in serum may be detected during mycoplasma infections by a variety of techniques, the most sensitive of which are radioimmunoprecipitation, complement-dependent mycoplasmacidal and ELISA tests. Generally, the first antibodies produced are of the IgM class; later IgG predominates. Humoral antibodies, however, do not fully protect against infection or disease, since infection and development of pneumonia may occur despite high titers of, for example, mycoplasmacidal antibodies to *M. pneumoniae* in the serum. Furthermore, natural or experimental respiratory tract infection of animals may produce only low titers of serum antibodies, yet such local infection provides greater resistance to reinfection than parenteral inoculation of organisms, which produces high titers of serum antibody. This suggests that local factors are crucial to resistance. Indeed, resistance of adult volunteers to *M. pneumoniae* has been related to the presence of specific IgA antibody in respiratory secretions. This antibody may function as the first line of defense by preventing the attachment of organisms to the respiratory epithelial cells. On the other hand, development of a cell-mediated immune response, which is detectable by lymphocyte transformation and macrophage migration inhibition, does not seem to be important in resistance.

In field trials, inactivated *M. pneumoniae* vaccines have prevented disease in only about half of those vaccinated. The inability of these and other killed mycoplasma vaccines to protect completely may be due to their failure to stimulate sufficient local antibody production. With this in mind, live but attenuated temperature-sensitive mutants of *M. pneumoniae* have been developed that multiply at the temperature of the upper respiratory tract but not at that of the lower tract. Some of the mutants have produced pulmonary infection both in the hamster and in human volunteers without causing disease and have induced resistance to challenge with virulent wild-type *M. pneumoniae*. However, assuring that such mutants are sufficiently stable and attenuated for large-scale use as a human vaccine is a problem. Furthermore, permanent protection seems unlikely because naturally acquired *M. pneumoniae* infection does not provide lifelong immunity. Reinfection occurs with appreciable frequency, and second attacks of *M. pneumoniae* pneumonia also occur.

LABORATORY DIAGNOSIS. Mycoplasmas grown in vitro are gram-negative. However, individual mycoplasma organisms are too small and do not take up the safranin counterstain well enough to be recognized on microscopic examination of gram-stained clinical specimens. The laboratory diagnosis depends, therefore, on cultural identification and on serologic tests. Details of these techniques are considered elsewhere (Razin and Tully, 1983; Tully and Razin, 1983).

The medium for primary isolation of *M. pneumoniae* consists of PPLO agar or broth, 20 per cent horse serum and 10 per cent vol/vol fresh yeast extract (25 per cent wt/vol). To enhance detection of *M. pneumoniae*, the medium is supplemented with thallium acetate and penicillin to inhibit bacteria and fungi, methylene blue to inhibit other human mycoplasmas, and glucose with phenol red as a pH indicator to detect acid produced by *M. pneumoniae*. A vial of diphasic medium (broth over agar) is inoculated with sputum or a pharyngeal swab and incubated at 37° C. A color change from purple to yellow-green, which usually occurs within 4 to 21 days, signals the fermentation of glucose with production of acid and the consequent change in color of the phenol red to yellow on a background of methylene blue. This presumptive positive identification is confirmed by subculturing to agar medium and demonstrating inhibition of colony development with commercial disks impregnated with specific antiserum. Hemadsorption and rapid hemolysis of guinea pig red cells by colonies of *M. pneumoniae* on agar are also used to help in presumptive identification. The hemadsorption occurs because of neuraminic acid receptors on red cells.

A similar strategy, utilizing the metabolism of arginine or urea, has been employed to design media that select for and presumptively identify, respectively, *M. hominis* and *U. urealyticum* in specimens from the genitourinary tract.

The most readily available serologic test for *M. pneumoniae* is the complement fixation test, for which reagents can be obtained commercially. It is positive in about 80 per cent of cases as indicated by a fourfold or greater rise in antibody titers between acute and convalescent specimens. However, the possibility of cross-reactivity with *M. genitalium* should be considered. The cold agglutinin test depends on nonspecific agglutination of O Rh-negative red blood cells at 4° C by antibodies to I antigen that arise in *M. pneumoniae* infection. The test is positive in only about 50 per cent of patients, usually those with more severe disease. Several serologic tests will detect antibody to *M. hominis* and *U. urealyticum* but the ELISA test may prove the most useful.

DRUG SUSCEPTIBILITY. Since the mycoplasmas lack a cell wall, they are resistant or indifferent to the penicillins, cephalosporins, and other antimicrobials that act on the cell wall. In contrast, mycoplasmas are generally sensitive to antimicrobials that inhibit protein synthesis. At clinically achievable concentrations, tetracycline is inhibitory for *M. pneumoniae, M. hominis*, and *U. urealyticum*. Whereas erythromycin has marked inhibitory activity against *M. pneumoniae*, it is only moderately active against *U. urealyticum* and is inactive against *M. hominis*. Both genital mycoplasmas, *U. urealyticum* and *M. hominis*, are sensitive to spectinomycin. Despite the sensitivity of *M. pneumoniae* to tetracycline and erythromycin and the good clinical responses to therapy that occur with these drugs, about 50 per cent of treated patients continue to harbor *M. pneumoniae* in the posterior pharynx for one to three months.

EPIDEMIOLOGY. Infections with *M. pneumoniae* apparently occur world-wide and account for approximately 20 per cent of all cases of pneumonia in some cities (Clyde, 1979). The disease is endemic with periodic epidemics. Spread of the organism, which occurs by aerosol transmission, is slow. Therefore, most infections occur in small groups of people who have frequent close contact such as families, military units, and college fraternities. The incubation period is two to three weeks. The disease is usually introduced into the family by a small child and moves from person to person over a period of months with an attack rate of greater than 50 per cent. Pneumonia is most frequent in persons aged 5 to 20 years. Thereafter, pneumonia occurs less frequently but is generally more severe as the patient's age increases.

Ureaplasmas are acquired at birth by up to 30 per cent of infants. Colonization of the genital tract is most common but is usually transient. The organisms are found again after puberty, and antibody is first detectable at this time. Thereafter, the frequency of occurrence is related to sexual activity; recovery rates of about 60 per cent and 80 per cent have been observed for men and women, respectively, attending venereal disease clinics (Taylor-Robinson and McCormack, 1980). The occurrence of ureaplasmas in apparently healthy persons has posed a problem in attributing a pathogenic role to them. However, the results of several studies, including the intraurethral inoculation of human volunteers with ureaplasmas, suggest that they cause some cases of nongonococcal urethritis.

M. hominis is acquired at birth by about 6 per cent of infants. Most of these individuals lose these strains but become colonized later in life when sexual activity commences. *M. hominis* is unlikely to play a role in nongonococcal urethritis, but it is sometimes a cause of acute pyelonephritis and causes a variety of pelvic infections. It has been isolated from the blood in the absence of other microorganisms in 8 per cent of women with fever after normal delivery or abortion.

Acute septic arthritis may occur in conjunction with infection by *M. pneumoniae, M. hominis*, or *U. urealyticum*, especially in hypogammaglobulinemic or other immunosuppressed patients. The frequent causation of chronic arthritis and neurologic diseases by different mycoplasmas in various animal species has suggested that they might cause such diseases in humans. In animals the susceptibility to mycoplasma-induced chronic arthritis is associated with the presence on host cells of certain histocompatibility antigens (Cassell and Cole, 1981). Despite the continued search for mycoplasmas in rheumatoid arthritis and other human diseases of unknown etiology, there is no firm evidence for their involvement.

References

Cassell, G. H., and Cole, B. C.: Mycoplasmas as agents of human disease. N Engl J Med 304:80, 1981.

Clyde, W. A., Jr.: *Mycoplasma pneumoniae* infections of man. In Tully, J. G. and Whitcomb, R. F. (eds.): The Mycoplasmas, Vol. 2. New York. Academic Press, 1979, p. 275.

Fernald, G. W. Immunologic actions between host cells and mycoplasmas: An introduction. Rev Infect Dis 4:S201, 1982. (This Supplement issue provides a good update.)

Hayflick, L. (ed.): The Mycoplasmatales and the L-Phase of Bacteria. New York, Appleton-Century-Crofts, 1969.

Hu, P. C., Collier, A. M., and Baseman, J. B.: Surface parasitism by *Mycoplasma pneumoniae* of respiratory epithelium. J Exp Med 145:1328, 1977.

Lynch, R. E., and Cole, B. C.: Mycoplasma pneumoniae: A prokaryote which consumes oxygen and generates superoxide but which lacks superoxide dismutase. Biochem Biophys Resh Comm 96:98, 1980.

McGee, Z. A., Rogul, M., and Wittler, R. G.: Molecular genetic studies of relationships among mycoplasma, L-forms and bacteria. Ann N Y Acad Sci 143:21, 1967.

Razin, S.: The mycoplasmas. Microbiol Rev 42:414, 1978.

Razin, S., and Tully, J. G. (eds): Methods in Mycoplasmology. Vol. 1. Mycoplasma characterization. New York, Academic Press, 1983.

Taylor, G., and Taylor-Robinson, D.: The part played by cell-mediated immunity in mycoplasma respiratory infections. Develop Biol Stand 28:195, 1975.

Taylor-Robinson, D., and McCormack, W. M.: The genital mycoplasmas. N Engl J Med 302:1003 and 1063, 1980.

Tully, J. G., and Razin, S. (eds.): Methods in Mycoplasmology. Vol. 2. Diagnostic mycoplasmology. New York, Academic Press, 1983.

Tully, J. G., Taylor-Robinson, D., Cole, R. M., and Rose, D. L.: A newly discovered mycoplasma in the human urogenital tract. Lancet 1:1288, 1981.

58

CELL WALL—DEFECTIVE BACTERIA

ZELL A. MCGEE, M. D.

Susceptible bacteria that are exposed to penicillin or other substances that damage the bacterial cell wall are usually killed. Under certain conditions, however, bacteria can survive with damaged cell walls and multiply as organisms with markedly altered morphology, physiology, and cultural characteristics (Dienes and Weinberger, 1951; Gutman et al., 1967; Hayflick, 1969). These wall-defective bacteria are undetectable by routine cultural techniques, are not affected by penicillin and other cell wall-active antimicrobials, and may revert to the intact bacterium if the cell wall-active antibiotic is removed. These characteristics of elusiveness, indifference to the most frequently administered antimicrobials, and morphologic versatility have stimulated interest in the possibility that wall-defective bacteria may play a role in various chronic, recurrent, or culture-negative infections of humans (Clasener, 1972; Guze, 1967).

MORPHOLOGY AND PHYSIOLOGY. The pliable bacterial cytoplasmic membrane is encased in a rigid peptidoglycan layer, which gives the bacterial cell its coccal or rod shape. In gram-negative bacteria, the intracellular osmotic pressure is 300 to 400 milliosmoles per kilogram water (mOsm/kg), and in gram-positive bacteria, it is 900 mOsm/kg or greater. When bacteria are suspended in serum or most bacteriologic media (270 to 300 mOsm/kg), the higher internal osmotic pressure of the bacteria favors the flow of water into their cytoplasm, but there cannot be a net gain of water because the peptidoglycan layer restricts any increase in volume. If the peptidoglycan layer is removed, water moves freely into the cytoplasm with increasing distention of the cytoplasmic membrane and dilution of the cytoplasm until the concentration of molecules inside the membrane equals the concentration outside. Before this equalization occurs, however, the cytoplasmic membrane usually ruptures, and the organism is killed. This seems to be the way that bacteria die when their cell walls are damaged by penicillin.

If the concentration of molecules that do not freely cross the cytoplasmic membrane is increased in the environment so that it balances the concentration within the bacterium, removal of the peptidoglycan may result in a change of shape (e.g., from a rod to a spherical shape), but the organism will not rupture (see Fig. 1a,b). Bacteria with damaged or absent cell walls can survive in environments with osmolalities lower than their intracellular osmotic pressure if their cytoplasmic membranes are stabilized intrinsically by divalent cations or polyamines, or by an adaptive change to a higher ratio of saturated to unsaturated fatty acids in the membrane (Leon and Panos, 1976).

When bacteria are exposed to penicillin in a hypertonic medium (strictly, a medium with an osmolality greater than

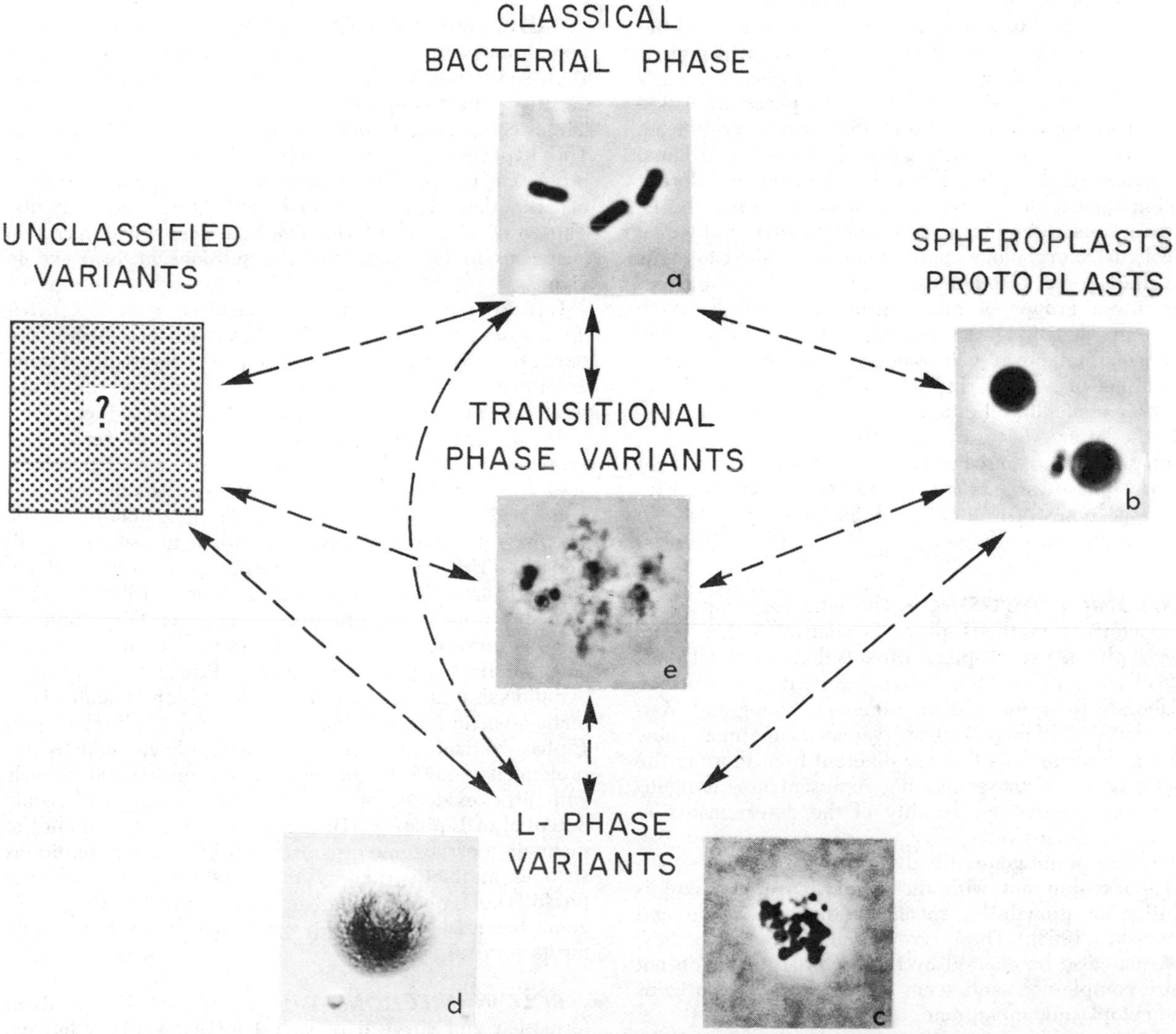

Figure 1. Schematic representation of the transition of a bacterium to different variant phases. Photos *a*, *b*, and *c* demonstrate the contrasting morphology of the classic bacterial phase, spheroplast phase, and a clump of L-phase variants of *Proteus mirabilis* in identical media (900 mOsm/kg) and at the same magnification (phase contrast, × 3400). Photo *d* shows a "fried egg" colony of L-phase variants of *Proteus mirabilis* (× 150). Photo *e* shows a clump of transitional phase variants of *Staphylococcus albus* from the blood culture of a patient with an infected prosthetic heart valve (phase contrast, × 1600). (From McGee, Z. A., Wittler, R. G., Gooder, H., and Charache, P.: J Infect Dis 123:433, 1971.)

that of human serum [290 mOsm/kg] but conventionally, about 900 mOsm/kg), they may simply round up to become *spheroplasts* (which have partial loss of the cell wall) or *protoplasts* (which have complete loss of the cell wall) (Fig. 1a,b). Since bacteria in the spheroplast or protoplast phase cannot multiply and are lysed at physiologic osmolalities, they are unlikely to play a role in human infections. Bacteria may also undergo a more fundamental change, however, either directly or by further transition from spheroplasts or protoplasts to L-phase variants or L-forms (Fig. 1c,d) (L stands for the Lister Institute in London where they were first described in 1935). Some bacteria, such as *Neisseria gonorrhoeae* and *Bacteroides fragilis*, can undergo this transition to the L-phase spontaneously; others require the presence of penicillin, lysozyme, or other cell wall-active substances. Bacteria in the L-phase can replicate serially as nonrigid cells that are spherical or pleomorphic and vary in size from "large bodies," larger than some human cells, to elementary bodies, which may be as small as some viruses. On solid media, L-phase variants produce tiny colonies composed of a central core, which grows into the agar, and a superficial growth around the core, which gives them a "fried egg" appearance (Fig. 1d). L-phase variants that cannot revert to the classic bacterial phase are called "stable" L-phase variants. Bacteria that have reverted from the L-phase may be indistinguishable from the original bacteria, except that when exposed to the same or different inducing agents, they enter the L-phase more readily. L-phase variants resemble mycoplasmas in their individual and colonial morphology, but studies have failed to show any immunologic, biochemical or genetic relationship between these groups of microorganisms (Hayflick, 1969; McGee et al., 1971). In many cases determination of whether an unknown cell wall-less microorganism is a mycoplasma or a stable L-phase variant can be made by testing for penicillin-binding proteins which are only present in the latter (Martin et al., 1980).

L-phase variants and bacteria undergoing transition to or from L-phase variants (*transitional phase variants*, Fig. 1e) are the types of wall-defective bacteria most likely to play a role in human disease.

ANTIGENIC COMPOSITION. The antigenic composition of a bacterium in the L-phase is similar to that of its bacterial phase. Even L-phase variants that completely lack cell-wall antigens on their external surface may continue to elaborate them into the environment (Yeung and Mattingly, 1983). Although L-phase variants sometimes show antigenic determinants that are different from those of the parental bacteria, these may not represent new antigens but merely greater accessibility of the determinants to antibody-producing cells.

One type of antigen-antibody reaction that occurs with the L-phase but not with the classic bacterial phase is inhibition of growth by specific antibody (Braude and Siemienski, 1968). These growth-inhibiting antibodies, which may also be elicited by the bacterial phase, do not require complement and seem to be directed at antigens of the cytoplasmic membrane.

METABOLISM. Transition to the L-phase is sometimes accompanied by loss of the ability to carry out certain metabolic reactions such as fermentation of a particular sugar or production of a hemolysin. The L-phase variants of a few bacterial species, such as *Salmonella typhi*, require anaerobic conditions, whereas the parental bacterium can grow aerobically. Nevertheless, L-phase variants generally carry out metabolic reactions and generate products characteristic of the bacteria from which they were derived, although they may do so at a slower rate.

HOST DEFENSES. A number of factors make the human body a potentially adverse environment for L-phase variants: (1) the osmolality of human serum and tissue fluid is approximately 290 mOsm/kg, well below the osmolality at which wall-defective variants of some bacteria undergo osmotic rupture; (2) normal human serum contains an antibody-complement system that rapidly disrupts the cytoplasmic membranes and kills L-phase variants of a variety of gram-positive and gram-negative pathogens; (3) growth-inhibiting antibodies may be elicited by L-phase variants or their parental bacteria; and (4) L-phase variants can be phagocytized by polymorphonuclear and mononuclear phagocytes.

PATHOGENIC PROPERTIES. None of the defenses mentioned above precludes the survival and multiplication of L-phase variants in humans. L-phase variants of both gram-negative and gram-positive bacteria can survive at osmolalities comparable to those of serum or purulent exudates. The hypertonic milieu of the kidney provides osmotic protection and inactivates the antibody-complement system in serum that might otherwise be lethal to L-phase variants. These variants can be formed and can persist within certain host cells under experimental conditions in vitro and in vivo.

L-phase variants of toxigenic bacteria, such as *Clostridium tetani* or *Vibrio* species, also produce toxins and might thereby be pathogenic. The L-phase variants of some gram-negative bacteria elaborate endotoxin and can evoke the localized Shwartzman reaction. Infection of the urinary tract of experimental animals with L-phase variants of *Proteus mirabilis*, which produce urease, has been associated with formation of bladder stones (Braude and Siemienski, 1968). L-phase variants of group A beta-hemolytic streptococci have been shown to adapt to osmotic conditions like those in human tissues and to invade and kill human heart cells in tissue culture (Leon and Panos, 1976). Antigens from the L-phase variants of certain strains of these streptococci, when used to immunize mice of particular genetic types, produce myocarditis and electrocardiographic abnormalities similar to those seen in acute rheumatic fever in humans (Matsunaga et al., 1982). However, L-phase variants of some other bacteria have persisted for prolonged periods in the tissues of experimental animals with little evidence of damage. The greatest pathogenic potential of L-phase variants may reside in their ability to maintain a pathogenic organism in a host under conditions such as antibiotic therapy that might kill the bacterial phase. The L-phase variant may then revert to the pathogenic bacterial phase when conditions become favorable for its survival.

ROLE IN INFECTIONS. Despite the varied methods of formation and survival of wall-defective variants in vivo under experimental conditions, it has been most difficult to prove that wall-defective variants play a role in human diseases. Koch's postulates have not been helpful in approaching this problem because they do not allow for a significant change in the nature of an organism during the course of an infection.

There are many reports of pyelonephritis, osteomyelitis, endocarditis, and other acute and chronic infections in which wall-defective variants were isolated on hypertonic but not on routine media. However, only a few of these studies provide evidence that L-phase variants were actually present in the patient and not merely induced on the media in the laboratory.

Microscopic examination of the urine from patients with pyelonephritis has revealed spheroplasts and other atypical bacteria during periods of antimicrobial therapy but only classic rod-shaped bacteria when therapy was not being administered. In one series of patients, the presence of viable cell-wall defective bacteria in the urine of 11 (16 per cent) of 57 patients with chronic pyelonephritis was documented by filtering the specimens to remove bacteria and isolating L-phase variants from the filtrates on hypertonic but not on isotonic media. In three patients, who had only wall-defective variants in their urine and were not receiving antibiotics, the variants were apparently either induced by autolytic bacterial enzymes, by host factors or both.

One patient, a 10-year-old girl (described by Gutman et al., 1967), had recurrent bouts of urinary tract infection characterized by urgency, chills, fever, and more than 10^5 *P. mirabilis* per ml. of urine. During ampicillin therapy, the patient's symptoms decreased and routine cultures became sterile, but L-phase variants of the *Proteus* were recovered from filtered urine cultured on hypertonic media. After therapy was discontinued, bacterial phase *P. mirabilis* returned, and cultures for L-phase variants became negative. The bacterial phase was sensitive to ampicillin but resistant to erythromycin. The L-phase variant was resistant to ampicillin but sensitive to erythromycin. After ampicillin therapy was begun, routine cultures became negative, but cultures for L-phase variants became positive. When erythromycin was added to the regimen, cultures for L-phase variants became negative within three days. After completion of 12 days of combined therapy, all cultures remained negative and the patient was free of urinary tract infection for a follow-up period of 18 months.

Wittler and colleagues (1960) described the five-year course of a young girl with similar changes of symptoms and culture results during periods of penicillin therapy for *Corynebacterium* endocarditis. When penicillin was administered, she became asymptomatic and cultures on routine media became negative, but wall-defective variants were recovered on hypertonic media. The bacterial phase returned when penicillin was discontinued. This study was more convincing because the variants were visualized microscopically in peripheral blood cells when variants were recovered from hypertonic culture media and because penicillinase was used in the cultures to decrease the likelihood of producing variants in vitro.

These and a few other careful clinical studies as well as data from experimental animals strongly suggest that L-phase variants may be produced and persist in vivo. It is not clear whether such organisms are of clinical significance in other than rare cases.

LABORATORY DIAGNOSIS. Cultures for wall-defective organisms can be performed by the laboratory on two different levels: (1) the laboratory may routinely use media that are appropriate for recovering wall-defective variants but will not determine whether organisms isolated were present in the patient as typical bacteria or as L-phase variants; or (2) the laboratory may perform on highly selected patients the specialized procedures necessary to isolate and identify wall-defective variants that do not revert on their first passage in vitro, determine their antimicrobial susceptibility, and establish whether the organism existed in a wall-defective form in the patient. The details of these procedures have recently been reviewed (McGee, 1977). Either or both approaches may be adopted, but the second requires experienced personnel, complex media, and a large commitment of time.

DRUG SUSCEPTIBILITY. Bacteria undergoing transition to the L-phase always lose susceptibility to penicillins, cephalosporins, and other agents that act on the cell wall. Conversely, gram-negative bacilli, such as *Pseudomonas aeruginosa* become more susceptible to erythromycin, tetracycline, and other agents that act within the bacterial cytoplasm but are normally excluded by the gram-negative cell wall. These changes in susceptibility provide a rationale for the therapy of infections involving bacterial variants.

Therapy of infections with cell wall-defective variants has generally consisted of a combination of two drugs: (1) a cell wall-active agent such as penicillin that either kills residual bacteria or makes them wall-defective, and (2) an antimicrobial such as erythromycin or gentamicin that acts within the bacterial cell. Although this approach has been effective in controlled studies of infected experimental animals, reports of its success in human infections are anecdotal. Currently, the use of such therapy seems justified only in highly selected and closely monitored patients whose clinical specimens contain wall-defective variants (McGee, 1977).

References

Braude, A. I., and Sieminski, J.: Production of bladder stones by L-forms. Trans Assn Amer Phys 81:323, 1968.

Clasener, H.: Pathogenicity of the L-phase of bacteria. Ann Rev Microbiol 26:55, 1972.

Dienes, L., and Weinberger, H. J.: The L-forms of bacteria. Bacteriol Rev 15:245, 1951.

Gutman, L. T., Schaller, J., and Wedgwood, R. J.: Bacterial L-forms in relapsing urinary-tract infection. Lancet 1:464, 1967.

Guze, L. B. (ed.): Microbial protoplasts, spheroplasts and L-forms. Baltimore, Williams and Wilkins, 1967.

Hayflick, L. (ed.): The mycoplasmatales and the L-phase of bacteria. New York, Appleton-Century-Crofts, 1969.

Leon, O., and Panos, C.: Adaptation of an osmotically fragile L-form of *Streptococcus pyogenes* to physiological osmotic conditions and its ability to destroy human heart cells in tissue culture. Infect Immun 13:252, 1976.

Martin, H. H., Schilf, W., and Schieffer, H. G.: Differentiation of mycoplasmatales from bacterial protoplast L-forms by assay for penicillin-binding proteins. Arch Microbiol 27:297, 1980.

Matsunaga, K., Katoh, K., Takahashi, T., Sakamoto, H., Tani, K., Okuda, K., Tadokoro, I., and Kitamura, H.: The experimental myocarditis of mice immunized with group A streptococcal cytoplasmic membrane fraction extracted from L-forms. Japan J Exp Med 52:267, 1982.

McGee, Z. A.: Cell-wall deficient bacteria. In von Graevenitz, Alexander (ed.): CRC Handbook Series in Clinical Laboratory Science, Section E: Clinical Microbiology, Vol. I. Cleveland, CRC Press, Inc., 1977, p. 367.

McGee, Z. A., Wittler, R. G., Gooder, H., and Charache, P.: Wall-defective microbiol variants: terminology and experimental design. J Infect Dis 123:433, 1971.

Wittler, R. G., Malizia, W. F., Kramer, P. E., Tuckett, J. D., Pritchard, H. N., and Baker, H. J.: Isolation of a corynebacterium and its transitional forms from a case of subacute bacterial endocarditis treated with antibiotics. J Gen Microbiol 23:315, 1960.

Yeung, M. K., and Mattingly, S. J.: Biosynthesis of cell wall peptidoglycan and polysaccharide antigens by protoplasts of type III group B *Streptococcus*. J Bacteriol 154:211, 1983.

5. Viruses

DNA VIRUSES

59

ADENOVIRUS

LENNART PHILIPSON, M.D., DR. MED. SCI.

Adenoviruses constitute a family of viruses originally isolated from the respiratory tract of man and other animals. They were discovered in 1953. They are nonenveloped icosahedral viruses with DNA genomes of intermediate size (20 to 30 $\times$ 10^6 daltons). The adenovirus family has been subdivided into two genera, mastadenovirus and aviadenovirus, referring to viruses isolated from mammalian and avian hosts respectively (Norrby et al., 1976). There is no cross-reacting antigen between these two genera. The mastadenovirus comprises at least 80 different serotypes, of which 33 have been isolated from human sources. The aviadenovirus contains 14 distinct serotypes.

Precise biochemical tools to characterize adenovirus genomes have become available during recent years, including separated strands of the DNA, restriction enzyme fragments, and liquid hybridization methods to detect the viral transcription products. The structural and nonstructural proteins encoded by the adenovirus genome have also been extensively characterized with regard to both structure and function. The adenoviruses have therefore become a model virus to investigate the complex control mechanism involved in macromolecular synthesis in mammalian cells. Studies of the molecular biology of these viruses may help to elucidate mechanisms for transcription, processing of the transcripts to messenger RNA, and control mechanisms for protein synthesis in mammalian cells. The molecular biology of the adenoviruses has been reviewed in the last decade (Philipson et al., 1975; Wold et al., 1978), but the role of these viruses in human infections has not been evaluated during recent years. Several earlier reviews may provide a more detailed insight into the clinical aspects of adenovirus infections (Sohier et al., 1965; Potter, 1967; and Rose, 1969). This chapter will focus on some properties of adenoviruses and their role in infectious diseases in man.

THE STRUCTURE OF THE VIRION

Morphology. The adenoviruses are nonenveloped viruses with a diameter of 65 to 80 nm. The capsid has 252 capsomers arranged into an icosahedron with 20 triangular facets and 12 vertices, as schematically shown in Figure 1. Two hundred forty of the 252 capsomers have six neighbors, and they are called *hexons*; whereas the 12 capsomers at the vertices have five neighbors, and are therefore called *pentons*. Each penton unit consists of a penton base anchored in the capsid and a rod-like projection with a knob attached at the distal end. The rod-like portion is referred to as the *fiber*. Two types of hexons may be defined: (1) those 60 located in juxtaposition to the pentons, *peripentonal hexons* that have the penton base as one of their six neighbors, and (2) those 180 that form the triangular facets and the edges of the icosahedron. The latter may be released from the virions in aggregates of nine hexons, *ninemers*, which form a defined structure with threefold rotational symmetry. Inside the capsid there is a core with a diameter of 40 to 45 nm, which contains the DNA and additional proteins. It can be revealed by electron microscopy of thin sections of particles stained with uranyl acetate. A circular protein-DNA complex was observed after degradation of virions with guanidine, suggesting that the two termini of the DNA in the virion are linked to each other by proteins.

Chemical Composition. The human adenovirus type 2 (ad2), which has been studied in detail, has an estimated particle weight of 175 $\times$ 10^6 daltons. It contains 13 per cent DNA corresponding to 23 $\times$ 10^6 daltons, and the additional components are all proteins. Unlike most other viruses the adenoviruses have capsid units that are soluble in nondenaturing solvent, which has facilitated the purification and characterization of the virus components. Methods have been developed for sequential disintegration of the virion. The pentons alone or together with peripentonal hexons can be selectively removed by dialysis at low pH. The release of pentons is accompanied by the release of additional antigens probably located in the peripentonal region. After treatment of the virus particle with sodium dodecyl sulfate (SDS), urea, or pyridine, the capsid is disrupted and the hexons from the triangular facets are released as ninemers. The polypeptide composition of adenoviruses has been studied by SDS-polyacrylamide electrophoresis. The virion of ad2, ad7, and ad12 contains a minimum of nine polypeptides that range in size from 7500 to 120,000 daltons. Eight of these are antigenically distinct and reside in different structures after sequential degradation of the virion. Five of the polypeptides are integral parts of the capsomers or the core. Thus, polypeptide II is the only polypeptide that is detected in purified hexons from infected cells. Polypeptide III resides in the penton base, IV, in the fiber, and polypeptide V and VII are associated with the core. The remaining polypeptides have been tentatively localized in the virion structure as indicated in Figure 2. The structural units observed in the virion as hexon, penton, and fiber are multimers of the integral polypeptide. Hexon contains three polypeptides, penton also three, and fiber contains two polypeptides, and each unit must therefore be assembled independently.

The DNA of human adenoviruses has been extensively characterized. There is a difference in base composition between the different subgroups of the human adenoviruses (Table 1). In addition, there is considerable homology of the DNA sequence within each subgroup but only 10 to 20 per cent homology between DNA of members of different subgroups, regardless of whether filter hybridization or electron microscopic analysis of heteroduplexes was used

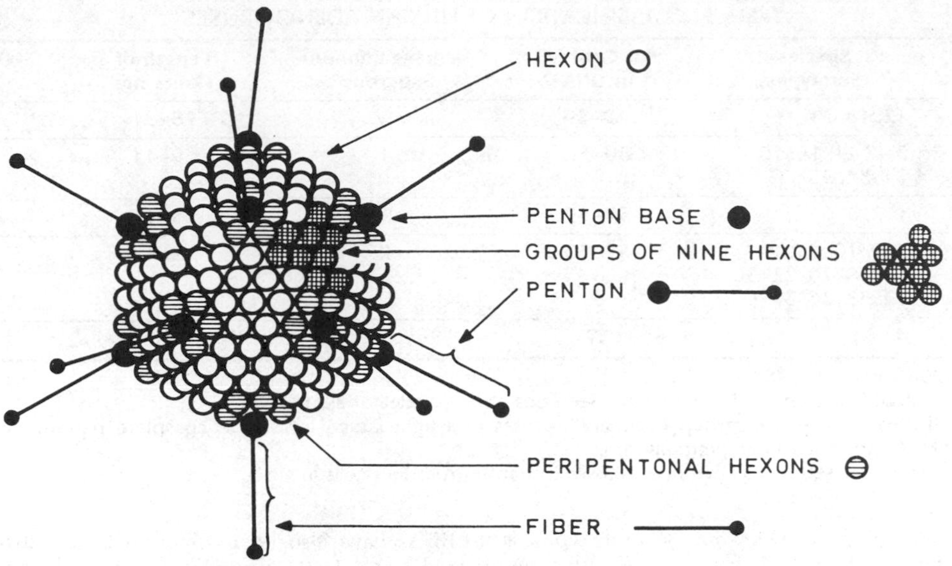

Figure 1. Structure of the adenovirus capsid. Schematic drawing showing the icosahedral outline of the adenovirus capsid and the location of various components. (Reprinted from Philipson et al., 1975.)

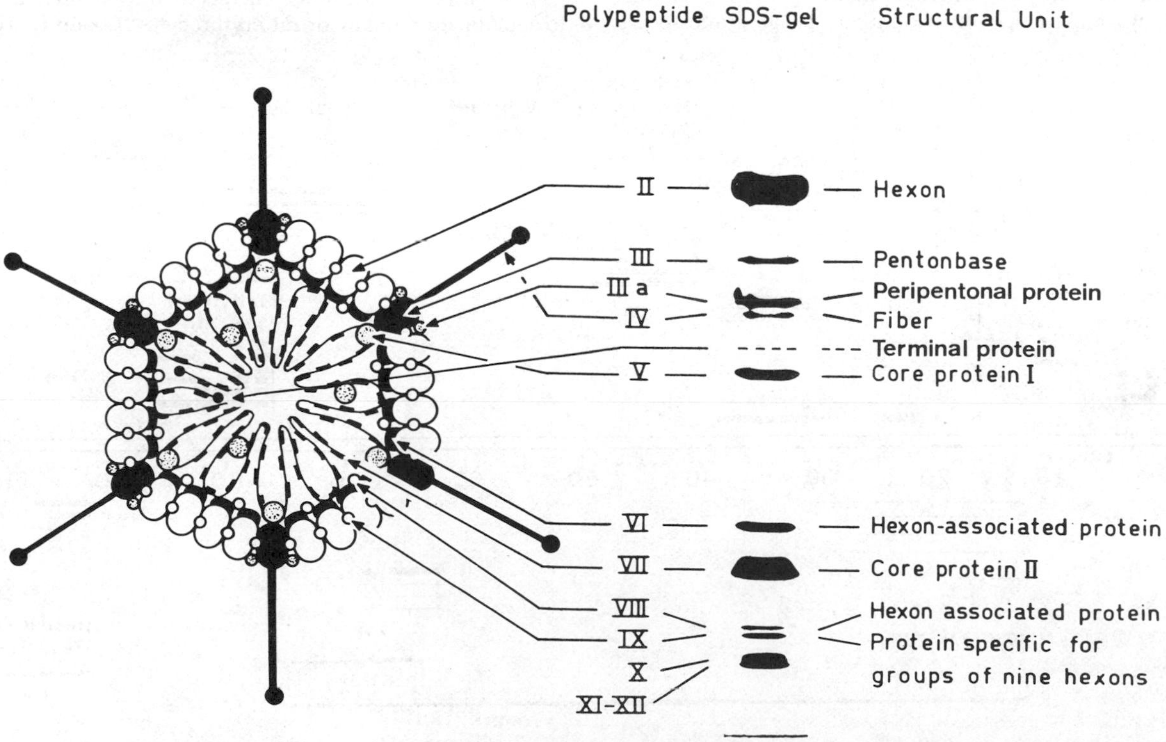

Figure 2. A tentative model of the location of different proteins in the ad2 virion. The core protein V may be located inside at the vertices, since it is partially released with the peripentonal region. It has been estimated that core protein VII may neutralize about 50 per cent of all phosphate residues in the DNA. The molar ratio between polypeptide VI and the hexon polypeptide is about 2, and the native protein VI exists as a dimer. Protein VI is not iodinated in intact virions, which suggests that protein VI is located at the inner surface of the hexons. Peripentonal hexons also possess this protein. Protein IX appears to be the cementing substance between hexons from the facets, since it is associated with groups of nine hexons. Protein VIII is also associated with the hexons and may reside at the inner surface of the triangular facets, since it is not iodinated in intact virions. Polypeptide IIIa is located in the peripentonal region. The localization of proteins X–XII is unknown. The polypeptide composition of the virion proteins as identified in a stained exponential (10 to 16 per cent) SDS-polyacrylamide gel are also shown. (From Philipson et al., 1975.)

Table 1. CLASSIFICATION OF HUMAN ADENOVIRUSES[a]

Subgenus[b] (Subgroup)	Species (Serotypes)	Per Cent GC in DNA	Hemagglutination Subgroup[c]	Length of Fibers nm	Oncogenicity in vivo[d]
A	12, 18, 31	47–49	IV	28–31	High
B	3, 7, 11, 14, 16, 21, 34, 35	50–52	I	9–11	Weak
C	1, 2, 5, 6	57–59	III	23–31	None
D	8, 9, 10, 13, 15, 17, 19, 20, 22–30, 32, 33, 36, 37	57–60	II	12–13	None
E	4	57	III	17	None

[a]Adapted from Wigand et al., 1982.
[b]Two additional subgenera, F and G, have recently been described (Wadell et al., 1980).
[c]Group I agglutinates monkey and group II rat erythrocytes in a tight lattice forming a complete pattern. Groups III and IV agglutinate rat erythrocytes in an incomplete pattern.
[d]Almost all nononcogenic serotypes have been shown to transform rodent cells in vitro.

to measure homology. The DNA for several types is infectious but the specific infectivity is at least 10^6 times lower than for virions measured as number of infectious units/μg of DNA. The protein associated with the termini of the viral DNA appears to enhance the infectivity of viral DNA. Specific fragments of DNA representing around 8.11 per cent of the total genome can transform cells. The DNA has been cleaved by several restriction enzymes and fragment maps have been established. The fragments have been used to map the position of transcripts and messenger RNA by nucleic acid hybridization. Isolated messenger RNAs have also been analyzed by in vitro translation in order to map the position of most of the gene products on the viral genome. The majority of the mRNA has been mapped on the viral DNA (Fig. 3) and the total DNA sequence of the human ad2 genome comprising 35,000 basepairs has recently been determined.

CLASSIFICATION OF HUMAN ADENOVIRUSES. Human adenoviruses have been separated into seven subgenera based among other characteristics on their ability to agglutinate monkey or rat erythrocytes. Group I viruses

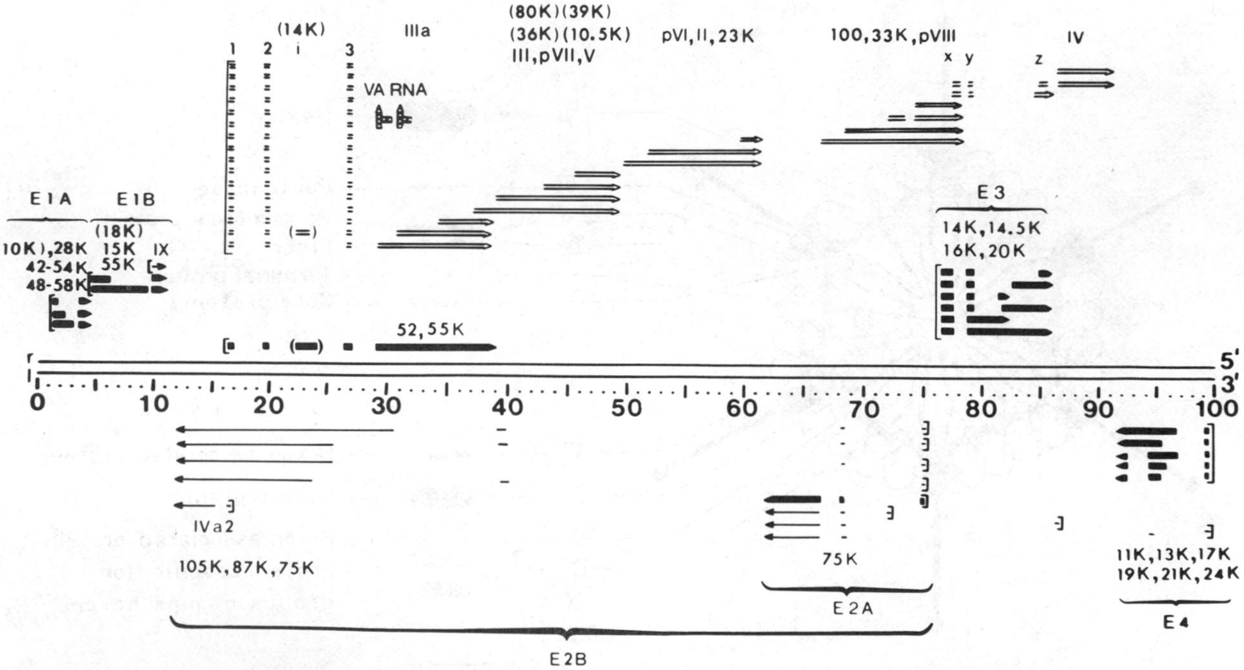

Figure 3. A genomic map of ad2-coded proteins and their mRNAs. The mRNAs shown in heavy lines can be detected at early times of infection in the absence of protein synthesis. Thin lines indicate intermediate mRNAs that can be expressed in the absence of viral DNA replication, but they are most easily detected at late times. *Arrowheads* show the 3′ end, and tentative promotor sites are indicated with *brackets.* Proteins unequivocally identified in an early region are also indicated. Minor species are given in *parentheses.* All late mRNAs shown with double lines originate from the major promotor at coordinate 16.3 and they contain tripartite leader segments derived from coordinates 16.4, 19.6, and 26.6 joined to the body of each mRNA. The late transcripts belong to five different families having coterminal 3′ ends *(arrowheads).* A fraction of all late mRNA also contains a fourth leader segment, the i leader. The polypeptides located in the virion are designated with Roman numerals and non-virion proteins with mol. weight × 10^{-3} (K). From Persson and Philipson, 1982.

cause complete agglutination of monkey erythrocytes, group II complete agglutination of rat erythrocytes, group III incomplete agglutination of rat erythrocytes, and group IV viruses, which were originally reported to lack hemagglutinin, agglutinate rat erythrocytes with an incomplete pattern similar to group III viruses. Members of each subgroup have fibers of a characteristic length (Table 1). A classification based on oncogenicity has also been proposed, which also correlates well with the DNA homology. Not all species within each subgenus have been studied with regard to DNA homology or biologic parameters.

ANTIGENIC COMPOSITION. Most of the antigens of adenoviruses reside in the outer capsid (Table 2). The hexons contain at least two different antigenic determinants, one is group specific (α) and the other type specific (ε). The penton base contains a dominant group-specific antigenic determinant (β). The fiber contains a type-specific determinant (γ) residing in the distal knob, which probably serves to anchor the virus to the cell at infection. An intrasubgroup determinant (δ) is also present in the proximal part of the fiber of subgroups A, C, and D.

All human types of adenovirus display hemagglutinating capacity. The type-specific part of the fiber interacts with the red cell surface. Since the intact virion carries several vertex projections, they can establish a bridge between the erythrocytes and give a complete hemagglutination pattern. Multimers of pentons and fibers can in the same way give rise to hemagglutination. Monomers of penton and fiber can establish only a monovalent link with the cell and agglutination can be detected only when antibodies are used to bridge the fibers anchored with their type-specific moiety on the erythrocyte. Heterotypic antibodies must be used to link the group-specific determinants available on the surface of the cells. The short fibers of subgroup B viruses therefore cannot agglutinate, since they only contain type-specific determinants. This method to reveal adenovirus hemagglutination by heterotypic antisera has been called *hemagglutination enhancement*. Antibodies directed toward the fiber can be assayed by *hemagglutination inhibition*.

Adenoviruses carry a mosaic of antigenic specificities on their surface. Since, by definition, all types are distinct by neutralization, type-specific antigens should induce neutralizing antibodies. Both the fiber (γ) and the hexon (ε) contain type-specific antigenic determinants and both have been claimed to induce neutralizing antibodies. The mechanism for adenovirus neutralization is still a matter of controversy. Antisera against crude hexon preparations induce neutralizing antibodies, and purified hexons from subgroup B and D viruses give rise to neutralizing antibodies, but hexons against subgroup C virions contain no or few exposed such determinants. Antisera against fibers from subgroup C viruses do not contain neutralizing activity when measured with the plaque assay. On the other hand, when neutralization is scored by the fluorescent focus assay, fiber antisera contain high titers of neutralizing activity. In general antisera prepared against disrupted virions are more efficient in neutralization than antisera against purified capsid components. The neutralizing antigen of adenoviruses may therefore have escaped detection.

SUSCEPTIBLE HOST CELLS. All adenoviruses of human origin produce cytopathic changes (CPE) when propagated in primary or continuous cell lines of human origin, such as diploid cells of human embryonic lung or kidney, HeLa, KB, or Hep-2 cells. Characteristic CPE manifests itself as rounding, enlargement, increased opacity, and aggregation of the cells into irregular clusters. The rapidity with which CPE occurs is a function of the dose of virus in the inoculum but the lower numbered types ad1 to ad7 produce CPE faster than the other types. Monkey cells support the early and most of the late expression of human adenovirus genomes but virions fail to assemble. The block may be overcome by concurrent infection with SV 40 virus. Hamster cells are permissive for ad2 and ad5. Ad12, on the other hand, can express early products but fails to replicate its DNA and express late genes. Ad12, nevertheless, can induce CPE. Rat cells are semipermissive for ad2 in the sense that single cells may support replication but most cells do not.

The lytic cycle of adenoviruses has been studied mostly in suspension cultures of KB or HeLa cells. The time course of the infection with ad2 is shown in Figure 4. When the cells are infected at high multiplicity (500 to 1000 PFU/cell), a synchronous response is observed with

Table 2. ANTIGENS ASSOCIATED WITH THE MAJOR STRUCTURAL PROTEINS

Protein	Corresponding Polypeptide (See Fig. 2)	Designation	Antigen Specificity	Remarks
Hexon	II	α	Group	Oriented toward the inside of the virion
		—	Inter- and intrasubgroup	
		ε	Type	Available at the surface of the virion from serotypes belonging to subgroups B and D
Penton base	III	β	Group	Carries toxin activity
		—	Inter- and intrasubgroup	
Fiber	IV	γ	Type	Reacts with HI-antibody
		—	Intersubgroup	Shared between members of subgroups C and D
		δ	Intrasubgroup	At the proximal part of the fiber present only in subgroups A, C and D

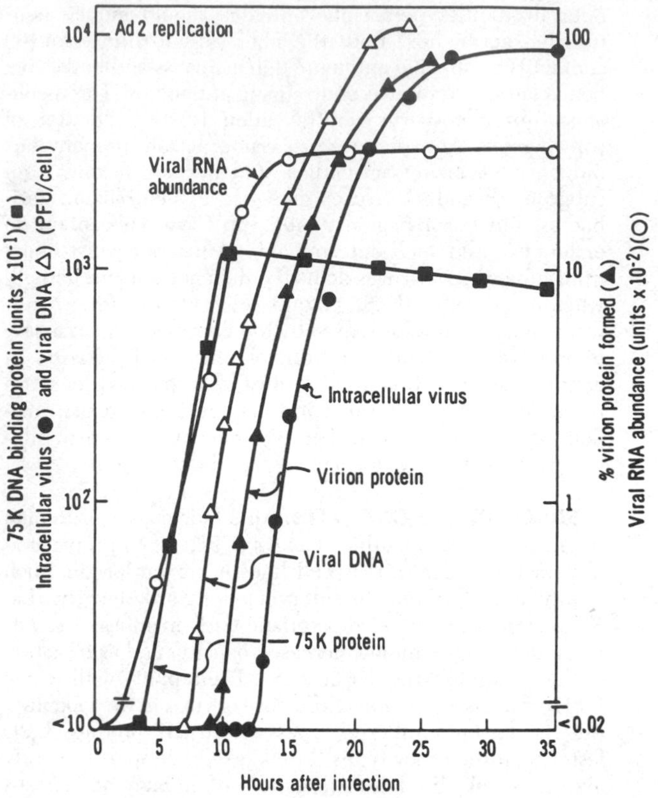

Figure 4. The replication cycle of adenovirus type 2. Time course of synthesis of viral RNA, early viral 75K protein, viral DNA, virion protein, and intracellular virus. (From Wold, W. S. M., Green, M., and Büttner, W.: Adenoviruses. In Nayak, D. P. (ed.): The Molecular Biology of Animal Viruses. New York, Marcel Dekker, Inc., 1978. With permission.)

two functionally different phases of the infectious cycle. During the early phase that precedes viral DNA replication, about 40 per cent of the viral genome is expressed, exemplified with the 75K DNA-binding protein, which is one of the early proteins. In the late phase, beginning with the onset of viral DNA synthesis about six hours after infection, approximately, 90 per cent of the genome is expressed, and the amount of viral RNA increases about ten-fold. At about 14 hours postinfection the synthesis of host cell protein is, to a large extent, replaced by fabrication of viral products, mostly viral structural proteins. New virus particles begin to appear at 15 hours, and the infectious cycle for ad2 and ad5, both members of subgroup C, is completed within 20 to 25 hours. Similar time courses have been obtained with other serotypes although the growth cycle of group A viruses is longer than for ad2. The growth cycle in primary cells is prolonged at least for 12 to 15 hours even for group C viruses.

One system for subdivision of human adenovirus into subgroups A to D (Table 1) was originally based on the frequency with which newborn hamsters develop tumors after inoculation with virus. Several human adenoviruses as well as adenoviruses from other species can, in addition, transform cells in vitro, regardless of their oncogenic capacity in vivo. Cells that are nonpermissive for virus replication are more susceptible to transformation. The events leading to transformation may therefore occur also in permissive cells but it escapes detection because infected cells do not survive. The frequency of transformation is in all cases low for adenoviruses with only one transforming focus per 10^6 cells or more. Only 4 to 8 per cent of the genome of ad5 is required for transformation, as revealed by transformation with DNA fragments. Accordingly, several cells transformed with ad2 and ad5 contain a limited amount of the viral DNA integrated into the host cell genome. With ad12, on the other hand, most of the viral genome appears to be integrated into the host genome of the transformed cell.

PATHOGENIC PROPERTIES. The human adenoviruses are almost exclusively pathogenic for man. A single type of adenovirus may cause different clinical syndromes and, conversely, more than one type may be responsible for the same clinical pattern. Four different syndromes of respiratory infection have been associated with adenoviruses.

1. *Acute febrile pharyngitis* is perhaps the most common clinical manifestation, especially in infants and children. It is difficult to distinguish the disease in individual cases from infections caused by influenza and parainfluenza viruses, respiratory syncytial virus, certain enteroviruses, and members of the rhinovirus group. It appears that subgroup C viruses are mainly responsible for infection in early life. Most children show serologic evidence of prior exposure to one or more of these antigenic types by the time they reach school age.

2. *Pharyngeal-conjunctival fever* is an infection usually observed in children and it may occur in epidemic form. It is an acute febrile pharyngitis with concurrent conjunctivitis. Ad3 has been most frequently implicated as the etiologic agent, although ad7 and ad14 have also been involved. All belong to subgroup B. Subgroup C viruses may also cause this syndrome in exceptional cases.

3. *Acute respiratory disease (ARD)* is prevalent in military recruits, and other institutionalized young adults of

similar age. Ad4 and ad7 are most frequently associated with this syndrome in recruit populations, but other types within subgroup B may periodically be involved as the responsible agent.

4. *Adenovirus pneumonia* is usually a complication of ARD in patients infected with ad4 or ad7. The clinical course resembles that of pneumonia caused by *Mycoplasma pneumoniae* but the disease does not respond to antibiotics. Pneumonia may also be observed occasionally in infants and several adenovirus types have been isolated from fatal cases in infants.

Adenovirus may also cause acute follicular conjunctivitis. It is mainly seen in adults and principally is caused by ad3 and ad7, although other types have also been incriminated. Ad8 is the major cause of epidemic keratoconjunctivitis of the classic type with corneal infiltrates, but conjunctivitis may be caused by several adenovirus types. Adenoviruses may also be associated with gastroenteritis without respiratory disease and intussusception in infants and young children. Acute mesenteric lymphadenitis is thought to be caused by adenoviruses, although a causal relationship has not been established. Systemic infection with adenoviruses with involvement of several organs has mostly been observed in infants or young children.

IMMUNITY. Susceptibility or resistance to most clinical infections by adenovirus appears to be correlated directly to the absence or the presence of circulating neutralizing antibodies. The adenoviruses are exceptionally good antigens for development of vaccines. One dose of vaccine apparently gives almost maximal antibody response. Several studies have demonstrated a reduction of 85 to 90 per cent in the attack rate of adenovirus infection in immunized groups. The low incidence of adenovirus infection in the civilian population, however, raises questions concerning the advisability of the indiscriminate use of adenovirus vaccines. It has been estimated from the incidence of adenovirus infections among civilians that a vaccine that completely prevented infection would lower by only 6 per cent the number of common respiratory illnesses experienced by an average child during the first 10 years of life. Since adenoviruses can transform cells and can be oncogenic to hamsters, adenovirus vaccines were abandoned. More recently, adenovirus vaccines that only contain purified protein components from infected cells have been reintroduced. Purified hexon or fiber preparations induce high levels of neutralizing antibodies in volunteers and a vaccine produced from these components was effective in a field trial. A vaccine of this type could be used for high risk military recruits. Successful vaccination has also been achieved by oral administration of live virus in capsules that decompose in the intestine.

LABORATORY DIAGNOSIS. For virus isolation, throat and fecal samples are inoculated into primary cell cultures of human origin. Rapid diagnosis by immunofluorescence has also been used (Gardner and McQuillin, 1974). Aspirated cells from the nasopharynx are fixed and stained with group-specific immunofluorescent antibodies.

The complement fixation test is the most useful procedure for serologic diagnosis of infection. One antigen detects antibodies to all human adenovirus strains and these antibodies increase in titer four-fold or greater in the sera of adult patients within two weeks after onset of infection. The antigen may be prepared by propagating any virus type in cultures of human embryonic kidney, HeLa or KB cells, and purifying the hexon component. After primary isolation adenovirus is classified into groups by determining if the isolate will agglutinate monkey or rat red blood cells. Hemagglutination inhibition and virus neutralization tests with type-specific rabbit antisera can establish the virus type. To establish the type-specific serologic response in the patient, both hemagglutination inhibition and neutralization tests should be performed on acute phase and convalescent sera. In general, heterologous reactions occur more frequently in hemagglutination inhibition than in neutralization. The heterologous reactions observed with the neutralization test appear to be based on the presence of overlapping intertypic antigenic determinants more than on an anamnestic antibody response.

EPIDEMIOLOGY. Adenoviruses exist in nearly all parts of the world. At least 33 antigenic types have been recovered from human sources, but not all are proven agents of disease. Serologic surveys indicate that most children become infected with one or more of the adenovirus types before the age of six years, but adenoviruses are probably responsible only for 2 or 3 per cent of acute febrile respiratory illness. The incidence may rise to 5 to 10 per cent of cases that require hospitalization. There is a general problem with estimating the incidence or significance of infections with adenoviruses, since infection leading to antibody response is not necessarily associated with clinical overt disease. Therefore, the recovery of the adenovirus from the respiratory tract or intestinal tract and a serologic response does not in itself permit the assumption that the virus is related to the observed disease. In general, adenoviruses do not cause more than 5 to 8 per cent of all cases of acute respiratory disease. Only sporadic cases have been observed in children and adults, but localized outbreaks may be encountered in boarding schools, summer camps, or colleges. Interestingly enough, the highest attack rates have been observed among military recruits where ad3, ad4, and ad7 have been responsible for major outbreaks. Ad14 and ad21 may also cause outbreaks among this population. The exceptional susceptibility of military recruits to these viruses is unexplained.

References

Gardner, P. S., and McQuillin, J.: Rapid Virus Diagnosis. Application of Immunofluorescence. London, Butterworth and Co., Ltd., 1974, p. 181.

Norrby, E., Bartha, A., Boulanger, P., Dreizin, R. S., Ginsberg, H. S., Kalter, S. S., Kawamura, H., Rowe, W. P., Russell, W. C., Schlesinger, R. W., and Wigand, R.: Adenoviridae. Intervirology 7:117, 1976.

Persson, H., and Philipson, L.: Regulation of adenovirus gene expression. In Current Topics in Immunology and Microbiology, 97:157, 1982.

Philipson, L., Pettersson, U., and Lindberg, U.: Molecular Biology of Adenoviruses. Virology Monographs, Vol. 14. Vienna and New York, Springer Verlag, 1975.

Potter, C. W.: Modern Trends in Medical Virology. Vol. 1., 1967, p. 162.

Roberts, R. J.: Restriction endonucleases. CRC Crit Rev Biochem 4:123, 1976.

Rose, H. M.: Adenoviruses. In Lennette, E. H., and Schmidt, N. J. (eds.): Diagnostic Procedures. 4th ed. American Public Health Association Inc., 1969, p. 205.

Sohier, R., Chardonnet, Y., and Prunieras, M.: Adenoviruses. Status of current knowledge. In Melnick, J. L. (ed.): Progress in Medical Virology, Vol. 7., New York, Karger Basel, 1965, p. 1.

Wadell, G., Hammarskjöld, M. L., Winberg, G. Varsanvi, T., and Sundell, G.: Genetic variability of adenoviruses. Ann NY Acad Sci 354: 16, 1980.

Wigand, R., Bartha, A., Dreizin, R. S., Esche, H., Ginsberg, H. S., Green, M., Hierholzer, J. C., Kalter, S. S., McFerran, J. B., Pettersson, U., Russell, W. C., and Wadell, G.: Adenoviridae, second report. Intervirology 18:169, 1982.

Wold, W. S. M., Green, M., and Büttner, W.: Adenoviruses. In Nayak, D. P. (ed.): The Molecular Biology of Animal Viruses. Marcel Dekker, Inc., 1978, p. 673.

60 THE HERPESVIRUSES

JOSEPH S. PAGANO, M.D.
STANLEY M. LEMON, M.D.

Few viruses have greater medical importance than the herpesviruses. These similar yet very different viruses are ubiquitous, infecting virtually everyone; they are all potentially pathogenic; and together they are responsible for a wide variety of diseases. Some of these viruses, especially the Epstein-Barr virus, have a special importance for developing nations. Once infection has taken place, these viruses or their genomes persist for life, usually silently. However, these latent infections are subject to reactivation, which may cause serious illness, especially in immunosuppressed patients who receive modern therapies ranging from organ transplants to cancer chemotherapy.

Although over 70 viruses of the herpes group infect many different animal species, there are only five distinct herpesviruses that commonly infect humans: herpes simplex virus (HSV) Types 1 and 2, varicella-zoster virus (VZV), cytomegalovirus (CMV), and Epstein-Barr virus (EBV). As a group these viruses are marked by both unity and diversity. All the herpesviruses resemble each other structurally and have biologic properties in common, particularly the hallmarks of latency and reactivation. However, pathogenetically and clinically they exhibit a spectrum of effects. On the molecular level the arrangement of genetic information is structured in herpesvirus genomes in a unique way.

All of these viruses may reactivate at any time during life upon natural or iatrogenic provocation. Curiously, the clinical manifestations of reactivated infection may be quite different from disease caused by primary infection. Finally, a most important property of these viruses is their oncogenic potential: Epstein-Barr virus is well known for its ability to "transform" or alter the growth potential of infected cells, and it is closely associated with at least two different human malignancies.

VIRUS STRUCTURE. HSV, VZV, CMV, and EB virus particles are indistinguishable by electron microscopy. They are among the largest of viruses, with a diameter of approximately 150 to 200 nm. An inner core consisting of DNA intertwined with protein is surrounded by a protein capsid of symmetrical structure composed of 162 capsomeres. This nucleocapsid is covered by a loose amorphous envelope that is derived from the nuclear and plasma membrane of the host cell (Fig. 1). The nucleocapsid is assembled in the cell nucleus and is enveloped as it exits from the nucleus. Loss of this envelope greatly reduces virus infectivity. There are at least 33 polypeptides involved in the structure of the HSV virion including some that are included in the envelope. Other polypeptides are in the core of the virion intimately associated with the viral DNA and may affect regulation of viral gene expression. These viruses do not appear to contain polypeptides with enzymatic activities as part of their structure. They do code for several virus-specific enzymes, including DNA polymerases and thymidine kinases that are distinct from those found in mammalian cells.

Herpesvirus genomes consist of linear double-stranded DNA ranging from approximately 90 $\times$ 10^6 daltons for certain EBV strains to 150 $\times$ 10^6 daltons for CMV. Herpesvirus genomes possess terminal and internal stretches of repeated sequences. That is, in addition to the unique sequences, some of the nucleotide sequences found at the ends of the genome are also situated internally in the genome. The general structure of the herpesvirus genome is shown in Figure 2. A variety of such arrangements, ranging from simple to complex permuted structures, exist in the herpes group of viruses. Such sequence arrangements, the significance of which is unknown, appear to exist only in herpesvirus genomes and not in other genomes, viral or nonviral. These novel arrangements may relate to the generation of defective genomes.

Defective or incomplete virus particles are common among the herpesviruses. These virions possess less than the full complement of viral DNA. For example, in the case of CMV many more virions contain only 100 $\times$ 10^6 daltons of DNA than the full genome complement of 150 $\times$ 10^6 daltons. Herpes simplex virions may possess a genome that is of normal unit length but is still defective in that many of the unique sequences are missing and are replaced by reiterations of a single segment of the genome. These defective forms may be important in some of the biologic effects of the herpesviruses such as persistent infection.

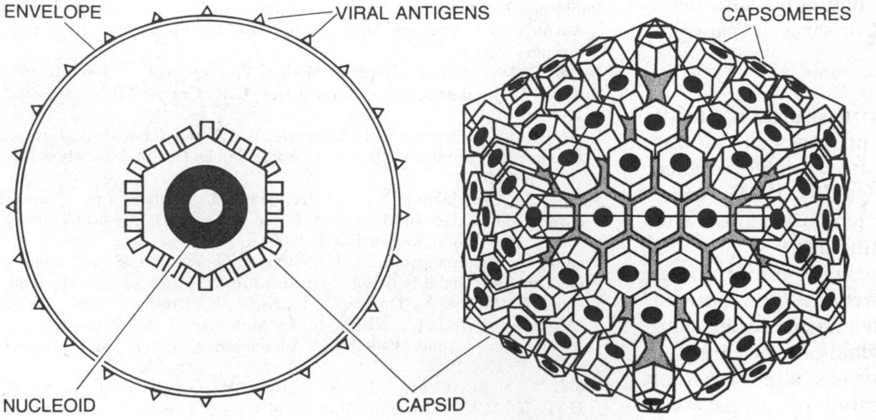

Figure 1. Structure of herpes group viruses. The virion consists of a central core, or nucleoid, which contains the viral DNA; a capsid, which is icosahedral in shape and made of tubular protein subunits called capsomeres; and an envelope derived from cellular membranes. The envelope contains viral proteins or antigens. (From Henle, W., Henle, G., and Lennette, E. T.: The Epstein-Barr virus. Sci Am 24:48, 1979.)

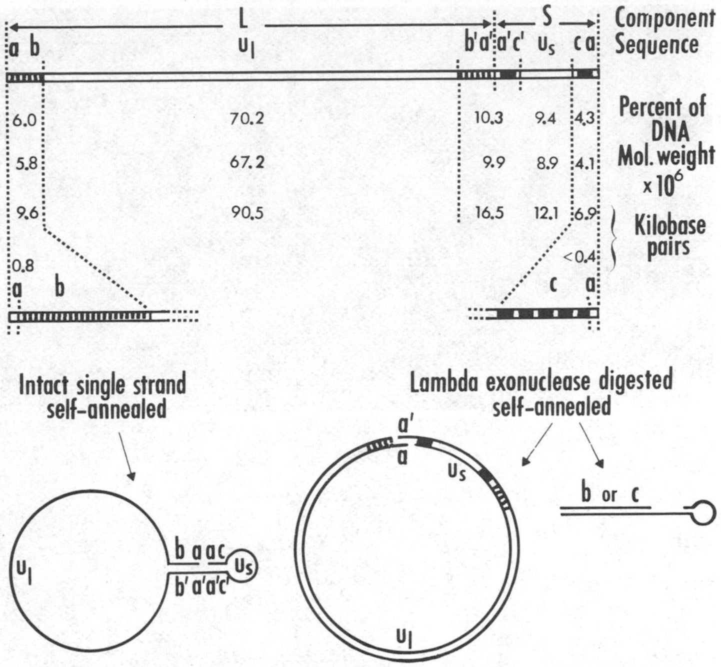

Figure 2. Sequence arrangement in herpes simplex type 1 DNA. The HSV genome is divided into a long (L) and a short (S) segment. At the ends of the genome are nucleotide sequences that are also repeated within the genome at the junction of the L and S segments. The terminal sequences *ab* and *ca* of single strands anneal to their inverted repeats (b′ a′ and a′ c′) to produce the barbell structure on the lower left. The digestion of the DNA with a progressive exonuclease allows it to circularize. Most if not all members of the herpes group exhibit similar although not identical structural arrangements. (From Roizman, B.: The structure and isomerization of herpes simplex genomes. Cell 16:481, 1979.)

In addition to the linear form, the EBV genome can assume an entirely novel closed circular form within the cell. This supercoiled genome, called the EBV episome or plasmid, is not encapsulated by virion structural protein (Fig. 3). It is found in the nuclei of latently infected cells within a nucleosomal structure similar to that of cellular chromatin. During latency the EBV episome is replicated as if it were a cellular constituent by host-cell DNA polymerase. This is the only episomal or plasmid DNA form known to exist in eukaryotic cells save for certain yeasts. Other herpesvirus genomes may be able to assume a similar episomal form, but thus far such closed circular genomes have been detected only in cells infected with an oncogenic herpesvirus of monkeys, *Herpesvirus samiri.* In the laboratory, however, linear HSV genomes can be circularized by exonuclease digestion of the ends of the DNA strands (Fig. 2). This digestion exposes homologous nucleotide sequences at either end of the genome, thereby permitting circularization. Some EBV DNA may also be directly integrated by covalent bonding into cellular DNA in latently infected cells.

With the exception of HSV Type 1 and HSV Type 2, the genomes of the human herpesviruses are completely or almost completely different as shown by cross-hybridization experiments. HSV Type 1 and HSV Type 2 share approximately 50 per cent of their genome content. A lesser degree of homology between, for example, the Epstein-Barr virus and cytomegalovirus—in the range of 5 *per cent or less*—has not yet been excluded. With the exception of certain simian EBV-like agents, the many herpes-group viruses of other animal species bear little if any genetic homologous relation to human herpes-group viruses. A few of the animal herpesviruses can infect man—herpes simiae and perhaps simian CMV—but do so rarely.

Sequence homology of DNA virus genomes can be analyzed by digestion with restriction endonucleases. These nucleases digest only at certain sites on different genomes, and thus generate specific DNA fragments which when examined by electrophoresis show characteristic patterns of sizes. Such patterns are a direct and precise reflection of virus strain differences that may be difficult to detect otherwise. HSV and CMV and to a lesser extent EBV and VZV genomes isolated from various sources exhibit great diversity, especially in some regions of the genomes. Such analyses have demonstrated epidemiologic usefulness in tracing transmission of specific strains of virus.

ANTIGENIC COMPOSITION. The relatively large herpesvirus genome contains sufficient genetic information to encode probably more than 100 different proteins, placing the herpesviruses among the most complex viruses of man. Many of these proteins, some of which are nonstructural (that is, not present in the intact virion), serve as efficient antigens. However, despite the identical morphologic appearance of the herpesviruses, there is little antigenic relatedness among most members of this group.

Among the human herpesviruses only HSV Type 1 and HSV Type 2 share a significant degree of antigenic relatedness. Although these two viruses are clearly separable by several different serologic techniques, antigenically related polypeptides common to both HSV Type 1 and HSV Type 2 have been identified by immunoprecipitation in gel-diffusion studies. This is not surprising in view of the high degree of nucleic acid homology (approximately 50 per cent) between these viruses. Heterologous neutralizing antisera are cross-reactive, which indicates that related antigenic sites exist on the envelope surface. Such cross-reactions appear to be clinically relevant inasmuch as previous HSV Type 1 infection modifies the severity of disease with subsequent HSV Type 2 infection. Cross-reacting internal and nonstructural antigens have been identified as well. Antigenic diversity in HSV is not restricted to differences between Type 1 and Type 2 viruses, however; there is also considerable variation among strains of the same type. Such variation sometimes leads to the identification of an HSV strain as "intermediate" between Type 1 and Type 2.

Unlike strains of HSV, VZV isolates are relatively ho-

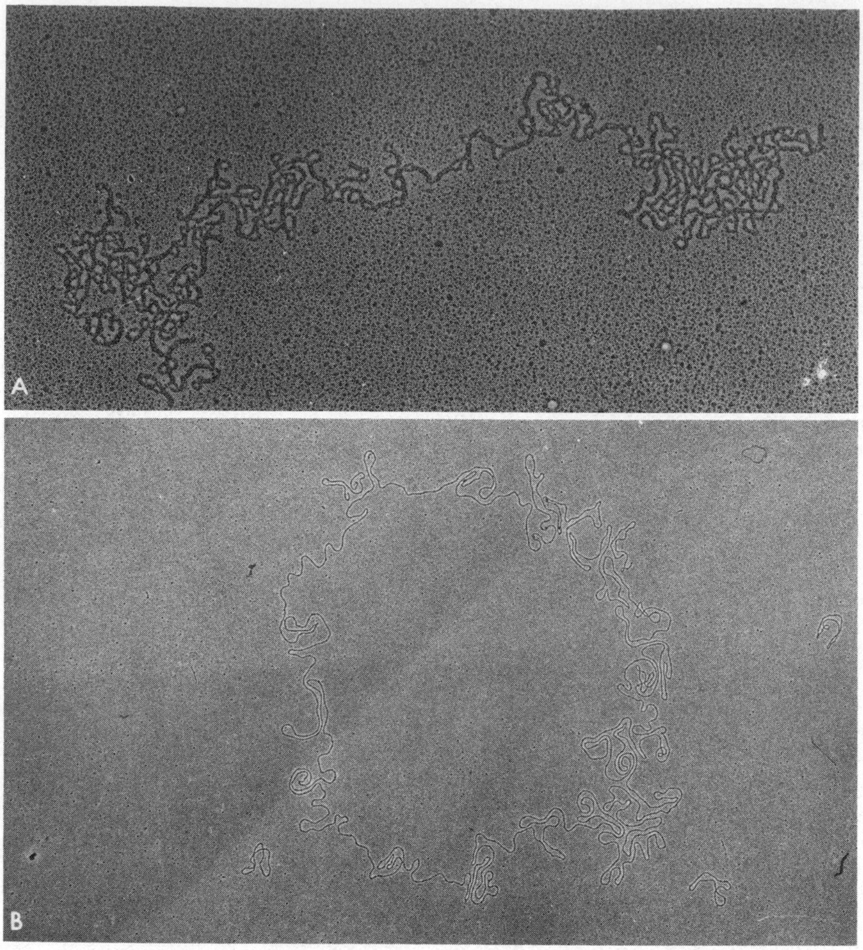

Figure 3. The Epstein-Barr Virus Episome. The episomal or plasmid form of the EBV genome is a closed-circular, supercoiled double-stranded DNA molecule of molecular weight 100 × 10^6 daltons. The EBV episome is found intracellularly, organized as part of the nucleosomal structure of chromosomes. It is replicated by host-cell enzymes. *A,* the closed-circular form; *B,* the open-circular form of a similar molecule. (Courtesy of J. E. Shaw, B. Colby, C. Moore, and J. Griffith; from J. S. Pagano, The Epstein-Barr Virus Plasmid, ICN-UCLA Symposium on Extrachromosomal DNA, Academic Press, 1979.)

mogeneous in terms of their antigenic composition. There is no demonstrable cross-reactivity between VZV and HSV antigens despite the heterologous antibody rises that are occasionally observed following infection with one of the viruses.

Human cytomegalovirus strains are antigenically unrelated to other human herpesviruses, although they are related to CMV-like agents isolated from nonhuman primates. As with HSV, strains of CMV demonstrate considerable antigenic diversity when analyzed either by neutralization kinetics or complement fixation. However, no definitive grouping of strains on the basis of antigenic differences has yet emerged. Recent studies have identified "early" nonstructural CMV antigens that are distinct from "late" CMV antigens including virion components. Early and late refer to approximate time of appearance in the viral replicative cycle, with "early" antigens being synthesized before, and "late" antigens after, viral DNA synthesis.

Several distinct antigens have been associated with EBV. None of these cross-reacts in any way with the other human herpesviruses, reflecting the general lack of nucleic acid homology among these agents. By the fluorescent antibody technique, viral capsid antigen (VCA) activity has been recognized as part of the virion structure. However, additional antigenic activities have been identified that are nonstructural. EBV "early" antigen (EA) is found in cells that are abortively infected with virus and unable to produce mature infectious virions. "Membrane" antigen (MA) appears on the surface of some EBV-producing cells grown in vitro from neoplasms associated with EBV. Such cells as well as latently infected cells also contain EBV nuclear antigen (EBNA), the function of which is still unknown. Because of the superficial similarity between EBNA and the T-antigens of the smaller DNA-containing tumor viruses, SV40 and adenovirus, there is a suspicion that EBNA may be involved in the transforming function of EBV. The appearance of antibodies to each of these distinct EBV antigens follows a characteristic temporal sequence after primary infection with the virus, and they are therefore of diagnostic significance.

SUSCEPTIBLE HOST CELLS AND PATHOGENESIS. Many different types of cells become infected with herpesviruses. The type of cell susceptible to infection is to some extent dependent upon age, since infants seem to have a broader cellular susceptibility than adults. The broader range of cellular susceptibility in infants might be related to specific differences in cellular permissiveness to the virus, or possibly an immature and inadequate immunological response to the infection. Primary infection, latency, and reactivation may involve different cell types even with the same virus. To add to the complexity, despite a common tendency to infect epithelial cells, each of the herpesviruses exhibits its own unique cellular interactions. Disease production may be linked directly to virus-caused cell death, or it may occur secondarily in relation to the immune response.

Both HSV Type 1 and Type 2 infect epithelial cells primarily. Type 1 virus is classically associated with oropharyngeal lesions, whereas Type 2 infects the genital mucosa and adjacent skin sites. Such territorial or organ-specific localization, while not absolute, is typical of herpes-group viruses. In severely affected infants and adults, HSV is found in the respiratory and gastrointestinal epithelium, the skin, and the parenchymal organs such as the liver. Such patients often have underlying immunocompromising conditions. HSV secondarily infects nervous tissue; Type 1 causes a latent infection in the trigeminal ganglion, and Type 2 infects the sacral ganglia. Reactivated infection occurs in mucosa and skin that the virus reaches from the ganglion by axonal spread. In addition to these silent ganglionic infections both viruses cause neurologic disease. In the United States, HSV Type 1 is the leading cause of sporadic and often fatal encephalitis. Whether the principal route of infection of the brain is directly from the trigeminal ganglion or through a cell-associated viremia is uncertain. However, it does seem likely that encephalitis can be produced not only by primary infection but also by reactivated infection. This view is supported by the occurrence of the condition at all ages. HSV Type 2 more commonly causes a benign aseptic meningitis, however, and meningitis may occur in 25 per cent of patients with primary, genital, Type 2 infections. Such infections may thus be generalized and systemic. Herpes neonatorum is usually caused by Type 2 infections contracted during birth from active genital lesions in the mother. The majority of primary and reactivated infections with HSV are probably asymptomatic.

Varicella-zoster virus primarily infects the respiratory epithelium, in which replication of the virus is for the most part asymptomatic. In adults who are infected for the first time with VZV, however, there is a high probability that a serious viral pneumonia will develop. The virus spreads to the skin by way of a cell-associated viremia. Virus may also spread to organs such as the liver in severe reactivated infection as well as in primary infection. Large amounts of infectious virus are replicated in the vesicles of chickenpox, but the virus seems to be transmitted primarily in respiratory aerosols. In the course of the infection peripheral sensory nerves in most parts of the body become infected asymptomatically. Here the virus persists for life, later to be reactivated in the form of herpes zoster, or "shingles." By all available criteria the viruses associated with varicella and with zoster are indistinguishable.

Cytomegalovirus replicates in the epithelial cells of the respiratory tract, salivary glands, and kidney; in the kidney the tubular cells shed virus for prolonged periods. In addition, CMV is frequently present in cervical secretions, especially late in pregnancy. Virus may also be found in the semen in CMV mononucleosis after its disappearance from other sites. Homosexual men have an especially high prevalence of CMV infection, as virus has been identified in the semen of up to 30 per cent of asymptomatic homosexual males. The exact site of replication in the male genital tract is uncertain. However, CMV has recently been discovered in spermatozoa by electron microscopy and CMV-specific nucleic acid cytohybridization. As with other herpesviruses, spread via the bloodstream is accomplished by a cell-associated viremia, the virus being associated with both lymphocytes and polymorphonuclear leukocytes. Cell susceptibility to human CMV is strikingly affected by age. Infections in utero result in devastating destruction of the central nervous system, whereas encephalitis from postnatal CMV infection is exceedingly rare. CMV infection acquired later in life is usually asymptomatic, but occasionally it results in a mononucleosis-like syndrome with liver involvement. Cytomegalovirus infection exemplifies the different clinical forms infection may take upon reactivation. In patients who have received bone-marrow transplants CMV appears to cause an interstitial pneumonitis, whereas pneumonic involvement in primary CMV infection is virtually unknown. However, in recipients of renal allografts fever, leukopenia, and mild hepatitis may occur both in primary and in reactivated infection. Such infections appear to be more severe if they are primary.

CMV has recently been associated with endemic Kaposi's sarcoma in central Africa as evidenced by the presence of the viral genome within tumor cells. Viral DNA has been found as well in Kaposi's sarcoma in homosexual men with the acquired immunodeficiency syndrome. In such patients, Kaposi's sarcoma appears to be a secondary "opportunistic" process.

Epstein-Barr virus probably replicates initially in the epithelial cells of the oropharynx and parotid gland. Subsequently, B lymphocytes are infected. Infected B lymphocytes do not appear to be a source of freely replicating virus in vivo, but they do harbor the episomal form of EBV DNA. Although symptoms of EBV infection arise from many organs, including the throat, lymphatic tissue, liver, and both the peripheral and central nervous systems, there is no direct evidence that the virus actually infects cells in parenchymal organs or the nervous system. Involvement of these organs may result from an intense immunologic response to the presence of EBV-bearing B lymphocytes and not from cellular invasion and destruction by virus itself.

In East and West Central Africa, EBV infection is closely associated with the development of Burkitt's lymphoma, a B-lymphocytic malignancy. Cells taken from African but not usually from the rarer North American Burkitt's lymphomas uniformly contain latent EBV DNA in its episomal form. In these areas of Africa, EBV infection takes place early in life. During the first year of life virtually 90 per cent of the children become infected, apparently asymptomatically, with EBV. This early exposure may be an important factor in the development of Burkitt's lymphoma. Persistently high EBV antibody titers early in life are predictive of the later development of Burkitt's lymphoma. Other factors, such as chronic infection with malaria, may be involved.

Several lines of evidence associate EBV with a second human malignancy, undifferentiated nasopharyngeal carcinoma. From a pathogenetic standpoint this association is especially interesting because this malignancy is epithelial in origin and points to the primary target cell of EBV replication. Although certain ethnic groups, especially Cantonese Chinese, Alaskan Eskimos, and those living in regions of North Africa are at high risk of developing this tumor, the association of the tumor with the virus is worldwide.

In addition, EBV has been linked to life-threatening, diffuse polyclonal B cell proliferation in renal transplant recipients. Such B cell proliferation regresses in some patients upon stopping immunosuppressive therapy. In other patients, polyclonal proliferation undergoes a monoclonal transformation resulting in fatal lymphoma. EBV remains a prime candidate human tumor virus.

LABORATORY DIAGNOSIS. HSV infection produces multinucleate giant cells and Cowdry type A intranuclear inclusion bodies. In cervical cytologic smears, such changes correlate well with isolation of virus but are less sensitive. Similar cytologic changes occur with VZV infection (see Fig. 2 in Chap. 235), and the examination of Giemsa-stained smears of cells scraped from the floor of fresh vesicles is helpful in the diagnosis of vesicular disease due to these two herpesviruses. Intracytoplasmic as well as intranuclear inclusions occur with CMV infection. Cytologic examination of exfoliated cells in urine may lead to the diagnosis of cytomegaloviruria. In general, however, as a diagnostic method cytologic examination is much less sensitive than virus isolation. Infection with other viruses, adenovirus and measles, for example, produce inclusion bodies and may cause confusion in the diagnosis.

HSV strains are easily isolated in a variety of cell cultures and can be recovered from the oropharynx, cervix, vesicular and ocular lesions, brain, and other tissues. Cytopathic effects caused by these virus strains develop rapidly and are usually obvious within 24 to 48 hours after inoculation of cell monolayers. VZV is less readily recovered but can be isolated from fresh vesicles (less than four days old) when fluid is inoculated into primary or diploid human cells. Cytopathic effects develop more slowly, and, unlike HSV, the virus remains tightly cell-associated. CMV can be recovered from urine, the cervix, semen, the oropharynx, and peripheral blood leukocytes. Replication of this virus in vitro is restricted to human diploid fibroblasts, despite the obvious presence of CMV within epithelial cells in vivo. Characteristic cytopathic effects may take several weeks to develop, and blind passage of infected cells may even be necessary. Final identification of these agents rests on fluorescent antibody tests or other immunologic procedures.

An in vitro cell system fully permissive for EBV replication has yet to be found. EBV biologic activity can, however, be detected by in vitro transformation assays with human cord-blood lymphocytes. Transforming EBV, found in oropharyngeal washings and parotid gland secretions, alters the growth potential of these lymphocytes so that they proliferate indefinitely in culture. Such transformed or "immortalized" lymphocytes contain EBNA. Transformation assays for EBV are complex and laborious, and are restricted to research laboratories. Clinical diagnosis depends on serologic techniques.

Antibodies to the herpesviruses can be detected by several methods. Serum neutralization tests have been developed for each virus and are both sensitive and specific. Following infection, neutralizing antibodies generally persist for the life of the individual. Neutralization tests are, however, time-consuming and expensive and are not suited for general clinical use. For detecting HSV antibodies the complement fixation technique is a useful alternative because it is widely available, and complement-fixing antibodies to HSV are generally long-lasting. Significant antibody titer changes take place following many but not all severe recurrent infections as well as during primary infections. Because of the strong degree of antigenic relatedness between HSV Type 1 and HSV Type 2, however, complement fixation is not able to distinguish type-specific antibodies unless special modifications are made.

Complement-fixing antibodies to VZV are short-lived, usually declining to undetectable levels within a year of infection. Antibodies to VZV antigen expressed on the membrane of infected cells may be detected by a fluorescent antibody technique. This assay is preferable for indicating immunity. IgM antibody to VZV occurs in both primary and reactivated infections.

As with VZV, complement-fixing antibodies to CMV may disappear following primary infection only to reappear after reactivation or reinfection. Antibody detected by the fluorescent antibody technique is more persistent and correlates better with neutralization test results. Detection of IgM antibody to CMV is important in the diagnosis of congenital infection.

Serodiagnosis of EBV infection depends on the detection of both virus-specific and heterophile antibodies. Paul-Bunnell-Davidsohn heterophile antibodies are predominantly IgM and are directed to surface antigens of erythrocytes from sheep and certain other animal species. These antigens do not cross-react with known EBV virion antigens. The reason for their occurrence in up to 90 per cent of cases of infectious mononucleosis due to EBV is unknown. In any case, such antibodies are highly suggestive of primary EBV infection. Indirect fluorescent antibody techniques may detect antibody to each of the several EBV-associated antigens. Antibodies to VCA and EA develop shortly after primary infection. VCA antibodies persist for life, whereas EA antibodies usually fall to low or undetectable levels within several months of infection. IgM antibody to VCA, although difficult to detect, is probably the best marker of acute primary EBV infection. EBNA antibodies do not appear until one to three months after infection, but then they persist for life. This kind of antibody interplay is helpful in diagnosing and roughly dating EBV infection. Furthermore, the measurement of certain antibodies associated with malignancies related to EBV infection (such as IgA antibody to EA, which may herald the development of nasopharyngeal carcinoma) provides diagnostic and prognostic information.

The promise of effective chemotherapy for some herpesvirus infections makes critical the need for rapid diagnostic procedures. The success of adenine arabinoside (Vidarabine) treatment of HSV encephalitis is highly dependent on how promptly therapy is begun. The most promising methods for rapid diagnosis of herpesvirus infections are based on the detection of virus antigen. A variety of techniques can be used to demonstrate virus antigens directly in fresh specimens. The techniques make use of virus-specific antibody labeled with fluorescein (direct and indirect IF tests), with radioisotopes (radioimmunoassays), or with enzymes (ELISA tests). Fluorescent antibody techniques may demonstrate HSV antigens in brain-biopsy material and may shorten the time required to document cytomegaloviruria. Rapid diagnosis of congenital CMV infection also is possible with electron microscopy of urine specimens. Nucleic acid hybridization techniques also have shown promise in the rapid diagnosis of infections due to herpesviruses.

A major problem in diagnosis is the tendency of herpesvirus to cause latent infection and the frequency with which reactivation of virus occurs. Many stimuli, including stress, fever, and immunosuppression, may lead to reactivation. For example, in patients with meningoencephalitis, the recovery of HSV from superficial mucosal sites does not correlate with its presence or absence in the brain. In severe or atypical herpesvirus infections the actual demonstration of virus in the affected organ is essential. Even then, the isolation of a herpesvirus must fit with the histopathologic findings and overall clinical pattern before an etiologic association can be made.

IMMUNITY. Immunity to the herpesviruses is the result of a complex interplay between humoral and cell-mediated immune systems. Infection with the herpesviruses does not necessarily produce permanent immunity either to exogenous reinfection or to reactivation of endogenous virus. By and large the presence of circulating antibodies to EBV and VZV prevents full-fledged reinfection with these viruses, whereas the antibodies conferred by previous infection with CMV and HSV may modify disease but do not prevent reinfection, which may recur repeatedly. Reinfection from exogenous sources with HSV Type 1, HSV Type 2, and cytomegalovirus is common. Reinfection may in part be permitted by virus-strain differences inasmuch as some strains of HSV and CMV differ enough antigenically that there is suboptimal cross-protection. In recipients of renal transplants, the presence of CMV antibody before transplantation seems to reduce the risk of symptomatic CMV disease following transplantation. Probably more important, however, is the ability of these viruses to establish infection in local areas that are sheltered from immunologic response mechanisms because of their superficial location. There is some epidemiologic evidence to suggest that exogenous reinfection with VZV may occasionally occur as well, although it is clear that most cases of zoster are due to reactivation of latent virus. There is no evidence for reinfection with EBV.

Cell-mediated immune mechanisms are crucial for preventing or limiting reactivated infection and probably also limit primary infection once it is underway. Depressed or absent cellular immune responses to HSV and VZV correlate with the risk of reactivation of these viruses in recipients of organ transplants. Also, CMV reactivation occurs in transplant recipients with defective cellular immunity despite the presence of high complement-fixing or neutralizing antibody titers. Asymptomatic reactivation of EBV can also be detected in such patients. Thus, with each of the herpesviruses, intact humoral immunity is not by itself a deterrent to reactivation of endogenous virus. Although depressed cellular immunity certainly predisposes to reactivation, the common syndrome of reactivated oral or genital herpes is probably linked more to environmental effects that act as local triggers than to immunologic factors. Exposure to ultraviolet light, stress, fever, and local irritation are provocative factors. Pregnancy also seems to increase susceptibility to HSV and CMV infections.

Cellular immune mechanisms probably limit the extent of primary herpesvirus infections. For example, the proliferation of infected B lymphocytes that occurs during acute infectious mononucleosis appears to be held in check by a cytotoxic T lymphocytic response; this response is most intense shortly after primary infection. In heavily immunosuppressed transplant recipients, however, EBV may induce a polyclonal proliferation of B lymphocytes, which may only respond to a reduction in immunosuppressive therapy. On the other hand, in patients with infectious mononucleosis, the cytotoxic cell-mediated response may be broadly reactive and may play a significant role in the production of disease. Thus, the atypical lymphocytosis that characterizes infectious mononucleosis is composed mainly of T lymphocytes responding to new antigens generated on the surface of B lymphocytes infected with EBV, although a nonspecific so-called killer cell (lymphocytic) response is also evoked.

EPIDEMIOLOGY. Virtually everyone is infected with HSV Type 1, CMV, VZV, and EBV before middle life. There is a significant difference in the epidemiology of these viruses in developing and industrialized countries, however, in that infections occur considerably earlier in life in poorly developed areas. This difference in age-related incidence of infection is striking in the case of EBV in Kenya and Uganda, where virtually every inhabitant has acquired antibodies to EBV by the end of the first year of life. In contrast, only about 40 per cent of students entering college in the United States have antibodies to EBV, although lower socioeconomic groups living in crowded conditions are more likely to be infected with EBV at an earlier age. Infectious mononucleosis is generally a manifestation of EBV infection acquired in the second or third decade of life, and it is therefore a disease that is virtually limited to the more highly developed nations.

Another epidemiologic difference is the striking incidence of Burkitt's lymphoma in endemic fashion in the so-called lymphoma belt of Africa. The pattern of occurrence of this tumor, including such features as its age-related incidence, geographic distribution according to elevation, and case-clustering in families and in districts, suggests a transmissible etiology. African Burkitt's lymphoma appears to be declining in incidence for unknown reasons. In the United States Burkitt's lymphoma is much rarer and is only occasionally associated with EBV infection.

The very consistent association of EBV with nasopharyngeal carcinoma holds true both in populations with a genetic predisposition to this malignancy and in other groups without such a predisposition. There appears to be an association of nasopharyngeal carcinoma and an HLA-2 subtype in genetically susceptible groups.

Among the herpesviruses, only CMV regularly infects the fetus in utero. CMV differs also in causing rather frequent perinatal infections. Thereafter the incidence of infection is related to age and socioeconomic status much like EBV infection. HSV Type 1 and VZV infections largely occur in childhood. HSV Type 2 and genital CMV infections occur mostly in late adolescence and early adulthood.

HSV Type 1 is spread primarily by exchange of oral secretions from person to person but also by direct contact with skin or mucous membranes infected with the virus. The disposition of HSV Type 1 to infect the mouth and lips and of HSV Type 2 to infect the genital region is by no means absolute. Both HSV Types 1 and 2 may be sexually transmitted. At least 10 per cent of initial episodes of genital herpes are due to HSV Type 1. Compared with genital infection with HSV Type 2, however, Type 1 infections are less likely to lead to recurrent, reactivated episodes of genital herpes. HSV is found not only in lesions of the external genitalia but also in cervical secretions where it may or may not be associated with cervicitis. The virus may be transmitted to infants during vaginal delivery and may cause disseminated neonatal infections. Cesarean section is usually recommended when there is active herpes genitalis.

Varicella is one of the most contagious of all human

diseases. VZV infects children (or the rare adult who has escaped infection earlier in life) primarily by the respiratory route, although vesicular fluid is also infectious. Children incubating varicella are infectious for several days before the rash develops. Patients with herpes zoster are also a source of infection for susceptible children and adults.

Cytomegalovirus resembles HSV in that it is probably spread primarily from person to person by direct contact and exchange of secretions such as saliva. Sexual transmission also occurs because the virus is found in both semen and vaginal fluids. Women with other venereal infections are much more likely to have CMV antibodies. Direct contact with virus results during the passage of an infant through an infected birth canal. Transplacental transfer of virus early in parturition is unfortunately all too common and frequently results in severe damage to the fetus. The presence of antibodies to CMV does not prevent reactivation of infection, nor do antibodies prevent reinfection with exogenous strains of CMV. Consequently, a mother who has given birth to one infant with congenital CMV infection may, rarely, deliver a second child who has been infected in utero. With the same virus strain, however, the second infection is likely to be asymptomatic. Virus may be present in milk and be transmitted to the infant via breast feeding. Last, leukocyte-associated CMV can be transmitted by transfusion of fresh blood and result in mild hepatitis with or without a mononucleosis-like syndrome.

EBV infection is also thought to spread primarily by close contact with exchange of oral secretions containing infectious virus. The virus is shed from the throat intermittently for long periods—certainly for several months and often for a year or longer. The period of contagiousness is unknown; estimates of the incubation period are imprecise and range from two to four weeks.

PREVENTION AND TREATMENT. There are as yet no widely accepted herpesvirus vaccines. The use of varicella hyperimmune globulin to ameliorate symptoms of VZV infection is well established, particularly in leukemic children who incur high mortality and morbidity. Experimental vaccines against cytomegalovirus and varicella-zoster virus, which are presumed to be attenuated by virtue of passage in vitro in tissue cultures, are now under study. Immunization against VZV with such an attenuated vaccine has been extensively evaluated in Japan. These are live virus vaccines, and the virus is expected to persist in a latent form just as in natural infection. Inactivated vaccines, including so-called herpes simplex virus "subunit" vaccines, are also under investigation; these preparations consist of disrupted virus with the viral DNA removed. Preparations of this type require large amounts of virus, which are hard to obtain with the other herpes-group viruses, but they will not produce infection, either active or latent. The success of such vaccines is difficult to predict given the fact that serum-neutralizing antibody is not necessarily protective against disease. Although herpesvirus vaccines present complicated and novel problems, their continued development is important, especially for the prevention of infections such as congenital CMV infection that elude early diagnosis and treatment.

Several specific HSV infections can be modified by available antiviral compounds. Iododeoxyuridine (IUdR) is of proven efficacy in herpes simplex keratitis. This is the only use for which IUdR is indicated.

Although both IUdR and cytosine arabinoside are either ineffective or even harmful in the treatment of HSV encephalitis, adenine arabinoside (Vidarabine) given intravenously early in the course of the illness reduces mortality and improves the likelihood of survival without serious neurological sequelae. The drug is now licensed for this use within the United States. Adenine arabinoside may also cause improvement in VZV infections in immunocompromised adults. Exogenous human interferon is of potential benefit in such cases of VZV infections because it tends to decrease the risk of dissemination. One striking feature of studies of these agents in VZV infection, however, is the surprisingly benign course of untreated disease in immunocompromised individuals. Interferon may also suppress CMV infection when administered prophylactically after renal transplantation.

Success in the treatment of a range of herpes simplex infections has been achieved with acyclovir (9-(2) hydroxyethoxymethyl guanine), a drug that represents a novel class of antiviral agents. The mechanism of action of acyclovir in HSV infections requires that it first be phosphorylated in vivo to its mono-, di-, and triphosphorylated forms before it will act. The initial phosphorylation reaction requires the virus-induced thymidine kinase enzyme, and thus phosphorylation (activation) of the drug is confined to the infected cell. The triphosphorylated derivative of acyclovir then specifically inhibits virus-induced DNA polymerase activity and also may become inserted into DNA, acting as a terminator of DNA chain elongation. In laboratory tests the drug is highly specific for infected cells; it appears to derive this specificity from the requirement that the drug be phosphorylated by the virus-coded thymidine kinase. A second level of specificity relates to the drug's selective inhibition of virus-induced DNA polymerase and relative lack of effect on normal host cellular DNA polymerases. Strains of HSV that have lost their ability to induce thymidine kinase are resistant to acyclovir yet may retain some degree of virulence.

Acyclovir is effective in the treatment of genital herpes simplex infections. In initial (but not recurrent) episodes of herpes genitalis, the use of 5 per cent topical acyclovir reduces the period of viral shedding and significantly shortens local symptomatology. There is no substantial clinical effect when acyclovir is applied topically to recurrent genital herpetic or orolabial herpetic infections. Intravenous acyclovir also has been used in severe cases of primary herpes genitalis and results in dramatically decreased periods of viral shedding, shortened time of crusting and healing of lesions, as well as diminished systemic symptoms. Given intravenously, the drug may also prevent complications of herpes genitalis such as sacral autonomic nervous dysfunction. No regular effect on the rate of subsequent recurrent (reactivated) disease has yet been demonstrated however, and it should be emphasized that acyclovir has no effect whatever upon latent HSV infections. At present, clinical trials with oral preparations are in progress, as is a comparison of intravenous acyclovir and adenine arabinoside in the treatment of herpes encephalitis. Except for transient reversible azotemia, little toxicity has been associated with clinical use of this compound.

Acyclovir has also shown promise in the treatment of VZV infections, although VZV is generally significantly less sensitive than either HSV Type 1 or HSV Type 2 viruses. In vitro the drug does not appear to be effective against human cytomegalovirus; this relative insensitivity may be because CMV does not seem to induce the appearance of a new viral thymidine kinase in infected cells. In vitro the drug also has an effect against the freely replicating form of EBV but not against the latent episomal form of EBV. EBV DNA polymerase is especially sensitive to the phosphorylated drug in vitro.

References

Corey, L., Adams, H. G., Brown, Z. A. and Holmes, K. K.: Genital herpes simplex virus infections: Clinical manifestations, cause and complications. Ann Intern Med 98:958, 972, 1983.

Epstein, M. A., and Achong, B. G.: Recent progress in Epstein-Barr virus research. Ann Rev Microbiol 31:421, 1977.

Henle, W., Henle, G. E., and Horwitz, C. A.: Epstein-Barr virus specific diagnostic tests in infectious mononucleosis. Human Pathol 5:551, 1974.

Huang, E. S., and Pagano, J. S.: Comparative diagnosis of cytomegaloviruses. New approach. In Kurstak, E. (ed.): Comparative Diagnosis of Viral Diseases. New York. Academic Press, 1977.

Kaplan, A. S. (ed.): The Herpesviruses. New York, Academic Press, 1973.

Nahamias, A. J., and Roizman, B.: Infection with herpes-simplex viruses 1 and 2. N Engl J Med 289:667, 719, 781, 1973.

Pagano, J. S.: Diseases and mechanisms of persistent DNA virus infection: Latency and cellular transformation. J Infect Dis 132:209, 1975.

Pagano, J. S., and Shaw, J. E.: Molecular probes and genome homology. In Epstein, M. A., and Achong, B. G. (eds.): The Epstein-Barr Virus. New York, Springer-Verlag, 1979.

Sixbey, J. W., and Pagano, J. S.: New perspectives on the Epstein-Barr virus in the pathogenesis of lymphoproliferative disorders. In Remington, J., and Swartz, M. (eds.): Current Clinical Topics in Infectious Diseases. New York, McGraw-Hill, 1984, pp. 146–176.

Weller, T. H.: The cytomegaloviruses: Ubiquitous agents with protean clinical manifestations. N Engl J Med 285:203, 267, 1971.

Weller, T. H.: Varicella-herpes zoster virus. In Evans, A. S. (ed.): Viral Infections of Humans, New York, Plenum Medical Book Company, 1976, p. 457.

61

POXVIRUSES

ABRAHAM I. BRAUDE, M.D., PH.D.

The poxviridae are a family of viruses composed of two subfamilies: (1) the Chordopoxvirinae, which produce pox lesions or benign tumors of invertebrates (Table 1), and (2) the Entomopoxvirinae, which infect insects. They have a similar morphology, a common nucleoprotein antigen, and the ability to recombine genetically. With the exception of ectromelia and myxoma viruses, the poxviruses are one of the most resistant groups of viruses. They are stable in storage under adverse conditions and remain infective in dried exudates and tissues for remarkably long periods.

Most poxviruses produce skin lesions. In man, the most virulent was smallpox virus until it was eliminated from the face of the earth. It produced a mortality rate up to 50 per cent. Variola minor (alastrim) produced a mortality less than 10 per cent and a milder illness with pustular rash. Infection with vaccinia virus was used to prevent smallpox and was responsible for eradication of the disease. Present-day strains of vaccinia virus are no doubt changed from the original strain of cowpox virus used by Jenner to prevent smallpox.

Table 1. THE GENERA OF CHORDOPOXVIRINAE

Genus	Primary Hosts	Disease
Orthopoxvirus	Man	Variola, vaccinia, alastrim
	Cows	Cowpox[a]
	Mice	Ectromelia
	Rabbits	Rabbitpox
	Monkeys	Monkeypox[a]
Capripoxvirus	Ungulates	Sheep-pox, goatpox
Leporipoxvirus	Rabbits and squirrels	Myxoma, fibroma
Parapoxvirus	Sheep	Orf[a]
	Cows	Papular stomatitis
	Cows	Milkers nodules[a]
Avipoxvirus	Birds	Fowlpox, canarypox
Suipoxvirus	Swine	

[a]Also produce human infections

VIRAL STRUCTURE. The poxviruses have the greatest size and the most complicated structure of any animal virus. The double-stranded DNA virus has a molecular weight of approximately 150×10^6, the largest of any animal virus. It is enclosed in a dense, dumbbell-shaped core, which is covered by a closely adherent lipoprotein inner membrane. Two oval masses of obscure function known as lateral bodies fill the concavity of the dumbbell. A second outer membrane covers the entire structure. The resulting particle is oblong, and the surface is covered with ridges (see Chapter 7, Fig. 8). In contrast to other viral envelopes, the outer membrane of the virion is not derived from the cytoplasmic membrane of the infected cell but is synthesized by the virus. This difference in origin of the poxvirus envelopes accounts for a difference in sensitivity of the viruses to ether. Many poxviruses (ortho and poxviruses) are resistant to ether, whereas other enveloped viruses are inactivated by ether. Vaccinia virions measure 300×240 nm, whereas the parapoxvirus particles (Orf, papular stomatitis, and milker's nodes) are 260×160 nm.

In addition to DNA, poxviruses contain neutral lipid, phospholipid, protein, and carbohydrate. There are at least 75 proteins, but the function of most has not been identified. The core contains at least 17 structural proteins or polypeptides, and the inner membrane has two structural glycoproteins. Five other proteins are located at the surface of the viral particle. Seven enzymes have been identified in the core that are involved in RNA synthesis. One of these is a DNA-dependent RNA polymerase, the first to be demonstrated in any virion. The other enzymes are deoxyribonuclease, a protein kinase, a DNA relaxing enzyme (nicking-closing), a polyadenylic acid polymerase, a guanyltransferase for mRNA, and methyltransferases for mRNA. All the phospholipid in the virion is located in the outer membrane. The predominant phospholipid is lecithin. Poxvirus DNA ranges from 80 to 100 nm in length. Its guanine plus cytosine content of 35 to 40 per cent is the lowest of any vertebrate virus.

Table 2. MAJOR POXVIRUS ANTIGENS

Category	Antigen	Composition	Size	Protective
Structural	NP	6% DNA + core proteins	50% of virion mass	0
	Surface antigens	Probably protein	?	+
Soluble	LS	Protein	MW 240,000	±
	Hemagglutinin	Lipoprotein	65 nm	0

ANTIGENIC COMPOSITION. In addition to the nucleoprotein antigen common to all members of the family, poxviruses contain a number of antigens derived from the structural components of the virion (structural antigens) and others known as soluble antigens (Table 2). The complex nucleoprotein antigen (NP), which is obtained by extraction with dilute alkali, constitutes over half the substance of the viral particle. NP contains 6 per cent DNA as well as certain core proteins. The structural antigens are demonstrated by chemical disruption of the virion or by neutralization of infectivity. At least 20 antigens are found in agar gel precipitin tests after virion disruption, of which four have been localized to the core and one outside the core beneath the outer membrane. Two surface antigens have been identified by neutralization of infectivity. The antigens that produce neutralizing antibody are the basis for division of the poxvirus family into the genera listed in Table 1.

The soluble antigen known as LS is identified by complement fixation. It is found in virus-free extracts of tissue infected by vaccinia virus and appears to be a complex protein with a molecular weight of 240,000. The protein has both a heat-labile and a heat-stable antigen designated L and S, respectively. The L antigen is inactivated at 60°C and the S antigen is resistant to 100°C. The LS antigen seems to be derived from the viral surface because it stimulates neutralizing antibodies; it does not, however, immunize animals against vaccinia infection of the skin, and absorption with LS does not remove neutralizing antibody from protective sera obtained after vaccinia infection. Thus, it does not appear to be related to the protective structural surface antigens that delineate the orthopoxviruses. Another soluble antigen agglutinates chicken red cells. This hemagglutinin is a lipoprotein and is inactivated by lecithinase. In contrast to hemagglutinin inhibition antibodies against influenza virus, antibodies that block hemagglutination of a poxvirus cannot neutralize infection by that virus. For this reason, the poxvirus hemagglutinin does not appear to be a structural unit of the viral surface.

SUSCEPTIBLE HOST CELLS. Besides the primary hosts listed in Table 1, each poxvirus can infect other animals. The most extensive studies on the range of susceptibility of different animal tissues have been carried out with vaccinia virus. Calves, sheep, and rabbits can be infected with vaccinia virus and are used for the production of a smallpox vaccine composed of virus harvested from the skin lesions. Monkeys, rats, mice, guinea pigs, and hamsters are susceptible to vaccinia infection but less so than rabbits. Chick embryos are used to prepare smallpox vaccine by propagation of virus on the chorioallantoic membrane. Chick embryos can also be infected by inoculation of the amniotic cavity or yolk sac. Repeated propagation of vaccinia strains on the chorioallantoic membrane or in chick embryo tissue culture tends to lessen the virulence of vaccinia strains for man (Downie, 1965).

In contrast to their susceptibility to vaccinia virus, most animals other than primates are resistant to variola virus. It has not been possible to propagate variola virus serially in rabbits, guinea pigs, calves, sheep, and goats. Although smallpox virus can produce in rabbits a keratitis with the formation of Guarnieri bodies (intracytoplasmic spherical eosinophilic inclusions) and a local skin lesion, the virus cannot be propagated further in the rabbit skin. Variola virus is also less virulent than vaccinia virus upon intranasal inoculation of adult mice, but it kills suckling mice after intraperitoneal inoculation. On the chorioallantoic membrane, the pocks produced by variola virus are smaller and less heat-tolerant than those of vaccinia virus; variola pocks do not occur in embryos incubated at 39°C or above, whereas vaccinia pocks develop even at 41°C with some strains. Monkeypox virus shows the restricted host range of variola virus (Ho and Wenner, 1973), whereas the host range of cowpox virus resembles that of vaccinia virus.

Serial passage of poxviruses establishes an affinity for certain tissues, a phenomenon known as tropism. Passage of vaccinia virus, for example, in rabbit or calf skin creates dermatotropic strains that have scant neurotropic properties. On the other hand, certain poxviruses are naturally neurotropic or become so after cerebral passage. Rabbitpox, cowpox, and vaccinia virus have all become neurotropic. The dermatotropism of fowlpox virus is evident from the extensive benign hyperplasia it produces in epithelial cells of the skin. Fibroma viruses have connective tissue tropism and produce benign connective tissue tumors in rabbits and squirrels.

Poxviruses multiply in cultured cells from many different tissues derived from rabbits, mouse, monkey, man, fowl, and cow. Variola virus, for example, can be propagated in HeLa, Hep 2, bovine kidney, bovine skin, human embryo skin, human embryo muscle, and L-cell cultures.

REPLICATION AND PATHOGENIC PROPERTIES. In poxvirus infections, the cell dies after its ability to synthesize proteins is blocked during viral replication. From studies with vaccinia virus, it has been learned that the virion enters the cell by phagocytosis. The outer viral membrane and lateral basal bodies are degraded within the phagocytic vacuole so that the core is released into the cytoplasm. It is clear that this early step of removing the outer coat is carried out by constitutive enzymes of the cell because all of the phospholipid in the virion and half of the virion protein are released in a soluble form (Joklik, 1966). The inner viral core membrane, on the other hand, is degraded by viral enzymes. The DNA-dependent RNA polymerase within the core synthesizes mRNAs which are extruded into the cytoplasm by a mechanism that requires ATP (McAuslan, 1979). The mRNAs are translated on the ribosomes of the infected cell into proteins that direct the release of virus DNA from the core. One of these proteins is an uncoating enzyme that degrades the viral core membrane and allows the naked DNA to leave the core and enter the cytoplasm. This requirement by poxviruses for a newly synthesized protein for uncoating makes them unique among animal viruses. The DNA-dependent RNA polymerase is heat-sensitive, so that poxviruses can be inactivated by heat. The heat-inactivated virus can be reactivated, however, by a viable poxvirus of any genus because all poxviruses appear to contain the RNA polymerase in their cores.

After the viral DNA leaves the core, viral growth begins with synthesis of viral DNA, virion enzymes, and structural proteins of the virion. This late phase of synthesis begins about 90 minutes after infection and lasts for about four hours. In contrast to other DNA viruses, the synthesis of poxvirus DNA takes place entirely in the cytoplasm in foci ("factories") that are composed of dense granules and random fine threads and are independent of mitochondria or other cytoplasmic organelles. During this phase of viral growth, the virus blocks the ability of the host cell to transport RNA from its nucleus or to manufacture protein. The synthesis of early virus proteins is also prevented. The ability of poxviruses to synthesize their DNA in the cytoplasm of infected cells is most clearly demonstrated by their ability to carry out most of their life cycle in enucleated cells (Prescott et al., 1971).

Viral assembly begins after replication of viral DNA is completed and takes place on the cytoplasmic foci where viral DNA is synthesized. The virus synthesizes its own membrane, which encloses the viral DNA to form an "immature particle." These particles mature into the complex virion with its dumbbell-shaped core, lateral bodies, and outer membrane.

An interesting fluctuation in cell metabolism is seen in infections with rabbit fibroma virus. When cells are infected with this virus, cell DNA synthesis may be stopped for long periods, but the cells survive and DNA synthesis resumes after the virion matures (Tompkins et al., 1969).

From studies with other poxviruses, it has been proposed that in human infections variola virus first replicates at the portal of entry in the cells of the upper respiratory tract (Lancaster et al., 1966; Roberts, 1962). After spreading through the lymphatics, it multiplies in the regional lymphatic tissue and then enters the bloodstream. Virus is cleared from the blood by the reticuloendothelial system, where further multiplication occurs. A second viremia occurs about 12 days after infection begins, marking the end of the incubation period. This viremia carries the infection to the skin and mucous membranes, where the virus first infects capillary endothelium and then epithelial cells. It has been suggested that the virus localizes in the skin because its lower temperature during fever is more conducive to viral replication than the temperature of visceral organs. Multiplication of virus in epithelial cells causes cytolysis, intradermal fluid accumulation, release of lysosomal enzymes, hydrolysis of matrix proteins, and the development of vesicles. An inflammatory reaction to the infection and to cell necrosis delivers polymorphonuclear leukocytes into the lesions, converting the vesicles to sterile pustules.

The pathogenesis of infection with monkeypox virus, another orthopoxvirus, is probably the same as smallpox, because the clinical features of monkeypox in human beings are almost identical to those of smallpox. The parapoxviruses, which infect sheep and cows primarily, can also be transmitted to people. The pathogenesis of infection with these viruses differs somewhat from that of orthopoxvirus infections, in that the parapoxviruses cause benign, hyperplastic reactions. In orf, the virus of "scabby mouth" in sheep (contagious pustular dermatitis) produces papules, rapidly evolving into hemorrhagic bullae at the sites of abrasions on the patient's hand or face. In lambs, the hyperplasia is evident in the watery papillomatous lesions of the mouth, lips, and cornea. In patients with milker's nodules, transmitted through human skin abrasions after contact with vesicular lesions of the skin of cattle, the virus produces flat papules that become vascular nodules, resembling warts. The leporipoxviruses of rabbits and squirrels also cause benign hyperplastic lesions in the form of myxomas and fibromas.

IMMUNITY. Observations on immunity were made in antiquity, when it was known that recovery from smallpox prevented another attack. Much later, a popular notion developed in Gloucestershire, England, that dairy maids who caught cowpox were afterwards immune to smallpox. The validity of this folklore was established by Jenner, who proved that vaccination of people with living cowpox virus produced solid immunity to smallpox (Fig. 1). Jenner had no idea of the mechanism of protection, let alone the nature of the material he was using, but he managed to discover the phenomenon of delayed hypersensitivity and its connection to smallpox immunity. This discovery was recorded in his description of the accelerated inflammatory reaction that occurred when smallpox material was injected into the skin of Mary Barge, who had once had cowpox. He wrote: "It is remarkable that variolous matter, when the system is disposed to reject it, should excite inflammation more speedily than when it produces the smallpox. It seems as if a change which endures had been produced in the action, or disposition to action, in the vessels of the skin" (Jenner, 1798). His observation that immunity to smallpox is related to a reaction that we recognize as delayed hypersensitivity has been substantiated and elaborated.

Contemporary observations on the response to smallpox vaccination have also given important insight into the mechanism of immunity in poxvirus infections. The relative importance of humoral and cellular immunity has been examined after vaccinating patients who have immune deficiency diseases. Most patients with severe deficiencies in gamma globulin respond normally to smallpox vaccination and recover from it completely. On the other hand, vaccination of patients who have depressed cellular immunity but normal humoral antibody (autosomal recessive lymphopenia, or Nezelof's syndrome) usually causes disseminated vaccinia (Fulginiti et al., 1968). This finding in patients is supported by experiments that showed that administration of antithymocyte serum to mice markedly increased mortality from mousepox, even though humoral antibody levels were the same as those in controls (Blanden, 1970). Furthermore, immunity against mousepox was restored by transfer of immune T cells (Blanden, 1971).

These observations by themselves would imply that cellular immunity is more important than humoral immunity in vaccinia and mousepox. Other observations indicate that antibody may also contribute to protection against poxviruses. The most compelling of these is simply that passive immunity to pox infection can be transferred with

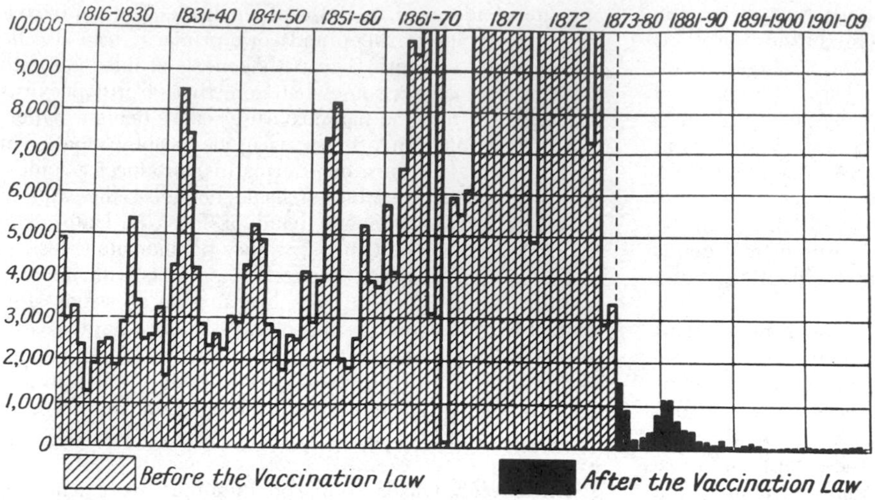

Figure 1. The chart shows smallpox mortality during a period of a century in Germany. Vaccination was made compulsory in April, 1875, and in that year the total deaths from smallpox dropped to about 1500 compared with totals exceeding 10,000 in each of the years 1871 and 1872. Thereafter, the death totals fell nearly to zero. (After Jockmann: Pocken und Vaccinationlehre, Berlin, 1913.)

virus-neutralizing antibody that develops after natural infection or after immunization with live virus. Neutralizing antibody can prevent skin lesions in animals and fatal encephalitis in mice.

LABORATORY DIAGNOSIS. Now that smallpox has disappeared and vaccination is no longer a standard practice, the laboratory diagnosis of smallpox or vaccinia should be confirmed in one of the few centers at which rapid reliable tests are available. Specimens from a suspected case of smallpox, vaccinia, and monkeypox should be examined by the electron microscope, inoculated into chick embryos and tissue cultures, and tested for pox antigens against specific antiserum by agar gel precipitin tests (Nakano and Bingham, 1974). Virus can be isolated earliest from heparinized blood during the pre-eruptive stage, and later from vesicular fluid and crusts. The vesicular fluid should be collected in capillary tubes and the crusts in screw-capped vials. Preparations of vesicle fluid or ground crusts are scanned in the electron microscope at a magnification of 13,500 to 25,000, and the virion is examined in detail at 76,000 to 184,000. The brick-shaped smallpox virus is readily distinguishable from the enveloped icosahedrons of varicella virus. Variola virus must also be distinguished from nonviral particles and from herpes viruses, which can produce similar vesicles and crusts.

Examination of smears by light microscopy is less reliable. Smears are made by scraping material from the base of a vesicle or from papules with a scalpel blade and spreading it on a glass slide. After washing carefully with distilled water and ether, the smears are fixed with 95 per cent methyl alcohol and stained with a mixture of equal parts of 1 per cent gentian violet and 2 per cent sodium bicarbonate. The staining mixture is filtered onto the smeared slide and steamed for five minutes. The stained preparation is then examined for the characteristic elementary bodies of smallpox.

Isolation of the virus is carried out in fertile chicken eggs that have been incubated at 38 to 39°C for 11 to 13 days (World Health Organization, 1969). The chorioallantoic membrane (CAM) can be inoculated with plasma or buffy coat from blood samples or with vesicular fluid or scab material diluted in a buffered solution containing penicillin and streptomycin. The eggs are incubated at 35°C for 48 to 72 hours and the CAM examined for pocks. The pocks from vaccinia, variola, and monkeypox are differentiated from each other, and from those of herpesviruses by their appearance (Dumbell, 1968).

Tissue cultures are also used for poxvirus isolation because the CAM method fails occasionally. Variola, vaccinia, and monkeypox viruses can all produce cytopathogenic effects in Vero (African green monkey kidney) cells within one to three days after inoculation.

Human poxvirus antigens in crusts or vesicle fluid can be detected in nearly 80 per cent of cases by agar gel precipitation. Antivaccinia antiserum is placed in the central well and the test specimens in outer wells. Upon incubation at 35°C, precipitin bands appear in a few hours between the wells containing antiserum and those containing pox antigen (Fig. 2). Antigens of smallpox, vaccinia, and human monkeypox viruses all react with vaccinia antiserum.

Serologic tests are of no practical value in smallpox because the antibody response is too slow for diagnostic help during the illness.

EPIDEMIOLOGY. Man was the only host or reservoir of smallpox. He transmitted the infection only when he had an outspoken illness in the active stage of the disease. Even in patients with partial immunity after vaccination, the attenuated infection still produced enough symptoms to identify the patient as a sick person so that direct contact with him was avoided. These features, and the absence of asymptomatic carriers, made smallpox easier to control than most other epidemic infections.

At first the eradication of smallpox was attempted through universal vaccination and revaccination. This approach was not entirely successful, however, because in many countries it was possible to vaccinate only three-fourths of the population. This might be enough with other epidemic infections such as poliomyelitis, but not with smallpox because its relatively low infectivity did not generate herd immunity. Small pockets of smallpox were able to persist in villages and spread by close contact in families to susceptible individuals who had escaped natural immunization or vaccination. These characteristics made

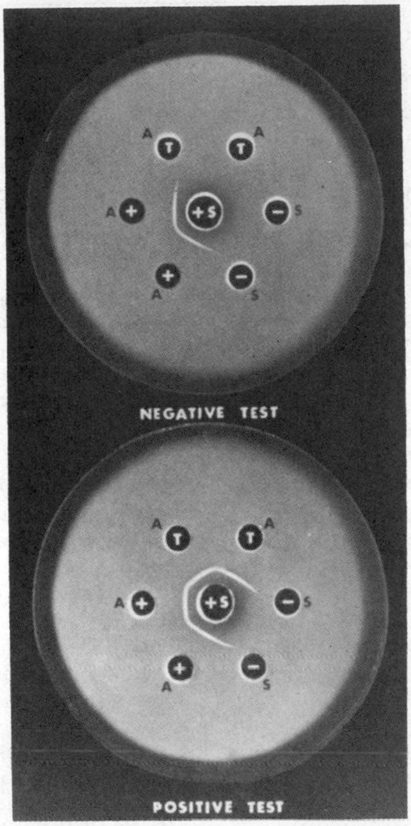

Figure 2. +S (center wells): Positive rabbit antivaccinial serum; TA (top wells): test antigen made from material taken from the skin lesions of a case of smallpox; +A (left): positive antigen prepared from the crusts of a known case of smallpox; −S (right): Normal rabbit serum from an animal known to be devoid of antibodies to variola.

Above, A negative test. There is no precipitation between the test antigen (TA) and the positive serum (+S). The only lines of precipitation are between the positive serum and the positive control antigen (+A).

Below, A positive test. The lines of precipitation between the positive serum (+S) and the test antigen (TA) join the lines between the positive control antigen (+A) and the positive serum (+S). (From Swain, R., and Dodds, T.: Clinical Virology. Baltimore, The Williams & Wilkins Company, 1967, p. 106.)

smallpox susceptible to control by surrounding each new case with a ring of immunized subjects (World Health Organization, 1968).

This change in approach from universal to selective (or strategic) vaccination came about in 1967 and involved two stages: First, the source of each outbreak was determined, and the chain of transmission was traced. Then the remaining susceptibles along the route of transmission were identified and vaccinated. When this surveillance-containment program began, cases of smallpox were reported from 44 countries, and smallpox was endemic in 33 of these (Arita, 1979). The program was so successful that smallpox was eradicated from all parts of the world by October 1977, when the last naturally occurring case was seen in Merkatown, Somalia.

References

Arita, I.: Virological evidence for the success of the smallpox programme. Nature 2:293, 1979.

Blanden, R. V.: Mechanisms of recovery from a generalized viral infection: Mousepox. I. The effects of antithymocyte serum. J Exp Med 132:1035, 1970.

Blanden, R. V.: Mechanisms of recovery from a generalized viral infection: Mousepox. II. Passive transfer of recovery mechanisms with immune lymphoid cells. J Exp Med 133:1074, 1971.

Downie, A. W.: Poxvirus group. In Horsfall, G., and Tamm, I. (eds.): Viral and Rickettsial Diseases of Man. Philadelphia, J. B. Lippincott Company, 1965, p. 932.

Dumbell, K. R.: Laboratory aids to the control of smallpox in countries where the disease is not endemic. Progr Med Virol 10:388, 1968.

Fulginiti, V., Kempe, C., Hathaway, W., Pearlman, D., Seeber, O., Eller, J., Joyner, J., and Robinson, A.: Progressive vaccinia in immunologically deficient individuals. In Bergema, D. (ed.): Immunologic Deficiency Diseases in Man. Washington, D.C., The National Foundation, 1968, p. 128.

Ho, T., and Wenner, H. A.: Monkeypox virus. Bacterial Rev 37:1, 1973.

Jenner, E.: An inquiry into the causes and effects of the variolae vaccinae, a disease discovered in some of the western counties of England, particularly Gloucestershire, and known by the name of the cowpox. London, Sampson Low, 1798.

Jochmann, G.: Pocken and Vaccinationslehre, Vienna, Alfred Hölder, 1913.

Joklik, W. K.: The poxviruses. Bacteriol Rev 30:33, 1966.

Lancaster, M., Boulter, E., Westwood, J., and Randles, J.: Experimental respiratory infection with poxviruses. II. Pathological studies. Br J Exp Pathol 47:466, 1966.

McAuslin, B. R.: The biochemistry of poxvirus replication. In Levy, H. B. (ed.): Biochemistry of Viruses. New York, Dekker Publishing Company, p. 360, 1969.

Nakano, J., and Bingham, P.: Smallpox, vaccinia, and human infections with monkeypox viruses. In Lennette, E., Spaulding, E., and Truant, J. (eds.): Manual of Clinical Microbiology. Washington, D.C., American Society of Microbiology, 1974, p. 782.

Prescott, D., Kabes, J., and Kirkpatrick, J.: Replication of vaccinia virus DNA in enucleated L-cells. J Mol Biol 59:505, 1971.

Tompkins, G., Gelehter, T., Granner, D., Martin, D., Samuels, H., and Thompson, E.: Control of specific gene expression in higher organisms. Science 166:1474, 1969.

World Health Organization: Smallpox Eradication. Report of a WHO Scientific Report Group. Technical Report Series No. 393, Geneva, World Health Organization, 1968.

World Health Organization: Guide to the Laboratory Diagnosis of Smallpox for Smallpox Eradication Programmes. Geneva, World Health Organization, 1969.

62
PAPOVAVIRUSES

MICHAEL N. OXMAN, M.D.
PETER M. HOWLEY, M.D.

Papovaviruses are small DNA-containing viruses that characteristically produce latent and chronic infections in their natural hosts. When adequately tested, most papovaviruses appear to be capable of inducing neoplasms in at least some animal species. The name papovavirus is derived from the first two letters of the names of the viruses first placed in the group: rabbit *pap*illoma virus, mouse *po*lyoma virus, and simian *va*cuolating virus (Melnick, 1962). The Papovavirus Family has been divided into two groups or genera, papillomaviruses and polyomaviruses (Table 1), primarily on the basis of the size of the viral genome (Melnick et al., 1974; Matthews, 1982).

The polyomavirus genus includes a number of viruses that appear to be harmless in their natural hosts (Table 1). Most seem to inhabit the urinary tract, where they establish persistent or latent infections. Although polyomaviruses are usually oncogenic when injected into susceptible laboratory animals, none has yet been demonstrated to be responsible for naturally occurring malignancies. Simian vacuolating virus (simian virus 40, SV40) and mouse polyomavirus, members of the polyomavirus genus that can cause tumors in experimental animals and transform cells in vitro, have been used extensively as models for the study of viral oncogenesis and for the analysis of the expression and regulation of eukaryotic genes. Thus, we now possess an enormous amount of information about their structure, replication, genetics and interactions with animal cells (Enders, 1965; Eddy, 1969; Ponten, 1971; Howley, 1980; Eckhart, 1981; Tooze, 1981; Norkin, 1982; Griffin and Dilworth, 1983).

Table 1. PAPOVAVIRUSES

Papillomavirus Genus
Human papilloma (wart) viruses
Shope rabbit papilloma virus (CRPV)
Rabbit oral papilloma virus
Bovine papilloma viruses
Canine papilloma virus
Papilloma viruses of horses, sheep, deer, and other species
Polyomavirus Genus
Mouse polyomavirus
Simian vacuolating virus (SV40)[a]
Mouse K virus
Rabbit kidney vacuolating virus
Human BK virus
Human JC virus
Papovavirus of chacma baboons (SA12)
Hamster polyomavirus
Bovine polyomavirus[b]
Monkey lymphotropic papovavirus (LPV)

[a]Includes two SV40-like viruses isolated from patients with progressive multifocal leukoencephalopathy (PML) that appear to be SV40 variants (Weiner et al., 1972).

[b]The polyomavirus previously characterized as stumptailed macaque virus (STMV) has now been shown to be of bovine origin (Parry et al., 1983).

Interest in the potential role of polyomaviruses in human disease was aroused in the early 1960s by the discovery that SV40 produced a latent infection of rhesus monkey kidneys and consequently was a common but unrecognized contaminant of viral vaccines which had been produced in rhesus monkey kidney cell cultures and administered to millions of people (Sweet and Hilleman, 1960; Melnick and Stinebaugh, 1962; Shah and Nathanson, 1976). This became more worrisome when it was discovered that SV40 could induce tumors in newborn hamsters and transform human cells in vitro (Eddy et al., 1962; Shein and Enders, 1962).

In 1965, particles resembling papovavirus virions were found within glial nuclei in the brains of patients with a rare demyelinating disease, progressive multifocal leukoencephalopathy (PML) (Zu Rhein and Chou, 1965; Silverman and Rubinstein, 1965; Howatson et al., 1965). In 1971, Padgett and her colleagues (Padgett et al., 1971) isolated a papovavirus, JCV, from the brain of a patient with PML. The same virus has now been isolated from many additional cases, indicating that JCV is the principal etiologic agent of PML (Walker and Padgett, 1983a).

In the same year Gardner and her associates (Gardner et al., 1971) isolated another papovavirus, BKV, from the urine of a renal allograft recipient. BKV has now been isolated from the urine of many additional immunosuppressed patients, but it has not yet been etiologically associated with any disease. JCV and BKV are both members of the polyomavirus genus. They are distinct from each other and from any previously recognized papovavirus. Serologic evidence indicates that both viruses infect the majority of the human population during childhood, causing asymptomatic but persistent infections (Takemoto, 1978; Howley, 1980; Walker and Padgett, 1983a and 1983b).

The papillomavirus genus includes the human papilloma (wart) viruses, the Shope rabbit papilloma virus, and a number of other species-specific viruses that usually cause benign skin papillomas or warts in their natural hosts (Rowson and Mahy, 1967). Human warts were one of the first neoplasms shown to be caused by a transmissible agent with the properties of a virus (Rowson and Mahy, 1967; Ciuffo, 1907). However, little is known about the multiplication of papillomaviruses or about their interactions with animal cells because there is no satisfactory tissue culture system for their propagation (Rowson and Mahy, 1967; Butel, 1972; zur Hausen, 1977). Nevertheless, the application of polyacrylamide gel electrophoresis, restriction endonuclease mapping, and recombinant DNA technology to the analysis of virions extracted directly from human and animal papillomas has led to the identification of many new members of the genus and has greatly expanded our knowledge of papillomavirus structure, molecular biology, and genome organization (zur Hausen, 1977; Danos et al., 1982; Howley, 1983a and 1983b). The results of these studies indicate that, despite their structural similarities, polyomaviruses and papillomaviruses are really unrelated. Consequently, we will deal separately with each genus.

POLYOMAVIRUSES

VIRUS STRUCTURE AND COMPOSITION. Polyomaviruses are small, nonenveloped, icosahedral DNA viruses that replicate in the nuclei of susceptible vertebrate cells. All members of the genus are similar in physical structure

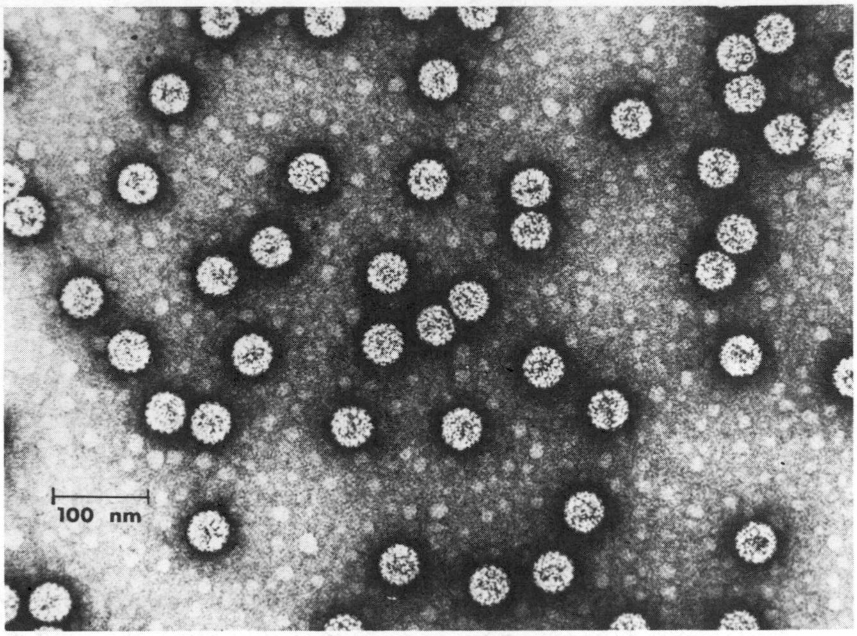

Figure 1. Electron micrograph of purified SV40 virions negatively stained with sodium phosphotungstate (Bar = 100 nm).

and chemical composition. Virions are 40 to 45 nm in diameter and are composed of 12 per cent DNA and 88 per cent protein. They have no essential lipid or carbohydrate. Complete (infectious) virions consist of a single molecule of double-stranded circular DNA enclosed within a spherical protein coat or capsid. The capsid is an icosahedral structure composed of 72 morphologic subunits or capsomeres (Fig. 1). It contains three virus-coded proteins. The major capsid protein, VP-1, has a molecular weight of 40,000 to 43,000 and accounts for about 75 per cent of the total virion protein. The 60 capsomeres on the triangular faces of the icosahedral capsid are each composed of 6 molecules of VP-1, and disulfide bridges within and between these capsomeres bind the VP-1 monomers together to form a very stable structure. Two minor structural proteins, VP-2 and VP-3, with molecular weights of 35,000 to 39,000 and 23,000 to 27,000, respectively, appear to make up the 12 vertex capsomeres. Within the capsid is a single molecule of covalently-closed circular double-stranded DNA approximately 5200 base pairs long, associated with cellular histones in a structure resembling the chromatin of eukaryotic cells. (Tooze, 1981; Reddy and Weissman, 1983).

Polyomaviruses are resistant to inactivation by lipid solvents (e.g., ether and chloroform) because they have no envelope; they are relatively resistant to heat and irradiation, and are stable over a wide range of pH. These properties are exploited in extracting and purifying polyomaviruses. Polyomaviruses are also resistant to inactivation by formalin, which explains the survival of SV40 in early batches of formalin-inactivated ("killed") poliovirus vaccine. Treatment with 0.1 per cent beta-propriolactone inactivates the infectivity of BK virus without destroying its hemagglutinating properties (Pitko et al., 1975). Thus noninfectious BK virus hemagglutinin can be prepared for use in serologic tests. When purified polyomavirus virions are gently disrupted with mild alkali, the viral DNA can be isolated in the form of a DNA-protein complex. This complex, the viral "minichromosome," consists of a circular molecule of viral DNA associated with octomers of cellular histones (H2A, H2B, H3, and H4) to form a set of nucleosomes. In the electron microscope, the viral "minichromosome" resembles a chain of beads and appears similar in structure to cellular chromatin; the number of nucleosomes per viral genome varies between 21 and 26 (Christiansen et al., 1977; Tooze, 1981).

When viral DNA is extracted free of protein from virions or from infected cells, two species are generally found. Most of the viral DNA is in the form of a covalently closed circular duplex molecule (DNA I), which in SV40 contains 26 negative superhelical turns. A small portion of the viral DNA is in the form of an open circular duplex molecule (DNA II), which is generated from DNA I by the rupture of one phosphodiester bond in either strand. Both forms of DNA are infectious. The degree of base sequence homology between various isolates has been studied by nucleic acid hybridization. Bacterial restriction endonucleases, which recognize specific nucleotide sequences in duplex DNA and cleave both strands at these sites, have been used to construct physical maps of polyomavirus genomes, and the genomes of several of the polyomaviruses have now been sequenced (see Soeda et al., 1980; Howley, 1980; Tooze, 1981; Frisque, 1983). These techniques have enabled us to compare different polyomaviruses and, in conjunction with studies of viral mutants, to analyze the expression and function of specific regions of polyomavirus genomes. An example of a physical map of the SV40 genome is shown in Figure 2.

VIRUS REPLICATION AND CELL TRANSFORMATION. When a polyomavirus infects the cells of its natural host, the usual result is a lytic (productive) infection characterized by extensive virus replication and cell lysis. Cells that support such a productive infection are termed "permissive" cells. Polyomaviruses can also infect cells of other species that do not support a complete cycle of virus replication. Infection of such "nonpermissive" cells results in an incomplete or abortive infection, in which only a part of the viral genome is expressed. Some abortively infected cells may be transformed to a malignant phenotype, a process that requires the persistence and expression of at least one viral gene. Much of our knowledge of polyoma-

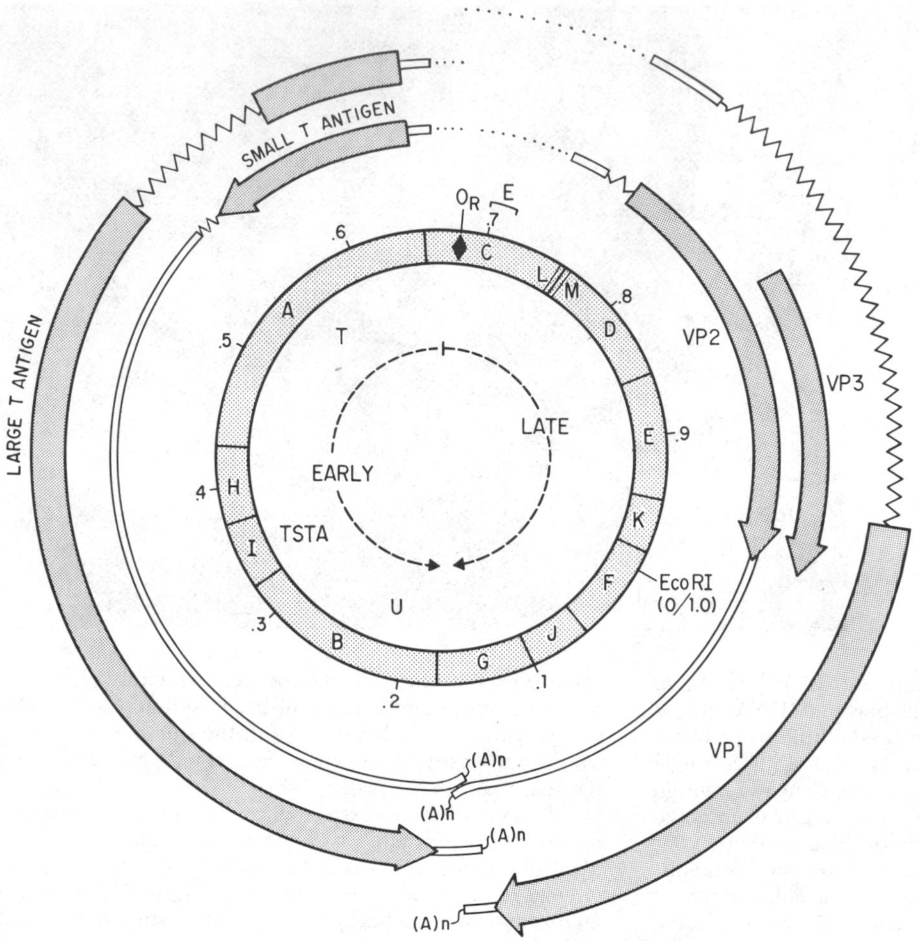

Figure 2. Principal features of the SV40 Genome. The stippled circle represents the *Hind* II/III restriction endonuclease map of the SV40 genome oriented with the origin of replication (O_R) at the top. Numbers outside the circle are map coordinates relative to the single *Eco* RI cleavage site at 0/1.0. Letters refer to the *Hind* II/III fragments. Inner dashed lines indicate regions transcribed into early and late SV40 RNA and the direction of transcription. The letters T, U, and TSTA indicate regions of the genome that appear to be critical determinants of these early SV40 antigens. Enhancer sequences (see Fig. 6) are indicated by the bracket labeled "E." Outer arcs represent RNA transcripts; the wider stippled portions correspond to sequences coding for the indicated viral protein, and the arrowheads point in the 5′→3′ direction. Sawtooth single lines correspond to sequences removed from the primary transcript by splicing. Poly (A) tracts are indicated by (A)n. (Prepared from information summarized in Tooze, 1981; Patch et al., 1979; and Khoury and Gruss, 1983.)

virus replication and transformation has come from studies of SV40 and mouse polyomavirus. Since the human polyomaviruses, BKV and JCV, are more closely related to SV40 than to mouse polyomavirus, we will use SV40 to illustrate polyomavirus replication and transformation. Monkey cells are permissive for SV40, and mouse cells are nonpermissive.

Productive infection begins with the adsorption of virus to receptors on the cell surface. In the case of mouse polyomavirus, and probably other hemagglutinating polyomaviruses such as BKV and JCV, adsorption can be prevented by treating cells with neuraminidase, which destroys sialic acid-containing cell receptors (SV40 does not hemagglutinate and its adsorption is not affected by neuraminidase). After adsorption, the virus penetrates the cell membrane and is transported to the cell nucleus, where it is uncoated (Salzman and Khoury, 1974; Diacumakos and Gershey, 1977; Tooze, 1981).

The replication cycle that follows is temporally regulated and can be divided into two phases: *early* and *late*. During the early phase, which precedes viral DNA replication (Fig. 3A), early viral RNA is transcribed from approximately one half of one strand of the viral DNA, i.e., from the E strand, counterclockwise from 0.66 to 0.15 on the map of the SV40 genome (Fig. 2). Transcription of early RNA, which can be detected as early as six hours after infection, is followed by synthesis of early viral proteins and by the appearance in the infected cells of virus-specific early antigens. Two of these, SV40 T antigen and SV40 U antigen, accumulate in the cell nucleus, where they can be detected by fluorescent antibody (FA) staining beginning about eight hours after infection (Fig. 4). A third early antigen, tumor-specific transplantation antigen (TSTA), can be detected on the surface of infected cells (Tevethia and Tevethia, 1976; Anderson et al., 1977). This antigen mediates cellular immune responses that render animals immune to tumors induced by the injection of SV40 virus or SV40 transformed cells.

The late phase of the cycle begins with the onset of viral DNA replication, 12 to 15 hours after infection (Fig. 3B). DNA replication proceeds bidirectionally from a unique origin located at about 0.67 on the restriction endonuclease map of the SV40 genome (Fig. 2). Replication terminates when the two replication forks meet, about 180° from the origin; there is no specific termination site or signal. Initiation of each round of viral DNA replication requires functionally active large T protein, which binds to the viral DNA at specific sites at the origin of replication (Tooze, 1981). In addition to initiating viral DNA replication, the binding of the large T protein to viral DNA also initiates the transcription of late viral RNA. Late viral RNA is transcribed from the remaining half of the genome (Fig. 2), its template being the opposite strand of the viral DNA from that involved in early RNA synthesis (i.e., the L strand). Late structural viral proteins, VP-1, VP-2, and VP-3, are then synthesized and transported to the nucleus,

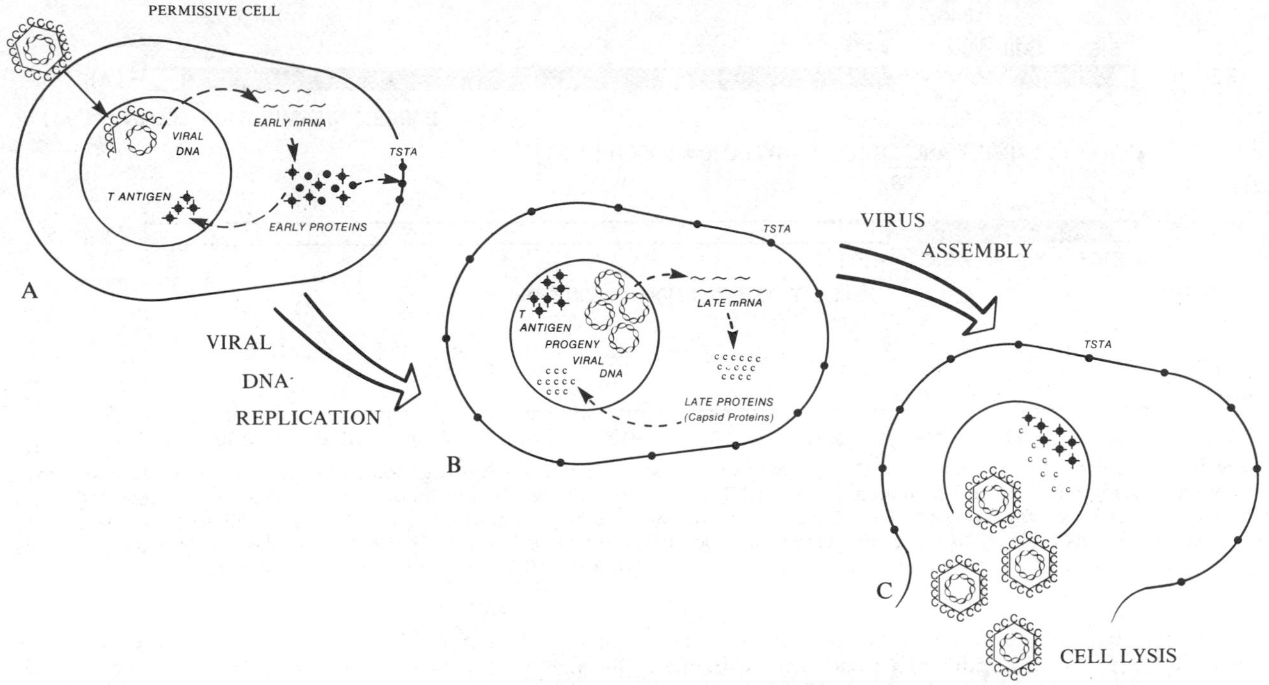

Figure 3. Productive polyomavirus infection as exemplified by SV40 infection of primary African green monkey kidney (AGMK) cells.

where they can be detected by FA staining by about 15 hours after infection. Progeny virions assemble in the nucleus beginning about 18 hours after infection and accumulate for a prolonged period, usually for at least 40 hours, before cell lysis occurs.

Two proteins are encoded by the SV40 early region: large T antigen with a molecular weight of about 82,000 and small T antigen with a molecular weight of about 20,000. The large T and small T proteins are immunologically related, share amino-terminal amino acids and have several common methionine-tryptic peptides (Paucha et al., 1978; Simmons and Martin, 1978). The synthesis of each of these early proteins is directed by a distinct cytoplasmic 19S mRNA, but both mRNAs are derived from the same primary early RNA transcript. This is accomplished by a process called *splicing*, which removes specific segments of RNA from the primary transcript. The RNAs for large T and small T both span almost the entire *early* region, from approximately 0.66 counterclockwise to 0.15 on the map of the SV40 genome (Fig. 2). However, while the same initiation codon at approximately 0.65 map units (SV40 nucleotide 5163) is used for both proteins, the two mRNAs differ in the size and location of deleted intervening sequences (Berk and Sharp, 1978; Crawford et al., 1978; Tooze, 1981). The mRNA coding for large T lacks a 346-nucleotide intervening sequence between 0.60 and 0.53, corresponding to SV40 nucleotides 4572 through 4917 (Fig. 5). Since termination codons located at about 0.54 map units are deleted, the entire mRNA can be translated into the 82,000 molecular weight large T protein. The mRNA for small T lacks a 66-nucleotide intervening sequence between 0.54 and 0.53, corresponding to SV40 nucleotides 4572 through 4637 (Fig. 5). However, a termination codon remains at about 0.54 (nucleotide 4641) just 5′ to the deleted sequences, and thus only that portion of the mRNA from 0.65 to 0.54 can be translated. This yields the 20,000 molecular weight small T protein, which is identical to large T in the region encoded by sequences from 0.65 to 0.60 (corresponding to nucleotides 5163 to 4918) in the SV40 genome.

The stable cytoplasmic late mRNAs, which direct the synthesis of VP-1, VP-2, and VP-3, are similarly formed by the splicing out of intervening sequences present in pri-

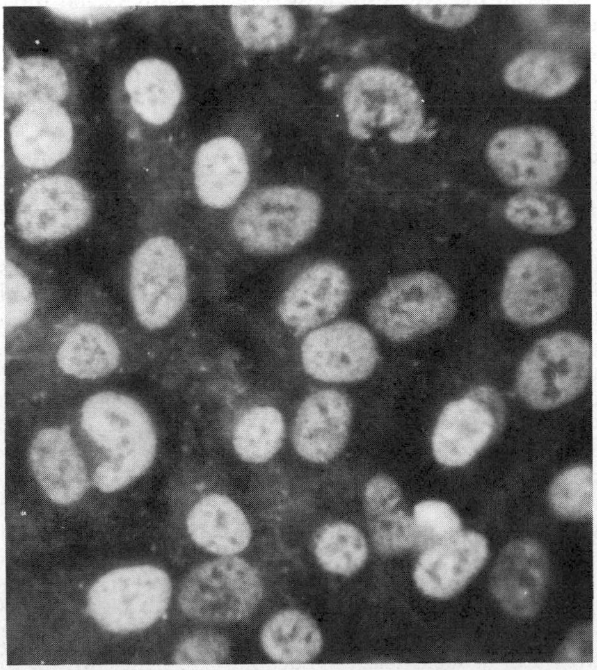

Figure 4. SV40 T antigen demonstrated by fluorescent antibody staining of SV40 transformed cells. Note the finely granular staining confined to the nucleus and exhibiting characteristic nucleolar sparing (1000 ×).

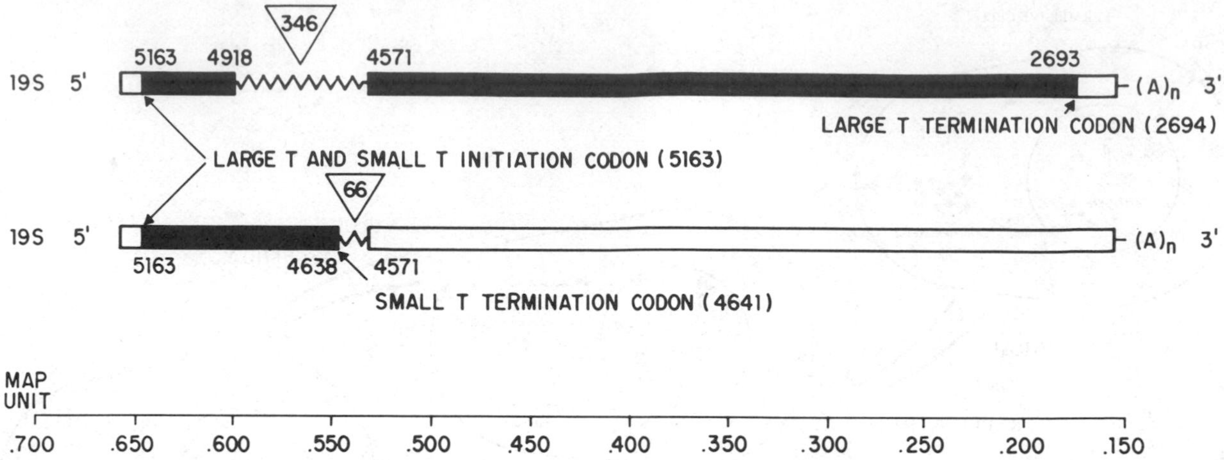

Figure 5. The structure of SV40 early mRNAs. The map of the early region of the SV40 genome is shown counterclockwise below. The regions coding for the large T antigen and the small T antigen are indicated by the shaded areas within the bars that define the two early 19S mRNAs. The sawtooth lines indicate regions of the primary transcript that are spliced out to form the mature polyadenylated cytoplasmic mRNAs, and the number of nucleotides removed is indicated within the triangles. The four-digit numbers adjacent to the bars are SV40 nucleotide numbers. (Modified from Howley, 1980 with information from Tooze, 1981.)

mary transcripts of the late region of the viral genome. VP-2 and VP-3 are encoded within the same reading frame and share carboxy-terminal amino acids. In fact, VP-3 corresponds to the carboxy-terminal two-thirds of VP-2 (Fig. 2). VP-1 is encoded in a different reading frame and, although the same DNA sequence that codes for its amino-terminal end also codes for the carboxy-terminal ends of VP-2 and VP-3, the amino acids specified are different. Similar patterns of splicing occur with the other members of the genus, including the human representatives, BKV and JCV. In the case of mouse polyomavirus, splicing of RNA transcribed from the early region of the genome results in the synthesis of three early mRNAs and three early proteins: an 88,000 molecular weight large T antigen, a 50,000 molecular weight middle T antigen, and a 23,000 molecular weight small T antigen. A single reading frame is used for the amino-terminal domains of all three of these T antigens, but three different reading frames are used for the carboxy-terminal portions that are specified by mRNA sequences distal to the splice sites (Tooze, 1981; Eckhart, 1983).

The discovery that identical primary transcripts are processed by the splicing out of different intervening sequences into different mRNAs, thus permitting the same region of the polyomavirus genome to code for more than one unique protein, resolved a troublesome dilemma. Without such a mechanism, polyomavirus genomes do not have sufficient coding capacity to specify all of the proteins known to be virus-coded.

The exact relationship between the three virus-specific early antigens (T, U, and TSTA) detected in infected cells, and the early SV40 proteins (large T and small T) continues to be the subject of active investigation. Several lines of evidence indicate that SV40 T antigen, U antigen, and TSTA are all specified by regions of genome that code for the large T protein. Analysis of a series of adenovirus-SV40 hybrid viruses containing segments of the early region of the SV40 genome that extend from 0.15 map units (3′ to the carboxy-terminus of large T) for varying distances toward the amino-terminus at 0.65 map units has demonstrated that the carboxy-terminal one-third of large T is sufficient for U antigen activity, that a somewhat larger fragment is required for TSTA activity, and that the amino-terminal portion is required for T antigen activity (Fig. 2) (Patch et al, 1979). However, more than one region of the large T protein may be involved in each of these antigenic activities, and the antigen specified may be determined, at least in part, by the cellular structure with which the large T protein is associated (Anderson et al., 1977; Deppert, 1979; Deppert and Walter, 1982). U antigen appears to correspond to a fraction of the large T protein within the nucleus that is bound to the nuclear matrix, whereas unbound large T protein in the nucleus exhibits T antigen activity. TSTA appears to correspond to another fraction of large T protein that is associated with the plasma membrane.

Polyomaviruses, being among the smallest animal viruses, have relatively little genetic information with which to carry out all of the functions required for their replication. Consequently, in addition to such devices as RNA splicing, the use of alternate reading frames and the synthesis of overlapping proteins, which enable one segment of the viral genome to specify more than one protein, polyomaviruses make extensive use of the host cell in their replication. For example, host cell RNA polymerase II is used for transcription, host cell pathways are used for the 5′ capping and 3′ polyadenylation of viral mRNA, host cell DNA polymerase is used for the synthesis of progeny viral DNA, and host cell histones are associated with polyomavirus DNA to form the viral "minichromosome." Perhaps because of this extreme dependence upon host cell metabolism, polyomavirus infection of permissive cells does not result in the early inhibition of host cell synthetic functions seen with many other viruses. Rather, there is an induction of host cell DNA, RNA, and protein synthesis during the early phase of infection, as well as a large increase in the activity of many host cell enzymes involved in DNA replication. There are also changes in the surface properties of infected cells. These include increased uptake of sugars, enhanced agglutinability by plant lectins, and the appearance of new surface antigens, including TSTA. Most of these changes depend upon the expression of the early portion of the viral genome, and in the case of SV40, upon the synthesis of large T antigen. Large T antigen is required for productive infection. It is responsible for the initiation of viral DNA replication and late viral mRNA synthesis, as well as for the induction of host cell DNA, RNA, and protein synthesis (Tooze, 1981). The large T protein contains an ATPase activity and binds specifically to SV40 DNA at the origin of replication. This is probably responsible for its effects upon the synthesis of viral DNA and RNA. It may act by locally unwinding a portion of the duplex DNA, allowing polymerases to bind and initiate replication. The large T protein also binds to host cell chromosomes, and this may mediate many of its effects upon host cell metabolism. However, since the SV40 large T protein also appears to have protein kinase activity (Tjian and Robbins, 1979), some of its biological effects may be mediated by the modification of cellular proteins. Large T antigen is also required for the initiation and maintenance of transformation in nonpermissive host cells.

Attempts to understand the regulation of SV40 early gene expression have uncovered a series of control or "promoter" elements located upstream from the early mRNA cap site in a stretch of about 200 nucleotides on the "late" side of the origin of DNA replication (Fig. 2). These sequences, which encode no viral protein, begin with an AT-rich region that includes a Goldberg-Hogness or TATA sequence typical of eukaryotic genes transcribed by RNA polymerase II (Fig. 6). This region appears to determine the precise site at which the transcription of early SV40 RNA is initiated. To the late side of the TATA sequence are three GC-rich 21 base pair repeats that appear to be involved in RNA polymerase binding. Finally, to the late side of the 21 base pair repeats, there is a 72 base pair tandem repeat that has been characterized as an *enhancer* element for early SV40 gene expression (Benoist and Chambon, 1981, Gruss et al, 1981). Deletion of this element reduces early gene expression (i.e., SV40 T antigen synthesis) by more than 100-fold and renders the virus nonviable. Similar enhancers have been found in this location in the genomes of mouse polyomavirus, BKV and JCV. They have also been found in papillomaviruses, adenoviruses, and retroviruses, and comparable enhancer elements have been identified in several cellular genes (Yaniv, 1982; Khoury and Gruss, 1983; Rosenthal et al., 1983). These enhancer elements are not gene- or promoter-specific; they can exert their effect when artificially joined to heterologous genes. To do so, they must be covalently linked to the gene, but they can be located several kilobases upstream or downstream from its transcription initiation site and can function in either orientation (Yaniv, 1982; Khoury and Gruss, 1983; Rosenthal et al., 1983). Although there is no extended base sequence homology among these different enhancer elements, a 7-12 base pair consensus or "core" sequence has been identified in a number of enhancers, and deletions or mutations in this core sequence abolish enhancer activity. The enhancer elements associated with cellular genes appear to be a major determinant of the cell and tissue specificity of cellular gene expression (e.g., immunoglobulin enhancers activate expression of adjacent genes to high levels only in lymphoid cells) whereas the viral enhancers are important determinants of virus host range and tissue tropism, probably because of their capacity to interact with cellular factors normally involved in controlling the activity of cellular genes (Laimins et al., 1982; Chatis et al., 1983; Rosenthal et al., 1983 and references therein). Thus mutations or substitutions in the enhancer sequences have been shown to alter markedly the host range and tissue specificity of polyomaviruses and retroviruses. For example, a viable mutant of BKV with a small deletion and insertion in this region induces insulinomas in hamsters, a type of tumor that is not induced by wild-type BKV (Uchida et al., 1979; Watanabe et al., 1979). It is noteworthy that the primate polyomaviruses (SV40, BKV, and JCV), which are identical in their genetic organization and share more than 70 per cent of their nucleotide sequences, differ markedly only in the noncoding region to the "late" side of the replication origin, i.e., in their enhancer sequences (Howley, 1980; Rosenthal, et al., 1983; Frisque, 1983 and references therein). This suggests that, rather than having evolved from a common viral ancestor, the enhancer elements of viruses may have been derived from the genomes of their host cells. This notion is supported by the recent identification of a homolog of the BKV enhancer in human cellular DNA (Rosenthal et al., 1983).

Productive SV40 infection results in characteristic cytopathic effects (Sweet and Hilleman, 1960; Hsiung and Gaylord, 1961). In unstained monolayer cultures these cytopathic effects (CPE) consist of cell rounding and enlargement with the development of extensive cytoplasmic vacuolization (Fig. 7). This extensive cytoplasmic vacuolization led to the original designation of SV40 as "simian vacuolating virus." Polyomavirus CPE is clearly visible when infected monolayer cultures are fixed and stained with hematoxylin and eosin. At about 24 hours after infection there is nuclear swelling, some clumping of chromatin, and the appearance of irregular patches of eosinophilic material within the nucleus. By about 48 hours after infection the nuclei show margination of chromatin and large basophilic Feulgen-positive intranuclear inclusions that, when examined by electron microscopy, are found to be composed of papovavirus virions. At about this time the extensive cytoplasmic vacuolization develops (Fig. 7). The fully developed intranuclear inclusions produced by mem-

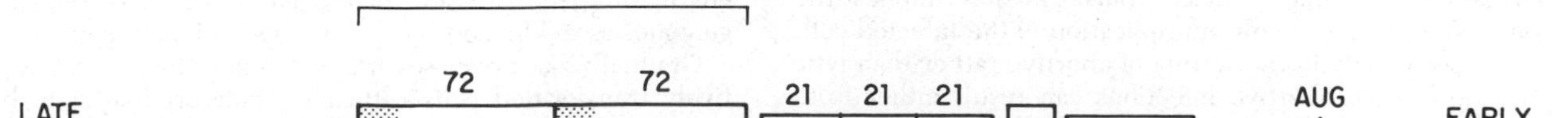

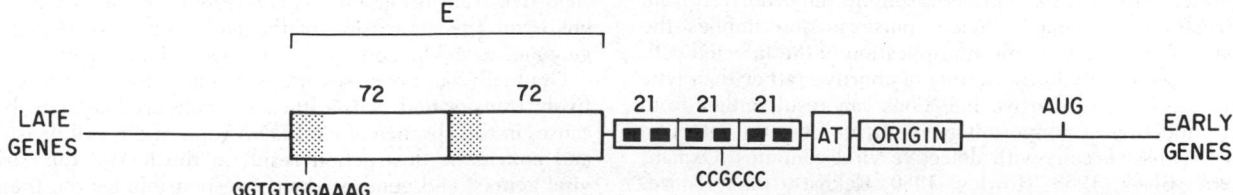

Figure 6. Promoter elements for early SV40 transcription located upstream from the early RNA cap site on the late side of the origin of replication. The Goldberg-Hogness or TATA sequence (AT) is preceded by three 21 base pair repeats, each containing two copies of the hexanucleotide CCGCCC (shaded blocks). These are preceded by an enhancer element (E) consisting of a 72 base pair tandem repeat. The stippled areas correspond to the consensus or "core" sequence (GGTGTGGAAAG). (Modified from Khoury and Gruss, 1983.)

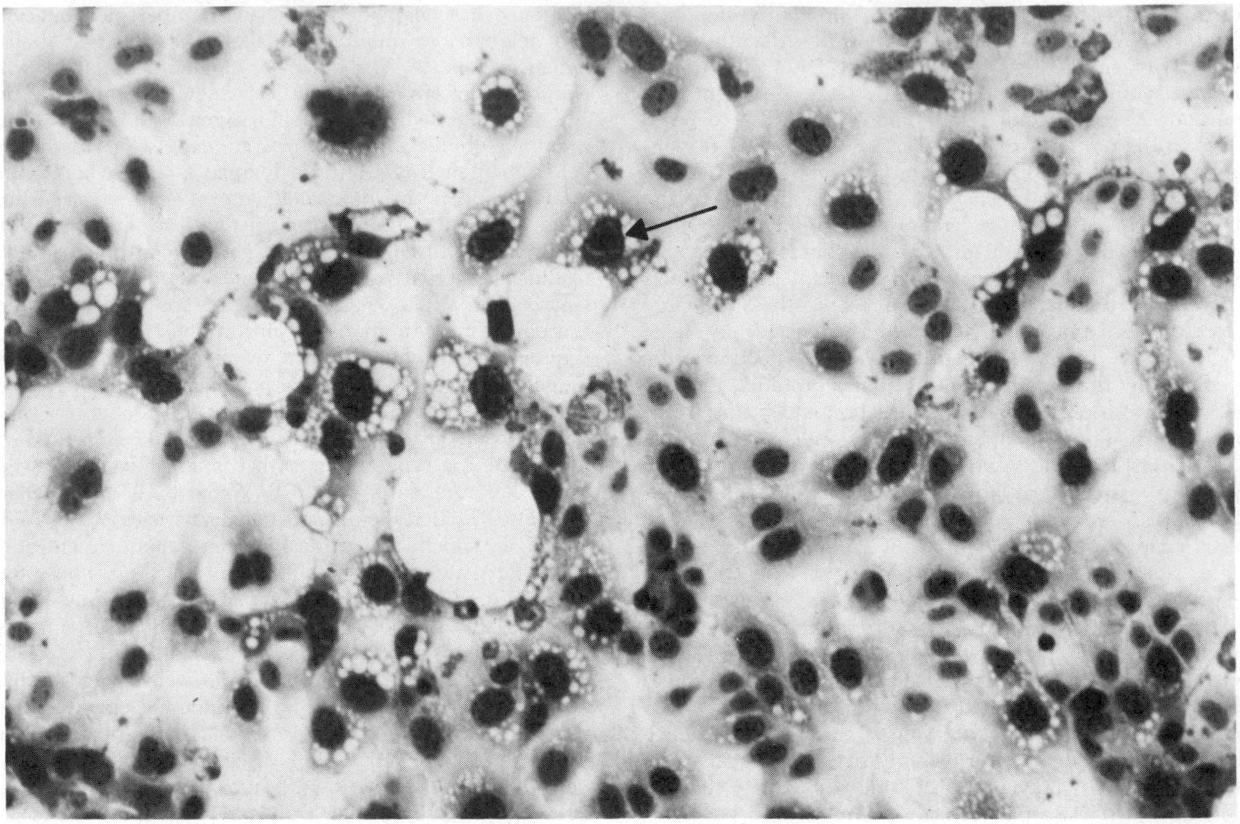

Figure 7. SV40 infection of permissive African green monkey kidney (AGMK) cells. Monolayer cultures were fixed and stained with hematoxylin and eosin 3 days after infection with a multiplicity of approximately 5 plaque-forming units per cell. Note the extensive cytoplasmic vacuolization. The arrow indicates a cell with a typical basophilic intranuclear inclusion body (350 ×).

bers of the polyomavirus genus may be basophilic, amphophilic, or eosinophilic, depending upon the virus strain, cell type, and method of fixation. Although productive infection results in cell lysis, progeny virions are not always efficiently released. This is especially true of mouse polyomavirus and the hemagglutinating human papovaviruses, BKV and JCV, which remain associated with cells and cell debris. To achieve good yields of these viruses it is necessary to disrupt the infected cells mechanically and use neuraminidase to free the virions from sialic acid-containing cell receptors.

Perhaps the most significant biologic property of the polyomaviruses is their capacity to transform normal cells into tumor cells. Although members of the polyomavirus genus are not associated with spontaneous tumors in their natural hosts, they regularly produce tumors experimentally. Moreover, they can transform normal cells in tissue culture into cells that closely resemble those derived from virus-induced tumors. Since transformation implies the survival and subsequent multiplication of the infected cell, it can occur only in the setting of abortive rather than lytic infection. Such abortive infections can result either from the infection of nonpermissive cells, or from the infection of permissive cells with defective viral genomes (Oxman, 1967; Black, 1968; Howley, 1980; Eckhart, 1981; Tooze, 1981; Norkin, 1982). The common denominator appears to be the persistence and continued expression of early viral genetic information in the absence of virus replication.

When polyomaviruses infect nonpermissive cells, e.g., when SV40 infects mouse 3T3 cells, the early phase of infection is similar to that described for infection of permissive cells. Virus adsorption, penetration, and uncoating occur, the early region of the viral genome is transcribed into early mRNA, and the early viral proteins (large T and small T) are synthesized. The cells express early virus-specific antigens (T, U, and TSTA), their surface properties are altered, and cellular DNA, RNA, and protein synthesis are stimulated (Fig. 8). However, the late phase of the virus replication cycle does not occur. There is little or no viral DNA replication, no synthesis of viral capsid proteins (V antigens), and no production of virions. Such abortively infected cells are stimulated to divide and behave for a few generations like transformed cells, i.e., they become insensitive to the controls that regulate the multiplication of normal cells. This transient abnormal behavior, called "abortive transformation," is coincident with and dependent upon the expression of the early region of the viral genome, as evidenced by the synthesis of T antigens.

Gradually, and over several cell generations, most abortively transformed cells return to their original state because, in the absence of viral DNA replication, cell division and enzymatic destruction result in the loss of the early viral gene(s) and gene product(s) responsible for the transformed phenotype (Oxman, 1967; Sambrook, 1972). However, abortive transformation is not the only possible outcome of abortive infection. Some of the infected cells

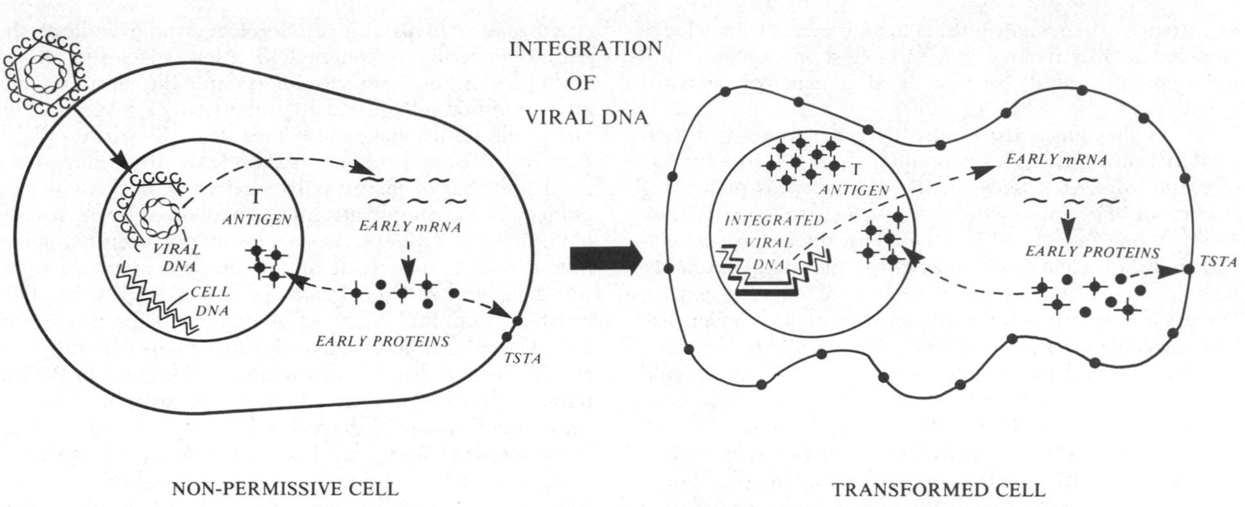

Figure 8. Cell transformation by polyomaviruses as exemplified by SV40 transformation of mouse 3T3 cells.

are permanently transformed. These cells and their progeny continue to express early polyomavirus gene(s) and never lose the transformed phenotype. The critical difference between the permanently and the abortively transformed cells is the integration of the polyomavirus genome (or at least the early region of the viral genome) into cell DNA in the permanently transformed cells. This event ensures the persistence and expression of the early viral genetic information that is responsible for the transformed phenotype (Fig. 8). Thus, permanently transformed cells contain polyomavirus DNA covalently linked to cell DNA, as well as early viral mRNA and early viral proteins (Enders, 1965; Oxman, 1967; Sambrook, 1972; Howley, 1980; Eckhart, 1981; Tooze, 1981; Griffin and Dilworth, 1983). Moreover, although they contain no infectious virus, transformed nonpermissive cells usually contain one or more integrated copies of the whole viral genome, and infectious virus can be rescued from them by fusion with uninfected permissive cells (Gerber, 1966). It should be noted that polyomavirus transformation (i.e., permanent transformation) is a very inefficient process; 10^4 to 10^5 infectious virions are required per transforming event (Sambrook, 1972).

The use of virus mutants and recombinant DNA technology has permitted more detailed analysis of the transformation process. It now appears that tumor induction in vivo and neoplastic transformation of primary cells in culture both involve two separate viral functions, one responsible for the immortalization of cells that would otherwise have a finite lifespan, and the other responsible for the structural and behavioral changes that constitute the transformed phenotype. The SV40 large T protein appears to be able to carry out both of these functions. However, in the case of mouse polyomavirus, these functions are mediated by different early proteins (Eckhart, 1981; Rassoulzadegan, et al., 1983). The mouse polyomavirus large T protein (which is located in the nucleus) can immortalize primary cells, but these cells remain phenotypically normal. The middle T protein (which is associated with the plasma membrane) can transform established (already immortal) cell lines, but cannot normally transform primary cells or induce tumors in vivo. Thus, for mouse polyomavirus, large T seems to be responsible for immortalization and middle T for the structural and behavioral changes that constitute the transformed phenotype. It has been shown for both viruses that the amino-terminal portion of the large T protein is sufficient to induce immortalization (see Rassoulzadegan et al., 1983 and references therein). Perhaps with SV40, the fraction of large T that is associated with the cell membrane is functionally analogous to mouse polyomavirus middle T, while that localized to the nucleus is responsible for immortalization. Post-translational modifications, e.g., phosphorylation, may be important in determining the cellular localization, and thus the specific function, of early polyomavirus proteins.

Polyomavirus transformation is of considerable importance to students of human disease. Because they contain early viral proteins, cells transformed by polyomaviruses are extremely useful sources of antigens for serologic tests to detect antibodies to these viral gene products. Moreover, the capacity of the human polyomaviruses, BKV and JCV, to induce malignancies in animals, together with the high frequency with which both agents produce infections in childhood, raises the important question of the possible role of these viruses in human cancers, especially those occurring in immunologically compromised individuals. To date, however, there is no convincing evidence implicating SV40, BKV, or JCV in the etiology of human malignancies (Padgett and Walker, 1976; Takemoto, 1978; Howley, 1980; Padgett, 1981; Howley, 1983a; Johnson, 1983).

BIOLOGIC BEHAVIOR AND PATHOGENIC PROPERTIES. Most members of the polyomavirus genus inhabit the urinary tract and produce harmless but persistent infections in their natural hosts. Human infection by polyomaviruses appears to be limited primarily to the human polyomaviruses, BKV and JCV (Walker and Padgett, 1983b) and to virus(es) similar or identical to the African green monkey lymphotropic papovavirus, LPV (Takemoto and Segawa, 1983). In addition, humans may be infected accidently with SV40, (Brown et al., 1975; Shah and Nathanson, 1976). Although the discussions that follow will focus primarily on the human polyomaviruses, we will also briefly discuss mouse polyomavirus and SV40, because of their historical importance, their contribution to our current knowledge of polyomavirus biology and virus-host interactions, and their potential utility as models of human polyomavirus infection.

Mouse Polyomavirus. Mouse polyomavirus was discovered by Ludwig Gross, as a contaminant in cell-free extracts of tissue from AKR mice, in the course of his pioneering studies of the transmission of murine leukemia (Gross, 1953). When inoculated into newborn mice, the contaminant induced adenocarcinomas of the parotid gland rather than leukemia. It was easily separated from the murine leukemia agent (a retrovirus) because of its smaller size and resistance to heating at 65°C. The parotid tumor agent was later named mouse "polyomavirus" because it could induce a wide variety of tumors when injected into newborns of several species (Eddy, 1969). Rowe and his colleagues showed that mouse polyomavirus infection is widespread among wild and laboratory mice; transmission is normally horizontal through saliva and urine, resulting in a generalized infection with virus replication in many organs, but without the production of overt disease. Thereafter, virus persists silently in the kidneys, becoming more difficult to detect with increasing passage of time postinfection (Rowe et al., 1960; 1961). In addition to its extensive use as a model for the study of viral oncogenesis and eukaryotic gene expression (Tooze, 1981), mouse polyomavirus infection in vivo has been studied as a model of human polyomavirus infection (McCance, 1983). These studies have shown that when previously infected mice with low or undetectable levels of virus in their kidneys are immunosuppressed, levels of virus in the kidney are markedly increased and urinary excretion can be detected. Pregnancy has a similar effect, with virus titers increasing during the latter part of gestation (McCance and Mims 1979). DNA hybridization reveals nonintegrated viral DNA in the kidneys of persistently infected mice, and small amounts of nonintegrated viral DNA are also found in the brains of a small percentage of these animals (McCance, 1983). Since virus is known to replicate in the brain during the acute infection, this DNA may simply reflect the presence of small amounts of residual virus not detectable in brain homogenates by infectivity assay because of the presence of neutralizing antibody. The long-term persistence of virus in the brains of a small fraction of infected mice has important implications with respect to the pathogenesis of PML in humans (vide infra).

Mouse polyomavirus is similar in genome organization to the primate polyomaviruses, SV40, BKV, and JCV. However, while there is considerable homology between the predicted amino acid sequences of the early and late proteins of the mouse and primate viruses (Soeda et al., 1980) there is no detectable immunologic cross-reactivity, except for a genus-specific antigenic determinant on the major capsid protein, VP-1, which is not exposed in intact virions (Shah et al., 1977a). There is no serologic or other evidence of human infections with mouse polyomavirus.

Simian Virus 40 (SV40). SV40 was discovered in 1960 in cultures of renal tissue from apparently normal rhesus and cynomolgus monkeys that were used for the preparation of poliovirus and adenovirus vaccines (Sweet and Hilleman, 1960). The virus replicated in these cultures without causing cytopathic effects (CPE) and thus its presence remained unsuspected until Sweet and Hilleman discovered that it produced easily recognized CPE when inoculated into cultures of renal cells from African green monkeys (*Cercopithecus aethiops*) (Fig. 7). Serologic studies indicate that natural infection is confined to a few species of Asiatic macaques. In these animals, for example the rhesus monkey (*M. mulatta*), only a small proportion of juveniles, but nearly all adults, have antibodies to SV40 (Shah and Nathanson, 1976 and references therein). Natural infection is similar to that of mouse polyomavirus in mice, with generalized but asymptomatic infection followed by persistence of virus in the kidneys. As seen in the persistently infected mouse and human (vide infra), immunosuppression can result in viral recrudescence and disease. SV40 has been isolated from the brains of rhesus monkeys dying with progressive multifocal leukoencephalopathy (Holmberg et al., 1977). The disease, which appears identical to PML in humans, has been observed only in presumably immunosuppressed animals with chronic infections or malignancies; these monkeys appear to have had the simian equivalent of the acquired immune deficiency syndrome (AIDS). Polyomavirus particles were demonstrated in glial nuclei in areas of demyelination in 9 of 10 cases examined, and SV40 was isolated from both cases subjected to virologic examination. FA staining of brain tissue confirmed the presence of SV40 T and V antigens in inclusion-bearing glial nuclei in areas of demyelination, and antisera specific for JCV and BKV gave negative reactions. In addition to providing an interesting parallel to PML in humans, the SV40-rhesus monkey system provides a potential model with which to study the pathogenesis and treatment of PML. SV40 has also been identified as the cause of fatal interstitial pneumonia and renal tubular necrosis in a rhesus monkey; the cells involved were primarily pneumocytes in the lung and tubular epithelial cells in the kidney (Sheffield et al., 1980). The monkey was a juvenile that appeared to have an immune deficiency, and the disease described may reflect the consequence of primary SV40 infection in an immunodeficient host. This is particularly interesting in view of the recent report of tubulo-interstitial nephritis in a BKV-infected child with a primary immunodeficiency (vide infra).

Human exposure to SV40 has been limited primarily to millions of recipients of SV40 contaminated vaccines and to individuals with significant exposure to monkeys (mainly workers in animal colonies and laboratories). Early batches of live attenuated poliovirus vaccine were also contaminated, but these were only administered to several thousand individuals. Parenteral administration of SV40 contaminated killed vaccines induced moderately high levels of antibodies to SV40, which persisted for years, suggesting that systemic infection with SV40 had occurred and raising the possibility of virus persistence (Shah and Nathansan, 1976). The discovery that SV40 could induce tumors in hamsters (Eddy et al, 1962) and transform human cells in tissue culture (Shein and Enders, 1962) raised concern that SV40 might cause malignancies in humans. A number of retrospective epidemiologic studies carried out to assess this possibility have shown no differences between the incidence or types of cancer in recipients of potentially contaminated vaccines and unvaccinated controls (Shah and Nathanson, 1976; Mortimer et al, 1981). However, two studies have suggested that children born to mothers vaccinated during pregnancy with potentially contaminated killed poliovirus vaccines might have had an increased incidence of neural tumors (Heinonen et al., 1973; Farwell et al., 1979). Many investigators have sought evidence that SV40 might play a role in the etiology of tumors, particularly brain tumors. While there are numerous reports of the detection of "polyomavirus-like particles," SV40 T antigens and SV40 DNA or RNA in tumor cells or in cell lines derived from tumors, most of these lack adequate controls and several careful studies have failed to confirm these observations (Greenlee et al., 1978; Shah et al., 1978; Howley, 1980; Johnson, 1983 and references therein).

Although there is little solid evidence implicating SV40 in the etiology of human malignancies, the observation that 2 to 4 per cent of the U.S. population with no known exposure to SV40 have low levels of neutralizing antibody to the virus, and the isolation of SV40 from two patients with PML (Weiner et al., 1972) suggest that SV40 might occasionally infect humans under natural conditions, cause a silent but persistent infection, and reactivate in the face of immunologic impairment to cause opportunistic infections, including PML. However, antibodies to SV40 in the sera of individuals who have not had contact with monkeys or exposure to contaminated vaccines appear in most, *but not all,* cases to be the result of infection with BKV or JCV (Brown et al., 1975). Furthermore, more than 60 cases of PML have been thoroughly evaluated since the reported isolation of SV40 from two patients with the disease in 1972; JCV has been identified as the agent involved in every one of these well-studied cases (Padgett and Walker, 1983; Walker and Padgett, 1983a and 1983b; D. L. Walker, personal communication). Thus, if SV40 does cause natural infections in humans, it does so rarely, and it does not appear to be a significant cause of human disease.

JC Virus. JC virus (JCV) was first isolated in 1971 by Padgett et al. from brain tissue of a case of PML that occurred in a 38-year-old man with Hodgkin's disease. Papovavirus virions were observed by electron microscopy in the nuclei of oligodendrocytes in the diseased tissue. The virus was isolated in primary human fetal glial (PHFG) cell cultures that had been inoculated with extracts of brain tissue.

JCV grows and produces CPE only in PHFG cell cultures that contain a high proportion of spongioblasts. Even in these cells the virus grows slowly, the CPE is subtle, and the majority of progeny virions remain cell-associated. It can take a month or more before the CPE is recognized. Once isolated, JCV can be grown in serial passage in cultures of PHFG cells containing a high proportion of spongioblasts. Although developing much more slowly, JCV CPE resembles that produced by SV40 in the same cells (Shein, 1967). About 10 to 14 days after JCV inoculation, spongioblasts enlarge, lose their characteristic spindle shape, and develop intranuclear inclusion bodies. Most of the infected spongioblasts are eventually destroyed. Astrocytes in the cultures are not destroyed, but enlarge and develop greatly enlarged and distorted nuclei. Electron microscopy reveals large numbers of virions in spongioblast nuclei, but few if any in the nuclei of astrocytes. JCV grows very slowly; at the same multiplicity of infection, its replication cycle seems to be at least 5 times longer than that of SV40. As with other polyomaviruses, passage of JCV in culture usually results in heterogeneity in the size of the viral DNA (due to the accumulation of defective virions), but such heterogeneity is not found in viral DNA extracted directly from diseased brain tissue (Frisque et al., 1979). Neither the restricted host range nor the slow growth of JCV can be explained by the presence of defective interfering particles (Grinnell et al., 1982). Temperature sensitivity also fails to explain these phenomena. In fact, JCV grows better at 39°C than at 37°C (Padgett and Walker, 1983).

Many human and animal cells have been tested in search of a better culture system (Padgett and Walker, 1976; Padgett et al., 1977a; Walker and Padgett, 1983a). JCV grows only in cells of human origin; virus replication has been documented in cells of adult brain, amnion, umbilical vein endothelium, and embryonic kidney. However, none are fully permissive, and none are suitable for the primary isolation of JCV. Epithelial cells derived from the urine of newborn infants have recently been reported to support the efficient replication of JCV, but these cells are not as sensitive as PHFG cells for primary isolation (Beckmann et al., 1982).

Primary hamster brain cells have been transformed by each of four isolates of JCV and by purified JCV DNA (Frisque et al, 1980). These cells, which synthesize JCV T antigen and induce tumors in hamsters, closely resemble hamster brain cells transformed by SV40.

With the exception of tumors that arise after inoculation of newborn hamsters, owl monkeys, and squirrel monkeys (Padgett, 1981) no acute or chronic disease attributable to JCV has been found in any of a variety of species inoculated by multiple routes and observed for months to years (Padgett and Walker, 1976). The animals tested include rabbits, guinea pigs, hamsters, mink, and rhesus monkeys. Newborn rhesus monkeys inoculated by several routes apparently become infected because they developed antibodies to JCV T antigens and V antigens. However, no disease or tumors have been recognized. JCV is highly oncogenic in newborn hamsters, especially following intracerebral inoculation, when it produces tumors, usually multiple malignant gliomas. Subcutaneous and intraperitoneal inoculation of JCV produces multiple sarcomas in visceral organs (Padgett, 1981). JCV also causes malignant tumors of the brain in owl monkeys and in squirrel monkeys (London et al., 1978; Rieth et al. 1980). This observation is particularly interesting in the light of a report of multiple gliomas in the brain of an 18-year-old immunodeficient patient with PML (Castaigne et al., 1974). However, careful studies have failed to implicate JCV in the etiology of human cerebral neoplasms (Greenlee et al., 1978; Johnson, 1983).

JCV is identical in size, structure, and genome organization to the other members of the polyomavirus genus. In fact, the JCV genome shares more than 70 per cent of its nucleotide sequences with the genomes of SV40 and BKV, differing markedly only in the noncoding region to the "late" side of the replication origin, i.e., in the enhancer sequences (Frisque, 1983). This region also seems to be the site of minor sequence variations in the genomes of different JCV isolates (Grinnell et al., 1983b). It is possible that characteristics of the JCV enhancer sequences account for the slow growth and narrow host range of the virus. Furthermore, variations in this region may explain the observation that one JCV isolate (MAD-2) induces only cerebellar medulloblastomas in newborn hamsters, whereas another isolate (MAD-4) induces tumors of the pineal gland as well (Padgett et al., 1977b). In addition to the minor variations in sequences on the "late" side of the replication origin that distinguish individual JCV isolates, restriction endonuclease mapping of JCV DNA cloned directly from brain tissue in each of 10 cases of PML suggests that there are two subtypes of JCV circulating in the human population (Grinnell et al., 1983b).

In view of the restricted host range of JCV, it is not surprising that earlier attempts to isolate virus from brain tissue of patients with PML failed, in spite of the inoculation of multiple cell types and animals (Padgett and Walker, 1976). However, since the original isolation of JCV, this virus has been identified in brain tissue from more than 60 patients with PML (Padgett and Walker, 1983; D. L., Walker, personal communication). The consistent finding of JCV in the diseased brains of patients with progressive multifocal leukoencephalopathy (PML) and the localization of JCV virions in the abnormal oligodendrocytes that are the hallmark of the disease provide strong evidence that JCV is the cause of PML.

PML is a subacute progressive demyelinating disease that usually develops in patients with long-standing systemic illnesses that are associated with impaired cellular immunity (Astrom et al., 1958; Richardson, 1961). Although most of the early cases of PML occurred in middle-aged or elderly patients with chronic lymphocytic leukemia or Hodgkin's disease (Astrom et al., 1958; Richardson, 1961), PML is now also being seen in a wide variety of immunosuppressed individuals, including organ allograft recipients, children with congenital immunodeficiency syndromes, and patients with the acquired immune deficiency syndrome (AIDS) (Padgett and Walker, 1983; Reichert et al., 1983).

The onset of PML is usually insidious, with symptoms and signs that indicate multifocal disease of the cerebral hemispheres. Abnormalities of speech and vision and alterations in mental function are frequent early signs. Once these appear, the disease is usually relentlessly progressive in the absence of fever or abnormalities in the cerebrospinal fluid. Paralysis, cortical blindness, and progressive mental deterioration are common, followed by coma and death, which usually occurs within three to six months of onset. However, some 25 per cent of patients survive for longer periods and about 10 per cent undergo remission or stabilization (Hedley-Whyte et al., 1966; Price et al., 1983; Padgett and Walker, 1983 and references therein). Thus, PML is not invariably fatal, and there is some indication that prolonged survival may be correlated with less severe immunosuppression.

The lesions in the central nervous system constitute the truly distinctive feature of PML (Zu Rhein and Chou, 1965; Silverman and Rubinstein, 1965; Howatson et al., 1965). They consist of multiple foci of demyelination varying in size from less than one mm to 2 or 3 cm in diameter. The lesions are most abundant in subcortical white matter, and early foci appear to enlarge and coalesce into confluent lesions which may eventually involve the white matter of entire lobes (Fig. 9A). Lesions are most common in the

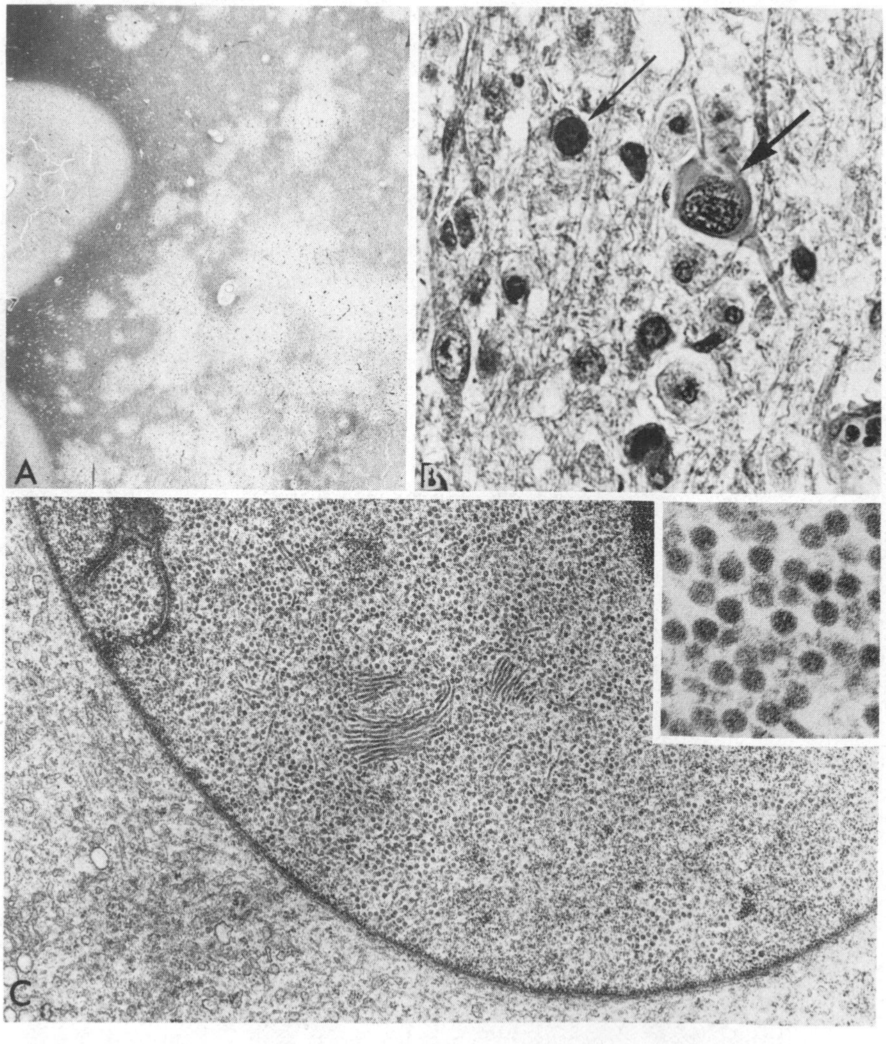

Figure 9. The brain in a typical case of progressive multifocal leukoencephalopathy. *A,* Patchy demyelination unrelated to vessels merging into confluent lesions. Stained with Luxol fast blue (8 ×). *B,* The enlarged oligodendroglial nucleus showing margination of chromatin and effacement of nuclear structure by an intranuclear inclusion body *(small arrow)* and the hypertrophic astrocyte with a bizarre, giant nucleus *(large arrow)* are characteristic light microscopic findings. Stained with hematoxylin and eosin (350 ×). *C,* Oligodendrocyte with enlarged nucleus filled with spherical and filamentous virus particles (20,000 ×) that are enlarged in the inset (80,000 ×). (Courtesy of Dr. Peter W. Lampert.)

cerebrum, sometimes occur in the cerebellum and brain stem, and only rarely involve the spinal cord. The histopathology of the lesions is characterized by two "unusual and striking" cytopathologic abnormalities (Astrom et al., 1958). The pathognomonic feature of PML is the presence of altered oligodendrocytes in and around the early foci of demyelination and at the periphery of the more advanced lesions. These oligodendrocytes are enlarged with markedly enlarged nuclei that are intensely basophilic, show effacement of their nuclear structure, and frequently contain irregular inclusion bodies (Fig. 9B). These changes are followed by cell necrosis, and thus oligodendrocytes are generally absent from the central portions of more advanced lesions. In spite of the presence of virus particles, viral proteins and cell necrosis, there is usually little or no inflammatory response. This is generally attributed to the immunologic impairment present in most patients with PML. In the few patients with PML who do not have severe immunologic impairment, survival time is often prolonged and examination of brain tissue frequently reveals perivascular cuffing with lymphocytes and plasma cells (Walker and Padgett, 1983a).

The other distinctive cytopathologic feature of PML is the presence, in the more advanced lesions, of giant astrocytes with bizarre hyperchromatic nuclei that resemble the malignant astrocytes of pleomorphic glioblastomas. These cells also resemble astrocytes that have been transformed in vitro by SV40 (Shein, 1967). These changes, and especially the presence of inclusions in the nuclei of oligodendrocytes, led Cavanagh et al. (Cavanagh et al., 1959) and Richardson (Richardson, 1961) to suggest that PML might represent an opportunistic viral infection involving oligodendrocytes in patients with impaired immunity. The demonstration in 1965 (Zu Rhein and Chou, 1965; Silverman and Rubinstein, 1965; Howatson et al., 1965) that nuclei of the affected oligodendrocytes in lesions of PML were packed with virus particles resembling papovavirus virions (Fig. 9C) lent strong support to this concept and set the stage for the subsequent isolation of JCV by Padgett et al. in 1971 (Padgett et al., 1971). It is now clear that PML is due to an opportunistic infection by JCV of persons with impaired immunity, and that demyelination occurs because JCV produces a lytic infection of the oligodendrocytes (Itoyama et al., 1982; Johnson, 1983; Padgett and Walker, 1983; Walker and Padgett, 1983a).

Although PML is a rare disease, JCV infection is ubiquitous. Primary infection is common in childhood and antibody to the virus is present in 65-90 per cent of adults in most populations (Walker and Padgett, 1983b). As is the case when other members of the polyomavirus genus infect their natural hosts, primary JCV infections seem to be asymptomatic, but they are accompanied by viremia and followed by long-term persistence of virus in the urinary tract. Subsequent immunosuppression in persistently infected individuals results in reactivation (or amplification) of the renal infection, with virus shedding in the urine. However, even when immunosuppression is severe and prolonged, it is only the rare individual who develops PML. This raises the question of whether PML is a consequence of the reactivation of latent JCV infection in an immunosuppressed individual or only results when primary JCV infection occurs in an immunocompromised host. The occurrence of PML in several children with combined immunodeficiency since birth suggests that, at least in these patients, PML developed in the course of a primary JCV infection. This view is supported by the detection of nonintegrated JCV DNA in the liver, lungs, lymph nodes, and spleen, as well as in the kidneys and brain, in two such patients (Grinnell et al., 1983a). However, most cases of PML have occurred in adults, many of whom can be expected to have had a primary infection in childhood. Serologic studies in many of these patients, although inconclusive, are more consistent with reactivation than with primary infection (Walker and Padgett, 1983a). At least one patient had serum antibodies to JCV before renal transplantation and did not develop PML until more than 16 months after surgery (Padgett and Walker, 1983).

In those cases of PML that do result from reactivation of persistent JCV infection, when and how does the virus reach the brain? Does it invade the central nervous system during primary infection and persist silently for years until reactivated by immunosuppression, or does it reach the brain, presumably by viremia, following immunosuppression-induced reactivation of persistent infection at a distant site (e.g., the kidney)? Analogy with mouse polyomavirus infection, in which virus does reach the brain during primary infection and persists in some animals, as well as the absence of JCV or JCV DNA from organs other than the brain and kidney in most adult cases of PML examined (Grinnell et al., 1983a) favor reactivation of virus that has persisted in the brain since primary infection. Furthermore, the development of neutralizing antibody after primary JCV infection, and its presence at normal levels in the serum of patients with PML (Walker and Padgett, 1983a; Willoughby et al., 1980) makes viremic spread to the brain from an extraneural site of JCV reactivation less likely. Although JCV DNA has not yet been detected in normal or diseased brain tissue except in cases of PML (Chesters et al., 1983; Grinnell et al., 1983a; McCance, 1983), the sensitivity of the assays employed (about 0.1 copy of viral DNA per cell) is not sufficient to permit detection if JCV persists in only a very tiny fraction of the cells.

BK Virus. BK virus (BKV) was first isolated in 1971 by Gardner et al. from the urine of a 39-year-old man receiving immunosuppressive therapy following a renal allograft. His urine contained abnormal epithelial cells with basophilic intranuclear inclusions. Electron-microscopic examination revealed papovavirus virions in the nuclei of these inclusion-bearing cells, as well as extracellular virions in the urine. Papovavirus virions were also detected in the nuclei of epithelial cells bordering the lumen of the donor ureter after its removal because of obstruction. BKV was isolated in the VERO monkey cell line after prolonged incubation, but primary human cells are much more susceptible to BKV than monkey cells, and thus human cells have been used to obtain most subsequent isolates (Padgett and Walker, 1976; Gardner, 1977; Takemoto, 1978; Howley, 1980; Gibson and Gardner, 1983). BKV grows very well in human embryonic kidney, human fetal fibroblast, human fetal brain and newborn human urinary epithelial cell cultures, and produces a CPE like that produced by SV40 in African green monkey kidney (AGMK) cells (Fig. 7). However, even in these human cells, primary isolation of BKV may be difficult and CPE may not appear for a month or more after inoculation. BKV grows more rapidly than JCV but more slowly than SV40 (Howley, 1980; Tooze, 1981).

BKV can transform cultured cells from a variety of species, including hamster, rat, mouse, rabbit, and monkey (Howley, 1980; Tooze, 1981; Howley, 1983a). BKV DNA has also been used to transform rat and hamster cells. These BKV transformed cells are similar to SV40 transformed cells in growth properties, morphology, and social behavior, and they usually induce tumors when inoculated into suitable animals. BKV transformed cells generally contain one or more copies of the viral genome integrated into cellular DNA and express early, but not late, viral genes. Thus they contain intranuclear BKV T antigens but no V antigens or infectious virus. Infectious BKV can be rescued from many BKV transformed cells by co-cultivation and fusion with permissive cells (Tooze, 1981; Howley, 1983a). BKV is also capable of establishing persistent infections in cultures of primary human embryonic kidney and human fetal brain cells (Takemoto et al., 1979; Purchio and Fareed, 1979). These persistently infected cells shed infectious BKV, express BKV T and V antigens, and contain nonintegrated episomal BKV DNA. Such persistently infected cell cultures provide a model for the persistence of BKV in vivo.

Large doses of BKV administered by various routes have produced no recognizable disease or tumors in newborn mice, rats, guinea pigs, or rabbits (Takemoto, 1978). Five newborn rhesus monkeys inoculated intracerebrally and intraperitoneally with large doses of purified BKV remained healthy during a 30-month period of observation, although infection was present, as evidenced by the development of antibodies to both BKV T and V antigens (Takemoto, 1978). BKV is less oncogenic in hamsters than JCV. However, injection of newborn hamsters results in a variety of malignant tumors, depending upon the strain of BKV, the route of inoculation and the dose of virus. These include ependymomas, choroid plexus papillomas, osteosarcomas, fibrosarcomas, and adenocarcinomas (Tooze, 1981; Howley, 1983a). A viable mutant of BKV with a small deletion and insertion in the enhancer region to the "late" side of the replication origin (Fig. 2) induces malignant insulinomas, a type of tumor not caused by wild-type BKV (Uchida et al., 1979; Watanabe et al., 1979). This appears to be another example of the importance of enhancer sequences in determining virus host range and tissue tropism.

BKV is identical in size, structure, and genome organization to other members of the polyomavirus genus. The BKV genome shares more than 70 per cent of its nucleotide sequences with the genomes of SV40 and JCV, differing markedly only in the enhancer sequences to the "late" side of the replication origin. Like SV40 and JCV, BKV has 3 capsid proteins and induces a large T and a small T protein, which can be detected in the nuclei of cells infected or transformed by BKV. The BKV T antigens and capsid proteins share 75 to 80 per cent amino acid sequence homology with the corresponding proteins of SV40 (Soeda et al., 1980; Howley, 1980; Tooze, 1981). In fact, early BKV gene products can substitute functionally for those of SV40. For example, BKV can complement an early temperature-sensitive mutant of SV40 (TsA58), allowing it to replicate at the nonpermissive temperature (Mason and Takemoto, 1976). Moreover, like SV40, the early region of the BKV genome can provide the "helper" function required to enable human adenovirus 2 to replicate in primary African green monkey kidney cells. BKV is also a hemagglutinating virus with a surface hemagglutinin similar to that of JCV and mouse polyomavirus; BKV agglutinates human, chicken, and guinea pig erythrocytes at 4°C (Padgett and Walker, 1976) and hemagglutination-inhibition tests are widely used to measure antiviral antibodies.

Since 1971, a number of investigators have isolated and identified BKV in the urine of renal and bone marrow allograft recipients, children and adults receiving chemotherapy for malignancies, and children with congenital immunologic disorders, including severe combined immunodeficiency, primary deficiences in antibody production, and Wiskott-Aldrich syndrome (Padgett and Walker, 1976; Gardner, 1977; Takemoto, 1978; Hogan et al., 1980a; O'Reilly et al., 1981; Rziha et al., 1981; Hogan et al., 1983; Gibson and Gardner, 1983). BKV has also been found in the urine in a small number of immunologically competent individuals and in 1 to 2 per cent of healthy pregnant women (Coleman et al., 1980; Gibson and Gardner, 1983). In the majority of these individuals, urinary excretion of BKV does not represent primary infection. Rather, it is a manifestation of the reactivation of latent BKV infection in the kidneys. Nonintegrated BKV DNA can be detected in isolated foci of cells in the kidneys of more than 50 per cent of the adult population (Heritage et al., 1981: Chesters et al., 1983). Most primary BKV infections occur in childhood. They are generally asymptomatic and, in immunocompetent individuals, they are virtually always benign and self-limited. That this may not be true in severely immunocompromised patients is suggested by the recent report of acute tubulo-interstitial nephritis and massive BKV viruria in a six-year-old child with congenital dysgammaglobulinemia (Rosen et al., 1983). Extensive BKV infection of the kidneys, as well as spread of virus to other organs, was clearly documented in this ultimately fatal infection. BKV reactivation has been associated with ureteral stricture in some renal allograft recipients, and with transient mild disturbances in hepatic function in some bone marrow transplant recipients.

In spite of the oncogenic capacity of BKV in hamsters and its long-term persistence in the human urinary tract, BKV does not appear to be etiologically associated with human malignancies (Israel et al., 1978; Shah et al., 1978; Greenlee et al., 1978; Howley, 1980 and 1983a; Johnson, 1983).

AS Virus (ASV). A new human polyomavirus (ASV) has recently been isolated, together with JCV, from the urine of a healthy pregnant woman in England (Gibson and Gardner, 1983). Although ASV is a hemagglutinating virus with in vitro growth properties that resemble those of BKV, it is distinct from both JCV and BKV in its serologic reactions and its restriction endonuclease cleavage pattern.

Lymphotropic Papovavirus (LPV). A new member of the polyomavirus genus was recently isolated from a B-lymphoblastoid cell line derived from an African green monkey (zur Hausen and Gissman, 1979). The virus has a very narrow host range, growing only in certain continuous lines of monkey and human B-lymphoblasts (Brade et al., 1981; Takemoto et al., 1982). This virus, which will not even replicate in mitogen-stimulated primary lymphocyte cultures, has been designated as African green monkey lymphotropic papovavirus (AGM-LPV or LPV). The structure and biochemical properties of LPV are typical of members of the polyomavirus genus, and the restriction endonuclease map of its genome is colinear with that of SV40 and BKV. However, homology with SV40 DNA can only be detected by hybridization at very low stringency (Tm-50°C). No homology is detected at intermediate stringency (Tm-36°C), conditions under which the DNAs of SV40, BKV, and JCV show extensive homology with each other throughout the early and late regions of the genome (Kanda et al., 1983). LPV, like other members of the polyomavirus genus, specifies three capsid proteins and a large T protein (Segawa and Takemoto, 1983). Monospecific antisera to purified JCV, BKV, SV40 and mouse polyomavirus all fail to react with LPV-infected lymphoblasts, and antisera to JCV, BKV, SV40 and mouse polyomavirus T antigens are also nonreactive (Takemoto and Segawa, 1983). LPV does possess the genus-specific antigenic determinant on its major capsid protein, but this is not exposed on intact virions. In limited studies, LPV has not yet been shown to induce tumors in vivo or to transform any of a variety of primate and rodent cells in vitro.

Antigenic Relationships

Viron Antigens. Hyperimmune rabbit antisera to SV40, BKV, JCV, and ASV all show minor reciprocal cross-reactions at low dilutions. Neutralization and FA staining appear to be the most sensitive techniques for detecting these cross-reacting virion antigens. There is a genus-specific antigenic determinant on the major capsid protein, VP-1, which is shared by all members of the polyomavirus genus, but it is not exposed on intact virions.

Nonvirion Antigens. Like SV40, BKV, JCV, ASV and LPV induce T antigens that are detectable by FA staining in the nuclei of acutely infected and transformed cells. Hamsters bearing tumors induced by these viruses develop anti-T antibodies (Padgett and Walker, 1976; Takemoto, 1978, Dougherty, 1976; Howley, 1980; Takemoto and Segawa, 1983). The T antigens induced by SV40, JCV and BKV have been shown to be immunologically similar (Padgett and Walker, 1976; Takemoto, 1978; Dougherty, 1976; Howley, 1980; Tooze, 1981). This is not unexpected, because they have some, but not all, of their methionine-tryptic peptides in common and have approximately 75 per cent amino acid sequence homology. The T antigen of LPV does not appear to be immunologically related to the T antigens of SV40, BKV, JCV, or mouse polyomavirus.

IMMUNITY. The human polyomaviruses are well-adapted parasites with very little virulence for their natural hosts. Primary infection normally induces virus-specific humoral and cell-mediated immunity, and in the immunocompetent host, neither the primary infection nor the persistent renal infection that follows appear to cause discernable disease. With both JCV and BKV, pregnancy and immunosuppression frequently result in recrudescence of the persistent renal infection, as evidenced by viruria and/or a rise in serum antibody titer (Coleman et al., 1980; Hogan et al., 1980a; O'Reilly et al., 1981; Hogan et al., 1983; Andrews et al., 1983). However, this is rarely associated with disease or with evidence of viremic spread to other organs, probably because most of these individuals have virus-neutralizing antibodies in their serum before reactivation.

Although relatively few patients with PML have been thoroughly studied, circumstantial evidence indicates that it is a deficiency in cellular immunity that determines susceptibility to the disease. When immune responses have been examined in patients with PML, humoral responses and antibody levels have been variable, but rarely profoundly depressed. Cell-mediated immunity has been consistently impaired (Walker and Padgett, 1983a and references therein). The most extensive analysis of immunologic function in PML is that of Willoughby et al. (1980) who studied seven patients with the disease. All exhibited a general impairment in cell-mediated immunity, as evidenced by a reduction in their lymphoproliferative response to mitogens, although their mitogen-induced production of lymphokines (as measured by production of leukocyte migration inhibitory factor, LIF) was relatively normal. Cell-mediated immunity to JCV, assessed by LIF production, was absent in all patients with PML despite the presence of relatively normal levels of serum antibody to JCV. This contrasted with positive LIF responses to JCV in all seropositive normal individuals and patients with other diseases. The specificity of the defect was indicated by the observation that three PML patients, although lacking LIF production in response to JCV, had a normal LIF response to varicella-zoster virus. Reactivation of persistent BKV infection is similarly associated with impaired cell-mediated immunity.

The prevalence of serum antibody to JCV, which would limit viremic spread to the brain from extraneural sites of virus replication, may explain the rarity of PML, even in those patients with prolonged and severe impairment of cellular immunity in whom reactivation of renal infection and viruria are common. The importance of antibody is also suggested by the apparent absence of transplacental transmission of JCV and BKV to the fetus when these viruses are reactivated in the kidney and shed in the urine during pregnancy (Coleman et al., 1980; Shah et al., 1980; Daniel et al., 1981; Andrews et al., 1983), by the greater frequency of active JCV and BKV infections in seronegative than seropositive recipients of renal allografts from seropositive donors (Andrews et al., 1982 and 1983), and by the fact that widespread visceral dissemination of JCV and BKV have only been observed in patients with defects in both humoral and cellular immunity (Grinnell et al., 1983a; Rosen et al, 1983; Walker and Padgett, 1983a).

EPIDEMIOLOGY. The human polyomaviruses appear to be worldwide in distribution, infecting most normal persons during childhood or adolescence and remaining latent in healthy adults. Since the human polyomaviruses are difficult to isolate, much of the available information about their epidemiology has come from serologic studies. The hemagglutination-inhibition (HI) test has been the technique most frequently employed to detect and quantitate antibodies to these viruses. It is rapid and relatively easy to perform, and HI titers correlate well with those obtained with virus neutralization assays.

JCV. Serologic studies indicate that JCV infection is ubiquitous throughout the world, except for a few small and isolated populations (Brown et al., 1975; Padgett and Walker, 1976; Gardner, 1977; Walker and Padgett 1983a and 1983b). Infection is most frequently acquired in childhood, and HI antibodies to JCV are found in 60 to 65 per cent of children aged 10 to 14 years. Primary infections are less frequent thereafter, but acquisition of antibody continues well into middle age, by which time 70 to 75 per cent of persons of both sexes have serum antibodies to the virus. There is little information about the route(s) of transmission or the characteristics of the primary infection, but the rapid acquisition of antibodies during childhood suggests efficient child-to-child transmission. Excretion in the urine or from the respiratory tract, and infection via the oral or respiratory route seems likely in view of the epidemiology of other polyomaviruses, such as mouse polyomavirus and SV40. However, such transmission has yet to be demonstrated in normal children. Although probably asymptomatic in most cases, the primary infection must progress to a viremia to account for the distribution of JCV to the kidneys and brain.

Serologic evidence of JCV infection and virus shedding

in the urine are common in immunosuppressed patients and pregnant women. Twelve to 30 per cent of renal allograft recipients develop serologic evidence of JCV infection, and JCV viruria has been observed in nearly 20 per cent (Hogan et al., 1980a and 1980b; Andrews et al., 1983; Walker and Padgett, 1983b). At least half of these appear to be primary JCV infections. Comparable observations have been made in immunosuppressed patients with malignancies (Hogan et al., 1983). Although the source of virus in most of these primary JCV infections is obscure, recent evidence implicates the transplanted kidney in at least some renal transplant recipients; seronegative renal transplant recipients are twice as likely to acquire JCV infection if the kidney donor is seropositive than if the donor is seronegative (Andrews et al., 1982 and 1983).

Three to 15 per cent of pregnant women show serologic evidence of active JCV infection during pregnancy, and at least 2 per cent shed virus in their urine, especially during the third trimester (Coleman et al., 1980; Daniel et al., 1981; Andrews et al., 1983). However, in contrast to organ allograft recipients and immunosuppressed patients with malignancies, none of the JCV infections observed in pregnant women have been primary infections. The absence of primary JCV infections in the pregnant women studied may explain the absence of any evidence of transplacental transmission and congenital infection with JCV (Andrews et al., 1983; Walker and Padgett, 1983b). In the mouse, congenital infection is only observed when primary polyomavirus infection occurs during pregnancy; it does not occur in the course of reactivation (McCance and Mims, 1977 and 1979). Except for PML, no identifiable disease has been clearly associated with either primary or recrudescent JCV infections in normal individuals, pregnant women or immunosuppressed patients.

Restriction endonuclease analysis has made it possible to characterize each isolate of JCV, and the application of this technique to JCV DNA isolated from brain tissue of patients with PML has provided data suggesting that there are two subtypes of JCV circulating in humans (Grinnell et al., 1983b). Padgett and Walker have recently observed an isolate (MAD-11) that is serologically distinguishable from the prototype strain and from most other isolates (Padgett and Walker, 1983). While these differences provide additional epidemiologic tools, their biologic significance remains to be determined.

The highly restricted host range of JCV makes a nonhuman reservoir of infection very unlikely. Furthermore, Padgett et al. (Padgett et al., 1977b) examined sera from a wide variety of animals for antibody to JCV and found that no species other than man had antibody to this virus. Thus, JCV appears to be a strictly human virus.

BKV. Serologic surveys indicate that BKV infection is common throughout the world; in fact BKV is even more ubiquitous than JCV (Brown et al., 1975; Gardner, 1977; Walker and Padgett, 1983b). BKV infection is most frequently acquired in childhood and occurs at an earlier age than JCV infection; thus HI antibody to BKV is found in 70 to 80 per cent of children by age 6 years and reaches its maximum prevalence of more than 80 per cent by early adolescence. As in the case of JCV, there is little information about the route(s) of BKV transmission or the nature of the primary infection. However, the observation of seroconversions to BKV in children with acute upper respiratory tract disease, the isolation of BKV from the urine in one of these children, and the detection of nonintegrated BKV DNA in tonsillar tissue from 5 of 12 children with recurrent upper respiratory tract infections (Goudsmit et al., 1982) suggests that BKV may cause acute upper respiratory infections in children and spread in early childhood by the respiratory route. In any case, like JCV, primary BKV infection must progress to a viremia to account for the distribution of BKV to the kidneys.

As in the case of JCV, serologic evidence of BKV infection and viruria are common in immunosuppressed patients and pregnant women. Twenty to 40 per cent of organ allograft recipients develop serologic evidence of BKV infection and up to one-third may have viruria (Lecatsas et al., 1973; Hogan et al., 1980a and 1980b; O'Reilly, et al., 1981; Andrews et al, 1983; Walker and Padgett, 1983b). Comparable observations have been made in immunosuppressed patients with malignancies (Hogan et al, 1983). In contrast to JCV, the majority of these BKV infections are not primary, but represent immunosuppression-induced recrudescence of persistent BKV infection in the kidneys of previously infected seropositive individuals. Although the source of most of the primary BKV infections in these patients remains obscure, it appears to be the transplanted kidney in many renal allograft recipients (Andrews et al., 1982 and 1983). Seronegative recipients of kidneys from seropositive donors have a 43 per cent incidence of primary BKV infection, as compared with a 10 per cent incidence in recipients of kidneys from seronegative donors.

Approximately 5 per cent of pregnant women show serologic evidence of active BKV infection, and some shed BKV in their urine (Coleman et al, 1980; Shah et al, 1980; Andrews et al, 1983; Walker and Padgett, 1983b). Although there have been reports of BKV-specific IgM in umbilical cord sera, the preponderance of data presently available argues against congenital transmission of BKV (Coleman et al., 1980; Shah et al, 1980: Andrews et al., 1983; Walker and Padgett, 1983b and references therein). Since the BKV infections observed in pregnant women have not been primary infections, transmission to the fetus would not be expected (vide supra). Although BKV infection has been associated with an increased frequency of transplant-related complications and ureteral stricture in renal transplant recipients, and with transient disturbances of hepatic function in bone marrow transplant recipients, most instances of recrudescent BKV infection are not associated with identifiable disease.

Analysis of clinical isolates of BKV reveals that the genomes of individual strains differ slightly, primarily as a result of small deletions or alterations in nucleotide sequences in the enhancer region. Several varients of BKV have been isolated that exhibit differences in the restriction endonuclease cleavage patterns of their DNA and in their serologic reactions (Howley, 1980; Gibson and Gardner, 1983). While these differences may occasionally be correlated with differences in biological behavior in cell culture and experimental animals (vide supra), no clinical differences have yet been recognized.

Like JCV, BKV appears to be a strictly human virus. The human population seems to be the natural reservoir for BKV, and there is no evidence that BKV is transmitted to people from animals.

ASV. This newly discovered hemagglutinating human polyomavirus is distinct from both JCV and BKV in its serologic reactions and restriction endonuclease cleavage pattern. Studies of the prevalence of antibody to ASV in England show a distribution similar to that of antibody to

JCV; antibody to ASV is acquired more slowly than antibody to BKV, and only about one-half of adults in England are seropositive (Gibson and Gardner, 1983).

LPV. Serologic studies indicate that infection with LPV, or a closely related virus, is widespread among Old and New World primates. The presence of antibodies that neutralize LPV infectivity in 30 per cent of human sera indicates that humans are also infected with LPV or a closely related virus (Takemoto and Segawa, 1983). However, the putative human LPV has yet to be isolated.

LABORATORY DIAGNOSIS. Primary isolation of the human polyomaviruses is a formidable undertaking. Although primary cultures of several human cell types can be used for the propagation of tissue culture-adapted strains of JCV, only primary human fetal glial (PHFG) cell cultures rich in spongioblasts are suitable for primary isolation of this virus, and CPE may not appear until 1 or 2 months after inoculation (Padgett et al., 1977a; Beckman and Shaw, 1983 and references therein). BKV and ASV can be isolated in primary cultures of human embryonic kidney, human embryonic lung, and newborn urinary epithelial cells, as well as in PHFG cell cultures. However, CPE may not appear until a month or more after inoculation and the possibility that JCV may be present in the material being studied will necessitate the use of PHFG cells in most situations. Thus the isolation of human polyomaviruses requires an enormous investment of time and effort, as well as the use of a cell culture that is not widely available.

Fortunately, tissues and body fluids suspected of containing human polyomaviruses can be examined for virus directly. Tissue sections or cytologic preparations from urine or other body fluids may be fixed and stained with hematoxylin and eosin or Papanicolaou stain and examined by light microscopy for the presence of cells with typical intranuclear inclusion bodies (Hogan et al., 1980b and references therein). These same preparations may be examined by immunofluorescent (FA) or immunoperoxidase staining by using cross-reactive and type-specific antisera to detect and identify viral antigens. The two approaches are complementary and have proven to be both sensitive and specific for the detection of viruria in immunosuppressed patients and pregnant women (Hogan et al., 1980a and 1980b; Coleman et al., 1980). However, it is important when using serologic techniques to employ appropriate controls, including antisera to more than one human polyomavirus. For example, formalin fixation may denature virion proteins, destroying type-specific antigenic determinants and exposing group- or genus-specific antigens (D. L. Walker, personal communication). Thus a formalin fixed specimen may react with antiserum to SV40, even though it is actually infected with JCV. Without proper controls, this can lead to misdiagnosis. The routine use of antisera to several different polyomaviruses will also permit detection of the simultaneous excretion of more than one human polyomavirus, a fairly common occurrence in immunosuppressed patients and pregnant women. Tissue sections, cytologic preparations, and urine or other body fluids may also be examined by electron microscopy in search of polyomavirus virions. When these are observed, they may be identified by using monospecific antisera and immune electron microscopy (Narayan et al., 1973). However, this is more cumbersome and less sensitive than the use of FA staining.

Polyomavirus DNA may be detected in suspect tissues by hybridization with radiolabeled or biotin-labeled nucleic acid probes prepared from prototype viruses. Restriction endonuclease digestion plus Southern blot analysis can then be used to examine the relationship between viral and cellular DNA (Chesters et al., 1983, Grinnell et al., 1983a). The DNA can be extracted from the specimen, or viral DNA can be detected directly in tissue sections or cytologic preparations by in situ hybridization. Viral DNA can also be cloned directly from infected tissues, obviating the need for culture and virus isolation (Rentier-Delrue et al., 1981; Grinnell et al., 1983b). This cloned DNA can then be analyzed by nucleic acid hybridization and restriction endonuclease cleavage.

The HI test has been extensively used to detect and quantitate antibodies to JCV, BKV and ASV in human serum (Walker and Padgett, 1983a and 1983b; Gibson and Gardner, 1983). Despite the problems posed by the presence of nonspecific inhibitors of polyomavirus hemagglutination in serum (Padgett et al., 1977a) and the need for more practical assays for polyomavirus-specific IgM antibodies, the HI test is well suited to serodiagnosis and seroepidemiology. The most pressing need at present is to employ it more widely to define better the natural history of human polyomavirus infections.

PREVENTION AND THERAPY. Except for the etiologic role of JCV in PML, there is no clear evidence linking human polyomavirus infections to human disease. Thus, there is no incentive to develop means (e.g., vaccines) to prevent infection in the general population. It would be theoretically possible to prevent those cases of PML that result from primary JCV infection of immunosuppressed seronegative patients by immunization before immunosuppression (e.g., with a vaccine containing JCV capsid proteins). However, the rarity of PML, even in high-risk patients, makes this approach impractical.

Treatment of PML presents many difficulties. The diagnosis is rarely established until there has been considerable damage to brain tissue. Moreover, many patients with PML are severely and irreversibly immunosuppressed, and in the absence of host resistance even a nontoxic drug capable of inhibiting JCV replication might not be able to eradicate infection in the brain. Thus reduction or elimination of immunosuppression, when possible, is essential in any patient with PML. The recognition that PML is a progressive polyomavirus infection has lead to the use of nucleoside analogs in an attempt to inhibit virus replication. Unfortunately, these therapeutic attempts have involved single cases without controls, and have employed the same drugs that have been used in attempts to treat herpes simplex virus (HSV) encephalitis (Walker and Padgett, 1983a and references therein). Idoxuridine seems to have been ineffective when used in several cases of PML. Vidarabine (adenine arabinoside), which selectively inhibits HSV DNA polymerase, has also been reported to be ineffective in cases of PML. Cytarabine (cytosine arabinoside) has been reported to induce marked improvement in several patients with PML, but has failed in other cases (Walker and Padgett, 1983a and references therein). Since occasional patients with PML undergo spontaneous remission or stabilization (Padgett and Walker, 1983) it is impossible to evaluate the significance of the positive reports. It should also be recognized that while HSV codes for several enzymes involved in the replication of its DNA, including an HSV-specific DNA polymerase and a thymidine kinase, polyomaviruses utilize host-cell enzymes for the transcription and replication of their genomes. Thus, drugs such as vidarabine and acyclovir (acycloguanosine), which selectively inhibit HSV replication because they interact specifically with HSV-coded enzymes, would not be expected to be effective in inhibiting polyomavirus replication.

Interferon, which has been shown to selectively inhibit SV40 replication in cell culture (Oxman and Black, 1966; Oxman and Takemoto, 1969) is another potential candidate for the therapy of PML. Unfortunately, preliminary studies in cell culture by Walker and his colleagues (D. L. Walker, personal communication) suggest that JCV may be relatively resistant to interferon, as are mouse polyomavirus and BKV (Oxman and Takemoto, 1969; Cheeseman et al., 1980). Nevertheless, interferon (perhaps in combination with cytarabine or another inhibitor of polyomavirus DNA replication) appears, at present, to offer the most promise for the treatment of PML.

In spite of the difficulties posed by the sporadic and infrequent occurrence of PML, every effort should be made to initiate multi-hospital placebo-controlled randomized studies to evaluate the therapeutic efficacy of cytarabine, interferon, and combinations of these two agents in biopsy-proven cases of PML. The most promising candidates for such therapeutic trials would be patients receiving immunosuppressive therapy after renal allograft or for various rheumatologic diseases; a reduction in immunosuppressive therapy in conjunction with the administration of antiviral agents would offer the best chance of halting the progression of PML.

PAPILLOMAVIRUSES

The papillomaviruses are widespread in nature and induce benign squamous epithelial tumors (papillomas or warts) in many higher vertebrates, including man (Table 1). Despite the fact that Shope described the first papillomavirus, the cottontail rabbit papillomavirus (CRPV), half a century ago, this group of viruses has remained refractory to study by standard virologic techniques (Shope, 1933). However, the availability of virus-containing papilloma tissue has permitted the extraction of sufficient quantities of virus to allow an analysis of papillomavirus DNA and capsid proteins. Restriction endonuclease mapping and nucleic acid hybridization of papillomavirus DNA, together with immunologic and electrophoretic analysis of papillomavirus proteins, has led to the identification of many new members of the genus. To date, more than two dozen different papillomaviruses have been recognized as the etiologic agents of a variety of cutaneous and mucosal squamous epithelial lesions in humans (Table 2), and there is every indication that the number of human papillomaviruses (HPV) will continue to expand.

VIRUS STRUCTURE AND COMPOSITION. Papillomaviruses are small, nonenveloped, icosahedral DNA viruses that replicate in the nuclei of squamous epithelial cells. Their virions consist of a single molecule of double-stranded circular DNA, approximately 8,000 base pairs in size, enclosed in a spherical protein coat or capsid composed of 72 morphologic subunits or capsomeres. The capsids of papillomaviruses are 52 to 55 nm in diameter and appear to be composed of one major protein that represents 60 to 80 per cent of the total viral protein and has an estimated molecular weight of approximately 55,000 (Gissmann et al., 1977). Within the capsid, the papillomavirus genome appears to be associated with cellular histones.

Each of the 26 different HPV genotypes (Table 2) has been distinguished on the basis of its lack of significant nucleic acid homology with the other types; specifically, each shares less than 50 per cent nucleic acid homology with the other types when assayed under stringent hybridization conditions.

VIRUS REPLICATION AND CELL TRANSFORMATION. The papillomaviruses have not yet been successfully propagated in tissue culture. This failure may be due in part to the fact that papillomavirus-productive functions, including

Table 2. HUMAN PAPILLOMAVIRUS TYPES

Type	Associated Lesion	Reference
HPV-1	Plantar warts	(Favre et al., 1975; Gissmann & zur Hausen, 1976)
HPV-2	Common warts	(Orth et al., 1977)
HPV-3	Flat warts and macular lesions in E.V.[a]	(Orth et al., 1978; Kremsdorf et al., 1983)
HPV-4	Plantar warts	(Gissmann et al., 1977; Heilman et al., 1980)
HPV-5[b]	Macular lesions in E.V.[a]	(Orth et al., 1980; Kremsdorf et al., 1982)
HPV-6	Condyloma acuminata	(De Villiers et al., 1981)
HPV-7	Common warts in meat handlers	(Orth et al., 1981)
HPV-8[b]	Macular lesions in E.V.[a]	(Kremsdorf et al., 1983)
HPV-9	Macular lesions in E.V.[a]	(Kremsdorf et al., 1982)
HPV-10	Flat warts	(Kremsdorf et al., 1983)
HPV-11	Laryngeal papillomas; flat cervical warts	(Gissmann et al., 1983)
HPV-12	Macular lesions in E.V.[a]	(Kremsdorf et al., 1983)
HPV-13	Focal oral epithelial hyperplasia	(Pfister et al., 1983)
HPV-14	Macular lesions in E.V.[a]	(Orth., G., personal communication)
HPV-15	Macular lesions in E.V.[a]	(Orth, G., personal communication)
HPV-16[b]	Bowenoid papulosis; cervical carcinoma	(Durst et al., 1983; Crum et al., 1984)
HPV-17	Macular lesions in E.V.[a]	(Orth, G., personal communication)
HPV-18[b]	Cervical carcinoma	(Boshart, M., Gissmann, L., & zur Hausen, H., personal communication)
HPV-19-26	Macular lesions in E.V.[a]	(Orth, G., personal communication; Pfister, H.; personal communication)

[a]Epidermodysplasia verruciformis
[b]Associated with malignant transformation

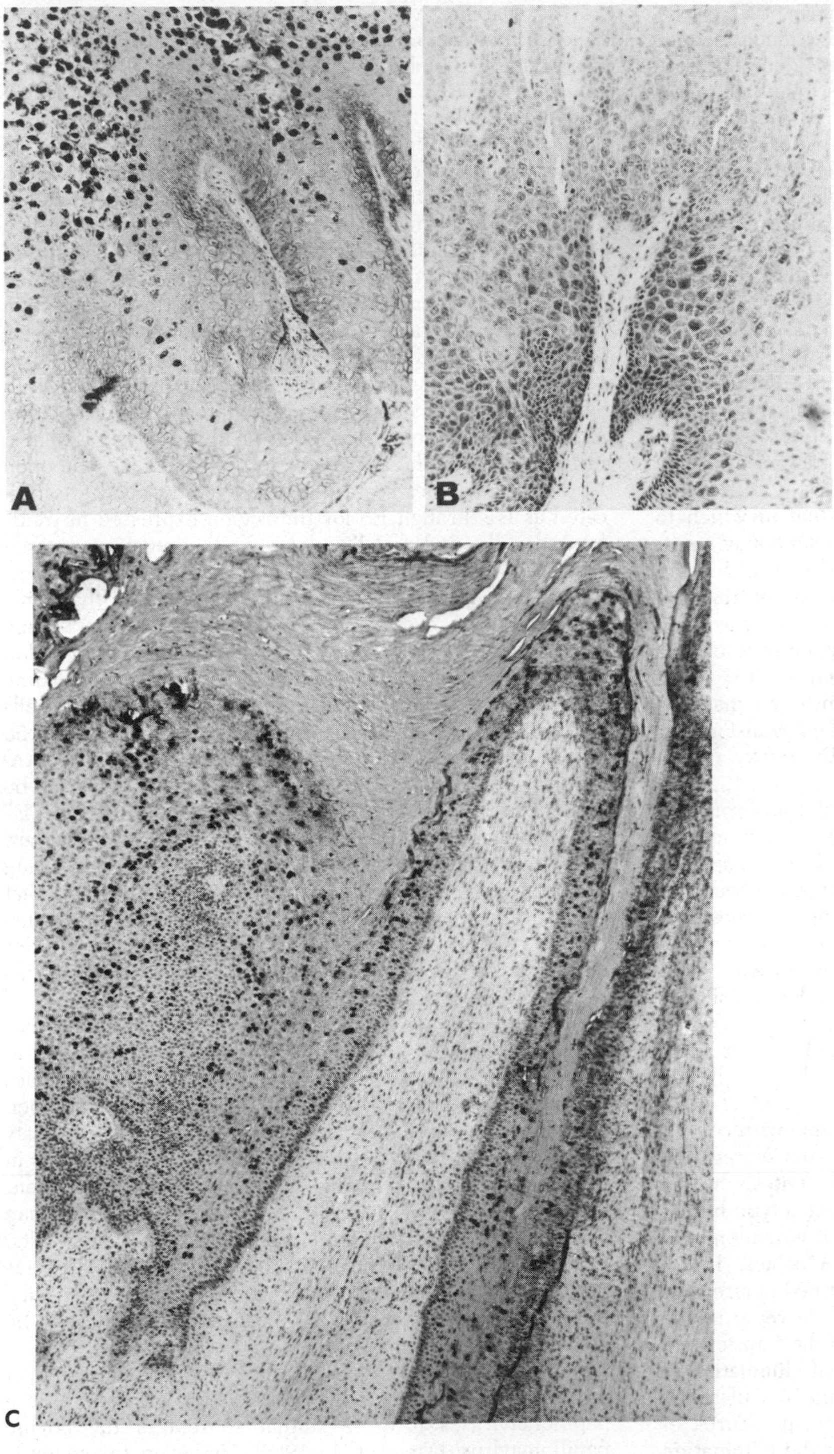

Figure 10. Detection of papillomvirus structural proteins and DNA in papilloma tissue. *A,* Papillomavirus structural proteins in cells in the stratum granulosum of a human plantar wart. Indirect peroxidase-antiperoxidase-DAB staining, using rabbit antiserum to SDS-disrupted HPV virions, which reacts with the genus-specific HPV capsid antigen. The black nuclei in the stratum granulosum are positive for large amounts of HPV capsid antigen. *B,* Normal rabbit serum control. The tissue was fixed in neutral formalin and counterstained with Mayer's hematoxylin. *C,* In situ hybridization to detect papillomavirus DNA. Radioautograph of a section of a bovine fibropapilloma hybridized with a radiolabeled BPV-1 DNA probe. The black nuclei in the outer portion of the stratum spinosum and in the stratum granulosum are positive for large amounts of BPV-1 DNA, indicating vegetative viral DNA synthesis. Cells in the basal layer of the epidermis and in the dermis are negative. (*A* and *B* reproduced with permission from Howley, P. M.: Search for evidence of possible association with human cancer. In Viruses Associated with Human Cancer [ed. Phillips, L. A.]. Marcel Dekker, New York, 1983, pp. 253–306. *B* Reproduced with permission from Howley, P. M.: The molecular biology of papillomavirus transformation. Am J Pathol 113:44, 1983.)

vegetative viral DNA synthesis, synthesis of capsid proteins, and virion assembly, occur only in differentiating squamous epithelial cells. Vegetative viral DNA synthesis has been detected by in situ hybridization in the squamous epithelial cells of papillomas, but only in the cells of the stratum spinosum and the stratum granulosum, not in the basal layer (Fig. 10C). Synthesis of the major capsid protein and assembly of virions has been detected in epidermal cells of the upper stratum spinosum, the stratum granulosum and the stratum corneum (Fig. 10A). To date, attempts to use epidermal cell culture systems that express some differentiated functions for the in vitro replication of papillomaviruses have been unsuccessful.

The lack of a permissive in vitro cell culture system has severely limited our capacity to study the molecular biology of the papillomaviruses. Recently, however, modern recombinant DNA technology has enabled investigators to clone the complete genomes of human papillomaviruses, the Shope rabbit papillomavirus (CRPV), and many of the bovine papillomaviruses into *Escherichia coli,* using the bacterial plasmid vector, pBR322 (Heilman et al., 1980; Howley et al., 1980). This has permitted the standardization of papillomavirus reagents and has provided sufficient quantities of purified papillomavirus DNA to initiate meaningful studies of the molecular biology of these unique viruses.

Certain papillomaviruses are capable of inducing fibroblastic tumors when inoculated into hamsters and are capable of transforming rodent tissue culture cell lines. The most thoroughly studied of the transforming papillomaviruses is bovine papillomavirus type 1 (BPV-1), which causes cutaneous fibropapillomas in cattle. This virus can also induce fibroblastic tumors in hamsters, rabbits and pikas, and is one of the agents associated with a naturally occurring fibroblastic tumor of horses, called equine sarcoid (Lancaster and Olson, 1982). Studies demonstrating the ability of BPV to transform cells in tissue culture date back to 1963 when Black et al. reported the transformation of bovine cells in tissue culture by BPV (Black et al., 1963).

In the absence of a tissue culture system in which to study the full replicative cycle of the papillomaviruses, papillomavirus-induced transformation of susceptible rodent cells has provided a biologic system permitting the study of at least some aspects of papillomavirus gene expression and virus-cell interactions. Bovine papillomavirus has been the most thoroughly studied for this transforming property, and it has been demonstrated that molecularly cloned BPV DNA is also capable of transforming mouse and rat cells in tissue culture (Dvoretzky et al., 1980; Howley et al., 1980).

In contrast to other well-studied viral transformation systems, including those of the polyomaviruses described earlier in this chapter, papillomavirus-induced neoplastic transformation and tumorigenicity are not associated with integration of the viral genome into the host chromosome. Instead, the viral genome or the segment of the genome that specifies the malignant phenotype is present as an extrachromosomal element, consisting of molecules of double-stranded, closed, circular DNA (Law et al., 1981). The extrachromosomal viral genome (or plasmid) is present in multiple copies (10 to 200 copies per diploid host cell) and the copy number in the cells of any individual BPV transformed cell line remains relatively stable with continued passage. It is not yet known whether the segregation of this extrachromosomal viral DNA during mitosis, which insures the inheritance of the malignant phenotype by the daughter cells, is controlled, or whether it is random and effectively insured by the multiple DNA copies. It has been shown that treatment of BPV transformed mouse cells with mouse interferon leads to a gradual decrease in the number of plasmid copies of BPV DNA in the transformed cells, and can eventually result in the total elimination of the viral genome. Cells thus "cured" of their BPV plasmids regain the normal (nontransformed) phenotype (Turek et al., 1982). It is this observation, i.e., that the elimination of the BPV genome from transformed cells by interferon results in the reversion of the cells to the normal phenotype, which has established that the continued presence of the viral genome (and presumably its expression) is required to maintain papillomavirus transformation.

The molecular cloning of papillomavirus genomes has also permitted a systematic evaluation of their genomic organization. To date, the genomes of four papillomaviruses have been completely sequenced: the BPV-1 genome (Chen et al., 1982), the HPV-1 genome (Danos et al., 1982), the HPV-6B genome (Schwarz et al., 1983), and the CRPV genome (Yaniv et al., unpublished information). Since BPV transformation of rodent cells has been unique in providing a biologic system with which to study papillomaviruses, BPV is the prototype for the study of the molecular biology of members of the genus. The organization of the BPV-1 genome has been deduced from the analysis of its nucleotide sequence, in conjunction with transcriptional data (Heilman et al., 1982; Engel et al., 1983). All of the major open reading frames greater than 380 bases in length are located on the same DNA strand (Fig. 11). The region transcribed in BPV-1 transformed cells contains open reading frames in all three translation frames, whereas the region transcribed only in productively infected bovine fibropapillomas is characterized by two large open reading frames (L1 and L2) partitioned by a single translation stop codon. A schematic representation of the BPV-1 genome derived from this analysis is shown in Figure 11. In the upper portion of the figure, the open reading frames located on the transcribed strand are indicated as E1 through E8 for the region expressed in transformed cells, and as L1 and L2 for the region expressed only in productively infected warts. The black lines superimposed on these bars indicate the positions of the translation initiation codon, ATG. The single slash separating L1 and L2 indicates the position of the single stop codon located in frame, which partitions the two open reading frames. The five transcripts detected in transformed cells by Heilman et al. (1982) are those with arrowheads at 0.53 map units. There is a polyadenylation site (AATAAA) located at base 4180. Promoter elements appear to be present in a 1000 base pair segment located 5′ to the "E" open reading frames, and potential TATAAA sequences are located at base 7108 and at base 58 in this noncoding segment. From the sequence analysis, it seems likely that the mRNA species that have been detected in BPV transformed cells are generated by differential splicing. Leader sequences for these RNAs have also been mapped to this region (Ahola et al., 1983).

Multiple BPV-1-specific polyadenylated RNA species have been identified in bovine fibropapillomas induced in vivo by BPV-1 (Engel et al., 1983). All of the RNA species are transcribed from the DNA strand containing the open reading frames; each of the five RNA species previously identified in BPV-1 transformed cells are also present in productively infected bovine fibropapillomas. In addition, four other RNA species with 3′ co-termini at 0.90 map units (Fig. 11) are found in productively infected warts, but not in BPV-1 transformed cells. Like the RNA species with their 3′ co-termini at 0.53 map units, the wart specific transcripts with co-termini at 0.90 map units appear to be generated by differential splicing.

From the sequence data that have been accumulated, it is clear that the genomic organization of each of the papillomaviruses is quite similar to that of the bovine papillomavirus (Danos et al., 1982). However, the genomic organization of the papillomaviruses is entirely different from that of the polyomaviruses. In addition, at the level of third base mismatch, there is no significant sequence homology between the coding and noncoding regions of the papillomaviruses and the polyomaviruses. Thus there is every indication that these two groups of viruses are evolutionarily unrelated.

PATHOGENIC PROPERTIES AND ANTIGENIC RELATIONSHIPS. Until the mid-1970's, it was generally believed that there was a single HPV and that the clinical and

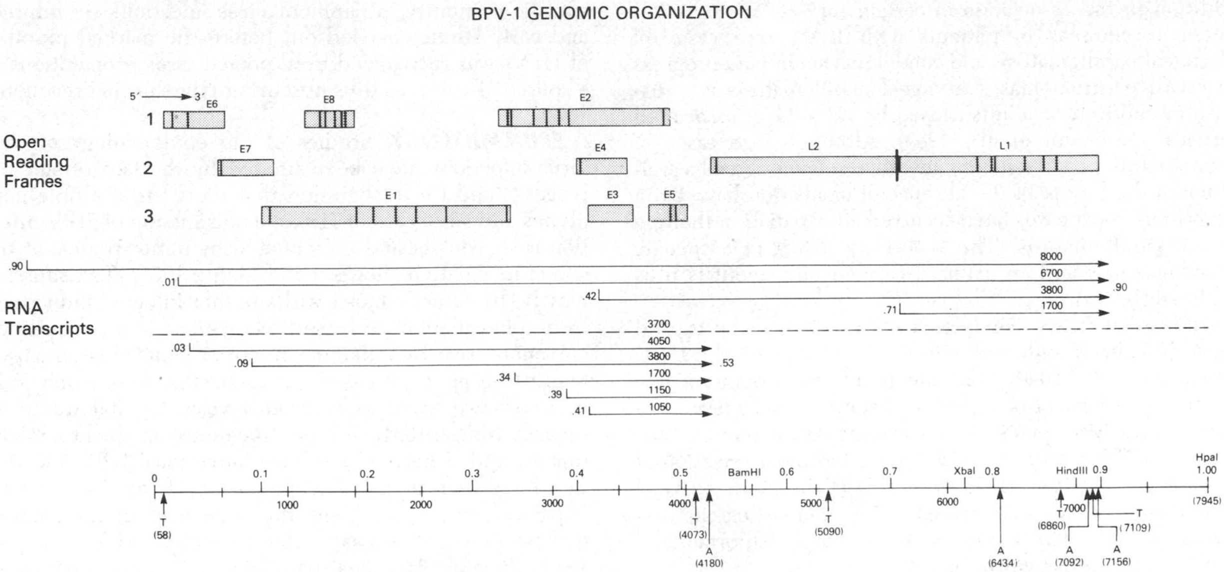

Figure 11. Genomic organization of a papillomavirus: translational and transcriptional map of the full molecule (7945 base pairs) of BPV-1 DNA. The genome is marked off in map units and bases at the bottom of the figure, beginning with the unique *Hpa* site (0/1.00). Potential adenylation sites (A) and potential TATA promoter elements (T) are indicated. The bodies of the BPV-1 specific polyadenylated transcripts and their sizes in bases are drawn immediately above. The horizontal stippled bars represent open reading frames and thus potential regions encoding BPV-1 specific proteins in each of the three translation frames. The vertical black lines mark the positions of inframe translation initiation codons, ATG. Open reading frames within the transforming region have been designated E1 to E8. The two open reading frames within the region not required for transformation, L1 and L2, are partitioned by a single stop codon. (Modified from Engel et al., 1983.)

pathologic differences among warty viral lesions were a function of the nature of the squamous epithelium at the site of the lesion. Currently, however, with the multitude of different HPVs that have already been recognized, and with the likelihood that additional HPVs will be described in the future, it is apparent that distinct HPVs can cause distinct pathologic lesions. The human papillomaviruses listed in Table 2 have been associated with a variety of benign papillomatous lesions of the skin and squamous mucosa, including common and plantar warts, flat warts, anal and genital condyloma acuminata, cervical flat warts, oral papillomas, bowenoid papulosis, juvenile laryngeal papillomas, and macular pityriasis-like lesions in patients with epidermodysplasia verruciformis (E.V.). Although histologically, different types of human warts can be readily distinguished, they share certain features. There is thickening of the epidermis with hyperplasia and acanthosis in the stratum spinosum, parakeratosis with kerato-hyalin granules in the stratum granulosum, and at least some degree of hyperkeratosis. Basophilic intranuclear inclusion bodies can often be seen in the upper stratum spinosum and stratum granulosum, and the nuclei of these cells often contain virions. Virus aggregates may also be seen in cells in the stratum corneum. The basement membrane is intact and the basal layer of the epidermis is histologically normal. Interestingly, different lesions vary in the amount of virus that they contain. Plantar warts, for instance, contain large amounts of virus, whereas laryngeal papillomas and condyloma acuminata usually contain very little virus.

Certain papillomavirus-induced lesions may progress to squamous cell carcinomas. Viruses associated with such a malignant progression include the Shope papillomavirus (CRPV), the bovine alimentary tract papillomavirus, and some of the HPVs associated with the flat macular lesions in epidermodysplasia verruciformis and with human genital papillomavirus-induced lesions (Rous and Beard, 1935; Jarrett et al., 1978; Orth et al., 1980; Durst et al., 1983; Syrjanen, 1984). One characteristic of the progression of a benign papillomavirus-induced lesion to a carcinoma is that this is usually associated with synergistic external carcinogenic factors. Squamous cell carcinomas in cottontail rabbits develop in Shope papillomas painted with tar or methylcholanthrene. Bovine alimentary tract carcinomas associated with esophageal papillomatosis occur in cattle that feed on bracken fern, which is known to contain a mitogenic substance. Similarly, the cutaneous carcinomas in patients with epidermodysplasia verruciformis (E.V.), which develop in the virus-associated pityriasis-like macular lesions, usually occur in areas exposed to UV light (Jablonska et al., 1972).

E.V. is a rare, life-long disease that usually begins in infancy or childhood and is characterized by disseminated polymorphic skin lesions that resemble flat warts or appear as reddish macules, sometimes referred to as "pityriasis-like lesions." One remarkable feature of E.V. is the occurrence of skin carcinomas, both of the in situ and of the invasive squamous cell types, in approximately one-third of the patients. Although HPVs have been found associated with the benign flat warts and the pityriasis-like lesions of patients with E.V. (see Table 2), no virus particles are found associated with the carcinomas (Orth et al., 1980; Kremsdorf et al., 1982). However, HPV DNA has been detected in both primary and metastatic malignant lesions, in the form of nonintegrated plasmids (Orth et al., 1980; Ostrow et al., 1982).

Most HPV-associated lesions, including common, plantar and flat warts, are entirely benign and are not clinically associated with malignant transformation. However, several HPVs are occasionally associated with subsequent development into squamous cell carcinomas (Syrjanen, 1984). In addition to the association of certain rare HPVs and cutaneous carcinomas in patients with E.V., rare cases of laryngeal papillomatosis and condyloma acuminata progress to invasive carcinomas. Laryngeal papillomatosis is a disease in children or adults caused by HPV-11 or associated viruses (Gissmann et al., 1983). Although rare cases of spontaneous progression to invasive squamous cell carcinoma of the larynx in the absence of irradiation have been described, most cases have occurred after radiation therapy of the papillomatosis. The synergistic effect of a specific papillomavirus and an external carcinogenic agent is thus again suggested.

Anogenital warts (condyloma acuminata) can be caused by a number of different HPVs (De Villiers et al., 1981; Krzyzek et al., 1980), and the literature contains a few anecdotal reports of progression of some of these lesions to locally invasive squamous cell carcinomas. Recently, zur Hausen and his colleagues have reported the association of two specific HPVs, HPV-16 and HPV-18, with cervical carcinomas, vulvar carcinomas, and penile carcinomas (Durst et al., 1983). However, the etiologic importance of this association has yet to be established.

In recent years an additional papillomavirus-associated entity has been recognized, which had previously been interpreted as mild to moderate cervical dysplasia in women. These lesions have been referred to by a variety of terms including cervical flat warts and cervical intraepithelial neoplasia (CIN) (Meisels et al., 1977 and 1982; Read et al., 1980; Laverty et al., 1978). These lesions are associated with koilocytotic atypia and dyskeratosis, which is recognizable on smears stained by the Papanicolaou method, and in tissue sections from cervical biopsies (Meisels et al., 1982). Koilocytes are large round cells in the upper layers of the lesion that have a large area of perinuclear cavitation surrounded by a ring of dense amphophilic cytoplasm. The nuclei of koilocytes often contain papillomavirus virions. HPV-specific antigens have been detected with a cross-reactive genus-specific antiserum in 50 per cent of the cervical lesions interpreted as dysplasia (Kurman et al., 1981). Papillomavirus DNA sequences can be demonstrated in even a higher proportion of these lesions. The association of these lesions with HPV infection is of particular significance because of the clear epidemiologic association of cervical dysplasia with carcinoma in situ and invasive cervical carcinoma (Kessler, 1976, Reid et al., 1982). The presence of HPV-16 has been associated with the presence of abnormal mitotic figures in cervical flat warts (Crum et al., 1984), but the etiologic role, if any, of specific HPVs in this progression has yet to be elucidated.

IMMUNITY. Immunity to papillomavirus infection is mediated by humoral as well as cellular mechanisms. Wart infections are common in children and young adults, and usually regress spontaneously after variable periods. Regression is often total and simultaneous in patients with multiple warts, and is usually associated with mononuclear cell infiltration of the upper dermis and involved epidermis. Immunosuppressed patients, such as those treated with immunosuppressive drugs after renal transplantation, often develop multiple non-regressing warts (Spencer and Andersen, 1979). Patients with cell-mediated immune deficiencies secondary to Hodgkin's disease or chronic lymphocytic leukemia are more prone to develop HPV infections than patients with humoral immune deficiencies (Pfister, 1983). Studies dealing with the role of HPV-specific immunity in papillomavirus infections are limited, and early studies carried out before the marked plurality of HPVs was recognized used pooled virus preparations as a source of antigen, thus obscuring type-specific reactions.

EPIDEMIOLOGY. Studies of the epidemiology of wart virus infections have been limited by the lack of suitable reagents and the recognition that there are multiple genotypes and serotypes of HPVs. Transmission of HPV infection is by contact and is facilitated by minor trauma at the site of inoculation (Rowson and Mahy, 1967). Transmission may be by direct contact with another infected individual, by autoinoculation, or by indirect contact (e.g., acquisition of plantar warts by walking barefoot). The incubation period before the appearance of a recognizable lesion may vary from two weeks to more than a year. Genital warts are sexually transmitted, and their incidence appears to exceed that of genital herpes. Evidence of cervical HPV infection can be found in 1 to 2 per cent of routine cervical Papanicolaou smears, and the incidence of infection is highest in young sexually active women (Meisels et al., 1982). Juvenile laryngeal papillomatosis appears to result, at least in many cases, from infection acquired during delivery through an HPV infected birth canal.

Molecular cloning of HPV DNAs provides nucleic acid hybridization reagents that could be used in epidemiologic studies. More useful will be synthetically prepared antigenic reagents that can be synthesized in bacteria as fusion proteins or in vitro as oligopeptides. Such reagents, which can be either group-specific or type-specific, should eventually permit detailed seroepidemiologic studies of HPV infections.

DIAGNOSIS. Most papillomavirus infections are clinically recognizable and are seldom misdiagnosed. Histologic examination can establish the diagnosis in cases of doubt. Immunologic identification of the genus-specific capsid antigen (Jensen et al., 1980; Lack et al., 1980) in the differentiated epithelial cells of a suspected lesion establishes its papillomavirus etiology (Fig. 10A). However, this antigen may be undetectable in 25 per cent or more of HPV-induced lesions. Immunologic diagnosis of the specific HPV type will certainly be possible when type-specific antisera are available, perhaps elicited by synthetic antigens. In situ hybridization with radiolabeled or biotinylated nucleic acid probes (Fig. 10C) provides another approach to specific diagnosis.

PREVENTION AND THERAPY. Most warts regress spontaneously. However, patients will seek treatment for cosmetic reasons, discomfort, or disability. Pregnant women, children with recurrent warts, immunosuppressed patients, and patients with epidermodysplasia verruciformis pose difficult therapeutic problems. At present, there is no generally effective treatment for all warts. In fact, the efficacy of any form of therapy may be difficult to assess without well-controlled studies, because of the tendency for spontaneous regression. Caustic agents are frequently applied directly to the lesions, e.g., podophyllin for genital warts and salicylic acid (often together with curettage) for plantar warts and common warts. Cryotherapy with liquid nitrogen or "dry ice" is often used for genital warts and heavily keratinized skin warts. Since warts generally regress spontaneously, every effort should be made to avoid scarring. Surgical therapy and cautery are utilized when other treatment modalities have failed or are not applicable (e.g., juvenile laryngeal papillomas; malignant condylomata acuminata). However, recurrences are frequent in these situations, and this may be explained by the recent report of HPV DNA in normal appearing tissue adjacent to lesions and in previously involved areas during periods of remission (Steinberg et al., 1983).

The episomal nature of the viral DNA in human papillomas and BPV transformed cells suggests that interferon might be an effective form of therapy for papillomavirus infections. In contrast to cells transformed by members of the polyomavirus genus, in which the integration of the viral DNA into the host cell chromosome renders viral gene expression refractory to interferon (Oxman, 1967), cells transformed by papillomaviruses appear to contain episomal viral genomes that retain their sensitivity to interferon. Since prolonged treatment with interferon can "cure" BPV-transformed cells in vitro (Turek et al., 1982) prolonged administration of interferon might be expected to cure HPV infections in humans. In fact, good clinical responses have been reported when human interferon has been administered to patients with juvenile laryngeal papillomatosis (Haglund et al., 1981), condyloma acuminata (Einhorn et al., 1983; Schonfeld et al., 1984) and extensive cutaneous warts (Pazin et al., 1982). However, lesions often recurred when interferon therapy was discontinued. Though far from conclusive, the results obtained to date are sufficiently encouraging to warrant the initiation of large, well-designed, placebo-controlled clinical trials in immunosuppressed patients with severe and intractable HPV infections. Such trials are now under way.

References

Ahola, H., Stenlung, A., Moreno-Lopez, J., and Petterson, U.: Sequences of bovine papillomavirus type 1 DNA: Functional and evolutionary implications. Nucleic Acids Res 11:2639, 1983.

Anderson, J. L., Martin, R. G., Chang, C., Mora, P. T., and Livingston, D. M.: Nuclear preparations of SV-40. Transformed cells contain tumor-specific transplantation antigen activity. Virology 76:420, 1977.

Andrews, C., Shah, K. V., Rubin R., Hirsch, M.: BK papovavirus infections in renal transplant recipients: contribution of donor kidneys. J Infect Dis 145:276, 1982.

Andrews, C. A., Daniel R. W., and Shah, K. V.: Serologic studies of papovavirus infections in pregnant women and renal transplant recipients. in *Polyomaviruses and Human Neurological Diseases*. (eds. Sever, J. L. and Madden, D. L.) Liss, New York, 1983. Prog Clin Biol Res 105:133.

Astrom, K. E., Mancall, E. L., and Richardson, E. P., Jr.: Progressive multifocal leuko-encephalopathy: A hitherto unrecognized complication of chronic lymphatic leukemia and Hodgkin's disease. Brain 81:93, 1958.

Beckmann, A. M., and Shah, K. V.: Propagation and primary isolation of JCV and BKV in urinary epithelial cell cultures. in *Polymaviruses and Human Neurological Diseases*. (eds. Sever, J. L. and Madden, D. L.) Liss, New York, 1983. Prog Clin Biol Res 105:31.

Beckmann, A. M., Shah, K. V. and Padgett B. L.: Propagation and primary isolation of papovavirus JC in epithelial cells derived from human urine. Infect Immun 38:774, 1982.

Benoist, C., and Chambon, P.: The SV40 early promoter region: sequence requirements in vitro. Nature (London) 290:304, 1981.

Berk, A. J., and Sharp, P. A.: Spliced early mRNAs of simian virus 40. Proc. Natl. Acad. Sci. U.S.A., 75:1274, 1978.

Black, P. H.: The oncogenic DNA viruses. A review of *in vitro* transformation studies. Annu Rev Microbiol 22:391, 1968.

Black, P. H., Hartley, J. W., Rowe, W. P., and Huebner, R. J.: Transformation of bovine tissue culture cells by bovine papilloma virus. Nature 199:1016, 1963.

Brade, L., Vogl, W., Gissmann, L., and zur Hausen, H.: Propagation of B-lymphotropic papovavirus (LPV) in human B-lymphoma cells and characterization of its DNA. Virology 114:228, 1981.

Brown, P., Tsai, T., and Gajdusek, D. C.: Seroepidemiology of human papovaviruses: Discovery of virgin populations and some unusual patterns of antibody prevalence among remote peoples of the world. Am J Epidemiol 102:331, 1975.

Butel, J. S.: Studies with human papilloma virus modeled after known papovavirus systems. J Natl Cancer Inst 48:285, 1972.

Castaigne, P., Rondot, P., Escourolle, R., Dumas, J. L. R., Cathala, F., and Hauw, J. J.: Leucoencephalopathie multifocale progressive et "gliomes" multiples. Rev Neurol 130:379, 1974.

Cavanagh, J. B., Greenbaum, D., Marshall, A. H. E., and Rubinstein, L. J.: Cerebral demyelination associated with disorders of the reticuloendothelial system. Lancet 2:525, 1959.

Chatis, P. A., Holland, C. A., Hartley, J. W., Rowe, W. P., and Hopkins, N.: Role for the 3′ end of the genome in determining disease specificity of Friend and Moloney murine leukemia viruses. Proc Natl Acad Sci USA 80:4408, 1983.

Cheeseman, S. H., Black, P. H., Rubin, R. H., Cantell, K., and Hirsch, M. S.: Interferon and BK papovavirus—clinical and laboratory studies. J Infect Dis 141:157, 1980.

Chen, E. Y., Howley, P. M., Levinson, A. D., and Seeburg, P. H.: The primary structure and genetic organization of the bovine papillomavirus (BPV) type 1 genome. Nature 299:529, 1982.

Chesters, P. M., Heritage, J., and McCance, D. J.: Persistence of DNA sequences of BK virus and JC virus in normal human tissues and in diseased tissues. J Infect Dis 147:676, 1983.

Christiansen, G. T., Landers, T., Griffith, J., and Berg, P.: Characterization of components released by alkali disruption of simian virus 40. J Virol 21:1079, 1977.

Ciuffo, G.: Innesto positivo con filtrato di verruca volgare. Giorn Ital Mal Venereol 48:12, 1907.

Coleman, D. V.: Recent developments in the papovaviruses: the human polyomaviruses (BK virus and JC virus). Recent Adv Clin Virology 2:89–110, 1980.

Coleman, D. V., Wolfendale, M. R., Daniel, R. A., Dhanjal, N. K., Gardner, S. D., Gibson, P. E., and Field, A. M.: A prospective study of human polyomavirus infection in pregnancy. J Infect Dis 142:1, 1980.

Crawford, L. V., Cole, C. N., Smith, A. E., Paucha, E., Tegtmeyer, P., Rundell, K., and Berg, P.: Organization and expression of early genes of simian virus 40. Proc. Natl. Acad. Sci. U.S.A., 75:117, 1978.

Crum, C. P., Ikenberg, H., Richart, R. M., and Gissmann, L.: Human papillomavirus type 16 and early cervical neoplasia. N Engl J Med 310:880, 1984.

Daniel, R., Shah, K., Madden, D., and Stagno, S.: Serological investigation of the possibility of congenital transmission of papovavirus JC. Infect Immun, 33:319, 1981.

Danos, O., Katinka, M., and Yaniv, M.: Human papillomavirus 1a complete DNA sequence: A novel type of genome organization among Papovaviridae. EMBO Journal 1:231, 1982.

Deppert, W.: Simian virus 40 T- and U-antigens: Immunological characterization and localization in different nuclear subfractions of Simian virus 40-transformed cells. J Virol 29:576, 1979.

Deppert, W., and Walter, G.: Domains of Simian virus 40 large T-antigen exposed on the cell surface. Virology 122:56, 1982.

De Villiers, E. M., Gissmann, L., and zur Hausen, H.: Molecular cloning of viral DNA from human genital warts. J Virol 40:932, 1981.

Diacumakos, E. G., and Gershey, E. L.: Uncoating and gene expression of simian virus 40 in CV-1 cell nuclei inoculated by microinjection. J Virol 24:903, 1977.

Dougherty, R. M.: A comparison of human papovavirus T antigens. J Gen Virol 33:61, 1976.

Durst, M., Gissmann, L., Ikenberg, H., and zur Hausen, H.: A papillomavirus DNA from a cervical carcinoma and its prevalence in cancer biopsy samples from different geographic regions. Proc Natl Acad Sci USA 80:3812, 1983.

Dvoretzky, I., Shober, R., and Lowy, D. R.: Focus assay in mouse cells for bovine papilloma virus. Virology 103:369, 1980.

Eckhart, W.: Polyoma T antigens, Adv Cancer Res, 35:1, 1981.

Eckhart, W.: Role of polyoma T antigens in malignant cell transformation. Prog Nucleic Acid Research and Molecular Biology 29:119, 1983.

Eddy, B. E.: Polyoma Virus. in *Virology Monographs*. vol 7. (eds. Gard, S., Hallauer C., and Meyer K. F.) Springer-Verlag, New York, 1969, pp. 1-113.

Eddy, B. E., Borman, G. S., Grubbs, G. E., and Young, R. D.: Identification of the oncogenic substance in rhesus monkey cell cultures as simian virus 40. Virology 17:65, 1962.

Einhorn, N., Ling, P., and Strander, H.: Systemic interferon alpha treatment of human condylomata acuminata. Acta Obstet Gynecol Scand 62:285, 1983.

Enders, J. F.: Cell transformation by viruses as illustrated by the response of human and hamster renal cells to simian virus 40. Harvey Lectures 59:113, 1965.

Engel, L. W., Heilman, C. A., and Howley, P. M.: Transcriptional organization of the bovine papillomavirus type 1. J Virol 47:516, 1983.

Farwell, J. R., Dohrmann, G. J., Marrett, L. D., Meigs, J. W.: Effect of SV40 virus-contaminated polio vaccine on the incidence and type of CNS neoplasms in children: A population-based study. Trans Am Neurol Assoc 104:261, 1979.

Favre, M., Orth, G., Croissant, O., and Yaniv, M.: Human papillomavirus DNA: physical map. Proc Natl Acad Sci USA 72:4810, 1975.

Frisque, R. J.: Nucleotide sequence of the region encompassing the JC virus origin of DNA replication. J Virol 46:170, 1983.

Frisque, R. J., Martin, J. D., Padgett, B. L., and Walker, D. L.: Infectivity of the DNA from four isolates of JC virus. J Virol 32:476, 1979.

Frisque, R. J., Rifkin, D. B., and Walker, D. L.: Transformation of primary hamster brain cells with JC virus and its DNA. J Virol 35:265, 1980.

Gardner, S. D.: New human papovaviruses: Their nature and significance. in *Recent Advances in Clinical Virology.* vol 1. (ed. Waterson, A. P.) Churchill-Livingstone, Edinburgh, 1977, pp. 93–115.

Gardner, S. D., Field, A. M., Coleman, D. V., and Hulme, B.: New human papovavirus (B.K.) isolated from urine after renal transplantation. Lancet 1:1253, 1971.

Gerber, P.: Studies on the transfer of subviral infectivity from SV40-induced hamster cells to indicator cells. Virology 28:501, 1966.

Gibson, P. E., and Gardner, S. D.: Strain differences and some serological observations on several isolates of human polyomaviruses. in *Polyomaviruses and Human Neurological Diseases.* (eds. Sever, J. L., and Madden, D. L.) Liss, New York, 1983. Prog Clin Biol Res, 105:119.

Gissmann, L., and zur Hausen, H.: Human papillomavirus: physical mapping and genetic heterogeneity. Proc Natl Acad Sci USA 73:1310, 1976.

Gissmann, L., Pfister, H., and zur Hausen, H.: Human papillomavirus (HPV). Characterization of four different isolates. Virology 76:569, 1977.

Gissmann, L., Wolnik, L., Ikenberg, H., Koldovsky, U., Schnurch, H. G., and zur Hausen, H.: Human papillomavirus types 6 and 11 DNA sequences in genital and laryngeal papillomas and in some cervical carcinomas. Proc Natl Acad Sci USA 80:560, 1983.

Goudsmit, J., Wertheim-van Dillen, P., van Strien, A., and van der Noorda, J.: The role of BK virus in acute respiratory tract disease and the presence of BKV DNA in tonsils. J Med Virol 10:91, 1982.

Greenlee, J. E., Becker, L. E., Narayan, O., and Johnson, R. T.: Failure to demonstrate papovavirus tumor antigen in human cerebral neoplasms. Ann Neurol 3:479, 1978.

Griffin, B. E. and Dilworth, S. M.: Polyoma virus—An overview of its unique properties. Adv Cancer Res 39:183, 1983.

Grinnell, B. W., Martin, J. D., Padgett, B. L., and Walker, D. L: Is progressive multifocal leukoencephalopathy a chronic disease because of defective interfering particles or temperature sensitive mutants of JC virus? J Virol 43:1143, 1982.

Grinnell, B. W., Padgett, B. L., and Walker, D. L.: Distribution of nonintegrated DNA from JC papovavirus in organs of patients with progressive multifocal leukoencephalopathy. J Infect Dis 147:669, 1983a.

Grinnell, B. W., Padgett, B. L., and Walker, D. L.: Comparison of infectious JC Virus DNAs cloned from human brain. J Virol 45:299, 1983b.

Gross, L.: A filterable agent, recovered from AK leukemic extracts, causing salivary gland carcinomas in C3H mice. Proc Soc Exp Biol Med 83:414, 1953.

Gruss, P., Dhar, R., and Khoury, G.: Simian virus 40 tandem repeated sequences as an element of the early promoter. Proc Natl Acad Sci USA 78:943, 1981.

Haglund, S., Lundquist, P-G., Cantell, K., and Strander, H.: Interferon therapy in juvenile laryngeal papillomatosis. Arch Otolaryngol 107:327, 1981.

Hedley-Whyte, E. T., Smith, B. P., Tyler, H. R., and Peterson, W. P.: Multifocal leukoencephalopathy with remission and five-year survival. J Neuropathol Exp Neurol 25:107, 1966.

Heilman, C. A., Engel, L., Lowy, D. R., and Howley, P. M.: Virus-specific transcription in bovine papillomavirus transformed mouse cells. Virology 119:22, 1982.

Heilman, C. A., Law, M. -F., Israel, M. A., and Howley, P. M.: Cloning of human papillomavirus genomic DNAs and analysis of homologous polynucleotide sequences. J Virol 36:395, 1980.

Heinonen, O. P., Shapiro, S., Monson, R. R., Hartz, S. C., Rosenberg, L., and Slone, D.: Immunization during pregnancy against poliomyelitis and influenza in relation to childhood malignancy. Int J Epidemiol 2:229, 1973.

Heritage, J., Chesters, P. M., and McCance, D. J.: The persistence of papovavirus BK DNA sequences in normal human renal tissue. J Med Virol 8:143, 1981.

Hogan, T. F., Borden, E. C., McBain, J. A., Padgett, B. L., and Walker, D. L.: Human polyomavirus infections with JC virus and BK virus in renal transplant patients. Annals Int Med 92:373, 1980a.

Hogan, T. F., Padgett, B. L., Walker, D. L., Borden, E. C. and McBain, J. A.: Rapid detection and identification of JC virus and BK virus in human urine by using immunofluorescence microscopy. J Clin Microb 11:178, 1980b.

Hogan, T. F., Padgett, B. L., Walker, D. L., Borden, E. C., and Frias, Z.: Survey of human polyomavirus (JCV, BKV) infections in 139 patients with lung cancer, breast cancer, melanoma, or lymphoma. in *Polyomaviruses and Human Neurological Diseases.* (eds. Sever, J. L. and Madden, D. L.) Liss, New York, 1983. Prog Clin Biol Res 105:311.

Holmberg, C. A., Gribble, D. H., Takemoto, P. M., Howley, C., Espana, C., and Osburn, B. I.: Isolation of simian virus 40 from rhesus monkeys (Macaca mulatta) with spontaneous progressive multifocal leukoencephalopathy. J Infect Dis 136:593, 1977.

Howatson, A. F., Nagal, M., and Zu Rhein, G. M.: Polyoma-like virions in human demyelinating brain disease. Can Med Assoc J 93:379, 1965.

Howley, P. M.: Molecular biology of SV40 and the human polyomaviruses BK and JC. in *Viral Oncology.* (ed. Klein, G.) Raven Press, New York, 1980, pp. 489–549.

Howley, P. M.: Papovaviruses: Search for evidence of possible association with human cancer. in *Viruses Associated with Human Cancer.* (ed. Phillips, L. A.) Marcel Dekker, New York, 1983a, pp. 253–306.

Howley, P. M.: The molecular biology of papillomavirus transformation. Am J Pathol 113:414, 1983b.

Howley, P. M., Law, M. -F., Heilman, C. A., Engel, L. W., Alonso, M. C., Lancaster, W. D., Israel, M. A., and Lowy, D. R.: Molecular characterization of papillomavirus genomes. in *Viruses in Naturally Occurring Cancers.* (eds. Essex, M., Todaro, G., and zur Hausen, H.) Cold Spring Harbor Laboratory, Cold Spring Harbor, N.Y., 1980, pp. 233-247.

Hsiung, G. D., and Gaylord, W. H., Jr.: The vacuolating virus of monkeys. I. Isolation, growth characteristics, and inclusion body formation. J Exp Med 114:975, 1961.

Israel, M. A., Martin, M. A., Takemoto, K. K., Howley, P. M., Aaronson, S. A., Solomon, D., and Khoury, G.: Evaluation of normal and neoplastic human tissue for BK virus. Virology 90:187, 1978.

Itoyama, Y., Webster, H. deF., Sternberger, N. H., Richardson, E. P., Jr., Walker, D. L., Quarles, R. H., and Padgett, B. L.: Distribution of papovavirus, myelin-associated glycoprotein, and myelin basic protein in progressive multifocal leukoencephalopathy lesions. Ann Neurol 11:396, 1982.

Jablonska, S., Dabrowski, J., and Jakubowicz, K.: Epidermodysplasia verruciformis as a model in studies on the role of papovaviruses in oncogenesis. Cancer Res 32:583, 1972.

Jarrett, W. F. H., McNeil, P. E., Grimshaw, W. T. R., Selman, I., and McIntyre, W.: High incidence area of cattle cancer with a possible interaction between an environmental carcinogen and a papillomavirus. Nature 274:215, 1978.

Jenson, A. B., Rosenthal, J. D., Olson, C., Pass, F., Lancaster, W. D., and Shah, K.: Immunologic relatedness of papillomaviruses from different species. J Natl Cancer Inst 64:495, 1980.

Johnson, R. T.: Evidence for polyomaviruses in human neurological diseases. in *Polyomaviruses and Human Neurological Diseases.* (eds. Sever, J. L. and Madden, D. L.) Liss, New York, 1983. Prog Clin Biol Res 105:343.

Kanda, T., Yoshiike, K., and Takemoto, K. K.: Alignment of the genome of monkey B-Lymphotropic papovavirus to the genomes of Simian virus 40 and BK virus. J Virol 46:333, 1983.

Kessler, I. I.: Human cervical cancer as a venereal disease. Cancer Res 36:783, 1976.

Khoury, G., and Gruss, P.: Enhancer elements. Cell 33:313, 1983.

Kremsdorf, D., Jablonska, S., Favre, M., and Orth, G.: Biochemical characterization of two types of human papillomavirus associated with epidermodysplasia verruciformis. J Virol 43:436, 1982.

Kremsdorf, D., Jablonska, S., Favre, M., and Orth, G.: Human papillomavirus associated with epidermodysplasia verruciformis. II. Molecular cloning and biochemical characterization of human papillomavirus 3a, 8, 10, and 12 genomes. J Virol 48:340, 1983.

Krzyzek, R. A., Watts, S. L., Anderson, D. L., Faras, A. J., and Pass, F.: Anogenital warts contain several distinct species of human papillomavirus. J Virol 36:236, 1980.

Kurman, R. J., Shah, K. H., Lancaster, W. D., and Jenson, A. B.: Immunoperoxidase localization of papillomavirus antigens in cervical dysplasia and vulvar condylomas. Am J Obstet Gynecol 140:931, 1981.

Lack, E. E., Jenson, A. B., Smith, H. G., Healy, G. B., Pass, F., and Vawter, G. F.: Immunoperoxidase localization of human papillomavirus in laryngeal papillomas. Intervirol 14:148, 1980.

Laimins, L. A., Khoury, G., Gorman, C., Howard, B., and Gruss, P.: Host-specific activation of transcription by tandem repeats from simian virus 40 and Moloney murine sarcoma virus. Proc Natl Acad Sci USA 79:6543, 1982.

Lancaster, W. D., and Olson, C.: Animal papillomavirus. Microbiol Rev 46:191, 1982.

Laverty, C. R., Russell, P., Hills, E., and Booth, N.: The significance of noncondylomatous wart virus infection of the cervical transformation zone. Acta Cytol 22:195, 1978.

Law, M. -F., Martin, J. D., Takemoto, K. K., and Howley P. M.: The colinear alignment of the genomes of papovaviruses JC, BK, and SV40. Virol 96:576, 1979.

Law, M. -F., Lowy, D. R., Dvoretzky, I., and Howley, P. M.: Mouse cells transformed by bovine papillomavirus contain only extrachromosomal viral DNA sequences. Proc Natl Acad Sci USA 78:2727, 1981.

Lecatsas, G., Prozesky, O. W., and Scheepers, F.: The cytopathology and development of a human polyoma virus (BK). Arch Ges Virusforsch 44:319, 1974.

London, W. T., Houff, S. A., Madden, D. L., Fucillo, D. A., Gravell, M., Wallen, W. C., Sever, J. L., Padgett, B. L., Walker, D. L., Zu Rhein, G. M., and Ohashi, T.: Brain tumors in owl monkeys following inoculation with a human polyomavirus (JC virus). Science 201:1246, 1978.

Mason, D. H., Jr., and Takemoto, K. K.: Complementation between BK human papovavirus and a simian virus 40 tsA mutant. J Virol 17:1060, 1976.

Matthews, R. E. F.: Classification and Nomenclature of Viruses: *Fourth report of the International Committee on Toxonomy of Viruses.* Intervirology 17:1, 1982.

McCance, D. J.: Persistence of animal and human papovaviruses in renal and nervous tissues. in *Polyomaviruses and Human Neurological Diseases.* (eds. Sever, J. L. and Madden, D. L.) Liss, New York, 1983. Prog Clin Biol Res 105:343.

McCance, D. J., and Mims, C. A.: Transplacental transmission of polyoma virus in mice. Infect Immun 18:196, 1977.

McCance, D. J. and Mims, C. A.: Reactivation of polyoma virus in kidneys of persistently infected mice during pregnancy. Infect Immun 25:998, 1979.

Meisels, A., Fortin, R., and Roy, M.: Condylomatous lesions of the cervix: II. Cytologic, colposcopic and histopathologic study. Acta Cytol 78:379, 1977.

Meisels, A., Morin, C., and Casas-Cordero, M.: Human papillomavirus infection of the uterine cervix. Int J Gynecol Pathol 1:75, 1982.

Melnick, J. L.: Papova virus group. Science 135:1128, 1962.

Melnick, J. L., Allison, A. C., Butel, J. S., Eckhart, W., Eddy, B. E., Kit, S., Levine, A. J., Miles, J. A. R., Pagano, J. S., Sachs, L., and Vonka, V.: Papovaviridae. Intervirology 3:106, 1974.

Melnick, J. L., and Stinebaugh, S.: Excretion of vacuolating SV-40 virus (papovavirus group) after ingestion as a contaminant of oral poliovaccine. Proc Soc Exp Biol Med 109:965, 1962.

Mortimer, E. A., Lepow, M. L., Gold E., Robbins, F. C., Burton, G. J., and Fraumeni, J. F.: Long-term follow-up of persons inadvertently inoculated with SV40 as neonates. N Engl J Med 305:1517, 1981.

Narayan, O., Penney, J. B., Jr., Johnson, R. T., Herndon, R. M., and Weiner, L. P.: Etiology of progressive multifocal leukoencephalopathy. N Engl J Med 289:1278, 1973.

Norkin, L. C.: Papovaviral persistent infections. Microbiolog Rev 46:384, 1982.

O'Reilly, R. J., Lee, F. K., Grossbard, L. E., Kapoor, N., Kirkpatrick, D., Dinsmore, R., Stutzer, C., Shah, K. V., and Nahmias, A. J.: Papovavirus excretion following marrow transplantation: Incidence and association with hepatic dysfunction. Transplant Proc 13:262, 1981.

Orth, G., Favre, M., and Croissant, O.: Characterization of a new type of human papillomavirus that causes skin warts. J Virol 24:108, 1977.

Orth, G., Jablonska, S., Favre, M., Croissant, O., Jarzabek-Chorzelska, M., and Rzesa, G.: Characterization of two types of human papillomavirus in lesions of epidermodysplasia verruciformis. Proc Natl Acad Sci USA 75:1537, 1978.

Orth, G., Favre, M., Breitburd, F., Croissant, O., Jablonska, S., Obalek, S., Jarzabek-Chorzelska, M., and Rzesa, G.: Epidermodysplasia verruciformis: A model for the role of papilloma viruses in human cancer. Cold Spring Harbor Confer Cell Prolif 7:259, 1980.

Orth, G., Jablonska, S., Favre, M., Croissant, O., Obalek, S., Jarzabek-Chorzelska, M., and Jibard, N.: Identification of papillomavirus in butcher's warts. J Invest Derm 76:97, 1981.

Ostrow, R. S., Bender, M., Niimura, M., Seki, T., Kawashima, M., Pass, F., and Faras, A. J.: Human papillomavirus DNA in cutaneous primary and metastasized squamous cell carcinomas from patients with epidermodysplasia verruciformis. Proc Natl Acad Sci USA 79:1634, 1982.

Oxman, M. N.: Some behavioral studies of simian virus 40 (SV40). Arch Ges Virusforch 22:171, 1967.

Oxman, M. N., and Black, P. H.: Inhibition of SV40 T antigen formation by interferon. Proc Natl Acad Sci USA 55:1133, 1966.

Oxman, M. N., and Takemoto, K. K.: Comparative interferon sensitivity of SV40 and polyoma virus. Proc Symposium on Interferon, Lyon, France, 1969. In *L'Interferon,* Les Colloques de L'I.N.S.E.R.M. No. 6, pp. 429-442, 1969.

Padgett, B.: Human papovaviruses. in *DNA Tumor Viruses.* Molecular Biology of Tumor Viruses, (ed. Tooze, J.) 2nd Edition, Part 2 Revised. Cold Spring Harbor Laboratory, Cold Spring Harbor, N.Y., 1981. pp. 339-370.

Padgett, B. L., and Walker, D. L: New human papovaviruses. Prog Med Virol 22:1, 1976.

Padgett, B. L., and Walker, D. L.: Virologic and serologic studies of progressive multifocal leukoencephalopathy. In *Polyomaviruses and Human Neurological Diseases.* (eds. Sever, J. L. and Madden, D. L.) Liss, New York, 1983. Prog Clin Biol Res 105:107.

Padgett, B. L., Walker, D. L., Zu Rhein, G. M., Eckroade, R. J., and Dessel, B. H.: Cultivation of papova-like virus from human brain with progressive multifocal leucoencephalopathy. Lancet 2:1257, 1971.

Padgett, B. L., Walker, D. L., Zu Rhein, G. M., Hodach, A. E., and Chou, S. M.: JC papovavirus in progressive multifocal leukoencephalopathy. J Infect Dis 133:686, 1976.

Padgett, B. L., Rogers, C. M., and Walker, D. L.: JC virus, a human polyomavirus associated with progressive multifocal leukoencephalopathy: Additional biological characteristics and antigenic relationships. Infect Immun 15:656, 1977a.

Padgett, B. L., Walker, D. L. ZuRhein, G. M., and Varakis, J. N.: Differential Neurooncogenicity of strains of JC virus, a human polyoma virus, in newborn Syrian hamsters. Cancer 37:718, 1977b.

Parry, J. V., Lucas, M. H., Richmond, J. E., and Gardner, S. D.: Evidence for a bovine origin of the polyomavirus detected in fetal rhesus monkey kidney cells, FRhK-4 and -6. Arch Virol 78:151, 1983.

Patch, C. T., Levine, A. S. and Lewis, A. M., Jr.: The adenovirus SV40 hybrid viruses. in *Comprehensive Virology.* vol 13. (eds. Fraenkel-Conrat, H., and Wagner, R. R.) Plenum, New York, 1979, pp. 495-542.

Paucha, E., Mellor, A., Harvey, R., Smith, A. E., Hewick, R. M., and Waterfield, M. D.: Large and small tumor antigens from simian virus 40 have identical amino termini mapping at 0.65 map units. Proc Natl Acad Sci USA 75:2165, 1978.

Pazin, G. J., Ho, M., Haverkos, H. W., Armstrong, J. A., Breinig, M. C., Wechsler, H. L., Arvin, A., Merigan, T. C., and Cantell, K.: Effects of Interferon-alpha on human warts. Interferon Res 2:235, 1982.

Pfister, H.: Biology and biochemistry of papillomaviruses. Rev Physiol Biochem Pharm 99:111, 1983.

Pfister, H., Hettich, I., Runne, U., Gissmann, L., and Chilf, G. N.: Characterization of human papillomavirus type 13 from focal epithelial hyperplasia Heck lesions. J Virol 47:363, 1983.

Pitko, V. M., Pyokari, P., Nase, L., and Mantyjarvi, R.: Effect of β-propiolactone on infectivity and haemagglutinin of the BK virus. Acta Pathol Microbiol Scand [B] 83:141, 1975.

Ponten, J.: Spontaneous and virus induced transformation in cell culture. in *Virology Monographs.* vol 8. (eds. Gard, S., Hallauer, C., and Meyer, K. F.) Springer-Verlag, New York, 1971, pp. 1-253.

Price, R. W., Nielsen, S., Horten, B., Rubino, M., Padgett, B. L., and Walker, D.L.: Progressive multifocal leukoencephalopathy: A burnt-out case. Ann Neurol 13:485, 1983.

Purchio, A. F., and Fareed, G. C.: Transformation of human embryonic kidney cells by human papovavirus BK. J Virol 29:763, 1979.

Rassoulzadegan, M., Naghashfar, Z., Cowie, A., Carr, A., Grisoni, M., Kamen, R., and Cuzin, F.: Expression of the large T protein of polyoma virus promotes the establishment in culture of "normal" rodent fibroblast cell lines. Proc Natl Acad Sci USA 80:4354, 1983.

Reddy, V. B. and Weissman, S. M.: The structure of papovaviruses. in *Viruses Associated with Human Cancer* (ed. Phillips, L. A.) Marcel Dekker, New York, 1983, pp. 195-251.

Reichert, C. M., O'Leary, T. J., Levens, D. L., Simrell, C. R., and Macher, A. M.: Autopsy pathology in the acquired immune deficiency syndrome. Am J Pathol 112:357, 1983.

Reid, R., Laverty, C. R., Coppleson, M., Isarangkul, W., and Hills, E.: Noncondylomatous cervical wart virus infection. Obstet Gynecol 55:476, 1980.

Reid, R., Stanhope, C. R., Herschman, B. R., Booth, E., Phibbs, G. D., and Smith, J. P.: Genital warts and cervical cancer. Evidence of an association between subclinical papillomavirus infections and cervical malignancy. Cancer 50:377, 1982.

Rentier-Delrue, F., Lubiniecki, A., and Howley, P. M.: Analysis of JC virus DNA purified directly from human progressive multifocal leukoencephalopathy brains. J Virol 38:761, 1981.

Richardson, E. P., Jr.: Progressive multifocal leukoencephalopathy. N Engl J Med 265:815, 1961.

Rieth, K., DiChiro, G., London, W., Sever, J., Houff, S., Kornblith, P., McKeever, P., Buonomo, C., Padgett, B., and Walker, D.: Experimental glioma in primates: A computed tomography model. J Comput Assist Tomogr 4:285, 1980.

Rosen, S., Harmon, W., Krensky, A. M., Edelson, P. J., Padgett, B. L., Grinnell, B., Rubino, M. J., and Walker, D. L.: Tubulo-interstitial nephritis associated with polyomavirus (BK type) infection. N Engl J Med 308:1192, 1983.

Rosenthal, N., Kress, M., Gruss, P. and Khoury, G: BK viral enhancer element and a human cellular homology. Science 222:749, 1983.

Rous, P., and Beard, J. W.: The progression to carcinoma of virus-induced rabbit papilloma (Shope). J Exp Med 62:523, 1935.

Rowe, W. P., Hartley, J. W., Estes, J. D., and Huebner, R. J.: Growth curves of polyoma in mice and hamsters. Natl Cancer Inst Monogr 4:189, 1960.

Rowe, W. P., Heubner, R. J., and Hartley, J. W.: Ecology of a mouse

tumor virus. in *Perspectives in Virolog*. vol II. (ed. Pollard, M.) Rutgers Univ Press, New Brunswick, N.J. 1961, pp. 177-194.
Rowson, K. E. K., and Mahy, B. W. J.: Human papova (wart) virus. Bacteriol Rev 31:110, 1967.
Rziha, H. -J., and Belohradsky, B. H.: BK virus infections in children with various primary immunodeficiencies and in related healthy household contact persons. Infect 9:137, 1981.
Salzman, N. P., and Khoury, S.: Reproduction of papovaviruses. in *Comprehensive Virology*. vol 3. (eds. Fraenkel-Conrat, H., and Wagner, R. R.) Plenum Press, New York, 1974, pp. 63–141.
Sambrook, J.: Transformation by polyoma virus and simian virus 40. Adv Cancer Res 16:141, 1972.
Schonfeld, A., Schattner, A., Crespi, M., Levavi, H., Shoham, J., Nitke, S., Wallach, D., Hahn, T., Yarden, O., Doerner, T., and Revel, M.: Intramuscular human interferon-β injections in treatment of condylomata acuminata. Lancet 1:1038, 1984.
Schwarz, E., Durst, M., Demankowski, C., Lattermann, O., Zech, R., Wolfsperger, E., Suhai, E., and zur Hausen, H.: DNA sequence and genome organization of genital human papillomavirus type 6B. EMBO Journal 2:2341, 1983.
Segawa, K. and Takemoto, K. K.: Identification of B-lymphotropic papovavirus-coded proteins. J Virol 45:872, 1983.
Shah, K.: Biological and immunological relationships of papovaviruses of the simian virus 40-polyoma subgroup. in *Microbiology*, (ed. Schlessinger, D.) American Society for Microbiology, Washington, D. C. 1978, pp. 439-442.
Shah, K., and Nathanson N.: Human exposure to SV40: Review and comment. Am J Epidemiol 103:1, 1976.
Shah, K. V., Ozer, H. L., Ghazey, H. N., and Kelly, T. J., Jr.: Common structural antigen of papovaviruses of the simian virus 40-polyoma subgroup. J Virol 21:179, 1977a.
Shah, K. V., Rangan, S. R. S., Reissig, M., Daniel, R. W., Beluhan, F. Z.: Congenital transmission of a papovavirus of the stump-tailed macaque. Science 195:404, 1977b.
Shah, K. V., Daniel, R. W., Stone, K. R., and Elliott, A. Y.: Investigation of human urogenital tract tumors for papovavirus etiology: brief communication. J Natl Cancer Inst 60:579, 1978.
Shah, K., Daniel, R., Madden, D., and Stagno, S.: Serological Investigation of BK papovavirus infection in pregnant women and their offspring. Infect Immun 30:29, 1980.
Sheffield, W. D., Strandberg, J. D., Braun, L., Shah, K., and Kalter, S. S.: Simian virus 40-associated fatal interstital pneumonia and renal tubular necrosis in a rhesus monkey. J Infect Dis 142:618, 1980.
Shein, H. M.: Transformation of astrocytes and destruction of spongioblasts induced by a simian tumor virus (SV40) in cultures of human fetal neuroglia. J Neuropath Exp Neurol 26:60, 1967.
Shein, H. M., and Enders, J. F.: Transformation induced by simian virus 40 in human renal cell cultures. I. Morphology and growth characteristics. Proc Natl Acad Sci USA 48:1164, 1962.
Shope, R. E.: Infectious papillomatosis of rabbits. J Exp Med 58:607, 1933.
Silverman, L., and Rubinstein, L. J.: Electron microscopic observations on a case of progressive multifocal leukoencephalopathy. Acta Neuropathologica 5:215, 1965.
Simmons, D. T., and Martin, M. A.: Common methionine-tryptic peptides near the amino-terminal end of primate papovavirus tumor antigens. Proc Natl Acad Sci USA 75:1131, 1978.
Soeda, E., Arrand, J. R., Smolar, N., Walsh, J. E., and Griffin, B. E.: Coding potential and regulatory signals of the polyoma virus genome. Nature 283:445, 1980.
Spencer, E. S., and Andersen, H. K.: Viral infections in renal allograft recipients treated with long-term immunosuppression. British Med J 2:829, 1979.
Steinberg, B. M., Topp, W. C., Schneider, P. A., and Abramson, A. L.: Laryngeal papillomavirus infection during clinical remission. N Engl J Med 308:1261, 1983.
Sweet, B. H., and Hilleman, M. R.: The vacuolating virus, SV40. Proc Soc Exp Biol 105:420, 1960.
Syrjanen, K. J.: Current concepts of human papillomavirus infections in the genital tract and their relationship to intraepithelial neoplasia and squamous cell carcinoma. Obstet Gynecol Survey 39:252, 1984.
Takemoto, K. K.: Human papovaviruses. Int Rev Exp Pathol 18:281, 1978.
Takemoto, K. K., and Segawa, K.: A new monkey lymphotropic papovavirus: Characterization of the virus and evidence of a related virus in humans. in *Polyomaviruses and Human Neurological Diseases*. (eds. Sever, J. L. and Madden, D. L.) Liss, New York, 1983. Prog Clin Biol Res 105:87.
Takemoto, K. K., Furuno, A., Kato, K., and Yoshiike, K.: Biological and biochemical studies of African green monkey lymphotropic papovavirus. J Virol 42:502, 1982.
Takemoto, K. K., Linke, H., Miyamura, T., and Fareed, G. C.: Persistent BK papovavirus infection of transformed human fetal brain cells. J Virol 29:1177, 1979.
Taguchi, F., Kajioka, J., and Miyamura, T.: Prevalence rate and age of acquisition of antibodies against JC virus and BK virus in human sera. Microbiol Immunol 26:1057, 1982.
Tevethia, M. J., and Tevethia, S. S.: Biology of SV40 transplantation antigen (TrAg). I. Demonstration of SV40 TrAg on glutaraldehyde-fixed SV40-infected African green monkey kidney cells. Virology 69:474, 1976.
Tevethia, M. J., and Tevethia, S. S.: Biology of simian virus 40 (SV40) transplantation antigen (TrAg). III. Involvement of SV40 gene A in the expression of TrAg in permissive cells. Virology 81:212, 1977.
Tjian, R., and Robbins, A.: Enzymatic activities associated with a purified simian virus 40 T antigen-related protein. Proc Natl Acad Sci USA 76:610, 1979.
Tooze, J.: (ed) *DNA Tumor Viruses*. Molecular Biology of Tumor Viruses, 2nd Edition, Part 2 Revised. Cold Spring Harbor Laboratory, Cold Spring Harbor, N.Y., 1981.
Turek, L. P., Byrne, J. C., Lowy, D. R., Dvoretzky, I., Friedman, R. M., and Howley, P. M.: Interferon induces morphologic reversion with elimination of extrachromosomal viral genomes in bovine papillomavirus-transformed mouse cells. Proc Natl Acad Sci USA 79:7914, 1982.
Uchida, S. S., Watanabe, S., Aizawa, T., Furuno, A., and Muto, T.: Polyoncogenicity and insulinoma-inducing ability of BK virus, a human papovavirus, in Syrian golden hamsters. J Natl Cancer Inst 63:119, 1979.
Walker, D. L., and Padgett, B. L.: Progressive multifocal leukoencephalopathy. in *Comprehensive Virology*. Vol 18. (eds. Fraenkel-Conrat, H., and Wagner, R. R.) Plenum Press, New York, 1983a, pp. 161-193.
Walker, D. L. and Padgett, B. L.: The epidemiology of human polyomaviruses. in *Polyomaviruses and Human Neurological Diseases*. (eds. Sever, J. L. and Madden, D. L.) Liss, New York, 1983b. Prog Clin Biol Res 105:99.
Watanabe, S., Yoshuke, K., Nozawa, A., Yausa, Y., and Uchida, S.: Viable deletion mutant of human papovavirus BK that induces insulinomas in hamsters. J Virol 32:934, 1979.
Weiner, L. P., Herndon, R. M., Narayan, O., Johnson, R. T., Shah, K., Rubinstein, L. J., Preziosi, T. J., and Conley, F. K.: Isolation of virus related to SV40 from patients with progressive multifocal leukoencephalopathy. N Engl J Med 286:35, 1972.
Willoughby, E., Price, R. W., Padgett, B. L., Walker, D. L., and Dupont, B.: Progressive multifocal leukoencephalopathy (PML): *In vitro* cell-mediated immune responses to mitogens and JC virus. Neurology, 30:256, 1980.
Yaniv, M.: Enhancing elements for activation of eukaryotic promoters. Nature 297:17, 1982.
zur Hausen, H.: Human papillomaviruses and their possible role in squamous cell carcinomas. Curr Top Microbiol Immunol 78:1, 1977.
zur Hausen, H., and Gissmann, L.: Lymphotropic papovaviruses isolated from African green monkey and human cells. Med Microbiol Immunology, 167:137, 1979.
Zu Rhein, G. M., and Chou, S. M.: Particles resembling papova viruses in human cerebral demyelinating disease. Science 148:1477, 1965.

RNA VIRUSES

63
ORTHOMYXOVIRUSES: THE INFLUENZA VIRUSES

DOUGLAS D. RICHMAN, M.D.

DEFINITION. Influenza is a highly contagious, acute respiratory disease that afflicts people of all ages. Influenza is a major cause of morbidity and mortality, which in some years may occur in worldwide epidemics. Our understanding of the influenza virus, from its structure and replication to its worldwide epidemiology involving animal reservoirs, has been accumulating rapidly.

The term myxovirus (Gr. *myxo,* mucus) has been applied to two families of enveloped RNA viruses, the *Orthomyxoviridae* and *Paramyxoviridae,* which share a number of characteristics. These viruses are transmitted via the respiratory route. The members of both families possess a single-stranded genome enclosed in a helical array of nucleoprotein. The viral RNA polymerase associated with this ribonucleoprotein structure transcribes viral messenger RNA from the virion RNA. Electron micrographs demonstrate virions to be pleomorphic ellipsoids or filaments possessing a lipid envelope with surface glycoprotein projections that bind to host cell receptors. Glycoproteins in the two families share homologous structural characteristics and amino acid sequence homology. Despite these common characteristics, these viruses have been separated into two families on the basis of a fundamental difference in their genome structure. The genome of the orthomyxoviruses is segmented and the genome of the paramyxoviruses is not.

STRUCTURE AND REPLICATION. Influenza virions are most frequently 80 to 120 nm in diameter (Figs. 1 and 2). Although generally spheroid, the virions may exhibit great variation in length; long filamentous forms are frequently observed. The virions have a buoyant density of 1.23 g/cm^3 and a composition of approximately 1 per cent RNA, 73 per cent protein, 20 per cent lipid, and 6 per cent carbohydrate. Influenza A and B virions contain seven structural proteins (Table 1). Three large proteins (PB1, PB2, and PA) associated with the virion RNA are responsible for RNA transcription and replication. The nucleoprotein (NP) is associated with the virion RNA in the ribonucleoprotein structures. The matrix (M) protein underlies the lipid envelope of the virion. Two glycoproteins, the hemagglutinin (HA) and the neuraminidase (NA) are inserted into the lipid envelope. The HA is a trimer of a glycoprotein with a molecular weight of 77,000 daltons; the NA is a mushroom-shaped tetramer of a 56,000-dalton glycoprotein. These glycoproteins attach to this lipid envelope by short sequences of hydrophobic amino acids. This hydrophobic attachment site occurs at the carboxyl terminus of the HA polypeptide and the amino terminus of the NA polypeptide. The amino acid sequences of many antigenic variants of the influenza virus glycoproteins have been reported, and the structures of the crystallized HA and NA glycoproteins of influenza A/Hong Kong/68 (H3N2) have been determined by X-ray diffraction.

The genomes of influenza A and B viruses consist of eight separate segments of single-stranded RNA with a total molecular weight of 5×10^6 daltons (Table 2). Influenza C virus contains seven segments, thus differing from types A and B in this characteristic, in the lack of neuraminidase activity, and in the presence of only one surface glycoprotein. Except where explicitly mentioned, the information in this chapter refers only to influenza A and B viruses. The segments of RNA are each associated with NP to form eight separate ribonucleoprotein structures with a diameter of 9 nm and a buoyant density of 1.34 g/cm^3. When a cell is coinfected by two different influenza viruses of the same type, the parental gene segments are assembled in a nonlinked manner in the progeny virions (Figure 3). This property, termed *genetic reassortment,* permits major single step changes in surface antigens and host susceptibility. This property carries major implications, both for the epidemiology of the disease and for vaccine development.

A single proteolytic cleavage of the HA glycoprotein by a cell or serum protease is necessary to activate the HA and thus to render the influenza virion infectious. This post-translational cleavage yields two polypeptide chains (HA1 and HA2) joined by a single disulfide bond. The replicative cycle of influenza is initiated by attachment of the virion HA to a sialyloligosaccharide receptor on a host cell membrane. Both uncleaved and cleaved HA will mediate attachment; however, only virions possessing HA in the cleaved form can infect the host cell. Two mechanisms of penetration have been proposed: fusion of viral and cell membranes, and receptor-mediated endocytotic ingestion of the virus by the cell (viropexis).

Influenza viruses are "negative-stranded" RNA viruses; the (−) virion RNA is complementary to (+) mRNA. RNA synthesis in the early hours of infection is mediated by the virion polymerase resulting in the production of 5′-capped 3′-polyadenylated mRNA. In addition to the synthesis of mRNAs for the seven structural proteins coded by segments 1–7, segments 7 and 8 code for at least 3 nonstructural peptides (Table 1). The M2 and NS2 mRNAs represent spliced transcripts and use different reading frames than the M1 and NS1 mRNAs. The functions of these nonstructural proteins are unknown.

Subsequent RNA synthesis represents the production of (+) RNA that is neither capped nor polyadenylated and serves as a template for the synthesis of (−) RNA for the assembly of new virions. The precise location, sequence, and control of influenza RNA and protein synthesis are still being investigated; nevertheless, the unusual requirement for the participation of the cell nucleus in influenza RNA replication is well recognized. In contrast to most other

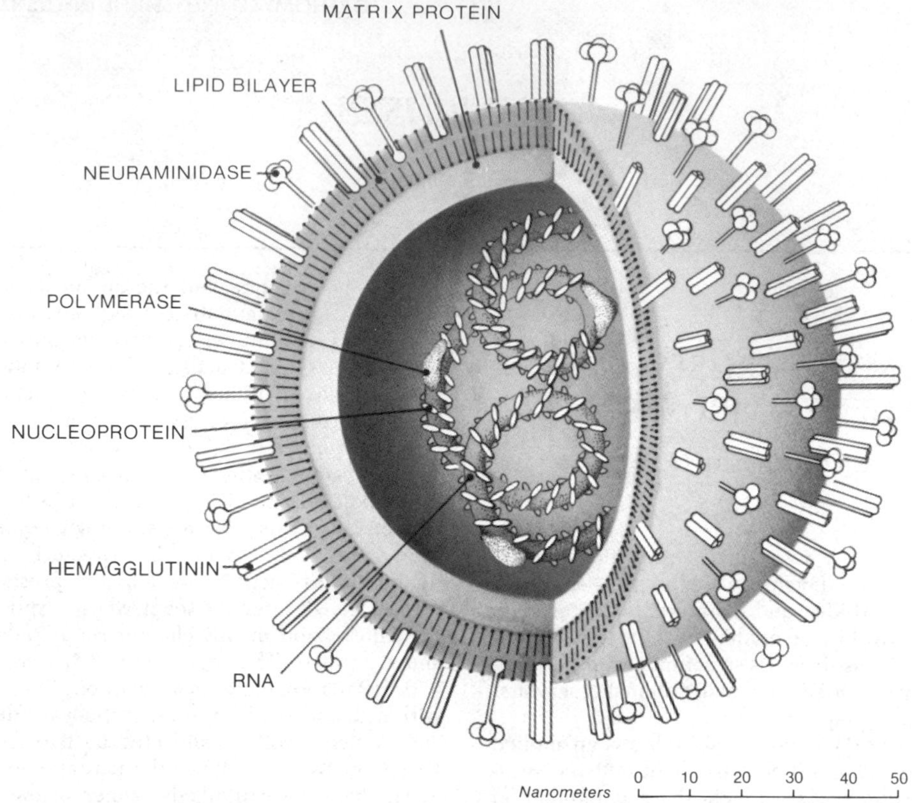

Figure 1. Cutaway diagram of influenza virion structure.

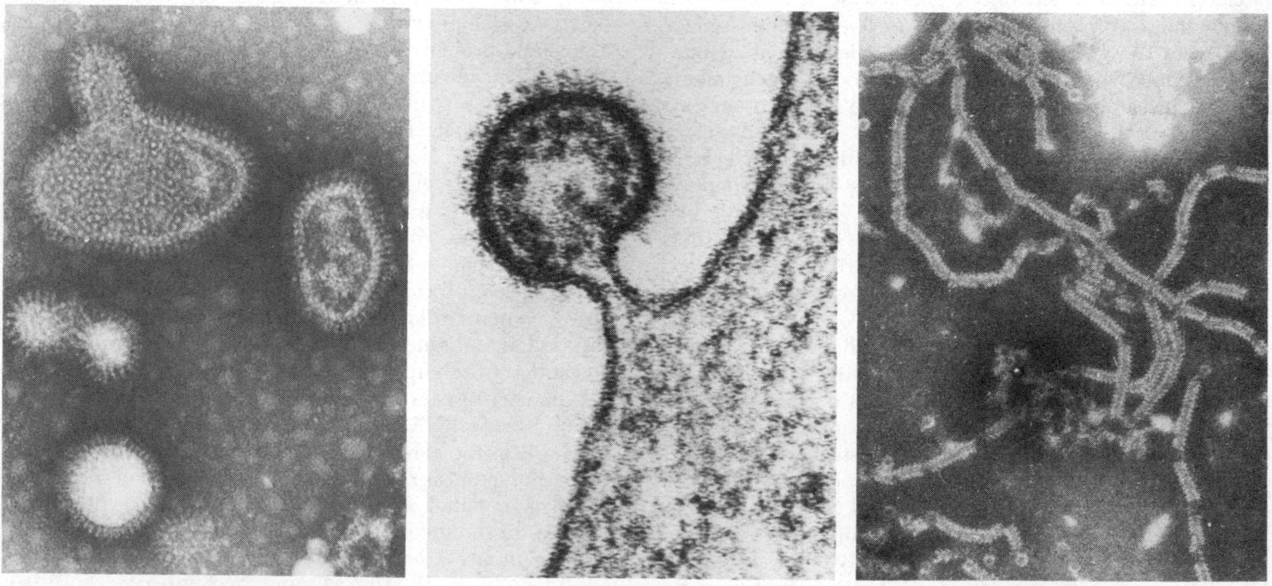

Figure 2. *Left,* Purified influenza A/Hong Kong/68 (H3N2). Note pleomorphic shapes, variable size, and glyco-protein projections covering the virion surface. Electron-photomicrograph kindly provided by A. R. Kalica, Ph.D. Laboratory of Infectious Diseases, NIAID National Institutes of Health, Bethesda, Maryland. (182,000 ×).

Center, Respiratory syncytial virus budding from the surface of an infected HeLa cell in culture. Electron-photomicrograph from Kalica, Wright, Hetrick, and Chanock electron microscopic studies of respiratory syncytial temperature sensitive mutants. Arch fur die ges Virusf 41:248, 1973, with permission. (132,000 ×).

Right, Purified nucleocapsids from mumps virus. Note helical array of ribonucleoproteins to form the nucleocapsid structure with an 18 nm diameter. This nucleocapsid contains an apparent hollow "core," which is apparent on both transverse and end-on views. Electron-photomicrograph from Huppertz, Hall and ter Meulen. Polypeptide composition of mumps virus. Med Microbiol Immunol 163:25, 1977, with permission. (142,025 ×).

Table 1. INFLUENZA VIRUS GENOME RNA SEGMENTS AND CODING ASSIGNMENTS*

RNA Segment	Length (Nucleotides)	Encoded Polypeptide: Designation	Nascent polypeptide length (a.a.)	Molecular weight by gel electrophoresis	Approx. no. of molecules per virion
1	2341	PB2	759	96,000	15–60
2	2341	PB1	757	87,000	15–60
3	2233	PA	716	85,000	15–60
4	1778	HA	566	77,000	500
5	1565	NP	498	56,000	1,000
6	1413	NA	453	56,000	100
7	1027	M1	252	28,000	3,000
		M2	96	15,000	0
8	890	NS1	230	26,000	0
		NS2	121	14,000	0

*Table adapted with permission from Lamb and Choppin (1983). The values for segment length are determined for A/PR/8/34(H1N1). The molecular weights of the HA subunits are approximately 48,000 for the HA_1 of which 24 per cent is carbohydrate and 27,000 for the HA_2 of which 5 per cent is carbohydrate. The molecular weights of the two glycoproteins, HA and NA, are for the glycosylated monomeric polypeptides.

RNA viruses, such as picornaviruses and parainfluenza viruses, whose cytoplasmic replication is independent of the cell nucleus, influenza virus replication requires the presence and function of the cell nucleus, which contains both viral RNA and protein during influenza replication. Enucleation of the host cell or treatment of it with sublethal doses of UV irradiation, actinomycin D, or α-amanitin will prevent influenza virus replication. None of these inhibits parainfluenza virus replication. Studies using cells resistant to the action of α-amanitin suggest that the host cell RNA polymerase II is essential for influenza virus replication. The viral ribonucleoprotein complex, consisting of RNA and the NP, PB1, PB2, and PA proteins, generates primed capped viral mRNA by appropriating the capped methyl guanosine-containing primers from heterologous cellular mRNAs which are synthesized by the RNA polymerase II.

The viral RNA and proteins are transported to the cell periphery by an undetermined mechanism. The processes of assembly of these viral components and of budding of virions from the host cell are also incompletely understood. The first evidence of a budding site is the accumulation of the HA and NA glycoprotein projections in a limited region of the cell outer membrane. A layer of the hydrophobic M protein then appears subjacent to the host membrane lipid bilayer in this region, which is to be incorporated into the budding virion. Ribonucleoprotein segments can then be seen by electron microscopy attached to these localized regions of altered cell membrane, which then progressively pouch out and finally bud off from the cell surface. The mechanism for packaging the eight RNA segments within the virion is unknown. Less than 10 per cent of most influenza virions are infectious, perhaps because they lack a complete set of eight gene segments. Release of new virions from the host cell surface requires hydrolysis by the virion NA of the N-acetylneuraminic acid-containing receptors that normally are present in the host cell membrane.

Table 2. SUBTYPES OF HUMAN TYPE A INFLUENZA VIRUSES*

Period of Prevalence	Subtype	Representative Antigenic Variants
1890–1900	H2N8	
1900–1918	H3N8	
1918–1957	H1N2	A/PR/8/34
		A/FM/1/47
1957–1968	H2N2	A/Japan/305/57
1968–present	H3N2	A/Hong Kong/1/68
		A/Texas/1/77
1977–present	H1N1	A/USSR/90/77

*The conclusions for the period before 1933 are based on immunologic recapitulation (seroarcheology) as described in the text.

ANTIGENIC COMPOSITION. Two internal structural proteins, the NP and the M protein, are used in typing influenza viruses. The RNA sequences and antigenicity are highly conserved within each of the three influenza types. Moreover, these proteins exhibit no antigenic cross-reactivity among the types. Consequently, whole virus or purified preparations of NP (previously called the soluble [S] antigen) or M protein are used in complement fixation or immunodiffusion tests to type influenza virus isolates as A, B, or C. In addition, these tests are used in the type-specific, but not subtype-specific or antigenic strain-specific, serodiagnosis of infection. Antibody to the NP or M proteins, which are not exposed on the virion, does not protect against infection.

The two surface glycoproteins, HA and NA, are the important antigens for host immunity, for antigenic variation of influenza viruses, and for serodiagnosis of influenza. The HA binds to sialyloligosaccharide residues, which are present in all eukaryotic cell membranes. Thus, the virus will probably bind to any cell, including both susceptible host cells and erythrocytes. Attachment to erythrocytes causes hemagglutination. Inhibition of this reaction by antibody, termed hemagglutination inhibition (HI), is the assay used most for measuring antibody against influenza viruses. This technique is also used to characterize antigenic variants of virus. Much of the antibody to the HA neutralizes the infectivity of influenza viruses in vitro and in vivo. By determining amino acid sequence changes in naturally occurring antigenic variants and in those selected by monoclonal antibodies in vitro, four antigenic sites (epitopes) have been mapped on the HA molecule.

The NA enzyme facilitates the release of free virus during the budding process and may also help virions reach the

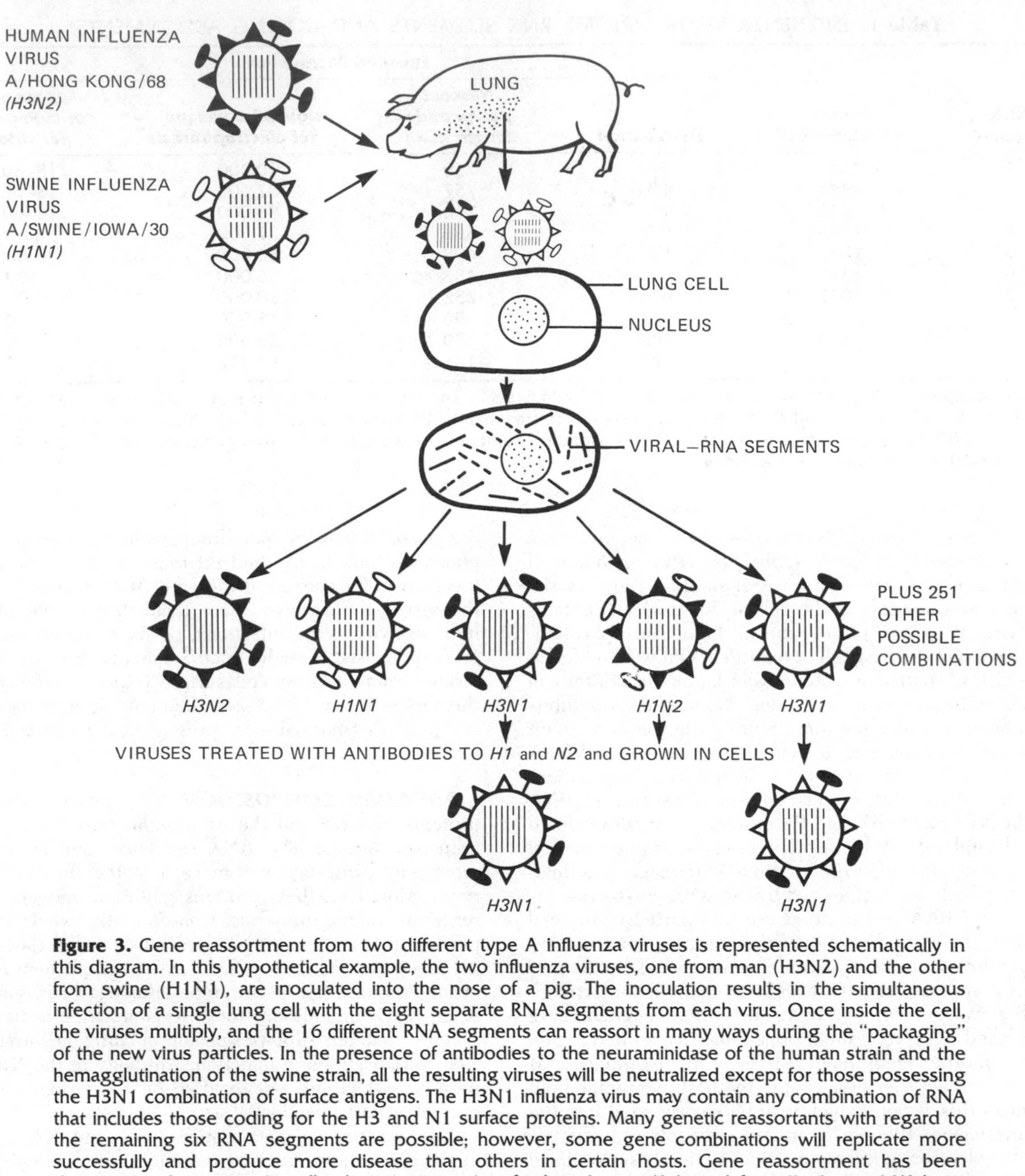

Figure 3. Gene reassortment from two different type A influenza viruses is represented schematically in this diagram. In this hypothetical example, the two influenza viruses, one from man (H3N2) and the other from swine (H1N1), are inoculated into the nose of a pig. The inoculation results in the simultaneous infection of a single lung cell with the eight separate RNA segments from each virus. Once inside the cell, the viruses multiply, and the 16 different RNA segments can reassort in many ways during the "packaging" of the new virus particles. In the presence of antibodies to the neuraminidase of the human strain and the hemagglutination of the swine strain, all the resulting viruses will be neutralized except for those possessing the H3N1 combination of surface antigens. The H3N1 influenza virus may contain any combination of RNA that includes those coding for the H3 and N1 surface proteins. Many genetic reassortants with regard to the remaining six RNA segments are possible; however, some gene combinations will replicate more successfully and produce more disease than others in certain hosts. Gene reassortment has been demonstrated to occur in cell culture, eggs, swine, fowl, and man. (Adapted from Kaplan and Webster 1977.)

respiratory epithelium, by hydrolyzing the protective layer of mucus with its rich content of glycoproteins containing N-acetylneuraminic (sialic) acid that bind to the virus. NA activity is measured by a colorimetric assay of N-acetylneuraminic acid released by the enzymatic hydrolysis of a substrate such as fetuin. Antibody to NA is measured by inhibition of this activity when serum and virus are mixed. This neuraminidase-inhibiting (NI) antibody appears to restrict the spread of virus from infected cells. In monolayers of cell cultures infected with influenza virus, HI antibody reduces the number of plaques formed (neutralization of inoculum virus), but the plaques that do appear are of normal size. Except in extremely high concentration, NI antibody does not reduce plaque number, but does reduce plaque size (restriction of spread of virus from infected to adjacent susceptible cells). In both animal models and in human studies, NI antibody tends to reduce severity of disease but not to prevent the acquisition of infection.

Influenza virus has the unique capability of changing the antigenic identity of its HA and NA. Antigenic changes occur in the HA and NA polypeptides with a frequency not observed in other viruses or in other influenza virus proteins. The resulting antigenic variants have a selective advantage over the parental antigenic strain in the presence of antibody to the original strain. All three types of influenza virus undergo minor changes in their HA and NA glycoprotein antigens termed *antigenic drift*. When the antigenic change in either HA or NA is large enough to remove immunologic cross-reactions with the original HA or NA, they are given a distinct subtype designation. Such HA and NA subtypes have been identified only with influenza type A. The appearance of a new subtype is termed *antigenic shift.* Antigenic drift and shift have profound epidemiologic implications, which will be considered below.

NOMENCLATURE. In recognition of the vast array of antigenic variants, combinations of HA and NA subtypes and hosts of origin, a World Health Organization committee has devised a systematic nomenclature for influenza viruses. The schema includes *(1) the type; (2) the host species, if not human: (3) geographic origin; (4) strain number for the year; and (5) year of isolation (H and N subtype, if type A).* Consequently, the human isolate of the swine-like influenza virus was designated A/New Jersey/6/76 (H1N1). One of the earliest swine isolates of influenza virus is designated A/swine/Wisconsin/15/30 (H1N1). This nomenclature supersedes the old terminology of A_0, A_1, and A_2, which ignores the independent variation of the HA and NA proteins and the animal reservoir of influenza. The influenza A subtypes that have circulated since the first human isolation in 1933 by Smith, Laidlaw, and Andrewes are indicated in Table 2. In addition, as of 1983, 13 HA subtypes and 9 NA subtypes in more than two dozen different combinations have been recognized in swine, horses, seals, and birds.

PATHOGENESIS AND CLINICAL MANIFESTATIONS. Deposition of influenza virus in droplet nuclei or by contact with contaminated hands or surfaces on almost any portion of the respiratory epithelium can initiate infection. Virus shedding precedes symptoms, which are first noticed one to three days after exposure. Typical symptoms are sneezing, chills, fever, headache, myalgia, nasal obstruction and discharge, sore throat, and nonproductive cough. These symptoms usually subside in two to four days with little residua after one week. Coincident with the onset of symptoms, the ciliated epithelium desquamates. Symptoms and local pathology usually lag out of phase with virus shedding, which usually diminishes rapidly within a day of the onset of symptoms, and rarely persist more than one week in adults and two weeks in children. The epithelium regenerates, passing through a series of stages from a transitional basal layer to stratified squamous to hyperplastic cuboidal until the normal ciliated columnar epithelium is reestablished in one to two weeks.

The pneumonia that can occur in the course of influenza infection can be viral, secondary bacterial, or a mixture of the two. Pure viral pneumonia causes focal alveolar exudation and hemorrhage, denuded alveolar walls, capillary thrombosis, and necrosis. The increased susceptibility of lungs infected with influenza virus to secondary bacterial invasion has been well documented and is attributed to loss of ciliary clearance, adherence to infected cells via antibody and protein A, a rich bacterial growth medium in the alveolar exudate, and injury to leukocytes by influenza virus infection. *Staphylococcus aureus, Streptococcus pneumoniae,* and *Hemophilus influenzae* are the most frequent secondary pathogens. The bacterial infection may often be difficult to distinguish from the viral on clinical grounds. The course may be biphasic with an interval of partial recovery between the viral syndrome and the bacterial pneumonia, or it may present as a bacterial pneumonia with only epidemiologic, serologic, or cultural evidence to indicate viral infection. Even in patients without clinically or radiologically apparent pneumonia, influenza increases bronchial reactivity and peripheral airway resistance that persists for weeks.

Severe myalgia is common in influenza, and serum creatinine phosphokinase is often elevated. The pathogenesis of this muscle involvement, which can be severe enough to cause myoglobinuria and renal failure, has not been explained. Myocarditis and encephalitis have also been associated with epidemic influenza. Children are more likely than adults to experience severe lower respiratory tract disease, high fever and febrile convulsions, gastrointestinal disturbances, and otitis media. In addition, Reye described a syndrome in 1963 of hepatic failure and encephalopathy in children shortly after one of several viral infections—including influenza A on occasion, but most frequently type B. In spite of sporadic claims of virus isolation from blood, there has been as yet no systematic documentation of extrarespiratory viral infection in humans with influenza virus.

It is important to note that only one half of infected individuals, as determined by antibody responses or viral isolation, develop clinical disease. It is not clear to what extent site of inoculation, inoculum size, and host susceptibility factors contribute to disease severity. Nevertheless, lethal complications are significantly more frequent at the extremes of age, in pregnancy, and in patients with underlying cardiopulmonary disease such as mitral stenosis or emphysema.

IMMUNITY. Antibody to the HA and NA prevents reinfection or reduces the severity of the disease. HI antibody plays the major role, although NI antibody alone in high titer can also prevent disease. Protection is correlated with both serum antibodies and IgA secretory antibodies in the respiratory tract. At the same level of serum HI antibody, respiratory infection provides most protection, parenteral vaccination with killed virus provides less, and passive parenteral immunization gives the least protection of the three methods. Multiple factors are thus important in immunity. The relative contributions of serum antibody, secretory antibody, and cell-mediated immunity are being delineated. Studies with the mouse and ferret models of influenza suggest that local secretory antibody correlates more with resistance to infection, while serum antibody correlates with the modification of disease in the lower respiratory tract. In mice and humans, influenza viral antigen-specific, HLA-restricted T-cell cytotoxicity correlates poorly with susceptibility to infection but does correlate with clearance of virus from the respiratory tract.

Immunity to a newly emerged antigenic variant is a function both of the degree of immunity to the previously circulating variant and the antigenic relatedness of the two strains. The three types of influenza share no antigenic relatedness and thus induce no cross-protection. Cross-protection becomes more complicated within a type, however. Thus, with a minor antigenic drift, a person with enough immunity for full protection against the older strain might develop a subclinical infection or mild disease with the newer strain; a person with partial protection against the older strain might develop severe influenza with the newer strain. Antibody levels correlate with protection on a statistical basis in a population, but not with the severity of individual responses to virus infection, which exhibit tremendous variation, in keeping with the multifactorial basis of resistance, including perhaps, nonimmune factors in disease response such as genetics and nutrition. The multiple infections a population experiences with influenza viruses that possess varying antigenic coats often make vaccine studies or immunodiagnosis unreliable and difficult to interpret.

Induction of immunity against mankind's last great infectious plague is a prime goal of modern medicine. Intramuscular injection of the standard vaccine, composed of inactivated egg-grown virus protects 70 per cent of adults against infection with an antigenically identical strain. Children respond with less antibody and more adverse effects to killed vaccine than do adults. With current purification of inactivated vaccine, adverse effects appear to correlate directly with the dose of virion components. An increased incidence of Guillain-Barré syndrome (approximately 1 in 10^5 versus the normal incidence of 1 in 10^6) followed immunization with the swine influenza vaccine in 1976–1977 but not with other inactivated influenza vaccines.

One contribution to influenza vaccine production has been Kilbourne's (1975) proposal to recombine high-yielding egg-adapted laboratory strains of influenza with each newly circulating epidemic virus. Reassortants possessing the surface antigens of the new virus and high-yield growth characteristics of the laboratory strain have cut costs and increased speed of production of killed vaccines. Nevertheless, the relative inefficacy of the inactivated influenza vaccine, when compared with polio or measles virus vaccines, for example, demands improvement. Among newly proposed approaches to immunoprophylaxis are the use of purified glycoprotein subunits prepared with cloned HA genes expressed in a bacterium or eukaryotic cell, and the use of synthetic oligopeptide sequences of the HA molecule that can induce protection.

Several approaches to live attenuated vaccine have been pursued. One approach proposed recombination between an older strain attenuated by multiple passages in eggs and an antigenically new epidemic strain. Unfortunately, the reassortants with the new antigens appear to have unpredictable levels of attenuation. A second method that may be combined with the first method selects for mutants that are resistant to nonimmunoglobulin serum inhibitors of the HA, thus resulting in strains that, for unknown reasons, are less pathogenic.

A more predictable approach involves the use of a master strain of donor virus that contains non-surface antigen genes that specify a desired level of attenuation. By reassortment, a specified level of attenuation could then be transferred by a rapid, single-step process to a virus containing the prevalent glycoprotein surface antigens. The precise genetic composition of the reassortant with regard to contribution from the two parental strains can now be ascertained with high resolution electrophoretic or hybridization techniques. Three sources of attenuating genes have been proposed. In one, genes containing temperature-sensitive mutations proved to have excellent phenotypic markers for attenuation that appeared effective and predictable. This approach was abandoned when reversion to virulent, wild-type virus in seronegative child recipients was observed. Two other sources of attenuating genes for live virus vaccines appear promising and are being investigated further. One is from viruses attenuated by multiple passages in cell cultures at ambient temperature (cold-adapted mutants); the other is from avian influenza A viruses that are poorly adapted to replicate and to produce disease in man.

LABORATORY DIAGNOSIS. Because the clinical characteristics of viral respiratory syndromes can be produced by dozens of different agents, the diagnosis of influenza requires isolation of the virus from the patient, identification of viral components (antigens or RNA) in patient's tissues, or documentation of a specific serologic response by the patient. The original technique for influenza virus isolation was growth in embryonated chicken eggs after allantoic or amniotic inoculation. Subsequently types A and B virus were isolated in primary kidney cell cultures, especially those from human embryos and rhesus monkeys. With the diminishing availability of these sources of primary kidney tissue, a reliable tissue culture substrate that could be propagated continuously was seriously needed. Laboratory strains of virus have been adapted to continuous cell lines; however, as is common with many viruses, the growth requirements of primary isolates are often fastidious. The Madin Darby canine kidney (MDCK) cell line along with trypsin in the culture medium to cleave and activate the HA glycoprotein now appears to be a readily available continuous cell line that is as sensitive as eggs or primary kidney cell cultures for the isolation of influenza viruses.

The best specimens for isolation are nasal washings obtained within the first few days of the onset of symptoms. The presence of virus in allantoic or tissue culture fluid is identified by hemagglutinating activity. The viral antigens can then be characterized with known antisera with an HI test. Alternatively, tissue culture monolayers can be identified as infected by the hemadsorption of erythrocytes, and the antigenic specificity of the agent can be determined by inhibiting the hemadsorption reaction with specific antisera (hemadsorption inhibition). More recently, specific immunofluorescent or immunoperoxidase staining has been used to identify infected cell cultures.

The rapid and specific identification of viral antigen in exfoliated nasopharyngeal cells using immunofluorescence or ELISA has also yielded good results when carefully performed with the proper reagents and controls. These approaches are neither as sensitive as virus isolation, nor do they yield an isolate which can be characterized for epidemiologic purposes. A more recently introduced approach for rapid viral diagnosis is the detection of influenza RNA in clinical specimens by hybridization with probes of cloned DNA complementary to influenza genes.

Although a fourfold rise in a virus-specific antibody has been used as a diagnostic standard of infection, this approach contains many pitfalls, especially for influenza virus infections. Any of the various influenza antibody measurements available may not reveal a rise in titer in some individuals with documented infection. Consequently, the failure to demonstrate an immune response by using appropriate acute and convalescent sera and a single reliable assay like the HI test does not exclude the diagnosis of influenza.

The complement-fixation test measures antibody to the NP and M proteins. This antibody usually falls to undetectable levels over a period of months so that an elevated convalescent serum complement-fixation titer has been considered indicative of a recent infection. Unfortunately, children, especially upon primary exposure, usually develop little or no complement-fixing antibody. With repeated influenza exposure this antibody response increases both in magnitude and duration so that elderly adults will often sustain elevated complement-fixation antibody levels for years.

The HI antibody response is generally considered the most reliable serologic indicator of infection. Caution is warranted, however, in using the HI antibody response to determine the antigenic identity of the infecting influenza virus because minor antigenic cross-reactions may occur between subtype antibodies and antibodies to unrelated, previously experienced subtype antigens (termed original antigenic sin). Consequently, knowledge of the antigenic composition of the prevalent viruses and use of potentially cross-reacting antigens as controls are helpful when performing the interpreting HI tests. Additional and potentially more rapid or less complicated methods, such as radial hemolysis, radial immunodiffusion, radioimmunoassay, indirect immunofluorescence, and immunoenzymatic assays, are currently under investigation.

EPIDEMIOLOGY. Although structurally similar, the three influenza types vary immensely in epidemiologic impact. Influenza C causes sporadic infections with mild upper respiratory tract disease; it does not cause epidemic influenza. Influenza B causes epidemics and can produce serious pneumonitis in adults. More importantly, it is associated with Reye's syndrome in children and is responsible for pneumonitis and croup in infants. The notoriety of influenza A stems from its capacity to produce pandemics.

Because numerous agents can cause similar syndromes, influenza must be detected either by laboratory surveillance for virus isolates and seroconversions, by excessive absenteeism in schools, or by excess pneumonia and mortality. By comparing the number of deaths or cases of pneumonia in a selected population with the baseline levels for previous years, the magnitude of the excess can be calculated. This measurement correlates well with the circulation of influenza in the population. Infants, the elderly, and those with underlying cardiopulmonary impairment are most susceptible to the complications of influenza. Young children also represent important vectors of influenza transmission.

The incidence of influenza peaks in the winter months. In tropical climates influenza remains an important disease, but it tends to occur over longer periods with dampened epidemic peaks. The mechanism of "overwintering"—that is, the maintenance of the agent in the population between epidemics has not been completely determined; nevertheless, surveillance of large populations during the summer indicates that the virus remains endemic in the population as determined by sporadic infrequent virus isolations and seroconversions, which often are associated with subclinical infection.

Influenza infection usually induces protective immunity to rechallenge with the homologous virus. The periodic recurrence of influenza in populations with previous experience with the virus results from the capacity of influenza virus to change surface antigens. Both in vitro and in vivo, the presence of partially protective levels of antibody gives a selective advantage to viruses with surface antigens that react less avidly with the antibody. After the population develops immunity to the circulating influenza strain, an antigenic drift occurs in either or in both of the surface antigens, resulting in a relatively more susceptible population. Peptide analysis ("fingerprinting") of the hemagglutinin polypeptide and nucleotide sequencing of its gene reveal that one or a few amino acid substitutions are responsible for an antigenic drift. Thus, antibody pressure provides a selective advantage for the growth of certain missense mutants. Such missense mutants can also be selected in vitro by use of subneutralizing concentrations of antisera or monoclonal antibodies. Both the naturally occurring and laboratory "drifted" antigenic variants have undergone missense mutations at restricted domains of the polypeptide (four in number for the HA) that result in a functionally unimpaired glycoprotein that is antigenically modified.

Although all three types of influenza virus exhibit antigenic drift, influenza A is the most virulent and influenza C the least virulent at given levels of immunity in the population. The progressively increasing sensitivity of the replication of types A, B, and then C to temperatures above body temperature has been proposed as an explanation for the observed gradient in virulence. Regardless of the intrinsic virulence of the different types, one additional property provides influenza A with the capacity to produce pandemic disease. Every 10 to 30 years, one or both of the surface antigens of human isolates of influenza A virus changes subtype, rendering a previously immune population completely susceptible. This antigenic shift is qualitative rather than the quantitative one characteristic of antigenic drift. Rather than a limited amino acid change typical of antigenic drift, the new subtype polypeptide contains multiple changes in its amino acid sequence that are not explicable on the basis of a few missense mutations. An accumulating body of circumstantial evidence suggests that antigenic shifts occur as a consequence either of rapid adaptation to man by an animal influenza A virus or of genetic reassortment during coinfection with influenza A viruses derived from man and animal.

Influenza A occurs in animals and man, whereas types B and C appear to be restricted to man, except for a report in 1983 of the isolation of influenza C from swine in China. The influenza A strains circulating in animals may provide a source of new antigenic subtypes of human influenza A viruses, thus accounting for antigenic shift. One species can transmit its influenza A virus to susceptible members of another species. The phenomenon of influenza virus infection with virus from another host species has been well described on swine farms with the exchange going in either direction between man and pig. Such exchange has also been observed on several occasions between migratory and domestic fowl. Influenza A viruses that have identical surface antigens but were isolated from different species replicate better and cause more disease in the homologous species. Nucleotide sequences of the NP gene suggest that there are equine, avian, and human-swine NP subgroups of influenza A that are independent of subtype and correlate with host species adaptation.

In 1979–1980, an epidemic killed approximately 20 per cent of the harbor seals (*Phoca vitulina*) of the northeast coast of the United States. The responsible virus, A/seal/Mass/1/80 (H7N7), was closely related to the fowl plague virus, A/FPV/Dutch/27 (H7N7), which had been isolated from several avian species but never from mammals. There had been no previous evidence of any seal influenza. The new seal H7N7 virus replicated well in mammals but not birds. This episode and a similar episode in seals caused by an H4N5 virus in 1983 suggests that the rapid introduction and adaptation of influenza virus to a new species is a possible mechanism for antigenic shift resulting in epidemic influenza.

Evidence documenting antigenic shift resulting from genetic reassortment of influenza A viruses is more available. Experimental studies with pigs and turkeys have demonstrated that genetic reassortment occurs in vivo after coinfection with two viruses (Fig. 3). Moreover, the selection of particular combinations of antigenic subtypes can be manipulated by adjusting the preinfection antibody levels present in the animal. These recombinants are then transmissible.

Ducks have been suspected as likely vectors of interspecies exchange of influenza viruses. High concentrations of influenza virus are found in duck feces and infectious virus persists in bodies of cold water. Such virus in lakes and rice paddies would then be available for transmission to other wild or domestic fowl or even swine, seals, and humans.

The subtypes of influenza A virus known to have circulated in humans are summarized in Table 2. The period of circulation of the subtype antigens that circulated before the original human isolate in 1933 have been deduced with a technique termed "immunologic recapitulation" or "seroarcheology," in which HI titers against numerous HA subtypes are determined with the sera from numerous age cohorts. These studies demonstrate that HI antibody to the H1 antigenic variant that was previously called Hswine is present in almost everyone born before 1918 and disappears in people born after 1927. Thus the 1918–1919 pandemic has been attributed to the abrupt introduction into the human population of the H1N1 subtype. This process of immunologic recapitulation indicates that the 1890 epidemic was probably caused by the H2N8 subtype and the 1900 epidemic by the H3N8 subtype. The H1N1 subtype circulated in humans from 1917 until 1957. Antigenic drift of this virus was so substantial that three subtypes (Hswine, H0, and H1) were thought to have circulated during this period until more precise serologic testing and nucleotide sequencing demonstrated these variants to be drifted members of the one subtype. In 1957, the H2N2 (Asian) influenza appeared. These 1957 isolates possessed new genes for the surface glycoproteins, but the remaining six genes were essentially the same as those that had been circulating with the previous H1N1 strains. In 1968 a shift to H3N2 virus resulted in the "Hong Kong" pandemic. H3N2 isolates from 1968 contained seven genes with sequences virtually identical to the recently circulating H2N2 strains and a HA gene quite unrelated to the H2 gene and almost identical in nucleotide sequence to the HA gene from H3N8 isolates from fowl and horses made in 1963 (A/duck/Ukraine/63 and A/equine/2/Miami/63). These isolates may have been descendents of the human strains presumably circulating from 1900 to 1918. In 1977, while H3N2 variants continued to circulate, a H1N1 virus reemerged that appeared to be identical in all eight genes to an antigenic variant that circulated in 1950. The origin of this virus, which caused disease primarily in individuals born since the disappearance of the H1N1 subtype in 1957, remains open to speculation. In 1978 and 1979, during simultaneous epidemics of H1N1 and H3N2 viruses in the same locale, several H3N2 isolates were shown to contain several nonglycoprotein genes identical to the circulating H1N1 strains.

There is thus documentation both for the abrupt introduction of new subtypes into animals and man and for the genetic reassortment of different subtypes of influenza A in animals and man. The reservoirs, frequencies, and mechanisms by which such antigenic shifts occur represent the subject of much exciting ongoing research, which ranges from worldwide wildlife ecology to nucleotide sequencing.

References

Couch, R. B., and Kasel, J. A.: Immunity to influenza in man. Annu Rev Microbiol 37:529, 1983.

Kaplan, M. M., and Webster, R. G.: The epidemiology of influenza. Sci Am 237:88, 1977.

Kilbourne, E. D. (ed.): The Influenza Viruses and Influenza. New York, Academic Press, 1975.

Lamb, R. A., and Choppin, P. W.: The gene structure and replication of influenza virus. Ann Rev Biochem 52:467, 1983.

Laver, W. G. (ed.): The Origin of Pandemic Influenza Viruses. New York, Elsevier Science Publishing Company, 1983.

Murphy, B. R., and Webster, R. G.: Orthomyxoviruses. In Fields, B. N. (ed.): Virology. New York, Raven Press (in press).

Stuart-Harris, C. H., and Schild, G. C.: Influenza: The Viruses and the Disease. Littleton, Massachusetts, Publishing Sciences Group, 1976.

Varghese, J. N., Laver, W. G., and Colman, P. M.: Structure of the influenza virus glycoprotein antigen, neuraminidase, at 2.9 A resolution. Nature 305:35, 1983.

Ward, C. W.: Structure of influenza virus hemagglutinin. Current Topics in Microbiology and Immunology. 94/95:1, 1981.

Webster, R. G., Laver, W. G., Air, G. M., and Schild, G. C.: Molecular mechanisms of variation in influenza viruses. Nature 296:115, 1982.

64

PARAMYXOVIRUSES

Douglas D. Richman, M.D.

CLASSIFICATION. The paramyxoviruses are enveloped, single-stranded, RNA viruses that are transmitted via the respiratory route. They include the most important respiratory viruses of infants (respiratory syncytial virus and the parainfluenza viruses) and two of the most important contagious diseases of childhood (measles and mumps). Properties of these viruses are delineated in Table 1. The family *Paramyxoviridae* has been divided into three genera. The genus *Paramyxovirus* includes parainfluenza virus types 1, 2, 3, 4a, 4b, and mumps virus. These viruses possess two surface glycoproteins, one with both hemagglutinating and neuraminidase enzyme activities and one with cell fusion and hemolysin activities. These viruses are all antigenically related. Sendai virus (mouse parainfluenza virus type 1), simian virus 5, and Newcastle disease virus of fowl belong to this genus. The genus *Morbillivirus* includes measles, canine distemper, and bovine rinderpest viruses, which are antigenically related, but do not cross-react immunologically with paramyxoviruses of the other two genera. These viruses lack neuraminidase activity and they hemagglutinate only red blood cells of old world monkeys. The genus *Pneumovirus* includes respiratory syncytial virus

(RSV) and pneumonia virus of mice. These agents have a smaller nucleocapsid and lack the hemagglutinating, neuramidinase, and hemolysin activities characteristic of the surface glycoproteins of the members of the other two genera.

STRUCTURE. *Paramyxovirus* virions are usually spheroids 150 to 250 nm in diameter, although preparations often show variant forms with dimensions ranging from 100 to 700 nm. These virions have a buoyant density of 1.19 to 1.22 g/cm³ and a sedimentation coefficient of 1000 to 1100S. Their genetic material is a linear, single-stranded RNA molecule that has a sedimentation coefficient of 50S and weighs approximately 5×10^6 daltons. This RNA represents 0.91 per cent of the total virion weight. The remainder of the virion is composed of 73 per cent protein, 20 per cent lipids, and 6 per cent carbohydrate.

The structural proteins of the paramyxoviruses appear to be in large part analogous to those of influenza A and B viruses. Several large proteins, including two designated P and L, and a nucleoprotein (NP) are associated with the virion RNA and participate in RNA transcription and replication. The NP surrounds the RNA in a helical array forming a ribonucleoprotein (RNP) structure (Figure 2 in preceding chapter). This structure has a buoyant density of 1.27 to 1.30 g/cm³ and a length of 1 μm. A hydrophobic matrix (M) protein underlies the host cell membrane during virion assembly and the lipid envelope of the budded virion. The M protein has an affinity for the NP, for lipid, and for the virion glycoproteins and may thus be important in virion assembly.

Inserted in the lipid envelope are projections consisting of two different glycoproteins, the activities of which distinguish the three genera of the paramyxovirus family. The parainfluenza and mumps viruses possess a glycoprotein (HN) with both hemagglutinin and neuraminidase activities and a glycoprotein (F) with both membrane fusion and hemolysin activities. The HN protein alone serves the two functions of host cell attachment and release served by the two glycoproteins (HA and NA) of the influenza viruses. As in the case of the influenza viruses, sialyloligosaccharide present in host cell and red blood cell membranes serve as the receptor and the substrate for the HN activities. Analogous to the influenza virus NA glycoprotein, the HN glycoprotein is a tetramer. Monoclonal antibodies to the HN glycoprotein of parainfluenza 1 virus segregate into four sets, one of which inhibits neuraminidase activity and the others inhibit the hemagglutinin. The F glycoprotein is analogous in several respects to the influenza virus HA glycoprotein and may in fact have evolved from a common ancestor. The F glycoprotein is derived from a precursor polypeptide (F_0) with a molecular weight of 65,000. The proteolytic cleavage of an 8000 to 10,000 dalton polypeptide is required to convert the F_0 to F and activate the fusion and hemolytic functions. This renders the virion infectious. The cleavage step is accomplished by a host-cell protease that represents one, if not the major, determinant of cell permissiveness in vitro. This host cell characteristic may also represent a critical factor in host range and tissue tropism in vivo. The product of this proteolytic cleavage is a glycoprotein consisting of two glycopeptides (F1 and F2) joined by a disulfide bond. F1, like HA2 of influenza virus, inserts into the lipid envelope at the carboxy terminus. The enzymatically active sites that are formed by this proteolytic cleavage, are generated at the amino termini of the F1 and the HA2 glycopeptides. Moreover, the amino acid sequences at the amino termini of these glycopeptides from these two virus families have been extensively conserved.

Measles virus possesses a similar F glycoprotein; however, the second glycoprotein does not contain hemagglutinin or neuraminidase activities. Measles virus does, however, agglutinate old world monkey red blood cells. This characteristic has some diagnostic utility, but presumably has no biologic relevance. This glycoprotein (H) is responsible for host cell attachment, although the receptor site is not N-acetylneuraminic (sialic) acid. Respiratory syncytial virus may also possess an F protein analogous to its relatives; however, with the exception of its well-documented fusion activity, the precise structure and function of the two RSV glycoproteins are unknown.

The virion RNA of the *Paramyxoviridae* has (−) sense and is transcribed by virion enzymes. The resulting mRNA thus is not dependent host protein synthesis. Subsequent viral RNA replication requires host cell translation and processing. The replication of the parainfluenza viruses and RSV is unaffected by inhibitors of cellular DNA synthesis such as actinomycin D or by irradiation or enucleation of the host cell. Synthesis of both measles virus RNA and protein is inhibited by such manipulations; however, it has not yet been determined whether such manipulations are affecting a specific requirement for nuclear RNA polymerase II (as with influenza virus) or whether such manipulations result in less specific disruptions of replication. Large amounts of measles virus ribonucleoprotein are found in nuclear inclusions found in cells both in acute measles and SSPE; however, it has not been determined whether these were synthesized in the nucleus or in the cytoplasm with subsequent transport to the nucleus.

ANTIGENIC COMPOSITION

Parainfluenza Viruses and Mumps Virus. There are four serotypes of the human parainfluenza viruses, which are distinct by neutralizing, hemagglutination inhibiting (HI), and complement-fixing antibody (CF) assays. Types 1, 2, and 3 are each antigenically homogeneous and stable as is mumps virus. Type 4 is composed of two subtypes, 4a and 4b, which are distinguishable by neutralization and HI, but not by CF. Antibody to the HN glycoprotein can inhibit adsorption and neutralize infectivity. This antibody can inhibit the HA and NA activities. Monoclonal antibodies can discriminate epitopes on the HN glycoprotein corresponding to these two enzymatic activities. Antibody to the F glycoprotein has no effect on adsorption or on the HA and NA activities. Anti-F antibody can neutralize infectivity and virus-induced hemolysis. CF utilizes the soluble (S) antigen associated with the nucleocapsid. Although these antigens are distinct for each type, hyperimmunization will stimulate cross-reactive antibody to the other types, to mumps virus, and to Newcastle disease virus. This phenomenon occurs with neutralizing, HI, and CF antibody responses. Humans are exposed to most of these agents during childhood and are repeatedly infected with the parainfluenza viruses; this accounts for the heterotypic antibody responses to infection often observed in humans, especially in older people.

Measles Virus. Measles virus is antigenically homogeneous and stable as determined with polyclonal antisera. It is antigenically related to distemper and rinderpest viruses. CF antibody is detected by utilizing the nucleo-

Table 1. HUMAN ORTHOMYXOVIRUSES AND PARAMYXOVIRUSES

	Virion Diameter (nm)	Genome Size (daltons × 10^6)	Number of Gene Segments	Diameter of Ribonucleo-protein	Nuclear Requirement for Replication	Enzyme Activities: RNA Polymerase
Orthomyxoviridae						
Influenza A & B	80–170	5	8	9	+	+
Influenza C	80–170	5	7	9	+	+
Paramyxoviridae						
Parainfluenza 1–4b	150–250	5	1	18	−	+
Mumps	150–250	5	1	18	−	+
Measles (Rubeola)	150–250	5	1	18	− (?)	+
Respiratory syncytial virus	90–180	5	1	13	−	+

capsid protein (soluble [S] antigen). Neutralizing and HI antibody is directed against the H glycoprotein. Anti-F antibody acts as with the parainfluenza viruses.

Respiratory Syncytial Virus. RSV isolates cannot be distinguished by CF; however, several minor antigenic variants have been detected by neutralization tests with early postinfection sera. Convalescent human sera appear to be unable to make this distinction. Monoclonal antibodies appear to be useful for discriminating these variants. Whether this antigenic variation has any biologic significance has not been determined.

SUSCEPTIBLE HOST CELLS. These agents all initiate their infections on the respiratory epithelium. The susceptibility of epithelial cells to these agents probably accounts for the value of primary human and primate kidney cell cultures for their laboratory isolation (Table 1). The respiratory pathogens (the parainfluenza viruses and RSV) are restricted to the respiratory tract. Measles and mumps disseminate from the respiratory tract via the bloodstream to various target organs as discussed below.

PATHOGENIC PROPERTIES. All paramyxoviruses are transmitted by inhalation of droplet aerosols or by inoculation of respiratory secretions (by hand, for example) onto the respiratory mucosa. The nature of the resulting infection then depends both on host factors, such as age and immune status, and on the specific agent.

Parainfluenza Viruses. The replication of these agents is restricted to the respiratory tract. No extrapulmonary replication has been well documented, although viremia has been reported. These agents cause only upper respiratory infections (the common cold syndrome) except in a proportion of infants who develop laryngotracheobronchitis (croup), bronchiolitis or pneumonitis during their primary infection.

Mumps. Mumps infection causes parotitis after an incubation period of 15 to 18 days following exposure to an infected individual. The incubation period has been reported to range from the extremes of 7 to 23 days. Early in the incubation period, after replication in the respiratory epithelium, viremia disseminates virus throughout the parotid duct secretions for two to three days before the onset of symptoms. The presence of virus in saliva before symptoms, the variable incubation period, and the numerous asymptomatic but still infectious cases, account for the difficulty in controlling transmission. Fever, malaise, myalgia, and coryza usually initiate the clinical disease. Parotitis usually follows within a day. Virus can be isolated from Stensen's duct or from the saliva for another five to seven days. Parotitis may be bilateral, unilateral, or absent. Other organs are involved, either singly or in a variety of combinations, even in the absence of parotitis. Most frequently recognized is infection of other salivary glands, testes, ovaries, pancreas, breasts, and meninges. Rare reports of thyroiditis and arthritis need confirmation. Myocarditis has been documented but fetal mumps infection as a cause of endocardial fibroelastosis remains controversial. Mumps virus is shed in the urine for ten days or longer after the onset of symptoms, even in the absence of orchitis. In addition, hematuria, proteinuria, and a reversible reduction in creatinine clearance also suggest that nephritis may be common, although neither viral replication in the kidneys nor immune complex disease has been documented.

Prior to the vaccine, mumps meningoencephalitis caused about 10 per cent of all cases of aseptic meningitis. The frequency of subclinical meningitis is unknown; however, an abnormal electroencephalogram (EEG) is uncommon with mumps parotitis in contrast to its frequency in uncomplicated measles. The cerebrospinal fluid in mumps meningitis tends to have lower sugars and higher polymorphonuclear leukocyte counts than in most other viral meningitides. Parotitis is absent in 25 to 50 per cent of cases of mumps meningoencephalitis, but when present, usually occurs three to ten days before CNS symptoms. Although parotitis occurs with equal frequency in both sexes, CNS mumps occurs three times more frequently in males. Sequelae are unusual after CNS mumps; the mortality from encephalitis is 1 per cent. Deafness due to auditory neuritis has been described, and may even occur without encephalitis.

Measles. After replication in the respiratory mucosa, measles virus is transported to lymphoid tissues, where it multiplies further, and then spreads via the bloodstream in leukocytes. During this asymptomatic incubation period,

Table 1. *(Continued)*

Enzyme Activities				Cultivation of Primary Isolates		
Hemagglutinin	***Neuraminidase***	***Hemolysin***	***Membrane Fusion***	***Embryonated Egg***	***Primary Human or Monkey Kidney***	***Continuous Cell Lines***
+	+	−	−	+	+	MDCK
+	−	−	−	+	−	MDCK
+	+	+	+	−	+	Some types only: MDCK, HeLa, HEp-2, WI-38
+	+	+	+	+	+	Vero, HeLa, LLC-MK2
+	−	+	+	+	+	HeLa, HEp-2, LLC-MK2
−	−	−	+	−	+	Hep-2, HeLa WI-38

cytolysis, tissue necrosis, and inflammation are not manifest; the only histologic sign of local replication is multinucleate giant cells with intranuclear inclusions (Warthin-Finkeldey cells). Just before or during the prodrome, these are seen in the lymph nodes, tonsils, appendix, and exfoliated nasal mucosa. The usual incubation period of 10 to 12 days terminates with the onset of coryza, conjunctivitis, dry cough, sore throat, lymphadenopathy, headache, fever, and Koplik's spots. Koplik's spots are tiny erythematous patches with bluish-white apices on the buccal mucosa along the molar bite line. These spots contain the giant cells with eosinophilic intranuclear inclusions that are composed of measles virus-specific proteins as determined by immunofluorescence and viral nucleocapsids as determined by electron microscopy. The exanthem usually appears on the second day, beginning on the head, then spreading to the trunk, and finally to the extremities. The incubation period is usually two to three days shorter when the usual respiratory portal of entry is bypassed by parenteral inoculation with either the wild-type virus experimentally or the live attenuated vaccine. The incubation period is prolonged up to 3 weeks, especially in older people or in recipients of measles antiglobulin.

During the prodrome, virus is present in tears, nasal secretions, throat, urine, and blood. The viremia disappears with the onset of the rash, which is followed within two to three days by the appearance of serum antibody. A causal relationship between the appearance of immunoglobulins and the onset of symptoms has been proposed. Although the cutaneous and upper respiratory involvement is most easily recognized, viremia carries the virus elsewhere throughout the body. Respiratory complications include otitis media, croup, and pneumonitis with or without secondary bacterial pneumonia. An acute abdomen, easily mistaken for appendicitis, may precede the exanthem. Myocarditis and thrombocytopenic purpura are other rare complications.

Although EEG aberrations are detectable in most patients with measles, clinically apparent encephalitis occurs in only one of every 1000 cases. The encephalitis results in a 15 per cent mortality and 25 per cent residual morbidity. Most cases of encephalitis occur on about day six and usually within 2 weeks of the onset of the rash. Despite its temporal relationship to the rash, the pathology in encephalitis differs from that in other organs, in that inclusion bodies and giant cells are not common. Instead, a perivascular mononuclear infiltrate, demyelination, petechial hemorrhages, and microglial proliferation are seen. The overall mortality from measles can approach 10 per cent in malnourished populations, primarily because of secondary bacterial pneumonia. Infants and the elderly are most susceptible and mortality in them may exceed 25 per cent. In affluent societies the mortality rate approximates 0.1 per cent.

Subacute sclerosing panencephalitis (SSPE) is a rare (1 per 100,000 cases) but intriguing expression of measles infection. It causes an insidious intellectual, behavioral, and motor deterioration, which progresses to convulsions, coma, and death usually within a year of onset. Victims of SSPE manifest a characteristic EEG pattern, markedly elevated serum and CSF measles antibodies, and typical histologic findings distinct from the acute encephalitis of measles. Measles antigen is readily demonstrable in SSPE brains, although virus isolation usually requires extensive effort, including cocultivation techniques. SSPE occurs with a median latent period of 7 years after typical measles, but at a younger age and in a more rural area than average. Immune defects and virus variants have been proposed to explain the pathogenesis of SSPE. There is evidence that infected cells in SSPE are defective in synthesis of M protein, which presumably is integral to the process of virion assembly.

Respiratory Syncytial Virus. The incubation period of RSV infection is four to five days. RSV replication appears to be restricted to the respiratory mucosa. It produces bronchiolitis, pneumonitis, and, less frequently, croup and apnea. These severe infections usually occur in children less than 6 months old who are experiencing their first RSV infection. Although most nonprimary RSV infections involve the upper respiratory tract, lower respiratory tract disease in older children and adults has been reported (see Immunity below).

IMMUNITY

Parainfluenza Viruses. Severe life-threatening infection occurs in infants experiencing their first infection. Passively acquired antibody appears to reduce the risk of severe disease in infants. IgA-neutralizing antibody appears in the nasal secretions after infection. The presence of this secretory antibody correlates well with protection from reinfection but it disappears in one to six months, leaving the child susceptible to reinfection despite substantial levels of serum neutralizing antibody. Past experience with the virus, however, does provide some protection; repeat infections are limited to the upper respiratory tract.

Life-threatening bronchiolitis and pneumonitis due to parainfluenza type 3, as with RSV, occur in infants, many of whom have maternally derived serum antibody. In contrast to RSV, administration of an inactivated vaccine (in one study) did not predispose to more severe disease, although it also failed to provide protection. Maternal antibody seems to give some protection from types 1 and 2 infection to infants in their first 4 months. Croup is seen after infection by these two viruses in some infants but also occurs in primary infection of older children.

Mumps Virus. CF antibody to the nucleocapsid protein (S antigen) is usually apparent at 1 week and peaks at 2 weeks postinfection; it is thus useful for laboratory diagnosis of recent infection. Antibody to the hemagglutinin glycoprotein (V antigen), as measured by hemagglutination inhibition or neutralization of viral infectivity, appears at 2 to 3 weeks and peaks at 3 to 4 weeks. This antibody is the best indicator of immunity because it is neutralizing antibody and because it is measurable for much longer than CF antibody. Reinfection is extremely rare; however, because asymptomatic infections are common and because other viruses may also cause parotitis, neither a history of parotitis nor its absence is useful in determining previous experience with mumps virus. In addition to mumps virus, parainfluenza viruses, enteroviruses, and influenza A virus have all been implicated as etiologic agents of parotitis.

The live attenuated mumps vaccine is grown in chick embryo cells. The vaccine causes an inapparent infection, seroconversion, and protection from mumps infection in over 95 per cent of seronegative recipients. The vaccine, which is inoculated subcutaneously, stimulates all commonly measured antibody responses but with lower mean titers than does natural infection. This vaccine does not produce detectable virus in saliva, viremia, viruria, or spread to contacts; however, vaccine virus has been isolated from an aborted placenta 10 days postinoculation of the mother. The vaccine was licensed in the United States in 1967, too recent for the long-term duration of immunity to be determined. However, studies to date are very encouraging. Killed mumps vaccines protect only for short durations. The efficacy of passive immunization with convalescent serum or pooled γ-globulins has not been demonstrated.

Measles. Infection confers lifelong protection. The presence of CF, HI, or neutralizing antibody indicates immunity. Passive immunization with pooled IgG is usually effective if given within 1 week of exposure. It is indicated for pregnant women, neonates, and immunosuppressed patients who are exposed and susceptible. Although it prevents reinfection, serum antibody does not appear to be essential for recovery from primary infection or the sole defense against reinfection because immunoglobulin-deficient patients recover from measles normally and resist reinfection. In contrast, patients with defective cellular immunity suffer serious complications of measles infection. Enders demonstrated that the syndrome of giant cell pneumonia without the usual morbilliform rash was a consequence of measles infection in such patients.

Modified measles is an abbreviated and milder form of ordinary measles, often with a prolonged incubation period. Modified measles is seen in children passively immunized with prophylactic IgG or with transplacental IgG. *Atypical measles* results from infection with either wild type or vaccine measles virus at least 2 years after immunization with formalin-inactivated measles vaccine. It is characterized by fever, pneumonitis, pleural effusion, edema of extremities, and an atypical rash. The rash has a predilection for the extremities and tends to be discrete, often with an urticarial, petechial, or vesicular component in contrast to the typical blanching, erythematous, maculopapular, morbilliform rash of ordinary measles. Norrby has proposed that atypical measles infection is a consequence of the inability of the killed vaccine to stimulate antibody to the F (hemolysin-fusion) protein as does natural or live attenuated vaccine infection. The production of killed vaccine by virus inactivation preserves the antigenicity of the H glycoprotein but not the F. Choppin has demonstrated that in the presence of antibody to H, free virus will be neutralized but the cell-to-cell spread of infection (via fusion) and the subsequent elaboration of antigen will occur in vitro. In vivo, this antigen could generate immune complexes or cell-mediated immune responses that could mediate atypical measles.

The live attenuated vaccine, grown in chick embryo fibroblasts at reduced temperature, has supplanted the killed vaccine. The live vaccine is >95 per cent effective. Failures have been attributed to vaccine inactivation and to administration to infants with residual transplacental immunity, usually in infants less than 1 year old. Ten per cent of vaccine recipients have a fever or a mild rash 10 days postinoculation. There is little, if any, vaccine virus excretion and no transmission has been documented. Mean antibody titers tend to be lower after vaccination than with natural infection; however, many vaccinees subsequently exposed to measles appear to have asymptomatic antibody boosts. The measles vaccine is administered in one dose subcutaneously. It can be given in combination with the mumps and rubella live attenuated vaccines with no apparent reduction in the efficacy of any of the three components. Serum antibody following live measles immunization may fall below detectable levels in standard HI assays. Immunity can be confirmed using more sensitive assays such as the large well ("macro") HI assay, microneutralization assays or enzyme immunoassays.

Respiratory Syncytial Virus. Newborns enjoy relative freedom from infection for two to four weeks, perhaps because exposure is limited or immunity is transmitted transplacentally. For the next six months, with a peak in month two, susceptibility to life-threatening infection is extremely high. The level of antibody in the cord blood correlates directly with the age of first infection. Moreover, infants with higher levels of passively acquired antibody tend to have milder disease. Secretory neutralizing antibody protects from infection. This secretory antibody is not long-lasting; however, immunity from previous RSV infection usually restricts reinfection to the upper respiratory tract.

The relative roles of antibody and components of cell-mediated immunity in conferring protection and in mediating some of the severe expressions of RSV infection are not known. Formalin-inactivated virus not only fails to protect, but places children as old as two years at risk for life-threatening bronchiolitis, a syndrome usually not seen after the sixth month in unimmunized children. Live attenuated vaccines have not yet proven effective. One vaccine, a temperature-sensitive mutant, was over-attenuated and replicated poorly in recipients. Another vaccine prepared by serial passage in cell culture and administered parenterally was immunogenic but not protective.

LABORATORY DIAGNOSIS

Parainfluenza Viruses. When respiratory tissue or secretions are inoculated into cell cultures, the presence of parainfluenza virus may be recognized by cell death or syncytium formation; however, hemadsorption or specific immunofluorescence is more sensitive because isolates in early passage may produce little or no visible cell injury. The parainfluenza virus isolate can be typed by hemadsorption inhibition with type-specific antiserum, by HI or CF characterization of progeny virus from the tissue culture supernatant, or by immunofluorescence of infected tissue culture cells. Rapid diagnosis by identification of specific viral antigen in exfoliated nasopharyngeal cells by immunofluorescence or ELISA is possible; however, highly specific immune reagents and appropriate controls are required. These assays are not as sensitive as virus isolation. Primary human embryonic or simian kidney cell cultures are the most sensitive cell lines for isolation of human parainfluenza viruses. Persistent infection with simian virus 5 (related to type 2) in simian cell cultures, and of that virus or Sendai virus (related to type 1) in rodent cultures may be a common source of error. HeLa, HEp2, and WI-38 cell lines are also effective for types 2 and 3. A continuous monkey kidney cell line, LLC-MK2, along with trypsin in the culture medium to cleave and activate the F glycoprotein, is a sensitive line for the isolation and propagation of parainfluenza viruses. CF antibody responses may not occur in mild disease; neutralization, HI, or ELISA are more sensitive assays for antibody responses. Interpretation of parainfluenza virus serology must take into account the occurrence of cross-reactive rises of antibody to different types that occur in reinfection.

Mumps. Although the typical syndrome of parotitis has also been attributed to parainfluenza viruses, coxsackieviruses, and influenza A virus, laboratory diagnosis is indicated only when complications occur. Virus can be isolated in the first few days of illness from saliva, parotid duct secretions, urine, or cerebrospinal fluid if meningitis is present. Viruria may persist for over two weeks. Although the virus was originally isolated by inoculation into the amniotic cavity of eight day old embryonated chicken eggs, primary or continuous human and primate cell lines are more sensitive. Cell rounding and syncytia are seen in infected cell monolayers, but hemadsorption and immunofluorescence are more sensitive indicators of infection. Prompt inoculation of a specimen is important because mumps virus infectivity is unstable both at room temperature and at 4°C. As discussed in the section on immunity, the CF antibody response is more prompt but less durable than the HI, neutralization, and ELISA antibody responses.

Measles. Measles usually produces a distinct syndrome even when the typical exanthem cannot be easily recognized—for example, in dark-skinned people. Confirmation is indicated in the atypical or complicated case. In the United States and other areas where eradication programs have reduced the incidence of measles, confirmation of all suspected cases is important for epidemiologic purposes. Diagnosis can be accomplished by isolation of virus from respiratory secretions, blood, or urine with embryonated eggs or cell culture. The virus is excreted in the respiratory secretions, tears, and urine during the prodrome and for about two days after the appearance of the rash. The virus is also present in blood leukocytes, lymph nodes, spleen, kidney, skin, and lungs. Measles isolation in cell culture, first reported by Enders and Peebles in 1954, provided the technology for the most sensitive isolation technique, and thus enabled us to obtain the data that underlie our current concepts of measles immunology, pathogenesis, and epidemiology. Cell cultures of primary human embryo, rhesus monkey kidney, or LLC-RMK2 using trypsin to activate the F glycoprotein are the most sensitive; cytopathic effects appear in one to two weeks. Isolation may require holding cell cultures for a month with "blind" passaging to permit adaptation of the isolate to cell culture. The classic cytopathology—multinucleate giant cells and intranuclear inclusions—may develop only with passaging. Earlier detection of infected cell cultures is possible with specific immunofluorescence or hemadsorption with monkey erythrocytes.

As mentioned, immunity in adults, especially recipients of live vaccine, may be difficult to assess with standard antibody assays. The antibody response following the onset of disease is sufficiently prompt and great, however, that any of the antibody assays (CF, neutralization, HI, ELISA) will diagnose measles, assuming that an acute serum is obtained early enough. A valid assay for IgM antibody to measles might permit the diagnosis of measles with a single serum.

Respiratory Syncytial Virus. RSV can be isolated from the respiratory secretions by using susceptible host cell cultures, such as primary monkey or bovine kidney, HeLa, HEp-2, or WI-38. Syncytia and eosinophilic cytoplasmic inclusions are produced, but specific confirmation is accomplished by CF of progeny virus or immunofluorescence of infected cells. Detection of RSV antigen with ELISA or immunofluorescence of exfoliated respiratory epithelial cells is effective for rapid diagnosis of RSV infection. Because RSV is extremely labile, isolation is improved by collecting good quantities of respiratory secretions—for example, nasopharyngeal washings rather than swabs, and by promptly inoculating cell cultures without prior storage of the specimen. Infants suffering primary infection may shed virus for four to six weeks, even after apparent recovery.

CF is the most available and least cumbersome serologic test. However, the neutralization test is more sensitive, with plaque reduction being slightly more sensitive than end-point neutralization of cytopathic effect. ELISA methods for measuring antibody also appear to be specific and sensitive.

EPIDEMIOLOGY

Parainfluenza Viruses. As with most respiratory agents, the risk of infection increases in those with contact with young children. Thus, high risk situations include large families, child care centers, schools, and pediatric wards of hospitals. Type 3 is the most prevalent of the parainfluenza types. Fifty per cent of children have serologic evidence of infection during their first year and 95 per cent by age six. Type 3 infections occur endemically throughout the year, whereas type 1 and, to a lesser extent, type 2 occur in epidemics during the fall or winter, often in a biannual pattern. Only respiratory syncytial virus exceeds type 3 in frequency as a cause of tracheobronchitis, bronchiolitis, and pneumonitis in infants. Type 1 and, to a lesser extent, type 2 are largely responsible for croup (acute laryngotracheobronchitis) infants.

Mumps. Mumps is not as contagious as measles or varicella; consequently, there is a fair proportion of seronegative young adults, perhaps 10 per cent. This percentage is increased in isolated areas; for example, more than 80 per cent of certain populations of Alaskan Eskimos may be seronegative. Infection is endemic throughout the year with a peak in the late winter and early spring in nontropical climates. Epidemics occur where children and young adults congregate, especially schools and military situations.

The incidence of encephalitis is 2.5 per 1000 cases of reported mumps; the incidence of fatal mumps is approximately 0.25 cases per 1000 cases of reported mumps. Mumps infections are probably underreported, however, because approximately one third of all infections are subclinical. The age incidence of encephalitis correlates well with the age incidence of parotitis; however, fatalities are disproportionately increased in infants and older adults. The incidence of mumps and its complications have diminished dramatically since the introduction of live, attenuated vaccine.

Measles. Measles is ideal for epidemiologic study because it is highly contagious, there is a low proportion of subclinical infection, infection confers immunity to reinfection, and there is no evidence that the virus is heterogeneous with regard to antigens or virulence. There is no apparent animal reservoir. Consequently, the virus is best maintained in populous, developing areas, where annual late winter and early spring epidemics are seen, with cases detectable throughout the year. Epidemics occur with lower attack rates and at longer intervals in less populous and more economically developed areas. The virus disappears periodically from sparsely populated and isolated areas, which are subject to outbreaks when the virus is reintroduced from the outside after a critical number of nonimmune individuals have accumulated.

Measles is usually contracted by preschool children in populous, developing areas. In developed countries the disease is most common in elementary school children. In a remote Eskimo village, measles occurs at the age at which the virus is introduced from the outside. Thus, before measles vaccine, children rarely reached adulthood without measles infection except in remote and sparsely populated areas. Since the introduction of measles vaccine—in the United States, for example—the incidence of measles has fallen below 1 per cent of its previous incidence and the disease is occurring in somewhat older people. Infection is occurring in older individuals because unvaccinated children tend to be older and because there are fewer susceptibles to maintain annual epidemics. The vaccination program in the United States may eradicate endemic measles in the 1980s.

Respiratory Syncytial Virus. RSV consistently produces annual winter epidemics between January and March in temperate climates in the northern hemisphere. Epidemics during the rainy summer season have been described in Trinidad. These epidemics attack approximately one third of seronegative children, so that by age five, 95 per cent of children are seropositive. The mechanism of "overwintering," the maintenance of the virus between epidemics, is an enigma. Low rates of endemic infection between epidemics have not been documented as has been done with influenza. In primary infection, virus is often excreted for one or two months after symptoms resolve; however, prolonged excretion after reinfection of either children or adults has not been documented. Reinfection occurs in up to 20 per cent of children and adolescents annually, diminishing to an annual rate of 3 to 5 per cent in adults. The risk of infection is highest in nurseries, institutions, and pediatric wards of hospitals where there are high concentrations of infants. Such epidemic transmission may result more from contact with infected hands and surfaces than from aerosols.

References

Choppin, P. W., and Compans, R. W.: Reproduction of paramyxoviruses. In Fraenkel-Conrat, H., and Wagner, R. R. (eds.): Comprehensive Virology. New York, Plenum, 1975, p. 95.

Choppin, P. W., and Scheid, A.: The role of viral glycoproteins in adsorption, penetration, and pathogenicity of viruses. Rev Infect Dis 2:40, 1980.

Evans, A. S. (ed.): Viral Infections of Humans, Epidemiology and Control. 2nd edition. New York, Plenum, 1982.

Hall, C. B.: The nosocomial spread of respiratory syncytial viral infections. Ann Rev Med 34:311, 1983.

Henderson, F. W., Collier, A. M., Clyde, W. A., Jr., and Denny, F. W. Respiratory syncytial virus infections, reinfections and immunity: a prospective, longitudinal study in young children. N Engl J Med 300:530, 1979.

Rima, B. K.: The proteins of morbilliviruses. J Gen Virol 64:1205, 1983.

Wechsler, S. L., and Meissner, H. C.: Measles and SSPE viruses: Similarities and differences. Prog Med Virol 28:65, 1982.

65
PICORNAVIRUSES

NATHANIEL A. YOUNG, M.D.*

PICORNAVIRUS STRUCTURE AND COMPOSITION. Picornaviridae is a large family of animal viruses named for their diminutive size, 22 to 30 nm, and nucleic acid type, RNA (Cooper et al., 1978, Matthews, 1982). Picornavirus particles (virions) are icosahedral and consist of two structural moieties: (1) an outer protein shell, or capsid, comprising 70 per cent of the mass, and (2) an inner strand of RNA, which is 30 per cent of the mass. Lacking a lipid envelope, the "naked" virions are not affected by ether, alcohol, or other lipid solvents, although they are readily inactivated by phenol, formaldehyde, or ionizing radiation, which damage the capsid or the enclosed nucleic acid.

The picornavirus capsid consists of 60 identical subunits, or capsomeres, each of which has a molecular mass of 88,000 to 100,000 daltons and is composed of four nonidentical virion polypeptides, VP1-4. Three of these polypeptides are large (molecular mass 24,000 to 41,000 daltons, depending upon the polypeptide and the particular picornavirus), and the fourth is small (5000 to 14,000 daltons). The capsids of picornaviruses are very stable structures that resist digestion by proteases that can hydrolyze dissociated capsomeres and virion polypeptides.

The RNA of picornaviruses is a linear, single-stranded, nonsegmented molecule with a molecule mass of about 2.6 million daltons (approximately 7500 nucleotides). Virion RNA has the polarity of viral messenger RNA (mRNA), i.e., it is positive (+) stranded. Thus it is infectious and can also be translated in vitro. Like cellular mRNA, the RNA of picornaviruses is polyadenylated at its 3′ terminus. However, its 5′ terminus is highly unusual (Kitamura et al., 1981). It does not contain a methylated guanosine cap like cellular mRNA, but has a small protein (VPg) covalently linked to its 5′-terminal phosphate (Fig. 1). VPg is a virus-coded, water-insoluble, basic oligopeptide consisting (in the case of poliovirus type 1) of only 22 amino acids. It is linked to the virion RNA by a phosphodiester bond between the 5′-terminal uridine and a tyrosine residue in VPg [VPg(tyr-0)-pUUAAAACAG. . .]. VPg may play a role in the initiation of RNA replication, and it may also be involved in virion assembly (Nomoto et al., 1977; Kitamura et al., 1981).

PICORNAVIRUS REPLICATION. The picornavirus capsid serves three important functions: it protects the RNA genome from nucleases in the environment; it mediates the attachment of virions to susceptible host cells, a process dependent upon the binding of a virion attachment site on the capsid surface to a specific receptor site on the plasma membrane; and it delivers the virion RNA into the host cell's cytoplasm as a result of its interaction with the plasma membrane. The attachment of picornaviruses to cell membrane receptors is specific, and there are different receptors for different members of the picornavirus family. For example, the three polioviruses compete for a common receptor, which is distinct from the receptor that binds group B coxsackieviruses; other unique receptors exist for group A coxsackieviruses, for echoviruses and for human rhinoviruses (Campbell and Cords, 1983; Crowell and Landau, 1983). Attachment sites on the surface of picornavirus capsids are determined by the viral genome, whereas receptors on the plasma membrane are under host cell genetic control, e.g., the information for poliovirus receptor formation is located on human chromosome 19 (Miller et al., 1974). The presence of appropriate receptors is a prerequisite for cell susceptibility to picornavirus infection: cells lacking receptors are invariably resistant, whereas cells possessing them are usually susceptible (Crowell and Landau, 1983). Thus the picornavirus-receptor interaction is a major determinant of virus host range and tissue tropism, and consequently an important factor in the pathogenesis of infections by specific picornaviruses. For example, the presence of receptors for polioviruses on human motor neurons accounts for the capacity of polioviruses to produce paralytic disease in man, and the absence of such receptors on mouse cells accounts for the resistance of mice, as well as cultured mouse cells, to poliovirus infection.

Initial attachment of picornaviruses to susceptible cells is loose and reversible, governed primarily by electrostatic forces. It soon becomes much tighter and essentially irreversible, perhaps because of the lateral migration of receptor molecules in the plasma membrane and their binding to additional attachment sites on the capsid. This irreversible step is accompanied by a modification of the capsid, evidenced by the loss of VP4 and the development of susceptibility to digestion by proteases. The modified virion may then be taken into the cell and uncoated, or be intercalated into the plasma membrane with the concomitant release of the viral RNA into the cytoplasm. Fifty to 80 per cent of attached virions are subsequently eluted or "sloughed" from the cell surface. These eluted virions (called "A particles") still contain intact viral RNA, but they lack VP4, are no longer infectious, and cannot attach to cell receptors. These "A particles" differ antigenically from native virions. They also sediment more slowly in velocity gradients, are more lipophilic (which may facilitate penetration of or intercalation into the plasma membrane) and are susceptible to digestion by proteases (Lonberg-Holm and Whiteley, 1976; Crowell and Landau, 1983).

After its release into the cytoplasm, the virion RNA first functions as messenger RNA (mRNA), making use of cellular ribosomes and other host cell synthetic components. Polyribosome-associated picornavirus mRNA lacks VPg, which is apparently removed by an enzymatic activity present in both infected and uninfected cells (Fig. 2). Translation of the viral mRNA begins (in the case of poliovirus type 1) at an AUG codon 741 nucleotides from the 5′ terminus and continues for 6621 nucleotides to a UAG codon 72 nucleotides from the 3′-terminal poly(A) tract (Fig. 1). This results in the synthesis of a 2207 amino acid (approximately 247,000 dalton) polyprotein precursor, which contains the amino acid sequences for all of the viral structural and nonstructural proteins. The individual viral polypeptides are produced by proteolytic processing of this large polyprotein precursor (Fig. 1). The picornavirus genome, and thus the polyprotein precursor, is organized into three regions. The 5′ (amino-terminal) region contains the sequences of the 4 capsid proteins, the middle region contains the sequences of polypeptides (e.g., "X") of un-

*Deceased. Chapter revised by M. N. Oxman, who is grateful to Dr. Roland R. Rueckert for advice and assistance.

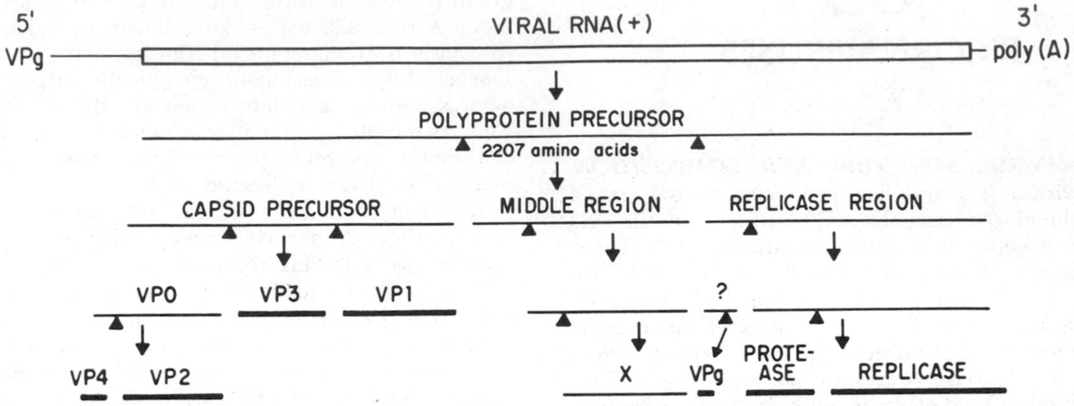

Figure 1. Translation of poliovirus RNA and proteolytic processing. The top line shows the genomic RNA with a single line representing untranslated regions at the 5′ and 3′ ends and the open box representing the coding sequences. Products of translation and processing are indicated below. Triangles indicate cleavage sites and heavy lines indicate final protein products. (Modified from Strauss, E. G., and Strauss, J. H., 1983.)

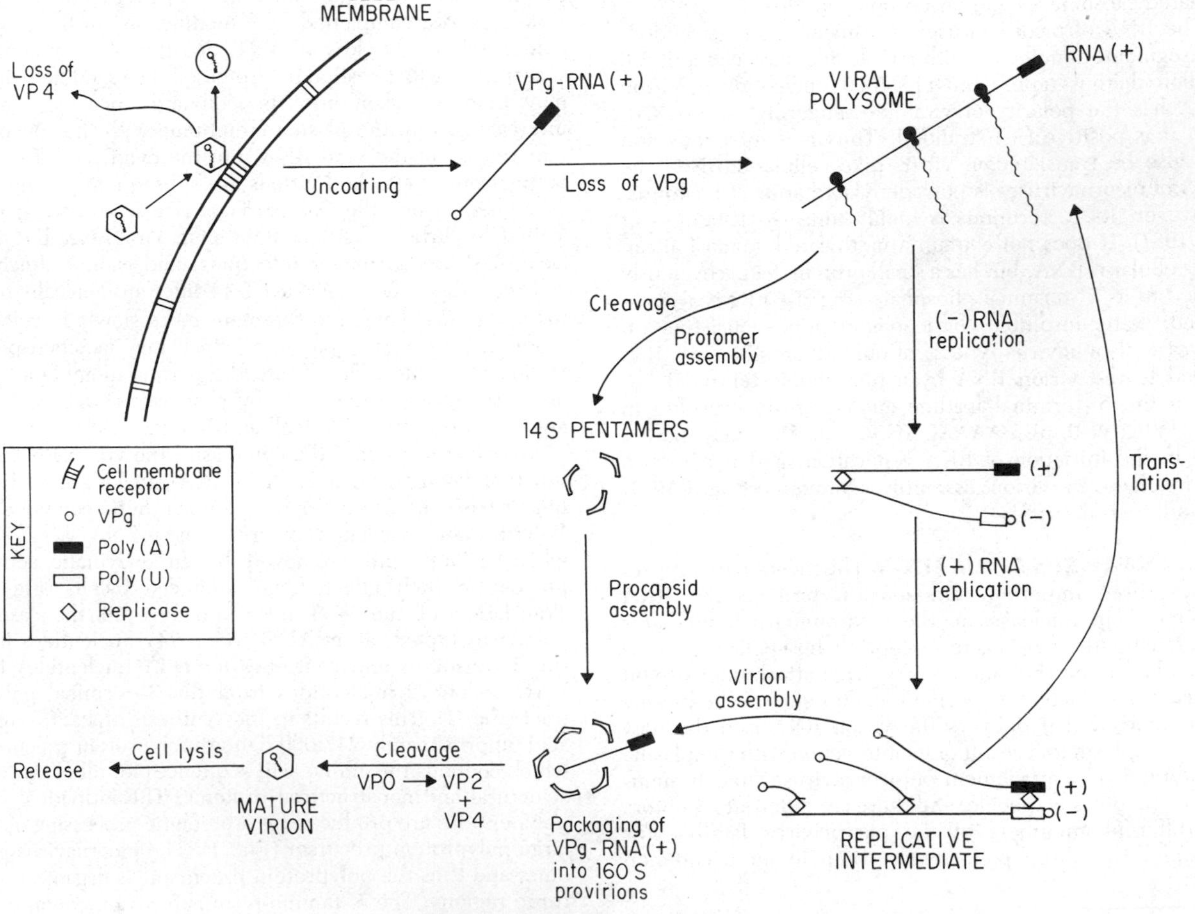

Figure 2. Picornavirus replication.

known function, and the 3′ (carboxy-terminal) region contains the sequences of VPg, the viral replicase, and the viral protease (a 20,000 dalton polypeptide responsible for most or all of the proteolytic processing). The protease is also active when still a part of its own precursor polypeptides, and this accounts for the autocatalytic cleavage of the replicase precursor to yield a precursor of VPg, a protease, and a protein required for the transcription of the plus-strand (+) RNA to form complementary minus-strand (−) RNA. Since eukaryotic ribosomes cannot initiate protein synthesis at multiple internal initiation codons on mRNA (i.e., cellular mRNA is monocistronic) the synthesis and subsequent cleavage of this large polyprotein precursor provides a mechanism by which the polycistronic picornavirus RNA can function as a monocistronic messenger RNA and still specify its multiple protein products.

After initially functioning as an mRNA, the virion RNA serves as a template for (−)RNA replication (Fig. 2). The newly synthesized (−)RNA strands then serve as templates for the synthesis of new (+)RNA strands, forming a partially double-stranded structure called the "replicative intermediate" (Fig. 2). The newly synthesized (+)RNA strands may function as messenger RNAs or as templates for the synthesis of (−)RNA strands, which then form additional replicative intermediates. This process results in an exponential increase in the production of picornavirus proteins and (+)RNA.

VPg is found covalently linked to the 5′ termini of newly synthesized (−)RNA strands, to the 5′ termini of the (−)RNA strands in replicative intermediates, and to the 5′ termini of the nascent (+)RNA strands being transcribed in replicative intermediates (Fig. 2). These observations suggest that VPg may function as a primer for the initiation of both (+) and (−) strand RNA synthesis. The rate of removal of VPg from newly synthesized (+)RNA may also control the relative rate of viral protein and (−)RNA synthesis.

When the concentration of capsid proteins is sufficiently high, immature capsomeres (or protomers), each composed of three proteins (VP0, VP3 and VP1) produced by cleavage of the capsid precursor protein (Fig. 1), assemble into 14S pentamers (Fig. 2). The pentamers then assemble around newly synthesized VPg-(+)RNA genomes to form provirions (Fig. 2), which are rapidly converted into mature infectious virions by the cleavage of VP0 to VP2 plus VP4. The cleavage of VP0 triggers a conformational change in the capsid, which results in a marked increase in its stability (Putnak and Phillips, 1981). Virion assembly may be initiated by the interaction of pentamers with the VPg of nascent viral polyribonucleotide chains, and this interaction may also protect the 5′-terminal VPg from cleavage, thus insuring that the newly synthesized (+)RNA is used for virion assembly rather than as mRNA. Progeny virions accumulate in the cytoplasm, often forming large crystalline arrays. They are released with lysis of the infected cell.

Shortly after infection, many picornaviruses inhibit host cell protein synthesis by inhibiting the translation of capped mRNAs. This inhibition, which requires translation of viral mRNA but not new viral RNA synthesis, appears to be caused by the inactivation of an initiation factor (Hansen et al., 1982). In addition to freeing host cell ribosomes and other components for use in the translation of viral mRNA, this inhibition of host cell protein synthesis contributes to the cytopathic effects (CPE) of picornavirus infection. It is interesting in this regard that human hepatitis A virus, which fails to inhibit host-cell macromolecular synthesis, also replicates in cell culture without producing CPE (Locarnini et al., 1981).

The growth of picornaviruses in susceptible cell monolayers is generally associated with a characteristic CPE. Infected cells retract, round up, and become refractile. They exhibit shrinkage and marked nuclear pyknosis, and eventually degenerate and detach from the glass or plastic substrate. Hematoxylin and eosin staining reveals an eosinophilic cytoplasmic mass that increases in size, eventually displacing the pyknotic nucleus and remaining cytoplasm to the cell periphery. Electron microscopy reveals large cytoplasmic aggregates of virus particles, often in crystalline arrays.

Several excellent reviews provide more detailed information on picornavirus structure, replication, classification and epidemiology (Rueckert, 1976; Sanger, 1979; Agol, 1980; Melnick, 1982; Gwaltney, 1982; Crowell and Landau, 1983; Melnick, 1983; Strauss and Strauss, 1983).

CLASSIFICATION OF PICORNAVIRUSES. Picornaviruses are subdivided into four genera—*Enterovirus*, *Cardiovirus*, *Rhinovirus*, and *Aphthovirus*—primarily on the basis of sensitivity to acid, buoyant density of the virion in CsCl, and clinical manifestations (Cooper et al., 1978, Matthews, 1982) (Table 1). The family also includes a number of other picornaviruses not yet assigned to genera. Only enteroviruses and rhinoviruses are major human pathogens.

Enteroviruses multiply throughout the alimentary tract and cause a variety of infections, which range in severity from asymptomatic to fatal. Among their distinctive properties are a buoyant density in CsCl of 1.33 to 1.35 g/cm^3 and maintenance of infectivity at a pH as low as 3. Because of their acid stability, enteroviruses that have undergone limited replication in the oropharynx survive transit through the stomach and implant in the lower intestinal tract, where they undergo more extensive multiplication. Enteroviruses are also relatively resistant to thermal inactivation at ambient temperatures, especially in the presence of 1 M $MgCl_2$. This chemical is therefore added to live poliovirus vaccines to enhance their stability, especially under field conditions or in tropical regions lacking refrigeration.

Rhinoviruses inhabit the upper respiratory tract and are the principal recognized etiologic agents of the common cold. Unlike enteroviruses, rhinoviruses are acid labile. They begin to lose infectivity at pH 6 and are completely unstable at pH 3. They are further distinguished from enteroviruses by their optimal temperature of replication (33° C) and by their higher buoyant density in CsCl. Preferential replication at lower than body temperature probably reflects their adaptation to the nasal passages.

Cardioviruses, examples of which include encephalomyocarditis virus and Mengo virus, have been recognized only rarely as causes of human diseases (Gajdusek, 1955; Tesh, 1978). Although they have been recovered chiefly from rodents, their natural host(s) is uncertain (Tesh, 1978; Tesh and Wallace, 1978). Their buoyant density and optimal temperature of replication are similar to those of enteroviruses. However, although they are usually stable over the broad range of pH 4 to 10, they differ from enteroviruses in being unstable at pH 5–6 in the presence of 0.1 M halide ion.

Aphthoviruses, named for the vesicular lesions that they

Table 1. THE PICORNAVIRUS FAMILY[a]

Genus	Number of Immunotypes (Species)	*Members*	Distinctive Properties: *Infectivity at pH 3*	*pH6*	*Density in CsCl g/cm³*	*Optimal Growth Temperature*
ENTEROVIRUS	3	Human polioviruses 1–3				
	23	Human coxsackieviruses A1-22, A24[b,c]				
	6	Human coxsackieviruses B1-6				
	32	Human echoviruses 1-9,11-27,29-34[d]	+	+	1.33–1.34	37°C
	4	Human enteroviruses 68–71				
	1	Human hepatitis A virus (= human enterovirus 72)				
	18	Simian enteroviruses 1-18				
	7	Bovine enteroviruses 1-7				
	11	Porcine enteroviruses 1-11				
	1	Murine poliovirus (Theiler's virus, TO, FA, GD7)				
CARDIOVIRUS	1	Encephalomyocarditis virus (EMC), mengovirus, murine encephalomyelitis virus (ME)	+	−[e]	1.33–1.34	37°C
RHINOVIRUS	>113	Human rhinoviruses 1-113	−	±[f]	1.38–1.42	33°C
	2	Bovine rhinoviruses 1-2				
APHTHOVIRUS	7	Foot-and-mouth disease viruses 1-7 (serotypes A,C,O, SAT 1,2,3, Asia 1)	−	±[g]	1.43–1.45	37°C
UNASSIGNED	>3	Equine rhinoviruses 1,2, Cricket paralysis virus, Drosophilia C virus, Gonometa virus				

[a]After Matthews (1982).

[b]Coxsackieviruses are named after Coxsackie, New York, the town in which the initial isolates were made. Coxsackievirus A23 has been reclassified as echovirus 9.

[c]Vacated numbers are now unused.

[d]Echo is an acronym for enteric cytopathic *h*uman orphan. Echovirus 10 has been reclassified as reovirus 1 and echovirus 28 as rhinovirus 1A.

[e]Cardioviruses are stable at pH 4-10, but in the presence of 0.1 M halide they are unstable at pH 5-6.

[f]Rhinoviruses are borderline stable at pH 6 and unstable at lower pH.

[g]Aphthoviruses are unstable below pH 7 at low ionic strength, but stable at pH 5-6 at high ionic strength.

produce in cloven-footed animals, are an important cause of economic loss in the cattle industry. Apthoviruses are among the densest of the picornaviruses when banded in CsCl (Table 1). They resemble rhinoviruses in their instability in acid, but they are relatively stable at pH 5 to 6 in solutions of high ionic strength.

Species of the four picornavirus genera are distinguished immunologically, usually by the ability of specific antiserum to neutralize only the homotypic virus. Sixty-nine human enterovirus species (immunotypes) and more than 113 human rhinoviruses have been identified (Table 1).

ANTIGENIC STRUCTURE OF PICORNAVIRUSES. Enteroviruses and rhinoviruses exhibit two distinct antigenic reactivities, C and D, associated with different physical forms of the virus particle (Roizman et al., 1958; Hughes et al., 1974). Empty capsids are C antigenic and give rise to group-specific reactions detectable by complement fixation (CF) or immunoprecipitin reactions. Intact infectious virions exhibit D antigenicity and elicit type-specific neutralizing antibodies. After infection, serum contains antibodies to both C and D antigens, but when the serum is absorbed with empty capsids it retains only D-specificity. Mild denaturing conditions, such as heating at 50° C or ultraviolet irradiation, convert the reactivity of virions from D to C. When enteroviruses are completely disrupted or when rhinoviruses are subjected to acidity (pH 3), the integrity of both C and D antigens is lost.

D and C antigenic reactivities are explained by changes in the conformation and molecular architecture of the virion. VP4 is essential for D reactivity (Breindl, 1971). The conformational change associated with the formation of "A particles" (vide supra) is similar to that involved in C particle formation. When virions are heated, converting their reactivity from D to C, they lose VP4 and RNA and become noninfectious. Empty capsids, consisting of VP1 and VP3 (and some VP2), retain C antigenicity, but this reactivity is also lost when capsids are further disrupted into their constituent capsomeres (Katagiri et al., 1971).

SUBCLASSIFICATION AND HOST RANGE OF PICORNAVIRUSES

Enteroviruses. Historically, human enteroviruses have been subclassified into polioviruses, coxsackieviruses, and echoviruses based upon antigenic relationships, differences in host range, and types of disease produced. *Polioviruses*, the first to be recognized, produce characteristic lesions when inoculated into the central nervous system of primates (see Chapter 185) and replicate only in primates or primate cell cultures. In contrast, most *coxsackieviruses* are only occasionally neuropathogenic for monkeys and are not readily isolated in cell cultures. However, they cause paralysis and death when inoculated into suckling mice. This property was responsible for their detection and differentiation from polioviruses in 1958, when they were first recovered from the feces of children with a poliomyelitis-like syndrome in the village of Coxsackie, New York (Dalldorf and Sickles, 1948). Shortly after their discovery, it was recognized that some coxsackieviruses, designated group A, produced widespread skeletal muscle lesions and flaccid paralysis in mice, whereas others, designated group B, produced only focal myositis but more widespread visceral lesions involving the heart, fat, pancreas, and central nervous system, which resulted in spastic paralysis. Moreover, the group B coxsackieviruses, unlike most of those of group A, could be propagated in primate cell cultures (Melnick, 1954). The discovery that polioviruses could be isolated and propagated in cultures of nonneural human or monkey cells, in which they produced characteristic cytopathic effects (Enders et al., 1949), led to the discovery of many additional picornaviruses. Further attempts to recover viruses from the feces of healthy children led to the discovery of agents that produced cytopathic effects in primate cell cultures but failed to cause disease in suckling mice or in the central nervous system of primates (Melnick and Agren, 1952; Melnick, 1954; Ramos-Alverez and Sabin, 1954). These agents, initially considered "orphan" viruses because they were unrelated to any disease, were called *echoviruses* (*e*nteric *c*ytopathic *h*uman *o*rphan).

During the thirty-five years that have elapsed since techniques for detecting enteroviruses were developed, three immunotypes of polioviruses have been recognized, as well as 23 group A coxsackieviruses, 6 group B coxsackieviruses, and 32 echoviruses. Many enteroviruses cannot be subclassified unambiguously. For example, some have the host range of a coxsackievirus but are antigenically related to echoviruses. Therefore, new agents are now designated simply as *enteroviruses* with serial numbers (Rosen et al., 1970). Since adoption of this simplified taxonomic scheme five new immunotypes, enteroviruses 68 to 72, have been recognized. However, because of established precedent, the first 67 immunotypes are still subclassified as polioviruses, coxsackieviruses, or echoviruses. Enterovirus 72 is the causative agent of hepatitis A and will continue to be referred to as human hepatitis A virus (Table 1).

Rhinoviruses. There are now 113 numbered species of human rhinoviruses, and additional immunotypes are awaiting formal recognition. Human rhinoviruses are infectious only for primates or primate cell cultures, and many can be propagated in vitro only in human embryonic fibroblasts. A few fastidious strains grow only in organ cultures of embryonic human tracheal epithelium. Rhinoviruses have been classified as H or M strains according to their growth in cells of human or monkey origin, but this subdivision has little clinical or epidemiologic significance.

RELATIONSHIPS AMONG PICORNAVIRUSES. Although each immunotype is distinct, human enteroviruses and rhinoviruses are related genetically and immunologically. Genetic relationships among enteroviruses are shown by reciprocal hybridization of their nucleic acids (Young, 1973), by oligonucleotide "fingerprinting" (Frisby et al., 1976), or by direct comparison of nucleotide sequences (Strauss and Strauss, 1983). Different immunotypes within a major group, such as the three species of poliovirus, share 30 to 50 per cent of their nucleotide sequences, whereas homologies among viruses of different groups, such as group A coxsackieviruses and echoviruses, are generally less than 20 per cent. At least 5 per cent of the RNA sequences are common to all human enteroviruses. On the other hand, less than 4 per cent homology has been found among the RNA of three rhinovirus species, suggesting that they are genetically very diverse (Yin et al., 1973).

D antigens of each enterovirus immunotype stimulate type-specific neutralizing antibodies, but immunologic cross-reactions are elicited by the C antigens of related viruses. Heterotypic reactions are most readily demonstrated in the serum of individuals who have previously experienced sequential infections with other enteroviruses. For example, a child whose first coxsackievirus infection is with immunotype B5 usually elaborates neutralizing and CF antibodies that react only or predominantly with homotypic antigens; on the other hand, if he has previously been infected by another group B coxsackievirus, titers of CF antibodies against all six group B coxsackieviruses may rise, even though the homotypic neutralizing antibody response will be the greatest. Such heterotypic serologic responses are common between certain pairs of viruses, such as polioviruses 1 and 2, coxsackieviruses A3 and A8, and echoviruses 6 and 30. Furthermore, a distant immunologic relationship between human enteroviruses and rhinoviruses can be demonstrated in immunoprecipitin reactions or by immune electron microscopy with undiluted human serum (Hughes et al., 1977). The weak cross-reaction of enteroviruses and rhinoviruses probably reflects the broadened antibody response resulting from multiple picornavirus infections, because no cross-reaction can be demonstrated with serum from animals hyperimmunized with a single picornavirus antigen.

PATHOGENESIS

Enteroviruses. The pathogenesis of poliovirus infections has been extensively studied and is discussed in Chapter 185. Data for other enteroviruses, meager because there are no readily available experimental models, indicate a basic similarity of the major pathogenetic events, excluding those involving the central nervous system. Briefly recapitulated, these events are as follows.

Infection is primarily a result of ingesting fecally contaminated material. In individuals lacking type-specific antibodies, enteroviruses implant and replicate in susceptible tissues of the gut, which probably include mucosal epithelial cells and lymphoid tissue of the lamina propria. Pathologic lesions are not apparent in these sites. Although most enteroviruses multiply in both the oropharynx and the distal small bowel or colon, evidence favors the view that replication in the lower gut is far more efficient (Ogra and Karzon, 1971): (1) Large doses of oral polio vaccines result in virus shedding in both oropharyngeal secretions and feces, whereas with small doses only fecal shedding occurs; (2) virus titers are substantially higher in feces, often 10^6 infectious units per gram; (3) virus can be recovered from the oropharynx only for several days, rarely for as long as three weeks, whereas fecal excretion of virus is more sustained, often continuing for five to six weeks or longer; (4) although some enteroviruses—for example, group B coxsackieviruses—may be recovered from both ends of the alimentary canal, echoviruses are commonly recovered only in the feces (Kogon et al., 1969).

After multiplying in the submucosal lymphatic tissues, enteroviruses reach the cervical and mesenteric lymph nodes. From these sites small quantities of virus escape into the bloodstream ("minor viremia") and are disseminated to reticuloendothelial tissues, such as the liver, spleen, and bone marrow. None of the replicative events up to this point produce symptoms, and in most individuals the infection is contained by host defense mechanisms without further progression. However, in a few infected persons, additional replication in reticuloendothelial tissues produces heavy, sustained shedding of virus into the bloodstream ("major viremia"). This event is temporally associated with the "minor illness" of poliomyelitis, and probably with the nonspecific febrile illnesses caused by other enteroviruses. Sustained viremia is also responsible for dissemination of virus to target organs, such as the meninges, skin, and heart. In these tissues the virus produces inflammatory lesions, often accompanied by necrosis. Although spread within the central nervous system occurs along neural pathways, the major route of entry into the central nervous system appears to be via the blood stream, with direct invasion through capillary walls (Nathanson and Bodian, 1962).

Rhinoviruses. Rhinoviruses implant and replicate in epithelial cells of the nasal mucosa, producing hyperemia and edema of the mucous membrane and a seromucinous exudate. A scant infiltrate of neutrophils, eosinophils, and mononuclear inflammatory cells is present beneath the epithelium, and mucin secretion by goblet cells is increased. Columnar epithelial cells exhibit impaired mucociliary clearance, become necrotic, and slough. Rhinovirus replication can be detected within 24 hours after implantation, often several days before the onset of symptoms, and reaches a peak in two to three days. Excretion generally ceases by seven days, but in a few individuals it persists for up to two weeks (Douglas et al., 1966; Kettler et al., 1969). Rhinoviruses are shed principally from the nose, and the concentration of virus in the nasal mucus is 10- to 100-fold higher than it is in saliva or oropharyngeal secretions (Hendley et al., 1973). The precise anatomic extent of rhinovirus infection has not been defined; it has not been established whether infection extends beyond the nose or whether virus in the oropharynx comes principally from contamination from the nose. In normal individuals, as well as in patients with chronic bronchitis, rhinovirus infections have been associated with abnormalities of pulmonary function (Cate et al., 1973), but this may be a consequence of reflex bronchoconstriction rather than of direct viral invasion of the lower respiratory tract.

Although rhinoviruses usually implant in the nose, infection can be initiated experimentally by dropping virus on the conjunctiva. Oropharyngeal inoculation is much less efficient (Hendley et al., 1973), and rhinoviruses are unable to replicate in the lower intestinal tract, even when the acidic environment of the stomach is bypassed and virus is artificially introduced into the small bowel (Cate et al., 1967). Among the possible reasons for failure to replicate in the intestine are lack of appropriate viral receptors on mucosal epithelial cells and the higher temperature at this site compared with the nasal passages. Neither viremia nor dissemination of rhinoviruses beyond the respiratory tract has been documented.

IMMUNITY. Type-specific neutralizing antibodies in the serum and in mucosal secretions are the main factors responsible for acquired immunity against picornaviruses. Cell-mediated immunity has not been thoroughly studied.

In the nasopharynx and the intestinal tract, secretory IgA antibodies directed against specific immunotypes of polioviruses and rhinoviruses are elicited by the initial infection with these agents (Ogra and Karzon, 1971; Cate et al., 1966; Gwaltney, 1982). Depending on the titer of secretory antibodies, either reinfection by the same immunotype is prevented or the outcome of infection is modified. High titers of IgA antibodies prevent implantation and replication of virus in the gut and pharynx. In contrast, reinfection is possible when antibody titers are low or when the virus challenge is massive. Reinfections are unaccompanied by illness and result only in transient excretion of virus (Kogon et al., 1969). IgA antibodies to poliovirus may also be acquired passively in milk by breastfed infants whose mothers are immune; these antibodies interfere with a "take" by live, oral poliovirus vaccines (OPV) and may also protect against natural infection during early infancy (Warren et al., 1964).

IgM and IgG neutralizing antibodies to enteroviruses begin to appear in the serum as early as one to three days after infection (Ogra and Karzon, 1971). IgA antibodies are usually not detected in serum until two to six weeks; they are generally of low titer and do not develop in all individuals. IgM antibodies usually persist for two to three months, but serum-neutralizing antibodies of the IgG and IgA classes are present for many years, possibly for life. Although serum-neutralizing antibodies do not prevent alimentary infection by enteroviruses, they effectively block viremia and hematogenous dissemination to target organs such as the meninges, skin, liver, and heart. Parenterally administered pooled immune serum globulin (ISG) produces trace levels of serum antibodies to poliovirus that protect against paralysis if given before exposure (Stevens, 1959). Protection against paralytic poliomyelitis is also afforded by either OPV or parenterally administered inactivated polio vaccine (IPV) because both types of vaccine stimulate serum-neutralizing antibodies in a high proportion of recipients. However, OPV has the additional advantage of interrupting the transmission of wild polioviruses in the community because the attenuated viruses replicate in the alimentary tract and stimulate secretory immunity, thereby preventing subsequent reinfection as well as central nervous system illness (Melnick, 1978, 1982). ISG also contains antibody to human hepatitis A virus, and this accounts for the prophylactic efficacy of ISG in individuals exposed to hepatitis A virus infection.

Rhinoviruses, like enteroviruses, stimulate neutralizing antibodies in both the serum and the nasopharyngeal secretions of up to 80 per cent of infected individuals. Antibody responses at these sites are closely linked, even after nasal or parenteral immunization with inactivated virus. It has not been established unequivocally, therefore, whether secretory or circulating antibodies are more important in type-specific immunity to the common cold (Gwaltney, 1982). Because antibodies in serum or nasal secretions may not be detected until approximately two weeks after infection, when virus shedding has already ceased, it is likely that recovery from acute infection is mediated by other mechanisms, possibly interferon.

Complement-fixing antibodies stimulated by enteroviruses or rhinoviruses are detectable for one to five years after infection. They do not appear in all individuals, and it is unclear whether they are protective.

LABORATORY DIAGNOSIS. Appropriate specimens for isolation of enteroviruses include, depending on the clinical syndrome, throat washings or swabs, feces, cerebrospinal fluid, vesicle fluid from skin lesions, pericardial fluid, conjunctival swabs (acute hemorrhagic conjunctivitis), and autopsy tissues such as brain, spinal cord, and myocardium. Isolation of an enterovirus from one or more of these sites is usually convincing evidence of an etiologic relationship to illness, but isolation from feces or pharyngeal secretions, especially in infants during the summer months when enteroviruses are prevalent, may be only circumstantial evidence of such a relationship because etiologically unrelated intercurrent infection may be present. Isolation of a rhinovirus from nasopharyngeal secretions likewise must be interpreted with regard to the possibility that another, unidentified respiratory pathogen may be present and be responsible for the illness.

Specimens for enterovirus isolation should be transported, on wet ice (0° C) if possible, to the virus laboratory, where they should be inoculated into human or primate cell cultures, such as rhesus monkey kidney or human embryonic kidney. For the diagnosis of illness due to group A coxsackieviruses, infant mice must also be inoculated. Rhinoviruses can usually be isolated in human diploid fibroblast cell cultures, such as WI 38, although the expense of this procedure is rarely warranted in patients with the common cold. Specimens that cannot be inoculated until many hours after their collection should be frozen, preferably at −70° C or lower. However, the characteristic stability of enteroviruses sometimes permits their recovery even from unrefrigerated specimens that have been mailed to the laboratory. Characteristic cytopathic effects in cell cultures are commonly observed after two to five days and permit a presumptive diagnosis of picornavirus infection. The specific immunotype is identified by the use of polyvalent immune sera in an "intersecting pool" scheme (Lim and Benyesh-Melnick, 1960).

For serodiagnosis, the acute phase serum should be collected as soon after onset of illness as possible, and the convalescent serum should be collected approximately two to three weeks later.

In the individual patient, the diagnosis of enterovirus or rhinovirus infection is made most conveniently by virus isolation. Rising titers of neutralizing antibodies in paired acute and convalescent sera are confirmatory, but serologic diagnosis generally cannot substitute for virus isolation. The reason is that group-reactive antigens encompassing all immunotypes are lacking, and it is not practical to perform serologic tests with type-specific antigens individually for the more than 60 enteroviruses or 100 rhinoviruses. The physician should therefore not expect the virus diagnostic laboratory to perform antibody "screens" unless a virus has been isolated from the patient, the particular epidemic immunotype is known or suspected, or the type of clinical illness suggests only a limited number of probable immunotypes. For example, serologic diagnosis of sporadic cases of aseptic meningitis or the common cold is not feasible, but it may be reasonable to measure antibodies to the three poliovirus immunotypes in paralyzed individuals or to coxsackieviruses, B1-B5 in patients with myocarditis. The direct detection of enterovirus RNA in infected tissues and body fluids is now possible by use of nucleic acid hybridization probes prepared from regions of the genome that are common to all enteroviruses (Rotbart et al., 1984).

EPIDEMIOLOGY. Most enteroviruses and rhinoviruses are distributed worldwide. Seasonal variation in prevalence and patterns of transmission of these two virus groups are dissimilar (Melnick, 1982; Gwaltney, 1982).

Enteroviruses. In temperate climates, enteroviral infections are most common in the summer and early autumn, whereas in tropical climates infection occurs year round. Virus is spread chiefly by the fecal-oral route directly from person to person or by fomites, although spread by respiratory secretions may play a lesser role. In economically developed countries, usually only one or two immunotypes are prevalent in the community each season; in contrast, children living in urban areas with low standards of sanitation are often multiply infected. Approximately 50 to 80 per cent of enteroviral infections are asymptomatic, and many of the remainder are characterized by undifferentiated febrile illnesses lasting only a few days, often accompanied by upper respiratory tract symptoms. The so-called "characteristic" enterovirus syndromes—such as aseptic meningitis, myopericarditis, and exanthems—are in fact unusual manifestations of infection. Enteroviruses are most efficiently disseminated by infected children less than 2 years old. Introduction of virus into the household by one family member results in high rates of infection among others lacking type-specific neutralizing antibodies; secondary attack rates of approximately 92 per cent for polioviruses, 75 per cent for coxsackieviruses, and 50 per cent for echoviruses have been observed in family surveillance studies in the city of New York (Kogon et al., 1969).

Although the epidemiology of most enteroviruses is basically similar, patterns of infection with some immunotypes are distinctive. Improved standards of hygiene and widespread use of poliovirus vaccines have resulted in striking changes in the epidemiology of poliomyelitis, discussed in Chapter 185. Enterovirus 70 and coxsackievirus A24, the principal etiologic agents of acute hemorrhagic conjunctivitis, are probably transmitted from hand to eye by conjunctival secretions; replication of these viruses in the alimentary tract, if it occurs at all, appears to be limited. Coxsackievirus A21 also is shed primarily from the upper respiratory tract, where it produces a rhinovirus-like illness.

Hepatitis A virus (enterovirus 72) is an important cause of human hepatitis. It continues to be endemic in developing countries, where infection is universal in childhood and nearly all young adults have antibody. In industrialized nations, infection is less frequent and a large proportion of the adult population is susceptible to infection. Since there appears to be only a single immunotype of hepatitis A virus, control by immunization is feasible. The recent propagation of hepatitis A virus in cell culture (Provost and Hilleman, 1979) has opened the way for the development of experimental live attenuated vaccines (Provost et al., 1983). Molecular cloning of hepatitis A virus complementary DNA (Ticehurst et al., 1983) may allow the in vitro synthesis of immunogenic hepatitis A virus polypeptides.

Control of other nonpolio enterovirus infections is best effected by hygienic measures and improvements in sanitation. Isolation of patients with enteroviral illnesses is generally not helpful in controlling epidemics because of the simultaneous existence of a large reservoir of unidentified, asymptomatically infected individuals who excrete virus. Because nonpolio enteroviral illness is rarely life-threatening and because there are so many immunotypes, control by vaccines is not practical.

Rhinoviruses. The peak incidence of rhinovirus infections in temperate climates occurs in the colder months, especially the early autumn and spring. In the tropics, peak activity occurs in the rainy season. Crowding indoors and the return of children to school are believed to be among the factors that account for this periodicity. Contrary to popular belief, there is no evidence that susceptibility to the common cold is enhanced by chilling of the body during the winter months. Rhinovirus infections experimentally induced at cold ambient temperatures do not occur with greater frequency or severity (Douglas et al., 1968).

Rhinovirus infections spread primarily in the home and in the classroom. As with enteroviruses, secondary attack rates of 50 to 80 per cent are common among susceptible family members, especially young children. Transmission of the common cold occurs with two to five day intervals between cases, and is most efficient when there is close contact between individuals. Although it has long been assumed that rhinoviruses are disseminated by respiratory droplet nuclei, recent data suggest that spread may occur more commonly by transfer of nasal mucus to the hands of infected individuals, who transmit virus via fomites or hand contact to others, who in turn autoinoculate the nose or conjunctiva (Gwaltney et al., 1978; Gwaltney, 1982).

Multiple rhinovirus immunotypes often circulate concurrently. Antibody prevalence rates increase with age, beginning in early childhood and peaking in young adults, who commonly have serum antibodies to approximately half of the recognized rhinovirus immunotypes. Most infections are symptomatic, the ratio of apparent to inapparent infections being approximately 3:1.

Practical measures for the control of rhinovirus infections have not been established. Transmission occurs primarily from hand to nose rather than by inhalation of respiratory droplets (Gwaltney, 1982) and thus handwashing or avoidance of hand contact with individuals with colds may reduce contagion. Interferon administered intranasally has shown prophylactic efficacy against experimental rhinovirus challenge (Hayden and Gwaltney, 1983) but specific chemotherapeutic agents are not available. Control by vaccines is not practical because of the large number of immunotypes.

References

Agol, V. .I: Structure, translation and replication of piconaviral genomes. In Melnick, J. L. (ed.): Progress in Medical Virology, vol. 26, Basel, S. Kargel, 1980, p. 119.

Breindl, M.: VP4, the D-reactive part of poliovirus. Virology 46:962, 1971.

Campbell, B. A., and Cords, C. E.: Monoclonal Antibodies that Inhibit Attachment of Group B Coxsackieviruses. J Virol 48:561, 1983.

Cate, T. R., Douglas, R. G., Jr., Johnson, K. M., Couch, R. B., and Knight, V.: Studies on the inability of rhinovirus to survive and replicate in the intestinal tract of volunteers. Proc Soc Exp Biol Med 124:1290, 1967.

Cate, T. R., Roberts, J. S., Russ, M. A., and Pierce, J. A.: Effects of common colds on pulmonary function. Am Rev Respir Dis 108:858, 1973.

Cate, T. R., Rossen, R. D., Douglas, R. G., Jr., Butler, W. T., and Couch, R. B.: The role of nasal secretion and serum antibody in the rhinovirus common cold. Am J Epidemiol 84:352, 1966.

Cooper, P. D., Agol, V. I., Bachrach, H. L., Brown, F., Ghendon, Y., Gibbs, A. J., Gillespie, J. H., Lonberg-Holm, K., Mandel, B., Melnick, J. L., Mohanty, S. B., Povey, R. C., Rueckert, R. R., Schaffer, F. L., and Tyrrell, D. A. J.: Picornaviridae: Second report. Intervirology 10:165, 1978.

Crowell, R. L. and Landau, B. J.: Receptors in the initiation of picornavirus infections. In H. Franekel-Conrat and R. R. Wagner (eds.), Comprehensive Virology, vol. 18, New York, Plenum Press, 1983. p. 1.

Dalldorf, G., and Sickles, G. M.: An unidentified, filtrable agent isolated from the feces of children with paralysis. Science 108:61, 1948.

Douglas, R. G., Jr., Cate, T. R., Gerone, P. J., and Couch, R. B.: Quantitative rhinovirus shedding patterns in volunteers. Am Rev Respir Dis 94:159, 1966.

Douglas, R. G., Jr., Lindgren, K. M., and Couch, R. B.: Exposure to cold environment and rhinovirus common cold: Failure to demonstrate effect. N Engl J Med 279:743, 1968.

Enders, J. F., Weller, T. H., Robbins, F. C.: Cultivation of the Lansing Strain of poliomyelitis virus in cultures of various human embryonic tissues. Science 109:85, 1949.

Enders, J. F., Weller, T. H., Robbins, F. C.: Alterations in pathogenicity for monkeys of Brunhilde strain of poliomyelitis virus following cultivation in human tissues. Fed Proc 11:467, 1952.

Frisby, D. P., Newton, C., Carey, N. H., Fellner, P., Newman, J. F. E., Harris, T. J. R., and Brown, F.: Oligonucleotide mapping of picornavirus RNAs by two-dimensional electrophoresis. Virology 71:379, 1976.

Gajdusek, D. C.: Encephalomyocarditis virus infection in childhood. Pediatrics 16:902, 1955.

Gwaltney, J. M., Jr.: Rhinoviruses. In Viral Infections of Humans, Epidemiology and Control. Alfred S Evans (ed.): New York, Plenum Medical Book Company, 1982, p. 491.

Gwaltney, J. M., Jr., Moskalski, P. B., and Hendley, J. O.: Hand-to hand transmission of rhinovirus colds. Ann Intern Med 88:463, 1978.

Hansen, J., Etchison, D., Hershey, J. W. B. and Ehrenfeld, E.: Association of cap-binding protein with eucaryotic initiation Factor 3 in initiation factor preparations from uninfected and poliovirus-infected HeLa cells. J of Virol 42:200, 1982.

Hayden, F. G., and Gwaltney, J. M. Jr.: Intranasal interferon-alpha$_2$ for prevention of rhinovirus infection and illness. J Infect Dis 148:543, 1983.

Hendley, J. O., Wenzel, R. P., and Gwaltney, J. M., Jr.: Transmission of rhinovirus colds by self-inoculation. N Engl J Med 288:1361, 1973.

Hughes, J. H., Chema, S., Lin, N., Conant, R. M., and Hamparian, V. V.: Acid lability of rhinoviruses: Loss of C and D antigenicity after treatment at pH 3.0. J Immunol 112:919, 1974.

Hughes, J. H., Gnau, J. M., Hilty, M. D., Chema, S., Ottolenghi, A. C., and Hamparian, V. V.: Picornaviruses: Rapid differentiation and identification by immune electronmicroscopy and immunodiffusion. J Med Microbiol 10:203, 1977.

Jacobson, M. F., and Baltimore, D.: Polypeptide cleavages in the formation of poliovirus proteins. Proc Natl Acad Sci USA 61:77, 1968.

Katagiri, S., Aikawa, S., and Hinuma, Y.: Stepwise degradation of poliovirus capsid by alkaline treatment. J Gen Virol 13:101, 1971.

Kettler, A., Hall, C. E., Fox, J. P., Elveback, L., and Cooney, M. K.: The virus watch program: A continuing surveillance of viral infections in metropolitan New York families. VIII. Rhinovirus infections: Observations of virus excretion, intrafamilial spread and clinical response. Am J Epidemiol 90:244, 1969.

Kitamura, N., Semler, B. L., Rothberg, P. G., Larsen, G. R., Adler, C. J., Dorner, A. J., Emini, E. A., Hanecak, R., Lee, J. J., van der Werf, S., Anderson, C. W. and Wimmer, E.: Primary structures, gene organization and polypeptide expression of poliovirus RNA. Nature 291:547, 1981.

Kogon, A., Spigland, I., Frothingham, T. E., Elveback, L., Williams, C., Hall, C. E., and Fox, J. P.: The virus watch program: A continuing surveillance of viral infections in metropolitan New York families. VII. Observation on viral excretion, seroimmunity, intrafamilial spread and illness association in coxsackievirus and echovirus infections. Am J Epidemiol 89:51, 1969.

Lim, K. A., and Benyesh-Melnick, M. L.: Typing of viruses by combinations of antiserum pools. Applications to typing of enteroviruses (Coxsackie and ECHO). J Immunol 84:309, 1960.

Locarnini, S. A., Coulepis, A. G., Westaway, E. G. and Gust, I. D.: Restricted replication of human hepatitis A virus in cell culture: Intracellular biochemical studies. J Virol 37:216, 1981.

Lonberg-Holm, K., and Whiteley, N. M.: Physical and metabolic requirements for early interaction of poliovirus and human rhinovirus with HeLa cells. J Virol 19:857, 1976.

Matthews, R. E. F.: Classification and nomenclature of viruses. Fourth report of the International Committee on Taxonomy of Viruses. Intervirology 17:1, 1982.

Melnick, J. L.: Application of tissue culture methods to epidemiological studies of poliomyelitis. Am J Public Health 44:571, 1954.

Melnick, J. L.: Advantages and disadvantages of killed and live poliomyelitis vaccines. Bull W H O 56:21, 1978.

Melnick, J. L.: Enteroviruses. In Evans, A. S. (ed.): Viral Infections of Humans, Epidemiology and Control. New York, Plenum Medical Book Company, 1982, p. 187.

Melnick, J. L.: Portraits of viruses: the Picornaviruses. Intervirology 20:61, 1983.

Melnick, J. L., and Agren, K.: Poliomyelitis and Coxsackie viruses isolated from normal infants in Egypt. Proc Soc Exp Biol Med 81:621, 1952.

Miller, D. A., Miller, O. J., Dev, V. G., Hashmi, S., Tantravahi, R., Medrano, L., and Green, H.: Human chromosome 19 carries a poliovirus receptor gene. Cell 1:167, 1974.

Nathanson, N., and Bodian, D.: Experimental poliomyelitis following intramuscular virus infection. III. The effect of passive antibody on paralysis and viremia. Bull Johns Hopkins Hosp 111:198, 1962.

Nomoto, A., Detjen, B., Pozzatti, R., and Wimmer, E.: The location of the polio genome protein in viral RNAs and its implication for RNA synthesis. Nature 268:208, 1977.

Nomoto, A., Kitamura, N., Golini, F., and Wimmer, E.: The 5′-terminal structures of poliovirion RNA and poliovirus mRNA differ only in the genome-linked protein VPg. Proc Natl Acad Sci USA 74:5345, 1977.

Ogra, P. L., and Karzon, D. T.: Formation and function of poliovirus antibody in different tissues. Progr Med Virol 13:156, 1971.

Provost, P. J., and Hilleman, M. R.: Propagation of human hepatitis A virus in cell culture in vitro. Proc Soc Exp Biol Med 160:213, 1979.

Provost, P. J., Conti, P. A., Giesa, P. A., Banker, F. S., Buynak, E. B., McAleer, W. J., and Hilleman, M. R.: Studies in chimpanzees of live, attenuated hepatitis A vaccine candidates. Pro Soc Exp Biol Med 172:357, 1983.

Putnak, J. R., and Phillips, B. A.: Picornaviral structure and assembly. Microbiol Reviews 45:287, 1981.
Ramos-Alvarez, M., and Sabin, A. B.: Characteristics of poliomyelitis and other enteric viruses recovered in tissue culture from healthy American children. Proc Soc Exp Biol Med 87:655, 1954.
Roizman, B., Mayer, M. M., and Rapp, H. J.: Immunochemical studies of poliovirus. III. Further studies on the immunological and physical properties of poliovirus particles produced in tissue culture. J Immunol 81:419, 1958.
Rosen, L., Melnick, J. L., Schmidt, N. J., and Wenner, H. A.: Subclassification of enteroviruses and ECHO virus type 34. Arch Ges Virusforsch 30:89, 1970.
Rotbart, H. A., Levin, M. J., and Villarreal, L. P.: Use of subgenomic poliovirus DNA hybridization probes to detect the major subgroups of enteroviruses. J Clin Microbiol 20:1105, 1984.
Rueckert, R. R.: On the structure and morphogenesis of picornaviruses. In Fraenkel-Conrat, H., and Wagner, R. R.: *Comprehensive Virology*, vol 6. New York, Plenum Press, 1976, p. 131.
Sanger, D. V.: The replication of picornaviruses. J Gen Virol 45:1, 1979.
Stevens, K. M.: Estimate of molecular equivalent of antibody required for prophylaxis and therapy of poliomyelitis. J Hyg (Camb) 57:198, 1959.
Strauss, E. G., and Strauss, J. H.: Replication of the single stranded RNA viruses of eukaryotes. Curr Top Microbiol Immunol 105:1, 1983.
Tesh, R. B.: The prevalence of encephalomyocarditis virus neutralizing antibodies among various human populations. Am J Trop Med Hyg 27:144, 1978.
Tesh, R. B., and Wallace, G. D.: Observations on the natural history of encephalomyocarditis virus. Am J Trop Med Hyg 27:133, 1978.
Ticehurst, J. R., Racaniello, V. R., Baroudy, B. M., Baltimore, D., Purcell, R. H., and Feinstone, S. M.: Molecular cloning and characterization of hepatitis A virus cDNA. Proc Natl Acad Sci USA 80:5885, 1983.
Warren, R. J., Lepow, M. L., Bartsch, G. E., and Robbins, F. C.: The relationship of maternal antibody, breast feeding, and age to the susceptibility of newborn infants to infection with attenuated polioviruses. Pediatrics 34:4, 1964.
Yin, F. F., Lonberg-Holm, K., and Chan, S. P.: Lack of a close relationship between three strains of human rhinoviruses as determined by their RNA sequences. J Virol 12:108, 1973.
Young, N. A.: Polioviruses, coxsackieviruses, and echoviruses. Comparison of the genomes by RNA hybridization. J Virol 11:832, 1973.

66

TOGAVIRUSES

MARIAN C. HORZINEK, D.V.M., PH.D.

The family Togaviridae includes the genera *Alphavirus*, *Flavivirus*, *Rubivirus*, and *Pestivirus*. Members of the family are characterized by spherical virions, 40 to 70 nm in diameter, that consist of a lipoprotein envelope with cellular lipids and virus-specified glycopeptides surrounding a spherical nucleocapsid of icosahedral symmetry. The virus contains one molecule of single-stranded RNA (molecular weight about 4×10^6) with positive polarity that is infectious when extracted and assayed under appropriate conditions. Togaviruses multiply in the cytoplasm and mature by budding (Fenner, 1976).

All species of the genus *Alphavirus* and most flaviviruses multiply in arthropods as well as in vertebrates and constitute the classic arthropod-borne viruses (formerly termed arbo-A and arbo-B viruses, respectively). Arboviruses are viruses that are maintained in nature principally, or to an important extent, through biologic transmission between susceptible vertebrate hosts by hematophagous arthropods (WHO Study Group, 1967). Essential to this ecologic definition is the term "biologic" (as opposed to mechanical) transmission, by which is meant that an "extrinsic incubation period" (5 to 12 days) elapses between the moments when the arthropod vector becomes infected after a blood meal and when it can transmit the virus to a new vertebrate host. Biologic transmission is not confined to the above mentioned togavirus genera: Members of the Reoviridae and Rhabdoviridae families and most Bunyaviridae are also arthropod-borne. On the other hand, members of the Rubivirus (Rubellavirus) and Pestivirus genera (hog cholera, bovine diarrhea viruses) as well as mouse lactic dehydrogenase virus and equine arteritis virus are nonarbotogaviruses (Horzinek, 1981). The following chapter will cover only togaviruses of medical importance—namely, a number of alphaviruses and flaviviruses (Tables 1 and 2) and rubella virus (RUV).

STRUCTURE. Togaviruses are the smallest enveloped animal viruses; alphaviruses and RUV are about 60 nm in diameter, and flaviviruses are smaller, about 45 nm. The size differences as determined by negative staining and thin section electron microscopy are reflected by the sedimentation coefficients, which range between 240 and 300S for the former group and 170 and 220S for the latter group. The buoyant densities of infectious virions depend on the substance used for building the gradient for analysis; values vary between < 1.18 g/ml for sucrose and 1.24 for cesium chloride and other salts.

In the electron microscope, togavirions appear as spherical particles consisting of an envelope and an isometric core. The envelope shows unit membrane characteristics and carries glycoprotein surface projections that are organized in a regular (icosahedral) surface lattice (Fig. 1); they are the substrate for a pH-dependent hemagglutinating activity. Organic solvents or detergents inactivate infectivity of virions by disintegrating the envelope, leading to hemagglutinating membrane fragments and to liberation of the nucleocapsid (30 to 40 nm in diameter for alphaviruses and RUV, and 20 to 30 nm for flaviviruses). The togavirion has a shape and substructure suggestive of icosahedral symmetry. In contrast to naked animal viruses, however, isolated togavirus capsids are nonrigid and susceptible to RNAase, which degrades the viral genome to small fragments. Since this treatment has no effect on intact virions, the envelope protects the viral RNA from enzymatic attack.

Consistent data of overall chemical analysis have been obtained only for alphaviruses, since these grow to high titers in tissue culture and can be obtained as suspensions of sufficient purity and concentration. The reported proportions of RNA: protein:lipid:carbohydrate (in glycoprotein) are about 6:61:27:6. The RNA of togaviruses is a single-stranded, colinear molecule that has an average molecular weight of 4.4×10^6, which corresponds to about 13,000 nucleotides, and sedimentation coefficients of 42 to 49S in sucrose gradients. Studies with alphaviruses have indicated that there is a significant degree of secondary structure in extracted RNA, which is necessary for infectivity. Polyadenylic acid sequences located near the 3′ terminus have been demonstrated; these, together with the

Table 1. ALPHAVIRUSES

		Isolated from												Isolated in					Human Disease	
		Arthropods				Vertebrates														
		Mosq.																		
Virus	Abbreviation	Culicine	Anopheline	Culicoides	Other	Man	Other Primates	Rodents	Birds	Bats	Marsupials	Other	Sentinels	Africa	Asia	Australasia	Europe	North America	South America	Natural Infection	Lab Infection
Aura	AURA	+																	+		
Bebaru	BEB	+													+						
Cabassou	CAB	+							+	+	+		+						+		
Chikungunya	CHIK	+				+	+		+	+			+	+	+					+	+
Eastern equine enc.	EEE	+	+	+	+	+	+	+	+		+	+			+		+	+	+	+	+
Everglades	EVE	+	+					+			+							+		+	
Fort Morgan	FM				+				+									+			
Getah	GET	+	+									+			+	+					
Highlands	HL	+							+				+					+			
Kyzylagach	KYZ	+													+						
Mayaro	MAY	+			+	+						+							+	+	+
Middleburg	MID	+												+							
Mucambo	MUC	+				+		+	+		+		+						+	+	+
Ndumu	NDU	+												+							
O'nyong-nyong	ONN		+			+							+	+						+	
Pixuna	PIX	+	+					+											+		
Ross River	RR	+				+					+					+				+	
Sagiyama	SAG	+												+							
Semliki Forest	SF	+	+						+			+	+								+
Sindbis	SIN	+	+		+	+			+				+	+	+	+				+	
Tonate	TON	+	+			+			+				+						+	+	
Una	UNA	+	+									+	+					+	+		
Venezuelan equine enc.	VEE	+	+			+		+		+	+	+						+	+	+	+
Western equine enc.	WEE	+	+		+	+		+	+			+	+				?	+	+	+	+
Whataroa	WHA	+														+					

From Berge, T. O. (ed.): International Catalogue of Arboviruses. Washington, D.C., U.S. Department of Health, Education, and Welfare, update 1982.

absence of a virion-associated polymerase, indicated that togaviral RNA is plus-stranded and might serve as the initial messenger molecule during infection. These assumptions have been confirmed by the demonstration of parental virion RNA in polysomes of infected cells and by its translation into virus-specific polypeptides in cell-free systems. Like other mRNAs from eukaryotic systems, viral RNAs contain methylated "capped" structures at their 5′ termini, which in alphaviruses are of the form 7mG (5′) pppAp.

A minimum of three structural polypeptides have been identified in togaviruses, one of them associated with the nucleocapsid; in alphaviruses and RUV this protein has a molecular weight of 30,000 to 35,000, and in flaviviruses the molecular weight ranges from 13,000 to 14,000. Amino acid analyses have shown that the alphavirus capsid protein has an *N*-terminal lysine and is relatively hydrophilic, a property consistent with its extensive and rapid interaction with viral RNA.

Two glycosylated envelope proteins have been identified in RUV (50,000 and 63,000 mw) and in most alphaviruses (E1 and E2, 45,000 to 59,000 mw) by SDS polyacrylamide gel electrophoresis. Using chromatographic techniques, three envelope proteins (52,000, 49,000, and 10,000 mw) were isolated from SFV (for abbreviations see Tables 1 and 2). In flaviviruses only one envelope (E) protein (50,000 to 60,000 mw) is glycosylated, whereas the other (M or matrix protein, 8000 to 9000 mw) seems to be buried in the lipid bilayer and may have a bridging function between the peripheral glycoprotein and the capsid. In alphaviruses both the E1 and the E2 proteins occupy a superficial position because they can be stripped away by treatment with proteolytic enzymes and can be demonstrated by enzymatic iodination of undisrupted virions. They penetrate the lipid bilayer and interact directly with the capsid.

Togaviral lipid is confined to the envelope; in alphaviruses it has been found that 25 to 31 per cent (by weight) is neutral lipid, predominantly cholesterol. Most of the remaining lipids are represented by phosphatidylethanolamine, phosphatidylserine, sphingomyelin, and phosphatidylcholine, which is the principal phosphatide. Of the viral fatty acids, oleic, palmitic, and stearic acids predominate. In general, the composition of togaviral lipids reflects that of the host cell membranes, as shown by a comparative analysis of SFV grown in BHK (baby hamster kidney) and *Aedes albopictus* cells, respectively (Pfefferkorn and Shapiro, 1974).

ANTIGENIC COMPOSITION. A togavirus is assigned to the alphagenus or flavigenus on the basis of immunologic cross-reactions. Virion surface antigens responsible for adsorption to susceptible cells and erythrocytes can be identified and compared by neutralization (NT) and hemagglutination inhibition (HI) tests. By using solvent-detergent-extracted antigens in complement fixation, gel diffusion, or radioimmunoassays, the total of antigen-antibody reactions can be measured, including those with the capsid protein. Capsid protein has been described as carrying group-reactive determinants, similar to the common nucleoprotein (gs) antigen of the orthomyxoviruses. These capsid determinants may mean that all alphaviruses are related (Dalrymple et al., 1976).

By using sera from animals that have been immunized by one inoculation of virus, it is possible to divide alphaviruses into subgroups and to make specific serologic identifications. Within the alphavirus genus the EEE subgroup only contains this virus, which has at least two geographic variants. WEE, SIN, WHA, AURA, MID, and NDU viruses form the second subgroup, of which the last two are only distantly related to the other members. The largest subgroup includes VEE with its very close relatives EVE, MUC, and PIX as well as BB, BEB, GET, RR, SAG, MAY, and UNA; also SF virus with its closely related CHIK and ONN viruses are in this subgroup. Geographic variants have also been found for WEE (≥3), SIN (3), and VEE (5), (Casals and Reeves, 1959; Karabatsos, 1975; Porterfield, 1980). The following flavivirus subgroups have been recognized by using plaque neutralization: (1) the tick-borne flaviviruses (Table 3) with the exception of POW; (2) APOI, CR, DB, ENT, KAD, MOD, and RB; (3) ALF, JE, KOK, KUN, MVE, SLE, STR, USU, and WN; (4) SPO and ZIKA; (5) IT, NTA, and TMU; (6) BAN, EH, and UGS; and (7) the four DEN type viruses. No relationships to any other flavivirus could be demonstrated with BUS, ILH, MML, POW, WSL, and YF (de Madrid and Porterfield, 1974). RUV is unrelated to any other animal virus and has been classified as a togavirus exclusively for structural reasons. It is the only representative of the *Rubivirus* genus.

It has been possible to determine the antigenic function of the respective alphavirion surface polypeptides. The E1 glycoprotein of SIN carries the complete hemagglutinating activity, whereas E2 appears to be important to infectivity because only antiserum directed against this molecular

Table 2. MOSQUITO-BORNE FLAVIVIRUSES

		Isolated from													Isolated in						Human Disease	
		Arthropods					*Vertebrates*															
		Mosq.		*Ticks*																		
Virus	**Abbreviation**	*Culicine*	*Anopheline*	*Ixodid*	*Argasid*	*Other*	*Man*	*Other Primates*	*Rodents*	*Birds*	*Bats*	*Marsupials*	*Other*	*Sentinels*	*Africa*	*Asia*	*Australasia*	*Europe*	*North America*	*South America*	*Natural Infection*	*Lab Infection*
Alfuy	ALF	+							+								+					
Bagaza	BAG	+													+							
Banzi	BAN	+					+							+	+						+	
Bouboui	BOU	+	+					+							+							
Bussuquara	BSQ	+					+		+					+					+	+	+	
Dengue-1	DEN-1	+					+								+	+	+				+	+
Dengue-2	DEN-2	+					+	+							+	+	+			+	+	+
Dengue-3	DEN-3	+					+									+	+			+	+	+
Dengue-4	DEN-4	+					+									+	+				+	
Edge Hill	EH	+	+														+					
Ilheus	ILH	+					+			+				+					+	+	+	+
Japanese enceph.	JE	+	+				+			+	+		+			+					+	+
Jugra	JUG	+									+					+						
Kokobera	KOK	+															+					
Kunjin	KUN	+					+			+							+					+
Murray Valley enceph.	MVE	+					+										+				+	
Naranjal	NJL	+												+						+		
Ntaya	NTA	+													+							
Rocio	ROC	+					+			+				+						+	+	+
Sepik	SEP	+															+				+	
St. Louis enceph.	SLE	+	+			+	+			+	+		+						+	+	+	+
Spondweni	SPO	+					+								+						+	+
Stratford	STR	+															+					
Tembusu	TMU	+	+													+	+					
Uganda S	UGS	+								+				+	+							
Usutu	USU	+							+	+					+							
Wesselsbron	WSL	+	+				+		+				+		+	+					+	+
West Nile	WN	+	+	+	+		+		+	+	+		+	+	+	+		+			+	+
Yellow fever	YF	+					+	+				+			+					+	+	+
Zika	ZIKA	+					+						+	+	+						+	+

From Berge, T. O. (ed.): International Catalogue of Arboviruses. Washington, D.C., U.S. Department of Health, Education, and Welfare, update 1982.

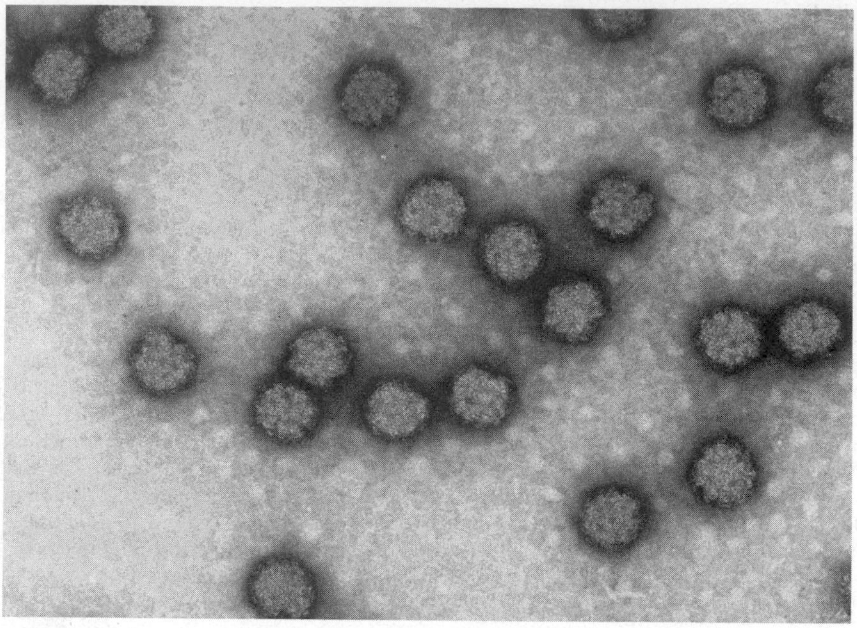

Figure 1. Sindbis virus, a member of the genus *Alphavirus* of the Togaviridae. Note the regular pattern on the virion surface. Negatively stained preparation (uranyl acetate, after fixation with glutaraldehyde). (Courtesy of Dr. D. J. Ellens, CDI Lelystad, The Netherlands.)

species effectively neutralized the virus. Glycoprotein E1 appears to be cross-reactive with antiserum to the closely related WEE and may therefore carry the determinant(s) responsible for defining the serologic complexes; E2 appears to be virus-specific (Dalrymple et al., 1976). By studying nucleotide sequence homologies between the nucleic acids of different alphaviruses, it was demonstrated that the closely related viruses of CHIK and ONN have only 13 per cent of the base sequences in common, whereas ≤1 per cent of RNA-RNA homologies occur between the other viruses of this genus. These rather low homologies can be reconciled with the established serologic relationship by assuming that the antigenic sites are composed of only a small number of amino acids and/or that the degeneracy of the genetic code allows a much larger homology to be present in the protein sequences than in corresponding RNA base sequences (Wengler et al., 1977). The E protein of flaviviruses appears to be a strongly variable glycoprotein at its antigenically active (genus-, subgroup-, type-, strain-specific) sites. By using monoclonal antibodies, eight epitopes of TBE have been identified, seven of which were partially linked and clustered in two domains, each of which contained constituents with different serological specificities and functions (Heinz et al., 1983).

Because of the simplicity of the test system, the hemagglutinating antigen has been studied most extensively (Clarke and Casals, 1958). For diagnostic purposes, alkaline aqueous extracts, fluorocarbon, ether-acetone, sucrose-acetone, or Tween 80–ether extracts of infected tissues (mostly mouse brain material for alpha- and flaviviruses) are used. Treatment with protamine sulfate results in precipitation of host material and improvement in the HA patterns. In contrast to most other viruses, the demonstration of HA by togaviruses is dependent on the ionic environment; in general, alphaviruses show optimal activity at pH 5.8 to 6.2 and flaviviruses at 6.2 to 6.4. RUV requires Ca^{++} ions for HA. Dependence on the ionic environment indicates that a specific conformation of the envelope glycoproteins is essential; for example, it has been shown that the isoelectric point of SIN virus E1 protein is the same as the pH that is optimum for HA.

REPLICATION. Adsorption of alphaviruses to susceptible cells occurs within a few minutes. Because it is dependent on the salt concentration (divalent cations inhibit attachment) and pH but independent of temperature, electrostatic forces are probably involved. The enhancing effect of DEAE-dextran, a polycation, further supports this assumption. Since alphaviruses can grow in a variety of cells from phylogenetically unrelated species including mammalian, avian, reptilian, amphibian, piscine, and arthropod, they may have a broad range of receptors. For SFV these are the major histocompatibility antigens HLA-A and HLA-B on human cells and H2-K and H2-D antigens on mouse cells. Penetration of adsorbed virus is dependent on temperature (optimum at 37°C) but independent of the ionic environment and follows first order kinetics. The virion is engulfed by a pinocytotic vacuole and subsequently uncoated.

Replication of viral RNA requires a new protein, a virus-specific RNA-dependent RNA polymerase. For its synthesis, the input parental RNA serves as a messenger; its 5′-terminal two-thirds code for the enzyme. The polymerase is bound to smooth cytoplasmic membranes, where it catalyzes the synthesis of so-called replicative intermediates. These consist of partially double-stranded RNA molecules containing one polynucleotide species serving as a template and a second species of complementary strandedness made up of nascent chains of varying length that are partially base-paired to the template. The major species of alphaviral RNA synthesized in infected cells is not virion RNA (4.2×10^6) but a subgenomic RNA species of 26S (1.6×10^6) that has the same polarity as virion RNA but contains only one third of its nucleotide sequences. It serves as the mRNA for the structural proteins of the virion. Studies in SFV-infected cells and with cell-free synthesizing systems have shown that the 5′→3′ gene order in 26S RNA is C, E3, E2, and E1 and that these proteins are synthesized as a polyprotein of about 130,000 daltons from a single initiation site. By a sequence of nascent and post-translational proteolytic cleavages, this molecule is processed to give the structural virion polypeptides.

The remaining coding capacity corresponding to protein

of about 300,000 daltons is used for nonstructural viral polypeptides. Since the 42S RNA is infectious, some, if not all, of these are likely to be components of the viral polymerase. The nucleotide sequence of the 26S RNA is located inward from the 3′ end of the 42S RNA, which implies that the genes coding for the nonstructural proteins must be situated in the two thirds of the genome near the 5′ terminal. Their synthesis is initiated at a single site near the 5′ end and is terminated internally before the structural protein genes. Also, the nonstructural polypeptides are synthesized as a giant precursor molecule, which is subsequently processed by proteolytic cleavage.

The alphavirus capsid is assembled in the cytoplasm of the infected cell around the RNA and then attaches to the inner surface of the host cell plasma membrane after that membrane has been modified by the insertion of the virus-specified glycoproteins. The membrane at this stage contains the definite E1 protein and a precursor to the second glycoprotein. The envelopment of the nucleocapsid takes place as it is progressively wrapped into the modified membrane while moving from the cytoplasm to a position physically outside the cell. During the terminal stages of this "budding" process, the precursor polypeptide is cleaved to form the E2 glycoprotein.

Intracytoplasmic vacuoles are the first evidence of subcellular alteration associated with virus replication. Alphaviruses and flaviviruses differ with respect to their morphogenesis; the former envelop their capsids by budding preferentially from the marginal membrane, whereas the latter emerge from internal vacuolar membranes. The general picture for RUV resembles that of alphaviruses. Only in alphavirus-infected cells may assembled capsids be detected around cytoplasmic vacuoles.

Different togaviruses vary in the intensity of their cytopathic action, which may depend on the cell species on the one hand and on environmental conditions (medium, pH, temperature, virus dose) on the other. In vertebrate cells growth of alphaviruses is rapid. Only a few hours after infection, newly formed virus is released. Virus production continues at a constant linear rate for up to 10 or 12 hours, approaching 1000 infectious units per cell. Flaviviruses show a latent period of about 12 hours, and a further 10 to 20 hours are required to achieve maximal titers of extracellular virus (Mussgay et al., 1975; Pfefferkorn and Shapiro, 1974).

PATHOGENIC PROPERTIES

Alphaviruses and Flaviviruses. The animal classes from which the arthropod-borne togavirus types have been isolated are listed in Tables 1 to 4. Additional information on susceptibility to infection of experimental hosts can be obtained from the *International Catalogue of Arboviruses* (Berge, 1975). In man, infections range in severity from completely subclinical but immunizing ones to rapidly fatal illness. Similar syndromes may be produced by immunologically different viruses, and completely different disease pictures can be caused even by strains of a virus that are immunologically identical.

A tendency to a biphasic temperature curve has been noted, in which the peaks may follow each other without an afebrile interval; this "saddle back" curve is considered typical for YF and DEN infections. However, in infections caused by the tick-borne encephalitis viruses (Table 3) there may be a period of 6 to 14 afebrile days between the two fever peaks. With the first rise in temperature—which may be mild and is often overlooked (in infections with

Table 3. TICK-BORNE FLAVIVIRUSES

		Isolated from											Isolated in						Human Disease	
		Arthropods			*Vertebrates*															
		Ticks																		
Virus	**Abbreviation**	*Ixodid*	*Argasid*	*Other*	*Man*	*Other Primates*	*Rodents*	*Birds*	*Bats*	*Marsupials*	*Others*	*Sentinels*	*Africa*	*Asia*	*Australasia*	*Europe*	*North America*	*South America*	*Natural Infection*	*Lab Infection*
[a]Absettarov	ABS	+			+						+					+			+	+
[a]Hanzalova	HAN	+			+											+			+	
[a]Hypr	HYPR	+			+		+	+	+		+					+			+	+
Kadam	KAD	+											+							
Karshi	KSI		+											+						
[a]Kumlinge	KUM	+			+		+	+			+					+			+	+
[a]Kyasanur Forest dis.	KFD	+	+	+	+	+	+	+	+		+			+					+	+
Langat	LGT	+												+						
[a]Louping ill	LI	+			+		+	+			+					+			+	+
[a]Omsk hem. fev.	OMSK	+			+		+				+			+		?			+	+
[a]Powassan	POW	+			+		+				+						+		+	
Royal Farm	RF		+											+						
[a]Russian spring summer enceph.	RSSE	+			+		+	+						+		+			+	+
Saumarez Reef	SRE	+	+												+					
Tyuleniy	TYU	+												+			+			

[a]Encephalitis in man has been observed after infection with the indicated viruses.

From Berge, T. O. (ed.): International Catalogue of Arboviruses. Washington, D.C., U.S. Department of Health, Education, and Welfare, update 1982.

Table 4. OTHER FLAVIVIRUSES, NO ARTHROPOD VECTOR DEMONSTRATED

		Isolated from								Isolated in						Human Disease	
		Vertebrates															
Virus	Abbreviation	Man	Other Primates	Rodents	Birds	Bats	Marsupials	Others	Sentinels	Africa	Asia	Australasia	Europe	North America	South America	Natural Infection	Lab Infection
Apoi	APOI			+							+						+
Aroa	AROA								+						+		
Carey Island	CI			+							+						
Cowbone Ridge	CR			+										+			
Dakar bat	DB	+				+				+							
Entebbe bat	ENT					+				+							
Israel turkey meningo.	IT				+						+						
Jutiapa	JUT			+										+			
Koutango	KOU			+						+							
Modoc	MOD			+										+			
Montana myotis leuko.	MML					+								+			
Negishi	NEG	+									+					+	+
Phnom-Penh bat	PPB					+					+						
Rio Bravo	RB					+								+		+	+
Saboya	SAB			+						+							
Sal Vieja	SV			+										+			
San Perlita	SP			+										+			
Sokoluk	SOK					+					+						

From Berge, T. O. (ed.): International Catalogue of Arboviruses. Washington, D.C., U.S. Department of Health, Education, and Welfare, 1982.

WEE, SLE, and JBE, for example)—systemic infection occurs and virus can be isolated from the blood. The second febrile period is associated with more serious clinical manifestations. During this phase, it is often impossible to isolate virus from the blood, and antibodies are usually already demonstrable. During the first febrile attack, virus multiplies in the internal organs and leukopenia is usually observed. Leukocytosis is often associated with later, more severe manifestations such as encephalitis. No consistent clinical picture is associated with arbo-togavirus infections. An influenza-like syndrome is observed in mild infections with accompanying headache, nausea, fever, gastrointestinal disturbances, myalgia, and joint pains. Encephalitis in humans and domestic animals is known to be caused by the alphaviruses EEE, VEE, and WEE; the flaviviruses that at times produce central nervous conditions are SLE, JBE, MVE, WN, members of the tick-borne flaviviruses, and possibly ILH. Hepatitis is a typical manifestation of YF in man and has also been observed after infection with KFD. Maculopapular rashes with lymphadenopathy are common in DEN infections and have also been reported for WN, CHIK, and ONN infections. Hemorrhages of varying severity are observed in some DEN epidemics and in OMSK and KFD infections. The black vomit ("vomito negro") of YF is the result of gastric hemorrhages.

The DEN hemorrhagic fever and a newly recognized DEN shock syndrome (which occurs with significant mortality, especially in children in Asia) are known to be immunologic diseases. The four DEN serotypes do not confer a high level of cross-protection; nevertheless, there is a rapid serologic response when an individual who has recovered from an attack of DEN caused by one serotype is infected with another. The secondary antibody response coincides with viremia owing to the superinfecting DEN type; circulating immune complexes are then formed, and complement depletion occurs. The immune complexes are deposited in the vessel walls, and hemorrhagic fever and shock result (Theiler and Downs, 1973). Immune enhancement of alpha- and flavivirus infections of macrophages in vitro by antibody has been established experimentally.

Rubella Virus. Primates appear to be the natural hosts of RUV; in monkeys (rhesus and African monkeys), infection occasionally causes symptoms but is mostly inapparent. Ferrets, hamsters, guinea pigs, rabbits, and newborn mice also have been found to support multiplication of RUV in vivo and display no clinical signs. Infection in pregnant rats can cause teratogenic damage to the offspring that is similar to that seen in human infants with congenital rubella.

Postnatal infection in an adult man frequently starts with mild fever, headache, malaise, and respiratory symptoms some days before the appearance of a maculopapular rash associated with lymphadenopathy. The latter symptom is a prominent feature of the disease, whereas the rash may be absent, especially in younger individuals. Although postnatal infection usually follows a benign course, arthritis, thrombocytopenic purpura, and encephalitis may occur as complications.

The pathogenic significance of RUV lies in its teratogenic properties. About 10 to 15 per cent of living infants born to mothers with apparent or inapparent rubella during the first trimester of pregnancy show evidence of infection that is recognizable at birth or during the first year of life. The consequences of in utero infection include spontaneous abortion, stillbirth, and live birth with moderate to severe abnormalities as well as completely normal infants. The congenital rubella syndrome consists of neurologic and developmental defects such as hearing loss, eye lesions (pearly cataract, glaucoma, chorioretinitis, microphthalmia, corneal clouding), cardiovascular defects, hepatosplenomegaly, thrombocytopenic purpura, anemia, interstitial pneumonia, metaphyseal bone lesions, and intrauterine growth retardation. Any combination of anomalies may occur in an individual infant.

IMMUNITY. In infected or vaccinated individuals, togaviral antigens cause a pronounced immune response that can be measured in vitro; like most viruses that produce systemic disease with a viremia, togavirus infection is controlled primarily by circulating antibody. Lifelong immunity after a togavirus attack has been observed. For instance, yellow fever antibodies have been found persisting for 75 years in the absence of reexposure. A specific aspect of alphavirus and flavivirus infections is the antibody response of individuals after multiple exposures to antigenically related viruses. In general, with repeated immunizations there is a broadening of the specificity of the antibodies produced and a heightened reaction to the original virus rather than to the virus responsible for reinfection. Thus, sequential infection of humans with two flaviviruses induced neutralizing antibodies that cross-reacted with a third flavivirus to which the subjects had never been exposed. Unfortunately, the existence of cross-reactive antibodies does not necessarily provide resistance to infection. Otherwise, vaccination with a series of carefully selected antigenically related viruses would produce a broad immunity that might be effective against all viruses of this genus. However, this cannot be achieved because of the "original antigenic sin" phenomenon: The immunologic response of a person to a togavirus is dominated throughout his life by his first experience with a virus of that type.

Vaccines against the epidemic and endemic arthropod-borne togavirus infections have been developed for human (medical personnel, laboratory workers, military forces) and veterinary use. Of the inactivated vaccines, formalin-treated TBE virus preparations have been in wide use in the U.S.S.R. Experimental vaccines against other flaviviruses (JBE, SLE, and KFD) have been tested. The accumulated evidence suggests that potent inactivated vaccines can be prepared. The substrate for virus production must be carefully selected, first for its ability to produce virus in high titer and second for the absence of undesirable components, such as the encephalitogenic factor in brain tissue. A vaccination regime of two initial doses followed by a yearly booster injection has been recommended (Smith, 1969). The immunizing potency of an experimental SFV virion subunit vaccine obtained after different solvent/detergent treatments has been tested in animals. Its efficiency depended on the size of the envelope fragments produced; large fragments (e.g., after Tween 80–ether treatment) offered the best protection (Mussgay et al., 1973).

Of the attenuated live virus vaccines, the YF strains 17D (prepared in chick embryo) and FN (mouse embryo) strains are in common use. The seed virus has to be strictly defined, since loss of immunogenicity has been observed at higher passage levels. The 17D vaccine has been one of the most innocuous and effective vaccines; the first fatality (in a 3-year-old child) was reported after the administration of some 34 million doses and 25 years of use. A number of other live attenuated viruses have given satisfactory antibody responses in human volunteers and experimental animals. Heterotypic immunization using LGT virus, a naturally occurring tick-borne virus from Malaya, against tick-borne viruses highly pathogenic to man (see Table 3) has been successful. When heterotypic vaccinations are used, the above-mentioned hazard of immunologic aggravation of diseases must be recognized.

After natural RUV infection, persistent levels of nasopharyngeal IgA, which play an important role in preventing reinfection of adults, have been detected at the portal of entry; cell-mediated immunity has also been demonstrated in tonsillar lymphoid tissue. If fetal infection is to be prevented, adequate and persistent levels of serum antibody, especially IgG, must be present in the mother's plasma. Several attenuated vaccine strains have been developed by serial passages of RUV in vervet monkey kidney cells (HPV 77) followed by passage in primary rabbit kidney (Cendehill) and primary guinea pig kidney cells (the Japanese strain To-336) or in human embryonic kidney cells and WI 38 fibroblasts (RA27/3). Administration of these strains resulted in seroconversion of 95 per cent of susceptible recipients, although antibody levels were often lower than those following naturally acquired disease. Reinfection of convalescent or vaccinated individuals does occur and may in fact be responsible for maintaining adequate levels of immunity in a community. In contrast to measles and poliomyelitis, however, the aim of RUV vaccination is not so much to protect the vaccinee herself against a relatively mild disease but to prevent infection of the fetus. Fetal infection is likely to occur only if maternal viremia develops, and viremia has not been observed in immune individuals after either natural or experimental challenge (Banatvala, 1977).

LABORATORY DIAGNOSIS

Alphaviruses and Flaviviruses. Suckling mice are considered the universal host system for virus isolation; they are inoculated intracerebrally with sera from patients, postmortem specimens, or extracts from pools of trapped arthropods. The mice become ill, and frequently have hind limb paralysis, usually two to three days or longer after injection. Affected mice are then sacrificed. Isolation of virus is confirmed by passage of brain suspension material to other suckling mice. For primary isolation, cell cultures of chicken fibroblasts and hamster kidney cells are commonly used; as for continuous lines, Vero (green monkey) and BHK-21 (hamster) cells are routinely employed. Not all cell-virus systems show cytopathic effects after viral multiplication. To isolate virus it is important to inoculate unknown specimens at two or more dilutions, since high concentrations of defective interfering particles may restrict or completely mask the signs of infection.

An isolated agent is usually identified by neutralization tests employing mice or cell cultures. The most sensitive animal method is the intraperitoneal inoculation of infant mice with serum-virus mixtures. The reproducibility of this assay is improved by the addition of complement, which in the presence of antibody causes lysis of the viral membrane and inactivation of its genome by RNAase. In a neutralization test for virus identification, the amount of serum is kept constant and incubated with serial tenfold virus dilutions. By comparing the neutralization indices (the difference in log virus titers in the presence and absence of antibodies) of the virus in question with homologous virus-serum mixtures, type identification can be made. By using this procedure, it is also possible to determine the extent of antigenic cross-relationship between viruses within one genus.

In general, cross-reactions between related viruses are more pronounced by hemagglutination inhibition (HI) and complement fixation (CF) tests than by neutralization. From studies on the HI antibody response of experimental animals, the following conclusions can be drawn:

1. Each virus, after primary infection, produces a distinctive HI pattern. The reaction may be entirely specific, such that the serum reacts only with the homologous antigen. When cross-reactions occur, they are always significantly lower in titer than the homologous reactions. Cross-reactions are highest with antigens prepared from viruses that are closely related to the immunizing antigen.

2. When animals are inoculated repeatedly with the same virus, the sera are more broadly cross-reactive and titers are higher, but the basic pattern remains the same.

3. Animals immunized to two different viruses of the same genus produce sera that are very widely cross-reactive; their cross-reactivity is always more marked than that observed with sera obtained from animals after two inoculations of the same virus. Anti-flavivirus sera tend to show more pronounced intragenus cross-reactivity than anti-alphavirus sera. Many of the problems encountered with conventional antisera can be eliminated by using (mixtures of) monoclonal antibodies with defined epitope specificity.

Sera contain nonspecific inhibitors for togavirus HA in high titer; they are lipoproteins and are removed by acetone extraction or adsorption to acid-washed kaolin. In addition, many sera show hemagglutinating activity for goose red blood cells (RBC), which is eliminated by adsorption to erythrocytes before the serum is titrated. Goose RBC are used in many laboratories to test HA, but chicken and pigeon cells (RBC) are also suitable. Optimal temperature is 25° to 37° C for alphaviruses; some flaviviruses and RUV require 4° C. Spontaneous elution does not occur.

From the foregoing it is clear that serologic tests for determining the type identity of alphavirus or flavivirus antibodies can be inconclusive, particularly when the sera are collected from patients in endemic areas. In these cases, the mere demonstration of a rise in antibody to a given virus by whatever test is not sufficient evidence that the infection is attributable to the virus used in the test. Only primary infection in individuals not previously exposed to any alphavirus or flavivirus can be reliably diagnosed by means of serology (Theiler and Downs, 1973).

Rubella Virus. Throat swabs or washings, acute phase blood, cerebrospinal fluid, urine, amniotic fluid, and placental or fetal tissues can be used for isolation in cultures of primary African green monkey kidney, human amnion, RK13 (rabbit), BHK-21 cells, and others. In established cell lines rubella virus may produce a CPE that is markedly influenced by environmental variables (e.g., serum concentration), whereas in primary cells CPE is often absent and virus multiplication must be demonstrated by interference with a challenge virus. For instance, primary African green monkey kidney cells show no evidence of CPE after infection with rubella virus but lose their ability to support growth of added echovirus type 11, coxsackievirus A9, or Newcastle disease virus. From fetal specimens RUV can be best isolated by explanting tissue fragments or trypsinizing fetal tissue; infected cells and media thus obtained can be used for virus identification. Since no antigenic cross-reactions occur between RUV and other togaviruses, unequivocal identification can be made by neutralization of the interfering or cytopathic effect by using a specific antiserum. A more rapid method consists of the application of indirect immunofluorescent antibody staining. In this method, acetone-fixed infected cells on coverslips are incubated with known immune rabbit sera and subsequently with fluorescein-conjugated goat anti-rabbit globulin prep-

Table 5. SUGGESTED TESTING FOR RUBELLA ANTIBODIES IN DIFFERENT SITUATIONS

	Source of Serum	Choice of Serologic Test 1st	2nd	3rd	Interpretation
A	Patient with rash less than 1 week previously. Convalescent serum 14 to 21 days posteruption	HI	FA	CF	Fourfold rise proves recent infection
B	Patient with rash more than 1 week previously. Convalescent serum 21 to 28 days posteruption	CF	FA	HI[a]	Fourfold rise proves recent infection
C	Subject in whom immunity is to be determined or pregnant women exposed to rubella	HI	Nt	FA	Presence of antibody at any titer shows immunity
D	Possible rubella-syndrome infant older than 6 months	HI	Nt	FA	Presence of antibody suggests congenital infection if child has not been exposed to rubella
E	Possible rubella-syndrome infant younger than 6 months	HI	Nt	FA	Presence of antibody suggests congenital infection if titer significantly higher than mother's or if contained in IgM fraction

[a]Determination of IgM rubella antibody may assist in the diagnosis.

From Plotkin, S. A.: In Lenette, E. H., and Schmidt, N. J. (eds.): Diagnostic Procedures for Viral and Rickettsial Infections. New York, American Public Health Association, 1969.

arations. The specificity of the cytoplasmic fluorescence must be verified by including preimmune rabbit serum and uninfected cells as controls.

For the determination of RU antibodies, HI, CF, and indirect immunofluorescence are mostly used; the reagents are commercially available. The suggested serologic tests and their interpretations are summarized in Table 5 (Plotkin, 1969). In general, the HI test gives the highest titer levels; CF antibodies tend to fade quickly and are often absent when other tests are still positive. For indirect immunofluorescence a fluorescein isothiocyanate-conjugated anti-human globulin preparation must be used as a second antibody. If this preparation is IgM-specific, it can be employed for the diagnosis of congenital infection (see case E in Table 5). After disease, precipitating antibodies directed against two viral antigens (ϑ and ι) may be detected in gel double diffusion tests. Anti-ϑ antibodies usually parallel those detected by HI, whereas anti-ι antibodies appear to correlate with resistance to reinfection.

EPIDEMIOLOGY. For an epidemiologic cycle to occur in nature, the following conditions must be met: A critical minimal amount of virus is necessary to establish infection of the arthropod vector. This threshold value is characteristic for every arthropod-virus combination and implies that the virus must circulate in the vertebrate host in sufficient quantities. The susceptibility of a given vector to a given virus can be either inferred from material collected in nature under endemic or epidemic conditions or determined by experimental infection of the arthropod (feeding on or inoculation with virus-containing material). For the virus to be transmitted by the vector, it must pass from the lumen of the arthropod's intestinal tract to susceptible cells, multiply, and reach the salivary glands in quantities adequate to inoculate an infectious dose by bite. This process determines the transmitting efficiency of the vector. Epidemiologically, climate conditions are critical. Thus, the extrinsic incubation period in the vector is shortened by increased temperature. Rainfall may favor breeding conditions for mosquitoes. Climate may control the geographic distribution of arboviruses by providing the ecologic conditions for vectors and hosts. Since each species of blood-sucking arthropod has an affinity for a vertebrate species or group of species, detailed knowledge of vector-host preferences or dependencies is essential to the epidemiology and control of arthropod-borne virus diseases. Infection chains and reservoirs (animal species in which virus is maintained and can be disseminated for a prolonged period) have been established for many arthropod-borne togaviruses (Theiler and Downs, 1973).

Rubella virus transmission occurs through droplet infection. The portal of entry is the lymphoid tissue of the pharynx and possibly the conjunctiva. Sources of infection are virus-excreting individuals with or without clinical symptoms. Children with chronic infection are an important source of infection. Rubella has a worldwide distribution. Infections in the northern hemisphere increase during March to May, and more extensive epidemics occur at regular intervals of 5 to 10 years (Norrby, 1969).

References

Banatvala, J. E.: Rubella vaccines. In Recent Advances in Clinical Virology. Edinburgh, London, New York, Churchill-Livingstone, vol. 1, 1977, p. 171.

Berge, T. O. (ed.): International Catalogue of Arboviruses. Washington, D. C., U. S. Department of Health, Education and Welfare, 1982.

Casals, J., and Reeves, W. C.: Arthropod-borne animal viruses. In Rivers, T. M., and Horsfall, F. L. (eds.): Viral and Rickettsial Infections of Man. London, Pitman Medical Publishing Company, 1959, p. 269.

Clarke, D. H., and Casals, J.: Techniques for hemagglutination and hemagglutination-inhibition with arthropod-borne viruses. Am J Trop Med Hyg 7:561, 1958.

Dalrymple, J. M., Schlesinger, S., and Russell, P. K.: Antigenic characterization of two Sindbis envelope glycoproteins separated by isoelectric focusing. Virology 69:93, 1976.

Fenner, F.: Classification and nomenclature of viruses. Intervirology 7:44, 1976.

Heinz, F. X., Berger, R., Tuma, W., and Kunz, C.: A topological and functional model of epitopes on the structural glycoprotein of TBE virus defined by monoclonal antibodies. Virology 126:525, 1983.

Horzinek, M. C.: Nonarthropod-borne togaviruses. London, Academic Press, 1981.

Karabatsos, N.: Antigenic relationship of group A arboviruses by plaque reduction neutralization testing. Am J Trop Med Hyg 24:527, 1975.

de Madrid, A. T., and Porterfield, J. S.: The flaviviruses (group B arboviruses). A cross-neutralization study. J Gen Virol 23:91, 1974.

Mussgay, M., Weiland, E., Strohmaier, K., Ueberschär, S., and Enzmann, P. J.: Properties of components obtained by treatment of Semliki Forest virus with Tween-80 and tri(N-butyl) phosphate. J Gen Virol 19:89, 1973.

Mussgay, M., Enzmann, P. J., Horzinek, M. C., and Weiland, E.: Growth cycle of arboviruses in vertebrate and arthropod cells. Progr Med Virol 19:257, 1975.

Norrby, E.: Rubella Virus. New York, Springer Verlag, 1969, p. 115.

Pfefferkorn, E. R., and Shapiro, D.: Reproduction of togaviruses. In Fraenkel-Conrat, H., and Wagner, R. R. (eds.): Comprehensive Virology, vol. 2. New York, Plenum Publishing Corporation, 1974, p. 171.

Plotkin, S. A.: Rubella virus. In Lenette, E. H., and Schmidt, N. J. (eds.): Diagnostic Procedures for Viral and Rickettsial Infections. New York, American Public Health Association, 1969, p. 364.

Porterfield, J. S.: Antigenic characteristics and classification of togaviridae. In Schlesinger, R. W. (ed.): The Togaviruses. New York, Academic Press, 1980.

Smith, C. E., Gordon: Arbovirus vaccines. Br Med Bull 25:142, 1969.

Theiler, M., and Downs, W. G.: The Arthropod-Borne Viruses of Vertebrates. New Haven, Yale University Press, 1973.

Wengler, G., Wengler, G., and Filipe, A. R.: A study of nucleotide sequence homology between the nucleic acids of different alphaviruses. Virology 78:124, 1977.

World Health Organization Study Group: Arboviruses and human disease. WHO Technical Report Series No. 369, 1967.

67
ARENAVIRUSES

FRITZ LEHMANN-GRUBE, M.D.

The group of arenaviruses comprises at present ten members, of which four are pathogenic for man, causing lymphocytic choriomeningitis, Lassa fever, Argentine hemorrhagic fever, and Bolivian hemorrhagic fever. The latter three illnesses are severe and of public health importance. Arenaviruses are of special interest for investigating virus-host relationships such as pathologic immune phenomena in virus diseases and persistent virus infections.

CLASSIFICATION. The lymphocytic choriomeningitis (LCM) virus was the first arenavirus to be discovered (Table 1). During serial transfers in monkeys of materials from a fatal case of the 1933 St. Louis epidemic of encephalitis, a virus was encountered that differed from the other isolates of that outbreak. The true origin of this first strain of LCM virus was never determined.

Between 1956 and 1958 the Tacaribe virus was isolated in Trinidad from bats and mosquitoes and shortly thereafter the Junin virus in Argentina from people suffering from Argentine hemorrhagic fever. Tacaribe virus and Junin virus were antigenically related, as was Machupo virus, recovered from cases of Bolivian hemorrhagic fever in 1963. These three agents formed the Tacaribe complex, soon to be joined by Amapari virus, Tamiami virus, Parana virus, Pichinde virus, and Latino virus (Johnson et al., 1973).

Similarities between Machupo virus and LCM virus were noted early, but it was their striking morphologic resemblance that led to the proposal to form a taxonomic entity comprising LCM virus and the viruses of the Tacaribe complex. In 1969 the agent causing Lassa fever was isolated from patients with the disease in Nigeria. Its relatedness with the LCM virus was recognized, and a new virus group was defined containing LCM, Lassa, and the Tacaribe complex viruses. The proposed name was arenoviruses (from the Latin word *arenosus*, meaning sandy)—later changed to arenaviruses—which was to reflect the characteristic granules seen by electron microscopy in ultrathin sections of infected cells (Rowe et al., 1970). This virus group has been given the status of a genus named *Arenavirus* belonging to the family *Arenaviridae*; type species is the LCM virus (Matthews, 1982). Whether the Flexal (BeAn 293022) virus (Pinheiro et al., 1977), the Lassa virus-related Mozambique virus (Wulff et al., 1977), and two further different but related agents isolated in Zimbabwe and the Central African Republic by Johnson et al. (1981) and Gonzales et al. (1983), respectively, are distinct arenaviruses has not been decided.

MORPHOLOGY AND BIOCHEMICAL PROPERTIES. Of the many features that the arenaviruses have in common, the morphology of virus particles is salient (Murphy and Whitfield, 1975). Arenavirus particles are round or pleomorphic with diameters of 50 to 300 nm (average 120 nm). In vivo and in vitro they are released from the infected cell by budding (Fig. 1). The viral envelopes are formed from plasma membranes: the density of both layers as well as the width of the intermediary zone increase, and club-shaped surface projections, approximately 10 nm long, are inserted often forming well-delineated margins. In their interior, arenavirus particles characteristically contain variable numbers of electron-dense granules that resemble cellular ribosomes. They are usually randomly distributed,

Table 1. ISOLATION HISTORY AND NATURAL OCCURRENCE OF VIRUSES PRESENTLY RECOGNIZED AS ARENAVIRUSES

Virus	First Isolation		Natural Occurrence	
	Reference	Source	Principal Host	Geographic Distribution
LCM	Armstrong and Lillie (1934)	Monkey (?)	*Mus musculus*	America, Europe
Lassa	Buckley and Casals (1970)	Man	*Mastomys natalensis*	Africa (Sierra Leone, Nigeria; other parts)
Amapari	Pinheiro et al. (1966)	*Oryzomys* sp. *Neacomys guianae*	*Oryzomys capito* *Neacomys guianae*	South America (Brazil)
Junin	Parodi et al. (1958)	Man	*Calomys laucha** *Akodon azarae*	South America (Argentina)
Latino	Webb et al. (1973)	*Calomys callosus*	*Calomys callosus*	South America (Bolivia, Brazil)
Machupo	Johnson et al. (1965)	Man	*Calomys callosus*	South America (Bolivia)
Parana	Webb et al. (1970)	*Oryzomys buccinatus*	*Oryzomys buccinatus*	South America (Paraguay)
Pichinde	Trapido and Sanmartín (1971)	*Oryzomys albigularis* *Thomasomys lugens*†	*Oryzomys albigularis*	South America (Colombia)
Tacaribe	Downs et al. (1963)	*Artibeus lituratus*‡ *Artibeus jamaicensis* Mosquitoes	?‡	Central America (Trinidad)
Tamiami	Calisher et al. (1970)	*Sigmodon hispidus*	*Sigmodon hispidus*	North America (Florida)

*Predominantly *C. laucha musculinus.*
†Subspecies *T. lugens fuscatus.*
‡Isolated between March 1956 and December 1958 from 11 bats and one pool of mosquitoes, but never since.

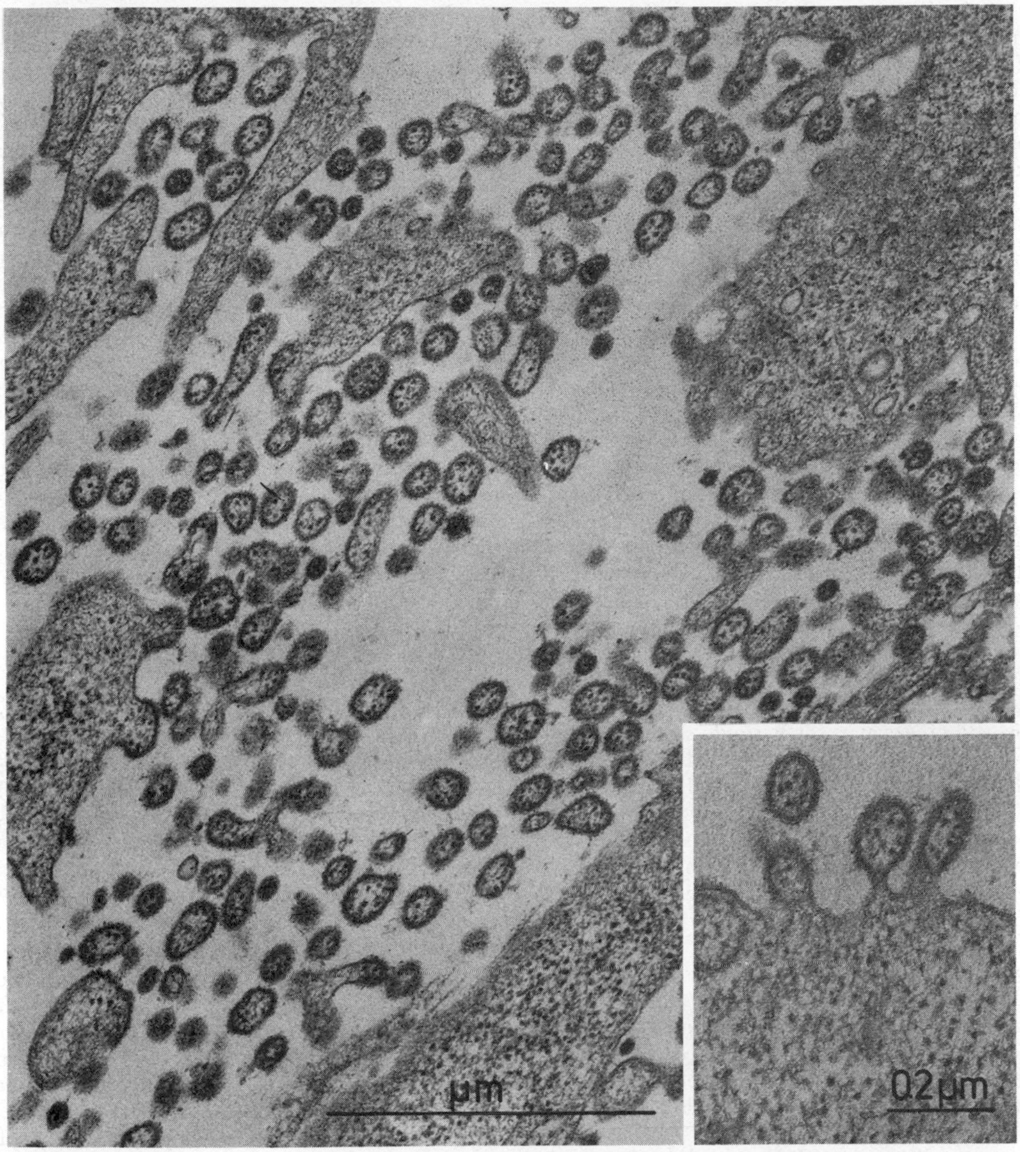

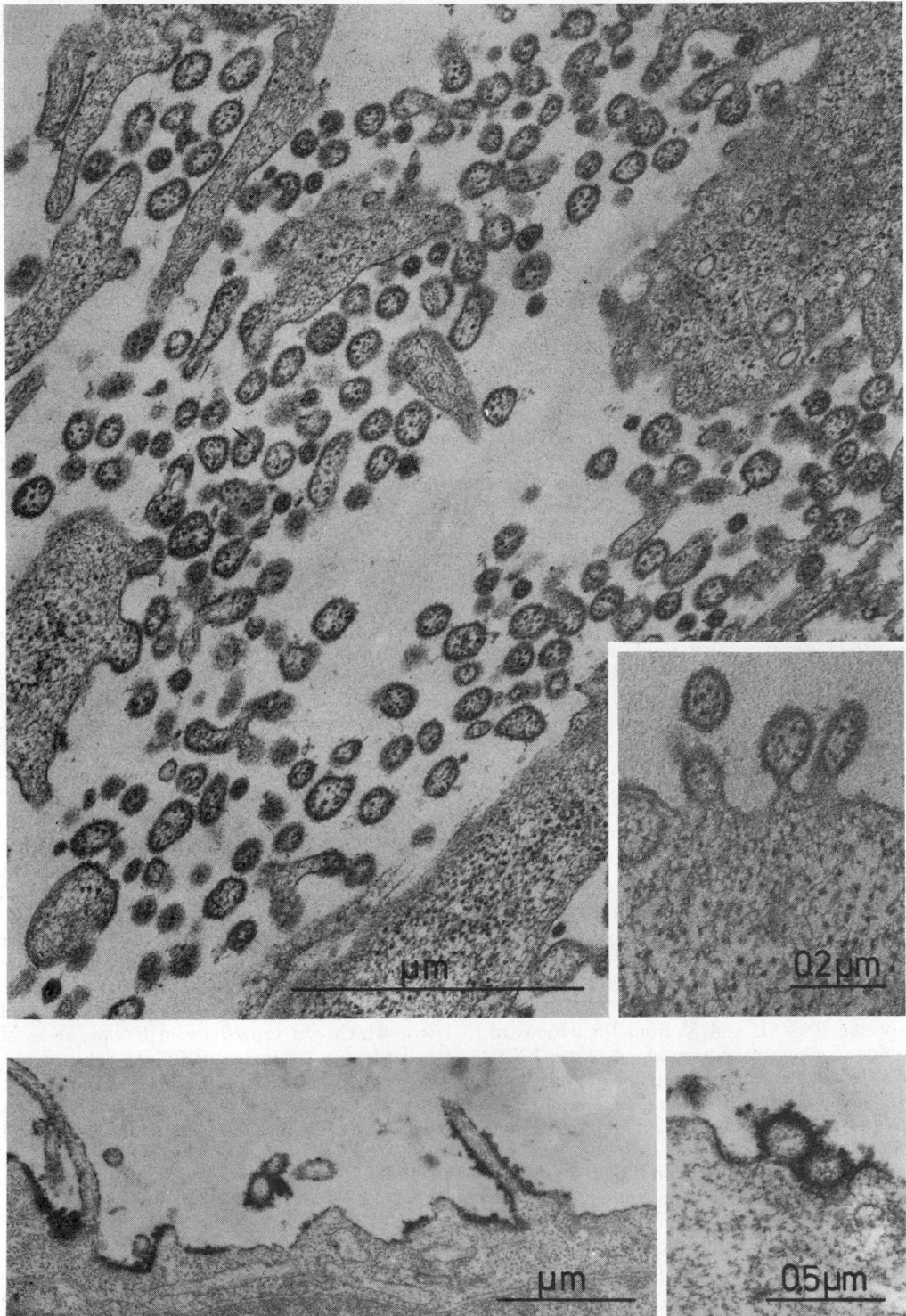

Figure 1. Thin section electron micrographs of LCM virus-infected cultivated mouse (L) cells. *Above,* Multiple arenavirus particles are seen either released from the plasma membrane or still budding. *Below,* Demonstration by means of the immunoperoxidase method of LCM virus-specific antigen(s) in association with budding virus particles and in distinct areas of the plasma membrane that are not otherwise visibly altered. Photographs kindly supplied by Dr. K. Mannweiler, Hamburg.

but sometimes they are arranged beneath the envelope in a circular pattern. A recently performed electron microscopic study of purified infectious LCM virus has led to results indicating that these granules represent fragmented virus cores (Müller et al., 1983), but other investigators assume that they are host cell ribosomes, which, however, are not essential for infectivity (Rawls and Leung, 1979).

Nucleocapsid cores have never been observed in arenavirus particles by thin section electron microscopy of infected cells. Such structures have been visualized, however, in purified preparations after removal of the viral envelopes with detergent. The fine structure of the interior of Pichinde virus was analyzed with the electron microscope by Young and Howard (1983). The results suggest that the nucleocapsid is built of nucleosomes, which appear to be individual nucleoprotein molecules. Their primary arrangement is that of linear arrays, which are coiled helically and supercoiled and twisted into more or less spherical forms consisting of viral nonglycosylated proteins and RNA.

Many determinations of the size of the infectious unit by various physical methods have given greatly divergent results, not only between different arenaviruses but also for one virus with different methods. Immuno-electron microscopy has shown (Fig. 1) that the characteristic particles budding from infected cells contain viral antigen(s). However, whether they are all virions and potentially infectious is unknown. The diameter of the infectious unit of LCM virus appears to be around 100 nm (Blechschmidt and Thomssen, 1976; Lehmann-Grube et al., 1983).

The nucleic acid of arenaviruses is single stranded RNA consisting of two distinct components called "L" and "S" with molecular weights 2.1 to 3.2 $\times$ 10^6 and 1.1 to 1.6 $\times$ 10^6, respectively. Usually, although not always, virus preparations contain further RNA species having sedimentation coefficients of 28S and 18S. Small molecules with 4 to 6S have also been identified, and a 15S species has been resolved in Pichinde virus but not yet in other arenaviruses. According to present evidence, the L and the S RNA contain the viral genetic information, while the 28S and 18S components originate from host cell ribosomes. As has been pointed out (see above), the association of the latter with the virions is still uncertain. The small RNA species resemble host cell transfer RNA with respect to both size and methylation ratio (Pedersen, 1979; Rawls and Leung, 1979; Harnish et al., 1983).

The virus-specific RNA (L and S) from the virions of Pichinde virus does not have properties of messenger RNA. Polysomal RNA, however, from virus-infected cells does have properties of messenger RNA and, furthermore, is complementary to the virion RNA. These findings, together with the demonstration of an association of RNA-dependent RNA polymerase with the virion, strongly suggest that the Pichinde viruse RNA—and by analogy the RNA of the other arenaviruses—is negative stranded (Rawls and Leung, 1979). This conclusion would explain why attempts to prepare infectious RNA from virions of LCM virus were unsuccessful (Welsh et al., 1975).

Structural proteins have been identified for LCM virus, Lassa virus, Junin virus, Machupo virus, Pichinde virus, Tacaribe virus, and Tamiami virus (Gangemi et al., 1978; Rawls and Leung, 1979; Buchmeier et al., 1980; Boersma et al., 1982; Harnish, et al., 1983; Bruns et al., 1983b; Clegg and Lloyd, 1983). For some time it appeared established that all arenaviruses are built of one major nonglycosylated protein with apparent molecular weight ranging from 63 to 72 $\times$ 10^3 and either one or two major glycoproteins with molecular weights ranging from 35 to 72 $\times$ 10^3. Further protein components were often detected but usually in low quantities. More recent findings, however, indicate that the composition of at least some of the arenaviruses is more complex. Thus, a large component ("L") with molecular weight 200 $\times$ 10^3 has been determined in the virions of Pichinde virus (Harnish et al., 1983), and our own studies suggest that the LCM virus is formed by not fewer than seven distinct proteins (including one with molecular weight 200 $\times$ 10^3) (Bruns et al., 1983b). Whether the protein composition of these agents is more diverse than had been assumed, or whether the differences between members of the group have a methodological basis can at present not be decided. Further proteins were detected in infected cells. Of these, one glycoprotein has been identified as a nonstructural precursor of at least two glycoproteins of the virion.

The arenaviruses disintegrate rapidly in the presence of lipid solvents and detergents, indicating that lipids are needed for their structural integrity. By analogy with other budding viruses, these lipids probably are derived from the host cell membrane forming part of the viral envelope. The glycoproteins are situated on or close to the surface of the virion, probably in the spikes. The one nonglycosylated major protein has always been found in association with the RNA and is probably part of the ribonucleoprotein complex.

The buoyant densities of the infectious units of different arenaviruses vary between 1.16 and 1.18 when determined in sucrose and between 1.18 and 1.23 when determined in CsCl (Rawls and Leung, 1979; Lehmann-Grube et al., 1983). Gschwender et al. (1975) arrived at values for LCM virus of 1.22 in CsCl and 1.14 in a gradient formed of iodinated organic compounds.

During replication of LCM virus, in addition to fully infectious (standard) virus, particles are produced that cannot multiply by themselves but reduce the infectious yield and, if the standard virus is cytolytic, abolish cytopathic effects. These interfering particles are slightly less dense and relatively resistant to ultraviolet light, neutral red, and heat (Welsh et al., 1975; Lehmann-Grube et al., 1983). Although these properties are characteristic for defective interfering (DI) particles, there are essential differences. "By definition DI particles are defective virions, which can grow only in the presence of a helper standard virus" (Huang, 1973). In contrast, LCM virus-interfering particles multiply predominantly in cells infected by standard virus alone rather than in cells dually infected with standard virus and interfering particles. Furthermore, both entities differ in their chemical composition (Lehmann-Grube et al., 1983). Interfering virus has also been detected in association with several other arenaviruses (Pfau, 1977).

ANTIGENIC COMPOSITION. Serologic relationships between arenaviruses have been demonstrated by complement-fixation tests (Casals et al., 1975) and immunofluorescence procedures (Wulff et al., 1978). In the case of Tacaribe complex viruses, the viral component responsible for cross-reactivity is the nucleoprotein (Buchmeier and Oldstone, 1978). As a rule, serologic relationships cannot be demonstrated by use of the neutralization test with one notable exception: guinea pigs infected with Tacaribe virus develop protective immunity against Junin virus and also

Junin virus-neutralizing antibody (Weissenbacher et al., 1975/76), and infection with Tacaribe virus protects marmosets against Junin virus, even though in these animals Junin virus-neutralizing antibody cannot be detected at the time of challenge infection (Weissenbacher et al., 1982).

The immunogen that induces complement-fixing antibody has been characterized for LCM and Pichinde viruses (Smadel et al., 1940; Gschwender et al., 1976; Buchmeier et al., 1977). It is produced in abundance in infected cells and is also a structural component of the virion; it is not, however, represented on the surface of either the virion or the infected cell and is distinct from the antigen combining with neutralizing antibody. Although serologically indistinguishable, the complement-fixing antigen from infected cells differs chemically from the antigen that is associated with the virion.

By necessity, the immunogen leading to the formation of neutralizing antibody is on the surface of the virion. In the case of LCM virus it is a glycoprotein with molecular weight 44×10^3 (Bruns et al., 1983a).

In double immunodiffusion tests in agar using extracts of LCM or Pichinde virus-infected cells and the respective antisera one line of precipitation is consistently formed. Its antigenic component is heat-stable and pronase-resistant, and corresponds to the complement-fixing antigen just mentioned. A second line is weaker and less regularly observed; its antigenic component is heat-labile and susceptible to the activity of the enzyme (Bro-Jørgensen, 1971; Buchmeier et al., 1977).

In the cytoplasm of LCM virus-infected cells two types of antigens can be distinguished by immunofluorescence (Rutter and Gschwender, 1973). One consists of coarse granules with bright fluorescence; serologically it is identical with the complement-fixing antigen mentioned above. The other antigen has a fine dust-like distribution; its relationship with viral structures is not known.

Several methods detect new antigens on the surfaces of LCM virus-infected cells. Letting the viable cell interact with fluorescein-labeled antibody and inspecting it with an immunofluorescence microscope is one, and incubating the infected cell with antiserum plus complement and watching for lysis is another (Rutter and Gschwender, 1973). New antigens on the surface of LCM virus-infected cells have been localized by immuno-electron microscopy (Mannweiler and Lehmann-Grube, 1973; Bruns et al., 1983a). Not surprisingly, budding viruses are thus labeled. In addition, virus-specific antigen is found in areas of the plasma membrane where morphologic alterations are not apparent (Fig. 1). Some viral antigen, together with a cell surface structure, forms the target for cytotoxic T lymphocytes (see below), and skin transplants from LCM virus carrier mice are rejected by nominally syngeneic recipients just like allografts (Holtermann and Majde, 1971), a phenomenon called skin heterogenization.

VIRUS-HOST RELATIONSHIPS. The host range of LCM virus is so wide that no mammalian species is known to resist infection. Virus strains differ in pathogenic properties. As a rule, disease signs are moderate or not detected; but there are exceptions. The adult mouse responds with a severe illness to infection with LCM virus (see below). Clinical signs also develop in humans and monkeys. One widely employed virus strain ("WE") is absolutely lethal for guinea pigs; in other words, one guinea pig infectious dose of WE strain virus is identical with one lethal dose. In vitro, too, cells from most mammalian species can be infected with LCM virus and respond with replication of infectious virus. Whether virus multiplication is accompanied by cytopathic effects depends on the strain of virus and its previous passage history as much as on origin and properties of the host cells. For instance, passage of LCM virus through mouse brains selects for cytolytic variants, whereas prolonged replication in the mouse spleen results predominantly in noncytopathogenic virus (Popescu and Lehmann-Grube, 1976). Cytopathic effects are blocked by interfering particles (see above).

The LCM virus does not damage vital tissues of the mouse, at least not enough to impair functions (Lehmann-Grube et al., 1983). Nonetheless, infection of an adult mouse with LCM virus results in severe, sometimes lethal disease. The explanation is that the immune response may kill the host; the LCM disease of the adult mouse is an immunopathologic phenomenon (Hotchin, 1962; Lehmann-Grube and Löhler, 1981). The antigen (allergen) that induces an allergic reaction is virus, which, however, is recognized as foreign only in conjunction with a self component contributed by the cell surface. It is well established that the cellular element that thus restricts the immunologic reaction is encoded by the major histocompatibility complex, but its spatial association with virus is still uncertain (Zinkernagel and Doherty, 1979). The immune response of the mouse leading to disease and even death is entirely cell-mediated; T lymphocytes play an essential role (Cole and Nathanson, 1974; Johnson et al., 1978). It is postulated that they damage virus-infected cells of mouse tissue just as the cytotoxic T lymphocytes damage virus-infected target cells in vitro (Zinkernagel and Doherty, 1979), but it should be stressed that the mechanism of the immunopathologic illness of LCM virus-infected adult mice is not yet fully understood. Indeed, recent findings of Thomsen et al. (1983) indicate that delayed-type hypersensitivity is involved.

Pathologic immune phenomena have also been observed with other arenavirus-host combinations, for instance LCM virus in the rat and Junin virus, Tamiami virus, and Tacaribe virus in the suckling mouse.

Most arenaviruses multiply with cytopathic effects in Vero cells; other cell lines widely employed are L and BHK21. The principal hosts in nature of these agents are listed in Table 1. Infection with Lassa virus of *Saimiri scirreous, Macaca mulatta*, and guinea pig, with Machupo virus of *M. mulatta, M. fascicularis, Saguinus geoffroyi*, strain C-13 guinea pig, suckling hamster, and suckling mouse, and with Junin virus of *Callithrix jacchus*, guinea pig, and suckling mouse leads to disease signs that often resemble human Lassa fever, Bolivian hemorrhagic fever, and Argentine hemorrhagic fever, respectively (Eddy et al.,1975; Walker et al., 1975; Webb et al., 1975; Weissenbacher et al., 1975; Jahrling et al., 1980; 1982; Carballal et al., 1981; Walker et al., 1982; Weissenbacher et al., 1982).

Arenaviruses have attracted much attention by their propensity to establish prolonged infections in rodents but there is no reason to assume that prolonged infection is restricted to these animals. The best studied example is the persistent infection of *Mus. musculus* with LCM virus. When a mouse is infected with LCM virus in utero or shortly after birth, it becomes a lifelong carrier, meaning that the virus is not eliminated and that it multiplies in all organs without causing overt disease (Traub, 1939) (Fig. 2). Carrier mice respond normally to most antigens, but

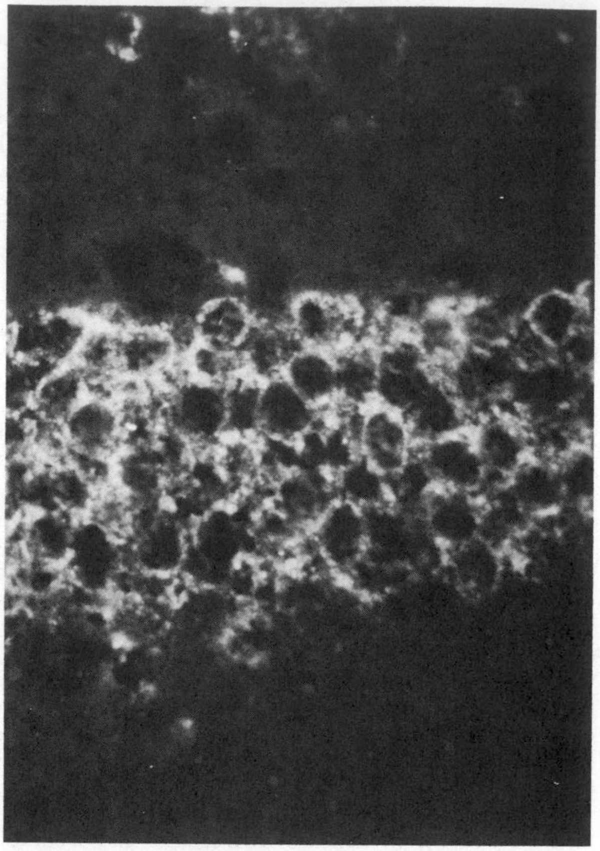

Figure 2. Brain of an LCM virus carrier mouse (stratum granulosum areae dentatae of the hippocampal region). Infected cells, primarily neurons, are visualized by the immunofluorescence procedure. Photograph kindly supplied by Dr. J. Löhler, Hamburg.

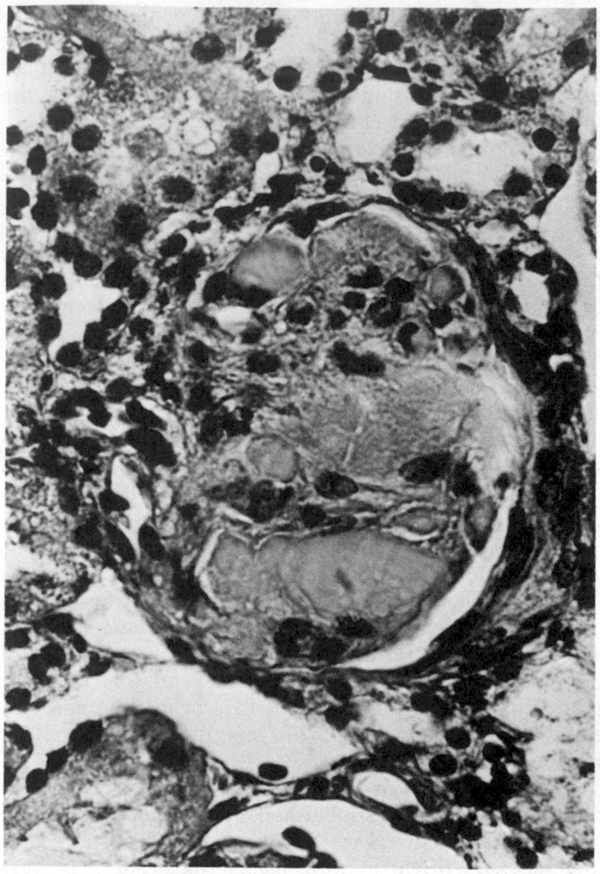

Figure 3. Final stage of glomerulonephritis of an LCM virus carrier mouse as part of late onset disease. Note the marked hyalinization of the glomerulum. Photograph kindly supplied by Dr. J. Löhler, Hamburg.

LCM virus-specific cell-mediated immunity is conspicuously absent. Since immune elmination of LCM virus is mediated by T lymphocytes and is readily accomplished by mice infected when adult, failure of virus elimination by a mouse infected congenitally or neonatally is attributed to LCM virus-specific immunologic tolerance. Antibodies directed against the LCM virus are formed, however (Oldstone, 1979); hence, tolerance in carrier mice is confined to the T cell compartment (Lehmann-Grube et al., 1983).

In carrier mice, replication of the virus is regulated so as to replenish losses due to natural decay, but not allow uninhibited increase. The mechanism of virus control is probably very complex and presumably involves interfering particles (Lehmann-Grube et al., 1983).

The type of virus-host relationship exemplified by LCM virus-*M. musculus* has been termed persistent tolerant infection (Hotchin, 1962); its salient features are lifelong duration, lack of a specific immune response, and absence of disease signs. Vertical transmission is also characteristic of the LCM virus-mouse relationship, but not a *conditio sine qua non* for designating an infection persistent tolerant.

The statement that mice persistently infected with LCM virus remain healthy requires qualification. In certain mouse strain-virus strain combinations aging carrier mice develop a "late onset disease" (Hotchin and Collins, 1964) characterized by runting and shortened life span. Many organs are affected, but a mesangioproliferative glomerulonephritis is prominent (Fig. 3). The evidence that the pathogenic mechanism is formation and deposition of immune complexes (Fig. 4) is impressive (Oldstone, 1979).

With the exception of Tacaribe virus all arenaviruses have been isolated from rodents with prolonged infections. However, only for LCM virus persisting in *M. musculus* has the pattern of infection been fully established. Reduced virus-specific immune responsiveness has been documented in several instances, especially well for *Callomys callosus* infected with Machupo virus (Justines and Johnson, 1969), but it is uncertain whether other arenavirus-host combinations (listed in Table 1) are persistent tolerant infections or merely unusually prolonged, in which case they should be termed chronic.

A better understanding of prolonged infection has been obtained by analyzing persistent infections of cell cultures with LCM virus in L cells and LCM virus, Parana virus, and Pichinde virus in BHK21 cells (Pfau, 1977). It appears that regulation of these infections, which go on for years, depends on an intricate interplay involving cells, virulent standard virus, attenuated standard virus, and interfering particles (Lehmann-Grube et al., 1983).

EPIDEMIOLOGY. The LCM virus has been found throughout Europe and America; whether it is distributed worldwide, as often stated, is doubtful (Lehmann-Grube, 1982). All other members of this group occur in small areas in South and Central America and in Africa. With the exception of the Tacaribe virus, arenaviruses are main-

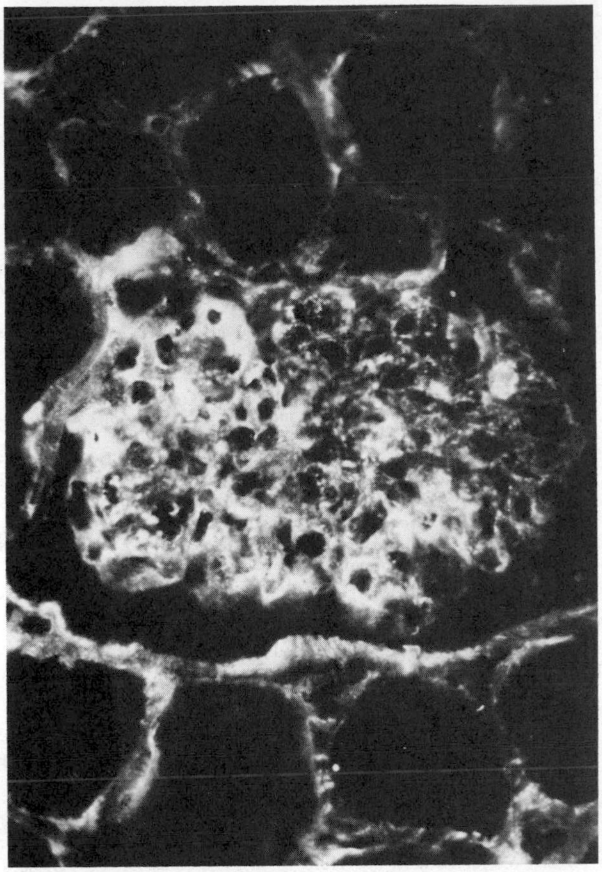

Figure 4. Deposition of immune complexes in the kidney of an LCM virus carrier mouse. Host immunoglobulin in the subendothelial space of capillaries and basement membrane of Bowman's capsule of a glomerulus and in the basement membranes of tubuli is visualized by immunofluorescence procedure. Photograph kindly supplied by Dr. J. Löhler, Hamburg.

tained in nature by rodents, and rodents are the principal source for infections of other animals and man. The mode of spread is not known with certainty, but the high virus concentrations in nasal secretions, saliva, and urine suggest that the virus is disseminated either by direct contact or via fomites and food. Airborne transmission is a further possibility. Arthropod vectors have never been convincingly incriminated.

The principal host for LCM virus is the persistently infected grey house mouse (*M. musculus*) (Armstrong et al., 1940). More recently, the Syrian hamster (*Mesocricetus auratus*) has also been identified as an important source for human infections (Ackermann, 1973; Maetz et al., 1976). Probably this animal is not a natural host of LCM virus but is infected from house mice that invade the hamsteries (Skinner and Knight, 1979). Transmission among members of mammalian species other than *M. musculus* and *M. auratus* is rare. In only one instance has man-to-man infection been documented; the circumstances were unusual (Smadel et al., 1942). Lassa virus is indigenous to certain areas of Africa where it is maintained by *Mastomys (Praomys) natalensis*. Unlike infections with other arenaviruses, Lassa virus may be transmitted from person to person and several hospital-centered outbreaks with usually one index case and secondary infections of medical personnel and visitors have been described. Outbreaks have also occurred in communities (Buckley and Casals, 1978). Sources for human infections with Machupo and Junin viruses, etiologic agents of Bolivian and Argentine hemorrhagic fevers, are rodents of the genera *Calomys* and *Akodon* (Johnson et al., 1973; Sabattini et al., 1977). As the names indicate, these diseases occur in Bolivia and Argentina, where they cause considerable health problems.

References

Ackermann, R.: Epidemiologic aspects of lymphocytic choriomeningitis in man. In Lehmann-Grube, F. (ed.): Lymphocytic Choriomeningitis Virus and Other Arenaviruses. Berlin, Heidelberg, New York, Springer-Verlag, 1973, p. 233.

Armstrong, C., and Lillie, R. D.: Experimental lymphocytic choriomeningitis of monkeys and mice produced by a virus encountered in studies of the 1933 St. Louis encephalitis epidemic. Public Health Rep 49:1019, 1934.

Armstrong, C., Wallace, J. J., and Ross, L.: Lymphocytic choriomeningitis. Gray mice, *Mus musculus*, a reservoir for the infection. Public Health Rep 55:1222, 1940.

Blechschmidt, M., and Thomssen, R.: Electron-microscopic identification of infectious particles of lymphocytic choriomeningitis. Med Microbiol Immunol 162:193, 1976.

Boersma, D. P., Saleh, F., Nakamura, K., and Compans, R. W.: Structure and glycosylation of Tacaribe viral glycoproteins. Virology 123:452, 1982.

Bro-Jørgensen, K.: Characterization of virus-specific antigen in cell culture infected with lymphocytic choriomeningitis virus. Acta path microbiol scand, Sect B 79:466, 1971.

Bruns, M., Cihak, J., Müller, G., and Lehmann-Grube, F.: Lymphocytic choriomeningitis virus. VI. Isolation of a glycoprotein mediating neutralization. Virology 130:247, 1983a.

Bruns, M., Martínez Peralta, L., and Lehmann-Grube, F.: Lymphocytic choriomeningitis virus. III. Structural proteins of the virion. J Gen Virol 64:599, 1983b.

Buchmeier, M. J., Gee, S. R., and Rawls, W. E.: Antigens of Pichinde virus. I. Relationship of soluble antigens derived from infected BHK-21 cells to the structural components of the virion. J Virol 22:175, 1977.

Buchmeier, M. J., and Oldstone, M. B. A.: Identity of the viral protein responsible for serologic cross reactivity among the Tacaribe complex arenaviruses. In Mahy, B. W. J., and Barry, R. D. (eds): Negative Strand Viruses and the Host Cell. London, New York, San Francisco, Academic Press, 1978, p. 91.

Buchmeier, M. J., Welsh, R. M., Dutko, F. J., and Oldstone, M. B. A.: The virology and immunobiology of lymphocytic choriomeningitis virus infection. Adv Immunol 30:275, 1980.

Buckley, S. M., and Casals, J.: Lassa fever, a new virus disease of man from West Africa. III. Isolation and characterization of the virus. Am J Trop Med 19:680, 1970.

Buckley, S. M., and Casals, J.: Pathobiology of Lassa fever. Int Rev Exp Pathol 18:97, 1978.

Calisher, C. H., Tzianabos, T., Lord, R. D., and Coleman, P. H.: Tamiami virus, a new member of the Tacaribe group. Am J Trop Med 19:520, 1970.

Carballal, G., Cossio, P. M., Laguens, R. P., Ponzinibbio, C., Oubiña, J. R., Meckert, P. C., Rabinovich, A., and Arana, R. M.: Junin virus infection of guinea pigs: immunohistochemical and ultrastructural studies of the hemopoietic tissue. J Inf Dis 143:7, 1981.

Casals, J., Buckley, S. M., and Cedeno, R.: Antigenic properties of the arenaviruses. Bull WHO 52:421, 1975.

Clegg, J. C. S., and Lloyd, G.: Structural and cell-associated proteins of Lassa virus. J Gen Virol 64:1127, 1983.

Cole, G. A., and Nathanson, N.: Lymphocytic choriomeningitis. Pathogenesis. Progr Med Virol 18:94, 1974.

Downs, W. G., Anderson, C. R., Spence, L., Aitken, T. H. G., and Greenhall, A. H.: Tacaribe virus, a new agent isolated from *Artibeus* bats and mosquitoes in Trinidad, West Indies. Am J Trop Med 12:640, 1963.

Eddy, G. A., Scott, S. K., Wagner, F. S., and Brand, O. M.: Pathogenesis of Machupo virus infection in primates. Bull WHO 52:517, 1975.

Gangemi, J. D., Rosato, R. R., Connell, E. V., Johnson, E. M., and Eddy, G. A.: Structural polypeptides of Machupo virus. J Gen Virol 41:183, 1978.

Gonzales, J. P., McCormick, J. B., Saluzzo, J. F., Herve, J. P., Georges, A. J., and Johnson, K. M.: An arenavirus isolated from wild-caught rodents (*Praomys* species) in the Central African Republic. Intervirology 19:105, 1983.

Gschwender, H. H., Rutter, G., and Lehmann-Grube, F.: Lymphocytic

choriomeningitis virus. II. Characterization of extractable complement-fixing activity. Med Microbiol Immunol 162:119, 1976.
Gschwender, H. H., Rutter, G., and Popescu, M.: Use of iodinated organic compounds for the density gradient centrifugation of viruses. Arch Virol 49:359, 1975.
Harnish, D. G., Dimock, K., Bishop, D. H. L., and Rawls, W. E.: Gene mapping in Pichinde virus: assignment of viral polypeptides to genomic L and S RNAs. J Virol 46:638, 1983.
Holtermann, O. A., and Majde, J. A.: An apparent histoincompatibility between mice chronically infected with lymphocytic choriomeningitis virus and their uninfected syngeneic counterparts. Transplantation 11:20, 1971.
Hotchin, J.: The biology of lymphocytic choriomeningitis infection: virus-induced immune disease. Cold Spr Harb Symp Quant Biol 27:479, 1962.
Hotchin, J., and Collins, D. N.: Glomerulonephritis and late onset disease of mice following neonatal virus infection. Nature 203:1357, 1964.
Huang, A. S.: Defective interfering viruses. Ann Rev Microbiol 27:101, 1973.
Jahrling, P. B., Hesse, R. A., Eddy, G. A., Johnson, K. M., Callis, R. T., and Stephen, E. L.: Lassa virus infection of rhesus monkeys: pathogenesis and treatment with ribavirin. J Inf Dis 141:580, 1980.
Jahrling, P. B., Smith, S., Hesse, R. A., and Rhoderick, J. B.: Pathogenesis of Lassa virus infection in guinea pigs. Inf Immunity 37:771, 1982.
Johnson, E. D., Monjan, A. A., and Morse, H. C.: Lack of B-cell participation in acute lymphocytic choriomeningitis disease of the central nervous system. Cell Immunol 36:143, 1978.
Johnson, K. M., Taylor, P., Elliott, L. H., and Tomori, O.: Recovery of a Lassa-related arenavirus in Zimbabwe. Am J Trop Med Hyg 30:1291, 1981.
Johnson, K. M., Webb, P. A., and Justines, G.: Biology of Tacaribe-complex viruses. In Lehmann-Grube, F. (ed.): Lymphocytic Choriomeningitis Virus and Other Arenaviruses. Berlin, Heidelberg, New York, Springer-Verlag, 1973, p. 241.
Johnson, K. M., Wiebenga, N. H., Mackenzie, R. B., Kuns, M. L., Tauraso, N. M., Shelokov, A., Webb, P. A., Justines, G., and Beye, H. K.: Virus isolations from human cases of hemorrhagic fever in Bolivia. Proc Soc Exper Biol Med 118:113, 1965.
Justines, G., and Johnson, K. M.: Immune tolerance in *Calomys callosus* infected with Machupo virus. Nature 222:1090, 1969.
Lehmann-Grube, F.: Lymphocytic choriomeningitis virus. In Foster, H. L., Small, J. D., and Fox, J. G. (eds): The Mouse in Biomedical Research, Vol. II, Diseases. New York, London, Paris, San Diego, San Francisco, São Paulo, Sydney, Tokyo, Toronto, Academic Press, 1982, p. 231.
Lehmann-Grube, F., and Löhler, J.: Immunopathologic alterations of lymphatic tissues of mice infected with lymphocytic choriomeningitis virus. II. Pathogenetic mechanism. Lab Invest 44:205, 1981.
Lehmann-Grube, F., Martínez Peralta, L., Bruns, M., and Löhler, J.: Persistent infection of mice with the lymphocytic choriomeningitis virus. Compr Virol 18:43, 1983.
Maetz, H. M., Sellers, C. A., Bailey, W. C., and Hardy, G. E.: Lymphocytic choriomeningitis from pet hamster exposure: a local public health experience. Am J Public Health 66:1082, 1976.
Mannweiler, K., and Lehmann-Grube, F.: Electron microscopy of LCM virus-infected L cells. In Lehmann-Grube, F. (ed.): Lymphocytic Choriomeningitis Virus and Other Arenaviruses. Berlin, Heidelberg, New York, Springer-Verlag, 1973, p. 37.
Matthews, R. E. F.: Classification and nomenclature of viruses. Fourth report of the International Committee on Taxonomy of Viruses. Intervirology 17:1, 1982.
Müller, G., Bruns, M., Martínez Peralta, L., and Lehmann-Grube, F.: Lymphocytic choriomeningitis virus. IV. Electron microscopic investigation of the virion. Arch Virol 75:229, 1983.
Murphy, F. A., and Whitfield, S. G.: Morphology and morphogenesis of arenaviruses. Bull WHO 52:409, 1975.
Oldstone, M. B. A.: Immune responses, immune tolerance, and viruses. Compr Virol 15:1, 1979.
Parodi, A. S., Greenway, D. J., Rugiero, H. R., Rivero, S., Frigerio, M., de la Barrera, J. M., Mettler, N., Garzón, F., Boxaca, M., de Guerrero, L., y Nota, N.: Sobre la etiología del brote epidémico de Junín. Día méd (B.A.) 30:2300, 1958.
Pedersen, I. R.: Structural components and replication of arenaviruses. Adv Virus Res 24:277, 1979.
Pfau, C. J.: The role of defective interfering (DI) virus in arenavirus infections. Medicina (B.A.) 37 Suppl 3:32, 1977.
Pinheiro, F. P., Shope, R. E., Paes de Andrade, A. H., Bensabath, G., Cacios, G. V., and Casals, J.: Amapari, a new virus of the Tacaribe group from rodents and mites of Amapa Territory, Brazil. Proc Soc Exper Biol Med 122:531, 1966.
Pinheiro, F. P., Woodall, J. P., Travassos da Rosa, A. P. A., and Travassos da Rosa, J. F.: Studies on arenaviruses in Brazil. Medicina (B.A.) 37 Suppl 3:175, 1977.
Popescu, M., and Lehmann-Grube, F.: Diversity of lymphocytic choriomeningitis virus: variation due to replication of the virus in the mouse. J Gen Virol 30:113, 1976.
Rawls, W. E., and Leung, W.-C.: Arenaviruses. Compr Virol 14:157, 1979.
Rowe, W. P., Murphy, F. A., Bergold, G. H., Casals, J., Hotchin, J., Johnson, K. M., Lehmann-Grube, F., Mims, C. A., Traub, E., and Webb, P. A.: Arenoviruses: proposed name for a newly defined virus group. J Virol 5:651, 1970.
Rutter, G., and Gschwender, H. H.: Antigenic alteration of cells in vitro infected with LCM virus. In Lehmann-Grube, F. (ed.): Lymphocytic Choriomeningitis Virus and Other Arenaviruses. Berlin, Heidelberg, New York, Springer-Verlag, 1973, p. 51.
Sabattini, M. S., González de Ríos, L. E., Díaz, G., y Vega, V. R.: Infección natural y experimental de roedores con virus Junín. Medicina (B.A.) 37 Suppl 3:149, 1977.
Skinner, H. H., and Knight, E. H.: The potential role of Syrian hamsters and other small animals as reservoirs of lymphocytic choriomeningitis virus. J Small Anim Pract 20:145, 1979.
Smadel, J. E., Green, R. H., Paltauf, R. M., and Gonzales, T. A.: Lymphocytic choriomeningitis: two human fatalities following an unusual febrile illness. Proc Soc Exper Biol Med 49:683, 1942.
Smadel, J. E., and Wall, M. J.: A soluble antigen of lymphocytic choriomeningitis. III. Independence of anti-soluble substance antibodies and neutralizing antibodies, and the rôle of soluble antigen and inactive virus in immunity to infection. J Exp Med 72:389, 1940.
Thomsen, A. R., Bro-Jørgensen, K., and Volkert, M.: Fatal meningitis following lymphocytic choriomeningitis virus infection reflects delayed-type hypersensitivity rather than cytotoxicity. Scand J Immunol 17:139, 1983.
Trapido, H., and Sanmartín, C.: Pichindé virus. A new virus of the Tacaribe group from Colombia. Am J Trop Med 20:631, 1971.
Traub, E.: Epidemiology of lymphocytic choriomeningitis in a mouse stock observed for four years. J Exp Med 69:801, 1939.
Walker, D. H., Johnson, K. M., Lange, J. V., Gardner, J. J., Kiley, M. P., and McCormick, J. B.: Experimental infection of rhesus monkeys with Lassa virus and a closely related arenavirus, Mozambique virus. J Inf Dis 146:360, 1982.
Walker, D. H., Wulff, H., Lange, J. V., and Murphy, F. A.: Comparative pathology of Lassa virus infection in monkeys, guinea-pigs, and *Mastomys natalensis*. Bull WHO 52:523, 1975.
Webb, P. A., Johnson, K. M., Hibbs, J. B., and Kuns, M. L.: Parana, a new Tacaribe complex virus from Paraguay. Arch ges Virusforsch 32:379, 1970.
Webb, P. A., Johnson, K. M., Peters, C. J., and Justines, G.: Behavior of Machupo and Latino viruses in Calomys callosus from two geographic areas of Bolivia. In Lehmann-Grube, F. (ed.): Lymphocytic Choriomeningitis Virus and Other Arenaviruses. Berlin, Heidelberg, New York, Springer-Verlag, 1973, p. 313.
Webb, P. A., Justines, G., and Johnson, K. M.: Infection of wild and laboratory animals with Machupo and Latino viruses. Bull WHO 52:493, 1975.
Weissenbacher, M. C., Coto, C. E., and Calello, M. A.: Cross-protection between Tacaribe complex viruses. Presence of neutralizing antibodies against Junin virus (Argentine hemorrhagic fever) in guinea pigs infected with Tacaribe virus. Intervirology 6:42, 1975/76.
Weissenbacher, M. C., Coto, C. E., Calello, M. A., Rondinone, S. N., Damonte, E. B., and Frigerio, M. J.: Cross-protection in nonhuman primates against Argentine hemorrhagic fever. Infect Immun 35:425, 1982.
Weissenbacher, M. C., de Guerrero, L. B., and Boxaca, M. C.: Experimental biology and pathogenesis of Junin virus infection in animals and man. Bull WHO 52:507, 1975.
Welsh, R. M., Burner, P. A., Holland, J. J., Oldstone, M. B. A., Thompson, H. A., and Villarreal, L. P.: A comparison of biochemical and biological properties of standard and defective lymphocytic choriomeningitis virus. Bull WHO 52:403, 1975.
Wulff, H., Lange, J. V., and Webb, P. A.: Interrelationships among arenaviruses measured by indirect immunofluorescence. Intervirology 9:344, 1978.
Wulff, H., McIntosh, B. M., Hamner, D. B., and Johnson, K. M.: Isolation of an arenavirus closely related to Lassa virus from Mastomys natalensis in south-east Africa. Bull WHO 55:441, 1977.
Young, P. R., and Howard, C. R.: Fine structure analysis of Pinchinde virus nucleocapsids. J Gen Virol 64:833, 1983.
Zinkernagel, R. M., and Doherty, P. C.: MHC-restricted cytotoxic T cells: studies on the biological role of polymorphic major transplantation antigens determining T-cell restriction-specificity, function, and responsiveness. Adv Immunol 27:51, 1979.

68

REOVIRIDAE PATHOGENIC FOR MAN

NEVILLE F. STANLEY, D. SC.

Reoviridae viruses are of interest to molecular biologists because all of them have a double-stranded RNA genome. Because of their great ubiquity in infecting plants, arthropods, and vertebrates, there still exist taxonomic problems that have not yet been resolved owing to paucity of data with some of these viruses. Our concern in this chapter will be with human infections with viruses belonging to three genera within this family: Reovirus, Orbivirus, and Rotavirus. The Plant-insect genera (Phytoreovirus, Fijivirus, and Cytoplasmicpolydrosis) do not infect man. Table 1 sets out some of the better known viruses that have been sufficiently well described to include them in the family, but only those appropriately marked infect humans and will form the basis for discussion in this brief review. A reevaluation of the taxonomic status of Colorado Tick Fever virus is required in view of its possessing 12 genes as opposed to 10.

Most of the orbiviruses and plant-insect viruses replicate in arthropods, whereas there is no evidence to show that reoviruses or rotaviruses replicate in arthropods, although the former have been isolated from mosquitoes (Stanley, 1977).

REOVIRUSES

The properties, comparative biology, pathogenesis, and diagnostic procedures have been described in a number of reviews (Hassan and Cochran, 1966; Stanley, 1967, 1974, 1977; Rosen, 1968) that are useful for further reference. The viruses were originally discovered by isolation in infant mice when they were called *hepatoencephalomyelitis* viruses (Stanley et al., 1953, 1954). Later these agents were named *reoviruses*, which derives from *r*espiratory *e*nteric *o*rphan (Sabin, 1959). The double-stranded RNA core is surrounded by an inner and an outer protein shell. The outer shell has a diameter of between 60 and 75 nm and is icosahedral (5:3:2 symmetry).

ANTIGENIC STRUCTURE. All mammalian strains of reovirus fall into three serotypes, known as 1, 2, and 3. Hemagglutination-inhibition and neutralization tests have been primarily used for this differentiation, although a common antigen is detected by complement-fixation or by immuno-diffusion. It has not been possible to distinguish antigenic differences between human and animal isolates. All three serotypes produce hemagglutinins to erythrocytes of humans and other animals.

SUSCEPTIBLE CELL LINES. All three types produce a distinctive cytopathic effect in many cell lines. Those cells that have been used for isolation or replication studies comprise *Macaca* kidney, *Cercopithecus* kidney, primary human kidney, human amnion, HELA and mouse L, as well as cells from marsupials, dogs, cats, guinea pigs, rabbits, dolphins, calves, and chick embryos (Stanley, 1977). The reovirus cytoplasmic inclusions are recognized in the perinuclear areas by staining or electron microscopy. Persistent infection with some cells has been reported and plaques useful for assays and replication studies have been produced with murine and simian cell lines. The main effects on host cell function are inhibition of DNA and protein synthesis and interferon induction.

CLINICAL DISEASE

Human. The association of any of three serotypes with disease in man is uncertain because of great virus ubiquity and the absence of clinical manifestations after infection. Outbreaks of mild clinical illness, supported by virus isolation, occur mainly in children with respiratory and gastrointestinal tract involvement. Only four fatal cases

Table 1. REOVIRIDAE

Properties of Well-Defined Members

- Capsid of 60–80 nm diameter
- Icosahedral symmetry (with inner and outer capsid)
- Genomes of 10–12 molecules of ds Ma
- Virion contains transcriptase
- Cytoplasmic replication
- Resistant to lipid solvents

Reovirus	***Orbivirus****	***Rotavirus***	***Plant-Inset Viruses****
3 Mammalian†	Many members, including:	Infantile diarrhea†	Several members in at least three genera including:
5 Avian	Bluetongue	Nebraska calf scours	Wound tumor
Simian	African horse sickness	Simian virus SA 11	Rice dwarf
Canine	Colorado tick fever†	EDIM§	Maize rough
	Corriparta	Pig enteritis	Sugarcane gall
	Eubenangee	"O" virus	
	EHD‡	Foal diarrhea	
	Kemerovo†		

*Natural arthropod transmission.
†Infects humans.
‡Epizootic hemorrhagic disease of deer.
§Epizootic diarrhea of infant mice.

have been recorded, and all of these appear to have had a disseminated infection with lesions in brain, heart, lung, or liver (Stanley, 1977).

Animal. Ubiquity of the reoviruses also poses similar difficulties with natural animal infections, although there is little doubt that reovirus 3 produces spontaneous disease in some mouse colonies, and reovirus 2 causes upper respiratory tract infection in laboratory-housed chimpanzees. A considerable amount of useful information has been derived from experimental murine models exploited by Australian workers (Stanley, 1974, 1977). These have developed our knowledge of virus pathogenesis in three areas: reovirus 1—hydrocephalus; reovirus 3—chronic active hepatitis and lymphoma; and reovirus 3—chronic biliary obstruction (Morecki et al., 1982). In addition to mice, experimental infections have been established in rats, guinea pigs, hamsters, rabbits, ferrets, dogs, swine, cattle, and nonhuman primates. Little is known about humoral or cell-mediated immunity in reovirus infections. More recently it has become clear that the pattern of virulence is determined by the three outer capsid proteins and that temperature-sensitive mutants are associated with persistent infection and specific clinicopathologic syndromes (Fields, 1982; Fields and Greene, 1982).

LABORATORY DIAGNOSIS. This is based on the isolation and indentification of the virus by cell cultures or infant mouse inoculation, the detection of the virus or its antigens, the presence of specific cellular changes and/or the development of a specific, significant, serologic response. Standard and detailed techniques have been published (Lennette et al., 1974). When cell cultures are used, primary *Macaca* kidney or human kidney are adequate. Intraperitoneal inoculation of newborn mice is a useful adjunct to cell culture for virus isolation, but the mouse colony should be demonstrated to be free from reovirus. Immunofluorescence and immunoperoxidase techniques have been developed for the detection of reovirus antigens. Serologic diagnosis is not helpful because of the early acquisition of antibody in most populations.

Four serologic tests are currently used for antibody estimation: hemagglutination-inhibition, complement-fixation, neutralization, and immunodiffusion.

EPIDEMIOLOGY. Antibodies to the three serotypes are widely distributed and antibody conversion rates show that infection is acquired early in life (Stanley et al., 1954, 1964; Stanley, 1961, 1967, 1974, 1977; Stanley and Leak, 1963; Rosen, 1968). The virus is usually isolated from the feces of children. Although the three mammalian types of reovirus have been isolated from large numbers of many vertebrates, an even greater ubiquity is indicated by the widespread occurrence of naturally occurring antibody. It would appear that the following, in addition to man, are frequently infected: nonhuman primates, cattle, horses, sheep, dogs, cats, rats, mice, rabbits, hares, guinea pigs, marsupials, reptiles, poultry, wild birds, and bats (Stanley, 1977).

The epidemiologic patterns indicate fecal-oral transmission, but infection via the respiratory tract has yet to be substantiated. It is possible that animal strains infect man and that human strains may infect animals. Their physical properties enable reoviruses to survive in the environment and they may, therefore, contaminate some ecosystems. It has been suggested (Stanley, 1977) that they be used as a virus marker for bird, animal, or human fecal pollution of water. All types have been isolated from stagnant water, river water, or raw sewage, and sometimes in higher concentrations than enteroviruses. The high rate of isolation from raw sewage (34 per cent) does not correlate with the low isolation rate (0.2 per cent) from human feces. Reoviruses may be recovered more consistently from sewage than most other viruses (England, 1972). Other evidence for gross contamination of the environment is the isolation of reoviruses from mosquitoes.

Although reoviruses then are not to be considered as serious producers of human disease, their involvement in congenital virus infection should be considered (Stanley, 1977).

ORBIVIRUSES

Borden et al. (1971) suggested the name *orbivirus* (from *orbis* [L], ring or circle) for a distinctive group of viruses equal in hierarchy to the reoviruses. They may be divided into antigenic subgroups, but do not share a common antigen (see Table 1). Although reoviruses are stable at pH 3.0, orbiviruses are inactivated at this pH. By thin section and negative-stain electron microscopy, Murphy et al. (1971) were able to distinguish orbiviruses from togaviruses and reoviruses. The surface architecture of bluetongue virus suggests that this virus with 32 morphologic units has an icosahedral structure, distinct from reoviruses. The virion is smaller than that of reoviruses and possesses large capsomeres with the appearance of rings. The outer layer covering the inner icosahedral capsid is frequently indistinct (see Fig. 1).

Although most members are transmitted by and multiply in arthropods they frequently cause viremia in the vertebrate hosts. The best known and perhaps the most important of the animal pathogens are bluetongue (20 serotypes) and African horse sickness (9 serotypes). One human pathogen in this subdivision is Colorado tick fever, which is spread to man through the bite of an infected tick. Only one antigenic type is known and an infection usually produces effective long-lasting immunity. With the exception of one fatal case, the disease is benign with headache, ocular pain, muscle and joint pains, lumbar pains, nausea, and vomiting. The pathogenesis is not clearly understood. Leukopenia is common. Patients have a persistent circulating erythrocyte-associated viremia and the disease has been transmitted by blood transfusion. Electron microscopy studies suggest that the virus infects early-stage hematopoietic cells with movement of virus to the circulating blood cells (Emmons et al., 1972).

The major distribution of the human disease confined to North America has followed the distribution of the wood tick, *Dermacentor andersoni*, which is primarily found in Colorado, Oregon, Utah, Idaho, Montana, and Wyoming. Infected rodents act as reservoirs for the immature tick. Recent studies have indicated endemic areas in California, where 205 cases have occurred since 1954. It has been estimated that more than 2000 cases occur annually in Colorado. The virus has also been found in an area where *D. andersoni* is absent. This suggests a maintenance cycle different from the chipmunk-ground squirrel *D. andersoni* cycle. The virus has recently been isolated from Ixodid and Argarid ticks (for further reference see Emmons et al., 1972; Oshiro, et al., 1978).

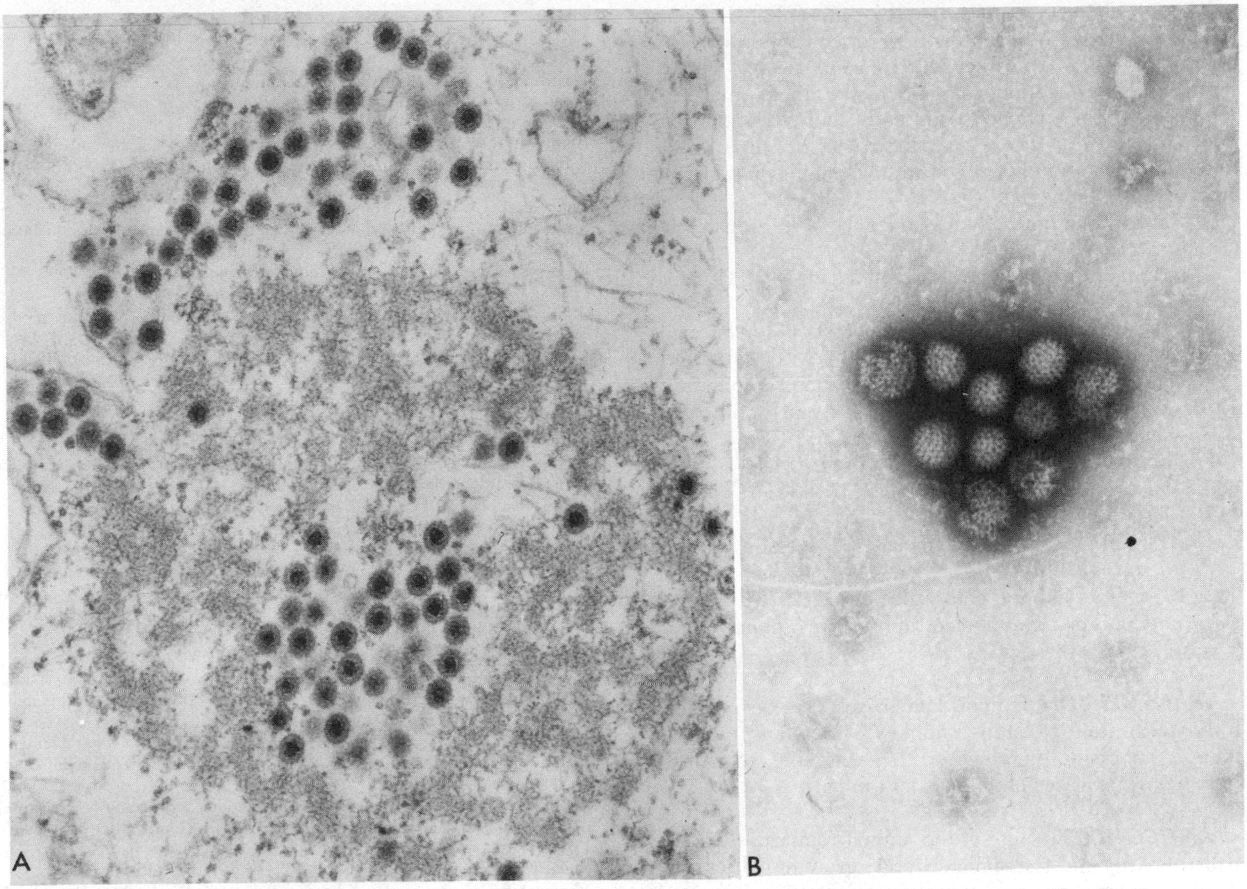

Figure 1. Electron micrographs of bluetongue (an orbivirus) grown in baby hamster kidney cells. (Supplied through the courtesy of Dr. Frederick A. Murphy, Center for Disease Control, Atlanta, Georgia, USA.) (A) × 109,000, (B) × 174,000.

Other orbiviruses that are tick-borne and known to infect humans are in the Kemerovo subgroup (Kemerovo, Tribec and Lipovnik). Kemerovo virus produced an outbreak of encephalitis in the USSR in 1962 (Stanley, 1977).

ROTAVIRUSES

These viruses are the most common cause of infantile enteritis—a disease now known to be widespread throughout the world and usually with a seasonal winter peak. Until agreement has been reached on nomenclature the term *rotavirus* will be used. It is synonymous with *duovirus* used by the Australian workers and some others (Holmes et al., 1975; Davidson et al., 1975). The disease and the virus are currently under extensive study and many of the observations relate to direct electron microscopy of human fecal material. New methods are now being employed and a chapter of this nature will need consistent modification as more precise information becomes available, particularly with the use of antisera against other nonhuman rotaviruses such as calf diarrhea.

CLINICAL AND EPIDEMIOLOGIC CHARACTERISTICS. Vomiting and significant dehydration are consistently associated with rotavirus diarrhea. The highest incidence is in children between the ages of 7 and 24 months. Most hospitalized children present with high fever between the second and fifth days after the diarrhea and vomiting. There may be involvement of the upper respiratory tract. The mean duration of uncomplicated cases is between one and two weeks, but coincident pathogenic enterobacterial infection may increase the severity and extend the time of the disease. The incubation period appears to be about two to three days. There is little doubt about the high winter incidence but no completely satisfactory explanation has yet been offered to explain this epidemiology. This epidemiology is not worldwide, since it is not commonly observed in tropical areas. Although adults associated with children with rotavirus diarrhea are usually not infected (serologic estimate), there have been reports of up to 41 per cent of adult contacts being infected (Kim et al., 1977). Nearly all adult contact infections were subclinical. In an interesting epidemiologic study by Murphy et al. (1977), in an examination of 628 newborn babies in Sydney hospitals in Australia, it was found that 49 per cent had rotavirus in their stools. Although none of the one day neonates were positive, many commenced excreting virus within three or four days after birth. Most of these were symptom free. Since there was no seasonal variation observed, it appears that rotaviruses may persist in some Sydney hospital nurseries and are spread between neonates.

DIAGNOSIS. It is important to differentiate rotavirus infantile diarrhea from enteritis produced by other microorganisms. Although direct electron microscopy, after differential centrifugation, has been the main and initial technique, other effective methods and variations have been introduced. These may be virus or virus antigen detection (by antibody rise) or both. The following methods are currently being explored:

1. Free viral immunofluorescence assay in human stools (Yolken et al., 1977b)
2. Enzyme-linked immunosorbent assay (ELISA) (Yolken et al., 1977a)
3. Fluorescent virus precipitation test (Peterson et al., 1976)
4. Cell culture plus immunofluorescence (Woode et al., 1974; Wyatt et al., 1974, 1976; Banatvala et al., 1975; Albrey and Murphy, 1976; Bryden et al., 1977)
5. Complement-fixation (Kapikian et al., 1975; Tufvesson and Johnsson, 1976a)
6. Electrophoresis:
   a. Immunoelectroosmophoresis (Tufvesson and Johnson, 1976b)
   b. Polyacrylamide gel (Kalica et al., 1976)
   c. Counter-immunoelectrophoresis (Spence et al., 1977)

TRANSMISSION. Human rotaviruses have been successfully transmitted to lambs, monkeys, dogs, and pigs. This is not surprising in view of the antigenic relationship between rotaviruses of animals and infants.

ANTIGENICITY. Some of the animal rotaviruses, notably calf rotavirus and the simian SA 11, grow in cell cultures. These viruses cross-react with human rotavirus by complement-fixation, immunofluorescence, and immuno-electron microscopy. In addition, the rotaviruses derived from pigs and mice (EDIM) also cross-react with the human strains. So far, all known members share a common antigen, but antigenic differences have yet to be explored. As the simian rotavirus (SA 11) replicates easily in primary cell culture it is being examined for use in the serodiagnosis of human infections (Schoub et al., 1977).

MORPHOLOGY. It is impossible to distinguish between rotaviruses from simian, porcine, equine, murine, or human origin by electronmicroscopy. Particles with and without outer capsids have been found in each animal species and their diameter varies between 50 and 68 nm depending on the presence of the outer capsid. When the outer layer is lost the inner capsomeres projecting from the surface give the particles a rough appearance around the edge. Sometimes flattened tubules with hexagonally packed subunits are observed.

For further reading see Flewett et al., 1973; Rodriguez et al., 1977; Middleton, 1977).

References

Albrey, M. B., and Murphy, A. M.: Rotavirus growth in bovine monolayers. Lancet 1:753, 1976.

Banatvala, J. E., Totterdell, B., Chrystie, I. L., and Woode, G. N.: In-vitro detection of human rotaviruses. Lancet 2:821, 1975.

Borden, E. C., Shope, R. E., and Murphy, F. A.: Physicochemical and morphological relationships of some arthropod-borne viruses to bluetongue virus—a new taxonomic group. Physicochemical and serological studies. J. Gen Virol 13:261, 1971.

Bryden, A. S., Davies, H. A., Thouless, M. E., and Flewett, T. H.: Diagnosis of rotavirus infection by cell culture. J Med Microbiol 10:121, 1977.

Davidson, G. P., Bishop, R. F., Townley, R. R. W., Holmes, I. H., and Ruck, B. J.: Importance of a new virus in acute sporadic enteritis in children. Lancet 1:242, 1975.

Emmons, R. W., Oshiro, L. S., Johnson, H. N., and Lennette, E. H.: Intra-erythrocytic location of Colorado tick fever virus. J Gen Virol 17:185, 1972.

England, E.: Concentration of reovirus and adenovirus from sewage and effluents by protamine sulfate (salmine) treatment. Appl Microbiol 24:510, 1972.

Fields, B. N.: Molecular basis of reovirus virulence. Arch Virol 71:95, 1982.

Fields, B. N., and Greene, N. I.: Genetic and molecular mechanisms of viral pathogenesis: implications for prevention and treatment. Nature 300:19, 1982.

Flewett, T. H., Bryden, A. S., and Davies, H. A.: Virus particles in gastroenteritis. Lancet 2:1947, 1973.

Hassan, S. A., and Cochran, K. W.: Teratogenicity of reo and poliovirus in mice. Bact Proc 42:115, 1966.

Holmes, I. H., Ruck, B. J., Bishop, R. F., and Davidson, G. P.: Infantile enteritis viruses: morphogenesis and morphology. J. Virol 16:937, 1975.

Kalica, A. R., Garon, C. F., Wyatt, R. G., Mebus, C. A., van Kirk, D. H., Chanock, R. M., and Kapikian, A. Z.: Differentiation of human and calf reoviruslike agents associated with diarrhea using polyacrylamide gel electrophoresis of RNA. Virology 74:86, 1976.

Kapikian, A. Z., Cline, W. L., Mebus, C. A., Wyatt, R. G., Kalica, A. R., James, H. D., Jr., van Kirk, D., and Chanock, R. M.: New complement-fixation test for the human reovirus-like agent of infantile gastroenteritis. Nebraska calf diarrhea virus used as antigen. Lancet 1:1056, 1975.

Kim, H. W., Brandt, C. D., Kapikian, A. Z., Wyatt, R. G., Arrobio, J. O., Rodriguez, W. J., Chanock, R. M., and Parrott, R. H.: Human reovirus-like agent infection. Occurrence in adult contacts of pediatric patients with gastroenteritis. JAMA 238:404, 1977.

Lennette, E. H., Spaulding, E. H., and Truant, J. P. (eds.): Manual of Clinical Microbiology. 2nd ed. Washington, American Society for Microbiology, 1974.

Middleton, P. J.: Rotavirus: clinical observations and diagnosis of gastroenteritis. In Kurstak, E., and Kurstak, C. (eds.): Comparative Diagnosis of Viral Diseases, vol. 1, Human and Related Viruses, part A. New York, San Francisco, London, Academic Press, 1977, p. 423.

Morecki, R., Glaser, J. H., Cho, S., Balistreri, W. F., and Horwitz, M. S.: Biliary atresia and reovirus type 3 infection. New Engl J Med 307:481, 1982.

Murphy, A. M., Albrey, M. B., and Crewe, E. B.: Rotavirus infections of neonates. Lancet 2:1149, 1977.

Murphy, F. A., Borden, E. C., Shope, R. E., and Harrison, A.: Physicochemical and morphological relationships of some arthropod-borne viruses to bluetongue virus—a new taxonomic group. Electron microscopic studies. J Gen Virol 13:273, 1971.

Oshiro, L. S., Dondero, D. V., Emmons, R. W., and Lennette, E. H.: The development of Colorado tick fever virus within cells of the haemopoietic system. J Gen Virol, 39:73, 1978.

Peterson, M. W., Spendlove, R. S., and Smart, R. A.: Detection of neonatal calf diarrhea virus, infant reovirus-like diarrhea virus, and a coronavirus using the fluorescent virus precipitin test. J Clin Microbiol 3:376, 1976.

Rodriguez, W. J., Kim, H. W., Arrobio, J. O., Brandt, C. D., Chanock, R. M., Kapikian, A. Z., Wyatt, R. G., and Parrott, R. H.: Clinical features of acute gastroenteritis associated with human reovirus-like agent in infants and young children. J Pediat 91:188, 1977.

Rosen, L.: Reoviruses. In Monographs in Virology, 1. Wien, New York, Springer-Verlag, 1968, p. 73.

Sabin, A. B.: Reoviruses. Science 130:1387, 1959.

Schoub, B. D., Lecatsas, G., and Prozesky, O. W.: Antigenic relationship between human and simian rotaviruses. J Med Microbiol 10:1, 1977.

Spence, L., Fauvel, M., Petro, R., and Bloch, S.: Comparison of counter-immunoelectrophoresis and electron microscopy for laboratory diagnosis of human reovirus-like agent-associated infantile gastroenteritis. J Clin Microbiol 5:248, 1977.

Stanley, N. F.: Reovirus—a ubiquitous orphan. Med J Aust 2:815, 1961.

Stanley, N. F.: Reoviruses. Br Med Bull 23:150, 1967.

Stanley, N. F.: The reovirus murine models. In Hotchin, J. (vol. ed.), Melnick, J. L. (ser. ed.): Progress in Medical Virology: Slow Virus Diseases, vol. 18. Basel, Karger, 1974, p. 257.

Stanley, N. F.: Diagnosis of reovirus infections: comparative aspects. In Kurstak, E., and Kurstak, C. (eds.): Comparative Diagnosis of Viral Diseases, vol. 1, Human and Related Viruses, part A. New York, San Francisco, London, Academic Press, 1977, p. 385.

Stanley, N. F., Dorman, D. C., and Ponsford, J.: Studies on the pathogenesis of a hitherto undescribed virus (hepato-encephalomyelitis) producing unusual symptoms in suckling mice. Aust J Exp Biol Med Sci 31:147, 1953.

Stanley, N. F., Dorman, D. C., and Ponsford, J.: Studies on the hepatoencephalomyelitis virus (HEV). Aust J Exp Biol Med Sci 32:543, 1954.

Stanley, N. F., and Leak, P. J.: The serologic epidemiology of reovirus infection with special reference to the Rottnest Island quokka *(Setonix brachyurus)*. Am J Hyg 78:82, 1963.

Stanley, N. F., Leak, P. J., Walters, M. N-I., and Joske, R. A.: Murine infection with reovirus. II. The chronic disease following reovirus type 3 infection. Br J Exp Path 45:142, 1964.

Tufvesson, B., and Johnsson, T.: Occurrence of reo-like calf viruses in young children with acute gastroenteritis. Diagnoses established by electron microscopy and complement fixation, using the reo-like virus as antigen. Acta Path Microbiol Scand(B) 84:22, 1976a.

Tufvesson, B., and Johnsson, T.: Immunoelectroosmophoresis for detection of reo-like virus: methodology and comparison with electron microscopy. Acta Path Microbiol Scand(B) 84:225, 1976b.

Woode, G. N., Bridger, J. C., Hall, G., and Dennis, M. J.: The isolation of a reovirus-like agent associated with diarrhoea in colostrum-deprived calves in Great Britain. Res Vet Sci 16:102, 1974.

Wyatt, G. B., Hocking, B., Bishop, R., and Wyatt, J. L.: Duovirus infection as a cause of infantile gastro-enteritis in Port Moresby. Papua New Guinea Med J 19:134, 1976.

Wyatt, R. G., Kapikian, A. Z., Thornhill, T. S., Sereno, M. M., Kim, H. W., and Chanock, R. M.: In vitro cultivation in human fetal intestinal organ culture of a reovirus-like agent associated with nonbacterial gastroenteritis in infants and children. J Infect Dis 130:523, 1974.

Yolken, R. H., Kim, H. W., Clem, T., Wyatt, R. G., Kalica, A. R., Chanock, R. M., and Kapikian, A. Z.: Enzyme-linked immunosorbent assay (ELISA) for detection of human reovirus-like agent of infantile gastroenteritis. Lancet 2:263, 1977a.

Yolken, R. H., Wyatt, R. G., Kalica, A. R., Kim, H. W., Brandt, C. D., Parrott, R. H., Kapikian, A. Z., and Chanock, R. M.: Use of a free viral immunofluorescence assay to detect human reovirus-like agent in human stools. Infect Immun 16:467, 1977b.

69

RHABDOVIRUS

Bosko Postic, M.D.
Tadeusz J. Wiktor, D.V.M.

The rhabdoviruses are a group of bullet-shaped viruses that infect vertebrates, invertebrates, and plants. An electron micrograph of a rabies virion, a member of the rhabdovirus group, is shown in Figure 1. Most rhabdoviruses measure 180 × 75 nm. Short particles measuring 70 to 100 nm and longer ones measuring up to 400 nm are also seen. Plant rhabdoviruses appear to have a similar conformation but are usually longer and bacilliform in shape.

Out of some twenty animal rhabdoviruses only the vesicular stomatitis virus (VSV) and the rabies virus subgroup are pathogenic for humans and domestic animals. In addition, several rhabdoviruses can cause economically important diseases of fish.

The central helical core of a rhabdovirus consists of a single-stranded RNA genome and various structural proteins forming the nucleocapsid, which is surrounded by a lipid envelope and an outer surface of glycoprotein spikes. Purified rabies virus consists of 22 per cent lipids, 3 per cent carbohydrate, 1 per cent RNA, and 74 per cent protein. Four major polypeptide components of different molecular sizes form the protein moiety of rabies virus; a nucleoprotein, a glycoprotein, and two membrane proteins. Recently, Rose and coworkers (1982) compared the computer-predicted aminoacid sequences of glycoproteins of VSV and rabies virus. They found homology, including the positioning of one glycosylation site. Lipid solvents can inactivate the infectivity of rhabdoviruses.

ANTIGENIC COMPOSITION. By means of virus neutralization, complement fixation, antibody binding, or fluorescent antibody staining rhabdoviruses can be classified into several antigenic groups.

In the VSV group containing some seven known strains, two major serotypes (VSV Indiana and VSV New Jersey) can be distinguished; other strains of VSV are related to major serotypes.

The rabies group contains rabies virus and five other viruses that share antigens with rabies virus. These are the Lagos bat, Mokola, Duvenhage, Obodhiang, and Kotonkan viruses, but only two, the Mokola and Duvenhage viruses, may be associated with human disease.

Two antigens of rabies virus have been obtained in pure form: (1) The glycoprotein induces virus-neutralizing antibody and is therefore important in immunity. Antibody to glycoprotein plus complement can produce lysis of cultured cells infected by rabies virus. (2) Antibody stimulated by the viral nucleocapsid does not neutralize virus or cause lysis, but does fix complement (CF). The CF antibody can identify the intracytoplasmic inclusions known as Negri bodies, which consist mostly of rabies virus ribonucleoprotein.

By means of cross-neutralization, a limited relationship has been detected between rabies, Mokola, and Lagos bat

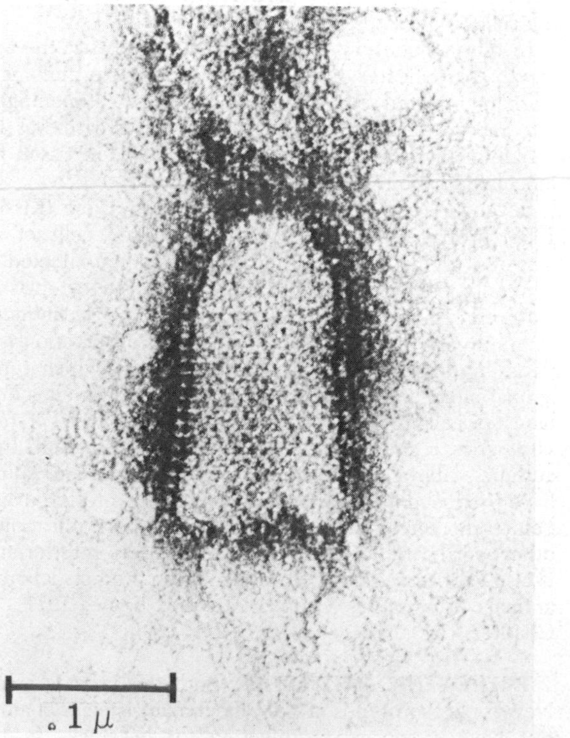

Figure 1. Electron micrograph of a rabies virion.

viruses. In CF tests and fluorescent antibody (FA) assays, there is considerable antigenic similarity between these viruses (Shope et al., 1970). Immunization of mice with Mokola or Lagos virus was not protective against challenge with rabies virus. On the other hand, mice immunized with attenuated rabies virus (high egg passage [HEP], Flury strain) resisted challenge with Lagos bat virus and, to a lesser degree, with Mokola virus (Tignor and Shope, 1972).

Rabies-related viruses, Mokola and Lagos bat, have been little more than biological curiosities. Recently, however, Mokola virus caused a rabies-like epidemic in dogs and cats in Bulawayo, Zimbabwe. Since current rabies vaccines do not protect against Mokola infection, a public health and veterinary threat exists in southeastern Africa, and a vaccine that protects against this virus is now needed.

Seven Mokola virus isolates of the Bulawayo epidemic were analyzed with monoclonal antibodies and cross-protection tests. Monoclonal, neutralizing antibodies against rabies virus glycoprotein were inactive against Mokola strains. Mokola virus was, however, neutralized by monoclonal antibodies produced in mice immunized with the homologous antigen. A potent rabies vaccine, protective against homologous challenge, failed to protect against Mokola infection in mice. No cross-reactivity between Mokola and rabies viruses was seen with cytotoxic T lymphocytes. (Wiktor et al. 1983).

SUSCEPTIBLE HOST CELLS. Vesicular stomatitis virus possesses great virulence for many cell cultures, causing a rapid cytopathic effect that is usually complete by 48 hours after infection. Plaques are also formed in cell cultures of several species. This virus is extremely sensitive to the action of interferon and is used for titration of interferon. Under certain experimental conditions, truncated virus particles are produced. These can interfere with the production of standard VSV particles in vivo and in vitro (see the section on Interference in Chapter 12).

In the last century, Louis Pasteur found that the agent of rabies replicates in the nerve tissue. He and his co-workers injected saliva from rabid dogs submeningeally into rabbits (Pasteur et al., 1884). The disease was then serially transmitted with suspensions of brain tissue from inoculated rabbits.

Seventy years later, Kissling and co-workers (Kissling, 1958) propagated rabies virus in cultured cells of non-nervous origin. A wide variety of cells can be infected, but generally no cytotoxicity is observed. The cytoplasm of cultured cells was shown to contain rabies virus antigen by staining with fluorescent antibody. This observation is the basis for diagnostic tests in tissue culture, which replace animal inoculations (see Chapter 179). A continuous line of hamster cells BH-21, is particularly supportive of rabies virus growth and can be used for plaque formation. In the authors' laboratories, rabies virus-infected cell cultures have produced interferon, and conversely, interferon added before inoculation of virus suppressed its replication. In other words, rabies virus not only induces interferon but is also suppressed by it. Interferon also protects laboratory animals from rabies virus (Postic and Fenje, 1971). (See Chapter 12.)

PATHOGENIC PROPERTIES. Both the Indiana and the New Jersey serotypes of VSV affect many species of animals but have a special predilection for livestock. In these animals vesicular stomatitis is characterized by vesicles on the oral mucosa, especially on the tongue. Vesicles and ulcers may also occur on the udders of cows and mares, and linear necrotic lesions have been observed on the corium and heels of horses and cattle. Over 95 per cent of animals survive the natural infection. The illness in cattle resembles foot-and-mouth disease, but vesicular stomatitis is milder. Both types of VSV can produce illness in man. Most outbreaks occur through professional exposure to animals and are due to the New Jersey serotype. The illness in humans is acute, self-limited, and similar to influenza. Fields and Hawkins (1967) described eight cases of vesicular stomatitis in persons exposed to animals naturally infected with the Indiana serotype. Three of these patients had oral lesions: vesicles on the gum, buccal, and pharyngeal mucosa, or a herpes-like lip lesion. All patients were febrile, and half of them complained of myalgia. Headache, nausea, vomiting, and pharyngitis were also prominent. Recovery occurred in all patients after a course of illness lasting from two to seven days.

Rabies can affect all warm-blooded animals either naturally or experimentally. It is discussed in Chapter 179. Rabies-related viruses were all isolated in Africa. They appear to play some role in human disease. Their pathogenicity for animals is suggested by the sources of isolation. Lagos bat virus was isolated from the pooled brains of an African frugivorous bat. Experimentally, mice, dogs, and monkeys could be infected by the intracerebral route. Negri bodies were not seen in these animals. Mokola virus was isolated from shrews and from two Nigerian patients experiencing a central nervous system infection. One had a fatal poliomyelitis-like disease, and the second patient had a nonfatal febrile illness with convulsions. The pathogenicity of Mokola virus for animals is similar to that of Lagos bat virus. Negri bodies were found in infected animals. Duvenhage virus was isolated in South Africa from the brain of a patient bitten by a bat.

Obodhiang and Kotonkan viruses were isolated from mosquitoes by inoculating homogenized pools into baby mice. According to serologic results, infection by Kotonkan virus may be prevalent in livestock and rodents.

IMMUNITY. The reader is referred to Chapter 179 for the immunologic aspects of rabies.

Antibodies to VSV appear in infected animals in the 1st week after infection. Antibody determinations to the Indiana or New Jersey serotypes are carried out by a plaque neutralization technique using the homologous virus as indicator. Neutralizing antibodies mediate immunity to the homologous virus in experimental infections.

The immunologic relationship of the rabies-related viruses to rabies virus is discussed under Antigenic Composition and in Chapter 179 on Rabies.

LABORATORY DIAGNOSIS. As in all virus diseases, the laboratory methods used for rhabdovirus can be subdivided into: (1) tissue diagnosis (see Chapter 179), (2) virus isolation, and (3) serology.

VSV can be cultured from a variety of samples (serum, vesicle fluid, throat swab) by the intracerebral inoculation of baby mice; since viral replication appears to be brief in humans, most cases are diagnosed serologically by the plaque neutralization test.

Rabies and rabies-related viruses are isolated by the mouse inoculation method from the brains and other tissues of infected animals. Identification of isolates is accomplished by virus neutralization, and vaccination challenge tests. The vaccination challenge appears to be the most discriminating of the conventional tests. The identification of isolates with monoclonal antibodies has obvious diagnostic implications (see Chapter 179 on Rabies).

EPIDEMIOLOGY. VSV has been isolated from a variety of naturally infected animals, mostly livestock. The virus has also been isolated from arthropods, such as *Phlebotomus* sandflies and *Aedes* sp. mosquitoes. The role of these arthropods in transmitting the disease is not clear. A prolonged vesicular stomatitis viremia has not been observed naturally or experimentally in a vertebrate. Thus, an infective blood meal for arthropods is probably not readily available in nature.

In humans VSV infection is most commonly acquired in the virus laboratory. Humans who processed animals from an epizootic have also been infected. The route by which VSV infects man is not known in most instances. Inhalation of aerosol, inoculation into the conjunctiva, and entry through abrasions of the skin are equally plausible portals of entry. Human-to-human transmission of vesicular stomatitis is unlikely.

Rabies is primarily a disease of domestic and wild animals. In areas where animal control programs are not extensively developed, dogs or cats account for most rabid animals and cause most human exposures to rabies. In such areas 90 per cent or more of human cases result from exposure to rabid dogs or cats. Effective domestic animal rabies control programs in these areas reduced sharply the numbers of rabid dogs and cats as illustrated by the decrease in the United States in the period 1950 to 1960 (Fig. 2). In the United States since 1960 the vast majority of cases of animal rabies occurred in wild animals, and most of the human rabies cases were secondary to bites by rabid wild animals. Where no wild animal reservoirs exist, as in the United Kingdom, eradication of dog rabies can eliminate rabies.

The epidemiology of human rabies closely follows the epizootiology of animal rabies. Human rabies has been reported from all continents except Australia and the Antarctic, although most cases occur in countries where control of domestic animal rabies has not been well developed. About 700 rabies deaths are reported each year to the World Health Organization, a number that is probably only a fraction of the actual number of cases. Human rabies is most common in persons under age 15, with about 40 per cent of cases occurring in children age 5 to 14. All age groups are susceptible. Most rabies victims are male, since they are more likely to be in contact with infected animals.

Rabies epidemics in humans follow two patterns. In one, a single rabid dog or wolf may attack and bite several people. In the other type of outbreak, human cases result from an increase of rabies in the domestic or wild animal population. Thus Central and Eastern Europe experienced a threat from rabies "fallout" from a major epizootic of rabies in foxes. The geographic distribution of rabies in wildlife is variable. In the USA, rabies reservoirs are found in wildlife: skunks, foxes, raccoons, and insectivorous bats. In South and Central America, dog and cattle rabies is prevalent; vampire bats there are an important reservoir as well as vectors. In Southeast Asia, dog rabies is enzootic except in Japan and Taiwan, which are rabies-free. European fox rabies has already been noted. North Africa abounds in dog rabies, whereas in sub-Saharan regions other *Canidae* (jackal) and *Felidae* genera also participate in forming the reservoir of enzootic rabies.

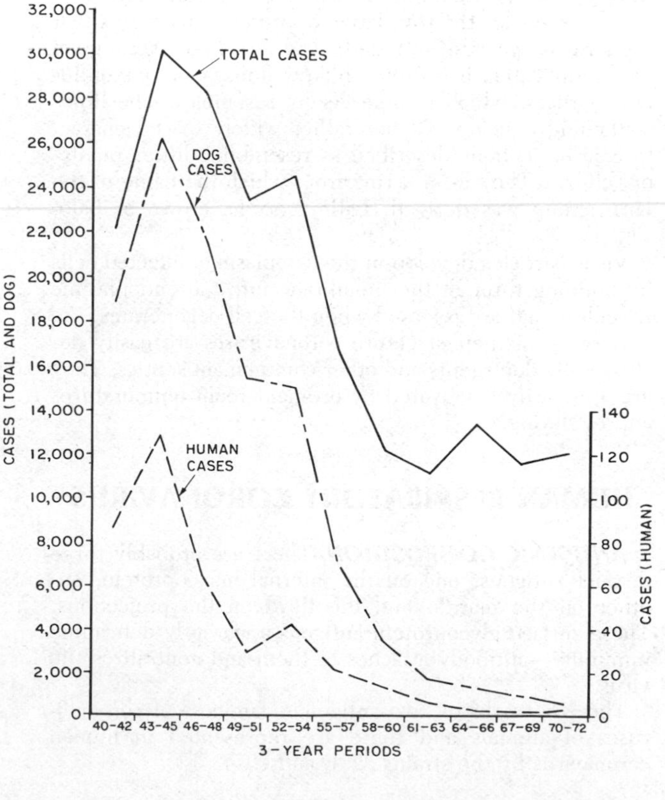

Figure 2. Rabies cases by 3-year periods, United States, 1940–1972. (Source: Wiktor and Hattwick, New York, Academic Press, Rhabdoviruses, *In* Kurstak, E. and C., Comparative diagnosis of viral diseases, Vol. I, Part A, p. 775, 1977.)

The epidemiology of rabies-related viruses is largely unexplored. As noted previously, these viruses only occasionally involve man. Their main medical significance lies in differentiation of them from rabies virus upon isolation from animals, or rarely, a human.

References

Fields, B. N., and Hawkins, K.: Human infection with the virus of vesicular stomatitis during an epizootic. N Engl J Med 277:989, 1967.

Kissling, R. E.: Growth of rabies virus in non-nervous tissue culture. Proc Soc Exp Biol Med 98:223, 1958.

Pasteur, L., Chamberland, M. M., and Roux, E.: Nouvelle communication sur la rage. C. R. Acad Sci (D) (Paris) 98:457, 1884.

Postic, B., and Fenje, P.: Effect of administered interferon on rabies in rabbits. Appl Microb 22:428, 1971.

Rose, J. K., Doolittle, R. F., Anilionis, A., Curtis, P. J., and Wunner, W. H.: Homology between the glycoproteins of vesicular stomatitis virus and rabies virus. J Virol 43:361, 1982.

Shope, R. E., Murphy, F. A., Harrison, A. K., Causey, O. R., Kemp, G. E., Simpson, D. I. H., and Moore, D. L.: Two African viruses serologically and morphologically related to rabies virus. J Virol 6:690, 1970.

Tignor, G. H., and Shope, R. E.: Vaccination and challenge of mice with viruses of the rabies serogroup. J Infect Dis 125:322, 1972.

Wiktor, T. J., and Hattwick, M. A. W.: Rhabdoviruses: Rabies and rabies related viruses. In Kurstak, E., and Kurstak, C. (eds.): Comparative Diagnosis of Viral Diseases. New York, Academic Press, Inc., 1977.

Wiktor, T. J., MacFarlan, R. I., Foggin, C. M., Koprowski, H.: Antigenic analysis of rabies and Mokola virus from Zimbabwe using monoclonal antibodies. Developments in Biologic Standardization, 1983, in press.

70
CORONAVIRIDAES

D. A. J. Tyrrell

The family of viruses known as the *Coronaviridae* affects primarily various species of animals, but there are also coronaviruses that affect humans and cause mild but frequent diseases. Laboratory diagnosis is usually impossible, but it is important for the physician to know about these organisms so that he may understand better the nature of the disease he encounters clinically.

VIRUS STRUCTURE. The virus particles vary in size and shape but are generally spherical with a diameter of 60 to 200 nm. The internal nucleic acid is RNA, which functions as messenger for the translation of protein; this means that the virus is "positive stranded," and thus in the strategy of its multiplication it is quite unlike influenza and parainfluenza viruses, which it superficially resembles. The lipid-containing envelope carries rather widely spaced characteristic projections described as resembling little "petals" or "clubs". They form a ring from which the name of the virus group was derived (Latin, *corona*, crown or halo, Fig. 1).

Virus particles develop in the cytoplasm of infected cells by budding through the membrane into the endoplasmic reticulum and are released when the cell degenerates.

Because of their structure coronaviruses are easily destroyed by detergents and other common antiseptics. They are also easily inactivated by ordinary room temperatures and by drying.

HUMAN RESPIRATORY CORONAVIRUS

ANTIGENIC COMPOSITION. There are probably three distinct antigens, one on the internal nucleoprotein, another on the matrix, and the third on the projections. These surface glycoprotein antigens apparently determine immunity—antibody attaches to them and neutralizes the virus.

There seem to be two antigenic "families" of coronaviruses of animals and these are represented in human coronavirus by the strains 229E and OC43.

SUSCEPTIBLE HOST CELLS. The viruses grow in a very limited range of human cells; in fact, many of them were originally isolated only by inoculating them into organ cultures of human fetal trachea or nasal epithelium. Of these viruses, OC43 and OC38, which proved to be identical, were found to produce disease in suckling mice and were then adapted to monkey cells in culture, but this has not been done with other viruses. A number of other coronaviruses have been isolated by inoculating clinical specimens into cultures of human embryo fibroblasts; these viruses have all proved to be antigenically related to the first one cultivated in this way, strain 229E. The virus may cause little obvious damage in organ cultures of respiratory epithelium, but it destroys susceptible strains of fibroblasts.

PATHOGENIC PROPERTIES. As might be expected, the human coronavirus is infectious when inoculated into the upper respiratory tract. After an incubation period of two to five days it produces a disease characterized by profuse nasal discharge, with nasal obstruction and sneezing. Constitutional upset is mild. There is little or no evidence of an effect on the lower respiratory tract, and the illness clears up rapidly and completely. It may be characterized

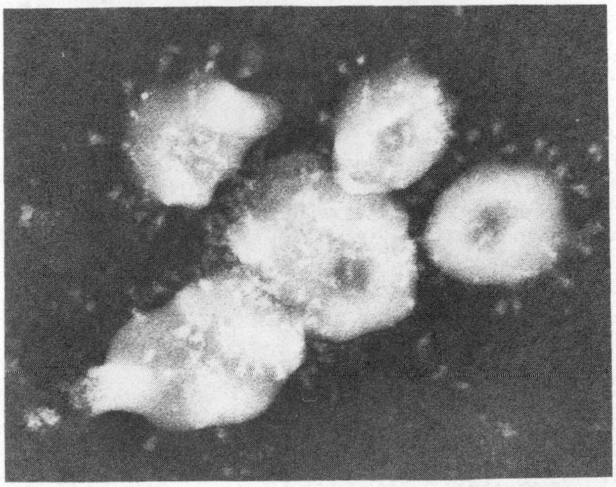

Figure 1. A group of five coronavirus particles visualized by negative contrast electron microscope. The particles are pleomorphic and show the typical surface projections. (Courtesy of Mrs. Heather Davies.)

as a typical streaming cold. In some cases, particularly children, there may be lower respiratory symptoms including wheezing. The virus seems to have no tendency to cause pneumonia or to predispose to bacterial infections but may precipitate exacerbations of chronic respiratory disease.

IMMUNITY. Only about one-third of experimentally inoculated subjects become infected. Circulating and secretory antibodies can be detected but do not completely explain resistance. Cell-mediated immunity has not been studied. Resistance to reinfection may last several years.

LABORATORY DIAGNOSIS. The virus is found in respiratory secretions and can be isolated from nasal or throat swabs or from nasal washings. At present the test is strictly a research procedure and requires special virus-sensitive cells and facilities for organ culture and electron microscopy. Rapid diagnosis by immunofluorescence has been attempted but is not available at the moment.

Infections have been diagnosed by complement fixation tests and by hemagglutination inhibition (OC43 only) on paired sera. Enzyme-linked immunosorbent assay (ELISA) with tissue culture antigens is now available and is more convenient and sensitive.

EPIDEMIOLOGY. Reliable figures are difficult to obtain, but coronaviruses are probably the second most frequent cause of the common cold, after rhinoviruses, and most likely cause about one case in five. They infrequently precipitate attacks of wheezing and asthma in children. They are usually prevalent during the coldest months of the year, January to April, in the northern temperate zones. There appear to be epidemic waves that can be recognized by laboratory tests but not by any distinctive clinical feature of the disease. These waves may affect cities and sometimes a whole country in a short period of time.

Although some of the coronaviruses of animals are related antigenically to those that infect man—mouse hepatitis virus is an example—there is no evidence that the viruses actually cross from one species to another.

HUMAN ENTERIC CORONAVIRUS-LIKE PARTICLES

There are reports of coronavirus-like particles in the feces of patients with or without diarrheal disease, particularly from developing countries. There is no proof that these are indeed virus particles, and if they are, they are unrelated to coronaviruses. However, since coronaviruses cause acute gastrointestinal infections and systemic disease, hepatitis, and nervous system disease in animals, it remains possible that human equivalents of these infections may be discovered one day.

References

ter Meulen, V., Sidell, S., and Wege, H. (ed.): Biochemistry and Biology of Coronaviruses. New York, Plenum Publishing Corporation, 1981.

Tyrrell, D. A. J., et al.: Coronaviridae: a second report, Intervirology 10:321, 1978.

71

MARBURG VIRUS AND EBOLA VIRUS

RUDOLF SIEGERT, M.D.

MARBURG VIRUS

VIRAL STRUCTURE. Like the closely related Ebola virus, Marburg virus exhibits unique morphologic features. Electron microscopy of infected organs and tissue cultures shows cylindrical particles with bizarre shapes, the most frequently found being staffs and long filaments with one rounded end and the other often coiled (Peters et al., 1971; Almeida et al., 1971). In addition, U-shaped, 6-shaped, and annular structures are found (Fig. 1 *A-C*).

The length of Marburg virus is also unusual. According to electron microscope measurements the average length is 665 nm but can be as much as 12,000 nm. The particles consist of a core with helical symmetry and an envelope with surface projections. The membranous material surrounds the inner cylindrical structure, which is considered to be the nucleocapsid.

The physicochemical composition of Marburg virus is largely unknown; from a few indirect tests, it was concluded that the genetic material is RNA. Experiments with lipid solvents and enzymes indicate that the infectious virion contains lipoprotein.

The morphogenesis of the virus takes place in cytoplasmic inclusion bodies in the infected cells. They consist of an aggregation of tubular structures (which may be nucleocapsids). These structures are provided with a coat from the cytoplasmic membrane during a budding process

ANTIGENIC COMPOSITION. Virus-specific antigen has been demonstrated in infected cells by immunofluorescence and immunoelectron microscopy. Infectiousness can be neutralized by specific antisera. A specific antigen for complement fixation has been prepared from infected Vero-cell cultures. It is antigenically distinct from other viruses.

SUSCEPTIBLE CELLS. Many cell-culture systems have been examined for their suitability for growing Marburg virus (Siegert, 1978). Primary monkey kidney cells, Vero cells, human amnion, and guinea pig fibroblasts are most suitable. Although in some cases considerable virus concentrations have been obtained, complete cytopathic effects have developed only in vervet monkey kidney cells after serial passages. In the absence of cell destruction, the propagation of the virus can be recognized by the development of cytoplasmic inclusion bodies as revealed by immunofluorescence (Fig. 2 *A, B*).

PATHOGENIC PROPERTIES. Marburg virus is pantropic. Its pathogenicity depends upon virulence and upon the nature of the host (Siegert, 1978).

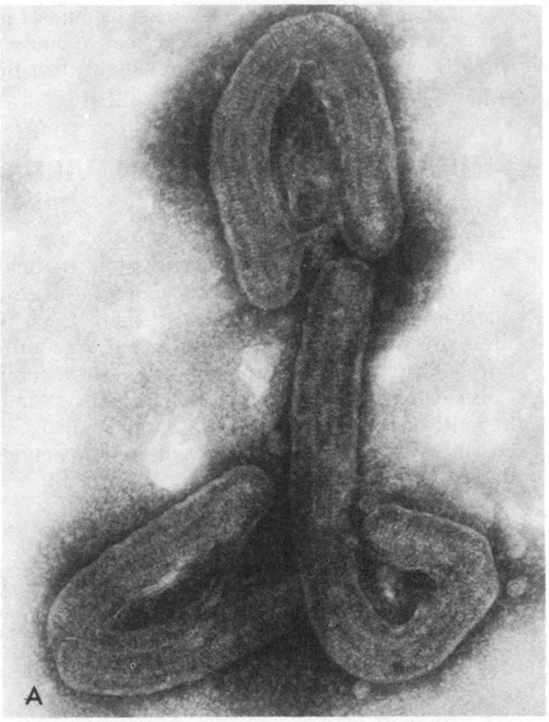

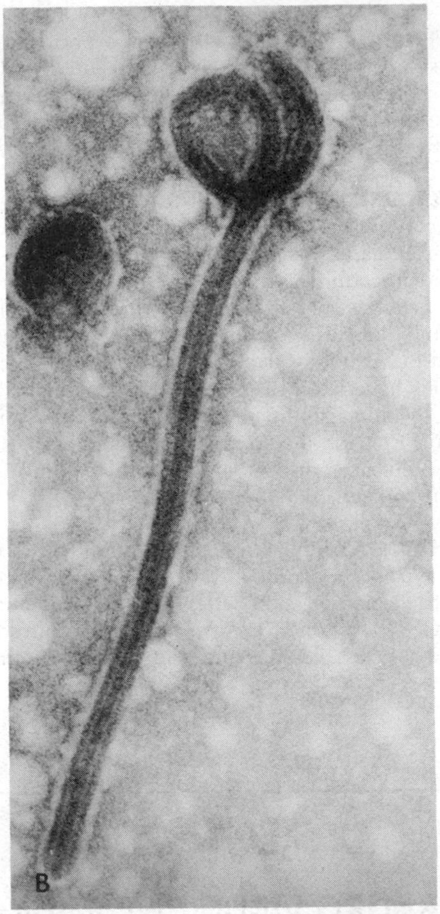

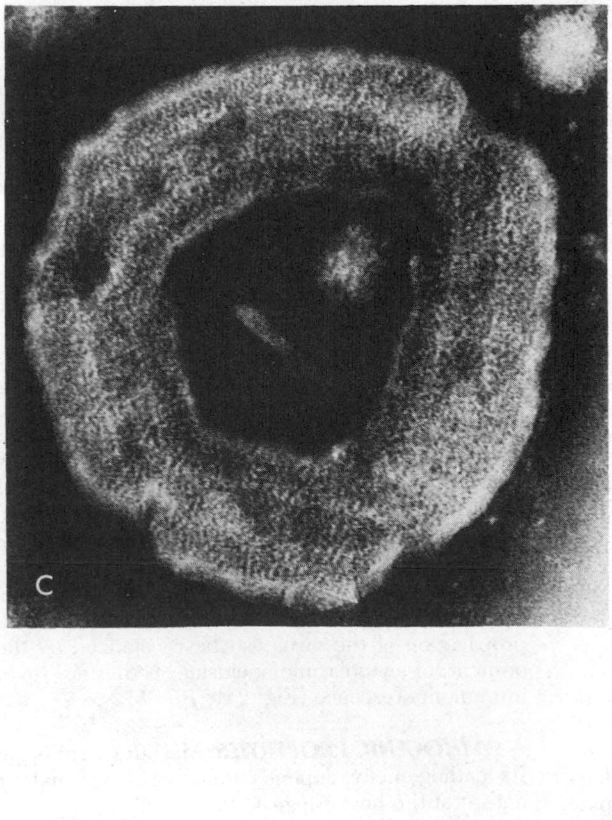

Figure 1. Marburg virus, which has been centrifuged directly onto a grid from guinea pig plasma. Fixed in glutaraldehyde and formaldehyde. Negative contrast. *A,* Three particles—two of normal length and one of longer length. Note membrane, periodicity and central core (× 66,000). *B,* Particularly long particle (about 2 to 4 μm) (× 46,000). *C,* Circular form with visible internal component, fixed in formaldehyde, negative contrast (× 300,000). (*A* and *B* electron micrographs by D. Peters and G. Müller, Hamburg. In Siegert, R.: The Marburg virus (vervet monkey agent). In Heath, R. B., and Waterson, A. P. (eds.): *Modern Trends in Medical Virology.* Vol. II. Butterworth Pub. Inc., 1970, p. 204, London. *C* electron micrograph by Dr. J. D. Almeida, Beckenham, England. In Siegert, R.: Marburgvirus-Krankheit. In Röhrer, H. (ed.): Handbuch der Virusinfektionen bei Tieren, Bd. VI, VEB Gustav Fischer Verlag, Jena 1978, p. 579.)

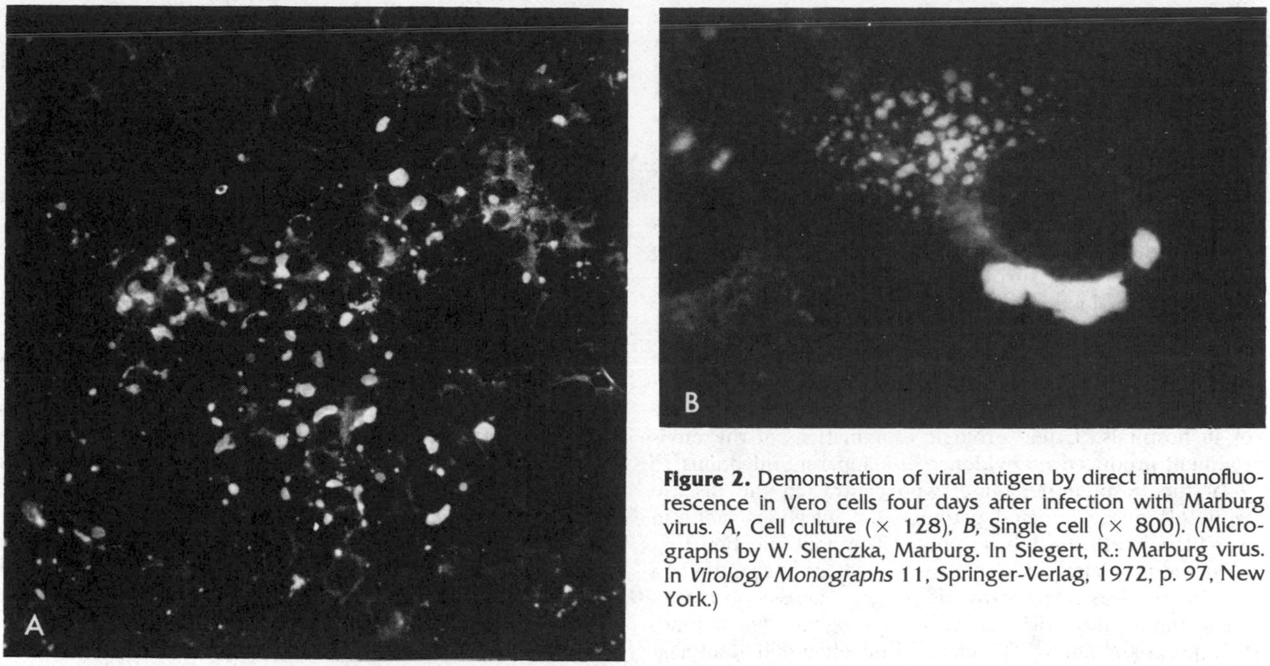

Figure 2. Demonstration of viral antigen by direct immunofluorescence in Vero cells four days after infection with Marburg virus. *A,* Cell culture (× 128), *B,* Single cell (× 800). (Micrographs by W. Slenczka, Marburg. In Siegert, R.: Marburg virus. In *Virology Monographs* 11, Springer-Verlag, 1972, p. 97, New York.)

Experimentally infected monkeys always died, regardless of the virus dose or the route of infection. Observable symptoms are scanty but resemble those found in humans suffering from the same infection (fever, anorexia, petechial exanthema, hemorrhagic diathesis).

Guinea pigs infected intraperitoneally developed fever for several days, as well as certain nonspecific symptoms (anorexia, loss of weight, dyspnea, conjunctivitis). The animals almost always survived the first passage, but after several passages they usually died.

We were able to adapt Marburg virus to hamsters and mice, and we found that newborn animals were more susceptible than adults. In contrast, chick embryos were not susceptible.

IMMUNITY. Infection with Marburg virus induced antibodies in all patients (Slenczka et al., 1970). With indirect immunofluorescence, antibodies could be demonstrated during the second week of the disease. They reached a peak one to two weeks later, then declined slowly, and were clearly demonstrable eight years later. Complement-fixing antibodies developed more slowly and declined faster, so that only very low titers were present two years later. The persistence of the antibodies indicates that immunity is long-lasting. Maternal antibodies transmitted transplacentally disappeared within three months in newborn infants. Nothing is known about cellular immunity during the disease.

LABORATORY DIAGNOSIS. Samples for laboratory examination should be transported in unbreakable plastic containers with screw-on lids. The World Health Organization recommends sending the material to the high-security laboratories (Class III facilities) of the Center for Disease Control in Atlanta, Georgia, or to the Microbiological Research Establishment in Porton, England.

Marburg virus can be demonstrated most reliably in whole blood, serum, and organ specimens obtained during the febrile period (Siegert, 1978). Virus concentrations in throat washes or urine were much lower. In one case the virus was demonstrated in semen, and in another it was found in the anterior chamber of the eye, but all the stool samples were negative.

The high concentrations of virus in the blood and organs in the acute phase of the disease permit rapid demonstration under the electron microscope (Siegert and Slenczka, 1971). Viral particles in serum or plasma can be sedimented directly upon the grid. Their size and shape are sufficiently characteristic to allow a diagnosis. Virus-specific antigen can be demonstrated in autopsy specimens by immunofluorescence.

Virus isolation should always be attempted in case the concentration of virus is too low to be seen by the electron microscope. Vero cells are most suitable for this purpose. Virus multiplication can be recognized a few days after inoculation by the appearance of a virus-specific antigen. Likewise, under an electron microscope, the virus can be demonstrated intracellularly and in the culture fluid. Lassa and yellow fever viruses, which are important for purposes of differential diagnosis, can also be propagated in Vero cells. Antigenic differentiation from Ebola virus is important.

Guinea pigs that become febrile after infection are also suitable for virus isolation. During the febrile phase, the virus can be demonstrated in the serum by electron microscopy and the antigen can be revealed in cell inclusions of organ specimens by immunofluorescence.

For serodiagnosis, blood from the acute and convalescent phases of the disease must be examined in order to detect a decisive rise in the antibody titer. However, the methods of choice are immunofluorescence or radioimmunoassay, owing to its greater sensitivity.

EPIDEMIOLOGY. Only three outbreaks of Marburg virus disease have been reported, with a total of 36 patients. The episodes differed considerably in basic epidemiology. In 1967, 31 persons in Marburg and Frankfurt (Federal Republic of Germany) and in Belgrade (Yugoslavia) became ill almost simultaneously; seven of them died. The epidemiologic situation was puzzling at first, but it was soon noted that the first victims all worked in institutes in which live poliomyelitis vaccines are produced and tested (Hennessen et al., 1968). It was then learned that all the primary cases had had contact with blood and organs of African green or vervet monkeys (*Cercopithecus aethiops*), which had been imported from Uganda by air freight via London. Those persons who ran the greatest risk were individuals involved in the actual surgical removal of organs from the animals. This is not surprising, since the virus concentrations in the blood and tissues of infected monkeys are particularly high and the measures taken to protect the workers were incomplete. The incidence was lower in persons working with cultures of monkey kidney cells. The remaining cases in contact with patients were in the family or in hospitals. Later serologic examinations of the environment produced no evidence of inapparent infections.

In the hospital personnel who contracted the disease while attending infected patients, the infectious medium was blood from the febrile phase. The only infection that occurred in a family was in a woman whose husband was a carrier; she was infected by his semen. There is no reason for assuming the existence of oral, aerogenic, or conjunctival portals of entry. The chain of infection ended after at most two human passages.

A second outbreak of the disease, with only three cases, took place in 1974 in Johannesburg (South Africa) (Gear et al., 1975). The first victim was an Australian who had traveled through Zimbabwe shortly before becoming ill. The woman accompanying him then contracted the disease, and the third case was the nurse who had attended the Australian before his death. During the latter's journey, he had had no direct contact with animals. The third known outbreak of Marburg fever occurred in 1980. The index patient acquired the infection in Western Kenya. It was a French electrician in a sugar factory who died in a hospital of Nairobi. A doctor developed the illness through contact (Smith et al., 1982). There was no further evidence of dissemination of the agent in this area.

In spite of extensive field studies, the natural reservoir of the virus has not yet been ascertained. Its presence in Uganda, Zimbabwe and Kenya indicates that it is more widespread in East Africa than was originally assumed. It is probable that monkeys, like humans, were only coincidental hosts. Although Marburg virus has been propagated in intrathoracically inoculated *Aedes aegypti* mosquitoes, no attempt has yet been made to transmit the virus from infected mosquitoes.

EBOLA VIRUS

VIRAL STRUCTURE. Ebola virus was isolated in 1976, following an epidemic of hemorrhagic fever in central Africa; it is named after a river in Zaire. In size, shape, and ultrastructure the virus is strikingly analogous to Marburg virus (Bowen et al., 1977; Johnson et al., 1977; Pattyn et al., 1977). Because of their special morphologic position, these two viruses may be considered the first representatives of a new group recently named *Filiviridae* (Kiley et al., 1982).

Biological data as well as oligonucleoside mapping of virion, RNA and an analysis of the structural polypeptides indicate that Ebola viruses from Sudan and from Zaire are different subtypes (Buchmeier et al., 1983). The genetic stability within each of both biotypes is noteworthy.

Ebola virus is constructed of preformed nucleocapsids that develop in the cytoplasm of the host cells and are coated by the plasma membrane during the budding process.

ANTIGENIC COMPOSITION. Antigenic analysis by a sensitive radioimmunoassay showed that the virus strains isolated from Sudan and Zaire were two different serotypes.

SUSCEPTIBLE CELLS. Of the numerous primary and permanent cells of varying origin that have been tested, Vero cells are the most suitable for propagation of Ebola virus. A cytopathic effect develops according to the culture medium used and increases with the number of passages made. The virus can be demonstrated in the cell-culture fluid before the cytopathic effect is apparent. Numerous intracytoplasmic antigen inclusions appear in the infected cells.

PATHOGENIC PROPERTIES. The range of the natural hosts of Ebola virus is not known. As with Marburg virus, monkeys are highly susceptible in experiments. Rhesus (*Macaca mulatta*) and vervet (*Cercopithecus aethiops*) monkeys become ill a few days after intraperitoneal infection, with symptoms of fever, maculopapular rash, diarrhea, and hemorrhages; they die after a short time.

In addition, Ebola virus is pathogenic for guinea pigs, which develop fever for several days but no other striking symptoms. Mortality is low after the first passages. Newborn and suckling mice die after intracerebral or intraperitoneal infection. The Zaire strains are biologically more virulent than those of Sudan for humans and for a variety of mammals.

IMMUNITY. In patients and infected guinea pigs, antibodies were demonstrated by means of indirect immunofluorescence, the complement fixation reaction, the neutralization test and radioimmunoassay. It is still too early to evaluate the persistence of the antibodies. There is no cross-immunity with Marburg virus.

LABORATORY DIAGNOSIS. Diagnostic examinations are based on the same principles as those used for diagnosis of Marburg virus (Emond et al., 1977). In every case, a rapid diagnosis should be attempted, with direct electron microscope demonstration of the virus in serum or plasma during the febrile phase and in ultra-thin sections of autopsy liver tissue. In addition, virus isolation should be attempted in Vero cells and guinea pigs. Zaire agents were much easier to isolate in cell cultures and in suckling mice than Sudan strains. The isolated virus must then be identified by means of serologic methods. Ebola virus was found regularly in serum samples taken during the febrile phase and also in the semen of one patient, but could not be demonstrated in throat washings, urine, or feces.

The method of choice for serodiagnosis is the radioimmunoassay.

EPIDEMIOLOGY. From August to November of 1976 there were epidemics of a hemorrhagic fever with high mortality in the southern Sudan and simultaneously in northern Zaire, around 850 km away. In the Sudanese towns of Nzara and Maridi there were 70 and 229 cases, respectively; of these almost one half died. In Maridi, 76 of 230 hospital employees became ill, and 41 of them died. After transfer of the patients to other hospitals, contact infections occurred in the personnel as well. In Zaire, at least 43 villages within a radius of 50 km around the missionary station at Yambucu were affected; 237 patients were registered, and 211 of them died. Here too there were nosocomial transmissions. In Porton, England, a laboratory technician infected himself accidentally with an injection needle.

The morbidity rates during the two epidemics varied considerably. In the Sudan, the rate was listed as 3.5 to 15.3/1000, and as less than 1 to 8/1000 in Zaire. The number of secondary cases is said to have been approximately 15 per cent in Zaire, whereas in the Sudan there were reports of 13 per cent secondary, 14 per cent tertiary, and 9 per cent quaternary cases. Direct transmissions from man-to-man could be demonstrated through a chain of at least 12 members.

It is still not known how the virus is eliminated from the organism or transmitted. Person-to-person infections require extremely close contact. Exposure was greatest among hospital personnel. In them, contamination with blood and other body fluids played an important part, and transmission was favored by skin and mucous lesions as well as by insufficiently sterilized instruments. Airborne droplet infections appear to play only a minor role, if any.

No arthropods or mammals have been demonstrated to be carriers or hosts. The different subtypes in Zaire and Sudan and the lack of established communications leads to the conclusion that the two epidemics were completely independent events except in time.

References

Marburg Virus

Almeida, J. D., Waterson, A. P., and Simpson D. I. H.: Morphology and morphogenesis of the Marburg agent. In Martini, G. A., and Siegert, R. (eds.): Marburg Virus Disease. New York, Springer Verlag, 1971, p. 84.

Gear, J. S. S., Cassel, G. A., Gear, A. J., Trappler, B., Clausen, L., Meyers, A. M., Kew, M. C., Bothwell, T. H., Sher, R., Miller, G. B., Schneider, J., Koornhof, H. J., Gomperts, E. D., Isaacson, M., and Gear, J. H. S.: Outbreak of Marburg virus disease in Johannesburg. Br Med J. 1:489, 1975.

Hennessen, W., Bonin, O., and Mauler, R.: Zur Epidemiologie der Erkrankung von Menschen durch Affen. Dtsch Med Wochenschr 93:582, 1968.

Peters, D., Müller, G., and Slenczka, W.: Morphology, development, and classification of the Marburg virus. In Martini, G. A., and Siegert, R. (eds.): Marburg Virus Disease. New York, Springer Verlag, 1971, p. 68.

Siegert, R.: Marburgvirus-Krankheit. In Röhrer, H. (ed.): Handbuch der Virusinfektionen bei Tieren, Bd. 6. Jena, Gustav Fischer Verlag, 1978, p. 579.

Siegert, R., and Slenczka, W.: Laboratory diagnosis and pathogenesis. In Martini, G. A., and Siegert, R. (eds.): Marburg Virus Disease. New York, Springer Verlag, 1971, p. 157.

Siegert, R., Shu, H. L., Slenczka, W., Peters, D., and Müller, G.: Zur Ätiologie einer unbekannten, von Affen ausgegangenen menschlichen Infektionskrankheit. Dtsch Med Wochenschr 92: 2341, 1967.

Slenczka, W., Siegert, R., and Wolff, G.: Nachweis komplementbindender Antikörper des Marburg-Virus bei 22 Patienten mit einem Zellkultur-Antigen. Arch Virusforsch 31:71, 1970.

Smith, D. H., Isaacson, M., Johnson, K. M., Bagshaire, A., Johnson, B. K., Siranapoel, R., Kiley, M., Tarap Siongok, Koinange Keruga, H.: Marburg-virus disease in Kenya. Lancet 1:816, 1982.

Ebola Virus

Bowen, E. T. W., Lloyd, G., Harris, W. J., Platt, G. S., Baskerville, A., and Vella, E. E.: Viral haemorrhagic fever in southern Sudan and northern Zaire. Lancet 1:571, 1977.

Buchmeier, M. J., DeFries, R. U., McCormick, J. B., and Kiley, M. P.: Comparative analysis of the structural polypeptides of Ebola viruses from Sudan and Zaire. J Infect Dis 147:276, 1983.

Emond, R. T. D., Evans, B., Bowen, E. T. W., and Lloyd, G.: A case of Ebola virus infection. Br Med J 2:541, 1977.

Johnson, K. M., Lange, J. V., Webb, P. A., and Murphy, F. A.: Isolation and partial characterisation of a new virus causing acute haemorrhagic fever in Zaire. Lancet 1:569, 1977.

Kiley, M. P., Bowen, E. T. W., Eddy, G. A., Isaacson, M., Johnson, K. M., McCormick, J. B., Murphy, F. A., Pattyn, S. R., Peters, D., Prozesky, D. W., Regnery, R. L., Simpson, D. I. H., Slenczka, W., Sureau, P., van der Groen, G., Webb, P. A., and Wulff, H.: Filoviridae: taxonomic home for Marburg and Ebola viruses? Intervirology 18:24, 1982.

Pattyn, S., van der Groen, G., Jacob, W., Piot, P., and Courteille, G.: Isolation of Marburg-like virus from a case of haemorrhagic fever in Zaire. Lancet 1:573, 1977.

HEPATITIS VIRUSES

72
HEPATITIS VIRUSES

SHALOM Z. HIRSCHMAN, M. D.

Many viruses, such as cytomegalovirus, measles virus, Epstein-Barr virus, and yellow fever virus, attack the liver during systemic infection. However, in this chapter we will examine the viruses whose only known organ of tropism is the liver. These viruses are the hepatitis A virus, the agent causing infectious hepatitis (short incubation hepatitis), and the hepatitis B virus, the cause of serum hepatitis (transfusion hepatitis, long incubation hepatitis).

Two classic epidemiologic patterns of transmission of viral hepatitis were recognized early and formed the basis for classification of viral hepatitis into two major clinical types. The more common variety of viral hepatitis, which often involved many people and exhibited a shorter incubation period, was termed infectious hepatitis. Hepatitis following blood transfusions or needle wounds, which had a longer incubation period, was called serum hepatitis. Only recently have the virologic differences between these two types of viral hepatitides been established in the laboratory.

The morphologic, biophysical, and biochemical properties of the newly identified hepatitis A and B viruses will be discussed here. The salient characteristics of the two viruses are summarized in Table 1. Pathogenesis and pathology are covered in Chapter 154.

Table 1. CHARACTERISTICS OF HEPATITIS A AND B VIRUSES

Characteristic	Virus A	Virus B	Virus Non-A, Non-B
Epidemiology	Endemic and epidemic, water-borne and food-borne epidemics	Endemic	Endemic
Transmission	Fecal-oral	Direct inoculation, ? venereal	Direct inoculation ? other
Incubation period	2–7 weeks	4 weeks to 6 months	2–8 weeks
Disease	Acute	Acute and chronic	Acute and chronic
Size of virus	27 nm	42 nm (27 nm core)	?
Coat protein	−	+	?
Nucleic acid	RNA	Open circular DNA (partially single-stranded; molecular weight $\sim 2.1 \times 10^6$)	?
DNA polymerase	−	+	?
Cell culture system	+	−	−
Animal infection	Marmosets, chimpanzees	Chimpanzees Gibbon	Chimpanzees
Chronic carrier	−	+	+
Vaccine	−	Purified coat protein	−
Passive immunity with immune globulin	+	+	?+

HEPATITIS A VIRUS

EPIDEMIOLOGY. Early epidemiologic studies conducted almost three decades ago and studies with stool filtrates fed to human volunteers suggested a fecal-oral route of transmission for the virus causing infectious hepatitis. Indeed, many water- and food-borne outbreaks of disease have been reported. The infection is more common in countries with low standards of living, and in these countries it infects the population at a younger age.

ISOLATION AND DETECTION OF VIRUS. The modern study of hepatitis A virus (HAV) began a decade ago with attempts to transmit this virus to marmosets (*Sanguinus mystax*) (Dienhardt et al., 1967). These studies were brought to practical fruition when strain CR326 of HAV was isolated in Costa Rica from the blood of a child with typical infectious hepatitis by serial passage in marmosets. Neutralizing antibody to CR326 developed in patients with hepatitis A infection. Use of viral antigen (now called hepatitis A antigen [HAAg]) derived from marmoset liver allowed the development of specific complement fixation, immune adherence, and radioimmunoassay tests for detection of antibody, thus providing sensitive serologic tests for viral infection (Krugman et al., 1975). At the same time, the virus was identified by immune electron microscopy in stool extracts of volunteers infected with virus by the oral route (Feinstone et al., 1973). Viral particles found in stool extracts were clumped by antibody present in convalescent serum.

HAV has been purified from human and chimpanzee stool extracts, from infected marmoset and chimpanzee livers, and from bile of infected chimpanzees (Dienstag et al., 1975). The purification techniques have included precipitation by polyethylene glycol (PEG), gel filtration on Sepharose 2B columns, and isopyknic ultracentrifugation on cesium chloride density gradients in sundry combinations (Bradley et al., 1976).

MORPHOLOGY AND BIOCHEMISTRY. The immunoreactive particles have a diameter of 27 nm (Fig. 1) (Provost et al., 1975). Electronmicroscopic observations with positive staining of the particles showed that many particles have a dense core that is presumably composed of nucleoprotein (Fig. 1). The viral particles are clumped by specific antibody (Fig. 2). Infectious virus bands at a density of 1.32 to 1.34 g/ml on cesium chloride density gradients; the sedimentation coefficient is approximately 160S. The infectivity of purified virus is destroyed by heating at 100°C for five minutes but is only partially reduced by heating at 60°C for one hour. Infectivity can be reduced by exposure to ultraviolet light. Purified virus is totally inactivated by treatment with 1:4000 formalin for three days at 37°C. The virus is acid stable. Electronmicroscopic study of marmoset liver showed that the virus was localized in small vesicles in cytoplasm but was absent in the nucleus. Preliminary studies suggested that hepatitis A virus may contain RNA. Acridine orange staining of purified concentrates of CR326 spread on slides gave an orange-red color characteristic of RNA staining, and partial inactivation of viral infectivity, beyond that produced by heat alone, was obtained by reacting the virus with pancreatic RNAse for one hour at 60°C.

Hepatitis A virus has been propagated in primary explant cell cultures of marmoset livers and in a fetal rhesus kidney cell line (Provost and Hilleman, 1979). Four structural viral polypeptides with molecular weights of 34,000; 25,500; 23,000; and 14,000 daltons have been identified (Coulepis

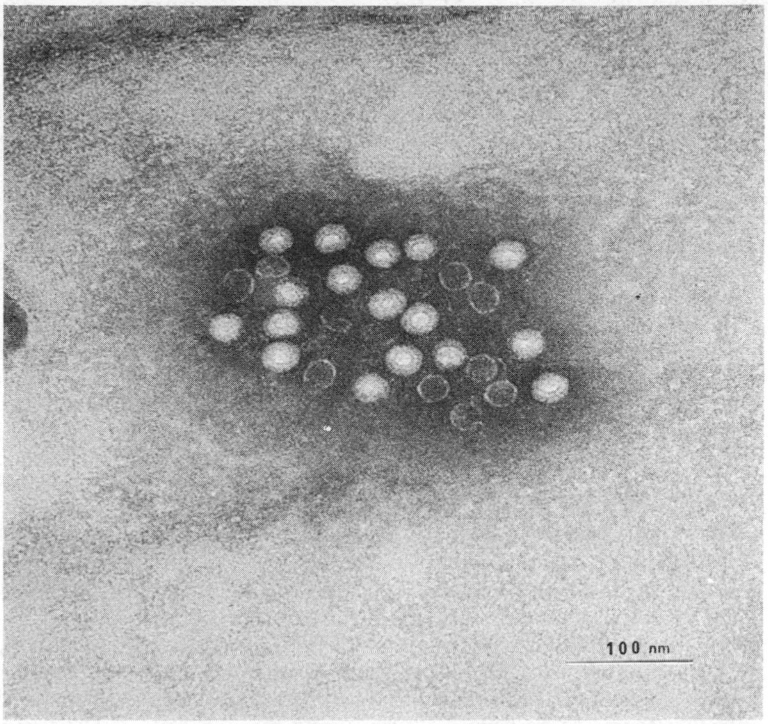

Figure 1. Electron micrograph of HAV particles extracted from HAV-infected marmoset liver showing electron dense cores (× 328,600; Prepared by Mr. E. H. Cook, Jr., and provided by courtesy of Dr. Daniel W. Bradley).

et al., 1980). Single-stranded RNA sedimenting at 35S has been isolated from the virions (Siegl and Frosner, 1978; Coulepis et al., 1981; Ticehurst et al., 1983). These properties of HAV have led to its classification as a member of the genus *Enterovirus* within the family *Picornaviridae*.

ANIMAL TRANSMISSION AND IMMUNITY. Hepatitis A virus has been successfully transmitted to chimpanzees (Pantroglodytes) by fecal extracts from infected patients administered either orally or intravenously. The chimpanzees developed lassitude and anorexia, accompanied by biochemical abnormalities such as elevation of serum glutamic oxaloacetic transaminase (SGOT) within two to five weeks. Viral 27-nm particles appeared in stools during the second week after inoculation and disappeared by the fifth week. Antibody appeared by the third week and remained

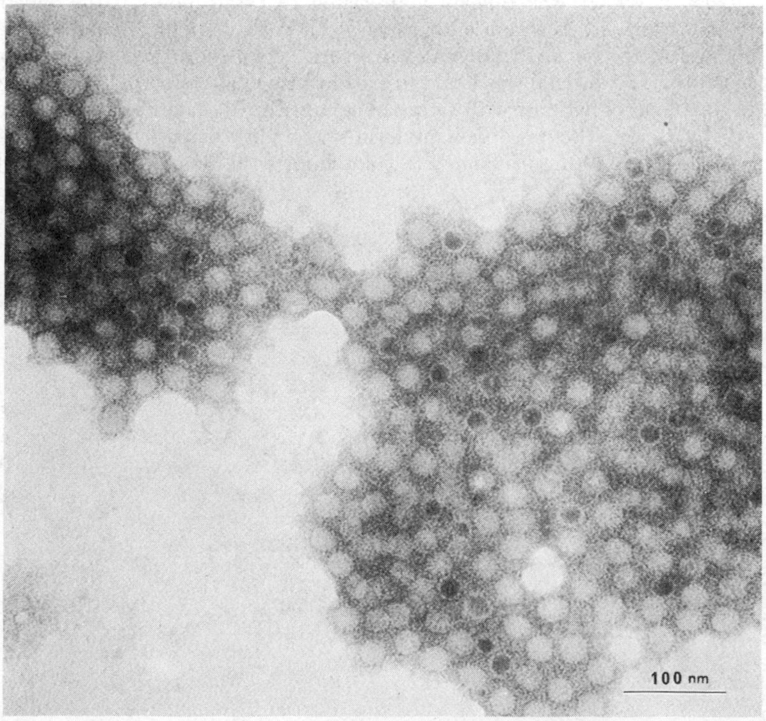

Figure 2. Highly purified HAV from pre-acute phase chimpanzee stool aggregated by anti-HAV (× 256,300; Prepared by Mr. E. H. Cook, Jr., and provided by courtesy of Dr. Daniel W. Bradley).

elevated. Although IgG and IgA immunoglobulins remained unchanged, there was a rise in the level of IgM with the onset of clinical illness. Highly purified HAV derived from extracts of acute phase feces of infected chimpanzees has transmitted typical clinical hepatitis when inoculated into previously uninfected chimpanzees. Thus, it has been established that the 27-nm particles containing HAAg derived from extracts of acute phase feces from both humans and chimpanzees are infectious and provoke a specific antibody response in inoculated chimpanzees. A tissue culture system for propagation of HAV has recently been developed.

Infection with HAV provokes a prolonged antibody response, and immunity appears to be lifelong. Passive protection with immunoglobulin appears both to prevent and ameliorate disease. There is still no vaccine for hepatitis A infection.

HEPATITIS B VIRUS

EPIDEMIOLOGY. A second form of viral hepatitis is associated with blood transfusions or direct needle inoculation and has a rather prolonged incubation period. In Western Europe and North America cases of serum hepatitis usually appear singly. However, in Asia large segments of the population have been found to be infected. Indeed, infection seems to be acquired even during the neonatal period. Mosquitoes can carry the virus, but it has not been established whether mosquitoes are important in transmitting the infection. Bedbugs can also harbor the virus and may possibly transmit disease from person to person in close family quarters.

BIOCHEMISTRY. The first biochemical trace of the hepatitis B virus was discovered when a new antigen was found in the blood of an Australian aborigine. This antigen formed a precipitin line with serum from a patient with hemophilia who had received multiple blood transfusions (Blumberg et al., 1967). It was quickly appreciated that this new antigen, termed Australia antigen (also called SH-antigen and hepatitis-associated antigen), was associated with serum hepatitis. The antigen was found to exist in particulate form in the blood of patients with serum hepatitis (Fig. 3) (Bayer et al., 1968). The predominant form was a disk-shaped particle 18 to 20 nm in diameter. Tube forms with diameters of 20 nm and lengths of 50 to 500 nm, and showing cross-striations with a periodicity of 3 nm also were observed in sera from most patients. A larger particle 40 to 42 nm in diameter, with a double shell and an inner core resembling a viral nucleoid, was also found in sera of patients with antigenemia (Dane et al., 1970). It was suggested that the larger particles represented the complete virion and that the other morphologic forms were excess coat protein. This suggestion was given experimental foundation when the internal component of the larger particle, also called the Dane particle, was released by treating the particles with 0.5 per cent Tween-80 (polysorbate) in phosphate-buffered saline (PBS) (Almeida et al., 1971). The internal component had a diameter of 27 nm and seemed to be morphologically identical to particles found in the nuclei of hepatocytes of patients with serum hepatitis. Thus, the coat protein of the Dane particle was called hepatitis B surface antigen (HBsAg), and the core particle was called hepatitis B core antigen (HBcAg). The long tube forms of HBsAg could be converted to the disk forms by exposure to mildly acidic buffers. Antibody directed against the internal component of the Dane particle, which was different from antibody to HBsAg, was found during acute attacks of hepatitis.

DNA polymerase is present in preparations of hepatitis B antigen containing Dane particles. The enzyme is associated with the core of the Dane particle. The core of the Dane particle contains covalently closed, open circular, mainly double-stranded DNA (Robinson et al., 1974, Summers et al., 1975; Delius et al., 1983), but has single-stranded regions comprising 30 to 60 per cent of the nucleotides, of molecular weight of 2.1×10^6 (Fig. 4). The base composition of this DNA is approximately 49 per cent guanosine plus cytosine. In the test tube, the DNA polymerase appears to function as a repair enzyme for the region of single-stranded DNA. Much information on the biology of the hepatitis B virus has been gleaned by cloning the viral genome (Tiollais et al., 1981).

Two populations of Dane particles can be identified in the electron microscope by using positive stains. One population, usually the minor one, shows densely staining cores, whereas the other population, usually the major one, shows lightly staining cores. The densely staining population of Dane particles contains very high DNA polymerase activity, while much less enzyme activity is found in the lightly staining particles. The densely staining

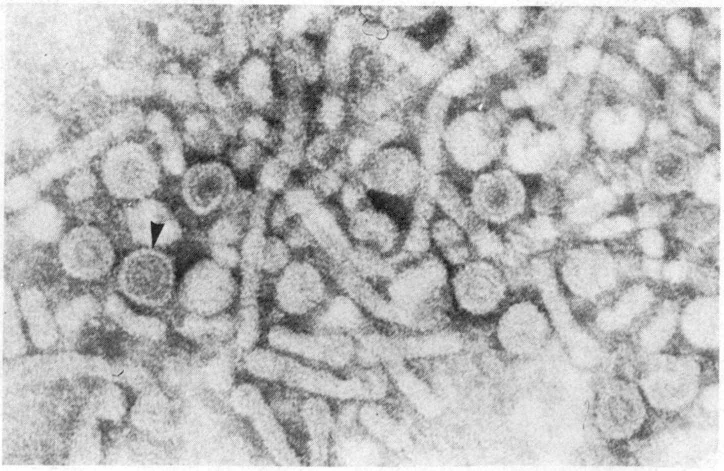

Figure 3. Electron micrograph of particulate Australia antigen (hepatis B surface antigen) showing 18 to 20 nm discs, long tubular forms and 42 nm Dane particles (arrow) (× 250,000; electron micrograph taken by Dr. Michael Gerber).

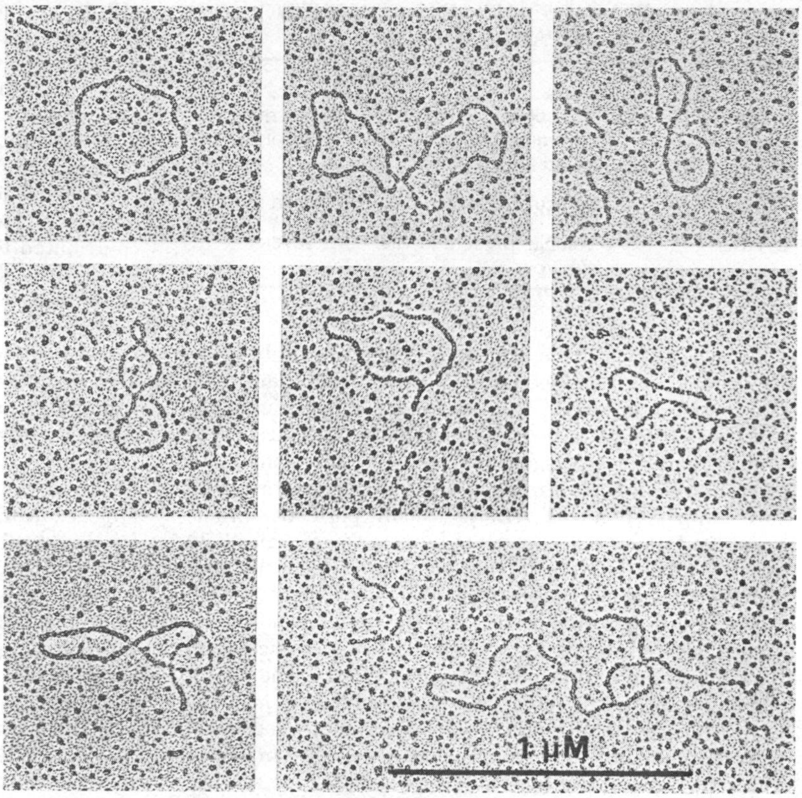

Figure 4. Electron micrograph of DNA extracted from Dane particles purified from human plasma showing open circles. (Provided by courtesy of Dr. Lacy R. Overby.)

particles sediment faster in sucrose. Core particles isolated from the heavier Dane particles band at densities of 1.36 to 1.34 gm/ml in cesium chloride, while core particles from the lighter Dane particles band at 1.33 to 1.30 gm/ml. It has been suggested that the densely staining core particles are complete, containing a full complement of both DNA and DNA polymerase, while the lightly staining core particles may not contain DNA. Core particles of density 1.30 to 1.32 gm/ml have been isolated from purified nuclei of hepatocytes infected by HBV (Fig. 5); although they contained linear double-stranded DNA, these particles did not show DNA polymerase activity. Core particles with DNA polymerase activity have been isolated from total

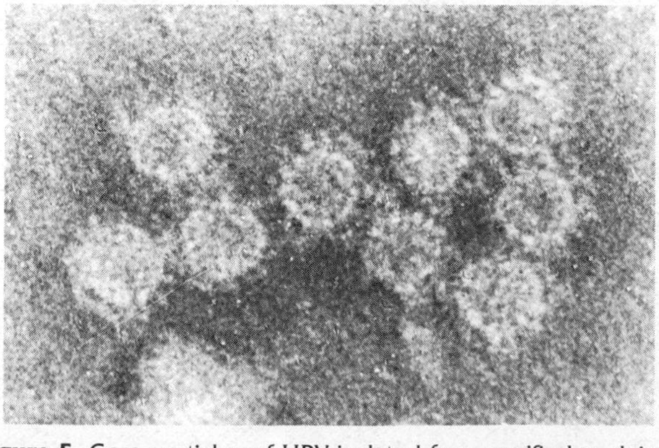

Figure 5. Core particles of HBV isolated from purified nuclei of infected human liver. The diameter of the core particle is 27 nm and the particle contains HBcAg (× 286,000; electron micrograph taken by Dr. Michael Gerber).

homogenates of both human and chimpanzee liver infected with HBV.

The core particle-associated DNA polymerase is active in very high concentrations of both salts of monovalent cations and magnesium chloride in which other known bacterial, mammalian, and viral DNA polymerases are inhibited (Hirschman and Garfinkel, 1977). This singular property of the core particle DNA polymerase forms the basis for a differential assay of the hepatitis B enzyme in reaction mixtures with ≥0.4 M KCl and ≥0.04 M $MgCl_2$. Hepatitis B DNA polymerase is inhibited by $MnCl_2$ and most other divalent cations. Nonionic detergents such as Nonidet P-40 enhance the DNA polymerase reaction of Dane particles, perhaps by removing the coat of HBsAg, thus allowing freer access of precursor deoxyribonucleotides to the viral core. The activity of core particle-associated DNA polymerase increases with rising concentrations of both salts of monovalent cations and $MgCl_2$. Hepatitis B DNA polymerase is not activated by linear or circular single- or double-stranded exogenous DNAs, suggesting specificity of the enzyme for its own DNA or inability of the exogenous templates to reach the active site of the enzyme.

Particles 27 nm in diameter containing HBcAg have been purified from infected human and chimpanzee liver. Double-stranded DNA has been isolated from these particles. Hepatitis B DNA appears to be integrated into the nuclear DNA of infected liver cells, especially in chronic infections.

A soluble antigen, called e antigen (HBeAg), is also found in sera of patients with hepatitis B virus infection. The antigen appears during acute infection and then usually disappears, but can be carried chronically in patients with chronic hepatitis B antigenemia and chronic hepatitis. The

Table 2. MAJOR ANTIGENS COMPRISING HEPATITIS B VIRUS

Antigen	Characteristic
Surface; HBsAg	Particulate; viral coat protein; has major and minor antigenic subdeterminants; found in cytoplasm
Core; HBcAg	Particulate; viral nucleoid; found in nucleus
e; HBeAg	Soluble; present in viral core; several subtypes

e antigen appears to be a protein of approximately 15 × 10^3 daltons, but the exact nature of this antigen is unknown (Takahashi et al., 1983). At present, three major antigenic subtypes, HBe_1Ag, HBe_2Ag, and HBe_3Ag are recognized. The presence of e antigen appears to be associated with the presence of Dane particles. Along with hepatitis B core antigen, persistence of HBeAg usually portends chronic hepatitis. HBeAg also appears to be a marker for infectivity of HBsAg positive blood. The major component antigens of HBV are summarized in Table 2.

The human hepatitis B virus was the prototype of similar viruses now described in woodchucks, Peking ducks, and Beechey ground squirrels (Summers, 1981). The woodchuck hepatitis virus serves as a model of human infection in that it causes acute and chronic infection in woodchucks with subsequent development of hepatocellular carcinoma. The properties of the hepatitis B-like viruses are summarized in Table 3. The duck hepatitis virus DNA appears to be synthesized by reverse transcription from an RNA intermediate (Summers and Mason, 1982).

The recently described delta agent appears to be an RNA virus that requires HBV as helper virus (Tiollais et al., 1981). Delta RNA is encased by HBsAg coat protein. Infection with delta agent enhances the likelihood that fulminant hepatitis will develop and that chronic hepatitis will be more severe in patients with hepatitis B.

IMMUNOLOGY

Assay of HBAg. The first method used to detect hepatitis B surface antigen in the laboratory was the rather insensitive method of immunodiffusion; this test was followed by the more sensitive counter-immunoelectrophoresis. Newer, more sensitive procedures for detecting HBsAg include the techniques of complement fixation, hemagglutination, and radioimmunoassay. The most commonly used test is radioimmunoassay. Hepatitis B core antigen can be detected both by complement fixation and radioimmunoassay, but the latter is preferred and more widely used. Unfortunately, HBeAg is still determined by immunodiffusion although radioimmunoassays have recently been developed. The wide use of radioimmunoassay, with its greater accuracy in detecting HBsAg, has certainly contributed to the great decrease of transmission of hepatitis B from the blood of commercial donors.

Subtypes of HBsAg. HBsAg contains a common immunologic determinant, a, and several major subdeterminants that are specified by the viral genome (LeBouvier, 1971). The subdeterminants can be detected by the presence of spurs in immunodiffusion tests with various antisera. Eight distinct categories and two of mixed subtype have been recognized (Table 4). These consist of various combinations of the subdeterminants d/y and w/r. The subdeterminants appear to comprise two groups composed of d/y on the one hand and w1, w2, w3, w4, and r on the other. The two mixed subtypes are very rare and may have been due to phenotypic or genotypic mixing of immunologic markers during simultaneous infection with viruses associated with more than one subtype of HBsAg. Several minor antigenic subdeterminants have been described, including q, x, f, p, j, n, and g; g has been found with w2. Antigenic types ayw2 and ayw3 appear to be more common in Africa and the Middle East. The subdeterminant r appears to predominate in the Far East and is very common in Japan. The antigenic type adw2 is common in the United States. In experiments in which chimpanzees were infected with different strains of HBV carrying distinct antigenic determinants it was found that the viral strains breed true with respect to the antigenic determinants. Purified hepatitis B surface antigen appears to share cross-antigenicity with some normal human proteins. Both lipid and carbohydrates are associated with purified HBsAg. The carbohydrate content appears to vary from 3.6 to 6.5 per cent, and antigenic activity is lost after mild periodate oxidation. The lipids associated with HBsAg include phosphatidylcholine, sphingomyelin, lysophosphatidylcholine, and glycosphingolipid.

HBsAg of adw and ayw subtypes appears to differ in both biophysical and biochemical characteristics. The buoyant density of HBsAg in cesium chloride is 1.21 g/cc. The

Table 3. HEPATITIS B-LIKE VIRUSES

Virus Subgroup	Host	Other Experimental Hosts	DNA in Nature Core	Surface Antigens Polypeptides (Daltons)	Disease
Hepatitis B virus	Humans	Chimpanzee Gibbon	Partially single-stranded open circle	29,000 25,000	Acute hepatitis Chronic hepatitis Hepatoma
Woodchuck hepatitis virus	Marmota monax	None	As above	27,000 23,000	As above
Ground squirrel hepatitis virus	Spermophilus beecheyi	Tree squirrel	As above	27,000 23,000	?
Duck hepatitis B virus	Peking and other ducks	None	Mainly double-stranded open circle	?	?

Table 4. ANTIGENIC SUBDETERMINANTS OF HEPATITIS B SURFACE ANTIGEN

Major	Minor
aywl	q
ayw2	x
ayw3	f
ayw4	t
ayr	j
adw2	n
adw4	g
adr	
adwy	
adyr	

molecular weight of adw preparations of HBsAg is 3.7×10^6. HBsAg of ayw subtype has an average molecular weight of 4.6×10^6. The acidic isoelectric point (pI) of HBsAg is due to a high proportion of acidic amino acid residues relative to basic amino acids. HBsAg contains high levels of cysteine, proline, leucine, and phenylalanine. Reduction and alkylation destroy the antigenic activity of HBsAg. Nine separate polypeptides have been found in preparations of the ayw subtype of HBsAg and only seven in the preparations of the adw subtype. The polypeptides appear to vary in antigenic activity. Much less is known about the chemical composition of hepatitis B core antigen, but preliminary studies indicate that this antigen has a much simpler composition than that of the surface antigen.

It is thus evident that HBV is a unique virion that contains not only partly single-stranded circular DNA but also a DNA polymerase. The virus contains many antigens that may not all be coded for by the small DNA in the virus (unless one postulates proteins composed of similar subunits and perhaps also overlapping DNA codons). Much further work will be required to delineate the replicative cycle, especially the role of the curious DNA polymerase, of this fascinating virus in the hepatocyte.

Antibodies to HBAg. After infection with hepatitis B virus, antibodies to HBcAg (anti-HBc) usually appear when liver disease becomes evident. Antibodies to HBsAg (anti-HBs) usually appear during convalescence and coincide with disappearance of circulating HBsAg. Both animal and human studies indicate that anti-HBc tends to decrease gradually and may become undetectable after one to two years. Anti-HBs lasts much longer and indeed may be present throughout life. Antibody to HBsAg seems to bestow immunity to further infection with HBV. In the chronic carrier state, with persistence of HBsAg, a high level of anti-HBc, but not anti-HBs, is usually found in serum. Anti-HBe appears with onset of overt liver disease in acute hepatitis and is considered a good prognostic sign.

Vaccines. The thesis that HBsAg represents excess coat protein of the complete hepatitis B virion led to the conclusion that vaccines of purified HBsAg would be protective but not infectious. Preliminary studies with such vaccines composed of purified HBsAg appeared to bear out this hypothesis (Melnick et al., 1976). An effective commercially produced vaccine for hepatitis B consisting of HBsAg purified from human serum recently became available (Szmuness et al., 1980). In attempts to avoid possible cross-reactions of HBsAg vaccines with normal human proteins and to ensure safety, much effort is being expended on the study of protein subunit vaccines and vaccines based on HBsAg synthesized by recombinant DNA techniques. Small antigenic peptides have been purified from HBsAg.

OTHER HEPATITIS VIRUSES

Evidence has been accumulating from epidemiologic studies that there may be at least two hitherto unrecognized viral agents causing acute hepatitis. The first such evidence came from epidemiologic and serologic studies of transfusion-associated hepatitis. In these studies it was found that half of the cases that occurred following transfusion were not due to either hepatitis A or B virus and were not caused by other recognizable viral agents such as Epstein-Barr virus or cytomegalovirus. Similar evidence for the presence of other hepatitis viruses has been deduced from a study of patients with multiple attacks of acute viral hepatitis. Some of the patients had four attacks of acute hepatitis, two of which could be accounted for by hepatitis A and hepatitis B infection. Thus it was presumed that the other two attacks may have been caused by other hitherto unrecognized hepatitis viruses. Now that infections of HAV and HBV can be determined serologically, much evidence is accumulating that non-A, non-B hepatitis is a prevalent infection (Feinstone et al., 1975; Prince, 1983). Non-A, Non-B infection is now the most common hepatitis transmitted by blood transfusion.

References

Almeida, J. D., Rubinstein, D., and Stott, E. J.: New antigen-antibody system in Australia-antigen-positive hepatitis. Lancet 2:1225, 1971.

Barker, L. F., Chisari, F. V., McGrath, P. P., Dalgard, D. W., Kirschstein, R. L., Almeida, J. D., Edgington, T. S., Sharp, D. G., and Peterson, M. R.: Transmission of type B viral hepatitis to chimpanzees. J Infect Dis 127:648, 1973.

Bayer, M. E., Blumberg, B. S., and Werner, B.: Particles associated with Australia antigen in the sera of patients with leukemia, Down's syndrome and hepatitis. Nature 318:1057, 1968.

Blumberg, B. S., Gerstley, B. J. S., Hungerford, D. A., London, W. T., and Sutnick, A. I.: A serum antigen (Australia antigen) in Down's syndrome, leukemia and hepatitis. Ann Int Med 66:924, 1967.

Bradley, D. W., Hollinger, F. B., Hornbeck, C. L., and Maynard, J. E.: Isolation and characterization of hepatitis A virus. Am J Clin Pathol 65:876, 1976.

Coulepis, A. G., Locarnini, S. A., and Gust, I. D.: Iodination of hepatitis A virus reveals a fourth structural polypeptide. J Virol 35:572, 1980.

Coulepis, A. G., Tannock, G. A., Locarnini, S. A., and Gust, I. D.: Evidence that the genome of hepatitis A virus consists of single-stranded RNA. J Virol 37:473, 1981.

Dane, D. S., Cameron, C. H., and Briggs, M.: Virus-like particles in serum of patients with Australia antigen associated hepatitis. Lancet 1:695, 1970.

Delius, H., Gough, N. M., Cameron, C. H., and Murray, K.: Structure of hepatitis B virus genome. J Virol 47:337, 1983.

Dienhardt, F., Holmes, A. W., Capps, R. B., and Popper, H.: Studies on the transmission of human viral hepatitis to marmoset monkeys. J Exp Med 125:673, 1967.

Dienstag, J. L., Feinstone, S. M., Purcell, R. H., Hoofnagle, J. H., Barker, L. E., London, W. T., Popper, H., Peterson, J. M., and Kapikian, A. Z.: Experimental infection of chimpanzees with hepatitis A virus. J Infect Dis 132:532, 1975.

Feinstone, S. M., Kapikian, A. Z., and Purcell, R. H.: Hepatitis A: Detection by immune electron microscopy of a viruslike antigen associated with acute illness. Science 182:1026, 1973.

Feinstone, S. M., Kapikian, A. Z., Purcell, R. H., Alter, H. J., and Holland, P. V.: Transfusion-associated hepatitis not due to viral hepatitis type A or B. N Engl J Med 292:767, 1975.

Hirschman, S. Z.: Integrator enzyme hypothesis for replication of hepatitis B virus. Lancet 2:436, 1975.

Hirschman, S. Z., and Garfinkel, E.: Ionic requirements of the DNA polymerase associated with serum hepatitis B antigen. J Infect Dis 135:897, 1977.

Krugman, S., Friedman, H., and Lattimer, C.: Viral hepatitis, type A.

Identification by specific complement fixation and immune adherence tests. N Engl J Med 292:1141, 1975.
LeBouvier, G. L.: The heterogeneity of Australia antigen. J Infect Dis 123:671, 1971.
Melnick, J. N., Dreesman, G. R., and Hollinger, F. B.: Approaching the control of viral hepatitis type B. J Infect Dis 133:210, 1976.
Prince, A. M.: Non-A, Non-B hepatitis viruses. Ann Rev Microbiol 37:217, 1983.
Provost, P. J., and Hilleman, M. G.: Propagation of human hepatitis A virus in cell culture in vitro. Proc Soc Exp Biol Med 160:213, 1979.
Provost, P. J., Wolanski, B. S., Miller, W. J., Ittensohn, O. L., McAleer, W. J., and Hilleman, M. R.: Physical, chemical and morphologic dimensions of human hepatitis. A virus strain. Proc Soc Exp Biol Med 148:532, 1975.
Robinson, W. S., Clayton, D. A., and Greenman, R. L.: DNA of a human hepatitis B virus candidate. J Virol 14:384, 1974.
Siegl, G., and Frosner, G. G.: Characterization and classification of viral particles associated with hepatitis A. II. Type and configuration of nucleic acid. J Virol 26:48, 1978.
Summers, J.: Three recently described animal virus models for human hepatitis B virus. Hepatology 1:179, 1981.
Summers, J., and Mason, W. S.: Replication of the genome of a hepatitis B-like virus by reverse transcription of an RNA intermediate. Cell 29:403, 1982.
Summers, J. A., O'Connell, A., and Millman, I. Genome of hepatitis B virus: restriction enzyme cleavage and structure of DNA extracted from Dane particles. Proc Natl Acad Sci USA. 72:4597, 1975.
Szmuness, W., Stevens, C. E., Harley, E. J., Zang, E. A., Oleszko, W. R., William, D. C., Sadovsky, R., Morrison, J. M., and Kellner, A.: Hepatitis B vaccine: demonstration of efficacy in a controlled clinical trial in a high risk population in the United States. N Engl J Med 303:833, 1980.
Takahashi, K., Machida, A., Funatsu, G., Nomura, M., Usuda, S., Aoyagi, S., Tachibana, K., Miyamoto, H., Imai, M., Nakamura, T., Miyakawa, Y., and Mayumi, M.: Immunochemical structure of hepatitis B e antigen in the serum. J Immunol 130: 2903, 1983.
Ticehurst, J. R., Racaniello, V. R., Baroudy, B. M., Baltimore, D., Purcell, R. H., and Feinstone, S. M.: Molecular cloning and characterization of hepatitis A virus cDNA. Proc Natl Acad Sci USA 80:5885, 1983.
Tiollais, P., Charnay, P., and Vyas, G.: Biology of the hepatitis B virus. Science 213:406, 1981.

6. Fungi

73
CRYPTOCOCCUS

Charles E. Davis, M. D.

Cryptococcus neoformans is a round, yeast-like fungus that produces urease and forms a large heteropolysaccharide capsule in infected tissues. It is abundant in the feces of healthy pigeons but occurs throughout the world, even in areas where pigeons are rare or absent. While it is ordinarily a saprophyte, *C. neoformans* is an important cause of fatal meningitis in certain susceptible individuals. It was classified for many years as an asporogenous yeast in the Cryptococcaceae family of the Fungi Imperfecti, but Kwon-Chung (1975) has demonstrated two perfect (sexual) states among different serotypes of *C. neoformans*. The perfect forms, which appear to be related to the rust and smut pathogens of higher plants, have been named *Filobasidiella neoformans* var. neoformans and *F. neoformans* var. bacillospora or gattii (Kwong-Chung et al., 1982, and Vanbreuseghem and Takashio, 1980).

Several other species of encapsulated, round, yeast-like fungi that produce urease also belong to the cryptococcal genus. They look and behave biochemically like *C. neoformans*, except that they grow poorly or not at all at 37°C. This growth limitation probably explains why they cannot cause natural or experimental disease in mammals. Little is known about their activities in the environment, but they are important to the medical mycologist, who must differentiate them from *C. neoformans*.

MORPHOLOGY. Colors of cryptococci are white or creamy and typical of yeasts. They become yellowish or light tan with age. The colonies are entire without pseudomycelia, and convex and mucoid because of the capsular polysaccharide. Colonies that produce abundant capsule on artificial media may flow to the bottom of agar slants. All strains of *C. neoformans* form capsules in mammalian tissue, but some produce little or no capsule on artificial media. Others lose part or all of their capsule on serial passage in culture. Colonies of unencapsulated cryptococci are dry and glabrous.

Individual cryptococci are round and 3.5 to 7 μ in diameter. They are surrounded by a capsule of 1 to 30 μ. Reproduction is accomplished by the formation of one or two daughter cells connected to the parental cell by a narrow isthmus. Buds may break off when quite small and cause considerable variation in the size of these round yeasts. Part of the parental wall is broken by the emerging bud.

The cell wall of *C. neoformans* has at least two layers (Fig. 1): an outer, electron-transparent layer and an inner electron-dense, lamellar layer (Cassone et al., 1974). The capsule is just outside the electron-transparent layer, which contains 20-nm particles (Takeo et al., 1973). These particles, which have not been observed in unencapsulated yeast, are excreted into the capsule when cryptococci are grown in vivo (Fig. 2) and are thought to be involved in assembly and transport of capsular polysaccharide (Takeo et al., 1973).

When *C. neoformans* reproduces, part of the bud wall (the electron-transparent layer) is synthesized in the parental cell wall, while the electron-dense, lamellar wall is a direct continuation of the parental wall. This process breaks up the parental wall, which is repaired by formation of a septum (Fig. 3). Shadomy (1971) has shown clamp connections between the parental and daughter cells in two strains of *C. neoformans*.

The electron-dense wall structure, the rupture of the parental wall by the newly emerging bud, and the presence of clamp connections all support the classification of the cryptococci among the basidiomycetes. In the basidiomycetes, two nuclei of mated cells travel to the newly formed cell by different routes, fuse, and form hyphae that bear a club-shaped structure called a basidium. In cryptococci (Filobasidiella) four post-meiotic nuclei give rise to four long chains of basidiospores. These characteristics were the

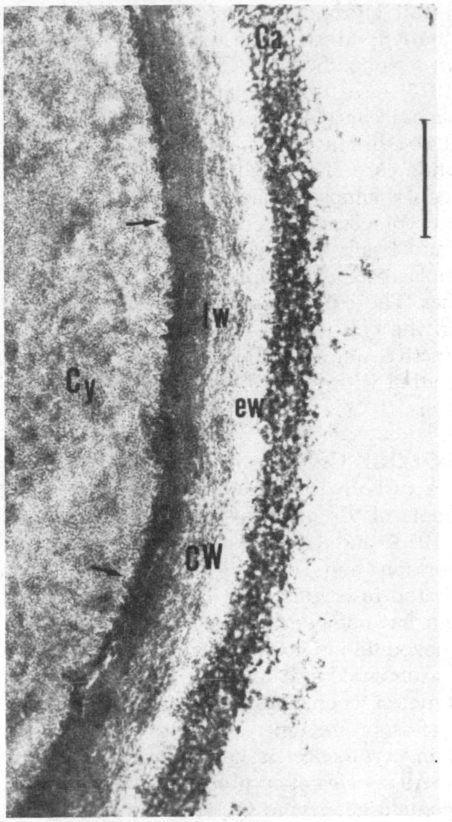

Figure 1. Cell wall of *C. neoformans.* Ca, capsule; CW, cell wall; Cy, cytoplasm; ew, electron-transparent layer; lw, electron-dense lamellar layer. The arrows point to the cytoplasmic membrane. The bar corresponds to 0.2 μ. (From Cassone, A. Simonetti, N., and Strippoli, V.: Arch Microbiol 95:205, 1974.)

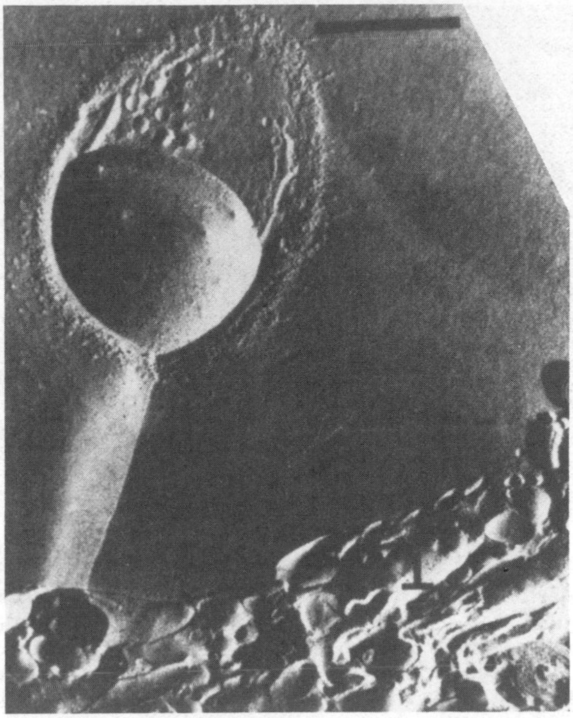

Figure 2. *Cryptococcus* in brain tissue. Wall particles appear to be excreted into inner portion of capsule. Bar corresponds to 1 μm. (From Takeo, K., Ueasaka, I., Uehina, K., and Nishiura, M.: J Bacteriol 113:1449, 1973.)

basis for Kwon-Chung's discovery (1975) that the sexual stage of *C. neoformans* was related to the rust and smut pathogens of plants and strengthened the suspected analogy between the budding of basidiomycetous yeasts and the germination of some fungal spores (Marchant and Smith, 1968). Figure 4 shows the hyphal form of *C. neoformans (Filobasidiella)* with clamp connections and a basidium. Basidiospores (Fig. 5) that are produced from the basidium complete the sexual cycle and become budding yeasts (Erke, 1976). The yeast forms have also been separated into two varieties, *C. neoformans* var. *neoformans* and *C. neoformans* var. *gattii*, depending on the variety of the parental sexual stage.

During the yeast (asexual) cycle, cryptococci do not form germ tubes, chlamydospores, or hyphae, either in vitro or in vivo. Although they are always encapsulated during infection, cryptococci in the environment are often shrunken and unencapsulated. Hyperosmolarity has been shown to be at least one of the factors that suppress capsule formation (Dykstra et al., 1977). There appear to be surface receptors for capsular polysaccharide in the outer wall of *C. neoformans*, since purified capsule adheres to unencapsulated *C. neoformans* but not to other yeasts or to heat-killed *C. neoformans* (Kozel, 1977).

The nonpathogenic species of cryptococci cannot grow at or above 37°C because an apparent imbalance of growth develops between the cytoplasmic contents and the cell wall. Growth of the cell wall is inhibited and bizarre-shaped spheroplasts and protoplasts emerge, probably from the site of bud formation (Dabbagh et al., 1974). These cells lyse almost immediately unless the experiment is carried out in hypertonic media.

ANTIGENIC COMPOSITION. The capsule of *C. neoformans*, which is a polymer of mannose, xylose, and glucuronic acid, can be divided into four serotypes (A, B, C, or D) by agglutination or fluorescent antibody testing with

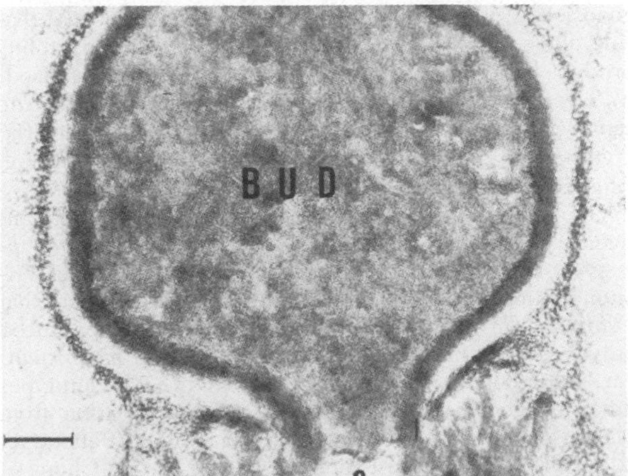

Figure 3. Late cryptococcal bud with septum. Note the broken remnants of the electron-dense layer of the parental wall covered by the electron transparent layer and the capsule. S, septum; bar, 0.2 μ. (From Cassone, A., Simonetti, N., Strippoli, V.: Arch Microbiol 95:205, 1974.)

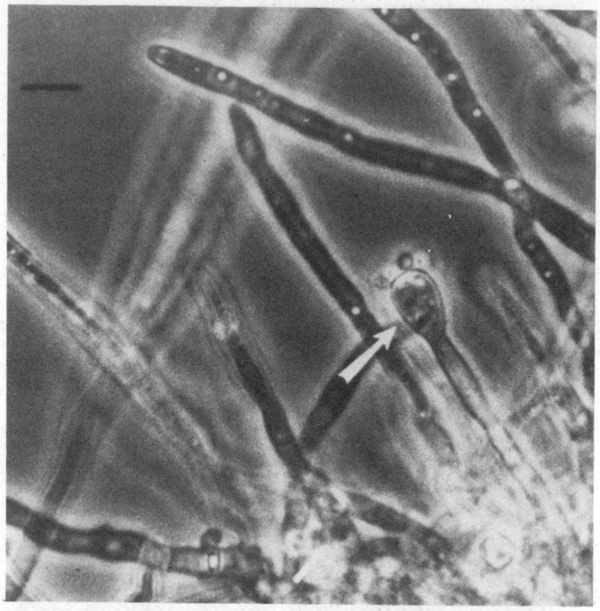

Figure 4. Sexual stage of C. (Filobasidiella) *neoformans.* The arrow points to a basidium with four basidiospores still attached. A clamp connection can be seen four bar lengths to the right; bar length 12 μm. (From Erke, K. H.: J Bacteriol 128:445, 1976.)

hyperimmune sera. The capsular polysaccharide usually elicits only a minimal humoral antibody response in man or experimental animals during infection, possibly because most of the antibody is adsorbed by the abundant capsular polysaccharide in the tissues. During the treatment of cryptococcosis, a good prognosis is associated with falling levels of cryptococcal polysaccharide in the serum; these falling levels are sometimes accompanied by rising levels of cryptococcal antibody.

Another possible explanation for the poor or absent antibody response to *C. neoformans* is that the capsule inhibits the immune response. Cryptococcal capsular polysaccharide causes immunologic paralysis in mice unless the dose is carefully monitored (Breen et al., 1982). Mice form good levels of antibody if given small doses of polysaccharide along with adjuvants or protein carriers, and rabbits produce high titers of antibody if they are hyperimmunized. Antisera to *C. neoformans* capsule cross-reacts with the capsule of Types 2 and 14 pneumococci. Like bacteria, cryptococci undergo a Quellung reaction (capsular swelling) when suspended in homologous antiserum.

The physicochemical differences responsible for the antigenic variations in the four capsular serotypes are unknown, but this grouping appears to have important taxonomic implications. Kwon-Chung originally found that *Filobasidiella neoformans* var. *neoformans* was produced only by mating Serotype A or D strains, and *F. neoformans* var. gattii only by mating Serotypes B and C. The serotypes differ in geographic distribution, ráte of isolation from pigeon droppings, and biochemical activities (Bennett et al., 1977, 1978). Because later studies by Kwong-Chung et al. (1982) and Schmeding et al. (1981) showed that viable bacillospores could sometimes be produced by crosses between the mating types, it seems reasonable to consider A and D serotypes and B and C serotypes as varieties of the same species.

Because of the prominence of the cryptococcal capsule, the cell-wall glycopeptides of cryptococci have received little attention. Most of the work has been done with *C. laurentii*, a nonpathogenic *Cryptococcus* species. Raizada et al. (1975) have isolated a glycopeptide that consists of three oligosaccharide side chains bound by O-glycosidic linkages to threonyl and seryl residues in a common polypeptide core. The oligosaccharides are α and β linked polymers of mannose, galactose, and xylose. Like *Candida* species, cryptococci also contain glucans in their cell wall (Meyer and Phaff, 1977). *C. neoformans* can be converted to protoplasts or spheroplasts by the action of certain glucanases. These polymers of mannose, glucose, and other sugars in the cell wall of cryptococci may be responsible for protective antibody that can be raised in mice by immunization with either live or killed unencapsulated *C. neoformans*.

PHYSIOLOGY. Cryptococci are nonfermentative aerobes that attack carbohydrates and other substrates oxidatively. Components of the electron-transport chain (Yamada and Kondo, 1973) and alpha-keto components of the Krebs cycle (Norkrans and Tumblad-Johannson, 1977) have been demonstrated in cryptococci. The complete electrontransport chain has not been worked out, but detailed studies of the benzoquinone coenzymes (coenzyme Q) have been used as taxonomic keys.

The type of coenzyme (categorized according to the number of isoprene units attached to the benzoquinone nucleus) in cryptococci is homogeneous and differs from *Candida*. All species of cryptococci except one saprophytic variant contain coenzyme Q_{10} (Yamada and Kondo, 1973). This coenzyme generally occurs in urease-positive yeasts with a high guanine plus cytosine content.

C. neoformans can acquire nitrogen from peptones, urea, and creatinine but cannot reduce nitrate. Among the saprophytic species, only *C. albidus* and *C. terreus* can obtain nitrogen from nitrate, but all can utilize peptones and urea as nitrogen sources.

C. neoformans synthesizes phenol oxidases that produce melanin-like pigments from phenols. The color of the

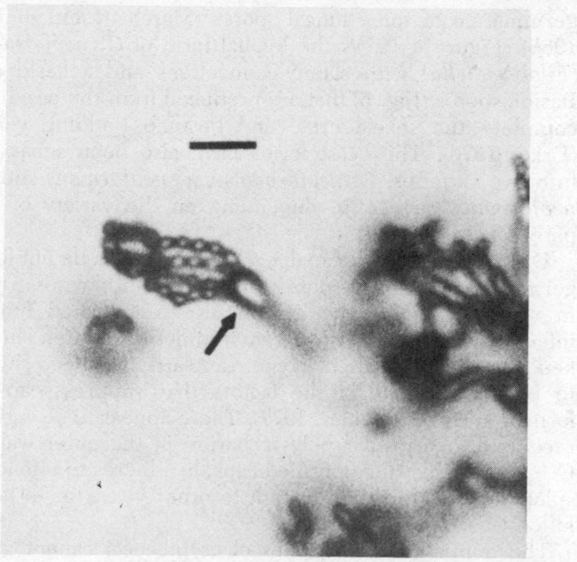

Figure 5. Basidium of *F. neoformans* with four chains of basidiospores. Bar 16 μm. (From Erke, K. H.: J Bacteriol 128:445, 1976.)

pigment depends on the substrate. Staub (1962) found that colonies of *C. neoformans*, but not nonpathogenic cryptococci or *Candida*, were brown if extracts from seeds of *Guizotia abyssinica*, a common weed, were included in the growth medium (nigerseed agar). Caffeic acid is the phenolic compound in *Guizotia* that is converted to a brown, melanin-like pigment. The phenoloxidase activity of *C. neoformans* is located in the cell wall and produces pigment in the colonies that does not diffuse into the medium (Shaw and Kapica, 1972). This observation has led to the production of several selective and differential media that have been useful for the isolation and identification of *C. neoformans*. Other species of cryptococci can produce pigment from certain aminophenol and diaminobenzene compounds, and can be presumptively identified by the substrates from which they produce pigment (Chaskes and Tyndall, 1978).

IMMUNITY. The natural resistance of people to *Cryptococcus neoformans* is so strong that cryptococcosis is sometimes referred to in Europe as "malade signal" because it is frequently a sign of underlying disease. About 50 per cent of patients with cryptococcal meningitis are found to have another disease, most frequently a lymphoid malignancy such as Hodgkin's disease. This association and the persistence of abnormal cell-mediated immunity to the cryptococcus in otherwise normal individuals after successful treatment suggests that cell-mediated immunity is the critical line of defense against cryptococcosis. Skin reactivity, lymphocyte transformation, and production of migratory-inhibition factor often show impaired response to cryptococcal antigens and sometimes to other antigens as well (Graybill and Alford, 1974; Schimpff and Bennett, 1975). Recently, Henderson et al. (1982) have shown that patients who have recovered from cryptococcal meningitis and have no known immunologic abnormality make normal antibody in response to pneumococcal polysaccharide but fail to respond to cryptococcal capsule.

Abnormal phagocytes and humoral reactions have not been definitely linked to susceptibility to cryptococcosis. There is no question, however, that human neutrophils and macrophages can ingest and kill *C. neoformans* in vitro. In pulmonary infections of mice and other experimental animals, neutrophils clear most of the cryptococci from early infiltrates, and monocytes remove the remainder in the later stages. Although human macrophages do not kill *C. neoformans* very efficiently (Diamond and Bennett, 1973), macrophages that have been activated by sensitized lymphocytes appear to make experimental animals resistant to cryptococcosis. The major opsonizing antibody is IgG, but in the presence of lymphokines, macrophages can ingest cryptococci that are coated only with C3b (Griffin, 1981). Delayed hypersensitivity and resistance to infection can be adoptively transferred by T lymphocytes from the animals resistant to *C. neoformans* (Lim et al., 1980), but lymph node cells from animals inoculated with cryptococcal capsule inhibit the afferent limb of delayed hypersensitivity (Murphy et al., 1982).

Nevertheless, two observations suggest that the quantity of the inflammatory response may be more important than the capacity of individual cells to ingest and kill cryptococci. First, many encapsulated cryptococci are probably too large for phagocytes to ingest. Second, there is evidence that white cells can surround cryptococci and kill them by nonphagocytic mechanisms. Whole cryptococci generate C5a from unheated human serum and attract neutrophils and monocytes (Diamond and Erickson, 1982). Monocytes and macrophages may kill cryptococci by release of hydrolases (Kalina et al., 1974); neutrophils, monocytes, and lymphocytes may be cryptococcicidal in the presence of specific antibody (Diamond and Allison, 1976).

Natural humoral substances that inhibit the growth of cryptococci are present in normal serum, saliva, and spinal fluid (Howard and Bolande, 1966; Reiss et al., 1975). Estrogens and other steroids may damage *C. neoformans* and promote phagocytosis (Mohr et al., 1974). There is little evidence that acquired antibody prevents infection. Immunization of mice with an appropriate concentration of capsule plus adjuvant or live unencapsulated cryptococci provides some protection against experimental infection but the mechanism of this resistance is unknown.

It is surprising that the relative importance of the various aspects of immunity against *C. neoformans* have not been defined because it is the only fungus with a definite pathogenic factor. The capsule is essential to the pathogenicity of *C. neoformans*. Stable acapsular mutants of *C. neoformans* that cannot form a capsule do not cause disease. When the capsule of cryptococci is phenotypically lost through manipulation of growth media, the capsule is regained after inoculation because these cryptococci kill mice and have capsules in the tissues (Dykstra et al., 1977). The capsular polysaccharide has so many effects on the immune response that it is hard to determine the most important. It inhibits phagocytosis (Bulmer and Sans, 1968), decomplements serum by activation of the classical and alternative pathway (Diamond and Erickson, 1982 and Macher et al., 1978); and adsorbs or neutralizes opsonins and other protective antibodies. In small concentrations it stimulates antibody synthesis and mixed lymphocyte responses; in high concentrations it inhibits these responses (Breen et al., 1982) and blocks the chemotaxis of neutrophils and monocytes (Diamond and Erickson, 1982). These various effects of the capsule and the numerous immune responses that are activated by experimental cryptococcosis suggest that a normal person has several lines of resistance against the cryptococcus. Nevertheless, the great predilection for cryptococcal infections in patients with the acquired immunodeficiency syndrome and other disorders of cell-mediated immunity implies that this immunologic defense is of critical value in resisting this infection.

C. neoformans probably synthesizes other pathogenic factors. One likely candidate is phenoloxidase, an iron-coating membrane-bound enzyme that catalyzes the oxidation of diphenols to melanin polymers. This property is exploited in certain screening tests for *C. neoformans* (see *Diagnosis* section below). Mutants that have lost the capacity to produce phenoloxidase are less virulent for mice (Kwong-Chung et al., 1982).

Another property of *C. neoformans* that enables it to infect humans and other animals is its ability to grow at 37°C. The other encapsulated cryptococci grow poorly if at all at 37°C and do not cause disease. Rabbits with a body temperature of 39.6°C are much more resistant than mice to infection, and the only recorded infection of a pigeon (body temperature 42°C) was in superficial tissues that were cooler than the core temperature (Ensley et al., 1979). Cryptococci do not grow above 39°C in vitro but survive temperatures up to 44°C. A fascinating and important corollary to these observations is that cryptococcal meningitis does not cause fever.

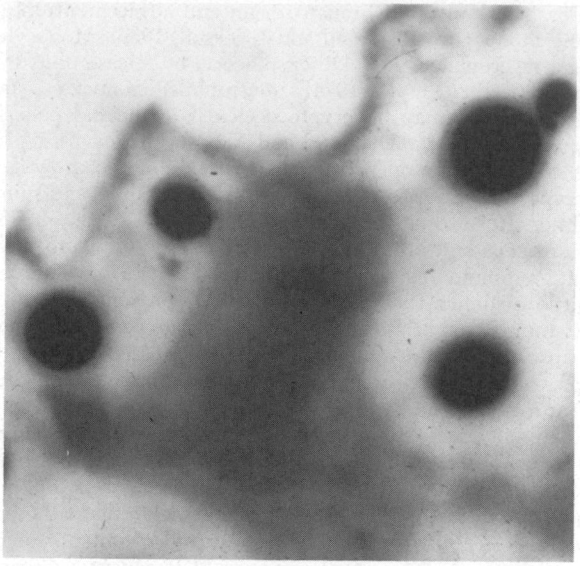

Figure 6. Gram stain of *C. neoformans* in cerebrospinal fluid at × 1000. Note the large capsules in this stain.

LABORATORY DIAGNOSIS. Identification of *C. neoformans* in wet mounts and smears of infected material and cultivation from these specimens are the cornerstones of the diagnosis of cryptococcal infection. This large, round, encapsulated yeast is most easily identified in gram-stained smears of spinal fluid, respiratory secretions, or other infected material. The yeast cell (3.5 to 7.0 μ) retains the crystal violet and is easily differentiated from surrounding leukocytes because of the large (up to 30 μ), lightly safranin-stained capsular halo (Fig. 6). Virtually the entire slide can be examined under × 100 power, and suspicious structures can be visualized in more detail under the oil immersion lens. The India ink preparation, prepared by mixing a few drops of the spinal fluid, spinal fluid sediment, or other specimens with a drop of India ink, is also a popular means of detecting cryptococci (Chapter 167), but there is a danger of confusing lymphocytes, tissue cells, fat droplets, aggregated particles of India ink, or even yeast contaminants of the India ink with cryptococci. If CSF (cerebrospinal fluid) is to be examined by India ink, the presumptive diagnosis of cryptococcosis should not be made without observing the typical small single or double bud and confirming the presence of the organism by Gram stain. Specimens of body fluids may be sedimented by centrifugation at 5,000 g or more before microscopic examination and cultivation, but care must be taken to avoid contamination during the process. Alternatively, a small portion of the fluid can be sedimented for microscopic examination and the remainder cultivated on as many different slants of media as required. Either a portion of the whole fluid or the supernatant from the sedimented fluid should be retained for antigen detection. The larger the volume of spinal fluid cultivated, the greater the chance of isolating the organism, and clinicians should be encouraged to submit as much spinal fluid as possible. We request 15 to 20 ml if the patient does not have increased CSF pressure.

If pulmonary or brain tissue is submitted for culture, impression smears should be made for Gram and special stains and the tissue carefully macerated with a scalpel. Before culture, smears should be made from the macerated tissue, and a portion should be mixed with 1 or 2 ml of 15 per cent potassium hydroxide and incubated at 37° C for 30 minutes before examination as a wet mount with and without India ink. The potassium hydroxide digests cells and artifacts that could be confused with cryptococci.

The histologic examination of tissue should include special stains as well as the routine hematoxylin and eosin stain. Cryptococci can be readily seen on hematoxylin and eosin stain, but the capsule does not stain and can be confused with a space containing a round yeast. Periodic-acid Schiff and Gomori methenamine silver stains are excellent screening stains and often permit visualization of the capsule as an unstained halo surrounding the round budding yeast, but Mayer's mucicarmine technique is the definitive stain because it stains the cryptococcal capsule. In addition to their large capsule, cryptococci differ from *Blastomyces* because the cryptococcal wall is thinner, and the buds are attached to the parent cell by a narrow isthmus. They can be distinguished from *Candida* because cryptococci are round instead of oval and form no pseudohyphae or hyphae. The spherules of *Coccidioides immitis* contain endospores and do not bud.

In patients with meningitis, the respiratory secretions, CSF, urine, blood, and any tissue obtained by biopsy should be examined microscopically and cultured, at least on Sabouraud's agar. It is helpful, especially if the specimen is contaminated, to cultivate a portion of the specimen on nigerseed agar and on media that contain antibacterial antibiotics. Some cryptococci are sensitive to cycloheximide (Actidione), and media containing this antibiotic should be avoided. As many slants as possible should be inoculated and incubated at room temperature or 25 to 30°C. Some tubes may also be placed at 37°C for quick differentiation from saphrophytic cryptococci. Growth often appears within 48 to 72 hours but may be delayed for seven days or more if the inoculum is small. For this reason, cultures should be kept for six weeks before being discarded as negative, and tubed media should be used to avoid drying.

When colonies appear, they are usually convex, mucoid, cream-colored to light tan, or very rarely a light pink. Individual cells are more round than oval, have at least a small capsule in India ink, and do not produce hyphae. In practice, every round yeast, encapsulated yeast, or urease producing yeast should be subjected to a complete work-up to exclude *C. neoformans*. The cultural identification of *C. neoformans* can be definitely established by three properties: growth of subcultures at 37°C, mouse pathogenicity, and urease production. If mice are inoculated intracerebrally, intravenously, or intraperitoneally with 10^5 to 10^7 *C. neoformans*, a rapid, progressively fatal infection follows within one to three weeks. One or two mice should be sacrificed at weekly intervals up to one month and the brain cultured and examined microscopically for the presence of round encapsulated yeast. Mouse pathogenicity, brown growth on nigerseed agar (Fig. 7), and the capacity to grow at 37°C separate *C. neoformans* from other cryptococci. The saprophytic cryptococci that occasionally grow at 37°C usually produce small, poorly developed colonies. We have also found the *C. neoformans*, but not the saprophytes, grows at 39°C. Rapid tests for phenyloxidase activity and cornmeal agar are used as screening tests in some laboratories (Kauffman and Merz, 1982).

In addition to these major characteristics, *C. neoformans* does not produce pseudohyphae, chlamydospores, or germ tubes; does not reduce nitrate; does not ferment (produce gas from) any sugars; and always assimilates inositol. Al-

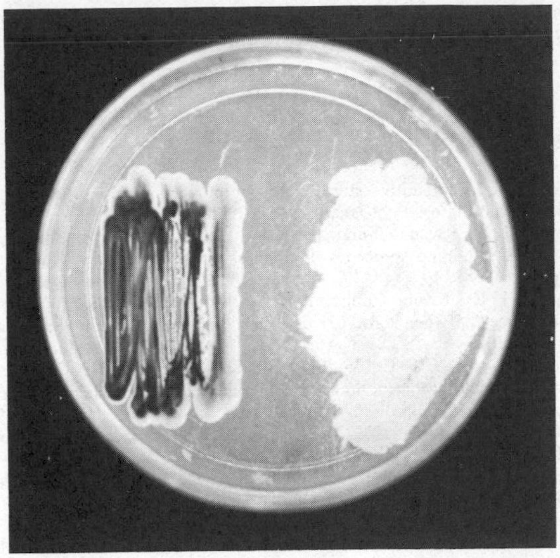

Figure 7. The darkly pigmented growth of *C. neoformans* on nigerseed agar clearly differentiates it from the white or cream-colored growth of *Candida albicans* on the other half of the agar plate.

though these properties can separate *C. neoformans* from any other fungus, the assimilation tests shown in Table 1 are usually performed. Mouse pathogenicity, failure to produce deep salmon-pink pigment, and assimilation of inositol separate *C. neoformans* from *Rhodotorula* species, which have similar sugar assimilation patterns.

Although the perfect state of *C. neoformans* has been described (see earlier sections on Morphology and Epidemiology), and several strains have produced hyphae in the laboratory, this is an unusual phenomenon and does not ordinarily occur without special techniques and media (Kwon-Chung, 1975). If hyphae are observed, they resemble the forms shown in Figures 4 and 5. *Filobasidiella (Cryptococcus) neoformans* var. gattii (Serotypes B and C) assimilates malic, fumaric, and succinic acids, while *F. (Cryptococcus) neoformans* var. *neoformans* (Serotypes A and D) does not (Bennett et al., 1978).

C. neoformans var. gattii can be separated from *C. neoformans* var. *neoformans* on canavanine-glycine-bromthymal blue agar (CGB) (Kwong-Chung et al., 1982). Canavanine, an arginine analog, inhibits all Serotype D strains and 33 per cent of Serotype A. All B and C Serotypes are resistant to canavanine and make acid from 1 per cent glycine. Neither Serotype A nor D strains can utilize 1 per cent glycine as the sole source of carbon and nitrogen. Thus, *C. neoformans* var. gattii (B and C serotypes) grow on CGB agar and turn the media blue. *C. neoformans* var. neoformans (A and D serotypes) is either completely inhibited or grows without changing the color of the agar.

The only useful serologic technique for identifying patients with cryptococcal infection is the agglutination of latex particles that are coated with antibody raised against the cryptococcal capsule. This test measures cryptococcal capsular antigen in the serum or spinal fluid of infected patients; the capsular polysaccharide reacts with the antibody on the latex and agglutinates the particles. False-positive tests are unusual unless the patient produces rheumatoid factor that also agglutinates the antibody-coated latex. A control to rule out rheumatoid factor should be performed in every test and is provided in the commercial test kits. Of several techniques to eliminate false-positive agglutination due to rheumatoid factor or other interfering substances, pretreatment of the sample with 1 per cent pronase-protease seems to be the most effective (Stockman and Roberts, 1982). The latex-agglutination test is very sensitive and is positive in the spinal fluid of most patients with cryptococcal meningitis but in a lower percentage of the serum of patients with isolated pulmonary disease. Although false-positive tests are rare, *C. neoformans* is usually easy to grow, and the diagnosis of cryptococcal infection should always be confirmed by culture. Tests for detection of cryptococcal antibody are not useful in the diagnosis of cryptococcal infection because some normal people have antibody and most patients with cryptococcal infection do not. During the course of successful treatment, the titer of cryptococcal polysaccharide should fall, but this may or may not be accompanied by the development of cryptococcal antibody. While this combination of serologic events is probably a good prognostic sign, some patients recover without developing antibody. Furthermore, dead cryptococci may be seen by microscopic examination of the spinal fluid for many weeks or months after successful treatment. If these organisms cannot be cultivated, their presence should not be taken as a bad prognostic sign.

Cryptococcal skin test preparations are useful for epidemiologic surveys but are of no value for diagnosis.

EPIDEMIOLOGY. Unlike many other fungi that can cause life-threatening infections in apparently normal, nonhospitalized patients, *C. neoformans* is widely distributed throughout the world. It can be isolated from fruit skins and juice, milk, and soil but is most often associated with pigeon dung. It is not part of the normal flora of man or other animals. Although the most common manifestation

Table 1. CHARACTERISTICS OF *CRYPTOCOCCUS NEOFORMANS**

Species	Mouse Virulence	Growth at 37° C	Pigment on Nigerseed Agar	Urease Activity	Assimilations						
					KNO_3	*Inositol*	*Sucrose*	*Lactose*	*Melibiose*	*Cellobiose*	*Raffinose*
C. neoformans	+	+	+	+	−	+	+	−	−	+	+
C. laurentii	−	+ or −	−	+	−	+	+	+	+	+	+
C. terreus	−	+ or −	−	+	+	+	−	rare	−	+	−
C. gastricus	−	−	−	+	−	+	−	−	−	+	−
C. uniguttulatus	−	−	−	+	−	+	+	−	−	− or +	+
C. luteolus	−	−	−	+	−	+	+	−	+	+	−
C. albidus var. *albidus*	−	rare	−	+	+	+	+	+ or −	− or +	+	+
C. albidus var. *diffluens*	−	− or +	−	+	+	+	+	−	+ or −	+	+

*Modified from Widra and Long, 1970, and Bennett et al., 1978.

of cryptococcal infection is meningitis, the primary lesion almost certainly occurs in the lung from inhalation of infective particles. Only 200 to 300 cases of cryptococcal meningitis are reported each year in the United States, but it is estimated that more than 15,000 subclinical respiratory infections occur annually in New York City alone (Ajello, 1969).

Although the capsule of *C. neoformans* is an essential virulence factor, its large size would appear to prevent cryptococci from reaching the terminal bronchioles and causing parenchymal disease. This paradox has probably been solved by two observations. First, in the hyperosmolar, alkaline environment of pigeon feces, *C. neoformans* is unencapsulated and shrunken in size, so that a small percentage of the yeast population has a diameter of 1 μ or less and could easily reach the alveoli (Powell et al., 1972). Second, the sexual stage of *C. neoformans, Filobasidiella*, produces basidiospores that are also about 1 μ in diameter. A role for the sexual stage in dissemination of cryptococci has not been proven but is an attractive possibility.

Cryptococci can reach numbers as high as 5×10^7 in pigeon feces and can be recovered in large numbers from the accumulated filth of pigeon roosts, attics, barn lofts, and cornices. They are often the predominant organism in this alkaline, hyperosmolar environment, with its rich content of creatinine and other nitrogen-containing compounds, but may disappear when the bird droppings are mixed with soil. They are infrequently isolated from organically enriched soil. Direct exposure to sunlight also inhibits their growth. In shaded, moist, or desiccated pigeon feces, they may persist for as long as two years or more. The fungi survive better if relative humidity is increased (Ishaq, et al., 1968).

Since *Cryptococcus neoformans* is a stable, soil dwelling organism in its sexual stage, it is possible that *C. neoformans* was infrequently isolated from soil because it converted to *Filobasidiella* and was not recognized. In fact, only *C. neoformans* Serotypes A and D are isolated from pigeon droppings. The ecologic site of Types B and C is unknown. Most clinical infections in the United States are caused by Serotype A strains except in southern California, where 51 per cent of infections are caused by Serotypes B and C (Bennett et al., 1977). The ecologic characteristics of the organism undoubtedly explain this interesting difference in the geographic distribution of infections.

C. neoformans infects many animals, but transmission from animal to man or man to man has never been documented. Ingestion of cryptococci has never been implicated as the portal of entry in human infection, even after exposure to large numbers of cryptococci in unpasteurized milk from cows with cryptococcal mastitis.

The reasons why cryptococci do not compete well with other organisms in the soil are unknown but may involve biological control mechanisms. For example, *Acanthamoeba palestensis* can phagocytize and kill *C. neoformans*, mites and sow bugs are fungivorous, and *Pseudomonas aeruginosa* and *Bacillus subtilis* produce inhibitory substances (Ruiz *et al.*, 1982). *Acanthamoeba polyphaga*, another free-living ameba, can phagocytose and kill up to 99 per cent of *C. neoformans* in mixed cultures (Bunting et al., 1979). One ameba can ingest and kill as many as 84 cryptococci per day. Interestingly, some of the surviving yeast cells develop into colonies containing hyphae. These forms may be a biological "escape hatch" and suggest the possibility that *C. neoformans* survives the hostile environment of the soil by conversion into the sexual stage.

References

Ajello, L.: A comparative study of the pulmonary mycosis of Canada and the United States. Publ Health Rep 84:869, 1969.

Bennett, J. E., Kwong-Chung, K. J., and Howard, D. H.: Epidemiological differences among serotypes of *Cryptococcus neoformans*. Am. J. Epidemiol 10:582, 1977.

Bennett, J. E., Kwong-Chung, K. J., and Theodore, T. S.: Biochemical. differences between serotypes of *Cryptococcus neoformans*. Sabouraudia 16:167, 1978.

Breen, J. F., Lee, I. C., Vogel, F. R. and Friedman, H.: Cryptococcal capsular polysaccharide-induced modulation of murine immune responses. Infect Immun 36:47, 1982.

Bulmer, G. S., and Sans, M. D.: *Cryptococcus neoformans*. III. Inhibition of phagocytosis. J Bacteriol 95:5, 1968.

Bunting, L. A., Neilson, J. B., and Bulmer, G. S.: *Cryptococcus neoformans*: Gastronomic delight of a soil amoeba. Sabouraudia 17:225, 1979.

Cassone, A., Simonetti, N., and Strippoli, V.: Wall structure and bud formation in *Cryptococcus neoformans*. Arch Microbiol 95:205, 1974.

Chaskes, S., and Tyndall, R. L.: Pigment production by *Cryptococcus neoformans* and other cryptococcus species from aminophenols and diaminobenzenes. J Clin Microbiol 7:146, 1978.

Dabbagh, R., Conant, N. F., Nielsen, H. S., and Burns, R. O.: Effect of temperature on saprophytic cryptococci: Temperature-induced lysis and protoplast formation. J Gen Microbiol 85:177, 1974.

Diamond, R. D., and Bennett, J. E.: Growth of *Cryptococcus neoformans* within human macrophages *in vitro*. Infect Immun 7:231, 1973.

Diamond, R. D., and Allison, A. C.: Nature of the effector cells responsible for antibody-dependent cell-mediated killing of *Cryptococcus neoformans*. Infect Immun 14:716, 1976.

Diamond, R. D., and Erickson, N. F. III: Chemotaxis of human neutrophils and monocytes induced by *Cryptococcus neoformans*. Infect Immun 38:380, 1982.

Dykstra, M. A., Friedman, L., and Murphy, J. W.: Capsule size of *Cryptococcus neoformans*: Control and relationship to virulence. Infect Immun 16:129, 1977.

Ensley, P. K., Davis, C. E., Anderson, M. P., and Fletcher, K. C.: Cryptococcosis in a male Beccari's Crowned Pigeon. J Am Vet Med Assoc 175:992, 1979.

Erke, K. H.: Light microscopy of basidia, basidiospores, and nuclei in spores and hyphae of *Filabasidiella neoformans (Cryptococcus neoformans)*. J Bacteriol 128:445, 1976.

Graybill, J. R., and Alford, R. H.: Cell-mediated immunity in cryptococcosis. Cell Immunol 14:12, 1974.

Griffin, F. M., Jr.: Roles of macrophage Fc and C3b receptors in phagocytosis of immunologically coated *Cryptococcus neoformans*. Proc Natl Acad Sci USA 78:3853, 1981.

Henderson, D. K., Bennett, J. E., and Huber, M. A.: Long-lasting, specific immunologic unresponsiveness associated with cryptococcal meningitis. J Clin Investig 69:1185, 1982.

Howard, J. I., and Bolande, R. P.: Humoral defense mechanisms in cryptococcosis. Substances in normal human serum, saliva, and cerebral spinal fluid affecting the growth of *Cryptococcus neoformans*. J Infect Dis 116:75, 1966.

Ishaq, C. M., Bulmer, G. S., and Felton, F. G.: An evaluation of various environmental factors affecting the propagation of *Cryptococcus neoformans*. Mycopathol Mycol Appl 35:81, 1968.

Kalina, M., Kletter, Y., and Aronson, M.: The interaction of phagocytes and the large-sized parasite *Cryptococcus neoformans:* Cytochemical and ultrastructural study. Cell Tiss Res 152:165, 1974.

Kauffman, C. S. and Merz, W. G.: Two rapid pigmentation tests for identification of *Cryptococcus neoformans*. J Clin Microbiol 15:339, 1982.

Kozel, T. R.: Non-encapsulated variant of *Cryptococcus neoformans* II. Surface receptors for cryptococcal polysaccharide and their role in inhibition of phagocytosis by polysaccharide. Infect Immun 16:99, 1977.

Kwong-Chung, K. J.: A new genus, *Filobasidiella*, the perfect state of *Cryptococcus neoformans*. Mycologia 67:1197, 1975.

Kwong-Chung, K. J., Polacheck, I., and Bennett, J. E.: Improved diagnostic medium for separation. I. *Cryptococcus neoformans* var. *neoformans* (serotypes A and D) and *Cryptococcus neoformans* var. *gattii* (serotypes B and C). J Clin Microbiol 15:535, 1982.

Kwong-Chung, K. J., Polacheck, I., and Popkin, T. J.: Melanin-lacking mutants of *Cryptococcus neoformans* and their virulence for mice. J Bacteriol 150:1414, 1982.

Kwong-Chung, K. J., Bennett, J. E., and Rhodes, J. C.: Taxonomic studies

of *Filobasidiella* species and their anamorphs. Antonie Van Leeuwenhoek 48:25, 1982.
Lim, T. S., and Murphy, J. W.: Transfer of immunity to Cryptococcosis by T-enriched splenic lymphocytes from *Cryptococcus neoformans*-sensitized mice. Infect Immun 30:5, 1980.
Macher, A., Bennett, J., Gadek, J., and Frank, M. M.: Complement depletion in cryptococcal sepsis. J Immunol 120:1686, 1978.
Marchant, R., and Smith, D. G.: Bud formation in *Sacchoromyces cerevisiae* and a comparison with the mechanism of cell division in other yeasts. J Gen Microbiol 53:163, 1968.
Meyer, M. T., and Phaff, H. J.: Survey for alpha-(1-3) glucanase activity among yeasts. J Bacteriol 131:702, 1977.
Mohr, J. A., Muchmore, H. G., and Tacker, R.: Stimulation of phagocytosis of *Cryptococcus neoformans* in human cryptococcal meningitis. J. Reticuloendothel Soc 15:149, 1974.
Murphy, J. M. and Moorhead, J. M.: Regulation of cell-mediated immunity in cryptococcosis. I. Induction of specific afferent T-suppressor cells by cryptococcal antigen. J Immunol 128:276, 1982.
Norkrans, B., and Tumblad-Johannson, I.: Cellular contents of the Krebs cycle keto acids in yeasts grown on different nitrogen sources including hydroxylamine. Arch Microbiol 115:127, 1977.
Powell, K. E., Bernhoff, A., Dahl, A., Weeks, R. J., and Tosh, F. E.: Airborne *Cryptococcus neoformans:* Particles from pigeon excreta compatible with alveolar deposition. J Infect Dis 125:412, 1972.
Raizada, M. K., Schutzbach, J. S., and Ankel, H.: *Cryptococcus laurentii* cell envelope glyco-protein. J Biol Chem 250:3310, 1975.
Reiss, F., Szilagyi, G., and Mayer, E.: Immunological studies of the anti-cryptococcal factor of normal human serum. Mycopathologia 55:175, 1975.
Ruiz, A., Neilson, J. B., and Bulmer, G. S.: Control of *Cryptococcus neoformans* in nature by biotic factors. Sabouraudia 20:21, 1982.
Schimpff, S. C., and Bennett, J. E.: Abnormalities in cell-mediated immunity in patients with *Cryptococcus neoformans* infection. J Allergy Clin Immunol 43:430, 1975.
Schmeding, K. A., Jong, S. C., and Hugh, R.: Sexual compatibility between serotypes of *Filobasidiella neoformans (Cryptococcus neoformans).* Curr. Microbiol 5:133, 1981.
Shadomy, H. J.: Clamp connections in two strains of *Cryptococcus neoformans.* Recent trends of yeast research. Atlanta Research Articles, School of Arts and Sciences, Georgia State University, 1971.
Shaw, C.E., and Kapica, L.: Production of diagnostic pigment by phenoloxidase activity of *Cryptococcus neoformans.* Appl Microbiol 24:842, 830, 1972.
Staub, F.: *Cryptococcus neoformans* and *Guizotia abyssinica* (syn. G. oleifera D.C. (Z Hyg 148:446, 1962.
Stockman, L. and Roberts, G. D.: Specificity of the latex test for cryptococcal antigen: a rapid simple method for eliminating interference factors. J Clin Microbiol 16:965, 1982.
Takeo, K., Ueasaka, I., Uehina, K., and Nishiura, M.: Fine structure of *Cryptococcus neoformans* grown *in vivo* as observed by freeze etching. J Bacteriol 113:1449, 1973.
Vanbreuseghem, R. and Takashio, M.: An atypical strain of *Cryptococcus neoformans* (San Felice) Vuillemin 1894. II. *Cryptococcus neoformans* var. *gattii* var. nov. Ann Soc Belge Med Trop 50:695, 1980.
Widra, A., and Long, I.: Taxonomic studies on cryptococci and related yeasts. Mycopathol Mycol Appl 40:89, 1970.
Yamada, Y., and Kondo, K.: Coenzyme Q system in the classification of the yeast genera *Rhodotorula* and *Cryptococcus*, and the yeast-like genera *Sporobolomyces* and *Rhodosporidium.* J Gen Appl Microbiol 19:59, 1973.

74
CANDIDA

ABRAHAM I. BRAUDE, M.D., PH.D.

Members of the genus *Candida* are indigenous human yeasts that colonize the skin and mucous membranes of normal people but produce infection only when natural resistance is compromised. *Candida glabraba* was formerly regarded as a separate genus and known as *Torulopsis glabrata.* A careful reappraisal of these yeasts disclosed that the differences between them and established members of the genus *Candida* were not enough to retain *Torulopsis* as a separate genus (Yarrow and Meyer, 1978). In this chapter, however, *C. glabrata* is discussed separately because its clinical significance differs from most of the other seven species of the genus *Candida.*

The most important of these is *Candida albicans,* but *Candida tropicalis* has become a serious cause of disseminated infection in patients undergoing treatment for hematologic malignancies or receiving bone marrow transplantation (Table 1) (Wingard et al., 1979). The other five species encountered in human disease are designated *C. krusei, C. guilliermondi, C. parapsilosis, C. pseudotropicalis,* and *C. stellatoidea.*

MORPHOLOGY. Members of the genus *Candida* characteristically develop both as yeast cells and as pseudohyphae. *C. albicans,* the principal pathogenic member of the genus, also produces true hyphae. Pseudohyphae are chains of budding cells that fail to detach, so that they develop into a branching network that resembles true hyphae. Colonies composed of pseudohyphae have the soft, white character of yeasts in contrast to the cottony or woolly growth of true mycelia. The yeast cells of *C. albicans* are oval and gram-positive; they vary in size from 2×3 μ to 8.5×14 μ. Less frequently, elongated cells may be seen after incubation at room temperature. On cornmeal agar, a nutritionally deficient medium composed only of cornmeal and water, *C. albicans* reproduces in four different forms: (1) true mycelia, (2) pseudomycelia, (3) blastospores, and (4) chlamydospores. The blastospores grow in round clusters at intervals along the pseudomycelia. Terminal chlamydospores (macroconidia) growing at the end of the hyphae are the most distinctive feature of *C. albicans* and are rarely produced by any other species of *Candida.* The chlamydospores are large (8 to 12 μ) and round and have a thick wall (Fig. 1). They are particularly adapted for maintaining vitality during starvation and other adverse conditions. Their large size is due to the storage of reserve nutritional substances, and their thick wall protects them from an unfavorable environment. The thick wall has two layers, of which the outer is polysaccharide (beta 1:3 glucan) and the inner, protein. There is also a high lipid content (Jansons and Nickerson, 1970). The poor nutritional quality of cornmeal agar causes the yeast cells to differentiate into the well-provisioned chlamydospores. Formation of chlamydospores is a test for distinguishing between *C. albicans*

Table 1. FREQUENCY OF ISOLATION OF DIFFERENT SPECIES OF *CANDIDA* FROM BLOOD CULTURES

Species	Number of Patients with Positive Blood Cultures
C. albicans	68
C. tropicalis	18
C. parapsilosis	12
C. glabrata	2

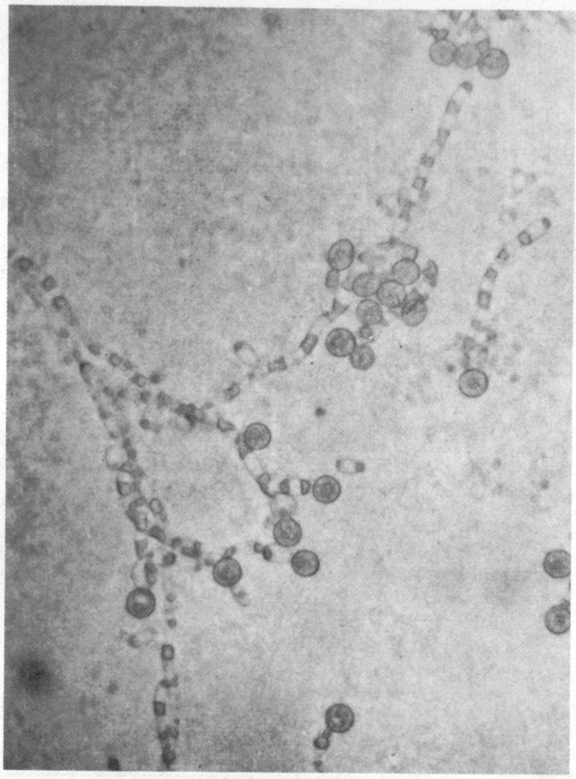

Figure 1. Chlamydospores of *C. albicans* after growth on cornmeal agar. The chlamydospores are the sharply defined large round bodies at the tips of the hyphae.

and those species of *Candida* that do not develop into these forms.

Perhaps the most interesting form is the germ tube (Reynolds and Braude, 1956). When yeast cells of *C. albicans* are suspended in serum and incubated at 37°C, they produce within two to four hours a short filament measuring $1.5 \times 15\ \mu$ and having the appearance of a bean sprout (Fig. 2). Because germ tubes develop so quickly, they are used as a rapid test for *C. albicans*. Some of the morphologic features of *C. albicans* are sometimes seen with *C. stellatoidea*, which can also produce blastospores, pseudohyphae, germ tubes, and rarely, chlamydospores. Since the two are also similar in antigenic structure, *C. stellatoidea* is regarded by some students of yeast taxonomy as an avirulent variant of *C. albicans* (Pollack and Benham, 1957). *C. tropicalis* also produces pseudohyphae, true mycelia and chlamydospores rarely, but not germ tubes. In broth cultures, *C. tropicalis* tends to form a thin film that can trap gas bubbles. The film of *C. tropicalis* is in contrast to that of *C. krusei*, which is much thicker and crawls up the side of the broth culture tube. The flat, dry, dull colonies of *C. krusei* on agar and its cylindrical cell morphology in broth are additional distinctive characteristics. These cells vary considerably in size, and elongated forms may look like crossed matchsticks. The cells of *C. pseudotropicalis* are also elongated in broth cultures but fall apart and lie parallel to each other.

The morphologic differences and species of *Candida* are summarized in Table 2.

ANTIGENIC COMPOSITION. The various species of *Candida* have been classified into six antigenic groups on the basis of slide agglutination tests with monospecific absorbed rabbit sera (Table 3). Each of 22 species of *Candida* were grouped according to their content of seven heat-stable and three heat-labile antigens. In this system of classification, both *C. stellatoidea* and *C. tropicalis* are closely related antigenically to *C. albicans*. Although all *Candida* species share a common antigen, the antigenic structures of *C. pseudotropicalis*, *C. krusei*, *C. parapsilosis*, and *C. guilliermondi* are distinctly different from *C. albicans*. These antigenic relationships have been largely substantiated by means of immunoelectrophoresis of soluble yeast extracts (Biguet et al., 1965). The important antigenic determinants in *Candida* appear to be surface polysaccharides, such as mannans and glucans. Mannan forms the outer layer and glucan the inner layer of the cell wall of *C. albicans*. The two sugars appear to occur naturally as complexes of polysaccharide-protein linked together by *N*-acetylglucosamine. The antigenic specificity of the mannans depends on the lengths of the polysaccharide side branches and the type of glycosidic linkages present in them. The mannans are polymers of mannose that, in the main chain or backbone of *C. albicans*, are connected by alpha 1 to 6 linkages. In the side chains, the linkages are alpha 1 to 2 or rarely, alpha 1 to 3, and there are six mannose units or less. Two serotypes of *C. albicans* have been described whose antigenic distinction may depend on the number and position of the linkages.

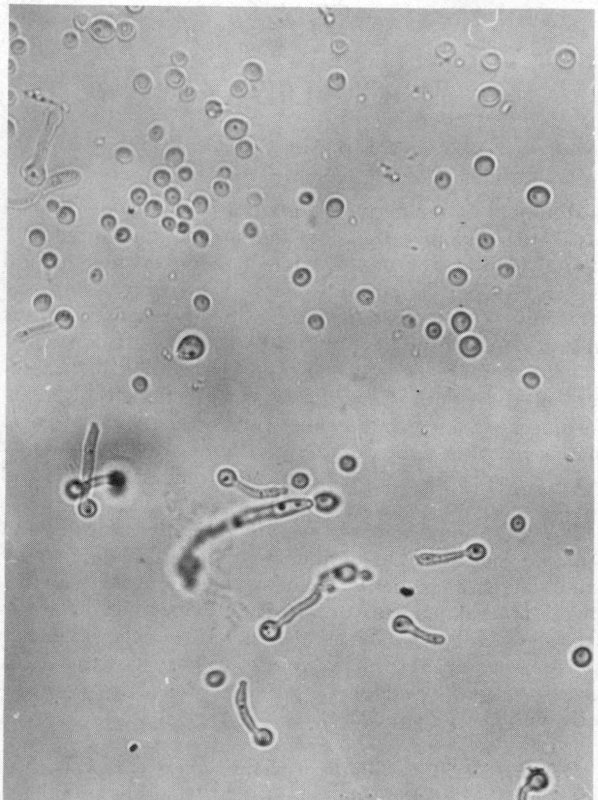

Figure 2. Germ-tube formation in *C. albicans*. Germ tubes are short filaments that protrude from yeast cells within two to four hours after incubation in serum at 37° C. (Reynolds, R., and Braude, A. I.: Clin Res Proc 4:40, 1956.)

Table 2. GROSS AND MICROSCOPIC APPEARANCE OF THE DIFFERENT SPECIES OF *CANDIDA*

Species	Colonies on Agar[a]	Film[b]	Yeast Cell Morphology	Germ Tubes	Chlamydospores
C. albicans	Creamy	0	Ovoid	+	+
C. stellatoidea	Creamy	0	Ovoid	±	Rare
C. tropicalis	Creamy	Thin, traps bubbles	Ovoid	0	0
C. krusei	Flat, dull, dry	Thick, climbs tube	Cylindrical, elongated cells arranged as crossed matchsticks	0	0
C. pseudotropicalis	Soft, smooth, white	0	Elongated cells lying parallel like logs in a stream	0	0
C. guilliermondi	Thin, flat, glossy	0	Ovoid or cylindrical	0	0
C. parapsilosis	Creamy	0	Ovoid, sometimes giant cells	0	0

[a]Three days' growth on Sabouraud's dextrose agar at 25° C.
[b]Three days' growth on Sabouraud's dextrose broth at 25° C.

PHYSIOLOGY. The metabolism of *Candida* is the same as that of other aerobic eukaryotic cells. They are capable of both aerobic glycolysis via the hexose monophosphate pathway and of anaerobic glycolysis through the Embden-Meyerhof pathway. They also have Krebs cycle enzymes and the mitochondrial enzymes for oxidative phosphorylation. Oxidative phosphorylation in *Candida* involves mainly cytochromes a, a_3, b, c, and c_1.

Protein synthesis also resembles that in eukaryotes. *C. albicans* has 80S ribosomes, which dissociate into 60S and 38S subunits (Yamaguchi and Iwata, 1970).

Little is known of the physiologic changes associated with or responsible for the development of hyphae or chlamydospores. Temperature is one important factor; relatively high temperatures (37°C) promote hyphae and blastospores, whereas lower temperatures (<25°C) seem to favor chlamydospores. Mycelial formation is accompanied by a suppression of the pentose phosphate pathway and the diversion of hexoses for cell wall biosynthesis.

PATHOGENIC PROPERTIES. Members of the genus *Candida* cannot infect healthy people, but cause serious infections in patients with disturbances of natural resistance. These disturbances may represent changes in endocrine function, normal microbial flora, or cell-mediated immunity. The two most prominent endocrine disturbances related to candidiasis are diabetes and hormonal changes related to pregnancy and the use of oral contraceptives. In diabetes the high glucose content of the urine promotes growth of *C. albicans* in the skin around the urethra, in the vagina, the groin, and the urinary tract. In pregnancy and in patients using oral contraceptives there is increased susceptibility to vaginitis, possibly because the estrogens stimulate growth of the yeast. Elimination of normal flora by antibiotics also promotes vaginal candidiasis, apparently because the yeast cells normally resident on the skin or mucosa are resistant to the drugs and overgrow the surfaces vacated by the inhibited bacteria. The mouth and pharynx also become the site of candidiasis (thrush) after antibiotic therapy. Disseminated candidiasis is usually seen when intravenous lines become infected. The kidney and brain bear the brunt of hematogenous infections, especially those associated with endocarditis, and renal failure or *Candida* encephalitis can be the cause of death.

There is reason to believe that germ-tube formation contributes to pathogenicity of *C. albicans*. Thus, *C. albicans*, the only species of *Candida* (with one exception) that produces germ tubes, is the most virulent and invasive. The relationship of virulence to germ-tube formation is demonstrated when *C. albicans* yeast cells are ingested by polymorphonuclear leukoyctes. Germ tubes of ingested yeast puncture through the wall of the phagocyte and allow the yeast to escape.

Table 3. ANTIGENIC GROUPING OF *CANDIDA* SPECIES OF MEDICAL IMPORTANCE

Group	Species	Thermostable Antigens	Thermolabile Antigens
I	*C. albicans*	1, 2, 3, 4, 5, 6, 7	
	C. tropicalis	1, 2, 3, 4, 5, 6	
II	*C. stellatoidea*	1, 8, 10	a
	C. pseudotropicalis	1, 2, 3, 4, 5, 10	
III	*C. krusei*	1, 2, 5, 11	b
IV	*C. parapsilosis*	1, 2, 3, 5, 13, 14, 15	c
V	*C. guilliermondi*	1, 2, 3, 4, 9	
VI	None of medical importance		

IMMUNITY. Cell-mediated immunity is thought to be more important than humoral immunity in resistance to *Candida* infection. At least in chronic infections of the skin due to *C. albicans*, there are often disturbances of T-cell function. Since there is a familial tendency for mucocutaneous candidiasis to occur in children who have abnormal T lymphocytes it would seem that the disturbance in these cells may sometimes be genetic in origin (see Chapter 211). There is some evidence that candidiasis occurs because the T cell cannot recognize the antigen or produce migration inhibition factor (MIF). There is also suggestive evidence that macrophage chemotaxis is depressed. Despite universal delayed sensitivity to *Candida* antigens in healthy people, those with chronic candidiasis are often anergic to its antigens, and transformation of their lymphocytes by *Candida* antigen is sometimes depressed. B lymphocytes and circulating antibodies, on the other hand, are normal. The importance of abnormal T cells as the cause of impaired immunity to *Candida* is suggested by the tendency of mucocutaneous candidiasis to occur in patients who have frank thymic disorders such as thymomas and congenital thymic aplasia (DiGeorge syndrome). Mucocutaneous candidiasis is also a serious problem in patients with the

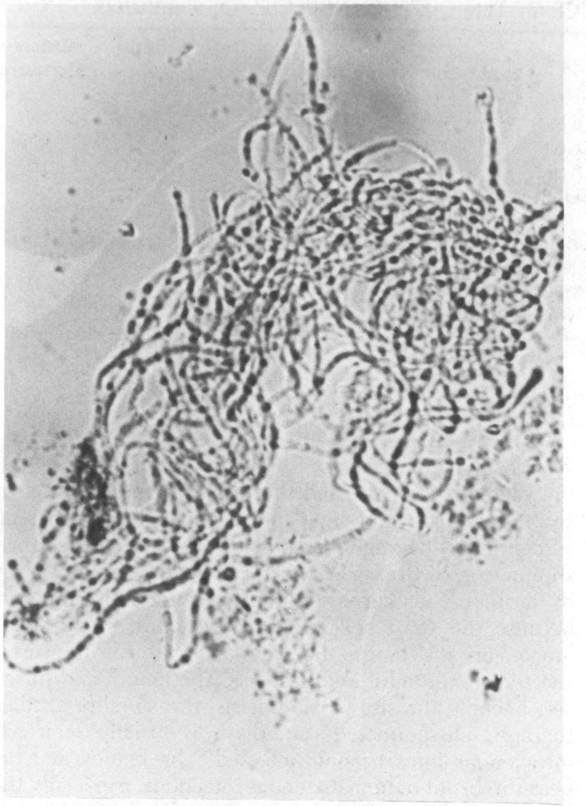

Figure 3. Wet mount of *C. albicans* in skin lesion from girl with chronic mucocutaneous candidiasis. The skin scraping had been treated with potassium hydroxide to digest away the epithelial cells and debris before microscopic examination. Note predominance of hyphae.

acquired immunodeficiency syndrome (AIDS), in which the ratio of T-helper cells to T-suppressor cells is decreased.

Abnormalities of humoral immunity, such as agammaglobulinemia, hypogammaglobulinemia, and multiple myeloma have not displayed a special susceptibility to *Candida* infection. Furthermore, the ability of humoral antibody to prevent experimental candidiasis after active or passive immunization has been inconsistent and unimpressive (Hurd and Drake, 1953).

The natural immunity of healthy persons to *Candida* infection is probably generated early in life when the alimentary tract becomes colonized with *C. albicans*. The surface glycoproteins (mannoproteins and glucoproteins) are thought to stimulate both humoral and cellular immunity. Thus, normal people develop antibodies and delayed hypersensitivity to *Candida* culture filtrates, which contain glycoprotein and polysaccharide antigens.

LABORATORY DIAGNOSIS

Morphologic and Cultural Methods. *C. albicans* infection of the skin, urinary tract, mouth, vagina, esophagus, and other tissues is easily recognized by microscopic examination of wet mounts (Fig. 3) or gram stains (Fig. 4) of the lesions. The material is taken for examination by scraping the skin or mucous patches (thrush) and smearing the infected scrapings on a microscope slide for gram staining. Yeast and mycelial forms of *Candida* are strongly gram-positive. Both superficial and deeper hematogenous *Candida* infections of the skin can be recognized by microscopic examination of smears made from skin scrapings. *C. albicans* is also cultured without difficulty from lesions on any conventional solid or liquid medium. It may appear overnight at 37°C on blood agar or nutrient agar and seldom needs more than 48 hours to grow out. Although less important for diagnosis than smears, culture is necessary for identifying the species of *Candida* and for testing sensitivity to drugs to which *C. albicans* can become resistant.

Culture of *Candida* from blood is more difficult than direct culture from infected tissues. The organism may not appear in culture for several days after onset of candidemia, if at all. Blood must be cultured aerobically to get an optimum recovery of *Candida* organisms. The speed of cultural isolation is also accelerated if blood is cultured in pour plates (1.0 ml heparinized blood added to 9 ml warm molten nutrient agar). If candidemia is secondary to contaminated intravenous lines, the diagnosis can also be made by smear and culture of the catheter tip after it is removed from the vein.

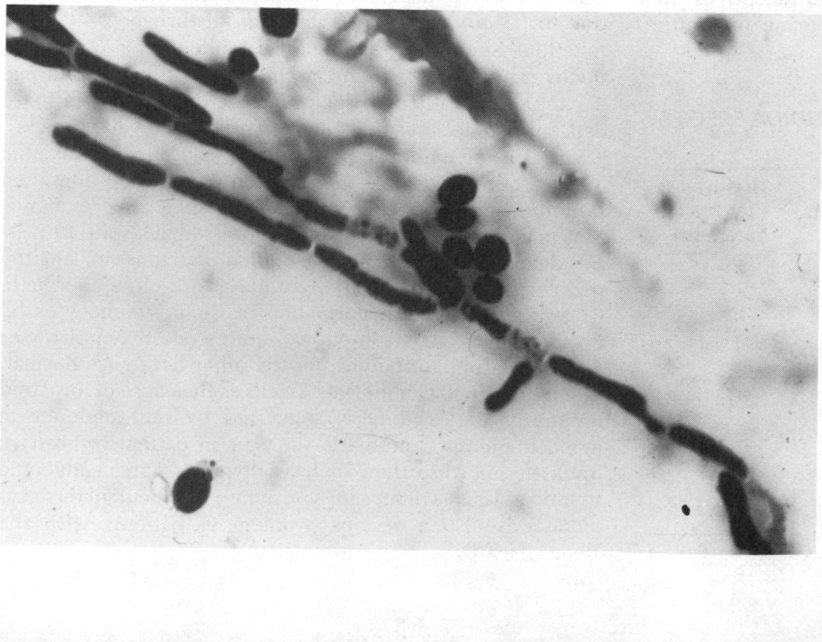

Figure 4. Gram stain of smear made from embolus to femoral artery in a patient with *Candida* endocarditis. *C. albicans* is strongly gram-positive. Both hyphae and blastospores appear to be growing in the embolus.

The first step in species identification is to test for germ tubes by suspending the yeast in serum and incubating it at 37°C for two to four hours. A presumptive diagnosis of *C. albicans* can be made if germ tubes are produced, and a final diagnosis is made by sucrose assimilation. *C. stellatoidea*, which can also produce germ tubes, can be excluded if sucrose is fermented and assimilated. The other species of *Candida* are also identified by fermentation and assimilation tests.

Assimilation tests are used to determine the ability of a yeast to use a given substance as the sole source of carbon or nitrogen. The test can be done either with solid or liquid media. In the test on solid medium, organisms are dispersed throughout warm agar, which is then poured into a plate before it solidifies. The seeded agar is prepared so that it lacks the specific sugar or nitrogen source under test, and small amounts of the test substance are placed at various points on the surface. The ability to assimilate a given substance is determined by the presence of growth at room temperature in the region where the test substance is applied. The test can also be done by streaking the surface and applying filter paper disks containing test substrate, or by inoculating the surface of agar slants containing each of the individual sugars to be examined. Bromcresyl blue is used as a pH indicator, and each tube is watched for growth and for a change in color from blue to yellow as acid is produced by fermentation. The same media can be used in liquid form for broth assimilation tests. Each broth tube contains one sugar as the test substrate and is inoculated with a suspension of organisms grown for 48 hours in the basal medium to deplete the cells of stored substrate. The tubes are incubated at room temperature, and growth is determined by the development of turbidity. In the nitrate assimilation test, a carbon base is inoculated with 0.078 per cent potassium nitrate in order to determine if this substrate can be used as the sole source of nitrogen.

Fermentation tests determine the ability of yeasts to ferment individual sugars in media that support their growth even in the absence of the test sugar. These media contain peptone, yeast extract (the water-soluble portion of autolyzed bakers' or brewers' yeast that is rich in B vitamins), and a pH indicator. Observations are made on production of both acid and gas. As recorded in Table 4, the yeasts cannot ferment to gas all sugars that they can assimilate. Examples of sugars that are assimilated but not fermented to gas are galactose by *C. stellatoidea* and sucrose by *C. parapsilosis*. It should also be noted that all species of *Candida* of medical importance assimilate and ferment glucose, and all except *C. krusei* assimilate galactose and xylose. Lactose, on the other hand, is assimilated and fermented only by *C. pseudotropicalis*, and inositol by none of them.

In contrast to certain cryptococci, no species of *Candida* in Table 4 can use nitrate as a sole source of nitrogen. Even more important, no species of *Candida*, except certain strains of *C. krusei*, has urease activity. The urease test is thus important for distinguishing *C. albicans* and other species of *Candida* from *Cryptococcus neoformans*, which does have urease activity.

Serologic Methods. Attempts to diagnose candidiasis by tests for antibody or circulating antigen are not yet reliable. Attempts have been made to find antibody in sera from patients by testing them for their ability to agglutinate *C. albicans* yeast cells, or to precipitate antigens from disrupted *C. albicans* in tubes or in gel diffusion plates. These tests have seldom been useful clinically because patients who develop disseminated candidiasis are often suppressed immunologically and cannot generate a specific immune response. Moreover, disseminated candidiasis is a disorder that requires recognition long before antibody can make its appearance. For this reason, efforts are being made to detect circulating *Candida* antigens by immunologic or chemical methods in order to make a diagnosis of systemic candidiasis in patients with negative blood cultures (Miller et al., 1974).

EPIDEMIOLOGY. In contrast to the other fungi that cause human infection, members of the genus *Candida* are not inhabitants of the soil but rather indigenous members of the normal flora of the human alimentary tract and skin. *C. albicans* is also widely distributed among animals and is responsible for oral, esophageal, genital, skin, and disseminated hematogenous infections in domesticated mammals or fowl. For example, *C. albicans* has caused epidemic venereal disease among geese and many cases of esophagitis in pigs (Beemer et al., 1973; Kadel et al., 1969). Despite its wide prevalence in these animal reservoirs, the source of human infections by *C. albicans* is endogenous, arising from carriage sites on the patient himself. About 10 per cent of healthy people carry *C. albicans* in their mouth, and 15 per cent carry it in the rectum. Carriage in the mouth and rectum can reach 40 per cent or more in patients and tends to increase with age and antibiotic treatment (Berdon and Seita, 1971; Chitale and Bhende, 1965). Vaginal carriage is highest normally in the child-bearing age, when it may reach 10 per cent. *C. albicans* is found less frequently on the skin than on mucous membranes; the skin isolation rate seldom exceeds 5 to 8 per cent even in hospitalized patients. *C. tropicalis* is found occasionally in the mouth and feces, and *C. parapsilosis* in feces but in much fewer numbers than *C. albicans*.

The normal residence of *C. albicans* in the vagina, bowel, mouth, and skin is significant in at least two respects. First, cultural isolation of this yeast from materials passing through the mouth or vagina does not constitute proof of infection. This must be kept in mind especially in the case of sputum, because pulmonary infection due to *C. albicans* is extremely rare, if it ever occurs, and positive candidal cultures of sputum almost always represent contamination of pulmonary secretions by the oral resident yeast flora. The second significant point about the normal carriage sites of *C. albicans* is that they represent foci for transmission. For example, *C. albicans* can spread from the vagina or rectum to cause intertriginous candidiasis of the groin in diabetics; from the vagina to the infant during passage through the birth canal to cause oral thrush in the newborn; and from the skin via intravenous catheters or from the gut via mucosal ulcers to the circulating blood. Transmission of infection from environmental sources of *C. albicans* occurs in exceptional circumstances but is far less important than transmission from normal carriage sites in the patient (Malmatinis et al., 1968; Cremer and DeGroot, 1967.

DRUG SENSITIVITY. The minimal inhibitory concentrations (μg/ml) of antifungal drugs against *C. albicans* are 0.2 to 0.8 for amphotericin B, 0.05 to 12.5 for 5-fluorocytosine, 0.1 to 10 for clotrimazole, and 0.1 to 3.0 for ketoconazole. These inhibitory drug levels can be reached in the body fluids of patients.

Table 4. ASSIMILATION AND FERMENTATION REACTIONS OF DIFFERENT SPECIES OF *CANDIDA*

	Assimilation Results												Fermentation (Gas Production)				
	Glucose	**Maltose**	**Sucrose**	**Lactose**	**Galactose**	**Melibiose**	**Cellobiose**	**Inositol**	**Xylose**	**Raffinose**	**Trehalose**	**Dulcitol**	**Glucose**	**Maltose**	**Sucrose**	**Lactose**	**Galactose**
C. albicans	+	+	+	0	+	0	0	0	+	0	+	0	+	+	A*	0	+
C. stellatoidea	+	+	0	0	+	0	0	0	+	0	+	0	+	+	0	0	0
C. tropicalis	+	+	+	0	+	0	+	0	+	0	+	0	+	+	+	0	+
C. parapsilosis	+	+	+	0	+	0	0	0	+	0	+	0	+	0	0	0	+
C. krusei	+	0	0	0	0	0	0	0	0	0	0	0	+	0	0	0	0
C. pseudotropicalis	+	0	+	+	+	0	+	0	+	+	0	0	+	0	+	+	+
C. guilliermondi	+	+	+	0	+	+	+	0	+	+	+	+	+	0	+	0	+
C. glabrata	+	0	0	0	+	0	0	0	0	0	+	0	+	0	0	0	0

*A, acid, no gas

CANDIDA GLABRATA (TORULOPSIS)

The yeast *C. glabrata* shares with *C. albicans* all of the first seven heat-stable antigens of Tsuchiya except antigen 4. Like *C. albicans*, it is also a member of the resident flora and forms ovoid cells. In contrast to other members of the genus *Candida*, *C. glabrata* does not form mycelia or pseudomycelia. In this respect, it resembles four other yeasts (*Candida pintolopesii*, *Saccharomyces tellustris*, *Candida bovina*, and *Candida sloofii*), from which it can be differentiated by the fact that *C. glabrata* can ferment trehalose, whereas the other four yeasts cannot. This one fermentation is important because all five species have otherwise identical fermentation and assimilation patterns.

It is also important to differentiate this yeast from *Cryptococcus neoformans*, which also forms no mycelia. The quickest way to differentiate them is to test for urease activity, which is present in *C. neoformans* but not in *C. glabrata*. Another differential point is that *C. neoformans* has a capsule but *C. glabrata* has none. Failure to assimilate inositol also distinguishes *C. glabrata* from cryptococci. The most common clinical source of *C. glabrata* is the urine, but occasionally it has been cultured from the blood (Table 1) and spinal fluid. When inoculated intraperitoneally in mice, it produces small granulomas and has an intracellular appearance in them that resembles that of *Histoplasma capsulatum*.

C. glabrata is sensitive to nystatin, amphotericin B, and 5-fluorocytosine in concentrations that can be achieved in human infections.

References

Beemer, A., Kutten, E., and Katz, Z.: Epidemic veneral disease due to *Candida albicans* in geese in Israel. Avian Dis 17:639, 1973.

Berdon, J., and Seita, C.: The incidence of *Candida albicans* in hospital patients. J Oral Med 26:123, 1971.

Biquet, J., Tran Van Ky, P., Andrieu, S., and Degaey, R.: Étude immunoelectrophorétique de la nature et de l'ordre d'apparition des anticorps précipitants du sérum de lapins en fonction de leur mode d'immunisation contre *Candida albicans*. Sabouraudia 4:148, 1965.

Chitale, A., and Bhende, Y.: The incidence of *Candida albicans* in throat and feces of healthy persons and patients on antibiotic therapy. J Postgrad Med 11:30, 1965.

Cremer, G., and DeGroot, W. P.: An epidemic of thrush in a premature nursery. Dermatologia 135:107, 1967.

Hurd, R., and Drake, C.: *Candida albicans* infections in actively and passively immunized animals. Mycopathologia 6:290, 1953.

Jansons, V., and Nickerson, W.: Chemical composition of chlamydospores of *Candida albicans*. J Bacteriol 104:922, 1970.

Kadel, W., Kelly, D., and Coles, E.: Survey of yeastlike fungi and tissue changes in esophagogastric region of stomachs of swine. Am J Vet Res 30:401, 1969.

Malamatinis, J., Mattniller, E., and Westphal, J.: Cutaneous moniliasis affecting varsity athletes. J Am Coll Health Assoc 16:294, 1968.

Miller, G., Witwer, M., Braude, A., and Davis, C.: Rapid identification of *Candida albicans* septicemia by gas-liquid chromatography. J Clin Invest 54:1235, 1974.

Pollack, J., and Benham, R.: The chlamydospores of *Candida albicans*: Comparison of three media for their induction. J Lab Clin Med 50:313, 1957.

Reynolds, R., and Braude, A. I.: The filament-inducing property of blood for *Candida albicans*: Its nature and significance. Clin Res Proc 4:40, 1956.

Rippon, J. W.: Medical Mycology, 1st ed. Philadelphia, W. B. Saunders Co., 1974.

Tsuchiya, T., Fukazawa, Y., and Kawakita, S.: Serologic classification of the genus *Candida*. In Tokyo Research Committee of Candidiasis: Studies of Candidiasis in Japan. Tokyo, Education Ministry of Japan, 1961, p. 34.

Wingard, J., Nierz, W., and Sarah, R.: *Candida tropicalis*: A major pathogen in immunocompromised patients. Ann Intern Med 91:539, 1979.

Yamaguchi, H., and Iwata, K.: *In vitro* and *in vivo* protein synthesis in *Candida albicans*. 2. Dissociation properties in ribosomes. Sabouraudia 8:189, 1970.

Yarrow, D. and Meyer, S.: A proposal for the amendment of the diagnosis of the genus *Candida*. Berkhout nom, cons. Int J Syst Bacteriol 28:611, 1978.

75

SPOROTHRIX SCHENCKII

FRANÇOIS MARIAT, D. SC.
R. G. GARRISON, PH.D.

Sporothrix schenckii is the etiologic agent of sporotrichosis, a chronic mycotic disease of man and animals. The fungus is a dimorphic, pathogenic hyphomycete that occurs naturally on vegetation or as a soil saprophyte. Traumatic introduction of the fungus into the skin causes ascending lymphangitis of the extremities after development of the primary lesion at the site of inoculation. Sporotrichosis may occur in other clinical forms and may be severe (Lavalle and Mariat, 1983).

The morphologic and cultural characteristics of this fungal pathogen were first described by Schenck in 1898. In the same publication, E. F. Smith suggested its inclusion in the genus *Sporotrichum*. In 1900, Hektoen and Perkins described a new human case of sporotrichosis and proposed the name *S. schenckii*. A black variety of the fungus was isolated in Europe in 1903 by de Beurmann and Ramond and was described under the name *Sporotrichum beurmanni*. In less than ten years, these authors observed more than 200 cases of sporotrichosis in France and published two classic studies: "Les sporotrichum pathogènes" in 1911 and "Les sporotrichoses" in 1912. Epidemics of sporotrichosis occurred in South Africa in 1927 and especially from 1941 to 1943. *S. schenckii* is reviewed by Nicot and Mariat (1973), Rippon (1974), Mariat (1977) and Travassos and Lloyd (1980).

TAXONOMY. The binomial *Sporothrix schenckii*, as proposed by Hektoen and Perkins, was long ignored and the fungus was classified in the genus *Sporotrichum*. At first, two species were recognized on the basis of pigment: *Sporotrichum beurmanni* (brown to black colonies) and *S. schenckii* (non-pigmented colonies). Other species created on the basis of different cultural characteristics were later consolidated into a single taxon, *S. schenckii*. Carmichael and Nicot and Mariat have established the validity of the binomial *S. schenckii*. The fungus is provisionally classed as Deuteromycotina (Fungi Imperfecti), Hyphomycetes, sympodulosporae, amerosporae.

The perfect state of *S. schenckii* has not been precisely established. On the basis of ecologic, morphologic, physiologic, immunologic, and biochemical properties, it has been speculated that *S. schenckii* is closely related to the ascomycetous fungi of the genus *Ceratocystis*. Mariat (1977) has reviewed the taxonomic problems concerned with the *Sporothrix-Ceratocystis* complex and pointed out the possible phylogenetic relationship of *S. schenckii* to *C. stenoceras* as well as other species of *Ceratocystis*.

Synonymy. *Sporothrix schenckii* Hektoen and Perkins 1900 = Sporotrichum sp. = *Sporotrichum beurmanni* = *Sporotrichum asteroides* = *Sporotrichum equi* = *Sporotrichum jeanselmei* = *Sporotrichum councilmani* = *Sporotrichum grigsby* = *Sporotrichum oculare* = *Sporotrichum biparasiticus* = *Sporotrichum tropicale* = *Rhinocladium beurmanni.*

Possible perfect stage: *Ceratocystis stenoceras* (Robak) Moreau or another *Ceratocystis* species with a *Sporothrix* mode of conidiogenesis.

MORPHOLOGY

The Saprophytic Mycelial Phase. The colonial morphology of *S. schenckii* varies with the strain when grown at 20 to 30°C on Sabouraud dextrose agar. It may be smooth, glabrous or velvety, folded or wrinkled, and sometimes moist with or without erect coremia. The colony varies from yellowish white to black. The consistency is always membranous and resistant. Sectorial variation is frequent.

The microscopic characters are relatively constant (Fig. 1). The thin, septate, mycelial filaments (1.5 μm in diameter) branch and bear mononucleate, hyaline conidia, which measure 1.5 to 2.5 by 2.5 to 5.5 μm. The ovoid to elongate conidia are borne directly on the vegetative filament by short sterigmata (radulaspores), or in clusters or bouquets at the top of fertile erect branches. In the latter case, the spores appear successive (sympodulospores). Many strains of *S. schenckii* produce a thick-walled, pigmented spore that is spherical to conical and characteristically triangular in contour. These spores measure from 2.5 to 4.0 μm in diameter. They are borne on the filament in the same fashion as the hyaline conidia but the sterigmata are larger. These conidia may be interpreted as "macrospores" and are considered specific for *S. schenckii.*

Yeast Phase in Vitro. *S. schenckii* is dimorphic. The saprophytic state is filamentous when grown at 20 to 30°C, whereas the parasitic form is yeastlike. The unicellular yeastlike form is obtained when grown at 37°C under CO_2 on a blood agar base (brain heart infusion agar, for instance) or in liquid shaker culture. Yeastlike colonies grown on a blood agar base resemble bacterial colonies and are creamy. The surface is moist, smooth, and off-white in color.

Yeastlike cells from cultures differ in morphology from those seen in vivo. The cells are ovoid to globose to elongate and measure 2.5 to 5.0 by 3.5 to 6.5 μm. Mycelial to yeast transformation occurs by direct budding from the conidium, the mycelium or by the formation of oidial yeastlike cells within the interior of the same filament (Garrison et al., 1975, 1982).

Ultrastructure of S. schenckii. Studies of yeastlike and mycelial phase cells of *S. schenckii* indicate that the cytoplasm of both forms contains typical fungal organelles (Lane *et al.*, 1969). The septal area of the mycelial phase cell is typical of that of an ascomycetous fungus. Cells of both phases are usually mononucleate and contain numerous mitochondria, an endoplasmic reticulum with ribosomes, and scattered vacuoles of varying size. Membrane-bound, osmiophilic structures thought to be involved in lipid storage may be observed in young cells of both phases (Garrison et al., 1977). A thickened, electron-dense layer of microfibrillar material is seen at the outer surface of the yeastlike cell wall. This material may be composed in part of an acid mucosubstance and represent portions of an extracellular capsular or slime layer.

PHYSIOLOGY. Physiologic characteristics are of little importance for the recognition of the species. All cultures isolated from cases of sporotrichosis require the pyrimidine moiety of thiamine for growth. A study of 15 strains showed that xylose, glucose, fructose, galactose, maltose, starch, and glycerol are readily utilized, but that acetate, citrate, and tartrate are not. Utilization of sucrose, lactose, and arabinose is strain variable.

The precise physiologic conditions necessary for the development of the yeastlike form are not known, although the presence of CO_2 appears important. It is interesting that the RNA/DNA ratio of mycelial phase cells is significantly higher than that of yeastlike cells.

LABORATORY DIAGNOSIS

Direct Examination. Smears of pus or sputum may be examined by the Gram stain or Giemsa stain. The parasitic yeastlike form of *S. schenckii* is observed very rarely on staining of clinical materials. However, in some cases they may be abundant. The yeastlike cells are small (2 to 3 by 3 to 6 μm) and spherical to ovoid to cigar-shaped, and may possess one or two buds. The cells are gram variable and are often surrounded by a clear halo. Staining by the fluorescent antibody method of Kaplan and González Ochoa or pretreatment of smears with diastase as proposed by Fetter may help demonstrate the yeastlike forms.

Histopathology. The cutaneous lesion is an irregular or papillomatous acanthosis with intradermal microabscesses containing lymphocytic and plasmocytic infiltrates. There are frequent giant cells and peripheral fibrosis. The granuloma may have three concentric zones: central suppurative, intermediate tuberculoid, and peripheral syphiloid. However, these zones are often indistinguishable. These pathologic features are not specific.

The parasitic yeastlike forms are very difficult to see in stained histologic sections of clinical materials. When present, the yeastlike cells are readily stained by the PAS or Gomori-Grocott methods. The cellular morphology resembles that of cells from pure cultures.

In many cases, and especially in chronic sporotrichosis, asteroid bodies may be readily seen on staining with hematoxylin-eosin. These structures are spherical to ovoid, large (3 to 10 μm in diameter), thick-walled cells that may bud. The cell is surrounded by eosinophilic projections in an irregular pattern. This eosinophilic material is thought to result from precipitation of an antigen-antibody complex (the Hoeppli-Splendore phenomenon). The diameter of the complete asteroid body may reach about 30 μm.

Cultures. *S. schenckii* may be isolated readily from clinical materials on various routine culture media. The mycelial phase is obtained in three to five days when grown on Sabouraud dextrose agar at room temperature. The fungus is resistant to cycloheximide and chloramphenicol. Thus, the addition of 0.5 g/liter cycloheximide and 0.1 g/liter chloramphenicol to the medium before sterilization helps isolate the fungus in pure culture. The yeastlike form may be obtained by inoculation on brain-heart infusion blood agar and then incubation at 37°C under CO_2. Mycelial to yeastlike cell transformation is important for specific identification of *S. schenckii.*

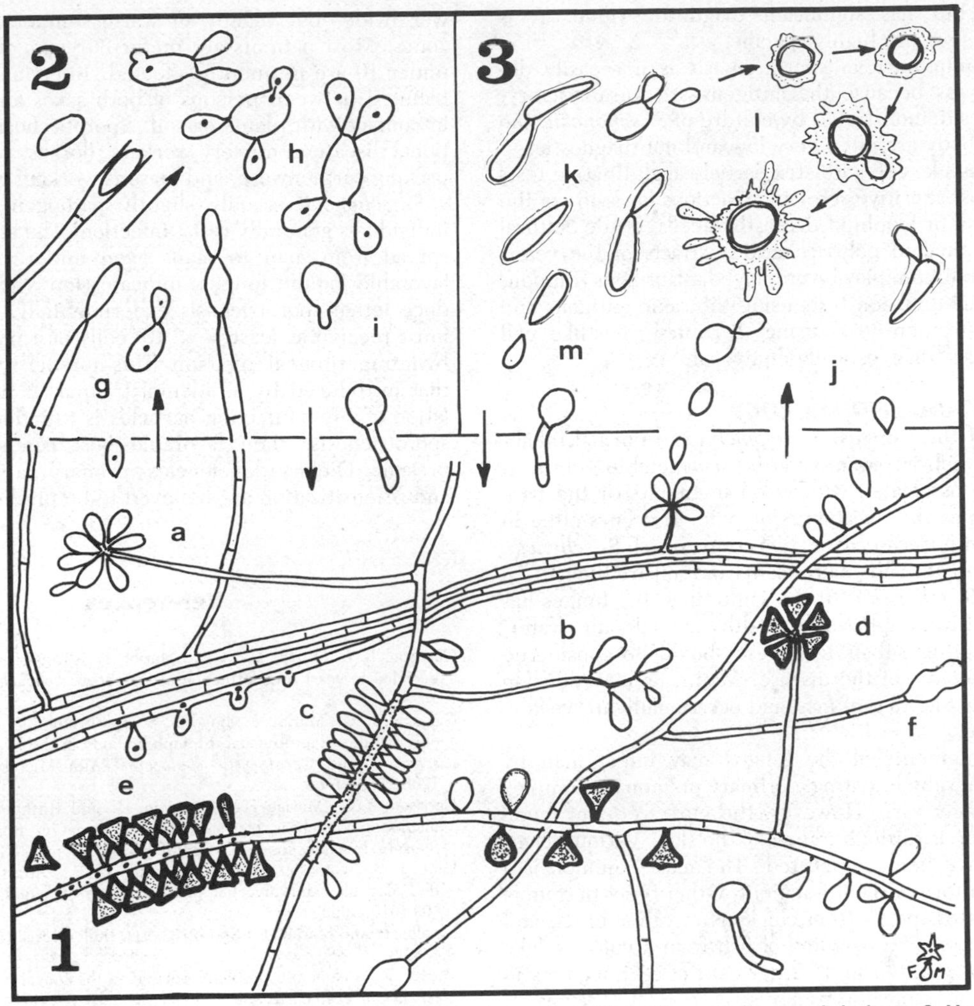

Figure 1. Diagrammatic representation of the life cycle of *Sporothrix schenckii.* 1, Saprophytic mycelial phase. 2, Yeastlike phase in vitro. 3, Parasitic yeastlike phase in vivo. a, Hyaline conidia in clusters. b, Conidia in sympodium. c, Conidia in radula. d, Triangular pigmented macrospores in clusters. e, Macrospores in radula. f, Chlamydospores. g, Mycelial (M) to yeast (Y) transformation in vitro. h, Yeastlike budding cells in vitro. i, Y→M transformation. j, M→Y transformation in vivo. k, Yeastlike budding cells in vivo. l, Asteroid bodies. m, Y→M transformation.

Laboratory Animal Inoculations. Intraperitoneal inoculations may be made in male mice or male rats, although male hamsters are the animals of choice. Characteristic disease is produced in two to three weeks, with involvement of the spleen, liver, and testes. Sections of these organs stained by the PAS, Gomori-Grocott or Gram method reveal abundant intracellular yeastlike forms. Asteroid bodies are usually frequent in histologic sections of the testes. Yeastlike forms are much easier to demonstrate in experimental infections than in naturally acquired disease. They are gram positive and resemble large rods.

ANTIGENIC COMPOSITION. Protein and lipid fractions from extracts of *S. schenckii* have been studied, but cell-wall glycoproteins are the most active antigens.

Comparative studies done by Toriello and Mariat have shown that polysaccharides synthesized by *S. schenckii* contain mannose and rhamnose as the main sugars, although appreciable amounts of galactose and traces of glucose and hexosamine occur. It is noteworthy that rhamnose is not frequently found in fungi. A protein moiety containing 1.1 to 1.9 per cent nitrogen is bound strongly to the polysaccharides.

The structure of the polysaccharides as peptido-rhamnomannans has been defined by Lloyd et al., Travassos et al., and Gorin et al., quoted by Mariat (1977) and Travassos and Lloyd (1980).

IMMUNITY. *S. schenckii* is ubiquitous in the environment, and natural resistance to infection is high. In endemic areas, hypersensitivity is noted in individuals with no clinical signs of disease. In such individuals, this state of hypersensitivity may affect the course of the infection.

Hypersensitivity may be determined by intradermal skin tests with cellular sporotrichin (a suspension of heat and/or chemically killed spores or yeastlike cells containing about 5×10^7 cells/ml). A positive skin test to cellular sporotrichin occurs in persons having immunosensitizing contact with *S. schenckii.* Clinical signs may or may not occur. Sporotrichin prepared from crude polysaccharide or purified peptido-rhamno-mannan extracts from the culture fluid of yeastlike phase *S. schenckii* is epidemiologically less interesting, but has significant diagnostic value. It is strongly reactive and highly specific.

Humoral immunity in sporotrichosis is not easily detected, perhaps because the antigens are unsatisfactory. Even in cases demonstrated by culture of *S. schenckii*, the titers of antibody are often very low and not diagnostic.

Whole yeastlike cell and latex particle agglutination tests seem the most sensitive serologic reactions for study of the disease. Fresh or lyophilized yeastlike cells, crude cultural extracts, or purified polysaccharide extracts of the yeastlike cultural medium may be employed as antigens (Rippon, 1974). Immunodiffusion tests using the same antigens and complement-fixation tests using disrupted yeastlike cell suspensions are diagnostically equivocal.

ECOLOGY AND EPIDEMIOLOGY

Ecology of the Fungus. *S. schenckii* is a normal inhabitant of soils rich in organic matter or vegetable debris. It is frequently associated with wood fragments or the bark of trees such as the eucalyptus or pine. It occurs often in association with *Ceratocystis stenoceras*, which *S. schenckii* closely resembles. Thus, both plants and soil are the natural reservoir of *S. schenckii*. At the same time, the fungus has been isolated from apparently healthy animals, air, water, and various other substrates; these should be considered as possible vectors of the disease. Mammals may develop sporotrichosis like that of man and occasionally are vectors of the disease.

Mycelial elements of the fungus may infect man by inhalation, thereby initiating a primary pulmonary complex that is no longer rare. However, the most frequent mode of transmission is through trauma of the skin. Various forms of trauma have been implicated. The most common is a prick from a thorn or plant fragment. Other types of trauma are animal bites, pecks from chickens or other birds, and stings of insects. The handling of fish from a volcanic lake in Guatemala resulted in 43.3 per cent of 53 infections in this endemic area of sporotrichosis.

The presence of *S. schenckii* and *C. stenoceras* in the same ecologic site is to be emphasized. *C. stenoceras* is widespread in nature, and its morphologic, biochemical, and antigenic characteristics are very similar, if not identical, to those of *S. schenckii*. It may play an important role in the epidemiology of sporotrichosis.

Epidemiology of Sporotrichosis. The disease occurs worldwide, but mainly in warm temperate and tropical zones. Most patients are under 30 years old and children under 10 are frequently affected. Infection is equally distributed between persons of both sexes and mainly those in contact with plants or soil. Sporotrichosis is an occupational disease of nursery workers, florists, potters, workers packing earthenware, and masons working with raw bricks.

S. schenckii is only slightly pathogenic, and healthy individuals generally resist infection. The absence of direct spread from man to man, even under conditions most favorable for the fungus, indicates low virulence. To produce lethal sporotrichosis experimentally, male hamsters must receive at least 5×10^6 cells of a pathogenic strain by intraperitoneal injection. This number is far higher than that introduced by accidental trauma. If traumatic inoculation of a few infecting particles is to induce spontaneous sporotrichosis, then favorable host conditions must be present. Dietary deficiencies, primary pathologic defects, and resensitization are believed to be predisposing factors.

References

Garrison, R. G., Boyd, K. S., and Mariat, F.: Ultrastructural studies of the mycelial to yeast transformation of *Sporothrix schenckii*. J Bact 124:959, 1975.

Garrison, R. G., Mariat, F., Boyd, K. S., and Fromentin, H.: Ultrastructural observations of an unusual osmiophilic body in the hyphae of *Sporothrix schenckii* and *Ceratocystis stenoceras*. Ann Microbiol (Inst Pasteur) 128B:275, 1977.

Garrison, R. G., Mariat, F., Fromentin, H., and Mirikitani, F. K.: Electron microscopic analysis of yeastlike cell formation from the conidia of *Sporothrix schenckii*. Ann Microbiol (Inst Pasteur) 133B:189, 1982.

Lane, J. W., Garrison, R. G., and Field, M. F.: Ultrastructural studies of the yeast-like and mycelial phases of *Sporotrichum schenckii*. J Bact 100:1010, 1969.

Lavalle, P. and Mariat, F.: Sporotrichosis. Bulletin Institut Pasteur, 81:295, 1983.

Mariat, F.: Taxonomic problems related to the fungal complex *Sporothrix schenckii/Ceratocystis spp*. In Iwata, K. (ed.): Recent Advances in Medical and Veterinary Mycology. Baltimore, University Park Press, 1977, p. 265.

Nicot, J., and Mariat, F.: Caractères morphologiques et position systématique de *Sporothrix schenckii*, agent de la sporotrichose humaine. Mycopath Mycol Applic 49:53, 1973.

Rippon, J. W.: Medical Mycology. The Pathogenic Fungi and the Pathogenic Actinomycetes. Philadelphia, W. B. Saunders Company, 1982.

Travassos, L. R., and Lloyd, K. O.: *Sporothrix schenckii* and related species of *Ceratocystis*. Microbiol Rev 44:683, 1980.

76

HISTOPLASMA CAPSULATUM

HOWARD W. LARSH, PH.D.

NANCY K. HALL, PH.D.

The etiologic agent of histoplasmosis, *Histoplasma capsulatum*, was mistakenly identified in 1906 by Darling as a protozoan *(Leishmania)*. Later, the infectious agent was proved to be a fungus with a pathogenic yeast stage and a saprophytic mycelial stage. Histoplasmosis varies from a mild or unnoticed respiratory infection to a widely disseminated lethal disease. African histoplasmosis caused by *H. capsulatum* var. duboisii rarely infects the lung but attacks the skin and bones. It is also known as histoplasmosis duboisii.

MORPHOLOGY. *Histoplasma capsulatum* is a dimorphic fungus. In its natural habitat in soils and at room temperature on agar, it grows as a mold. The colony on agar is usually fluffy and either white or buff-brown. Two types of spores are formed by most strains: small spherical aleuriospores (microconidia) that are 2 to 4 μ in diameter and larger macroaleuriospores (macroconidia) that measure 8 to 14 μ in diameter. Both micro and macro spores are found at the end of narrow aleuriophores that arise at right angles from vegetative mycelia. With time, the surface of the macroaleuriospores may become covered with evenly spaced spines ("tubercles"), which gives them a character-

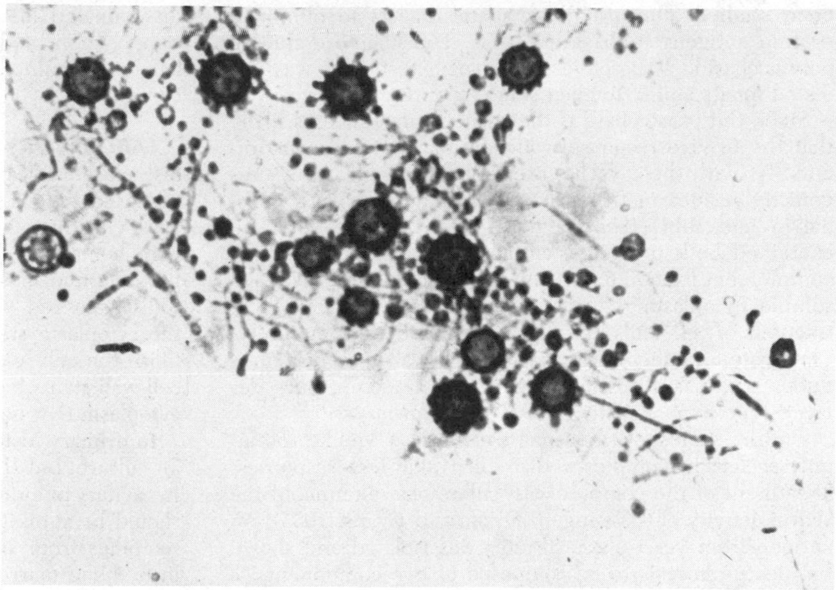

Figure 1. Macroaleuriospores (macroconidia) of *Histoplasma capsulatum* covered with spines or "tubercles."

istic appearance (Fig. 1). These structures are not absolutely diagnostic, however, since a saprophytic mold *Sepedonium* also produces tuberculate spores.

When *H. capsulatum* grows in tissue, it transforms into a small oval yeast. The yeast phase can also be propagated in vitro on blood agar media. Colonies are white and moist. Individual yeast are 2 to 4 μ long and reproduce by budding at their narrow end (Fig. 2). The pore that connects mother and daughter cells is narrow and fragile and therefore may break prematurely, producing marked variation in the size of individual cells. The cell wall is thin. When stained, the cytoplasm shrinks away from the cell wall, creating a halo that has been mistaken for a capsule. Each cell contains only one nucleus, which may be hard to see in stained preparations.

The perfect stage of *H. capsulatum* has been described. It is heterothallic and is therefore classified in the family Gymnoascaceae of the Ascomycetes.

In lesions, the *duboisii* strains of African histoplasmosis resemble the double-contoured yeast cells of blastomycosis with diameters up to 15 μ. In culture, the morphology is identical grossly and microscopically to *H. capsulatum*.

ANTIGENIC COMPOSITION. Four major antigenic preparations are now used for investigative, clinical, and epidemiologic studies of histoplasmosis: extracts of mycelial and yeast-phase cells of *H. capsulatum* and culture filtrates of the two morphologic types. The classic mycelial culture filtrate antigen (histoplasmin) is prepared from a synthetic broth culture incubated at room temperature.

The active components of mycelial culture filtrates have been identified by using column chromatography and polyacrylamide disk gel electrophoresis (Sprouse et al., 1969). Two antigenic fractions were found in a five-month asparagine medium preparation, the more potent being a high molecular weight protein that elicits a skin-test reaction in guinea pigs with experimental histoplasmosis.

By using an ammonium sulfate precipitation and Pevikon block electrophoresis, crude histoplasmin has also been separated into two main fractions, a protein that elicits a positive skin test and a less reactive fraction rich in polysaccharide (O'Connell et al., 1967). No increase in skin sensitivity was observed with either fraction.

Many techniques have been used to isolate and characterize a reactive component from the mycelial phase cells themselves. Alkali-extracted mycelium yielded a galactomannan protein complex that is separable into polysaccharide and glycoprotein complexes by ion-exchange chromatography (Reiss et al., 1974). The galactomannan did not elicit a skin-test response, but it elicited a cell-mediated reaction (production of migration-inhibition factor) from sensitized lymphocytes.

Polysaccharide antigens of mycelial *H. capsulatum* have

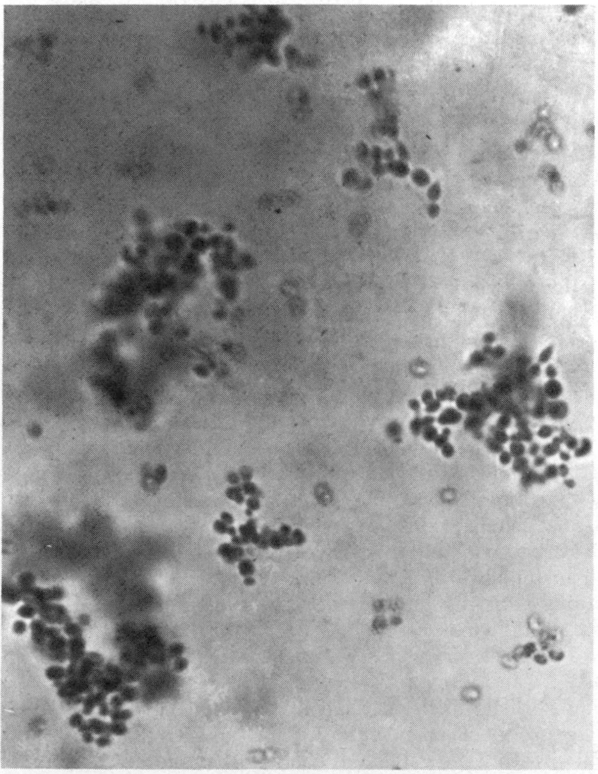

Figure 2. Yeast phase of *H. capsulatum* grown in vitro. Individual yeast are 2 to 4 μ long and reproduce by budding.

been studied after using enzymatic digests to eliminate protein antigens (Kobayashi, 1971). The mannose-glucose polysaccharide was active in serologic tests but was not tested for its ability to elicit skin responses.

Since the yeast phase is the tissue form, it seems likely that the in vivo response would be to yeast-cell constituents. As with the mycelial preparations, most of the antigenicity resides in the protein-rich moiety of yeast cells. Salvin and Ribi (1955) demonstrated that the cell wall contained both protective antigens and antigens used for complement fixation tests. Domer and Ichinose (1977) used soluble cytoplasmic substances and ethylenediamine extractions of cell walls in assays of cell-mediated immunity. The protein moiety of the isolated cell-wall glycoprotein is under study as a possible antigen for detecting pure delayed-type hypersensitivity to *H. capsulatum.*

Culture fluids of yeast-phase cells also yield protein-polysaccharide complexes that elicit skin-test responses. Treatment of the complex with chloroform eliminated the skin reactivity of the antigen (Dyson and Evans, 1955). An antigen from yeast-phase filtrates was isolated and shown by electrophoresis to be composed of two components, a skin-test reactive protein and a less reactive polysaccharide. Increased specificity has not been achieved.

A purified, specific antigen capable of standardization is being sought in mycelium, mycelial culture filtrates, yeast, and yeast-phase culture filtrates.

IMMUNITY. Immunity to *H. capsulatum* correlates with the development of delayed hypersensitivity. In experimental animals, immunity is transferable with T-lymphocytes. Macrophages from immunized mice inhibit the growth of ingested macrophages, presumably due to activation by lymphokines (Howard and Otto, 1977). The antigen(s) responsible for eliciting a cellular immune response has not been identified. Antibody to the fungus is produced regularly in response to infection but does not result in immunity.

PATHOGENESIS. The source of human infection is soil containing spores of *H. capsulatum* (see Epidemiology). The fungus has been isolated from soil in areas occupied by chickens, other birds, and bats. Contamination of caves with *H. capsulatum* may lead to outbreaks of "cave fever." City dwellers are often exposed to the fungus grown in soil under trees that shelter starlings or blackbirds. The portal of entry is the lung, where a primary complex may be formed by extension of infection from the pulmonary focus to the regional lymph nodes. Most primary infections undergo benign self-limited dissemination, as evidenced by hepatic and splenic calcifications.

The basic pathologic process is multiplication of *H. capsulatum* in reticuloendothelial cells of the liver, lymph nodes, lung, spleen, adrenal glands, intestine, and marrow. The adrenals, which are involved in nearly all disseminated infections, are often massively enlarged. Least resistance to histoplasmosis is encountered in young infants and in adults after the fifth decade, when most cases of disseminated infection occur.

The portal of entry of *H. duboisii* is unknown, but might also be the lung. It rarely causes disease there, however, and spreads to the skin, lymph nodes, or bone where it may produce a single chronic localized granulomatous mass filled with huge giant cells containing numerous yeast cells (Cockshott and Lucas, 1964). It may also cause rapidly fatal disseminated histoplasmosis with multiple lesions in the skin, lymph nodes, bones, and abdominal viscera. In laboratory animals, *H. duboisii* is less virulent than *H. capsulatum.*

LABORATORY DIAGNOSIS. A definitive diagnosis of histoplasmosis can be made by culturing the fungus from tissue secretions or excretions, or by demonstrating the yeast cells histologically. *H. capsulatum* stains very poorly with hematoxylin-eosin and is usually evident only as a protoplasmic mass surrounded by a halo. The yeast cell walls stain red with periodic acid-Schiff stains, although the cytoplasm stains poorly. With silver stains (e.g., Gomori) the cell wall is black. Organisms appear larger with cell-wall stains because the artifactual shrinkage of the cell cytoplasm that occurs during fixation is not evident.

In primary histoplasmosis, sputum is often not produced for culture, but *H. capsulatum* may be cultured from urine. In cavitary pneumonias, sputum or gastric lavage specimens should be submitted for culture. In disseminated disease, scrapings from surface lesions, tissue biopsies (especially liver, bone marrow, and lymph nodes), blood, urine, and sputum may yield positive cultures.

Specimens for microscopic examination of secretions are fixed and air-dried on a microscope slide and then stained using either the Giemsa or Wright method. The yeast appear in histiocytes and macrophages as small oval cells, 2 to 5 μ in diameter. If rupture of the phagocytic cells occurs, it may be difficult to differentiate the extracellular *H. capsulatum* from other yeasts. Nevertheless, their small size, the budding from the narrow end, and the narrow attachment to the mother cells are distinguishing characteristics.

The use of test tubes or Petri dishes for inoculation of sputum is debatable. The organism is an obligate aerobe, and Petri dishes allow more inoculum to be spread on the surface of the medium, but unsealed Petri dishes may present a hazard to laboratory personnel. The specimens suspected of harboring pathogenic fungi should be cultured in a bacteriologic safety hood.

Sputum as well as all other secretions and excretions should be treated with antibiotics to suppress contaminating bacteria. To ensure that the specimens are well homogenized, they may be diluted with sterile cysteine-saline and shaken in a mechanical shaker for 30 minutes to an hour. One-half milliliter of sputum, urine, gastric, or bronchial lavage is added to the following media, and the plates incubated for at least four weeks: (1) Emmon's modified Sabouraud's agar pH 7 without antibiotics; (2) Emmon's modified Sabouraud's agar (1 per cent Neopeptone, 2 per cent glucose, 2 per cent agar) pH 7 with penicillin, streptomycin, and Actidione or the same medium with chloramphenicol and Actidione; (3) blood agar base with 5 per cent defibrinated blood with gentamicin and Actidione, or blood agar base with 5 per cent defibrinated blood with gentamicin, carbenicillin, and Actidione. At least one medium should contain no Actidione, since *Cryptococcus neoformans, Petriellidium boydii, Aspergillus* sp., and other fungi that may cause pulmonary disease are inhibited by the antifungal agent.

Another medium using a soil extract has been routinely used in our laboratories for the past five years. The medium accelerates growth so that it appears as early as one to three days. The number of tuberculated macroaleuriospores in cultures grown on soil extract agar is greater than the number routinely found on screening media.

Sterile tissue grinders are used to prepare tissues for plating. The homogenates are diluted and one-half milliliter is spread on the media listed above. Spinal fluids and other aseptic specimens are plated directly on the media without addition of antibiotics.

Most isolates of *H. capsulatum* do not grow well at 37°C, since it is near the maximal growth range of this fungus. If the yeast stage is to be obtained from infected tissue, an enriched medium containing blood should be used and incubated at 30°C. Mycelium can be converted without difficulty to the pathogenic yeast stage by inoculating tissue cultures (e.g., Hela cells).

Periodic examination of the cultures after 7 to 10 days usually reveals growth. From "typical" cultures, lactophenol preparations can be made of the mycelia that reveal microaleuriospores and macroaleuriospores.

In the patient with chronic histoplasmosis, an isolate of *H. capsulatum* frequently is "atypical." Neither microaleuriospores nor macroaleuriospores are produced, and the cultures may be neither white nor brown. These isolates must be inoculated into mice or tissue culture to obtain the yeast form of the fungus. Mice often survive the infection and should be autopsied two to four weeks after inoculation to demonstrate the yeast cells in liver and spleen. Sputum, or other material contaminated with bacteria, should be treated with antibiotics before injection. Alternatively, *H. capsulatum* can be identified by detecting serologically specific exoantigens in broth culture supernatants of the mold (Standard and Kaufman, 1976).

In ecologic studies, mice are usually used to isolate *H. capsulatum* from soils, bird feces, and other highly contaminated specimens. The samples must be treated with antibiotics before inoculation intraperitoneally. In addition, antibiotics may be added to the drinking water and a second injection of antibiotic administered after 24 hours.

The antibody response to *H. capsulatum* is complex. Immunodiffusion of histoplasmin against *Histoplasma* antisera results in six distinct precipitin bands (Heiner, 1958). These bands correlate with the clinical condition of the patient: H-band is associated with infection; M-band appears after skin tests with mycelial antigen or infection; c-band indicates exposure to skin testing with histoplasmin, coccidioidin, or blastomycin; n-band is nonspecific, and x- and y-bands are of unknown significance.

The complement fixation antigens in common use are whole yeast-phase cells or histoplasmin. Due to the unpredictability of the individual patient response, both antigens should be used; for example, sera may react with only one antigen or with both antigens in variable titer (Campbell, 1960). Complement fixation titers normally appear soon after onset of clinical symptoms and may persist for months or years after infection. Titers usually parallel the course of the disease. Titers are low or negative at first (and may remain so in asymptomatic infections), rise during the acute illness, and disappear slowly after several months. In the progressive form of the disease, titers remain high for a long time.

Recently, the sensitivity of serologic tests was reassessed after a large urban epidemic (Wheat et al., 1982). M or H bands were as specific for infections as a yeast phase CF titer of 1:32 or greater. However, 15–20 per cent of patients had negative precipitin tests. Only 3 per cent of nonimmunosuppressed patients had CF titers of 1:8 or less, using both the yeast and mycelial antigens.

A particulate agglutination test is also used to demonstrate antibodies to *H. capsulatum*. Histoplasmin is adsorbed to collodion particles, to sheep erythrocytes, or to latex particles to serve as antigen. Whole yeast-phase cells can also be used successfully (Cozad and Larsh, 1960).

EPIDEMIOLOGY. The growth of *H. capsulatum* in soils enriched with bird or bat droppings is the source of human and animal exposure. Disturbances of the environment in which the fungus is growing produce aerosols containing aleuriospores that may be inhaled and cause primary infections. The specific role of feces in large bird roosts in the epidemiology of the disease is clear. The birds themselves do not contract histoplasmosis as a natural infection, since the blood temperature of birds is too high to support growth of the fungus. The fungus is not communicable from person to person, animal to person, or animal to animal. Each species acquires a natural infection by inhalation of spores. The fungus is also associated with bat guano, and some caves are heavily contaminated. Bats can develop histoplasmosis. The urban brown bat may be another source of histoplasmosis in urban areas.

H. capsulatum is an aerobic organism that grows in the upper 1 to 3 centimeters of soil or other enriched materials. Although there is controversy about whether or not this fungus has been isolated from dry pigeon droppings, it is conceded that pigeon droppings will enrich the ability of the soil to support the growth of *H. capsulatum* (Ajello, 1964). It is important to understand that although birds are not naturally infected, their droppings provide an enriched medium for the growth of *H. capsulatum*, whereas certain bats have the disease and their droppings can likewise support the growth of the fungus (Emmons, 1958).

The distribution of *H. capsulatum* in the soil is not uniform, even in highly endemic areas. Frequently *H. capsulatum* can be isolated from soil at the site of a point-source epidemic, but the soil only a few inches away will be negative. It is very difficult to disinfect contaminated soil.

The fungus has a worldwide distribution. Highly endemic areas have been identified by serologic and skin-test surveys with histoplasmin. In highly endemic areas such as the Ohio and Mississippi River valleys in the United States, up to 90 per cent of residents react to histoplasmin. However, the fungus does exist outside these areas where it can be cultured from soil and from native animals (Ajello, 1958; Edwards, 1971). In these areas, such as the eastern seaboard of the United States, skin-test surveys do not reveal the presence of the fungus because only isolated areas of soil are contaminated, and the rate of infection is consequently low.

African histoplasmosis is limited almost exclusively to the region where trypanosomiasis is endemic between the latitudes 15 degrees north and 10 degrees south of the equator. Unlike the deserts to the north and south, some areas of this part of Africa have much rain and humidity. Like American histoplasmosis, the *duboisii* type may be acquired upon exposure to chicken and bat excretion.

References

Ajello, L.: Geographic distribution of *Histoplasma capsulatum*. Mykosen 1:147, 1958.

Ajello, L.: Relationship of *Histoplasma capsulatum* to avian habitats. Pub Health Rep 79:266, 1964.

Campbell, C. C.: The accuracy of serologic methods in diagnosis. Ann NY Acad Sci 89:163, 1960.

Cockshott, W. P., and Lucas A. O.: Histoplasmosis duboisii. Quart J Med 33:223, 1964.
Cozad, G. C., and Larsh, H. W.: A capillary tube agglutination test for histoplasmosis. J Immunol 85:387, 1960.
Darling, S. T. A.: A protozoon general infection producing pseudotubercles in the lungs and focal necroses in the liver. JAMA 46:1283, 1906.
Domer, J. E., and Ichinose, H.: Cellular immune responses in guinea pigs immunized with cell walls of *Histoplasma capsulatum* prepared by several different procedures. Infect Immun 16:293, 1977.
Dyson, J. E., and Evans, E. E.: Delayed hypersensitivity in experimental fungus infection. J Lab Clin Med 45:449, 1955.
Edwards, P. Q.: Histoplasmin sensitivity patterns around the world. In Histoplasmosis. Proceedings of the Second National Conference. Springfield, Ill., Charles C Thomas, 1971.
Emmons, C. W.: Association of bats with histoplasmosis. Pub Hlth Rept 73:590, 1958.
Goodman, N. L., Sprouse, R. F., and Larsh, H. W.: Histoplasmin potency as affected by culture age. Sabouraudia 6:273, 1968.
Heiner, D. C.: Diagnosis of histoplasmosis using precipitin reactions in agar gel. Pediatrics 22:616, 1958.
Howard, D., and Otto, V.: Experiments on lymphocyte-mediated cellular immunity in murine histoplasmosis. Infect Immunity 16:226, 1977.
Kaufman, L., and Standard, P.: Improved version of the exoantigen test for identification of *Coccidioides immitis* and *Histoplasma capsulatum*. J Clin Microbiol 8:42, 1978.
Kobayashi, G. S.: Isolation and characterization of polysaccharide of *Histoplasma capsulatum*. In Histoplasmosis. Proceedings of the Second National Conference. Springfield, Ill., Charles C Thomas, 1971.
O'Connell, E. J., Hermans, P. E., and Markowitz, H.: Skin reactive antigens of *Histoplasma capsulatum*. Proc Soc Exp Biol Med 124:1015, 1967.
Reiss, E., Mitchell, W. O., Stone, S. H., and Hasenclever, H. F.: Cellular immune activity of a galactomannan-protein complex from mycelia of *Histoplasma capsulatum*. Infect Immun 10:802, 1974.
Salvin, S. B., and Ribi, E.: Antigens from yeast phase of *Histoplasma capsulatum*. Proc Soc Exp Biol Med 108:498, 1955.
Sprouse, R. F., Goodman, N. L., and Larsh, H. W.: Fractionation, isolation and chemical characterization of skin test active components of histoplasmin. Sabouraudia 7:1, 1969.
Thor, D. E., and Dray, S.: A correlation of human delayed hypersensitivity: Specific inhibition of capillary tube migration of sensitized human lymph node cells by tuberculin and histoplasmin. J Immunol 101:51, 1968.
Wheat, J., French, M. L., Kohler, R. B., et al.: The diagnostic laboratory tests for histoplasmosis. Analysis of experience in a large urban outbreak. Annals Int Med 97:680, 1982.

77

COCCIDIOIDES IMMITIS

HENRY A. WALCH, PH.D.

MORPHOLOGY

Dimorphic Growth Cycle. *Coccidioides immitis* is a dimorphic fungus that reproduces asexually by the formation of arthroconidia in the saprophytic stage and a spherule-endospore form in infected tissues.

The arthroconidia are formed within fertile hyphae alternating with an intercalary cell. Separation and secession of the matured arthroconidium occurs following autolysis and wall collapse of the intercalary cell (Huppert et al., 1982).

Infection of man and other animals usually occurs through inhalation of arthroconidia into the lungs (Fig. 1). The arthroconidia, 2 to 3 μ in diameter and 3 to 10 μ in length, undergo a rounding up and enlargement (Fig. 2) to form the parasitic or spherule form, 20 to 80 μ in diameter, (Fig. 3). The multinucleate cytoplasm of the spherule is eventually transformed to a multitude of uninucleate endospores 2 to 3 μ in diameter (Fig. 4). This endosporulation results from a progression of segmentation planes originating from the inner spherule wall (Huppert et al., 1982). Within the body the released endospores continue the parasitic cycle by developing into mature spherules. A clinical specimen containing spherules and endospores that is cultured to a routine medium will produce the mycelium-arthroconidium colony or saprophytic stage (Fig. 5) as a result of germination of endospores and immature spherules.

It is historically pertinent to note that the spherule-endospore tissue form led the original students of this disease (1892–1896) to conclude that it was of protozoan (coccidioidal) etiology and to speciate it as *Coccidioides immitis* (not mild), since the few known human cases were all fatal.

Classification. No sexual stage has been demonstrated. However, the studies of Kwon-Chung (1969), demonstrating ultrastructural characteristics of hyphae, and those of Hupert et al. (1982), showing a simple septal pore and Woronin bodies, are mutually supportive of an ascomycetous relationship.

Cell Wall Composition. The chemical composition of the cell wall is apparently similar to that of other fungi. Chitin is present in the wall of the three morphologic forms. Other carbohydrate polymers are also present such as β-1–3 glucans, mannans, or possible glucomannans as major cell wall components. Protein is present also, and differences in amino acid composition have been found in the different morphologic forms (Wheat et al., 1977). Studies concerned specifically with the mature spherule wall have shown a structure consisting of multiple layers. The layer nearest the cell membrane appears to consist of chitin and

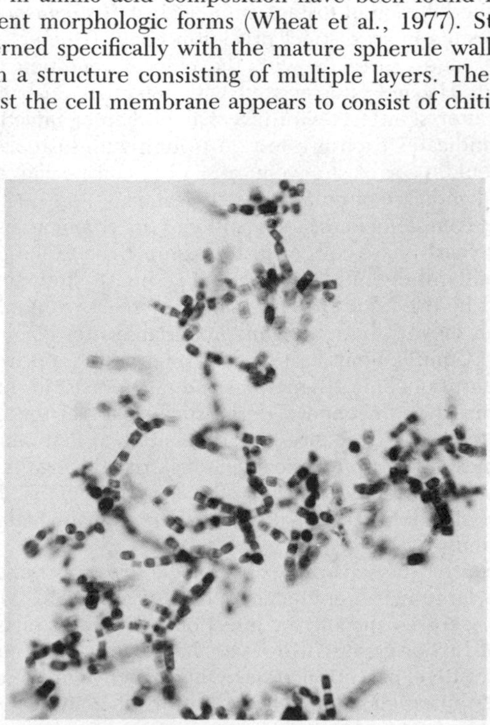

Figure 1. Arthrospores of *Coccidioides immitis* (approximately 600 ×).

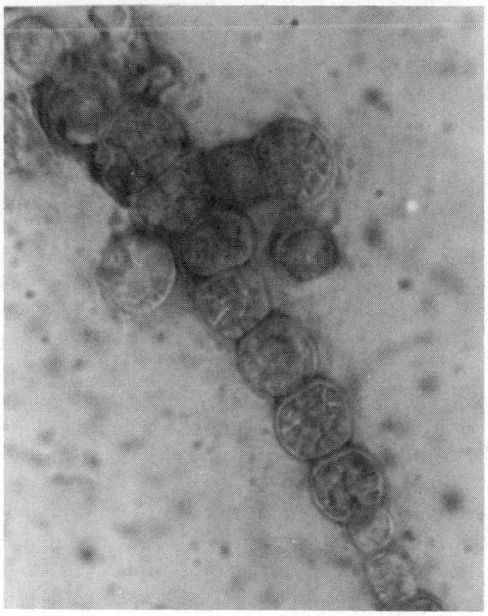

Figure 2. Chain of arthrospores of *Coccidioides immitis* undergoing spherulation in vitro (approximately 1200 ×)

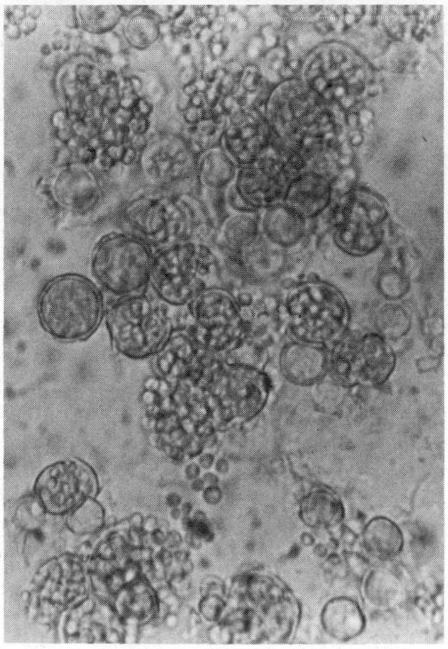

Figure 4. Mature in vitro formed spherules of *Coccidioides immitis* showing large numbers of released endospores (approximately 1200 ×).

β-1–3 glucan. The outer most layer consisted largely of α-1–3 glucan. Interspersed throughout the wall appears to be a mannan-protein complex that may serve to hold the layers together (Hector and Pappagianis, 1981).

ANTIGENIC COMPOSITION

Immunologic Test Antigens. Mycelial coccidioidin is made from a filtrate of an aging (two months) and autolyzing stationary broth culture, or a pool of broth cultures of different strains to allow for possible antigenic variability. This type of coccidioidin was originally used as a successful serologic and skin test antigen beginning in the early 1940 period (Smith et al., 1950). Because of the extensive past and continued record of use and commercial availability, it serves as a standard of comparison for test antigens. Another type of mycelial coccidioidin is a toluene-induced lysate of a young (two to three day) shaken culture (Pappagianis et al., 1961a). This has been used in immunodiffusion testing and in experimental applications. These coccidioidins can be dialyzed without loss of activity. Heat treatment by autoclaving does not impair the activity of antigens involved in precipitin testing or skin test reactivity. Complement-fixing antigen activity is destroyed, however, by heating at 60°C for 30 minutes.

Spherule coccidioidin (available commercially as spherulin) is a lysate of a washed, water suspension of in vitro

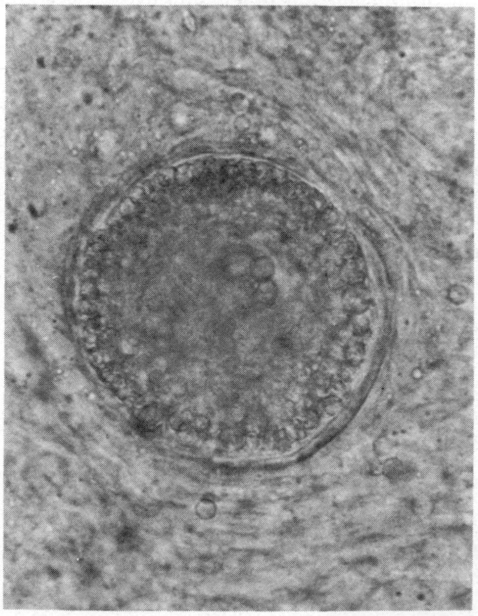

Figure 3. Large, mature spherule of *Coccidioides immitis,* unstained in tissue cleared with sodium hydroxide solution (approximately 1200 ×).

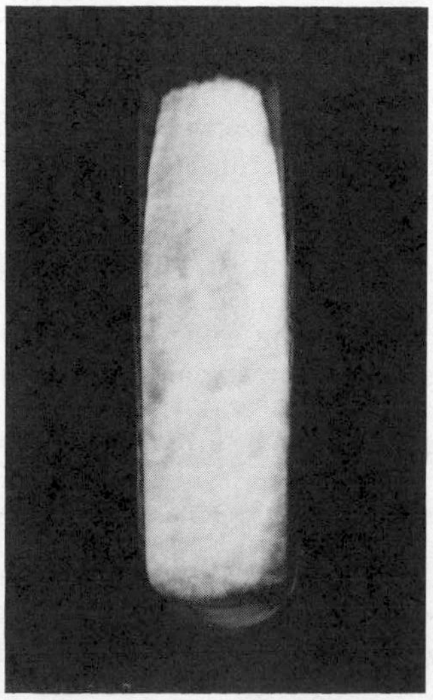

Figure 5. Mature culture of *Coccidioides immitis* showing typical aerial mycelium.

cultured, mature, endosporulating spherules (Levine et al., 1969). In common with the mycelial coccidioidins, the active portion is nondialyzable. In contrast to mycelial coccidioidin, its skin testing potency is definitely impaired by heating at 60°C for 20 minutes.

Analysis of these two complex test antigens by two-dimensional immunoelectrophoresis demonstrated at least 26 antigens for mycelial coccidioidin (as a toluene-induced lysate) and 12 for spherulin. Ten antigens were in common, two were unique to the spherule, and 16 to the mycelial derived antigens (Huppert et al., 1978).

Spherulin is more reactive and sensitive for cutaneous hypersensitivity testing than mycelial coccidioidin, and is probably more specific (Levine et al., 1973; Stevens, 1974; Levine et al., 1975). It has also been more effective as an antigen when used in the lymphocyte transformation test (Deresinski et al., 1974). Use as a complement-fixing antigen, in comparison with the mycelial coccidioidin, has shown that spherulin provided a higher titer (Scalarone et al., 1974). The results of comparing the reactivity of the two antigens with sera from noncoccidioidal mycoses, however, showed that spherulin was considerably less specific (Huppert et al., 1977).

Recent studies have reported the use of two different experimental antigens. One of these is an alkali-soluble, water-soluble extract from either mycelium or spherule walls. The mycelial extract has demonstrated a broad range of immunological reactivity and has the advantage of reproducibility of the extraction technique. Fractionation and immunoelectrophoresis has shown this antigen to comprise four components (Cox, 1981). The other antigen preparation is a supernatant filtrate of a spherule culture medium. This "endosporulation" antigen has a human lymphocyte transformation potency (at the optimal test dilution) that is 500 times greater, on a weight basis, than spherulin (Brass et al., 1982).

Antigen Standardization. Coccidioidins, as mixtures of antigens, are subject to variability of reactivity between different lots produced at different times even though conditions of culture are uniformly maintained. Because of this antigenic heterogeneity and variability, standardization by weight or chemical analysis is not useful. Also, no comparative laboratory animal testing system for biologic reactivity and potency testing is available. Therefore, standardization for serologic or cutaneous hypersensitivity testing must be done by different procedures. Details of these procedures are considered by Huppert (1970), Kobayashi and Pappagianis (1970) and Huppert et al. (1974). In summary, skin test standardization requires human subjects of known cutaneous hypersensitivity and a reference antigen. Serologic standardization requires both a reference serum and antigen and strict adherence to the prescribed test procedure.

Chemical Composition. Attempts have been made to identify the skin test-active components of mycelial coccidioidin. Pappagianis et al. (1961b) showed it was a polysaccharide composed primarily of mannose associated with some amino acids. Later studies have demonstrated that 3–0-methylmannose was a notable component (Andersen et al., 1971 and Porter et al., 1971).

Recent studies by Cox and coworkers (1981), using an alkali-soluble, water-soluble extract of mycelial cell walls in guinea pigs, showed the antigenically active component to be a polysaccharide-protein complex containing 3–0-methyl-mannose.

IMMUNITY

Infection and Immunity. The extensive human case studies of Smith and his associates (1957) provided evidence that immunity resulted from primary coccidioidomycosis. In addition, asymptomatic infection with conversion to skin test reactivity also seems to induce immunity.

The immune experience of the host begins with a transitory exposure to arthroconidia. Infecting arthroconidia possess, in addition to their own enterothallically formed wall, an attached remnant portion of the hyphal outer wall (Drutz and Huppert, (1983). Conversion of the arthroconidia to the spherule-endospore stage, and incidental exposure to the cytoplasm of these structures engenders, through multiple antigens, either humoral antibodies or the cell-mediated immune response.

Cell-Mediated Immunity. Immunity to *C. immitis* is of the cell-mediated type. Infection is accompanied by cutaneous delayed hypersensitivity, lymphocyte transformation, and macrophage migration inhibition through the use of mycelial and spherule coccidioidins. The role of T cells is implied by the resistance of normal mice to infection after receiving an intravenous inoculation of spleen cells from spherule-vaccinated mice (Beaman et al., 1977), and transfer of delayed hypersensitivity in mice (Rifkind et al., 1976).

The intactness of the mechanisms of cell-mediated immunity is of major importance, since patients who maintain or recover skin test reactivity to coccidioidin or spherulin seem to have better clinical outcomes than those who remain anergic (Drutz and Catanzaro, 1978).

Immunization. A vaccine composed of formalin-killed mature spherules has provided for increased survival and reduced pathologic involvement in mice (Levine et al., 1960; 1965). The spherule wall was the most effective immunogenic component of this vaccine (Kong et al., 1963). This monotype mature spherule-endospore vaccine protects against subsequent challenge with typical and atypical strains of established virulence, indicating a similarity of immunizing antigens among different isolates of the fungus (Huppert et al., 1967).

Immunization trials with human volunteers has begun (Pappagianis and Levine, 1975; Walker, 1981). In general, side effects have been local and minimal. Conversion to a positive skin test does not regularly occur as a result of vaccination. This lack of conversion may not, as is the case with experimental animals, correlate with any lack of immune protection.

The problem with human immunization with the whole spherule vaccine is that the quantity tolerated as a single intramuscular injection is, on a body weight basis, only 1/400 of the dose needed to immunize mice. In order to overcome this problem Pappagianis and coworkers (1979) have used particulate and supernatant extracts of spherule walls to provide protection of mice at dry weights significantly below that of the whole spherule vaccine.

LABORATORY DIAGNOSIS

Fungus Growth and Confirmation. Those who identify cultures of *C. immitis* must consider that arthroconidia are found in a number of saprophytic fungi (Sigler and Carmichael, 1976; Emmons, 1967); that atypical strains occur (Huppert et al., 1967); and that the fungus grows on cycloheximide-containing culture media, making the growth of any doubtful isolate on such a media suspicious of *C. immitis*.

In vivo confirmation is done by injection of mice intraperitoneally and guinea pigs intratesticularly in order to demonstrate spherule-endosporulation capability. Allowance must be made for the fact that virulence for mice varies considerably for different strains of the fungus. Also, the mere culture of the suspected fungus from the tissues of an injected animal is not confirmatory since nonpathogenic fungi may persist in tissues of the injected animal without any pathologic effect.

Two convenient in vitro confirmatory identification methods are available. With the method of Sun et al. (1976) arthrospores convert to spherules in three to five days. The method of Standard and Kaufman (1977) uses immunodiffusion for detecting antigens in a fluid culture supernatant and is particularly useful for atypical nonsporulating cultures.

Immunologic Diagnosis. The two serologic tests that have been most extensively documented and serve as the standards for comparison with other methods are the tube precipitin and the complement-fixation tests. Strict adherence to prescribed procedures and the use of a standardized antigen are required for diagnostic use. Details for the performance of the precipitin test are provided by Kaufman (1976). The complement-fixation procedure using the full volume test is described in the Pan American Health Organization Manual, part II (1974); for the micro complement-fixation test technique consult the United States Public Health Service Publication Number 1228 (1965). Critical evaluations of these complement-fixation methods are contained in the publications of Huppert et al. (1970) and of Kaufman et al. (1970).

Precipitating antibodies (probably IgM) occur transiently in the serum and may appear as early as the first week of illness during primary disease. Precipitins are usually not detected in the cerebrospinal fluid (Pappagianis and Crane, 1977). Serum complement-fixing antibodies (probably IgG) generally are not evident as early as precipitin antibodies, but they remain detectable for a longer period of time.

Serologic diagnosis and prognosis depend on the testing of subsequent serum samples to determine changes of the complement-fixing antibody titer. The titer usually rises in proportion to severity of disease and declines with improvement of the patient. The generally accepted interpretation of these titers in relation to the disease process is based on the studies of Smith and his associates (1950, 1956). Titers 1:16 or above indicate possible dissemination. Lower titers, 1:8 or less, may indicate early, stable residual or meningeal coccidioidomycosis or may be false positives. Negative results do not exclude disease, however, since about 40 per cent of chronic residual pulmonary disease cases are nonreactive. About 25 per cent of patients with coccidioidal meningitis give negative results when the spinal fluid is used for complement fixation but a positive complement-fixation test of cerebrospinal fluid is a valid test for the diagnosis of coccidioidal meningitis. If, however, the spinal fluid is allowed to bind complement overnight in the cold (4°C), only 5 per cent of the meningitis cases tend to be negative (Pappagianis and Crane, 1977). Other body fluids—pleural, ascitic, joint—can contain CF antibody but the titers are generally lower than simultaneously obtained serum (Pappagianis, 1980).

Alternative immunologic procedures have been studied for routine screening or supplementary test systems. Huppert and his associates (1968) have recommended a combination of the latex particle agglutination test (in place of the tube precipitin test) and the immunodiffusion test that correlates with the complement-fixation test) (IDCF) as a rapid and reliable primary test system. The ID test in conjunction with the microcomplement-fixation test is recommended by Kaufman and Clark (1974), since a positive immunodiffusion test and a low complement-fixation titer indicates active or recent disease.

EPIDEMIOLOGY

Geographic Distribution. Coccidioidomycosis is endemic only in limited areas of North, Central, and South America. In Southwestern United States, annual infection rates have been estimated at 35,000 to 100,000. These have been predominantly from Arizona and California, with fewer from Texas. New Mexico is of low endemicity and in Nevada and Utah skin test surveys give the only indication of the disease.

Mayorga and Espinoza (1970) reviewed the distribution of coccidioidomycosis in Mexico and Central America. Although most of the reported cases in Mexico are from hospitals in the states of Sonora, Neuvo Leon, and Coahuila, a more extensive occurrence of the disease is indicated by the skin test surveys of Gonzalez-Ochoa (1967). In Central America disease has been reported only from Guatemala, with eight, and Honduras, with two cases. The Guatemala endemic area, however, has a skin test reactor rate of 42.5 per cent.

At the time of Campins' report (1970) Argentina and Venezuela had 27 and 35 cases respectively, and Paraguay and Colombia 2 each. Recent soil isolations have been reported from Argentina (Borghi et al., 1977).

Transmission to Humans. The incidence of infection is directly related to occupations that break up soil. Incidental infection in an endemic area depends on proximity to areas of soil disturbance, prevailing and seasonal wind conditions, and weather patterns affecting growth of the fungus in the soil.

About 60 per cent of humans infected will be asymptomatic and the remainder will have symptoms ranging from those of a mild respiratory condition to prolonged severe illness. A small number of the primary infections will disseminate to bones, joints, internal organs, or meninges. Disseminated disease occurs in approximately 1.0 per cent of white males and 10 per cent or more of black males and an even higher percentage of Filipinos. Pregnancy may also contribute to an increased incidence of dissemination (Pappagianis, 1980). A possible interrelationship of human sex hormones as a predisposing factor to dissemination in pregnancy has been shown by two recent studies (Drutz et al., 1981; Drutz and Huppert, 1983).

Ecology. In the United States and elsewhere the fungus has been most frequently isolated from the soil in semiarid areas from sea level to a few hundred feet elevation, which have mild winters and hot summers, with a yearly rainfall total of 5 to 20 inches occurring in one or two seasonal periods. There are exceptions to these usual geographic areas of disease endemicity. In Mexico, two small tropical areas are apparently endemic. One of these, comprising Colima and Michoacan border areas, has recorded two disseminated cases in children. The other is a limited area in the state of Guerrero where skin test reactivity indicates low endemicity (González Ochoa, 1967). In the United States, from California, soil isolations have been made from a mediterranean woodland region, from areas as high as 3200 feet and from sites where occasional snow and freezing temperatures occur during winter months (Swatek, 1975).

There is no association with the macroflora (Lacy and Swatek, 1974). The fungus has been isolated from the environs and even the burrows of rodents, but there is no evidence that such sites are regular ecologic niches. The chemical and physical conditions in the soil that favor the fungus are not known beyond the general association with alkaline, sandy soil types with a high content of salts.

References

Anderson, K. L., Wheat, R. W. and Conant, N. F.: Fractionation and composition studies of skin test active components of sensitins from *Coccidioides immitis*. Appl Microbiol 22:294, 1971.

Beaman, L., Pappagianis, D., and Benjamini, E.: Significance of T cells in resistance to experimental murine coccidioidomycosis. Infect Immun 17:580, 1977.

Borghi, A. L., Rossi de Benetti, M. S., and Corallini de Bracalenti, B. J.: *Coccidioides immitis:* Su Aislamiento de Muestras de Suelos de las Provincias de San Luis Y Mendoza. Sabouraudia 15:51, 1977.

Brass, C., Levine, H. B. and Stevens, D. A.: Stimulation and suppression of cell-mediated immunity by endosporulation antigens of *Coccidioides immitis*. Infect Immun 35:431, 1982.

Campins, H.: Coccidioidomycosis in South America. A review of its epidemiology and geographic distribution. Mycopath et Mycologia Appl 40:1, 1970.

Cox, R. A., Mead, C. G. and Pavey, E. F.: Comparisons of mycelia- and spherule-derived antigens in cellular immune assays of *Coccidioides immitis*-infected guinea pigs. Infect Immun 31:687, 1981.

Deresinksi, S. C., Levine, H. B., and Stevens, D. A.: Soluble antigens of mycelia and spherules in the in vitro detection of immunity to *Coccidioides immitis*. Infect Immun 10:700, 1974.

Drutz, D. J., and Huppert, M.: Coccidioidomycosis: Factors affecting the host-parasite interaction. J Infect Dis 147:372, 1983.

Drutz, D. J., Huppert, M., Sun, S. H., and McGuire, W. L.: Human sex hormones stimulate the growth and maturation of *Coccidioides immitis*. Infect Immun 32:897, 1981.

Drutz, D. J., and Catanzaro, A.: Coccidioidomycosis: State of the art (in two parts). Am Rev Resp Dis 117:727, 1978.

Emmons, C. W.: Fungi which resemble Coccidioides immitis. In Ajello, L. (ed.): Proceedings of Second Coccidioidomycosis Symposium. University of Arizona Press, Tucson, 1967, p. 333.

González-Ochoa, A.: Coccidioidomycosis in Mexico. In Ajello, L. (ed.): Proceedings of Second Coccidioidomycosis Symposium. Tucson, The University of Arizona Press, 1967, p. 293.

Hector, R., and Pappagianis, D.: Structure of Coccidioides immitis spherule wall. Proceedings of the 26th annual Coccidioidomycosis. Study Group Meeting, California Thoracic Society, Sacramento, Calif., 1981.

Huppert, M.: Standardization of immunological reagents. Proceedings—International Symposium on Mycoses. Scientific Publication PAHO No. 205, 1970, p. 243.

Huppert, M., Chitjian, P. A., and Gross, A. J.: Comparison of methods for coccidioidomycosis complement fixation. Appl Microbiol 20:328, 1970.

Huppert, M., Krasnow, I., Vukovich, K. R., Sun, S. H., Rice, E. H., and Kutner, L. J.: Comparison of coccidioidin and spherulin in complement fixation tests for coccidioidomycosis. J Clin Microbiol 6:33, 1977.

Huppert, M., Levine, H. B., Sun, S. H., and Peterson, E. T.: Resistance of vaccinated mice to typical and atypical strains of *Coccidioides immitis*. J Bact 94:924, 1967.

Huppert, M., Peterson, E. T., Sun, S. H., Chitjian, P. A., and Derrevere, W. J.: Evaluation of a latex particle agglutination test for coccidioidomycosis. Am J Clin Path 49:96, 1968.

Huppert, M., Spratt, N. S., Vukovich, K. R., Sun, S. H., and Rice, E. H.: Antigenic analysis of coccidioidin and spherulin determined by two-dimensional immunoelectrophoresis. Infect Immun 20:541, 1978.

Huppert, M., Sun, S. H., and Vukovich, K. R.: Standardization of mycological reagents. Proceedings: International Conference on Standardization of Diagnostic Materials. U.S. Dept. HEW, CDC, Atlanta, 1974, p. 187.

Huppert, M., Sun, S. H., and Bailey, J. W.: Natural variability in *Coccidioides immitis*. In Ajello, L. (ed.): Proceedings of Second Coccidioidomycosis Symposium. University of Arizona Press, Tucson, 1967, p. 323.

Huppert, M., Sun, S. H., and Harrison, J. L.: Morphogenesis throughout saprobic and parasitic cycles of Coccidioides immitis. Mycopath 78:107, 1982.

Kaufman, L.: Serodiagnosis of fungal diseases. In Manual of Clinical Microbiology. American Society of Microbiology, 1976, p. 363.

Kaufman, L., and Clark, M. J.: Value of the concomitant use of complement fixation and immunodiffusion tests in the diagnosis of coccidioidomycosis. Appl Microbiol 28:641, 1974.

Kaufman, L., Hall, E. C., Clark, M. J., and McLaughlin, D.: Comparison of macrocomplement and microcomplement fixation techniques used in fungus serology. Appl Microbiol 20:579, 1970.

Kobayashi, G. S., and Pappagianis, D.: Preparation and standardization of antigens of *Histoplasma capsulatum* and *Coccidiodes immitis*. Mycopath et Mycolog Appl 41:139, 1970.

Kong, Y. M., Levine, H. B., and Smith, C. E.: Immunogenic properties of undisrupted and disrupted spherules of *Coccidioides immitis* in mice. Sabouraudia 2:131, 1963.

Kwon-Chung, K. J.: *Coccidioides immitis*: Cytological study on the formation of the arthrospores. Canad J Genet Cytol 11:43, 1969.

Lacy, G. H., and Swatek, F. E.: Soil ecology of *Coccidioides immitis* at Amerindian middens in California. Appl Microbiol 27:379, 1974.

Levine, H. B., Cobb, J. M., and Scalarone, G. M.: Spherule coccidioidin in delayed dermal sensitivity reaction of experimental animals. Sabouraudia 7:20, 1969.

Levine, H. B., Cobb, J. M., and Smith, C. E.: Immunity to coccidioidomycosis induced in mice by purified spherule, arthrospore and mycelial vaccines. Trans N Y Acad Sci 22:436, 1960.

Levine, H. B., González-Ochoa, A., and Ten Eyck, D.: Dermal sensitivity to *Coccidioides immitis*. Am Rev Resp Dis 107:379, 1973.

Levine, H. B., Kong, Y. M., and Smith, C. E.: Immunization of mice to *Coccidioides immitis*: dose regimen and spherulation stage of killed spherule vaccines. The J Immun 94:132, 1965.

Levine, H. B., Restrepo, M. A., Ten Eyck, D. R., and Stevens, D. A.: Spherulin and coccidioidin: cross reactions in dermal sensitivity to histoplasmin and paracoccidioidin. Am J Epidem 101:512, 1975.

Mayorga, R. P., and Espinoza, H.: Coccidioidomycosis in Mexico and Central America. Mycopath et Mycol Appl 40:13, 1970.

Pan American Health Organization. Manual of standardized serodiagnostic procedures for systemic mycoses. Part II. Complement fixation tests. Washington, D.C., Pan American Health Organization, 1974.

Pappagianis, D., and Crane, R.: Survival in coccidioidal meningitis since introduction of amphotericin B. In Ajello, L. (ed.) Coccidioidomycosis. Miami, Symposia Specialists, 1977, p. 223.

Pappagianis, D., Smith, C. E., Kobayashi, G. S., and Saito, M. T.: Studies of antigens from young mycelia of *Coccidioides immitis*. J Infect Dis 108:35, 1961a.

Pappagianis, D., Putman, E. W., and Kobayashi, G. S;: Polysaccharide of *Coccidioides immitis*. J Bact 82:714, 1961b.

Pappagianis, D.: Serology and serodiagnosis of coccidioidomycosis. In D. A. Stevens (ed.). Coccidioidomycosis: A text. Plenum Medical Book Co., New York, 1980, p. 97.

Pappagianis, D., Hector, R., Levine, H. B., and Collins, M. S.: Immunization of mice against coccidioidomycosis with a subcellular vaccine. Infect Immun 25:440, 1979.

Pappagianis, D., and Levine, H. B.: The present status of vaccination against coccidioidomycosis in man. Am J Epidem 102:30, 1975.

Porter, J. F., Scheer, E. C., and Wheat, R. W.: Characterization of 3 0-methylmannose from *Coccidioides immitis*. Infect Immun 4:660, 1971.

Rifkind, D., Frey, J. A., Davis, J. R., and Petersen, E. A.: Delayed hypersensitivity to fungal antigens in mice. I. Use of the intradermal skin and foot pad swelling tests as assays of active and passive sensitization. J Infect Dis 133:50, 1976.

Scalarone, G. M., Levine, H. B., Pappagianis, D., and Chaparas, S,: Spherulin as a complement fixing antigen in human coccidioidomycosis. Am Rev Resp Dis 110:324, 1974.

Sigler, L., and Carmichael, J. W.: Taxonomy of Malbranchea and some other hyphomycetes with arthroconidia. Mycotaxon 4:349, 1976.

Smith, C. E., Pappagianis, D., and Saito, M.: The public health significance of coccidioidomycosis. U.S. Public Health Service Publication No. 575, 1957, p. 3.

Smith, C. E., Saito, M. T., Beard, R. R., Kepp, R. M., Clark, R. W., and Eddie, B. V.: Serological tests in the diagnosis and prognosis of coccidioidomycosis. Amer J Hyg 52:1, 1950.

Smith, C. E., Saito, M. T., and Simons, S. A.: Pattern of 39,500 serologic tests in coccidioidomycosis. JAMA 160:546, 1956.
Standard, P. G., and Kaufman, L.: Immunological procedure for the rapid and specific identification of *Coccidioides immitis* cultures. J Clin Microbiol 5:149, 1977.
Stevens, D. A., Levine, H. B., and Ten Eyck, D. R.: Dermal sensitivity to different doses of spherulin and coccidioidin. Chest 65:530, 1974.
Sun, S. H., Huppert, M., and Vukovich, K. R.: Rapid in vitro conversion and identification of *Coccidioides immitis*. J Clin Microbiol 3:186, 1976.
Swatek, F. E.: The epidemiology of coccidioidomycosis. In Al-Doory, Y. (ed.): The Epidemiology of Human Mycotic Diseases. Springfield, Charles C Thomas Publishers, 1975, p. 74.
United States Public Health Service. Standardized diagnostic complement fixation method and adaption to micro test. U. S. Public Health Service Publication No. 1228, 1965.
Walker, J.: The Vaccine Study Group. Progress report on coccidioidomycosis vaccine trial (Abstract no. 8). In D. A. Stevens (ed.). Proceedings of the 26th Annual Coccidioidomycosis Study Group Meeting. Calif. Thoracic Society, Sacramento, Calif. 1981.
Wheat, R. W., Tritschler, C., Conant, N. F., and Lowe, E. P.: Comparison of *Coccidioides immitis* arthrospore, mycelium and spherule cell walls, and influence of growth medium on mycelial cell wall composition. Infect Immun 17:91, 1977.

78

BLASTOMYCES AND PARACOCCIDIOIDES

SMITH SHADOMY, PH. D.
DENNIS M. DIXON, PH.D.

Blastomyces dermatitiditis and *Paracoccidioides brasiliensis* are important causes of pulmonary infections in the Western Hemisphere. Blastomycosis due to *B. dermatitiditis* was once called North American blastomycosis because the disease had only been recognized in North America, but in recent years there are reports of infections throughout the world. *P. brasiliensis*, on the other hand, is limited in its distribution to areas of Central and South America, where it causes a disease known as Paracoccidioidomycosis (formerly South American blastomycosis). *B. dermatitiditis* has a marked tendency to spread from the lung to the skin, bones, and the urogenital tract, but all viscera may become involved. *P. brasiliensis* may occasionally cause disseminated visceral disease of the spleen, adrenals, and liver, but the most common sites of extrapulmonary infection in paracoccidioidomycosis are the mouth, pharynx, bowel, regional lymph nodes, and skin. Amphotericin B is active against both fungi in vitro and in patients. The imidazoles, miconazole and ketoconazole, are very effective at controlling infections due to *P. brasiliensis*.

MORPHOLOGY. *Blastomyces (Ajellomyces) dermatitidis* and *Paracoccidioides brasiliensis* are dimorphic fungi that grow in tissue as budding yeasts and in culture at room temperature as molds. The two fungi are morphologically similar and share antigens. Despite its name, *P. brasiliensis* is now considered to be in the genus *Blastomyces*.

Yeast cells of *B. dermatitidis* range from 8 to 15μ in size. In wet mounts or when stained with lactophenol cotton blue, the cell wall appears as a highly refractile structure (Fig. 1). The thick nature of the cell wall has led various authors to describe the fungus as doubly rounded or doubly contoured as if delimited by two cell walls. Yeast phase cells of *B. dermatitidis* produce single buds that are characterized by a wide pore, approximately one-half the width of the parent cell, between the parent cell and bud. The wall of the bud is initially thinner than that of the parent cell. These features distinguish *B. dermatitidis* from the other human fungal pathogens.

Yeast cells of *P. brasiliensis* are from 2 to 30μ in diameter and have thinner cell walls than *B. dermatitidis*. Additionally, *P. brasiliensis* is differentiated by the production of multiple buds from a single cell. This gives rise to the familiar "Mickey Mouse hat" appearance when three such buds are involved, or the "pilot's wheel" when multiple buds are produced around the circumference of the parent cell (Fig. 2). Also, pores between the parent cell and buds are narrower than those with *B. dermatitidis*.

In culture, *B. dermatitidis* grows as a whitish buff-colored mold with a yellow-brown underside. Colonies may be floccose or glabrous, furrowed or smooth. Microscopically, one sees fine, septate hyphae that have characteristic pyriform conidia measuring 2 to 10μ. The conidia are borne on short lateral or terminal branches (conidiophores) and

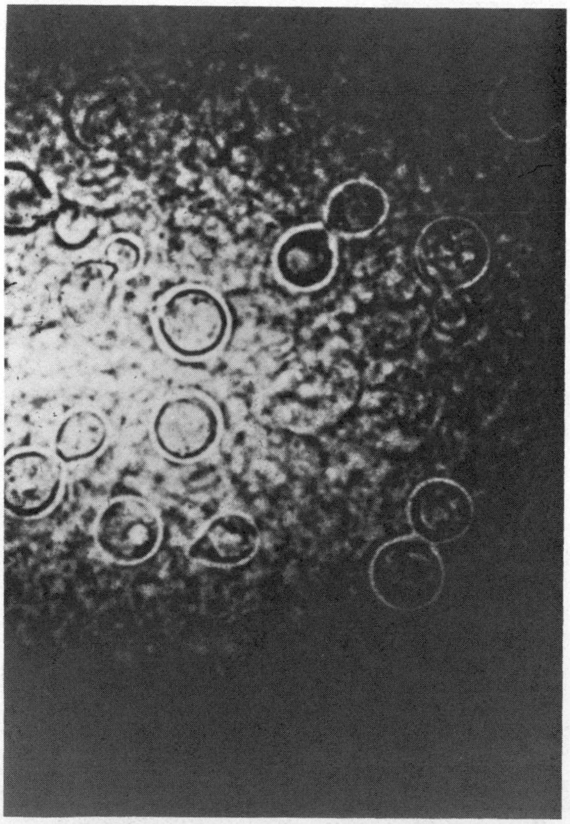

Figure 1. Yeast cells of *Blastomyces dermatitidis* in pus. Note thick cell wall and single buds. Compare with multiple buds of *Paracoccidioides brasiliensis* in Figure 2. (× 1200)

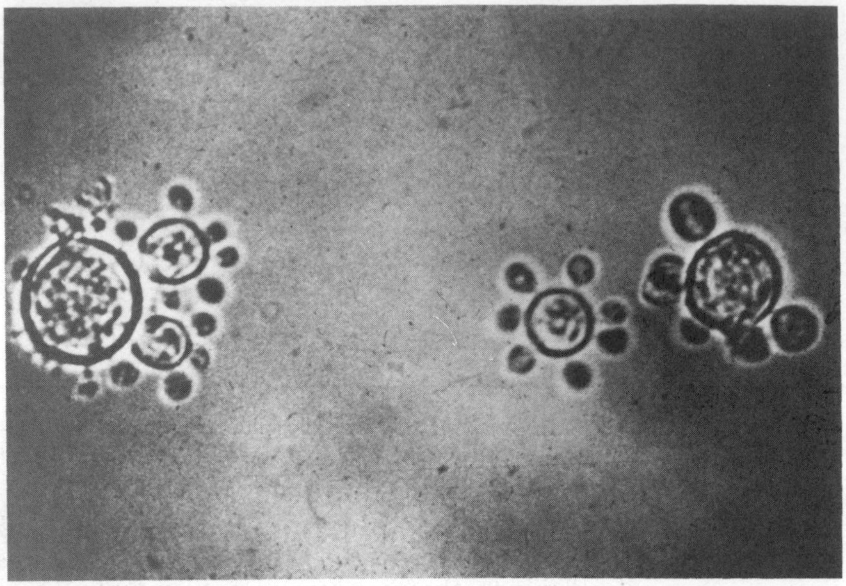

Figure 2. Yeast cells of *Paracoccidioides brasiliensis*. Note thinner cell wall than those of *B. dermatitidis* in Figure 1, and multiple buds in a single cell (pilot's wheel). (× 1500)

typically have a truncated base that can be more clearly seen after their separation from the parent conidiophore (Fig. 3). Such conidia are commonly termed aleurioconidia or aleuriospores and may be confused with the smooth-walled conidia of *Histoplasma capsulatum* and certain saprophytic *Chrysosporium* species. *B. dermatitidis* and *H. capsulatum* can be differentiated on the basis of yeast phase morphology. *Chrysosporium* species do not grow as a yeast in vitro.

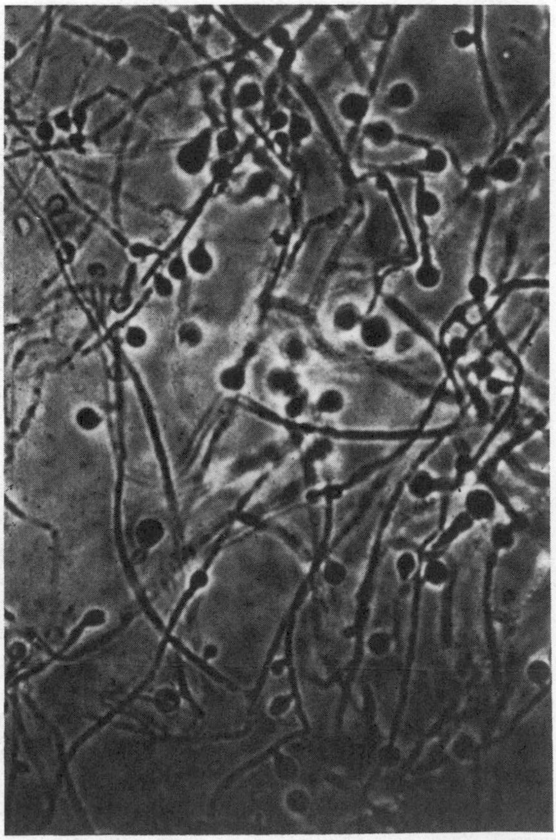

Figure 3. Filamentous growth of *Blastomyces dermatitidis* showing spherical or pyriform spores. Note short pedicles that attach spores to hyphae.

P. brasiliensis is essentially indistinguishable from *B. dermatitidis* in the mycelial phase and often does not produce conidia. When present, the conidia are aleurioconidia measuring 2 to 4μ in diameter. Arthroconidia, produced by disarticulation of the vegetative hyphae, and intercalary chlamydospores, or thick-walled swollen cells, have been reported. For both fungi, media such as potato dextrose agar or yeast extract agar usually enhance the production of conidia while limiting the growth of vegetative hyphae.

On Sabouraud's agar at room temperature, both *B. dermatitidis* and *P. brasiliensis* appear as slow-growing molds and are indistinguishable from each other. Colonies are generally apparent after one week of incubation, but maximum growth may not be attained for three or more weeks. Colonies typically are white-buff to brown with a yellow-brown reverse and may be floccose to glabrous, furrowed or smooth. *B. dermatitidis* and *P. brasiliensis* occasionally produce tufts of aerial hyphae (coremia) that are most distinctive in young cultures; otherwise, the colonies are similar in appearance to *H. capsulatum*. Microscopically, *B. dermatitidis* consists of fine, septate hyphae and characteristic pyriform conidia measuring from 2 to 10μ.

On brain-heart infusion blood agar at 37°C, both *B. dermatitidis* and *P. brasiliensis* grow as cream-colored, wrinkled, heaped colonies. Growth rates are similar to those of mycelial phase cultures, but the colonial growth is more restricted than the mycelial growth that may cover the agar surface.

B. dermatitidis has a sexual stage, *Ajellomyces dermatitidis*. The sexes are separate (heterothallism), and opposite mating types (+ and −) are required to obtain fertile cultures of *A. dermatitidis*. When the two mating types are cultured at 25°C on appropriate media, specialized rounded structures (cleistothecia) are produced. Within these are sac-like structures, or asci, each of which contains eight ascospores. The fungus is therefore classified as an *Ascomycete*. The ascospores are somewhat smaller than the asexual conidia and are infectious. A sexual stage has not been described for *P. brasiliensis*.

ANTIGENIC STRUCTURE. Blastomycin and paracoccidioidin are concentrates that have been prepared from filtrates of mycelial phase cultures. They are used as the antigens for serodiagnosis of infection with these fungi as well as antigens for in vivo skin tests. These materials are heterogenous mixtures of antigens that lack both sensitivity and specificity, and, to compound the problem, they are poorly standardized. Work is under way to isolate antigens that will be both specific and sensitive for serodiagnosis (Cox and Larsh, 1974a, b). Cell-wall proteins are believed to be the antigens responsible for skin-test reactions. An alkaline-stable, water-soluble extract of yeast cell walls appears to contain a skin-test antigen that is both sensitive and specific (Lancaster and Sprouse, 1976). Restrepo and others have isolated specific antigens from yeast cells that can be used for serodiagnosis of paracoccidioidomycosis (Restrepo, 1966; Kaufman, 1972).

IMMUNITY. Cell-mediated immunity is a more significant factor than humoral immunity in most of the mycoses, and blastomycosis and paracoccidioidomycosis are not exceptions. Although circulating antibodies can generally be detected at some point in the course of the diseases, they do not appear to be protective. In contrast, cell-mediated immune responses show a positive correlation with the host's ability to overcome the infections. Poor clinical progress is generally correlated with impairment in some aspect of cell-mediated immunity (Mok and Greer, 1977; Musatti et al., 1976). Whether there is a causal relationship between lymphocyte responses and immunity remains to be determined; however, it has been suggested that paracoccidioidomycosis leads to impairments in cell-mediated immunity. Various parameters of cell-mediated immunity should be examined closely in order to assess their roles in determining the clinical manifestations and outcome in these and other systemic fungal infections.

LABORATORY DIAGNOSIS. *B. dermatitidis* and *P. brasiliensis* bear striking mycologic similarities. Both are dimorphic, existing as molds at room temperature and as yeasts in infected tissues and in vitro at 37°C on enriched media. While *B. dermatitidis* and *P. brasiliensis* are virtually indistinguishable in the mycelial phase, both have certain characteristic morphologic differences in the yeast phase.

While unequivocal diagnosis of any mycosis requires isolation of the causative fungus in vitro, a presumptive diagnosis can be made by direct microscopic observation of the fungus in clinical materials. Samples of cerebrospinal fluid and urine are first sedimented by centrifugation and the sediment taken for direct examination and culture. Tissue must be homogenized by using a small amount of physiologic saline and a glass tissue grinder or mortar and pestle. The tissue homogenate is then subject to both culture and direct microscopic examination. Viscous materials are digested by adding a drop of 10 per cent KOH to the material on a microscope slide and covering it with a coverslip while still wet.

The morphologies of *B. dermatitidis* and *P. brasiliensis* in infected tissues are the same as those of the yeast phases when grown in vitro. Histopathologic staining of infected tissue can therefore be a useful adjunct to laboratory diagnosis. Sections of involved tissue should be stained with methenamine silver, periodic acid–Schiff (PAS), and hematoxylin and eosin (H & E). Yeasts that were viable at the time of fixation are discernible with H & E stain, but they are most easily located with methenamine silver, which stains them black. With the Gomori's stain, they appear slightly enlarged due to the impregnation effect of the silver. More details of cell morphology can be resolved with PAS and H & E.

The presence of thick-walled cells producing single buds with a broad base of attachment represents presumptive histopathologic evidence of infection with *B. dermatitidis*. There may be superficial resemblance to *Histoplasma duboisii* (the etiologic agent of African histoplasmosis), but this latter fungus buds with narrow pores. Also, *H. duboisii* is uninucleate, whereas *B. dermatitidis* is typically multinucleate. With PAS and H & E stain, the cytoplasm of B. dermatitidis shrinks away from the cell wall, leaving a clear space. This appearance should not be confused with the capsule of *Cryptococcus neoformans* which stains red with both PAS and Mayer's mucicarmine stains and which produces buds through narrow pores. (*B. dermatitidis* stains poorly at best with mucicarmine.) Single cells of *B. dermatitidis* have been mistaken for spherules of *Coccidioides immitis*. In some cases, it may be difficult to distinguish small intracellular yeast cells of *B. dermatitidis* from *H. capsulatum*. The former may have multiple nuclei that are visible with H & E stain, while the latter has only a single nucleus per yeast cell. In some cases, it may not be possible to exclude a dual infection by histologic criteria alone.

The morphology of *P. brasiliensis* in tissues is like that of the yeasts grown in vitro. Small forms of *P. brasiliensis* with single buds can be differentiated from *B. dermatitidis* on the basis of pore size. Single yeast cells of *P. brasiliensis* can be differentiated from *C. neoformans* and *C. immitis* by using the same criteria that are used for *B. dermatitidis*.

Materials for culture are prepared as described above for direct observation and are streaked in duplicate on both Sabouraud's agar and brain-heart infusion blood agar. Agar media may be used that contain both chloramphenicol, to inhibit bacterial contaminants, and cycloheximide (Actidione), to inhibit saprophytic fungal contaminants. However, such media should not be the sole media employed because certain opportunistic fungal pathogens as well as *Cryptococcus neoformans* are also inhibited by cycloheximide. One set of plates should be incubated at room temperature, or 30°C if possible, and one set at 37°C. Plates should be kept for four weeks before discarding, but growth should be observable after one week of incubation.

B. dermatitidis and *P. brasiliensis* can be grown in vitro on a variety of media. The nutritional requirements of both fungi are quite similar, and no special growth factors or vitamins are required. Both fungi are slow growing, with mean generation times of 12 hours or more, and both fungi grow as molds at room temperature as well as at 30°C. Temperature is the primary stimulus for dimorphism, and culturing on an enriched medium such as brain-heart infusion blood agar with incubation at 35° or 37°C will result in conversion of the fungi to their parasitic yeast phases. Colonies of yeast cells should appear within five days; if they do not, subsequent transfers may be necessary.

The preparations are stained with lactophenol cotton blue and examined microscopically for the charactistic aleurioconidia. For confirmation, yeast phase conversion should be demonstrated. Production of the characteristic budding yeasts differentiate *B. dermatitidis* from *P. brasiliensis* and from the saprophytic *Chrysoporium* species. Cottonseed agar may be more efficient for conversion of *B. dermatitidis* mold to its yeast phase than brain-heart infusion blood agar. Not all isolates convert to the yeast phase. Inoculation of mice intraperitoneally with mycelia of *B. dermatitidis* produces (after four weeks) local infections that will contain yeasts.

The yeast forms of *B. dermatitidis* and *P. brasiliensis* can be rapidly identified in cultures and in smears of clinical materials by specific fluorescent antibody.

EPIDEMIOLOGY. Recent studies of the epidemiology of blastomycosis have shown that the disease is not limited to North America as believed earlier. Rather, autochthonous infections have been reported in Europe and throughout Africa. The majority of cases, however, do come directly or indirectly from North America, where the disease is endemic to several geographic regions, including the Mississippi, Ohio, and Missouri River basins, as well as the Great Lakes region on the western shore of Lake Michigan.

Paracoccidioidomycosis is limited to Central and South America. In the case of infections reported from other countries, travel to known endemic areas usually can be documented. Highly endemic regions include both humid tropical forests and humid or very humid subtropical forest zones. Most cases have been reported from the state of São Paulo, Brazil.

Both blastomycosis and paracoccidiodomycosis are reported more commonly from rural than from urban areas. With both infections, similar occupational patterns are seen among the patients who are often laborers, farmers, and tree cutters. A unique epidemic of blastomycosis occurred in Bigfork, Minnesota, where members of four families were infected during the clearing of forest undergrowth and construction of a cabin (Tosh et al., 1974).

Neither blastomycosis nor paracoccidioidomycosis is naturally transmissible from man to man or from animal to man. The infections are acquired from some as yet poorly defined sources in nature, probably by inhalation of infectious conidia. The natural habitats of these fungi are assumed to be soil; however, only a few reports of isolation of these organisms from soil have been recorded. Isolation studies employing bird and bat manure have ruled out these materials as natural sources.

Blastomycosis and paracoccidioidomycosis occur in all age groups, but the preponderance of cases occurs in the 20- to 50-year-old age group. Males are more commonly affected than females in ratios of approximately 9 to 1. This is probably a reflection of hormonal as well as sociologic and occupational differences. There is no clear-cut predilection with respect to race as is seen in coccidioidomycosis.

References

Cox, R. A., and Larsh, H. W.: Isolation of skin test-active preparations from yeast-phase cells of *Blastomyces dermatitidis*. Infect Immun 10:42, 1974a.

Cox, R. A., and Larsh, H. W.: Yeast and mycelial-phase antigens of *Blastomyces dermatitidis:* Comparison using disc gel electrophoresis. Infect Immun 10:48, 1974b.

Kaufman, L.: Evaluation of serological tests for paracoccidioidomycosis: Preliminary report. In Pan American Health Organization: Paracoccidioidomycosis. Proceedings of the First Pan American Symposium. Geneva, World Health Organization, 1972, pp. 221-223.

Lancaster, M. V., and Sprouse, R. F.: Isolation of a purified skin test antigen from *Blastomyces dermatitidis* yeast-phase cell wall. Infect Immun 14:623, 1976.

Mok, P. W. Y., and Greer, D. L.: Cell-mediated immune responses in patients with paracoccidioidomycosis. Clin Exp Immunol 28:89, 1977.

Musatti, C. C., Rezkallah, M. T., Mendes, E., and Mendes, N. F.: *In vivo* and *in vitro* evaluation of cell-mediated immunity in patients with paracoccidioidomycosis. Cell Immunol 24:365, 1976.

Restrepo, A.: La prueba de immunodiffusion en el diagnostico de la paracoccidioidomicosis. Sabouraudia 4:223, 1966.

Tosh, F. E., Hammerman, K. J., Weeks, R. J., and Sarosi, G. A.: A common source epidemic of North American blastomycosis. Am Rev Resp Dis 109:525, 1974.

79

THE ASPERGILLI

Abraham I. Braude, M.D., Ph.D.

The aspergilli are a group of versatile fungi belonging to the class Hyphomycetes and the family Moniliaceae. As noted in Chapter 14, *Aspergillus fumigatus* and *Aspergillus flavus* differ from most nonzygomycete fungi in the ability of these two organisms to grow deep in tissue in mycelial form.

A sexual stage occurs among several pathogenic species of *Aspergillus* when they reproduce by forming ascospores in asci containing 8 spores. Once sexual reproduction is demonstrated, the fungi are given a second name to meet the classification provisions of the International Code of Botanical Nomenclature. *Sartorya fumigata,* for example, is the name for the sexual (ascomycetous) state of *Aspergillus fumigatus,* the most important cause of human disease among the aspergilli.

The name for this group of fungi is taken from the word aspergillum, which means a brush used for sprinkling holy water. This brush has a remarkable resemblance to the microscopic appearance of the fungus *Aspergillus niger* (Fig. 1).

MORPHOLOGY. In order to appreciate the structure of the brushlike portion of the aspergilli, it is necessary to be familiar with *four* components: the conidiophore, the vesicle, the sterigmata, and the spores. These are identified in Figure 2, where it can be seen that the handle of the brush consists of the unbranched conidiophore, which has a swollen end, the vesicle. A number of little stalks, shaped like a bottle, radiate from the vesicle and are arranged in one or two rows (Fig. 2A or 2B). Chains of spores arise from the tips of these stalks, or sterigmata, in the outer row.

The spores (or conidia) develop from the tips of the fertile sterigmata. The first stage in spore formation is a constriction of an elongated portion of the sterigma; the second stage is the development of a septum that separates the spore from the sterigma. Chains of attached spores evolve as the cutting process continues at the tip of the sterigma. The compact mass of spores around the vesicle is called a conidial head and corresponds to the portion of a brush in which the bristles are set.

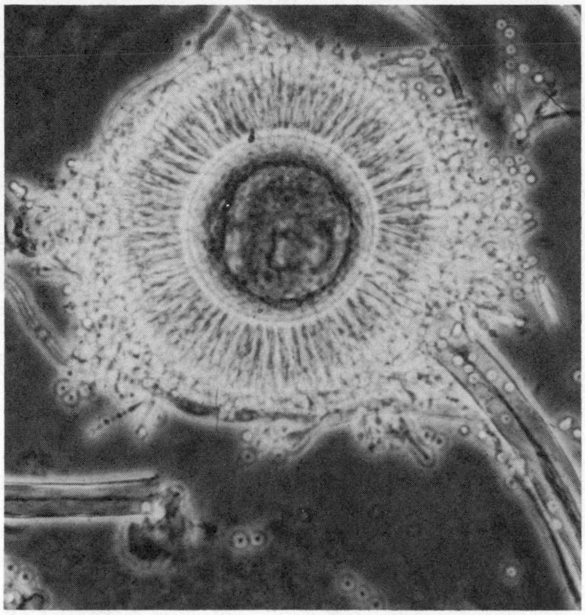

Figure 1. *Aspergillus niger* bears a remarkable resemblance to the aspergillum, a brush used for sprinkling holy water.

At its opposite end, the conidiophore arises from a foot cell, an enlarged thick-walled cell of the segmented mycelium. The conidiophore is borne as a stalk perpendicular to the long axis of the foot cell (Fig. 2).

The morphologic classification of all species of the genus *Aspergillus* is enormously complex and is beyond the scope of this chapter. Those members of medical importance, however, are relatively few and can generally be recognized by their color, the shape of their vesicle, and the arrangement of their sterigmata and spores. The groups of *Aspergillus* species that cause human disease are listed in Table 1 and can be arranged according to the following classification.

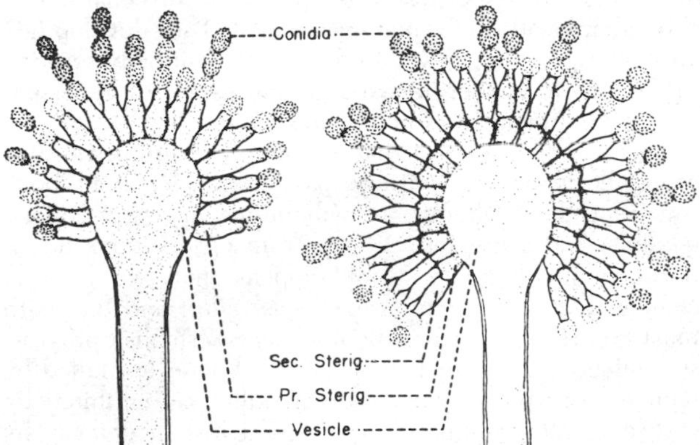

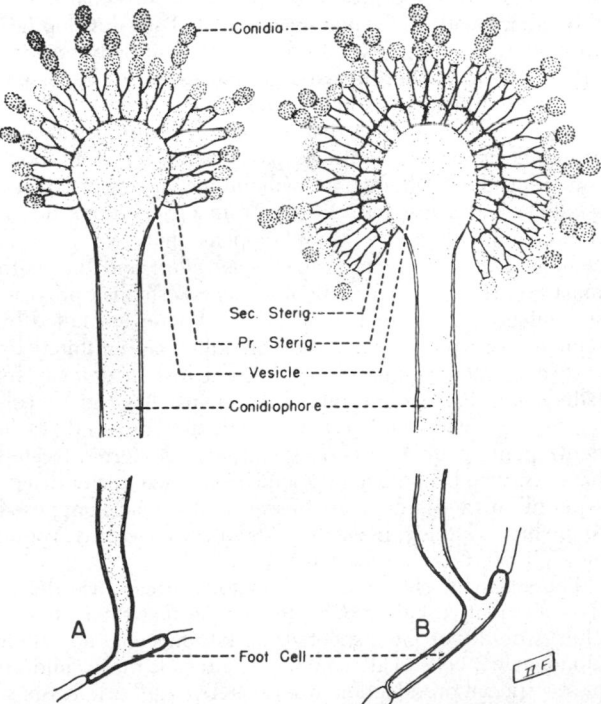

Figure 2. Diagram of two different morphologic types of aspergilli showing one row of sterigmata (uniseriate) in *A* and two rows (biseriate) in *B*. (From Roper, K. B., and Fennel, D. I.: The Genus Aspergillus. Baltimore, The Williams & Wilkins Company, 1965.)

I. Green colonies
 A. Sterigmata arranged in single rows (uniseriate)
  1. *Conidial heads are split* (clavate) into two or more divergent columns of compact chains of spores; they have swollen ends. Vesicles are also split and appear as an elongated, gradually swelling portion of the end of the conidiophore. They are fertile over their entire surface and are blue-green *(A. clavatus)*.
  2. *Conidial heads are compact, not split;* vesicles are fertile in their upper half so that sterigmata arise from the upper half only. Sterigmata are arranged parallel to each other and to the long axis of the conidiophore, pointing upward; they are green to dark green in color. (*A. fumigatus*, Fig. 3).
  3. *Conidial heads are not split;* interspersed among the green conidial heads are abundant bright yellow cleistothecia (round bodies containing multiple asci, which are sacs of sexual spores). Cleistothecia are about equal in size to conidial heads (*A. glaucus*).
 B. Sterigmata are arranged in two rows (biseriate): purple cleistothecia and orange-red ascospores *(A. nidulans)*.

II. Black colonies. Sterigmata are in either one row or two rows, depending on the species, and arise from the entire surface of the globular vesicle (*A. niger*, Fig. 1).

III. Yellow colonies. A mixture of uniseriate or biseriate sterigmata occur in the same culture or even on the same vesicle; vesicles are globular and are sometimes split. They are fertile over most of their surface *(A. flavus)*.

IV. Orange-brown or cinnamon colonies. There are two rows of sterigmata; the vesicles are hemispherical *(A. terreus)*.

ANTIGENIC COMPOSITION. Most immunologic reactions in *Aspergillus* infections have been studied with crude

Table 1. DISEASES CAUSED BY DIFFERENT SPECIES OF ASPERGILLI

Type of Aspergillosis	Species of Aspergillus
Invasive pulmonary	*fumigatus*
Allergic bronchopulmonary	*fumigatus*
	flavus
	niger
	terreus
	clavatus
Pulmonary aspergilloma	*fumigatus*
	niger
Otomycosis	*niger*
Sinusitis	*flavus*
Disseminated	*fumigatus*
	flavus
Mycetoma	*glaucus*
	nidulans

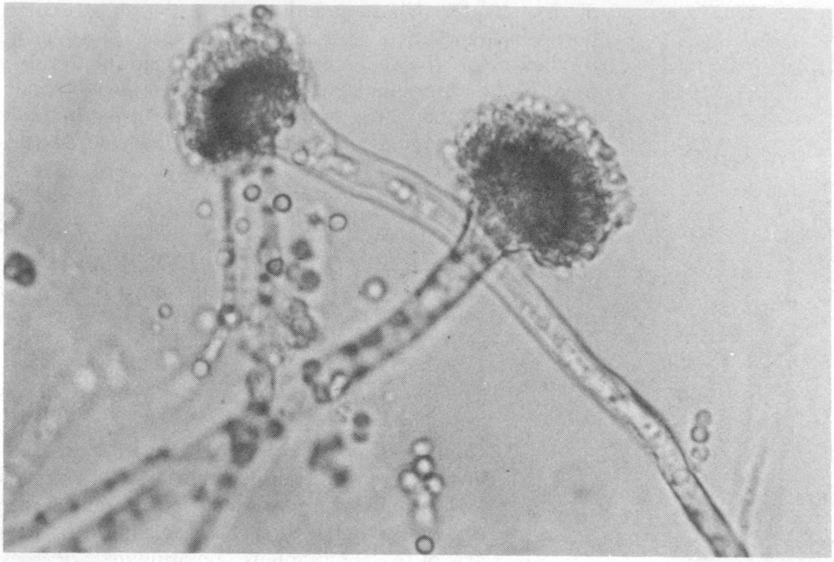

Figure 3. Wet mount of *Aspergillus fumigatus* cultured from ethmoid sinus (× 400). Note following diagnostic features typical of *A. fumigatus*: (1) compact (unsplit) conidial head; (2) single row of sterigmata; (3) sterigmata arise from upper half of vesicle only; (4) sterigmata are arranged parallel to each other and to the long axis of the conidiophore.

filtrates of *Aspergillus* cultures grown for several weeks at room temperature in Sabouraud broth. These contain countless unidentified antigens that can give up to 20 precipitin lines when examined by immunodiffusion against hyperimmune rabbit serum. Both protein and carbohydrate antigens have been identified in these *Aspergillus* culture filtrates, and some of the proteins are enzymes (oxoreductases, hydrolases, proteases). One of the polysaccharides reacts with C-reactive protein. C-reactive protein appears during the acute phase of various infections and other inflammatory processes and reacts with the somatic polysaccharide (C substance) of the pneumococcus. Its reaction with an antigen from *Aspergillus* suggests that this fungal polysaccharide may have properties that are similar to the pneumococcal C polysaccharide. Since the reaction with C-reactive protein clouds the specificity of immunodiffusion reactions with *Aspergillus* filtrates, it is necessary to eliminate the C-reactive substance by incorporating sodium citrate in the gel (Longbottom and Pepys, 1964).

The antigens in different species of *Aspergillus* cross-react in serologic tests with each other and with antigens of other fungi. These cross-reactions occur mainly between polysaccharide antigens and may occur not only with dermatophytes and *Cladosporium* but also with nematodes, trematodes, cestodes, and vegetable dusts. All of these cause immediate reactions to skin tests in patients with *Aspergillus* hypersensitivity and precipitin reactions with sera from some patients with pulmonary aspergilloma (Pepys, 1969). Galactomannans are prominent polysaccharide antigens in aspergilli as in other fungi, and they may be partly responsible for the cross-reactions observed between different species of *Aspergillus* and between aspergilli and other fungi.

IMMUNITY. At least two types of antibody are important in the pathogenesis of aspergillosis. IgE antibody is responsible for bronchospasm and asthma, whereas IgG seems to cause Arthus-type reactions in the walls of bronchi that progress to bronchiectasis, or alveolitis (hypersensitivity pneumonitis). If the respiratory tract becomes colonized with aspergilli, it releases the multiple antigens described in the previous section, and these sensitize certain patients with inherited hypersensitivity to aspergilli. These atopic patients produce IgE antibody to *Aspergillus* antigens and develop immediate hypersensitivity reactions in the respiratory tree when they are re-exposed to inhaled *Aspergillus* spores. They also develop high serum levels of IgG antibody, which precipitates *Aspergillus* antigens around the vessels in the alveoli and bronchial walls. The ensuing Arthus inflammatory reaction (Chapter 89) is thought to cause transient pneumonitis and a progressive injury to the bronchial wall that culminates in the characteristic bronchiectasis of allergic bronchopulmonary aspergillosis (Golbert and Patterson, 1970).

Nonatopic persons may be immunized to *Aspergillus* antigens by heavy exposure to spores and mycelial debris through inhalation of contaminated dust. They develop IgG antibodies, but not IgE, and the antigen-antibody reaction in the lung to further inhalation of spores causes hypersensitivity pneumonitis six hours later.

There is no evidence that antibody can protect against aspergillosis; on the contrary, passive transfer of antibody can reproduce allergic bronchopulmonary aspergillosis (Golbert and Patterson, 1970). From observations in experimental animals, it would appear that two lines of cellular defense operate against *Aspergillus* and that both must be breached before the fungus can establish progressive infection (Schaffner et al., 1982). Spores are killed by mononuclear phagocytes, and this killing is inhibited by cortisone. Neutrophils form a second line of defense by killing mycelia. Natural immunity against *Aspergillus* collapses only when both types of cells are impaired, as in neutropenic patients receiving steroids. In steroid-treated patients, who become neutropenic from leukemia or drugs, aspergilli invade pulmonary vessels and spread unopposed to the brain, kidney, liver, thyroid, and other organs (Young et al., 1970; Gerson et al., 1984).

Patients with chronic granulomatous disease are defective in oxidative killing (Chapter 87), so that their neutrophils would not be expected to kill mycelia nor their mononuclear cells to kill conidia. As a result, these children have a special predilection to serious *Aspergillus* infections.

The importance of mechanical clearing processes, which prevent colonization of the respiratory or alimentary tract by pathogenic organisms, is illustrated by the types of aspergillosis that develop in the lung and esophagus when these mechanisms are lost. Structural damage to the lung and bronchopulmonary tree by any form of bronchiectasis or lung cavity interferes with the ability of cilia and cough to remove inhaled aspergillus spores and allows them to proliferate in the defenseless cavities in which they grow as aspergillomas (or fungus balls). Similarly, when esophageal motility and swallowing is disturbed by severe debilitating illness, aspergilli are propelled less effectively into the acid gastric juice. Instead, they colonize the esophagus and can produce severe invasive esophagitis. Thus, loss of natural immunity through impaired protective mechanical processes may be among the most important disturbances responsible for defective resistance to aspergillosis.

Acquired resistance after infection with aspergillus has been observed experimentally only in limited studies in mice. Mice are normally resistant to aspergillus infection but become susceptible to pulmonary, renal, and fatal disseminated aspergillosis after treatment with cortisone. If they are injected first with viable aspergillus spores but not cortisone, they are no longer susceptible to progressive aspergillosis when rechallenged with aspergilli plus cortisone. The mechanism or specificity of this immunity is unknown; neither antibodies nor cellular immunity has been examined carefully enough to indicate its relative contribution to this important phenomenon. Although patients with disseminated aspergillosis have no antibodies to *A. fumigatus* antigens, a loss of humoral immunity cannot be blamed for susceptibility to this infection because the patients are also subject to suppression of cellular immunity by the chemotherapy given for their hematologic malignancies (Young and Bennett, 1971).

LABORATORY DIAGNOSIS

Mycologic Examination. Aspergilli are frequently cultured as contaminants in specimens from patients, but may be difficult to recover from patients with certain forms of

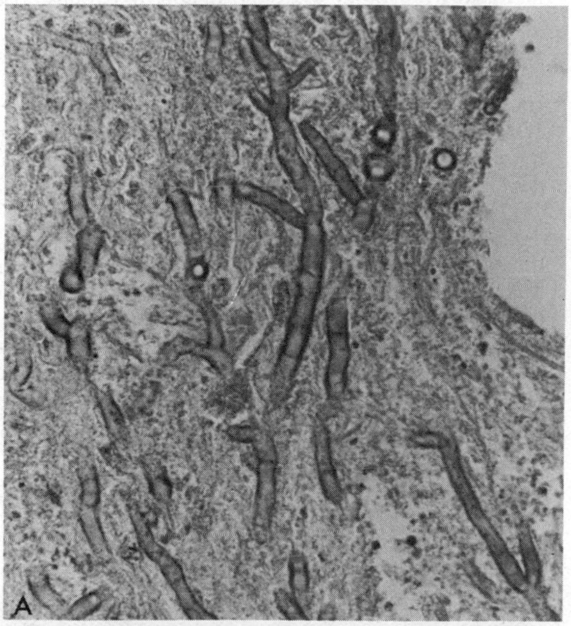

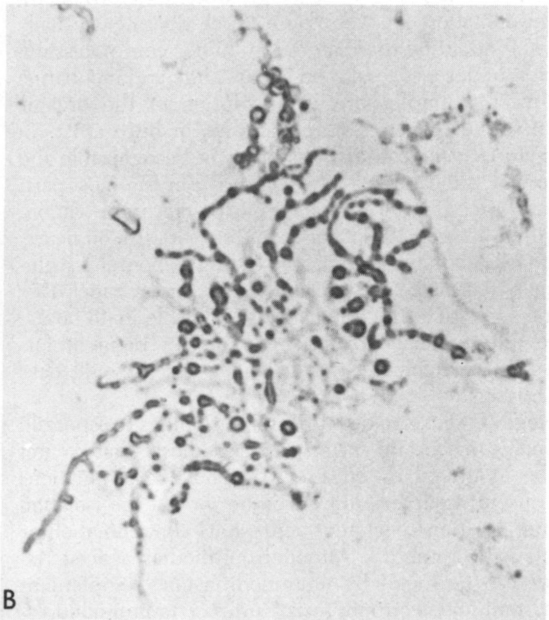

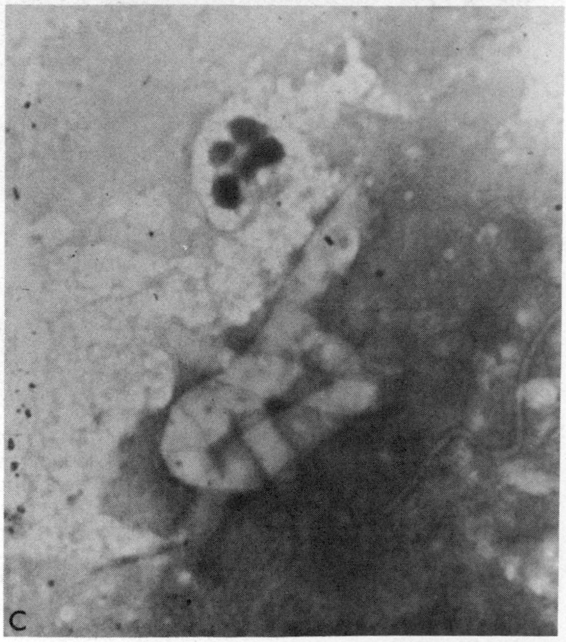

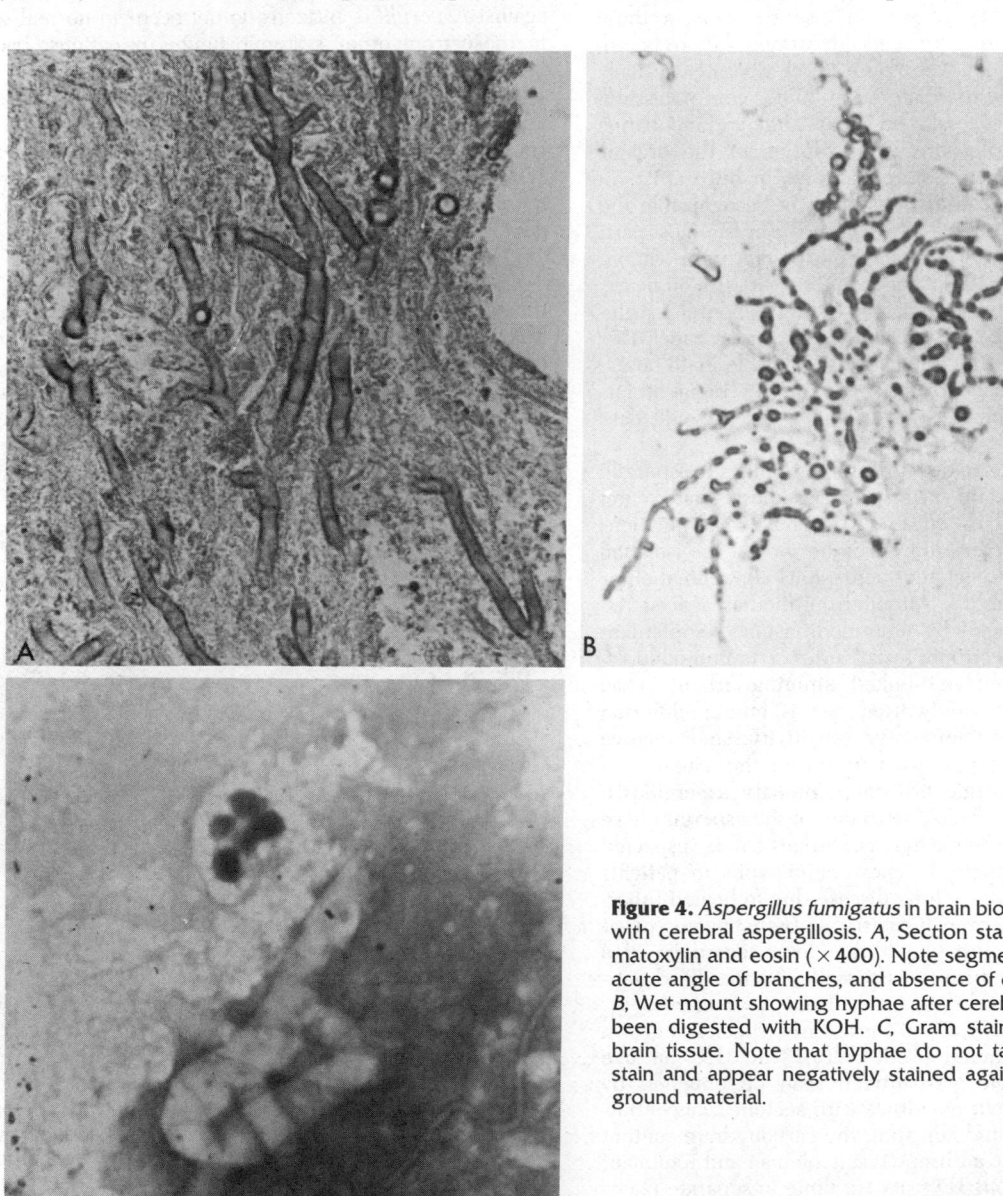

Figure 4. *Aspergillus fumigatus* in brain biopsy of patient with cerebral aspergillosis. *A,* Section stained with hematoxylin and eosin ($\times 400$). Note segmented hyphae, acute angle of branches, and absence of conidial head. *B,* Wet mount showing hyphae after cerebral tissue has been digested with KOH. *C,* Gram stain of smeared brain tissue. Note that hyphae do not take the Gram stain and appear negatively stained against the background material.

invasive aspergillosis. Thus, it is unusual to recover aspergilli from the sputum of patients with pulmonary aspergilloma or invasive *Aspergillus* pneumonias, and the fungus is rarely found in blood cultures of patients with disseminated aspergillosis. The organism can be isolated most readily in invasive disease of the lung, brain, sinuses, orbit, or skin when the infected tissue is obtained by biopsy (Fig. 4). In such tissues, the mycelial elements are usually found easily in histologic sections stained with hematoxylin and eosin or the methenamine-silver method; they appear in 24 to 48 hours in culture after aerobic incubation at 35°C on any standard medium. The only nonbiopsied specimens from which aspergilli are easily cultured are the sputa of patients with allergic bronchopulmonary aspergillosis, the pleural fluids in *Aspergillus* empyema, the exudates of burns infected with aspergilli, and the discharges from ears of patients with *A. niger* infection of the external auditory canal. Characteristic hyphae can also be seen in these specimens but may require special treatment before microscopic examination of a wet mount. Such treatment usually consists of mounting the material in 20 per cent potassium hydroxide under a coverslip on a glass slide and incubating at 37 or 56°C until there is dissolution of the organic material in the bronchial plug, ear wax, or burn crust. In some materials, the conidial head may be recognizable and will allow identification of *A. fumigatus*. For the most part, however, exact identification depends on cultural isolation. Aspergilli grow well at 37°C or room temperature on nearly all standard laboratory media, including Sabouraud's glucose agar, brain heart infusion agar, and Czapek-Dox medium. Growth of the fungus is often visible in 48 hours, but the differential characteristics, such as pigment formation and arrangement of sterigmata, take several days longer to develop.

Serologic Tests. Serologic tests for antibodies to aspergilli are valuable in certain forms of aspergillosis that cannot easily be identified by culture. Antibody determinations are also useful in determining whether or not the isolation of the fungus from specimens represents contamination or infection with aspergilli. Although antibodies against *Aspergillus* can be found by immunodiffusion, complement fixation, immunoelectrophoresis, indirect immunofluorescence, and the enzyme-linked immunosorbent assay (ELISA), the most widely used test is immunodiffusion (ID) because of its simplicity, sensitivity, and relative reliability. The ID test is most useful for the diagnosis of fungus ball and allergic bronchopulmonary aspergillosis. Patients with fungus balls due to one of the aspergilli have positive reactions. The diagnosis of fungus ball is suspected by characteristic lesions in chest radiographs in patients with underlying cavitary lung disease due to healed tuberculosis, sarcoidosis, bronchiectasis, or bronchogenic carcinoma, and an ID test should be done regardless of a negative sputum culture for aspergilli. Standardized antigen preparations should be made from *A. fumigatus*, *A. niger*, and *A. flavus*. Each of these three species is grown separately in Sabouraud broth cultures at 31°C for five weeks. Reproducible test antigens can be obtained by precipitating them out of culture with acetone, concentrating them eightfold and adjusting the carbohydrate content to 1000 μg/ml by the anthrone test (Coleman and Kaufman, 1972). If simultaneous ID tests are done in separate plates with each of the three antigens, precipitins will be found in over 90 per cent of patients with fungus balls and 70 per cent of those with allergic bronchopulmonary aspergillosis. The test is controlled with positive reference sera, and the diagnostic precipitin lines are recognized by their fusion with the reference lines (Fig. 5). Nonspecific lines produced by C-reactive substance are identified by their failure to fuse with the reference lines and their fuzzy appearance. They are greatly minimized by using antigens prepared from five week old cultures and eliminated by soaking the agar with 5 per cent sodium citrate for 45 minutes before reading the test. At least three specific precipitin bands are produced by antibody to *A. fumigatus* and one or more by antibody to *A. niger* or *A. flavus*. The precipitating antibodies belong to the IgG class of immunoglobulin (Warnock and Eldred, 1975). When multiple lines of identity occur with those of reference sera, a diagnosis of *Aspergillus* infection should be very seriously considered. Cross-reactions with antibody to fungi other than aspergilli are not likely to give multiple lines of identity, and clinical experience indicates that precipitins against *Aspergillus* antigens do not occur in normal sera or in those from other systemic fungus infections, bacterial infections, or cancer.

In contrast to patients with allergic bronchopulmonary aspergillosis, those with *Aspergillus* asthma do not have IgG precipitins for *Aspergillus* antigens and give negative ID reactions. Instead, the asthma cases can be identified by positive reactions for specific IgE antibodies against *Aspergillus* antigens by ELISA (Sepulveda et al., 1979).

EPIDEMIOLOGY. Aspergilli are found everywhere "from the winds of the Sahara to the snows of the Antarctic." They grow on soil, dead vegetation, any kind of organic debris, and laboratory reagents. They are extremely hardy and can withstand extremes of temperature, pH, and salt concentration. They are frequently encountered in farm houses, stables, barns, and grains, and infections have been acquired through inhalation of spores by farmers, millers,

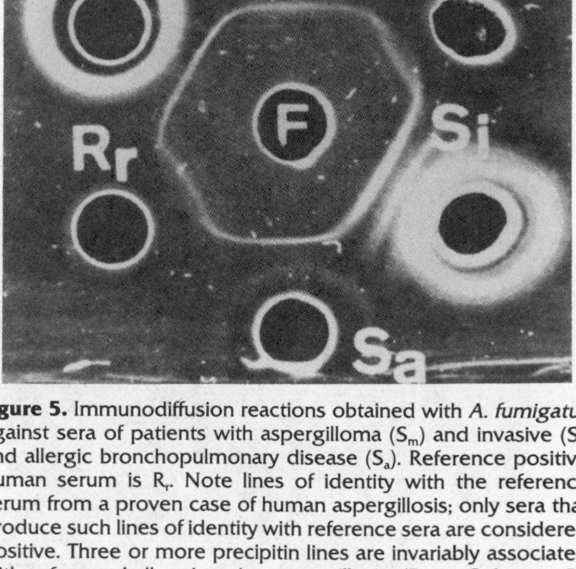

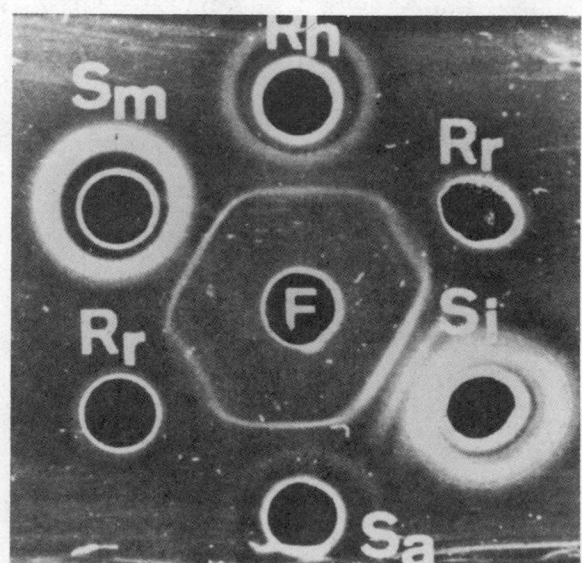

Figure 5. Immunodiffusion reactions obtained with *A. fumigatus* against sera of patients with aspergilloma (S_m) and invasive (S_i) and allergic bronchopulmonary disease (S_a). Reference positive human serum is R_r. Note lines of identity with the reference serum from a proven case of human aspergillosis; only sera that produce such lines of identity with reference sera are considered positive. Three or more precipitin lines are invariably associated with a fungus ball or invasive aspergillosis. (From Coleman, R., and Kaufman, L.: Appl. Microbiol 23:301, 1972.)

and gardeners. The most pathogenic species, *A. fumigatus*, is thermophilic—i.e., it can grow at the high temperatures that develop in compost piles from bacterial decomposition of wet leaves and wood chips. Enormous numbers of spores are produced, and, if inhaled by susceptible gardeners, they can produce pulmonary aspergillosis. The same phenomenon accounts for the heavy growth of *A. fumigatus* in stored hay or grains. Grain is an important source of infection in herds and livestock. Epidemics of aspergillosis involving the air sacs or lungs of birds have been traced to feeding on moldy grain. Horses, cattle, and sheep also get pulmonary aspergillosis by inhaling spores from their feed. Many years ago, infected squabs were thought to be a source of human aspergillosis. These pigeons were fattened by persons known as "gaveurs de pigeons" who used their tongues to force chewed grain into the bird's esophagi (Renon, 1897). It is also possible that the infection was acquired from the grain rather than from the squab.

Among patients newly admitted to sanatoriums in the south central United States, the incidence of aspergillosis was reported in 1970 to be nearly as great as that of chronic pulmonary histoplasmosis (Parker et al., 1970). Since then, it is likely that more cases of aspergillosis have developed in patients after admission to the hospital. These are debilitated patients who have been given immunosuppressive drugs for treatment of hematologic malignancy or for prevention of renal transplant rejection. Air ducts contaminated by bird droppings have been incriminated as a source of exposure for immunosuppressed patients (Kyriakides et al., 1976), and some observations suggest that the acquisition of pulmonary aspergillosis in the hospital might be eliminated if all incoming hospital air were filtered, properly vented, and not recirculated (Rose, 1972).

Aflatoxins, the mycotoxins produced by *A. flavus*, are a potential epidemiologic problem because they are found in the ground peanuts that are heavily consumed by certain African tribes afflicted with a high incidence of hepatoma. A direct etiologic relationship between cancer and aflatoxin has not been established, however, although aflatoxin can cause hepatomas in experimental animals. The epidemiologic problems related to mycotoxin are fully covered in Chapter 15.

References

Coleman, R., and Kaufman, L.: Use of the immunodiffusion test in the serodiagnosis of aspergillosis. Appl Microbiol 23:301, 1972.

Gerson, S. L., Talbot, G. H., Hurwitz, S., Strom, B. L., Lusk, E. J., and Cassileth, P. A.: Prolonged granulocytopenia: the major risk factor for invasive pulmonary aspergillosis in patients with acute leukemia. Ann Intern Med 100:345, 1984.

Golbert, T., and Patterson, R.: Pulmonary allergic aspergillosis. Ann Intern Med 72:395, 1970.

Kaufman, L.: Value of immunodiffusion tests in the diagnosis of systemic mycotic diseases. Ann Clin Lab Sci 3:141, 1973.

Kyriakides, G., Zinneman, H., Hall, W., Arora, V., Lifton, J., Dewolf, W., and Miller, J.: Immunologic monitoring and aspergillosis in renal transplant patients. Am J Surg 131:246, 1976.

Longbottom, J. L., and Pepys, J.: Pulmonary aspergillosis: Diagnostic and immunologic significance of antigens and C-substance in *Aspergillus fumigatus*. J Pathol Bacteriol 88:141, 1964.

Parker, J., Sarosi, G., Doto, I., and Tosh, F.: Pulmonary aspergillosis in sanatoriums in the South Central United States. Am Rev Resp Dis 101:551, 1970.

Pepys, J.: Hypersensitivity diseases of the lung due to fungi and organic dusts. In Kallos, P., Goodman, H., Hasek, M., Inderbitzin, T., and Waksman, B. (eds.): Monographs in Allergy, Vol. 4. Basel, S. Karger, 1969.

Renon, L.: Etude sur l'Aspergillose Chez les Animaux et Chez l'homme. Paris, Masson et cie, 1897.

Rose, H. D.: Mechanical control of hospital ventilation and aspergillus infections. Am Rev Resp Dis 105:306, 1972.

Schaffner, A., Douglas, H., and Braude, A.: Selective protection against conidia by mononuclear and against mycelia by polymorphonuclear phagocytes in resistance to *Aspergillus*. J Clin Investig 69:617, 1982.

Sepulveda, R., Longbottom, J., and Pepys, J.: Enzyme linked immunosorbent assay (ELISA) for IgG and IgE antibodies to protein and polysaccharide antigens of *Aspergillus fumigatus*. Clin Allergy 9:359, 1979.

Warnock, D., and Eldred, G.: Immunoglobulin classes of antibodies to *Aspergillus fumigatus* in patients with pulmonary aspergillosis. Sabouraudia 13:204, 1975.

Young, R., Bennett, J., Vogel, C., Carbone, P., and DeVita, V.: Aspergillosis. The spectrum of the disease in 98 patients. Medicine 49:147, 1970.

Young, R., and Bennett, J.: Invasive aspergillosis. Absence of detectable antibody response. Am Rev Resp Dis 104:710, 1971.

80

THE ZYGOMYCETES

ABRAHAM I. BRAUDE, M.D., PH.D.

The Zygomycetes are the only medically important class belonging to the group of primitive fungi known as Phycomycetes. The various members of the class Zygomycetes have in common the production of sexual spores known as zygospores. The Zygomycetes produce two entirely different human infections: (1) Mucormycosis is a malignant infection of cerebral, pulmonary, and abdominal blood vessels due to Mucorales, the bread molds. The Mucorales are unique among the pathogenic fungi because they have no septa in their hyphae (Zycha et al., 1969). (2) Tropical subcutaneous phycomycosis and nasal phycomycosis (or rhinoentomophthoromycosis) are benign chronic infections due to the insect fungi known as Entomophthorales. These curious fungi can shoot off their conidia forcibly.

MORPHOLOGY. The three important pathogenic genera of the order Mucorales are known as *Mucor, Rhizopus,* and *Absidia.* All three are characterized by white or gray woolly growth on food or agar. Under the microscope, the woolly growth consists of mycelium that is not divided into individual cells by septa, so that the entire mass of mycelium forms one large cell containing multiple nuclei. This nonseptate mycelium is called coenocytic, which means *common cell* in Greek.* In all genera of Mucorales, the mycelia give rise to specialized branches known as conidiophores. At the tip of the conidiophores are sacs filled with asexual spores. These sacs, called sporangia, measure 20 to 115 μ and are seen with the naked eye as dark dots scattered throughout the woolly colony (Fig. 1). In *Rhizopus* and *Absidia,* other specialized branches arise from the mycelium that allow them to spread rapidly over the surface of the agar, climb the sides of the culture plate, and fill it

*Since certain green algae are also coenocytic, these nonseptate fungi are also called Phycomycetes, or algae-like fungi.

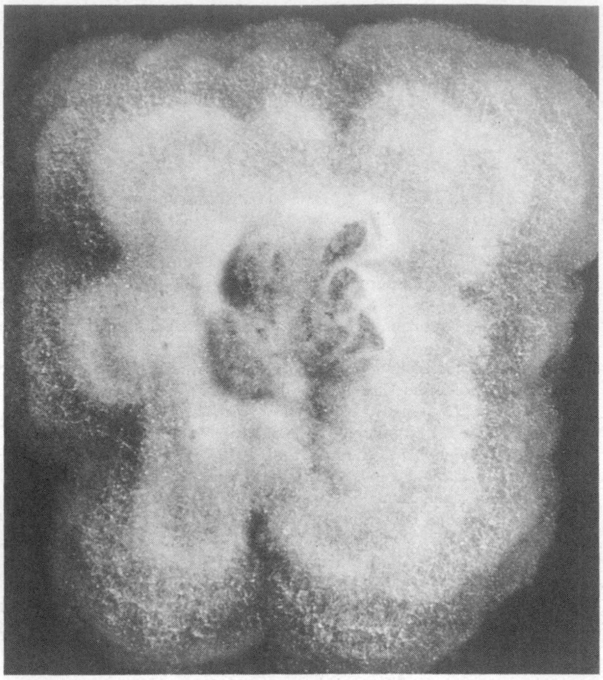

Figure 1. *Rhizomucor pusillus* isolated from blood of patient. Note dots scattered throughout the woolly colony. These dots represent sporangia.

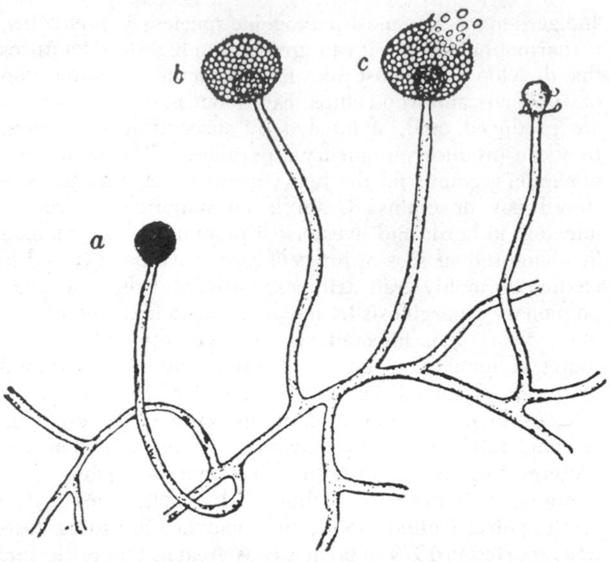

Figure 2. Diagram of *Mucor* sp. showing young sporulating head (a), mature sporangium (b and c), and columella after scattering of spores (d). Note that in contrast to *Rhizopus* and *Absidia* (Fig. 4) the sporangiophores arise from all parts of the thallus, and no stolons or rhizoids are produced. (From Waksman, S. A., and Starkey, R. L.: The Soil and the Microbe. New York, John Wiley and Sons, 1931.)

with aerial mycelium. One of these structures is the stolon (or "runner"). It is a filament of mycelium that extends out into the air from the point at which the sporangiophore branches from the mycelium. The newly extended runner then produces a "hold-fast," or rhizoid, which anchors the filament to the surface of the agar, the side of the plate, or its cover. In *Rhizopus,* the rhizoid is found at a node opposite the origin of the conidiophore. In *Absidia,* on the other hand, the sporangiophore arises from the arch of the stolon at a point between the nodes where the rhizoids branch off. In contrast to *Rhizopus* and *Absidia, Mucor* has neither stolons nor rhizoids and consequently fills the culture dish less rapidly and does not adhere to the lid. In some species *(Rhizomucor pusillus* and *Rhizopus rhizopodoformis)* rhizoids are scant and poorly developed. These relationships are shown in Figures 2, 3, and 4.

In addition to the asexual spores in the sporangia, the Mucorales also produce sexual spores, but they are rarely seen on routine agar cultures. The sexual spores are designated zygospores and result from the fusion of hyphae from two neighboring thalli, a process known as heterothallic conjugation. Despite the implication that two different sexes participate in this conjugation, the conjugating hyphae cannot be distinguished from each other. When

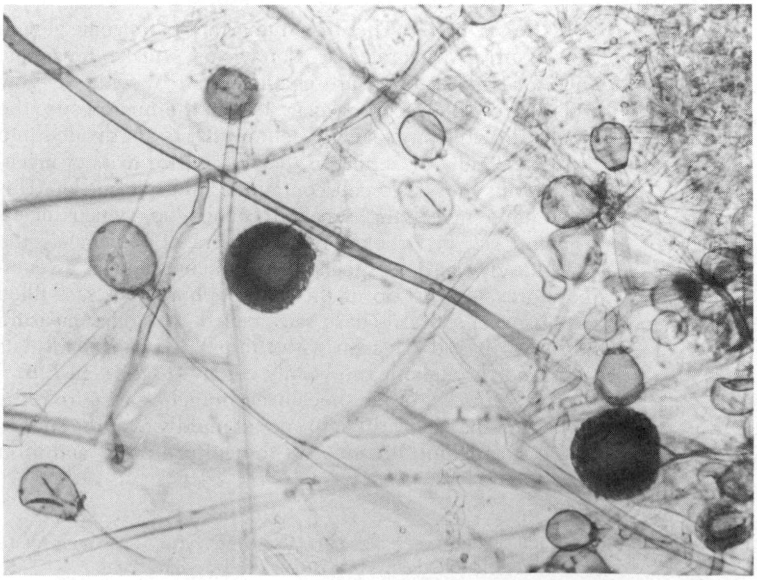

Figure 3. Culture mount of *Rhizomucor pusillus* from blood of fatal case of pulmonary mucormycosis. Note nonseptate mycelium, sporangiophore, and sporangium filled with asexual spores. The tip of the sporangiophore appears within the sporangium as a round swelling known as the columella. (Identification confirmed by J. J. Ellis, Research Mycologist, United States Department of Agriculture Research Service, Peoria, Illinois, Accession #NRRLA 12, 299.)

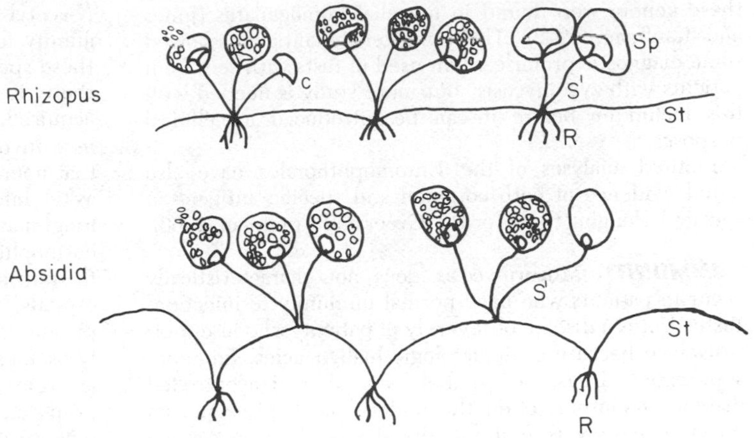

Figure 4. Diagram of structural relationships of stolons (ST), rhizoids (R), sporangiophore (S), columella (C), and sporangium (SP) in *Rhizopus* and *Absidia*. Note that the sporangiophores of *Rhizopus* arise from the point at which the rhizoids are formed, whereas in *Absidia* the sporangiophores come off from the arched stolons. Also note the hemispherical shape of the columella in *Rhizopus* and the pear-shaped columella in *Absidia*.

two hyphae conjugate, their tips come together and become separated from the rest of the mycelium by a cross-wall, the only septum that characteristically occurs in these otherwise nonseptate fungi. As the tips fuse, the walls separating them dissolve, so that the multinucleated masses of protoplasm in the two cells can run together, and the nuclei fuse. The wall of the fused cell becomes very thick.

In contrast to the prolific woolly colonies of the Mucorales, those of the Entomophthorales are flat and are covered by short, white mycelial fuzz. In further contrast, the mycelia of the Entomophthorales are septate. The two main pathogenic genera of Entomophthorales are known as *Entomophthora* and *Basidiobolus*.

Basidiobolus haptosporus, the organism that causes tropical subcutaneous phycomycosis, grows rapidly at room temperature and produces three kinds of spores: conidia, zygospores, and chlamydospores. The conidia are actually uninucleate sporangia that are carried at the end of a short sporangiophore. These sporangia (or conidia) are discharged forcibly onto the glass surface of the culture tube or lid of the petri dish. The fragment of sporangiophore (or "basidium") immediately adjacent to the ejected sporangium is carried along with it. The sporangium is a smooth, globular structure measuring 16 to 45 μ in length. The zygospores are the most distinctive spores. They are spherical, have a thick, smooth wall, and measure 20 to 40 μ in diameter. Two "conjugation breaks" protrude from the zygospore (Fig. 5) as remnants of the hyphal ends (copulation tubes) that fuse during conjugation. The third spore, the chlamydospore, differentiates from other cells within the septate mycelium by developing a markedly thickened cell wall. Production of chlamydospores continues to increase as the culture ages and the relative number of zygospores and sporangia declines.

Entomophthora coronata, which causes African nasal phycomycosis (rhinoentomophthoromycosis), also produces many chlamydospores. In contrast to *Basidiobolus*, however, *E. coronata* rarely has any zygospores and has only sparse septa in the mycelium. The organisms contain numerous conidia, which are shot off from their short individual conidiophores, but the expelled conidia do not carry a fragment of conidiophore (or "basidium") as do the conidia of *Basidiobolus*. The discharged conidia of *E. coronata* have the unique property of producing small secondary conidia that may form a crown around the parent (hence the name "coronata"). These secondary conidia are carried on short conidiophores that emerge from the primary conidium. Instead of secondary conidia, degenerating conidia may produce at their periphery many hairlike appendages that resemble flagella.

ANTIGENIC COMPOSITION. The Zygomycetes have not been subject to the extensive antigenic analysis carried out with other pathogenic fungi, and no serologic test has been standardized for the diagnosis of mucormycosis, subcutaneous phycomycosis, or rhinoentomophthoromycosis. In preliminary studies using immunodiffusion, common antigens shared by *Absidia*, *Mucor*, and *Rhizopus* have been found in culture filtrates, and antigens specific for each of

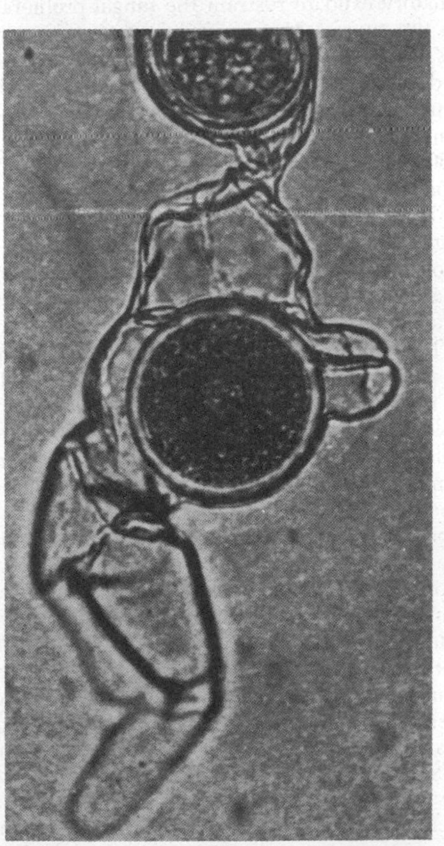

Figure 5. Zygospore of *Basidiobolus haptosporus*. The two conjugation beaks that protrude from the zygospore are remnants of the hyphal ends that fuse during conjugation. (From Burkitt, D. P., Wilson, A., and Jelliffe, D.: Br Med J 1:1669, 1964.)

these genera were found in mycelial homogenates (Jones and Kaufman, 1978). The homogenate antigens showed some diagnostic promise when used in tests with sera from patients with zygomycosis, but more study is needed with this technique before it can be introduced for clinical purposes.

Limited analyses of the Entomophthorales have also found evidence of both common and specific antigens in species belonging to this order (Greer and Friedman, 1966).

IMMUNITY. Mucormycosis does not characteristically occur in patients who have normal immunity to infection. Instead, it is a disease of severely ill patients who lose their resistance because of hematologic malignancies, immunosuppressive drugs, or metabolic disorders. Uncontrolled diabetes mellitis is often the underlying disease, and an infection closely resembling the disease in man can be produced in rabbits with acute alloxan diabetes, but not in metabolically normal rabbits. The hyperglycemia in both human and experimental diabetes probably stimulates the growth of the fungus and at the same time impairs phagocytosis. In experimental diabetes, the polymorphonuclear (PMN) leukocytes respond vigorously to invasion by *Rhizopus oryzae,* but the PMN leukocytes uniformly show nuclear pyknosis and karyorrhexis (Bauer et al., 1956). It is also known that high glucose levels impair phagocytosis of other pathogenic organisms (Chernew and Braude, 1962). The importance of normal leukocytes in preventing mucormycosis is evident when normal rabbits are inoculated with spores of *R. oryzae;* the leukocytes in the acute inflammatory exudate restrain the fungal proliferation and destroy the spores. Moreover, in neutropenic animals or patients, there is less resistance to mucormycosis. Most reported cases of phycomycosis in nondiabetics have occurred in leukemic patients with severe neutropenia (Parkhurst and Vlahides, 1967; Meyer et al., 1972; McBride et al., 1960). Other cases have occurred in burn wounds in which phagocytosis is impaired.

If leukocytes and other immune factors cannot restrain the fungus, it invades vessels and infarcts tissues. The usual portal of entry appears to be the nasal turbinates or paranasal sinuses; from there, the organism extends along the invaded vessels to the retroorbital tissues and cerebrum. Thrombosis of arteries and veins causes multiple infarcts throughout the brain, but only a minimal inflammatory response is found because the inflammatory cells are depleted or their function is impaired. If spores of the Mucorales are inhaled or ingested, they may invade the walls and vessels of bronchi, stomach, or intestine of neutropenic patients.

In contrast to the Mucorales, the Entomophthorales produce infection in apparently normal people. Like mucormycosis, rhinoentomophthoromycosis also invades the nasal mucosa but stops short of the vessels, and there is no tendency to infarct the tissues. The affinity of spores from both Mucorales and Entomophthorales for the human nasal mucosa is a striking phenomenon, but its mechanism is mysterious. Normally, the cilia of the nose carry foreign particles to the posterior pharynx, where they are swallowed. Since other fungal spores are not arrested in the nose, it is possible that those of the Zygomycetes can impair ciliary action and inactivate this important means of natural resistance to nasal infection. A second possibility is that the nasal mucosa has receptors that hold the spores to the cell surfaces. Finally, it has been suggested that the *N*-acetyl neuraminic acid in nasal mucin has a specific affinity for spores of the Zygomycetes. Although none of these speculations on natural resistance has been verified, there is more solid information on the mechanism of acquired immunity. It appears that immunity to *E. coronata* involves eosinophils through a mechanism similar to that operating in schistosomiasis, filariasis, and other parasitic infections. The inflammatory exudate around the fungi may be composed almost entirely of eosinophils, and eosinophil granules are aggregated in close apposition to the fungal cell walls (Williams et al., 1969). Charcot-Leyden crystals, which are derived from eosinophils, are also present. In addition to the eosinophil granules and crystals, lysosomes, mitochondria, vacuoles, and pinocytic vesicles are released by cell necrosis. For this reason it has been proposed that the fungi lyse the eosinophils and other inflammatory cells so that their cytoplasmic and nuclear contents are released. These form an eosinophilic precipitate or "sleeve" around the fungus, called the Splendore-Hoeppli phenomenon, like that seen around schistosome ova. The adjacent granulomatous infiltrate is composed of macrophages, lymphocytes, and plasma cells. If current concepts on cellular immunity to worms can be translated into immunity against fungi, these histologic observations in enterophthoromycosis imply that IgE interacts with macrophages and eosinophils so that both cells can kill *E. coronata.* The tissue reaction in subcutaneous phycomycosis due to *Basidiobolus haptosporus* is identical, producing an eosinophilic sheath around the hyphae and showing no invasion of vessels. The cellular immune reaction of eosinophils and macrophages appears to be effective because both infections are benign and may even regress spontaneously (Burkitt et al., 1964). Since the infection by *B. haptosporus* occurs almost exclusively in childhood, it would seem that immunity acquired then protects adults.

LABORATORY DIAGNOSIS. In cerebral mucormycosis, the fungus can be found in sections and cultures of the infarcted nasal turbinate or paranasal sinus. In pulmonary mucormycosis, it can be found in lung biopsies or in metastatic skin lesions. For mysterious reasons, the etiologic agent of cerebral mucormycosis has rarely if ever been cultured from the brain or spinal fluid, even when fresh tissues known to harbor the characteristic mycelium were subjected to expert mycologic techniques. The fungus most frequently isolated in mucormycosis is *Rhizopus oryzae.* Other species have been identified as *Rhizopus arrhizus, Rhizopus rhizopodiformis, Absidia corymbifera,* and *Rhizomucor pusillus.* Two other Mucorales, *Cunninghamella bertholetiae* and *Saksenaea vasiformis,* have also caused opportunistic human infection of the lung *(C. bertholetiae)* and brain *(S. vasiformis)* on rare occasions. *Cunninghamella* is easily separated from the other Mucorales because it has no sporangium and its conidia arise from a vesicle like that found in *Aspergillus.* Both *Cunninghamella* and *Sakesenaea* resemble *Mucor* in their rapidly growing gray colonies and coenocytic hyphae. *Saksenaea* produces a unique flask-shaped sporangium but only after prolonged incubation under special cultural conditions (Ajello et al., 1976). A third genus involved in some human infections is *Mortierella,* which is characterized by the absence of a columella and branched, tapering sporangiophores.

It is impossible to distinguish among the species of Mucorales in the tissues of patients with mucormycosis, but they can be differentiated from other fungi that produce hyphae in tissues. In contrast to the hyphae of *Aspergillus* and *Candida*, those of the Mucorales are nonseptate, branch irregularly, and stain deeply with hematoxylin and eosin or silver-methenamine but poorly with the periodic acid-Schiff (PAS) stain. *Aspergillus* is septate, stains better with PAS than hematoxylin, and branches with great regularity. The various genera of Mucorales are identified by the characteristics in Figures 2, 3, and 4. Special guides must be consulted for identification of species (Ellis and Hesseltine, 1966; Zycha, 1935).

The Entomophthorales, *B. haptosporus* and *E. coronata*, are also identified by biopsy and culture. As noted in the previous section, the two produce identical histologic changes that strongly suggest the diagnosis without culture. In contrast to those of the Mucorales, the hyphae of the Entomophthorales take up hematoxylin poorly and are usually septate. The poorly stained hyphae may appear as circular spaces surrounded by a cuff of amorphous eosinophilic material representing the Splendore-Hoeppli phenomenon. Large numbers of eosinophils are also present in acute exudates. The hyphae may be surrounded by epithelioid cells and ingested by giant cells. The poorly staining walls of the hyphae and the absence of cytoplasm in subcutaneous phycomycosis give the impression of tunnels through subcutaneous inflammatory tissue. Because of the prominent eosinophils, these tunnels were thought at one time to be the track of an unidentified worm larva (Burkitt et al., 1964).

If tiny fragments of tissue are incubated on Sabouraud's medium at 37°C, the fungi grow rapidly, and the characteristic radially folded, wax-colored colonies appear in three days. The diagnostic zygospores are seen after one or two weeks in cultures of *B. haptosporus* but do not develop in *E. coronata*.

DRUG SUSCEPTIBILITY. The zygomycetes are uniformly susceptible to amphotericin B, which is effective in treatment if started early in the infection. The minimal inhibitory concentration of amphotericin B ranges from 0.8 to 1.6 μg/ml. These organisms are usually resistant to 5-fluorocytosine and miconazole.

EPIDEMIOLOGY. The Mucorales are ubiquitous thermotolerant molds that thrive in any organic material. *Rhizopus* is an important cause of spoilage in fruits and sweet potatoes. The disease in strawberries is known as leak because of drippings from the softened fruit. The mucors are also found frequently on stale, moist breads ("bread molds") and can hydrolyze starch to sugar. Yet despite their wide prevalence in food and other organic materials, the Mucorales are not commonly encountered in hospital environments where susceptible diabetics, leukemics, and burn patients are likely to be exposed. Recent outbreaks of skin and subcutaneous mucormycosis were reported in hospitals using contaminated commercial elastic dressings (Elastoplast tapes), but cultures of the environment over a ten year period in the same institution have not grown Mucorales (Gartenberg et al., 1978). Their absence in the hospital despite their frequent presence in food is puzzling and might indicate that Mucorales in food can infect debilitated patients without spreading to the hospital environment. This puzzle, and the mysterious failure to culture the fungus from the brains of patients with histologically proven cases of mucormycosis, imply that pathogenic Mucorales may sometimes lose their ability to grow on environmental or laboratory substrates but not in certain tissues.

The epidemiology of infection by the Entomophthorales is also puzzling because infections by these fungi are remarkably infrequent for such ubiquitous fungi. It has been suggested that environmental temperatures limit the period during which *B. haptosporus* can be infectious. The fungus grows poorly at 15°C, so that in temperate climates it can be disseminated only during the few warm months from its reservoir in the gastrointestinal tracts of insectivorous reptiles (Clark, 1968). This factor also explains why nearly all cases of subcutaneous phycomycosis occur in tropical areas such as Uganda, Kenya, Sudan, the Cameroons, Indonesia, India, and parts of Southeast Asia. It has not been reported from the Western Hemisphere. Infections with *B. haptosporus* occur mainly in children, who probably acquire them from minor trauma or insect bites. It is a fungus of low pathogenicity and is seldom able to cause infection in adults, who seem to acquire immunity from clinical or subclinical exposure earlier in life.

The epidemiology of rhinoentomophthoromycosis due to *E. coronata* differs in two main respects from that of subcutaneous phycomycosis caused by *B. haptosporus*. First, *E. coronata* infections are probably transmitted by spore inhalation rather than insect bites, since the portal of entry is the nose. Second, it is a disease of adult agricultural workers, especially men exposed to the fungus growing in the soil or vegetation of tropical rain forests in Africa. It has also been reported from similar regions such as Colombia, Brazil, India, and Puerto Rico.

References

Ajello, L., Dean, F., and Irwin, R.: The zygomycete *Saksenaea vasiformis* as a pathogen of humans with a critical review of the etiology of zygomycosis. Mycologia 68:52, 1976.

Bauer, H., Flanagan, J., and Sheldon, W.: The effects of metabolic alterations on experimental *Rhizopus oryzae* (mucormycosis) infection. Yale J Biol Med 29:23, 1956.

Burkitt, D. P., Wilson, A., and Jelliffe, D.: Subcutaneous phycomycosis: A review of 31 cases seen in Uganda. Br Med J 1:1669, 1964.

Chernew, I., and Braude, A.: Depression of phagocytosis by solutes in concentrations found in the kidney and urine. J Clin Invest 41:1945, 1962.

Clark, B.: The epidemiology of phycomycosis. In Wolstenholme, G., and Porter, R. (eds.): Symposium on Systemic Mycoses. Boston, Little, Brown & Company, 1968, p. 179.

Ellis, J., and Hesseltine, C.: Species of *Absidia* with ovoid sporangiospores. Sabouraudia 5:59, 1966.

Gartenberg, G., Bottone, E., Keusch, G., and Weitzman, I.: Hospital-acquired mucormycosis *(Rhizopus rhizopodiformis)* of skin and subcutaneous tissues: Epidemiology, mycology and treatment. N Engl J Med 299:1115, 1978.

Greer, D., and Friedman, L.: Antigenic relationships between the fungus causing subcutaneous phycomycosis and saprophytic isolates of *Basidiobolus meristosporus* and *B. ranarum*. Sabouraudia 5:7, 1966.

Jones, K., and Kaufman, L.: Development and evaluation of an immunodiffusion test for diagnosis of systemic zygomycosis (mucormycosis): Preliminary report. J Clin Microbiol 7:97, 1978.

McBride, R., Corson, J., and Dammin, G.: Mucormycosis: Two cases of disseminated disease with cultural identification of *Rhizopus:* Review of literature. Am J Med 28:832, 1960.

Meyer, R., Rosen, P., and Armstrong, D.: Phycomycosis complicating leukemia and lymphoma. Ann Intern Med 77:871, 1972.

Parkhurst, G., and Vlahides, G.: Fatal opportunistic disease. JAMA 202:279, 1967.

Waksman, S. A., and Starkey, R. L.: The Soil and the Microbe. New York, John Wiley and Sons, 1931.

Williams, A., Lichtenberg, F., Smith, J., and Martinson, F.: Ultrastructure of phycomycosis due to entomophthora, basiodiobolus, and associated "Splendore-Hoeppli" phenomenon. Arch Pathol 87: 495, 1969.

Zycha, H., Siepman, R. and Linnemann, G.: Mucorales. Verlag von J Cramer, Lehre Federal Republic of Germany, 1969.

81

DEMATIACEAE: AGENTS OF CHROMOMYCOSIS AND PHAEOHYPHOMYCOSIS

YOUSEF AL-DOORY, PH.D
GERALD E. WAGNER, PH.D

The dematiaceous fungal agents of chromomycosis encompass several genera of genetically related pigmented fungi. All of these fungi contain a cytoplasmic, melanin-like pigment that appears to have ecological significance by decreasing the susceptibility of these organisms to physical and chemical antifungal agents. Traditionally, five species of dematiaceous fungi have been considered to be the etiologic agents of chromomycosis on the basis of their repeated isolation from diseased tissue. The clinical appearance of chromomycosis, a chronic disease of skin and subcutaneous tissue, does not differ with respect to the species of fungus isolated. These fungi produce nodules or plaques on the legs, arms, face, and trunk of adults living in rural areas throughout the world.

The taxonomy of the dematiaceous fungi is complex and confusing. The names used in this chapter are those proposed by McGinnis (1980). The four principal fungi of chromomycosis are: *Fonsecaea pedrosoi*, *Fonsecaea compacta*, *Phialophora verrucosa*, and *Cladosporium carrionii*. As a group these fungi are characterized by an abundance of dry aerial hyphae on culture media. *Wangiella dermatitidis*, formerly considered a cause of chromomycosis, shows a second type of growth consisting of dark, soft, moist colonies that undergo a yeast-like phase during the course of their development.

A few other dematiaceous fungi occasionally have been reported as the etiologic agents of human disease. For example, *Cladosporium bantianum* (synonymous with *Cladosporium trichoides*) has been described as the causative agent of phaeohyphomycosis, formerly considered to be cerebral chromomycosis by some workers (Al-Doory, 1972). It produces thick-walled brain abscesses or meningitis. Species of the genera *Wangiella*, *Exophiala*, and *Phialophora* may cause subcutaneous phaeohyphomycosis, in which cystic granulomas develop in the subcutis of the extremities.

MORPHOLOGY. All of the etiologic agents of chromomycosis grow slowly on standard mycological culture media producing darkly colored colonies that appear black when viewed from the reverse side of the culture medium. However, individual strains of these fungi show considerable variation in color, rate of growth, and colonial morphology. *F. pedrosoi* colonies are flat and covered with short, feltlike aerial hyphae that are dark green to brown or black. *F. compacta* colonies, on the other hand, are heaped, brittle, and covered with coarse aerial hyphae. Colonies of *C. carrionii* may appear smooth or irregular with a defined margin bordered by darker submerged hyphae. *P. verrucosa* is characterized by dark brown to black colonies with olive to gray aerial hyphae. *W. dermatitidis* matures from a moist, glistening olive to black colony to one showing feathery strands of submerged, tightly compressed hyphae radiating outward from the margin. These hyphae eventually give rise to olive-gray aerial mycelia (Fig. 1).

Microscopically, these species of fungi reveal dark conidia and pigmented hyphae with three types of conidiophores (Fig. 2). The phialophora-type, found mainly in *P. verrucosa*, is a distinct conidiophore formed either terminally or along the hypha. It generally is flask-shaped with an oval or elongated base, constricted neck, and an opening that may or may not have a flaring collarette and lip. The conidia form semi-endogenously and extrude through the neck.

The cladosporium-type conidiophore is found principally in *C. bantianum*. This is a simple conidiophore that is slightly enlarged at the distal end. The conidia form at the tip of this type of conidiophore and a few may bud, forming secondary conidia. A continuation of this budding process produces long branching chains of conidia.

The third type of conidiophore is the fonsecaea-type, which was formerly and erroneously referred to as the acrotheca-type. The two species of *Fonsecaea* associated with chromomycosis commonly are characterized by this type of conidiophore, although the other two types also may be found occasionally in *Fonsecaea* species. This structure resembles vegetative hyphae with conidia forming irregularly at the tip and along the sides of the conidiophore.

In tissue taken from a case of chromomycosis, pigmented spherical sclerotic bodies are observed. These characteristic cells are 4 to 12 μm in size and exhibit muriform transverse sections (Fig. 3). Phaeohyphomycosis is characterized by irregular masses of darkly pigmented hyphae in the tissue.

ANTIGENIC COMPOSITION. Few studies of the antigenic composition and relatedness of the various etiologic agents of chromomycosis have been reported. The cell walls of *F. pedrosoi*, *P. verrucosa*, and *C. carrionii* are composed of 17 to 31 per cent glucose, 8 to 14 per cent mannose, 6 to 8 per cent glucosamine, and 29 to 42 per cent protein (Szaniszlo et al., 1972).

Complement fixation, agglutination, agglutination-absorption, and precipitation tests have been described (Martin et al., 1936; Seeliger et al., 1959; Seeliger, 1968). Furthermore, patients with chromomycosis have circulating antibodies (Buckley and Murray, 1966). Cross-precipitation tests show that *F. pedrosoi*, *F. compacta*, and *P. verrucosa* are related and antigenically distinct from *C carrionii* (Buckley and Murray, 1966). *C. carrionii* can be differentiated by fluorescent antibody from *C. bantianum*, which causes phaeohyphomycosis (cerebral chromomycosis) (Al-Doory and Gordon, 1963; Gordon and Al-Doory, 1965).

No consistent antigenic patterns have been found to describe firmly and delineate antigenically the various species of chromomycotic fungi. Similarly, there is no serologic test with diagnostic significance for patients in whom the disease is suspected.

METABOLISM. Major studies on the metabolism of the chromomycotic fungi have not been reported. They produce neither exotoxins nor endotoxins, and lack the proteolytic enzymes that peptonize milk. They cannot liquefy Loeffler's coagulated-serum medium or gelatin (Fuentes and Bosch, 1960).

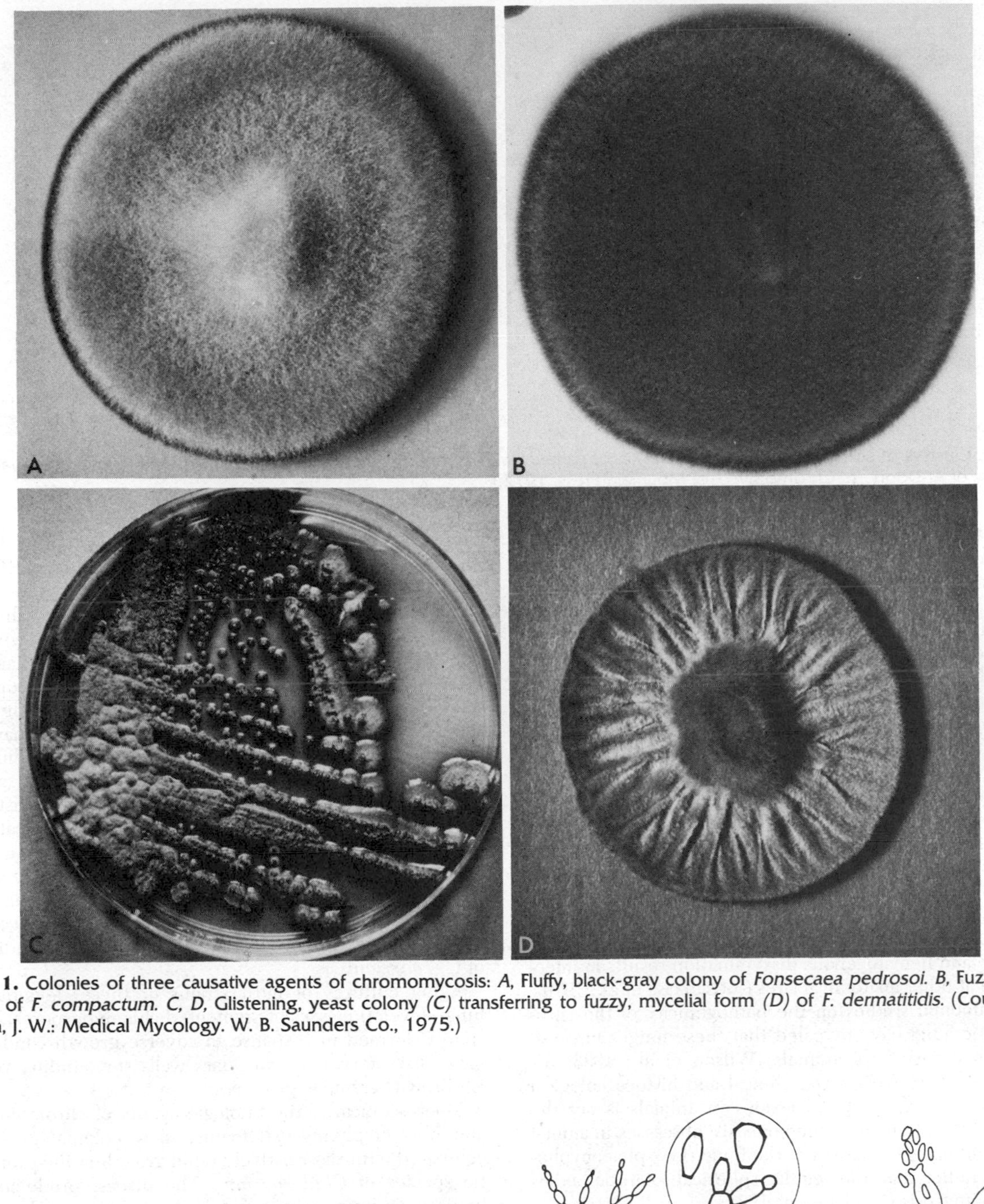

Figure 1. Colonies of three causative agents of chromomycosis: *A,* Fluffy, black-gray colony of *Fonsecaea pedrosoi. B,* Fuzzy, black colony of *F. compactum. C, D,* Glistening, yeast colony *(C)* transferring to fuzzy, mycelial form *(D)* of *F. dermatitidis.* (Courtesy of Rippon, J. W.: Medical Mycology. W. B. Saunders Co., 1975.)

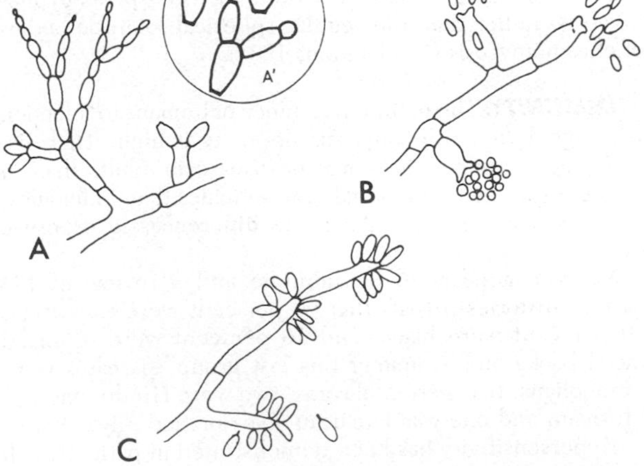

Figure 2. Sporulation types in the causative agents of chromomycosis. *A,* Cladosporium-type. Note the thickened sacs or disjunctors *(A').* *B,* Phialophora type. *C,* Fonsecaea type. (Courtesy of Rippon, J. W.: Medical Mycology. W. B. Saunders Co., 1975.)

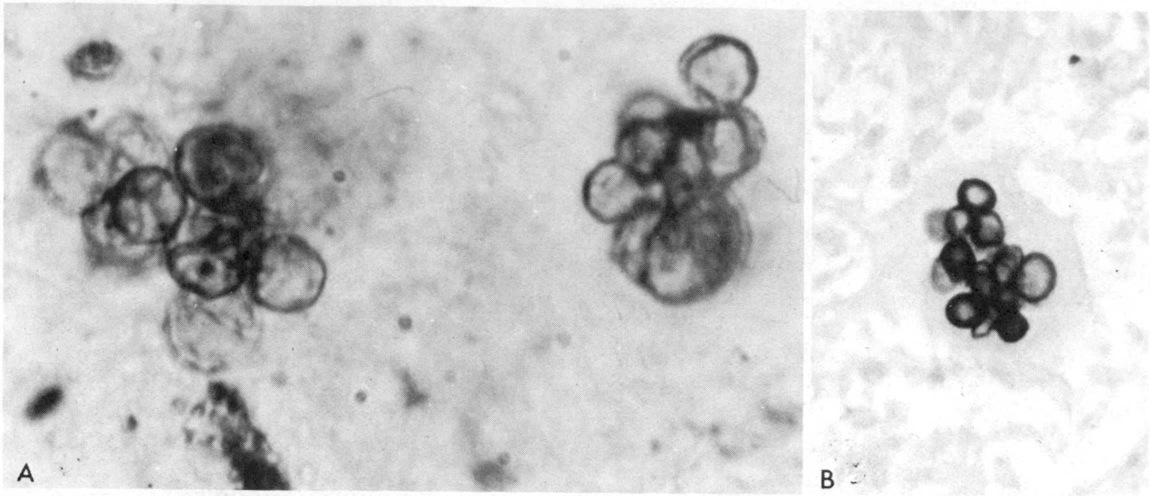

Figure 3. Clusters of sclerotic fungal cells from skin of patients with chromomycosis. Note internal septa in *A* and thick walls in *B*. (Courtesy of Al-Doory, Y.: Chromomycosis. Mountain Press, 1972.)

PATHOGENIC PROPERTIES. The chromomycotic fungi are found in soil, organic debris, and on certain plants. Therefore, infection is from an exogenous source and actual implantation of the fungus occurs through a break in the skin and/or subcutaneous tissue. It is believed that these fungi are not highly pathogenic because it appears that repeated exposure is required for the fungi to overcome the natural barriers and normal resistance of the human body. Accordingly, chromomycosis is a noncontagious disease and transmission from human to human never has been reported.

The chromomycotic fungi can affect organ systems and tissues other than those at the site of inoculation, resulting in systemic or cerebral involvement. A review of the available medical histories of patients with chromomycosis provides evidence that, in addition to localized foci of infection on the extremities, aerosolization of the fungus can cause primary pulmonary lesions. Subsequent lymphangitic and hematogenous dissemination results in infectious foci at other anatomical sites (Jotisankasa et al., 1970).

Experimental studies on the pathogenicity of the chromomycotic fungi have revealed that these fungi can cause lesions in a variety of animals (Wilson et al., 1933; Al-Doory, 1972). However, the clinical and histopathological appearance of experimental lesions in animals is not the same as that in human chromomycosis; abscesses in animal tissue yield mycelial masses of the fungi (i.e., phaeohyphomycosis) rather than the regular spherical sclerotic bodies of chromomycosis (MacKinnon, 1934).

IMMUNITY. The natural resistance of humans to infection with agents of chromomycosis normally is high. There is, however, a greater incidence of disease in adults than in younger (preteen) individuals and in males than in females, but this may be due, in part, to differences in exposure rates.

No race appears to be immune and a review of 124 patient histories reveals that 60 per cent were Caucasian, 30 per cent were black, and 10 per cent were of mixed racial backgrounds; among this last group, six cases were Mongolians, two were Malayans, two were Hindu, one was Mexican, and one was Jamaican (Carrion and Silva, 1947).

Hypersensitivity has been demonstrated in patients with chromomycosis; this response diminishes after clinical recovery. However, the relationship between this finding and resistance to reinfection is unknown (Rippon, 1982).

LABORATORY DIAGNOSIS. The appearance of the chromomycotic fungi in tissue or pus as spherical, thick-walled, chestnut-brown sclerotic bodies is a significant diagnostic feature in histopathology (Fig. 3). In the microscopic examination of culture material, the presence of the three types of conidiophore formations is an important characteristic of *Fonsecaea* species although the ratio of conidiophore types varies depending upon species, strain, and growth environment. Additionally, the appearance of moist, glistening, yeast-like colonies that grow at 40°C indicates *W. dermatitidis*, while subglobose conidia borne in a tight, compact chain indicates *F. compacta*. The presence of only phialophora-type conidiophores in the culture is characteristic of *P. verrucosa* and the cladosporium-type conidiophores with extremely long chains of conidia is indicative of *C. caorrionii*.

Aging cultures of most strains of these dematiaceous fungi develop masses of pigmented chlamydospores. These spores, formed in response to adverse growth conditions, have characteristic coarse, dark walls surrounding yellowish-brown, granular protoplasm.

Macroscopically, the etiologic agents of chromomycosis and phaeohyphomycosis feature slow colonial growth as compared with the relatively rapid growth of the saprophytic species of *Cladosporium*. The disease-producing dematiaceous fungi cannot hydrolyze starch, coagulate milk, or liquefy gelatin, Loeffler's medium, or any other proteinaceous substance. The saprophytic species, on the other hand, are proteolytic (Fuentes and Bosch, 1960).

DRUG SENSITIVITY. The chromomycotic fungi are insensitive to antibiotics employed in the treatment of bacterial infections. In addition, aggressive therapy with currently available antifungal compounds only occasionally results in clinical remission. Amputation of the affected limb often is the eventual cure for chromomycosis and disseminated phaeohyphomycosis usually is fatal.

Amphotericin B is the drug of choice in most subcutaneous and systemic mycoses. However, large quantities of this polyene antibiotic are required to inhibit in vitro growth of the dematiaceous fungi. Dixon et al. (1978)

reported a mean MIC of 21 μg/ml for 13 dematiaceous fungi including *Cladosporium*, *Phialophora*, and *Fonsecaea* species. The average attainable serum level of amphotericin B is only 1.0 μg/ml.

The imidazole antifungal compounds have shown greater activity in vitro. The mean MIC for miconazole was reported to be 1.0 μg/ml and for an experimental imidazole it was 5 μg/ml (Dixon et al., 1978). Dixon et al. (1978a) also have reported an average MIC of 4 μg/ml for ketoconazole. Sufficient in vivo trials have not been conducted to establish the therapeutic efficacy of the imidazoles in chromomycosis.

5-Fluorocytosine appears to have minimal therapeutic efficacy in chromomycosis and phaeohyphomycosis although it has been used in combination with other drugs. The mean MIC was 60 μg/ml in a study of 14 dematiaceous fungi (Wagner et al., 1975). Among other chemotherapeutic agents inhibitory levels of thiabendazole (2-[4′-thiazoyl] benzimidazole) were in the range of 0.75 μg/ml for these fungi. The growth of *F. pedrosoi* was inhibited by sulfamerazine (Deeney et al., 1944), stilbamidine, propamidine, and pentamidine (Bocobo et al., 1953), and deamidines (Al-Doory, 1972). Potassium iodide, sodium iodide, and copper sulfate also inhibit their growth.

EPIDEMIOLOGY. Although reported from every continent, chromomycosis is most frequently encountered in the tropical and subtropical regions. It also appears that specific species of the dematiaceous fungi show geographic endemicity.

C. carrionii usually has been isolated from patients in South Africa, Venezuela, and Australia; *F. pedrosoi* from patients in the tropical and subtropical areas of Brazil, Costa Rica, and Cuba. *P. verrucosa* is considered to be the major cause of chromomycosis in cooler climates, including the United States.

The number of reported cases of chromomycosis is not an accurate representation of the distribution of these fungi due, in part, to the lack of accuracy and completeness in the reporting procedure. There is, however, no other guide available and Brazil has most reported cases of chromomycosis. In decreasing order, Madagascar, Costa Rica, Dominican Republic, Australia, Cuba, Colombia, Mexico, South Africa, and Paraguay also report a high incidence of the disease. Occupation, repeated exposure to the fungi with trauma, personal hygienic habits, and environmental conditions are important factors in the epidemiology of chromomycosis and may influence the geographic distribution of the fungi.

References

Al-Doory, Y.: Chromomycosis, Missoula, Mont., Mountain Press, 1972.

Al-Doory, Y.: The Epidemiology of Human Mycotic Diseases. Springfield, Ill., Charles C Thomas, 1965.

Al-Doory, Y., and Gordon, M.: Application of fluorescent-antibody procedures to the study of pathogenic dematiaceous fungi. I. Differentiation of *Cladosporium carrionii* and *Cladosporium bantianum*. J Bacteriol 96:332, 1963.

Blank, H., and Rebell, G.: Thiabendazole activity against the fungi of dermatophytosis, mycetomas and chromomycosis. J Invest Dermatol 44:219, 1965.

Bocobo, F. C., et al.: *In vitro* fungistatic activity of stilbamidine, propamidine, pentamidine and diethylstilbestrol. J Invest Dermatol 21:149, 1953.

Buckley, H. R., and Murray, I. G.: Precipitating antibodies in chromomycosis. Sauboraudia 5:78, 1966.

Carrion, A. L., and Silva, M. L.: Chromoblastomycosis and its etiologic fungi. Ann Cryptogamid Phytopathol 6:20, 1947.

Dixon, D., et al.: *In vitro* comparison of the antifungal activities of R34,000, miconazole and amphotericin B. Chemotherapy 24:364, 1978.

Dixon, D., et al.: Comparison of the *in vitro* antifungal antivity of miconazole and a new imidazole, R41,000. J Infect Dis 138:245, 1978a.

Fuentes, C. A., and Bosch, Z. E.: Biochemical differentiation of the etiological agents of chromoblastomycosis from nonpathogenic *Cladosporium* species. J Invest Dermatol 34:419, 1960.

Gordon, M. A., and Al-Doory, Y.: Application of fluorescent-antibody procedures to study the pathogenic dematiaceous fungi. II. Serological relationships of the genus *Fonsecaea*. J Bacteriol 89:551, 1965.

Jotisankasa, V., et al.: *Phialophora dermatitidis:* Its morphology and biology. Sabouraudia 8:98, 1970.

Mackinnon, J. E.: Estudio del primer casa Uruguayo de chromoblastomycosis y revista critica sobra el enfermedad. Arch Urug Med Cir Esep 5:201, 1934.

McGinnis, M. R.: Recent taxonomic developments and changes in medical mycology. Ann Rev Microbiol 34:109, 1980.

Martin, D. S., et al.: A case of verrucous dermatitis caused by *Hormodendrum pedrosoi* (chromoblastomycosis) in North Carolina. Am J Trop Med 16:593, 1936.

Rippon, J. W.: Medical Mycology: The Pathogenic Fungi and the Pathogenic Actinomycetes, 2nd ed. Philadelphia, W. B. Saunders Company, 1982.

Seeliger, H. P. R.: In The Fungi, vol. 3. New York, Academic Press, 1968.

Seeliger, H. P. R., et al.: Identification of fungi by serologic tests. Further serologic studies with dematiaceous fungi. Proceedings of the Sixth International Congress of Tropical Medicine. Malaria 4:636, 1959.

Szaniszlo, P. J., et al.: Chemical composition of the hyphal walls of three chromomycosis agents. Sabouraudia 10:94, 1972.

Wagner, G., et al.: New method for susceptibility testing with antifungal agents. Antibicrob Ag Chemother 8:107, 1975.

Wilson, S. J., et al.: Chromomycosis in Texas. Arch Dermatol 27:107, 1933.

82 FUSARIUM

Lynn A. Lancaster, M.D.

Molds of the genus *Fusarium* are distributed in soil throughout the world. They cause vascular wilt and cortical rot in numerous important plants, and recently have been recognized as the cause of keratomycosis and superficial nail and wound infections in normal people, and rarely of serious disseminated infection in immunocompromised patients.

Fusaria belong to the family Moniliaceae in the class *Hyphomycetes* of the *Fungi Imperfecti*. Asexual reproduction occurs through production of characteristic fusiform macroconidia, microconidia, and chlamydospores. Many species undergo sexual reproduction with formation of brightly colored perithecia. These specialized hyphal structures enclose packets (asci) of sexually derived spores called ascospores. Known perfect phases belong to the genera *Gibberella*, *Nectria*, *Calonectria*, and *Hyphomyces*. For further information see Nelson, Toussoun, and Cook (1981).

MORPHOLOGY. Fusaria produce fuzzy or wooly colonies on laboratory media. Colony pigmentation is highly variable in both color and intensity, and shades of every color (including white) are found.

Microscopically these molds consist of tangled masses of nonpigmented septate hyphae. Macroconidia are typically slightly curved with one or more septae dividing the spore into multiple cells (Fig. 1). Slight differences in the shapes of the apical and basal cells, the number of septae, the overall size, and the degree of curvature of the walls are important in distinguishing certain species. Microconidia may be pear shaped, oval, kidney shaped, or spindle shaped. In some species they may be divided by a septum. Conidia are born on simple or complex modifications of the hyphae called phialides. Chlamydospores, present in many species, are thick walled modifications of hyphae. They have refractile walls and are slightly larger than the surrounding hyphae. Chlamydospores are either born terminally at the end of a hyphal branch or are intercalated between vegetative hyphae.

PATHOGENIC PROPERTIES. Fusaria produce dozens of toxins, pigments, antibiotics, and other compounds. Many of these compounds have been extracted, purified, and well characterized. Some make farm animals ill when ingested as contaminants of cereal grains. Trichothecene toxins are suspected of causing toxic alimentary aleukia (see Chapter 15).

Tissue invasion by fusaria virtually never occurs in normal people with intact epithelium. Moist ulcerated skin in burn patients, diabetics, and patients with stasis ulcers may be colonized but usually without serious effect (English et al., 1971). However, fatal dissemination has been reported in severely burned patients (Wheeler et al., 1981; Abramonsky et al., 1974).

Cellular immunity and granulocytes prevent deep infection and dissemination from colonized sites, so that deep soft tissue infection in patients with soil-contaminated wounds is rare. Most disseminated infections have occurred in patients who possess readily recognized defects in cellular immunity or granulocyte function. In such patients, hyphae invade vessels and disseminate hematogenously. They plug end arteries and infarcts that become heavily

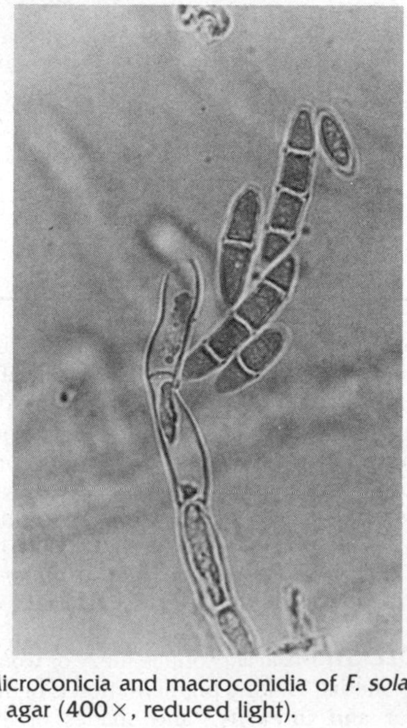

Figure 1. Microconicia and macroconidia of *F. solani* grown on Sabourands agar (400×, reduced light).

colonized by the fungus. The histological reaction is variable and ranges from almost no inflammatory cell infiltrate to suppuration and granuloma formation.

Fusarium causes serious infections of the cornea in healthy patients without recognizable defects in immunity (Forster and Rebell, 1975). Apparently, minor corneal abrasions can disrupt the protective epithelium. Inoculated spores can rapidly initiate mycelial growth and invade the corneal stroma. Untreated corneal infections almost always progress to perforation and blindness, perhaps because the avascular corneal stroma cannot deliver inflammatory cells. Strains isolated from the cornea are reported to grow well at 37°C, whereas strains from colonized leg wounds grow best at lower temperatures (English, 1972).

LABORATORY DIAGNOSIS. Hyphae of fusaria can be seen in smears by Gram, Geimsa, periodic acid–Schiff, and methenamine silver stains. The septate hyphae have parallel walls and branches that angle at 45 to 90°. Occasional swollen, rounded hyphal forms may be seen. Hyphae are well visualized in tissue sections by any of the methenamine silver stains.

Fusaria grow rapidly on most laboratory media used for primary isolation of fungi and bacteria. Media containing cycloheximide is inhibitory. Growth is usually visible after 24 to 48 hours' incubation on blood agar at 35°C and Sabouraud's agar incubated at room temperature. Characteristic macroconidia are easily visualized in tape mounts or tease preparations of the fungus soon after growth is visible.

A number of systems for speciation of the genus have been proposed. The more complex schemes recognize over 50 species (Booth, 1971; Nelson, Toussoun, and Cook, 1981). Medical mycologists prefer the nine species system of Snyder and Hansen in which species are distinguished largely by the morphology of the conidia. Accurate identification is difficult and requires careful microscopy with comparison of the observed morphology to drawings or photographs. Excellent pictoral guides for such purposes are available (Booth, 1971; Toussoun and Nelson, 1966; and Booth, 1977).

DRUG SUSCEPTIBILITY. Susceptibility of fusaria to amphotericin B has been reported to vary widely among strains isolated from wounds and disseminated disease, from minimum inhibitory concentrations less than 1.0 μg/ml to greater than 100 μg/ml (Bourguignon et al., 1976; Wheeler et al., 1981). Rebell (1981) states that *F. solani* isolates from cases of keratomycosis are usually susceptible to 1.25 μg/ml of amphotericin B, and 2.5 μg/ml natamycin (pimaricin) when tested at 37°C. Natamycin, a polyene antibiotic of smaller molecular weight than amphotericin B, appears to be very effective in treatment of keratomycosis due to fusaria (Forster and Rebell, 1975). Strains tested against 5 fluorocytosine have shown high level resistance. Two of four strains were inhibited by less than 1.56 μg/ml miconozole (Wheeler et al., 1981).

EPIDEMIOLOGY. Fusaria cause over half the reported cases of keratomycosis in many parts of the world, and *F. solani* is the species isolated in the vast majority. Less frequently isolated species include *F. dimerum*, *F. episphaeria*, *F. nivale*, *F. oxysporum*, and *F. moniliforme* (Rebell, 1981). Cuero (1980) showed that *F. solani* isolated from human eyes was similar to *F. solani* isolated in the local environment. Environmental sampling recovered more isolates in rural than urban areas. This correlates well with the increased incidence of trauma from plant or other outdoor material in patients with keratomycosis.

White onychomycosis, usually caused by *Trichophyton mentagrophytes,* is occasionally caused by *F. oxysporum* (Zaias, 1966). Deep localized soft tissue infections and osteomyelitis in normal persons are extremely uncommon. One case of osteomyelitis followed a thorn injury (Bourguignon et al., 1976), and another occurred postoperatively (Page et al., 1982). *F. oxysporum* and *F. solani* occasionally colonize burn wounds and stasis ulcers. Demonstration of tissue invasion by biopsy distinguishes potentially serious infection from colonization in burn wounds (Wheeler et al., 1981). Disseminated infections are rare in burn patients but potentially fatal. Although widespread in soil, fusaria are not common laboratory contaminants and deserve careful attention when recovered from burn wounds (Abramowsky et al., 1974). Disseminated infection has been reported rarely in leukemia, lymphoma, granulocytopenia, graft versus host disease, and other conditions (Cho et al., 1973; Young et al., 1979; and Mutton et al., 1980). An unusual case of brain abscess and meningitis occurred in a patient with chronic Epstein-Barr virus infection (Steinberg, 1983). *F. solani, F. oxysporum,* and *F. moniliforme* are the species most often recovered in disseminated infection. Mortality is high despite systemic antifungal therapy.

References

Abramowsky, C. R., Quinn, D., Bradford, W. D., and Conant, N. F.: Systemic infection by *Fusarium* in a burned child. J Pediatr 84:561, 1974.

Booth, C.: The Genus *Fusarium.* Kew, England; Commonwealth Mycological Institute, 1971.

Booth, C.: *Fusarium,* Laboratory Guide to the Identification of the Major Species. Kew, England, Commonwealth Mycological Institute, 1977.

Bourguignon, R. L., Walsh, A. F., Flynn, J. C., Baro, C., and Spinos, E.: *Fusarium* species osteomyelitis. J Bone Jt Surg 58-A:722, 1976.

Cho, C. T., Vats, T. S., Lowman, J. T., Brandsberg, J. W., and Tosh, F. E.: *Fusarium solani* infection during treatment for acute leukemia. J Pediatr 83:1028, 1973.

Cuero, R. G.: Ecological distribution of *Fusarium solani* and its opportunistic action related to mycotic keratitis in Cali, Colombia. J Clin Microbiol 12:455, 1980.

English, M. P., Smith, R. J., and Harman, R. R.: The fungal flora of ulcerated legs. Br J Dermatol 84:567, 1971.

English, M. P.: Observations on strains of *Fusarium solani, F. oxysporium* and *Candida parapsilosis* from ulcerated legs. Sabouraudia 10:35, 1972.

Forster, R. K, and Rebell, G.: The diagnosis and management of keratomycoses. I. Cause and diagnosis. Arch Opthalmol 93:975, 1975.

Forster, R. K. and Rebell, G.: The diagnosis and management of keratomycoses. II. Medical and surgical management. Arch Opthalmol 93:1134, 1975.

Mutton, K. J., Lucas, T. J., and Harkness, J. L.: Disseminated *Fusarium* infection. Med J Aust 2:624, 1980.

Nelson, P. E., Toussoun, T. A. and Cook, R. J. (eds.): *Fusarium:* Diseases, Biology, and Taxonomy. University Park, Pennsylvania State University Press, 1981.

Page, J. C., Friedlander, G., and Dockerg, G. L.: Postoperative *Fusarium* osteomyelitis. J Foot Surg 21:174, 1982.

Rebell, G. E.: *Fusarium* infections in human and veterinary medicine. In Nelson, P. E., Toussoun, T. A., and Cook, R. J. (eds.): *Fusarium:* Diseases, Biology, and Taxonomy. University Park, Pennsylvania State University Press, 1981.

Steinberg, G. K., Britt, R. H., Enzmann, D. R., Finlay, J. L., and Arvin, A. M.: *Fusarium* brain abscess. J Neurosurg 58:598, 1983.

Toussoun, T. A. and Nelson, P. E.: A Pictorial Guide to the Identification of *Fusarium* species. University Park, Pennsylvania State University Press, 1968.

Young, N. A., Kwon-Chung, K. J., Kubota, T. T., Jennings, A. E., and Fisher, R. I.: Disseminated infection by *Fusarium moniliforme* during treatment for malignant lymphoma. J Clin Microbiol 7:589, 1978.

Wheeler, M. S., McGinnis, M. R., Schell, W. A., and Walker, D. H.: *Fusarium* infection in burned patients. Am J Clin Path 75:304, 1981.

Zaias, N.: Superficial white onychomycosis. Sabouraudia 5:99, 1966.

83

MISCELLANEOUS FUNGI: THE AGENTS OF MYCETOMA AND RHINOSPORIDIUM

ABRAHAM I. BRAUDE, M.D., PH.D.

AGENTS OF MYCETOMA

Mycetoma is a clinical syndrome (Chapter 252) produced either by soil bacteria, the *Actinomycetes,* or by certain soil fungi that enter the tissues after trauma to the skin. They produce a chronic destructive inflammatory disease of skin and bones, converting the limb to a useless mass of tissue full of sinuses exuding granules of the infecting organism. The most common site of infection is the foot (Taralakshmi et al., 1977; Reddy et al., 1972), and the most common fungi causing mycetoma are *Pseudallescheria boydii, Madurella mycetomatus* and *Acremonium* sp. Among the less common causes are *Madurella grisea, Leptosphaeria senegalensis, Pyenochaeta romeroi, Exophiala jeanselmei,* and *Neotestudina rosatti.* Descriptions are provided here of *P. boydii, M. mycetomatus* and *Acremonium* sp. The properties of the others are summarized in Chapter 252.

Pseudallescheria boydii. This fungus, known as *Sadosporium apiospermum* in the asexual state, is the most common cause of mycetoma in the United States and Europe. It produces on any medium a rapidly spreading, fluffy white colony that turns gray and resembles the fur of mice. The most distinctive feature is the manner in which the conidia are attached to the mycelium. These asexual spores are usually borne singly at the tips and sides of single conidiophores but may sometimes occur in small groups (Fig. 1). The spores are egg- or lemon-shaped, measure 4 to 8 by 5 to 15 μ, and have a brown color.

Sexual reproduction is homothallic, i.e., the sexual spores, or ascospores, result from the fusion of cells from the same mycelial mat or thallus. Groups of eight ascospores are contained in sacs known as asci, which measure 8 to 20 μ in diameter. After a couple of weeks, the asci become enclosed in a protective hollow globe known as an ascocarp or perithecium. The ascocarps are dark brown and have a thin wall composed of one layer of modified hyphal cells. Ascocarps are not seen in many cultures but when present can be found in the agar or in the mycelium

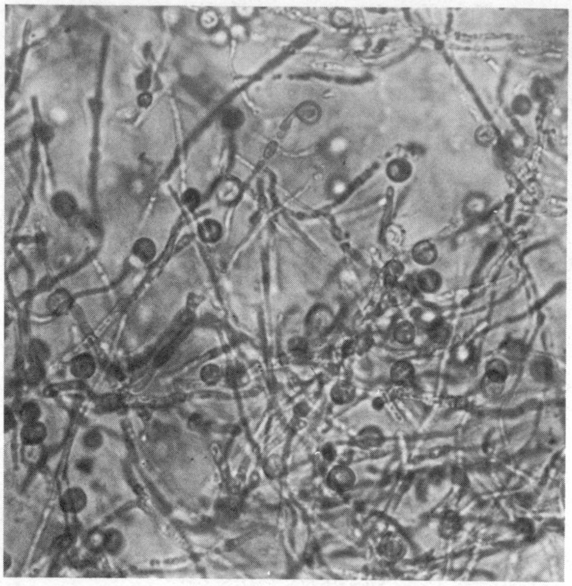

Figure 1. Hyphae and asexual spores of *Pseudallescheria boydii.* The asexual spores are borne singly at the tips and sides of single conidiophores.

near the edge of the colony. When they reach maturity, the thin wall of the ascocarp ruptures and releases the ascospores (Fig. 2).

In infected fistulas, colonies of the fungus take the form of white or yellow grains. In wet preparations or stained smears of crushed granules, a mycelial mass is seen. The mycelium measures 2 to 4 μ in diameter and swells peripherally to 10 μ. The periodic acid-Schiff stain or the Gomori methenamine silver stain may sometimes bring out details of the organism that are not visible in wet mounts.

In addition to mycetomas, the fungus can sometimes be cultured from *Pseudallescheria* infections of the lung, cornea, ear, paranasal sinuses, eye, and meninges. The infection can be introduced or disseminated by surgery and other invasive therapeutic procedures. Thus, chronic meningitis due to *P. boydii* has followed spinal anesthesia (Benham and George, 1948), and disseminated infection to the spine and long bones has occurred after lung biopsy performed at the time of heart surgery. A syndrome due to *P. boydii* that resembles lymphocutaneous sporotrichosis has also been reported (Conti-Diaz, 1980). Ketoconazole has been the most effective drug for treating infections with this fungus. The fungus is usually resistant to amphotericin B and may be sensitive (<1.0 μg/ml) to miconazole and ketoconazole.

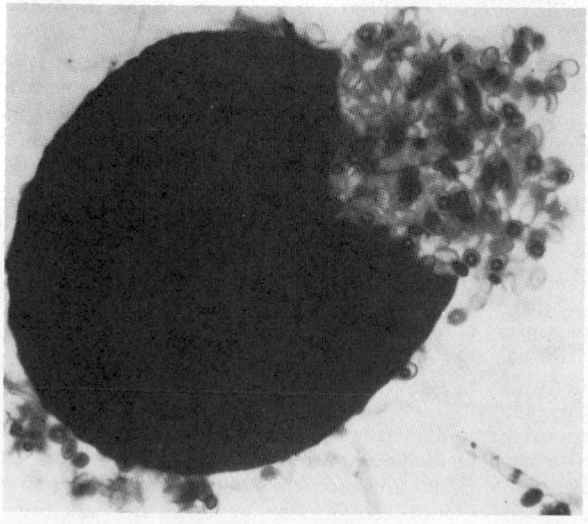

Figure 2. Ascospores of *P. boydii* escaping from perithecium (ascoscarp). (From Parker, J. C., and Klintworth, G. F.: In Baker, R. D. (ed.): Human Infections with Fungi, Actinomycetes, and Algae. New York, Springer-Verlag, 1971.)

M. mycetomatis. This fungus is probably the most common cause of eumycotic mycetoma and is found in Asia, Africa, and South America. In India, for example, it is isolated at least ten times more often from mycetoma than *P. boydii* (Taralakshmi et al., 1977). *M. mycetomatis* varies in colonial appearance from strain to strain, from case to case, and from one geographic area to another. In general, *M. mycetomatis* grows well at 37°C, producing in several days a white mycelium that soon turns brown. The growth is compact and has a wrinkled leathery surface, which becomes covered with a powdery down. Diffusible brown pigments stain the reverse side of the agar.

The hyphae are 3 to 4 μ in width and segmented. Spores are rare but, when present, take two forms: pyriform conidia and phialospores. The pyriform conidia are carried on short conidiophores, and the phialospores are extruded from short bottle-shaped stalks known as phialides.

In tissues, the hyphae form round masses that issue from draining fistulas as hard, black granules measuring 0.5 to 5 mm. The hyphal mass in the dense type is held together by a brownish cement that is homogenously distributed throughout the granule. In the vesicular type of granule, the cement is located around its periphery.

Acremonium Species (Cephalosporium Species). The characteristic feature of this genus is the balls of conidia (Fig. 3). The conidia are borne one at a time at the tips of short erect conidiophores that branch from the aerial hyphae. Successive conidia push the others aside so that they form clusters or small balls held together by a sticky exudate. The conidia are nonpigmented and elongated.

The fungus grows rapidly at room temperature and produces cottony white colonies with mycelia measuring 2 to 3 μ in diameter. In the tissues, it produces white oval granules less than 1 mm in size. The granules contain in their center a dense matt of mycelium with eosinophilic clubs at the periphery. There is no cement. They resemble the granules of *A. boydii*.

RHINOSPORIDIUM

The fungus *Rhinosporidium seeberi* produces small tumor-like masses usually in the nose (Fig. 4) and nasopharynx, but sometimes in the eye. The endosporulating fungus is seen in the tissues but cannot be cultured on laboratory media. It is placed in the class Phycomycetes (Ashworth, 1923) and in the family Coccidioidaceae because characteristic giant sporangia develop in the tissues (Fig. 5). These thick-walled, endospore-filled sporangia resemble the spherules of *Coccidioides immitis*.

Almost 90 per cent of reported cases have been from India and Sri Lanka. In the western hemisphere, rhinosporidiosis occurs mainly in Argentina, Brazil, and Mexico. The disease involves animals, especially horses, as well as humans.

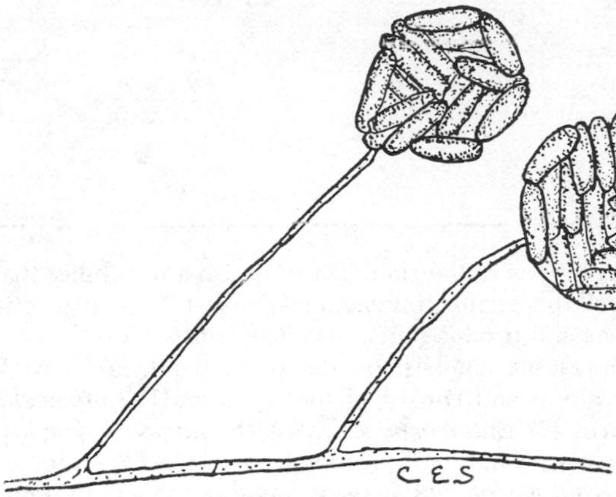

Figure 3. *Cephalosporium* species. The conidia form small balls at the tips of the conidiophores. (Drawing by C. E. Skinner from Skinner, C. E., Emmons, C. W., and Tsachiya, H. M.: Molds, Yeasts, and Actinomycetes. New York, John Wiley and Sons, 1947.)

The nasal disease is probably acquired by bathing or diving in infected water. In India, where rhinosporidiosis reaches epidemic proportions, its rarity in women is attributed to social taboos that prohibit women from bathing in open places. The characteristic lesion is a vascularized papillomatous proliferation of the nasal or pharyngeal mucous membrane containing sporangia in various stages of maturity. Red blood cells, inflammatory pus cells, and extruded endospores fill the interstitial tissues. As sporangia enlarge, they compress the columnar epithelium of the pharynx and allow endospores to escape and reinoculate the adjacent tissue. Ocular infection occurs in dry, dusty regions and may be transmitted in dust storms. In Texas, half the cases of rhinosporidiosis are ocular.

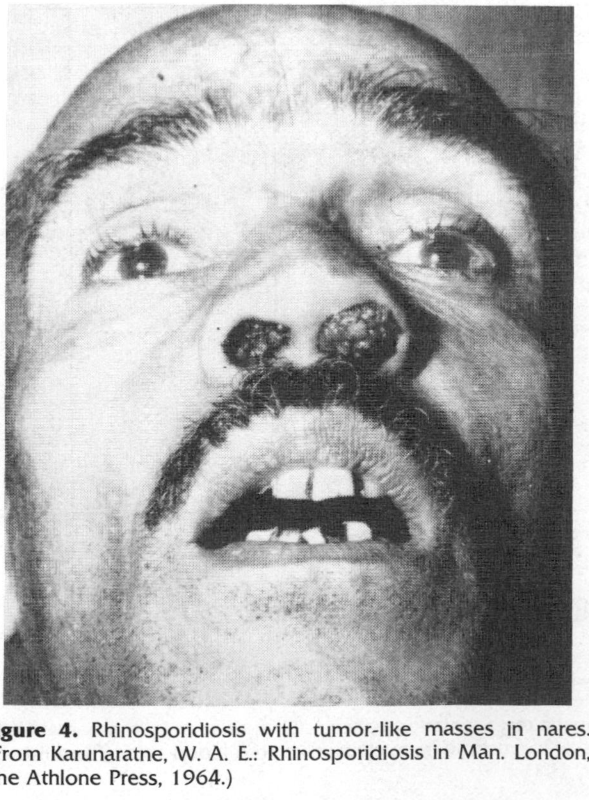

Figure 4. Rhinosporidiosis with tumor-like masses in nares. (From Karunaratne, W. A. E.: Rhinosporidiosis in Man. London, The Athlone Press, 1964.)

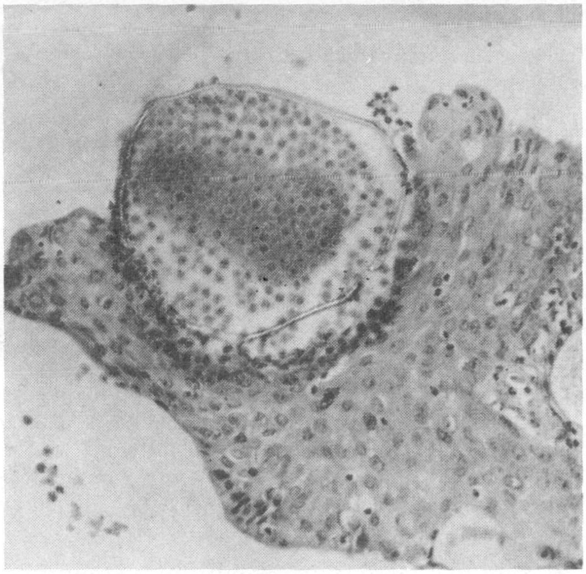

Figure 5. A sporangium is embedded in the epithelium, which is attempting to encircle it; the sporangium is filled with endospores. (From Karunaratne, W. A. E.: Rhinosporidiosis in Man. London, The Athlone Press, 1964.)

The vascularized papillomas produce single or multiple pedunculated, fleshy, red masses in the nares or pharynx and cause rhinitis, epistaxis, and nasal obstruction. In exceptional cases, hoarseness may develop from laryngeal infection. The conjunctiva of the lids is predominantly affected in the ocular form, which tends to be unilateral and remarkably free of pain. Although usually confined to the eye or nose, the infection may infrequently be seen in the vagina, rectum, male urethra, and bronchi. Generalized rhinosporidiosis and visceral involvement have also been reported.

The lesions can be completely removed by surgery or electrocautery. Electrocautery is preferred, because surgery leaves open incisions in which spores can be implanted and produce recurrences (Chitravel and Sundoram, 1981).

References

Ashworth, J. H.: On *Rhinosporidium seeberi* (Wernicke, 1903) with special reference to its sporulation and affinities. Trans R Soc Edin 53:301, 1923.

Benham, R., and George, L.: *Allescheria boydii*, causative agent of a meningitis. J Invest Dermatol 10:99, 1948.

Chitravel, V. B. M., Sundoram, B., et al.: Recurrent rhinosporidiosis in man: case reports. Mycopathologia 73:79, 1981.

Conti-Diaz: Micetomas Y procesos premicetomatoses en el Uruguay. Mycopathologia 72:59, 1980.

Karunaratne, W. A. E.: Rhinosporidiosis in Man. London, The Athlone Press, 1964.

Parker, J. C., and Klintworth, G. K.: Miscellaneous uncommon diseases attributed to fungi and actinomycetes. In Baker, R. D. (ed.): Human Infections with Fungi, Actinomycetes, and Algae. New York, Springer-Verlag, 1971, p. 958.

Reddy, C., Sundareschwar, B., Pattabni Rama Rao, A., and Reddy, S.: Mycetoma: Histopathologic diagnosis of causal agents in 50 cases. Indian J Med Sci 26:733, 1972.

Skinner, C. E., Emmons, C. W., and Tsuchiya, H. M.: Molds, Yeasts, and Actinomycetes. New York, John Wiley and Sons, 1947, p. 109.

Taralakshmi, V. V., Pankajalakshmi, V. V., Paramaswan, C. N., Shetty, B. M. V., and Subramanian, S.: Mycetomas in Madras. Sabouraudia 15:17, 1977.

7. Parasites

84
THE PROTOZOA

Joseph H. Miller, M.S., Ph.D.

In this presentation the parasitic protozoa of man are grouped as follows: 1. The Tissue and Intestinal Amebas; 2. The Intestinal and Atrial Flagellates; 3. An Intestinal Ciliate; 4. The Coccidia (including malaria); 5. Blood and Tissue Trypanosomes; 6. Tissue Leishmania.

1. The Tissue and Intestinal Amebas

Members of this group include free-living soil/water amebas that are opportunistic parasites of man and the amebic parasites of man's large intestine and mouth.

Two genera of soil amebas—*Naegleria*, and *Acanthamoeba*—are known to cause meningoencephalitis in man. In all cases, when culture was possible, *Naegleria fowleri* was isolated. However, *Acanthamoeba* sp. has been identified morphologically in a few cases in which the disease has been less fulminant. Other species of *Acanthamoeba* are associated with corneal ulceration and chronic granulomatous lesions of the skin. There is also a possibility that species of the genus *Hartmannella* may be opportunistic pathogens and produce meningoencephalitis.

The intestinal amebas, on the other hand, are a well-defined group and consist of five species: (1) *Entamoeba histolytica*, (2) *Entamoeba coli*, (3) *Dientamoeba fragilis*, (4) *Endolimax nana*, and (5) *Iodamoeba bütschlii*. Another species, *Entamoeba gingivalis*, is found in the mouth. Only *Entamoeba histolytica* is an important pathogenic species, although *Dientamoeba fragilis* may cause chronic but mild intestinal symptoms. The comparative morphology of these six parasitic species in humans is presented in Figure 1. Another species, occasionally found in the intestine, is *Entamoeba hartmanni*, a commensal very similar to, but smaller than, *E. histolytica*.

Naegleria fowleri

MORPHOLOGY. This species, most often associated with meningoencephalitis in man, has an ameboid stage, 10–35 μm, in which broad pseudopodia form eruptively. The endoplasm and ectoplasm are well defined, and there is one contractile vacuole. The nucleus has a large central karyosome (Fig. 2). A biflagellate form develops in water. A smooth walled cystic stage also occurs.

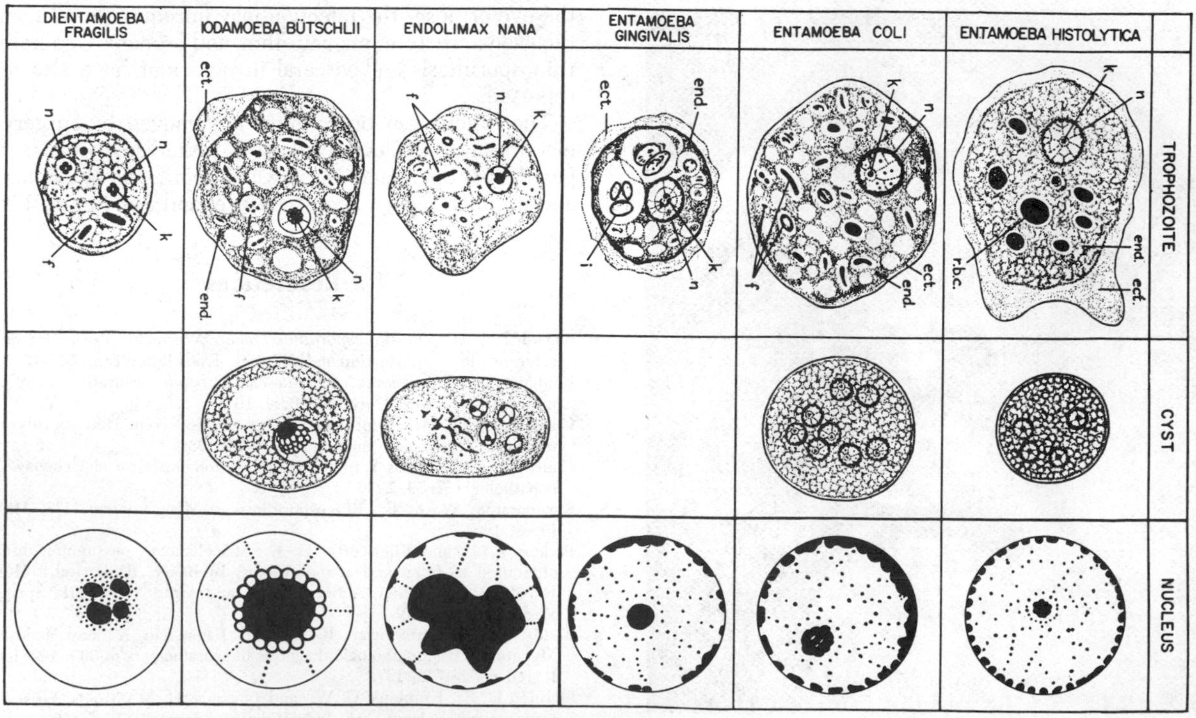

Figure 1. Comparative morphology of the amebae of man and schematic representation of their nuclei as seen in iron-hematoxylin stains. ect., ectoplasm; end., endoplasm; f, food vacuoles; i, inclusions; k, karyosome; n, nucleus; r.b.c., red blood cells. (From Brown, H. W.: Basic Clinical Parasitology. Appleton-Century-Crofts, New York, 1975.)

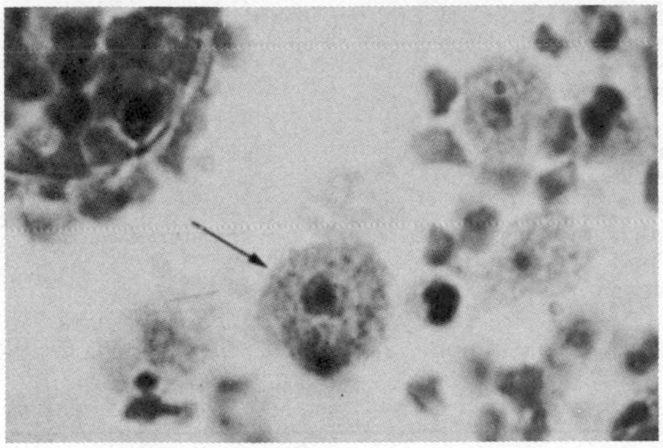

Figure 2. Section of a brain from a patient who died of primary amebic meningoencephalitis. The *arrow* indicates an amoeba. ×390. (Courtesy of Dr. R. Hays.)

EPIDEMIOLOGY. Most cases have occurred in young healthy adults after swimming in fresh water lakes or pools. These water-borne amebas may traverse the nasal mucosa, penetrate the cribriform plate, and multiply in the gray matter of the brain, and cause death within 72 hours after onset of symptoms.

LABORATORY DIAGNOSIS. The cerebral spinal fluid should be examined for the presence of progressively motile amebas with broad pseudopods. Preparations stained with Giemsa will show the characteristic large central karyosome. Organisms can be cultured on plates containing 1.5 per cent non-nutrient agar spread with a lawn of *Enterobacter aerogenes* or *Escherichia coli*. Amebas placed in sterile distilled water produce flagellate forms (Visvesvara, 1980).

DRUG SUSCEPTIBILITY. Amphotericin B is effective against experimental *Naegleria* infections. Tetracycline, in association with the former, has shown promising results in vivo and in vitro but has not been tried in humans (Dorsch et al., 1983).

IMMUNITY. Experimental animals have been protected to 88 per cent from nasal challenge with *N. fowleri* by immunization with nonpathogenic *N. gruberi*. In nature, man's exposure to the common *N. gruberi* may afford some protection against lethal exposures to *N. fowleri* (John, 1982).

Acanthamoeba sp.

MORPHOLOGY. Several species of *Acanthamoeba* (e.g., *A. culbertsoni, A. castellanii, A. polyphaga, A. astronyxis*) are considered pathogenic. These amebas are larger than *Naegleria* (15–45 μm), share the same nuclear characteristics, but produce fine, tapering, hyaline pseudopodia (acanthopodia), and do not possess a flagellate stage. Cysts have a wrinkled outer wall.

LIFE CYCLE/EPIDEMIOLOGY. *Acanthamoeba* are found in soil. The exact route of infection in man is unknown, but cysts may be contaminants of the skin, conjunctiva, and nasal epithelium. In immunocompromised hosts there may be hematogenous spread to any organ with the production of abscesses.

LABORATORY DIAGNOSIS. Amebas in cerebral spinal fluid demonstrate acanthopodia and are easily cultured with the same technique as for *Naegleria*. Amebas will not produce flagellate forms when placed in sterile distilled water.

DRUG SUSCEPTIBILITY. *Acanthamoeba* are sensitive to sulfadiazine in experimental infections.

IMMUNITY. Complement fixation and precipitin antibodies have been demonstrated in infected patients.

Entamoeba histolytica

MORPHOLOGY. *E. histolytica* may exist as a trophozoite, precyst, or cyst in feces (Fig. 3). The trophozoite is usually 15 to 25 μm in length. The clear ectoplasm is sharply demarcated from the granular endoplasm, which may contain ingested red cells. Its single nucleus appears ringlike when stained with iodine in fresh feces. Iron hematoxylin or other permanent staining techniques demonstrate a fine nuclear membrane encrusted with a layer of minute chromatin granules. A small punctiform karyosome is centrally located. The trophozoite is usually extremely active and exhibits progressive motility until it is cooled below body temperature. The precystic stage is a rounded, nonmotile trophozoite, devoid of inclusions. It is smaller than a trophozoite but usually larger than a cyst. The cysts are round-to-oval hyaline bodies, 5 to 20 μm in size, with smooth, refractile walls. Immature cysts are uninucleate with a large ringlike nucleus. As nuclear division occurs, individual nuclei decrease in size until the quadrinucleate mature cyst forms. In immature cysts glycogen is usually diffuse, and sausage-shaped chromatoid bodies may be seen. In unstained preparations chromatoid bodies are highly refractile, whereas in iron hematoxylin stains, they are uniformly dark. The chromatoid bodies,

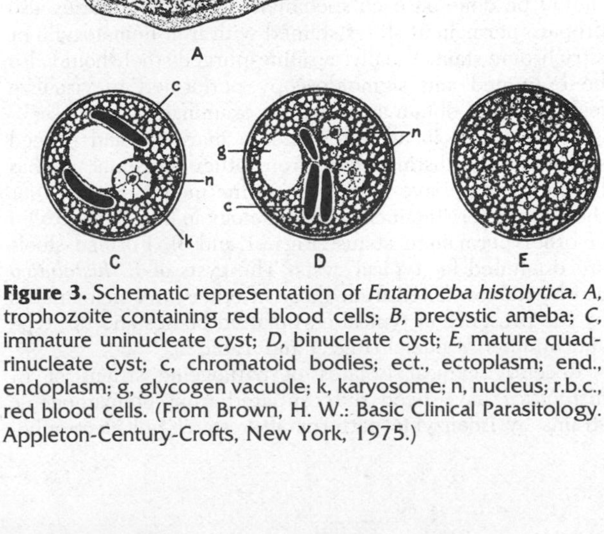

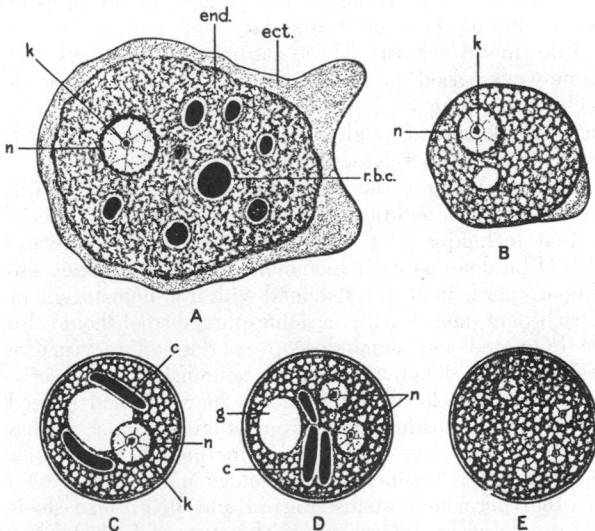

Figure 3. Schematic representation of *Entamoeba histolytica. A,* trophozoite containing red blood cells; *B,* precystic ameba; *C,* immature uninucleate cyst; *D,* binucleate cyst; *E,* mature quadrinucleate cyst; c, chromatoid bodies; ect., ectoplasm; end., endoplasm; g, glycogen vacuole; k, karyosome; n, nucleus; r.b.c., red blood cells. (From Brown, H. W.: Basic Clinical Parasitology. Appleton-Century-Crofts, New York, 1975.)

Table 1. KEY FOR DIFFERENTIATION OF AMEBIC TROPHOZOITES IN WET MOUNTS

Unstained saline smear of fresh feces	
A. Trophozoites usually medium or large sized (except for small strains of *Entamoeba histolytica*)	
1. Progressive motility with cytoplasm flowing into pseudopod; motile forms have slug-like shape; may or may not contain ingested red cells; nucleus usually not visible without stain	*E. histolytica*
2. No progressive motility; cytoplasm does not flow into pseudopod; blunt pseudopodia extended and retracted; ring-like nucleus frequently visible unstained	*Entamoeba coli*
B. Trophozoites usually small or medium sized; ordinarily motility is sluggish	
1. Pseudopodia often blunt or round, resembling a yeast budding	*Endolimax nana*
2. Pseudopodia angular (triangular or tent-like), rectangular or lobulated; outline of non-motile trophozoites perfectly round or cyst-like	*Dientamoeba fragilis*
3. Pseudopodia blunt; resemble small *E. coli* trophozoites	*Iodamoeba bütschlii*

which contain ribonucleic acid, disappear as nuclear division occurs in the cyst.

LIFE CYCLE/EPIDEMIOLOGY. Cysts in feces are the infective stage. Persons are infected through food or drink contaminated by infective feces, flies, or the unwashed hands of food handlers. Cross-connections between sewage and water lines have been responsible for waterborne epidemics. Excystation occurs when the mature cyst reaches the lower small intestine. A four-nucleate ameba is released, which divides into small trophozoites. These amebas move downward and establish themselves at areas of stasis in the large intestine. They may feed in the lumen and invade the mucosa. Multiplication occurs by binary fission. Cysts are produced and passed in the feces. Trophozoites are seen in diarrheic and dysenteric stools, but they are not resistant to environmental conditions and do not spread the infection. Man is the principal host and source of infection, although natural infections of monkeys, dogs, hogs, and rats with amebas indistinguishable from *E. histolytica* have been reported.

LABORATORY DIAGNOSIS. The laboratory diagnosis rests on the identification of the parasite in the feces or tissues and on serologic studies.

Intestinal Amebiasis. Three naturally passed stools over a one-week period should be examined by the direct smear technique, using fresh saline and iodine preparations (1 per cent potassium iodide saturated with iodine crystals). Because cysts are released intermittently, three stool examinations increase the likelihood that the infection will be detected. In addition to direct examination, a concentration technique (e.g., formalin-ether or ethyl acetate) should be done on each specimen. Many laboratories also prepare permanent slides stained with iron-hematoxylin or a trichrome stain. Finally, a saline-purged stool should also be examined and sigmoidoscopy performed to visualize lesions and to obtain aspirates for examination.

Trophozoites in aspirates and in diarrheic and purged stools may be distinguished from other intestinal amebas by their progressive motility in saline mounts (Table 1) or their characteristic nuclear morphology in iron hematoxylin or other permanent stains (Figs. 1 and 3). Formed stools are examined for typical cysts. The cysts of *E. histolytica* can be differentiated from those of other intestinal amebas by the presence of typical chromatoid bodies and the type and number of nuclei (Fig. 4 and Table 2).

Recently clinical isolates of pathogenic strains of *E. histolytica* have been differentiated from nonpathogenic strains by isoenzyme patterns after starch-gel electrophoresis. Strains causing clinical disease could be characterized into one of seven zymodemes, whereas nonpathogenic strains were distributed among 11 completely different zymodemes (Sargeaunt et al., 1982).

Extraintestinal Amebiasis. All extraintestinal amebiasis originates from a primary intestinal infection, and evidence of such infection should be sought. Extraintestinal amebiasis without demonstrable concurrent intestinal infection

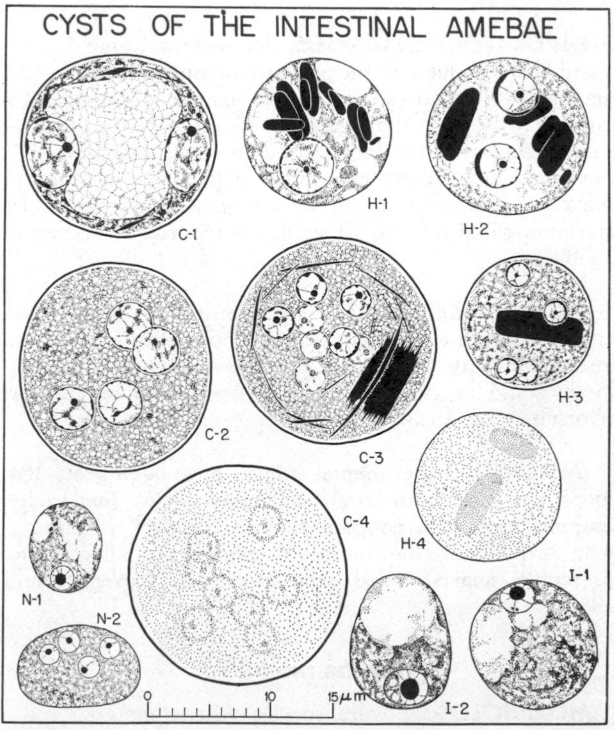

Figure 4. C-1, Iron-hematoxylin-stained immature binucleate cyst of *Entamoeba coli.* C-2, Iron-hematoxylin-stained immature quadrinucleate cyst of *E. coli.* C-3, Iron-hematoxylin-stained mature cyst of *E. coli.* C-4, Unstained mature cyst of *E. coli.* H-1, Iron-hematoxylin-stained immature uninucleate cyst of *Entamoeba histolytica.* H-2, Iron-hematoxylin-stained immature binucleate cyst of *E. histolytica.* H-3, Iron-hematoxylin-stained mature cyst of *E. histolytica.* H-4, Unstained cyst of *E. histolytica* with chromatoid bodies. N-1, Iron-hematoxylin-stained uninucleate cyst of *Endolimax nana.* N-2, Iron-hematoxylin-stained mature cysts of *E. nana.* I-1, I-2, Iron-hematoxylin-stained mature cysts of *Iodamoeba bütschlii.* (From Hunter, G. W., Swartzwelder, J. C., and Clyde, D. F.: Tropical Medicine. W. B. Saunders Co., Philadelphia, 1976.)

Table 2. KEY FOR THE DIFFERENTIATION OF AMEBIC CYSTS IN WET MOUNTS

I. Unstained saline smear of fresh feces	
A. Presence of rod-like or sausage-shaped chromatoid bars (in some but not in all infections)	*Entamoeba histolytica*
B. Absence of chromatoid bars	II
II. Iodine-stained smear of fresh feces (and of formalin-ether concentrate)	
A. Presence of ring-like nuclei	1
1. Medium sized or small cyst with one to four nuclei	*E. histolytica*
2. Large cyst with five or more nuclei	*Entamoeba coli*
B. Absence of ring-like nuclei	3
3. Small, round, or oval cyst with nuclei appearing as vacuole-like areas	*Endolimax nana*
4. Medium sized cyst with large dark brown mass sharply delimited from cytoplasm	*Iodamoeba bütschlii*

is common, however. Serologic methods (complement fixation, immunodiffusion, and indirect hemagglutination) are sensitive and important diagnostic aids for confirming the clinical diagnosis of extraintestinal amebiasis. Many tests are available commercially in kit form. Microscopic examination of aspirates for motile trophozoites as well as cultural procedures are helpful.

DRUG SUSCEPTIBILITY. *E. histolytica* is susceptible to many drugs. Metronidazole is now the treatment of choice for all forms of amebiasis. However, either diiodohydroxiquin, tetracycline, paromomycin, or diloxanide furoate can be used after metronidazole treatment to assure removal of luminal forms. Any of the former may be used alone for the treatment of the asymptomatic cyst passer. Patients with severe intestinal amebiasis who are too ill to take oral medication may be successfully treated with dehydroemetine. The combination of dehydroemetine and chloroquine may also be needed for treatment of the occasional liver abscess caused by metronidazole-resistant *E. histolytica*.

IMMUNITY. Invasive amebiasis elicits the production of antibody to many different antigens of *E. histolytica*. Neither these antibodies nor other immune mechanisms are known to prevent either extraintestinal invasion or reinfection. Recently it was found that pathogenic strains were resistant to complement-mediated lysis by human serum that would permit their hematogenous spread to extra intestinal sites (Reed et al., 1983).

2. The Intestinal and Atrial Flagellates

Three intestinal and two atrial flagellates are common in humans. The nonpathogenic species include *Chilomastix mesnili* and *Trichomonas hominis* of the intestine (Fig. 5) and *Trichomonas tenax* of the mouth. *Giardia lamblia* in the small intestine and *Trichomonas vaginalis* in the urogenital tract of humans are the pathogenic species. The species can be differentiated on the basis of habitat and by the morphologic comparison shown in Figure 5. *Blastocystis hominis*, a commensal yeast found in the intestine of humans, may be confused with the cysts of these flagellates and intestinal amebic cysts.

Giardia lamblia

MORPHOLOGY. *Giardia lamblia* is a worldwide parasite of the upper small intestine of humans. It has two stages in its life cycle: the trophozoite, which multiplies by binary fission, and the infective cyst, which is passed in the feces. The trophozoite is a pear-shaped, bilaterally symmetrical flagellate, 12 to 15 μm long, with a broad rounded anterior surface and a tapering posterior extremity (Fig. 5). The dorsal surface is convex. Most of the anterior ventral surface assumes a rigid bilobed concavity (ventral disk) in which a negative pressure is created by the beating of a pair of specialized ventral flagella. The organism is thus able to adhere to the brush border of the duodenal mucosa. Anteriorly, two large nuclei contain karyosomes. Two axostyles between the nuclei pass into the posterior extremity. Three pairs of trailing flagella are located dorsally. The ellipsoid cyst is 9 to 12 μm long and has a well-defined wall. The mature cyst contains four nuclei and the remnants of organelles found in the trophozoite. Because mitosis

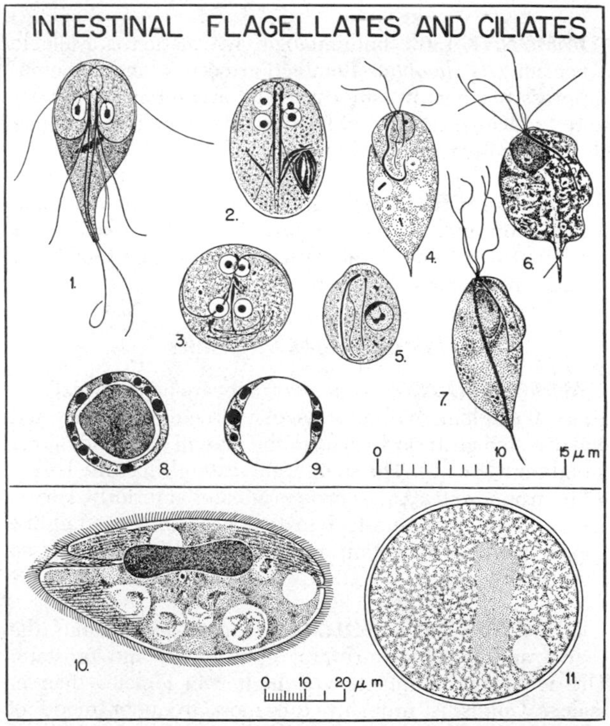

Figure 5. 1, Iron-hematoxylin-stained trophozoite of *Giardia lamblia*. 2, Iron-hematoxylin-stained cyst of *G. lamblia*. 3, Iron-hematoxylin-stained cyst of *G. lamblia*, end-view. 4, Iron-hematoxylin-stained trophozoite of *Chilomastix mesnili*. 5, Iron-hematoxylin-stained cyst of *C. mesnili*. 6, Iron-hematoxylin-stained trophozoite of *Trichomonas hominis*. 7, Iron-hematoxylin-stained trophozoite of *Trichomonas vaginalis*. 8, Iron-hematoxylin-stained *Blastocystis hominis*. 9, Unstained *B. hominis*. 10, Trophozoites of *Balantidium coli*. 11, Unstained cyst of *B. coli*. (From Hunter, G. W., Swartzwelder, J. C., and Clyde, D. F.: Tropical Medicine. W. B. Saunders Co., Philadelphia, 1976.)

occurs in the cyst, two trophozoites are produced during excystation.

LIFE CYCLE/EPIDEMIOLOGY. Infected persons, children more frequently than adults, pass cysts in the feces intermittently. Watery stools occasionally contain trophozoites, but they are not infective. Excystation of cysts ingested through fecal contamination of food or drink occurs in the small intestine and establishes the infection. Water-borne epidemics have occurred when drinking water was contaminated by feces containing cysts from human and animal reservoirs (e.g. dogs, beavers, mule-deer). The cysts are resistant to normal chlorination but seem to be destroyed by iodine compounds in concentrations recommended for water purification (Wolfe, 1975).

LABORATORY DIAGNOSIS. The diagnosis may be made by finding the characteristic cysts in iodine and saline mounts of fresh feces (Fig. 5). Motile trophozoites may also be distinguished by their characteristic morphology and jerky motility in watery stools. Fecal smears, stained with trichrome stain, are also useful to distinguish *G. lamblia* especially since organisms are brightly stained in contrast to fecal debris (Thornton et al., 1983). Concentration techniques should always be used. The string method (Entero-Test) of recovering trophozoites from duodenal samples is simple and useful when stool findings are negative and symptoms persist.

IMMUNITY. Little immunologic information is available concerning *G. lamblia*. Reinfection occurs, and immunosuppressive therapy can cause an asymptomatic carrier state to change rapidly into active infection. Hypogammaglobulinemia predisposes to acute infection.

DRUG SUSCEPTIBILITY. *G. lamblia* is sensitive to atabrine, metronidazole, and furazolidone. Paromomycin is used in treating pregnant patients as the safety of other drugs is not assured in this condition.

Trichomonas vaginalis

MORPHOLOGY. *T. vaginalis* is a pear-shaped flagellate, 10 to 30 μm long, with four flagella directed anteriorly and one directed posteriorly to form the margin of an undulating membrane (Fig. 5). The membrane extends half the length of the trophozoite. An axostyle originates anteriorly, curves about the nucleus, and terminates posteriorly as a tail-like appendage. Multiplication is by binary fission. There is no cyst stage.

LIFE CYCLE/EPIDEMIOLOGY. *T. vaginalis* inhabits the vagina and the male urethra, epididymis, and prostate. The incidence of infection is higher in females than in males. Coitus is probably the most frequent mode of infection, but the exchange between women of toilet articles contaminated with vaginal discharge is also a common cause of infection.

LABORATORY DIAGNOSIS. The examination of fresh vaginal discharge material in a drop of saline will disclose motile *T. vaginalis*. The erratic jerky motility of the organism is characteristic. The rippling wave-like motion of the undulating membrane can be visualized clearly when specimens begin to dry. Permanently stained specimens may also be prepared and examined for the undulating membrane and flagella.

Examination of prostatic secretions obtained by prostate massage is the best method for diagnosing infections of men. The secretion should be examined for motile trophozoites with undulating membranes. Smaller numbers of trophozoites may also be found in the first few mls of a urine sample.

For practical purposes, *Trichomonas* spp. may be differentiated on the basis of the source of infected material: *T. tenax* is found in material from the oral cavity, *T. hominis* from feces, and *T. vaginalis* from vaginal discharge, prostatic fluid, or urine.

DRUG SUSCEPTIBILITY. Oral metronidazole is highly effective in eliminating the infection in either sex. No other systemic drug is effective.

3. An Intestinal Ciliate

Balantidium coli

MORPHOLOGY. *B. coli* is the only ciliated pathogen of man (Fig. 5). This large ovoid trophozoite, measuring 50 to 70 μm by 30 to 60 μm, is enclosed by a pellicle covered with longitudinal spiral rows of cilia. The beating cilia account for the smooth gliding motility of the organism in fresh fecal preparations. At the anterior end is a funnel-shaped peristome lined by long cilia. A large kidney-shaped macronucleus with a small rounded micronucleus lying in its concavity is usually centrally located. There are two contractile vacuoles. At the posterior end is a cytopyge for the discharge of solid waste material. The rounded trophozoites secrete a double cyst wall. Cysts measure 50 to 65 μm. The macronucleus, contractile vacuoles, and cilia are visible within the cyst.

LIFE CYCLE/EPIDEMIOLOGY. *B. coli* trophozoites inhabit the lower ileum and large intestine, where they may penetrate the mucosa and multiply by binary fission. Conjugation has been observed. Infective cysts are passed in the feces. Trophozoites do not survive the extracorporeal environment. Each cyst ingested in fecally contaminated food or drink produces a single trophozoite.

Morphologically identical forms of *B. coli* in monkeys, hogs, guinea pigs, and rats do not seem to play a major role in human infections. Instead, infection seems to result primarily from man-to-man transmission via fecal contamination.

LABORATORY DIAGNOSIS. A number of fecal specimens should be examined because the number of parasites may vary from specimen to specimen. Large, motile trophozoites with gliding motility may be found in diarrheic stools. Less frequently, typical large cysts are found in formed stools (Fig. 5). Sigmoidoscopy with aspiration of visible lesions may be helpful.

DRUG SUSCEPTIBILITY. *B. coli* is most sensitive to oxytetracycline or diiodohydroxyquin.

4. The Coccidia

Taxoplasma gondii

MORPHOLOGY. *T. gondii* is an obligate intracellular sporozoan parasite of man and animals with worldwide distribution. Recent studies of its life cycle and morphology reveal a taxonomic relationship to the Eimeriidae, order

Coccidia. Tachyzoites, the rapidly multiplying forms in acute infection, are cresent shaped, 6 to 7 μm long by 2 to 4 μm wide, and contain an oval nucleus (Fig. 6). Intracellular multiplication occurs by endodyogeny, with two daughter cells forming within the pellicle of the parent. Cysts formed in chronic infections are 20 to 100 μm in diameter, oval to round, and contain numerous bradyzoites, the slowly multiplying forms. Oocysts containing eight sporozoites are passed in the feces of infected felines, primarily the domestic cat.

LIFE CYCLE/EPIDEMIOLOGY. Many animals, both wild and domestic, are infected with *T. gondii*. Man becomes infected primarily by eating poorly cooked or raw meat containing cysts. Contamination of food or drink with oocysts from cat feces also occurs but probably plays only a minor role in human transmission. The ingestion of cysts or oocysts by humans gives rise to a schizogonic or proliferative phase with rapidly multiplying tachyzoites in many tissues. Eventually, as a resting stage, cysts containing many bradyzoites develop. A schizogonic and gametogenic cycle occurs in the intestinal epithelium of felines with production of oocysts. In the acute stage in humans, the organisms may be transferred transplacentally. The life cycle is presented in Figure 7.

LABORATORY DIAGNOSIS. The demonstration of cysts via biopsy specimens does not establish a causal relationship for clinical illness because cysts are found in both acute and chronic infections. Demonstration of organisms in brain impression smears of a newborn infant at necropsy establishes the diagnosis of toxoplasmosis. Animal passage is difficult. Test animals must be tested serologically and then killed and examined for parasites. Four serologic tests are in use: the Sabin-Feldman dye test, complement fixation test, indirect fluorescent antibody test, and indirect hemagglutination test. The indirect fluorescent antibody test is most widely used. The titer suggests whether the infection is acute or chronic. However, because of the wide occurrence of *T. gondii* antibody in the general population, the diagnosis is based on a significant increase in titer upon subsequent testing. The presence of IgM antibody in a child less than 6 months old suggests acute disease because maternal IgM does not cross the placenta. Commercial kits are available for indirect fluorescent antibody testing.

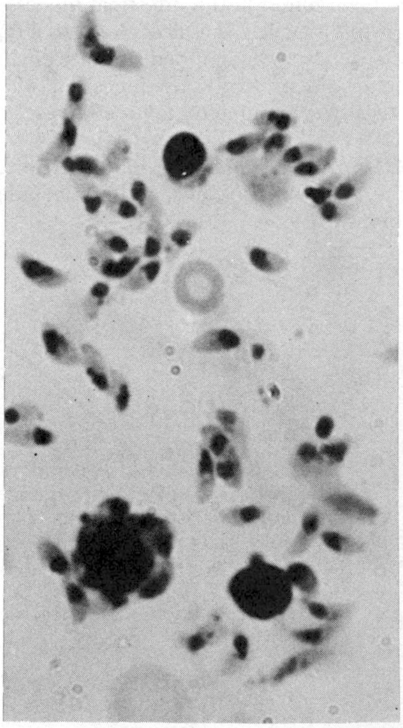

Figure 6. Mouse peritoneal fluid demonstrating tachyzoites freed from cells (1000 ×). (From Hunter, G. W., Swartzwelder, J. C., and Clyde, D. F.: Tropical Medicine. W. B. Saunders Co., Philadelphia, 1976.)

DRUG SUSCEPTIBILITY. Experimental and natural infections with toxoplasma are most responsive to the combination of pyrimethamine and trisulfapyrimidines.

IMMUNITY. Humoral and cellular immunity develop during the lymphoreticular phase, and the number of tachyzoites rapidly diminishes. Antibodies against several antigens of toxoplasma can be demonstrated, and immune mononuclear cells no longer support the intracellular multiplication of *Toxoplasma* organisms. The development of immunity coincides with the transformation of toxoplasmosis into the chronic, cyst-forming stage. Cysts are isolated from the immune processes, and reactivation can occur during natural or artificial immunosuppression.

Pneumocystis carinii

MORPHOLOGY. *P. carinii* is believed to be a coccidian; however, its exact taxonomic status is unknown. The most easily recognizable stage is the cyst, which is 5 to 12 μm in diameter and contains eight ovoid or crescent-shaped parasites (sporozoites) with eccentric nuclei. Cysts are found in a honeycombed exudate in the alveoli.

LIFE CYCLE/EPIDEMIOLOGY. The life cycle of *P. carinii* is unknown. The infection was first reported in endemic form from Europe, but sporadic cases have been reported worldwide. *P. carinii* is widespread in animals, both wild and domestic, but host specificity seems high, and transmission from animals to humans seems unlikely. Aerosol dispersion of respiratory tract secretions may be involved in epidemics. Sporadic cases are thought to result from latent infections that become activated by immunosuppression.

LABORATORY DIAGNOSIS. Silver or Giemsa stains of tissue from open lung biopsy or needle aspirates have been most productive (Fig. 8). Sputum, tracheal smears, and hypopharyngeal material do not routinely show evidence of the parasite, but bronchial brushings are sometimes useful. Experimental serologic tests are of unproven value.

DRUG SUSCEPTIBILITY. Trimethoprim-sulfamethoxazole and pentamidine isethionate are the only useful drugs.

IMMUNITY. Active infection occurs in neonates and in adults with disturbances of either immunoglobulins or cell-mediated immunity. Normal adults do not develop disease but are probably infected frequently. The prominence of infection in patients with the acquired immunodeficiency syndrome has established the importance of acquired immunity.

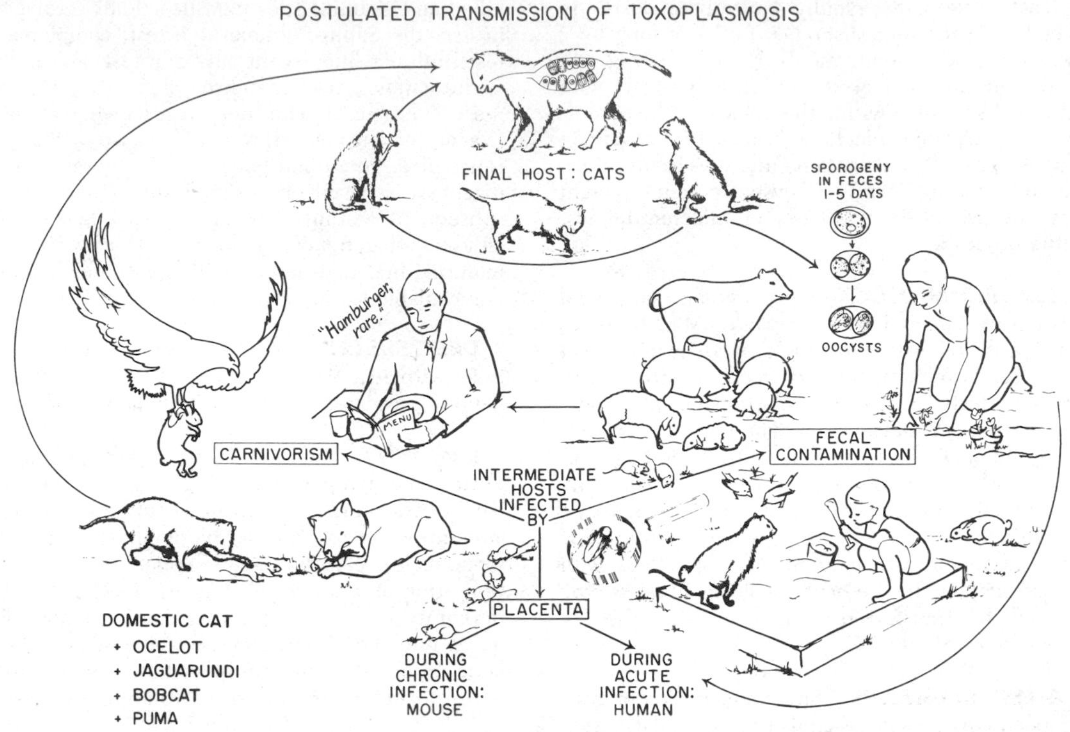

Figure 7. Life cycle and transmission of *Toxoplasma.* Cats and certain other felines are shown as final hosts, and other animals and humans as intermediate hosts. Flies and cockroaches can serve as transport hosts. At right, infection with oocysts is shown. At left, transmission by carnivorism is indicated. Below, the transplacental route of transmission is indicated. (Modified slightly from Frenkel, J. K.: Toxoplasmosis. *In* Marcial-Rojas, R. A. (ed.): Pathology of Protozoal and Helminthic Diseases. Williams & Wilkins, Baltimore, 1971.)

Isospora belli

MORPHOLOGY. *I. belli* is a rare coccidian parasite of man. Unsporulated, unicellular, ovoidal oocysts, 25 to 30 by 12 to 16 μm, are passed in the feces. The granular cytoplasm is surrounded by a smooth colorless double-layered wall. Division into two sporoblasts, each surrounded by a cyst wall and producing four sporozoites, ensues after fecal passage (Fig. 9).

LIFE CYCLE/EPIDEMIOLOGY. Asexual as well as sexual stages have been found in the intestinal mucosa. Thus it is thought that the life cycle is a direct fecal-oral type without intermediate hosts and confined to intestinal epithelial cells. Infection is probably by ingestion of sporulated oocysts in fecally contaminated food or water.

DIAGNOSIS. Oocysts may be found in fecal samples, sporocysts in duodenal aspirates, and intracellular stages in intestinal biopsies.

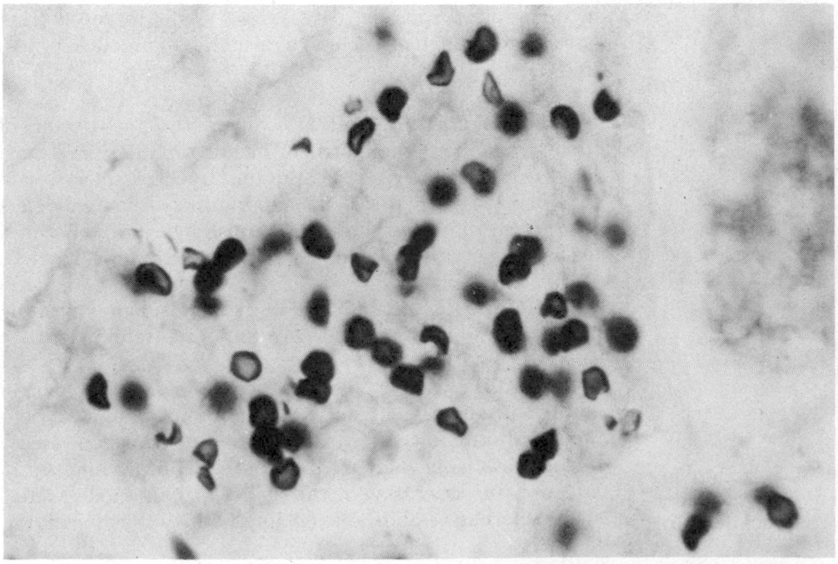

Figure 8. Cysts of *Pneumocystis carinii* in alveolar exudate. Note round, crescentic, and other-shaped cysts with collapsed walls; silver methenamine-fast green stain, 1000 ×. (From Hunter, G. W., Swartzwelder, J. C., and Clyde, D. F.: Tropical Medicine. W. B. Saunders Co., Philadelphia, 1976.)

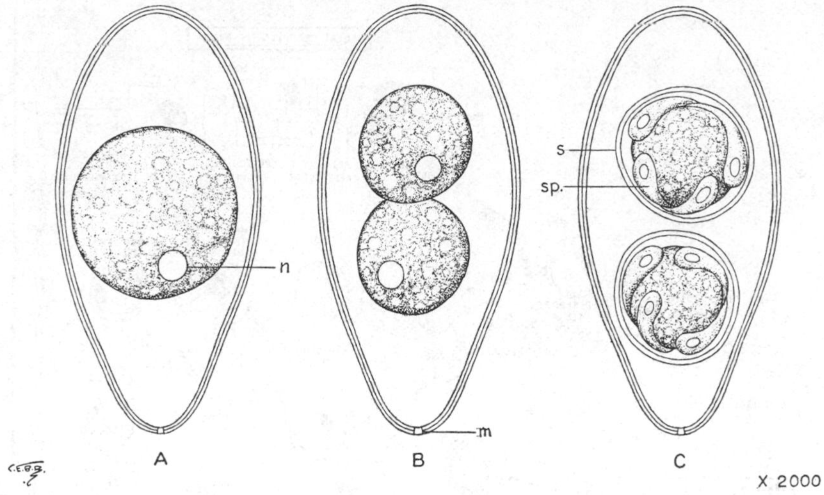

Figure 9. *Isospora belli. A,* Unicellular oocyst. *B,* Oocyst with two sporoblasts. *C,* Oocyst with two spores, each containing four sporozoites. m, micropyle; n, nucleus; s, spore; sp., sporozoite. (From Brown, H. W., and Niva, N. A.: Basic Clinical Parasitology. 5th ed., Appleton-Century-Crofts, New York, 1983.)

TREATMENT. Combined pyrimethamine and sulfadiazine seem to elicit a specific response.

Cryptosporidium sp.

MORPHOLOGY. *Cryptosporidium* spp. are parasites causing enterocolitis and malabsorption in a wide variety of vertebrates, including man. Spherical to subspherical oocysts (4 to 6 μm) are passed in the feces. They are smooth and thin-walled with a prominent internal granule and lesser granules. Some oocysts may contain four sporozoites when passed in fresh feces. Others will sporulate when mixed half and half with 2 per cent potassium dichromate and aerated for 5 to 7 days at room temperature. Phase contrast optics aid the visualization of sporozoites.

LIFE CYCLE/EPIDEMIOLOGY. The life cycle in man is unknown but can be inferred from the cycle in calves, which is probably of the same species. Asexual and sexual forms are found in the brush border of crypt epithelial cells in the small and large intestine. Such endogenous forms are round encapsulated and 2 to 4 μm in diameter. Oocysts are formed, detached, and passed in the feces. The infection is acquired from the ingestion of oocysts in fecally contaminated food and water. Such contamination may be from human or animal origin as present investigation seems to indicate a lack of host-specificity for the genus *Cryptosporidium* (Tzipori et al., 1980).

DIAGNOSIS. Human diagnosis has been accomplished by intestinal or rectal biopsies with the demonstration of asexual and sexual stages in the brush border. Concentration techniques commonly used for detection of ova and parasites in fecal samples, e.g., sugar and zinc sulfate flotation, formalin-ether, and formalin-ethylactate sedimentation, all give excellent oocyst recovery (Anderson, 1983). However, most laboratory technicians are unfamiliar with the appearance of the oocysts, and their small size (about the size of a red cell) and lack of characteristics make identification difficult (Fig. 10). Acid-fast staining of fecal films stains oocysts red against unstained fecal debris.

DRUG SUSCEPTIBILITY. At the present time no compound has been found with activity.

IMMUNITY. The infection runs a self-limited two-week course in normal individuals; however, in individuals who are immunologically deficient such as acquired immune deficiency syndrome (AIDS) patients or those under drug suppression, the course of the infection may be extended indefinitely with severe symptomatology.

Malaria Parasites

The malarial parasites of man are species of the genus *Plasmodium* in which schizogony (asexual cycle) takes place in human liver and erythrocytes and sporogony (sexual cycle) takes place in mosquitoes of the genus *Anopheles.* All species have similar life cycles with variations in the length of the liver stage and with fine morphological differences in the erythrocytic stages (Fig. 11). The species involved are *Plasmodium falciparum, P. vivax, P. malariae,* and *P. ovale.*

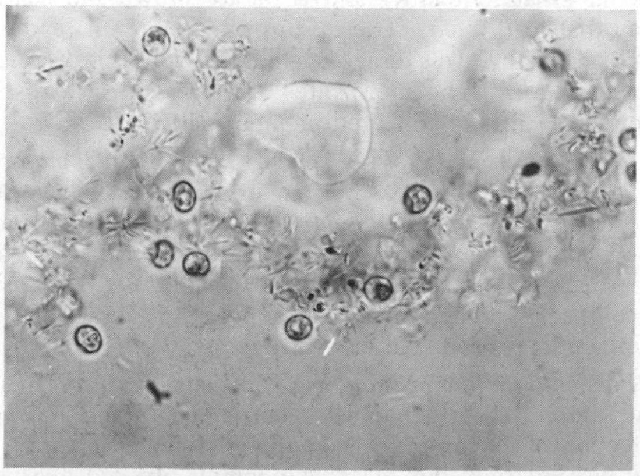

Figure 10. Sheather's sugar flotation preparation of cryptosporidial oocysts from a 12-day-old calf. Slight halo may be due to mucoid material on the capsule or other refraction. Oocysts are pink in color, which makes them easy to find (× 1280). Cryptosporidial oocysts are acid-fast and readily seen after staining by the Ziehl Neelsen method or with a fluorochrome stain.

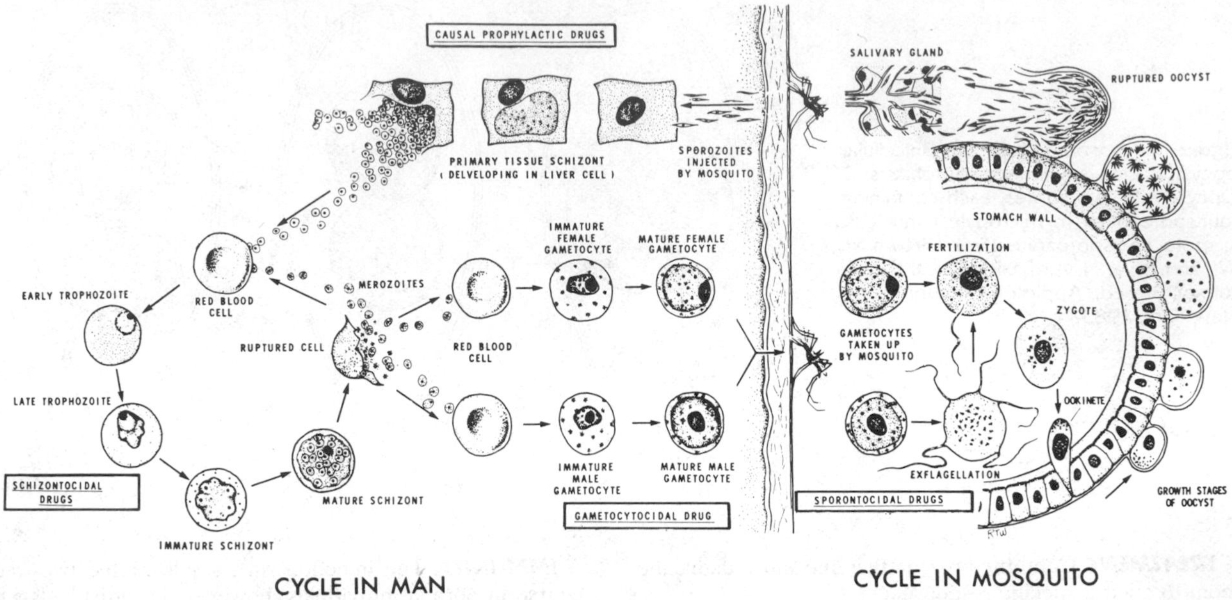

Figure 11. Schematic representation of typical malaria life cycle. (Modified from Hunter, G. W., Swartzwelder, J. C., and Clyde, D. F.: Tropical Medicine. W. B. Saunders Co., Philadelphia, 1976.)

MORPHOLOGY

Plasmodium vivax (Fig. 12). Young trophozoites appear in Giemsa-stained blood films as delicate rings of blue cytoplasm. Each contains one red nucleus and is about one third the size of the red cell. As the trophozoite grows, it becomes actively motile and its outline becomes extremely irregular. Granules of yellowish-brown pigment develop in the cytoplasm of the parasite. The erythrocyte becomes enlarged, and bright red diffuse stippling, Schüffner's dots, may be seen in some cases. Large trophozoites undergo schizogony, producing an average of 16 merozoites.

Plasmodium malariae. (Fig. 12). The ring stage is identical to that of *P. vivax.* Mature trophozoites are more compact than those of *P. vivax* and may extend as bands across the infected erythrocyte. Pigment appears earlier and in greater quantity and is darker brown and coarser than that in *P. vivax.* The erythrocyte is not enlarged and stains normally. An average of eight merozoites is produced by schizogony. The merozoites are arranged in a rosette around a centrally collected pigment mass.

Plasmodium ovale. This species resembles *P. malariae* in many ways, but the infected erythrocytes behave like those infected with *P. vivax.* Erythrocytes, which may show Schüffner's dots, are oval, slightly enlarged, and pale. The margin is often crenated. The trophozoite of *P. ovale* is compact and band forms may appear. An average of eight merozoites is produced by schizogony.

Plasmodium falciparum. (Fig. 12). Ring forms are smaller and more delicate than those of *P. vivax* and multiple infection of erythrocytes is common. Infected erthrocytes are not enlarged but may have comma-like red markings (Maurer's clefts) in the cytoplasm. The plasmalemma of infected erythrocytes becomes altered and erythrocytes adhere to the endothelial lining of small blood vessels and thus are removed from the peripheral circulation. Further development and schizogony are accomplished in such cells in the capillaries of the viscera. Therefore, intermediate and mature forms of the schizogonic cycle are not usually seen in the peripheral circulation. Crescentic gametocytes, however, may be seen in the peripheral circulation. Their shape differs from that of the rounded gametocytes of *P. vivax, P. malariae,* and *P. ovale.*

LIFE CYCLE/EPIDEMIOLOGY. Malaria generally occurs between the latitudes 45 degrees north and 40 degrees south. *P. vivax* infections are the most widely distributed; *P. malariae* infections are comparatively rare. *P. falciparum* occurs predominantly in tropical regions, and *P. ovale* is mostly limited to Africa.

The sexual cycle in certain anopheline mosquitoes begins with the ingestion of mature gametocytes (Fig. 11). In the mosquito stomach the microgametocyte produces microgametes (flagella-like structures) that detach (exflagellation) and migrate to the macrogamete (female cell), which was formed by maturation of the macrogametocyte. Fertilization takes place, and the zygote elongates and becomes motile (ookinete). It penetrates the mosquito stomach wall and grows into an oocyst beneath the outer layer. Many filamentous sporozoites are produced by rapid multiplication, which results finally in rupture of the oocyst. Sporozoites move to the salivary glands and are injected at the next feeding.

The asexual cycle begins with the entry of sporozoites into human hosts. They rapidly enter the parenchymal cells of the liver and undergo multiplication (exoerythrocytic stage). The rate of development and certain morphologic characteristics vary with the species of *Plasmodium.* Finally, infected parenchymal cells rupture, releasing myriads of merozoites that invade erythrocytes, producing ring stages. Schizogony occurs in parasitized erythrocytes, and their eventual rupture frees merozoites to invade other erythrocytes and repeat the cycle. The schizogony is usually synchronous in all species except *P. falciparum.* Eventually some merozoites invading erythrocytes produce gametocytes to perpetuate the cycle.

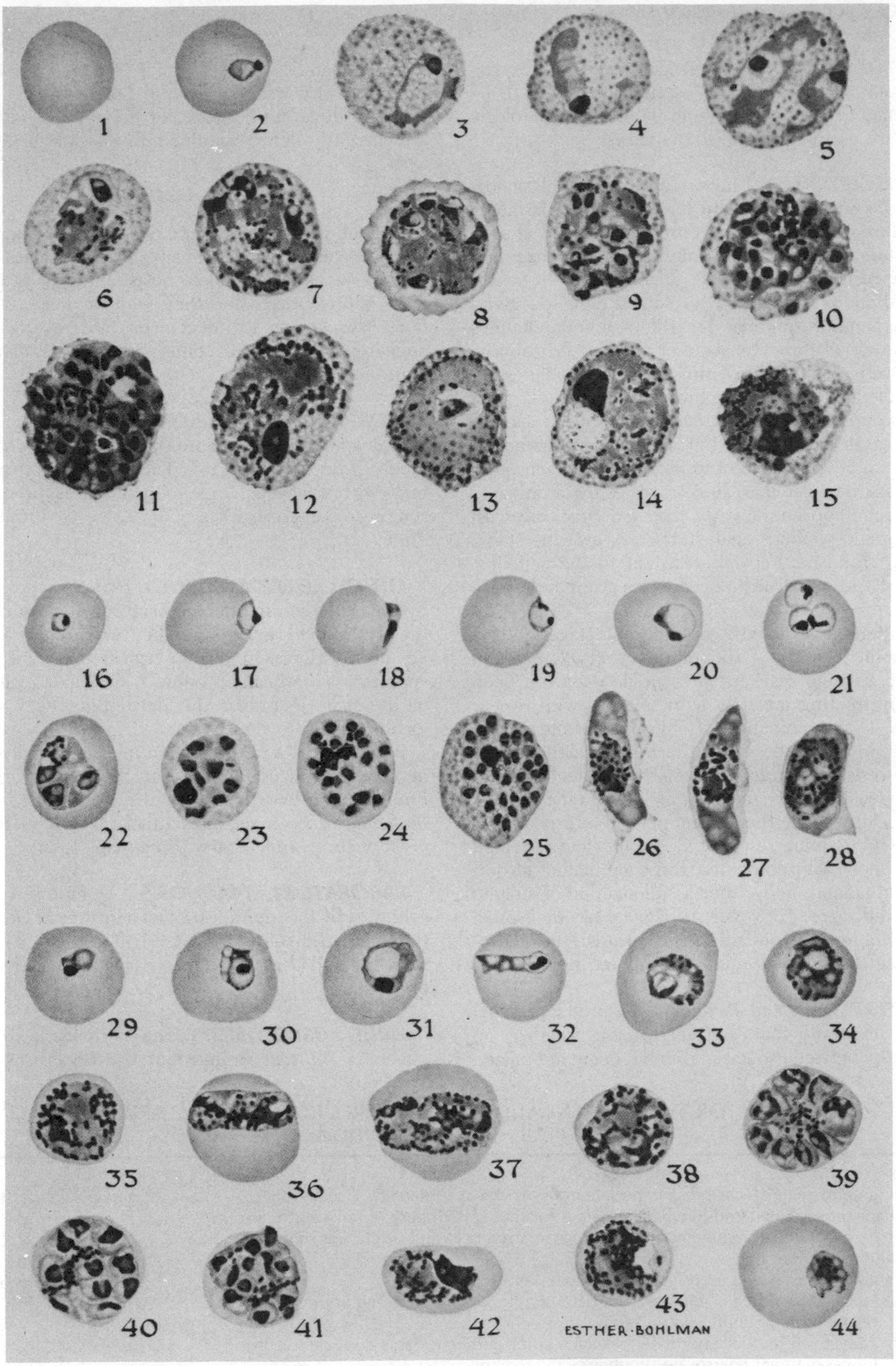

Figure 12. Malarial Parasites of Man. 1. Uninfected red cell; 2–15, *Plasmodium vivax;* 16–28, *P. falciparum;* 29–43, *P. malariae.* Magnification ×2,000. Drawn by E. Bohlman. 2. Ring stage of trophozoite. 3, 4. Ameboid uninucleate trophozoites. 5. Double infection with uninucleate trophozoites. 6. Uninucleate trophozoite. 7. Ameboid schizont. 8, 9. Schizonts. 10, 11. Segmenters. 12, 14. Macrogametocytes. 13, 15. Microgametocytes. 16, 17. Young "ring" stages. 18. Uninucleate trophozoite. 19, 20. Binucleate trophozoites. 21. Multiple infection with rings. 22, 23. Schizonts, *from placental smears.* 24, 25. Segmenters, *from placental smears.* 26, 27. Macrogametocytes (crescents). 28. Microgametocyte (crescent). 29, 30, 31. Uninucleate trophozoites. 32. "Band" form of trophozoite. 33, 34. Older uninucleate trophozoites. 35. Schizont. 36, 37. "Band" forms of schizont. 38. Schizont. 39. Segmenter in "rosette" form. 40, 41. Segmenters. 42. Macrogametocyte. 43. Microgametocyte. 44. Uninfected red cell with superimposed blood platelet. All stages from peripheral blood except 22–25, which are from placental smears.

LABORATORY DIAGNOSIS. Definitive diagnosis depends on identifying plasmodia in thick and thin blood smears stained with Giemsa stain (Table 3). Serologic techniques are useful as an aid to diagnosis.

DRUG SUSCEPTIBILITY. The susceptibility of plasmodia to drugs varies with the stage in the life cycle. Plasmodia in the erythrocytic stage are most sensitive to the 4-aminoquinoline drugs, chloroquine and amodiaquine. Chloroquine-resistant strains of *P. falciparum* from Southeast Asia and South America have retained their sensitivity to quinine. Neither quinine nor the 4-aminoquinolines eradicate the exoerythrocytic stage of malaria. Primaquine is the most active drug against this stage of the life cycle. The dihydrofolate reductase inhibitors, proqunil, pyrimethamine, and trimethoprim, show only weak activity against the erythrocytic stage but are sporontocidal; that is, they prevent development of sporozoites in the mosquito and in humans inoculated with sporozoites by an infected mosquito. Trimethoprim, however, acts synergistically with sulfonamides and sulfones against the erythrocytic stage. *Plasmodium* organisms become resistant to the sulfones, sulfonamides, and dihydrofolate reductase group if they are used alone.

The variation in sensitivity of different stages in the *Plasmodium* life cycle and the tendency of *Plasmodium* organisms to become resistant to a single drug has been countered by treating most forms of malaria with two or more drugs. The combination of chloroquine and primaquine results in radical cure of all forms of malaria except chloroquine-resistant *P. falciparum* malaria. Infections with chloroquine-sensitive *P. falciparum* are eradicated by chloroquine alone, since there is no persistent exoerythrocyte cycle. Chloroquine-resistant *P. falciparum* is treated with two or more schizontocides; the combination of quinine, pyrimethamine, and either a sulfonamide or sulfone is especially effective. However, resistance has developed to pyrimethamine plus sulfadiazine (Fansidar) in chloroquine-resistant *P. falciparum* in Thailand and Brazil.

IMMUNITY. *P. vivax* and *P. falciparum* produce partial homologous immunity that is strain-specific. There is no cross-immunity between species. Man has been immunized with irradiated sporozoites of *P. falciparum* and *P. vivax*, but immunity was short-lived. Stages in the erythrocytic cycle produce antibodies, and these forms of the parasite are currently being examined for possible use in vaccines.

Babesia sp.

Various species of the genus *Babesia* are parasitic in the erythrocytes of many domestic and wild mammals. Ixodid ticks serve as intermediate hosts. Infected ticks may inoculate sporozoites when they feed on man. Only *Babesia bovis* was known to infect man until recent case reports appeared of human infections with *Babesia microti*, a strain found in rodents.

MORPHOLOGY. *Babesia* spp. form tiny (1.5 to 5 μm) pear-shaped, ovoid, ellipsoid, ring- or rod-shaped bodies in erythrocytes (Fig. 13). The number, shape, and size vary with each species. No pigment is produced. Their staining characteristics are the same as those of *Plasmodium*.

LIFE CYCLE/EPIDEMIOLOGY. *Babesia* species reproduce by binary fission in infected erythrocytes. During division, the erythrocyte ruptures and new erythrocytes are invaded. Sexual development takes place in the arthropod. When sporozoites are finally produced, they invade all the tissues of the tick, including the developing eggs and salivary glands.

Babesiosis is a rare infection in man, but it may be fatal in splenectomized patients or those who are otherwise immunologically compromised. An epidemic involving *Babesia microti* occurred on Nantucket Island off the northeast coast of the United States (Spielman, 1976).

LABORATORY DIAGNOSIS. Definitive diagnosis is achieved by the identification of parasites in Giemsa-stained thick and thin blood smears. Differentiation of species is difficult, and the species are easily confused with malaria organisms.

DRUG SUSCEPTIBILITY. The antimalarial drugs have no effect on *Babesia* strains, but the organisms show some

Table 3. KEY FOR THE DIFFERENTIATION OF THE THREE COMMON MALARIA SPECIES IN PERIPHERAL BLOOD FILMS

Thin Films	
1. No intermediate stages present (no late trophozoites or schizonts). Usually only characteristic rings (rod-like nucleus; rings located at periphery of red cell; binucleate rings; small rings; frequently multiple rings in a red cell) and/or cresent-shaped gametocytes present	*P. falciparum*
2. Intermediate stages present (late trophozoites and schizonts)	*P. vivax* or *P. malariae*
A. Parasitized red cells enlarged and pale; trophozoites with irregular outlines; pigment fine; Schüffner's dots may be present	*P. vivax*
B. Parasitized red cells normal in size and color; growing forms compact or "band" forms; pigment coarse; no stippling of the red cells	*P. malariae*
Thick Films	
1. No intermediate stages present. Usually only characteristic *rings* (rings, exclamation marks, swallows, comets, etc.) and/or cresent-shaped gametocytes present	*P. falciparum*
2. Intermediate stages present	*P vivax* or *P. malariae*
A. Trophozoites with irregular cytoplasmic outline	*P. vivax*
B. Trophozoites with compact cytoplasm or "band" forms	*P. malariae*
Note: Schüffner's dots are not always present in *P. vivax* infection. Crescents are not always present in *P. falciparum* infection. Band forms are not always present in *P. malariae* infection.	

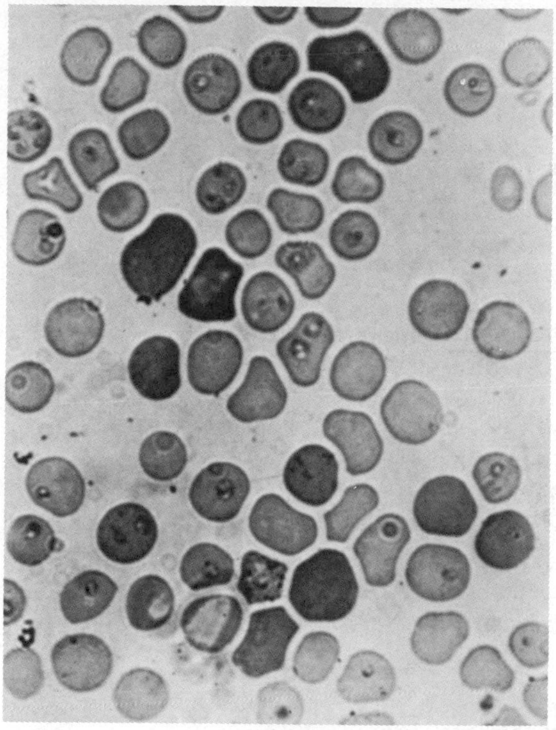

Figure 13. Red blood cells infected with *Babesia microti.* ×1,000. (From Katz, M., et al.: Parasitic Diseases. New York, Springer-Verlag, 1982.)

sensitivity to the antitrypanosomal drugs 4,4′-diazoaminobenzamidine and pentamidine isethionate, but parasitemia recurs after treatment. Despite the limited response, these three drugs should be used in the immunocompromised patient because infections under these circumstances are often fatal (Miller et al., 1978).

IMMUNITY. There is serologic cross-reactivity between *B. bovis, Plasmodium falciparum,* and *P. vivax,* but cross-immunity between *Babesia* and *Plasmodium* has not been investigated.

5. The Trypanosomes

Three species of hemoflagellates of the genus *Trypanosoma,* family Trypanosomatidae, are pathogenic for man: *Trypanosoma gambiense* and *T. rhodesiense* in Africa and *T. cruzi* in America. The life cycle of each is carried out partly in humans or another mammal and partly in an insect intermediate host, in which cyclic development occurs. *T. gambiense* and *T. rhodesiense* are extracellular trypomastigote parasites of the blood, lymph, or cerebrospinal fluid, whereas *T. cruzi* occurs as trypomastigote forms in the blood and amastigote forms in the tissue.

Trypanosoma gambiense

MORPHOLOGY. *T. gambiense* trypomastigotes in the blood of humans are polymorphic. They may be either typical slender flagellates with a pointed anterior end, a blunt posterior extremity, and a long flagellum, or short stumpy forms with or without a short flagellum. Only the long slender form replicates in the mammal; the short stumpy is the form that infects the tsetse fly. The flagellum of the slender form, 8 to 30 μm in length, projects from the anterior end after passing along the edge of the undulating membrane (Fig. 14). A large, oval nucleus is centrally located. A kinetoplast is located posteriorly at the base of the flagellum. The cytoplasm contains minute refractile volutin granules. Motility is wavy and spiraling. Trypomastigotes multiply by binary longitudinal fission.

LIFE CYCLE/EPIDEMIOLOGY. Although *T. gambiense* and *T. brucei* are morphologically identical, they are very different organisms. *T. brucei* is a parasite of wild and domestic animals that does not infect man, whereas *T. gambiense* is primarily a human parasite, without an important reservoir in animals. *T. gambiense* is transmitted from man to man by tsetse flies of the *Glossina palpalis* group. It is limited by the habitat of its vectors to forest belts, especially along rivers in tropical West and Central Africa. Trypanosomes that have been ingested by the fly during a blood meal undergo reproduction in the midgut. Long slender forms finally appear and move anteriorly through the proventriculus to the salivary glands and ducts, where epimastigote forms are produced. Eventually, metacyclic trypanosomes are derived and pass through the channel in the hypopharynx into the bite wound when the fly feeds. During epidemics, a tsetse fly may transmit trypanosomes directly ("flying needle") from an infected person, if the blood meal is interrupted. Congenital infections are rare.

LABORATORY DIAGNOSIS. Diagnosis is made by finding trypanosomes in the blood, lymph node aspirates, or bone marrow in early disease, and in centrifuged cerebrospinal fluid in late disease. Preparations are examined wet for motile organisms or stained with Romanowsky stains. The hematocrit tube-centrifuge technique is valuable in the diagnosis of *T. gambiense* infections (Lumsden, 1977). Small laboratory animals are less susceptible to *T. gambiense* than to the Rhodesian form. Culture of *T. gambiense* is difficult and not useful in diagnosis. Presumptive diagnosis is possible by monitoring serum IgM levels, which are greatly elevated. Serologic techniques include the complement fixation and indirect immunofluorescent tests.

DRUG SUSCEPTIBILITY. Suramin sodium, pentamidine isethionate, and lomidine methanesulfonate are effective in the treatment of the early stages of infection before the central nervous system is involved. In the late stages, synthetic arsenicals or antimony analogs of the melarsen group, which cross the blood-brain barrier, are used for treatment. Of these drugs, *T. gambiense* is most sensitive to tryparsamide, melarsoprol (Mel B), and MSbB. *T. gambiense* may become resistant to these compounds, which are frequently used in combination with suramin.

IMMUNITY. *T. gambiense* can escape the immune response of the host by antigenic variation. The variant antigens are glycoproteins, which are the major components of the surface coat (glycocalyx) of the trypanosome. This phenomenon has delayed immunologic approaches to prevention (Doyle, 1977).

Trypanosoma rhodesiense

MORPHOLOGY. The morphology of this species is identical with that of *T. gambiense.*

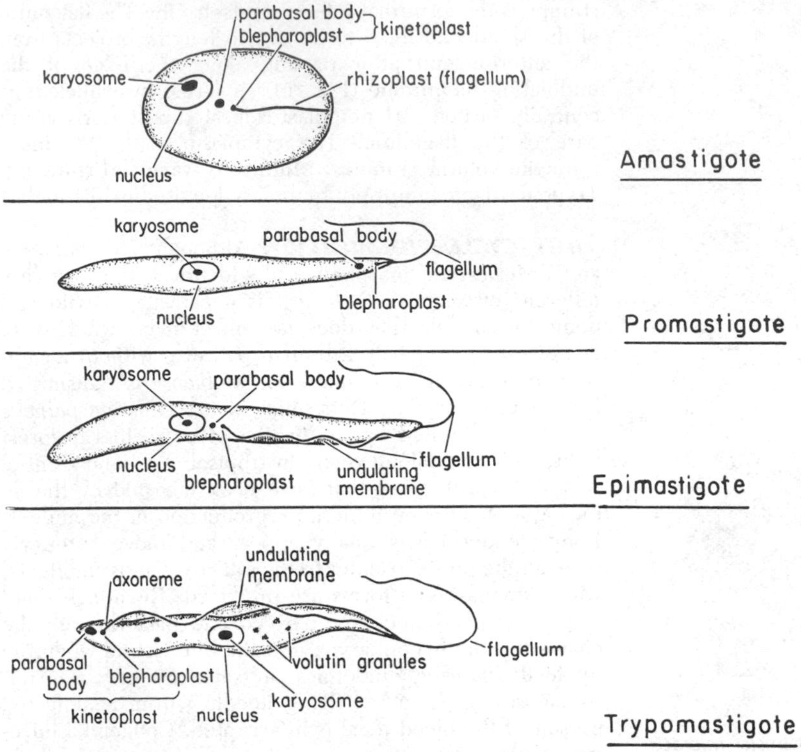

Figure 14. The developmental stages in the family Trypanosomatidae. (From Hunter, G. W., Swartzwelder, J. C., and Clyde, D. F.: Tropical Medicine. W. B. Saunders Co., Philadelphia, 1976.)

LIFE CYCLE/EPIDEMIOLOGY. *T. rhodesiense* is confined to East Africa in savannah areas in which cattle are raised. Its incidence and the occurrence of epidemics are lower than those for *T. gambiense. T. rhodesiense* has a large reservoir in wild animals, and the vectors *Glossina morsitans, G. pallidipes,* and *G. swynnertoni* feed primarily on ungulates and only infrequently on man. The life cycle is the same as that of *T. gambiense.*

LABORATORY DIAGNOSIS. The same procedures for *T. gambiense* infections are used for *T. rhodesiense* infections. Parasites are usually more numerous in the blood during Rhodesian trypanosomiasis, and small laboratory rodents are easily infected by intraperitoneal inoculation of whole blood that contains trypanosomes.

DRUG SUSCEPTIBILITY. The same drugs used to treat *T. gambiense* infections are used against *T. rhodesiense.*

IMMUNITY. Immunologic response is the same as that of *T. gambiense.*

Trypanosoma cruzi

MORPHOLOGY. *T. cruzi* is a pleomorphic hemoflagellate that infects the blood and tissue of mammals in most countries of the Western Hemisphere. Man is less frequently infected than smaller mammals. The trypomastigote in the blood is about 20 μm long. In some cases, stumpy forms about 15 μm long may be observed. In stained blood smears the organism is usually U- or S-shaped and has a large kinetoplast near its posterior end. A flagellum arises in this area, passes through the margin of the undulating membrane, and proceeds free anteriorly for about one third of the body length. The organism does not multiply in the trypomastigote form. The amastigote form is found in various tissue cells. It is a small oval body 3 to 5 μm in diameter, containing a nucleus and a small rodlike kinetoplast (Fig. 14). In this stage the parasite divides rapidly and forms many amastigotes.

LIFE CYCLE/EPIDEMIOLOGY. *T. cruzi* is transmitted to small mammals by many species of blood-feeding triatomids that serve as intermediate hosts. Man becomes infected when susceptible species of triatomids become domesticated. Human infections are common in South America and rare in the United States, because domestic triatomes usually live in thatched roofs or cracks in adobe walls in the former location where they can easily feed on man. Trypomastigotes are ingested by triatomids during a blood meal and undergo cyclic development in the gut of the insect. Amastigotes form in the foregut, epimastigotes in the midgut, and infective trypomastigotes in the hindgut. Trypomastigote forms are deposited on the skin with the feces during feeding. The feces is rubbed either into the bite wound or onto the conjunctiva, since the insect often feeds on the human face during sleep. Trypomastigotes invade local reticuloendothelial cells and multiply rapidly as amastigotes. Trypomastigote forms are produced and appear in the blood. They circulate to various tissues, where amastigote forms are again produced intracellularly. After an acute phase in man, the parasitemia subsides, but amastigotes may continue to multiply, which may lead to serious consequences years later as the chronic stage.

Nondomestic species of triatomids live in the nests of various mammals and carry on the cycle in nature by fecal contamination or by being eaten by certain mammals. In the latter case, infective stages may be passed across the mucous membranes of the mouth. Various modifications of the life cycle are presented in Figure 15.

Significant human disease is found only in areas in which the triatomid is domesticated and defecates while feeding.

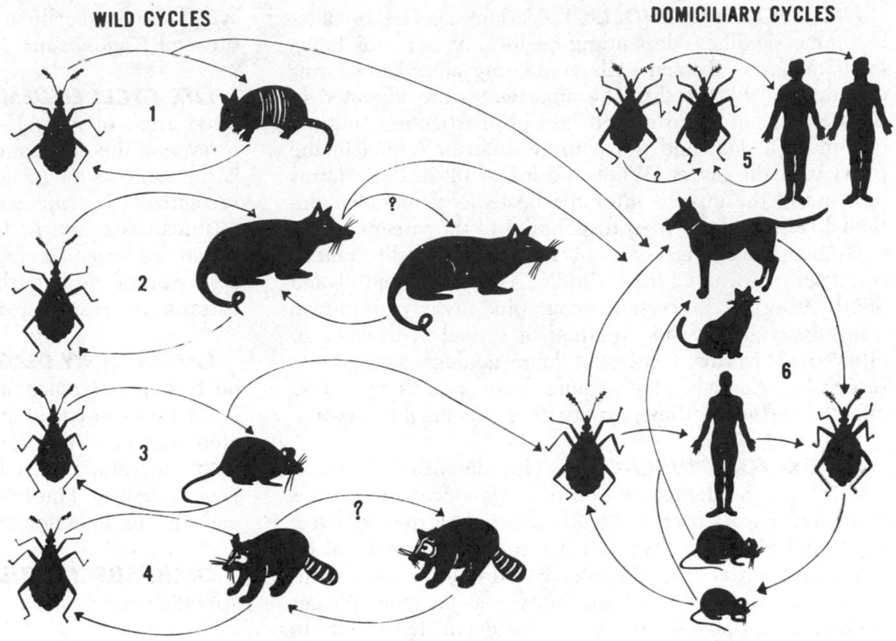

Figure 15. Wild and domestic cycles of Chagas' disease—modalities and relationships. 1, *Panstrongylus geniculatus* is often associated with armadillos: adults enter houses, attracted by light. 2, Opposums (*Didelphis* spp.) are associated with several triatomines and both marsupials and insects visit human dwellings. 3, Rats and other rodents are associated with insects that also fly to houses. 4, Raccoons may be associated with triatomines but, as with opossums, they may transmit *T. cruzi* among themselves without participation of the insect. 5, In the absence of domestic animals there is a cycle between insect and man. Transmission from one insect to another has been suggested, and transmission from man to man is a fact, both transplacentally and transfusionally. 6, Other domestic animals might participate in the cycle and some of them may become infected by eating small rodents. (From Zeledón, R. *In* Trypanosomiasis and Leishmaniasis with specific reference to Chagas' disease. Ciba Foundation Symposium 20, new series, 1974. Published by Elsevier. Excerpta Medica. North-Holland, Associated Scientific Publishers, Amsterdam.)

Dogs and cats are important reservoirs in endemic areas. Asymptomatic infections with *T. cruzi* occur and have been documented primarily in geographic areas in which triatomid species do not live in close association with humans. Nonpathogenic strains of *T. cruzi* may be responsible for some of these cases.

Congenital transmission has been reported.

LABORATORY DIAGNOSIS. The laboratory diagnosis depends on finding the organism in blood or tissue. Thick and thin blood films prepared during the acute stage, stained and unstained, may exhibit trypanoform stages. Parasites are never plentiful, however, because they do not multiply in peripheral blood. Concentration of large volumes of blood is helpful. Biopsies may reveal amastigote forms. Blood and bone marrow aspirates cultivated on diphasic blood agar media yield epimastigote forms in about 30 per cent of patients with positive serology. In xenodiagnosis, parasite-free triatomids are allowed to feed on the patient. Two weeks later, the intestinal contents of the triatomids are examined for hemoflagellates. This method of detecting the acute and chronic stages of the disease is not used outside of Latin America. Finally, sensitive serologic techniques (complement fixation, indirect hemagglutination, and indirect fluorescent antibody) are available for establishing a presumptive diagnosis. Many are available commercially as kits (Kagan, 1980).

T. rangeli, a nonpathogenic species of trypanosome, is found in Central and South America in humans and other mammals. It can be differentiated from *T. cruzi* by its smaller kinetoplast and by the presence of dividing forms in stained blood smears. It does not invade tissue cells.

DRUG SUSCEPTIBILITY. A nitrofuran derivative (nifurtimox, Lampit) can cause a radical cure by eliminating the blood forms in the acute disease. However, no known agent is effective against the intracellular amastigote stage.

IMMUNITY. *T. cruzi* is strongly immunogenic. The highest titers of antibodies are found during the acute stage. When the parasitemia drops, the titers also decrease. Cell-mediated immunity plays an important role in resistance to *T. cruzi* but may also be responsible for the tissue damage in chronic infections.

Antigenic variation does not occur with *T. cruzi*, and there is cross-immunity between heterologous strains. Vaccination confers only partial protection.

6. The Leishmania

The genus *Leishmania*, family Trypanosomatidae, includes four species—*Leishmania donovani*, *L. tropica*, *L. mexicana*, and *L. braziliensis*—all of which occur as intracellular amastigotes in man and promastigotes in phlebotomine sandfly intermediate hosts and in cultures (Fig. 14). All species are morphologically identical, and serologic separation has not been entirely satisfactory, although recent use of isoenzyme patterns appears promising. They have been separated primarily by their tendency to cause visceral, cutaneous, or mucocutaneous involvement in humans.

Leishmania donovani

MORPHOLOGY. In this species the organism is located in the viscera, in the reticuloendothelial cells of the spleen, liver, bone marrow, and lymph glands. *L. donovani* is a small, round, or ovoid intracellular amastigote, 2 to 5 μm in diameter. It contains a rodlike kinetoplast and a peripheral nucleus.

LIFE CYCLE/EPIDEMIOLOGY. Various species of phlebotomine sandflies, depending on locality, serve as intermediate hosts. Human cells containing amastigote forms are ingested by the fly. The amastigotes are liberated in the insect's gut, transformed into promastigotes, multiply by binary fission, and move to an anterior station in the pharynx of the insect. When the insect bites, these forms pass out of the insect, enter the host's local reticuloendothelial cells, and are then distributed to the viscera.

Human infections occur in India, the Mediterranean countries, Africa, China, Middle Asia, and Central and South America. In certain geographic areas man-to-man transmission is the sole method of spread of disease. In other areas, jackals, foxes, and domestic dogs may serve as reservoirs. Animals may acquire leishmaniasis by eating infected carcasses, thus perpetuating an animal reservoir.

LABORATORY DIAGNOSIS. The definitive diagnosis depends on the demonstration of *L. donovani* amastigotes in stained smears from material collected by splenic, liver, or sternal puncture (Fig. 16). Culture of the material on NNN medium is also valuable. Blood culture and examination of stained films of the buffy coat for macrophages containing amastigote forms will yield positive results in most cases. The complement fixation test is usually positive. The formol-gel test is a useful screening technique. When 1 drop of commercial formalin is added to 1 ml of serum from a patient with kala-azar, the serum solidifies and becomes opaque within 3 to 30 min.

DRUG SUSCEPTIBILITY. *L. donovani* is sensitive to two groups of compounds: (1) pentavalent antimony derivatives, including sodium antimony gluconate, neostibosan, and urea stibamine; and (2) certain aromatic diamidines, including hydroxystilbamidine and pentamidine isethionate.

IMMUNITY. *Leishmania* organisms are protected from antibodies by their location inside macrophages where they thrive. Humans have been successfully vaccinated with promastigotes from a rodent strain.

Leishmania tropica

MORPHOLOGY. *L. tropica* invades mononuclear and polymorphonuclear leukocytes and epithelial cells of the skin. The intracellular amastigote forms are identical to those of *L. donovani.*

LIFE CYCLE/EPIDEMIOLOGY. Infection is prevalent in large areas of Asia, the countries around the Mediterranean, and the north and west coasts of Africa. Transmission is the same as for *L. donovani.* Two subspecies have been recognized: *L. tropica major,* which causes "moist" or rural leishmaniasis, and *L. tropica minor,* the cause of "dry" or urban leishmaniasis. Gerbils are a primary extrahuman reservoir of rural leishmaniasis, and dogs are a primary extrahuman reservoir of urban leishmaniasis.

LABORATORY DIAGNOSIS. Diagnosis is made by demonstrating *L. tropica* amastigotes in cells of stained smears obtained from curettage or needle aspiration of the indurated margin of the dermal lesion. Culture of aspirates on NNN medium, with bacterial growth controlled, yields promastigotes. The leishmanial skin test becomes positive early in the infection and remains positive for life.

DRUG SUSCEPTIBILITY. Pentavalent antimony (sodium stibogluconate) is the most effective drug.

IMMUNITY. Infection results in life-long immunity to homologous strains. Therefore, children are often deliberately inoculated intradermally with material from lesions.

Leishmania braziliensis

MORPHOLOGY. Like *L. tropica, L. braziliensis* invades cells of the skin but may also spread to the mucous membranes. The amastigote stage is identical with that of *L. donovani.*

LIFE CYCLE/EPIDEMIOLOGY. Infections with *L. braziliensis* are widely distributed as a zoonosis in the forests of Central and South America, with the exception of Chile and Argentina. Rodents serve as reservoirs. Man is infected by phlebotomine sandflies of the genus *Lutzomyia.*

LABORATORY DIAGNOSIS. The demonstration of *T. braziliensis* amastigotes from skin lesions (see *L. tropica*) is comparatively easy in early infections because the parasites are numerous. In older infections, culture on NNN

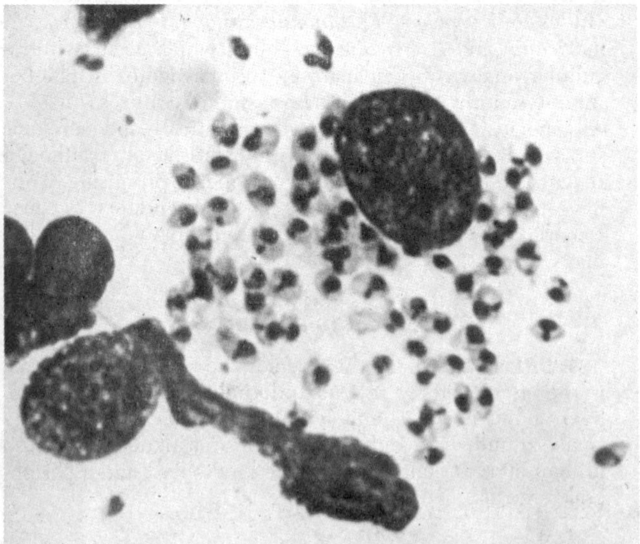

Figure 16. *Leishmania donovani* in stained smear from spleen puncture. (From Hunter, G. W., Swartzwelder, J. C., and Clyde, D. F.: Tropical Medicine. W. B. Saunders Co., Philadelphia, 1976.)

medium may be successful. The Montenegro skin test, which employs antigen from cultured promastigotes, is specific and sensitive, and remains positive for life.

DRUG SUSCEPTIBILITY. *L. braziliensis* is sensitive to pentavalent antimonials, cycloguanil pamoate, and amphotericin B.

IMMUNITY. Infection produces only strain specific immunity. Experimental work suggests that immunity may be induced by vaccination with epimastigotes from culture.

Leishmania mexicana

MORPHOLOGY. *L. mexicana* amastigotes invade cells of the skin and are identical with those of *L. donovani*.

LIFE CYCLE/EPIDEMIOLOGY. Infections occur in Mexico, Belize, and northern Guatemala. However, the organism is believed to be present throughout the forests of Central and northern South America. Like *L. braziliensis*, it is also a forest zoonosis maintained in wild rodents with phlebotomine sandflies of the genus *Lutzomyia* as vectors.

LABORATORY DIAGNOSIS. Amastigote forms of *L. mexicana* are easy to find in smears of early lesions. In late infections they are difficult to find and isolate. A skin test using refined antigen is helpful (Zeledón and Ponce, 1974).

DRUG SUSCEPTIBILITY. *L. mexicana* is sensitive to pentavalent antimonials and cycloguanil pamoate.

IMMUNITY. Immunity against reinfection occurs with *L. mexicana*, but little cross-immunity occurs between strains.

References

Anderson, B. C.: Cryptosporidiosis. Lab Med 14:55, 1983.

Brook, M. M., and Melvin, D. M.: Intestinal and urogenital protozoa. In Lennette, E. H. (ed.): Manual of Clinical Microbiology, 3rd ed. Washington, D.C., American Society of Microbiology, 1980, p. 1044.

Dorsch, M. M., Cameron, A. S., and Robinson, B. S.: The epidemiology and control of primary amoebic meningoencephalitis with particular reference to South Australia. Trans R Soc Trop Med Hyg 77:372, 1983.

Doyle, J. J.: Antigenic variation in the salivarian trypanosomes. In Miller, L. H., Pinto, J. A., and McKelvey, Jr., J. J. (eds.): Immunity to Blood Parasites of Animals and Man. (Advances in Experimental Medical Biology, vol. 93), New York, Plenum Press, 1977, p. 321.

John, D. T.: Primary amebic meningoencephalitis and the biology of *Naegleria fowleri*. Ann Rev Microbiol 36:101, 1982.

Kagan, I. G.: Serodiagnosis of parasitic diseases. In Lennette, E. H. (ed.): Manual of Clinical Microbiology, 3rd ed. Washington, D.C., American Society of Microbiology, 1980, p. 1044.

Lumsden, W. H. R.: Field diagnosis of trypanosomiasis. Trans R Soc Trop Med Hyg 71:8, 1977.

Miller, L. H., Neva, F. A., and Gill, F.: Failure of chloroquine in human babesiosis (*Babesia microti*). Ann Intern Med 88:200, 1978.

Reed, S. L., Sargeaunt, P. G., and Braude, A. I.: Resistance to lysis by human serum of pathogenic *Entamoeba histolytica*. Trans R Soc Trop Med Hyg 77:248, 1983.

Sargeaunt, P. G., Jackson, T. F. H. G., and Simjee, A.: Biochemical heterogeneity of *Entamoeba histolytica* isolates, especially those from liver abscess. Lancet i: 1386, 1982.

Spielman, A.: Human babesiosis on Nantucket Island: Transmission by nymphal Ixodes ticks. Am J Trop Med Hyg 25:784, 1976.

Thornton, F. A., West, A. H., DuPont, H. L., and Pickering, L. K.: Comparison of methods for identification of *Giardia lamblia*. Am J Clin Path 80(6):858, 1983.

Tzipori, S., Angus, K. W., Campbell, I., and Grey, E. W.: Cryptosporidium: Evidence for a single-species genus. Infect and Immun 30:884, 1980.

Visvesvara, G. S.: Free-living pathogenic amoebae. In Lennett, W. H. (ed.): Manual of Clinical Microbiology, 3rd ed. Washington, D.C., American Society of Microbiology, 1980, p. 1044.

Wolfe, M. S.: Giardiasis. JAMA 233:1362, 1975.

Zeledón, R., and Ponce, D.: Parasitological and immunological diagnosis of cutaneous leishmaniasis. Proceedings of the Third International Congress of Parasitology 3:239, 1974.

85
NEMATHELMINTHES (ROUNDWORMS)

A. O. ANYA, Ph.D.

The name Nemathelminthes was first used by Gegenbaur in 1859 to describe the roundworms. In his conception, the roundworms included three zoologically distinct groups of animals: the acanthocephalans, the nematodes, and the gordiaceans (nematomorphs). Although most zoology texts include rotifers, gastrotrichs, kinorhynchs, nematodes, and nematomorphs in this designation, the zoologic affinities of these groups are not clear, and Hyman (1951) prefers to regard each as an independent entity of phyletic status. Most modern authors have preferred this arrangement. Because the nematodes are the only Nemathelminthes of medical importance, the following discussion will concentrate on this group.

FUNCTIONAL MORPHOLOGY. Nematodes are generally small, spindle-shaped, unsegmented, bilaterally symmetric organisms. The digestive and reproductive systems lie more or less freely in the fluid-filled body cavity, which is a pseudocoelom (Figs. 1 and 2).

Within the body cavity may also be found two, four, or six ovoid or many-branched cells called pseudocoelomocytes of unknown function. Organs of respiration and circulation are absent, and the "excretory" organs are unlike those of other invertebrates. An often-quoted characteristic of nematodes is the absence of cilia or flagella. The electron microscope, which has opened up a new era in nematode morphology and anatomy, has demonstrated typical flagella in the intestine of a free-living nematode *Eudorylaimus* sp and modified flagella in the sense organs of many nematodes including parasitic species (Zmoray and Guttekova, 1972; McLaren, 1976).

The body surface is covered by a living, thin, relatively inelastic but flexible cuticle made of modified collagen (Anya, 1966). The cuticle lines part of the inner surface of the main body openings of the digestive and reproductive systems. Fine striations and annuli may be present on the cuticular surface.

The cuticle, which is a three-layered structure consisting of cortical, median, and basal layers, is often delimited by a basement lamella from the hypodermis. The latter may be either syncytial or cellular tissue. It projects into the body cavity along the middorsal, midventral, and lateral lines, giving rise to four ridges or chords (Fig. 3). When

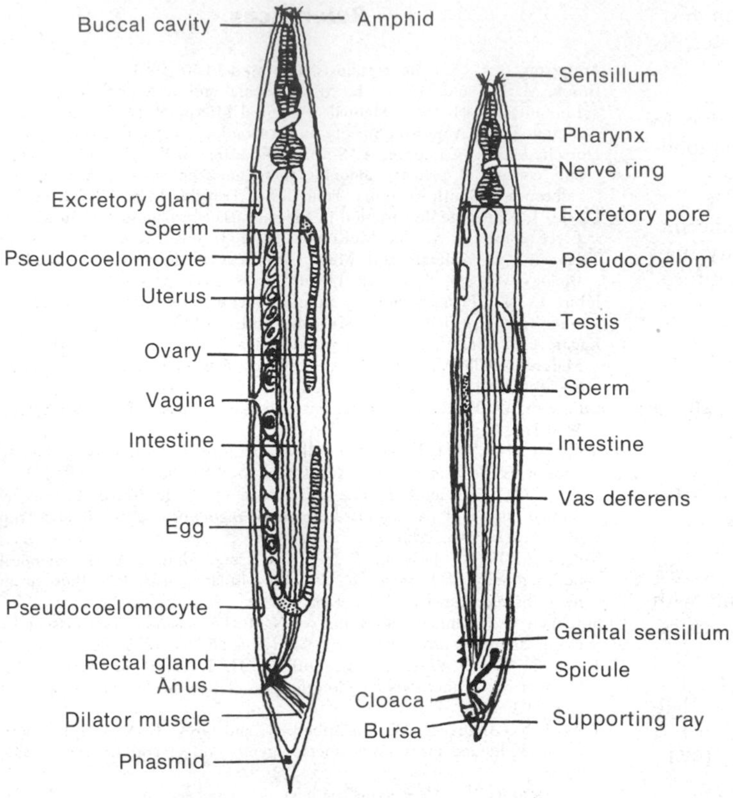

Figures 1 and 2. Diagram of a hypothetical nematode: female (left) and male (right).

excretory canals are present, they are embedded in the tissues of the lateral chords. The main nerves run in the middorsal and midventral hypodermal chords.

The muscle layer lies beneath the hypodermis and consists of unique, spindle-shaped, and elongated cells oriented only in the longitudinal direction. There are no circular muscles. The muscle cells are characteristically divided into contractile and noncontractile portions (Fig. 4) and are obliquely striated with the filaments of actin and myosin restricted to the basal contractile portion of the cell. The noncontractile part of the muscle cell contains the main cell organelles, such as the nucleus and mitochondria, as well as stores of glycogen and fat. The nerve processes extend from the muscle cells to make synaptic contact with the longitudinally oriented nerve trunks in the middorsal and midventral hypodermal chords. Thus, unlike the situation in other organisms, the muscle cells transmit innervation impulses to the nerve tissue.

The fluid-filled body cavity is notable for its high but variable turgor pressure, which ensures that its incompressible fluid content acts as a hydrostatic skeleton that is antagonistic to the longitudinal muscle layer. The efficiency of this arrangement is assured by the special arrangement of the fibers in the nematode cuticle. In *Ascaris lumbricoides*, for example, the fiber layers consist of a meshwork of spiral and relatively inelastic fibers that run counter to one another in a trellis or lattice fashion. This may best be visualized as a series of parallelograms subtending an angle (Q) that will vary within defined limits (Fig. 5). Anisometric extension of the cuticle is thus possible, and the angle Q defines the critical position from which the length and diameter of the cylindrical nematode can change without altering the volume. It has been shown mathematically that as long as Q is larger than 55 degrees, an increase in length of the worm compensates for a slight decrease in diameter, and, in such an arrangement, the muscles must be oriented longitudinally. Measurements of fixed preparations of the cuticle of *Ascaris* give a value of 75 degrees 30′ for Q (Harris and Crofton, 1957). The interaction of pressure changes with the cuticle and the muscle maintain static equilibrium during variations in body volume, permitting the ingestion or expulsion of fluid despite the high pressure in the body cavity. This system may explain the relative invariability of nematode structure.

The alimentary system includes a mouth, buccal cavity, pharynx (esophagus), intestine, rectum, and anus (Fig. 1). The mouth is usually surrounded by lips arranged according to a hexamerous triradiate arrangement. In the male nematode, the distal section of the reproductive system also opens into the rectal region, converting the rectum into a cloaca. The buccal cavity, like the pharynx, is lined by cuticle, which may be modified into teeth or cutting plates. The triradiate pharynx is a highly muscular organ that may be divisible into muscular and glandular regions. Alternatively, it may contain three glands that open into the lumen at different points along its length. The intestine is lined by microvilli and may be demarcated functionally from the pharynx and rectum (or cloaca) by a valve or sphincter that controls the entry or exit of materials in the alimentary system.

Nematodes are generally bisexual and show sexual dimorphism in that males are usually smaller. The female reproductive system consists of two tubes whose diameters vary in different regions. Each tube differentiates into

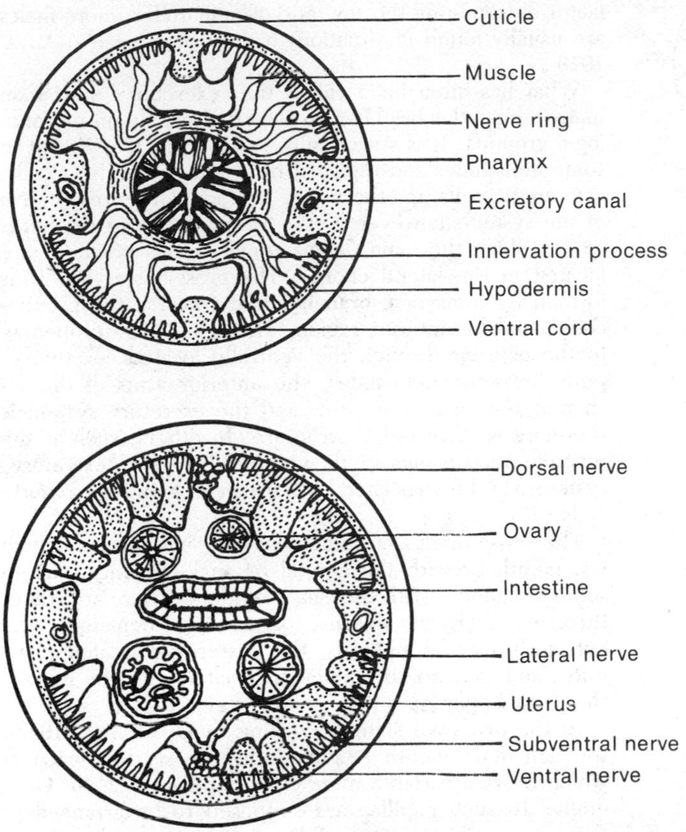

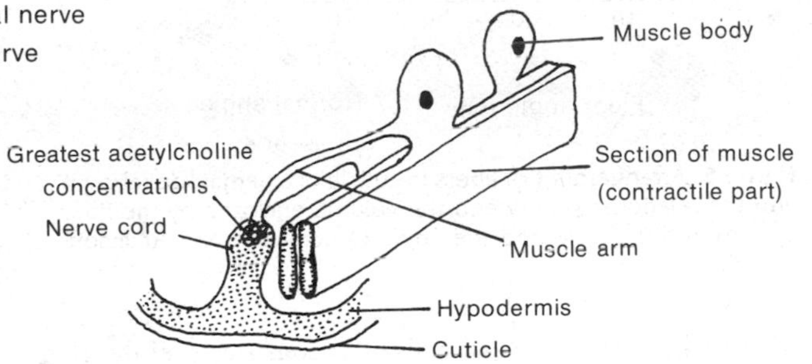

Figure 3. Transverse sections through a female nematode in the pharyngeal region (above) and in the midregion (below).

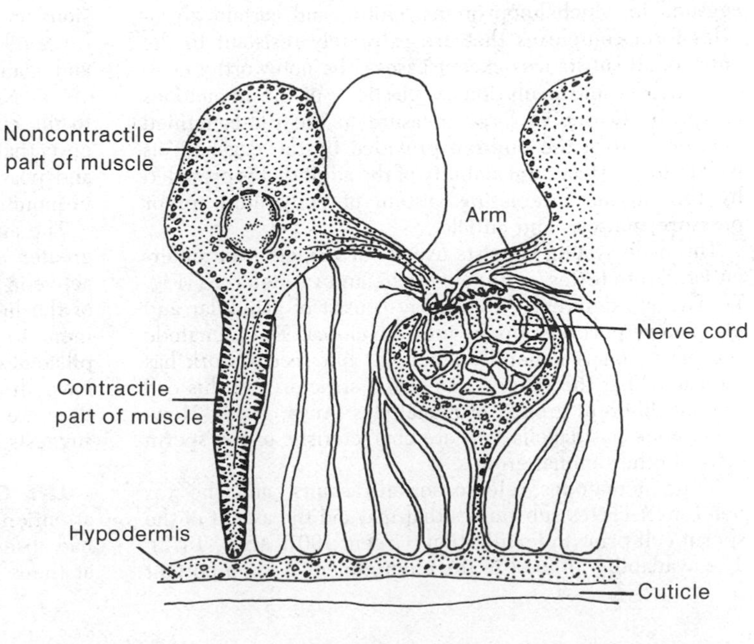

Figure 4. The muscle cells in nematodes. Longitudinal aspect of two muscle cells (above) and muscle cells at myoneural junction, transverse section (below).

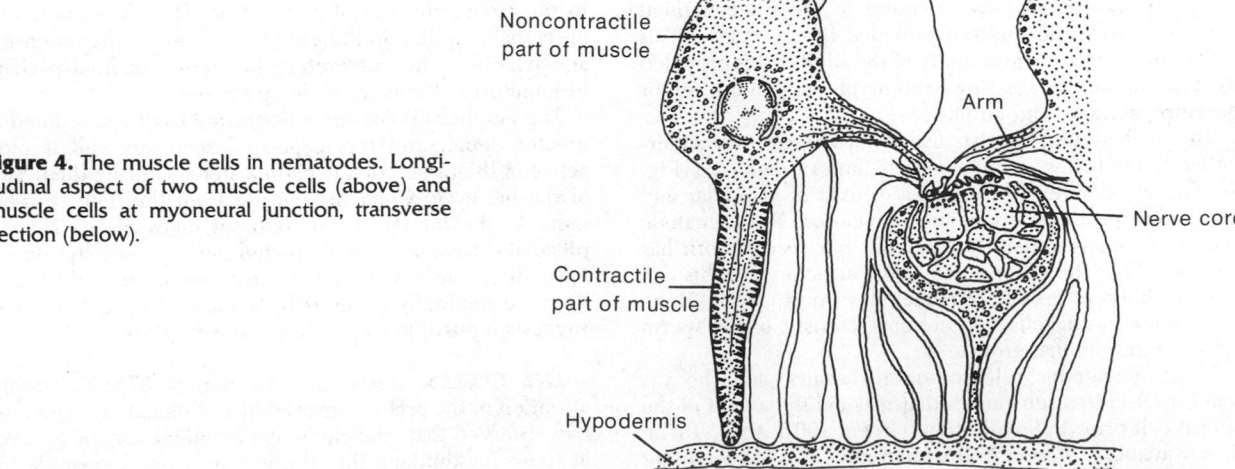

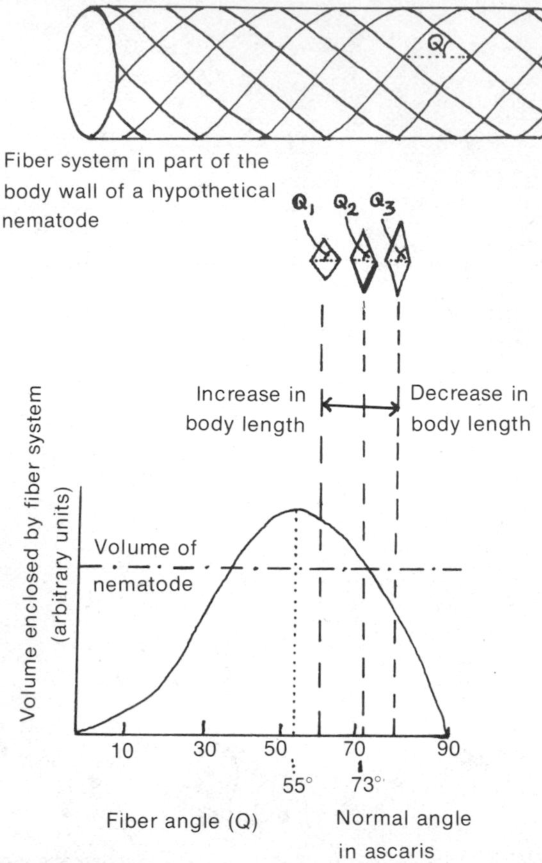

Figure 5. Arrangement of fibers in cuticle of a nematode (above) and the relationship between the volume enclosed by the fiber system in the cuticle and the angle Q (after Lee and Atkinson, 1976).

ovary (where the germinal cells at various stages of development are found), oviduct, seminal receptacle, and uterus. The two uteri may be joined to form a vagina uterina that leads to the exterior through the vulva (Fig. 6). The nematode egg is covered by a highly resistant three-layered eggshell in which lipoproteins, chitin, and certain glycosides form complexes that are extremely resistant to the entry of all substances except gases. The noteworthy ecologic success and evolutionary plasticity of the nematodes are probably due in large measure to the self-contained environment of the embryo provided by the eggshell, as well as to the structural stability of the adult that is provided by the unique interacting system of body fluid turgor pressure, muscle, and cuticle.

The male system consists usually of a single tube differentiated into testes, seminal vesicle, and vas deferens (Fig. 7). The vas deferens, which may consist of glandular and ejaculatory portions, opens into the cloaca. The nematode spermatozoon is generally ameboid, but recent work has indicated that the shapes, sizes, and structures of this cell vary in different groups of nematodes (Anya, 1976). However, none has flagella that are characteristic of the sperm cells of other animal groups.

Some nematodes release sex attractants, and the vas deferens secretes substances that may aid the ascent of the sperm cell prior to fertilization (Green, 1967; Anya, 1973). The availability of food in the environment is an important factor determining the sex ratio of nematodes; more males are usually found in situations of nutritional stress (Anya, 1976).

What has often been called the "excretory" system in many nematodes has been so regarded purely on morphologic grounds. It is structurally variable, as it is absent in some nematodes and replaced by a pair of glandular cells, the renette cells, in others. The best known representative of the system, however, is the H type seen in *Rhabditis* sp, in which the main (longitudinal) trunks of the H are located in the lateral chords. The cross-bar of the H is formed by transverse branches that traverse the pseudocoelom in the anterior region. These join before opening to the exterior through the ventrally located "excretory" pore. In some nematodes, the anterior arms of the H-shaped system may be lost, and the excretory system is therefore an inverted U structure. In others, such as the juvenile *Ancylostoma* sp, the inverted U type of "excretory" system may be associated with a pair of glandular renette cells.

The sense organs of nematodes may be associated with the mouth or with the genital or anal openings (and in some nematodes with the caudal region). There are, then, three main groups of sense organs in a nematode: the anteriorly located amphids, the posteriorly located phasmids, and the various papillae associated with the mouth, the genital opening, or the caudal region.

In the primitive state, according to De Conick (1942), the nematode mouth is surrounded by six lips, each of which bears a variable number of papillae (Fig. 8). Generally, 16 such papillae are supposed to be arranged in three concentric circles as follows: an inner and an outer circle of labial papillae on each lip and four cephalic papillae situated behind the lips. The amphids are located on either side of the head region. The pair of phasmids is located posteriorly, one on either side of the ventral median line, behind the anal opening in the female. The male nematode may bear (also in the posterior region) several pairs of genital or caudal papillae. The papillae are usually supported by an expansion of the caudal cuticle called alae or bursae, depending on the structure or the degree of cuticular inflation and the nematode group.

The amphids and the phasmids are cuticle-lined depressions on the body surface. Recent ultrastructural work has revealed that these depressions are associated with receptor and glandular cells with ciliated nerve axons (McLaren, 1976). Nerve processes from these cells have been traced to the circumpharyngeal nerve ring. This association suggests that amphids and phasmids may have a chemosensory and possibly a neurosecretory function, essential perhaps in monitoring the external environment.

The amphid of *Necator americanus* has been studied in greater detail, and the associated secretory cell is most active in the production of cholinesterase during the period of the life cycle when the change from the lung environment to the intestinal environment takes place. The papillae also have associated ciliated nerve axons, but do not have direct access to the external environment because they are generally covered by a rather thin cuticle. This suggests a possible role as mechanoreceptors.

LIFE CYCLES. Harris and Crofton (1957), in drawing attention to the relative invariability of nematode structure, had observed that "the elementary student may be forgiven at times for thinking that there is only one nematode but

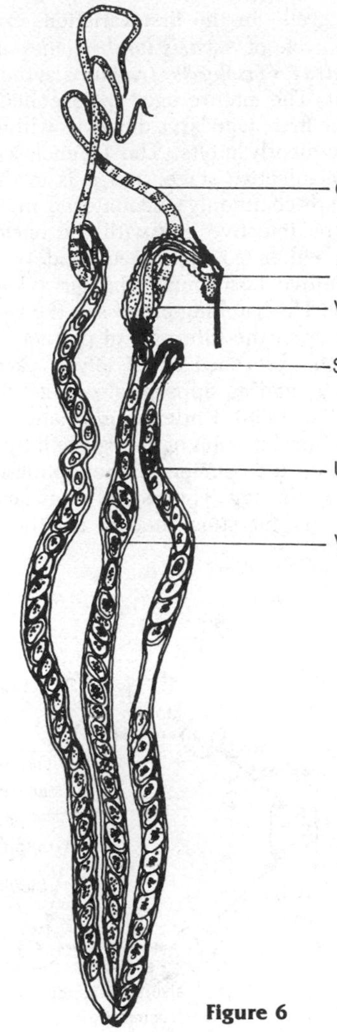

Figure 6

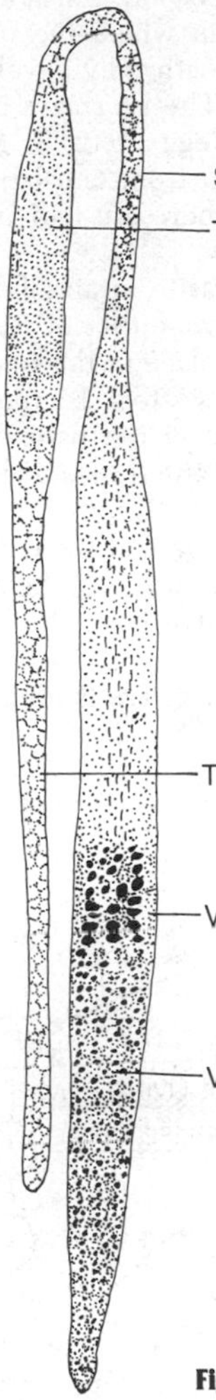

Figure 7

Figures 6 and 7. Reproductive system of the parasitic nematode, *Aspiculuris tetraptera*: female (left) and male (right). (Figure 6 from Spencer, F. M., and Monroe, L. S.: The Color Atlas of Intestinal Parasites. 2nd ed, 1982. Courtesy of Charles C Thomas, Publisher, Springfield, Illinois.)

that the model comes in different sizes and with a great variety of life histories." The apparent uniformity of nematode structure is meaningful if interpreted in the context of the unique structural relations of cuticle, muscle, and body pressure changes. The apparent variety of life cycle patterns is equally logical (and reducible to basic types) if

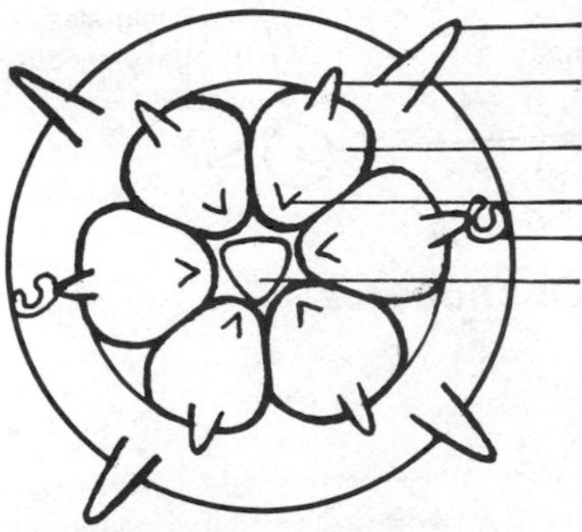

Figure 8. En-face view of the hypothetical primitive nematode (after De Conick, 1942).

it is seen as an ecologic adaptive strategy for parasitic life and against the background of the evolutionary history of parasitism among the nematodes. For parasitism as a way of life has evolved independently several times among these organisms.

Moreover, it must be remembered that parasites occur as a population of organisms within an *individual* member of a host population. The regular infection of *other* members of the host population often dictates a period of sojourn in the environment outside the host. A parasite must therefore be capable of surviving in the very different environments *within* and *outside* a host; alternatively, it must develop a stage or stages in its life cycle adapted to survive best in each of these environments. Nematodes have chosen the latter strategy. The dispersive phase of the life cycle is either the resistant egg, in which a developing embryo or larva is often enclosed, or a specially adapted, hardy, and resistant infective larval stage, generally the third stage larva.

It is best to begin a consideration of the life cycle of the parasitic nematodes from the basic patterns of the nonparasitic, free-living members in the aquatic and soil environment. In these, there are an egg and five stages of growth and development: the first, second, third, and fourth larval stages and the fifth stage, in which the organism attains final maturity or adulthood with fully developed and functional reproductive organs. The six stages in this cycle are represented in Fig. 9 as E (egg), 1, 2, 3, 4 (larval), and A (adult) stages. The transition from one larval stage to the next is marked by a molt: there are four molts in the life cycle of a nematode.

The host in which a parasite attains full development and production is called the *definitive* or *final* host. Earlier stages of development take place in the *intermediate* host, which may also serve as a vector. Temporary hosts that transport the infective stage of the parasite to a suitable environment are often called the *transport* host. Life cycles that involve direct contact between the infective agent (whether egg or infective larva) and the definitive host are called *direct*. If development of any of the stages occurs in a host other than the definitive host, the life cycle is said to be *indirect*.

In the parasitic species, there are five main variations in this basic life cycle. In the first variation, exemplified by the direct life cycle of *Ascaris lumbricoides* and *Trichocephalus trichiurus (Trichuris trichiura)*, the egg is the infective agent. The mature eggs are expelled in the feces of the host. The first-stage larva develops within the *Ascaris* egg and subsequently molts. The L_2 enclosed within the eggshell is the infective stage, and it is in this stage that the parasites are commonly encountered in contaminated soils. When the infective egg with the enclosed larva is swallowed in either contaminated food or water by a potential definitive host, man, the larva hatches in the small intestine. The hatching process in the gastrointestinal tract depends upon the interplay of physiocochemical factors, chiefly the presence of dissolved carbon dioxide, reducing agents, and an appropriate range of pH (Rogers and Sommerville, 1968). Under appropriate conditions, the larva hatches after digestion of the eggshell by the enzymes chitinase, lipase, and leucine aminopeptidase, which are produced within the egg. The second-stage larva now molts and penetrates the intestinal mucosa as a third-stage larva,

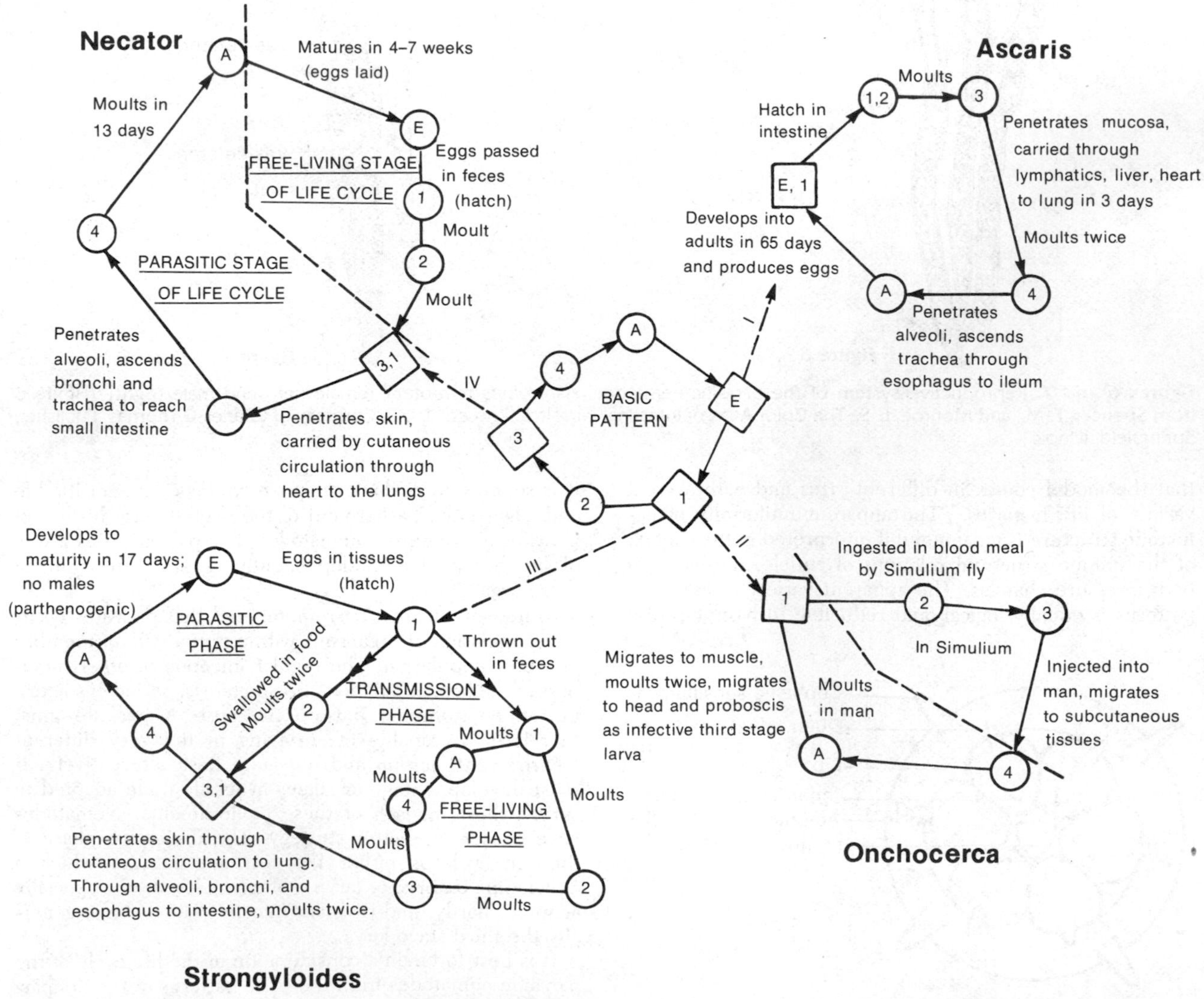

Figure 9. Diagrammatic representation of the basic pattern and four of the five variations of life cycle patterns in nematodes (see text).

which is carried through the lymphatics to the liver, heart, and finally to the lungs within one to three days. During these wanderings (the histotrophic phase), it molts two more times to transform itself into the young adult that breaks through the lung alveoli, ascends the trachea, migrates to the esophagus, and finally descends to the ileum, where the young adult worm reaches egg-producing maturity in about 65 days from the original infection. When evacuated in the feces, the eggs repeat the cycle.

The life cycle is similar in *Trichocephalus trichiurus (Trichuris trichiura)*. The only difference is that the first-stage larvae do not wander as extensively as *Ascaris* larvae. They merely penetrate the villi for a brief sojourn of about a week before returning to the lumen of the cecum to continue their development to full maturity, which takes about three months.

The second pattern, an indirect life cycle, is characteristic of the order Spirurida and is exemplified by the filarial worm of the subcutaneous tissues of man, *Onchocerca volvulus*. Adult females produce eggs that give rise to microfilariae enclosed in the inner membrane of the egg while still within the adult females. When released into the cutaneous circulation, these microfilariae reinitiate the cycle with the next insect bite.

The sequence, summarized in Figure 9, II, is as follows. When an insect vector, usually *Simulium damnosum* in the West African region, bites an infected human, the microfilariae are ingested with the blood meal. The microfilariae migrate to the thoracic muscles of the insect, molt twice, and, as the third-stage larvae, finally come to rest in the head and proboscis region of the insect. When an infected *Simulium* fly bites the next human victim, the infective larva is reinjected into the cutaneous circulation. This larva molts, migrates to the subcutaneous tissues of the host, and molts once more before reaching maturity. Thus, the infective stage for human infection is the third-stage larva, but the first-stage larva is infective for the *Simulium* intermediate host.

The life cycle is essentially the same in all the spirurids with minor variations in the intermediate host or vector that influence the mode of entry into the human host. The intermediate hosts of *Wuchereria bancrofti* are mosquitoes of the genera *Anopheles*, *Aedes*, and *Culex*. *Anopheles* is the major vector in West Africa, while *Culex pipiens fatigans* is predominant in Southeast Asia. The vector of *Loa loa* is the day-biting tabanid fly, *Chrysops* sp. Aquatic crustaceans of the genus *Cyclops* are the intermediate hosts of *Dracunculus medinensis*. Man is infected by drinking contaminated water. *Culicoides* sp is the vector of *Dipetalonema streptocerca* in Africa and *Mansonella ozzardi* in South America, where *Simulium* sp may also transmit mansonelliasis.

The third variation that may be considered unique is found in the Rhabditida and exemplified by *Strongyloides stercoralis*. Adult female worms live in the small intestine of the definitive host. Eggs are released in the intestine, where they hatch and give rise to first-stage larvae that reach the soil in the feces. In the soil, two paths of development are open to these larvae. They may follow a free-living, nonparasitic pattern of development in which adult males and females develop from four molts, which give rise to four larval stages and finally adult males and females. The females produce eggs that repeat the cycle.

Alternatively, the first-stage larvae can undergo two successive molts and produce infective third-stage larvae that penetrate the skin of humans, reach the cutaneous circulation, migrate to the lungs, break through the alveoli, ascend the bronchi and trachea to the esophagus, and descend to the intestine. During migration, the parasitic larvae molt twice and reach maturity in about 17 days. There are no males, and egg production is through parthenogenesis. The essential elements of this cycle are summarized in Figure 9, III. The parasitic phase is an example of a direct life cycle, although a free-living phase regularly alternates with this parasitic phase. During the free-living phase, some third stage larvae may also become infective and participate in the parasitic phase by penetrating into the definitive host (Nigon, 1947).

The fourth pattern, also direct, is characteristic of most of the Strongylidae, including *Necator americanus*. When eggs are excreted in the feces of the host, the first-stage larvae emerge, feed, and molt into second-stage larvae, which develop into infective third-stage larvae. The latter do not feed. They are enclosed in the uncast sheaths derived from the molted cuticle of the second-stage larva. The survival of third-stage larvae depends upon the reserves of lipids built up in their tissues during the feeding phase of second-stage larvae. Recent work in our laboratories has shown that the infectivity of *Necator americanus* varies with the lipid level, activity, and age of the larva. Under the tropical conditions of Nsukka, the viability and infectivity of the larva in contaminated fields are maintained for up to 21 days (Udonsi, unpublished observations).

On contact with a person, infective larvae penetrate the skin, are carried in the circulation through the heart to the lungs, molt within 24 hours, break through the alveoli, ascend the bronchi and trachea, and descend the esophagus to arrive at the small intestine. Here they molt again, usually within 13 days, and the female adults produce eggs in four to seven weeks. There are thus a free-living and a parasitic stage in the life cycle of each *Necator* nematode. The pattern is summarized in Figure 9, IV.

This pattern is essentially the same in other members of the Strongylidae except that most of the trichostrongylids do not infect the host by penetrating the skin. Infective larvae are swallowed with food or water. *Ancylostoma* may also develop by an identical life cycle.

The fifth pattern of the life cycle is exemplified by *Trichinella spiralis* (Fig. 10, I). First-stage larvae are encysted in the muscles of pigs or carnivores such as foxes and wolves. When infected meat is eaten raw or undercooked by another carnivore or human, the cyst walls are digested in the stomach, and the first-stage larvae are released. These larvae invade the mucosa of the duodenum and jejunum and undergo four molts. Some authorities insist that each larva undergoes only three molts within the mucosa, an earlier molt having taken place in the cyst. According to this view, the encysted larva is a second-stage larva.

Immature worms are found in the intestinal lumen within 24 hours of the ingestion of cysts. Adult females are ovoviviparous—i.e., first-stage larvae are released from the uterus rather than eggs. These larvae penetrate the intestinal mucosa, migrate through lymphatics and blood vessels to the skeletal muscles, penetrate the sarcolemma, and form the cyst. The life cycle is completed when the host is eaten by another carnivore (Fig. 10, I). Under normal circumstances, human infections represent a biologic dead end for the parasite. Transmission of the parasite is made possible by the zoonotic maintenance of reservoir hosts in wild carnivores. The nature of the available reservoir host in each locality introduces local variations in the life cycle in different geographic regions (Fig. 10, II to IV).

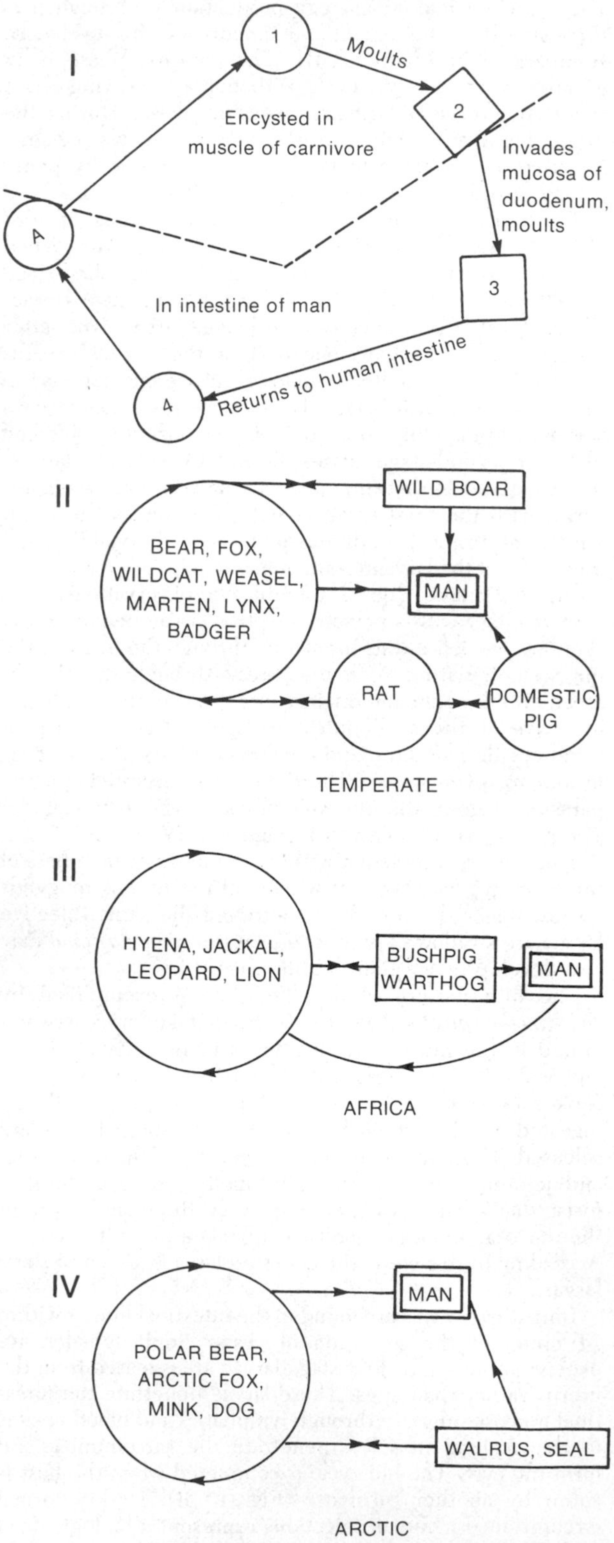

Figure 10. The life cycle pattern of *Trichinella spiralis* (the fifth pattern) and the pattern of zoonotic relationship in different geographic regions: temperate, tropical (Africa), and arctic.

IMMUNITY. The relationship between a helminth and its host is complex and influenced by physiologic, biochemical, genetic, nutritional, immunologic, and other biologic mechanisms. Host specificity, which is common in vertebrate-helminth interactions, may arise from natural resistance mediated by any of these factors. Acquired immunity, on the other hand, follows the general principles elucidated in studies of viral and bacterial infections. Progress in our understanding of the principles of immunity to helminths was relatively slow until recently.

One explanation for the complexity of helminth immunology is the fact that helminths are collections of different populations of cells with different biochemical, metabolic, and antigenic characteristics. Nevertheless, studies of various experimental systems such as *Nippostrongylus braziliensis* and *Trichuris muris* in mice (Ogilvie and Jones, 1973; Selby and Wakelin, 1973; Wakelin and Lloyd, 1976), *Ascaris suum* and *Toxocara cati* in rats and mice (Larsh and Race, 1975), *Ancylostoma caninum* in dogs (Miller, 1964), and *Onchocerca volvulus* in man (WHO, 1976) have shed considerable light on the essential features and mechanisms of helminth immunogenicity.

The immune response to helminth infections can be mediated through either circulating antibodies or delayed hypersensitivity (cell-mediated immunity) involving lymphoid cells (Larsh and Race, 1975; Muller, 1975). For example, circulating antibodies of the complement-fixing IgG and IgM classes have been detected in onchocerciasis, while *Ascaris* has stimulated the production of IgM, IgA, and IgG. *Trichinella spiralis* elicits predominantly reaginic IgE antibodies. An increase in the serum level of IgE from about 100 ng/ml to 1000 ng/ml encourages the view that IgE is an important line of immunologic defense in these infections. Indeed, a generalized eosinophilia, whose significance is at present uncertain, and these reaginic antibodies are becoming the characteristic indicators of vertebrate host-helminth interactions, especially when the association of parasite with host tissue can be regarded as close, e.g., with *Trichinella spiralis* and *Nippostrongylus braziliensis*.

Another feature of helminth immunity is the inability of killed helminth material or purified extracts of helminth excretions or secretions to afford long-lasting protection. Rather, protection has been secured in some cases by the regular and persistent release of antigens. Thus, live vaccines of irradiated larvae by x-rays have provided significant protection against *Dictyocaulus viviparus* bronchitis in cattle and the canine hookworm. Understandably, live vaccines have not been used in humans.

It is now generally accepted that any of the typical host reactions associated with the immune response, namely anaphylaxis, immune complex disease, and delayed hypersensitivity may occur in nematode infections. For example, the so-called self-cure of *Haemonchus contortus* infections characterized by the expulsion of preexisting adult worms on the entry of new infective larvae, is explicable on the basis of anaphylaxis. It is suggested that the release of molting fluid (and thus antigens) by third-stage infective larvae results in an anaphylactic reaction brought about by the production of pharmacologically active substances such as histamine, serotonin (5-HT), and kinins, which render the intestinal mucosa unsuitable for the continued existence of the adult worms. However, recent studies in Kenya have attempted to explain the self-cure phenomenon, not on the basis of local intestinal anaphylaxis but on nutritionally induced unsuitability of the intestine for the adult worms. In *Nippostrongylus braziliensis* infections of rats and *Haemonchus placei* infections of cattle, on the other hand, it has been shown that the immune reaction leads to structural changes in the intestinal cells of the nematodes, characterized by extreme vacuolation and the accumulation of lipids. These nematodes are unable to maintain their normal position in the hosts' intestine because of this interference with their normal metabolism.

After treatment of *Onchocerca volvulus* infections the histologic appearance of tissues suggests that antigens released from dying larvae form complexes with circulating antibodies in and around blood vessels. These immune complexes induce infiltration and degranulation of polymorphonuclear leukocytes. Immune complex formation in the eye or the testes may lead to blindness or infertility, respectively (WHO, 1976).

The importance of cell-mediated immunity in infections with *Trichinella, Nippostrongylus, Trichostrongylus, Trichocephalus (Trichuris),* and *Capillaria* has been demonstrated by protecting animals with immune cells from lymph nodes, spleen, and previously sensitized thymic lymphocytes.

Thus immune phenomena are associated with nematode infections, but the manifestations and modulation of the host responses are complicated by the biologic and functional complexity of the parasites. This complexity limits the effectiveness of helminth-induced antibodies and increases the helminth's chances of adaptation to immunologically induced changes in its environment (Ogilvie and Jones, 1973). Progress in the utilization of immunologic mechanisms for the control of nematode infections has been limited and may remain so, but continued research should provide additional approaches, such as the regulation of parasite reproduction.

SYSTEMATICS AND LABORATORY DIAGNOSIS. The Nematoda are broadly divided into two taxonomic classes depending upon whether or not they possess the ventrally and posteriorly located female sense organ, the phasmid. Nematodes that possess the phasmid belong to the class Phasmidia (Secernentea) and those without it belong to the class Aphasmidia (Adenophorea). Because the phasmid is not an easy structure to identify, other characteristics such as the structure of the pharynx and excretory system or the life history have often been utilized. The assignment of nematodes into the various orders varies from authority to authority and is of little practical use to the nonspecialist. For example, nematodes may be divided into 11, 16, or 18 orders depending upon the classification scheme adopted (Chabaud, 1974; Crofton, 1966; Maggenti, 1976). Nematodes parasitic in vertebrates and hence of potential medical significance are found in the following orders:

Phylum:	Nematoda (Cobb, 1919)
Class:	Phasmidia (Secernentea) (Dougherty, 1958)
1. Order:	Rhabditida (Chitwood, 1933)—e. g., *Strongyloides*
2. Order:	Ascaridida (Railliet and Henry, 1925)—e.g., *Ascaris, Enterobius, Toxocara, Anisakis, Toxoascaris*
3. Order:	Strongylida (Diesing, 1815)—e.g., *Ancylostoma, Necator, Syngamus, Oesophagostomum, Trichostrongylus, Angiostrongylus*
4. Order:	Spirurida (Chitwood, 1933)—e.g., *Wuchereria, Brugia, Loa, Onchocerca, Dracunculus, Dipetalonema, Mansonella, Dirofilaria, Gnathostoma, Habronema*
Class:	Adenophorea (Aphasmidia) (Chitwood, 1958)
5. Order:	Trichocephalida (Skryabin and Schultts, 1938)—e. g., *Trichocephalus (Trichuris), Trichinella, Dioctophyma, Capillaria*

The important and obligate parasites of man are summarized in Table 1. An outline of the life cycles with characteristics of diagnostic relevance is presented in Table 2, while an identification key generally based on the features of the life cycle, morphology, and anatomy is presented in Table 3. Table 4 and Figure 11 present aids for the identification of nematodes in tissue sections.

In addition to the adult characteristics indicated in Tables 1 through 4, three main methods are used to identify parasitic nematodes in the laboratory. These are (1) fecal examination for eggs or culture of feces for the infective larval stages; (2) examination of blood, tissue fluid, or skin snips for microfilariae; and (3) immunologic techniques.

Fecal Examination. The simplest method for the detection of helminth eggs in feces is direct examination under the microscope of about 5 mg of feces diluted with tap water or saline and smeared on a slide with a coverslip. Only heavy infections are usually detected by this method. The typical appearance of some of the more common nematode ova is shown in Figure 12.

Modifications of this simple method such as Kato's thick smear technique are also useful. In this method, about 50 mg of a fecal sample is placed on a microscope slide, and a 30 × 22 mm piece of cellophane soaked in a mixture of 100 ml of glycerine, 100 ml of water, and 1 ml of 3 per cent aqueous malachite green is placed over it. The specimen is pressed down and examined after 20 to 30 minutes at 37° C. The feces has cleared by this time, and the relatively uncleared eggs are seen in bolder relief.

Various methods for the estimation of the intensity of infection by egg counts have been developed. The best known is the Stoll dilution egg counting technique and the McMaster technique. These methods rely upon concentration techniques such as the formol-ether method or the zinc-sulfate centrifugal flotation technique (Muller, 1975). Unfortunately, efforts to relate the egg production of a female worm to the number of eggs recovered from feces have so far proved unreliable. For example, it is becoming increasingly clear that while the number of eggs laid by an individual female worm may vary from time to time and may also vary between individuals, the total egg output of a given worm population is fairly constant and is related to the nutritional status of the host (Michel, 1974). Thus, until we understand the biology of egg production in nematodes, predictions of population size from egg counts continue to be of doubtful validity.

The best known method for the differential diagnosis of nematode infections by culturing larvae in fecal matter is the Harada-Mori test tube and filter paper method (Muller, 1975). Larvae can be identified by the characteristics summarized in Table 5.

Examination of Blood, Tissue, or Skin Snips for Microfilariae. The easiest method for the diagnosis of the various filariae is to make a wet preparation from a drop of blood with a coverslip. Microfilariae can be easily detected moving under low-power magnification. Light infections are often missed by this method. However, diethylcarbamazine has improved the sensitivity of wet preparations immeasurably, especially in periodic filariasis. When this drug is administered, the microfilariae may be found with ease in

Table 1. SUMMARY OF OBLIGATE PARASITES OF MAN BELONGING TO THE NEMATODA

Phylum	Class	Order	Superfamily	Genus and Species
Nematoda	Phasmidia (Secernentea)	Rhabditida	Rhabditoidea	1. *Strongyloides stercoralis*
		Ascaridida	Ascaridoidea	2. *Ascaris lumbricoides*
			Oxyuroidea	3. *Enterobius vermicularis*
		Strongylida	Strongyloidea	4. *Ancylostoma duodenale*
				5. *Necator americanus*
				6. *Syngamus*[a] sp
			Trichostrongyloidea	7. *Trichostrongylus*[a] sp
				8. *Oesophagostomum*[a] sp
			Metastrongyloidea	9. *Angiostrongylus*[a] sp
		Spirurida	Spiruroidea	10. *Habronema*[a] sp
				11. *Gnathostoma spinigerum*
			Dracunculoidea	12. *Dracunculus medinensis*
			Filarioidea	13. *Brugia*[a] sp
				14. *Wuchereria bancrofti*
				15. *Dipetalonema perstans*
				16. *Onchocerca volvulus*
				17. *Dirofilaria immitis*
	Aphasmidia (Adenophorea)	Trichocephalida	Trichuroidea	18. *Trichocephalus* sp (*Trichuris*)
				19. *Capillaria philippinensis*
			Trichinelloidea	20. *Trichinella spiralis*
			Dioctophymoidea	21. *Dioctophyma*[a] *renale*

[a]Not obligate parasites of man but of other vertebrates; these have, however, been found often enough in man to deserve consideration as human parasites.

Table 2. SUMMARY OUTLINE OF NEMATODE LIFE CYCLES OF DIAGNOSTIC RELEVANCE

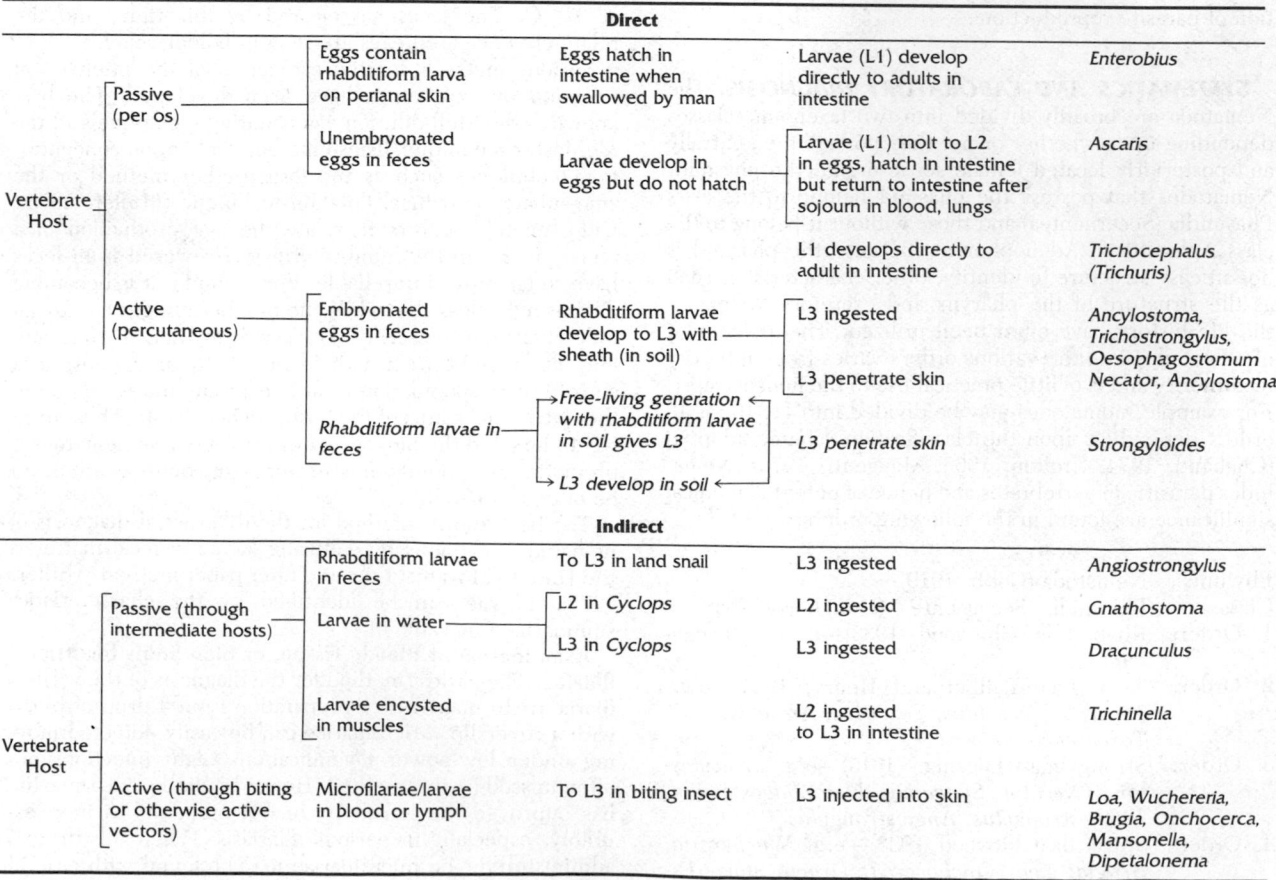

Direct					
Vertebrate Host	Passive (per os)	Eggs contain rhabditiform larva on perianal skin	Eggs hatch in intestine when swallowed by man	Larvae (L1) develop directly to adults in intestine	*Enterobius*
		Unembryonated eggs in feces	Larvae develop in eggs but do not hatch	Larvae (L1) molt to L2 in eggs, hatch in intestine but return to intestine after sojourn in blood, lungs	*Ascaris*
				L1 develops directly to adult in intestine	*Trichocephalus (Trichuris)*
	Active (percutaneous)	Embryonated eggs in feces	Rhabditiform larvae develop to L3 with sheath (in soil)	L3 ingested	*Ancylostoma, Trichostrongylus, Oesophagostomum*
				L3 penetrate skin	*Necator, Ancylostoma*
		Rhabditiform larvae in feces	*Free-living generation with rhabditiform larvae in soil gives L3* / *L3 develop in soil*	*L3 penetrate skin*	*Strongyloides*
Indirect					
Vertebrate Host	Passive (through intermediate hosts)	Rhabditiform larvae in feces	To L3 in land snail	L3 ingested	*Angiostrongylus*
		Larvae in water	L2 in *Cyclops*	L2 ingested	*Gnathostoma*
			L3 in *Cyclops*	L3 ingested	*Dracunculus*
		Larvae encysted in muscles		L2 ingested to L3 in intestine	*Trichinella*
	Active (through biting or otherwise active vectors)	Microfilariae/larvae in blood or lymph	To L3 in biting insect	L3 injected into skin	*Loa, Wuchereria, Brugia, Onchocerca, Mansonella, Dipetalonema*

Modified from Muller, 1975.

Table 3. KEY TO NEMATODES PARASITIC IN MAN

1.	Filiform anterior and spindle-shaped posterior; pharynx is either a stichosome that consists of a single row of cells with a centrally located fine tube or a long and narrow structure slightly dilated posteriorly; male with or without copulatory bursa	2
	Regular spindle-shaped, relatively stout or filiform worms with muscular pharynx that may be cylindrical or rhabditiform— i.e., having a posterior bulb that has a valvular apparatus	3
2.	Male has muscular copulatory bursa without supporting rays; pharynx is long and narrow, not a stichosome; vulva is located anteriorly	Trichocephalida (Dioctophymoidea) *Dioctophyma* sp
	Filiform anterior and spindle-shaped posteror; male without bursa; pharynx a stichosome; female vulva located at junction of anterior and posterior positions; eggs with characteristic opercular (polar) plug	Trichocephalida (Trichuroidea) *Trichocephalus (Trichuris) trichiura*
	Filiform anterior; male without bursa; pharynx a stichosome; female ovoviviparous with larvae in uterus	Trichocephalida (Trichinelloidea) *Trichinella spiralis*
3.	Relatively stout round worms with muscular pharynx; cylindrical or with valvular posterior bulb	4
	Filiform worms with cylindrical pharynx	5
4.	Relatively stout but small worms; muscular pharynx with valvular posterior bulb; male with genital papillae; female with pointed tail; eggs embryonated and slightly flattened on one side	Ascaridida (Oxyuroidea) *Enterobius vermicularis*
	Relatively stout large worms; mouth usually with three lips; muscular pharynx more or less cylindrical, not dilated posteriorly and without valvular apparatus	Ascaridida (Ascaridoidea) *Ascaris, Toxocara*
5.	Filiform worm with cylindrical pharynx; no parasitic males; parasitic female parthenogenetic; small buccal capsule without teeth; larvae always found alongside adult females	Rhabditida (Rhabditoidea) *Strongyloides stercoralis*
	Filiform worm with cylindrical pharynx that is muscular anteriorly and glandular posteriorly; not usually intestinal	6
	Filiform worm with cylindrical pharynx, muscular throughout its length; copulatory bursa in males with muscular rays	7
6.	Usually two lateral lips; cuticle of buccal capsule particularly toughened; vulva in middle of female body or posterior; characteristc and spiny head bulb; parasite of alimentary canal, respiratory system, or orbital, nasal, or oral cavity	Spirurida (Spiruroidea) *Gnathostoma* sp
	Usually without lips; no buccal capsule; vulva in region of pharynx; parasites of circulatory, lymphatic, or serous cavities, not intestinal; females not more than three times longer than males	Spirurida (Filarioidea) *Loa, Wuchereria, Onchocerca, Mansonella, Dipetalonema*
	Females much longer than males; atrophied vulva in gravid female	Spirurida (Dracunculoidea) *Dracunculus* sp
7.	Parasites of alimentary canal, very rarely found in kidney tissue	8
	Parasites of respiratory system	9
8.	Buccal capsule very feebly developed or absent; thread-like worms	Strongylida (Trichostrongyloidea) *Trichostrongylus* sp
	Buccal capsule well developed with ventral teeth; anterior end more or less straight	Strongylida (Ancylostomoidea) *Ancylostoma duodenale*
	Buccal capsule well-developed with cutting plates; anterior end characteristically recurved	Strongylida (Ancylostomoidea) *Necator americanus*
9.	Buccal capsule without teeth or cutting plates but mouth surrounded by characteristic leaf crown	Strongylida (Trichostrongyloidea) *Oesophagostomum* sp
10.	Well-developed, toughened, and cuticular buccal capsule; male often attached to female	Strongylida (Strongyloidea) *Syngamus laryngeus*
	Buccal capsule rudimentary or absent; filiform	Strongylida (Metastrongyloidea)

Table 4. IDENTIFICATION KEY FOR SECTIONS OF NEMATODES

1. A.	Hypodermal chords (few to many) arranged asymmetrically. Lateral excretory canals absent. In the ovaries and testes the germinal region extends the entire length of the gonad, and gametes at various stages of development can be found at any level. Esophagus nonmuscular.	Trichurids (*Trichinella, Trichocephalus [Trichuris] Capillaria)*
B.	Hypodermal chords (two to four) arranged symmetrically. Excretory canals in lateral chords except at extremities. In the ovaries and testes the germinal region is confined to the proximal extremity of the gonad, and gametes at uniform stage of development can be found at any one level.	2
2. A.	Intestine composed of a few large multinucleate cells, rarely with more than two cells in a cross-section. Anterior paired excretory gland cells present.	Strongylids (hookworms, *Trichostrongylus, Ternidens, Oesophagostomum)*
B.	Intestine composed of few to many, small, uninucleate cells; excretory glands single, paired, or absent	3
3. A.	Somatic muscle cells few, large and flat. Lateral alae present or absent.	4
B.	Many somatic muscle cells, U-shaped in cross-section. Lateral alae usually absent.	5
4. A.	Lateral alae present. Vagina long and muscular. Esophagus has posterior bulb. Many eggs in uterus. Excretory gland cells absent.	*Enterobius*
B.	Lateral alae absent. Vagina very short. Ova large. Viviparous, with eggs developing into larvae. Excretory cells single or paired. Very small and often larvae (or eggs) in tissues.	*Strongyloides*
5. A.	Somatic musculature divided by large lateral chords (often very wide and flattened) into two crescent-shaped folds.	6
B.	Somatic musculature divided into four fields	7
6. A.	Females often contain microfilariae and uterus double. Diameter less than 0.5 mm.	Filariids *(Wuchereria, Brugia, Dipetalonema, Dirofilaria, Onchorcerca, Loa)*
B.	Females contain larvae with long pointed tails, uterus single, diameter more than 1 mm.	*Dracunculus*
7. A.	Lateral chords very large and stalked and project into body cavity; frequently unequal in size.	Spirurids *(Thelazia, Gnathostoma)*
B.	Lateral chords large and project into body cavity but not stalked; usually equal in size.	Ascarids (Ascaris, *Toxocara, Toxoascaris, Anisakis)*

Table 5. THE DIFFERENTIATION OF INFECTIVE FILARIFORM LARVAE FOUND IN CULTURES FROM HUMAN FECAL SPECIMENS

	Strongyloides[a]	**Trichostrongylus**	**Ancylostoma**	**Necator**	**Ternidens**
Length (microns)	500	750	660	590	680 (630–730)
Sheath	Absent	Present	Sheath 720 microns, striations not clear	Sheath 660 microns, striations clear at tail end	Present
Length of esophagus as proportion of total body length	1:2	1:4	1:3	1:3	1:3
Intestine	Straight	Intestinal lumen zigzagged	Anterior end narrower in diameter than esophageal bulb. No gap between the esophagus and the intestine.	Anterior end as wide as the esophageal bulb. Gap between the esophagus and the intestine.	Following esophagus is a pair of sphincter cells. Intestinal lumen somewhat zigzagged.
Tail	Divided into three at the tip	End of tail knob-like	Blunt	Sharply pointed	Pointed
Head	—	—	Blunt	Rounded	—
Mouth	—	—	Mouth spears not very clear and parallel	Mouth spears clear and divergent	—

[a]Free-living adults and first-stage (rhabditiform) larvae likely to be present as well.

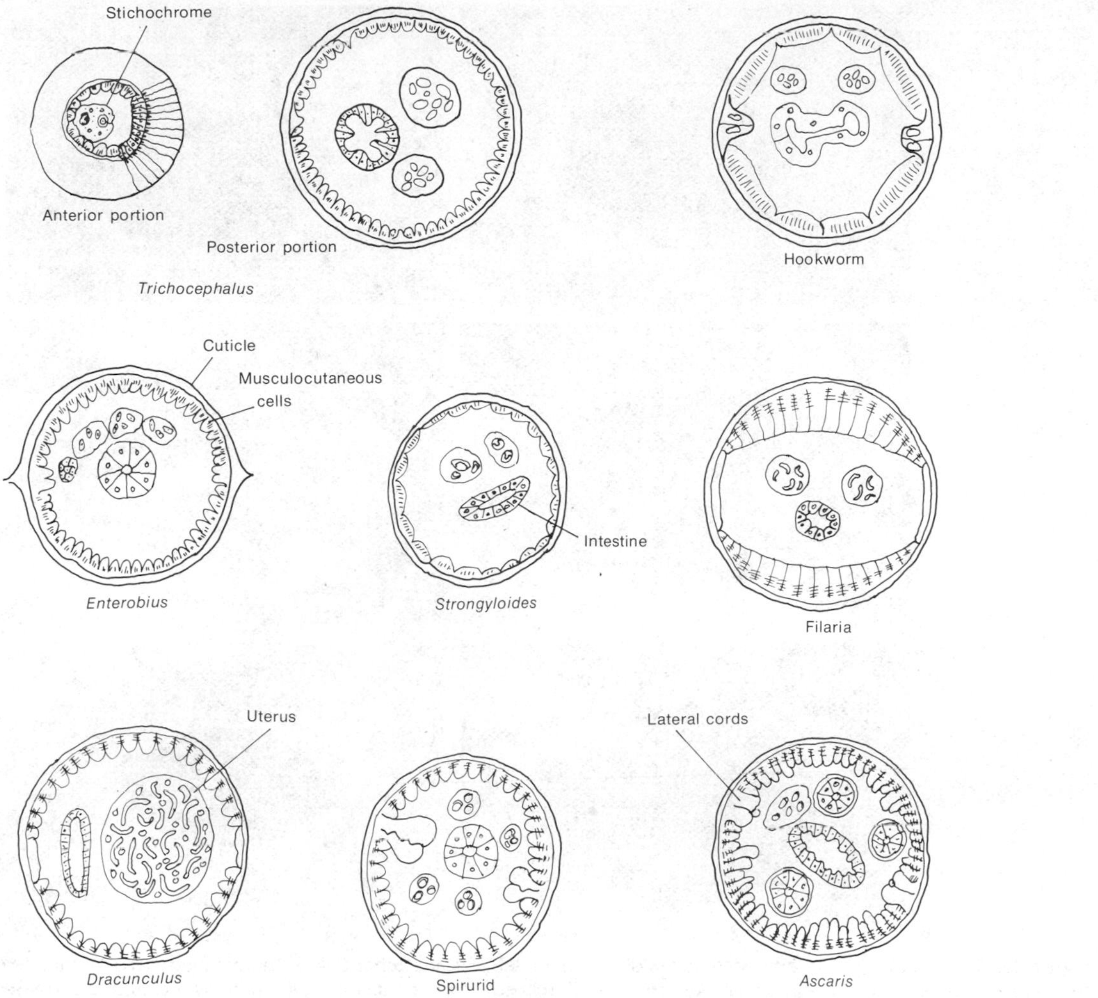

Figure 11. Transverse sections of females of various nematodes (from Muller, 1975; after Chitwood and Lichtenfels, 1972).

the peripheral and cutaneous circulation. When microfilariae are identified, thick blood smears should be stained with hematoxylin or Giemsa stain. Differential diagnosis of the various microfilariae such as *Onchocerca, Brugia, Loa, Dirofilaria, Wuchereria, Dipetalonema,* and *Mansonella* is then possible. Finally, membrane filtration techniques using nucleopore or millipore membrane filters (pore size 5 μm) fitted to hypodermic syringes with an adaptor have considerably improved diagnostic accuracy in filariasis.

In tropical Africa, the most important filarial nematode is *Onchocerca volvulus,* whose microfilariae are easily recognized by their larger size (270 to 320 μm long compared with *Dipetalonema* or *Mansonella*) and their characteristic head and pointed tail. The most common diagnostic procedure in *Onchocerca* infections is examination of skin snip biopsies for emerging larvae. Alternatively, dermal juices obtained after scarification of the skin can be examined after staining. This procedure may pick up not only *Onchocerca* but also *Dipetalonema* and even malarial parasites.

The best site for obtaining skin snips may depend upon the geographic strain of the parasite. Skin snips can be taken with a razor blade, sharp scissors, or a scleral punch such as the Holth model. The snips are then examined for living microfilariae in water or saline, with or without teasing. The number of emerging microfilariae is usually counted after 10 to 30 minutes. Examination of emerging larvae in water is preferred, especially under dry conditions, although emergence tends to take longer.

In large-scale epidemiologic surveys, reasonably good results can be obtained by placing individual snips in a drop or two of saline in wells of an agglutination tray. The microfilariae emerge over a 24-hour period and are then preserved in the wells by the addition of a drop of 10 per cent formol-saline. The trays are sealed with a transparent plastic sealer, and the preserved material can then be examined at leisure.

Immunodiagnostic Techniques. As emphasized earlier, an individual nematode is a complex population of cells and the source of a complex assortment of antigens. This fact is the source of the two main problems with immunodiagnostic detection of nematode infections. These problems are the lack of specific, well-characterized antigens (this introduces an element of uncertainty in diagnosis) and the high level of cross-reactivity that confuses many positive results. Except in such situations as visceral larva migrans, in which the absence of adult parasites precludes easy detection of the causative agent, parasitologic diagnosis is

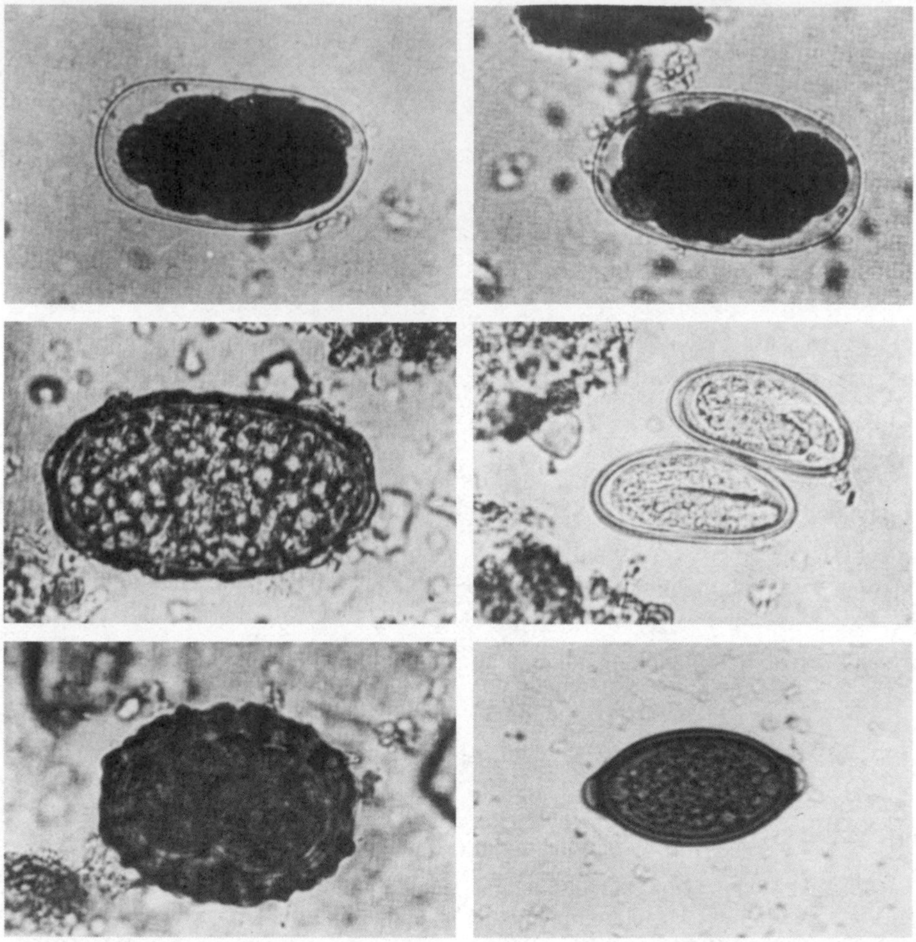

Figure 12. Top panels, *Nector americanus;* middle panel on left, *Ascaris lumbricoides* (unfertilized); middle panel on right, *Enterobius vermicularis;* lower panel on left, *Ascaris lumbricoides* (fertilized); lower panel on right, *Trichuris trichiura.* (From Spencer and Monroe, 1977.)

more reliable at the present time. Nevertheless, many standard immunologic techniques have been used with good, variable, or indifferent results.

Standard serologic procedures such as precipitation tests have been used for the detection of a wide variety of nematodes and other helminths. Serologic procedures have been useful in diagnosing hookworm and *Trichinella* infections, but success often depends on a continuing challenge of the immune system with living parasites. For example, in hookworm infections, there is a lack of correlation between immunologic reactions and the presence of eggs in the feces.

Complement fixation tests (CFT) have been used for the detection of many nematode infections but particularly for visceral larva migrans. Its reproducibility and sensitivity for some nematode infections are questioned, and anticomplementary activity in sera collected in field studies of onchocerciasis has been a problem (WHO, 1976).

The immunofluorescent antibody test (IFA) has gained wide support, especially for the diagnosis of onchocerciasis. Using frozen sections of the adult worm as antigen, up to 90 per cent of positive cases can be identified by this procedure. Titers of between 1:20 and 1:40 are considered significant. There is good correlation between this test and the results of skin biopsies in surveys of onchocerciasis.

The latest addition to the serologic diagnosis of helminth infections is the enzyme-linked immunosorbent assay (ELISA). This test utilizes the enzymes alkaline phosphatase or peroxidase, labeled with anti-immunoglobulin, in antigen-coated tubes or microtiter plates. This promising technique is as sensitive as the IFA test and is easier to perform.

Other serologic and immunologic diagnostic procedures have been attempted, but results have been so variable that no further consideration will be given to them here.

DRUG SUSCEPTIBILITY. The search for new and effective drugs against human helminthiasis has underscored the need for a greater understanding of the physiologic basis of anthelmintic action. An ideal anthelmintic should combine extreme toxicity against the parasite with complete inaction against the host tissue. Generally, action is directed against a target tissue or physiologic process whose special position in the overall physiology of the organism guarantees that if the target is rendered nonoperational, the parasite will die. With nematodes, four main targets have been identified: neuromuscular function, energy metabolism, lipoproteins, and hemoproteins. Effective anthelmintics presently in use affect one or the other of these targets.

Table 6 summarizes the anthelmintics of choice for the various human nematodes. The twelve anthelmintics listed represent the best of the newer drugs, many of which have come into use in the last decade or so. In addition to these twelve, diphetarsone (an arsenical), suramin (a urea derivative), and metriphonate (an organophosphorus compound) are also used, particularly for the treatment of filariasis. Of the older drugs, such as carbon tetrachloride and tetrachloroethylene, the latter is still used occasionally for the treatment of hookworms.

Of the newer drugs, the *piperazine* derivatives, piperazine adipate or citrate and diethylcarbamazine citrate, have been particularly popular for the treatment of ascariasis and filariasis, respectively. These drugs are anticholinergic and cause hyperpolarization of the neuromuscular junction. The parasite is expelled as a result of the consequent paralysis. *Thiabendazole* is an effective broad-spectrum anthelmintic that is active against *Ascaris, Strongyloides, Enterobius, Dracunculus, Trichinella,* and larva migrans, among others. It is an inhibitor of fumarate reductase, an important enzyme of energy metabolism in nematodes. *Tetramisole* and *Levamisole* among the newer drugs also act by selective enzyme inhibition. In this case, succinic dehydrogenase, which acts as a fumarate reductase in nematode mitochondria, is also inhibited (Davis, 1973). *Mebendazole,* one of the most useful newer anthelmintics, inhibits glucose and amino acid uptake of a wide variety of nematodes, including *Ascaris, Necator, Ancylostoma, Trichocephalus, Strongyloides, Enterobius, Trichinella,* and *Capillaria.*

Bephenium, which is often given as the hydroxynaphthoate, is active against hookworms, *Trichostrongylus,* and larva migrans. The mode of drug action is not well understood, but it is assumed to have a blocking action on the neuromuscular junction. It is more effective against mucosal than luminal helminths.

EPIDEMIOLOGY. Epidemiologic techniques may be expected to provide the basis for planning and evaluating preventive health care, defining the major patterns and distribution of parasitic disease, and describing and classifying these conditions. The determinants of the distribution and maintenance of human parasitic disease, especially in the tropics, have received scant attention. Ultimate control of the major nematodes such as the hookworms and filariae, however, depends on our understanding of these factors.

The maintenance of a parasitic population in a community depends upon a complex series of interrelated factors (including host behavior) that regulate the number of parasites within individuals as well as the population size of the community. These factors may determine the level and frequency of contact between individual members of the two populations and thus the incidence and intensity of infection. The life cycle of the parasite is important in these considerations because it indicates whether one or two hosts (as distinct populations) are involved, as well as whether one or more parasitic stages should be considered in the total epidemiologic situation. It is usual to express the dynamics of such a host-parasite system in a flow chart such as that indicated in Figure 13 for *Ascaris* and *Trichuris* (direct life cycle) and the hookworms (direct life cycle with a stage consisting of free-living organisms). Although these life cycles of *Ascaris* and *Trichuris* are fairly simple, they involve three distinct populations of organisms, namely, the host, the adult parasite, and the protected but free-living egg population. Any factor that changes the numbers of any of these populations will alter the infection rate and hence the epidemiologic parameters of the equilibrium between host and parasite. For the hookworm, four distinct populations are involved. In each population, such factors

Table 6. SUMMARY OF DRUGS OF CHOICE WITH NEMATODE PARASITES OF MAN

Nematode Species	1 Thiabendazole (Mintezol)	2 Mebendazole (Telmin)	3 Levamisole (Ketrax)	4 Piperazine Adipate (Antepar)	5 Bephenium Hydroxynaphthoate (Alcopar)	6 Pyrantel Embonate (Combantrin)	7 Pyrvinium Embonate (Vanquin)	8 Dichlorvos	9 Bitoscanate	10 Diethylcarbamazine (Hetrazan)	11 Dithiazanine Iodide
Ascaris lumbricoides		++++	++++	++++		++++					++
Trichocephalus (Trichuris trichiura)	++	+++						++			++
Ancylostoma duodenale		+++			+++	++					
Necator americanus		+++				+++					
Strongyloides stercoralis	++++	++					++				+++
Enterobius vermicularis	+++	+++		+++		++++					++
Trichostrongylus	+++				+++	+++					
Larva migrans	++	++			++				+		
Dracunculus	++									+++(mf)	
Trichinella	++	+++									+
Wuchereria (mf)										+++	
Brugia (mf)										+++	
Onchocerca (mf)										+++	
Loa										++	

Also diphetarson, suramin, metriphonate.

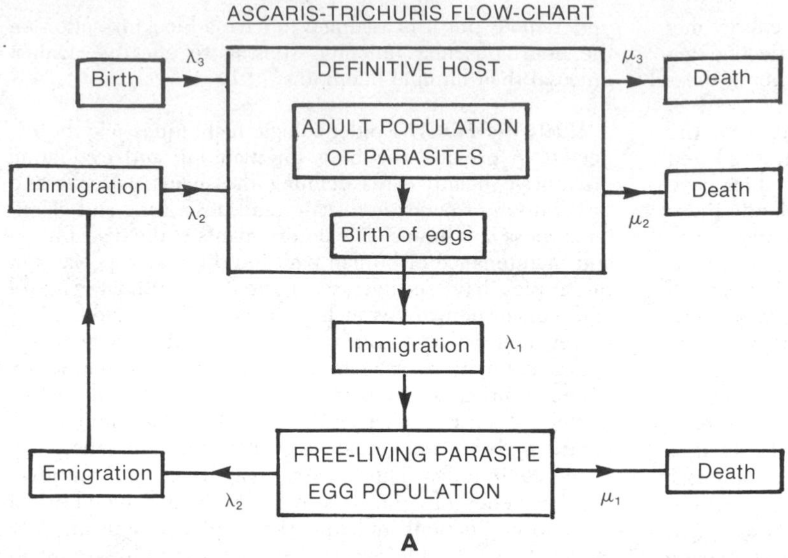

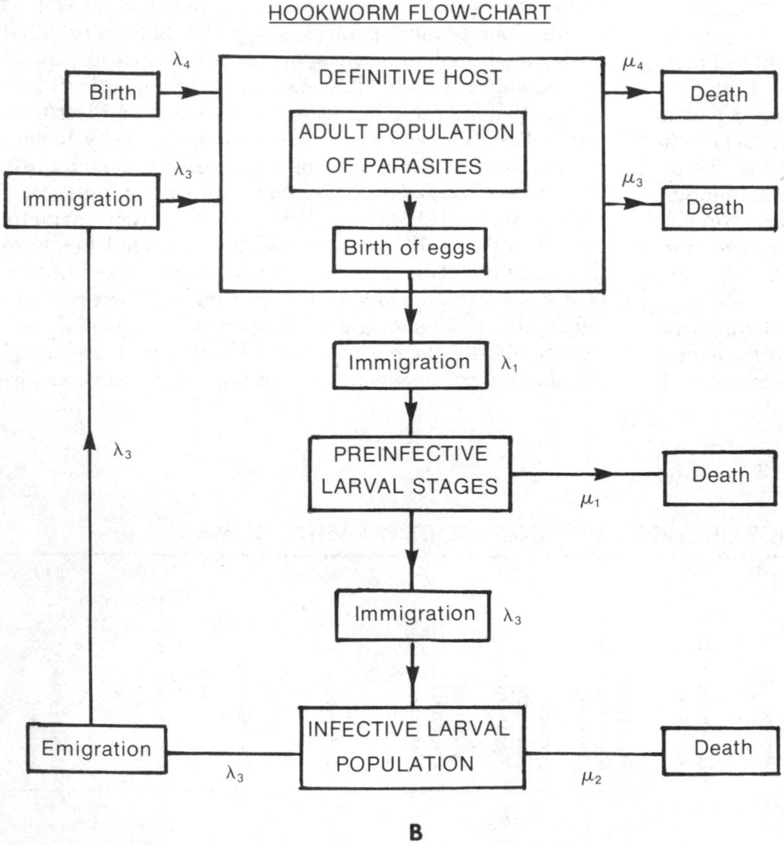

Figure 13. Diagrammatic representation (as a flow-chart) of the direct life cycle of *Ascaris/Trichuris (A)* and the Hookworm *(B)*. The population (rate) parameters indicated in the charts determine the flow of parasites through the system and are defined as rates per parasite per unit of time (based on Anderson, 1976).

as age, physiology, and ecology will determine population size, contact between the populations, and, ultimately, the infection pressure (Udonsi, 1980). In recent years, the introduction of mathematical models in the analysis of host-parasite systems has increased our understanding of the epidemiologic characteristics of some parasitic diseases (Bradley, 1974; Anderson, 1976).

In our laboratories in Nsukka, this approach has been used in an epidemiologic study of parasitic infections, particularly hookworms. As can be seen from Figure 14, which represents a study of a defined rural community, a small proportion of the population (the 5- to 20-year-olds, 19.5 per cent of the population) harbors a major proportion of the community worm burden. A notable seasonality in the pattern of these hookworm infections has been observed (Nwosu and Anya, 1980). This has given rise to the concept of a target time/target population approach to the control of these helminths. The basic idea is to concentrate mass chemotherapy efforts on that segment of the population with the preponderance of the worm burden during those months that are unfavorable to transmission of the parasites. Thus, the worm population would be depressed below the

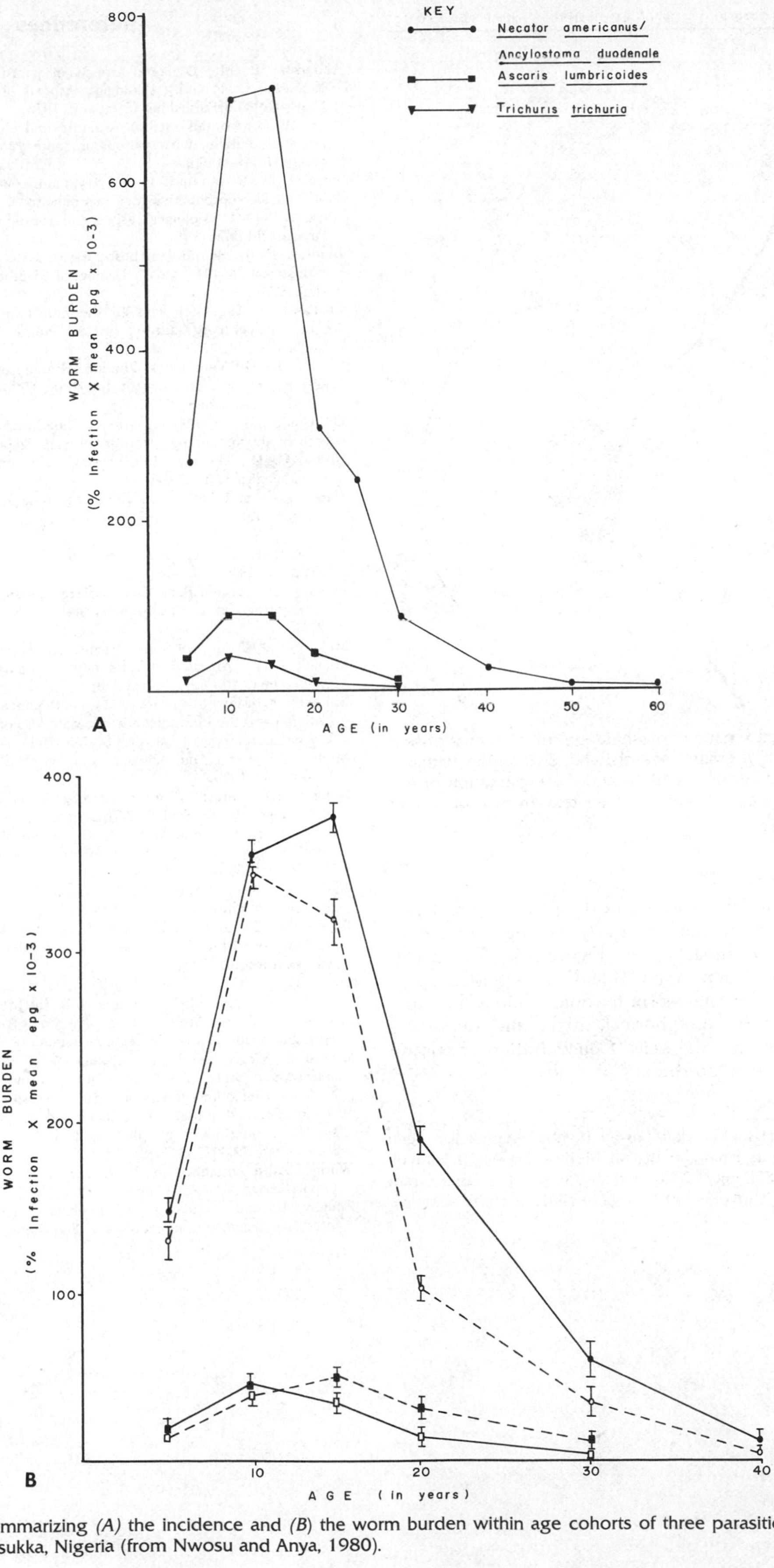

Figure 14. Graphs summarizing *(A)* the incidence and *(B)* the worm burden within age cohorts of three parasitic nematodes in a rural community in Nsukka, Nigeria (from Nwosu and Anya, 1980).

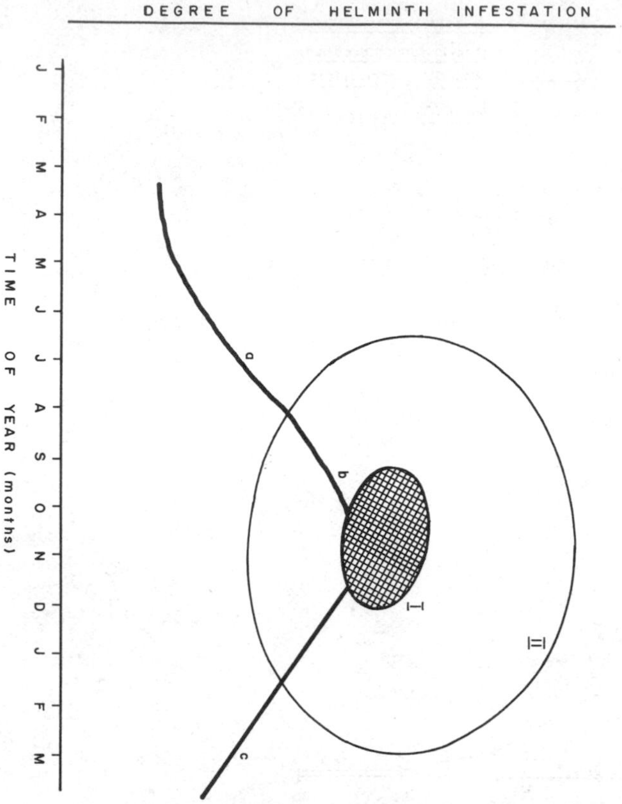

Figure 15. Diagrammatic representation of the relationship between infection pressure, season, and distribution within a community of nematode infections and the exploitation of this relationship in control procedures (see text–from Nwosu and Anya, 1980).

threshold level for maintenance of the parasite population (within the host population) at a fraction of the normal cost. The concept is summarized in Figure 15. The circles represent the total population (I) and the segmental population (II) with the high worm burden, while a, b, and c represent the periods of normal, high, and depressed infection rates during the year. Concentration of control efforts on II and c is the strategy of choice.

Some of the original work reported in this chapter has been supported by grants from the British Medical Research Council (ODM Research Scheme R2836) and the Senate Research Grant Committee of the University of Nigeria to whom grateful acknowledgment is made.

References

Anderson, R. M.: Dynamic aspects of parasite population ecology. In Kennedy, C. R. (ed.): Ecological Aspects of Parasitology. Amsterdam, North-Holland Publishing Company, 1976.

Anya, A. O.: Studies on the structure and chemical composition of the nematode cuticle. Observations on some oxyuroids and *Ascaris*. Parasitology 56:179, 1966.

Anya, A. O.: Serotonin (5-hydroxytryptamine) and other indolealkylamines in the male reproductive tract of a nematode. Int J Parasitol 3:573, 1973.

Anya, A. O.: Physiological aspects of reproduction in nematodes. Adv Parasitol 14:267, 1976.

Bradley, D. J.: Stability in host-parasite systems. In Usher, M. B., and Williamson, M. H., (eds.): Ecological Stability. London, Chapman and Hall, 1974.

Chabaud, A. G.: CIH keys to the nematode parasites of vertebrates. Commonwealth Agricultural Bureau, No. 1. Slough, Buckinghamshire, England, 1974.

Crofton, H. D.: Nematodes. London, Hutchinson, 1966.

Davis, A.: Drug Treatment in Intestinal Helminthiasis. Geneva, World Health Organization, 1973.

De Conick, L.: De symmetrie—verhoudingen aan het vooreinde der vrijlevende Nematoden. Natuurwetench. Tijdschr (Ghent) 24:29, 1942.

Green, C. D.: The attraction of male cyst nematodes by their females. Nematologica 13:172, 1967.

Harris, J. E., and Crofton, H. D.: Structure and function in the nematodes: Internal pressure and cuticular structure in *Ascaris*. J Exp Biol 34:116, 1957.

Hyman, L. H.: The Invertebrates, Vol. 3. New York, McGraw-Hill Book Company, 1951.

Larsh, J. E., Jr., and Race, G. J.: Allergic inflammation as a hypothesis for the expulsion of worms from tissues: A review. Exp Parasitol 37:251, 1975.

McLaren, D.: Nematode sense organs. Adv Parasitol 14:195, 1976.

Michel, J. F.: Arrested development of nematodes and some related phenomena. Adv Parasitol 12:279, 1974.

Miller, T. A.: Effect of x-irradiation upon the infective larvae of *Ancylostoma caninum* and the immunogenic effect in dogs of a single infection with 40 kr-irradiated larvae. J Parasitol 50:735, 1964.

Muller, R.: Worms and Disease. London, William Heinemann Medical Books Ltd., 1975.

Nigon, V.: Le determinisme du sex et la pseudogamie chez un nematode parthenogenetique. Bull Biol Fr Belg 81:1947.

Nwosu, A. B. C., and Anya, A. O.: Seasonality in human hookworm infection in an endemic area of Nigeria, and its relationship to rainfall. Tropenmed Parasit 31:(1980).

Ogilvie, B. M., and Jones, V. E.: Immunity in the parasitic relationship between helminths and hosts. Prog Allergy 17:93, 1973.

Rogers, W. P., and Sommerville, R. I.: The infectious process and its relationship to the development of early parasitic stages of nematodes. Adv Parasitol 6:327, 1968.

Selby, G. R., and Wakelin, D.: Transfer of immunity against *Trichuris muris* in the mouse by serum and cells. Int J Parasitol 3:717, 1973.

Spencer, F. M., and Monroe, L. S.: The Color Atlas of Intestinal Parasites. Springfield, Ill., USA, Charles C. Thomas, 1977.

Udonsi, J. K.: Studies on the ecology of the infective larvae of *Necator americanus* (Stiles, 1902) in relation to the epidemiology of human hookworm infections. Ph.D. Thesis, University of Nigeria, 1980.

Wakelin, D., and Lloyd, M.: Accelerated expulsion of adult *Trichinella spiralis* in mice given lymphoid cells and serum from infected donors. Parasitology 72:307, 1976.

World Health Organization: Epidemiology of Onchocerciasis. Technical Report Series No. 597. Geneva, 1976.

Zmoray, I., and Guttekova, A.: Ecological aspect of the study of the intestinal structure of nematodes. Z Parasitenk 39:127, 1972.

86

PLATYHELMINTHES

ZBIGNIEW S. PAWLOWSKI, M.D.

Some of the platyhelminthes (flat worms) are free-living animals (for example, Turbellaria), but most are exclusively parasitic and belong to the classes Trematoda (flukes) and Cestoda (tapeworms). Only a few of the Trematoda and Cestoda are parasites of man (Tables 1 and 6); the others are parasites of other vertebrates.

Trematoda (Fluke Worms)

The trematodes parasitizing man can be classified according to morphologic criteria, localization in the human host, and specificity for the human host (Table 1).

Trematodes are usually classified by their anatomic location, because each family largely localizes in a certain anatomic site of the body; for example: (1) blood flukes—family Schistosomatidae; (2) liver flukes—family Opisthorchiidae and Dicrocoeliidae, Fasciolidae, except Fasciolopsis; (3) intestinal flukes—Fasciolopsis and family Heterophyidae, Echinostomatidae; and (4) lung flukes—family Troglotrematidae.

The host-specificity of trematodes correlates well with their prevalence and medical importance. For example, there are four different degrees of specificity for man among the Schistosoma: (1) man is the main definitive host of *Schistosoma haematobium*, *Schistosoma intercalatum*, and *Schistosoma mansoni;* (2) man shares *Schistosoma japonicum* with a wide range of mammals; (3) man is only an occasional definitive host of *Schistosoma matthei* and *Schistosoma rhodhaini;* and (4) man can be invaded by other trematodes, such as Gigantobilharzia and Trichobilharzia, which cannot complete their development in man and can cause only skin lesions. The trematodes of groups 1 and 2 are of greater medical importance than the occasional or atypical parasites of groups 3 and 4 (Table 1).

MORPHOLOGY AND LIFE CYCLES

Blood Flukes—Schistosomatidae. Schistosomatidae are exceptional among trematodes in that they are dioecious (sexes separated). The female worm has a cylindric body and the male a canoe-shaped body with a gynecophoral canal in which the adult female spends most of her time. The main species of the schistosomes of man are morphologically distinct (Figs. 1 and 4).

The life cycle of *S. haematobium* is shown in Table 2. *S. mansoni* requires a shorter time of development in the snail (four to five weeks) and in man (25 to 28 days) before first egg production. *S. japonicum* has a shorter time of development in man, but a longer one in the snail (over seven weeks). It also produces many more eggs (3500 per day per female). *S. intercalatum* and *S. mekongi* have been newly recognized as the separate species.

Liver Flukes. *Clonorchis (Opisthorchis) sinensis, Opisthorchis felineus,* and *Opisthorchis viverrini* are common liver flukes (Komiya, 1966). All have a flat lanceolate body between 10 and 20 mm in length. The testes of *Opisthorchis* spp. are lobed, whereas those of *C. sinensis* are in a dendritic arrangement. The differences between *O. felineus* and *O. viverrini* are biologic rather than morphologic.

The life cycles of *C. sinensis*, *O. felineus*, and *O. viverrini*

Table 1. TREMATODES PARASITIZING MAN: HABITAT AND HOSTS

Species	Habitat in Man	Definitive Hosts Other Than Man	Snails as First Intermediate Hosts	Other Intermediate Hosts (or Plants Involved in Transmission)
Schistosoma haematobium	Vesical and pelvic venous plexuses	—	*Bulinus*	—
S. intercalatum	Mesenteric veins	—	*Bulinus*	—
S. mansoni	Mesenteric veins	Baboon, rodents	*Biomphalaria*	—
S. japonicum	Mesenteric veins	Many domesticated and wild animals	*Oncomelania*	—
Clonorchis (Opisthorchis) *sinensis*	Bile ducts	Dog, cat, pig	*Bulinus, Paraphossalurus*	Cyprinid fishes
Opisthorchis felineus	Bile ducts	Cat, dog, pig, fox	*Bithynia*	Cyprinid fishes
Opisthorchis viverrini	Bile ducts	Civet cat	*Bithynia*	Cyprinid fishes
Fasciola hepatica, Fasciola gigantica	Bile ducts	Sheep and other herbivores	*Lymnaea*	Watercress and grass
Fasciolopsis buski	Small intestine	Pig	*Segmentina, Planorbis*	Water caltrop and water chestnut
Heterophyes heterophyes	Small intestine	Dog, cat, fish-eating wild carnivores	*Pirenella, Cerithidia*	Mullet and tilapia fishes
Metagonimus yokogawai	Small intestine	Dog, cat, pig, fish-eating birds	*Semisulcospira*	Different fresh water fishes
Gastrodiscoides hominis	Coecum, colon	Pig	*Helicorbis*	Water caltrop
Paragonimus westermani	Lungs	Cat, tiger, leopard, dog, pig, monkey	*Semisulcospira, Thiara, Oncomelania*	Fresh water crabs and crayfish

Table 2. SCHISTOSOMA HAEMATOBIUM: LIFE CYCLE

Host and Habitat	Time	Stage and Activity	Number
Man	2–25 years	EGGS fully embryonated expelled in urine (and feces)	20–260 per worm per day
Water	16–32 hrs	MIRACIDIUM hatches in water and penetrates snail	1
Snails *Bulinus* spp.	5–6 weeks	PRIMARY SPOROCYST produces SECONDARY SPOROCYSTS, which produce CERCARIAE, which leave the snail host for months	1 n n^m = ca 250,000
Water	Up to 8 hrs	cercaria swimming in water and penetrating skin	1
Man lungs, liver, venous plexuses	6–12 weeks	preadult SCHISTOSOMULA migrating and developing in lungs and liver into ADULT worm situated finally in pelvic and vesical venous plexuses and producing eggs	1 1

are similar, but the snail and fish hosts and the geographic distribution differ (Tables 1 and 3, Figs. 2 and 3).

Dicrocoelium dendriticum, an unusual parasite of man, completes its strange life cycle on the ground by using terrestrial snails and ants as hosts. *Fasciola hepatica* is not uncommon in some countries (France, Algeria, Peru, and Cuba). It has a life cycle similar to that of Fasciolopsis (see below), but encysts on watercress, lettuce, and radishes.

Intestinal Flukes. The most important intestinal fluke is *Fasciolopsis buski,* the largest fluke of man (up to 70 mm long and 20 mm wide). It has no second intermediate host (Table 4, Figs. 2 and 3).

The remaining intestinal flukes (*Heterophyes, Metagonimus,* and *Echinostoma*) are small parasites, 2 to 8 mm long. Fish are the second intermediate hosts (Table 1, Figs. 2 and 3).

Lung Flukes. *Paragonimus westermani* is the common representative of the family of Troglotrematidae (Yokogawa, 1965). Unlike other trematodes, it has an oval, thick body with a ventral sucker in the middle. Its life cycle includes two intermediate hosts (Table 5, Figs. 2 and 3).

IMMUNOLOGY. Natural resistance to trematodes depends on many biochemical, physiologic, genetic, and nutritional factors, and is low in man. Acquired immunity against trematodes rarely prevents infection but can limit its intensity. For example, new invading schistosomulae are rapidly destroyed by hosts who are already infected with adult worms. However, seven days after infection, preadult schistosomulae are no longer recognized by the host as foreign, probably owing to the incorporation of host antigens or continuous turnover of the surface membrane. Living adult worms are usually not attacked by immunologic reactions but provoke a reaginic (IgE) response, releasing pharmacologic mediators of anaphylaxis. These hypersensitivity reactions are stage-specific and are intensive against eggs and cercariae. For example, schistosome eggs swept back from the mesenteric veins into the liver cause antibody-mediated reactions (Hoeppli phenomenon) first, and then a cell-mediated delayed hypersensitivity reaction producing eosinophilic granulomas. The skin reaction against penetrating cercariae is also of the cell-mediated type. Antigen-antibody complex diseases occur in schistosomiasis as glomerulonephritis (*S. mansoni*) or Katayama syndrome (*S. japonicum*), which resembles serum sickness with gastroenteritis.

There is no immunization against trematode infection. It is possible, however, that infection or immunization with some less pathogenic, but highly immunogenic, animal schistosomes might partially protect man against human schistosomes.

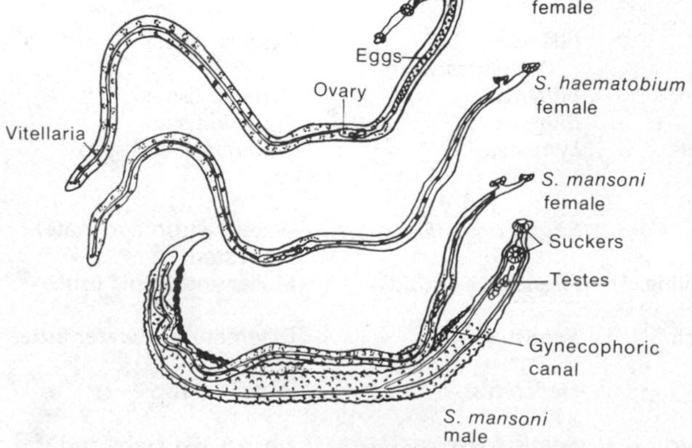

Figure 1. Adult schistosomes. Diagram of morphologic characteristics.

LABORATORY DIAGNOSIS. The symptoms or signs of human infections with trematodes are rarely pathognomonic. Therefore, the diagnosis is usually made by finding the eggs (Fig. 4) of the trematode in feces (most species), urine (*S. haematobium*), duodenal contents (*Clonorchis, Opisthorchis, Fasciola*), liver and rectal biopsies (*Schistosoma*), or sputum (*Paragonimus*). The flotation coprologic techniques are less effective than sedimentation or thick smear because the eggs are relatively heavy. Before eggs are produced it is difficult to make the diagnosis. The intradermal test, as well as the complement fixation, indirect hemagglutination, indirect fluorescent antibody, and precipitin tests, is of limited help in the early stages of infection with *Schistosoma, Clonorchis, Opisthorchis,* and *Paragonimus.*

DRUG SUSCEPTIBILITY. Intestinal flukes are susceptible to many anthelminthics including praziquantel. Liver,

TABLE 3. CLONORCHIS (OPISTHORCHIS) SINENSIS: LIFE CYCLE

Host and Habitat	Time	Stage and Activity	Number
Man, dog, cat, pig	Up to 20–30 years	EGGS fully embryonated in bile and feces	1000 per worm per day
Water	Up to 3 months	Eggs survive in water	
Snail *Bulimus* spp. *Parafossalurus* spp. *Semisulcospira* spp.	 3–4 weeks	MIRACIDIUM hatches from egg ingested by snail SPOROCYST procudes REDIAE, which produce CERCARIAE; these actively leave snail-host for months	1 1 n n^m
Water	1–2 days	cercaria, free-swimming, penetrating second intermediate host	1
Cyprinid fish	3 weeks	METACERCARIA encysts in tissue and survives for many months	1
Man, dog, cat, pig	3–4 weeks	Metacercaria excysts in duodenum and PREDADULT migrates through ampulla of Vater to bile ducts and develops into an ADULT worm, producing eggs	1 1

Table 4. FASCIOLOPSIS BUSKI: LIFE CYCLE

Host and Habitat	Time	Stage and Activity	Number
Man, pig	6 months	EGGS undeveloped, expelled in feces	21,200–28,000 per worm per day
Water	3–7 weeks Few hours	egg embryonates in water and hatches as MIRACIDIUM which penetrates snail	1 1
Snail *Segmentina* spp. *Planorbis* spp.	Few weeks	SPOROCYST produces REDIAE of first generation, which produce REDIAE of second generation; these produce CERCARIAE, which actively leave snail	1 n n^m $(n^m)^p$
Water (Water chestnut) (Water caltrop)	Several months	cercaria shortly encysts on water vegetation and becomes METACERCARIA, which survives several months	1 1
Man, pig	3–4 months	Metacercaria excysts in duodenum and PREADULT developes into an ADULT worm	1 1

Table 5. PARAGONIMUS WESTERMANI: LIFE CYCLE

Host and Habitat	Time	Stage and Activity	Number
Man, various mammals	6–20 years	EGGS expelled in sputum or feces	?
Water	3 weeks	egg develops into MIRACIDIUM, which hatches in water and penetrates snail in 24 hrs.	1 1
Snail *Semisulcospira* spp. *Thira* spp. *Oncomelania* spp.	3 months	SPOROCYST in snail tissue produces REDIAE I generation, which emerges as REDIAE II generation; Rediae II produce CERCARIAE, which actively leave snail	1 n n^m $(n^m)^p$
Water	24–48 hrs	cercaria, free-swimming and penetrating crabs	1
Crabs	Several months	METACERCARIA encysted in crab tissue	1
Man	 20 days 5–6 weeks	Ingested by definitive host; hatches in duodenum, as PREADULT migrates through gut wall, abdominal and pleural cavities, and lung tissue ADULT, produces eggs in lung cysts	 1 1

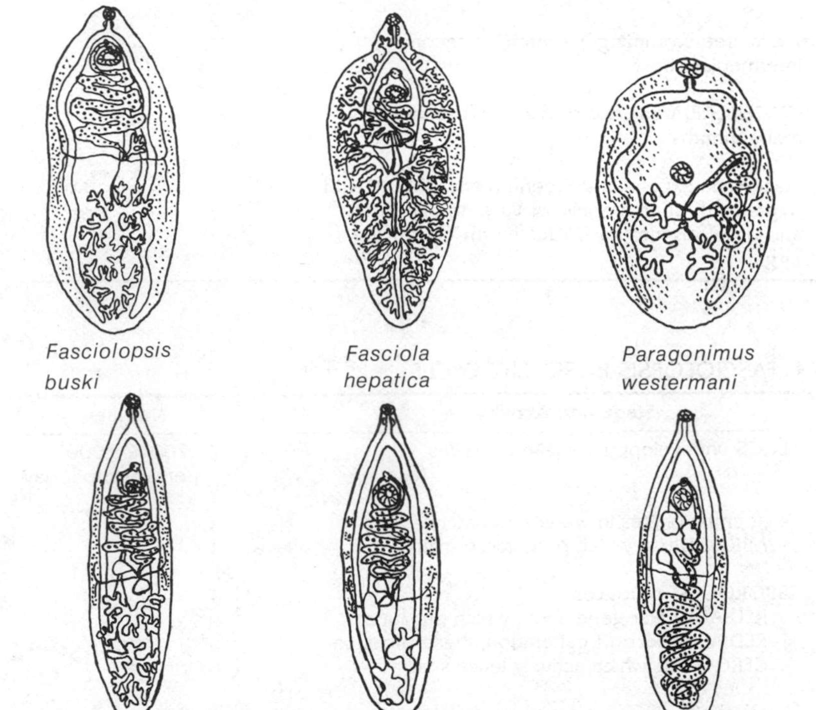

Figure 2. Adult trematodes (except the schistosomes). Diagram of morphologic characteristics.

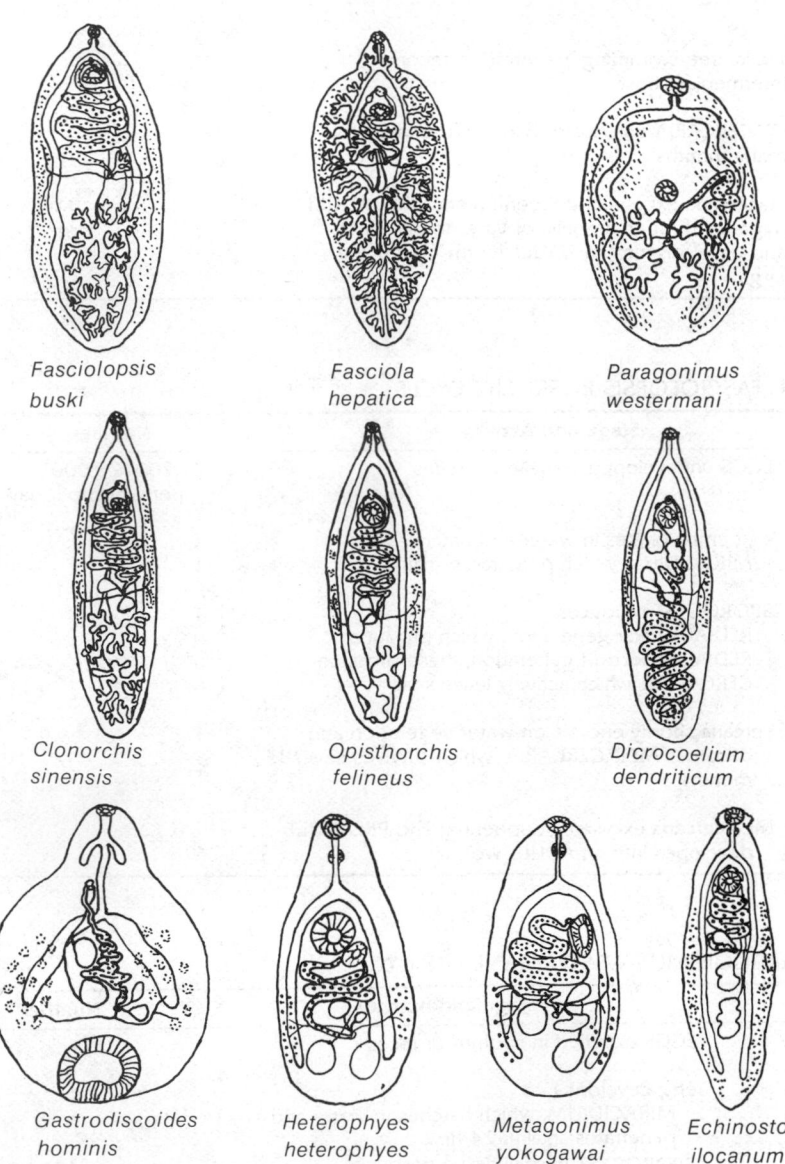

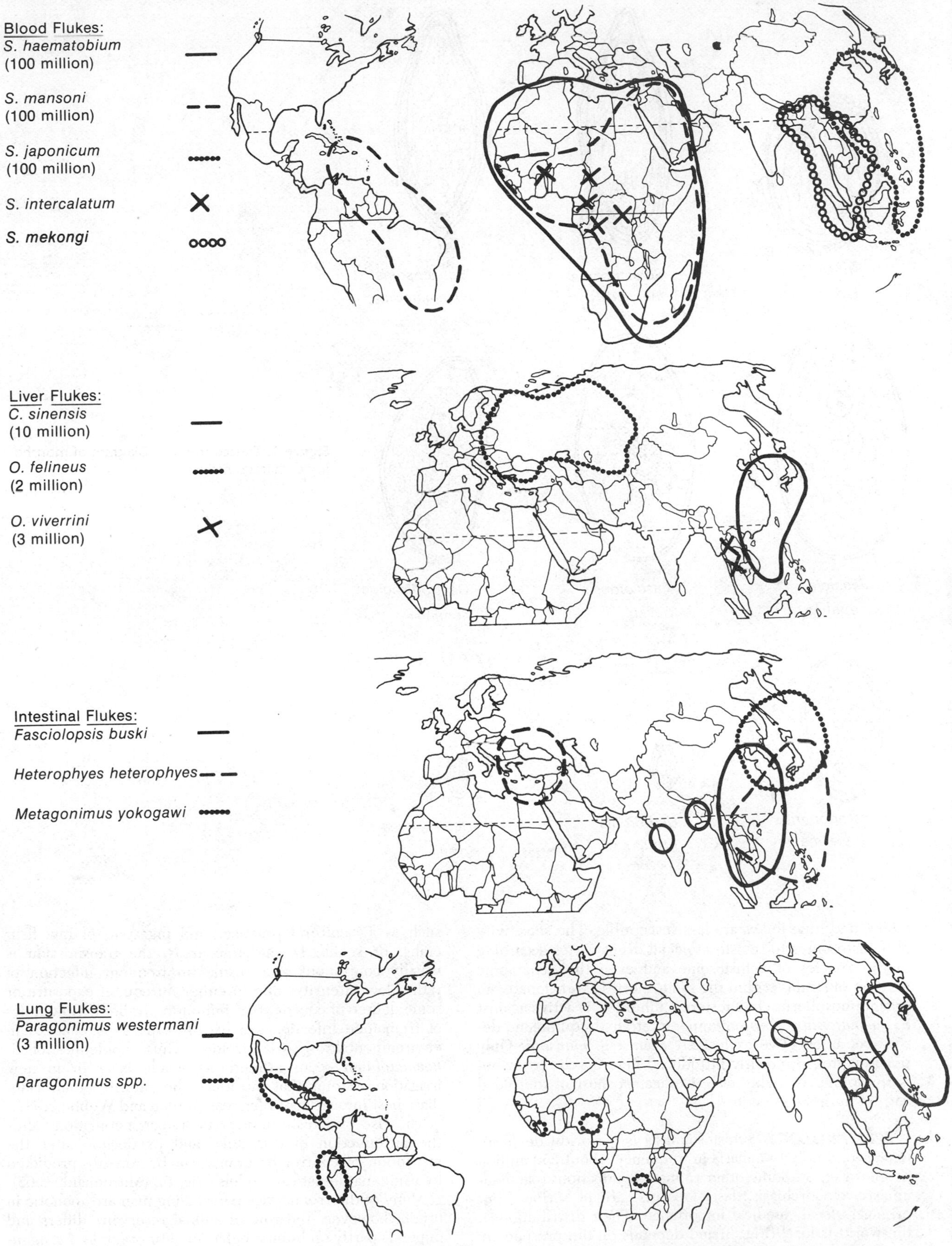

Figure 3. Geographic distribution of flukes.

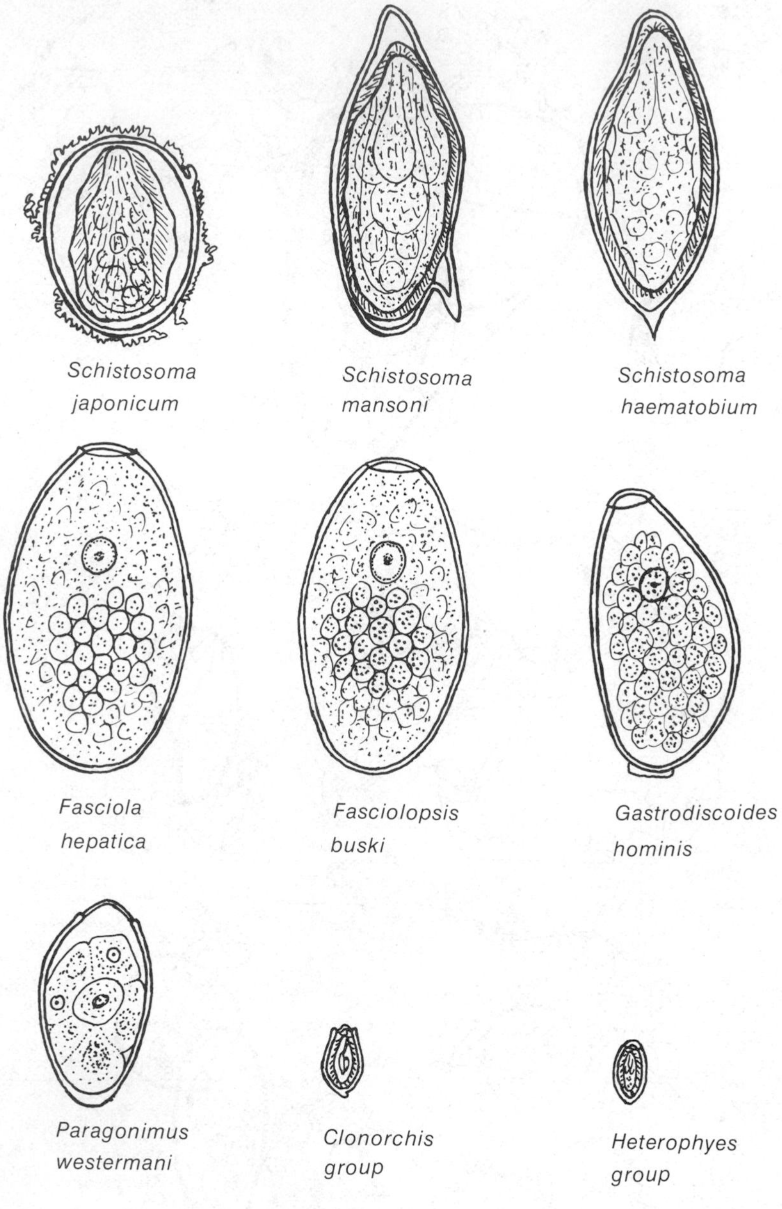

Figure 4. Trematode ova. Diagram of morphologic characteristics.

blood, and lung flukes are less susceptible. The sensitivity of Schistosomes to schistosomicidal drugs varies according to the species of Schistosome and even the geographic location of strains within the same species. Metrifonate, an organophosphorus cholinesterase inhibitor, is active against *S. haematobium.* Oxamniquine, a tetrahydroquinolene derivative, is effective exclusively against *S. mansoni.* Only praziquantel, a recently introduced heterocyclic pyrazinoisoquinoline, is highly effective against most of the blood and tissue fluke infections.

EPIDEMIOLOGY. Schistosomiasis is a worldwide problem second only to malaria in frequency (about 250 million people; Fig. 3). Some other trematode infections (paragonimiasis, clonorchiasis, fasciolopsiasis) are of serious, but primarily local, medical importance. Their distribution in the world is focal (Fig. 3) and depends on the presence of a suitable species of snail and certain local behavior factors, such as agricultural practices and ingestion of raw fish, crabs, or snails. In endemic areas, the transmission is usually continuous and results in frequent infection of rather low intensity, due to either infrequent exposure or some degree of concomitant immunity, or both. Epidemics of trematode infection are usually caused by changes in environmental or social factors. Thus, epidemics of *S. haematobium* occur around man-made lakes or in new irrigation systems that introduce the parasite or intermediate host into susceptible areas (Jordan and Webbe, 1982).

The rise of schistosomiasis in human populations after the introduction of this fluke and its decline after the institution of control programs can be roughly predicted by using mathematical models (Fig. 5), (Macdonald, 1965).

Many of the trematodes parasitizing man are zoonotic in origin; however, the role of animal reservoirs differs and depends partly on human behavior. For example, *Paragonimus africanus* is a zoonotic infection in Nigeria and Ca-

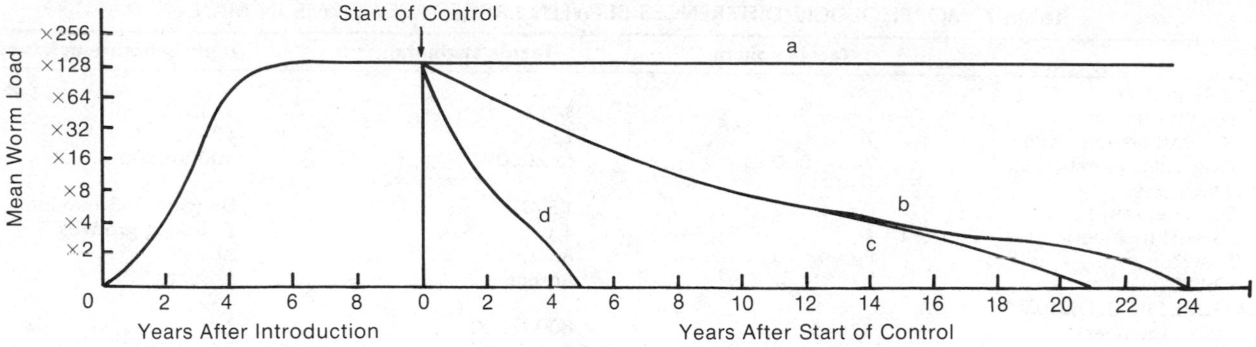

Figure 5. Diagram of the rise and fall of the mean load of schistosomes in human populations as predicted by the mathematical model of Macdonald (1965). *a* = reduction of water contamination to 1/15 of the original by improvement of sanitation; *b* = reduction of snail population to 1/15 original; *C* = reduction of exposure to water to 1/5 by public education; *d* = reduction of longevity of worms to 1/15 by chemotherapy plus reducing *b* and *c* to 1/3 of their original values.

meroon, whereas the transmission of *P. westermani* in China, Japan, and Korea is probably independent of animals. In Indonesia, Malaysia, and Ceylon, the infections occur exclusively in animals.

Community control measures require education about transmission, sanitary disposal of feces and urine, and installation of safe water supplies. Mass-control programs are based primarily on improved irrigation and agricultural practices, on using molluscicides, and on mass treatment of infected people (schistosomiasis).

Personal protection is enhanced by using cercarial repellents; avoiding contaminated water for bathing, washing, and drinking (schistosomiasis); cooking fish, crabs, and crayfish (clonorchiasis, opisthorchiasis, heterophyiasis, paragonimiasis); and immersing water plants in boiling water before ingestion (fasciolopsiasis).

Cestoda (Tapeworms)

Tapeworms parasitizing man belong to the order Cyclophyllidea (families Taeniidae and Hymenolepididae) and Pseudophyllidea (*Diphyllobothrium* spp. and *Spirometra* spp.). All the adult tapeworms are intestinal parasites of their definitive vertebrate host; some are human tissue parasites in their larval stage (Table 6).

For some tapeworms (*T. saginata, T. solium*) man is the only definitive host. For a few species (*Diphyllobothrium* spp.) man is one of many vertebrate definitive hosts. For a larger number, man is an occasional definitive or an intermediate host (Pawlowski and Schultz, 1972) (Table 6).

MORPHOLOGY AND LIFE CYCLE. There are three large (4 to 15 m) tapeworms parasitizing man: *Taenia solium, T.*

Table 6. CESTODES PARASITIZING MAN: HOSTS, HABITAT, AND DISTRIBUTION

Taxonomic Classification	Habitat in Man: *Adult Worm*	Habitat in Man: *Larval Stage*	Definitive Hosts Other Than Man	Intermediate Hosts	World Distribution
Order Cyclophyllidea*					
Taeniidae					
Taenia saginata	Small intestine (jejunum)	No	No	Cattle and other Boviidae	Cosmopolitan
Taenia solium	Small intestine (jejunum)	CYSTICERCUS in muscle and internal organs (brain, eye)	No	Pig, man, and many other mammals	Central and South America, Mexico, South Africa, India, Southeast Asia, USSR
Taenia multiceps	—	COENURUS in brain, eye, skin	Dog and wild canidae	Sheep, other ruminants, and rabbits	Several areas in the world
Echinococcus granulosus	—	ECHINOCOCCUS in liver, lungs, brain	Dog and wild carnivora	Sheep, cattle, pig, horse, camel, goat, and many wild mammals	Cosmopolitan
E. multilocularis	—	Alveolar ECHINOCOCCUS in liver	Fox, dog, cat, and wild canidae	Wild rodents	Northern hemisphere
Hymenolepididae					
Hymenolepsis nana	Ileum	Intestinal villi	Full development in man only		Cosmopolitan, warm countries
H. diminuta	Small intestine (jejunum)	No	Rats, mice, wild rodents	Fleas, flour beetles	Cosmopolitan
Order Pseudophyllidea					
Diphyllobothrium latum†	Small intestine (jejunum)	—	Cat, dog, and fish-eating carnivora	Planktonic copepoda (*Cyclops* and *Diaptomus*) and freshwater fish	Lakes, rivers, and deltas in Finland, Siberia, Canada, USA, Chile, Argentina

*Some other Cyclophyllidea occasionally invade man: e.g., the common dog tapeworm *Dipylidium caninum*.

†Several other species of Diphyllobothrium have been found in man in North and South America. Occasionally in the Far East plerocercoid larvae of *Sparganum proliferum* or *Spirometra mansoni* invade human tissues.

Table 7. MORPHOLOGIC DIFFERENCES BETWEEN LARGE TAPEWORMS IN MAN

	Taenia solium	Taenia saginata	Diphyllobothrium latum
ENTIRE BODY			
Length (m)	1,5–8	4–12	3–15
Maximal breadth (mm)	7–10	12–14	10–12
Proglottids (number)	700–1000	ca 2000	3000–4000
SCOLEX			
Diameter (mm)	0,6–1	1,5–2	Elongate 2–3 mm long
Suckers (number)	4	4	2 sucking grooves
Rostellum	Present	Absent	Absent
Hooks (number)	22–32	Absent	Absent
MATURE PROGLOTTIDS			
Testes (number)	375–575	800–1200	?
Ovary (number of lobes)	3	2	2
Uterus as	Blind tube	Blind tube	Coiled with a pore
Vaginal sphincter	Absent	Present	?
Genital atrium at	Lateral margin	Lateral margin	Ventral surface
GRAVID PROGLOTTIDS			
Uterus (number of branches each side)	7–12	18–32	None
Way of leaving host	In groups, passively	Single, spontaneously	

saginata, and *Diphyllobothrium latum*. Their morphologic characteristics are listed in Table 7 and Figure 6. *Hymenolepis diminuta* and *Dipylidium caninum* are of medium size (20 to 60 cm) and only *Hymenolepis nana* (dwarf tapeworm) is small (15 to 40 mm). The morphology and life cycle of *H. nana* is presented in Figure 7.

The larval stages of the tapeworms parasitizing man are as follows: (1) cysticercus (*T. solium*); (2) cysticercoid (*H. nana*); (3) coenurus (*T. multiceps*); (4) echinococcus (*Echinococcus granulosus* and *Echinococcus multilocularis*); and (5) sparganum, a plerocercoid-type larva (*Diphyllobothrium erinacei, Spirometra mansoni*). The first four are bladderworms of different sizes and different macroscopic and microscopic structures (Table 8, Fig. 8).

Human tapeworms have three basic types of life cycles: (1) The first type has water as an environment, aquatic copepoda (crustaceans) as the first intermediate hosts, fish as the second, and many vertebrates as definitive hosts (*Diphyllobothrium*, Table 9); (2) The second type uses various herbivorous vertebrates as intermediate hosts and carnivorous vertebrates as definitive hosts (*Taenia, Echinococcus*, Table 10); (3) The third type requires only one host because the larval stages develop in the intestinal villi of the definitive host (*H. nana*) (Fig. 7). Those tapeworms (*H. diminuta, Dipylidium*) with insects (fleas, beetles) as intermediate hosts rarely parasitize the intestine of man.

IMMUNOLOGY. The natural resistance of man against cestodes is low. Acquired immunity has been confirmed only in experimental *H. nana* infections. Adults are more resistant than children to human hymenolepiasis, and general immunity and nutrition are the major influences on the course of infection. Living taeniid larvae usually cause no local cellular reaction, but dead parasites invoke a strong response that produces a certain degree of resistance to reinfection. Migrating oncospheres seem to be the most immunogenic stage.

Adult *T. saginata* tapeworms frequently cause a rise in

Table 8. MORPHOLOGIC DIFFERENCES BETWEEN TENIID LARVAE PARASITIZING MAN

	Taenia solium	Taenia saginata	Taenia multiceps	Echinococcus granulosus	Echinococcus multilocularis
TYPE OF BLADDER	Cysticercus	Cysticercus	Coenurus	Echinococcus	Alveolar Echinococcus
MACROSCOPIC STRUCTURE					
number of bladders	1	1	1	One primary cyst, many brood capsules	Many
maximum size (mm)	20	8	30	200	2
number of scolices in a bladder	1	1	100 if fertile	Many thousands if fertile	Few or none
MICROSCOPIC STRUCTURE					
hooks on scolex	Present	Absent	Present	Present	Present
surface	Cuticle	Cuticle	Cuticle	Stratified hyaline membrane	Thin membrane
make-up of wall	Wortlike processes	Rugae	Smooth and also rugae	Smooth	Smooth
superficial protuberances					
height (μm)	15–27	23–27	15–22	No	No
width at base (μm)	27–38	50–70	28–46	No	No

Table 9. DIPHYLLOBOTHRIUM LATUM: LIFE CYCLE

Host and Habitat	Time	Stage and Activity	Number
Man and many mammals	Up to 30 years	EGGS undeveloped, expelled in feces	Up to 1,000,000 per day
Water	at least 12 days 1–2 days	egg embryonates in water, and hatches free-swimming coreciolium CORACIDIUM is ingested by copepoda	1 1
Fresh water copepoda (crustaceans) *Diaptomus* spp. *Cyclops* spp.	2–3 weeks	PROCERCOID develops in body cavity; ingested by fish transforms into plerocecoid	1
Fresh-water plankton-eating fish (lota, perch)	4 weeks	PLEROCERCOID, which develops in muscle or connective tissues, invades mammals or fish when ingested	1
Fresh-water carnivorous fish (pike) as transport host	Months	plerocercoid	1
Man and many fish-eating mammals (dog, cat, bear)	3–5 weeks	PREADULT and ADULT tapeworm in small intestine, produces eggs	1 1

blood IgE but allergic reactions are rare in taeniasis. However, fatal anaphylactic shock may follow rupture of a cyst of *E. granulosus*.

LABORATORY DIAGNOSIS. Stool examination is useful in the diagnosis of diphyllobothriasis and hymenolepiasis, but has some limitations in taeniasis. Eggs occur in the feces irregularly and those of *T. solium* and *T. saginata* are identical (Fig. 9). The correct differential diagnosis between *T. solium* and *T. saginata* is based on the morphology of scolices (hooks), mature segments (ovarian lobes), and gravid segments (vaginal sphincter, uterine branches) (Table 7). Laboratory identification of intestinal tapeworms is not possible until they start producing eggs and/or excreting proglottids. Differentiation of larval stages usually requires macroscopic and microscopic examination (hooks, protuberances; Table 8).

Immunodiagnostic tests are useful in cysticercosis and echinococcosis. Biopsy is of diagnostic value in the identification of subcutaneously localized larvae (cysticercosis, sparganosis).

DRUG SUSCEPTIBILITY. The intestinal tapeworms are susceptible to several taeniacides (niclosamide, praziquantel, paromomycin, Atabrine). Recently, some drugs (praziquantel, mebendazole) have been found that are effective against the larval stages of cestodes.

EPIDEMIOLOGY. Except for hymenolepiasis, cestode infections are zoonoses involving mainly domesticated animals. Their distribution depends chiefly on agricultural and pastoral practices (taeniasis, echinococcosis, coenurosis). When man is the only definitive host (*T. solium, T. saginata*), he is responsible for contamination of the environment with teniid eggs and proglottids of species invasive for the intermediate host (pig, cattle). Man rarely acquires infection from tapeworms circulating in feral (wild animal) cycles (*D. latum, E. multilocularis, T. multiceps, H. diminuta*).

Table 10. TAENIA SOLIUM: LIFE CYCLE

Host and Habitat	Time	Stage and Activity	Number
Man only	Up to 30 years	EGGS, fully developed, expelled in feces	50,000 per one proglottid
External environment	Months (years ?)	egg survives in water or soil	1
Pig; rarely in sheep dog, cat, and man	30 minutes 60–75 days	ONCOSPHERE hatches in small intestine, migrates mainly to muscle tissue, and develops into CYSTICERCUS, a bladder larva, which lives for months	1 1
Man only	5–12 weeks	Ingested cysticercus evaginates and transforms into ADULT worm, which produces proglottids and eggs	1

T. saginata develops slower in cattle (10–12 weeks) and in man (12 weeks) and produces more proglottids (6–9 per day) and eggs (80,000) per one proglottid.

	Taenia solium	*Taenia saginata*	*Diphyllo–bothrium latum*	*Hymenolepis diminuta*	*Dipylidium caninum*	*Hymenolepis nana*
Scolex	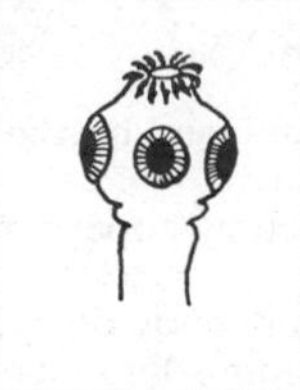	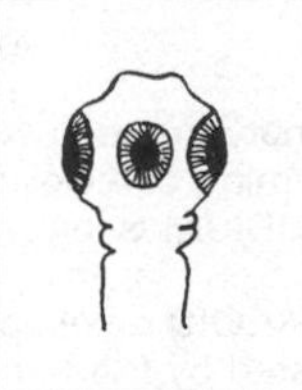	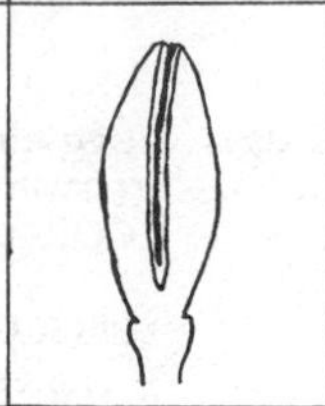	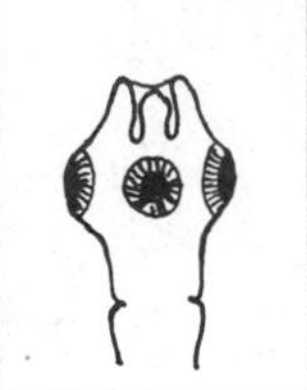	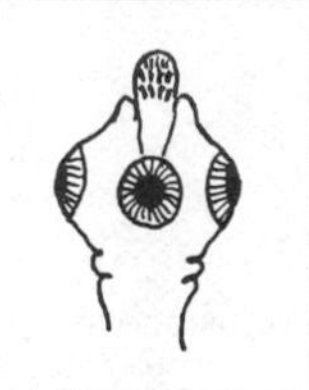	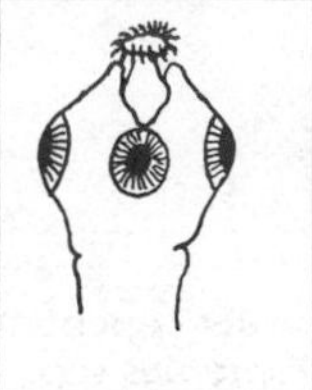
Gravid proglottid	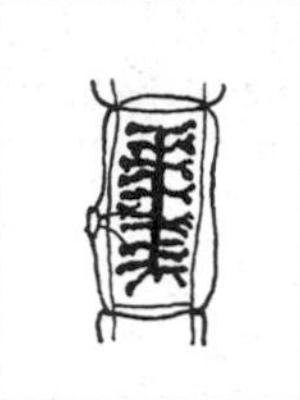	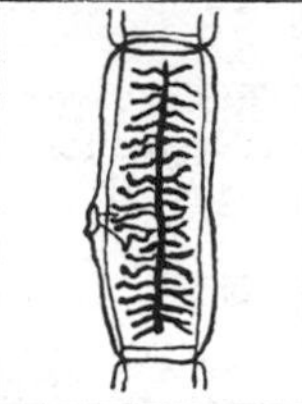	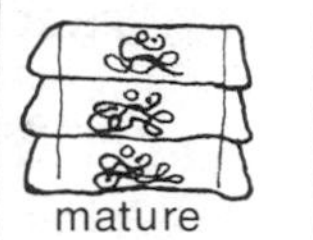 mature proglottids only	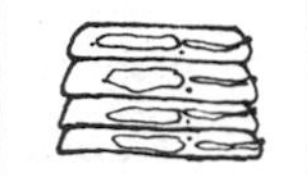	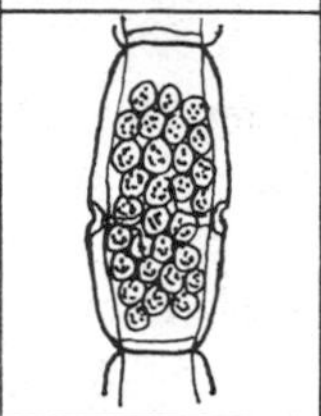	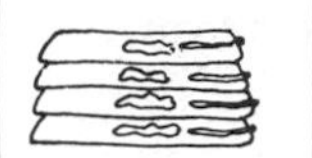
Number of proglottids	700–1000	ca 2000	3000–4000	800–1000	60–175	ca 200
Length of strobila (cm)	150–800	400–1200	300–1500	30–60	20–40	1½–4

Figure 6. Cestodes of man. Diagram of morphologic characteristics.

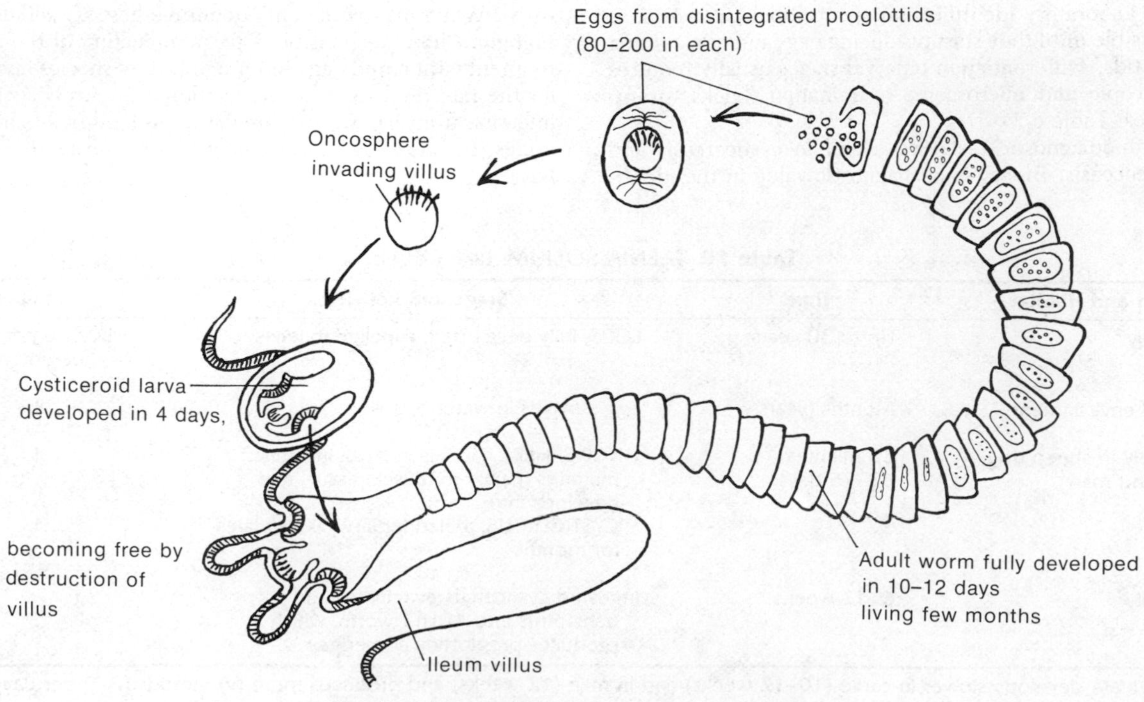

Figure 7. *Hymenolepis nana.* Diagram of life cycle.

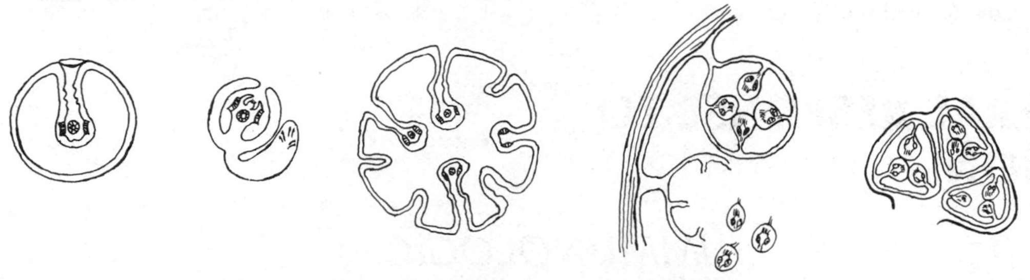

Figure 8. Larval cestodes. Diagram of morphologic characteristics.

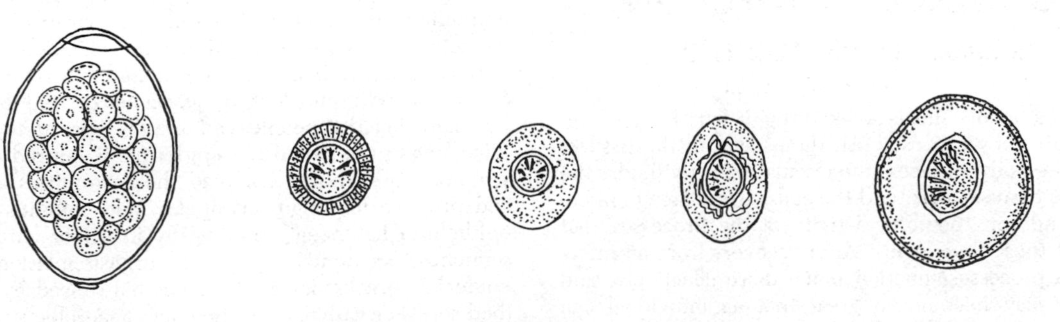

Figure 9. Cestode ova.

Hands and food contaminated with cestode eggs play an essential role in transmission of infections with *E. multilocularis*, *T. solium* (cysticercosis), and *H. nana*. Autoinfection is rare in *T. solium* taeniasis, but is common in hymenolepiasis and is responsible for the continuation of infection for many years. National programs for the control of echinococcosis in Ireland, Cyprus, and New Zealand were based on education, control of the dog population, mass diagnosis and treatment of dogs, and sanitary practices of sheep slaughter and carcass inspection.

T. solium infections usually disappear spontaneously with improved sanitation and modern pig husbandry (Europe). Contamination of the environment by increased numbers of human *T. saginata* carriers makes the control of this taeniasis difficult, in spite of meat inspection that helps to identify and destroy many of the cysticerci.

Personal protection against cestode infections is effected by personal hygiene and avoiding the consumption of raw meat.

References

Jordan, P., and Webbe, G.: Human Schistosomiasis. London, Heinemann 1982.

Komiya, Y.: Clonorchis and clonorchiasis. In Ben Dawes (ed.): Advances in Parasitology. New York and London, Academic Press, 1966, vol. 4, pp. 53.

Macdonald, G.: The dynamics of helminth infections with special reference to schistosomes. Trans R Soc Trop Med Hyg 59:489, 1965.

Pawlowski, Z., and Schultz, M. G.: Taeniasis and cysticercosis (Taenia saginata). In Ben Dawes (ed.): Advances in Parasitology. New York and London, Academic Press, 1972, vol. 10, p. 269.

Yokogawa, M.: Paragonimus and paragonimiasis. In Ben Dawes (ed.): Advances in Parasitology, New York and London, Academic Press, 1965, vol. 3, p. 99, and 1969, vol. 7, p. 375.

C. GENERAL RESPONSE TO INFECTION

IMMUNOLOGIC

87

MECHANISMS OF NATURAL RESISTANCE TO INFECTION

ABRAHAM I. BRAUDE, M.D., PH.D.

Infectious agents must break through four lines of defense before they can establish themselves in the tissues, namely, the body surfaces, the circulating body fluids, the connective tissue matrix, and the cells. Resistance to infection depends on the joint activity of the processes that operate at these four levels. After recovery from an infection these processes function much more effectively, and resistance may become so great that an individual can withstand heavy exposure to the same infection with no sign of illness. This enhanced resistance is designated acquired immunity, as distinguished from the weaker native resistance or natural immunity.

AT BODY SURFACES

Mechanical Factors. The mechanical barrier offered by the epithelial surface of the skin and mucous membranes is probably the most important natural means of preventing infection.

Squamous epithelium is a more effective barrier because several layers of cells connected by desmosomes block the route of invading organisms. Not only is the single layer of columnar epithelium a weaker barrier but also the cells ingest bacteria and thus facilitate their progress to the underlying tissue. Intracytoplasmic microbes have been observed in many studies on the columnar intestinal epithelium. These consist of protozoa, *Escherichia coli, Salmonella, Shigella,* and enteroviruses. Most of these organisms penetrate the epithelial cell through the microvilli on its brush border, but *Entamoeba histolytica* trophozoites pass through the intracellular junctions between two adjoining cells (Takeuchi, 1975). Rupture of the dermal epithelium by trauma, ischemia, or viruses (especially varicella) is complicated by infection with *Staphylococcus aureus*, group A or B streptococci, and anaerobic bacteria. *S. aureus* and group A streptococci are carried in the nose by many healthy people and readily spread to establish infections of the face if the epidermis is injured. Group A streptococci may also colonize the extremities and trunk and produce impetigo, erysipelas, and cellulitis after the epithelium has been ruptured by insect or animal bites, scratches, accidental injury, or surgical incisions. If the epidermis breaks down after ischemia caused by pressure (bed sores) or vascular insufficiency, anaerobic streptococci and *Bacteroides fragilis* invade the tissues and produce ischemic ulcers.

The bacteria of the mouth and colon also invade broken epithelium but less readily than after injury to the skin. In the mouth, the anaerobic streptococci, *Bacteroides,* and fusobacteria frequently produce infection of necrotic gums and adjacent mucous membranes in persons suffering from poor oral hygiene. The fetid odor of these mouth infections reflects the activity of these anaerobes.

In addition to the epithelial barrier, other mechanical factors enable the body surfaces to resist infection. In the mouth, infectious particles are drawn backward by suction currents that converge at the base of the tongue and bypass the tonsils and posterior pharynx (Bloomfield, 1922). Bacteria transported through the mouth in this fashion are swallowed and exposed to the bactericidal gastric juice. Resident bacteria, however, remain firmly entrenched. These suction currents are set up by movements of the lips and tongue and by swallowing, and are mediated by saliva. Normally they remove particles in 15 to 30 minutes but weaken or disappear if saliva dries up from dehydration or if swallowing is disturbed by paralysis or weakness. Thrush and other oral infections occur in weak or paralyzed patients who lose these oral suction currents.

Cilia provide another means of sweeping mucous membranes free of pathogenic organisms. The bacteria and viruses that are carried on dust particles into the nose may be arrested by the hairs in the nares, but if the particles penetrate beyond this barrier, they are carried backward by cilia to the posterior nasopharynx and then join the oral bacteria swept to the base of the tongue. In the trachea and bronchi, currents of mucus are moved at a rate of 1 to 3 cm/hour by the ciliated epithelium and carry inspired bacteria from the small bronchioles back up to the pharynx where they can be swallowed. The cilia are moved by microtubules that are straight hollow cylinders, 24 nm in diameter. Nine pairs of cylinders project from the cytoplasm of the cell into the periphery of each cilium. Dynein arms connect the microtubules to each other and control the sliding movements of adjacent microtubules. The cilia beat at a rate of approximately 1000 per minute and receive their energy from ATP or ADP. The cilia can be bypassed when infectious agents are carried on small particles. Thus particles carrying tubercle bacilli cause more infection experimentally if they are only 3 μ in diameter than those measuring 10 to 12 μ even though there are more bacilli on the larger particles. The larger particles are preferentially deposited in the upper airway where they are removed by cilia, whereas the smaller particles are able to pass beyond the cilia.

Particle size is also important in carrying viruses beyond the cilia. Those hygroscopic particles that are discharged in coughs shrink to 1.5 μ after they leave the nose or mouth and lose moisture, and then swell to 2 μ in the nose. These particles are small enough to pass beyond the cilia and reach the alveolar ducts, where they swell more by absorption of water from the moist air of the lung and become trapped in the narrow (0.6 μ) alveolar ducts. Larger particles will land on the ciliated respiratory epithelial cells, which have receptors for rhinoviruses, influenza viruses, and *Mycoplasma pneumoniae*. These agents may then initiate infection in the bronchial epithelium. Both influenza and *M. pneumoniae* impair mucociliary transport, so that increased susceptibility to secondary bacterial infection would be expected. Such secondary infection is prominent in influenza but does not occur in *Mycoplasma* infections, possibly because the impaired clearance is more severe in influenza.

Ciliary motion can also be reduced by cigarette smoke and alcohol. The amount of alcohol required for ciliary inhibition approaches the lethal dose and is not the important factor responsible for increased susceptibility of alcoholics to pneumonia. Formaldehyde, cyanide, and acetone are the ingredients in cigarette smoke that retard ciliary movement. When ciliary activity is damaged, the impaired ciliary clearance can be replaced by coughing. Patients with mucoviscidosis, for example, clear radioactive aerosols normally because their cough can compensate for the loss of mucociliary clearance. On the other hand, patients who suffer from congenital immotility of cilia are victims of chronic airway infections despite adequate coughs (Eliasson et al., 1977). The lack of motility in such cilia is due to an absence or abnormality of the dynein arms of the microtubules (Afzelius, 1976).

In the small intestine, bacteria are moved along by the action of mucosal villi, which free themselves of adherent particles by causing them to stick to the extensive lacy film of mucus that lines the bowel. The mucus is propelled along in the form of small balls by peristalsis. The absence of this protective mechanism may explain the greater tendency for *Shigella* and enteropathogenic *E. coli* to attack the colon, which has no villi. Peristalsis may be even more important than villous movement in protecting the small bowel from disease. In disorders of small bowel motility in which peristalsis is deficient, as in scleroderma, neurogenic disorders, or surgical blind loops, the colonic bacteria ascend and overgrow the small bowel. A major consequence of this bacterial overgrowth in the small bowel is deconjugation of bile salts by *B. fragilis*, the most populous member of the intestinal flora. The fall in concentration of conjugated bile salts and the corresponding rise in free bile acids (cholic, deoxycholic, and chemodeoxycholic) interfere with fat absorption and produce steatorrhea. Antibiotics that are active against *B. fragilis* will overcome the malabsorption problem. Further evidence of the importance of peristalsis is found in experiments that show that in order to infect guinea pigs with *Shigella*, it is necessary to inhibit intestinal motility with opiates. Opiates or belladonna drugs also impair resistance to human shigellosis. By restricting intestinal motility, these drugs produce more severe infection of the bowel.

Expectoration is a key process for transporting pathogenic bacteria from the respiratory tract, and the flushing action of tears, saliva, and urine removes infectious materials. Flushing the urethra by urinating after coitus will prevent cystitis in women. A sneeze or cough may contain 40,000 or more particles carrying bacteria. This reflex, as well as the epiglottis reflex, which prevents gross aspiration from reaching the pharynx, may be less efficient in adults than in children. If a contrast medium (iodized oil) is placed in the mouth of sleeping patients, chest x-rays will show the medium in the lungs of adults but not in children the following morning (Amberson, 1954). Alcohol, deep anesthesia, and exposure to cold all prevent closure of the glottis and allow aspiration pneumonia to occur.

Chemical Factors. Body surfaces also owe their freedom from infection to nonmechanical processes. The chemicals secreted by sebaceous and sweat glands inhibit bacterial growth on the skin surface. The sweat glands provide lactic, uric, and amino acids, and sebaceous glands contribute triglycerides, free fatty acids, and alcoholic waxes to the antimicrobial action of the film over the skin (Stoughton, 1959). Some of these depend on the action of mucin, a disaccharide of acetylneuraminil-acetylglucosamine attached to a peptide. Because these disaccharides are hydrophilic the mucin is hydrated. The negatively charged neuraminil residues repel each other and expand the hydrated molecule to form a moist lubricating blanket that moves on the surface of cilia and intestinal villi. Mucin granules can adsorb myxoviruses in mucus cells and reexcrete them as unincorporated virus into the moving mucus sheet. Susceptible cells are protected by this mechanism from infection. In a similar process, the mucin-secreting goblet cells of intestinal crypts respond to an inflammatory stimulus by rapidly discharging organisms that could infect the bowel. The *N*-acetyl neuraminic acid residue on mucin is a receptor for the hemagglutinins on myxoviruses and theoretically, at least, may prevent attachment of myxoviruses to cells by acting as a competitor for cell receptors. Should attachment occur, however, the viral neuraminidase could still free the virus from the mucin.

Acid kills most bacteria that reach the stomach and is the most important natural barrier to infection by intestinal pathogens (Garrod, 1937). *Brucella, Salmonella, Shigella,* and *Vibrio cholera* die quickly on exposure to gastric juice. In patients whose stomachs have been removed, the incidence of salmonellosis rises 3.3-fold, and the disease is more severe. The same applies to cholera; in a small epidemic in 1971 it was found that 25 per cent of cholera victims had had gastric resections. This association was predictable from the early experiments in 1885 of Robert Koch, who could produce infection in guinea pigs only if cholera organisms were given orally with sodium bicarbonate to neutralize the gastric juice. Bacteria are not the only agents affected by gastric acid. Although many viruses are killed by acid, the acid resistance of enteroviruses, hepatitis viruses, reoviruses, and adenoviruses is important in their ability to infect the bowel and be excreted in the feces. Among patients who get giardiasis, 42 per cent have achlorhydria. Normally the acid pH keeps the stomach and small bowel sterile or nearly so. Not until the pH approaches neutrality in the ileum do the intestinal flora assume a rich and varied character.

The low pH of normal urine may also be important in killing bacteria. Urines of pH 6 or below inhibit growth of *E. coli* and kill gonococci. This phenomenon may help prevent *E. coli* urinary infections and may also explain why the urethras of most men resist infection after exposure to gonorrhea, and why gonorrhea never spreads to the bladder or kidney (McCutchan et al., 1977).

Peroxide (H_2O_2) is another bactericidal factor found on mucous membranes. Alone or in conjunction with salivary peroxidase and thiocyanate, H_2O_2 kills various pathogenic bacteria, presumably through its powerful oxidizing ability. Peroxidase catalyzes the oxidation of thiocyanate to produce hypothiocyanite ion, which inhibits or kills bacteria (Thomas and Aune, 1978):

$$\underset{\text{Thiocyanate}}{SCN^-} + \underset{\text{Peroxide}}{H_2O_2} \xrightarrow{\text{peroxidase}} \underset{\text{Hypothiocyanite}}{OSCN^-} + H_2O_2$$

The $OSCN^+$ radical appears to kill bacteria by oxidation of their sulfhydryls to sulfenyl thiocyanate. The thiocyanate-peroxidase-H_2O_2 system is found both in the mouth and in milk.

Peroxide is elaborated by streptococci and other catalase-deficient bacteria in the mouth, bowel, and vagina. H_2O_2 from mouth bacteria correlates well with the ability of these normal resident flora to inhibit the diphtheria bacillus. These and other resident bacteria undoubtedly defend the body surfaces against infection by various mechanisms. In addition to H_2O_2, *Streptococcus mitis, Streptococcus salivarius,* and *Streptococcus mutans* elaborate antibiotics that range in molecular weight from 200 to 12 million and inhibit growth of most gram-negative and gram-positive cocci, including the pneumococcus and meningococcus (Sanders, 1982). One of these, known as enocin, is produced by *S. salivarius* and inhibits group A streptococci by interfering with the utilization of pantothenate. This antibiotic could offer protection against streptococcal pharyngitis. On the other hand, pneumococci that are carried in the throat are usually not inhibited by the resident streptococcal flora, possibly because resistant pneumococci are selected for implantation or acquire resistance afterwards (Johanson et al., 1970). The normal pharyngeal flora also prevent colonization by the gram-negative bacilli that overgrow the pharnyx of persons given penicillin and other antibiotics (Saene et al., 1983). These antibiotics can suppress the streptococci that predominate among inhibitory strains in the pharyngeal flora.

Normal Flora. In the bowel, *E. coli* is antagonistic to enteric pathogens. *Shigella,* for example, cannot be implanted in germ-free guinea pigs if *E. coli* is introduced first, but can cause experimental shigellosis more readily in conventional animals after suppression of the normal bowel flora by antibiotics. Similarly, the infective dose of *Salmonella typhosa* was reduced from 100,000 to 1000 bacteria in volunteers who swallowed streptomycin, a drug that inhibits intestinal *E. coli* but not the anaerobic bacteria of the bowel (Hornick et al., 1970). Colicines, the peptide antibiotics elaborated by *E. coli,* can kill *Salmonella* and *Shigella* and may help prevent intestinal infection by these bacteria. There is also evidence that colicines contribute to recovery from shigellosis. *E. coli* and other intestinal bacteria also produce acetic and butyric acids, which can inhibit growth of virulent enteric pathogens.

Antagonists of potential clinical significance have also been found among vaginal flora. *Candida albicans,* a common inhabitant of the vagina, inhibits most gonococci. *Staphylococcus epidermidis,* nonhemolytic streptococci, and *Pseudomonas* are also potent inhibitors of gonococci among vaginal flora. Other bacteria in the vagina can stimulate growth of the gonococcus; the stimulators are gram-positive and predominantly lactobacilli. The inhibition, which is thought to enhance natural resistance to gonorrhea in women, is mediated by acid production (killing of gonococci progressively increases as pH falls below 7.0), and by antibiotics produced by the normal flora. Stimulation of gonococci, which occurs by unknown mechanisms, might be important in promoting infection (Braude et al., 1977).

Surface Immunoglobulins. Immunoglobulins (Ig) A, M, G, and E all appear on normal mucous membranes and probably contribute to natural resistance. Secretory IgA is probably the most important of these because it is not only most abundant but also resistant to denaturation and hydrolysis by enzymes and chemicals in intestinal and other external secretions. Secretory IgA is a dimer of IgA molecules with a sedimentation coefficient of 11S. Secretory IgA is produced in submucosal plasma cells in close contact with the overlying glandular epithelium. The IgA monomers appear to be linked together by the glycopeptide J chains into stable dimers within the plasma cells. After secretion by the plasma cell, the IgA dimer forms a complex with a protein known as secretory-component. This secretory-component is manufactured by epithelial cells and from its position on the cell membrane is believed to function as a receptor protein that carries the IgA dimer into the cell and then out onto the surface of the mucous membrane (Hauptman and Tomasi, 1978). Secretory piece also appears to facilitate transport of locally synthesized IgM onto mucous membranes.

Local production of all immunoglobulins is stimulated on mucous surfaces by direct contact of B lymphocytes with microbial antigens during subclinical infection or with cross-reacting antigens present in food or in the normal microbial flora. Secretory IgA and other immunoglobulins seem to adhere to epithelial cell surfaces by sticking to the overlying mucus and provide an "antiseptic paint" that can block adherence of pathogenic agents to epithelial cells and neutralize their toxins. IgA has a limited ability, if any, to participate in reactions involving complement and, therefore, in promoting lysis or phagocytosis of bacteria. Furthermore, gonococci, meningococci, and certain streptococci produce a proteolytic enzyme that inactivates IgA1, which constitutes approximately 40 per cent of secretory IgA. Despite these limitations, the surface immunoglobulins undoubtedly contribute to natural resistance by preventing the initial attachment stage of infection by *Salmonella, Shigella,* pathogenic *E. coli,* gonococci, meningococci, *V. cholera,* group A streptococci, polio and other enteric viruses, various respiratory viruses, and certain protozoa. The importance of IgA in preventing intestinal infection is emphasized by the unique susceptibility of patients with hypogammaglobulinemia and selective IgA deficiency to giardiasis. Similarly, the presence of secretory IgA in colostrum and human milk may explain the lower incidence of gastrointestinal infections in breast-fed infants, and their resistance to infection with polioviruses (Winberg and Wessner, 1971). In the respiratory tract, the IgA in mucus can inhibit the neuraminidase activity of influenza virus on the neuraminic acid moiety of mucin and thereby block penetration of the mucin barrier by the virus.

IN EXTRACELLULAR FLUIDS

After infectious organisms pass beyond the body surfaces into the subepithelial tissues, their survival depends on their ability to withstand the environment of the extracellular fluids until taken up by phagocytic cells. They may elicit inflammatory reactions that confine them to the point of invasion, or they may pass into the lymphatic channels, travel to the lymph nodes, and eventually enter the general circulation. After phagocytosis they may escape from the cells and reappear in the body fluids.

Extracellular fluids are an ideal culture medium for certain organisms, as shown by the value of human blood, serum, and ascitic fluid for the isolation and growth of some organisms in the diagnostic laboratory. On the other hand, fresh human blood may inhibit the growth of meningococci, gonococci, coliform bacteria, *Brucella, Haemophilus influenzae,* and coagulase-negative staphylococci. Survival of an infectious agent in the body fluids depends on the temperature, pH, Eh (oxidation-reduction potential), osmolality, antibodies, complement, enzymes, electrolytes, and other metabolically active substances of the given fluid.

Temperature. The oral temperature of the normal human is about 37° C; that of the internal organs is 1 to 2° C higher. Most pathogenic organisms grow well in this temperature range, but *Sporothrix schenckii* and *Mycobacterium marinum* are exceptions. These do not grow well at 37° C or higher and are the cause of infections that usually remain confined to the extremities, where the temperature is lower. As might be expected from these temperature restrictions, external heat is useful for treating sporotrichosis and *M. marinum* infections. Among viruses, rhinovirus often grows best at 33° C on primary isolation, a property that fits with the reported prevalence of rhinovirus infections in colder weather when the temperature of the nasopharynx might be lowered by cold air. Yet rhinoviruses cause widespread infection in the warm temperatures of the tropics. In any case, the failure of rhinoviruses to replicate well at body temperature probably confines them to the respiratory tract and prevents infection of the warmer internal organs.

The normal body temperature has been important in recovery from transfusion reactions with blood contaminated by psychrophilic ("cold-loving") bacteria that grow well in the refrigerator but die at 37° C. Among cryptococci, only *Cryptococcus neoformans* can grow at 37° C, and it is the only cryptococcus that is pathogenic. *C. neoformans* cannot, however, withstand temperatures above 39° C, a fact that might explain clinical improvement during malaria and other febrile disorders in patients with cryptococcosis (Kligman and Weidman, 1949). On the other hand, artificial fever therapy has been useless in the treatment of cryptococcosis. Experiments in rabbits infected with *Pasteurella multocida* suggest that fever may help control infection by lowering the plasma iron level below that needed for survival of infecting bacteria (Kluger and Rothenburg, 1979).

Acidity. Homeostatic mechanisms maintain pH of extracellular fluids within such a narrow range that even under the most extreme conditions there is not enough change to influence the reproduction of pathogenic microbes. The only exception is urine, which can become sufficiently acid (pH 4.9 to 5.8) to inhibit or kill *E. coli,* gonococci, and other bacteria (McCutchan et al., 1977).

Redox Potential. The relatively high oxidation-reduction potential (Eh) of the extracellular fluids helps prevent infection by anaerobic bacteria. Eh is a measure in millivolts of the tendency to give up electrons, or the potential that would exist between the body fluids and a hydrogen half-cell at pH 0. Eh of extracellular fluids is a function not only of their inherent reducing tendency but also of their hydrogen ion concentration, and it becomes more negative as hydrogen ion concentration diminishes. The importance of Eh was first brought out in the case of tetanus by Fildes (1929), who showed that tetanus spores will not germinate readily at an Eh more oxidizing than +10 millivolts (mv) at pH 7.0 to 7.6. In living animal tissues he found the Eh to be approximately 120 mv at the prevailing pH 7.4. If the Eh is kept down by electrical methods, clostridia will grow even if a stream of air is passed through the culture (Hanke and Bailey, 1945). If the pH is kept in the acid range (6.4 to 6.8), *Clostridium perfringens* will grow at an Eh of 160 or more. In ischemic tissues, the anoxia lowers the Eh and lactic acid accumulation lowers the pH, so that anaerobic bacteria proliferate at Eh levels that are too high for their growth at the normal pH of 7.4. Since acidosis enhances proteolysis and accumulation of amino acids, the pH falls even more. Anaerobic infections do not occur unless the redox potential is lowered by one of the following disorders: (1) impairment of local blood supply by arterial occlusion; (2) pressure of foreign bodies such as sutures, clothing, dirt, and metal; (3) contamination of wounds with ionized calcium salts commonly present in fertile soil from farmlands, a powerful cause of tissue necrosis; (4) destruction of tissue by trauma, infection, or injection of quinine or epinephrine; (5) growth of aerobic or facultative bacteria in the tissues. The aerobic growth of the group A *Streptococcus* in a medium having an initial Eh of 300 mv induces a fall in redox potential to 150 to 200 mv.

Natural Antibodies and Complement. In the absence of any detectable previous antigenic stimulus, immunoglobulins appear in human sera that destroy pathogenic organisms in the presence of complement, promote their phagocytosis, or neutralize their toxins. These "natural" immunoglobulins, or antibodies, have been examined mainly for their action against meningococci, *E. coli.*, *Salmonella*, *H. influenzae*, pneumococci, staphylococci, and diphtheria bacilli. The importance of natural antibody in preventing disease was first appreciated in diphtheria. By demonstrating antitoxin with the Schick test, it has been possible to show a good correlation between resistance to diphtheria and the presence of antitoxin in people who have had no clinical history of diphtheria or active immunization. The most likely stimulus for natural antitoxin is inapparent infection.

The importance of inapparent infection in natural resistance has also been established for the meningococcus. Natural immunity against meningococci can result from antibodies that are stimulated by asymptomatic colonization of the throat with these bacteria (Goldschneider et al., 1969). The protective antibody appears to be directed against the meningococcal capsule. Natural antibodies against the capsule also prevent infection by *H. influenzae* and the pneumococcus, but these antibodies are more likely generated by stimuli from antigenically related organisms than from subclinical infection with the specific agents of influenzal and pneumococcal disease. Infants and children develop natural anticapsular antibody and immunity to *H. influenzae* type b, despite a very low colonization rate of their nasopharynx with *H. influenzae* type b. The same is true in laboratory animals that have high levels of serum antibodies to type b without having been colonized by that organism. *E. coli* K100 appears to be one of the important cross-reacting bacteria for producing *H. influenzae* type b immunity. The K100 antigen is a potent antigen for stimulating type b antibody when the whole bacteria are fed to children, and *E. coli* K100 colonizes their bowel naturally. The acidic polysaccharides in the K100 capsule appear to have the cross-reacting determinants for the type b capsule. Various other bacteria of the bowel cross-react with the *H. influenzae* type b capsule, including gram-positive bacteria with polyribitol phosphate in their cell wall teichoic acid. Ribitol is a component of the type b capsular polysaccharide antigen of *H. influenzae*.

The production of natural protective antibody against the pneumococcus is more complicated because many types of pneumococci are virulent, whereas only type b is virulent among *H. influenzae*. Nevertheless, there is enough exposure to cross-reacting antigens in bacteria and foodstuffs to provide good protection against pneumococcal infection by an early age. This is illustrated by the fact that 80 per cent of babies at the age of 1 year have antibody to type 7 pneumococcus, even though the carrier rate is only 1 per cent. The type 7 antibody response results from exposure to cross-reacting surface antigens in *S. viridans*. A partial list of other important cross-reactions with pneumococci is shown in Tables 1 and 2. These cross-reactions help explain how a broad spectrum of natural antibodies against pneumococcal infection is acquired early in life, long before subclinical infection with each of these types would be possible. Children with congenital hypogammaglobulinemia who are unable to make this natural antibody suffer from repeated pneumococcal infections of the same or different types (Bruton, 1952). The attacks of pneumococcal pneumonia and septicemia begin at 6 months after disappearance of the maternal immunoglobulins derived by transplacental passage, and affect mainly boys because the disorder is usually X-linked. The protective value of natural IgG antibody against pneumococcal infections in infancy and childhood is demonstrated by the effectiveness of commercial gamma globulin when given prophylactically to boys with hypogammaglobulinemia. Commercial gamma globulin is prepared from the blood of healthy people who have not been given pneumococcal vaccines, so that the protective IgG is naturally acquired antibody. The same susceptibility to overwhelming recurrent pneumococcal infections is seen in adults who lose their natural antibody when they develop the specific immunoglobulin disorders of multiple myeloma or acquired hypogammaglobulinemia.

Table 1. CROSS-REACTIONS BETWEEN PNEUMOCOCCI AND VARIOUS MICROORGANISMS OR PLANTS

Pneumococcus Type	Source of Cross-Reacting Antigens
1	Coliform bacilli Plant hemicelluloses (Felton et al., 1955)
2	Yeast polysaccharides Gum arabic (Heidelberger et al., 1929) Gum acacia (Marrack and Carpenter, 1938) Cherry gums *K. pneumoniae* polysaccharide B *S. typhi* *S. paratyphi* B Plant hemicelluloses
3	Gum arabic (Heidelberger et al., 1929) Gum acacia Cherry gums (Marrack and Carpenter, 1938) Meningococcus Gonococcus Plant hemicelluloses
14	Group A human red cells (Beeson and Goebel, 1939) Anthrax bacillus somatic polysaccharide
29,34,35	*H. influenzae* type b

Although natural antibody seems to be important against both pneumococci and *H. influenzae*, its mode of action against the two is different. Natural antibody against the pneumococcus (and other gram-positive bacteria) acts exclusively as an opsonin to promote phagocytosis, whereas natural antibody to *H. influenzae* can be both opsonic and bacteriolytic. Both IgM and IgG participate in opsonization, but IgM requires complement. The Fc portion of IgG attaches to the neutrophils and the Fab portion to the pneumococcal capsule. This opsonic bridge between leukocyte and pneumococcus does not require complement for phagocytosis to proceed. Complement becomes involved in a different opsonic process when Fab of either IgG or IgM reacts with capsular polysaccharide to form a complex that activates the classic complement pathway through the sequence C1, C4, C2, and C3. Activation of C3 makes it opsonic, so that it becomes the bridge between the pneumococcus and the phagocytic cell. Complement can also be opsonic for the pneumococcus when the cell wall activates C3 through the alternative pathway, which does not involve the participation of antibody. The generation of pneumococcal opsonins by the alternative pathway

Table 2. DISTRIBUTION OF IMMUNIZING ANTIGEN AGAINST PNEUMOCOCCAL INFECTION IN MICE AMONG HEMICELLULOSES FROM COMMONLY "EDIBLE" PLANTS[a]

Source of Hemicellulose	Immunity Against 10^3 LD		
	Pn I	*Pn II*	*Pn III*
Melon, honeydew (rind)	+++	+++	+++
Collard greens	+++	+++	++
Sunflower seed	+++	+++	+
Pumpkin pulp	+++	++	+
Squash (fruit)	+++	+++	0
Peanut meal	+++	++	0
Tomato (fruit)	++	++	+++
Watermelon rind	++	++	++
Green bean (fruit)	++	++	++
Parsnip greens	++	++	+
Pomegranate (fruit)	++	+	++
Wheat germ	++	+++	0
Cucumber	++	++	0
Kale greens	++	++	0
Soybean meal	++	++	0
Rape greens	++	+	0
Lettuce	++	0	0
Rutabaga (root)	++	0	0
Nutmeg powder	+	+++	++
Onion bulb	+	+++	0
Lima bean	+	++	0
Potato, white	+	+	+
Barley	+	0	0
Sugar cane	+	0	0
Yeast (baker's)	+	0	0
Apple, Winesap	0	+++	0
Grapefruit rind	0	+++	0
Irish moss (carrageen)	0	+++	0
Oatmeal	0	+++	0
Rhubarb, leaves	0	+++	0
Green pepper (fruit)	0	++	++
Cabbage	0	++	0
Coconut	0	+	++
Cinnamon powder	0	0	++
Carrot	0	0	+
Broccoli greens	0	0	0
Swiss chard greens	0	0	0
Eggplant (fruit)	0	0	0
Orange (rind)	0	0	0
Pear (fruit)	0	0	0
Pectin	0	0	0
Radish root	0	0	0
Rice (polished)	0	0	0

[a] + + + indicates immunity with 0.0005 mg or 0.005 mg of hemicellulose; + + indicates immunity with 0.05 or 0.5 mg; + indicates immunity with 1.0 or 5.0 mg.

Modified from Felton, L., et al.: J. Bacteriol 69:519, 1955.

Pn indicates pneumococcus type, I, II, or III.

does not seem to be important in clinical medicine because it does not protect patients who lack gamma globulin from developing overwhelming pneumococcal infections. On the other hand, complement activation via the classic pathway is important for the opsonic activity of nonimmune human serum because most natural antibody against the pneumococcus is IgM. Because C1 and C2 are inactivated by heating at 56° C, the opsonic activity of nonimmune serum is often referred to as heat labile to distinguish it from the heat-stable, complement-independent, opsonic activity of hyperimmune antipneumococcal serum whose opsonins are IgG.

The natural antibodies against the meningococcus and *H. influenzae* are also opsonic, but in addition, they kill these two gram-negative bacteria by lysis in the absence of phagocytes. Bacteriolysis by natural antibody is a reaction between the bacterial surface antigens (polysaccharide capsules), IgM, and complement. As in opsonization, the reaction may follow either the classic or the alternative pathway of complement. After IgM attaches via the Fab to the capsular polysaccharide antigen, the first step in the classic pathway is attachment of C1 through its subunit C1q to a binding site on the Fc portion of IgM. This interaction with antibody globulin activates C1 and catalyzes the assembly of C4 and C2. Together ($C\overline{42}$) they function as the enzyme C3 convertase. This enzyme cleaves C3 into two fragments, C3a and C3b, where it can function either as an opsonin (as described for pneumococcus), or mediate lysis of gram-negative bacteria. C3b attaches to receptors on the bacterial cell. After attachment to the bacteria cell, C3b combines with neighboring $C\overline{42}$ and apparently modifies the specificity of the latter enzyme so that it can now cleave C5 into C5a and C5b. The large fragment C5b then attaches to the cell membrane, binding in turn C6 and C7 to form the trimolecular complex $C\overline{567}$, which then becomes tetramolecular when C8 is incorporated. The terminal complex of C activation becomes complete when C9 fixes to binding sites on $C\overline{5678}$. The large complex of the five individual terminal C proteins is essential for killing susceptible gram-negative bacteria. This bactericidal activity is far more effective when it is generated via the classic pathway, but it can operate through the alternative pathway (also known as the properdin pathway). The lipopolysaccharide (LPS) in gram-negative bacteria can activate the alternative pathway by reacting directly with a noncomplement protein, C3 proactivator (properdin B) (C3PA). Upon reacting with LPS, C3PA splits into at least two fragments: One has the electrophoretic mobility of gamma globulin (mw 60,000), and a second consists of an acidic peptide (mw 20,000). The larger fragment, known as C3 activator, splits C3 into C3a and C3b (properdin A), and thereby initiates the terminal sequences of complement activation.

In addition to complement, lysozyme, calcium, and magnesium are important components of extracellular fluids that are required for killing gram-negative bacteria. Ca^{++} and Mg^{++} ions are essential for initiation of the classic complement sequence, and lysozyme is needed for disrupting the cell wall peptidoglycan. Lysozyme splits the 1–4 glycosidic linkages between *N*-acetyl muramic acid and *N*-acetylglucosamine in the peptidoglycan so that complement may have greater access for its attack on the cytoplasmic membrane. The electron microscope (Figs. 1 and 2) discloses dramatic disturbances of bacterial morphology in cells that have been killed by serum. Both cell walls and cytoplasmic membranes are ruptured.

In contrast to gram-positive bacteria, which are all resistant to lysis by complement, all species of gram-negative bacteria are susceptible to lysis by the classic or alternative pathway. This difference in susceptibility to killing by complement is best explained by the concept that the cell wall of gram-positive bacteria is a barrier that hinders access of complement to the cytoplasmic membrane. This concept is reinforced by the fact that protoplasts of gram-positive bacteria whose cell walls are removed are killed

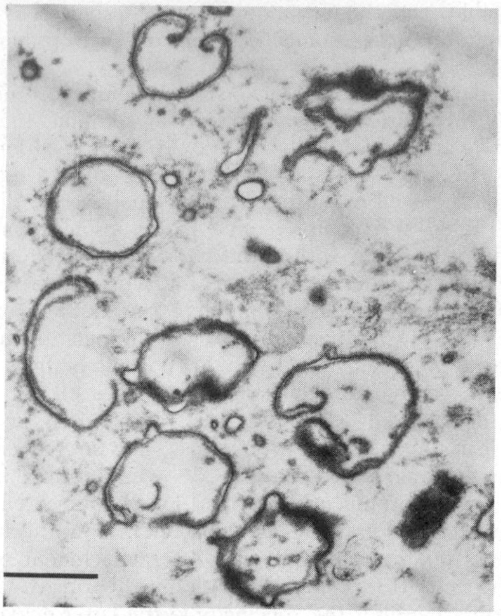

Figure 1. Representative electron micrographs of markedly serum-sensitive *E. coli* bacteria incubated with undiluted fresh normal serum. Note that both cell walls and cytoplasmic membrane are ruptured by the bactericidal action of fresh serum. Compare this with Figure 2, which shows appearance of same bacteria in serum after inactivation of complement. × 16,000 (From Olling, S.: Scand J Infect Dis (Suppl), 1977.)

by complement. The thicker peptidoglycan and the absence of LPS could explain how the cytoplasmic membrane enjoys a sanctuary in gram-positive bacteria from complement. In many gram-negative bacteria, LPS is the key intermediate factor in killing because it activates complement by either pathway. Each of the three primary structural components of LPS—O antigens, core sugars, and lipid A—can activate the classic pathway by reacting with natural antibody (Fig. 3). In the absence of antibody, lipid A can activate either the classic pathway by direct reaction with C1q or the alternate pathway. For unknown reasons, virulent enteric gram-negative bacteria often resist complement-mediated bacteriolysis, survive in the extracellular fluids, and cause bacteremia. The importance of complement in natural resistance to infection is also seen in patients who share a familial deficiency of C6, C7, and C8 and are subject to severe recurrent attacks of bacteremia due to gonococci and meningococci. Phagocytosis of these bacteria is normal because opsonins can be generated through C3, but the serum of these patients cannot kill pathogenic *Neisseria* because the terminal complex of complement is not formed.

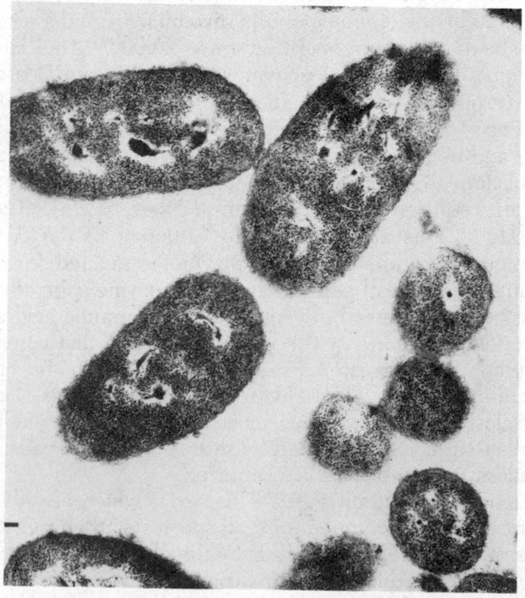

Figure 2. Same as Figure 1 except that serum has been heated to inactivate complement. In the absence of complement the bactericidal system is inoperative and does not injure the bacterial cell. × 16,000 (From Olling, S.: Scand J Infect Dis (Suppl), 1977.)

Aside from gram-negative bacteria, certain protozoa, trematodes, and leptospiras undergo lysis in nonimmune serum in the presence of complement. Resistance to such lysis seems to be correlated with virulence. For example, the blood from nearly every person kills members of the *Trypanosoma brucei* group in vitro and protects experimental animals. The only trypanosomes of the *T. brucei* group that resist being killed by human serum are *T. gambiense* and *T. rhodesiense,* which can infect human beings and cause sleeping sickness. *Trypansoma cruzi,* the cause of Chagas' disease, also resists killing by human serum. Such a relationship also seems to exist for highly pathogenic *Schistosoma mansoni*. High dilutions of human serum will lyse cercaria of many trematodes within a few minutes but not those of *S. mansoni* unless the serum is from a patient infected with *S. mansoni* (Culbertson, 1951). Similarly, virulent leptospiras resist killing by normal human serum, which destroys nonpathogenic leptospiras and some avirulent lines of pathogenic leptospiras (Johnson and Harris, 1967).

Beta-lysin. Although not killed by antibody and complement, most gram-positive bacteria are killed by beta-lysin, a relatively heat-stable cationic protein with a molecular weight of 6,000 (Donaldson, 1975). With the exception of streptococci, most gram-positive bacteria are killed by beta-lysin, but gram-negative bacteria, molds, yeasts, viruses, and mycoplasmas are not killed. Beta-lysin does not require complement to kill and, unlike bactericidal antibody, is present in higher concentrations in serum than in plasma because it is released from platelets when blood clots. It is also present in inflammatory exudates. The bacterial cell membrane is thought to be the primary site of action of beta-lysin.

Acute Phase Substances. During a variety of unrelated acute illnesses, substances suddenly and promptly appear that react with streptococci. One of these kills group A streptococci, and the other combines with the group-specific polysaccharide C-substance of *S. pneumoniae* (C-reactive protein). Neither is an antibody. The C-reactive protein (CRP) is normally present in trace amounts in human serum but increases rapidly in infection and inflammation as a consequence of increased synthesis in hepatocytes (Kushner and Feldmann, 1978). It was first discovered in pneumococcal pneumonia but later observed in other acute infections, rheumatic fever, cancer, arthritis, serum sickness, ulcerative colitis, myocardial infarction, and various forms of tissue injury. CRP is composed of five subunits in cyclic symmetry and its chemical structure is similar to that of C1t, a serum protein that may be involved in regulation of complement (C1) function. Despite the ability to react with pneumococcal C polysaccharide and to fix

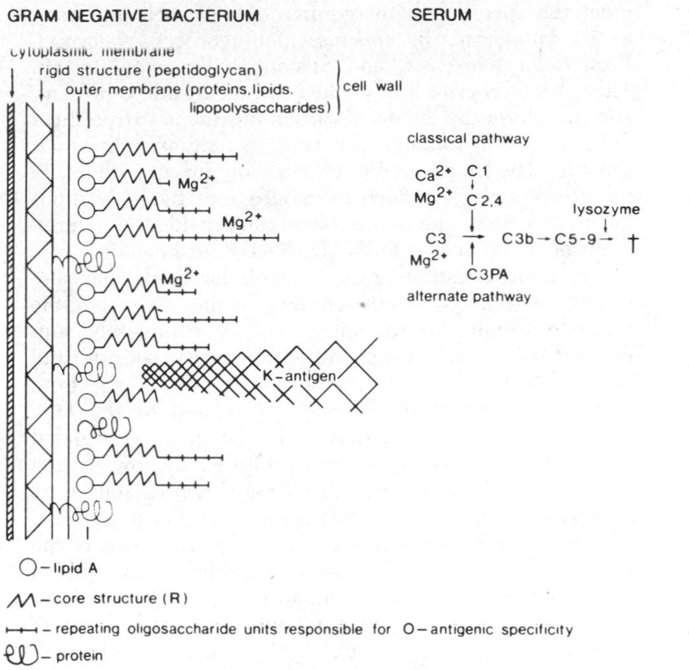

Figure 3. Proposed model for the structure of the surface layers of gram-negative bacteria and the serum factors involved in bacterial killing. Each of the three primary structural components of LPS—O antigens, core sugar, and lipid A—can activate the classic pathway by reacting with natural antibody. Reactions between K antigen or other capsular antigens and antibody can probably also activate the classic pathway. In the absence of antibody, lipid A can activate either the classic or the alternate pathway. Activation of complement by either pathway kills the cell. This may occur either because holes are punched in the outer membrane, so that lysozyme can hydrolyze the mucopeptide and produce spheroplasts that rupture from osmotic forces, or because activated complement may cause lethal damage to the cytoplasmic membrane. (From Olling, S.: Scand J Infect Dis (Suppl), 1977.)

complement with it, CRP has no demonstrable antimicrobial activity except for weak opsonic properties for various pathogenic bacteria. Its protective properties seem to depend instead on its ability to modulate inflammatory and immune responses by inhibiting platelet aggregation and mediator release and by suppressing lymphocyte stimulation and lymphokine production after binding to T-cells (Mortenson et al., 1977).

Both acute-phase substances were discovered by W. S. Tillett (1937), and the bactericidal factor is known as Tillett factor. Its ability to kill streptococci separates it from beta-lysin; Tillett factor is also unusual in that its activity is abolished under anaerobic conditions or in the presence of reducing agents. Both CRP and Tillett factor differ from antibody in their time of appearance and the nonspecificity of their stimuli. The two acute-phase substances are most active in the most active periods of disease, and disappear during convalescence when specific antibody usually begins to increase. For this reason, it has been suggested that acute-phase substances provide a means of body defense against bacterial invasion that is uniquely different from that of the complement-antibody apparatus and the phagocytic system.

Interferons. Various tissues can react with viruses to elaborate proteins that inhibit infection by the same or different viruses. These inhibitors, designated interferons by Isaacs and Lindenmann (1957), enhance the resistance of cells to infection by viruses. Interferon produced by one type of cell is active against a wide variety of viruses; for example, an interferon produced by treatment of cells with influenza virus will prevent infection not only by various influenza viruses but also by vaccinia viruses, togaviruses, and others. Moreover, interferon produced in cells of different organs shows no tissue specificity, so that interferon produced during a pulmonary infection, for example, might inhibit viral growth in the brain. Because interferon has been found in tissues during recovery from viral infection, it has been suggested that this viral inhibitor might depress viral multiplication before specific antibody reaches effective levels. (Interferon is fully discussed in Chapter 12.)

Tuftsin. This tetrapeptide of splenic origin stimulates phagocytosis and it occupies the location 289–292 in the amino acid sequence of all the IgG subclasses. Tuftsin is freed from the gamma globulins by two enzymes: 1) tuftsin endocarboxypeptidase (found in the spleen) and a surface enzyme on PMN leukocytes. Its formula is L-threonyl-L-lysyl-L-prolyl-L-arginine. It has a high positive charge that allows it to bind to negatively charged groups (e.g., sialic acid) on the neutrophil surface. An enzyme in the membrane of neutrophils splits tuftsin from a gamma globulin known as leukokinin. Deficiencies of tuftsin occur as a rare familial disorder (Constantopoulos et al., 1972) and apparently after splenectomy. The susceptibility to overwhelming pneumococcal infection in splenectomized patients is thought by some to be a consequence of tuftsin deficiency.

Enzymes, Electrolytes, and Other Metabolites. The peculiar susceptibility of the poorly controlled diabetic to infections by *Klebsiella pneumoniae*, tubercle bacilli, *Mucor*, *Rhizopus*, and *Candida albicans* suggests that chemical abnormalities of the extracellular fluids may enhance the capacity of these microorganisms to establish infection. At least 0.3 per cent glucose is necessary in culture media for the formation of well-encapsulated *K. pneumoniae* (Hoogerheide, 1939). This concentration of glucose in the tissue fluids in poorly controlled diabetes might enable these bacteria to produce larger capsules and enhance their virulence by enabling them to resist phagocytosis. High concentrations of glucose also favor growth of *Mucor*, *Rhizopus*, and *C. albicans*. Although there is no evidence that variations in the concentration of glucose in vivo affect the survival of tubercle bacilli, the stimulating effect of keto acids at the acid pH of inflammatory exudates may enhance the growth of these bacteria in human tuberculosis during uncontrolled diabetes (Dubos, 1954).

In normal persons, the body fluids are well suited to

meet the special growth requirements of such organisms as *H. influenzae*, *B. abortus*, meningococci, gonococci, *Francisella tularensis*, and *Streptobacillus moniliformis*. These bacteria grow better when carbon dioxide is present, and the physically dissolved carbon dioxide in extracellular fluid (about 3 volumes per cent) is optimum for their growth. The requirement of cysteine for growth of *F. tularensis* and *H. influenzae* is also met by body fluids during infection, and human blood can provide the requirement of *H. influenzae* for NAD, NADP, or hematin.

The same constituents of extracellular fluids may also inhibit bacterial growth or activity of toxins. Growth of the tubercle bacilli, for example, may be completely suppressed by excessive concentrations of carbon dioxide, and the beneficial effects on tuberculosis of lung collapse from therapeutic pneumothorax may be related to the high concentration of carbon dioxide in the poorly ventilated lung. Tubercle bacilli are also inhibited by low oxygen tension, and their disappearance from closed caseous areas is attributed in part to local anoxia. In sharp contrast, where an open bronchus permits good oxygenation of the cavity, tubercle bacilli flourish, and conditions are optimal for growth of drug-resistant mutants.

Iron and iron-containing compounds appear to have an important influence on virulence of bacteria. Although hematin is essential for the growth of *H. influenzae*, it may be toxic for certain gram-positive bacteria even in minute amounts. Heme is lethal for staphylococci in concentrations of 0.0003 per cent at pH 7.0 (Dubos, 1954). For the most part, however, iron or heme compounds promote virulence and growth in vivo. Virulence for mice is markedly enhanced, and disseminated lethal infections occur when gonococci are suspended in a mixture of hemoglobin and mucin, the same menstruum in which they exist during menstruation when they most commonly disseminate hematogenously in women. If elemental iron is used in place of hemoglobin the virulence of gonococci is not increased. Under other circumstances, however, iron alone will enhance and iron deprivation will lower bacterial virulence. This correlation of virulence with available iron seems to parallel the ability of iron to stimulate microbial growth. Staphylococci, clostridia, *Listeria*, mycobacteria, various enteric bacteria, *Pseudomonas*, *Pasteurella*, *Yersinia*, *Vibrio*, *Aeromonas*, *Candida*, and plasmodia are among the genera of bacteria, fungi, and protozoa whose members are stimulated by excess iron to grow in body fluids (Weinberg, 1978). This growth stimulation by iron in serum and other body fluids is thought to depend on saturation of transferrin, a nonheme iron-binding protein with a molecular weight in the range of 75,000 to 80,000. It binds reversibly two ferric ions/molecule through tyrosyl and histidyl residues. Under normal conditions human transferrin is only 25 to 35 per cent saturated, so that the amount of free ionic iron in plasma is at least 100 million-fold less than that required for bacterial growth (0.4 to 4.0 μM). If circulating transferrin is saturated by injecting iron intravenously, intraperitoneally, or intramuscularly, there is an increased mortality rate of animals with experimental candidiasis, tuberculosis, staphylococcal infections, salmonellosis, and meningococcal infections. By saturating transferrin, the injection of iron makes available enough free iron to meet microbial growth requirements. Impaired resistance to infection is not limited to experimental animals treated with iron, since impaired resistance has been reported in human beings after exposure to excess iron. Thus, the incidence of serious gram-negative infections has increased in newborn infants after intramuscular injection of iron (Barry and Reeve, 1977). It should be noted that transferrin can also be saturated if its concentration falls in relation to iron, as occurs in patients with kwashiorkor whose nutritional disorder damages their ability to make iron-binding proteins. The plasma obtained from kwashiorkor victims supports growth of *S. aureus* and is bacteriostatic upon addition of transferrin. Lactoferrin, an iron-binding protein in human milk, has been given credit, along with antibodies, for the lower incidence of gastroenteritis in breast-fed compared with formula-fed infants (Weinberg, 1977). For this reason the practice of supplementing infant formulas with iron has been questioned.

In addition to lactoferrin, human milk contains a lipase that is involved in rapid killing of the protozoan *Giardia lamblia*. Killing of *Giardia* by the lipase requires that the enzyme be stimulated by bile salts. Human milk may thus protect breast-fed infants against this protozoan (Gillin et al., 1983).

Constituents of body fluids can further influence pathogenicity by affecting bacterial toxins. The virulence of staphylococci is correlated, for example, with coagulase production. Coagulase is generated from staphylococcal procoagulase by an activator in the body fluids, and coagulase converts fibrinogen to fibrin. The tendency for staphylococci to produce extensive thrombosis in the lung and other tissues and to cause severe intravascular coagulation suggests that coagulase activator has an important place in the pathogenesis of staphylococcal infection. Its importance is further implied by the greater resistance to staphylococcal infections among certain animals whose plasma lacks coagulase activator. Staphylokinase, another staphylococcal toxin, acts through plasminogen, a constituent of normal plasma. Both staphylokinase and streptokinase convert plasminogen to plasmin, which can digest fibrin clots and prevent clotting. Both enzymes are elaborated in human infections and stimulate antibodies that neutralize their activity. Staphylokinase is thought to initiate lysis of infected thrombi and the release of septic emboli to the lung during staphylococcal septicemia; streptokinase could explain the poor localization of streptococcal cellulitis by preventing fibrin deposition around an infected focus.

The chemical environment of body fluids may disturb normal immune processes, especially in the renal medulla. Within the range found in the normal kidney and urine, high concentrations of sodium, urea, and hydrogen ion inhibit phagocytosis of human leukocytes (Chernew and Braude, 1962). These observations help explain why the kidney is uniquely susceptible to invasion by *E. coli*, *Proteus*, and other bacteria that possess little capacity to establish infection elsewhere.

In the genital tract, infection can be increased in severity by hormonal manipulation. Oral contraceptives, which increase the levels of progestins and estrogens in the body fluids, promote *Candida* and chlamydial infections of the genital tract of women (Catterall, 1971). Estradiol has a similar effect in enhancing the severity of experimental chlamydial infections of the genital tract (Rank et al., 1982). The mechanism of these endocrine effects is unknown, but might be due to stimulation of the infecting organism or to suppression of local immunity. Fluctuations in estrogen levels could thus explain the increased susceptibility to infection at certain stages of the menstrual cycle and pregnancy. Menstruation, for example, is accompanied by more susceptibility to *Herpes simplex* and gonococcemia, whereas pregnant women are more susceptible to disseminated infections with the gonococcus, tubercle bacilli, and *Coccidioides immitis*.

IN CELLS

Transport by Lymphatics. When organisms reach the tissue fluids they may be phagocytized by neutrophils or macrophages, or carried by the lymphatics to the right or left subclavian vein. During the course of this passage to the general circulation they may be trapped in lymph nodes and phagocytized by macrophages. If they get beyond the lymph nodes and into the blood they will then be ingested by circulating neutrophils or by histiocytes in the liver, spleen, bone marrow, adrenal, or pituitary. It is unlikely that any microorganism can enter blood capillaries directly because these vessels are impermeable to substances with a molecular weight of greater than 20,000. Lymph capillaries, on the other hand, easily become permeable to particles as large as red cells, even though they appear to be closed completely by endothelium and have no direct opening into the tissues. Passage through the lymph vessels is an important process in natural immunity because infectious particles are carried to potent fixed phagocytic cells. By itself, however, the lymph has limited protective ability because it contains almost no phagocytic cells and its content of antibodies is less than that of the blood (Braude and Carlson, 1908). The impotence of lymph against gram-positive bacteria can be observed when type III pneumococci are injected intravenously. These bacteria can be cultured promptly from the lymph after intravenous injection because they migrate passively through the walls of blood capillaries into tissue fluid and then through the lymphatic capillaries. Upon intravenous injection of type III pneumococcal antiserum, the blood becomes sterile but pneumococci are still found in the lymph seven hours later (Field et al., 1937). In the absence of phagocytic cells, pneumococci can multiply in the lymph even in the presence of antibody. The meningococcus, *H. influenzae*, and other gram-negative bacteria, on the other hand, would not survive in lymph because antibody and complement can kill these bacteria without phagocytic cells. This difference accounts for the tendency of certain gram-positive bacteria to remain dormant in the lymphatics and produce recurrent infection. The best known example of this phenomenon is recurrent erysipelas, an infection in which the lymph vessels of the skin are filled with streptococci (Fehleisen, 1886).

The flow of lymph depends on body movement, massage, or the increase in tissue pressure that occurs during inflammation. The network of fibers attached to the outer wall of the lymphatic vessels is stretched by increased tissue pressure so that the lymphatics are opened and can accommodate the larger volumes of lymph that flow during inflammation (Pullinger and Florey, 1935). The importance of adequate lymph flow in the removal of organisms for the prevention of infection is obvious after the lymphatics become obstructed, when the resulting elephantiasis becomes the focus of repeated infections. The remarkable filtering capacity of lymph nodes depends for its efficiency on a network of trabeculae that fills the sinusoids. The histiocytes lining the sinuses can then ingest and destroy the trapped organisms.

Transport by Blood. Microorganisms carried by the lymphatics to the subclavian veins may be phagocytized in the blood by neutrophilic leukocytes, which are then sequestered in the capillaries of the lung and liver. Many organisms are also removed by the Küpffer cells of the liver and the macrophages in the spleen. Bacteria, fungi, protozoa, and viruses can be taken out of the circulation by both the circulating phagocytes and the macrophage (reticuloendothelial) system. The route of viruses is illustrated by mousepox (Fenner, 1949). After multiplying in the skin, mousepox virus passes within eight hours to the regional lymph node. After multiplication in the node, the virus is carried into the blood and removed by phagocytes in the liver and spleen. Multiplication in the liver may lead to another viremia with secondary spread to the skin, where the characteristic eruption appears. During viremia, pox virus is associated with lymphocytes and monocytes; in lymphocytic choriomeningitis, Rift Valley fever, and Colorado tick fever the virus is adsorbed to erythrocytes. Others, like the togaviruses and the enteroviruses, circulate free in the plasma. After removal by the macrophages in the liver, some viruses (poxviruses, yellow fever virus) multiply in these cells and then infect the hepatic cells. Some pass directly into hepatic cells without multiplication in Küpffer cells (Rift Valley fever virus), and others, such as vaccinia and influenza viruses, are rapidly destroyed within the Küpffer cells (Fenner et al., 1974).

Virulent bacteria may also multiply in the liver and spleen and reenter the circulation to cause bacteremia or fungemia. The ability of the human liver to clear some, but not all, bacteria was discovered in patients with endocarditis when it was shown that hepatic venous blood always contained many fewer colonies of streptococci than blood from arteries or other veins (Beeson et al., 1945). Bacteria may also establish a sustained bacteremia by penetrating the wall of a capillary or venule and producing an infected thrombus. This thrombus may discharge a continuous stream of organisms at a rate that exceeds the ability of phagocytic cells to remove them. Such a bacteremia, often observed with staphylococci and *Bacteroides*, is dominated by lung abscesses.

Fungi and protozoa are no exceptions to the clearance of circulating organisms by the reticuloendothelial system. Perhaps the most dramatic example of phagocytosis by tissue macrophages is the tremendous number of *Histoplasma* organisms present in these phagocytes during human infection. Similarly, malaria illustrates the prominent phagocytosis of protozoa by the reticuloendothelial cells in liver, spleen, and bone marrow. Malaria is unique, however, in that the parasitized red cells are phagocytized but not the parasite alone.

Mode of Entry into Phagocytic Cells. The contact between phagocytic cell and infectious particle in the blood and tissue is made either through chance collision or through a positive attraction between phagocytes and microorganisms known as chemotaxis. In chemotaxis experiments in vitro, phagocytes can be seen to crawl by ameboid motions toward the particle to be ingested. Chemotaxis in vivo has often been difficult to demonstrate, but a striking example can be found in coccidioidomycosis. In the infected tissues, the fungus *Coccidioides immitis* has the form of a thick-walled spherule containing numerous endospores. The intact spherule is surrounded by mononuclear cells, but when it begins to rupture and release its endospores, there is a chemotactic rush of neutrophilic leukocytes to the point on the spherule where the endospores will

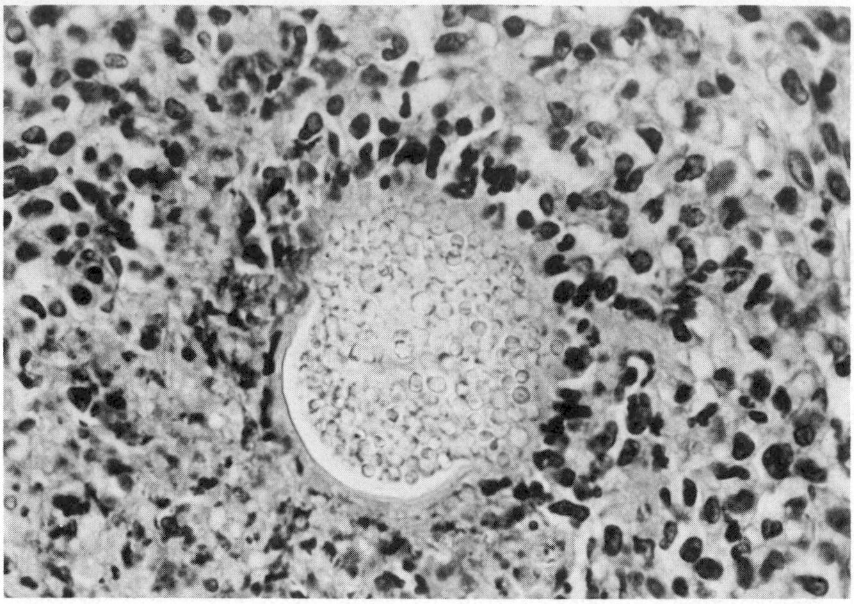

Figure 4. Chemotactic rush of neutrophilic leukocytes to the point where the endospores emerge from the rupturing spherule of *Coccidioides immitis.* Notice absence of neutrophils at lower left margin of spherule where its cell wall is intact.

emerge (Fig. 4). The attraction by the contents of the spherule is so great that neutrophils pour into the empty shell and seem to attack the inner wall even after the endospores are gone. The mechanism of this chemotaxis is not known, but in other infections chemotaxis results from the activation of complement by microbial antigens. This activation may occur via the classic or alternative pathway and generates chemotactic properties in the small peptides C3a and C5a, and in the trimolecular complex $\overline{C567}$. Bacterial proteases and proteases released from neutrophil granules can also attack C3 and C5 to produce chemotactic derivatives. In addition to complement factors, chemotactic products of a low molecular weight are elaborated by certain bacteria. Chemotactic factors, regardless of origin, probably create a concentration gradient that directs the phagocyte to its target. It is also possible that chemotactic factors bind to specific receptors on neutrophil or monocyte membranes and activate their contractile apparatus. Synthetic chemotactic peptides, which require a formyl group for chemotactic activity, attach to a specific formyl peptide receptor on the neutrophil membrane. Bacteria also produce N-formylated peptides (mol wt ~1000), which induce chemotaxis of neutrophils and monocytes (Ward and Kunkel, 1983). Anaerobic glycolysis appears to be the major energy source for chemotaxis in neutrophils because inhibitors of the glycolytic pathway depress chemotaxis but inhibitors of oxidative metabolism do not. Chemotaxis of leukocytes probably results from movements of actin and myosin, the contractile proteins of muscle, which are also present in phagocytes. Actin polymers in phagocytes form a tangled meshwork whose filaments are cross-linked by myosin and by actin-binding protein. It has been suggested that the cross-linked meshwork forms a rigid gel at the periphery of the cell ("cortical gel"), which provides the conditions for firm contractility that would be needed in pseudopods during chemotaxis and phagocytosis. The direction of movement of the phagocytic cell is thought to be determined by calcium concentrations greater than 2×10^{-7}M, which dissolve actin gel by activating a protein known as gelsolin. Calcium would thus create a gradient of actin gelation that controls directionality of movement (Yin and Stossel, 1982). This theory of phagocytic motility would take into account glycolysis as the energy source for chemotaxis, since ATP is required for movements of myosin and actin during contraction. It would also fit with the observation that cytochalasin B, which dissolves actin gels, inhibits phagocytosis by polymorphonuclear leukocytes and macrophages (Stossel, 1978).

After phagocytes reach their target and make contact, a microbe will be taken into the cell if their surfaces are properly attached. This attachment may depend partly on the hydrophobic character of the organism (Van Oss, 1978). Among the gram-negative bacteria, for example, smooth organisms with complete hydrophilic O polysaccharides are more resistant to phagocytosis than their rough hydrophobic mutants that are deficient in these surface sugars. Similarly, the hydrophilic polysaccharide capsules of pneumococci, *H. influenzae,* and *Klebsiella pneumoniae* make these bacteria more difficult for phagocytes to ingest than their unencapsulated variants. The opsonic activity of complement and specific antibody may also depend on their ability to make hydrophilic bacteria more hydrophobic. The Fc portion of IgG, which protrudes from the opsonized bacterial cell, is reported to be hydrophobic so that it can attach to the surface of the phagocytic cell. The surface protein (protein A) of *Staphylococcus aureus,* on the other hand, binds IgG by attaching to its Fc portion so that the hydrophilic Fab fragment protrudes. As a result, the opsonic property of IgG is subverted by virulent staphylococci and used instead to enhance their virulence by opposing phagocytosis.

Phagocytosis by both neutrophils and macrophages begins when proper contact is made with the microbial agent. The ingested particle is encircled by the phagocytic cell membrane through a process that combines invagination of the membrane and extrusion of pseudopods around the particle. The encirclement of the particle probably requires the participation of the contractile proteins (actin and myosin) and energy from ATP, as well as close adherence between particle and cell membrane and a sticky surface (Stossel, 1977). The sticky surface helps explain particle ingestion as well as why leukocytes stick to each other in clumps during phagocytosis and how the ends of pseudopods fuse to complete the encirclement. In neutrophils, the energy for engulfment comes primarily from anaerobic glycolysis. There are very few mitochondria in polymorphonuclear leukocytes, and Krebs cycle activity provides less than 20 per cent of ATP during glucose catabolism. Peritoneal and lung macrophages, on the other hand, have numerous mitochondria, and ATP is produced mainly from oxidative phosphorylation. Thus, inhibitors of oxidative metabolism (cyanide, dinitrophenol) inhibit ingestion by macrophages but not neutrophils, whereas inhibitors of glycolysis (iodoacetate, NaF) block phagocytosis by neutrophils but not macrophages.

Killing Within Phagocytes. Fusion of the pseudopods at their poles completes the encirclement of the particle by neutrophils and creates a phagocytic pouch, or vacuole, which separates from the cell membrane and moves centrally, accumulating cytoplasmic granules at its periphery (Fig. 5). The granules fuse to the membrane of the phagocytic vacuole and dissolve so that their contents empty into the vacuole. The azurophilic granules (purple color in Wright's stain), which have a dense appearance in the electron microscope, are actually lysosomes and release nucleases, lipases, acid phosphatase, elastase, collagenase, proteases, and other hydrolytic enzymes that digest dead organisms but are not bactericidal. The heme protein, myeloperoxidase (mw 150,000), and the mucopeptidase known as lysozyme are the important bactericidal enzymes released from azurophilic granules. Although neither kills pathogenic bacteria by itself, both help in such killing, as

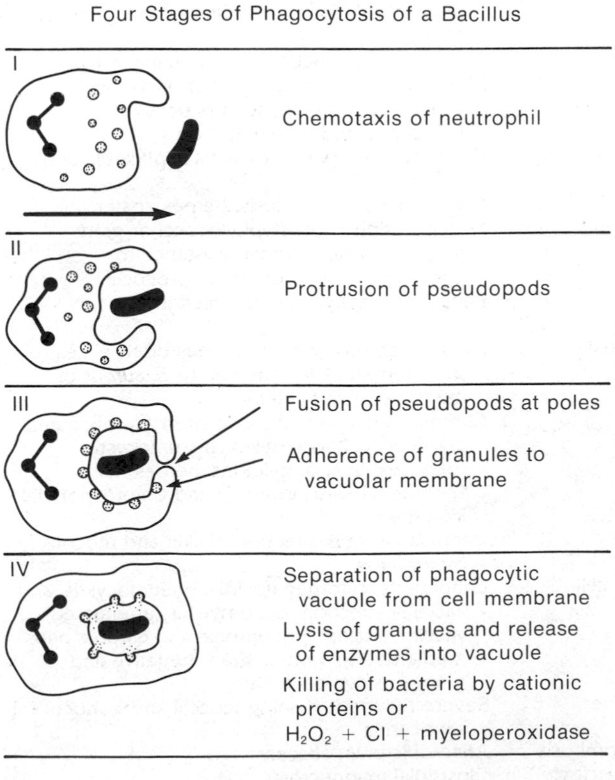

Figure 5. Phagocytosis.

described elsewhere. In the Chediak-Higashi syndrome there are giant lysosomal-like abnormal azurophilic granules in leukocytes that cannot degranulate properly, so that killing by phagocytes is defective and repeated staphylococcal infections occur in the lungs, skin, and upper respiratory tract. A second group of granules of lower density is known as secondary granules because they appear second in granulocyte maturation. They contain lactoferrin, a bacteriostatic iron-binding protein that resembles transferrin in depriving bacteria of iron. Another group of antibacterial proteins, known as cationic proteins because of their basic charge, is also present in secondary granules. These basic proteins attach to the negatively charged surface of bacteria and kill them through unknown mechanisms.

Another group of bactericidal substances is produced through a series of metabolic phenomena known as the "respiratory burst" (Babior, 1978). Phagocytosis is undiminished in the absence of oxygen, but killing of the ingested organism does not occur unless there is a sharp increase in oxygen uptake, which is the first event in the respiratory burst. This rise in leukocyte oxygen uptake is stimulated by opsonized bacteria and other particles and by C5a within 30 to 60 seconds after contact with the cell membrane. The immediate consequence of this sudden utilization of oxygen is the production of superoxide (O_2^-) by the one-electron reduction of oxygen in the following reaction: and activation of a membrane-bound oxidase that catalyzes the reduction of oxygen by NaDPH.

$$2O_2 + NADPH \longrightarrow 2O_2^- + NADP^+ + H^+$$

The enzyme superoxide dismutase then converts superoxide to hydrogen peroxide (H_2O_2):

$$2O_2^- + 2H^+ \xrightarrow[\text{dismutase}]{\text{superoxide}} O_2 + H_2O_2$$

The hydrogen peroxide then acts with myeloperoxidase and a halide to kill the bacteria in the phagocytic vesicle where the myeloperoxidase has been released upon lysis of the azurophilic granules. Although hydrogen peroxide can kill bacteria, its bactericidal activity is greatly increased in the presence of myeloperoxidase (Klebanoff, 1973). Myeloperoxidase, like other peroxidases, catalyzes oxidation by hydrogen peroxide. In the bactericidal reaction, Cl^+ appears to be the main substrate; it is oxidized to hypochlorite as follows:

$$Cl^- + H_2O_2 \xrightarrow[\text{myeloperoxidase}]{} ClO^- + H_2O$$

I^- and Br^- can also be oxidized in this reaction, which incorporates the halide in the bacterial cell. Halogenation of the bacteria is not entirely responsible for their death, however, and other unknown mechanisms must also be involved in the bactericidal effect of myeloperoxidase.

One of the key reactions in the metabolic burst is the hexose monophosphate shunt (HMP), which is the major source of NADPH, the reducing agent needed for production of superoxide. The first step in the shunt produces NADPH by the following reaction:

$$\text{Glucose-6-phosphate} + NADP^+ \xrightarrow[\text{G-6-PD}]{} \text{6 phosphogluconic acid} + NADPH$$

The reaction is catalyzed by G-6-PD (glucose-6-phosphate dehydrogenase). In the second HMP reaction more NADPH is produced as follows:

$$\text{6 phosphogluconic acid} + NADP^+ \xrightarrow[\text{dehydrogenase}]{\text{6-phosphogluconate}} NADPH + CO_2 + \text{ribulose-5-phosphate}$$

In patients whose leukocytes are deficient in G-6-PD, inadequate amounts of NADPH are generated after phagocytosis. The deficiency in NADPH results in less production of superoxide and, in turn, insufficient hydrogen peroxide for killing certain bacteria. This metabolic disturbance gives rise to increased susceptibility to pyogenic infections by *E. coli*, *K. pneumoniae*, and *S. aureus*.

The importance of hydrogen peroxide in killing bacteria is also evident from infections encountered in boys with chronic granulomatous disease (CGD), a disorder in which the respiratory burst and the production of hydrogen peroxide in leukocytes are selectively deficient. Their leukocytes kill streptococci but not staphylococci, so that they are prone to severe staphylococcal but not streptococcal infections. This difference is explained by the absence of catalase in streptococci and its presence in staphylococci. Catalase is needed to destroy hydrogen peroxide, so that hydrogen peroxide accumulates in streptococci and replaces the deficiency in peroxide within CGD neutrophils. In other words, streptococci provide the missing reagent that is needed for their own destruction by the bactericidal effect of myeloperoxidase-Cl-H_2O_2. Staphylococci possess catalase and thus protect themselves against this reaction by destroying the peroxide component.

The phagocytic cell protects itself from its own H_2O_2 by a glutathione-dependent detoxifying system (Voetman et al., 1980). This system, which consists of glutathione (GSH) plus the coupled enzymes glutathione peroxidase and glu-

Table 3. DEFICIENCY DISEASES AND OTHER DISORDERS OF NATURAL RESISTANCE TO INFECTION

Disorder	Immune Defect	Predominant Type of Infection
Immotile cilia	Loss of respiratory mucociliary clearance	Chronic airway infection
Achlorhydria	Loss of gastric bactericidal activity	Cholera, salmonellosis, shigellosis, giardiasis
Intestinal blind loop syndrome	Loss of small bowel motility	Overgrowth of small bowel with *B. fragilis* and deconjugation of bile salts causing malabsorption
Bruton's disease	Sex-linked agammaglobulinemia	Recurrent sinusitis, otitis, pneumonia, septicemia, and meningitis due to *Pneumococcus* and *H. influenzae;* also echovirus infections and encephalomyelitis
Acquired hypogammaglobulinemia (adult men and women)	Deficient specific antibody responses	Pneumococcal and *H. influenzae* sinusitis, conjunctivitis, pneumonia, and bacteremia; giardiasis
Selective IgA deficiency	IgA less than 5 mg per cent	Recurrent infections of sinuses, bronchi, and lung (esp. middle lobe) with viruses and bacteria; giardiasis
Multiple myeloma	Absence of specific antibody globulin	Pneumococcal pneumonia and bacteremia
Wiskott-Aldrich syndrome	Low serum IgM; inability to respond to immunization with polysaccharide antigens	Meningitis, otitis media, pneumonia, and septicemia due to pneumococcus, *H. influenzae,* and meningococcus
Tuftsin deficiency (congenital or after splenectomy)	Defective phagocytosis	Overwhelming pneumococcal septicemia and meningitis
Hodgkin's disease	Depressed cellular immunity	Cryptococcosis, listeriosis, herpes zoster
Chronic granulomatous disease	Inability to generate H_2O_2 in leukocytes	Fatal infections with staphylococci or gram-negative bacilli; normal resistance to pneumococci and other streptococci
Chediak-Higashi syndrome	Abnormal azurophilic leukocyte granules	Recurrent staphylococcal infection
Profound G-6-PD deficiency (< 5% of normal G-6-PD)	Deficient hexose-monophosphate-shunt activity	Same as chronic granulomatous disease, i.e., granulomatous lesions due to *S. aureus* or gram-negative bacteria
Acquired immunodeficiency syndrome (AIDS) and congenital thymic aplasia or hypoplasia	Depressed T-cell function	Chronic candidiasis; disseminated mycobacterial, cryptococcal, aspergillus, pneumocystis, toxoplasma, strongyloides, herpes (esp Cytomegalovirus in AIDS) and Cryptosporidial infections.
Chronic mucocutaneous candidiasis	Defective T-cell function	*Candida albicans* infection of skin and mucous membranes
Combined immunodeficiency (including Swiss-type, X-linked, or adenosine deaminase deficiency)	Complete absence of T and B cells	Candidiasis; cytomegalovirus, pneumocystis, and vaccinia infection; poliomyelitis (attenuated vaccine strains); pneumonia and chronic otitis media due to various gram-negative and gram-positive bacteria
Familial complement deficiency (C6, C8)	Loss of serum bactericidal power	Severe recurrent meningococcal and gonococcal septicemia
Cyanotic congenital heart disease	Polycythemia and cerebral thrombosis	Anaerobic brain abscess
Arteriosclerosis obliterans	Low redox potential of leg muscles	Clostridial myonecrosis

tathione reductase, reduces H_2O_2 to water by NaDPH via the following reactions:

$$2GSH + H_2O_2 \xrightarrow[\text{peroxidase}]{\text{glutathione}} GSSH + 2H_2O$$

$$GSSH + NADPH \xrightarrow[\text{reductase}]{\text{glutathione}} 2GSH + NADP$$

It must be emphasized that other systems for microbial killing exist within phagocytes and that the absence of peroxide-mediated killing does not necessarily promote infection. Alveolar macrophages, for example, have no peroxidase but kill ingested bacteria and fungal spores (Schaffner et al., 1983). Chickens and other birds have no peroxidase in their PMN leukocytes, but these cells kill bacteria and the birds are as resistant to infection as other animals. More important, patients with myeloperoxidase deficiency, in striking contrast to those with chronic granulomatous disease, are rarely troubled by infections (Babior, 1978).

It is also important to point out that in addition to PMN leukocytes, oxygen-dependent killing also appears to occur in mononuclear phagocytes. When these cells are activated, they respond with a respiratory burst and H_2O_2 generation during phagocytosis of some pathogenic organisms, but not all. Killing by macrophages depends on whether or not the ingested organisms initiate the respiratory burst, and are susceptible to killing by H_2O_2 and other reactive oxygen intermediates (Nathan, 1983).

DISEASES SECONDARY TO DISTURBANCES IN NATURAL RESISTANCE

A number of infections have been discussed in this chapter in relation to specific disturbances in natural resistance. These are summarized in Table 3. The disturbances in acquired cellular immunity described in the next chapter are also listed.

References

Afzelius, B.: A human syndrome caused by immotile cilia. Lancet 193:317, 1976.

Amberson, J. B.: A clinical consideration of abscesses and cavities of the lung. Bull Johns Hopkins Hosp 94:227, 1954.

Babior, B.: Oxygen-dependent microbial killing by phagocytes. N Engl J Med 298:659, 1978.

Barry, D., and Reeve, A.: Increased incidence of gram-negative neonatal sepsis with intramuscular iron administration. Pediatrics 60:908, 1977.

Beeson, P., and Goebel, W.: The immunological relationship of the capsular polysaccharide of type XIV pneumococcus to the blood group A substance. J Exp Med 70:239, 1939.

Beeson, P., Brannon, E. S., and Warren, J. V.: Observations on the sites of removal of bacteria from the blood of patients with bacterial endocarditis. J Exp Med 81:9, 1945.

Bloomfield, A. L.: The dissemination of bacteria in the upper air passages. I. The circulation of foreign particles in the mouth. Am Rev Tuberc 5:903, 1922.

Braude, B., and Carlson, A. J.: The influence of lymphagogues on the relative concentration of bacterioagglutinins in serum and lymph. Am J Physiol 21:221, 1908.

Braude, A., Corbeil, L., Levine, S., Ito, J., and McCutchan, J.: Possible influence of cyclic menstrual changes on resistance to the gonococcus. In Brooks, G., Gotschlich, E., Holmes, K., Sawyer, W., and Young, F. (eds.): Immunobiology of Neisseria Gonorrhoeae. Washington, D.C., American Society of Microbiology, 1978, p. 328.

Bruton, O.: Agammaglobulinemia. Pediatrics 9:722, 1952.

Catteral, R.: Influence of gestogenic contraceptive pills on vaginal Candidiasis. Br J Vener Dis 47:45, 1971.

Chernew, I., and Braude, A.: Depression of phagocytosis by solutes in concentrations found in the kidneys and urine. J Clin Invest 41:1945, 1962.

Constantopoulos, A., Najjar, V., and Smith, J.: Tuftsin deficiency: A new syndrome with defective phagocytosis. J Pediatr 80:564, 1972.

Culbertson, J. T.: Immunologic mechanisms in parasitic infections. In Most, H. (ed.): Parasitic Infections in Man. New York, Columbia University Press, 1951.

Donaldson, D.: Beta-lysin. In Schlesinger, D. (ed.): Microbiology, 1975. Washington, D.C., American Society Microbiology, 1975, p. 223.

Dubos, R. J.: Biochemical Determinants of Microbial Diseases. Cambridge, Mass., Harvard University Press, 1954.

Eliasson, R., Mossberg, B., Camner, P., and Afzelius, B.: A congenital ciliary abnormality as an etiologic factor in chronic airway infections and male sterility. N Engl J Med 297:1, 1977.

Fehleisen, F.: On erysipelas. In Cheyne, W. W. (ed.): Microparasites in Disease. London, New Sydenham Society, 1886, p. 261.

Felton, L., Prescott, B., Kauffmann, G., and Ottinger, B.: Antigens of vegetable origin active in pneumococcus infections. J Bacteriol 69:519, 1955.

Fenner, F.: Mouse-pox (infectious etromelia of mice): A review. J Immunol 63:341, 1949.

Fenner, F., McAuslan, B., Mims, C., Sambrook, J., and White, D.: The Biology of Animal Viruses, 2nd ed. New York, Academic Press, 1974, p. 363.

Field, M. E., Shaffer, M. F., Enders, J. F., and Drinker, C. K.: The distribution in the blood and lymph of pneumococcus type III injected intravenously into rabbits, and the effect of treatment with specific antiserum on the infection of the lymph. J Exp Med 65:469, 1937.

Fildes, P.: Tetanus: IX. The oxidation-reduction potential of the subcutaneous tissue fluid of the guinea pig: Its effect on infection. Br J Exp Pathol 10:197, 1929.

Garrod, L. P.: The susceptibility of different bacteria to destruction in the stomach. J Pathol Bacteriol 45:473, 1937.

Gillin, F., Reiner, D., and Wang, C.: Human milk kills parasitic intestinal protozoa. Science 221:1290, 1983.

Goldschneider, I., Gotschlich, E., and Artenstein, M.: Human immunity to the meningococcus. II. Development of natural immunity. J Exp Med 129:1385, 1969.

Hanke, M., and Bailey, J.: Oxidation-reduction potential requirements of *C. welchii* and other clostridia. Proc Soc Exp Biol Med 59:163, 1945.

Hauptman, S., and Tomasi, B.: The secretory immune system. In Fudenberg, H., Stites, D., Caldwell, J., and Wells, J. (eds.): Basic and Clinical Immunology, 2nd ed. Los Altos, Lange, 1978, p. 205.

Heidelberger, M., Avery, O., and Goebel, W.: A "soluble specific substance" derived from gum arabic. J Exp Med 49:847, 1929.

Hoogerheide, J. C.: Studies on capsule formation 1 conditions under which *Klebsiella pneumoniae* (Friedländer's bacteria) forms capsules. J. Bacteriol., 38:367, 1939.

Hornick, R., Greisman, S., Woodward, T., DuPont, H., Dawkins, A., and Snyder, M.: Typhoid fever. I. Pathogenesis and immunologic control. N Engl J Med 283:686, 1970.

Isaacs, A., and Lindenmann, J.: Virus interference. I. The interferons. Proc R Soc B147:258, 1957.

Johanson, W., Blackstock, R., Pierce, A., and Sanford, J.: The role of bacterial antagonism in pneumococcal colonization of the human pharynx. J Lab Clin Med 75:946, 1970.

Johnson, R., and Harris, V.: Antileptospiral activity of serum. II. Leptospiral virulence factors. J Bacteriol 93:513, 1967.

Klebanoff, S.: Myeloperoxidase-halide-hydrogen peroxide antibacterial system. J Bacteriol 95:2131, 1968.

Kligman, A., and Weidman, F.: Experimental studies on treatment of human torulosis. Arch Dermatol Syph 60:726, 1949.

Kluger, M., and Rothenburg, B.: Fever and reduced iron: Their interactions as a host defense response to bacterial infections. Science 203:374, 1979.

Kushner, I., and Feldman, G.: Control of the acute phase response: Demonstration of C-reactive protein synthesis and secretion by hepatocytes during acute inflammation in the rabbit. J Exp Med 148:466, 1978.

McCutchan, J., Wunderlich, A., and Braude, A.: The role of urinary solutes in natural immunity to gonorrhea. Infect Immun 15:149, 1977.

Marrack, J., and Carpenter, B.: The cross-reactions of vegetable gums with type II antipneumococcal serum. Br J Exp Pathol 19:53, 1938.

Mortenson, R., Braun, D., and Gewurz, H.: Effects of C-reactive protein on lymphocyte functions. III. Inhibition of antigen-induced lymphocyte stimulation and lymphokine production. Cell Immunol 28:59, 1977.

Nathan, C.: Mechanisms of macrophage antimicrobial activity. Trans Roy Soc Trop Med and Hyg 77:620, 1983.

Olling, S.: Sensitivity of Gram-negative bacilli to the serum bactericidal activity: A marker of the host-parasite relationship in acute and persisting infections. Scand J Infect Dis (Suppl), p. 8, 1977.

Pullinger, B. D., and Florey, H. W.: Some observations on the structure and functions of lymphatics: Their behaviour in local edema. Br J Exp Pathol 16:49, 1935.

Rank, R., White, H., Hough, A., Posley, J., and Barron, A.: Effect of estradiol on chlamydial genital infection of female guinea pigs. Infect and Imm 38:699, 1982.
Saene, H., Willems, F., and Zweens, J.: Influence of amoxycillin and cefaclor on the colonization resistance of the oropharynx. Scand J Inf Dis Suppl 39:97, 1983.
Sanders, W. E.: Interactions between streptococci and other bacteria in the throat. In Schlesinger, D. (ed.): Microbiology, 1975. Washington, D.C., American Society of Microbiology, 1975.
Sanders, C., and Sanders, W.: Enrocin: an antibiotic produced by *Streptococcus salivarius* that may contribute to protection against infections due to Group A streptococci. J Inf Dis 146:683, 1982.
Schaffner, A., Douglas, H., Braude, A., and Davis, C.: Killing of *Aspergillus* spores depends on the anatomical source of the macrophage. Infect Immun 42:1109, 1983.
Stossel, T.: How do phagocytes eat? Ann Int Med 89:398, 1978.
Stossel, T.: Phagocytosis. In Greenwalt, T., and Jamieson, G. (eds.): The Granulocyte in Function and Clinical Utilization. New York, Alan R. Liss, Inc., 1977, p. 87.
Stoughton, R. B.: Relation of the anatomy of normal and abnormal skin to its protective function, in Rothman, S.: The Human Integument, Washington, D.C., Am Assn Adv Sci 1959, p. 7.
Takeuchi, A.: Electronmicroscope observations on penetration of the gut epithelial barrier by *Salmonella typhimurium*. In Schlesinger, D. (ed.): Microbiology, 1975. Washington, D.C., American Society of Microbiology, 1975, p. 174.
Thomas, E., and Aune, T.: Lactoperoxidase, peroxide, thiocyanate antimicrobial system: Correlation of sulfhydril oxidation with antimicrobial action. Infect Immun 20:456, 1978.
Tillitt, W. S.: The bactericidal action of human serum on hemolytic streptococci. I. Observations made with serum from patients with acute infections and from normal individuals. J Exp Med 65:147, 1937.
Van Oss, C.: Phagocytosis as a surface phenomenon. Ann Rev Microbiol 32:19, 1978.
Voetman, A., Loos, J., and Roos, D.: Changes in the levels of glutathione in phagocytosing human neutrophils. Blood 55:741, 1980.
Ward, P. A., and Kunkel, S. L.: Bacterial virulence and the inflammatory system. Rev Inf Dis 5:5793, 1983.
Weinberg, E.: Iron and infection. Microbiol Rev 42:45, 1978.
Winberg, J., and Wessner, G.: Does breast milk protect against septicemia in the newborn? Lancet 1:1091, 1971.
Yin, H., and Stossel, T.: The mechanism of phagocytosis. In Karnovsky, M., and Bolis, L.: Phagocytosis - Past and Future, New York, Academic Press, 1983, p. 19.

88

MECHANISMS OF ACQUIRED RESISTANCE TO INFECTION

ABRAHAM I. BRAUDE, M.D., PH.D.

Untreated patients do not recover from an infection unless their resistance increases enough to overcome the infecting agent or its toxins. This state of increased resistance may be manifested in the following ways:

1. The person remains well upon re-exposure to the same pathogenic organism during epidemics with high attack rates. The solid life-long immunity to measles, chickenpox, rubella, and mumps illustrates the permanence of this acquired resistance against highly contagious viral infections.
2. The patient's blood inhibits the growth of the corresponding organism in vitro. This characteristic is typical of blood from patients who have recovered from streptococcal sore throats or pneumococcal pneumonia.
3. The patient's serum will protect laboratory animals from the infectious agent. This protection is found with serum obtained after infections by bacteria (Group A streptococci, pneumococci, diphtheria bacilli, *Klebsiella pneumoniae*, leptospiral organisms, and *Treponema pallidum*), all rickettsiae, all viruses, and certain parasites (*Toxoplasma gondii*).
4. The patient's serum will prevent infection of tissue cultures by the virus that caused the disease.
5. The patient's serum will damage the responsible microorganism (lysis of leptospira, meningococci, and *Hemophilus influenzae;* immobilization of *T. pallidum;* capsular swelling of pneumococci, *K. pneumoniae,* and *H. influenzae;* and distortion of toxoplasmas).

These signs of resistance are specific: The activity of the serum or blood and the resistance of the patient are directed only against the species or serologic type of infectious agent responsible for the illness. They are mediated by specific antibodies that are generated during the early stages of infection and increase as the patient recovers from the illness. In some infections lymphocytes and macrophages are also thought to be involved in acquired immunity to infection.

ACQUIRED HUMORAL IMMUNITY. As in any type of primary immune response, whether to living or dead antigens, the early humoral response to infection is predominantly IgM. Within ten days, however, IgG begins to appear and thereafter exceeds and outlasts IgM. IgM, which is heavier (M.W. 900,000, sedimentation coefficient 19S), tends to remain within the blood vessels and does not cross the placenta. IgG is smaller (M.W. 146,000, sedimentation coefficient 7S) and is actively transported across the placenta. Thus, IgG is responsible for the long-term immunity against many systemic infections and prevents many bacterial and viral infections in the newborn, whose immune system is undeveloped.

Opsonins. The mechanism of protection by IgG varies with the organism. As noted in the previous chapter, IgG is opsonic and protects against infections by pneumococci, *H. influenzae*, *K. pneumoniae*, group B *Streptococcus*, *Escherichia coli*, and certain other gram-negative bacilli by combining through its Fab portion with the capsular or K antigens. The Fc portion of the IgG attaches at the same time to surface receptors on neutrophilic leukocytes, so that an opsonic bridge occurs between bacterial cell and phagocyte. IgG, as well as IgM, can also promote phagocytosis after combining with bacterial antigens by activating complement via the classic pathway, so that opsonin is generated in the form of activated C3. Opsonins are also important in acquired resistance to *Streptococcus* group A, but they do not react with the streptococcal capsule. The reason for this is that the capsule of group A streptococci is composed of hyaluronic acid, a normal constituent of connective tissues, so that antibody is not produced against it. Instead, opsonins for the group A *Streptococcus* are directed against its M protein, which is carried on fimbria. Since the fimbria extend beyond the capsule, the overlying M protein antigen can react with specific anti-M IgG and thwart the antiphagocytic effect of the capsule.

Antitoxins. Most bacteria are pathogenic by virtue of their exotoxins, and antibody must neutralize these toxins to provide protection. Recovery from diphtheria is accompanied by the production of antitoxin, which appears to prevent the attachment of toxin to cells. The evidence supporting this mode of protection by antitoxin comes from observations with fragments A and B of diphtheria toxin. Fragment A has the enzymatic (or toxic) activity and fragment B is necessary for attachment and transport into the susceptible cell. When separate antisera that are specific for either the A or the B fragment are prepared, only the antibody against the B fragment will neutralize the toxin, apparently by interfering with its attachment to cells. In addition to blocking the attachment of toxin to substrate, antibody can accelerate the clearance of the toxic antigen from the circulation before it reaches susceptible cells. Recovery from diphtheria is accompanied by the production of antitoxin, which protects against toxin elaborated in the later stages of infection. Early in the infection, toxin combines with cells before antibody is produced and probably becomes inaccessible to neutralization. After recovery from diphtheria, the active production of diphtheria antitoxin gives protection for years, and its concentration in the body is probably increased periodically as a result of subclinical exposure to the diphtheria bacillus. With the Schick test, antitoxin can be demonstrated by its ability to neutralize the small amount of toxin that is injected into the skin.

Recovery from streptococcal infections is likewise accompanied by the development of antibodies against streptococcal toxins, but none of these antitoxins are known to bring about recovery. Antibodies against streptococcal hemolysin (streptolysin O), fibrinolysin (streptokinase), deoxyribonuclease (streptodornase), and hyaluronidase may all rise in titer as the streptococcal infection subsides but contribute little if anything to protection against the diseases caused by group A streptococci. Thus, sera containing high titers of antistreptolysin O cannot protect animals against *Streptococcus* group A unless antibody to M protein is also present. Antibody to streptococcal erythrogenic toxin will prevent the rash of scarlet fever but not streptococcal infections.

Aside from diphtheria there is no evidence that infection by toxin-producing bacteria produces a protective antitoxin or subsequent immunity. Second attacks of tetanus have occurred because the disease is produced by quantities of toxin that are too small to be antigenic. The lethal dose of botulinus toxin, which is even more potent than tetanus toxin, is also less than the antigenic dose. Protective antisera against the clostridial toxins can be prepared, however, by immunizing with toxoids made from the toxins of *C. botulinum*, *C. tetani*, and *C. perfringens*.

The endotoxins of gram-negative bacteria also produce protective antitoxins (i.e., antiendotoxins) after immunization with the lipopolysaccharide (LPS) or the whole bacterial cell. The LPS from smooth bacteria stimulates primarily antibody to the O antigenic side chains, and LPS from rough bacteria stimulates antibody to the core (see Chapter 6). Antibody to either O or core antigens of endotoxin can prevent all toxic manifestations of endotoxin, including the local Shwartzman reaction, generalized Shwartzman reaction, and death. Antibody to endotoxin can also protect experimental animals from bacteremias due to gram-negative bacteria. The protection by O antibody is specific and is limited to homologous endotoxins or bacteria, whereas that by core antibody gives broad protection against a wide range of different bacteria and their endotoxins (Braude et al., 1977). Antibody against endotoxin also protects against gram-negative bacteremia in patients. Antigens prepared by vaccinating human subjects with a rough mutant of *E. coli* neutralized the toxicity of LPS in animals and lowered the mortality from severe gram-negative bacteremia by 50 per cent (Ziegler et al., 1982).

Lysins. In addition to preparing the pathogen for phagocytosis or neutralizing its toxin, antibody may destroy it by uniting with its antigens. Destruction of a microorganism, however, is not a universal feature of antibody activity; it is observed with certain gram-negative bacteria, spirochetes, leptospiras, protozoa, and viruses but not with gram-positive bacteria or fungi. Even when antibodies protect against infection by gram-positive bacteria, the antibodies are not lethal to them in vitro.

As noted in the preceding chapter, lysis of gram-negative bacteria by IgG or IgM requires the participation of complement. Perhaps the most important examples of protection by *acquired* bacteriolytic antibodies are those against the meningococcus and *H. influenzae*. In both cases, the bacteriolytic antibody acquired through infection is specifically directed against the capsules. In addition to bacteria, trypanosomes are susceptible to immune lysis. In studying this phenomenon in rats infected with *T. lewisi*, Taliaferro (1938) noted that the infected animal resorts to three mechanisms for disposing of the parasite: lysis, phagocytosis, and inhibition of reproduction. The power of reproduction was lost near the sixth day of infection, and soon afterward the parasites were killed by lysis and phagocytosis. The lysis was caused by the action of antibody plus complement, and was manifested by a precipitous fall in the number of trypanosomes in the blood after the tenth day. Despite these dramatic effects of antibodies, they soon become impotent because the surface antigens of trypanosomes are changed at each succeeding cycle of infection. Although these new antigenic variants are removed by the specific antibody they later stimulate, the next cycle of trypanosomal variants will not be susceptible to existing antibody. As many as 100 successive variants may occur, thus enabling the trypanosome to keep one step ahead of the antibody response. This phenomenon could explain why large amounts of IgM are produced in the serum and cerebrospinal fluid of patients with trypanosomiasis. Most of this immunoglobulin does not react with the trypanosome, possibly because it was stimulated by variants with different antigenic specificities.

Antiparasitic. In malaria a different mechanism seems to bring recovery from infection. In this disease, recovery and protection are best correlated with antimerozoite IgG, which probably blocks the invasion of red cells by the parasite. The antibody is primarily strain-specific but also offers some protection against other strains of the same species. The antimalarial IgG persists for relatively long periods and protects newborns and infants by passing the placental barrier and by appearing in breast milk. These antibodies develop slowly, and several infections are sometimes required before immunity to malaria occurs. There are at least three reasons for this sluggish immune response: (1) Malaria suppresses immunity (Williamson and Greenwood, 1978). Humoral immunity is affected more than cellular immunity, probably because macrophages no longer process antigens normally. Immunity to both malaria and other infections is probably suppressed. (2) Immunity is stage-specific, so that different antigens determine immunity for each extrahepatic stage in the cycle of parasitic development. Thus, specific antibody is needed against the sporozoite introduced by the mosquito bite, against the merozoites present in red cells, and against the gametocytes that transmit the parasites to the blood-feeding mosquito (Deans and Cohen, 1983). (3) In certain forms of malaria, variation can occur among surface antigens as in trypanosomiasis (Brown and Brown, 1965).

Immunity also develops to worms. A study by Taliaferro and Sarles (1939) of immunity to nematodes in rats demonstrated that *Nippostronglyus muris* may become exposed to lethal antibody by penetrating the intestinal wall and feeding on blood and tissue fluids. Antibody in these fluids forms a precipitate around the mouth of the parasite and seals the genital pore so that egg production is prevented. Unable to obtain nourishment or reproduce, the adult worm may be dislodged by peristalsis.

Humoral antibody is probably involved in immunity to other nematodes. Antibodies act in conjunction with eosinophils to protect against *Trichinella spiralis* by attacking adult worms in the gut and larvae en route or in the muscle. The immune response, which is elicited by products secreted by both larvae and adults, can reduce fertility of the adult, eliminate the adult before it engages in maximum production of larvae, or prevent the establishment of larvae in muscle. In other words, immunity reduces the number of larvae that can reach muscle and thus reduces the severity of the disease (Despommier, 1977). The role of eosinophils in controlling trichinosis in mice was convincingly demonstrated by eliminating these cells with antiserum against eosinophils. Treatment of mice with this antiserum, which depletes eosinophils selectively and affects no other leukocytes, caused a rise in tissue larvae to twice the number found in control mice (Ellner and Mahmoud, 1982).

Antibody and eosinophils also operate together in killing schistosomules, the first stage in development of *Schistosoma mansoni* infection after penetration of the skin by cercariae. In the presence of IgG antibody from infected patients, both eosinophils and macrophages kill schistosomules. This process, called *antibody-dependent cell-mediated cytotoxicity*, works differently for different cells and immunoglobulins. For example, IgG can behave like any opsonin, attaching via the Fab portion to the target and via Fc to the killer cell. IgE, on the other hand, can bind to the surface of macrophages and activate them so that they kill schistosomules. This type of macrophage activation may involve complexes composed of schistosome antigens with IgE antibody and is specific; that is, other parasites are not injured by these macrophages. Immune serum containing high levels of IgE-immune complexes can protect against experimental schistosomiasis (Capron et al., 1977).

Antiviral. Opsonization and immune-lysis are also involved in acquired resistance to virus infections after intravenous injection. Opsonic activity was demonstrated by Mims (1964), who injected complexes of mousepox virus and antibody intravenously and found that they were taken up by macrophages in the liver. Virus alone entered hepatic parenchymal cells and multiplied there, whereas virus injected with antibody disappeared after ingestion by macrophages. Immune lysis by antiviral antibody plus complement has been observed with enveloped viruses such as rubella and influenza viruses. Under electronmicroscopy, holes have been seen that appear to be punched through the envelope by complement (Almeida and Lawrence, 1969). Other structural changes have been identified in viruses after neutralization and exposure to complement. For example, studies with equine enteritis virus have shown that ribonucleases can penetrate the injured virus membrane after neutralization by antibody plus complement, and release the RNA from within the nucleocapsid (Radwan and Crawford, 1974). Although antibody on the surface of a virus particle can simply block viral attachment and penetration of susceptible cells, many exceptions to this process have been noted. There is good evidence, in fact, that the reverse may sometimes occur—namely, that antibody may help entry of virus particles into such cells. When particles of certain viruses such as vaccinia, poliovirus, and Newcastle disease virus are taken into cells in the presence of neutralizing antibody, the cells may not be infected and the virus is degraded (Doles and Kajiola, 1964; Silverstein and Marcus, 1964). Even though the target cells are not "professional" phagocytes (such as polymorphonuclears or macrophages), they confine the ingested virus to the phagocytic vesicle where nucleases and other lysosomal enzymes can degrade it. Thus, under some circumstances antibody seems to prevent the type of penetration by viruses that would enable them to appropriate the biosynthetic apparatus of the cell, and instead produces opsonization, phagocytosis, and destruction of virus particles by cells that are not customarily regarded as phagocytic.

Antibody may also prevent attachment of viruses to susceptible target cells by changing the viral surface charge and shape, by blocking critical sites for attachment of virus to cell, and by clumping virus particles so that many are sequestered within the aggregate. Autoaggregation, or clumping, of virus particles in the absence of antibody may have the reverse effect, that is, prevention of neutralization because the virus in the center of the clump is protected from antibody. Neutralization also depends on the number of immunoglobulin molecules and the fractions of complement. Many immunoglobulin molecules must attach to each virus particle to neutralize its infectivity; one antibody molecule is not enough. Complement is an important accessory factor in neutralization of viruses and can help to coat the virus surface, agglutinate the particles, or induce lysis of the virion. Studies with herpes simplex virus show that C1 is ineffective but sequential incubation with C4, C2, and C3 contributes to neutralization by coating the viral surface rather than by virolysis (Daniels, 1975). The lysis of enveloped viruses described earlier requires the terminal components (C5 through C9). Antibodies on the viral surface may not be able to neutralize infectivity if they are too few or are bound to sites that are not critical for infection. These antibody-viral complexes may circulate and remain infectious, as in experimental infection with lymphocytic choriomeningitis virus. Viral-antibody complexes can be neutralized, however, through the participation of antiglobulins such as rheumatoid factor. One of the rheumatoid factors is a large globulin (M.W. 900,000) of the IgM class that attaches to the Fc portion of IgG. Upon combining with IgG-virus complexes, rheumatoid factor itself does not reduce infectivity but allows complement to do so. Since antiglobulins appear during convalescence from cytomegalovirus, Epstein-Barr, hepatitis B, rubella, and influenza virus infection, it is possible that they contribute to recovery by participating in viral neutralization.

The exact contribution of specific antibody to recovery from viral infection in patients is not easy to identify in many cases because cell-mediated immunity can also protect against viruses. Patients with X-linked agammaglobulinemia, for example, have recurrent bacterial infections but usually respond normally to viral infections. The exceptions are the picornaviruses, especially echovirus, coxsackievirus, and poliovirus, which produce severe progressive infections in agammaglobulinemic persons (Cooper et al., 1983). Echovirus depresses cell-mediated immunity so that agammaglobulinemics are left with no defense against this virus and die from progressive meningoencephalitis and dermatomyositis (Mease et al., 1981). The key role of antibody against this disease is brought out by its cure with specific intravenous immune globulin.

ACQUIRED SECRETORY IMMUNITY. The agents of most infectious diseases enter the body through mucous surfaces where secretory rather than humoral antibody may be important in recovery from and protection against infection. The importance of secretory IgA in natural resistance to infection is discussed in the preceding chapter. Its role in acquired resistance was discovered by Burrows in studies with experimental cholera (Burrows et al., 1947). He demonstrated that protection against infection after cholera vaccination was correlated with fecal antibody rather than with serum antibody. The ability of cholera vaccine to protect as many as 60 per cent of humans against cholera shows the significance of Burrow's experimental findings in clinical medicine. Furthermore, protection against cholera by vaccines that contain killed vibrios shows that antibacterial rather than antitoxic immunity can produce acquired resistance. Much evidence suggests that secretory immunity against cholera vibrios is mediated primarily by antibody that blocks their attachment to the intestinal mucosa rather than by complement-mediated reactions such as bacteriolysis or opsonization by neutrophils. IgA cannot fix C1 (Ishizaka et al., 1966), and its bactericidal activity via the alternative complement pathway has been observed only under special conditions that would not exist in the anticomplementary milieu of the gut. The idea that IgA blocks attachment of vibrios is supported by Freter's report (1969) that coproantibodies (fecal antibodies) sharply reduced the number of vibrios that adhered either to the mucosa in isolated loops of rabbit intestine or to viable slices of rabbit ileum. Coproantibody also inhibited the growth of *V. cholera* in the presence of viable mucosal cells, but the mechanism of such growth inhibition is unknown.

Other pathogenic bacteria adhere selectively to certain mucosal surfaces. Thus group A streptococci attach to human pharyngeal cells much better than *E. coli*, whereas *E. coli* adhere to bladder mucosa much better than group A streptococci (Gibbons, 1977). Similarly, gonococci and group B streptococci adhere to vaginal epithelial cells in larger numbers than *E. coli*, *Bacteroides fragilis*, fusobacteria, and lactobacilli (Mardh and Westrom, 1976). Adherence to intestinal epithelium likewise appears to determine the virulence of various enteric pathogens such as *Shigella* and enteropathogenic *E. coli*. This selective adherence of bacteria to certain epithelial cells seems to parallel their relative ability to produce infection in tissues or organs covered by these cells. The surface components of bacteria that are responsible for adherence seem to vary with the organisms and the mucosal surface. There is evidence, for example, that the following surface components are involved in adherence: lipoteichoic acid and surface fibrils for group A streptococci (Beachey, 1975); pili for gonococci, *E. coli*, and *Proteus;* and flagella for *V. cholerae* (Jones and Freter, 1972). The surface components of epithelial cells responsible for adherence seem to be primarily glycoproteins (Gibbons, 1977). Similar glycoproteins are abundant in the mucus that bathes these cells and can apparently block adherence of pathogenic bacteria by competing for attachment sites on the surface of these organisms. The increased flow of mucus during respiratory, intestinal, and genital infections could thus interrupt their spread by delivering two proteins, IgA and glycoprotein, that might block further adherence of pathogenic bacteria to the diseased mucosa. Because secretory IgA is also antitoxic it may contribute to recovery from diphtheria, cholera, and diarrhea caused by the enterotoxins of *E. coli* (Stoliar et al., 1976). Thus, acquired secretory immunity might be both antitoxic and antibacterial. These attractive hypotheses, however, need more critical experimental support. Indirect support for the protective property of secretory IgA comes from the observation that certain pathogenic bacteria are armed with proteases that split IgA1 by attacking a heavy-chain hinge region (Plaut, 1983). As a result the Fab and Fc regions are separated from each other and are no longer functional. Since these IgA proteases are elaborated only by pathogenic bacteria, which initiate infection by attaching to epithelial membranes, but not by nonpathogenic organisms on mucous membranes, they strongly imply that a protective property of IgA must be overcome in order for these organisms to initiate infection. Gonococci, meningococci, *Hemophilus influenzae*, pneumococci, and *Streptococcus sanguis* all produce IgA protease, but closely related genera in the same species, which are nonpathogenic, are IgA protease negative.

There is more convincing evidence that immunity against virus infections is acquired by the local production of secretory IgA on mucosal surfaces. This antibody, however, may be more important in providing immunity against reinfection than in recovery from infection. In influenza, for example, IgA appears in nasal washings early during the infection, but its antiviral activity is directed against strains of influenza virus that produced outbreaks in the past. This early IgA seems to be antibody stored in epithelial cells and has been found in both the respiratory and the intestinal mucosa (Kaur et al., 1972). It has no activity against the virus causing the infection and contributes nothing to recovery. Specific secretory IgA with activity against the infecting virus does not appear until two to three weeks after the onset of infection and long after the infection has ended (Alford et al., 1967). For this reason, other processes such as interferon production or cell-mediated immunity are thought to bring about recovery.

The presence of secretory antibody on mucous surfaces acquired after local infection or local inoculation of vaccines can be correlated with resistance to infection by rhinovirus, influenza virus, parainfluenza virus, and polioviruses. The IgA response to local inoculation of living viruses is better than the response to inactivated viruses, and live virus may also produce a systemic humoral immune response. The ability of local antibody to protect against mucosal viral infection was shown by studies in which local inoculation of inactivated viruses gave protection when local but not systemic antibody was elaborated. Two striking differences have been noted between local and systemic immunization. For one thing, local immunization of mucous membranes tends to produce a very localized IgA response, which is restricted to the immunized or infected site and does not appear on other mucous membranes. Second, local immunization does not seem to evoke a secondary or booster type of secretory IgA response. Studies on the secondary IgA response are limited, but local vaccination by intranasal instillation of inactivated poliovaccine produced no difference in the quantity or duration of poliovirus antibody after primary and secondary immunization. The absence of a booster effect indicates that the secretory IgA response to poliovirus may be devoid of immunologic memory, and that long-lasting protection after primary immunization may result from continued local antibody synthesis in response to prolonged stimulation by persistent antigen (Ogra et al., 1975).

NONPROTECTIVE ANTIBODY ACQUIRED DURING INFECTION. Not all antibodies acquired after infection or vaccination can protect against infection, despite their specificity for antigens in the infectious agent. These nonprotective antibodies react with antigens that are not responsible for virulence and are often released from beneath the surface of the infecting agent. The C polysaccharide of streptococci, the structural components of virions, the teichoic acids of staphylococci, the nucleoprotein of *Brucella*, the cell-wall polysaccharide of *B. anthracis*, and the polysaccharides of mycobacteria are examples of antigens that generate specific but nonprotective antibodies during infection. Nonprotective antibodies also develop to viral enzymes that participate in the manufacture of structural proteins and nucleic acids. In fact, antibodies that develop during viral infection may be directed against antigens that are elaborated during viral synthesis but are never incorporated into the virion. The various antibodies that have no role in protection are identified by complement fixation, agglutination, or precipitation and are often useful for diagnosis.

ACQUIRED CELLULAR IMMUNITY. The increased resistance observed after certain infections, such as those caused by mycobacteria and fungi, is not always accompanied by protective antibody in the blood or body fluids. Persons who have overcome the infection are more resistant to exogenous infection than previously uninfected persons. Although precipitins and complement-fixing antibodies may be present at some stage in these infections, many healthy persons who have recovered from all clinical signs of the disease possess no detectable antibodies for the infectious agent. This type of acquired resistance without demonstrable antibody is manifested by an intense local inflammatory response to the living organisms or to their products. The local reaction is more intense and appears more rapidly than that in the nonimmune individual and prevents the extension of the organism to the regional lymph nodes. Because this reaction is marked by an intense infiltration of inflammatory cells, it is sometimes spoken of as *cellular immunity*, a term that implies a specific increase in the capacity of the cells themselves to resist infection.

Although cellular immunity has been regarded as the basis of acquired resistance to infection in various bacterial, fungal, viral, and parasitic infections, the most important original discoveries in this field were made by Robert Koch (1891) in his studies of experimental tuberculosis. Koch described his discovery of the altered response to tuberculous reinfection in the following manner:

> If a normal guinea pig is inoculated with a pure culture of tubercle bacilli, the wound, as a rule, closes and in the first few days seemingly heals. After ten to fourteen days, however, there appears a firm nodule which soon opens, forming an ulcer that persists until the animal dies. Quite different is the result if a tuberculous guinea pig is inoculated with tubercle bacilli. For this purpose it is best to use animals that have been infected four to six weeks previously. In such an animal, also, the little inoculation wound closes at first, but in this case no nodule is formed. On the next, or second day, however, a peculiar change occurs at the inoculation site. The area becomes indurated and assumes a dark color, and these changes do not remain limited to the inoculation point, but spread to involve an area 0.5 to 1.0 cm in diameter. In the succeeding days it becomes evident that the altered skin is necrotic. It finally sloughs, leaving a shallow ulcer which usually heals quickly and permanently, and the regional lymph nodes do not become infected. The action of tubercle bacilli upon the skin of a normal guinea pig is thus entirely different from their action upon the skin of a tuberculous one. This striking effect is produced not only by living tubercle bacilli but also by dead bacilli, whether killed by prolonged low temperature, by boiling, or by certain chemicals.

This remarkable observation by Koch brought out two essential features of the immune response in tuberculosis:

1. *A hypersensitivity reaction to the tubercle bacillus.* The effect of hypersensitivity is to produce an accelerated inflammatory response upon reinfection. This accelerated reaction was actually first described by Jenner with cowpox when he vaccinated people who had recovered from smallpox.

2. *Increased resistance to tuberculosis.* The bacteria are confined to the site of inoculation. In contrast to primary infection, they do not spread to the regional lymph nodes or beyond.

The hypersensitivity reaction in tuberculosis is called "delayed" hypersensitivity because it is not noticed until after 24 hours. It differs from the immediate type of hypersensitivity in anaphylaxis, which elicits tissue reactions within minutes after the antigen is injected. Delayed hypersensitivity is also different from the Arthus reaction, which begins in a few hours after challenge with antigen. These two rapid forms of hypersensitivity require a reaction between antigen and antibody, but delayed hypersensitivity does not. Delayed hypersensitivity is seen in all forms of infection but has special significance in those diseases in which immunity is not acquired through circulating antibody. This is true in all fungus infections; in such bacterial infections as leprosy, brucellosis, tularemia, lymphopathia venereum, and syphilis; in smallpox and certain other virus infections; and in various parasitic infections, including cutaneous leishmaniasis and schistosomiasis.

Because acquired immunity develops simultaneously with hypersensitivity in these diseases, because the two phenomena share the same inflammatory reaction, and because humoral antibody provides no resistance against these infections, it is generally assumed that delayed hypersensitivity can produce this form of acquired resistance. The inflammatory cells in delayed hypersensitivity are those that are important in resistance to infection. When a moderate or large dose of organisms or their antigens is injected into an infected individual, many polymorphonuclear cells appear, followed by mononuclear phagocytes (macrophages), which tend to arrange themselves in sheetlike aggregates and in tubercles. When a very small concentration of organisms is inoculated, only mononuclear phagocytes may appear. These polymorphonuclear and mononuclear cells can kill bacteria and other organisms, and their accelerated delivery to the site of infection in delayed hypersensitivity is associated with a more rapid disappearance of organisms than in controls.

In addition to this accelerated migration, reinfection stimulates macrophages to greater phagocytosis and killing.

Because of these increased activities, they have been designated "activated" macrophages. Activation generally occurs after infection by organisms that reside within macrophages. Once activated by such infection, macrophages provide increased resistance against infections caused by other unrelated organisms. This increase in nonspecific resistance is accompanied by greater nonspecific killing of injected organisms. For example, macrophages from animals infected with either *Listeria monocytogenes* or *Salmonella typhimurium* can kill *S. typhimurium* equally well (Blanden et al., 1966). The increased antimicrobial properties of activated macrophages are accompanied by other functional and morphologic changes. They are larger than normal macrophages, spread out more and adhere better to glass, and have more cytoplasmic granules. They also utilize more glucose through the hexose monophosphate shunt and have more activity of certain enzymes, such as the membrane enzyme adenylate cyclase and the cytoplasmic enzyme lactic dehydrogenase. They also have more lysosomes with their hydrolytic enzymes.

Lymphocytes also play an important part in cellular immunity by regulating macrophage activity. Soon after reinfection occurs with the intracellular bacteria that induce delayed hypersensitivity, specifically sensitized T lymphocytes react with the bacterial antigens and release substances, known as lymphokines, into the infected tissues. These lymphokines, which are chemotactic, attract macrophages to the infection and activate them. The specifically sensitized T lymphocytes have long lives and can provide long-lasting specific resistance to reinfection by reactivating macrophages. The macrophages, on the other hand, lose their activation within a few weeks. Generally speaking, humoral antibody is involved in these reactions only under exceptional circumstances such as trichinosis and schistosomiasis. Experimental studies indicate that acquired immunity in these parasitic infections results from a form of cellular immunity that is dependent on antibody. The role of humoral antibody in rejecting the invading larvae (schistosomules) has been established by passive transfer of immunity with immune serum. The antibody involved is IgE, which interacts with both macrophages and eosinophils, so that both cells then kill the parasite (Capron et al., 1977).

The importance of lymphocytes in resistance to protozoa has become obvious in the acquired immunodeficiency syndrome, or AIDS (Fauci et al., 1984) (Chapter 273). Patients with this disorder suffer from severe recurrences of cerebral toxoplasmosis, pneumocytis pneumonia, and cryptosporidiosis of the small bowel (Wong et al., 1984; Payne et al., 1983). Since the basic immune disturbance in these patients is a defect in T lymphocyte function, their unique susceptibility to these protozoal infections is undoubtedly a consequence of this lymphocyte disorder. In addition to these intracellular protozoa, other intracellular organisms, such as mycobacteria, cytomegalovirus, Herpes simplex virus, and varicella-zoster virus are prominent causes of disease in AIDS.

The mechanisms of cellular immunity in virus infections are still obscure, even though delayed hypersensitivity was first described with inoculation of vaccinia virus by Jenner in 1798. One reason for the difficulty in identifying the cell-mediated component of antiviral immunity is that humoral antibody usually affords prominent protection and may overshadow cellular immune processes. According to current evidence, antibody functions mainly by preventing viral infection and limiting its extracellular spread, and cell-mediated immunity functions by eliminating virus-infected cells. In patients suffering from diseases or receiving drugs that would be expected to lower cellular immunity, there is a predilection for infection with four viruses that acquire their envelope from nuclear or cytoplasmic membranes of infected cells: measles, cytomegalovirus, varicella-zoster, and herpes simplex. These viruses cause severe recurrent infections in patients given immunosuppressive therapy, and children with congenital immunodeficiencies. Since the antigens of these membrane-associated viruses are incorporated in the membrane of the infected cell, they are available on the cell surface for reactions with the inflammatory cells involved in delayed hypersensitivity. This idea gains support from the fact that infections by all membrane-associated viruses are followed by delayed hypersensitivity reactions to the specific viral antigens (Bloom and Rager-Zisman, 1975).

At least three mechanisms have been postulated to explain how cell-mediated reactions could work against virus infections. One is by a reaction of T cells against virus-infected cells. Purified T lymphocytes can lyse target cells containing specific membrane antigens (Henney, 1973). A second potential mechanism involves interferon production by activated lymphocytes. Viral antigens can cause blast cell transformation of specifically immune lymphocytes and the secretion of lymphokines, including interferon. The secretion of lymphokines with chemotactic activity could attract macrophages that can inactivate viruses, including viruses that have combined with antibody. Because macrophages have receptors for the Fc portion of IgG molecules, virus-antibody complexes can be attacked, ingested, and degraded. In the third mechanism, infected cells containing viral antigens in their membranes would be recognized as foreign and rejected by a cell-mediated reaction.

Each of these theoretical processes for mediating cellular immunity in virus infections has been demonstrated in systems examined in vitro. Until these have been found to operate in vivo as well, the mechanisms of cell-mediated immunity in human viral infections will continue to be speculative.

References

Alford, R., Rossen, R., Butler, W., and Kasel, J.: Neutralizing and hemagglutination-inhibiting activity of nasal secretions following experimental human infection with A_2 influenza virus. J Immunol 98:724, 1967.

Almeida, J., and Lawrence, G.: Heated and unheated antiserum on rubella virus. Am J Dis Child 118:101, 1969.

Beachey, E.: Binding of group A streptococci to human oral mucosal cells by lipoteichoic acid. Trans Assoc Am Phys 88:285, 1975.

Blarden, R., Mackaness, G., and Collins, F.: Mechanisms of acquired resistance in mouse typhoid. J Exp Med 124:585, 1966.

Bloom, B., and Rager-Zisman, B.: Cell-mediated immunity in viral infections. In Notkins, A. (ed.): Viral Immunology and Immunopathology. New York, Academic Press, 1975, p. 113.

Braude, A., Ziegler, E., Douglas, H., and McCutchan, J.: Protective properties of antisera to R core. In Schlesinger, D. (ed.): Microbiology, 1977. Washington, D.C., American Society for Microbiology, 1977, p. 253.

Brown, K., and Brown, I.: Immunity to malaria: Antigenic variation to chronic infections of *Plasmodium knowlesi*. Nature 208:1286, 1965.

Burrows, W., Elliott, M., and Havens, I.: Studies on immunity to asiatic cholera. IV. The excretion of coproantibody in experimental enteric cholera in the guinea pig. J Infect Dis 81:261, 1947.

Capron, A., Dessaint, J., Joseph, M., Torpier, G., Capron, M., Rousseaux, R., Santoro, F., and Bazin, H.: IgE and cells in schistosomiasis. Am J Trop Med Hyg 26:39, 1977.

Cooper, J., Prall, W., English, B., and Shearer, W.: Coxsackievirus B3 producing fatal meningoencephalitis in a patient with X-linked agammaglobulinemia. Am J Dis Child 137:82, 1983.
Dales, S., and Kajioka, R.: The cycle of multiplication of vaccinia virus in Earle's strain L cells. 1. Uptake and penetration. Virology 24:278, 1964.
Daniels, C.: Mechanism of viral neutralization. In Notkins, A. (eds.): Viral Immunology and Immunopathology. New York, Academic Press, 1975, p. 79.
Deams, J., and Cohen, S.: Immunology of malaria. Ann Rev Microbiol 37:25, 1983.
Despommier, D.: Immunity to *Trichinella spiralis*. Am J Trop Med (Suppl.) 26:part 2, 68, 1977.
Ellner, J., and Mahmoud, A.: Phagocytes and worms: David and Goliath revisited. Rev Inf Dis 4:698, 1982.
Fauci, A., Hocher, A., Longo, D., et al.: Acquired immunodeficiency syndrome: epidemiologic, clinical, immunologic, and therapeutic considerations. Ann Int Med 100:92, 1984.
Freter, R.: Studies of the mechanism of action of intestinal antibody in experimental cholera. Tex Rep Exp Biol Med 27 (Suppl 1):299, 1969.
Gibbons, R.: Adherence of bacteria to host tissue. In Schlesinger, D. (ed.): Microbiology, 1977. Washington, D.C., American Society for Microbiology, 1977, p. 395.
Henney, C.: On the mechanics of T cell mediated cytolysis. Transplant Rev 17:37, 1973.
Ishizaka, T., Ishizaka, K., Borsos, T., and Rapp, H.: C'1 fixation by human isoagglutinins: Fixation of C'1 by γG and γM but not γA antibody. J Immunol 97:711, 1966.
Jones, G., and Freter, R.: Adhesive properties of *Vibrio cholerae:* Nature of the interaction with isolated rabbit brush border membranes and human erythrocytes. Infect Immun 6:918, 1972.
Kaur, J., McGhee, J., and Burrows, W.: Immunity to cholera: The occurrence and nature of antibody-active immunoglobulins in the lower ileum of the rabbit. J Immunol 108:387, 1972.
Koch, R.: Further communication on a remedy for tuberculosis. Dtsch Med Wochenschr 17:101, 1891.
Mardh, P., and Westrom, L.: Adherence of bacteria to vaginal epithelial cells. Infect Immun 13:661, 1976.
Mease, P., Ochs, H., and Wedgwood, R.: Successful treatment of Echovirus meningoencephalitis and Myositis-fasciitis with intravenous immune globulin therapy in a patient with X-linked agammaglobulinemia. N Engl J Med 304:1278, 1981.
Mims, C.: Aspects of the pathogenesis of virus diseases. Bacteriol Rev 28:30, 1964.
Ogra, P., Morag, A., and Motti, L.: Humoral immune response to viral infections. In Notkins, A. (ed.): Viral Immunology and Immunopathology. New York, Academic Press, 1975, p. 57.
Payne, P., Lancaster, L., Heinzman, M., and McCutchan, J. A.: Identification of Cryptosporidium in patients with the acquired immunodeficiency syndrome. N Engl J Med 309:613, 1983.
Plaut, A.: The IgA1 proteases of pathogenic bacteria. Ann Rev Microbiol 37:603, 1983.
Radwan, A., and Crawford, T.: The mechanism of neutralization of sensitized equine arteritis virus by complement components. J Gen Virol 25:229, 1974.
Silverstein, S., and Marcus, P.: Early stages of Newcastle disease virus-Hela cell interaction: An electron microscopic study. Virology 23:370, 1964.
Stoliar, O., Kaniecki-Green, E., Pelley, R., Klaus, M., and Carpenter, C.: Secretory IgA against enterotoxins in breast milk. Lancet 1:1258, 1976.
Taliaferro, W. H.: Ablastic and trypanocidal antibodies against *Trypanosoma duttoni*. J Immunol 35:303, 1938.
Taliaferro, W. H., and Sarles, M.: The cellular reactions in the skin, lungs, and intestine of normal and immune rats after infection with *Nippostrongylus muris*. J Infect Dis 64:157, 1939.
Williamson, W., and Greenwood, B.: Impairment of the immune response to vaccination after acute malaria. Lancet 1:1328, 1978.
Wong, B., Gold, J., Brown, A., et al.: Central nervous system toxoplasmosis in homosexual men and parenteral drug abusers. Ann Int Med 100:36, 1984.

89
MECHANISMS OF IMMUNOLOGIC INJURY IN INFECTIOUS DISEASES

ABRAHAM I. BRAUDE, M.D., PH.D.

Microbial antigens may injure cells or tissues during infection by the eight mechanisms listed in Table 1.

These mechanisms may operate independently or simultaneously, and some may involve both antibodies and mononuclear cells (lymphocytes and macrophages). The first three also require complement.

Table 1. MECHANISMS OF IMMUNOLOGIC INJURY IN INFECTIONS

Mechanism	Example of Infectious Agents
Antibody-mediated cytolysis	Enveloped virus
Complement-mediated chemotaxis	Pyogenic bacteria
Immune complex vasculitis	Agents of endocarditis, viral hepatitis, leprosy, and quartan malaria
Intravascular coagulation	Meningococcus and other gram-negative bacteria
Anaphylaxis	Worms and aspergilli
T cell-mediated cytolysis	Lymphocytic choriomeningitis virus
Antibody-dependent cell-mediated cytotoxicity	Influenza virus
Delayed hypersensitivity	*M. tuberculosis, Brucella, Histoplasma,* vaccinia virus

ANTIBODY-MEDIATED CYTOLYSIS. Lysis of cells may result from the interaction of antibody, complement, and microbial antigens on the surface of infected cells (Porter, 1971). This type of injury has been observed almost exclusively in cells infected with viruses that have envelopes such as poxviruses, herpesviruses, paramyxoviruses, arenaviruses, togaviruses, and rhabdoviruses (Rawls and Tompkins, 1975). Viral antigens appear on the surface of infected cells after RNA viruses pass through the cellular cytoplasmic membrane during the release of the nucleocapsid from the infected cell by the process of "budding." The virus picks up its envelope from the cytoplasmic membrane and at the same time deposits viral antigen on the surface of the membrane (Rawls and Tompkins, 1975). A DNA virus such as herpes simplex picks up its envelope by budding through the nuclear membrane, but herpes antigens also appear at the cell surface. The union of IgG or IgM antibodies with viral antigen on the cell surface activates complement via the classic pathway, and cell lysis ensues through the same mechanism as that described for bacterial lysis in Chapter 87. After reacting with antibody and antigenic sites on the cell membrane, C1 is activated to react with C4 and C2. This generates C3 convertase, which splits C3 into two fragments, the larger (C3b) remaining attached to the cell membrane. The protease activity of C3b binds C5, 6, and 7, thus building a complex on the cell surface composed of C1 through C7. Damage to the cell membrane is initiated when C8 is bound to the C1 through C7 complex. Cytolysis is accelerated when C9 becomes incorporated (Kolb and Müller-Eberhardt, 1975).

This type of cytolysis is a theoretical mechanism not only for eliminating virus infections but also for injuring the infected organ. The effectiveness of the process in producing cytolysis depends on the type of cell and on the number of antigenic sites that appear on the cell surface (Kibler and Ter Meulen, 1975). For example, during persistent infection in tissue culture by measles virus, relatively few surface antigens appear compared with acute measles infections, and few if any cells undergo lysis. This finding correlates with the absence of necrotic foci in subacute sclerosing panencephalitis, a form of persistent measles infection of the brain.

COMPLEMENT-MEDIATED CHEMOTAXIS AND SUPPURATION. When the classic complement pathway is activated by union of antibody with microbial antigen, or the alternative pathway by bacterial lipopolysaccharides, the chemotactic factors C3a and C5a are produced. These chemotactic factors attract inflammatory cells that not only attack microbial cells and virus-infected cells but also injure the infected tissues. The chemotactic factors C3a and C5a can also stimulate the release from mast cells of histamine, which in turn increases the permeability of vessels for leukocytes. The heavy influx of granulocytes during inflammation causes the characteristic tissue damage of suppuration by release of proteolytic enzymes from neutrophil granules. These enzymes can destroy both connective tissue proteins (collagenase and elastase) and cells (Williams et al., 1977).

IMMUNE COMPLEX VASCULITIS (ARTHUS REACTION). When microbial antigens unite with antibody, the infectivity of the organism may be inactivated so that the infection is terminated. But if the antigen is discharged from organisms protected within a "privileged sanctuary" that cannot be eliminated by immune processes, the steady supply of antigen may form soluble complexes with its antibody. Such complexes can develop from antigens released upon microbial lysis by antibody and complement or as a by-product of microbial growth. These soluble complexes can circulate in the blood until they are deposited in the tissues by phagocytosis or trapping. Phagocytosis by reticuloendothelial (RES) cells removes large complexes preferentially so that the small complexes formed in antigen excess remain in the circulation. If the large complexes contain infectious virus or toxic microbial antigens that persist within the Küpffer cells, they may impair phagocytic clearance by the RES and promote the circulation of complexes (Oldstone and Dixon, 1975). As RES clearance fails and the concentration of complexes mounts in the circulation, the complexes pass through permeable vessels and are deposited in the tissues. The permeability of these vessels is apparently increased when the antigen in the complexes reacts with IgE that is adherent to basophils or mast cells. The antigen thus causes mast cell or basophilic granules to release certain factors that can increase vascular permeability and others that cause platelets to clump and in turn release vasoactive amines. The combined effect of such basophilic and platelet permeability factors on blood vessels permits the leakage of immune complexes and their deposition in the tissue along the vessel walls (Cochrane and Koffler, 1973). In addition, glomerular capillaries have normal endothelial fenestrations that favor leakage of complexes and help explain the unique susceptibility of glomeruli to immune-complex deposition. Immune complexes with a density in the range of 19S or larger are most likely to be deposited along vessels and damage them (Cochrane and Koffler, 1973); complexes with a density of less than 19S not only fix complement poorly but are also cleared slowly from the blood.

One important mechanism for vessel injury requires fixation of complement by the immune complexes (Cochrane and Koffler, 1973). Activation of the complement system generates C3a and C5a, which increase permeability of vessels and attract granulocytes. The accumulation of granulocytes (neutrophilic leukocytes) is followed by the release of their lysosomal enzymes, which destroy the elastic laminae of small arteries and injure the basement membrane of glomerular capillaries. The consumption of complement by these complexes is reflected in the diminished concentration of C3 and other complement components in the serum and by the presence of complement components at the site of immune complex deposition. If complement and polymorphonuclear leukocytes are depleted in experimental animals with immune complex disease, the arterial lesions are prevented, but glomerular injury can still occur (McCluskey and Klassen, 1974) through mediators other than complement.

In bacterial endocarditis, quartan malaria, lepromatous leprosy, syphilis, and viral hepatitis B, the occurrence of immune complex disease is well established (Bayer et al., 1976; Kohler et al., 1974; Gamble and Reardon, 1975). Each of these is a subacute or chronic infection in which a bacterial, protozoan, or viral antigen is released constantly into the bloodstream at a time when high levels of antibody are already present. The immune complexes that result from the union of circulating antigen with antibody produce granular deposits along the glomerular basement membrane. These complexes, containing immunoglobulin plus antigen plus complement, produce electron-dense deposits in the glomerular basement membrane and diffuse proliferative glomerulonephritis. Those infections that have been implicated in the production of immune complex glomerulonephritis are listed in Table 2. In most of these, the specific microbial antigens have been demonstrated in the glomerular deposit. In the immune complex glomerulonephritis of syphilis, schistosomiasis, infected ventriculoatrial shunts, and quartan malaria, the clinical syndrome has usually been that of the nephrotic syndrome.

In viral hepatitis B and lepromatous leprosy there have been prominent clinical features attributed to immune complex deposition outside the kidney. In chronic carriers of hepatitis B virus, for example, hepatitis B surface antigen immune complexes were identified in vascular lesions in periarteritis nodosa. In other cases of viral hepatitis B, immune complexes do not necessarily contain viral antigens. In these immune complexes the antigen is usually IgG and the antibody is IgM (Levo et al., 1977). It appears that some of the IgG generated in various chronic infections can become antigenic itself and stimulate a form of autoimmunity to the patient's own immunoglobulin. Perhaps the antigenic groups of IgG that react with IgM antibody are normally buried within the IgG molecule and become exposed when IgG molecules unfold after union with the specific microbial antigen. Activation of the classic complement pathway by these complexes of IgG and IgM results in systemic vasculitis involving the skin, kidneys, and joints and producing vascular purpura, glomerulonephritis, and arthritis. These immune complexes composed of IgG and IgM have the distinctive property of precipitating at cold

Table 2. INFECTIOUS DISEASES UNDERLYING THE PRODUCTON OF IMMUNE COMPLEX GLOMERULONEPHRITIS

Underlying Disease	Organisms
Subacute bacterial endocarditis	*Staphylococcus aureus, Streptococcus viridans*, enterococcus, *Coxiella burnetii*
Ventriculoatrial shunt infections	*S. epidermidis*
Malaria	*Plasmodium malariae* and *falciparum*
Lepromatous leprosy	*Mycobacterium leprae*
Syphilis	*Treponema pallidum*
Hepatitis	Hepatitis B virus
Pneumococcal pneumonia	Type 14 pneumococcus
Streptococcal pyoderma or pharyngitis	Group A streptococci
Typhoid fever	*Salmonella typhosa*
Shistosomiasis	*Schistosoma mansoni*
Toxoplasmosis	*Toxoplasma gondii*

temperatures and are known as cryoglobulins.* They occur in leprosy, endocarditis, cytomegalovirus infections, and infectious mononucleosis, and can produce vascular lesions in these conditions. The most dramatic of these occur in lepromatous leprosy and take the form of painful red papules known as erythema nodosum leprosum. They may be accompanied by arthritis and glomerulonephritis.

INTRAVASCULAR COAGULATION. Tissue injury from intravascular coagulation in human infection is best illustrated by the hemorrhagic skin necrosis and renal cortical necrosis of meningococcemia. The hemorrhagic skin necrosis in meningococcemia is an example of the dermal Shwartzman reaction (Davis and Arnold, 1974), and renal cortical necrosis is typical of the generalized Shwartzman reaction. As noted in Chapter 6, either phenomenon can be produced experimentally by giving rabbits two injections of the lipopolysaccharide (LPS) antigen from any gram-negative bacteria. Two intravenous injections of LPS, given 24 hours apart, invariably produce severe disseminated intravascular coagulation (DIC) culminating in bilateral renal cortical necrosis. This dramatic form of kidney damage (Sanarelli-Schwartzman reaction) results from glomerular deposits of fibrin. The dermal Shwartzman reaction is also produced by two separate injections of LPS, the first intradermally and the second intravenously 24 hours later. Soon after the cutaneous dose, the site of the intradermal injection undergoes hemorrhagic necrosis secondary to local thrombosis and infarction. The first injection causes an Arthus-like inflammation about the skin vessels, and the intravenous dose initiates coagulation and thrombosis that are limited to the inflamed vessel.

The essential role of coagulation is illustrated by the prevention of both reactions by heparin and other anticoagulants. In the generalized Shwartzman reaction, the first dose of LPS triggers intravascular conversion of fibrinogen to fibrin by the mechanisms discussed in Chapter 6, but the reticuloendothelial system (RES) clears the fibrin before it can be deposited in the glomerular capillaries and other vessels (Lee and Stetson, 1965). The first dose of LPS seems to condition the RES so that its clearance activity is blocked by the second dose. As a result, the fibrin aggregates produced by the second dose are no longer cleared from the blood; instead, they are filtered out by the glomeruli, where they occlude the capillaries and produce infarction of the renal cortex. DIC consumes clotting factors such as fibrinogen, platelets, and prothrombin. In addition, DIC activates fibrinolysis so that fibrin degradation products are released. These fragments prevent clotting by inhibiting proteolysis of fibrinogen by thrombin and blocking polymerization of fibrin monomer to form a clot. The anticoagulant effect of these degradation products can cause serious bleeding in patients whose clotting factors are depleted by DIC, not only aggravating hemorrhages into the necrotic lesions of the skin and kidneys but also producing hemorrhages in other tissues not affected by the Shwartzman lesions.

Although meningococcemia is the most dramatic and consistent example of the two Shwartzman reactions, severe bacteremias with any gram-negative bacteria can cause DIC. One of the most devastating examples is the DIC that occurs in *E. coli* bacteremia of pregnancy. This condition is characterized by hemorrhagic lesions in the skin and by fatal renal cortical necrosis. For obscure reasons, pregnancy appears to prepare for the generalized Shwartzman reaction so that only one intravenous dose of LPS is required to evoke DIC and renal cortical necrosis.

Although gram-negative bacteria, including rickettsiae, are the primary cause of DIC because of their LPS, infections by gram-positive bacteria, viruses, fungi, and protozoa can also cause intravascular coagulation. These organisms can initiate clotting by various mechanisms such as the release of tissue factor, a lipoprotein contained in the plasma membrane of endothelial cells and monocytes. When tissue factor is liberated by damage of these cells, it can initiate clotting by complexing with Factor VII and calcium ions to activate Factor X. Bacteria can also initiate clotting through their proteolytic enzymes that break down fibrinogen. But the most relevant immunologic mechanism is the initiation of coagulation or of platelet aggregation by circulating immune complexes composed of microbial antigens and antibody. Such complexes can accelerate fibrin formation in vitro, but only in cell-rich plasma, presumably because tissue-factor is released. Similarly, soluble antigen-antibody complexes can initiate clotting in vivo by substituting for the provocative injection of LPS in the dermal Shwartzman reaction. The intravenous injection of antigen into specifically immunized rabbits also produces DIC and the generalized Shwartzman reaction (Lee, 1963).

*These cryoglobulins in chronic infections are composed of polyclonal IgM and IgG. They are designated Type III cryoglobulins and must be distinguished from Type I and Type II (mixed monoclonal-polyclonal) cryoglobulins that are produced in certain noninfectious diseases.

ANAPHYLAXIS. Anaphylactic antibodies occur primarily in worm and fungus infections. These antibodies belong mainly to the IgE class and act through attachment via the Fc receptor to the surface of tissue mast cells and basophils. When a divalent antigen from worms or fungi combines with two IgE molecules to form a bridge, the antibody becomes distorted. This distortion of IgE on the cell surface causes the discharge of intracellular granules, which release histamine and serotonin and other mediators such as SRS-A. SRS-A is a mixture of extremely potent agents of smooth muscle contraction and vasodilation, the leukotrienes. Leukotrienes are metabolites of arachidonic acid, and are at least 100 times more potent than histamine in causing bronchial smooth muscle contraction and in increasing vascular permeability. Histamine and SRS-A cause bronchospasm and pulmonary edema when released into the lung during anaphylaxis. The eosinophil chemotactic factor of anaphylaxis is released from mast cell granules and attracts eosinophils to the site of anaphylaxis. Eosinophils appear to check the allergic reaction by ingesting the antigen-antibody complexes and by inactivating histamine and SRS-A through the release of histaminase and arylsulfatase B, respectively (Goetzl and Austen, 1977). Worms induce very high levels of IgE and eosinophils and various manifestations of anaphylaxis. *Ascaris* worms are especially potent causes of anaphylactic hypersensitivity when they invade the tissues and especially when they migrate through the lungs. They produce the syndrome of eosinophilic pneumonia, an allergic pneumonitis with a prominent asthmatic component. Eosinophilia is also prominent in strongyloidiasis, visceral larva migrans, trichinosis, certain types of filariasis, and acute schistosomiasis. *Angiostrongylus cantonensis*, a nematode that invades the central nervous system, causes eosinophilic meningitis. Systemic fatal anaphylactic shock can occur in echinococcosis upon rupture of a hydatid cyst and release of echinococcal antigen into the peritoneum, where high levels of IgE are delivered from the circulation. A more benign systemic reaction, known as Katayama fever, occurs at the onset of egg production in schistosomiasis, but the role of IgE is debatable in the induction of this reaction.

Among fungus diseases, pulmonary allergic aspergillosis is the most important example of a hypersensitivity disorder mediated by IgE (Golbert and Patterson, 1970). After colonization of the bronchial mucous secretions with aspergilli, these patients develop asthma, eosinophilia, and migratory pulmonary infiltrates suggestive of allergic pneumonitis. IgG also participates in the allergic bronchial reaction by producing an Arthus-type reaction.

CYTOLYSIS MEDIATED BY T LYMPHOCYTES. T lymphocytes can kill infected cells in the absence of antibody if three requirements are met: (1) antigen of the infecting virus must appear on the surface of the cell; (2) the T cells must have immune-specificity for the virus; and (3) the T cells must be histocompatible with the target cell. In other words, virus-immune T lymphocytes can cause lysis of infected cells only if the T cell reacts with the viral antigen on the surface of a cell that is recognized as nonforeign. The recognition of a cell as nonforeign, or "self," is thought to involve a reaction between the lymphocyte and the histocompatibility antigen on the target cell. Thus, the attacking T lymphocyte would require two receptors to kill the infected cells: one for the viral antigen and the other for the histocompatibility antigen (Zinkernagel, 1978). T cell-mediated cytolysis may be important in infections by viruses that do not themselves destroy the infected cell. One example is lymphocytic choriomeningitis (LCM) virus. In intracerebral LCM virus infection of mice, the disease is caused by T cells rather than by the virus. The severity of this infection depends on when the T cells reach the target cells: if they reach the target cells early, they can eliminate the virus infection by destroying the cells before the virus replicates and spreads. At this point the damage to cells would be relatively insignificant. On the other hand, a cytolytic attack by T cells on advanced infections could kill the animal. In lymphocytic choriomeningitis, the choroid plexus is heavily infected, and cytolytic damage to this structure destroys the blood-brain barrier so that lethal cerebral edema occurs. A similar attack by T lymphocytes on liver tissue has been postulated as a mechanism for liver injury in viral hepatitis because the virus is assumed not to be cytotoxic. Hepatitis B surface antigen (HBsAg) can be found in the membrane of liver cells, and T cell-mediated cytotoxicity against HBsAg has been demonstrated in both acute and chronic hepatitis B (Hirschman, 1979).

From these observations and others, it has been suggested that killer lymphocytes can be beneficial only in infections with highly cytopathic viruses, because the infected cells must be sacrificed to ward off more extensive damage by the virus itself. In infections by viruses with slight cytopathic potential, on the other hand, the onslaught of T cells may cause more tissue injury than the virus (Zinkernagel, 1978).

ANTIBODY-DEPENDENT CELL-MEDIATED CYTOTOXICITY (ADCC). Peripheral blood lymphocytes from persons recovering from influenza will injure cells infected with influenza virus (Greenberg et al., 1979). In contrast to lysis by T cells, described in the preceding section, this cytotoxicity produced by blood lymphocytes against cells infected with influenza virus is mediated by non-T lymphocytes secreting antibody. The cell damage can also be produced by free antibody in the presence of lymphocytes and other leukocytes. Antibody appears to act as a bridge that attaches by the Fc portion to lymphocytes and by the Fab component to viral antigens expressed on the surface of infected cells (Hashimoto et al., 1983). Since neutrophils and monocytes also have Fc receptors for IgG, they can also mediate cytotoxicity against cells infected with influenza virus. Except for the bridging phenomenon mediated by IgG, the steps involved in cell damage are unknown.

Since the cytotoxic T-cell reaction has also been implicated in influenza, both processes can contribute to tissue damage and recovery from that infection.

DELAYED HYPERSENSITIVITY. This form of hypersensitivity has been most extensively studied in tuberculosis and is also known as the "tuberculin" type of hypersensitivity. When living or dead tubercle bacilli are injected into the tissues of an animal or patient with tuberculosis, the inflammatory reaction does not begin until after a few hours; it progresses to its maximum size and intensity within 24 to 48 hours. This delay in onset and peak intensity of the reaction, compared with the anaphylactic and Arthus types of inflammatory response, is responsible for the term *delayed hypersensitivity*. The concept that this reaction represents hypersensitivity is based on the fact that in nontuberculous animals, the injection of living bacilli produces no reaction for a week or more (until sensitization has time to develop), and dead bacilli may produce no reaction at any time. The intact bacillus is not required because antigenic tuberculous proteins can also elicit the phenomenon. The same delayed response to antigenic fractions of the infecting organism is seen in many other infections. The response is specific, occurring only when the organisms or antigens causing the infection are injected.

Because delayed hypersensitivity is characterized by necrosis at the injection site if large doses of dead organisms or antigen are used, this reaction is considered to be responsible for necrosis of tissues in natural infection after immune hypersensitivity has developed. In pulmonary tuberculosis, for example, the bacilli multiply slowly in mononuclear phagocytes that aggregate undamaged at the portal of entry until hypersensitivity develops. Then the cells are killed, the tissues undergo necrosis, and tubercle bacilli are discharged by the ulcerating focus into the lumen of the bronchioles (Canetti, 1954, 1958).

Necrosis is thought to be mediated by the lymphocytes that dominate the inflammatory reaction. A few lymphocytes and monocytes first accumulate around vessels in the area into which antigen or bacteria are injected. These specifically sensitized T lymphocytes react with the antigen to release mediators that attract and hold other mononuclear cells in the inflammatory focus. One of these mediators is a chemotactic factor, which attracts macrophages, and the other is migratory inhibitory factor (MIF), which holds them in place. In the meantime, lymphocytes themselves proliferate in situ upon stimulation by specific antigen and release a mitosis-stimulating factor that causes other lymphocytes to multiply. These reactions and others amplify the cellular response and produce the characteristic heavy infiltration of mononuclear cells that is the hallmark of delayed hypersensitivity. Polymorphonuclear leukocytes are seen very early in the inflammatory response but soon disappear before the delayed response is underway. Antibody also seems to be unimportant, because delayed hypersensitivity can be transferred by the mononuclear cells but not by serum.

At least three mechanisms have been proposed to explain cell necrosis by mononuclear cells. First, T lymphocytes attack target cells directly. They can be seen to kill cells in tissue culture, and the amount of killing can be measured by the radioactivity released from target cells labeled with ^{51}Cr. The second mechanism of killing by lymphocytes is lymphocytotoxin, a mediator released from lymphocytes after reaction with specific antigen. This cytotoxic factor is a protein-like substance with a molecular weight in the range of 85,000 and the capacity to kill a wide variety of different cells (Williams and Granger, 1973). A third process of possible importance in the production of necrosis involves macrophages. In response to lymphocyte mediators and other stimuli, macrophages release hydrolytic enzymes such as cathepsins, hyaluronidase, and collagenases, which can injure the matrix that supports the cells, the vessels that supply them, and the cells themselves.

Killing of cells by T lymphocytes can be specific or nonspecific. Specific cytolysis is carried out by T lymphocytes that have immune specificity for the antigens on the surface of the target cell, as described in the preceding section on cytolysis by T lymphocytes. The surface antigens can be derived from the viruses infecting the cells or from other microbial antigens that adhere to the cytoplasmic membrane of the target cell. Cytolysis is nonspecific when the killer lymphocytes are a product of the mitosis that follows blast transformation. This blast transformation in T cells may be induced either by specific antigen or by lymphocytic mediators released from other lymphocytes.

References

Bayer, A., Theofilopoulos, A., Eisenberg, R., Dixon, F., and Guze, L.: Circulating immune complexes in infective endocarditis. N Engl J Med 295:1500, 1976.

Canetti, G.: The Tubercle Bacillus in the Pulmonary Lesion of Man. New York, Springer Publishing Company, 1954.

Canetti, G.: Pathogenesis of tuberculosis in man. Ann NY Acad Sci 154:13, 1968.

Cochrane, C., and Koffler, D.: Immune complex disease in experimental animals and man. Adv Immunol 16:186, 1973.

Davis, C., and Arnold, K.: Role of meningococcal endotoxin in meningococcal purpura. J Exp Med 140:159, 1974.

Gamble, C., and Reardon, J.: Immunopathogenesis of syphilitic glomerulonephritis. N Engl J Med 292:449, 1975.

Goetzl, E., and Austen, K.: Cellular characteristics of the eosinophil compatible with a dual role in host defense in parasitic infections. Am J Trop Med Hyg 26:142, 1977.

Golbert, T., and Patterson, R.: Pulmonary allergic aspergillosis. Ann Int Med 72:395, 1970.

Hirschman, S.: Virologic, immunologic, and clinical correlations in viral hepatitis. Seminars Infect Dis 2:48, 1979.

Kibler, R., and Ter Meulen, V.: Antibody-mediated cytotoxicity after measles virus infection. J Immunol 114:93, 1975.

Kohler, P., Cronin, R., Hammond, W., Olen, D., and Carr, R.: Chronic membranous glomerulonephritis caused by hepatitis B antigen-antibody immune complexes. Ann Intern Med 81:448, 1974.

Kolb, W., and Müller-Eberhard, H.: The membrane attack mechanism of complement. J Exp Med 141:724, 1975.

Lee, L.: Antigen-antibody reaction in the pathogenesis of bilateral renal cortical necrosis. J Exp Med 117:365, 1963.

Lee, L., and Stetson, C.: The local and generalized Shwartzman phenomenon. In Zweifach, B., Grant, L., and McClusky, R. (eds.): The Inflammatory Process. New York, Academic Press, 1965, p. 791.

Levo, Y., Gorevic, P., Kassab, H., Zucker-Franklin, D., Gigli, I., and Franklin, E.: Mixed cryoglobulinemia: Immune complex disease often associated with hepatitis B virus infection. Trans Assoc Am Phys 90:167, 1977.

McCluskey, R., and Klassen, J.: Immunologically mediated glomerular, tubular, and interstitial renal disease. N Engl J Med 288:564, 1973.

Oldstone, M., and Dixon, F.: Immune complex disease associated with viral infections. In Notkins, A. (ed.): Viral Immunology and Immunopathology. New York, Academic Press, 1975, p. 341.

Porter, D. D.: Destruction of virus-infected cells by immunological mechanisms. Ann Rev Microbiol 25:283, 1971.

Rawls, W., and Tompkins, A.: Destruction of virus-infected cells by antibody and complement. In Notkins, A. (ed.): Viral Immunology and Immunopathology. New York, Academic Press, 1975, p. 99.

Williams, T., and Granger, G.: Lymphocyte in vitro cytotoxicity: Mechanism of human lymphotoxin-induced target cell destruction. Cell Immunol 6:171, 1973.

Williams, T., Lyons, J., and Braude, A.: In vitro lysis of target cells by rat polymorphonuclear leukocytes isolated from acute pyelonephritic exudates. J Immunol 119:671, 1977.

Zinkernagel, R. M.: Major transplantation antigens in host responses to infection. Hospital Practice 13(7):83, 1978.

90

IMMUNOPROPHYLAXIS AND IMMUNOTHERAPY

STEPHEN A. SPECTOR, M.D.

In the spring of 1796, Edward Jenner took some fluid from a large cowpox vesicle on the hand of dairymaid Sarah Nelmes and inoculated it at two sites on the arms of 8-year-old James Phipps (Creighton, 1889; Parish, 1965, 1968). The boy developed typical cowpox lesions, and 2 months later, when Jenner inoculated him with smallpox, no disease developed. Less than 200 years later, on October 26, 1977, Ali Maow Maalin, a cook in Merka, Somalia, became the "last reported case" of endemic variola. The global eradication of smallpox must be considered a major accomplishment of modern science and a triumph for immunizations. The elimination of this dreaded disease, as with most immunization programs, was not without setbacks and risks to vaccinees. Prophylactic inoculation against variola (variolation) was practiced in China, India, Persia, and elsewhere for centuries before it was popularized in England by Lady Mary Wortley Montagu in the early 18th century. The practice of variolation was far from safe, and possibly 2 to 3 per cent so vaccinated died of smallpox. This fatality rate was tenfold less than that from naturally occurring smallpox, and the artificial inoculation of variola was widely practiced until Jenner developed his "improved vaccine." The concept of intentionally exposing an individual to either live or killed immunogens to prevent disease, combined with the principle of passive transfer of antibody to prevent and ameliorate infections, serves as the cornerstone of present day immunoprophylaxis.

PRINCIPLES OF PASSIVE IMMUNIZATION. Short-term immunity to many infections may be conferred by administering preformed antibody as immune serum or gamma globulin prepared from it (Stiehm, 1979). Two types of gamma globulin preparations are available: standard human immune globulin (IG), previously called immune serum globulin (ISG), for general use, and special human immune serum globulins with known antibody content for specific illnesses. Certain diseases may also be ameliorated or prevented by the use of animal sera and antitoxins.

IgG is produced primarily in plasma cells that have evolved from B-lymphocytes. Destruction of IgG-coated bacteria occurs following phagocytosis in the granulocytes of the reticuloendothelial system and in the gastrointestinal tract. IgG crosses the placenta and provides passive protection to the newborn infant for approximately six months. These passively acquired IgG antibodies may inhibit an infant's immune system and prevent an adequate response to certain vaccines.

IG is prepared by alcohol fractionation of pooled human sera by Cohn's alcohol fractionation procedure, which removes most other serum proteins and hepatitis viruses. IG is composed of 95 per cent IgG at 165 mg per ml (16.5 per cent solution), along with trace quantities of IgM and IgA globulins and other serum proteins. IgG has a mean half-life of 22 days. Metabolism of IgG is directly controlled by its level in serum; there is an increase in the breakdown of IgG with elevated plasma levels and a decrease in catabolism with decreased levels.

IG until recently was available only for intramuscular injection. In vitro, it has been shown to aggregate into large molecular weight complexes that can activate spontaneously the complement system. These aggregates are probably responsible for the occasional systemic reactions to IG that occur in approximately 2 per 1000 injections (Ellis and Henney, 1969). The incidence of reactions is increased with repeated injection of IG and with intravenous administration. Approximately 20 per cent of patients receiving repeated intramuscular doses of gamma globulin can be expected to experience mild reactions including dyspnea, tightness in chest, faintness, hypotension, flushing, facial swelling, and anxiety (Squire et al., 1969). Recently intravenous preparations of gamma globulin have been developed that eliminate most anticomplementary activity. These IV preparations may prove useful in severe infections when large amounts of antibody must be administered over a short period of time.

Human gamma globulin is frequently used without proven indications. Patients with certain defined immune defects or with documented exposure to one of the infections listed in Table 1 are good candidates for passive prophylaxis. There is no evidence suggesting that the child with an apparent overabundance of upper respiratory infections without documented immunologic deficits benefits from short or prolonged treatment with gamma globulin. Similarly, special human immune serum globulins are in limited supply and should be administered only when

Table 1. INDICATIONS FOR THE USE OF HUMAN IMMUNE GLOBULIN (IG)

Disorder	Purpose	Dose (I.M.)	Comment
	Proved Value		
Antibody deficiency disease (agammaglobulinemia, hypogammaglobulinemia)	Treatment	0.6 ml/kg every 3–4 wk	Maximum dose is 20–30 ml; double dose at onset of therapy
Measles	Modification Prevention	0.05 ml/kg 0.25–0.5 ml/kg	Give immediately after exposure
Viral hepatitis type A (HAV)	Prevention: single exposure continuous exposure	 0.02 ml/kg 0.06 ml/kg, repeat in 5–6 mo	Give as soon as possible after exposure
Viral hepatitis type B (HBV)	Prevention	0.12 ml/kg	Use when hepatitis B immune serum globulin is not available

Table 2. PASSIVE IMMUNIZATION

Disease	Source of Antibody	Indication	Dose	Adverse Reactions	Comment
Bacterial					
Diphtheria	Horse serum (antitoxin)	Prevention and treatment	10,000–80,000 units (I.M. and I.V.) depending on type of involvement and age of patient	Hypersensitivity, serum sickness, anaphylaxis	
Pertussis	Human pertussis immune globulin (PIG)	Treatment	<1 year old; 1.25 ml >1 year old; 2.5 ml I.M.	Pain and tenderness at injection site	Doubtful efficacy
Botulism	Horse serum against types A, B, and E	Treatment	1 vial I.V.; 1 vial I.M. Repeat in 2–4 hours if symptoms continue	Hypersensitivity, serum sickness, anaphylaxis	Has not been helpful in infantile botulism Effectiveness uncertain
Tetanus	Human tetanus immune globulin (TIG)	Prevention and treatment	Prevention: 250–500 U—half I.M., half locally Treatment: 3000–6000 U—half I.M., half locally	Pain and tenderness at injection site	If TIG unavailable tetanus antisera from horse serum (TAT) may be used
Viral					
Hepatitis B	Human hepatitis B immune globulin (HBIG)	Prevention (see text)	0.06 ml/kg I.M.; repeat after 28 days	Pain and tenderness at injection site	See text
Varicella-zoster	Human varicella-zoster immune globulin (VZIG)	Prevention (see text); should be given within 96 hours of exposure	1 complete vial per 10 kg up to 5 vials I.M.	Pain and tenderness at injection site	If VZIG unavailable, VZIP 10 ml/kg I.V. may be used Not indicated for active chickenpox or zoster
Rabies	Human rabies immune globulin (RIG)	Prevention	20 units/kg, half into wound and half I.M.	Pain and tenderness at injection site	If RIG not available, equine rabies immune serum should be used
Mumps	Human mumps immune globulin	Prevention and treatment in adult men	20 ml I.M.	Pain and tenderness at injection site	Questionable efficacy in preventing orchitis in postpubertal males
Smallpox	Human vaccinia immune globulin (VIG)	Within 24 hours after known exposure	0.3 ml/kg I.M.	Pain and tenderness at injection site	Not indicated with active infection

I.V., intravenous
I.M., intramuscular

patients are likely to benefit from their use (Table 2). Animal antisera and antitoxins particularly should be used only when there are definite indications (Table 2). Refined and concentrated horse sera are still the only effective prophylaxis for diphtheria, gas gangrene, and botulism once exposure has occurred. Animal serum against tetanus and rabies should only be used when special human gamma globulin is unavailable. The use of animal sera may be associated with acute febrile reactions, serum sickness, or anaphylaxis. Febrile reactions following injections of animal serum are usually mild but may be severe, requiring vigorous antipyretic therapy. Serum sickness occurs in from 10 to 40 per cent of recipients of some animal sera and consists of rash, urticaria, arthritis, adenopathy, and fever appearing hours or several days after a second injection, or 7 to 12 days after a first injection. Anaphylaxis occurs in approximately 1 per cent of individuals receiving animal antisera. Since anaphylactic reactions are life-threatening, an intracutaneous skin test, preceded by a scratch or eye test, should be performed on every patient before any injection of animal serum. Since intradermal skin tests have resulted in fatal reactions, a skin test should never be performed unless a syringe containing 1 ml of 1:1000 epinephrine is immediately available. If the skin test is positive or a patient has a strong allergic history, desensitization of the patient should be carried out under close medical supervision if the prophylactic use of animal antiserum is strongly indicated.

A new human antiserum has been developed which attempts to protect patients from death due to gram-negative bacteremia. The antiserum is made by immunizing volunteers against a stable mutant of *Escherichia coli* that lacks the ability to form the O antigenic side chains. The antibody thus formed is against the common lipopolysaccharide core of gram-negative bacteria and in animal studies has been highly effective in protecting against lethal gram-negative bacteremic shock and disseminated intravascular coagulation (Braude et al., 1977). In a randomized controlled trial, patients given human antiserum to the lipopolysaccharide core had significantly fewer deaths from gram-negative bacteremia than controls given nonimmune serum (Ziegler et al., 1982).

ACTIVE IMMUNIZATION. Active immunization is the induction of immunity by inoculation of a specific organism or some fragment or toxin associated with that organism. Although passive immunizations have prevented some diseases, there are clearly many advantages to active vaccination. Some active immunizations give lifelong protection and thus do not require knowledge of exposure to be effective. Additionally, the immunity conferred during active immunizations frequently approaches 100 per cent, whereas passive protection is often substantially less successful. The cost of preparing immune sera is often more expensive than preparing vaccines.

Most immunogens used for active immunizations are crude fractions of an organism, or killed or live whole bacteria or viruses. The most notable exceptions to this are the vaccines against tetanus and diphtheria, which contain preformed inactivated toxins as immunogens.

Inactivated "killed" vaccines may be produced by three techniques. The first of these consists of whole organisms that are killed by heat or chemicals (e.g., formaldehyde). Examples of such killed vaccines are pertussis, typhoid, cholera, inactivated poliomyelitis, and influenza. These vaccines generally do not confer lasting immunity and frequently are only partially effective. Killed measles vaccine is no longer licensed because it not only offers less protection than attenuated live measles vaccine but also sensitizes individuals to future challenge with live measles, so that infections are more severe. The killed poliomyelitis vaccine, however, has been extremely useful. Although it has been generally replaced by the attenuated Sabin vaccine, the killed Salk vaccine was effective in substantially reducing the number of clinical cases of paralytic polio in the United States before the introduction of the live polio vaccine. The killed vaccine has virtually eradicated the disease in Scandinavia, where the live vaccine has not been used.

The second method of preparing inactivated vaccines is by using extracted cellular fractions that have been shown to induce immunity in man. Vaccines prepared from the polysaccharide capsules of the meningococcus and the pneumococcus appear to be effective and safe in adults and children above the age of two years (Lepow et al., 1977; Peltola et al., 1977; Klein and Mortimer, 1978; Cowan et al., 1978; Center for Disease Control, 1978; Wilkins and Wehrle, 1979).

Immunizations with toxoids are prepared by inactivating large amounts of toxin with formalin rather than formalinizing the organisms themselves. The antibodies induced by these vaccines are active in neutralizing the toxin produced during infection. This third method of preparing inactivated vaccines has been extremely useful in the prevention of diphtheria and tetanus.

The major disadvantages of inactivated vaccines lie in their inability to confer lasting and local immunity. Multiple doses and boosters are required for continued protection, and local IgA fails to develop from the parenteral injection. As a result, protection against respiratory and gastrointestinal infections is suboptimal.

Live attenuated vaccines are prepared by serial passage of organisms in tissue culture or embryos so that the vaccine strain organism loses virulence. Local secretory IgA production may be stimulated by administration of the vaccine at the site of entry in the gut or the respiratory tract (Rothberg et al., 1973). This method of immunization produces the strongest and most durable immunity.

Active immunization may also be achieved by inducing an infection with a nonpathogenic organism that cross-reacts with a virulent organism. For example, Bacillus Calmette-Guérin (BCG), a strain of bovine tuberculosis, is used to induce immunity to human tuberculosis (Eickhoff, 1977). Similarly, protection against smallpox has been achieved by immunization with cowpox or vaccinia (Creighton, 1889).

PROBLEMS ASSOCIATED WITH IMMUNIZATIONS. Associated with the desired benefits of vaccines are many real and potential problems. Live attenuated viral vaccines may revert to more virulent viruses and result in severe disease. In general, however, reversion has not been a problem, and serious reactions usually reflect abnormal host response rather than virus alteration. Contacts of vaccines given live viruses may be at risk of developing an infection with the vaccine strain organism. Unfortunate cases of paralytic poliomyelitis have been well documented to occur rarely in both normal and immunosuppressed individuals following immunization or exposure to a recently immunized family member (Davis et al., 1977). Contaminating viruses or other organisms undetected in continuous cultures may lead to acute or chronic diseases and conceivably could result in malignancies in vaccine recipients (Fraumeni et al., 1963). Since many viruses cause latent or persistent infections and may produce slow viral diseases, concern has been expressed that certain vaccines may promote the development of these infections. To date, these concerns have not been substantiated. In fact, the incidence of subacute sclerosing panencephalitis (SSPE) in children following measles vaccine is nine times less common than in children with a history of naturally acquired measles (Modlin et al., 1977). The presence of unsuspected passenger viruses has been found in both live and killed vaccines. Simian viruses 40 (SV40), present in monkey cells, contaminated the polio cultures of both the Salk and Sabin vaccines and were injected with many of the original polio as well as adenovirus vaccines. Avian leukosis viruses are present in most flocks of chickens and their eggs and are subsequent contaminants of any virus grown in chick embryo cells.

Sensitization of individuals either to the organism to which immunity is desired or to the cellular antigens or antibiotics used to grow the organism has been observed. Severe reactions to vaccine prepared with chick or duck embryos are well described. In addition, repeated immunization of experimental animals with large doses of antigen has resulted in conditions similar to amyloidosis and multiple myeloma in man (White et al., 1974).

NATURALLY ACQUIRED PASSIVE IMMUNITY. Newborn infants receive many antibodies from the mother. Placental transfer of antibody depends on the quantity of antibodies in the maternal circulation, as well as the molecular size.

Table 3. TRANSPLACENTAL TRANSFER OF MATERNAL ANTIBODY IN NEWBORN INFANTS

Good Passive Transfer	Poor Passive Transfer	No Passive Transfer
Diphtheria antitoxin Tetanus antitoxin Antierythrogenic toxin Antistaphylococcal antibody Salmonella flagellar (H) antibody Antistreptolysin All the antiviral antibodies present in maternal circulation (rubeola, rubella, mumps, poliovirus) VDRL antibodies	*Haemophilus influenzae,* *Bordetella pertussis,* *Shigella flexneri,* *Streptococcus*	Enteric somatic (O) antibodies (*Salmonella, Shigella, E. coli*) Heterophile antibody

Only IgG with its low molecular weight passes readily. IgA and IgM are not placentally transmitted. Viral antibodies present in high amounts are equally present in maternal and infant serum, while macroglobulins (e.g., heterophil antibody) are excluded (Table 3). Passively acquired antibody clearly protects against some diseases. Neonatal tetanus, for example, may be completely eliminated by administering at least two doses of tetanus toxoid to pregnant women. Previously immune pregnant women provide sufficient antibodies to their infants to protect them from neonatal tetanus.

Passively acquired antibody may interfere with a newborn's ability to respond adequately to immunizations. Several studies have confirmed that maternally acquired antibody to diphtheria and pertussis may actually inhibit antibody formation following active immunization. Placentally transmitted antibody may neutralize the virus in live vaccines, thus rendering the vaccine ineffective. How long passively acquired antibody may interfere with an infant's ability to respond to certain vaccines is uncertain. Low levels of maternal antibody to measles have been found to persist beyond the twelfth month of life (Albrecht et al., 1977). Several studies have shown that children vaccinated before 12 months of age have a lower seroconversion rate than those immunized after 1 year (Shelton et al., 1978; Wilkins and Wehrle, 1979). Until this question is resolved, it is recommended that children be immunized against measles at 15 months of age. Prolonged acquisition of passive antibody through breast feeding may play a role in those 5 to 10 per cent of normal children who fail to respond adequately to one dose of the live measles vaccine, and certainly may interfere with the success of live polio virus immunization.

CURRENT IMMUNIZATION SCHEDULES. At present, seven immunizations are recommended for routine use in the United States. The schedule outlined in Table 4 is the suggested sequence outlined in the Red Book, 1982, as recommended by the Committee of Infectious Diseases (American Academy of Pediatrics, 1982). The American Public Health Association and the Advisory Committee on Immunization Practices (ACIP) of the United States Public Health Service also publish recommended immunization schedules. Although there is usually consistency among the three organizations, occasionally recommendations may vary slightly.

The combined vaccines recommended for routine use have been shown to be just as efficacious without increased side effects when given concomitantly as when given individually (Centers for Disease Control, 1980). Single live virus vaccines should be given one month apart, since interference with the immune response to the second vaccine has been demonstrated with some immunizations. Two weeks and preferably four weeks should separate administration of killed vaccines with another inactivated or live virus vaccine.

Most immunizations may be associated with various side effects. Local reactions consist of mild induration and tenderness at the injection site. Repeat dosages of tetanus toxoid or typhoid vaccine have been associated with severe local reactions including marked edema, induration, erythema, and tenderness. If there is a severe reaction, subsequent immunization with the offending antigen should be avoided unless there are extremely compelling reasons for repeating the immunization. In such cases, fractional doses should be administered under close medical supervision.

Severe febrile reactions associated with irritability, malaise, headaches, and chills may follow the use of inactivated vaccines and usually subside within 48 hours. Mild febrile reactions are much more common and are easily controlled with antipyretics. Fever and rashes associated with the measles and rubella vaccines usually appear one to several weeks after immunization and persist for one to three days. Arthralgias associated with attenuated rubella vaccines follow a similar time sequence. The persistent arthritic symptoms occasionally associated with rubella vaccines have not been shown to represent vaccine complications and at present are felt to represent coincidental disease.

Table 4. RECOMMENDED SCHEDULE FOR ACTIVE IMMUNIZATION OF NORMAL INFANTS AND CHILDREN

2 mo	DTP	TOPV
4 mo	DTP	TOPV
6 mo	DTP	TOPV (optional)
1 yr		Tuberculin test
15 mo	Measles, rubella	Mumps (MMR)
1½ yr	DTP	TOPV
4–6 yr	DTP	TOPV
14–16 yr	Td—repeat every 10 years	

DPT, diphtheria-tetanus-pertussis vaccine
Td, tetanus-diphtheria vaccine
TOPV, trivalent oral polio vaccine
MMR, measles-mumps-rubella vaccine
From American Academy of Pediatrics: Report of the Committee on Infectious Diseases, 19th ed., 1982

IMMUNIZATIONS FOR INDIVIDUALS OUT OF STEP. Interruption of the recommended immunization schedule does not interfere with the final immunologic outcome (Phillips, 1975). It is not necessary to resume the series regardless of the time between discontinuation and reinstitution of immunizations. The schedule for primary immunization of children not immunized in infancy is shown in Table 5. Children less than 7 years old are immunized with the standard DTP triple antigens by using three dosages at intervals of four to eight weeks. Pertussis vaccine is not recommended for children older than 6 years. In addition, children older than 6 years should receive the adult-type diphtheria-tetanus toxoid. The standard DT preparation contains 7 to 25 Lf (flocculating units) and may cause severe reactions in older children and adults. The adult type of combined diphtheria-tetanus toxoid (Td) with adjuvant contains, at most, 2 Lf of diphtheria toxoid and is recommended for all adults and children older than 6 years.

CONTRAINDICATIONS TO IMMUNIZATIONS. The decision to immunize an individual with a given vaccine should be based on the belief that the benefits accrued by that person and society outweigh the potential risks of vaccination. During the acute febrile phase of an illness, immunization should be deferred. Minor illnesses without fever, however, should not be considered contraindications. Patients with malignancies or receiving immunosuppressive therapy including chemotherapy, radiation therapy, and corticosteroids should not receive live vaccines. Similarly, individuals with immunodeficiency disorders may develop overwhelming infections when immunized with live vaccines and should not be vaccinated. Individuals allergic to eggs, chickens, or ducks should not receive vaccines grown in duck or chick embryos. Vaccines grown in fibroblast cultures derived from chicks or ducks do not contain egg albumin or yolk components and are not contraindicated in individuals with known hypersensitivity to ducks and chickens.

Individuals with neurologic disorders present considerable controversy regarding immunization. Current recommendations are that children with static neurologic disorders should generally be immunized following the usual vaccine schedules. But the child with an evolving neurologic problem should not receive immunizations likely to cause fever or to be associated with central nervous system (CNS) complications.

PREGNANCY AND IMMUNIZATIONS. In general, the use of attenuated vaccines should be avoided during pregnancy (Levine, 1974). Theoretically, immunization with live virus may be harmless to the pregnant woman and yet be hazardous to her unborn child. It is recommended, therefore, that before any woman of childbearing potential is vaccinated, she should be shown to be serosusceptible and not pregnant. In addition, adequate contraception should be provided for three months following immunization.

Table 5. RECOMMENDED IMMUNIZATION SCHEDULES FOR INFANTS AND CHILDREN NOT INITIALLY IMMUNIZED AT USUAL RECOMMENDED TIMES IN EARLY INFANCY

	Recommended Schedules				
		Alternatives			
Timing	***Preferred Schedule***	*#1*	*#2*	*#3*	**Comments**
First visit	DTP #1, OPV #1, Tuberculin test (PPD)	MMR, PPD	DTP #1, OPV #1, PPD	DTP #1, OPV #1, MMR, PPD	MMR should be given no younger than 15 mo old.
1 mo after first visit	MMR	DTP #1, OPV #1	MMR, DTP #2	DTP #2	
2 mo after first visit	DTP #, OPV #2	—	DTP #3, OPV #2	DTP #3, OPV #2	—
3 mo after first visit	(DTP #3)	DTP #2, OPV #2	—	—	In preferred schedule, DTP #3 can be given if OPV #3 is not to be given until 10–16 mo.
4 mo after first visit	DTP #3 (OPV #3)	—	(OPV #3)	(OPV #3)	OPV #3 optional for areas for likely importation of polio (e.g., some southwestern states.)
5 mo after first visit	—	DTP #3 (OPV #3)	—	—	
10–16 mo after last dose	DTP #4, OPV #3 or OPV #4	DTP #4, OPV #3 or OPV #4	DTP #4, OPV #3 or OPV #4	DTP #4, OPV #3 or OPV #4	—
Preschool	DTP #5, OPV #4 or OPV #5	DTP #5, OPV #4 or OPV #5	DTP #5, OPV #4 or OPV #5	DTP #5, OPV #4 or OPV #5	Preschool dose not necessary if DTP #4 or #5 given after fourth birthday.
14–16 yr old	Td	Td	Td	Td	Repeat every 10 years.

Alternative #1 can be used in those more than 15 months old if measles is occurring in the community.
Alternative #2 allows for more rapid DTP immunization.
Alternative #3 should be reserved for those whose access to medical care is compromised by poor compliance.
From American Academy of Pediatrics. Report of the Committee on Infectious Diseases, 19th ed. 1982.

It occasionally becomes necessary, because of plans to travel, to immunize a pregnant woman against anticipated high-risk exposures. Under these unavoidable circumstances immunization against yellow fever and poliomyelitis may be warranted. Since in these settings immediate prophylaxis is required for protection against polio, the live oral vaccine is recommended. Generally, all other live vaccines are discouraged during pregnancy. Inactivated vaccines, however, may be used when specifically indicated. Tetanus and diphtheria toxoids (adult Td) may be given routinely to update pregnant women during their antepartum care.

A pregnancy in the family should not alter the immunization schedules of any family members or contacts of the pregnant woman. Specifically, rubella vaccination of children need not be avoided when their mother is pregnant. A woman who is seronegative for rubella during pregnancy should be given the attenuated rubella vaccine postpartum. Similarly, breastfeeding is not a contraindication to the immunization of a mother or her baby.

IMMUNIZATION FOR TRAVELERS. With increased foreign travel, it has become important that physicians be able to recommend proper immunizations to their patients to protect their health while traveling (Barrett-Connor, 1979; Medical Letter on Drugs and Therapeutics, 1979). Necessary vaccinations include not only those recommended for protection of the traveler but also those required specifically by individual nations. Detailed information is available in *Health Information For International Travel*, prepared by the Center for Disease Control and obtainable from the Superintendent of Documents, US Government Printing Office, Washington, D.C. 20402. Table 6 summarizes some of the present recommendations for foreign travelers. More detailed and up-to-date information can be obtained from the above CDC publication. Other prophylactic measures should be explored as well before the trip is begun, with particular emphasis on medications for the prevention of gastroenteritis and malaria. When children or adolescents travel, their immunization records should be reviewed and routine immunizations updated if necessary. International travelers must have their vaccinations against yellow fever and cholera documented on an approved version of the International Certificate of Vaccination or Revaccination. These certificates, approved by the World Health Organization, are usually available at local health departments and passport offices.

CONTROVERSIES IN IMMUNIZATIONS. Many of the vaccines currently available are widely accepted as effective and worthwhile (Table 7). Virtually no vaccine, however, has been developed and used without eliciting controversy as to its efficacy, indications, target population, and side effects (Fulginiti, 1976). Some of the major controversies involving passive and active immunizations are discussed below. The reader is encouraged to review specific chapters for more detailed descriptions of immunizations available and those currently being developed for individual infectious diseases (Table 8).

Meningococcal Disease. Four meningococcal polysaccharide vaccines are licensed in the United States. They are prepared as monovalent group A, monovalent group C, bivalent groups A and C, and quadravalent groups A,

Table 6. IMMUNIZATION FOR FOREIGN TRAVEL

Disease	Areas Where Indicated or Required	Comments
Bacterial		
Cholera	Only where required	Risk to tourist small, vaccine of limited efficacy
Plague	Southeast Asia or frequent contact with rodents in S. America, Asia, Africa	For most tourists not necessary
Tetanus, diphtheria	All persons every 10 years regardless of travel	
Tuberculosis	Developing countries	BCG or INH prophylaxis in areas with high risk; otherwise skin test every six months
Typhoid	Countries with poor sanitation	Frequently associated with fever and sore arm for one to two days. Requires two doses four weeks apart
Rickettsial		
Typhus	Mountainous, highland, or cold areas with louse infestation in Ethiopia, Rwanda, Burundi, Mexico, Ecuador, Bolivia, Peru, and Asia	Vaccine no longer available in U.S.
Viral		
Hepatitis A	≥ 3 months in tropical areas and developing countries	IG immunization close to departure
Poliomyelitis	Rural developing countries	If previously immunized: one dose of TOPV; if no previous immunization: primary series of TOPV or inactivated vaccine; altered immune status: inactivated vaccine
Rabies	Only where exposure to rabid animals is a constant threat	HDCV is immunization of choice
Smallpox	No longer required	
Yellow fever	Rural S. America, tropical Africa; most countries require vaccine if traveler is coming from area with reported case of yellow fever within six days of arrival	Should be included by traveler who might change itinerary to include areas with endemic yellow fever. Immunocompromised persons should not be vaccinated

C, Y and W-135. As with all polysaccharide vaccines, they are type-specific and offer little protection against other serotypes. The recommended dosage of each polysaccharide is 50 μg administered subcutaneously, although recent evidence suggests that there may be no advantage to using doses exceeding 5 μg in young adults for groups Y and W-135 (Griffiss et al., 1982). The vaccines are safe but of variable efficacy. Field trials in Egypt, the Sudan, and Finland have demonstrated that group A vaccine results in protection against group A meningococcal disease in 90 per cent of individuals, and suggest that children as young as 3 months of age may be immunized successfully. The group C vaccine has also been successful in protecting 90 per cent of adults against disease. Young children, however, do not fare as well, since the C vaccine is only 65 per cent protective in children 2 to 3 years old and provides virtually no protection to children less than 2 years of age. Persistence of antibody is also superior for the type A vaccine. Eighty per cent of children older than 2 years of age when immunized against group A have protective antibody against A disease after four years, while only 40 per cent of children immunized with group C polysaccharide will have antibody against C disease (Lepow et al., 1977; Peltola et al., 1977; Wilkins and Wehrle, 1979).

The incidence of meningococcal disease in the United States has remained low with groups B and C accounting for most disease. However, the emergence of group Y and group W-135 *N. meningitidis* as relatively common causes of disease, particularly in military recruits, has stimulated the development of capsular polysaccharides for use in vaccines (Griffiss et al., 1981). The quadravalent A/C/Y/W-135 vaccine is currently given to American military recruits.

An effective vaccine for group B *N. meningitidis* is not available since group B capsular polysaccharide is insufficiently immunogenic to provide protection. However, recent attempts to combine the capsular group B polysaccharide with the outer membrane protein may provide a better immunogen (Peppler and Frasch, 1982).

The current meningococcal vaccines are not recommended for routine use in civilians unless an epidemic of meningococcal disease due to serogroups A, C, Y or W-135 necessitates immunizing susceptible individuals. The vaccine should be considered for travelers visiting countries having an epidemic caused by one or more of the four strains, or as an adjunct to antibiotic prophylaxis for household contacts of cases infected with susceptible strains.

Pertussis. In the United States, immunization against pertussis is routinely begun at 2 months of age along with vaccination against diphtheria and tetanus (Center for Disease Control, 1977). Although some physicians in the United States have expressed doubts about the efficacy and overall benefits of the current pertussis vaccine, the raging debate occurring in Europe has been largely avoided (Grady and Wetterlow, 1978; Manclark, 1979; Mathias, 1978; Pittman, 1979). In England, the major reservation to the pertussis vaccine is the high incidence of severe reactions (Enrengut, 1978; Stewart, 1977; Lister, 1977). Reactions to the vaccine have been reported in the United States, but they have not been of the frequency or the severity of the British experience. Estimates of severe neurologic reaction to the pertussis vaccine have ranged from 1:2500 to 1:500,000 children. The adverse reactions described include: high fever; collapse sometimes associated with a shock-like state; prolonged periods of screaming during which the infant cannot be comforted; convulsions with or without fever; frank encephalopathy with changes in the level of consciousness, focal neurologic signs, and convulsions; and thrombocytopenic purpura. Although the incidence of these severe reactions is uncertain, mild reactions including low grade fever and pain and induration at the injection site may occur in as high as 90 per cent of vaccine recipients. Rarely, permanent neurologic sequelae have been described.

The true risk-benefit ratio remains to be established (Koplan et al., 1979). Many British physicians have argued that the current risk of contracting a serious pertussis infection is less than the risk of acquiring permanent neurologic sequelae including mental retardation from the vaccine. Proponents of the vaccine contend that the severe complications and high mortality from pertussis in infancy are major reasons for immunization early in life. They point to the dramatic decline in pertussis since routine vaccination was begun. Opponents of the vaccine, however, vehemently emphasize that the incidence of pertussis was decreasing before routine immunization was begun, and that overall cases with subsequently lower morbidity could have been predicted without the use of pertussis vaccine. The most convincing evidence for vaccine efficacy has come recently from Japan and England, where immunization rates have dropped to 10 per cent and 40 per cent, respectively. Both countries have encountered serious outbreaks of pertussis, and interest has renewed in immunizing children. In underdeveloped nations, pertussis remains a serious health problem, and immunization is the only currently viable method for control of disease.

Over the past 40 years, studies of vaccine efficacy have given results varying from 0 to 90 per cent protection. The full series of pertussis vaccinations presently confers immunity in 76 to 92 per cent of recipients (Church, 1979; Grob et al., 1981). Protection is not longlasting, however, and after 10 years only approximately 50 per cent of vaccinees have detectable protective antibody. Pertussis immunization is recommended for children from age 6 weeks up to their seventh birthday. Since most cases occur in infants and young children, and two thirds of pertussis deaths occur in infants less than 1 year of age, immunization should be instituted in infancy as part of the DPT vaccine.

Children who have experienced severe reactions within 48 hours following pertussis-containing vaccines should not receive further pertussis immunizations. These severe reactions include collapse or shock, persistent screaming, temperature of 40.5° C (105° F) or higher, seizures, severe alterations of consciousness, generalized and/or focal neurologic signs, or systemic allergic reactions (Centers for Disease Control, 1984). Static neurologic conditions in infants are not reasons for deferring immunizations against pertussis. In evolving neurologic conditions, however, pertussis immunization should not be used because of the theoretical concern of exacerbating the disorder. There is no convincing evidence that pertussis immune globulin is effective in preventing or treating pertussis, and its use is not recommended.

A new pertussis vaccine is being investigated in Japan (Oda et al., 1983). This acellular vaccine is enriched in two proteins, the lymphocytosis-promoting factor hemagglutinin (LPF-HA) and the filamentous hemagglutinin (F-HA). The vaccine protects as well as the whole cell pertussis vaccine in a mouse model, and may prove to be an acceptable alternative to the current pertussis vaccine.

Pneumococcus. *Streptococcus pneumoniae* (pneumococ-

Table 7. CURRENTLY AVAILABLE IMMUNIZATIONS

Disease	Immunizing Agent	Indication	Administration: *Primary*	Administration: *Booster*	Administration: *Route*	Efficacy[a]	Adverse Reactions	Comments
Bacterial								
Anthrax	Cell-free, alum-concentrated inactivated protein antigen of *Bacillus anthracis*	High-risk > 6 mo old	0.5 ml for three doses given two to three weeks apart	0.5 ml annually	S.Q.[b]	+ + + +	Local erythema, induration; fever	
Cholera	Phenol-inactivated *Vibrio cholerae*	Travel to or residence in countries with cholera	Intradermal >5 yr, 0.2 ml; S.Q. or I.M. 6 mo—4 yr, 0.2 ml; 5–10 yr, 0.3 ml; > 10 yr, 0.5 ml in two doses at least one wk apart	Every 6 mo or just before cholera season	As indicated	+	Pain, erythema, and induration at injection site; fever, malaise, and headache	
Diphtheria, tetanus, pertussis (DTP)	Alum-precipitated or absorbed toxoids of diphtheria and tetanus D 7 to 25 LF, killed *B. pertussis*	All persons < 7 yr old	See tables 4 and 5			+ + + + + + − + + +	See text	See text
Tetanus, diphtheria (Td)	T—as above d—≤ 2 LF	All persons > 7 yr old	See tables 4 and 5; booster every 10 yr for life			+ + + +	Local pain and induration and mild fever	
Meningococcus types A, C, Y, and W-135	Capular polysaccharide of *Neisseria meningitidis* types A, C, Y, W-135	> 2 yr old in epidermic or high-risk setting	50 μ of each polysaccharide 0.5 ml of vaccine		S.Q.	+ + +	Local erythema and pain	Vaccine ineffective against other types of *N. meningitidis*
Plague	Formaldehyde-inactivated *Yersinia pestis*	High-risk	Three doses: first two doses 0.5 ml at least 4 wk apart; third dose 0.2 ml 4 to 12 wk after second dose (see comments)	Same amount as third dose at 6-month intervals to total of five doses (3 primary and two boosters)	I.M.[c]	+ + + +	Mild pain, erythema, and local induration with repeated doses; headache, malaise	Adjust dosage for age: < 1 yr, one fifth adult dose: 1–4 yr, two fifths adult dose; 5–10 yr, three fifths adult dose
Pneumococcus	Capsular polysaccharide of 23 types	Persons > 2 yr old with high risk of pneumococcal infections	25 μg of each polysaccharide 0.5 ml of vaccine	Unknown	S.Q.	+ + +	Local erythema, induration and pain; fever	See text
Tuberculosis	BCG (an attenuated strain of *Mycobacterium bovis)*	Any age: (1) high risk for continued exposure; (2) populations	Newborns: 0.05 ml; > 1 mo old: 0.1 ml	Give full dose to newborn at 1 yr if risk still present; all	S.Q. or multiple percutaneous	+ − + +	Ulceration, lymphadenitis, osteomyelitis, dissemination, and death	Vaccine should be repeated at two to three months

		where skin test conversion > 1% per yr		others not recommended (see comments)				after vaccination if skin test is negative
Typhoid	Acetone-killed *Salmonella typhi*	Close contact to typhoid carrier or traveler to high-risk areas	6 mo–10 yr old: 0.25 ml; > 10 yr old: 0.5 ml Two doses divided by four or more weeks	Every three years	S.Q.	+ + − + + +	Local erythema and pain; fever, malaise, headache	See text
Rickettsiae								
Typhus	Formaldehyde-inactivated Rickettsia *prowazekii* grown in chick embryos	Travel to or residence in area with known typhus and medical personnel and laboratory workers in frequent contact with *R. prowazekii*	Two doses four or more weeks apart	Every 6–12 months	S.Q.	Unknown	Local pain, induration and erythemia; fever and malaise	See text Vaccine no longer available in U.S.
Viruses								
Hepatitis B	Suspension of inactivated, alum-absorbed 22-nm surface antigen particles purified from human sera inactivated with 8 M urea, pepsin at pH-2 and 1:4,000, formalin	Exposure or high-risk (see text)	Adult: 3 doses 1.0 ml (20 μg/ml) repeated at 1 and 6 months < 10 yrs old: 3 similarly spaced doses 0.5 ml (10 μg/ml)	Unknown	I.M.	+ + + +	Local erythema and swelling	See text
Influenza	Formalin-inactivated influenza virus grown in chick embryos; usually trivalent preparations of influenza viruses expected to be prevalent	All persons ≥ 6 mo old at increased risk of adverse consequences from infections of lower respiratory tract	One to two doses annually depending on age and past exposure; doses four or more weeks apart 6–35 mo old, 0.25 ml; ≥ 3 yr old, 0.5 ml		S.Q.	+ + − + + +	Local pain, induration and erythema; fever, malaise, allergic hypersensitivity Guillain-Barré syndrome < 1/100,000 doses	Live vaccine currently being extensively studied
Measles	Live attenuated Edmonston B measles virus from chick embryos	All persons > 15 mo old	One dose 0.5 ml	Unknown	S.Q.	+ + + +	Fever, rare encephalitis and encephalopathy	See text

[a]Efficacy:
50–65% = +
65–80% = + +
80–90% = + + +
> 90 % = + + + +

[b]S.Q., subcutaneous

[c]I.M., intramuscularly

Table 7. CURRENTLY AVAILABLE IMMUNIZATION *Continued*

Disease	Immunizing Agent	Indication	Administration: *Primary*	*Booster*	*Route*	Efficacy[a]	Adverse Reactions	Comments
Mumps	Live attenuated Jeryl-Lynn strain of mumps virus grown in chick embryo cells	All children > 15 mo old (see text)	One dose 0.5 ml	Unknown	S.Q.	+ + + +	Uncommon parotitis, allergic reactions, rash, pruritus, purpura	See text
Poliomyelitis	OPV (oral polio vaccine)—live attenuated poliovirus of types 1, 2, and 3	All children ≥ 6 wk to 18 yr; adults when indicated	Two doses at least 6 weeks apart followed by dose 8 to 12 months later	At 4 to 6 years old or before travel to endemic areas	Oral	+ + + +	Rare paralysis in normal individuals	Absolutely contraindicated in any immunocompromised person (see text)
	IPV (formalin) inactivated polio vaccine) of three serotypes grown in monkey cell cultures	≥ 6 week old in selected instances (see text)	Three doses 4 to 8 weeks apart with fourth dose 6 to 12 months following third dose	Every 5 yr until age 18 yr	S.Q.	+ + + +	Local pain	See text
Rabies	HDCV (human diploid cell vaccine) rabies virus grown in human diploid cell cultures and inactivated by N-tributyl phosphate and beta propiolactone or beta propiolactone only	Person at high risk of rabies virus following wild animal bites except rodents, or laboratory exposure	Pre-exposure: Two 1 ml doses 1 wk apart followed by 3rd dose 2–3 wks later Post-exposure: Five 1 ml doses on days 0, 3, 7, 14 and 28 (6th dose on day 90 recommended by WHO)	1.0 ml every 2 years	I.M.	+ + + +	Local swelling erythema, induration and pain	Post-exposure prophylaxis should always include 1 dose of RIG 20 IU/Kg given ½ into wound and ½ I.M. except in individuals previously vaccinated. For pre-exposure: 0.1 ml intradermal doses may be given at same schedule.
Rubella	Live attenuated rubella virus RA 27/3 grown in human diploid fibroblast cells	See text	One dose 0.5 ml	Unknown (see text)	S.Q.	+ + + +	Rash, lymphadenopathy, joint pain	See text
Smallpox	Live attenuated vaccinia virus in lyophilized or glycerinated vaccine	Laboratory workers studying smallpox (see text)	1 drop	1 drop every three years	Multiple pressure, multiple puncture, jet injection	+ + + +	Fever, pain, malaise, lymphadenopathy, rare dissemination, encephalitis	No longer available for civilian use
Yellow fever	Live attenuated yellow fever virus strain 17D grown in chick embryo cells	Traveling or residing in high-risk area or laboratory worker studying yellow fever	0.5 ml	Every 10 years	S.Q.	+ + + +	Headache, myalgia, and fever	Dakar strain associated with 0.5% incidence of meningo-encephalitis and is not recommended

Table 8. SOME DISEASES FOR WHICH IMMUNIZATIONS ARE CURRENTLY BEING INVESTIGATED OR ARE OF LIMITED AVAILABILITY

Adenovirus
Botulism
Cytomegalovirus
Gonorrhea
Haemophilus influenzae type B
Hepatitis A
Herpes simplex 1 and 2
Influenza
Malaria
Mycoplasma pneumoniae
Neisseria meningitidis type B
Parainfluenza 1–3
Pseudomonas
Q fever
Respiratory syncytial virus
Rotavirus
Streptococci
Syphilis
Trachoma
Tularemia
Varicella

cus) remains a common bacterial cause of otitis media, pneumonia, and meningitis in infants and children. Patients who have undergone splenectomy and individuals with sickle-cell disease, nephrotic syndrome, chronic liver disease, malignancy, or primary immunodeficiency are at increased risk of developing severe pneumococcal infections.

Recently a new 23-valent pneumococcal vaccine composed of purified, capsular polysaccharide antigens has been approved to replace the 14-valent formulation. Under the Danish system of nomonclature the 23 types of Streptococcus pneumoniae included in the vaccine are 1, 2, 3, 4, 5, 6B, 7F, 8, 9N, 9V, 10A, 11A, 12F, 14, 15B, 17F, 18C, 19A, 19F, 20, 22F, 23F and 33F. Each dose of the vaccine contains 25 μg of each of the 23 polysaccharides that account for approximately 87 per cent of bacteremic pneumococcal disease in the United States. Nasopharyngeal acquisition of the pneumococcal types included in the vaccine is reduced in vaccinees, and there is no evidence that immunized individuals have any greater risk of acquiring diseases caused by other microorganisms. The duration of protection is unknown, but elevated antibody has been found to persist for at least three to five years for the 14-valent vaccine (Centers for Disease Control, 1981).

Despite the promising findings with the presently licensed pneumococcal vaccine, several problems remain (Artenstein, 1973; Hirschmann and Lipsky, 1981). A vaccine that is protective against 87 per cent of the disease-causing pneumococci and that is 80 per cent effective can reduce pneumococcal disease by at most 70 per cent. In addition, the current vaccine is ineffective in children less than 2 years old (Klein and Mortimer, 1978) and more recent studies indicate that the immune response to the most common pediatric serotypes, 6A, 14, 19F and 23F, is poor in children less than four or five years old (Douglas et al., 1983; Lawrence et al., 1983). This is particularly unfortunate for children with sickle-cell disease, who are at greatest risk of pneumococcal infection during infancy (Ammann et al., 1977; Ahonkhai et al., 1979).

Pneumococcal vaccine is not recommended for healthy people. Special populations including residents of nursing homes and institutions, and localized populations experiencing outbreaks may be considered for pneumococcal vaccination. Those over 2 years of age with sickle-cell disease or other splenic dysfunction including splenectomy, or with chronic illnesses or conditions including diabetes mellitus, chronic cardiorespiratory disease, renal disease, hepatic dysfunction, or old age, may all benefit from pneumococcal vaccination. Caution must be advised, however, against totally relying on the present pneumococcal vaccine to prevent serious *Streptococcus pneumoniae* infections, particularly in children with sickle-cell disease (Ahonkhai, 1979; Ammann et al., 1977). Since the vaccine at best can be expected to prevent 70 per cent of pneumococcal disease, penicillin prophylaxis of children with sickle-cell disease should be continued despite vaccination until the children are 6 years old, when the risk of pneumococcal infection is markedly decreased and prophylaxis may not be necessary.

The current recommendations of the Advisory Committee on Immunization Practice are that the pneumococcal vaccine should be given only once to adults, since local and systemic reactions are more frequent and more severe after revaccination. Additionally, persons who have received the 14-valent pneumococcal vaccine need not receive the 23-valent vaccine since the additional protection provided by the new vaccine does not warrant the risk of adverse reactions.

Tuberculosis. The World Health Organization has credited the BCG vaccine with playing a major role in reducing worldwide morbidity owing to tuberculosis (Eickhoff, 1977). Controlled trials, however, have found extremely variable immunity in vaccine recipients. In fact, despite the use of BCG since 1921, there is still debate about whether the vaccine is effective.

BCG is derived from a strain of *Mycobacterium bovis* that was attenuated at the Pasteur Institute in Lille, France, by Calmette and Guérin. All BCG vaccines available today were derived from the original strain. Differences in production, methods and routes of vaccination, and characteristics of the populations and environments in which the vaccine has been used have resulted in great variation in immunogenicity, efficacy, and reactogenicity among the daughter strains. At present, most laboratories producing BCG vaccine maintain production strains in a lyophilized state in an attempt to minimize genetic variation. The production strains are usually named by the city in which they are produced (e.g., BCG-London, BCG-Copenhagen). In the United States, the Bureau of Biologics, Food and Drug Administration, has specified that each freeze-dried BCG strain used for vaccination must have specified characteristics of safety and potency and be capable of inducing tuberculin sensitivity in guinea pigs and humans (Center for Disease Control, 1979). Unfortunately, induced tuberculin sensitivity has never been proved to be related to immunity.

The rationale behind the use of the BCG vaccine to prevent tuberculosis is to confer cell-mediated immunity against an attenuated, immunologically similar strain of mycobacteria. It is known that most hosts, upon primary infection with tubercle bacilli, are able to mount an immunologic response sufficient to localize the infection and thus establish a latent or dormant infectious state. The inactive infection may continue for life or may reactivate frequently but not invariably during times of altered host cell-mediated immunity. There is evidence that the BCG vaccine prevents the establishment of a latent infection when the vaccinee is challenged with live tubercle bacilli, thus preventing not only primary tuberculosis but also the breakdown or reactivation disease.

The lyophilized vaccines have demonstrated substantial protection in animals and are being tested in India. Field trials, all conducted before 1955 with liquid vaccines, showed protection ranging from 0 to 80 per cent. Some argued that the potencies of the BCG strains used in these studies were sufficiently different to account for the contradictory findings. Another possibility is that populations showing little protection from BCG had a large prior exposure to atypical mycobacterial infections. These previous infections may have induced enough immunity to tuberculosis to mask any contribution made by BCG immunization. Interestingly, field trials performed where there is a relatively high incidence of tuberculosis in the control group have tended to show a high efficacy for the BCG vaccine, whereas areas with a low incidence of tuberculosis in the unvaccinated group have shown little benefit from BCG. Continual mycobacterial challenges may be necessary, therefore, to maintain the immunity conferred by BCG vaccination.

The most recent trial organized by the Indian Council for Medical Research, the World Health Organization, and the U.S. Public Health Service in 1968 in Southern India was intended to document the efficacy of BCG in preventing tuberculosis. After a 7-½ year followup, the number of pulmonary tuberculosis cases in the vaccine and placebo groups was approximately the same (Madras: Trial of BCG vaccine in the South India). The methodology of this study has been challanged, however, because of apparent surveillance and diagnostic-testing bias (Clemens et al., 1983). This trial, therefore, has done little to settle the issue, and other studies will be needed before the usefulness of BCG is known.

In the United States, it is recommended that BCG should be "seriously considered" for patients such as infants who are tuberculin skin-test-negative but who can be expected to have repeated exposure to individuals with sputum-positive pulmonary tuberculosis. In addition, BCG vaccination should be considered for groups in which the skin-test conversion rates exceed 1 per cent annually and in which the usual surveillance and treatment programs have failed or are not feasible. In developing countries where tuberculosis is epidemic and short-term INH prophylaxis or skin-test screening is not possible, BCG is indicated to attempt tuberculosis control.

In the United States, where the current annual infection rate among 6-year-olds is approximately 3 per 100,000, BCG is rarely indicated. Infants tolerate two to three months of INH prophylaxis extremely well and thus can allow time for sufficient screening and treatment of family contacts, eliminating the need for BCG vaccination. In addition, tuberculin skin tests are rendered less valuable, since it is usually impossible to distinguish between a tuberculin reaction caused by a virulent supra-infection and one resulting from persistent postvaccination sensitivity. After the immediate postvaccination period, however, caution is advised in attributing a positive skin test to BCG, and tuberculosis should always be considered a possible diagnosis.

BCG should be used only in individuals who are skin-test-negative to 5 tuberculin units of tuberculin purified protein derivative (PPD). The dosage is indicated by the manufacturer in the package insert. Infants less than 28 days old should receive one half the usual dose. If the need for immunization persists, these children should receive a full dose at 1 year of age. The World Health Organization recommends that BCG be given by intradermal injection to provide for a uniform and reliable dose. In the United States, however, both intradermal and percutaneous vaccines are licensed, and vaccination should only be by the route indicated in the package labeling (Center for Disease Control, 1979). Individuals receiving BCG should have a tuberculin skin test two to three months after immunization. If that skin test is negative and the indications for BCG remain, a second dose of vaccine should be administered.

Adverse reactions to BCG have included severe or prolonged ulceration at the vaccination site, lymphadenitis, osteomyelitis, lupoid reactions, disseminated BCG infection, and death (Passwell et al., 1976). Ulceration and lymphadenitis occur in 1 to 10 per cent of vaccinees; osteomyelitis may occur in 1 per million vaccine recipients but may be as high as 5 per 100,000 in newborns. Disseminated BCG infection and death occur in 1 to 10 per 10 million vaccinees and are seen almost exclusively in children with impaired immunity. BCG should, therefore, not be given to anyone with impaired immune status. Although no harmful effects of BCG on the fetus have been observed, immunization should be avoided during pregnancy unless there is an immediate excessive and unavoidable exposure to infectious tuberculosis.

Typhoid. Typhoid fever remains a major world health problem, particularly in developing countries, where poor sanitation and ingestion of inadequately cooked food are common. Killed typhoid vaccines have been used since the late 19th century, although their efficacy was not established until the 1960s. The Yugoslav Typhoid Commission in 1962 showed that a heat-killed, phenol-preserved vaccine gave considerable protection against typhoid fever for at least three years, whereas an alcohol-killed, alcohol-preserved vaccine was ineffective. Subsequent field trials in Guyana showed the heat-phenol and acetone-inactivated vaccines to be 65 to 90 per cent effective in preventing typhoid fever (Ashcroft et al., 1967). Although typhoid fever usually confers lifelong immunity, the nature of protection is unknown. The titers of antibodies against O, H, and Vi antigens have not been connected with protection. Naturally occurring sources of *Salmonella typhosa* usually contain 10^5 or less organisms, resulting in infection of 25 per cent of unvaccinated individuals. Following typhoid fever or immunization, most individuals are protected against a challenge of 10^5 organisms. Volunteer studies indicate, however, that vaccine-acquired immunity can be easily overcome with a challenge of 50 per cent infectious dose (10^7) of *S. typhosa* organisms (Hornick et al., 1970). The effectiveness of paratyphoid A and B vaccines has never been established, and they are not recommended for use either individually or in combination with typhoid vaccine.

Typhoid vaccine in the United States is not recommended for general use (Center for Disease Control, 1978). Persons with intimate exposure to a documented typhoid carrier or travelers to areas where there is a high risk of exposure to typhoid because of poor food or water sanitation should receive typhoid vaccine. In the United States vaccination is not indicated for use in controlling outbreaks from a common source or natural disasters such as floods.

Primary immunization of adults and children 10 years or older consists of two doses of 0.5 ml of vaccine injected subcutaneously, three or more weeks apart, or three doses at weekly intervals. Children 6 months to 10 years old should receive 0.25 ml of vaccine following one of the same schedules. Revaccinations are recommended every three years if there is continuing exposure, with a single booster given intradermally (0.1 ml of vaccine into the flexor surface of the forearm) or subcutaneously (0.5 ml of vaccine in individuals older than 10 years or 0.25 ml in children less than 10 years old). The acetone-killed vaccine should not be given intradermally. If more than three years have elapsed since the last vaccination only one booster is still required. Reactions including local pain, malaise, headache, and fever are common.

A new live attenuated oral typhoid vaccine is currently being tested. This vaccine uses a mutant (Ty 21a) of *Salmonella typhi* that lacks the enzyme uridine 5′-diphosphate-glucose-4-epimerase. The vaccine, when grown in brain-heart infusion broth in the presence of 0.1 per cent galactose, showed great promise in early investigations (Gilman et al., 1977). More recently, a controlled field trial of the Ty 21a oral vaccine was conducted among 32,388 children in Alexandria, Egypt (Wahdan et al., 1982). The incidence of typhoid fever was 4.9 cases per 10,000 children per year in the control group and 0.2 cases per 10,000 children per year in the vaccine group. The estimated protection afforded by the vaccine was 95 per cent. These results strongly suggest that the Ty 21a oral vaccine is safe and effective in controlling typhoid fever and could lower the morbidity associated with typhoid fever throughout the world.

Cytomegalovirus. Cytomegalovirus (CMV) is the most common congenital infection resulting in mental retardation and deafness. Primary CMV infection and reactivation disease are often responsible for severe illness and the death of immunocompromised patients; they may also be associated with renal allograft rejection. Pneumonia, hepatitis, encephalitis, atypical lymphocytosis, and leukopenia are all clinical manifestations of CMV infections.

It is likely that everyone develops a persistent CMV infection after primary exposure. Immunization against CMV ideally, therefore, would prevent primary as well as reactivated disease. In order to prevent transplacental transmission of CMV, a vaccine should also prevent reinfection viremia. Several theoretical problems must be faced before people are immunized against CMV. The capability of CMV to transform normal cells has stimulated concern that a vaccine might be oncogenic. Additionally, if a persistent infection is established after CMV immunization, reactivation of the vaccine virus may result in more severe disease than natural infection. Moreover, CMV strains are so heterogeneous that it is unclear if enough cross-reactivity exists for a vaccine made from one strain to establish broad protection.

Two live attenuated CMV vaccines are being investigated in renal transplant patients. Preliminary studies indicate that both the Towne-125 strain vaccine and the AD-169 strain vaccine can induce CMV-specific cellular immunity in previously seronegative recipients (Just et al., 1975; Plotkin et al., 1976; Glazer et al., 1979; Fleisher et al., 1982). Although the vaccines have not been shown to prevent CMV infections, reactivation of the vaccine strain virus has not been demonstrated. The effect of immunization of seronegative women with the CMV vaccines and the subsequent incidence of infants born with congenital CMV is unknown. Additional work is being done on a specific CMV immune globulin and immune plasma in an attempt to ameliorate or possibly prevent primary CMV infections (Winston et al., 1982; Meyers et al., 1983). Cautious investigation seems warranted to determine the risks and benefits of these approaches to immunoprophylaxis of CMV infections in selected populations.

Hepatitis. Standard IG is effective for the prevention or modification of hepatitis A infection (Krugman et al, 1960; Center for Disease Control, 1981; Woodson and Clinton, 1969). When administered within one to two weeks after exposure to hepatitis A, it prevents illness in 80 to 90 per cent of individuals exposed. IG should be given as soon after close contact with an infected person as possible and is not indicated if more than 2 weeks have elapsed since exposure or if clinical illness is present. Preexposure prophylaxis should be used for those at high risk of hepatitis A exposure and repeated every four to six months when risk continues. Frequently it is not necessary to continue prophylaxis in individuals with continued high contact over one year, since subclinical disease will often develop within that time.

All sexual contacts and household contacts of persons with hepatitis A should receive IG. Staff, children and all members of households where children attending a day care center are in diapers should receive IG if hepatitis A is being transmitted in the center. Contacts in schools where older children attend, however, usually do not require prophylaxis unless a documented outbreak is occurring there. Prophylaxis also may be indicated in institutional settings when hepatitis A outbreaks occur. IG is not indicated for casual contacts in office or hospitals. Transmission of hepatitis A through foodhandling is a risk and exposed kitchen employees should receive IG. In order to protect exposed diners, they must receive IG within two weeks of exposure.

Both IG and specific hepatitis B immune globulin (HBIG) contain anti-HBsAg, and since 1977 IG has contained anti-HBsAg at a titer of at least 1:100 by radioimmunoassay while HBIG has a titer of at least 1:100,000 (Centers for Disease Control, 1981). Administration of immune globulins prevent approximately 75 per cent of hepatitis B following exposure (Seeff et al., 1978; Hoofnagle et al., 1979). The advantage of HBIG over IG for percutaneous or mucous membrane exposure to blood containing HBsAg is unknown, but HBIG is preferred for such exposures. The benefit of globulin given beyond 7 days of exposure is unclear, and every effort should be made to administer either IG or HBIG as soon after exposure as possible. The cost of HBIG is approximately 20 times that of IG. Decision to use HBIG depends upon the potential risk of hepatitis B transmissions following exposure. Percutaneous or mucous membrane exposure to known HBsAg positive blood is justification for immediate administration of HBIG followed 1 month later by a second dose. In high-risk exposure situations where the HBsAg status of the source is unknown, IG should be administered provided test results of the hepatitis B status of the source can be obtained within 7 days. If HBsAg test cannot be known within 7 days, HBIG is indicated. One of the most important uses of HBIG is its administration to infants born to HBsAg positive mothers. In a large clinical trial in Taiwan, HBIG given within 30 hours of birth (usually in the delivery room) was 75 per cent effective in preventing the HBV carrier state in infants of mothers who were both HBsAg positive and HBeAg positive (Beasley et al., 1981). In this study infants were given HBIG at delivery, 3 months and 6 months. In order to use HBIG in the delivery room, however, it is necessary to know before delivery that the mother is HBsAg positive. The following women are at increased risk of being HBsAg positive and are candidates for hepatitis B screening before delivery of their infant (Oxman et al., 1983): Those with acute or chronic liver disease; those rejected as blood donors; women of Asian, Pacific Islands, native Alaskan (Eskimo), Haitian, or sub-Saharan African descent; women who work or whose spouses work in a renal dialysis unit; women who work or reside in an institution for the retarded; women with a history of percutaneous drug abuse; women who live in a household with persons with acute or chronic hepatitis B; women who receive multiple blood transfusions; women with frequent occupational exposure to blood; and prostitutes.

A hepatitis B virus vaccine prepared as a suspension of inactivated, alum absorbed 22-nm surface antigen particles purified from human plasma has been licensed in the United States (Centers for Disease Control, 1982). The vaccine is inactivated by treatment with 8M urea, pepsin at pH-2 and 1:4,000 formalin. Each of these processes inactivate not only hepatitis B virus, but representative viruses in all known groups. The vaccine administered with three intramuscular doses produces antibody in over 90 per cent of recipients (Francis et al., 1982; Szmuness et al., 1980) and has an efficacy of 80 to 95 per cent. Reactions to the vaccine have been limited to soreness and redness at the injection site and no cases of hepatitis B or nonA/non-B hepatitis have been associated with the vaccine. In addition, there is no increased risk of developing the acquired immune deficiency syndrome in recipients of the vaccine.

The question of who should receive pre-exposure hepatitis B vaccination is controversial. The following should be considered for such immunization: health-care workers; hospital staff; clients and staff of institutions for the mentally retarded; hemodialysis patients; homosexually active males; illicit injectable drug users; recipients of large amounts of blood products; household and sexual contacts of hepatitis B carriers; inmates of long-term correctional facilities; and other special high-risk populations.

The vaccine potentially can have its greatest impact when used for infants born to HBsAg positive mothers. Although HBIG can successfully prevent most infants born to chronic HBsAg carrier mothers from becoming chronic carriers themselves, infants who do not develop their own protective antibody will be continuously exposed to hepatitis B during their childhood. It is recommended, therefore, that infants born to mothers who are chronic carriers be immunized. Although the optimum schedule for these infants is unknown, it is likely that immunization can begin immediately after birth. Until further information is available, it is recommended that infants receive 0.5 ml HBIG intramuscularly and 10 μg of hepatitis B vaccine immediately at delivery, followed at 1 and 6 months by 10 μg of hepatitis B vaccine intramuscularly. Other individuals who may benefit from post-exposure prophylaxis include household contacts of hepatitis B cases, and healthcare workers exposed to needle sticks from HBsAg positive individuals.

Measles (Rubeola). Measles is a frequently severe illness associated with encephalitis in 1 of 1000 cases and commonly resulting in permanent neurologic sequelae including mental retardation. Respiratory or neurologic complications result in death in approximately 1 of 1000 cases. At present, a highly effective live vaccine is available (Center for Disease Control, 1982). The degree of measles control depends primarily on the extent to which a given population is immunized. The current further-attenuated Edmonston B strain vaccine has been so effective that the major controversies revolve around how best to immunize as many susceptible persons as possible. It is available in monovalent form (measles only) and in combination with rubella (MR) and mumps and rubella (MMR) vaccines. Follow-up studies indicate that durable immunity is achieved in 95 per cent of individuals older than 15 months of age given the live measles vaccine. Children immunized before 12 months of age have significantly lower seroconversion rates following immunization (Wilkins and Wehrle, 1978). Conflicting data exist for children between 12 and 14 months old, but it appears that these children respond adequately to measles immunization. However, because of this uncertainty, it is currently recommended that children receive their primary measles immunization at 15 months of age. Whenever there is high risk of exposure to natural measles, infants should be immunized at 6 months of age and then revaccinated when they are 15 months old. Children who have been vaccinated with live measles vaccine before 12 months of age should be revaccinated after they are 15 months old (Centers for Disease Control, 1982).

Despite the widespread use of measles vaccine in the United States, epidemics have continued to occur, albeit to a much lesser extent than in prevaccine years (Orenstein et al., 1978; Weiner et al., 1977; Shasby et al., 1977; McCormick et al., 1977; Modlin et al., 1977). Laws requiring primary immunizations for children entering school have had a great influence in lowering the incidence of measles in the United States where an attempt is being made to eliminate indigenous measles. The effects of revaccination have become important with the increasing number of public schools requiring all children to have documented immunization histories before entrance (Deseda-Tous et al., 1978). Fortunately, revaccination has not been associated with any increase in complications in children who have previously received live measles vaccines or who have had natural measles. Increased reactions including local induration, pain, edema, and fever have occurred in over 50 per cent of individuals given live measles vaccine who had previously received killed vaccine (Krause et al., 1978). The risk of atypical measles in these young adults is sufficient, however, to warrant vaccination.

Exposure to measles is not a contraindication to vaccination (Ruuskanen et al., 1978). If given within 72 hours of exposure, evidence suggests that immunization may provide protection. Measles may be prevented or modified by administration of IG within six days of exposure. Live measles vaccine should not be given until three months after administration of IG. Measles outbreaks are best controlled by vaccination of susceptible individuals. Widespread use of IG in these situations is not recommended.

Mumps. Clinical mumps is generally a benign disease associated with parotid swelling, tenderness, and fever. Meningoencephalitis or meningitis occurs in 0.5 to 10 per cent of all mumps cases. Although death is rare, morbidity may be severe. Bilateral orchitis occurs in approximately 2 per cent of cases in men, but sterility is uncommon. Unilateral deafness following endolymphatic labyrinthitis occurs in 2 per 10,000 cases. Arthritis, nephritis, subacute thyroiditis, pancreatitis, myocarditis, and hepatitis are all uncommon complications of mumps infections.

A highly effective, live attenuated mumps vaccine has been available in the United States since 1967 (Center for Disease Control, 1982; Hayden et al., 1978). The Jeryl-Lynn strain of mumps virus is used for immunization following attenuation of virulence in embryonated hens' eggs, and in tissue culture. Antibody appears in 95 per cent of vaccine recipients older than 12 months of age, and protection lasts for at least 15 years. The development of the combined measles-mumps-rubella (MMR) vaccine has greatly accelerated the rate of mumps immunization. Well over 55 million doses of mumps vaccine have been administered since it was licensed and have clearly shown the vaccine to be efficacious with few side effects. Uncommon adverse reactions include parotitis, low-grade fever, rash, and pruritus. Severe CNS complications following immunization are rare, occurring in 1 per million individuals immunized. Individuals with anaphylactic reactions to egg ingestion should receive mumps vaccine only with extreme caution. Other less serious egg allergies are not a contraindication to receiving the mumps vaccine. Additionally, since the mumps vaccine contains trace amounts of neomycin, individuals who have experienced anaphylactic reaction to neomycin should not receive the vaccine.

Mumps vaccine is recommended for all children over 12 months of age. As part of general well-child care, it is best given to a child as the MMR at 15 months. Mumps vaccination is of particular value to susceptible preadolescent males who have no evidence of previous infection, and they should be the target population in countries where the vaccine is not widely available.

Poliomyelitis. Poliovirus vaccines have been widely used for over 25 years. From 1955 to 1965, the inactivated vaccine was the only widely available polio immunization, and it dramatically reduced the incidence of paralytic poliomyelitis in countries where it was extensively used. Although both the IPV (formalin-inactivated polio vaccine) and the OPV (oral polio vaccine) are effective, the OPV has become the vaccine of choice in the United States (Centers for Disease Control, 1982). Countries that prevent poliomyelitis with IPV are generally homogeneous populations that are able to maintain very high vaccination rates. In Sweden and Finland, where only IPV is used, intensive poliovirus surveillance has shown that not only is paralytic disease rare but circulation of the virus is virtually absent. This and animal studies suggest that blocking antibodies produced by IPV can prevent virus implantation despite failure to produce local IgA. In areas with endemic or epidemic poliovirus, however, the populations are best immunized with the live virus vaccine. OPV not only provides intestinal immunity with subsequent prevention of fecal growth of wild virus and decreases circulating virus in the community but also establishes active infections in the nasopharynx and gastrointestinal tract of vaccinees. The virus that is shed following immunization with OPV spreads to susceptible contacts, resulting in inapparent immunizing infections. Additionally, individuals who have received IPV should be reimmunized every five years until the age of 18 years, whereas over 90 per cent of those receiving OPV have neutralizing antibodies to the three types of poliovirus after eight years. It should be noted that problems have occurred in attempting to immunize effectively some populations in tropical and semitropical areas. Viral interference by infection with other enteroviruses at the time of vaccination with OPV may play some role in reducing "take" rates to 50 per cent in these areas. There is also some evidence that 10 to 20 per cent of children in these populations have an inhibitory substance in their saliva that may prevent poliovirus replication. Probably most important in these vaccine failures is inadequate storage of the OPV, which results in inactivation of virus and decreased response rates. Repeated immunization of target populations, however, can eliminate paralytic disease, as has been demonstrated in Cuba and Puerto Rico.

In countries such as the United States where the use of OPV has made paralytic poliomyelitis uncommon, the use of IPV in certain specific situations is warranted. Current estimates indicate that less than one in three million doses of OPV distributed has been associated with paralytic disease in vaccine recipients or their close contacts. Administration of IPV should be oriented toward minimizing the chance of high-risk individuals developing paralytic poliomyelitis from OPV. IPV should be provided to persons with increased susceptibility to infections, including immunodeficient children, and other immunocompromised individuals and their household contacts. Adults undergoing initial vaccination who have the time and are committed to a full course of inoculations are also candidates for IPV since they have a slightly higher risk of developing paralysis. Adults should receive OPV if possible poliomyelitis exposure is to occur before two doses of IPV four weeks apart can be administered. If OPV is inadvertently administered to a household contact of an immunocompromised person, the patient should be isolated from the immunized person for at least two to three weeks after vaccination. Any child born to a family with a history of immunodeficiency disorders should not be given OPV until the immune status of the child is found to be normal.

Regardless of which immunization is used, the goal of polio immunization programs should be to immunize over 90 per cent of the population. When this is achieved, virtual elimination of paralytic poliomyelitis can be expected.

Rubella. Rubella is usually a mild childhood disease with rare complications. It was not until 1964, when a major epidemic in the United States caused more than 20,000 damaged children born of pregnancies complicated by rubella infection, that the need for a rubella vaccine was clearly established. Control of rubella by vaccination presents a unique problem, since it is the only immunization program that attempts to protect a distant fetus by preventing maternal infection during pregnancy. Two immunization strategies have been used in an attempt to decrease the number of congenitally infected infants. The "United States Program" has instituted routine immunization of all prepubertal children, boys and girls, and the selective immunization of postpubertal girls and women of childbearing age documented to be susceptible to rubella infection (Centers for Disease Control, 1981; Modlin et al., 1975). The goal is to induce a high degree of herd immunity, which will prevent circulation of the agent and thus prevent susceptible pregnant women from acquiring rubella. By immunizing young children, the most likely sources of disseminating the infection are in theory eliminated. The "British Program" routinely immunizes girls 11 to 14 years of age and selectively immunizes women of childbearing potential. Thus, it attempts to prevent maternal infection without reducing circulation of the wild-type virus in the remainder of the population.

The two immunization strategies appear to have yielded

different results. In the United States, the incidence of rubella has declined fourfold. Proponents argue that the expected epidemic in the mid-1970s was avoided by massive immunization. Along with the reduction in disease, more importantly, the number of reported cases of congenital rubella in the United States has also declined. In England, on the other hand, only approximately 70 per cent of girls have received the rubella vaccine, and the incidence of congenital rubella has changed little. It is estimated that at least 90 per cent of prepubertal girls would need to be immunized for the incidence of congenital rubella to decline using the "British Program." This approach at best would require a 10-year lag period before the immunized girls became the major portion of the women of childbearing potential, thus affecting the occurrence of congenital rubella.

Questions have been raised concerning the duration of immunity to the rubella vaccines (Wilkins and Wehrle, 1979; Fogel et al., 1978). Of youngsters immunized with the HPV77 DE5 vaccine, between 4 and 36 per cent lack HAI antibodies three to five years after immunization. In addition, children immunized before 12 months of age have significantly lower antibody responses to rubella as well as to measles, probably secondary to persistence of passively transferred maternal antibody. Two other rubella vaccines previously licensed in the United States but now withdrawn had lower overall failure rates. The HPV77 DK12 vaccine, available from 1969 to 1973, had a failure rate of less than 1 per cent, and a 1 to 11 per cent serologic failure rate had been noted for the Cendehill vaccine, which was available from 1970 to 1976. The RA27/3 vaccine, which has been extensively used in Europe and since 1979 has been the only rubella vaccine licensed for use in the United States, is highly immunogenic (Plotkin et al., 1973) and has primary and secondary failure rates of less than 3 per cent.

Rubella reinfection is typically an inapparent infection characterized by the absence of viremia, no or minimal transient pharyngeal virus shedding, and a prompt fourfold or greater rise in rubella HAI antibody. Subclinical reinfection has occurred more frequently after HPV77 or Cendehill immunizations than has been observed with the RA27/3 vaccine or following natural immunity. The potential risks of these subclinical reinfections are unknown but are probably small.

What to do about children, particularly girls, who were immunized with the HPV77 or Cendehill vaccines remains controversial. Revaccination of all prepubertal girls who have previously received these vaccines has been suggested by some (Balfour, 1979). Another approach is premarital screening of all women and immunization with RA27/3 of all seronegative women once adequate precautions are taken to ascertain that they are not pregnant and will not conceive for at least three months after immunization.

A major concern regarding the rubella vaccine has been the inadvertant vaccination of pregnant women, particularly within the 3 months before or after conception. Although rubella virus has been isolated from products of conception of some aborted fetuses (Fleet et al., 1974; Wyll and Hermann, 1973), no newborn has had abnormalities compatible with congenital rubella syndrome after rubella vaccination of 730 pregnant women reported to the Centers for Disease Control (1982). Nevertheless no woman should be given the rubella vaccine who is pregnant or is intending to become pregnant within 3 months. Since the risk of developing congenital rubella syndrome after vaccination is negligible, rubella vaccination of a pregnant woman should not in itself be an indication for abortion. A final decision, however, should rest with the patient and her physician.

Smallpox. The live vaccinia virus vaccine, which is a stable hybrid of both smallpox and cowpox, is no longer available for civilian use. At present, only the few individuals actively involved in doing research using the smallpox virus should be immunized. The vaccine may be obtained only from the Centers for Disease Control (1983). The vaccine at any time is strongly contraindicated in individuals with any impairment of immunity or persons with eczema; individuals with active skin lesions including burns, poison ivy, and impetigo; and pregnant women.

Varicella-Zoster. While varicella has a low incidence of serious complications and sequelae in normal individuals, immunocompromised patients are at high risk of developing serious and potentially fatal infections. These high-risk individuals have been the impetus for the development of means to prevent or ameliorate varicella infections. Varicella-zoster immune globulin (VZIG) prepared from outdated donor blood, or zoster immune globulin (ZIG) obtained from individuals with varicella-zoster infections has been shown to modify or prevent varicella in susceptible children when given within 96 hours of exposure (Brunell and Gershon, 1973; Center for Disease Control, 1979; Gershon et al., 1974; Judelsohn et al., 1974). At present, VZIG is available in the United States through distribution centers for those meeting the criteria outlined in Table 9 (Centers for Disease Control, 1981). Varicella-zoster immune plasma (VZIP), obtained from patients with active zoster, has also been shown to modify varicella infections in high-risk individuals (Balfour and Groth, 1979; Balfour et al., 1977; Geiser et al., 1975). There is no evidence that VZIG or VZIP has any benefit in individuals with active chickenpox or zoster and neither should be used in these situations.

An experimental varicella vaccine has been extensively studied in Japan and is currently under investigation in the United States (Asano et al., 1977; Takahashi et al., 1974). The vaccine protected all of 26 healthy children for at least

Table 9. FIVE CRITERIA FOR RELEASE OF VARICELLA-ZOSTER IMMUNE GLOBULIN (VZIG) FOR THE PROPHYLAXIS OF VARICELLA

I. One of the following underlying illnesses or conditions
   A. Leukemia or lymphoma
   B. Congenital or acquired immunodeficiency
   C. Under immunosuppressive medication
   D. Newly born of mother with varicella
II. One of the following types of exposure to varicella or zoster patient
   A. Household contact
   B. Playmate contact (>1 hour play indoors)
   C. Hospital contact (in same two- to four-room bedroom or adjacent beds in a large ward)
   D. Newborn contact (newborn whose mother contracted varicella less than five days before delivery or within 48 hours after delivery)
III. Negative or unknown prior disease history
IV. Age of less than 15 years
V. Treatment can be initiated within 96 hours of exposure

From Center for Disease Control: Varicella-zoster immune globulin. Morbid Mortal Weekly Rep 30:22, 1981.

5 years (Asano et al., 1983). A similar live attenuated varicella vaccine prepared from the KMcC strain is being investigated in the United States (Arbeter, 1983).

The potential of preventing varicella and its complications in childhood and the misery of herpes zoster in adult life has made some researchers believe that the varicella vaccine may be widely used. Controversy remains, however, about the eventual target population for such a vaccine. Some argue that normal children are at little risk from chickenpox and are not suitable candidates. The risk that more frequent or serious herpes zoster infections will follow vaccination, or that initial infection with varicella will be postponed from childhood when it is mild to adulthood when it is more often severe makes routine immunization against varicella potentially unattractive. High-risk, immunocompromised children are considered to be the group most likely to benefit from a varicella vaccine. This population, however, is the group in which live vaccines are usually avoided and which is most likely to respond inadequately to immunizations. Preliminary studies in Japan have indicated that children with leukemia, neuroblastoma, retinoblastoma, and others with chronic illnesses receiving steroid therapy can be successfully immunized. Clearly, further research will be necessary before benefits and risks of the live varicella vaccines are fully evaluated.

Rickettsial Diseases. The incidence of Rocky Mountain spotted fever (RMSF) continues to increase in the United States. Laboratory workers are at high risk of developing disease while working with *Rickettsia rickettsii*, the causative agent in RMSF. The first RMSF vaccine developed in 1924 was a phenol and formalin-inactivated preparation obtained from infected tick tissue. Since the 1940s, a killed vaccine produced in infected yolk sacs of embryonated eggs had been used. Although early findings in guinea pigs and human field trials suggested vaccine efficacy, after over 30 years of use studies have clearly shown the yolk sac vaccine to be ineffective in preventing infections in humans after laboratory exposure or direct challenge. Since 1970, a new formalin-inactivated vaccine, prepared from *R. rickettsii* grown in tissue culture of chick embryo fibroblasts and purified by sucrose density gradient, has been studied (Kenyon and Pedersen, 1975; Kenyon et al., 1975). The vaccine proved to be highly immunogenic and protective in guinea pigs and rhesus monkeys. (Ascher et al., 1978). A recent clinical trial in volunteers, however, found that the vaccine provided only partial protection against Rocky Mountain spotted fever but ameliorated the illness (Clements et al., 1983). At present, no effective vaccine for RMSF is available.

Louse-borne typhus remains a major problem in rural or remote highland areas of Ethiopia, Rwanda, Burundi, Mexico, Guatemala, Ecuador, Bolivia, Peru, and the mountanous areas of Asia. A formalin-inactivated vaccine which was prepared from *Rickettsia prowazekii* grown in embryonated eggs is no longer being produced (Centers for Disease Center, 1980).

At present, there is no effective vaccine against Q fever. A formalin-inactivated preparation prepared from *Coxiella burnetii* is relatively effective at eliciting an immunogenic response and providing protection in humans but is associated with an unacceptably high incidence of sterile abscesses at injection sites. A live attenuated vaccine utilizing *C. burnetii* strain M-44 initially appeared promising, but guinea pig studies showing microscopic evidence of myocarditis and hepatitis following vaccination suggest that the vaccine will require further attenuation before human use can be recommended (Johnson et al., 1976, 1977; Robinson and Hasty, 1974).

IMMUNIZATIONS FOR DEVELOPING COUNTRIES. Issues concerning immunizations in developed industrial countries often have little relevance for the over three billion people living in less developed nations who suffer from a multitude of infectious diseases. Preventing congenital rubella, avoiding mumps, meningoencephalitis, and orchitis, and protecting immunocompromised individuals from overwhelming varicella infections are medical luxuries shared only by inhabitants of wealthy developed nations. The collective state of ill health in these underdeveloped countries at present, unfortunately, makes comprehensive primary health care an impossibility. Selective primary health care that chooses priorities for disease control is currently the only reasonable goal (Walsh and Warren, 1979). Water and sanitation programs associated with vector control and improved nutrition must be combined with educational campaigns if infectious diseases are to be controlled. Selective immunization for children up to 3 years old and women of childbearing age should at least include vaccination against measles, diphtheria, pertussis, and tetanus. Further immunizations including those against poliomyelitis, tuberculosis, and typhoid could make a large impact on the general state of health in developing countries. The cost of these programs would be substantial and would require a worldwide commitment in order to be successful.

References

General

Artenstein, M. S.: The current status of bacterial vaccines. Hosp Prac 8:49, 1973.

Barrett-Connor, E.: Advice for young travelers. Pediatr Rev 1:25, 1979.

Center for Disease Control: Recommendation of the Immunization Practices Advisory Committee (ACIP): General recommendations on immunization. Morbid Mortal Weekly Rep 29:83, 1980.

Collins, F. M.: Vaccines and cell-mediated immunity. Bacteriol Rev 38:371, 1974.

Fraumeni, J. F., Ederer, F., and Miller, R. W.: An evaluation of the carcinogenicity of simian virus 40 in man. JAMA 185:713, 1963.

Fulginiti, V. A.: Controversies in current immunization policy and practices: One physician's viewpoint. Curr Probl Pediatr 66:3, 1976.

Harrison, H. R., and Fulginiti, V. A.: Bacterial immunizations. Am J Dis Child 134:184, 1980.

Krugman, S., and Katz, S. L.: Childhood immunization procedures. JAMA 237:2228, 1977.

Levine, M. M.: Live-virus vaccines in pregnancy risks and recommendations. Lancet 2:34, 1974.

Marks, J. S., Halpin, T. J., Irvin, J. J., Johnson, D. A., and Keller, J. R.: Risk factors associated with failure to receive vaccinations. Pediatrics 64:304, 1979.

Medical Letter on Drugs and Therapeutics: Immunizations for travelers. 21:57, 1979.

Mortimer, E. A.: Immunization against infectious disease. Science 200:902, 1978.

Phillips, C. F.: Children out of step with immunization. Pediatrics 55:877, 1975.

Rand, K. H., and Merigan, T. C.: Can immunization eradicate viral diseases? Arch Intern Med 137:723, 1977.

Rothberg, R. M., Sumner, C. K., and Michalek, S. M.: Systemic immunity after local antigenic stimulation of the lymphoid tissue of the gastrointestinal tract. J Immunol 111:1906, 1973.

Walsh, J. A., and Warren, K. S.: Selective primary health care: An interim strategy for disease control in developing countries. N Engl J Med 301:967, 1979.

White, C. S., Adler, W. H., and McGann, V. G.: Repeated immunization: Possible adverse effects. Ann Intern Med 81:594, 1974.

Passive Immunization

Braude, A. I., Ziegler, E. J., Douglas, H., and McCutchan, J. A.: Antibody to cell wall glycolipid of gram-negative bacteria: Induction of immunity to bacteremia and endotoxemia. J Infect Dis 136:S167, 1977.

Ellis, E. F., and Henney, C. S.: Adverse reactions following administration of human gamma globulin. J Allergy 43:45, 1969.

Squire, J. R., et al.: Hypogammaglobulinaemia in the United Kingdom. Lancet 1:163, 1969.

Stiehm, E. R.: Standard and special human immune serum globulins as therapeutic agents. Pediatrics 63:301, 1979.

Stiehm, E. R., and Fudenberg, H. H.: Antibodies to gamma-globulin in infants and children exposed to isologous gamma-globulin. Pediatrics 35:229, 1965.

Ziegler, E. J., McCutchan, J. A., Fierer, J., Glauser, M. P., Sadoff, J. S., Douglas, H., and Braude, A. I.: Treatment of gram-negative bacteremia and shock with human antiserum to a mutant Escherichia coli. N Engl J Med 307:1225, 1982.

Cytomegalovirus

Fleisher, G. R., et al.: Vaccination of pediatric nurses with live attenuated cytomegalovirus. Am J Dis Child 136:294, 1982.

Glazer, J. P., et al.: Live cytomegalovirus vaccination of renal transplant candidates. Ann Intern Med 91:676, 1979.

Just, M., Buergin-Wolff, A., Emoedi, G., and Hernandez, R.: Immunization trials with live attenuated cytomegalovirus, Towne 125. Infection 3:111, 1975.

Meyers, J. D., et al.: Prevention of cytomegalovirus infection by cytomegalovirus immune globulin after marrow transplantation. Ann Intern Med 98:442, 1983.

Plotkin, S. A., Farquhar, J., and Hornberger, E.: Clinical trials of immunization with the Towne 125 strain of human cytomegalovirus. J Infect Dis 134:470, 1976.

Winston, D. J., et al.: Cytomegalovirus immune plasma in bone marrow transplant recipients. Ann Intern Med 97:11, 1982.

Diphtheria, Pertussis, Tetanus

Barkin, R. M., and Pichichero, M. E.: Diphtheria-pertussis-tetanus vaccine: Reactogenicity of commercial products. Pediatrics 63:256, 1979.

Centers for Disease Control: Diphtheria and tetanus toxoids and pertussis vaccine. Morbid Mortal Weekly Rep 26:401, 1977.

Centers for Disease Control: Supplementary statement of contraindications to receipt of pertussis vaccine. Morbid Mortal Weekly Rep 33:169, 1984.

Church, M. A.: Evidence of whooping-cough-vaccine efficacy from the 1978 whooping-cough epidemic in Hertfordshire. Lancet i:188, 1979.

Enrengut, W.: Whooping cough vaccination. Lancet 1:370, 1978.

Grady, G. F., and Wetterlow, L. H.: Pertussis vaccine: Reasonable doubt. N Engl J Med 298:966, 1978.

Grob, P. R., Crowder, M. J., Robbins, J. F.: Effect of vaccination on severity and dissemination of whooping cough. Brit Med J 282:1925, 1981.

Kendrick, P. L.: Can whooping cough be eradicated? J Infect Dis 132:707, 1975.

Koplan, J. P., et al.: Pertussis Vaccine—An analysis of benefits, risks, and costs. N Engl J Med 301:906, 1979.

Linneman, C. C., et al.: Use of pertussis vaccine in an epidemic involving hospital staff. Lancet 2:540, 1975.

Lister, J.: The care of children—Pertussis vaccination. N Engl J Med 296:984, 1977.

Manclark, C. R.: Summary of an international symposium on pertussis. J Infect Dis 140:129, 1979.

Mathias, R. G.: Whooping cough in spite of immunization. Can J Public Health 69:130, 1978.

Oda, M., Izumiya, K., Sato, Y., Hirayama, M.: Transplacental and transcolostral immunity to pertussis in a mouse model using acellular pertussis vaccine. J Infect Dis 148:138, 1983.

Peebles, T. C., et al.: Tetanus-toxoid emergency boosters. N Engl J Med 280:575, 1969.

Pittman, M.: Pertussis toxin: The cause of the harmful effects and prolonged immunity of whooping cough. Rev Infect Dis 1:401, 1979.

Stewart, G. T.: Vaccination against whooping cough. Lancet 1:234, 1977.

White, W. G., et al.: Duration of immunity after active immunization against tetanus. Lancet 2:95, 1969.

Hepatitis

Beasley, R. P., et al.: Hepatitis B immune globulin (HBIG) efficacy in the interruption of perinatal transmission of hepatitis B virus carrier state. Lancet ii:388, 1981.

Centers for Disease Control: Hepatitis B virus vaccine safety: Report of an inter-agency group. Morbid Mortal Weekly Rep 31:465, 1982.

Centers for Disease Control: Immune globulins for protection against viral hepatitis. Morbid Mortal Weekly Rep 30:423, 1981.

Centers for Disease Control: Inactivated hepatitis B virus vaccine. Morbid Mortal Weekly Rep 31:317, 1982.

Francis, D. P., et al.: The prevention of hepatitis B with vaccine. Ann Intern Med 97:362, 1982.

Hoofnagle, J. H., et al.: Passive-active immunity from hepatitis B immune globulin. Ann Intern Med 91:813, 1979.

Krugman, S., Ward, R., Giles, J. P., Jacobs, A. M.: Infectious hepatitis: Studies on the effect of gamma globulin and on the incidence of inapparent infection. JAMA 174:328, 1960.

Oxman, M. N., Richman, D. D., Spector, S. A.: Management at delivery of mother and infant when herpes simplex, varicella zoster, hepatitis, or tuberculosis have occurred during pregnancy. Current Clinical Topics in Infectious Diseases. (ed.) J. S. Remington, M. N. Swartz. New York p. 224, 1983.

Seeff, L. B., et al.: Type B hepatitis after needle-stick exposure: Prevention with hepatitis B immune globulin. Ann Intern Med 88:285, 1978.

Szmuness, W., et al.: Hepatitis B vaccine: demonstration of efficacy in a controlled clinical trial in a high-risk population in the United States. N Engl J Med 303:833, 1980.

Woodson, R. D., Clinton, J. J.: Hepatitis prophylaxis abroad. JAMA 209:1053, 1969.

Measles

Albrecht, P., Ennis, F. A., Saltzman, E. J., and Krugman, S.: Persistence of maternal antibody in infants beyond 12 months: Mechanism of measles vaccine failure. J Pediatr 91:715, 1977.

Center for Disease Control: Measles prevention. Morbid Mortal Weekly Rep 27:427, 1978.

Deseda-Tous, J., et al.: Measles revaccination. Am J Dis Child 132:287, 1978.

Krause, P. J., et al.: Revaccination of previous recipients of killed measles vaccine: Clinical and immunologic studies. J. Pediatr 93:565, 1978.

Landrigan, P. J., and Witte, J. J.: Neurologic disorders following live measles-virus vaccination. JAMA 223:1459, 1973.

Marks, J. S., Halpin, T. J., and Orenstein, W. A.: Measles vaccine efficacy in children previously vaccinated at 12 months of age. Pediatrics 62:955, 1978.

McCormick, J. B., Halsey, N., and Rosenberg, R.: Measles vaccine efficacy determined from secondary attack rates during a severe epidemic. J Pediatr 90:13, 1977.

Modlin, J. F., Jabbour, J. T., Witte, J. J., and Halsey, N. A.: Epidemiologic studies of measles, measles vaccine, and subacute sclerosing panencephalitis. Pediatrics 59:505, 1977.

Orenstein, W. A., et al.: Current status of measles in the United States, 1973–1977. J Infect Dis 137:847, 1978.

Ruuskanen, O., Salmi, T. T., and Halonen, P.: Measles vaccination after exposure to natural measles. J Pediatr 93:43, 1978.

Shasby, D. M., et al.: Epidemic measles in a highly vaccinated population. N Engl J Med 296:585, 1977.

Shelton, J. D., et al.: Measles vaccine efficacy: Influence of age at vaccination vs duration of time since vaccination. Pediatrics 62:961, 1978.

Weiner, L. B., et al.: A measles outbreak among adolescents. J Pediatr 90:17, 1977.

Wilkins, J., and Wehrle, P. F.: Additional evidence against measles vaccine administration to infants less than 12 months of age: Altered immune response following active/passive immunization. J Pediatr 94:865, 1979.

Wilkins, J., and Wehrle, P. F.: Evidence for reinstatement of infants 12 to 14 months of age into routine measles immunization programs. Am J Dis Child 132:162, 1978.

Meningococcus

Centers for Disease Control: Meningococcal polysaccharide vaccines. Morbid Mortal Weekly Rep 27:327, 1978.

Griffiss, J. M., et al.: Safety and immunogenicity of group Y and group W135 meningococcal capsular polysaccharide vaccines in adults. Infect Immun 34:725, 1981.

Griffiss, J. M., Brandt, B. L., Broud, D. D.: Human immune response to various doses of group Y and W135 meningococcal polysaccharide vaccines. Infect Immun 37:205, 1982.

Lepow, M. L., et al.: Persistence of antibody following immunization of children with groups A and C meningococcal polysaccharide vaccines. Pediatrics 60:673, 1977.

Peltola, H., et al.: Clinical efficacy of meningococcus group A capsular polysaccharide vaccine in children three months to five years of age. N Engl J Med 297:686, 1977.

Peppler, M. S., Frasch, C. E.: Protection against group B Neisseria meningitidis disease: Effect of serogroup B polysaccharide and polymyxin B on immunogenicity of serotype protein preparation. Infect Immun 37:264, 1982.

Wilkins, J., and Wehrle, P. F.: Further characterization of responses of infants and children to meningococcal A polysaccharide vaccine. J Pediatr 94:828, 1979.

Mumps

Biedel, C. W.: Recurrent mumps parotitis following natural infection and immunization. Am J Dis Child 132:678, 1978.

Center for Disease Control: Mumps vaccine. Morbid Mortal Weekly Rep 31:617, 1982.

Hayden, G. F., Preblud, S. R., Orenstein, W. A., and Conrad, J. L.: Current status of mumps and mumps vaccine in the United States. Pediatrics 62:965, 1978.

Hosai, H., et al.: Studies on live attenuated mumps virus vaccine. Biken J 13:121, 1970.

Lerner, A. M.: Guide to immunization against mumps. J Infect Dis 122:116, 1970.

Yamanishi, K., et al.: Studies of live attenuated mumps virus vaccine: Biological characteristics of the strains adapted to the amniotic and chorioallantoic cavity of developing chick embryos. Biken J 13:127, 1970.

Yamauchi, T., Wilson, C., and St. Geme, J. W.: Transmission of live, attenuated mumps virus to the human placenta. N Engl J Med 290:710, 1974.

Pneumococcus

Ahonkhai, V. I., et al.: Failure of pneumococcal vaccine in children with sickle-cell disease. N Engl J Med 301:26, 1979.

Ammann, A. J., et al.: Polyvalent pneumococcal polysaccharide immunization of patients with sickle-cell anemia and patients with splenectomy. N Engl J Med 297:897, 1977.

Center for Disease Control: Pneumococcal polysaccharide vaccine. Morbid Mortal Weekly Rep 30:410, 1981.

Cowan, M. J., et al.: Pneumococcal polysaccharide immunization in infants and children. Pediatrics 62:721, 1978.

Douglas, R. M., Paton, J. C., Duncan, S. J., Hansman, D. J.: Antibody response to pneumococcal vaccination in children younger than five years of age. J Infect Dis 148:131, 1983.

Fikrig, S. M., et al.: Antibody response to capsular polysaccharide vaccine of *Streptococcus pneumoniae* in patients with nephrotic syndrome. J Infect Dis 137:818, 1978.

Hirschmann, J. V., Lipsky, B. A.: Pneumococcal vaccine in the United States: A critical analysis. JAMA 246:1428, 1981.

Klein, J. O., and Mortimer, E. A.: Use of pneumococcal vaccine in children. Pediatrics 61:321, 1978.

Lawrence, E. M., et al.: Pneumococcal vaccine in normal children: Primary and secondary vaccination. Am J Dis Child 137:846, 1983.

Minor, D. R., Schiffman, G., and McIntosh, L. S.: Response of patients with Hodgkin's disease to pneumococcal vaccine. Ann Intern Med 90:887, 1979.

Poliomyelitis

Centers for Disease Control: Poliomyelitis prevention. Morbid Mortal Weekly Rep 31:22, 1982.

Davis, L. E., et al.: Chronic progressive poliomyelitis secondary to vaccination of an immunodeficient child. N Engl J Med 297:241, 1977.

John, T. J., et al.: Effect of breast-feeding on seroresponse of infants to oral poliovirus vaccination. Pediatrics 57:47, 1976.

Krugman, R. D., et al.: Antibody persistence after primary immunization with trivalent oral poliovirus vaccine. Pediatrics 60:80, 1977.

Melnick, J. L.: Vaccines and vaccine policy: The poliomyelitis example. Hosp Pract 13:41, 1978.

Nightingale, E. O.: Recommendations for a national policy on poliomyelitis vaccination. N Engl J Med 297:249, 1977.

Rousseau, W. E.: Persistence of poliovirus neutralizing antibodies eight years after immunization with live, attenuated-virus vaccine. N Engl J Med 289:1357, 1973.

Rabies

Centers for Disease Control: Rabies prevention. Morbid Mortal Weekly Rep 29:265, 1980.

Nicholson, K. G., Turner, G. S., and Aoki, F. Y.: Immunization with a human diploid cell strain of rabies virus vaccine: Two year results. J Infect Dis 137:783, 1978.

Plotkin, S. A., and Wiktor, T.: Vaccination of children with human cell culture rabies vaccine. Pediatrics 63:219, 1979.

Rickettsial Diseases

Ascher, M. S., et al.: Initial clinical evaluation of a new Rocky Mountain spotted fever vaccine of tissue culture origin. J Infect Dis 138:217, 1978.

Centers for Disease Control: Production of typhus vaccine discontinued in the United States. Morbid Mortal Weekly Rep 29:465, 1980.

Clements, M. L., et al.: Reactogenicity, immunogenicity, and efficacy of a chick embryo cell-derived vaccine for Rocky Mountain spotted fever. J Infect Dis 148:922–930. 1983.

Johnson, J. W., Eddy, G. A., and Pedersen, C. E.: Biological properties of the M-44 strain of *Coxiella burnetii*. J Infect Dis 133:334, 1976.

Johnson, J. W., et al.: Lesions in guinea pigs infected with *Coxiella burnetii* strain M-44. J Infect Dis 135:995, 1977.

Kenyon, R. H., and Pedersen, C. E.: Preparation of Rocky Mountain spotted fever vaccine suitable for human immunization. J Clin Microbiol 1:500, 1975.

Kenyon, R. E., Sammons, L. C., and Pedersen, C. E.: Comparison of three Rocky Mountain spotted fever vaccines. J Clin Microbiol 2:300, 1975.

Robinson, D. M., and Hasty, S. E.: Production of a potent vaccine from the attenuated M-44 strain of *Coxiella burnetii*. Appl Microbiol 27:777, 1974.

Rubella

Balfour, H. H.: Rubella reimmunization now. Am J Dis Child 133:1231, 1979.

Boue, A., Nicolas, A., and Montagnon, B.: Reinfection with rubella in pregnant women. Lancet 1:7712, 1971.

Center for Disease Control: Rubella prevention. Morbid Mortal Weekly Rep 30:37, 1981.

Center for Disease Control: Rubella vaccination during pregnancy—United States, 1971–1981. Morbid Mortal Weekly Rep 31:477, 1982.

Fleet, W. F., et al.: Fetal consequences of maternal rubella immunization. JAMA 227:621, 1974.

Fogel, A., et al.: Response to experimental challenge in persons immunized with different rubella vaccines. J Pediatr 92:26, 1978.

Horstmann, D.: Controlling rubella: Problems and perspectives. Ann Intern Med 83:412, 1975.

Medical Letter on Drugs and Therapeutics: The new rubella vaccine. 21:53, 1979.

Modlin, J. F., et al.: A review of five years' experience with rubella vaccine in the United States. Pediatrics 55:20, 1975.

Plotkin, S. A., Farquhar, J. D., and Ogra, P. L.: Immunologic properties of RA27/3 rubella virus vaccine. JAMA 225:585, 1973.

Schoenbaum, S. C., et al.: Benefit-cost analysis of rubella vaccination policy. N Engl J Med 294:306, 1976.

Wilkins, J., and Wehrle, P. F.: Further evaluation of the optimum age for rubella vaccine administration. Am J Dis Child 133:1237, 1979.

Wyll, S. A., and Herrmann, K. L.: Inadvertent rubella vaccination of pregnant women. JAMA 225:1472, 1973.

Smallpox

Centers for Disease Control: Smallpox vaccine available for protection of at risk laboratory workers Morbid Mortal Weekly Report 32:543, 1983.

De Vries, R. P., Kreeftenberg, M., Loggen, H., and Van Rood, J. J.: In vitro immune responsiveness to vaccinia virus and HLA. N Engl J Med 297:692, 1977.

Tuberculosis

Centers for Disease Control: BCG vaccines. Morbid Mortal Weekly Rep 28:241, 1979.

Clemens, J. D., Chuong, J. H., Feinstein, A. R.: The BCG controversy: A methodological and statistical reappraisal. JAMA 249:2362, 1983.

Eickhoff, T. C.: The current status of BCG immunization against tuberculosis. Annu Rev Med 28:411, 1977.

Passwell, J., et al.: Fatal disseminated BCG infection. Am J Dis Child 130:433, 1976.

Tuberculosis Prevention Trial, Madras: Trial of BCG vaccine in South India for tuberculosis prevention. Indian J Med Res 70:349, 1979.

Typhoid

Ashcroft, M. T., et al.: A seven year field trial of two typhoid vaccines in Guyana. Lancet 2:1056, 1967.

Centers for Disease Control: Typhoid vaccine. Morbid Mortal Weekly Rep 27:231, 1978.

Gilman, R. H., et al.: Evaluation of a UDP-glucose-4-epimeraseless mutant of *Salmonella typhi* as a live oral vaccine. J Infect Dis 136:717, 1977.

Hornick, R. B., et al.: Typhoid fever: Pathogenesis and immunologic control. N Engl J Med 283:686, 739, 1970.
Wahdan, M. H., Serie, C., Cerisier, Y., Sallam, S., Germanier, R.: A controlled field trial of live Salmonella typhi strain Ty 21a oral vaccine against typhoid: Three year results. J Infect Dis 145:292, 1982.

Varicella

Arbeter, A. M., et al.: Live attenuated varicella vaccine: The KMcC strain in healthy children. Pediatrics 71:307, 1983.
Asano, Y., et al.: Protection against varicella in family contacts by immediate inoculation with live varicella vaccine. Pediatrics 59:3, 1977.
Asano, Y., et al.: Five-year followup study of recipients of live varicella vaccine using enhanced neutralization and fluorescent antibody membrane antigen assays. Pediatrics 72:291, 1983.
Balfour, H. H., and Groth, K. E.: Zoster immune plasma prophylaxis of varicella: A follow-up report. J Pediatr 94:743, 1979.
Balfour, H. H., Groth, K., McCullough, J., Kallis, J., Marker, S., Nesbit, M., Summons, R., and Najarian, J.: Prevention or modification of varicella using zoster immune plasma. Am J Dis Child 131:693, 1977.
Brunell, P. A., and Gershon, A. A.: Passive immunization against varicella-zoster infections and other modes of therapy. J Infect Dis 127:415, 1973.
Centers for Disease Control: Varicella-zoster immune globulin. Morbid Mortal Weekly Rep 28:589, 1979.
Centers for Disease Control: Varicella-zoster immune globulin—United States. Morbid Mortal Weekly Rep 30:15, 1981.
Geiser, C. F., et al.: Prophylaxis of varicella in children with neoplastic disease: Comparative results with zoster immune plasma and gamma globulin. Cancer 35:1027, 1975.
Gershon, A. A., Steinberg, S., and Brunell, P. A.: Zoster immune globulin. N Engl J Med 290:243, 1974.
Judelsohn, R. G., et al.: Efficacy of zoster immune globulin. Pediatrics 53:476, 1974.
Takahashi, M., Otsuka, T., and Okuno, Y.: Live vaccine used to prevent the spread of varicella in children in hospital. Lancet 2:1288, 1974.
Uduman, S. A., Gershon, A. A., and Brunell, P. A.: Should patients with zoster receive zoster immune globulin? JAMA 234:1049, 1975.

Other Articles

Balfour, H. H., and Amren, D. P.: Rubella, measles and mumps antibodies following vaccination of children. Am J Dis Child 132:573, 1978.
Beachey, E. H., Stollerman, G. H., and Bisno, A. L.: A strep vaccine: How close? Hosp Pract 14:49, 1979.
Center for Disease Control: Plague vaccine. Morbid Mortal Weekly Rep 27:255, 1978.
Center for Disease Control: Cholera vaccine. Morbid Mortal Weekly Rep 27:173, 1978.
Center for Disease Control: Yellow fever vaccine. Morbid Mortal Weekly Rep 27:268, 1978.
Horstmann, D. M.: Viral vaccines and their ways. Rev Infect Dis 1:502, 1979.
Krugman, S.: Present status of measles and rubella immunization in the United States: A medical progress report. J Pediatr 90:1, 1977.
Melnick, J. L.: Viral vaccines: New problems and prospects. Hosp Pract 13:104, 1978.
Sato, H., et al.: Transfer of measles, mumps and rubella antibodies from mother to infant. Am J Dis Child 133:1240, 1979.
Stumpf, D. A., and Frost, M.: Immunity after rubella and measles viral vaccines. Am J Dis Child 132:748, 1978.
Weibel, R. E., et al.: Long-term follow-up for immunity after monovalent or combined live measles, mumps and rubella virus vaccines. Pediatrics 56:380, 1975.

Books

American Academy of Pediatrics: Report of the Committee on Infectious Disease, 19th ed., Evanston, Illinois, 1982.
Creighton, C.: Jenner and Vaccination: A Strange Chapter of Medical History. London, Suvan Sonnen Schein & Company, 1889.
Parish, H. J.: A History of Immunization. London, E. & S. Livingstone Ltd., 1965.
Parish, H. J.: Victory with Vaccines. London, E. & S. Livingstone Ltd., 1968.
Voller, A., and Friedman, H.: New Trends and Developments in Vaccines, Baltimore, University Park Press, 1978.

METABOLIC

91
FEVER

SHELDON M. WOLFF, M.D.

Fever has been recognized as a major manifestation of a large variety of diseases since antiquity. Although clinicians and investigators have been interested in the mechanisms of production of fever in the intact human for decades, it has been only during the past 30 years that significant progress has been made. It is not known if this commonest of all clinical symptoms is of any value in host defenses or whether it is a nonspecific response. Recent work suggests that in certain species fever can play a protective role against bacterial infections (Kluger, Ringler, Anver, 1975).

Normal body temperature follows a very reproducible circadian rhythm, with the maximum temperature ordinarily occurring in the late afternoon or early evening and then gradually falling to its low point in the morning. Normal temperature can be influenced by a variety of stimuli such as exercise, menstrual cycle, and environmental temperature changes, but it generally follows the same circadian pattern in a given individual. Thirty-seven degrees centigrade (98.6° F) is generally accepted as the "normal" temperature. These are mean values derived from old studies. When interpreting a temperature reading, there are a number of variables to be considered. Among these are how it was obtained (i.e., from which orifice), time of day, and whether the subject had just participated in strenuous physical activity. An isolated temperature reading in a patient is usually of little value, since so many factors can influence body temperature. Fever is a symptom of disease, and it is rare for it to be the sole sign of an illness. Normal individuals may have temperatures that occasionally rise above 38° C in the evening, and, unless multiple readings are taken, or a careful history obtained and a physical examination done, one would be incorrect in calling such an isolated reading a fever. All of the preceding facts emphasize that a temperature reading may be of no value unless it is considered merely as part of a more detailed evaluation of the patient as a whole.

Regardless of the cause of fever, most of the physiologic processes that occur when body temperature rises follow similar patterns. It is well established that the thermoregulatory center resides in the anterior hypothalamus in the floor of the third ventricle. The development of fever depends upon an intricate set of interrelated events involving heat loss, heat production, and peripheral vasoconstriction. Some of these events are mediated by agents such as prostaglandins, but the exact role of such substances in the febrile response in human beings is unclear. When a patient first develops a fever, he or she may have a chill, which is accompanied by an increase in metabolic activity as measured by such things as oxygen consumption. The severity and length of the chill depend on the stimulus. Concomitant with or shortly after the increased metabolic activity, core temperature begins to rise. Peripheral vasoconstriction occurs with the chill and is associated with a decrease in heat loss, which is maximal over the more peripheral areas of the body. The increase in metabolic activity persists during the fever. With the dissipation of the fever, peripheral vasodilatation occurs, and heat loss ensues. Depending on the height of the fever, the rate of heat loss, and the rapidity of the lowering of the temperature, sweating (i.e., diaphoresis) may occur.

Certain clinical findings accompany fever in human beings regardless of the cause. The presence or absence and the magnitude of such findings depend on the severity and duration of the febrile reaction. Headache, myalgias, arthralgias, nausea, vomiting, backache, and feelings of warmth are some of the more common complaints heard from patients with fever. Tachycardia is usual, although in certain infectious diseases a relative bradycardia may be seen. Tachypnea, widening of the pulse pressure, and flushing are additional signs that are usually noted in febrile human beings.

Fever can be a prominent symptom of all infectious and inflammatory diseases. It is also seen in a wide variety of neoplastic and metabolic illnesses. The agents that cause fever are called pyrogens, and the list of pyrogenic substances continues to increase. For example, most bacteria, viruses, and fungi are pyrogenic. Exogenous pyrogens also include the endotoxins of gram-negative bacteria, antigens in previously sensitized subjects (Root and Wolff, 1968), antigen-antibody complexes (formed either in vivo or in vitro), and some synthetic polynucleotides. Certain C-19, C-21, and C-24 steroids of endogenous human origin that share the 5-β-H configuration are potent pyrogens. The best known of these is etiocholanolone (Wolff et al., 1967). Some hormones, such as progesterone, have also been shown to be pyrogenic. What role, if any, is played by these pyrogenic steroids in human disease is not known.

It is generally accepted that the basic series of events put into motion by any exogenous pyrogen is the same. In addition, as noted above, the febrile response is similar. In other words, there is a "final common pathway" that results in fever regardless of the cause. The basic hypothesis states that pyrogens activate host cells, which in turn release an endogenous pyrogen (or leukocytic pyrogen); this endogenously produced substance then stimulates the thermoregulatory centers in the brain, resulting in fever. Much of the information that resulted in this hypothesis has been obtained from experimental animals, but during the past few years information gained from investigations on human cells has become available. Despite the recent rapid advances, considerably more work needs to be done before we can define in exact terms the pathogenesis of fever in man (Dinarello and Wolff, 1978).

It was originally suggested that the neutrophil was the blood leukocyte that was responsible for endogenous pyrogen production (Wood, 1958). However, it was later demonstrated that blood leukocytes from patients with severe granulocytopenia or monocytic leukemia produced large quantities of endogenous pyrogens when stimulated in vitro. The blood monocyte has been established as a potent source of endogenous pyrogen, and this finding provided an explanation for the presence of fever in patients without circulating granulocytes. Certain tumors, namely hypernephromas, which are often associated with febrile episodes, have been shown to release endogenous pyrogens spontaneously in vitro. Kupffer's cells in the liver, splenic macrophages, alveolar macrophages, and peritoneal lining cells are sources of endogenous pyrogen in rabbits and most likely are potent producers of this mediator substance in humans. It is clear that only phagocytic cells derived from bone marrow precursors produce endogenous pyrogen. Furthermore, it is now apparent the mononuclear phagocytes are the predominant, if not the sole, source of endogenous pyrogen (Hanson, Murphy, Windle, 1980). Lymphocytes are not a source of endogenous pyrogen.

When blood leukocytes are incubated with inhibitors of protein synthesis such as puromycin or cycloheximide during the activation process, the subsequent production of endogenous pyrogen is prevented (Nordlund et al., 1970). Neither cycloheximide nor puromycin prevents phagocytosis. Hence, the activation process is unaffected by these drugs. Actinomycin, which prevents the transcription of DNA into messenger RNA, also prevents the production of endogenous pyrogen in vitro. It is clear that the process of activation of mononuclear phagocytes to make endogenous pyrogen begins with the repression of the genome for endogenous pyrogen and that new messenger RNA must be synthesized.

Considerable progress has been made recently in the characterization of human leukocytic pyrogen (Dinarello and Wolff, 1982). The major portion of human leukocytic pyrogen is a protein with a molecular weight of 15,000 and an isoelectric point of 6.9. A second molecule with a molecular weight of 45,000 and an isoelectric point of 5.1 is also produced. Antibodies to these molecules have been produced and a radioimmunoassay developed. These advances should lead to the measurement of this mediator protein in various disease states. Such measurements will undoubtedly improve our ability to diagnose and to treat specifically febrile states.

The preoptic region of the anterior hypothalamus appears to control body temperature. The hypothalamus also contains the monoamines that are critical for normal thermoregulation. When tumors or vascular accidents have involved this center in patients, hypothermia or, rarely, hyperthermia has occurred. Moreover, the circadian temperature rhythm may be lost in such patients.

The preoptic anterior hypothalamus contains the neurons that respond when endogenous pyrogen is injected in animals, and it seems likely that the same area contains pyrogen-sensitive neurons in man. The mechanism by which endogenous pyrogen causes thermosensitive neurons to increase their firing rate is unknown; however, it has been suggested that prostaglandins have a critical role in the production of fever. Mounting evidence suggests that endogenous pyrogen induces synthesis of prostaglandins in the hypothalamus, in which they function as central transmitters in initiation of fever; furthermore, the well-known ability of aspirin and similar drugs to reduce fever appears to be directly related to their ability to block prostaglandin synthesis. Aspirin and other salicylate-like antipyretics do not affect either the production of endogenous pyrogen by leukocytes or the pyrogenicity of the endogenous-pyrogen molecule. The ability of an antipyretic to reduce fever is proportional to its ability to inhibit prostaglandin synthesis. In addition, antipyretics do not lower body temperature in human beings unless fever is present; thus, they do not affect the body temperature of subjects in whom the normal daily temperature is above the mean or exhibits a wide circadian range.

It has become apparent lately that endogenous pyrogen probably plays a broad role in modulating the inflammatory response, in addition to its function in mediating fever. For example, endogenous pyrogen induces the release of products from the specific granules of neutrophils and increases levels of certain acute phase proteins. Certain monokines, such as lymphocyte activating factor, have been demonstrated to be either the same or closely related to endogenous pyrogen. In fact, most investigators now believe that interleukin I and endogenous pyrogen are one and the same molecule. (Dinarello, 1984).

References

Dinarello, C. A., and Wolff, S. M.: Pathogenesis of fever in man. N Engl J Med 298:607, 1978.

Dinarello, C. A., Wolff, S. M.: Molecular basis of fever in humans. Am J Med 72:800, 1982.

Dinarello, C. A.: Interleukin I. Rev. Inf. Dis. 6:51, 1984.

Hanson, D. F., Murphy, P. A., Windle, B. E.: Failure of rabbit neutrophils to secrete endogenous pyrogen when stimulated with staphylococci. J Exp Med 151:1360, 1980.

Kluger, M. J., Ringler, D. H., Anver, M. R.: Fever and survival. Science 188:166, 1975.

Nordlund, J. J., Root, R. K., and Wolff, S. M.: Studies on the origin of human leukocytic pyrogen. J Exp Med 131:727, 1970.

Root, R. K., and Wolff, S. M.: Pathogenetic mechanisms in experimental immune fever. J Exp Med 128:309, 1968.

Wolff, S. M., Kimball, H. R., Perry, S., Root, R. K., and Kappas, A.: The biological properties of etiocholanolone. Ann Intern Med 67:1268, 1967.

Wood, W. B., Jr.: Studies on the cause of fever. N Engl J Med 258:1023, 1958.

92

SHOCK IN INFECTIOUS DISEASES

HERBERT S. HEINEMAN, M.D.

Shock is a syndrome of generalized metabolic failure resulting from prolonged inadequacy of tissue perfusion. Its early clinical manifestations reflect malfunction of those organs most dependent on uninterrupted blood flow, particularly the brain, as well as compensatory adjustments designed to maintain adequate arterial pressure. As these adjustments fail, urinary output decreases and biochemical indices of distorted metabolism are detectable; specifically nonoxidative glycolysis with low yield of high energy chemical bonds testifies to the widespread nature of the disorder. In the end, it is the failure of energy production rather than damage to a particular organ that leads to death.

Other terms, such as "circulatory collapse," "circulatory failure," and "hypoperfusion," have been substituted for "shock" in an attempt to pinpoint the specific nature of the derangement. When it occurs as a specific complication of infection, it is referred to as "infectious shock," "septic shock," "bacteremic shock," and even "endotoxin shock." The last three terms specifically implicate bacterial infection and are therefore too restrictive. Because "infectious shock" is sufficiently broad as well as concise, this term will be used in the present chapter.

ETIOLOGY. Shock may occur in the course of almost any severe infection, but it is particularly characteristic of bacteremia due to gram-negative bacilli. In fact, although gram-negative bacteremia is a common event in seriously ill patients, shock occurs in only a small minority, and the proximate factors leading to this complication have not been identified. The importance of endotoxin, the lipopolysaccharide composing part of all gram-negative cell walls, is readily apparent because it produces a similar syndrome in experimental animals. Partly because of the extensive use of endotoxin as an investigative tool, endotoxin shock is commonly regarded as the prototype of infectious shock. Care must be taken not to use the terms interchangeably, because to do so could lead to incorrect therapy for shock of other causes.

Besides gram-negative bacilli, some of the better known etiologic agents associated with circulatory collapse are meningococci, clostridia, and staphylococci. Shock in meningococcemia is unique because of the hemorrhagic syndrome so commonly associated with it. In the case of clostridia and staphylococci, which contain no endotoxin, protein exotoxins that produce the syndrome in animals and may play an important role in human shock have been identified. The issue is complicated by the production of numerous distinct exotoxins by the same organism. For example, clostridial alpha-toxin, or phospholipase C, appears to be implicated in both hemolysis and progressive tissue destruction and has been identified in the blood during clostridial septicemia (Moore et al., 1976); however, vascular collapse does not correlate with hemolysis, and a role for one of the many other exotoxins made by *C. perfringens* seems likely.

Shock also occurs in infections due to fungi, rickettsiae, and viruses. Fungal endotoxins with varying effects in experimental animals have been described, but their role in humans is speculative.

PATHOGENESIS AND PATHOLOGY. The feature that distinguishes infectious shock from shock of other causes (cardiac, hemorrhagic, neurogenic) is the occurrence of widespread circulatory collapse without preceding loss of intravascular fluid or identifiable damage to a critical organ. In this connection, it must be emphasized that many infections do cause damage to specific organs, and this may result in vascular collapse just as if the damage had been inflicted by a noninfectious agent. The detailed mechanisms of shock in such cases will not be described here, but their various causes are listed in Table 1. Recognition of the many distinct mechanisms that produce shock is essential for proper patient evaluation because of the different therapeutic measures appropriate to each.

Understanding of the pathogenesis of true infectious shock in humans has been hampered, first, by the absence of any characteristic pathologic changes that could localize the primary insult; second, by interspecies differences among animals that make extrapolation of experimental

Table 1. CLASSIFICATION OF SHOCK ASSOCIATED WITH INFECTION

Mechanism of Shock	Diseases in Which Mechanism Is Operative
I. Shock Secondary to Identifiable Factors	
A. Loss of blood volume	
1. Fluid loss due to capillary damage	Gas gangrene; anthrax; hemorrhagic fever; allergic reaction to antibiotic
2. Fluid loss due to malfunction in fluid regulation	
a. Severe diarrhea	Cholera; staphylococcal enteritis
b. Adrenal insufficiency	Tuberculosis; histoplasmosis
c. Uncontrolled diuresis	Salt-losing pyelonephritis
d. Peritoneal exudation	Peritonitis
B. Impaired cardiac function	
1. Myocardial failure	
a. Myocarditis	Diphtheria; infective endocarditis; influenza; rickettsial infections; trichinosis; toxoplasmosis; trypanosomiasis (Chagas' disease)
b. Myocardial infarction	Coronary embolism in infective endocarditis
c. Myocardial abscess	Infective endocarditis; septicemia
d. Acute valvular insufficiency	Infective endocarditis
2. Cardiac tamponade	
a. Pericardial effusion	Pericarditis
b. Hemopericardium	Ventricular rupture, as in tuberculous myocarditis
3. Mechanical outflow obstruction	
a. Intraventricular blockage	Intraventricular rupture of echinococcus cyst
b. Pulmonary embolism	Myocarditis with mural thrombosis
C. Loss of arteriolar tone	
1. Destruction of vasomotor center	Bulbar poliomyelitis
2. Anaphylaxis	Rupture of echinococcus cyst; allergic reaction to antibiotic
II. True Infectious Shock	
Maldistribution of blood	Gram-negative bacillary infection; meningococcemia; clostridial infections; staphylococcal and other gram-positive coccal septicemia; influenza; rickettsial infection; systemic candidiasis

observations to humans hazardous; and third, by overlapping but apparently distinct syndromes associated with different infections.

Common to all forms of infectious shock is a maldistribution of blood. Repeated observations and measurements have shown that hypotension and diminished tissue perfusion occur in the presence of normal blood volume. Furthermore, central venous pressure is typically low at the onset, and fluid overloading is often well tolerated, indicating that cardiac decompensation does not play a primary role. By exclusion, this places the functional deficit in the vascular system. On the basis of cardiac output measurements, two kinds of infectious shock have been described, low resistance ("hot dry") and high resistance ("cold clammy"), with features shown in Table 2. Terminally, all patients pass through the cold clammy stage, which represents compensatory sympathetic vasomotor activity.

Table 2. TWO TYPES OF INFECTIOUS SHOCK

Characteristic	Low Resistance	High Resistance
Arterial blood pressure	Low	Low
Tissue oxygenation	Decreased	Decreased
Cardiac output	High	Low
Peripheral vascular resistance	Low	High
Venous sequestration	Absent	Present
Arteriovenous shunting	Present	Absent
Arteriovenous oxygen difference	Low	High

Low resistance dynamics may be seen in the early stages of shock caused by any bacterial infection, but they are particularly characteristic of shock due to gram-positive cocci. In this stage, hot dry skin is evidence of hyperkinetic circulation, and hemodynamic measurements may reveal a markedly lowered peripheral resistance and a cardiac output well above normal. Despite this, the patient is hypotensive and obtunded, and oxygen extraction by the cells is disproportionately decreased. For a given cardiac index, variation in arteriovenous oxygen difference has been found to reflect the severity of shock and to correlate with ultimate survival (Nishijima et al., 1973). This finding suggests a specific defect in oxygen extraction at the tissue level independent of central hemodynamics. The most widely proposed mechanism is arteriovenous shunting, although it is not clear whether such shunting is truly anatomic or whether normal gas exchange in the capillary bed simply does not take place, thus creating a purely physiologic shunt (Archie, 1976; Seyfer et al., 1977).

High resistance dynamics eventually supervene in patients dying in shock. In this stage, there is a marked increase in peripheral resistance on the arterial (resistance) side of the circulation, but central venous pressure remains low until cardiac decompensation sets in, indicating pooling of blood in a dilated venous (capacitance) bed. In different animal species, particular venous beds (for example, splanchnic or pulmonary) have been implicated. In humans, specific localization has not been demonstrated, and the defect is believed to be generalized. Venous pooling leads in turn to diminished venous return to the heart, diminished cardiac output, and compensatory arteriolar constriction. Resembling hemorrhagic shock, it is manifested by cold clammy skin, tachycardia, thready pulse, mental obtundation, and oliguria.

In addition to measurable parameters of altered circulatory dynamics, several indices of altered metabolism can be detected. One of these is disseminated intravascular coagulation, most dramatically seen in meningococcemia, in which there is widespread deposition of fibrin thrombi may occur in small vessels. Because coagulation factors are consumed faster than they can be replaced, the blood may become virtually incoagulable, and this results in hemorrhages into the skin (ecchymoses) and viscera. The adrenal glands are frequently the site of visceral hemorrhage, which results in the so-called Waterhouse-Friderichsen syndrome. Adrenal hemorrhage was originally thought to explain infectious shock on the basis of adrenal insufficiency. However, this explanation is rendered invalid by the inconsistency of pathologic findings in patients dying of infectious shock, the presence of a normal concentration of adrenocortical steroids in the blood, and the failure of physiologic doses of steroids to reverse the course.

The mechanism of disseminated intravascular coagulation is poorly understood. Endotoxins from gram-negative bacteria are capable of activating Factor XII (Hageman factor), which could initiate the clotting cascade. However, this leaves unexplained the occurrence of the same phenomenon in infections due to organisms that do not contain endotoxin.

Whether intravascular coagulation actually plays a role in circulatory collapse is debatable. Although the fibrin thrombi can occlude vessels, the extent of thrombosis seen at autopsy is highly variable, and in many cases of shock studied during life it is not possible to demonstrate significant consumption of coagulation factors. Finally, even though abnormal coagulation can be arrested by the administration of heparin, clinical trials have failed to show improvement in prognosis as a result. Rather than being part of the fundamental process of shock, intravascular coagulation may be only one of its complications.

Along similar lines, several vasoactive substances appear in the blood of endotoxin-shocked animals—for example, catecholamines, histamine, serotonin, and prostaglandins. Also, animals may become abnormally reactive to adrenalin. However, from all these observations it has not been possible to construct a comprehensive sequence of events that explains exactly how endotoxin or any other microbial product leads to circulatory collapse in infection.

Recent work suggests a possible role for endorphins in shock due to endotoxin (and other causes). In shocked animals, hypotension was dramatically reversed by naloxone, an opiate antagonist (Faden and Holaday, 1980).

Whatever the mechanism of infectious shock, the end result is metabolic failure at the cellular level, involving carbohydrate, fat, and protein (Siegel, 1981). It is usually assumed that the critical substance of which cells are deprived is oxygen, and indeed, one of the universal consequences of shock is anaerobic metabolism, which can be demonstrated by increased concentrations of lactate in the blood. However, other metabolic effects not readily linked to oxygen utilization have been described—for example, failure of gluconeogenesis in the face of increased glucose utilization (Archer et al., 1976; Garcia-Barreno and Balibrea, 1978). The basic biochemical lesion has been traced to the inner mitochondrial membrane, whose transport function is believed to be inhibited by products of lipolysis (Jones, 1977).

CLINICAL MANIFESTATIONS. In most patients suffering from infectious shock, this complication occurs in a setting in which the infection is already recognized. However, vascular collapse may be the first or only sign of severe infection, especially in elderly debilitated patients who may not demonstrate fever or local symptoms.

Gram-negative bacillary (endotoxin) shock is seen most frequently in patients with urinary infection, when trauma to the infected tissues (for example, cystoscopy) induces a sudden burst of bacteremia. The effects closely resemble those in experimental animals infused with endotoxin. Within a few hours of the traumatic event, the patient suddenly has shaking chills followed by a steep rise in temperature to 39° C or higher with corresponding tachycardia. The blood pressure may begin to fall within less than an hour or several hours later, and this is accompanied by prostration, apprehension, vomiting, and confusion. Examination at first may reveal hot dry skin, systolic pressure of less than 80 mm Hg, and diastolic pressure that is barely recordable. Hyperventilation to the point of respiratory alkalosis is typical of this stage. If the condition is untreated or unresponsive to treatment, peripheral vasoconstriction sets in with cold clammy cyanotic extremities, further diminution in pulse pressure, continued hyperventilation as metabolic acidosis ensues, and oliguria. Various therapeutic measures may prolong life for several days without reversal of shock, until death supervenes.

A similar sequence of events, likewise associated with gram-negative bacteremia, occurs following septic delivery or abortion. It has been observed that, except for pregnant women, patients under 40 infrequently develop shock from gram-negative bacillary infections (Weil, 1977). On the other hand, shock due to meningococcemia is typically a syndrome of children and young adults, because of the age distribution of meningococcal infection. The full-blown syndrome of meningococcemia is easily recognized, but this infection should be suspected even in the absence of meningitis or cutaneous manifestations whenever fever and shock occur in a previously healthy young person.

The clinical syndromes of shock in gram-positive infections differ chiefly in the settings in which they occur. The best recognized pathogens are the histotoxic clostridia—that is, those with the capacity for progressive and destructive tissue invasion—and coagulase-positive staphylococci. Shock is a typical concomitant of clostridial myonecrosis (gas gangrene), a syndrome easily recognized by the presence of large areas of edematous, often crepitant, discolored, and exquisitely tender muscle tissue. Invasion of muscle appears to be a prerequisite, as clostridial cellulitis sparing the muscle is generally not associated with this degree of systemic toxicity (MacLennan, 1962). However, shock does occur in the absence of myonecrosis when clostridia invade the blood stream from such foci as the large intestine and the uterus. In the latter cases, jaundice, hemoglobinemia, and hemoglobinuria may develop because of intravascular hemolysis, a feature that is usually absent in clostridial myonecrosis.

Shock may occur in staphylococcal septicemia with or without evidence of focal infection. The prototype of shock without focal infection was manifested in a disastrous outbreak in Bundaberg, Australia (Kellaway et al., 1928), following injection of a contaminated diphtheria toxin-antitoxin mixture. Shock and death occurred too rapidly to be explained by widespread staphylococcal infection and was probably caused by exotoxin. More recently, the staphylococcal "toxic shock syndrome" has received much attention because of its epidemic occurrence in women using highly absorbent vaginal tampons during menstruation (National Academy of Sciences, 1982). A protein exotoxin of low molecular weight is apparently released from staphylococci in the vagina and causes shock. In more typical situations, shock occurs during the course of severe staphylococcal infection, such as pneumonia.

A wide variety of other infections may be complicated by shock (Heineman and Braude, 1961), with clinical manifestations basically reflecting the underlying cause. Finally, it must be remembered that shock may be caused by damage or malfunction of specific organs (see Table 1)—for example, myocarditis, adrenal insufficiency, pulmonary embolism, and massive diarrhea. Alertness to these possibilities is especially important because of their unique therapeutic implications.

Laboratory Tests. Hematologic findings are variable, more often reflecting the underlying infection than any characteristic of shock as such. Depending on the state of endotoxemia, for example, either leukopenia or leukocytosis may be present. Hemoglobin concentration may be normal, elevated (for example, hemoconcentration in cholera), or depressed (for example, intravascular hemolysis in clostridial septicemia). More specifically associated with shock is thrombocytopenia, which is one of the manifestations of disseminated intravascular coagulation. In such a case, other evidence of coagulopathy is also found, such as prolongation of prothrombin time and partial thromboplastin time and the presence of fibrin split products in the blood (Hardaway, 1976.)

Findings specific for shock regardless of its cause relate to the deterioration of oxidative metabolism by the tissues—for example, decreased arteriovenous oxygen gradient, metabolic acidosis, and increased serum lactate concentration.

In shock due to bacterial or fungal sepsis, the causal organisms can usually be recovered from the blood. However, blood cultures are more often negative than positive in clostridial myonecrosis and may be so even in gram-negative bacillary shock, emphasizing the role of bacterial toxins apart from the presence of replicating organisms.

Arterial hypoxia has been noted in some patients with infectious shock. Radiologically visible pulmonary infiltrates may be present that resemble those of pulmonary edema. However, they occur in the absence of heart failure and are generally ascribed to "shock lung" or "adult respiratory distress syndrome." In this condition, increased capillary permeability leads to interstitial edema and eventually hyaline membrane formation, with resultant block of alveolocapillary oxygen diffusion.

COMPLICATIONS AND SEQUELAE. The mortality in infectious shock is high, its incidence generally being quoted at about 70 per cent. A lower incidence is found in series involving predominantly younger patients, specifically women with complications of pregnancy, for in this age group the prognosis is better than in elderly debilitated patients, in whom infectious shock occurs most frequently.

The road to recovery may be marked by acute renal failure due to shock or hemoglobinuria, or by infarction of organs such as the myocardium or brain, rendered vulnerable to ischemia through occlusive arterial disease of old age. Peripheral gangrene may be seen even in young subjects with shock-related coagulative disorders, as in meningococcemia.

In addition, there may be sequelae related to damage done by the infection itself or by heroic therapeutic measures, such as surgery, corticosteroids, and toxic antibiotics.

DIAGNOSIS. The diagnosis of infectious shock is easy in the typical case, and it can be made by an alert observer before serious damage is done. There are two diagnostic signs: (1) presence of infection, and (2) falling blood pressure without hemorrhage or cardiac failure. These easily recognized signs are emphasized because if a patient has already been in shock for several hours before his hypotensive state is noticed, damage to cellular metabolic functions may have already been done and such damage will be progressively harder to reverse. On the other hand, since hypotension occurs very early in the course, close monitoring of vital signs in patients with severe infections, and especially in those who have just undergone manipulation of infected pelvic organs, is the key to early diagnosis and eventual recovery.

Besides hypotension, patients in shock may exhibit hyperventilation, confusion, apprehension, prostration, and vomiting. Depending on the type of circulatory derangement, the skin may be hot and dry or cold and clammy.

Circulatory insufficiency at the tissue level is recognized most easily by oliguria (hourly urine output of less than 20 ml) and subsequent increases in concentrations of blood urea and creatinine and a decrease in bicarbonate. Excess lactate will be found in the serum (more than 16 mg/dl), specifically indicating inadequate tissue oxygenation.

TREATMENT. The aims of treatment in infectious shock are control of the infection and correction of the circulatory disturbance. On the basis of the relative roles of the infecting organism, their toxins, and the availability of specific therapy, patients may be divided into five groups.

Group 1: Specific antibiotic treatment for the infection is available; for example, shock cases due to bacteria, rickettsiae, and fungi. Infection and shock must be treated simultaneously.

Group 2: Specific antibiotics are available to combat the organism but not its toxins; for example, gas gangrene and diphtheria. Amputation of the gangrene and administration of antitoxin may be indicated, although the value of antitoxin in the treatment of shock has not been proved in either gas gangrene or diphtheria.

Group 3: No specific antibiotic treatment for the infection is available; for example, shock cases due to viruses. The objective of therapy is to sustain life long enough to allow the host to control the infection.

Group 4: Specific antibiotic treatment is available but not critical, since invasion of tissues by the infecting organism is not a significant feature of the illness; for example, cholera.

Group 5: The potential for shock continues to exist even after the infection is under control; for example, pulmonary embolism from myocarditis, coronary embolism from endocarditis, chronic sequelae of poliomyelitis, and tuberculous adrenal insufficiency.

When it is recalled that, in addition to the foregoing possibilities, some infections can cause shock in more than one manner, the necessity for an accurate appraisal of the situation becomes obvious.

TREATMENT OF INFECTION. The urgency of treatment of patients in shock necessarily will modify the approach to selection of antibiotics. However, since the object of antibiotic therapy should always be to eliminate the infection, the guiding principle here, as in less desperate situations, should be to identify the etiologic organism as soon as possible and to prescribe an optimal antibiotic regimen to which it is sensitive. Unfortunately, there is no time to withhold treatment, so that other guides to the selection of the proper drugs must be employed. The history is often helpful in this regard. For example, a sudden temperature elevation and shock occurring in a patient with an indwelling urethral catheter is presumptive evidence of bloodstream invasion by an organism originating in the urinary tract. If the results of a recent urine culture are available, one may assume that the same organism is responsible for infection of both urine and blood. Physical examination occasionally is so typical of a specific infection that antibiotic therapy can be chosen on this basis alone. A good example is the child or young adult with an acute illness characterized by fever, nuchal rigidity, purpura, and shock. Meningococcemia should be suspected and treated with large intravenous doses of potassium penicillin G or, in the case of penicillin allergy, chloramphenicol sodium succinate.

Sometimes the smear from a lesion is sufficiently characteristic to allow positive identification, as in gas gangrene, meningococcal infection (spinal fluid or exudate from a punctured petechia), and staphylococcal pneumonia. In the infrequent cases of septicemia that occur without an obvious focus of infection, it is wise to use a combination of antibiotics that can be expected to cover most possibilities, such as a cephalosporin and an aminoglycoside. An anti-*Pseudomonas* beta-lactam antibiotic may be indicated in patients susceptible to *Pseudomonas* infection, as in leukemia or severe burns.

When shock is due to mechanical factors, as in pulmonary embolism from a mural thrombus, myocardial infarction from coronary embolism in bacterial endocarditis, or Addisonian crisis in tuberculosis of the adrenals, the infection itself generally demands less urgent treatment, since it is not the immediate presence of the bacteria that causes circulatory collapse.

TREATMENT OF SHOCK. The prognosis in shock could probably be improved if it were possible to address the basic cellular lesions that underlie collapse of normal energy metabolism. Unfortunately, these lesions are only beginning to be understood, so that there is still no foundation for the development of a specific therapeutic strategy. Based on present knowledge, the only rational objective of therapy can be to restore the circulation. The agents employed, listed in order of importance, are (1) fluids, (2) vasoactive drugs, (3) adrenal corticosteroids, and (4) digitalis. Additional measures include assisted ventilation and, questionably, anticoagulation and opiate antagonism.

Fluids. Replenishment of the venous bed is always the first consideration and is frequently all that is needed. It is understood, of course, that the need for extra fluid is created not by dehydration (except in fluid-losing conditions such as cholera) but by an abnormal increase in the capacity of the vascular bed owing to loss of venous tone. In the early stages, simply ensuring an adequate venous return to the right atrium will result in adequate cardiac output. However, myocardial depression may limit the ability of the heart to handle the volume of fluid necessary to reverse shock, at which point further fluid loading would result in pulmonary edema. To avoid this, the pre-load of the heart should be carefully monitored. The simplest measurement is that of central venous pressure, which is done by means of a catheter opening in the superior vena cava just outside the right atrium. As long as the pressure does not exceed 10 cm saline, infusion of fluids can safely be continued; above 15 cm saline, there is danger of overloading the heart. However, since the real danger to life is pulmonary edema, many authorities feel that a more appropriate measurement is that of the left atrial filling pressure, which can be closely approximated by the pulmonary wedge pressure. The latter is obtained through a balloon-tipped catheter passed through the right cardiac chambers and pulmonary artery as far as it will go, at which point the pulmonary venous pressure is reflected back into it. Continued infusion is safe as long as the pulmonary wedge pressure is less than 15 mm Hg; above 20 mm Hg, there is danger of pulmonary edema.

The fluid most commonly used for replenishment, when there has been no extravascular fluid loss, is normal saline. If there has been exudation of fluids through capillary leakage, as in gas gangrene or peritonitis, or through inflammatory diarrhea, as in shigella dysentery, it is rational to use a colloid such as 5 per cent human serum albumin.

If the maximum tolerated amount of fluid does not reverse the shock state, the rate of infusion must be reduced to the minimum necessary to maintain patency of the access line, and therapeutic efforts are continued with vasoactive agents.

Vasoactive Drugs. In contrast to fluid loading, which simply fills the vascular bed to its exaggerated capacity, the aim of vasoactive drugs is to alter the capacity of the vessels selectively to overcome specific abnormalities of blood distribution. In theory, this should be the obvious first line of approach, but the fact is that no drug with the right selectivity has been identified. It must be remembered that the two recognized defects of distribution are dilatation of the venous bed and arteriovenous shunting. Defects in cardiac output and arteriolar tone are not primary in most cases, yet all vasoactive drugs in use affect cardiac performance and arteriolar tone predominantly. The only advance made in the past several decades has been identification of effective beta-adrenergic drugs, such as isoproterenol and dopamine, that raise the blood pressure by increasing the cardiac output while decreasing peripheral resistance, thereby increasing total blood flow. Their vasomotor effect is opposite from that of alpha-adrenergic drugs, such as noradrenalin and metaraminol, whose antihypotensive action is based primarily on increase in peripheral resistance; these drugs may actually decrease tissue perfusion, so that the metabolic insult is aggravated at the same time that central arterial pressure is increased.

Isoproterenol has been used successfully but nowadays is not favored because of its tendency to increase ventricular irritability and bring about potentially dangerous arrhythmias, to increase myocardial oxygen demand, and to shunt blood from the viscera to skeletal muscle. Dopamine lacks these adverse cardiac effects and shunts blood to the viscera, a specific distributive effect aptly termed "dopaminergic" (Reid and Thompson, 1975). This drug is administered by intravenous drip at an initial rate of 2 to 20 μg/kg body weight/minute, then titrated to the desired response (see Monitoring section below).

Adrenal Corticosteroids. Steroids are considered by

many to be useful therapeutic agents in treatment of infectious shock, although their action, unlike that of fluids and vasoactive drugs, is not immediately reflected in hemodynamic measurements. It is not clear whether their mechanisms of action involve their anti-inflammatory effect (Cline and Melmon, 1966), a direct effect on the circulation (Sambhi et al., 1965), or some as yet undetected property, although the need for superpharmacologic doses suggests mechanisms distinct from those involved in other applications of these agents. Methylprednisolone and dexamethasone in respective loading doses of 30 mg/kg and 3 mg/kg, followed by fractional doses every 4 to 6 hours for up to 48 hours, illustrate the order of magnitude of the dosage used. Significant reduction in mortality was found in a prospective double-blind, controlled study with these drugs (Schumer, 1976). The possibility that steroids might impair resistance to infections is generally considered of secondary importance in these desperate situations, especially since antibiotic coverage is provided. Because their effect is delayed by several hours, the loading dose of steroids should be given as soon as it is clear that fluid loading alone is insufficient.

Digitalis. Myocardial depression can occur in sepsis, and failure of cardiac output to increase in response to increasing pulmonary wedge pressure has been shown to correlate with mortality (Weisel et al., 1977). It seems appropriate, therefore, to digitalize a patient in whom central venous or pulmonary wedge pressure rises rapidly during fluid infusion without satisfactory clinical response. Caution is necessary in patients with myocarditis or myocardial anoxia because these states heighten susceptibility to the toxic effects of digitalis, and dangerous arrhythmias may result.

Assisted Ventilation. In certain patients, arterial hypoxemia complicates shock, possibly because of intrapulmonary arteriovenous shunting or alveolocapillary block due to "shock lung." In these patients, oxygen administered by intermittent positive pressure or positive end-expiratory pressure may be helpful (Ledingham and McArdle, 1978).

Oxygen under pressure has been advocated for the treatment of severe clostridial infections because of its proposed inhibition of toxin production. Although opinion regarding its true value and potential hazards is divided, it has been used in centers equipped with hyperbaric chambers (Darke et al., 1977).

Other Measures. The consumption of clotting factors in disseminated intravascular coagulation can usually be reversed by heparin, with normalization of corresponding laboratory values. However, clinical trials have failed to demonstrate reversal of the shock state, and anticoagulation is not generally recommended.

Naloxone, an opiate antagonist, has been tried with inconsistent results. The place of this approach, based on the postulated role of endorphins in the etiology of shock, is not established.

Promising results have been obtained in gram-negative infectious shock with antiserum to endotoxin. When the core polysaccharide is used as the immunizing antigen, bacterial specificities due to the oligosaccharide side chains are circumvented and the resulting antiserum is effective in shock due to a broad range of gram-negative bacteria (Ziegler et al., 1982).

MONITORING THERAPY IN THE SHOCK PATIENT. Since the two most important therapeutic measures, namely, fluids and vasoactive drugs, are titrated on an hour-to-hour or minute-to-minute basis, and overtreatment may have serious adverse effects, it is important to monitor the response accurately and quantitatively. Measurement of blood pressure, which is so useful in the initial diagnosis, has only limited usefulness once vasoactive drugs are used, since central arterial pressure may correlate very poorly with tissue blood flow. A more relevant criterion of response is one that measures end-organ performance. The most readily available is urine output, increase in which is usually taken as indicative of increased renal perfusion. Less readily measured on a continuing basis but valuable as an indicator of anaerobic metabolism is serum lactate, which should decrease as the shock state is reversed.

PROPHYLAXIS. Since shock is a complication of severe infection, its prevention lies in the timely and effective treatment of infection when this is possible. One approach is carefully selected antibiotic prophylaxis for invasive procedures likely to be complicated by local infection or bacteremia, for example, surgery on the urinary tract (Sullivan et al., 1973), gastrointestinal and biliary tracts (Stone et al., 1976), and pelvic organs (Roberts and Homesley, 1978).

References

Archer, L., Benjamin, B., Lane, M. D., and Hinshaw, L. B.: Renal gluconeogenesis and increased glucose utilization in shock. Am J Physiol 231:872, 1976.

Archie, J. P., Jr.: Systemic and regional arteriovenous shunting in endotoxic and septic shock in dogs. Surg Forum 27:55, 1976.

Cline, M. J., and Melmon, K. L.: A possible explanation of the anti-inflammatory action of cortisol. Science 153:1135, 1966.

Darke, S. G., King, A. M., and Slack, W. K.: Gas gangrene and related infection: Classification, clinical features and aetiology, management and mortality. A report of 88 cases. Br J Surg 64:104, 1977.

Faden, A., and Holaday, J.: Experimental endotoxin shock: The pathophysiologic function of endorphins and treatment with opiate antagonists. J Infect Dis 124:229, 1980.

Garcia-Barreno, P., and Balibrea, J. L.: Metabolic responses in shock. Surg Gynecol Obstet 146:182, 1978.

Hardaway, R. M., III: Gram-negative shock. Antibiot Chemother 21:208, 1976.

Heineman, H. S., and Braude, A. I.: Shock in infectious diseases. Disease-a-Month, October, 1961.

Jones, G. R. N.: The basic biochemical lesion in shock. Biochem Soc Trans 5:213, 1977.

Kellaway, C. H., MacCallum, P., and Tebbutt, A. H.: Report of the Royal Commission of Enquiry into the Fatalities at Bundaberg. Med J Austral 2:2, 38, 1928.

Ledingham, I., and McArdle, C. S.: Prospective study of the treatment of septic shock. Lancet 1:1194, 1978.

MacLennan, J. D.: The histotoxic clostridial infections in man. Bacteriol Rev 26:177, 1962.

Moore, A., Gottfried, E. L., Stone, P. H., and Coleman, M.: Clostridium perfringens septicemia with detection of phospholipase C activity in the serum. Am J Med Sci 271:59, 1976.

National Academy of Sciences: The Toxic Shock Syndrome (Conference). Ann Int Med 96:831, 1982.

Nishijima, H., Weil, M. H., Shubin, H., and Cavanilles, J.: Hemodynamic and metabolic studies on shock associated with Gram negative bacteremia. Medicine 52:287, 1973.

Reid, P. R., and Thompson, W. L.: The clinical use of dopamine in the treatment of shock. Bull Johns Hopkins Hosp 137:276, 1975.

Roberts, J. M., and Homesley, H. D.: Low-dose carbenicillin prophylaxis for vaginal and abdominal hysterectomy. Obstet Gynecol 52:83, 1978.

Sambhi, M. P., Weil, M. H., and Udhoji, V. N.: Acute pharmacodynamic effects of glucocorticoids. Cardiac output and related hemodynamic changes in normal subjects and patients in shock. Circulation 31:523, 1965.

Schumer, W.: Steroids in the treatment of clinical septic shock. Ann Surg 184:333, 1976.

Seyfer, A. E., Zajtchuk, R., Hazlett, D. R., and Mologne, L. A.: Systemic

vascular performance in endotoxic shock. Surg Gynecol Obstet 145:401, 1977.
Siegel, J. H.: Relations between circulatory and metabolic changes in sepsis. Ann Rev Med 32:175, 1981.
Stone, H. H., Hooper, C. A., Kolb, L. D., Geheber, C. E., and Dawkins, E. J.: Antibiotic prophylaxis in gastric, biliary and colonic surgery. Ann Surg 184:443, 1976.
Sullivan, N. M., Sutter, V. L., Mims, M. M., Marsh, V. H., and Finegold, S. M.: Clinical aspects of bacteremia after manipulation of the genitourinary tract. J Infect Dis 127:49, 1973.
Weil, M. H.: Current understanding of mechanisms and treatment of circulatory shock caused by bacterial infections. Ann Clin Rev 9:181, 1977.
Weisel, R. D., Vito, L., Dennis, R. C., Valeri, C. R., and Hechtman, H. B.: Myocardial depression during sepsis. Am J Surg 133:512, 1977.
Ziegler, E. M., McCutchan, J. A., Fierer, J., Glauser, M. P., Sadoff, J. C., Douglas, H., and Braude, A. I.: Treatment of Gram-negative bacteremia and shock with human antiserum to a mutant *Escherichia coli*. N Engl J Med 307:1225, 1982.

93
METABOLIC EFFECTS OF INFECTION

WILLIAM R. BEISEL, M.D.*

Mechanisms that protect the host against infection include the inflammatory, phagocytic, and immunologic responses. In addition, cells throughout the body undergo predictable changes in their metabolic function during a generalized infection. These metabolic responses account for some of the clinical features of infectious illness.

The predictable metabolic changes during infection can be considered physiologic or homeostatic responses, because they appear to contribute to survival. Because metabolic responses are similar during infections caused by widely different microorganisms, the responses are said to be generalized or nonspecific. The magnitude and duration of generalized metabolic responses are governed by the severity and persistence of an infectious process rather than by its cause. Thus, generalized infectious illnesses are accompanied by fever, increased oxygen consumption, the need to generate additional carbohydrate fuels, redistribution within the body of amino acids, lipids, electrolytes, and minerals, increased utilization of vitamins, and hepatic synthesis of enzymes and "acute phase" serum proteins.

Other metabolic changes, superimposed upon the broad group of physiologic ones, are secondary to localization of an infectious process within a major organ. For example, pneumonia can interfere with gas exchange in the lungs, pyelonephritis can cause uremia, and diarrhea can cause a loss of intestinal fluids and electrolytes. Localized infections can thus produce both generalized illness and single organ dysfunction. In some instances, the metabolic consequences of these combinations can reach life-threatening severity.

METABOLIC COSTS OF INFECTION. Certain daily costs must be met in order to maintain host resistance mechanisms. These costs can be expressed in metabolic terms, since they are based on a need for energy-producing substrates and precursor nutrients for producing new cells and products essential to host resistance. For example, new phagocytes, lymphocytes, and epithelial cells must be produced each day; immunoglobulins and other molecules with unique roles in host defense must also be synthesized. Malnourished patients become increasingly susceptible to infection if they cannot meet the nutritional requirements for maintaining resistance mechanisms.

Because fever causes metabolic rates to increase, additional costs are incurred by the patient with fever. These costs must be met either by using fuels already present in body stores or by increasing the intake of calories and other nutrients.

Because a loss of appetite is common during acute febrile illness, metabolic costs are generally met by mobilizing substrates from tissue stores. This mobilization process can be recognized by measurable losses from the body of nitrogen and the other principal intracellular elements (potassium, phosphorus, magnesium, sulfur, and zinc), and by a loss of body weight and muscle mass. Other metabolic costs are met by changing the patterns of cellular metabolism by using biochemical pathways already available within different tissues. Some of these pathways must be augmented by manufacturing additional enzymes. If an infection is not rapidly controlled, its metabolic costs can deplete body stores of vital nutrients.

Metabolic costs of a curable infection continue to increase until after fever has disappeared, and complete recovery from the metabolic consequences of an infection may require additional weeks or months. Depleted nutritional stores make the convalescing patient extremely susceptible to a superimposed infection by new microorganisms. Until stores can be replenished, metabolic losses can initiate a vicious cycle of recurring infections and progressive malnutrition.

IMPORTANCE OF HOST METABOLIC RESPONSES DURING INFECTION. Clinicians should understand the biochemical, metabolic, and hormonal events that lead to loss of body nutrients and altered cellular functions. If the clinician can predict the most likely time of onset, magnitude, and duration of important metabolic responses, he should be able to plan optimal supportive care as an adjunct to antimicrobial drug therapy. It is important to anticipate and recognize the special metabolic complications of infection that are immediate threats to survival.

INCREASED DEMANDS FOR METABOLIZABLE ENERGY. One of the principal metabolic effects of a febrile infection is the increase in oxygen consumption. The basal metabolic rate increases about 13 per cent for each degree (Centigrade) rise in body temperature. The demand for cellular energy increases at the same time that anorexia causes less food intake.

During simple starvation in the absence of infection, tissues get energy chiefly from lipids. These include free fatty acids obtained from adipose tissue and ketones synthesized from fatty acid precursors within the mitochondria of liver cells. Because the use of glucose is curtailed, less

*The views of the author do not purport to reflect the positions of the Department of the Army or the Department of Defense.

is manufactured. These metabolic adjustments to simple starvation allow the body to conserve protein and amino acid stores and to minimize nitrogen losses.

Infectious illnesses are generally accompanied by a reduction in food intake, but the usual metabolic adjustments to simple starvation are not made. Rather, glucose production is stimulated and ketone body production is inhibited. During infection, readjustments take place in metabolic pathways of individual cells and tissues, especially in muscle and liver cells. The endogenous metabolism of body fats, carbohydrates, and proteins are all involved in this process. While free fatty acids continue to be used as major sources of fuel, most of the extra requirements for cellular energy are supplied by glucose. Glucose production is speeded up within the liver by using amino acids as major additional substrates. Amino acids move more rapidly than usual from serum into liver cells. At the same time, large quantities of additional glucose-producing free amino acids, namely, alanine and glutamine, are manufactured and released by skeletal muscle for transport via plasma into the liver. Skeletal muscle contains the largest source of "labile" body protein—protein that can be degraded rapidly during an infection to yield free amino acids for use in other tissues. Some of the newly released branched-chain amino acids (leucine, isoleucine, and valine) are oxidized in situ and used for fuel in muscle cells. Nitrogen groups released by this process are used within muscle for the synthesis of alanine and glutamine. The body initiates mechanisms, to degrade the proteins in skeletal muscle and other somatic tissues to release free amino acids to maintain visceral organ functions, generate energy, and manufacture new cells and proteins.

All the sugar-regulating hormones help stimulate or modulate the increased production and release of glucose by the liver. Plasma concentrations of glucagon, insulin, glucocorticoids, catecholamines, and growth hormone increase. Thyroid hormones are also used more rapidly.

The increased hepatic output of glucose leads to high blood glucose values and a larger glucose pool. A speedier turnover of glucose within this larger pool is caused by its increased use as a cellular fuel.

Severe hypoglycemia, accompanied by a fall of body temperature to subnormal values, can occur if the liver fails to maintain its output of glucose. Hepatic glucose production generally fails because (1) substrates are depleted or (2) the mechanisms for glucose production fails (hepatic cell failure).

Substrate depletion accounts for severe hypoglycemia during bacterial sepsis in newborns. Because infants have little skeletal muscle, their stores of "labile" protein are too limited to support a prolonged need for glucose production.

Failure of hepatic cells is usually caused by direct injury to the cells by viruses, such as hepatitis or yellow fever viruses, or by bacterial products such as endotoxin. Liver cells may also fail to synthesize glucose during the terminal stages of overwhelming infections.

ALTERATIONS IN LIPID METABOLISM. In addition to producing more glucose during acute infections, liver cells accelerate lipid metabolism. The hepatocellular uptake of plasma free fatty acids is increased. Production of triglycerides within liver cells is accelerated and more triglycerides move into the plasma. Some triglycerides may also accumulate as droplets in liver cells and cause fatty metamorphosis.

On the other hand, less free fatty acid is used for the synthesis of ketone bodies than would normally be expected during fasting. Increased release of insulin from the pancreas, a common secondary manifestation of generalized infection, and the lipogenic action of insulin on hepatic cells account for this curtailment in production of ketone bodies. As a result, fewer ketone bodies are available to meet energy requirements. Curtailment of ketone body production is thus a physiologic hormonal response during infection rather than a pathologic breakdown of biochemical pathways.

According to evidence obtained with isotope tracers, the liver, in addition to increasing its output of triglycerides, produces and releases more cholesterol and phospholipids during infection. Since these lipids are all released into plasma as lipoproteins, the liver must produce lipid transport proteins, but little is known about the mechanisms that regulate the rates of lipid release into plasma. However, changes in plasma lipid concentrations are controlled by the rates of lipid removal (or utilization) and by changes in the rates of lipid production. Plasma cholesterol, phospholipid, free fatty acid, and triglyceride values vary individually during different infections or even during different stages of a single infection. A massive accumulation of triglycerides is consistently observed during gram-negative sepsis and may give the plasma a milky appearance. Triglycerides accumulate because of increased hepatic production and decreased activity of the lipolytic enzymes that initiate cellular removal of triglycerides from plasma.

CHANGES IN PROTEIN AND AMINO ACID METABOLISM. All aspects of protein metabolism are affected by infection. Every host defense mechanism depends on the presence or function of some kind of body protein, whether it is a cellular enzyme, a structural protein, a cell membrane receptor, an immunoglobulin, an interferon, a transport protein, a component of the complement, kinin, or coagulation systems, or some other plasma protein. Infection causes cells to speed up the production of some proteins, to slow the production of others and at the same time to break down "labile" body proteins into free amino acids.

During acute infections, plasma albumin values decline. Skeletal muscle proteins are catabolized faster than they are produced and more free amino acids are released into plasma. Despite the entry of more free amino acids into plasma, there is a still greater increase in uptake of amino acid by the liver. As a result, plasma concentrations of most free amino acids decline, especially the branched-chain group.

Free amino acids are used to produce phagocytic and lymphoid cells and to maintain the functional and structural integrity of other tissues. The liver also increases production of certain enzymes and the "acute phase" plasma proteins. These include C-reactive protein, haptoglobin, $alpha_1$-antitrypsin, ceruloplasmin, fibrinogen, and others.

Before amino acids are used for producing glucose, their amino nitrogen must be removed from the carbon skeleton. This nitrogen is converted into urea within the hepatic cells and excreted in the urine. Increased free tryptophan in liver cells is shunted into the serotonin pathway or degraded via the kynurenine pathway for excretion as urinary diazo-positive reactants.

Because of the increased use of amino acids to produce glucose and urea, losses of nitrogen in the urine are high during the acute stages of most febrile infections. Additional nitrogen is lost by sweating, by vomiting or diarrhea, or by nasal secretion and sputum production during respiratory tract infections. The diminished intake of nitrogen-containing foods in combination with continued losses causes negative nitrogen balance.

Nitrogen balance does not become negative during the incubation period of an infection, but begins to be negative soon after the onset of fever. Losses of body nitrogen may reach 10 to 15 g per day if fever is high; cumulative total losses may exceed 100 g during the course of an acute illness. Large daily losses of nitrogen cannot be sustained indefinitely. If an infection becomes subacute or chronic, the body again approaches a state of nitrogen equilibrium, but at a cachectic level.

After recovery, nitrogen balance should become strongly positive as degraded proteins are resynthesized. Nitrogen stores can be rebuilt faster by eating more high quality protein foods, especially during early convalescence.

CHANGES IN MINERAL METABOLISM. Principal body minerals undergo complex changes during acute infection. Large amounts of some minerals are lost from the body, while others are either redistributed or sequestered in certain tissues. Minerals of soft tissue are lost during acute infections roughly in parallel with the losses of body nitrogen. Negative balances are caused by the combination of diminished dietary intake plus losses in the urine or feces of magnesium, phosphorus, potassium, sulfur, and zinc. Change in calcium stores is generally minimal unless immobilization is prolonged, as in poliomyelitis. Similarly, deficits of body phosphorus appear to reflect losses from soft tissue rather than bone.

Although negative phosphorus balance generally parallels that of nitrogen, phosphorus losses during the period of early symptoms are also influenced by changes in acid-base balance. When fever occurs, respiratory rates become faster. The increased loss of carbon dioxide causes respiratory alkalosis accompanied by a transient disappearance of phosphorus from sweat and urine. During severe or protracted infectious diarrhea, potassium ions escape by way of the intestine. This loss of potassium may be enough to produce the vacuolar changes in kidney tubules and myocardial cells characteristic of potassium deficiency.

Each of the three most widely studied essential trace minerals—iron, zinc, and copper—are redistributed abruptly within the body during infectious illnesses. These changes are under physiologic control mechanisms and are stimulated by inflammation and activation of phagocytic cells. The concentrations of iron and zinc abruptly decline in the plasma as they are taken up by the liver. These two minerals become physiologically "sequestered" within cellular storage sites. Iron is held as hemosiderin or ferritin, while zinc is bound within liver cells to newly synthesized metallothionein. Copper, on the other hand, is secreted by the liver into plasma as a component of newly synthesized ceruloplasmin.

A rapid decline in plasma iron and zinc concentrations may precede the onset of fever, while the increase in plasma copper follows soon afterward. Since only the "loosely bound" fractions of plasma zinc move into the liver, plasma values of zinc rarely fall more than 50 per cent. In contrast, plasma iron may fall to undetectable values, leaving the iron-binding capacity of plasma almost entirely unsaturated. At the same time, plasma copper and ceruloplasmin values may double or triple.

Physiologic sequestration inhibits the incorporation of iron into hemoglobin and eventually causes the "anemia of infection." This process cannot be reversed by oral or parenteral iron. In addition to temporary sequestration of zinc within the liver, it may be lost in the urine. The redistribution of iron, zinc, and copper are reversed after recovery from infection. Little is known about the responses of other trace minerals.

CHANGES IN ELECTROLYTE AND WATER METABOLISM. Fluid and electrolyte responses vary greatly during different infections. Imbalances can cause death, either from severe dehydration or from fluid overload.

In most acute infections, an increased adrenal output of aldosterone during fever causes reabsorption by renal tubular cells of sodium and chloride, their virtual disappearance from urine, their retention in body fluids, and a secondary increase in the extracellular fluid volume. Recovery from an acute period of fever may be followed by diuresis in early convalescence.

Retention of body water can also be caused by "inappropriate" secretion of antidiuretic hormone from the posterior pituitary. This phenomenon is common in infections of the central nervous system and may occur during severe generalized infections. Some severe infections may also be complicated by the accumulation and sequestration of sodium within cells so that plasma sodium concentrations drop. Attempts to correct low sodium values with intravenous isotonic NaCl solutions may lead to acute cardiac failure or cerebral edema. If low plasma sodium values during severe infections cannot be explained by losses from the patient, fluid and sodium intake should be restricted until the urine volume consistently increases.

On the other hand, diarrhea may produce massive loss of extracellular fluids and electrolytes. In cholera or severe enterotoxic diarrhea, fluid loss may lead to hypovolemic shock and death. Therapy requires prompt resuscitation with iso-osmotic saline and correction of concomitant acidosis and potassium deficiency.

ACID-BASE DISTURBANCES. A wide variety of acid-base abnormalities occur during different kinds of infections. Rapid deep breathing during fever causes excessive loss of dissolved carbon dioxide from the blood and a transient period of uncompensated respiratory alkalosis. In contrast, impairment of ventilatory exchange of pulmonary gases by pneumonia leads to oxygen deficits and carbon dioxide retention with respiratory acidosis. Respiratory acidosis can also result from acute poliomyelitis or tetanus, both of which can prevent breathing.

Increased cellular generation of organic acids may produce metabolic acidosis. Septic shock or localized capillary-bed stasis can lead to cellular hypoxia, which increases lactic acid production and the severity of metabolic acidosis. Acute intestinal loss of bicarbonate during severe diarrhea can also produce acute metabolic acidosis. On the other hand, the cumulative loss of body potassium that accompanies protracted diarrhea causes chronic metabolic alkalosis.

ENDOCRINE RESPONSES. Whereas hormones affect salt and water metabolism and energy-generating responses during infection, thyroid and parathyroid hormones, certain pituitary trophic hormones, and the gonadal steroids have no clearly defined role.

The adrenal glucocorticoid hormones serve a central but largely "permissive" role. These steroids are necessary to allow some molecular mechanisms to function in hepatic cells. The adrenal secretion of cortisol increases several fold early in the course of fever. This increase in cortisol secretion is accompanied by smaller increases in the adrenal output of ketosteroids and pregnanetriol. These increases do not persist beyond the onset of recovery. Increased adrenal output is never of sufficient magnitude or duration to produce negative nitrogen balances or the other physiologic changes known to accompany the administration of pharmacologic doses of synthetic glucocorticoid hormones.

Failure of hepatic enzyme systems during overwhelming infections may permit the plasma concentration of cortisol to reach unusually high levels. Conversely, destruction of the adrenals by infection prevents steroid production and leads to death unless this complication is recognized and treated. If an infection becomes subacute or chronic, steroid output also falls below normal.

Substances released by phagocytes and lymphocytes also have hormone-like functions. These include prostaglandins, lymphokines, enzymes, and endogenous mediators, which initiate fever, mobilize neutrophils, cause trace mineral redistribution, and speed muscle protein catabolism.

SUMMARY. Generalized infectious illnesses are accompanied by a broad group of metabolic, biochemical, and endocrinal responses. Although caused by many different molecular mechanisms, generalized metabolic changes occur in relatively predictable patterns related to the onset, severity, and duration of fever. These changes include the catabolism of skeletal muscle proteins, acceleration of hepatic gluconeogenesis, ureagenesis and lipogenesis, inhibition of ketogenesis, retention of extracellular salt and water, loss of major intracellular elements, and redistribution within the body of certain trace minerals. Additional metabolic changes develop if an infection becomes localized in a major organ. Some metabolic consequences of infection, which include hypoglycemia, hypovolemia, fluid overload, and failure of various key organs, are life-threatening.

References

Beisel, W. R.: Mediators of fever and muscle proteolysis. N Engl J Med 308:586, 1983.

Beisel, W. R., Blackburn, G. L., Feigin, R. D., Keusch, G. T., Long, C. L., and Nichols, B. L. (eds.): Symposium on Impact of Infection on Nutritional Status of the Host. Am J Clin Nutr 30:1203, 1439, 1977.

Suskind, R. M. (ed.): Malnutrition and the Immune Response. New York, Raven Press, 1977.

94

MALNUTRITION AND INFECTION

GERALD T. KEUSCH, M.D.

Sorrow may be fated, but to survive and grow is an achievement all its own.

R. COLES

Children of Crisis, 1964

Malnutrition of the affluent as well as the poor, whether because of excess, insufficiency, or inappropriate choice of foods, is a common malady throughout the world. In developing countries, the most common clinical forms of malnutrition are due either to insufficiency of food per se, or to inadequacy of specific nutrients in the diet such as protein, vitamin A, or iron. However, single nutrient inadequacies rarely exist; most malnutrition is caused by a lack of both protein and energy, for which the term protein-energy malnutrition (PEM) will be used. Upon this base of PEM is engrafted specific nutrient inadequacies that differ in type from one country to the next. Clinically, PEM spans a spectrum from wasting of fat and lean body mass with relative sparing of plasma proteins (marasmus) to more pronounced protein deficiency and hypoalbuminemia with edema (kwashiorkor). Underlying chronic malnutrition of the marasmic type often develops into the more severe kwashiorkor, usually ushered in by an acute infectious episode.

In developing nations, the youngest in society are the principal targets of PEM (Mata, 1978). In industrialized nations, adults are at greatest risk, developing PEM secondary to debilitating chronic diseases, neoplasms, alcoholism, inflammatory bowel disease, or renal failure. Recently, adult PEM has also been recognized in hospitalized patients who are maintained on the routine, semistarvation regimens of parenteral fluid and electrolytes during the treatment of many acute medical and surgical illnesses (Bistrian et al., 1974; Bistrian et al., 1976). In both situations, malnutrition may greatly exaggerate both the susceptibility to infectious agents and the severity of the illnesses they produce (Keusch, 1979). Because infection itself causes losses of nutrients by a number of mechanisms, the interaction of infection and malnutrition may lead to progressive debilitation and increased mortality. Although this interaction has been termed "synergistic," it is difficult to precisely define this synergism (Scrimshaw et al., 1968). Longitudinal observations demonstrate that malnutrition and infection occur in cyclic fashion, which inexorably progresses in a downhill spiral to severe or fatal conditions unless the cycle is interrupted. The minimum consequence in young children is impaired growth that may result in permanent stunting and failure to achieve optimal intellectual potential. In adult PEM, the analogous end of the spectrum may be impaired wound healing or infection that prolongs hospitalization. In both age groups, the other end of the spectrum is death. In developing countries, the overall mortality rate in childhood from birth to age 7 often reaches 50 per cent, primarily because of the combined forces of infection and malnutrition (Chen et al., 1980).

Several important points have emerged from recent studies in developing countries. First, malnutrition and infectious diseases must be understood as ecologic problems that are interrelated, not only to each other but also to cultural, sociological, political, and economic factors, for which long-term corrective measures are required. The ultimate solution to these problems lies neither in a simple nutritional supplement nor in a vaccine, for example, but in the complex and difficult process of national development. Second, PEM is usually caused by a succession of insults, most often infections, over an extended period of time rather than by a single problem at a particular time

(Keusch, 1979). Third, intrauterine events, both nutritional and infectious, may impair in utero development, birth weight, and postnatal growth, and increase postnatal morbidity and mortality from infectious agents (Mata, 1978).

The purpose of this chapter is to examine the interaction between malnutrition and infection in sufficient detail to permit the physician to make rational medical decisions for his patients in the short term. To accomplish this, we will separately consider the effects of infections on nutrition and effects of nutrition on infections via alterations in host defense mechanisms.

EFFECT OF INFECTIONS ON NUTRITION

DEFINITION OF MALNUTRITION. To attempt a definition of malnutrition is not a simple task, perhaps because it is so difficult to describe good nutrition. To be adequate, a diet must supply enough protein, energy, and essential vitamins and minerals to maintain all body tissues, to permit growth in children, and to allow a wide range of physiological processes and functions to proceed normally. This entails not only day-to-day needs, but, in addition, sufficient reserves to deal with increased needs during periods of exogenous stress (infections, injury, other diseases) or normal processes such as pregnancy or lactation. The most simple model looks at the quantitative intake of a given nutrient and some quantifiable result such as body size, composition, or nutrient levels in blood or tissues (Calloway, 1982). Requirements for a nutrient are considered to be met when the chosen indicator reaches a defined standard under stipulated conditions (age, sex, physiological state, etc.) (Calloway, 1982). Acceptable levels for dietary components are thus arbitrary. They account for individual variability only in being set high enough to cover the needs of nearly everyone in a population. To improve the validity of the standards, efforts are being made to define needs in terms of functional capacity within several domains including disease response, reproductive competence, cognitive function, work output, and social and behavioral habits (Calloway, 1982). For the present, we remain dependent on anthropometry, body composition, and biochemical assessments. Unfortunately, biochemical indices usually do not show change until malnutrition is far advanced, while body composition studies are technically demanding. The most practical measures to assess protein and energy status are, therefore, anthropometric. These rely upon body weight, height, skinfold thickness to assess stores of subcutaneous fat, and limb circumference (corrected for subcutaneous tissues) to assess muscle mass. Age-specific standards are derived from "healthy" populations and currently are based on data from the U.S. National Center for Health Statistics (NCHS) as a reference (U.S. Department of Health, Education, and Welfare, 1977). An arbitrary grading system is generally employed (Table 1). However, this has practical utility, especially for growing children, and allows separation of current PEM (relative deficit in weight greater than height = wasting) from past effects (deficit in height relative to expected growth at a particular age = stunting) (Waterlow, 1976). Criteria for diagnosis of PEM in adults have also been defined for well-nourished populations, using "ideal body weights" for age derived from actuarial tables such as those published by the Metropolitan Life Insurance Co. (Keusch, 1979).

Simple biochemical studies such as serum albumin and/or transferrin levels as indicators of the ability of the individual to maintain visceral protein synthesis improve the assessment of malnutrition, and help in the classification of marasmus and kwashiorkor. In order to measure lean body mass (i.e., the protein stores), a more complex assessment, the creatinine-height index (CHI) is used (Viteri and Alvarado, 1970). This involves determination of daily total urinary creatinine, which is proportional to lean body mass. The value is compared to expected standards derived from well-nourished normal controls matched for sex and height. When urinary collections are complete, the CHI serves as an excellent and sensitive indicator of lean body mass.

Definition of vitamin or mineral malnutrition is based on measurement of actual nutrient (or in some cases, metabolite or nutrient dependent enzyme activity) levels in appropriate tissues. Standards are based on correlations of levels with clinical status in patients, results of treatment, and small numbers of experimental volunteers during depletion-repletion protocols. In developing countries such data are usually not available for individuals, but rather are obtained in samples of the population as surveillance data for specific nutrient status in that population.

THE METABOLIC EFFECTS OF FEVER AND LEUKOCYTIC PYROGEN. Fever is one of the cardinal manifestations of infection and is due to a regulated change in the thermostatic set point in the hypothalamus under the influence of a mediator released primarily from monocytic cells called leukocytic pyrogen (Dinarello, 1984). This monokine appears to be identical to interleukin 1 (IL-1), an important regulator of the immunologic network. As a pyrogen, IL-1 acts to release arachidonic acid and increases synthesis of prostaglandin E_2 (PGE_2) in the thermoregulatory center in the hypothalamus (Dinarello, 1984). This, in turn, alters the balance between heat production and heat loss, resulting in elevated body temperature. The benefits of fever during infection are not certain, but may relate to temperature inhibition of microbial growth or virulence factors at elevated temperature and improved function of host defenses, so that survival from infection improves (Dinarello, 1984; Roberts, 1979). The metabolic costs of fever are more clear; energy utilization increases on the average of 13 per cent per °C increase in temperature, and resting metabolic expenditures may be raised by 35 to 40 per cent during sepsis. Because anorexia commonly accompanies fever,

Table 1. CLINICAL GRADING OF MALNUTRITION BY ANTHROPOMETRY

	Grade (Per cent of NCHS Standards)			
		Clinical Grade		
Anthropometric Measure	*Normal*	*Mild*	*Moderate*	*Severe*
Weight for height	90–110	80–89	70–79	<70
Height for age	95–105	90–94	85–89	<85

intake of energy falls (Mata et al., 1977), and the patient must turn to body stores to sustain life.

Energy is stored as carbohydrate and lipids. However, the carbohydrates are primarily in the form of limited glycogen deposits in the liver and are perhaps sufficient for 24 hours (Keusch, 1979). In contrast to simple starvation in which the body's extensive fat stores are utilized, release of IL-1 elevates the levels of circulating insulin, glucagon, and growth hormone that interfere with efficient utilization of fat (Rayfield et al., 1977). These hormonal changes appear to mandate an increase in gluconeogenesis in the liver from amino acid precursors such as alanine or glutamine derived from contractile proteins in muscle (Long, 1977). Catabolism of muscle proteins is stimulated by local PGE_2 production, also under the influence of IL-1 (Baracos et al., 1983), and it is considerably augmented at elevated temperature. The overall result is a pseudodiabetic state with an increase in the glucose pool size, fasting hyperglycemia, abnormal glucose disappearance curves after a glucose load, and augmented glucose turnover and oxidation rates (Rayfield et al., 1973; Long et al., 1976). Because of peripheral insulin resistance, energy in muscle is obtained from oxidation of branched-chain amino acids released from catabolized contractile protein (O'Donnell et al., 1976). Deamination of gluconeogenic precursor amino acids and conversion to urea and other metabolites results in nitrogen loss, while the carbon skeleton in the form of newly synthesized glucose is oxidized to CO_2 and blown off in the lungs. Thus the entire structure of the amino acid is lost from the body and the muscle mass melts away (Keusch, 1979).

Nonreutilizable amino acids released from muscle such as 3-methylhistidine and phenylalanine are excreted in increased amounts in urine; the rest are taken up by the liver for new protein synthesis. At least some of this new protein synthesis is directed by IL-1; the production of some hepatic acute phase proteins (e.g., serum amyloid A component) is under direct control of IL-1 (Sztein et al., 1981). At the same time, synthesis of normal plasma proteins such as albumin and transferrin decreases. Albumin also appears to be used as a labile pool of amino acid for new protein synthesis (Powanda, 1977), and if infection is prolonged, especially if nutritional status is marginal, serum levels of these proteins decrease. Significant hypoalbuminemia results in the edema of kwashiorkor.

OTHER ANABOLIC RESPONSES IN INFECTION. In addition to the synthesis of acute-phase proteins, amino acid substrates are utilized for increased synthesis of cells and circulating proteins involved in host defense responses. Thus, turnover of phagocytic cells and lymphocytes from bone marrow increases, complement proteins are consumed and synthesized in increased amounts, and immunoglobulin production is turned on (Keusch, 1979). If the infection damages tissues, the repair process consumes additional substrates for new protein synthesis. All of this occurs primarily at the expense of endogenous proteins, which are broken down to provide amino acids for the protein anabolic response.

IL-1 EFFECTS ON MINERALS. Dramatic decreases in plasma iron and zinc concentration associated with the onset of fever are also triggered by IL-1 (Keusch, 1979; Beisel and Pekarek, 1974; Kampschmidt and Pulliam, 1978). Iron taken up by hepatic mononuclear cells is sequestered in nonmetabolically active forms such as ferritin and hemosiderin. The mechanism for this may be IL-1–induced degranulation of neutrophils with release of the iron transport protein, lactoferrin, and uptake of the lactoferrin-Fe complex (Klempner et al., 1978). Reduced circulating iron deprives microorganisms of free iron. This appears to curtail microbial growth, particularly at elevated body temperature (Mackowiak, 1981).

When IL-1 is released, hepatic cells take up zinc secondary to new synthesis of cellular zinc-binding proteins, metallothienines (Sugarman, 1983). The reduction in circulating zinc levels may activate phagocytosis, because neutrophil function is inhibited at physiological concentration of the metal (Sugarman, 1983). In addition, uptake of zinc into lymphoid cells could prime them for the proliferative response so essential to lymphocyte function as immune effector cells since many of the enzymes involved in nucleic acid synthesis are zinc metalloenzymes. Indeed, enhanced proliferative responses of T cells to mitogens have been observed in both in vitro and in vivo zinc supplementation studies (Sugarman, 1983).

The cost of iron sequestration is the anemia of infection, because the amounts of iron available for heme synthesis are reduced. Administration of iron supplements does not correct the anemia so long as the stimulus for the sequestration, release of IL-1, remains (Beisel, 1977). The cost of zinc sequestration is less clear. Whereas long-term zinc deficiency impairs development and maturation of T cells and T cell–mediated immune responses (Keusch et al., 1983), it is not obvious that the acute hypozincemia of infection has any similar effect.

Coincidental with shifts in iron and zinc, copper levels in plasma increase (Beisel, 1977). This is because ceruloplasmin, the binding protein for copper, is an acute-phase protein. Increased hepatic synthesis of ceruloplasmin results in entry of copper-ceruloplasmin in plasma. This may serve a beneficial role by increasing the efficiency of iron transfer in heme synthesis by means of the ferroxidase activity of copper-ceruloplasmin.

EFFECTS OF NUTRITION ON HOST DEFENSES

T LYMPHOCYTES AND CELL-MEDIATED IMMUNE RESPONSES. Before the role of the thymus gland in the maturation of T lymphocytes was discovered, it was observed that PEM resulted in lymphocyte depletion in thymus, spleen, and lymph nodes (Keusch et al., 1983). This cellular depletion is principally from T cell regions of these lymphoid tissues and is accompanied by a reduction in the number and per cent of mature circulating T cells with an associated increase in immature T cells. These changes are accompanied by altered T lymphocyte–dependent and cell-mediated immune responses (reviewed in Keusch et al., 1983).

Most of our understanding of these alterations is derived from study of circulating lymphocytes, since blood is the only tissue we can readily sample in humans during life. In patients with PEM, the number of E-rosetting T lymphocytes decreases, the number of surface immunoglobulin (Ig^+)–bearing B cells is unchanged, and the number of null cells with neither B nor T cell surface markers is increased. These changes are more pronounced in kwashiorkor patients compared to marasmics. The null cells are responsive to thymic hormonal factors, and, under their influence in

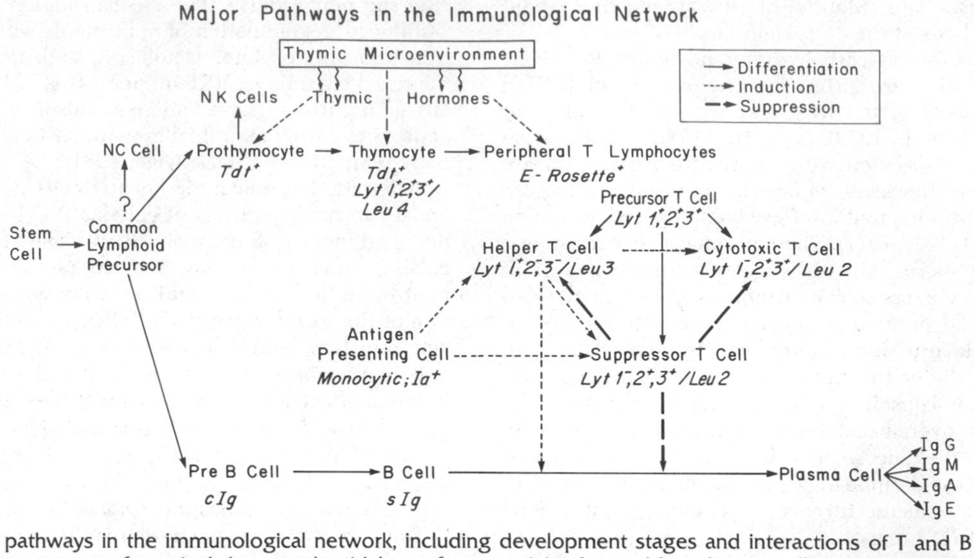

Figure 1. Major pathways in the immunological network, including development stages and interactions of T and B lymphocytes. Tdt⁺ signifies the presence of terminal deoxynucleotidyl transferase activity; Lyt and Leu denote cell surface differentiation markers detected by monoclonal antibodies for murine and human T lymphocytes, respectively; cIg and sIg indicate the presence of cytoplasmic or surface immunoglobulin on B lymphocytes. (Reproduced with permission from Keusch, G. T., Wilson, C. S., Waksal, S. D., Nutrition, host defenses and the lymphoid system. In Gallin, J. I., and Fauci, A. S. (eds): Advances in Host Defense Mechanisms, Volume 2, N.Y., Plenum, 1982.)

vitro will mature to E-rosetting T cells. Impaired maturation of T cells in PEM may not only be due to abnormal thymic influences, but may also be at prethymic levels of maturation. This is based on the fact that natural killer (NK) cells, which are believed to be prethymic T cells (Keusch et al., 1983), do not increase in number as expected with the loss of thymic function and are refractory to gamma interferon, a known regulator of NK cell function (Salimonu et al., 1982).

The functional consequences of maturational arrest of T lymphocytes are a decreased ability to proliferate in response to antigens and to produce lymphokine regulators of the immunologic network (Fig. 1). This results in major impairment of T lymphocyte–dependent, cell-mediated immune responses, such as delayed tuberculin type hypersensitivity skin-test responses, and production of antibodies that require T lymphocyte helper functions. Physiologically, this may be due to disproportionate loss of helper compared to suppressor cells. In addition, serum from kwashiorkor patients has been found to suppress in vitro proliferative responses, apparently due to a lack of needed, but unidentified, small molecular weight growth factors (Keusch et al., 1983).

Clinically, these changes are reflected in increased morbidity and mortality due to infections that are normally combatted by cell-mediated immune responses. These include measles, tuberculosis, and *Pneumocystis carinii* infection, among others (Keusch, 1984).

B LYMPHOCYTES AND ANTIBODY RESPONSES. As already noted above, B cell regions of spleen and lymph nodes, and the number of circulating surface Ig⁺ B lymphocytes, remain relatively normal in PEM patients. Indeed, Ig levels in serum are normal to elevated (Keusch, 1979; Keusch et al., 1983). IgE levels are usually elevated several-fold as a result of frequent helminthic infection and, probably, a loss of T lymphocyte regulatory function.

In contrast to elevated Ig levels in serum, secretory IgA concentrations are reduced in external body fluids (saliva, nasopharyngeal washings, tears). Other proteins in these secretions are reduced much less, indicating a more profound effect of PEM on the secretory immune system.

More important than Ig levels, however, are functional antibody responses. Results using vaccines to probe the antibody response have been highly variable (Keusch et al., 1983). These depend in part on the nature of the antigen, the adjuvant (if any), the dose and time of sampling, and the presence or absence of infection at the time of immunization. Deficient responses in serum and/or secretions have been observed most consistently with polio, measles, or yellow fever viruses, and with typhoid O antigen, but usually not with tetanus toxoid. These results cannot be simply explained on the basis of inadequate T cell help. Since tetanus is a T-dependent antigen, whereas *Salmonella typhi* O polysaccharide should be a relatively T-independent antigen, one would expect the opposite results. Nevertheless, animal experiments, which permit a more careful and quantitative analysis of the antibody response, indicate that B cells remain functionally responsive to antigenic stimulus, and that failure of T help and/or macrophage presentation of antigen is primarily responsible for decreased B cell function.

Clinically, these antibody defects adversely alter responses to mucosal infections of the gastrointestinal, respiratory, or urinary tracts, and may also affect the course of suppurative skin infections and systemic invasion by pyogenic or gram-negative enteric bacteria (Keusch, 1984).

PHAGOCYTOSIS AND INTRACELLULAR MICROBICIDAL SYSTEMS. For normal phagocytosis, the size of the pools of polymorphonuclear neutrophils (PMNs) and mononuclear phagocytic (MNPs) cells as well as capacity of bone marrow to mobilize additional cells must be adequate. Then, the capacity of cells to ingest and kill microorganisms will determine the outcome of the interaction of host cell and invading pathogen.

Many, but not all, of these aspects of phagocytosis have been studied in PEM patients. While pool sizes have not been measured, the bone marrow response to endotoxin administration has been impaired (Chandra et al., 1977). In vivo studies have demonstrated delayed mononuclear cell mobilization into abraded skin windows, while in vitro studies have shown delayed chemotactic movement of PMNs through milipore filters in response to normal chemotactic factors (Keusch, 1979). Alterations in PMN adherence to nylon wool fibers occur with normal cells exposed to chemotactic factors. However, the expected decrease in adhesiveness is not observed with PEM cells incubated with either endotoxin-generated chemotactic factors or chemotactic oligopeptides (Anderson et al., 1983). This correlates with impaired chemotactic migration in vitro in response to bacterial factors or zymosan-activated serum. The data are consistent with activation of PMNs in vivo, which may be observed in several clinical situations in which in vivo activation of complement occurs (Craddock et al., 1979).

Once phagocytic cells have been mobilized and have migrated to the site of infection, the next step is ingestion of the offending microorganism. In the presence of normal humoral factors for phagocytosis (Ig- or complement-derived opsonins), there is no evidence for impaired particle ingestion in PEM, and degranulation of lysosomes appears to be normal as well (Keusch, 1979). The membrane perturbations during phagocytosis initiate biochemical changes leading to activation of microbicidal systems. In spite of normal phagocytosis and degranulation, however, these microbicidal related reactions are blunted in PEM cells. The oxidative reactions that generate microbicidal compounds are not turned on as much as expected, including oxygen consumption, hexose monophosphate shunt activity, and iodination of bacteria by myeloperoxidase (Keusch, 1979; Schopfer and Douglas, 1976). Consistent with these results, diminished microbicidal activity for *E. coli*, *S. aureus*, and *C. albicans* has been observed (Keusch, 1979; Schopfer and Douglas, 1976). These studies have generally utilized normal serum for opsonization and therefore measure only cellular function. Because of opsonic defects in PEM patients, microbial uptake may be restricted in vivo, further inhibiting microbicidal activity. This is clinically reflected in the frequency of gram-negative sepsis in kwashiorkor patients, an often fatal infectious problem (Keusch, 1979).

COMPLEMENT, CHEMOTAXIS, OPSONIZATION, AND CELLULAR LYSIS. Activation of the complement system by either the classical or alternative pathways generates biologically active byproducts of importance to host defense. These include C5a, the most potent host-derived chemotactic factor; C3a, which enhances migration of phagocytic cells through small vessels; C3b, which is deposited on microbial surfaces where it acts as an opsonin when recognized by C3b receptors on phagocytic cell surfaces; and C789, the membrane attack complex that mediates hemolysis of target erythrocytes or bacterial lysis of susceptible microbes. Complement appears to be activated in vivo in PEM, for activation-breakdown products are present in serum. There is a concomitant reduction in circulating levels of all components except C4, and diminished hemolytic complement activity by both the classical and alternative pathways (Keusch, 1979; Keusch et al., 1984). Functionally, this decrease in residual functional complement is translated into decreased generation of chemotactic factors and of heat-labile serum opsonins (Keusch et al., 1984; Keusch et al., 1981). Functional deficiencies in the complement system act synergistically in vivo with cellular defects to produce a more severe microbicidal defect. It is this combined depression of phagocytic host defenses that undoubtedly underlies the susceptibility of PEM patients to systemic gram-negative infections.

THE ARENA OF THE INTERACTION OF MALNUTRITION AND INFECTION

Malnutrition and infection must be considered together because, as documented in the previous discussion, they interact in cyclic fashion. Both factors are invariably present in the populations of the developing world, and both contribute to the excessive morbidity and mortality among these populations, especially preschool children (Chen et al., 1980). To improve the situation, it will be necessary to address both the undernutrition and the overexposure to infection. The factors underlying undernutrition are exceedingly complex, and include poverty, landlessness, market forces, inadequate technology, and undereducation. Ill use of available food resources, the decline in prevalence and duration of breast feeding, physiologically inappropriate cultural responses to the presence of infection (withdrawal of food or substitution of nonnutritious "bland" diets), and lack of knowledge of convalescent needs all serve to worsen the underlying nutritional state, and are directly related to a lack of education and training. Inadequate facilities for sanitary disposal of feces, unavailability of water of good quality and in sufficient quantity, lack of appropriate food preparation or storage areas in the household, inability to reduce or remove insects or other vectors of disease transmission, and a dearth of accessible basic health care and preventive medicine all contribute to the high burden of infectious diseases. These issues must be addressed in some orderly fashion consistent with available resources in order to make progress. Of fundamental importance in this process is to ensure that the practice of medicine incorporates nutritional considerations into the care and prevention of infectious diseases. Concern for convalescent care and total nutritional rehabilitation becomes a part of proper therapy when this approach is taken, and physicians become promoters of health as well as alleviators of disease.

References

Anderson, D. C., Krishna, G. S., Hughes, B. C., Mace, M. L., Mintz, A. A., Smith, C. W., and Nichols, B. L.: Impaired polymorphonuclear leukocyte motility in malnourished infants: relationship to functional abnormalities of cell adherence. J Lab Clin Med 101:881, 1983.

Baracos, V., Rodemann, H. P., Dinarello, C. A., and Goldberg, A. L.: Stimulation of degradation of muscle proteins during fever. A mechanism for the increased degradation of muscle proteins during fever. N Engl J Med 308:553, 1983.

Beisel, W. R.: Magnitude of the host nutritional responses to infection. Am J Clin Nutr 30:1236, 1977.

Beisel, W. R., and Pekarek, R. S.: The impact of infectious disease on trace element metabolism of the host. In: Hockstra, W. G., Suttie, J. W., Gauther, H. E., and Mertz, W. (eds.): Trace Element Metabolism in Animals. Baltimore, University Park Press, 1974, p. 217.

Bistrian, B. R., Blackburn, G. L., Hallowell, E., and Heddle, R.: Protein status of general surgical patients. JAMA 238:858, 1974.
Bistrian, B. R., Blackburn, G. L., and Vitale, J. J.: Prevalence of malnutrition in general medical patients. JAMA 235:1567, 1976.
Calloway, D. H.: Functional consequences of malnutrition. Rev Infect Dis 4:736, 1982.
Chandra, R. K., Seth, V., and Chandra, S. Polymorphonuclear leukocyte function in malnourished Indian children. In Suskind, R. M., (ed.): Malnutrition and the Immune Response. New York, Raven Press, 1977, p. 259.
Chen, L. C., Chowdry, A. K. M. A., and Huffman, S. L.: Anthropometric assessment of energy-protein malnutrition and subsequent risk of mortality among preschool aged children. Am J Clin Nutr 33:1838, 1980.
Craddock, P. R., Hammerschmidt, D. E., Moldow, C. F., Yamada, O., and Jacobs, H. S.: Granulocyte aggregation as a manifestation of membrane interactions with complement: possible role in leukocyte margination, microvascular occlusion and endothelial damage. Semin. Hematol. 16:140, 1979.
Dinarello, C. A.: Interleukin-1. Rev Infect Dis 6:51, 1984.
Kampschmidt, R. F., and Pulliam, L. A.: Effect of human monocyte pyrogen on plasma iron, plasma zinc, and blood neutrophils in rabbits and rats. Proc Soc Exp Biol Med 158:32, 1978.
Keusch, G. T.: Nutrition as a determinant of host response to infection and the metabolic sequelae of infectious diseases. Seminars in Infectious Diseases. Weinstein, L. and Fields, B. A. (eds.): Stratton Intercontinental Book Corp., New York, 1979, p. 265.
Keusch, G. T.: Nutrition and infection. In Remington J. D., and Swartz, M. (eds.): Current Clinical Topics in Infectious Diseases. Vol. 5. New York, McGraw-Hill, 1984, pp. 106–123.
Keusch, G. T., Urrutia, J. J., Guerrero, O., Castaneda, G., and Smith, H., Jr.: Serum opsonic activity in acute protein-energy malnutrition. Bull WHO 59:923, 1981.
Keusch, G. T., Wilson, C. S., and Waksal, S. D.: Nutrition, host defenses, and the lymphoid system. In Fauci, A. S., and Gallin, J. I. (eds.): Advances in Host Defense Mechanisms. Vol. 2. New York, Raven Press, 1983, p. 275.
Keusch, G. T., Torun, B., Johnston, R. B. III, and Urrutia, J. J.: Impairment of hemolytic complement activation by both classical and alternative pathways in serum from patients with kwashiorkor. J Pediatr 105:434, 1984.
Klempner, M. S., Dinarello, C. A., and Gallin, J. I.: Human leukocytic pyrogen induces release of specific granule contents from human neutrophils. J Clin Invest 61:1330, 1978.
Long, C. M.: Energy balance and carbohydrate metabolism in infection and sepsis. Am J Clin 30:1301, 1977.
Long, C. M., Kenney, J. M., and Geiger, J. W.: Non-suppressability of gluconeogenesis by glucose in septic patients. Metabolism 25:193, 1976.
Mackowiak, P. A.: Direct effects of hyperthermia on pathogenic microorganisms: teleologic implications with regard to fever. Rev Infect Dis 3:508, 1981.
Mata, L. J.: The Children of Santa Maria Cauque. Cambridge, MA, MIT Press, 1978.
Mata, L. J., Kronmal, R. A., and Urrutia, J. J.: Effect of infection on food intake and the nutritional state: perspectives as viewed from the village. Am J Clin Nutr 30:1215, 1977.
O'Donnell, T. F., Jr., Clowes, G. H. A., Jr., Blackburn, G. L., Ryan, N. T., Benotti, P. N., and Miller, J. D. B.: Proteolysis associated with a deficit of peripheral energy fuel substrates in septic man. Surgery 80:192, 1976.
Powanda, M. C.: Changes in body balances of nitrogen and other key nutrients: description and underlying mechanisms. Am J Clin Nutr 30:1254, 1977.
Rayfield, E. J., Curnow, R. T., George, D. T., and Beisel, W. R.: Impaired carbohydrate metabolism during a mild viral illness. N Engl J Med 298:618, 1973.
Rayfield, E. J., Curnow, R. T., Reinhard, D., and Kochicheril, N. M.: Effects of acute endotoxemia on glucoregulation in normal and diabetic subjects. J Clin Endo Metab 45:513, 1977.
Roberts, N. J.: Temperature and host defenses. Microbiol Rev 43:241, 1979.
Salimonu, L. S., Ojo-Amaize, E., Williams, A. I. O., Cooke, A. R., Adekunle, F. A., Alm, G. V., and Wigzell, H.: Depressed natural killer cell activity in children with protein-calorie malnutrition. Clin Immunol Immunopathol 24:1, 1982.
Schopfer, K., and Douglas, S. D.: Neutrophil function in children with kwashiorkor. J Lab Clin Med 88:450, 1976.
Scrimshaw, N. S., Taylor, C. E., and Gordon, J. E.: Interactions of Nutrition and Infection. Geneva, World Health Organization, Monograph Series 57, 1968.
Sugarman, B.: Zinc and infection. Rev Infect Dis 5:137, 1983.
Sztein, M. B., Vogel, S. N., Sipe, J. D., Murphy, P. A., Mizel, S. B., Oppenheim, J. J., and Rosenstreich, D. C.: The role of macrophages in the acute phase response: SAA inducer is closely related to lymphocyte activating factor and endogenous pyrogen. Cell Immunol 63:164, 1981.
United States Department of Health, Education, and Welfare: NCHS growth curves for children from birth to 18 years. Hyattsville, MD, DHEW Publication PHS 78:1650, 1977.
Viteri, F., and Alvarado, J.: The creatinine-height index: its use in the estimation of the degree of protein depletion and repletion in protein-calorie malnourished children. Pediatrics 46:696, 1970.
Waterlow, J. C.: Nutrition in Preventive Medicine. In Beaton, G. H., and Bengoa, J. M. (eds.): Classification and Definition of Protein-Energy Malnutrition. Geneva, World Health Organization 1976, p. 530.

Clinical Infectious Diseases II

A. UPPER RESPIRATORY AND ORAL INFECTIONS

95

STREPTOCOCCAL PHARYNGITIS AND TONSILLITIS

Hans A. Valkenburg, M.D., Ph.D.

ETIOLOGY. The most important cause of sore throat, because of the possibility of serious suppurative and non-suppurative sequelae, is *Streptococcus pyogenes* (group A beta-hemolytic streptococcus; see Chapter 24). Occasionally, groups C and C beta-hemolytic streptococci are responsible, particularly in tropical areas. *Corynebacterium diphtheriae* (see Chapter 90) is still an important cause of pharyngitis in some countries. These bacterial pathogens typically cause an infection that is characterized by tonsillar exudate or a membrane. *Neisseria gonorrhoeae* and *Candida* can also cause exudative pharyngitis. Other bacteria, such as *Neisseria meningitidis* and *Hemophilus influenzae* type B, undoubtedly cause nasopharyngeal infections, but these are either asymptomatic or too nondescript to be recognized as clinical entities.

Most pharyngeal infections are nonbacterial. Of patients with nonbacterial pharyngitis, adenovirus can be recovered from about 25 per cent. Other viruses that are often isolated include herpes simplex, coxsackievirus A, and the echovirus group. Primary herpes infection is often manifest as pharyngitis associated with gingivitis; otherwise herpes does not cause pharyngitis. Coxsackieviruses usually cause herpangina (Chapter 106); echovirus pharyngitis may be associated with exanthems, which can simulate rubeola, rubella, or even meningococcemia. Epstein-Barr virus, the agent of infectious mononucleosis, often causes a sore throat. Unlike most other viral infections, it is typically exudative. *Mycoplasma pneumoniae* may also cause a sore throat, although this is usually only one manifestation of a more generalized respiratory infection. Isolated pharyngitis has been produced in volunteers.

PATHOGENESIS AND PATHOLOGY

Streptococcal Pharyngitis. Infection is usually spread by droplets sprayed from air passages, but the organism can also be transmitted by dust or fomites or from skin lesions. Epidemics of tonsillitis or scarlet fever can also originate from contaminated milk or food. The source of infection can be either a carrier or a patient; children are more likely to transmit infection than adults. Nasal carriers are less common than throat carriers but shed large numbers of bacteria and are more infectious (Holmes and Williams, 1958). Convalescent carriers are more likely to harbor M-typable group A streptococci than chronic carriers. M protein confers virulence to the organism (see Chapter 24).

Organisms harboring M protein are more virulent, and most epidemic strains are M-typable. In the presence of high antibacterial immunity, that is, antibody to the particular M protein, the streptococcus may fail to become established or may be confined to the surface of the mucosa or skin of the host. When antibacterial resistance is low or the streptococcus is highly virulent, colonization results in tonsillitis or impetigo and suppurative complications, such as lymphadenitis or septicemia. If the invading organism produces large amounts of erythrogenic toxin and antitoxic immunity is also low, the patient may develop scarlet fever. Eradication of a streptococcal infection by antibiotics may permit reinfection with the same M type at a later time owing to insufficient development of type-specific antibodies (Valkenburg et al., 1963). Children who have had tonsillectomies have a lower incidence of symptomatic streptococcal pharyngitis but not of asymptomatic infection nor of nonstreptococcal pharyngitis.

Little is known about the pathology of streptococcal pharyngitis and tonsillitis. Generalized pharyngeal erythema and edema is characteristic, and a discrete or patchy exudate due to polymorphonuclear cell infiltrates often appears after 12 to 36 hours. Deep-seated cellulitis develops in streptococcal upper respiratory tract infections and involves tonsillar and peritonsillar tissues. Spread to regional (cervical) lymph nodes with suppurative lymphadenitis is common. In young children the lymphadenitis may be confused with mumps.

Nonbacterial pharyngitis is usually caused by respiratory viruses that are spread by droplet or direct contact. The viruses multiply locally in the respiratory epithelium. Adenovirus is remarkable because it apparently can remain latent within lymphoid tissue in the oropharynx. Coxsackievirus A is primarily an enterovirus, but large numbers of virus particles can be found in nasal and pharyngeal secretions of patients with herpangina.

CLINICAL MANIFESTATIONS. The clinical manifestations of streptococcal pharyngitis are determined by the patient's age, immune status, the virulence of the organism, and the presence of tonsils. In *infants* there is usually only a mucopurulent nasal discharge and fever. This illness, which lasts about one week, cannot be distinguished from a common cold except by culture. *Young children,* up to the age of about 3 years, react to infection with mild constitutional symptoms including anorexia, vomiting, fever to 103° F, and listlessness. Purulent coryza is characteristic but nonspecific. Anterior cervical adenitis is usual, and the subacute illness may persist for as long as four to eight weeks.

In *older children* and *adults,* streptococcal pharyngitis characteristically begins abruptly with fever, sore throat, vomiting (sometimes with abdominal pain), headache, and malaise. Throat symptoms may not appear for up to 24 hours from onset. If the infectious organism produces erythrogenic toxin and the patient lacks antitoxin, the erythematous punctiform exanthem of *scarlet fever* develops 12 to 48 hours later.

It must be recognized, however, that a definitive diagnosis of streptococcal pharyngitis cannot be made on clinical grounds. No single characteristic, even tonsillar exudate, has a diagnostic sensitivity of greater than 50 per cent. The combination of fever, moderate to marked pharyngeal erythema, and anterior cervical adenitis (with or without tonsillar exudate) is associated with a positive throat culture for group A streptococci in 75 per cent of cases. If there are also palatal petechiae, the diagnostic accuracy approaches 90 per cent. Unfortunately, only a minority of patients with streptococcal pharyngitis have these specific signs. (Stollerman and Bernstein, 1961). The remainder of patients have an illness that cannot be differentiated from nonbacterial pharyngitis. In fact, close to 90 per cent of patients with sore throats have so few complaints that they do not even consult physicians. Many of these sore throats are due to streptococcal infections. Both streptococcal and nonstreptococcal sore throats are self-limited infections that resolve within four to five days. Therefore, the response to empiric therapy does not differ either. Even the most severe streptococcal sore throat resolves by 10 days without treatment.

Diphtheria, when it involves the tonsils and pharynx, usually begins insidiously. The membrane develops after 24 hours and varies in extent from a small patch to a complete tonsillar blanket. It is smooth, white or gray, and adherent. The underlying tissues bleed if the membrane is removed. There is a variable amount of reactive adenitis, which may be dramatic ("bull neck"). In mild cases the membrane sloughs in 7 to 10 days, and the patient recovers. In severe cases, the fever and toxemia increase and progress to stupor, coma, and death within 7 to 10 days.

In *Candidiasis* the exudate consists of small localized white spots with little swelling or redness in between.

Viral pharyngitis can mimic streptococcal pharyngitis, including the presence of a tonsillar exudate. There are a few distinct syndromes, however. The punctate vesicles in the soft palate, anterior tonsillar pillars, and uvula are typical and characteristic of herpangina (coxsackievirus A). Infectious mononucleosis is usually associated with generalized lymphadenopathy, splenomegaly, and atypical lymphocytosis. Other viral infections are less characteristic.

COMPLICATIONS AND SEQUELAE

Suppurative Complications. The most common suppurative complication of pharyngitis or tonsillitis is peritonsillar abscess. The incidence varies between 1.5 and 4 per cent of all cases of pharyngitis, increases with age, and occurs in men 1.5 times more often than in women. The incubation period is between two and nine days after the onset of the sore throat. Retropharyngeal abscess and otitis media are less frequent complications (each occurs in less than 0.5 per cent of cases); otitis occurs in children. In about half the cases with peritonsillar abscess or otitis, the condition is already present at the time of the first visit to the doctor and therefore could not have been prevented. Tonsillectomy reduces the risk of peritonsillar abscess by approximately 90 per cent.

Erysipelas is now a rare suppurative complication of streptococcal upper respiratory tract infection (see Chapter 220). It is more common in older people with degenerative skin changes in whom it usually involves the face or legs. Erysipelas starts abruptly with generalized symptoms after an incubation period of about a week. Sensations of burning and tightness develop at the site of invasion, followed by rapidly spreading erythema. The spreading edge is sharply defined and elevated. There is a marked tendency for recurrences in the same location.

Suppurative lymphadenitis, sinusitis, osteomyelitis of the frontal bone, and thrombophlebitis are rare complications due to local spread of streptococci. Bacteremia is extremely rare.

Nonsuppurative Sequelae. The most prominent complications of streptococcal pharyngitis and pyoderma are rheumatic fever and glomerulonephritis. Acute rheumatic fever never follows impetigo, but acute glomerulonephritis can be preceded by either streptococcal pharyngitis or pyoderma.

The attack rates for rheumatic fever during an epidemic of a rheumatogenic strain can be as high as 3 per cent in a closed (e.g., school) population but are considerably lower in sample studies of open populations. The attack rates of acute nephritis after infection with a known nephritogenic strain are around 10 to 15 per cent, regardless of the site of the primary infection. The stricter the definition one uses for streptococcal infection, the higher the attack rates for the late sequelae. In patients with characteristic clinical signs and symptoms from whom group A streptococci are isolated and who develop antibodies to streptolysin O, the attack rate for rheumatic fever is 0.95 to 1.70 per cent. For glomerulonephritis, it is 0.19 to 3.40 per cent.

Scarlet Fever. Scarlet fever results from skin or throat infection with an erythrogenic strain of streptococcus. It starts suddenly with fever, sore throat, and vomiting, although the latter two symptoms may be absent. The exanthem follows within 24 to 36 hours and evolves from above downwards, becoming generalized within 24 hours. It is a red punctate rash that blanches on pressure and spares the area around the mouth (circumoral pallor). The rash is more intense in folds (axilla, groin, and neck).

During the first days, the tongue is covered with a thick white "fur," which peels from the tip and edges in a few days to develop into the typical red and white strawberry tongue. Exanthems and petechiae may be found on the palate. The petechiae may mimic the exanthem of meningococcal septicemia. Typical scarlet fever resembles sunburn, drug rash, or the exanthem seen in viral infections, such as rubella and echovirus. Desquamation begins on the face as fine scales at the end of the first week spreading gradually over the next two weeks to the trunk and finally to the hands and feet. It may persist for weeks if the rash is severe.

GEOGRAPHIC VARIATION IN DISEASE. In temperate climates more than 60 per cent of all people have at least one attack of sore throat annually, but only 2 per cent of the total population consult their doctor for this complaint. In half of these patients, *S. pyogenes* is isolated. Based on sample studies, 14 per cent of the general population suffers from a streptococcal sore throat annually. Twenty to 25 per cent of people over 5 years of age carry group A streptococci in their throat, but only 10 per cent of these have a simultaneous sore throat. Available data suggest that in any country 10 to 15 serotypes of *S. pyogenes* circulate.

In subtropical and tropical areas the incidence of pharyngitis and tonsillitis is not known. However, scarlet fever is rarely observed, and tonsillectomy is seldom performed. On the other hand, skin infections are common and are probably the major source of epidemics of acute nephritis. Carrier studies in schoolchildren suggest that streptococcal infections are about as common in subtropical climates as in temperate zones. This finding corresponds with the high attack rate of rheumatic fever among children in North America.

In tropical Africa, carriage of group A streptococci in the throat is low (about 2 per cent) but is three times higher in the skin. Streptococcal pharyngitis is rare (occurring in less than 0.5 per cent of young schoolchildren), but skin infections occur in more than 7 per cent. Ninety per cent of these skin infections are caused by *S. pyogenes.* The course of streptococcal pharyngitis and diphtheria may be modified by immunity acquired during previous skin infections with these bacteria (Franz et al., 1964).

Crowding and poor socioeconomic conditions contribute to the spread of streptococci, regardless of race or the site of infection. Tonsillectomy reduces carrier rates for streptococci but not the incidence of clinical upper respiratory tract disease (Matanoski, 1972).

Although the attack rates for rheumatic fever and glomerulonephritis are still high in some developing areas of the world, this problem has decreased considerably in the more developed countries over the past 30 years. The reason for this is not the disappearance of streptococcal infections or even the liberal application of antibiotics. More likely explanations are that the virulence of the streptococcus has changed or that the relation between the organism, host, and environment has changed as a result of improved socioeconomic, hygienic, and nutritional conditions.

According to hospital admissions records, rheumatic fever and rheumatic heart disease are still common in poor countries (Strasser, 1978).

DIAGNOSIS. Because streptococcal pharyngitis and tonsillitis cannot be diagnosed from clinical signs and symptoms only, a throat culture has to be done to establish the cause. One throat culture can identify about 90 per cent of cases of streptococcal pharyngitis if it is obtained by vigorously swabbing the tonsils and pharynx, inoculating onto a rich agar base with 5 per cent sheep red blood cells, and incubating in a 5 per cent carbon dioxide atmosphere. More than a twofold rise or fall in antibody titers between two serum samples taken at least 3 weeks apart is also absolute evidence for a recent infection. One should be cautious in interpreting titers from a single specimen. In children high ASO (antistreptolysin O) titers (e.g., over 1:400 Todd units) may be observed long after a streptococcal infection has occurred. The most common antibodies measured are those against streptolysin O, DNAase-B, and hyaluronidase. Both ASO and anti-DNAase-B antibodies can be found after uncomplicated streptococcal pharyngitis. Leukocytosis is usually present in streptococcal pharyngitis but is often absent in streptococcal pyoderma and impetigo.

TREATMENT. Controlled trials of therapy for streptococcal pharyngitis have shown that clinical recovery is similar in cases with and without antibiotic treatment (Haverkorn et al., 1971). Eradication of *S. pyogenes* is most successful after parenteral administration of penicillin. Oral penicillin is less effective because the patients do not take the drug for the obligatory period of 10 days. Persistent carriage of the same type of streptococcus in over 70 per cent of the patients is observed after treatment with sulfonamides or aspirin.

Eradication of group A streptococci from the throat can be achieved by one injection of long-acting benzathine benzylpenicillin G (1.2 million units in persons over 12 years; 600,000 units in children). When treatment is started within a few days after the onset of symptoms, the frequency of secondary infections such as acute otitis and peritonsillar abscess is reduced. Penicillin instituted within the first week is effective prophylaxis for rheumatic fever but reduces the incidence of acute nephritis by only about 50 per cent. Patients who are allergic to penicillin can be treated successfully with oral erythromycin (50 mg/kg/day). Tetracyclines should not be used because some group A streptococci are resistant to them.

Most of the questions about treatment of streptococcal pharyngitis and pyoderma are related to identifying subclinical infection, differentiating true infection from the carrier state, and defining the risk of rheumatic fever and acute nephritis. Scarlet fever and suppurative complications should be treated with adequate doses of penicillin.

PROPHYLAXIS. In developed countries with a moderate or cold climate, most patients with (mild) pharyngitis and tonsillitis do not consult the doctor and hence cannot be protected from the complications of streptococcal infection. However, the risk of contracting rheumatic fever or acute nephritis is low in these countries under nonepidemic conditions.

In general, penicillin should be given to patients with suspected streptococcal infection, especially if there is a history of rheumatic fever, chorea, or acute glomerulonephritis. If a throat culture can be obtained, it is justified to await the results of the culture before instituting antibiotic therapy. Sequelae can be prevented even if treatment is delayed for one week.

In epidemic situations, contacts of patients with scarlet fever, rheumatic fever, or acute nephritis should be treated with penicillin. In closed communities, such as boarding schools, outbreaks of streptococcal infections should be aborted by the administration of benzathine penicillin to the entire community. Immunization against group A streptococci is not yet possible.

Recurrent attacks of rheumatic fever can be prevented successfully by monthly injections of benzathine penicillin in a dose of 1.2 million units. This prophylaxis should be continued as long as contacts with streptococcal reservoirs are likely to occur. Prophylaxis for recurrences of acute nephritis is less successful, probably because of differences in the pathogenesis of this (auto)immunologic disease.

References

Franz, K. H., Muller, A. S., Rienmeijer, B. J., Bynum, G., and Nolan, G.: Results of Dick and Schick tests in Liberian children. Trans R Soc Trop Med Hyg 58:68, 1964.

Haverkorn, M. J., Valkenburg, H. A., and Goslings, W. R. O.: Streptococcal pharyngitis in the general population. I. A controlled study of streptococcal pharyngitis and its complications in the Netherlands. J Infect Dis 124:339, 1971.

Holmes, M. C., and Williams, R. E. O.: Streptococcal infections among children in a residential home. I. Introduction and definitions; the incidence of infection. J Hyg 56:43, 1958.

Matanoski, G. M.: The role of the tonsils in streptococcal infections: A comparison of tonsillectomized children and sibling controls. Am J Epidemiol 95:278, 1972.

Maxted, W. R., and Potter, E. V.: The presence of Type 12 M-protein antigen in Group G streptococci. J Gen Microbiol 49:119, 1967.

Moffet, H. L., Siegel, A. C., and Doyle, H. K.: Nonstreptococcal pharyngitis. J Pediat 73:51, 1968.

Stollerman, M., and Bernstein, S. H.: Streptococcal pharyngitis: Evaluation of clinical syndromes in diagnosis. Am J Dis Child 101:476, 1961.

Strasser, T.: Rheumatic fever and rheumatic heart disease in the 1970s. WHO Chronicle 32:18, 1978.

Valkenburg, H. A., Goslings, W. R. O., Bots, A. W., De Moor, C. E., and Lorrier, J. C.: Attack rate of streptococcal pharyngitis, rheumatic fever and glomerulonephritis in the general population. II. The epidemiology of streptococcal pharyngitis in one village during a two-year period. N Engl J Med 268:694, 1963.

Valkenburg, H. A., Haverkorn, M. J., Goslings, W. R. O., Lorrier, J. C., De Moor, C. E., and Maxted, W. R.: Streptococcal pharyngitis in the general population. II. The attack rate of rheumatic fever and acute glomerulonephritis in patients not treated with penicillin. J. Infect Dis 124:348, 1971.

96
DIPHTHERIA

Richard V. McCloskey, M.S., M.D.

Diphtheria is an acute communicable disease caused by *C. diphtheriae,* which infects the upper respiratory tract and skin. The cardinal signs and symptoms are a membrane in the pharynx, sore throat, fever, nausea, vomiting, headache, and chills. Death results from respiratory obstruction or myocarditis. Myocarditis is caused by an exotoxin elaborated only by strains of *C. diphtheriae* lysogenic for specific bacteriophages (Barksdale and Arden, 1974; Groman, 1955).

EPIDEMIOLOGY AND GEOGRAPHIC VARIATIONS. Modern epidemics of diphtheria disrupt community life in every respect. Morbidity and death from diphtheria may exhaust the community's medical resources and disorganize its facilities for delivering health care. Intimate contact with infected persons is required for the spread of diphtheria, usually by way of infected droplets or nasopharyngeal secretions. Infective skin exudate is also involved in man-to-man spread. Transmission may also occur by way of animals, fomites, or milk. Carriers are persons harboring a toxinogenic strain of *C. diphtheriae* in the nasopharynx or skin. If the carrier remains asymptomatic he can be detected only by culture of the nasopharynx or skin. Attention is often directed toward these persons when their close associates, siblings, or marital partners develop diphtheria. A carrier state may exist for several days before onset of symptoms. A convalescent carrier state occurs after symptoms subside. The duration of a convalescent carrier state is greatly shortened by treatment of diphtheria with penicillin or erythromycin. These carriers constitute the reservoir from which the disease spreads to susceptible patients. Recent surveys of diphtheria carriers show that 88 per cent have completed or partially completed a course of diphtheria immunization.

In developing countries, for example, India, the highest death rate occurs in infancy and between 5 and 14 years of age (Udani et al., 1975). Tonsillar and pharyngeal localizations are the most common presentations of diphtheria in India, the United States, Canada, Iran, and Gambia (Heyworth et al., 1973; Zamiri et al., 1972). The disease may be more often manifest on the skin in tropical and subtropical areas than in the respiratory tract. It has been suggested that skin infections are important in maintaining endemicity of *C. diphtheriae* infections in tropical and subtropical areas. Skin infections, because of greater contagiousness, result in higher environmental carrier levels of *C. diphtheriae* than respiratory tract diphtheria (Koopman and Campbell, 1975; Belsey and Le Blanc, 1975). As the incidence of skin infections increases, so do the reservoir, acquisition, and transmission of *C. diphtheriae.* Such mechanisms have been thought to be important in instituting respiratory tract diphtheria in tropical and, more recently, in temperate climates (Belsey, 1969; Zalma et al., 1970).

Diphtheria affects mainly poor persons living under crowded conditions and having poor access to health care (Heath and Zusman, 1962; McLeod, 1950). The tragedy of such outbreaks is that morbidity and mortality are highest in children under 14 years. In the United States, attack rates are highest in blacks and Mexican Americans between 5 and 14 years old (Brooks, 1969). Attack rates among unimmunized household members and contacts are higher than in fully immunized persons. More people develop diphtheria when susceptible children congregate in schools and households. In the past decade, diphtheria in the United States has been a disease of urban populations rather than of rural populations.

Epidemiologists use several techniques to classify toxin-producing *C. diphtheriae* in order to identify the epidemic strain and disrupt its method of spread. Three types, *mitis, intermedius,* and *gravis,* are identified by colony morphology and biochemical properties (McLeod, 1943). This classification does not necessarily imply that disease caused by an *intermedius* strain is invariably less severe than that produced by a *gravis* strain. *Mitis* strains, however, have produced less severe disease than the other two biotypes.

Gravis types have produced epidemics in unimmunized persons previously experiencing disease due to *mitis* or *intermedius* strains. Well-immunized populations more often experience disease caused by *mitis* types. Each type can cause epidemic diphtheria.

C. diphtheriae strains can also be classified by patterns of bacteriophage lysis into at least 35 types (Saragea and Maximescu, 1966). Each bacteriophage type is stable and specific. This powerful epidemiologic tool has revealed that a particular lysotype may persist in the throats of healthy carriers for years and that in a given geographical area a single lysotype may be obtained from both patients and asymptomatic carriers. Some bacteriophage types are confined to or more frequently found in certain countries, suggesting that the lysotyping scheme may reflect the adaptability of *C. diphtheriae* to selected populations. The ease with which a strain of *C. diphtheriae* can be induced to liberate the identifying bacteriophage virus into the surrounding medium (lysogenicity) may be directly correlated with high toxin production and high capacity to spread among a population.

Recent urban epidemics of diphtheria in the United States have been difficult to control, even though hundreds of thousands of persons completed diphtheria immunization. Immunization with diphtheria toxoid of susceptible persons must be combined with a program that identifies carriers of diphtheria and terminates the carrier state by antibiotic treatment. Quarantine is not effective in an open urban society.

ETIOLOGY. The only cause of diphtheria is *C. diphtheriae*, a gram-positive bacillus that is pleomorphic, unencapsulated, and nonmotile. Smears prepared with differential stains (Albert's stain) may reveal metachromatic granules. The organism may be arranged in palisades, L or V forms, or in groups resembling "Chinese characters" when examined in stained preparations. Growth is aerobic on ordinary media, although media containing potassium tellurite, or coagulated serum (Loeffler's medium) promote growth. Colonies of *Corynebacterium* species (as well as streptococci and staphylococci) growing on tellurite-containing media develop a grayish black color. *C. diphtheriae* characteristically produces both a brown-gray halo and a garlic odor when growing on Tinsdale's agar. *C. diphtheriae* cohabitates the mucous membranes of man with other morphologically similar saprophytic diphtheroids from which it must be distinguished (see Chapter 25).

Myocarditis and neuritis are caused by the toxin elaborated by *C. diphtheriae* and absorbed by the infected patient. The toxin is an acidic globular protein with a molecular weight of 62,000 to 63,000 (Gill and Pappenheimer, 1973). It is characterized by extreme potency, a cellular site of activity, and a latent period before inhibition of cellular protein synthesis is manifest. Strains of *C. diphtheriae* infected by a lysogenic bacteriophage produce the toxin in the presence of a critical concentration range of iron in the surrounding medium. Protein synthesis by host cells is terminated by a unique chain of events (Bowman, 1970; Collier, 1967; and Gill et al., 1973) described in Chapter 5. Nontoxinogenic *C. diphtheriae* elaborates a physicochemically similar but immunochemically dissimilar and biologically innocuous protein. Therefore, identification of toxin production in vitro by *C. diphtheriae* (toxinogenicity) is of paramount importance. This is usually accomplished by demonstrating immunoprecipitation lines produced by a strain of *C. diphtheriae* growing on agar upon which is placed a filter paper strip containing a diluted, highly purified diphtheria antitoxin (Elek's test) (see Chapter 25). Spreading factor (substance B or hyaluronidase) (O'Meara et al., 1947) contributes to local edema, necrosis, and hemorrhage. It was produced by essentially all *C. diphtheriae* organisms isolated from clinical infections in Ireland during 1947 and may be of importance in producing "hypertoxic" diphtheria (see below) and diphtheria occurring among immunized persons. Other biologically active extracellular products of *C. diphtheriae* play some role in the production of diphtheria because nontoxinogenic *C. diphtheriae* may cause clinical diphtheria, although milder than that produced by toxinogenic organisms.

SYMPTOMS AND CLINICAL MANIFESTATIONS. Diphtheria may be symptomless or a rapidly fatal hypertoxic disease that devastates the heart and lungs (McCloskey et al., 1969). The primary determinants of diphtheria are the patients' immunity toward diphtheria toxin, the virulence and toxinogenicity of the infecting strain of *C. diphtheriae*, and the anatomic location of the infection (Edward and Allison, 1951). Additional characteristics that may influence the symptoms elicited are age, co-existing systemic disease, and pre-existing local nasopharyngeal disease. The incubation period is usually two to six days. Most patients, excluding those with the mildest of nasal or skin infections, present to the physician after several days of systemic illness. The speed of onset is variable. Some authors describe an abrupt onset. More often there is no dramatic deterioration in health. Younger patients may be desperately ill in the face of deceptively modest malaise and fatigue. The temperature gradually rises, seldom exceeding 102°F except in those most severely ill. Children are less likely than adults to complain of sore throat, which at any age is not usually the initial complaint. Other signs and symptoms depend on the extent of the local diphtheritic lesion.

Anterior Nasal Diphtheria. These patients may be minimally inconvenienced while producing a thick mucopurulent nasal discharge which may irritate the external nares and upper lips. A creamy yellowish membrane, with or without crusting, may be seen in the nose. Severe intoxication from nasal diphtheria is not common.

Tonsillar (Faucial) Diphtheria. The membrane begins as a glary thin mucilaginous structure on one or both tonsils. It is not confined to tonsillar crypts. By the time medical advice is sought, usually there is a characteristic graying green color of some area of the membrane. The membrane, which is several millimeters thick, may be difficult to dislodge with a swab and often leaves a bleeding surface on the tonsil when torn off (Fig. 1). Sometimes the membrane crosses anatomic borders and may spill over the anterior pillar of the tonsil, which is often enlarged. The five most common complaints during an outbreak in Texas were sore throat (85 per cent), pain on swallowing (23 per cent), nausea and vomiting (25 per cent), and headache (18 per cent) (McCloskey et al., 1971). The most common sign was fever (85 per cent). Moderately tender lymph nodes 1 to 2 cm in diameter can usually be palpated in the anterior triangle of the neck.

Pharyngeal Diphtheria. Outside the palatine tonsil the membrane spreads to the uvula, the soft palate, and the pharyngeal wall. The marked swelling of the tonsils at this

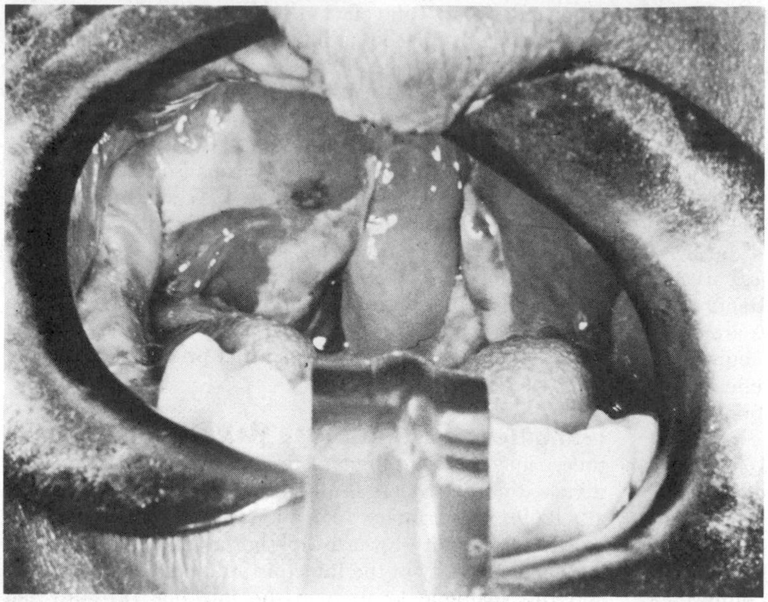

Figure 1. Pharynx of a 39-year-old woman with bacteriologically confirmed diphtheria. Photograph taken four days after the onset of fever, malaise, and sore throat. Hemorrhage is apparent in one area where membrane was removed by swabbing.

point often obscures large areas of membrane on the posterior aspect of the tonsil. The nasal mucosa may be involved and may bleed profusely. The greenish character of the membrane is more prominent. There may be necrotic black patches in older areas of the membrane. The so-called diphtheritic fetor is of little diagnostic value because it is also observed in infectious mononucleosis and Vincent's infection. A hot tender edema (bull neck) of the anterior part of the neck may obscure the angle of the jaw, the border of the sternocleidomastoid muscle, the clavicle, and enlarged lymph nodes, which become more prominent as the edema subsides. The child with pharyngeal diphtheria is pathetically weak, limp, unresisting, pale, and exhausted. Bleeding from the upper airway is a grave prognostic sign.

Laryngeal and Bronchial Diphtheria. The membrane may extend downward or involve the larynx exclusively and cause hoarseness, inspiratory and expiratory stridor, dyspnea, and cyanosis (Dobie and Tobey, 1979). The accessory muscles of respiration are used. Casts of the major bronchi can be formed by the membrane (Fig. 2). If not removed by bronchoscopy, this membrane may cause death by hypoxia.

DIFFERENTIAL DIAGNOSIS. The diagnosis must rest on clinical grounds alone, since treatment cannot await bacteriologic confirmation. Diphtheria must be considered whenever a membrane is present in the throat, especially if the uvula is involved. In infectious mononucleosis the membrane is confined to the tonsils and remains creamy white without necrotic patches for a longer time than the diphtheritic membrane. Streptococcal pharyngitis causes fiery redness of the throat and white exudate. Severe throat pain and faucial distortion are not seen in uncomplicated diphtheria. The foul necrotic exudate complicating leukemia may be impossible to distinguish from diphtheria. Vincent's angina may involve the gums and is identified by Gram's stain of the exudate. Simultaneous infection with streptococci (32 per cent in a recent outbreak) does not alter the physical findings suggestive of diphtheria. The laboratory findings in diphtheria are nonspecific and include moderate leukocytosis, and transient albuminuria.

PROGNOSIS AND COMPLICATIONS. The outcome depends on (1) the location and extent of the membrane; (2) amount of toxin absorbed; and (3) patient's immunity status. Myocarditis and cardiac arrhythmia may be seen from the

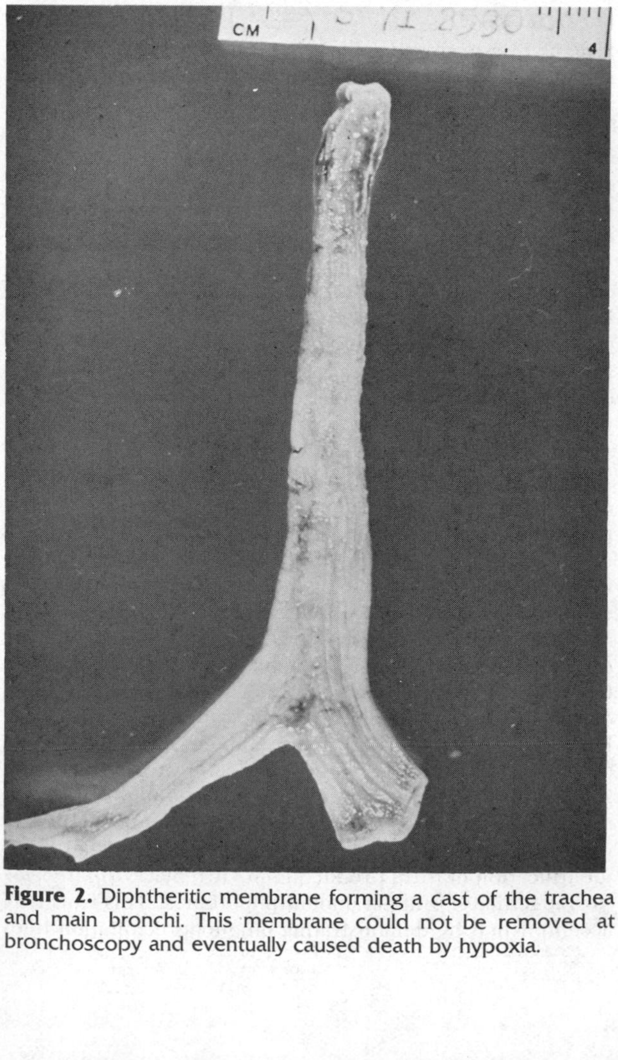

Figure 2. Diphtheritic membrane forming a cast of the trachea and main bronchi. This membrane could not be removed at bronchoscopy and eventually caused death by hypoxia.

second to the sixth week. ST-T wave changes and abnormalities occur in 40 per cent of the electrocardiograms but are not always accompanied by signs of congestive heart failure.

Myocarditis. There is a correlation between delayed conduction velocity of the median, ulnar, and common peroneal nerves and myocardial conduction system disturbances (Burkhardt et al., 1938; Kazemi et al., 1973). Moreover, the delayed peripheral nerve conduction velocity precedes clinical evidence of myocarditis and myocardial conduction system abnormalities. The determination of peripheral nerve conduction delay may be used to predict the appearance of myocarditis and cardiac arrhythmias.

Most of the electrocardiographic abnormalities appear during the first week of illness. ST-T wave changes that are destined to improve usually do so within 10 days of appearance of the abnormalities. The severity of the illness and the toxemia are roughly related to the severity of EKG abnormalities and acute circulatory failure. Acute circulatory failure is practically never seen with nasal diphtheria but may occur in 9 per cent of patients with pharyngeal-laryngeal infection, largely as a consequence of the greater amount of toxin that is produced by the more extensive deeper respiratory infections. Acute circulatory failure appears with a sudden onset of pallor, hypotension, collapsed peripheral pulses, and profuse perspiration. The EKG in acute failure may be normal. Muffled heart sounds, murmurs, embryocardia, pulse rate, and pulse pressure are not always associated with well-defined electrocardiographic abnormalities.

Nevertheless, diphtheria with ST-T wave changes has a significantly higher mortality rate (28 per cent) than diphtheria without EKG changes (6 to 10 per cent). Serial tests of serum glutamic oxalacetic transaminase (SGOT) levels will identify most patients with myocarditis (Naiditch and Bower, 1954).

Early identification of diphtheritic myocarditis is important in reducing morbidity and mortality. Since clinical examination of the heart is not reliable for diagnosis of myocarditis, patients with EKG abnormalities during diphtheria should be monitored in specialized units equipped with all support facilities, which can offer effective treatment of the more serious arrhythmias and conduction disturbances that may occur. Atrioventricular (AV) block and left bundle branch block (LBBB) are ominous signs, associated with mortality of 60 to 100 per cent. Recent case reports have shown that electrical pacing with temporary transvenous pacing electrodes or myocardial demand pacemakers can resolve AV block and LBBB produced by diphtheritic myocarditis (Matisonn et al., 1972). Treatment regimens usually include salt restriction, careful fluid balance, and short-acting digitalis preparations if congestive heart failure is marked. Antiarrhythmic agents, such as procaine amide, lidocaine, and isoproterenol are used when indicated to suppress or control specific arrhythmias. High doses of adrenal steroids are often given with the aim of reducing edema and fibrosis of the myocardium or conducting system, but there is no firm evidence that steroids accomplish these objectives.

Since myocarditis represents severe intoxication, the physician should expect other toxic manifestations. Intensive nursing care may be needed to support respiration and to prevent permanent complications of peripheral neuritis. Thrombocytopenia also occurs in malignant diphtheria. Active platelet destruction may complicate the myocarditis and warrant platelet transfusions.

A rare cardiac complication of diphtheria is infective endocarditis due to *C. diphtheriae* (Davidson et al., 1976). Blood cultures may contain toxinogenic or nontoxinogenic *C. diphtheriae*. The infection can be established on normal or previously deformed valves. This unusual complication may occur in the absence of clinical diphtheria when signs of endocarditis are present. The reported mortality rate is 70 per cent.

Patients with hypertoxic diphtheria may develop peripheral circulatory failure, hypotension, thrombocytopenia, and skin hemorrhages in the first week (Fisher and Cobb, 1948). They usually die with evidence of bleeding into the vascular endothelium, tracheobronchial mucosa, and adrenals. Palatal paralysis, the most common and often the only paralysis, appears in the third week, often after myocarditis. Paralysis of respiratory muscles, pharynx, and larynx appears six to eight weeks after onset. There may be a deceptively symptom-free interval before the patient is unable to swallow and develops aspiration pneumonia. Late-appearing tachycardias may cause death at this time. A Guillain-Barré-like peripheral neuritis may also appear as a late complication.

TREATMENT AND PREVENTION. A patient with tonsillar or nasopharyngeal diphtheria requires isolation in the hospital at bed rest for 10 to 14 days. The early use of adequate amounts of diphtheria antitoxin (DAT) remains the most important specific mode of treatment. Every patient with diphtheria merits DAT therapy, even a week or more after the onset. Since DAT is composed of horse serum, intradermal and/or conjunctival tests should be performed before administration. If either is positive, desensitization is justifiable even though it is time-consuming and hazardous because DAT is the only specific treatment available. DAT prepared from human serum would obviate some of these problems. The dose of DAT need not be complicated. If the membrane does not extend beyond the tonsil it may be treated by intramuscular administration of 20,000 units if there is no thrombocytopenia. More extensive membrane requires 80,000 to 100,000 units, preferably intravenously. The minimum amount of DAT necessary to prevent complications is unknown. Penicillin or erythromycin is used to eliminate the organism from the upper respiratory tract and to terminate the carrier state. If the patient cannot swallow, treatment with parenteral penicillin produces less pain upon injection than does parenteral erythromycin. Tetracycline, rifampin, clindamycin, and ampicillin are effective in vitro against *C. diphtheriae* but cephalexin, oxacillin, and lincomycin are not. Both benzathine penicillin and erythromycin therapy can terminate the carrier state (McCloskey et al., 1974). Myocarditis, congestive failure, and arrhythmias require intensive cardiac care and strict bed rest. Cardiac pacemakers can control arrhythmia. Unless congestive heart failure appears, digitalization is unnecessary. Airway obstruction requires tracheostomy. Bronchoscopy may be performed to remove membrane from the larger bronchi.

The complications of diphtheria can be prevented by active immunization beginning in childhood, with booster immunizations every 10 years thereafter. Active immunization and early treatment of carriers are both necessary for control of the disease. Immunization with DPT (diphtheria-pertussis-tetanus vaccine) should be administered to infants at 6 weeks of age. Three 0.5-ml injections of DPT are given at monthly intervals, with a booster dose of 0.5 ml at 6 months or 1 year. Children who have received this primary series should receive a booster dose before entering school. For older children, primary immunization may be accomplished by two doses of pediatric diphtheria-tetanus (DT) vaccine of 0.5 ml each, six weeks apart with a booster dose six months to one year later. Persons over 12 years should be primarily immunized on the same schedule, but adult-type diphtheria-tetanus vaccine (dT) should be used. Schick tests are unnecessary before adult immunizations. Persons who are heavily exposed (physicians, nurses, hospital workers) to diphtheria should receive a booster 0.5 ml dose of dT every five years (McCloskey, 1969). All others should receive 0.5 ml of dT at 10-year intervals. Exposure to a suspected case dictates administration of a 0.5 ml dT booster dose to those exposed who have been immunized previously but have not had booster immunization within 10 years.

References

Altshuler, S. S., Hoffman, K. M., and Fitzgerald, P. J.: Electrocardiographic changes in diphtheria. Am J Med 29:294, 1948.

Barksdale, L., and Arden, S. B.: Persisting bacteriophage infections, lysogeny, and phage conversions. Ann Rev Microbiol 28:265, 1974.

Belsey, M. A.: *Corynebacterium diphtheriae* skin infections in Alabama and Louisiana. A factor in the epidemiology of diphtheria. N Engl J Med 280:135, 1969.

Belsey, M. A., and LeBlanc, D. R.: Skin infections and the epidemiology of diphtheria. Am J Epidemiol 102:179, 1975.

Bonventre, P. F.: Diphtheria Microbiology, 1975. Washington, D.C., American Society of Microbiology. 1975, pp. 272–277.

Bowman, G. C.: Studies on the mode of action of diphtheria toxin III. Effect on subcellular components of protein synthesis from the tissues of intoxicated guinea pigs and rats. J Exp Med 131:659, 1970.

Brooks, G. F.: Recent trends in diphtheria in the United States. J Infect Dis 120:500, 1969.

Burkhardt, E. A., Eggleston, C., and Smith, L. W.: Electrocardiographic changes and peripheral nerve palsies in toxic diphtheria. Am J Med Sci 195:301, 1938.

Collier, R. J.: Diphtheria toxin: Mode of action and structure. Bacteriol Rev 39:54, 1975.

Davidson, S., Rotem, Y., Bozkowski, B., and Rubenstein, E.: *Corynebacterium diphtheriae* endocarditis. Am J Med Sci 271:351, 1976.

Dobie, R. A., and Tobey, D. N.: Clinical features of diphtheria in the respiratory tract. JAMA 242:219, 1979.

Edward, D. G., and Allison, V. D.: Diphtheria in the immunized with observations on diphtheria-like disease associated with nontoxinogenic strains of *Corynebacterium diphtheriae.* J Hyg 49:205, 1951.

Gill, D. M., Pappenheimer, A. M., Jr., and Uchida, T.: Diphtheria toxin protein synthesis and the cell. Fed Proc 32:1508, 1973.

Groman, N. B.: Evidence for the active role of bacteriophage in the conversion of nontoxinogenic *Corynebacterium diphtheriae* to toxin production. J Bacteriol 69:9, 1955.

Heath, C. W., and Zusman, J.: An outbreak of diphtheria among skid-row men. N Engl J Med 267:809, 1962.

Heyworth, B., and Ropp, M.: Diphtheria in the Gambia. J Trop Med Hyg 76:61, 1973.

Kazemi, B., Tahernia, A. C., and Zandian, K.: Motor nerve conduction in diphtheria and diphtheritic myocarditis. Arch Neurol 29:104, 1973.

Koopman, J. S., and Campbell, J.: The role of cutaneous diphtheria infections in a diphtheria epidemic. J Infect Dis 131:239, 1975.

Matisonn, R. E., Mitha, A. S., and Chesler, E.: Successful electrical pacing for complete heart block complicating diphtheritic myocarditis. Br Heart J 38:423, 1976.

McCloskey, R. V.: Diphtheria antitoxin titers in hospital workers after a single dose of adult type diphtheria tetanus toxoid. Am J Med Sci 258:209, 1969.

McCloskey, R. V., Eller, J. J., Green, M., Mauney, C. U., and Richards, S. E. M.: The 1970 epidemic of diphtheria in San Antonio. Ann Intern Med 75:495, 1971.

McCloskey, R. V., Green, M. J., Eller, J., and Smilack, J.: Treatment of diphtheria carriers: Benzathine penicillin, erythromycin, and clindamycin. Ann Intern Med 81:788, 1974.

McLeod, J. W.: The types mitis, intermedius, and gravis of *Corynebacterium diphtheriae.* Bacteriol Rev 7:1, 1943.

McLeod, J. W.: A survey of the epidemiology of diphtheria in northwest Europe and North America in the period of 1920–1946. J Pathol Bacteriol 62:137, 1950.

Moffat, R. C.: Diphtheritic heart block. Angiology 10:609, 1972.

O'Meara, R. A. Q., Baker, R. S. W., and Balch, H. H.: Production of substance B by *Corynebacterium diphtheriae.* Lancet 1:212, 1947.

Saragea, A., and Maximescu, P.: Phage typing of *Corynebacterium diphtheriae.* Bull WHO 35:681, 1966.

Tahernia, A. C.: Electrocardiographic abnormalities and serum transaminase levels in diphtheritic myocarditis. J Pediatr 75:1008, 1969.

Udani, P. M., and Kumbhat, M. M., Bhat, U. S., Nadkarni, M. S., Bhave, S. K., Ezuthachan, S. G., and Kamath, B.: Diphtheria. Some epidemiological observations in Bombay: A clinical and bacteriological study of 320 and autopsy study of 5 children. Prog Drug Res 19:423, 1975.

Zalma, V. M., Older, J. J., and Brooks, G. F.: The Austin, Texas diphtheria outbreak. Clinical and epidemiological aspects. JAMA 211:2125, 1970.

Zamiri, I., McEntegart, M. G., and Saragea, A.: Diphtheria in Iran. J Hyg (Camb) 70:619, 1972.

97

VINCENT'S INFECTION

LYNN A. LANCASTER, M.D.

HOWARD ROBERT ATTEBERY, D.D.S.

Acute necrotizing ulcerative gingivitis (ANUG) is an ulcerative necrosis of the interdental papillae and the marginal gingivae. The acute stage is characterized by sudden onset and severe pain. The chronic form shows interproximal destruction of the periodontal tissues with alveolar bone loss.

The term ANUG is restricted to disease of the gingivae. If the disease spreads to other oral structures the term acute necrotizing ulcerative mucositis (ANUM) or Vincent's stomatitis is used. Vincent's angina is acute pseudomembranous involvement of the pharynx or tonsils. ANUG, ANUM, and Vincent's angina are all classified as Vincent's disease or Vincent's infection. ANUG is also known as trench mouth, Plaut-Vincent's infection, fusospirochetosis, and ulceromembranous gingivitis.

ETIOLOGY. The etiology is unknown. One or more predisposing factors and a limited number of oral bacteria, commonly referred to as the fusospirochetal complex, seem to be needed to cause the disease. Poor oral hygiene, local irritation from food impaction or poor dental restoration, excessive smoking, erupting teeth, and third molar tissue flaps are important local factors. Malnutrition, fatigue, emotional or physical stress, endocrine dysfunctions, and metabolic disturbances are among the predisposing systemic factors. Depressed polymorphonuclear leukocyte phagocytosis and chemotaxis have been reported in otherwise healthy individuals with ANUG (Cogen et al., 1983). Since the lesions of ANUG always contain a predominantly gram-negative fusospirochetal complex, and since the disease is rapidly brought under control with antibiotics, the consensus reigns that the disease is bacterial. However, it is not clear whether the bacteria initiate the disease or are secondary invaders. No single organism or combination of organisms has yet proved to be the causative factor. The fusiform most often identified from the necrotic material is *Fusobacterium nucleatum*, an anaerobic member of the normal oral flora.

PATHOGENESIS AND PATHOLOGY. Evidence for involvement of fusobacteria and spirochetes comes from microscopic examination of plaque from lesions and from pathologic studies of the diseased sites. Electron microscopic studies show that ANUG lesions have four distinct strata all occupied by spirochetes. Spirochete invasion of normal tissue occurs below the necrotic zone (Listgarten, 1965; Heylings, 1967). These spirochetes have not been cultured. Listgarten (1967) also showed by electron microscopy that necrotic areas form around these large spirochetes.

Attempts to culture the diseased sites using modern anaerobic techniques have been limited. Loesche and colleagues (1982) cultured 22 ulcerated areas in eight patients and examined plaque samples microscopically. A constant flora composed of *Bacteroides melaninogenicus* ssp. *intermedius* and *Fusobacterium* sp. was isolated from all patients. A variable flora composed of a heterogeneous collection of species was also present. Spirochetes and spirilla-like organisms identified as *Selemonas* were the dominant organisms in the accompanying smears. Successful therapy with metronidazole, reduced the number of spirochetes, *B. melaninogenicus* ssp *intermedius*, and *Fusobacterium* sp. in plaque samples. The numbers of these bacteria remained low for at least two to three months. Such studies suggest that these organisms contribute to the disease process but do not prove that they initiate the condition.

Necrotizing ulcerative gingivitis has been studied in beagle dogs. The disease occurs naturally in these animals and is similar to that of humans. Microscopic examination of plaque from diseased and disease-free sites reveals the same predominance of spirochetes. Mikx and van Campen (1982 and 1982a) induced NUG by application of debris from lesions of diseased dogs to the gingiva of healthy beagles pre-treated with systemic glucocorticoids. The lesions contained more spirochetes and fewer fusobacteria compared with samples of plaque from controls. In addition, a spirillum type A was present in the lesions of inoculated dogs but rarely found in controls. The organism, which resembles a spirochete, has bipolar lophotrichous flagella. Isolation and further characterization of the organism has not been reported. Mikx and van Campen's demonstration of transmissibility in animals, although preliminary, may stimulate re-examination of the widely held belief that the human disease is not transmissible.

Since a large number of gram-negative bacteria are present in the ANUG lesion, endotoxin may be involved in this inflammatory disease. One investigation of biopsies failed to demonstrate immune complexes (Dolby, 1972).

Kardachi and Clark in 1974 postulated that the disease starts as an aseptic necrosis secondary to capillary stasis, due largely to stress, smoking, and poor oral hygiene. Stress and smoking stimulate epinephrine and norepinephrine release. Nicotine and epinephrine infusions reduce gingival arterial flow in rabbits (Clarke et al., 1981). Poor oral hygiene might also contribute to stasis by the release of bacterial products from the accumulating dental plaque.

CLINICAL MANIFESTATIONS. The disease may begin suddenly with gingival bleeding, fetid odor, and pain. These symptoms are accompanied by necrosis of interproximal papillae, pseudomembranes, lymphadenopathy, and excess salivation. The incidence of gingival bleeding is 96 per cent, pain 86 per cent, and fetid odor 84 per cent (Barnes, Bowles, and Carter, 1973). Patients often complain of a metallic taste and loss of the tactile sense in their teeth. Fever, anorexia, and other gastrointestinal symptoms may also occur.

COMPLICATIONS AND SEQUELAE FROM ANUG. The disease may spread to other mucosae from the gingivae to cause stomatitis and tonsillitis or gangrenous stomatitis or angina. The most serious oral complication is noma. Noma usually begins in the corner of the mouth or cheek and rapidly involves the entire thickness of the lips and cheeks, with conspicuous necrosis and complete sloughing of tissue. The disease may also spread to the lungs and produce pulmonary fusospirochetosis. Transient bacteremia or septicemia may occur from the mass of bacteria at bleeding sites. Meningitis has been reported after Vincent's disease. Genital fusospirochetosis may occur after contact with infected saliva (Von Hamm, 1938). Oral surgical procedures or any other gingival manipulation should be postponed until the disease has subsided.

GEOGRAPHIC VARIATIONS IN THE DISEASE. ANUG afflicts adolescents and adults throughout the world. Few data are available on comparative prevalences for vast areas of the world. Vincent's disease is severe in populations in which protein and calorie malnutrition is common in children (Russell, 1967).

ANUG is rarely seen in children in the United States, Canada, or Europe, but is common in children in other parts of the world (Jiminez, 1969). Affected children are usually from the lower socioeconomic groups who suffer from lack of protein. In Nigerian villages ANUG and noma occurs in children as young as three or four years (Emslie, 1963; Sheiham, 1965).

DIAGNOSIS. A gingival disease with sudden onset accompanied by pain, blunted papillae, and fetid odor is ANUG. Herpetic gingivitis does not start at the papillae and there is no fetid odor. Lymphadenopathy appears before the oral lesions of herpes and after the lesions of ANUG.

ANUG will not be confused with secondary syphilis of the mouth if the characteristics described above are kept in mind. The oral lesions of leukemia, infectious mononucleosis, granulocytopenia, and other blood dyscrasias may be a diagnostic problem and require blood counts and smears for differentiation.

It was once a common procedure to stain a smear of the oral lesion with 2 per cent methyl violet or with carbol fuchsin for microscopic examination; large numbers of fusiform bacteria and spirochetes were characteristic of Vincent's disease. The clinical symptoms are so widely appreciated today that microscopic examinations are seldom used to confirm the clinical picture. Furthermore, a positive smear without the clinical picture is meaningless because fusobacteria and spirochetes are present in every mouth.

TREATMENT. Antibiotics should be used for severe infections. Procaine penicillin, 600,000 units, is given intramuscularly twice daily for three to seven days. Metronidazole is given orally, 200 mg, three times daily for three to seven days. The alternate drug of choice is tetracycline, given orally 250 mg every four hours (Braude, 1976).

Oral rinses of a 3 per cent hydrogen peroxide solution diluted 1 part to 3 parts of water should be used at least every two hours while awake. If possible the diet should be rich in protein and calories and contain soft or liquid nonirritating foods. Three days after starting treatment, when the mouth is comfortable, the dentist can debride the lesions, curette, do minor scaling, and clean the teeth. Instructions should now be given on oral hygiene procedures so that the patient can institute an effective home treatment program. In addition, a list of predisposing factors should be discussed with a view to removing or avoiding them. When the necrotizing ulcerative gingivitis has subsided and the gingivae have stabilized, a dentist should be consulted to determine if a recontouring surgical procedure is needed.

ANUG tends to recur if treatment and oral hygiene are stopped and if predisposing factors are neglected. If severe ANUG does not improve rapidly with treatment the possibility of a blood dyscrasia should be investigated. Successful treatment of ANUG in immunosuppressed children with hematopoietic malignancies may be difficult. Relapse and neutropenia are associated with poor responses (Ryan et al., 1983).

The treatment of ANUM is the same as for ANUG. However, for noma (gangrenous stomatitis) the antibiotic treatment should be prolonged, nutrition restored, and the underlying disease corrected (Uohara, 1967).

PROPHYLAXIS. ANUG is not proven or widely believed to be contagious. The high incidence of disease among individuals living in close proximity is thought to be due to a common environmental predisposing factor or factors. Many of the large outbreaks attributed to ANUG have actually been caused by herpetic gingivostomatitis.

To prevent either the initial encounter with ANUG or its recurrence, the predisposing factors have to be eliminated or diminished. The avoidance of stress, nicotine, and fatigue, good oral hygiene, and good nutritional practices are the major factors in the prevention of Vincent's infection.

References

Barnes, P. B., Bowles, W. F., III, and Carter, H. G.: Acute necrotizing ulcerative gingivitis: a survey of 218 cases. J Perio 44:35, 1973.

Braude, A. I.: Antimicrobial Drug Therapy. Philadelphia, W. B. Saunders Company, 1976.

Clarke, N. G., Shephard, B. C., and Hirsch, R. S.: The effects of intra-arterial epinephrine and nicotine on gingival circulation. Oral Surg 52:577, 1981.

Cogen, R. B., Stevens, A. W., Jr., Cohen-Cole, S., Kirk, K., and Freeman, A.: Leukocyte function in the etiology of acute necrotizing ulcerative gingivitis. J Perio 54:402, 1983.

Dolby, A. E.: Acute ulcerative gingivitis: Immune complex. J Dent Res 51:1639, 1972.

Emslie, R.: Cancrum oris. Dent Practit 13:481, 1963.

Heylings, R. T.: Electron microscopy of acute ulcerative gingivitis (Vincent's type) Br Dent J 122:51, 1967.

Jiminez, L. M., Ramos, J., Garrington, G., and Baer, P.: The familial occurrence of acute necrotizing gingivitis in children in Colombia, South America. J Perio 40:414, 1969.

Kardachi, B. J., and Clarke, N. G.: Aetiology of acute necrotising ulcerative gingivitis: a hypothetical explanation. J Perio 45:830, 1974.

Listgarten, M. A.: Electron microscopic observations on the bacterial flora of acute necrotizing ulcerative gingivitis. J Perio 36:328, 1965.

Listgarten, M. A., and Lewis, D. W.: The distribution of spirochetes in the lesion of acute necrotizing ulcerative gingivitis: An electron microscopic and statistical survey. J Perio 38:379, 1967.

Loesche, W. J., Syed, S. A., Laughon, B. E., and Stoll, J.: The bacteriology of acute necrotizing ulcerative gingivitis. J Perio 53:223, 1982.

Mikx, F. and van Campen, G. J.: Preliminary evaluation of the microflora in spontaneous and induced necrotizing ulcerative gingivitis in the beagle dog. J Peridontal Res 17:460, 1982.

Mikx, F., and van Campen, G. J.: Microscopical evaluation of the microflora in relation to necrotizing ulcerative gingivitis in the beagle dog. J Peridont Res 17:576, 1982a.

Russell, A. L.: Epidemiology of periodontal disease. Int Dent J 17:282, 1967.

Ryan, M. E., Hopkins, K., and Wilbur, R. B.: Acute necrotizing ulcerative gingivitis in children with cancer. Am J Dis Child 137:592, 1983.

Sheiham, A.: An epidemiological study of oral diseases in Nigerians. J. Dent Res 44:184, 1965.

Uohara, G. I., and Knapp, M. J.: Oral fusospirochetosis and associated lesions. Oral Surg Oral Med and Oral Path 24:113, 1967.

Von Hamm, E.: Venereal fuso-spirochetosis. Am J Trop Med 18:595, 1938.

98

PARANASAL SINUSITIS

PAUL B. VAN CAUWENBERGE, M.D.

Sinusitis is an inflammation of the mucous membranes of the paranasal sinus cavities. Acute sinusitis is less than 3 weeks' duration. Subacute sinusitis has a duration of 3 weeks to 3 months, and chronic sinusitis lasts longer than 3 months. This subdivision is important because of the different histopathology and consequently different treatment of acute, subacute, and chronic sinusitis.

ETIOLOGY. Sinusitis results from the spread of an infection in the surrounding tissues, e.g., nasal and dental infections, but especially from an obstruction of the ostium of the sinus. Closure or narrowing of the natural ostium impairs ventilation and causes transudation from the mucous membrane. Because of the obstructed ostium, fluid stagnates in the sinus and provides a rich bacterial culture medium.

In cases of dentogenous sinusitis, infection starts at the floor of the maxillary sinus and results from the spread or rupture of an apical abscess, a granuloma, or a dental cyst. This is the origin of an ascending inflammation of the mucosal lining. Infrequently, the ostium is completely closed by this type of infection.

A brief review of anatomy is necessary to understand the etiology and natural history of paranasal sinusitis. The nasal sinuses are cavities of varying sizes that develop from the nasal chambers. They consist of four paired structures: the maxillary, frontal, ethmoidal, and sphenoidal sinuses (Figs. 1 and 2). Only the maxillary and ethmoidal sinuses are present at birth, while the sphenoidal sinus is very small and the frontal sinus is absent at birth.

The ostia of the frontal, ethmoidal, and maxillary sinuses are situated at the lateral nasal wall, in the middle meatus. The sphenoidal ostium is found at the anterior wall of this sinus.

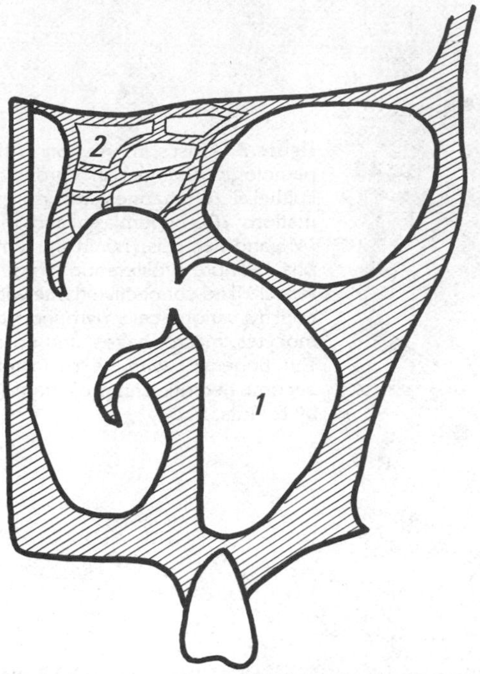

Figure 1. Diagram of a frontal cross-section of the skull, showing the left maxillary sinus *(1)* with its ostium and the ethmoidal cells *(2)*.

MICROBIOLOGY. Whereas the viral etiology of rhinitis is well documented (rhinoviruses, coronaviruses, RSV and others), the role of viruses in sinusitis is obscure except for the important role of parainfluenza virus type 3 (Saito et al. 1981). In most sinus secretions obtained by direct puncture, a rich bacterial flora is found. In acute sinusitis, the pneumococcus, *Hemophilus influenzae* and *Branhamella catarrhalis* are the most frequently involved bacteria. *Staphylococcus aureus* and *epidermidis* and *Streptococcus pyogenes* are less important. Gram-negative rods are almost never encountered in acute sinusitis (van Cauwenberge et al., 1976). Although we found anaerobes in 34 per cent of the secretions sampled in acute sinusitis (mainly Peptococcus and Veillonella), their pathogenic role is probably less important than in chronic sinusitis. In chronic sinusitis the bacteriological picture is different. Although the pneumococcus and *H. influenzae* are also the most frequently encountered aerobic bacteria, gram-negative rods like *Pseudomonas* and *Proteus* are only cultured occasionally. Most purulent heavily infected secretions have a heavy growth of bacteria, almost always including anaerobic bacteria. (Frederick and Braude, 1974; van Cauwenberge et al., 1977; Verschraegen and van Cauwenberge, 1982). These purulent cases usually contain anaerobic gram-negative rods (*Bacteriodes oralis* and *melaninogenicus, Fusobacterium* and less often *B. fragilis*) and sometimes anaerobic gram-positive cocci (especially *Peptostreptococcus* and *Peptococcus*). In view of the histopathologic changes in sinusitis, it is not surprising to find this high incidence of anaerobes. The decreased mucosal blood flow, the increased intrasinal pressure, the occasional angiitis and the presence of viscid secretions provoke a low oxygen tension and a low pH, providing the low oxidation–reduction potential that is necessary for anaerobic proliferation.

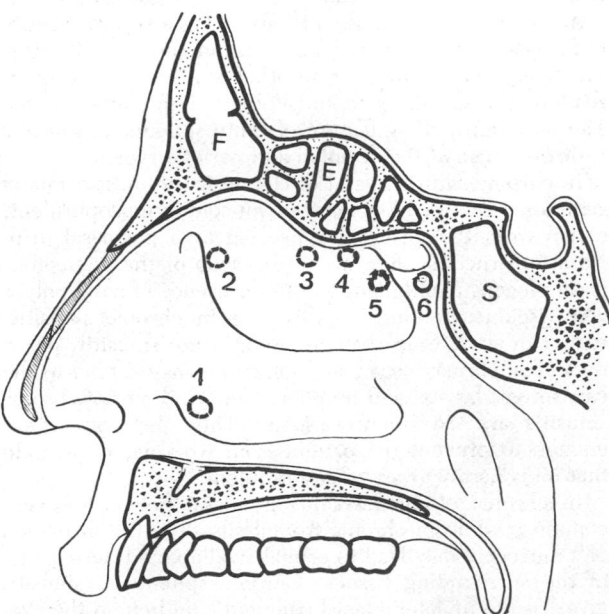

Figure 2. Diagram of a sagittal cross-section of the skull, showing the frontal *(F)*, ethmoidal *(E)*, and sphenoidal *(S)* sinuses with projection of their ostia: *(1)* distal end of the nasolacrimal duct, *(2)* frontal sinus ostium, *(3)* ostium of the anterior ethmoidal cells, *(4)* maxillary sinus ostium, *(5)* ostium of the posterior ethmoidal cells, and *(6)* sphenoidal sinus ostium. (Drawing by A. Derycke, M.D.)

Yeasts and molds are rarely reported as etiologic agents in sinusitis. Occasionally, aspergillosis and mucormycosis (see below) of the sinuses occur.

PREDISPOSING FACTORS. Any condition impairing ostial function and thus impairing ventilation of the sinus can give rise to sinusitis. The most important factors are septal deviation, a narrow bony sinus ostium, choanal atresia, cleft palate, nasal infection, allergic and vasomotor rhinopathy, benign and malignant tumors, adenoidal hypertrophy, and intranasal foreign bodies.

In systemic conditions such as cystic fibrosis, the production of abnormal sinus secretions facilitates bacterial growth. Immune deficiencies, such as hypo- or agammaglobulinemia and neutropenia, also promote sinusitis. In the immotile cilia syndrome, sinusitis is nearly always present. Sinusitis is also always present in the APA-syndrome, characterized by asthma, nasal polyposis, and aspirin-intolerance.

PATHOGENESIS AND PATHOLOGY. Acute sinusitis is purulent. The lamina propria is edematous and shows a polymorphonuclear infiltrate, while the periosteum and bone remain intact except for dentogenous sinusitis.

In subacute sinusitis there is a striking proliferation of young connective tissue.

Chronic sinusitis should be considered to be the result of an unhealed acute form. Histopathologic examinations show two important findings: proliferation and necrosis (Fig. 3). The mucosal lining undergoes polypoid changes, metaplasia into a pseudostratified squamous form, and necrosis of the epithelium. In the lamina propria young, well-vascularized connective tissue proliferates and lymphocytes, plasmocytes, macrophages, and eosinophils infiltrate. Edema also occurs as a result of angiitis, with

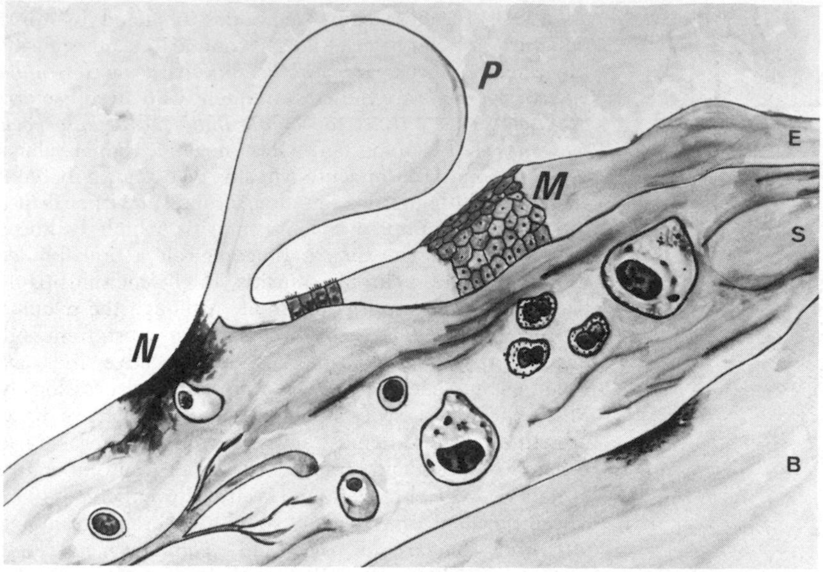

Figure 3. Artist's impression of the histopathologic changes in chronic sinusitis. Epithelial *(E)* changes are: polypoid formations *(P)*, hyperplasia and metaplasia *(M)*, and necrosis *(N)*. In the lamina propria *(S)*, note proliferation of young, well-vascularized connective tissue with infiltration by various cells (lymphocytes, plasmocytes, macrophages, and eosinophils). The bone *(B)* with its periosteum may become necrotic and proliferate. (Drawing by L. Vidts, M.D.)

secondary venous and lymphatic obstruction. Occasionally, the bone and its periosteum become necrotic and proliferate.

CLINICAL MANIFESTATIONS. In acute sinusitis, pain is the most important symptom. It is mostly intense, gnawing, and compressing, and increases on stooping and jarring. It localizes to the involved sinuses. Nasal obstruction, mucoid or mucopurulent discharge, disturbed smell, and epistaxis may also be present. There may be fever, but other symptoms of systemic illness are seldom found. The ascent or descent of the sinus infection may lead to hearing problems, because of involvement of the eustachian tube, and to sore throat, coughing, and hoarseness.

In acute maxillary sinusitis, pain is intense and referred to the area overlying the nasal sinus, the root of the nose, and the upper premolars and molars. Because of the obstruction of the nasofrontal duct and the consequent negative pressure in the frontal sinus, vacuum headache pain is usually present. The pain may also spread to the temporal and retroauricular regions. In dentogenous sinusitis, the characteristic symptomatology of pulpitis or dental abscess is added to the sinusitis symptoms. Nasal obstruction is always present.

In the early stages of an acute maxillary sinusitis, the patient complains of a seromucous nasal discharge, associated with a viral infection. Secondary bacterial invasion transforms the secretions into a mucopurulent or purulent nasal discharge or postnasal drip. A swelling over the affected cheek is rare in uncomplicated maxillary sinusitis of nasal origin, although it may occur in children. It is, on the other hand, a common finding in dentogenous sinusitis.

Acute frontal sinusitis is mostly associated with ethmoidal or maxillary sinusitis. It is very rare as an isolated infection. A very intense, sharp pain is felt in the supraorbital region. Nasal obstruction and discharge are usually present. Because of the intimate relationship with the orbit, edema of the upper eyelid often accompanies an acute frontal sinusitis.

Acute ethmoidal sinusitis, like frontal sinusitis, is seldom found as an isolated phenomenon but usually accompanies maxillary and frontal sinusitis. The ethmoidal cells are the best developed sinuses at birth and are the most frequently involved sinuses in acute sinusitis in children.

Because the ethmoidal cells are separated from the orbital contents only by an extremely thin bony lamella (the lamina papyracea), orbital symptoms and complications are common. The orbital symptoms may be lacrimation, edema of the eyelids, and even impairment of visual acuity. Pain is severe, is located along the inner canthus of the eye, and may spread to the infraorbital and temporal region. Nasal obstruction and discharge are usually present.

Acute sphenoidal sinusitis is unusual as a separate entity but may accompany acute ethmoidal and maxillary sinusitis. The symptoms of infection in other sinuses tend to overshadow any specific symptomatology of the sphenoiditis. The only outstanding feature of acute sphenoidal sinusitis is distinct pain at the occipital and parietal regions.

In chronic sinusitis nasal discharge is the most common symptom. The secretions may be mucoid or mucopurulent, blown from the nose, or appearing as a postnasal drip. Nasal obstruction often occurs because of the edematous nasal mucous membranes and the presence of nasal polyps and viscid secretions. Pain is rare in chronic sinusitis, except in acute exacerbations. As in acute sinusitis, disorders of smell may occur, and infections may extend to the ear, throat, larynx, and bronchi. The symptoms of chronic sinusitis are extremely variable. They may be severe enough to prevent the patient from working, or so mild that he is hardly aware of any problem.

In chronic ethmoidal sinusitis, nasal polyps are very common, while in chronic frontal sinusitis, the formation of a mucocele may lead to orbital swelling and destruction of the surrounding tissues. Chronic sphenoidal sinusitis gives rise to unilateral facial pain and pain behind the eye, and headaches referred to the occipital and parietal regions are also characteristic.

Sinusitis in Children. Because of the marked fall in the incidence of sinusitis in children in the antibiotic era and the improvement in public health, there is no longer a special problem with sinusitis in children (Bernstein, 1971). It is of interest, however, that the nasal sinuses are evaginations of the mucous membrane of the nasal cavities, so that sinusitis often accompanies rhinitis and adenoiditis in children. The symptoms are identical to acute rhinitis in the early stages of infection, e.g., purulent nasal secretions, nasal obstruction, cough, and sneezing. As the disease advances, local symptoms become more evident, especially the mucopurulent discharge. It is extremely difficult to elicit symptoms referable to any particular sinus in small children, unless there are complications like those in acute ethmoiditis.

COMPLICATIONS AND SEQUELAE. Ascending infection of the eustachian tube and middle ear and descending infection of the pharynx, larynx, and bronchi often accompany sinusitis. These complications are usually not dangerous and disappear with proper treatment of the infection. More serious complications arise when infections spread from the paranasal sinuses to adjacent intracranial structures or to the orbit (Litton, 1971).

Acute ethmoiditis may progress to acute meningitis in children. Before the era of antibiotics, this infection was often a fatal one. In adults, frontal, ethmoidal, and sphenoidal sinusitis may be complicated not only by meningitis, but also by epidural and subdural abscesses, brain abscesses, and cavernous sinus thrombosis. Orbital cellulitis and abscesses are common as a complication of ethmoiditis in children, and of ethmoidal and frontal sinusitis in adults, especially in cases of frontal mucocele. Osteomyelitis of the walls of the sinus may develop in chronic sinusitis and less often in acute sinusitis, and occasionally it may produce fistulas.

Maxillary sinusitis seldom leads to severe complications.

GEOGRAPHIC VARIATIONS. These depend on nutrition, air pollution, and access to antibiotics. Poor standards of public health and general living conditions, along with nutritional deficiencies, favor the development of sinusitis, especially in children (Takahashi, 1977). In areas of air pollution, the occurrence of sinusitis is much higher than in rural areas. Hot, dry or cold, moist climates also promote sinusitis. It must be stressed that in areas deprived of antibiotics, the incidence of sinusitis and its complications is higher than in the more privileged countries.

DIAGNOSIS. Inspection of the nose and pharynx is the most important examination. Anterior rhinoscopy may reveal edema and erythema of the nasal mucosa, especially of the inferior turbinate. In suppurative sinusitis, mucoid and mucopurulent secretions are noticed (Fig. 4). The localization of these secretions aids in the determination of which sinuses are involved. While in frontal sinusitis secretions are visible anteriorly at the inferior turbinate, maxillary and ethmoidal secretions appear over the posterior end of the inferior turbinate. One must also look for nasal polyps, nasal septum deviations, and malignant processes. A posterior rhinoscopy and inspection of the oropharynx may also reveal redness, edema, and drainage of mucoid and mucopurulent secretions. In cases of sphenoidal sinusitis, the pus is mainly visible at the posterior wall of the nasopharynx. Palpation may reveal tenderness over the involved sinuses, and the condition of the teeth should be inspected.

Transillumination can be useful in the diagnosis of everyday acute sinusitis. It requires a completely darkened room and a bright light source. The maxillary sinuses are illuminated by placing the light in the patient's mouth. The patient is asked to close his lips tightly around the covered light source. In normal maxillary sinuses, the light is transmitted to the anterior wall of the antrum so that a bright crescent zone is seen in the infraorbital region. The pupil is also lighted. Another method is to place the light source on the maxillary sinus roof. It can then be seen through its floor, the palate. Illumination of the frontal sinus is obtained by placing a covered light source against the frontal sinus floor. The diagnostic value of transillumination has considerable limitation, however. It is much less accurate than x-ray, especially in bilateral sinusitis, in patients with a dense bony structure, in children, and after previous operation upon the sinuses.

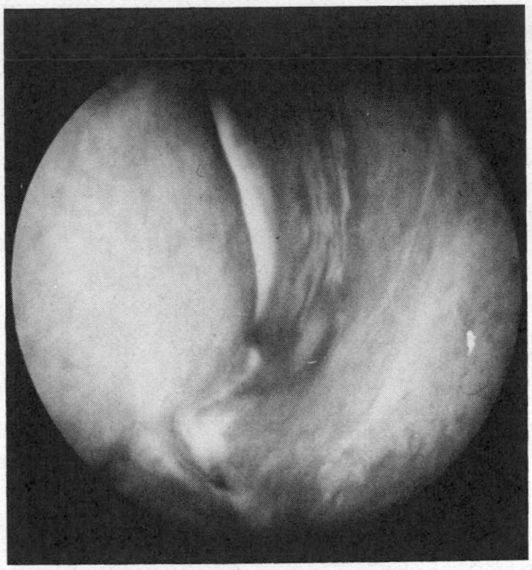

Figure 4. Purulent secretion in the middle meatus in a case of maxillary sinusitis, as seen in anterior rhinoscopy.

Radiography is indispensable in the exact diagnosis of sinusitis. The standard paranasal sinus examination consists of the Waters view (occipitomental position), the Caldwell view (occipitomental position), the profile view (lateral position), and the basal view (Bowen, Hirz, submentovertical position). Observations are made on the presence of thickening of the mucous membrane, an air-fluid level, polypoid tumors, and bony destruction. Complete sinus opacification may be the result of a marked mucous membrane thickening or a complete filling of the sinus by transudate, exudate, or blood, and neoplasia should not be overlooked (Fig. 5). Tomography is necessary to give a more precise diagnosis. It is advisable to add 3 or 4 tomographic views in a frontal plane to standard radiography. Computed tomography is valuable in diagnosis of malignancies or fractures, and in the work-up of chronic sinusitis. (Fig. 7). Panoramic tomography is a very useful examination in sinusitis of dental origin (Fig. 6).

Endoscopic examination of the maxillary sinus permits direct vision of the antral mucosa. With this method, biopsy of the lesions is also possible while the broad naso-sinusal opening (4-mm diameter) created by the sinoscope helps in ventilating the sinus.

Diagnosis of Mucormycosis. This rare sinus infection occurring in diabetic patients in acidosis is caused by phycomycetes. It leads to an angiitis in the nasal and paranasal regions resulting in thrombosis and hemorrhagic infarction. Early clinical manifestations are a black and bloody unilateral rhinorrhea. Rhinoscopy and inspection of

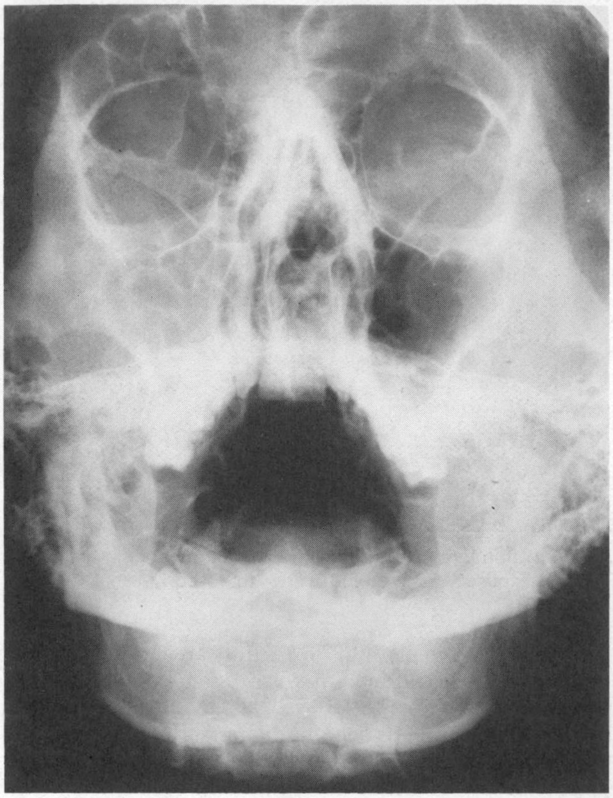

Figure 5. X-Ray of the maxillary sinuses (Water's view) showing a complete opacification of the right maxillary sinus of acute maxillary sinusitis.

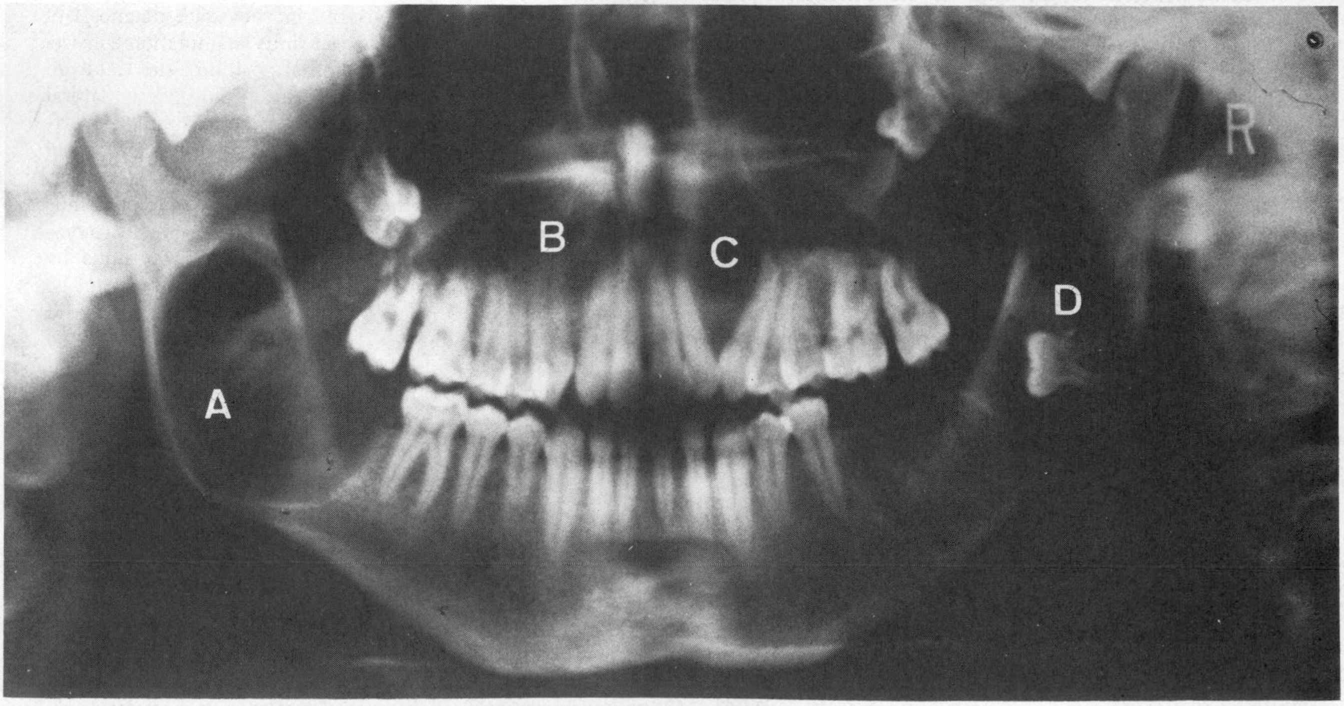

Figure 6. Panoramic tomography showing two dental cysts *(B, C)* causing maxillary sinusitis. Note also two mandibular cysts *(A, D)*. (Courtesy of Prof. R. van Clooster, M.D.)

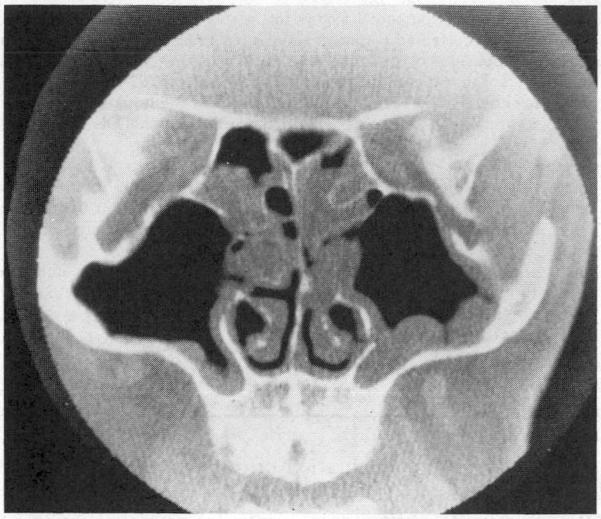

Figure 7. Computed tomography of the maxillary and ethmoidal sinuses. Note the important mucosal swelling in both ethmoidal sinuses, the polypoid mucosal changes at the base of the left maxillary sinus, and the less pronounced swelling at the base of the right maxillary sinus. (Courtesy of Prof. P. A. R. Clement, M.D.)

the mouth reveal a black inferior turbinate sometimes accompanied by a necrotic perforation of the nasal septum and the hard palate. Orbital and endocranial extension is common. Radiography of the sinuses reveals involvement of the maxillary, frontal, and ethmoidal sinuses, showing a homogeneous sinus opacification. Mucormycosis of the sinuses is a lethal disease. Only with early diagnosis and adequate treatment do some patients survive (Chapter 103).

TREATMENT AND PROPHYLAXIS. There are three difficult factors in sinusitis treatment: (1) the sinuses are contained within rigid bony walls, (2) the clearance of the secretions depends on normal ciliary activity, and (3) drainage for the sinus cavity requires an unobstructed orifice.

Acute Sinusitis. An uncomplicated acute sinusitis will heal without any medication in 80 per cent of the cases (Mann et al., 1981), except for analgesics to control the severe headache. Nevertheless, antibiotics are recommended as standard treatment to prevent progression of the 20 per cent subacute and chronic disease, to shorten the course, and to prevent serious complications. Local or systemic vasoconstricting compounds may help restore ventilation of the sinus. The antimicrobial agent must be active against *H. influenzae, S. pneumoniae,* and the anaerobic *Peptostreptococcus.* Also, the antibiotic must penetrate sufficiently into the infected mucous membrane and produce few side effects. Accordingly, any of the following drugs are recommended in the treatment of uncomplicated sinusitis (peroral administration): amoxycillin (500 mg four times daily in adults), bacampicillin (800 mg twice daily), doxycycline (100 mg once or twice daily), cotrimoxazol (160 mg trimethoprim and 800 mg sulfamethoxazole twice daily), and cefaclor (250 mg four times daily). In severe or complicated cases intravenous administration of antibiotics is recommended: 4 g ampicillin + 2 g dicloxacillin or doxycycline (200 mg daily). If the complicated sinusitis is caused by betalactamase-producing *Haemophilus influenzae,* chloramphenicol should be given intravenously (4 g daily).

Subacute Sinusitis. The suppuration in these cases may be reversible with medical treatment alone, or with simple repetitive irrigation; or it may go on to chronicity, with irreversible tissue damage. In cases of maxillary sinusitis, an antral irrigation is performed. After administration of a local anesthetic, the puncture needle penetrates the medial wall of the maxillary sinus (lateral nasal wall) under the inferior turbinate.

The sinus is washed out with sterile water at body temperature, and antibiotics with corticosteroids may be introduced. This irrigation is repeated every 2 to 4 days until the rinsing water is free of pus.

Chronic Sinusitis. In many cases, patients with chronic sinusitis do not have many complaints and are sometimes not aware of their disease. In these cases, no medical interference is warranted. On the contrary, when the patient is suffering from severe mucopurulent or purulent nasal discharge or nasal obstruction, or when complications are likely to occur or are already present, surgery must be performed in order to drain pus, ventilate air-containing cavities, and remove irreversibly damaged mucoperiosteum.

In cases of maxillary sinusitis, an intranasal antrostomy can cure the moderately diseased sinus by restoring sinus ventilation. If this rather conservative surgical procedure turns out to be unsuccessful, a radical Caldwell-Luc procedure should be performed. Ethmoidal sinusitis can be approached by transantral, intranasal, or external ethmoidectomy, of which the last is the most effective and safe technique but leaves an external scar. Subacute frontal sinusitis can be cured by trephination, while chronic frontal sinusitis requires definitive frontal surgery in the form of a nonobliterative or an obliterative procedure. The sphenoid sinus may be approached through the ethmoidal labyrinth after an external ethmoidectomy, through the nasal septum, or transantrally.

Sinusitis in Children. Sinusitis in children should be handled in a more conservative manner than in adults. A supplementary aid in the medical treatment is the Proetz displacement (aspiration and irrigation of the nose and sinuses). It is imperative, prior to undertaking a sinus irrigation, to have adequate radiographs to show the size of the sinus, its position, and its relationship to other structures. If surgical intervention is necessary, it should be minimal; e.g., in chronic maxillary sinusitis, the Caldwell-Luc procedure should be avoided if possible, and the intranasal antrostomy is recommended. The recommended antibiotics in children are amoxycillin, bacampicillin, and a combination of erythromycin and sulfa.

Mucormycosis. First, it is necessary to treat the underlying disease, usually diabetes. In addition, surgical debridement of the affected tissues, and drainage and curettage of the sinus, orbit, and nasal fossa should be performed. Amphotericin B is given intravenously in doses of 50 mg daily for a total of 2.2 g.

PROPHYLAXIS. Predisposing factors, such as nasal septal deviation and allergy, should be treated. Adequate treatment of acute and subacute sinusitis should prevent the development of a chronic form. Complications of sinusitis have become rare since the era of antibiotics. Proper surgical management of chronic sinusitis, with restoration of normal sinus ventilation and removal of all irreversibly damaged tissues, should prevent relapses.

References

Bernstein, L.: Pediatric sinus problems. Otolaryngol Clin North Am 4:127, 1971.

Brorson, J. E., Axelsson, A., and Holm, S. E.: Studies on Branhamella catarrhalis with special reference to maxillary sinusitis. Scand J Infect Dis 8:151, 1976.

Frederick, J., and Braude, A. I.: Anaerobic infection of the paranasal sinuses. New Engl J Med 290:135, 1974.

Litton, W. B.: Acute and chronic sinusitis. Otolaryngol Clin North Am 4:25, 1971.

Mann, W., Pelz, K., Gobel, U., and Jonas, I.: Therapeutic considerations in sinusitis. Rhinology, Suppl 1:227, 1981.

Saito, H., Takenaka, H., Hoshino, A., and Mizukoshi, O.: Antiviral defense mechanisms of the nasal mucosa. Rhinology, Suppl 1:19, 1981.

Takahashi, R.: Environmental factors in the development of infection and allergy of the nose and paranasal sinuses. *In* Proceedings of the International Symposium of Infection and Allergy of the Nose and Paranasal Sinuses. Tokyo, Scimed Publications, Inc., 1977, pp. 21–26.

van Cauwenberge, P., Verschraegen, G., and Van Renterghem, L.: Bacteriologic findings in sinusitis (1963–1975). Scand J Infect Dis Suppl 9:72, 1976.

van Cauwenberge, P., Van Renterghem, L., Verschraegen, G., and Kluyskens, P.: Bacteriology in sinusitis with special reference to the role of the anaerobes. *In* Proceedings of the International Symposium of Infection and Allergy of the Nose and Paranasal Sinuses. Tokyo, Scimed Publications, Inc., 1977, pp. 151–155.

Verschraegen, G., and van Cauwenberge, P.: The role of anaerobes in sinusitis. In Advances in Sinusitis (P. van Cauwenberge and C. Ekedahl, eds.). Gent, Scient Soc Med Inf, 1982, p. 27.

99

OTITIS MEDIA AND OTITIS EXTERNA

BURT R. MEYERS, M.D.,
WILLIAM LAWSON, M.D., D.D.S.

OTITIS MEDIA

DEFINITION; ETIOLOGY; PATHOGENESIS. Otitis media is an acute and chronic inflammatory state of the middle ear which may be suppurative or nonsuppurative. Acute otitis media is primarily a disease of infants and children, whereas the chronic form and its complications generally arise in later life. Although most infections are bacterial, other agents (including viruses and mycoplasma) may produce an acute syndrome with serous effusion.

The eustachian tube has a cardinal role in the development of otitis media. In acute suppurative otitis media the occurrence of a viral upper respiratory tract infection produces hyperemia and edema of the nose and nasopharynx with partial occlusion of the eustachian tube orifice. This impairment of middle ear ventilation results in the transudation of fluid from the negative pressure produced by the continuous resorption of gases by the hyperemic middle ear mucosa. This, coupled with copious mucoid secretions and frequent sneezing, coughing, and swallowing, permits pathogenic organisms such as *Streptococcus pneumoniae* and *Hemophilus influenzae,* which normally colonize the nasopharynx, to enter the eustachian tube and middle ear, where they produce inflammation, exudation, and finally suppuration. Many of the viral exanthems are often followed by middle ear infections, probably as a result of the same mechanisms. Certain systemic bacterial infections, such as pneumococcal pneumonia and meningococcal meningitis, may be associated with otitis media; however, it is not clear if these represent local extension from the oropharynx or are secondary to hematogenous seeding.

Epidemiologic data seem to support this concept of the pathogenesis of acute bacterial otitis media. First, there is a seasonal variation in its incidence; it is more common during the winter months when viral respiratory infections are frequent. Attacks accompany or follow viral infections and the offending bacteria are those normally found in the nasopharynx. Anatomic predisposing factors in young children include the configuration of the eustachian tube and lymphoid hyperplasia of Waldeyer's ring. The great frequency of acute otitis media in infants and young children may be related to the relatively short and straight course of the eustachian tube in this age group, permitting direct access from the nasopharynx to the middle ear.

The role of immunologic factors in the etiology of otitis media is unclear. In chronic serous and acute purulent otitis media the fluid present in the middle ear space contains antibodies of all immunoglobulin classes. However, the high titer of secretory IgA in serous otitis indicates that the fluid is not entirely produced by transudation but contains constituents produced locally. Patients with either hypo- or agammaglobulinemia are prone to bacterial infections including otitis media. Opsonization is necessary for phagocytosis of the microorganisms most responsible for this infection, and the lack of gamma globulins may account for their increased virulence in this group of patients.

High levels of interferon have been demonstrated in the middle ear fluid of patients with bacterial otitis media without detectable virus infection (Howie et al., 1982).

Macrophages are the predominant cellular element in middle ear effusions. These cells appear to induce a hyporesponsiveness of lymphocytes in the middle ear, as well as the peripheral blood and adenoid tissue (Yamanaka et al., 1982). This suppressive activity appears to be mediated by low molecular weight substances produced by these macrophages (Yamanaka et al., 1983).

There may be ethnic and social factors operative in the susceptibility to otitis. There appears to be a propensity for otitis media in certain races; both American Indians and Asians have a higher incidence of infection. It has been suggested but not proven that economically depressed groups may be more prone to infection.

In chronic otitis media there is persistent obstruction of the eustachian tube, produced by a variety of factors such as chronic nasal and pharyngeal infection, lymphoid hyperplasia, allergy, or cleft palate. Atopic allergy, exposure to cigarette smoke, and recurrent otitis have been reported as high risk factors in children with persistent middle ear effusions (Kraemer et al., 1983). With recurrent infection the middle ear mucosa may undergo alterations with metaplasia and an increase in goblet cells or irreversible changes with the formation of polyps, granulations, and tympanosclerosis. The tympanic membrane may become atrophic, sclerotic, or perforated, with ingrowth of epithelium and formation of a secondary cholesteatoma. Persistent infection may also result in destruction of the ossicles. Extension of the infection into the mastoid may cause sclerosis with limited pneumatization, osteitis, or osteomyelitis of the bone, possibly with the formation of a sequestrum. The hyaline submucosal plaques of tympanosclerosis may calcify, producing immobility of the tympanic membrane, fixation of the ossicles, and partial obliteration of the tympanic cavity. From persistent negative pressure due to eustachian tube dysfunction, fluid may accumulate and thicken, producing an adhesive otitis. This may result in immobilization of the ossicular chain and retraction of the tympanic membrane, with progressive conductive hearing loss. In some cases, continuous retraction of the pars flaccida produces a primary acquired cholesteatoma.

Bacteriology. Bacteriologic studies on the etiology of acute otitis media have been best described in children. When tympanocentesis was performed and the fluid examined it was noted that *S. pneumoniae*, *H. influenzae* (nontypable strains), and *Streptococcus pyogenes* were responsible for 90 per cent of positive culture specimens. *S. aureus* and *Branhamella catarrhalis* are also isolated not infrequently. Though studies vary, most find rates of 50 per cent *S. pneumoniae* and 20 to 30 per cent *H. influenzae*, and *S. pyogenes* in the remainder. *H. influenzae* type B isolates may cause cellulitis. Since anaerobic cultures are less frequently performed, it appears they are not responsible for acute infection.

S. pneumoniae is the most common cause of otitis media in the adult, accounting for more than 80 to 90 per cent of the isolates. *S. pyogenes*, *Staphylococcus aureus*, and *H. influenzae* comprise the other pathogens. In the adult with chronic otitis media, with a history of acute exacerbation, the usual pathogens are *S. pneumoniae*, *H. influenzae*, and *S. aureus*. In chronic otitis media associated with aural drainage, gram-negative microorganisms including *Proteus* sp., *Pseudomonas* sp., *Escherichia coli*, or *S. aureus* have been isolated. Recent reports have found anaerobes in mixed cultures from 50 per cent of specimens obtained by tympanocentesis. Bacterial isolates from the complications of chronic otitis, such as brain abscesses, are often anaerobic, suggesting a causal relation.

Mycoplasma pneumoniae, adenovirus, influenza virus, and respiratory syncytial virus have been isolated from middle ear aspirates.

Countercurrent immunoelectrophoresis on middle ear fluid is of limited diagnostic value for identifying the infectious organism and seems useful only as a screening procedure (Ostfeld and Altman, 1980).

CLINICAL FEATURES; DIAGNOSIS. In acute bacterial otitis media the presenting symptom is pain. In infants this may be communicated by crying and tugging at the ears. It may be accompanied by high fever. Otoscopy may reveal only injection over the handle of the malleus, or diffuse redness and loss of anatomic landmarks, or even bulging of the entire eardrum. Insufflation with a pneumatic otoscope may help in revealing a bulging drum by its immobility. If a significant amount of a fluid accumulates in the middle ear there is also a decrease in hearing acuity. With continued suppuration there may be spontaneous perforation of the tympanic membrane with the development of a purulent discharge and lessening of the pain. These perforations tend to heal with resolution of the infection. However, in a small number of cases, infection with β-hemolytic streptococci produces an early and extensive necrotizing otitis with loss of the pars tensa and portions of the ossicular chain.

Viral otitis media may also accompany upper respiratory infections. In this condition the dominant symptom is fullness and mild hearing loss; pain is uncommon and generally signifies secondary bacterial infection. Otoscopy usually reveals only dullness and either mild retraction or fullness of the drumhead, depending on the quantity of fluid produced. Impedance audiometry may reveal a persistent negative pressure in the middle ear space or a pattern of decreased compliance suggestive of fluid. Treatment is directed toward improvement of eustachian tube function and aeration of the middle ear space by the use of decongestants and the Valsalva maneuver. Viral infections, especially influenza and occasionally mycoplasma, may attack the tympanic membrane itself, causing bullous myringitis. The syndrome produces intense pain lasting 1 or 2 days. Otoscopy reveals hemorrhagic blebs over the drumhead, which often spontaneously rupture, producing bleeding in the ear canal or fullness in the tympanic cavity. This condition is self-limiting, requiring only analgesics or anodyne eardrops for a few days. Persistent pain signifies secondary bacterial infection and requires systemic antibiotics.

COMPLICATIONS. Acute mastoiditis is now an uncommon complication of acute suppurative otitis media and results from incomplete or inappropriate antibiotic treatment or an immunologically deficient host. It usually is associated with chronic otitis media and cholesteatoma. Severe inflammation in the middle ear space may result in attic block with accumulation of pus in the mastoid air cells and the dissolution of the bony septa between them. The patient may then develop fever and mastoid pain. Otoscopy may reveal an intact eardrum with sagging of the posterosuperior canal wall or an actively draining perforation. The mastoid area may show tenderness or swelling or outward displacement of the pinna if a subperiosteal abscess develops. Radiographs will show clouding and coalescence of the mastoid air cells and blurring of the bony margins. Simple mastoidectomy may be required if infection does not resolve after a few days of systemic antibiotic therapy.

Acute petrositis classically is characterized by Gradenigo's syndrome, in which diplopia caused by a sixth cranial nerve palsy and ocular pain accompany aural discharge. It occurs most commonly in patients with chronic otitis media, some of whom have undergone a prior simple mastoidectomy. Failure of resolution with high-dose intravenous antibiotic therapy requires surgical drainage of the petrous apex.

Serous or suppurative labyrinthitis may complicate acute otitis media, producing vestibular (vertigo, nystagmus, nausea, vomiting) or cochlear (neurosensory hearing loss) symptoms. Inflammation of the labyrinth may occur through the middle ear (round or oval window) or secondary to meningitis. With serous labyrinthitis the symptoms are generally mild and self-limiting and respond to intravenous antibiotics and drainage of the middle ear space by myringotomy. With suppurative labyrinthitis, there is complete loss of hearing, severe vertigo, absent caloric response, and the danger of intracranial extension. If meningeal symptoms develop and cerebrospinal fluid abnormalities are found, surgical drainage of the labyrinth is necessary; otherwise intravenous antibiotics are usually adequate to control the infection.

Facial nerve paralysis may occur in acute or chronic otitis media from edema of the nerve in response to suppuration extending through a dehiscence in the tympanic portion of its bony canal. It almost invariably responds completely to high-dose antibiotic therapy and prompt myringotomy. Some authors also advocate steroid therapy (prednisone, 60 to 80 mg daily) and surgical decompression, which is reserved for only those few cases that go on to show evidence of degeneration of the nerve.

Intracranial Complications. The development of meningitis, epidural or brain abscess, otitic hydrocephalus, and lateral sinus thrombosis may follow middle ear infection. These may extend intracranially directly through a bony dehiscence or surgical defect, or by thrombophlebitis of emissary veins or Haversian systems, or via the labyrinth. Continued fever, pain, toxicity, the development of headache, somnolence, irritability, or nausea and vomiting despite antibiotic therapy signal extension of the infection. There may be continued aural drainage through a perforation, or an intact inflamed or even normal eardrum found on otoscopy. Radiographs may or may not reveal bone destruction. Examination of the cerebrospinal fluid, ophthalmoscopy for the detection of papilledema, and blood cultures are mandatory with this clinical picture. These patients should also have a detailed neurologic examination and be observed closely for the development of signs of meningeal irritation. If a brain abscess is suspected, bone and brain scanning and computerized axial tomography may define the lesion. Management includes intense antibiotic therapy initially and, when the patient's condition warrants, definitive surgery. Surgery is generally required since these complications usually accompany chronic otitis media and mastoiditis, often with cholesteatoma. Meningitis can be managed primarily with antibiotics, but recurrent otogenic meningitis suggests chronic mastoiditis, a condition that often requires radical mastoidectomy for exploration and removal of diseased bone and granulation tissue. Craniotomy may be needed for drainage of a brain abscess.

TREATMENT. Studies in children have been carried out to determine the level of antibiotic present in the middle ear during an infection. Antibiotic levels have been calculated by tympanocentesis and comparisons to the serum level, minimum inhibitory concentration (the least amount of antibiotic which inhibits growth in the test tube), and response of the patient determined. The following compounds have been found in the middle ear in concentrations adequate to inhibit *S. pneumoniae* strains isolated: penicillins G and V, amoxicillin, erythromycin estolate, triple sulfonamide, cefaclor, trimethoprim, sulfamethoxazole, and others. The levels of penicillin found in one study would not have inhibited 75 per cent of *H. influenzae* isolated. In other studies, levels of 4 μg/ml were found after penicillin V and these were inhibitory and efficacious. Erythromycin estolate would have been effective against only 60 per cent of these strains.

The treatment of choice for an adult with uncomplicated otitis media is penicillin. This may be administered orally as phenoxymethyl penicillin, or may be given once intramuscularly in a dose of 1.2 million units. Procaine and benzathine penicillin (Bicillin), 1.2 million units, is especially effective. In adults allergic to penicillin, erythromycin, 250 mg, should be given orally every 6 hours for 7 to 10 days. Oral cephalosporins have also been proven effective but their cost may be prohibitive for developing nations. Tetracycline hydrochloride should not be used, because resistant *S. pneumoniae*, *S. pyogenes*, and *S. aureus* strains have been reported. The use of tetracycline in children under 8 years is contraindicated because of staining of the permanent dentition. These recommendations for antimicrobial drugs are made even though any form of treatment, including antibiotics alone, or antibiotics plus myringotomy or myringotomy alone gave results in children that were no better than those in untreated controls in a double blind study (Van Buchen et al., 1981). Antimicrobial drug therapy is recommended to prevent the complications of otitis media.

In the patient with a history of chronic suppurative otitis with exacerbations, treatment directed against *S. aureus* (presumed penicillin-resistant) and *H. influenzae* is necessary if material for culture is unavailable. A penicillinase-resistant penicillin like dicloxacillin is recommended for *S. aureus* infection and ampicillin for *H. influenzae*, both at a dose of 250 mg every 6 hours. Increasing numbers of *H. influenzae* strains are being isolated that are resistant to ampicillin because of β-lactamase production. In those patients, trimethoprim-sulfamethoxazole amoxycillin/clavulonic acid or an oral cephalosporin such as cefaclor would be efficacious.

The use of an antihistamine or decongestant in conjunction with antibiotic therapy for acute otitis media is controversial, at least in children. In a double blind randomized trial of 553 patients suffering from otitis media with effusion, a placebo was compared to an oral decongestant-antihistamine combination. There proved to be no difference in resolution of effusion in either unilateral or bilateral disease between treated and placebo groups (Cantekin et al., 1983). For an acute episode in which severe pain is accompanied by a bulging tympanic membrane, myringotomy will provide rapid relief. In prolonged or repeated episodes of acute otitis media or hearing loss accompanied by an abnormal eardrum, fluid in the middle ear space must be presumed and myringotomy, generally with the insertion of a ventilating tube, is indicated. In young children with recurrent otitis media, adenoidectomy may also be performed in an attempt to clear the eustachian tube orifices of the obstructing lymphoid tissue. Attention must also be directed to the elimination of other etiologic factors such as chronic nasal or sinus infection and allergy.

The treatment of chronic otitis media in the adult requires not only a systemic but also a topical antibiotic in order to control the otorrhea. A variety of otic preparations have been devised that are directed primarily against the offending gram-negative flora (e.g., gentamicin, colimycin, chloromycetin, and polymyxin eardrops). The definitive management of chronic otitis media and its complications, including tympanic membrane perforation, cholesteatoma, conductive hearing loss, and mastoiditis, are primarily surgical and are detailed in standard textbooks of otology (e.g., Shambaugh and Glasscock: *Surgery of the Ear.*)

TUBERCULOUS OTITIS. Tuberculous involvement of the middle ear occurs in both adults and children, although more commonly in the latter. Congenital cases have been reported. *M. tuberculosis* is generally the causative organism, producing secondary involvement of the temporal bone. The proposed routes of infection are via the eustachian tube, by hematogenous spread, or, on rare occasions, directly through the auditory canal.

Characteristically, there is painless aural discharge through multiple tympanic membrane perforations. Later in the disease these coalesce into one large opening with exuberant granulations and extensive destruction in the middle ear space. There is also severe hearing loss (generally conductive) early in the disease. Occasionally there is bilateral involvement. The middle ear infection rapidly involves the mastoid, and complications develop, including facial paralysis, labyrinthine fistula, subperiosteal and cervical abscess, meningitis, cutaneous fistula, and formation of a sequestration of bone. Unlike other forms of chronic otitis media in which x-rays of the mastoid bones reveal sclerosis, in tuberculous otitis they are generally extensively pneumatized.

Diagnosis may be established by biopsy of middle ear tissue revealing caseating epithelioid granulomas. Cultures are positive in only a small number of cases. Tuberculin skin tests are usually positive and chest x-rays may reveal old or acute tuberculous changes. Tuberculous mastoiditis should be suspected in any patient with painless otitis media accompanied by severe hearing loss, profuse granulations in the middle ear space, and evidence of coalescent mastoiditis in a well-pneumatized mastoid.

The treatment of this condition is primarily with antituberculous therapy, principally isoniazid and rifampin or ethambutol. Surgery, primarily radical mastoidectomy, is reserved for those cases that are refractory to treatment or develop the complications of otitis media.

PROPHYLAXIS. Since viral syndromes of the upper respiratory tract often precede otitis media, their prevention might decrease bacterial invasion. At present immunization is effective against the viral exanthems but a "cold" vaccine is not available. The use of prophylactic antibiotics in proved viral infections has not been of value and is not recommended. Intermittent administration of antibiotics to patients with a history of chronic suppurative or serous otitis has been carried out but proof of its efficacy is lacking. Pneumococcal vaccine has been given to prevent otitis media in children, but in controlled trials, the mean number of bouts of infection was not significantly different in those vaccinated from the number in controls (Teele and Klein, 1981; Mäkela et al., 1981). γ-Globulin should be administered to patients with either congenital or acquired agammaglobulinemia.

OTITIS EXTERNA

DEFINITION; ETIOLOGY; PATHOGENESIS. Otitis externa is an inflammatory condition of any portion of the skin of the external auditory canal. It has been classified by Senturia and Marcus (1967) as an infectious disease, neurogenic eruption, allergic dermatosis, traumatic lesion, and disease of unknown etiology. This reflects the multiplicity of causative factors in the pathogenesis of this condition. The most important factors are high humidity and temperature, trauma or excoriation of the skin, and allergy to hair sprays and dyes. The significance of climatic conditions is seen in the popular names used for description, such as swimmer's ear, hot-weather ear, or Hong Kong or Singapore ear. The incidence of this disease has been estimated at 3 to 10 per cent of the general population, and as high as 50 per cent of otologic cases. This increased prevalence is especially notable in tropical and subtropical zones.

The most commonly encountered form of this condition is diffuse otitis externa, either acute or chronic, arising from bacterial infection. Otitis externa results from disruption of the physiologic defense mechanisms operative in the external auditory canal. The most important of these is the local pH, whereby the acidity of the secretions of the skin, sweat, and sebaceous glands is bacteriostatic or bactericidal to organisms that would flourish in an alkaline medium (Goffin, 1963). Other protective factors include the secretion of lysozyme by sweat glands. The antimicrobial action of unsaturated fatty acids derived from lipids secreted by sebaceous glands may be active against gram-negative bacteria and certain fungi. The water-repellent coating of waxes secreted by the apocrine glands and the clearing action of the lateral migration of keratin through the ear canal also play a protective role (Cassisi et al., 1977).

While the sigmoid configuration of the external canal limits the entry of exogenous material, it also promotes the entrapment of water to form a skin-lined culture tube. The presence of exostoses, whose growth is encouraged by cold-water swimming, further enhances the retention of moisture. Prolonged exposure to moisture produces maceration of the epithelial lining with swelling of the surface keratin and blockage of the ducts of the glands, which in turn are penetrated by endogenous nonpathogenic organisms. This produces a low-grade inflammation and promotes the invasion by exogenous, primarily gram-negative organisms (Senturia, 1957). This is further aggravated by the development of an itch-scratch cycle.

Bacteriology. Studies of the flora of the normal external auditory canal show that *Staphylococcus epidermidis* and diphtheroids are the predominant organisms. *S. aureus* is only occasionally and *Pseudomonas* sp. rarely isolated. However, in chronic otitis externa *Pseudomonas* sp. becomes the predominant organism cultured, followed by *S. aureus*. Cassisi et al. (1977) found, on study of 232 ears with a positive culture, a single organism in 63 per cent, two organisms in 31 per cent, and three organisms in 5 per cent. Of these, 59 per cent were gram-positive. *Pseudomonas* sp. constituted 66 per cent of the first group; the remainder were primarily *Proteus*, *Enterobacter*, *Klebsiella*, and *E. coli*. Of the gram-positive organisms, *S. aureus* comprised 30 per cent and *Streptococcus* strains only 12 per cent. Fungal forms were isolated in a very small number of the cases with acute diffuse otitis externa.

CLINICAL FEATURES; DIAGNOSIS. The clinical manifestations of the commonly encountered acute diffuse form of otitis externa vary widely in intensity. The dominant symptoms are itching and pain. The pain may be mild to extremely severe because of progressive swelling in a confined space. There may be an accompanying exudate which may be thin and watery or purulent. With continued swelling and exudate in the canal the patient may describe or present with hearing loss. On clinical examination canal wall edema and erythema are the most common findings. The swelling may progress to the point of total closure of the canal, preventing visualization of the eardrum. Examination of the tympanic membrane is mandatory since otitis externa may be secondary to suppurative middle ear disease. Aural drainage and excoriation of the canal lining also occur frequently. Pain on manipulation of the pinna, periauricular edema, and regional lymphadenopathy accompany severe attacks. Constitutional symptoms are unusual and represent bacterial invasion of the surrounding soft tissues. The chronic diffuse form, common in humid climates, is characterized also by itching and fullness of the ears. In this condition, *Aspergillus niger*, *Actinomyces*, or yeasts produce a chronic superficial infection. Otoscopy reveals erosion and desquamation of the epithelial lining, with formation of a membrane and a musty-smelling exudate. Occasionally a fungus ball may fill the canal. Eczematoid and seborrheic changes in the external auditory canal, meatus, concha, or remainder of the pinna represent allergic and dermatologic conditions, respectively, rather than infectious processes. Rarely, in uncontrolled chronic otitis externa, extensive hyperkeratosis and subcutaneous fibrosis produce stenosis of the external auditory canal.

TREATMENT. Treatment is directed to symptomatic relief and control of the infectious organisms. A topical preparation containing antibiotics effective against *Pseudomonas* (e.g., polymyxin B or colistin) and staphylococci (e.g., neomycin) in a mildly acidified hygroscopic vehicle (e.g., propylene glycol) along with an anti-inflammatory agent (hydrocortisone) produces relief in the vast majority of cases of acute diffuse otitis externa. The skin swelling may be so severe that a small gauze wick may have to be inserted to permit entry of the drops into the canal. This may be combined with the use of an astringent such as Thiersch's solution. Supplemental analgesics may also be required for the control of pain until the edema subsides. Systemic antibiotics directed against gram-positive cocci (penicillin, ampicillin, cephalosporin, erythromycin) are indicated only when there is evidence of perichondritis or periauricular swelling or regional lymphadenopathy. With chronic otitis externa and after the severe inflammation has subsided in the acute form, cleansing, drying, and acidification of the canal are necessary. Debris may be removed by irrigation or aspiration, followed by the use of Burow's solution or acidified alcohol (2 to 4 per cent boric or acetic acid in 70 per cent ethanol). These latter agents are also very effective against fungal organisms commonly present in the chronic form. Systemic antifungal therapy has no role in the treatment of chronic otitis externa or otomycosis. When stenosis of the external auditory canal occurs, treatment consists of total excision of the hypertrophic lining, widening of the bony canal, and skin grafting of the defect.

PROPHYLAXIS. Patients with recurrent and chronic otitis externa must keep the external auditory canal dry. This includes the exclusion of moisture by earplugs when swimming or bathing and the periodic use of alcohol eardrops if water enters or itching occurs.

MALIGNANT OTITIS EXTERNA

Malignant otitis externa is an infection caused by *Pseudomonas aeruginosa* which begins in the external auditory canal and extends into the temporal bone; it may invade the base of the skull, contiguous soft tissues, and the brain. It occurs primarily in elderly diabetics but has also been reported with blood dyscrasias (e.g., chronic lymphocytic leukemia, granulocytopenia). In a series of 72 patients, all but 4 patients were diabetic. Of these 68 cases, 6 had only chemical diabetes and 27 were insulin-dependent. The pathogenicity of the *Pseudomonas* organism appears to be its ability to produce a vasculitis, with accompanying thrombosis and ischemic necrosis of tissue; however, the reason for its invasiveness in this select group is unclear. In the early stages of infection there is a thick layer of degenerating collagen that extends from the cartilage to the dermis. Some believe that bacteria, notably *Pseudomonas aeruginosa*, invade this tissue, which loses its vitality secondary to vascular insufficiency (Ostfeld et al., 1981).

The infection spreads through skin and cartilage to cause mastoiditis or osteomyelitis of the skull, cranial nerve palsies, sinus thrombosis, meningitis, and death. The mastoid may be destroyed by direct extension without middle ear involvement. One of the most characteristic symptoms of this condition is intense local pain. Facial nerve paralysis generally results from infection of the nerve within the soft tissues and is a poor prognostic sign. In one series, this occurred in 32 per cent of patients; half of the survivors were left with permanent nerve damage. The development of paralysis of the cranial nerves that pass through the jugular foramen generally signifies thrombosis of the jugular bulb and sigmoid sinus.

The disease should be suspected in any case of a refractory otitis externa, especially if granulations are present in the canal along with persistent purulent discharge, particularly in a diabetic. If there is no history of diabetes a glucose tolerance test should be performed. Fever may or may not be prominent, but the erythrocyte sedimentation rate is generally elevated. Cultures of the aural discharge will reveal *Pseudomonas* sp. Cerebrospinal fluid (CSF) analysis reveals mild pleocytosis, with normal glucose and a negative gram stain. When meningitis develops, polymorphonuclear leukocytes will increase and a low CSF sugar will be found. Radionuclide scanning and computerized axial tomography may be used to define the areas of the involvement.

After appropriate cultures are taken, initial therapy with either carbenicillin, ticarcillin, azlocillin, or piperacillin coupled with an aminoglycoside should be instituted. This combination has produced synergistic effects in the laboratory. Carbenicillin in a dose of 5 g every 4 to 6 hours, ticarcillin at one half the dose or piperacillin 12 to 18 g/day, all given intravenously. Both ticarcillin and carbenicillin have approximately 5 meq of sodium per gram, and in the elderly who may be in congestive heart failure, the amount of sodium delivered is a limiting factor. For these reasons piperacillin, a monosodium salt, which is 5 to 10 times more potent, is preferable. For the aminoglycoside, tobramycin 1 mg/kg given every 8 hours is a more logical choice than gentamicin because of its greater effect in vitro against *Pseudomonas* sp. and the smaller dose necessary to achieve synergism with carbenicillin or ticarcillin. We have cautiously administered these drugs from 4 to 15 weeks to 11 patients. Five of 11 required surgery other than local debridement, and 7 recovered. Five had cranial nerve palsies that improved only slightly. Monitoring of the eighth nerve is mandatory in patients receiving aminoglycosides for a prolonged time.

Cefsulodin, a narrow-spectrum antipseudomonal cephalosporin, is another drug studied in this infection. In a clinical trial with this agent alone, we successfully treated 7 of 11 elderly diabetic patients (Mendelson et al., 1984). This compared favorably with combination antibiotic therapy. Treatment of concomitant infections (if they occur), adequate fluid replacement, and nutritional balance hasten recovery.

Antibiotic treatment should be continued for as long as improvement continues, usually 6 to 12 weeks. Surgery should be reserved until symptoms progress; intervention consists of radical mastoidectomy with debridement of all necrotic soft tissue and bone. Sinus thrombosis may be an indication for mandatory surgery. Hyperbaric oxygen has been used but no controlled trials have been done.

CT scanning is of limited value in assessing the therapeutic response because the osseous structures rarely return to normal; however, continued bone destruction signifies active and progressive disease (Lucente et al., 1982). The technetium bone scan remains positive after resolution of the infection. but the gallium scan may better reflect response to therapy.

References

Cantekin, E., Mandel, E., Bluestone, C., et al.: Lack of efficiency of decongestant-antihistamine combination for otitis media with effusion (secretory otitis media) in children. N Eng J Med 308:297, 1983.

Cassisi, N., Cohn, A., Davidson, T., and Witten, B. R.: Diffuse otitis externa. Clinical and microbiologic findings in the course of a multicenter study on a new otic solution. Ann Otol Suppl 39:1–16, 1977.

Chandler, J. R.: Malignant external otitis: Further considerations. Ann Otol 86:417–428, 1977.

Goffin, F. B.: pH as a factor in external otitis. New Engl J Med 268:287–289, 1963.

Howie, V., Pollard, R., Kleyn, K., Lawrence, B., Peskuric, T., Paulker, K., and Baron, S.: Presence of interferon during bacterial otitis media. J Inf Dis 145:811, 1982.

Kraemer, M., Richardson, M., Weiss, N., and Furukawa, L.: Risk factors for persistent middle ear effusions: otitis media, catarrh, cigarette smoke exposure, and atopy. JAMA 249:1022, 1983.

Lucente, F., Parisier, S., Som, P., and Arnold, L.: Malignant external otitis: a dangerous misnomer. Otolaryngol Head Neck Surg 90:266, 1982.

Mäkela, P., Leinonen, M., Pukander, J., and Karma, P.: A study of the pneumococcal vaccine in prevention of clinically acute attacks of otitis media. Rev Inf Dis 3:5124, 1981.

Mendelson, M., Meyers, B., Hirschman, S. Z., et al.: Treatment of invasive external otitis with cefsulodin. Rev Inf Dis 6:Suppl. 3S698–704, 1984.

Ostfeld, E., and Altmann, G.: Evaluation of countercurrent immunoelectrophoresis as a diagnostic tool in bacterial otitis media. Ann Oto-Rhinol Laryngol Supp 68:110, 1980.

Ostfeld, E., Segal, M., Czernofils, B.: Malignant external otitis: early histopathologic changes and pathogenic mechanism. Laryngoscope 9:965, 1981.

Senturia, B. H.: Diseases of the External Ear. Springfield, Ill., Charles C Thomas, 1957.

Senturia, B. H., and Marcus, M. D.: Diseases of the external ear. Minn Med 50:837–838, 1967.

Shambaugh, G. E., and Glasscock, M. E., III: Surgery of the Ear. 3rd ed. Philadelphia, W. B. Saunders Co., 1980.

Teele, D., and Klein, J.: Greater Boston collaborative otitis media study group. Use of pneumococcal vaccine for prevention of recurrent acute otitis media in infants in Boston. Rev Inf Dis 3:5113, 1981.

Van Buchen, F., Dunk, T., Vanthof, M.: Therapy of acute otitis media: myringostomy, antibiotics, or neither? A double blind study in children. Lancet 2:883, 1981.

Yamanaka, T., Cumella, J., Parker, C., Bernstein, J., and Ogra, P.: Immunologic aspects of otitis media with effusion: characteristics of lymphocyte and macrophage reactivity. J Inf Dis 145:824, 1982.

Yamanaka, T., Cumella, J., Parker, C., Bernstein, J., and Ogra, P.: Immunologic aspects of otitis media with effusion. II. Nature of cell-mediated immunosuppressive activity in middle ear fluid. J Inf Dis 147:794, 1983.

100

EPIGLOTTITIS AND PSEUDOCROUP

PAULA BRANEFORS-HELANDER, M.D., PH.D.,
OLLE NYLÉN, M.D.,
TERESA LAGERGÅRD, PH.D.

In the laryngeal region there are two diseases caused by infections: acute epiglottitis and pseudocroup (laryngitis subglottica). Both processes affect mainly children. Acute epiglottitis is a rare disease. Pseudocroup is more than 10 times as common. Because they have some clinical signs in common, acute epiglottitis is often mistaken for pseudocroup. It is, however, of the utmost importance to differentiate these two entities, since epiglottitis is a hyperacute and potentially fatal bacterial infection. Pseudocroup is generally of viral origin and only rarely constitutes a threat to life.

Acute epiglottitis is an inflammation of the supraglottic region and may affect not only the epiglottis, but also the aryepiglottic folds and even the prevertebral soft tissue. The pharynx is usually only slightly affected, and the true vocal cords and the subglottic tissue are seldom involved.

Pseudocroup is characterized by marked swelling of the tissue just below the vocal cords—the subglottic region—which is the narrowest part of the upper airway in small children.

ETIOLOGY. As already mentioned, acute epiglottitis is of bacterial origin. The most common cause is *Haemophilus influenzae* type b. In children, blood cultures are nearly always positive for *H. influenzae* type b, and nose and throat cultures also yield *H. influenzae* in most cases. Blood cultures from adults are less likely to be positive. A greater proportion of adults than children have infections due to bacteria other than *H. influenzae.* Betahemolytic group A streptococci, *Streptococcus pneumoniae, Staphylococcus aureus,* and nonencapsulated *H. influenzae* have been isolated from pharyngeal swabs and on occasion from blood cultures. In a substantial number of pediatric and adult patients, throat cultures yield only a mixed flora of commensal bacteria.

Pseudocroup, on the other hand, is caused most commonly by parainfluenzae types 1, 2, and 3. Other viruses that are isolated less often are influenza A, respiratory syncytical virus, and, occasionally, members of the enterovirus group such as coxsackie and echoviruses. Allergy may predispose to pseudocroup in certain children.

The incidence of pseudocroup is highest in children from the age of 6 months to 3 years, while acute epiglottitis is most common in children 2 to 7 years old. It is important, however, to be aware of the fact that acute epiglottitis may occur at any age, in newborns as well as in old people. Some individuals may have a hereditary predisposition for pseudocroup, which is twice as common in boys as in girls. A child may have several attacks of pseudocroup before age 3, whereas recurrences of epiglottitis are extremely rare.

PATHOGENESIS AND PATHOLOGY. The generally clear-cut distinction between the manifestations of supraglottic and subglottic infections (epiglottitis and psuedocroup) is due to differences in the anatomy of the two regions. At the level of the true vocal cords, the mucosa is firmly attached to the underlying cartilage. In contrast, the supra- and subglottic mucosa and submucosa are quite loosely connected to the underlying tissue. Therefore, when infected, these tissues tend to become very swollen, which may lead to a life-threatening obstruction of the air passages (Fig. 1). In most cases of acute epiglottitis, the inflammatory edema is most pronounced in the epiglottis, which may become several times larger than normal. Occasionally the epiglottis is only slightly inflamed, while other parts of the supraglottic region show more pronounced inflammatory edema.

In acute epiglottitis, the submucosa is edematous and enormously infiltrated with polymorphonuclear and mononuclear cells. Interstitial hemorrhage and thrombosis of the small vessels in the submucosa are prominent. The mucosa, especially over the epiglottis, is markedly edematous, hemorrhagic, and sometimes even necrotic (Kissane and Smith, 1967). Abscesses may also develop.

The pathogenesis of the intense inflammatory changes that occur in acute epiglottitis, especially when they are caused by *H. influenzae* type b, has not yet been clarified. The epiglottic region is probably the route of entry for the bacteria. As such, there may be local accumulation of *H. influenzae* endotoxin with induction of the local Shwartzman phenomenon. In addition, it may be that sensitization to the causative organism must be present before the clinical picture of acute epiglottitis can develop, since patients with acute epiglottitis are in an age group in which specific antibodies against *H. influenzae* capsular polysaccharide can be demonstrated in most individuals. In acute epiglottitis, an allergic reaction of the Arthus type might also contribute to the pronounced pathologic changes (Branefors-Helander and Jeppsson, 1975).

The pathogenesis of the respiratory obstruction associated with epiglottitis appears to be related to the anatomy of the area. The considerable edema swells the epiglottis, which curls posteriorly and inferiorly. In combination with the edema of the other supraglottic tissues, the airway is

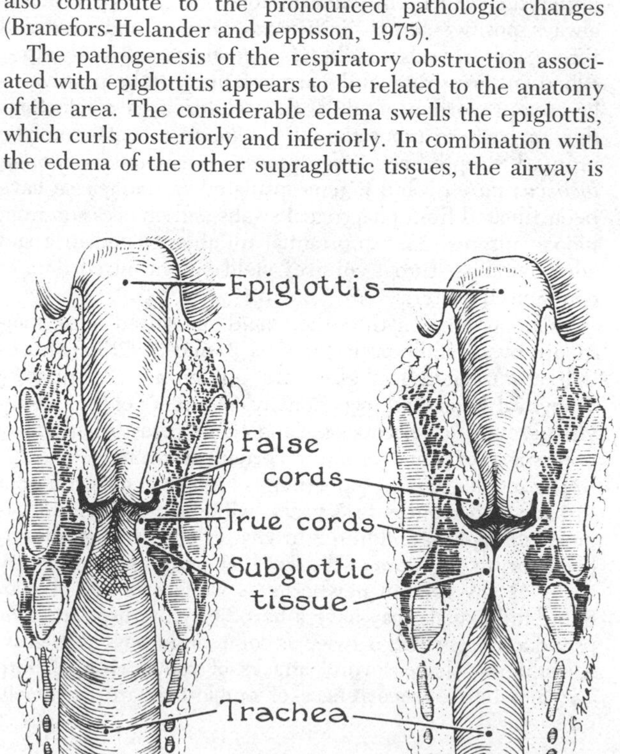

Figure 1. Larynx and trachea. Compare the normal anatomy on the left with the typical changes of pseudocroup on the right. (From Krugman and Ward: Infectious Diseases of Children. 4th ed. St. Louis, C. V. Mosby Company, 1968.)

narrowed, especially during inspiration when the tissues are forced downward, creating a ball-valve effect. As a result, hypoxia ensues but not hypercarbia, since expiration can continue normally. Sitting up, leaning forward, and breathing slowly appear to maximize the airway lumen.

The pathologic findings in fatal cases of pseudocroup are edema and a predominantly mononuclear infiltrate. The bronchi may be plugged with a thick, gummy exudate that accumulates as a result of the inflammation and the ineffectual cough. This exudate can cause atelectasis and further respiratory distress.

CLINICAL MANIFESTATIONS. Acute epiglottitis is a true medical emergency because in children, sudden respiratory obstruction may occur without warning at any time, even during early stages of the infection. The onset is usually sudden, although slight symptoms such as a sore throat and vomiting may have preceded the symptoms of croup for one or two days. In children, the interval from apparent health to severe symptoms may be as short as 2 to 3 hours and is usually less than 24 hours. In adults, the onset is often more insidious and the symptoms less severe, but hyperacute courses may also occur. Children have a high fever (around 39° to 40° C) more commonly than adults. Throat pain is often severe. High fever accompanies *H. influenzae* type b septicemia. Patients, especially children, often have a toxic appearance; a pale, ashen color is more typical than true cyanosis. Patients with advanced illness have respiratory distress with slow, difficult breathing, and they may have inspiratory stridor (a harsh, rasping sound on respiration). Accessory respiratory muscles may be used, and there is retraction of the suprasternal notch and intercostal muscles. Because of pain the patient refuses to eat and drink and often has difficulty swallowing the saliva. Therefore, drooling is a common sign of acute epiglottitis. The patient refuses to lie down but prefers to sit up with head forward, neck extended, and with open mouth. Small children may be in a state of fatigue and lie down quietly (a late ominous sign).

An attack of pseudocroup is usually preceded by symptoms of a slight upper respiratory tract infection. In some cases, however, the child is apparently healthy when he goes to sleep but awakens in the night with stridor, a hollow, barking cough, and a hoarse voice. In severe cases the patient displays marked dyspnea and loud inspiratory stridor. The child uses the accessory respiratory muscles, and breathes with intercostal, supraclavicular, and epigastric retractions. The child with pseudocroup has no sore throat and no difficulty swallowing. The temperature in pseudocroup is normal or only slightly elevated, rarely above 38.5° C. An attack may last for only a few hours, although a duration of one or two days is more common. Some children may have several attacks of pseudocroup during the winter months.

COMPLICATIONS. Most patients with acute epiglottitis have an uneventful recovery, provided that the correct diagnosis is made early and adequate treatment is started immediately. The severest course of acute epiglottitis involves sudden respiratory obstruction leading to cardiac arrest and death. The respiratory obstruction may be caused either by secretions or by the edematous epiglottis. A relatively common complication of acute epiglottitis is pneumonia. A more unusual complication is acute *H. influenzae* type b meningitis, a consequence of the septicemia.

DIAGNOSIS. Patients with acute epiglottitis are often admitted to the hospital with an incorrect diagnosis, most commonly pseudocroup. The diagnosis of acute epiglottitis is established by the clinical symptoms. Dysphagia with refusal to eat and drink and inability to swallow the saliva is pathognomonic. The child with pseudocroup, on the other hand, has the typical hollow barking cough and an inspiratory stridor, but no difficulty swallowing. The diagnosis of acute epiglottitis may sometimes be confirmed by rapid direct inspection of the pharynx. A bright red cherry-like epiglottis may be seen. The importance of minimizing disturbance and avoiding attempts at visualization of the epiglottis in the absence of a skilled team cannot be overemphasized because improper examination can cause laryngeal spasm, total obstruction of the air passage, and cardiac arrest. Further, the patient should be in a sitting position when examined. Respiratory distress is a late sign in acute epiglottitis and necessitates urgent action. In all cases of suspected epiglottitis, the patient should immediately be sent to the nearest emergency unit or ENT department. If possible, the physician should accompany the patient to the hospital and be prepared to try mouth-to-mouth resuscitation if respiration ceases.

At the hospital, the diagnosis may be confirmed by indirect laryngoscopy if equipment for immediate intubation is available. The clinical picture is so characteristic that there is no need for diagnostic studies like x-ray, which may delay the adequate treatment, i.e., to ensure an open airway. In pseudocroup, a narrowed air passage below the larynx is visible in radiographs, which may also help to exclude the possibility of a foreign body in the air passages or the esophagus. A foreign object is one of the common causes of sudden respiratory distress with cough in small children and must be excluded before intubation is performed.

Another differential diagnosis to bear in mind in patients with respiratory distress and stridor is allergic edema of the larynx (angioneurotic edema). In these cases, a history of previous allergic manifestations is generally obtained. Although it is now a rare disease, diphtheritic croup must also be considered. The onset in diphtheria is generally more insidious, and the diphtheritic membranes may be seen on the pharynx as well. A peritonsillar abscess may cause severe pain, dysphagia, and a muffled voice, but does not usually cause rapidly developing airway obstruction. Retropharyngeal abscess must also be considered, but pain is not usually as severe. Tonsillar and retropharyngeal infections are usually accompanied by cervical swelling due to edema and adenitis, while patients with epiglottitis usually have normal cervical nodes, probably because of the hyperacute onset. In adults, the possibility of a laryngeal tumor should also be considered.

GEOGRAPHIC VARIATIONS. Both diseases are illnesses of the temperate zones of the world. There are great variations in the frequency of acute epiglottitis from year to year as well as from season to season. Cases may occur any time of the year, although they are most common during the winter months. In areas where acute epiglottitis is comparatively common (e.g., Scandinavia), cases tend to occur in small groups, probably reflecting the epidemiologic situation in the community. Pseudocroup is most common during the cold season.

TREATMENT. An artificial airway must be provided in most children with acute epiglottitis and sometimes in adults. Tracheostomy or intubation should be performed. Most literature today favors nasotracheal intubation but we feel that both methods can be used with low complication rates if properly managed (Kinnefors and Olofsson, 1983). In pseudocroup an artificial airway is seldom necessary.

In addition to these measures, the patient with epiglottitis is to be treated with antibiotics. Earlier, the drug of choice was ampicillin. However, high rates of β-lactamase-mediated ampicillin resistance of *H. influenzae* strains have been reported (USA 20 to 25 per cent, Canada 13 per cent, and Sweden 5 to 7 per cent). This fact indicates that ampicillin may no longer be used routinely as the drug of choice. We recommend as a reliable alternative a β-lactamase-resistant cephalosporin in the treatment of a potentially fatal infection such as acute epiglottitis. It is advisable to take samples for bacterial cultivation both from the blood and the epiglottic region, if possible, in order to investigate the drug resistance pattern. Antibiotics are not indicated in pseudocroup, but steroids may be efficacious. A humid atmosphere with increased oxygen is beneficial for patients with either acute epiglottitis or pseudocroup. Dehydration should be avoided by the administration of parenteral fluids.

References

Branefors-Helander, P., and Jeppsson, P.-H.: Acute epiglottitis. A clinical, bacteriological and serological study. Scand J Infect Dis 7:103, 1975.

Kinnefors, A., and Olofsson, J.: Acute epiglottitis in children: Experiences with tracheotomy and intubation. Clin Otolaryngol 8:25, 1983.

Kissane, J. M., and Smith, M. G.: Pathology of Infancy and Childhood. 2nd ed. St. Louis, C. V. Mosby Company, 1967.

101

LUDWIG'S ANGINA

BURT R. MEYERS, M.D.

In 1836, Wilhelm Frederick von Ludwig, a Stuttgart physician, read a detailed report to the local medical society describing five cases of infections involving the floor of the mouth (von Ludwig, 1836). This clinical condition was known as morbus strangulatorius, garotillo (Spanish after the hangman's loop), angina maligne, and cynanche (dog choking), all referring to the respiratory obstruction so prominent in this syndrome. Ludwig's original description of a rapidly spreading cellulitis or phlegmon, brawny in character, originating in the area of the submaxillary gland and extending by continuity without involving the lymph nodes, has been only slightly modified by subsequent investigators. The infection may start in either the sublingual or the submaxillary space (Fig. 1), but must involve both in order to meet the criteria of Ludwig's syndrome. Involvement of only the submaxillary space with suppuration has been called pseudo-Ludwig's angina.

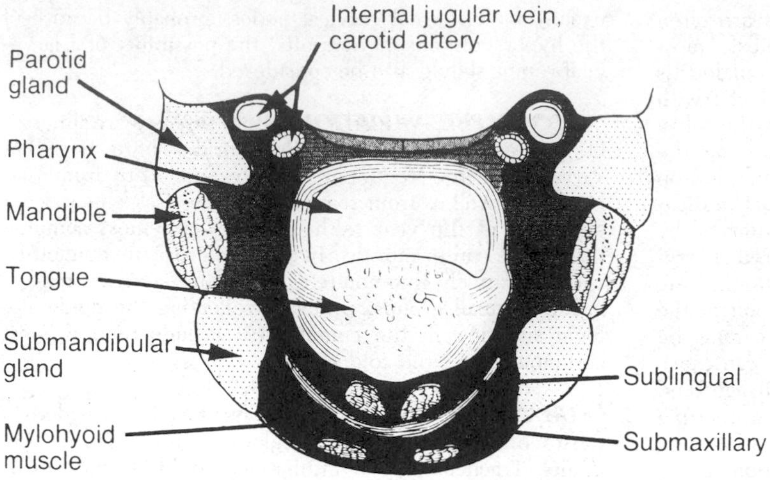

Figure 1. Oblique section of top of neck shows continuity of sublingual and submaxillary spaces and potential for spread of infection from one to another. (From Johnson and Tucker, 1976.)

ETIOLOGY. From 51 to 90 per cent of the cases are related to a dental extraction. Ludwig's angina has also followed lacerations of the floor of the mouth, mandibular fractures, foreign bodies, and peritonsillar abscess. Systemic disease may play a role because cases have occurred in patients with acute and chronic glomerulonephritis, systemic lupus erythematosus, diabetes mellitus, hypersensitivity states, malnutrition, and aplastic anemia, and in those who are immunosuppressed. In the author's experience, patients are frequently chronic alcoholics who engage in a drinking bout after dental extraction.

The bacteria responsible for the infection are believed to originate from the oral flora. The earlier investigators found predominantly streptococci, both hemolytic and nonhemolytic. Staphylococci, including *S. aureus* and *S. epidermidis*, have also been isolated, although the role of the latter is not clear. Fusiform bacillae and spiralla-like forms have been seen on smear, and in some cases foul-smelling pus has been described. Although references were made earlier to the possibility that anaerobes were involved, no anaerobic cultures were obtained until recently, when case reports of anaerobic infection have appeared (Maki and Agger, 1977; Gross, 1976).

Gram-negative aerobic bacteria, including *Escherichia coli*, *Pseudomonas aeruginosa*, and *Haemophilus influenzae*, have been noted. In many cases, however, mixed cultures were recovered.

PATHOLOGY AND PATHOGENESIS. Infection occurs primarily in the submandibular space, an area that extends from the mucous membranes of the floor of the mouth superiorly to the muscle and facial attachment of the hyoid bone below. The mylohyoid muscles divide the space horizontally into the sublingual space superiorly and the submaxillary space inferiorly.

Extractions of the second and third molar teeth are implicated in the pathogenesis of this syndrome because the position of their root apices beneath the mylohyoid ridge and the relative thinness of the mandibular alveolar bone lingually give dental infections ready access to the submaxillary space (Fig. 2). Following extraction, hairline fractures may occur in the lingual cortex of the mandible,

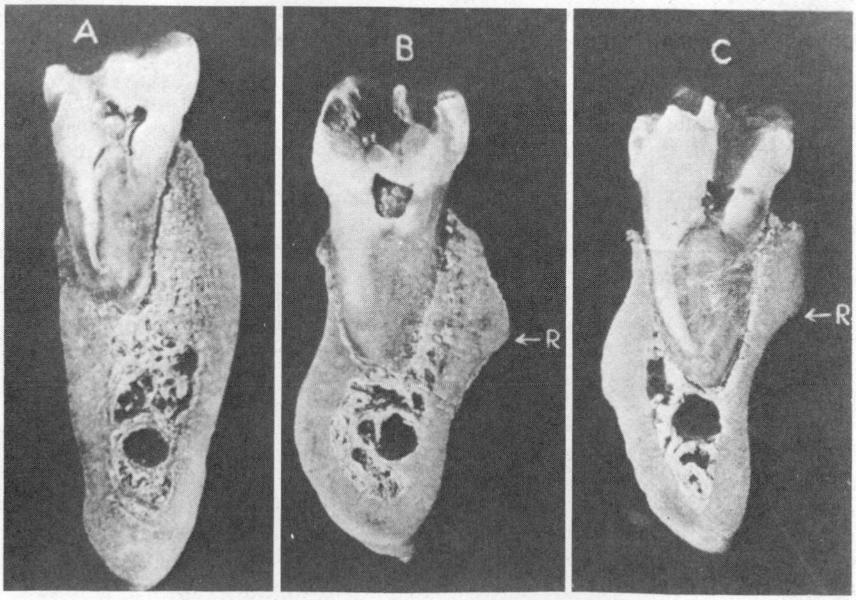

Figure 2. Cross-sections through to mandible: *A*, first molar tooth; *B*, second molar tooth; *C*, third molar. Note the difference in the relation of the mylohyoid ridge (R) to the apices of the teeth. The second and third molar teeth have roots below the mylohyoid ridge and are more likely to cause submaxillary cellulitis. The first molar is more likely to cause sublingual infection. (From Tschiassny, K., 1943.)

and these, coupled with pulp infections, may explain the egress of bacteria. The apices of the premolars and often the first molar are superior to the mylohyoid ridge, and when infections occur, they enter the sublingual space. When the sublingual space is infected, edema, swelling, and elevation of the tongue develop. As this space becomes progressively involved, the tongue is displaced, and the supraglottic larynx becomes edematous and distorted, compromising the airway.

Following the fascial planes, the infection may dissect into the parapharyngeal or pharyngeomaxillary space, giving it access to the carotid sheath. The internal carotid may form a mycotic aneurysm and its erosion may cause massive hemorrhage. Further extension may result in thromboses of the internal jugular vein or cavernous sinus thrombosis. Dissection into the superior mediastinum, involving the pericardium and pleural space, has been observed by the author.

In most cases the involved areas are brawny, indurated, and edematous and are involved with a spreading cellulitis that may be gangrenous. The salivary glands and lymph nodes are usually spared. However, in some cases drainage of the tooth sockets or abscess formation in the neck has been described.

CLINICAL MANIFESTATIONS. Most patients present with painful swelling of the face and neck. There is usually a history of dental extraction, recent dental pain, infection, or some intraoral problem such as gingivitis (Maki and Agger, 1977). Fever and tachycardia are usually present. Depending on the extent of tongue involvement, the patient will complain of dysphagia, drooling, and dyspnea. Signs of dehydration may develop. Trismus occurs when the internal pterygoid muscles are involved, and this implies that the infection has spread to the pharyngomaxillary space.

Oral, facial, cervical, and even supraclavicular swelling may be found on examination. The neck may have a bull-like appearance. The involved areas are indurated, painful, and usually not fluctuant. The tongue may enlarge and protrude from the mouth. The tongue is often edematous and elevated, touching the roof of the mouth. There is swelling of the submental and submaxillary spaces, often bilaterally. The lymph nodes and submaxillary glands are not involved. A recent extraction site or carious tooth may be noted. Respiratory obstruction causes stridor and cyanosis. Massive hemoptysis may follow vascular erosion. When the mediastinum is involved, anterior chest pain signifies pericarditis. Pleuritic chest pain and pleural effusion suggest mediastinal extension. Patients may have patchy aspiration pneumonia.

DIAGNOSIS. Facial swelling, a swollen tongue, and thickening of the floor of the mouth suggest the diagnosis of Ludwig's angina. The patient may present with respiratory distress (Meyers, 1972). The oral cavity must be examined and any areas of suppuration aspirated for Gram stain and culture, both aerobically and anaerobically. Gram stain of the aspirate may reveal mixed flora, and a fetid odor indicates anaerobic infection. Blood cultures should also be performed.

TREATMENT. The mainstay of therapy is to ensure an adequate airway. Since respiratory obstruction occurs very rapidly, patients must be constantly observed for this development. At the first signs of respiratory embarrassment, early tracheostomy under local anesthesia is mandatory. Since swallowing is often impaired and aspiration a possibility, a cuffed tracheostomy tube is recommended. Because of the distortion of the upper airway, direct laryngoscopy and intubation are potentially dangerous, for they may result in laryngospasm and sudden death. Fiberoptic laryngoscopy and intubation can secure an airway and avoid tracheostomy.

In the severely ill patient, antibiotic coverage at first should be directed at four possible groups of bacteria: (1) penicillinase-producing staphylococci, (2) gram-negative enteric organisms, (3) streptococci, and (4) anaerobes. Though most oral anaerobes are sensitive to penicillin, recent isolates of *Bacteroides melaninogenicus* that produce a beta lactamase have been reported (Murray, 1977). A dose of clindamycin 600 mg every six hours I.V. and oxacillin 2.0 g every three hours I.V. should be given along with gentamicin or tobramycin in doses adjusted for age and renal function. Third generation cephalosporins, which are beta-lactamase stable, may be used as alternate therapy. When culture and sensitivity reports are available, therapy may be adjusted accordingly.

In the pre-antibiotic era various drainage procedures through submandibular and intraoral incisions were performed. The rationale was to decompress the submandibular space; however, in one report suppuration was found in only 1 of 51 cases. Incision and drainage should be performed only in the presence of fluctuation. If the infection extends into the parapharyngeal space, drainage of this deep neck infection is usually required by an external approach.

References

Gross, B. D.: Ludwig's angina due to bacteroides. J Oral Surg 34:456, 1976.

Johnson, J. T., and Tucker, H. M.: Recognizing and treating deep neck infection. Postgrad Med 59:95, 1976.

Maki, D., and Agger, W. A.: Morbid Mortal Weekly Report 26:199, 1977.

Meyers, B. R., Lawson, W., and Hirschman, S. Z.: Ludwig's angina. Case report, with review of bacteriology and current therapy. Am J Med 53:257, 1972.

Murray, P. R., and Rosenblatt, J. E.: Penicillin resistance and penicillinase production in clinical isolates of Bacteroides melaninogenicus. Antimicrob Agents Chemother 11:605, 1977.

Tschiassny, K.: Ludwig's angina. An anatomic study of the role of the lower molar teeth in its pathogenesis. Arch Otolaryngol 38:485.

von Ludwig, F. W.: Eine neue Art von Halsentzeundung. Med Cor Bl Württemb arztl Ver 6:21, 1836.

102
ACTINOMYCOSIS

ABRAHAM I. BRAUDE, M.D., PH.D.

Actinomycosis is a noncontagious infection produced by an anaerobic organism normally resident in the mouth, bowel, and female genital tract. The disease is characterized by chronic inflammatory induration and sinus formation.

ETIOLOGY. The causative agent is *Actinomyces israelii*, a branching gram-positive filamentous organism. Another actinomycete, *Arachnia propionica*, may produce chronic abscesses and draining sinuses.

Intolerance of free oxygen and failure to grow on Sabouraud's medium distinguish *A. israelii* from *Nocardia* and other actinomycetes. On blood agar, colonies require 4 to 6 days of anaerobic incubation at 37° C to reach a size of 1 to 2 mm. Although most strains require anaerobic conditions for isolation, some can be subcultured aerobically in 10 to 20 per cent carbon dioxide. *Actinomyces israelii* has never been found outside human beings or animals, and case-to-case transmission is unknown. *Ar. propionica* resembles *A. israelii* in oxygen intolerance, colonial morphology, and microscopic appearance. Distinction is based on the ability of *Ar. propionica* to produce large amounts of propionic acid and the presence of diaminopimelic acid in its cell wall (Brock et al., 1973).

PATHOGENESIS. The oxidation-reduction potential of normal tissues is probably too high for multiplication of *A. israelii* but dead tissues allow it to reproduce and spread. The frequency of actinomycosis of the face and neck may be explained by the greater population of *A. israelii* on teeth, in carious teeth, and in tonsillar crypts, and by trauma from eating, dental procedures, or infection with oral bacteria. Anaerobic conditions also prevail in atelectatic areas of the lung after aspiration of *A. israelii* so that pulmonary actinomycosis can develop. It is also conceivable that pulmonary actinomycosis may arise hematogenously from an infected focus in the mouth. Mediastinal actinomycosis probably spreads from the esophagus into the superior or posterior mediastinum, quickly involving the pleura to produce early pleural effusion or empyema, and then tending to attack the adjacent ribs and vertebral bodies. Eventually mediastinal actinomycosis produces abscesses that point in the paravertebral region. Ileocecal actinomycosis is the most common intestinal form, occurring after appendiceal rupture and the escape of actinomycetes to form an inflammatory mass in the right iliac fossa. The liver is the solid abdominal viscus most frequently attacked by actinomycosis. Grossly the lesions resemble large metastatic tumor masses, which undergo necrosis and abscess formation. The abscesses become loculated and the liver takes on a honeycombed appearance (Cope, 1952). *A. israelii* is a frequent member of the normal flora in the genital tract of women and can invade the surrounding tissues when they are traumatized by intrauterine devices (Grice and Hafiz, 1983).

From foci in the jaw, lung, or intestine, actinomycosis may spread by contiguity or through the bloodstream to the liver, spine, brain, kidneys, genitalia, spleen, and subcutaneous tissues. Lymphatic spread is rare and actinomycosis of lymph nodes probably never occurs (Colebrook, 1921).

The inflammatory reaction to *A. israelii* is characterized by three features: (1) chronic suppuration, (2) extensive necrosis, and (3) intense fibrosis. The so-called "sulfur granules" in the inflammatory lesion are composed of intertwined mycelial filaments, or colonies, of *A. israelii*.

CLINICAL MANIFESTATIONS. The essential feature of actinomycosis is a painful, indurated swelling. This lesion may appear over the jaw a week or more after such trauma as tooth extraction or compound fracture of the mandible. As it increases in size, points of suppuration—the openings of fistulas—appear on the bluish red surface of the edematous skin. Trismus is prominent early. Cervical lymphadenopathy is rare.

The lower lobes of the lung are frequently affected, and the disease suddenly becomes evident when the pleura and chest wall are involved by direct extension from the lung. Physical examination at this time reveals a diffuse, tender, indurated swelling of the chest wall with pulmonary consolidation and empyema. Until then the patient may notice only fever, cough, and expectoration. In fact, the symptoms may be so mild that they are thought to be those of mild bronchitis. When fever and severe cough occur, a chest x-ray may be taken and consolidation found (Fig. 1); frequently the diagnosis is not made until the chest wall is invaded.

Abdominal actinomycosis is often mistaken for appendicitis, carcinoma of the cecum, tuberculosis, or amebiasis. Patients with abdominal actinomycosis are subjected to surgery for drainage of a supposed appendiceal abscess, and the true nature of the disease may be recognized only when an indurated draining sinus stubbornly refuses to heal.

Actinomycosis may also be mistaken for tumor of the reproductive organs in women or for tuberculous psoas abscess. The ovary and fallopian tube have frequently been the seat of actinomycosis after extension from an appendiceal focus. Lately tubo-ovarian actinomycosis has been associated with intrauterine devices (Hager and Majmudar, 1979). There is nothing pathognomonic that would distinguish the clinical features of genital actinomycosis in women from those of chronic pelvic inflammatory disease, and the diagnosis is often made by examination of a tube or ovary after surgical removal. Sometimes diagnostic pus can be obtained from an abscess pointing through the skin of the groin or buttock, or bulging into the posterior vagina. Rarely, peritonitis develops. Actinomycosis involving the perianal region can cause recurrent multiple draining sinuses and fistulas in ano (Brewer et al., 1974).

Spread to the liver can occur from any abdominal focus via the portal vein. Sometimes the primary focus is inapparent clinically and hepatic actinomycosis appears as an isolated disease. It begins then with fever, sweats, weight loss, and hepatomegaly with or without palpable nodules on the liver surface.

In the rare case of hematogenously disseminated actinomycosis, lesions appear in all parts of the body. Painful indurated nodules or abscesses under the skin of the legs, arms, back, and scalp are prominent, and nonsuppurative effusions of the pleura or pericardium develop. The primary focus for dissemination is usually the lung (Varkey et al., 1974).

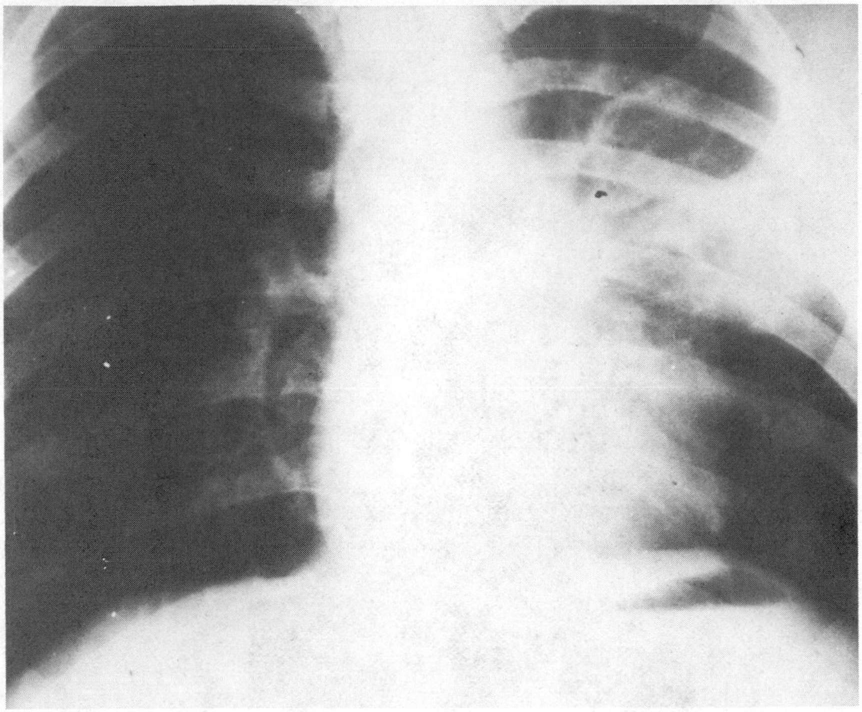

Figure 1. Actinomycosis of the lung. The diagnosis was made when the infection broke through the chest wall and *A. israelii* was found in the pus by gram stain and culture.

The kidneys may be infected during the course of disseminated actinomycosis, or may be the only detectable site of disease. Solitary actinomycosis of the kidney is usually a chronic suppurative process resembling a renal carbuncle. Fever, sweats, and weight loss may precede any sign of renal disease, so that actinomycosis of the kidney may be the source of an unexplained (or cryptic) fever. Eventually tenderness and pain over the kidney and a palpable renal mass will develop.

COMPLICATIONS. The chief complications of all forms of actinomycosis result from direct invasion by contiguous spread into neighboring structures. Thoracic actinomycosis may extend retroperitoneally downward through the diaphragm, medially through the psoas to the vertebrae, or down into the pelvis (Cope, 1952). Hepatic actinomycosis may also rupture through the diaphragm into the lung or through the anterior abdominal wall. Mediastinal actinomycosis attacks adjacent ribs, pericardium, or vertebrae. Actinomycotic osteomyelitis almost always results from contiguous, rather than hematogenous, spread.

The most serious hematogenous complication is actinomycotic brain abscess, which usually spreads from pulmonary actinomycosis.

GEOGRAPHIC VARIATIONS IN DISEASE. Actinomycosis occurs everywhere and anyone may have *A. israelii* as a normal inhabitant of the mouth or bowel. Variations in frequency of actinomycosis will depend on geographic differences in dental hygiene. The old idea that actinomycosis was a disease of farmers because they chewed straws is absurd. The reason some farmers get actinomycosis is that they have bad teeth.

DIAGNOSIS. The disease is easily recognized by detecting *A. israelii* in pus obtained from sinuses, empyema fluid, or abscess cavities. The significance of actinomycetes in sputum is difficult to interpret because the organisms are normal inhabitants of the mouth. Sulfur granules vary in size from several microns to 3 mm in diameter. Large granules are found if a thorough search is made by diluting the pus with saline solution and filtering through gauze. They are white, yellow, or brown and stand out sharply against the background of blood-tinged pus. Gram-positive branching filaments or bacilli that fail to grow aerobically are key findings (Fig. 2). Granules of other organisms (staphylococci, nocardias, monosporia), fragments of caseous material, and clumps of pus cells or fibrin may be confused with actinomycotic granules. Sabouraud's medium will not support the growth of *A. israelii.* Cultural isolation of *A. israelii* is not difficult if anaerobic methods are used. A small gram-negative bacillus, *Actinobacillus actinomycetemcomitans,* is often associated with *A. israelii* in actinomycosis. Anaerobic streptococci, *Bacteroides,* and other anaerobes are also present frequently. Hence actinomycosis is characteristically a mixed anaerobic infection.

Biopsy may suggest the diagnosis if the actinomycotic colony ("ray fungus") is observed microscopically, but cultural proof is necessary for absolute diagnosis. The gram-positive branching rods of *Nocardia asteroides* closely resemble those of *A. israelii* in tissue sections and can be distinguished by the weakly acid-fast properties of *Nocardia.* Cultural differentiation between the two is easy because *N. asteroides* grows well aerobically on Sabouraud's agar and most conventional media. Demonstration of the organism may be difficult, requiring careful search of many sections.

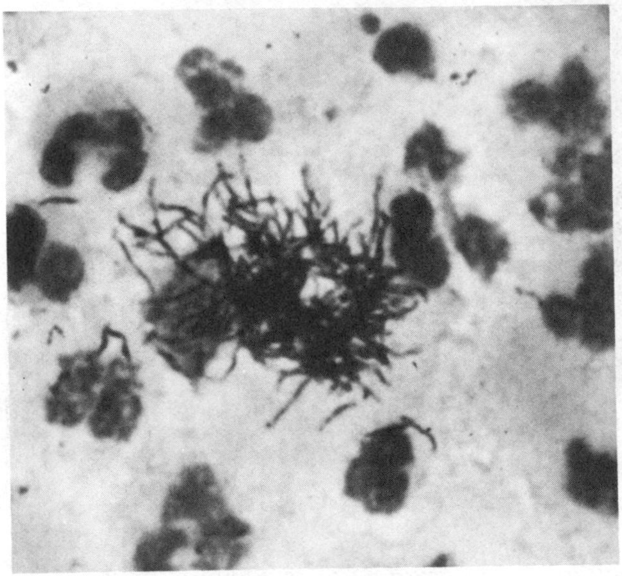

Figure 2. Gram stain of pus from sinus in chest wall of patient in Figure 1. The gram-positive branching filaments were found to be *A. israelli* on culture.

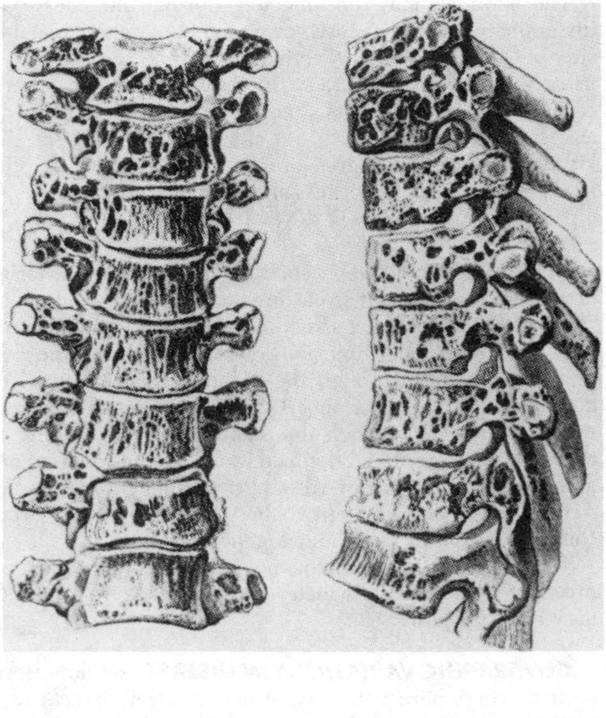

Figure 3. Effect of actinomycosis on the vertebrae. The slow absorption and formation of new bone allow the vertebral body to retain its strength, so that vertebral collapse is rare. The intervertebral disks are also spared, for the most part. Thus spinal actinomycosis differs markedly from tuberculosis, which causes vertebral collapse and disk destruction. In actinomycosis the spine takes on the appearance of a coarse sieve. (From Cope, V. Z.: Human Actinomycosis. London, William Heinemann, Ltd., 1952.)

Intradermal or serologic tests with *A. israelii* or its fractions are of no diagnostic aid. Radiologic examination may suggest actinomycosis if consolidation of the lungs and periosteal proliferation of the ribs are found, because this combination rarely occurs in other conditions (Flynn and Felson, 1970). The appearance of the spine in lateral views may be almost pathognomonic, because the areas of absorption and newly formed bone give a picture of a coarse sieve not seen in any other vertebral disease (Fig. 3).

TREATMENT. Penicillin and the tetracycline antibiotics are so effective that the disease is disappearing through the wide use of these drugs prophylactically after dental extraction and in other conditions that might evolve into actinomycosis. When either is administered in large doses over long periods of time, remarkable improvement may be expected even when the purulent foci are inaccessible to surgical drainage. Many reports indicate that tetracycline is superior to penicillin. When tetracycline is given in doses of 500 mg every 6 hours there is a reduction in pain and swelling within a few days as well as gain in strength, increase in weight, and prompt defervescence. In view of the tendency for actinomycosis to relapse, treatment should be continued for several weeks after the patient appears cured. Because penicillin is no more effective than the tetracyclines and because it requires repeated intramuscular or intravenous injection of large doses for long periods of time, it should be reserved for patients who cannot tolerate tetracycline drugs. The optimum dose of penicillin is not known, but at least 4 million units daily should be given parenterally.

Surgical drainage is a valuable adjunct to chemotherapy and may occasionally lead to spontaneous cure (Colebrook, 1921). Older treatments such as iodides, irradiation, and the sulfonamides have no place in the treatment of actinomycosis, and amphotericin B is of no value.

References

Brewer, N., Spencer, R., and Nichols, D.: Primary anorectal actinomycosis. JAMA 228:1397, 1974.

Brock, D. W., George, L., Brown, J., and Hicklin, M.: Actinomycosis caused by *Arachnia propionica*. Am J Clin Pathol 59:66, 1973.

Colebrook, L.: A report on 25 cases of actinomycosis with special reference to vaccine therapy. Lancet T:893, 1921.

Cope, V. Z.: Human Actinomycosis. London, William Heinemann, Ltd., 1952.

Flynn, M. W., and Felson, B.: The roentgen manifestations of thoracic actinomycosis. Am J Roentgenol 110:707, 1970.

Grice, G., and Hafiz, S.: Actinomyces in the female genital tract. Br J Ven Dis 59:317, 1983.

Hager, W., and Majmudar, B.: Pelvic actinomycosis in women using intrauterine devices. Am J Obst Gynecol 156:60, 1979.

Varkey, B., Landis, F., Tang, T., and Rose, H.: Thoracic actinomycosis: Dissemination to skin, subcutaneous tissue, and muscle. Arch Int Med 134:689, 1974.

103

PHYCOMYCOSIS (ZYGOMYCOSIS)

FRANCIS D. MARTINSON, M.D., CH.B. (ED), F.R.C.S. (ENG & ED)

The term phycomycosis should refer to all infections caused by fungi of the large group Phycomycetes, but it has, by clinical usage, been restricted to those caused by species of two orders, Mucorales and Entomophthorales. Since both belong to Zygomycetes, one of the six classes into which the Phycomycetes have been divided (Ainsworth, 1973), "zygomycosis" is considered a more appropriate collective name, the infections being subdivided into "mucormycosis" and "entomophthoromycosis" (Clark, 1968) according to the order of fungi involved (Fig. 1).

MUCORMYCOSIS

ETIOLOGY. The fungi identified so far include several species of the genera *Rhizopus, Absidia, Mucor, Mortierella, Cunninghamella,* and *Saksenaea*. Like other zygomycetes they are ubiquitous and normally saprobic to man, but these become pathogenic in patients whose resistance has already been compromised by diabetes and other prolonged acidoses, leukemia, kwashiorkor, severe diarrheas, lymphomas, congenital defects of IgA production, and prolonged cytotoxic, steroid, or immunosuppressive therapy. The mucormycoses are therefore described as "opportunistic infections" or more recently as "Asthenomycoses" (Vanbreuseghem and Larsh, 1977). Very occasionally the predisposing factor eludes detection.

PATHOGENESIS AND PATHOLOGY. The fungi penetrate the mucosa of the respiratory or digestive tract or gain entry through lacerations, burns, and occasionally surgical incisions, inducing a granulomatous reaction. They have a propensity for penetrating blood vessels, thereby causing thromboses, infarcts, and hemorrhages, and being disseminated to all organs. Secondary infection often supervenes.

On microscopy large numbers of neutrophils but very few eosinophils are seen; very occasionally lymphocytes and plasma cells may predominate. There are scattered areas of infarcts and hemorrhages. Fungi are easily identified with hematoxylin-eosin stains but less so with Grocott's methenamine silver. They are often seen penetrating vascular walls. Fibrosis is rarely present except in those granulomas occasionally seen at the site of prolonged intravenous infusion lines, or in the rare sclerosing orbital lesion in which the tuberculoid giant cell granuloma may also be present. Also rare is the circumfungal eosinophilic mantle often seen in entomophthoromycosis (vide infra).

CLINICAL MANIFESTATIONS. The disease affects any age and either sex. The clinical features vary according to the sites of commencement or main activity of the granuloma. These sites are the head and neck, bronchopulmonary region, digestive tract, superficial tissues, and other deep-seated foci. Infection from any of these may at any stage become disseminated.

Head and Neck Infection. Various self-explanatory names such as rhino-orbital, rhinocerebral, orbital, orbitocerebral, facial and nasal, and rhinomucormycosis have

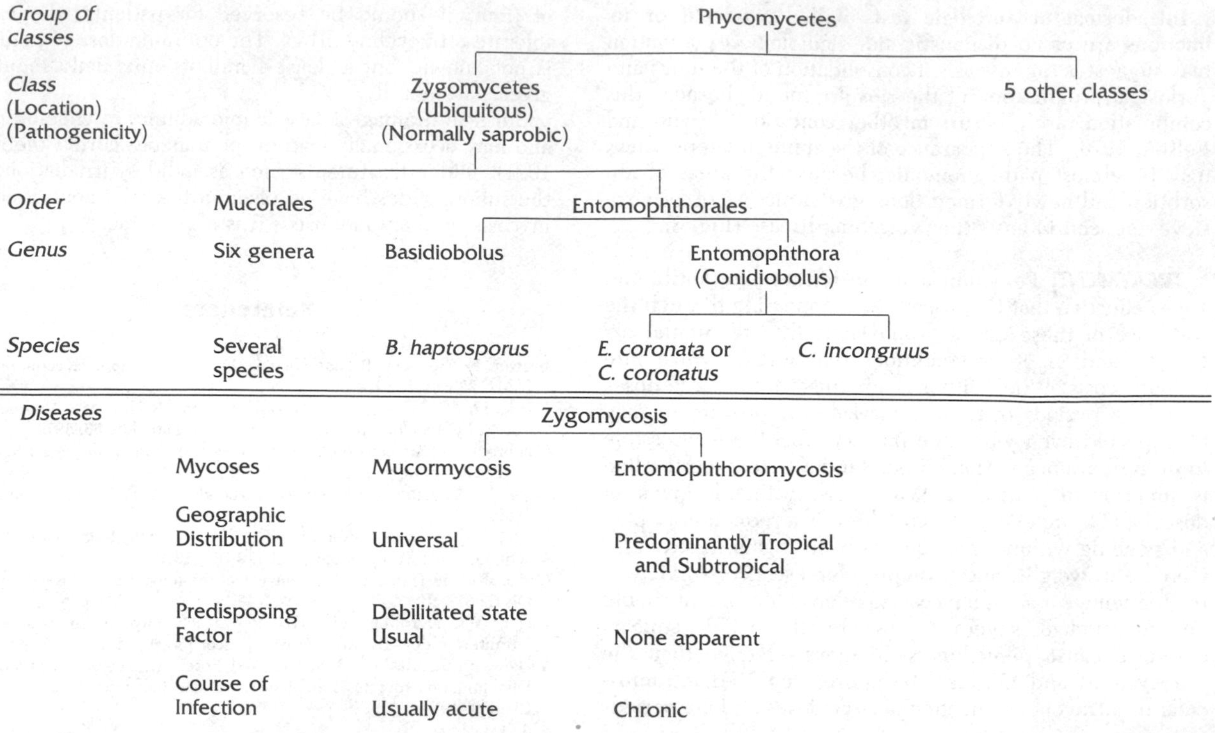

Figure 1. Classification of Phycomycetes and human zygomycoses.

been used to indicate the site of involvement. The infection almost invariably starts in the nose or paranasal sinuses. On inspection the granuloma is covered by black or brown crusts and foul, blood-stained discharge. Subsequent progress depends on the direction and rate of local or vascular spread. There may be swelling of the nose and cheek, followed by ulceration through to the face or palate. Spread to the orbit produces orbital edema, proptosis, ophthalmoplegia, loss of vision, deep pain, and anesthesia of the face around the eye. Intracranial spread direct from the nose or via the orbit produces evidence of meningitis, cerebral infarct or hemorrhage, or cavernous sinus thrombosis. Vascular dissemination may be early or late, commonly spreading to the lung first.

Diagnosis. Radiographic appearances are nonspecific and may resemble those of sinusitis or malignancy.

Biopsy is taken for both histopathologic examination and mycologic culture. A predisposing factor or a history of administration of immunosuppressives should arouse suspicion.

Conditions simulated are acute sinusitis, osteomyelitis, carbuncle, rhinitis caseosa, malignant tumors, cancrum (noma), orbitoethmoidal aspergilloma, midline lethal granuloma, and Burkitt's lymphoma.

Bronchopulmonary Infection. This is due to inhalation of infected material from the upper respiratory tract or to vascular dissemination from another site. Symptoms consist of dyspnea, cough, hemoptysis, and sometimes progressive or sudden chest pain. Later the lesions may spread to the mediastinal viscera (esophagus or pericardium) or outward to the chest wall or may disseminate further.

Diagnosis. Here also radiologic features are not specific and, like the symptoms, may suggest pneumonia, tuberculosis (with or without cavitation), neoplasm, or pulmonary embolism. Examination of the sputum often does not reveal the fungus. The true diagnosis is usually made after pneumonectomy and histopathologic examination of the specimen, and at this stage it is often too late.

Digestive Tract Lesions. These may be due to ingestion of infected material, direct spread to the esophagus from the lungs, or vascular spread. Ulcers, usually multiple in the stomach, form in the wall of the viscus, or a nutrient vessel may be thrombosed, leading to local gangrene. Hematemesis, melena, and perforation with peritonitis are late signs which also suggest various intra-abdominal emergencies; hence the correct diagnosis is made occasionally after laparotomy but more often at necropsy.

Focal Infection. This may, uncommonly, occur in other intra-abdominal organs, for example, the kidney, spleen, or liver, sometimes without evidence of the mode of entry; hence diagnosis is made only after surgical intervention and histopathologic examination of the diseased viscus.

Superficial Lesions. Superficial lesions may be acute, presenting as a spreading necrosis from a deep-seated lesion or commencing in a laceration, burn, or surgical wound. There is usually an obvious predisposing factor. They may present also as a chronic ulcer or, rarely, a granuloma at the site of prolonged intravenous infusion. There is often no predisposing factor and in some cases the infection may be self-limiting.

Infections may appear disseminated almost from the start or may become so as a complication originating from one of the sites previously mentioned.

TREATMENT. Most patients die because diagnosis is too late, but a few patients, diagnosed before dissemination or irreversible damage, have been successfully treated by a combination of medical therapy and excision of the affected organ. Occasionally early infection may resolve spontaneously after cure or control of the underlying disease, especially diabetes.

The predisposing disease must first be identified and controlled or cured if treatment is to succeed. In a diabetic, for example, the hyperglycemia and acidosis must be corrected rapidly. Second, affected tissue must be excised if possible, or surgical drainage carried out. Third, intravenous amphotericin B, the specific drug for this infection, should be given in doses of 50 mg intravenously daily for a total dose of approximately 2.2 g.

ENTOMOPHTHOROMYCOSIS

There are three known clinical syndromes caused by fungi that are normally saprobic yet become pathogenic without apparent predisposing adverse host conditions.

Basidiobolomycosis (Syn. Entomophthoromycosis basidiobolae)

This name was coined by Vanbreuseghem (1966) for the disease first described by Lie Kian Joe and his colleagues in 1956 under the name subcutaneous phycomycosis.

ETIOLOGY. The disease is caused by *Basidiobolus haptosporus (meristosporus).*

PATHOGENESIS AND PATHOLOGY. The infection follows traumatic implantation of the fungus. It begins and spreads as a subcutaneous granuloma, often infiltrating muscle but never bone. Regional lymph glands may occasionally undergo reactive hyperplasia but do not become infected except occasionally when engulfed and infiltrated by the advancing granuloma. The blood picture is not affected.

The granuloma is tough and creamy pink. Its cut surface is homogeneous or streaky and studded with occasional small abscesses. If cut up, digested in potassium hydroxide, teased out, and examined microscopically, the hyphae are easily recognized. They usually show up poorly in sections stained with hematoxylin and eosin but well with Grocott's methanamine silver. In the former they often exhibit the "Hoeppli-Splendore phenomenon" (Fig. 2), a strongly eosinophilic mantle considered by Williams and colleagues (1969) to be antigen-antibody reaction. Eosinophils are numerous but fibrosis predominates in older areas. Microabscesses may be seen with fungi in them or within multinucleate giant cells (Fig. 3). Tuberculoid giant cell granulomas are present. Reported vascular penetration is atypical and very rarely observed.

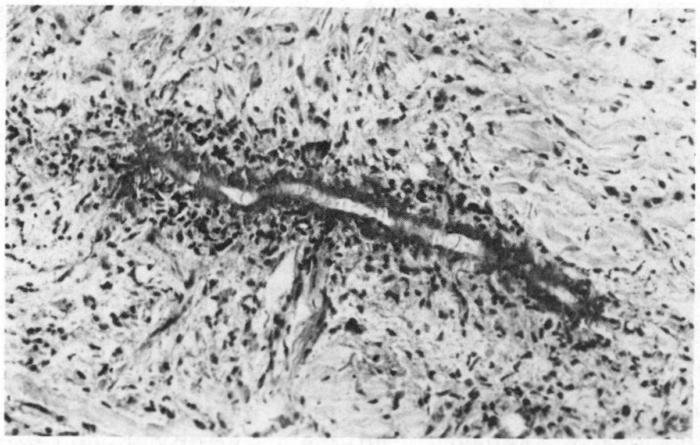

Figure 2. Fungus cut longitudinally surrounded by amorphous mantle, the "Hoeppli-Splendore phenomenon," and chronic inflammatory reaction. (From Martinson, F. D.: Rhinophycomycosis. J Laryng 77:691, 1963.)

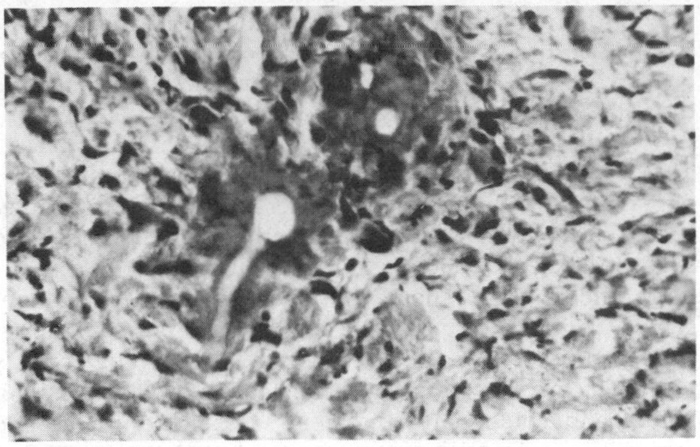

Figure 3. Hyphae cut across and longitudinally, lying in microabscess. (From Martinson, F. D.: Rhinophycomycosis. J Laryng 77:691, 1963.)

CLINICAL MANIFESTATIONS. About 80 per cent of all patients are under 10 years old. Males outnumber females by about 3:1. The lesion commences anywhere on the body but commonly the lower half and sometimes simultaneously at more than one site. It enlarges slowly to become a painless smooth or lobulated mass, characteristically very firm with palpably discrete borders—a diagnostic feature—and is freely movable over underlying muscles until it invades them. It may become enormous after several months and cross anatomic regional boundaries. The penis, vulva, and scrotum are not spared. There are no constitutional disturbances. The overlying skin does not usually ulcerate unless traumatized, and then secondary bacterial or other fungal infection may occur.

COMPLICATIONS AND SEQUELAE. Infiltrating perineal muscles, the granuloma enters the pelvis and obstructs the rectum, ureter, or sometimes the iliac vessels, or in the neck may involve the perilaryngeal muscles, causing obstruction. Very extensive and longstanding involvement of an arm has been followed by muscle atrophy. Deaths are rare and usually due to secondary fungal or bacterial infection, including tetanus. Also rare are totally resistant lesions that eventually require amputation of the affected part. Spontaneous arrest of spread is uncommon and spontaneous resolution of the granuloma is rare except in a few early cases. Complete cure can be achieved but disfigurement and malfunction due to extensive fibrosis in older areas of the lesion may often persist. It is uncertain whether reinfection can occur after cure.

DIAGNOSIS. Radiography will rule out upper respiratory tract involvement, bony lesions, and calcified parasitic infections. Biopsy should be taken from the growing edges where the typical granuloma and viable culturable fungi are usually found. Mycologic culture is imperative for accurate diagnosis.

DIFFERENTIAL DIAGNOSIS. In the head and neck, cervical adenitis, neoplasm, facial onchocerciasis, and rhinoentomophthoromycosis should be excluded. In the foot the absence of discharging sinuses and bony involvement rules out mycetoma. Lymphedema is much less firm, has no discrete edge, and usually extends distally to the toes.

TREATMENT. Between 1.5 and 3.5 g of potassium iodide, depending on the age of the patient, is given three times a day. The combination of trimethoprim, 160 mg, and sulfamethoxazole, 800 mg, orally twice a day is usually more effective and should be given first trial. Treatment should continue for at least a month after the swellings have completely subsided because one cannot judge exactly when the fungi have been adequately controlled or eliminated, and inadequate treatment leads to resistance and apparent recurrence. As long as treatment is adequate in dosage and duration, a successful outcome can be anticipated in cases that are uncomplicated by secondary infection or not unduly neglected before treatment is sought.

Rhinoentomophthoromycosis (Syn. Rhinophycomycosis entomophthorae; Rhinophycomycosis; Entomophthoromycosis conidiobolae)

Various names have been given to this disease but this one coined by Clark (1968) is generally accepted.

ETIOLOGY. The causative organism, *Entomophthora coronata (Conidiobolus coronatus),* was first identified in nasal granulomas in horses by Emmons and Bridges in 1961, and in human infection by Bras and co-workers in 1965. Infection follows traumatic implantation of the spores by an insect or a fingernail.

PATHOGENESIS AND PATHOLOGY. The granuloma commences in the submucosa, usually of the inferior turbinate, and spreads without ulcerating to the nasopharynx or paranasal sinuses and externally through interosseous sutures and foramina without eroding bone (Fig. 4). In the face it soon invades muscle and becomes closely applied to the skin but does not ulcerate it.

Histopathologic features are identical to those of basidiobolomycosis previously described. Differentiation is therefore by mycologic culture.

CLINICAL MANIFESTATIONS. About 80 per cent of all cases occur in adolescents or adults, with a male to female ratio of about 8:1. The inferior turbinate is large and nonulcerated. There is nasal obstruction and occasionally epistaxis. Externally the firm granuloma spreads over the dorsum to the glabella, forehead, cheek, eyelids, alae nasi, and upper lip and, unlike basidiobolomycosis, usually restricts itself to the central part of the face above the level of the angle of the mouth. It rarely spreads further unless there has been trauma or surgical intervention at these limits (Figs. 5*A* and 6). There is no pain, fever, or glandular infection, and no constitutional upset unless caused by secondary infection.

DIAGNOSIS. Radiography excludes bony disease and shows the extent of sinus and pharyngeal involvement (Cockshott et al., 1968). Biopsy should be taken from the nasal cavity or through the buccal sulcus if possible to avoid a visible facial scar. Culture should be performed to confirm the diagnosis.

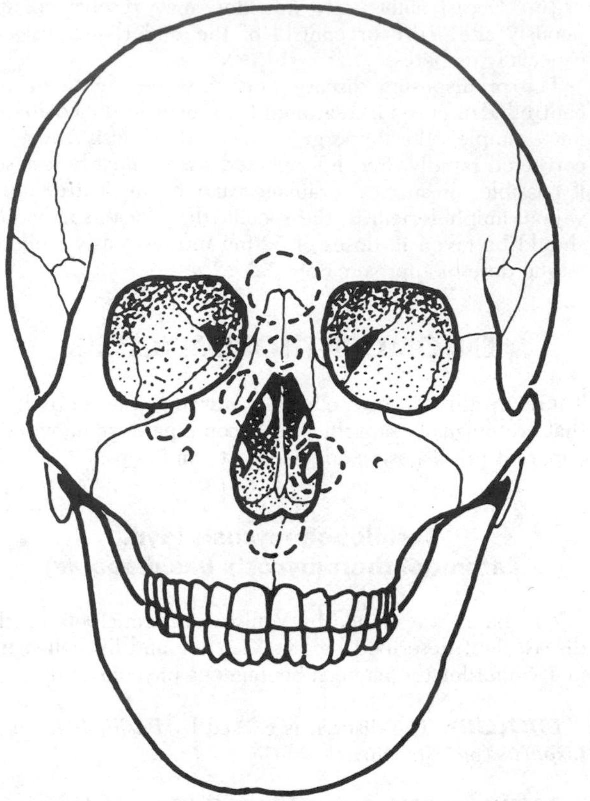

Figure 4. Dotted circles indicate sites through which granulomas usually emerge from the nasal cavity. (From Martinson, F. D.: Rhinophycomycosis. J Laryng 77:691, 1963.)

Pharyngeal and nasal neoplasms, hypertrophic rhinitis, rhinoscleroma, fibrous dysplasia, dental cyst, angioneurotic edema, nodular leprosy, goundou, facial onchocerciasis and African histoplasmosis, and chronic forms of mucormycosis must be excluded.

COMPLICATIONS AND SEQUELAE. Secondary bacterial paranasal sinus infection is not a serious problem. Rarely the pharyngeal granuloma may spread downward to obstruct the larynx. Spontaneous arrest of spread may occur but spontaneous resolution is rare. Complete cure can be achieved and the face returns to its normal appearance and texture (Fig. 5*B*). No deaths due to proven infection have been recorded.

TREATMENT. This is identical with that of basidiobolomycosis.

Pulmonary Infection by *Conidiobolus incongruus*

Only one case of this, the third entomophthoromycosis, has been reported. It occurred in the United States in 1970. Unlike previously described infections, it affected the lung of a previously healthy 15-month-old child and caused signs of respiratory obstruction and later heart failure. Radiography showed areas of increased density in one lung and the mediastinum. The diagnosis of Entomophthorales infection was made following thoracot-

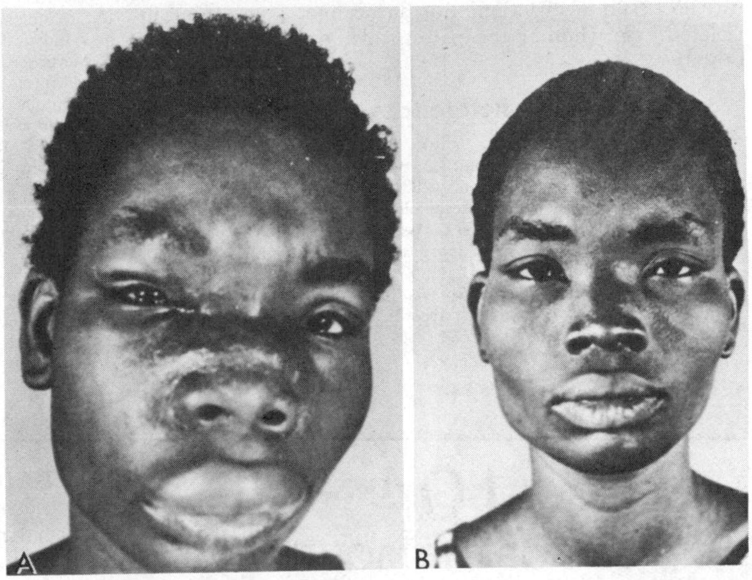

Figure 5. *A*, Involvement of dorsum of nose, glabella, upper lid, cheek, and upper lip before treatment. *B*, Same patient after treatment. (From Martinson, F. D.: Clinical, epidemiological and therapeutic aspects of entomophthoromycosis. Ann Soc Belg Med Trop 52:339, 1972.)

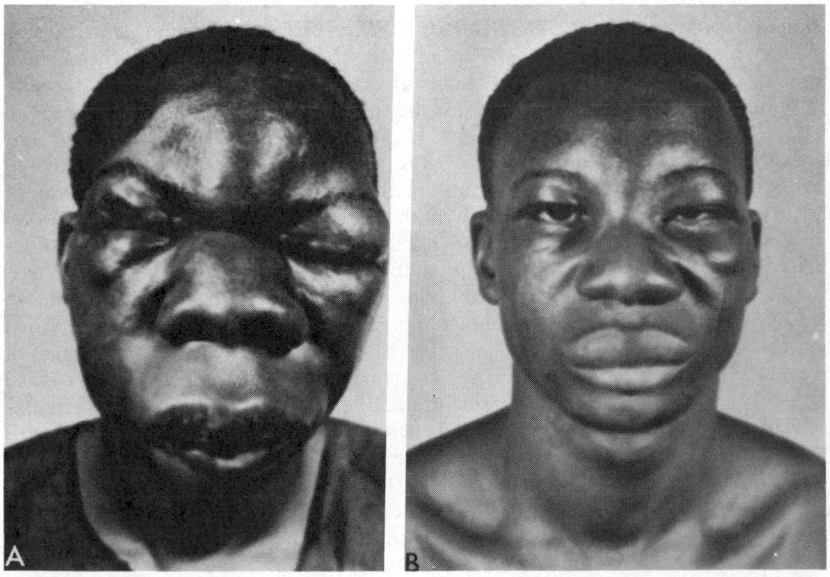

Figure 6. *A*, Severe extensive lesion involving eyelids, glabella, dorsum of nasal alae, and upper lip (lower lip not involved). *B*, Same patient halfway through treatment. (From Martinson, F. D.: Upper respiratory infection due to Conidiobolus coronatus: "Rhino-entomophthoromycosis" ISIAN 170–174: 1976.)

omy and biopsy of the granuloma, which involved the lung, mediastinum, and pericardium. Inhalation of an insect was considered the probable mode of infection.

Treatment with amphotericin B led to complete recovery and no apparent sequelae. Culture by King and Jong in 1976 showed the fungus to be *Conidiobolus incongruus*. In this sole case, as in other entomophthoromycoses, there was no tissue destruction. But one cannot assess from an isolated case whether the pattern of the disease is representative.

References

Ainsworth, G. C.: Introduction and keys to higher taxa. In Ainsworth, G. C., Sparow, F. K., and Sussman, A. S. (eds.): The Fungi: An Advanced Treatise. Vol. IVA. New York, Academic Press, 1973, pp. 1–7.

Bras, G., Gordon, C. C., Emmons, C. W., Prendegast, K. M., and Sugar, M.: A case of phycomycosis in Jamaica. Infection with Entomophthora coronata. Am J Trop Med 14:141, 1965.

Clark, B. M.: Epidemiology of phycomycosis. In Wolstenholme, G. E. W., and Porter, R. (eds.): Systemic Mycoses. London, J. & A. Churchill, Ltd., 1968, pp. 179–192.

Cockshott, W. P., Clark, B. M., and Martinson, F. D.: Upper respiratory infection due to Entomophthora coronata. Rhinoentomophthoromycosis. Radiology 90:1016, 1968.

Emmons, C. W., and Bridges, C. H.: Entomophthora coronata, the etiological agent of a Phycomycosis in horses. Mycologia 53:307, 1961.

King, D. S., and Jong, S. O.: Identity of the etiological agent of the first deep entomophthoraceous infection of man in the United States. Mycologia 68:181, 1976.

Lie Kian Joe, Njo-Injo Tjoel Eng, Pohan, A. and van der Meulen, H.: Basidiobolus ranarum as a cause of a subcutaneous phycomycosis in Indonesia. Arch Derm 74:378, 1956.

Martinson, F. D.: Rhinophycomycosis. J Laryngol 77:691, 1963.

Martinson, F. D.: Clinical epidemiological and therapeutic aspects of entomophthoromycosis. Ann Soc Belge Med Trop 52:329, 1972.

Vanbreuseghem, R.: Guide pratique de mycologie médical et vétérinaire. Paris, Masson et Cie, 1966.

Vanbreuseghem, R., Larsh, H. W.: Conclusions to the round table on the global problems due to opportunistic fungi. In Iwata, K. (ed.): Recent Advances in Medical and Veterinary Mycology, p. 253 (University of Tokyo Press, Tokyo 1977).

Williams, A. O., Von Lightenberg, F., Smith, J. H., and Martinson, F. D.: Ultrastructure of phycomycosis due to Entomophthora and Basidiobolus species and associated "Splendore-Hoeppli" phenomenon. Arch Path 87:459, 1969.

104

THRUSH OF THE MOUTH AND ESOPHAGUS

JOHN E. EDWARDS, JR., M.D.

Although the term thrush has been used to refer to infection caused by organisms of the genus *Candida* in any anatomic site (usually mucosal), the word thrush is most appropriately applied to a specific form of oral candidiasis classified by Lehner (1966) as acute pseudomembranous moniliasis. The condition is characterized by creamy-white, curd-like patches on the tongue or other oral mucosal surfaces. The patches are removable by scraping, which leaves a bleeding, raw, and painful surface.

Lehner, in 1966, expanded upon his classification of the several forms of oral candidiasis; this classification remains an excellent framework for organization and discussion of these diseases (Table 1).

Esophageal candidiasis, recognized with increased frequency in recent years, is characterized by mucosal invasion of *Candida* hyphae, usually in the distal two-thirds of the esophagus. The patchy plaque formation can be visualized at endoscopy.

Table 1. CLASSIFICATION OF ORAL CANDIDIASIS*

Acute
Acute Pseudomembranous Moniliasis (Thrush)
Acute Atrophic Moniliasis (Antibiotic Sore Mouth)
Chronic
Chronic Atrophic Moniliasis (Denture Sore Mouth)
Chronic Hyperplastic Moniliasis
Chronic Oral Candidosis (*Candida* Leukoplakia)
Endocrine Candidosis Syndrome
Chronic Localized Mucocutaneous Candidosis
Chronic Diffuse Candidosis

*(From Lehner, 1966)

ETIOLOGY. Thrush of the mouth and esophagus is caused by yeasts of the genus *Candida*, constituents of the flora of normal individuals (Odds, 1979). The clinical and pathologic manifestations are a result of direct tissue invasion by the yeasts and the ensuing inflammatory response.

Among the numerous species of Candida, only seven have been recovered commonly from man, including patients with thrush. These species are *C. albicans, C. guilliermondi, C. krusei, C. parapsilosis, C. stellatoidea, C. tropicalis,* and *C. pseudotropicalis*. They vary in pathogenicity in the mouth and elsewhere, and *C. albicans* is considered the most pathogenic (Howlett, 1976).

PATHOGENESIS AND PATHOLOGY. *Candida* organisms are normal commensals of low pathogenicity; the normal defense mechanisms are usually compromised for the organism to invade the tissues and cause disease. The compromise may be at a local or systemic level, or both. An example of local level compromise is the mucosal damage associated with ill-fitting dentures and the resultant trauma to the oral mucosa. A second example is oral candidiasis associated with inhalation of steroid beclomethasone dipropionate in the treatment of asthma (Vogt, 1979). Recent studies have demonstrated that *Candida* adheres to both acrylics used in dentures and to normal oral epithelial cells (King et al., 1980). The importance of this adherence in pathogenesis is under study. Topical antibiotics, xerostomia, heavy smoking, cessation of smoking (acute period), and radiation of the head and neck also lower local resistance to thrush.

The same factors that compromise systemic immunity and predispose to oral and esophageal candidiasis also predispose to disseminated candidiasis. They include systemic antibiotics, immunosuppressive agents, hyperalimentation fluids, plastic catheters, pressure monitoring devices, heroin abuse, organ transplantation, extensive abdominal surgery, and placement of prosthetic cardiac valves.

In newborns, thrush has been related to maternal vaginal candidiasis during delivery.

Approximately 50 per cent of esophageal candidiasis

occurs without oral candidiasis (Grieve, 1964). Although *Candida* esophagitis has been reported without underlying illnesses, it is much more commonly associated with hematopoietic or lymphatic malignancy or with the acquired immunodeficiency syndrome (AIDS) (Gottlieb et al., 1981).

Discussion of the pathology of oral and esophageal candidiasis is facilitated through the classification of Lehner, found in Table 1.

Acute Pseudomembranous Candidiasis. A pseudomembrane composed of desquamated epithelial cells, keratin and necrotic tissue, food debris, leukocytes, and bacteria forms the curd-like patches visualized clinically. The membrane is attached to the epithelium by *Candida* hyphae. Although the inflammatory reaction in the epithelium is usually minor, microabscesses may be present.

Acute Atrophic Candidiasis. The epithelium of the tongue undergoes atrophy, presumably as a sequel to acute pseudomembranous candidiasis and detachment of the pseudomembrane. Lehner has also suggested that the condition occurs de novo and that some cases of "antibiotic sensitive tongue" are this form of candidiasis. An inflammatory edema is the predominant reaction and is responsible for the smooth appearance of the tongue.

Median rhomboid glossitis may be a result of *Candida* infection rather than a congenital anomaly as previously thought (Wright, 1981). Although "black hairy tongue" was once considered to be due to *Candida*, it is now thought to be secondary to changes in oral bacterial flora that cause hypertrophy of the tongue papillae. The role of *Candida* in tongue fissures is doubtful because invasion of tissue has not been established by biopsy.

Chronic Atrophic Candidiasis. This condition is "denture sore mouth" and is characterized by chronic inflammation, edema, and thinning of the epithelium in areas under the dental plate. The masses of hyphae recovered from the involved area do not generally invade the tissue. Inflammation occurs predominantly under the maxillary denture and is rare under the mandibular plate. An interesting postulate for the maxillary localization is that the negative pressure caused by the weight of the maxillary denture keeps the area dry and deficient in salivary antibodies. Since individuals without denture stomatitis may also have hyphae in large numbers under the denture plate (Olsen and Birkeland (1977) and Budtz-Jörgensen et al. (1975), the specificity of *Candida* as the agent causing denture sore mouth has been questioned. Yeasts were found in 98 per cent of individuals with denture sore mouth. *C. albicans* was isolated in pure or mixed culture with other yeast species in 86.5 per cent and other yeast species such as *Trichosporon*, *Torula*, *Saccharomyces*, and *Rhodotrula*, were isolated in pure culture in 6.5 per cent.

Angular cheilitis is frequently associated with denture stomatitis. *Candida* has been considered the specific cause of this chronic inflammatory reaction at the corners of the mouth. However, in patients with angular cheilitis, an infective etiology has been found in only 68 per cent, *Staphylococcus aureus* in pure or mixed culture in 79 per cent, *Candida* species alone in 44 per cent, and beta-hemolytic streptococci alone in 15 per cent (MacFarlane and Helnarska, 1976). Thus, *Candida* species were not the most common, nor the only significant infective agent causing angular cheilitis. Noninfective factors also appear responsible for angular cheilitis; these are loss of vertical dimension of mouth, drooling of saliva, vitamin deficiencies, and allergy to denture-base materials or cleansing agents.

Chronic Hyperplastic Candidiasis

Chronic Oral Candidiasis (Candida leukoplakia). This condition is a firm white plaque of the cheek, lips, and tongue. The lesion consists of parakeratosis, acanthosis, pseudoepitheliomatous hyperplasia, microabscess formation, edema of the superficial layers of epithelium and chronic inflammatory cell infiltration of varying intensity of the cornium. Hyphae are always present, but only in the superficial part of the epithelium.

Endocrine Candidiasis Syndrome—Chronic Localized Mucocutaneous Candidiasis and Chronic Diffuse Candidiasis. These syndromes are discussed in Chapter 224. The histopathology is not different from other forms of chronic *Candida* infection.

Candida Esophagitis. Both acute and chronic inflammation are present. There is associated hyperkeratosis, pseudokeratosis, acanthosis, proliferation of the rete ridges, ductal squamous metaplasia, lymphoid nodule and lymphoid follicle formation, ductal dilatation, and focal oncocytic hyperplasia. In addition, a pseudomembrane may form similar to that of thrush, which can cause intraluminal protrusions and result in partial esophageal obstruction. Intraluminal diverticulosis may also be present; however, these diverticulae may more frequently be related to mucosal hyperplasia, and pseudodiverticulae may be a more accurate term. *Candida* esophagitis usually affects the lower two-thirds of the esophagus. As a result of a chronic inflammation and/or abscess formation, segmental narrowing may occur with shoulder defects. Fistulas may form and achalasia may occur.

CLINICAL MANIFESTATIONS. *Acute pseudomembranous candidiasis* (thrush) is characterized by bluish-white to white, adherent, milk curd-like patches on the oral mucosa (Fig. 1). They are relatively nonpainful and are not easily removed. When freed from their base, however, the exposed surface is painfully raw and bleeds easily. The patient may be relatively asymptomatic despite extensive involvement. A metallic taste or loss of taste may precede the infection. In contrast, *acute atrophic candidiasis* is characterized by considerable pain, smoothness of the tongue, and a generalized glossitis. *Chronic atrophic candidiasis* (denture stomatitis) causes inflammation of the denture-bearing area. These lesions may be white and cause a burning sensation. There is a high incidence of angular cheilitis. *Chronic hyperplastic candidiasis (Candida* leukoplakia) is characterized by white, firm, and persistent plaques, most commonly involving the cheek, tongue, palate, and lips and resembles leukoplakia. These lesions may have a protracted course, lasting for years.

The most common symptoms of *Candida* esophagitis are painful difficult swallowing, substernal chest pain, nausea, and vomiting. Lack of normal peristalsis may result in aspiration. The denervation, in its most extensive form, may result in true achalasia. On the other hand, some patients have had extensive disease with minimal or no symptoms. In patients with severe *Candida* esophagitis, the pain may subside as the infection progresses through the esophageal wall and causes denervation (Jones, 1980). *Candida* esophagitis may resemble thrush in appearance with white patches over the esophageal mucosa (Fig. 2).

COMPLICATIONS AND SEQUELAE. In the neonate, elderly, or immunocompromised host, pain during eating may interfere with nutrition. Thrush may extend contiguously from the mouth to the bronchopulmonary tree

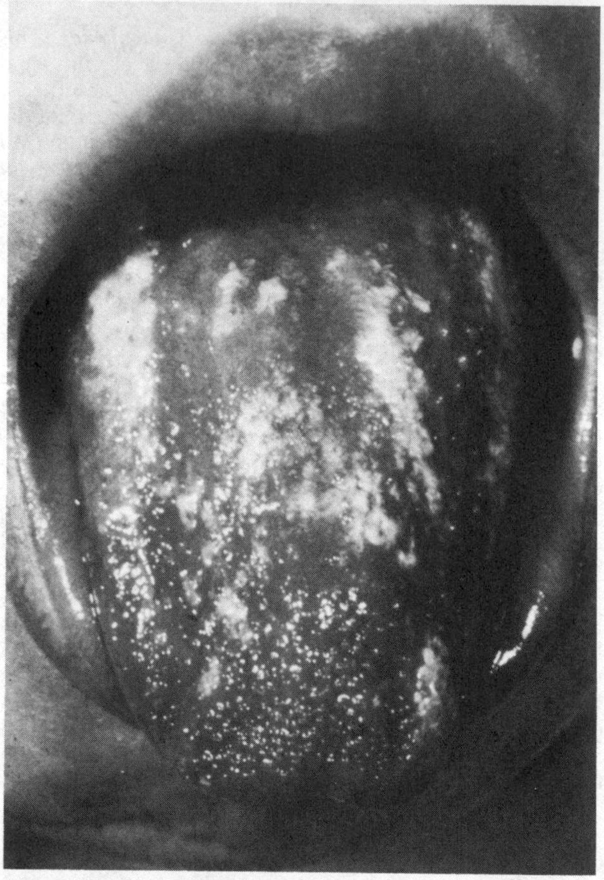

Figure 1. Typical mild to moderate oral thrush with white, mild-curd patches over tongue surface.

(including larynx) into the esophagus or into bone and cause osteomyelitis of the palate. Limited data suggest that *Candida* leukoplakia may rarely be precancerous. Although it would seem that esophageal candidiasis results from extension of oral candidiasis, only half of the cases have been associated with oral disease. Candidiasis may disseminate hematogenously from the mouth.

The complications of esophageal candidiasis are fistula formation, ulceration, luminal obstruction, loss of peristalsis, achalasia, diverticulae, aspiration, pneumonia, bleeding, and presumably dissemination. Esophageal perforation secondary to *Candida* esophagitis is rare.

DIAGNOSIS. The only method to diagnose definitively any form of *Candida* infection is by biopsy of the involved tissue and demonstration of *Candida* invasion by hyphae or pseudohyphae. Because of the presence of *Candida* as part of the normal oral flora, simply recovering the organism from saliva or from a swab does not prove *Candida* infection. However, it is not always necessary to make a tissue-proven diagnosis of oral or esophageal *Candida* infection in order to manage patients. For instance, the typical milk curd, white exudate that shows multiple pseudohyphae or hyphae on either Gram stain or potassium hydroxide preparation can be presumed to be thrush and treated. More aggressive biopsy procedures should be reserved for refractory or atypical situations.

Oral infections with several different bacteria, including staphylococci, streptococci, lactobacilli, neisseria, and coliforms may occur in immunocompromised patients and may resemble thrush. Efforts should be made to rule out other organisms causing lesions resembling thrush (Tyldesley et al., 1976).

The diagnosis of esophageal candidiasis can be made by biopsy during endoscopy. The cobblestone appearance of the esophageal mucosa and the x-ray appearance with contrast studies are helpful in the presumptive diagnosis. X-ray of the esophagus shows a shaggy outline of the mucosa (Fig. 3), loss of mucosal folds, deep ulceration, and nodular filling defects that may be secondary to either mucosal edema, ulceration, or pseudomembrane formation. On fluoroscopy, peristalsis is diminished or absent and contrast media may be seen entering the lungs. Segmental narrowing may occur and contrast media may adhere to the esophageal wall. Large filling defects may resemble esophageal varices. It is important to point out that radiologic examination may be negative in cases of *Candida* esophagitis proved at endoscopy or postmortem examination.

In immunocompromised patients it is possible to have concomitant *Candida* and herpetic esophagitis. Dual infection must be considered when diagnostic features are atypical or therapeutic response is inadequate.

TREATMENT. The most important facet of the treatment of any *Candida* infection is elimination of predisposing factors, including antibiotics, steroids, cytotoxic agents, ill-fitting dentures or any of the others listed under *Pathogenesis.*

The main drug for thrush is nystatin, which is available in oral suspension at concentration of 100,000 units per cc; as vaginal suppositories containing 100,000 units of nystatin

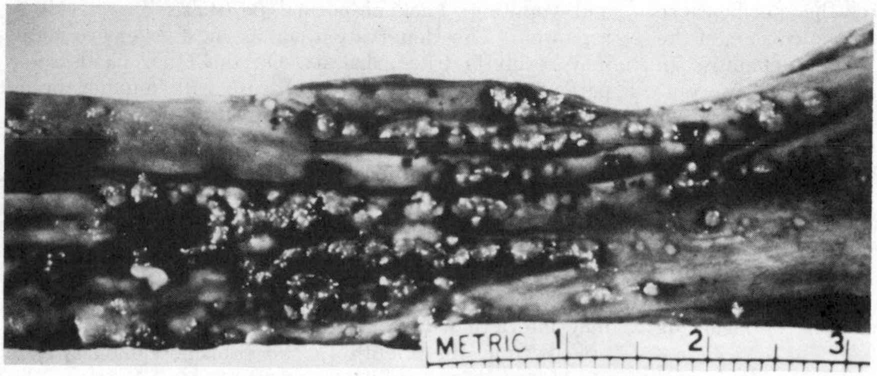

Figure 2. *Candida* esophagitis visualized at autopsy. Note resemblance to oral thrush.

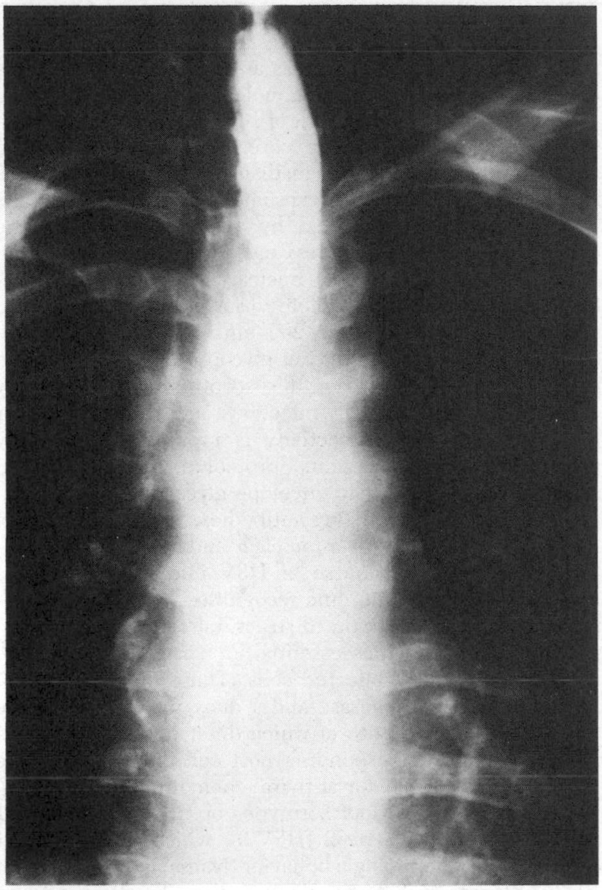

Figure 3. X-ray appearance of *Candida* esophagitis. Note irregularity of right border of esophagus compared with normal-appearing left border.

with lactose, ethyl cellulose, stearic acid, and starch; or as tablets containing 500,000 units. The dose of the suspension for infants is 1 ml in each side of the mouth, four times per day (one-half that amount in premature and low birth weight infants) and 4 to 6 ml, four times per day, in adults with half the dose in each side of the mouth. The tablets can be sucked four times daily. Because of the unpleasant taste of the tablets and oral suspension, some patients prefer the vaginal suppositories, which are more palatable and are used identically to the oral tablets.

Alternatives to nystatin are gentian violet, which may be disadvantageous because of its staining, amphotericin B oral suspension, and amphotericin B troches, which are available in the United Kingdom. Clotrimazole troches are also effective. Acute pseudomembranous candidiasis generally resolves within seven to ten days of therapy but occasionally longer courses are necessary. Treatment should be continued for 48 hours after clinical resolution.

Denture sore mouth requires the treatment for thrush, in addition to correction of ill-fitting dentures and their removal, if possible, until healing occurs. Dentures should be meticulously cleaned. A 2 per cent concentration of amphotericin B in an adhesive paste or powder or incorporation of nystatin into modified soft denture liners is also effective. The angular cheilitis associated with denture sore mouth is treated with topical nystatin or 3 per cent amphotericin B cream or ointment applied four times per day. In addition, defects in the denture design, which may help cause skin folds at the mouth corners, must be corrected. Management of the chronic hyperplastic candidiasis syndromes will be discussed in Chapter 224.

Candida leukoplakia is treated with a longer course of nystatin and surgical removal in refractory cases.

Candida esophagitis is usually more difficult to treat than oral thrush. In some patients, pain or swallowing may be so severe that oral nystatin cannot be delivered to the esophagus and amphotericin B must be given intravenously in doses of 30 mg on alternate days for a total of 750 to 1000 mg (or less if there is rapid clinical improvement). Clotrimazole, 5-fluorocytosine, intravenous miconazole, and oral ketoconazole may also prove useful.

References

Budtz-Jörgensen, E., Stenderup, A., and Gabrowsky, M.: An epidemiologic study of yeasts in elderly denture wearers. Community Dent-Oral Epidemiol 3:115, 1976.

Gottlieb, M. S., Schroff, R., Schauber, H. M., et al.: Pneumocystis carinii pneumonia and mucosal candidiasis in previously healthy homosexual men. New Eng J Med 305:1425, 1981.

Grieve, N. W. T.: Monilial oesophagitis. Brit J Radiol 37:551, 1964.

Howlett, J. A.: The infection of rat tongue mucosa in vitro with five species of Candida. J Med Microbiol 9:309, 1976.

Jones, J. M.: Necrotizing Candida esophagitis. Failure of symptoms and roentgenographic findings to reflect severity. JAMA 244:2190, 1980.

King, R. D., Lee, J. C., Morris, A. L.: Adherence of Candida albicans and other Candida species to mucosal epithelial cells. Infect Immun 27:667, 1980.

Lehner, T.: Classification and clinico-pathological features of Candida infections in the mouth. In Winner, H. I., and Hurley, R. (eds.): Symposium on Candida Infections. Edinburgh and London, E. & S. Livingstone, Ltd., 1966, p. 119.

MacFarlane, T. W., and Helnarska, S. J.: The microbiology of angular cheilitis. Brit Dent J 140:403, 1975.

McCourtie, J., Douglas, L. J.: Relationship between cell surface composition of Candida albicans and adherence to acrylic after growth on different carbon sources. Infect Immun 32:1234, 1981.

Odds, F. C.: Candidosis of the oropharynx. In Odds, F. C.: Candida and Candidosis. Baltimore, University Park Press, 1979, p. 93.

Olsen, I., and Birkeland, J. M.: Denture stomatitis—yeast occurrence and the pH of saliva and denture plaque. Scand J Dent Res 85:130, 1977.

Tyldesley, W. R., Rotter, E., and Sells, R. A.: Bacterial thrush-like lesions of the mouth in renal transplant patients. Lancet 1:485, 1976.

Vogt, F. C.: The incidence of oral candidiasis with use of inhaled corticosteroids. Ann Allergy 43:205, 1979.

Wright, B. A. and Fenwick, F.: Candidiasis and atrophic tongue lesions. Oral Surg Oral Med & Oral Path 51:55, 1981.

General References

Cawson, R. A.: Chronic oral candidiasis, denture stomatitis and chronic hyperplastic candidiasis. In Winner, H. I., and Hurley, R. (eds.): Symposium on Candida Infections. London, E. & S. Livingstone, Ltd., 1966, p. 138.

Jones, J. M.: The recognition and management of Candida esophagitis. Hospital Practice, April 1981, p. 64.

Kods, B. E., Wickremesinghe, P. C., Kozinn, P. J., Iswara, K., and Goldberg, P. K.: Candida esophagitis. A prospective study of 27 cases. Gastro 71:715, 1976.

105
HERPES STOMATITIS

MICHAEL N. OXMAN, M.D.

Herpes stomatitis (acute herpetic gingivostomatitis) is an acute inflammatory infection of the mucous membranes of the mouth caused by herpes simplex virus (HSV). It is the result of primary HSV infection of a susceptible person and occurs mainly in children under 5 years of age. The disease is normally self-limited, and symptoms generally disappear in 12 to 14 days. In the newborn or immunosuppressed patient, infection may disseminate to the liver, lungs, adrenal glands, and other viscera. In young adults, primary oropharyngeal HSV infections more often produce acute pharyngitis and tonsillitis, without lesions in the anterior part of the mouth. In this age group, primary HSV infection is an important cause of acute pharyngotonsillitis, and its clinical manifestations are often indistinguishable from those of β-hemolytic streptococcal infection. Although gingivostomatitis and pharyngotonsillitis are the most common clinical manifestations of primary oropharyngeal HSV infection, they are seen in only a minority of infected individuals. Most primary HSV infections are asymptomatic.

Symptomatic or not, primary HSV infection of the oropharyngeal mucosa is followed by lifelong persistent infection. For the most part, the virus remains silent or *latent*, but reactivation occurs periodically, with reappearance of virus and recurrence of disease at the site originally infected. The recurrent infection is different in location and character from the primary infection. It usually presents as *herpes labialis*, the well-known "cold sore" or "fever blister," on or adjacent to the vermilion border of the lip. Herpes labialis is far more common than acute herpetic gingivostomatitis or pharyngotonsillitis; it afflicts 30 to 50 per cent of the world's adult population.

The term *herpes*, derived from the Greek word meaning "to creep" has been used to describe herpes labialis since the time of Hippocrates (Juel-Jensen and MacCallum, 1972). The infectious nature of herpes labialis was established as early as 1912, when Grüter produced keratitis in rabbits with material from human herpetic lesions (Grüter, 1920). Several investigators reasoned that herpes labialis must represent the reactivation of a latent HSV infection previously initiated by an earlier primary infection of the oral mucosa (Goodpasture, 1929), but the nature of that primary infection was not recognized until 1938. In the United States, Dodd et al. (1938) showed that HSV was the cause of acute gingivostomatitis in infants and young children. Burnet and Williams (1939), in Australia, confirmed that observation and, in addition, showed that acute herpetic gingivostomatitis was always a manifestation of primary HSV infection.

ETIOLOGY. Herpes simplex virus (herpesvirus hominis) is a member of the herpesvirus family (Chapter 60), which includes three other human herpesviruses, varicella-zoster virus (VZV), cytomegalovirus (CMV), and Epstein-Barr virus (EBV). These herpesviruses are morphologically indistinguishable and share a number of properties, including a remarkable propensity for establishing lifelong latent infections. The HSV virion has an internal core that contains the viral genome, a linear molecule of double-stranded DNA with a molecular weight of 100 million, together with several viral proteins. The core is enclosed within an icosahedral capsid 100 nm in diameter, composed of 162 identical protein subunits (capsomers). This structure, the *nucleocapsid*, is surrounded by a layer of protein (the *tegument*) of variable thickness and, finally, by a lipoprotein envelope derived from the nuclear membrane of the infected host cell. The complete virion is roughly spherical with a diameter of 150 to 200 nm. The virus envelope contains radially-oriented viral glycoproteins that mediate the attachment of the virion to susceptible host cells. Only enveloped virions are fully infectious, and this accounts for the lability of HSV; infectivity is rapidly destroyed by organic solvents, detergents, proteolytic enzymes, heat, and extremes of pH. The envelope glycoproteins are antigenic and elicit neutralizing antibodies. The appearance of these viral glycoproteins on nuclear and cytoplasmic membranes early in the course of HSV infection provides a mechanism for host-immune recognition and lysis of HSV-infected cells. In addition to structural components of the virion, certain enzymes essential for virus replication are synthesized in HSV-infected cells. These include a virus-specified DNA polymerase and a deoxypyrimidine kinase (thymidine kinase), both of which differ in substrate specificity from the corresponding host cell enzymes and are thus potential targets for antiviral chemotherapy.

There are two distinct serotypes of HSV, HSV Type 1 (HSV-1) and HSV Type 2 (HSV-2), which differ in their clinical and epidemiologic behavior (Nahmias and Roizman, 1973; Nahmias and Josey, 1982) and can be distinguished on the basis of antigenic, biologic, and biochemical differences (Table 1). The two serotypes of HSV also differ in their mode of transmission (Nahmias and Josey, 1982). HSV-1 is transmitted primarily by nonsexual routes, usually involving contact with infected saliva. HSV-2 is transmitted sexually or from a maternal genital infection to the newborn. Acute herpetic gingivostomatitis is caused by HSV-1, which is also the serotype responsible for most cases of HSV pharyngotonsillitis, and for most cutaneous lesions above the waist. HSV-1 is also responsible for herpes simplex keratitis (Chapter 245) and for herpes simplex encephalitis (Chapter 180). HSV-2 is responsible for most cases of herpes genitalis, for cutaneous lesions below the waist, and for the majority of neonatal HSV infections. HSV-2 infection has also been associated epidemiologically with carcinoma of the cervix, although this disease appears to be more closely associated with human papillomavirus infection (see Chapter 62).

It should be recognized, however, that the classical clinical and epidemiological features of HSV-1 and HSV-2 infections are changing as a result of improving socioeconomic conditions, changing sexual practices, and advances in medicine, such as organ transplantation and cancer chemotherapy, which are increasing the number of immunocompromised patients.

HSV-1 and HSV-2 have many common antigens; their genomes share about 40 per cent of their nucleotide sequences, are colinear with respect to the arrangement of genetic loci, and can undergo recombination to yield multiple viable intertypic recombinants (Honess and Watson,

Table 1. DIFFERENCES BETWEEN HERPES SIMPLEX VIRUS TYPE 1 (HSV-1) AND TYPE 2 (HSV-2)

Characteristics	HSV-1	HSV-2
Clinical		
Manifestations of Primary Infection		
Acute herpetic gingivostomatitis	+[a]	−[b]
Acute herpetic pharyngotonsillitis	+	−[c]
Acute herpetic keratoconjunctivitis	+	−
Neonatal herpes simplex infections	±[d]	+
Manifestations of Recurrent Infection		
Herpes labialis	+	−
Herpes keratitis	+	−
Manifestations of Primary or Recurrent Infection		
Cutaneous herpes		
Skin above waist	+	−
Skin below waist	−	+
Hands or arms	+	+
Herpetic whitlow	+	+
Eczema herpeticum	+	−
Herpes genitalis	±[e]	+
Herpes simplex encephalitis	+	−
Herpes simplex meningitis	±[f]	+
Epidemiologic		
Transmission	Non-sexual	Sexual
Epidemiologic association with carcinoma of the cervix	−	+
Latency		
Trigeminal and cervical sensory ganglia	+	−
Sacral ganglia	−	+
Biochemical		
DNA guanine + cytosine	67%	69%
Homology between viral DNAs	approximately 40%	
Stability of virus-specific thymidine kinase at 40° C	+	−
Biologic		
Neurotropism in mice on peripheral inoculation	less neurotropic	more neurotropic
Pock size on chick chorioallantoic membrane	small	large
Plaque formation in chick embryo cell monolayer culture	−	+
Temperature sensitivity of replication (40° C)	−	+
Heparin sensitivity	+	−
Inhibition of replication by thymidine	−	+
Other		
HSV-1 and HSV-2 can be unequivocally differentiated by serologic techniques, by DNA:DNA hybridization, by restriction endonuclease fingerprinting of viral DNA, and by electrophoretic analysis of virus-specified proteins.		

[a]+ = frequent or predominant cause.
[b]− = infrequent cause (except under special epidemiologic circumstances).
[c]HSV-2 is frequently isolated when pharyngotonsillitis is associated with orogenital sexual contact.
[d]HSV-1 is isolated from 15 to 30 per cent of cases, reflecting the increasing frequency with which HSV-1 causes genital herpes (in the mother), as well as some cases of postnatal infection acquired from individuals shedding HSV-1.
[e]HSV-1 is now being isolated from 10 to 40 per cent of patients with genital herpes. Herpetic vulvovaginitis in infants is generally caused by HSV-1, acquired from adults or by autoinoculation of infected saliva.
[f]Some cases reported, but insufficient data to estimate frequency.

1977; Morse et al., 1978; Roizman and Tognon, 1983). Nevertheless, they each have type-specific antigenic determinants that permit them to be differentiated unequivocally by a variety of serologic techniques (Rawls, 1979; Plummer et al., 1974; Spear, 1980). In addition, HSV-1 and HSV-2 can be readily distinguished by nucleic acid hybridization, by electrophoretic analysis of virus-specified proteins, and by restriction endonuclease fingerprinting of the viral DNA (Honess and Watson, 1977; Lonsdale et al., 1979; Roizman and Tognon, 1983). The latter technique, which can also distinguish between different strains of the same serotype, has been particularly useful for epidemiologic studies (Roizman and Tognon, 1983).

Unlike other human herpesviruses, HSV has a wide host range. HSV can infect many experimental animals, including rats, mice, hamsters, guinea pigs, rabbits, nonhuman primates, chick embryos, and a wide variety of cell cultures from human and animal tissues. In cell cultures, HSV causes cytoplasmic edema (so that cells become enlarged and round), acidophilic Cowdry Type A intranuclear inclusion bodies, and fusion of cells into multinucleated giant cells. The same cytopathology is seen in cutaneous and visceral lesions in vivo. These changes are identical to those produced by varicella-zoster virus. However, in tissue culture, the cytopathic effect of VZV remains focal because progeny virus remains cell-associated, whereas the cytopathic effect of HSV quicky spreads to involve the entire culture because HSV-infected cells release large amounts of progeny virus into the culture medium.

PATHOLOGY AND PATHOGENESIS. HSV infection is usually cytolytic, and the resulting pathology is a consequence of necrosis of infected cells together with local inflammation. In immunosuppressed patients, the herpetic lesions may be atypical and difficult to recognize clinically. The skin and mucous membrane lesions of HSV-1 and HSV-2 are the same and resemble those produced by VZV. The characteristic cytopathology, which can be observed in vivo as well as in tissue culture, consists of "ballooning degeneration" of individual infected cells, the production of Cowdry Type A intranuclear inclusion bodies, and the formation of multinucleated giant cells. Individual infected cells become greatly enlarged with pale, vacuolated cytoplasm. The nuclei exhibit margination of chromatin and contain inclusion bodies. These are initially homogeneous and slightly basophilic, and often fill the nucleus. However, they rapidly condense and evolve into sharply demarcated acidophilic inclusion bodies that are separated from the deeply basophilic ring of marginated chromatin at the nuclear membrane by a clear zone or halo (Fig. 1). Multinucleated giant cells are formed primarily by cell fusion, a process associated with the appearance of HSV-specified glycoproteins on the membranes of infected cells. Fusion of infected cells with adjacent uninfected cells provides an efficient method for the cell-to-cell spread of HSV infection, even in the presence of antibody capable of neutralizing extracellular virions.

HSV infection of the skin and mucous membranes causes intraepidermal vesicles. The virus, usually acquired by contact with infected saliva, replicates locally in the cells of the stratum spinosum. Infected cells undergo ballooning degeneration with loss of intercellular bridges, and are soon separated by intercellular edema. At this early stage, the lesions are papular and contain a few small multinucleated giant cells. Typical intranuclear inclusion bodies are

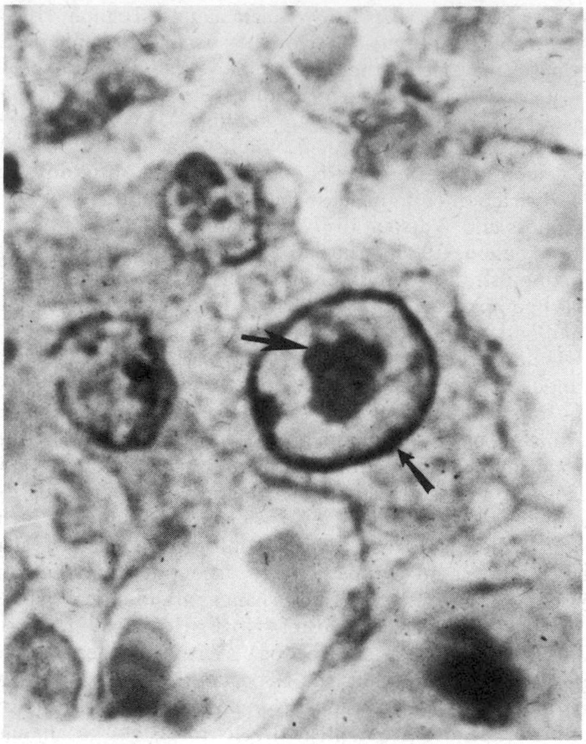

Figure 1. Herpes simplex, intranuclear inclusion body. A section of liver from a malnourished child who died with disseminated herpes simplex virus infection. A parenchymal cell shows a typical eosinophilic Cowdry type A intranuclear inclusion body (large arrow), which is separated from the basophilic ring of marginated chromatin at the nuclear membrane (small arrow) by a clear zone or halo. Hematoxylin and eosin. Magnification 2000 ×.

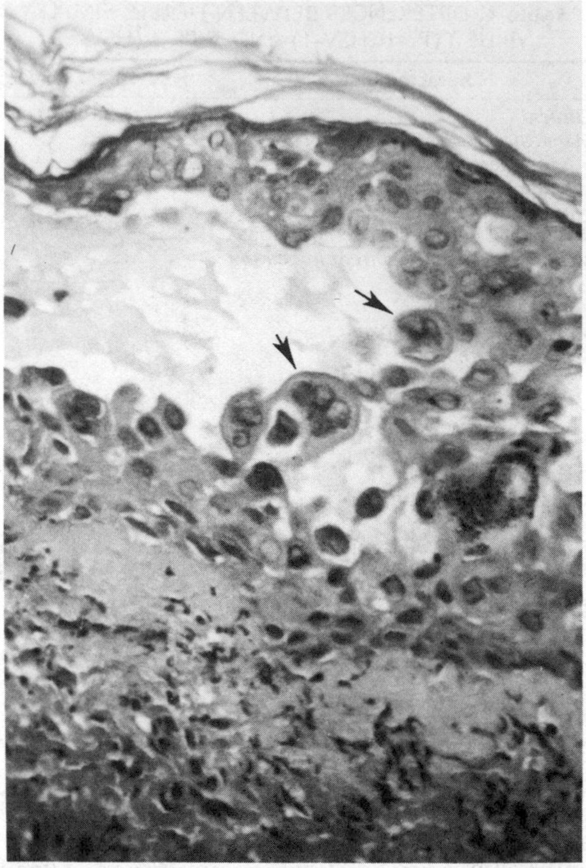

Figure 2. Herpes simplex, early vesicle. Intraepidermal vesicle produced by herpes simplex virus infection of the skin. Infected epithelial cells show "ballooning degeneration" with the formation of multinucleated giant cells (arrows). Edema fluid has elevated the overlying stratum corneum. The underlying dermis shows edema and mononuclear cell infiltration. Hematoxylin and eosin. Magnification 200 ×. (Courtesy Dr. R. J. Barr.)

already present. The papular lesions rapidly evolve into intraepidermal vesicles as a result of the infection and degeneration of more epithelial cells and the continuing influx of edema fluid, which elevates the uninvolved stratum corneum to form a delicate clear vesicle (Fig. 2). The vesicle fluid contains fibrin, degenerating epithelial cells, multinucleated giant cells, and a large amount of cell-free virus. In the underlying dermis or lamina propria, capillary dilatation and infiltration by inflammatory cells is pronounced, but necrosis is absent. The inflammatory cells soon invade the vesicle, the fluid becomes cloudy, and the vesicle is transformed into a pustule. When the vesicle is in the skin, the fluid is absorbed, leaving a flat adherent crust that becomes detached when subjacent epithelial cells grow back. The lesions heal without scars. Lesions in the mucous membranes develop in the same way, but the thin roof of the vesicle quickly breaks down, leaving a shallow ulcer.

During primary infection (for example, acute herpetic gingivostomatitis) there is usually spread to regional lymph nodes and probably viremia (Ruchman and Dodd, 1950). In the normal person, both nonspecific and specific defense mechanisms combine to localize the infection and eventually terminate virus replication. They also limit HSV replication at any sites of viremic spread. These mechanisms include the antiviral and cytotoxic activities of activated monocytes and macrophages, nonspecific killer (NK) cells, HSV-specific cytotoxic T lymphocytes, antiviral antibody plus complement, antibody-dependent cell-mediated cytotoxicity (ADCC). and interferons (Chapters 12 and 88). It is also noteworthy that peripheral blood mononuclear cells from normal individuals do not support HSV replication. However, when activated by mitogens or allogeneic stimulation, adult T and B lymphocytes replicate HSV, as do peripheral blood leukocytes from some newborns and organ allograft recipients (Kleinman et al., 1972; Hammer et al., 1982; Braun et al., 1984). This may contribute to the occurrence of disseminated HSV infections in neonates and immunocompromised patients. When these defenses are deficient, as they are in newborns, malnourished children, and immunosuppressed children and adults, primary HSV infection may spread to the liver, adrenal glands, lungs, and brain. Individuals with defects in cellular immunity are particularly vulnerable. In visceral lesions (for example, in the liver) there is usually coagulation necrosis of parenchymal cells, stroma, and blood vessels. Cells containing typical intranuclear inclusion bodies are generally found at the periphery of the necrotic areas.

Early in the course of acute herpetic gingivostomatitis or asymptomatic primary oropharyngeal HSV-1 infection, virus invades local nerve endings in the mucous membranes of the mouth and ascends within axons to reach the trigeminal ganglion. There it establishes a latent infection in sensory neurons that persists for the life of the host (Goodpasture, 1929; Stevens, 1975, Wildy et al., 1982). Despite the host's immunity, this latent virus can be reactivated by various stimuli. The reactivated HSV may then travel within axons from the neuronal soma to the periphery and infect the perioral skin or mucous membranes. Replication and cell-to-cell spread in epithelial cells produce an intraepidermal vesicle indistinguishable from that produced by primary HSV infection. It is noteworthy that during recurrent HSV infections, there are inflammatory changes in the portion of the corresponding sensory ganglion that contains neurons that provide sensation to the skin at the site of the recurrent lesion (Howard, 1905). Humoral and cellular immune mechanisms normally limit this local virus replication and spread, so that recurrent HSV infections are less severe, less extensive, and of shorter duration than primary infections. In fact, many recurrences are asymptomatic, resulting only in the shedding of virus in saliva.

HSV-1 is a remarkably successful parasite. Primary infection usually occurs during childhood but rarely causes severe disease. In fact, it is most often asymptomatic (Fig. 3). After primary infection, HSV, in contrast to many other viruses, does not disappear and leave behind a solid immunity to reinfection. Instead, it persists for the life of the host, who, in spite of the presence of HSV-specific humoral and cellular immunity, is subject to recurrent attacks of HSV infection. This persistence of HSV is in the form of a latent infection that is completely asymptomatic most of the time. However, a variety of provocative factors, such as fever, emotional stress, sunlight, menstruation, or trauma, can reactivate the virus and produce a brief, self-limited episode of recurrent infection during which HSV is shed into the environment. When symptomatic, these episodes of recurrent HSV-1 infection usually present as herpes labialis. But they are often asymptomatic and detectable only by the presence of HSV-1 in the saliva. HSV-1 infections rarely produce severe disease in the normal person, and persistence of the virus does not interfere with long-term survival or reproductive capacity. Thus most infected individuals remain in the community as lifelong carriers of HSV. The periodic reactivation of latent HSV infection provides ample opportunity for the transmission of HSV to susceptible children before the adult carriers succumb to old age or to other diseases. In this regard, it is probably no accident that herpes labialis is frequently brought on by the fever associated with severe and life-threatening bacterial infections. The deathbed kiss provides one last opportunity for HSV to be transmitted to the next generation. The remarkable degree to which HSV is adapted to man, its natural host, is underlined by its behavior in other species. For example, in rabbits or mice, HSV-1 infections are generally severe and often fatal. Similarly, *Herpesvirus simiae* causes severe and usually

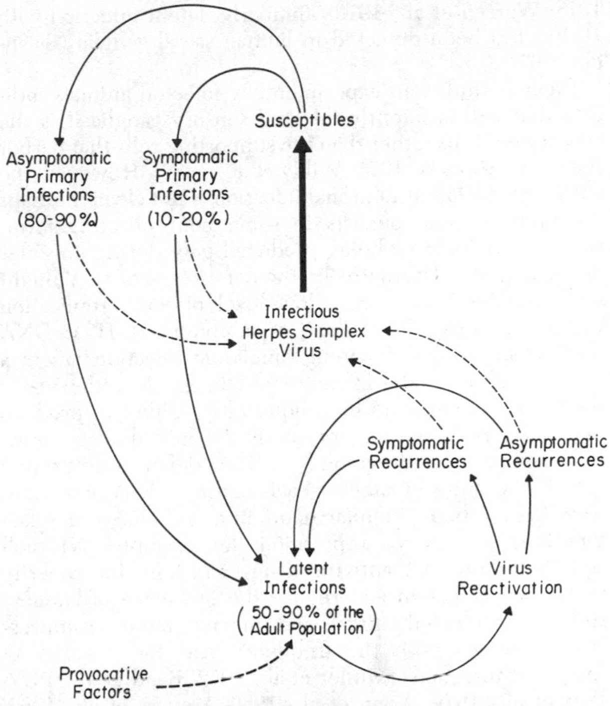

Figure 3. The ecology of herpes simplex virus. The 50 to 90 per cent of adults with latent infections are the reservoir of herpes simplex virus. New susceptibles (usually children) are infected when adults shed virus during recurrences (for example, episodes of herpes labialis). After their primary infection (which is usually asymptomatic), the children develop latent infections and join the pool of lifelong virus carriers.

fatal encephalitis in man, whereas in its natural host, it produces a mild or asymptomatic infection that is followed by lifelong latency analogous to HSV-1 in humans (Chapter 181).

It is clear from studies in humans and experimentally infected animals that latent HSV is harbored in sensory ganglia innervating the site of primary HSV infection (Baringer, 1975; Stevens, 1975; Wildy et al, 1982). Thus lesions of recurrent HSV-1 are usually within the distribution of the second or third division of the trigeminal nerve, and only rarely in areas of skin innervated by the first division. This implies that latent HSV infections in neurons have little tendency for horizontal spread to other neurons within the ganglion. Recurrent infections—i.e., herpes labialis or asymptomatic shedding of HSV-1 in saliva—are regularly induced by section or manipulation of the sensory root of the trigeminal ganglion (Carton and Kilbourne, 1952; Pazin et al., 1978). The appearance of recurrent herpetic lesions in the skin depends upon the integrity of the peripheral sensory nerve. Local denervation by section of the branches of the sensory nerve prevents the subsequent recurrence of HSV in the denervated skin, but not in adjacent skin with intact sensation. Latent infection has not been demonstrated in the skin itself at sites of recurrent lesions (Rustigian et al., 1966), but HSV-1 has been detected by explantation and cocultivation techniques in human trigeminal, superior cervical, and vagus ganglia (Bastian et al., 1972; Baringer and Swoveland,

1973; Warren et al., 1978). Similarly, latent infection with HSV-2 has been detected in human sacral ganglia (Baringer, 1974).

Elegant studies in experimentally infected animals indicate that within latently infected sensory ganglia it is the sensory neurons rather than the supporting cells that harbor the virus (Stevens, 1975; Wildy et al., 1982). However, the nature of the latent neuronal infection is not clear. Perhaps the viral genome persists in some nonreplicating form, with infectious virus being produced only during episodes of reactivation. Alternatively, the persistence of HSV might be maintained by a very low level of virus replication within neurons. The failure of inhibitors of HSV DNA replication to abolish latent ganglionic infection favors a nonreplicating model of neuronal latency. In either case, the neuron appears to be unique in its ability to produce infectious HSV (either constantly or only during recurrences) without undergoing lysis. Host defenses determine the course and outcome of each phase of HSV infection. Antiviral antibody, cellular immunity, and nonspecific factors that limit virus replication (for example, NK cell activity, interferon, antiviral drugs) can limit the severity of primary infection and reduce the incidence of latency. In latently infected animals and humans, immunosuppression increases both the frequency and the severity of recurrent infections (Muller et al., 1972; Rand et al., 1977; Pass et al., 1979; Arvin et al., 1980; Meyers et al., 1980; Siegel et al., 1981; Rand et al., 1982; Wade et al., 1982; Pollard et al., 1982). Both humoral and cellular immunity also seem to be important in maintaining latency, but the mechanisms involved are unclear. Perhaps the capacity of the latently infected neuron to replicate HSV is modulated by the interaction of antibody or sensitized cells with virus-induced antigens on the cell membrane (Lehner et al., 1975). Even more obscure, at present, is the mechanism by which such diverse stimuli as fever, sunlight, emotional stress, physical trauma, and menstruation can induce the reactivation of latent HSV infections.

In addition to host factors, viral genes must also play an important role in determining the nature and severity of HSV infections. No specific "high pathogenicity" strains of HSV have yet been isolated from human infections. For example, restriction endonuclease analysis of isolates from a cluster of cases of HSV encephalitis, thought possibly to represent local spread of an "encephalitogenic" strain of HSV, revealed instead that each patient was infected with a different, epidemiologically unrelated, strain of HSV-1 (Hammer et al., 1980). Nevertheless, studies in animal models demonstrate that genetic differences can markedly affect the virulence of HSV strains and the nature of the diseases they produce (Thompson et al., 1983, Dix et al., 1983; Centifanto-Fitzgerald et al, 1982). While selective pressure has been in the direction of a benign HSV-human interaction, it seems possible that uncommon severe infections, such as HSV encephalitis, might be associated with some alteration in one or more specific HSV gene. The report of Chaney et al. (1983) of similarities in the distribution of restriction endonuclease sites in HSV isolates from cases of HSV encephalitis may represent the first step in identifying genetic determinants of HSV pathogenicity for humans.

CLINICAL MANIFESTATIONS. The clinical manifestations of HSV infection are determined by the nature of the infection, that is, whether it is a primary or a recurrent infection; the portal of entry of the virus; the serotype and the amount of virus initiating the infection; and by such host factors as age, immune status, nutritional status, immunocompetence, and the presence or absence of conditions like eczema or burns that alter the resistance of the skin. The major clinical syndromes produced by HSV infection are listed in Table 1. Herpes simplex encephalitis and meningitis are discussed in Chapter 180, and HSV infections of the eye in Chapter 245. Genital herpes and neonatal HSV infection, which are caused predominantly by HSV-2, are discussed in Chapter 163. The remaining syndromes, which are caused most often by HSV-1, are discussed below. Because they often differ, the clinical manifestations of primary and recurrent HSV-1 infections are discussed separately.

The designation of HSV infections as *primary* or *recurrent* fails to reflect the true complexity of the situation because HSV-1 and HSV-2, though antigenically distinct, have common antigenic determinants that can induce cross-reactive humoral and cellular immune responses. These immune responses provide some protection against heterotypic infection in vivo. Thus, HSV infection in someone who has never been infected with either HSV serotype (for example, genital herpes in a patient with no antibody to HSV-1 or HSV-2) is not equivalent to infection with that HSV serotype in an individual previously infected with the heterologous serotype (for example, genital herpes in a patient with a history of herpes labialis and preexisting antibody to HSV-1). The initial HSV-2 infection is usually less severe in a person already immune to HSV-1 than in someone without any prior HSV infection. Although both types of *initial* HSV-2 infection are ordinarily described as *primary* genital herpes (primary HSV-2 infections) they should actually be termed *initial primary* and *initial non-primary*, respectively. The distinction may be relevant among people living under better socioeconomic conditions in whom the acquisition of HSV-1 infection is delayed so that most children reach sexual maturity without having been infected with HSV-1. Their initial HSV-2 infections will be *primary* rather than *initial non-primary*, and are likely to be more severe. The term *recurrent* infection, as generally used, refers to the recurrence of infection by the same serotype at the same anatomic site. The source of virus responsible for the recurrence may be endogenous (for example, the typical case of herpes labialis) or exogenous (for example, an episode of genital herpes caused by exogenous HSV-2 in someone with a history of recurrent herpes genitalis caused by HSV-2). It is clear from restriction endonuclease fingerprinting of viral DNA that, while most episodes of recurrent genital herpes are due to the reactivation of endogenous HSV-2 latent in sacral ganglia, a recurrence may occasionally represent a sexually acquired exogenous reinfection with a new HSV-2 strain (Buchman et al., 1979).

Primary Infections

Acute Herpetic Gingivostomatitis. Acute herpetic gingivostomatitis is the most common herpetic infection of childhood. It occurs primarily in children between 6 months and 5 years of age, but it may also be seen in older children and adults (Black, 1938; Dodd et al., 1938; Burnet and Williams, 1939; Scott et al., 1941; Buddingh et al., 1953). The source of infection is usually an adult with herpes labialis or with an asymptomatic recurrence who is shedding HSV-1, but it may be another infected child, especially in a household or institutional epidemic (Juretić,

1966). The incubation period is usually 4 to 6 days, with a range of 2 days to 2 weeks. The illness begins with the abrupt onset of fever (usually to 102° to 104° F), anorexia, and listlessness; the infant soon becomes restless, irritable, and unwilling to eat or drink. The mouth usually becomes sore 12 to 96 hours after the onset of constitutional symptoms, but before oral lesions appear. Gingivitis is the most constant and striking lesion of the disease, occurring in every case. The gums are first hyperemic and then become markedly swollen (sometimes almost covering the teeth), reddened, friable, and exquisitely tender. They bleed easily and sometimes spontaneously, and there is a bright red line along the dental margin (Fig. 4). In most patients, vesicular lesions also develop on the oral mucous membranes. They first appear as tiny vesicles on a red base, but quickly rupture, leaving very tender, round, 1 to 3 mm, shallow, yellowish-gray, indurated ulcers or plaques. They often run together and are surrounded by a thin red halo. These lesions may occur anywhere on the mucous membranes of the mouth or pharynx, but they are most common on the tongue, the inner surface of the lips, and the buccal and sublingual mucosa. Lesions occur less frequently on the soft palate and on the gums themselves, occasionally in the pharynx, and rarely in the larynx. The submandibular and anterior cervical lymph nodes are almost always enlarged and tender. The breath is usually fetid owing to the overgrowth of oral anaerobic bacteria. Salivation and drooling are marked. Herpetic lesions readily develop in areas of skin contaminated with infected saliva, which contains large amounts of infectious HSV. Thus, many patients develop herpetic vesicles in the perioral skin (Fig. 5), and herpetic paronychia are seen in finger suckers. Cutaneous vesicles may also appear at more distant sites, and autoinoculation occasionally results in herpetic vulvovaginitis and HSV infection of the eye.

Although self-limited in normal children, and without sequelae, the disease varies considerably in severity and duration. An occasional infant may be extremely ill with high fever, systemic toxicity, and severe and extensive mucosal lesions that prevent adequate drinking. Fortunately, most symptomatic cases are mild, and, of course, most primary HSV-1 infections are asymptomatic. Symptoms subside after an average of 12 to 14 days. The acute phase generally lasts for 5 to 7 days, after which the temperature returns to normal, the soreness in the mouth disappears, and the oral lesions begin to heal. The herpetic ulcers usually heal in 4 to 7 days, but the gingivitis often resolves more slowly, and the adenopathy may persist for several weeks.

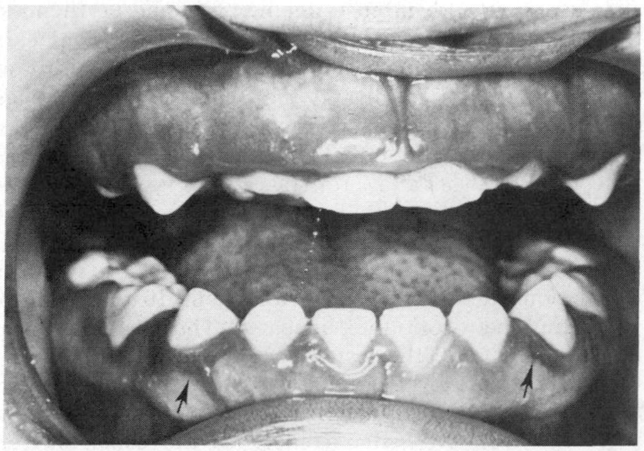

Figure 4. Acute herpetic gingivostomatitis. Gingivitis in a child with acute herpetic gingivostomatitis. The gums are tender, swollen, and hyperemic, and there is a bright red line along the dental margin (arrows).

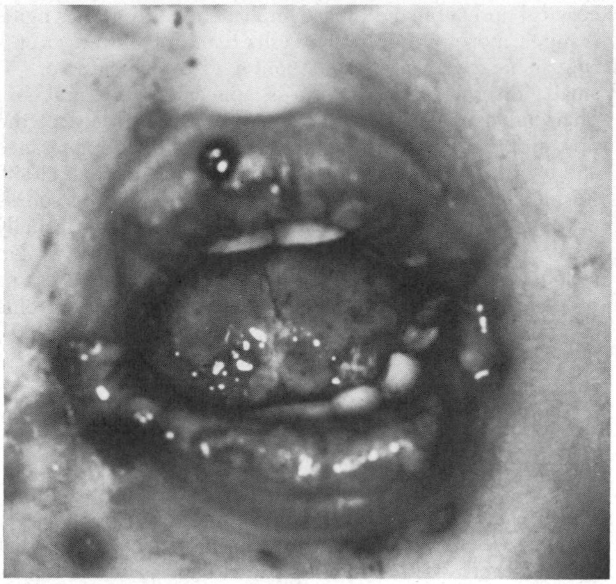

Figure 5. Acute herpetic gingivostomatitis. In addition to having vesicles on the oral mucosa, palate, and tongue, this child with acute herpetic gingivostomatitis has herpetic vesicles on the lips and perioral skin.

HSV-1 can be readily isolated from saliva and stool during the active disease. Furthermore, although neutralizing antibodies appear in the first week of illness and reach maximum levels by the third week, most of the children excrete virus for many weeks after recovery, without clinical evidence of infection (Scott et al., 1941; Buddingh et al., 1953). Eventually, shedding of HSV-1 in the saliva becomes intermittent, but this intermittent shedding continues indefinitely, both in those who are and those who are not subject to recurrent herpes labialis (Cesario et al., 1969; Douglas and Couch, 1970). Although rarely documented, viremia probably occurs in many cases of uncomplicated HSV gingivostomatitis.

The incidence of symptoms varies markedly from one study to another. Surveillance of many normal children indicates that primary HSV-1 infection causes manifest disease in anywhere from 1 per cent to over 15 per cent (Scott, 1957; Juretić, 1966). The most thorough study has yielded the highest incidence (Juretić, 1966). In family and orphanage epidemics, the incidence of overt disease is higher, often approaching 100 per cent (Hale et al., 1963; Juretić, 1966). These variations may be explained by differences in the dose of virus transmitted, the age of the infected children, the general health and nutritional status of the children studied, the intensity of surveillance, and the diagnostic criteria used.

HSV-1 causes primary acute herpetic gingivostomatitis in adults as well as children. In adults, the disease begins with malaise; soreness in the mouth and throat; pain on swallowing; swollen, tender, bleeding gums; and anterior cervical and submandibular lymphadenopathy. Pharyngitis is much more prominent in adults than in children, occurring in nearly every case. About 1 to 3 days after onset, small, discrete, round vesicles appear on the oral and pharyngeal mucosa, the tongue, the inner surface of the lips, and the palate. These are identical in their appearance and evolution to those seen in children (Rogers et al., 1949; Farmer, 1956; Sheridan and Herrmann, 1971). The course of the disease in adults is like that in children, but usually less severe. Drooling is not a problem, and perioral skin lesions are rare in patients over 16 years of age. Lesions produced by autoinoculation—namely, herpetic paronychia or whitlows, skin lesions at sites distant from the mouth, ocular infections, and vulvovaginitis—are also rare in adults.

Acute Herpetic Pharyngotonsillitis. In adults, primary oropharyngeal HSV-1 infection causes pharyngitis and tonsillitis much more frequently than gingivostomatitis. The illness begins with fever, malaise, headache and sore throat. Tiny vesicles appear on the tonsils and posterior pharynx, but they quickly break down to form shallow ulcers that run together. A grayish-yellow exudate forms on the tonsils and posterior pharynx in over one-half of the patients. Lesions of the anterior mouth or lips are seen in only 10 per cent of adults with herpetic pharyngitis and tonsillitis, and the disease is usually indistinguishable from the pharyngitis and tonsillitis caused by the β-hemolytic streptococci (Evans and Dick, 1964; Glezen et al., 1975). In college and university students, 70 per cent or more of whom have no antibody to HSV-1 or HSV-2, acute herpetic pharyngotonsillitis is a significant illness. In a 6-year study, 10 per cent of susceptible college and graduate students developed primary HSV infection each year. Although fewer than 3 per cent of these infections resulted in clinically recognized disease, primary HSV infections accounted for 12 per cent of the acute respiratory illness in students admitted to the student infirmary (Glezen et al., 1975). In this age group, HSV caused more cases of pharyngitis and tonsillitis than did the Group A streptococcus. Although most cases appear to be caused by HSV-1, HSV-2 is now being isolated with increasing frequency, especially when pharyngotonsillitis is associated with orogenital sexual contact.

Acute Herpetic Vulvovaginitis. In infants, acute herpetic vulvovaginitis may result from autoinoculation during primary oropharyngeal HSV-1 infection or from contact with an adult shedding HSV. It is a rare manifestation of primary HSV-1 infection. There is fever and malaise, and the perineal area is red, edematous, and studded with tiny vesicles that rapidly evolve into shallow, yellowish-white ulcers 2 to 4 mm in diameter. These are extremely painful, and dysuria may lead to urinary retention. Lesions coalesce to form larger ulcers, and the inguinal lymph nodes are enlarged and tender. Fever and constitutional symptoms subside in a week, and healing is complete without scarring in 12 to 18 days.

Primary Herpetic Infections of the Skin. In contrast to mucous membranes, the intact skin is resistant to HSV infection. Consequently, primary cutaneous HSV infections are relatively uncommon in healthy individuals. When they do occur, they are usually associated with heavy virus exposure and trauma to the skin. Most primary cutaneous infections occur in the course of acute herpetic gingivostomatitis or herpes genitalis. Sometimes it is viremia that brings the virus from the primary oral or genital focus of infection to the skin, but more often the skin lesions result from autoinoculation. The lesions begin as erythematous papules, develop into vesicles, and progress through pustules to crusts over several days. In primary infections, the vesicles tend to be discrete rather than grouped. They generally heal without scarring in 7 to 14 days.

Traumatic Herpes. On occasion, primary cutaneous herpes appears in a normal person without oropharyngeal or genital infection. Such lesions result from the direct exogenous infection of skin rendered susceptible by trauma. This can occur when a parent who is shedding HSV-1 in saliva "kisses away" the pain of a child's abrasion. A diaper rash can be the site of primary cutaneous HSV-1 infection in infants (Juel-Jensen and MacCallum, 1972). Primary cutaneous herpes has also been reported among wrestlers ("herpes gladiatorum"). Presumably, traumatized skin is infected with virus shed in saliva (Selling and Kibrick, 1964). In addition to the local lesions, which are generally confined to the area of traumatized skin, there is usually regional lymphadenopathy and often symptoms of systemic illness. Cutaneous HSV infections are often severe and life-threatening when they occur in patients with disorders of the skin, such as eczema or burns, which permit more extensive local virus replication and spread, and facilitate visceral dissemination.

Herpetic Whitlow (Herpetic Paronychia). Primary HSV infections of the fingers are relatively uncommon except when individuals are heavily exposed to the virus. As noted above, this may occur in acute herpetic gingivostomatitis as a result of finger sucking. It also occurs in primary herpes genitalis, presumably as a result of a similar exposure to infected vaginal secretions. However, the most common form of herpetic whitlow is that which occurs among physicians, nurses, respiratory therapists, and dental personnel. Stern et al. (1959) reported a series of 54 cases of herpetic whitlow occurring in nurses, most of whom were caring for tracheostomy patients in a neurosurgical unit. HSV was present in the saliva of only 1.2 per cent of patients on hospital admission, but it could be isolated from the bronchial secretions of 6.5 per cent of tracheostomy patients. Only nurses without antibody to HSV were afflicted, although it is now clear that herpetic whitlow can also occur in individuals with antibody to HSV-1 or HSV-2 induced by earlier oropharyngeal or genital HSV infections. The whitlow begins 2 to 7 days after exposure with intense itching, pain and erythema in the infected finger. Within a day, a deep vesicle appears, usually in the terminal segment of one digit. Soon other vesicles appear (Fig. 6) and then coalesce. The process continues, destroying considerable tissue. Many cases seem to have pus under the cuticle, but incision discloses only a little clear fluid or, at a later stage, thick, yellow, necrotic debris. Intense local pain is always present. Systemic symptoms and epitrochlear or axillary lymphadenopathy are common, and lymphangitis and neuralgia may occur. The lesions tend to progress for about 10 days, during which time pain continues unabated. There is then abrupt improvement, and the lesions begin to dry. Resolution is usually complete by 18 to 20 days. If the lesion is incised, secondary bacterial infection may occur, prolonging the period of disability. Recurrences at the same site are common, but are usually less severe than the primary infection and are rarely accompanied by constitutional symptoms. Most of the herpetic whitlows that occur in medical and paramedical personnel are caused by HSV-1.

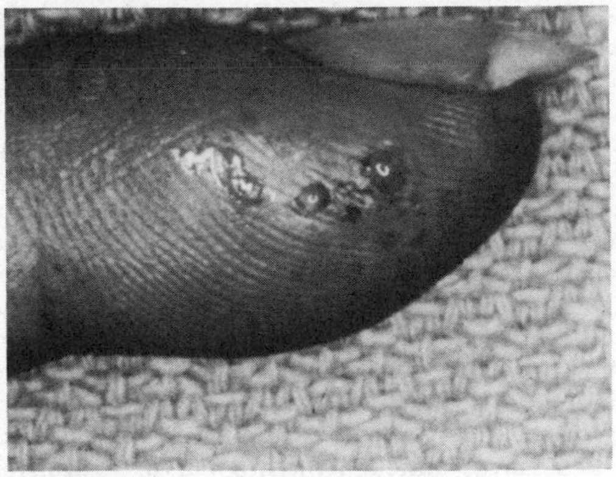

Figure 6. Herpetic whitlow. The terminal segment of the index finger of a respiratory therapist is exquisitely painful, swollen, and erythematous, with multiple deep and superficial herpetic vesicles. Herpes simplex virus type 1 was isolated from vesicle fluid.

A history of trauma is uncommon, but contact with oral or respiratory secretions is almost universal (Greaves et al., 1980). The thumb or index finger is most often affected, and involvement of more than one finger is uncommon.

Herpetic Infections of the Eye. Primary herpetic infection of the eye may occur alone or by autoinoculation during acute herpetic gingivostomatitis. It is usually manifest as a unilateral follicular conjunctivitis with preauricular adenopathy, and is often accompanied by fever and constitutional symptoms. Blepharitis with vesicles on the lid margin is common, and vesicles may also occur on the periorbital skin. Superficial corneal involvement, if present, is characterized by dendritic ulcers. Healing is spontaneous and is usually complete in 2 to 3 weeks. Ocular herpetic infections are discussed in detail in Chapter 245.

Recurrent Infections

Herpes Labialis. Herpes labialis (cold sore, fever blister) is the most common manifestation of recurrent HSV-1 infection. It occurs in 30 to 50 per cent of adults (Embil et al., 1975; Grout and Barber, 1976; Young et al., 1976b). In most patients (60 to 80 per cent), the recurrence has a prodrome of pain, burning, tingling, or itching at the site of the subsequent eruption. This usually lasts for 6 hours or less (but occasionally for 24 to 48 hours) and is followed by a small cluster of raised erythematous papules that rapidly develop into tiny thin-walled intraepidermal vesicles (Fig. 7). These quickly become pustular and then either burst or dry, with the formation of a scab. If the scab is removed shortly after its formation, it leaves a shallow ulcer. Left undisturbed, the scab is soon displaced by the regrowth of epidermis. The evolution of the lesion is generally rapid, with the papular stage lasting for only a few hours and vesicles crusting within 2 days (Spruance et al., 1977). Lesion area (usually <100 mm^2) and pain are maximal during the vesicular stage and decline rapidly thereafter. Healing is completed, with loss of the scab and without scarring, within 6 to 10 days. Patients sometimes have local lymphadenopathy, but not constitutional symptoms.

The most common site of herpes labialis is the vermilion border of the lip (95 per cent), usually the outer third, and more often the lower lip than the upper. Other sites are the nose, the chin, the cheek, and, rarely, the oral mucosa. HSV is not the cause of recurrent aphthous ulcers, which afflict many persons with no history of HSV infection and no antibody to HSV (Blank et al., 1950, Ship et al., 1967). Most people subject to herpes labialis suffer 1 to 2 episodes per year, but some have recurrences at intervals of a month or less. In a given person, the lesions generally recur at the same site, and the provoking factor may also be stereotyped. In some, it is exposure to sunlight; in others, menses; and in others, emotional stress induced by school examinations.

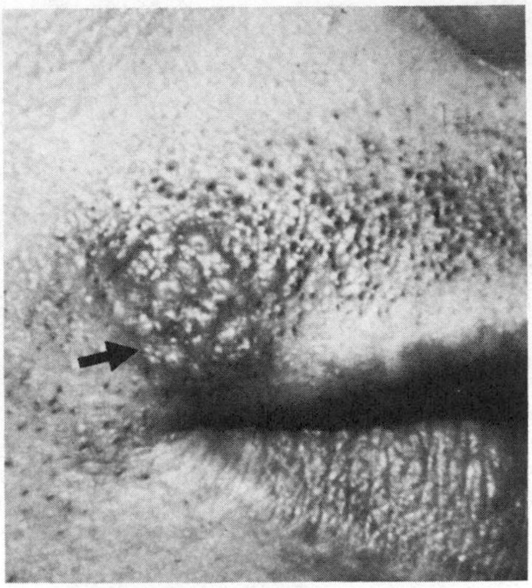

Figure 7. Herpes labialis. Following a 12-hour prodrome of localized itching and burning, this medical student developed a small group of erythematous papules that quickly evolved into a typical cluster of tiny vesicles on an erythematous base (arrow).

The virus titer is highest ($>10^5$ infectious doses per ml of vesicle fluid) during the first 24 hours, when the lesions are vesicular, and it decreases steadily thereafter. HSV is rarely recovered after 5 days. HSV is usually present in the saliva during episodes of herpes labialis; it has been recovered from the saliva of 25 to 85 per cent of patients tested while lesions of herpes labialis were present (Douglas and Couch, 1970; Spruance et al., 1977; Pazin et al., 1978). HSV can also be recovered from 1 to 5 per cent of saliva samples obtained from adults when they are free of herpes labialis, but the concentration of virus is considerably lower. Repeated sampling reveals asymptomatic salivary shedding of HSV-1 at some time by most seropositive individuals. Intraoral lesions are rarely present, and virus is not recovered from parotid secretions. Thus, the source of HSV in the saliva is a mystery.

Recurrent Ocular Herpes. Ocular herpes may recur in the form of keratitis, blepharitis, or keratoconjunctivitis, as discussed in detail in Chapter 245. Many patients suffer multiple recurrences of herpes keratitis, and this may cause considerable disability and even permanent visual loss. Asymptomatic virus shedding also occurs, and HSV can be isolated from the conjunctivae and tears in the absence of clinical disease.

Recurrent Cutaneous Herpes. Primary HSV infection results in a latent infection in the corresponding sensory ganglia. Thus, it is often followed by recurrent herpetic infections at or near the site of the initial lesion. Because the virus originates in sensory ganglia and is transported to the skin by sensory nerves, the lesions of recurrent cutaneous herpes may assume a segmental or dermatomal

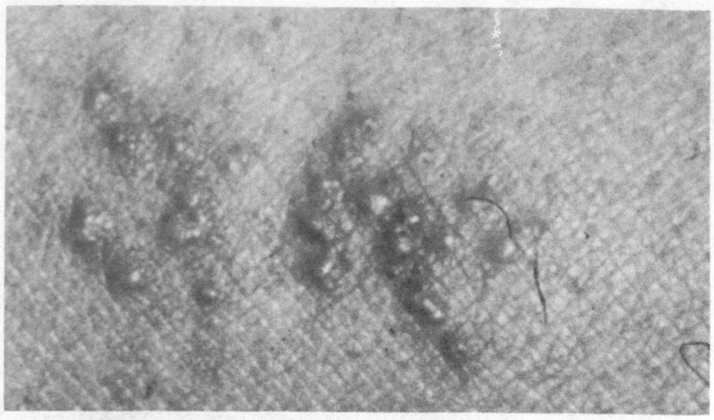

Figure 8. Recurrent cutaneous herpes simplex. A young woman who had cutaneous lesions on her arm during an episode of primary herpetic gingivostomatitis (the results of autoinoculation) has subsequently suffered periodic recurrences. They appear as a typical patch of grouped vesicles on an erythematous base.

distribution that resembles herpes zoster (Slavin and Ferguson, 1950). However, the lesions of recurrent herpes simplex are usually confined to a smaller area of the skin within the dermatome than is herpes zoster; perhaps, because the primary cutaneous infection is more circumscribed in herpes simplex than in varicella, HSV establishes latency in fewer sensory neurons within the ganglion. The lesions of recurrent herpes simplex occur most often on the face, on the hands and arms, and on skin innervated by the sacral ganglia. They generally appear as grouped vesicles rather than the individual vesicles seen in primary infections (Fig. 8). They also tend to recur repeatedly, usually at the same site. In contrast, herpes zoster rarely recurs, and when it does, it usually involves a different dermatome. Nevertheless, the appearance, evolution, and histopathology of the skin lesions are the same in herpes zoster and recurrent herpes simplex, and it is often impossible to distinguish between them without laboratory identification of the etiologic agent. A prodrome of pain, burning, itching, or tingling often precedes the herpetic lesions by 1 to 3 days. The lesions begin as grouped erythematous papules that progress to vesicles, pustules, and crusts over several days. They heal without scarring in 6 to 10 days. Regional lymphadenopathy is sometimes present, but constitutional symptoms are rare. Recurrent cutaneous herpes is sometimes associated with severe local neuralgia, and recurrences on extremities may be accompanied by local edema and lymphangitis (Nicolau and Poincloux, 1924; Slavin and Ferguson, 1950; Behrman and Knight, 1954; Juel-Jensen and MacCallum, 1972; Layzer and Conant, 1974).

Recurrent Herpetic Whitlow. Primary herpetic whitlows are frequently followed by multiple recurrences. While unaccompanied by constitutional symptoms and of somewhat shorter duration, the recurrent whitlow is often as painful as the primary lesion. It is frequently accompanied by swelling and edema of the hand, by regional adenopathy, and by severe neuralgic pain in the arm (Nicolau and Poincloux, 1924; Stern et al., 1959; Juel-Jensen and MacCallum, 1972). It may also be accompanied by lymphangitis.

COMPLICATIONS AND SEQUELAE. In the normal person (beyond the neonatal period), HSV infections are usually asymptomatic. Even symptomatic infections are almost always benign and self-limited. The only major exception is HSV encephalitis, a rare complication of primary and recurrent HSV-1 infection that accounts for most cases of sporadic acute necrotizing encephalitis in the Western World. Herpes simplex encephalitis is discussed in Chapter 180.

The newborn infant seems unable to limit the replication and spread of HSV. Thus neonatal HSV infections have a mortality of over 50 per cent, with severe sequelae in many survivors. Most infections are acquired during passage through the birth canal of a mother with genital herpes and thus most are caused by HSV-2. A minority may be acquired post partum by nosocomial spread from other infants in the nursery or by contact with an adult shedding HSV-1 in saliva. Although the oropharynx is probably an important portal of entry, the infected neonate rarely has gingivostomatitis.

Acute herpetic gingivostomatitis is rarely complicated by bacterial infection. In severe cases, the painful lesions in the mouth may prevent drinking and cause dehydration and acidosis. Occasionally, oropharyngeal or genital herpes in adults or children is complicated by clinically significant viremia with cutaneous or visceral dissemination. This may result in a varicelliform eruption difficult to distinguish from chickenpox, in fatal HSV hepatitis or hepatoadrenal necrosis with disseminated intravascular coagulation (DIC), in HSV esophagitis, in HSV arthritis, in HSV cystitis, or in HSV meningitis (Naraqui et al., 1976; Long et al, 1978; Anuras and Summers, 1976; Keane et al., 1976; Taylor et al., 1981; Walker et al., 1981; Fishbein et al., 1979; Buss and Scharyj, 1979; Shortsleeve et al., 1981; Craig and Nahmias, 1973; Remafedi and Muldoon, 1983). While these complications occur most often in immunocompromised patients, they may also occur in apparently normal individuals (Auch Moedy et al., 1981; Bastian and Kaufman, 1982; Connor et al., 1979; Deprew et al., 1977; Owensby and Stammer, 1978; Remafedi and Muldoon, 1983). Moreover, they may even occur during an otherwise asymptomatic infection—in the absence of signs or symptoms of disease at the portal of entry (Auch Moedy et al., 1981; Connor et al., 1979; Pazin, 1978; Bastian and Kaufman, 1982).

A variety of compromised hosts are at increased risk of developing severe, even fatal, HSV infections. These include malnourished children, pregnant women, patients who are immunosuppressed by disease or therapy (especially patients with deficient cellular immunity) and patients with disorders of the skin such as eczema or burns. Severe and fatal disseminated HSV infections are frequent in malnourished children (Becker et al., 1968). The disease begins with acute herpetic gingivostomatitis, which is followed by a sustained viremia with dissemination of infection to the liver, adrenal glands, lungs, and other viscera. There is also extensive infection of the esophagus and intestinal mucosa, due either to viremia or to large amounts of swallowed virus. Disseminated HSV infection with fatal hepatitis and encephalitis has also been observed in pregnant women with primary oropharyngeal or genital herpes and in older adults, often in association with corticosteroid therapy (Juel-Jensen and MacCallum, 1972; Goyette et al., 1974; Young et al., 1976a; Keane et al., 1976).

Both the frequency and the severity of HSV infections are markedly increased in patients with hematologic malignancies, in patients with acquired immune deficiency syndrome (AIDS), and in renal, cardiac and bone marrow transplant recipients, particularly in the first 2 to 3 months after transplantation, when immunosuppression is greatest (Berg, 1955; Logan et al., 1971; Muller et al., 1972; Montgomerie et al., 1969; Korsager et al., 1975; Rand et al., 1977; Schneidman et al., 1979; Pass et al., 1979; Arvin et al., 1980; Meyers et al., 1980; Siegel et al., 1981; Rand et al., 1982; Wade et al., 1982; Pollard et al., 1982). These infections occur mainly in patients with pre-existing antibody to HSV and thus generally reflect the reactivation of latent infection. Most seropositive transplant recipients shed HSV, and, while this is sometimes asymptomatic, it is usually associated with severe and persistent mucocutaneous infections. Chronic atypical mucocutaneous HSV infections involving the perioral or anogenital regions are a major cause of morbidity in severely immunosuppressed patients. The lesions begin as typical herpes labialis, but they enlarge, become necrotic, ulcerate, and extend to deeper tissues. Satellite lesions develop and mucous membrane involvement is often extensive with ulcerative, sometimes nodular, lesions on the lips, buccal mucosa, tongue and palate. Pain and chronicity are hallmarks of this disease; lesions may persist for 10 weeks or more, during which time saliva and involved tissues contain large amounts of virus. However, while local extension is a major problem, these lesions are rarely associated with HSV dissemination (Montgomerie et al., 1969). HSV is also reactivated during postchemotherapy mucositis. Rand et al. (1982) documented persistent HSV excretion in 85 per cent of seropositive patients who developed stomatitis after cancer chemotherapy. Reactivation of oropharyngeal HSV in this setting can result in spread to the esophagus and trachea. This is facilitated by mucosal damage secondary to radiation, chemotherapy, or intubation (Nash and Ross, 1974; Buss and Scharyj, 1979). Herpes esophagitis, in particular, is a common but generally unrecognized manifestation of HSV infection in immunologically compromised and debilitated patients, especially in the presence of a nasogastric tube (Nash and Ross, 1974). There are typical herpetic ulcers of the esophageal mucosa that may become confluent in the lower third. Herpetic esophagitis can lead to viremia with involvement of the liver and other viscera. It is often also a focus for superinfection by *Candida*, which may further obscure the diagnosis. Herpetic esophagitis is thought to result from the direct extension of infection from the oropharynx. However, it may sometimes be a recurrent infection resulting from reactivation of virus latent in the vagus ganglia (Warren et al., 1978). The lungs may also be infected with HSV, either by direct extension from the oropharynx, or hematogenously (Ramsey et al., 1982; Graham and Snell, 1983). Direct extension is facilitated by injury to the respiratory epithelium, e.g., by endotracheal intubation, burn injury, chemotherapy or radiation. This probably explains the 10 per cent incidence of HSV tracheobronchitis in hospitalized burn victims, and the frequency of HSV infection in patients intubated for adult respiratory distress syndrome (Nash and Foley, 1970; Tuxen et al., 1982). In these settings, most patients have focal or multifocal pneumonia, and concurrent HSV esophagitis is common (Herout et al., 1966). There is usually evidence of active oral HSV infection long before the onset of pneumonia. Immunosuppressed patients can also develop diffuse interstitial pneumonia from hematogenous HSV dissemination; their liver, adrenals, and other internal organs are often infected concurrently.

In patients with atopic eczema, the skin is especially susceptible to HSV infection and appears deficient in its capacity to limit virus replication and spread. When they (or patients with certain other skin disorders, such as Darier's disease, Sézary syndrome, pemphigus, and burns) are exposed to HSV, they develop a severe and sometimes fatal infection (eczema herpeticum, Kaposi's varicelliform eruption), which was initially described by Kaposi as a complication of eczema in children (Brain, 1956; Wenner, 1944; Ruchman et al., 1947). Eczema herpeticum is usually a primary infection in which the eczematous skin is the portal of entry. The source of virus is most often an adult with herpes labialis. The disease begins acutely with high fever (104 to 105° F), irritability, and restlessness, and with the appearance of numerous small vesicles, primarily on the eczematous skin (Fig. 9). Individual lesions resemble those of varicella and quickly become umbilicated. They may appear in crops, with new lesions continuing to appear for a week or more. Individual lesions evolve from vesicle to pustule to crust over a few days. The largest numbers are found in the eczematous skin, where they may be confluent, but smaller numbers also appear on adjacent intact skin. The affected skin is edematous, and there is always regional or generalized lymphadenopathy. Fever and constitutional symptoms usually subside by the tenth day, and lesions heal in 2 to 3 weeks. Eczema herpeticum varies in severity from a mild to a rapidly fatal infection. When the cutaneous lesions are extensive, large areas of skin may be denuded of epithelium, with severe loss of fluid, electrolytes and protein, and marked susceptibility to bacterial superinfection. Mortality in children may be as high as 10 to 15 per cent, and is often associated with visceral dissemination and infection of the liver, lungs, adrenal glands, gastrointestinal tract, and brain. Recurrences are common, and, while they are generally less severe and of shorter duration than primary infections, they may still result in severe, even fatal, disease. Enormous quantities of virus are present in the skin of patients with eczema herpeticum, and care must be taken lest they be the source of hospital epidemics and infections—for example, herpetic whitlows—in hospital personnel.

Burned patients resemble patients with eczema in their vulnerability to HSV infection (Foley et al., 1970). Areas

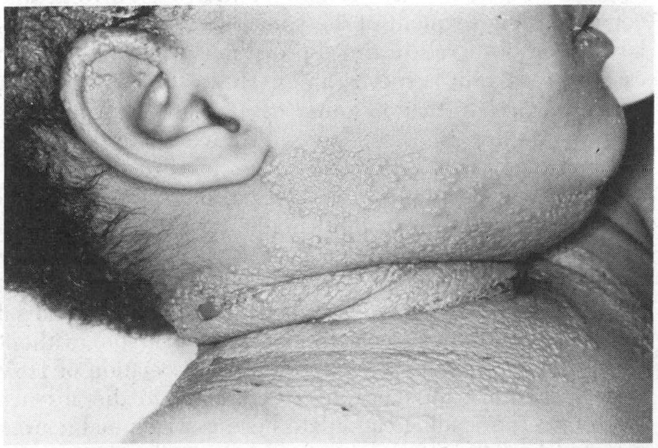

Figure 9. Eczema herpeticum. An infant with atopic eczema developed fever, irritability, and numerous tiny vesicles that quickly became umbilicated. His mother had developed herpes labialis four days earlier. A Tzanck smear from the base of a vesicle showed multinucleated giant cells and eosinophilic intranuclear inclusion bodies. Herpes simplex virus type 1 was isolated from vesicle fluid.

of healing second-degree burns are easily infected and appear to provide ideal conditions for HSV replication. The resulting infection resembles eczema herpeticum, with multiple small vesicles and erosive lesions in areas of healing partial-thickness injury. The HSV infection may contribute to mortality by interfering with healing, increasing the extent of cutaneous damage, promoting bacterial superinfection, and disseminating to produce infection of the liver, lungs, adrenal glands, gastrointestinal tract, urinary bladder, and other viscera. These patients shed enormous quantities of HSV and are thus potential sources of nosocomial infection.

The intimate association of HSV with neurons has led many observers to implicate this virus in the pathogenesis of various neurologic syndromes of unknown etiology, including trigeminal neuralgia, atypical pain syndromes, idiopathic facial paralysis (Bell's palsy), temporal lobe epilepsy, recurrent psychosis, and multiple sclerosis (Juel-Jensen and MacCallum, 1972; Nahmias and Roizman, 1973; Finelli, 1975; Mertens et al., 1982). However, the ubiquity of HSV, its lifelong latent residence in seropositive individuals, and its frequent reactivation by a variety of stimuli minimize the etiologic significance of any temporal association between the occurrence or recurrence of HSV infection and the onset of another disease. Of all of these associations, the best supported is that of HSV with atypical pain syndromes, including trigeminal neuralgia. Recurrent cutaneous HSV infections are sometimes associated with a prodrome of severe neuralgic pain that may continue for several days after the eruption has appeared (Slavin and Ferguson, 1950; Layzer and Conant, 1974). However, the pain almost never persists after the cutaneous lesions have healed, and, in spite of numerous recurrences in the same site, there is rarely any evidence of permanent neurologic impairment. This is in marked contrast to herpes zoster, which rarely recurs but which may often be associated with prolonged postherpetic neuralgia, as well as sensory loss and signs of lower motor neuron damage. These sequelae may be explained by the pathologic changes observed in herpes zoster; there is acute inflammation and subsequent fibrosis of the sensory nerve and ganglion corresponding to the involved area of skin. This process, the direct result of virus infection, may extend centrally to involve the corresponding segment of the spinal cord. Similar changes have been observed in the sensory nerve and ganglion in cases of recurrent herpes simplex (Howard, 1905). Thus, it is not surprising that in some cases in which cutaneous herpes simplex is associated with severe neuralgia, repeated attacks over a period of years have resulted in the development of chronic pain and permanent sensory and motor deficits (Behrman and Knight, 1954; Juel-Jensen and MacCallum, 1972; Krohel et al., 1976). Furthermore, the well-documented occurrence of zoster sine herpete (that is, the reactivation of latent varicella-zoster virus in a dorsal root ganglion with associated neuralgic pain but without skin lesions) provides a model for the association of HSV with unilateral pain syndromes that occur in the absence of a rash. The leading candidate here is trigeminal neuralgia, which almost always involves pain in the distribution of the second and third divisions of the trigeminal nerve, the same region involved in most cases of recurrent facial or labial herpes simplex. The association is supported by serologic studies (Juel-Jensen and MacCallum, 1972), by the association of some cases of trigeminal neuralgia with recurrent cutaneous herpes in the same area (Behrman and Knight, 1954), and by the almost invariable occurrence of facial herpes in the denervated skin following section of the trigeminal sensory root for the relief of trigeminal neuralgia (Carton and Kilbourne, 1952). These observations indicate that sensory neurons in the trigeminal ganglion, which mediate the pain of trigeminal neuralgia, may also harbor latent HSV, but they do not prove that the virus is responsible for the recurrent episodes of pain. Moreover, the absence of antibody to HSV in some patients with trigeminal neuralgia indicates that even if HSV does cause this syndrome, it is not the only cause. The association of HSV with idiopathic facial paralysis (Bell's palsy) is based primarily upon serologic studies and is tenuous at best (Adour et al., 1975; Finelli, 1975). The association of HSV with the other neurologic syndromes may only be coincidental, for it is based upon virus isolations, serologic studies, and observed temporal relationships between attacks of recurrent herpes and the neurologic syndrome in very few cases.

Recurrent HSV infections may be associated with allergic cutaneous and mucocutaneous disorders, especially erythema multiforme (Nasemann, 1964; Shelley, 1967; Britz and Sibulkin, 1975; Kazmierowski et al., 1982). In 10 to 15 per cent of cases, erythema multiforme is preceded by a symptomatic attack of recurrent herpes simplex. Furthermore, the disease has been induced by the intradermal inoculation of inactivated HSV antigen in patients who suffer erythema multiforme in association with recurrent herpes simplex, but not in individuals with a history of uncomplicated recurrent herpes simplex (Nasemann, 1964; Shelley, 1967). The erythema multiforme usually begins 3 to 10 days after the appearance of the herpetic lesions and varies in severity from mild disease with typical target (iris) lesions on the extremities (erythema multiforme minor) to severe and extensive disease with lesions over the entire body, including the palms and soles (Fig. 10), and painful bullous-erosive lesions on the mucous membranes of the eyes, nose, oropharynx, genitalia, and anus (erythema multiforme major or Stevens-Johnson syndrome). Although the mucosal lesions may be confused with lesions caused directly by HSV infection, their histopathology is quite distinct (Lever, 1975). They are vasculitic in origin, and vesicles, when present, are subepidermal. Their formation represents an allergic response, presumably to circulating HSV antigens or HSV antigen-antibody complexes (Kazmierowski et al., 1982) and is not the result of virus replication in the skin. Thus, they do not contain inclusion bodies or multinucleated giant cells, and almost never yield HSV when cultured.

GEOGRAPHIC VARIATION IN DISEASE AND EPIDEMIOLOGY. Herpes simplex viruses are worldwide in distribution. Although many experimental animals can be infected, humans are the only natural reservoir, and no vectors are involved in transmission. The principal mode of transmission is by contact with infected secretions.

Geographic variations in the pattern of diseases caused by HSV (for example, the occurrence of fatal disseminated HSV-1 infections in African children) reflect differences in the conditions of host populations and in the age of acquisition of infection, and not variations in the parasite. There is no evidence of differing racial or sexual susceptibility to HSV.

There are two distinct serotypes of HSV, HSV-1 and HSV-2, which can be distinguished on the basis of anti-

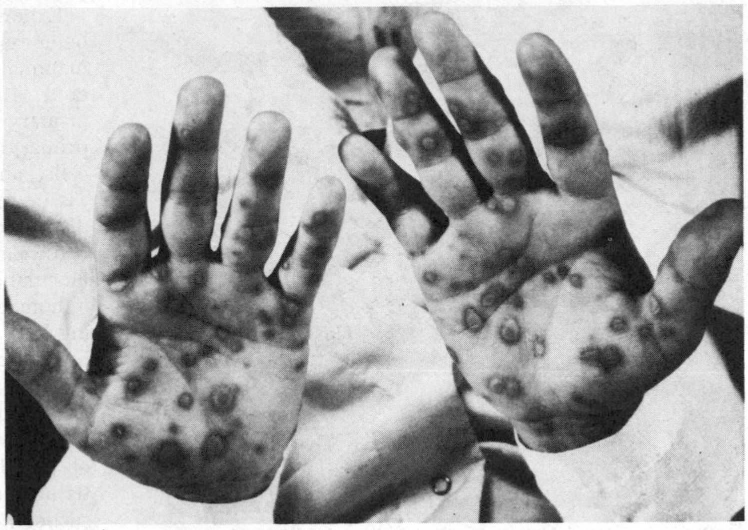

Figure 10. Recurrent erythema multiforme associated with recurrent herpes simplex. A young man with recurrent herpes simplex involving a small patch of skin over the left scapula regularly develops erythema multiforme 3 to 5 days after the onset of each herpetic recurrence. The rash, which consists of characteristic target (iris) lesions, involves primarily the skin of the trunk and extremities, including the palms and soles. Herpes simplex virus type 1 is regularly isolated from the herpes lesion, but it is not present in the target lesions, and no inclusion bodies or multinucleated giant cells were detected when the lesions of erythema multiforme were biopsied.

genic, biologic, and biochemical differences (Nahmias and Dowdle, 1968; Nahmias and Roizman, 1973; Honess and Watson, 1977; Nahmias and Josey, 1982; Roizman and Tognon, 1983). However, the greatest difference between HSV-1 and HSV-2 is probably their epidemiology. HSV-1 is transmitted mainly by nongenital routes, as a result of contact with infected saliva. HSV-2 is transmitted sexually or from a mother's genital infection to her newborn. These differences are reflected by differences in the age of acquisition and in the anatomic sites of infection (Table 1). Since HSV-2 is transmitted by sexual activity, most primary HSV-2 infections occur after puberty, and involve the genitals and other body sites below the waist. The epidemiology of HSV-2 infection is discussed in Chapter 163.

Primary infection with HSV-1 occurs most frequently in children, causing acute herpetic gingivostomatitis in a few, and asymptomatic infections in most. Whether or not it produces symptoms, the primary infection results in a latent infection that persists indefinitely, and in the production of antibodies and cell-mediated immunity that help to keep the endogenous HSV-1 in the latent state and render the host moderately resistant to exogenous reinfection. The presence of antibody is evidence of prior HSV-1 infection and identifies latently infected individuals. These antibody-positive individuals are subject to periodic reactivation of their latent HSV-1, and this results in symptomatic disease (herpes labialis) or asymptomatic shedding of HSV-1 in saliva (Fig. 3). It is the latently infected adults, 1 to 5 per cent of whom are shedding virus in their saliva at any given time, who are the major source of the virus that produces primary infections in susceptible children. This pattern of lifelong latent infection with periodic reactivation and virus shedding ensures the survival of HSV, even in populations too small and isolated to support the continuous circulation of such epidemic diseases as measles and influenza (Black, 1975). Thus, HSV-1 is endemic in every human society throughout the world. However, the rate of infection is related to the degree of exposure, and this is greatly influenced by population density, housing conditions, and hygiene. Crowding and poor hygiene promote the transmission of HSV-1, and, accordingly, the frequency of HSV-1 infection is inversely related to socioeconomic status (Burnet and Williams, 1939; Juel-Jensen and MacCallum, 1972; Nahmias and Josey, 1982). Thus, while nearly 100 per cent of Bantu children in Cape Town acquire antibody to HSV-1 by the age of 4 years, only about one-third of English and American university students have antibody to the virus. Age-specific differences in the response to HSV-1 infection (for example, gingivostomatitis in young children vs. pharyngitis and tonsillitis in adults) and the increased severity of HSV-2 infections in persons without prior HSV-1 infection, result in different patterns of symptomatic HSV infection in different societies or even in the same society at different stages in its development.

DIAGNOSIS. HSV infections are identified by their characteristic clinical picture and a positive laboratory diagnosis. Although a presumptive diagnosis can often be made on clinical grounds alone (for example, herpes labialis), HSV infections are often confused with other diseases, and laboratory confirmation of the clinical diagnosis is usually necessary. For example, diagnostic studies have revealed that many herpetic eruptions on the buttocks and legs that were thought to be herpes zoster are actually zosteriform herpes simplex. They have also demonstrated that some cases of typical eczema herpeticum are actually caused by varicella-zoster virus. The availability of specific antiviral chemotherapy (vide infra) now places an especially high premium on early and reliable diagnosis.

The histopathology of the skin and mucous membrane lesions caused by HSV provides a rapid and practical means of diagnosis. Multinucleated giant cells and epithelial cells containing eosinophilic intranuclear inclusion bodies distinguish the lesions of HSV from those produced by almost all other agents. Only measles and varicella-zoster virus produce multinucleated giant cells and eosinophilic intranuclear inclusion bodies. The rash of measles is normally not vesicular, the disease does not resemble HSV infection clinically or epidemiologically, and the skin lesions of measles are histopathologically distinct from those of HSV. The characteristic cytologic changes induced by HSV (and varicella-zoster virus) can be easily demonstrated in Tzanck smears prepared at the bedside (Fig. 11). Cells are scraped from the base of an early vesicle in the skin (mucous membranes, conjunctivae), spread gently on a glass micro-

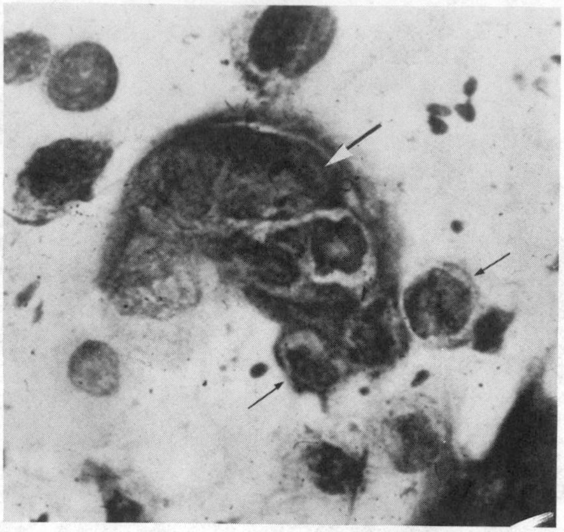

Figure 11. Tzanck smear. Cells scraped from the base of a herpetic vesicle were smeared on a glass slide and Giemsa stained. The multinucleated giant cell contains a dense clump of nuclei (large arrow). Two adherent cells (small arrows) are probably in the process of fusing with the giant cell.

scope slide, and stained with hematoxylin-eosin, Giemsa's, Papanicolaou's or Paragon Multiple stain (Blank et al., 1951; Barr et al., 1977; Rawls, 1979). Punch biopsies provide more reliable material for histologic examination, especially when lesions are secondarily infected with bacteria or fungi. Biopsy also facilitates diagnosis in the prevesicular stage. Biopsy should be obtained from edges of lesions and should be fixed in Bouin's or another acid fixative to demonstrate best intranuclear inclusion bodies. Scrapings, vesicle fluid, and biopsy specimens can also be examined for virus particles by electron-microscopy. However, neither electron-microscopy nor histopathologic examination can distinguish HSV from VZV infection. This can be done only by virus isolation or by the direct detection and identification of HSV antigens or nucleic acids in tissue or vesicle fluid.

Rapid detection and identification of HSV antigens or nucleic acids in clinical specimens is now a reality (Olding-Stenkvist and Grandien, 1976; Schmidt et al., 1980; Moseley et al., 1981; Richman et al., 1984). Immunofluorescent or immunoperoxidase staining of cellular material obtained by scraping or biopsy can identify viral antigens and, in skilled hands, provide a rapid and specific diagnosis. Highly specific antisera or monoclonal antibodies can differentiate HSV from VZV, and HSV-1 from HSV-2 (Rawls, 1979; Balachandran et al., 1982b; Richman et al., 1982; Goldstein et al., 1983). A number of other approaches to the rapid detection and identification of viral antigens are under investigation, including solid-phase radio-immunoassays, enzyme-linked immunosorbent assays (ELISA), and solid-phase enzyme immunoassays (Cleveland et al., 1982; Richman et al, 1984). Nucleic acid hybridization with radiolabeled or biotinylated probes can detect HSV nucleic acids in clinical specimens (Redfield et al., 1983) and promises rapid diagnosis at least as sensitive and specific as antigen detection. At present, however, virus isolation is the most sensitive and specific method for the diagnosis of HSV infections (Cho and Feng, 1978; Richman et al., 1984).

Experimental animals and embryonated eggs have now been replaced in most laboratories by tissue cultures of mammalian cells for isolation of HSV (Rawls, 1979; Landry et al., 1982). The most sensitive cells for HSV isolation are primary human embryonic kidney, primary human amnion, primary guinea pig embryo, and primary rabbit-kidney cells, and diploid human lung and foreskin fibroblasts. Tissue for virus isolation should be finely minced and/or dispersed with collagenase or trypsin, washed with tissue culture medium, and inoculated into tissue cultures. The inoculation of viable cells rather than a clarified suspension of homogenized tissue will increase the likelihood of isolating HSV from specimens containing small amounts of virus, especially if antibody is also present. Vesicle fluid should be aspirated from fresh vesicles and inoculated directly into tissue cultures. Since the titer of virus in vesicle fluid is usually maximal during the first 24 to 48 hours (Spruance et al., 1977), patients should be cultured then. Other tissues and body fluids should also be cultured when suspect. These include blood, spinal fluid, urine, stool, saliva, throat washings or swabs, urethral swabs, seminal fluid, and vaginal and cervical secretions. Many require special preparation before inoculation (Rawls, 1979). All specimens for virus isolation should be carried to the virology laboratory on ice and processed immediately. They may be held at 0°C for several hours (never in the freezer compartment of a refrigerator or in an ordinary −20°C freezer) but if tissue cultures cannot be inoculated within 12 to 18 hours, specimens should be stored at −70°C or lower. Typical cytopathic effects are usually apparent within 24 to 48 hours if the specimen contains much virus, but cultures should be observed for at least 2 weeks before being considered negative. Virus isolates can be identified as HSV and typed as HSV-1 or HSV-2 by a variety of serologic techniques (Nahmias and Dowdle, 1968; Plummer, 1973; Plummer et al., 1974; Rawls, 1979; Richman et al., 1982; Goldstein et al., 1983), by nucleic acid hybridization, by restriction endonuclease analysis of viral DNA (Roizman and Tognon, 1983) or by electrophoretic analysis of viral proteins (Cassai et al., 1975; Londsdale et al., 1979). Restriction endonuclease analysis of viral DNA or electrophoretic analysis of viral proteins can also distinguish between different strains of the same HSV serotype. HSV-1 and HSV-2 can also be differentiated by biologic and biochemical characteristics (Table 1; Kelman et al., 1975; Marks-Hellman and Ho, 1976; Nordlund et al., 1977), but these methods are less definitive than serotyping or analysis of viral DNA.

The differential diagnosis of HSV infection depends upon the anatomic site involved. Acute herpetic gingivostomatitis can usually be recognized clinically, but it may sometimes be confused with herpangina (caused by Coxsackie A viruses), Stevens-Johnson syndrome, aphthous ulcers, or oral candidiasis. The vesicular lesions of herpangina are clinically indistinguishable from those caused by HSV, but they are usually confined to the soft palate and posterior pharynx. Gingivitis, which is invariably present in acute herpetic gingivostomatitis, does not occur in herpangina. The oral lesions of Stevens-Johnson syndrome may look the same as those of acute herpetic gingivostomatitis, but the rash is characteristic (see Fig. 10). The histopathology of the lesions of Stevens-Johnson syndrome (and of herpangina and aphthous ulcers) is totally different from that of the lesions induced by HSV. Varicella usually produces a few lesions in the mouth, but the typical rash on the trunk develops rapidly, making the diagnosis obvious.

Acute herpetic pharyngotonsillitis may be confused with acute exudative tonsillitis caused by β-hemolytic streptococci, diphtheria, or infectious mononucleosis. When vesicular lesions are absent, microbiologic cultures, blood smears, serologic tests, and virus isolation may be required to make the diagnosis.

Acute herpetic vulvovaginitis may sometimes be confused with ammoniacal dermatitis (diaper rash), impetigo, candidiasis, or gonococcal infection. The diseases may be differentiated by smears and cultures. Autoinoculation with vaccinia may be hard to distinguish from herpetic vulvovaginitis, but this can be done by histopathologic examination and confirmed by immunologic studies or virus isolation. The eradication of smallpox and cessation of routine vaccination should eliminate this complication.

Eczema herpeticum must be differentiated from eczema vaccinatum, varicella-zoster virus infection of the eczematous skin, and from secondary bacterial infection. A careful epidemiologic history is often helpful, but the diagnosis must be established by histopathologic examination of the involved tissue, and by direct detection of HSV antigens or nucleic acids, or by virus isolation. The herpetic lesions may be very atypical and are often superinfected with bacteria. This is especially true in burn patients, in whom the diagnosis often depends upon a high index of suspicion and laboratory examination of suspect tissues. Biopsy at the edge of the involved area and examination of satellite lesions is helpful.

HSV hepatitis usually occurs during an obvious primary HSV infection, along with other evidence of dissemination and often complicated by DIC. Early diagnosis requires a high index of suspicion and, in some cases, a liver biopsy. Herpetic esophagitis is usually unrecognized or confused with *Candida* esophagitis, with which it frequently coexists. Esophagoscopy with multiple biopsies from the margins of ulcers will usually yield the diagnosis, revealing typical multinucleate giant cells and intranuclear inclusions. CMV may also be present, but the cytopathology differs from that of HSV, and direct identification of viral antigens or nucleic acids will provide an unequivocal diagnosis.

Traumatic herpes may be confused with herpes zoster, contact dermatitis, and bacterial superinfection of the traumatized site. Examination of the involved tissue for HSV antigens or nucleic acid, or virus isolation may be required to establish the diagnosis.

Herpetic whitlow is often mistaken for a bacterial infection, treated with antibiotics, and, when there is no improvement, incised. The presence of vesicles (Fig. 6) may suggest herpetic infection, but the diagnosis is made by aspiration, with cytologic examination of the exfoliated cells, and assay for HSV antigens or nucleic acid, or virus isolation.

Herpetic keratoconjunctivitis may be confused with infections of the eye caused by adenoviruses and enteroviruses, and also with bacterial, chlamydial and mycobacterial conjunctivitis. Histopathologic examination of conjunctival scrapings, assay for HSV antigens or nucleic acid, and virus or bacterial isolation, are required for diagnosis.

Recurrent cutaneous herpes simplex may be confused with herpes zoster. However, herpes simplex characteristically recurs repeatedly at the same site, whereas herpes zoster rarely recurs in the same dermatome. The lesions caused by the two viruses are indistinguishable histologically, but they may be easily differentiated by direct assay for HSV antigens or nucleic acid, and virus isolation. The lesions may also be confused with contact dermatitis.

Disseminated cutaneous lesions occurring in the course of primary or recurrent HSV infections cannot be distinguished from the lesions of varicella or disseminated herpes zoster, except by virus isolation or direct detection of HSV antigens or nucleic acid.

A number of serologic assays have been developed to detect and quantitate antibodies to HSV (Nahmias and Dowdle, 1968; Plummer, 1973; Nahmias and Josey, 1982; Rawls, 1979). They have been valuable for epidemiologic surveys and can give a retrospective diagnosis of primary HSV infection. However, their diagnostic value is limited by the need to obtain a convalescent serum in order to demonstrate seroconversion. Neither a rising titer of antibody to HSV (as opposed to the acquisition of antibody by a seronegative individual) nor the presence of HSV-specific IgM antibody is diagnostic of primary infection because recurrent HSV infections may also occasionally be associated with a fourfold or greater increase in antibody titer and often result in the synthesis of IgM antibody to HSV. The diagnostic value of serologic assays is also limited by the antigenic cross-reactivity of HSV and VZV (heterotypic anamnestic responses to VZV may occur in individuals infected with HSV, and vice versa) and by the fact that HSV-1 and HVS-2 share many antigens. Antibodies produced in response to infection by either of the two serotypes react with both HSV-1 and HSV-2, although the response to the homologous virus is generally greater. A number of techniques have been developed to detect type-specific responses (Plummer, 1973; Plummer et al., 1974; Rawls, 1979), but they often fail to give clear-cut results. In the future, the use of type-specific HSV antigens and type-specific monoclonal antibodies should permit the development of practical type-specific serologic assays (Eberle and Courtney, 1981).

TREATMENT. In normal persons, primary infections with HSV-1 are usually asymptomatic. Most symptomatic infections are self-limited and relatively brief, so that treatment is chiefly supportive. Attempts at specific therapy have focused upon severe infections, such as herpes simplex encephalitis (Chapter 180), neonatal HSV infections (Chapter 163), mucocutaneous infections in immunocompromised patients, and recurrent infections, which account for significant morbidity because of their frequency and prevalence.

Progress has been made in the development, evaluation, and application of specific antiviral agents for the therapy of severe HSV infections, and many important lessons have been learned. These include the realization (a) that anecdotal experience, case reports, and uncontrolled trials can lead to the false impression of efficacy and can encourage both physicians and patients to use ineffective and harmful remedies; (b) that in diseases such as those caused by the herpesviruses, the efficacy and toxicity of an antiviral agent can be evaluated only by randomized, double-blind, placebo-controlled studies involving *proven* cases; and (c) that antiviral drugs that act by direct inhibition of virus multiplication can be effective only if administered at a time when progression of disease is dependent upon continuing virus replication. Thus, therapeutic efficacy in herpes labialis in the normal person will be difficult to demonstrate, since virus replication is maximum during the first 24 hours and, even without therapy, declines rapidly thereafter (Spruance et al., 1977). In contrast, it is much easier to assess therapeutic efficacy in mucocutaneous herpes simplex in severely immunosuppressed patients, since HSV replicates continuously for two weeks or more in this disease (Wade et al., 1982).

The most promising chemotherapeutic agents for severe HSV infections are nucleoside derivatives that interfere with HSV DNA synthesis, and interferon. Two of the former, 5′-iodo-2′-deoxyuridine (idoxuridine, IUdR) and 1-β-D-arabinofuranosylcytosine (cytosine arabinoside, ara-C) are ineffective and toxic when administered systemically. A third, 9-β-D-arabinofuranosyladenine (adenine arabinoside, vidarabine), is effective for therapy of herpes simplex encephalitis (Whitley et al., 1977), for neonatal HSV infections (Whitley et al., 1980), and for VZV infections in immunocompromised patients (Whitley et al., 1982; Hirsch and Schooley, 1983). However, administered intravenously at 10 mg/kg/day for 7 days in a placebo-controlled crossover study involving 85 immunocompromised patients with mucocutaneous HSV infections, vidarabine failed to alter significantly the clearance of virus from lesions or the time to healing, except in a subgroup of older patients infected with HSV-1 (Whitley et al., 1984b). More encouraging is the advent of a new generation of antiviral drugs designed to take advantage of two HSV-specific enzymes, deoxypyrimidine (thymidine) kinase and DNA polymerase. The first to be evaluated clinically is acyclovir [9-(2-hydroxyethoxymethyl) guanine, acycloguanosine], a guanosine analogue that is selectively phosphorylated by HSV deoxypyrimidine kinase, but is a poor substrate for cellular thymidine kinases. As a result, the concentration of acyclovir monophosphate in HSV-infected cells is 30 to 100 times greater than in uninfected cells. Cellular enzymes convert acyclovir monophosphate to acyclovir triphosphate, which is a selective inhibitor of HSV DNA polymerase (Elion, 1982). In addition, any acyclovir incorporated into DNA causes chain termination. Acyclovir is a highly effective and nontoxic inhibitor of HSV replication in tissue culture and in animal models of HSV infection. At therapeutic concentrations, it has no observable effects on hematopoietic precursor cells or on the immune system (Hirsch and Schooley, 1983). Acyclovir has been safe and effective in a number of clinical trials and is being compared with vidarabine for treatment of HSV encephalitis, neonatal HSV infections, and disseminated VZV infections in immunosuppressed patients.

A double-blind placebo-controlled trial of intravenous acyclovir (250 mg/m^2 each 8 hours for 7 days) for treatment of mucocutaneous HSV infection in bone marrow transplant recipients showed a beneficial response in 13 of 17 acyclovir recipients, compared with 2 of 17 placebo recipients (Wade et al., 1982). Acyclovir reduced the average duration of virus shedding from 17 to 3 days, the average duration of pain from 16 to 10 days, the average time to crusting of all lesions from 14 to 7 days, and the average time to complete healing from 28 to 14 days. There was no observable toxicity, but recurrences occurred earlier in acyclovir than in placebo recipients. Similar controlled treatment studies have been carried out in cardiac transplant recipients and in other immunosuppressed patients (Chou et al., 1981; Mitchell et al., 1981; Meyers et al., 1982) with comparable results. Uncontrolled trials in immunocompromised patients with mucocutaneous HSV infections suggest that orally administered acyclovir is also effective (Straus et al., 1982) and controlled trials are underway. Uncontrolled trials in several patients with eczema herpeticum suggest that both intravenous and oral acyclovir are also effective in this disease (Swart et al., 1983; Woolfson, 1984). Topical acyclovir (5 per cent acyclovir in polyethylene glycol ointment) administered 6 times daily in a double-blind placebo-controlled study in immunocompromised patients accelerated the healing of mucocutaneous lesions caused by HSV-1 when these lesions were accessible to the application of the ointment (Whitley et al., 1984a). No attempt was made to treat intraoral lesions, and these did not resolve more rapidly in acyclovir recipients. Taken together, these data indicate that acyclovir, administered intravenously, is a safe and effective drug capable of inhibiting HSV replication in severely immunocompromised patients and, presumably in normal individuals as well. Preliminary observations, as well as the results of placebo-controlled trials in patients with genital herpes (Chapter 163), suggest that acyclovir is also effective when administered orally.

On the basis of the information discussed above, intravenous acyclovir (250 mg/m^2 or 5 mg/kg each 8 hours for 7 to 10 days) is recommended for treatment of mucosal and cutaneous HSV infections in immunocompromised patients when their infection or underlying disease is severe enough to warrant hospitalization. Oral acyclovir (200 mg 5 times daily for 10 days) appears to be a reasonable alternative, especially for patients who are not hospitalized. When accessible to application, mucocutaneous HSV infections in immunocompromised patients can often be successfully treated with topical acyclovir (5 per cent acyclovir ointment) applied 4 to 6 times daily for 10 to 14 days or until cultures for HSV are negative or the lesions have crusted. Immunosuppression should be reduced if possible.

Acute herpetic gingivostomatitis, even when severe, is self-limited. Therapy should reduce pain and maintain nutrition. Cold, bland liquids and semisolids (for example, ice cream) are usually well tolerated. Frequent bland mouthwashes (for example, with a solution of sodium bicarbonate) may reduce pain and improve oral hygiene. Systemic analgesics also help. A topical anesthetic (for example, viscous Xylocaine) relieves pain and promotes eating and drinking. Infants must be carefully observed for dehydration and acidosis, and if oral intake cannot be maintained, they should receive parenteral fluids and electrolytes in the hospital. Antibiotics have no effect, and corticosteroids are contraindicated. Acute herpetic pharyngotonsillitis is are also treated symptomatically with systemic analgesics and warm saline or tap water gargles. The local pain of acute herpetic vulvovaginitis may be relieved by warm sitz baths and systemic analgesics. Pain and local edema may cause urinary retention, and this may require catheterization. Herpetic whitlows are treated with systemic analgesics. Elevation of the affected hand often helps to reduce pain. The lesion should not be incised. Although firm recommendations must await the results of appropriate clinical trials, it appears reasonable to treat initial HSV infections in normal patients that are severe enough to warrant hospitalization with intravenous acyclovir (250 mg/m^2 or 5 mg/kg every 8 hours for 5 to 7 days). Oral acyclovir (200 mg 5 times daily for 10 days) provides an attractive alternative, especially in patients who do not require hospitalization.

It was hoped that by reducing virus replication at the portal of entry, effective antiviral therapy of primary HSV infections would reduce the quantity of virus reaching the sensory ganglion and thereby reduce the number of latently infected neurons; this, in turn, would reduce the frequency of subsequent attacks of recurrent herpes simplex. Unfortunately, studies in animal models and experience with the treatment of primary genital herpes (Chapter 163) suggest that neuronal latency is established very early in primary HSV infection; therapy begun when lesions appear can reduce the duration and severity of illness, but does not appear to reduce the frequency or severity of recurrences.

In eczema herpeticum and HSV infections of burns, a major concern is bacterial superinfection and fluid and electrolyte balance. Silver nitrate (0.5 per cent), aluminum acetate, sulfamylon, silver sulfadiazine, or povidone-iodine dressings may be employed, and frequent surveillance for bacterial infection is essential. Because of their severity and propensity for dissemination, these HSV infections should be treated with intravenous acyclovir (250 mg/m^2 or 5 mg/kg each 8 hours) for 7 to 10 days or until serial cultures are negative for HSV. Oral acyclovir (200 mg 5 times daily) may provide a reasonable alternative.

Human immune serum globulin contains antibody to HSV-1 and HSV-2. It is of unproven value, but in view of the efficacy in mice of antibody administered within 48 hours of primary infection (Oakes and Rosemond-Hornbeak, 1978; McKendall et al., 1979; Balachandran et al., 1982a) it seems reasonable to administer it in relatively large amounts (10 to 40 ml) to patients early in primary eczema herpeticum, to HSV-infected burn patients and, perhaps, to other compromised hosts with primary HSV infections.

Severe cases of erythema multiforme or Stevens-Johnson syndrome, which usually begin as the lesions of recurrent herpes with which they are associated are resolving, may respond to a short, tapering course of parenteral corticosteroids. However, care must be taken that the skin and mucosal lesions do not represent HSV dissemination. Administration of acyclovir (250 mg/m^2 or 5 mg/kg each 8 hours for 5 to 7 days) at the outset of each recurrence (during the neuralgic prodrome, if possible) may reduce the incidence or severity of HSV-associated erythema multiforme, and would certainly alleviate concerns about HSV dissemination during corticosteroid therapy.

Herpetic infections of the eye should be treated by an ophthalmologist. Corticosteroids (local or systemic) are contraindicated. They facilitate progression and local extension of infection and should be avoided in undiagnosed conditions that might prove to be herpetic. HSV infections in the eye are amenable to topical treatment with several different nucleoside derivatives and human interferons. Active nucleoside derivatives include idoxuridine, vidarabine, trifluorothymidine, and acyclovir (Pavan-Langston, 1982). Corneal infections are uniquely susceptible to antiviral therapy, and responses in the eye are easily evaluated. Therefore, it was no accident that herpes keratitis was the first infection for which the efficacy of antiviral chemotherapy was established (Chapter 245).

Although generally regarded by the unafflicted as little more than a common nuisance, herpes labialis and other recurrent mucocutaneous HSV infections frequently cause physical and emotional distress. Thus, many patients with recurrent herpes seek medical advice and receive some form of treatment. These treatments have ranged from psychotherapy and vitamins to smallpox vaccination, the local application of corticosteroids, x-irradiation, and photodynamic inactivation with neutral red and light. A variety of substances have been used in an attempt to increase immune responses to HSV and thereby reduce the frequency and severity of herpetic recurrences. These have included smallpox vaccinations (Kern and Schiff, 1959); levamisole (Mehr and Albano, 1977); Bacillus Calmette-Guerin (BCG) (Bierman, 1976); and a number of live and inactivated HSV "vaccines" (Wise et al., 1977). When subjected to controlled trials, none of these treatments have altered the frequency or severity of herpetic recurrences (Overall, 1979). Furthermore, the rapidity with which each new therapy is embraced by physicians and their patients testifies to the lack of efficacy of the methods previously in vogue. Because many of these forms of therapy are hazardous and ineffective (for example, x-irradiation, corticosteroids, smallpox vaccinations), it is important that any new treatment be carefully evaluated before being accepted for general use. All regimens involving the topical application of agents designed to limit virus replication for the treatment of recurrent mucocutaneous herpes simplex have been ineffective in controlled studies (Overall, 1979). They include idoxuridine (Kibrick and Katz, 1970); vidarabine (Adams et al., 1976); vidarabine monophosphate (Spruance et al., 1979); photodynamic inactivation with neutral red and light (Myers et al., 1975); and ether (Corey et al., 1978).

Several problems are encountered in attempting to treat recurrent herpes simplex with agents that inhibit HSV replication. During recurrent infections, HSV multiplication usually reaches its peak shortly after the onset of visible lesions, and thus, unless therapy is initiated very early, it is too late to have any impact on the course of the disease. The cornified layer of the epidermis is impenetrable to many compounds and may prevent drugs that are applied to the surface from reaching the deeper layers of the epidermis in which HSV replicates. Recurrent herpes simplex results from the reactivation of HSV that is latent in the corresponding sensory ganglion, and thus it seems unlikely that local therapy applied to the skin will alter the latent HSV infection at this distant ganglionic site. Therefore, even if topical therapy were to succeed in decreasing the duration and severity of an individual recurrence, it is unlikely to alter the frequency of subsequent recurrences (Myers et al., 1975). Topical acyclovir (5 per cent in polyethylene glycol) has recently been evaluated for treatment of herpes labialis in normal individuals and for treatment of mucocutaneous HSV infections in immunocompromised patients. Topical acyclovir (5 per cent and 10 per cent in polyethylene glycol ointment) had no effect on recurrent orolabial HSV infections (herpes labialis) in normal individuals (Spruance et al., 1982 and 1984). However, while less effective than intravenous acyclovir, topical acyclovir did shorten the period of virus shedding, halt progression, reduce pain and accelerate healing in immunocompromised patients with mucocutaneous HSV-1 infections (Whitley et al., 1982 and 1984a). Acyclovir cream appears to be more effective than acyclovir ointment; it has some clinical efficacy in herpes labialis (Yeo and Fiddian, 1983).

The efficacy of acyclovir for the treatment and prophylaxis (vide infra) of HSV infections, especially in immunocompromised patients, suggests that this drug (and other similar compounds presently being evaluated) will soon be widely used. This poses two potential problems: (1) the emergence of drug resistant mutants of HSV and (2) depressed immunity to HSV infection as a consequence of drug therapy, which might result in more frequent or more severe recurrences.

Acyclovir and other promising antiviral agents depend for their selective antiherpes activity upon their specific interaction with HSV deoxypyrimidine (thymidine) kinase (TK) and HSV DNA polymerase. Mutants of HSV affecting these enzymes occur in nature and can be selected by growing virus in the presence of acyclovir (Parris and Harrington, 1982; Coen and Schaffer, 1980; Schnipper and Crumpacker, 1980; Field, 1983; Balfour, 1983). The most common mutation is one characterized by total or partial absence of HSV TK synthesis. Such mutants, which are relatively resistant to acyclovir and similar inhibitors, have already been recovered from immunocompromised patients during or following courses of acyclovir therapy (Crumpacker et al., 1982; Sibrack et al., 1982). Fortunately, TK-deficient mutants of HSV appear to be relatively nonvirulent, at least in some animal models (Field, 1983). A second class of acyclovir-resistant mutants produce an HSV TK with altered substrate specificity. Such mutants may not be less virulent than wild-type HSV. A third class of mutants are resistant to acyclovir because they synthesize an altered DNA polymerase. Such mutants are often resistant to many other inhibitors, including vidarabine, and do not appear to be significantly less virulent than wild-type HSV. To date, almost all clinical isolates of acyclovir-resistant HSV have been of the TK-deficient variety, but it will only be a matter of time before we are faced with the emergence of mutants of the other two classes. Clearly, careful surveillance is warranted in patients being treated with acyclovir, especially immunocompromised patients receiving repeated courses of therapy. Moreover, efforts must be made to prevent the clinical abuse of acyclovir and other antivirals to avoid widespread drug resistance.

In bone marrow transplant patients with mucocutaneous HSV infections and in normal individuals with primary genital HSV, early treatment with parenteral or oral acyclovir diminishes the humoral and cell-mediated immune responses to HSV (Ashley and Corey, 1984; Wade et al., 1984). This does not seem to be due to any direct immunosuppressive effect of acyclovir, but appears to be related to reduced antigenic stimulation resulting from inhibition of HSV replication (the desired therapeutic effect). Treated patients with such reduced immune responses tended to have earlier and more severe recurrences than untreated controls who suffered unmodified infection. This potential problem, as well as the failure of treatment initiated after the onset of symptoms to prevent the establishment of neuronal latency, will have to be considered as we develop strategies for the use of antiviral drugs in various clinical situations.

PROPHYLAXIS. Disease associated with primary HSV infection can be prevented, at least in theory, by avoiding exposure to the virus; by using something to prevent HSV replication, and thus infection, in exposed individuals (e.g., early post-exposure administration of VZIG to prevent varicella; Chapter 235); or by modifying host resistance so that exposure produces either no infection or an attenuated infection unaccompanied by disease. Since much of the morbidity associated with HSV is the result of recurrent infections, prophylaxis, to be effective, would have to prevent the establishment of latent infections or at least greatly reduce the frequency and severity of their subsequent reactivation. Once latency has been established, prevention of disease can be accomplished by preventing reactivation of HSV in latently infected neurons, by blocking the intra-axonal transport of reactivated virus to the periphery, or by preventing the peripheral replication of HSV in the skin or mucous membranes.

The ubiquity of HSV infection and the frequency of asymptomatic virus shedding make avoidance of exposure impractical except under very special circumstances. For example, medical and dental personnel can reduce their risk of acquiring herpetic whitlows by wearing gloves when using tracheal catheters or when working with their fingers in patients' mouths. Patients with eczema herpeticum or HSV-infected burns (who shed enormous quantities of HSV) should be isolated. Individuals with symptomatic herpes labialis (who shed virus in saliva more frequently and in larger quantities than they do when they are asymptomatic) should avoid contact with particularly vulnerable individuals—for example, newborns or children with eczema. Men and women with genital herpes should avoid intercourse when lesions are present (Chapter 163). The incidence of neonatal herpes may be reduced by monitoring high-risk pregnant women for genital herpes during pregnancy and delivering infants whose mothers have genital herpes at term by cesarean section, in order to avoid exposure to virus during passage through the infected birth canal (Chapter 163).

Since recurrent herpes occurs in immunologically normal individuals with high levels of neutralizing antibody, both as a consequence of reactivation of latent endogenous HSV and following exogenous re-exposure (Roizman and Tognon, 1983) passive immunization would not be expected to provide solid protection. However, results obtained in animal models (Oakes and Rosemond-Hornbeck, 1978; McKendall et al., 1979; Balachandran et al., 1982a) and analogy with post-exposure prophylaxis of varicella (Chapter 235) suggest that, if available, immunoglobulin preparations with high titers of antibody to HSV might modify, if not prevent, primary HSV infections. In addition, the successful use of acyclovir to prevent recurrences of HSV infection in immunocompromised patients (vide infra), as well as studies in experimental animals, suggest that immediate post-exposure administration of acyclovir might prevent, or at least modify, primary HSV infections. Studies addressing this possibility are underway with oral acyclovir in individuals with sexual exposure to HSV.

Successful immunization against most virus infections induces virus-specific neutralizing antibodies and cell-mediated immune responses that mimic those induced by natural infection. However, we do not understand the nature of immunity to HSV infection, and this poses a major problem when we seek to design and evaluate safe and effective HSV vaccines. Host defenses against HSV are multifaceted and many components appear to be interdependent. Under some circumstances, an increase in the activity of one component may be able to compensate for a deficiency in another. Yet we have not identified the critical determinants of resistance to HSV infection. Studies of susceptible immunocompromised patients should be revealing, but immunosuppressive diseases and treatments often affect multiple components of the host defense. Thus, even when the results of an in vitro assay correlate with in vivo resistance and susceptibility, the particular mechanism identified may not be among those directly responsible. Recurrent infections occur in the presence of high titers of neutralizing antibody. In fact, the level of antibody to HSV appears to reflect the level of continuing antigenic stimulation. Thus, in renal transplant recipients, HSV reactivation occurs most often in patients with the highest pretransplantation titers of antibody to HSV (Pass et al., 1979). Moreover, while an increased frequency of HSV reactivation is associated with the period of maximal immunosuppression in organ transplant recipients, and is correlated with a depressed lymphocyte response to HSV antigens (Rand et al., 1977; Arvin et al., 1980), many normal individuals with recurrent herpes have cell-mediated immunity to HSV that appears normal when assayed by current techniques. Thus there are serious questions as to the biologic relevance of presently available assays of cell-mediated immunity to HSV. More detailed analysis of HSV proteins (Braun et al., 1983) may eventually lead to the development of more valid in vitro tests of host resistance to HSV infection, and thus to a better understanding of immunity. Although live and inactivated HSV vaccines (including nucleic acid–free vaccines) can protect experimental animals from lethal primary HSV infections, and can reduce the incidence of latent ganglionic infection in animal models, the demonstration that normal individuals with recurrent herpes can be superinfected with virus of the same serotype suggests that while HSV vaccines may reduce the probability of infection they will not prevent it (Roizman and Tognon, 1983). Experimental HSV vaccines, including live attenuated and nucleic acid-free subunit vaccines, are being developed and evaluated, but many questions remain to be answered before any HSV vaccine will be readily accepted for general use in humans (Allen and Rapp, 1982).

We do not understand how fever, sunlight, emotional stress, and menstruation induce the reactivation of latent HSV. Thus, it is not surprising that no means has been developed to prevent reactivation of HSV in latently infected neurons. Some people are convinced that they can prevent recurrent episodes by avoiding the provocative events (for example, by the local application of a sunscreen containing derivatives of para-amino-benzoic acid). However, the efficacy of this approach is unproven.

Acyclovir has been tested for prophylaxis of HSV infections in patients undergoing bone marrow transplantation and remission induction chemotherapy for acute leukemia. Reactivation of latent HSV infection is a major cause of illness in these profoundly immunosuppressed patients; 60 to 90 per cent of seropositive patients develop HSV infections following transplantation. None of 20 bone marrow transplant recipients treated with intravenous acyclovir developed HSV infections during two studies, whereas HSV infections occurred in 60 per cent (12 of 20) of the placebo recipients (Saral et al., 1981; Hann et al., 1983). Similarly, only 6 per cent (2 of 33) of the leukemic patients treated with intravenous acyclovir developed HSV infections, compared with 60 per cent (21 of 35) of the placebo recipients (Saral et al., 1983; Hann et al., 1983). No hematologic, renal, or hepatic toxicity was observed, although neurologic symptoms have been reported in bone marrow transplant recipients treated with acyclovir (Wade and Meyers, 1983). Comparable results were reported in patients given prophylactic oral acyclovir (200 mg every 6 hours) from 8 days before until 35 days after bone marrow transplantation (Gluckman et al., 1983). None of 20 patients treated with oral acyclovir developed HSV infections during the study, whereas HSV infections developed in 68 per cent (13 of 19) placebo recipients. No toxicity was observed. Unfortunately, acyclovir prophylaxis does not eliminate latent HSV infection, and many of the acyclovir recipients in all of these studies developed symptomatic HSV infections after the drug was stopped.

Pazin et al. (1979) have demonstrated that parenteral human leukocyte interferon administered perioperatively can reduce the frequency of reactivation of latent HSV infection induced by surgical manipulation of the trigeminal sensory root. In this placebo-controlled study, the incidence and severity of herpetic lesions and the frequency of asymptomatic salivary shedding of HSV were both reduced in recipients of interferon.

HSV vaccination has also been considered for preventing frequent recurrent HSV infections (Allen and Rapp, 1982). However, individuals with this problem appear already well immunized, and while there is some evidence that patients with frequent recurrence may have defects in HSV-specific lymphocyte transformation and γ interferon production (Pollard et al., 1982; Cunningham and Merigan, 1983) there is no evidence that HSV vaccination will alter these responses.

References

Adams, H. G., Benson, E. A., Alexander, E. R., Vontver, L. A., Remington, M. A., and Holmes, K. K. Genital herpetic infection in men and women: Clinical course and effect of topical application of adenine arabinoside. J Infect Dis 133:Suppl.:A151, 1976.

Adour, K. K., Bell, D. N., Hilsinger, R. L, Jr.: Herpes simplex virus in idiopathic facial paralysis (Bell palsy). JAMA 233:527, 1975.

Allen, W. P., and Rapp, F.: Concept review of genital herpes vaccines. J Infect Dis 145:413, 1982.

Anuras, S., and Summers, R.: Fulminant herpes simplex hepatitis in an adult: report of a case in a renal transplant recipient. Gastroenter 70:425, 1976.

Arvin, A. M., Pollard, R. B., Rasmussen, L. E., and Merigan, T. C.: Cellular and humoral immunity in the pathogenesis of recurrent herpes viral infections in patients with lymphoma. J Clin Invest 65:869, 1980.

Ashley, R. L., and Corey, L.: Effect of acyclovir treatment of primary genital herpes on the antibody response to herpes simplex virus. J Clin Invest 73:681, 1984.

Auch Moedy, J. L., Lerman, S. J., and White, R. J.: Fatal disseminated herpes simplex virus infection in a healthy child. Am J Dis Child 135:45, 1981.

Balachandran, N., Bacchetti, S., and Rawls, W. E.: Protection against lethal challenge of BALB/c mice by passive transfer of monoclonal antibodies to five glycoproteins of herpes simplex virus type 2. Infect Immun 37:1132, 1982a.

Balachandran, N., Frame, B., Chernesky, M., Kraiselburd, E., Kouri, Y., Garcia, D., Lavery, C., and Rawls, W. E.: Identification and typing of herpes simplex viruses with monoclonal antibodies. J Clin Microb 16:205, 1982b.

Balfour, H. H., Jr.: Resistance of herpes simplex to acyclovir. Ann Intern Med 98:404, 1983.

Baringer, J. R.: Recovery of herpes simplex virus from human sacral ganglions. N Engl J Med 291:828, 1974.

Baringer, J. R.: Herpes simplex virus infection of nervous tissue in animals and man. Prog Med Virol 20:1, 1975.

Baringer, J. R., and Swoveland, P.: Recovery of herpes-simplex virus from human trigeminal ganglions. N Engl J Med 288:648, 1973.

Barr, R. J., Herten, R. J., and Graham, J. H.: Rapid method for Tzanck preparations. JAMA 237:1119, 1977.

Bastian, F. O., Rabson, A. S., Yee, C. L., and Tralka, T. S.: Herpesvirus hominis: Isolation from human trigeminal ganglion. Science 178:306, 1972.

Bastian, J. F., and Kaufman, I. A.: Herpes simplex esophagitis in a healthy 10-year-old boy. J. Pediatr 100:426, 1982.

Becker, W. B., Kipps, A., and McKenzie, D.: Disseminated herpes simplex virus infection. Am J Dis Child 115:1, 1968.

Behrman, S., and Knight, G.: Herpes simplex associated with trigeminal neuralgia. Neurology 4:525, 1954.

Bierman, S. M.: BCG immunoprophylaxis of recurrent herpes progenitalis. Arch Dermatol 112:1410, 1976.

Black, W. C.: Acute infectious gingivostomatitis ("Vincent's stomatitis"). Am J Dis Child 56:126, 1938.

Black, F. L.: Infectious diseases in primitive societies. Science 187:515, 1975.

Blank, H. Burgoon, C. F., Coriell, L. L., and Scott, T. F. M.: Recurrent aphthous ulcers. JAMA 142:125, 1950.

Brain, R. T.: The clinical vagaries of the herpes virus. Br Med J 1:1061, 1956.

Braun, D. K., Pereira, L., Norrild, B., and Roizman, B.: Application of denatured, electrophoretically separated, and immobilized lysates of herpes simplex virus-infected cells for detection of monoclonal antibodies for the studies of the properties of viral proteins. J Virol 46:103, 1983.

Braun, R. W., Teute, H. K., Kirchner, H., and Munk, K.: Replication of herpes simplex virus in human T lymphocytes: characterization of the viral target cell. J Immun 132:914, 1984.

Britz, M., and Sibulkin, D.: Recurrent erythema multiforme and herpes genitalis (Type 2). JAMA 233:812, 1975.

Buchman, T. G., Roizman, B., and Nahmias, A. J.: Demonstration of exogenous genital reinfection with herpes simplex virus type 2 by restriction endonuclease fingerprinting of viral DNA. J Infect Dis 140:295, 1979.

Buddingh, G. J., Schrum, D. I., Lanier, J. C., and Guidry, D. J.: Studies of the natural history of herpes simplex infections. Pediatrics 11:595, 1953.

Burnet, F. M., and Williams, S. W.: Herpes simplex: a new point of view. Med J Aust 17:637, 1939.

Buss, D. H., and Scharyj, M.: Herpesvirus infection of the esophagus and other visceral organs in adults. Incidence and clinical significance. Am J Med 66:457, 1979.

Carton, C. A., and Kilbourne, E. D.: Activation of latent herpes simplex by trigeminal sensory-root section. N Eng J Med 246:172, 1952.

Cassai, E. N., Sarmiento, M., and Spear, P. G.: Comparison of the virion proteins specified by herpes simplex virus types 1 and 2. J Virol 16:1327, 1975.

Centifanto-Fitzgerald, J. M., Yamaguchi, T., Kaufman, H. E., Tognon, M., and Roizman, B.: Ocular disease pattern induced by herpes simplex virus is genetically determined by a specific region of viral DNA. J Exp Med 155:475, 1982.

Cesario, T. C., Poland, J. D., Wulff, H., Chin, T. D. Y., and Wenner, H. A.: Six years experience with herpes simplex virus in a children's home. Am J Epidemiol 90:416, 1969.

Chaney, S. M. J., Warren, K. G., and Subak-Sharpe, J. H.: Variable restriction endonuclease sites of herpes simplex virus type 1 isolates from encephalitic, facial and genital lesions and ganglia. J Gen Virol 64:2717, 1983.

Cho, C. T., and Feng, K. K.: Sensitivity of the virus isolation and immunofluorescent staining methods in diagnosis of infections with herpes simplex virus. J Infect Dis 138:536, 1978.

Chou, S., Gallagher, J. G., and Merigan, T. C.: Controlled clinical trial of intravenous acyclovir in heart-transplant patients with mucocutaneous herpes simplex infections. Lancet 1:1392, 1981.

Cleveland, P. H., Richman, D. D., Redfield, D. C., Disharoon, D. R., Binder, P. S., and Oxman, M. N.: Enzyme immunofiltration technique for rapid diagnosis of herpes simplex virus eye infections in a rabbit model. J Clin Microb 16:676, 1982.

Coen, D. M., and Schaffer, P. A.: Two distinct loci confer resistance to acycloguanosine in herpes simplex virus type 1. Proc Natl Acad Sci 77:2265, 1980.

Connor, R. W., Lorts, G., and Gilbert, D. N.: Lethal herpes simplex virus type 1 hepatitis in a normal adult. Gastroenterol 76:590, 1979.

Corey, L., Reeves, W. C., Chiang, W. T., Vontver, L. A., Remington, M., Winter, C., and Holmes, K. K.: Ineffectiveness of topical ether for the treatment of genital herpes simplex virus infection. Medical Intelligence 299:237, 1978.

Craig, C. P., and Nahmias, A. J.: Different patterns of neurologic involvement with herpes simplex virus type 1 and type 2: isolation of herpes simplex virus type 2 from the buffy coat of two adults with meningitis. J Infect Dis 127:365, 1973.

Crumpacker, C. S., Schnipper, L. E., Marlowe, S. I., Kowalsky, P. N., Hershey, B. J., and Levin, M. J.: Resistance to antiviral drugs of herpes simplex virus isolated from a patient treated with acyclovir. Med Intelligence 306:343, 1982.

Cunningham, A. L., and Merigan, T. C.: γ Interferon production appears to predict time of recurrence of herpes labialis. J Immunol 130:2397, 1983.

Deprew, W. T., Prentice, R. S. A., Beck, I. T., Blakeman, J. M., and DaCosta, L. R.: Herpes simplex ulcerative esophagitis in a healthy subject. Am J Gastroenterol 68:381, 1977.

Dix, R. D., McKendall, R. R., and Baringer, J. R.: Comparative neurovirulence of herpes simplex virus type 1 strains after peripheral or intracerebral inoculation of BALB/c mice. Infect Immun 40:103, 1983.

Dodd, K., Johnston, L. M., and Buddingh, G. J.: Herpetic stomatitis. J Pediatr 12:95, 1938.

Douglas, R. G., and Couch, R. B.: A prospective study of chronic herpes simplex virus infection and recurrent herpes labialis in humans. J Immunol 104:289, 1970.

Eberle, R., and Courtney, R. J.: Assay of type-specific and type-common antibodies to herpes simplex virus types 1 and 2 in human sera. Infect Immunol 31:1062, 1981.

Elion, G. B.: Mechanism of action and selectivity of acyclovir. Am J Med 73(1A):7, 1982.

Embil, J. A., Stephens, R. G., and Manuel, F. R.: Prevalence of recurrent herpes labialis and aphthous ulcers among young adults on six continents. CMA J 113:627, 1975.

Evans, A. S., and Dick, E. C.: Acute pharyngitis and tonsillitis in University of Wisconsin students. JAMA 190:699, 1964.

Faden, H. S., Bybee, B. L., Overall, J. C., and Lahey, M. E.: Disseminated herpesvirus hominis infection in a child with acute leukemia. J Pediatr 90:951, 1977.

Farmer, E. D.: Diseases of the mouth caused by the herpes simplex virus. Proc R Soc Med 49:640, 1956.

Field, H. J.: Acquired resistance to acyclovir: laboratory phenomenon or clinical problem? J Infect 6:11, 1983.

Finelli, P. F.: Herpes simplex virus and the human nervous system: Current concepts and review. Milit Med 140:765, 1975.

Fishbein, P. G., Tuthill, R., Kressel, H., Friedman, H., and Snape, W. J.: Herpes simplex esophagitis: A cause of upper-gastrointestinal bleeding. Am J Digestive Dis 24:540, 1979.

Foley, F. D., Greenawald, K. A., Nash, G., and Pruitt, B. A.: Herpesvirus infection in burned patients. N Engl J Med 282:652, 1970.

Glezen, W. P., Fernald, G. W., and Lohr, J. A.: Acute respiratory disease of university students with special reference to the etiologic role of herpesvirus hominis. Am J Epidemiol 101:111, 1975.

Gluckman, E., Devergie, A., Melo, R., Nebout, T., Lotsberg, J., Zhao, X. M., Gomez-Morales, M., and Mazeron, M. C.: Prophylaxis of herpes infections after bone-marrow transplantation by oral acyclovir. Lancet 2:706, 1983.

Goldstein, L. C., Corey, L., McDougall, J. K., Tolentino, E., and Nowinski, R. C.: Monoclonal antibodies to herpes simplex viruses: use in antigenic typing and rapid diagnosis. J Infect Dis 147:829, 1983.

Goodpasture, E. W.: Herpetic infection, with special reference to involvement of the nervous system. Medicine 8:223, 1929.

Goyette, R. E., Donowho, E. M., Hieger, L. R., and Plunkett, G. D.: Fulminant herpesvirus hominis hepatitis during pregnancy. Obstet Gynecol 43:191, 1974.

Graham, B. S., and Snell, J. D., Jr.: Herpes simplex virus infection of the adult lower respiratory tract. Medicine 62:384, 1983.

Greaves, W. L., Kaiser, A. B., Alford, R. H., and Schaffner, W.: The problem of herpetic whitlow among hospital personnel. Infect Control 1:381, 1980.

Grout, P., and Barber, V. E.: Cold sores—an epidemiological survey. J R Coll Gen Pract 26:428, 1976.

Grüter, W.: Experimentelle und klinische Untersuchungen über den sogenannten Herpes corneae. Ber Dtsch Ophthalmol Ges 42:162, 1920.

Hale, B. D., Rendtorff, R. C., Walker, L. C., and Roberts, A. N.: Epidemic herpetic stomatitis in an orphanage nursery. JAMA 183:1068, 1963.

Hammer, S. M., Buchman, T. G., D'Angelo, L. J., Karchmer, A. W., Roizman, B., and Hirsch, M. S.: Temporal cluster of herpes simplex encephalitis: investigation by restriction endonuclease cleavage of viral DNA. J Infect Dis 141:436, 1980.

Hammer, S. M., Carney, W. P., Iacoviello, V. R., Lower, B. R., and Hirsch, M. S.: Herpes simplex virus infection of human T-cell subpopulations. Infect Immunol 38:795, 1982.

Hann, I. M., Prentice, H. F., Blacklock, H. A., Ross, M. G. R., Brigden, D., Rosling, A. E., Burke, E., Crawford, D. H., Brumfitt, W., and Hoffbrand, A. V.: Acyclovir prophylaxis against herpes virus infections in severely immunocompromised patients: randomised double blind trial. British Med J 287:384, 1983.

Herout, F., Vortel, V., and Vondrackova, A.: Herpes simplex involvement of the lower respiratory tract. Am J Clin Pathology 46:411, 1966.

Hirsch, M. S., and Schooley, R. T.: Treatment of herpesvirus infections. N Engl J Med 309:963 and 309:1034, 1983.

Honess, R. W., and Watson, D. H.: Unity and diversity in the herpesviruses. J Gen Virol 37:15, 1977.

Howard, W. T.: Further observations on the relation of lesions of the gasserian and posterior root ganglia to herpes, occurring in pneumonia and cerebrospinal meningitis. Am J Med Sci 136:165, 1905.

Juel-Jensen, B. E., and MacCallum, F. O.: Herpes Simplex Varicella and Zoster. Philadelphia, Lippincott, 1972.

Juretić, M.: Natural history of herpetic infection. Helv Paediatr Acta 4:356, 1966.

Kazmierowski, J. A., Peizner, D. S., and Wuepper, K. R.: Herpes simplex antigen in immune complexes of patients with erythema multiforme: Presence following recurrent herpes simplex infection. JAMA 247:2547, 1982.

Keane, J. T., Malkinson, F. D., Bryant, J., and Levin, S.: Herpesvirus hominis hepatitis and disseminated intravascular coagulation. Arch Intern Med 136:1312, 1976.

Kelman, A. D., Capozza, F., and Kibrick, S.: Differential action of deoxynucleosides on mammalian cell cultures infected with herpes simplex virus types 1 and 2. J Infect Dis 131:452, 1975.

Kern, A. B., and Schiff, B. L.: Smallpox vaccinations in the management of recurrent herpes simplex: A controlled evaluation. J Invest Derm 33:99, 1959.

Kibrick, S., and Katz, A. S.: Topical idoxuridine in recurrent herpes simplex. Ann NY Acad Sci 173:83, 1970.

Kleinman, L. F., Kibrick, S., Ennis, F., and Polgar, P.: Herpes simplex virus replication in human lymphocyte cultures stimulated with phytomitogens and anti-lymphocyte globulin. PSEBM 141:1095, 1972.

Korsager, B., Spencer, E. S., Mordhorst, C.-H., and Andersen, H. K.: Herpesvirus hominis infections in renal transplant patients. Scand J Infect Dis 7:11, 1975.

Krohel, G. B., Richardson, J. R., and Farrell, D. F.: Herpes simplex neuropathy. Neurology 26:596, 1976.

Landry, M. L., Mayo, D. R., and Hsiung, G. D.: Comparison of guinea pig embryo cells, rabbit kidney cells, and human embryonic lung fibroblast cell stains for isolation of herpes simplex virus. J Clin Microbiol 15:842, 1982.

Layzer, R. B., and Conant, M. A.: Neuralgia in recurrent herpes simplex. Arch Neurol 31:233, 1974.

Lehner, T., Wilton, J. M. A., and Schillitoe, E. J.: Immunological basis for latency, recurrences, and putative oncogenicity of herpes simplex virus. Lancet 2:60, 1975.

Lever, W. F.: Histopathology of the Skin, 5th ed. Philadelphia, Lippincott, 1975.

Linnemann, C. C., Buchman, T. G., Light, I. J., Ballard, J. L., and Roizman, B.: Transmission of herpes-simplex virus type 1 in a nursery for the newborn: Identification of viral isolates by D.N.A. "fingerprinting." Lancet 1:964, 1978.

Logan, W. S., Tindall, J. P., and Elson, M. L.: Chronic cutaneous herpes simplex. Arch Dermatol 103:606, 1971.

Long, J. C., Wheeler, C. E., and Briggaman, R. A.: Varicella-like infection due to herpes simplex. Arch Dermatol 114:406, 1978.

Lonsdale, D. M.: A rapid technique for distinguishing herpes-simplex virus type 1 from the type 2 by restriction-enzyme technology. Lancet 1:849, 1979.

Lonsdale, D. M., Brown, S. M., Subak-Sharpe, J. H., Warren, K. G., and Koprowski, H.: The polypeptide and DNA restriction enzyme profiles of spontaneous isolates of herpes simplex virus type 1 from explants of human trigeminal, superior and vagus ganglia. J Gen Virol 43:151, 1979.

MacCallum, F. O., and Juel-Jensen, B. E.: Herpes simplex virus skin infection in men treated with idoxuridine in dimethyl sulphoxide: Results of a double-blind controlled trial. Br Med J 2:805, 1966.

Marks-Hellman, S., and Ho, M.: Use of biological characteristics to type herpesvirus hominis types 1 and 2 in diagnostic laboratories. J Clin Microbiol 3:277, 1976.

McKendall, R. R., Klassen, R., and Baringer, J. R.: Host defenses in herpes simplex infections of the nervous system: effect on disease and viral spread. Infect Immun 23:305, 1979.

Mehr, K. A., and Albano, L.: Failure of levamisole in herpes simplex. Lancet 2:773, 1977.

Mertens, T., Thomas, J. P., Zippel, C., and Eggers, H. J.: Peripheral facial palsy and viral infections—findings and problems. Med Microbiol Immunol 171:77, 1982.

Meyers, J. D., Flournoy, N., and Thomas, E. D.: Infection with herpes simplex virus and cell-mediated immunity after marrow transplant. J Infect Dis 142:338, 1980.

Meyers, J. D., Wade, J. C., Mitchell, C. D., Saral, R., Lietman, P. S., Durack, D. T., Levin, M. J., Segreti, A. C., and Balfour, H. H.: Multicenter collaborative trial of intravenous acyclovir for treatment in the immunocompromised host. Am J Med 73(1A):229, 1982.

Mitchell, C. D., Gentry, S. R., Boen, J. R., Bean, B., Groth, K. E., and Balfour, H. H.: Acyclovir therapy for mucocutaneous herpes simplex infections in immunocompromised patients. Lancet 1:1389, 1981.

Montgomerie, J. Z., Becroft, D. M. O., Croxson, M. C., Doak, P. B., and North, J. D. K.: Herpes-simplex-virus infection after renal transplantation. Lancet 2:867, 1969.

Morse, L. S., Pereira, L., Roizman, B., and Schaffer, P. A.: Anatomy of herpes simplex virus (HSV) DNA X. mapping of viral genes by analysis of polypeptides and functions specified by HSV-1 X HSV-2 recombinants. J Virol 26:369, 1978.

Moseley, R. D., Corey, L., Benjamin, D., Winter, C., and Remington, L. M.: Comparison of viral isolation, direct immunofluorescence, and indirect immunoperoxidase techniques for detection of genital herpes simplex virus infection. J Clin Microbiol 13:913, 1981.

Muller, S. A., Herrmann, E. C., and Winkilmann, R. K.: Herpes simplex infections in hematologic malignancies. Am J Med 52:102, 1972.

Myers, M. G., Oxman, M. N., Clark, J. E., and Arndt, K. A.: Failure of neutral-red photodynamic inactivation in recurrent herpes simplex virus infections. N Engl J Med 293:945, 1975.

Nahmias, A. J., and Dowdle, W. R.: Antigenic and biologic differences in herpesvirus hominis. Prog Med Virol 10:110, 1968.

Nahmias, A. J., and Josey, W. E.: Herpes simplex viruses 1 and 2. In Evans, A. S. (ed.): *Viral Infections of Humans*. Plenum Publishing Corp., New York, 1982, pp. 351–372.

Nahmias, A. J., and Roizman, B.: Infection with herpes simplex viruses 1 and 2. N Engl J Med 289:667, 719, 781, 1973.

Naraqi, W., Jackson, G. G., and Jonasson, O. M.: Viremia with herpes simplex type 1 in adults: Four nonfatal cases, one with features of chicken pox. Ann Intern Med 85:165, 1976.

Nasemann, T.: Ueber das postherpetische Erythema exsudativum multiforme. Hautarzt 15:346, 1964.

Nash, G., and Foley, F. D.: Herpetic infection of the middle and lower respiratory tract. A.J.C.P. 54:857, 1970.

Nash, G., and Ross, J. S.: Herpetic esophagitis: A common cause of esophageal ulceration. Hum Pathol 5:339, 1974.

Nicolau, S., and Poincloux, P.: Etude clinique et experimentale d'un cas d'herpès récidivant du doigt. Ann Inst Pasteur 38:977, 1924.

Nordlund, J. J., Anderson, C., Hsiung, G. D., and Tenser, R. B.: The use of temperature sensitivity and selective cell culture systems for differentiation of herpes simplex virus types 1 and 2 in a clinical laboratory. Proc Soc Exp Biol Med 155:118, 1977.

Oakes, J. E., and Rosemond-Hornbeak, H.: Antibody-mediated recovery from subcutaneous herpes simplex virus type 2 infection. Infect Immun 21:489, 1978.

Olding-Stenkvist, E., and Grandien, M.: Early diagnosis of virus-caused vesicular rashes by immunofluorescence on skin biopsies. Scand J Infect Dis 8:27, 1976.

Overall, J. C., Jr.: Dermatologic diseases. In Galasso, G. J., Merigan, T. C., and Buchanan R. A. (eds.): Antivirals in Man. New York, Raven Press, 1979.

Owensby, L. C., and Stammer, J. L.: Esophagitis associated with herpes simplex infection in an immuno-competent host. Gastroenterol 74:1305, 1978.

Parris, D. B., and Harrington, J. E.: Herpes simplex virus variants resistant to high concentrations of acyclovir exist in clinical isolates. Antimicrobiol Agents Chemoth 22:71, 1982.

Pass, R. F., Whitley, R. J., Whelchel, J. D., Diethelm, A. G., Reynolds, D. W., and Alford, C. A.: Identification of patients with increased risk of infection with herpes simplex virus after renal transplantation. J Infect Dis 140:487, 1979.

Pavan-Langston, D.: Herpetic diseases. In Smulin, G., and Thoft, R. (eds.): The Cornea: Scientific Foundations and Clinical Practice. Boston, Little, Brown, 1982, pp. 178–195.

Pazin, G. J.: Herpes simplex esophagitis after trigeminal nerve surgery. Gastroenterol 74:741, 1978.

Pazin, G. J., Ho, M., and Jannetta, P. J.: Reactivation of herpes simplex virus after decompression of the trigeminal nerve root. J Infect Dis 138:405, 1978.

Pazin, G. J., Armstrong, J. A., Tai Lam, M., Tarr, G. C., Jannetta, P. J., and Ho, M.: Prevention of reactivated herpes simplex infection by human leukocyte interferon after operation on the trigeminal root. N Engl J Med 301:225, 1979.

Plummer, G.: A review of the identification and titration of antibodies to herpes simplex viruses type 1 and type 2 in human sera. Cancer Res 33:1469, 1973.

Plummer, G., Goodheart, C. R., Miyagi, M., Skinner, G. R. B., Thouless, M. E., and Wildy, P.: Herpes simplex viruses: discrimination of types and correlation between different characteristics. Virology 60:206, 1974.

Pollard, R. B., Arvin, A. M., Gamberg, P., Rand, K. H., Gallagher, J. G., and Merigan, T. C.: Specific cell-mediated immunity and infections with herpes viruses in cardiac transplant recipients. Am J Med 73:679, 1982.

Ramsey, P. G., Fife, K. H., Hackman, R. C., Meyers, J. D., and Corey, L.: Herpes simplex virus pneumonia: Clinical, virologic, and pathologic features in 20 patients. Ann Intern Med 97:813, 1982.

Rand, K. H., Rasmussen, L. E., Pollard, R. B., Arvin, A., and Merigan, T. C.: Cellular immunity and herpesvirus infections in cardiac-transplant patients. N Engl J Med 296:1372, 1977.

Rand, K. H., Kramer, B., and Johnson, A. C.: Cancer chemotherapy associated symptomatic stomatitis. Role of herpes simplex virus (HSV). Cancer 50:1262, 1982.

Rawls, W. E.: Herpes simplex virus types 1 and 2 and herpesvirus simiae.

In Lennette, E. H., and Schmidt, N. J. (eds.): Diagnostic Procedures for Viral, Rickettsial and Chlamydial Infections, Washington, D.C., American Public Health Association, p. 309, 1979.

Redfield, D. C., Richman, D. D., Albanil, S., Oxman, M. N., and Wahl, G. M.: Detection of herpes simplex in clinical specimens by DNA hybridization. Diagn Microbiol Infect Dis 1:117, 1983.

Remafedi, G., and Muldoon, R. L.: Acute monarticular arthritis caused by herpes simplex virus type 1. Pediatr 72:882, 1983.

Richman, D. D., Cleveland, P. H., and Oxman, M. N.: A rapid enzyme immunofiltration technique using monoclonal antibodies to serotype herpes simplex virus. J Medical Virology 9:299, 1982.

Richman, D. D., Cleveland, P. H., Redfield, D. C., Oxman, M. N., and Wahl, G. M.: Rapid viral diagnosis. J Infect Dis 149:298, 1984.

Rogers, A. M., Coriell, L. L., Blank, H., and Scott, T. F. M.: Acute herpetic gingivostomatitis in the adult. N Engl J Med 241:330, 1949.

Roizman, B., and Tognon, M.: Restriction endonuclease patterns of herpes simplex virus DNA: Application to diagnosis and molecular epidemiology. In *Current Topics in Microbiology and Immunology*, Vol. 104, Springer-Verlag, New York, 1983, pp. 273–286.

Ruchman, I., Welsh, A. L., and Dodd, K.: Kaposi's varicelliform eruption: Isolation of the virus of herpes simplex from the cutaneous lesions of three adults and one infant. Arch Derm & Syph 56:846, 1947.

Rustigian, R., Smulow, J. B., Tye, M., Gibson, W. A., and Shindell, E.: Studies on latent infection of skin and oral mucosa in individuals with recurrent herpes simplex. J Invest Dermatol 47:218, 1966.

Saral, R., Ambinder, R. F., Burns, W. H., Angelopulos, C. M., Griffin, D. E., Burke, P. J., and Lietman, P. S.: Acyclovir prophylaxis against herpes simplex virus infection in patients with leukemia. Ann Intern Med 99:773, 1983.

Saral, R., Burns, W. H., Laskin, O. L., Santos, G. W., and Lietman, P. S.: Acyclovir prophylaxis of herpes-simplex-virus infections. A randomized, double-blind, controlled trial in bone-marrow-transplant recipients. N Engl J Med 305:63, 1981.

Schmidt, N. J., Gallo, D., Devlin, V., Woodie, J. D., and Emmons, R. W.: Direct immunofluorescence staining for detection of herpes simplex and varicella-zoster virus antigens in vesicular lesions and certain tissue specimens. J Clin Microbiol 12:651, 1980.

Schneidman, D. W., Barr, R. J., and Graham, J. H.: Chronic cutaneous herpes simplex. JAMA 241:592, 1979.

Schnipper, L. E., and Crumpacker, C. S.: Resistance of herpes simplex virus to acycloguanosine: role of viral thymidine kinase and DNA polymerase loci. Proc Natl Acad Sci 77:2270, 1980.

Scott, T. F. M.: Epidemiology of herpetic infections. Am J Ophthalmol 43:134, 1957.

Scott, T. F., Steigman, A. J., and Convey, J. H.: Acute infectious gingivostomatitis. JAMA 117:999, 1941.

Selling, B., and Kibrick, S.: An outbreak of herpes simplex among wrestlers (herpes gladiatorum). N Engl J Med 270:979, 1964.

Shelly, W. B.: Herpes simplex virus as a cause of erythema multiforme. JAMA 201:153, 1967.

Sheridan, P. J., and Herrmann, E. C.: Intraoral lesions of adults associated with herpes simplex virus. Oral Surg Oral Path 32:390, 1971.

Ship, I. I., Brightman, V. J., and Laster, L. L.: The patient with recurrent aphthous ulcers and the patient with recurrent herpes labialis: A study of two population samples. JADA 75:645, 1967.

Shortsleeve, M. J., Gauvin, G. P., Gardner, R. C., and Greenberg, M. S.: Herpetic esophagitis. Radiology 141:611, 1981.

Sibrack, C. D., Gutman, L. T., Wilfert, C. M., McLaren, C., St. Clair, M. H., Keller, P. M., and Barry, D. W.: Pathogenicity of acyclovir-resistant herpes simplex virus type 1 from an immunodeficient child. J Infect Dis 146:673, 1982.

Siegal, F. P., Lopez, C., Hammer, G. S., Brown, A. E., Kornfeld, S. J., Gold, J., Hassett, J., Hirschman, S. Z., Cunningham-Rundeles, C., Adelsberg, B. R., and Parham, D. M.: Severe acquired immunodeficiency in male homosexuals, manifested by chronic perianal ulcerative herpes simplex lesions. New Engl J Med 305:1439, 1981.

Slavin, H. B., and Ferguson, J. J.: Zoster-like eruptions caused by the virus of herpes simplex. Am J Med 8:456, 1950.

Spear, P. G.: Herpesviruses. In Blough, H. A., and Tiffany, J. M. (eds.): Cell Membrane and Viral Envelopes. Academic Press, London, 1980, pp. 709–750.

Spruance, S. L., Overall, J. C., Kern, E. R., Krueger, G. G., Pliam, V., and Miller, W.: The natural history of recurrent herpes simplex labialis: Implications for antiviral therapy. N Engl J Med 297:69, 1977.

Spruance, S. L., Crumpacker, C. S., Haines, H. H., Bader, C., Mehr, K., MacCalman, J., Schnipper, L. E., Klauber, M. R., Overall, J. C., and the Collaborative Study Group: Ineffectiveness of topical adenine arabinoside 5′-monophosphate in the treatment of recurrent herpes simplex labialis. N Engl J Med 300:1180, 1979.

Spruance, S. L., Schnipper, L. E., Overall, J. C., Kern, E. R., Wester, B., Modlin, J., Wenerstrom, G., Burton, C., Arndt, K. A., Chiu, G. L., and Crumpacker, C. S.: Treatment of herpes simplex labialis with topical acyclovir in polyethylene glycol. J Infect Dis 146:85, 1982.

Spruance, S. L., Crumpacker, C. S., Schnipper, L. E., Kern, E. R., Marlowe, S., Arndt, K. A., and Overall, J. C., Jr.: Early patient-initiated treatment of herpes labialis with topical 10% acyclovir. Antimicrob. Agents Chemother. 25:553, 1984.

Stern, H., Elek, S. D., Millar, D. M., and Anderson, H. F.: Herpetic whitlow: A form of cross-infection in hospitals. Lancet 2:871, 1959.

Stevens, J. G.: Latent herpes simplex virus and the nervous system. Curr Top Microbiol Immunol 70:31, 1975.

Straus, S. E., Smith, H. A., Brickman, C., de Miranda, P., McLaren, C., and Keeney, R. E.: Acyclovir for chronic mucocutaneous herpes simplex virus infection in immunosuppressed patients. Ann Intern Med 96:270, 1982.

Swart, R. N. J., Vermeer, B. J., van Der Meer, J. W. M., Enschede, F. A. J., and Versteeg, J.: Treatment of eczema herpeticum with acyclovir. Arch Dermatol 119:13, 1983.

Taylor, R. J., Saul, S. H., Dowling, J. N., Hakala, T. R., Peel, R. L., and Ho, M.: Primary disseminated herpes simplex infection with fulminant hepatitis following renal transplantation. Arch Intern Med 141:1519, 1981.

Thompson, R. L., Wagner, E. K., and Stevens, J. G.: Physical location of a herpes simplex virus type-1 gene function(s) specifically associated with a 10 million-fold increase in HSV neurovirulence. Virology 131:180, 1983.

Tuxen, D. V., Cade, J. F., McDonald, M. I., Buchanan, M. R. C., Clark, R. J. and Pain, M. C. F.: Herpes simplex virus from the lower respiratory tract in adult respiratory distress syndrome. Am Rev Respir Dis 126:416, 1982.

Wade, J. C., and Meyers, J. E.: Neurologic symptoms associated with parenteral acyclovir treatment after marrow transplantation. Ann Intern Med 98:921, 1983.

Wade, J. C., Newton, B., McLaren, C., Flournoy, M. S., Keeney, R. E., and Meyers, J. D.: Intravenous acyclovir to treat mucocutaneous herpes simplex virus infection after marrow transplantation. Ann Intern Med 96:265, 1982.

Wade, J. C., Day, L. M., Crowley, J. J., and Meyers, J. D.: Recurrent infection with herpes simplex virus after marrow transplantation: Role of the specific immune response and acyclovir treatment. J Infect Dis 149:750, 1984.

Walker, D. P., Longson, M., Lawler, W., Mallick, N. P., Davies, J. S., and Johnson, R. W. G.: Disseminated herpes simplex virus infection with hepatitis in an adult renal transplant recipient. J Clin Path 34:1044, 1981.

Warren, K. G., Brown, S. M., Wroblewska, Z., Gilden, D., Koprowski, H., and Subak-Sharpe, J.: Isolation of latent herpes simplex virus from the superior cervical and vagus ganglions of human beings. N Engl J Med 298:1068, 1978.

Wenner, H. A.: Complications of infantile eczema caused by the virus of herpes simplex: Description of the clinical characteristics of an unusual eruption and (b) identification of an associated filtrable virus. Am J Dis Child 67:247, 1944.

Whitley, R., Barton, N., Collins, E., Whelchel, J., and Diethelm, A. G.: Mucocutaneous herpes simplex virus infections in immunocompromised patients. A model for evaluation of topical antiviral agents. Am J Med 73(1A):236, 1982.

Whitley, R. J., Soong, S.-J., Dolin, R., Galasso, G. J., Ch'ien, L. T., Alford, C. A., and the Collaborative Study Group: Adenine arabinoside therapy of biopsy-proved herpes simplex encephalitis. N Engl J Med 297:289, 1977.

Whitley, R. J., Nahmias, A., Soong, S. J., Galasso, G. J., Fleming, C. L., and Alford, C. A.: Vidarabine therapy of neonatal herpes simplex virus infections. Pediatrics 66:495, 1980.

Whitley, R. J., Spruance, S., Hayden, F. G., Overall, J., Alford, C. A., Gwaltney, J. M., and Soong, S.-J.: Vidarabine therapy for mucocutaneous herpes simplex virus infections in the immunocompromised host. J Infect Dis 149:1, 1984b.

Whitley, R. J., Levin, M., Barton, N., Hershey, B. J., Davis, G., Keeney, R. E., Whelchel, J., Diethelm, A. G., Kartus, P., and Soong, S-J.: Infections caused by herpes simplex virus in the immunocompromised host: Natural history and topical acyclovir therapy. J Infect Dis 150:323, 1984a.

Wildy, P., Field, H. J., and Nash, A. A.: Classical herpes latency revisited. In Mahy, B. W. J., Minson, A. C. and Darby, G. K. (eds.): Virus Persistence. Cambridge University Press, 1982, pp. 133–167.

Wise, T. G., Pavan, P. R., and Ennis, F. A.: Herpes simplex virus vaccines. J Infect Dis 136:706, 1977.

Woolfson, H.: Oral acyclovir in eczema herpeticum. Br Med J 288:531, 1984.

Yeo, J. M., and Fiddian, A. P.: Acyclovir in the management of herpes labialis. J Antimicrob Chemother 12, Suppl. B:95, 1983.

Young, E. J., Killam, A. P., and Greene, J. F.: Disseminated herpesvirus infection: Association with primary genital herpes in pregnancy. JAMA 235:2731, 1976a.

Young, S. K., Rowe, N. H., and Buchanan, R. A.: A clinical study for the control of facial mucocutaneous herpes virus infections. Oral Surg 41:498, 1976b.

106

HERPANGINA

DAVID I. MINKOFF, M.D.
JAMES CONNOR, M.D.

Herpangina was first described by Zahorsky in 1920 as an acute febrile disease in children characterized by vesicular and ulcerative lesions on the anterior tonsillar pillars, tonsils, soft palate, and posterior buccal mucosa (Zahorsky, 1924). His description of the illness in 82 patients referred to "herpetic sore throat," but he later renamed the clinical complex "herpangina" in his 1924 report.

ETIOLOGY. In 1951 Huebner and his co-workers isolated Coxsackie A virus from stools of children with the clinical syndrome and serum neutralizing antibody rise to that virus was demonstrated. Since then the clinical syndrome has been associated with different viral serotypes, including Coxsackie A viruses 1 through 10, 16, and 22, Coxsackie B 1 through 5, and ECHO 9, 16, and 17 (Cherry and Jahn, 1965).

CLINICAL MANIFESTATIONS. The original clinical description of herpangina by Zahorsky remains accurate today:

> The disease begins suddenly as an acute febrile movement. The temperature often rises to 104° F. A convulsion may occur. Vomiting is often present. Anorexia and prostration are marked. The throat and posterior part of the mouth show minute vesicles, or if these have ruptured, small punched-out ulcers. They occur on the anterior pillar of the fauces, the tonsils, the pharynx, and the edges of the soft palate. The number of lesions varies from two to twenty. Dysphagia is often marked. The general and local symptoms disappear in a few days. The disease may be easily confused with ulcerative stomatitis which sometimes begins in the throat. The disease usually occurs in the summer months, in an epidemic manner, and children are most frequently affected.

After an incubation period of 4 to 10 days the enanthem begins as small papules and progresses to vesicles within 24 hours. They rupture, leaving ulcers surrounded by an inflammatory areola ranging in size from 1 to 5 mm with erythematous borders. These ulcers then become covered by a thin gray-white membrane. The appearance is quite different from erosions of ulcerative stomatitis. Although clinical symptoms diminish in 2 to 3 days, the ulcers persist 4 to 6 days, leaving a slight hypopigmented scar at the site.

Since multiple types of Coxsackie A, B, and ECHO viruses have been associated with the clinical entity herpangina, some patients have had additional signs common to enterovirus infection, including parotitis, aseptic meningitis, paralytic poliolike illness, exanthem, and pleurodynia.

EPIDEMIOLOGY. As stated by Zahorsky, the disease tends to be epidemic in nature during the summer months. Its highest incidence is in the 3- to 10-year age group and occurs only in persons without preexisting, type-specific neutralizing antibody. The prevalent strains produce clinical illness in 30 to 50 per cent of infected persons. The virus is isolated from 85 per cent of patients, 60 per cent of neighborhood contacts, 40 per cent of family contacts, and 3.5 per cent of others. The disease has only recently been reported in newborn infants.

DIAGNOSIS. The laboratory may confirm a specific virologic diagnosis, but the clinical syndrome is usually obvious. The white blood counts tend to be normal with a relative lymphocytosis. Stool is the richest source of virus and is positive in 85 per cent of cases; anal (57 per cent) and throat swabs (58 per cent) also have good yield.

The differential diagnosis must rule out herpes gingivostomatitis. A diagnosis of herpes is favored if there are fetor oris, hyperemia, hypertrophy, or hemorrhage of gingivae, cervical adenopathy or involvement of tongue, lip, or eye. These are common in herpes and rare to unheard of in herpangina. Another distinguishing feature is that most Coxsackie virus enanthemata occur in the posterior half of the oropharynx, and herpetic lesions are mainly anterior.

TREATMENT. There is no specific treatment. Symptoms are mild and all patients recover.

References

Cherry, J. D., and Jahn, C. L.: Herpangina: The etiologic spectrum. Pediatr 36:632, 1965.

Huebner, R. J., Cole, R. M., Beeman, E. M., et al.: Herpangina: Etiologic studies of a specific infectious disease. JAMA 145:628, 1951.

Zahorsky, J.: Herpangina (a specific disease). Arch Pediatr 41:181, 1924.

107
BACTERIAL PAROTITIS

DONALD L. LEAKE, A.B., M.A., D.M.D., M.D.

Bacterial parotitis is an acute or chronic inflammation of bacterial origin of one or both parotid salivary glands. Suppurative parotitis, pyogenic parotitis, and septic parotitis are synonyms. In postoperative surgical patients, it is sometimes described as surgical parotitis.

ETIOLOGY. Bacterial parotitis is most often caused by *Staphylococcus aureus* (Petersdorf, 1958), although the infecting organisms may be quite varied, reflecting the oral flora (Burnett and Scherp, 1968; Speirs and Mason, 1972; Spratt, 1961). There may be one organism, or a mixed infection.

In newborns, staphylococci are most commonly implicated (Leake and Leake, 1970). *Pseudomonas aeruginosa*, streptococci, especially viridans and pneumococci, and *Escherichia coli* occasionally are found. In a study of suppurative parotitis in older children, one third of the infections were caused by *S. aureus*, approximately one third resulted from streptococci, and the final third were distributed among *Haemophilus*, beta-hemolytic streptococci, and combinations of alpha-hemolytic streptococci, and *S. aureus* or pneumococci.

In another series of still older patients, studied in the 1950s, viridans streptococci accounted for 65 per cent of the cases and pneumococci for another 20 per cent. Streptococci, *Proteus*, *E. coli*, and diptheroids may be either normally or transiently found in the oral cavity.

PATHOGENESIS AND PATHOLOGY

Acute Bacterial Parotitis. Acute bacterial parotitis usually occurs in debilitated patients, and dehydration is a common predisposing condition (Petersdorf et al., 1958). In the very young patient, only moderate dehydration is necessary to produce salivary stasis (Leake and Leake, 1970; Leake et al., 1971). Infection may then take place by bacteria ascending the duct. Infection of the gland also may result from septicemia. Occasionally caused by staphylococci, hematogenous parotitis is more often caused by gram-negative organisms such as *E. coli* or *Pseudomonas*.

The parotid is almost purely a serous gland and is very susceptible to infection secondary to stasis. By contrast, the submaxillary gland is a mixed gland that produces both mucous and serous secretions. It is thought that mucus is bacteriostatic and that the submaxillary salivary glands tend to become infected only when the duct is occluded as by a sialolith.

Decreased host resistance, dehydration, and poor oral hygiene predispose to acute bacterial parotitis. With dehydration from any cause, commonly diarrhea or vomiting, inadequate fluid replacement, or severe diaphoresis, there may be a concomitant reduction of salivary flow. Anticholinergics, antihistamines, some tranquilizers, and diuretics also may decrease salivary flow.

Bacterial parotitis occasionally occurs in patients who are otherwise healthy (Leake and Leake, 1970). Obstruction from a sialolith, stricture, or a mucous plug should be sought. While rare in the parotid gland, stones do occur and may occlude or partially obstruct Stensen's duct. This causes stasis of salivary flow and predisposes the gland to infection. Palpation with thumb and index finger usually establishes the presence of a stone in the duct. It can be confirmed by x-ray in most cases. Mucous plugs sometimes can be expressed during palpation. Strictures can be determined by gentle probing with a lacrimal duct probe or by sialography.

Obstruction of salivary flow may cause irreversible tissue damage to the gland parenchyma. There is a marked polymorphonuclear leukocyte infiltration in the stroma, the parenchyma, and the ducts. Chronic inflammation is marked by increasing numbers of lymphocytes and plasma cells. Fibrosis may replace portions of the gland or, if the inflammation is reversed, there may be regeneration of glandular and ductal elements.

Recurrent Parotitis. The pathogenesis of recurrent parotitis in children is unknown. It has been proposed that the episodes are the sequelae of acute infections, congenital sialoangiectasis with some degree of stasis, or autoimmune disease. Boys are affected more often than girls.

Recurrent parotitis is more common in women than in men and seems often to be associated with Sjögren's syndrome. This symptom complex includes keratoconjunctivitis sicca, xerostomia, and a collagen disease, particularly rheumatoid arthritis.

The histopathology of chronic parotitis is better known than is the pathogenesis. Hyperplasia of the duct epithelium, periductal lymphocytic infiltration, acinar atrophy, and fibrosis ultimately progress to loss of acini and replacement by fibroadipose tissue.

CLINICAL MANIFESTATIONS. In acute parotitis there is a sudden onset of swelling with purulent drainage from Stensen's duct (Krippaehne et al., 1962; Leake and Leake, 1970; Leake et al., 1971; Petersdorf et al., 1958). It is usually unilateral, although as many as 25 per cent of the cases may be bilateral. The swelling is diffuse and involves the whole gland. The area is firm, smooth, and extremely tender to palpation. The entire side of the face may be swollen. Often there is trismus. Generally, there is a low-grade fever and moderate leukocytosis. Malaise and loss of appetite are common. With antibiotic therapy and adequate hydration, the swelling subsides over a period of a week.

The course of recurrent parotitis is variable (Pearson, 1961; Rose, 1954). Painful attacks are often intensified by eating. Secretions are generally flocculent and turbid in contrast to the free-flowing saliva of the normal parotid. Attacks last from two to seven days and may occur as often as every few months. Usually the onset is unilateral, but it may become bilateral. Occasionally both sides are involved simultaneously. The gland may be somewhat more prominent than normal between attacks. In many patients, the recurring painful swellings ultimately resolve, undoubtedly because of the replacement of functioning acini by fibrosis. Chronic recurrent parotitis in children usually subsides by the middle teens, suggesting a hormonal association.

COMPLICATIONS AND SEQUELAE. In the pre-antibiotic era, bacterial parotitis was a serious and often fatal postoperative complication, particularly in elderly patients. Bacterial parotitis also poses a threat in patients with severe underlying diseases such as poorly controlled diabetes mellitus, carcinoma, leukemia, Hodgkin's disease, or renal failure, and in those who have just experienced cerebral vascular accidents. Septicemia, resulting in septic shock, may be the terminal event. In children as in adults, underlying diseases contribute to susceptibility. Myelogenous leukemia, dysautonomia (Riley-Day syndrome), acute glomerulonephritis, hypothyroidism with immunologic deficiency, cystic hygroma, and hemangiomas have been implicated. The occurrence of bacterial parotitis in a sick, hospitalized patient is a poor portent, but many mild cases are treated successfully without hospitalization.

Adequate antibiotic therapy based on culture and sensitivity findings and attention to fluid and electrolyte balance have decreased the mortality figures reported from 90 per cent in 1920 to approximately 20 per cent since the 1960s. Bacterial parotitis may be an incidental feature of a terminal disease.

As the inflammatory process invades the parenchyma, multiple abscesses form and sometimes coalesce. If the pus penetrates the capsule and invades the surrounding tissue, it may dissect into the deep fascial planes of the neck, flow posteriorly to the external auditory canal, or drain from the fistulae through the overlying skin.

Sialography (the instillation of radiopaque contrast material via Stensen's duct) in recurrent parotitis will show sialoangiectasis, a dilation of the ducts and a decrease in their number. Small, cystic dilatation of the terminal radicals reflects loss of acini. Sialography is contraindicated in acute parotitis.

DIAGNOSIS. The diagnosis of bacterial parotitis is usually made readily on the basis of visible suppuration at the parotid duct orifice (Krippaehne et al., 1962; Leake and Leake, 1970; Leake et al., 1971; Petersdorf et al., 1958). If pus is not spontaneously draining from the duct, it can be expressed by placing the thumb of the examining hand just inside the mouth anterior to the parotid orifice and the fingers of the same hand placed externally over the parotid gland anterior to the ear. A gentle milking of the gland by moving the fingers forward will produce a specimen. Inspissated saliva may form a plug in the duct and obstruct the flow of saliva in the patient with a dry mouth. After expelling an inspissated plug, the character of the pus can be determined. In acute parotitis the flow generally is copious. In chronic or recurrent parotitis, the pus may be turbid or flocculent (Pearson, 1961). A specimen should be used to prepare a stained smear, and bacteriologic culture and antibiotic sensitivity should be determined. When no exudate can be expressed, it is possible to cannulate the duct with a fine catheter or a blunt-end abscess needle to irrigate the gland and thus obtain a specimen for culture.

In the history, the onset of swelling, the duration and frequency, particularly if recurrent, and precipitating factors such as food or juice should be noted. Acute swelling, secondary to an obstruction, may occur immediately after eating or drinking. A stone or calculus in the parotid salivary duct often can be palpated. When a sialolith is suspected, a periapical dental film can be placed intraorally under the suspected area and an x-ray taken with a dental x-ray machine.

There is a moderate to marked polymorphonucleocytosis and low grade fever (100° to 101° F). The gland is swollen and tender. The patient may be dehydrated or may be receiving medications that contribute to dryness.

The differential diagnosis of salivary gland swelling includes tumors that often involve only a part of the gland. Lymphadenopathy in the parotid and buccinator area may be due to adjacent inflammation in the mouth, teeth, facial skin, eyes, or external auditory canal, or it may be caused by neoplastic disease (Banks, 1968). Cat scratch fever may produce lymphadenopathy in the parotid or buccinator node areas. Other causes of salivary gland swellings include mumps, amyloidosis, sarcoidosis (Heerfordt's syndrome), disseminated lupus erythematosus, lymphoma, leukemia, and such granulomatous diseases as tuberculosis, atypical mycobacterial infection and actinomycosis (Waldman, 1982). Chronic parotid swelling has been reported as a finding in pediatric AIDS (Ammann, 1983). Asymptomatic or slightly tender swellings of the parotids may occur after ingesting iodine, for example, supersaturated potassium iodide (SSKI), with the thiouracils or following intravenous urography (Alexander et al., 1968; Nakadar and Harris-Jones, 1971). Guanethidine, an antihypertensive agent, may result in salivary gland enlargement also. Toxic parotitis has also been reported secondary to copper, lead, or mercury poisoning.

Bilateral, nontender parotid swelling may be found with chronic alcoholism and malnutrition as in Laennec's cirrhosis. In older women Sjögren's syndrome is commonly associated with bacterial parotitis (Bloch et al., 1965).

Parotid swelling and fever, sometimes associated with lacrimal adenitis and uveitis (Mikulicz's syndrome), occurs in patients with chronic disease such as tuberculosis, leukemia, Hodgkin's disease, or lupus erythematosus (Morgan and Castleman, 1953). The onset often is sudden, although the course is long and usually painless. Salivary gland enlargement has also been observed in Waldenström's macroglobulinemia.

Benign bilateral hypertrophy of the masseter muscles due to habitual clenching of teeth may be confused with painless parotid swelling.

The differential diagnosis of acute facial swellings, aside from intrinsic salivary gland disease, includes cellulitis, sometimes associated with unerupted third molars and mandibular cysts.

A rare cause of parotitis is that associated with Reiter's syndrome (a triad of arthritis, conjunctivitis, and urethritis). Rarer still is the parotitis secondary to lipoidproteinosis infiltrating the parotid duct and causing stenosis.

In areas of the world where hydatid disease is endemic, cysts in the parotid area due to *Echinococcus granulosa* may cause swelling that simulates parotitis. Other exotic causes of parotitis include yaws and aspergillosis.

Sialography may be helpful in distinguishing tumors from other chronic parotid swellings. With tumors, the parotid gland tends to be displaced laterally. Sjögren's syndrome almost always reveals sialoangiectasis by sialographic examination and may present parotid swelling without suppuration. Recurrent sialoadenitis also shows sialoangiectasis when studied by sialography (Calcaterra et al., 1977).

A patient may very occasionally present with a history of recurrent swelling in the parotid or submaxillary area. Radiographs may show small radiopacities suggesting sialolithiasis. These small concretions in vessel walls are phleboliths. Sialography will reveal them to be outside the parotid gland (Dempsey and Murley, 1970).

Sialography may be therapeutic for recurrent parotitis. Sialoadenitis often is improved after sialography.

Because as many as 20 per cent of sialoliths are radiolucent, standard radiographic examinations may fail to reveal their presence. Sialography usually shows the point of obstruction when there is a sialolith.

Radionuclide scans may provide useful information in the differential diagnosis of swellings of the parotid area. More recently, scintigraphy has been proposed and still greater promise is held for Emission Computed Axial Tomography (ECAT) as an aid in the differential diagnosis of salivary gland disease (Ohrt and Shafer, 1982).

TREATMENT. Antibiotics and adequate hydration are essential to the treatment of acute bacterial parotitis. Analgesics often are necessary in acute parotitis.

Staphylococcal parotitis is treated with 1.0 g oxacillin intravenously every six hours in the adult if the organism produces penicillinase; otherwise, 1.0 million units of benzylpenicillin is given every six hours intravenously. After the infection is controlled, intravenous drugs are stopped and oral dicloxacillin is given in a dose of 500 mg every six hours.

Patients with recurrent parotitis should be given antibiotics, although many patients do equally well without treatment, and recovery occurs in a week.

Incision and drainage may be helpful for abscesses, although the parotid duct provides a built-in mechanism for drainage. Irradiation is no longer recommended in acute parotitis because of the effectiveness of antibiotics. Chronic parotitis is less responsive to radiation, and it is mentioned only to be condemned.

For chronic recurrent painful parotitis, ligation of the parotid duct will produce autoparotidectomy without associated hazard to the facial nerve (Diamont, 1958).

PROPHYLAXIS. Protection against bacterial parotitis depends on adequate hydration, hygiene, and appropriate supportive measures, including avoidance of drugs that decrease salivary flow.

References

Alexander, W. D., Harden, R. M., and Shimmins, J.: The concentration of iodide, pertechnetate and bromide in human saliva and gastric juice. J Physiol 194:89, 1968.

Ammann, A. J.: Is there an acquired immune deficiency syndrome in infants and children? (Commentaries) Pediatrics 72:430, 1983 (Table).

Banks, P.: Nonneoplastic parotid swellings: A review. Oral Surg Oral Med Oral Pathol 25:732, 1968.

Bloch, K. S., Buchanan, W. W., Wohl, M. J., and Bunim, J. J.: Sjögren's syndrome, a clinical, pathological, and serological study of sixty-two cases. Medicine 44:187, 1965.

Burnett, G. W., and Scherp, H. W.: The microbial flora of the oral cavity. In Oral Microbiology and Infectious Disease. Baltimore, Williams & Wilkins Company, 1968, p. 273.

Calcaterra, T. C., Hemenway, W. G., Hansen, G. C., et al.: The value of sialography in the diagnosis of parotid tumors. Arch Otolaryngol 103:727, 1977.

Dempsey, E. F., and Murley, R. S.: Vascular malformations simulating salivary disease. Br J Plast Surg 23:77, 1970.

Diamont, H.: Ligation of the parotid duct in chronic recurrent parotitis. Acta Otolaryngol 49:375, 1958.

Krippaehne, W. W., Hunt, T. K., and Dunphy, J. E.: Acute suppurative parotitis. Ann Surg 156:251, 1962.

Leake, D. L., and Leake, R. C.: Neonatal suppurative parotitis. Pediatrics 46:203, 1970.

Leake, D. L., Krakowiak, F. J., and Leake, R. C.: Suppurative parotitis in children. Oral Surg Oral Med Oral Pathol 31:174, 1971.

Morgan, W. S., and Castleman, B.: A clinicopathologic study of "Mikulicz's disease." Am J Pathol 29:471, 1953.

Nakadar, A. S., and Harrison-Jones, J. N.: Sialadenitis after intravenous pyelography. Br Med J 3:351, 1971.

Ohrt, H. J., and Shafer, R. B.: An atlas of salivary gland disorders. Clin Nucl Med 7:370, 1982.

Pearson, R. S. B.: Recurrent swellings of the parotid gland. Gut 2:210, 1961.

Petersdorf, R. G., Forsyth, B. R., and Bernanke, D.: Staphylococcal parotitis. N Engl J Med 259:1250, 1958.

Rose, S. S.: A clinical and radiological survey of 192 cases of recurrent swellings of the salivary glands. R Coll Surg Engl Ann 15:374, 1954.

Speirs, C. F., and Mason, D. K.: Acute septic parotitis: Incidence, aetiology and management. Scot Med J 17:62, 1972.

Spratt, J. S., Jr.: The etiology and therapy of acute pyogenic parotitis. Surg Gynecol Obstet 112:391, 1961.

Waldman, R. H.: Tuberculosis and the atypical mycobacteria. Otolaryngol Clin North Am 15:581, 1982.

108
MUMPS

Melvin I. Marks, M.D.

Mumps is an acute, communicable viral infection most commonly manifest as parotitis. Mumps virus may also infect the central nervous system, other salivary glands (i.e., submandibular, sublingual), and other organs, including the pancreas, testes, and ovaries. Although often occurring together, parotitis or infection of one or more other organs may be present independently. As many as one half of mumps infections are asymptomatic.

ETIOLOGY. Mumps was first described as a clinical entity by Hippocrates in the 5th century BC. The condition, characterized by nonsuppurative swelling of the parotid glands, was successfully reproduced in monkeys in 1934 by Johnson and Goodpasture. These experiments provided evidence that the syndrome was caused by a filterable (i.e., virus-like) agent that could be passed from human to animal by injection of infected saliva. In 1945, the virus was grown in hens' eggs, and the viral property of hemagglutination described. Some of the host's responses were also defined, including the development of complement-fixing antibody and the acquisition of dermal hypersensitivity. The virus was attenuated in the 1960's, and the contemporary live mumps virus vaccine was prepared in chick embryo tissue culture by Bunyak and Hilleman in 1966.

Mumps virus is a paramyxovirus (Chapter 63). It is neurotropic in experimental animal infections. Two other paramyxoviruses, influenza and parainfluenza viruses, can cause infections resembling mumps.

PATHOGENESIS AND PATHOLOGY. Man is apparently the only reservoir for mumps virus, and person-to-person contact is essential for spread. Prospective study of normal subjects with respiratory infections and appropriate controls has provided evidence that mumps virus is often associated with upper (e.g., common cold syndrome and pharyngitis) and lower (e.g., bronchopneumonia, croup, and bronchiolitis) respiratory symptoms, and attests to the initial respiratory colonization in mumps infection. Virus attaches to and invades respiratory epithelial cells and elicits local immune responses, including secretion of IgA (Freidman, 1981), edema, lymphocytic infiltration, and increased vascular permeability. The immune subject has no symptoms or may have some respiratory discomfort associated with the successful containment of mumps virus infection to the surface epithelium.

In susceptible hosts, virus multiplies in the upper respiratory tract, and occasionally in the conjunctiva, before entering the circulation. Viremia is followed by infection of many organs, including the central nervous system.

Infection with mumps virus stimulates humoral and secretory antibody, as well as cell-mediated immune responses. The latter can be measured by cutaneous hypersensitivity, lymphocyte proliferation in response to mumps antigen, and the specific immune release of radioactivity from mumps-infected tissue culture cells (Chiba et al., 1976). Thus, the immunopathogenesis of mumps infection in humans involves direct virus infection, interaction of virus with local IgA antibodies, and cell-mediated and humoral immune responses. Immunoglobulin G and M antibodies against mumps virus and interferon have also been demonstrated in the cerebrospinal fluid in patients with mumps meningitis (Ukkonen et al., 1981). Postinfectious tissue injury, manifest as recurrent encephalomyelitis or orchitis, is occasionally observed, and may be mediated by antigen-antibody complexes and/or complement.

Parotid swelling is caused by interstitial edema. There are varying degrees of degeneration of duct epithelium and polymorphonuclear cell infiltration in the early stages of parotitis. A periductal and perivascular mononuclear cell infiltrate follows. There is usually minimal necrosis and scarring (Fig. 1).

Changes in the brain may be those of postinfectious encephalomyelitis or, more commonly, of acute viral meningoencephalitis. These include neuronal destruction by intracellular virus and inflammation. Postinfectious perivascular demyelinization, lymphocytic infiltration, and gliosis may occur later. It is assumed that most cases of mumps meningoencephalitis have a transient inflammatory response secondary to vasculitis, perivascular edema, and glial reaction followed by complete recovery. Only rare cases progress to more severe perivascular edema, hemorrhage, and anoxia secondary to the vasculopathy. Encephalomyelitic changes and/or hypoxic damage may contribute to the clinical observations of late-onset encephalitis and prolonged cerebrospinal fluid pleocytosis (Vaheri et al., 1982).

Certain pathologic features suggest that mumps meningoencephalitis may cause aqueductal stenosis and hydrocephalus in rare instances. Viral nucleocapsid-like material is present in ependymal cells in the cerebrospinal fluid of patients with mumps meningitis but not in enteroviral meningitis (Herndon et al., 1974). It is postulated that scarring occurs after ependymal cell necrosis and leads to narrowing and obstruction of the aqueduct of Sylvius. These changes have been reproduced in hamsters experimentally infected with mumps virus.

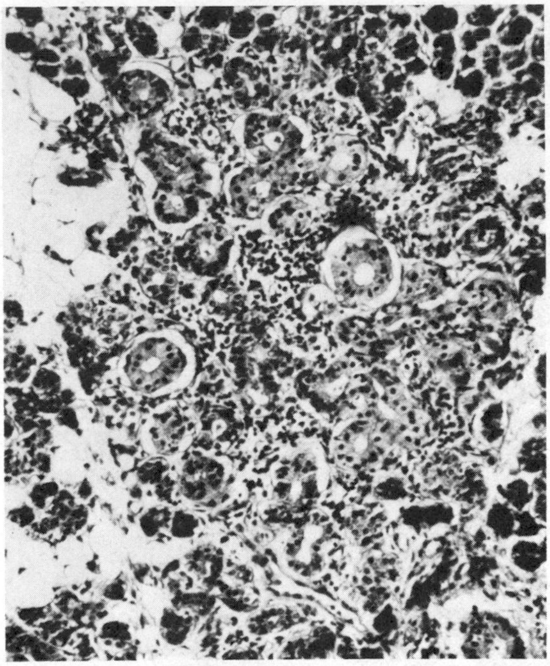

Figure 1. Mumps parotitis. There is marked periductular infiltration of mononuclear cells. These inflammatory cells extend outward between acini. This is associated with atrophy, degeneration, and necrosis of acinar cells. H & E. 100 ×. (Courtesy of Robert P. Bolande, M.D.)

In orchitis there are massive interstitial edema and perivascular lymphocytic exudate, which may be followed by focal hemorrhage and destruction of germinal epithelial cells (Fig. 2). The spermatic cord and tunica vaginalis are usually involved as well. Epithelial breakdown products, cellular inflammatory debris, and fibrin may obstruct the tubules. There are also focal tubular lesions and deposition of collagen in areas of hemorrhage and necrosis. These lead to scarring and atrophy in the final stages. It must be emphasized that these changes are focal, involve both testes in only 10 to 20 per cent of cases, and are extremely variable in degree. Complete destruction of germinal tissue and/or loss of tubular function is very rare. Epididymitis accompanies orchitis in approximately 85 per cent of cases and is characterized by dense lymphocytic inflammation of the connective tissue, usually with sparing of the epithelial components. Occasionally, a hydrocele may develop.

Acute interstitial (occasionally necrotizing) pancreatitis (Fig. 3) and thyroiditis are less common features. Endolymphatic labyrinthitis is an extremely rare but serious form of mumps infection. Clinical features of tinnitus, vertigo, vomiting, and deafness are caused by inflammation of the stria vascularis with subsequent permanent degeneration of the involved cochlear receptors.

The consequences of intrauterine mumps infections have been the subject of much investigation and speculation. It has been suggested that endocardial fibroelastosis, a myocardiopathy of young infants, and aqueductal stenosis with subsequent hydrocephalus are conditions closely related to intrauterine mumps infection. There are several immunologic, epidemiologic, and animal studies that support these contentions (London et al., 1979). Mumps virus is partic-

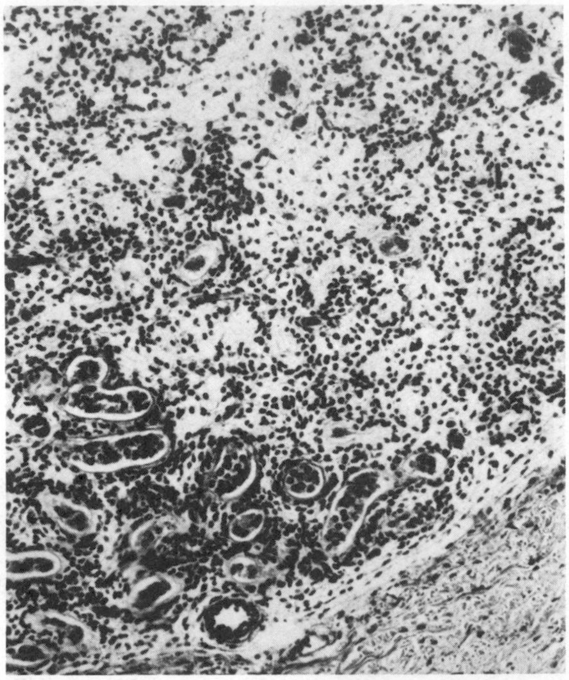

Figure 2. Mumps orchitis. There is marked interstitial edema and mononuclear cell infiltrate of the testis obliterating many seminiferous tubules. A few can be still identified at the bottom adjacent to the tunica albuginea. H & E. 100 ×. (Courtesy of Robert P. Bolande, M.D.)

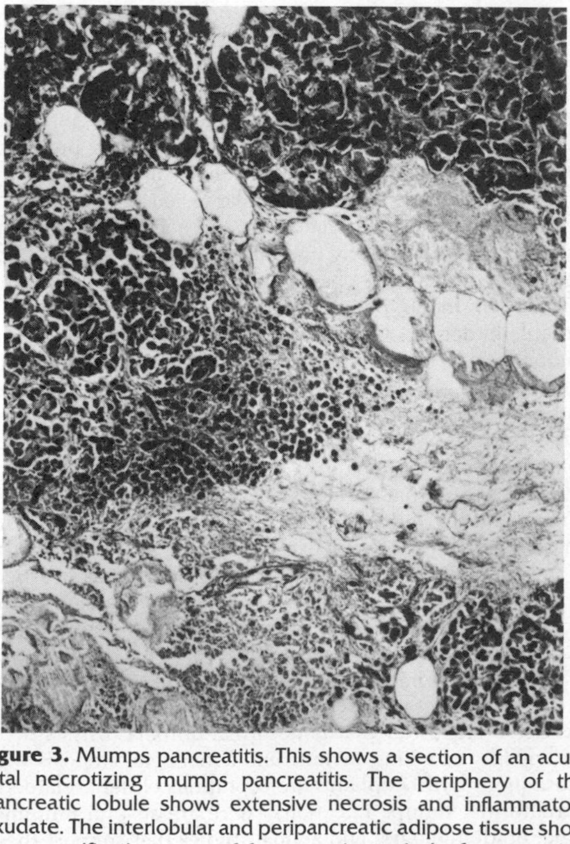

Figure 3. Mumps pancreatitis. This shows a section of an acute fatal necrotizing mumps pancreatitis. The periphery of this pancreatic lobule shows extensive necrosis and inflammatory exudate. The interlobular and peripancreatic adipose tissue show the saponification type of fat necrosis, typical of pancreatitis. H & E. 100× (Courtesy of Robert P. Bolande, M.D.)

ularly destructive to myocardial tissue in chick embryos and is also neurotropic in suckling hamsters. Patients with endocardial fibroelastosis usually have cutaneous hypersensitivity to mumps antigen but do not have circulating mumps antibody. Experimental infections in chick embryo and clinical observations in the offspring of patients with documented intragestational mumps suggest that this "split immune response" is also characteristic of intrauterine mumps infection (Aase et al., 1972). The absence of humoral antibody in the presence of lymphocyte sensitization and cutaneous mumps hypersensitivity persists well into childhood.

CLINICAL MANIFESTATIONS. The most common form of mumps infection is parotitis (Fig. 4). Usually only one parotid gland swells in the first 2 days of infection but then both swell in approximately 70 per cent of cases. The incubation period is frequently 17 to 21 days; however, cases have been reported as early as 12 days after exposure and as late as 35 days. In more severe cases, a mild prodrome of fever, malaise, headache, chills, sore throat, earache, and parotid tenderness may precede parotid swelling by 2 to 3 days. Exanthems and enanthems have also been described. Orchitis and/or meningitis may precede parotitis or maybe occur as the sole manifestations of mumps. As many as one half of children under 5 years are asymptomatic; others may have a respiratory syndrome. These children are important in the spread of mumps.

The parotid gland is variably enlarged, tense, and tender, and there may be pain on movement of the jaw. Local heat

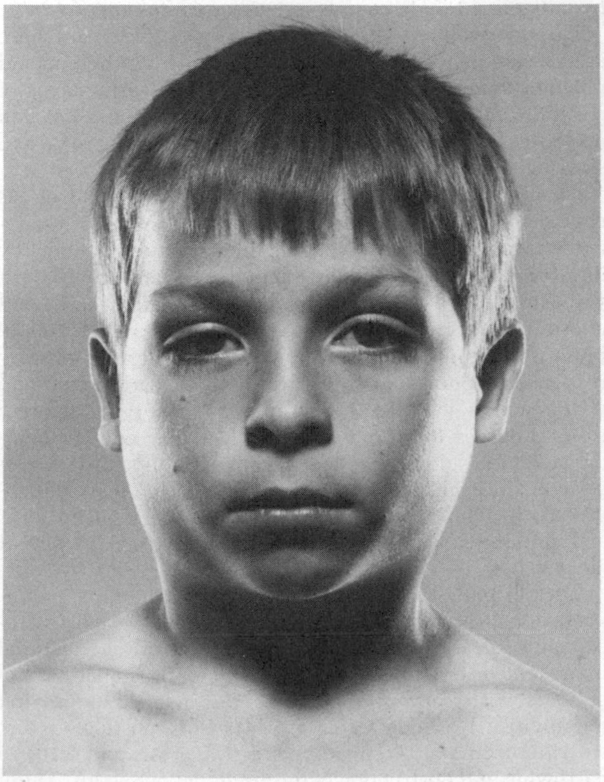

Figure 4. Mumps parotitis. Bilateral parotid enlargement in an 8-year-old boy, more marked on right side. (Courtesy of G. Ahronheim, M.D.)

and erythema are absent. Swelling, which often obliterates the hollow between the mastoid process and the ascending ramus of the lower jaw, is usually maximal over a 2- to 3-day period and disappears by 7 to 10 days. Swelling of the sublingual and submaxillary salivary glands is frequently present as well. Because salivary gland ducts may be partly occluded by inflammation, pain can be experienced upon exposure to acid drinks and other stimulation of salivary secretion. The papillae at the opening of Stensen's or Wharton's duct may be reddened, but this is an inconsistent finding.

Most patients with parotitis are mildly febrile, but this rarely lasts longer than 5 days. Symptoms are mild in children and often absent in the youngest patients. The disease is usually not seen under 6 to 9 months of age owing to the presence of passively acquired (maternal) immunity; however parotitis and pneumonia have been noted in newborns exposed to perinatal maternal mumps infection (Jones et al., 1980). Adults are more likely to develop constitutional symptoms and extraparotid lesions such as orchitis. They commonly have a prodrome of fever, headache, and chills as well.

Although sometimes considered complications of mumps, central nervous system (CNS) involvement, orchitis, and other manifestations can occur without parotitis and represent primary infection by mumps virus. As many as one half of patients with mumps have cerebrospinal fluid pleocytosis, and one quarter have signs of meningeal involvement. Mumps is the most common cause of endemic aseptic meningitis in North American children. Wilfert (1969) reviewed the clinical features of 45 children with mumps meningoencephalitis and found that 13 had no evidence of parotitis. In most cases, CNS signs became evident 1 to 6 days after the onset of parotitis; however, in three patients, the signs of meningitis preceded those of parotid gland involvement by 3 days. Occasionally, several weeks ensue between the onset of parotitis and the appearance of meningoencephalitis. The majority of patients with CNS involvement have meningoencephalitis; nevertheless, the clinical syndrome may be predominantly that of aseptic meningitis or, alternatively, encephalitis. Although the criteria for encephalitis are arbitrary, pure mumps encephalitis has been estimated to occur in approximately 8 per cent of patients with CNS involvement. Meningoencephalitis is more frequent in males (3:1); however, mumps infection shows no sex predilection.

Other manifestations of mumps infection include conjunctivitis, dacryoadenitis, pancreatitis, oophoritis, thyroiditis, and arthritis. These are discussed in more detail under complications. Approximately 6 per cent of patients develop presternal pitting edema, probably due to obstruction of anterior chest wall lymphatics by swollen lymph nodes and salivary glands. This complication requires no treatment and is seen between days 5 and 8 after the onset of parotitis.

COMPLICATIONS. An outline of some of the reported complications of mumps infection is presented in Table 1. Many of these have been associated with mumps and have not been proven to be due to the virus.

Recurrent idiopathic parotitis may follow mumps parotitis. Inflammation of Stensen's duct may lead to sialectasis and a predisposition to obstruction, secondary infections, and/or stricture.

Seizures occur in as many as 18 per cent of patients with mumps encephalitis. Coma, disturbances of sensorium, ataxia, and transient or, rarely, permanent paralysis of ocular or facial muscles have also been described. Labyrinthitis and nerve deafness, complications of CNS mumps infection, may be preceded by tinnitus, vertigo, nausea, and vomiting. A rare complication of mumps is a paralytic poliomyelitis-like syndrome of transient asymmetric flaccid paralysis of the lower extremities, frequently accompanied by myalgia and intact sensation. Urinary sphincter dysfunction and extensor plantar responses may also be present. Guillain-Barré syndrome has also been reported (Pollack et al., 1981).

Atrophy of the testicles occurs in as many as one half of patients with mumps orchitis, but this is focal and sterility after mumps is extremely rare. In a study of 132 men with orchitis, 47 developed some degree of atrophy, but this was bilateral in only 2 (Beard et al., 1977). One of these men subsequently fathered a child, and the other was lost

Table 1. COMPLICATIONS OF MUMPS

Neurologic:
- Meningoencephalitis
- Guillain-Barré syndrome
- Myelitis
- Neuropathies
- Deafness
- Labyrinthitis
- Hydrocephalus
- Diabetes insipidus

Ocular:
- Conjunctivitis
- Scleritis
- Keratitis
- Optic neuritis
- Iritis
- Iridocyclitis
- Dacryoadenitis

Genitourinary:
- Orchitis
- Epididymitis
- Oophoritis
- Nephritis
- Priapism
- Bartholinitis
- Prostatitis

Hematologic:
- Thrombocytopenia
- Hemolysis
- Leukemoid reaction
- Paroxysmal cold hemoglobinuria
- Splenomegaly

Other:
- Pancreatitis
- Thyroiditis
- Mastitis
- Hepatitis
- Polyarthritis
- Myocarditis
- Pericarditis
- Laryngitis
- Psychosis
- Teratogenicity (microcephaly, hydrocephalus, endocardial fibroelastosis, abortion)

to follow-up. Two patients in this cohort subsequently developed testicular neoplasms. The association of testicular or mammary neoplasia with mumps has been noted in the past, although the pathogenesis is unknown. There has been no evidence of congenital malformations in any children fathered by men with a history of mumps orchitis.

Oophoritis is difficult to diagnose, although ovarian enlargement may be palpable in some patients. It occurs in approximately 7 per cent of patients with mumps and is manifest by lower quadrant or back pain. Sterility after oophoritis has not been reported.

Pancreatitis occurs in less than 10 per cent of patients with mumps and is usually associated with vomiting and severe epigastric pain. Abdominal muscular spasm may be present and the clinical syndrome may suggest appendicitis. This is also true of patients with mumps of the right ovary. Epidemiologic and serologic correlations between mumps pancreatitis and juvenile diabetes mellitus have been reported. Genetic predisposition and other factors are also important.

The virus has been isolated from the thyroid during acute mumps thyroiditis. It has been estimated that as many as one half of the patients with subacute thyroiditis have a history of recent mumps infection.

Arthritis has been reported in approximately 0.4 per cent of patients with mumps. Knees, ankles, shoulders, and wrists are most frequently involved, but any joint in the body may be affected. Most patients with the polyarthritis syndrome are adults, and the condition usually has its onset 10 days to 2 weeks after the onset of parotitis. Arthritis usually lasts only a few days, although several cases have persisted for as long as 3 months. The migratory nature of the disease may confuse the differential diagnosis.

Thrombocytopenic purpura may occur in children after natural disease and with mumps vaccination. Other hematologic changes are outlined in Table 1. Myocarditis is rare, but can be fatal (Brown et al., 1980).

In addition to endocardial fibroelastosis and aqueductal stenosis, mumps virus infection in the first trimester of pregnancy has also been associated with abortion (Garcia et al., 1980); imperforate anus; spina bifida; microcephaly; and auditory, optic, and urogenital deformities, although a cause-and-effect relationship has not been demonstrated. In addition, lenticular cataracts have been produced in chick embryos infected early in embryonic development.

The case fatality ratio is approximately 0.1 to 0.4 per 100,000 cases of mumps. There is no sex predilection among those fatally infected, and 38 per cent of the deaths occur in patients over the age of 40 years.

GEOGRAPHIC VARIATIONS IN DISEASE. Mumps infections occur throughout the world and in all seasons, although there is some increase in incidence during the winter and spring months. Most (85 to 90 per cent) infections occur in children under 14 years of age. Epidemics of mumps affecting all ages occur in populations with little exposure to the virus. Such "virgin" populations have been described in the St. Lawrence and St. George Islands in Alaska (Reed et al., 1967). High attack rates for clinical (65 per cent) and subclinical (20 per cent) disease are noted in these populations. Evidence of life-long immunity was provided by 13 patients in these communities who had their previous exposure to mumps 58 years before the reported epidemics. None of these patients developed clinical illness, although 6 of the 10 tested seroconverted upon reexposure to the virus.

Public health surveys of mumps infection in the continental United States report an incidence of approximately 7 to 10 cases per 100,000 population per year. A prospective study performed in 1968 revealed approximately 2000 cases per 100,000 population per year (Levitt and Casey, 1970). The difficulty of frequency estimates in this disease is compounded by the frequent occurrence of subclinical infection and by the fact that physicians rarely see more than 40 per cent of clinical cases. Secondary attack rates in families of children with mumps range from 14 to 46 per cent.

DIAGNOSIS. The diagnosis of mumps is usually based on the presence of parotitis and a history of contact with the illness. Other viral causes of mumps include parainfluenza and influenza viruses (Brill and Gilfillan, 1977). A differential diagnosis of parotid swelling is included in Table 2 and should be considered when a history of exposure is not provided or the illness is atypical.

Table 2. PAROTID SWELLING—DIFFERENTIAL DIAGNOSIS

Infectious:
Mumps
Parainfluenza
Influenza
Cytomegalovirus
Coxsackie virus
Lymphocytic choriomeningitis
Echovirus
Suppurative (bacterial)
Actinomyces
Mycobacteria
Cat scratch disease
Noninfectious:
Drug hypersensitivity (thiouracil, phenothiazines, thiocyanate, iodides, copper, isoprenaline, lead, mercury, phenylbutazone)
Sarcoidosis
Tumors, mixed
Hemangioma, lymphangioma
Sialectasis
Sjögren's syndrome
Mikulicz's syndrome (scleroderma, mixed connective tissue disease, systemic lupus erythematosis)
Recurrent idiopathic parotitis
Pneumoparotitis
Trauma
Sialolithiasis
Foreign body
Cystic fibrosis
Malnutrition (marasmus, alcohol cirrhosis)
Dehydration
Diabetes mellitus
Waldenström's macroglobulinemia
Reiter's syndrome
Amyloidosis
Nonparotid Swelling:
Hypertrophy of masseter muscle
Lymphadenopathy
Rheumatoid mandibular joint swelling
Tumors of jaw
Infantile cortical hyperostosis

Unlike bacterial parotitis, there is little heat and redness over the parotid in mumps (see Chapter 107). Approximately 6 per cent of patients with sarcoidosis have chronic parotid swelling due to granulomatous changes.

Parotid and, occasionally, submandibular swelling may be an allergic reaction to drugs. Eosinophils in the glandular secretions support this diagnosis. Iodides are often responsible, and isoprenaline parotitis has been reproduced in rats; other drugs are listed in Table 2. Adrenal corticosteroid therapy may help in this condition.

Malnutrition, alcoholism, and diabetes mellitus all may be associated with parotid enlargement. The term "nutritional mumps" has been used in these cases and suggests a common pathogenesis that is related to fatty infiltration of the gland, acinar swelling, and increase in zymogen granules. Parotitis has also been produced in rats by protein deprivation.

Curious noninfectious etiologies for parotid swelling include papillary hypertrophy secondary to cheek biting and the trauma of poorly fitting dentures. "Wind parotitis," also called pneumoparotitis, is the name given to parotid swelling due to the introduction of air into the gland. This may be secondary to trauma or surgery or self-induced. It has also been reported in musicians playing wind instruments, glassblowers, and persons who have performed strenuous inflation of rubber balloons. Occasionally, crepitation may be detected along the course of Stenson's duct in these patients.

Laboratory findings are nonspecific in uncomplicated mumps parotitis. The white blood cell count is usually within the normal range although there may be a relative lymphocytosis. A polymorphonuclear leukocytosis (15,000 to 20,000/mm^3) is common with extraparotid manifestations. This is also true of the erythrocyte sedimentation rate, which, normal or slightly elevated with mumps parotitis, is markedly elevated with arthritis and orchitis. The serum amylase is above normal in mumps and can be used to differentiate nonparotid from parotid swelling, but not pancreatitis from parotitis.

Cerebrospinal fluid (CSF) pleocytosis is usually in the order of 100 to 500 cells/mm^3. This may be predominantly polymorphonuclear in the early stages; however, a mononuclear cell reaction is characteristic thereafter. The CSF protein is normal or slightly elevated, and the glucose concentration may be decreased in 2 to 20 per cent of cases. Persistence of pleocytosis for 3 to 4 days in most cases, and for as long as 15 weeks in occasional cases, has been reported. Similarly, increased CSF protein concentration has been observed for as long as 29 days. Late inflammatory changes in the CSF may be the hallmark of postinfectious encephalomyelitis.

A specific viral diagnosis can be made by inoculation of primary Rhesus monkey (or other appropriate cell line) with saliva, urine, blood, or CSF from patients with mumps and/or mumps meningoencephalitis. Saliva may contain virus from 7 days before the onset of parotitis to 8 days after. In exceptional cases, virus has been cultured up to 14 days after the onset of parotitis despite the absence of clinical disease at the time. The virus has also been isolated directly from parotid, testicular, and thyroid tissue. A characteristic cytopathic effect appears in tissue culture 5 to 7 days after inoculation, and the hemadsorption test with guinea-pig red blood cells is positive. The virus is further identified by neutralization of this hemadsorption with specific antisera. More rapid experimental approaches have been used for the diagnosis of mumps infection, including direct fluorescent antibody staining of epithelial cells in the saliva and hemagglutination by saliva, urine, and CSF.

Serologic diagnosis of mumps infection is based upon demonstration of one of several humoral antibody responses. Two complement-fixing mumps antigens have been described. The viral (V) hemagglutinin antigen is found on the surface and the soluble (S) nucleocapsid antigen in the core. Antibody directed against the soluble antigen rises significantly over the first 2 to 6 weeks of illness and then begins to fall. Viral-associated antigen stimulates a slower antibody response that persists for 6 months to a year. Because of the earlier rise and fall of the antibody against soluble antigen, a high S/V ratio of complement-fixing antibody may indicate recent infection. Similarly, complement-fixation titers over 1/200 suggest recent infection because such antibody concentrations are present in less than 2 per cent of adults. The short duration of these antibodies makes the complement-fixation test less satisfactory for detection of long-term immunity. Hemagglutination inhibition or, preferably, neutralizing antibody is a more sensitive test for this purpose. Neutralizing-antibody titers of greater than 1:2 correlate with immunity. At least a fourfold antibody titer rise accompanies acute infection. Heterologous serologic responses to parainfluenza virus have been documented with mumps infection.

The mumps skin test has occasionally been used as an indicator of immunity. Preparations of this material are extremely variable in their antigenic potency, and false-positive and false-negative results are common. If the test is done, a tissue-culture control antigen should be administered intradermally in the contralateral forearm. One-tenth milliliter of the test and control antigen materials is administered intradermally, and the results are recorded at 24 and 48 hours. A transverse diameter of erythema around the test antigen of 10 mm or more than around the control is used to define positivity. The skin test may boost humoral antibody in patients with preexisting titers.

The differential diagnosis of meningoencephalitis in the absence of parotitis includes enteroviral, herpes simplex, and tuberculous infections. A low CSF sugar concentration in the presence of a lymphocytic cellular reaction may suggest meningeal tuberculosis. Orchitis in the absence of parotitis may be due to Coxsackie viruses types A and B, echoviruses, and lymphocytic choriomeningitis virus. Noninfectious causes of testicular hypertrophy need to be excluded as well.

TREATMENT AND PROPHYLAXIS. Mumps is usually a benign and self-limited infection that requires little treatment. Antipyretics and rest may be used, but there is no specific antiviral therapy.

Patients with mumps meningoencephalitis may have severe headache and require aspirin or codeine. This should be used with caution in patients with encephalitis, in which masking of the symptoms and signs may be dangerous. The headache in this condition is often relieved by lumbar puncture.

Patients with orchitis may require more potent analgesics such as meperidine or morphine. Support for the scrotum and warm or cold compresses are often useful. The patient's subjective response to this treatment can be used as a guide. A controlled study demonstrated no benefit from adrenocorticosteroid therapy in orchitis. Patients should be reassured that sterility after orchitis is extremely rare.

Other modalities such as diethylstilbestrol, injection of the spermatic cord with local anesthetics, incision of the tunica albuginea, and oxyphenbutazone seem useless.

Mumps vaccine (5000 $TCID_{50}$/dose) is immunogenic in 93 to 98 per cent of subjects and has a protective efficacy of about 95 per cent. Neutralizing antibody persists for at least 10 years. Immunity is also durable after mumps immunization combined with measles and rubella vaccines (Weibel et al., 1980). Although antibody titers are lower than after natural infection, they are still protective. Adverse effects after vaccination are mild and extremely rare. These include parotitis, low-grade fever, rash, pruritus, and purpura; serum amylase concentrations are not usually elevated. Central nervous system problems have followed vaccination but usually not with greater incidence than expected in the normal population. Thus, approximately one case of CNS illness per million doses of vaccine has been reported in the United States. These problems include cranial neuropathies (diplopia, Bell's palsy) that usually occur within 8 days after vaccination and encephalopathy (meningoencephalitis, febrile convulsions) most often noted 3 weeks after immunization.

The live attenuated virus vaccine (Jeryl Lynn strain) produces a noncommunicable, subclinical infection, and the virus has been isolated from vaccinees only in rare instances. The vaccine is contraindicated in patients allergic to egg protein or neomycin, which are present in the preparation. In view of possible teratogenicity, it is also contraindicated in pregnancy. The vaccine virus has infected the placenta of susceptible women (although viremia has not been demonstrated after vaccination). As with other live virus vaccines, administration to immunosuppressed and/or debilitated patients is contraindicated.

The vaccine should be used to prevent mumps in all children over the age of 13 months. Seroconversion rates probably will be highest after this age. Simultaneous administration of mumps and measles virus vaccines at 13 to 15 months of age is safe and effective. Mumps and mumps vaccination is followed by a period of diminished cutaneous tuberculin sensitivity. Skin testing should, therefore, be carried out before, or simultaneous with, vaccination.

Prophylaxis for family contacts and containment of epidemic spread are difficult to achieve via isolation or vaccination. Isolation is ineffective because the virus is present in the saliva for as long as a week before the onset of symptoms, and many patients are asymptomatic. Use of respiratory droplet isolation procedures (mask and handwashing) may be indicated in certain situations (e.g., admission of a patient with mumps to hospital). Materials in contact with patient secretions and urine should be disinfected. Vaccine-induced antibody may develop slowly (14 to 28 days) and may, therefore, not prevent infection during the first few weeks following vaccination. Skin tests cannot be relied upon to predict susceptibility. There is no contraindication to vaccination of seropositive individuals with mumps vaccine, and indeed, this procedure often boosts humoral antibody without adverse effects.

In an effort to study the efficacy of mumps hyperimmune globulin, 56 serologically susceptible subjects received this material during a mumps epidemic. The attack and complication rates were not altered (Reed et al., 1967). Use of immunoglobulin to prevent mumps orchitis in adult males is also not supported by these data.

Although mumps is generally a mild and self-limited illness, there are occasional deaths from it. Patients with severe parotitis and neurologic or testicular involvement may also suffer greatly. Now that an effective vaccine is available, such cases need no longer occur (Koplan et al., 1982).

References

Aase, J. M., Noren, G., Reddy, D., and St. Geme, J., Jr.: Mumps-virus infection in pregnant women and the immunologic response of their offspring. New Engl J Med 286:1379, 1972.

Beard, C. M., Benson, R. C., Kelalis, P. P., Elveback, L. R., and Kurland, L. T.: The incidence and outcome of mumps orchitis in Rochester, Minnesota, 1935 to 1974. Mayo Clin Proc 52:3, 1977.

Brill, S. J., and Gilfillan, R. F.: Acute parotitis associated with influenza Type A, New Engl J Med 296:1391, 1977.

Brown, N. J., and Richmond, S. J.: Fatal mumps myocarditis in an 8-month-old child. Brit Med J 281:356, 1980.

Chiba, Y., Dzierba, J. J., Morag, A., and Ogra, P. L.: Cell-mediated immune response to mumps virus infection in man. J Immunol 116:12, 1976.

Friedman, M. G.: Salivary IgA antibodies to mumps virus during and after mumps. J Infect Dis 143:617, 1981.

Garcia, A. G. P., Pereira, J. M. S., Vidigal, N., Lobato, Y. Y., Pegado, C. S., and Branco, J. P. C.: Intrauterine infection with mumps virus. Obstet & Gynecol 156:756, 1980.

Herndon, R. M., Johnson, R. T., Davis, L. E., and Descalgi, L. R.: Ependymitis in mumps virus meningitis. Arch Neurol 30:475, 1974.

Jones, J. F., Ray, C. G., and Fulginiti, V. A.: Perinatal mumps infection. J Pediatr 96:912, 1980.

Koplan, J. P., and Preblud, S. R.: A benefit-cost analysis of mumps-vaccine. Am J Dis Child 136:362, 1982.

Levitt, L. P., and Casey, H. L.: Mumps in a general population. Am J Dis Child 120:134, 1970.

London, W. T., Kent, S. G., Palmer, A. E., Fucillo, D. A., Houff, S. A., Saini, N., and Sever, J. L.: Induction of congenital hydrocephalus with mumps virus in rhesus monkeys. J Infect Dis 139:324, 1979.

Pollack, S., Bar-On, E., and Enat, R.: Guillain-Barré syndrome; Association with mumps. NY State J Med 5:795, 1981.

Reed, D., Brown, G., Merrick, R., Sever, J., and Feltz, E.: A mumps epidemic on St. George Island, Alaska. JAMA 199:113, 1967.

Ukkonen, P., Granstrom, M-L., Rasanen, J., Salonen, E-M., and Penttinen, K.: Local production of mumps IgG and IgM antibodies in the cerebrospinal fluid of meningitis patients. J Med Virol 8:257, 1981.

Vaheri, A., Julkunen, I., and Koskiniemi M-L.: Chronic encephalomyelitis with specific increase in intrathecal mumps antibodies. Lancet 2:685, 1982.

Weibel, R. E., Buynak, E. B., McLean, A. A., and Hilleman, M. R.: Persistence of antibody in human subjects for 7 to 10 years following administration of combined live attenuated measles, mumps, and rubella virus vaccines. Proc Soc Exp Biol Med 165:260, 1980.

Wilfert, C. M.: Mumps meningoencephalitis with low cerebrospinal fluid glucose, prolonged pleocytosis, and elevation of protein. New Engl J Med 280:855, 1969.

109
INFLUENZA

R. GORDON DOUGLAS, JR., M.D.

Influenza is an acute infectious disease caused by influenza A or B virus. It occurs in outbreaks, usually in the winter months in temperate climates, and produces symptoms of fever, cough, headache, and myalgias. The disease is usually self-limited, but pulmonary complications develop in a few cases. Infection with influenza viruses may also produce pharyngitis, croup, tracheobronchitis, bronchiolitis, pneumonia, or even common colds. Conversely, other respiratory viruses such as rhinoviruses, adenoviruses, or enteroviruses may produce sporadic cases of acute, self-limited, febrile illness that mimic those produced by influenza viruses.

ETIOLOGY. Influenza viruses are members of the Orthomyxoviridae family. Influenza virus type A and influenza virus type B are two genera within this family. The third type of influenza virus, type C, probably represents another genus, although it has not been officially so classified. Influenza viruses are medium-sized (80 to 100 nm) enveloped viruses containing a helical nucleocapsid that is segmented into eight separate pieces. A total of eight gene products (proteins) has been identified. The most important antigenic determinants are the two surface glycoproteins known as the hemagglutinin (H) and the neuraminidase (N), named after certain biological functions possessed by these proteins. The H and N project as spikes from a lipid envelope that is derived from host cell membrane. Changes in the antigenicity of these surface proteins are thought to be important determinants of the unusual epidemiologic behavior of influenza virus. Both surface proteins undergo relatively minor changes that occur frequently, that is, almost every year. These are referred to as "antigenic drift," and they result from point mutations resulting in alterations of one or more amino acids. More dramatic changes in the antigenicity of either or both proteins are referred to as "antigenic shift." Antigenic shift is thought to occur most often from genetic reassortment that occurs when two influenza viruses simultaneously infect a single cell (Webster et al., 1982). As a result of the presence of a segmented genome, random reassortment of the eight RNA segments from each parent results in creation of new virions with varying characteristics of either parent. In this way, progeny virus that retain the virulence factors of one parent but also contain "new" H or N or both develop. To date, three hemagglutinins (H1, H2, H3) and two neuraminidases (N1, N2) have been recognized.

Influenza A viruses are named by their H and N to identify the subtype (e.g., H3N2, H1N1), and by site of origin and year to recognize strain variation within a subtype (e.g., A/Hong Kong/68 H3N2, A/England/42/72 H3N2, A/Texas/77 H3N2 [Table 1]).

EPIDEMIOLOGY. Influenza A and B virus infections characteristically occur in epidemics (Glezen et al, 1982). In a given community or region they begin rather abruptly, reach a sharp peak in two to three weeks, and last five to six weeks. During these epidemics, the number of people with febrile respiratory disease increases, school and industrial absenteeism rises, and hospital admissions for pneumonia, chronic obstructive pulmonary disease, croup, and congestive heart failure all increase. There are also more deaths.

Such epidemics may be localized to a community or region, or they may involve countries or continents or occur worldwide, in which case they are called pandemics. Epidemics do not occur everywhere simultaneously; rather, sequential spread from one area to another over several months is usual. Epidemics occur during October through April in the northern hemisphere and May through September in the southern hemisphere.

PATHOGENESIS AND PATHOLOGY. Influenza viruses are transmitted from person to person via the respiratory route, predominantly by small particle aerosols (<10μ mass median diameter). It is also possible that some spread occurs from closer contact transmission including hand-to-hand contact, or fomites, or by direct deposition of large droplets of respiratory secretions containing infectious virus (Douglas, 1975).

Virus is deposited on the mucosal epithelium of the respiratory tract where it may be neutralized by specific secretory IgA antibody and nonspecific mucoproteins or removed by the mucociliary blanket or cough reflex. If it is not neutralized or removed, virus adsorbs to and penetrates a columnar epithelial cell, where it initiates the viral replication cycle. As infectious virus is released from cells, it spreads to adjacent cells where the replication cycle is repeated. Within a relatively short time many cells in the respiratory tract are infected. Such replication eventually kills the cell. The incubation period from deposition of virus to onset of illness (usually one to two days) varies from 18 to 72 hours, depending in part on the size of the inoculum dose. Virus is shed from the respiratory tract just before the onset of illness. Virus titers in nasal or tracheal secretions peak within 24 hours, remain elevated for 24 to 48 hours, and then rapidly decrease. As virus titers fall, interferon is detected in the respiratory secretions and may be responsible for recovery from illness. Viral replication is the major determinant of illness, since neither antibody nor cell-mediated responses can be detected at this time in unprimed subjects. The occurrence of systemic symptoms and fever suggests that virus disseminates hematogenously, but infectious virus has only rarely been recovered from blood.

Table 1. ANTIGENIC SHIFTS OF INFLUENZA A

Year	Subtype Designation	Common Name
1889	H3N2	—
1918	H1N1	Swine
1957	H2N2	A_2, Asian
1968	H3N2	Hong Kong
1977	H1N1	Russian

During acute uncomplicated influenza, ciliated columnar epithelial cells commonly desquamate into the lumen of the bronchus. Individual cells show shrinkage, pyknotic nuclei, and loss of cilia. In fatal influenza viral pneumonia, extensive hemorrhage, hyaline membrane formation, and few polymorphonuclear cells are found in the lung.

Neutralizing, hemagglutination-inhibiting (HAI), neuraminidase-inhibiting (NI), complement-fixing (CF) ELISA and immunoflourescent antibodies develop in the serum of patients experiencing primary infection with influenza virus. They are first detected the second week after exposure and reach peak titers by four weeks. In patients who have been primed by previous infection, the antibody response is more brisk. HAI, NI, and neutralizing antibodies persist for months to years and gradually decline thereafter. Neutralizing and HAI tests distinguish among strains as well as among subtypes of influenza. CF antibody is directed against the ribonucleoprotein and is type-specific, so that all strains and subtypes within the influenza A type cross-react in CF tests.

Secretory antibodies, predominantly IgA, develop in the respiratory tract after influenza infection. Their peak titers are reached 14 days after the onset of infection. They are found in saliva, nasal secretions, sputum, and tracheal washings by neutralization tests. Secretory antibodies do not persist as long as serum antibodies, usually only several months.

Substantial levels of antibody protect against infection. Serum HAI titers of 1:40 or greater or neutralizing titers of 1:8 or greater are commonly associated with protection against infection. Similarly, most persons with nasal neutralizing antibody titers of 1:4 or greater are protected against infection.

Antibody also modifies the course of illness. That is, if antibody is present in lower titers in serum, or is present in serum and not in nasal secretions, the subject may become infected but will experience a milder illness than someone who has no antibody. In addition, antibody that is directed against neuraminidase or against a heterotypic strain may prevent severe illness but not infection.

CLINICAL FINDINGS IN UNCOMPLICATED INFLUENZA. Influenza characteristically starts abruptly. Many patients can pinpoint the hour of onset. At first systemic symptoms such as feverishness, chilliness or frank shaking chills, headache, myalgias, malaise, and anorexia predominate. The temperature usually rises rapidly to a peak of 38 to 40° C or higher within 12 hours of onset. Usually myalgias and headache are the most troublesome symptoms, and their severity is related to the height of the fever. Myalgias may involve the extremities or the long muscles of the back, and arthralgias are commonly observed. Systemic symptoms usually persist for three days, the usual duration of fever.

When present, ocular symptoms such as photophobia, tearing, burning, and pain on moving the eyes are helpful diagnostically. Respiratory symptoms, particularly dry cough and nasal discharge, are usually present also at the onset but are overshadowed by the systemic symptoms. Nasal obstruction, hoarseness, and dry or sore throat may also be present. These symptoms tend to become more prominent as the disease progresses.

Fever is usually continuous but may be intermittent, especially if antipyretics are administered. On the second and third days of illness, the temperature elevation is usually 0.5 to 1.0 degree lower than on the first day. The duration of fever is three days commonly, but it may last from one to five or more days.

Early in the illness the patient appears toxic with flushed face and hot moist skin. The eyes are watery and reddened and clear nasal discharge is common. The mucous membranes of the nose and throat are hyperemic, but exudate is not observed. Small, tender cervical lymph nodes are often present. Transient scattered ronchi or localized areas of rales are found in less than 20 per cent of cases.

Respiratory symptoms and signs usually persist for three to four days after fever subsides. Cough, lassitude, and malaise commonly persist for one to two or more weeks.

The above description of illness occurs with any type, subtype, or strain of influenza A or B virus. In contrast, influenza C infection causes afebrile common colds and rarely if ever produces the influenza syndrome. It also does not occur in epidemics.

Maximal temperatures tend to be higher among children, and cervical adenopathy is more frequent among children than adults. Among elderly persons, fever remains a frequent finding, although the height of the febrile response may be lower than among children and young adults.

COMPLICATIONS AND SEQUELAE

Pulmonary Complications. Three pulmonary complications of influenza are well recognized: primary influenza viral pneumonia, secondary bacterial infection, and mixed viral and bacterial pneumonias.

Primary Influenza Viral Pneumonia. This complication has occurred primarily in persons with underlying cardiovascular, pulmonary, renal, or other chronic disease, although cases occur in every large outbreak in young healthy adults. Pregnancy has been implicated as a risk factor in some epidemics. Following a typical onset of influenza there is rapid progression of fever, cough, dyspnea, and cyanosis. Physical examination and chest x-ray reveal bilateral findings but no consolidation. Blood gas studies show marked anoxia. Sputum culture reveals normal flora, whereas viral cultures yield high titers of influenza A virus. Such patients do not respond to antibiotics and mortality is high.

Milder forms of influenza viral pneumonia involving only one lobe or segment have been described. They are not invariably lethal and are more likely to be confused with pneumonia due to *Streptococcus pneumoniae* than with pneumonia produced by viral infection. Pneumonia and/or bronchiolitis occurs in children but is less common than in adults.

Secondary Bacterial Pneumonia. Patients who are elderly or have chronic pulmonary, cardiac, metabolic, or other diseases have a classic influenza illness followed by a period of improvement lasting one to four days. Recrudescence of fever is associated with symptoms and signs of bacterial pneumonia such as cough, sputum production, chest pain, and an area of consolidation seen on physical examination and chest roentgenogram. Gram stain and culture of sputum reveal predominance of a bacterial pathogen, most often *S. pneumoniae, Staphylococcus aureus,* or *Haemophilus influenzae.* Such patients usually respond to specific antibiotic therapy.

Mixed Viral-Bacterial Pneumonias. During an outbreak of influenza many cases are observed that do not clearly fit the description of primary influenza or secondary bacterial pneumonias. The disease does not progress relentlessly, yet the fever pattern is not biphasic. These patients may have primary viral, secondary bacterial, or mixed viral and bacterial infection of the lung and many respond to antibiotics.

Croup. Significant numbers of cases of croup occur in influenza A and B outbreaks. Such cases associated with influenza A virus are more severe but less frequent than those associated with parainfluenza virus types 1, 2, or 3, or respiratory syncytial virus.

Exacerbation of Chronic Obstructive Pulmonary Disease. In adults with chronic obstructive pulmonary disease, infection with influenza A or B virus may result in acute exacerbation of chronic bronchitis, a syndrome associated with other respiratory viruses and bacteria as well. Such infections may result in permanent loss of pulmonary function.

Although the majority of patients with influenza do not have clinically detectable pneumonia, abnormalities in gas exchange and peripheral airway resistance frequently occur in nonpneumonic influenza infections and persist well beyond the period of clinical illness (Little et al., 1978). These findings suggest that viral invasion of the lower respiratory tract is common in influenza and may help to explain the relatively long convalescence. Lower respiratory tract disease is found by auscultation or roentgenogram in about 10 per cent of patients. The rate is lower in children and young adults but rises rapidly after age 50.

Nonpulmonary Complications

Myositis. Myositis and myoglobinuria with tender leg muscles and elevated serum creatinine phosphokinase (CPK) levels have been reported in children after influenza B and less commonly influenza A infection. The pain may be severe enough to prevent walking.

Cardiac Complications. Both myocarditis and pericarditis have been associated with influenza A and B virus infections. However, neither myocarditis nor pericarditis is observed commonly at autopsy among those dying of primary influenza viral pneumonia.

Central Nervous System Complications. Guillain-Barré syndrome has been reported to occur after influenza A infection, as it has after numerous other infections, but no definite etiologic relationship has been established. In addition, cases of transverse myelitis and encephalitis have occurred rarely.

Reye's Syndrome. Reye's syndrome, first described in 1963, is now a frequently recognized hepatic and central nervous system complication of influenza B, influenza A, and varicella zoster virus infection. Pathologic examination reveals a liver that is pale yellow due to the presence of multiple small droplets of lipids uniformly distributed throughout hepatocytes. Neither the brain nor the liver shows inflammatory changes. The urea-cycle mitochondrial enzymes in the liver are transiently abnormal.

The syndrome occurs only in children between the ages of 2 and 16 years, and its mortality has fallen from 40 per cent to 10 per cent as milder cases have been diagnosed and therapy has become standardized (Consensus Conference, 1981). Because of the epidemic nature of influenza, Reye's syndrome also occurs epidemically as well as endemically. Most of the large outbreaks have resulted from influenza B virus infection. An association with ingestion of aspirin for fever during influenza and subsequent development of Reye's syndrome has been claimed and challenged (Daniels et al., 1983).

Reye's syndrome usually starts with nausea and vomiting several days after a typical upper respiratory, gastrointestinal, or chickenpox infection. Within one or two days mental changes are noted. The manifestations range from lethargy to delirium, obtundation, seizures, and respiratory arrest. The children are usually afebrile and have hepatomegaly but not jaundice. Mortality is related to stage of coma on admission to the hospital, and appears to be decreasing with earlier recognition and hospitalization. Lumbar puncture reveals increased intracranial pressure and normal protein values and cell counts, confirming the presence of encephalopathy rather than meningoencephalitis. The most frequent laboratory abnormality is elevation of the blood ammonia value, which occurs in almost all patients. Hypoglycemia is present more often in patients with antecedent varicella or gastrointestinal illness than in those with upper respiratory illness. Serum glutamic oxaloacetic transaminase (SGOT), serum glutamic pyruvic transaminase (SGPT), bilirubin, and prothrombin values are commonly elevated, as are CPK and lactic dehydrogenase (LDH) levels.

DIAGNOSIS. Specific viral diagnosis is made by virus isolation, serology, and epidemiology. Detection of infectious virus or viral antigen in respiratory secretions is optimal for clinical purposes, since serologic tests, although sensitive and specific, are still negative during the acute illness. Virus can be isolated readily from nasal swab specimens, throat swab specimens, nasal washes, and sputum. Sputum is the best specimen, but if it is not produced, a combined nose and throat swab specimen or a nasal wash is ideal. Such swabs should be thrust into containers of viral transport medium and brought to the laboratory at once. Specimens for diagnosis of influenza are inoculated onto Madin-Darby canine kidney (MDCK) or cynomologous kidney cell cultures, and virus replication is detected by cytopathic effect and/or hemadsorption. About two thirds of the positive cultures can be detected within three days of inoculation and the remainder by seven days. Many hospital or regional viral diagnostic laboratories can recover influenza virus by these cell culture techniques or by inoculation of embryonated hens' eggs.

Complement-fixing antibody tests are most commonly used for serologic diagnosis. Serum specimens from the acute and convalescent periods (obtained 10 to 20 days after the acute phase serum) should be submitted for testing. Fourfold or greater rises or falls in titer are considered diagnostic of infection, and a high convalescent titer, when only one convalescent specimen is available, suggests recent infection.

Diagnosis can also be made on epidemiologic grounds. For example, when influenza virus is confirmed in a region or community by the local or state health department, or by the Centers for Disease Control, persons presenting with fever, muscle aches, and cough most likely have influenza.

TREATMENT

Uncomplicated Influenza. Amantadine is approved in the United States for treatment of influenza. It shortens the duration of signs and symptoms of clinical influenza by approximately 50 per cent. Its major drawback is minor reversible central nervous system side effects such as insomnia, dizziness, and difficulty in concentrating, which occur in about 5 per cent of subjects. However, in controlled studies the reduction of influenza symptoms is greater than the occurrence of drug side effects, resulting in net benefit to patients. The usual dose is 200 mg orally daily for three to five days. Recent studies indicate that 100 mg per day of amantadine or 200 mg of rimantadine are just as effective as 200 mg per day of amantadine (Van Voris et al., 1981). Amantadine is superior to aspirin for relief of symptoms (Younkin et al., 1983).

Acutely ill, febrile patients should rest in bed and take enough fluids. Acetylsalicylic acid 0.6 to 0.9 g every three to four hours reduces headache, fever, and myalgias but should not be used in those less than 16 years of age. Nasal obstruction may be relieved by phenylephrine or oxymetazoline hydrochloride nasal sprays or drops, and cough may be reduced by cold water vaporization or guaifenesin cough syrup containing dextromethorphan, 1 to 3 teaspoons every three to four hours.

Pulmonary Complications. Because there have been no controlled studies of amantadine treatment of influenza viral pneumonia, its use in this condition is based on extrapolation from cases of uncomplicated influenza, anecdotal case reports of benefit, and the effect of amantadine on peripheral airway resistance in uncomplicated influenza. Supportive care is important, including fluid and electrolyte management, supplemental oxygen, intubation, tracheostomy, assisted ventilation, and use of positive end expiratory pressure. For patients with proven or suspected bacterial superinfection, antibiotics should be administered. Because of the rapidly advancing nature of many cases of pneumonia that occur during an influenza epidemic, therapy to cover the potential pathogens, most importantly *S. aureus*, *S. pneumoniae*, and *H. influenzae*, is indicated if a clearcut diagnosis cannot be made from Gram stain of the sputum or transtracheal aspirate. Cephamandole, 12 g/day I.V. in divided doses, might be a reasonable choice in this situation because it has good in vitro activity against the three most common organisms, including ampicillin-resistant *H. influenzae*. Alternatively, a semisynthetic penicillinase-resistant penicillin such as methicillin or nafcillin, 12 g/day I.V. in divided doses, and ampicillin, 8 to 12 g/day I.V. in divided doses, could be used. If ampicillin-resistant *H. influenzae* is suspected, chloramphenicol may be substituted for ampicillin. If there is a suspicion of gram-negative rod pneumonia due to organisms other than *H. influenzae*, cephamandole, cefazolin, or an aminoglycoside such as gentamicin, tobramycin, or amikacin could be considered. For penicillin-allergic patients, vancomycin for *S. aureus*, chloramphenicol for *H. influenzae* and *S. pneumoniae*, or clindamycin for *S. aureus* and *S. pneumoniae* may be considered.

Other Complications. There is no specific therapy for cardiac, central nervous system, or other complications, including Reye's syndrome.

PREVENTION. The mainstay for prevention of influenza in the United States is inactivated virus vaccines. In some other countries, live virus vaccines are used. Vaccines are safe and effective in preventing influenza, but several problems are worthy of mention. Most studies indicate that vaccines have a protective efficacy of about 70 per cent. Mild local side effects occur in 25 per cent of vaccine recipients, and systemic side effects, including fever, occur in 1 to 2 per cent. Guillain-Barré syndrome (GBS) occurred in 1 in 100,000 patients, and 5 per cent of those with GBS died during the 1976 Swine Influenza Immunization Program in the United States. GBS has not occurred with influenza vaccines since 1976. Warfarin or theophylline toxicity is not a problem in patients receiving these drugs who are vaccinated.

The Immunization Practices Advisory Committee in the United States, the World Health Organization, and other governmental bodies make recommendations annually with regard to the composition of the vaccine. In general, the vaccines have contained both an A type and a B type virus (bivalent), usually the types isolated in the previous winter's influenza season. In some years, two A types have been included in addition to a B type (thus, trivalent) because both A types have circulated in the previous winter and because the type of influenza to be encountered cannot be reliably predicted.

Inactivated vaccines have recently been purified and their antigenic mass standardized. One dose of 15 μg of antigen is enough to elicit serum HAI titers of 1:40 or greater in 90 per cent of persons who have previously been exposed to the antigen. Two doses are necessary to achieve comparable levels in unprimed subjects.

The only contraindication to vaccination is hypersensitivity to hens' eggs. If an individual can eat eggs or egg-containing products, the vaccine is safe. In the United States, vaccine is recommended for persons at increased risks of dying from pulmonary complications of influenza (Barker et al., 1982). Highest priority for vaccination is given to persons with chronic heart or pulmonary disease requiring medical attention and to residents of nursing homes and other chronic care facilities. Next, medical personnel who have extensive contact with high risk patients and finally persons of 65 years of age and over and those with chronic underlying disease should be considered. Antibody responses are usually good or only slightly diminished in these chronic conditions and additional harmful effects have not been observed in groups of patients with renal disease, systemic lupus erythematosus, or multiple sclerosis. Pregnancy is not a contraindication to vaccination.

Chemoprophylaxis. Amantadine is an approved prophylactic agent against influenza (Dolin et al., 1982). It is as effective as vaccine and adds to vaccine efficacy. Because two 100 mg capsules are required each day for five to six weeks, and because of cost, side effects, and the need for a surveillance program to detect the onset of an epidemic, vaccine is preferred to amantadine for routine prophylaxis. However, there are certain situations in which the prophylactic use of amantadine may be important. Persons who have not received vaccine at the time of an influenza outbreak should be given vaccine together with amantadine 100 mg twice daily for 10 to 14 days. Persons with egg hypersensitivity, who cannot receive influenza vaccine, may be given amantadine for the duration of the outbreak. Household contacts of an index case may be given amantadine. Staff and patients in hospitals or institutions may be given amantadine to prevent an outbreak.

References

Barker, W. H., Mulloohy, J. P.: Pneumonia and influenza deaths during epidemic: Implications for prevention. Arch Intern Med 142:85, 1982.

Consensus Conference: Diagnosis and treatment of Reye's syndrome. JAMA 246:2441, 1981.

Daniels, S. R., Greenberg, R. S., and Ibrahim, M. A.: Scientific uncertainties in the studies of salicylate use and Reye's syndrome. JAMA 249:1311, 1983.

Dolin, R., Reichman, R. C., Madore, H. P., et al.: A controlled trial of

amantadine and rimantadine in the prophylaxis of influenza A infection. N Engl J Med 307:580, 1982.
Douglas, R. G., Jr.: Influenza in man. In Kilbourne, E. D. (ed.): Influenza Viruses and Influenza. New York, Academic Press, 1975, p. 395.
Glezen, W. P., Payne, A. A., Synder, D. N., and Downs, T. D.: Mortality and influenza. Jour Infec Dis 146:313, 1982.
Little, J. W., Hall, W. J., Douglas, R. G., et al.: Airway hyperreactivity and peripheral airway dysfunction in influenza A infection. AM Rev Resp Dis 118:295, 1978.
Van Voris, I. P., Betts, R. F., Hayden, F. G., et al.: Successful treatment of naturally occurring influenza A/USSR/77 H1N1. JAMA 245:1128, 1981.
Webster, R. G., Laver, W. G., Air, G. M., and Schild, G. C.: Molecular mechanisms of variation in influenza viruses. Nature, London 296:115, 1982.
Younkin, S. W., Betts, R. F., Roth, R. K., et al.: Reduction in fever and symptoms in young adults with aspirin or amantadine. Antimicrobial Agents Chemother 23:577, 1983.

110
PERTUSSIS

JAMES D. CONNOR, M.D.

Pertussis is an acute disease of the respiratory tract usually characterized by progressive, repetitive, paroxysmal coughing, mild systemic complaints, and lymphocytosis. Because the hallmark of the clinical disease is an inspiratory whoop, it is commonly referred to as whooping cough. Pertussis occurs throughout the world in immunized and unimmunized populations, usually causing sharp outbreaks or epidemics of disease in cycles of two to four years. The disease is caused by *Bordetella pertussis*, a minute bacillus that was first isolated from children with the disease by Bordet and Gengou in 1906. Although infection may occur at any age, clinical disease is most frequent in older infants and children. The morbidity is associated with the severity of coughing paroxysms and is especially marked in infants under 1 year of age (Buchanan and Broohn, 1970). The incidence has continued to decline throughout the era of active immunization, and the mortality rate has declined markedly in both immunized and unimmunized populations in developed countries.

ETIOLOGY. *B. pertussis*, originally known as the Bordet-Gengou bacillus, was assigned to the genus *Haemophilus* along with *Haemophilus influenzae*. After it was recognized that the pertussis bacillus did not require hemin and NAD (see Chapter 36) for growth, it was placed in a separate genus (see Chapter 35) that now also includes *B. parapertussis* and *B. bronchiseptica* (formerly *Brucella bronchiseptica)*. In optimal liquid or semisolid medium, *B. pertussis* is a highly uniform, minute coccobacillus measuring approximately 0.5 μ in length. It stains faintly pink with the Gram stain. The bacilli are encapsulated but nonmotile. Under suboptimal conditions, the bacilli become pleomorphic and produce long rod forms mixed with *coccoid* and *ovoid* organisms. This change in appearance is accompanied by defects in the antigenic structure, including the loss of the antigen that induces protection in animals and humans. *B. pertussis* produces several other antigens, including agglutinogens, which are used to identify different antigenic types in the genus *Bordetella* as well as individual clinical strains of *B. pertussis.* Eldering and Kendrick (1957) identified agglutinogen Types 1 through 6 among various strains of *B. pertussis,* with Types 2, 3, and 5 being major agglutinogens for *B. pertussis*, and Types 4 and 6 were minor. Type 7 is common to the genus; Type 12 is species-specific for *B. bronchiseptica* and Type 14 for *B. parapertussis* (Eldering et al., 1957). Therefore, it is possible to differentiate the three members of the genus antigenically by agglutination with immune sera. Although there are common antigens among the genus, no cross-immunity has been recognized. Other antigens of *B. pertussis* include IAP (islet-activating protein), adenylcyclase, histamine-sensitizing factor, hemagglutinins, and lymphocyte-promoting factor (Munoz, 1963; Pittman, 1970). The last is the factor responsible for the characteristic lymphocytosis that appears during the paroxysmal stage of the disease and after immunization with whole killed bacilli (Welsh et al., 1959). Pertussis adenylcyclase reduces phagocytic bactericidal activity (Confer and Eaton, 1982) and is important in the pathogenesis of the disease.

INCIDENCE. In relatively isolated, unimmunized populations, pertussis occurs in sharp outbreaks and epidemics. During epidemics the incidence of the characteristic acute disease is highest among infants and young children. This age group is at highest risk because it was born after the preceding epidemic. The primary attack rate in this group may be as high as 40 to 60 per cent, with a secondary attack rate among family members of 70 to 90 per cent. In immunized populations, the attack rate varies between 16 and 50 per cent in different countries, probably depending on the type of surveillance, the potency of the vaccine, and the age of those immunized. Very young infants as well as older children and adults may account for most cases in outbreaks among well-immunized populations, since older infants and younger children have relatively greater protection from more recent immunization. There is no recognized carrier state; infants that are considered index cases in families may actually have been infected by an adult family member with unrecognized disease. The manner in which the endemic reservoir of infection is maintained is unknown. The disease usually occurs in late spring or summer and persists throughout the fall and early winter. Outbreaks among susceptible hospital personnel may be particularly inconvenient and jeopardize critical health care services (Kurt et al., 1972).

The mortality rate has fallen remarkably over the last three decades, even among the youngest infants, in whom it has always been highest (Buchanan and Broohn, 1970). A great reduction in the incidence of protein-calorie malnutrition may be the most important reason for this decline. Since antibiotics do not alter the morbidity or duration of the primary disease, it is unlikely that they influence the mortality of the primary disease. However, the mortality from secondary infectious complications, such as bacterial pneumonia, probably has been reduced by antibiotics.

Primary nursing care and supportive measures may also be responsible for the reduced mortality.

The reduction in incidence clearly began before the introduction of general immunization in the United States, but the wide use of potent killed bacillary vaccines has certainly contributed to the continuing fall in incidence. The diagnosis is also often missed or unconfirmed because most laboratories cannot isolate or identify *B. pertussis*, and young physicians may never have seen the clinical disease. The present low incidence among highly immunized populations is unlikely to fall further unless effective methods are found to immunize susceptible adults and infants under 3 to 4 months of age.

In contrast to most childhood infections, the mortality of pertussis is higher among females. At one time, 90 per cent of cases with characteristic clinical disease occurred in children under the age of 9 years (Ipsen and Bowen, 1955), but now most cases occur among the very young who are either unimmunized or incompletely immunized.

PATHOLOGY AND PATHOGENESIS. Three types of lesions predominate in the respiratory tract. In early paroxysmal and midparoxysmal stages of the disease, peribronchitis and peribronchiolitis may develop. Dense accumulations of lymphocytes, mast cells, and plasmocytes infiltrate the supporting tissues of smaller bronchi and bronchioles. At either this stage or later, endobronchiolitis and endobronchitis may occur. These lesions are characterized by accumulation of debris within the bronchial lumen and infiltration of the bronchial wall by mononuclear cells. Clusters of bacilli may be found either on the ciliated epithelial cells or mixed with debris, but not in peribronchial tissues. Atelectasis may accompany these changes. In prolonged or severe disease, alveolar lesions consisting of thickening of the wall, mononuclear cell infiltration, and accumulation of fibrinous debris have been described. Peribronchial lymphadenopathy commonly accompanies the peribronchial lesion. In late disease, dysplasia and thickening of the bronchial epithelium is associated with replacement of columnar cells by squamous cells. Although the pathology of the disease is well established, the pathogenesis of the changes has not been determined. During infection, bacterial replication is essentially confined to the respiratory mucous membrane, with no bacillemia. The induction of lymphocytosis by the lymphocyte-promoting factor demonstrates that antigenemia occurs; thus, the immune response of the host is probably generated both through local and humoral mechanisms.

CLINICAL MANIFESTATIONS. The clinical syndrome of pertussis has been divided into several stages, beginning with the early and most communicable period called the catarrhal or preparoxysmal stage. The catarrhal stage begins at the end of the incubation period, or about five to ten days after exposure. Generally, the manifestations are those of any early upper respiratory infection, with irritation of the mucous membranes, hacking cough, and fever. The catarrhal stage lasts usually seven to ten days, and is generally not recognized as pertussis.

The paroxysmal stage begins at the end of the catarrhal stage when fever usually subsides. The disease is usually first recognized during the paroxysmal stage. Particularly in older infants and children, this stage is marked by crescendo development of inexorable paroxysmal coughing. Ultimately, the paroxysms may be induced by any stimulus (e.g., speech, swallowing, movement, tracheal pressure), and they occur with increasing frequency, severity, and duration as the paroxysmal stage progresses. Each paroxysm may consist of several bouts separated by momentary intervals insufficient for inspiration, until hypoxia and partial asphyxia occur. The end of the paroxysmal episode may be marked by a massive single inspiratory stroke causing the whoop of inspiratory stridor. During severe paroxysms, the patient may become plethoric or cyanotic, with bulging eyes and anxious or frantic countenance; it may appear that the patient's life is threatened. After severe episodes, the immediate post-tussive period may be marked by apparent respiratory arrest. In infants, the post-tussive period may also be marked by exhaustion and lethargy during which the usual environmental stimuli fail to bring about a typical response. In the most severely affected infants, this state may merge into the next paroxysm on awakening. Vomiting occurs frequently at the end of a paroxysm. Paroxysmal coughing may last from seven days to a month and may vary from mild uncomplicated episodes to severe protracted episodes requiring hospitalization and acute supportive care.

The greatest morbidity of the disease is due to repetitive paroxysmal coughing that is inexorable, fatiguing, and at times pernicious. In the very young, individual paroxysms may present with frightening signs of hypoxia (cyanosis), asphyxia (pallor, limpness, post-tussive cyanosis), recurrent vomiting, and overt signs of mucous impaction of the trachea or larynx. These cases require intensive supportive care for a minimum of five to seven days.

During the most severe period, fatigue, weakness, pallor, anorexia, and somnolence may characterize the intervals between paroxysms. As the frequency, duration, and severity of attacks decrease, the morbidity is recognized only during an attack. Following the early paroxysmal stage, nighttime attacks may continue to occur over a prolonged period, sometimes for one to five months following the acute illness, with disruption of the rest patterns of adults in the household. Bacilli are recovered from the nasopharynx most frequently during the catarrhal (preparoxysmal) and early paroxysmal stages. This correlates with the period of highest communicability. In rare cases, the infection is transmitted during the later stages and bacilli are isolated for prolonged periods.

Infants, particularly those under 6 months of age, may not develop typical paroxysms and thus may go undiagnosed. The typical whoop may not be a part of the clinical syndrome in young infants. Instead, recurrent periods of apparent strangling and asphyxia may occur and lead to a variety of presumptive diagnoses other than pertussis.

Between attacks, quiet breathing usually occurs without abnormal auscultatory findings. The abnormal chest x-ray shows minimal peri-bronchial inflammatory changes (Barnhard, 1960), but the chest x-ray is frequently normal. Pertussis pneumonia rarely occurs; it is characterized by an unusual course with fever, auscultatory rales, and a "shaggy cardiac border" indicative of intense interstitial pneumonitis.

In most cases (estimated to be 80 per cent in unimmunized older infants and children) hyperleukocytosis and lymphocytosis develop during the paroxysmal stage; their presence is helpful in making the diagnosis. The total white blood cell count may exceed 100,000/mm^3; commonly the count is in the range of 25,000 to 40,000/mm^3 with a predominance of small mature lymphocytes. These cells are discharged from the marginal pool into the circulation under the influence of the lymphocyte-promoting factor of *B. pertussis*. Again, hyperleukocytosis may not be present in infants under 6 months of age, but relative lymphocytosis usually is present (Brooksaler and Nelson, 1967).

The convalescent stage is usually characterized by a return to normal activity and development without complications. In most patients, immunity is conferred by one attack.

COMPLICATIONS AND SEQUELAE. Complications and sequelae are steadily declining among infants and children in developed countries (White et al., 1964). Bronchiectasis is no longer a complication of pertussis in the United States. Likewise, central nervous system complications, such as seizures or encephalopathy, are very uncommon even in severe outbreaks. Less serious complications include epistaxis and hemorrhage into the conjunctivae and soft tissues about the eyes due to the high venous pressure that accompanies paroxysms. Occasionally, hemorrhage from the tracheobronchial tract may accompany or follow the paroxysm; usually these hemorrhagic episodes do not cause serious complications or marked blood loss. Rarely, intracranial hemorrhage may occur, causing neurologic damage, but the symptoms and signs of intracranial hemorrhage commonly resolve during the decline of the paroxysmal stage. Otitis media and purulent pneumonia were once important and frequent complications; the use of antibiotics to eradicate *B. pertussis* from the tracheobronchial tree is probably responsible for the disappearance of these complications. Other mechanical complications include anal prolapse, hernia, and trauma to the frenulum of the tongue (Zamora et al., 1962).

GEOGRAPHIC VARIATION. Before the great increase in international travel, isolated populations such as those in the Faroe Islands and Iceland responded to the introduction of pertussis with isolated epidemics that occurred at intervals of five to seven years, with no cases between epidemics. All susceptibles were infected within a moderate period of time (usually about one year), and the infection disappeared until a new generation of susceptibles appeared and pertussis was reintroduced. With the new ease of movement within urban societies and across international boundaries, the characteristics of the epidemics have changed to that of waves that occur on a base of relative subepidemic or endemic infection. Thus, it is likely that cases will occur throughout a given outbreak period with relative frequency, then subside to a lower endemic frequency and recur seasonally each year.

In most recent outbreaks in the United States, the great majority of cases have occurred in children under 5 years of age, with over 50 per cent in infants under 1 year. In other countries in which general immunization is practiced, most cases also occur within the first 10 years of life, with the majority within the first 5 years. The morbidity rate (cases reported per 100,000 population) has continued to decline throughout most of the world; in the United States, it had declined to 4.2 cases per 100,000 population by 1970. In other countries in which immunization is the rule, the morbidity rate is also declining. However, it still exceeds 80 per 100,000 population in some countries. These differences probably relate to the percentage of susceptibles that are vaccinated and to the reliability of the vaccines. In countries yet to establish effective vaccine programs, the morbidity rate varies from 100 to 500 per 100,000 population.

The mortality rate among immunized and unimmunized populations has continued to decline more rapidly than the morbidity rate. The decline in mortality is probably related to adequate nutrition, literacy and the accessibility of medical care for acute cases. The case-fatality ratio in the United States for all cases fell to 0.3 per cent or less during the 1960s and may be below 0.1 per cent now. In some countries in continental Europe, England, and Scandinavia, mortality has reached a nadir, with no calculable rate. Thus, various factors have provided satisfactory solutions to the problems of mortality in these countries. The incidence of disease may not decline further until more effective means of inducing and maintaining immunity are found. In contrast, in Central America the case-fatality rate was 18 per cent in the 1960s, and remains high in other countries in which the populations are predominantly rural, the literacy rates are low, and access to emergency medical care is limited.

DIAGNOSIS. It is easy to make a clinical diagnosis of pertussis in an infant or young child who presents in the paroxysmal stage with an antecedent history that is compatible with the catarrhal stage. Other causes of paroxysmal cough must be considered, however.

The differential diagnosis includes other infections that give rise to tracheobronchial lymphadenopathy, a foreign body in the bronchial airway, necrotizing bronchiolitis caused by adenovirus, interstitial pneumonitis caused by respiratory syncytial virus, parainfluenza virus, and *H. influenzae* Type B bronchitis; any of these may cause a paroxysmal cough. Some of the viral infections result in frequent vomiting with the paroxysms. Both *B. parapertussis* and *B. bronchiseptica* infections may cause a mild clinical syndrome (parapertussis) that is indistinguishable from mild to moderate pertussis.

Adenoviruses especially have been associated with pertussis. The frequency of virus isolation is remarkably high, both in proven *B. pertussis* infection and in cases of clinical disease without bacterial isolation (Connor, 1970; Nelson et al., 1975). However, there is no proof that adenoviruses can cause pertussis. All cases should be regarded as Bordetella infections and a thorough search should be made for the bacterium, regardless of viral isolation (Keller et al., 1980).

The specific diagnosis of pertussis is established by isolating the bacillus from the nasopharynx or identifying it in smears of the nasopharynx by immunofluorescence techniques. The medium and the principles that are important in the isolation and identification of *B. pertussis* were originally described by Bordet and Gengou. Bordet-Gengou (B-G) culture medium, with minor modifications, is still preferred. Commercial preparations from which a final complete medium is prepared are usually satisfactory. If properly prepared, adequately stored, and appropriately used, B-G medium will result in frequent isolations of *B. pertussis* from nasopharyngeal swabs of individuals with clinical disease (Miller et al., 1943). The isolation rate depends upon a concentration of whole blood in the final medium higher than that usually utilized in diagnostic bacteriology. For that reason, 20 to 30 per cent whole, defibrinated sheep blood is incorporated into appropriately prepared Bordet-Gengou medium. The medium may be stored in sealed plastic sleeves for two weeks or longer. The agar surface should be glistening, moist, and cherry-red.

After inoculation with material from nasopharyngeal swabs, B-G plates should be incubated in a humidified environment at 35°C for five to seven days. Minute, milky-white, convex colonies may be found as early as 72 hours or as late as five to six days. The isolation rate may be improved by inoculating two B-G plates, one containing 0.25 IU of penicillin G per milliliter of agar and the other containing no penicillin (Bradford et al., 1946). Overgrowth of nasopharyngeal microflora may be controlled by the penicillin, but some strains of *B. pertussis* are also sensitive to this concentration. Microscopic examination of a Gram stain of a single colony from the isolation plate reveals minute, lightly stained, gram-negative coccoid and ovoid bacteria. If the medium is inadequate, pleomorphism may be noted, with long rod forms mixed with coccobacillary forms. Final identification is established immunologically. Macroscopic agglutination occurs when a moderate suspension of bacteria is mixed with specific immune serum against *B. pertussis*. The suspension is prepared by swabbing the surface of a plate with confluent growth and immersing the swab in several drops of saline on a glass slide or plate; diluted serum is added to the slide suspension. With slow agitation and mixing, agglutination occurs in five to ten minutes. Macroscopic agglutination firmly establishes a final identification of the *Bordetella* genus. Alternatively, a similar slide preparation of the bacilli may be air-dried and reacted with fluorescein-conjugated immune globulin specific against *B. pertussis*. Bright specific fluorescence under the ultraviolet microscope establishes the identification of *B. pertussis*. *B. pertussis* and *B. parapertussis* can be differentiated by using commercially prepared immunofluorescence reagents against each bacillus.

The immunofluorescence technique can also be used to obtain an immediate specific diagnosis by examining nasopharyngeal swabs for *B. pertussis* (Holwerda and Eldering, 1963). Nasopharyngeal swabs are used to make several smears on clean glass slides. After air-drying, the fluorescent globulin is applied to the smears and the excess stain is removed by appropriate washing. Under the ultraviolet microscope, the minute coccoid or ovoid bacteria are highly fluorescent. Properly applied, the direct immunofluorescence method results in a frequency of bacteriologic diagnosis that equals or exceeds that of the culture method. By either method, study of unimmunized cases in the paroxysmal stage of the disease should result in a specific diagnosis in 70 to 90 per cent of cases. In contact cases and immunized cases, a laboratory diagnosis is established less frequently.

Differentiation by bacteriologic characteristics is also practical. In contrast to *B. pertussis*, both *B. parapertussis* and *B. bronchiseptica* will form colonies on infusion agar, without blood, during subcultivation. *B. parapertussis* colonies have a characteristic light chocolate pigment (Bradford and Slavin, 1937), whereas *B. pertussis* colonies remain pearly white. Biochemical differences are also found among the species and may also be used in differentiation.

Some of the serologic methods used to make a retrospective diagnosis of pertussis are used in public health laboratories; none is in general use (Ross et al., 1970). The agglutination test has been the most widely applied, but most commonly to evaluate responses to immunization, rather than the natural infection, since agglutinating antibody may be absent in human or animal serum that has protective antibody. Thus, after natural infections of infants, agglutinins may be present in only 30 to 50 per cent of cases, in contrast to protective antibody, which is present in 90 to 100 per cent of cases.

A simple, inexpensive gel precipitin method demonstrates precipitating antibody against extracted *B. pertussis* antigens (Aftandelians and Connor, 1973). Between 80 and 90 per cent of patients with the clinical syndrome develop gel precipitins during convalescence; 25 to 30 per cent of immunized patients also develop these antibodies. The gel precipitin test may have application in the routine diagnosis of an infection in an unimmunized patient or in the identification of an outbreak. In the latter case, it has been found that 80 to 90 per cent of clinical cases will have precipitin antibody in convalescent serum, in contrast to 25 to 30 per cent of newborns, immunized children, and healthy adults.

IMMUNITY. Immunity is probably conferred through a variety of host factors, but none has been identified as being of singular importance in solid protection (Pittman, 1970). Agglutinins and complement-fixing antibody correlate with the immune state when they are present in high serum concentrations after immunization or unrecognized infection, but immunity may be present in their absence. Bactericidal antibody develops after infection or immunization of animals without the development of protective antigen. Mouse-protecting antibody correlates best with protective immunity. It is considered to be present when convalescent serum protects the mouse against a lethal intracerebral infection with a mouse-virulent strain of pertussis. However, the presence of protective antibody in serum correlates with immunity only after active infection or intensive (complete) immunization. In the latter case, immunity wanes rapidly, so that adults or children who are five years or more away from the last immunizing injection, even if they have detectable mouse-protective antibody, are liable to an attack rate of 35 to 95 per cent when they are exposed in families in which there is an index case. On the other hand, naturally acquired immunity is highly effective, with an estimated recurrence rate of approximately 2 per cent. Undoubtedly, there are factors of importance other than protective antibody, and these are probably present on surface membranes as well as at the initial site of infection within the respiratory tract. Immune serum enhances phagocytosis and also contains antiadherence factors. These and other factors limit or control the loci of early infection. When inflammation develops at the site of infection on the respiratory membranes, the organisms may also be exposed to immune serum containing protective antibody and the complement-dependent bactericidal antibody. Much work is still required to define the mechanisms of immunity to pertussis.

TREATMENT. Small infants with frequent, severe paroxysms, especially if complicated by post-tussive exhaustion and spells of unresponsiveness, should be hospitalized for supportive care. In well-nourished, well-developed infants, the height of the paroxysmal stage may be reached and passed in a period of five to seven days, and the need for hospitalization then declines. Intravenous hydration is infrequently required. Oxygenation is usually not required; although the inspiratory volume is ineffective during a paroxysm, the respiratory exchange is adequate between paroxysms. Repetitive seizures require both anticonvulsive therapy and strong supportive measures. In the most severe cases in infants, transient respiratory arrest following an extensive paroxysm may require resuscitation. Endotracheal suction by direct or indirect methods is infrequently required, since compacted endobronchial mucus is usually expelled at the end of a paroxysm. However, during episodes of post-tussive cyanosis, moderate suctioning may be needed to remove mucus from the upper airway and trachea. Antitussive medications and heavy sedation are to be avoided.

Malnourishment may develop in severe, prolonged cases owing to exhaustion, lack of intake, and frequent vomiting. Small, repetitive feedings are usually tolerated immediately after paroxysms (or after vomiting), when the cough reflex is suppressed. Likewise, a feeding may be repeated directly after the loss of the previous meal. In the hospital, strict isolation is required to reduce contact with susceptible children, visiting adults, and hospital employees.

As measured by clinical response, the benefit of antibiotic chemotherapy has never been proved in comparison with placebo controls. However, erythromycin for five to seven days may eradicate infection of the tracheobronchial membrane and reduce spread. Ampicillin also has been recommended. Pure cultures of pertussis bacilli have been isolated from pharyngeal swabs of some patients after treatment with either drug. Since corticosteroids modify the clinical course compared with placebo controls, severe cases may benefit from cortisone for three to five days. Corticosteroids are not recommended for mild or moderate cases. Like antibiotics, pertussis hyperimmune globulin has not proved to be effective during the paroxysmal stage. Nevertheless, some physicians recommend hyperimmune globulin for severely affected infants under 6 months of age, since earlier studies reported moderate benefit.

PROPHYLAXIS. The standard method of active immunization against pertussis utilizes three primary injections of a highly concentrated suspension of killed whole *B. pertussis* organisms in a repository vehicle combined with diphtheria and tetanus toxoids (DPT) (Felton, 1957). Slow absorption from the repository injection site provides an adjuvant effect on the immune response; thus, the combined form of immunization against the three diseases is preferable to injections of individual antigens. Since there is no effective immunity against pertussis in the newborn period, immunization is started as soon as the immune response mounted by the infant can provide protection. For this reason, the primary injection series usually begins at 2 to 3 months of age and is completed by 4 to 5 months of age. Immunity against pertussis is not developed until some time after the second injection; the magnitude of protection is extended by the third injection. A booster is given at 1 year of age and is repeated one or two times before school age. Studies of fully immunized children who have had intimate contact with the naturally occurring disease (Preston, 1972) and other studies indicate that 12 to 50 per cent of immunized children may develop pertussis. The greatest protection is observed during the first 36 months after completion of the series or after a booster. Immunity wanes remarkably after three years. Lambert's study of an epidemic in Kent County, Michigan, indicated that seven years after the last immunization the attack rate was 47 per cent. After 12 years or more, the rate was 95 per cent among contacts exposed to index cases in families (Lambert, 1965).

Up to 25 per cent of infants receiving second or third injections of DPT vaccine may have a local or systemic response, or both, consisting of swelling and tenderness at the injection site and moderate fever beginning 12 to 24 hours after the injection and declining sharply within 24 hours. Earlier in the vaccine era, evidence of encephalitis following second or third injections of DPT in infants was seen with a frequency of 1 case per 200,000 vaccine doses; however, this complication is now rare (1 case in 1 million doses in the United States). Latest statistics comparing the morbidity of immunization with the morbidity of disease continue to demonstrate the benefit of general immunization against pertussis.

A booster injection may re-establish immunity in a previously immunized family contact, but active immunization during the incubation period or during active disease is neither effective nor desirable. The effectiveness of commercially prepared hyperimmune globulin for preventing pertussis in contacts has not been proved. However, it is sometimes used for attempted prophylaxis, particularly in small infants for whom the risk of moderate or severe morbidity is high. Chemoprophylaxis should be attempted in infant or child contacts, preferably with erythromycin for five to seven days. If the disease does not develop after the full incubation period, the exposed individual should then be immunized appropriately. Disease in exposed adults is usually moderate, and it may be either mild or uncharacteristic. Since the attack rate is very high in adults of families with index cases, it may be appropriate in the future to consider prophylactic treatment and immunization of the older age group as well as infants and children.

PARAPERTUSSIS. Parapertussis is an acute disease of the respiratory tract caused by infection with *B. parapertussis* (Miller et al., 1941). The characteristics of the clinical syndrome are indistinguishable from those of a mild or moderate case of pertussis. During an outbreak, the diagnosis is evident clinically in only 5 per cent of infected persons. *B. parapertussis* organisms are coccobacillary, gram-negative, nonmotile bacilli that are usually indistinguishable from *B. pertussis* on primary isolation. They were first described by Eldering and Kendrick in the United States in 1937 and later during the same year by Bradford and Slavin, who called attention to pigment changes that are useful in the laboratory differentiation of *B. parapertussis* and *B. pertussis*. On Bordet-Gengou medium, *B. parapertussis* grows more rapidly than *B. pertussis*. Otherwise, the colonies may be identical until a pigment change occurs that lends a light chocolate hue to the colonies of the parapertussis bacilli. Transfer to regular infusion agar can usually be accomplished from the isolation plate, which quickly distinguishes it from *B. pertussis*. *B. parapertussis* shares antigens (agglutinogens) with both *B. pertussis* and *B. bronchiseptica* and reacts lightly with immunofluorescent serum against *B. pertussis* owing to common antigen or antigens.

Recent evidence suggests that *B. parapertussis* are merely strains of *B. pertussis* that have lost a toxigenic bacteriophage (Pereverzev et al., 1981); in theory, then, parapertussis outbreaks could be caused by non-toxigenic forms of *B. pertussis (B. parapertussis)* (Granstrom and Ashelof, 1982). Further study is needed before this unitarian hypothesis is acceptable.

The incidence of parapertussis is estimated to be 2 to 10 per cent that of pertussis (Eldering and Kendrick, 1952). In Denmark, parapertussis occurs in four-year cycles. A distinct wave or outbreak rising above the endemic level of disease in urban environments occurs between pertussis outbreaks (Lautrop, 1971). As with pertussis, it is assumed that the most contagious period is during the catarrhal stage, before the onset of paroxysms. Single cases can be moderately severe, but the infection is usually mild. Death is certainly rare; however, fatal cases have been reported in which *B. parapertussis* was isolated from the trachea at postmortem examination (Zuelzer and Wheeler, 1946). Most cases are unrecognized, even during an outbreak, because the clinical course is mild compared to pertussis. More severe cases are often misdiagnosed as pertussis. It is presumed that the infection proceeds in the same manner as pertussis, but it is more difficult to distinguish clearly separate stages because the total period of the clinical disease is usually shorter and the severity less than in pertussis. However, when paroxysms develop they are characteristic of pertussis, and typical whoops may be heard.

The pathology of parapertussis in the human has not been well described because of the mildness of the disease. In animals, mononuclear cell inflammation surrounding and within bronchi and bronchioles closely resembles the pathologic pattern seen in pertussis. There is no cross-immunity between parapertussis and pertussis. As with pertussis, immunity following disease is solid, and a second attack is rare. *Immunization against pertussis does not protect against para-pertussis.* The disease is not preventable by any currently available means. Treatment is usually not required, although supportive care may be justified in moderately severe cases.

References

Pertussis

Aftandelians, R. A., and Connor, J. D.: Immunologic studies of pertussis. Development of precipitins. J Pediatr 83:206, 1973.

Barnhard, H. J., and Kniker, W. T.: Roentgen findings in pertussis. Am J Roentgenol Radium Ther Nucl Med 84:445, 1960.

Bradford, W. L., Day, E., and Bery, G. P.: Improvement of the nasopharyngeal swab method of diagnosis in pertussis by the use of penicillin. Am J Public Health 36:468, 1946.

Brooksaler, F., and Nelson, J. D.: Pertussis: A re-appraisal and report of 190 confirmed cases. Am J Dis Child 114:389, 1967.

Buchanan, T. M., and Broohn, G. F.: Pertussis in the US. J Infect Dis 122:123, 1970.

Connor, J. D.: Evidence for an etiological role of adenoviral infection in pertussis syndrome. N Engl J Med 283:390, 1970.

Eldering, G., Hornbeck, C., and Baker, J.: Serological study of *Bordetella pertussis* and related species. J Bacteriol 74:133, 1957.

Felton, H. M.: Pertussis: Current status of prevention and treatment. Pediatr Clin North Am 4:271, 1957.

Holwerda, J., and Eldering, G. D.: Culture and fluorescent antibody methods in the diagnosis of whooping cough. J Bacteriol 86:449, 1963.

Ipsen, J., and Bowen, H. E., Whooping cough trends in age-specific attack rates. Am J Public Health, 45:312, 1955.

Keller, M. A., Aftandelians, R. A., and Connor, J. D.: Etiology of pertussis syndrome. Pediatrics 66:50, 1980.

Kurt, T. L., Yeager, A. S., Guerette, S., and Dunlop, S.: Spread of pertussis by hospital staff. JAMA 221:264, 1972.

Lambert, H. J.: Epidemiology of a small pertussis outbreak in Kent County, Michigan. Pub Health Rep 80:365, 1965.

Miller, J. J., Jr., Leach, C. W., Saito, R. M., et al.: Comparison of the nasopharyngeal swab and the cough plate in the diagnosis of whooping cough and *Hemophilus* pertussis carriers. Am J Public Health 33:839, 1943.

Munoz, J. J.: Symposium on relationship of structure of microorganisms to the immunological properties. I. Immunological and other biological activities of *Bordetella pertussis* antigens. Bacterial Rev 27:325, 1963.

Nelson, K. F., Gavitt, F., Batt, M. D., et al.: The role of adenoviruses in the pertussis syndrome. J Pediatr 86:335, 1975.

Pittman, M.: *Bordetella pertussis*—bacterial and host factors in the pathogenesis and prevention of whooping cough. In Mudd, S. (ed.): Infectious Agents and Host Reactions. Philadelphia, W. B. Saunders Company, 1970, p. 239.

Preston, N. W., and Stanbridge, T. N.: Efficacy of pertussis vaccines: A brighter horizon. Br Med J 3:448, 1972.

Ross, C. A., Calder, M. C., Cruickshank, R., et al.: Diagnosis of whooping cough: Comparison of serological tests with isolation of *Bordetella pertussis*. A combined Scottish study. Br Med J 4:637, 1970.

Welsh, J. D., Denny, W. F., and Bird, R. M.: The incidence and significance of the leukemoid reaction in patients hospitalized with pertussis. South Med J 52:643, 1959.

White, R., Finberg, L., and Tramer, A.: The modern morbidity of pertussis in infants. Pediatrics 33:705, 1964.

Zamora, A. F., Chiozza, A., and Alonso, A. T.: Complications of whooping cough in 500 cases. Rev Assoc Med Argent 76:121, 1962.

Parapertussis

Bradford, W. L., and Slavin, B.: An organism resembling *Hemophilus pertussis:* With special reference to color changes produced by its growth upon certain media. Am J Public Health 27:1277, 1937.

Bradford, W. L., and Slavin, B.: Parapertussis. Lancet 75:232, 1955.

Confer, D. L., And Eaton, J. W.: Phagocyte impotence caused by invasive bacterial adenylate cyclase. Science 217:948, 1982.

Eldering, G., and Kendrick, P. L.: Incidence of parapertussis in diagnostic culture. Am J Public Health 42:27, 1952.

Granstrom, M., and Ashelof, P.: Parapertussis: An abortive pertussis infection? Science 217:1249, 1982.

Lautrop, H.: Epidemics of parapertussis. Lancet 1:1195, 1971.

Miller, J. J., Jr., Saito, T. M., and Silverberg, R. J.: Parapertussis: Clinical and serological observations. J Pediatr 19:229, 1941.

Pereverzev, N. A., Lapaeva, I. A., Abdyrasulov, S. A., Siniashina, I. N., and Mebel', S. M. Ul'trastrukturnaia organizatsiia bakteriofaga, vydelennogo iz Bordetella pertussis. Zh. Mikrobiol Epidemiol Immunobiol 5:54, 1981. (Eng Abstr)

Zuelzer, W. W., and Wheeler, W. E.: Parapertussis pneumonia. Report of two fatal cases. J Pediatr 29:493, 1946.

B. Pleuropulmonary Infections

111

COMMON PNEUMONIAS DUE TO PYOGENIC COCCI

W. G. JOHANSON, JR., M.D.
GARY D. HARRIS, M.D.

Bacterial pneumonia is an inflammatory process of the lung characterized by alveolar consolidation due to the presence of pathogenic bacteria. It is almost always acute and abrupt in onset.

ETIOLOGY. The "pyogenic cocci," *Streptococcus pneumoniae* (pneumococcus), *Streptococcus pyogenes*, and *Staphylococcus aureus*, are the most common etiologic agents of bacterial pneumonia. The pneumococcus is by far the most important, causing perhaps 80 per cent of all bacterial pneumonias. Of the many types of pneumococci (over 80), only 14 capsular types (1, 2, 3, 4, 6, 8, 9, 12, 14, 19, 23, 25, 51, and 56) are responsible for about 80 per cent of bacteremic pneumococcal pneumonias (Centers for Disease Control, 1978), a fact that makes preventive vaccination against pneumococcal infection feasible.

PNEUMOCOCCAL PNEUMONIA

PATHOGENESIS AND PATHOLOGY. Pneumococci enter the body via the respiratory tract. Although 30 to 40 per cent of healthy persons may harbor pneumococci in their upper respiratory secretions, such carrier organisms are usually not the capsular types that produce pneumonia. Highly virulent strains are passed from person to person, including both asymptomatic carriers and persons with evident infection. Non-human reservoirs of the organism are not important in the epidemiology of human pneumococcal infections. Whether transmission among humans is airborne or by personal contact is not settled; however, pneumococcal pneumonia is probably due not to direct inhalation of the organism into the lungs but to aspiration of upper respiratory secretions. Several observations support the view that the lung possesses remarkably effective defenses against airborne bacteria (Green, 1970). Large (>10 μm) airborne particles impinge on the mucosa of the upper respiratory tract by inertial impaction, are carried to the oropharynx by ciliary action, and are swallowed. Smaller particles may land on ciliated airways; the cross-section of the branching airway system expands markedly so that flow becomes progressively slower as inhaled particles pass into the airways, causing them to be deposited by gravitational settling. Particles that land on ciliated airways are rapidly removed by ciliary action; the time needed for removal depends on the site of deposition but may be as rapid as 30 minutes for particles deposited in major airways. Particles that reach the alveolar spaces are cleared from the lung much more slowly, and, in the case of infectious agents, phagocytosis and in situ killing of the organisms become the critical elements of defense. The alveolar macrophage normally performs this function without the participation of either polymorphonuclear leukocytes or serum factors. This process is so efficient that normal lungs contain no bacteria and few or no PMNs, despite the daily inhalation and aspiration of infectious agents. Early investigators were unable to cause pneumonia in normal experimental animals by exposing them to airborne bacteria despite deposition of organisms in the lungs. Infection could be produced only if the animals were manipulated, for example, by the administration of alcohol. More recent studies using quantitative bacteriologic techniques have shown that most bacterial species, including the pyogenic cocci, are rapidly killed in the lungs of normal animals following exposure to contaminated aerosols and that an initial inoculum of as many as 10^5 bacteria causes no disease.

In contrast to the lower airways, organisms are present in enormous numbers in upper respiratory secretions. Saliva may contain 10^8 to 10^9 aerobic bacteria per ml. Bacteria that persist following inoculation into the upper respiratory tract multiply and may subsequently gain access to the lungs via aspiration; even normal persons aspirate oropharyngeal secretions during sleep (Huxley et al., 1978). Aspiration of only small quantities can infect the lung. As little as 0.01 ml would deliver a large bacterial load to a small region of lung, in contrast to the diffuse deposition that occurs with airborne organisms. Pneumococci implanted in the noses of experimental animals reach the lungs within a few minutes, and pneumonia can be readily produced in experimental animals by an inoculum of 10^4 pneumococci delivered in a small fluid bolus into the airways.

These experimental observations illustrate several important features of the pathogenesis of pneumococcal pneumonia. First, pneumococcal pneumonia is uncommon among healthy people; at least 75 per cent of patients with pneumococcal pneumonia have underlying diseases (Sullivan et al., 1972). Second, pneumonia is likely to occur in people who handle upper respiratory secretions poorly, owing to either increased volume of secretions as with viral infection or impaired laryngeal reflexes during sleep or coma. Third, pneumonia is likely to occur in patients whose pulmonary antibacterial defenses are impaired, as in chronic obstructive lung disease or congestive heart failure (Winterbauer et al., 1969).

Pneumococcal pneumonia develops in the absence of swift phagocytosis of organisms on the alveolar surface. Pneumonia is initiated by bacterial multiplication and an outpouring of protein-rich edematous fluid and erythrocytes into alveolar spaces. Edema is followed by an influx of neutrophils that phagocytose bacteria and eventually fill the alveolar spaces. Pneumococcal pneumonia is thus a spreading process characterized by capillary congestion, alveolar hemorrhage, edema, and rapid bacterial proliferation at the leading edge ("red hepatization"), and dense consolidation due to leukocytes and organizing exudates ("gray hepatization") at the center. Pneumococci invade the pulmonary lymphatics early, presumably in the edematous regions; bacteremia occurs when the hilar lymph nodes do not remove enough bacteria from the lymph draining the lung.

The inflammatory process spreads from acinus to acinus via the pores of Kohn and from lobe to lobe by spilling of contaminated materials into the airways. Its progress tends to be checked by the pleura or its interlobular extensions, although involvement of the pleura itself may cause pleural effusion. Empyema results if organisms pass through the pleura.

Despite the intense inflammation and the enormous number of bacteria present, necrosis of lung tissue rarely occurs in pneumococcal pneumonia. Healing is initiated by an influx of macrophages, probably derived in large part from circulating blood monocytes. These cells ingest alveolar debris, consisting of dead organisms and PMNs, strands of fibrin, and erythrocytes, and the architecture of the lung is preserved. Normal function returns within a few weeks. The lack of tissue destruction is apparently due to two factors. Pneumococci, with the possible exception of type 3, do not possess necrotizing extracellular enzymes. Destruction of lung tissue by leukocytic proteases is apparently prevented by the abundant exudation of plasma, containing the protease inhibitors alpha-1-antitrypsin and alpha-2-macroglobulin, into the lung.

CLINICAL MANIFESTATIONS. Most patients have rhinorrhea, pharyngitis, and cough for several days before the onset of pneumococcal pneumonia. Although these symptoms suggest a preceding viral illness, proof of this association has been scanty except in the case of influenza A. These prodromal symptoms are overshadowed by the abrupt occurrence of fever, typically 102° F, pleuritic chest pain, and at least one shaking chill. Repeated rigors are uncommon in pneumococcal pneumonia and suggest another bacterial cause. Cough may intensify, although sputum production is frequently scant in the first few days. The sputum is typically "rusty" in color due to alveolar hemorrhage. The severity of these symptoms and the accompanying prostration cause most patients to seek medical attention within 48 hours of onset. Elderly patients may present only with fever and depressed consciousness. In patients with chronic heart or lung disease, the principal symptom may be only worsening dyspnea, although signs of infection can also be found.

On physical examination the patient is warm to touch, perspiring, tachycardic, and tachypneic. Cool vasoconstricted skin, with or without hypotension, is a manifestation of impending cardiovascular collapse and is ominous. The signs of pneumonia will vary with its stage. The earliest sign consists of fine, inspiratory crackles (rales) that appear before consolidation is evident by x-ray or by auscultation as altered breath sounds with increased transmission of tracheal sounds to the chest wall. The intensity of the breath sounds may be increased, normal, or decreased. Over consolidated lung served by a patent bronchus, breath sounds are "tubular." Altered transmission of sound to the chest wall should be sought with several techniques. Increased transmission of the whispered voice ("whispered pectoriloquy") is easiest for most examiners to appreciate and is elicited by having the patient whisper "one, two, three." Increased tactile fremitus can be detected by placing the palm over the consolidated area while the patient says loudly "ninety-nine." "Egophony," or the "E to A" sign, is more difficult to detect, although it is striking when present. Each sign depends upon the presence of two factors: consolidated lung and a patent bronchus in the immediate vicinity. Dullness on percussion will be present if the volume of consolidated lung is sufficient and is adjacent to the region of chest wall being percussed. The major value of percussion and examination for fremitus is detection of the flatness and diminished fremitus of pleural effusion. It is important to remember that bronchial obstruction with distal pneumonia or atelectasis may produce exactly the same signs as a pleural effusion.

During treatment, fine rales may disappear while signs of consolidation increase. This stage is followed by the appearance of coarse rales and even rhonchi, usually associated with abundant sputum production as the alveolar process begins to resolve.

Dense consolidation extending from one pleural surface to another, the pattern of lobar consolidation, is distinctly uncommon on radiography. Most often the areas of increased roentgenographic density are patchy and frequently multiple, with lack of respect for segmental boundaries. An air bronchogram is usually present, a finding that confirms that the abnormal shadow is due to consolidation, at least in part. With preexisting lung disease, especially emphysema, the pattern of radiographic abnormality may be markedly altered, varying from multiple cavitary infiltrates to poorly defined, hazy peribronchial densities (Ziskind et al., 1970). Pleural effusions, usually small, are present in 10 per cent of patients with pneumococcal pneumonia at the time of initial presentation.

The blood leukocyte count is most often 15,000 to 30,000 per mm^3, although very high or very low values may be found, especially in alcoholics with folate deficiency. Regardless of the total count, an increased percentage of PMNs is immature. The BUN may be slightly elevated, usually due to prerenal factors. A BUN over 50 mg/100 ml has been associated with a lower rate of survival in patients with pneumococcal pneumonia. Evidence of glomerulitis, including protein, casts, and erythrocytes in the urine, is uncommon, usually transient, and apparently caused by circulating pneumococcal capsular material, possibly complexed to immunoglobulin. Jaundice may result from hepatocellular damage or hemolysis, the latter particularly in G-6-PD-deficient patients.

Arterial blood gas analysis is an important facet of the evaluation of many patients with pneumococcal pneumonia. Cyanosis is unreliable, and its apparent absence should not dissuade the examiner from obtaining arterial blood for study. Patients with extensive disease, respiratory distress, compromised cardiopulmonary function, or an altered mental state should have such studies. Patients with pneumonia are typically hypoxemic with hypocarbia and acute respiratory alkalosis. The degree of hypoxemia does not correlate well with the extent of disease as judged radiographically in that some patients with apparently small and usually scattered infiltrates will be severely hypoxemic. The mechanism of hypoxemia is the continued perfusion of regions of lung in which ventilation has been impaired by alveolar filling. This abnormality leads to regions with low ventilation-to-perfusion ratios and intrapulmonary shunts; to the extent that the latter is responsible, the arterial oxygen tension will fail to rise with supplemental oxygen therapy. Hypocarbia and respiratory alkalosis are due to tachypnea and increased alveolar ventilation.

DIAGNOSIS. The diagnosis of pneumococcal pneumonia depends on the establishment of two facts: that the patient's symptoms are the result of pneumonia and that the pneumonia is due to the pneumococcus. The former is usually straightforward, while the latter finding is frequently difficult to establish with certainty. Purulent sputum and a radiographic infiltrate are found in conjunction with an appropriate history and physical findings. Common sense will help sort out most of the more difficult problems in differential diagnosis. For example, patients with congestive heart failure may have infiltrates, leukocytosis, and perhaps even low-grade fever, but they certainly do not have chills or purulent sputum unless a complicating infection is present.

Confirmation of the etiologic role of the pneumococcus in pneumonia may require examination of several types of specimens. By far the most valuable specimen for culture is the blood, because contaminating organisms are not present and the results can be readily interpreted. About one third of patients with pneumococcal pneumonia have demonstrable bacteremia (Austrian and Gold, 1964; Tilghman and Finland, 1937). Since a similar fraction of patients with other common bacterial pneumonias are bacteremic, blood cultures should be obtained on all patients suspected of having bacterial pneumonia. Pleural fluid is present in few patients with pneumococcal pneumonia on admission, but the organism can be demonstrated in about one half of such fluids. Since the presence of pleural fluid strongly suggests other bacterial causes for the pneumonia, specimens of such fluid should always be obtained and examined by stain and culture before therapy is instituted.

Cultures of expectorated nasopharyngeal sputum and swabs may be seriously misleading in the evaluation of patients with pneumococcal pneumonia because many sputum or pharyngeal cultures contain bacteria other than pneumococcus. Further, since pneumococci can be recovered from sputum in at least 30 per cent of patients without pneumonia, its presence in sputum does not confirm the diagnosis of pneumococcal pneumonia (Barrett-Connor, 1971). Microscopic examination of gram-stained, expectorated sputum is more useful than culture in establishing the diagnosis of pneumococcal pneumonia (Heineman et al., 1977). The cellular content of the smear should be determined first, since specimens that contain numerous squamous epithelial cells are not representative of lower respiratory tract flora. The finding of typical lancet-shaped, encapsulated, gram-positive diplococci in association with macrophages or PMNs and in the absence of other bacteria strongly supports the diagnosis.

Contamination by the oropharyngeal flora can be minimized by transtracheal aspiration, in which a specimen is collected via a catheter passed through the cricothyroid membrane into the trachea. This technique increases the yield of pneumococci from patients with pneumonia and reduces the number of contaminating agents. False-positive cultures are obtained in 20 to 30 per cent of patients, but false-negative results occur in less than 1 per cent of patients in the absence of antimicrobial therapy (Bartlett, 1977). In chronic lung disease with persistent colonization of the lower airways, the specificity of transtracheal aspirates is diminished. Complications of the procedure, consisting principally of hemorrhage and subcutaneous emphysema, are infrequent, but fatalities have occurred. Transtracheal aspiration should not be performed in small children, in patients with hemorrhagic diathesis, or in uncooperative patients. Performed carefully by experienced personnel, this technique may provide valuable diagnostic information in patients with pneumonia.

Specimens for smear and culture may be obtained from the distal lung by bronchoscopy, using either flexible or rigid instruments. The flexible are better tolerated by acutely ill patients and can sample more peripheral regions under direct vision. Unless special precautions are taken, bronchoscopically obtained specimens are routinely contaminated by oropharyngeal organisms. However, it is possible to collect secretions with sterile bronchial brushes that are protected from contamination during introduction by encasement within a sterile catheter. This procedure is useful in patients with complicated pneumonias or in whom the diagnosis is uncertain and unlikely to be resolved by simpler techniques.

Material may be aspirated directly from the lung with a thin (20-gauge) needle inserted through the chest wall. Although the needle track crosses the pleural space, empyema following transthoracic aspiration of pneumonia is exceedingly uncommon. Pneumothorax occurs in 5 to 22 per cent of patients but rarely requires treatment. This procedure has been used widely in children but relatively infrequently in adult patients. The rate of false-negative results is reported to range from 16 to 28 per cent. Transthoracic aspiration of the lung is probably underutilized as a technique of obtaining diagnostic material in patients with pneumonia and may be especially useful when fiberoptic bronchoscopy is not readily available. However, the procedure should not be performed by inexperienced operators or when complete resuscitative support is not available.

To summarize the foregoing, the diagnosis of pneumococcal pneumonia is assured when pneumococci are recovered from the blood, pleural fluid, or transthoracic lung aspirate. Isolation from a sterile swabbing of the involved lung segment or from a transtracheal aspirate is strong supporting evidence, while isolation of pneumococci from culture of expectorated sputum has less diagnostic value, although it may support a diagnosis of pneumococcal pneumonia made on clinical grounds.

Using these bacteriologic criteria, including recovery of pneumococci from expectorated sputum in conjunction with an illness and response to therapy that are compatible with pneumococcal pneumonia, recent investigators have found that *S. pneumoniae* is responsible for 60 to 70 per cent of bacterial pneumonias among adults (Dorff et al., 1973; Sullivan et al., 1972). If patients are included in whom no bacterial agent was recovered but who responded to penicillin therapy, the proportion of adult pneumonias that are probably due to pneumococci approaches 80 per cent.

DIFFERENTIAL DIAGNOSIS. Pneumonias caused by other pyogenic cocci or by aerobic bacilli may closely mimic pneumococcal pneumonia clinically, and their differentiation depends largely on bacteriologic findings. Lung abscess due to anaerobic bacteria may simulate pneumococcal pneumonia, although the typical illness associated with abscess formation is subacute and protracted; cavitation is rare with pneumococcal infection, and putrid sputum does not occur. Mycoplasma pneumonia is usually associated with a prominent cough, but sputum production is scanty and organisms are infrequent in tracheobronchial secretions; typically, patients with mycoplasmal infection complain of headache, myalgias, and malaise for several days, while the patient with pneumococcal pneumonia experiences an abrupt onset of fever, cough, and sputum production.

Pulmonary embolism may cause difficulty in differential diagnosis. Such patients rarely have temperatures over 101° F or leukocyte counts over 12,000/mm^3. Arterial blood gases show similar changes in pneumonia and embolism, namely, hypoxemia and hypocarbia. The hemoptysis of pneumococcal pneumonia usually consists of rusty sputum or streaks of blood within purulent sputum, whereas that associated with embolism is often gross blood without purulent sputum. However, in some patients, the distinction between pulmonary embolism and pneumococcal pneumonia cannot be made with confidence on clinical findings alone, and additional studies are required. In most cases, a perfusion (or ventilation and perfusion) lung scan will suffice. It must be remembered that perfusion will always be diminished in the region of lung consolidation, and no useful information will be gained in this area. However, if the scan fails to demonstrate perfusion defects in other lung regions, pulmonary embolism is highly unlikely, since nearly all such patients demonstrate multiple perfusion defects.

Carcinoma of the lung may present as pneumococcal pneumonia. In some patients, associated symptoms of weight loss, hoarseness, or prior hemoptysis may suggest the proper diagnosis. In others, the chest radiograph reveals a mass lesion or hilar adenopathy that can never be attributed to pneumococcal pneumonia in an adult. In some patients, the only clue to the presence of a tumor is the failure of the pneumonic process to resolve with therapy. All patients with pneumonia should be followed until resolution is complete clinically and radiographically.

TREATMENT. Penicillin is the treatment of choice for pneumococcal pneumonia. There is no evidence that the dose of penicillin should be titered against the severity of the pneumonia. Administration of more than 2.4 million units per day increases the incidence of superinfection, usually by gram-negative bacilli, and does not reduce the mortality or morbidity of the initial infection. For hospitalized patients, treatment should be initiated with procaine penicillin, 600,000 units intramuscularly every eight hours. Ambulatory patients can be treated with an oral penicillin such as phenoxymethyl penicillin, 250 mg every six hours. Patients who are allergic to penicillin can be effectively treated with erythromycin or clindamycin. Tetracycline is contraindicated in certain localities where as many as 25 per cent of isolates of *S. pneumoniae* have been resistant to it. Such resistance is usually found in less than 5 per cent of isolates. Antimicrobial treatment should be continued for seven days.

Unfortunately, these recommendations for therapy may need modification in the near future. Penicillin-resistant pneumococci have caused recent outbreaks of serious disease in several hospitals in South Africa (Jacobs et al., 1978) and have been isolated from humans in many parts of the world. Although the emergence of resistant strains appears to follow antibiotic usage, these strains do not produce beta-lactamase, and the mechanism of microbial resistance is unknown.

Supplemental oxygen, intravenous fluids, and analgesics for relief of pleuritic pain may also be required. Evacuation of tracheobronchial secretions is best ensured by maintaining systemic hydration, and parenteral fluids should be used if needed. Inhalation of bland aerosol mists and positive pressure breathing treatments are unnecessary in most patients but may be of benefit in patients with underlying airway obstruction and in those with an ineffective cough for other reasons. Postural drainage may assist in the evacuation of secretions from involved regions of the lung.

COMPLICATIONS AND SEQUELAE

Initial Complications. Shock is present in 5 to 10 per cent of patients admitted with pneumococcal pneumonia. Circulatory collapse is more likely to occur in bacteremic patients and in patients who show dense lobar consolidation radiographically. Not surprisingly, these findings are more common among patients who delay seeking medical attention for several days after the onset of symptoms. Hypotension usually responds promptly to intravenous fluids; dopamine may be used initially as a temporary measure but is usually unnecessary when the intravascular volume has been repleted with isotonic solutions. Cardiac output in patients with sepsis due to gram-positive organisms is usually high, and myocardial-stimulating drugs are not required. In patients with underlying heart disease, diffuse pulmonary infiltrates, or physical findings suggesting left ventricular failure, the treatment of shock can be undertaken safely only when left ventricular performance is monitored via a balloon catheter positioned in a pulmonary artery. Volume expansion of patients in left ventricular failure is obviously catastrophic.

Empyema is present in about 5 per cent of patients with pneumococcal pneumonia. Pleural disease should be sought as a part of the initial evaluation of all patients with pneumonia. Of the 10 per cent of patients with pneumococcal pneumonia who have effusions, half will have sterile exudates while in the others the fluid will contain organisms. The nature of these fluids varies from mild exudates to gross pus. Untreated empyemas always become grossly purulent and entrap the lung with an extensive pleural "peel" consisting of organizing proteinaceous exudate and loculated abscesses. This reaction is much more common with pleural infection due to gram-negative bacilli, hemolytic streptococci, *S. aureus*, and anaerobic bacteria but occurs following pneumococcal infection if untreated. Although penicillin in the usual doses sterilizes the pleural space, the pleural reaction may continue. Therefore, the key principle underlying treatment of pleural effusion in association with pneumonia is drainage. In the presence of pneumococcal infection, fluid that is clear or slightly turbid should be aspirated at the time of the initial thoracentesis; recurrence is usually slight in the presence of penicillin therapy. If the initial fluid is grossly purulent, chest tube drainage should be instituted promptly to prevent loculation. The pH of the pleural fluid helps predict which patients will require tube drainage; fluids with pH values greater than 7.3 rarely need drainage, while those with values less than 7.1 usually do. Institution of such drainage early can shorten morbidity from the pleural process. Young children have a greater propensity to clear extensive pleural reactions and require mechanical drainage less often.

Extrapulmonary pneumococcal infections occur rarely in patients with pneumonia and are usually evident shortly after admission. Meningitis must be considered in any patient with pneumonia who manifests depressed consciousness, stiff neck, or severe headache. Endocarditis, pericarditis, and septic arthritis are rare complications of pneumococcal pneumonia.

Late Complications. Effusion during treatment occurs typically on the third or fourth day of illness and is associated with pleural pain and continuing fever. Thoracentesis reveals slightly turbid fluid with 5000 to 10,000 leukocytes per mm^3, predominantly PMNs. The organisms cannot be seen by gram stain or recovered in culture. Treatment consists of needle aspiration of the bulk of the fluid. Such "sterile empyemas" are by far the most common cause of persistent fevers beyond three or four days of starting penicillin therapy. Some patients present in this stage of illness, i.e., pleural effusion, chest pain, and fever, usually after having taken antimicrobial agents. Since the underlying pneumonia may no longer be readily apparent radiographically or on physical examination, the diagnosis may be obscure; examination of the pleural fluid for pneumococcal capsular polysaccharides by counterimmunoelectrophoresis may identify the cause of such parapneumonic effusions.

Lung abscess does not follow pneumococcal pneumonia, except possibly with infection due to type 3 organisms. Occasionally, air-fluid levels appear in one or more areas on the chest radiograph during resolution of the illness. Such cavities are usually pre-existing lesions, the result of emphysema or remote chronic infection, which have filled with fluid during the course of pneumonia. Treatment should be gauged by the patient's clinical course, and endobronchial drainage should be encouraged. No treatment may be indicated if the patient has become afebrile and is steadily improving.

Pneumococcal pneumonia should resolve completely radiographically (Jay et al., 1975). The rate of resolution is much slower in elderly patients and in those with chronic lung disease or alcoholism (Fig. 1). Consolidative changes should disappear in all patients within ten weeks; evidence of volume loss may persist somewhat longer. There is no reason, as a general rule, to follow patients with weekly radiographs after discharge from the hospital; however, all patients should have a radiograph ten weeks after discharge, and patients with persistent abnormalities should undergo more extensive evaluation to rule out bronchial obstruction or other regional lung dysfunction.

PREVENTION. Immunization with polyvalent pneumococcal vaccines reduces the occurrence of pneumococcal disease in susceptible populations (Austrian et al., 1976). The feasibility of this approach rests on the continued demonstration that only a few of the over 80 pneumococcal types are responsible for most of clinical infections. A commercial vaccine contains purified capsular polysaccharides from 14 types (types 1, 2, 3, 4, 6, 8, 9, 12, 14, 19, 23, 25, 51, and 56) that account for 80 per cent of bacteremic pneumococcal infections in the United States. Immunization is recommended for patients with sickle cell anemia, azotemia, chronic cardiopulmonary disease, diabetes, liver disease, and the aged, especially those confined to institutions. Patients who develop one pneumococcal infection are at increased risk of another and should be immunized after recovery from the first episode. Mild pain and erythema may occur at the injection site for a day. Only one immunization is recommended because the duration of protection is unclear and local reactions are more frequent upon revaccination. Pneumococcal vaccine may be given with influenza and other vaccines.

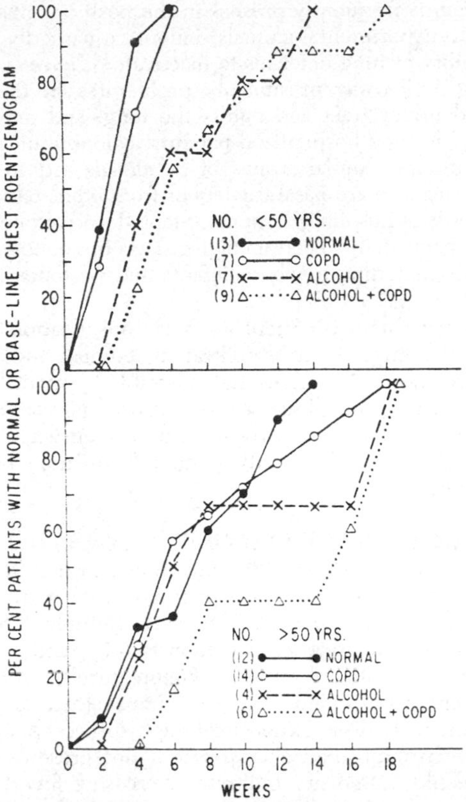

Figure 1. Effects of age on the radiographic resolution of *Streptococcus pneumoniae* pneumonia in patients without underlying disease (normal), with chronic obstructive pulmonary disease (COPD), with acute alcoholism (Alcohol), and with both (Alcohol + COPD).

Note that radiographic resolution was more rapid in patients less than 50 years of age in all groups. The presence of COPD or alcoholism prolonged resolution in patients under and over 50 years of age. The presence of COPD and alcoholism resulted in markedly delayed radiographic resolution, especially in patients over 50 years of age (Jay et al., 1975).

PNEUMONIA DUE TO STAPHYLOCOCCI

PATHOGENESIS AND PATHOLOGY. Staphylococcal pneumonia tends to occur in three situations: following epidemic influenza, among hospitalized patients, and in persons who inject unsterile materials into their veins. In the first two circumstances, colonization of the upper respiratory tract by *Staphylococcus aureus* usually precedes the development of pneumonia. About one third of healthy adults harbor *S. aureus* in their upper respiratory tracts; the anterior nares is the most common site, but the organism is frequently present in the posterior pharynx as well. In experimental animals, influenza markedly impairs the ability of lung defenses to inactivate *S. aureus*. In this setting *S. aureus* presumably proliferates in the virus-injured upper tract and enters the lung, and pneumonia results. Among hospitalized patients, colonization may occur with nosocomial strains of *S. aureus* acquired from personnel who are nasal carriers or from other patients via the hands of hospital personnel. Staphylococcal pneumonia occurs principally in certain high-risk groups of hospitalized patients including newborn infants and postoperative patients.

Autopsy shows confluent areas of consolidation characterized by intense PMN infiltration, edema, and hemorrhage. Clumps of cocci are demonstrable by special stains. Tissue necrosis and abscesses ranging from microscopic foci to enormous cavities are regular features. Airways may be occluded by sloughed epithelium, inflammatory exudate, and mucus.

CLINICAL MANIFESTATIONS. Staphylococcal pneumonia usually starts with shaking chills and high fever. In hematogenous staphylococcal pneumonia the radiographic features are characteristic. There are multiple 1 to 2 cm nodules, which undergo cavitation rapidly, and early development of pleural effusion. Pneumatoceles, which are expanding thin-walled cysts, are unusual in adults but common in children. Nosocomial staphylococcal pneumonia has no distinguishing characteristics but presents with a nonspecific pulmonary infiltrate, increasing fever, leukocytosis, and purulent tracheobronchial secretions. Staphylococcal pneumonia complicating influenza tends to occur in two forms: as a lobar or segmental process occurring five to seven days after the onset of influenza symptoms or as a diffuse process that appears virtually concurrently with the onset of influenza (Louria et al., 1959). The diffuse form may be difficult to distinguish from viral pneumonia, and its mortality approaches 70 per cent. The mortality of localized forms of staphylococcal pneumonia after influenza is equal to that in the absence of influenza.

DIAGNOSIS. As with pneumococcal pneumonia, the diagnosis of staphylococcal pneumonia depends on culture from blood, pleural fluid, or, least reliably, tracheobronchial secretions. The presence of staphylococci in Gram-stained specimens of tracheobronchial secretions in one of the above clinical settings strongly suggests the diagnosis of staphylococcal pneumonia and demands prompt treatment with an agent resistant to penicillinase.

TREATMENT. Since most isolates of *S. aureus* are resistant to penicillin, treatment should be with a penicillinase-resistant drug such as methicillin, oxacillin, or nafcillin in doses of 200 mg/kg/day. intravenously (I.V.). The daily dose should be divided into six portions and each given at 4-hour intervals. Patients allergic to penicillin should be treated with these doses of cefazolin. Vancomycin in doses of 500 mg every 6 hours I.V. is also effective in patients allergic to penicillin. Parenteral or oral therapy should be continued for at least 10 to 14 days and not stopped until the pulmonary infiltrates have cleared or stabilized.

COMPLICATIONS. Staphylococcal pneumonia may be complicated by abscess, empyema, pyopneumothorax, and obstruction of major airways by intensely purulent exudate and sloughed epithelium. These complications occur so often that each must be considered in all patients with staphylococcal pneumonia to prevent delay of their recognition and treatment. Lung abscess will usually resolve with the same antibiotics given for staphylococcal pneumonia. Empyema requires drainage with an indwelling tube.

PNEUMONIA DUE TO STREPTOCOCCUS (PYOGENES)

CLINICAL FEATURES. Pneumonia due to *Streptococcus pyogenes* is rare, accounting for less than 5 per cent of bacterial pneumonias, and pneumonia due to other streptococci is even less common. Streptococcal pneumonia has occurred in near-epidemic proportions as a complication of viral infection in closed populations. High rates of upper respiratory streptococcal carriage and an epidemic viral illness, usually influenza or measles, provide the necessary conditions for such an outbreak. Streptococcal pneumonia now occurs sporadically, principally among young people.

The infection starts abruptly with shaking chills, fever, and frequently pleural pain. Radiographs of the chest reveal consolidation of varying extent and, in 30 to 50 per cent of cases, pleural effusion. The tendency to cause early and frequently extensive pleural disease is the only feature that distinguishes this pneumonia from that due to the pneumococcus.

DIAGNOSIS AND TREATMENT. Isolation of *S. pyogenes* from blood or pleural fluid establishes the diagnosis, but isolation from expectorated sputum alone is of less certain significance because this organism may be carried in the upper respiratory tracts of healthy individuals. Treatment with procaine penicillin, 600,000 units twice daily intramuscularly for seven days, is effective. Erythromycin stearate, 500 mg orally four times daily for seven days, is a suitable alternative for penicillin-sensitive patients.

The major complication is empyema, which may result in a patient with an extensive exudative pleural reaction. In adults prompt drainage of the empyema via a thoracostomy tube will usually avoid the need for later decortication; procrastination in effecting adequate drainage frequently leads to a long and complicated hospital course. Because pleural disease in children more often resolves with antibiotics and needle aspiration of the pleural space, placement of intercostal drainage tubes can be postponed.

MENINGOCOCCAL PNEUMONIA

Meningococcal pneumonia occurs as an occasional consequence of meningococcemia, usually with meningitis, and as a primary pneumonia without extrathoracic disease. Primary pneumonia may follow influenza and perhaps adenoviral respiratory infection (Ellenbogen et al., 1974). Meningococcal pneumonias have been documented most often in groups in which there is a high proportion of upper respiratory tract carriage of the organism, such as military populations (Irwin et al., 1975). The incidence of meningococcal pneumonia probably has been underestimated in the past, at least in certain populations. Because the meningococcus is encapsulated, the pathogenesis of meningococcal pneumonia is presumably similar to that described for the pneumococcus.

CLINICAL MANIFESTATIONS AND DIAGNOSIS. The clinical features of meningococcal pneumonia do not differentiate it from other bacterial pneumonias. The occasionally positive blood culture confirms the diagnosis. *N. meningitidis* has been difficult to recover from expectorated sputum in many reported cases, whereas transtracheal aspirates or transthoracic lung aspiration reveals the organism (Ellenbogen et al., 1974; Irwin et al., 1975). These observations suggest that the meningococcus fares poorly in competition with other organisms during cultivation on artificial media and, further, that *N. meningitidis* might be incriminated more often in pneumonia if invasive culturing techniques were employed routinely.

TREATMENT. Procaine penicillin in a dose of 600,000 units every 12 hours for seven days is given for meningococcal pneumonia not complicated by meningitis. Chloramphenicol (500 mg orally or 1.0 g intravenously every six hours) is a suitable alternative for penicillin-sensitive individuals.

References

Austrian, R., Douglas, R. M., Schiffman, G., Coetzee, A. M., Koornhof, H. J., Hayden-Smith, S., and Reid, R. D. W.: Prevention of pneumococcal pneumonia by vaccination. Trans Assoc Am Physicians 89:184, 1976.

Austrian, R., and Gold, J.: Pneumococcal bacteremia with special reference to bacteremic pneumococcal pneumonia. Ann Intern Med 60:759, 1964.

Barrett-Connor, E.: The nonvalue of sputum culture in the diagnosis of pneumococcal pneumonia. Am Rev Resp Dis 103:845, 1971.

Bartlett, J. G.: Diagnostic accuracy of transtracheal aspiration bacteriologic studies. Am Rev Respir Dis 115:777, 1977.

Centers for Disease Control: Morbidity and Mortality Weekly Report 27 (4), January 27, 1978.

Dorff, G. J., Rytel, W., Farmer, S. G., and Scanlon, G.: Etiologies and characteristic features of pneumonias in a municipal hospital. Am J Med Sci 266:349, 1973.

Ellenbogen, C., Graybill, J. R., Silva, J., Jr., and Homme, P. J.: Bacterial pneumonia complicating adenoviral pneumonia: A comparison of respiratory tract bacterial culture sources and effectiveness of chemoprophylaxis against bacterial pneumonia. Am J Med 56:169, 1974.

Green, G. M.: The Amberson Lecture: In defense of the lung. Am Rev Respir Dis 102:691, 1970.

Heineman, H. S., Chawla, J. K., and Lofton, W. M.: Misinformation from sputum cultures without microscopic examination. J Clin Microbiol 6:518, 1977.

Huxley, E. J., Viroslav, J., Gray, W. B., and Pierce, A. K.: Pharyngeal aspiration in normal adults and patients with depressed consciousness. Am J Med 64:564, 1978.

Irwin, R. S., Woelk, W. K., and Coudon, W. L., III: Primary meningococcal pneumonia. Ann Intern Med 82:493, 1975.

Jacobs, M. R., Koornhof, H. J., Robins-Browne, R. M., et al.: Emergence of multiple resistant pneumococci. N Engl J Med 299:735, 1978.

Jay, S. J., Johanson, W. G., Jr., and Pierce, A. K.: Radiographic resolution of *Streptococcus pneumoniae* pneumonia. N Engl J Med 293:798, 1975.

Louria, D. B., Blumenfeld, H. L., Ellis, J. T., et al.: Studies on influenza in the pandemic of 1957-1958. II. Pulmonary complications of influenza. J Clin Invest 38:213, 1959.

Sullivan, R. J., Jr., Dowdle, W. R., Marine, W. M., and Hierholzer, J. C.: Adult pneumonia in a general hospital: Etiology and host risk factors. Arch Intern Med 129:935, 1972.

Tilghman, R. C., and Finland, M.: Clinical significance of bacteremia in pneumococci pneumonia. Arch Intern Med 59:602, 1937.

Winterbauer, R. H., Bedon, G. A., and Ball, S. W. C., Jr.: Recurrent pneumonia: Predisposing illness and clinical patterns in 158 patients. Ann Intern Med 70:689, 1969.

Ziskind, M. M., Schwarz, M. I., George, R. B., et al.: Incomplete consolidation in pneumococcal lobar pneumonia complicating pulmonary emphysema. Ann Intern Med 72:835, 1970.

112

COMMON GRAM-NEGATIVE BACILLARY PNEUMONIAS

W. G. JOHANSON, JR., M.D.
GARY D. HARRIS, M.D.

ETIOLOGY. The gram-negative bacilli that produce pneumonia in humans are principally *Klebsiella pneumoniae, Escherichia coli, Pseudomonas aeruginosa,* and *Haemophilus influenzae* (Tillotson and Lerner, 1966). A variety of other gram-negative organisms produce pneumonia occasionally.

PATHOGENESIS AND PATHOLOGY. Bacterial pneumonia of all types is uncommon among healthy individuals; this is especially true of pneumonias due to gram-negative bacilli. Only about 10 per cent of bacterial pneumonias acquired in the community are due to these organisms, and affected patients virtually always have serious underlying diseases. *K. pneumoniae* is responsible for most community-acquired bacillary pneumonias, followed by *E. coli, Proteus,* and other organisms. *P. aeruginosa* is rarely the cause of pneumonia acquired outside the hospital but is a common cause of nosocomial pneumonia.

In Chapter 111 the concept that bacterial pneumonia results from aspiration of upper respiratory secretions was developed. This concept applies particularly well to pneumonia due to gram-negative bacilli. These organisms are found in the oropharynx of only 2 to 6 per cent of healthy people. Hospital personnel who are exposed to patients with infections due to bacilli may acquire these hospital strains in their gastrointestinal tracts, but the organisms are excluded from their upper respiratory tracts. Gram-negative bacilli instilled into the upper respiratory tracts of healthy subjects are rapidly removed, and persistent colonization does not occur. Thus, it appears that highly effective mechanisms prevent colonization of the upper respiratory tracts of healthy individuals by gram-negative bacilli (Johanson et al., 1969).

The incidence of oropharyngeal colonization with gram-negative bacilli rises dramatically in patients with acute or chronic illness, approaching 50 per cent of subjects in most studies. The organisms that colonize are those that cause pneumonia. Colonization of the upper respiratory tract with gram-negative bacilli markedly increases the risk of subsequent pneumonia among seriously ill hospitalized patients; in one study of 213 patients admitted to an intensive care unit, pneumonia occurred in 23 per cent of colonized patients compared to 3 per cent of noncolonized patients (Johanson et al., 1972). Thus, patients who are already ill with other diseases are most likely to develop oropharyngeal colonization with gram-negative bacilli; the organisms probably reach the lungs by aspiration of small quantities of oropharyngeal secretions, and pneumonia develops when the organisms multiply more rapidly than they are killed by intrinsic defenses.

In experimental animals exposed to aerosolized bacilli or to purified endotoxin, polymorphonuclear leukocytes (PMNs) appear promptly in the walls of airways and alveoli and, to a lesser degree, in alveolar spaces. On the other hand, the cellular reaction of patients dying of bacillary pneumonia is occasionally only mononuclear, suggesting that failure of the PMN response may have played a critical role in the outcome. The greater frequency of gram-negative bacillary pneumonias in leukemics and other neutropenic patients supports the importance of PMN deficiency in pathogenesis.

Microscopically, in bacillary pneumonias necrosis of lung tissue and, especially with *P. aeruginosa* infections, fibrinoid necrosis of pulmonary arteries and veins are characteristic. It is not clear whether lung necrosis results from these vascular lesions or from destruction of alveolar walls by bacterial collagenases and elastases. Bacillary pneumonia may be peribronchial initially but may coalesce to a lobar consolidation and extensive abscess formation. Resolution usually leaves persistent disturbances in lung structure and function.

CLINICAL MANIFESTATIONS. Pneumonia due to aerobic bacilli, when community-acquired, is usually a catastrophic, prostrating, acute infection. The pneumonia may be somewhat obscured by the underlying disease. However, chills, fever, cough productive of purulent or bloody sputum, and chest pain are common symptoms. Excessively mucoid sputum containing blood ("currant jelly sputum") is occasionally seen with *K. pneumoniae* pneumonia but is a nonspecific finding. Hypotension, frank shock, and delirium are more common with this type of pneumonia than with pneumococcal pneumonia.

Rales and signs of consolidation may be present, depending on the extent of involvement and the stage of the process. Pleural effusion and empyema are much more common than with pneumococcal pneumonia, and evidence of pleural disease must be sought carefully by clinical and radiographic techniques. Cavitation of the lung parenchyma is common but can rarely be detected on physical examination.

Radiographic changes are nonspecific. Infiltrates range from scattered peribronchial disease to dense unilobar consolidation, most often involving an upper lobe. Edema, hemorrhage, and tissue necrosis of the involved lobe may increase its volume so that fissures bulge in pneumonia due to *K. pneumoniae*. Pleural disease is frequent. Air-fluid levels may be seen with abscess formation, varying from multiple nodular lesions to entire lobes or even one lung.

Nosocomial (hospital-acquired) pneumonia may be difficult to detect. At least 75 per cent of such pneumonias are due to gram-negative bacilli. However, the patients usually have complicated illnesses or are postoperative, and the signs and symptoms of their underlying processes obscure the onset of nosocomial pneumonia. The combination of leukocytosis, fever, new or progressing infiltrates on radiographs and the presence of purulent secretions are reliable signs of pulmonary infection in this setting if the patient's underlying disease does not involve the lungs. In patients with pulmonary edema of various causes, the presence of a superimposed bacillary pneumonia may be manifested only as worsening of the patient's overall condition; oxygenation, mental state, renal function, and hematopoietic parameters are commonly affected (Andrews et al., 1981).

DIAGNOSIS. The presence of pneumonia is usually readily apparent in nonhospitalized patients but may be difficult to ascertain among critically ill patients who may have radiographic infiltrates due to other causes. About 25 per cent of patients with gram-negative bacillary pneumonias have positive blood cultures that establish the bacteriologic etiology of the pulmonary disease. Pleural fluid, when present, usually contains the responsible bacteria and should always be aspirated for diagnostic purposes. A major diagnostic problem is presented by patients whose upper respiratory tracts have been colonized by gram-negative bacilli and who then develop signs and symptoms of lower respiratory infection. Several approaches have been proposed to distinguish colonization from significant infection, including washing of sputum to remove surface contaminants and quantitative cultures of the sputum. Neither technique clearly distinguishes colonization from infection in our experience. Transtracheal aspiration may be helpful, although in this patient population multiple pathogenic species are frequently recovered from the trachea. Gram stain of material recovered by this technique is far more valuable than culture in determining whether or not infection is present. In especially difficult situations, transthoracic lung aspiration or bronchoscopic procedures are indicated to determine the cause of progressing lung infiltrates.

COMPLICATIONS AND SEQUELAE. Overall, about 50 per cent of patients with pneumonia due to gram-negative bacilli die (Pierce and Sanford, 1974). Among intensive care patients, the mortality of nosocomial *P. aeruginosa* pneumonia approaches 80 per cent. The causes of death are multifactorial, including the underlying disease, shock, lung necrosis, and acute respiratory failure. Lung abscess and empyema are early complications. Lung abscess may require repeated bronchoscopy to promote endobronchial drainage; the temptation to aspirate intrapulmonary collections of pus transthoracically via needle or chest tube should be resisted, since such procedures violate the pleural space and may add the complication of bronchopleural fistula to an already desperate situation. Massive hemoptysis and pyopneumothorax secondary to pleural rupture are major complications.

Pleural effusions developing during bacillary pneumonia usually contain infecting bacteria. At first the fluid is free-flowing and easily aspirated, but it loculates if removal is delayed, and adequate drainage via needle or chest tube may not be possible. Decortication, the débridement of the pleural space, should be considered in patients with extensive pleural disease who still have fever after seven days of tube drainage and adequate antimicrobial therapy.

TREATMENT. Antimicrobial therapy of these infections must be guided by in vitro susceptibility testing. At least two antimicrobial drugs should be used and selected on the basis of known in vitro sensitivities of the gram-negative bacilli isolated from these patients before the development of pneumonia. A combination of piperacillin and amikacin are active against the important pathogenic gram-negative bacilli causing pneumonia and are synergistic. This combination can be used until drug susceptibility is known. The dose is 40 mg piperacillin per kg every 4 hours and 5 mg amikacin per kg every 8 hours intravenously. Ticarcillin can also be used (with amikacin) in place of piperacillin; and in patients allergic to penicillin, moxalactam, cefotaxime, or trimethoprim-sulfamethoxazole can be given with amikacin in place of piperacillin or ticarcillin. Clearing of secretion from the tracheobronchial tree is especially important because respiratory failure is a common cause of death and may be due to obstruction of airways by tenacious secretions.

PROPHYLAXIS. Contaminated respiratory therapy equipment has been responsible for many nosocomial bacillary pneumonias, and continued awareness of this potential hazard and rigorous enforcement of preventive measures are indicated (Pierce et al., 1970). Medications, parenteral solutions, and even hand lotions are also potential sources of contamination. Further, it is likely that colonization occurs in many patients following transport of the organisms from other patients on the hands of their attendants. This mode of transmission is especially common in critical care areas where susceptible patients are concentrated in relatively small spaces.

Attempts to reduce the susceptibility of the patient to colonization by gram-negative bacilli have not been highly successful. Topical instillation of bactericidal agents into the oropharynx tends to promote drug resistance and does not lower the incidence of pneumonia. Systemic antibacterial therapy increases the tendency of sick people to sustain colonization with gram-negative bacilli.

PNEUMONIA DUE TO HAEMOPHILUS INFLUENZAE. Although serious infection with *Haemophilus influenzae* occurs predominantly among children less than 3 years of age, pneumonia due to *H. influenzae* may also occur in adults (Quintiliani and Hymans, 1971; Tillotson and Lerner, 1968). These pneumonias are either a localized (lobar or segmental) consolidation or a diffuse bronchopneumonia. Both types occur mainly in patients with serious underlying illnesses, especially chronic obstructive lung disease. Patients with localized consolidation have an illness similar to pneumococcal pneumonia; and upper respiratory tract illness usually precedes the onset of chills, pleuritic chest pain, and purulent sputum. Pleural effusion is common. Chest radiography reveals a consolidating process, most often in the right lower lobe, with or without evidence of effusion. Cavitation may develop but is not common at first.

Patients with the bronchopneumonia form of *H. influenzae* pneumonia usually have a less acute illness; increased cough, sputum production, and low-grade or intermittent fever may have been present for days or even weeks. Radiographs of the chest reveal multiple, small, ill-defined densities scattered throughout both lungs. Pleural effusion is rare with this type of illness.

In both types of pneumonia numerous small, pleomorphic gram-negative bacilli and many polymorphonuclear leukocytes are seen in smears of the sputum. Culture of *H. influenzae* requires special attention. Heat-labile inhibitors in fresh human and sheep blood agar interfere with isolation, but these are inactivated by the heating process that is used for making chocolate agar. Both chocolate agar and Fildes peptic digest agar provide the X factor (heme) and the V factor (nicotinamide adenine nucleotide) required for growth and primary isolation of *Haemophilus* influenzae. Blood cultures and demonstration of capsular antigen by counterimmunoelectrophoresis are also important for diagnosis.

Encapsulated strains, especially Type b, cause most if not all pneumonias due to *H. influenzae*. The pathogenicity of nonencapsulated and nontypable strains is controversial. These organisms may be found in the upper respiratory tracts of healthy individuals and are commonly present in the tracheobronchial secretions of persons with chronic bronchitis. Evidence of the pathogenicity of the nontypable strains in chronic bronchitis rests largely on the higher frequency of its isolation in purulent secretions compared with nonpurulent secretions; however, many investigators have found nontypable strains of *H. influenzae* in the sputum of as many as 25 to 50 per cent of bronchitic patients during stable periods without purulent exacerbations, and the role of this organism in causing episodes of purulent bronchitis is uncertain.

The treatment of choice for pneumonia due to *H. influenzae* is ampicillin, 0.5 g intravenously every four to six hours. Chloramphenicol in doses of 500 mg orally every four hours or 1.0 g intravenously every six hours is used in patients who are allergic to penicillin or from whom penicillinase-producing *H. influenzae* are recovered. A rapid penicillinase test permits the choice of antibiotics upon isolation of the organism. If the diagnosis is seriously suspected before the culture is positive, both antibiotics can be used until the penicillinase test is completed, and then one of the drugs is stopped. Treatment of the underlying chronic pulmonary disease usually expedites symptomatic recovery.

References

Andrews, C. P., Coalson, J. J., Smith, J. D., and Johanson, W. G., Jr.: Diagnosis of nosocomial bacterial pneumonia in acute, diffuse lung injury. Chest 80:254, 1981.

Johanson, W. G., Jr., Pierce, A. K., and Sanford, J. P.: Changing pharyngeal bacterial flora of hospitalized patients: Emergence of gram-negative bacilli. N Engl J Med 281:1137, 1969.

Johanson, W. G., Jr., Pierce, A. K., Sanford, J. P., and Thomas, G. D.: Nosocomial respiratory infections with gram-negative bacilli. Ann Intern Med 77:701, 1972.

Pierce, A. K., and Sanford, J. P.: Aerobic gram-negative bacillary pneumonias. Am Rev Respir Dis 110:647, 1974.

Pierce, A. K., Sanford, J. P., Thomas, G. D., and Leonard, J. S.: Long-term evaluation of decontamination of inhalation therapy equipment and occurrence of necrotizing pneumonia. N Engl J Med 282:528, 1970.

Quintiliani, R., and Hymans, P. J.: The association of bacteremic *Haemophilus influenzae* pneumonia in adults with typable strains. Am J Med 50:781, 1951.

Tillotson, J. R., and Lerner, A. M.: Pneumonias caused by gram-negative bacilli. Medicine 45:625, 1966.

Tillotson, J. R., and Lerner, A. M.: *Hemophilus influenzae* bronchopneumonia in adults. Arch Intern Med 121:428, 1968.

113
MELIOIDOSIS

MICHAEL BROWN, MB, FRCP, FRCPE, DTM&H
ROBERT NICOL THIN, M.D., FRCPE

Melioidosis is an uncommon disease that is due to the gram-negative bacillus *Pseudomonas pseudomallei.* The main endemic areas of the world are Southeast Asia and Northern Australia, and a few cases have originated in other places between the 20° north and south parallels of latitude, such as Ecuador and Panama (Howe et al., 1971). The disease may present as an acute, acute fulminating septicaemic (often fatal), subacute, or chronic illness. It may also be a mild self-limiting unexplained fever or subclinical (diagnosed only by the results of serological tests).

ETIOLOGY. Melioidosis was first recognized in 1911 by Whitmore in Rangoon at an autopsy examination. The causative organism, *P. pseudomallei,* has been called by a variety of names, including *Pfeifferella whitmori, Loefflerella whitmori,* and *Malleomyces pseudomallei.* Surveys have shown that this organism occurs naturally in the soil and surface water in Northern Australia, East and West Malaysia, Singapore, and Vietnam.

P. pseudomallei is a small, motile, gram-negative, non-acid-fast, non-spore-bearing bacillus that shows characteristic bipolar staining. It grows on ordinary media, although it may be overgrown by other organisms. In suspected cases, specimens from all septic lesions, and blood in acute cases, should be cultured. Nutrient agar, incorporating 3 per cent glycerol and 1:200,000 crystal violet, is a useful selective medium on which smooth colonies, deeply tinted by the dye, are visible after 24 hours' incubation. They enlarge to a maximum diameter of 7 mm after 14 days' incubation when they have a dry, wrinkled, beaten aluminium appearance. A characteristic pungent, yeasty odor is given off by fresh cultures, and this may be a useful clue to the presence of this organism. Twenty-four hours' incubation in nutrient broth produces an even turbidity and surface pellicle. The organism is pathogenic for most laboratory animals, and in animals, melioidosis resembles glanders. In male guinea pigs a characteristic acute orchitis is produced (Strauss reaction); a similar reaction occurs in guinea pigs infected with *Actinobacillus mallei* (the glanders bacillus). Serologic tests assist in diagnosis; the polysaccharide hemagglutination test is more sensitive and specific than the simple agglutination, or complement-fixation, tests, which are limited by cross-reactions with *A. mallei, Escherichia, Aerobacter, Klebsiella,* and *Salmonella* species (Alexander et al., 1970; Strauss et al., 1969). An indirect IgM immunofluorescent test for circulating human antibodies to *P. pseudomallei* appears to be useful for the diagnosis of active clinical disease, and monitoring its persistence and treatment (Ashdown, 1981).

PATHOGENESIS AND PATHOLOGY. The disease affects both sexes but has been reported more often in men due to large studies on nonindigenous servicemen such as those from the conflicts in Southeast Asia. Even in local surveys from Malaysia and northern Australia this difference, although less, still shows a male predominance.

P. pseudomallei is found in a wide variety of animals, including rats, rabbits, guinea pigs, sheep, goats, pigs, and horses. At one time, it was thought that man was infected by direct contact with diseased animals or by ingestion or inhalation of infected material from them. It is now believed that infection is most commonly acquired directly from infected soil and surface water. *P. pseudomallei* enters the body either through pre-existing skin lesions, contaminated penetrating wounds or burns, or by inhalation of the organism from dust or droplets (Editorial, Lancet, 1975; Rode et al., 1981; Moore, 1982). It is possible that organisms enter the body by ingestion, but it seems unlikely that they survive in the normal stomach. One case of probable sexual transmission of melioidosis has been reported and this is the only well-documented case of person-to-person transmission (McCormick et al., 1975).

Unrecognized chronic infections may flare up after decline of host resistance. Debilitating conditions such as diabetes, alcoholism, drug addiction, malnutrition, leprosy, and pregnancy predispose to acute melioidosis (Rode et al., 1981; Moore, 1982; Ashdown et al., 1980). Previously healthy individuals are more likely to develop subacute or chronic melioidosis.

The lesions of melioidosis occur most commonly in the lungs, but they are also found in the joints, liver, spleen, kidney, and bone marrow. Less often, lesions occur in the adrenal glands and lymph nodes, but any organ can be affected, including the heart and brain. Patients with acute illness of short duration have small abscesses, whereas those with longer illnesses tend to have larger abscesses.

Lesions start as microscopic foci that develop into inflammatory nodules, and multiple nodules coalesce to form abscesses. The lesions have a characteristic histology (Piggot and Hochholzer, 1970). They start as collections of polymorphonuclear neutrophils surrounded by zones of congestion. When larger, they have centers of necrotic caseous material containing nuclear debris, surrounded by a narrow zone of lymphocytes and histiocytes, and outside this a thin layer of fibrous tissue may form. At the periphery, intensely congested dilated capillaries form a distinctive collar, sharply demarcating the lesion from the surrounding tissue.

At autopsy in fulminating cases, *P. pseudomallei* may be cultured from the heart blood and abscesses (Thin et al., 1970) and can be seen in histologic sections, stained by the Gram method or by immunofluorescence.

CLINICAL MANIFESTATIONS. The incubation period is unknown, but is almost certainly very variable. The clinical manifestations of melioidosis vary greatly and there are no specific diagnostic features (Editorial, *Lancet,* 1975; Moore, 1982).

The acutely ill patient has a high fever; chills, a cough often productive of blood-stained mucopurulent sputum, diarrhea, and abdominal pain. Physical examination may reveal pneumonia, empyema, and lung abscess, mild jaundice, hepatomegaly, splenomegaly, acute or subacute arthritis, and septic pustules. There may be overwhelming septicemia and the patient's condition can rapidly worsen with increased confusion, tremor, profuse watery diarrhea that may resemble cholera, and a pustular rash, until he becomes comatose and dies in septicemic shock.

In the subacute case, pulmonary features often predominate. There is fever, cough productive of mucopurulent sputum that may be streaked with blood, signs of pneumonia, lung abscess, and, occasionally, pleural involvement. Joint pains may occur; there may also be a sparse pustular rash and hepatosplenomegaly. Subacute or chronic illness may precede or follow the acute disease, or may develop in the absence of acute illness. Pneumonitis may occur alone and the clinical features may resemble tuberculosis.

Chronic forms are very variable. Osteomyelitis, lung abscess, psoas or subcutaneous abscesses, liver or spleen abscesses, and lymphadenopathy occur (Prevatt and Hunt, 1957). Fistulas may appear. There may be a long latent period (up to 24 years has been recorded) between exposure and the diagnosis of melioidosis. Chronic melioidosis may persist for many months.

Melioidosis may also take the form of a mild, self-limiting febrile illness without any specific features. It must be considered among the many causes for short-term "fever of undetermined origin" among people who are in or who have visited endemic areas. This form of melioidosis will be diagnosed only by serologic tests. Surveys have shown raised serum antibody titers among those living in, and those who have visited, endemic areas. Raised antibody titers have been found in a higher proportion of those surveyed than would be expected from the comparatively few recorded clinical cases. Unsuspected or subclinical infection is therefore more prevalent than was realized at one time.

Cases have been reported in which, initially, there has been an unremarkable skin lesion, often traumatic in origin, with or without localized infection, lymphangitis or lymphadenitis, followed by progression to systemic melioidosis.

COMPLICATIONS AND SEQUELAE. The main problem with melioidosis is that however mild the condition is at first, there may be rapid progression to a severe fulminating illness in which the patient's condition deteriorates until he dies. Therefore, it is vital that all suspicious cases be carefully investigated. Occasional chronic cases may be left with deformities, such as flexion contractures, which are probably more common in local populations than is generally realized. Residual pulmonary changes may persist, including linear radiologic scars, cavities, and emphysema.

In adequately treated cases, there will be no sequelae but prolonged treatment is vital, as will be emphasized later, and a long, careful, follow-up after treatment is important.

GEOGRAPHICAL VARIATIONS. As already noted, melioidosis takes many forms, but no relation has been reported between the place where the organism was acquired and the course of the disease.

DIAGNOSIS. Melioidosis may be suspected at the bedside, but the diagnosis can be confirmed only in the microbiologic laboratory (Editorial, *Lancet*, 1975; Moore, 1982). Simple laboratory investigations are of little value; some cases have a polymorphonuclear leukocytosis and a high erythrocyte sedimentation rate. The chest radiograph frequently shows infiltration resembling pulmonary tuberculosis and cavities are common. Like tuberculosis, pulmonary melioidosis usually affects the upper lobes and this may cause confusion. Sometimes, many cavities are present, resembling staphylococcal pneumonia, and segmental consolidation may also occur.

P. pseudomallei can be easily cultured. In acute cases, blood should always be cultured and the presence of bipolar rods in blood cultures from these patients, after 24 hours' incubation, may be the first microbiologic indication of the diagnosis. The organism is easily isolated from pus and has been found in almost all body fluids except feces. Physicians must be acutely aware of the possibility of melioidosis and send specimens to the laboratory from all septic lesions. The laboratory staff should be informed that melioidosis is a possible diagnosis so that appropriate culture media may be used from the beginning. The diagnosis of melioidosis should be considered in all patients who are in, or who have returned from, endemic areas with fever of undetermined origin, pulmonary disease, or pyogenic lesions, and in all patients in whom the diagnosis is obscure. It must be remembered that in some reported cases there has been a very long latent period between return from endemic areas and the development of melioidosis. This is especially important in the present modern era of air travel, and in the movement of refugees. This is well documented in a study of Asian refugees in the United States, and has earned the title of "Time Bomb Disease" for melioidosis (Coleman et al., 1981).

This condition must be differentiated from a wide variety of other diseases. The acute fulminating form must be distinguished from other causes of septicemia, typhoid fever, malaria, leptospirosis, typhus, plague, and mycoses. Pulmonary forms must be differentiated from tuberculosis, lung abscess, and pneumonia, particularly staphylococcal pneumonia, and pulmonary mycoses. Confusion with pulmonary tuberculosis has often occurred in the past. Jaundice and hepatomegaly, due to melioidosis, may mimic hepatitis A and B, infectious mononucleosis, and cytomegalovirus disease. Chronic forms resemble osteomyelitis due to other causes, and tuberculous and other chronic abscesses. Simple febrile illness must be differentiated from other causes of fever of undetermined origin.

TREATMENT. Disc sensitivity tests usually indicate that *P. pseudomallei* is sensitive to tetracycline, chloramphenicol, sulphonamides, kanamycin, and novobiocin, and resistant to penicillins. No information is available on the new cephalosporins. Quantitative assays show more complex patterns; colonies from one specimen may show different sensitivities, and sensitivity may vary between consecutive specimens taken from one patient. Careful laboratory investigations are essential for good antibiotic treatment; the ideal regimen for treating acute melioidosis is controversial. Combined regimens of large doses of chloramphenicol, novobiocin, kanamycin, and sulphonamides have cured fulminating cases but have shown marked toxicity with cases of bone marrow depression, ototoxicity, nephrotoxicity, and hepatotoxicity. Furthermore, the response is unpredictable in spite of full in vitro sensitivity (Moore, 1982). Antagonism occurs in vitro between kanamycin and chloramphenicol, tetracycline and kanamycin, and sulphadiazine and chloramphenicol.

In all but the most severe acute cases, tetracycline is the drug of choice. The daily dose should be 40 mg/kg/day (3 g daily for a 70 kg adult), and this should be continued until serial cultures are negative for a month and the chest radiograph has cleared or stabilized with minimal residual change.

In the severe fulminating or septicemic case a combined regimen using chloramphenicol 40 to 80 mg/kg/day with tetracycline 40 mg/kg/day, intravenously, should be started, together with trimethoprim 4 mg/kg/day and sulphamethoxazole 20 mg/kg/day, orally (Coleman et al., 1981).

In less acute cases intravenous tetracycline or intravenous doxycycline (200 mg twice daily) with trimethoprim and sulphamethoxazole has been used successfully (Ashdown et al., 1980). During the acute stages, the patient's vital functions should be carefully monitored, and supportive measures instituted. Correction of any underlying debilitating disease such as diabetes is mandatory. Accessible abscesses should be drained surgically.

Prolonged treatment is most important in all clinical forms of melioidosis; 3 to 6 months' therapy may be necessary in some cases (Howe et al., 1971). If therapy is stopped prematurely, relapse is likely. Serial cultures should be sent until all lesions are healed, and the patient followed up for a prolonged period after treatment is discontinued to ensure remission is maintained.

PROPHYLAXIS. No vaccine is available against melioidosis. The best method of prevention is to avoid undue exposure to soil and surface water in endemic areas, especially after the start of heavy rain, since organisms are particularly prevalent in surface water at this time. Improved drainage for poorly drained areas will also help to reduce exposure.

CONCLUSIONS. Melioidosis is more prevalent in endemic areas than is generally realized. The main endemic area, Southeast Asia, is an important tourist and trading area. With air travel, patients suffering from melioidosis may present anywhere in the world, with any clinical form of melioidosis, and a long latent period may elapse between exposure and illness. A large number of United States servicemen, and servicemen of other countries, were exposed to infection in endemic areas in the late 1960s and early 1970s (Moore, 1982). This form of delayed melioidosis may continue to be a problem in such individuals for some years to come. To make a rapid diagnosis, physicians must be alert to the possibility of this condition, take appropriate specimens for microbiologic examination, and inform their laboratory colleagues if they suspect melioidosis. Antibiotic treatment should be vigorous and prolonged, and careful follow-up is important to ensure a satisfactory cure.

References

Alexander, A. D., Huxsoll, D. L., Warner, A. R., Shepler, V., and Dorsey, A.: Serological diagnosis of human melioidosis with indirect hemagglutination and complement fixation tests. Appl Microbiol 20:825, 1970.

Ashdown, L. R.: Relationship and significance of specific immunoglobulin M antibody response in clinical and subclinical melioidosis. J Clin Microbiol 14: 4:361, 1981.

Ashdown, L. R.: Demonstration of human antibodies to *Pseudomonas* pseudomallei by indirect fluorescent antibody staining. Pathology 13:597, 1981.

Ashdown, L. R., Duffy, V. A., Douglas, R. A.: Melioidosis. Med J Aust 1: 314, 1980.

Coleman, D. L., Root, R. K.: Pulmonary infections in South East Asian refugees. Clinics in Chest Medicines 2:1:133, 1981.

Editorial: Melioidosis. Lancet 2:962, 1975.

Howe, C., Sampath, A., and Spotnitz M.: The pseudomallei group, a review. J Infect Dis 124:598, 1971.

John, J. F.: Trimethoprim-sulphamethoxazole therapy of pulmonary melioidosis. Am Rev Respir Dis 114:1021, 1976.

McCormick, J. B., Sexton, D. J., McMurray, J. G., Carey, E., Hayes, P., and Feldman, R. A.: Human to human transmission of *Pseudomonas pseudomallei.* Ann Intern Med 83:512, 1975.

Moore, W. L.: Melioidosis. Internal Medicine in Vietnam Vol. 2: 197 Medical Department, United States Army, Office of the Surgeon General and Center of Military History, United States Army, Washington, D.C., 1982.

Piggot, J. A., and Hochholzer, L.: Human melioidosis. A histopathologic study of acute and chronic melioidosis. Arch Pathol 90:101, 1970.

Prevatt, A. L., and Hunt, J. S.: Chronic systemic melioidosis. Review of literature and report of a case, with a note of visual disturbance due to chloramphenicol. Am J Med 23:810, 1957.

Rode, J. W., Webling, D. D'A.: Melioidosis in Northern Australia. Med J Aust 1:181, 1981.

Strauss, J. M., Alexander, A. D., Rapmund, G., Gan, E., and Dorsey, A. E.: Melioidosis in Malaysia III. Antibodies to *Pseudomonas pseudomallei* in the human population. Am J Trop Med Hyg 18:703, 1969.

Thin, R. N. T., Brown, M., Stewart, J. B., and Garrett, C. J.: Melioidosis—a report of ten cases. Q J Med 153:115, 1970.

Thin, R. N. T., Groves, M., Rapmund, G., and Mariappan, M.: *Pseudomonas pseudomallei* in the surface water of Singapore. Singapore Medical Journal 12:181, 1971.

114
MYCOPLASMA PNEUMONIA

MAURICE A. MUFSON, M.D.

Mycoplasma pneumonia (formerly atypical or Eaton agent pneumonia), caused by *Mycoplasma pneumoniae,* is an acute infection of the lower respiratory tract that exhibits the following characteristics: (1) usually involves the dependent lobes of the lung, (2) lasts 14 to 21 days in untreated cases, (3) stimulates the formation of specific antibodies during convalescence, (4) stimulates the production of cold agglutinins or other nonspecific antibodies in more severely ill individuals, (5) responds to treatment with erythromycin or tetracycline and its analogues, and (6) almost always heals without sequelae.

ETIOLOGY. *Mycoplasma pneumoniae* (formerly known as PPLO or the Eaton agent organism), which belongs to the class Mollicutes, order Mycoplasmatales, family Mycoplasmataceae, and genus *Mycoplasma,* is the etiologic agent of mycoplasma pneumonia (syn. *Mycoplasma pneumoniae* pneumonia) (Tully, 1978). Mycoplasmas are the smallest (0.3 nm in diameter) free-living microorganisms capable of replicating in cell-free media. On appropriate media they form microscopic colonies of 50 to 250 nm in diameter (see Fig. 2, Chapter 57). Individual mycoplasmas may be coccobacillary or filamentous. They contain DNA and RNA and possess a lipophilic, triple-layered limiting membrane, but they lack a cell wall. *M. pneumoniae* ferments glucose, produces peroxide, and hemolyzes erythrocytes layered over colonies on agar media. These characteristics differentiate it from other mycoplasmas (see Table 3, Chapter 57). Unlike bacteria, *M. pneumoniae* incorporates, although it does not synthesize, sterols into its cell membrane.

PATHOGENESIS AND PATHOLOGY. The respiratory tract is the primary target of *M. pneumoniae*; infections occur at all anatomic levels including the oropharynx, trachea, bronchi, and lungs. Clinical pneumonia develops in 3 to 10 per cent of infected individuals in "open" populations and in 50 per cent of infected individuals in the family environment. Mycoplasma infection is endemic throughout the world, but superimposed epidemics occur every four or five years. Infrequently, involvement of other organs such as the central nervous system, pancreas, joints, skin, heart, and pericardium may be associated with *M. pneumoniae* infection. The mode of spread to these organs has not been documented, although it is probably hematogenous.

M. pneumoniae spreads by infectious droplets from person to person. Aerosol particles less than 5 nm in diameter reach the lower respiratory tract directly, but larger particles deposit on the nasal and upper respiratory tract passages. Colonization of the respiratory tract occurs readily and persists for days or weeks.

The effect of *M. pneumoniae* infection on the respiratory tract seems to involve multiple factors whose importance and interrelations are unresolved (Archer, 1979). *M. pneumoniae* attaches to neuraminic acid residues on ciliated epithelial cells and stops ciliary activity with subsequent destruction of cilia and cell surfaces. Attachment may be mediated by glycoproteins in the membrane of the mycoplasma. The infection is superficial (see Fig. 1 in Chapter 57); intracellular organisms have not been observed by electron microscopy. *M. pneumoniae* does not produce endotoxin or exotoxins; it produces hydrogen peroxide, which may be toxic to cells if a sufficient concentration of peroxide is maintained at the cell surface by close association of the mycoplasma and the cell. The organism is motile, although it lacks flagella, and this property may enhance its pathogenic potential. An actin-like protein, which has been extracted from *M. pneumoniae*, may be involved in motility of this organism.

While antibody to *M. pneumoniae* appears to mediate recovery from infection and resistance to reinfection, cellular immune responses also may be involved, since *M. pneumoniae* stimulates lymphocyte transformation and production of macrophage migration inhibition factor (Whittlestone, 1976). Peribronchial mononuclear infiltrates that characterize *M. pneumoniae* infection support this thesis. IgA secretory antibody in nasal secretions and complement-mediated lysis may play a prominent role in preventing infection. C1 is membrane-bound by *M. pneumoniae*. Circulating antibody to *M. pneumoniae* correlates with protection from infection, but this protection wanes and reinfections can occur five years after the first infection.

Multiple autoantibodies develop during *M. pneumoniae* infections including anti-red cell (cold agglutinins), anti-brain, antilung, and antiliver antibodies. Antibodies also develop to other bacteria including streptococcus MG and reagin-like antibody that yields false-positive tests for syphilis. These nonspecific, that is, nonmycoplasma-reactive, antibodies may contribute to the pathogenicity of disease through autoimmune mechanisms. The pneumonia caused by *M. pneumoniae* may be influenced by antigen-antibody reactions in the lung. Infection in childhood may sensitize the child so that subsequent infections with *M. pneumoniae* are more severe. Circulating immune complexes have been detected and may contribute to some of the extrapulmonary manifestations of this infection. Immune mechanisms may be involved in the pathogenesis of central nervous system disease. *M. pneumoniae* has not been isolated from brain tissue of patients with central nervous system involvement, except in one case.

M. pneumoniae causes a patchy, interstitial pneumonia with acute and chronic inflammation and swollen alveolar lining cells. The bronchiolar walls are thickened by congestion and edema. There is an intraluminal exudate of polymorphonuclear leukocytes, epithelial cells, and proteinaceous debris. Perivascular and peribronchial cuffing by lymphocytes may be prominent (see Fig. 3A, Chapter 57). In experimental infections of hamsters, the histopathologic changes develop slowly in primary infections and rapidly in reinfection.

CLINICAL MANIFESTATIONS. Characteristically, the onset of *M. pneumoniae* pneumonia is insidious. A nonproductive cough is the most common first symptom (Mufson and Zollar, 1975). Later, the cough produces white and watery or mucoid sputum. Blood-tinged or blood-streaked sputum is infrequent and frank hemoptysis is rare. Fever of 100 to 103° F develops in nearly all patients. Fever and the physical findings of pneumonia last for one to two weeks in untreated patients. Headache is prominent and may be intensified during high fever.

Other common findings include chills, malaise, rhinorrhea, chest pain, and generalized myalgia. Most of these symptoms develop in at least half of the patients. Rales and rhonchi can be detected in three fourths of the patients with pneumonia but often are not evident until after the first few days of illness. Early in the course, the patient frequently appears much more ill than the physical findings indicate, but the pulmonary findings increase after a few days. Although these clinical features are characteristic of mycoplasma pneumonia, they do not differentiate it from other nonbacterial pneumonias.

Tympanitis occurs in 10 per cent of patients with mycoplasma pneumonia. Bullous myringitis, which develops less often, is characterized by large hemorrhagic bullae on the tympanic membrane that heal without scarring. *M. pneumoniae* can be isolated from the bullae.

Mycoplasma pneumonia usually occurs unilaterally in the lower lobe. Bilateral infiltration occurs in about one fourth of cases; upper lobe involvement is less frequent. The radiographic appearance of mycoplasma pneumonia (Fig. 1) is diffusely reticulonodular, segmental, or lobar (Putnam et al., 1975). The infiltrate often radiates from the hilum to the base of the lung. Radiographically, mycoplasma pneumonia cannot be distinguished from other nonbacterial pneumonias. Unilateral or bilateral pleural effusions occasionally occur, but they are usually very small and almost always resolve completely.

Routine laboratory examinations are consistent with any nonbacterial infection. Leukocytosis occurs in only 15 per

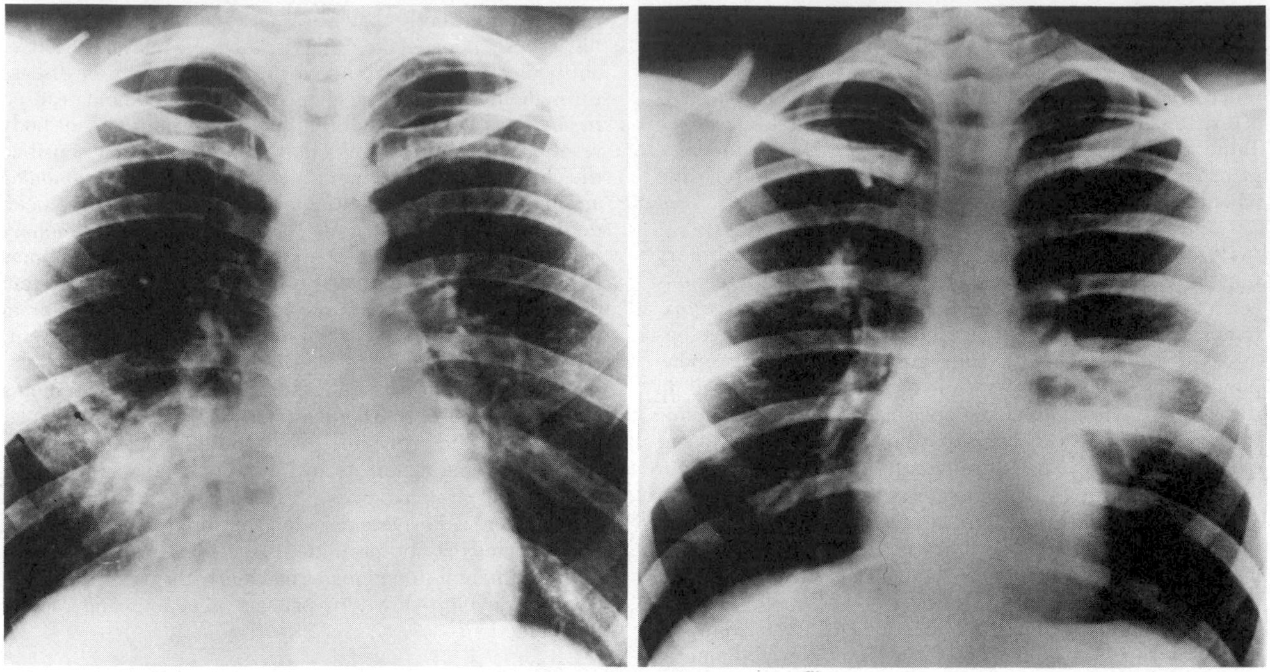

Figures 1A and 1B. Mycoplasma pneumonia in two patients illustrating segmental infiltrate radiating from hilum.

cent of the clinically evident cases, and the erythrocyte sedimentation rate is elevated in only about one third of cases.

Cold agglutinins develop in one half of all patients with mycoplasma pneumonia, but in a higher percentage of severely ill individuals. A titer greater than 1:40 can be detected in a single serum specimen obtained early in the course of the illness, and cold agglutinin antibodies rise fourfold or more during convalescence. Cold agglutinins represent a nonspecific antibody response, and this finding by itself is not diagnostic of *M. pneumoniae* infection. Rising titers of type-specific *M. pneumoniae* antibodies appear during convalescence (see Diagnosis). When high levels of specific IgM *M. pneumoniae* antibody develop early after the onset of illness, especially in children and young adults, they suggest recent infection with *M. pneumoniae*.

COMPLICATIONS AND SEQUELAE. Most patients with mycoplasma pneumonia recover without sequelae or complications. Symptoms and signs of pneumonia usually abate within 10 to 14 days. Antibiotics hasten recovery. Radiographic findings usually resolve within three to four weeks in untreated patients, but nearly one in five may have persistent infiltrates for as long as four months. Even these late-resolving pneumonias usually heal without sequelae.

Lung abscess occurs rarely in mycoplasma pneumonia (Cherry and Welliver, 1976). In these exceptional cases of cavity formation, which have been recognized in both adults and children, one or several small cavities form in areas of segmental consolidation and heal completely or with minimal scarring.

Rarely, mycoplasma pneumonia may present with lobar consolidation of one or more lobes. Except for the lobar involvement, the clinical features in these cases resemble those of atypical pneumonia, rather than a bacterial pneumonia (Cockroft, 1981).

Although an occasional pleural effusion develops in patients with mycoplasma pneumonia, residual pleural abnormalities are rare. Other rare sequelae include severe respiratory failure, adult respiratory distress syndrome, and disseminated pulmonary disease. Widespread pulmonary involvement is more common in children and adolescents. More severe pneumonia occurs in individuals with underlying autoimmune disorders.

In a few cases, mycoplasma pneumonia is complicated by involvement of other organs. These complications include myocarditis or pericarditis or both, the Stevens-Johnson syndrome, nonspecific exanthems, hemolytic anemia, arthritis, and central nervous system manifestations (Murray et al., 1975). The number of cases described with each of these complications is fewer than 200. No reliable data are available that permit calculation of complication rates. Considering the high incidence of *M. pneumoniae* infection (and pneumonia) and the few reports of cases with other manifestations, the rate of complications in mycoplasma pneumonia is probably less than one in several thousand cases.

In myocarditis, pericarditis, or perimyocarditis, fever, chest pain, pericardial friction rub, and an enlarged heart occur. Electrocardiographic examination indicates epicardial injury, nonspecific ST-T wave abnormalities, and arrhythmias. Deaths are rare.

Hemolytic anemia, another uncommon complication, is accompanied by cold agglutinin titers of 1:1000 or higher and occurs late in the course of the illness, when the cold agglutinin titers reach peak levels and the pneumonia begins to resolve. The hemolysis can vary from mild to marked. It is self-limiting, and complete recovery ensues in several weeks. The pathogenesis of the hemolytic anemia is autoimmune; 19S cold agglutinins formed in response to *M. pneumoniae* infection are specific antibodies to the I antigen of the red blood cell membrane as demonstrated by their failure to react with cord blood or fetal erythrocytes, which lack the I antigen. Anti-I cold agglutinins might be expected to form if *M. pneumoniae* contains antigens that cross-react with red blood cells. Although direct evidence that *M. pneumoniae* contains an I antigen (or an antigenic configuration similar to I antigen) is lacking, absorption experiments with antibody to this organism and I red blood cells suggest that possibility.

The central nervous system manifestations of *M. pneumoniae* infection span the spectrum of possible nervous tissue infection: aseptic meningitis, meningoencephalitis, cerebellar ataxia, hemiplegia, transverse myelitis, polyradiculitis, and psychosis. More than half of patients with central nervous system disease caused by *M. pneumoniae* also have had prior or simultaneous pulmonary involvement. The case fatality rate overall with central nervous system involvement is approximately 10 per cent.

GEOGRAPHIC VARIATIONS. Mycoplasma pneumonia occurs worldwide in both temperate and tropical climates. It has been recognized in all countries where specific tests for its identification have been employed.

DIAGNOSIS. Specific laboratory procedures must be used for the definitive diagnosis of mycoplasma pneumonia (Clyde, 1979). The organism can be recovered on special supplemented media (see Chapter 57) from sputa, throat swabs, pleural fluids, or tissues. The specimen is inoculated directly onto agar plates or into a diphasic broth. Small colonies appear on the agar in 10 to 12 days (longer in some instances). They can be identified as *M. pneumoniae* by metabolic characteristics and by growth neutralization tests using antibody-impregnated disks. Similarly, in 10 to 12 days spherules and acid production appear in the diphasic medium. Growth in diphasic media can be confirmed by subculturing the organism onto agar, and specific identification can be established by disk neutralization tests. Guinea pig erythrocytes suspended in buffer will rapidly adsorb to colonies of *M. pneumoniae* but not to other *Mycoplasma* organisms. If the red cells are added in an agar overlay, hemolysis around the colonies can be seen with the naked eye within a day or two.

A fourfold or greater rise in specific antibody during convalescence is also diagnostic of mycoplasma infection. IgM cold agglutinins develop in half of all cases and in a greater percentage of the more severely ill.

Antibody responses to *M. pneumoniae* can be measured by any of several procedures: indirect immunofluorescence, complement fixation, metabolic inhibition, tetrazolium reduction inhibition, indirect hemagglutination, mycoplasmacidal assay, enzyme-linked immunosorbent assay (ELISA), and radioimmunoprecipitation. The individual antibody assays differ significantly in sensitivity, ease of performance, and cost. Immunofluorescence, mycoplasmacidal assay, and radioimmunoprecipitation tests are very sensitive, but they are complex and are used mainly for research purposes. The ELISA is sensitive and easy to perform. The other tests are only moderately sensitive, but they are easier to perform and are less expensive. Of the tests applicable for the diagnostic laboratory, the complement fixation and metabolic inhibition tests have been used most widely; the ELISA may become more widely used as a routine diagnostic test since it is easily performed and both IgG- and IgM-specific *M. pneumoniae* antibodies can be determined using this test. In less than 2 per cent of cases, the presence of rheumatoid factor may interfere with the detection of IgM-specific *M. pneumoniae* antibody by ELISA (Dussaix, 1983). Since antibody to *M. pneumoniae* can be measured by using the standard complement-fixation procedure, most diagnostic laboratories use this test for antibody determinations. The test can be done with either the lipid antigen of *M. pneumoniae* or the whole organism. The lipid antigen provides a more sensitive antigen and yields higher antibody levels. However, it shares similarities with galactolipids of plants (vegetables), and nonspecific antibody may be measured in individuals sensitized to these galactolipids.

Specific antibody to *M. pneumoniae* becomes detectable within the first two weeks after the onset of infection, reaches peak levels in two to six months, and may persist for four or more years. By contrast, cold agglutinins develop in the first few days after *M. pneumoniae* infection but usually disappear within six months, as is generally true of IgM antibodies. There is no cross-relationship between specific *M. pneumoniae* antibody and cold agglutinin antibody. If tests for specific *M. pneumoniae* antibody are not available, high titers of cold agglutinins are strong presumptive evidence of infection with *M. pneumoniae* and justifies specific antibiotic treatment.

TREATMENT. Tetracycline, 2 g daily in four divided doses, or erythromycin, 1 to 2 g daily in four divided doses, for 10 days will effectively treat the disease, lessen the severity of symptoms and signs, and shorten the course of the illness (Mufson and Zollar, 1975). (The analogues of tetracycline are also effective in appropriate dosages.) Although the severity and duration of disease are reduced by treatment with these antibiotics, shedding of *M. pneumoniae* usually continues for some time after therapy has been discontinued. In addition to antibiotic treatment, the usual supportive measures for pneumonia are helpful: bed rest, adequate diet, abundant liquids, antipyretics for fever, antitussives, and bronchodilators.

PROPHYLAXIS. Immunoprophylaxis for high-risk populations is under investigation. Inactivated and live attenuated vaccines have been tested experimentally in volunteers. Inactivated vaccines that were tested for efficacy in large groups of volunteers proved only marginally effective. Although they stimulated antibody production, their protective efficacy was relatively low. Live attenuated *M. pneumoniae* vaccines may provide a better means of protection, but they are still being developed. Temperature-sensitive mutants, organisms attenuated by multiple passages, and *M. pneumoniae* polysaccharide vaccines are under investigation.

References

Archer, D. B.: Pathogenic mechanisms of mycoplasmas. Nature 277:268, 1979.

Cherry, J. D., and Welliver, R. C.: *Mycoplasma pneumoniae* infections of adults and children (medical progress). West J Med 125:47, 1976.

Clyde, W. A., Jr.: *Mycoplasma pneumoniae* infections of man. In Tully, J.

G., and Whitcomb, R. F. (eds.): The Mycoplasmas. Vol. II, Human and Animal Mycoplasmas. New York, Academic Press, 1979, p. 275.

Cockroft, D. W. and Stilwell, G. A.: Lobar pneumonia caused by *Mycoplasma pneumoniae*. Can Med Assoc J 124:1463, 1981.

Dussaix, E., Slim, A. and Tournier, P.: Comparison of enzyme-linked immunosorbent assay (ELISA) and complement-fixation test for the detection of *Mycoplasma pneumoniae* antibodies. J Clin Path 36:228, 1983.

Mufson, M. A., and Zollar, L. M.: Non-bacterial respiratory infections. DM November, 1975.

Murray, H. W., Masur, H., Senterfit, L. B., and Roberts, R. B.: The protean manifestations of *Mycoplasma pneumoniae* infection in adults. Am J Med 58:229, 1975.

Putnam, C. E., Curtis, A. M., Simeone, J. F., and Jensen, P.: Mycoplasma pneumonia. Clinical and roentgenographic patterns. Am J Roentgenol 91:560, 1975.

Tully, J. G.: Biology of the mycoplasmas. In McGarrity, G. J., Murphy, D. G., and Nichols, W. W. (eds.): Mycoplasma infection of cell cultures. New York, Plenum Publishing Company, 1978, p. 1.

Whittlestone, P.: Immunity to mycoplasmas causing respiratory diseases in man and animals. Adv Vet Sci Comp Med 20:277, 1976.

115
PSITTACOSIS

Stanley D. Freedman, M.D.

Psittacosis is a disease of birds that is transmissible to humans. There is a variable pattern of disease in the avian species, with either minor illness and prolonged excretion of the causative agent or severe rapidly evolving disease. Mortality rates may be over 60 per cent. Similarly, in humans the disease ranges from subclinical cases to fulminant infections with mortality rates in some epidemics of 20 per cent. At first only psittacine birds (parrots, parakeets, cockatiels, macaws, and other birds of the order Psittaciformis) were regarded as sources of human infection, but now the disease is known to affect many other species of birds such as pigeons, turkeys, chickens, ducks, canaries, sea gulls, egrets, and chaparral birds. Thus the more inclusive term ornithosis was suggested for this disease. The causative agent is *Chlamydia psittaci;* therefore, the generic term psittacosis is preferred for human disease.

ETIOLOGY. The agent responsible for psittacosis belongs to the genus *Chlamydia*, formerly called *Bedsonia*. The chlamydiae have been placed in their own order, the Chlamydiales, because of a unique developmental cycle described in Chapter 56. Earlier, they were considered to be large viruses because of their size and obligatory intracellular parasitism. Over the years the differences from viruses and the similarities to bacteria have been delineated (Moulder, 1964; Manire, 1977). Chlamydiae contain both DNA and RNA, and divide by binary fission. They appear on light microscopy as gram-negative bacilli about one third the size of *E. coli*, and, in fact, their cell walls are structurally and chemically analogous to those of gram-negative bacteria. They have ribosomes that are similar in size to those of bacteria. As would be expected *C. psittaci* is susceptible to antibiotics. There may be multiple serotypes of *C. psittaci* because multiple infections in individual patients have been documented.

PATHOGENESIS. Psittacosis in humans develops after exposure to discharges of infected birds and is therefore a true zoonosis. Affected birds demonstrate nonspecific signs of disease. Chlamydiae infect most of the organs and are shed in secretions from the eyes and nostrils as well as in the feces. In addition, the organism remains viable in dried feces, and can be cultured from bird feathers and dust in the vicinity of the infected birds. The agent can be shed for prolonged periods by asymptomatic birds or by birds who have recovered from infection. One should consider all avian species as potential sources. Human-to-human transmission is rare but has occurred and is a problem for hospital personnel. Disease acquired by this route is considered more severe than that acquired directly from an avian source.

Latent infections and the carrier state are recognized in birds (Manire, 1977). In parrots and parakeets persistently high antibody levels are associated with latent psittacosis infection (usually in the spleen). These birds show some degree of resistance to reinfection, but they are prone to relapses when environmental conditions are adverse. Australian budgerigars, a common host, excrete large amounts of chlamydiae through the alimentary canal during egg laying and hatching. Their nestlings are then infected, and a chain of latent infection is established. When infected birds are introduced into aviaries, susceptible contacts more frequently develop latent or subclinical infections with repeated relapses than lethal infections. These features explain the persistence of *C. psittaci* in birds.

The route of entry into humans is the respiratory tract in nearly all cases, but infection may occur after a bite from an infected bird. After inhalation, the organism spreads hematogenously to the reticuloendothelial system, where it matures before clinical illness develops. It is unclear if the subsequent pulmonary involvement represents progressive pneumonitis originating at the site of implantation of the droplet nuclei or if the lung is infected hematogenously, as are the other organ systems.

Antibody develops between the third and fifth week of infection and gradually wanes thereafter. Cellular immunity is thought to be important, since reinfection is rare. However, prolonged illness and carrier states with shedding of the agent in the respiratory secretions have been described, suggesting modulation of the immune response (Lammert, 1981).

PATHOLOGY. The initial inflammatory reaction in the lungs begins with a polymorphonuclear infiltrate, and this intra-alveolar cellular exudative process resembles a bacterial infection. Later this changes to a lymphocytic and mononuclear cell reaction in the alveoli and interstitium. Both prominent alveolar pneumocytic hyperplasia with sloughing and erythroleukophagocytosis have been noted. Abundant fibrin is present. Varying degrees of edema, necrosis, and hemorrhage occur. Pulmonary macrophages containing basophilic cytoplasmic inclusion bodies, if present, characterize the disease as psittacosis. These inclusion bodies have been called LCL bodies after the independent discoverers, Levinthal, Coles, and Lillie (Coles, 1930; Levinthal, 1930). Unlike influenza, the tracheobronchial epithelium is spared (Yow, 1959). Grossly, lobular pneumonia is most commonly seen. Hepatic inflammation with intralobular focal necrosis occurs, and elementary bodies can be found in Kupffer cells. Inflammatory changes in other organ systems, notably the pericardium and myocardium, have been described, and the basophilic inclusion bodies may be seen in these tissues as well. Direct central nervous system involvement is distinctly unusual; meningeal exudate containing the inclusions has been reported (Walton, 1954).

CLINICAL MANIFESTATIONS. It is important to stress that the signs and symptoms of psittacosis vary greatly, and this accounts for the difficulties of diagnosis. The clinical course ranges from subclinical to fatal infections. The incubation period is 7 to 14 days but may be longer. The early symptoms are sore throat, anorexia, weakness, malaise, myalgia, and headache. Photophobia, nausea, and vomiting are less often reported. Chills are common; true rigors are not. A nonproductive cough is characteristic of the disease but, rarely, may be absent. Hemoptysis is unusual, and chest pain due to pleuritis or pericardial inflammation is infrequent. Epistaxis occurs in up to one fourth of the cases. Confusion and mild disorientation are the most common sensorial changes. Of the many symptoms, diffuse headache is almost always present and is so intense that it may dominate the clinical picture. In fact, the presentation of profound headache and weakness with only minimal pulmonary signs or symptoms is typical for psittacosis.

Fever is the most constant sign, reaching 39 to 40° C at the height of illness, and is sometimes accompanied by a relative bradycardia. A faint macular eruption reminiscent of rose spots is described (Horder's spots). Pharyngitis and cervical adenopathy may be present. Tachypnea and fine crepitant rales are the usual pulmonary findings and often occur late in the course of the disease. Percussion flatness, altered tactile fremitus, egophony, and whispered pectoriloquy are frequently absent, although consolidation can occur. Hepatosplenomegaly is common, not unexpectedly, considering the pathogenesis of this infection. The finding of splenomegaly with pneumonia should alert one to the diagnosis of psittacosis. Signs of meningeal irritation and focal central nervous system involvement are extremely rare. Icterus, cyanosis, signs of congestive heart failure, and coma are manifestations of fulminant infections and fortunately are uncommon.

Inflammatory heart disease may be part of *C. psittaci* infection. Myocarditis, frequent in some avian species, is the most commonly reported manifestation; pericarditis is rare (Sutton, 1967; Kundu, 1979). Endocarditis has been reported from two continents, and the presentation is subacute (Jones, 1982). This is an important consideration in cases of culture-negative endocarditis.

The similarity of these signs and symptoms with those of other diseases is evident. The differential diagnosis includes encephalitis, influenza, typhoid fever, mycoplasmal pneumonia, Q fever, bacterial pneumonia, Legionnaires' disease, primary coccidioidomycosis, and tuberculosis. A history of bird exposure is obviously important.

Psittacosis acquired from parrots or parakeets is usually more serious than that from pigeons or turkeys. Mild disease, if not treated, usually subsides within two to three weeks with the fever and pneumonia running a parallel course. More chronic illness is recognized. With therapy, there is prompt clinical response within 24 to 72 hours.

COMPLICATIONS AND SEQUELAE. Clinical relapse is recognized but is quite unusual. Thrombophlebitis of the lower extremities occurs during convalescence, and pulmonary infarction is feared (Jörgensen and Steffensen, 1956). Psittacosis does not predispose to secondary bacterial infections (Yow, 1959). Sequelae due to permanently altered organ systems are not recognized except that epidemiologic studies suggest that heart infection may damage valves (Ward, 1978). Disseminated intravascular coagulation has been described.

GEOGRAPHIC VARIATIONS IN DISEASE. Since this is a true zoonosis acquired from birds, the distribution of cases is widespread. It was first recognized as a disease in Switzerland and later in France and Germany. Soon thereafter cases were reported in many different countries. Psittacine birds everywhere have been recognized as the source. When they are shipped from one country to another there are outbreaks of infection among the birds. High rates of infection among birds are associated with the adverse conditions that occur during shipping. Some variations in incidence and severity are noted in the disease transmitted from other species of birds. In the United States psittacosis is an occupational disease seen most commonly in processing plants; the reservoir is the turkey. In eastern Europe the duck is an important source.

DIAGNOSIS. Clinical signs and symptoms are not diagnostic. The importance of the epidemiologic history has been stressed. Similarly, routine laboratory studies are not helpful. Leukopenia may be present early in the disease in about 25 per cent of patients. Leukocytosis develops during convalescence. The sedimentation rate is usually normal. Mild proteinuria may be present early. Cold agglutinins are absent. Although headache and mild sensorial changes may dominate the clinical picture, the cerebrospinal fluid is normal (mild pleocytosis is the exception). The x-ray findings vary widely; the most common pattern is a patchy infiltrate in the lower lobes. Pleural effusions are very uncommon, although there is pleural involvement pathologically.

Early in the disease *C. psittaci* can be isolated from the blood and sputum, and it persists in the sputum during convalescence (Meyer and Eddie, 1951). The chlamydiae are isolated from infected material by inoculating the material intraperitoneally into mice, into the yolk sac of embryonated hen's eggs, or into tissue cultures. A tissue culture technique using irradiated or IUDR-treated McCoy cells has recently been reported to increase the yield of chlamydiae. Such isolation procedures are not generally available, and the yield remains low in human infections.

The serologic test most widely used is the complement fixation test. This uses a heat-stable chlamydial group antigen prepared from infected chick embryos. With this antigen, the complement fixation antibody reaches a maximum titer that ranges from 1:32 to 1:256 during the third to fifth week of illness, and slowly diminishes thereafter. A fourfold rise in titer can be demonstrated between acute and convalescent serum specimens. The rise in titer may be delayed by therapy. Problems with anticomplementary sera and the presence of chlamydial antibodies in certain lots of normal guinea pig complement have led to some of the difficulties with this technique. The antigen used for CF tests is a group-specific antigen that measures antibody response to all chlamydiae and is therefore not specific for psittacosis. A radioisotope precipitation technique and an indirect fluorescent antibody test have been used in special laboratories. Recently, the enzyme-linked immunosorbent assay method has been adopted for chlamydial infections and may become the preferred serologic procedure.

TREATMENT. Tetracycline is the treatment of choice. The usual adult dose is 500 mg orally every six hours; it is usually continued for 12 to 14 days to prevent relapse. This treatment causes defervescence and clinical improvement within 24 to 72 hours. Intravenous fluids, oxygen, and other supportive measures may be necessary. Intravenous penicillin in a dose of one million units every four hours can be used as an alternate form of therapy. Experience with erythromycin and rifampin is limited. The mortality rate may reach 20 per cent with no treatment.

PROPHYLAXIS. There is no human vaccine, and vaccines for psittacine birds have not been generally effective. However, chlamydial infections in psittacines and poultry are effectively controlled by the incorporation of chlortetracycline in the feed during quarantine. Properly administered and supervised programs should eliminate the reservoir for human psittacosis, but this treatment program does not always eliminate the infection in birds. Unfortunately, the disease remains an important occupational hazard of poultry workers (Schacter, 1978).

References

Coles, A. C.: Micro-organisms in psittacosis. Lancet 1:1011, 1930.

Jones, R. B., Priest, J. B., and Kuo, C.: Subacute chlamydial endocarditis. JAMA 247:655, 1982.

Jörgensen, M., and Steffensen, K.: Ornithosis: An analysis of 44 human cases with positive complement fixation tests. Dan Med Bull 3:20, 1956.

Kundu, C. R., and Scott, M.E.: Pericardial effusion complicating psittacosis infection. Br Heart J 42:603, 1979.

Lammert, J. K., and Wyrick, P. B.: Modulation of the host immune response as a result of *Chlamydia psittaci* infection. Infect and Immun 35:537, 1982.

Levinthal, W.: Die Atiologie der Psittacosis. Klin Wochen Schr 9:654, 1930.

Manire, G. P.: Biologic characteristics of chlamydiae. In Hobson, D., and Holmes, K. (eds.): Nongonococcal Arthritis and Related Infections. Washington, D.C., American Society of Microbiology, 1977, p. 167.

Meyer, K., and Eddie, B.: Human carrier of the psittacosis virus. J Infect Dis 88:109, 1951.

Moulder, J. W.: The psittacosis group as bacteria. In Ciba Lectures in Microbial Biochemistry, New York, John Wiley & Sons, 1964.

Schacter, J.: Psittacosis: The reservoir persists. J Infect Dis 137:44, 1978.

Sutton, G. C., Morrissey, R. A., Tobin, J. R., and Anderson, T. O.: Pericardial and myocardial disease associated with serologic evidence of infection by agents of the psittacosis-lymphogranuloma venereum group (chlamydiaceae). Circulation 36:830, 1967.

Walton, K. W.: The pathology of a fatal case of psittacosis showing intracytoplasmic inclusions in the meninges. J Pathol Bacteriol 68:565, 1954.

Ward, C.: "Rheumatic" heart disease, psittacosis and the importance of epidemiology. Am Heart J 95:266, 1978.

Yow, E.: The pathology of psittacosis: A report of two cases with hepatitis. Am J Med 27:739, 1959.

116

Q FEVER

WALTER P. G. TURCK, M.B., F.R.C.P., F.R.C.P (EDIN.)

Q fever is a rickettsial zoonosis of sudden onset with influenza-like symptoms of fever, sweating, and severe headache. Over half the patients have a pneumonitis resembling that found in viral pneumonias. Usually a self-limited acute disease, it may be subacute or chronic (see Chapter 207). In the United States it is considered to be one of the three rickettsial diseases of greatest importance (Woodward, 1973).

It differs from other rickettsial diseases as follows: a rash may occur but does not form part of the typical picture; propagation of the disease does not depend on an arthropod vector; the etiological agent is filterable, more resistant to physical and chemical factors, and does not produce agglutinins against the X strains of *Proteus vulgaris* that are responsible for the Weil-Felix reaction. For these reasons the organism was assigned to a separate genus, *Coxiella*, in honor of Cox, who had described it in the United States, with the qualification *burnetii* retained for Burnet, who had recognized it almost simultaneously in Australia. The name "Q (for query) fever," adopted by Derrick as a temporary expedient until further knowledge allowed a better name, has persisted. In the French literature the name "la maladie de Derrick et Burnet" exists as an alternative.

ETIOLOGY. The etiologic agent is *Coxiella burnetii*, a pleomorphic rod that is between 0.3 and 0.7 μ long and is occasionally plump or coccoid in shape—an appearance consistent with that of rickettsiae. It is an obligate, intracellular parasite that grows in the cytoplasm but not in the nuclei of endothelial and serosal cells, where it may be present in large, closely packed masses. It is transmissible to guinea pigs and mice, and may be grown and maintained in the yolk sac of the chick embryo by serial passage. In the guinea pig it induces a fever that lasts for four to six days when it circulates in the blood, but it does not cause a tunica or scrotal reaction. Guinea pigs that develop fever become immune to further infection. Many organisms are found in the liver and spleen of infected mice.

C. burnetii can undergo a host-controlled variation (phase variation) that is in many ways similar to the rough-smooth variations of *Streptococcus pneumoniae*. Rickettsial suspensions prepared from the yolk sac of chick embryos infected with recent isolates from patients, animals, or arthropods will not fix complement with convalescent phase sera from patients with Q fever. After serial passage in the chick embryo, most strains alter and will then fix complement with these sera. The original nonreactive state and the reactive state induced by passage in the chick embryo are called, respectively, phase I and phase II. Rickettsiae in phase II can be made to revert to phase I by passage through guinea pigs, mice, or hamsters (Stoker and Fiset, 1956). This definition of phase variation by complement fixation has been questioned, and other serologic methods of determining the phase of *C. burnetii* have been proposed. Since a transition phase, similar to a pure phase II serologically but more virulent, has been recognized, the phase state of a strain may be determined by other criteria based on its physicochemical characteristics, susceptibility to nonspecific phagocytosis by polymorphonuclear leukocytes, and ability to multiply in the mouse spleen and in cell cultures (Brezina, 1978).

Strains of *C. burnetii* also vary in virulence and in sensitivity of detecting antibody in human and guinea pig sera.

EPIDEMIOLOGY

Incidence and Distribution. Q fever is a disease of men rather than of women because of occupational exposure, and usually affects those between 20 and 60 years of age. Symptomatic infection in childhood is rare, but subclinical infection, which is usually acquired by ingestion of milk, is not uncommon. In areas of high Q fever endemicity, human fetal infection has been demonstrated, but whether such fetal infection has any later effect on the developing child is unknown.

Abattoir workers, farm workers, shepherds, dairy workers, veterinary personnel, wool sorters, and tanners are particularly liable to infection, as are newcomers to any community that has already acquired immunity from previous exposure.

In many regions a seasonal variation in incidence occurs, related in most cases to farming activity. Higher incidences are to be expected at times of calving, lambing, or shearing. Dry summers encourage airborne propagation.

Q fever is found throughout the world with the exception of Sweden, Norway, Iceland, and New Zealand. The few reported Scandinavian patients were probably infected while traveling or working in the Mediterranean region, where Q fever is common.

Transmission. One reason for the success of *C. burnetii* has been its ability to grow equally well in the intestine of ticks, the reproductive tract of cows or sheep, and the respiratory tract of humans (Marmion, 1953).

The organism has been found in at least 30 species of ticks, and since transovarian transmission occurs in many of these, an arthropod reservoir may be recognized (Fig. 1). The tick facilitates a wildlife cycle in which the participating animal varies in different parts of the world. The bandicoot and kangaroo in Australia and the merion in North Africa are typical examples. A similar relationship may exist between some argasid ticks and birds. Although these reservoirs maintain *C. burnetii* in the world, they are of little direct relevance to Q fever in man, for whom livestock represents a more important reservoir. However,

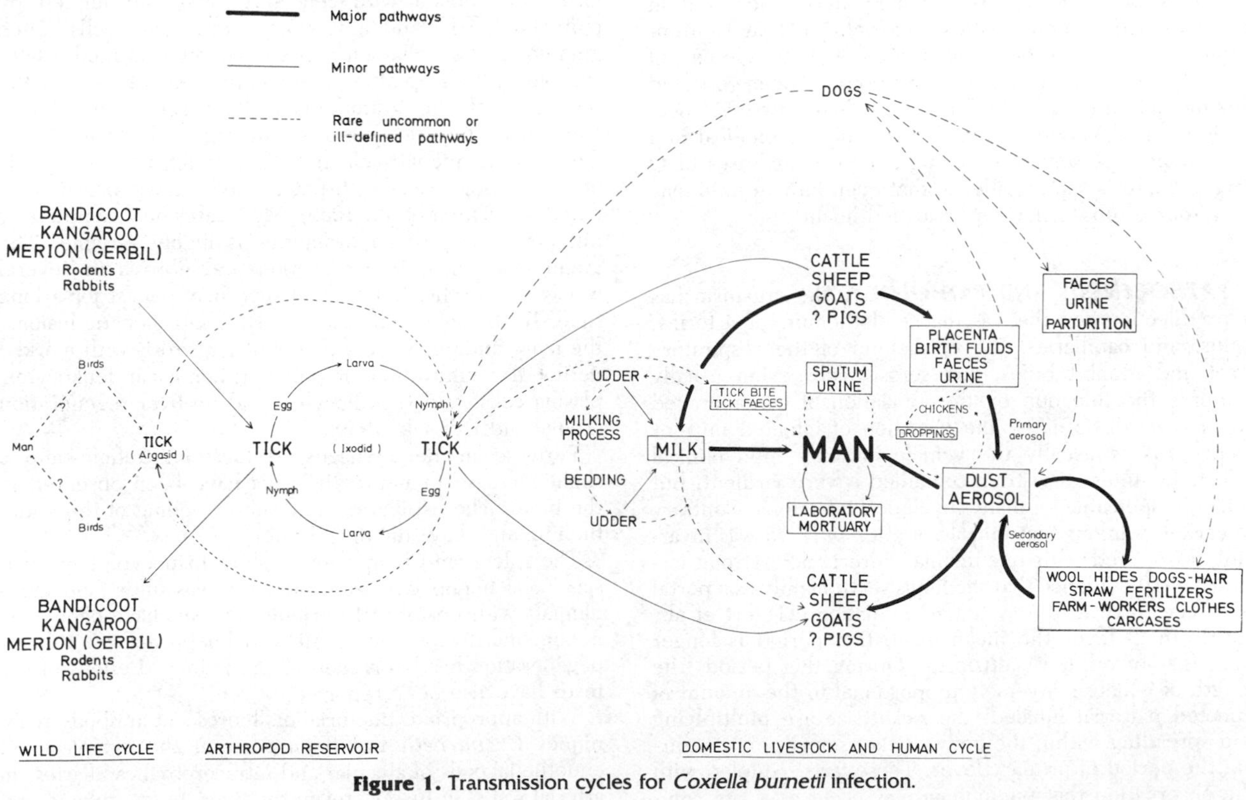

Figure 1. Transmission cycles for *Coxiella burnetii* infection.

on rare occasions a connection between the two cycles may be established, as when the infection is transmitted to sheep by ticks that have previously fed on kangaroos, or when infectious tick feces are inhaled by man. Man rarely gets Q fever from a tick bite.

C. burnetii infection is widespread among cattle, sheep, and goats. The organism may be present in high concentrations in the placental and birth fluids and in the feces and urine of these animals.

Human Q fever is acquired by inhalation of infected aerosols. *C. burnetii* may be disseminated as a primary aerosol after parturition by an infected animal. Alternatively, because the organism is resistant to heat, drying, and sunlight, a *C. burnetii*–laden dust often forms from contaminated birth fluids, blood, feces, or urine. Such dusts may be disseminated by dry and windy weather or carried on fomites such as wool, hides, farmworkers' clothing, straw, and packing materials, to be released later as secondary aerosols in other environments. Farm dogs, particularly if fed on infected placentas, and farmyard chickens may contribute their own excreta to this part of the cycle.

Lower but significant concentrations of the organism are found in the udders and milk of infected cows. Drinking infected raw milk accounts for most sporadic cases. The protective or neutralizing properties of whey antibody in infected milk are a possible explanation for the low incidence of clinical Q fever arising from this mode of transmission.

Within the herd or flock the infection is probably maintained by inhalation of infected dusts and aerosols. In some herds the organism may be transferred from udder to udder by the milking process or by animal bedding.

Man-to-man infection is extremely uncommon, but in rare instances patients with *C. burnetii* in their sputum, urine, or placenta have been identified as sources of infection. A high incidence of infection has been reported among laboratory workers handling infected tissues, specimens, and laboratory animals, and among medical and paramedical personnel attending autopsies on cases of Q fever. There is some evidence that even human milk may be a source of infection for breast-fed infants.

PATHOGENESIS AND PATHOLOGY. The organism has a predilection for the vascular endothelium of arteries, veins, and capillaries, the epithelium of the respiratory tract and renal tubules, and serosal cells. Man usually acquires the infection by the inhalation of contaminated aerosols or dusts or by the ingestion of infected milk or food. Milk is usually the vehicle for only mild clinical infections unless the strain contained is very virulent, but milk is responsible for many subclinical infections. Contrary to earlier opinions that inhalation of *C. burnetii* was invariably associated with pneumonia there is now strong circumstantial evidence that the lungs serve mainly as a portal of direct entry to the systemic circulation (Tiggert et al., 1961). In Q fever the mean incubation period is longer than that of other rickettsioses. During this period, the length of which is inversely proportional to the amount of infected material inhaled, the rickettsiae are multiplying and spreading within the body. Rickettsemia persists during the period of primary fever. These facts, coupled with the observation that pneumonia may occur as a late complication, indicate that Q fever is essentially a systemic infection (Derrick, 1973).

Acute Q fever is seldom fatal in otherwise healthy persons, but rare deaths have occurred from fulminating pneumonia or massive hepatic necrosis. Histopathologic studies of pneumonia in man are scarce because of limited autopsy material, but the hepatic lesion has become clarified through biopsies.

In fatal cases of severe pneumonia the consolidated areas may contain foci of suppuration and hemorrhage. The interlobar fissures and pleural surfaces may contain fibropurulent exudate and be associated with pleural effusions. The bronchi may be hyperemic and edematous. Microscopically, there has been severe focal necrotizing hemorrhagic intra-alveolar pneumonia with associated necrotizing bronchitis and bronchiolitis (Urso, 1975). The intra-alveolar infiltrate is fibrinous, and histiocytes, lymphocytes, and plasma cells predominate. Alveolar septa are swollen with monocytic infiltrates, but hyaline membranes are absent. A peribronchial interstitial infiltrate is often seen. The bronchi contain a similar fibrinocellular exudate with necrosis in the mucosa and desquamation of epithelium in the bronchioles. Pneumonitis of such severity is never seen in other rickettsial disease—apart from the more florid cases of scrub typhus. In surviving patients the organizing segmental pneumonia may present as a pseudotumor.

In the liver, abnormalities may be observed microscopically as early as the late incubation period (Dupont et al., 1971) and are invariably present once the disease is fully established (Powell, 1961). The earliest lesions are numerous small foci of histiocytes with fewer lymphocytes, polymorphonuclear leukocytes, and eosinophils, and no reticulin. Small areas of liver cell necrosis also occur as in viral hepatitis. A nonspecific progressive inflammatory infiltrate is seen in the portal triads. The histiocytic foci enlarge to form granulomata with central necrosis surrounded by epithelioid cells and a few Langhans' giant cells. Such granulomata are characteristically centered around a fatty vacuole with a ring of fibrin fibers present within or at the periphery of the granulomata (Pellegrin et al., 1980). Uninvolved hepatic cells may undergo mild to moderate focal cytoplasmic fatty change. Thickening and eosinophilia of the sinusoid walls with patchy necrosis are occasionally noted (Bernstein et al., 1965). Most cases heal completely, but persistence of abnormalities is highly variable. The granulomata heal by absorption and fibrosis in several weeks or months, but fatty change may persist for a long time. In the sole fatal case reported with hepatic lesions, the main findings were a panlobular necrosis with marked perilobular infiltration of polymorphonuclear leukocytes, plasma cells, and lymphocytes, and no liver regeneration (Tonge and Derrick, 1959).

Perivascular hemorrhages, cellular infiltration, and a slight increase in neuroglial cells have been observed in the brain. The capillaries may show swelling of the endothelium and may contain thrombi.

The spleen and lymph nodes show histiocytic hyperplasia. Focal hypoplasia, frank necrosis, vasculitis, and granulomata with peripheral fibrinoid deposits have been seen in bone marrow, and focal interstitial nephritis with tubular degeneration has been seen in the kidney. Lesions of the testis have also been reported.

With appropriate tinctorial or fluorescent antibody techniques *C. burnetii* has been seen in the cytoplasm of endothelial cells of alveolar and intracerebral capillaries, in arterial walls, in histiocytes in the liver, lungs, spleen, and testes, and in the neuroglial cells of the brain.

There may be a relative lymphocytosis in the blood and

elevation of the sedimentation rate. Rarely, an absolute lymphocytosis mimicking infectious mononucleosis may occur. Thrombocytopenia with increased numbers of megakaryocytes in the marrow smear has also been reported. Abnormal cephalin-cholesterol flocculation and thymol turbidity tests reflect increases in serum gamma globulin and IgM. Elevations of serum alkaline phosphatase and aminotransferases are common, but increases in the latter are invariably moderate.

CLINICAL FEATURES. The incubation period ranges from 11 to 26 days but is usually 18 to 20 days. Massive doses, as may be acquired in laboratory infections, may be associated with much shorter periods, whereas prolonged incubation probably represents minimal dosage.

The onset is sudden, with fever that rises progressively over two to four days to 39 to 40° C. At this point there may be marked prostration and delirium. High fever persists for another four to seven days and then falls by lysis to normal temperature within 15 days. Accompanying the fever is a severe retro-orbital or occipital headache. Arthralgias and muscular aches and pains in the calves and lumbar region are usual. Profuse sweats, chills, and occasional rigors also occur. There is general malaise, often accompanied by anorexia, nausea, diarrhea, or constipation. In milder cases the fever may occur in the evening only and be accompanied by no other symptoms.

The most striking physical finding is a relative bradycardia. The pharynx and tonsils may be hyperemic. The constant rash seen in other rickettsial diseases does not occur, but evanescent exanthems resembling those of measles, rubella, scarlet fever, or urticaria, and distributed over the shoulders, thorax, or trunk, have been described in 5 to 10 per cent of cases. Purpura is rare.

As described so far, the infection resembles influenza, and in many patients no further symptoms develop. In others there is pulmonary or hepatic involvement. Pneumonia occurs in just over half the patients. Cough due to bronchitis is common. On the third to fifth day there may be moderate dyspnea and a sense of constriction around the chest. The sputum may become purulent or slightly blood-stained. The physical signs vary from those of consolidation to small patches of basal crepitant rales. Poorly defined lobar or segmental infiltrates are seen in the x-ray. These infiltrates have hazy outlines and a ground glass appearance, are frequently multiple, and are usually in the lower lobes, often in association with linear atelectasis. They persist for 10 to 30 days and may recur.

Liver involvement is more common than originally thought. Moderate hepatomegaly may be detected in up to two thirds of patients, but jaundice is uncommon (Powell, 1961). Clinically, the picture may be very similar to that of viral hepatitis (Alkan et al., 1965).

Headache with neck stiffness is common, and the cerebrospinal fluid findings may be those of a mild aseptic meningitis. Febrile convulsions and encephalitis have occurred in childhood Q fever, but usually the infection is mild or inapparent at this age.

COMPLICATIONS AND SEQUELAE. In most patients the illness lasts up to 15 days, but fever may be prolonged in a continuous or intermittent form with persistent malaise for as long as eight weeks (Derrick, 1973). The more severe forms, found mostly in patients over the age of 40 or in those with liver involvement or impaired immune mechanisms, have a slow convalescence.

Complications are not rare. Thrombophlebitis, sometimes with pulmonary embolism or infarction, has been noted. Intermittent claudication has been attributed to Q fever arteritis. Myocarditis and pericarditis may occur separately or together and pericardial pain may dominate the clinical picture. Orchitis, epididymitis, parotitis, thyroiditis, and pancreatitis may be associated with Q fever. Pleural effusions are not uncommon, but ascites is rare. Arthritis, acute nephritis, and thrombocytopenia have been reported as separate complications. Nonimmune hemolytic anemia has been reported (Spelman, 1982). Encephalitis and encephalomyelitis may occur late in the disease. Other neurologic complications include neuritis, Guillain-Barré syndrome, extrapyramidal disease, dementia, toxic confusional states, and manic psychosis. Visual disturbances may be caused by retinal vasculitis, chorioretinitis, or uveitis. Abortion and sudden infant death syndrome may have been a complication of Q fever infection in a few instances (Ellis et al., 1983).

Recovery from acute Q fever is the rule, but infection with *C. burnetii* may become latent and persist for long periods. For fuller discussion of this subject and the clinical manifestations of the whole spectrum of chronic Q fever, including endocarditis, the reader is referred to Chapter 207.

Death from acute Q fever is extremely rare and usually occurs only in elderly and diseased patients.

Following recovery from acute Q fever, most patients enjoy life-long immunity, but rare cases of reinfection have been reported.

GEOGRAPHIC VARIATIONS IN DISEASE. Although the influenza-like symptoms are found in most outbreaks throughout the world, the pneumonic form of Q fever has been particularly common in Europe and America. In Southern Africa, hepatic manifestations are more common (Gear, 1980). Significant variations have occurred within smaller geographic limits. In Australia, the hepatic form predominates in Queensland, while most cases in Victoria have pneumonic features. In California, hepatic complications were rare in the south but relatively frequent in the north. A difference in the infecting strain possibly accounts for this phenomenon.

DIAGNOSIS. The diagnosis of Q fever should be considered whenever a patient with a fever of unknown origin, especially if accompanied by severe headache, is discovered to have the appropriate epidemiologic background. Such a background includes veterinary work; employment in an abattoir; laboratory work with infected material or infected sheep and goats; contact with wool, hides, or farm products; work or home near farms or in areas where sheep, cattle, or goats graze; or military deployment in areas with primitive animal husbandry. The diagnosis should be suspected in patients with hepatitis, particularly if the serum alkaline phosphatase is elevated and a liver biopsy shows granulomata. If pneumonitis is present, Q fever must be considered along with viral and mycoplasmal pneumonias and psittacosis.

Serologic tests confirm the diagnosis. The complement fixation test with the phase II antigen is the most frequently used test and gives clear results. Complement-fixing antibodies rise in the second week of illness, reach their peak at the end of the third week, and may persist for many months. Two specimens of serum are required, an early one and another after 12 to 20 days. A fourfold rise in antibody titer is taken as evidence of recent infection. For retrospective diagnosis in the convalescent period, an isolated titer of at least 1:32 strongly suggests recent acute Q fever, but the demonstration of circulating Q fever–specific IgM globulin may establish the diagnosis more convincingly (Murphy and Hunt, 1981). Strain variation in virulence and ability to detect antibody must be taken into account. Early effective antibiotic treatment may slow the rise in titer.

Failure to recognize a prozone phenomenon may allow false-negative results to be recorded in the complement-fixation test in sera with high antibody titers. Positive sera for Q fever may give false-positive serologic tests for syphilis. Q fever complement-fixing antibody has been found in adenovirus 7 and 27 infections, psittacosis, and Rocky Mountain spotted fever, but the Q fever titers have been low and have not risen significantly. Anamnestic responses have been recorded in *Mycoplasma pneumoniae* infections.

The newer technique of detection of antibody by fluorescent immunoassay (FIAX) may produce more rapid results (Ascher et al., 1983). Agglutination tests have also been used in Q fever. Agglutinins rise and peak approximately one week earlier than complement-fixing antibody. Microagglutination and the radioisotope precipitation techniques are more sensitive and useful for population surveys.

C. burnetii may be isolated from blood by guinea pig inoculation during the febrile period, and also from sputum, urine, cerebrospinal fluid, milk, placenta, and postmortem tissues. Frequent infections among laboratory staff make serologic methods preferable in routine situations.

TREATMENT. The only drugs of proven value for acute Q fever are tetracycline and chloramphenicol. Neither is rickettsicidal. The small but definite risk of marrow toxicity from chloramphenicol makes tetracycline the drug of choice. Tetracycline should be given in a dose of 2 grams per day in divided doses for at least two weeks. On this regimen the fever falls within two days in most cases, but if fever is slow to respond, the antibiotic must be continued until 48 hours after fever disappears. Premature withdrawal of the antibiotic is usually followed by relapse. If fever recurs after the standard regimen, a second course of tetracycline should be given. When the patient presents with the features of severe atypical pneumonia, erythromycin may be effective (Ellis and Dunbar, 1982).

PROPHYLAXIS. Ideally all workers in occupations where the risk of Q fever is high should be immunized. Vaccines are prepared from *C. burnetii* grown in the yolk sac. The protective polysaccharide antigen seems to be present in the rickettsial cell wall, and is present in larger amounts in extracts of *C. burnetii* in phase I than in phase II. A killed Q fever vaccine, injected subcutaneously and capable of protecting man against airborne infection, has been available for many years. Local and general reactions may be avoided by use of vaccine of adequate purity and by skin testing of prospective vaccine recipients for immune hypersensitivity. Vaccination may thus be restricted to skin test–negative persons. In Czechoslovakia and Romania, vaccines prepared from a trichloracetic acid extract of soluble phase I antigenic components produced a satisfactory antibody response with minimal local or systemic reactions (Kazár et al., 1982).

Vaccination can reduce infection rates in cattle and sheep (Sádecký and Brezina, 1977), but it is an expensive procedure, and since Q fever causes little or no illness in livestock, there is little economic incentive for this type of control. Vaccination of sheep and goats used in long-range research would prevent shedding of *C. burnetii* in milk, but whether it would prevent the organisms being shed in placental or fetal tissues is still unknown.

In endemic areas, milk from cattle or goats should be pasteurized or boiled. A change in location and timing of lambing and calving, in housing and density of animals, and in other conditions of animal husbandry may alter the pattern of human infection. Flocks should be monitored with regard to both antibody prevalence and individual antibody titer. In cases admitted to hospital, sputum and urine should be disinfected by autoclaving. Persons attending postmortem examinations of cases of Q fever, and undertakers handling such cases, should wear masks and protective clothing and take specimens with precautions to minimize aerosol formation (Andrews and Marmion, 1959). In institutions in which sheep are used as experimental animals, similarly strict precautions are recommended (Curet and Paust, 1972). Personnel involved in research should be serotested at regular intervals.

References

Alkan, W. J., Evenchik, Z., and Eshchar, J.: Q fever and infectious hepatitis. Am J Med 38:54, 1965.

Andrews, P. S., and Marmion, B. P.: Chronic Q fever. 2. Morbid anatomical and bacteriological findings in a patient with endocarditis. Br Med J 2:983, 1959.

Ascher, M. S., Horwith, G. S., Thornton, M. F., Greenwood, J. R., and Berman, M. A.: A rapid immunofluorescent procedure for serodiagnosis of Q fever in mice, guinea pigs, sheep, and humans. Diagn Immunol 1:33, 1983.

Bernstein, M., Edmondson, H. A., and Barbour, B. H.: The liver lesion in Q fever. Arch Intern Med 116:491, 1965.

Brezina, R.: Phase variation phenomenon in *Coxiella burnetii.* In Kazár, J., Ormsbee, R. A., and Tarasèvich, I. N. (eds.): Rickettsiae and Rickettsial Diseases. Bratislava, Veda, 1978, p. 221.

Curet, L. B., and Paust, J. C.: Transmission of Q fever from experimental sheep to laboratory personnel. Am J Obstet Gynecol 114:566, 1972.

Derrick, E. H.: The course of infection with *Coxiella burnetii.* Med J Aust 1:1051, 1973.

Dupont, H. L., Hornick, R. B., Levin, H. S., Rapoport, M. I., and Woodward, T. E.: Q fever hepatitis. Ann Intern Med 74:198, 1971.

Ellis, M. E., and Dunbar, E. M.: In vivo response of acute Q fever to erythromycin. Thorax 37:867, 1982.

Ellis, M. E., Smith, C. C., and Moffat, M. A. J.: Chronic or fatal Q fever infection: A review of 16 patients seen in North East Scotland (1967–80). Q J Med 52:54, 1983.

Gear, J. H. S.: Q fever. S Afr J Hosp Med 6:244, 1980.

Kazár, J., Brezina, R., Palanova, A., Tvrdá, B., and Schramek, Š. Bull WHO 60:389, 1982.

Marmion, B. P.: World-wide Q fever. Lancet 2:616, 1953.

Murphy, A. M., and Hunt, J. G.: Retrospective diagnosis of Q fever in a country abattoir by the use of specific IgM globulin estimations. Med J Aust 2:326, 1981.

Pellegrin, M., Delsol, G., Auvergnat, J. C., Familiades, J., Faure, H., Guin, M., and Voigt, J. J.: Granulomatous hepatitis in Q fever. Hum Pathol 11:51, 1980.

Powell, O. W.: Liver involvement in Q fever. Aust Ann Med 10:52, 1961.

Sádecký, E., and Brezina, R.: Vaccination of naturally infected ewes against Q fever. Acta Virol (Praha) 21:89, 1977.

Spelman, D. W.: Q fever. A study of 111 consecutive cases. Med J Aust 1:547, 1982.

Stoker, M. G. P., and Fiset, P.: Phase variation of the Nine Mile and other strains of *Rickettsia burnetii.* Can J Microbiol 2:310, 1956.

Tiggert, W. D., Benenson, A. S., and Gochenour, W. S.: Airborne Q fever. Bacteriol Rev 25:285, 1961.

Tonge, J. I., and Derrick, E. H.: A fatal case of Q fever associated with hepatic necrosis. Med J Aust 1:594, 1959.

Urso, F. P.: The pathologic findings in rickettsial pneumonia. Am J Clin Pathol 64:335, 1975.

Woodward, T. E.: A historical account of the rickettsial diseases with a discussion of unresolved problems. J Infect Dis 127:583, 1973.

117

VIRAL PNEUMONIA

RICHARD E. BRYANT M.D.

Viral pneumonia is an inflammation of lung parenchyma caused by a virus that reaches the lung hematogenously or by inhalation. The inflammatory response is usually mononuclear and interstitial. A high incidence of pneumonia occurs in immunosuppressed patients with viruses that rarely cause pneumonia in otherwise healthy people.

ETIOLOGY. The incidence of viral pneumonia depends on the age, immunologic status, and environmental circumstances of the population being considered. During an eight-year period, Foy and co-workers (1973) documented pneumonia in a large prepaid medical group at a rate of 10 cases/1000 patient years. Children under 5 had a rate of 42 cases/1000 patient years. Infection rates of viral pneumonia per 1000 patient years were as follows: influenza A, 0.2; influenza B, 0.2; parainfluenza, 0.8; respiratory syncytial virus, 1.2; and adenovirus, 0.4. Less common causes of viral pneumonia include herpesviruses, rhinoviruses, rubeola, echoviruses, coronaviruses, and coxsackieviruses. Rare cases have been reported with reovirus type 3, lymphocytic choriomeningitis, variola, vaccinia, and rabies viruses.

Respiratory syncytial virus is the most common cause of viral penumonia in children under 5 years of age and causes infection most frequently in midwinter to spring. This virus can also cause pneumonia in elderly or immunocompromised patients.

Influenza A and adenovirus deserve special consideration because of their epidemic potential and the mortality, morbidity, and long-term sequelae associated with these infections. Adenoviruses are a common cause of pneumonia in military recruits and have been recognized as an important cause of chronic pulmonary disease in infants and young children.

Pneumonia caused by herpesviruses often represents a complication of depressed immunity. Primary varicella pneumonia rarely occurs in normal children. However, 90 per cent of cases of varicella pneumonia occur in adults or in patients with depressed resistance. Varicella pneumonia is a dreaded complication of pregnancy or of disseminated zoster following chemotherapy of leukemia or lymphoma. Cytomegalovirus pneumonia is usually seen in patients with impaired defenses. This virus may cause primary pneumonia or may be associated with polymicrobic pulmonary infection.

Bacterial superinfection has been characteristically associated with influenza A virus infection during the third trimester of pregnancy, in the elderly, and in patients with rheumatic heart disease, mitral stenosis, or chronic bronchopulmonary disease. There is an increased frequency of bacterial superinfection in children with measles or chickenpox and in recruits with adenoviral infection, and patients with primary cytomegalovirus infection.

PATHOLOGY. Bronchiolitis, interstitial pneumonitis, and exudation of fluid into alveoli are present to a variable degree in all forms of viral pneumonia.

Influenza viral pneumonia is characterized by ulcerative and destructive bronchitis and by development of diffuse hemorrhagic necrotizing pneumonitis with marked pulmonary edema.

Respiratory syncytial virus, parainfluenza virus, and adenovirus cause necrotizing bronchitis, bronchiolitis, and interstitial pneumonia. Intranuclear inclusions may be seen in tissues of patients with varicella-zoster pneumonia, cytomegalovirus pneumonia, *Herpesvirus hominis* pneumonia, and early in the course of adenoviral pneumonia. Multinucleated giant cells, intranuclear inclusions, intracytoplasmic inclusions, and hyperplasia of distal bronchial cells are pathologic features of rubeola pneumonia.

EPIDEMIOLOGY AND PATHOPHYSIOLOGY. Many respiratory viruses are spread from person to person by inhalation of material aerosolized during coughing or sneezing (Knight, 1973). This is probably the primary mechanism of transmission of adenovirus and influenza virus infection. Rhinovirus infection may be transmitted primarily by direct contact with infected secretions. It is likely that both mechanisms are responsible for transmission of many viral respiratory infections. After implantation and replication in the respiratory cells, viruses are released and spread down the respiratory tract in mucus, by cell-to-cell transmission, or by lymphatic or systemic routes.

A number of defense mechanisms are impaired during viral infection. Ciliated cells are destroyed and bronchial clearance mechanisms disrupted during influenza. Increased mucous secretion and post-nasal discharge help deliver both virus and bacteria to the lower respiratory tract. Influenza A and adenoviral infection may cause dysfunction of phagocytic cells. Impairment of delayed hypersensitivity during viral pneumonia has been attributed to virus mediated lymphocyte dysfunction. Structural damage of bronchi, bronchioles, and alveolar epithelium, direct toxicity of viruses to alveolar macrophages, and the presence of increased alveolar fluid during a viral infection probably all enhance susceptibility of patients to bacterial superinfection.

Pulmonary function may be severely impaired in viral pneumonia. Injury to type 2 alveolar epithelial cells can cause loss of surfactant and collapse of alveoli. Alternatively, bronchiolitis can trap air and cause hyperinflation of involved segments. The pathologic findings of increased tissue fluid, capillary thickening and induration, and exudation of fluid into alveoli may present clinically as decreased lung compliance, increased work of breathing, dyspnea, and cyanosis. Hypoxia results primarily from abnormalities of ventilation and perfusion. The acute changes of viral pneumonia, which include increased tissue fluid with minimal alveolar exudation, account for the discrepancy between the radiologic and the auscultatory findings. There is rarely enough alveolar fluid to produce auscultatory signs of pulmonary consolidation.

Varicella pneumonia is usually more severe than other forms of primary viral pneumonia. This infection frequently involves both upper and lower lobes bilaterally. Nodular lesions throughout the lung coalesce and cause severe hypoxia. Vesicular lesions on the pleura appear to cause the pleuritic pain that is frequent in varicella pneumonia.

CLINICAL PRESENTATION

Influenza A Viral Pneumonia. This is the most common

cause of viral pneumonia in adults. Symptoms of influenza usually begin abruptly with severe headache, myalgia, prostration, chills, and fever of 39 to 40° C. Many patients are dizzy. Rhinorrhea, nasal congestion, and sore throat are frequent complaints. Hoarseness and photophobia occur less commonly. Gastrointestinal symptoms are rare.

Cough, tachypnea, dyspnea, and persistently high fever are prominent features of primary influenza viral pneumonia. Sputum is usually scanty but may become bloody as the disease progresses. Chest pain is substernal and nonpleuritic. Auscultatory findings are usually limited to rales and rhonchi. Chest x-rays show diffuse, often bilateral, bronchopneumonia.

The white blood cell count is frequently greater than 10,000 per mm^3 during the acute phase of infection and does not distinguish between primary viral pneumonia and secondary bacterial infection. Differential counts of the peripheral blood smear may reveal a marked "left shift." A mild leukopenia and lymphocytosis may occur late in the course of infection. Although of little value clinically, the sedimentation rate is more likely to be normal in patients with primary viral pneumonia than in those with bacterial superinfection. Changes in pO_2, pCO_2, and pH provide important but nonspecific evidence of the severity of infection. Hypoxemia ($pO_2 < 60$ mm Hg) and hypercarbia are ominous prognostic signs.

Diagnosis is established by culture and/or demonstration of a fourfold rise in complement fixation titer. Patients with viral influenza during the third trimester of pregnancy or in association with mitral stenosis, chronic lung disease, or immunodeficient or immunosuppressed states are especially susceptible to secondary bacterial pneumonia. Bacterial superinfection characteristically occurs one to five days after onset of viral illness when the patient appears to be getting well. Alternatively, patients may present with a concomitant viral pneumonia and bacterial pneumonia caused by *Staphylococcus aureus, Streptococcus pneumoniae, Haemophilus influenzae,* or *Streptococcus pyogenes* (Louria, 1959). Purulent sputum or physical findings of consolidation suggest the presence of bacterial superinfection.

The place of amantadine in therapy of influenza A viral pneumonia is unproved. Pulmonary function test abnormalities associated with influenza A viral disease of the lower respiratory tract have been shown to improve with amantadine (Little et al., 1976). Unfortunately, there are no controlled studies documenting the beneficial effects of amantadine in naturally occurring influenza viral pneumonia. For the present, it seems advisable to use amantadine in patients thought to have pneumonia caused by, or associated with, influenza, especially during an influenza A epidemic. Amantadine may be given orally to adults in doses of 100 mg every six to eight hours (Knight and Kasel, 1973). Recent studies by (Knight et al., 1981 and McClung et al., 1983) showed that ribavirin aerosol therapy caused significant symptomatic improvement and reduction of virus shedding from patients with influenza A or influenza B viral infection, and may be of value in treating primary influenza A viral pneumonia.

Pathologic changes associated with influenza A viral pneumonia include destruction of ciliated epithelial cells and disruption of goblet cells and mucous glands that may extend to the basement membrane. Bronchioles become thickened, distended, and infiltrated with mononuclear cells into interlobular septa. Necrotizing bronchiolitis and ulceration may be marked, and capillary thrombosis and necrosis may lead to necrotizing hemorrhagic pneumonitis. Exudation of fluid into the alveolar spaces may have a hyaline appearance and a variable composition of fibrin, red blood cells, or white blood cells, depending on the extent of hemorrhagic pulmonary edema. Severe inflammatory edema is often the outstanding feature of influenza pneumonia and appears to be reversible with positive end expiratory pressure (PEEP) (Fig. 1).

Adenoviral Pneumonia. Adenoviral pneumonia is usually seen in military recruits and is caused by type 3, 4, or 7. Adenoviral pneumonia is rare in civilian adults. Children may have severe or fatal pneumonia caused by type 1, 2, 3, or 7. Complications of bronchiectasis or chronic pulmonary disease after adenoviral infection are seen only in children. Symptoms and physical findings of patients with adenoviral pneumonia are shown in Tables 1 and 2.

There are few features that help to distinguish adenoviral pneumonia from pneumococcal pneumonia. Sore throat, nausea, or vomiting occurs more frequently in patients with adenoviral infection. Pharyngitis, rhinitis, and rales occur commonly in patients with adenoviral infection but bronchophony and egophony are rare (Bryant and Rhoades, 1967). Myringitis and conjunctivitis are infrequent. Herpes labialis was seen in only one patient with adenoviral infection. There are few laboratory findings suggestive of adenoviral pneumonia. Leukocyte counts may range from

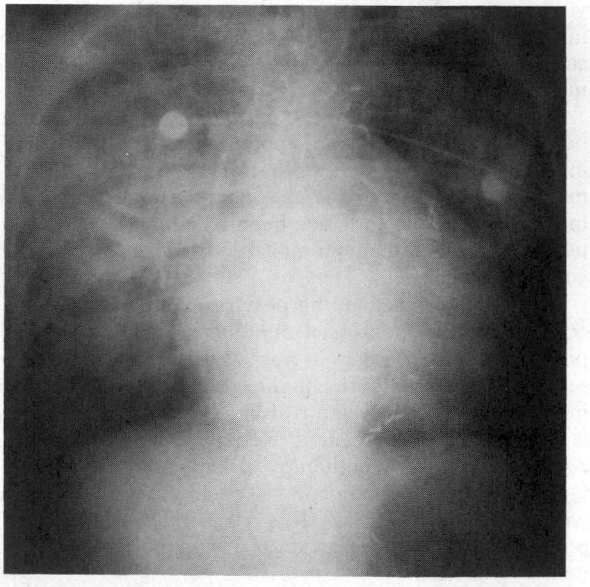

Figure 1. Severe influenza pneumonia in a 57-year-old diabetic white man with atherosclerotic cardiovascular disease. He was intubated and 15 cm of positive end expiratory pressure (PEEP) was instituted. Four days later the chest x-ray was remarkably clear, but infiltrates returned when PEEP was stopped. The chest cleared again when PEEP was reinstituted and patient recovered. Influenza A virus was isolated from sputum on admission. This case illustrates predisposition of patients with heart disease to influenza pneumonia and the value of PEEP in reversing the characteristic picture of adult respiratory distress syndrome in that infection. (Courtesy John Ryan, Dept. of Medicine, Yale University and New Haven Veterans Administration Hospital.)

Table 1. SYMPTOMS OF PATIENTS WITH PNEUMONIA

	Adenoviral—12 Patients (%)	Pneumococcal—25 Patients (%)
Cough	100	96
Sore throat	92	28
Nausea	75	28
Vomiting	58	28
Diarrhea	25	8
Rhinorrhea	75	48
Chest pain	67	80
Chills	33	52
Headaches	33	56
Myalgia	33	28

Table 2. PHYSICAL FINDINGS OF PATIENTS WITH PNEUMONIA

	Adenoviral—12 Patients (%)	Pneumococcal—25 Patients (%)
Pharyngitis	92	64
Rhinitis	75	44
Conjunctivitis	33	44
Myringitis	25	28
Herpes labialis	8	12
Rales and rhonchi	92	96
Bronchophony and/or egophony	8	48

5000 to 30,000 cells per mm^3. Two thirds of patients will have less than 10,000 cells per mm^3. When present, leukocytosis usually declines rapidly during the first week. Sputum is scanty but may be purulent or bloody. Skin test reactivity may be transiently suppressed. Characteristic roentgenographic features of adenoviral pneumonia may include: (1) irregular reticular infiltrates that may appear mottled or may coalesce in some areas; (2) indistinct segmental margins; (3) predilection for lower lobes; (4) occasional hilar enlargement (Fig. 2). Infiltrates may decrease in some segments while increasing in others. Pleural effusions are very rare. Roentgenograms usually clear by the second or third week. There is no effective therapy for adenoviral pneumonia. Diagnosis is usually established by sequential complement-fixation testing or by culture. Pathologic lesions of adenoviral pneumonia consist of bronchiolitis, interstitial pneumonitis, and intranuclear inclusions in alveolar cells in necrotic areas.

Rubeola (Measles) Pneumonia. Pneumonia is said to occur in 7 to 50 per cent of patients with rubeola. It is usually observed in children under 6 years of age and occurs within five days of the development of the rash. The signs and symptoms of patients with rubeola pneumonia differ little from those of patients without pneumonia except for findings of rales and rhonchi on chest examination and x-ray evidence of an interstitial pneumonia. Lower lobes are frequently involved, and signs of consolidation or pleural effusions occur rarely unless secondary bacterial infection is present.

Exacerbation or persistence of fever or leukocytosis suggests the presence of bacterial superinfection. *S. pneu-*

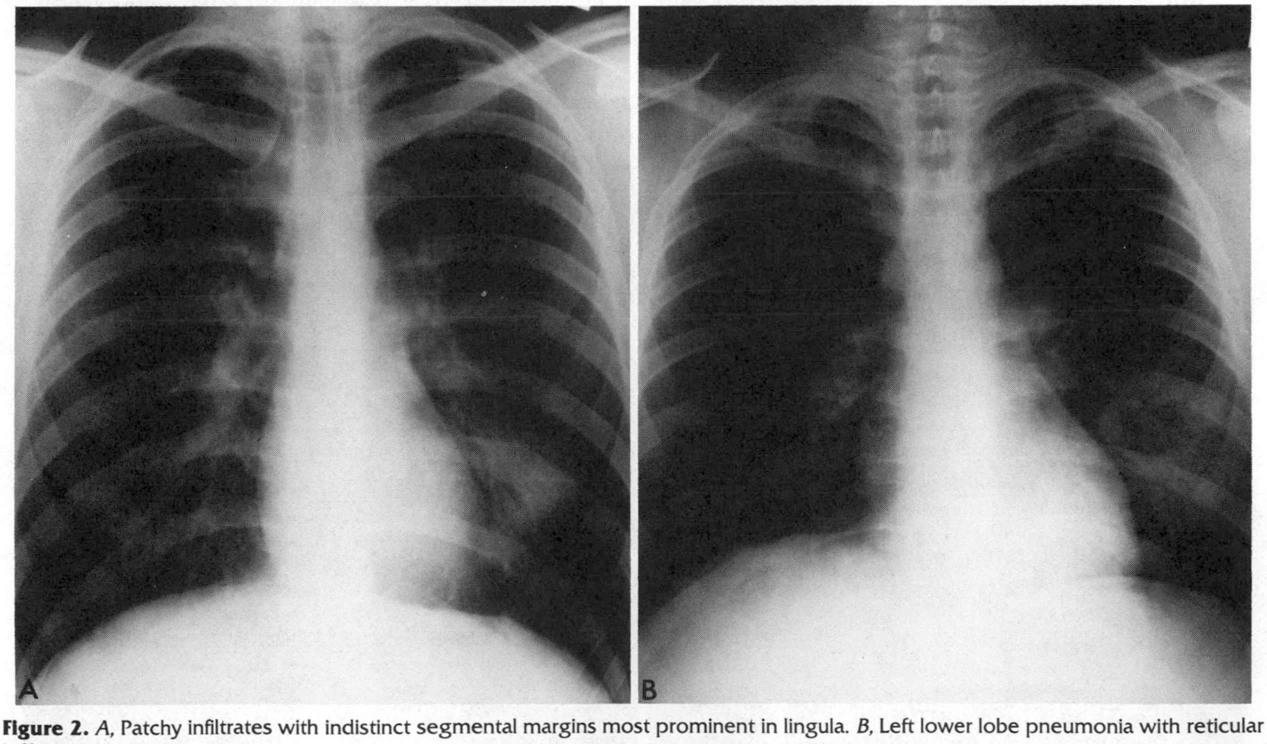

Figure 2. *A,* Patchy infiltrates with indistinct segmental margins most prominent in lingula. *B,* Left lower lobe pneumonia with reticular infiltrates.

Right hilar enlargement subsided after parenchymal lesion began to clear on left. Both patients were young healthy adults who recovered promptly from their adenoviral penumonia.

moniae, *S. pyogenes*, *S. aureus*, and *H. influenzae* are the most common bacterial pathogens causing superinfection. Secondary bacterial pneumonia occurs more often in immature or debilitated children and accounts for most severe or fatal complications of measles. Bacterial superinfection can also occur in healthy young adults. Olson and Hodges (1975) identified secondary bacterial infection in 10 of 16 naval recruits. Diagnosis was established by transtracheal aspiration culture and prompt response to antibiotic therapy. *Neisseria meningitidis*, serogroup Y, was the only species of bacteria isolated from six patients.

Primary measles pneumonia is an interstitial pneumonia characterized by multinucleated giant cells with nuclear and cytoplasmic inclusions. Measles pneumonia in the immunocompromised patient is an especially virulent disease. It may occur without rash and is usually fatal. Immunodeficient patients should not receive live attenuated measles vaccine because it can cause giant cell pneumonia in them.

When people who are partially immunized against rubeola acquire measles naturally, they may have an atypical rash and pneumonia characterized by hilar adenopathy, pleural effusion, and peripheral eosinophilia. Nodular infiltrates may persist after this disease subsides.

Varicella (Chickenpox) Pneumonia. Primary varicella pneumonia is largely an adult disease. Ninety per cent of patients are more than 20 years of age. In children, primary varicella pneumonia usually represents a complication of neonatal infection, immunodeficiency, debilitation, or drug-induced suppression of host defenses. Varicella pneumonia usually occurs within one to six days after onset of the typical vesicular rash. Symptoms frequently increase in severity over a one- to three-day period with severe cough, pleuritic chest pain, dyspnea, tachypnea, and hemoptysis.

Adults with varicella pneumonia characteristically have a nonproductive cough and dyspnea. Approximately 40 per cent of patients are cyanotic and 20 per cent complain of chest pain.

The characteristic generalized papulovesicular eruption of chickenpox is present in all patients with varicella pneumonia. Mucosal lesions occur in 26 per cent of patients with pneumonia. Rales and rhonchi are heard in only 50 to 60 per cent of patients. Hyperresonance or decreased breath sounds may be present. Tachypnea and labored breathing may be the most prominent findings.

Roentgenographic characteristics of varicella pneumonia are diffuse bilateral nodular infiltrates with peribronchial distribution. Nodules rarely exceed 5 mm but may coalesce in the hilus or lung bases. Nodular and reticular infiltrates may become dense enough to obscure the lung markings (Fig. 3).

Intranuclear inclusions may be seen in skin scrapings or in sputum cytologic examination. Leukocytosis is present in one third of patients. Thrombocytopenia is rare. Hypoxia is common in patients with varicella pneumonia who have the adult respiratory distress syndrome.

Sputum examination is especially important in children with varicella pneumonia because of their susceptibility to superinfection of the lungs. Criteria for distinguishing bacterial superinfection from primary varicella pneumonia are shown in Table 3.

There is controversy over the value of zoster-immune globulin or plasma, and of adenine arabinoside in therapy of varicella pneumonia. Both may be of value in the critically ill patient with severe immunodeficiency. Although direct clinical trials have not been completed, acyclovir is probably the drug of choice for primary varicella pneumonia. Acyclovir should be given intravenously in three divided doses at 1500 mg/M^2 or 30 mg/Kg/per day

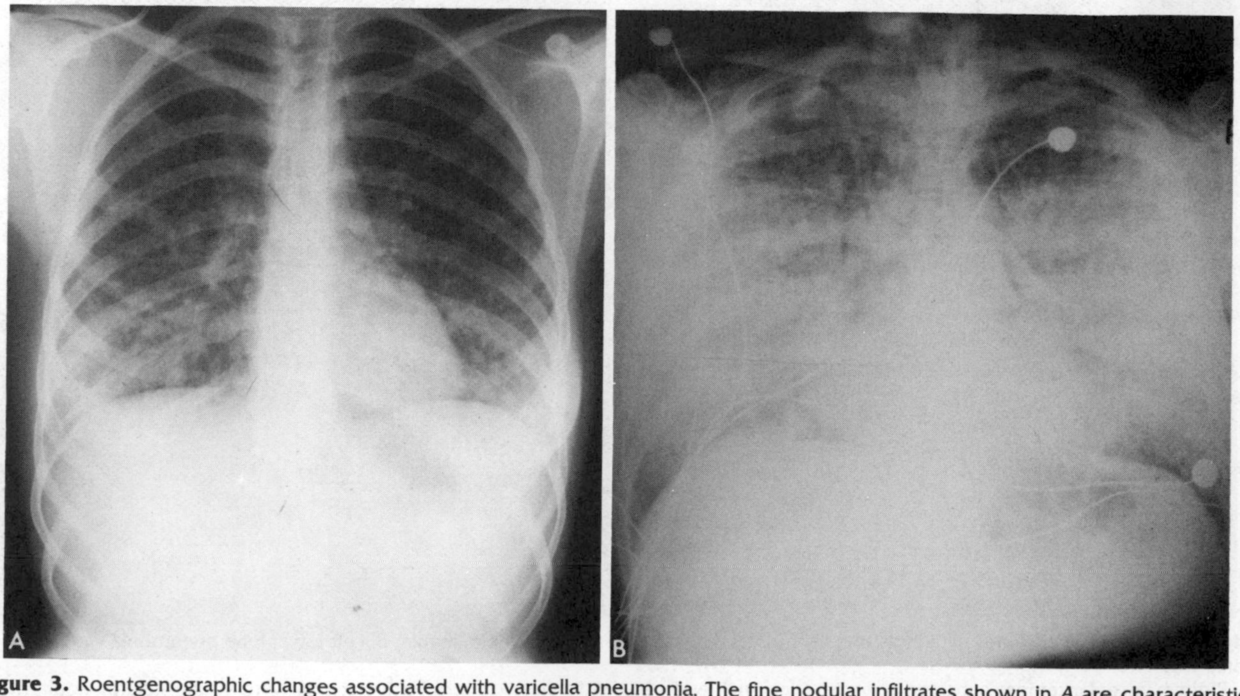

Figure 3. Roentgenographic changes associated with varicella pneumonia. The fine nodular infiltrates shown in *A* are characteristic of the diffuse bilateral changes seen in early varicella pneumonia. More extensive involvement with coalescence of nodular densities is shown in *B*. Both patients were adults without secondary infection.

Table 3. DIFFERENTIAL CHARACTERISTICS BETWEEN PRIMARY VARICELLA PNEUMONIA AND VARICELLA WITH SECONDARY BACTERIAL PNEUMONIA

Varicella Pneumonia	Bacterial Pneumonia
Adults	Usually children less than 7 years of age
Usually early in course with marked paucity of physical findings	Late in course with secondary rise in temperature
Normal to slightly increased white blood cell count	Elevated white blood cell count and "left shift" of differential
Negative blood and sputum cultures	Positive blood and sputum cultures
Diffuse nodular infiltration, usually without true consolidation	Symmetric distribution on x-ray with segmental or lobar consolidation

From Triebwasser, J. H., et al.: Medicine 46:409, 1967.

for varicella-zoster infections. Dosage must be reduced in the presence of renal failure and in the extremely obese patient. (See chapters 235 and 236 for discussion of acyclovir therapy of varicella-zoster infection.) Exogenous interferon has been considered as possible therapy, but its value is unproved.

Immunoprophylaxis with zoster-immune globulin (ZIG) or varicella-zoster immune globulin (VZIG) is beneficial to the nonimmune patient with compromised host defenses who is treated within 72 hours of exposure to infection. Circumstances or disease states appropriate for ZIG immunoprophylaxis include leukemia, lymphoma, congenital or acquired immunodeficiency, and immunosuppression or steroid therapy. Use of ZIG immunoprophylaxis is also appropriate in newborns of mothers with varicella. Use of ZIG is reviewed succinctly in the 1982 Medical Letter. Inquiries concerning local acquisition of ZIG should be made to the Eastern Massachusetts Red Cross (617-731-2130) or may be found in the 1982 Medical Letter. Inquiries from outside the U.S. should be directed to 617-449-0073.

The pathology of varicella pneumonia is characterized by vesicles on pleural and tracheobronchial surfaces and by interstitial pneumonitis that extends in a peribronchiolar distribution. Focal areas of hemorrhagic consolidation occur in the lung parenchyma. Alveoli and bronchi are filled with hyaline material containing fibrin, red blood cells, and monocytes. Capillary endothelium undergoes swelling, cell necrosis, and mononuclear perivascular infiltration. Intranuclear inclusions may be found in septal cells, giant cells, fibroblasts, capillary endothelium, and tracheobronchial epithelial cells. Healing of focal areas of necrosis after varicella pneumonia can lead to a miliary pattern of pulmonary calcification.

Cytomegalovirus (CMV) Pneumonia. This infection often occurs in patients with leukemia, lymphoma, or tissue transplantation. The virus may cause primary pneumonia in the neonate or immune deficient adult, or may occur as part of a mixed pulmonary infection (Abdallah et al., 1976). Patients with acquired immunodeficiency syndrome are especially susceptible to CMV pneumonia. It is often difficult to identify the precise role that CMV plays in a patient's illness.

There are few distinguishing features of CMV pneumonia. The best clue is a slowly progressive viral pneumonia syndrome in an immunosuppressed patient. Cytomegalovirus infection is further suggested by a finding of chorioretinitis. Roentgenograms usually show reticular, bilateral, and ill-defined densities. There is no specific therapy for CMV pneumonia. Experience with acyclovir therapy was disappointing (Wade et al., 1982), and combined therapy with vidarabine and leukocyte interferon was shown to be both toxic and ineffective (Meyers et al., 1982).

Two forms of CMV infection occur in transplant patients. The first is reactivation of CMV infection, which causes a relatively mild disease with brisk antibody response. The second is primary CMV pneumonia, which in immunodeficient patients is often fatal. The primary CMV infection syndrome begins with spiking fever, leukopenia, prostration, and orthostatic hypotension and hypoxemia without initial x-ray evidence of pneumonia (Simmons et al., 1977). Patients have dyspnea and nonproductive cough. Hypoalbuminemia, thrombocytopenia, and lymphopenia are often present. Antibody response to CMV is minimal as the disease progresses with worsening of pulmonary, hepatic, and cerebral function. Myalgia, arthralgia, muscle wasting, abdominal distention, and tenderness are prominent features of the relentless three- to four-week course of this disease.

Chest radiographs usually show diffuse bilateral interstitial or alveolar infiltrates. Despite extensive viremia, viruria, and high titers of virus in most tissues, acute rejection is not seen on renal biopsy. Most patients with hypoxia due to CMV pneumonia die.

Successful therapy requires recognition of this disorder and rapid reduction of immunosuppressive therapy. Preliminary studies suggest that use of a live attenuated CMV vaccine before tissue transplantation may protect patients from lethal primary CMV pneumonia after transplantation (Glazer et al., 1978).

Isolation of CMV from lung tissue of patients with pneumonia is clearly a more sensitive means of detecting virus than is the morphologic demonstration of intranuclear inclusions (Abdallah et al., 1976). Lung biopsy will show interstitial pneumonia in most instances, but only a third of culture-positive biopsies will show intranuclear inclusions. Specific immunofluorescent stains of biopsy tissue for CMV may be especially useful as a diagnostic method in the future. Serologic evidence of CMV or herpesvirus infection is not an acceptable criterion for diagnosing viral pneumonia because of the variability of such titers and the ubiquity of the viruses. However, positive viral cultures from blood, urine, or sputum, or demonstration of multinucleated giant cells in urine or sputum is strong circumstantial evidence that CMV is one of the pathogens causing pneumonia in the compromised patient. Patients with CMV pneumonia may have concomitant infection with *Pneumocystis carinii,* fungi, mycobacteria, gram-negative bacilli, or a variety of bacteria or viruses.

Respiratory Syncytial Virus Pneumonia. This infection may occur in the elderly but is most serious in the very young. Bronchiolitis occurs most frequently in children less than 1 year old and bronchopneumonia most often in 4- to 5-year-old children. Bronchiolitis and pneumonia may be present in the same patient. Dyspnea, fever, and wheezing are prominent symptoms. Intercostal retraction with wheezing respiration may be marked. Cough may or may not be present. Sputum is scanty. Affected children are usually irritable and tachypneic. Rales and rhonchi are present. Chest radiographs show bilateral bronchopneumonia. Hyperlucency from air trapping may be present in bronchiolitic areas. Leukocyte counts are nondiagnostic. A needle aspiration culture may be necessary to establish the diagnosis of viral disease and exclude bacterial superinfection in the severely ill child. Use of immunofluorescent microscopic techniques to demonstrate virus in respiratory secretions will become more important when effective chemotherapeutic agents are discovered in the future. In the past, therapy of respiratory syncytial viral pneumonia was limited to supportive measures, maintenance of ventilation, and removal of secretions interfering with respiration. Aerosolized ribavirin has been shown to reduce the severity of illness of infants hospitalized with lower respiratory tract infection caused by respiratory syncytial virus (Hall et al., 1983). Toxic side effects or development of drug resistance were not observed during trials of therapy. Aerosolized ribavirin appears to represent a promising new therapy for respiratory syncytial virus infection.

Immunization against respiratory syncytial (RS) virus is harmful because the vaccinated children get a more severe disease.

COMPLICATIONS AND ADVERSE SEQUELAE OF VIRAL PNEUMONIA. Complications of viral pneumonia may be immediate or delayed. Patients with fulminant infection may develop acute respiratory insufficiency indistinguishable from the adult respiratory distress syndrome. Concomitant encephalitis, myocarditis, hepatitis, nephritis, or a hemorrhagic diathesis may be unusual clinical features of viral pneumonia. Abortion or fetal wastage has been documented best in association with varicella pneumonia in the third trimester of pregnancy.

A high mortality occurs at the extremes of age or with pre-existing heart disease, lung disease, or immunodeficiency. Adenoviral pneumonia in the very young has been reported to have an 8 to 10 per cent mortality. Varicella pneumonia in the adult is lethal in 10 to 30 per cent of patients, but the death rate may reach 40 per cent in pregnant women (Triebwasser et al., 1967).

Respiratory syncytial virus infection in the elderly can be complicated by bacterial superinfection. This complication may also occur in children who have a lower respiratory tract infection with rubeola or varicella. *S. aureus* frequently causes infection under these circumstances.

Pulmonary function defects will probably persist in most patients with severe varicella pneumonia or with viral infection presenting as the adult respiratory distress syndrome. Subtle changes in pulmonary function attributable to less severe involvement will continue to elude detection until prospective studies are done.

The most severe delayed complications of viral pneumonia in children follow adenoviral infection. These consist of obliterative bronchiolitis, severe bronchiectasis, lobar collapse, unilateral hyperlucent lung, post-inflammatory vascular disease, and residual pulmonary fibrosis. Long-term complications associated with respiratory syncytial viral disease may be more subtle than those with adenovirus. Kattan and co-workers (1977) observed a high frequency of hyperinflation, abnormal gas exchange, and small airway disease in patients examined 10 years after an episode of bronchiolitis during their first 18 months of life. The high incidence of wheezing observed in patients with a history of respiratory syncytial virus infection in childhood raises the possibility of a participatory role of respiratory syncytial virus in the pathogenesis of asthma in some patients.

GEOGRAPHIC VARIATION IN DISEASE. Age-specific death rate of rubeola in Greenland was three- to fivefold higher than that in the United States in a comparable period. Developing nations in Africa may have an even higher mortality. Most deaths from rubeola in children less than 2 years old are associated with pneumonia. Varicella pneumonia also has a high mortality in such populations, but it is not clear whether primary viral pneumonia or a greater frequency of bacterial superinfection is responsible for the excess mortality. Similarly, it is not known whether age, malnutrition, anemia, lack of herd immunity, underlying disease, or genetic or environmental factors affect the adverse course of such populations.

Excess mortality and morbidity have been reported with adenoviral pneumonia in Polynesian, Auckland, and Manitoba Eskimo populations. Lang and co-workers (1969) reported a 20 per cent incidence of bronchiectasis and a 40 per cent incidence of other types of chronic pulmonary disease in New Zealand children convalescing from severe adenoviral pneumonia.

DIAGNOSIS. With the exceptions noted for certain entities, the clinical presentation and roentgenographic findings of viral pneumonia are not specific (Table 4). Primary influenza A viral pneumonia, varicella pneumonia, and rubeola pneumonia usually present with bilateral involvement. Infants with respiratory syncytial infection may have bilateral disease or involvement of the right upper lobe. Most patients with viral pneumonia have involvement of lower lobes. Infiltrates are usually reticular, feathery, or mottled. Segmental margins are indistinct. Late in the course of infection, exudation of fluid into alveoli is associated with development of an acinar pattern of radiodensity in addition to an overall reticular pattern. Segmental atelectasis may occur in a small percentage of cases. During the course of infection, hilar adenopathy may develop and new reticular infiltrates may appear as infiltrates in other areas of the lungs disappear. With more severe involvement, the infiltrates may coalesce. Pleural effusions are uncommon, and lobar consolidation is so rare that when it does occur it suggests the presence of bacterial superinfection. Similarly, rapid progression of pneumonia over a few hours suggests the presence of bacterial infection. Radiographic differentiation of bacterial and viral pneumonia is accurate in only two thirds of cases (Tew et al., 1977).

Laboratory proof of viral infection is obtained by culture of nasal or oropharyngeal swabs, gargle, or sputum and demonstration of a fourfold rise in antibody titers to the specific virus in the absence of evidence of bacterial infection. Rigorous proof of viral pneumonia is provided by cultural or ultramicroscopic demonstration of virus in diseased lung tissue obtained by biopsy or needle aspiration. Strict criteria for demonstrating viral growth from pulmonary tissue that is sterile by conventional bacterial cultures are rarely met. Diagnosis may be suggested by demonstration of viral antigens in exfoliated cells from the nose or oropharynx by immunofluorescent microscopic techniques. This method has been used with respiratory syncytial virus, parainfluenza virus, influenza A virus, and cytomegalovirus.

It is important to differentiate viral pneumonia from the primary atypical pneumonia syndrome caused by *Mycoplasma pneumoniae*, psittacosis, Q fever, tularemia, or *Legionella pneumophila*. A careful history and physical examination demonstrating splenomegaly due to psittacosis; or hemolytic anemia; bullous myringitis, an erythema mul-

Table 4. CLINICAL FINDINGS SUGGESTING CAUSE OF PNEUMONIA

Cause	Epidemiologic	Symptoms	Physical Examination	Laboratory	Chest X-ray
Influenza A	Epidemic or pandemic period, history of exposure, susceptible host	"Flu"-like symptoms, chills, fever, myalgia, headache, rhinorrhea, photophobia, sore throat, scanty sputum may become bloody	Prostration, rhinitis, conjunctivitis, pharyngitis, rales, and rhonchi	WBC is nondiagnostic, lymphocytosis late, few bacteria or neutrophils in sputum. Hypoxia or hypercarbia is an ominous prognostic sign	Bilateral bronchopneumonia with reticular pattern. Effusions rare
Adenovirus	Increased risk of exposure — military recruits, children, nursery epidemic	Relatively nonproductive cough, sore throat, nausea, vomiting, rhinorrhea	Rhinitis, pharyngitis, rales, and rhonchi. Otitis in children	Leukocytosis early, scanty sputum, rarely purulent or bloody	Interstitial bronchopneumonia of lower lobes
Respiratory syncytial virus	Extremes of age. Peak age 4 to 5 years old	Dyspnea, wheezing, and cough	Fever, tachypnea, cyanosis, wheezing respiration, rales, and rhonchi	Scanty sputum	Interstitial pneumonia may have hyperinflation in some areas
Cytomegalovirus	Compromised host	Depends on immune status	Chorioretinitis otherwise dependent on secondary pathogens	Demonstration of CMV in tissue or sputum by immunofluorescent microscopy or culture. Presence of giant cells on lung biopsy	Interstitial pneumonia
Varicella-zoster (chickenpox)	History of exposure of a susceptible patient (see Table 3)	Rash followed by cough, dyspnea, and pleurisy	Papulovesicular rash. Tachypnea cyanosis, rales, and rhonchi	Intranuclear inclusion in skin scraping or sputum	Diffuse bilateral nodular infiltrates. Infiltrates may coalesce
Rubeola (measles)	History of exposure of susceptible patient	Measles prodrome, cough, and sputum production usually within first five days of rash	Persistence of exacerbation of fever exanthem and enanthem of measles. Rales and rhonchi	Leukocytosis suggests bacterial superinfection	Lower lobe interstitial pneumonia
Bacterial superinfection of viral respiratory disease	More frequent in children with varicella or lung disease, compromised host with CMV pneumonia	Exacerbation of fever, cough, and hypoxia. Purulent sputum	Pleural effusion. Signs of pulmonary consolidation. Rapidly worsening course	Leukocytosis. Purulent sputum	Lobar pneumonia. Pleural effusion, coalescence of infiltrates
Chlamydia (in infants)	Neonates	Progressive increase in respiratory symptoms from 2 to 6 weeks. Protracted course	Afebrile-mucoid nasal discharge, tachypnea. Conjunctivitis (50 per cent). Middle ear abnormalities (50 per cent). Distinctive staccato cough. Good breath sounds. Rales	Eosinophilia, two- to four-fold rise in serum IgG, IgM, and IgA levels. Culture and/or serology	Hyperexpansion with diffuse interstitial and patchy alveolar infiltrates. Clears slowly

tiforme-like rash or a neuropathy due to mycoplasma pneumonia; or a skin lesion of tularemia may be helpful, but most often it is necessary to treat the patient empirically on the basis of epidemiologic, clinical, and laboratory evidence that is imprecise.

It is mandatory that the physician distinguish viral pneumonia from bacterial pneumonia or bacterial superinfection of viral disease. The diagnosis of bacterial infection is favored by recurrent chills, abrupt onset of hypotension, physical or radiologic evidence of pulmonary consolidation, and compromised defense mechanisms that predispose to bacterial infection. Diagnosis is confirmed by microscopic demonstration of bacteria in purulent sputum obtained by having the patient cough, or by performing fiberoptic bronchoscopy, endotracheal aspiration, or transtracheal aspiration techniques. The former may be misleading because of contamination of sputum by bacteria in the mouth. Transtracheal aspiration specimens are less apt to be contaminated, but the procedure is contraindicated in the presence of severe hypoxia or bleeding diathesis, or in uncooperative patients. Thoracotomy may be required for diagnosis in special circumstances. X-ray evidence of lobar infiltrates, pneumatoceles, cavitation, or pleural effusion is evidence of bacterial infection. Pleural fluid should be examined and cultures of blood and other body fluids should be performed. Direct needle aspiration of infected lung tissue has been used extensively to document bacterial pneumonia in children.

TREATMENT. With the exceptions discussed previously under Influenza A, respiratory syncytial virus, or varicella pneumonia, treatment of viral pneumonia is for the most part nonspecific. Unfortunately, studies documenting efficacy of the new antiviral agents are for the most part anecdotal and incomplete. Most patients with viral pneumonia have minimal involvement and require only supportive therapy. Patients with fulminant infection presenting as the adult respiratory distress syndrome (ARDS) require heroic efforts to improve oxygenation. It has been suggested that alveolar exudation of fluid, decreased lung compliance, and increased interstitial fluid can be managed best by the use of positive end expiratory pressure (PEEP) or continuous positive airway pressure (CPAP) (Taylor et al., 1976). Either method is usually performed in an intensive care unit in association with intubation, mechanical control of ventilation, and high concentrations of oxygen. Airway pressure must be regulated to optimize ventilation and minimize impairment of venous return. This frequently permits reduction of the concentration of inspired oxygen to a level less likely to be harmful to the lung (i.e., $\leqq$ 50 per cent FiO_2). Additional measures for treating patients with ARDS include corticosteroids, intentional dehydration with diuretics, and other methods that attempt to reduce lung water (O'Brien and Sweeney, 1973). Severe hypoxia in patients with ARDS has been treated with hyperbaric oxygen or extracorporeal membrane oxygenation devices. Both procedures are still experimental and results have been surprisingly poor.

In seriously ill patients with pneumonia, therapy must be started before the diagnosis is proved conclusively. Differentiation of primary viral pneumonia from antibiotic responsive pneumonia may be difficult. Bacterial pneumonia or superinfection requires precise diagnosis and appropriate antimicrobial therapy. In critically ill patients with pneumonia of undetermined origin, it is usually wisest to perform appropriate diagnostic procedures, treat appropriately for suspected microbial pathogens, and stop antibiotics when the clinical course, cultures, biopsy, or serologic studies confirm the absence of antibiotic responsive pathogens.

References

Abdallah, P. S., Mark, J. B. D., and Merigan, T. C.: Diagnosis of cytomegalovirus pneumonia in compromised hosts. Am J Med 61:326, 1976.

Balfour, H. H., Bean, B., Laskin, O. L., et al.: Acyclovir halts progression of herpes zoster in immunocompromised patients. NEJM 308:1448, 1983.

Bryant, R. E., and Rhoades, E. R.: Clinical features of adenoviral pneumonia in Air Force recruits. Am Rev Resp Dis 96:717, 1967.

Crane, L. R., Kish, J. A., Ratanatharathorn, V., et al.: Fatal syncytial virus pneumonia in a laminar airflow room. JAMA 246:366, 1981.

Foy, H. M., Cooney, M. K., McMahan, R., and Grayston, J. T.: Viral and mycoplasma pneumonia in a prepaid medical care group during an eight year period. Am J Epidemiol 97:93, 1973.

Glazer, J. P., Friedman, H. M., Grossman, R. A., et al.: Cytomegalovirus vaccination and renal transplantation. Lancet 1:90, 1978.

Hall, C. B., McBride, J. T., Walsh, E. E., et al.: Aerosolized ribavirin treatment of infants with respiratory syncytial viral infection. A randomized double-blind study. New Engl J Med 308:1443, 1983.

Kattan, M., Keens, T. G., Lapierre, et al.: Pulmonary function abnormalities in symptom-free children after bronchiolitis. Pediatrics 59:683, 1977.

Knight, V.: Airborne transmission and pulmonary deposition of respiratory viruses. In Knight, V. (ed.): Viral and Mycoplasma Infections of the Respiratory Tract. Philadelphia, Lea & Febiger, 1973, p. 1.

Knight, V., and Kasel, J. A.: Influenza viruses. In Knight, V. (ed.): Viral Mycoplasma Infections of the Respiratory Tract. Philadelphia, Lea & Febiger, 1973, p. 108.

Knight, V., Wilson, S. Z., Quarles, J. M., et al.: Ribavirin small-particle aerosol treatment of influenza. Lancet 31:945, 1981.

Lang, W. R., Howden, C. W., Laws, J., et al.: Bronchopneumonia with serious sequelae in children with evidence of adenovirus type infection. Br Med J 1:73, 1969.

Little, J. W., Hall, W. J., et al.: Amantadine effect of peripheral airways abnormalities in influenza. Ann Intern Med 85:117, 1976.

Louria, D. B., Blumenfeld, H. L., Ellis, J. T., et al.: Studies on influenza in the pandemic of 1957–1958. II. Pulmonary complications of influenza. J Clin Investig 38:213, 1959.

McClung, H. W., Knight, V., Gilbert, B. E., et al.: Ribavirin aerosol treatment of influenza B virus infection. JAMA 249:2671, 1983.

Meyers, J. D., McGuffin, R. W., Bryson, J. J., et al.: Treatment of cytomegalovirus pneumonia after marrow transplant with combined vidarabine and human leukocyte interferon. J Infect Dis 146:80, 1982.

O'Brien, T. G., and Sweeney, D. F.: Interstitial viral pneumonitis complicated by severe respiratory failure. Successful management using intensive dehydration and steroids. Chest 63:314, 1973.

Olson, R. W., and Hodges, G. R.: Measles pneumonia, bacterial superinfection as a complicating factor. JAMA 232:363, 1975.

Simmons, R. L., Motas, A. J., Rattazzii, L. C., et al.: Clinical characteristics of the lethal cytomegalovirus infection following renal transplantation. Surgery 82:537, 1977.

Taylor, G. J., Brenner, W., and Summer, W. R.: Severe viral pneumonia in young adults. Therapy with continuous positive airway pressure. Chest 69:6, 1976.

Tew, J., Calenoff, L., and Berlin, B. S.: Bacterial or nonbacterial pneumonia: Accuracy of radiographic diagnosis. Diag. Radiol. 124:607, 1977.

Triebwasser, J. H., Harris, R. E., Bryant, R. E., and Rhoades, E. R.: Varicella pneumonia in adults. Medicine 46:409, 1967.

Varicella-zoster immune globulin. Medical Letter on Drugs and Therapeutics 24:51, 1982.

118

BACTERIAL LUNG ABSCESS, NOCARDIAL LUNG ABSCESS, AND ASPIRATION PNEUMONIA

S. J. D. Brooks, M.D.
Abraham I. Braude, M.D., Ph.D.

BACTERIAL LUNG ABSCESS

A lung abscess results when necrosis and liquefaction occur in an area of suppurative pneumonitis. When the liquefied material is discharged into a bronchus, air enters and a cavity with an air-fluid level remains.

ETIOLOGY. Aspiration lung abscess is due to a mixed anaerobic infection (Bartlett et al., 1973). Anaerobes outnumber aerobes 10 to 1 in the mouth, and the ratio is greatly increased in dental or gum disease. A concentration of 10^{11} bacteria/ml of saliva occurs in these diseases. Bacteria proliferate in tonsillar crypts, chronic sinusitis, and dead tissues of the mouth, all of which can be foci for delivering infection to the lungs by aspiration. Aspiration abscess acquired outside the hospital is caused by a mixed anaerobic infection, whereas in hospitals it is invariably a mixed infection with aerobes plus anaerobes (Lorber and Swenson, 1974). Among the anaerobic organisms isolated from lung abscesses are the gram-negative bacteria *Bacteroides melaninogenicus*, *Bacteroides fragilis*, *Fusobacteria* sp, *Bacteroides corrodens*, and *Veillonea* sp.

The anaerobic gram-positive organisms are the *Peptococcus* and *Peptostreptococcus* sp, *Eubacterium*, and *Propionibacterium* sp. *Actinomyces israelii* and *Arachnia propionica* are anaerobic gram-positive bacilli that can cause lung abscess. These are discussed in Chapter 48.

The aerobic organisms most commonly isolated from lung abscess are *Staphylococcus aureus* and the gram-negative bacilli *Klebsiella pneumoniae*, *Escherichia coli*, *Pseudomonas aeruginosa*, and *Pseudomonas pseudomallei*. *Legionella pneumophila*, *L. micdadei* (Dowling et al., 1983) (Chapter 119) and *Francisella tularensis* (Chapter 257) are fastidious organisms that cause severe pulmonary suppuration. *Streptococcus pyogenes S. pneumoniae* (Yangco et al., 1980) *Neisseria meningitidis*, *Pasteurella multocida*, *Yersinia enterocolitica*, *Listeria monocytogenes*, *Haemophilus influenzae*, and *Campylobacter fetus* are occasionally reported in association with lung abscess.

PATHOGENESIS. Bacteria reach the lung either by aspiration from the upper respiratory tract, hematogenous spread, inhalation, or contiguous spread from infected adjacent organs. Pus may spread from one site to another within the lung via the bronchi, a process known as internal bronchoembolism.

Aspiration is prevented by the cough and gag reflexes. Although some aspiration occurs at night, these reflexes protect the lung from large or frequent aspirations. They are compromised in patients whose level of consciousness is depressed by alcoholic stupor, narcotics, overdose, fits, anesthesia, or brain injury; in patients with myasthenia gravis neuromuscular diseases complicated by bulbar or pseudobulbar palsy or laryngeal palsy. Esophageal diseases with abnormal peristalsis, obstruction, or a fistula into the lungs and with gastrointestinal lesions that cause vomiting and reflux or disturb the integrity of the gastroesophageal junction also predispose to aspiration.

Aspirated material carries with it the bacterial flora of the oropharynx. Solid materials such as pus, dental tartar, tissue fragments (from tonsils, adenoids, or malignant tissue), and food particles are especially hazardous because they cause areas of atelectasis in which bacteria can multiply. Brock (1952) called this aspirated, infected material a bronchoembolus and showed that its destination in the lung varied according to its size, the posture of the patient, and the direction of gravitational flow at the time of aspiration (Figs. 1 and 2). If the patient is lying on his back, the bronchoembolus lodges more frequently in the right lung because the right bronchus is wider and at a lesser angle to the trachea. The first dependent bronchial orifice in its floor is that leading to the apical segment of the lower lobe of the right lung, which turns out to be the most common location for an aspiration abscess. If the patient is lying on his right side, the embolus enters the bronchus to the right superior lobe and then, according to the degree of anterior or posterior tilt of the body, the anterior, apical, or posterior branches of the bronchus. The posterior segment is most commonly affected. With the patient in the left lateral position, the apicoposterior is favored. When the patient is upright, the embolus enters the lower lobe branches. A similar course of events occurs if it enters the left lung. The middle lobe and lingula are rarely affected, because aspiration must take place in the prone or semiprone positions, as when someone vomits in the bent-forward position or after near drowning. The latter is more common in males because they float in the prone position.

Septic emboli from the heart or peripheral veins may also cause a lung abscess. Endocarditis of the right side, due to infection of a congenitally deformed valve or to intravenous drug addiction, showers emboli into the lungs. *S. aureus* is responsible for 85 per cent of cases, but a wide range of organisms cause the remaining 15 per cent. Septic emboli may come also from phlebitis in the pelvic veins or in more peripheral veins after intravenous cannulation. Pelvic thrombophlebitis results from colonic or gynecologic disease and follows surgery, childbirth, and abortions. *Bacteroides* spp. are especially likely to invade these venous channels, but streptococci, staphylococci, and gram-negative organisms have been isolated from abscesses caused by such emboli. Intravenous cannulation is an important iatrogenic cause of phlebitis, and lung abscess has been reported in association with intravenous drips, cardiac pacemakers, ventriculovenous shunts, hemodialysis shunts, and hyperalimentation. *S. aureus* causes 50 per cent of these infections, and the rest are caused by a great variety of opportunistic organisms. A fibrin clot forms where the vein is pierced, and this acts as a bacterial trap. Inflammation causes the clot to enlarge, and septic emboli result from clot fragmentation. Burn patients develop *Pseudomonas* thrombophlebitis. Septic emboli may also come from inflammatory areas in bone, pharynx, or kidney.

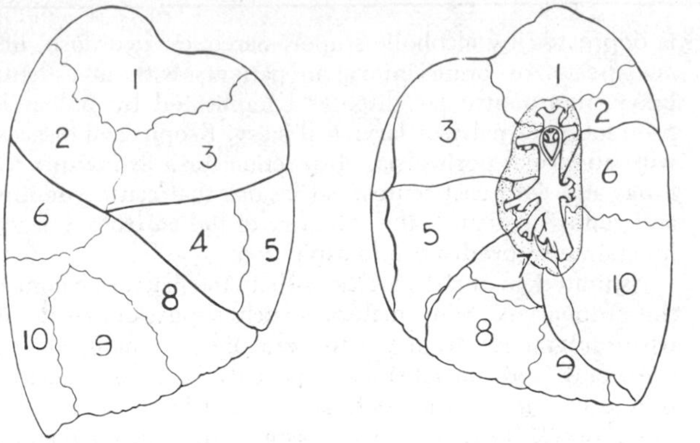

Figure 1. The segments of the right lung. The posterior segment (No. 2) of the upper lobe is most vulnerable to bronchoembolism when patient is on his right side, and the apical segment (No. 6) of the lower lobe is most vulnerable when he is on his back. (From Brock, R. C.: Lung Abscess. Springfield, Ill., Charles C Thomas, 1952.)

Infected particulate matter may pass directly into the lungs after intravenous injection by addicts. Less than 5 per cent of bland infarcts become infected from within the lung.

When bacteria reach the lung, the infection is controlled or arrested by polymorphonuclear leukocytes, macrophages, and IgG, unless there is neutropenia, neutrophil dysfunction, or any breach in the integrity of the T and B cell system, which is essential to the formation and efficient function of IgA, IgG, and macrophages. This occurs in congenital agammaglobulinemia, Hodgkin's disease, multiple myeloma, and chronic lymphatic and lymphocytic leukemias. Steroids, immunosuppressives, and antineoplastic drugs increase susceptibility. Chronic disease of the heart, lung, kidney, and liver depress immunity in the lung, as do diabetes mellitus, hypoxia, alcohol, and hypothermia.

Many who develop pneumonia with abscess formation have their lung defenses compromised by one or more of these disturbances. The most common organisms responsible for these pneumonias are *S. aureus* and the gram-negative *bacilli.* They colonize the oropharynx in long-stay hospital inpatients, and they reach the lung by inhalation or aspiration.

S. aureus infections may follow influenza. Infants under 1 year old and pregnant women are also vulnerable to staphylococcal pneumonia. Alcoholism, chronic lung disease, immunosuppression, and diabetes mellitus play an important debilitating role in gram-negative infections. *Pseudomonas* spp. proliferate in antiseptic solutions and creams and in the nebulizers of ventilators. This organism is a particular hazard to those on ventilators, to burn patients, and to infants with congenital heart disease.

Abscesses can also be formed in or from existing pathology. Anaerobic abscesses may develop from aspirated material trapped distally to an obstructing bronchial carcinoma (Fig. 3). Bronchogenic cysts are infected via the bronchus or the bloodstream, but dermoid cysts and sequestered lobes are always infected hematogenously. Bronchiectasis, bronchogenic cysts, and infected carcinomas may spread by internal bronchoembolism to set up secondary abscesses. Rarely, infections may spread from the spine, the esophagus, or beneath the diaphragm to invade the lung.

PATHOLOGY

Aspiration Lung Abscess. When the aspirated bronchoembolus obstructs the bronchus, it causes atelectasis, which provides the ideal environment for anaerobes. The infection is usually confined to the bronchopulmonary segment served by that bronchus so the abscess is unilobar and unilateral. A localized pneumonitis and consolidation is followed 10 to 14 days later by necrosis. The affected segment or subsegment always extends to the visceral pleura, but the pleura itself, along with a small layer of subjacent lung, does not become necrotic because its blood supply is from a subpleural vascular plexus. As a result, pleurisy and effusion occur, but empyema is unusual. Granulation tissue lines the cavity, which contains liquefied pus, tissue sloughs, debris, and organisms. Pneumonitis surrounds the granulation tissue. Ultimately, the abscess ruptures into a bronchus, pus drains into the bronchial tree, air enters the cavity, and an air-fluid level results. The slough prevents complete emptying by exerting a ball-valve effect. Without treatment, the abscess becomes chronic and is filled with thick gluelike material. Satellite abscesses are scattered through its thick fibrous walls, which become adherent to the pleura. Chronic pneumonitis is present, and the lung becomes honeycombed by fistulous tracks. Erosion of large blood vessels may cause hemoptysis, and septic thrombosis of the pulmonary veins results in septic emboli to the brain.

Inhalational Lung Abscess. Staphylococcal pneumonia begins in the airways following inhalation. There is an intense granulocyte response. The alveoli are destroyed and peritracheal abscesses form. Because air can enter these abscesses but cannot escape, the weakened tissue becomes distended and creates thin-walled cavities that

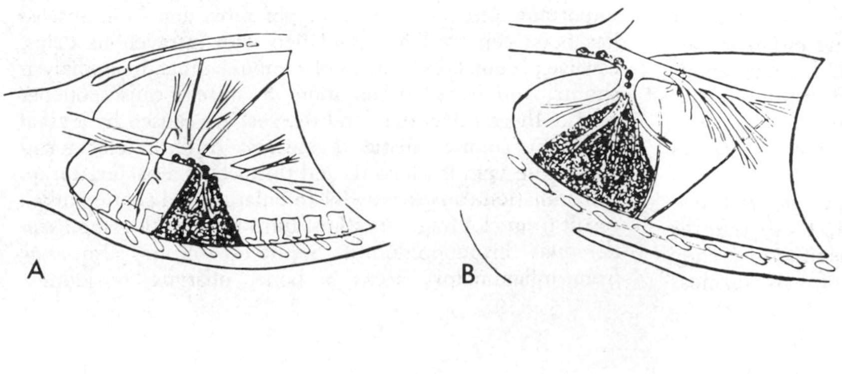

Figure 2. Influence of position on segmental localization of lung abscess. *A,* With the patient on his back, the apical segment of the lower lobe is the most dependent site for localization of bronchoemboli. *B,* The posterior segment of the upper lobe is most vulnerable when the patient is lying on his side. (From Brock, R. C.: Lung Abscess. Springfield, Ill., Charles C Thomas, 1952.)

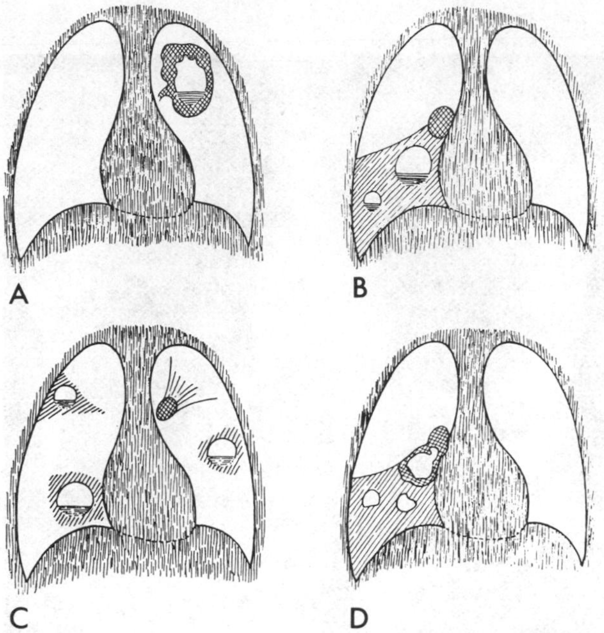

Figure 3. Formation of lung abscess in patients with bronchogenic carcinoma. *A*, Abscess after necrosis of central portion of tumor. *B*, Abscess due to infection of lobe obstructed by tumor (usually two or more). *C*, Spillover abscesses from primary carcinoma in left upper lobe. *D*, Combination of A and B. (From Brock, R. C.: Lung Abscess. Springfield, Ill. Charles C Thomas, 1952.)

contain a small amount of pus. These pneumatoceles may become very large. They occur especially in children and are virtually pathognomonic of staphylococcal pneumonia. The alveoli are filled with proteinaceous material, bacteria, debris, and neutrophils. Multiple thick-walled abscesses occur as well, and bronchopleural fistulas and empyema result. A fulminant hemorrhagic *Staphylococcus* pneumonia follows influenza A. The lungs are plum-colored, engorged, and heavy. The cut surfaces show multiple tiny abscesses.

Pseudomonas pneumonia is characterized by peribronchial abscesses and alveolar necrosis (Fetzer et al., 1967). Yellow-brown, necrotic, umbilicated nodules form that contain myriads of bacteria arranged around large blood vessels. The alveolar septa are intact, and there is a minimal inflammatory response in which lymphocytes and monocytes predominate. *E. coli* causes a hemorrhagic pneumonia. Mononuclear cells infiltrate the interstitium, and proteinaceous exudate fills the alveoli. Areas of atelectasis and emphysema are prominent.

In glanders, the abscess consists of nodules in which neutrophils are surrounded by a zone of congestion. Extensive nuclear degeneration causes small foci of deeply staining debris. Later, the abscess consists of epithelioid cells around a central core of necrosis. Melioidosis causes thin-walled abscesses in the upper lobes; if the lower lobes are affected, it is via the bloodstream. The abscesses contain a core of debris and multinucleated giant cells surrounded first by a layer of neutrophils and then by a layer of hemorrhage. In chronic infections, a core of caseation necrosis is surrounded by granulation tissue, plasma cells, and mononuclear cells.

Hematogenous Lung Abscess. Septic emboli (in contrast to bronchoemboli) occlude branches of the pulmonary artery and cause gangrenous infarction. The infarction progresses rapidly to cavity formation, pleural effusion, and empyema. *S. aureus* is by far the most common organism isolated, but *B. fragilis*, other *Bacteroides*, peptostreptococci, and gram-negative organisms are also responsible.

CLINICAL MANIFESTATIONS

The Clinical Setting. An accurate diagnosis can be made on the basis of the history, clinical findings, and setting in which the infection occurred. In aspiration lung abscess, there may be a history of alcoholic stupor or an epileptic fit in a patient with gingival disease; the symptoms of pulmonary infection have a subacute onset with the production of copious foul sputum. In hospitals, the precipitating event is likely to be a neurologic illness, esophageal disease, or anesthesia; and a mixed aerobic/anaerobic infection is present.

Septic emboli typically occur in a young male addict and cause a disease of dramatic suddenness because of pulmonary infarction and fulminant pulmonary infection. Occasionally, it occurs among patients hospitalized for intestinal or gynecologic disease (Griffith et al., 1977) or in those given intravenous cannulation.

Gram-negative bacterial pneumonia and lung abscesses may occur outside the hospital, but most are nosocomial infections in patients already very ill with chronic debilitating illnesses or immunosuppression. Superinfection with *Klebsiella* and other gram-negative bacteria may cause lung abscess in patients receiving penicillin therapy for pneumococcal pneumonia (Fig. 4). *Pseudomonas* spp. have a propensity to attack patients with burns or on ventilators.

Staphylococcal pneumonia occurs after influenza A and is a common cause of sepsis in infants. Pneumatoceles and empyema are pathognomonic of staphylococcal disease at that age. It may also occur in the same context as the gram-negative pneumonias and is a leading cause of septicemia, endocarditis, pneumonia, and lung abscess in patients with intravenous catheters.

Aspiration Abscess. Occasionally, a patient may willfully conceal part of the history, especially when it concerns alcoholic stupor, epilepsy, or criminal head injuries. Men outnumber women at least 4 to 1 among patients with aspiration abscesses. It is virtually unknown in edentulous patients unless there is a previous history of stupor. Malaise, fever, nonproductive dry cough, chills, and pleuritic pain or a dull, deep-seated ache in the chest begin three to four days after aspiration. After bronchial communication occurs, the contents of the entire abscess may be expectorated, but usually the amount of sputum steadily increases, and the abscess is only partially drained. The pus is foul in about 50 per cent of cases; only certain obligate anaerobes produce the foul odor, which takes about one week to develop and is quickly abolished by penicillin. Physical signs are minimal before and after abscess formation. There may be dullness, reduced breath sounds, and fremitus, and few rales, if any. These findings differ from those of lobar pneumonia because in lung abscess the lobe does not have the firmness of pneumococcal hepatization. Instead, it is a poorly ventilated, wet, sodden spongy lobe, heavy with pus and undergoing disintegration (Amberson, 1954). A pleural effusion may be found. Spontaneous cure is rare without treatment. If clubbing of the fingers is

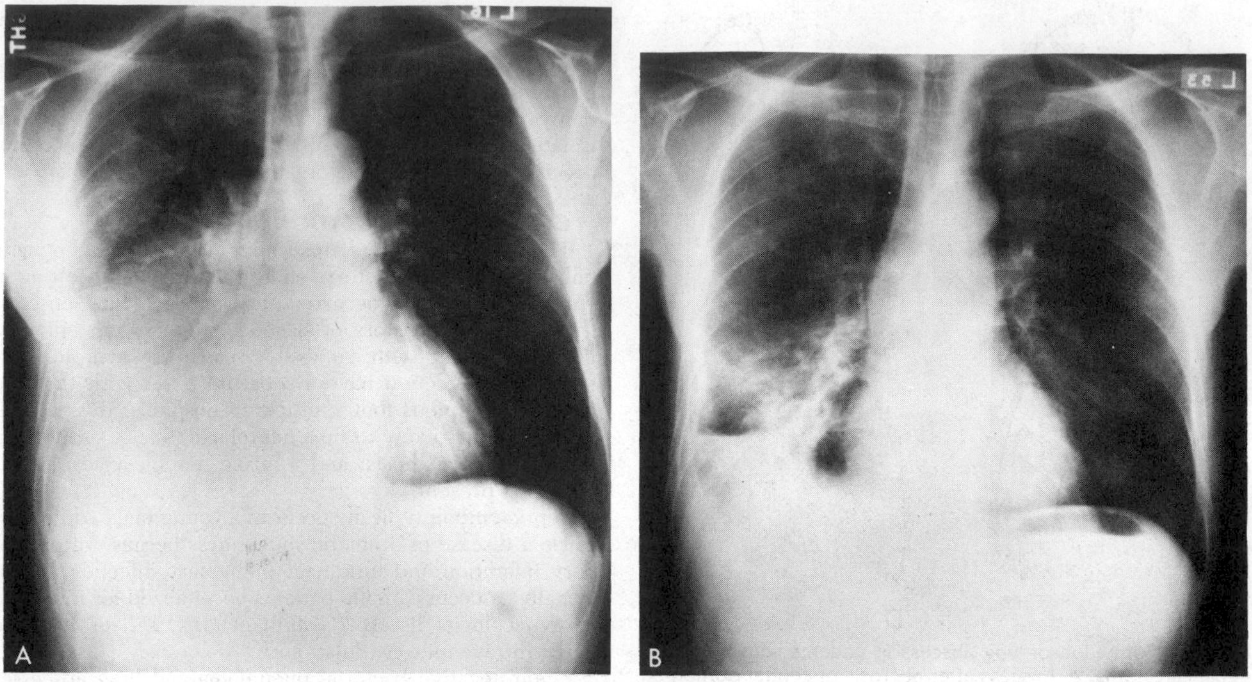

Figure 4. Superinfection lung abscess due to *Klebsiella pneumoniae* in patient treated with 800,000 units penicillin G daily for pneumococcal pneumonia. *A,* Chest x-ray showing pneumonia before lung abscess. *B,* Chest x-ray showing *Klebsiella* lung abscess.

found in a patient with an acute abscess, bronchogenic carcinoma should be suspected.

With chronic abscess, the patient becomes wasted, ill, and toxic; and he has a persistent cough and sputum. His fingers are clubbed, and there is weight loss, anemia, and low-grade fever. Brain abscess and severe hemoptysis may occur. Rarely, a chronic abscess can be clinically silent.

Embolic Lung Abscess. When lung abscess is due to septic emboli, the signs and symptoms are tachypnea, tachycardia, dyspnea, chest pain, hemoptysis, and syncope. They may be preceded by chills, fever, and rigors. Less than 20 per cent of cases of tricuspid endocarditis have cardiac signs and this condition must be suspected on the basis of intravenous drug addiction, septicemia, and pulmonary infarction. Drug addiction is recognized by the needle tracks and microabscesses in the skin. Emboli from the heart cause multiple lesions in the lower lobes with pleural effusion. Cavitation occurs in 25 per cent of lesions, but empyema is rare. Positive blood cultures in endocarditis of the right side are to be expected, in contrast to aspiration abscesses in which positive blood cultures are rare.

Emboli from peripheral veins are larger than those from endocarditis, and approximately 50 per cent of lesions cavitate. A solitary abscess occurs in half the cases. Over 80 per cent have leukocytosis and positive blood cultures. Pleural effusion and empyema are common. The external condition of a vein is not a reliable guide to the presence of thrombophlebitis even though it is inflamed, because a vein may be the source of emboli long after a cannula has been removed. In women, thrombosed veins may be palpated in a vaginal fornix. Sometimes soft tissue infections have resolved, and an infected contiguous vein remains as a source of emboli.

Pneumonic Lung Abscess. Cavities that occur in pneumonia are overshadowed by the signs and symptoms of the pneumonia. Many of the signs and symptoms are common to all the pneumonias (Chapters 111 and 112), including fever, breathlessness, pleurisy, tachypnea, and purulent, blood-stained sputum. Cavitation occurs in approximately 50 per cent of pneumonias due to gram-negative bacteria. Staphylococcal pneumonia carries a high mortality after influenza A and in infancy. Pneumatocele may be associated with mediastinal shift and symptoms of lung compression. Empyema occurs early and in 90 per cent of children, and metastatic infections of the skin occur in 15 per cent of cases.

DIAGNOSIS. A provisional diagnosis can often be made on the basis of the history and clinical findings. Severe alcoholism is prominent in 70 per cent and dental caries in nearly 100 per cent of aspiration abscesses. A putrid (fetid) sputum is diagnostic of an anaerobic infection. Culture of bronchial secretions accurately reflects the responsible organisms, but when expectorated, such secretions are contaminated by mouth organisms. Because of this, specimens should also be taken from blood, pleural fluid, empyema fluid, discharging sinuses, and the tips of intravenous cannulas, which are less likely to be contaminated. When this is not possible, transtracheal aspiration should be considered for obtaining a specimen (Bartlett and Finegold, 1972). The front of the neck is cleaned, and local anesthetic is infiltrated in the area of the thyroid cartilage. With the neck hyperextended, a 16-gauge intracatheter is passed through the cricothyroid membrane and threaded into the trachea, and the needle is pulled back. Secretions are sucked into a syringe or into a Lukens trap by a constant suction apparatus. This procedure should not be done on anyone with bleeding disorders, cardiac arrhythmias, uncontrolled cough, or hypoxia. The procedure may be complicated by bleeding from an aberrant artery, local and mediastinal emphysema, and an infection along the needle track. If squamous cells are present, the specimen is discarded because it indicates that the catheter passed into the mouth.

Aspiration abscess results from an infection by several species of bacteria; and the Gram stain should show numerous polymorphonuclear leukocytes, gram-positive fusiform beaded bacilli with tapered or cigar-shaped ends, streptococci, gram-negative rods resembling *Bacteroides* spp., and a variety of pleomorphic gram-negative rods. In a specimen that is not contaminated by mouth flora, spirochetes are virtually diagnostic of anaerobic infection.

The presence and exact position of an abscess can only be determined by examining both posteroanterior and lateral chest x-rays. Aspiration abscesses almost always occur in the apical segment of a lower lobe or the posterior segment of an upper lobe. They are usually solitary and have thick walls with a ragged lining. Empyema occurs with 30 per cent of all embolic abscesses. Their walls are also thick and their lining ragged. Staphylococcal pneumonia has no lobe predilection; and in children, pneumatoceles, pneumothorax, and pyopneumothorax are diagnostic. *Klebsiella,* and occasionally *Pseudomonas,* cause pneumonias that affect predominantly the upper lobes. All cause thick-walled abscess with ragged linings. The lower lobes are affected by *Pseudomonas, E. coli, N. asteroides,* and *A. israelii* infection. *Proteus, Klebsiella, Nocardia,* and *F. tularensis* all cause radiographic appearances that can mimic *M. tuberculosis.*

Ordinary lung abscesses must be differentiated from carcinomatous abscesses, which are thick-walled and have eccentric cavities. They should be suspected if the abscess is located in a segment that is not dependent during aspiration; in other words, abscesses in the anterior segment, lingula, or middle lobe should raise the question of carcinoma. Sputum cytology makes the diagnosis in 90 per cent of cases (Wallace et al., 1979). It should be kept in mind that one third of lung cavities are due to underlying bronchogenic carcinoma in patients over 45 (Brock, 1952). Bronchogenic cysts are thin-walled, occur in the medial third of the lower lobes, and remain after the infection has been cured. Sequestrated segments have thin walls also and usually occur in the lower lobes. Dermoid cysts are found in the anterior mediastinum. *Entamoeba hystolytica* and *Echinococcus granulosus* affect the lower lobes. In the latter, air between the endocyst and ectocyst creates a halo effect, and, where the lining membrane falls into the cavity fluid, the "water lily" sign results.

Tuberculosis, atypical mycobacterial infections, coccidioidomycosis, histoplasmosis, and blastomycosis produce cavitary disease and are important in the differential diagnosis in endemic areas. All may be acquired by visitors to these areas.

COMPLICATIONS AND SEQUELAE. Aspiration abscess has few complications or sequelae, surgery is rarely required, and mortality is low. With any large abscess there is a risk of asphyxiation from sudden rupture and discharge of pus through both lungs. Since chronic abscesses are unusual, severe hemoptysis, bronchopleural fistulas, and empyemas are not common. After successful treatment, the cavity may persist for one or more years, but eventually it closes spontaneously. A bronchogram may reveal residual asymptomatic bronchiectasis.

Septic emboli cause infarction, septicemia, and fulminant pulmonary infection, any of which may be lethal. Empyema occurs with 30 per cent of emboli from peripheral sites. If the primary source is promptly and adequately treated, there should be few sequelae.

Bacteremia and shock are important complications in staphylococcal and gram-negative pneumonias. Often the prognosis is that of the underlying disease, but it is difficult to control infections in those with marked neutropenia. Pleural effusion and empyema are common. Dissemination of abscesses to other organs may occur in staphylococcal pneumonia. There is a high mortality when the pneumonia complicates influenza or occurs in infancy. Pneumatoceles may cause mediastinal compression, but usually the air spontaneously reabsorbs. Gram-negative organisms may cause fibrosis, shrinkage, and chronic cavitation.

GEOGRAPHIC VARIATION. In Africa, aspiration abscess is still a dangerous disease with a high mortality (Adebonojo et al., 1979; Atherstone and Gelfand, 1972). It often presents in the chronic stage, and hemoptysis is frequent and requires immediate surgery. The maximum incidence is in the fourth decade of life when bronchiectasis, lobar pneumonia, and esophageal stricture are common causes. Its severity is attributed to late presentation for medical care, sickle cell disease, and poor nutrition. In Zimbabwe, there is also a high incidence in the fourth decade of life. However, it is a much milder disease and has a low mortality. Again, lobar pneumonia figures prominently in the etiology. The incidence and pattern of the disease in India and Japan seem to mirror those in Western countries (Kaltreider, 1976; Shinoi, 1960).

Glanders is seen only in Africa, Asia, and South America. Melioidosis is endemic in Southeast Asia and occurs sporadically in the surrounding nations. Tularemia is endemic in Europe, Asia, Texas, Oklahoma, Louisiana, and Arkansas. All these diseases may affect travelers to endemic areas.

TREATMENT

Anaerobic Lung Abscess. Penicillin is the treatment of choice in aspiration abscess even in the presence of penicillinase-producing *B. fragilis.* (Abernathy, 1968; Bartlett and Gorbach, 1975). Penicillin is effective whether given orally or parenterally. Although clindamycin may be somewhat more effective, it has remained a second line drug because it can cause life threatening colitis, neutropenia and liver function disturbance. The dose of penicillin G is one million units every six hours, intravenously, or penicillin V, 750 mg, orally, every 6 hours. Clindamycin is given every 4 hours, intravenously, in a dose of 300 mg, or 450 mg, orally, every 6 hours. A theoretical reason for the effectiveness of clindamycin is its concentration in alveolar macrophages and leukocytes and therefore within abscesses (Hand and King-Thompson, 1982.)

In a recent multicenter prospective study of lung abscess, patients treated with clindamycin had fewer days of fever and fetid sputum, compared to those given penicillin. Also, they were less likely to have radiologic extension of their lesions, and they had fewer relapses either late in their treatment, or after it was discontinued (Levison et al., 1983). A single-center retrospective study of lung abscess showed no difference between children treated with penicillin or clindamycin (Brook, 1981).

These results may reflect the changing sensitivity of anaerobes in different parts of the United States. Twenty per cent of isolates of *B. melaninogenicus* now have plasmid-mediated resistance to penicillin (Bawdon et al., 1982; Bartlett 1983). *B. melaninogenicus* is isolated from about 40 per cent of lung abscesses (Bartlett and Finegold 1974). Newly recognized pathogenic anaerobes such as *B. ureolyticus* and *B. ruminicola* (subspecies *brevis*) are penicillin resistant.

Conjugative resistance to clindamycin is present in about 2 per cent of isolates of *B. fragilis*. In some hospitals there is clustering of isolates that are resistant to clindamycin, cefoxitin, and piperacillin. Up to 20 per cent of isolates of peptococci, and *Clostridia* are now clindamycin resistant. The differences in resistance patterns may lead to a wider use of sensitivity tests as a guide to treatment of anaerobic infections.

Where the patient is seriously ill, clindamycin may be preferable to penicillin, but in most cases, penicillin should remain the drug of first choice, unless contraindicated by penicillin allergy, poor response to treatment, or penicillin resistance in the isolated anaerobes (Bartlett, 1982).

Metronidazole has good activity against strict anaerobes, but there have been conflicting reports about its effectiveness in lung abscess.

Postural drainage is important adjunctive therapy. Surgical resection is used only for severe hemoptysis (Thoms and Arbula, 1970), or for the few abscesses that do not respond to antibiotics. With adequate treatment all patients are afebrile, and cavities shrink by 10 days. At 6 weeks, 70 per cent are healed. Clinical recovery is accompanied by decreased production, and less purulence of sputum, an increase of weight and appetite, a fall in leukocyte count, and disappearance of fever. Failure of response should raise the question of bronchogenic carcinoma.

Embolic Lung Abscess. The source of septic emboli must be identified early and treated vigorously in order to minimize the need for heparin and to prevent a fatal embolus. All intravenous cannulas should be removed and abscesses drained. Veins suspected of being the source of emboli may need exploration, ligation, or excision. Because a wide variety of organisms cause phlebitis at intravenous drip sites, the initial antimicrobial drug therapy may have to be based on Gram stain of the cannula tip. Clindamycin or metronidazole should be used for septic emboli of pelvic origin because *B. fragilis* is likely to be involved there. If tricuspid endocarditis cannot be controlled with high doses of antimicrobials because of drug resistance, it should be excised early.

Staphylococcal pneumonia and lung abscesses are treated with oxacillin or nafcillin in a dose of 1.0 g, intravenously, every 3 hours. If penicillin allergy is present, the treatment is intravenous cefazolin in a dose of 1.0 g every 6 hours. If pneumatoceles cause respiratory embarrassment, they should be aspirated. Pneumothorax and pyopneumothorax must be drained. Gram-negative organisms are treated on the basis of sensitivity tests. Until these results are known, a combination of amikacin and piperacillin will cover most gram-negative bacteria that produce lung abscess. The dose is 15 mg/kg amikacin every 8 hours, intravenously. Ticarcillin can be used (with amikacin) in place of piperacillin. In patients allergic to penicillin, moxalactam, cefotaxime, or trimethoprim-sulfamethoxazole can be given with amikacin instead of piperacillin. Immunosuppressive drugs may be reduced in dosage, if necessary, until the infection can be controlled.

PREVENTION. Lung abscesses will continue to be a problem among intravenous drug addicts and alcoholics. In all vulnerable groups, oropharyngeal sepsis should be eradicated before surgery or dental procedures and after fracture of the jaw in order to reduce the risk of aspiration abscess. *Staphylococcus* lung abscess can be minimized by influenza vaccination because primary *Staphylococcus* lung abscess in adults is almost exclusively a complication of influenza. The development of a pneumococcal vaccine that reflects African serotypes may have an important role to play in Nigeria, since abscess commonly follows lobar pneumonia there.

The biggest reduction may occur as a result of better control of iatrogenic nosocomial infection (Stein and Pruitt, 1970). Intravenous cannulation should be kept to the absolute minimum. Intravenous drip sites and the delivery tubing should be changed frequently. In hemodialysis, those shunts with the lowest infection rate, such as the Cimino shunt, should be used. Respirator ventilators should be sterilized and constantly monitored for *Pseudomonas* sp. *L. pneumophila* should be eradicated from the cooling towers of air conditioning systems, especially in hotels and hospitals (Dondero et al., 1980). Patients with dangerous organisms resistant to many antibiotics should be placed in isolation from debilitated or immunosuppressed individuals.

NOCARDIOSIS

Nocardiosis, an infection caused by an aerobic actinomycete, may produce lung abscesses and spread to the brain and elsewhere, or it may appear as a chronic deforming granulomatous infection limited to the foot (mycetoma, Chap 252).

ETIOLOGY. Pulmonary and disseminated nocardiosis usually results from infection with *Nocardia asteroides*. This organism is relatively acid-fast, and its bacillary form resembles the tubercle bacillus, but *N. asteroides* is easily differentiated from the tubercle bacillus by rapid growth on Sabouraud's medium or 10 per cent blood agar at room temperature, and by the presence in exudates of long-branched, gram-positive mycelial forms.

PATHOGENESIS. *Nocardia asteroides* can be recovered readily from soil. Nocardiosis appears, therefore, to be an exogenous infection usually having its portal of entry in the lungs. In almost every patient with nocardiosis (other than maduromycosis), the earliest and most extensive lesions are acute pulmonary suppurative foci (Weed et al., 1955). A well-defined wall is absent, a fact that probably accounts for the marked tendency of nocardial abscesses to spread to the brain and to a lesser extent to the spleen, skin, peritoneum, and kidney. Occasionally, noncaseating granulomas are found. Susceptibility to nocardiosis is increased in Cushing's syndrome, in pulmonary alveolar proteinosis, and in some patients with lymphomas or leukemia after antitumor chemotherapy (Andriole et al., 1964; Danowski et al., 1962).

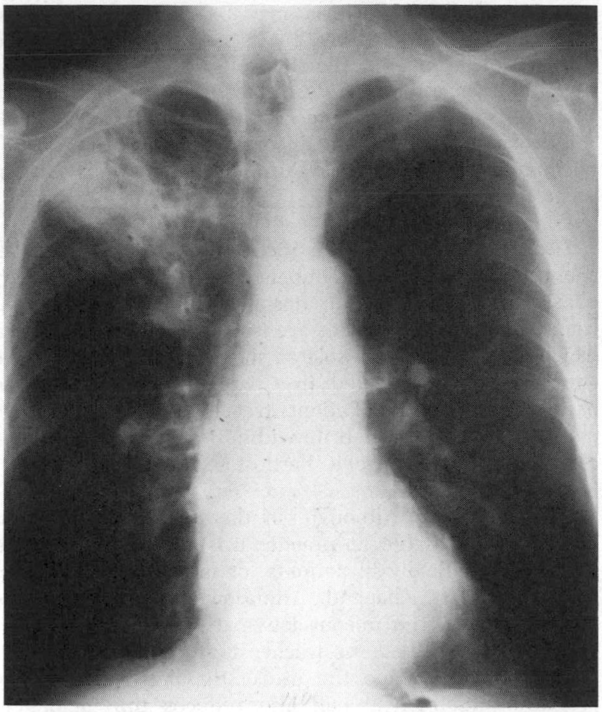

Figure 5. Nocardial lung abscess resembling tuberculosis.

CLINICAL MANIFESTATIONS. The chief symptom is cough, usually productive of a thick, sometimes bloody, sputum. Chest pain and dyspnea are common, as are fever, sweats, chills, leukocytosis, weakness, anorexia, and weight loss. The illness may be prolonged and present the picture of chronic pulmonary tuberculosis, lung abscess (Fig. 5), or unresolved suppurative pneumonia. This syndrome can be interrupted suddenly by the acute neurologic changes of metastatic brain abscess. At this time, the patient may have severe headache and focal sensory or motor disturbances. The protein concentration, cells, and pressure of the spinal fluid are increased, but the concentration of glucose is not reduced unless the meninges are also infected. Occasionally, brain abscess is the first clinical manifestation of nocardiosis, especially in Cushing's syndrome secondary to adrenal steroid therapy. Infection of the skin is frequent and produces numerous scattered abscesses or single draining sinuses of the hand, chest wall, or buttocks.

The disease is usually fatal after months to years, if not treated.

DIAGNOSIS. Because patients with nocardiosis are suspected of having tuberculosis, their sputa are examined for tubercle bacilli. The usual methods for concentrating tubercle bacilli often kill *N. asteroides. N. asteroides* may also be overlooked in smears stained by the Ziehl-Neelsen method because it is less resistant than the tubercle bacillus to decolorization by alcohol. Killing the organism can be avoided by concentrating with trisodium phosphate, and overdecolorizing can be avoided by using 1 per cent sulfuric acid.

Although sulfur granules are not found in pulmonary or disseminated nocardiosis, the gram-positive filamentous organisms in nocardial exudates often resemble *Actinomyces israelii*. The two pathogens can be distinguished, however, by the ease with which *N. asteroides* is cultivated on Sabouraud's medium or blood agar aerobically and by its acid-fast staining characteristics. In biopsy material, the nongranulomatous and minimally fibrotic character of the nocardial suppurative reaction also helps to distinguish it from infections due to *A. israelii*. The absence of tubercles is valuable in differential diagnosis from tuberculosis.

TREATMENT. Administration of sulfadiazine is sometimes successful treatment. Penicillin and tetracycline appear to be ineffective, and resistance of nocardiosis to these drugs may be used in distinguishing it from actinomycosis due to *A. israelii* and from other pulmonary infections that respond to these antibiotics. Patients with nocardiosis should receive 8 to 12 g of sulfadiazine daily. The successful treatment of nocardiosis with the combination of trimethoprim-sulfamethoxazole is attributed to the sulfamethoxazole. Cycloserine shows promise for patients allergic to sulfonamides.

ASPIRATION PNEUMONIA

Aspiration pneumonia is an inflammatory lesion of the lung parenchyma due to the aspiration of bacteria-laden secretions from the oropharynx. It may be a stage in the development of aspiration lung abscess, and many of the etiologic, pathogenic, and clinical features described for such abscesses also pertain to aspiration pneumonia. Its true incidence is unknown, but it is probably underdiagnosed because it resembles other bacterial pneumonias (Bartlett, 1979). Also it is obscured by a wide range of underlying medical problems, and not every hospital has the facilities to diagnose anaerobic infections of the lung.

Aspiration pneumonia is one of the aspiration syndromes, each of which is defined by the material aspirated (Table 1). It is the commonest of these syndromes, but has a lower mortality, tends to be subacute or chronic (as well as acute)

Table 1. ASPIRATION SYNDROMES

Substances	Onset	Sequela	Mortality
Gastric Acid, pH< 2.4.	Within 2 hours	Hypoxia. Respiratory failure. Superimposed infection.	High
Fluids: Hypertonic, Hypotonic	Instantaneous	Hypoxia. Severe electrolyte and fluid problems. Superimposed infection.	May be high
Fluids: Isotonic		Hypoxia	Low
Particulate Matter	Instantaneous. Small particles may be silent.	Apnea. Chronic chemical inflammation, Superimposed infection.	High with large particles
Oropharyngeal Secretions	Seldom less than 24 hours	Depends upon the extent and severity of infection.	Low for aspiration pneumonia

and never occurs with the dramatic suddenness associated with the other syndromes. There are important microbiological differences related to whether the aspiration occurs in hospital or in the community. Thus 91 per cent of aspiration pneumonias in the community are due to anaerobes, and pure aerobic aspiration pneumonia in community-acquired cases are less than 10 per cent of the total. In the hospital, by contrast, over a third of cases of aspiration pneumonia appear to be pure aerobic infections.

PATHOGENESIS. The pathogenesis of aspiration pneumonia is the same as that described above for aspiration lung abscess. Aspiration pneumonia may be due to aspiration of normal or abnormal flora. Colonization of the oropharynx with abnormal flora occurs in many illnesses, and certain environments predispose the sick to develop such colonization (Johanson et al., 1972, Mackowiak et al., 1978; Valenti et al., 1978). Among these predisposing factors are alcoholism, bladder incontinence, deteriorating clinical states, terminal illness, diabetes mellitus, the bedridden state, chronic lung disease, cardiac or neoplastic disability, acidosis, and intubation. Spread to the oropharynx is believed to be by the fecal-oral route, but there is some evidence that the stomach, especially if hypochlorhydric, may act as a reservoir for these organisms (Du Moulin et al., 1982, Atherton and White 1978).

Anaerobic pneumonia is the commonest of the pleuropulmonary anaerobic diseases. Occasionally, it progresses to form an acute necrotizing pneumonia in which multiple abscesses occur, but in 20 per cent of cases, it will progress to lung abscess (Bartlett and Finegold, 1974).

CLINICAL FEATURES. This pneumonia may not differ in its presentation from other bacterial pneumonias, except that shaking chills do not occur. The clue to its diagnosis should be the presence of an illness predisposing to aspiration and a new shadow in a gravity dependent segment. Alcoholism, epilepsy, and drug addiction predispose to community-acquired infections. The majority have bad teeth and gums, but toothlessness is not protective. Putrid sputum is rare (Lorber and Swenson 1974, Bartlett et al., 1974).

RADIOLOGIC DIAGNOSIS. Aspirated material lodges in the gravity-dependent segments of the lung, especially the anterior and posterior segments of the upper lobes, and the superior and basilar segments of the lower lobes (Bartlett and Finegold 1974). Where infection occurs in a nondependent segment, a neoplasm should be considered. Resolution should begin in the first week of treatment, although deterioration may be apparent in the first few days.

LABORATORY DIAGNOSIS. Because of oropharyngeal contamination, culture of expectorated sputum is unreliable in both aerobic and anaerobic infections. The diagnosis can be made by transtracheal aspiration, or directly from the lesion by fiberoptic bronchoscope. The former is safe in experienced hands and gives a 1 per cent false negative result, and a 20 per cent false positive result. False positives rarely occur with anaerobic infections. A gram stain of the aspirate is 90 per cent reliable for preliminary identification. The use of a protected catheter or brush with the fiberoptic bronchoscope permits quantitative counts, and immunofluorescent techniques to be applied to the bacteria so that colonizing bacteria may be differentiated from pathogenic bacteria. Few patients have positive blood cultures or empyema (Bartlett, 1977). The commonest anaerobes isolated are *Peptostreptococcus sp.*, *Peptococcus sp.*, microaerophilic streptococci, *B. melaninogenicus*, *B. fragilis* and *F. nucleatum*. The commonest aerobes are *S. pneumoniae*, *S. aureus*, *Klebsiella sp.*, and *Enterobacteriaceae sp.*

TREATMENT. Penicillin is the treatment of choice in all community-acquired pneumonias from which *any* anaerobes are isolated, and for hospital acquired pneumonias from which *only* anaerobes are isolated. Pneumonias from which only aerobes are isolated should be treated with the antibiotics recommended in Chapters 111 and 112 on bacterial pneumonias. Patients treated correctly for anaerobic pneumonia are afebrile within 3 days, and radiologic clearing occurs by 1 week (Bartlett and Gorbach, 1975).

PROPHYLAXIS. Although, in theory, aspiration pneumonia is preventable, in practice it is not because it often occurs in terminally ill patients, or in those whose social habits cannot be changed. Attention to the principles of nursing care in the unconscious patient reduces its incidence and the need for tracheostomy (Atkinson, 1970). Skilled anesthesia and the use of the high volume, low pressure endotracheal cuff also reduces the incidence. Attention to some of the conditions that predispose to gram-negative colonization may also help.

References

Abernathy, R. S.: Antibiotic therapy of lung abscess. Dis Chest 53:292, 1968.

Adebonojo, S. A., Osinowo, O., and Adebo, O.: Lung abscess. A review of three years' experience at the University College Hospital, Ibadan. J Nat Med Assoc 71:39, 1979.

Amberson, J. B.: A clinical consideration of abscesses and cavities of the lung. Bull Johns Hopkins Hosp 94:227, 1954.

Andriole, V. T., et al: The association of nocardiosis and pulmonary alveolar proteinosis. Ann Intern Med 60:266, 1964.

Atherstone, N., and Gelfand, M.: Lung abscess in Africans admitted to the Medical Unit, Harare Hospital. Cent Afr J Med 18:49, 1972.

Atherton, S. T., and White, D. J.: Stomach as a source of bacteria colonizing respiratory tract during artificial ventilation. Lancet 2:968, 1978.

Atkinson, W. J.: Posture of the unconscious patient. Lancet 1:404, 1970.

Bartlett, J. G., and Finegold, S. M.: Anaerobic pleuropulmonary infections. Medicine 51:413, 1972.

Bartlett, J. G., and Gorbach, S. L.: Treatment of aspiration pneumonia and primary lung abscess. Penicillin G vs clindamycin. JAMA 234:939, 1975.

Bartlett, J. G., Rosenblatt, J. E., and Finegold, S. M.: Percutaneous transtracheal aspiration in the diagnosis of anaerobic pulmonary infection. Ann Intern Med 79-535, 1973.

Bartlett, J. G.: Anti-anaerobic antibacterial agents. Lancet 2:478, 1982.

Bartlett, J. G.: Recent developments in the management of anaerobic infections. Reviews of Infectious Diseases 5:2:235, 1983.

Bawdon, R. E., Crane, L. R., Palchaudhuri, S.: Antibiotic resistance in anaerobic bacteria: molecular biology and clinical aspects. Reviews of Infectious Diseases 4:6:1075, 1982.

Brock, R. C.: Lung Abscess. Springfield, Ill., Charles C Thomas, 1952.

Brook, I.: Aspiration pneumonia in institutionalized children. A retrospective comparison of treatment with penicillin G, clindamycin and carbenicillin. Clinical Pediatrics 20:2:117, 1981.

Danowski, T. S., et al.: Cushing's syndrome in conjunction with *Nocardia asteroides* infection. Metabolism 11:2, 1962.

Dondero, T. J., et al.: An outbreak of Legionnaire's disease associated with a contaminated air conditioning cooling tower. N Engl J Med 302:365, 1980.

Dowling, J. N., Kroboth, F. J., Karpf, M., Yee, R. B., Pasculle, A. W.: Pneumonia and multiple lung abscesses caused by dual infection with *Legionella micdadei*, and *Legionella pneumophila*. Am Rev Respir Dis 127:121, 1983.

Du Moulin, G. C., et al.: Aspiration of gastric bacteria in antacid-treated patients. A frequent cause of post-operative colonization of the airway. Lancet 1:247, 1982.
Fetzer, A. E., Werner, A. S., and Hagstrom, J. W. C.: Pathologic features of pseudomonal pneumonia. Am Rev Resp Dis 96:1121, 1967.
Flavell, G.: Lung abscess. Br Med J 1:1032, 1966.
Griffith, G. L., Maull, K. I., and Sachatello, C. R.: Septic pulmonary embolization. Surg Gynecol Obstet 144:105, 1977.
Hand, W. L., King-Thompson, N. L.: Membrane Transport of clindamycin in alveolar macrophages. Antimicrob Agents Chemother 21:241, 1982.
Johanson, W. G., et al.: Nosocomial respiratory tract infections with gram-negative bacilli. The significance of colonization of the respiratory tract. Ann. Intern. Med. 77:701, 1972.
Kaltreider, H. B.: Expression of the immune mechanism in the lung. Am Rev Resp Dis 113:347, 1976.
Levison, M. E., Mangura, C. T., Lorber, B., Abrutyn, E., Pesanti, E. L., Levy, R. S., Macgregor, R. R., Schwartz, A. R.: Clindamycin compared with penicillin for the treatment of anaerobic lung abscess. Ann Intern Med 98:466, 1983.
Lorber, B., and Swenson, R. M: Bacteriology of aspiration pneumonia. Ann Intern Med 81:329, 1974.
Murray, P. R., Weber, C. J.: Rapid detection of clindamycin resistance in *Bacteroides spp.* J Clin Micr 18:1001, 1983.
Stein, J. M., and Pruitt, B. A.: Suppurative thrombophlebitis. A lethal iatrogenic disease. New Engl J Med 282:1452, 1970.
Thoms, N. W., and Arbulu, A.: Significance of hemoptysis in lung abscess. J Thorac Cardiovasc Surg 59:5, 1970.
Valenti, W., Trudell, R., and Bentley, D.: Factors predisposing to oropharyngeal colonization in the aged. N Engl J Med 298:1108, 1978.
Wallace, R., Cohen, A., Aeve, R., Greenberg, D., Hadlock, F., and Park, S.: Carcinomatous lung abscess. Diagnosis by bronchoscopy and cytopathology. JAMA 242:521, 1979.
Weed, L. A., et al.: Nocardiosis: Clinical, bacteriologic, and pathologic aspects. N Engl J Med 253:1138, 1955.
Yangco, B. G., Deresinski, S. C.: Necrotizing or cavitating pneumonia due to *Streptococcus pneumoniae*. Medicine 59:6:449, 1980.

119

LEGIONELLOSIS (LEGIONNAIRES' DISEASE AND PONTIAC FEVER)

JEFFREY D. BAND, M.D.
DAVID W. FRASER, M.D.

Legionellosis is an acute bacterial infection of humans caused by members of the genus *Legionella (L. pneumophila, L. micdadei, L. bozemanii, L. dumoffii, L. gormanii, L. longbeachae, L. jordanis, L. oakridgensis, L. wadsworthii,* and *L. feeleii),* recently described, fastidious aerobic gram-negative bacilli. Two distinct clinicoepidemiologic syndromes have been observed: Legionnaires' disease, a multisystem illness characterized by pneumonia and a high case-fatality ratio, and Pontiac fever, a nonpneumonic, self-limited, acute nonfatal, febrile illness. Legionellosis occurs both sporadically and in explosive clusters such as the epidemic at the American Legion Convention in Philadelphia in 1976 (Fraser et al., 1977). Although *L pneumophila* was initially identified by McDade in late 1976 (McDade et al., 1977), subsequent investigation has shown that disease caused by *Legionella* is not new. The earliest documented cases occurred in the 1940's *(L. micdadei,* 1943; *L. pneumophila,* 1947; *L. bozemanii,* 1959), and at least six outbreaks of respiratory illness of previously undefined etiology that preceded the 1976 Philadelphia outbreak have now been shown to have been caused by *L. pneumophila*. Search for *L. pneumophila* in cases of pneumonia of uncertain cause has recently led to the discovery of other fastidious pneumonia-causing bacteria, many of which are still being classified and are the subject of intensive research.

ETIOLOGY. Members of the genus *Legionella* are faintly staining, thin, pleomorphic gram-negative bacilli that do not grow on most commonly used bacteriologic media. There are currently 10 distinct species of *Legionella* (Fig. 1). Ultrastructurally, the *Legionella* resemble other typical gram-negative rods with a double envelope of unit membrane and an extremely thin cell wall (Fig. 2). Vacuoles may be seen within the organism that stain with Sudan black B. *Legionella* can be stained with the Wolbach modification of the Giemsa stain or a modification of the Dieterle silver impregnation stain, although neither reaction is specific. In tissue, these organisms are typically found within macrophages or free in the alveoli. Direct immunofluorescent staining with conjugated rabbit antiserum is a more specific method of identification. The organisms have primarily been isolated from respiratory secretions, pleural fluid, and lung tissue, as well as from several environmental sites, such as water within heat rejection systems (cooling towers, evaporative condensers), rivers, lakes, ponds, riparian soil and more recently from municipal potable water systems, showerheads, and water

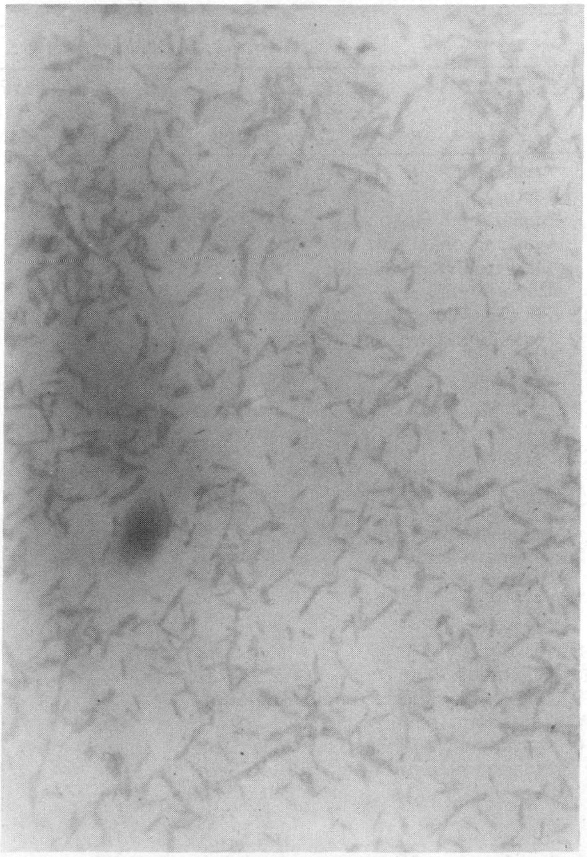

Figure 1. Gram-stain of *Legionella pneumophila* isolated from lung of a patient with LD. Courtesy of R. Weaver.

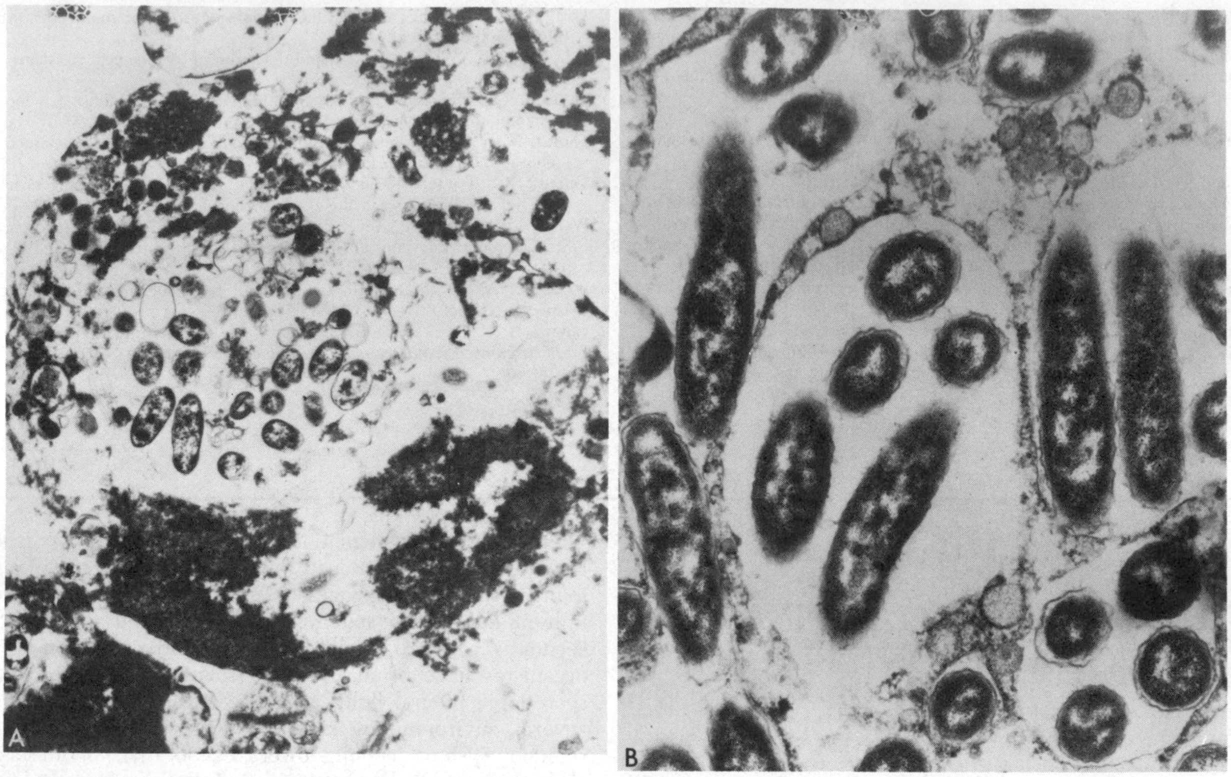

Figure 2. Electron micrograph of *L. pneumophila. A,* Within phagosome of alveolar macrophage from patient. Note both intact and degenerating organisms are present. 21,300× *B,* In yolk-sac membrane of embryonic hen's egg, organisms are intracellular and enclosed by a double envelope, each composed of a triple-layered unit membrane. 47,400× Courtesy of F. W. Chandler.

Table 1. SUMMARY OF 33 OUTBREAKS OF LEGIONELLOSIS

Location	Date	No. of Cases	Estimated Attack Rate (%)	Incubation Period	Syndrome	Case-Fatality Ratio (%)	Source of Organism
1. Austin, MN Factory	June-Aug 1957	78	—	—	LD	3	?
2. St. Elizabeth Hospital Washington, D. C.	July-Aug 1965	81	1.4	—	LD	17	Suspect excavation site
3. Oakland County Health Department Pontiac, Michigan	July-Aug 1968	144	95	5-66 hours (mean 36 hours)	Pontiac fever	0	Evaporative condenser
4. Hotel Benidorm, Spain	July 1973	8	—	—	LD	38	—
5. James River, Virginia	July 1973	10	100	17–43 hours (mean 37 hours)	Pontiac fever	0	Suspect turbine condenser
6. Odd Fellow Convention Philadelphia, Pennsylvania	Sept 1974	11	2.9	1–9 days	LD	10	Associated with grand ballroom of hotel
7. American Legion Convention Philadelphia, Pennsylvania	July-Aug 1976	221	4.0	2–10 days	LD	15	Associated with lobby of hotel and street in front of hotel
8. Hospitals Columbus, Ohio	July-Sept 1977	15	—	—	LD	13	—
9. Community and Hospital Kingsport, Tennessee	Aug-Sept 1977	33	0.2	—	LD	19	—
10. Community and Hospital Burlington, Vermont	May–Dec (Aug-Sept peak) 1977	69	—	—	LD	25	Hyperendemic
11. Hospital Los Angeles, California	1977→ (peak, late fall)	106	0.5	—	LD	26	Nosocomial outbreak

Table continued on opposite page

in whirlpool spas. Successful isolation techniques include intraperitoneal inoculation of guinea pigs with subsequent culturing of infected tissue in embryonic hens' eggs and on solid agar medium and, more recently, direct plating of specimens on solid agar medium that contains supplementary L-cysteine and ferric salts and activated charcoal. Examples of media used for isolation are Mueller-Hinton agar base with 0.04 per cent L-cysteine and 0.25 per cent ferric pyrophosphate (FG agar) and charcoal yeast-extract (CYE) agar with or without Aces buffer.

L. pneumophila grows slowly (3 to 10 days) on FG agar, producing small, glistening gray colonies with discoloration of the surrounding agar by brown soluble pigment. A yellow fluorescence of both the colonies and the surrounding medium is demonstrable under longwave (366 μm) ultraviolet light. L-tyrosine or L-phenylalanine seem to be important for production of the brown soluble pigment. On CYE agar, colonies appear earlier (2 to 4 days) and are more numerous than on FG agar. Growth appears optimal on CYE agar at pH 6.8 to 6.9 and at 35° C. The organism is a strict aerobe, but growth on FG and CYE media may be stimulated by 2.5 per cent carbon dioxide. The other members of the genus *Legionella* initially grow poorly if at all on FG agar and appear to grow best when CYE agar is buffered with ACES buffer (BCYE agar). BCYE agar does not require incubation in CO_2 (Pasculle et al., 1980).

Table 1. SUMMARY OF 33 OUTBREAKS OF LEGIONELLOSIS *(Continued)*

Location	Date	No. of Cases	Estimated Attack Rate (%)	Incubation Period	Syndrome	Case-Fatality Ratio (%)	Source of Organism
12. Hotel Bloomington, Indiana	1978→ (peak, summer-fall)	56	0.1 – 0.2	4–12 days	LD	12	Hyperendemic
13. Country Club Atlanta, Georgia	July 1978	8	1.5	—	LD	0	Evaporative condenser?
14. Garment district New York, New York	Aug-Sept 1978	38	—	—	LD	8	—
15. Hospital Memphis, Tennessee	Aug-Sept 1978	39	2.8	2–10 days	LD	13	Cooling tower condenser
16. Veterans of Foreign Wars Convention Dallas, Texas	Aug-Sept 1978	18	0.2	2–10 days	LD	6	—
17 Community and Hospital Norwalk, Connecticut	1978 (peak, summer-fall)	28	0.7	—	LD	36	Hyperendemic area
18. Eau Claire, WI Hotel	June-July 1979	13	0.3	2–9	LD	31	Cooling tower condenser
19. Jamestown, NY Factory	July 1979	7	0.7	—	LD	14	?
20. Pittsburgh, PA Hospital	1979	28	—	—	LD	—	?
21. Vasteras, Sweden	Aug-Sept 1979	58	—	—	LD	2	?
22. San Francisco, CA Office Building	Feb-March 1980	6	—	—	LD	33	? Cooling tower condenser
23. Burlington, VT Hospital & Community	June-Sept 1980	86	—	—	LD	—	? Cooling tower condenser
24. Benidorm, Spain Hotel	July 1980	20	—	—	LD	5	?
25. Leiden, Netherlands Hospital		8	—	—	LD	0	?
26. Como, Italy Hotel	July-Oct 1980	17	—	—	LD	6	?
27. England Hospital	Dec-July 1979–80	12	—	—	LD	—	? Cooling tower condenser ? Potable water
28. Windsor, Canada Factory	August 1981	395	—	—	Pontiac fever	—	Industrial grinder condenser
29. Iowa City, Iowa Hospital	March-Dec 1981	24	—	—	LD	46	? Potable water
30. Paris, France Hospital	July-Aug 1981	6	—	—	LD	—	? Potable water
31. Virgin Islands Hotel	1979–82	27	< 5%	—	LD	—	?
32. Rochester, MI Health Club	May 1982	14	100%	3–38 hours	Pontiac fever	0	Whirlpool
33. Vermont Inn	March 1982	34	46%	0–2 days	Pontiac fever	0	Whirlpool

Table 2. COMPARATIVE EPIDEMIOLOGIC AND CLINICAL FEATURES OF THE ATYPICAL PNEUMONIAS

Epidemiologic Features	Legionnaires' Disease	Mycoplasma Pneumonia	Psittacosis	Q Fever	Tularemia	Viral Pneumonia[a]	Histo-plasmosis	Coccidioido-mycosis
Incubation period (days)	2–10	12–21	7–14	14–38	1–8	1–3	3–21	7–28
Seasonality	Summer	Fall-winter	Year-round ? summer peak	Year-round ? spring peak	Year-round ? summer peak	Fall-winter	? Winter nadir	Summer-fall
Patient age	Middle-age elderly	Children and young adults	Adult	Adult	Adult	Children, young adult, elderly	All	All
Sex ratio	M>F	M=F	M≥F	M≥F	M>F	M=F	M=F	M=F
Exposure to animals	0	0	Psittacine birds, turkeys, pigeons	Livestock	Rodents, rabbits, ticks	0	Starlings, chickens, bats	0
Exposure to other infective sources	Construction sites/recent travel	0	Pet shop	Contaminated milk, fomites (hay)	0	0	Great river valleys—N. Am., S. Am., Africa, S. Asia; construction sites	Southwest U.S., Chaco district Argentina, esp. construction sites
Person-to-person transmission	0	+	rare	0	0	+	0	0
Underlying chronic diseases	+	0	0	0	0	+/−	+/−	0
Smoking/alcohol abuse	+	0	0	0	0	+/−	+/−	0
Clinical Features								
Rapidity of onset	Abrupt or insidious	Insidious	Abrupt or insidious	Abrupt	Abrupt	Abrupt	Abrupt	Abrupt
Myalgias, malaise, headache	+	+	+	+	+	+	+	+
Unproductive to minimally productive cough	+	+	+	+	+	+	+	+
Upper respiratory symptoms	0	+	+/−	0	+/−	+	+/−	+/−
Rigors	+ (Recurrent)	Rare	Rare	Rare	+	Rare	Rare	+
Diarrhea	+	Infrequent	Infrequent	Infrequent	Infrequent	Infrequent	0	0

Temperature ≥39° C	+	+	+	Rare	+	+	+	+
Other focal signs	Confusion	Bullous myringitis, rash, pharyngitis, arthritis, myocarditis, CNS signs	Hepatosplenomegaly, rash, myopericarditis	Hepatomegaly, tender liver, endocarditis	Lymphadenopathy, hepatosplenomegaly, rash, ocular findings	Pharyngitis, conjunctivitis	Mucous membrane lesions, erythema-nodosum, lymphadenopathy	Rash (erythema nodosum), meningitis, lymphadenopathy
WBC per mm³	5,000–20,000	5,000–20,000	10,000–20,000	10,000–20,000	15,000–20,000	10,000–25,000	10,000–20,000	10,000–20,000
Unexplained hematuria	+	Rare	0	0	0	Rare	Rare	0
Abnormal liver and renal function	+	Occasional	Occasional	Occasional		Occasional	Occasional	Occasional
Chest radiographs								
Character of infiltrate	Patchy bronchopneumonia	Perihilar bronchopneumonia	Interstitial or lobar pneumonia	Interstitial pneumonia	Diffuse broncho- or lobar pneumonia	Perihilar bronchopneumonia	Patchy bronchopneumonia	Patchy bronchopneumonia
Hilar adenopathy	0	Rare	Rare	Rare	+	Rare	+	+
Pleural effusion	20–30% (small)	10–25% (small)	Rare	Rare	+	Rare	Rare	Common
Cavitation/calcification	Rare/0	0/0	0/0	0/0	0/0	0/0	Occasional/+	+/+
Diagnostic serologic tests	IFA[b]	Cold agglutinins CF[c]	CF	CF	Agglutinins	HI[d] CF	CF ID[e]	CF ID
Case-fatality ratio (%)	15–20	<0.1	15–20 5 (treated)	<1	30–40 (untreated)	?	<1	<1
Treatment	Erythromycin	Erythromycin or tetracycline	Tetracycline	Tetracycline	Streptomycin	–	Amphotericin B—if progressive disseminated, or cavitary	

[a]Influenza, parainfluenza, adenovirus; [b]IFA, indirect fluorescent antibody; [c]CF, complement fixation; [d]HI, hemagglutination inhibition; [e]ID, immunodiffusion

Biochemically, *L. pneumophila* and the other *Legionella* are largely inert except for catalase, oxidase, and gelatinase production. None ferment carbohydrates (other than starch), reduce nitrate, or degrade urea. Most produce beta-lactamase, with a notable exception being *L. micdadei*. Gas-liquid chromatographic measurements have shown that more than 60 per cent of the organism's fatty acids have branched chains, a distinctively unusual pattern for gram negative bacteria. Further studies of the biochemical characteristics, molecular weight of the genome, guanine-cytosine content, and DNA homology have not demonstrated relatedness with any other known family of bacteria.

At least nine distinct serogroups of *L. pneumophila* have been identified by immunofluorescence studies (McKinney et al., 1979). Most of the clinical isolates belong to serogroup 1 (type strain Philadelphia 1). Two distinct serogroups of *L. longbeachae* have been observed. Serogroup-specific antigens from strains of *L. pneumophila* and *L. longbeachae* have been isolated and partially characterized. Other antigens seem to be shared by all nine serogroups of *L. pneumophila*, or the two serogroups of *L. longbeachae*. The other species of *Legionella* also appear to contain common antigens as well as specific antigens.

L. pneumophila can survive for months in distilled water and for over a year in tap water. Most of the *Legionella* have been isolated from diverse environmental sites including natural bodies of water, riparian soil, water in heat-rejection systems, and potable water. The organism has not been isolated from natural animal reservoirs.

EPIDEMIOLOGY. Legionnaires' disease occurs sporadically, endemically, and in explosive point-source outbreaks that last for several days to a few weeks. An incubation period of 2 to 10 days has generally been observed (mean of 5.5 days). Attack rates have ranged between 0.1 and 4.0 per cent of those exposed. Thus far, all outbreaks of Legionnaires' disease have been caused by *L. pneumophila*, although sporadic cases of Legionnaires' disease have been caused by other species of *Legionella*. In sharp contrast, Pontiac fever (nonpneumonic short-incubation-period legionellosis) has been recognized only in epidemic form and is characterized by an incubation period of 5 to 66 hours (mean of 36 hours), and attack rates of up to 100 per cent have been reported. Four of the five outbreaks of Pontiac fever that have been described have been due to *L. pneumophila*. One outbreak was caused by *L. feeleii* (Herwaldt et al., 1982). Outbreaks of legionellosis have occurred in the United States and in at least seven other countries (Table 1) and have ranged in size from 6 to more than 200 cases. Most of the outbreaks have been associated with buildings or institutions such as hotels, hospitals, or factories or business establishments. Recurrent outbreaks at the same institution and continuing occurrence of endemic disease at high rates have been reported.

Sporadic cases have been identified in every state in the United States, and nearly every country has had documented disease caused by *Legionella* when sought. Data from several serologic surveys in the United States suggest that exposure to *L. pneumophila* may vary widely from region to region. In most studies, the prevalence of antibody titers of ≥ 128 to serogroup 1 by immunofluorescence testing is 1 to 4 per cent (Storch et al., 1979). However, in some areas considered hyperendemic for *L. pneumophila* serogroup 1, antibody titers of ≥ 128 have been found in 5 to 25 per cent. The incidence of legionellosis in the United States or other countries is unknown. Between 0.5 and 4.5 per cent of otherwise undiagnosed pneumonia cases have now been confirmed as Legionnaires pneumonia by immunofluorescence testing, suggesting an incidence of 2 to 16 cases/100,000 population per year in the United States. In a study of the incidence of community-acquired pneumonia in Seattle, Washington, 1 per cent of the patients with pneumonia of uncertain etiology had a fourfold rise in antibody titer to *L. pneumophila*, representing an incidence of 12 cases/100,000 population per year (Foy et al., 1979). Legionellosis may also occur as a sporadic nosocomial infection and may account for 5 per cent of fatal nosocomial pneumonias. Many cases of Legionnaires' disease caused by other *Legionella* species besides *L. pneumophila* have occurred in the hospital.

A summer seasonality has been observed both for point-source outbreaks and for sporadic cases, although cases occur in all months. Most cases have occurred in middle-aged or elderly persons; the mean age of patients is about 55 years. Few cases have been identified in children. Persons with the nonpneumonic form of legionellosis are generally younger than persons with Legionnaires' disease. The distribution by sex of cases of Legionnaires' disease demonstrates a striking male predominance in outbreaks and for sporadic cases (male: female ratio of 2 to 3:1). Other risk factors for illness are underlying chronic disease states such as renal insufficiency or malignancy, use of corticosteroids or immunosuppressive agents, cigarette smoking, heavy alcohol consumption, construction work, living near ongoing excavation or construction, and recent travel (Table 2).

Airborne transmission of *Legionella* has been the only documented natural mode of spread of legionellosis, although in most outbreaks and in sporadic cases the mode of spread has not been proved. Secondary cases of Legionnaires' disease have never been identified, and to date there has been no documented instance of person-to-person spread. In several outbreaks, heat-rejection systems have been implicated as the vehicles of spread. Water in these systems is commonly contaminated with bacteria and as heat is exchanged from water to air through evaporation, as in cooling towers or evaporative condensers, an aerosol is generated that would disseminate the bacteria. Infection likely occurs through inhalation of these bacteria as droplet nuclei.

Other outbreaks have occurred at sites without air-conditioning or heat-rejection systems. In a large study of sporadic cases, no association was observed between acquisition of disease and the use of air conditioning, heating, humidifying, or dehumidifying systems, although disease did occur more frequently in construction workers and in individuals living near ongoing construction or excavation sites (Storch et al., 1979). In recent years, several observations have suggested that the *L. pneumophila* may be waterborne: clusters of hospitalized patients have been observed in centers with contaminated potable water and these clusters have stopped when measures were taken to eradicate *Legionella* from the water (Cordes et al., 1981; Shands et al., 1980). Two recent outbreaks of Pontiac fever occurred at health clubs. Epidemiologic evidence suggested that illness was associated with whirlpool use. The other species of *Legionella* have all caused sporadic cases of community-acquired or nosocomial pneumonia. The modes of spread and incubation periods are unknown.

PATHOGENESIS AND PATHOLOGY. Studies on the pathogenesis of legionellosis are limited. The portal of entry appears to be the respiratory tract, since the only consistent changes observed in patients with Legionnaires'

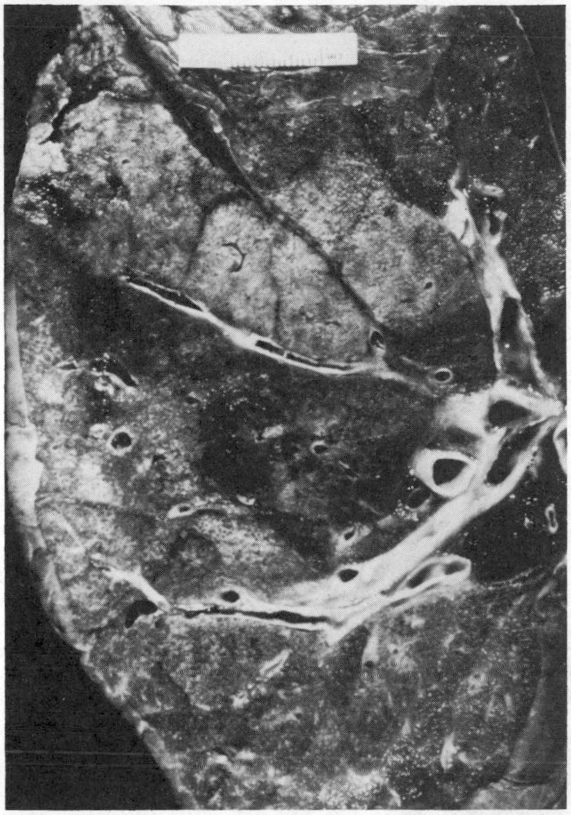

Figure 3. Macroscopic appearance of lung tisse obtained from a fatal case of Legionnaires' disease pneumonia. Note circumscribed peripheral nodular pneumonia. Several similar nodules were present in other lobes. From Winn, W. C., Jr.: Arch Pathol 102:347, 1978.

disease are in the lungs (Fig. 3). Characteristically, the lesion produced is an acute fibrinopurulent bronchopneumonia with acute diffuse alveolar damage. The intra-alveolar infiltrate consists of many neutrophils admixed with macrophages and fibrin (Fig. 4). Desquamation of alveolar epithelium may be prominent, and small focal areas of necrosis may be observed. Cavity formation is uncommon and, when observed, is often in an immunocompromised patient or in a person with a concomitant gram-negative bacterial superinfection. Pathologic changes affect the terminal bronchioles, but spare large airways. Bacilli can be demonstrated in the exudate with a modification of Dieterle silver impregnation stain or the Wolbach modification of the Giesma stain, but rarely with the Brown-Brenn or Brown-Hopps modification of the Gram stain. Organisms may be seen within macrophages and neutrophils and extracellularly. Although hilar lymph nodes are rarely enlarged, the organism has been observed within the hilar lymphatic tissue by direct immunofluorescent staining techniques. The direct immunofluorescent stain (DFA) is more sensitive and specific for *Legionella* with the highest yield observed in lung tissue scrapings. The Gimenez stain is useful for impression smears and frozen sections but not for paraffin-embedded tissue. In some patients pneumonia does not resolve completely; varying degrees of interstitial inflammation and fibrosis may be found months to years later.

Bacteremia has been documented in Legionnaires' disease, but whether the multisystem manifestations frequently observed in these patients are due to direct bacterial invasion or to other mechanisms is unknown. *Legionella* have rarely been identified in other organs, and no consistent histopathologic findings have been noted. Although *L. pneumophila* can lyse guinea pig red cells and has certain properties of endotoxin (cell suspensions induce gelation of *Limulus* amebocyte lysate and are pyrogenic to rabbits), the role of toxins or enzymes in producing human disease is not known.

The pathogenesis of Pontiac fever is not known. No histopathologic studies have been done in humans because the disease is uniformly benign and self-limited.

Humoral immunity to *L. pneumophilia* may be important in humans. A cell membrane fraction containing protein, carbohydrate, and lipid induces an antibody response in experimental animals and protects them against subsequent challenge with homologous live organisms (Wong et al., 1979). Complement and bactericidal antibodies appear to play important roles in mediating resistance. The organism can be ingested by monocytes and human alveolar macrophages. Activated macrophages slow the growth or even destroy the organism, suggesting an important role for cell-mediated immunity.

The pathogenosis of Pontiac fever is unknown. No differences have been observed in the strains capable of causing Pontiac fever or Legionnaires' disease, and no differences have been observed in the source or modes of spread to explain the clinical or epidemiologic differences between Pontiac fever and Legionnaires' disease.

CLINICAL MANIFESTATIONS OF DISEASE CAUSED BY LEGIONELLA

Disease caused by *Legionella* can be associated with a wide range of clinical presentations, ranging from an asymptomatic infection to fulminant pneumonia. At least two distinct clinicoepidemiologic syndromes have been described: Pontiac fever and Legionnaires' disease.

Legionnaires' Disease. Legionnaires' disease has a broad range of manifestations from a mild grippe to a fulminant multisystem disease (Tsai et al., 1979). After an incubation period of 2 to 10 days (mean of 5.5 days), the patient may have a prodrome of malaise, diffuse myalgias, headache, and fever often accompanied by rigors. Cough, dyspnea, and chest pain are also common early manifestations. Upper respiratory symptoms including sore throat, nasal congestion, and coryza are infrequently reported. Chest pain is usually pleuritic rather than musculoskeletal in nature and at times may be incapacitating. Diarrhea (without mucus, blood, or pus) may be present in up to 40 per cent of the patients, and mental confusion or delirium is common. Over the next several days, the fever usually persists unremittingly (up to 41° C), and the patient may continue to have recurrent rigors. Respiratory symptoms may progress, and in nearly 50 per cent of the patients the cough becomes productive usually of a small amount of mucoid rather than mucopurulent sputum. The patient often appears severely ill, tachypneic, and diaphoretic, and in respiratory distress. The temperature is above 38.9° C in half of the patients, and respiratory rates are over 25/min in 40 per cent. Although tachycardia is frequently observed, the heart rate is often slower than would be expected for the amount of fever. Additional findings have been largely confined to the lungs and include moist inspiratory rales, rhonchi, and, for <25 per cent of the patients, evidence of consolidation. Skin rash, mucous membrane lesions, lymphadenopathy, and hepatosplenomegaly are not typical of Legionnaires' disease. On occasion, transient neurologic deficits have been observed. There are a normal or moderately elevated white blood cell count ($\leq 20{,}000$ wbc/mm^3)

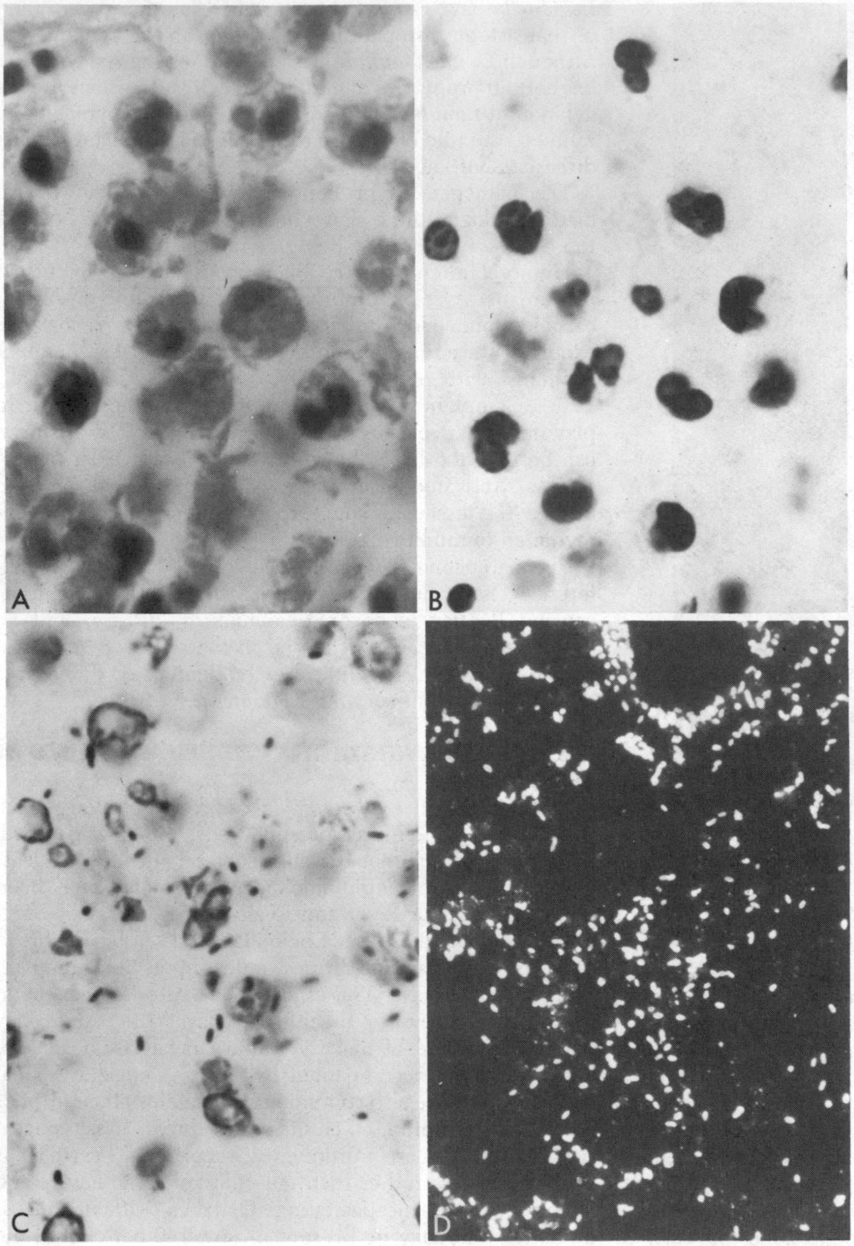

Figure 4. Microscopic appearance of Legionnaires' disease pneumonia. *A,* Intra-alveolar exudate consisting of fibrin, polymorphonuclear leukocytes, and macrophages. Note necrosis of inflammatory exudate. Hematoxylin and eosin, 600 × *B,* Gram-stained smear of lung tissue. Note paucity of visualized organisms. *C,* Myriads of small pleomorphic intracellular and extracellular bacilli. Dieterle silver impregnation stain, 600× *D,* Fluorescent-antibody stains of scraping of formalin-fixed lung tissue from a patient with fatal pneumonia caused by *L. pneumophila.* Courtesy of F. W. Chandler and W. B. Cherry.

with an increase in band cells, an elevated erythrocyte sedimentation rate, and mild abnormalities in liver and renal function. Proteinuria and microscopic hematuria may be present. Thrombocytopenia and disseminated intravascular coagulation have been observed. Hyponatremia, possibly due to inappropriate antidiuretic hormone secretion and hypophosphatemia, may also be seen in some patients. Sputum, if obtainable, generally has few polymorphonuclear cells and no predominant bacterial species. A pleural exudate or transudate, usually scant, may be seen in up to 40 per cent of patients. Radiographic findings include poorly defined infiltrates that may start in one lung but generally progress to bilateral patchy or nodular alveolar involvement (Fig. 5). Lobar consolidation is seen in less than 25 per cent of patients with pneumonia. Cavitation and abscess formation are uncommon (Fig. 6). Serologic tests such as cold and febrile agglutinins are either negative or not found in significant titers.

Pontiac Fever. Pontiac fever is an acute, self-limited, febrile illness with an incubation period of 5 to 66 hours (mean of 36 hours) (Glick et al., 1978). It starts abruptly with diffuse myalgias, headache, and fever. Upper respiratory symptoms may be present. A mild unproductive cough, nausea, and dizziness are additional features. Fever up to 41° C, tachypnea, and tachycardia also occur. Examination of the chest is unremarkable. Leukocyte counts have ranged from normal levels to 25,000 wbc/mm^3. Chest x-rays do not reveal pulmonary infiltrates.

Other Infections. Patients with confirmed legionellosis have had only diarrhea and fever without pneumonia, prolonged fever alone, endocarditis, or other extrapulmonary localized disease such as pyelonephritis, wound infection, myocarditis, and perirectal abscess. Not all confirmed infections require hospitalization, and asymptomatic seroconverters have been documented. Mild illness without radiographic evidence of pneumonia occurred in 28 of 142

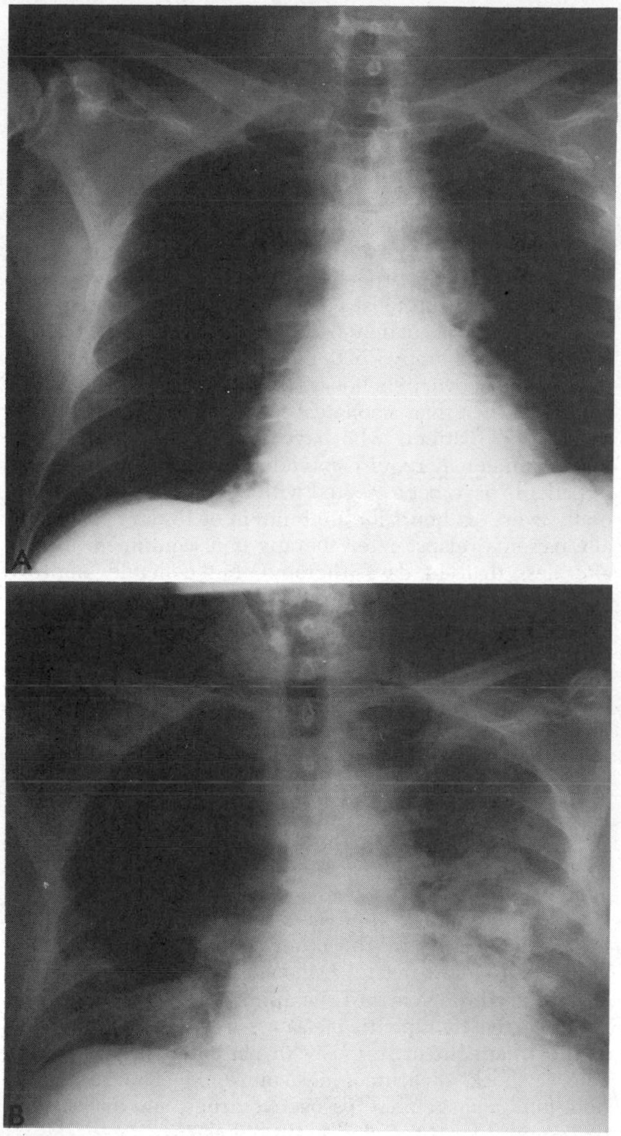

Figure 5. Legionnaires' disease in a middle-aged male with cough and fever. *A,* Note stringy, poorly defined left perihilar infiltrate on admission. *B,* Five days after admission. Note progression of bronchopneumonia with bilateral patchy involvement. From Tsai, T. F.: Ann Intern Med 90:510, 1979.

patients who had chest x-rays in the 1976 Philadelphia outbreak. The total clinical spectrum of infection with *Legionella* is unknown.

COMPLICATIONS AND SEQUELAE. Patients recover from Pontiac fever in two to five days without treatment. No deaths or long-term sequelae have been noted with this syndrome. Patients with Legionnaires' disease, however, may suffer respiratory failure. During the 1976 Philadelphia outbreak, 16 per cent of hospitalized patients needed assisted ventilation. Acute renal failure, disseminated intravascular coagulation, and shock may also complicate the illness. The overall case-fatality ratios observed for outbreak settings and for sporadic cases are between 10 and 20 per cent. These rates are higher for older individuals and for individuals with underlying disease problems or receiving immunosuppressants. Death usually is a result of pulmonary insufficiency or shock. Without correct treatment, fever continues until the infection resolves on the seventh to twelfth day. Roentgenographically, the pneumonia resolves slowly, sometimes over several months. Recovery is usually complete, although pulmonary diffusion capacity has been impaired years after the acute illness. Whether patients with *Legionella* infection are protected from reinfection or whether infection can reactivate during immunosuppressant therapy is not known.

DIAGNOSIS. Legionnaires' disease can resemble other bacterial pneumonias or infections caused by *Mycoplasma pneumoniae, Chlamydia psittaci* (psittacosis), *Coxiella burnetti* (Q fever), *Francisella tularensis* (tularemia), influenza and other respiratory viruses, cytomegalovirus, *Histoplasma capsulatum, Coccidioides immitis, Toxoplasma gondii,* and *Pneumocystis carinii.* Noninfectious illnesses that may resemble Legionnaires' disease include the hypersensitivity pneumonitides, collagen vascular disorders with pulmonic involvement, drug reactions, and a few toxins. Legionnaires' disease occurs predominantly in middle-aged and elderly men and has a peak incidence in the summer, incubation period of 2 to 10 days, no history of exposure to animals, and no person-to-person spread. It occurs in individuals with a history of underlying chronic disease states, heavy cigarette smoking or alcohol use, and recent travel or exposure to construction or excavation. An explosive common-source outbreak of pneumonia in the summer within 10 days of suspected exposure and with no evident person-to-person spread would be highly suggestive of Legionnaires' disease. Specific clinical features that may also assist in the diagnosis are watery diarrhea, altered states of consciousness, high unremitting fever with repeated rigors, relative bradycardia, lack of preceding upper respiratory symptoms, abnormal liver and renal function, including an active urinary sediment, and negative sputum and blood cultures on conventional media. Legionnaires' disease has no exanthem or enanthem, pharyngitis, lymphadenopathy, or hepatosplenomegaly.

Definitive diagnosis requires the isolation of the organism from clinical specimens, demonstration of the organism or

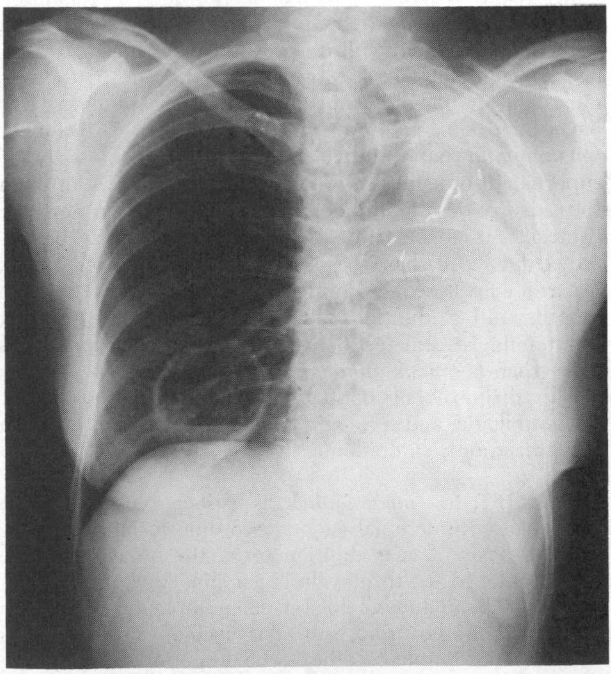

Figure 6. Large pulmonary abscess that developed in the right lung of a patient with Legionnaires' disease who had previously had left pneumonectomy for carcinoma. Gump, D. W.: Ann Intern Med 90:539, 1979.

its antigens in tissue or body fluids, or documentation of ≥ fourfold rise in specific antibodies. *Legionella* have been recovered from respiratory secretions, pleural fluid, and lung tissue by using special culture media. For contaminated specimens, the isolation of *Legionella* may be aided by the incorporation of cefamandole or vancomycin, polymyxin B, and anisomycin in the agar to inhibit other organisms (Edelstein et al., 1981). However, growth may take several days.

The organism has been visualized in respiratory secretions (both expectorated and obtained by transtracheal aspiration), pleural fluid, and lung tissue and other tissues and body fluid with various staining procedures. Direct immunofluorescent staining appears to be quite specific, although occasional strains of *Pseudomonas*, other gram-negative aerobic bacteria, and *Bacteroides fragilis* may also stain brightly. Recent experience suggests that direct immunofluorescent smears are positive in up to 71 per cent of the cases if multiple samples of sputum are obtained from the same patient. *L. pneumophila* antigen can be demonstrated in urine of patients with Legionnaires' disease by an enzyme-linked immunosorbent assay (ELISA), latex agglutination, or radioimmunoassay, and may persist for several weeks. The most commonly used method for the diagnosis of Legionnaires' disease caused by *L. pneumophila* is serology by indirect immunofluorescent (IFA) staining, hemagglutination, hemagglutination inhibition, microagglutination, or ELISA. The IFA test has been the serologic method most widely applied to date. A ≥ fourfold increase of antibody (to a titer of ≥128) during convalescence is considered diagnostic; this increase is usually observed within three weeks of onset of illness but may not occur until the sixth week of illness. The sensitivity of the IFA can be estimated from well-defined outbreaks that have shown 75 to 85 per cent of persons with clinical and epidemiologic compatible illness to have ≥ fourfold increase of antibody to a titer of ≥128. Antibody is generally specific for the serogroup causing infection, but patients with broadly reacting sera have been observed (Wilkinson et al., 1979). Rising titers to *L. pneumophila* have been seen in patients with culture-proved plague and tularemia, and concomitant increases in antibody to other pathogens including *M. pneumoniae, C. psittaci*, and influenza virus have been documented. The specificity of IFA for *L. pneumophila* may improve when sera are mixed with the supernatant of a culture of *E. coli* 013, apparently through the adsorption of antibodies to common gram-negative bacterial antigens. Titers to *L. pneumophila* may be detected for more than 10 years, but typically, after a peak in early convalescence, titers drop 1 to 2 dilutions after 6 months and 2 dilutions after 18 months. The indirect immunofluorescent test is not well standardized for strains other than *L. pneumophila*.

The diagnosis of Pontiac fever is made on clinical, epidemiologic, and serologic grounds and has thus far been recognized only in epidemic form.

THERAPY. *L. pneumophila* is susceptible to a wide variety of antimicrobial agents according to in vitro tests. On the basis of agar dilution tests, the organisms were susceptible to erythromycin, rifampin, the aminoglycosides, the penicillins, cefoxitin, chloramphenicol, trimethoprim-sulfamethoxazole, and doxycycline. The organism was not susceptible to other cephalosporins, tetracycline, clindamycin, or vancomycin. Only erythromycin and rifampin were markedly effective in prophylaxis and in treatment of infected embryonic hens' eggs and guinea pigs.

Although a randomized prospective trial of antimicrobial therapy of Legionnaires' disease has not been done, clinical observations suggest that erythromycin may be effective against *L. pneumophila* infection in humans. Retrospective analysis of the 1976 Philadelphia, 1977 Vermont, and 1977 Los Angeles outbreaks showed that case-fatality ratios were lowest for those patients treated with erythromycin. In the Vermont outbreak, the case-fatality ratio for patients treated with erythromycin was 5 per cent, significantly lower than the ratio of 24 per cent for patients not treated with erythromycin (Broome et al., 1979). The dose, route, and duration of the most effective therapy are not known. For seriously ill patients and for patients who cannot tolerate oral therapy, 500 to 1000 mg of erythromycin intravenously every six hours (15 mg/kg every six hours for children other than neonates) for at least 14 days is recommended. Patients who have a lung abscess due to *L. pneumophila* may require extended therapy. Less seriously ill patients have been treated with 500 mg of erythromycin orally every six hours for a minimum of 14 days. Occasionally patients relapse after therapy is discontinued (usually after less than 14 days' therapy), but generally improve when erythromycin therapy is resumed. There is little clinical experience with rifampin as therapy for Legionnaires' disease. It is recommended that rifampin be reserved for combined therapy with erythromycin for those patients not responding to high-dose intravenous erythromycin therapy alone and possibly for those patients with documented lung abscess. For patients with severe hepatic insufficiency, although few data are available, it is generally recommended that the dose of erythromycin be decreased by at least 25 per cent. Intravenous erythromycin is extremely irritating to the veins and needs to be diluted and administered slowly.

Erythromycin also appears to be the antibiotic of choice for disease caused by the other species of *Legionella*. In vitro tests suggest that all *Legionella* are highly susceptible to both erythromycin and rifampin.

Supportive therapeutic measures are of major importance in the treatment of seriously ill patients with respiratory failure, shock, or acute renal failure. Mechanical ventilation, fluid management, vasoactive drugs, and dialysis may be required for these clinical problems.

Specific therapy is probably not needed for the Pontiac fever syndrome.

PREVENTION AND CONTROL. The environmental reservoir and distribution in nature of the *Legionella* have not been defined nor has the mode of spread in sporadic cases and most outbreaks of legionellosis. In settings in which spread has been demonstrated to be due to aerosolized droplet nuclei from heat-rejection devices, stopping the production of the aerosols and eliminating the organism from the contaminated system may prevent further cases. Whether chemical treatment and other preventive maintenance of these systems can prevent some outbreaks is not known. Outbreaks traced to contaminated potable water have been controlled by either hyperchlorination or by raising the temperature of the hot water to at least 55° C. A vaccine is currently being tested in animal models. Hospitalized cases do not need to be placed in respiratory isolation; secretion precautions alone should suffice. Laboratory workers should exercise care in handling cultures and potentially contaminated specimens so as not to generate aerosols. Work with the organism that may lead to production of infectious aerosols should be done with appropriate precautions for containment.

References

General References

Balows, A., and Fraser D. W. (eds) International Symposium on Legionnaires' Disease. Ann Intern Med 90:489, 1979.

Jones, G. L., and Herbert, G. A. (eds): Legionnaires': The Disease, the Bacterium and Methodology. Center for Disease Control Laboratory Manual, Atlanta, CDC, 1979.

Thornsberry, C., Feeley, J. C., Jakubowski, W., and Balows, A. (eds): Proceedings of Second International Symposium on *Legionella*. Am Soc Microbiol, 1983.

Specific References

Brenner, D. J., Steigerwalt, A. G., and McDade, J. E.: Classification of the Legionnaires' disease bacterium: *Legionella pneumophila*, genus novum, species nova, of the family *Legionellaceae*, family nova. Ann Intern Med 90:656, 1979.

Broome, C. V., Goings, S. A. J., Thacker, S. B., Vogt, R. L., Beaty, H. N., Fraser, D. W., and the Field Investigation Team: The Vermont epidemic of Legionnaires' disease. Ann Intern Med 90:573, 1979.

Cordes, I. G., Wiesenthal, A. M., Gorman, G. W., Phair, J. P., Sommers H. M., Brown, A., Yu, V. L., Magnussen, M. H., Meyer, R. P., Wolf, J. S., Shands, K. N., and Fraser, D. W.: Isolation of *Legionella* pneumophila from hospital shower heads. Ann Intern Med 94:195, 1981.

Edelstein, P. H., Meyer, R. D., Reingold, S. M.: Laboratory diagnosis of Legionnaires' disease. Am Rev Respir Dis 121:317, 1980.

Edelstein, P. H.: Improved Semiselective Medium for Isolation of *Legionella pneumophila* from contaminated clinical and environmental specimens. J Clin Micro 14:298, 1981.

Foy, H. M., Broome, C. V., Hayes, P. S., Allan, I., Cooney, M. K., and Tobe, R.: Legionnaires' disease in a prepaid medical-care group in Seattle 1963-1975. Lancet 1:767, 1979.

Fraser, D. W., Tsai, T. F., Orenstein, W., Parkin, W. E., Beecham, H. J., Sharrar, R. G., Harris, J., Mallison, G. F., Martin, S. M., McDade, J. E., Shepard, C. C., Brachman, P. S., and The Field Investigation Team: Legionnaires' disease: A description of an epidemic of pneumonia. N Engl J Med 297:1189, 1977.

Glick, T. H., Gregg, M. B., Berman, B., Mallison, G. F., Rhodes, W. W., Jr., and Kassanoff, I.: Pontiac fever: An epidemic of unknown etiology in a health department. I. Clinical and epidemiologic aspects. Am J Epidemiol 107:149, 1978.

Herwaldt, L. A., Gorman, G., Hightower, A. W., Brake, B., Wilkinson, H., Boxer, P. A., McCrath, T., Brenner, D., Moss, C. W., and Broome, C. V.: Pontiac fever in an engine assembly plant. Proceedings of the 22nd Interscience Conference on Antimicrobial Agents and Chemotherapy, Abstract 100, 1982.

Horowitz, M. A., and Silberstein, S. C.: Intracellular multiplication of Legionnaires' disease Bacteria *(Legionella pneumophila)* in human monocytes is reversibly inhibited by erythromycin and rifampin. J Clin Investig 71:15, 1983.

McDade, J. E., Shepard, C. C., Fraser, D. W., Tsai, T. F., Redus, M. A., Dowdle, W. R., and the Laboratory Investigation Team: Legionnaires' disease: Isolation of a bacterium and demonstration of its role in other respiratory disease. N Engl J Med 297:1197, 1977.

McKinney, R. M., Thacker, L., Harris, P. P., Lewallen, K. R., Herbert, G. A., Edelstein, P. H., and Thomason, B. M.: Four serogroups of Legionnaire's disease bacteria defined by direct immunofluorescence. Ann Intern Med 90:490, 1979.

Muder, R. R., Yu, V. L., and Zuravleff, J. J.: Pneumonia due to the Pittsburgh pneumonia agent: new clinical perspective with a review of the literature. Medicine 62:120, 1983.

Pasculle, A. W., Feeley, J. C., Gibson, R. J., Cordes, L. G., Myerowitz, R. L., Patton, C. M., Gorman, G. W., Carmack, C. L., Ezzell, J. W., and Dowling, J. N.: Pittsburgh pneumonia agent: direct isolation from human lung tissue. J Infect Dis 141:727, 1980.

Shands, K. N., Ho, J. L., Meyer, R. D., and Fraser, D. W.: Potable water: possible role in epidemic Legionnaires' disease (LD). Proceedings 20th Interscience Conference Antimicrob Agents and Chemotherapy, Abstract 501, 1980.

Storch, G., Baine, W. B., Fraser, D. W., Broome, C. V., Clegg, H. W., II, Cohen, M. L., Goings, S. A. J., Politi, B. D., Terranova, W. A., Tsai, T. F., Plikaytis, B. D., Shepard, C. C., and Bennett, J. V.: Sporadic community Legionnaires' disease in the United States. A case-control study. Ann Intern Med 90:596, 1979.

Storch, G., Hayes, P. S., Hill, D. L., and Baine, W. B.: Prevalence of antibody to Legionnaires' disease bacterium in middle-aged and elderly Americans. J Infect Dis 140:748, 1979.

Tsai, T. F., Finn, D. R., Plikaytis, B. D., McCauley, W., Martin, S. M., and Fraser, D. W.: Legionnaires' disease: Clinical features of the epidemic in Philadelphia. Ann Intern Med 90:509, 1979.

Wilkinson, H. M., Fikes, B. J., and Cruce, D. D.: Indirect immunofluorescence test for serodiagnosis of Legionnaires' disease: Evidence for serogroup diversity of Legionnaires' disease bacterial antigens and for multiple specificity of human antibodies. J Clin Microbiol 9:379, 1979.

Wilkinson, H. W., Reingold, A. L., Blake, B. J., McGibboney, D. L., Gorman, G. W., and Broome, C. V.: Reactivity of serum from patients with suspected Legionellosis against 20 antigens of Legionellaceae and *Legionella*-like organisms by indirect immunofluorescence assay. J Infect Dis 147:23, 1983.

Wong, K. H., Schalla, W. O., Arko, R. J., Bullard, J. C., and Feeley, J. C.: Immunochemical, serologic, and immunologic properties of major antigens isolated from the Legionnaires' disease bacterium. Observations bearing on the feasibility of a vaccine. Ann Intern Med 90:634, 1979.

120
TUBERCULOSIS

WILLIAM LESTER, M.D.

Tuberculosis is usually acquired by inhalation of *Mycobacterium tuberculosis,* which causes nodular, caseating granulomas (called tubercles) that fibrose, ulcerate, or calcify. The disease is confined to the lungs in most patients but may spread to almost any part of the body, especially the meninges, kidneys, bones, and lymph nodes. Sensitized T cell lymphocytes participate in the development of delayed hypersensitivity and the formation of caseating granulomas, whereas humoral antibodies play a minimal role in the disease. Clinical manifestations of the disease may appear soon after the start of infection when tuberculin sensitivity develops, and especially if the inoculum is large; or they may arise after a variable period of dormancy (years to decades), particularly when immunity has been compromised. Tuberculosis has an inverse relationship to the standard of living within a society and increases dramatically during times of social catastrophe. Tuberculosis invariably decreases as the standard of living and nutrition improve.

ETIOLOGY. Tuberculosis is caused by *M. tuberculosis.* Popular convention also has included disease caused by *M. bovis* but not by other mycobacteria. This causes confusion, since other mycobacteria produce disease that clinically, roentgenographically, and pathologically is identical to that produced by *M. tuberculosis.* Infections caused by *M. kansasii* and the *M. avium-intracellulare* complex are examples and can be differentiated from tuberculosis only upon the cultural recovery of the organism. Thus, if cultures are unavailable, for whatever reason, the term tuberculosis is applied to all cases of mycobacterial disease except that caused by *M. leprae.*

The tubercle bacillus *(M. tuberculosis)* is aerobic, nonmotile, non-spore-forming, high in lipid content, and acid- and alcohol-fast (Barksdale and Kim, 1977). It grows slowly and differs from other mycobacteria by its ability to produce niacin. Unless modified by drug resistance, tubercle bacilli are virulent for man and most laboratory animals, especially guinea pigs. Colonies of tubercle bacilli are slow-growing, buff in color, rough and eugonic in appearance, and they usually require 10 to 21 days' incubation on complex media for their recognition and identification.

PATHOGENESIS AND PATHOLOGY. The clinical manifestations and pathologic findings in patients with tuberculosis are the result of the interplay between delayed hypersensitivity and cellular immunity, on the one hand, and the extent and virulence of the tuberculous infection on the other. The complexity of this interaction explains the fact that the pathologic findings can vary from acute to subacute to chronic, depending upon the immune state of the patient and the extent and nature of disease, as well as the time in the natural history of the disease (Youmans, 1979).

Most cases of tuberculosis are acquired by the inhalation of tubercle bacilli dispensed into the air from an active case by coughing, singing, and similar activities. Airborne particles measuring 1 to 5 μ and containing tubercle bacilli are inhaled into the airways and deposited in the alveoli. The tubercle bacilli are ingested by the alveolar macrophages and multiply intracellularly, and an acute exudative reaction results. At this time, delayed hypersensitivity has not yet been developed, and the multiplying tubercle bacilli spread by lymphohematogenous routes to other parts of the lung, to lymph nodes, and, ultimately, to such remote locations as bone marrow, meninges, and kidneys. However, shortly after the initiation of infection, cellular immunity and delayed hypersensitivity begin to develop and become manifest 4 to 6 weeks later. The macrophages are then increasingly lethal for tubercle bacilli and the tuberculoprotein released into the tissue causes platelet thrombi and vascular occlusion, so that local lesions become necrotic and caseation necrosis is seen in its classic form. This phenomenon greatly diminishes the risk of dissemination, but at the cost of irreversible damage to the lung.

Thus, in the previously uninfected patient, the initial lesions of tuberculosis are those of an acute pneumonitis that spreads to the hilar lymph nodes, and the combined process is called a Ghon complex. At this time necrosis is minimal, the tubercle bacilli multiply without restraint, and they may disseminate either scantily or in large numbers, depending on the size of the original inoculum and the patient's resistance. This is a dangerous period for the patient, because fatal dissemination may occur as a consequence of impaired immunity or overwhelming infection.

Most patients infected with tubercle bacilli never have clinical manifestations of the disease but show delayed hypersensitivity to tuberculoprotein and are designated positive tuberculin reactors. However, tubercle bacilli survive in their tissues for the rest of their lives and can multiply and spread whenever immunity decreases as a result of malnutrition, diabetes mellitus, or immunosuppression. Most of these reactivated cases show only pulmonary involvement, but in about 10 per cent, tuberculosis appears in the lymphatics, kidneys, pleura, bones, and meninges. This small proportion of extrapulmonary cases is important because, if not diagnosed and treated, the meningeal, miliary, and renal forms of the disease are invariably fatal.

The pathogenesis of tuberculosis depends on the social and economic environment. In populations living in very primitive and crowded conditions, tuberculosis causes a high infant and child mortality, and a second peak in early adult years. In societies with better nutritional support and higher standards of living, the disease becomes more common in older people, as more and more children grow up without ever being exposed to tuberculosis. By the same token, tuberculosis is more acute, and dissemination more likely, when the disease is epidemic in an undeveloped society than in Western Europe or much of North America.

Transmission depends on the excretion of large numbers of viable tubercle bacilli in the sputum. Most extrapulmonary foci are dangerous only to the patient and do not disseminate infectious tubercle bacilli into the environment. However, once an area of caseating granulomatous disease erodes into a bronchus and sloughs its liquid contents into the air passage, the classic tuberculous cavity is developed. At this time, the growth rate of tubercle bacilli located in the necrotic wall of the cavity is greatly stimulated, and large numbers of virulent tubercle bacilli are discharged into the draining bronchus. These tubercle bacilli spread through the bronchi to other parts of the lung, causing an acute tuberculous pneumonia and, at the same time, spread by coughing into the environment, where they infect others. The extending necrotizing inflammation can cause a pulmonary hemorrhage by eroding a blood vessel. Cavitary pulmonary tuberculosis increases the risk of infection for other patients and also impairs the prognosis for the individual patient. For these reasons, early identification and treatment of sputum-positive patients is an important element in the control of tuberculosis.

CLINICAL MANIFESTATIONS. Although many clinical manifestations of tuberculosis are possible, most patients present as cases of pulmonary tuberculosis with fever, asthenia, cough, weight loss, and pulmonary hemorrhage. These symptoms vary, depending on the stage at which the patient's condition is first diagnosed. Thus, in patients encountered early in their disease, clinical findings and evidences of toxicity are few; such patients have little fever or constitutional signs and their disease is evident only in a chest roentgenogram, a positive tuberculin reaction, and low bacillary counts in their sputum. However, in patients identified late in their disease, constitutional signs are pronounced: high, hectic fever; weight loss; cachexia; advanced findings on physical examination; anemia and hemoptysis; and high bacillary counts in their sputum. Once a patient becomes symptomatic, the disease is in an advanced state, so that every effort should be made to recognize the disease at the earliest possible stage when it can be treated most effectively and before irreversible tissue damage can occur.

As already indicated, tuberculosis may involve areas of the body other than the lungs. Miliary tuberculosis is caused by the discharge of variable numbers of viable tubercle bacilli into the bloodstream and dissemination of the infection throughout the body. Untreated, it is invariably fatal. It occurs most commonly shortly after initial infection with an overwhelming inoculum, or late in life with decline in immunologic competence. In both instances, the patient cannot resist infection, and the prognosis is very poor unless the condition is promptly recognized and vigorously treated.

As might be expected, the clinical manifestations of miliary tuberculosis are extremely variable, since they depend on the stage at which the process is recognized. The very early case, most often seen in infants, may have only low-grade fever, failure to thrive, and little or no roentgenographic abnormalities. At the other end of the scale, the disease is most extensive, giving rise to extreme dyspnea that is unresponsive to oxygen therapy and producing massive roentgenographic abnormalities that represent the replacement of alveoli with innumerable tubercles. The diagnosis usually is easy in the advanced case but can be made only by biopsies of the liver, marrow, or lung in the early stages of miliary tuberculosis.

Miliary tuberculosis may be acute or protracted. The acute form is much more common in children, but still an important cause of fulminant lethal disease in adults. In about 1 to 3 weeks after the sudden onset of fever, miliary lesions can just be seen in the chest film. In most cases there are no respiratory symptoms or physical findings, but patients who develop acute exudative tubercles throughout the lung may suffer from the respiratory distress syndrome, as a result of injury to the alveolar capillary membrane. Respiratory distress may begin suddenly after a brief illness of only a few days or may come on after several weeks of low grade systemic symptoms. In adults, this syndrome tends to occur in middle age, and most reported cases have been black patients (Murray et al., 1978). Chest x-ray shows bilateral reticulonodular infiltrates that progress rapidly to pulmonary opacification. A few cases survive if treated promptly with corticosteroids and isoniazid. The spleen, liver, and lymph nodes are often enlarged (50 per cent of children). Most children (50 per cent) have positive tuberculin tests; in adults the frequency of negative tuberculin tests is higher. Two peripheral lesions help in the diagnosis: choroidal tubercles and papulonecrotic tuberculids of the skin. Neither is common nor numerous.

In protracted miliary tuberculosis, tubercle bacilli are presumably released into the blood repeatedly. In addition to fever, in children and adults there is very prominent lymphadenopathy of the superficial, mediastinal and abdominal nodes, pleural and peritoneal effusion and successive crops of papulonecrotic tuberculids, and uniformly positive skin tests. Marked leukocytosis is a characteristic feature and leukemoid reactions occur. Tubercles with acute lesions are mixed with tubercles containing fibrosis or calcification, as would be expected with episodic protracted infection.

An important group with generalized tuberculosis is composed of anergic elderly patients who are being studied for tumors, renal failure, blood malignancies, or alcoholism. They usually have an unexplained fever, but no signs of pulmonary tuberculosis, and the spleen may not be palpable even though it is full of tubercles. Peripheral adenopathy and pulmonary lesions are frequently absent. Even cultures of sputum, urine, and gastric washings are negative for tubercle bacilli. Hence, it is important to consider the diagnosis of miliary tuberculosis in any wasting febrile illness and to perform liver and marrow biopsy in order to demonstrate tubercles (Slavin et al., 1980). Both alcoholism and end-stage renal failure are commonly associated with miliary tuberculosis.

Meningeal tuberculosis, described in Chapter 166, may occur as part of a miliary or hematogenous process after a tuberculoma erodes into the meningeal space.

Renal tuberculosis is also fatal, if it is not recognized and is allowed to progress. It may occur in conjunction with other forms of tuberculosis, or it may be the only manifestation of the disease. Renal tuberculosis usually arises from the erosion of a tuberculoma through a papilla into the renal pelvis, so that viable tubercle bacilli are discharged into the urinary tract. The infection tends to spread to other parts of the kidney, ureters, bladder, and testicles. Healing often causes ureteral obstruction and obstructive nephropathy. Far-advanced cases are complicated by renal calculi, and in the end-stages, multiple perineal and inguinal urinary fistulae create a life of torture. Therefore, it is important to diagnose renal tuberculosis as early as possible in order to minimize irreversible tissue damage and preserve as much renal function as possible. In the early stages, the only finding is a persistent, low-grade pyuria, and the lesions are too small to demonstrate by pyelography. It can be diagnosed only by cultures of urine on medium appropriate for the growth of tubercle bacilli.

Genitourinary tuberculosis in men presents a characteristic picture. It is a disease of young and middle-aged adults with no recent history of tuberculosis elsewhere and no systemic symptoms. The complaints of dysuria, hematuria, or flank pain are reported in only 70 per cent of patients and 20 per cent are entirely asymptomatic. Over 90 per cent have an abnormal urinalysis, positive urine cultures for tubercle bacilli, abnormal intravenous pyelogram and positive tuberculin tests. Asymptomatic tuberculous masses occur in the scrotum in every case of cavitary renal tuberculosis, and in half of those with non-cavitary caseous renal lesions (Simon et al., 1977). Both kidneys are infected in three-fourths of cases.

Other extrapulmonary manifestations of tuberculosis are less threatening to life but still represent extensive spread of the disease; these result from pleural, osseous, lymph node, pericardial, intestinal, or peritoneal involvement. Tuberculosis may infect the bowel through the blood or by direct extension from the pelvic organs, but most often by swallowing infected sputum. The ileum is the most frequent location of tuberculous enteritis, but not necessarily the ileocecal region. The diagnosis is made by finding granulomatous enteritis in patients with pulmonary tuberculosis. Caseating granulomas and positive smears for acid-fast bacilli are found in the bowel wall (Sherman et al., 1980).

Since the clinical manifestations of pulmonary tuberculosis are quite variable, it is important to emphasize that in many cases the diagnosis will be first suspected from abnormal roentgenographic findings in patients who have nondescript or ill-defined complaints. The essential roentgenographic features of tuberculosis are granulomas with varying degrees of calcification, pneumonic areas undergoing necrosis; cavity formation, often with air-fluid levels; and usually significant volume loss in the lobe or segment involved. All of these are superimposed upon fibrosis. The roentgenographic findings of pulmonary tuberculosis vary as widely as the clinical findings. They range from small or large closed lesions with or without calcification (tuberculomas) to fibrocavitary involvement. The fibrocavitary disease is usually in the apical posterior segments of the upper lobe or the superior segment of the lower lobe. All of these lesions may be accompanied by pleural fibrosis, and they

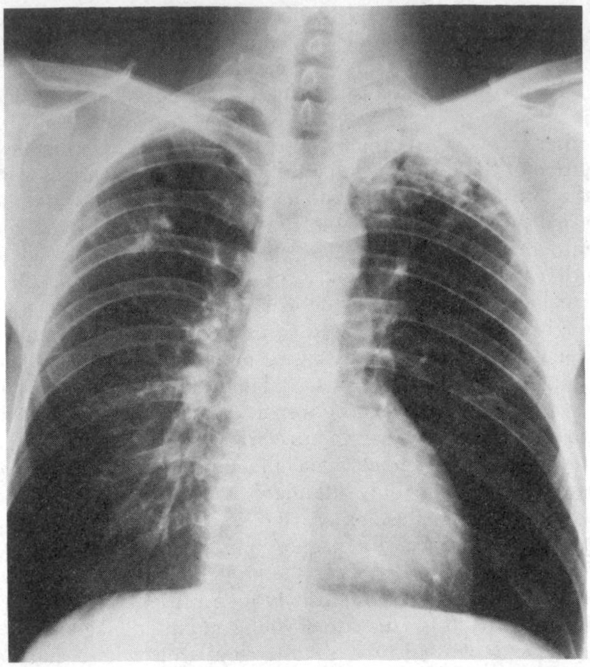

Figure 1. Typical roentgenographic findings in adult pulmonary tuberculosis. The cardinal features are caseonodular granulomatous disease with necrosis and cavitation, fibrosis and volume loss, and hilar retraction to the affected area. Note left upper lobe fibrocavitary disease with nodular spread to anterior segment right upper lobe.

may occur singly or together. As can be seen in Figures 1 and 2, the usual upper lobe fibrocavitary process is highly suggestive of granulomatous infection but may not be pathognomonic of tuberculosis, since histoplasmosis and other fungal diseases may produce a similar process. In addition, although it is less common, acute tuberculous pneumonia may resemble a pneumococcal or *Klebsiella* infection roentgenographically.

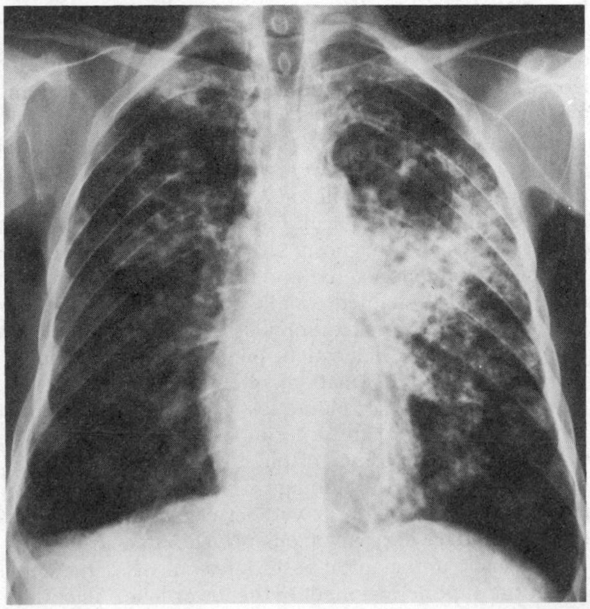

Figure 2. Bilateral upper lobe fibrocavitary tuberculosis with extensive bronchogenic spill.

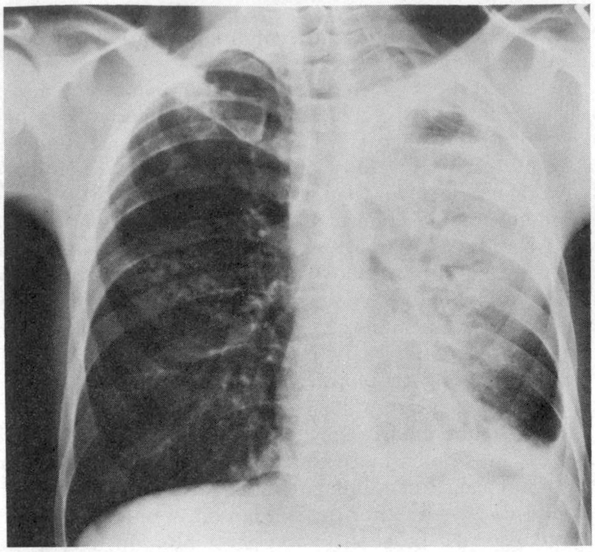

Figure 3. Destroyed left lung with large apical tuberculous cavity and air-fluid level.

Far-advanced cases of pulmonary tuberculosis often present with the picture of a destroyed lung (Fig. 3), usually the left, bronchopleural fistula, and empyema. This finding is highly suggestive of tuberculosis, especially in a young person.

Ideally, the diagnosis of miliary tuberculosis should be made before significant roentgenographic findings appear, since chemotherapy is most effective at the early stage. However, in practice, many patients are not seen until the process is well established. In such cases, the earliest roentgenographic finding is a ground-glass haziness of definition in the chest film that is best recognized by comparison with earlier films. Later, innumerable pinpoint alveolar densities appear uniformly distributed throughout the chest, go on to coalesce, and terminally become confluent (Fig. 4). By the time the process has become confluent and massive, it usually is irreversible and the prognosis is poor, in spite of vigorous antituberculosis chemotherapy.

COMPLICATIONS AND SEQUELAE. Most people infected with tubercle bacilli never develop clinical disease but only demonstrate delayed hypersensitivity to tuberculoprotein in the form of a positive tuberculin reaction. Among the minority who develop clinical disease, it may become apparent shortly after infection has started, especially if the infecting dose is massive or the patient has impaired immunity. In others, the disease may become clinically apparent at any later time because tubercle bacilli can survive in infected tissue for a lifetime, and, if the general health of the individual is impaired, the subclinical stable lesions may break down and the infection may spread. Thus, the most common complication of tuberculous infection is activation whenever the patient's resistance is decreased. For this reason, the development of pulmonary tuberculosis in older patients, known to be positive tuberculin reactors, can be regarded as a late complication

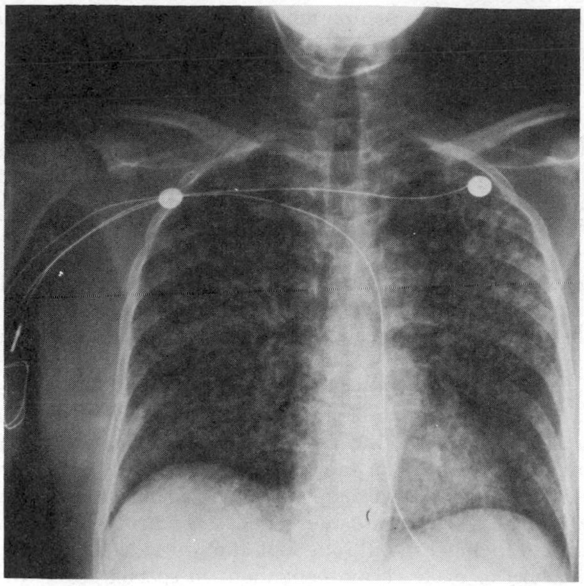

Figure 4. Fatal case of massive miliary tuberculosis.

of tuberculous infection. The same can be said for extrapulmonary manifestations.

If diagnosis is made late in the course of the disease, there is massive destruction of organs such as lung or kidney by necrosis and fibrosis. If diagnosis is made in the early stages of involvement, tissue destruction is minimal if effective treatment is started promptly. Thus, in one sense, significant organ destruction from tuberculosis can be considered a sequel of the disease, which can be avoided with proper treatment.

GEOGRAPHIC VARIATIONS. There are wide geographic variations in the incidence of tuberculosis throughout the world. In Western Europe in the 18th and 19th centuries A.D., tuberculosis was so common and severe that it was called "The Captain of the Men of Death," and the disease came close to destroying Western society. Today, the disease has decreased markedly in incidence and severity in developed societies but remains a major problem in many areas of the world, especially those in which malnutrition, overcrowding, and poverty are common denominators. Wars and social upheavals only accentuate this difference. It is clear that the impact of tuberculosis on the Western World was decreasing markedly before any effective treatment was available. Hence, the decline in incidence and severity occurred as a result of improvements in diet, living conditions, and personal hygiene. Similar improvement can be anticipated if the standard of living can be raised in those areas of the world today in which tuberculosis remains a major threat. In addition, the decline in the disease today should become even more rapid because of effective antituberculosis chemotherapy.

Tuberculosis also has been called a disease of social pathology, because it tends to be a disease of the poor and underprivileged within any society and is increasingly rare among the more fortunate. Even in countries such as the United States, tuberculosis remains a significant problem in the inner-city ghettos and among the poor. Since this is a worldwide phenomenon, it means that case-finding and treatment facilities must be made available for everybody, but especially for those populations who are least exposed to modern medical practice and have the greatest difficulty in understanding what it comprises.

DIAGNOSIS. The key to the diagnosis of tuberculosis is a high index of suspicion for the disease and the prompt utilization of appropriate diagnostic procedures. Ideally, all cases should be confirmed by culturing tubercle bacilli. In practice, however, this is not possible for much of the world, and simpler procedures are all that can be used. Thus, sputum specimens should be obtained and stained for acid-fast bacilli by the Ziehl-Neelsen, Kinyoun, or fluorochrome techniques. The latter technique has the advantage of greater sensitivity and speed but requires a fluorescence microscope.

Because most cases of tuberculosis present as pulmonary disease, which is the most infectious, diagnostic efforts should be concentrated on patients with active pulmonary tuberculosis. Mass radiography helps identify suspect cases, and all symptomatic patients should be sent for chest roentgenograms. At the same time, appropriate sputum specimens should be obtained for smear and, if possible, culture. Sputum induction by inhaled saline aerosols is of value for patients who cannot produce adequate sputum specimens, but such procedures should not be done in nonventilated areas. Bronchial brushing and lavage to obtain secretions for smear and culture is effective in many patients with low bacillary output, but should be done only if conventional sputum studies have been negative. Miliary tuberculosis usually requires transbronchial, liver, or marrow biopsy for diagnosis.

Many different media are available throughout the world for the cultivation of tubercle bacilli, and the choice of one or several depends, to an extent, on the resources of each facility. The most commonly used medium in the United States today is the Middlebrook-Cohn 7H11. This has the advantage of being transparent, thus permitting earlier recognition of colonies, but it has the disadvantage of requiring 5 per cent CO_2 in the incubator. A significant advantage of the 7H11 medium is that it is easily adapted to drug susceptibility studies. Traditional Lowenstein-Jensen medium also is commonly used for initial isolation of tubercle bacilli.

Because of the great variability of the extrapulmonary manifestations of tuberculosis, all biopsy specimens of chronic inflammatory or suppurative disease should be submitted for culture of tubercle bacilli in addition to histologic examination. A common error is for a biopsy specimen such as necrotic lymph node or fistula tract to be excised, not cultured, and placed in formalin for fixation. This renders the procedure valueless for the diagnosis of tuberculosis.

The tuberculin test should be a definite part of the evaluation of all suspect cases of tuberculosis. As with any biological test, 100 per cent correlation with disease does not occur, but a positive tuberculin reaction is demonstrated in more than 95 per cent of patients with tuberculosis. Thus, a negative tuberculin test makes the diagnosis of tuberculosis unlikely, but does not rule it out in any absolute sense. Tuberculin testing for diagnostic purposes should be done by the intradermal or Mantoux techniques. Only carefully standardized tuberculin, such as PPD-S or its equivalent, should be used at a concentration of 5 tuberculin units injected intradermally into the medial aspect of the skin of the forearm and read at 48 to 72 hrs. The reading consists of the measurement of the greatest diameter of induration recorded in millimeters. Thus, a properly recorded tuberculin test specifies the material injected (PPD-S), its strength in tuberculin units, and the millimeters of induration observed at 48 to 72 hrs. The result should not be recorded as positive or negative because these standards have changed from time to time; if recorded in millimeters, the result can always be interpreted in terms of current standards. At present, induration 10 mm or greater in diameter is considered a positive reaction, while that between 6 and 10 mm is deemed indeterminate, and less than 6 mm is negative.

Tuberculin testing is of great value in identifying the people at risk of developing tuberculosis within a population. Present experience in the United States today shows that more than 90 per cent of all new active cases come from known positive tuberculin reactors, even though they comprise less than 8 per cent of the total population. Thus, tuberculin testing provides a means of detecting potential cases that can be protected by chemoprophylaxis. It is prudent to tuberculin test all patients with diseases that in the future might require steroid therapy or immunosuppression before such treatment is initiated. Such therapy depresses tuberculin hypersensitivity and therefore gives rise to a false negative response, and it is well known that patients with positive tuberculin reactions are at risk of developing active tuberculosis when they are immunosuppressed.

Pleural effusion is a fairly common manifestation of tuberculosis and is often misdiagnosed if the proper studies are not initiated at the time of diagnostic thoracentesis. It arises most commonly in the early months or years after infection has occurred and hypersensitivity is at its peak. The pathogenesis of tuberculous pleural effusion involves a subpleural focus of active infection that erodes into the pleural space and actively seeds it with tubercles, or the leakage of tuberculoprotein into adjacent tissues so that an exudative inflammatory response is evoked. The fluid that is produced usually is serofibrinous in nature and has the characteristics of an exudate. Early in its formation, acute inflammatory cells (polymorphonuclear leukocytes) prevail; as the process matures, round cell pleocytosis becomes apparent. The fluid usually resolves with treatment but may produce pleural fibrosis and restriction of thoracic movement. For this reason, as much of the fluid as possible should be removed at the time of thoracentesis.

Today, in most parts of the world, tuberculosis is a diminishing cause of pleural effusion; lung cancer, viral infections, congestive heart failure, and pulmonary embolism are more common causes. Therefore, at the time the thoracentesis is done, proper diagnostic studies should be initiated on the pleural fluid. These include determinations of specific gravity, protein concentration, glucose, and lactic dehydrogenase (LDH). At the same time, serum determinations should be obtained for glucose and LDH. In addition, the cells in the pleural fluid should be counted and a cell block made for cytologic study. Whenever practicable and when there are no contraindications (low or absent platelets, prolonged bleeding time), pleural biopsy should be done at the time of initial thoracentesis and appropriate sections stained for acid-fast bacilli. If an adequate pleural specimen is obtained, caseating tubercles are often seen. In addition, pleural fluid and biopsy always should be cultured for tubercle bacilli. If these procedures are done routinely at the time of diagnostic thoracentesis, the role of tuberculosis is accurately delineated. If they are not done, and the pleural fluid is examined casually, many cases of tuberculous pleurisy are missed.

TREATMENT. Modern antituberculosis chemotherapy is so effective today that no patient should die of the disease if they can survive the first 30 days of treatment (Johnston and Wildrick, 1974). The problem is to identify the patients needing treatment and make certain that they actually take their medications as ordered. Because of the way in which tuberculosis remains endemic in the lower social strata, many of the patients are poorly motivated to cooperate in their treatment. However, the important thing is to deliver the most effective treatment possible rather than wasting time denigrating the patients. More ingenuity is needed to provide effective rewards for cooperative patients.

The ultimate aim of antituberculosis chemotherapy is *tissue sterilization* (the elimination of all viable tubercle bacilli in the body of the infected patient). Twenty years ago, attainment of this aim was thought unlikely; today, it is a reality. There are now at least 12 drugs of varying efficacy being used throughout the world, and it is not practical to make recommendations in specific terms that are applicable worldwide. However, the basic principles of antituberculosis chemotherapy are universal.

Tissue sterilization is best achieved by an early intensive treatment regimen utilizing the best three drugs available followed by a longer period of maintenance therapy comprising the two most effective drugs of the initial program. In this way, the early intensive period reduces the bacterial population most rapidly and thereby renders the emergence of drug resistance least likely. The longer period of maintenance therapy ensures the ultimate destruction of any of the persisting, slowly metabolizing tubercle bacilli.

The 12 antituberculosis drugs available are listed in Table 1 with their recommended dosages and major toxic reactions. It should be emphasized that hypersensitivity varying from mild symptoms to major anaphylactic reaction can occur from any of these drugs. Practical considerations dictate specific choices as to drug regimens because of factors of cost and availability. For a variety of reasons, the best oral drugs are isoniazid (INH), rifampin (RM), ethambutol (EM), and pyrazinamide (PZA). The best aminoglycoside is streptomycin (SM). Thus, these five drugs provide the basis for modern chemotherapy regimens. The remaining seven drugs should be used only in special situations.

At the time antituberculosis chemotherapy is initiated, the status of the patient should be carefully evaluated. Every effort should be made to determine whether or not the patient has undergone any previous antituberculosis treatment. If so, the possibility of drug resistance should be considered, and an initial four-drug regimen set up until the results of drug susceptibility studies are available. If there is no history of previous treatment, the patient can be committed to the usual initial triple-drug regimen, unless the patient comes from an area known to have significant rates of drug resistance, in which case a four-drug regimen might well be justified.

The basic regimen recommended consists of daily SM for 30 to 60 days, plus INH, EM, RM, or PZA in a double oral drug program for 10 to 12 months. Current studies are being reported that indicate that the previous recommendations for duration of therapy for 18 to 24 months are no longer justified. It may well be that 12 months is unnecessarily long. It is very probable that the most effective regimen is SM-INH-RM; however, the other

Table 1. DRUG TREATMENT OF TUBERCULOSIS

Major Oral Drugs	**Dosage**	**Major Toxic Effects**
Isoniazid	300 mg daily	Hepatotoxicity, polyneuritis
Ethambutol	15 mg/kg daily	Decrease in visual acuity
Rifampin	600 mg daily	Hepatotoxicity
Pyrazinamide	2 to 3 g daily	Hepatotoxicity, hyperuricemia
Ethionamide	1.0 g daily	Gastrointestinal intolerance
Less Effective Oral Drugs		
Cycloserine	1.0 g daily	Convulsion, depression
Aminosalicylic acid	12 to 15 g daily	Gastrointestinal intolerance, hepatotoxicity
Thiacetazone	150 mg daily	Hepatotoxicity
Aminoglycosides (parenteral administration) in order of preference: Streptomycin, Kanamycin, Capreomycin, Viomycin	1.0 g or 15 mg/kg daily during initial phase of therapy	Audiovestibular injury, renal damage

possible combinations are so effective that it would require controlled studies involving many thousands of patients to get a satisfactory answer as to which is best.

In addition to changing concepts as to the duration of treatment, it now is clear that, after the early initial intensive period of treatment, twice-weekly intermittent administration of drugs is highly effective and can be maintained within a framework of 6 to 12 months. Such programs have been shown to be comparable in efficacy to programs based on daily drug administration of equal duration, and they obviously produce great economies in terms of time and effort (Fox and Mitchison, 1974; Dutt et al., 1979). It is hoped that such savings can be invested in greater care in making certain that the drugs are taken as prescribed and, in many instances, supervised administration becomes quite practical. The drug dosages for the twice-weekly regimens are determined by multiplying the daily dose by seven and dividing by two, except for RM, which is best given in a dose of 600 mg twice weekly.

As antituberculosis chemotherapy was developing 20 to 25 years ago, surgery was thought to be a valuable adjunct to treatment. Collapse procedures were developed for control of disease in drug-resistant, therapy-failure cases, and pulmonary resections were recommended for the removal of irreversibly damaged tissue (cavities, destroyed lobes or segments, and areas of bronchiectasis). However, with the passing of time and the improvement of the efficacy of antituberculosis chemotherapy, these indications for surgical treatment of tuberculosis have become obsolete and no longer applicable. Today, there is one remaining problem in tuberculosis for which a skilled and experienced thoracic surgeon can be helpful, and that is in the management of bronchopleural fistula and empyema. Open drainage in such cases in conjunction with optimal chemotherapy may be life-saving but requires careful teamwork; fortunately, such cases are rare. Therefore, the investment of money, facilities, and personnel required to support an active surgical program for tuberculosis treatment is unjustified, and such resources are used much better if they are put into the support of the chemotherapy program and appropriate public health facilities.

The addition of steroid therapy to effective antituberculosis chemotherapy is of little or no value in the usual case of tuberculosis and has some risk, especially if drug-resistant infection is a possibility. However, the combination of prednisone 30 to 40 mg daily for 4 to 6 weeks plus intensive antituberculosis chemotherapy is justified in the following cases: (1) hypertoxic patients who may otherwise not survive long enough for chemotherapy to become effective (usually 3 weeks), (2) patients with meningeal tuberculosis who appear to be developing acute cerebral edema or spinal block and (3) patients with massive miliary disease who have major diffusion defects and cannot maintain adequate oxygen levels. Fortunately, the latter two categories are not common; therefore, steroids are most frequently used in patients of the first category.

One of the valuable by-products of the lengthy chemotherapy trials evaluated in the treatment of tuberculosis was an experience and understanding of the role of adverse drug reactions in the outcome of chemotherapy. The commonly used antituberculosis drugs (SM, INH, EMB, and RM) fortunately have few adverse reactions, although, when they occur, they may be highly significant. On the other hand, the less commonly used antituberculosis drugs have a wide variety of adverse side effects, some of which can be life-threatening. Therefore, when a physician assumes responsibility for antituberculosis chemotherapy, he should acquaint himself in detail with the pharmacology of the drugs he is using and adequately monitor his patients in order to protect them against serious adverse drug reactions.

In general, there are four major types of adverse drug reactions: hypersensitivity, toxic action, side effects, and idiosyncrasy. Of these, only hypersensitivity is life-threatening, and its recognition is of paramount importance. Any patient receiving antituberculosis chemotherapy who unexpectedly develops fever, rash, purpura, or marked vasomotor reactions after parenteral injections should be considered as possibly developing hypersensitivity to one or more of the drugs included in the regimen. These findings should lead to a cessation of the treatment program until all have disappeared. The continuance of drugs in the presence of developing hypersensitivity is dangerous and may lead to a life-threatening reaction. Hypersensitivity may develop to any drug.

Toxic effects are dose-related and are a reflection of the molecular nature of the drug. If ignored, they can be dangerous but can usually be controlled easily by the experienced physician by appropriate reductions in dosage. An example is the neurotoxicity of isoniazid.

Side effects are related to the nature of the drug and the size of the dose. The usual effect is nausea and vomiting, as seen when para-aminosalicylic acid is prescribed. Although a nuisance factor, side effects are rarely dangerous and usually can be controlled by the competent physician.

Idiosyncratic reactions are unpredictable and represent peculiar and illogical responses to any particular drug. They are rarely dangerous but may produce sufficient symptoms to warrant replacement of the offending drug.

Antituberculosis drugs must be used cautiously in pregnant women because of the risk of teratogenicity. Isoniazid can be given in pregnancy in the usual dosage because careful studies of many cases disclose no evidence that fetal abnormalities are increased by its administration (Snider et al., 1980). Ethambutol also appears to be a safe drug in pregnant women, but rifampin appears to cause fetal limb abnormalities, central nervous system lesions, and bleeding tendencies. Streptomycin should not be used in pregnancy because it produces ototoxicity in the fetus.

Today, there exist at least 11 major antituberculosis drugs. Therefore, if any one produces major problems, an appropriate alternative usually can be found. If a drug must be stopped because of adverse reactions in the early weeks of treatment, it usually can be replaced by another drug. If, however, a drug must be stopped in the third or later months of treatment, it should be replaced with two other drugs until it is certain that the patient has acquired negative culture status and drug resistance has not emerged.

PROPHYLAXIS. With the advent of INH, chemoprophylaxis of tuberculosis became feasible, and many studies confirmed its value. The drug was safe, economical, and effective when given for 1 year in a daily dose of 300 mg to known positive tuberculin reactors. Since most cases of tuberculosis arise in patients with positive tuberculin reactions, it was easy to identify the population at risk by tuberculin testing.

Carefully designed double-blind studies have shown that the use of INH chemoprophylaxis in positive tuberculin reactors with no evidence of disease for 1 year reduces the rate of tuberculous disease by 70 to 80 per cent during the year of drug ingestion, and the long-term reduction remains in the 60 to 70 per cent range. It is also clear that certain positive tuberculin reactors are obviously at greater risk than others. Infants, known recent converters, silicotics, diabetics, and immunosuppressed patients are at greater risk than adult or elderly patients with no associated risk factors. Therefore, each facility should evaluate its population in terms of priority. Hepatotoxicity of INH is strongly age-dependent, occurring in about 0.2 per cent of children below the age of 15 and 2.0 per cent or more of individuals over 55. Therefore, each patient should be evaluated individually in terms of the risk-benefit ratio. When properly used, INH chemoprophylaxis is very valuable for the reduction of tuberculosis.

Vaccination with BCG (Bacille Calmette-Guérin) has significant value in control of tuberculosis, especially in areas of the world in which case rates are high and tuberculosis mortality is centered in the very young. The vaccine is made from a strain of bovine tubercle bacilli that was made avirulent over a period of years by Calmette and Guérin. It has been grown all over the world and is very difficult to standardize. For these and other reasons, controversy exists as to the overall efficacy of BCG vaccination. As previously indicated, at this time BCG vaccination is worthy of consideration in a society with high and unchanging rates of tuberculosis, especially when the infant mortality for the disease remains elevated. It markedly reduces the early infant mortality if newborn infants are immunized. However, for much of the world, BCG vaccination no longer is recommended.

Tuberculosis is an infectious disease of major public health significance for much of the world today. Therefore, it is of critical importance to find the patients capable of spreading the infection, eliminate their infectiousness by effective treatment, and, at the same time, identify the persons whom they have infected. Those individuals capable of transmitting tuberculosis, for all practical purposes, are those patients with active pulmonary disease excreting large numbers of viable tubercle bacilli in their sputum; patients with extrapulmonary tuberculosis are not disseminators of the disease but are victims of it.

The individuals at risk of acquiring tuberculosis are the household and occupational contacts of the infectious or "index" case. Such contacts ideally should be evaluated by tuberculin testing, chest radiography of all positive reactors, and initiation of either curative or prophylactic antituberculosis treatment. If no disease is detectable, prophylactic drug therapy is given, but full chemotherapy is indicated for the positive tuberculin reactor contact who has detectable pulmonary disease. It should be emphasized that among household contacts, infants and small children are most likely to be the first and most seriously infected. However, as the standard of living improves, the age distribution of tuberculosis shifts increasingly to the older age groups, and, in this circumstance, the identification and prophylactic treatment of positive tuberculin reactors becomes an important element in the prevention of late breakdowns of the disease. Mass radiography is not a practical solution for this problem.

References

Barksdale, L., and Kim, K.-S.: Mycobacterium. Bacteriol Rev 41:217, 1977.

Dutt, A. K., Jones, L., and Stead, W.: Short-course chemotherapy for tuberculosis with largely twice-weekly isoniazid-rifampin. Chest 75:441, 1979.

Fox, W., and Mitchison, D. A.: Short-course chemotherapy for tuberculosis. Lung Disease: State of the Art 1974–75. American Lung Association, p. 176.

Johnston, R. F., and Wildrick, K. H.: The impact of chemotherapy on the care of patients with tuberculosis. Lung Disease: State of the Art 1974–75. American Lung Association, p. 147.

Murray, H., Tuazon, C., Kirmani, N., and Sheagren, J.: Adult respiratory distress syndrome associated with miliary tuberculosis. Chest 73:37, 1978.

Sherman, S., Rohwedder, J., Raukrishnan, K., and Weg, J.: Tuberculous enteritis and peritonitis: Report of 36 General Hospital cases. Arch Int Med 140:506, 1980.

Simon, H. B., Weinstein, A. J., Pasternak, M. S., Swartz, M. N., and Kunz, L. J.: Genitourinary tuberculosis: clinical features in a general hospital population. Am J Med 63:410, 1977.

Slavin, R., Walsh, T., and Pollack, A.: Late generalized tuberculosis: analysis and comparison of 100 cases in preantibiotic and antibiotic eras. Medicine (Baltimore) 59:352, 1980.

Snider, D., Layde, P., Johnson, M., and Lyle, M.: Treatment of tuberculosis during pregnancy. Am Rev Respir Dis 122:65, 1980.

Youmans, G. P.: Tuberculosis. Philadelphia, W. B. Saunders Company, 1979.

121
NONTUBERCULOUS MYCOBACTERIAL INFECTIONS

WILLIAM LESTER, M.D.

Nontuberculous mycobacterial infections may be clinically, pathologically, and radiologically identical to tuberculosis but are caused by mycobacteria that have primary drug resistance, diminished virulence for guinea pigs, and distinct cellular and colonial morphologic differences from tubercle bacilli. At first these organisms were classified as atypical, anonymous, or unclassified mycobacteria, but now they have achieved species designation, and the term nontuberculous mycobacteria is more appropriate.

The genus *Mycobacterium* is one of the most widely distributed bacterial genera in nature and ranges from saprophytes to such important pathogens as *M. tuberculosis* and *M. leprae*. Classically, the term tuberculosis long has been applied to infections caused by *M. tuberculosis* and *M. bovis*. This discussion will be restricted to human mycobacterial infections caused by bacteria other than *M. tuberculosis, M. bovis,* or *M. leprae*.

Nontuberculous mycobacterial infections may present clinical manifestations that are indistinguishable from those of tuberculosis and can be recognized only by cultural recovery of the etiologic agent. Such infections may disseminate to many organs, especially in patients with impaired immunity. At the other extreme, they may cause only self-limited localized lymph node suppuration. In many other instances, however, they may produce pulmonary involvement that is indistinguishable from that seen in classic tuberculosis. Finally, they may produce isolated extrapulmonary lesions—bone and joint, renal, or skin lesions—somewhat like those seen in tuberculosis (Chapman, 1977; Lester, 1966; Lincoln and Gilbert, 1972).

ETIOLOGY. It is convenient to separate the nontuberculous mycobacteria into the four groups originally proposed by Runyon (1959) on the basis of simple morphologic characteristics that usually are easily recognized in initial cultures. These four groups are:

I. Photochromogens. These form a yellow carotene pigment on exposure to light. Colonies grown in the dark are buff colored and become yellow on exposure to light.

II. Scotochromogens. Colonies are pigmented when grown either in the dark or the light.

III. Nonphotochromogens. The buff (or occasionally light yellow color) of these colonies does not change on exposure to light.

IV. Rapid growers. The rapid growth of these organisms makes mature colonies visible in four to six days when they are incubated at 37° C, whereas most other mycobacteria require one to two weeks.

All four groups are resistant to drugs on initial isolation (primary resistance). However, photochromogens are less resistant to routine antituberculosis agents—isoniazid, ethambutol, and rifampin—than the mycobacteria in groups II, III, and IV.

Table 1 is a general summary of the taxonomy and characteristics of mycobacteria, especially those considered to be nontuberculous. Although this classification is by no means final, it is noteworthy that the original classification proposed by Runyon, which was based on simple colonial characteristics of the mycobacteria, has held up in the face of biochemical studies, serologic analysis, and patterns of mycobacteriophage susceptibility.

Certain generalizations are suggested from Table 1 that should alert the clinician to the possibility of nontuberculous mycobacterial infection. First, as mentioned previously, all the mycobacteria in the four Runyon groups are characterized by significant primary drug resistance. Thus, any resistant isolate obtained from a patient with a clear history of *no* prior antituberculosis treatment should be viewed as a potential nontuberculous mycobacterium. Second, a negative niacin test on a drug-resistant mycobacterium greatly enhances the likelihood that it is nontuberculous. Finally, a resistant culture with a negative niacin test and a strong catalase reaction almost certainly will be a nontuberculous mycobacterium.

Table 1 also emphasizes that the nontuberculous mycobacteria produce syndromes that are indistinguishable from classic tuberculosis. Since there is no evidence that these infections are transmitted from one case to another, they will most likely not diminish in frequency in the future as has tuberculosis. Thus, the proportion of nontuberculous mycobacterial infections will probably increase as infections due to *M. tuberculosis* decline.

Since these organisms are widespread and many can occur as contaminants, a single isolation may have no etiologic significance. Multiple specimens should be obtained for culture, and these will usually be positive if the patient has a nontuberculous mycobacterial disease. The isolation of nontuberculous mycobacteria from a single specimen, especially if the colony count is low, is not diagnostic, and treatment should not be started until further efforts to recover the organism succeed and confirm the diagnosis.

PATHOGENESIS. The pathogenesis and epidemiology of nontuberculous mycobacterial disease are poorly understood. Transmission from one patient to another has not been demonstrated, and all authorities agree that individual cases represent no public health threat. Many of the etiologic organisms can be recovered from soil, water, or organic debris and may be ingested or inhaled in dust particles or, like *M. marinum,* introduced into the skin through abrasions.

Since the nontuberculous mycobacteria have diminished virulence and cause a low rate of disease among infected patients, those individuals who have severe disseminated infections with these organisms may well have abnormal immune responses. Thus, these infections are being recognized more frequently in immunosuppressed patients who have organ transplants or are being treated for leukemia and cancer, and they should be kept in mind in all patients undergoing immunosuppressive therapy for any reason. In line with this concept is the recent observation that patients suffering from the acquired immune deficiency syndrome (AIDS) have an unusually high incidence of disseminated infection caused by nontuberculous mycobacteria, especially *M. avium intracellulare* (Greene et al., 1982; Zakowski et al., 1982).

Skin test preparations similar to PPD-S (tuberculin from *M. tuberculosis*) have been prepared from various nontu-

Table 1. NOMENCLATURE AND CHARACTERISTICS OF MYCOBACTERIA

Organism	Relative Pathogenicity for Man	Clinical Manifestations	Niacin Production	Catalase Production
M. tuberculosis	+ + + +	Human tuberculosis	+	+ +
M. bovis	+ + + +	Human tuberculosis	Variable	+
M. africanum	+ + +	Pulmonary	Variable	+
M. ulcerans	+ + + +	Cutaneous	−	+ + + +
Group I				
M. kansasii	+ + +	Pulmonary, extrapulmonary, disseminated	−	+ + + +
M. marinum	+ + +	Extrapulmonary, cutaneous	Variable	+
M. simiae	+ +	Pulmonary	+	+ + + +
Group II				
M. flavescens	0	None	−	+ + + +
M. gordonae	0	None	−	+ + + +
M. scrofulaceum	+ +	Pulmonary, extrapulmonary, lymphadenitis	−	+ + + +
Group III				
M. avium	+ + +	Pulmonary, extrapulmonary, disseminated	−	+
M. gastri	0	None	−	+
M. terrae	Rare	Extrapulmonary, disseminated	−	+ + + +
M. triviale		Extrapulmonary, arthritis	−	+ + + +
M. intracellulare	+ + +	Pulmonary, extrapulmonary, lymphadenitis, disseminated	−	+ + +
M. xenopi	+	Cutaneous	−	+
Group IV				
M. chelonei	+	Pulmonary, extrapulmonary, abscesses, lymphadenitis	−	+ + + +
M. fortuitum	+	Pulmonary, extrapulmonary, disseminated, abscesses	−	+ + + +

berculous mycobacteria. PPD-Y, prepared from *M. kansasii*, and PPD-B, prepared from *M. intracellulare*, are the most useful. These preparations, applied and read like PPD-S, have demonstrated striking epidemiologic differences in reactivity. In areas where *M. kansasii* and *M. intracellulare* are endemic, many positive reactions to PPD-Y and PPD-B will be found. Such studies also indicate that the disease-infection ratio for such organisms is low. However, because of common or shared antigens with other mycobacteria, the results of such skin tests alone are not diagnostic in any individual case. PPD-Y and PPD-S are closely related antigenically, whereas PPD-B is less likely to cross-react with PPD-Y. Thus, a patient with a large reaction to PPD-B and little or no reaction to PPD-S has probably been infected with *M. intracellulare*. Results of differential skin tests may therefore be of epidemiologic importance, but the exact diagnosis in any individual case depends on the recovery of the specific organism in cultures.

Among nontuberculous mycobacterial infections, most reported cases of pulmonary disease have been caused by *M. kansasii* or *M. intracellulare-avium* complex. Both infections are concentrated in relatively small geographic areas with sharp differences in local frequency. Comparative skin testing with mycobacterial sensitins also shows sharp differences in frequency of reactions in adjacent areas. Such differences cannot be explained on the basis of climatic or environmental factors and raise the possibility that food, water, milk, or other routes of transmission may be responsible. Although the role of these latter possibilities has not been established, it is likely that different mechanisms of transmission apply to various environments, since these organisms are largely ubiquitous.

Another unexplained feature of pulmonary disease caused by *M. kansasii* or the *M. intracellulare-avium* complex is that approximately two thirds of cases occur in males. There is no documented occupational exposure related to these infections. However, *M. kansasii* disease is more common in urban patients, whereas that caused by *M. intracellulare-avium* complex is more frequent in rural areas.

Isolated cervical lymph node disease is a very common manifestation of nontuberculous mycobacterial infection, especially in young children; it suggests that the oropharyngeal route may be a major portal of infection. The striking infrequency with which pleural effusions are caused by these organisms suggests that inhalation may not be a common route of infection.

PATHOLOGY. The gross and microscopic features of nontuberculous mycobacterial disease are identical to those characteristic of *M. tuberculosis*. The most characteristic finding is that of caseating granulomas with varying proportions of Langhans' giant cells, epithelioid cells, and acid-fast bacilli. The amount of fibrosis and caseation necrosis is related to the chronicity and extent of the lesion. Disseminated infections in immunosuppressed patients often do not show the classic caseating granulomas, usually because the lesions have not had time to mature. Because the granulomas are not diagnostic, the diagnosis depends on the cultural isolation and identification of the organism. In AIDS cases, enormous numbers of acid-fast bacilli pack the macrophages in the bone marrow, spleen, liver, lung, and gastrointestinal tract so that the cells resemble lepra cells.

CLINICAL MANIFESTATIONS. Nontuberculous mycobacterial infection varies widely in its manifestations. It can be an isolated, self-limited, lymph node infection, usually cervical, which improves spontaneously or after resection of the infected tissue. On the other hand, it may be a rapidly progressive, overwhelming disseminated infection with massive lymphohematogenous invasion of all major organs and little chance for survival. Fortunately, such disseminated cases are rare. They usually are associated with massive infection, very poor host resistance, or both.

A significant number of patients have a fibrotic, fibrocavitary, or pneumonic pulmonary disease that is roentgenographically indistinguishable from tuberculosis. The disease often progresses more slowly than tuberculosis, but fresh pneumonic lesions and acute toxicity are encountered in some individuals. The pulmonary disease will show progression, fever, toxicity, hemorrhage, weight loss, and cachexia similar to tuberculosis. Most patients with pulmonary disease due to nontuberculous mycobacteria will have infections caused by either *M. kansasii* or *M. intracellulare-avium* complex. In both instances, but especially in the latter, primary drug resistance is prominent. If it is not recognized and the patient is erroneously given drugs of minimal efficacy, therapy will fail and the probability of response to a retreatment regimen will be diminished. Thus, although the disease in general may be more indolent than tuberculosis, it is more refractory to treatment and requires meticulous attention to the selection of an optimally effective chemotherapeutic regimen. Failure is associated with progression of the disease, and spontaneous remissions do *not* occur.

Pulmonary disease due to groups II and IV mycobacteria is rare. Unfortunately, no one has encountered more than a few such cases, and little is known of their natural history or prognosis. They are often infections superimposed on old pulmonary processes—bullous or cystic disease, fibrosis, bronchiectasis, or old tuberculosis. In a recent report of 24 pulmonary infections due to rapidly growing mycobacteria, 12 (50 per cent) cases had previously normal lungs and the others had underlying predisposing conditions (Wallace et al., 1983). Most of these infections were caused by *M. chelonei* subspecies *abscessus* and involved mainly women. Patchy unilateral lung infiltrates were much more common than cavities. Patients excreting either group II or group IV organisms must be carefully studied to determine if the organism isolated is a commensal or a pathogen.

COMPLICATIONS AND SEQUELAE. Rapid progression of obstructive lung disease occurs in adult patients who may at the time of initial diagnosis show relatively limited lung involvement and good overall pulmonary function. The condition of such patients, even though effectively treated so that infection is controlled, may deteriorate rapidly and may progress to incapacitating obstructive lung disease. Thus, whenever pulmonary disease caused by nontuberculous mycobacteria is encountered, all possible measures should be introduced to diminish the progression of obstructive lung disease. The one measure that may be most helpful in diminishing the progress of obstructive lung disease is the elimination of cigarette smoking. The reason for this association between pulmonary infection with nontuberculous mycobacteria and obstructive lung disease is unknown. More than 50 per cent of patients with pulmonary disease caused by *M. kansasii* or *M. intracellulare-avium* complex will have coexisting obstructive pulmonary disease. It is possible that defects in alveolar and mucociliary clearance may play a role.

GEOGRAPHIC VARIATIONS IN DISEASE. It is difficult to discuss the geographic variations in disease caused by nontuberculous mycobacteria because facilities for their proper recognition and identification are not available in much of the world. Despite limited facilities and the tentative state of classification, these mycobacteria are known to be worldwide in distribution. If all biopsy specimens were cultured appropriately for mycobacteria as well as for bacteria and fungi, our understanding of the regional or local basis of these infections would be greatly augmented.

Human disease due to *M. kansasii* is often strikingly localized within a large community, suggesting a focal exposure. However, evidence of case-to-case transmission, including household contact spread, is absent.

Human disease due to *M. intracellulare-avium* complex also tends to show certain focal epidemiologic characteristics. Although it was once more common in the southeastern area of the United States, it is most frequently encountered in California (Good and Snider, 1982). Isolated cases are seen throughout the world. Human cases of *M. avium* infection are seen more frequently in farming populations of central Europe, but little is known of their distribution elsewhere.

There is a well-known association of *M. marinum* infection with swimming pool granulomas in swimmers and aquarium-keepers.

The extent to which nontuberculous mycobacteria are responsible for chronic skin ulcers in humid tropical countries is not well known or understood. Probably they are more closely related than is presently recognized. Once again, the availability of reliable facilities for culturing appropriate specimens would help to increase our knowledge of these organisms.

DIAGNOSIS. Because the clinical spectrum of disease caused by these organisms is nonspecific, it has not been possible to develop reliable clinical, pathologic, or radiologic criteria for specific diagnosis. Only bacteriologic diagnosis is reliable, and cultures from sputum, gastric contents, purulent secretions, tissue biopsy, and urine must be planted on Loewenstein-Jensen or Middlebrook-Cohn 7 H 10 or 7 H 11 culture media. The demonstration of acid-fast organisms in stained preparations of the specimens is not adequate for diagnosis but should alert the physician to the necessity of culturing on such media. The isolation of nontuberculous mycobacteria in only a single specimen or with a very sparse colony count should be viewed with suspicion. In patients afflicted with nontuberculous mycobacterial disease the organisms are usually found in multiple cultures and in large numbers.

In many instances nontuberculous mycobacteria produce such lesions as suppurative adenitis, skin ulcers, or a localized nodule. A common error is to overlook culturing the excised specimen and do only histologic studies, resulting in a report to the clinician of caseating granulomas with demonstrable acid-fast organisms that have not been cultured. Once the node is fixed in formalin, the only opportunity to make a specific diagnosis is lost. A possible exception is *M. intracellulare*, which is said to be the only *Mycobacterium* that stains with the periodic acid–Schiff

Table 2. PARENTERAL ANTITUBERCULOSIS DRUGS

	Normal Adult Daily Dose	Duration of Administration	Toxicity
Streptomycin	1.0 gm 15 mg/kg body weight	30–90 days	Vestibular, auditory, renal
Viomycin	1.0 gm	30–90 days	Vestibular, auditory, renal
Kanamycin	1.0 gm	30–90 days	Auditory, vestibular, renal
Capreomycin	1.0 gm	30–90 days	Vestibular, auditory, renal

(PAS) method, and may be recognizable in tissues by that property.

Relatively simple routine laboratory studies and procedures will lead to recognition of most cases of nontuberculous mycobacterial infections. Incubators should be dark, and cultures should be checked weekly and examined under a dissecting microscope. If drug susceptibility studies and catalase and niacin tests were done on all initial isolates, the finding of primary drug resistance in niacin-negative, highly positive catalase cultures would almost certainly identify the organisms as one of the nontuberculous mycobacteria. Whenever possible all questionable cultures should be sent to an appropriate reference laboratory for full evaluation.

TREATMENT. Isolated lymph node involvement without dissemination probably is handled best by excision and does not require intensive chemotherapy unless the patient has impaired immunity. Such lymph node involvement is seen most commonly in the neck, and by deep extension may encroach upon vital structures such as the jugular vein and facial nerve. Since the extent and depth of the involvement cannot be determined accurately before biopsy-excision, the procedure should be done by a surgeon who is experienced in the anatomic relationships of the area. It is best to remove the involved tissue as completely as possible.

Disseminated infection and pulmonary disease require chemotherapy (Tables 2 and 3). *M. kansasii* is resistant to the conventional antituberculosis drugs streptomycin, isoniazid, and ethambutol but usually only to low concentrations of these agents. The organism is very sensitive to rifampin. Thus, adult patients with pulmonary or disseminated *M. kansasii* infection are best treated with an intensive drug regimen consisting of streptomycin, isoniazid, and rifampin daily. If rifampin is not available, ethambutol or paraaminosalicylic acid can be substituted. The streptomycin should be continued daily until there is a satisfactory clinical response and cultures become negative. The two oral drugs should then be continued for 24 months. Such a program, especially if rifampin is included, should result in success rates approaching 100 per cent. If this therapy fails or if the patient had been inadequately treated in the past, a triple drug retreatment regimen based on another aminoglycoside such as capreomycin, viomycin, or kanamycin plus two oral drugs selected from pyrazinamide, ethionamide, or cycloserine may be used.

The results of chemotherapy in patients with *M. intracellulare-avium* infections are not as good as those in disease caused by *M. kansasii*. The *M. intracellulare-avium* complex is characterized by primary drug resistance to all of the available antituberculosis drugs and to higher concentrations of these agents than are readily attainable in the body at the usual dosages. For this reason, only 20 to 30 per cent of patients with *M. intracellulare* infections respond to the conventional drug regimens used in the treatment of tuberculosis. If untreated, the pulmonary or disseminated form of this infection is fatal; therefore, every effort should be made to treat these cases effectively and in specialized facilities.

Although it is not ideal, the most effective treatment for *M. intracellulare* infections consists of a six-drug regimen—one given parenterally, selected from among streptomycin, capreomycin, viomycin, or kanamycin, and five oral agents, chosen from among isoniazid, rifampin, ethambutol, pyrazinamide, ethionamide, cycloserine, or para-aminosalicylic acid. Such a regimen obviously requires expert and intensive monitoring for side effects and adverse reactions and should be used only in patients with life-threatening disease who have no other therapeutic options. Every effort should be made to continue the six-drug regimen until satisfactory clinical response and negative culture status have been obtained. Thereafter, the parenteral drug can be stopped, and every effort is made to continue the five-drug oral program for a total of 24 months. Such a regimen will succeed in approximately 80 per cent of cases, except in elderly or debilitated patients, who respond less well. It should not be used casually or without careful evaluation

Table 3. ORAL ANTITUBERCULOSIS DRUGS

	Normal Adult Daily Dose	Duration of Administration	Toxicity
Isoniazid	300 mg	18–24 months	Neuropathy, hepatic signs
Ethambutol	15 mg/kg body weight	18–24 months	Optic signs
Rifampin	600 mg	18–24 months	Hepatic signs
Pyrazinamide	2–3 gm	18–24 months	Hepatic signs, hyperuricemia
Ethionamide	1.0 gm	18–24 months	Gastrointestinal discomfort, depression, hypothyroidism
Cycloserine	1.0 gm	18–24 months	Depression, convulsions, psychosis
Para-aminosalicylic acid	12 gm	18–24 months	Hepatic signs, cutaneous reactions
Thiacetazone	150 mg	18–24 months	Hepatic signs

of each patient. The recent use of ansamycin and clofazamine for *M. intracellulare-avium* infections in AIDS suggests that these two drugs have greater potency against these mycobacteria and may change the outlook.

Usually pulmonary disease caused by *M. intracellulare-avium* complex is not recognized until it has become extensive and multifocal. In such cases surgical treatment is not practical. However, occasional patients will be encountered in whom the disease is circumscribed and limited to one lobe or one lung. Pulmonary resection can be curative in such cases even when sputa are positive at the time of surgery. Thus, although such patients are uncommon, they should be identified early in the course of their disease and should undergo resection at the earliest opportunity after chemotherapy has been initiated.

Experience is lacking in the treatment of disease caused by nontuberculous mycobacteria other than *M. kansasii* and *M. intracellulare-avium* complex. Therefore, although it is impossible to recommend specific regimens for these other infections, certain general principles can be stated. Skin ulcers may heal spontaneously; if they do not, they may require block excision and skin grafting. If lymph node involvement is progressive or disfiguring, it is best treated by excision by a surgeon experienced in dissecting an extensive process involving the deep structures of the neck or axilla. Although a palpable node is the only clinical sign of infection, the adjacent area may be deeply infiltrated by underlying disease.

References

Barksdale, L., and Kim, K.: Mycobacterium. Bact Rev 41:217, 1977.

Chapman, J. S.: The Atypical Mycobacteria and Human Mycobacteriosis. New York, Plenum Medical Book Company, 1977.

Good, R., and Snider, D.: Isolation of nontuberculous Mycobacteria in the United States, 1980. J Infect Dis 146:829, 1982.

Greene, J., Sidhu, G., Levin, S., et al.: *Mycobacterium avium-intracellulare*: A cause of disseminating life-threatening infection in homosexuals and drug abusers. Ann Intern Med 97:539, 1982.

Lester, W.: Unclassified mycobacterial diseases. Ann Rev Microbiol 17:351, 1966.

Lincoln, E. M., and Gilbert, L. A.: Disease in children due to mycobacteria other than *Mycobacterium tuberculosis*. Am Rev Respir Dis 105:683, 1972.

Runyon, E. H.: Anonymous mycobacteria in pulmonary disease. Med Clin North Am 43:273, 1959.

Wallace, R., Swenson, J., Silcox, V., Good, R., Tschen, J., and Stone, M.: Spectrum of disease due to rapidly growing Mycobacteria. Rev Infect Dis 5:657, 1983.

Zakowski, P., Gligel, S., Berlin, G., and Johnson, B. L.: Disseminated *Mycobacterium avium-intracellulare* infection in homosexual men dying of acquired immundeficiency. JAMA 248:2980, 1982.

122

PULMONARY CRYPTOCOCCOSIS

GERALD MEDOFF, M.D.

Pulmonary cryptococcal infection has been known for many years, but its true incidence, clinical manifestations, and course have come to light very slowly. It was not until 1968 (Tynes et al., 1968; Warr et al., 1968) that it was shown that the organism could be cultured from sputum frequently and that a saprophytic form of cryptococcosis that was distinct from the invasive form of the disease could exist.

ETIOLOGY. Pulmonary cryptococcal infection is caused by the single species *Cryptococcus neoformans*. It is an encapsulated yeast-like fungus, pathogenic for animals and man. Four serotypes, A, B, C, and D, have been described. Serotypes A and D appear to be most frequently associated with human disease. The organism is ubiquitous and is commonly found in nature.

PATHOGENESIS AND PATHOLOGY. The presence of *C. neoformans* in bird dung is well documented, but this association is best known in regard to pigeon droppings. Concentrations of fungi as high as 5×10^7/g of feces have been found in some samples. In most cases of cryptococcal infection the source cannot be discerned. The presence of the fungus in bird droppings and the great numbers of birds found in the environment suggest this route of transmission. However, direct epidemiologic evidence for this is lacking. Man-to-man transmission or direct animal transmission to man has not been documented.

Cryptococcal infection comes to medical attention most frequently as a central nervous system disease (see Chapter 167), but in almost all human infections the fungus enters the body through the respiratory tract by inhalation of infectious particles. Until recently, it was not clear how a heavily encapsulated yeast 3 to 10 μ in diameter could be aerosolized and reach the alveolar spaces in the lung. However, in laboratory studies yeasts with decreased capsules and 0.5 to 2 μ in diameter have been described; these small forms can colonize the alveoli and thereby initiate the disease. More recently, a description of the perfect states of the organism *Filobasidiella neoformans* (Kwon-chung, 1975) has implicated inhalation of the small, light basidiospores as another mode of contracting the infection.

Phagocytosis is important in the killing of *C. neoformans*, and both the classic and alternative complement pathways are required for optimal ingestion of the fungi (Diamond et al., 1974). It also seems that nonphagocytic mononuclear cells can kill *C. neoformans*, but only if anticryptococcal antibody is present (Diamond, 1974). In most cases the normal host response can deal with the infection, and only a small granulomatous cryptococcoma and perhaps minimal granulomatous cryptococcal lymphadenitis occur. However, in a few cases the infection produces diffuse cryptococcal pneumonia and lymphadenitis. Unlike other forms of cryptococcal infection, pneumonia occurs commonly in patients without apparent immune deficiency, although most patients with pulmonary cryptococcal infection appear to have underlying pulmonary disease of various types.

In routine hematoxylin and eosin stains, the organism is poorly demarcated. In tissue sections stained by the periodic acid-Schiff or Gomori methenamine silver method, round to oval budding cells are easily seen. The capsular polysaccharide stains a brilliant pink with Mayer's muci-

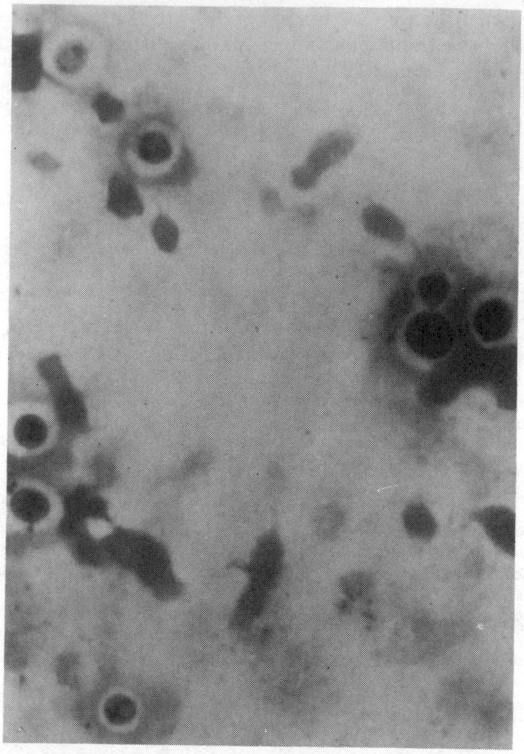

Figure 1. Cryptococci in bronchial brushings from patient with lingular cryptococcosis. Note budding and encapsulation. The yeast cells are gram positive (Gram stain ×500).

carmine stain, which differentiates this organism from other yeasts that do not possess a capsule. The yeast cell also takes the gram stain (Fig. 1).

CLINICAL MANIFESTATIONS. The cryptococcus seems to be considerably more prevalent in human sputum than is generally appreciated, but most of these infected people have no cryptococcal disease; hence, colonization with *C. neoformans* is probably the most common form of infection (Hammerman et al., 1973). Despite this, isolation of *C. neoformans* from respiratory secretions is rare enough to be taken seriously and pursued until localized or disseminated cryptococcosis is excluded.

Pulmonary cryptococcal infection presents no characteristic clinical picture. It appears to have a marked predilection for the white male and may start like influenza with cough and minimal pleuritic chest pain. Frequently patients have a history of prolonged respiratory infection with cough, low-grade fever, easy fatigability, and weight loss. An asymptomatic coin lesion on the chest radiograph may be the only manifestation of disease.

The cryptococcal lesions in the lungs may be solitary, multiple (Fig. 2), or disseminated, or may take the form of a tumor mass or diffuse pneumonitis. Cavities or mediastinal adenopathy are rare, but pleural effusion is not uncommon. The typical clinical course of pulmonary cryptococcal infection has not been well defined, but from a review of the accumulated experience of patients with cryptococcal pneumonia, it appears that most patients will recover without treatment. Cellular reactions may not occur, and large discrete cryptococcal masses may give the impression of a myxoma.

COMPLICATIONS AND SEQUELAE. Complications and sequelae of cryptococcal pulmonary infections are unusual. Pneumonia or diffuse pulmonary infection may be fatal or may damage the lung with permanent impairment of pulmonary function. Local lesions (a coin lesion or a mass) may require a thoracotomy to rule out a neoplasm. In a few patients pulmonary infection may disseminate to the central nervous system especially, but rarely to the bone, skin, eye, adrenals, spleen, or kidney.

GEOGRAPHIC VARIATIONS IN DISEASE. Cryptococcal infection in general occurs sporadically in all parts of the world without any significant geographic variation. Evidence from skin test surveys suggests that it probably has a higher incidence in people who have a significant exposure to birds. However, standardized skin test reagents are not available, and epidemiologic studies are limited in this regard.

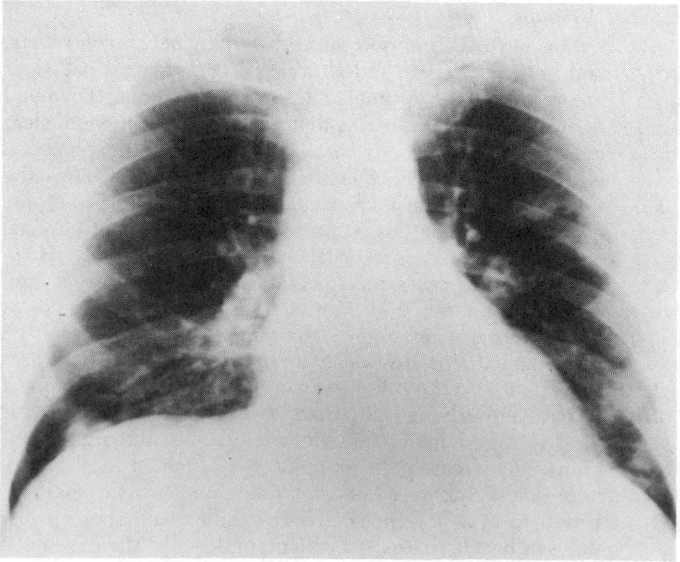

Figure 2. Cryptococcal infection of lung. There are multiple nodular lesions in both lungs.

There are four serotypes of *C. neoformans* labeled A through D. In a recent epidemiologic study, the most prevalent serotype isolated from the environment and from cases of clinical infection was serotype A. Serotypes B and C were infrequent causes of infection except in southern California. Interestingly, these serotypes were not isolated at all from environmental sources, indicating that the site or sites in nature where serotypes B and C exist are currently unknown and differ from those of serotypes A and D. Serotype D may be unusually prevalent both in the environment and in patients from Denmark and Italy (Bennett et al., 1977).

DIAGNOSIS. The presence of *C. neoformans* in the sputum or bronchial washings (Fig. 1) in the presence of an active pulmonary process is strong evidence of disease. The detection of cryptococcal polysaccharide antigen in the blood of patients with suspected infection is also a strong indication of active disease. It is important to note that patients with a positive rheumatoid factor may have a falsely positive result when blood is examined for cryptococcal antigen and appropriate controls should be included for correct interpretation. Unfortunately, one may have to resort to lung biopsy to make a definitive diagnosis. Diagnosis can be made by finding cryptococci in sections and upon culture. The mucicarmine stain helps identify the characteristic capsular substance in biopsy sections.

TREATMENT AND PROPHYLAXIS. The indications for treatment of pulmonary cryptococcal infection have not been defined. Recent evidence suggests that patients with underlying disease that results in significant immunosuppressions should be treated (Kerkerring et al., 1981). Most patients with normal immune response with cryptococcal pneumonia apparently recover without treatment, and dissemination to the CNS is quite rare. Total excision of localized lesions that are usually removed to rule out a tumor in an otherwise normal individual is probably sufficient and no additional medical therapy is required. The following management of patients whose sputum or lungs contain cryptococci is recommended by Hammerman et al., (1973) and appears reasonable:

1. Close observation for one to two months. If there is evidence of progression or if there is failure of the chest lesion to resolve, treatment should be instituted.
2. Evidence of dissemination from the lungs justifies a full course of therapy.

As with CNS infection, amphotericin B at a dosage of 0.3 to 1.0 mg/kg/day for six to ten weeks is recommended. A good index of response is the serum antigen, which should be negative when therapy is stopped. Some investigators use 5-fluorocytosine 150 mg/kg/day alone or added to the amphotericin B (see Chapter 154 for a further discussion of the combined regimen).

No prophylaxis is necessary for this disease except avoidance of unnecessary exposure to bird droppings.

References

Bennett, J. E., Kwon-Chung, K. J., and Howard, D. H.: Epidemiologic differences among serotypes of *Cryptococcus neoformans*. Am J Epidemiol 105:582, 1977.

Diamond, R. D.: Antibody-dependent killing of *Cryptococcus neoformans* by human peripheral blood mononuclear cells. Nature 247:148, 1974.

Diamond, R. D., May, J. E., Kane, M. A., Frank, M. M., and Bennett, J. E.: The role of the classical and alternate complement pathways in host defenses against *Cryptococcus neoformans* infection. J Immunol 112:2260, 1974.

Griffin, F. M.: Roles of macrophages Fe and C_3B receptors in phagocytosis of immunologically costed *cryptococcus neoformans*. Proc Natl Acad Sci 78:3853, 1981.

Hammerman, K. J., Powell, K. E., Christianson, C. S., Huggin, P. M., Larsh, H. W., Vivas, J. R., and Tosh, F. E.: Pulmonary cryptococcosis: Clinical forms and treatment. A Center for Disease Control mycoses study. Am Rev Resp Dis 108:1116, 1973.

Kerkerring, T. M., Duma, R. J., and Shadomy, S.: The evolution of pulmonary cryptococcus clinical implications from a study of 41 patients with and without compromising host factors. Ann Intern Med 94:611, 1981.

Kwon-Chung, K. J.: Description of a new genus *Filobasidiella*, the perfect state of *Cryptococcus neoformans*. Mycologia 67:1197, 1975.

Tynes, B., Mason, K. N., Jennings, A. E., and Bennett, J. E.: Variant forms of pulmonary cryptococcosis. Ann Intern Med 69:1117, 1968.

Warr, W., Bates, J. H., and Stone, A.: The spectrum of pulmonary cryptococcosis. Ann Intern Med 69:1109, 1968.

123

NORTH AMERICAN BLASTOMYCOSIS

ABRAHAM I. BRAUDE, M.D., PH.D.

Blastomycosis is a fungus infection of the skin, lungs, and other viscera caused by *Blastomyces dermatitidis*. It occurs primarily in North America. A similar disease is caused by *Paracoccidioides brasiliensis* in South America. Paracoccidioidomycosis is described in Chapter 124.

ETIOLOGY. In infected tissues, *B. dermatitidis* has the appearance of a yeast, forming single buds from 3 to 24 μ in diameter. Two features aid in recognition: (1) its thick wall, spoken of as "double-contoured," because the inner and outer margins can be seen; and (2) the wide opening between parent cell and bud at the base of attachment.

In culture, *B. dermatitidis* is dimorphic and appears as a wrinkled, waxy yeast form on blood agar incubated at 37° C or as a mold with branching hyphae on Sabouraud's agar at room temperature. On microscopic examination, the cultured yeast may be identical with that in the infected lesions or may have abortive mycelia. The mycelia give rise to oval or pear-shaped spores.

PATHOGENESIS AND PATHOLOGY. Although *B. dermatitidis* has seldom been cultured from the soil and soon disappears after inoculation into natural soil, soil is the most likely source of the fungus. Most infections occur in people who are in close contact with soil, especially in the Mississippi and Ohio River Valleys. Bird droppings must also be considered as a possible source of human infection because *B. dermatitidis* has been recovered from pigeon manure. A strong association between canine and human blastomycosis has been observed, but it is unlikely that the infection was transmitted from dogs to man; rather, both were probably exposed together to the same source in nature (Sarosi et al., 1979).

The lung is the major portal of entry for blastomycosis. Because of strong natural resistance to *B. dermatitidis*, most persons develop subclinical pulmonary infections recognizable only by skin tests. Heavy infection in healthy persons can cause multiple benign pulmonary lesions that heal spontaneously. Primary lesions may give rise to progressive disease, with or without a variable latent interval. The pulmonary lesion may enlarge and spread to other parts of the lung before dissemination to skin and bones; or systemic dissemination may occur from a small stationary pulmonary focus, sometimes after reactivation from a dormant stage. In patients with leukemia or other forms of depressed immunity, the infection can cause fulminant pulmonary dissemination (Onal et al., 1976).

The basic lesion in blastomycosis is the suppurative granuloma with Langhans and foreign-body giant cells. In the skin and mucous membranes, this combination of abscesses and epithelioid cell granulomas occurs in the midst of pseudoepitheliomatous hyperplasia. Characteristic cells of *B. dermatitidis*, with its single broad-based bud, can be seen in these lesions.

CLINICAL MANIFESTATIONS. The rare acute pulmonary form of North American blastomycosis varies from asymptomatic infection to a severe illness resembling acute histoplasmosis. Two clinical types of acute infection have been recognized. The first consists of fever, productive cough, and joint and muscle pains, with multiple nodular pulmonary densities in roentgenograms and budding yeast in the sputum. In the second type, pleuritic chest pain of variable severity and lasting only a few hours is the distinctive feature, but chest x-rays reveal no pleural effusions despite multiple pulmonary nodules. Both forms are benign, and the patient recovers without specific treatment.

In the typical case of progressive North American blastomycosis, the onset is insidious. The patient may seek medical attention because of a persistent "chest cold," low-grade fever, weight loss, or progressive disability. Physical examination and a roentgenogram of the chest disclose evidence of pneumonia, which may involve any segment or lobe of the lung. Cavitation is frequent, and mediastinal lymph nodes may be prominent. Hemoptysis, purulent sputum, chest pain, and dyspnea appear as the disease progresses. Although the pulmonary infection may subside spontaneously, extrapulmonary lesions of the skin, bones, joints, and viscera eventually call attention to dissemination. These metastatic suppurative lesions are accompanied by an increase in fever, sweats, chills, and weakness. Death in the untreated infection sometimes occurs in less than 6 months, but most patients live for 1 or 2 years. The overall mortality rate in systemic blastomycosis is said to be 92 per cent in patients whose cases have been followed for 2 years or longer without specific therapy.

COMPLICATIONS. Metastatic infections of the skin, bone, and genitourinary tract are the chief complications of pulmonary blastomycosis. The adrenal may also be infected.

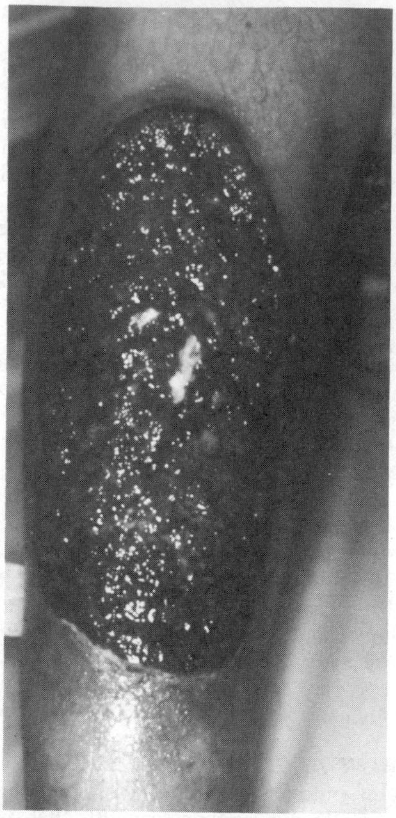

Figure 1. Blastomycosis of leg acquired in Arkansas by an engineer working for the telephone company in the Arkansas wilderness. The lesion healed completely with 30 mg amphotericin B daily.

Infection of the skin by *B. dermatitidis* is the most common form of extrapulmonary disease, occurring in as many as 80 per cent of patients with blastomycosis. It first appears on unclothed areas such as the hands, face, forearm, or lower leg (Fig. 1), but not the scalp, palms, or soles. The infection begins as a firm nodule surrounded by similar lesions that tend to coalesce. Suppuration in the center of the nodule is followed by partial healing and fibrosis as extension occurs peripherally. The hyperplastic epithelium gives these lesions a hard, raised, wartlike margin. When fully developed, blastomycosis of the skin presents the appearance of one or more ragged ulcers with partially healed centers and thick, raised margins.

Because blastomycosis of the skin is often the first clinical sign of the disease, it was previously thought to result from direct inoculation of the fungus into the site of the lesion. According to present concepts, direct inoculation is an extremely rare cause of cutaneous blastomycosis and produces an entirely different lesion than that seen in hematogenous infection of the skin. The primary cutaneous lesion resembles a chancre with its indurated ulcer and regional adenopathy (Wilson et al., 1955). It tends to appear on the fingers and remain there until it heals. It does not disseminate.

Osteomyelitis is the next most common hematogenous complication of pulmonary blastomycosis. As many as half the patients with blastomycosis have osteolytic skeletal lesions, sometimes as the only sign of the disease. Almost

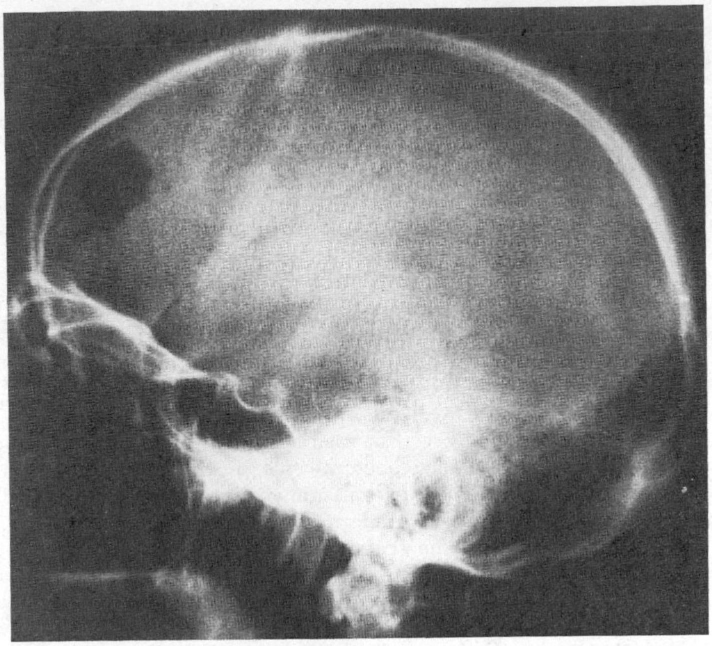

Figure 2. Osteomyelitis of the skull due to *Blastomyces dermatiditis.* Osteolytic lesion with irregular margins of the frontal bone is secondary to dissemination from the lungs. (From Bell, W., and McCormick, W.: Neurologic Infections in Children. Philadelphia, W. B. Saunders Company, 1975, p. 334.)

any bone may show hematogenous infection, but the vertebrae and ribs do so most frequently. Blastomycosis of the vertebrae may be indistinguishable from tuberculosis of the spine. In both diseases, the infection begins in the vertebral body, destroys the disk, and produces paraspinal or epidural abscesses that cause paraplegia by compressing the spinal cord (Greenwood and Voris, 1950). The brain may also suffer compression from intracranial extradural abscesses secondary to osteomyelitis of the skull (Fig. 2).

Direct hematogenous spread to the brain is less common than to bone. Primary blastomycosis of the nervous system may take the form of meningitis, single or multiple brain abscesses, and brain or cord granuloma (Fig. 3) (Fetter et al., 1967). In blastomycotic meningitis, there is headache, vomiting, confusion, and a stiff neck. The cerebrospinal fluid shows pleocytosis with either lymphocytes or neutrophils predominating, an elevation of the protein to 300 mg/ml or more, and a reduction in glucose. The meningitis causes a fibrinopurulent exudate that may spread diffusely through the subarachnoid space or become localized at the base of the brain, so that an obstructive hydrocephalus develops.

The third most common hematogenous complication is blastomycosis of the prostate, epididymis, and testis. The kidney and female genitalia, on the other hand, are rarely affected.

GEOGRAPHIC DISTRIBUTION. Most cases of blastomycosis have been reported from the Mississippi and Ohio River Valleys and the Southeastern United States. Outbreaks have occurred in connection with a peanut harvest in Enfield, North Carolina, canoeing in Hayward, Wisconsin, and a small cabin in the woods at Big Fork, Minnesota (Brewer et al., 1979; Furcolow et al., 1976; Tosh et al., 1974). The infection also occurs in Canada, Mexico, Central America, South America, and Africa. African cases were found in Zaire, Uganda, Tanzania, Gambia, Zambia, Rhodesia, Tunisia, Morocco, and South Africa (Bregant et al., 1973). The identity of the strains isolated from American and African cases of blastomycosis has not been established.

DIAGNOSIS. Pulmonary blastomycosis closely resembles tuberculosis, carcinoma of the lung, aspiration pneumonitis, actinomycosis, nocardiosis, and other fungus infections, including coccidioidomycosis, and histoplasmosis. Differentiation must be based on the recovery of the etiologic agent, because neither clinical nor epidemiologic features are specific.

It is usually possible to find *B. dermatitidis* by microscopic examination of biopsied material, sputum, or pus. The yeastlike forms can be observed if a drop of purulent material is first mixed on a slide with a drop of 10 per cent

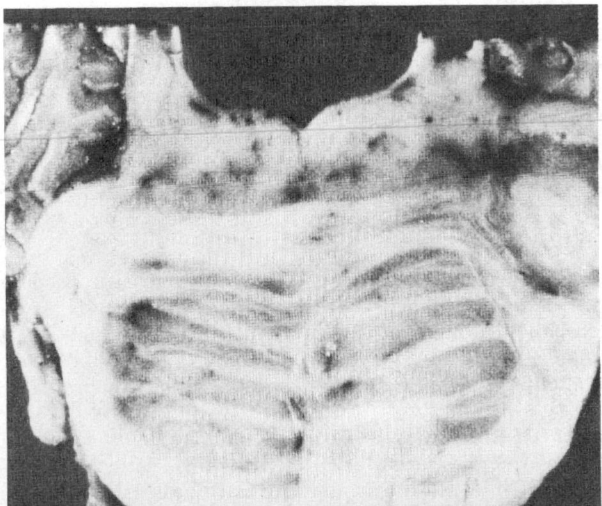

Figure 3. Blastomycosis of the brain. A solitary solid granuloma of the pons is located at the level of the trigeminal nerves. (From Bell, W., and McCormick, W.: Neurologic Infections in Children. Philadelphia, W. B. Saunders Company, 1975, p. 335.)

potassium hydroxide and kept at room temperature for 30 minutes. Buds of *B. dermatitidis* are connected to the parent cell by a wide communication. *Blastomyces dermatitidis* is isolated by culturing pus on Sabouraud's agar at room temperature and on blood agar at 37° C. *B. dermatitidis* can be identified rapidly in exudates by use of fluorescent antibody prepared in rabbits against the yeast form (Kaufman, 1980).

The diagnostic value of the skin test for blastomycosis is limited. The complement-fixation test in North American blastomycosis is positive in high titer with serums of patients who have systemic infections but has limited diagnostic value, because the antigens are neither specific nor sensitive (Kaufman, 1976). The immunodiffusion test, on the other hand, is specific and has a sensitivity of 80 per cent. Negative tests with either method do not exclude a diagnosis of blastomycosis (Kaufman et al., 1973); in fact, negative serologic tests have been the rule in certain acute outbreaks of non-disseminated blastomycosis (Brewer et al., 1979). The results of intradermal and serologic tests may be of prognostic value. Patients with marked dermal hypersensitivity and low serum titers of complement-fixing antibody are said to have a better prognosis in North American blastomycosis than those with negative skin tests and high complement-fixation titers.

TREATMENT. Amphotericin B can cure blastomycosis. Blastomycosis also responds but less favorably to 2-hydroxystilbamidine. Either drug is given daily or every other day by slow intravenous drip in increasing doses. The maximum adult daily dose of amphotericin B is 40 mg, and that of 2-hydroxystilbamidine is 250 mg. Blastomycosis should be treated with a total of 1.5 g amphotericin B; 7 to 8 g of 2-hydroxystilbamidine may be required. Anesthesia over the distribution of the trigeminal nerve is the main untoward reaction from 2-hydroxystilbamidine; it persists after treatment. Surgical excision of pulmonary cavities or destroyed tissues is sometimes necessary in addition to chemotherapy.

References

Bregant, S., Gigase, P., Bastin, J. P., and VanDePitte, J.: La blastomycose Norde-Américaine en République du Zaïre. Bul Soc Path Exot 66:77, 1973.

Brewer, N., Rhodes, R., Roberts, G., Rosenblatt, J., Van Scoy, R., Utz, J., and Davis, J.: Blastomycosis in canoeists in Wisconsin. Morbidity and Mortality Weekly Report 28:450, 1979.

Fetter, B., Klintworth, G., and Wilson, S.: Mycoses of the central nervous system. Baltimore, Williams & Wilkins Company, 1967.

Furcolow, M., Smith, C., Gallis, H., Hoag, L., Bradham, F., Freeman, J., Hines, M., and MacCormack, J.: Blastomycosis—North Carolina. Morbidity and Mortality Weekly Report 25:205, 1976.

Greenwood, R. C., and Voris, H. C.: Systemic blastomycosis with spinal cord involvement. J Neurosurg 7:450, 1950.

Kaufman, L.: Serodiagnosis of fungal diseases. In Rose, N., and Friedman, H. (eds): Manual of Clinical Immunology. Washington, D.C., Am. Soc. Microbiol., 1980, pp. 556 and 569.

Kaufman, L., McLaughlin, D., Clark, M., and Blumer, S.: Specific immunodiffusion test for blastomycosis. Appl Microbiol 26:244, 1973.

Onal, E., Lopata, M., and Lourenco, R.: Disseminated pulmonary blastomycosis in an immunosuppressed patient. Am Rev Resp Dis 113:83, 1976.

Sarosi, G., Echman, M., Davies, S., and Laskey, W.: Canine blastomycosis as a harbinger of human disease. Ann Int Med 91:733, 1979.

Tosh, F., Hammerman, K., Weekes, R., and Sarosi, G.: A common source of epidemic of North American blastomycosis. Am Rev Resp Dis 109:525, 1974.

Wilson, J., Cawley, E., Weidman, F., and Gilmer, W.: Primary cutaneous North American blastomycosis. AMA Arch Dermat Syph 71:39. 1955.

124

PARACOCCIDIOIDOMYCOSIS (SOUTH AMERICAN BLASTOMYCOSIS)

ALBERTO THOMAZ LONDERO, M.D.

Paracoccidioidomycosis is a systemic mycosis caused by the dimorphic fungus *Paracoccidioides brasiliensis*. Paracoccidioidal infection may be benign and self-limited or it may progress to involve virtually any organ. As a result, the clinical manifestations of the disease may be protean.

EPIDEMIOLOGY. Paracoccidioidomycosis is found in Latin America from Mexico to Argentina, with the exception of Chile, Nicaragua, and the Caribbean Islands. Cases reported in countries outside Latin America have involved patients who lived for some time in the endemic areas.

The infection primarily affects rural inhabitants and is acquired mostly between the ages of 15 and 19 years. Both sexes are infected at the same rate. Fifty-two per cent of cases of the progressive form of the disease are seen in patients between 30 and 50 years of age, with a male/female ratio of 14.7 to 1. The disease is rare in children. All races are susceptible, although European and Asian immigrants present very severe clinical pictures.

PATHOGENESIS AND PATHOLOGY. Like other agents of systemic mycoses, *P. brasiliensis* enters the human body by inhalation and causes a primary lymph node complex in the lung (Severo et al., 1979). Hematogenous dissemination to other organs can occur simultaneously. These disseminated lesions usually heal or become latent if immunity is normal. Rarely, the primary lesion progresses, disseminates, and causes very severe disease. This is presumed to occur in patients under 20 years of age (Restrepo, 1978).

The latent primary lesions may be reactivated many years later and thus occur in patients seen in nonendemic countries (Balabanov et al., 1964; Murray et al., 1974). The reactivation may be brought on by a deficiency in cell-mediated immunity and may occur either spontaneously without apparent cause or secondary to immunosuppressive disease and/or therapy (Londero and Severo, 1981). The reactivation of a latent lesion in the lung may cause a progressive pulmonary infection that sometimes disseminates hematogenously to other organs.

Mucocutaneous ulcers are the most common disseminated manifestation. These ulcers are secondary to inflammation of the underlying skeletal muscles. (Mackinnon, 1961). When *P. brasiliensis* is inoculated into the skin, a chancriform or sporotrichoid lesion is produced (Castro et al., 1975).

The gross pathology is similar to that of other systemic mycoses or tuberculosis. The most common reaction to *P. brasiliensis* is granulomatous. When there is no secondary infection, the granulomas are composed of epithelial cells and Langhans' foreign-body giant cells. Necrosis can occur in the center of the nodule. When the epithelioid nodule is not necrotic, it resembles a sarcoid. Regressing nodules become fibrotic or hyalinized. A mixed granulomatous and pyogenic reaction with microabscesses also occurs. Diffuse or extensive inflammation is rare.

Paracoccidioidal lesions contain areas of suppuration as well as macrophages, giant cells, caseation necrosis, and fibrosis. Only the presence of *P. brasiliensis* establishes the cause of the lesions, since the pathology resembles that of other mycoses.

CLINICAL MANIFESTATIONS. Clinical manifestations are so protean that the mycosis may simulate an enormous number of diseases. These manifestations may be grouped into four clinical forms: (1) primary pulmonary, (2) progressive pulmonary, (3) disseminated, and (4) acute juvenile.

Primary Pulmonary Form. The primary lesion in the lung is similar to Ghon's complex in tuberculosis. In the early stages, the disease is thought to be usually either asymptomatic or too mild to be differentiated from a slight bacterial or viral infection. The infection is not recognizable except for the immunologic response to *P. brasiliensis*, as shown by the skin test and precipitin test. However, the first case of primary pulmonary symptomatic disease was reported recently in a 9 year-old girl with a seven-month history of recurrent fever, cough, dyspnea, heavy sweats and weight loss. A chest x-ray on admission revealed alveolar consolidations in both lungs and enlargement of the hilum (Fig. 1). She was treated for tuberculosis, but six months later paracoccidioidomycosis was identified by lung biopsy. Parenchymal lesions had improved then but hilar lymphadenopathy persisted. Primary lesions usually heal but rarely with calcification (Melo and Londero, 1983). A radiologic picture of these lesions has not yet been characterized. Sometimes they are nodular or coin lesions—paracoccidioidoma (Angulo-Ortega, 1975; Restrepo et al., 1976). Early hematogenous spread may occur to other organs, where asymptomatic lesions develop. The metastatic foci usually heal but are rarely calcified, so that they are seldom found. Some foci of infection may remain quiescent (latent) in the lung and perhaps in other organs as well. Their reactivation would explain progressive cases diagnosed outside endemic areas.

Progressive Pulmonary Form. Approximately 30 per cent of patients manifest this form of the disease. The progressive pulmonary form results from a reactivation of a quiescent lesion or, rarely, the progression of a primary focus (Londero et al., 1978). Early progressive lung lesions may be asymptomatic. More rarely, patients present nonspecific respiratory symptoms. A small nodule or one or more small apical infiltrates are seen in radiographs (Fig. 2). After months or years, the lesions may spread throughout the lungs, and then symptoms appear. Patients present a history of a subacute or chronic (rarely acute) respiratory infection with a prolonged or recurrent course. A cough is always present that produces mucoid or mucopurulent sputum, later becoming bloody. Dyspnea and, less frequently, fever, thoracic pain, and weight loss follow. Physical signs vary according to the extent and localization of the lung lesions, but they are not specific. In the early stage of the disease radiographs are often not characteristic of paracoccidioidomycosis (Fig. 3), but in advanced stages they show suggestive bilateral, symmetric and polymorphic lesions (Londero and Severo, 1981). Patients with localized lesions have been observed for as long as 15 years without dissemination (Fig. 4). On the other hand, it has been reported that 7.6 per cent of these patients develop disseminated lesions (usually oral) within a short time.

Disseminated Form. About 65 to 70 per cent of patients undergo dissemination. Most have pulmonary lesions as well as disease elsewhere. The lung lesions may be overlooked because respiratory symptoms and physical signs are scarce, although radiologic lesions are extensive. More rarely, lesions are not evident on the chest radiograph.

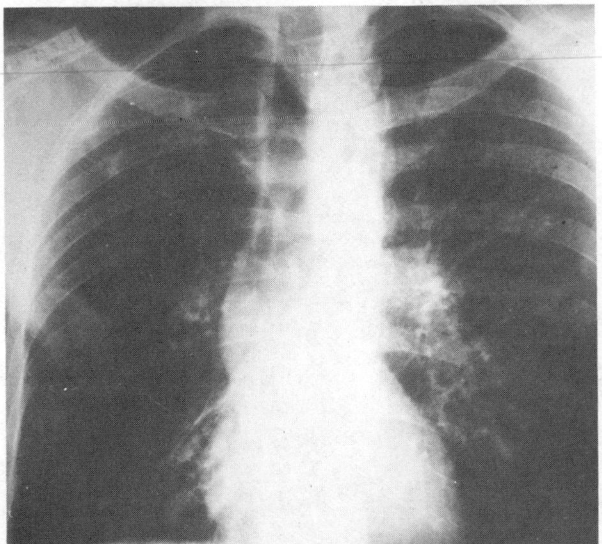

Figure 1. Chest radiograph showing primary pulmonary paracoccidioidal lesions in a child.

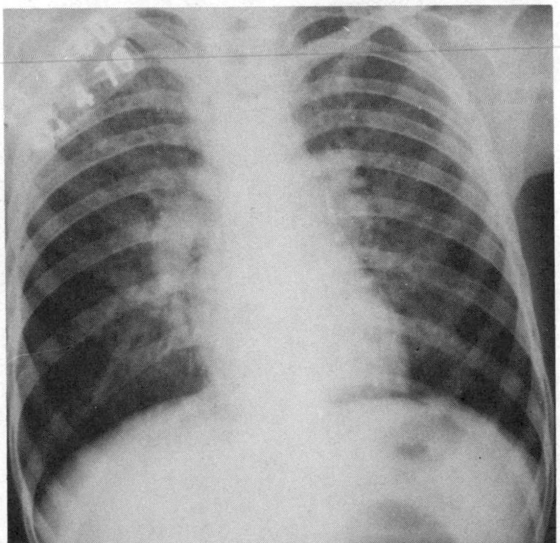

Figure 2. Chest radiograph showing small infiltrations in the right upper lobe—initial lesions of the pulmonary progressive form.

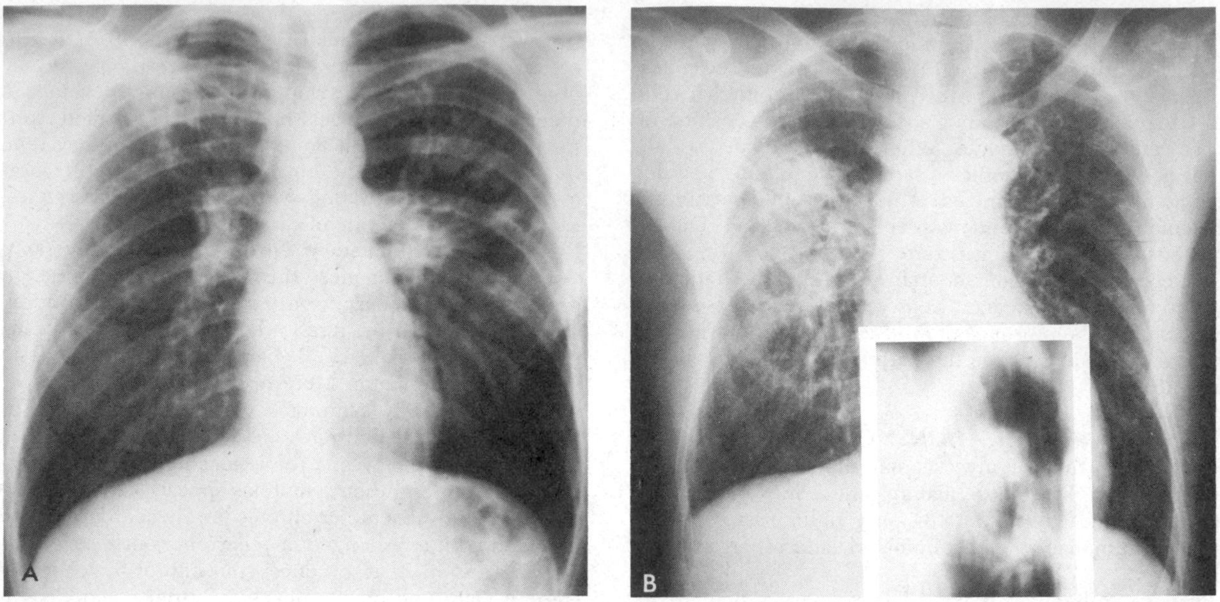

Figure 3. Chest radiographs showing consolidations and necrotic cavities simulating *(A)* tuberculosis and *(B)* bacterial abscess (*inset:* tomogram).

When there are no mucocutaneous manifestations, the pulmonary lesions may be misdiagnosed as tuberculosis. Extrapulmonary lesions in disseminated paracoccidioidomycosis are found most frequently in the mucous membranes, lymph nodes, skin, spleen, adrenal glands, intestine, and liver, and less frequently in the arteries, bones, brain, meninges, genitals, heart, kidney, and endocrine glands. The clinical presentation of the disseminated form is variable, depending on the site or sites and extent of involvement (Restrepo et al., 1976). The lesions may be generalized (affecting many organs or systems) or they may be confined to one organ.

Mucocutaneous and lymphatic lesions are the most frequent manifestations of hematogenous dissemination. They are the most obvious lesions and sometimes may be the presenting symptoms. Lesions are found most often on the mucosal surfaces of the lips, gums, palate, and tongue (Fig. 5) and may extend to the skin around the mouth. Sometimes the lesions originate in the pharynx or the larynx. They appear as ulcers with a granulomatous mulberry-like base. Painful ulcers are usually superficial and enlarge slowly at the periphery. In advanced cases they deepen and destroy the buccal structures. Sometimes a peculiar hard, deep infiltration of the lips may occur. Ulcerative

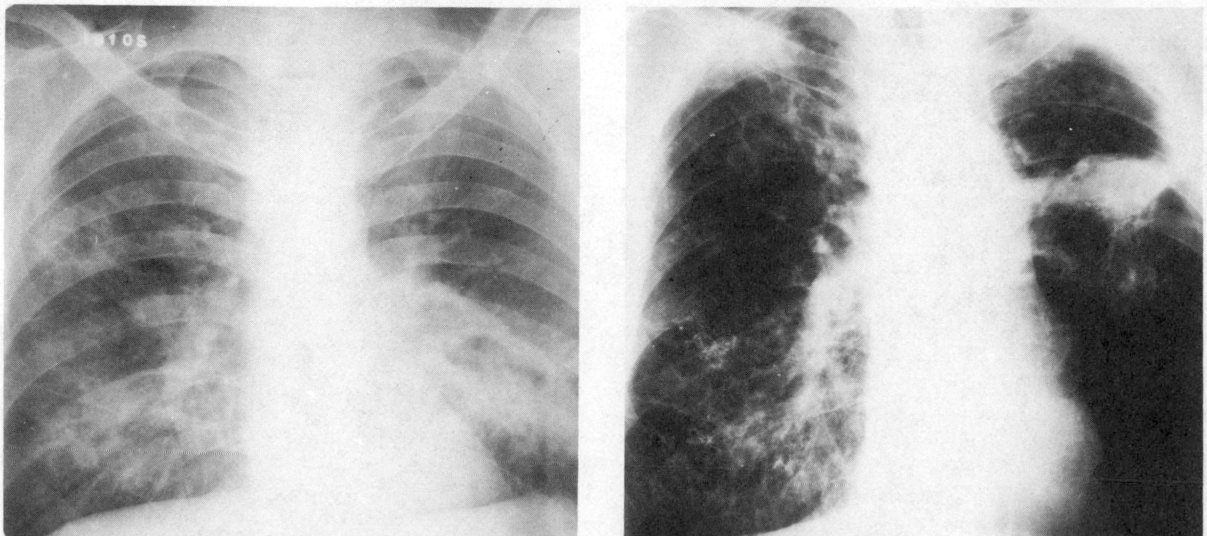

Figure 4. Chest roentgenograms of same patient in 1963 *(A)* and in 1978 *(B)*. On both occasions he was referred for mycologic examination. From 1963 through 1964, he was treated with sulfa drugs. From 1965 to 1978 the disease relapsed, and the patient presented with recurrent respiratory undifferentiated infections, which were treated as tuberculosis.

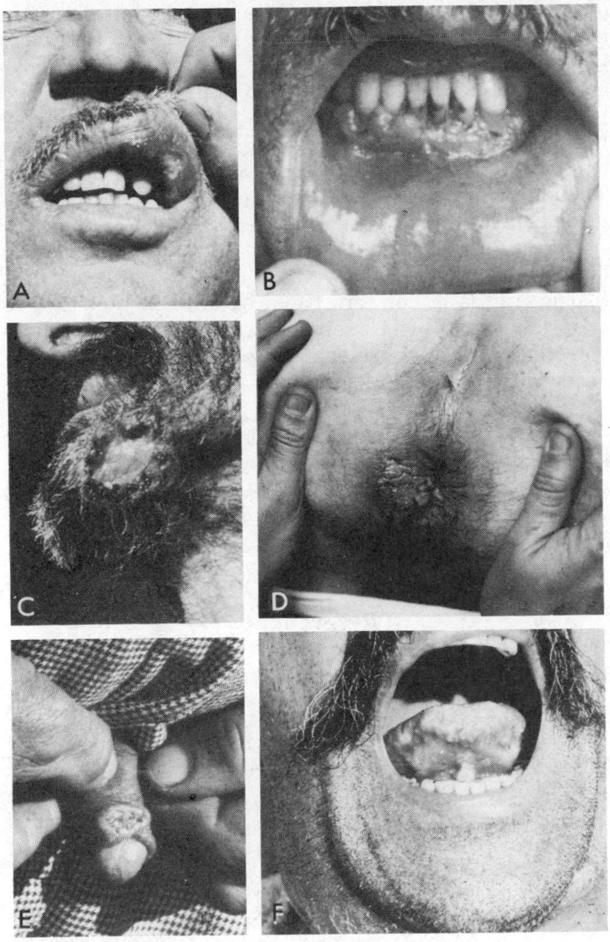

Figure 5. Mucocutaneous and lymphatic lesions: Ulcerations of the lips *(A)*, gums *(B)*, jaw *(C)*, and penis *(E)*. Granulomatous lesion of the perineum *(D)*. Lesion of the tongue and right submaxillary adenopathy *(F)*.

gingivitis may cause loss of teeth. Extensive disease of the oropharynx can interfere with eating, and destruction of the vocal cords may cause dysphonia or aphonia.

A great variety of skin lesions has been described. The crusting ulcer of the skin usually results from the extension of the buccal lesions at the mucocutaneous border of the lips. Solitary ulcerative or granulomatous lesions may occur in the anorectal region and elsewhere rarely (Fig. 5). Generalized polymorphic skin lesions are also rare.

Cervical lymph nodes are involved early and are discrete, firm, and hard. They may enlarge, become painful, suppurate, and drain. Massive cervical lymph nodes may be the only abnormality on physical examination.

When no mucocutaneous lesion or superficial lymph node involvement is present (in 5 to 20 per cent of patients with the disseminated form), the clinical picture of the mycosis may take many forms that vary according to the type of organ involved, the sequence of organ involvement, the severity of destruction, and the chronicity of the disease.

Visceral lymph node enlargement may cause intestinal obstruction or cholestatic jaundice. Intestinal paracoccidioidal lesions may produce symptoms of a mild enteritis, bowel tumor, or an acute abdomen. Lesions of the adrenal glands may be asymptomatic, but when they are severe, they may cause Addison's disease (Marsiglia and Pinto, 1966). Signs of brain tumor or leptomeningitis are the most common manifestation of central nervous system involvement (Raphael, 1966). Mild paracoccidiodal arteritis is very common, and aortitis or thrombotic occlusion of the mesenteric vessels may occur. All grades of hepatic and splenic involvement may develop. Paracoccidioidal osteomyelitis, epididymitis, and prostatitis have been reported. Cardiac, renal, and endocrine lesions (other than adrenal) are rare.

Acute Juvenile Form. In highly endemic areas this syndrome occurs in children and adolescents, probably soon after the primary lung infection. The disease runs an acute course.

The clinical picture of infantile paracoccidioidomycosis is very polymorphic. Almost all systems of the body are involved but symptoms may be more prominent in one or another system according to the age of the child. Under 9 years of age abdominal symptoms prevail with fever and weight loss. Abdominal pain, abdominal masses, diarrhea and vomitus are the usual complaints. Chest x-ray usually reveals hilar enlargement. At 10 to 12 years of age, signs of fungemia and osteoarticular manifestations, or generalized lymphadenopathy with signs of systemic involvement, are the most prominent features. Hilar enlargement is again common in these patients. In those 13 and 14 years of age generalized lymphadenopathy is the most conspicuous manifestation; hepatomegaly and splenomegaly, skin lesions and gastrointestinal involvement may occur also. The clinical picture of the infantile form may simulate that of acute abdominal conditions, osteomyelitis, rheumatic fever, tuberculosis, septicemia, leukemia or lymphoma (Londero and Melo, 1983).

COMPLICATIONS AND SEQUELAE. The most frequent sequelae result from therapeutic measures. Pulmonary fibrosis may cause "cor pulmonale." Aphonia and dysphonia may result from destructive lesions of the vocal cords. Tracheal or glottic stenosis and microstomy are complications of scar retraction.

GEOGRAPHIC VARIATIONS. Paracoccidioidomycosis is not uniformly distributed in Latin America. Climatic conditions help determine the extent of this disease throughout a geographic area.

Clinical manifestations of the mycosis present interesting geographic variations in Brazil. Cutaneous and lymphatic lesions are uncommon in the south but very frequent in the central and eastern parts of the country. Gastrointestinal manifestations of the disease are frequently reported in patients from the central Brazilian plateau, but they are very rare in the southern area. The reverse is true for the pulmonary lesions. The juvenile form of the disease and the osseous manifestations are almost entirely confined to patients in the states of Minas Gerais, Rio de Janeiro, and São Paulo.

DIAGNOSIS. The diagnosis must be based on the demonstration of *P. brasiliensis* in specimens taken from the lesions. The clinical diagnosis can only be suspected from suggestive mucocutaneous lesions. Paracoccidioidal lung lesions must be differentiated from tuberculosis, histoplasmosis, and nonspecific respiratory infections. The disseminated forms, especially when lesions are confined to a system or organ, present such variable manifestations that differential diagnosis is almost impossible. The juvenile form of the infection must be differentiated from septicemias and lymphomas.

Laboratory Diagnosis. Mycologic diagnosis is very sim-

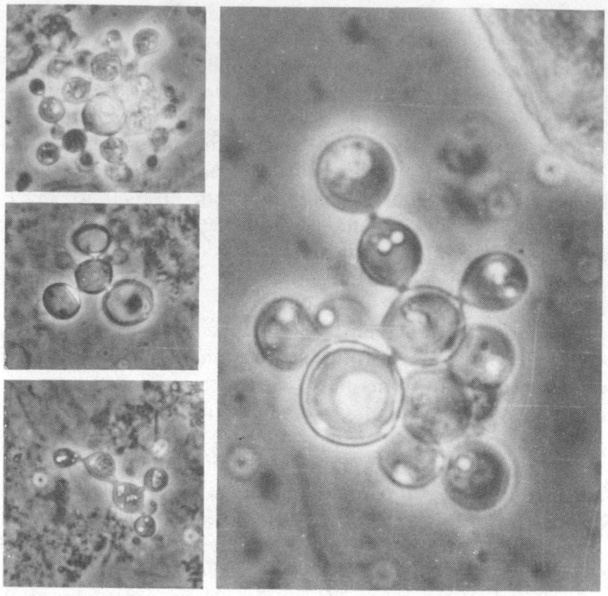

Figure 6. Multibudding forms of *P. brasiliensis* in sputum. ×250 and ×60

ple when there is easy access to such lesions as mucocutaneous ulcers, suppurating lymph nodes, and productive lung infection. Scrapings of mucocutaneous lesions, exudate, pus, sputum, bronchial washing, organic fluids, tissues taken for biopsy, and feces should be examined in a drop of 10 per cent potassium hydroxide. Before examination, organic fluids and sodium hydroxide-treated sputum can be centrifuged (Lopes, 1955). *P. brasiliensis* is a large, 10 to 40 μ, double-walled, round organism with multiple buds (Fig. 6).

Cultures. Pus, exudate, centrifuged body fluids, and tissues from biopsies should be incubated on Mycosel agar at both 25 and 35° C. Isolates of this fastidious fungus should be identified on the basis of the dimorphic forms seen at 25 and 35° C. Sputum and feces should be inoculated intratesticularly into guinea pigs, and the aspirated pus from the animal should then be cultured.

Serologic Diagnosis. Serologic tests are helpful in patients whose lesions are difficult to approach. The immunodiffusion test is the most useful because of its simplicity and specificity (Yarzabal et al., 1978; Restrepo, 1966). Immunoelectrophoresis and counterimmunoelectrophoresis give quicker results than immunodiffusion but are used in only a few laboratories. All these tests have high sensitivity and specificity when a good antigen is used. Recently, Restrepo and Moncada (1978) introduced the latex agglutination test. It can be used more widely, but its sensitivity is 70 per cent, and it gives cross-reactions with sera of patients with histoplasmosis. The complement fixation test is more useful for prognostic purposes.

TREATMENT. Three drugs are used in the treatment of paracoccidioidomycosis: sulfonamides, amphotericin B, and ketoconazole. Sulfonamides (sulfadiazine, sulfamethoxypiridazine, and sulfamethoxine) have been administered in the usual dosage for bacterial infections for months or even years. Presently they are recommended as a "supportive" therapy in cases of primary pulmonary regressive lesions, for 2 or 3 months. Amphotericin B has been used less often. It is given in a dose of 0.5 mg per kg intravenously every other day for a total dose of 1.5 to 2.0 g. However, ketoconazole is the first line drug for paracoccidioidomycosis. Treatment consists of one 200 mg tablet daily, two hours before a meal, for 6 to 12 months. This dosage may be increased to 400 mg a day in patients with severely disseminated disease. Ketoconazole may be used with amphotericin B in patients with central nervous system involvement.

The criteria of cure cannot be based on the clinical disappearance of lesions, because relapses can occur. Serologic criteria of cure are based on a fall in titer to zero or to low stable levels (serologic scar). It is important to note that clinical, radiologic, or serologic cure does not necessarily mean mycologic cure.

PROPHYLAXIS. Paracoccidioidomycosis is acquired by inhalation of the spores of *P. brasiliensis*, which lives in soil (Albornoz, 1971). Environmental conditions associated with its presence are still unknown; for this reason, prophylactic measures are unknown.

References

Albornoz, M. B.: Isolation of *Paracoccidioides brasiliensis* from rural soil in Venezuela. Sabouraudia 9:248, 1971.

Angulo-Ortega, A.: Lesiones numulares pulmonares de origen inflamatorio. Paracoccidioidomas. Torax (Caracas) 2:25, 1975.

Balabanov, K., Balabanoff, V. A., and Angelov, N.: Blastomycose sud-americaine chez un laboureur bulgare revenu depuis 30 ans de Brésil. Mycopathologia 24:265, 1964.

Castro, R. M., Cucé, L., and Fava-Netto, C.: Paracoccidioidomicose: Inoculação acidental in "anima nobili." Relato de um caso. Med Cutan Iber Lat Am 4:289, 1975.

Londero, A. T., and Melo, I. S.: Paracoccidioidomycosis in childhood. A critical review. Mycopathologia, 82:49, 1983.

Londero, A. T., Ramos, C. D., and Lopes, J. O.: Progressive pulmonary paracoccidioidomycosis. A study of 34 cases observed in Rio Grande do Sul (Brazil). Mycopathologia 63:53, 1978.

Londero, A. T. and Severo, L. C.: The gamut of progressive pulmonary paracoccidioidomycosis. Mycopathologia 75:65, 1981.

Lopes, O. S. S.: Descrição de uma técnica de concentração para pesquisa do *Paracoccidioides brasiliensis* no escarro. Hospital (Rio) 47:557, 1955.

Mackinnon, J. E.: Miositis en la blastomicosis suramericana y en la histoplasmosis. Mycopathologia 15:171, 1961.

Marsiglia, I., and Pinto, J.: Adrenal cortical insufficiency associated with paracoccidioidomycosis (South American blastomycosis). J Clin Endocrinol 26:1109, 1966.

Melo, I. S. and Londero, A. T.: Spontaneously resolving pulmonary lesions in paracoccidoidomycosis. Case report and review. Mycopathologia 82:57, 1983.

Murray, H. W., Littman, M. L., and Roberts, R. B.: Disseminated paracoccidioidomycosis (South American blastomycosis) in the United States. Am J Med 56:209, 1974.

Ramos, C. D., Londero, A. T. and Gal, M. C. L.: Pulmonary paracoccidioidomycosis in a nine year old girl. Mycopathologia 74:15, 1981.

Raphael, A.: Localização nervosa na blastomicose sul-americana. Arq Neuropsiquiatr 24:69, 1966.

Restrepo, A.: La prueba de immunodiffusion en el diagnostico de la paracoccidioidomicosis. Sabouraudia 4:223, 1966.

Restrepo, A.: Paracoccidioidomicosis. Acta Med Colombiana 3:33, 1978.

Restrepo, A., Gomez, I., Cano, L. E. et al.: Treatment of paracoccidioidomycosis with ketoconazole. A three-year experience. Am J Med (Supplement) January 24, 1983, Pp 48.

Restrepo, A., and Moncada, L. H.: Una prueba de latex en lamina para el diagnostico de la paracoccidioidomicosis. Bol Panam 84:520, 1978.

Restrepo, A., Robledo, M., Giraldo, R. et al.: The gamut of paracoccidioidomycosis. Am J Med 61:33, 1976.

Severo, L. C., Geyer, G. R., Londero, A. T., Porto, N. S., and Rizzon, C. F. C.: The primary pulmonary lymph node complex in paracoccidioidomycosis. Mycopathologia 67:115, 1979.

Yarzabal, L. A., Albornoz, M., Cabral, M., and Santiago, A. R.: Specific double diffusion microtechnique for the diagnosis of aspergillosis and paracoccidioidomycosis using monospecific antisera. Sabouraudia 16:55, 1978.

125 HISTOPLASMOSIS

GEORGE A. SAROSI, M.D.
SCOTT F. DAVIES, M.D.

Histoplasmosis is an infection by the fungus *Histoplasma capsulatum*. Exposure occurs by inhalation of organisms living in the soil. Although the primary infection is in the lung, *Histoplasma* may cause a wide variety of clinical manifestations because of its tendency to invade the bloodstream during the primary infection and its capacity to cause progressive disease in multiple sites.

Infection by the related fungus *Histoplasma duboisii* (African histoplasmosis) also probably occurs via respiratory exposure to the organism in the soil. The yeast form is much larger than that of *Histoplasma capsulatum*. Spread to bone and skin is common. The clinical features of this illness resemble North American blastomycosis more than histoplasmosis caused by *Histoplasma capsulatum* (Williams et al., 1971).

ETIOLOGY. *Histoplasma capsulatum* is a dimorphic fungus that grows on Sabouraud's medium at 25° C as a fluffy white mycelium bearing characteristic macroconidia ("tuberculate chlamydospores"). The term *capsulatum* is a misnomer because *H. capsulatum* has no capsule. The so called "capsule" is an artifact created by shrinkage of the protoplasm away from the cell wall so that an unstained capsule-like space is seen. The organism is free-living in nature in this mycelial phase. In contrast, at 37° C on blood agar and in infected mammalian tissue, the fungus grows as an oval budding yeast 2 to 4 microns in diameter. The organism is identified in the laboratory by conversion of the isolate from the mycelial to the yeast phase and by demonstration of typical tuberculate chlamydospores in microscopic mounts of the mycelial phase. Small laboratory animals can be infected by intraperitoneal injections of either clinical specimens (treated with penicillin) or suspensions of culture. The organism can be isolated from the spleen or liver of infected animals after sacrifice three to four weeks after infection.

H. duboisii, although different in its appearance and pathogenic features, is probably a variant of *H. capsulatum*. *H. duboisii* is also dimorphic, producing a mycelial growth at 25° C that has microconidia and tuberculate macroconidia exactly like those of *H. capsulatum*. The large yeast forms of *H. duboisii* measure about 10 μ in diameter, have thick walls, and many budding forms, some of which have a broad base like *B. dermatiditis*. One feature of the budding that distinguishes *H. duboisii* from *B. dermatiditis* is the delayed separation until it reaches the size of the parent cell. Since the bud and parent remain connected by a narrow "isthmus" they have an hour-glass configuration.

PATHOGENESIS AND PATHOLOGY. The concentration of *Histoplasma* in the soil varies widely from site to site even within a highly endemic area. Excrement of chickens, starlings, pigeons, and other wild birds provides an excellent growth medium, although birds are protected from infection by their high body temperature. Bat droppings also support the growth of *Histoplasma*.

In highly endemic areas infection is nearly universal in humans and is common in wild and domestic animals. A minor disturbance of contaminated soil is enough to scatter spores in the air. Inhalation of spores may cause patchy areas of interstitial pneumonitis. The spores undergo metamorphosis to yeast cells, which are engulfed by macrophages and multiply intracellularly with a generation time of 11 hours (Howard, 1965). The regional lymph nodes are quickly involved, and hematogenous spread occurs. The fungus is cleared from the blood by reticuloendothelial cells throughout the body. Specific lymphocyte-mediated cellular immunity develops after 14 days and rapidly limits the infection both in the lung and at distant foci where necrosis and granuloma formation occur (Howard et al., 1971). Humoral antibody also develops but is of little importance in limiting infection. Hyperimmune serum does not protect against experimental infection; hypogammaglobulinemic patients are not more prone to progressive infection.

The histology of the individual lesions depends on the adequacy of the immune response. In overwhelming infections, macrophages in the spleen, liver, lymph nodes, bone marrow, and adrenal are crowded with organisms with little surrounding tissue reaction and these organs are enlarged grossly. In contrast, when the primary disease is limited by normal defenses, pulmonary and reticuloendothelial granulomas are well developed with only rare organisms, central necrosis, and dense surrounding fibrosis (Straub and Schwarz, 1955). Multinucleated giant cells may be seen. Eventual calcification of individual foci may lead to characteristic small scattered calcifications in the liver, spleen, and lung (Fig. 1). The organisms seen with regularity on histopathologic examination of healed granulomas, can only rarely be cultivated from these lesions.

Like *H. capsulatum*, the African fungus *H. duboisii* probably uses the lung as the portal of entry. But unlike *H. capsulatum* it rarely produces pulmonary disease. Instead, it disseminates to skin, bones, joints, or abdomen. The tissue response is also different from that in classic histoplasmosis. In *duboisii* infections massive syncytial giant cells measuring up to 200 μ in diameter are filled with large yeasts that resemble *B. dermatiditis*. When these giant cells rupture they release masses of extracellular yeasts. Together with histiocytes filled with yeasts, these giant cells are part of the granulomatous tissue that forms in the infected skin, bones, lymph nodes, spleen, and liver. The skin is most commonly infected and the bones next. The granulomatous tissue in the skin tends to invade deeply into the subcutaneous tissue and to erode bone. The giant cell granulomas in the lymph nodes, spleen, and skull are sharply circumscribed and resemble tumor nodules.

CLINICAL MANIFESTATIONS. Infection with *Histoplasma capsulatum* was first described in 1906 by Samuel Darling, who found a disseminated infection of the reticuloendothelial organs with an organism that he thought to be protozoan at autopsy of a laborer working on the Panama Canal. Sporadic autopsy reports of similar cases followed. In 1934 the first premortem diagnosis of such a patient was made by finding the characteristic intracellular organisms on a peripheral blood smear. DeMonbreun isolated the infective agent from this patient and proved that it was a fungus. In 1945 Christie and Peterson and Palmer, using antigen derived from this first isolate, demonstrated the

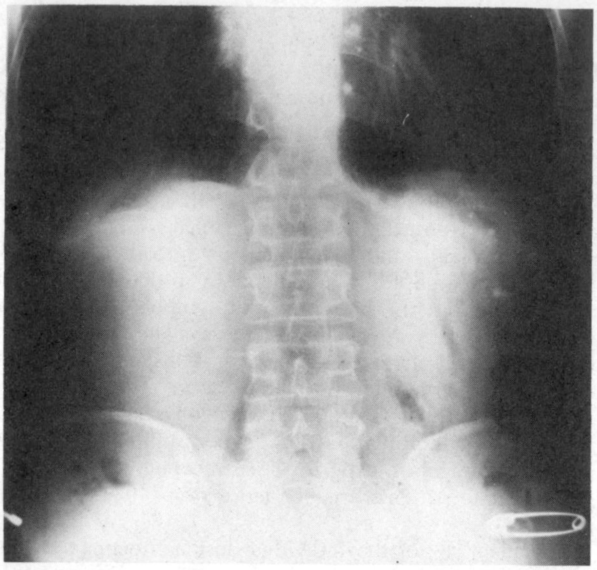

Figure 1. The abdominal flat film of a patient from an area endemic for *Histoplasma capsulatum* shows scattered calcifications in the liver, lung, and spleen. There was no history of previous symptomatic pulmonary or systemic infection. The calcifications reflect healing of primary lesions that were associated with a benign fungemia. They are not indicators of true dissemination.

totally unexpected finding that great numbers of asymptomatic people in the central United States had been previously infected with the fungus. Skin test reactions to the antigen correlated with the presence of pulmonary calcifications in individuals who did not respond to tuberculin skin tests.

Most of the histoplasmin skin test reactors in these early surveys had had asymptomatic primary infections. However, the retrospective discovery of a highly symptomatic but also self-limited form of pulmonary histoplasmosis soon followed. Small groups of patients exposed to high concentrations of organisms at a variety of point sources had been described in the earlier literature as victims of an unknown epidemic pulmonary illness. An epidemiologic investigation of one such outbreak in a military camp in 1944 demonstrated convincingly that *Histoplasma capsulatum* had been the offending pathogen. Follow-up six years after the outbreak revealed that 16 of 21 men had scattered punctate pulmonary calcifications on chest radiographs and that all had positive histoplasmin skin tests (Grayston and Furcolow, 1953). Furthermore, *Histoplasma capsulatum* was cultured from the storm cellar where the soldiers initially had been infected. Epidemiologic investigations of other outbreaks were similarly successful.

It had been believed for 40 years that histoplasmosis was a universally fatal illness. The discovery that it was a very common, usually benign, and remarkably self-limited infection opened the way for further understanding of its varied clinical manifestations. The known forms of the disease (Goodwin and DesPrez, 1978) are discussed below.

Primary Pulmonary Histoplasmosis. If exposure is light, pulmonary histoplasmosis may be totally asymptomatic. Nevertheless, chest roentgenograms, even in asymptomatic cases, may show patchy, nonsegmental areas of pneumonitis mainly involving the lower lobes. Hilar adenopathy is common and tends to be more prominent than in primary tuberculosis. Pleural effusions are distinctly uncommon.

A heavier exposure may cause a nonspecific influenza-like illness with fever, chills, myalgias, headache, and a nonproductive cough. Pleuritic pain occurs in a minority of patients. Symptoms, if present, follow exposure by one to two weeks. Regardless of the presence or absence of symptoms, it is at this time that primary fungemia generally occurs. Organisms can on occasion be recovered from the blood and bone marrow at this stage of infection without implying that there will be progressive dissemination. Following heavy exposure, more diffuse pulmonary involvement may occur, with an extensive micronodular infiltrate on the roentgenogram. In a normal person, the entire process usually resolves quickly. Rarely it may continue for weeks to months with a remitting and relapsing course. Calcified granulomas, the residue of the primary fungemia, are commonly demonstrated postmortem in spleens and livers of patients from endemic areas.

The chest roentgenogram usually returns to normal after the primary pulmonary infection. However, a variety of benign residual abnormalities can be seen. The initial infiltrates may "harden" and leave one or several nodules. These "histoplasmomas" may grow slowly over a period of months to years. Central necrosis may lead to a dense core of calcium (a "target" lesion), but this is not universal. Infrequently, alternate periods of activity followed by healing may result in characteristic concentric rings of calcium as the lesion slowly enlarges. Lymph node calcification, either in association with a histoplasmoma or as a solitary finding, is common. Finally, small, punctate, "buckshot" calcifications may be scattered over both lung fields, a pattern very characteristic of healed primary histoplasmosis (Fig. 2).

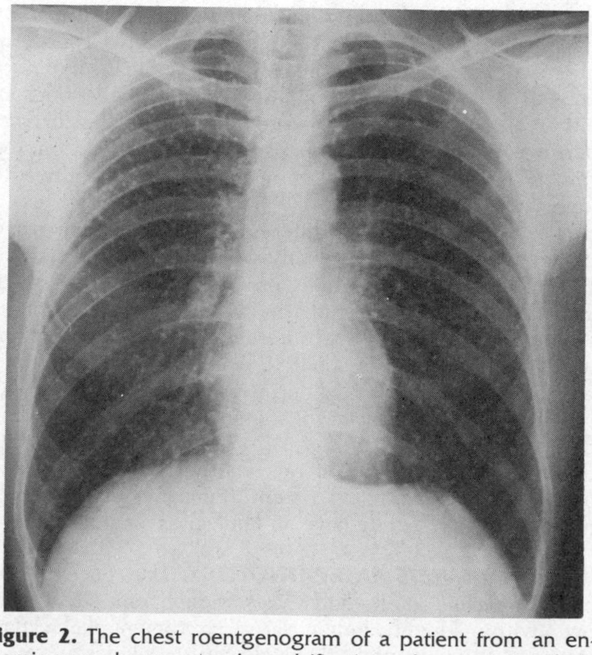

Figure 2. The chest roentgenogram of a patient from an endemic area shows extensive calcifications characteristic of old primary histoplasmosis. The exact time of the primary infection could not be determined by history, despite the striking residual roentgenographic abnormality.

Large epidemics have been associated with excavation of infected soil for construction of roads or buildings. The association of erythema nodosum and erythema multiforme with acute histoplasmosis was first appreciated during investigations of these epidemics. Careful follow-up studies of these patients have revealed that progressive dissemination after a primary respiratory infection is exceedingly rare. Only one case of disseminated disease was seen among more than 6000 cases in an urban epidemic. In a more recent urban outbreak of histoplasmosis over 10 per cent of the hospitalized patients developed disseminated disease. However, when calculated on the basis of total infections, 46 cases of disseminated histoplasmosis occurred among 100,000–200,000 infections, which is the same order of magnitude as the previous report. (Wheat et al., 1981).

Immunity is incomplete. Heavy exposure at a later date can result in a second illness with an earlier onset and a shorter symptomatic period. There has been some speculation that this shorter illness may have an allergic component. Serial studies of individuals in endemic areas demonstrate waxing and waning of both skin test positivity and the serologic titers, which suggests that periodic reexposure to the organism results in asymptomatic immunogenic infections.

Chronic Cavitary Histoplasmosis. Upper lobe cavitary histoplasmosis closely resembles reinfection tuberculosis in roentgenographic appearance. In fact, it was first described among sanitorium patients being treated for presumed tuberculosis (Furcolow and Brasher, 1956). However, the mechanism of infection is not endogenous reactivation, as it is in tuberculosis. Rather, cavitary histoplasmosis is the direct result of a progressive primary infection.

Cavitary histoplasmosis usually occurs in middle-aged male smokers with structural changes of centrilobular emphysema. In most cases, acute pulmonary histoplasmosis in this setting usually resolves without sequelae. In a minority of cases, infected air spaces persist and lead to a progressive, fibrosing cavitary process, which requires specific antifungal chemotherapy. Although bilateral upper lobe involvement is most characteristic, cavitary disease may occur in any part of the lung (Goodwin et al., 1976).

Chronic cough is a common clinical presentation, although patients may be asymptomatic. Constitutional symptoms increase as the illness progresses. Weight loss is usual in far advanced disease. Fever may not be present.

The coexistence of cavitary histoplasmosis with either tuberculosis or bronchogenic carcinoma is common. In one large retrospective study of cavitary histoplasmosis, 20 per cent of the cases simultaneously also had one of these other diseases (Parker et al., 1970).

Disseminated Histoplasmosis. Disseminated histoplasmosis refers to any progressive extrapulmonary infection with *Histoplasma capsulatum*. It may occur as an overwhelming postprimary spread with very little cellular inflammatory reaction despite the presence of massive numbers of organisms. This pattern has been seen most often in very young children and is called the infantile form. Among immunocompetent adults, dissemination is most common in the elderly. Adults usually demonstrate more of an inflammatory reaction with fewer organisms and definite granuloma formation. The disease in adults may follow a smoldering subacute course.

Disseminated histoplasmosis can present as an opportunistic infection in the immunosuppressed patient. High-dose glucocorticoid therapy is an important predisposing factor (Davies et al., 1977). In the immunosuppressed child, dissemination usually follows a primary pulmonary infection. In the immunosuppressed adult, there is usually no history of a preceding respiratory illness, and the mechanism of infection may be an endogenous reactivation. The degree of granulomatous response in the immunosuppressed patient may vary from almost none (the "infantile" form) to a considerable amount.

Glucocorticoids may also limit the ability of a normal patient to control a primary pulmonary infection. Patients who are not immunosuppressed initially but who are given glucocorticoids during an undiagnosed primary *Histoplasma* infection (often for a presumed diagnosis of sarcoidosis) may develop progressive systemic illness.

Only about half of patients with disseminated histoplasmosis present with cough, dyspnea, or other pulmonary symptoms. The chest roentgenogram may be normal or may show a diffuse interstitial infiltrate that suggests a hematogenous process. Although at least a third of patients with normal immunity will have a localized interstitial infiltrate on chest roentgenogram, such a finding is unusual in the immunosuppressed adult.

Other clinical features of disseminated histoplasmosis include high fever, hepatosplenomegaly, and lymphadenopathy. Skin lesions include mucocutaneous ulcerations that are often painful and subcutaneous nodules. Ulcerative lesions of the tongue, palate, epiglottis, and larynx are particularly characteristic. Since primary inoculation of the skin is most unusual, skin lesions nearly always imply dissemination.

Involvement of the adrenal glands in disseminated histoplasmosis must be emphasized; adrenal hypofunction is a significant cause of death (Sarosi et al., 1971). Adrenal granulomas are regularly found at autopsy in the more reactive forms of disseminated histoplasmosis.

Diarrhea secondary to involvement of the gastrointestinal tract is uncommon but can be a prominent symptom. Hemorrhage and perforation have occurred. The infection can mimic granulomatous colitis.

The clinical picture of disseminated histoplasmosis is extremely variable and nonspecific. Fever is the only constant finding. Diagnosis depends on demonstration of the organism in histopathologic material or on culture from clinical specimens. Early diagnosis is important because specific therapy is generally effective if the patient survives long enough to receive an adequate course.

Laboratory findings may include anemia, leucopenia, and thrombocytopenia. Liver function tests may be abnormal; an elevated alkaline phosphatase is most characteristic and represents granulomatous foci in the liver. Disseminated intravascular coagulation occurs rarely.

Other cases of progressive extrapulmonary histoplasmosis present with a more localized infection. These include central nervous system histoplasmoma, endocarditis, pericarditis, and isolated gastrointestinal histoplasmosis, usually involving the terminal ileum. These cases may represent instances of endogenous reactivation in which the inability to contain the organism is more focal.

Histoplasmosis duboisii. Single localized, or multiple disseminated lesions may occur. The localized infection usually takes the form of a papular or nodular skin lesion, which may regress and heal spontaneously. Single lesions of subcutaneous tissue and bones also occur. The disseminated disease is a progressive systemic illness with multiple lesions in skin, bones, lymph nodes, liver, and spleen. The disseminated skin granulomas start as flat papules that enlarge into nodules. Subcutaneous and bone lesions begin as painful swellings that liquefy and produce cold abscesses. The skull is frequently involved with multiple lesions resembling those of multiple myeloma on x-ray. Multiple lesions also appear in the jaw, spine, sternum, scapula, and extremities. This marked tendency to attack bones is not seen in *H. capsulatum* infections. Anemia is prominent in disseminated *duboisii* infection due to marrow destruction and bleeding from skin ulcers. Fever and weight loss are prominent and death occurs rapidly.

GEOGRAPHIC VARIATIONS IN DISEASE. *Histoplasma capsulatum* has been isolated from the soil in more than 50 countries. It is most common in temperate climates along river valleys and has been found in North, Central, and South America, India, and Southeast Asia. It is rare in Europe and in Australia.

However, it must be noted that despite a worldwide distribution, the Ohio and Mississippi River valleys in the central United States represent a unique area of heavy concentration of the fungus. In this region there are 500,000 pulmonary infections annually and a total of perhaps 40,000,000 persons with previous infection. More than 90 per cent of adults are skin-test positive, and the organism can be demonstrated at autopsy in more than 70 per cent of cases. A similar situation has not been demonstrated in any other area.

Histoplasma duboisii is apparently limited to Africa. Most reports have been from the West African nations of Nigeria, Zaire, and Senegal. *Histoplasma capsulatum* has also been found in Africa, but isolates have been very uncommon.

COMPLICATIONS AND SEQUELAE. A common sequela of primary histoplasmosis is the presence on chest roentgenogram of a "coin lesion," which must be differentiated from bronchogenic carcinoma. Central calcification or concentric rings of calcium are helpful; if present, these findings exclude malignancy. If there is no calcification, thoracotomy may be necessary, especially if old roentgenograms are not available or the lesion is enlarging.

Uncommon local complications within the chest due to direct extension of the active inflammatory process include fibrosing mediastinitis, which can cause the superior vena cava syndrome, and pericarditis, which can lead to pericardial calcification. The esophagus can also be involved by direct extension of the inflammatory process from adjacent lymph nodes causing dysphagia, traction diverticula, or even frank abscess.

Rarely, old inactive histoplasmosis can also lead to complications. Broncholiths may develop when calcified nodes erode into the bronchial tree. Hemoptysis is common in this setting.

Focal areas of posterior uveitis known as "histospots" are a significant ophthalmologic problem and may lead to blindness. They occur in areas endemic for histoplasmosis, but their precise pathogenesis is uncertain.

In the absence of active dissemination, healed granulomas involving the adrenals may sometimes be the cause of Addison's disease. The presentation is that of primary adrenal insufficiency, not infection.

DIAGNOSIS. The diagnosis of acute pulmonary histoplasmosis in an endemic area is suggested by a history of exposure to an aerosol of contaminated soil in a patient with compatible clinical and roentgenologic findings. A positive skin test and rising complement-fixing antibodies against yeast and mycelial antigens are confirmatory. Skin testing is performed with histoplasmin, a mycelial antigen. The skin test is generally positive two weeks after initial exposure and remains positive for years. Serologic titers against yeast and mycelial antigens are elevated at three to four weeks in most cases. They usually decrease over 3 to 12 months but occasionally remain high for many years. Nonetheless, titers against the yeast antigen of 1:16 or greater in the appropriate clinical setting are highly suggestive of recent infection. A rising titer is diagnostic. Unlike the situation in coccidioidomycosis (see Chapter 126), a high titer during primary infection is not a bad prognostic sign. The immunodiffusion test with histoplasma antigens ("H" and "M") becomes positive later than the complement fixation test, and it is less sensitive. Its main advantage is that it is easier to perform.

Chronic cavitary histoplasmosis is easier to diagnose. Skin tests and serologic titers are almost invariably positive, and the organism is routinely found in the sputum. However, the coexistence of tuberculosis or carcinoma is not uncommon.

Diagnosis of disseminated histoplasmosis depends on a high index of suspicion. Adult cases are not limited to endemic areas, suggesting endogenous reactivation as the mechanism of some infections. Skin tests and the complement fixation titers are negative in more than half the patients. Histoplasmosis must be included in the differential diagnosis of illnesses with hectic fever in immunosuppressed patients and of progressive systemic infections in infants who live in endemic areas. Organisms may be seen on smears of peripheral blood or grown from routine blood cultures if they are incubated for 10 to 15 days. Bone marrow aspirates yield organisms on direct smear or by culture in almost 70 per cent of patients. Biopsies of liver mucosal and skin lesions will show granulomas or diffuse infection of histiocytes with *H. capsulatum* cells. Urine cultures are occasionally positive. All tissue obtained should be stained specifically for fungus with Gomori's methenamine silver or the periodic acid-Schiff techniques. Yeast forms can be missed on routine hematoxylin and eosin sections.

Several diagnostic pitfalls must be noted. A histoplasmin skin test can stimulate the formation of antibody to histoplasma antigens, especially if the patient had unrecognized primary histoplasmosis in the past. This booster response peaks by the end of the second week following the skin test. The titer rise is greater to the mycelial antigen than to the yeast phase antigen. Although the titer is usually higher to the yeast phase in primary pulmonary infection, blood for serologic tests should be obtained before the skin test is placed.

Another significant problem is that of cross-reactivity between the antigens for *Histoplasma capsulatum, Blastomyces dermatitidis, Coccidioides immitis,* and other common fungi. Although the antibody response to the specific etiologic agent is usually more marked than the response to cross-reacting organisms, positive skin tests and serologic titers against other fungi can be expected.

THERAPY AND PROPHYLAXIS

H. capsulatum Infection. No treatment is required for the usual primary pulmonary infection. Amphotericin B may be used for severe primary infections in which exposure is unusually heavy or patients are febrile for longer than three weeks. A total course of 500 mg (given as 1 mg/kg every other day) may be adequate, but this has not been well studied. Very rarely, a massive primary exposure may result in acute respiratory failure with marked hypoxia. Oxygenation and ventilatory support may be required; the use of amphotericin B is mandatory. Isolation of patients with histoplasmosis is not necessary because human-to-human transmission does not occur.

No therapy is required after excision of a solitary pulmonary nodule that proves to be a histoplasmoma.

Progressive chronic cavitary histoplasmosis requires full therapy with amphotericin B. This can be given in a dose of 1 mg/kg (not to exceed 50 mg) every other day for a total dose of 35 to 40 mg/kg. It may be necessary to treat some patients longer (Parker et al., 1970).

Disseminated histoplasmosis must also be treated with a minimum dose of 40 mg/kg of amphotericin B over many weeks. The response is gratifying if therapy is started early (Sarosi et al., 1971). Ketoconazole, an oral alternative to amphotericin B., has been used with some success in patients with chronic cavitary histoplasmosis and in patients with slowly progressive disseminated histoplasmosis. The standard dose is 400 mg daily taken one-half hour before breakfast, but may be increased by 200 mg per day to a total of 800 mg per dose. The exact duration of treatment has not been determined; currently a six-month total course of treatment is recommended. Its use is limited by nausea, vomiting, and anorexia and occasionally hepatocellular damage. In addition, the agent is fungistatic, rather than fungicidal so that visible improvement is not seen before 3 weeks. For these reasons ketoconazole should not be used in critically ill patients.

There is no effective immunization against histoplasmosis. Efforts to decontaminate the soil are too expensive to be practical on a widespread basis. However, 3 per cent formaldehyde spray has been used successfully to sterilize localized areas.

H. duboisii Infection. Single lesions may be cured by excision. Disseminated disease responds to amphotericin B. given by the same dosage schedule used for *H. capsulatum* infections.

References

Christie, A., and Peterson, J. C.: Pulmonary calcification in negative reactors to tuberculin. Am J Pub Health 35:1131, 1945.

Darling, S. T.: Protozoan general infection producing pseudotubercles in the lungs and focal necrosis in liver, spleen and lymph nodes. JAMA 46:1283, 1906.

Davies, S. F., Khan, M., and Sarosi, G. A.: Histoplasmosis in immunologically suppressed patients. Occurrence in a non-endemic area. Am J Med 64:94, 1978.

DeMonbreun, W. A.: The cultivation and cultural characteristics of Darling's *H capsulatum*. Am J Trop Med 14:93, 1934.

Furcolow, M. L., and Brasher, C. A.: Chronic progressive (cavitary) histoplasmosis as a problem in tuberculosis sanitoriums. Am Rev Tuberc Pul Dis 73:609, 1956.

Goodwin, R. A., and DesPrez, R. M.: Histoplasmosis. State of the art. Am Rev Resp Dis 117:929, 1978.

Goodwin, R. A., Owens, F. T., Snell, J. D., Hubbard, W. W., Buchanan, R. D., Terry, R. T., and DesPrez, R. M.: Chronic pulmonary histoplasmosis. Medicine 55:413, 1976.

Grayston, J. T., and Furcolow, M. L.: Occurrence of histoplasmosis in epidemics: Epidemiological studies. Am J Pub Health 43:665, 1953.

Howard, D. H.: Intracellular growth of *Histoplasma capsulatum*. J Bacteriol 89:518, 1965.

Howard, D. H., Otto, V., Guptka, R. K.: Lymphocyte-mediated cellular immunity in histoplasmosis. Infect Immun 4:605, 1971.

Palmer, C. E.: Non-tuberculosis pulmonary calcification and sensitivity to histoplasmin. Pub Health Rep 60:513, 1945.

Parker, J. D., Sarosi, G. A., Doto, I. L., Bailey, R. E., and Tosh, F. E.: Treatment of chronic pulmonary histoplasmosis. A National Communicable Disease Center cooperative mycoses study. N Engl J Med 283:225, 1970.

Sarosi, G. A., Voth, D. W., Dahl, B. A., Doto, I. L., and Tosh, F. E.: Disseminated histoplasmosis: Results of a long-term follow-up. A center for Disease Control cooperative mycoses study. Ann Intern Med 75:511, 1971.

Silverman, R. N., Schwarz, J., Lahey, M. E., and Carson, R. P.: Histoplasmosis. Am J Med 19:410, 1955.

Straub, M., and Schwarz, J.: The healed primary complex in histoplasmosis. Am J Clin Pathol 25:727, 1955.

Wheat, L. G., Slama, T. G., Eitzen, H. E., Kohler, R. B., French, M. L. V., and Biesecker, J. L.: A large urban outbreak of histoplasmosis: clinical features. Ann Int Med 94:331, 1981.

Williams, A. O., Lawson, E. A., and Lucas, A. O.: African histoplasmosis due to *Histoplasma duboisii*. Arch Pathol 92:306, 1971.

126

COCCIDIOIDOMYCOSIS

THEO N. KIRKLAND, M.D.

Coccidioidomycosis is a pulmonary and disseminated infection of respiratory origin caused by the soil-resident fungus *Coccidioides immitis*. The infection occurs in man and animals and is endemic in arid regions of the Americas.

ETIOLOGY. The etiologic agent is the pathogenic fungus *C. immitis*, which inhabits the soil in the Lower Sonoran life zone of the Southwestern United States and in similar desert regions of Mexico (Gonzales-Ochoa, 1967), and Central and South America (Negroni, 1967). These geographic areas are characterized botanically by the presence of the creosote bush. *C. immitis* is adapted to the high salinity and alkaline pH of these soils.

The fungus is dimorphic, replicating in the soil in the mycelial phase and in tissue in the spherule phase. In the soil, the mycelium is composed of long hyphae 2 to 4 μ in diameter, which fragment into highly resistant barrel-shaped arthrospores.

During the summer months, the intensely hot air sterilizes the surface soil of *C. immitis*, but the fungus remains viable in the subsurface layer and in rodent burrows. After rainfall, surface growth of *C. immitis* is stimulated, and numerous arthrospores are formed. These arthrospores become airborne with winds or when the soil is disturbed during excavation or construction.

The airborne arthrospores are the infectious units of the fungus, and inhalation initiates the infection. Each arthrospore develops into a spherule, or sporangium, which may reach a diameter of 36 to 60 μ. Within the spherule numerous sporangiospores (endospores) of 2 to 5 μ diameter are formed. These spores are released when the spherules rupture, resulting in rapid growth of the organism within the host.

PATHOGENESIS AND PATHOLOGY. Infection almost invariably follows inhalation of arthrospores from soil. The organisms are phagocytosed by pulmonary macrophages and replicate within these host cells in the form of spherules. A few cases of percutaneous inoculation coccidioidomycosis, usually laboratory acquired, have been reported.

The basic host defense against *C. immitis* is cell-mediated immunity (delayed hypersensitivity). In most patients, such immunity appears within a few weeks of the onset of symptoms. Early in the infection, the fungus replicates unrestrictedly in the macrophages, until cell-mediated immunity appears. Then the macrophages become activated and kill the ingested fungi. This acquired immunity is reflected in a positive delayed hypersensitivity skin test to coccidioides skin-test reagent.

In a minority of patients, cell-mediated immunity to the fungus appears to be defective, delayed, or absent. In such cases, either active chronic pulmonary lesions persist, or hematogenous dissemination to other organs occurs. The immune response fails for obscure reasons. Genetic factors must be involved because blacks and Filipinos carry a much higher risk of dissemination than Caucasians (see below).

Seventy per cent of patients who develop disseminated coccidioidomycosis are anergic to *C. immitis* antigens but most patients retain delayed hypersensitivity to other antigens. Anergy to all antigens occurs only when the patient is gravely ill. In other assays, such as *C. immitis*-specific lymphocyte transformation or lymphokine production, T cells fail to react normally. Yet patients with disseminated coccidioidomycosis form granulomas indistinguishable from those in patients whose infection does not disseminate. Patients with disseminated coccidioidomycosis make a vigorous antibody response to the fungus, but it is not protective. In fact, a high titer of IgG antibody to *C. immitis* is a poor prognostic sign.

Not all patients with disseminated coccidioidomycosis lose their delayed hypersensitivity reactions to *C. immitis*. Dissemination in patients who react to a coccidioidin skin test shows that the skin test does not measure directly the ability of T lymphocytes to activate macrophages to kill the organism and suggests that these patients may lack the appropriate T cell function.

The basic pathologic response to coccidioidomycosis is the granuloma (Forbus and Bestebreurtje, 1946). Initially, polymorphonuclear leukocytes enter the site of infection, followed by monocytes and lymphocytes and occasional plasma cells. In lesions, the characteristic *C. immitis* spherules, both intact and ruptured, can be seen. As the spherule ruptures, polymorphonuclear cells swarm around the extruded endospores but are usually ineffectual and are replaced by the granuloma (Baker and Braude, 1956).

The disease is not contagious because the spherule and endospores released from lesions apparently cannot survive in the external environment. For this reason, isolation procedures during the treatment of patients with coccidioidomycosis are not required. However, transmission to hospital personnel via organisms that had reverted to the mycelial phase on a plaster cast in a patient with draining osteomyelitis was reported.

CLINICAL MANIFESTATIONS. Coccidioidomycosis usually starts as an acute to subacute pneumonia, which may be complicated by chronic pulmonary infection or dissemination to other sites and organs. The incubation period is one to four weeks. In military populations in endemic areas approximately 60 per cent of *C. immitis* infections were asymptomatic. Of the remaining 40 per cent, the clinical manifestations ranged from mild undifferentiated respiratory illness to severe pneumonia. The pulmonary infiltrate is usually found in one lower lobe, although multilobar disease also occurs. Fever is usually present. Cough is frequent although mild, and sputum is scanty and white. Hemoptysis is not common. Pleurisy is also a frequent manifestation of the disease and can be the presenting symptom.

In Caucasians, approximately 5 per cent of males and 24 per cent of females present with allergic manifestations such as rash and arthralgia. The rash ranges from a mild pruritic maculopapular eruption, usually on the chest and trunk, to erythema nodosum, usually on the legs. The arthralgia was originally termed "desert rheumatism," and the erythema nodosum was called "bumps" before their relation to coccidioidomycosis was discovered. Erythema nodosum is associated with vigorous delayed hypersensitivity and is a good prognostic sign.

The course of the primary infection may be protracted, with several weeks to months of debility in varying degrees. The pneumonia usually heals without residual effects, although characteristic thin-walled cavities or small nodules may persist.

COMPLICATIONS AND SEQUELAE. When the primary pulmonary infection fails to heal, either chronic pulmonary lesions or dissemination supervenes.

Approximately 5 per cent of patients develop cavities and nodules, which may be either inactive or active and resemble chronic pulmonary tuberculosis (Sarosi et al., 1970). These patients have a long history of cough, weight loss, fever, chest pain, and dyspnea, their sputum is filled with spherules, and their cell-mediated immune response to the fungus is depressed or absent, as reflected in the negative or weak skin test reaction.

Dissemination via the bloodstream occurs in 0.1 per cent of Caucasians and in up to 1 per cent of blacks and 10 per cent of Filipinos and Orientals. Dissemination in most cases is probably an early event, although it may not be recognized until several months after the onset of pulmonary infection. It is a particular hazard in those receiving cytotoxins, immunosuppressants, and corticosteroids. Renal transplant recipients who have diabetes mellitus have a uniquely high incidence of dissemination. Dissemination is more common in men than in women. Pregnancy also increases the risk of dissemination, although the fetus is usually unaffected (Smale and Waechter, 1970). The high levels of circulating estradiol and progesterone in pregnancy may contribute to disseminated infection because the growth of *C. immitis* is stimulated by these steroid hormones (Drutz and Huppert, 1983).

The clinical spectrum of disseminated coccidioidomycosis is very wide. In miliary coccidioidomycosis, there are high fevers, inanition, infection of almost every organ, and early death. At the other extreme, a single disseminated skin lesion is frequently not associated with systemic symptoms. Cases of disseminated coccidioidomycosis present at all points between these two extremes.

Dissemination to the central nervous system is the most ominous form of disease and carries a mortality rate of nearly 100 per cent in untreated patients. The infection presents with the insidious onset of fever, headache, and meningeal signs and runs a course of months to years. The leptomeninges are primarily involved, and only rarely are cerebral lesions such as pituitary abscesses produced. With extensive disease, the ventricles may also be infected.

The spinal fluid is under increased pressure and shows an elevated protein content of about 300 mg per 100 ml. The glucose concentration is usually but not invariably depressed to a level below 40 mg per 100 ml. Leukocytes are present in counts of several hundred/mm^3. The cells are usually mononuclear, although polymorphonuclear leukocytes may temporarily predominate with acute or exacerbated disease. The infecting organisms are rarely seen or cultured in the cerebrospinal fluid.

Hematogenous dissemination may also affect the lungs and may closely resemble miliary tuberculosis. The course may be chronic and progressively downhill or acute, fulminating, and rapidly fatal. Radiography shows diffuse nodular densities in both lungs, and hypoxia may be severe (Fig. 1). Diagnosis can be made in 60 per cent of the cases by liver biopsy, even though the liver is not enlarged and function tests are normal. Transbronchial biopsy may also produce diagnostic material.

Dissemination to the subcutaneous tissue produces large, fluctuant, usually cool, and painless nodules. These lesions are frequently multiple, occur on all parts of the body, and spontaneously drain a whitish, blood-tinged purulent exudate without a distinctive odor. Spherules are abundant in these exudates. Another characteristic skin lesion is the verrucous granuloma resembling that of blastomycosis (Fig. 2).

Osteomyelitis and arthritis are common. All bones are involved, most frequently the spine. The lesions are usually painless and may be associated with overlying subcutaneous lesions. Radiographically, osteomyelitis appears as punched-out areas of rarification with some reactive new bone formation if there is a healing component. Multiple lytic lesions of ribs and skull may resemble metastatic carcinoma or multiple myeloma (Bayer et al., 1976).

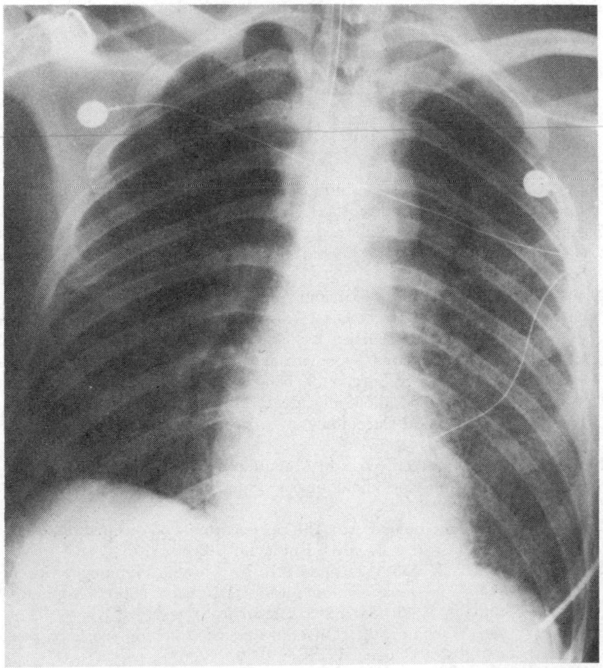

Figure 1. Fatal miliary coccidioidomycosis of lung.

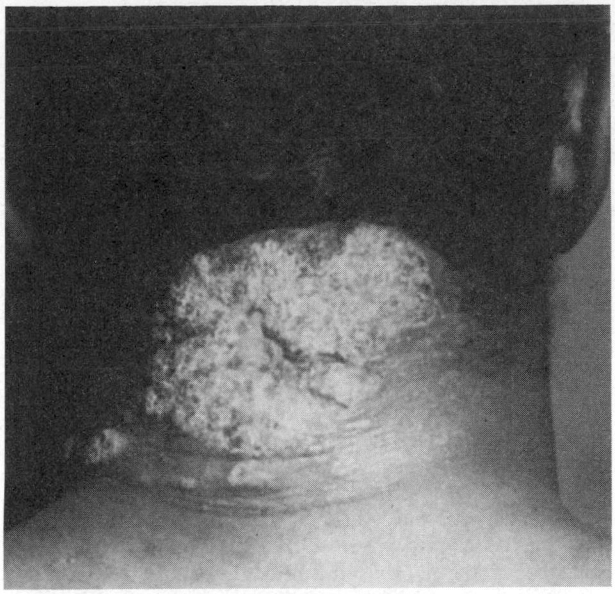

Figure 2. Verrucous skin lesion of coccidioidomycosis.

The joint infection may cause a chronic monoarticular arthritis (most frequently in the knee) without evidence of coccidioidomycosis elsewhere. The radiographic findings are minimal and usually show no bone involvement. Unless it is recognized and treated with synovectomy and intra-articular amphotericin, the disease will destroy the articular cartilage.

Dissemination to the liver, spleen, adrenals, eye, pituitary, kidneys, prostate, and seminal vesicles have all been reported.

DIAGNOSIS. The diagnosis of coccidioidomycosis is made by demonstrating *C. immitis* in exudates and tissues and measurement of the antibody and delayed hypersensitivity responses of the patient to the fungus.

The infecting spherules and endospores can be seen in simple wet mount preparations of sputum and exudates. In biopsy material the organisms are well stained by PAS and silver stains.

Culture of the organism can be accomplished on routine fungal media such as Sabouraud's agar, but growth is also abundant on blood agar and other routine bacteriologic media. Growth usually requires 5 to 10 days and occurs in the mycelial and arthrospore phase. Culture of the fungus in the spherule phase has been described with Converse medium at 40° C, but the procedure is not used in routine diagnosis. Because arthrospores develop on laboratory media, this organism poses a significant infection risk to laboratory personnel, and cultures must be manipulated with caution and in appropriate isolation equipment.

The delayed hypersensitivity skin-test response is useful in both the diagnosis and the assessment of the prognosis in coccidioidomycosis. The skin-test antigen, coccidioidin, is derived from a filtrate of the mycelial arthrospore phase-grown organisms. The standard dilution is 1:100. Also available is a 1:10 dilution, although this is of limited usefulness. In addition, a skin-test reagent prepared from spherule-phase organisms is available; this reagent is more sensitive for diagnosis than coccidioidin, but its prognostic significance is unknown (Stevens et al. 1975).

In patients with self-limited pulmonary infection, a positive delayed hypersensitivity skin-test response to coccidioidin develops within one to three weeks of the onset of symptoms and lasts for life. A positive skin-test on initial testing may represent only a past asymptomatic infection; however, a negative skin-test response followed a short time later by conversion to positivity is diagnostic. The skin-test response and immunity are of lifelong duration.

In 70 per cent of patients with dissemination or progressive pulmonary infection, the skin-test response to coccidioidin remains negative. The patients who recover from the severe complications of disseminated coccidioidomycosis may or may not develop a positive skin test. Some of these treated patients have a positive skin test to coccidioidin in the presence of residual disease.

In patients with coccidioidomycosis, precipitating 19S and complement-fixing 7S antibodies may develop. In about 75 per cent of patients with the self-limiting pulmonary infection, precipitating antibody is detectable. This antibody appears within the first two weeks of symptoms and persists for only three to six months. Complement-fixing antibody, however, appears in only about 25 per cent of patients with self-limited infection, and when it occurs it is present in titers of less than 1:32. This antibody declines over a period of months to a few years.

In the disseminated disease, precipitating antibody develops in about 50 per cent of patients and wanes within a few months. The complement-fixing antibody develops in most patients with disseminated disease and is present in titers greater than 1:32. This antibody indicates the status of dissemination. It persists and rises with progressive infection and declines with quiescence or response to treatment.

The cerebrospinal fluid complement-fixing antibody titer is of particular use both in diagnosing meningitis and in monitoring its course. This antibody is produced locally within the central nervous system and is not serum antibody that has passively diffused into the spinal fluid. The spinal fluid complement-fixing antibody may be the first laboratory sign of meningitis, appearing before any other marked abnormality of the spinal fluid. Sequential titers will reflect the natural course of the infection or the response to treatment, a declining titer is associated with a favorable course.

TREATMENT. Amphotericin B remains, after 25 years, the mainstay of antifungal chemotherapy in coccidioidomycosis. All strains of *C. immitis* are inhibited by amphotericin B, but the drug is not fungicidal in clinically achievable concentrations. In most cases of acute pulmonary infection, amphotericin B is not given because its side effects, particularly nephrotoxicity, are worse than the self-limited disease. Whether or not early treatment of pulmonary infection might decrease the incidence of chronic pulmonary disease or dissemination has not been evaluated. Nonetheless, it might be prudent to treat pulmonary infection in patients who have a high risk of progressive disease, such as blacks, orientals, or patients with underlying lymphoma or leukemia, or those who are receiving cytotoxic or corticosteroid drug therapy. The drug might also be indicated in pregnancy but only after the first trimester, because the effect of amphotericin on the fetus is unknown.

Amphotericin B is frequently used in patients with chronic active pulmonary infection, although this treatment usually only ameliorates symptoms, and repeated courses are required to maintain remission.

Amphotericin B is most clearly indicated for disseminated infections, but the response to treatment is poor. In patients with osteomyelitis with multiple lesions, intravenous amphotericin B may be helpful, while in those with single lesions, excision should be performed if possible. Subcutaneous lesions frequently drain spontaneously.

In chronic pulmonary disease, surgery may be employed, the usual criteria for such intervention being hemoptysis or an enlarging cavity with impending rupture. Because of the presence of occult satellite lesions, lobectomy rather than segmental resection is frequently necessary. Surgery may be complicated by bronchopleural fistulae with empyema and the appearance of new pulmonary lesions in contiguous segments. The use of amphotericin B in the intraoperative period for preventing surgical complications is debatable.

Ketoconazole, has also been used to treat coccidioidomycosis. Skin lesions respond better than bone and joint lesions, and usually show improvement but not cure. Not all patients improve with therapy and relapses are common. In chronic pulmonary coccidioidomycosis the symptoms of approximately half the patients treated with ketoconazole improve usually without eradication of the organism from the sputum. This drug has no use in meningitis because in the usual dose of 400 mg/day very little ketoconazole enters the CSF. Since ketoconazole has not been examined in primary coccidioidomycosis we do not know if it prevents progressive disease. Ketoconazole is much less toxic than amphotericin B and may be useful in ameliorating symptoms of chronic disseminated lesions. Patients with rapidly progressive disease or meningitis should be treated with amphotericin B.

PROPHYLAXIS. Prevention is based upon avoiding exposure to dust containing arthrospores. Planting fields with grass prevents aerosolization of arthrospores, as does wetting the soil with water or commercial dust retardants.

There is no commercial vaccine, although an experimental vaccine composed of inactivated cultured spherules is undergoing evaluation (Pappagianis and Levine, 1975).

References

Baker, O. and Braude, A.: A study of stimuli leading to the production of spherules in coccidioidomycosis. J Lab and Clin Med 47:169, 1956.

Bayer, A., Yoskikawa, T., Galkin, J., and Guze, L.: Unusual syndromes of coccidioidomycosis: Diagnostic and therapeutic considerations. Medicine 55:131, 1976.

Drutz, D. and Huppert, M.: Coccidioidomycosis: Factors affecting the host-parasite interaction. J Infect Dis 147:372, 1983.

Forbus, W., and Bestebreurtje, A.: Coccidioidomycosis: A Study of 95 Cases of the Disseminated Type with Special Reference to the Pathogenesis of the Disease. Mil Surgeon 99:653, 1946.

Gonzales-Ochoa, A.: Coccidioidomycsis in Mexico. In Coccidioidomycosis: Proceedings of Second Coccidioidomycosis Symposium. Tucson, University of Arizona Press, 1967.

Negroni, P.: Coccidioidomycosis in Argentina. In Coccidioidomycosis: Proceedings of Second Coccidioidomycosis Symposium. Tucson, University of Arizona Press, 1967.

Pappagianis, D., and Levine, H.: The present status of vaccination against coccidioidomycosis in man. Am J Epidemiol 102:30, 1975.

Sarosi, G., Parker, J., Doto, I., and Tosh, F.: Chronic Pulmonary Coccidioidomycosis: A National Communicable Disease Center Cooperative Mycosis Study. N Engl J Med 283:326, 1970.

Smale, L., and Waechter, K.: Disseminated coccidioidomycosis in pregnancy. Am J Obstet Gynecol 107:356, 1970.

Stevens, D., Levine, H., Deresinski, S. and Blaine, L.: Spherulin in clinical coccidioidomycosis. Chest 68:697, 1975.

127
ASPERGILLOSIS

George A. Sarosi, M.D.
Scott F. Davies, M.D.

Aspergillosis refers to an infection caused by one of the numerous members of the genus *Aspergillus*. The vast majority of human infections are caused by *Aspergillus fumigatus;* occasionally infections are caused by *Aspergillus niger, Aspergillus clavatus, Aspergillus flavus,* or *Aspergillus nidulans*. These fungi have low pathogenicity unless the normal defense mechanisms are weakened by illness or medication. Common sites of infection are the lung, external ear, orbit, and paranasal sinuses. In severely immunocompromised patients dissemination can occur.

ETIOLOGY. Members of the genus *Aspergillus* are ubiquitous in nature. In addition to their pathogenicity for man and other mammals, some species are infectious for birds, insects, or, more commonly, plants. In nature the fungus grows as an aerial mycelium that releases spores. When these are inhaled, they reach the lung or the upper airway. In the laboratory the fungus will grow well on most media, including Sabouraud's agar, and equally well at room temperature or 35° C. The colonies are fast growing and appear first as white filamentous surface growth on solid media. They quickly become green, yellow, or black as spores are produced. These colonies are composed of segmented mycelia. Expanded, knob-like swellings called conidiophores are located on the ends of specialized mycelia. These conidiophores, or spore-heads, are covered by multiple spores that become airborne when the mycelium is disturbed. Identification of the species of *Aspergillus* is based on the morphology of the conidiophores and their spore-bearing surfaces.

PATHOGENESIS AND PATHOLOGY. After becoming airborne, the infecting spore may settle on some external surface or may be inhaled into the lung. In external otitis caused by *Aspergillus*, there is no tissue invasion. On histopathologic examination the organism is seen in the superficial keratinized layer of the skin, evoking little or no inflammatory response. Occasionally, and usually in debilitated patients, superficial lesions invade the middle ear, paranasal sinuses, and orbit, evoking a mixed polymorphonuclear-macrophage inflammatory exudate with giant cells. Hyphae are scarce in routine hematoxylin-eosin stained sections, but are readily seen in silver stains. Speciation is difficult unless well-preserved conidiophores are seen in the section. Clinically significant involvement of the gastrointestinal tract below the oropharynx is rare, although isolation of *Aspergillus* species from the gut is not. *Aspergillus* may produce multiple deep esophageal or gastrointestinal ulcers that invade the muscularis and occasionally perforate.

In disseminated (or pyemic) aspergillosis, there is widespread necrosis of various organs. Multiple areas of bronchopneumonia occur in the lung where invasion of blood vessels causes thrombosis, infarction, and cavitation. Metastatic abscesses are common in the brain, liver, and heart. Despite this evidence of hematogenous spread, recovery of the organism from blood culture is rare.

Aspergillus endocarditis occurs, usually after cardiac surgery. The vegetations are large, bulky, and friable, and frequently cause distant emboli in major arteries.

Perhaps the most distinctive lesion produced by *Aspergillus* species is the intracavitary fungus ball that is often referred to erroneously as a "mycetoma." These matted masses of aspergilli grow in pre-existing cavities that communicate with bronchi. The fungus ball is composed of mycelia as well as necrotic debris, and the entire mass is often attached at one place to the underlying cavity. The cavity is lined by respiratory epithelium, but outside the fibrous capsule there is a varying amount of mononuclear cell infiltrate, liberally sprinkled with eosinophils. The cavity colonized by the fungus may be an inactive residual lesion that is secondary to tuberculosis, another fungal disease (such as histoplasmosis), sarcoidosis, carcinoma, or bronchiectasis (British Tuberculosis Association, 1968, 1970). The first sign of colonization by *Aspergillus* is usually thickening of the cavity wall, which can be seen in the chest roentgenogram.

Aspergillus is also a secondary invader in the pleural cavity. Thus, pleural aspergillosis occurs almost exclusively in established cases of empyema, usually tuberculosis, with a bronchopleural fistula (Krakowka et al., 1970). This form of aspergillosis is more common than the scarcity of publications on it would indicate.

In bronchial allergic aspergillosis the expectorated mucus plugs contain mycelia that are visible to the naked eye in the form of brown or tan flecks interspersed throughout the thick tenacious mucus. When these specks of mycelia are examined as a wet preparation, the characteristic septate hyphae are seen but not the spore-bearing conidiophores. The dilated bronchi contain inspissated mucus in the lumen. The hyphae in the mucus do not invade the bronchial wall. In addition to fungal elements the mucus also contains much eosinophilic debris. The walls of the bronchi are heavily infiltrated by eosinophils as well. In the surrounding pulmonary tissue some of the smaller bronchioles are obliterated by masses of granulation tissue, and the alveoli show focal eosinophilic pneumonia. A special feature of the bronchiectasis in allergic aspergillosis is the normal pattern of many small bronchi and bronchioles beyond the grossly dilated proximal bronchi (Scadding, 1967). Most other diseases causing bronchiectasis produce obliteration of the bronchioles so that the dilated bronchi end blindly and no longer communicate with their alveoli (Fig. 1). There is evidence that the bronchi are damaged by an Arthus-type reaction in which antigen-antibody precipitates are involved. The antigens are derived from the *Aspergillus* mycelium in the mucus plugs. The eosinophilic pneumonia is thought to depend on both reaginic and precipitating antibody for its development.

CLINICAL MANIFESTATIONS. External otitis usually causes pain, redness, and swelling of the ear. Invasion of a paranasal sinus produces local swelling and redness in the involved area. Marked tenderness in the area of induration suggests osteomyelitis. In the sinuses, nose, and palate the fungus grows as a large, bulky, soft tissue mass that can bleed profusely when touched.

In the syndrome of allergic bronchopulmonary aspergillosis, most of the early symptoms are related to underlying chronic asthma (Henderson, 1968; Hinson et al., 1952). Episodic dyspnea is common. Whereas not all patients with the syndrome have a distinct history of asthma, all

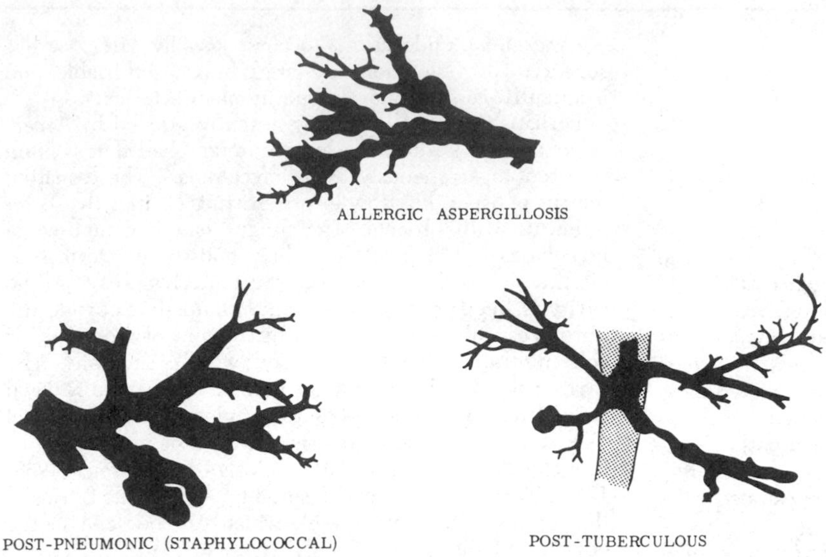

Figure 1. Comparison of bronchograms in different forms of bronchiectasis. In allergic aspergillosis, the dilated bronchi characteristically communicate with normal small bronchi and bronchioles beyond the grossly dilated primary bronchi. Conversely, in postpneumonic staphylococcal and posttuberculous bronchiectasis, the dilated bronchi usually end blindly. (From Scadding, J. G.: Scand J Resp Dis 48:372, 1967.)

have evidence of airway obstruction when carefully tested. As fungi proliferate in the thick asthmatic mucus, they bring on intermittent bouts of increased bronchial obstruction. When this happens, fever and cough are common, and active infiltrates are seen on the chest roentgenogram. Mucus plugs are frequently expectorated, and pleuritic chest pain and peripheral blood eosinophilia are common. Despite these episodes in the early stages of disease, the patients are relatively asymptomatic between acute exacerbations of bronchial plugging except for the symptoms of underlying asthma. Later, however, repeated attacks of bronchial plugging may result in gradual destruction of the bronchial mucosa, and saccular bronchiectasis may develop. If this occurs, the symptoms of infective bronchiectasis may dominate the clinical picture, with continuous production of purulent sputum even during the intervals between episodes of bronchial plugging. Hemoptysis occurs in about half of the patients and is almost always scanty; the blood comes from the bronchiectatic lesions.

The major clinical feature of intracavitary fungus balls is hemoptysis. Hemoptysis may sometimes be profuse and even life-threatening; aspiration of the blood into the uninvolved lung may occur, and exsanguination is possible. Otherwise, the main symptoms are related to the underlying chronic cavitary disease and are determined by the extent of pulmonary destruction that was present before the fungus ball appeared.

With the advent of antineoplastic drugs and organ transplantation, the pyemic or septicemic form of aspergillosis has become common in medical centers. Patients under treatment with large doses of glucocorticoids and cytotoxic agents are at risk. Frequently, the patients have been rendered granulocytopenic with therapy and have been ill and under treatment with antimicrobial agents for previous infections. The symptoms of this form of invasive aspergillosis are those of an acute pulmonary infection, with fever, cough, and tachypnea. Hemoptysis is common but seldom massive. The chest film may show rapidly cavitating infiltrates in any of the lung fields; because of intravascular growth of the fungus, the picture may resemble that of pulmonary infarction. Pleural extension of the infiltrate may cause chest pain. The fungus may disseminate from the necrotizing pulmonary infection. Common secondary sites are the central nervous system, heart, liver, and skin.

The division of pulmonary aspergillosis into allergic bronchopulmonary aspergillosis in certain asthmatics, colonizing aspergillomas in patients with pre-existing cavities, and invasive aspergillosis in profoundly immunosuppressed patients has never been quite adequate to encompass all forms of aspergillosis. The term chronic necrotizing pulmonary aspergillosis represents a group of patients with locally destructive pulmonary infection who do not fit well into any of the three standard categories (Binder et al., 1982).

In these patients *Aspergillus* does not colonize existing cavities but instead causes progressive tissue destruction. Patients may develop unilateral or bilateral upper lobe fibrocavitary disease suggestive of tuberculosis or chronic cavitary histoplasmosis. Large areas of lung may shell out and aspergillomas may develop in new cavities caused by *Aspergillus* infection itself, in contradistinction to the usual situation where aspergillomas colonize a cavity resulting from another destructive pulmonary process.

This form of *Aspergillus* infection tends to occur in middle-aged male smokers who presumably have some centrilobular emphysema. The abnormal airspaces in the damaged lung may predispose to proliferation of the fungus. Defects in mucociliary clearance may also be a factor. Many of these patients have other underlying diseases including malnutrition, diabetes mellitus, connective tissue disorders, or low dose corticosteroid therapy. However, they do not have the profound immune depression observed in leukemics, renal transplant recipients, or children with chronic granulomatous disease of childhood.

Chronic necrotizing aspergillosis is progressive over a period of a few months to several years. Patients may be chronically ill with cough, weight loss, fever, night sweats, and malaise. Acute episodes of purulent bronchitis may reflect bacterial superinfection. The process sometimes extends directly to the pleural space with formation of *Aspergillus* empyema (Hillerdal, 1981). There is little if any tendency to distant spread.

Aspergillus pneumonia is the commonest fungus infection in chronic granulomatous disease, a disorder in which phagocytes cannot kill ingested organisms (Chapter 87). The pneumonia in this condition is invasive and the infection extends to the ribs and vertebrae (Altman, 1977; Cohen et al., 1981).

COMPLICATIONS AND SEQUELAE. Once *Aspergillus* infection becomes established in paranasal sinuses, extension to the orbit and the central nervous system may occur. When the orbit is invaded, proptosis and ophthalmoplegia may be the dominant signs. A stroke indicates invasion of an intracranial vessel and hemorrhagic infarction. If the patient survives long enough, abscesses form.

The most important late complication of allergic bronchopulmonary aspergillosis is bronchiectasis, predominantly in the upper lobe, with resultant bronchial obstruction and fibrosis. Occasionally, the fungus will persist in the lumen of these dilated bronchi and produce an aspergilloma in situ.

Intracavitary fungus balls produce few late sequelae as a rule. Progressive breathlessness secondary to the underlying cavitary disease will continue, but the fungus ball will not invade to cause disseminated disease. Continuous low-grade hemoptysis is the main late complication, but exsanguination or fatal aspiration of blood can occur.

Septicemic aspergillosis carries a very poor prognosis. Very few patients will survive long enough to develop late sequelae. Occasionally, however, patients survive the acute necrotizing pneumonia and develop fungus balls in the residual necrotic cavities.

Chronic necrotizing aspergillosis shares many clinical features of other progressive fibrocavitary infections. Progressive destruction of lung parenchyma may cause respiratory failure, especially if there is underlying chronic obstructive lung disease. Intracavitary aspergillomas may develop in destroyed areas of the lung and cause hemoptysis. Bronchiectasis occurs as the lung scars and retracts.

GEOGRAPHIC VARIATION IN DISEASE. Allergic bronchopulmonary aspergillosis is common in Great Britain and northern Europe and considerably less common in North America (Henderson, 1968; Hinson et al., 1952; Longbottom and Pepys, 1964). The syndrome has been described from other continents, but its true incidence is difficult to ascertain.

Fungus balls appear to be common wherever healed cavitary tuberculosis is common; one would expect to find a high incidence of these patients where the incidence of cavitary tuberculosis remains high.

Invasive septicemic aspergillosis seldom occurs in immunologically normal people. Its frequency is highest in countries where aggressive cytotoxic and glucocorticoid therapy for the treatment of neoplastic disease is common and where organ transplantations occur frequently. Most cases have been reported from specialized centers in the United States dealing with neoplastic disease and renal transplantation.

Orbital aspergillosis predominates in localities with a warm and humid climate and most cases have been reported from Sudan, India, and the southern United States (Hedges and Leung, 1976).

DIAGNOSIS. Diagnosis of allergic bronchopulmonary aspergillosis requires the following criteria (Henderson, 1968; Hinson et al., 1952; Longbottom and Pepys, 1964):

1. Chronic asthma, or evidence of chronic airway obstruction.
2. More than two distinct episodes of transient pulmonary infiltration, separated by an asymptomatic interval confirmed by chest x-ray.
3. Precipitins to *A. fumigatus* antigens in serum.
4. Peripheral blood eosinophilia in excess of 500 eosinophils per cubic millimeter when the infiltrates are present.
5. Demonstration of *A. fumigatus* in sputum at least twice by culture or direct visualization of the fungus.
6. Dual skin-test results; immediate wheal and flare (type I) reaction, followed in five to six hours by a type III (Arthus) reaction after injection of *Aspergillus* antigens.

Patients with allergic bronchopulmonary aspergillosis (ABPA) can be separated from asthmatics without ABPA (who may meet many of the above criteria) by virtue of much higher levels of specific IgE and IgG antibodies directed against *Aspergillus fumigatus* (Wang, et al., 1978).

An important diagnostic feature is the discrepancy between the relatively mild clinical symptoms and the extensive pulmonary consolidation. This relationship helps in differentiating allergic aspergillosis from bacterial pneumonia in which a similar area of consolidation would produce severe symptoms. In the late stages of bronchopulmonary aspergillosis, when cavitation occurs or the upper lobes shrink, a diagnosis of pulmonary tuberculosis is often made erroneously.

Diagnosis of the other forms of aspergillosis is complicated by the fact that recovery of the fungus from expectorated sputum is often difficult in patient's with aspergillosis and common in patients without aspergillosis because aspergilli may colonize the normal mouth and upper airways. Hence, the most reliable diagnostic method is direct sampling of infected tissues.

In sino-orbital disease direct biopsies of the large friable masses of fungus should be performed, and care must be taken not to contaminate the instruments by passing them through the mouth and oropharynx.

The diagnosis of pleural aspergillosis is easily made by finding brown clumps of hyphae in the pleural pus (Young et al., 1970). Diagnosis of chronic necrotizing aspergillosis requires typical clinical and roentgenographic features, positive sputum cultures for *Aspergillus*, and careful exclusion of mycobacteria and pathogenic fungi. Transbronchial biopsy may demonstrate tissue invasion by *Aspergillus*.

In invasive pulmonary aspergillosis the chest roentgenogram is not diagnostic and may mimic lung abscess, carcinoma, pneumonia, or pulmonary infarction. In suspicious cases, fiberoptic bronchoscopy may be used to obtain biopsy material and brushings for culture and to show invasive fungal elements histopathologically. If bronchoscopy fails to confirm the diagnosis, early open biopsy should be done.

The chest radiograph helps in the diagnosis of intracavitary fungus balls. The appearance of a crescentic radiolucency surrounding a mass is highly suggestive (Monod's sign) (Figs. 2 and 3). Although other fungi, notably *Pseudallescheria boydii*, may produce a similar x-ray picture, the majority of such lesions indicates *Aspergillus* sp.

Agar diffusion tests for precipitins are positive in patients with allergic bronchopulmonary aspergillosis, fungus balls, and pleural aspergillosis. In contrast, positive serologic tests are infrequent in invasive disseminated aspergillosis because the immunosuppression of these patients prevents

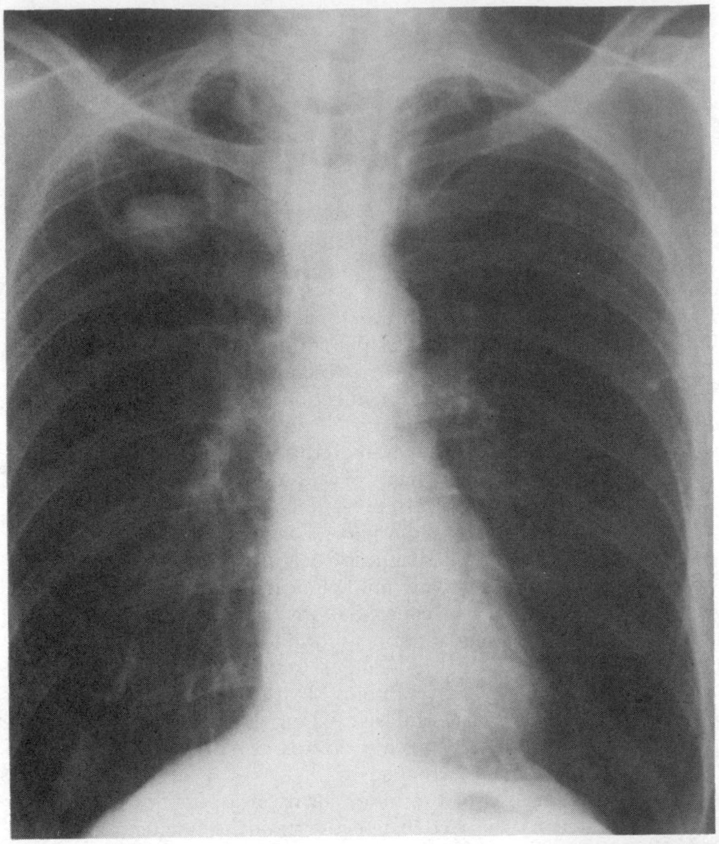

Figure 2. Fungus ball *(Aspergillus fumigatus)* in a residual old tuberculous cavity *(upright position).*

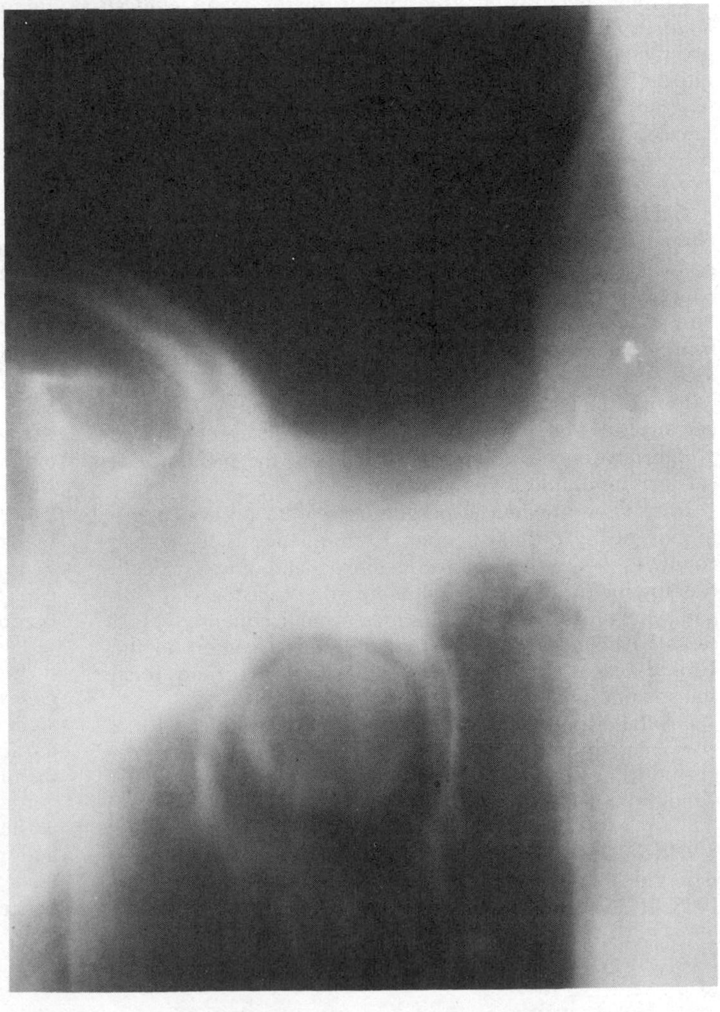

Figure 3. Tomogram of the same fungus ball seen in Figure 2. Patient is now lying down—note different position of the fungus ball.

a normal antibody response (de Repentigny and Reiss, 1984).

TREATMENT. Prednisone in a dose of 7.5 mg/day has been used successfully to treat allergic bronchopulmonary aspergillosis and to prevent recurrences. Nebulized amphotericin B and nystatin have also been used but are difficult to evaluate.

Surgical excision with wide débridement of the margins can be successful in sino-orbital disease.

In patients with aspergilloma, resection of the involved lobe has been curative when the underlying chronic pulmonary disease has not been too severe to prohibit such intervention. The fungus ball must be resected when hemoptysis threatens to kill the patient. Intravenous amphotericin B is probably of no value (Hammerman et al., 1974; Varkey and Rose, 1976). Successful treatment with endobronchial and intracavitary amphotericin B has been reported only in isolated cases and should be regarded as anecdotal, especially since fungus balls may lyse spontaneously or be expectorated.

In disseminated invasive aspergillosis intravenous amphotericin B is the treatment of choice. Even though such treatment often fails because of the severe underlying illness, it may be effective when used early in the course of the disease in an average daily dose of 0.6 mg/kg (Aisner et al., 1977; Pennington, 1976). Treatment for chronic necrotizing aspergillosis is difficult. Often the severity of the underlying lung disease precludes surgical resection of involved lung. Amphotericin B is not of proven benefit but may be tried in rapidly progressive cases. Episodes of purulent bronchitis should be treated with antibacterial agents.

PROPHYLAXIS. Since the fungus is ubiquitous in nature, it is impossible to avoid exposure to it during everyday living. Protection of immunologically incompetent patients in a hospital setting should include careful environmental monitoring and elimination of recognized foci of fungal growth. In the winter, when *A. fumigatus* spores are most prevalent, prednisone (7.5 mg/day) can prevent recurrent attacks of pulmonary consolidation and eosinophilia in patients with allergic bronchopulmonary aspergillosis (Safirstein et al., 1973).

References

Aisner, J., Schimpff, S. C., and Wiernik, P. H.: Treatment of invasive aspergillosis: Relation of early diagnosis and treatment to response. Ann Intern Med 86:539, 1977.

Altman, A.: Thoracic wall invasion secondary to pulmonary aspergillosis: A complication of chronic granulomatous disease of childhood. Am J Roentgenol 129:140, 1977).

Binder, R. E., Faling, L. J., Pugatch, R. D., Mahasaen, C., and Snider, G. L.: Chronic necrotizing pulmonary aspergillosis: A discrete clinical entity. Medicine 61:109, 1982.

British Tuberculosis Association: *Aspergillus* in persistent lung cavities after tuberculosis. Tubercle 49:1, 1968.

British Tuberculosis Association: Aspergilloma and residual tuberculous cavities—the results of a resurvey. Tubercle 51:227, 1970.

Cohen, M., Isturiz, R., Malech, A., Root, R., Wilfert, E., Gutman, L., and Buckley, R.: Fungal infection in chronic granulomatous disease. The importance of the phagocyte in defense against fungi. Am J Med 71:59, 1981.

de Repentigny, L., and Reiss, E.: Current trends in immunodiagnosis of candidiasis and aspergillosis. Inf Dis Rev 6:301, 1984.

Hammerman, K. J., Sarosi, G. A., and Tosh, F. E.: Amphotericin B in the treatment of saprophytic forms of pulmonary aspergillosis. Am Rev Resp Dis 109:57, 1974.

Hedges, T., and Leung, L.: Parasellar and orbital apex syndrome caused by aspergillosis. Neurology 26:117, 1976.

Henderson, A. H.: Allergic aspergillosis: Review of 32 cases. Thorax 23:501, 1968.

Hillerdal, G.: Pulmonary aspergillus infection invading the pleura. Thorax 36:745, 1981.

Hinson, K. F. W., Moon, A. J., and Plummer, N. S.: Bronchopulmonary aspergillosis. A review and a report of eight new cases. Thorax 7:317, 1952.

Krakowka, P., Rowenska, E., and Holweg, H.: Infection of the pleura by *Aspergillus fumigatus*. Thorax 25:245, 1970.

Longbottom, J. L., and Pepys, J.: Pulmonary aspergillosis: Diagnostic and immunological significance of antigens and C-substance in *Aspergillus fumigatus*. J Pathol Bacteriol 88:141, 1964.

Pennington, J. E.: Successful treatment of *Aspergillus* pneumonia in hematologic neoplasia. N Engl J Med 295:426, 1976.

Safirstein, B., D'Souza, M., Simon, G., Tai, E., and Pepys, J.: Five-year follow-up of allergic bronchopulmonary aspergillosis. Am Rev Resp Dis 108:450, 1973.

Scadding, J. G.: The bronchi in allergic aspergillosis. Scand J Resp Dis 48:372, 1967.

Varkey, B., and Rose, H. D.: Pulmonary aspergilloma. A rational approach to treatment. Am J Med 61:626, 1976.

Wang, J. L. F., Patterson, R., Rosenberg, M., Roberts, M., and Cooper, B. J.: Serum IgE and IgG antibody activity against *Aspergillus fumigatus* as a diagnostic aid in allergic bronchopulmonary aspergillosis. Am Rev Respir Dis 117:917, 1978.

Young, R. C., Bennett, J. E., Vogel, C. L., Carbone, P. P., and DeVita, V. T.: Aspergillosis. The spectrum of the disease in 98 patients. Medicine 49:147, 1970.

128
PULMONARY MUCORMYCOSIS

Burt R. Meyers, M.D.

Pulmonary mucormycosis is an infection of the lung by the nonseptate fungi known as *Phycomycetes*. The disease is characterized by pneumonia, invasion of pulmonary vessels, and infarction of the lung (Baker, 1956). It usually occurs in patients with diabetes, leukemia, or lymphoma.

ETIOLOGY. *Phycomycetes* are ubiquitous fungi of soil, fruits, vegetables, and moldy bread but have been isolated only rarely from the air in hospitals. Members of the order Mucorales, belonging to the genera *Mucor*, *Rhizopus*, and *Absidia*, have been isolated from rhinocerebral mucormycosis and other forms of human infection, but the exact genera causing most cases of pulmonary mucormycosis have not been identified. This is because diagnosis has been made not from culture but rather from the appearance of the nonseptate fungi in histologic sections of biopsies or postmortem tissues. In the few cases with positive cultures, the fungi have been identified as *Rhizopus pusillus* (see Chapter 80; Meyer et al., 1973), *Rhizopus* sp. (Record and Ginder, 1976) and *Absidia* sp. (Lombardi et al., 1970).

PATHOGENESIS AND PATHOLOGY. The spores of the Mucorales are inhaled through the nares into the nasal sinuses, bronchial tree, and lung parenchyma. An ulcer of the skin has also been proposed as a rare portal of entry from which the infection spreads to the lung. The hyphae invade blood vessels and cause pulmonary infarction, pulmonary hemorrhage, and gangrene of the lung. The bronchial walls and lymphatics may also be invaded. Pulmonary infarction may be secondary to thrombi that develop in the region of the fungus or to vascular occlusion by the mass of hyphal elements. The infarct may be large and fatal or small and nonprogressive; in the latter instance, it may produce a solitary nodule in the chest x-ray. The Mucorales also produce acute inflammation with a polymorphonuclear reaction unless the patient is severely neutropenic. The broad (4 to 20μ) nonseptate hyphae are surrounded by neutrophilic leukocytes. This inflammatory reaction gives a clinical picture of pneumonia or lung abscess. Thus, mucormycosis may be characterized by infarct, pneumonia, lung abscess, or a combination of the three processes.

Infection with *Phycomycetes* commonly occurs in compromised patients, including those with acute leukemia and lymphomas or recipients of kidney transplants. In most cases, the patients are receiving either corticosteroids, Cytoxan, or immunosuppressive agents. Diabetic patients, especially those in ketoacidosis, are also prone to mucormycosis.

CLINICAL PRESENTATION. Pulmonary mucormycosis may be acute and fulminant or subacute and slowly progressive. In the patient who is immunosuppressed or has an underlying malignancy, especially leukemia or lymphoma, the presence of chills, fever, and pulmonary infiltrates should rouse suspicion of infection with the Mucorales. Whereas bacterial, especially gram-negative, pneumonias are much more likely to cause this syndrome, the sudden development of chest pain (mainly pleuritic in nature), bloody sputum, pleural friction rub and the roentgenographic appearance of a pulmonary infarction should suggest mucormycosis. The usual picture, however, is that of a patchy, nonhomogeneous infiltrate that may progress despite antibiotic therapy to lobar consolidation with the development of a cavity. A hemorrhagic pleural effusion may also be found.

In diabetics, the disease may be less fulminant and produce a subacute pneumonitis with cavitation. Solitary pulmonary nodules, composed of a small mycotic infarct, have also been described (Gale and Kleitsch, 1972).

COMPLICATIONS. The three major complications of pulmonary mucormycosis are fatal hemorrhage, dissemination, and bacterial superinfection. Abrupt, massive, and fatal hemoptysis can occur if the pulmonary artery is eroded by the hyphae (Murray, 1975). Hematogenous dissemination reaches nearly every organ, including the heart, brain, kidney, thyroid, bone, pancreas, bowel and spleen (Meyer et al., 1973). Severe bacterial infections, especially with *Pseudomonas* or *Staphylococcus aureus*, may aggravate and obscure the fungus infection (Meyer et al., 1972).

DIAGNOSIS. The diagnosis must be suspected in a compromised patient with fever, pulmonary infarct, and an acute pneumonitis that does not respond to antibiotics (Fig. 1). *Phycomycetes* are rarely observed on Gram stain or isolated in sputum culture, and the specific diagnosis has most often been made post mortem or following open lung biopsy. Transbronchial biopsy of the lung parenchyma to obtain tissue for smears, culture, and pathologic sections may be useful if not contraindicated by thrombocytopenia. Platelet transfusions should be given before the procedure

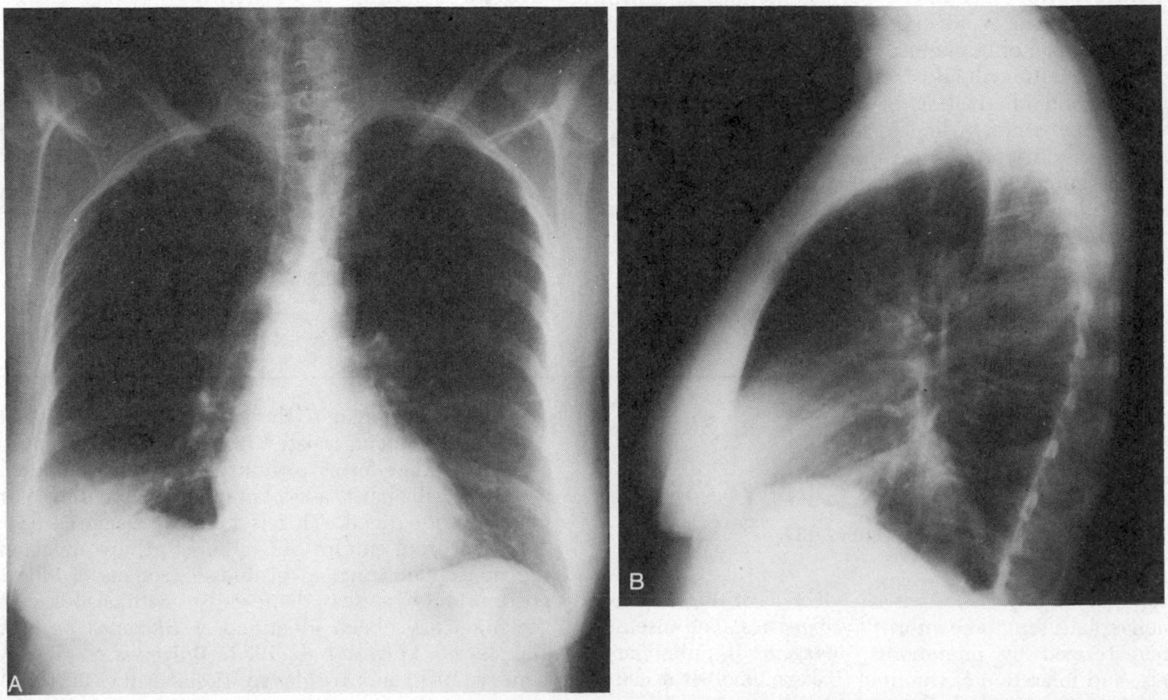

Figure 1. Mucormycosis of right lower lobe in patient with idiopathic pancytopenia. At autopsy there was invasion of the pulmonary artery and mediastinum by *Mucor.* A mycotic mural thrombus, 6 cm in length, of the abdominal aorta extended into the left renal artery where it produced necrotizing enteritis. *Mucor* was also isolated from skin lesions of the feet. The increased iron stores from transfusion for pancytopenia may have contributed to infection by saturating transferrin and thus making available adequate iron for growth of *Mucor* in the tissues.

in a thrombocytopenic patient. The presence of large, broad, nonseptate hyphae, sometimes with hyperacute, even right-angle, branching suggest that Mucorales are present. These fungi may be confused with aspergilli, though the latter are narrower and septate.

Clinical isolates should be grown on blood or Sabouraud's agar at 37° C. Growth usually appears at 1 to 2 days, though cultures should be kept for 10 to 14 days. The direct plating of biopsy material on agar has increased the yield of positive cultures. There are no reliable serologic tests for mucormycosis.

Differential diagnosis must take into account other microorganisms that produce pulmonary disease in the compromised patient. *Nocardia asteroides* may produce an acute necrotizing pneumonia, with a tendency to spread to the brain. The branching, gram-positive, partially acid-fast filamentous rods of *N. asteroides* are often seen in sputum smears of patients with pulmonary nocardiosis. *Pneumocystis carinii* infection and cytomegalic inclusion disease produce acute pneumonia in immunosuppressed patients, but often present as acute respiratory distress syndromes. The patients are dyspneic and hypoxic, and the roentgenograms reveal a diffuse interstitial pattern. Fiberoptic bronchoscopy with brushing and/or biopsy is necessary for the diagnosis of *Pneumocystis* infection. Cytomegalic inclusion disease may be diagnosed by serology or lung biopsy. The pulmonary vasculature is not invaded in either *Pneumocystis* or cytomegalovirus infections, and cavitation and pulmonary infarction are not found.

Aspergilli invade blood vessels and can produce a clinical picture identical to that of mucormycosis. *Aspergillus* pneumonia is more common in immunosuppressed patients, and aspergilli are the most common infectious agents found post mortem in patients with leukemia. Differentiation from mucormycosis must usually be made by transbronchial or open lung biopsy because aspergilli do not often appear in the sputum. If biopsy is impossible, amphotericin B therapy is warranted for patients who present the picture of mycotic pulmonary pneumonia with infarction.

TREATMENT. Prompt therapy is essential. Antileukemic and cancer chemotherapy should be regulated, if possible. Most cases of pulmonary mucormycosis have been terminal infections in debilitated patients with leukemia or lymphoma. Survival from pulmonary phycomycosis has been achieved, however, by treatment with Amphotericin B in a total intravenous dose of 1200 mg over 12 weeks in a patient with acute lymphocytic leukemia (Medoff and Kobayashi, 1972). The *Phycomycetes* are resistant to the imidazole derivatives. Surgical resection of infarcted lung has been performed successfully in some cases. It appears that pulmonary resection may be curative in patients without malignancy (Wright et al., 1980). The role of white blood cell transfusion in the leukopenic patient with these infections has not been determined. Without treatment, the infection is almost always lethal in patients with malignancies.

References

Baker, R. D.: Pulmonary mucormycosis. Am J Path 32:287, 1956.

Gale, A. M., and Kleitsch, W. E.: Solitary pulmonary nodule due to phycomycosis (mucormycosis). Chest 62:752, 1972.

Lombardi, D. L., Mason, J. O., and Hughes, R. K.: Pneumocystis and mucormycosis pneumonitis. Chest 57:318, 1970.

Medoff, G., and Kobayashi, G.: Pulmonary Mucormycosis. N Engl J Med 286:86, 1972.

Meyer, R., Kaplan, M., Ong., M., and Armstrong, D.: Cutaneous lesions in disseminated mucormycosis. JAMA 225:737, 1973.

Meyer, R., Rosen, P., and Armstrong, D.: Phycomycosis complicating leukemia and lymphoma. Ann Int Med 77:871, 1972.

Murray, H. W.: Pulmonary mucormycosis with massive fatal hemoptysis. Chest 68:65, 1975.

Record, N. B., Jr., and Ginder, D. R.: Pulmonary phycomycosis without obvious predisposing factors. JAMA 235:1256, 1976.

Wright, R. N., Saxena, A., Robin, A., and Thomas, P. A.: Pulmonary mucormycosis *(Phycomycetes)* successfully treated by resection. Ann Thorac Surg 2:166, 1980.

129

PARAGONIMIASIS

CHARLES E. DAVIS, M.D.

DEFINITION AND HISTORY. Paragonimiasis (endemic hemoptysis) is a lung infection of man and other mammals acquired by ingestion of fresh water crabs or crayfish infested with larvae of *Paragonimus*, the trematode lung fluke. Although it is widely distributed, the most important foci are in Southeast Asia and the Far East. It is often confused with tuberculosis because the adult worms are walled off in cystic cavities or "burrows" that cause hemoptysis when they erode into a bronchus. Nevertheless, it is a relatively benign disease unless the fluke localizes in ectopic foci like the brain.

Kerbert (1878) first described the adult fluke in the lungs of two Bengal tigers at the Amsterdam Zoo. He named the organism *Distoma* (two suckers—oral and ventral) *westermani* (after G. F. Westerman, who was the Director of the Amsterdam Zoo). In 1880, Ringer discovered an adult worm in the lung of a Formosan man at autopsy and forwarded it to Manson, who realized that its ova were identical to those in the bloody sputum of a Chinese patient that he was attending at the time. He also recognized that it was a distome and published these cases as human infections with *Distoma ringeri* (Manson, 1881). Manson subsequently studied the disease in Formosa while Baelz (1880) was making independent observations in Japan. When they exchanged specimens, they realized that "endemic hemoptysis" of Formosa and Japan were caused by the same parasite (Manson, 1883).

In 1889, Leuckhart concluded that the tiger and human lung flukes were identical. Braun (1899) first suggested the genus name of *Paragonimus*, but *Distoma* persisted for many years as an alternative name for *Paragonimus* and as the name for the Fasciola group of trematodes. "Pulmonary distomiasis" is still used occasionally as a synonym for paragonimiasis.

The life cycle of *Paragonimus* was worked out by Nakagawa (1916), who demonstrated larvae in the freshwater crab, S. Yokogawa (1915), who traced the migration of the fluke from the intestine to the lungs of the definitive host, and Ameel (1934), who described the developmental stages of *Paragonimus*.

Paragonimiasis is a major health problem in many parts of the world but is of far greater importance in Korea than in any other country. For this reason, the Korean War in the 1950s, which involved personnel from many countries, thrust this disease into international prominence.

ETIOLOGY. *Paragonimus* is a typical, hermaphroditic, leaf-like fluke that is thicker, broader, and more opaque than other flukes. It belongs to the family Troglotrematidae. The adult is red to brown and 7 to 12 mm long by 4 to 7 mm in width. External microscopic spines, a ventral and oral sucker of approximately equal size, and its ovoid, "fleshy" appearance help distinguish it from other trematodes (see Chapter 86). *P. westermani* (Fig. 1) is the chief human parasite.

Ova (Fig. 2) are operculated and undeveloped when they are excreted in the sputum or stool. Their size ranges from 80 to 120 μm in length by 50 to 60 μm in width. They are golden brown, broader at the operculated end, and form a thicker shell at the abopercular end.

Life Cycle. Ova are passed in the sputum or feces of the infected mammal. If they reach fresh water, they hatch within 17 to 28 days. The operculum opens to allow the free-swimming first larval stage (miracidium) to emerge. The miracidium penetrates various species of snails within 24 hours. The most important snail hosts in Asia are the species of *Semisulcospira* (Kobayashi, 1918), but other species serve as the first intermediate host in other geographic areas. During a three- to five-month developmental period in the snail, the larvae develop through two rediae stages to produce a stumpy-tailed, second larval stage called

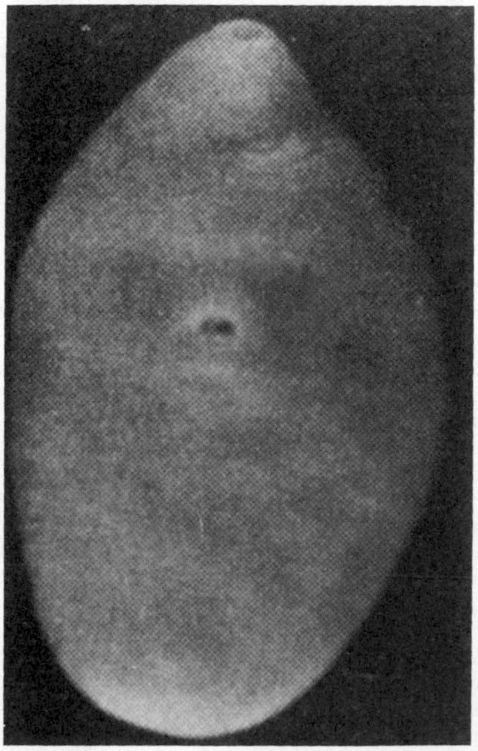

Figure 1. Adult *Paragonimus westermani.* × 5 (From Mitsuno et al.: J. Nerv Ment Dis 116:685, 1952.)

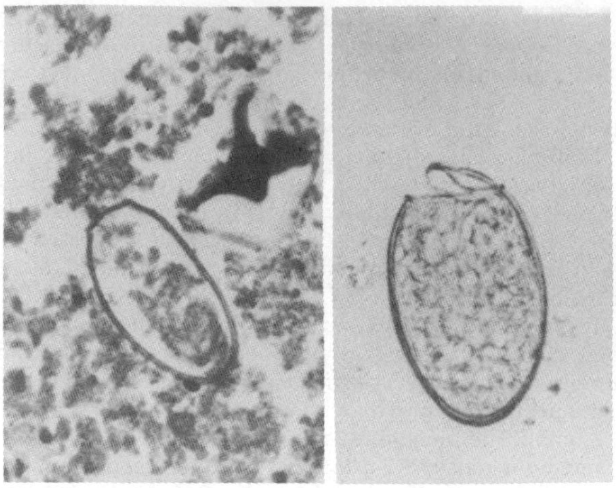

Figure 2. Ova of *P. westermani. Left,* typical appearance of egg in tissue section. The operculum is often missed because the section does not pass through the center of the ovum along its long axis. *Right,* typical ova with the operculum partly open. (From Mitsuno et al.: J Nerv Ment Dis 116:685, 1952.)

a cercaria. Freshwater crabs or crayfish either eat the digestive gland of the snails or are penetrated by free-swimming cercaria that have emerged from the tissues of the snail (Yokogawa, 1965). More than 11 different species of crayfish and crabs have been reported as second intermediate hosts of *P. westermani* alone. The distribution of *P. westermani* and the other species of *Paragonimus* is clearly dependent on the presence of the appropriate snail and freshwater crustacean.

Man is infected by eating raw, salted, or wine-soaked (drunken) fresh water crabs or crayfish. The disease is limited to areas where these crustaceans are eaten in this manner. Heating the crustaceans to 55° C kills the cercariae. However, Yokagawa (1965) has shown that infectious metacercariae that adhere to knives and strainers during the preparation of crabs for inclusion in soups and other cooked dishes can be transferred by these utensils and by hands to salads and other uncooked dishes. He suggests that this is probably the route of infection in geographic areas of Japan where crabs or crayfish are not ordinarily eaten raw. Another way that *Paragonimus* may be transmitted to people that do not ordinarily eat raw freshwater crustaceans is in folk medicines. Yun (1960) reported seven cases of paragonimiasis in children whose only exposure to raw crustaceans was the liquid from crushed, strained crayfish, which is a common folk remedy for measles in rural Korea.

More recently, it has been demonstrated that when wild boars ingest the metacercariae of *P. westermani,* the larvae do not migrate to the lungs. Instead, they encyst in the muscle. These encysted forms are immature and infectious for experimental animals and are probably the source of infection in some areas of Japan where raw freshwater crustaceans are not eaten (Miyazaki and Habe, 1976).

After man or other mammalian hosts ingest infected raw crabs or crayfish, the metacercariae encyst in the duodenum and migrate through the wall of the small intestine into the peritoneal cavity. Most reach the lungs by penetrating the diaphragm. Abnormal migration routes to ectopic sites are responsible for many of the bizarre and severe complications of paragonimiasis. The parasites are encapsulated by the host, develop into adults, and produce ova within four to six weeks. When the cyst erodes into a bronchus, ova are expectorated along with blood and purulent sputum. Swallowed ova are also excreted in the feces. When these ova reach fresh water, the life cycle begins again. The life span of adult *Paragonimus* varies, but some have lived at least 20 years (Yokogawa, 1965).

Speciation. For many years, the major issue in the speciation of *Paragonimus* was whether *P. westermani* was the only species that infected man. The criteria for speciation of *Paragonimus* progressed through two stages before the modern era. At first, each isolation of *Paragonimus* from a new host or a new geographic region was considered to be a new species. Later, most species were thought to be identical to *P. westermani*, which was assumed to be the only *Paragonimus* that infected man. Among the reasons for this confusion are the variation in the shape and size of ova produced by a single lung fluke and the fleshiness of adult flukes that makes it difficult to work out their internal morphology. Now, species are usually determined by the arrangement of the spines, the shape of the ovary and testes, the relative size of the oral and ventral suckers, and the properties of the ova. A lung fluke is usually not accepted as a new species, however, until the entire life cycle and each larval stage are described and characterized. Isoenzyme patterns may also be helpful (Zillman and Voelker, 1980).

Between 15 and 25 lung flukes from different mammalian hosts and geographic areas are thought to be distinct species by some investigators (Yokogawa, 1969). Of these, only a few have been isolated from man. *P. westermani* causes virtually all paragonimiasis in Asia and the Far East. *P. africanus* and *P. uterobilateralis* are newly recognized species that are probably responsible for West African paragonimiasis. *P. mexicanus* has caused autochthonous cases of human paragonimiasis in Mexico, Central America, and Peru. *P. ecuadoriensis* may be a distinct South American species. *P. kellicotti* is a well-defined species that has been isolated from many wild and domestic animals in the western hemisphere and has probably caused rare autochthonous human cases in the United States. *P. heterotremus* and *P. skrjabini* are rare causes of human paragonimiasis in China.

P. westermani is by far the most important cause of paragonimiasis in humans and may coexist with the other valid species in Central America, South America, and Africa. All species require snails as the first intermediate host and utilize crabs or crayfish as the normal second intermediate host. The species of snail or fresh-water crustacean may differ. The species that have been isolated from man are thought to cause identical diseases.

GEOGRAPHIC DISTRIBUTION AND HOST RANGE. The human species of *Paragonimus* are widely distributed over three land masses: Asia, Africa, and the western hemisphere. The most important foci of infection in Asia and the Far East are in China, Japan, Taiwan, Korea, the Philippines, Thailand, Laos, and Vietnam. There are major foci in many West African countries including Nigeria, Guinea, Liberia, the Ivory Coast, the Republic of Dahomey, Cameroon, and the Zaire Republic. Paragonimiasis occurs in Mexico and all of Central America, but Costa Rica has the highest prevalence. Cases have been documented from Peru, Ecuador, Venezuela, Brazil, and Colombia in South America (Yokogawa, 1969). The other species of *Paragonimus* that usually infect only wild and domestic animals are even more widely distributed. It is likely that the geographic distribution of human paragonimiasis is limited primarily by the eating habits of the population. Civil war in Nigeria from 1967 to 1970 caused massive population movements and short food and cooking supplies. As a result large numbers of people turned to improperly cooked freshwater crabs as a source of protein. This change in eating habits caused a hundred-fold increase in the number of recognized cases of paragonimiasis in some areas of Nigeria after the civil war (Nwokolo, 1972).

All species of *Paragonimus*, including *P. westermani*, infect wild and domestic animals. Paragonimiasis has been reported to infect almost every carnivorous animal, but members of the cat family, dog family, and pigs are among the most common hosts. Minks are commonly infected with *P. kellicotti* in the United States.

PATHOGENESIS AND PATHOLOGY. The pathologic manifestations of paragonimiasis are related to the migratory route of the larvae and the inflammatory response stimulated by the larvae and adult worms. In experimental infections, only a small percentage of ingested worms reach the lungs. Mild inflammatory changes occur at the site of penetration through the small intestine, but some young flukes do not penetrate. Instead, they encyst in the intestinal mucosa, develop into adults, and produce ova. Inflammation may progress to ulceration and excretion of ova in the stool. Parasites that localize in the abdominal cavity may provoke an abscess that simulates an intra-abdominal bacterial infection. Eosinophilia occurs during the migratory phase but usually subsides after the worms have encysted in the lung.

The typical manifestations of paragonimiasis occur in the lungs. Migration of the larvae across the pleural space into the lung parenchyma from the diaphragm can cause pneumothorax and pleural effusion. Intrapulmonary migration causes transient eosinophilia and polymorphonuclear infiltration that may resemble Löeffler's syndrome. After migration, the developing parasite elicits a polymorphonuclear response, necrosis of the parenchyma, and formation of a fibrous tissue capsule (Fig. 3). The necrosis in the center of the cyst or capsule is induced partly by the polymorphonuclear enzymes but may also be formed by arteriolar obstruction and infarction (Diaconita and Goldis, 1964). These cavities or "burrows" become walled off by fibrous transformation that is partly contributed by foreign body granulomas. These granulomas usually surround the cavity and encircle ova or egg shells. The egg tubercles consist of lymphocytes, plasma cells, eosinophils, fibroblasts, and histiocytes. Langhan's giant cells and multinuclear foreign body cells sometimes engulf the ova. Calcification of old lesions is usually in the vicinity of the eggs in these egg granulomas. Interstitial pneumonia and bronchopneumonia with peribronchitis and endobronchitis may occur during migration but also often accompany erosion of the cavities into bronchioles. After the rupture, the sputum consists of mixtures of polymorphonuclear leukocytes, lymphocytes, ova, and blood.

Grossly, the cavities are grayish-white nodules that vary from grape to plum size. On section they are irregular or uneven in shape. The cyst walls are thick and fibrosclerotic (Yokogawa, 1965). Microscopically, they consist of the egg granulomas described above. The adult fluke may be seen either grossly or microscopically within the cavities.

Hyperplasia of the bronchial epithelium and bronchial erosion and ulceration occur in the area of the cysts. The bronchiectasis that complicates chronic paragonimiasis is

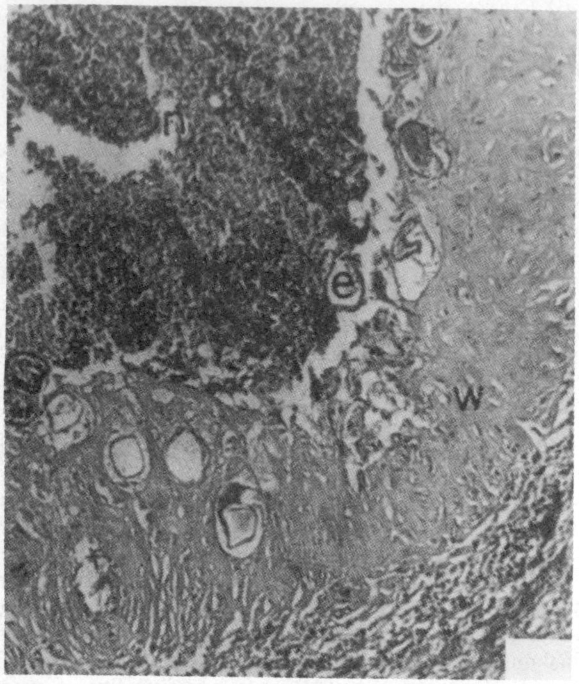

Figure 3. *Paragonimus* cyst. n = necrotic debris, e = ova, which are most concentrated along the inner aspect of the cyst wall, w = cyst wall composed of a dense layer of collagenous connective tissue and chronic inflammation. (From Mitsuno et al.: J Nerv Ment Dis 116:685, 1952.)

caused by bronchial obstruction secondary to *Paragonimus* cavities and bronchial inflammation and hyperplasia.

Toxins have not been isolated from *Paragonimus* and it seems likely that arteriolar inflammation and egg granulomas are elicited mechanically and by hypersensitivity. The gamma-globulin concentrations are high during this stage of the disease (Sadun and Buck, 1960), and fully developed tubercles develop alongside foreign body granulomas.

Ectopic paragonimiasis of the brain and other organs causes "burrows" or cavities and granulomas similar to those in the lung (Mitsuno et al., 1952). The lesions enlarge during the process of liquefaction, probably because fluid is imbibed, and cause brain damage and atrophy. Calcification of the abundant granulomas is common. Adult flukes are found less commonly in cavities in the brain than the lung. The reasons for this difference are not known, but it is possible that adult flukes migrate out of this abnormal site. Yokogawa (1921) found larvae in the loose connective tissue of the neck and suggested that the larvae migrate through the loose connective tissue along the blood vessels and nerve trunks through the jugular foramen into the brain. Experimentally, flukes migrated out of the brain into the pleural cavity by way of the cerebral sinuses, the internal jugular veins, and the pulmonary arteries (Yokogawa, 1921).

CLINICAL MANIFESTATIONS. The typical patient with pulmonary paragonimiasis presents to the physician with a history of chronic bronchitis and blood-tinged or reddish-brown sputum. In spite of a long history of disease, the general health is often unimpaired. Cough occurs predominantly in the early morning and produces gelatinous or blood-tinged sputum that is either streaked with blood or is a reddish-brown color. Among 270 Koreans who did not seek medical advice but had *Paragonimus* ova in their sputum, almost 25 per cent were asymptomatic (Sadun and Buck, 1960). The percentage of asymptomatic patients decreased with advancing years. Almost all patients over 30 years of age had pulmonary symptoms, and 72 per cent of the 270 had hemoptysis.

Hemoptysis occurs in 65 to 100 per cent of hospitalized patients. If blood-tinged sputum, brownish or red sputum, and frank hemoptysis are included in the definition of hemoptysis, 80 to 100 per cent of patients are affected (Table 1). Chest pain, occurring in about a third of patients, is usually pleuritic in nature and may be accompanied by pleural effusion or empyema. Fever at the time of admission to the hospital is common but may subside on bed rest. Loss of appetite and weight loss occur in about 10 per cent of patients.

Physical findings are sparse. Dullness and rales are distinctly uncommon and suggest the possibility of coexisting pulmonary tuberculosis or bacterial pneumonia. Clubbing of the fingers is uncommon unless the patient has developed full-blown bronchiectasis.

The white blood cell count may be slightly elevated early in the course of pulmonary involvement but returns to normal after the first year. Low-grade, peripheral eosinophilia is a uniform finding. Eosinophilia to 50 per cent may occur during the migratory phase of early infection. Elevation of the gamma globulins with a reduction in albumin and other globulins is a common finding.

Most patients have abnormal chest x-rays. Chien (1955) and Sadun and Buck (1960) described a typical pattern of changes progressing from the early active stages to late

Table 1. SYMPTOMS AND SIGNS OF PULMONARY PARAGONIMIASIS IN HOSPITALIZED PATIENTS[a]

Symptom or Sign	Per Cent	Comment
Cough	95	
Hemoptysis	80–100	blood-tinged, reddish-brown, and frank hemorrhage
Chest pain	36	
Fever and night sweats	33	
Weight loss	11	
Physical examination		
Dullness and rales	—	unusual
Laboratory examination		
Leukocytosis above 10,000/mm³	20	early infections
Eosinophilia 10 to 20 per cent	100	
Hypergammaglobulinemia	—	statistically significant difference between patients and controls
X-ray		
Abnormal chest x-ray	76–100	
Pleural effusion or empyema	13	

[a]Number of patients evaluated ranges from 63 to more than 250 depending on the symptom or sign. Data from series published by Sadun and Buck, 1960; Nwokolo, 1972; Iwasaki, 1955.

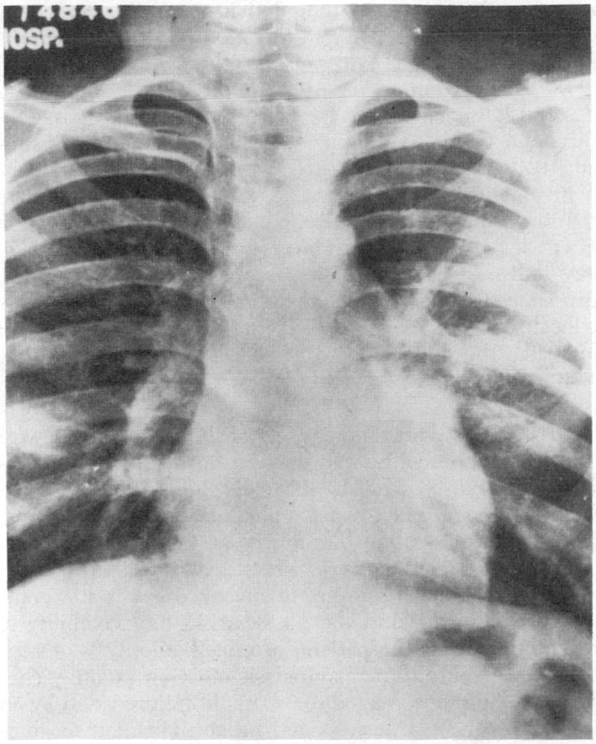

Figure 4. Infiltrative form of pulmonary paragonimiasis. No cysts or cavities could be detected on tomograms. (From Sadun, E., and Buck, A.: Am J Trop Med Hyg 9:562, 1960.)

residual stages after the parasites have died. A pulmonary infiltrate with the appearance of localized pneumonitis occurs in response to parenchymal migration. Cysts may or may not be present (Figs. 4 and 5). The infiltrate is

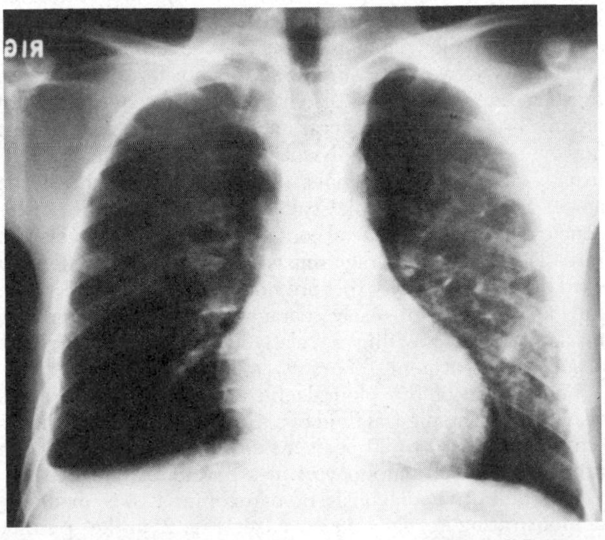

Figure 5. A 14-year-old Laotian with hemoptysis and *Paragonimus* ova in sputum and stool. Extensive reticular infiltrates with loss of volume are most prominent in the superior segment of the left lower lobe. There are no large cavities but lucencies within the infiltrate may represent *Paragonimus* cysts. Bilateral pleural disease is more prominent on the right. (From University of California at San Diego Medical Center, Case number 7511728-G.)

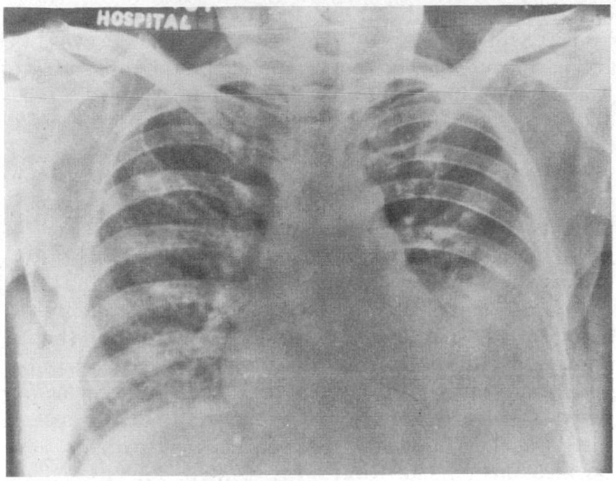

Figure 6. Disseminated nodular-cystic paragonimiasis with left empyema. (From Sadun, E., and Buck, A.: Am J Trop Med Hyg 9:562, 1960.)

replaced by isolated nodules that may cavitate because of air that has entered the nodules from the bronchioles. These nodules may be infraclavicular, basal, or disseminated (Fig. 6). One or two basal, round or elliptical nodules are easy to diagnose as possible paragonimiasis, but the disseminated form in which nodules of various densities are found in x-rays of both lungs is frequently confused with tuberculosis. The fact that the apex is usually spared, however, should cast doubt on the diagnosis of tuberculosis. The late stages of the disease are characterized by fibrosis and calcification that occur after the parasite dies. Fibrosis also occurs outside the nodular areas and may be extensive. Round or oval spots of calcification represent areas where cysts have been absorbed and replaced by calcification. Individuals who live in endemic areas are reinfected frequently and may have lesions in all stages.

Pleural reactions are common and are often bilateral. They range from small effusions to thickened, fibrotic pleura. The fibrotic tissue examined after decortication frequently contains ova.

COMPLICATIONS AND SEQUELAE. The major pulmonary complications include bronchiectasis, fibrosis, and chronic obstructive bronchopulmonary disease. Right heart failure occurs rarely. Superimposed pulmonary tuberculosis and pyogenic pneumonia are common complications.

The most dramatic complications of paragonimiasis occur, however, when the young flukes fail to reach the lung or migrate into ectopic foci. The worm often encysts widely in the abdomen and pelvis. The retroperitoneum, scrotum, kidneys, mediastinum, lymph nodes, and orbit are less frequently invaded (Mitsuno et al., 1952). By far the most common and most threatening extrathoracic localization, however, is in the brain. Of 143 patients with paragonimiasis studied by Sadun and Buck (1960), 22 (15 per cent) had extrathoracic lesions. The brain was invaded in 12 (8 per cent). Thus, in this series as well as in many others (Yokogawa, 1965), cerebral paragonimiasis accounts for about half the ectopic foci. It is more common in men than women and usually occurs in children and young adults (76 per cent under age 20) (Mitsuno et al., 1952). The age distribution probably represents the fact that most patients with cerebral paragonimiasis die before age 20. The frequency of reported cerebral foci in paragonimiasis varies from 0.8 per cent to 26 per cent (Oh, 1968; Yokogawa, 1965). Since 50 per cent of the population of some areas of Korea were estimated to have paragonimiasis in the 1950s and 1960s, it is very possible that 0.5 per cent or more of the population had cerebral paragonimiasis.

In the acute stage or in spinal cord localization, meningitis may be the presenting syndrome. More commonly, patients present with epilepsy, tumor syndromes, or organic brain syndromes. Headache, seizures, visual disturbances, and motor and sensory disorders are the most common symptoms. Mental deterioration, hemiplegia, hemihypesthesia, homonymous hemianopsia, and optic atrophy are the most common signs (Oh, 1968). Lumbar puncture reveals a pleocytosis of 3 to 125 leukocytes per mm^3, an elevated protein concentration, and a normal sugar level. More than 50 per cent of patients have calcifications on skull x-rays (Fig. 7) (Oh, 1968). Calcifications are usually found in clusters of a few to more than 50 more or less spherical elements ranging in size from a few to more than 30 mm (Galatius-Jensen and Uhm, 1965). Calcifications are most common in the occipital and parietal areas, slightly less common in the temporal lobes, and unusual in the frontal lobe. Without surgical intervention, the time from onset of symptoms to death varies from one to four years.

Ectopic lesions in other organs usually cause the symptoms of either abscess or tumor. Hematuria is a common presenting symptom of renal paragonimiasis. Paragonimiasis of the abdominal wall has simulated appendicitis.

GEOGRAPHIC VARIATIONS IN DISEASE. Oriental paragonimiasis caused predominantly by *P. westermani* has been more extensively studied than American infections with *P. mexicanus* or African infections with *P. africanus.* To date, there is no evidence that the syndromes caused by these major human parasites are different. *P. heterotremus* and *P. skrjabini* are rare causes of pulmonary paragonimiasis in China. Most patients have had migratory subcutaneous swellings with or without pulmonary involvement. Hepatic migration with severe liver damage is also a common manifestation of *P. skrjabini* infection (Hu et al., 1982). This high incidence of ectopic localization may indicate that these species are not well adapted to man, since the major human parasite, *P. westermani,* seems to localize in the muscle and subcutaneous tissue of unusual hosts like the hog, rat, and chicken (Miyazaki and Habe, 1976).

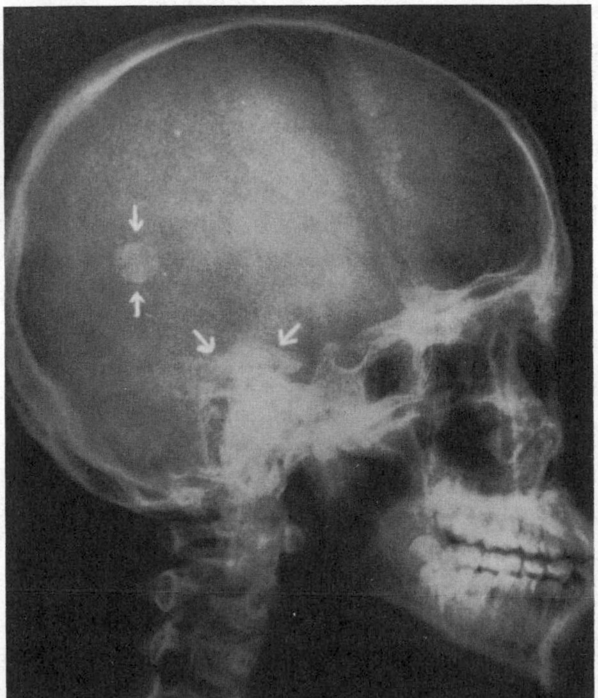

Figure 7. Intracerebral calcification of *Paragonimus* cysts in 18-year-old with Jacksonian epilepsy. (From Sadun, E., and Buck, A.: Am J Trop Med Hyg 9:562, 1960.)

DIAGNOSIS. Paragonimiasis is most often confused with pulmonary tuberculosis but may be misdiagnosed as aspiration lung abscess or, in the early infiltrative stage, as bacterial or viral pneumonia. Pulmonary fungal infections, like histoplasmosis and blastomycosis, could also be mistaken for paragonimiasis in areas where these diseases coexist. A history of exposure to uncooked freshwater crabs or crayfish should alert the physician to the possibility of paragonimiasis. If the patient also has hemoptysis or reddish-brown sputum, paragonimiasis must be carefully considered. Aspiration lung abscess should be preceded by an episode of unconsciousness and be accompanied by foul-smelling and tasting (fetid) sputum. The color of the sputum, frequent absence of fever (especially on bed rest), and the usual relative well-being of the patient with paragonimiasis help differentiate it from bacterial and viral pneumonias. Serologies and skin tests for pulmonary fungal infections and the color and nature of the sputum in paragonimiasis aid in the differentiation between these diseases.

Except for miliary lesions and extensive bronchopneumonia, almost all of the roentgenographic features of pulmonary tuberculosis may be mimicked by paragonimiasis. Furthermore, as many as 30 to 100 per cent of patients in areas endemic for paragonimiasis may have positive tuberculin tests (Nwokolo, 1972; Sadun and Buck, 1960). In these areas, patients may also have active disease with both organisms. There are several major radiologic differences, however, (Ogakwu and Nwokolo, 1973). Paragonimiasis usually affects the midzones of the lungs instead of the apices and causes "bubble" cavities, smooth-edged translucencies within an area of consolidation. Fluid levels are rare. The lesions of paragonimiasis are often poorly defined shadows of low density that are not very extensive. Finally, the appearance of early paragonimiasis may undergo marked changes within a relatively short period in the absence of treatment.

The nature of the pleural effusion in the two diseases also differs. The pleural fluid of patients with paragonimiasis often contains 80 to 90 per cent eosinophils instead of the predominance of lymphocytes in tuberculous effusions.

The definitive diagnosis of paragonimiasis is made by demonstrating *Paragonimus* ova (see Fig. 2) in the sputum. If three specimens are examined, the direct sputum is positive in about 80 per cent of patients with pulmonary paragonimiasis and pigmented sputum. Concentration of 24-hour sputum collection by techniques like those used for acid-fast bacilli will identify ova in an additional 12 to 15 per cent. Direct and concentrated stools will also reveal ova in a high percentage of patients because of the habit of swallowing sputum. Finally, surgical specimens should be examined grossly for the adult fluke (see Fig. 1) and sections carefully examined for the ova.

In patients with extrapulmonary paragonimiasis and some patients with pulmonary disease, ova may not be detected. In these cases the skin test and serologic tests are particularly valuable. The complement fixation test performed with a fractionated antigen from the adult worm (Sawada et al., 1968) is usually positive only in active disease. The skin test with purified antigens standardized to contain 10 mg of protein/100 ml was first widely used by Sadun and Buck (1960). It produces a wheal within 15 to 20 minutes that is at least twice the size of a control injection of buffered saline in virtually 100 per cent of patients with paragonimiasis. It also cross-reacts strongly with *Clonorchis sinensis* and remains positive after successful treatment or self-cure. Yokogawa (1969) found that in patients without demonstrable ova in the sputum, a positive complement fixation test correlated with improvement after specific treatment. Patients with a positive skin test and a negative complement fixation test did not improve. Counterimmunoelectrophoresis of the patient's serum against *Paragonimus* antigens may prove to be as reliable as the complement fixation test (Hu et al., 1982).

TREATMENT. Bithionol, 2,2' thiobis (4,6-dichlorophenol), was the treatment of choice for paragonimiasis for many years, but this effective parenteral drug may soon be replaced by oral praziquantel. Bithionol interferes with fumarate utilization by inhibiting fumarate reductase (Hamajima et al., 1979) and causes separation of the tegument from the basement membrane and deterioration of structures beneath the membrane.

A daily dosage of 30 to 40 mg/kg orally every other day for 10 to 15 doses cures more than 90 per cent of patients with paragonimiasis (Yokogawa et al., 1963). Ova usually disappear within ten days and the chest x-ray improves within two weeks. Only a few chest x-rays remain abnormal after 6 to 12 months. Relapses usually respond to retreatment.

Bithionol also acts on flukes in ectopic foci. Good results have been obtained in several patients with cerebral paragonimiasis. This is important because surgical management is difficult and often disappointing.

Diarrhea is the most common side effect. It may occur in as many as 50 per cent of patients but is usually transient and subsides within a few days after treatment is completed. Severely pruritic generalized urticarial or papular skin eruptions occur in about 15 per cent of patients about one to two weeks after beginning therapy. The rash is probably stimulated by allergic reactions to destroyed worms because it occurs most frequently in patients with very heavy infections. Headache and giddiness occur in about 10 per cent of patients.

Praziquantel, a heterocyclic pyrazinoisoquinoline, has broad-spectrum activity against trematodes and cestodes. It has few side effects at therapeutic doses and can be given in a single oral dose for some forms of schistosomiasis (See Chapter 145). It has been used successfully for the treatment of paragonimiasis in a dosage of 25 mg per kg three times a day for 2 days (Monson et al., 1983; Rim and Chang, 1980; and Vanijanonta et al., 1981). It has fewer side effects than niclofolan, an oral veterinary drug for fascioliasis, which has also been used successfully to treat African and Asian paragonimiasis at a single dose of 2 mg per kg (Rim and Chang, 1980).

Decortication with or without thoracoplasty has been used successfully to treat chronic, unresponsive empyema.

PROPHYLAXIS. Ova in the excreta of people with paragonimiasis are the major source of contamination of freshwater crustaceans. Wild and domestic animals are a minor reservoir (Yokogawa, 1965). Accordingly, Yokogawa (1965) and Kim (1970) have shown that mass therapy with bithionol is effective and causes the disease to die out slowly in the tested area. Now that praziquantel is available, single dose mass therapy with this oral agent is probably the prophylactic technique of choice. Eradication of the snail host is impractical, and hungry populations cannot be educated to avoid the use of night soil on their crops or to stop eating the abundant crustaceans. Efforts to teach the people to cook crayfish and crabs should be continued even though they have not been well accepted.

References

Ameel, D. J.: *Paragonimus,* its life history and distribution in North America and its taxonomy (Trematoda: Troglotrematidae). Am J Hyg 19:279, 1934.

Baelz, E.: Über parasitäre Häemoptoë (Gregarinosis pulmonum). Zentralbl Med Wissensch 18:721, 1880.

Braun, M.: Über clinostomum Leidy. Zool Anz 22:484, 1899.

Chien, M. H.: Roentgenological diagnosis of paragonimiasis. Chin M J 73:37, 1955.

Diaconita, G. H., and Goldis, G. H.: Investigations on pathmorphology and pathogenesis of pulmonary paragonimiasis. Acta Turberc Scand 44:51, 1964.

Galatius-Jensen, F., and Uhm, I. K.: Radiological aspects of cerebral paragonimiasis. Br J Radiol 38:404, 1965.

Hamajima, F., Fujino, T., Yamagami, K., and Eriguchi, N.: Studies of the *in vitro* effects of bithionol and menicholopholan on flukes of *Clonorchis sinensis, Metagonimus takahashii* and *Paragonimus miyazakii.* Int J Parasitol 9:241, 1979.

Hu, X., Feng, R., Zheng, Z., Liang, J., Wang, H., and Lu, J.: Hepatic damage in experimental and clinical paragonimiasis. Am J Trop Med Hyg 31:1148, 1982.

Iwasaki, M.: Clinical studies of paragonimiasis (in Japanese). Rinshō Naiko Shōnika 10:207, 1955.

Kerbert, C.: Zur trematoden Kenntnis. Zool Anz 1:271, 1878.

Kim, J.: Treatment of *Paragonimus westermani* infections with bithionol. Am J Trop Med Hyg 19:940, 1970.

Kobayashi, H.: Studies on the lung fluke in Korea. I. On the life history and morphology of the lung fluke. Mil Med Hochs Keijo 2:95, 1918.

Leuckhart, R.: Die parasiten des Menschen und die von ihnen herrührendra Krankheiten, 2nd ed. Leipzig, C. F. Winter, 1889.

Manson, P.: On endemic hemoptysis. Lancet I:532, 1883.

Manson, P.: *Distoma ringeri.* M Times Gaz 2:8, 1881.

Mitsuno, T., Siko, T., Inanaga, K., and Zimmerman, L. E.: Cerebral paragonimiasis, a neurosurgical problem in the Far East. J Nerv Ment Dis 116:685, 1952.

Miyazaki, I., and Habe, S.: A newly recognized mode of human infection with the lung fluke, *Paragonimus westermani* (Kerbert, 1878). J Parasitol 62:646, 1976.

Monson, M. H., Koenig, J. W., and Sachs, R.: Successful treatment of six patients infected with the African lung fluke: *Paragonimus uterobilateralis.* Am J Trop Med Hyg 32:371, 1983.

Nakagawa, K.: The mode of infection in pulmonary distomiasis. Certain fresh water crabs as intermediate hosts of *Paragonimus westermani.* J Infect Dis 18:131, 1916.

Nwokolo. C.: Endemic paragonimiasis in Eastern Nigeria. Clinical features of the recent outbreak following the Nigerian civil war. Trop Geogr Med 24:138, 1972.

Ogakwu, M., and Nwokolo, C.: Radiological findings in pulmonary paragonimiasis as seen in Nigeria: A review based on one hundred cases. Br J Radiol 46:699, 1973.

Oh, S. J.: Paragonimus meningitis. J Neurol Sci 6:419, 1968.

Rim, H. J., and Chang, Y. S.: Chemotherapeutic effect of niclofolan and praziquantel in the treatment of paragonimiasis. Korean Univ Med J 17:113, 1980.

Sadun, E., and Buck, A.: Paragonimiasis in South Korea—immunodiagnostic, epidemiologic, clinical, roentgenologic and therapeutic studies. Am J Trop Med Hyg 9:562, 1960.

Sawada, T., Takei, K., Sato, S., and Matsuyama, S.: Studies on the immunodiagnosis of paragonimiasis. 3. Intradermal skin tests with fractionated antigens. J Infect Dis 118:235, 1968.

Vanijanonta, S., Radomyos, P., Bunnag, D., and Harinasuto, T.: Pulmonary paragonimiasis with expectoration of worms: a case report. Southeast Asian J Trop Med Publ Hlth 12:104, 1981.

Yokogawa, M.: Paragonimus and paragonimiasis. Adv Parasitol 3:99, 1965.

Yokogawa, M.: Paragonimus and paragonimiasis. Adv Parasitol 7:375, 1969.

Yokogawa, M., Iwasaki, M., Shigeyasu, M., Hirose, H., Okura, T., and Tsuji, M.: Chemotherapy of paragonimiasis with bithionol. V. Studies on the minimum effective dose and changes in abnormal x-ray shadows in chest after treatment. Am J Trop Med Hyg 12:859, 1963.

Yokogawa, S.: On the migratory course of the human lung fluke in the final host (in Japanese). Taiwan Igakkwai Zasshi 152-153:685–728, 1915.

Yokogawa, S.: An experimental study of the intracranial parasitism of the human lung fluid, *Paragonimus westermani*. Am J Hyg 1:63, 1921.

Yun, D. J.: Paragonimiasis in children in Korea. J. Pediatr 56:736, 1960.

Zillman, U., and Voelker, J.: Species characterization of the lung fluke *Paragonimus ecuadoriensis* by isozyme electrophoresis. Tropenmed Parasitol 31:15, 1980.

130

INFECTION WITH PNEUMOCYSTIS CARINII

STEPHEN N. COHEN, M.D.

The protozoan *Pneumocystis carinii* is the most frequent cause of sporadic interstitial pneumonia in immunosuppressed patients, particularly among patients with the Acquired Immunodeficiency Syndrome (AIDS) and individuals who have received prolonged corticosteroid therapy for lymphoproliferative malignancy, organ transplantation, or collagen-vascular disease. Less frequent today, *Pneumocystis* also has presented as an endemic and intermittently epidemic illness in premature or malnourished infants. Ruskin and Hughes (1983) have authoritatively reviewed our knowledge of this infection.

ETIOLOGY. *Pneumocystis* was first detected in the lungs of guinea pigs and rats by the Brazilian investigators Chagas (1909) and Carini (1910), who considered it an unusual variant of the trypanosomes with which they had experimentally infected the rodents. Shortly thereafter, the Delanöes at the Institut Pasteur in Paris demonstrated these structures in the lungs of ordinary sewer rats and appreciated that they were a unique new microorganism, which they named *P. carinii* (Delanöe and Delanöe, 1912). Thirty years then elasped before *Pneumocystis* was definitely associated with human disease by Van der Meer and Brug in 1942, who described three cases of pneumonia caused by this organism.

Our limited ability to propagate *Pneumocystis* in vitro has prevented the fulfillment of Koch's postulates and seriously hampered the study of *P. carinii*. Many wild and domestic animals are naturally infected with *Pneumocystis*, but the organisms are ordinarily sparse and difficult to detect. Corticosteroids activate latent *Pneumocystis* infection of rodents, providing a model infection with a large number of organisms (Weller, 1956; Frenkel et al., 1966). Electronmicroscopic investigation of the organism's life cycle in animals (Campbell, 1972) and the response of experimental infection to treatment with classic antiprotozoal chemotherapy are the basis for characterizing *P. carinii* as a protozoan. The trophozoite is probably motile, may reproduce by binary fission, and invades the lung parenchyma. The trophozoite wall then thickens, and the organisms encyst. The cyst matures with the development of eight intracystic sporozoites or "daughter" bodies, which are liberated when the cyst wall ruptures and, in turn, develop into trophozoites (Fig. 1). Serologic studies and experimental cross-infection with morphologically identical human and animal strains of *P. carinii* demonstrate some species-specificity (Walzer and Rutledge, 1980), although the histologic features of the infections are similar.

PATHOGENESIS. Animal studies suggest that the usual mode of acquisition of *Pneumocystis carinii* is the airborne route (Hughes, 1982). Most infants involved in nursery epidemics are about 4 months old, an age that allows little environmental contact and coincides with the physiologic nadir of serum immune globulin levels. However, most infected infants are not hypogammaglobulinemic, and there is no consistent correlation between immunoglobulin levels per se and *Pneumocystis* infection in either infants or adults.

Unrecognized infection with *P. carinii* must be extremely common in infancy, one survey finding immunofluorescent antibody in 100 per cent of children two years of age (Meuwissen et al., 1977).

Sporadic *Pneumocystis* pneumonia is five times more common in the first year of life than at any other age, and over 25 per cent of sporadic illness occurs before age 5 years. Nursery outbreaks, which were common in Europe during the early post-World War II years, have become unusual there, but outbreaks have subsequently been reported from Korea, Vietnam, and Iran under similar conditions of crowding and malnutrition. The adult patients who are most likely to present with *Pneumocystis* infection frequently suffer as well from reactivation of a variety of latent infections (tuberculosis, cryptococcosis, varicella-zoster infection, cytomegalovirus [CMV], toxoplasmosis). Cell-mediated immune mechanisms are probably more important than humoral defenses against all of these infections, and are impaired in these patients.

A number of case reports, as well as serologic studies showing a greater prevalence of antibody to *Pneumocystis* in contacts of infected patients than in healthy adults, suggest that person-to-person spread of infection in hospital among immunosuppressed patients or in the family is possible, and airborne transmission of experimental infection has been unequivocally demonstrated (Hendley and Weller, 1971).

The pathogenesis of *Pneumocystis* infection probably begins with the excretion of trophozoites of *P. carinii* (or perhaps cysts, which might be hardier) in the fomites of individuals whose pulmonary infection is mild. The organisms are then aspirated and transformed, if initially encysted, into invasive trophozoites upon reaching the alveoli, and attach to type I pneumocytes, whereupon the normal host's leukocytes, primarily macrophages, rapidly phago-

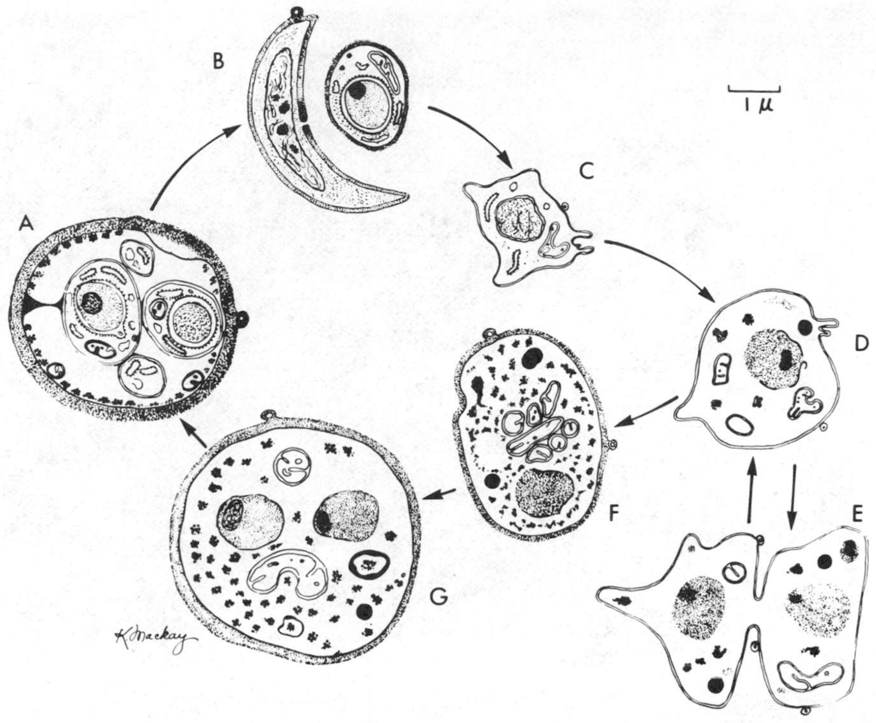

Figure 1. Probable life cycle of *Pneumocystis* within pulmonary alveoli. *A*, Mature cyst with intracystic bodies; *B*, empty cyst and recently escaped intracystic body; *C*, small trophozoite; *D*, larger trophozoite; *E*, possible budding or conjugating form; *F*, large trophozoite undergoing thickening of pellicle; *G*, precyst. (From Campbell, W. G. Jr.: Ultrastructure of pneumocystis in human lung. Arch Pathol 93:312, 1972.)

cytize and destroy most of them. Antibody and complement facilitate phagocytosis by macrophages (Masur and Jones, 1978), but are probably not directly lethal to the organism (Pesanti, 1980) and not critical in determining the outcome of infection. Clinical disease is either absent or mild. A small proportion of organisms encyst and escape destruction by the host defenses. These organisms persist in the tissues, possibly for the life of the host, but they may be intermittently released, like the periodic excretion of EB virus or CMV by the normal host, perhaps during intercurrent viral infection. In infants and children with defective cell-mediated immunity due to malnutrition, congenital deficiencies (usually lymphopenic hypogammaglobulinemias) or immunosuppression due to chemotherapy such as cyclophosphamide and/or corticosteroids, and very rarely in apparently normal persons, the primary infection develops into a severe interstitial pneumonia. Primary infection may also cause *Pneumocystis* pneumonia in immunologically depressed adults who will usually have been receiving corticosteroid therapy, but most pneumonia in the adult arises from the uncontrolled reactivation of latent infection. If the infection is not limited by the immune defenses, the organisms proliferate and attach to and occlude the alveolar surfaces, causing an alveolar-capillary block with hypoxia. The type I pneumocytes degenerate, with exudation of serum and tissue fluid into the alveolus, entry of the parasite into the interstitium, and further impairment of gas exchange (Yoneda and Walzer, 1980). Many episodes of *Pneumocystis* pneumonia arise as steroid therapy is being reduced, suggesting that the inflammatory reaction to infection contributes to the pulmonary disease.

PATHOLOGY. The lungs of a patient with severe, diffuse, interstitial pneumonia resemble liver tissue, are heavy, and are usually dark bluish-purple. Only the marginal areas may be aerated. Subpleural air blebs may rupture and presumably cause occasional spontaneous pneumothorax. There is rarely a pleural reaction or necrosis of the lung unless *Pneumocystis* infection is complicated by infection with other organisms. Less extensively involved lungs do not have so characteristic an appearance.

Microscopically, the alveoli of hematoxylin-eosin stained sections are filled with pinkish, foamy, honeycombed or vacuolated material, the clear areas often containing small dots (Figs. 2 and 3). The alveolar content is PAS-positive and consists largely of coalesced, desquamated macrophages whose digestive vacuoles contain degenerating organisms. Hyaline membranes may or may not be present. Giant cells and hypertrophied lining cells are often seen in the alveolar walls, sometimes with some lymphoid cells. Plasma cells have been prominent in the interstitial infiltrates of the infantile pneumonias seen in nursery outbreaks, and fluorescence studies demonstrate immunoglobulins bound to the intra-alveolar masses of *Pneumocystis* organisms. Plasma cells and globulins are not usually seen in tissues taken from immunosuppressed or congenitally lymphopenic patients. There are rare reports in which the dominant histologic elements are epithelioid-giant cell granulomas in the alveolar spaces. In cases of long duration, organization of the alveolar exudate with an appearance of fibroblasts, macrophages, and calcification may occur.

Cysts clumped within alveoli are best visualized with the methenamine silver stain (Grocott, 1955) (Fig. 4). They have thin, black capsules that are round or slightly wrinkled but often appear folded into a cup or crescent shape. The cysts are approximately 4 to 6 μ in diameter, or half the width of a red blood cell, with which they can be confused. The unfolded cysts often "contain" a pair of darkly staining structures 1 to 2 μ long and shaped like opposed parentheses; these structures (actually thickenings in the wall) are pathognomonic of the parasite. Budding is not seen. Cysts may also be visualized in tissue, though with less contrast against the background, by using the simpler and more rapid modified toluidine blue O stain (Chalvardjian and

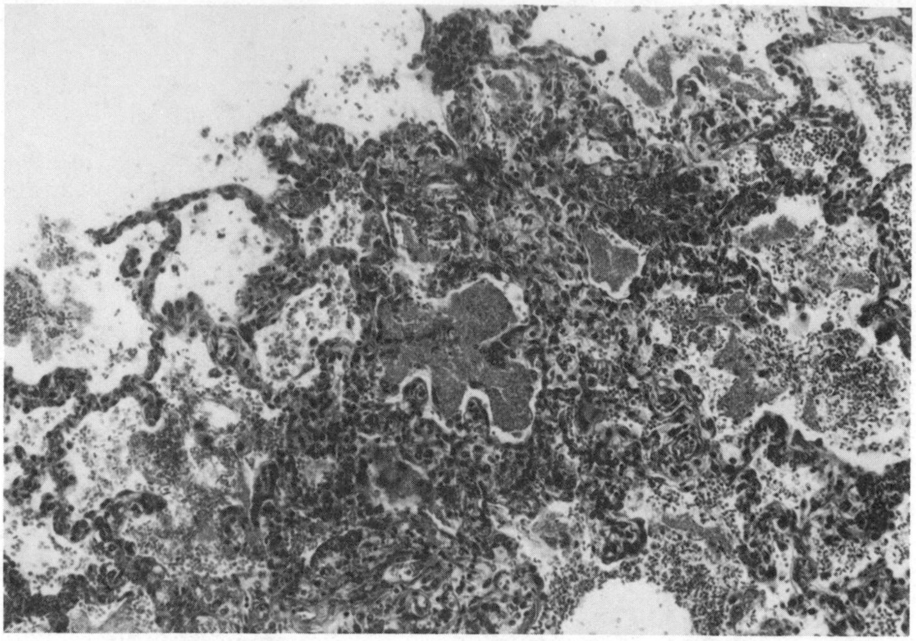

Figure 2. Section of lung tissue obtained at autopsy, showing extensive intra-alveolar deposition of eosinophilic, foamy material that is characteristic of untreated *Pneumocystis* infection. Few inflammatory cells are present, and discrete organisms are not recognizable. (Hematoxylin and eosin stain, ×100.)

Grawe, 1963). Giemsa (Blumenfeld et al., 1984), Gridley, and Gram-Weigert stains also have their enthusiasts. Cysts rapidly lose their "internal" structure, and organisms usually fragment and disappear from the sections within a few days of starting treatment, but may persist for 10 to 14 days or even longer, despite an apparent clinical response.

Although *Pneumocystis* infection seldom extends beyond the lung, local lymph nodes may be involved, and in rare instances organisms spread hematogenously and proliferate in the liver, spleen, marrow, myocardium, kidney, adrenal, thyroid, pancreas, colon, brain and other tissues, often with abscess formation.

In addition to the widespread histologic involvement in clinically severe *Pneumocystis* disease, similar microscopic findings may be restricted to focal areas in patients with inapparent *Pneumocystis* infections that are often associated with depressed immunity, radiation therapy, and malignancy.

CLINICAL MANIFESTATIONS AND LABORATORY FINDINGS. The mainstay of diagnosis is a high index of suspicion in the susceptible patient population, since there are no reliable indicators of the presence of *Pneumocystis* infection. *P. carinii* is responsible for one fourth to one half of all interstitial pneumonia in immunosuppressed patients, is diagnosed in approximately 50 per cent of patients afflicted with AIDS, and affects at least 1 per cent of all children with acute lymphocytic leukemia each year

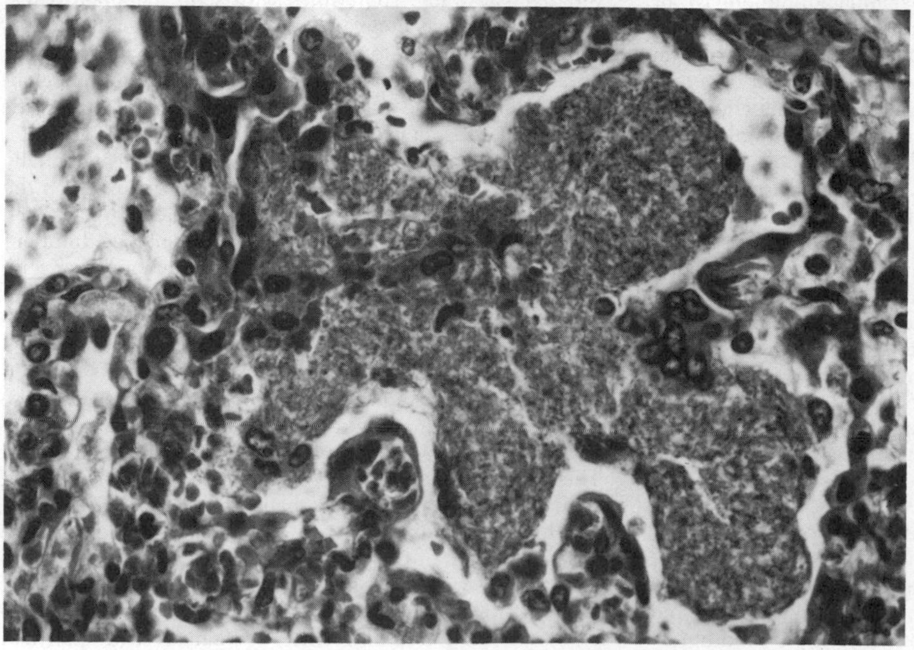

Figure 3. High-power view of the lung tissue of Figure 2. The eosinophilic intra-alveolar material may appear completely amorphous, but often closely packed vacuoles in this matrix contain a single off-center granule, which is highly suggestive of *P. carinii.* (Hematoxylin and eosin stain, ×400.)

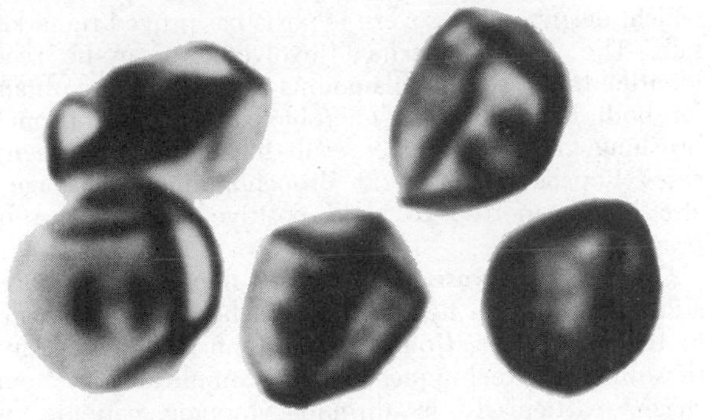

Figure 4. Biopsy imprint smear stained with methenamine silver from lung of patient with *Pneumocystis* pneumonia. The clustering, the slightly folded edges, and the cyst wall components, which appear as comma-shaped structures within the cysts, are characteristic. The organisms have a similar appearance in tissue sections, as well as in imprints or sections stained with toluidine blue O. (Grocott's methenamine silver stain, ×1000.)

(Walzer et al., 1974). Illness tends to occur as corticosteroid dosage is reduced.

The clinical presentation of *Pneumocystis* infection is highly variable and may depend upon the coexistence of infection with other organisms, which occurs in as many as 25 per cent of sporadic cases. Coinfection with CMV is frequent; it is unclear whether one infection predisposes to the other or whether their conjunction simply reflects a common predisposition. Illness among nursery infants is often insidious, characterized only by poor feeding and little or no fever for a few weeks. Gradually, the pneumonia worsens, and respiratory distress becomes manifest by tachypnea, nasal flaring and eventually by cyanosis.

However, illness in infants may be, and adult cases usually are, rapidly progressive, the patient appearing in extremis within a few days during which fevers of 39 to 40° C, often with shaking chills, are common. Cough, which is usually nonproductive, is present in less than half of the patients. The patient's only complaint may be shortness of breath, but at times the patient denies respiratory distress despite obvious tachypnea. Cyanosis may develop, but other physical signs are minimal, and auscultation of the chest is remarkable only for the absence of findings.

Chest radiographs usually reveal diffuse, bilateral granular infiltrates that spread from the hilus in a pattern similar to that of pulmonary edema and initially spare the periphery (Fig. 5). This picture may progress over several hours to complete opacification of the lungs with air bronchograms. An occasional patient with extreme dyspnea has a normal chest film, but extensive changes usually develop within the next 24 to 48 hours. The radiographs of clinically severe, biopsy-confirmed illness may rarely show lobar pneumonia, focal bronchopneumonia, or even pulmonary nodules, and spontaneous pneumothorax may occur.

Most laboratory studies are unrewarding. Lymphopenia and hypoalbuminemia are often present, but hypogammaglobulinemia is found only irregularly. The most consistent and diagnostically useful laboratory abnormalitiy is arterial hypoxemia, with pAO_2 commonly in the range of 35 to 45 mm Hg.

COMPLICATIONS AND SEQUELAE. The mortality of untreated *Pneumocystis* infection in nursery outbreaks before the introduction of specific chemotherapy was about 50 per cent, while that of sporadic cases was close to 100 per cent, there being only one report documenting recovery of an untreated patient with a predisposing illness. Death results from pulmonary insufficiency due to *Pneumocystis* infection or to the local and systemic effects of associated infection.

The pulmonary insufficiency resulting from the pneumonic process may be aggravated by pneumothorax or pneumomediastinum arising from the infection itself, from respiratory therapy at high inspiratory pressures, or from diagnostic sampling of the lung.

Patients who recovery from acute *Pneumocystis* pneumonia generally have little or no clinically significant residua of pulmonary damage, although pulmonary fibrosis has been described late in the acute stage of illness in fatal cases and in at least two long-term survivors. The frequency of this complication is difficult to ascertain because of a paucity of published reports with adequate follow-up, and because many of these patients also receive irradiation, potentially pneumotoxic drugs such as methotrexate, and prolonged high tension oxygen therapy. In one study, 80 per cent of 23 infected subjects age 7 to 18 years showed abnormal tests of pulmonary function, particularly of diffusing capacity, at the time of discharge from the hospital. Hypoxemia was due to intrapulmonary shunting rather than to impaired gas exchange, however, and all abnormalities disappeared within 6 months (Sanyal et al., 1981).

Involvement of organs other than the lung has not been recognized before death, possibly because it is overshadowed by overwhelming hypoxia. Cotton-wool exudates are frequently seen on direct opthalmoscopy of AIDS patients with *Pneumocystis* pneumonia, but whether these reflect *Pneumocystis* invasion of the eye is disputed.

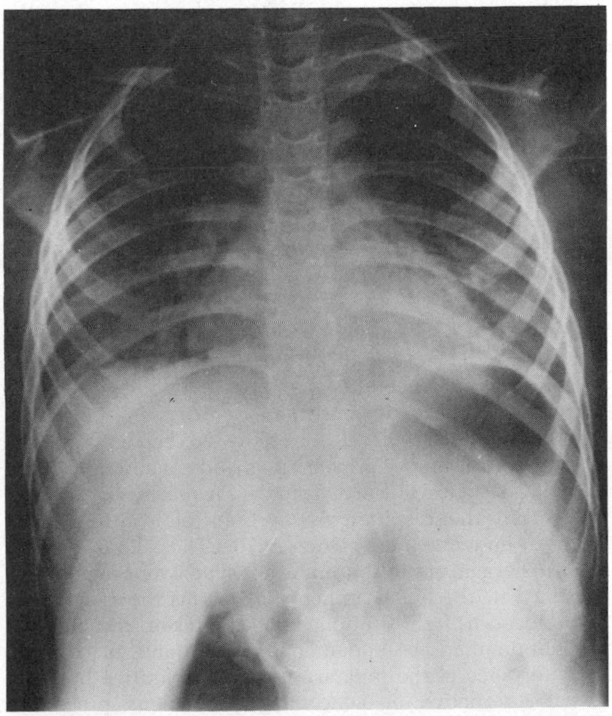

Figure 5. Chest x-ray of patient with bilateral, interstitial pneumonia due to *Pneumocystis* infection. The granular infiltrates are most prominent centrally and at the bases, with relative sparing of the periphery and apices. Air bronchograms are seen in the consolidated areas behind the cardiac shadow.

GEOGRAPHIC VARIATIONS. Sporadic *Pneumocystis* infections in immunosuppressed patients are worldwide in distribution. Nursery outbreaks, in contrast, are reported primarily in developing countries or impoverished areas of wealthy countries.

The identification of *Pneumocystis* infection in European nurseries and foundling homes after World War II may well have reflected the availability of antibiotics, which prevented the death of these malnourished children from acute bacterial infection (Dutz, 1970). As the nutritional status of Europe improved markedly in the decade following World War II, reports of illness in nurseries became uncommon. Episodes subsequently reported from Asia and Africa probably reflect similar socioeconomic conditions that provide antibiotic therapy and adequate diagnostic facilities in institutions but inadequate nutrition for many people. Malnutrition is the only experimental manipulation that activates latent *Pneumocystis* infection in animals as effectively as corticosteroid administration and has been unequivocally shown to impair the immune response, particularly cell-mediated reactions (Smythe et al., 1971; Hughes et al., 1974).

Since 1980, *Pneumocystis carinii* infections in the United States have increased greatly, primarily in those cities with a relatively large population of gay males, e.g., Los Angeles, New York, and San Francisco. A cluster of five cases was first recognized and described in detail by Gottlieb et al. (1981). All had concurrent infection with CMV, mucosal candidiasis, and an inversion of the normal T cell helper/suppressor ratio due to the virtual absence of the helper-inducer subset of T lymphocytes. Two of these five patients had died of *Pneumocystis* pneumonia despite prompt and appropriate therapy. Within a few months of the original report, an association with Kaposi's sarcoma, a vascular neoplasm common in Africa but unusual in the United States, was recognized.

Numerous publications since then have defined the Acquired Immunodeficiency Syndrome (AIDS), an epidemic that has predominantly affected young male homosexuals (including Haitians) and heterosexual drug addicts. These patients have an unusually high incidence of Kaposi's sarcoma, *Pneumocystis* pneumonia, CMV infection, and mucosal candidiasis and of lymphomas and other classically opportunistic infections due to viruses, fungi, protozoa, and mycobacteria (See Chapter 273).

DIAGNOSIS. Diagnosis of infection with *Pneumocystis* requires a demonstration of the organism in the lung. Despite the evidence of contagiousness by the respiratory route, attempts to demonstrate organisms in sputum or aspirated hypopharyngeal secretions succeed in less than 10 per cent of biopsy-proven cases and usually only serve to delay diagnosis. Furthermore, *Pneumocystis* may be present in the respiratory secretions of healthy infants living in endemic areas (Dutz, 1970). Thus, finding *Pneumocystis* organisms in sputum is not synonymous with their presence in the lung parenchyma, just as the isolation of pneumococcus from sputum cannot be taken as conclusive proof of pneumococcal pneumonia. Techniques that sample the substance of the lung are not only definitive but best reveal alternative or concomitant infectious processes. Transbronchial biopsy is probably the most popular diagnostic technique (Hodgkin et al., 1973) and, since pulmonary involvement is commonly diffuse, is usually successful; occasionally inadequate sampling may be a problem. Sampling problems are largely obviated by open lung biopsy, which, despite often severe hypoxia has proved remarkably safe. The area of maximal involvement can be readily identified, and adequate amounts of tissue can be obtained for both histologic and microbiologic studies. Bronchial brushing gives a positive result in 80 to 85 per cent of cases (Repsher et al., 1972). Bronchopulmonary lavage has also been reported to yield positive smears in a high proportion of cases.

One popular invasive technique is needle aspiration with a 22-gauge, 1-inch needle through the chest wall, usually in the right axilla (Johnson and Johnson, 1970). Any of these invasive techniques may be complicated by hemorrhage, particularly in thrombocytopenic patients, who should be given platelet transfusions preoperatively. Even when less extensive procedures than thoracotomy are employed, a complicating pneumothorax may further impair pulmonary function and require a chest tube.

The cut surface of the material obtained by biopsy should be rubbed firmly on several clean glass slides to prepare imprint smears or scraped with a scalpel blade and smears made of the scrapings. If aspirates have been obtained, a drop of the aspirate is placed on each slide. The air-dried slides are then stained. Homogenization of the infected lung and concentration of the organisms by centrifugation increased the number of organisms seen, but did not significantly improve the detection of infected animals beyond the number found by touch prep and/or tissue sections (Thomson et al., 1982). A portion of the tissue should also be fixed and submitted for histologic examination, including specimens prepared with PAS and methenamine silver stains. Smears are first examined with the toluidine blue O stain, which demonstrates the cyst wall and, usually, the comma-like structures. If organisms are not found, additional slides can be stained by the more tedious methenamine silver method, in which the gray-black organisms stand out most clearly against the counterstained green background. However, it is unusual for the silver stain to detect organisms missed by toluidine blue O. Experience is necessary for the proper interpretation of these smears, particularly from samples taken through the bronchi in which debris often stains artifactually. Particular confusion may arise with silver stains from red blood cells (which, however, usually stain yellow-orange), less often with the grayish nuclei of polymorphonuclear leukocytes or with yeast, both of which pick up both toluidine blue O and silver stains but lack the characteristic structure. The Giemsa stain (Blumenfeld et al., 1984) is also popular, and even the ordinary Gram stain (Macher et al., 1983) can be used; both of the latter stain trophozoites. The limitations of these and other stains are well discussed in reviews by Kim and Hughes (1973) and by Kagan and Norman (1977). Experimental fluorescent antibody (FA) reagents for direct staining have been developed and offer greater sensitivity, but false-positive results have also been reported with FA, which is no more rapid than the toluidine blue O method. Unlike the preceding methods, which detect cyst forms and have generally been most sensitive for diagnosis, acridine orange and Giemsa stains detect trophozoites and intracystic daughter forms.

Specimens examined for *Pneumocystis* should also be cultured and stained for bacteria, fungi, and mycobacteria. Viral cultures are desirable. As noted above, simultaneous infection with CMV is frequently detected, especially in AIDS patients. Its contribution to the pulmonary symptoms is often unclear since many patients improve with specific therapy directed at the protozoan infection alone.

Early reports of serial propagation of *Pneumocystis* (Latorre et al., 1977) have not been widely confirmed; it appears thus far that at best replication continues for a few generations before the organisms degenerate. Pesanti and Cox (1981) found that a suspension of organisms in tissue culture medium were able to take up vital dyes, to incorporate radio-labelled substrates into RNA and protein but not DNA, and to produce CO_2 from glucose.

Serologic diagnosis has been used in Europe and Asia, particularly in evaluating nursery outbreaks. Crude antigens are prepared from the infected lungs of patients or steroid-treated rats and are usually employed in a complement fixation test. Titers of $\geq$ 1:4 are usually considered positive, although each laboratory must standardize its own test procedure. Immunofluorescent tests upon fixed sections of human lung have also been studied extensively. European investigators found elevated CF titers in 75 to 100 per cent of nursery cases, but American investigators have found only about 15 per cent of sporadic cases positive for CF antibody. This discrepancy is probably not due to antigenic differences between strains nor to technique; similar results are obtained in all laboratories when the same sera are examined. The likely explanation for the seronegative American cases is the overwhelming preponderance in the U.S.A. of immunosuppressed patients, who fail to develop a normal antibody response. Serologic diagnosis is in any case only possible in retrospect, as antibody is absent during the acute onset of disease and requires several weeks to develop.

The absence of antibody during the acute stage of illness may be due to its reaction with an excess of circulating antigen, as titers are inversely proportional to the number of organisms seen in the lungs of cortisone-treated mice (Walzer and Rutledge, 1982).

Antigen detection has been unconvincingly reported to be a useful diagnostic test. It may be found in as many as 80 per cent (Pifer et al., 1982) or as few as 11 per cent (Maddison et al., 1982) of cases, and is also said to be present in 3 per cent of normal adults, afebrile patients with carcinoma of the lung or other malignancies, in 10 per cent of patients with non-pulmonary infection, with non-malignant lung disease or with pulmonary infections other than *Pneumocystis* pneumonia, and in 30 per cent of febrile patients with malignancy who have no evidence of *Pneumocystis* pneumonia (Pifer et al., 1982). It was detected as frequently in marrow-transplant patients who remain asymptomatic as in those who are acutely ill with *Pneumocystis* pneumonia (Meyers et al., 1979).

TREATMENT. Two antimicrobial agents have found wide acceptance in the therapy of *Pneumocystis* pneumonia: pentamidine, a drug long employed in both treatment and prophylaxis of Gambian sleeping sickness, and cotrimoxazole, or trimethoprim-sulfamethoxazole, a widely used antibacterial combination, which because of lesser toxicity and ready availability is now considered to be the treatment of choice.

Pentamidine. Pentamidine is an aromatic diamidine that was originally developed as a hypoglycemic agent. Since the discovery of its effectiveness against the early stages of *Trypanosoma gambiense* infection in 1941, the drug has been administered to millions of Africans with minimal toxicity. Successful treatment of *Pneumocystis* pneumonia was first reported by Ivady and Paldy in 1958, who employed pentamidine in nursery epidemics. Numerous investigators have subsequently confirmed their results. Pentamidine is supplied as the isethionate salt, a white powder that should be kept in a cool location until use and that must be dissolved in sterile distilled water for parenteral administration. The drug is poorly soluble in saline, which should not be used. If contamination is avoided, the solution can be kept refrigerated for five to seven days, when slight turbidity or crystalline deposits may develop. These do not denote a loss of activity, and the solution remans suitable for intramuscular, but not intravenous, injection. Pentamidine is not absorbed orally. The usual dosage is 4 mg of the salt per kg (or 100 to 150 mg/m^2 body surface area), given in a volume of no more than 3 ml, and administered intramuscularly once daily for 12 to 14 days. The anterior thigh is a useful injection site for pediatric patients with little muscle mass. Intravenous (IV) administration is not recommended unless the patient is severely thrombocytopenic; in that case, the drug should be diluted to 5 to 10 ml and given over a 5 to 10 minute interval, during which the IV fluid is kept running and blood pressure is monitored. Plasma levels are low; pentamidine is concentrated primarily in the kidneys and to a lesser extent in the liver. Excretion is prolonged, with most of the drug being recovered unchanged in the urine over a six- to eight-week period. It has been suggested from animal studies that the lungs may concentrate pentamidine that has been slowly released from other tissues.

A wide spectrum of complications has been reported in recipients of pentamidine, but many reports are difficult to assess because of severe underlying illness (Western et al., 1970). Side effects do not usually prevent completion of a full course of therapy. The most serious problem is pain and/or abscess formation at the injection site, which occurs in nearly 20 per cent of patients and may result in lethal superinfection. Azotemia develops during therapy in a similar proportion of patients but is generally mild and reversible when the drug is discontinued. Depression of blood glucose or of serum calcium is less common and usually asymptomatic, but should be considered in any patient who deteriorates neurologically. A recent report (Bouchard et al., 1982) suggests that the hypoglycemia may be caused by cytolytic release of insulin, followed by beta-cell destruction and the development of diabetes mellitus. Elevation of liver enzymes or bilirubin has also been reported but is usually slight and transient. Rare individuals develop rashes, and fatal erythema multiforme and toxic epidermal necrolysis with renal failure have been described. Thrombocytopenic purpura occurs uncommonly. "Herxheimer-like" reactions (exacerbation of illness with treatment) have been recognized in trypanosome-infected Africans but are very unusual with *Pneumocystis*. There is no evidence that the pulmonary fibrosis occasionally seen following *Pneumocystis* pneumonia is related to pentamidine treatment.

Trimethoprim-Sulfamethoxazole. Combination therapy with the antifolates pyrimethamine and sulfadiazine for the protozoan infections malaria and toxoplasmosis is well accepted. In 1966, Frenkel et al. reported that pentamidine and pyrimethamine-sulfadiazine were about equally potent in treating cortisone-induced *Pneumocystis* infection of rats. The slightly more rapid clearing of parasites by the diamidine was balanced by its greater toxcity, especially necrosis at the injection site. Subsequent uncontrolled clinical trials of pyrimethamine-sulfadiazine in *Pneumocystis*-infected humans gave mixed results.

A new antifolate combination, trimethoprim-sulfamethoxazole (TMP-SMX), was superior to pentamidine in treating *Pneumocystis* pneumonia induced in cortisone-fed rats. Accordingly, Hughes et al. (1975) administered TMP-SMX to immunosuppressed children who were moderately ill with *Pneumocystis* infection and obtained results equal to those expected with pentamidine. Adult cases have also responded well (Lau and Young, 1976). The clinical equivalence of these two regimens is interesting in light of the finding of Pesanti (1980) that pentamidine is lethal, whereas TMP-SMX is only inhibitory for organisms maintained in vitro, possibly because the latter can only kill replicating organisms.

The combination of trimethoprim-sulfamethoxazole is available as tablets containing 80 mg TMP and 400 mg SMX and also as double-strength tablets containing 160 mg TMP and 800 mg SMX, or as a suspension containing 40 mg TMP and 200 mg SMX per 5 ml. A parenteral preparation containing 80 mg TMP and 400 mg SMX in 5 ml ethanol with 1 per cent benzyl alcohol as a preservative is also available. Fluid overloading may be a problem with the parenteral product because of its relatively poor solubility, which requires 75–125 ml 5 per cent dextrose in water per 5 ml ampule (Winston et al., 1980). Doses have ranged as high as 20 mg TMP and 100 mg SMX/kg per day, divided into two to four doses and administered for 14 days.

Side effects of the antifolate combination are largely limited to occasional skin rashes and other allergic responses well known for sulfonamides. In patients with AIDS, such skin rashes, along with fever and leukopenia, appear in up to 60 per cent of patients 8 to 19 days after starting TMP/SMX, so that a change to pentamidine therapy then is almost the rule (Kovacs et al., 1984). Folate deficiency is uncommon with a short course of therapy. TMP has a poor affinity for mammalian dihydrofolate reductase, and sulfonamides do not function as antifolates in mammals, but in about 5 per cent of chronically treated patients, evidence of folate deficiency does develop (Harris et al., 1980). In such cases the patient can be given intramuscular folinic acid, a form of the vitamin that man can utilize but protozoans cannot. The combination of pyrimethamine and sulfadoxine (Fansidar) may prove to be a useful alternative in patients who cannot tolerate TMP-SMX prophylaxis (Gottlieb et al., 1984).

In a carefully controlled clinical comparison of pentamidine versus TMP-SMX, the drugs were found equally effective in treating *Pneumocystis* pneumonia, but TMP-SMX caused substantially fewer undesirable side effects (Hughes et al., 1978). Combined therapy with both pentamidine and TMP-SMX has not been evaluated in man but offered no significant advantage over administration of TMP-SMX in experimental infection of rats (Kluge et al., 1978).

Treatment other than antimicrobial chemotherapy is limited to respiratory support and oxygen therapy. Elevated levels of inspiratory oxygen are extremely important to the hypoxic patient in the few days before histologic improvement can occur. An occasional patient may survive only with the aid of a membrane oxygenator during this critical period. The clinician must follow these seriously ill patients closely for signs of the reactivation of other latent infections or of bacterial or fungal superinfection of their poorly aerated lungs. Acute pulmonary deterioration should also suggest the possibility of unrecognized pneumothorax or some mechanical complication of respiratory therapy. Although tapering of steroid dosage is often temporally associated with the onset of symptomatic *Pneumocystis* pneumonia, the administration of steroids does not appear to improve the outcome. Injections of immune serum globulin have also been without obvious effect in controlling *Pneumocystis* infection of immunosuppressed children.

Antimicrobial therapy has improved the survival rate of patients with *Pneumocystis* pneumonia. If the patient's pneumonia is due only to *Pneumocystis*, he usually becomes afebrile within one or two days and, within that time, notes first a halt to the progression of his shortness of breath, and then an improvement in this symptom. The chest film does not clear as rapidly but lags several days to weeks behind the symptoms except in the mildest cases. Although only 10 per cent or fewer patients fail to clear the infecting parasite from their tissues within a few days of instituting treatment, the mortality for sporadic cases remains in the range of 30 to 50 per cent. Deaths may result from associated pulmonary infections as well as from nonpulmonary complications in the immunosuppressed patient but are most frequently due to resiratory failure, particularly in the presence of pre-existing pulmonary disease or a delay in diagnosis. The response of *Pneumocystis* pneumonia in AIDS patients to antimicrobial therapy appears poorer, with frequent failure to clear the organisms despite a full course of treatment with one or both recommended drugs. In contrast, the introduction of pentamidine therapy has reduced the mortality of nursery epidemic disease, admittedly not always biopsy-proven, from about 50 per cent to 3 per cent. Improved survival from *Pneumocystis* pneumonia probably requires earlier diagnosis and better respiratory support rather than new antimicrobials.

It has not been possible to study the antimicrobial resistance of *Pneumocystis* strains from the small proportion of patients who fail to clear the organisms despite an appropriate dose and duration of treatment. Perhaps the organisms in these patients are not unusual but persist because the immune defect prevents a critical response of which recovered patients are capable. Furthermore, successful control of one clinical episode of *Pneumocystis* infection apparently cannot be relied upon to immunize or to eradicate organisms from the host. As noted earlier, asymptomatic infants in endemic surroundings carry *Pneumocystis* in their respiratory secretions for prolonged periods, and recurrent bouts of *Pneumocystis* are known to occur in both immunosuppressed patients and animals. Relapse and recurrence appear to be particularly common in AIDS.

PROPHYLAXIS. The evidence for respiratory transmission of *Pneumocystis* infection is sufficient to suggest that any patient with acute *Pneumocystis* pneumonia should be segregated from individuals known to be highly susceptible to severe *Pneumocystis* disease, i.e., patients with AIDS, and malnourished, steroid-treated, or otherwise immunologically incompetent patients.

Chemoprophylaxis against *Pneumocystis* pneumonia is effective. Hughes et al. (1977) protected cancer patients, mainly children with lymphatic leukemia, with 150 mg trimethoprim plus 750 mg sulfamethoxazole/M^2/day, given as two divided doses 12 hours apart. Prophylaxis was continued for two years, and the only untoward effect was a moderate increase in oral candidiasis. They recommend screening of blacks for glucose-6-phosphate dehydrogenase deficiency before employing this treatment. Unfortunately, prophylaxis does not eradicate carriage of latent infection (Hughes, 1979), which develops at the same rate as in untreated control patients after prophylaxis has been discontinued (Wolff and Baehner, 1978). The available evidence suggests that prophylaxis is necessary as long as the predisposing conditions exist. For example, Western et al. (1975) administered pentamidine for 14 days to cortisone-treated rats and delayed their death from *Pneumocystis* pneumonia for a mean of 13 days in comparison with controls, and Hughes et al. (1974) completely protected cortisone-injected rats by chronic administration of TMP-SMX. In the five years since he introduced routine TMP-SMX prophylaxis for high-risk patients, Hughes (1984) has essentially abolished *Pneumocystis* pneumonia as a complication of anticancer therapy in children.

Clinical reports from Hungary and Iran report similar success with pentamidine and with pyrimethamine-sulfadiazine. The toxicity of pentamidine excludes chronic administration, but the ease and safety of oral antifolate therapy is well suited to prophylaxis.

An effective vaccine might appear to be an even more attractive means of preventing *Pneumocystis* infection. One attempt to immunize rats against infection failed despite the development of high antibody titers before cortisone administration. Since a deficient immune response seems to be the sine qua non for clinically significant *Pneumocystis* infection, any vaccine may be doomed to failure. The passive administration of immune serum globulin is ineffective in preventing the development of *Pneumocystis* pneumonia in children with congenital hypogammaglobulinemia (although the product administered is deficient in IgM and IgA). Transfer of cell-mediated immunity with living cells cannot be attempted because of the hazard of graft-versus-host reaction in the immunosuppressed population most clearly at risk for infection.

References

Blumenfeld, W., Wagar, E., and Hadley, W. K.: Use of the transbronchial biopsy for diagnosis of opportunistic pulmonary infections in acquired immunodeficiency syndrome (AIDS). Am J Clin Pathol 81:1, 1984.

Bouchard, P., Sai, P., Reach, G., Caubarriere, I.,Ganeval, D., and Assan, R.: Diabetes mellitus following pentamidine-induced hypoglycemia in humans. *Diabetes* 31:40, 1982.

Campbell, W. G., Jr.: Ultrastructure of pneumocystis in human lung. Arch Pathol 93:312, 1972.

Carini, A.: Formas de eschizogonia do *Trypanosoma lewisii.* Soc Med Cir Sao Paolo, 16 Aout 1910.

Chagas, C.: Nova tripanozomiaze humana. Mem Inst Oswaldo Cruz 1:159, 1909.

Chalvardjian, A. M., and Grawe, L. A.: A new procedure for the identification of *Pneumocystis carinii* in tissue sections and smears. J Clin Pathol 16:383, 1963.

Delanöe, P., and Delanöe, M.: Sur les rapports des kystes de Carini du poumon des rats avec le *Trypanosoma lewisii.* C R Acad Sci (Paris) 155:658, 1912.

Dutz, W.: *Pneumocystis carinii* pneumonia. Pathol Annu 5:309, 1970.

Frenkel, J. K., Good, J. T., and Shultz, J. A.: Latent pneumocystis infection of rats, relapse and chemotherapy. Lab Invest 15:1559, 1966.

Gottlieb, M. S., Schroff, R., Schanker, H. M., Weisman, J. D., Fan, P. T., Wolf, R. A. and Saxon, A.: *Pneumocystis carinii* pneumonia and mucosal candidiasis in previously healthy homosexual men. New Engl J Med 305:1425, 1981.

Gottlieb, M. S., Groopman, J. E., Weinstein, W. M., Fahey, J. L., and Detels, R.: The acquired immunodeficiency syndrome. Ann Intern Med 99:208, 1983.

Gottlieb M. S., Knight S., Mitsuyasu, R., Weisman, J., Roth, M., and Young, L. S.: Prophylaxis of *Pneumocystis carinii* infection in AIDS with pyrimethamine-sulfadoxine. Lancet ii:398, 1984.

Grocott, R. G.: A stain for fungi in tissue sections and smears. Am J Clin Pathol 25:975, 1955.

Harris, R. E., McAllister, J. A., Allen, S. A., Barton, A. S., and Baehner, R. S.: Prevention of *Pneumocystis* pneumonia: use of continuous sulfamethoxazole-trimethoprim therapy. Amer J Dis Child 134:35, 1980.

Hendley, J. O., and Weller, T. H.: Activation and transmission in rats of infection with pneumocystis. Proc Soc Exp Biol Med 137:1401, 1971.

Hodgkin, J. E., Andersen, H. A., and Rosenow, E. C., III: Diagnosis of *Pneumocystis carinii* pneumonia by transbronchoscopic lung biopsy. Chest 64:551, 1973.

Hughes, W. T.: Limited effect of trimethoprim-sulfamethoxazole on *Pneumocystis carinii.* Antimicrob Agents Chemother 16:33, 1979.

Hughes, W. T.: Feldman, S., Chaudhary, S. C., Ossi, M. J., Cox, F., and Sanyal, S. K.: Comparison of pentamidine isethionate with trimethoprim-sulfamethoxazole in the treatment of *Pneumocystis carinii* pneumonia. J Pediatr 92:285, 1978.

Hughes, W. T.: Feldman, S., and Sanyal, S. K.: Treatment of *Pneumocystis carinii* pneumonitis with trimethoprim-sulfamethoxazole. Can Med Assoc J 112:475, 1975.

Hughes, W. T., Kuhn, S., Chaudhary, S., Feldman, S., Verzosa, M., Aur, R. J. A., Pratt, C., and George, S. L.: Successful chemoprophylaxis for *Pneumocystis carinii* pneumonia. N Engl J Med 297:1419, 1977.

Hughes, W. T., McNabb, P. C., Makres, T. D., and Feldman, S.: Efficacy of trimethoprim and sulfamethoxazole in the prevention and treatment of *Pneumocystis carinii* pneumonitis. Antimicrob Agents Chemother 5:289, 1974.

Hughes, W. T., Price, R. A., Sisko, F., Havron, W. S., Kafatos, A. G., Schonland, M., and Smythe, P. M.: Protein-calorie malnutrition. A host determinant for *Pneumocystis carinii* infection. Am J Dis Child 128:44, 1974.

Hughes, W. T.: Natural mode of acquisition for de novo infection with *Pneumocystis carinii.* J Infect Dis 145:842, 1982.

Hughes, W. T.: Five-year absence of *Pneumocystis carinii* pneumonitis in a pediatric oncology center. J Infect Dis 150:305, 1984.

Ivady, G., and Paldy, L.: Ein neues Behandlungsverfahren der interstitiellen plasmazelligen Pneumonie Frühgeborener mit fünfwertigen Stibium und aromatishen Diamidinen. Monatsschr Kinderheilkd 106:10, 1958.

Johnson, H. D., and Johnson, W. W.: *Pneumocystis carinii* pneumonia in children with cancer. JAMA 214:1067, 1970.

Kagan, I. G., and Norman, L.: The laboratory diagnosis of *Pneumocystis carinii* pneumonia. Health Lab Sci 14:155, 1977.

Kim, H., and Hughes, W. T.: Comparison of methods for identification of *Pneumocystis carinii* in pulmonary aspirates. Am J Clin Pathol 60:462, 1973.

Kluge, R. M., Spaulding, D. M., and Spain, A. J.: Combination of pentamidine and trimethoprim sulfamethoxazole in the therapy of *Pneumocystis carinii* pneumonia in rats. Antimicrob Agents Chemother 13:975, 1978.

Kovacs, J., Heimans, J., Macher, A., Stover, C., Murray, H., Shelhamer, J., Lane, H., Urmacher, C., Honig, C., Longo, D., Parker, M., Natanson, C., Parillo, J., Fauci, A., Pizzo, P. and Masur, H.: *Pneumocystis carinii* pneumonia: A comparison between patients with the Acquired Immunodeficiency Syndrome and patients with other immunodeficiencies. Ann Int Med 100:663, 1984.

Latorre, C. K., Sulzer, A. J., and Norman, L. G.: Serial propagation of *Pneumocystis carinii* in cell line cultures. Appl Environ Microbiol 33:1204, 1977.

Lau, W. K., and Young, L. S.: Trimethoprim-sulfamethoxazole treatment of *Pneumocystis carinii* pneumonia in adults. N Engl J Med 295:716, 1976.

Macher, A., Shelhamer, J., MacLowry, J., Parker, M., and Masur H.: *Pneumocystis carinii* identified by Gram stain of lung imprints. Ann Intern Med 99:484, 1983.

Maddison, S. E., Hayes, G. V., Slemenda, S. B., Norman, L. G., and Ivey, M. H.: Detection of specific antibody by enzyme-linked immunosorbent assay and antigenemia by counterimmunoelectrophoresis in humans infected with *Pneumocystis carinii.* J Clin Microbiol 15:1036, 1982.

Masur, H. and Jones, T. C.: The interaction in vitro of *Pneumocystis carinii* with macrophages and L-cells. J Exper Med 147:157, 1978.

Meuwissen, J. H. E., Tauber, I., Leeuwenberg, A. D. E. M., Beckers, P. T. A., and Sieben, M.: Parasitologic and serologic observations of infection with *Pneumocystis carinii* in humans. J Infect Dis 136:43, 1977.

Meyers, J. D., Pifer, L. L., Sale, G. E., and Thomas, E. D.: The value of *Pneumocystis carinii* antibody and antigen detection for diagnosis of *Pneumocystis carinii* pneumonia after marrow transplantation. Amer Rev Respir Dis 120:1283, 1979.

Pesanti, E.: In vitro effects of antiprotozoan drugs and immune serum on *Pneumocystis carinii.* J Infect Dis 141:775, 1980.

Pesanti, E., and Cox, C.: Metabolic and synthetic activities of *Pneumocystis carinii* in vitro. Infect Immun 34:908, 1981.

Pifer, L. L., Niell, H. B., Morrison, B. J., Freeman, J. M. and Counce, J. D., Jr.: Incidence of *Pneumocystis carinii* antigenemia in adults with infection, pulmonary disease, malignancy or homosexual life style. Abstract No. 21, Interscience Conference on Antimicrobial Agents and Chemotherapy, Miami, Florida, 1982.

Repsher, L. H., Schroter, G., and Hammond, W. S.: Diagnosis of *Pneumocystis carinii* pneumonitis by means of endobronchial brush biopsy. N Engl J Med 287:340, 1972.

Ruskin, J., and Hughes, W. T.: Pneumocystis carinii. In Remington, J. S., and Klein, J. O. (eds.): Infectious Diseases of the Fetus and Newborn Infant. 2nd ed., Philadelphia, W.B. Saunders Company, 1983.

Sanyal, S. K., Mariencheck, W. C., and Mackert, P. W.: Course of pulmonary dysfunction in children surviving *Pneumocystis carinii* pneumonitis (PCP): a prospective study. Pediat Res 15:620, 1981.

Smythe, P. M., Schonland, M., Brereton-Stiles, G. G., Coovadia, C. C., Grace, H. J., Loening, W. E. K., Mafoyane, A., Parent, M. A., and Vos, G. H.: Thymolymphatic deficiency and depression of cell-mediated immunity in protein-calorie malnutrition. Lancet 2:939, 1971.

Thomson, R. B., Jr., Smith, T. F., and Wilson, W. R.: Comparison of two methods used to prepare smears of mouse lung tissue for detection of *Pneumocystis carinii*. J Clin Microbiol 16:303, 1982.

Van der Meer, G., and Brug, S. L.: Infection par pneumocystis chez l'homme et chez les animaux. Ann Soc Belg Med Trop 22:301, 1942.

Walzer, P. D., Perl, D. P., Krogstad, D. J., Rawson, P. G., and Schultz, M. G.: *Pneumocystis carinii* pneumonia in the United States. Ann Intern Med 80:83, 1974.

Walzer, P. D., and Rutledge, M. E.: Comparison of rat, mouse, and human *Pneumocystis carinii* by immunofluorescence. J Infect Dis 142:449, 1980.

Walzer, P. D., and Rutledge, M. E.: Serum antibody responses to *Pneumocystis carinii* among different strains of normal and athymic mice. Infect Immun 35:620, 1982.

Weller, R.: Weitere Untersuchungen über experimentele. Rattenpneumocystose in Hinblick auf die interstitielle Pneumonie der Frühgeborenen. Z Kinderheilkd 78:166, 1956.

Western, K. A., Norman, L., and Kaufmann, A. F.: Failure of pentamidine isethionate to provide chemoprophylaxis against *Pneumocystis carinii* infection in rats. J Infect Dis 131:273, 1975.

Western, K. A., Perera, D. R., and Schultz, M. G.: Pentamidine isethionate in the treatment of *Pneumocystis carinii* pneumonia. Ann Intern Med 73:695, 1970.

Winston, D. J., Lau, W. K., Gale, R. P., and Young, L. S.: Trimethoprim-sulfamethoxazole for the treatment of *Pneumocystis carinii* pneumonia. Ann Intern Med 92:762, 1980.

Wolff, L. J., and Baehner, R. L.: Delayed development of *Pneumocystis* pneumonia following administration of short-term high-dose trimethoprim-sulfamethoxazole. Am J Dis Child 132:525, 1978.

Yoneda, K. and Walzer, P. D.: Interaction of *Pneumocystis carinii* with host lungs: an ultrastructural study. Infect Immun 29:692, 1980.

C. ABDOMINAL INFECTIONS

131
FOOD POISONING

SAM T. DONTA, M.D.

This chapter deals with diseases caused by bacterial toxins that are either ingested preformed or elaborated in the intestine by bacteria ingested in contaminated food. Most of the toxins affect the gastrointestinal tract directly. These intoxications are to be contrasted with gastrointestinal infections by bacteria ingested in contaminated food (Chapter 132). The distinction between infections and intoxications is somewhat arbitrary, since the pathogenesis of many enteric infections requires the elaboration of enterotoxins.

Approximately three-fourths of cases of food poisoning are due to contamination of food with microbes or their products. The three leading causes of bacterial food poisoning throughout the world are *Staphylococcus aureus*, *Clostridium perfringens*, and *Salmonella* sp. *Salmonella* causes a direct infection of the intestine, as does *Vibrio parahemolyticus*, which is the major etiologic agent in certain coastal areas. Less frequent causes include *Shigella* sp., *Bacillus cereus*, *Escherichia coli*, and *Clostridium botulinum*. Although other bacteria have been implicated in sporadic cases, their pathogenetic roles remain uncertain.

PATHOGENESIS. Some resistance to enteric bacteria or their toxins is provided by gastric acid, proteolytic enzymes, intestinal motility, secretory and humoral immune mechanisms, and the resident microflora itself; the role of cellular immunity has not been assessed.

Gastric acid is ineffective against the acid-stable enterotoxins of *Staphylococcus aureus* and the neurotoxins of *Clostridium botulinum*. Disease may result from acid-labile toxins or acid-susceptible bacteria if the amount of toxin or the number of bacteria ingested exceeds the inactivation potential of gastric acid, or if gastric acidity is reduced or absent. Patients with gastrectomies or who have achlorhydria are more susceptible to enteric diseases. Neutralization of gastric acid with food or with antacids probably enhances the potential to develop enteric disease (Donta, 1975).

STAPHYLOCOCCAL FOOD POISONING

ETIOLOGY. With rare exceptions, *Staphylococcus aureus* causes this clinical syndrome. *Staphylococcus epidermidis* has also been incriminated, but most of the implicated strains are not enterotoxigenic.

PATHOGENESIS. People are the major reservoir of the organism; up to 50 per cent of the population carry *S. aureus*, but not all strains are enterotoxigenic. Staphylococci multiply in food at rates that are temperature-dependent. Between 10 and 45° C, cells can divide as rapidly as every 20 minutes and, depending on the initial inoculum, total counts per gram of food can reach levels of 10^5 to 10^8 in a few hours.

As organisms reach their stationary phase of growth, enterotoxin is produced. Although the stimulus to enterotoxin synthesis is not known, toxin is probably elaborated in response to a still unidentified nutritional stimulus, and its synthesis is under some degree of catabolite repression. The ingestion of food contaminated with enterotoxin is responsible for staphylococcal food poisoning. In contrast, staphylococcal enterocolitis results from hematogenous seeding of the intestine during bacteremia or from intestinal overgrowth of staphylococci after administration of certain antibiotics or after abdominal surgery.

In epidemics of *S. aureus* food poisoning, ham products, cold meats, salads, and cream-filled desserts are commonly involved. Contaminated foods usually have no change in odor or flavor. Outbreaks are more common during the summer.

Five antigenically-distinct enterotoxins (A through E) have been identified. Although initially thought to be a new enterotoxin responsible for the toxic-shock syndrome, enterotoxin F appears to be identical to staphylococcal pyrogenic exotoxin C and is not enterotoxic. Most strains of *S. aureus* can produce one or more types of enterotoxin. All types have been implicated in outbreaks of food poisoning, although types A, B, and D are most common. The purified enterotoxins are single polypeptide chains of ~30,000 daltons and are stable to heat, acid, and several proteolytic enzymes. A plasmid regulates the synthesis of enterotoxin, but the structural genes are chromosomal (Dyer and Iandolo, 1981). The different enterotoxins may bind to the same receptor sites (Buxser et al., 1981).

Once 1 μg or more of toxin is ingested, a neural response is initiated that results in centrally activated, vagal-mediated emesis and hypermotility of the bowel (Elwell et al., 1975). The toxin does not act directly on the small bowel, and causes no fluid to accumulate in experimentally ligated intestinal loops; this is in contrast to the action of other enterotoxins. The delta-toxin of *S. aureus* is an exception; it does induce fluid secretion in small intestinal segments that may be of pathogenetic significance in staphylococcal enterocolitis (Kapral et al., 1976).

CLINICAL MANIFESTATIONS. One to six hours after the ingestion of enterotoxin-containing food, nausea and vomiting begin. Emesis continues at 15 to 30 minute intervals until the illness subsides. The illness lasts no longer than 24 hours and usually no more than a few hours after the onset of clinical symptoms. Abdominal cramping and diarrhea occur and can occasionally be severe enough to cause dehydration and prostration. Other symptoms are excessive salivation, sweating, headache, and chills. Fever is notably absent.

There are no complications or sequelae except those related to dehydration. In the very old and very young, circulatory collapse may ensue.

DIAGNOSIS. The sudden onset and short incubation period of the clinical illness suggests a staphylococcal etiology. Involvement of other persons and an incriminated food source lend further support to the diagnosis. The short incubation period and short duration of illness distinguish it from most other forms of bacterial food poisoning; chemical food poisoning has an even shorter incubation period.

Diagnosis is made by the detection of staphylococcal enterotoxin and/or $\geq 10^5$ staphylococci per g in food. Immunologic assays have replaced bioassays for the detection of toxin in foods but are not sufficiently sensitive to detect the toxin in body fluids. An antitoxin response can be found two to six weeks following the clinical illness.

TREATMENT. No specific therapy is available. Because the illness is not an infection, no antibiotics are needed. Supportive therapy should consist of bedrest and an abdominal heating pad to relieve cramping. Food and oral fluids should be avoided during the acute attack; they may only increase the possibility of aspiration pneumonitis. Occasionally, intravenous fluids may be indicated if dehydration develops, and phenothiazines may be needed to help control vomiting.

PROPHYLAXIS. Since the enterotoxins are very stable, all preventive measures must be directed toward the circumstances that permit contamination of food with staphylococci and subsequent multiplication of the organism. Food handlers with skin infections should not be permitted to work, and effective hand washing techniques should be encouraged. Disposable gloves should probably be worn by all commercial food handlers. Perishable items, especially those frequently implicated in staphylococcal food poisoning, should be kept under constant refrigeration at temperatures of less than 7° C.

Although an antitoxin response has been noted in experimental animals and in patients, its protective value for preventing future attacks is not known.

BOTULISM

ETIOLOGY. The causative agent is *Clostridium botulinum*, a spore-forming bacillus that can produce one of seven types of neurotoxins (A through G). The organism is widely distributed in nature, and, although a strict anaerobe, it grows well on a variety of media. Neutral or slightly alkaline conditions favor spore formation. The spores withstand boiling for up to 20 hours but are inactivated by autoclaving temperatures (120° C) after exposure for 20 or more minutes. The toxin is destroyed by temperatures of 100° C for 10 minutes or 80° C for 30 minutes, but is resistant to acid and proteolytic enzymes. Toxin production is probably governed by specific bacteriophages (Oguma and Iida, 1979).

PATHOGENESIS. The ubiquitous organism and its spores are found in animals and soil, so that a variety of foods are often contaminated. Because toxin formation requires strict anaerobic conditions, foods are rarely contaminated with toxin. When enough toxin is formed to produce symptoms, the vast majority of exposures involve raw, smoked, and fermented fish products and preserved foods or meat (especially home-cured ham) that have been standing at room temperature for several days. Improperly home-canned foods, especially vegetables, are responsible for more than 75 per cent of food-borne botulism. Whereas acidic vegetables (e.g., tomatoes) do not generally support the growth of *C. botulinum*, some tomatoes have a low content of acid and overripe tomatoes can lose their acidity.

Botulism can also result from contamination of wounds with the spores of *C. botulinum*, with subsequent germination, multiplication of organisms, and elaboration of toxin (Merson and Dowell, 1973). Types A and B have been recovered from patients with this form of botulism.

Infants between 3 and 26 weeks of age may develop botulism after ingestion of *C. botulinum* spores, intestinal infection with *C. botulinum* and absorption of toxin from the gut. Honey has been implicated as a contaminated food source, but it is likely that there are other sources of the bacteria. In California, where this syndrome was first identified, Types A and B organisms and toxin have been recovered from the stools of affected infants (Arnon et al., 1977). Since then a single case of Type F botulism has been reported. Animal models for the study of infant botulism have been developed (Sugiyama, 1979).

Following the ingestion of food containing nanogram quantities of toxin, the toxin is absorbed from the upper small bowel, eventually reaching its target tissue, cholinergic nerve endings. There the toxin binds to membrane receptors (gangliosides) and inhibits the release (exocytosis) of acetylcholine and perhaps other neurotransmitters. Neither the storage of acetylcholine nor the entry of calcium into the nerve terminals during depolarization is affected by the toxin.

The toxin is a large molecular weight complex (900,000 daltons) which, in type A toxin, has hemagglutinin activity. Type B and E toxins are secreted as inert protoxins that are activated by proteolysis. The toxin itself is approximately 150,000 daltons; the active fragment may be as small as 10,000 daltons (see Chapter 5).

CLINICAL MANIFESTATIONS. Symptoms begin as early as two hours or as late as three to eight days after the ingestion of toxin, with the usual interval being 12 to 36 hours. Earlier onset of symptoms is usually associated with more severe disease and a worse prognosis. Nausea, vomiting, and diarrhea can occur early in the disease, and are probably the result of disturbances mediated by factors other than neurotoxin. Symmetric involvement of cranial nerves and a descending pattern of weakness or paralysis are the hallmarks of botulism. Diplopia, dysarthria, and dysphagia are the most common symptoms; in severe cases, respiratory paralysis occurs. Cranial nerve involvement, especially nerve VI, may be the only neurologic manifestation. Cognitive and sensory functions remain intact. Symptoms referable to autonomic nervous system dysfunction include dry mouth and constipation.

Type A disease is usually more severe than type B or E disease, although all three have been fatal. Type E botulism seems to cause more gastrointestinal symptoms than others, and the recurrent neurologic symptoms seen with this type are apparently due to intestinal infection with *C. botulinum*, so that production and absorption of toxin are continuous. It is conceivable that the prolonged paralysis (weeks to months) that can occur in type A or B disease is also the result of continued infection and absorption of toxin from the colon.

The incubation period of 4 to 14 days in wound botulism probably reflects the length of time needed for infection to become established. Early gastrointestinal symptoms are not observed, but this form of botulism is otherwise identical to food-borne botulism.

The infant form of botulism is characterized by acute hypotonia, generalized muscle weakness, and a "floppy" appearance. Constipation and weak sucking are prominent, and ptosis, loss of neck muscle strength, and diminished gag reflex are common.

COMPLICATIONS AND SEQUELAE. Mortality in classic botulism varies from outbreak to outbreak. Case/fatality ratios vary from 2:1 to 25:1 in recent years. Ventilatory insufficiency is the most life-threatening aspect of botulism. There are no long-term sequelae in patients who survive.

GEOGRAPHIC VARIATION. Botulism occurs worldwide. The incidence varies with the eating habits of populations and the control exercised over commercial food processors rather than the distribution of *C. botulinum*. Cases due to ingestion of raw or lightly smoked fish are usually caused by Type E toxin and occur more commonly in the U.S.S.R., Scandinavia, Japan, and the Great Lakes region of the United States than elsewhere because of dietary preferences. In the United States, Types A and B poisoning are more common and are usually associated with home-canned vegetables, fruits, or prepared meats. In France, most cases occur after the patients have eaten home-cured hams and are usually due to Type B toxin. One outbreak in Kenya was associated with eating white ants.

Most cases of infant botulism have been diagnosed in California. Now that the syndrome has been publicized, cases are being recognized outside California and the United States.

DIAGNOSIS. The diagnosis should be made on the clinical presentation of a symmetric descending paralysis of the cranial nerves, extremities, and trunk whether or not a food source can be incriminated.

Myasthenia gravis and the Guillain-Barré syndrome are confused with botulism most frequently. In myasthenia gravis, weakness may not be symmetric and is accentuated by repetitive muscle use. The improvement in strength in myasthenia after injection of edrophonium chloride (tensilon) distinguishes it from botulism. The Guillain-Barré syndrome is distinguished by its ascending form of paralysis, frequent sparing of cranial nerves, sensory abnormalities, and abnormal cerebrospinal fluid. Electromyographic studies are often helpful and demonstrate potentiation (facilitation) of the action potential upon rapid repetitive stimulation and a depressed response to a single supramaximal stimulus. These findings most closely resemble those found in the myasthenic syndrome of Lambert and Eaton (carcinomatous neuropathy) and help to distinguish botulism from the Guillain-Barré syndrome. Other important disorders to be considered include poliomyelitis, drug toxicity (methyl alcohol, atropine, aminocyclitols), cerebrovascular accidents, multiple sclerosis, and diabetic neuropathy.

The definitive diagnosis is made by the detection of toxin in the serum for up to several weeks after the onset of symptoms. The finding of toxin and/or *C. botulinum* in patient feces or in a suspected food strongly supports the diagnosis. Immunologic assays are apparently less sensitive than the mouse toxin-neutralization test.

TREATMENT. The mainstay of therapy is trivalent (A, B, E) antitoxin, available in the United States from the Center for Disease Control. Each vial of equine antiserum contains 7500 IU Type A, 5500 IU of Type B, and 8500 IU of Type E antitoxin. Two vials are administered intravenously, and two more are injected four hours later. Desensitization may be necessary if the patient is allergic to horse serum. Repeated injections of antiserum may be needed if symptoms recur, as can happen in Type E botulism. Rare cases of botulism due to Types other than A, B, or E may not respond to trivalent antitoxin.

Supportive treatment, especially of respiration, can help reduce morbidity and mortality. Tracheostomy and mechanically assisted respiration should be employed early when indicated.

Emetics and cathartics for cleansing the gastrointestinal tract of toxin and organisms are probably of little value if antiserum is available and may precipitate aspiration pneumonia in patients who have dysphagia.

Although penicillin is probably not helpful in most patients with food-borne botulism, it should be considered for patients with Type E botulism who appear to have concomitant intestinal infection. In this situation, and in patients with infant botulism, however, penicillin may not be very effective because it may be inactivated by the β-lactamases present in the microflora of the colon. Penicillin is indicated in the management of patients with wound botulism, along with aggressive debridement. Antibiotic therapy need not be continued longer than one week.

The use of guanidine hydrochloride to counteract the

neurotoxic effects has been generally unsuccessful and is not routinely recommended, especially if antiserum and supportive therapy are available.

Without antitoxin therapy, the overall mortality can be as high as 70 per cent. With therapy, the mortality rate has been reduced to about 25 per cent.

PROPHYLAXIS. Education of the public on the dangers of home canning and processing (aging, smoking) of meat and fish should help to decrease the incidence of botulism. Pressure cooking should be used for all vegetables, including tomatoes, because reliance on acidity alone to inhibit toxin production is undependable. In the absence of pressure cooking, citric acid should be added to home-canned tomatoes.

Canned commercial products that are damaged or are under increased air pressure should not be consumed. Public health officials should be notified whenever botulism is suspected.

Although a formalinized toxoid is used to produce protective immunity in research workers, immunization of the public is not recommended because of the low incidence of botulism. Protective immunity apparently does not develop from botulism, probably because of the small quantities of toxin present.

CLOSTRIDIUM PERFRINGENS FOOD POISONING

ETIOLOGY. *Clostridium perfringens* is a spore-forming bacillus that is classified into five types (A through E) on the basis of its ability to produce various toxins. Only types A and C have been associated with food-borne disease, although type D has recently been shown to elaborate an enterotoxin that is immunologically and biologically identical to that produced by the other two types. *C. perfringens* causes approximately one third of cases of food poisoning throughout the world. Type C organisms produce a beta-toxin that may be responsible for an endemic necrotizing enteritis ("pig-bel") of the New Guinea highlands.

PATHOGENESIS. The organism is ubiquitous and can be isolated from soil and the intestinal tracts of man and other animals. Contaminated meat products, especially beef and gravy, constitute the majority of implicated food sources.

Several characteristics of *C. perfringens* are important in relation to food poisoning. Optimal temperature for growth in meat is 43 to 47° C, a temperature range that is frequently maintained inside a large piece of meat that is slowly cooling. The spores are sometimes quite heat-resistant and are activated at 75 to 80° C. Furthermore, heating the meat drives out sufficient air to make the meat anaerobic. Although these conditions promote growth of *C. perfringens,* they are not conducive to sporulation. Since toxin is produced during sporulation, it is unlikely that significant amounts of preformed toxin are absorbed from meat under most circumstances. Instead, sporulation and toxin production occur after the ingested bacteria reach the intestine. Administration of enterotoxin to volunteers does cause diarrhea when gastric acid is neutralized (Skjelkvåle and Uemura, 1977).

All the symptoms and signs of the illness can be attributed to an enterotoxin produced by *C. perfringens* types A, C, and D. The purified 35,000-dalton protein is heat-labile and acid-labile, and is inactivated by some proteolytic enzymes but not by trypsin. In ligated rabbit ileal loops, the absorption of glucose is inhibited, and the toxin induces a reversal of net transport, with resultant secretion of water, sodium, and chloride (Duncan and Strong, 1969). In addition, the epithelium of villous tips is denuded in the presence of toxin. This cytotoxic effect of the *C. perfringens* enterotoxin resembles that noted with *Shigella dysenteriae* toxin in tissue cultures and contrasts with the noncytotoxic effects of *V. cholerae* and *E. coli* enterotoxins (Keusch and Donta, 1975). The effects of the clostridial enterotoxin are not mediated through adenylate cyclase, although an intermediary role of prostaglandins has not been excluded. The ileum appears to be most sensitive to the toxin's effects (McDonel, 1974).

Pig-bel is due to *C. perfringens* type C infection. Bacteria ingested with a large amount of protein ("pork feasting") proliferate in the intestine and elaborate beta toxin, which is responsible for patchy gangrene of the jejunum and ileum. The natives may be deficient in intestinal proteases, since the beta toxin is very sensitive to proteolysis.

CLINICAL MANIFESTATIONS. The incubation period can be as short as two to four hours, but most patients have symptoms that begin 8 to 12 hours following the ingestion of contaminated food. Frequent episodes of watery diarrhea and cramping abdominal pain are the major complaints. Blood or mucus in the feces does not occur, except in the necrotizing enteritis form of type C disease. Fever is absent, and vomiting and nausea are rare. The illness is usually over in 24 hours.

Pig-bel is characterized by anorexia, severe abdominal pain, and bloody diarrhea. There can be intestinal obstruction due to sequential necrosis of the small intestine.

GEOGRAPHIC VARIATION. Clostridial food poisoning occurs worldwide. There are no reliable incidence figures for most of the world. Pig-bel is limited to the highlands of Papua New Guinea but could occur elsewhere.

DIAGNOSIS. The diagnosis is based on the clinical picture, an implicated food source, and the recovery of *C. perfringens* from the food source and the patient. As *C. perfringens* is normally found in feces, large numbers ($>10^5$ organisms/g) must be isolated from feces and food to confirm the diagnosis. Immunologic assays are used to detect enterotoxin in food and feces but are not sensitive enough to detect toxin in body fluids. Staphylococcal food poisoning causes more frequent and severe vomiting, and other enteric disorders can usually be distinguished by their longer duration of illness and the inflammatory signs and symptoms of invasive organisms such as *Salmonella* and *Shigella*.

TREATMENT. Because the illness is short, no treatment is needed. On occasion, oral or intravenous fluid replacement may be necessary to prevent dehydration in the elderly or newborn. Antibiotics are not indicated, and there are no known agents to counteract the effects of the enterotoxin. There is no effective therapy for pig-bel enteritis.

PROPHYLAXIS. Because it is nearly impossible to eradicate spores without pressure cooking, the public needs education on the dangers of allowing meat dishes to be kept at room temperature. Food should be served hot or kept refrigerated. Reheating of food destroys the heat-labile enterotoxin but may not destroy the organisms and spores themselves.

The role of humoral or local immunity is unknown. Repeat episodes of clostridial food poisoning have been reported. Pig-bel enteritis can be prevented by active immunization with beta toxoid from *C. perfringens* type C (Lawrence et al., 1979).

BACILLUS CEREUS FOOD POISONING

ETIOLOGY. Most strains of *Bacillus cereus* produce an enterotoxin that appears to be responsible for the clinical picture. The organism is a gram-positive, spore-forming rod, but, unlike the clostridia, it grows only under aerobic conditions.

PATHOGENESIS. The spores of *B. cereus* are heat-resistant, and, after the germination and multiplication process that occurs at temperatures of between 15 and 50° C, enterotoxin can be elaborated by the organisms. Typically, fried or boiled food has been allowed to stand at room temperature and is then reheated at temperatures too low to destroy the organisms or spores. The enterotoxin is destroyed by heating and is inactivated by acid pH. Enterotoxic activity appears to be distinct from the hemolysin and phospholipase produced by *B. cereus* and can elicit fluid accumulation in ligated rabbit ileal loops (Spira and Goepfert, 1975). Although the molecular mechanisms mediating enterotoxicity are unknown, it appears that direct stimulation of the adenylate cyclase system is not involved. The enterotoxin can cause cytotoxic changes in certain tissue cultures, but the relationship between these two activities has not been established.

It is likely that two disease phases, or even two syndromes, are possible: a short incubation illness associated with the ingestion of preformed toxin, and a longer incubation illness due to in vivo production of enterotoxin. Some authors have suggested the existence of two separate enterotoxins—one that is similar to staphylococcal enterotoxin and primarily induces vomiting, the other a diarrheagenic toxin. In volunteer studies in the 1950's, Hauge demonstrated that ingestion of approximately 10^{10} organisms in a vanilla sauce could reproduce the clinical disease.

CLINICAL MANIFESTATIONS. The incubation period can be as short as 30 to 120 minutes after the ingestion of preformed toxin that has escaped inactivation by gastric acid. An incubation period of 8 to 12 hours is also common, as was the case in Hauge's volunteer studies, and probably represents the period of time needed for in vivo production of enterotoxin. Watery diarrhea that is devoid of blood or mucus occurs at 15- to 30-minute intervals and is accompanied by abdominal cramping but not by fever. Nausea and vomiting can occur, especially in association with a shorter incubation period. The entire illness lasts 12 to 24 hours and usually leaves no sequelae.

GEOGRAPHIC VARIATION. The organism is common in soil and on vegetation, but no animal reservoir is known. It has been most commonly associated with starches and grain products, especially rice, instant mashed potatoes, and pasta, but other foods such as milk products, meat loaf, vegetable sprouts, green bean salad, and soups have been implicated as well. Although currently *B. cereus* accounts for less than 5 per cent of all cases of food poisoning in the United States, increasing awareness of the disorder and improved methods of detection may place its true incidence at a higher level. The illness occurs worldwide.

DIAGNOSIS. The diagnosis primarily rests on the clinical picture and an implicated food source. Demonstration of more than 10^5 organisms per g of food or feces lends strong support to the diagnosis. The enterotoxin has not yet been demonstrated in food or body fluids. Differentiation from staphylococcal or clostridial food poisoning may be difficult on clinical and epidemiologic grounds alone.

TREATMENT. As the disease is of short duration and is primarily an intoxication, no specific therapy is warranted. Rarely, parenteral fluid replacement and antiemetics may be needed.

PROPHYLAXIS. Public awareness of the epidemiology and pathogenesis of the disease is the most important preventive measure. Special attention needs to be given to the storage of rice after it is fried or boiled. Food processing firms, especially those concerned with grain products, must be made aware of the potential problems, and inspection procedures designed to minimize contamination.

References

Arnon, S. S., Midura, T. F., Clay, S. A., Wood, R. M., and Chin, J.: Infant botulism. Epidemiological, clinical, and laboratory aspects. JAMA 237:1946, 1977.

Buxser, S., Bonventre, P. F., and Archer, D. L.: Specific receptor binding of staphylococcal enterotoxins by murine splenic lymphocytes. Infect and Immun 33:827, 1981.

Donta, S. T.: Changing concepts of infectious diseases. Geriatrics 30:123, 1975.

Duncan, C. L., and Strong, D. H.: Ileal loop fluid accumulation and production of diarrhea in rabbits by cell-free products of *Clostridium perfringens*. J Bacteriol 100:86, 1969.

Dyer, D. W., and Iandolo, J. J.: Plasmid-chromosomal transition of genes important in staphylococcal enterotoxin B expression. Infect and Immun 33:450, 1981.

Elwell, M. R., Liu, C. T., Spertzel, R. O., and Beisel, W. R.: Mechanisms of oral staphylococcal enterotoxin B-induced emesis in the monkey. Pro Soc Exp Biol Med 148:424, 1975.

Kapral, F. A., O'Brien, A. D., Ruff, P. D., and Drugan, W. J., Jr.: Inhibition of water absorption in the intestine by *Staphylococcus aureus* delta-toxin. Infect Immun 13:140, 1976.

Keusch, G. T., and Donta, S. T.: Classification of enterotoxins on the basis of activity in cell culture. J Infect Dis 131:58, 1975.

Lawrence, T., Shaun, F., Freestone, D. S., and Walker, P. D.: Prevention of necrotizing enteritis in Papua New Guinea by active immunization. Lancet 1:227, 1979.

McDonel, J. L.: In vivo effects of *Clostridium perfringens* enteropathogenic factors on the rat ileum. Infect Immun 10:1156, 1974.

Merson, M. H., and Dowell, V. R., Jr.: Epidemiologic, clinical, and laboratory aspects of wound botulism. N Engl J Med 289:1005, 1973.

Oguma, K., and Iida, H.: High and low toxin production by a non-toxigenic strain of *Clostridium botulinum* type C following infection with Type C phages of different passage history. J Gen Microbiol 112:203, 1979.

Skjelkvåle, R., and Uemura, T.: Experimental diarrhoea in human volunteers following oral administration of *Clostridium perfringens* enterotoxin. J Appl Bacteriol 43:281, 1977.

Spira, W. M., and Goepfert, J. M.: Biological characteristics of an enterotoxin produced by *Bacillus cereus*. Can J Microbiol 21:1236, 1975.

Sugiyama, H.: Animal models for the study of infant botulism. Rev Infect Dis 1:683, 1979.

132

BACTERIAL ENTERITIS

HARVEY S. KANTOR, M.D.

I am poured out like water and all my bones are out of joint: my heart is like wax; it is melted in the midst of my bowels. Psalms 22:14

"It's this damned belly that gives a man his worst troubles." Homer, Odessey XV, 344, c. 850 B.C.

Inflammatory disease of the small intestine and colon as a consequence of bacterial infection is one of the most common afflictions of man throughout history. It is worldwide, and where malnutrition and crowded living conditions exist, enteric disease is a striking cause of morbidity and death.

SHIGELLOSIS

Shigellosis (bacillary dysentery) is an acute, self-limited infection of the intestinal tract caused by bacteria of the genus *Shigella*. The disease varies from the asymptomatic carrier to diarrhea or to frank dysentery characterized by fever, tenesmus, abdominal cramps, and diarrhea with stools containing mucus and blood. Man is the principal host of shigellae, and the infection is usually transmitted by the oral-fecal route.

ETIOLOGY. *Shigella* species belong to the family Enterobacteriacea and are gram-negative, nonmotile organisms. Strains of *Shigella* can be characterized by specific cell wall antigens, and there are four serologic groups responsible for disease in man. The clinically important species within the respective groups are *Sh. dysenteriae* (Shiga bacillus), *Sh. flexneri*, *Sh. boydii*, and *Sh. sonnei*. These species are also known as subgroups A, B, C, and D, respectively. They are distinguished from *Escherichia coli* by their failure to ferment lactose (*Sh. sonnei* ferments lactose slowly), from salmonellae by their inability to produce gas in glucose, and from *Salmonella typhi* by their lack of motility.

PATHOGENESIS AND PATHOLOGY. *Shigella* must adhere to the mucosal surface, penetrate epithelial cells, and multiply within the mucosa to cause disease. Otherwise, these organisms are rapidly cleared from the gut. The number (10 to 100) of invasive organisms needed to cause disease is much smaller than that required for the noninvasive toxigenic pathogens such as *Vibrio cholerae* and *E. coli* (10^8 organisms). Since shigellae invade the colon but not the jejunum, it may be necessary to postulate a site-specific receptor mechanism that selectively recognizes virulent bacteria and mediates bacterial penetration of the bowel. Evidence has been obtained that *Sh. dysenteriae* binds to a specific cell membrane receptor involving 1–4 linked *N*-acetyl-D-glucosamine oligomers. In addition, expression of the virulent phenotype, invasiveness, requires a specific plasmid. Strains in which the plasmid has been eliminated are avirulent and unable to penetrate epithelial cells.

After multiplication within epithelial cells, the bacteria may spread from cell to cell. In acute shigellosis, there is a distinct gradation of inflammation, diminishing from the luminal surface of the colon to the submucosa, which shows little reaction. The number of bacteria sharply decreases toward the submucosa and this may explain why bloodstream invasion is infrequent. In contrast, the luminal concentration of shigellae may reach 10^6 to 10^{10} organisms per gram of stool. The severe inflammation probably is an important factor in limiting the disease to the bowel wall and causes fever, cramps, tenesmus, inflammation, mucosal ulceration, microabscess formation, and fluid and electrolyte loss into the intestinal lumen. Colonic mucosal ulceration is a characteristic of *Shigella* infections not usually observed in *Salmonella* infections. This differential response may be due to a cytotoxin elaborated by shigellae and not salmonellae.

Shigellosis may cause three patterns of diarrhea: (1) classic dysentery, with multiple small liquid stools containing blood, mucus, or pus; (2) uncomplicated watery diarrhea; or (3) a combination of watery diarrhea and dysentery. Watery diarrhea frequently precedes the dysentery, signifying early involvement of the small intestine. The mechanisms of diarrhea are unknown but may involve an enterotoxin with effects like those of *V. cholerae* and *E. coli*. *Sh. dysenteriae* 1 elaborates a protein exotoxin that causes enterotoxicity (intestinal fluid-secreting activity), alteration in myoelectric activity, and stimulation of adenylate cyclase, resulting in increased intracellular cyclic AMP levels in the ligated rabbit ileal loop model, neurotoxicity in mice, cytotoxicity for HeLa cells, and inhibition of mammalian and bacterial protein synthesis. A toxin with similar biologic and antigenic properties has been found in *Sh. flexneri* 2a, and a cell-free cytotoxin has been isolated from *Sh. sonnei*.

The significance of toxin in the pathogenesis of shigellosis is unclear. Studies of Shiga dysentery using live bacterial challenge in humans and monkeys reemphasize the importance of tissue invasion, since nonpenetrating mutants that were toxin-producing failed to elicit overt signs of illness. These findings do not exclude a function for the toxins of these three species of Shigella because toxin elaborated after penetration could be a virulence factor. Sera from patients with shigellosis due to *Sh. flexneri*, *Sh. sonnei*, and *Sh. dysenteriae* 1 contained antibodies that neutralized *Sh. dysenteriae* 1 toxin in vitro, thus suggesting that toxin is produced in vivo.

CLINICAL MANIFESTATIONS. The most frequent presenting symptoms in patients with shigellosis are diarrhea, abdominal pain, and fever. The incubation period is about two to four days but may be as long as a week. In its classic form, shigellosis is a biphasic illness. The initial symptoms are fever, followed by abdominal pain and watery diarrhea without gross blood, usually lasting one to three days. The second phase is that of true dysentery; the character of the stool changes to small volume, bloody movements, and the patient complains of tenesmus, fecal urgency, and painful defecation. The initial phase may relate to the action of the enterotoxin. The second phase corresponds to invasion of the colonic epithelium and acute colitis (DuPont et al., 1969). Abdominal tenderness is most pronounced in the lower quadrants and hyperactive bowel sounds are common, but there is no peritoneal irritation.

COMPLICATIONS AND SEQUELAE. Most cases of shigellosis in well-nourished populations are mild and terminate without complications in a few days.

In severe infections, which occur especially in young children and elderly individuals, dehydration, acid-base disturbances, and shock may supervene early because of excessive loss of fluid and electrolytes; these are the most frequent serious complications of *Shigella* gastroenteritis. Other complications of shigellosis, found most often in children, are seizures, meningismus, pneumonia, a hemolytic-uremic syndrome associated with endotoxemia and circulating immune complexes, vaginitis, and, rarely, agranulocytosis. *Shigella* bacteremia occurs rarely and may produce metastatic septic foci. Reiter's syndrome—urethritis, conjunctivitis, and arthritis—may develop two to four weeks after the onset of *Shigella* dysentery; individuals with a specific histocompatibility antigen (HL-A B27) appear to be at much higher risk of this complication. Perforation of the intestine is rare despite considerable ulceration. Pyelonephritis, empyema, glomerulonephritis, and otitis media may develop (Barrett-Connor and Connor, 1970). A complication that apparently is peculiar to one strain of *Sh. dysenteriae* is peripheral neuropathy. Chronic bacillary dysentery may mimic ulcerative colitis. Mucosal ulceration produced by *Shigella* occasionally provides a portal of entry for other enteric bacteria to the bloodstream.

Shigellae, like other bacterial enteric pathogens, cause more subclinical than clinical cases, and short-term fecal excretion of organisms may persist for days to weeks. An asymptomatic carrier state beyond one year has been reported for *Sh. sonnei* and *Sh. flexneri* 2a.

GEOGRAPHIC VARIATIONS IN DISEASE. Shigellosis is worldwide, occurring in arctic, temperate, and tropical climates. Wherever acute diarrheal diseases are a major health problem, *Shigella* organisms cause most of the more severe diarrheal illnesses.

Over the past 10 years *Sh. sonnei* has accounted for most of the *Shigella* isolations in the United States, with *Sh. flexneri* second. A similar trend has been observed in Great Britain, Western Europe, Japan, and Korea. It has been suggested that *Sh. sonnei* predominates in countries with increasing industrialization, economic development, and a higher standard of living. In the United States, *Sh. flexneri* has predominated in states that are largely rural, sparsely populated, poorly industrialized, or that have a large American Indian population.

Sh. dysenteriae 1 has never been a frequent cause of diarrhea and dysentery in the Western Hemisphere. Shiga dysentery has been consistently present primarily in the Middle and Far East. After an absence of several decades, *Sh. dysenteriae* 1 reappeared in Central America and caused a pandemic with unusually severe dysentery from 1968 to 1972 that encompassed five countries.

DIAGNOSIS. *Shigella* infections should be considered in anyone with diarrhea, with or without fever. A positive diagnosis depends on isolating shigellae from the stools. Since a small percentage of initial stool cultures may not yield shigellae, several stool samples during the first 24 hours may increase the chances for isolating this organism. Although many shigellae are usually excreted during active disease, they often remain alive in the feces only briefly and must be cultured without delay. A rectal swab is excellent for culture. Specimens from intestinal ulcers, taken under direct vision through a sigmoidoscope, are most likely to contain the organisms.

Shigella dysentery has a more acute onset than amebic dysentery and is usually self-limited, whereas amebic dysentery may have spontaneous remissions and frequent relapses. Sigmoidoscopic examination may provide a further distinction—diffuse mucosal involvement with multiple, very superficial ulcers is characteristic of shigellosis, whereas undermined ulcers with raised edges and normal intervening mucosa are typical in amebiasis. Microscopic examination of stool in shigellosis shows discrete red cells, numerous intact polymorphonuclear leukocytes, scanty nonmotile microorganisms, and numerous macrophages; that of amebic infection contains clumped red cells, degenerate leukocytes, numerous motile microorganisms, and trophozoites of *Entamoeba histolytica*. The presence of fecal leukocytes appears to indicate a colitis with disruption of the distal intestinal mucosa. Fecal leukocytes may also be found in patients with salmonellosis, invasive *E. coli* colitis, and ulcerative colitis, but not in diarrheas caused by enterotoxins or viruses.

Other causes of diarrhea considered in the differential diagnosis include *Giardia lamblia*, viral agents, and staphylococcal and clostridial enterotoxins, none of which usually cause clinical dysentery. Shigellosis can be distinguished with certainty from acute ulcerative colitis only by bacteriologic studies.

Serologic tests have not been very useful for diagnosis of shigellosis.

TREATMENT. The role of specific antimicrobial therapy in the treatment of shigellosis is uncertain. In some studies, antibiotics shortened the duration of symptoms and the excretion of organisms but not in other studies. Furthermore, the repeated emergence of *Shigella* strains that are resistant to antibiotics that had been in common use at the time has made it difficult to choose a drug that is both effective and safe.

The primary treatment of shigellosis is supportive; in patients who are acutely ill, particularly young children or elderly persons, the main goal is restoration of fluids and electrolytes. It is reasonable to withhold antibiotics from patients who are moderately ill. In severe dysentery, antibiotics should be selected on the basis of sensitivity tests and the prevailing pattern of sensitivity in each community. Sulfonamides, formerly the drugs of choice, are no longer reliable. Ampicillin is the current drug of choice; it should be administered orally as 50 (adult) to 100 (children) mg/kg body weight/day in four equal doses for three to five days. When shigellae are resistant to ampicillin, they usually have multiple antibiotic resistance to tetracyclines, sulfonamides, and chloramphenicol. Under these circumstances, trimethoprim-sulfamethoxazole is the best choice; it is administered for 5 days in two divided oral doses of 20 to 25 mg/kg/dose of sulfamethoxazole and 4 to 5 mg/kg/dose of trimethoprim (Chang et al., 1977). In areas where antimicrobial susceptibility testing is not available, a single oral dose (2.5 g) of tetracycline may be the most practical therapy for adults with shigellosis. It may even be effective in treatment of resistant strains (Pickering et al., 1978).

Drugs that retard intestinal motility, such as paregoric or diphenoxylate hydrochloride with atropine (Lomotil), may prolong the clinical illness, the duration of the diarrhea, and excretion of shigellae and should therefore be avoided (Dupont and Hornick, 1973).

PROPHYLAXIS. Sanitary disposal of human feces so that they cannot contaminate water or food supplies is basic to prophylaxis in shigellosis. Attempts to develop a safe, effective vaccine have been hampered by the numerous serotypes of these organisms, the need for booster vaccinations, and the brief immunity.

SALMONELLOSIS

The term salmonellosis refers to infections caused by bacteria of the genus *Salmonella,* which consists of more than 2000 serotypes. Human salmonellosis can be divided into four syndromes: gastroenteritis ("food poisoning"), enteric fever (typhoid-like disease), bacteremia with and without focal extra-intestinal infection, and the asymptomatic carrier state (Black et al., 1960). Infection caused by *Salmonella typhi* (typhoid fever) is considered separately in Chapter 191.

ETIOLOGY. Salmonellae are gram-negative, facultatively anaerobic, and generally motile bacilli that do not ferment lactose and, with the exception of *S. typhi,* produce acid and gas from glucose. They are classified in three primary species: *S. typhi, S. choleraesuis,* and *S. enteritidis. S. typhi* and *S. choleraesuis* each consist of a single serotype. In contrast, over 2000 antigenically distinct serotypes of *S. enteritidis* have been defined. The serotype of each *Salmonella* depends both on its somatic or O antigens and on its H or flagellar antigens.

The salmonellae fall into divisions according to their host preference and the clinical syndromes they produce (Table 1). It should be noted that *Salmonella* serotypes that are not adapted to specific hosts constitute the vast majority of *Salmonella* species. These species cause over 80 per cent of current *Salmonella* infections in the United States, generally taking the form of acute gastroenteritis.

PATHOGENESIS AND PATHOLOGY. Only *Salmonella* strains that invade the ileal epithelium can cause enteritis or intestinal fluid secretion and subsequent diarrhea. Strains that do not penetrate cause no disease. These organisms have a predilection for villous epithelium, tend to spare crypt cells, and inflict far less damage on epithelium than do shigellae. The preferential attachment of these salmonellae to the tips of villi suggests a specific receptor on villi, and salmonellae do interact with mannose residues of the glycoprotein in intestinal epithelial surfaces. Salmonellae do not multiply in epithelial cells as shigellae do, and ulcer formation in salmonellosis is infrequent.

The biochemical lesion underlying intestinal fluid secretion and diarrhea in *Salmonella* enteritis remains elusive. In animal models infected with *S. typhimurium,* changes in ileal water and electrolyte transport, stimulation of adenylate cyclase, and elevation of intracellular cyclic AMP levels are qualitatively similar to those described in cholera and enterotoxigenic *E. coli* diarrhea. Mucosal invasion alone appears not to be a sufficient stimulus to cause transport abnormalities. Infection with strains of *S. typhimurium* that invade intestinal mucosa without causing associated secretion of intestinal fluid does not change sodium and chloride transport or adenylate cyclase activity.

S. typhimurium in monkeys elicits severe ileitis, but no histologic alterations in the jejunum. Yet fluid is secreted in both the jejunum and ileum, suggesting that enterotoxins may be responsible for jejunal fluid secretion. *S. typhimurium* produces small amounts of a heat-labile cholera-gen-like toxin that increases vascular permeability when injected into skin, increases intracellular levels of cyclic AMP and causes elongation of Chinese Hamster ovary cells. It is neutralized by cholera antitoxin and preincubation with G_{ml} ganglioside, and rabbits immunized with heated cholera toxin are protected against loss of fluid from ileal loops infected with live *S. typhimurium* (Peterson, 1980).

Within 24 hours most of the bacteria have passed through the epithelium into the lamina propria, where an intense reaction with inflammatory cells is evoked. It has been suggested (Sprinz, 1969) that the tissue response determines the clinical features. *Salmonella* species other than *S. typhi* and *S. paratyphi* elicit a polymorphonuclear

Table 1. RELATION OF SALMONELLA SPECIES AND REPRESENTATIVE SEROTYPES TO HUMAN DISEASE

Species	Representative Serotype	Natural Host	Human Disease
S. typhi	—	Man	Enteric fever
S. choleraesuis	—	Swine	Bacteremia or focal infection
S. enteritidis			
	paratyphi[a] schottmulleri[a] hirschfeldi[a]	Man	Enteric fever
	typhimurium		Gastroenteritis, bacteremia, and focal infection
	newport enteritidis and hundreds of related serotypes	No Host specificity	Gastroenteritis
	dublin	Cattle	Bacteremia and enteric fever
	pullorum gallinarium	Fowl	None
	abortus equi abortus ovis	Horses Sheep	

[a]These three salmonella serotypes were formerly designated *S. paratyphi* A, *S. paratyphi* B, and *S. paratyphi* C, respectively.
Adapted from Grady, G. F., and Keusch, G. T.: N Engl Med 285:831, 1971.

leukocyte response that quickly eliminates the organisms, and clinical illness is generally limited to gastroenteritis, although metastatic abscesses can occur. In typhoid and paratyphoid infections the predominant response is mononuclear, and the clinical syndrome is enteric fever. The Peyer's patches of the distal ileum are the primary site of bacterial penetration with infection spreading to the regional lymph nodes. Many *Salmonella* species will be successfully contained by mucosal and lymphatic barriers and restricted to the intestine. The more virulent serotypes spill into the thoracic lymph from the intestinal lymph nodes, reach the systemic circulation, and disseminate to the liver, spleen and other parts of the reticuloendothelial system.

Between 10^5 and 10^6 viable salmonellae must be swallowed by volunteers for clinical disease to occur, whereas a transient carrier state will follow ingestion of 10- to 100-fold fewer organisms. However, in retrospective investigations of human salmonellosis outbreaks, the actual doses ingested were calculated to be $<10^3$ organisms. Variations in vehicle and serotype may explain this discrepancy. Salmonellosis occurs most frequently in infants and the aged and often as a second illness in persons whose resistance has been lowered by another infection, neoplastic disease, or malnutrition. *Salmonella* infections complicate malaria, sickle cell anemia, and bartonellosis at a significantly higher frequency than that of other pathogens. Hemolysis is the common feature of the three diseases, and the free hemoglobin may block killing of *Salmonella* organisms by macrophages.

CLINICAL MANIFESTATIONS, COMPLICATIONS, AND SEQUELAE. Two thirds of all recognized diseases caused by *Salmonella* in man take the form of enteritis. Certain *Salmonella* serotypes are consistently associated with specific clinical syndromes (see Table 1). Despite this, every serotype can produce any of the varied clinical patterns of salmonellosis. The separation of human salmonellosis into four syndromes is useful for classification, but in practice the syndromes overlap.

Gastroenteritis. Although referred to as *Salmonella* food poisoning, the disease is actually an intestinal infection. No preformed toxin is involved as in staphylococcal food poisoning (see Chapter 131). In 1981, salmonellae were responsible for more outbreaks (26 per cent) of food-borne acute gastroenteritis of confirmed etiology in the United States than any other cause and the greatest number of deaths. The incubation period is 6 to 48 hours or longer. The first symptoms are nausea and vomiting, which subside within a few hours, followed rapidly by gripping abdominal pain. The most prominent symptom is usually diarrhea of variable severity, ranging from only one or two loose stools in mild cases, to profuse, bloody diarrhea in severe cases, to a cholera-like syndrome. The temperature is moderately elevated (less than 102° F) for 24 to 48 hours in most cases. In uncomplicated gastroenteritis in adults, bacteremia occurs in less than 4 per cent of patients. Bowel sounds are hyperactive and abdominal tenderness is moderate. In some patients the abdominal findings are severe enough to be confused with acute appendicitis or cholecystitis. The illness often subsides within five days but may last only one day or persist for weeks. If simultaneous infection by more than one serotype occurs, the clinical picture does not differ from that produced by a single strain. Microscopic stool examinations may disclose a few to moderate number of white blood cells, as compared to the sheets and clumps shed in shigella infections.

Although salmonellosis is usually regarded as a disease of the small intestine, the colon may also be involved. *Salmonella* colitis usually starts like ulcerative colitis, but a positive stool culture, a self-limited course, and deterioration with corticosteroids (perforation and septicemia) differentiate the two conditions.

Enteric Fevers. Although enteric fever is most often produced by *S. typhi* and the paratyphoid bacilli (*S. enteritidis*, serotypes *S. paratyphi*, *S. schottmuller*, and *S. hirschfeldi*), it may be caused by any serotype of *Salmonella*. Regardless of serotype, the manifestations of enteric fever are similar. When caused by serotypes other than *S. typhi*, the clinical picture is usually milder, but otherwise it is indistinguishable from typhoid fever. The clinical features of typhoid fever are described in Chapter 191.

Salmonella Bacteremia (Septicemia). Organisms may be present transiently in the blood of patients with *Salmonella* gastroenteritis. This occurs most commonly in children and is generally benign. Of greater importance is a syndrome of transient bacteremia and fever in adults with serious underlying illness (carcinoma, lymphoma, liver disease, collagen vascular disease) and no gastroenteritis. Their fatality rate with nontyphoidal bacteremia is about 13 per cent (Cherubin et al., 1974). The major significance of *Salmonella* in the blood is the high risk of development of metastatic infections. This risk is more important than the bacteremia, which has a low mortality compared with that of bacteremias due to other gram-negative organisms. *S. typhimurium* most often causes *Salmonella* bacteremia and is followed in frequency by *S. enteritidis* and *S. choleraesuis*.

Chronic *Salmonella* bacteremia has been associated with concomitant *Schistosoma mansoni* infection. Colonization of the ceca of the schistosomes by *Salmonella* may provide a continuing reservoir of *Salmonella* organisms.

Focal Infections. *Salmonellae* may cause localized tissue infections either accompanied by or after septicemia. Osteomyelitis, meningitis, and pneumonia are most common, followed by *Salmonella* pyelonephritis, endocarditis, and suppurative arthritis. Tissue anywhere in the body may be seeded, but damaged tissue is particularly susceptible to abscesses and chronic destructive lesions. Thus, metastatic infections may develop in hematomas, malignant tumors, bone infarcts, gall stones, or abnormal endovascular tissue. Twenty-five per cent of focal infections occur in structures connected to the gastrointestinal tract. Estimates of focal infections after prolonged or untreated bacteremia have ranged from 8 to 25 per cent of cases. After *S. typhi*, the serotypes that invade the bloodstream and produce focal infection most often are *S. cholerasuis* and *S. typhimurium*.

Carrier State. The transient asymptomatic carrier may be even more common than gastroenteritis. All individuals with *Salmonella* infections excrete the organisms for varying time periods and are referred to as convalescent carriers. In the early period of acute gastroenteritis as many as 10^6 to 10^9 salmonellae per gram of feces may be present. With recovery, the number of bacteria that can be recovered from stools gradually diminishes. By the third month, approximately 90 per cent of patients will have stopped excreting organisms. Individuals who excrete salmonellae for one year or more are considered to be chronic carriers.

The incidence of chronic carriers of S. *paratyphi* is about 3 per cent and of nontyphoidal serotypes less than 1 per cent. The severity of the initial infection has no relation to the duration of Salmonella carriage. Gallbladder disease predisposes to chronic carriage.

GEOGRAPHIC VARIATION. Salmonellosis is a common worldwide disease and is reported most extensively in North American and European countries. Ingestion of food contaminated directly or indirectly with *Salmonella*-infected feces of man and wild or domesticated vertebrates is the primary source of infection or disease. In the United States it is estimated that salmonellae are the causal agent of two million cases of human gastroenteritis annually but that only 1 per cent of the total is reported. Some *Salmonella* serotypes tend to demonstrate geographic patterns. *S. typhimurium* is an example of a serotype with a widespread distribution; it is the most common cause of human salmonella infections in the United States and Europe. Other species may have such a limited distribution in nature that their isolation from an infected person may be used to determine the source of infection. For instance, in 1980, *Salmonella* surveillance in the United States revealed that 96 per cent of isolates of S. *weltrevreden* were reported from Hawaii. However, mass production of foods coupled with a rapid transportation system can spread *Salmonella*-contaminated food great distances.

DIAGNOSIS. The diagnosis of salmonellosis on clinical grounds is difficult and must be considered in every case of diarrhea. The diagnosis can be established only by isolation of *Salmonella* from blood, stool, urine, or elsewhere. Agglutination tests are of little value.

TREATMENT. *Salmonella* gastroenteritis is usually a mild, self-limited illness. With careful attention to the management of fluids and electrolytes, recovery is generally uneventful. Antibiotic therapy does not shorten or help the illness. Some authors have suggested that specific antimicrobial therapy prolongs rather than shortens postconvalescent fecal excretion of *Salmonella.* More recently, a randomized prospective, double-blind study in infants showed oral antibiotic therapy had no significant effect on the duration of positive stool cultures. In addition, 53 per cent of patients who received antibiotics suffered bacteriologic relapse after therapy and in more than one-third of cases, this was associated with recurrence of diarrhea. Relapse did not occur after placebo therapy (Nelson et al., 1980). Drug therapy also promotes the acquisition of antibiotic-resistant strains. Occasionally antibiotics appear to convert gastroenteritis or simple carrier states to systemic disease with bacteremia. Antibiotics are indicated only for patients with *Salmonella* gastroenteritis with bacteremia or in neonates, the elderly, patients with lymphoproliferative, cardiovascular, or bone and joint disorders, and those with chronic hemolytic anemia. These are patients who are at high risk of developing bacteremia or metastatic infection. Agents that impair intestinal motility such as opiates and diphenoxylate hydrochloride with atropine (Lomotil) are often administered for symptomatic relief of abdominal cramps and diarrhea. When used excessively, they seem to delay convalescence, prolong fecal carriage of *Salmonella*, and rarely cause bacteremia.

For the treatment of the enteric fevers and *Salmonella* bacteremia, the drug of choice is chloramphenicol given only intravenously* in a dose of 4 g/day (in four equally divided doses every six hours) for three to four weeks. Ampicillin should be reserved for chloramphenicol-resistant, ampicillin-sensitive organisms and should be given intravenously in the range of 8 to 12 g/day. The trimethoprim-sulfamethoxazole combination is effective and should be given orally in doses of 160 mg trimethoprim and 800 mg sulfamethoxazole every 12 hours. Metastatic abscesses must be drained.

Antibiotic therapy is ineffective for eradication of salmonellae in the convalescent carrier. Chronic carriers with normal gallbladders are treated with 1.5 g ampicillin plus 0.5 g probenecid orally every six hours for 30 days. If cholelithiasis is present, cholecystectomy may also be necessary.

PROPHYLAXIS. The prevention and control of *Salmonella* infections is complicated by the ubiquitous distribution of these organisms in nature. They infect many species of animals and can survive for prolonged periods in the inanimate environment.

Man acquires salmonellosis primarily by ingestion of contaminated water, milk, and food. Food production, food processing, water supplies, and sewage systems must maintain a high level of sanitation. Acutely ill individuals who are excreting Salmonella organisms should be isolated. Asymptomatic carriers should practice high standards of personal hygiene and should not be employed as food handlers.

No effective immunization is available against nontyphoidal Salmonella species.

ESCHERICHIA COLI DIARRHEA

ETIOLOGY. Three groups of *Escherichia coli* cause diarrheal disease. They are enterotoxigenic *E. coli* (ETEC), which produce enterotoxins and are important causes of diarrhea in infants, young children, and adults in developing countries and travellers to these countries; enteropathogenic *E. coli* (EPEC), which have produced frequent outbreaks of epidemic infantile diarrhea in many parts of the world and belong to specific serotypes; and enteroinvasive *E. coli* (EIEC), which are invasive and evoke pathologic reactions like those of *Shigella* (Table 2).

PATHOGENESIS AND PATHOLOGY

Enterotoxigenic E. coli (ETEC). ETEC is a group of *E. coli* that do not belong to EPEC serotypes previously known to cause diarrhea in humans.

The first requirement for ETEC diarrhea is colonization of the upper small intestine by the pathogen after it is ingested in contaminated food and survives the acid barrier of the stomach. Pathogenic *E. coli* can colonize sites in the bowel where nonpathogenic *E. coli* normally do not survive. The ETEC colonize the epithelial surface of the small

*Chloramphenicol sodium succinate, when given by the intramuscular route, is of little value because of its slow rate of conversion to the active compound; oral administration of chloramphenicol should be avoided because almost all cases of bone marrow aplasia that have been recorded have occurred in patients receiving the drug by mouth.

Table 2. TYPES OF *E. COLI* INTESTINAL PATHOGENS

Common Name	Toxin	Mechanism
Enterotoxigenic (ETEC)	LT	Activates adenylate cyclase
	ST	Activates guanylate cyclase
Enteropathogenic (EPEC)	Shigella-like cytotoxin	Associated by serotype; entero-adhesive, destroys intestinal brush borders, no invasion
	Novel enterotoxin-like activity	Unknown
Enteroinvasive (EIEC)	—	Penetrates colonic epithelium

intestine without mucosal damage, tissue invasion, or bacteremia.

The initial step in colonization by ETEC involves attachment of the bacteria to small intestinal epithelium. Attachment is mediated by pili or fimbriae, which have also been termed "adherence or colonization factor antigens" (CFA). Two major human ETEC fibrial CFA's have been described: CFA/I and CFA/II. They are each produced by only certain ETEC serotypes. Neither CFA has ever been identified on a strain of nonentertoxigenic *E. coli* because both CFA/I and CFA/II are plasmid-determined products and the respective genes reside on enterotoxin (*ent*) plasmids. All of the known CFA fimbriae can cause hemagglutination (HA) of animal or human erythrocytes. HA mediated by these fimbriae is not inhibited by mannose, and thus the term mannose-resistant HA. The common fimbriae of *E. coli* that mediate nonspecific attachment to many different cell types are recognized by the inhibition of their HA by mannose. An HA-typing scheme has been developed as a rapid and simple presumptive test for CFAs and, thus, for ETEC (Evans and Evans, 1983). The antigenic structure of the adherence fimbriae determines the host specificity of the ETEC strains. For example, the adherence antigen for the pig, K88, will allow *E. coli* to adhere to porcine intestinal cells and not to bovine cells. The biochemical receptors for CFA/I and CFA/II have not been identified but there is some data to suggest the CFA/I receptor may be G_{M2}-type ganglioside.

In addition to adherence antigens, ETEC must produce enterotoxins to cause disease. Two types of enterotoxins are made by ETEC—heat labile (LT) and heat stable (ST). The heat-labile toxin is of large molecular weight and appears to be similar to cholera toxin both antigenically and in its mechanism of action. Both cholera toxin and the heat-labile toxin give rise to a noninflammatory secretory diarrhea by first binding to a G_{M1} ganglioside receptor on the intestinal mucosal cell surface, and then activating adenylate cyclase so that intracellular cyclic AMP is elevated. This results in anion hypersecretion, inhibition of sodium absorption, and ultimately, an outpouring of fluid from the gut and watery diarrhea.

The mechanism by which cyclic AMP mediates enhanced intestinal secretion is unknown. It has been proposed that cyclic AMP-dependent protein kinases are the molecular receptors for cyclic AMP and mediate the biologic effects of cyclic AMP by regulating phosphorylation of membrane protein. This hypothesis is supported by the recent finding that there is a direct correlation between intestinal secretion and activation of cyclic AMP-dependent protein kinase by cholera toxin (Kantor et al., 1981).

In contrast to the heat-labile toxin, the stable toxin is of low molecular weight and is antigenically unrelated to either the heat-labile toxin or to cholera toxin; it neither stimulates intestinal adenylate cyclase nor alters intracellular cyclic AMP levels. Recent work suggests that the diarrheagenic effect of the heat-stable toxin is mediated by guanylate cyclase stimulation and increased intestinal mucosal concentrations of cyclic GMP (Field et al., 1978).

There is increasing evidence that certain O:K:H: (somatic:capsular:flagellar) serotypes indicate a high probability of a strain being enterotoxigenic. There is also an association between serotype and enterotoxin type. Both enterotoxins are known to be genetically controlled by DNA residing in transferrable plasmids. This association between chromosomally mediated cell-wall antigens and plasmid-determined enterotoxin and fimbria production is not understood.

Enteropathogenic E. coli (EPEC). EPEC are diarrheagenic *E. coli* belonging to serogroups epidemiologically incriminated as pathogens but without LT, ST, or *Shigella*-like invasiveness (Edelman and Levine, 1983). The list of *E. coli* serogroups epidemiologically connected with infantile gastroenteritis includes about 15 members, of which 0 serogroups 26, 55, 111, 119, 125–128, and 142 are the most prevalent.

Recent in vitro and in vivo studies clearly identify a pathognomonic lesion associated with EPEC colonization consisting of intestinal brush border destruction and pedestal formation of intestinal epithelial cell plasma membranes at sites where EPEC are attached as seen by electron microscopy (Edelman and Levine, 1983).

There is evidence that EPEC can produce a cytotoxin that is biologically, antigenically, and biochemically indistinguishable from pure *Shigella dysenteriae* type 1 (Shiga) toxin. Like Shiga toxin, the EPEC toxin is enterotoxic for rabbits, and paralytic and lethal for mice, and inhibits protein synthesis in HeLa cells (O'Brien et al., 1982). These results suggest that like the cholera–*E. coli*–heat-labile toxin family, a family of Shiga-like toxins exist. In addition, EPEC may produce a second enterotoxin that is heat-stable and associated with the lipopolysaccharide.

Enteroinvasive E. coli (EIEC). Certain strains of *E. coli* may penetrate the cells of the intestinal epithelium and cause a syndrome similar to shigellosis. These strains do not produce an enterotoxin, and pili are not required to attach to and invade the mucosa. EIEC produce a keratoconjunctivitis in eyes of guinea pigs (positive Sereny test), which is identical to that of shigella. This test detects the invasiveness of such bacteria. Similarly, EIEC will penetrate monolayers of HeLa cells. Some of the invasive strains may possess somatic antigens related to one of the various *Shigella* serotypes. Like shigellae, the invasive *E. coli* strains multiply predominantly in the colon. Recently it has been shown that EIEC, and *Sh. flexneri* share a common plasmid of expression of cell penetration. The number of invasive *E. coli* necessary to produce diarrheal disease in volunteers is at least 10,000 times higher than the infectious dose for *Sh. flexneri* 2a. The massive infecting dose may be one of the reasons these organisms have been overlooked in the past.

E. coli species responsible for nosocomial urinary tract infections and bacteremias have rarely invaded the bowel or produced enterotoxin.

CLINICAL MANIFESTATIONS. Diarrheal disease caused by ETEC may vary from a mild one-day illness consisting of abdominal cramps, vomiting, loose stools, and a low-grade fever, to a severe secretory diarrhea resembling cholera. Profuse rice-water stools may cause hypovolemic shock. The illness caused by *E. coli* that produces heat-labile toxin cannot usually be distinguished from that due to heat-stable toxin producers. The incubation period in volunteers varies from 24 to 48 hours. Occasionally asymptomatic pharyngeal colonization occurs in patients with diarrhea.

Most persons will stop shedding ETEC within four to five days after recovery from diarrhea. However, in some individuals, particularly those living in endemic areas, asymptomatic excretion may be more persistant.

There is nothing distinctive about the clinical presentation of EPEC diarrhea. Although long associated with diarrheal outbreaks in newborn nurseries, volunteer studies have confirmed that these strains will produce diarrhea in adults or babies.

The clinical picture of EIEC infection is indistinguishable from shigellosis: high fever, chills, headache, myalgia, and abdominal cramps, followed by diarrhea and dysentery. Spontaneous recovery occurs with no specific antibiotic therapy.

GEOGRAPHIC VARIATION

ETEC. In general, ETEC are a common cause of diarrhea in developing countries and a relatively infrequent cause in the developed world, except in areas where sanitation is poor. From limited studies there seem to be geographic differences in the type of enterotoxin produced by ETEC; for example, in Mexico and Morocco LT/ST strains predominate, in Kenya LT strains are most common, and in Bangladesh ST strains are slightly more common than LT/ST strains and LT strains are less common. However, all three enterotoxin types have been found in all geographic areas. ETEC infections are particularly important in travelers going from North America and Northern Europe to areas of the world where diarrheal disease is prevalent. It is claimed that ETEC cause from 50 to 70 per cent of travelers' diarrhea.

EPEC. Evidence collected in the 1940's and 1950's demonstrated that EPEC strains were a globally important cause of serious nosocomial enteritis in neonates. During the past two decades they appear to be less frequent in North America and Europe. However, EPEC remain an important cause of sporadic diarrhea in developing countries.

EIEC. Little is known about the epidemiology of EIEC diarrhea with the exception of occasional reports of sporadic outbreaks in Central and Eastern Europe. A large multistate outbreak in the USA was attributed to imported French cheese.

DIAGNOSIS. *E. coli* diarrheal disease should be a primary diagnostic consideration in two clinical settings: (1) in any acute gastroenteritis in which a recognized enteric pathogen cannot be isolated, and (2) in an acute cholera-like dehydrating diarrhea in patients who have not been to an area endemic or epidemic for *V. cholerae* and in whom this organism cannot be recovered.

Laboratory identification of toxigenic and invasive *E. coli* is difficult. Stool cultures are of little value because *E. coli* normally inhabit the bowel. There are no assays for either type of *E. coli* that are readily adapted for routine diagnosis. The selection of *E. coli* colonies for virulence testing is random and insensitive; about 10^6 bacteria per gram of feces must be present for detection. Serum antitoxin titers to heat-labile toxins do not regularly rise after diarrheal illness except in heavily endemic areas, and serum antibodies to the heat-stable variety have not been recognized. A significant rise in titer of serum antibody to the somatic antigen of invasive *E. coli* has been documented in animal models. The application of this technique as a diagnostic tool in human infection has not yet been determined.

Enterotoxin is demonstrated by inducing diarrhea in the gut of laboratory animals such as the rabbit or suckling mouse. The rabbit test will detect both heat-labile and heat-stable toxin, while the mouse test is specific for the stable toxin. Another approach, which allows multiple specimens to be examined, is the use of tissue culture assays. Chinese hamster ovary cells or adrenal tumor cells will show characteristic morphologic changes only when exposed to the heat-labile toxin. Recent advances in technology have provided a newer generation of tests now being evaluated. Some involve the detection of binding of LT to specific antibody, or involve the direct identification by enzyme-linked immunosorbent assay. Others involve the direct identification of the enterotoxin-producing genes by DNA probes.

The detection of invasive *E. coli* relies on the development of keratoconjunctivitis in the eyes of guinea pigs inoculated with the test organism (Sereny test).

It should be noted that occasionally infection with toxigenic *E. coli* may simultaneously coexist with viral gastroenteritis.

TREATMENT. Rehydration is the main treatment of disease caused by enterotoxigenic *E. coli.* Oral glucose in a balanced electrolyte solution is a simple and effective alternative to intravenous fluid replacement. Antibiotics do not shorten the illness, and may cause harm. A single conjugative plasmid in *E. coli* carries the genes for both drug resistance and enterotoxin production, so that the indiscriminate use of antibiotics for enterotoxic diarrhea, which promotes antibiotic resistance in Enterobacteriaceae, may also promote the acquisition of plasmids mediating the production of enterotoxin. A nontoxic agent, bismuth subsalicylate,* rapidly relieves diarrhea, nausea, and abdominal pain when given orally in 30 to 60 ml amounts every 30 minutes for eight doses (Dupont et al., 1977).

Neither antibiotics nor drugs that retard intestinal motility have any established value for treatment of disease caused by invasive E. coli.

PROPHYLAXIS. Prevention of ETEC diarrhea has been attempted with various specific and nonspecific agents. Antimicrobial agents have been used in several successful prevention trials including phthalylsulphathiazole, neomy-

*Commercially available as Pepto Bismol.

cin, doxycycline and trimethoprim/sulfamethoxazole. Despite the obvious effectiveness of these drugs, there is considerable concern about the general application of antimicrobial agents for preventing ETEC diarrhea. Concerns about induction of antibiotic resistance in bacteria (see above) have led most authorities in this field to agree that such drugs should not be used routinely. Some evidence has also been presented that prophylactic antibiotics can promote salmonellosis among those taking the drug.

Another approach to prevention is to take bismuth subsalicylate in doses of 60 ml orally four times a day for three weeks.

The fact that persons in high risk areas are less susceptible to the illness that plague the travelers from a low risk area has encouraged research on immunoprophylaxis. Diarrhea due to ETEC does promote immunity as shown by volunteer studies wherein second exposures to the agent occurred experimentally.

No vaccine is available for use in man; however, vaccines against CFAs from ETEC strains have been highly effective in preventing disease in a number of animal species. Both food and water may be the vehicles for transmission of this disease. Attention to sources of water and food and food preparation is important in prevention of the disease, since ingestion of many organisms is required to produce illness in most people. Accordingly, protection will be afforded by eating only cooked food that is held at proper temperatures, and boiling inadequately treated water before drinking.

Healthy transient carriers are probably an important reservoir for the spread of these organisms, but they will remain undetected until a simple method for detecting them becomes available.

VIBRIO PARAHAEMOLYTICUS GASTROENTERITIS

Vibrio parahaemolyticus is a leading cause of acute, self-limited, food-borne gastroenteritis acquired by consumption of raw or processed seafood, usually in the summer (Blake et al., 1980).

ETIOLOGY. *V. parahaemolyticus* is a halophilic (salt-loving) anaerobic gram-negative rod found in marine life and coastal water throughout the world. The organism can be serotyped with specific somatic antisera. Serologic testing, although useful for epidemiologic purposes, has limited diagnostic value because of extensive cross-reactivity with other marine vibrios. *V. parahaemolyticus* will not grow on most routine laboratory enteric media unless these media have a high salt content.

PATHOGENESIS AND PATHOLOGY. The mechanism by which *V. parahaemolyticus* causes acute enteritis is not completely resolved. Using animal models and human volunteers, a strong correlation has been found between enteropathogenicity and a positive Kanagawa reaction (the production of a hemolysin by this organism on special high salt agar). Paradoxically, *V. parahaemolyticus* strains isolated from seafood that is epidemiologically linked with specific outbreaks of acute gastroenteritis are almost invariably Kanagawa-negative. The Kanagawa hemolysin has been purified but has not been clearly demonstrated to be enterotoxic. Direct bacterial invasion of ileal mucosa has been observed in some experimental models, whereas in others the viable organisms produce rapid cytotoxicity to epithelial cells without cellular invasion. Some strains produce a bacterial cell-associated, heat stable material, cytotoxic for HeLa cells and completely neutralized by antibody to purified *Sh. dysenteriae* 1 (Shiga)toxin (O'Brien et al., 1984). Like toxigenic *E. coli*, enteropathogenic strains of *V. parahaemolyticus* adhere to epithelial cell surfaces, but nonvirulent strains do not. Despite extensive study of the pathogenic mechanisms of *V. parahaemolyticus*, we do not yet understand how it causes gastrointestinal disease in man (Blake et al., 1980).

CLINICAL MANIFESTATIONS. *V. parahaemolyticus* gastroenteritis most commonly resembles *Salmonella* enterocolitis; explosive watery diarrhea is the cardinal manifestation, followed less frequently by abdominal cramps, nausea, and vomiting. Occasionally, some patients have chills or fever. The median incubation period ranges from 14 to 23 hours, and the illness lasts about three days.

Another *V. parahaemolyticus* syndrome resembles *Shigella* dysentery and is characterized by fever, abdominal pain, and bloody, mucoid stools.

Bacteremia and localized extraintestinal tissue infections are rare.

GEOGRAPHIC VARIATION. This disease has a worldwide distribution, appears primarily in areas adjacent to marine waters, and occurs exclusively in warm weather.

DIAGNOSIS, TREATMENT, AND PROPHYLAXIS. The diagnosis should be suspected when acute diarrhea develops following the ingestion of seafood. Confirmation depends on the recovery of the organism from stool and incriminated food.

Specific antimicrobial therapy is not indicated in most cases because of the limited severity and duration of the illness.

Prevention is best achieved through measures that ensure adequate cooking, hygienic preparation, and rapid refrigeration of seafood.

CAMPYLOBACTER ENTERITIS

Campylobacter (formerly known as *Vibrio fetus*), long recognized as a commensal and a pathogen of various domestic animals, has been increasingly implicated as an enteric pathogen of man over the past 30 years. *Campylobacter* may also be responsible for a wide variety of clinical syndromes, including bacteremia, phlebitis, arthritis, septic abortion, and meningitis.

ETIOLOGY. *Campylobacter* are gram-negative, motile, nonsporing, curved, spiral rods. All are microaerophilic and do not grow under aerobic or strict anaerobic conditions. They do not ferment carbohydrates and are distinguished from true vibrio species by differences in their DNA base-pair ratios. *C. jejuni* and *C. coli* are a major cause of diarrhea. Because *C. jejuni* and *C. coli* differ only slightly and *C. jejuni* is found more commonly in human beings, they will be referred to, collectively, as *C. jejuni*

(Blaser and Reller, 1981). *C. fetus* subsp. *fetus* is an opportunistic pathogen that sometimes causes septicemic illness in compromised hosts and recently has occasionally been isolated from stools of patients with diarrhea.

PATHOGENESIS AND PATHOLOGY. The pathogenesis and mode of transmission of human campylobacteriosis is poorly understood. Although the infection is a recognized zoonosis, there is no evidence that exposure to *C. jejuni* in its natural habitat—that is, the intestinal tract of domestic animals—immediately precedes human campylobacteriosis. That this pathogen of animals is a human enteric pathogen is based on the following observations: *C. jejuni* has been simultaneously recovered from feces and blood cultures of patients with diarrhea; the organism disappears from the stools during convalescence; significant specific rising serum antibody titers develop in patients with campylobacter enteritis; clustering of symptomatic cases occurs; a human volunteer who ingested *C. jejuni*, developed a typical clinical illness, and the organism was recovered from his feces; and treatment with an antibiotic to which the organism is sensitive in vitro leads to rapid disappearance of *C. jejuni* from feces and prompt resolution of symptoms.

The pathology of *C. jejuni* infections suggests that the disease should be considered an enterocolitis. Acute hemorrhagic necrosis of the jejunum and ileum has been observed at autopsy. The organism has been recovered from aspirates taken from different levels of the small bowel. The frequent occurrence of blood and polymorphonuclear leukocytes in the feces of affected individuals suggests that the large bowel is also commonly involved. Histologic sections show an acute colitis with inflammatory infiltrates of the lamina propria and crypt abscesses. These pathologic features are nonspecific and may also be seen in shigellosis, *Salmonella* colitis, amebiasis, Crohn's disease, and ulcerative colitis.

A heat-labile choleralike enterotoxin has been demonstrated in strains isolated from patients with *C. jejuni* infection and was associated with significant antibody response to autologous *C. jejuni* somatic antigen (Ruiz-Palacios et al., 1983). The clinical significance of enterotoxin production is unknown. The microorganism appears to penetrate the intestinal wall by an as yet undefined mechanism, perhaps similar to that observed with other pathogens, such as nontyphoidal salmonellae and yersiniae, which may cause similar clinical illnesses.

The survival of the organism in the bloodstream may be associated with a glycoprotein cell surface antigen that is antiphagocytic.

CLINICAL MANIFESTATIONS, COMPLICATIONS, AND SEQUELAE. Three reasonably distinct patterns of human *Campylobacter* infection can be delineated that correlate the bacterial species with the age, sex, underlying health of the host, the clinical presentation, and the outcome (Torphy and Bond, 1979).

The first, most frequent pattern of disease is enteritis. It is usually uncomplicated and due to *C. jejuni*. A typical incubation period is about 2 to 5 days. Although campylobacter enteritis affects all age groups, the incidence is highest in young children. The male:female ratio is about 3:2. The most common clinical features are fever, bloody diarrhea, and abdominal pain. Vomiting and dehydration are not common. Fever may be accompanied by several constitutional symptoms, such as malaise, headache, musculoskeletal pain, and occasionally rigors and delirium, which may be more prominent than the enteric symptoms. The severity of the illness is quite variable; in most cases it is brief, self-limited, and subsides within a week. In some cases, mild abdominal pain may persist for several weeks after the onset of symptoms and occasionally the illness is persistent or relapsing, mimicking ulcerative colitis or Crohn's disease. Cases of toxic megacolon, pseudomembranous colitis and a massive lower gastrointestinal hemorrhage have also been described. The incidence of asymptomatic fecal excretion of *C. jejuni* has been estimated at 1.3 per cent in Belgian children and 13 per cent in black South African children. Untreated children continue to excrete *C. jejuni* for about 4 to 5 weeks after the onset of symptoms.

A second form of disease consists of focal infections, often associated with vasculitis and/or chronic bacteremia. These infections are most often due to *C. fetus* ssp. *fetus* and occur in older, debilitated, or chronically ill adults, particularly men. To date, over 100 varieties of human infection caused by *C. fetus* ssp. *fetus* have been described, including meningitis, septic arthritis, pneumonia, empyema, peritonitis, hepatitis, pericarditis, endocarditis, mycotic aneurysm, and thrombophlebitis. In addition, *C. fetus* ssp. *fetus* infection has been associated with Reiter's syndrome as well as a reactive arthritis in an HLA-B27 positive patient. A vascular tropism has been proposed in that vascular sites are frequently infected by *C. fetus* ssp. *fetus*, vascular necrosis has been frequently reported in cases of endocarditis and pericarditis, and thrombophlebitis is commonly associated with *C. fetus* ssp. *fetus* bacteremia. In some, febrile episodes were prolonged and relapsing, reminiscent of brucellosis or malaria. The patient's age and underlying diseases appear to determine the severity of *C. fetus* ssp. *fetus* infections. Thus, these infections have been more common in patients with diabetes, malignancy, hepatorenal disease, and severe cardiovascular disease. In this respect, this organism can be considered an opportunistic pathogen.

A third pattern, perinatal infections, causing abortion, prematurity, neonatal sepsis, and meningitis, is the least frequent and usually due to *C. fetus* ssp. *fetus*. These infections are usually fatal to the fetus or infant, whereas the mothers survive the illness.

Venereal transmission, a common mode of spread of *Campylobacter* species in cattle, has been described in homosexual men in the form of infectious proctitis.

GEOGRAPHIC VARIATIONS IN DISEASE. *Campylobacter* enteritis is widely distributed in tropical as well as temperate areas of the world. *C. fetus* sspp. *jejuni* can be isolated in from 1.3 to 11 per cent of persons with diarrhea (when using selective culturing techniques). It appears to be one of the most common bacterial causes of enteritis in some areas of the world, such as the United Kingdom, The Netherlands, and Canada; *C. jejuni* is a common cosmopolitan enteric pathogen. For reasons that are unknown, the incidence of *C. jejuni* enteritis in Western Europe and North America is highest in the warmest months. The prevalence of *C. jejuni* infection in some of the developing countries may be as great as that in the industrialized countries. In studies in South Africa and Bangladesh, 40 per cent of children 9 to 24 months of age excreted *C. jejuni*. The high prevalence of excretion among healthy children makes the interpretation of isolations from children with diarrhea difficult. The geographic distribution of

C. fetus sspp. *fetus* is not yet known. In a serologic survey, antibody titers to *C. fetus* sspp. *fetus* were 4 times higher in preparations of commercial human γ-globulin obtained from South Africa than in batches from other parts of the world.

DIAGNOSIS. Diarrhea, abdominal pain, and constitutional symptoms, especially fever, are the predominant clinical features of *Campylobacter* enteritis. From the symptoms and natural history, the diagnosis may easily be confused with viral or other bacterial gastroenteritis, such as salmonellosis, shigellosis, or yersiniosis. The frequent occurrence of either gross or occult blood and leukocytes in the stools is an important diagnostic feature. The acute colitis that may be present can mimic acute ulcerative colitis.

A rapid presumptive diagnosis can be made by direct phase-contrast microscopy of stools and visualization of the motile curved spiral rods, resembling treponemes. Confirmation of the diagnosis is made by isolation of *Campylobacter* from stools cultured on selective medium containing antibiotics and grown under microaerophilic conditions. Cultures are usually positive after 48 hours. Serologic diagnosis is a research tool. Patients infected with *C. jejuni* acquire specific serum antibodies. It is not known whether these antibodies protect against reinfection by homologous or heterologous organisms.

TREATMENT. Most patients with *Campylobacter* enteritis will have a mild self-limited illness and do not require antimicrobial therapy. Fluid replacement may be needed in more severely ill patients. Uncontrolled reports suggest that antimotility agents, such as diphenoxylate hydrochloride (Lomotil), should be avoided in *Campylobacter* enteritis. A premature return to solid foods may precipitate a recurrence of symptoms. In a recent double-blind controlled clinical trial, erythromycin eradicated the organism from the stools but did not alter the natural course of uncomplicated acute *Campylobacter* enteritis (Anders et al., 1982). Nevertheless, erythromycin has been recommended as the preferred antibiotic for the treatment of severe enteritis given as 25 to 50 mg/kg/day in three divided doses for 7 to 10 days. Occasional reports of erythromycin-resistant strains of *C. fetus* warrant determination of antibiotic sensitivities of clinical isolates. Extraintestinal disease has been treated successfully with various antimicrobial agents depending on the site of infection. Gentamicin is the drug of choice for the treatment of septicemia, endocarditis, and other nonenteric *Campylobacter* disease when the antibiotic sensitivity is not known. For infections of the central nervous system, chloramphenicol is recommended. Treatment of systemic infections for 4 weeks has been suggested because relapse has occurred in a few cases after shorter treatment.

PROPHYLAXIS. The epidemiology of *Campylobacter* infection in man is obscure. At least six routes of transmission have been suggested: (1) direct contact with infected animals, (2) ingestion of contaminated food, (3) ingestion of contaminated water, (4) venereal transmission, (5) placental transfer or exposure at delivery, and (6) person-to-person spread by fecal-oral route (Taylor et al., 1979). To date, each one of these six modes of transmission appears to have occurred. This information comes from investigations of several outbreaks and case reports (Blaser and Reller, 1981). Additionally, *Campylobacter* has been suggested to be part of the normal indigenous flora. Awareness of the necessity for handwashing after contact with animals or animal products and the importance of proper cooking and storage of foods of animal origin are important in preventing *C. jejuni* infections. Pasteurization of milk, chlorination of water supplies, and thorough cooking of meat all readily kill *C. jejuni*.

References

Shigellosis

Barrett-Connor, E., and Connor, J. D.: Extraintestinal manifestations of shigellosis. Am J Gastroenterol 53:234, 1970.

Chang, M. J., et al.: Trimethoprim-sulfamethoxazole compared to ampicillin in the treatment of shigellosis. Pediatrics 59:726, 1977.

DuPont, H. L., et al.: The reponse of man to virulent *Shigella flexneri* 2a. J Infect Dis 119:296, 1969.

DuPont, H. L., and Hornick, R. B.: Adverse effect of lomotil therapy in shigellosis. JAMA, 226:1525, 1973.

Pickering, L. K., et al.: Single-dose tetracycline therapy for shigellosis in adults. JAMA 239:853, 1978.

Salmonella Enteritis

Black, P. H., et al.: Salmonellosis—a review of some unusual aspects. N Engl J Med 262:811, 1960.

Cherubin, C. E., et al.: Septicemia with non-typhoid salmonella. Medicine 53:365, 1974.

Nelson, J. D., et al.: Treatment of *Salmonella* gastroenteritis with ampicillin, amoxicillin, and placebo. Pediatrics 65:1125, 1980.

Peterson, J. W.: *Salmonella* toxin. Pharmac Ther 11:719, 1980.

Sprinz, H.: Pathogenesis of intestinal infections. Arch Pathol 87:566, 1969.

E. coli Diarrhea

DuPont, H. L., et al.: Symptomatic treatment of diarrhea with bismuth subsalicylate among students attending a Mexican University. Gastroenterology 73:715, 1977.

Edelman, R. and Levine, M. M.: Summary of a workshop on enteropathogenic *Escherichia coli*. J Infect Dis 147:1108, 1983.

Evans, D. J., and Evans, D. G.: Classification of pathogenic *Escherichia coli* according to serotype and the production of virulence factors with special reference to colonization-factor antigens. Rev Infect Dis 5:S692, 1983 (Supp 4).

Field, M., et al.: Heat-stable enterotoxin of *Escherichia coli*: In vitro effects on guanylate cyclase activity, cyclic GMP concentration and ion transport in small intestine. Proc Natl Acad Sci 75:2800, 1978.

Kantor, H. S., et al.: Cycloheximide-induced reversal of cholera toxin effects on protein-bound forms of cyclic AMP and cyclic AMP-dependent protein kinoses of ileal mucosa in vivo. Clin Res 29:728A, 1981.

O'Brien, A. D., et al.: Production of *Shigella dysenteriae* Type 1-like cytotoxin by *Escherichia coli*. J Infect Dis 147:763, 1982.

Vibrio parahaemolyticus Gastroenteritis

Blake, P. A., et al.: Disease of humans (other than cholera) caused by vibrios. Ann Rev Microbiol 34:341, 1980.

O'Brien, A. D., et al.: Environmental and human isolates of Vibrio cholerae and Vibrio parahaemolyticus produce a shigella dysenteriae 1 (Shiga)-like cytotoxin. Lancet I:77, 1984.

Campylobacter Enteritis

Anders, B. J., et al.: Double blind placebo controlled trial of erythromycin for the treatment of *Campylobacter* enteritis. Lancet 1:131, 1982.

Blaser, M. J., and Reller, L. B.: *Campylobacter* enteritis. N. Engl J Med 305:1444, 1981.

Ruiz-Palacios, G. M., et al.: Cholera-like enterotoxin produced by *Campylobacter jejuni*. Characterization and clinical significance. Lancet 2:250, 1983.

Taylor, P. R., et al.: *Campylobacter fetus* infection in human subjects: association with raw milk. Am J Med 66:779, 1979.

Torphey, D. E., and Bond, W. W.: *Campylobacter fetus* infections in children. Pediatrics 64:898, 1979.

133

ANTIBIOTIC-ASSOCIATED COLITIS DUE TO CLOSTRIDIUM DIFFICILE

HARVEY S. KANTOR, M. D.

A toxin or toxins produced by *Clostridium difficile* have been widely accepted as the most important cause of antibiotic-associated diarrhea. Such diarrhea is classified as pseudomembranous colitis when exudative colonic mucosal plaques or a pseudomembrane is detected, and it can be fatal. Many mild cases of antibiotic-associated colitis without pseudomembranes in which *C. difficile* is implicated are now detected. Therefore, the terms antibiotic-associated colitis and *C. difficile* colitis are preferred.

ETIOLOGY. *C. difficile* is a toxigenic gram-positive, spore-forming obligate anaerobic rod, which has been considered somewhat difficult to isolate and accounts for the original name, *"Bacillus difficilis."* It was described as early as 1935 as a normal component of the fecal flora of newborn infants and was considered nonpathogenic for humans until recently (Bartlett et al., 1978; Larson et al., 1978).

PATHOGENESIS AND PATHOLOGY. The etiologic role of *C. difficile* in antibiotic-associated colitis was discovered by several groups between 1976 and 1978 employing the hamster model. After hamsters were given an antibiotic, a hemorrhagic cecitis was produced that resembled antibiotic-associated colitis in humans. This was accompanied by quantitative increases in *C. difficile* and production of a fecal cytotoxin. Cell-free supernatants of stool from afflicted animals consistently transferred the disease upon intracecal injection into healthy animals. The active component could be neutralized with *Clostridium sordellii* antitoxin, suggesting a clostridial toxin. Since *C. difficile* produces a toxin that is neutralized by *C. sordellii* antitoxin, the two seem to be immunologically similar. This toxin was universally present in hamsters with lethal colitis following exposure to a variety of antimicrobial agents. The same toxin was found regardless of the drug used to induce the disease. The clinical relevance of these observations in animals became apparent when *C. difficile* and its cytopathic toxin were detected in patients with antibiotic-associated colitis.

Most isolates of *C. difficile* produce two toxins: one is enterotoxic and lethal for hamsters (toxin A) and the other is cytopathic in cell cultures and in vivo (toxin B). Although these toxins are presumed to cause the disease, their exact role in pathogenesis is not clear. Hamsters immunized against both toxins were protected from the disease, but vaccination with either toxin alone gave no protection.

The pathologic changes in the colons of patients with antibiotic-associated diarrhea range from an entirely normal mucosa to severe life-threatening pseudomembranous colitis. The most common findings with endoscopy are normal mucosa or evidence of mild erythema and edema. The most characteristic lesion, the pseudomembranous plaque or nodule is often loosely adherent to the mucosal surface. This plaque, which consists of fibrin, mucin, sloughed mucosal epithelial cells, and acute inflammatory cells, is often too thin to be seen with the naked eye, but may be visible microscopically. No particular bacterial type is predominant within the pseudomembrane, and there is no bacterial invasion of the colonic mucosa.

The diarrhea associated with the toxin of *C. difficile* has usually been associated with mucosal lesions and colitis. A purely secretory diarrhea has not yet been documented (Fekety, 1983).

CLINICAL MANIFESTATIONS. The one symptom in nearly all patients with *C. difficile* colitis is diarrhea. Diarrhea may begin within a week of starting antibiotics or up to four weeks to six weeks after stopping antibiotic(s) in one-third of patients. In some of these cases, the organism may have been acquired after therapy, or it could have been inhibited but not eradicated while antibiotics were given (Fekety, 1983).

The diarrhea of antibiotic-associated colitis usually consists of loose or watery stools, sometimes containing mucus but rarely with grossly evident blood. Fecal leukocytes are detectable in about 50 per cent of patients. The diarrhea ranges from a trivial, self-limited bout of loose stools to 30 stools per day for four weeks or longer. The average duration of diarrhea after discontinuation of the antibiotic is 10 to 12 days.

Most patients have abdominal cramps, lower quadrant tenderness, fever, and leukocytosis. These findings may suggest intraabdominal sepsis and occasionally lead to an unwarranted laparotomy. Other patients, however, simply have diarrhea with no evidence of systemic toxicity.

Nearly all antibiotics, except vancomycin and parenteral aminoglycosides, have been implicated as causes of antibiotic-associated colitis; some cancer chemotherapeutic agents have also been blamed. The most frequent antibiotics are ampicillin, clindamycin, and cephalosporins. There is no clear relationship between the dosage, duration of treatment, or even the route of administration of these drugs. Drugs with activity restricted to mycobacteria, fungi, and parasites do not appear to cause *C. difficile*-induced enteric disease.

COMPLICATIONS AND SEQUELAE. Occasionally, patients with antibiotic-associated colitis have fevers over 104 degrees F and some have leukemoid reactions with peripheral leukocyte counts exceeding 40,000/mm^3. Potentially serious complications reflect severe fluid, electrolyte, and albumin losses with dehydration, electrolyte imbalance, hypotension, and hypoalbuminemia, sometimes with anasarca. Cecal perforation may occur, particularly in granulocytopenic patients. Toxic megacolon is a risk when there has been a delay in diagnosis and after recent x-ray studies by the barium contrast technique. Polyarthritis involving large joints has been reported with circulating antibodies to *C. difficile* cytotoxin. *C. difficile* may be responsible for relapses of inflammatory bowel disease during antibiotic treatment.

GEOGRAPHIC VARIATION. *C. difficile* is second only to *Salmonella* as a bacterial agent of enteric disease in industrialized countries (Bartlett, 1983). The incidence of antibiotic-associated colitis throughout the world is not well delineated. Estimates of the frequency of *C. difficile* colitis following antibiotic treatment have varied widely among institutions. The true incidence of the disease nationwide is probably less than one per 1,000 treated patients, although much higher rates have been observed.

DIAGNOSIS. The diagnosis of antibiotic-associated colitis should be suspected in any patient with otherwise unexplained diarrhea that occurs during antibiotic therapy or up to 6 weeks after antibiotics have been stopped. Gross inspection of the colon typically reveals punctate, raised, yellowish-white plaques with "skip areas" of a normal mucosa or a mucosa showing erythema or edema. The plaques will vary in size from a few mm to 20 mm in diameter. Pseudomembranes are typically located throughout the distal colon so that sigmoidoscopy is generally adequate. However, up to 30 per cent or more of patients will have pseudomembranes restricted to the right colon requiring the use of colonoscopy as the most definitive study. Some cases are recognized only with histologic studies of biopsy specimens. Microscopic examination shows epithelial necrosis, goblet cells distended with mucus, and infiltration of the lamina propria with polymorphonuclear cells and eosinophilic exudate.

The diagnostic test for *C. difficile* is a tissue culture assay of stool to demonstrate a cytopathic toxin. Neutralization of toxicity with *C. difficile* or *C. sordellii* antitoxins is necessary to rule out false-positive cytotoxic effects. Although toxin titers do not correlate well with the severity of the illness in individual patients, the titers decline rapidly after initiation of appropriate therapy. Nearly all patients who have this toxin in the stool will also have *C. difficile* recovered on selective medium. However, 20 to 25 per cent of patients who receive antibiotics without any gastrointestinal complications will harbor *C. difficile*. Alternative methods to detect *C. difficile* toxin, such as counterimmunoelectrophoresis or enzyme-linked immunoabsorbent assays are too variable.

TREATMENT. Patients with mild antibiotic-associated colitis may not need to be treated with specific antimicrobial therapy. Often all that is needed is to discontinue antibiotics and give replacement or supportive therapy with fluids and electrolytes.

The best studied and most effective treatment for *C. difficile* colitis is oral vancomycin, 125 to 500 mg four times daily for 7–14 days. Except in very ill patients, the lowest dose is adequate. Vancomycin is active against virtually all strains of *C. difficile*, the levels in the colon with oral administration are extremely high, and systemic toxicity is rare because of poor absorption with oral administration even in the presence of an inflamed bowel. Patients treated with vancomycin usually show improvement within 24 to 48 hours, but cessation of diarrhea and defervescence may require a week or more. Vancomycin is bitter tasting, expensive, in relatively short supply, and unavailable in some parts of the world. *C. difficile* is also usually susceptible to bacitracin and metronidazole, which are alternatives to vancomycin. Approximately 20 per cent of those patients suffer a symptomatic relapse within a few weeks of treatment. Stool assays at the time of relapse show positive toxin assays, and cultures yield strains of *C. difficile* that are always sensitive to vancomycin. Patients with relapse will respond to another course of vancomycin but may be at risk for further relapse. One method that has been effective in achieving definitive cure is to give a course of vancomycin in the usual dose for 7–14 days followed by 2–3 weeks of cholestyramine treatment (Bartlett, 1983). The rationale for this approach is that vancomycin presumably provides optimal treatment for serious disease, and cholestyramine, an anion exchange resin, then provides satisfactory control while the normal flora becomes re-established.

PROPHYLAXIS. Prevention of spread of *C. difficile* from patients with the disease to others in the hospital who are receiving antibiotics may be achieved by careful handwashing by personnel and the use of enteric isolation precautions when patients have active *C. difficile* colitis.

References

Bartlett, J. G., et al.: Antibiotic-associated pseudomembranous colitis due to toxin producing clostridia. New Engl J Med 298:531, 1978.

Bartlett, J. G.: Recognition and treatment of antibiotic-associated colitis. Survey of Digestive Dis 1:54, 1983.

Fekety, R.: Recent advances in management of bacterial diarrhea. Rev Infect Dis 5:246, 1983.

Larson, H. E., et al.: *Clostridium difficile* and the aetiology of pseudomembranous colitis. Lancet 1:1063, 1978.

134

APPENDICITIS AND DIVERTICULITIS

O. J. A. GILMORE, M.S., F.R.C.S.(ENG.), F.R.C.S.(ED.)

The word *appendicitis* refers to inflammation occurring in the vermiform appendix. In infants, the appendix is a conical outpouching or diverticulum at the apex of the cecum. With differential growth of the cecum, the appendix eventually comes to arise medially and slightly posteriorly, just below the ileocecal valve. The base of the appendix lies where the teniae of the cecum converge, thus enabling the surgeon to find it at operation.

Diverticulitis refers to inflammation in an acquired colonic diverticulum. "Diverticulosis" implies that colonic diverticulae are present but are not inflamed. The term diverticular disease of the colon should now be used instead of diverticulosis or diverticulitis, which are misleading. Diverticula tend to develop where blood vessels penetrate the muscle and therefore are more common on the mesenteric border. They vary from a few millimeters to several centimeters in diameter, and their necks may be narrow or wide.

ETIOLOGY. There is no specific microbial cause of appendicitis or diverticulitis. Infection is caused by the bacteria that make up the autochthonous microflora. Since anaerobes make up 90 per cent of the fecal flora, these infections are polymicrobial and have the characteristics of anerobic infections. *Bacteroides* species, *Clostridia*, and peptostreptococci are the most frequently isolated anaerobes; *E. coli* and enterococci are the most commonly isolated aerobic bacteria either from the inflamed serosa or from an associated abscess.

PATHOGENESIS. The incidence of both appendicitis and

diverticular disease appears to be closely linked both historically and geographically with a low fiber diet and its associated excess of refined carbohydrates in the form of white flour and sugar (Cleave and Campbell, 1966; Burkitt, 1973). Such a diet results in an increase in inspissated feces and fecoliths, which may enter the appendix or a diverticulum and cause obstruction. In addition, the bacterial flora of the colon and the appendix change with such a diet. The number of *Bacteroides* and lactobacilli tend to increase, while the enterococci and Enterobacteriaceae decrease.

Pressure studies of the colon indicate that segmentation occurs, narrowing the colonic lumen at intervals. Thus, the colon acts not as a tube but as a series of "little bladders" whose outflow is temporarily obstructed at both ends. When this occurs, high pressures develop, sometimes in excess of 90 mm Hg, which can produce "blow-outs" or diverticula. People who throughout their lives take a high residue diet and produce a bulky stool have a colon of wide diameter and tend not to develop such high intracolonic pressures.

Appendicitis. Acute appendicitis results from obstruction of the lumen followed by infection. In children and teenagers obstruction is usually associated with hyperplasia of the lymphoid follicles, and in adults with inspissated feces or a fecolith. Other less common causes of obstruction are foreign bodies, strictures, worms, and tumors. The rate at which the inflammation proceeds depends upon the degree of obstruction and the virulence and number of the bacteria present. The most common aerobic organisms found in the appendix are *Escherichia coli* and the most common anaerobes are *Bacteroides* species.

The inflammatory process advances through catarrhal inflammation to acute inflammation with pus in the lumen and then to gangrene and perforation due to increasing intraluminal pressure that occludes the mural blood supply. Approximately 30 per cent of patients with acute appendicitis are found to have a gangrenous or perforated appendix at operation (Gilmore and Martin, 1974). If the pathologic process is relatively slow, adhesions form around the appendix between loops of bowel, the greater omentum, and the parietal peritoneum, thereby localizing the peritonitis should perforation occur. If appendicitis progresses rapidly to perforation and adhesions have not formed, general peritonitis then ensues, increasing both the morbidity and mortality of the disease.

Diverticulitis. Acute inflammation in a diverticulum, like appendicitis, is associated with obstruction that is usually due to a hard concretion or fecolith. In these cases acute diverticulitis may progress in a manner similar to that of appendicitis, and gangrene and perforation may result, causing local or generalized peritonitis depending on whether or not the inflamed area has become walled off by the adhesions. As in appendicitis, *E. coli* and *Bacteroides* species are the dominant organisms. Unlike appendicitis, however, the acute inflammatory process is not usually limited to a single diverticulum. This is because the adjacent bowel wall becomes inflamed and edematous, and thus neighboring diverticula become occluded so that the process spreads along the colon.

Chronic inflammation is much more common in diverticular disease. Bacteria cross the thin diverticulum wall and induce extramucosal inflammation. Granulation tissue forms, and this later becomes converted into fibrous tissue; as a result, a palpable mass may form, or the bowel lumen may become narrowed or obstructed.

CLINICAL MANIFESTATIONS

Appendicitis

Symptoms. Acute appendicitis has varied manifestations and may mimic many other acute abdominal conditions (Gilmore et al., 1975). In a typical case, the initial symptoms are central abdominal pain and anorexia. Some patients complain of nausea, and others vomit once or twice but not persistently. The initial pain is visceral and usually consists of a central ache but may be colicky, depending upon the degree of appendicular obstruction. Later, when the inflamed appendix irritates the parietal peritoneum, the pain increases and moves to the right iliac fossa. If the appendix is retrocecal or lying between loops of small bowel (retroileal) or in the pelvis, this localization may not occur or may be less marked. Some patients admit to constipation and others, especially young children and those with a pelvic appendix, to diarrhea.

Physical Signs. In classic acute appendicitis, the face is flushed, the tongue furred, and the patient has a temperature of about 38° C and an oral fetor. The temperature rarely goes much above 38° C unless perforation has occurred. The pulse rate is often normal, but there may be a mild tachycardia. Inspection of the abdomen may reveal reduced respiratory movements in the lower half if the symptoms have been present for more than a few hours. Gentle palpation reveals tenderness in the right iliac fossa that is often maximal around McBurney's point. Guarding is present and, in advanced cases, rigidity and rebound tenderness. Rebound tenderness should be elicited by gentle percussion, not by pressing the hands in at the site of maximum tenderness and suddenly removing them. This method only causes the patient unnecessary distress. Rovsing's sign (pain in the right iliac fossa when the left iliac fossa is pressed) is sometimes helpful, as is the psoas stretch sign. This consists of turning the patient on the left side and extending the right hip; if this causes increased discomfort it suggests that the appendix is retrocecal.

If symptoms have been present for more than 48 hours, the patient may have a mass in the right iliac fossa representing adherent ilium and omentum around the inflamed appendix.

Rectal examination is mandatory in every patient, and in women, when the diagnosis is doubtful, a vaginal examination is also necessary. Pelvic examination is undertaken to elicit tenderness in pelvic appendicitis and to exclude other lesions such as salpingitis or an ovarian cyst.

Laboratory Diagnosis. Acute appendicitis is a clinical diagnosis. Laboratory investigations are of secondary importance. A patient with the symptoms and signs of appendicitis deserves an appendectomy as soon as possible. In case of doubt, a raised leukocyte count with a shift to the left suggests appendicitis, but a normal count does not exclude the diagnosis. In appendicitis, there are no pathognomonic radiologic signs except for the presence of a fecolith. The urine should always be examined to exclude infection.

Diverticulitis

Symptoms. Uncomplicated diverticular disease is symptomless, but diverticulitis, like appendicitis, presents with pain. The initial pain consists either of a suprapubic ache or, more often, due to parietal peritoneal irritation, a left lower quadrant pain. Such patients often complain of alternating diarrhea and constipation. Nausea and anorexia are relatively uncommon and vomiting even less so. In very loose terms, diverticulitis can be considered as a left-sided appendicitis occurring in an older patient.

Some patients present with peritonitis after perforation of a diverticulum. A few complain of pneumaturia due to a ruptured diverticulum that causes a vesicocolic fistula. Massive rectal bleeding is an unusual presentation.

Physical Signs. In diverticulitis, like appendicitis, the patient may have a mild fever and tachycardia. The tongue may be furred, and there may be an oral fetor. Often, however, physical signs are limited to the abdomen. Examination reveals tenderness and guarding in the left iliac fossa. Rigidity and rebound tenderness indicate advanced pathology. The presence of a mass in diverticulitis, owing to the slower advancement of the inflammatory process, is much more common than in appendicitis. There may also be pelvic tenderness or even a pelvic mass.

In both conditions, when perforation occurs without localization, generalized peritonitis ensues, and the patient usually presents with fever of 39° C or more, a pulse rate of over 100, and a rigid abdomen.

Laboratory Investigations. In diverticulitis the leukocyte count is similar to that in appendicitis. Full sigmoidoscopy without anesthesia and with limited air insufflation should be undertaken. Sometimes a diverticulum is seen, but more commonly narrowing of the colon, spasm, or rigidity with increased mucus is noted. Perforation of a diverticulum may result in collections of extraluminal gas that can be seen on a plain film of the abdomen. Definitive diagnosis is based on barium enema examination but this must not be undertaken in patients with an acute attack because of the risk of causing perforation. In case of doubt, fiberoptic colonoscopy may be helpful but should not be undertaken if the patient is acutely ill.

DIFFERENTIAL DIAGNOSIS

Appendicitis. In children nonspecific mesenteric adenitis is the condition that most frequently mimics appendicitis. Constipation and tubo-ovarian disorders such as ruptured, twisted, or bleeding ovarian cysts and salpingitis constitute the main differential diagnoses in women (Gilmore, 1978). Other confusing conditions include acute pyelonephritis, ureteric colic, ectopic pregnancy, Meckel's diverticulitis, Crohn's disease, tuberculous ileitis, small bowel obstruction, intussusception, carcinoma of the cecum, gastroenteritis, acute pancreatitis, torsion of the omentum, perforated peptic ulcer, yersinia entercolitis and, very occasionally, basal pneumonia and myocardial ischemia.

Diverticulitis. Acute diverticulitis, in which a long sigmoid loop comes to lie in the right iliac fossa, may also present as appendicitis. The most common differential diagnosis to diverticulitis, however, is carcinoma of the colon.

COMPLICATIONS

Appendicitis. The most common complications of appendicitis are perforation, peritonitis, and abscess formation. Perforation may result in local or generalized peritonitis or in local abscess formation. General peritonitis in turn may result in a pelvic or subphrenic abscess. Portal pyemia, a suppurative thrombophlebitis of the portal system, is an unusual complication. Liver abscess can result.

Diverticulitis. Acute diverticulitis may result in similar complications. In addition, fistulous communications may develop between the colon and the bladder or between the colon and the small bowel. Intestinal obstruction occurs, usually because of excessive peridiverticular fibrosis and occasionally because of adhesions.

Both appendicitis and diverticulitis may kill the patient, especially the very young and the very old. The most common postoperative complication in both diseases is wound infection, and its likelihood increases if the appendix ruptures.

GEOGRAPHIC VARIATION. Appendicitis and diverticulitis appear to be diseases of western civilization. Both are more common in Europe and North America than in Asia and Africa. In western countries, about 5 to 8 per cent of people develop appendicitis, usually before age 20. Diverticular disease is the most common colonic pathology in developed countries. It is estimated that 10 per cent of people in their fifth decade and 60 per cent of people in their ninth decade have diverticula. In parts of Africa in which people still adhere to a traditional diet of grain, maize, and fruit, both appendicitis and diverticulitis are rarities. Like appendicitis, the incidence of diverticulitis is increasing in urban areas of developing countries (Archampong et al., 1978).

TREATMENT

Appendicitis. The treatment of appendicitis is appendectomy. Conservative treatment with antibiotics and intravenous fluid should be used only in the absence of anesthesia or a competent surgeon, or when the patient presents with an appendiceal mass. An aminoglycoside such as kanamycin or gentamicin for coliforms, and clindamycin or metronidazole for anaerobes are the antimicrobials of choice. If the mass increases in size or the patient's general condition deteriorates, the appendiceal abscess must be drained. In those patients with a mass who stabilize, an appendectomy is done two to three months later.

In the remainder, appendectomy should be carried out as soon as possible after adequate preoperative preparation and under general anesthesia. A right iliac fossa skin crease incision over the site of maximum tenderness is employed. The muscles are then split in the direction of their fibers. This gridiron incision is the incision of choice, since it is less liable to complications, including sepsis, than the paramedian incision (Gilmore and Sanderson, 1975). The appendix is then located at the base of the cecum, delivered into the incision, and removed. The mesentery of the appendix is divided between clamps, and the base of the appendix is then crushed, ligated, and inverted into the cecum by means of a purse-string suture.

Intravenous antibiotics as described above are indicated if the appendix is gangrenous or perforated or if there is an abscess. The first dose should be given at the time of operation and the course continued for two to three days. Drainage, preferably through the wound, is necessary if there is an abscess or excessive soiling of the peritoneum. In generalized peritonitis, the peritoneal cavity should be lavaged with 1 to 2 liters of warm normal saline until the effluent is clear. Postoperatively, the patient may start drinking as soon as the bowel sounds return and eat following the passage of flatus. In case of peritonitis, progress is slower, and the patient requires nasogastric aspiration and intravenous fluids until borborygmi are heard.

Diverticulitis. In contrast to appendicitis, diverticulitis is usually treated conservatively. In mild cases, an antispasmodic and a high residue diet suffice. In patients with signs of peritoneal irritation, nasogastric aspiration, intravenous (I.V.) fluids, and parenteral antibiotics—kanamycin (twice daily) or gentamicin (every 8 hours) with clindamycin (every 8 hours) or metronidazole (every 8 hours)—are indicated.

Surgery is reserved for patients with complications and for those with recurrent attacks that do not respond to medical treatment. The complications of diverticular disease often require urgent surgery and are associated with some morbidity and a significant mortality.

Perforation (30 to 40 per cent) is the most common complication and results in local or generalized peritonitis or abscess formation. These patients used to be treated by performing a transverse colostomy as the first stage of a three-stage procedure. This, however, is inadequate. One must also drain the perforation site or, preferably, exteriorize the colon at the site of perforation so that a stream of fecal material above the hole in the colon is avoided. Some surgeons advocate primary resection and anastomosis, even in the presence of pus, and claim a lower mortality. If this is done, it is prudent to carry out a covering transverse colostomy. The same antibiotics are given in perforations of the colon as in perforations of the appendix since the bacterial flora are similar.

Fistula formation, usually to the bladder and sometimes to the small bowel, vagina, skin, or hip joint, is the second most common complication (10 to 15 per cent). Barium enema examination shows diverticular disease, but the fistula is rarely demonstrated. Colovesical fistulas are best diagnosed from the symptoms of pneumaturia, foul-smelling urine, and a persistent or recurrent urinary tract infection due to mixed fecal organisms. The diagnosis is confirmed by cytoscopy. The majority of fistulas can be dealt with by a one-stage resection and anastomosis after careful preoperative preparation. Complex fistulas may require a three-stage procedure consisting of (1) performance of a transverse colostomy, (2) resection and anastomosis of the fistula(s), and (3) closure of the colostomy.

Obstruction (5 to 10 per cent) in diverticular disease is rarer than in carcinoma. Relief of obstruction from diverticular disease may require a one-, two-, or three-stage procedure, depending on the general condition of the patient and the severity of the obstruction.

Massive hemorrhage is an unusual but well-recognized complication of diverticular disease. Depending on the site and speed of the bleed, the blood presenting at the anus varies from brown to bright red in color. Selective mesenteric arteriography may locate the site of hemorrhage, and, if the bleeding does not cease, urgent resection is required. Local resection is adequate if the site of hemorrhage is known; if not, the patient should have a total colectomy. Ileorectal anastomosis can be done then or at a later stage, depending on the condition of the patient and the experience of the surgeon.

Patients with diverticulitis who have repeated attacks of pain and fail to respond to medical treatment should always be considered for elective surgery. Resection in these patients need not be as extensive as in carcinoma, since only the involved segment needs excision. Although anastomotic complications are common in diverticulitis, a one-stage procedure can be done. Many surgeons prefer a three-stage procedure.

PROPHYLAXIS. Africans who still adhere to their traditional way of life and consume a high residue diet containing a minimum of carbohydrates rarely develop either appendicitis or diverticulitis. If the rest of us adopted a similar diet from childhood, we would be less likely to develop appendicitis and very unlikely to get diverticulitis.

Postoperative wound infection after appendectomy and colon resection can be prevented by a short course of systemic metronidazole and kanamycin.

References

Archampong, E. Q., et al.: Third world diverticular disease. Ann R Coll Surg Engl 60:464, 1978.

Burkitt, D. P.: Some diseases characteristic of modern western civilization. Br Med J 1:274, 1973.

Cleave, T. L., and Campbell, G. D.: Diabetes, Coronary Thrombosis and the Saccharine Disease. Bristol, John Wright & Sons Ltd., 1966.

Gilmore, O. J. A.: Diagnostic error in acute appendicitis. Med Annual 1978. Bristol, John Wright & Sons Ltd., 1978.

Gilmore, O. J. A., Brodribb, A. J. M., Browett, J. P., Cooke, T. J. C., Griffin, P. H., Higgs, M. J., Ross, I. K., and Williamson, R. C. N.: Appendicitis and mimicking conditions. A prospective study. Lancet 2:421, 1975.

Gilmore, O. J. A., and Martin, T. D. M.: The aetiology and prevention of wound infection after appendectomy. Br J Surg 61:281, 1974.

Gilmore, O. J. A., and Sanderson, P. J.: Prophylactic interparietal povidone iodine in abdominal surgery. Br J Surg 62:792, 1975.

135

CHOLERA

CRAIG K. WALLACE, M.D.

Cholera is an acute, sometimes fulminant diarrheal disease resulting from an enterotoxin elaborated by *Vibrio cholerae* in the small intestine. It generally occurs in epidemics and may cause a rapid massive gastrointestinal fluid loss with extreme saline depletion, acidosis, and shock.

ETIOLOGY. *V. cholerae* is a short, slightly curved, rod-shaped, gram-negative bacterium that is rapidly motile by means of a single polar flagellum (see Chapter 32, Fig. 2). It grows aerobically on nutrient media at 37° C, preferably at an alkaline pH.

The common delta of the Ganges and Brahmaputra Rivers of India and Bangladesh has been a known focus of cholera since the 16th century. Until the 19th century, cholera was confined to Asia, almost exclusively to India; however, cholera spread along the trade routes over most of the globe in six pandemics between 1817 and 1923. Subsequently, cholera was again confined to the endemic regions of Southeast Asia except for one isolated epidemic in Egypt during 1947. The present seventh pandemic spread of disease extended from the Celebes in 1961 northward to Korea and through Southeast Asia, the Indian subcontinent, the Middle East, southern Europe, and Africa. Endemic foci in many of these recently involved areas, as well as isolated illness, have occurred since this pandemic reached its acme in 1971.

Since the discovery of the cholera vibrio by Robert Koch in 1884, a wide variety of hemolytic vibrios have been found in nature; true cholera vibrios were not hemolytic. This distinction seemed valid until 1906, when Gotschlich isolated hemolytic strains of cholera vibrios from dead pilgrims at the Eltor quarantine station in Egypt. There was no cholera epidemic then and the pathogenicity of this hemolytic cholera vibrio was not ascertained. In 1939, DeMoor described cholera in Sulawesi (Celebes), Indonesia, that was due to *V. cholerae* biotype Eltor. This Eltor vibrio is the etiologic agent in the present pandemic. Interestingly, the Eltor biotype of *V. cholerae* has lost its hemolytic characteristic in recent years and is now distinguished from the classical vibrio by resistance to Murkerjee's phage IV, resistance to polymyxin, and the ability to agglutinate chicken red blood cells (Wallace, 1969).

PATHOGENESIS AND PATHOLOGY. The cholera patient ingests viable *V. cholerae*. The organisms multiply in the small bowel and produce an enterotoxin, which stimulates the mucosal cells to secrete large quantities of isotonic fluid faster than the colon can reabsorb, so that a watery, isotonic diarrhea results. All strains of *V. cholerae* produce the same stool fluid-electrolyte losses that cause the physical findings and laboratory abnormalities seen in cholera. There is no evidence that the vibrio invades any tissue or that the enterotoxin directly affects any organ other than the small intestine. Cholera has the shortest incubation period of any infection; grave symptoms may occur within a few hours of infection.

Vibrio enterotoxin has a molecular weight of 84,000 and stimulates adenyl cyclase in the intestinal epithelial cells. The resultant increase in intracellular cyclic adenosine 3',5'-monophosphate leads to the secretion of isotonic fluids by all of the small intestine. This enterotoxin-induced electrolyte secretion occurs with no demonstrable histologic damage to intestinal epithelial cells or capillary endothelial cells of the lamina propria.

The cholera stool has little protein and is isotonic with plasma, having a remarkably predictable composition of approximately 135 mEq sodium, 15 mEq potassium, 105 mEq chloride, and 45 mEq bicarbonate per liter in adults (Watten et al., 1959). In children the electrolyte composition of the diarrheal fluid is different and contains approximately 100 mEq sodium, 25 mEq potassium, 75 mEq chloride, and 32 mEq bicarbonate per liter.

CLINICAL MANIFESTATIONS. Most infections with *V. cholerae* are asymptomatic or mild. The ratio of severe disease to mild and inapparent infections has been from 1:5 to 1:10 in classic cholera and only about 1:25 to 1:100 for cholera Eltor. The hospitalized cases of both forms of disease, therefore, represent extreme manifestation of disease, with most infections going undetected unless intensive bacteriologic or serologic studies are made.

The sudden onset of profuse, effortless diarrhea is the *sine qua non* of severe symptomatic cholera. The diarrheal stool initially may be bile-tinged and contain fecal particles, but shortly a "rice water stool" is seen. This is a continuous, light-gray, water diarrhea with flecks of mucous material, but no pus or blood, and an odor like amniotic fluid. A rare patient may have pooling in the gut without diarrhea (*cholera sicca*). Most patients, soon after the onset of diarrhea, have copious effortless vomiting that is precipitous but not persistent. Severe muscular cramps, most frequently located in the fingers, toes, and lower extremities, but which may be generalized, are present in 75 per cent of patients. Patients usually are not seen by a physician until 8 to 16 hours after onset of diarrhea. If not moribund, the patient is hoarse, reasonably alert, and oriented. Marked dehydration causes sunken eyes and cheeks, dry tongue and mucous membranes, poor skin turgor, shriveled feet, and "washer-woman's hands." The lips are cyanotic, skin is cold and clammy, temperature is subnormal, and respirations are rapid and shallow. There is tachycardia and hypotension or an imperceptible pulse and blood pressure. The abdomen is scaphoid, nontender, and the bowel sounds are not remarkable.

Children do not respond like adults. They frequently have fever, tetany or generalized convulsions, and pulmonary edema.

Laboratory studies reveal a metabolic acidosis and confirm the clinical findings of dehydration and hemoconcentration (Watten et al., 1959). The plasma electrolytes (mEq/liter of plasma water) are normal except for a low bicarbonate that averages from 7 to 18 mEq/liter.

Prompt fluid, electrolyte, and base replacement rapidly ameliorates all signs and symptoms except diarrhea. The illness may last from 12 hours to 7 days (Carpenter et al., 1966).

COMPLICATIONS AND SEQUELAE. There should be no complications or sequelae if cholera is treated promptly and correctly.

Cholera may, of course, be superimposed upon preexisting disease. Persistent circulatory failure will cause hypotensive shock, cyanosis, and anuria. Most patients are anuric upon admission and may remain oliguric for several days. If rehydration is not achieved rapidly and maintained, acute renal failure may ensue. Prolonged acidosis may cause persistent cramps and vomiting, increased dyspnea with rales and obvious pulmonary-myocardial failure. Acidosis is often intensified by infusion of abundant saline without alkali. Untreated hypokalemia may cause muscle weakness, ileus, cardiac arrhythmia, abdominal distention, and occasional central nervous system disturbances. The patient must be carefully monitored for overhydration. If it does occur, the hepatojugular reflux and slow full pulse usually give adequate warning before pulmonary edema.

Fetal mortality and abortion, especially in the third trimester, are frequent in pregnant women with cholera.

Pediatric cholera is especially severe; water exchange in proportion to body weight is far greater than in adults and fluid balances are more readily disturbed. A few children with prolonged diarrhea and impaired oral intake have premonitory drowsiness or convulsions as a result of hypoglycemia.

Under ideal conditions and with prompt and adequate fluid replacement, mortality and significant sequelae approach zero. Oral glucose-electrolyte therapy can be effective even under the most primitive conditions. Unfortunately, high death rates are still being reported especially at the start of an epidemic. This reflects the lack of both appropriate oral and pyrogen-free intravenous fluids in remote areas, as well as the difficulties of initiating prompt treatment to many patients under emergency conditions.

GEOGRAPHIC VARIATIONS IN DISEASE. The spectrum of cholera is identical throughout the world: most infections are asymptomatic and relatively few result in shock from marked dehydration.

Koch's discovery of the vibrio, although elucidating the

etiology of cholera, did not lead to clarification of the epidemiology and ecology of the disease. Why the cluster of infection has remained in the delta of the Ganges and Brahmaputra Rivers is unknown. With the exception of the present pandemic, all epidemics have originated from this endemic focus. We do not know why it is that from time to time at irregular intervals the disease has spread from country to country and from continent to continent (Politzer, 1959). All previous widespread epidemics lasted several years and then inexplicably abated.

What factors favor a new cholera epidemic and continental migration? As suggested by Jusatz (1977) the initial spread of disease continued only very slowly *overland,* not reaching central European countries and Great Britain until 1831. Since 1865, cholera has moved more rapidly by *sea;* especially pilgrims making their way to and from Mecca have carried cholera far and wide. A third phase became evident during the present, or seventh, cholera pandemic when *air* passengers provided a particularly fast transit mode for the vibrio to cholera-free areas in the space of hours. *Water* is the most frequent transport medium of cholera vibrios outside the human body. The type of water supply, the velocity of rivers, as well as the quality of water, its acidity or alkalinity, and degree of salinity are considered of great significance in accounting for the movement and distribution of cholera in different geographic areas. Deserts and water-poor areas are largely circumvented during cholera migrations. The influence of the *seasons* indicates that cold, snow, and frost are inhibiting factors. Other seasonal variations are seen, such as those in India and Bangladesh. In Calcutta, cholera always decreases with the onset of the annual monsoon, whereas in Dacca, less than 200 miles distant, the onset of the monsoon is coincident with an increase of cholera infections. Another predisposing factor is the *mass movement of people.* such as for religious and military events.

Of note, the classic *V. cholera* has not been involved in the post-1961 migrations, but rather the biotype Eltor has been identified in all countries invaded during the seventh pandemic. This variant causes disease identical to that caused by the so-called classic vibrio, but there are marked epidemiologic differences. The infection-to-case ratio is higher with Eltor. It is excreted over a longer period of time. The Eltor vibrio is generally hardier, surviving longer in the environment on infected foodstuffs, in water and feces, which makes it more easily detectable in surveys of water and night soil. The few chronic carriers of *V. cholerae* described in the literature have all been infected with biotype Eltor.

DIAGNOSIS. The clinical impression of typical cholera needs no laboratory confirmation for treatment purposes. Laboratory confirmation, however, is necessary to differentiate the sporadic case from other diarrheal diseases and to alert public health personnel. Although the epidemiologic and fulminant characteristics of cholera are suggestive, past experience has shown that diagnoses of the first few cases usually take too long because the laboratory is unprepared.

Direct plating of a cholera stool on bile salt, gelatin-tellurite-taurocholate (GTT), or thiosulfate-citrate-bile salt-sucrose (TCBS) agar is optimal for cultural diagnosis. On the first two media, *V. cholerae* appear as typical translucent colonies in 18 hours (see Chapter 32); oblique lighting makes it possible to identify one vibrio colony from among several hundred colonies of other organisms. On TCBS agar, *V. cholerae* appear at 24 hours as large, discrete yellow colonies. Cultural identification of large numbers of vibrios (10^7 to 10^9/ml) in the stools is relatively simple. In the patient with fewer vibrios, as in convalescence, recovery can be enhanced by enrichment for six hours in alkaline peptone water before subculture to solid media.

Rapid identification of vibrios in stools or primary culture is possible by observing immobilization of vibrios by type-specific antisera, by darkfield or phase microscopy, or by immunofluorescent methods.

Serologic diagnosis requires demonstration of rises in agglutinating or vibriocidal antibody titers. Significant rises in both titers are present by the seventh to tenth day of illness in over 90 per cent of patients with bacteriologically proven *V. cholerae* infection.

TREATMENT. Replacement of water and electrolytes lost in stool and vomitus is the basis of cholera therapy. This regimen has been used in many parts of the world with a mortality of less than 1 per cent. If the patient is conscious, an oral regimen is optimal; in very severe cholera, oral therapy is effective after hypovolemia has been corrected by rapid intravenous replacement.

Oral and Intravenous Fluids. A supply of preweighed salts and glucose for the preparation of an oral replacement solution should be available, preferably stored in double plastic bags, to be added to a specified volume of ordinary water before use. An acceptable composition is glucose 20 g/liter, sodium chloride 3.5 g/liter, sodium bicarbonate 2.5 g/liter, and potassium chloride 1.5 g/liter of drinking water.

An intravenous solution containing approximately 140 mEq/liter sodium, 10 mEq/liter potassium, 100 mEq/liter chloride, and 50 mEq/liter bicarbonate is simple to use but generally not available. Ringer's lactate is recommended as a single intravenous rehydration fluid by the World Health Organization and is readily available. This is especially satisfactory for children. Effective and available are two solutions given in a 2:1 ratio as isotonic saline: isotonic sodium lactate (1/6 molar) or isotonic sodium bicarbonate. If potassium is not given intravenously, it may be given orally and will be absorbed regardless of the stool volume or intestinal transit time. Ten milliliters of a solution containing 100 g each of potassium citrate, potassium acetate, and potassium bicarbonate in 1 liter of water given three times a day orally will balance the potassium losses in the average patient.

Treatment Centers. Predetermined treatment areas should be available to any potential patient within three hours after the onset of symptoms. Adequate glucose and salts for making up oral solutions, plastic oro- or nasogastric tubes, pyrogen-free intravenous fluids, intravenous administration tubing, large-gauge needles, scalp vein sets, and a scale should be available.

A number of cholera cots should be available. These are generally simple cots with a reinforced hole located in the center for the patient's buttocks and can be made of canvas on a wooden frame or more simply boards elevated upon supports. Any 2 to 3 gallon receptacle can be easily calibrated and when placed under the hole in the cot will be effective for collecting and measuring excreta. The time and amount of all infusions or oral fluids when initiated and the output when discarded must be carefully recorded at the bedside.

Management. The patient should be weighed; if a scale is not available, this may be estimated. The degree of dehydration may be assessed by clinical observation to determine the amount of replacement fluid needed. *Mild* dehydration (5 per cent body weight deficit) is indicated by only a slightly decreased skin turgor and tachycardia. *Moderate* dehydration (8 per cent body weight deficit) is indicated by markedly decreased skin turgor, tachycardia, and hypotension. *Severe dehydration* (10 per cent body weight deficit) has all the above plus cyanosis, stupor, or coma. By knowing the weight and approximating the volume deficit, the amount of fluid necessary for rehydration can be determined.

The comatose patient should receive intravenous fluid through an 18-gauge needle. A smaller-gauge needle or a scalp vein set is usually necessary for children. The femoral vein in adults or the external jugular vein in children may be utilized in patients with severe vascular collapse. Fluids may be given by holding the needle in place until the plasma volume expands enough to make superficial veins visible and the infusion can be easily transferred to a more suitable vein. Intravenous fluid should be started rapidly by giving at least 100 ml per minute to the collapsed adult patient until blood pressure is restored. After rehydration a slower rate of infusion should balance the measured diarrheal output and estimated insensible loss. An adult's insensible water loss is approximately 1 ml/kg per hour and should be replaced. The oral administration of this amount of water contributes to the patient's state of well-being. During the acute phase of disease, the vital signs should be checked at two-hour intervals. There can be no substitute for careful, constant clinical observation.

Initial rehydration and maintenance therapy solely by oral fluids is encouraged because of its safety, ease of administration, and general availability. The solution should be warmed to about 45° C before administration. Some prefer to give the solution through a thin plastic oro- or nasogastric tube connected to an infusion bottle. From 750 to 1500 ml per hour is given for the first four hours, depending upon the degree of admission dehydration. Thereafter, the measured output plus the calculated insensible loss during the preceding four-hour period indicates the volume of oral solution to be given. Allow further oral fluids upon demand and a soft diet as tolerated. Vomiting does not occur after initial correction of the dehydration and acidosis (Pierce and Hirschhorn, 1977).

Treatment of pediatric cholera is difficult in respect to initiating and maintaining intravenous fluids. Water loss in proportion to body weight is far greater, fluid balances are more readily disturbed, and the electrolyte losses are different from those of adults. Children should be closely followed with frequent clinical observations, including weight, to avoid overhydration. Children should never gain more than 10 per cent of their admission body weight. If possible, children should be treated in a separate pediatric area. Intravenous fluids as outlined above have been used with success; particular attention is advised to replacing insensible losses with oral glucose water. Children with prolonged diarrhea and impaired oral intake can have drowsiness or convulsions as a result of hypoglycemia. They respond dramatically to 50 per cent intravenous glucose solution, although fruit juice suffices in the conscious patient. Convulsions and coma unrelated to fever, hypoglycemia, hypocalcemia, hypernatremia, or overhydration may be seen. Intravenous magnesium sulfate succeeds occasionally when other methods fail to control convulsions.

Although adequate intravenous saline and alkali replacement alone results in rapid recovery of virtually all cholera patients, a dramatic reduction in duration and volume of diarrhea and early eradication of vibrios from the stool may be effected by antibiotic therapy. Oral tetracycline, 500 mg every six hours for adults and 10 mg/kg body weight every six hours for children for the first 48 hours, has been most successful. Other antibiotics, including chloramphenicol and furazolidone, are slightly less effective than tetracycline (Wallace et al., 1968).

Additional adjuncts of therapy (oxygen, cardiorespiratory stimulants, vasopressors, and antidiarrheal compounds) are not indicated and divert essential medical and financial resources.

Therapy is continued until the diarrhea has practically ceased and fluid electrolyte requirements can be met by oral fluids and a soft diet. Patients may be discharged as soon as they are ambulatory, eating, and have an adequate urinary output. The public health problems of unsuspected carriers and the rare convalescent who excretes vibrios are unsolved.

PROPHYLAXIS. The current cholera vaccines composed of classic or biotype Eltor strains are of limited value. In endemic area field trials, vaccines have been only about 50 per cent effective in reducing the incidence of clinical illness for a period of three to six months. They do not prevent transmission of infection.

Primary immunization with commercial vaccines, containing 10 billion organisms per milliliter, is given in two doses one week to one month or more apart, either subcutaneously or intramuscularly as follows: 0.2 ml from six months to four years of age, 0.3 ml five to ten years, and 0.5 ml over ten years. A booster immunization in a similar dosage may be given every six months for travel or to residents in highly endemic, unsanitary areas. When cholera occurs in an annual two or three month "season," protection is best if the booster dose is given at the beginning of the season. The primary series need not be repeated.

Field trials have shown that antibiotics like tetracycline and chloramphenicol prevent the transmission of infection among close contacts of cholera patients, but giving these drugs to both close and community contacts has not controlled cholera outbreaks. In any circumstance, the indiscriminate use of antimicrobial drugs is to be avoided. If chemoprophylaxis is considered at all, the drug chosen should be administered only with close supervision for contraindications and for follow-up of reactions.

Cholera can be eliminated only by improved standards of living, public health, and sanitation. In those parts of the world where water supply and sewage disposal are adequate, cholera no longer poses a problem.

References

Barua, D., and Burrows, W.: Cholera. Philadelphia, W. B. Saunders Company, 1974.

Carpenter, C. C. J. et al.: Clinical studies in Asiatic cholera, I–VI. Bull Johns Hopkins Hosp 118:165, 1966.

Jusatz, H.: Cholera. In Howe, G. M. (ed.): A World Geography of Human Diseases. London, New York, and San Francisco, Academic Press, 1977, p. 131.

Pierce, N. F., and Hirschhorn, N.: Oral fluid—a simple weapon against dehydration in diarrhoea. WHO Chronicle 31:87, 1977.

Pollitzer, R.: Cholera. Geneva, WHO Monograph Series, No. 43, 1959.

van Heyningen, W. E., and Seal, J. R.: Cholera: The American Scientific Experience, 1947–1980. Boulder, Colorado, Westview Press, Inc., 1983.

Wallace, C. K. et al.: Optimal antibiotic therapy in cholera. Bull WHO 39:239, 1968.

Wallace, C. K.: Cholera: A Continuing Threat and Challenge. In Lincicome, D. R., and Woodruff, D. W. (eds.): International Review of Tropical Medicine. New York and London, Academic Press, 1969, p. 159.

Watten, R. H. et al.: Water and electrolyte studies in cholera. J Clin Invest 38:1879, 1959.

136

YERSINIA ENTERITIS

GERALD T. KEUSCH, M.D.

DEFINITIONS AND HISTORY. Abdominal infections of man with *Yersinia enterocolitica* and *Y. pseudotuberculosis* cause a variety of syndromes, but enteritis and mesenteric adenitis are by far the most common. Typically, *Y. enterocolitica* causes an acute febrile watery diarrhea in children under 5 years of age. Mesenteric adenitis, which may imitate appendicitis, is most common in 5- to 15-year-olds and may be caused by either species of *Yersinia*. Reactive polyarticular arthritis is a late, noninfectious complication of *Yersinia* enteritis in adults. It occurs most commonly among those with HLA B27 type in Scandinavia.

Yersinia is a new genus that was created to accommodate *Y. pestis* (the plague bacillus), *Y. enterocolitica,* and *Y. pseudotuberculosis.* Although *Yersinia* organisms share many characteristics with *Francisella* and *Pasteurella* and were formerly classified with these bacteria, they fit the definition of Enterobacteriaceae and are now placed in this family. In the future, the species *Y. enterocolitica* may be subdivided into four distinct species.

Y. pseudotuberculosis was first isolated in 1883 from necrotizing granulomas in the livers, spleens, and lymph nodes of various mammals and birds. The disease was called pseudotuberculosis because of the nature of the lesions. Occasional cases of human septicemia were described early in this century, but acute mesenteric adenitis, the chief form of intestinal disease caused by this bacterium, was not reported until 1954. *Y. enterocolitica* was unknown until 1939 and was not recognized as a human pathogen until 1964. Since then, there has been a spectacular rise in the reported incidence of *Y. enterocolitica* enteritis. This has been due principally to heightened interest in the organism rather than recent pandemic spread.

MICROBIOLOGY. Members of the genus *Yersinia* have been reclassified into the Enterobacteriaceae family because they are facultatively anaerobic, oxidase-negative, gram-negative bacilli that ferment glucose and reduce nitrate. Motile species synthesize peritrichous flagella. *Y. enterocolitica* and *Y. pseudotuberculosis* may be coccobacillary but are usually relatively large bacilli, 0.5 to 1.0 by 1 to 2 μm. They must be differentiated from *Proteus* on the one hand and the plague bacillus (*Y. pestis*) on the other (Table 1). They may also be difficult to isolate from cultures of the stool.

When first recovered from the stool, *Y. pseudotuberculosis* is likely to be discarded as a *Proteus* species, a normal member of the fecal flora, because both are lactose-negative and urease-positive, and both produce an alkaline slant/acid butt reaction on triple sugar iron agar (TSI). *Y. enterocolitica* can ferment both sucrose and glucose in TSI and therefore produces the acid slant/acid butt characteristic of *Escherichia coli.* Because this pattern is typical of the nonpathogens, the organism is likely to be discarded. Newer media, devised to overcome these problems, contain arabinose, arginine, and lysine. *Y. enterocolitica* ferments arabinose but does not utilize arginine or lysine and the resulting acidification turns the medium red. Certain organisms that may be confused with *Y. enterocolitica* are differentiated by their inability to ferment arabinose (*Proteus*); or their fermentation of arginine, and ability to decarboxylate the other substrates (*E. coli*), generating alkaline products that neutralize the medium and preclude a color change. Once selected for further study, identification is quite straightforward. Failure to produce H_2S or deaminate phenylalanine and the absence of motility at 37° C are among the important reactions that differentiate *Yersinia* from the indole-negative *Proteus* spp. Motility when grown at 22° C but not at 37° C, and urease activity are important properties of the two organisms that distinguish them from *Y. pestis.* Ornithine decarboxylase activity, indole production, and sucrose fermentation are seen with *Y. pseudotuberculosis* but not *Y. enterocolitica* (Table 1). The biochemical identification can be confirmed by agglutination with specific typing sera.

Isolation of both organisms is enhanced by the cold enrichment technique, in which a 10 per cent suspension of feces (or other sample) in phosphate-buffered saline, pH7.6, is maintained at 4°C for serial subculture to enriched media after 7 to 28 days. *Yersinia,* but not other *Enterobacteriaceae*, preferentially multiply at this low temperature to give progressive enrichment of *Yersinia* in the buffer. It has been recommended that cultures be incubated at both room temperature and 37° C because primary isolation of some strains from clinical material might be achieved only at the lower temperature. In practice, however, isolation of typical (DNA group 1) *Y. enterocolitica* is not improved from patients with gastrointestinal disease, but recovery of *Yersiniae* from other sources, such as food,

Table 1. SELECTED MICROBIOLOGIC CHARACTERISTICS OF *YERSINIA*

Property	Y. Pseudotuberculosis	Y. Enterocolitica	Y. Pestis
TSI[a] reaction (slant/butt)	Alkaline/acid	Acid/acid	Alkaline/acid
H_2S production (TSI)	−	−	−
Indole	−	+ (except serotype 0:3)	−
Urease production (Christensen's)	+	+	−
Ornithine decarboxylase	−	+	−
Rhamnose fermentation	+	−	−
Sucrose fermentation	−	+	−
Lactose fermentation	−	−	−
Motility 22° C	+	+	−
37° C	−	−	−
Esculin hydrolysis	+	−	+

[a]TSI, Triple sugar iron agar. *Y. enterocolitica* produces an acid slant because it ferments sucrose.

Table 2. SEROEPIDEMIOLOGIC AND CLINICAL CLASSIFICATION OF *Y. ENTEROCOLITICA*

Serotype	Distribution	Clinical Pattern[a]
0:3/Biotype 4/phage type 8	Europe, Japan	Classic; also reactive arthritis
0:3/Biotype 4/phage type 9A	South Africa	Classic; reactive arthritis
0:3/Biotype 4/phage type 9B	Canada	Classic
0:5,27/Biotype 2/phage type 10	United States	Classic
0:8/Biotype 1/phage type 10[b]	United States	Classic
0:9/Biotype 2/phage type 10	Scandinavia	Classic; also reactive arthritis and erythema nodosum
0:12, 0:14, 0:16, NAG[c]	Worldwide	Diverse, atypical
0:17/Biotype 1/phage type 10	United States	Diverse, atypical

[a]See text.
[b]Phage type 10 includes all nontypable strains.
[c]Nonagglutinable with the 34 antisera currently available.

may be improved (Schiemann, 1982). Certain characteristics, such as the synthesis of peritrichous flagella and surface 0 antigens, are expressed only at temperatures less than 30° C.

Phage-typing systems have been developed to subtype isolates of several 0 serotypes. This is useful for epidemiological studies. The 20 flagellar H antigens are also helpful in this regard.

Most human illness due to *Y. entercolitica* has been caused by a few serogroups, including 0:3, 0:5, 0:8, and 0:9. Serogroups are not distributed uniformly throughout the world; rather, certain 0 groups predominate in different countries (Table 2). With the exception of serogroup 0:3, which is often found in pigs and may be part of the normal porcine oral flora, these strains are apparently adapted to people; the other strains appear to be adapted to animals. Attempts have been made to classify the organism by DNA hybridization techniques. Four different species are distinguished (Table 3) and it is proposed that only relatedness group 1 be called *Y. enterocolitica* (Brenner et al., 1980). This species contains the human adapted strains, which are uniform and typical with regard to microbiologic growth characteristics and biochemical, serologic, and phage-typing patterns. They are sucrose positive and negative for salicin, esculin, rhamnose, raffinose, melibiose, α-methylglucoside, and citrate. These strains tend to produce certain "classic" clinical syndromes, including acute enteritis, mesenteric adenitis, terminal ileitis, and septicemia, and they possess virulence markers that have been defined by in vitro and in vivo animal experiments. The other groups contain organisms usually recovered from the environment, a wide range of animal hosts, or foods. They are of different serotypes than the first group, are of different biotypes, and are biochemically atypical. They usually ferment rhamnose (and often raffinose and melibiose) at 22° C, and they may fail to ferment sucrose. These organisms are avirulent or have been responsible for less typical syndromes in people, including urinary tract infection, wound infection, localized skin abscesses, conjunctivitis, and mild diarrhea.

PATHOGENESIS AND PATHOLOGY. *Y. pseudotuberculosis* and *Y. enterocolitica* cause pseudotuberculosis in mammals and birds. Current evidence suggests that they are zoonotic bacteria that are transferred between human beings and animals, primarily through fecal contamination of food or water. Pseudotuberculosis is therefore not quasituberculosis nor is it transmitted like mycobacterial infection.

In all geographic areas, the organisms are isolated during the coldest months of the year. This seasonal incidence may partly reflect a cold enrichment phenomenon. Although previously it was believed that the organisms require low temperatures for the synthesis of virulence factors recent studies have identified virulence markers that are produced at 37° C (Carter et al., 1980; Portnoy et al., 1981; Schiemann and Devenish, 1982).

Y. enterocolitica and *Y. pseudotuberculosis* both synthesize endotoxins (O antigens) with biologic properties similar to those of the endotoxins of other gram-negative bacteria, but there is no evidence that these lipopolysaccharides contribute to the unique abdominal disease syndromes caused by *Yersinia*. *Y. enterocolitica* produce a heat-stable enterotoxin (Pai and DeStephano, 1982; Schiemann and Devenish, 1982) that could contribute to the symptoms of *Yersinia* enteritis but is not produced at 37° C and thus appears to be irrelevant.

Both *Yersinia* can invade mammalian cells. Cellular penetration correlates better than enterotoxicity with the pathology in animals and people (Pai and DeStephano, 1982; Schiemann and Devenish, 1982). Enteric infections cause ulcerations in the terminal ileum, involvement of Peyer's patches, and suppurative granulomatous lesions in the ileocecal lymph nodes. Pseudotuberculosis in animals and septicemia in man causes similar lesions in the liver, spleen, and other organs.

In addition to invasiveness, which is not sufficient for virulence, other traits have been associated with production of experimental diarrhea in rabbits and mice by *Y. enterocolitica* grown at 37° C. These properties include serum

Table 3. SUBCLASSIFICATION OF *Y. ENTEROCOLITICA* BY DNA RELATEDNESS CHARACTERISTICS (BRENNER ET AL., 1980)

DNA Relatedness Group	Proposed Species Name	Selected Biotype Features*	Clinical Pattern
1	*Y. enterocolitica*	$S^+R^-M^-C^-$	Classic
2	*Y. intermedia*	$S^+R^+M^+C^+$	Wounds, skin infection
3	*Y. fredericksenii*	$S^+R^+M^-C^\pm$	Wounds, skin infection
4	*Y. kristensenii*	$S^-R^-M^-C^-$	Avirulent (Environmental strains)

*S = sucrose, R = rhamnose, M = melibionate, C = citrate, $^+$ = fermentation, $^-$ = no fermentation.

resistance, calcium-dependent growth and autoagglutinability, and synthesis of *Y. pestis* V and W antigens and at least three outer membrane peptides in the presence of restricted calcium and high (20 mM) magnesium (Carter et al., 1980; Portnoy et al., 1981; Pai and DeStephano, 1982; Schiemann and Devenish, 1982). A class of 40–48 Mdal plasmids in various *Y. enterocolitica* serotypes appear to code for autoagglutination, Ca^{++} dependent growth, the three OM peptides and probably V and W antigens. The OM peptides and the latter antigens would likely be synthesized within invaded cells where the Ca^{++} and Mg^{++} concentrations are appropriate. Their function is not known at present.

The reactive polyarthritis that may follow infection with *Yersinia* is immunologic rather than infectious, although septic arthritis may develop during the course of septicemia (Spira and Kabins, 1976). The occurrence of reactive arthritis, most commonly in Scandinavia, suggests that strain specificity is responsible for joint localization. Arthritis, urethritis, and uveitis occur most commonly in patients with histocompatibility antigen HLA-B27 whereas erythema nodosum is not associated with B27 (Leirisalo et al., 1982). Alterations in in vitro cell-mediated immune responses have been demonstrated in patients with yersinial arthritis, along with a persistant IgA antibody response that is related to the severity of the joint manifestations, which supports an immunologic mechanism for this manifestation (Granfors et al., 1980; Goebel et al., 1982).

CLINICAL MANIFESTATIONS. *Y. pseudotuberculosis* and *Y. enterocolitica* both cause a variety of enteric illnesses. The frequency of each clinical syndrome varies with the agent (Table 4). The most common clinical presentation of infection with *Y. pseudotuberculosis* is acute mesenteric adenitis (pseudoappendicitis) while acute enteritis (watery diarrhea) is the most common presentation of infection with *Y. enterocolitica*. The portal of entry of both species is presumed to be the alimentary tract. Differences in the clinical manifestations are probably due to the degree of penetration of the organism into or through the intestinal mucosa, which is related to strain and inoculum size. In experimental oral infection of mice, very large numbers of *Y. enterocolitica* grown at room temperature cause septicemia, whereas lower inocula of the same organism cause only intestinal disease. The clinical manifestations of *Y. enterocolitica* are more protean than *Y. pseudotuberculosis* and are generally related to the age of the patient (Table 5). The reasons for these associations are not understood, and exceptions certainly occur.

Acute enteritis from *Y. enterocolitica* in a child less than 5 years old usually presents as acute, watery diarrhea without blood or mucus (Vantrappen et al., 1982). There is nothing to distinguish this illness from the many other causes of watery diarrhea in children. The manifestations are generally self-limited within 5 to 10 days. In a minority, blood is present in the stool and the presentation is like a dysentery. Diarrhea, abdominal pain, or fever may each appear alone as the only clinical manifestation of yersinia infection. *Y. enterocolitica* can also cause epidemic gastroenteritis, probably water- or food-borne. This illness may affect either children or adults and may resemble staphylococcal "food poisoning" (abrupt onset of nausea, vomiting, abdominal cramps, and watery diarrhea) except that one half to two thirds of patients with *Y. enterocolitica* gastroenteritis also have fever. The presence of blood, mucus, and leukocytes in the stools of many of these patients suggests that this illness is an invasive inflammatory enteritis. The other syndrome associated with acute epidemic gastroenteritis is a self-limited, 24-hour febrile diarrheal illness.

Table 4. INTESTINAL MANIFESTATIONS OF YERSINIOSIS

Clinical Presentation	Infecting Organism *Y. pseudotuberculosis*	*Y. enterocolitica*
Mesenteric adenitis	+ + + +[a]	+ +
Terminal ileitis	+	+
Acute enteritis	±	+ + + +

[a]Frequency of the manifestation from rare (±) to common (+ + + +).

Table 5. AGE-RELATED CLINICAL PRESENTATIONS OF *Y. ENTEROCOLITICA* INFECTION (LEINO AND KALLIOMAKI, 1974)

Age Group (Years)	Clinical Presentation
< 5	Acute diarrhea
5 to 15	Acute mesenteric adenitis ("pseudoappendicitis")
10 to 20	Acute terminal ileitis ("pseudo Crohn's disease")
Adults	Acute diarrhea and nongastrointestinal manifestations
Nongastrointestinal Manifestations	
Infants and adults more than 60 years	Septicemia
Compromised hosts	Septicemia
Adults (especially females)	Erythema nodosum
Adults	Polyarthritis

In children from 5 to 15 years of age, both *Y. pseudotuberculosis* and *Y. enterocolitica* are most likely to cause acute mesenteric adenitis, sometimes called "pseudoappendicitis." The illness often begins nonspecifically with headache, arthralgia, and fever but may begin with diarrhea when *Y. enterocolitica* is the etiologic agent. After a few days, the patient develops diffuse abdominal pain that localizes to the right lower quadrant after a variable interval of hours to days. There is often tenderness, particularly over McBurney's point, with localized rebound tenderness in this area and tenderness to the right on rectal examination. These signs are ordinarily less impressive than would be expected from the other clinical findings. Unless the patient has had an appendectomy or the examiner detects a mass, the diagnosis of acute appendicitis is made, and a laparotomy is performed. The appendix is either normal or only slightly reddened, but the mesenteric lymph nodes overlying the terminal ileum are markedly enlarged (2 to 8 cm in diameter), intensely inflamed, and usually matted together. The mesentery surrounding the nodes and the serosa of the adjacent terminal ileum and cecum are also inflamed. There is ordinarily a small quantity of free fluid in the peritoneal cavity. The surgeon usually performs an appendectomy and should also perform a biopsy on the involved nodes for culture and histology. Typically there are numerous cortical pyroninophilic large histiocytes with follicular hyperplasia and scattered microabscesses in the nodes. The illness resolves after a few days to two weeks.

In older adolescents and young adults, the inflammatory process may be mostly limited to the terminal ileum, with only minimal suppurative adenitis of the mesenteric nodes. This acute ileitis may be caused by either species of *Yersinia*. The clinical features may resemble acute mesenteric adenitis, but it can progress occasionally to a fatal hemorrhagic necrosis of the ileocecal area or even of the entire bowel. In some individuals, the illness begins with acute diarrhea and abdominal pain, which either persists or remits and exacerbates for weeks to months. Radiologic examination uniformly shows abnormalities of the terminal ileum that range from thickening of the mucosal folds or distortion of the mucosal pattern to nodular filling defects or even solitary or multiple ulcerations (Vantrappen et al., 1982). Barium enema is usually normal, but there may be spasm of the terminal ileum due to inflammation. The absence of fistulae or granulomas and the presence of longitudinally oriented discrete punched out or polypoid granular ulcerations with an overlying fibro-purulent exudate help to distinguish yersinial ileitis from Crohn's disease. Colonoscopy reveals lesions in about half the patients, usually small, 1 to 2 mm round apthous ulcers of uniform size and shape.

In adults, acute self-limited dysentery may be followed in one to six weeks by acute polyarthritis of the knees, ankles, and small joints of the hands or feet. The joint symptoms are usually polyarticular, migratory, and bilateral. Persistent activity in one or more joints for several months is common, and some patients may experience chronic rheumatoid arthritis-like symptoms for over a year. Joint manifestations have been noted principally in Scandinavia and are associated with the presence of histocompatibility locus HLA-B27. Other extraintestinal manifestations reported include erythema nodosum, erythema multiforme, urethritis, uveitis, Reiters syndrome, hepatitis, carditis, thyroiditis, and suppurative bone and joint infections (Vantrappen et al., 1982).

GEOGRAPHIC VARIATIONS. *Yersinia pseudotuberculosis* and *Y. enterocolitica* are probably distributed worldwide, but most cases have been identified in a few Scandinavian countries, Belgium, France, South Africa, and Canada, and more recently in the United States and Japan. The incidence is much higher in Scandinavia and other parts of Europe than in the rest of the world. The high prevalence in temperate and cold climates could be related to cold selection, but *Yersinia* can generally be found in any country if it is carefully sought clinically and bacteriologically.

In addition to this high prevalence of *Yersinia* in certain geographic areas, some specific serotypes exhibit a limited geographic range and association with specific clinical syndromes (Table 2). The high prevalence of certain serologic types in Scandinavia and the susceptibility of patients with histocompatibility type HLA-B27 to reactive arthritis and of non-B27 women to erythema nodosum suggests that this clinical selectivity is determined by bacterial strain characteristics as well as host genetics.

DIAGNOSIS AND DIFFERENTIAL DIAGNOSIS. Acute yersinial diarrhea can only be differentiated from diarrhea caused by other agents by culture and/or serology. The cold enrichment technique may be valuable, but the diligence of the laboratory in seeking this microorganism is probably more important. Plates for primary culture and subculture should always be held at 22 to 25° C, as well as at 37° C, to enhance recovery. Serologic diagnosis is useful but less reliable, because titers may not develop (certain serotypes) or disappear rapidly during convalescence. Rising titers of agglutinating antibody or sera with titers greater than 1:100 are indicative of yersinial infection. Furthermore, although *Y. pseudotuberculosis* and *Y. enterocolitica* are easily separated serologically, these organisms cross-react with other bacteria (Table 6). In regions in which *Brucella* infections are prevalent, absorptions of serum are necessary for the serodiagnosis of *Y. enterocolitica* 0:9. Fortunately, the seroreaction to *Y. pseudotuberculosis* type I, which accounts for 90 per cent of human infections with this organism, is quite specific. The cross-reactive type IV *Y. pseudotuberculosis* is rarely isolated from human sources.

Table 6. SEROLOGIC CROSS-REACTIONS BETWEEN *YERSINIA* SPECIES AND OTHER BACTERIA

Organism	Cross-Reacting Antigens
Y. enterocolitica 0:9	*Brucella* (smooth)
	Salmonella group N
Y. pseudotuberculosis type II	*Salmonella* group B
Y. pseudotuberculosis type IV	*Salmonella* group D
type IV_A	*E. coli* 0:17, 0:77
	Enterobacter cloacae
Y. pseudotuberculosis type VI	*E. coli* 0:55

Because acute mesenteric adenitis mimics appendicitis, the diagnosis is usually made at surgery. *Y. pseudotuberculosis* has a marked predilection for young boys, however, and the agglutinin titer may already be elevated on admission to the hospital. Therefore, for *Y. pseudotuberculosis*, but not *Y. enterocolitica*, which takes longer to cause an antibody response, it is at least theoretically possible to make a specific serodiagnosis shortly after admission and avert unnecessary surgery. When postpubertal females are affected, an important preoperative differential diagnosis is gynecologic disease, including ruptured or bleeding ovarian cysts, salpingitis, retrograde menstrual bleeding, or fibroid uterus. Diverticulitis, acute cholecystitis, and even urinary tract infection can also mimic this condition and should be considered, especially in adults.

Staphylococcus aureus and *Streptococcus pyogenes*, coxsackie viruses, and echoviruses have also been isolated from inflamed mesenteric nodes. The specific diagnosis can be made by isolation of the organism directly from the biopsied node. Therefore, resected tissues should be subjected to routine cultures, as well as cold enrichment and periodic subculture at 22° C and 37° C. The histologic changes of *Yersinia* adenitis are characterized by suppurative granulomas that resemble those of cat-scratch disease and lymphogranuloma venereum.

Francisella, *Salmonella typhi*, *Entamoeba histolytica*, and *Mycobacterium tuberculosis* can cause terminal ileitis like *Yersinia*. Microbiologic diagnosis is required. Initially, the illness may be indistinguishable from Crohn's disease. For this reason, ileal biopsy is not suggested because the development of fistulae is a common complication of Crohn's disease. Biopsy and culture of the mesenteric nodes in *Yersinia* infection does not cause fistulae and establishes the correct diagnosis. Subsequent radiologic study may be helpful if the patient does not improve because late fistulae, stenosis, pseudodiverticula, skip lesions, or marked persistent thickening of the bowel or mesentery do not occur following *Yersinia* infections.

THERAPY. *Y. enterocolitica*, especially serotypes 0:3 and 0:9, and *Y. pseudotuberculosis* exhibit similar antimicrobial sensitivity patterns. They are usually quite sensitive to the aminoglycosides, chloramphenicol, colistin, sulfonamides, tetracycline, and the combination of trimethoprim-sulfamethoxazole. Because it synthesizes broad-spectrum, constitutive and/or inducible beta-lactamases, *Y. enterocolitica* is resistant to penicillin, ampicillin, amoxicillin, and to first and second generation cephalosporins. In vitro data suggest that newer beta-lactam drugs (mecillinam, moxalactam, and cefotaxime) may be useful agents. *Y. pseudotuberculosis* is usually quite sensitive to penicillin, ampicillin, and the cephalosporins. Strains of either organism may become resistant to almost any antimicrobial by acquisition of a transferable drug-resistant plasmid.

There is, however, no evidence yet that antibiotics are useful in the therapy of any of the enteric *Yersinia* infections. These infections appear to run their course independent of surgery or antimicrobial therapy. Controlled clinical trials will be required to determine whether antimicrobials can shorten the usual course. The important measures are to rule out the presence of true surgical emergencies, replace fluids, and allow sufficient time for recovery. Antidiarrheal mixtures of any sort are not helpful in enteric infections and should be avoided.

When *Yersinia* septicemia develops, however, the situation is markedly altered. This is not a benign, self-limited condition. Many of these patients are immunocompromised, and the mortality is high. Correct antimicrobial therapy is essential. A parenteral aminoglycoside such as gentamicin in combination with one of the new beta-lactam drugs is a good initial choice while awaiting the results of sensitivities. Some septicemic patients may develop hepatic or splenic abscesses. Surgical drainage is desirable but may be impossible in the face of multiple lesions.

References

Brenner, D. J., Ursing, J., Bercovier, H., Steigerwalt, A. G., Fanning, R. G., Alonso, J. M., Mollaret, H. H.: Deoxyribonucleic acid relatedness in *Yersinia enterocolitica*. Curr Microbiol 4:195, 1980.

Carter, P. B., Zahorchak, R. J., Brubaker, R. R.: Plague virulence antigens from *Yersinia enterocolitica*. Infect Immun 28:638, 1980.

Goebel, K. M., Goebel, F. D., Baier, R.: Impaired cell mediated immunity among HLA-B27 related rheumatoid variants responding to yersinia antigen. J Clin Lab Immunol 8:75, 1982.

Granfors, K., Viljanen, M., Tiilikainen, A., Towanen, A.: Persistence of IgM, IgG, and IgA antibodies to *Yersinia* in yersinia arthritis. J Infect Dis. 141:424, 1980.

Leino, R., and Kalliomaki, J. L.: Yersiniosis as an internal disease. Ann Intern Med 81:458, 1974.

Leirisalo, M., Skylu, G., Kousa, M., Voipio-Pulkki, L. M., Suoranta, H., Nissila, M., Hvidman, L., Nielsen, E. D., Svejgaard, A., Tiilikainen, A., Laitinen, O.: Followup study on patients with Reiter's disease and reactive arthritis, with special reference to HLA-B27. Arthr Rheum 25:249, 1982.

Pai, C. H., DeStephano, L.: Serum resistance associated with virulence in *Yersinia enterocolitica*. Infect Immun 35:605, 1982.

Portnoy, D. A., Moseley, S. L., Falkow, S.: Characterization of plasmids and plasmid-associated determinants of *Yersinia enterocolitica* pathogenesis. Infect Immun 31:775, 1981.

Schiemann, D. A.: Development of a two-step enrichment procedure for recovery of *Yersinia enterocolitica* from food. Appl Environ Microbiol 43:14, 1982.

Schiemann, D. A., Devenish, J. A.: Relationship of HeLa cell infectivity to biochemical, serological, and virulence characteristics of *Yersinia enterocolitica*. Infect Immun 35:497, 1982.

Spira, T. J., and Kasins, S. A.: *Yersinia enterocolitica* septicemia with septic arthritis. Arch Intern Med 136:1305, 1976.

Vantrappen, G., Agg, H. O., Geboes, K., Ponette, E.: Yersinia enteritis. Med Clin N Amer 66:639, 1982.

137

AMEBIC DYSENTERY (INTESTINAL AMEBIASIS)

FRANCISCO BIAGI, M.D.

Amebic dysentery is a form of acute intestinal amebiasis characterized by a severe picture of tenesmus with passage of mucus and bloody stools; diarrhea (abundant liquid stools) usually accompanies the dysentery. Tenesmus is the sensation of urgent evacuation against resistance from spasm of the sphincter ani secondary to rectal ulcers. The evacuation is small and painful and leaves the feeling of a full rectum; in infants, tenesmus causes spasmodic bowel movements with mild rectal prolapse and is detected by inspection of the perineal region when the child cries.

Amebic dysentery is one of the clinical forms of amebiasis. If infections by *Naegleria* and *Acanthamoeba* are excluded, amebiasis is defined as infection by *Entamoeba histolytica*. According to epidemiologic, clinical, and autopsy observations, we may differentiate nine basic anatomoclinical types of amebiasis (Table 1). The term intestinal amebiasis comprises five different types.

ETIOLOGY. *E. histolytica* is a Sarcodina protozoan that moves and phagocytoses by pseudopods and reproduces as a trophozoite by binary fission. It has a nucleus with fine peripheral chromatin and a central endosome (Fig. 1). Within the intestinal lumen and under ill-defined conditions, it may become encysted and is excreted. The mature cysts have four nuclei.

In view of the limitations of most medical laboratories, the name *E. histolytica* is used here in the broad sense and includes *E. hartmanni*, small or large race, Laredo type, and other forms, which may be differentiated only through subtle features, such as isoenzyme patterns, by a few experts (Sargeaunt et al., 1978). *E. histolytica* can be differentiated from *Entamoeba coli, Iodamoeba bütschlii, Endolimax nana*, and *Dientamoeba fragilis* in any clinical laboratory (Biagi, 1976).

EPIDEMIOLOGY. The great majority of cases are caused by the ingestion of cysts and only rarely by direct implantation of trophozoites into the skin. The source of infection is the stool of human carriers. Since the cyst is killed by desiccation, fecal contamination must be recent in order for transmission to occur. The process of cyst transmission from carriers is called fecalism and involves dissemination of stools in the environment and transmission of cysts to the new host mainly by food handlers. Dissemination occurs by means of open air defecation, defective sewage disposal, irrigation with contaminated water, and filthy personal sanitation.

Once the cyst has arrived in the intestine, schizogony ends with hatching of eight trophozoites, and these establish a colony of trophozoites in the lumen of the bowel. This luminal colony disappears spontaneously in 50 per cent of cases within six months, but reinfections maintain the prevalence rate. The monthly incidence is about one twelfth of the prevalence rate. The larger number of clinical cases during the hot season suggests that the incidence of

Table 1. CLINICAL TYPES OF AMEBIASIS

<table>
<tr><th rowspan="2">Location of Parasite[a]</th><th rowspan="2">Clinical Type of Amebiasis</th><th rowspan="2" colspan="2">Forms of Amebiasis</th><th colspan="2">Diagnosis</th></tr>
<tr><th>PE[c]</th><th>Serology</th></tr>
<tr><td>Colonization of intestinal lumen</td><td>1. Carrier[b]</td><td rowspan="2">Intestinal</td><td>Luminal</td><td rowspan="2">+</td><td>—</td></tr>
<tr><td>Invasion of intestinal wall</td><td>2. Asymptomatic
3. Chronic intestinal
4. Acute intestinal
5. Ameboma</td><td rowspan="3">Invasive</td><td rowspan="3">+</td></tr>
<tr><td>Invasion of liver</td><td>6. Hepatitis
7. Liver abscess</td><td rowspan="2">Extraintestinal</td><td rowspan="2">—</td></tr>
<tr><td>Invasion of other organs and tissues</td><td>8. Cutaneous
9. Other locations</td></tr>
</table>

[a]A patient may present with disease in several locations at the same time.
[b]A patient of this type may later suffer an invasion of tissues by the parasite. Carriers can also result from satisfactory clinical treatment that does not include parasitologic cure, in which case serology might be positive for a period of time.
[c]PE, Parasitologic examination of feces.

infection may be variable throughout the year. Prevalence rates usually are between 0 and 10 per cent in temperate and developed areas of the world and 5 to 60 per cent in tropical developing areas. Within the same city, prevalence rates show big differences in diverse sociocultural groups. Generally speaking, prevalence is higher in communities with poor housing, inadequate excreta disposal, high population density, improper personal hygienic habits, and a tropical climate. The infection is seldom found during the first two weeks of life. Prevalence increases slowly throughout the first year, and then rapidly from the second to fourth year of age; thereafter it is sustained through adulthood with no sex difference. An infection does not generate protection against reinfections.

Serologic tests are the basis for estimating the frequency of invasive amebiasis. In the United States, positive serologic tests for amebiasis are found in 0.4 to 3.6 per cent of the population, so there may be approximately five million people with invasive amebiasis at a given time. In Mexico the average figure is 5 per cent. Amebiasis was the cause of death in 5 to 11 per cent of autopsies in different hospitals in Mexico City. In other Latin American countries, the figure ranges from 2 to 4 per cent. In the United States and Europe, only a few cases have been found at autopsy.

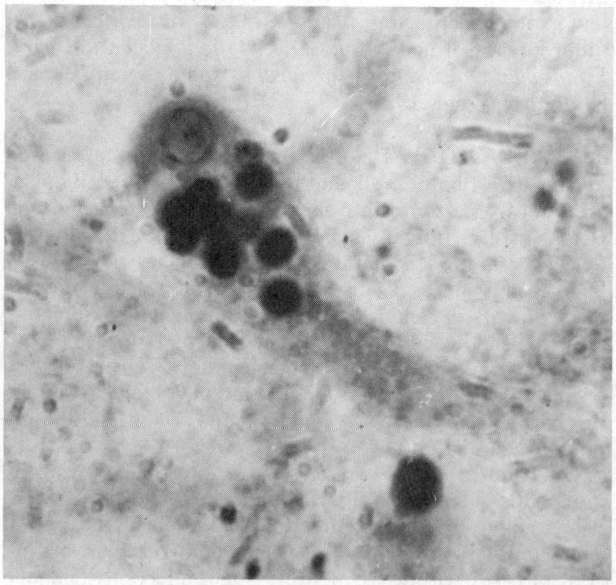

Figure 1. Trophozoite of *Entamoeba histolytica* in the feces; iron hematoxylin stain showing erythrocytes and the typical nucleolus.

PATHOGENESIS AND PATHOLOGY. The basic pathogenic mechanism is tissue lysis by *E. histolytica*. In the intestine and the skin, this lysis results in ulcers; in the liver, brain, and other organs it causes necrosis like that of abscesses.

After the infection has been established in the bowel lumen (luminal amebiasis), trophozoites sometimes invade the intestinal wall to the submucosa, where they produce necrosis and initiate invasive amebiasis (Biagi and Beltrán, 1969). First, a small ulcer opens into the lumen, forming a lesion known as a "bouton de chemise" because the large circular submucosal necrosis, with its small opening onto the surface, has the configuration of a button (Fig. 2). This early lesion quickly ulcerates the overlying mucosa and produces ulcers of variable form, size, and number (Fig. 3), ranging from a few tiny ulcers to ulceration of the whole colon. The size of the ulcers determines the severity and clinical type of intestinal amebiasis.

It is estimated in Mexico that of every 1000 persons with luminal amebiasis, 200 have invasion of the intestinal wall, and one develops liver abscess (Biagi, 1976; Brandt and Pérez-Tamayo, 1970). Each of these three stages is the result of multifactorial interactions. The establishment of *E. histolytica* in the gut lumen is favored by the presence of the normal intestinal flora, by ingestion of many cysts, and by a starch diet. Migration to the intestinal wall and the liver is promoted by cholesterol, steroid hormones, large numbers of trophozoites, and high virulence of the strain. Virulence or invasiveness is a function of isoenzyme patterns (Sargeaunt et al., 1978). Analysis of amebic phosphoglucomutase and hexokinase has shown that pathogenic strains of *E. histolytica* display characteristic mobility of isoenzymes that differentiate them from nonpathogenic

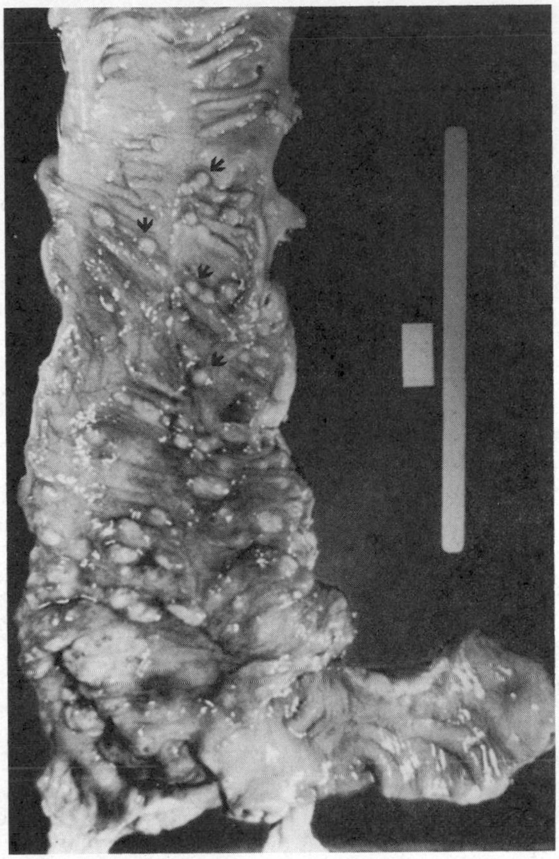

Figure 2. Small amebic ulcers (arrows) in "bouton de chemise" at the cecum.

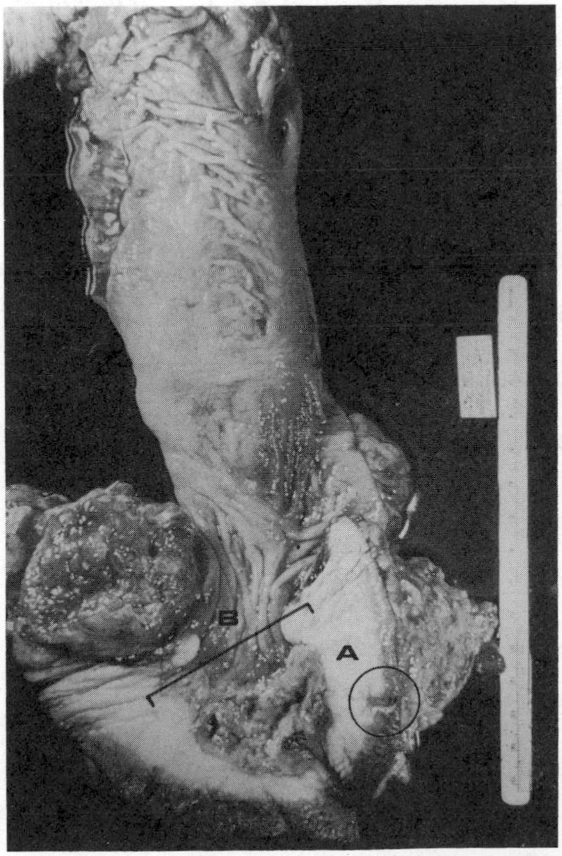

Figure 3. Larger amebic ulcer at the rectum *(B)* with a small cutaneus lesion *(A)* by fistula formation.

strains. These invasive strains are also characterized by resistance to complement-mediated lysis (Reed et al., 1983). According to experimental evidence, previous infections may also favor invasion because the trophozoites can digest antiameba immunoglobulin attached to their surface and thus use them for nutrition.

Another pathologic feature is the very mild or absent inflammatory reaction. It appears that chemotaxis is absent, and leukocytes making chance contact with *E. histolytica* are immediately lysed.

Intestinal amebiasis is more severe in infants than in adults. Intestinal amebiasis progresses faster in infants and preschool children, and intestinal perforation is the most common cause of death. The most common cause of death from amebiasis in adults is amebic liver abscess; 90 per cent of the cases are found in men and 10 per cent in women. There is an equal sex distribution of liver abscess in children, and 90 per cent of the cases have concurrent, usually severe, intestinal involvement. Among adults with liver abscess, only 30 per cent have intestinal involvement, and it is usually mild.

Geographic areas also show differences. Areas with a low transmission rate have few reinfections, low prevalence, few clinical cases, and very infrequent fatalities. In areas with high prevalence, by contrast, reinfections are frequent, clinical amebiasis is abundant, and large numbers of fatal cases are seen at autopsy.

CLINICAL MANIFESTATIONS AND DIAGNOSIS. The clinical picture of intestinal amebiasis is related to the size of the ulcers. The incubation period is not well known; it appears to be as short as two days in the newborn and may be as long as a few months. The prepatent period is equal to or shorter than the incubation period. Five clinical forms of intestinal amebiasis are recognized, as indicated in Table 2.

The amebiasis carrier state has neither symptoms nor antibody response because it is only a luminal infection. It accounts for 80 per cent of the cases and is the most common type of infection. Diagnosis can be made by positive fecal examinations with negative serology. It is the least dangerous clinical form because chemotherapy is very effective, and the prognosis is best.

Asymptomatic amebiasis, in contrast to the previous type, is characterized by tissue invasion and antibody formation. Small ulcers are found in the bowel at autopsy or rectosigmoidoscopy in persons with no intestinal complaints. This group has invasive amebiasis; even though clinically silent, it is the initial stage for severe illness like dysentery or liver abscess. In fact, two thirds of adults with amebic liver abscess do not recall intestinal complaints. The diagnosis is established by a positive fecal examination along with positive serology in an asymptomatic patient. This stage requires chemotherapy.

Chronic intestinal amebiasis includes a variety of clinical pictures secondary to intestinal ulcers causing mild symptoms that the patient tends to ignore. There are periods of remission and recrudescence. These patients very often medicate themselves so that parasitologic cure is seldom achieved.

The most common symptoms are meteorism; abdominal pain, often stimulated by eating; changes in bowel schedule and alternating periods of constipation and diarrhea; change in the stool consistency from formed at the beginning to liquid at the end of the same evacuation; fresh blood in the stools, varying from small strings to abundant hemorrhage; pyrosis; and headache, somnolence, and asthenia that are prominent enough to bring the patient to the physician. The illness may resemble bacterial enteric infections, intestinal tuberculosis, giardiasis, trichuriasis, hookworm disease, strongyloidiasis, ulcerative colitis, rectal abscess, regional enteritis, malignant tumors of the bowel, polyposis, diverticulosis, and megacolon. The precise diagnosis is very important because therapy and prognosis are different.

After a good clinical history, rectosigmoidoscopy is desirable, but the absence of ulcerations does not exclude the diagnosis because lesions may be present only in the cecum. When ulcers are found, they should be sampled at the edge for parasites. Rectoscopy alone is helpful and can be done with a simple plastic tube 2 × 15 cm attached to an otoscope if better equipment is not available.

If cysts are sought by a concentration method on three consecutive daily samples of formed stool, they are found in 85 per cent of the cases. Six examinations give 95 per cent accuracy. Diarrhea stools require direct microscopic examination while fresh if trophozoites are to be found. Serologic tests, such as indirect hemagglutination and

Table 2. DRUGS OF CHOICE IN AMEBIASIS

		Drugs and Amebicidal Concentration (μg/ml)					
Location of Parasites[a]	**Clinical Types of Amebiasis**	***Oxyquinolines (8)***	***Arsenicals (8)***	***Emetine (3)***	***Chloroquine (300)***	***Imidazole (3)***	***Dichloroacetamides (0.04–0.6)***
Intestinal lumen	1. Carrier	×	×				×
Intestinal wall	2. Asymptomatic	×	×				×
	3. Chronic intestinal	×	×			×	×
	4. Acute intestinal			×		×	×
	5. Ameboma			×		×	×
Liver	6. Amebic hepatitis			×	×	×	
	7. Amebic liver abscess			×	×	×	
Others	8. Cutaneous			×		×	
	9. Other locations			×		×	

[a]A patient may have infection in several locations.

immunodiffusion, are positive in approximately 98 per cent of the cases and at moderate titers (1:32 to 1:2048) (Healy and Kraft, 1972).

A carrier may have positive stool examinations for amebae when intestinal complaints have another cause. In order to establish the diagnosis of intestinal amebiasis, it is necessary to demonstrate ulcers in the bowel, *E. histolytica* in stools (cysts or trophozoites), and positive serologic tests with *E. histolytica* antigen (Healy and Kraft, 1972). If these studies are not available or reliable, a working diagnosis of chronic intestinal amebiasis may be made with less stringent criteria and a therapeutic trial with antiamebic drugs carried out, especially in patients living in or having traveled through areas where amebiasis is common and severe.

Acute intestinal amebiasis may take the form of amebic dysentery, episodes of bloody diarrhea, or so-called fulminant amebiasis. It may also be only a severe case of diarrhea with no blood or tenesmus. In all cases, the patient is severely ill and often needs hospitalization. Large ulcerated areas are found in the bowel, mainly at the cecum and rectosigmoid; in a few cases, ulcers are also found in the appendix or the terminal ileum.

Abdominal pain is prominent, and evacuations are multiple and usually scanty with mucus and blood. Tenesmus characterizes the dysentery syndrome. Water and electrolyte balance may be abnormal, especially in children, and fever is present in one third of the cases. The general status of the patient may undergo marked deterioration, and toxemia may be present. Signs of an acute abdomen may appear, due either to severe lesions in the wall of the colon or to intestinal perforation. Among children living in endemic areas, *E. histolytica* may be found in the stool in 5 per cent of cases with acute simple diarrhea, one third of cases with bloody diarrhea, and most of those with dysenteric syndrome. In children, severe cases may develop without previous intestinal complaints while in adults there are usually several recrudescences.

Rectosigmoidoscopy is hazardous in severe cases because the colon may be very fragile. Fresh blood on the stools suggests bowel ulcers. Flat x-ray of the abdomen is done to detect evidence of peritonitis. If there is hepatomegaly, which is found in nearly 40 per cent of children with acute intestinal amebiasis, a liver scan, ultrasound examination, or CAT scan should be done to look for liver abscesses.

Examinations of freshly passed stool demonstrate trophozoites, often with phagocytosed erythrocytes, in 90 per cent of the cases on the first examination; if a second stool sample is taken from the next evacuation, the diagnosis can be confirmed in almost all cases. Microscopic stool examinations should be performed before any specific therapy, because the first dose of an antiamebic drug or even an antibiotic may turn them negative, even though the parasite is still present and causing disease. Diagnosis is established after the finding of parasites in a patient with the clinical picture described above. If a reliable parasitologic examination is not available, or some therapy has been started and the patient is living in, or has traveled through, an area where amebiasis is common and severe, it is wise to complete full therapy because acute intestinal amebiasis is life-threatening. In contrast to bacterial or viral diarrheas in children in whom correction of fluid and electrolyte disturbances is usually sufficient therapy, amebiasis might go on to perforation with such treatment unless specific antiamebic therapy is given also.

Serologic tests are usually positive in adults with acute intestinal amebiasis but take more time to perform than fresh stool examination. In infants, the picture progresses so rapidly that one third do not have time to develop positive serology before hospitalization.

Acute intestinal amebiasis can resemble enteric bacterial or viral infections, balantidiasis, trichuriasis, rectal stenosis with ulcerations, malignant tumors of the bowel, and ulcerative colitis. A culture for enteric bacteria should always be performed, since differentiation on clinical grounds is not reliable. Fever, hepatomegaly, tenesmus, meteorism, or blood in the stools may be present in both parasitic and bacterial diarrhea. A few patients have a double etiology.

Ameboma, an uncommon inflammatory pseudotumor of the bowel wall, produces chronic changes in intestinal habits, bloody stools, meteorism, and abdominal pain. An abdominal mass is palpated and demonstrated by barium enema. It is rare in adults and almost never seen in children.

The finding of the parasite on fecal examination and a positive serology may confirm the diagnosis of ameboma but does not exclude neoplasm; diagnostic error in both directions has been confirmed at autopsy. The treatment consists of partial colectomy and antiamebic drugs.

COMPLICATIONS. The complications of intestinal amebiasis result from extension into surrounding organs and are life-threatening. If peritoneal and retroperitoneal extension occurs, bacterial infection becomes the most important problem. Fistula formation to the female genitalia usually involves invasion by the parasite. Cutaneous amebiasis is discussed in Chapter 233. Hepatic amebiasis is not considered to be a complication because spread to the liver is part of the natural history of the infection along the regular pathway of migration. Liver abscess is discussed in Chapter 138.

TREATMENT. The dichloroacetamides and oxyquinolines, which act only within the lumen of the bowel because their absorption is poor, are useful in treating intestinal amebiasis (Welling and Monro, 1970). The imidazoles, emetines, and chloroquines can act systemically against invasive amebiasis because they can be given parenterally or are fully absorbed from the small intestine. No drug can act against *E. histolytica* in all sites; some patients have luminal amebiasis only or tissue invasion alone, but others have parasites in the tissues and the lumen. Table 2 is presented as a guide to help select the type of drug for an individual case. The objective is to achieve both clinical and parasitologic cure. Sometimes a patient with intestinal amebiasis may only achieve clinical cure after imidazole or emetine therapy and may require dichloroacetamides or oxyquinolines for parasitologic cure.

The imidazoles are important because they are active in patients with chronic intestinal amebiasis and amebic liver abscess. Metronidazole was the first in use; tinidazole, ornidazole, and nimorazole are better tolerated and have longer half-lives. All can produce pyrosis, nausea, and vomiting; all have antabuse effect; and all are potentially mutagenic, but no cases of neoplasm have been attributed to them after more than 15 years of very extensive clinical use, perhaps due to the short courses of treatment. Although there is no evidence of teratogeny, use in the first trimester of pregnancy is not recommended. They cause a problem in nursing mothers because they pass into the milk and produce anorexia in the infant. In spite of these limitations, they are widely used and effective. Their dosage is 20 to 40 mg/kg body weight per day for 5 to 15 days (usually 10). Tinidazole may be used in adults at single doses of 2 g after dinner for 1 to 4 consecutive days.

Emetines are cardiotoxic on overdosage, but with careful administration are safe to use; their injection is painful. The dosage is 1 mg/kg body weight (not more than 60 mg) per day for 10 days.

Dichloroacetamides are very active and are almost nonabsorbed. Meteorism and loose stools are the most important side effects. Etichlordifene is ten times more active than teclozan. Dosage is 20 mg/kg body weight (up to one g) per day for 5 days.

Oxyquinolines have been in use for many years. In patients under very prolonged therapy, a few cases of optic neuritis have been described; mutagenic activity has also been found. Dosage is 30 mg/kg body weight for 10 to 20 days.

Acute intestinal amebiasis demands bed rest and proper control of fluids and electrolytes. Partial colectomy is sometimes necessary when the intestinal wall is extensively damaged or perforation has occurred; these cases have a high mortality. Diet should be bland during the first days; afterwards, vegetables should be introduced to regulate the bowel. In endemic areas in which patients have reinfections, the repeated episodes of amebiasis may leave in their wake a prolonged irregularity of bowel movements.

With proper treatment tenesmus should disappear and diarrhea should improve in 48 hours. The physician should be familiar with drug side effects in order to differentiate them from a persistence of the disease. About one week after treatment, all symptoms should have disappeared. Rectosigmoidoscopy shows improvement of ulcers on the third day and the healing of most of them by the seventh day of treatment. In all cases, three examinations for amebae should be done by a concentration method two weeks after treatment to assess parasitologic cure. Quantitative serology two months later is also useful to demonstrate a drop in titer; tests become negative in 2 to 24 months, depending on the initial titer. Thus, serology is not always diagnostic because a positive test may also represent a past infection.

PROPHYLAXIS. Good standards of urbanization, housing, personal hygiene, and food handling have no substitute; these require a good level of economic productivity and may be the result of individual attitudes and a positive community structure. In endemic areas, patients should be instructed to avoid food handled after cooking or uncooked food, such as fruit cocktails, hard-boiled eggs, and salads. Unfortunately, the most popular and tasty food in endemic areas is handled extensively. It is important to do fecal examinations and serologic tests as soon as intestinal complaints start, or every year in endemic areas.

Chemotherapy for control or prophylaxis has been documented as useful, even in open communities, on the basis of repeated mass therapy. It is effective, less expensive, and less dangerous than amebiasis; for this purpose, the best choice is the dichloracetamides because they act in the lumen of the intestine and are effective against diverse types of intestinal amebiasis, including the carrier state.

References

Biagi, F.: Enfermedades Parasitarias. 2nd ed. Prensa Med Mex, 1976.

Biagi, F., and Beltrán, F.: The challenge of amoebiasis: Understanding pathogenic mechanisms. Int Rev Trop Med 3:219, 1969.

Brandt, H., and Pérez-Tamayo, R.: Amebiasis. Prensa Med Mex, 1970.

Healy, G. R., and Kraft, S. C.: The indirect hemagglutination test for amebiasis in patients with inflammatory bowel disease. Am J Digest Dis 17:97, 1972.

Reed, S. L., Sargeaunt, P. G., and Braude, A. I.: Resistance to lysis by human serum of pathogenic *Entamoeba histolytica*. Trans Roy Soc Trop Med Hyg 77:248, 1983.

Sargeaunt, P. G., Williams, J. E., and Grene, J. D.: The differentiation of invasive and noninvasive *Entamoeba histolytica* by isoenzyme electrophoresis. Trans Roy Soc Trop Med Hyg 72:519, 1978.

Welling, P. G., and Monro, A. M.: The Pharmacological Basis of Therapeutics. 4th ed. New York, Macmillan Publishing Company, 1970, p. 1151.

138

AMEBIC LIVER ABSCESS

DAVID A. KATZENSTEIN, M.D.

Invasion of the hepatic parenchyma by trophozoites of *Entameba histolytica* results in focal necrosis and liquefaction of liver tissue. Formation of amebic liver abscess (ALA) causes a systemic illness characterized by fever, anorexia, and point tenderness over the liver. ALA is distinguished from pyogenic liver abscess by the absence of purulence and bacteria and the presence of trophozoites of *E. histolytica* at the margin of the lesion. In lieu of invasive procedures the diagnosis depends upon serologic evidence of invasive amebiasis, demonstration of cystic lesions in the liver by hepatic imaging, and response to specific amebicidal therapy.

ETIOLOGY. *E. histolytica* is a dimorphic protozoan parasite of man endemic to most tropical and subtropical regions. Fecal contamination of water used for drinking and food preparation disseminates the cyst form of *E. histolytica*. Ingestion of cysts is followed by multiplication of motile trophozoites in the large intestine. Amebas may colonize the bowel without disease (asymptomatic cyst passage) or cause local and extraintestinal disease, amebic dysentery, and liver abscess, respectively. Only a small percentage of patients excreting amebas will manifest disease and ALA often occurs without preceding evidence of dysentery.

The occurrence of dysentery or liver abscess in some cases of infection, as opposed to a greater number of patients with asymptomatic carriage, has not yet been explained. Early investigators proposed that variation in the outcome of infection by amebas might be explained by the existence of two morphologically identical species, one pathogenic, the other commensal. This hypothesis was confirmed in some animal models of invasive amebiasis in which the intracecal injection of cysts from cases of human disease produced cecal ulceration in rats while cysts from asymptomatic patients failed to cause disease in animals (Neal and Vincent, 1955). Recently, Sargeaunt and Williams have identified distinct patterns of certain isoenzymes (zymodemes) that distinguish pathogenic and nonpathogenic isolates of *E. histolytica* (Sargeaunt and Williams, 1979). On the basis of isoenzyme electrophoresis these workers could differentiate strains causing disease from those that result in asymptomatic cyst passage in patients from India, Mexico, South Africa, and Great Britain. Thus, it is likely that only certain strains of *E. histolytica*, which may be identified by zymodeme, are the etiologic agents of ALA.

PATHOLOGY AND PATHOGENESIS. Amebic abscess formation is a focal necrotic process in which trophozoites in the liver form discrete cysts by centrifugal destruction of liver tissue. In the hepatic parenchyma surrounding the abscess there is little inflammatory response or damage to cells beyond the perimeter of the lesion. One lesion in the right lobe of the liver is present in most cases, although the left lobe is affected in about a quarter of patients. Abscess cavities reach a volume over 2 liters. The abscess fluid is characteristically acellular, odorless, and may be straw colored, dark green, or brown. Usually bile or blood leaks into the lesion resulting in the characteristic "anchovy paste" or "chocolate sauce" appearance. Leukocytes and trophozoites are rarely seen in aspirated fluid and amebas are found only at the margin of the lesion in the thin rim of necrotic tissue that lies between the abscess cavity and healthy liver tissue.

Liver abscess is relatively unusual among the 10 to 50 per cent of individuals residing in an endemic area who are colonized by amebas. Invasive disease due to amebas, dysentery, and ALA occurs in less than 10 per cent of those with evidence of intraluminal gut infection. ALA may occur as a complication of overt amebic colitis, but, more commonly, hepatic amebiasis occurs without a history of dysentery. Cysts or trophozoites of *E. histolytica* are found in the stool of less than a quarter of patients who present ALA.

Two cytotoxic mechanisms have been described that may explain the ability of *E. histolytica* to penetrate host defenses. On their surface, amebas have a carbohydrate-binding glycoprotein (lectin), which causes the reversible rounding and detachment of tissue culture cells (Lushbaugh et al., 1979). In addition, a contact-dependent lysis of mammalian cells, mediated by functioning microfilaments in the ameba, takes place through direct interaction between the cells and the pseudopods of trophozoites (Ravdin et al., 1980). Pathogenicity in animal models of colonic and hepatic amebiasis has been found to correlate with some of these in vitro cytotopathogenic effects. In addition, trophozoites of *E. histolytica* overcome the first line of defense by rapid lysis of human polymorphonuclear leukocytes (Jarumilinta, 1964).

Humoral immunity, antibody, and complement may play a role in determining the outcome of amebic infection. Young patients who show a brisk, primary antibody response to the infection develop the acute form of ALA with rapid enlargement of the liver lesions and a systemic illness. In contrast, older patients develop an insidious chronic illness in which the rate of growth of the abscess is slow and serum antibody titers are stable. This suggests a role for preexisting antibody in limiting the rate of growth of ALA, although the occurrence of ALA in patients previously treated for amebiasis shows that antibody is unlikely to be protective. In vitro, immunoglobulin has little effect on amebas that "cap" and ingest serum antibodies without apparent damage to the protozoa. With respect to the role of complement, axenic amebas are lysed by normal human serum by activation of the alternative pathway (Ortiz-Ortiz, 1978). Recently, Reed, Sargeaunt and Braude have demonstrated that pathogenic strains of amebas survive in human serum whereas nonpathogenic strains are rapidly killed on exposure to human serum with intact complement. This resistance of specific strains of *E. histolytica* to complement-mediated lysis explains their capacity to survive in portal blood and thus cause liver disease.

Nutrition and sex influence susceptibility to ALA. The disease is almost 10-fold more frequent in men than women. This striking sexual difference remains unexplained; however, in animal models of amebiasis both iron and cholesterol appear to increase the virulence of axenic laboratory strains. The discovery that strains of *E. histolytica* that cause human disease have distinct isoenzyme patterns supports the concept that certain strains of amebas are intrinsically pathogenic.

CLINICAL MANIFESTATIONS. ALA is nearly 10 times more common in men than women and occurs predominantly in young adulthood and middle age. There is always a history of travel or residence in an endemic area, but, a history of diarrhea or dysenteric illness is elicited in less than a third of patients. Two divergent clinical presentations, acute and chronic ALA, have been recognized in patients with hepatic amebiasis (Klatskin, 1945, Lamont and Pooler, 1957). Patients with the acute form of ALA present shortly after the abrupt onset of a toxic illness manifest as high fever with rigors and abdominal pain. In contrast, chronic disease is characterized by the insidious onset of low grade fevers, weight loss, and anemia. In both types of ALA, life threatening complications, the rupture of an abscess into the peritoneal cavity, pleural space, or the pericardium, may be the event that signals the need for medical attention. The clinical presentation of acute and chronic ALA is distinct enough to merit separate consideration.

Acute ALA. In younger individuals ALA usually presents as an acute febrile illness accompanied by abdominal complaints ranging from mild right upper quadrant discomfort to general, severe, abdominal pain. Patients frequently complain of anorexia and nausea, but vomiting is unusual. The temperature is usually greater than 102° F accompanied by rigors, tachycardia, and diaphoresis. Although point tenderness over the liver is usual, the hepatic span is normal in two-thirds of patients with acute ALA. Thus, tenderness may only be elicited by palpation of the liver through the intercostal spaces. Findings on abdominal examination range from slight discomfort over the liver to a "surgical abdomen" with signs of peritoneal irritation including guarding, rebound tenderness, and absent bowel sounds. Depending on the location of the abscess, pain may be referred to the right or left shoulder, or the anterior chest. Involvement of the dome of the liver may result in sufficient diaphragmatic irritation to provoke cough or hiccough and pleural effusion is found in one-third of patients. The right diaphragm is often elevated and splinting results in atelectasis with rales particularly at the right base of the thorax.

Chronic ALA. Older patients are more likely to present

with several months of fever, sweats, and weight loss. Abdominal pain is less prominent in chronic ALA, whereas symptoms of malaise and fatigue due to anemia are more common. In contrast to acute ALA, the temperature is usually less than 100° F and a third of patients have only slight fever. Palpation of the liver will reveal an area of point tenderness in most patients and the liver is enlarged in all cases. Due to the increase in liver size, elevation of the right hemidiaphragm, pleural effusion, and right sided chest findings of rales and rhonchi are more prominent in patients with chronic ALA.

DIAGNOSIS. In endemic areas amebic liver abscess is frequently a cause of hepatic tenderness and enlargement. Physicians in these areas readily recognize patients with ALA and often the diagnosis is made by palpating the liver, locating a point of maximal tenderness, and aspirating the abscess. As world travel increases and amebiasis becomes less common in temperate regions, recognition of the laboratory findings of ALA become more important. The diagnosis of ALA in the context of the modern hospital can be confirmed by a positive serologic test for invasive disease due to *E. histolytica* and a liver imaging study that shows intrahepatic cystic lesions.

The most consistent laboratory abnormality in ALA is an elevated alkaline phosphatase, which may be detected in 90 per cent of patients with ALA. In some cases of acute disease the alkaline phosphatase is initially within the normal range, although an elevated value is often obtained after several days. Serum glutamic oxaloacetate transaminase (SGOT) is elevated in half of the patients with acute ALA. From studies in San Diego, it appears that an elevated SGOT (greater than 40 I.U) differentiates those patients with aggressive as opposed to a more benign form of ALA (Katzenstein, Rickerson, and Braude, 1982). Hyperbilirubinemia may occur in a few patients with aggressive disease, but jaundice (serum bilirubin greater than 3 mg/dl) is an ominous sign that often indicates the presence of superinfection or rupture.

Patients with acute ALA have leukocytosis (>10,000 white cells/cu mm) with a predominance of polymorphonuclear leukocytes and band forms. Dohle bodies and toxic granulations are frequently recognized on the peripheral smear. In chronic ALA the white count is less likely to be elevated; half of the patients will demonstrate fewer than 10,000 white cells/cu mm. The hemoglobin and hematocrit are normal or minimally depressed in patients with acute ALA whereas in chronic disease anemia is almost universal. The urine analysis is frequently abnormal in acute ALA, with proteinuria in half of the cases and red cells, white cells, and cellular casts in the urine in a few. Blood urea nitrogen and creatine are normal unless there is dehydration or a complication that results in shock.

Standard radiographic studies of the chest and abdomen may provide evidence of ALA. Chest x-ray often shows an elevated right hemidiaphragm, atelaectasis in the right lower lobe, and a pleural effusion. In some cases the chest x-ray showing a large pleural effusion may suggest pneumonia, tuberculosis, or metastases to the pleura. In chronic ALA the liver will usually be enlarged and this is appreciated on abdominal x-rays. Air fluid levels in the liver are not seen with uncomplicated ALA and suggest bacterial superinfection or pyogenic abscess.

Serologic tests that measure specific antibody directed against amebas are a key part of the laboratory evaluation for ALA. A wide range of test procedures are available including complement fixation (CF), immunohemagglutination (IHA), latex agglutination, agar gel diffusion (AGD), and counterimmune electrophoresis (CIE). All of these have a sensitivity that exceeds 90 per cent in cases of ALA, but their specificities vary. In the AGD test, a precipitin line between patient's sera and an antigen prepared from whole trophozoites is observed in up to 96 per cent of cases of ALA while false-positive tests are rare (Maddison, 1965). This contrasts with CF and indirect hemagglutination tests, which may be positive in asymptomatic cyst passers, persons who have resided in an endemic area, or in patients with a history of treated amebiasis (Kessel et al., 1965). False-negative serologic tests in ALA are seen in patients with acute disease and repeat testing yields a positive result within 7 days. When the AGD test is titered, patients with acute amebic liver abscess have positive tests only at relatively low dilutions of sera (less than 1:32 dilution). Patients with chronic ALA will always have a positive AGD test for amebiasis, with a titer usually over 1:64. CIE using the same antigen as the AGD may be slightly more sensitive in acute ALA and provide a more rapid result.

Hepatic imaging techniques, technetium sulfur colloid liver scans, ultrasound, and computed axial tomography are sensitive, noninvasive methods to detect ALA. Combined with serologic tests, hepatic imaging can substantiate or disprove the diagnosis. With ultrasound, amebic abscess is seen as an anechoic, fluid-filled cyst within the hepatic parenchyma (Monroe, 1971). Some internal echos may be observed within the cyst, but these will be less sharp and complex than in echinococcal cyst. Technetium liver scans show a focal area in the liver in which there is markedly diminished uptake of isotope, a "cold" spot. Ultrasound examination of patients with very early acute disease occasionally fails to demonstrate an abscess on initial examination and subsequent tests repeated after 3 to 7 days will demonstrate an abscess cavity. In some cases the liver scan will show a "cold" area, consistent with a liver abscess when ultrasound fails to detect the early abscess. Both techniques define the location and multiplicity of abscesses and are a sensitive means of detection. In a few cases gallium scans have demonstrated increased accumulation of isotope at the site of an abscess. Patients with acute ALA are more likely to have multiple small abscesses, (Fig. 1) whereas those with chronic disease more often have one large abscess of the right lobe.

COMPLICATIONS AND SEQUELAE. Amebic abscesses may rupture through the abdominal wall or into the peritoneum, pericardium, transverse colon, or the pleura (Adams and MacLeod, 1977). The dome of the liver is commonly involved by ALA and rupture of an abscess into the right pleural space is frequently observed. This results in a "pulmonary presentation" with pleural effusion, empyema, and drainage of the abscess into a bronchus. Rarely, hematogenous spread of amebas to the lung may result in focal, necrotizing lung abscesses. Rupture of the abscess into the peritoneum causes amebic peritonitis. Trophozoites invade the bowel causing multiple perforations and fistulae. Drainage into the pericardium results in pericarditis and may cause death due to rapid cardiac tamponade or constrictive pericarditis despite treatment. Patients with extrahepatic rupture of an ALA are more likely to demonstrate jaundice, an elevated SGOT, and signs of peritoneal

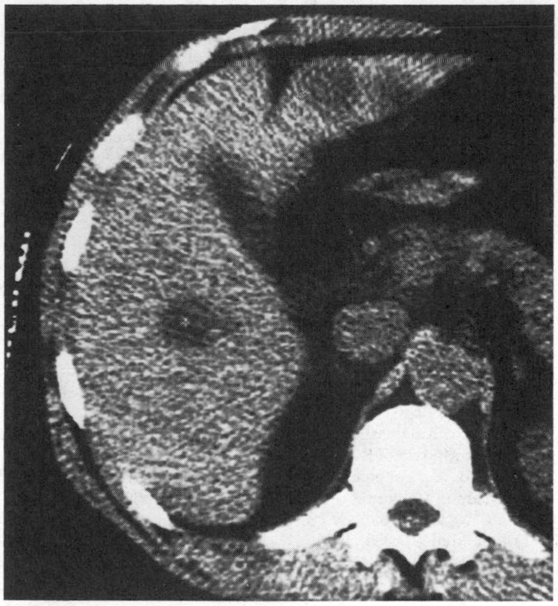

Figure 1. CT scan of the liver of a patient with multiple liver abscesses. (UCSD # 1014948; courtesy Radiology Department, University of California at San Diego Medical Center.)

irritation. In rare instances ALA may drain through the skin of the abdominal wall resulting in cutaneous amebiasis. This is more often a complication of surgery for an unsuspected ameboma.

The incidence of bacterial superinfection of ALA varies widely among series of patients (Crane et al., 1972; Knauer, 1969). Multiple percutaneous aspirations or surgical treatment appears to increase the risk of bacterial infection, although spontaneous superinfection may occur in 5 to 10 per cent of patients presenting with ALA (DeBakey and Oschsner, 1951). The bacteria most often cultured from amebic abscesses are *S. aureus, K. pneumonia, E. coli, Proteus sp.*, salmonellae and streptococci. In some cases, purulent foul smelling material has been obtained at aspiration, suggesting that anaerobic bacteria were the cause of secondary infection. Bacterial infection is suspected when blood cultures are positive, jaundice is present, or the patient fails to respond promptly to therapy for ALA. Aspiration of the liver abscess under these circumstances is vital to exclude superinfection or identify the bacteria involved. Treatment of superinfection requires drainage and parenteral antibiotics.

Treatment of uncomplicated ALA generally results in the rapid resolution of symptoms without long term sequelae. Despite the remission of pain and fever, an elevated alkaline phosphatase may persist for several months. Serial ultrasound studies will continue to demonstrate cystic lesions decreasing in size over six months to a year. Similarly, the titer of antibody as measured by AGD or CF will decline in the months after treatment. Liver abscess or amebic dysentery may recur after treatment of ALA.

TREATMENT. ALA can be cured without drainage by the administration of metronidazole, emetine, or chloroquine. Metronidazole is the safest and most effective therapy, and is given orally in a dose of 750 mg three times a day for 5 days. Several authors have successfully treated ALA with a single dose of 2.4 g of metronidazole (Powell et al., 1969), ornidazole, or tinidazole (Lasserre et al., 1983). Some patients, after surgery or intra-abdominal rupture may not absorb oral medications and require parenteral therapy. Emetine hydrochloride has been the most widely used parenteral agent in amebiasis, but dehydroemetine (available in the United States only as an investigational drug) appears to be effective and causes less cardiac and neurological toxicity. Dehydroemetine hydrochloride 65 mg/day or chloroquine 200 mg/day may be given as an intramuscular injection until oral metronidazole can be tolerated. Although there is little experience with parenteral metronidazole in ALA, the intravenous preparation now available is likely to be effective.

In most cases the response to metronidazole is dramatic, and aspiration of the abscess should not be considered unless patients do not respond after three days of metronidazole therapy. In these unresponsive patients, aspiration is indicated to exclude bacterial superinfection and to confirm the diagnosis of ALA. There have been rare cases of ALA in which metronidazole has failed to diminish symptoms and an increase in the size of the abscess has been noted during therapy. It is not clear whether these cases represent intrinsic resistance of *E. histolytica* to the drug or failure to absorb oral metronidazole. Patients who do not improve on metronidazole should be treated with a regimen combining chloroquine 250 mg twice daily for 2 weeks and dehydroemetine 65 mg/day for 10 days.

Rupture of the abscess into an adjacent structure does not require alteration of the chemotherapy of ALA. In amebic pericardial tamponade, aspiration of the material must be performed immediately. Pericardiectomy or a pericardial window may prevent the late sequelae of constrictive pericarditis. Although pleural effusion is common in ALA, chest tube drainage is not necessary unless bacterial superinfection has occurred. In patients with intra-abdominal rupture, ALA is often identified at laparotomy. In some cases there may be an associated perforation of the colon due to intestinal amebiasis. If there has not been perforation of the bowel with peritoneal soilage, the prognosis with amebicidal therapy is good. In patients with superinfection of the liver abscess, pleural effusion, or peritoneum, parenteral antibiotics and surgical drainage and debridement are vital additions to amebicidal therapy.

References

Adams, E. B. and MacLeod, I. N.: Invasive amebiasis II. Amebic liver abscess and its complications. Medicine 56:325, 1977.

Crane, P. S., Young, T. L., and Seel, D. J.: Experience in the treatment of two hundred patients with amebic abscess of the liver in Korea. Am J Surg 123:332, 1972.

DeBakey, M. E., and Oschner, A.: Hepatic amebiasis, a 20 year experience and analysis of 263 cases. Int Abstr Surg 92:209, 1951.

Jarumilinta, R. and Kradolfer, F.: The toxic effects of *E. histolytica* on leukocytes. Ann Trop Med Parasit 58:375, 1964.

Katzenstein, D. A., Rickerson, V. and Braude, A. I.: New Concepts of amebic liver abscess derived from hepatic imaging, serodiagnosis, and hepatic enzymes in 67 consecutive cases in San Diego. Medicine 61:237, 1982.

Kessel, J. F., Lewis, W. P., Pasquel, C. M., and Turner, J. A.: Indirect hemagglutination and complement fixation tests in amebiasis. Am J Trop Med Hyg 14:540, 1965.

Klatskin, G.: Amebiasis of the liver: classification, diagnosis and treatment. Ann Int Med 25:601, 1946.

Knauer, M. C.: Amebic abscess of the liver. Experience with 15 cases in 3½ years in California. Am J Dig Dis 14:253, 1969.

Lamont, N. and Pooler, N. R.: Hepatic Amoebiasis. A study of 250 cases. Q Jour Med 107:389, 1958.

Lasserre, R., Jaroonvesama, N., Kurathong, S., and Soh, C.-T.: Single-day drug treatment of amebic liver abscess. Am J Trop Med Hyg 32:732, 1983.

Lushbaugh, W. B., Kairalla, A. B., Cantey, J. R., Hofbauer, A. F., and Pittman, F. E.: Isolation of a cytotoxin-enterotoxin from *Entameba histolytica*. J Infect Dis 139:9, 1979.

Maddison, S. E.: Characterization of *Entameba histolytica* antigen-antibody reaction by gel diffusion. Exp Parisitol 16:224, 1965.

Monroe, L. S., Leopold, G. R., Brown, J. W., and Smith, J. L.: The ultrasonic scan in the management of amebic hepatic abscess. Dig Dis 16:523, 1971.

Neal, R. A. and Vincent, P.: Strain variation in *Entameoba histolytica* I. Correlation of invasiveness in rats with the clinical history and treatment of the experimental infections. Parasitol 45:152, 1953.

Ortiz-Ortiz, L., Capin, N. R., Sepulveda, B., and Zamacara, G.: Activation of the alternative pathway of complement by *E. histolytica*. Clin Exp Immunol 34:10, 1978.

Powell, S. J., Wilmot, A. J., and Elsdon-Dew, R.: Further trials of metronidazole in ameobic dysentery and amoebic liver abscess. Ann Trop Med Parasitol 63:139, 1969.

Ravdin, J. I., Croft, B. Y., and Guerrant, R. L.: Cytopathogenic mechanisms of *Entamoeba histolytica*. J Exp Med 152:377, 1980.

Reed, S. L., Sargeaunt, P. G., and Braude, A. I.: Resistance to lysis by humans serum of pathogenic *Entameoba histolytica*. Trans Roy Soc Trop Med Hyg 77:248, 1983.

Sargeaunt, P. G., Williams, J. E., and Grene, J. D.: The differentiation of invasive and non-invasive *Entamoeba histolytica* by isoenzyme electrophoresis. Trans Roy Soc Trop Med Hyg 72:519, 1978.

139

GIARDIASIS

LIISA JOKIPII, M.D.,
ANSSI M. M. JOKIPII, M.D.

Giardia lamblia in the upper small intestine causes either asymptomatic or symptomatic giardiasis. In acute giardiasis abdominal symptoms usually appear within 2 weeks after the acquisition of the parasite. The patient may recover spontaneously or the disease may continue for several years as chronic giardiasis. Endemic giardiasis differs in some features from travelers' giardiasis.

ETIOLOGY. Several other names have been used for *G. lamblia*, such as *Lamblia intestinalis*, *G. intestinalis*, *G. enterica*, *Megastoma enterica*, and *Cercomonas intestinalis*. *G. lamblia* is a worldwide flagellated protozoon, and its closest relatives are the Giardia parasites of other animals and the genus Trichomonas. Despite morphologic similarity, the giardiae of various species may be host specific. *G. lamblia* has been thought to be an obligate parasite of man, but the natural resistance of mice, rats, gerbils, beavers and dogs may be less than perfect. The vegetative form, the trophozoite, proliferates in the human small intestine. It is 10–20 μm long and has the stable shape of a split pear, two nuclei, four pairs of flagella, and a ventral sucking disk (Fig. 1), and it multiplies by binary fission. For unknown reasons, the motile trophozoites transform into oval 8–15 μm long immobile cysts, which means that the protozoon is surrounded by a wall (Fig. 2). *G. lamblia* divides once within the cyst, which thus usually contains four nuclei. The cysts are excreted in feces and they are the infective stage of the parasite. They are resistant to environmental factors, except drying and heating; for example, they survive many usual disinfectants and the chlorination of drinking water. The mode of transmission is the ingestion of fecally contaminated material, either through a vehicle, such as water, food, toys, or insects, through direct contact from one person to another, or as autoinfection. *G. lamblia* is highly contagious: 10 or 100 cysts may be enough to infect all recipients (Rendtorff, 1954).

PATHOGENESIS AND PATHOLOGY. Ingested cysts of *G. lamblia* are carried through the stomach and through excystation initiated by low pH liberate trophozoites, which settle in the small intestine and attach to the epithelium. The parasite inhabits the duodenum and the upper parts of the jejunum, but the caudal extent of its residence is unknown. It has been found in the gallbladder. Most *G. lamblia* trophozoites lie freely in the intestinal mucus, many adhere to the epithelial surface, and some may invade epithelial cells and penetrate as far as the lamina propria (Saha and Ghosh, 1977).

Giardiasis may present without detectable lesions of the small intestine, but either acute or chronic giardiasis may cause morphologic changes in the mucosa. Microvilli may be shortened and epithelial mitoses increased. Inflammation of the epithelium and lamina propria, edema, and inftration by neutrophils, eosinophils, lymphocytes, and plasma cells may be seen, and in advanced cases there may be elongation of crypts and changes in villous architecture, varying from mild blunting of the villi to subtotal villous atrophy. Parasitic tissue invasion or accelerated mucin production leading to plugging of crypts may be pathogenetic in some patients, but cell-mediated immune responses in the mucosa probably explain in a unifying manner the damage to innocent bystander tissues, the severity of symptoms, and the titers of systemic antibodies. The mucosal abnormalities are reversible upon eradication of the parasite.

A correlation between the degree of mucosal changes

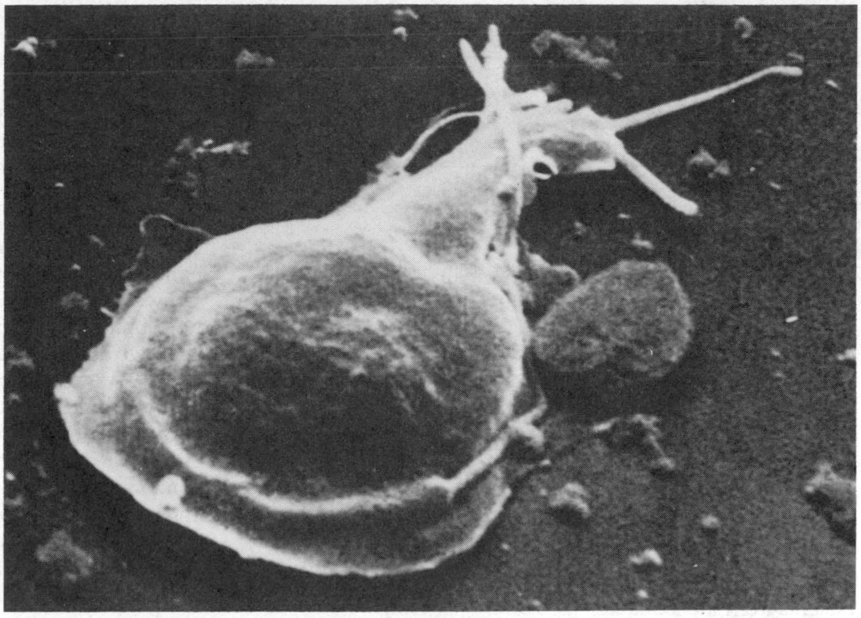

Figure 1. Trophozoite of *G. lamblia* (5000×; scanning electron microscopy by Dr. Ismo Virtanen).

and the severity of illness has been reported (Hoskins et al., 1967). In asymptomatic *G. lamblia* infections, mononuclear cells may be increased in the mucosa, and microvilli may be injured (Barbieri et al., 1970). In acute infections polymorphonuclear leukocytes predominate, and in chronic cases the cellular infiltrate is mainly mononuclear. The morphologic changes in children are the same as those in adults, although less severe and less common. In patients with hypogammaglobulinemia the mucosal changes of giardiasis are more severe, and are characterized by nodular lymphoid hyperplasia and the virtual lack of plasma cells.

G. lamblia infestation causes malabsorption of fat, vitamin A, folic acid, vitamin B_{12}, and xylose and disaccharidase deficiency. The ensuing steatorrhea and lactose intolerance may resemble those of celiac disease. Although more severe malabsorption is associated with greater morphologic changes (Wright et al., 1977), the latter are seldom sufficient to explain the malabsorption. The mechanical barrier created by numerous parasites adhering to the epithelium and competition for nutrients between the parasite and the patient may contribute to malabsorption.

CLINICAL MANIFESTATIONS. At least every fourth healthy individual exposed to *G. lamblia* by visiting an endemic area may become infected (Jokipii and Jokipii, 1974; Brodsky et al., 1974). The incidence depends on the number of cysts ingested (Rendtorff, 1954) and on the duration of exposure. Most healthy children entering an infected nursery acquire the parasite in a few months (Black et al., 1977). Another risk group with high prevalence of giardiasis is the male homosexual population (Most, 1968; Kean et al., 1979). Immunodeficiency and reduced gastric acidity predispose to giardiasis, but explain only a minority of cases. In outbreaks of giardiasis overt illness occurs in 50 to 90 per cent of persons with parasitic infestation after an incubation period of 1 to 2 weeks (Jokipii and Jokipii, 1974; Brodsky et al., 1974). Serum immunoglobulin levels are not below normal in unselected giardiasis patients (Jokipii and Jokipii, 1982a), and information about intestinal fluid immunoglobulins is contradictory.

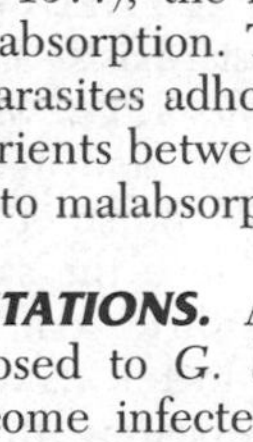

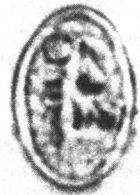

Figure 2. Iodine-stained cyst of *G. lamblia* (2000×).

The symptoms of giardiasis are predominantly abdominal, and those listed in Table 1 can occur alone or in various combinations. There are statistical differences between epidemic and chronic or endemic giardiasis, and children differ because of their growing and limited ability to describe symptoms. Asymptomatic intervals are typical of giardiasis. The disease is not life threatening, but a few deaths have been reported in infants (Ormiston et al., 1942), and giardiasis may contribute to the 5 million deaths annually caused by diarrheal diseases of children in developing countries.

The severity of acute giardiasis ranges widely from mild malaise to profuse watery diarrhea. It often begins with watery diarrhea that lasts for a few days and gives way to frequent loose stools. There is an urgency to defecate in the mornings and after meals. The stools may be offensive, frothy, and yellow or pale gray in color, and with prolonged diarrhea the patient loses considerable weight. A second group of patients suffer from abdominal pains without change in defecation. These vary from colicky cramps to mere discomfort, most frequently epigastric. In a third type of patient, giardiasis may present with flatulence in the absence of diarrhea or pain; in Table 1, flatus, borborygmus, belching, and abdominal distention are included in flatulence. Even small meals precipitate fullness and other symptoms leading to anorexia despite hunger. Acute

Table 1. SYMPTOMATOLOGY OF PARASITOLOGICALLY CONFIRMED GIARDIASIS

Symptom	Frequency of Symptom (Per Cent)		
	Outbreaks* *(acute)*	***Endemic**** *(chronic)*	***Children****
Diarrhea	87	55	53
Constipation	14	18	31
Blood in stool	0	6	7
Abdominal pain	75	61	37
Flatulence	70	44	NR†
Nausea	65	20	NR
Vomiting	23	16	30
Anorexia	68	16	28
Loss of weight	58	32	7
Failure to thrive	NR	NR	49
Anemia	NR	NR	23
Weakness	72	12	31
Fever	12	8	6
Nervousness	28	31	18
Urticaria	10	5	NR
No symptoms	9	12	17

*Based on 603 (outbreaks), 1548 (endemic), or 492 (children) patients from the literature.

†NR, not recorded sufficiently.

giardiasis may be self-limited or may last for 2 to 3 months, whereas more prolonged cases fit the description of chronic giardiasis.

The intermittent symptomatology of chronic giardiasis, or of repeated infections in endemic areas, is indistinguishable from, and is as nonspecific as, that of acute giardiasis in individual cases, but the average patient differs (Table 1). Chronic giardiasis may last for years or even decades, and intestinal malabsorption develops in many of the patients.

COMPLICATIONS AND SEQUELAE. Irreversible sequelae have not been associated with giardiasis, most complications are rare, and their causal relationship with giardiasis has not been proved. Aside from nonspecific symptoms, the malabsorption syndrome may include milk intolerance, meat intolerance, anemia, and steatorrhea. In a few instances *G. lamblia* has caused cholecystitis (Calder and Rigdon, 1935; Hartman et al., 1942), but the frequency of this association is not known. Infrequent manifestations suggesting immunologic sensitization, such as urticaria, arthritis, and uveitis, are probably caused by *G. lamblia*, since they subside with specific treatment.

GEOGRAPHIC VARIATIONS IN DISEASE. Heterogeneity in *G. lamblia* from various parts of the world has not been described, and each human race is susceptible to the infection. The parasite is worldwide, but owing to social conditions some aspects of giardiasis vary between countries. Its prevalence seems inversely related to the hygienic standard; in Scandinavia, for instance, persons with a history of traveling to endemic areas account for the 1 per cent prevalence of infestation. In such countries most cases of giardiasis are of the acute type, described as travelers' giardiasis, and occur in young adults. In endemic areas asymptomatic giardiasis is more common, the infections are of the chronic or recurrent type, and the prevalence is highest in children. Relatively high figures come from Eastern European countries and former colonial powers like Great Britain and the Netherlands, and the highest from tropical or subtropical areas in India, Southeast Asia, South America, and Africa. The geographic distributions of male homosexuality and AIDS (Acquired Immunodeficiency Syndrome) are not even. Attention was drawn to giardiasis in homosexuals in 1968 (Most, 1968), the prevalence figures were high in several urban areas a decade later (Kean et al., 1979), and giardiasis is one of the intestinal parasite infections in patients with AIDS (Pitchenik et al., 1983), which was described shortly thereafter. Growth retardation is associated with giardiasis in the developing world because of the prevalence in children, shortage of food, and malabsorption. In travelers' epidemics a high proportion of persons from nonendemic areas may acquire clinical giardiasis, whereas those coming from other endemic areas may be protected. Diet may affect the clinical picture, and the pathologic changes are more common and more severe in connection with strongly spiced food, as in India.

DIAGNOSIS. Giardiasis should be suspected in all cases of prolonged abdominal illness. Although in some geographic areas clinical history and epidemiologic information may reveal most cases of giardiasis, the demonstration of *G. lamblia* is the only way to establish the diagnosis. The usual procedure is to examine feces either immediately after defecation for cysts and trophozoites or after the concentration of a formalin-preserved specimen for cysts. In parasitologically confirmed cases of giardiasis, stool examination often gives a negative result during the first 3 weeks after infection—that is, there is a period of prepatency (Rendtorff, 1954; Jokipii and Jokipii, 1977)—and, later, cyst-passing is intermittent. Repeated examinations are therefore advisable. Trophozoites of *G. lamblia* should be looked for in duodenal or jejunal biopsy or aspirate when abdominal disease persists without diagnosis and fecal examinations have not been helpful. Simpler methods of duodenal sampling, such as swallowing and pulling back a nylon thread are convenient. Although there are several reports on serum antibody levels in giardiasis, their diagnostic value has not been established.

TREATMENT AND PROPHYLAXIS. Nitroimidazoles are the drugs of choice in giardiasis. A single dose of tinidazole (1.5 to 2 g) or ornidazole (1.5 g) will cure over 90 per cent of adult patients (Jokipii and Jokipii, 1979; Jokipii and Jokipii, 1982b). A 3-day course of metronidazole, 2 g once daily, is needed to achieve the same cure rate. Metronidazole, 200 or 250 mg thrice daily, or tinidazole, 150 mg twice daily, for seven to ten days produces cure rates of about 75 per cent. Repeating the course after a week's pause will cure more than 90 per cent. The oldest specific treatment, quinacrine (mepacrine), 100 mg thrice daily for seven to ten days, is also effective. The one-week courses of metronidazole or quinacrine have been used in infants at one-third the adult dosage, and furazolidone as a suspension is available and effective against giardiasis in children (Murphy and Nelson, 1983). Since asymptomatic carriers are potential sources of outbreaks, and since they may become ill later, it is advisable to treat them.

The drugs relieve the symptoms and eradicate the parasite from the feces in a few days in almost all cases. The success of therapy should be monitored clinically and by stool examination at 2, 4, and 8 weeks, since late relapses may occur. Treatment failures are more frequent in acute than in chronic giardiasis, and light infestations are more readily cured than heavy ones. After the eradication of *G. lamblia*, symptoms indistinguishable from giardiasis may continue in 10 per cent of the patients for up to a year (Jaremin et al., 1976; Jokipii and Jokipii, 1978). This has been termed postgiardiac syndrome.

No specific prophylaxis is available, and the way to escape giardiasis is to avoid all forms of unboiled water in endemic areas.

References

Barbieri, D., DeBrito, T., Hoshino, S., Nascimento F[a], O, B., Martins Campos, J. V., Quarentei, G., and Marcondes, E.: Giardiasis in childhood. Absorption tests and biochemistry, histochemistry, light, and electron microscopy of jejunal mucosa. Arch Dis Child 45:466, 1970.

Black, R. E., Dykes, A.C., Sinclair, S. P., and Wells, J. G.: Giardiasis in day-care centers: evidence of person-to-person transmission. Pediatrics 60:486, 1977.

Brodsky, R. E., Spencer, H. C., Jr., and Schultz, M. G.: Giardiasis in American travelers to the Soviet Union. J Infect Dis 130:319, 1974.

Calder, R. M., and Rigdon, R. H.: Giardia infestation of gall bladder and intestinal tract. Am J Med Sci 100:82, 1935.

Hartman, H. R., Kyser, F. A., and Comfort, M. W.: Infection of the gallbladder by Giardia lamblia. JAMA 118:608, 1942.

Hoskins, L. C., Winawer, S. J., Broitman, S. A., Gottlieb, I. S., and Zamcheck, N.: Clinical giardiasis and intestinal malabsorption. Gastroenterology 53:265, 1967.

Jaremin, B., Chmielewski, J., Zwierz, C., and Spiralska, I.: A "postgiardiac syndrome" (an analysis of the observed cases). Bull Inst Marit Trop Med Gdynia 27:93, 1976.

Jokipii, A. M. M., and Jokipii, L.: Prepatency of giardiasis. Lancet 1:1095, 1977.

Jokipii, A. M. M., and Jokipii, L.: Comparative evaluation of two dosages of tinidazole in the treatment of giardiasis. Am J Trop Med Hyg 27:758, 1978.

Jokipii, A. M. M., and Jokipii, L.: Serum IgG, IgA, IgM, and IgD in giardiasis: the most severely ill patients have little IgD. J Infect 5:189, 1982a.

Jokipii, L., and Jokipii, A. M. M.: Giardiasis in travelers: a prospective study. J Infect Dis 130:295, 1974.

Jokipii, L., and Jokipii, A. M. M.: Single-dose metronidazole and tinidazole as therapy for giardiasis: success rates, side effects, and drug absorption and elimination. J Infect Dis 140:984, 1979.

Jokipii, L., and Jokipii, A. M. M.: Treatment of giardiasis: comparative evaluation of ornidazole and tinidazole as a single oral dose. Gastroenterology 83:399, 1982b.

Kean, B. H., William, D. C., and Luminais, S. K.: Epidemic of amoebiasis and giardiasis in a biased population. Br J Vener Dis 55:375, 1979.

Most, H.: Manhattan: "A tropic isle?" Am J Trop Med Hyg 17:333, 1968.

Murphy, T. V., and Nelson, J. D.: Five v ten days' therapy with furazolidone for giardiasis. Am J Dis Child 137:267, 1983.

Ormiston, G., Taylor, J., and Wilson, G. S.: Enteritis in a nursery home associated with Giardia lamblia. Br Med J 2:151, 1942.

Pitchenik, A. E., Fischl, M. A., Dickinson, G. M., Becker, D. M., Fournier, A. M., O'Connell, M. T., Colton, R. M., and Spira, T. J.: Opportunistic infections and Kaposi's sarcoma among Haitians: evidence of a new acquired immunodeficiency state. Ann Intern Med 98:277, 1983.

Rendtorff, R. C.: The experimental transmission of human intestinal protozoan parasites. II. Giardia lamblia cysts given in capsules. Am J Hyg 59:209, 1954.

Saha, T. K., and Ghosh, T. K.: Invasion of small intestinal mucosa by Giardia lamblia in man. Gastroenterology 72:402, 1977.

Wright, S. G., Tomkins, A. M., and Ridley, D. S.: Giardiasis: clinical and therapeutic aspects. Gut 18:343, 1977.

140
CRYPTOSPORIDIOSIS

LIISA JOKIPII, M.D.,
ANSSI M. M. JOKIPII, M.D.

Cryptosporidiosis is a newly recognized enteric infection caused by *Cryptosporidium*. As a potentially fatal diarrhea in domestic animals, it is of considerable importance in veterinary medicine. Human cryptosporidiosis is a self-limiting gastrointestinal disease, sometimes a zoonosis, and a potentially life-threatening infection in immunocompromised patients.

ETIOLOGY. *Cryptosporidium* is a coccidian protozoal genus in the suborder *Eimeriina*, to which *Sarcocystis*, *Isospora*, and *Toxoplasma* also belong. It differs from other coccidia in being an extracellular parasite, having a rapid life cycle, and lacking host specificity to such a degree that it has been called a single-species genus (Tzipori et al., 1980); however, numerous species have been named in the past mainly according to over 30 host species among mammals, birds, fishes, reptiles, and arthropods. After ingestion the infectious form of *Cryptosporidium* produces trophozoites developing to eight-nucleated schizonts that liberate merozoites (Fig. 1). After a second schizogony, the second generation merozoites produce macrogametes and microgametes and thus, via sexual fusion, zygotes that develop to oocysts (Fig. 2), which are the infectious life-cycle stage found in feces. The endogenous stages invade the microvillous borders of enterocytes, do not enter the cytoplasm, but become completely surrounded by host cell membrane. The oocysts are nearly spherical and measure 4 to 6 μm; and the dimensions of the various endogenous stages vary between 2 and 6 μm. The fecal-oral route is thought to operate in the transmission of *Cryptosporidium* to man. The oocysts are resistant to environmental conditions and extremely so to various disinfectants. The infectious dose is unknown, and the oocysts are probably infective immediately after defecation (Moon and Bembrick, 1981).

PATHOGENESIS AND PATHOLOGY. The pathogenesis of human cryptosporidiosis is unknown. Work with animals has revealed no tissue invasion, toxic products, host reactions, or other mechanisms to explain the observed pathology. In cryptosporidiosis as seen in otherwise healthy patients, endogenous stages of *Cryptosporidium* attached to the surface epithelium, blunting and shortening of the villi, mild inflammatory changes, prominent Peyer's patches with germinal centers, and follicular hyperplasia of the draining lymph nodes have been described in the terminal ileum and extending to the cecum; the rest of the colon is unaffected (Fletcher et al., 1982; Babb et al., 1982). The anatomic distribution is consistent with that reported in animals. In immunocompromised patients the distribution is wider, ranging from the pharynx and rectum and including the gallbladder. The inflammatory changes may

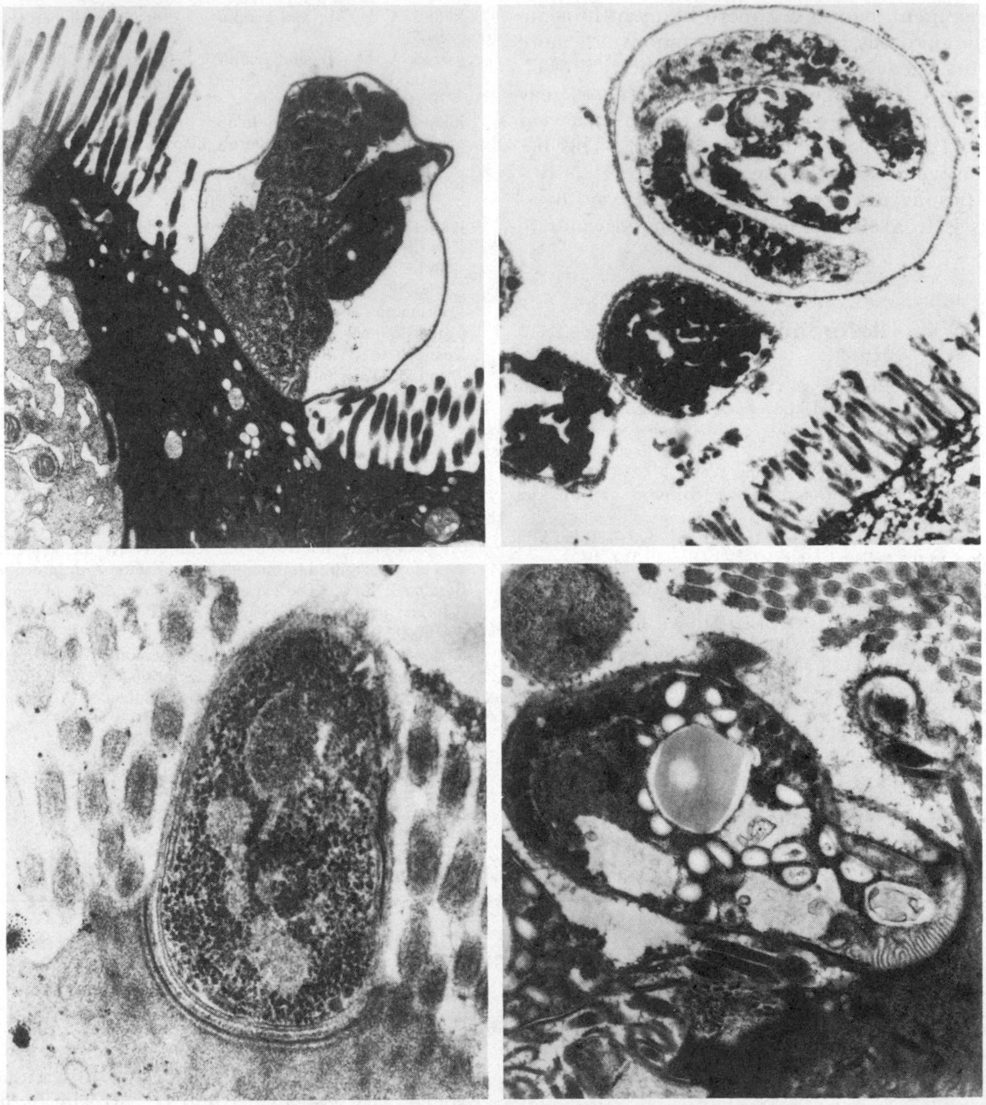

Figure 1. Electron microscopic appearance of cryptosporidia in various stages of development shown in jejunal biopsy specimen from a 9-year-old boy with congenital hypogammaglobulinemia. Upper left (20,700×) shows a trophozoite undergoing schizogony; upper right (7500×) shows trophozoites below and a schizont containing several merozoites; lower left (10,500×) is a merozoite penetrating a cell; cell in lower right (20,700×) illustrates macrogamete. (From original prints provided by K. Lasser and published by Lasser, K. H., et al.: Hum Pathol 10:234, 1979.)

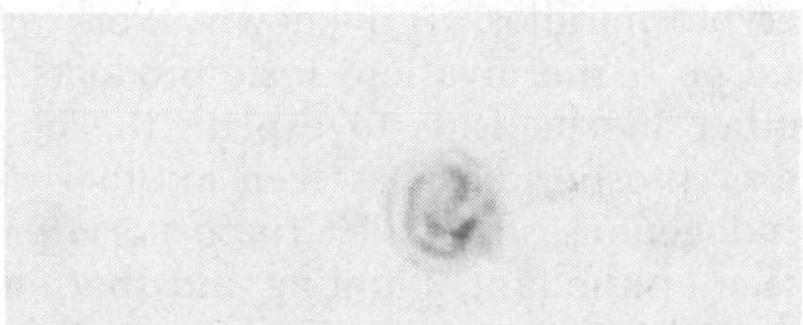

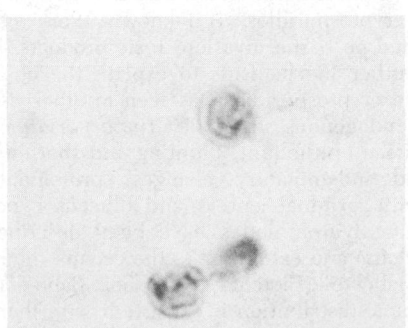

Figure 2. Oocysts of *Cryptosporidium* from human feces after formalin-ether concentration (modified Ziehl-Neelsen, 2000×).

be more severe, but these patients have other infections and malignancies in addition to cryptosporidiosis.

CLINICAL MANIFESTATIONS. In patients infected with *Cryptosporidium* gastrointestinal symptoms appear 4 to 12 days after contact with the apparent source of transmission and usually last for a few days to two weeks (Current et al., 1983; Jokipii et al., 1983). The symptoms are not different from those of various other gastrointestinal infections (Table 1). The evidence that *Cryptosporidium* causes the symptoms is circumstantial: accepted pathogens are not detected in the same patients, and the timing of oocyst shedding and clinical illness is the same.

The incidence of human cryptosporidiosis, the proportion of asymptomatic infections, and the prevalence of *Cryptosporidium* in the population are unknown.

Table 1. SYMPTOMS OF 25 PATIENTS INFECTED WITH *CRYPTOSPORIDIUM**

	No.	(%)
Diarrhea	23	(92)
Abdominal pain	19	(76)
Nausea	9	(36)
Vomiting	3	(12)
Anorexia	6	(24)
Weakness	5	(20)
Fever	8	(32)

*From the literature. Only symptomatic patients with no detectable underlying disease or other pathogens were included.

COMPLICATIONS AND SEQUELAE. Cryptosporidiosis is normally self-limiting. In immunocompromised patients more severe illness, including chronic, profuse, watery diarrhea and malabsorption continuing until the patient's death, has been ascribed to *Cryptosporidium.* This is one of the opportunistic infections frequently encountered in patients with AIDS (Acquired Immunodeficiency Syndrome) (Navin and Juranek, 1984).

GEOGRAPHIC VARIATIONS IN DISEASE. The fact that human cryptosporidiosis has been described in the U.S.A., U.K., Haiti, France, Finland, and Australia may reflect the distributions of medical and veterinary research and of AIDS. The prevalence of the infection elsewhere cannot be predicted until competent examiners look for it.

DIAGNOSIS. Oocysts can be identified as nearly round red bodies with thick walls and characteristic inner structures in concentrates of formalin-preserved feces stained with the modified Ziehl-Neelsen method (Fig. 2). When intestinal biopsy specimens are taken, those from the distal ileum are most likely to reveal endogenous stages of *Cryptosporidium,* but jejunal biopsy can also be used to demonstrate these stages as shown in Figures 1 and 3.

TREATMENT AND PROPHYLAXIS. No drug has been effective in treatment or prophylaxis, although more than 50 have been tried (Goldfarb et al., 1982; Tzipori, 1983). Most disinfectants are ineffective, but formaldehyde and ammonia destroy the infectivity of *Cryptosporidium* oocysts (Campbell et al., 1982). Since it is self-limiting, cryptosporidiosis in otherwise healthy persons is not a therapeutic problem in the light of present knowledge. However, the prevention of transmission to immunocompromised patients is important.

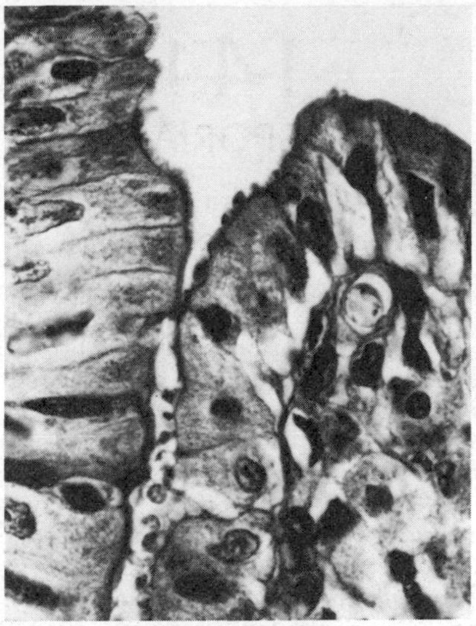

Figure 3. Cryptosporidia in jejunal biopsy specimen from case shown in Figure 1. The organisms are seen as a row of tiny spherical bodies attached to the brush border of columnar epithelium (hematoxylin-eosin, 1000 ×). (From original prints provided by K. Lasser and published by Lasser, K. H., et al.: Hum Pathol 10:234, 1979.)

References

Babb, R. R., Differding, J. T., and Trollope, M. L.: Cryptosporidia enteritis in a healthy professional athlete. Gastroenterology 77:833, 1982.

Campbell, I., Tzipori, S., Hutchison, G., and Angus, K. W.: Effect of disinfectants on survival of cryptosporidium oocysts. Vet Rec 111:414, 1982.

Current, W. L., Reese, N. C., Ernst, J. V., Bailey, W. S., Heyman, M. B., and Weinstein, W. M.: Human cryptosporidiosis in immunocompetent and immunodeficient persons. N Engl J Med 308:1252, 1983.

Fletcher, A., Sims, T. A., and Talbot, I. C.: Cryptosporidial enteritis without general or selective immune deficiency. Br Med J 285:22, 1982.

Goldfarb, J., Tanowitz, H., Grossman, R., et al.: Cryptosporidiosis: assessment of chemotherapy of males with acquired immune deficiency syndrome (AIDS). Morbid Mortal Weekly Rep 31:589, 1982.

Jokipii, L, Pohjola, S., and Jokipii, A. M. M.: Cryptosporidium: a frequent finding in patients with gastrointestinal symptoms. Lancet 2:358, 1983.

Lasser, K. H., Lewin, K. J., and Ryning, F. W.: Cryptosporidial enteritis in a patient with congenital hypogammaglobulinemia. Hum Pathol 10:234, 1979.

Moon, H. W., and Bembrick, W. J.: Fecal transmission of calf cryptosporidia between calves and pigs. Vet Pathol 18:248, 1981.

Navin, T. R., and Juranek, D. D.: Cryptosporidiosis: Clinical, epidemiologic, and parasitologic review. Rev Infect Dis 6:313, 1984.

Tzipori, S.: Cryptosporidiosis in animals and humans. Microbiol Rev 47:84, 1983.

Tzipori, S., Angus, K. W., Campbell, I., and Gray, E. W.: *Cryptosporidium*: evidence for a single-species genus. Infect Immun 30:884, 1980.

141
ISOSPORIASIS

LIISA JOKIPII, M.D.,
ANSSI M. M. JOKIPII, M.D.

Isosporiasis is a collective name for the enteric infections caused by those coccidian protozoa for which man, as the final host, provides the site for intracellular multiplication and completion of the sexual life-cycle stages in the intestinal mucosa. The best known among these organisms are *Isospora belli*, *Sarcocystis fusiformis*, and *Sarcocystis miescheriana*. Coccidiosis has been used as a synonym, but logically includes other coccidian infections besides isosporiasis. The taxonomically related *Sarcocystis* spp. and *Isospora (Toxoplasma) gondii* cause unrelated human diseases, sarcocystosis and toxoplasmosis, respectively, and fall outside the scope of isosporiasis.

ETIOLOGY. The coccidia, which are shed in the human feces as mature sporocysts without oocyst walls, were called *Isospora hominis*, until it was discovered that the larger form (13–17 × 8–11 μm) of these sporocysts was the end product of the intestinal life-cycle stages of *Sarcocystis fusiformis* found in cattle muscle, and that the smaller form (11–14 × 8–11 μm) was that of *S. miescheriana* found in swine muscle (Rommel and Heydorn, 1972). New names for these organisms, *S. bovihominis* and *S. suihominis*, respectively, have been proposed but not generally accepted (Tardos and Laarman, 1982), and also a new collective name, *S. hominis*, is being used. Man may become infected by eating raw beef or pork.

I. belli is released from the intestinal wall as immature oocysts, and further development occurs in the feces, which thus contains various oocyst stages (20–33 × 10–20 μm). (Fig. 1). Transmission seems to occur by ingestion of fecally contaminated material.

There are several isolated reports on other *Isospora*-like coccidia in human feces. Unequivocal classification of the etiological organism as *I. belli*, *S. hominis*, or another species is possible only in a minority of all published cases of human isosporiasis.

Little is known about the intestinal coccidian life-cycle stages in man. The schizogony of the obligately heteroxenous *Sarcocystis* takes place in the intermediate host's muscle while that of *I. belli*, which is found only in man, and the gametogony and oocyst formation of both genera, occur intracellularly in the human small intestinal wall.

PATHOGENESIS AND PATHOLOGY. In severe and fatal cases, endogenous stages of *Isospora* reside in the proximal small intestine within the epithelium or immediately below it, destroy the parasitized cells, and are rarely found also in the lamina propria and the submucosa (Brandborg et al., 1970). The pathology attributable to isosporiasis in its common self-limited form and in the absence of other intestinal pathogens or underlying diseases is virtually unknown. Biopsy of the upper jejunum of one patient with *I. belli* showed flattening of the villi, infiltration of the lamina propria with round and plasma cells, and intraepithelial lymphocytes (French et al., 1964). The invasiveness of *Isospora* and *Sarcocystis* is regarded as the pathogenetic mechanism of isosporiasis. Eosinophilia is common in *I. belli* infection and eosinophils have been seen in the cellular infiltrates in the mucosa.

CLINICAL MANIFESTATIONS. In experimental infections in volunteers *S. miescheriana* and *S. fusiformis* may cause symptoms in a variable proportion of exposed subjects, starting from one to a few days after the ingestion of raw pork or beef, and including fullness, nausea, vomiting, diarrhea, epigastric pain, headache and fever (Piekarski et al., 1978; Hiepe et al., 1979). The acute phase subsided in a day, some symptoms lasted for weeks, but the disease was self-limited in all cases. Naturally acquired isosporiasis caused by *S. hominis* is almost always asymptomatic, and rarely associated with symptoms like those of the experimental infections; its incubation period is not known.

Isosporiasis due to *I. belli* is usually associated with symptoms, such as diarrhea, abdominal pain, flatulence, vomiting, anorexia, weight loss and fever (Jarpa, 1966; Sagua et al., 1978). The incubation period is about one week. Eosinophilia is frequent. *I. belli* isosporiasis is also self-limited in otherwise healthy individuals, but rarely may persist for months; the role of autoinfection or reinfection in such persistent cases is not known.

COMPLICATIONS AND SEQUELAE. Isosporiasis by *I. belli* may cause malabsorption and steatorrhea. In compromised patients it may cause severe diarrhea lasting until death, and it is associated with the Acquired Immunodeficiency Syndrome or AIDS (Pitchenik et al., 1983).

GEOGRAPHIC VARIATIONS IN DISEASE. Isosporiasis, like diarrheal diseases in general, must be more severe in infants in the developing world than in other populations. *I. belli* and *S. hominis* are not rare in South America, and they are said to be relatively common in other tropical and subtropical regions as well. In developed countries, *I. belli* is rare and then usually imported or associated with extremely poor hygiene. Asymptomatic isosporiasis by *S. hominis* is common with prevalences of up to 10 per cent in the Netherlands, France, Germany, Poland, and possibly elsewhere, once looked for. Its prevalence is determined by the occurrence of sarcocystosis in cattle and pigs and the habit of eating incompletely cooked meat.

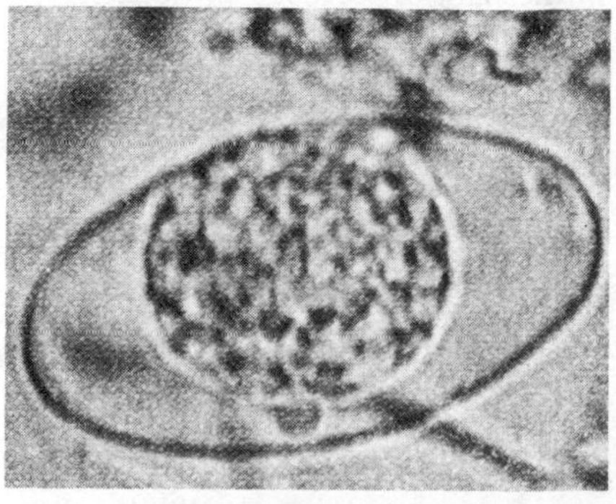

Figure 1. This oocyst of *Isopora belli* is the immature form usually found in freshly formed feces (2000×). (From Spencer, F., and Moore, L.: Color Atlas of Intestinal Parasites. Springfield, Ill., Charles C Thomas, 1977, p. 87.)

DIAGNOSIS. Isosporiasis can be diagnosed from feces or intestinal biopsies. Both *I. belli* oocysts (Fig. 1) and *Sarcocystis* sporocysts are found in small numbers and periodically in fecal samples, and although concentration methods increase findings, isosporiasis is difficult to diagnose. Most patients with *I. belli* also have fecal Charcot-Leyden crystals, whereas those with *S. hominis* do not. Clinical features are nonspecific, except for eosinophilia, which should suggest *I. belli.* With *S. fusiformis* and *S. miescheriana* there is a prepatent period of over a week, during which symptoms may be present in the absence of sporocyst excretion. In both *I. belli* and *S. hominis* isosporiasis, cyst excretion may continue for a week or two after the symptoms have subsided.

TREATMENT AND PROPHYLAXIS. No drug is of proven value. Because meat inspection ignores *Sarcocystis,* and there is no way to prevent sarcocystosis in livestock, human isosporiasis can be prevented only by avoiding the ingestion of raw meat or fecally contamined material.

References

Brandborg, L. L., Goldberg, S. B., and Breidenbach, W. C.: Human coccidiosis—a possible cause of malabsorption. N Engl J Med 283:1306, 1970.

French, J. M., Whitby, J. L., and Whitfield, A. G. W.: Steatorrhea in a man infected with coccidiosis *(Isospora belli).* Gastroenterology 47:642, 1964.

Hiepe, F., Hiepe, Th., Hlinak, P., Jungmann, R., Horsch, R., and Weidauer, B.: Experimentelle Infektion des Menschen und von Tieraffen (Cercopithecus callitrichus) mit Sarkosporidien-Zysten von Rind und Schwein. Arch Exp Veterinaermed 33:819, 1979.

Jarpa, A.: Coccidiosis humana. Biologica (Santiago) 39:3, 1966.

Piekarski, G., Heydorn, A. O., Aryeetey, M. E., Hartlapp, J.-H., and Kimmig, P.: Klinische, parasitologische und serologische Untersuchungen zur Sarkosporidiose (Sarcocystis suihominis) des Menschen. Immun Infekt 6:153, 1978.

Pitchenik, A. E., Fischl, M. A., Dickinson, G. M., Becker, D. M., Fournier, A. M., O'Connell, M. T., Colton, R. M., and Spira, T. J.: Opportunistic infections and Kaposi's sarcoma among Haitians: evidence of a new acquired immunodeficiency state. Ann Intern Med 98:277, 1983.

Rommel, M., and Heydorn, A.-O.: Beiträge zum Lebenszyklus der Sarkosporidien. III. Isospora hominis (Railliet und Lucet, 1891) Wenyon, 1923, eine Dauerform der Sarkosporidien des Rindes und des Schweins. Berl Muench Tieraerztl Wochenschr 85:143, 1972.

Sagua, H., Soto, J., Délano, B., Fuentes, A., and Becker, P.: Brote epidémico de isosporosis por *Isospora belli* en la ciudad de Antofagasta, Chile. Consideraciones sobre 90 casos diagnosticados en 3 meses. Bol Chile Parasit 33:8, 1978.

Spencer, F., and Monroe, L.: Color Atlas of Intestinal Parasites. Springfield, IL, Charles C Thomas, 1977, p. 87.

Tardos, W., and Laarman, J. J.: Current concepts on the biology, evolution and taxonomy of tissue cyst-forming eimeriid coccidia. Adv Parasitol 20:293, 1982.

142
BALANTIDIASIS

LIISA JOKIPII, M.D.
ANSSI M. M. JOKIPII, M.D.

Balantidiasis is the infection caused by *Balantidium coli* in the human colon; extraintestinal balantidiasis is rare. Balantidiasis is a zoonosis to which man is naturally resistant and it may cause no symptoms. Severe infections require predisposing host factors and are rare.

ETIOLOGY. The genus *Balantidium* parasitizes mammals, birds, reptiles, fishes, worms, and arthropods. The recognition of species is based on morphology and host origin. *B. coli* is worldwide and common in pigs and has been found in man, monkeys, and rats. *B. coli* is the largest protozoon and the only ciliated protozoon parasitizing man. Its life cycle has two stages, the trophozoite, measuring 30 to 200 × 30 to 70 μm, and the nearly round thick-walled cyst with a diameter of 40 to 65 μm containing one parasite. The trophozoite which is covered by cilia, has an anterior cytostome (mouth) and a posterior cytopyge (anus), contains a macronucleus and a micronucleus, and proliferates by transverse binary fission. Cysts are formed in feces and may survive for weeks outside the host. They are destroyed by drying, sunlight, and acidity and transmit balantidiasis when ingested by new hosts. The obvious source of natural human infections has been feces, mostly of pigs and sometimes of man and rats, but experimental transmission to human volunteers has failed. For man to become infected, it seems that a massive and repeated inoculation may be necessary, as may occur in primitive societies where people live in close contact with pigs or in mental institutions where personal hygiene is poor.

PATHOGENESIS AND PATHOLOGY. After the ingestion of cysts, trophozoites are liberated, settle in the large bowel, and start lysing the mucosa. The early lesions are small ulcers covered with mucus; there may be hemorrhagic areas, superficial abscesses, deep penetration and spread to the local lymphatics. The tissue reactions consist of edema and infiltration by mononuclear cells and eosinophils. Neutrophils predominate after secondary bacterial invasion. Colonic ulcers may develop without symptoms (Khamtsov, 1968).

CLINICAL MANIFESTATIONS. *B. coli* infections may be asymptomatic, chronic, acute, or fulminating. Most cases of overt balantidiasis are chronic and intermittent, and the main symptoms are diarrhea with watery, mucus-streaked, and sometimes blood-stained stools, abdominal pain and loss of weight. These may last for years. In acute balantidiasis, dysentery, cramps or colicky pains, nausea, anorexia and vomiting predominate; the patients lose weight and anemia may develop. Recovery may be spontaneous.

COMPLICATIONS AND SEQUELAE. The host's nutritional and immunological status determines the extent of tissue destruction, and rare deaths have been described due to perforation and peritonitis or hemorrhage and shock. Fulminating balantidiasis may lead to dehydration and renal insufficiency. There are rare findings of *B. coli* in the appendix, ileum, liver abscess, lung, vagina, and urinary tract.

GEOGRAPHIC VARIATIONS IN DISEASE. Balantidiasis has been described in all continents, and its incidence and severity is determined more by social and nutritional host factors and less by the climate, animal reservoirs, or other geographic variables. The main endemic areas are in Central and South America, some islands in the Pacific Ocean, New Guinea, the Philippines, Central Asia, and eastern Europe.

DIAGNOSIS. Balantidiasis is diagnosed by demonstrating trophozoites in wet preparations of fresh stool specimens or scrapings from ulcers at endoscopy. Cysts are found more rarely and then intermittently in formed stools in chronic infections. Concentration techniques do not increase the number of diagnoses (Walzer et al., 1973). Although *B. coli* can be cultured in vitro, the method is not used for diagnosis.

TREATMENT AND PROPHYLAXIS. The treatment of choice is said to be tetracycline, 500 mg four times daily for 10 days, and diiodohydroxyquin is an alternative. Metronidazole and nimorazole are active in vitro against *B. coli* and successful in symptomatic balantidiasis (Zrubec, 1967; Garcia-Laverde and de Bonilla, 1975; Nicholson, 1978; Delgado y Garnica et al., 1971), but may not eradicate *B. coli* in asymptomatic cases (Beasley and Walzer, 1972), Paromomycin has been clinically and parasitologically effective (Sotolongo et al., 1966). There is no specific prophylaxis, and prevention consists of recognizing and avoiding sources of infection.

References

Beasley, J. W., and Walzer, P. D.: Ineffectiveness of metronidazole in treatment of *Balantidium coli* infections. Trans R Soc Trop Med Hyg 66:519, 1972.

Delgado y Garnica, R., Brito Lugo, P., and Clark y Rodriquez Leal, R.: Balantidiasis en la ciudad de Mexico. Rev Invest Salud Publica 31:106, 1971.

Garcia-Laverde, A., and de Bonilla, L.: Clinical trials with metronidazole in human balantidiasis. Am J Trop Med Hyg 24:781, 1975.

Khamtsov, V. G.: Clinical evaluation of criteria of "healthy" carrier state of *Balantidium coli.* Med Parazitol (Mosk) 37:435, 1968.

Nicholson, N. W.: Case report of *Balantidium coli* infection. East Afr Med J 55:133, 1978.

Sotolongo, F., Otero, R., and Argudín, J.: La paromomicina en el tratamiento de la Balantidiasis. Rev Cubana Med Trop 18:103, 1966.

Walzer, P. D., Judson, F. N., Murphy, K. B., Healy, G. R., English, D. K., and Schultz, M. G.: Balantidiasis outbreak in Truk. Am J Trop Med Hyg 22:33, 1973.

Zrubec, J.: Balantidiáza u detí a jej Liečba metronidazolom. Bratisl Lek Listy 47:235, 1967.

143

INTESTINAL ROUNDWORMS

ELIZABETH BARRETT-CONNOR, M.D., D.C.M.T. (LONDON)

ASCARIASIS

Ascariasis, caused by the largest and most common roundworm of man, *Ascaris lumbricoides,* is found throughout temperate and tropical climates in most parts of the world.

ETIOLOGY. Infective eggs are chiefly transmitted from hand to mouth by children who have touched or eaten contaminated soil, or by ingestion of raw vegetables grown in infected soil. Larvae are released, penetrate the intestinal blood vessels, and are carried to the lungs. The larvae break out of the alveolar capillaries, migrate up the pulmonary tree, and are swallowed. They mature in the lumen of the small intestine, where they maintain their position by propulsive muscular activity. The adults produce eggs two to three months after infection is acquired and live an average of one year. They do not multiply in man. In soil, fertilized eggs become infective in about three weeks and can survive for years under appropriate conditions. Where sanitation is inadequate or where human feces are used as fertilizer, virtually everyone is infected. It is believed that one fourth of the world population has ascariasis. In some endemic areas the reinfection rate after deworming is as high as 30 per cent per month.

PATHOGENESIS AND PATHOLOGY. Larvae migrating through the lung can cause a patchy pneumonia, with focal hemorrhage, consolidation, and eosinophilia. Adult ascarids in the human intestine are usually found in the jejunum where they may cause roentgenographically identifiable coarsening of the mucosal folds. A less common but more serious complication is mechanical obstruction of a hollow viscus. For example, obstruction of the biliary tree can cause obstructive jaundice or ascending cholangitis. Obstruction of the pancreatic duct can cause pancreatitis. Obstruction of the upper airway can cause death from suffocation. Partial or complete small bowel obstruction, and occasionally volvulus or intussusception, may be caused by a mass of worms. Rarely, adults or ova are found outside the intestine in the liver, lung, or peritoneum, usually surrounded by granulomatous reaction.

CLINICAL MANIFESTATIONS. The pulmonary phase of larval migration, in the second week after ingestion of ova, usually passes unnoticed. However, in some cases migrating larvae cause Loeffler's syndrome; indeed, *Ascaris* is the commonest helminth reported as a cause of this disease (Spillman, 1975). Loeffler's syndrome is typically a one-week illness characterized by symptoms of tracheobronchitis and rapidly changing pulmonary infiltrates, followed by marked peripheral eosinophilia. The presence of a papular or urticarial rash in 15 per cent of cases, the greater frequency of the syndrome in adults rather than children in areas where *Ascaris* is acquired seasonally, the presence of eosinophilia, and studies of IgE all suggest that the pulmonary disease is due to a hypersensitivity reaction. In addition to Loeffler's syndrome attributed to migrating larvae, a relationship between allergic asthma and intestinal ascariasis has been postulated; evidence for this association is much more contradictory (Pawlowski, 1982).

Most patients with ascariasis are asymptomatic. The spontaneous passage of large worms from the mouth, nose, or anus may be the first indication of infection. The most serious consequence, which occurs in perhaps 2 in 1000 infections is obstruction caused by a bolus of worms or by the migration of a single adult *Ascaris*. Such complications, primarily in preschool children, include obstruction of the biliary or pancreatic ducts, appendicitis, volvulus, intussusception, intestinal perforation, and, most commonly, intestinal obstruction at the terminal ileum. Signs and symptoms of the obstructive complications are not specific for ascariasis. On occasion, an abdominal mass that contains a visible or palpable moving bolus of worms affords a preoperative diagnosis, but often the diagnosis is first made at surgery.

Ascariasis may cause malnutrition as a consequence of competition of parasites and host for limited nutrients in children who have a borderline diet and a heavy worm burden. Repeated worming results in a significant improvement in growth and development as compared with untreated infected controls (Gupta, 1977).

DIAGNOSIS. Except for a past history of worm passage, there are no diagnostic signs or symptoms of ascariasis. Diagnosis at the stage of larval migration is rarely possible, although transient patchy infiltrates and eosinophilia are suggestive. Occasionally, a diagnostic third-stage larva can be found in the sputum. Normal stools at the time of migration followed by the appearance of ova in the stools within three months establishes a probable retrospective diagnosis. (Serologic tests do not distinguish this illness from other larval migrations.) During the intestinal phase eosinophila is usually absent. Diagnosis is made by microscopic examination of unconcentrated stool. A few patients harbor only male *Ascaris*, no eggs are excreted, and the diagnosis is made after passage of a worm or by demonstration of ascarids on roengenographic examination of the abdomen.

TREATMENT. Because a single ascarid sometimes causes a serious complication, the goal of therapy is cure. Many drugs are effective for the treatment of ascariasis. The choice depends on availability, cost, and the necessity for single dose treatment in a given patient population. Piperazine citrate is an effective and inexpensive ascaricide used extensively over the years. A single oral dose of 75 to 100 mg/kg/body weight to a maximum of 3.5 g gives a cure rate of about 75 per cent, and a two-day course cures over 90 per cent of patients. Levamisole in a single dose of 2.5 mg/kg is as effective as piperazine. Pyrantel pamoate is more efficient, curing 90 to 100 per cent of patients after a single oral dose of 10 mg/kg. Other broad spectrum antihelmintics such as bephenium hydroxynaphthoate, thiabendazole, and mebendazole are also ascaricidal but are rarely as effective as pyrantel pamoate in a single dose.

Intestinal obstruction is treated by nasogastric suction. After vomiting is controlled, piperazine is given in the standard dosage by nasogastric tube, flushed through with saline, and the tube is then clamped for one or two hours. This process can be repeated every 8 to 12 hours for up to six doses until the obstruction is relieved. The symptoms usually improve in one or two days, but *Ascaris* organisms may not appear in the stool until four days after the initiation of therapy. In about one fifth of cases obstruction cannot be relieved and surgery is necessary.

PROPHYLAXIS. Improved sanitation, the building and use of latrines, and the prohibiton of the use of untreated human wastes as fertilizer all reduce the prevalence of ascariasis. In communities where such programs are not yet available, periodic mass worming of children has been recommended to prevent malnutrition and possibly reduce the risk of surgical complications of infection.

HOOKWORM INFECTION AND DISEASE

Hookworm infection is the presence of adult hookworms, *Ancylostoma duodenale* or *Necator americanus*, in the human intestine; hookworm disease occurs when the worms are present in sufficient numbers to cause iron deficiency anemia. Both *A. duodenale* and *N. americanus* are found in most parts of the world, although *N. americanus* is the predominant species in the Americas and Central Africa, and *A. duodenale* the prevailing species in coastal North Africa.

ETIOLOGY. Man is the principal host of *A. duodenale* and *N. americanus*. Hookworms are found wherever people go without shoes and defecate promiscuously into a warm, moist, and shaded soil suitable for the maturation of larvae. When eggs in feces are deposited on soil under optimal conditions, the ova hatch to rhabditiform larvae in one to two days, and molt to become infective filariform larvae within one week. Infective larvae may survive for as long as one year. On contact, the larvae penetrate skin or buccal mucosa, enter the circulation, and are carried to the lungs, where they pass from the capillaries to the alveoli. They ascend the respiratory tree, are swallowed, and mature to adults in the small intestine four to seven weeks after infection. Infection may also be established by ingestion of *A. duodenale* larvae. These organisms may remain dormant in the intestine or tissues for as long as nine months before ova are found in the stool (Banwell and Schad, 1978). The adult worms attach to the mucosa by buccal capsules and suck blood. Hookworms do not multiply in man. They survive two to ten years (average four years), although egg production decreases after two years. It is estimated that one fourth of the world population has hookworm infection, but most have a light infection, unassociated with disease.

PATHOGENESIS AND PATHOLOGY. Migration of larvae through the lungs may produce changes similar to those caused by *Ascaris* larvae. The attachment of worms to the wall of the intestine results in digestion of the distal villi. The intestinal mucosa between parasites appears normal. The major disorder produced by the hookworm is iron deficiency anemia, which is caused by the leeching of blood from the host. Bone marrow examination reveals absent iron stores. In advanced cases, cardiovascular changes consistent with severe anemia are seen.

CLINICAL MANIFESTATIONS. Skin penetration usually goes unnoticed but may cause "ground itch," with intense pruritus and papulovesicular rash at the site of larval entry. Larval migration through the lungs infrequently causes Loeffler's syndrome, as described under Ascariasis. Although massive infections can cause abdominal pain, diarrhea, and weight loss, intestinal symptoms are rare. The only significant consequence of hookworm infestation occurs when a heavy worm burden is coupled with an iron-poor diet. In this setting hookworm anemia, also called hookworm disease, is seen (Roche and Layrisse, 1966). Anemia is most apt to occur in women and children, owing to their greater iron needs. Anemia is also more common with *A. duodenale* infestation because it is a more efficient blood leech than *N. americanus*. A single *A. duodenale* sucks 0.15 ml per day compared with 0.03 ml by *N. americanus*. The signs and symptoms of anemia due to hookworm disease are those of any iron deficiency anemia. Although hookworms leech protein as well as iron, there is little evidence that hookworm increases the risk of malnutrition.

DIAGNOSIS. Diagnosis is rarely possible during the larval migration phase preceding the appearance of ova in the feces. Iron deficiency anemia and a slight eosinophilia in an individual with a history of soil contact in an endemic area should suggest hookworm disease, but eosinophilia may be absent. Occult blood is often found in the stool.

The diagnosis is confirmed by the demonstration of hookworm eggs in the feces. Any hookworm infection heavy enough to produce anemia is readily found on microscopic examination of a fecal smear without concentration. Unconcentrated smears will demonstrate eggs if the counts are greater than 1200 eggs/ml. (Egg counts of at least 2000/ml in feces from women and children and 5000/ml from men are usual in patents whose anemia is due to hookworm.) Quantitative techniques can be used to confirm the cause of anemia in patients with other possible causes of iron deficiency.

TREATMENT. Light infestations do not cause disease and require no treatment. For patients requiring treatment, a significant reduction in worm burden is an acceptable goal of therapy. Eradication of every worm is not necessary to prevent anemia and is impractical in populations with a high probability of reinfection.

A variety of agents has been used successfully. Reported cure rates differ according to hookworm species, geographic areas, and criteria for cure. The choice of agent should depend on the experience in a given area, the cost and availability of the drug, the likelihood of population compliance if multidose regimens are selected, the potential benefit of broad spectrum agents, and the frequency and severity of side effects. Tetrachlorethylene in a single dose of 0.12 ml/kg (maximum, 5 ml) cures approximately half of all patients and reduces the worm burden in most of the remainder. It is dependable and cheap. Purgatives are not required and indeed reduce the effectiveness and increase the toxicity of tetrachlorethylene. One dose of any of the following is also effective: 5 mg of bephenium hydroxynapthoate, 10 mg of pyrantel pamoate, or 25 mg/kg/body weight of levamisole. Mebendazole requires 100 mg twice a day for three days for effective treatment.

None of these anthelmintics are recommended for pregnant women, who should delay specific therapy until completion of pregnancy. Any patient with severe anemia should be treated first with iron therapy, which will promptly correct the anemia without affecting the worm load. Some authorities treat all patients who have hookworm anemia with iron as well as a vermifuge to hasten recovery from anemia.

PROPHYLAXIS. Shoes and latrines prevent hookworm infestation. Public health education must be coupled with attempts to improve sanitation. Otherwise, the newly built latrines are not used, and shoes are saved for special occasions.

TRICHOSTRONGYLIASIS

There are at least seven species of the genus *Trichostrongylus*, all of which are parasites of mammals that occasionally infect the intestinal tract of man. Human infection with *Trichostrongylus* is most common in Japan, Korea, Indonesia, and Iran, but is also found in other parts of Asia and in Africa (Ghadirian and Arfaa, 1975).

ETIOLOGY. Adult nematodes in the small intestine of ruminants lay eggs that are passed in feces. Infective larvae develop in suitable soil and infect man by skin penetration and pulmonary migration as in hookworm infection or, more often, by mouth as a result of ingestion of infected vegetation. When infection occurs by the oral route there is apparently no pulmonary migration, and the larvae mature to adults directly in the small intestine. Man usually acquires the infection from eating larvae on green vegetables or chewing contaminated grasses. Although human infections from this nematode are much less common than those caused by other intestinal nematodes, over two thirds of the population of some areas are infected.

PATHOGENESIS AND PATHOLOGY. Very little is known about this infection in man. Larvae are believed to mature while burrowed in the intestinal mucosa. The adults live attached to the duodenum and jejunum and suck blood in the manner of hookworms.

CLINICAL MANIFESTATIONS. *Trichostrongylus* infections are usually light, transient, and asymptomatic. Because most patients who have trichostrongyliasis also have other intestinal parasites, it is not possible to attribute symptoms directly to this infection.

DIAGNOSIS. Eggs are readily found in the stool and are easily confused with hookworm ova. Because *Trichostrongylus* infection is refractory to the usual anthelmintics, the discovery of ova in feces is not infrequently attributed to intractable hookworm infection.

TREATMENT. *Trichostrongylus* infection rarely, if ever, requires treatment. Because these nematodes lie protected in the intestinal mucosa, they are not eradicated by most of the broad spectrum anthelmintics. Thiabendazole and, less frequently, bephenium hydroxynapthoate have been used successfully. Thiabendazole, 25 mg/kg twice daily for two days, affords good cure rates but often causes nausea, dizziness, vomiting, and anorexia.

PROPHYLAXIS. Theoretically, prevention can be achieved by avoiding the consumption of raw plants grown in contaminated soil.

STRONGYLOIDIASIS

Strongyloidiasis, which is caused by the intestinal nematode *Strongyloides stercoralis*, has a patchy worldwide distribution. It often coexists with but is less common than hookworm.

ETIOLOGY. Like hookworm, *S. stercoralis* infects man by skin penetration. Within 48 hours the larvae migrate through the pulmonary capillaries. Some larvae may develop into adult worms in the lungs, but most pass from the respiratory tract to the duodenum and jejunum, where the females invade the mucosa and deposit eggs about one month after the initial infection. The larvae ordinarily hatch in the mucosa and bore into the intestinal lumen. Rhabditiform larvae are usually found in the feces. At times, the larvae may develop into the infective filariform stage in the intestine and penetrate the intestinal mucosa or perianal skin. This autoinfection is responsible for the heavy parasitism seen in some patients and for the persistence of infection long after the host has left an endemic area.

Strongyloides also has a free-living cycle. After leaving the host, rhabditiform larvae may develop into infective larvae either directly or indirectly through a generation of free-living males and females. Under appropriate conditions, the free-living cycle can be continued indefinitely.

PATHOGENESIS AND PATHOLOGY. Migration of larvae through the lungs may produce changes similar to those caused by *Ascaris*. The severity of the pulmonary process in strongyloidiasis is proportional to the number of parasites in the tissues, which reflects the level of autoinfection. Mechanical, lytic, and allergic mechanisms of lung damage have been proposed. In the small intestine adult females are anchored to the epithelium or deep in the mucosa. Small bowel biopsy usually shows eggs in crypts and submucosa, little inflammatory reaction, and flattening or atrophy of the villi. In patients with autoinfection, larvae may be seen migrating through the intestinal wall.

In fatal cases, adult worms, larvae, and eggs are found widely disseminated throughout the body. The heaviest parasitism occurs in the intestine and lungs. Hemorrhage, eosinophilia, and consolidation are seen in the alveoli. In the intestines, there is a variable amount of mucosal edema, necrosis, ulceration, and pseudopolyposis. A diffuse enteritis may progress to hemorrhagic enterocolitis and fibrosis. Dead and dying larvae presumably cause the most marked inflammatory response, which may be primarily granulomatous, lymphocytic, or eosinophilic. Other changes compatible with secondary bacterial infection are common.

CLINICAL MANIFESTATIONS. Most infections are asymptomatic. An itchy, maculoerythematous rash is sometimes noted at the site of skin penetration. Persons with chronic infection sometimes show recurrent urticaria, manifest as transient pruritic wheals and nodules. Acute pneumonitis is sometimes seen during the primary passage of the larvae through the lungs, but this is probably more often a consequence of autoinfection when larger numbers of larvae are migrating through the lungs. The most common complaints are watery, rarely bloody, diarrhea or symptoms suggestive of duodenal ulcer. In some patients, particularly, but not always, those with immunoglobulin deficiencies, a malabsorption syndrome may occur.

Disseminated strongyloidiasis is a serious and potentially fatal complication of massive autoinfection. This type of hyperinfection can occur in apparently heathy hosts but is much more common in patients who are immunocompromised owing to disease (malignancy, malnutrition, burns, chronic renal failure, tuberculosis, leprosy) or drugs (chemotherapy and corticosteroids). Symptoms and signs reflect the involved organ systems and are nonspecific. Clinical pictures suggestive of miliary tuberculosis, an acute abdomen, paralytic ileus, and granulomatous or ulcerative bowel disease have been observed. Secondary bacterial infection may result in gram-negative sepsis with fever, abdominal pain, and shock (Scowden et al., 1978).

DIAGNOSIS. Patients with pneumonia and eosinophilia should have a sputum examination for larvae. At the time of pulmonary migration, *Strongyloides* filariform larvae, each with a characteristic forked tail, often can be demonstrated in unstained or Papanicolaou-stained sputum.

The initial diagnosis of strongyloidiasis is usually attempted by stool examination. *Strongyloides* larvae can be found in only one-fourth of stool specimens from infected patients. (*Strongyloides* ova are rarely found in the stool, and hookworm larvae, which differ morphologically from those of *Strongyloides*, are not seen in stool unless there is a long interval between passage and examination.) The yield from stool examination can be increased by suspending approximately 100 g of fresh stool in fine surgical gauze over a glass, adding lukewarm water to the level of suspended stool, and waiting one hour for the larvae to migrate through the gauze to the bottom of the glass. The sediment is examined for larvae.

A duodenal or jejunal specimen yields the diagnosis in approximately 90 per cent of cases. Similar results can be achieved by examination of the bile-stained mucus that adheres to a nylon yarn, which is withdrawn several hours after being swallowed in a weighted gelatin capsule.

Peripheral eosinophilia is found in over 90 per cent of persons with strongyloidiasis. Unfortunately, only 20 per cent of patients with massive autoinfection and disseminated strongyloidiasis have peripheral eosinophilia as a clue to diagnosis.

Roentgenograms of the chest may show a miliary pattern, a lobular or lobar infiltrate, or cavities. Not infrequently, active tuberculosis coexists with pulmonary strongyloidiasis and may be responsible for part of the clinical and radiographic picture. Barium examination of the small intestine sometimes demonstrates duodenitis, small bowel dilatation, or a tubular rigid deformity of the small bowel; the latter is said to be strongly suggestive of chronic strongyloidiasis.

TREATMENT. The potential for autoinfection, illness, and even death supports the need for curative treatment. Patients who are candidates for immunosuppressive therapy should be systematically studied for strongyloidiasis and should receive specific therapy before corticosteroids or immunosuppressives are begun. Thiabendazole, 25 mg/kg twice daily for two days, is the preferred drug, although nausea, vomiting and bizarre neuropsychiatric symptoms including a sense of impending death are common side-effects (Grove, 1982). Approximately 10 per cent of patients will require a second course of therapy for cure; consequently some authorities routinely recommend a second course of treatment two weeks after the first. In disseminated strongyloidiasis, thiabendazole should be continued for at least five days. Total doses of as high as 50 g have been required for cure. Disseminated strongyloidiasis is fatal despite treatment in 50 per cent of patients. When possible, immunosuppressives should be discontinued until the parasite is eradicated.

PROPHYLAXIS. Preventive measures are the same as those used to control hookworm infection.

INTESTINAL CAPILLARIASIS

Human intestinal capillariasis is caused by the intestinal nematode *Capillaria philippinensis*. It is presently limited to specific coastal areas of the Philippines and one small focus in Thailand. Although there are over 200 nematodes of the genus *Capillaria*, only a few have been found in man and only *C. philippinensis* is an important cause of disease.

ETIOLOGY. Human intestinal capillariasis was first noted in the intestine of a severely wasted man who died in a Manila hospital in 1963. Three years later an epidemic of disease caused by this parasite affected over 1500 persons in northern Luzon, Philippines.

All stages of the parasite can be found in humans. Autoinfection and parasite multiplication are believed to be responsible for the very heavy infections seen in some patients. The high morbidity and mortality indicate that this parasite is new to humans. How this new infection was introduced remains a mystery. Although a marine fish or mammal is the suspected natural host, examinations of thousands of fish and other aquatic specimens have been negative. Infective larvae develop in the intestines of lagoon fish that are eaten raw in the affected communities; however, ingestion of raw fish is not new to this area. Feeding embryonated eggs to a variety of animals and humans in transmission experiments has failed to produce infection.

PATHOGENESIS AND PATHOLOGY. Unlike most intestinal nematodes, *C. philippinensis* can multiply within the intestinal tract of man. Dissemination of parasites may occur, but usually, even in fatal cases, the parasites are limited to the small intestine. At autopsy the small bowel is indurated, edematous, and distended with watery fluid. In some cases the ileal fluid contains from 10,000 to 200,000 larvae and adults per liter. Eggs, larvae, and adult worms are found in enormous numbers in the glands and lamina propria of the small intestine, particularly the jejunum where flattened or obliterated villi are also seen. There is a modest increase in the number of lymphocytes in the lamina propria, but no acute inflammatory reaction is present, nor is eosinophilia a consistent finding.

Altered absorption and intestinal protein loss result in chronic diarrhea and wasting. The cause of this effect is unknown; overwhelming numbers of parasites, a parasite-toxin, a parasite-allergin, or a parasite-induced deficiency of digestive enzyme(s) has been postulated as the pathogenic factor.

CLINICAL MANIFESTATIONS. The first symptoms are very characteristic loud gurglings in the stomach and diffuse abdominal pain. Two to three weeks later diarrhea, which is at first watery and then bulky and foul, appears. Severe muscle wasting, weakness, edema, and cardiopathy follow in the majority of cases. Early in the epidemic in 1966, virtually every person who had eggs in their stools became symptomatic, and nearly one quarter died two weeks to two months after the onset of illness, usually of heart failure or bacterial infection (Watten et al., 1972). Recently, there have been increasing numbers of asymptomatic persons with ova in their stools, and the severe form of the disease is less common. The reason for the lower pathogenicity of the disease is unknown. It may be that early recognition of the characteristic symptoms leads to earlier treatment.

DIAGNOSIS. In residents of an endemic area, the characteristic noisy stomach is practically diagnostic. Later steatorrhea, wasting, and eosinophilia suggest the diagnosis. Diagnosis is confirmed by stool examination. Eggs resemble those of *Trichuris trichiura* and are usually plentiful.

Other laboratory studies show anemia, hypoalbuminemia (with high values of alpha-2 and gamma-globulins compared with controls), and high IgE levels. Eosinophilia may be present. Marked electrolyte derangements, particularly hypokalemia, are usual. Increased fecal fat, impaired vitamin B_{12} absorption (Shilling test), and an abnormal D-xylose test are all characteristic of symptomatic intestinal infection with *C. philippinensis*. A severe protein-losing enteropathy can be demonstrated in persons with either symptomatic or asymptomatic infection.

TREATMENT. Previously thiabendazole for 30 to 40 days was the best treatment, but some patients relapsed and many had gastrointestinal side effects, dizziness, and weakness. Recently mebendazole has become the treatment of choice. Four hundred milligrams daily in divided doses for 20 to 30 days gives good cure rates without side effects. Diarrhea usually decreases and the patient feels better within 48 hours of initiation of treatment; in the interim, fluid and electrolyte replacement is important.

PROPHYLAXIS. No methods of control are known, although the avoidance of uncooked fish is recommended.

ENTEROBIASIS

Enterobiasis is infection of the intestinal tract of man with the pinworm *Enterobius vermicularis*. Pinworm infection is worldwide in distribution and vies with *Ascaris* for first place as the most common nematode of man. Unlike *Ascaris*, pinworm is equally common in developed and developing countries.

ETIOLOGY. This small roundworm lives in the cecum and adjacent portions of the gastrointestinal tract. Adult worms seldom live more than two months and do not multiply in man. The male is smaller than the female and is rarely seen. At night, the gravid female migrates from the anus to deposit thousands of eggs on the perianal or perineal skin. The embryonated ova are infective within a few hours and are transferred to the mouth of the same or another host by way of hands, bedclothes, and possibly aerosols. Man is the only known host. Owing to their personal hygienic habits, children are most often infected and reinfected. However, when a child brings the infection into a household, other members of all ages are often infected. It is estimated that 30 per cent of children and 15 per cent of adults have pinworm (Weller and Sorenson, 1941). For unknown reasons, enterobiasis is less prevalent in blacks.

PATHOGENESIS AND PATHOLOGY. Pinworms cause no recognized intestinal pathology. Some patients experience pruritus ani. This symptom leads to scratching and thus to direct anus-finger-mouth transmission, a highly efficient mechanism for parasite survival. Why some infected persons have severe pruritus ani and most have none is not known.

Occasionally adults, larvae, or ova are reported from unusual ectopic sites (Chandrasoma and Mendis, 1977). For example, pinworm migration into the female genital tract is a rare cause of pelvic granulomas. Although it is not infrequently found in the appendix, the association of pinworm infection with appendicitis seems to be coincidental rather than causal.

CLINICAL MANIFESTATIONS. The symptoms attributed to pinworm are legion and include anorexia, enuresis, masturbation, nausea, vomiting, abdominal pain, diarrhea, weight loss, and irritability. In controlled studies none of these symptoms, not even the single symptom generally attributed to pinworm infection—pruritus ani—is more common in infected than in uninfected children. Pruritus ani does, however, disappear with pinworm treatment and reappear with reinfection (Weller and Sorenson, 1941). Migration into the female urethra may be a cause of "night cries" in little girls and possibly of cystitis.

DIAGNOSIS. Pinworm is a noninvasive infection, and therefore neither eosinophilia nor elevations in serum IgE are found. Adult pinworms can be seen with the naked eye and may be brought to the physician for diagnosis. Under the microscope, the egg-laden female can be differentiated easily from artifacts and fibers. Pinworm eggs are not often found in the stool but can be demonstrated by the cellophane-tape test. In this procedure, the adhesive side of cellophane tape is pressed repeatedly against the perianal skin as soon as the patient awakens in the morning and before bathing. The tape is placed adhesive side down on a glass slide, with or without a drop of toluene, and the slide is examined microscopically for adherent ova. A single test will detect approximately half of all infections, three tests will diagnose 90 per cent of cases, and five tests are diagnostic of 100 per cent.

TREATMENT. In the absence of symptoms, there is no reason to treat this infection. Once the diagnosis is made, parents should be educated about the high prevalence and low pathogenic potential of pinworms. In societies in which worms are equated with a lack of personal cleanliness, parents should be advised that pinworm carries no such stigma and that the most rigidly applied sanitary measures, such as sterilization of bedclothes and two showers daily, have failed to control enterobiasis.

A high cure rate can be achieved with a variety of agents, several in single dose regimens. A single oral dose of mebendazole, 100 mg independent of body weight, or pyrantel pamoate, 11 mg/kg, or pyrvinium pamoate, 5 mg/kg to a maximum of 250 mg, will cure about 90 per cent of cases. A second course two weeks later is usually recommended. To prevent reinfection, some experts suggest that all other infected household members be treated, although there is no evidence that this measure significantly reduces reinfection.

PROPHYLAXIS. No effective control measures are known.

TRICHURIASIS

Trichuriasis, caused by the intestinal whipworm *Trichuris trichiura*, is worldwide in distribution, and is found particularly in rural areas with poor sanitation.

ETIOLOGY. Man, the principal host of *T. trichiura*, is infected by the ingestion of embryonated ova. Larvae hatch in the small intestine, and young worms develop to mature, egg-producing adults in one to three months. In very heavy infections whipworms may be found throughout the large intestine, but usually they remain in the cecum and ascending colon. Adult worms do not multiply in man but live for several years, producing characteristic eggs that embryonate in two to four weeks when deposited in moist shaded soil.

PATHOGENESIS AND PATHOLOGY. Adult *Trichuris* live with their thin anterior end inserted into the mucosa of the large bowel. The parasites are readily visible; rectal prolapse or sigmoidoscopy may disclose myriads of white worms on the mucosa. Manual detachment of the parasite leaves a small petechial hemorrhage at the site. In light infections there is remarkably little cellular response. In heavy infections the unparasitized mucosa is hyperemic, friable, and edematous. The mechanism of these changes and of the diarrhea or dysentery attributed to this nematode is unknown. Whipworm infection may coexist with amebic or balantidial dysentery.

CLINICAL MANIFESTATIONS. Most persons with trichuriasis have light infections of no medical importance. Heavy infections occur primarily in young children. Diarrhea, dysentery, and rectal prolapse are the only diseases attributable to heavy *T. trichiura* infection. In some cases dysentery is a consequence of amebiasis, which often coexists with trichuriasis.

DIAGNOSIS. The diagnosis is readily made by microscopic stool examination. A single unconcentrated stool specimen can lead to identification of as few as five worm pairs. Indeed, the prolific production of readily identifiable eggs ensures that this diagnosis is rarely missed by the laboratory.

TREATMENT. It is unnecessary to treat asymptomatic patients. When therapy is indicated, reduction in worm burden rather than cure is an acceptable goal. Until recently no safe, effective, and nontoxic oral drugs were available for treatment of trichuriasis. Now mebendazole in a dose of 100 mg twice a day for three days regardless of body weight yields a cure in over 75 per cent of cases and a reduction in worm burden in over 90 per cent, with no untoward effects (Peña Chavarría et al., 1973). Because mebendazole acts on contact with the worms, some patients with diarrhea may receive no benefit. The same treatment regimen can be repeated in three weeks, if necessary.

PROPHYLAXIS. The same control measures as those used for ascariasis are recommended.

ANISAKIASIS

Anisakiasis is caused by ingestion of one of several genera of larvae, commonly found in marine fish in Japan, Northern Europe, and North America. These include *Anisakis*, or herring-worm disease, *Phocanema*, or cod-fish disease, and *Contracaecum*.

ETIOLOGY. A fish-eating reptile, bird, or marine mammal is believed to be the definitive host, harboring the

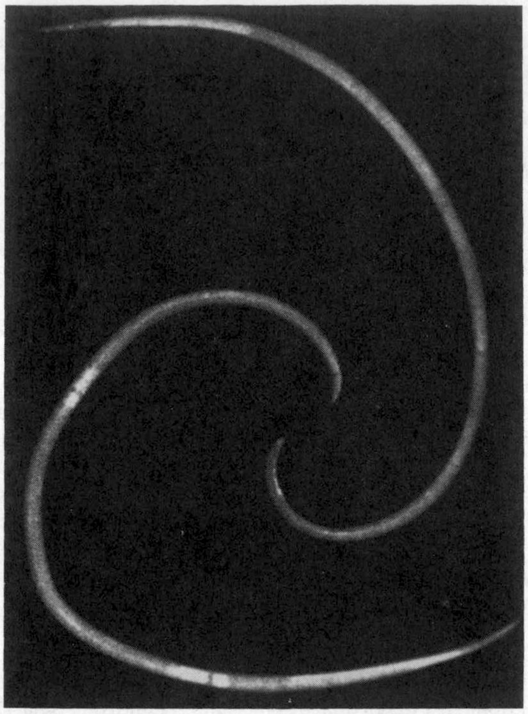

Figure 1. Anisakis larvae enlarged 3.3×. They must be differentiated from *Phocanema* and *Contracaecum,* the other anisakine larvae that are found in man. They can be differentiated by the absence of a cecum and appendix in the anisakis type. (Reproduced from Binford and Connor, Pathology of Tropical and Extraordinary Diseases Vol. 2, 1976).

adult nematode and excreting ova in its feces. Small crustaceans eat the larvae hatched from these eggs. Infective third stage larvae develop when these crustaceans are eaten by fish or squid. The larva cannot mature in man, who acquires the infection by eating raw, pickled, or lightly salted fish. The adult nematodes are large ascarids and human infections are caused by larvae belonging to the subfamily Anisakinae. The larvae may be 50 mm long and 1 mm wide.

PATHOGENESIS AND PATHOLOGY. In man the larva may remain in the lumen of the gastrointestinal mucosa. Incomplete early penetration of the gastric mucosa often is associated with local or generalized mucosal edema. Gastric edema may cause the typical acute abdominal pain, which often persists for several days after removal of the larva at endoscopy.

In other cases the larva invades the gastric or intestinal mucosa and sometimes penetrates into the mesentery or peritoneal cavity. In such cases the larva may be free in the peritoneal cavity or encapsulated in an abscess or granuloma located in the gastrointestinal wall, mesentery, or peritoneal cavity.

CLINICAL MANIFESTATIONS. Patients with luminal anisakiasis pass a larva from the mouth or rectum hours to days after the fish meal. Symptoms are limited to a tickling sensation and the unpleasant shock of seeing the worm. Acute gastric anisakiasis, the most common clinical manifestation, is characterized by acute cramping abdominal pain, with or without nausea, vomiting or abdominal distention, beginning 2 to 12 hours after a fish meal. Some patients also have urticaria. Chronic gastric, intestinal, or extraintestinal anisakiasis produces diverse abdominal complaints and is rarely diagnosed before laparotomy.

DIAGNOSIS. Diagnosis is made by demonstration of a thread-like filling defect on barium swallow or by direct visualization at endoscopy or laparotomy. Stool examination is useless, since larvae do not produce ova. Differentiation of the larva from *Ascaris,* which it resembles, as well as determination of the anisakine larval type, is based on the morphology of the larval gastrointestinal tract (Fig. 1).

TREATMENT. There is no specific therapy except removal of the larva. Many patients with acute gastric anisakiasis recover within a week after treatment with analgesics and antacid. When the pain is intolerable, the larva is removed at endoscopy with biopsy forceps. Other complications usually require surgical management.

PROPHYLAXIS. Human anisakiasis can be prevented by eating only well-cooked fish and squid, or by freezing fish intended for other uses at −20°C for 60 hours. Candling of fresh fish has been recommended to detect the presence of worms but is not always successful.

References

Banwell, J. G., and Schad, G. A.: Hookworm. Clinics in Gastroenterology 7:129, 1978.

Chandrasoma, P. T., and Mendis, K. N.: *Enterobius vermicularis* in ectopic sites. Am J Trop Med Hyg 26:644, 1977.

Ghadirian, E., and Arfaa, F.: Present status of trichostrongyliasis in Iran. Am J Trop Med Hyg 24:935, 1975.

Grove, D. I.: Treatment of strongyloidiasis with thiabendazole: an analysis of toxicity and effectiveness. Trans Roy Soc Trop Med & Hyg 76:114, 1982.

Gupta, M. C., Arora, K. L., Mithal, S., and Tandon, B. N.: Effect of periodic deworming on nutritional status of ascaris-infested preschool children receiving supplementary food. Lancet 2:108, 1977.

Olson, A. C. Jr, Lewis, M. D., and Hauser, M. L.: Proper identification of anisakine worms. Amer J Med Tech 49:111, 1983.

Pawlowski, Z. S.: Ascariasis: Host-pathogen biology. Rev Inf Dis 4:806, 1982.

Peña Chavarría, A., Swartzwelder, J. C., Villarejos, M., and Zeledón, R.: Mebendazole, an effective broad-spectrum anthelmintic. Am J Trop Med Hyg 22:592, 1973.

Roche, M., and Layrisse, M.: The nature and causes of "hookworm anemia." Am J Trop Med 15 (pt 2):1031, 1966.

Scowden, E. B., Schaffner, W., and Stone, W. J.: Overwhelming strongyloidiasis: an unappreciated opportunistic infection. Medicine 57:527, 1978.

Spillman, R. K.: Pulmonary ascariasis in tropical communities. Am J Trop Med Hyg 24:791, 1975.

Watten, R. H., Beckner, W. M., Cross, J. H., Gunning, J. J., and Jarimillo, J.: Clinical studies of capillariasis philippinensis. Trans R Soc Trop Med Hyg 66:828, 1972.

Weller, T. H., and Sorenson, C. W.: Enterobiasis: Its incidence and symptomatology in a group of 505 children. N Engl J Med 224:143, 1941.

144

CESTODIASES

Z. S. PAWLOWSKI, M.D.

Man can be infected with two classes of flatworms, the cestodes (tapeworms) and the trematodes (flukes). Adult tapeworms possess a scolex or head, a neck, and multiple hermaphroditic segments, or proglottids, that produce ova. Adults attach to the small intestine of the definitive host by suckers or hooklets on the scolex and only rarely cause serious disease. Larval forms are released from ingested ova and develop into bladderworms in the tissues of intermediate hosts, where they may produce severe and fatal diseases. The definitive host becomes infected after ingesting the larvae contained in the raw or rare flesh of the intermediate host. Man is thus the definitive host for tapeworms whose larval forms encyst in the flesh of the animals that comprise his sources of meat. He can be the intermediate host of some other tapeworms when he accidentally ingests ova excreted in the feces of domesticated or wild animals. Intestinal cestodiasis refers to tapeworm infections for which man is the definitive host. Somatic or tissue cestodiasis refers to the diseases that occur when man is the intermediate host of a cestode.

The most common causes of intestinal cestodiasis are *Hymenolepis nana*, the dwarf tapeworm; *Taenia saginata*, the beef tapeworm; and *Taenia solium*, the pork tapeworm. Less frequent causes are *Diphyllobothrium latum*, the broad or fish tapeworm; *Dipylidium caninum*, a dog tapeworm; and *Hymenolepis diminuta*, the rat tapeworm. Some other *Diphyllobothrium* spp, *Bertiella* spp, *Inermicapsifer* spp, *Raillietina* spp, and *Multiceps* spp are exceptionally rare and focally distributed causes of abdominal cestodiasis.

Somatic or tissue infections with the larval stages of cestodes may be caused by *T. solium*, *T. multiceps*, *Echinococcus granulosus*, *E. multilocularis*. *Diphyllobothrium erinacei*, *Sparganum proliferum*, *Mesocestoides* spp, and *Spirometra mansoni*.

HYMENOLEPIS NANA HYMENOLEPIDOSIS

H. nana, which mainly affects children, is the most common cause of intestinal cestodiasis in the world. The course of hymenolepidosis is greatly modified by immunity. Although widespread, these infections are usually mild and self-limited.

ETIOLOGY. Children are infected by ingesting *H. nana* eggs from the feces of human carriers. *H. nana* is a dwarf tapeworm that can grow to 4 cm and localizes in the ileum of man. Although the lifespan of adult tapeworms is only a few weeks, the intestinal population of tapeworms stays at hundreds to thousands for many years because *H. nana* can complete its life cycle in humans, who continually reinfect themselves with ova from their own feces and/or with larvae developing in their intestines.

Larvae hatch from ingested ova in the small intestine, penetrate a villus, and develop into small cysticercoids. After a few days, the young tapeworms break out of the villus, return to the intestinal lumen, attach to the mucosa, and develop into maturity within 10 days (Fig. 6, Chapter 86).

PATHOGENESIS AND PATHOLOGY. Lysis, desquamation, or necrosis of epithelial cells of the intestinal mucosa is caused by adult parasites and invading larvae. Larval stages may produce complete destruction of the invaded villi. Mechanical and toxic irritation of the intestinal mucosa by larval and adult worms causes enteritis in heavy infections. Intestinal absorption, especially in the ileum, may be disturbed.

CLINICAL MANIFESTATIONS. Symptoms depend on the intensity of the infection as modified by the individual's general nutrition and immunity. Most infections are asymptomatic. Abdominal discomfort, diarrhea, inanition, irritability, and urticaria have been ascribed to hymenolepidosis. Evaluation of sequelae is difficult because *H. nana* infection frequently coexists with malnutrition, protein deficiency, and other parasitic or bacterial infections of the intestine.

GEOGRAPHIC VARIATIONS. In arid and warm climates in populations with low standards of sanitation, 5 to 20 per cent of children may be infected with *H. nana*. Infection is especially common in Latin America, the Mediterranean countries, and the Indian subcontinent but occurs throughout the world. In adults infection either disappears spontaneously or continues at very low levels. Epidemics may occur in orphanages and other closed communities where fecal transmission is likely.

DIAGNOSIS. Infection is recognized by finding typical ova (Fig. 9, Chapter 86) in the feces. Ova can usually be detected by direct examination, but repeated examinations by flotation methods may be necessary after treatment or in light infections when the output of eggs is inconstant.

TREATMENT. Praziquantel (CESOL) given in a single dose of 25 mg/kg is the drug of choice. The alternative drug is niclosamide (YOMESAN) in a dose of 60 to 80 mg/kg, but not more than 2 g daily for five to seven days. Treatment with praziquantel or niclosamide cures over 90 per cent of infections. Heavy infections may require another course of treatment after two weeks. If these drugs are not available, paromomycin (45 mg/kg for five to seven days) may be used. Asymptomatic infections should be treated to reduce the spread of hymenolepidosis, especially in closed communities.

PROPHYLAXIS. Good personal hygiene and high levels of general sanitation diminish the exposure to infection. In epidemic situations mass treatment of the infected, isolation of the uninfected, long-term surveillance, and improvement of sanitation are important control measures.

TAENIA SAGINATA TAENIASIS

Man is the definitive host for *T. saginata*, the beef tapeworm, which causes a benign intestinal infection. When man ingests the larval form of *T. saginata*, the cysticercus, in raw beef, the tapeworm excysts, attaches to the small intestine, and matures into an adult.

ETIOLOGY. The adult beef tapeworm is between 4 and 12 meters long. Its scolex is usually localized in the upper jejunum, but its strobila may extend down to the terminal ileum. The parasite can live as long as its host and not uncommonly persists for 30 to 40 years.

PATHOGENESIS AND PATHOLOGY. *T. saginata* may cause subacute inflammation of the small intestinal mucosa but usually causes little pathology. Intestinal transit time and gastric acidity may decrease. Moderate eosinophilia may occur but is not correlated with a rise in serum IgE, which also occurs in some patients.

CLINICAL MANIFESTATIONS. Ninety-eight per cent of carriers feel some sensation in the perianal area when proglottids migrate out of the anus. Other symptoms are present in 76 per cent of patients, but many of these complaints may be related to the patients' knowledge that they harbor a large worm in their intestine. Abdominal pain, nausea, anorexia, weight loss, weakness, globus hystericus, vomiting, diarrhea or constipation, increased appetite, increased body weight, and allergic symptoms have all been reported. In fact, most patients are usually asymptomatic until they discover that they are parasitized. *T. saginata* tissue infection, or cysticercosis, of man has not been documented.

Appendicitis or cholecystitis may be caused by motile proglottids of *T. saginata* that stray into the appendix or bile ducts.

GEOGRAPHIC VARIATIONS. Geographic variations in the infection may occur; the natural transmission of *T. saginata* in the Philippines and Taiwan is not clear. Infections are common both in urban (Europe and the United States) and pastoral communities. East and central Africa, the south-central Asian republics of the U.S.S.R., and the Near East countries are areas with a high prevalence of infection.

DIAGNOSIS. *T. saginata* must be differentiated from *T. solium,* which causes cysticercosis. Finding *Taenia* eggs on anal swabs or during fecal examination confirms the diagnosis of taeniasis but does not differentiate *T. saginata* from *T. solium* because the ova are indistinguishable (Fig. 9, Chapter 86). Final species determination requires examination of either the scolex (unarmed in *T. saginata*) or the gravid proglottids (more than 15 uterine branches per side in *T. saginata*) (Fig. 6, Chapter 86). *T. saginata* gravid proglottids usually actively pass through the anus. Differentiation of *T. saginata* from *T. solium* is of critical clinical and epidemiologic importance.

TREATMENT. The drugs of choice are niclosamide (YOMESAN) and praziquantel (CESOL); both are effective in over 90 per cent of cases. Niclosamide is given in an early morning dose of 2 g in adults; purgation is usually not necessary. Praziquantel is given in a single dose of 5 to 10 mg/kg. The only contraindication to treatment with niclosamide or praziquantel is the first trimester of pregnancy, when any anthelmintic treatment is undesirable. Alternative drugs are paromomycin in a single dose of 4 g, metallic tin compounds (five-day treatment), and mepacrine. The efficacy of the treatment is evaluated either by finding the scolex (which is difficult after using niclosamide or praziquantel), or by negative examination for eggs and proglottids four months after treatment.

PROPHYLAXIS. For personal prophylaxis one should avoid eating raw or semiraw beef. Lightly infected beef carcasses may pass the routine meat inspection. Prophylaxis at the national level requires proper sanitation, meat inspection, and freezing of lightly infected carcasses.

TAENIA SOLIUM

Taenia solium taeniasis is a human intestinal infection caused by the adult pork tapeworm. *T. solium* cysticercosis is an infection with the larval stage, the cysticercus. *T. solium* cysticercosis may be fatal because the larvae frequently localize in the brain.

ETIOLOGY. Adult pork tapeworms do not differ very much from *T. saginata,* but they can be differentiated. The pork tapeworm is smaller (1½ to 8 m), the scolex is armed with hooks, and the proglottids have a three-lobed ovary and less than 15 lateral uterine branches on the side (Fig. 6, Chapter 86). The proglottids do not move actively and are usually expelled passively with feces in groups of three to five. The ova of *T. solium* are indistinguishable from those of *T. saginata.* The cysticercus is a larva, 5 to 20 mm in diameter, that consists of a bladder filled with fluid surrounding a scolex armed with hooks.

Man acquires intestinal infection (taeniasis) by ingesting undercooked pork infected with cysticerci and cysticercosis, the tissue form, by ingesting *T. solium* ova disseminated by a human carrier. Autoinfection with *T. solium* eggs is not uncommon. Although *T. solium* occurs focally throughout the world, it is highly prevalent in areas with poor sanitation where raw, uninspected pork is eaten. In seven countries of Central and South America cysticercosis is found in over 1 per cent of the pigs slaughtered. Other endemic foci include central and southern Africa as well as some countries of Southeast Asia. *T. solium* is nearly eradicated from Europe and North America.

T. SOLIUM TAENIASIS

The pathogenesis, pathology, and clinical manifestations of *T. solium* taeniasis are similar to those of *T. saginata.* Because of the risk of cysticercosis, early treatment of *T. solium* taeniasis is important for clinical and epidemiologic reasons. *T. solium* taeniasis usually responds better than *T. saginata* to taeniacides. The success of treatment should be evaluated by periodic examination of the feces by the laboratory and visual inspection of the feces for proglottids by the patient. Proglottids and eggs usually reappear within two months if treatment is unsuccessful.

T. SOLIUM CYSTICERCOSIS

PATHOGENESIS AND PATHOLOGY. Man may be parasitized by one to more than 1000 cysticerci. Muscular localization of cysticerci is frequently unnoticed unless calcified cysticerci are incidentally recognized by x-ray examination. Subcutaneous cysticerci produce detectable nodules that are easy to obtain for biopsy. Ocular and cerebral localizations of cysticerci cause the most serious damage, and cysticerci seem to have a predilection for the central nervous system. Localization in the hemispherical parenchyma or cortex and the subarachnoid space are most common. Less frequently, cysticerci localize in the ventricles, brain stem, cerebellum, and spinal cord. Meningitis, meningoencephalitis, ependymitis, and/or signs of focal damage occur, depending on the site of localization. Living cysticerci usually provoke a mild cellular response. Dead ones cause a foreign body granuloma and may become calcified.

CLINICAL MANIFESTATIONS. Injury from cysticercosis is of mechanical and/or inflammatory nature; the localization and number of cysticerci, as well as the host reaction, determine the symptoms and signs. There are four syndromes of cerebral cysticercosis: (1) Symptoms of a slow-growing intracranial tumor with focal neurologic deficits, epileptic seizures, and increased intracranial pressure. This presentation occurs mainly in adults with a single or few cysticerci. (2) Rapid development of increased intracranial pressure, loss of vision, and organic brain syndrome (occurs mainly in children with heavy infections). (3) Symptoms of leptomeningitis, ependymitis, and internal hydrocephalus; these symptoms occur when cysticerci localize at the base of the brain. (4) Sudden unexpected death when cysticerci affect vital centers of the brain (Flisser et al., 1982).

The symptoms of ocular cysticercosis vary according to the part of the eye affected. Cysticercosis often remains asymptomatic in other internal organs and tissues.

DIAGNOSIS. The diagnosis of cysticercosis is made by identification of the scolex and hooks or microscopic structures of the cysticercus wall in biopsied or autopsied material.

The presumptive diagnosis of cysticercosis may be based on the clinical findings of subcutaneous nodules, a cysticercus-like body in the eye, characteristic lesions in CT scans of the brain, calcified cysticerci on radiographs, and/or a high antibody titer against *Taenia* antigens by indirect hemagglutination, immunofluorescence, or bentonite flocculation.

The detection of *Taenia* eggs or proglottids from the patient or a close relative make the possibility of cysticercosis more likely.

TREATMENT. For many years the only effective treatment for cerebral or ocular cysticercosis has been surgery. The neurosurgical fatality rate is between 24 and 67 per cent, depending on the location and number of parasites. Recently praziquantel (CESOL) has been introduced into the treatment of in-patients with neuro-cysticercosis. In about 60 per cent of cases, chemotherapy is successful, but it is ineffective in some and contraindicated in others (e.g., ocular cysticercosis). Further studies of the chemotherapy of human cysticercosis are necessary to determine the optimal use of the available cysticercicides.

PROPHYLAXIS. *T. solium* infections are controlled by meat inspection, improvement of general sanitation, health education, and early treatment of human taeniasis. Personal prophylactic measures against cysticercosis are the same as those used in other fecal-borne infections. Early diagnosis and treatment of *T. solium* taeniasis is important.

DIPHYLLOBOTHRIASIS

Diphyllobothrium latum, the fish tapeworm, is the longest tapeworm of man (3 to 15 m). The strobila of *D. latum* resides in the small intestine and absorbs large quantities of vitamin B_{12}. If the parasite is located in the proximal portion of the jejunum, macrocytic, megaloblastic anemia may develop.

D. latum infection is easy to diagnose by fecal examination; a large number of characteristic operculated ova (Fig. 9, Chapter 86) are produced as early as three to five weeks after ingestion of an invasive plerocercoid larva in fish. Proglottids are also distinctive because of the rosette-shaped uterus that lies medially in each segment (Fig. 6, Chapter 86). Diphyllobothriasis is easily cured with niclosamide, praziquantel, or other taeniacides.

The infection is common in communities where freshwater fish are eaten raw or partly cooked, for example, among fishermen at river deltas or lakes in Finland, Siberia, Canada, and the United States. Infection can be prevented by avoiding raw or undercooked fish in endemic areas. Control of endemic diphyllobothriasis is difficult because of the traditional eating habits of the local population and the large reservoir of infection in wild, fish-eating animals.

OTHER INTESTINAL CESTODIASES

At least seven other species of *Diphyllobothrium* have been reported as sporadic causes of human disease in Alaska, Greenland, and Peru. Clinical and epidemiologic aspects of these are similar to *D. latum*.

Hymenolepidosis due to *H. diminuta* (the rat tapeworm) is not as rare in the world as was once believed. More than 1 per cent of children are infected in the New Guinea highlands and some villages in Iran, where human population have close contact with the parasite in rodents and the insects (fleas, beetles, *Myriapoda*) that serve as intermediate hosts. Clinical manifestations of *H. diminuta* infection are usually mild. The diagnosis is made by finding typical eggs in the feces. Infection can be easily eradicated by treatment with niclosamide or other taeniacides.

Dipylidium caninum is a common tapeworm of dogs and cats and incidentally of man. Most infections occur in children, who ingest fleas and flour beetles that are infected with cysticercoid larvae. Dipylidiasis only rarely causes diarrhea or allergic reactions. The diagnosis is made by finding the characteristic pumpkin seed-shaped proglottids or ova (Figs. 6 and 9, Chapter 86) in the feces. Taeniacides are very effective, and many infections probably clear spontaneously.

Rarely, man may be parasitized by the rat tapeworms, *Raillietina* spp. and *Inermicapsifer* spp., and the monkey tapeworm, *Bertiella studeri*. Little is known about the clinical, epidemiologic, and taxonomic features of these parasites.

ECHINOCOCCOSIS (HYDATID DISEASE)

Echinococcosis is a zoonotic human infection caused by the larval hydatid form of *Echinococcus granulosus*. Man acquires the infection by ingesting ova shed in the feces of infected dogs. The clinical course is that of a chronic, space-occupying lesion mainly in the liver or lungs. Patients may remain asymptomatic or die of complications, depending on the size and location of the hydatid cyst.

ETIOLOGY. In the traditional, pastoral life cycle, man is infected by close contact with his sheep dogs. In the natural cycle, the hydatid occurs in the organs of sheep (intermediate host), which, like man, are infected by ova disseminated in the feces of dogs. Dogs are infected when they eat the hydatids in the tissue of sheep or other domesticated herbivores. In the sylvatic cycle, wild carnivores and herbivores maintain the cycle in nature. Man is infected by ova from his hunting dogs, who are infected by eating larvae in the tissues of wild herbivores.

E. granulosus larvae in man consist of a primary cyst, which can continue to develop for years to a size of over 20 cm in diameter. Secondary (daughter) cysts are produced in the primary cysts or, rarely, outside the hydatid. Brood capsules containing tens to hundreds of invaginated protoscoleces may develop inside the primary and daughter cysts. Protoscoleces that are liberated from a cyst may develop into secondary cysts, for example, in the abdominal cavity.

PATHOGENESIS AND PATHOLOGY. Hydatid cysts develop most frequently in the liver (60 per cent) and lungs (20 per cent), rarely in the brain (3 per cent), eye, heart, bone, and other internal organs. The primary cyst in the liver is usually surrounded by a thick fibrous capsule produced by the host. Pathologic changes depend largely on the location and size of the cyst and are mainly due to pressure from the enlarging cyst. Complications include anaphylaxis from sudden rupture of a cyst, pyogenic abscesses in secondarily infected cysts, spontaneous fractures of infected bones, respiratory distress, liver damage, and severe ocular or CNS damage. Anaphylaxis can occur when cysts rupture spontaneously or at surgery because many individuals have become sensitized by leakage of small amounts of material from the intact cyst.

CLINICAL MANIFESTATIONS. Symptoms depend on the location and size of the cyst. Hepatic echinococcosis is usually asymptomatic until the cyst has become large. Even then, the symptoms are usually vague unless secondary pyogenic infection or pressure on blood vessels or bile ducts causes obstructive jaundice and portal hypertension. Echinococcosis of the lung may remain asymptomatic for years. Rupture into the pleural cavity or the bronchi, bacterial infection, or pressure on pulmonary vessels or bronchi may cause lung abscesses, bronchopleural fistulae, atelectasis, or pulmonary hypertension. Cerebral echinococcosis is often fatal because of the size of the growing cyst. In other internal organs, echinococcosis produces symptoms characteristic of slow-growing, benign tumors. Calcified cysts in the spleen or kidney, for example, may be found accidentally without any symptoms of disease.

GEOGRAPHIC VARIATION. Each strain of *E. granulosus* circulating in definite natural cycles (dog-sheep-dog, dog-pig-dog, dog-horse-dog, domesticated herbivora-wild carnivora-man) shows its own growth pattern in in vitro culture and different degrees of invasiveness for man. These differences may explain the occurrence of outbreaks of human echinococcosis in certain regions of the world; e.g., in the Turkana tribe in Kenya. Echinococcosis is endemic in many countries throughout the world where sheep, dogs, and man live in close contact.

DIAGNOSIS. The definitive diagnosis of *E. granulosus* depends on the identification of typical protoscoleces with hooks and morphology of the cysts on microscopic examination. Rarely, hooks are present in the sputum, duodenal contents, feces, urine, or peritoneal or pleural fluid. Radiographic, sonographic and CT (computerized tomography) examinations that show a cyst and positive serologic tests (hemagglutination, complement fixation, flocculation, and immunofluorescent antibody) strongly support the diagnosis.

TREATMENT. Some cases of human echinococcosis need no treatment (old calcified cysts, small hepatic cysts, some pulmonary cysts). Various surgical techniques such as total extirpation, marsupialization, and removal after opening have been developed to remove symptomatic hydatid cysts. The success of surgical intervention depends on proper diagnosis of the number, location, and size of the cysts, as well as on the skill of the surgical team. Surgical rupture of the cyst may cause anaphylactic shock or secondary echinococcosis unless its contents are sterilized with 15 or 20 per cent hypertonic saline. Chemotherapeutic methods of treatment with some benzimidazoles are still being investigated.

PROPHYLAXIS. Personal prophylaxis in endemic areas is based on avoiding contact with infected dogs and their feces. Some countries have developed public health programs for control of echinococcosis.

OTHER TISSUE CESTODIASES

Alveolar echinococcosis, caused by *Echinococcus multilocularis*, differs from *E. granulosus* infection in many respects. The distribution of *E. multilocularis* in man is limited to the northern hemisphere (southern Germany, southeast France, Switzerland, Siberia, China, Japan, central Canada, north central U.S. and Alaska). The parasite circulates naturally in wild Canidae and wild rodents. Man is incidentally infected when he ingests ova on the fur or in the feces of infected foxes or other Canidae. Domestic dogs and cats that catch and eat the flesh of wild rodents have been implicated as a source of human infection. *E. multilocularis* larvae usually develop in the liver. The larvae are alveolar and consist of hundreds or thousands of small vesicles (0.5 to 2 mm in diameter). Alveolar echinococcus may be necrotic in its center but may also spread, either by producing new vesicles peripherally or by metastasizing to other organs. The clinical manifestations of alveolar echinococcosis are similar to those of liver neoplasm, including protracted jaundice and emaciation. The prognosis is poor. Serologic tests (immunofluorescent antibody and hemagglutination) and the patient's history (possibility of exposure) are helpful. The final diagnosis is established at surgery or at autopsy by parasitologic and histopathologic examination of the lesions. Surgical treatment is sometimes successful. Recently, high doses of mebendazole have been used in human cases of alveolar echinococcosis with promising results.

Coenurosis in man is caused by bladder larvae of *T. multiceps*, a tapeworm that parasitizes dogs and sheep. Cerebral and ocular coenurosis produces symptoms similar to those of cerebral or ocular cysticercosis. The definitive diagnosis is usually possible only by parasitologic examination of larvae removed at surgery or autopsy.

Other tapeworm larvae that invade man include *Sparganum proliferum, Diphyllobothrium erinacei,* and *Spirometra mansoni,* which occur in the Far East and South America. The larvae usually invade the subcutaneous tissue or the eye, causing the disease called sparganosis. The infection is acquired by ingestion of raw frog or snake or by the use of their raw tissues as poultices. Treatment is surgical.

References

Flisser, A., et al.: Cysticercosis: Present State of Knowledge and Perspectives. New York, Academic Press, 1982.

Muller, R.: Worms and Disease. London, W. Heinemann Medical Books, 1975, p. 38.

Pawlowski, Z., and Schultz, M. G.: Taeniasis and cysticercosis (*Taenia saginata*). Adv Parasitol 10:269, 1972.

Slais, J.: The morphology and pathogenicity of the bladder worms *Cysticercus cellulosae* and *Cysticercus bovis.* Prague, Academia, 1970.

Smyth, J. D., and Heath, D. D.: Pathogenesis of larval cestodes in mammals. Helm Abstr 39:1, 1970.

WHO Guidelines for Surveillance, Prevention and Control of Echinococcosis Hydatidosis, VPH/81:28, WHO Geneva, 1981.

145

SCHISTOSOMIASIS

GUNTHER DENNERT, PH.D.

Human schistosomiasis is a water-borne, parasitic disease that presently afflicts at least 200 million people in Asia, Africa, the Caribbean, and Latin America. It was first recorded in Egypt about 4000 years ago. Schistosomiasis is caused by schistosomes or bloodflukes—digenetic trematodes from the superfamily of Schistosomatoidea. Unlike other trematodes, they are elongated and resemble roundworms, apparently as an adaptation to living in blood vessels. They have oral and ventral suckers and a nonmuscular pharynx. The female worm is held in the gynaecophoric canal of the male (the schist) and lays nonoperculate eggs. The eggs are excreted with human waste and release a free-swimming form that infects and multiplies in the intermediate host, a snail. A second free-swimming form is released from the snail and infects the definitive vertebrate host. Their geographic distribution (see Chapter 86) is limited by the availability of a suitable snail host.

ETIOLOGY AND LIFE CYCLE. Schistosomiasis is caused by one of three parasitic worms that live in one of several sets of veins. *S. mansoni* inhabits the inferior mesenteric veins and causes intestinal schistosomiasis. The eggs have a large lateral spine. The principal molluscan hosts are snails of the genus *Biomphalaria.* Among vertebrates besides man, rodents, insectivores, marsupials, and cattle can be infected, providing an animal reservoir for this parasite. *S. mansoni* occurs in most African countries, Saudi Arabia, the northern and eastern parts of South America, and some Caribbean islands. *S. haematobium* lives in the vesical venous plexus and causes urinary schistosomiasis. It is less adaptable to nonhuman hosts, but other primates and even some rodents can be infected. This species lays eggs with a large terminal spine and is endemic in Africa and some Middle Eastern countries. *S. japonicum* is found mostly in the superior mesenteric veins and causes intestinal schistosomiasis like that of *S. mansoni.* Its eggs have a tiny lateral spine. The principal snail host is the genus *Oncomelania. S. japonicum* is the least host-specific of the three schistosomes and infects many different domestic animals. It is found in the Philippines, Japan, the Chinese mainland, Thailand, and Indonesia. Recently, another species, *S. mekongi,* which closely resembles *S. japonica,* has been recognized in Laotian refugees (Nash et al., 1982).

The life cycle of schistosomes (Chapter 86) (Ansari, 1973; Jordan and Webbe, 1969) alternates between two generations. The sexual generation lives in the vertebrate and lays eggs from which a short-lived, free-swimming form (miracidium) hatches. The miracidium infects a freshwater snail and establishes the second, asexual generation. It becomes a mother sporocyst that gives rise to daughter sporocysts, which in turn produce numerous cercariae. The cercariae leave the snail, infect the vertebrate by skin penetration, migrate as schistosomula to the target tissue, and mature into adult worms.

The function of the spine on the eggs may be to anchor them so as to resist the flow of blood and to penetrate venules. Eggs release histiolytic substances as they pass through the tissues and during maturation of the miracidium. Most eggs (about 50 per cent) do not reach the lumen of the bladder or intestine but are trapped in tissues and cause serious tissue damage. Excreted eggs hatch at low osmotic pressure in water at temperatures of between 10 and 30° C. The miracidium (about 0.16 mm in length) is propelled by cilia on four rows of epidermal plates. It has a bilobed, probably nonfunctional gut and four flame cells that serve as the excretory system. The miracidium shows positive phototaxis and negative geotaxis and swims to the snail to which it attaches. Penetration is aided by glands that secrete lytic substances. The miracidium loses its ciliated coat after penetration and reforms into a nonmotile sac, the mother sporocyst, in which germinal cells differentiate to daughter sporocysts. This process takes about 10 to 15 days. The daughter sporocysts are motile and migrate to the hepatic and gonadal tissues while they grow. Cercariae differentiate from germinal cells in the daughter sporocysts, pass through the blood sinuses and tissues, and leave from the edge of the snail's mantle. The sporocysts regenerate and produce more cercariae. The output of cercariae is variable, but up to 100,000 cercariae can be released per snail. The life cycle in the snail takes about four to seven weeks.

The cercariae have a discrete head and a bifurcated tail that allows locomotion. The head carries small oral and ventral suckers, a nonfunctional gut, flame cells, and a primitive nervous system. Three or four pairs of unicellular glands close to the ventral sucker (posterior postacetabular glands) secrete mucilage that assists in attachment. The other glands (preacetabular glands) empty during penetration. If the cercariae fail to find a vertebrate host they will die after about 8 to 12 hours because their glycogen reserve is exhausted. After penetration, the cercaria, having emptied its glands and shed its tail and cercarial glycocalyx, is now called a schistosomulum (about 0.1 mm in length).

The trilaminate tegument is replaced within a few hours by a multilaminate one that is characteristic of the adult worm. There is evidence that the schistosomula take up host antigens, which may prevent immune attack by masking the foreign antigens. Within the next 48 hours the schistosomula penetrate the subcutaneous tissue and enter the venous blood vessels and peripheral lymphatics. During the next five to seven days, they are transported via the heart to the lungs.

The next stage of the migration is not well understood. The schistosomula either migrate via the blood vessels to the portal system or directly through the diaphragm, which takes about 10 to 20 days. The parasites mature and mate in the liver and then migrate to the veins of the vesical plexus or to the mesenteric veins, where egg production begins. The worms migrate as a pair with the female held in the schist of the male. When the caliber of the venules becomes small enough to restrict migration, the female often leaves the male and continues to migrate as far as the size of the smallest venules will permit. Between 300 and 3000 eggs can be released per day per worm and are found in the stool or urine as early as 30 to 40 days after infection. Schistosomes usually live 5 to 10 years but have also been reported to survive for more than 30 years. Adult parasites (Chapter 86) are between 6 and 28 mm long. Their most important energy source is carbohydrate that is incompletely degraded to organic acids such as lactic acid, acetic acid, and propionic acid. Erythrocytes are ingested, and a hematin-like pigment that is regurgitated by the parasites is phagocytosed by reticuloendothelial cells.

PATHOGENESIS AND PATHOLOGY. The pathology of schistosomiasis (Warren, 1973; von Lichtenberg et al., 1971; Sadun et al., 1970) can be divided into stages that are associated with the life cycle of the schistosome in the infected individual. The pathogenesis of most of the lesions and clinical manifestations are related to the host response to the invading cercariae, the migrating adult worms, and the ova. The fundamental lesion of schistosomiasis, the granuloma, is formed around the ova in response to antigens contained in the hatching fluid. The cercariae, schistosomula, and adult worms also sensitize the host not only to their own antigens but also to cross-reactive antigens in the ova. Although many ova are excreted in the body fluids of the patients, a large number remain in the mucosa of the bowel and bladder. Others are "swept back" in the portal circulation to the liver or to ectopic localization in the lungs or central nervous system (CNS). Granuloma formation around these retained ova account for the manifestations of established, chronic schistosomiasis.

Schistosome Dermatitis. Schistosome dermatitis occurs in response to cercarial skin penetration and migration. The cercaria cause minute areas of necrosis during penetration and early migration, but these mechanical effects cause no signs or symptoms. The dermatitis, which may range from transient urticaria to macules to a papular rash, is uncommon in natives of endemic areas. It occurs more commonly in visitors who have been sensitized recently but lack the relative immunity of local inhabitants with low-grade, established schistosomiasis. Penetration of cercariae disorganizes the squamous cells, and migration damages the transitional cells of the granular layer beneath the squames. Experimental studies suggest that unsensitized individuals develop edema and a polymorphonuclear infiltrate that is replaced by mononuclear cells within 48 hours. Sensitized individuals develop a more rapid and more intense polymorphonuclear response with more tissue damage. The accelerated reaction can be provoked either by serum or lymphoid cells (Colley et al., 1972; Stirewalt and Dorsey, 1974).

Acute Schistosomiasis (Katayama Syndrome). Schistosomula migration usually causes no symptoms, but inflammatory reactions in the lungs and liver may occasionally produce fever and cough. Maturation, migration of adults, and early egg production may cause an acute febrile illness called Katayama fever. It can occur in any form of schistosomiasis but is most common in infections with *S. japonicum*, probably because this schistosome produces the most ova. The majority of patients with schistosomiasis, however, never experience the acute phase of the disease. The acute syndrome is caused by local reactions to young schistosomes and ova and consists of local and general symptoms including abdominal pain, diarrhea, fever, weakness, myalgia, and headache. The pathogenesis is similar to that of serum sickness—that is, it appears to be an immune complex disease elicited by antibody production to the antigenic stimulus of cercariae, adult worms, and ova.

Established and Chronic Schistosomiasis. In established infections intensive ova production by adult worms and excretion of large numbers of ova by the patient has commenced. In late infections egg output is often decreased as the disease becomes chronic with portal hypertension or obstructive uropathy. The pathologic reaction of established and late schistosomiasis is essentially a series of chronic inflammatory lesions elicited primarily by ova but also by dead worms. Therefore, the severity of the disease is proportional to the severity of the infection—the relative burden of worms and ova. A heavy burden of worms and ova is necessary to produce significant disease because small vascular lesions are easily repaired. The pathologic manifestations of significant disease consist of progressive tissue destruction and formation of fibrous tissue in various organs, depending on the species of schistosome.

The Egg Granuloma. Severe pathologic manifestations of schistosomiasis (Warren, 1972) are to a large extent the result of an immunologic response of the host to the eggs. The eggs start eliciting a reaction when the encased miracidium matures (day 6). Histiolytic substances are secreted, leading to a focal granulomatous reaction (day 12). In acute schistosomiasis, a periovular area of necrosis is seen with or without deposition of a hyaline eosinophilic band (Hoeppli phenomenon), surrounded by an exudative cellular reaction consisting of many polymorphonuclear leukocytes, lymphocytes, and eosinophils. Later, the central necrosis and the perivascular eosinophilic material disappear, and the leukocytes are replaced by epithelioid cells. Foreign body giant cells surround and invade the dead egg, completing the formation of the pseudotubercle, which is the classic lesion of schistosomiasis (Fig. 1). The egg may become calcified or may disappear entirely. Healing may be complete or scarring may occur with thickening of the wall of the intestine or bladder or obstruction of the portal venules. Thus, the most serious lesions occur during early infection, so that a massive primary infection may lead later to severe clinical symptoms.

The pathogenesis of the egg granuloma has been studied mostly in mice. Eggs are isolated from mouse tissue and injected into the tail vein of recipient mice. Mice previously sensitized by intraperitoneal injection of eggs show an accelerated and augmented inflammatory response around

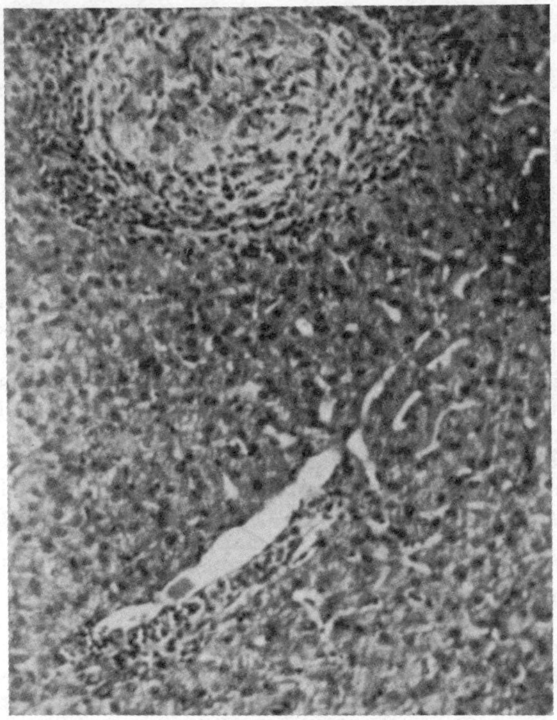

Figure 1. Liver biopsy with a typical schistosomal pseudotubercle surrounded by a halo of lymphocytes and eosinophils. The portal space is infiltrated by lymphocytes and eosinophils (×360). (From Diaz-Rivera, R. S. et al.: Ann Intern Med 47:1082, 1957.)

eggs in the lungs. The ability to respond in this fashion can be transferred to recipient mice by injecting lymphoid cells but not serum and can be inhibited in presensitized mice by antilymphocyte serum. This is in agreement with the contention that the granuloma formation is a kind of delayed type hypersensitivity (DTH) reaction. Sensitization can also be achieved by a cell-free extract from eggs (SEA), and granuloma formation can be induced by SEA-coated bentonite particles. Eggs depleted of SEA by incubation in tissue culture do not induce granulomas. Granuloma formation is inhibited by substances that inhibit DTH but not by humoral antibody synthesis. It is also suppressed in thymectomized, immuno-incompetent animals. The egg granuloma may benefit the infected animal to some degree by curtailing the diffusion of antigens. As mentioned above, mice that have passed the acute stage of infection regularly modulate their granulomas, so that lesions become smaller during the chronic phase of the disease. This modulation is probably caused by suppressor T cells that may act on the DTH effector cells (Colley, 1976). It is not known whether similar reactions occur in man.

S. mansoni and S. japonicum. Both schistosomes live in the mesenteric veins and therefore affect primarily the gastrointestinal tract and the liver. There is generalized lymphadenopathy, soft hepatomegaly, and soft splenomegaly in established infections. Eggs in the mucosa and submucosa of the colon and small intestine give rise to granulomas. The intestinal mucosa is reddened and edematous with yellowish papules, small hemorrhages, and occasional small ulcerations. Acute changes in the colon are confined to the lumen. Later, massive oviposition causes progression from the pseudotubercular stage to a diffuse transmural fibrosis. Massive intraluminal polypoid lesions are frequent in Egypt. Ova that are "swept back" by the portal venous current cause liver inflammation and damage. Hepatic granulomas induced by these ova may totally occlude the intrahepatic radials of the portal venules. Acute endophlebitis results in occlusion of other vessels by organized thrombi. Recanalized, newly formed blood vessels communicate through the wall of the vein with other vessels (Garcia-Palmieri and Marcial-Rojas, 1962). There is also a great increase in thin, straight arterial branches without evidence of obstruction. As shown in Figure 2, this increase in arterial branches is responsible for a large periportal vascular network that maintains normal blood flow to hepatic cells but contributes to portal hypertension. Eventually, there is a marked increase in fibrous tissue in the portal fields that surrounds and compresses the hepatic venules. These vascular and fibrotic changes in the portal areas cause them to be markedly broadened and lengthened, so that they stand out in cross-section. This appearance has given rise to the term "pipestem" fibrosis to describe this condition. The liver is enlarged, slightly nodular, and not hobnailed. The gross appearance is altogether different from that of Laennec's cirrhosis. The hepatic parenchymal cells do not show the degenerative or necrotic changes of Laennec's or post-hepatitis cirrhosis.

This unique type of liver pathology explains the development of severe portal hypertension with preservation of the function of hepatic parenchymal cells. Maintenance of

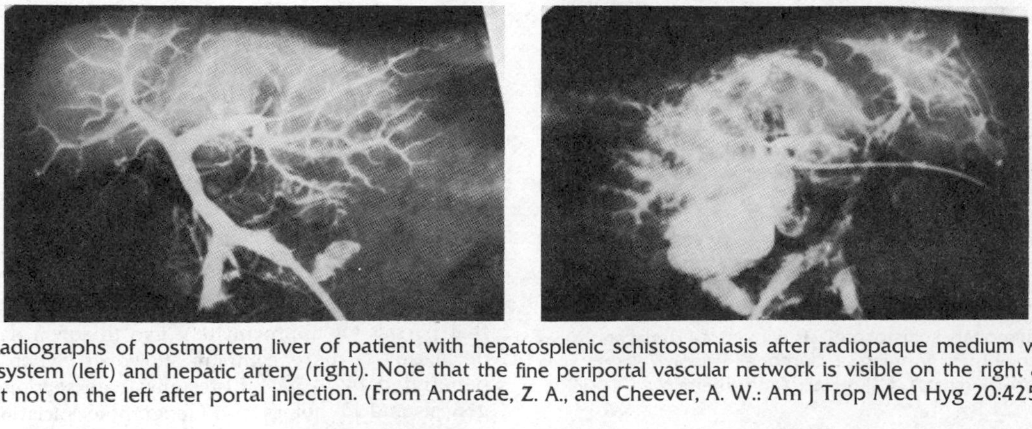

Figure 2. Radiographs of postmortem liver of patient with hepatosplenic schistosomiasis after radiopaque medium was injected into portal system (left) and hepatic artery (right). Note that the fine periportal vascular network is visible on the right after arterial injection but not on the left after portal injection. (From Andrade, Z. A., and Cheever, A. W.: Am J Trop Med Hyg 20:425, 1971.)

liver cell function may contribute to the capacity of patients with schistosomal portal hypertension to tolerate multiple episodes of bleeding from esophageal varices. Massive varices develop in patients with severe illness at a much younger age than is characteristic of patients with Laennec's cirrhosis.

Most patients do not develop severe hepatosplenic schistosomiasis. The pathologic findings vary from a few hepatic granulomas to fully developed pipestem fibrosis. Severely infected individuals may develop portal hypertension within a few months, but the pathologic process more commonly develops over a period of many years.

Embolization of ova into the pulmonary vasculature may result in multiple intravascular granulomas and arteritis, pulmonary hypertension, and cor pulmonale. The pathognomonic lesions are intra-arterial and para-arterial granulomas that form a dumbbell shape (Fig. 3). Pulmonary localization occurs much more frequently in patients with portal hypertension secondary to severe hepatosplenic disease. Significant, isolated pulmonary schistosomiasis is rare.

S. japonicum affects the same organs as *S. mansoni*, but there are pathologic differences. *S. japonicum* lays about 10 times more eggs than *S. mansoni*. These eggs are found in aggregates and tend to calcify. There is more infiltration of neutrophils and a larger, more exudative granuloma. *S. japonicum* pairs tend to stay in one location and produce large masses of eggs that cause intestinal obstruction and a higher frequency of ectopic localization.

Splenomegaly occurs in all patients with severe hepatosplenic schistosomiasis. At least two factors contribute to splenic enlargement, namely, passive congestion and cellular proliferation. In early infection, cell proliferation is

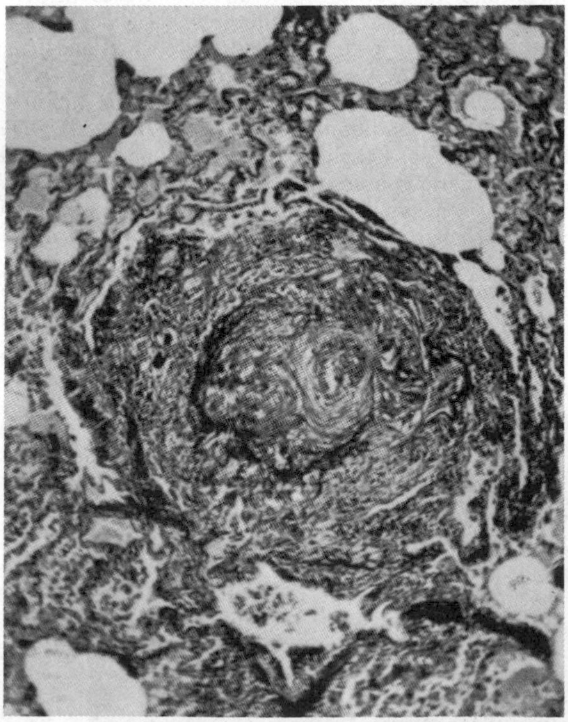

Figure 3. Pulmonary schistosomiasis with intra-arterial and para-arterial granulomas, forming a dumbbell shape (elastic stain ×80). (From Marchand, E. J. et al.: Arch Intern Med 100:965, 1957.)

prevalent in the red pulp and germinal centers of the lymphoid follicles. Later, a multifocal basophil proliferation is observed that coincides with elevated immunoglobulin levels in the serum. Distended venous sinuses and dense splenic cords are caused by portal hypertension. Giant follicular lymphoma may develop in affected spleens.

In addition to pipestem fibrosis, chronic parenchymal hepatitis occurs in some patients with hepatosplenic schistosomiasis. In this condition, inflammatory cells infiltrate the liver and destroy liver cells at the limiting plate. In early infection, even before oviposition, a diffuse infiltration of eosinophils can be seen. Later, this infiltration becomes more patchy and perivascular. In patients with decompensated hepatosplenic schistosomiasis, chronic hepatitis, which is characterized by septal fibrosis, active periportal inflammation, and bile duct proliferation, is more prominent than it is in patients with compensated hepatosplenic schistosomiasis. These histologic manifestations of the disease and their progression do not appear to be related to the intensity of the infection and egg production. Hepatitis B antigen has been reported in 4 per cent of the patients with hepatosplenic schistosomiasis compared with less than 1 per cent of uninfected controls.

S. haematobium. *S. haematobium* organisms lay as many eggs as *S. mansoni*, but they are released in aggregates and tend to calcify. Since the adult worms live in the veins of the vesical plexus, they affect primarily the urinary tract, and secondarily the lungs. The eggs are found in the mucosa and submucosa of the bladder and the lower part of the ureters. They give rise to granulomas that initially are very cellular and large (polypoid lesions) and may block the flow of urine and lead to hydronephrosis, a condition often seen in schoolage children. Later, the lesions, now called sandy patches, become relatively acellular and fibrous and contain calcified eggs. Calcified eggs may cause bladder calcification and deformation. Although sloughing of necrotic polypoid patches is detectable in the early active phases of the disease, chronic ulceration of the bladder occurs later at sites of very heavy egg burdens. Some active lesions may persist as polyps in the later, inactive stages of disease if the antecedent active infection was heavy. The rectum, seminal vesicles, prostate, ureter, and urethra may be involved. Eggs can be found in the lung and less often in the liver. If the CNS is involved, lesions are usually found in the spinal cord. In some geographic areas, mixed infections with *S. mansoni* are frequent.

CLINICAL MANIFESTATIONS. The host-parasite relationship is well balanced in schistosomiasis. The majority of infected people are asymptomatic or have mild, nonspecific symptoms. Only 5 to 10 per cent of infected populations have severe clinical symptoms, and the life expectancy of persons in an infected population is not significantly different from that of individuals in an uninfected one.

Acute Schistosomiasis Due to *S. mansoni* and *S. japonicum*. The disease is recognized infrequently at this stage because most patients are asymptomatic. This phase of the illness usually follows exposure to heavily contaminated streams or bodies of water. Immediate itching and urticaria occur in a small percentage of patients and may begin as soon as the film of water on the skin begins to dry. Schistosome dermatitis may develop into papular lesions that persist for approximately five to seven days. Papular dermatitis is more common, however, when the skin is penetrated by avian schistosomes (see sections on Pathogenesis and Pathology and Geographic Variations).

During the migration of the schistosomula, fever and cough may be experienced in association with mechanical and inflammatory changes in the lung and liver, but this stage is usually asymptomatic. In acute schistosomiasis the worms mature in the liver, migrate to the small venules, and begin egg production. The acute disease is similar in all three forms of schistosomiasis and has an explosive onset about 20 to 40 days after heavy exposure. Major symptoms include chills, spiking fever with afternoon elevations to 105° F, generalized weakness, myalgia, headache, anorexia, profuse diarrhea, and weight loss. Extensive urticaria may occur in large patches on various parts of the body. Nausea and vomiting are common and cough may be prominent. The fever usually lyses spontaneously 2 to 10 weeks after onset.

Physical findings are usually minimal but may include urticaria, patches of moist rales over both lung fields, generalized lymphadenopathy, and hepatosplenomegaly. Edema and purpura of the eyelids may occur.

On sigmoidoscopic examination the rectal mucosa is hyperemic and edematous with pinpoint yellowish elevations, minute hemorrhages, and shallow ulcerations (Garcia-Palmieri and Marcial-Rojas, 1962).

The leukocyte count may be normal or elevated, but eosinophilia, which may approach 70 per cent is always present. Levels of immunoglobulins E and G are elevated.

In Asia this disease is called Katayama fever. This syndrome, which resembles serum-sickness, occurs more frequently during acute infection with *S. japonicum*, which produces about 10 times more ova per female worm than *S. mansoni* or *S. haematobium*.

Chronic Schistosomiasis Due to *S. mansoni* and *S. japonicum*. Most patients with chronic schistosomiasis never experience acute symptoms. The classic pseudotubercle may be found in liver biopsies as early as 80 days after exposure, but symptoms or signs of chronic schistosomiasis usually take from months to many years after initial contact to appear. Multiple exposures are probably necessary to acquire enough egg granulomas to produce severe chronic disease.

Patients with chronic schistosomiasis usually go to the doctor because of gastrointestinal bleeding or hepatosplenomegaly. The most striking symptoms are melena and hematemesis. Abdominal discomfort and intermittent diarrhea may be prominent. Patients with schistosomal portal hypertension tolerate multiple episodes of esophageal bleeding better than patients with intrahepatic portal hypertension (Garcia-Palmieri and Marcial-Rojas, 1961). Jaundice is characteristically absent except in terminal illness.

The liver is usually large, firm, and nontender. The spleen is greatly enlarged in virtually all cases of severe schistosomiasis due to *S. mansoni* and *S. japonicum*. Other findings that accompany Laennec's cirrhosis such as ascites, spider nevi, peripheral edema, testicular atrophy, and feminization are characteristically absent. The healthy appearance and absence of the stigmata of liver disease in the usual patient with hepatosplenic schistosomiasis are shown in Figure 4. Decompensated hepatosplenic schistosomiasis, is unusual.

Thrombocytopenia accompanies the severe hypersplenism. There is also blood-loss anemia, reduced hepatic clearance, hyperglobulinemia, hypoalbuminemia in 25 per cent of cases, elevated serum alkaline phosphatase, and diminished prothrombin. The serum bilirubin and pyruvic and oxalacetic transaminases are normal or slightly elevated. Varices can usually be demonstrated by esophagram, esophagoscopy, or splenoportography.

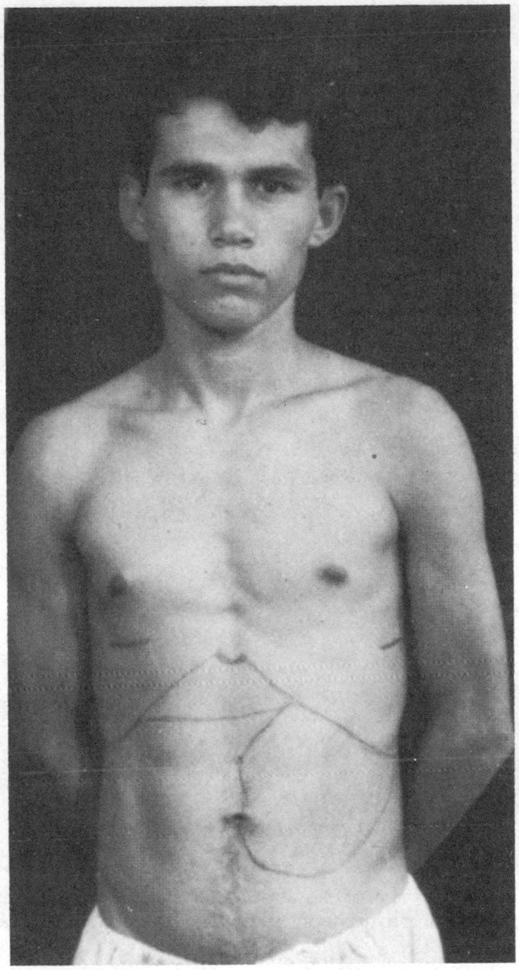

Figure 4. Typical patient with compensated hepatosplenic schistosomiasis. Despite major hepatosplenomegaly, the patient appears healthy and shows none of the secondary manifestations of severe liver disease. (From Reboucas, G.: Yale J Biol Med 48:369, 1975.)

Schistosomiasis Due to *S. haematobium*. All manifestations of acute schistosomiasis described above may occur during infections with *S. haematobium*. Although most worms migrate from the mesenteric to the pelvic veins and discharge their ova in the wall of the bladder, some ova are also deposited in the rectal mucosa.

Urinary frequency and dysuria are common early symptoms, but hematuria may be the first symptom. Microscopic hematuria progresses to frank bloody urine as the bladder mucosa ulcerates. Intermittent pain is usually referred to the suprapubic or perineal region. Bladder distention and hydronephrosis result from granulomas in the bladder wall, ureters, urethra, and prostate. Recurrent pyogenic urinary tract infections are common.

Cystoscopy discloses bleeding points, minute ulcers, and calcified sand-like excrescences in chronic cases. Pyelography reveals hydronephrosis, often with acute and chronic pyelonephritis, bladder calcification, and bladder-filling defects (Fig. 5).

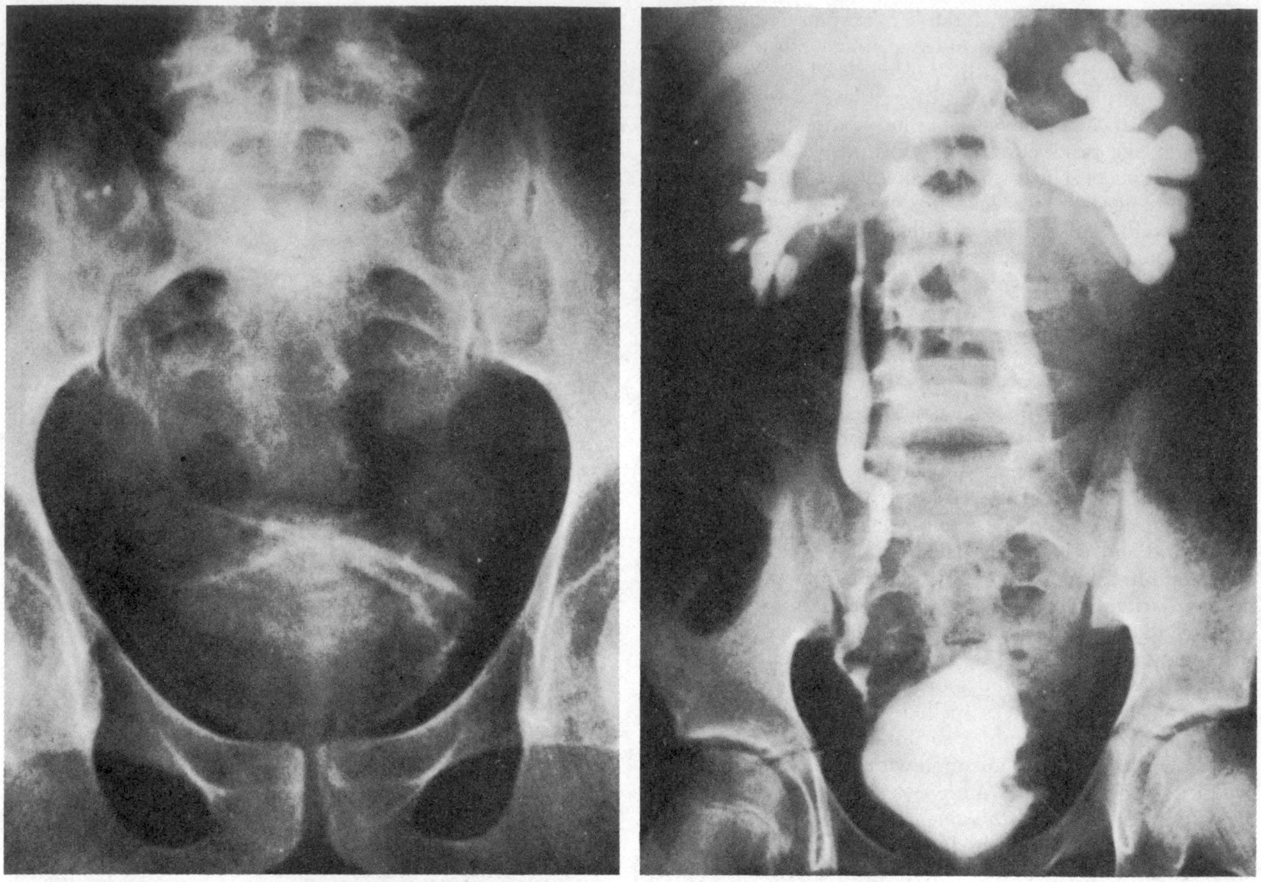

Figure 5. Plain film of the abdomen (left), showing calcification of the bladder, and intravenous pyelogram (right), showing left hydroureter and hydronephrosis, right ureteral deformity, and bladder filling defects. (From Lehman, J. et al.: Ann Intern Med 75:49, 1971.)

COMPLICATIONS AND SEQUELAE. The most common cause of death in hepatosplenic schistosomiasis is exsanguination from bleeding esophageal varices. Although rare, hepatic coma may occur after hemorrhage. In decompensated hepatosplenic schistosomiasis, chronic hepatitis with periportal inflammation and bile duct proliferation is more prominent than in compensated schistosomiasis. In Brazil 1 per cent of spleens removed from schistosomiasis patients contain giant follicular lymphoma.

Mesangioproliferative glomerulonephritis with immune complexes has been demonstrated in renal biopsies. Chronic glomerulonephritis unrelated to the granulomas of urinary schistosomiasis has been reported in as many as 12 per cent of severe, postmortem cases.

Obstructive uropathy, chronic pyelonephritis, and renal failure are major complications of urinary schistosomiasis. The association of bladder carcinoma and *S. haematobium* is well-known. A causal role has been ascribed to beta-glucuronidase, which is increased in the urine of infected patients and is known to hydrolyze inactive glucuronides into carcinogenic substances (Norden and Gelfand, 1972).

Ectopic deposition of ova is a common and potentially severe complication of schistosomiasis. Pulmonary lesions may vary from scattered, asymptomatic granulomas to massive perivascular fibrosis with secondary cor pulmonale. Ectopic granulomas may occur in the spinal cord or brain. Localization of *S. japonicum* in the brain is a major cause of epileptiform seizures in patients with schistosomiasis.

Salmonellosis is common in patients infected with *S. mansoni* and *S. haematobium*. Reduced hepatic clearance and urinary obstruction probably contribute to the occurrence and persistence of these infections, but salmonellae also infect the tegument and tissues of schistosomes (Young et al., 1973).

GEOGRAPHIC VARIATIONS. The manifestations of schistosomiasis vary with the geographic distribution of the different schistosomes. *S. japonicum* females produce about 10 times as many ova as the other schistosomes. Consequently, ectopic lesions and the early hypersensitivity manifestations of Katayama fever occur more commonly in Oriental schistosomiasis. Furthermore, the ova are deposited in aggregates, induce a more exudative response, and tend to calcify. For these reasons, and because of the greater number of ova, infections with *S. japonicum* are more fulminating and may progress to lethal pipestem cirrhosis within a year.

Within the geographic distribution of *S. mansoni*, severe hepatosplenic pathology is more common in Brazil, Egypt, and Puerto Rico than it is in the eastern, western, and southern parts of Africa. This difference has been ascribed to diet, but it is difficult to be certain that the differences are not due primarily to the degree of exposure and relative burden of ova and adult worms. Giant follicular lymphoma was found in 1 per cent of spleens removed from patients in Brazil, but further studies are necessary to establish the true comparative frequency of this complication.

Free-swimming cercariae of more than 20 non-human schistosomes are prevalent in many parts of the world. These parasites of birds and small mammals are distributed throughout the Americas, Europe, Australia, and New Zealand as well as Africa and Asia. Like the human schistosomes, they are limited by the distribution of a suitable snail host. Although these nonhuman schistosomes can penetrate human skin, the cercariae die in the skin or subcutaneous tissue. Unsensitized individuals may experience only a fleeting macular rash, but the sensitized patient can develop a papular eruption that persists for 7 to 10 days. The disease is self-limited and treatment is symptomatic.

Another species of schistosome, S. *intercalatum*, is found only in limited foci in West Central Africa and differs from S. *mansoni* in that the lateral spine is bent, the ova are acid-fast by Ziehl-Neelsen stain, and symptomatic disease is limited to the gastrointestinal tract (Wright, 1973). It is uncertain whether S. *intercalatum* is a separate species or a subspecies of S. *mansoni* or whether the morphology of the ova and the disease are merely altered by host defenses or other local environmental influences.

IMMUNITY. Protective immunity (Allison et al., 1974; Smithers and Terry, 1975) has been demonstrated only in experimental animals, and only after infection with living schistosomes. Good evidence indicates that the adults, not the eggs, provide the main stimulus for immunity in the rhesus monkey. Transfer of worms into rhesus monkeys induces protection to reinfection that is directed against the migrating schistosomula in the lungs. It is important to note that adult worms are protected from the immunity they provoke. Soon after penetration, the parasite absorbs host antigens onto its surface, including antigens from the major histocompatibility gene complex (Goldring et al., 1976; Sher et al., 1978) and A, B, and O blood group antigens. This coating masks the antigens of the parasite and probably makes it unrecognizable by the immune system of the host. Immunization of mice or rhesus monkeys with one schistosome species may convey immunity to another because of cross-reacting antigens. Unfortunately, immunity in animals that are good hosts for schistosomes, like man, is relatively weak, perhaps because the parasite and host share antigens or because the parasite surface is coated with host antigens. Smithers and Terry call this latter phenomenon "concomitant immunity." Some animals that develop protective immunity, for example, rats, can eliminate worms even when thymectomized. In this case, a delayed, yet efficient, elimination of parasites is observed (Cioli et al., 1980).

The evidence for immunity in man (Bradley and McCullough, 1973; Warren, 1973b) is circumstantial. In most endemic areas, most infections occur in the second decade of life, as reflected by peak egg output. This age prevalence could be due to a combination of two factors. One is the more frequent water contact in early life and the other is the spontaneous death of worms. Several studies support the importance of these factors. The prevalence in women in Sierra Leone, who have more water contact than men throughout life, falls only a little from the peak, as compared with the greater fall in men. However, a group of men in Brazil who moved from a nonendemic to an endemic area showed the highest prevalence and intensity of infection 15 to 19 years after they moved. Also, in areas of very high transmission in Sierra Leone and southern Rhodesia, the prevalence peak is reached before age 10, whereas it occurs in the second decade of life in nearby areas with low transmission rates. Furthermore, in areas of high transmission rates in southern Rhodesia and St. Lucia (West Indies), children show a much higher egg output than children in areas of low transmission rates. Among adults from these two areas, however, the egg output is similar and reduced. All these findings pointed to some regulatory suppressive mechanisms, possibly acquired immunity, 10 to 20 years after the initial infection.

During the last decade, investigators have concentrated on in vitro studies of the immune reactivity of lymphocytes to schistosome antigens. Early in the course of infection, lymphocyte blastogenic reactivity to parasite antigens develops but declines 3 to 4 months after the initial infection (Ottesen et al., 1978). The loss of lymphocyte reactivity during the chronic phase of the disease could be traced to various suppressor mechanisms including serum factors (Colley et al., 1977), mononuclear cells (Ottesen, 1979), and suppressor T cells (Rocklin et al., 1981). It appears that these suppressive mechanisms are reversible. Eight months after curative drug treatment, patients showed a rise in blastogenic responsiveness to schistosome antigens (Nash et al., 1982). Modulation of the humoral antibody response also occurs. In the acute phase of the infection, there is a dramatic increase in specific IgE antibody, which is sustained during the chronic phase. Little allogenic reactivity is observed, however, apparently due to the production of blocking antibodies that inhibit immediate hypersensitivity to schistosome antigens (Hofstetter et al., 1982). When the disease progresses from the acute to the chronic phase, circulating immune complexes increase significantly with a maximum at 2½ to 6 months after infection. In general, the levels of immune complexes correlated with the intensity of the infection and severity of symptoms (Lawley et al., 1979). Glomerulonephritis caused by immune complexes has been documented (Hoshino-Shimuzu et al., 1976). Differential susceptibility among patients to the development of hepatosplenic disease may be immunomediated and correlate with ABO blood groups and histocompatibility antigens (Abdel Salam et al., 1979; Camus et al., 1977; Pereira et al., 1979).

DIAGNOSIS. Schistosomiasis must be suspected in any patient with a possible exposure history who presents with any of the following symptoms: fever, eosinophilia, hepatosplenomegaly, hematuria, obstructive uropathy, urinary tract infection, pulmonary granulomas, melena, or cor pulmonale. Patients may even present with granulomatous lesions of the skin or convulsions secondary to ectopic localization of ova.

Demonstration of the parasite is still the only reliable way to diagnose schistosomiasis. Ova of S. *mansoni* and S. *japonicum* (Chapter 86) may be demonstrated directly by examination of fecal smears, but this technique is not very sensitive, and negative stools must be examined by a concentration technique. For concentration, stools are suspended in 0.5 per cent glycerol in water and the suspension washed, sieved, and either centrifuged or allowed to yield sediment. The formol-ether and merthiolate-iodine-formol methods (Allen and Ridley, 1970; Beer, 1972) may be used either directly or on the sediment to remove detritus, mucus, and fats. The Bell filtration method uses ninhydrin as the stain (Bell, 1963), and the Kato technique (Martin and Beaver, 1969) uses a solution of glycerol malachite green.

Urine collected near midday should be examined for *S. haematobium* ova, identified by sedimenting, filtering and examining the residue microscopically, with or without staining. The proportion of live eggs may be determined by suspending the ova in water, exposing them to light, and counting hatched miracidia. The number of viable ova measures the effectiveness of treatment.

Ova in stools must be repeatedly washed and concentrated before reliable viability tests may be performed. Rectal biopsy is the most successful method of diagnosing schistosomiasis when the stools are negative and the best way to assess the effectiveness of chemotherapy (Figs. 6 and 7). Biopsy material may be sectioned and processed like other tissue, but a squash preparation of the fresh tissue should always be examined as well. It is also important to verify that the eggs are viable since dead or calcified eggs are not necessarily an indication for treatment. Viability of the eggs can be tested by incubating the squashed biopsy material for 15 minutes in water.

Serologic tests are still not sufficiently sensitive or specific to identify active infection, although some progress has been made. Acutely infected patients typically have a marked increase in total IgM and a moderate increase in IgG and IgE, while chronically infected patients maintain elevated levels of IgG and IgE (Nash et al., 1978). To assay for specific antibody, two antigens, the gut associated proteoglycan (GASP) and a polysaccharide antigen (PSAP), extracted from adult worms, have been used in radioimmune or other assay techniques. Acutely infected patients had increased IgM and IgG antibody titers, mostly specific for GASP. Chronically infected patients had lower levels. Since anti-GASP antibodies are significantly elevated even in cases of low-grade infection, this assay system may detect early infection (Nash, 1978). In contrast, antibody titers to PSAP appear to correlate well with the intensity of infection (Nash et al., 1981) and may be more useful in assessing the severity of the disease.

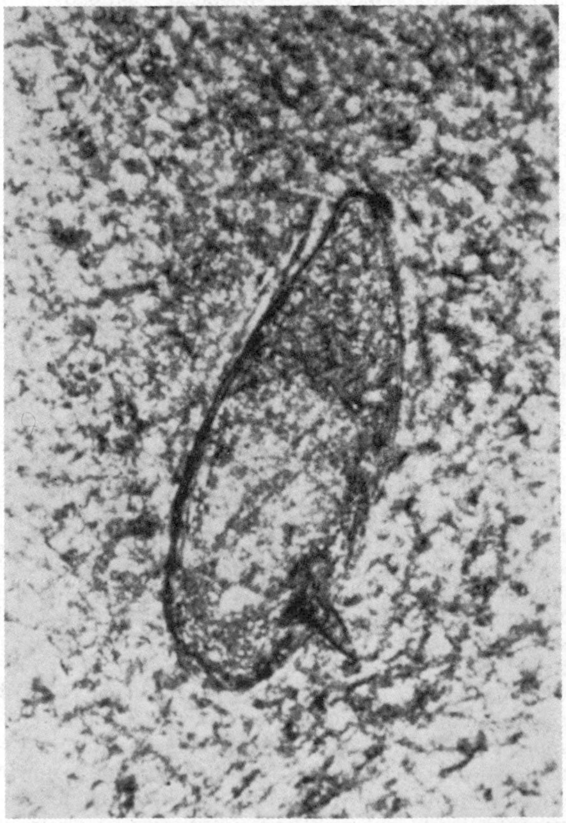

Figure 6. Rectal biopsy containing a mature, viable ovum of *S. mansoni* (× 425). (From Spingarn, C. L. et al.: New Engl J Med 256:290, 1957.)

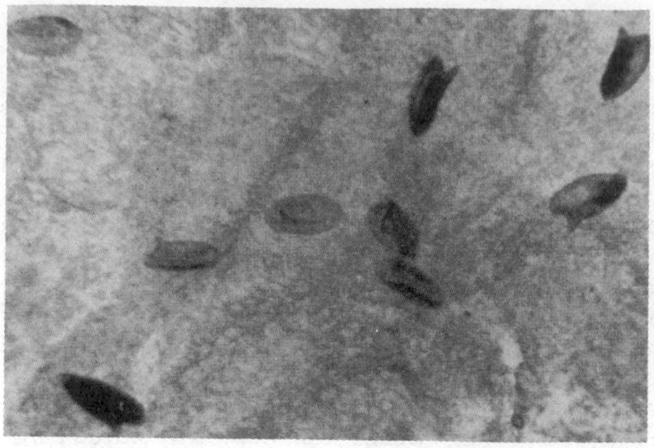

Figure 7. Rectal biopsy showing degenerating ova of *S. mansoni* after treatment (× 75). (From Spingarn, C. L. et al.: New Engl J Med 256:290, 1957.)

TREATMENT. Enormous progress has been made in the last few years due to the availability of safer drugs for the treatment of schistosomiasis. The first successful drugs were antimony compounds that were so toxic that they could not be used for mass therapy. In the 1940's, the miracil compound, lucanthone, was introduced. Although this drug could be taken orally, it was almost as toxic as the antimonial drugs. Niridazole and hycanthone were introduced in the 1960's. Both drugs are still in limited use throughout the world. They are less toxic and more effective than the antimonials, but there is concern about their mutagenicity and carcinogenicity (Batzinger and Bueding, 1977).

Niridazole, a nitrothiazole derivative, can be given orally and is therefore useful for mass therapy, particularly for children. The recommended dose is 25 mg/kg body weight in two daily doses for one week. The drug is very effective against *S. haematobium*, but less so against *S. mansoni* and produces cure in 20 to 100 per cent of patients depending on the dose. Vomiting, nausea, and diarrhea are common, and mental disturbances may occur. Experimentally, niridazole is anti-inflammatory (Riesterer et al., 1971) and suppresses delayed hypersensitivity as manifested by skin tests (Daniels et al., 1975) or formation of the egg granuloma (Mahmoud et al., 1975). This anti-inflammatory property may contribute to the effectiveness of niridazole against schistosomiasis.

Hycanthone is also suitable for mass therapy, since the total dose can be given in a single injection. The recommended dose has been 2.5 ± 0.5 mg/kg in one intramuscular injection. No deaths have been reported from the use of this drug, but vomiting and diarrhea are common. Ninety-seven per cent of patients with S. *mansoni* infections have been cured and the results with S. *haematobium* are probably equally as good. Several studies have indicated that half the recommended dose (1.5 mg/kg) achieves high cure rates. These studies (Warren et al., 1978; Rees et al., 1975) were based on the premise that elimination of all worms is not necessary for arresting the disease and that the preimmunity achieved by retaining a very low level of egg production may be useful in endemic areas.

Metrifonate, an organophosphate (Davis and Bailey, 1969), paralyzes the worm by blocking its acetyl cholinesterase. Clinical tolerance to the drug is good, although nausea, vomiting, and bronchospasm may occur in some people. The drug is only active against S. *haematobium*, but cure levels are in the range of 70 to 80 per cent. Unfortunately, the drug has to be given in three doses at intervals of two weeks. The dose is 7.5 to 10 mg/kg body weight. There are no contraindications to retreatment.

Oxamniquine is a tetrahydroquinoline that is active against S. *mansoni* in a single dose of 15 mg/kg body weight. Side effects are mild, especially when the drug is administered late in the day and after a meal. Seven to forty per cent of the patients experience mild dizziness of short duration. Patients with a history of seizures should be adequately controlled before oxamniquine treatment. In children below 30 kg, a higher dose of 20 mg/kg body weight may be more effective. Some African strains of S. *mansoni* are less sensitive to this drug (Omer, 1978; Kilpatrick et al., 1981) and a dose of up to 60 mg/kg body weight over a period of two days may be required to obtain satisfactory results. The drug has been used extensively in Africa and Brazil.

Praziquantel (Davis and Wegner, 1979; Davis et al., 1979; Katz et al., 1979; Ishizaki et al., 1979; Santos et al., 1979), a heterocyclic pyrazinoisoquinoline, is effective against S. *mansoni*, S. *hematobium*, S. *japonicum*, and S. *mekongi*. This new drug is probably the most important of all anti-schistosomes because it is not only effective against all schistosomes, but also against *Clonorchis sinensis*, *Opisthorchis viverrini*, *Paragonimus westermani*, *Metagonimus yokogawai*, *Hymenolepis nana*, and *Cysticercus cellulosae*. Praziquantel increases the permeability of the cell membrane to calcium ions, causing massive contraction and paralysis of the musculature, followed by disintegration of the tegumental layer. It is highly effective orally whether given as a single dose or in several doses on the same day. Cure rates between 75 and 95 per cent after six months have been obtained. A dose of 40 mg/kg body weight is effective for S. *mansoni* and S. *hematobium* infections, but S. *japonicum* and S. *mekongi* require 60 mg/kg body weight in three doses every 4 hours. No major toxic effects have been observed. Transient abdominal pain may occur, especially when the drug is given in a single dose. Dizziness and fever have been reported. The drug was not found to be mutagenic.

While drug treatment is now very effective in curing schistosomiasis, it is important to note that Symmer's fibrosis, portal hypertension, and serum sickness-like disease are not reversed by anti-schistosomal therapy.

Surgical treatment involves the correction of obstructive uropathy, resection of bladder polyps, resection of colonic polyps, and partial colectomy for severe gastrointestinal polyposis and fibrosis. Portal hypertension can be reversed by a distal splenorenal shunt (Wilson, 1976). Patients with active infections should be treated with praziquantel before surgery.

PROPHYLAXIS. Visitors to endemic areas can escape schistosomiasis by avoiding contact with fresh water. Because this is difficult or impossible for the local population, extermination of the intermediate snail host is the most practical method of control. Niclosamide appears to be the best molluscicide and has an excellent record in Rhodesia, the Philippines, Egypt, Tanzania, and South Africa. It is used in a concentration of 4 to 8 parts per million per hour (ppm/hr) in flowing water. The most active molluscicide is *N*-trityl-morpholine, which is used at 0.1 to 0.5 ppm/hr. Sodium pentachlorophenate has been relatively reliable in Japan, Egypt, Rhodesia, and Venezuela when used at 50 to 80 ppm/hr. Copper sulfate (20 to 30 ppm/hr) is used in Egypt and the Sudan.

The snail habitat should be destroyed by clearing weeds from waterways, increasing the flow of water in irrigation ditches, and lining ditches with concrete. Clean water must be provided for household use in endemic areas. Safe sewage disposal is needed to prevent live eggs from reaching fresh water.

Mass chemotherapy is another important method of control. The erection of new dams, extension of irrigation, and the use of freshwater ponds for commercial fish farming have complicated control efforts.

References

Abdel Salam, E., and Ishaac, S., Mahmoud A. A. F.: Histocompatibility-linked susceptibility for hepatosplenomegaly in human schistosomiasis mansoni. J Immunol 123:1829, 1979.

Allen, A. V. H., and Ridley, D. S.: Further observations on the formol-ether concentration technique for faecal parasites. J Clin Pathol 23:545, 1970.

Allison, A. C., et al.: Immunology of schistosomiasis. Bull WHO 51:533, 1974.

Andrade, Z. A., and Cheever, A. W.: Alterations of the intrahepatic vasculature in hepatosplenic schistosomiasis mansoni. Am J Trop Med Hyg 20:425, 1971.

Ansari, N.: Epidemiology and control of schistosomiasis (bilharziasis). Basel, S. Karger, 1973.

Batzinger, R. P., and Bueding, E.: Mutagenic activities of five antischistosomal compounds. J Pharmacol Exp Ther 200:1, 1977.

Beer, R. J. S.: A rapid technique for the concentration and collection of helminth eggs from large quantities of faeces. Parasitology 65:343, 1972.

Bell, D. R.: A new method for counting *Schistosoma mansoni* eggs in faeces, with special reference to therapeutic trials. Bull WHO 29:525, 1963.

Bradley, D. J., and McCullough, F. S.: Egg output stability and the epidemiology of *Schistosoma haematobium*. II. An analysis of the epidemiology of endemic *S. haematobium*. Trans R Soc Trop Med Hyg 67:491, 1973.

Camus, D., Bina, J. C., Carlier, Y., et al.: Grupos sanquineos A, B, O_e forman clinicas da esquistossomose mansonica. Rev Inst Med Trop Sao Paulo, 19:77, 1977.

Cioli, D., Malorni, W., De Martino, C., and Dennert, G.: A study of *Schistosoma mansoni* reinfection in thymectomized rats. Cell Immunol 53:246, 1980.

Colley, D. G., Magalhaes-Filho, A., and Barros Coelho, R.: Immunopathology of dermal reactions induced by *Schistosoma mansoni* cercariae and cercarial extract. J Trop Med Hyg 21:558, 1972.

Colley, D. G.: Adoptive suppression of granuloma formation. J Exp Med 143:696, 1976.

Colley, D. G., Hieny, S. E., Bartholomew, R. K., and Cook, J. A.: Immune responses during human schistosomiasis mansoni. III. Regulatory effect of patient sera on human lymphocyte blastogenic responses to schistosome antigen preparations. Am J Trop Med Hyg 26:917, 1977.

Daniels, J. C., Warren, K. S., and David, J. R.: Studies on the mechanism of suppression of delayed hypersensitivity by the antischistosomal compound niridazole. J Immunol 115:1414, 1975.

Davis, A., and Bailey, D. R.: Metrifonate in urinary schistosomiasis. Bull WHO, 41:209, 1969.

Davis, A., Biles, J. E., and Ulrich, A-M.: Initial experiments with praziquantel in the treatment of human infections due to *Schistosoma haematobium*. Bull WHO, 57:773, 1979.

Davis, A., and Wegner, D. H. G.: Multicenter trials of praziquantel in human schistosomiasis: design and techniques. Bull WHO 57:767, 1979.

Diaz-Rivera, R. S., Ramos Morales, F., Sotomayer, Z. R., Lichtenberg, F., Garcia-Palmieri, M. R., Cintron-Rivera, A. A., and Marchand, E. J.: The pathogenesis of Manson's schistosomiasis. Ann Intern Med 47:1082, 1957.

Garcia-Palmieri, M. R., and Marcial-Rojas, R. A.: The protean manifestations of schistosomiasis mansoni. A clinicopathological correlation. Ann Intern Med 57:763, 1962.

Goldring, O. I., Ceeg, J. A., Smithers, S. R., and Terry, R. J.: Acquisition of human blood group antigens by *Schistosoma mansoni*. Clin Exp Immunol 26:181, 1976.

Hofstetter, M., Poindexter, R. W., Ruiz-Tiben, E., and Ottesen, E. A.: Modulation of the host response in human schistosomiasis: III. Blocking antibodies specifically inhibit immediate hypersensitivity responses to parasite antigens. Immunology 46:777, 1982.

Hoshino-Shimuzu, S., Brito, T., Kanamura, H. Y., et al.: Human schistosomiasis: *Schistosoma mansoni* antigen detection in renal glomeruli. Trans R Soc Trop Med Hyg 70:492, 1976.

Ishizaki, T., Kamo, E., and Boehme, K.: Double-blind studies of tolerance to praziquantel in Japanese patients with *Schistosoma japonicum* infections. Bull WHO 57:787, 1979.

Jordan, P., and Webbe, G.: Human schistosomiasis. London, Heinemann, 1969.

Katz, M.: Anthelminthics. Drugs 13:124, 1977.

Katz, N., Rocha, R. S., and Chaves, A.: Preliminary trials with praziquantel in human infections due to *Schistosoma mansoni*. Bull WHO 57:781, 1979.

Kilpatrick, M. E., Farid, Z., Bassily, S., El-Masry, N. A., Trabolsi, B., and Watten, R. H.: Treatment of schistosomiasis mansoni with oxamniquine—five years' experience. Am J Trop Med Hyg 30:1219, 1981.

Lawley, T. J., Ottesen, E. A., Hiatt, R. A., and Gazze, L. A.: Circulating immune complexes in acute schistosomiasis. Clin Exp Immunol 37:221, 1979.

Lehman, J., Stauffer, Z. F., Bassily, S., and Kent, D. C.: Hydronephrosis, bacteriuria, and maximal urine concentration in urinary schistosomiasis. Ann Intern Med 75:49, 1971.

von Lichtenberg, F., et al.: Experimental infection with *Schistosoma japonicum* in chimpanzees: Parasitologic, clinical, serologic and pathological observations. Am J Trop Med Hyg 20:850, 1971.

Mahmoud, A. A. F., Mandel, M. A., Warren, K. S., and Webster, L. T.: Niridazole. II. A potent, long-acting suppressant of cellular hypersensitivity. J Immunol 114:279, 1975.

Marchand, E. J., Marcial-Rojas, R. A., Rodriguez, R., Polanco, G., and Diaz-Rivera, R. S.: The pulmonary obstruction syndrome in *Schistosoma mansoni* pulmonary endarteritis. Arch Intern Med 100:965, 1957.

Martin, L. K., and Beaver, P. C.: Evaluation of Kato thick-smear technique for quantitative diagnosis of helminth infections. Am J Trop Med Hyg 17:382, 1969.

Nash, T. E.: Antibody response to a polysaccharide antigen present in the schistosome gut: I. Sensitivity and specificity. Am J Trop Med Hyg 27:938, 1978.

Nash, T. E., Hofstetter, M., Cheever, A. W., and Ottesen, E. A.: Treatment of *Schistosoma mekongi* with praziquantel: a double blinded study. Am J Trop Med Hyg 3:977, 1982.

Nash, T. E., Lunde, M. N., and Cheever, A. W.: Analysis and antigenic activity of a carbohydrate fraction derived from adult *Schistosoma mansoni*. J Immunol 126:805, 1981.

Nash, T. E., Ottesen, E. A., and Cheever, A. W.: Antibody response to a polysaccharide antigen present in the schistosome gut: II. Modulation of antibody response. Am J Trop Med Hyg 27:944, 1978.

Norden, D. A., and Gelfand, M.: Bilharzia and bladder cancer. An investigation of urinary glucuronidase associated with *S. haematobium* infection. Trans R Soc Trop Med Hyg 66:865, 1972.

Omer, A. H. S.: Oxamniquine for treating *Schistosoma mansoni* infection in Sudan. Br Med J 2:163, 1978.

Ottesen, E. A.: Modulation of the host response in human schistosomiasis: I. Adherent suppressor cells which inhibit lymphocyte proliferative responses to parasite antigens. J Immunol 123:1639, 1979.

Ottesen, E. A., Hiatt, R. A., Cheever, A. W., Sotomayor, Z. R., and Neva, F. A.: The acquisition and loss of antigen-specific cellular immune responsiveness in acute and chronic schistosomiasis in man. Clin Exp Immunol 33:38, 1978.

Pereira, F. E. L., Bortolini, E. R., Carneiro, J. L. A., da Silva, C. R. M., and Neves, R. C.: A, B, O blood groups and hepatosplenic form of schistosomiasis mansoni (Symmer's fibrosis). Trans R Soc Trop Med Hyg 73:238, 1979.

Reboucas, G.: Clinical aspects of hepatosplenic schistosomiasis: A contrast with cirrhosis. Yale J Biol Med 48:369, 1975.

Rees, P. H., Bowny, H. N., Robert, J. M. D., and Thuku, J. J.: The treatment of schistosomiasis mansoni in Murang's District, Kenya: A double blind controlled trial of three hycanthone regimens and oxamniquine. Am J Trop Med Hyg 24:823, 1975.

Riesterer, L., Majer, H., and Jacques, R.: On the anti-inflammatory properties of the schistosomicide niridazole (Ambilhar). Experientia 27:546, 1971.

Rocklin, R. E., Tracy, J. W., and El Kholy, A. E.: Activation of antigen-specific suppressor cells in human schistosomiasis mansoni by fractions of soluble egg antigens nonadherent to Con A Sepharose. J Immunol 127:2314, 1981.

Sadun, E. H., et al.: Experimental infection with *Schistosoma haematobium* in chimpanzees: Parasitologic, clinical, serologic and pathological observations. Am J Trop Med Hyg 19:427, 1970.

Santos, A. T., Blas, B. L., Nosenas, J. S., et al.: Preliminary clinical trials with praziquantel in *Schistosoma japonicum* infections in the Philippines. Bull WHO 57:793, 1979.

Sher, A., Hall, B. E., and Vadas, M. A.: Acquisition of murine major histocompatibility complex gene products by schistosomula of *Schistosoma mansoni*. J Exp Med 148:46, 1978.

Smithers, S. R., and Terry, R. J.: The immunology of schistosomiasis. Adv Parasitol 13:41, 1975.

Spingarn, C. L., Edelman, M. H., Gold, T., Yarnis, H., and Turell, R.: Value of rectal biopsies in the diagnosis and treatment of *Schistosoma mansoni* infections. N Engl J Med 256:290, 1957.

Stirewalt, M. A., and Dorsey, C. H.: *Schistosoma mansoni:* Cercarial penetration of host epidermis at the ultrastructural level. Exp. Parasitol 35:1, 1974.

Warren, K. S.: The immunopathogenesis of schistosomiasis: A multidisciplinary approach. Trans R Soc Trop Med Hyg 66:417, 1972.

Warren, K. S.: The pathology of schistosome infections. Helminth abstracts series A 42:591, 1973a.

Warren, K. S.: Regulation of the prevalence and intensity of schistosomiasis in man: Immunity or ecology? J Infect Dis 127:595, 1973b.

Warren, K. S., Ouma, J. H., Arap Siongok, T. K., and Houser, H. B.: Hycanthone dose-response in *Schistosoma mansoni* infection in Kenya. Lancet 1:352, 1978.

Wilson, R. B.: Surgical implications of *Schistosoma mansoni* infestation. Mt Sinai J Med 43:657, 1976.

Wright, W. H.: Geographic distribution of schistosomas and their intermediate hosts. In Ansari, N. (ed.): Epidemiology and Control of Schistosomiasis (Bilharziasis). Baltimore, University Park Press, 1973, pp. 32–249.

Young, C. W., Higashi, G., Kamel, R., El-Abdin, A. Z., and Mikhail, I. A.: Interaction of salmonellae and schistosomes in host-parasite relations. Trans R Soc Trop Med Hyg 67:797, 1973.

146
VIRAL GASTROENTERITIS

RUTH BISHOP, D.SC.

Gastroenteritis is a common illness that occurs in epidemic and sporadic form throughout the world. The disease is most severe in infants and young children, and is one of the major causes of death in childhood, particularly in malnourished children. Gastroenteritis results from infection of the gastrointestinal tract by a variety of microorganisms, including viruses, and clinical symptoms are not a reliable guide to the identity of the microbial pathogen.

ETIOLOGY. Electron microscopy has identified two types of viral particles that do not grow readily in cell culture but are undoubtedly responsible for gastroenteritis in humans (Leading Article, 1975). Advances in knowledge of these agents are reviewed in detail by Schreiber et al., (1977) Kapikian et al. (1981) and Holmes (1983).

The Norwalk Group of Agents. This is a heterogeneous group of viruses (27 to 30 nm in diameter) associated with epidemics of gastroenteritis in children and adults. The particles have a variety of names, which usually indicate the geographic location of the outbreak and include Norwalk agent (Kapikian et al., 1972), Hawaii agent, Montgomery County agent, Ditchling agent, W agent and Cockle agent. These particles have been only partially characterized. They have similar morphologies and buoyant densities, but are antigenically distinct. The protein structure of Norwalk agent resembles caliciviruses. The source of this group of viruses can be contaminated shell food, drinking water, or swimming water. Person-to-person spread occurs during epidemics. One-third of family and community outbreaks of acute non-bacterial gastroenteritis in U.S.A. are due to Norwalk virus.

Norwalk Virus. This agent was first seen by immune electron microscopy of diarrheal feces from an experimentally infected adult volunteer (Fig. 1). Extracts of diarrheal feces, processed to remove contaminating bacteria and larger viruses, regularly produce acute gastroenteritis in 50 per cent of adult volunteers after oral ingestion. The incubation period is 18 to 48 hours, and symptoms last for 24 to 48 hours. Virus-like particles are detectable in feces for 72 hours from onset of symptoms and are absent from stools during convalescence. Seroconversion occurs during infection. There are two forms of clinical immunity. Short-term immunity appears to be serotype specific. Long-term immunity cannot be related to pre-existing antibodies and may be genetically pre-determined. Large scale epidemiologic surveys based on immune adherence hemagglutination assay (IAHA) or radioimmunoassay (RIA) show that infection with Norwalk agent (or serologically related agents) is worldwide. Children in developing countries acquire antibodies at an earlier age than children in developed countries. After 40 years of age, at least 50 per cent of adults show serologic evidence of past infection. Norwalk agent is not regarded as an important cause of severe gastroenteritis in young children in developed countries. Its importance in childhood diarrhea in developing countries remains to be determined.

Rotaviruses. First described in 1973 in epithelial cells of duodenal mucosa from children with acute gastroenteritis (Bishop et al., 1973), this virus was initially referred to by different names, including duovirus, rotavirus, orbivirus, infantile gastroenteritis virus (IGV), and human reovirus-like agent (HRVL). The name rotavirus now replaces all alternative names.

Rotavirus particles seen in diarrheal feces (Fig. 2) are double-stranded RNA viruses classified as members of a new genus within the family Reoviridae. The rotavirus genome consists of 11 ds RNA segments. This genus includes rotaviruses that cause diarrhea in the young of avian and mammalian species, including calves, pigs, lambs, foals, mice, and rabbits. These animal viruses are morphologically identical with human rotaviruses but differ antigenically from them and from each other.

Rotavirus infections are likely to be clinically more severe than infections due to other agents. Antibody prevalence surveys show that most individuals possess rotavirus antibodies by the end of the third year of life. Serum antibodies cannot be correlated with resistance to infection. Gut mucosal antibodies are difficult to measure but are probably a more accurate indication of immunity. Human rotaviruses can be classified into at least two sub-groups on the basis of antigens present on the inner coat of the particle, and into at least four serotypes representing antigenic differences on the outer coat. Sequential rotavirus infections due to different sub-groups or serotypes of the virus have been recorded in young children. Little is known about cross protection (if any) between different strains of rotavirus. The source of rotavirus infection is person-to-person spread, but contaminated water supplies may be important in initiating infection, particularly in developing countries.

Rotaviruses cause sporadic and epidemic disease in all age groups, but severity of disease and serologic response to infection differ.

Newborn Babies. Rotaviruses infect many newborn babies in obstetric hospital nurseries during the first weeks of life. Diarrhea can be severe but infection is often asymptomatic because of passive protection by maternal antibodies acquired transplacentally or through breast milk. Colostrum and breast milk contain rotavirus antibodies and breast feeding is associated with decreased incidence of rotavirus infection.

Virus particles are shed in feces before onset of symptoms, so isolating only symptomatic babies is unlikely to control spread of infection in a communal nursery. Seroconversion, measured by complement fixation or indirect immunofluorescence, seldom occurs after infection in the newborn. However, neonatal infection probably stimulates gut mucosal antibodies since post-neonatal infection is clinically less severe in children who have experienced neonatal infection (Bishop et al., 1983).

Infants and Young Children. Rotaviruses are the most commonly identified infectious agents in children aged three months to five years who require hospitalization for acute gastroenteritis. They have been identified in 50 to 60 per cent of children in developed countries and in 30 to 50 per cent of children in developing countries. The importance of rotavirus infection in causation of diarrhea not requiring admission to hospital is not known. In temperate countries rotavirus infection is seasonal with a peak incidence during winter months (Davidson et al., 1975). In

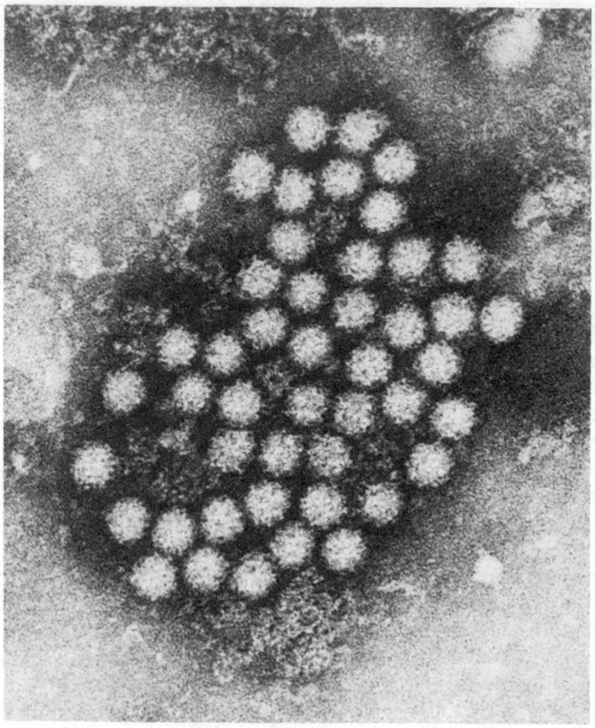

Figure 1. Immune aggregate of Norwalk agent in stool filtrate. (× 156,000) (From Kapikian, A. Z. et al.: J Virol 10:1075, 1972.)

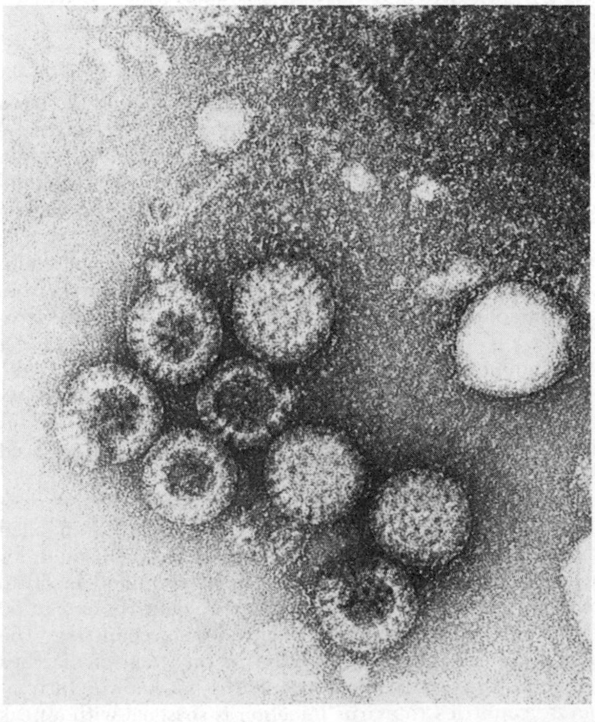

Figure 2. Rotavirus particles in extract of diarrheal stool. (× 132,000).

tropical countries the monthly incidence of rotavirus infection shows little variation throughout the year. The incubation period of the disease is 24 to 48 hours. Virus particles are usually shed in feces in detectable numbers for four to eight days after onset of symptoms. Rotaviruses may be persistently shed in feces from children with immune deficiencies. Nosocomial infection is common in children less than three years of age admitted to hospital with other illnesses. Most infants and young children with rotavirus diarrhea show no detectable levels of antibody at the onset of symptoms, and seroconversion occurs during the disease. The duration of immunity is not known.

Older Children and Adults. By the age of three to five years, most children possess CF antibodies to rotavirus (Blacklow et al., 1976; Gust et al., 1977), and infection is often asymptomatic. Epidemics of diarrhea have been documented in school children 6 to 12 years old and in adults. Fourfold or greater rises in rotavirus antibody occur in some adults with diarrhea, but rotavirus particles are not usually shed in feces in sufficient numbers to be detected by electron microscopy.

Other Viruses. A variety of virus particles has been observed by electron microscopy in diarrheal feces from newborn babies, children, and adults. Their relation to the etiology of diarrhea is uncertain, but some may prove to be pathogens following satisfaction of Koch's postulates as applied to viruses (Rivers, 1937).

Adenoviruses. Electron microscopy has revealed adenoviruses that are not cultivable by the usual cell culture techniques in 5 to 10 per cent of children with gastroenteritis and in nosocomial gastroenteritis. They are identified significantly more frequently from children with diarrhea than from control children (Flewett et al., 1975, Retter et al., 1979, Kapikian et al., 1981) and are excreted in temporal relationship with symptoms of disease. Noncultivable adenoviruses have been identified in children throughout the world, but their importance in developing countries and the age range of infection is not known. A radioimmunoassay to detect adenovirus in stool specimens should assist further studies of their importance in etiology of acute diarrhoea (Halonen et al., 1980).

Astroviruses. These viruses were first described in the United Kingdom in the stools of newborn babies with mild diarrhea and later associated with nosocomial gastroenteritis (Kurtz et al., 1977). The particles are 28 to 30 nm in diameter, exhibit a star-like appearance, and grow poorly, producing no cytopathogenic effects in human embryo kidney cells. Diarrheal illness has been induced and seroresponse to infection has been observed in adult volunteers given astrovirus particles orally. Studies of the prevalence of astrovirus antibodies show that 75 per cent of individuals tested in U.K. had astrovirus antibodies by the 10th year of life. (Kurtz and Lee, 1978). Astrovirus particles have been identified in Japanese children and adults with acute gastroenteritis. The geographic distribution throughout the world is unknown.

Coronaviruses. These agents may be enteric pathogens in man as they are in pigs, dogs, and calves (Kapikian, 1977). Coronavirus-like particles have been seen in an outbreak of gastroenteritis in the United Kingdom and in feces from Indian villagers, Australian aborigines, and residents of a training center for the intellectually retarded. They may not be associated with any specific disease but may contribute to intestinal morphologic abnormalities and malabsorption.

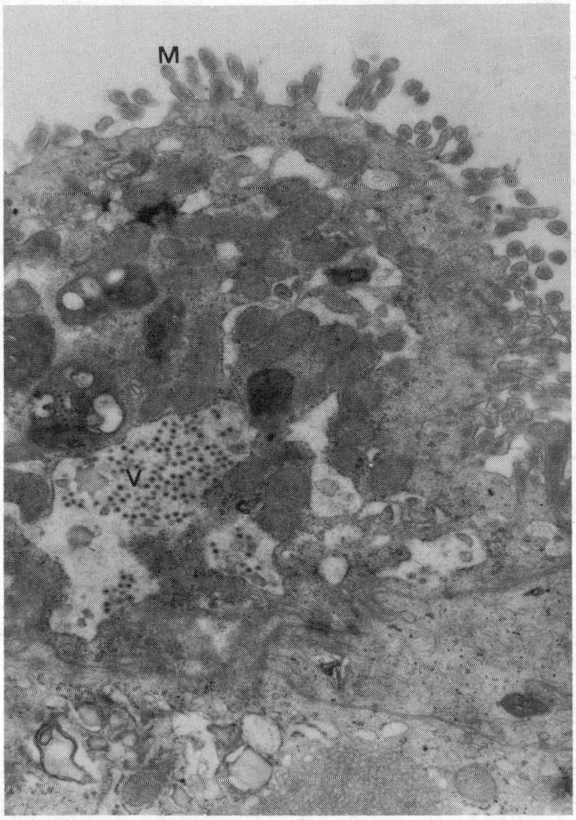

Figure 3. Portion of an epithelial cell of a duodenal villus infected with rotavirus. M, microvilli; V, rotavirus particles. (× 16,000)

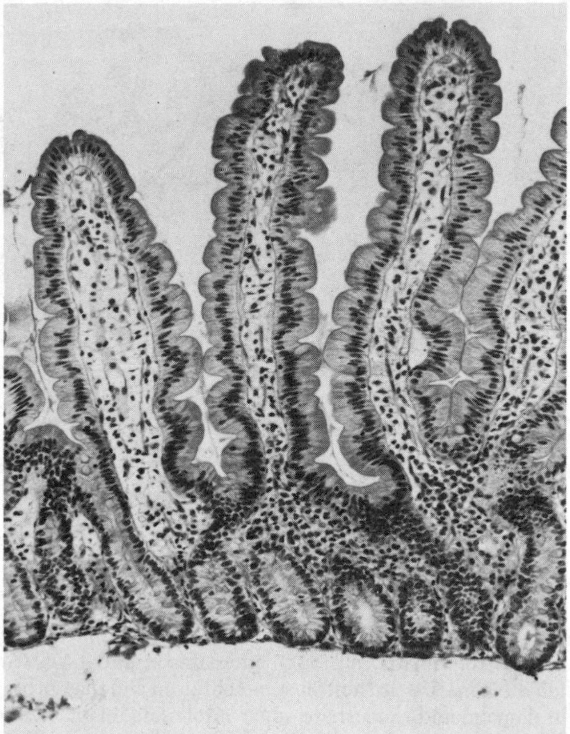

Figure 4. Normal duodenal mucosa from a 4-year-old child. (Hematoxylin and eosin, ×125)

Adenoviruses and echoviruses cultivable by routine cell culture have been isolated from occasional epidemics of diarrhea. Calicivirus particles have been described in the gut mucosa obtained at postmortem from one child with acute gastroenteritis. A variety of small virus-like particles 22 nm in diameter have been seen in human feces (Flewett et al., 1974). They may be bacteriophages or nonpathogenic viruses that infect human gut cells or are shed into the gut lumen from other tissues.

PATHOGENESIS AND PATHOLOGY. Infection with rotaviruses, Norwalk agent, and Hawaii agent results in similar nonspecific and reversible inflammatory changes in human gut mucosa.

The viruses multiply in mature epithelial cells lining the villi of the small intestine (Fig. 3). These cells show vacuolation of the endoplasmic reticulum, swollen mitochondria, increased numbers of cell lysosomes, and multivesicular bodies. Microvilli are irregular and shortened. The cells undergo lysis, leaving the villi denuded. The villi rapidly collapse and are covered by immature epithelial cells that migrate from the crypts.

The pathogenesis of diarrhea probably involves two stages. Initially, denudation of villi allows leakage of fluid and electrolytes into the gut lumen. Later, contraction of the denuded villi and replacement of mature epithelial cells by enzymatically immature cells are associated with the more severe stage of diarrhea (Davidson et al., 1977). This severe stage is probably due to a combination of factors that may include a decrease in the total absorptive surface of the small intestine, a decrease in activity of epithelial cell brush border enzymes including disaccharidases, and secretion by crypt-type cells. Glucose-coupled sodium transport is decreased during viral enteritis compared with infection due to enterotoxigenic bacteria (for example, *Vibrio cholerae* or *E. coli*), in which it is unaffected.

Infection with viral enteric pathogens seems to be restricted to the mucosa of the small intestine, although the stomach and rectal mucosa are mildly inflamed in some children. There is no proof of viremia in immuno-competent children, although rotaviruses have been detected in sera from children with cellular immune deficiencies. Histologically, the gut mucosa shows mild to moderate patchy inflammatory change in most patients (Figs. 4 and 5). Villi appear shorter and blunter and are lined by epithelial cells that are cuboidal and irregular in shape. The lamina propria is infiltrated with mononuclear cells and polymorphonuclear leukocytes. In some children the damage and loss of villi are severe enough to resemble celiac disease (Fig. 6).

It is not known to what extent the severity of clinical symptoms is correlated with the extent of infection along the small intestine. Infection in fatal cases has been seen to extend along the length of the small bowel.

Persistent histologic damage and depression of disaccharidase levels occur in some children, particularly those less than six months old, and may account for sugar intolerance after the symptoms of acute gastroenteritis have subsided. In most children and adults diarrhea is of short duration (one to three days), and the gut mucosa is histologically normal three to four weeks from onset of symptoms.

The bacterial flora of the upper small intestine remains

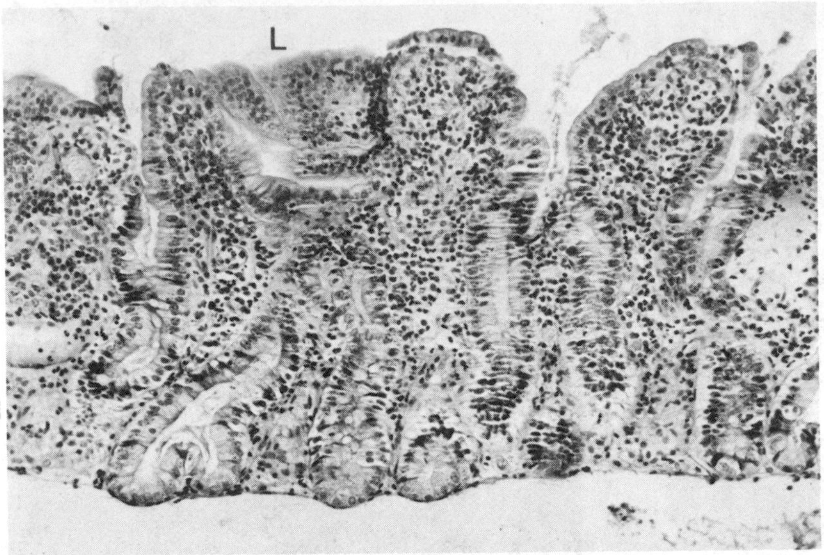

Figure 5. Moderately damaged duodenal mucosa from a 19-month-old child with rotavirus enteritis after two days of illness. Villi are shortened. There is cellular infiltration of the lamina propria and patchy epithelial damage. L, lumen. (Hematoxylin and eosin, ×125)

normal in well-nourished children and adults during acute viral gastroenteritis, although increased numbers of *Candida albicans* are present in some children and may prolong gut damage and exacerbate sugar intolerance. Colonization of the stomach and small intestine may be a consequence of acute gastroenteritis in malnourished children.

CLINICAL MANIFESTATIONS. Viral gastroenteritis has a sudden onset. The symptoms are watery diarrhea, fever, nausea and vomiting, and colicky abdominal pain. Vomiting and fever often precede diarrhea. Stools contain excess electrolytes and may also contain excess sugar (> 0.5 per cent) but blood or leukocytes are uncommon. An apparent upper respiratory tract infection with pharyngeal and tympanic membrane erythema may be present.

Loss of salt and water in stools has little systemic effect in older children and adults. In infants and children less than five years old such losses can lead rapidly to dehydration, electrolyte imbalance, acidosis, shock, and death. Early signs of dehydration are often difficult to detect, particularly in obese or malnourished children. The detectable signs of dehydration are dry mouth, sunken eyes, poor peripheral circulation, and sunken fontanelle. The child may be either irritable or lethargic. The skin loses its elasticity and, if pinched up on the abdominal wall, does not immediately spring back. Decreased urine output is often difficult to detect because bowel movements may be very watery.

The best guide to the degree of dehydration in well-nourished children is measured weight loss. Loss of 5 per cent of body weight (5 per cent dehydration) can just be detected clinically. Severe dehydration occurs when 10 per cent or more of body weight has been lost. This is equivalent to the total blood volume in an infant.

In most children salt losses equal water losses so that serum sodium levels change little. Some patients lose more

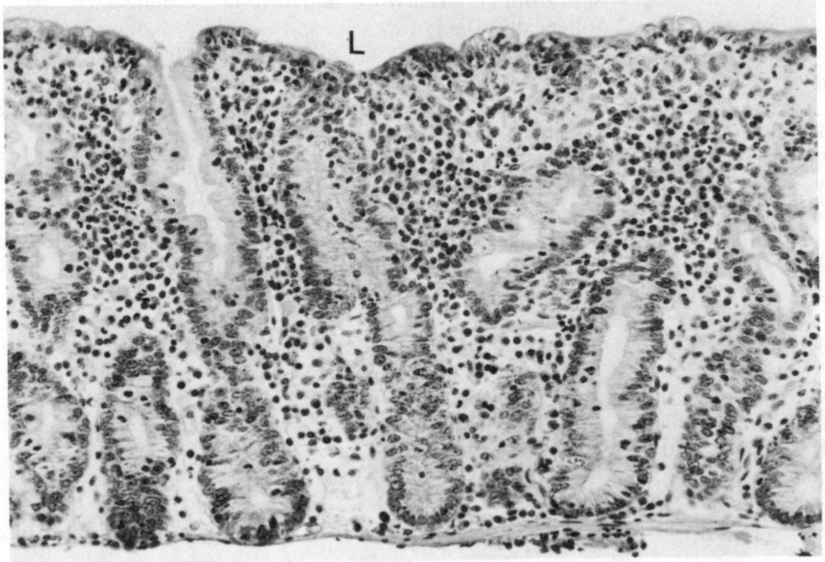

Figure 6. Duodenal mucosa from a 13-month-old child with celiac disease. (Hematoxylin and eosin, ×125)

water than salt and develop hypernatremia. Others become hyponatremic, a special problem in malnourished children. Severe hypokalemia may occur in enteritis associated with malnutrition.

COMPLICATIONS AND SEQUELAE. Viral gastroenteritis is usually self-limited, lasting less than a week. The complications are dehydration with peripheral circulatory failure and death, and hypernatremia (serum sodium >150 mmol/L), which may be associated with convulsions. Sequelae include a persistence of diarrhea, which is associated with sugar intolerance, exacerbation of existing malnutrition, and protracted diarrhea of infancy.

Approximately 1 per cent of children admitted to hospital in urban developed communities die from dehydration and fluid-electrolyte imbalance. Mortality rates among malnourished children for whom medical attention is not readily available can be as high as 30 per cent (Rohde and Northrup, 1976). The severity of diarrhea increases with the degree of malnutrition. Deaths due to viral gastroenteritis in India alone may approach 350,000 per year (Maiya et al., 1977).

Sequelae of viral gastroenteritis differ according to age and nutritional state. Well-nourished older children and adults usually recover quickly with no sequelae. In young children, particularly those less than six months old, diarrhea due to sugar intolerance, which is caused by depression of disaccharidase enzymes, can persist for months.

In malnourished children, the diarrheal episode leads to further malnutrition owing to decreased appetite and restriction of calorie intake. An infant or child given no food will lose approximately 1 per cent of his body weight per day. If the child is already on the borderline of malnutrition this weight loss is serious and can contribute to growth retardation.

DIAGNOSIS. Viral gastroenteritis cannot reliably be distinguished from gastroenteritis caused by other infectious agents on clinical evidence alone. Diagnosis is based on finding viral particles in stool or gut contents, or demonstration of a seroresponse to a viral antigen during infection.

Detection of Viral Particles. A variety of techniques of locating noncultivable viruses in diarrheal stools are available. These techniques vary in efficiency and in practicality. Most have been used only to detect rotaviruses. Feces should be obtained no later than four days after onset of symptoms and can be stored, preferably at +4° C or −70° C, until tested. All techniques are relatively insensitive compared with cell culture for isolation of cultivable viruses. Although human rotaviruses can now be isolated in cell culture (Sato et al., 1981) the technique is not suited to routine diagnosis of infection.

Electron Microscopy. This technique is simple, rapid, and efficient. It permits detection of a wide variety of morphologically different particles but is impractical for large-scale surveys. Fluid feces can be screened for virus particles after negative staining with sodium phosphotungstate or ammonium molybdate. Extracts free of cell debris can also be prepared by differential centrifugation in an ultracentrifuge (Bishop et al., 1974). Norwalk group of agents are detected by immune electron microscopy.

Counter Immunoelectro-osmophoresis. Stool suspensions and rotavirus antisera are placed in adjacent wells on an agarose slide and examined for precipitin lines after incubation and application of an electric current (Middleton et al., 1976). The technique is less sensitive and less specific than electron microscopy but easy to perform, inexpensive, and suitable for rapid screening of many specimens.

Enzyme-Linked Immunosorbent Assay (ELISA). Rotavirus antigen in stool extracts is detected by incubation in microtiter trays with rotavirus antisera, followed by the addition of enzyme-conjugated anti-immunoglobulins (Yolken and Stopa, 1979). The test is sensitive and specific and applicable to large-scale epidemiologic surveys.

Radioimmunoassay (RIA). After the reaction of crude unfiltered fecal suspensions with antisera in microtiter trays ^{125}I-labeled globulin is added. Rotaviruses (Kalica et al., 1977), Norwalk virus (Kapikian et al., 1981), and noncultivable adenoviruses (Halonen et al., 1980) can be detected in stools by using radioimmunoassay.

Immune Adherence Hemagglutination Assay. (IAHA) has been used to identify Norwalk virus in feces (Kapikian et al., 1981).

Detection of rotaviral ds RNA in stool. The rotaviral genome in diarrheal feces is solubilized and extracted and identified by separation of the 11 bands of RNA by gel electrophoresis (Herring et al., 1982). The technique is less sensitive than ELISA but is probably as sensitive as electron microscopy. A 'dot' hybridization assay (Flores et al., 1983) for detection of rotavirus in stools, using labeled RNA probes, may eventually replace many of these techniques.

Detection of Antibodies. The most practical and widely used technique for detection of rotavirus antibodies (adaptable to detection of class-specific antibodies) is ELISA, which uses simian rotavirus (SA11) as antigen (Ghose et al., 1978). Substitution of cultivable human rotaviruses of known serotype will enhance sensitivity and specificity of this test.

Antibody response to infection with Norwalk agent and related agents is demonstrated by immune electron microscopy, IAHA, or RIA.

TREATMENT. Antidiarrheal preparations and antispasmodics are of little value in treatment of viral gastroenteritis and may be dangerous for young children. Antiemetics may give relief in older children and adults when the main symptom is vomiting. Antibiotics are of no value in treatment of viral enteritis and in fact may cause further mucosal damage. When the etiologic agent is unknown, antibiotics are indicated only if there is clinical suspicion of septicemia or meningitis.

Childhood diarrhea is initially treated by oral rehydration at home. Although glucose-stimulated Na^+ absorption is decreased in viral gastroenteritis, it is possible that sufficient uninfected gut remains to allow some absorption of water, electrolytes, and glucose. It is extremely important to start rehydration early, because dehydration begins with the first diarrheal stool. The measures adopted for oral rehydration vary according to the state of nutrition of the child. Well-nourished children in developed countries are treated by temporary withdrawal of regular feeds, and oral feeding with isotonic carbohydrate solutions, such as soft drinks exhausted of carbonation, glucose, or corn syrup in boiled water (one tablespoon per liter). It is important not to give solutions containing large amounts of sodium since they may lead to, or worsen, hypernatremia.

In developing countries, rehydration is begun at home by using Oralyte packets (UNICEF), containing NaCl, $NaHCO_3$, KC1 and glucose. These are available at village stores or are distributed by local health workers. Contents of the package are diluted in one liter of clean water and given initially to assuage thirst. This is followed by one glass of prepared fluid for each stool passed (Rohde and Northrup, 1976). If the UNICEF packages are not available, a simple rehydration kit can be assembled locally (Cutting, 1976). Breast feeding, if established, should be continued.

Once moderate dehydration is evident, the patient should be hospitalized. Electrolyte and acid-base studies are not required routinely but are indicated if there is severe dehydration, disturbance of the conscious state, twitching, or convulsions. Intravenous fluid volumes are adjusted to replace fluid and electrolyte *deficit* with saline (40 mmol/L of sodium chloride and dextrose, 5 per cent). Once urine output is established, 40 mmol/L of potassium chloride is added. The deficit of fluid and electrolytes is usually replaced during the first 24 hours in the absence of hypernatremic dehydration. During the first 24 hours it is also necessary to administer *maintenance* fluid requirements and to replace *continuing losses* due to vomiting, diarrhea, and insensible losses. Maintenance fluid requirements adjusted for age are then continued until an oral diet is established.

Hypernatremic dehydration has special hazards including convulsions and other neurologic sequelae. Intravenous rehydration should be slow (e.g., replacement of deficit over 48 hours or more). This allows more time for electrolyte and water transport across cell membranes and decreases the likelihood of cerebral edema.

Peripheral circulatory failure occurs in severe dehydration (>10 per cent body weight loss). It is characterized by tachycardia, weak pulse, low blood pressure, and cold mottled skin over the extremities. The first priority is to restore circulation with isotonic fluids. In otherwise healthy children isotonic electrolyte solutions containing some bicarbonate (20 to 25 ml/kg given in 30 minutes) will suffice. In malnourished children hypoproteinemia may be present, so plasma or whole blood may be more appropriate. After circulation has been restored, rehydration and maintenance fluids are given as above.

Within 24 to 48 hours of the start of intravenous therapy, oral fluids can usually be reintroduced. Initially, glucose-electrolyte solutions are given as described above. In most patients the previous diet can be resumed a day or two later, but fruits and other foods that may cause loose movements in healthy children should be avoided. If diarrhea persists, stools should be checked for sugar content by the Clinitest method (Kerry and Anderson, 1964). A sugar concentration of greater than 0.5 per cent is abnormal. Glucose-containing milk substitutes can be used when available. Many children with lactose intolerance can tolerate sucrose feeds. It may be necessary to stop breast feeding temporarily; the mother should express breast milk meantime to maintain the flow. In malnourished children and infants under three months the primary concern after 48 to 72 hours should be reestablishment of an adequate nutrient intake, even at the expense of an increase in fecal output.

PROPHYLAXIS. Improvements in housing, environmental sanitation, and purity of water supplies should reduce the incidence of enteric disease in developing countries but may have little impact on viral gastroenteritis, since this remains a major health problem even in wealthy, developed, urban communities. Control of viral enteritis awaits understanding of the mechanisms of immunity and may be achieved eventually by oral vaccination, particularly against rotavirus; however, more immediate prophylactic measures against viral gastroenteritis are available and should be used.

Prevention of Gastroenteritis in Infants. Infection with rotaviruses in babies is often asymptomatic, probably due to passive protection by maternal antibody acquired transplacentally or in breast milk. In countries where nutrition of the small child is threatened by poverty and inadequate diet, breast feeding may be vital in protecting against viral enteric infection.

Prevention of Nosocomial Infection. This should be possible by attention to strict standards of hygiene in hospital wards. Design and staffing of wards must take into account the highly infectious nature of viral enteric pathogens. Hands must be washed carefully with soap and water between attending to patients, since rotavirus particles have been detected on the hands of ward attendants.

Prevention of Dehydration. This is of major importance in reducing deaths due to viral gastroenteritis and may be a key factor in preventing onset or exacerbation of malnutrition in infants in poor communities (Rohde and Northrup, 1976). It is necessary first to inform mothers that diarrhea is not a normal phase of growth but a life-threatening disease. Through health education, parents can be made to understand the need for early oral rehydration and can be given the means to do so with readily available cheap sources of glucose and electrolytes.

References

Bishop, R. F., Barnes, G. L., Cipriani, E. and Lund, J. S.: Clinical immunity after neonatal rotavirus infection: A prospective longitudinal study in young children. N Engl J Med 309:72, 1983.

Bishop, R. F., Davidson, G. P., Holmes, I. H., and Ruck, B. J.: Virus particles in epithelial cells of duodenal mucosa from children with acute non-bacterial gastroenteritis. Lancet 2:1281, 1973.

Bishop, R. F., Davidson, G. P., Holmes, I. H., and Ruck, B. J.: Detection of a new virus by electron microscopy of faecal extracts from children with acute gastroenteritis. Lancet 1:149, 1974.

Blacklow, N. R., Echeverria, P., and Smith, P. H.: Serological studies with reovirus-like enteritis agent. Infect Immun 13:1563, 1976.

Cutting, W. A. M.: In Acute Diarrhoea in Childhood. Ciba Foundation Symposium 42 (new series). Amsterdam, Elsevier Publishing Company, 1976, p. 361.

Davidson, G. P., Bishop, R. F., Townley, R. R. W., Holmes, I. H., and Ruck, B. J.: Importance of a new virus in acute sporadic enteritis in children. Lancet 1:242, 1975.

Davidson, G. P., Gall, D. G., Butler, D. G., Petric, M., and Hamilton, J. R.: Human rotavirus enteritis induced in conventional piglets: Intestinal structure and transport. J Clin Invest 60:1402, 1977.

Flewett, T. H., Bryden, A. S., and Davies, H.: Diagnostic electron microscopy of faeces. I. The viral flora of faeces as seen by electron microscopy. J Clin Pathol 27:603, 1974.

Flewett, T. H., Bryden, A. S., and Davies, H.: Epidemic viral enteritis in a long stay children's ward. Lancet, 1:4, 1975.

Flores, J., Boeggeman, E., Purcell, R. N., Sereno, M., Perez, I., White, L., Wyatt, R. G., Chanock, R. M., and Kapikian, A. Z.: A dot hybridisation assay for detection of rotavirus. Lancet, 1:555, 1983.

Ghose, L. H., Schnagl, R. D., and Holmes, I. H.: Comparison of an enzyme linked immunosorbent assay for quantitation of rotavirus antibodies with complement fixation in an epidemiological survey. J Clin Microbiol 5:268, 1978.

Gust, I. D., Pringle, R. C., Barnes, G. L., Davidson, G. P., and Bishop, R. F.: Complement-fixing antibody response to rotavirus infection. J Clin Microbiol 5:125, 1977.

Halonen, P., Sarkkinen, H., Arstila, P., Hjertsson, E., and Torfason, E.: Four-layer radioimmunoassay for detection of adenovirus in stool. J Clin Microbiol 11:614, 1980.

Herring, A. J., Inglis, N. F., Ojeh, C. K., Snodgrass, D. R. and Menzies, J. D.: Rapid diagnosis of rotavirus infection by direct detection of viral nucleic acid in silver-stained polyacrylamide gels. J Clin Microbiol 16:473, 1982.

Holmes, I. H. Rotaviruses, in Joklik, W. K. (ed.): The Reoviridae. Plenum Publishing Corp, N.Y. 1983, p. 350.

Kalica, A. R., Purcell, R. H., Sereno, M. M., Wyatt, R. G., Kim, H. W., Chanock, R. M., and Kapikian, A. Z.: A microtitre solid phase radioimmunoassay for detection of the human reovirus-like agent in stools. J Immunol 118:1275, 1977.

Kapikian, A. Z.: The Coronaviruses. In Oxford, J. S. (ed.): Chemoprophylaxis and Virus Infections of the Respiratory Tract, Vol. 2. CRC Press, 1977, p. 95.

Kapikian, A. Z., Greenberg, H. B., Kalica, A. R., Wyatt, R. G., Kim, H. W., Brandt, C. D., Rodriguez, W. J., Flores, J., Singh, N., Parrot, R. H., and Chanock, R. M.: New developments in viral gastroenteritis. In Holme, T., Holmgren, J., Merson, M. H., and Möllby, R. (eds.): Acute enteric infections in children, New prospects for treatment and prevention. Elsevier/North Holland Biomedical Press, 1981, p. 9.

Kapikian, A. Z., Wyatt, R. G., Dolin, R., Thornhill, T. S., Kalica, A. R., and Chanock, R. M.: Visualization by immune electron-microscopy of a 27 nm particle associated with acute infectious non-bacterial gastroenteritis. J Virol 10:1075, 1972.

Kerry, K. R., and Anderson, C. M.: A ward test for sugars in faeces. Lancet 1:981, 1964.

Kurtz, J. B., and Lee, T. W.: Astrovirus age distribution of antibody. Med Microbiol Immunol 166:227, 1978.

Kurtz, J. B., Lee, T. W., and Pickering, D.: Astrovirus associated gastroenteritis in a children's ward. J Clin Pathol 30:948, 1977.

Leading article: Rotaviruses of man and animals. Lancet 1:257, 1975.

Maiya, P. P., Pereira, S. M., Mathan, M., Bhat, P., Albert, M. J., and Baker, S. J. Aetiology of acute gastroenteritis in infancy and early childhood in Southern India. Arch Dis Child 52:482, 1977.

Middleton, P. J., Petric, M., Hewitt, C. M., Szymanski, M. T., and Tam, J. S.: Counter-immunoelectro-osmophoresis for the detection of infantile gastroenteritis virus (orbi-group) antigen and antibody. J Clin Pathol 29:191, 1976.

Retter, M., Middleton, P. J., Tam, J. S., and Petric, M.: Enteric adenoviruses: Detection, implication and significance. J Clin Microbiol 10:574, 1979.

Rivers, T. M.: Viruses and Koch's postulates. J Bacteriol 33:1, 1937.

Rohde, J. E., and Northrup, R. S.: Taking science where the diarrhoea is. In Acute Diarrhoea in Childhood. Ciba Foundation Symposium 42 (new series). Amsterdam, Elsevier Publishing Company 1976, p. 339.

Sato, K., Inaba, Y., Shinozaki, T., Fuji, R., and Matumoto, H.: Isolation of human rotavirus in cell cultures. Arch Virol, 69:155, 1981.

Schreiber, D. S., Trier, J. S., and Blacklow, N. R.: Recent advances in viral gastroenteritis. Gastroenterology 73:174, 1977.

Yolken, R. N., and Stopa, P. J.: Analysis of non-specific reactions in enzyme linked immunosorbent assay testing for human rotavirus. J Clin Microbiol 10:703, 1979.

147

CHOLECYSTITIS AND CHOLANGITIS

KAORU SHIMADA, M.D.

CHOLECYSTITIS

Cholecystitis, inflammation of the gallbladder, may be acute or chronic. Over 90 per cent of cases are associated with gallstones. Acute cholecystitis is usually superimposed on a chronic process, and is precipitated by obstruction of the cystic duct by a stone (or rarely, by invasion of resident organisms or edema in the absence of calculus).

ETIOLOGY. Gallbladder outlet obstruction is the common factor in the vast majority of cases of acute cholecystitis. The impacted calculus is the commonest cause for obstruction. Other possible causes of obstruction are malformation of the cystic duct; mucosal edema and fibrosis secondary to inflammatory changes at duct orifice; kinking and torsion of the cystic duct; stasis bile plugs; compression by adhesions or by enlarged lymph nodes; infiltration by neoplasm; and parasites, particularly *Ascaris lumbricoides*. Outlet obstruction by itself does not evoke acute cholecystitis, and additional factors are required to initiate inflammation. Bacterial infection was once regarded as the principal etiologic factor, but was not consistent with the fact that patients without cholecystitis sometimes had bacteria in the gallbladder and that, in the early stage of acute cholecystitis, sterile cultures were obtained by surgery from the bile or gallbladder wall. Experimentally bacteria alone cannot produce acute cholecystitis unless there is damage to the gallbladder or interference with its blood supply. From these findings the idea evolved that cholecystitis is caused by chemical action and that infection is superimposed upon the damaged gallbladder. Acute cholecystitis has been reproduced experimentally by injecting pancreatic juice or concentrated bile into the obstructed gallbladder. Lecithin, a phospholipid normally present in bile, is converted to lysolecithin by phospholipase, an enzyme in the pancreatic juice and liver. The toxicity of lysolecithin for membranes may be implicated, at least experimentally, in acute cholecystitis in the obstructed gallbladder. Thus, in some cases it is possible that reflux of pancreatic juice is responsible for acute cholecystitis. Bile acids are found conjugated with glycine or taurine in bile. The major human bile acids are cholic, chenodeoxycholic, and deoxycholic acids. Unconjugated bile acids are much more toxic than conjugated and deoxycholic acid produces the most marked reaction. Deconjugation of bile salts by bacteria may enhance the inflammatory reaction that the bile salts are thought to trigger. The infecting organisms most often recovered from acute cholecystitis are primarily enteric bacteria, such as *Escherichia coli, Klebsiella, Enterobacter, Proteus*, and streptococci, including the enterococcus. Recent studies revealed that anaerobes may be more frequently involved in biliary tract infections than had been appreciated. *Bacteroides fragilis* was the most common anaerobe, followed by *Clostridium perfringens*. Since *B. fragilis*, clostridia and *Streptococcus fecalis* can hydrolyze bile acid conjugates, it is possible that these bacteria produce more toxic bile salts in the gallbladder.

Infecting bacteria may reach the gallbladder via bile duct, blood, or lymphatics, or extension from neighboring organs. Severe systemic infection may be accompanied by cholecystitis. Salmonella infection of the gallbladder is frequently observed in patients who have a history of typhoid fever. Other possible factors are vascular (arteritis, arteriolitis, venous or lymphatic stasis), neural (imbalance between sympathetic and vagal action), and humoral (cholecystokinin). The etiologic factors of chronic cholecystitis are believed to be the same as those involved in acute cholecystitis. However, the details of its evolution remain obscure.

PATHOLOGIC ANATOMY AND PATHOGENESIS. In acute cholecystitis, the gallbladder is hyperemic, edematous, and enlarged. The lumen is tensely filled with a mixture of turbid bile, inflammatory exudate, and pus. The cystic duct may be obstructed owing to stone incarceration and/or dyskinesia of Oddi muscles or cell debris. Microscopically, inflammatory changes consist of vascular congestion, interstitial edema, and cellular infiltration. In severe cases, the mucosa may be gangrenous and frequently have ulceration that penetrates the wall of the bladder. The morphologic features of chronic cholecystitis vary with the stage of inflammation. The gallbladder is sometimes contracted and scarred, or normal in size, or enlarged, and may develop inflammatory adhesions to the surrounding tissues. Commonly, the wall shows fibrous thickening, or may be severely distended by obstruction. The contents are clear, turbid, or composed of mucoid bile and multiple gallstones. Histologically, the herniation of the epithelium into the smooth musculature, known as Rokitansky-Aschoff's sinuses, is recognized in up to 90 per cent of cases. Acute inflammatory changes are often superimposed on the chronically inflamed gallbladder.

At autopsy more than half of all adults have inflammatory changes in the gallbladder, of no clinical significance.

CLINICAL MANIFESTATIONS. Cholecystitis is prominent in those who are "female, fat, and forty." It occurs about three times as often in women and especially in obese persons. Although cholecystitis is seen at all ages, it is uncommon until the thirties, and most common in the fifth and sixth decades. Acute cholecystitis is frequently precipitated by overwork or a heavy meal. The most prominent symptom is severe right upper quadrant pain, which usually radiates to the right shoulder or infrascapular region. It may start with discomfort in the midepigastrium, increase in intensity as biliary colic develops, and soon becomes a continuous and unbearable pain in the right hypochondrium, accentuated by movement or deep inspiration. Breathing may be shallow and rapid to prevent intensifying the pain. The patients writhe or lie in a jackknife position. Nausea and vomiting are frequent. Fever (38° C to 39° C) and chills occur regularly. Most patients exhibit tenderness and muscle spasm in the right upper quadrant and epigastrium. An acutely inflamed gallbladder is palpable only at times. If the patient takes a deep, slow breath while the physician's fingers are hooked up deep beneath the right costal arch, there may be momentary interruption of breathing because of pain (Murphy's sign). The clinical manifestations of acute cholecystitis depend on the severity of inflammation. As inflammation progresses from serous to seropurulent, purulent, and phlegmonogangrenous, the manifestations become worse. Rebound tenderness in the right hypochondrium and midepigastrium occurs in suppurative cholecystitis with peritoneal inflammation. Persistent vomiting, the spread of tenderness, and rebound tenderness over the abdomen commonly indicate either perforation of the gallbladder or associated pancreatitis.

Leukocytosis is usually moderate. Leukocytosis over 20,000 raises the suspicion of gangrene or perforation. The serum bilirubin and alkaline phosphatase may be elevated mildly even in the absence of common duct obstruction, probably owing to inflammatory edema of the extrahepatic bile duct. Serum bilirubin over 5 mg/100 ml suggests concomitant common duct stone. Rise of serum amylase level reflects associated pancreatitis. Urobilinogen is usually increased in the urine, and decreases rapidly after the inflammation subsides.

Bile may be collected by duodenal intubation (Meltzer-Lyon test) but only after acute inflammation has fully subsided to avoid gallbladder contraction. Many pus cells and epithelial cells are observed. If concentrated gallbladder bile (B-bile) does not appear the cystic duct may be obstructed or the gallbladder nonfunctioning. A carefully collected specimen can be used for bacteriologic examination.

A plain film of the abdomen frequently shows gallstones. Intravenous cholecystocholangiography by drip infusion will not opacify the gallbladder if the cystic duct is obstructed or the gallbladder is unable to concentrate the dye. Excretion of contrast media may also fail in acute hepatitis or acute pancreatitis. Thus, a negative cholecystogram should be interpreted with caution. On the other hand, visualization of a gallbladder with normal shape and contractive properties rules out acute cholecystitis. Gallbladder scanning with HIDA (^{99}mTc dimethyl acetanilide iminodiacetic acid) is also used in the evaluation of cholecystitis. If no radioactivity accumulates in the gallbladder, usually within 90 minutes after injection, the bile duct may not be patent and inflammation is likely. Ultrasound shows calculi, sludge and a thick wall.

Chronic cholecystitis is almost invariably associated with gallstones. The manifestations of chronic cholecystitis fall into two categories: vague digestive complaints and recurrent biliary colic. The digestive complaints include postprandial belching and intolerance of fat. Although occasionally the attacks may not be clear-cut, the diagnosis is suggested by right hypochrondrium tenderness, indigestion after a fat meal, and inflammatory signs such as slight fever and positive test for C-reactive protein. On cholecystography, calculi are frequently demonstrated. The gallbladder is not visualized, or is opacified very faintly without contracting. Hydrops of the gallbladder or limy bile are radiologic findings compatible with chronic cholecystitis. Duodenal drainage may provide important information if the diagnosis is in doubt. Since chronic cholecystitis may cause a wide variety of nonspecific symptoms, the diagnosis is often misused as a wastebasket for functional indigestion in patients with no gallbladder disease. The term should be reserved for patients with recurrent attacks of acute cholecystitis in whom gallbladder function is abnormal on x-ray or in whom chronic inflammation is seen in the gallbladder on peritoneoscopy.

Many attacks of acute cholecystitis subside within one to three days, but in a few cases the inflammatory process does not abate and is progressive. Septicemia, cholangitis, pancreatitis, pylephlebitis, and perforation are complications of acute cholecystitis. Chronic cholecystitis with cholelithiasis is prone to relapse and recurrence.

DIAGNOSIS. Differential diagnosis includes perforated peptic ulcer, acute pancreatitis, appendicitis, mesenteric arterial occlusion, bowel strangulation, pyelonephritis, urolithiasis, acute salpingitis, pleurisy, right lower lobe pneumonia, and myocardial infarction. In cases with jaundice, one must also exclude acute hepatitis, hemolytic crisis, and malignancy of the extrahepatic biliary system. These diseases are easily differentiated from acute cholecystitis. Most errors in diagnosis occur in patients with pyelonephritis, urolithiasis, or pyonephrosis. In general back tenderness is more severe, fever is higher, leukocytosis is greater with an infected kidney, but none of these is specific or pathognomonic. Urinalysis will usually exclude renal infections.

A particularly difficult diagnostic problem is presented by acute pancreatitis, which tends to occur in alcoholic patients. Elevated levels of lipase in serum, and amylase level in both serum and urine suggest pancreatitis. However, pancreatitis and cholelithiasis often occur together. Patients with hepatic problems (acute hepatitis, hepatic congestion, or metastatic disease) may have severe pain and a mass in the right hypochondrium.

TREATMENT. It is generally accepted that symptomatic cholelithiasis is a surgical disease. The same applies to most patients with cholecystitis, since over 90 per cent have gallstones, but the time for operation is controversial. Some surgeons prefer early surgical treatment within 24 to 48 hours after the onset to avoid rupture of the gallbladder during the attack. The collected experiences indicate that for the acute attack, operative and nonoperative measures are equally effective in patients without coincident serious disease such as diabetes mellitus. It should be emphasized, however, that the patient must be managed medically if suitable operating facilities and experienced personnel are not available. Most patients, especially those under 50 can be treated conservatively until recovery from the acute attack. Elective cholecystectomy is recommended after several weeks.

Parenteral fluids, nasogastric suction, antispasmodics, analgesics, and antibiotics are used in acute cholecystitis. Nasogastric suction not only decompresses the stomach, but also reduces the stimulus to gallbladder contraction from gastrointestinal hormones. Meperidine 0.1 g and atropine sulfate 0.5 g every 4 to 6 hours, as needed, is given subcutaneously for moderate pain. For severe pain, a combination of opiates and atropine sulfate may prove satisfactory. Antibiotics are an essential part of therapy. One should choose a drug excreted in bile in high concentration and effective against coliform bacteria. Cefoperazone or moxalactam in doses of 1 g intravenously every eight hours fulfills these requirements. Cefoxitin (1 g intravenously every four to six hours) or ampicillin (1 g intravenously every six hours) is also recommended, but ampicillin is not effective against *Klebsiella* or *Enterobacter*, which are the next most common organisms in bile. The efficacy of the aminoglycosides in biliary tract infection is in doubt, since their biliary excretion is negligible. Over 80 to 90 per cent of patients respond to these medical measures within one to three days. Failure to improve would indicate a complication requiring emergency operation.

Aged patients with acute cholecystitis are less likely to respond to conservative therapy, especially when diabetic. Advanced age, arteriosclerosis and decreased resistance to infection together cause a high incidence of perforation with consequent infection. There is no place for prolonged medical treatment of acute cholecystitis in diabetics, and old age is no longer a contraindication for biliary surgery, even as an emergency operation. In a desperate situation, percutaneous biliary decompression may be life-saving.

Cholecystectomy is indicated for chronic cholecystitis if patients have biliary stones, or convincing evidence of gallbladder nonfunction. For patients whose diagnosis is questionable, who have minimal symptoms, or who refuse surgery, medical management is composed of a low fat diet and antispasmodics. Patients who complain of vague gastrointestinal symptoms with minor abnormalities on cholecystogram—that is, faint opacification and impaired contraction—are a difficult problem. Conservative treatment is better for these patients than surgery, since those who have a normal biliary tract at surgery are not relieved by cholecystectomy.

CHOLANGITIS

Cholangitis is an inflammation of intra- and extrahepatic bile ducts usually associated with bacterial infection, and characterized by the triad of Charcot (1877): spiking fever with chills, jaundice, and pain in the right upper abdominal quadrant. Obstruction of the common duct is an important etiologic factor. Cholangitis occurs primarily in elderly patients with choledocolithiasis or scarring at the choledochoduodenal junction. The incidence of cholangitis is low with biliary neoplasms. The same bacteria are found in the bile as in cholecystitis, and two or more organisms are often cultured.

Cholangitis comprises a variety of clinical syndromes depending on the degree of obstruction. The nonsuppurative form is most common. At the other extreme is the catastrophic picture of acute suppurative obstructive cholangitis (Welch and Donaldson, 1976). Nonsuppurative cholangitis subsides promptly after antibiotics without surgical therapy, probably because the obstruction is transient. Acute suppurative cholangitis appears to be related to complete obstruction of bile flow within the common duct in the presence of pathogenic bacteria. Its development after transhepatic or retrograde cholangiography, suggests that these procedures can elevate pressure in the bile duct and simulate sudden obstruction.

PATHOLOGY. Above the obstruction, the bile duct becomes distended and its wall shows inflammatory thickening. The liver is enlarged and in suppurative cholangitis there may be multiple microabscesses. There is the neutrophil infiltration within small ducts in periductal and portal areas, proliferation of ducts, and centrilobular bile stasis.

MANIFESTATIONS AND TREATMENT. Acute suppurative cholangitis starts abruptly, progresses rapidly, and is often fatal in a few hours or days. Patients suffer agonizing right upper quadrant pains, progressive obstructive jaundice, unremitting high fever, and circulatory collapse. Septicemia, shock, and mental confusion or delirium are common. Septic shock is thought to be the common cause of death. Antibiotics have no effect unless biliary obstruction is relieved. Only surgical decompression of the pus-filled duct is life-saving. Operative mortality approximates 40 to 50 per cent in patients with hypotension and septicemia, but is much lower if surgery is performed before septic shock develops. Therefore, surgery should be considered as an emergency procedure if patients deteriorate rapidly or do not improve within 24 to 36 hours. Fluid and electrolyte replacement is essential both pre- and postoperatively to prevent renal failure. It is also important to administer intravenously antibiotics effective against gram-negative bacteria and anaerobes, such as cefazolin and clindamycin in combination. A dose of 1 g cefoperazone and 600 mg clindamycin can be given every six hours.

RECURRENT PYOGENIC CHOLANGITIS

ETIOLOGY. Recurrent pyogenic cholangitis, also known as oriental cholangiohepatitis, intrahepatic pigment stone disease and biliary obstruction syndrome of the Chinese is found almost exclusively in China, Southeast Asia, Korea, and Japan. In Hong Kong, after acute appendicitis and perforated peptic ulcer, it is the third most common cause of acute abdominal emergencies admitted to hospitals. Sporadic cases reported in North America, Britain, Australia, and Ceylon usually occur in immigrants from these countries.

Since the liver fluke *Clonorchis sinensis* is endemic in China, infestation of the bile duct with *Clonorchis sinensis* was thought to be an etiologic factor, resulting in stone formation, biliary obstruction, stasis, and infection. *Clonorchis sinensis* ova were recognized in stools of 25 per cent of the patients in Hong Kong, and ova or dead adult worms could be found in the center of occasional stones. But this cannot be the cause outside the endemic area, as in Malaya where many patients with recurrent pyogenic cholangitis are seen, because *Clonorchis* infestation does not occur due to the absence of a suitable snail as intermediate host. Other possible etiologic factors include portal bacteremia, congenital or acquired biliary strictures, low protein and low saturated fat diet, and coliform and anaerobic bacterial infection in the biliary tract, producing β-glucuronidase, which deconjugates bilirubin to precipitate insoluble calcium bilirubinate. A combination of these probably causes most cases.

PATHOLOGY. The stones in this disease are usually multiple pigment stones that usually originate in the bile duct, in contrast with cholelithiasis in Western countries where cholesterol stones formed primarily in the gallbladder are predominant. The whole biliary system dilates secondary to multiple strictures filled with soft friable stones, mud, and debris. The bile duct walls are usually thickened by fibrosis. The gallbladder is enlarged, shows chronic inflammation, and contains stones in 10 to 20 per cent of the patients. The liver shows acute purulent cholangitis, and portal fibrosis with accompanying inflammatory infiltrates.

CLINICAL MANIFESTATIONS AND TREATMENT. Unlike biliary tract infections in Western countries, which are much more common in older women, recurrent pyogenic cholangitis usually occurs between 30 and 40 years of age with no sexual predilection. Manifestations are almost the same as those of other types of cholangitis with spiking fever, shaking chills, right upper quadrant pain, and jaundice. Each attack may subside in several days, or cause septicemia, shock, or miliary hepatic abscesses. Oral and intravenous cholecystography is usually unrevealing, but sonography shows dilated ducts and intrahepatic stones. Computerized tomography is also excellent for evaluating recurrent pyogenic cholangitis.

Antibiotics control many acute exacerbations, but recurrence is common. Removal of stones combined with a biliary drainage procedure such as choledochojejunostomy and sphincteroplasty is not entirely satisfactory, since intrahepatic stones cannot usually be extirpated. Stones and strictures recur after surgery and the relapsing clinical course sometimes terminates in hepatic failure. However, prolonged relief is achieved by external biliary drainage or duodenal intubation with administration of cholagogues and choleretics after removal of stones.

References

Charcot, J. M.: Lecon sur les maladies due Foie des Voies Filiares et des Reins, Paris, Faculte de Medecine de Paris, 1877.

Du Plessis, D. J., and Jersky, J.: The management of acute cholecystitis. Surg Clin North Am 53:1071, 1973.

Federle, M. P., Cello, J. P., Laing, F. C., and Jeffrey, Jr., R. B.: Recurrent pyogenic cholangitis in Asian immigrants. Use of ultrasonography, computed tomography, and cholangiography. Radiology 143:151, 1982.

Halasz, N. A.: Counterfeit cholecystitis, a common diagnostic dilemma. Am J Surg 130:189, 1975.

Saik, R. P., Greenburg, A. G., Farris, J. M., and Peskin, G. W.: Spectrum of cholangitis. Am J Surg 130:143, 1975.

Schein, C. J.: Acute Cholecystitis. New York, Harper & Row, 1972.

Shimada, K., Inamatsu, T., and Yamashiro, M.: Anaerobic bacteria in biliary disease in elderly patients. J Infect Dis 135:850, 1977.

Stock, F. E., and Fung, J. H.: Oriental cholangiohepatitis. Arch Surg 84:47, 1962.

Welch, J. P., and Donaldson, G. A.: The urgency and surgical treatment of acute suppurative cholangitis. Am J Surg 131:527, 1976.

148

LIVER AND SUBPHRENIC ABSCESS

EDWARD BROOK ROTHERAM, JR., M.D.

Liquefactive or suppurative lesions of the liver and subphrenic spaces are caused by *Entamoeba histolytica* or bacteria. A few of the species of bacteria are well-known pathogens but most are poorly virulent members of the normal intestinal flora. The latter are often recovered in mixed culture and many are strict anaerobes (Sabbaj et al., 1972).

PATHOGENESIS AND PATHOLOGY. Amebas reach the liver from the colon via the portal vein and often produce liver abscesses in the absence of symptomatic colitis. Inexplicably, men are afflicted far more often than women. As with all solitary abscesses of portal venous origin, the right hepatic lobe is involved much more often than the left lobe. Since blood from the splenic vein streams preferentially into the left lobe, the right lobe, already six times larger, receives an even larger proportion of the blood coming from the heavily colonized lower intestine.

Named for their ability to lyse living tissue, *E. histolytica* organisms do not incite a local granulocytic inflammatory response. Although strict anaerobes, they do not produce a foul odor. Thus, amebic abscess fluid, in the absence of bacterial superinfection, consists of liquefied liver tissue containing few if any granulocytes and no bacteria on gram stain or culture. Motile trophozoites are confined largely to the abscess wall, and their demonstration in the abscess fluid is difficult. The classic "anchovy paste" results from hemorrhage into the abscess cavity. If bleeding has not occurred, the fluid is yellow or green rather than red or chocolate brown.

Since bacteria produce cavities filled with granulocytes, the adjective "pyogenic" is applied to all liver abscesses of bacterial etiology. If the pus has a fetid odor, the presence of anaerobic bacteria is ensured whether or not aerobes are also recovered.

Bacteria can reach the liver by way of the biliary tree, the portal vein, the hepatic artery, a contiguous infection, or a penetrating wound. Bacterial colonization of the unobstructed biliary tract is well tolerated as illustrated by the chronic typhoid carrier. However, partial obstruction of the common bile duct by stone, benign stricture, or periampullary carcinoma leads to ascending cholangitis if the bile is infected. Abscesses secondary to ascending cholangitis are often multiple and caused by those bacteria associated with cholelithiasis (Table 1). Although strict anaerobes are relatively infrequent in ascending cholangitis, *Clostridium perfringens* must be considered. Since cholelithiasis and prior operations upon the biliary tract are associated with a high incidence of biliary tract infection, the obstructing lesion is often not neoplastic and prompt diagnosis can be rewarded by a full recovery.

Bacteremia of the portal vein (pylephlebitis) results from septic thrombophlebitis in tributary veins draining foci of infection in the gastrointestinal tract. (Thrombosis of the portal vein itself is rare.) Resulting liver abscesses are usually single, but two or three large abscesses or even multiple small abscesses can occur. Their bacterial flora is of lower intestinal origin and, hence, often polymicrobial and predominantly or exclusively anaerobic (Table 1). The failure to recover these anaerobic bacteria because of unsatisfactory culture methods accounts for the high incidence of sterile pyogenic liver abscesses reported in many series. Most liver abscesses for which no source can be found (cryptogenic abscesses) are presumed to arise from subclinical self-limited infections within the portal system, such as a colonic diverticular abscess. Blunt trauma to the abdomen can disrupt the bowel mucosa and allow bacterial seeding of a simultaneously induced hepatic hematoma. A liver abscess may present several weeks after the trauma. Although portal bacteremia is thought to be common in uncomplicated Crohn's disease and ulcerative colitis, liver abscess rarely occurs in the absence of intestinal perforation and local abscess formation. The liver's defense against infection is not easily breached by the portal route.

Invasion of the liver via the hepatic artery implies a systemic bacteremia often due to virulent bacteria, such as *Staphylococcus aureus* and *Streptococcus pyogenes*. The range of invasive microorganisms is greater in granulocytopenic and immunosuppressed patients and includes *Pseudomonas aeruginosa* and fungi such as *Candida albicans*. Resulting liver abscesses are usually multiple and small or microscopic in size, and similar abscesses are present in other organs. Foci of infection contiguous with the liver result from natural catastrophes such as a perforated peptic ulcer or surgical procedures. The invading bacterial flora may be simple or complex and of high or low intrinsic virulence. Careful examination of pus from an associated wound infection may permit identification of the bacteria

Table 1. BACTERIAL ETIOLOGY OF LIVER AND SUBPHRENIC ABSCESSES

A. Abscesses secondary to ascending cholangitis, biliary and upper intestinal tract surgery, and penetrating trauma.*

Microorganism	Approximate Incidence (%)
Escherichia coli	40
Klebsiella pneumoniae	20
Other Enterobacteriaceae	15
Enterobacter spp.	
Proteus spp.	
Citrobacter spp.	
Salmonella spp.	
Staphylococcus aureus	15
Clostridium spp.	10
Pseudomonas spp.	10
Enterococcal spp.	10
Other streptococcal spp.	10
Bateroides fragilis	5

B. Fetid abscesses secondary to pylephlebitis, appendiceal, colonic, and pelvic foci.†

Microorganism	Approximate Incidence (%)
Anaerobic streptococcal spp.	30
Streptococcus milleri	30
Bacteroides fragilis	25
Other *Bacteroides* spp.	15
Sphaerophorus spp.	10
Fusobacterium spp.	10
Actinomyces spp.	10
Escherichia coli	10
Other Enterobacteriaceae spp.	10
Enterococcal spp.	10
Other aerobic streptococcal spp.	10

*More than 25 per cent of cultures will yield two or more microbial species. The streptococci are particularly likely to appear in mixed culture.

†More than 50 per cent of cultures will yield two and often more microbial species.

involved. Liver abscesses resulting from penetrating trauma have much in common with those resulting from contiguous infection.

The term subphrenic abscess is applied to any intraperitoneal or retroperitoneal collection of pus occurring in the zone bounded by the diaphragm above and the transverse colon below. The massive right lobe of the liver suspended from the posterior aspect of the diaphragm (not from the dome as commonly taught) creates two large potential peritoneal spaces, one above the liver in contact with the diaphragm and one below the liver excluded from such contact. Both spaces easily become divided by pyogenic membranes, and abscesses are usually loculated anteriorly, posteriorly, or laterally, rather than occupying the entire potential space. The small left lobe of the liver creates no effective division of the left subphrenic space, in which only the lesser omental sac is a distinct anatomic subdivision. Abscesses in either of these two left-sided spaces are likely to produce diaphragmatic irritation.

Bacteria reach the subphrenic spaces by rupture of an underlying hepatic abscess or by spread of infected material within the peritoneal cavity. Venous and lymphatic channels play no direct role. Natural or surgical injury to organs within the subphrenic zone, such as the gallbladder, stomach, duodenum, and pancreas, is a common antecedent, and abscesses of the left lateral subphrenic space are often due to infection of a hematoma after splenectomy. However, subphrenic abscesses may also result from remote intra-abdominal foci, such as a perforated appendix. The potential spaces of the upper abdomen exhibit negative pressures characteristic of the intrapleural space above and so tend to aspirate peritoneal exudates. This mechanism is thought to explain the formation of subphrenic abscesses in the absence of a contiguous route of infection. The occurrence of isolated abscesses in remote recesses suggests that bacteria spread widely through the peritoneum after focal contamination. Since abscess formation is comparatively rare, the peritoneum must possess a high natural resistance to infection.

Retroperitoneal subphrenic abscesses may be secondary to infection in or around the kidneys, pancreas, duodenum, or vertebrae. Such abscesses usually point below the subphrenic zone, since the retroperitoneal pathway of least resistance leads inferiorly along the psoas muscle. Pseudocysts resulting from necrotizing pancreatitis may become secondarily infected, sometimes spontaneously and always after surgical drainage. Fever, bacteremia, and shock may result. Even so, infection remains secondary to autodigestion despite antibiotic treatment of a changing microbial flora.

Inflammatory edema from infection in the upper abdomen is cleared cephalad through a rich lymphatic network in the diaphragm. Overload of this system results in a sterile pleural effusion with the characteristics of an exudate. Lymphatic spread does not account for infected pus within the pleural space, since a direct communication through the diaphragm can almost always be demonstrated when pleural empyema complicates a subphrenic infection.

CLINICAL MANIFESTATIONS. The clinical manifestations of liver abscesses vary with respect to their microbial etiology, to their anatomic location in the liver, and to the type and pace of their underlying pathogenic mechanism (Barbour and Juniper, 1972; Rubin et al., 1974). Historical details, depending heavily upon the events that have led to the abscess, may be rich or meager. If the onset is insidious, weight loss and debility are prominent. Nausea and vomiting are unusual except in biliary tract obstruction. Fever is almost always present but may be low grade in an indolent process or high and spiking with chills in the presence of bacteremia or rapidly enlarging abscesses. Right subcostal pain, aggravated by percussion over the lower ribs, and a palpable tender liver are common, but many other findings depend upon the location of the abscess. Abscesses in the right or left lobes adjacent to the diaphragm mimic intrathoracic infection. The patient may complain of cough and pleuritic pain in the chest or shoulder. Protracted episodes of hiccough may occur. The involved hemidiaphragm may be elevated and fixed on inspiration, with rales and bronchial breathing heard in the adjacent lung as a result of compressive atelectasis. Abscesses in the posterior or lateral portions of the right hepatic lobe may produce a tender fullness with localized subcutaneous edema in the overlying rib spaces or in the costovertebral angle. An abscess in the left hepatic lobe often presents as a tender epigastric mass.

The clinical manifestations of the small abscesses associated with septicemia are overwhelmed by those of the systemic infection. Fortunately, treatment of the septicemia constitutes treatment of the liver infection. However, a liver abscess may also be obscured when a contiguous or remote intra-abdominal infection dominates the physician's attention. Prompt diagnosis in this circumstance is often life-saving.

Subphrenic abscess may be indistinguishable, clinically, from liver abscess, and indeed the two conditions may coincide (Harley, 1949). A common presentation is a low-grade or episodic fever in a patient recovering slowly and incompletely from abdominal surgery. An obvious infection elsewhere in the wound or abdomen may distract attention from the subphrenic zone. Thoracic symptoms and signs, as described for liver abscess, may occur when the infection contacts the diaphragm. Subhepatic abscesses tend to produce few or no localizing manifestations. Abscesses beneath the left hemidiaphragm may be missed by physicians unaware that one-quarter of subphrenic abscesses are on the left side.

Patients with isolated subphrenic abscesses have suffered vague pains, debility, fever, and anemia for more than ten years before diagnosis. Such indolence has given rise to an oft repeated paraphrase: "Pus somewhere, pus nowhere, pus under the diaphragm."

COMPLICATIONS AND SEQUELAE. Both amebic and pyogenic liver abscess may rupture to produce subphrenic abscesses and, occasionally, generalized peritonitis. Liver abscesses or subphrenic abscesses of either etiology may rupture through the diaphragm to produce empyema, pericardial effusion and tamponade, lung abscess, and bronchobiliary fistula. Interestingly, decompression through the bronchial tree is associated with a mortality rate lower than that observed in abscesses that do not drain spontaneously. Rarely, an abscess may point and drain through the skin. Bacteremia may be complicated by hypotensive shock and by metastatic abscesses in other organs. A persisting focus of infection may become reactivated months to years after apparent cure.

GEOGRAPHIC VARIATIONS IN DISEASE. Since one in ten patients with clinical amebiasis presents a liver abscess,

E. histolytica is by far the most common cause of liver abscess in endemic areas. Conversely, amebae account for a small fraction of liver abscesses in economically advanced countries of the temperate zones where a breakdown in sanitation produces epidemic amebiasis. The increasing travel to and from endemic regions, the existence of endemic foci within countries largely free of the disease, and the latency for which amebiasis is notorious are further reasons to consider an amebic etiology regardless of the patient's current residence.

Within any one geographic area, referral centers are more likely to see abscess resulting from biliary tract obstruction or contiguous infection in older patients suffering from cancer. Abscesses secondary to pylephlebitis in younger patients are likely to predominate in hospitals giving largely primary care.

DIAGNOSIS. A polymorphonuclear leukocytosis of over 15,000/mm³ is characteristic of both amebic and pyogenic liver abscesses. Leukemoid reactions may be seen. The degree of anemia correlates with the duration of the inflammatory process or with the amount of blood loss from associated lesions, such as amebic colitis or diverticulitis. The serum alkaline phosphatase is elevated in more than 90 per cent of all liver abscesses. The elevation may be slight and the accompanying bilirubin concentration normal when liver abscesses arise via the portal venous or hepatic arterial routes. In ascending cholangitis there is often a marked rise in the alkaline phosphatase and clinical jaundice. Other tests of liver function are variable and of little help in diagnosis.

Blood cultures are positive in at least 50 per cent of pyogenic liver abscesses. The high frequency of bacteremia in ascending cholangitis has long been known, but the renewed interest in anaerobic infections has led to an appreciation that systemic bacteremia is also common in pylephlebitis. A patient presenting with fever, chills, elevated alkaline phosphatase, and a continuous anaerobic bacteremia must be suspected of having pylephlebitis even though no evidence of a gastrointestinal focus can be found. An associated liver abscess must be ruled out. A liver or subphrenic abscess is also one cause of an obscure intermittent bacteremia.

Roentgenographic studies are often abnormal in hepatic and subphrenic abscesses. Either hemidiaphragm may be elevated and relatively immobile, often with a pleural effusion or pulmonary infiltrate above. A left subphrenic abscess may separate the gastric air bubble from the diaphragm in the erect posteroanterior view of the chest. An abscess in or around the left lobe of the liver may produce pressure deformities in the barium- or gas-filled stomach or colon. An air-fluid level proved to be outside the bowel and hence within liver tissue or a subphrenic space is virtually diagnostic of a pyogenic abscess. It must be remembered that free air within an uninfected peritoneum may be observed up to three weeks after surgery.

Imaging techniques using radioisotopes, ultrasound, and computed tomography have revolutionized the diagnosis of liver and subphrenic abscesses. Where these modalities are available, such infections are no longer common causes of prolonged unexplained fever.

Hepatic photoscans using technetium-99m sulfur colloid performed in anterior, posterior, and lateral projections will detect most liver abscesses larger than 2 cm in diameter. They appear as defects in an otherwise homogeneous uptake of radioactivity by the liver. Conversely, gallium-67 citrate is concentrated in a pyogenic abscess to produce an area of increased uptake on photoscan. Neither isotope will differentiate an abscess from primary or metastatic cancer. Although small abscesses are easily missed on hepatic angiography, this technique may show vessels or a venous blush within neoplastic lesions. Radioisotope scans are also valuable in demonstrating subphrenic abscesses. A combined liver-lung scan may show a cold area between the two organs when the abscess is suprahepatic. Large collections of pus within the abdomen can usually be demonstrated on gallium-67 scans but interpretation of the uptake may be difficult, especially in the postoperative patient, since the isotope collects in recent wounds, hematomas, and colonic feces as well as in abscesses and neoplasms.

Real-time gray-scale ultrasonography does not require the expense and availability of radioisotopes, but it does require careful and conservative interpretation. The interposition of fatty or air-filled organs between the transducer and the area of interest may prevent study of certain portions of the subphrenic zone. Vascular and biliary structures, especially when distorted by disease, may be misinterpreted. Nevertheless, the technique shows best those abscesses most accessible to percutaneous aspiration and drainage. A successful ultrasound study will give the precise location and depth of a fluid-filled cavity and even identify the tissues through which the exploring needle must pass to reach it.

The superb resolution of modern computed tomographic images allows the visualization of small lesions in areas inaccessable to other noninvasive techniques. Aspiration biopsy using a thin flexible needle often allows diagnosis of such lesions without surgical exploration.

As detailed in Chapter 138, the differentiation of amebic from pyogenic liver abscess can often be made on clinical, epidemiological, and serological grounds. Percutaneous aspiration may occasionally be needed.

TREATMENT AND PROPHYLAXIS. Decompression of the biliary tract is mandatory for liver abscesses secondary to ascending cholangitis. Although endoscopic and percutaneous techniques are being developed for biliary decompression in poor risk patients, surgery remains the procedure of choice when infection is present. Other pyogenic liver abscesses can often be cured by percutaneous drainage (guided by ultrasound or computed tomography) and intensive antibiotic treatment of the bacteria recovered from the pus (Gerzoff et al., 1981). Response to therapy can be followed by repeated noninvasive imaging. The morbidity of surgical drainage is thereby avoided. Multiple small abscesses have been healed by antibiotics alone. Aspiration of one of the abscesses will establish the microbial etiology.

Localized subphrenic abscesses may also yield to percutaneous drainage and precise antibiotic therapy (vanSonnenberg et al., 1982). However, complex multiloculated collections of pus (often associated with a perforated viscus) remain an indication for a thorough transabdominal surgical exploration of the subphrenic zone. Antibiotics have greatly reduced the danger of spreading infection during transperitoneal drainage.

Regardless of the drainage procedure employed, antibiotics must be given in full doses for three weeks or longer. Empirical treatment of all the bacteria implicated in abscesses of biliary, upper intestinal, and traumatic origin is unwieldy. A "third generation cephalosporin" such as cefotaxime or ceftizoxime, 2 g every six hours intravenously, plus intravenous gentamicin (dosage adjusted to body size and renal function) provides broad coverage but may not be adequate for *C. perfringens, B. fragilis, P. aerugenosa*, or the enterococci. Antibiotic therapy tailored to the microbes actually identified in culture is obviously superior to an empirical approach. With current aspiration and culture techniques, the physician should not long remain ignorant of the infecting flora.

Fetid anaerobic abscesses of colonic and pelvic origin are well treated by penicillin G, 20 million units a day intravenously, and either clindamycin, 600 mg every six hours intravenously, or metronidazole, 500 to 750 mg every six hours intravenously. Clindamycin and metronidazole are effective against *B. fragilis*, which is routinely resistant to beta-lactam antibiotics and sometimes resistant to the tetracyclines. An aminoglycoside such as kanamycin or gentamicin is also indicated until *Escherichia coli* and other facultative gram-negative rods are excluded by aerobic culture of the pus.

Occasionally, subphrenic abscesses associated with a perforated viscus stabilize into a gastro- or enterocutaneous fistula following drainage and antibiotic therapy. The fistula then slowly heals as the microbial content of the drainage changes to antibiotic-resistant species, often yeasts. If such patients show no evidence of invasive infection, antibiotic therapy can be terminated in two or three weeks and the new microbes need not be treated.

The treatment of amebic abscesses is described in Chapter 138.

Liver and subphrenic abscesses produce prolonged, expensive illnesses, and overall mortality rates continue to approach 50 per cent. However, the prompt diagnosis and treatment of patients without underlying neoplastic disease shifts the odds strongly in favor of survival. Antibiotics have not decreased the overall incidence of these infections. Here again, the gross statistics may be misleading, since these abscesses now occur less frequently in young people with benign underlying disease and more frequently in older people after extensive surgery for malignant disease. Given the high natural resistance of the liver and peritoneum to infection, antibiotic therapy of a primary contamination or overt infection must prevent the complication of hepatic and subphrenic abscess in many instances. When antibiotics fail to prevent such a complication, they are accused, with some justification, of suppressing its clinical manifestations and delaying its diagnosis. Successful prophylaxis goes unnoted.

References

Block, M. A., Schuman, B. M., Eyler, W. R., Truant, J. P., and DuSault, L. A.: Surgery of liver abscess. Arch Surg 88:602, 1964.

Gerzof, S. G., Robbins, A. H., Johnson, W. C., Birkett, D. H., and Nabseth, D. C.: Percutaneous catheter drainage of abdominal abscesses. A five year experience. N Engl J Med 305:653, 1981.

Harley, H. R. S.: Subphrenic abscess. Thorax 4:1, 1949.

Rubin, R. H., Swartz, M. N., and Malt, R.: Hepatic abscess: Changes in clinical, bacteriologic and therapeutic aspects. Am J Med 57:601, 1974.

Sabbaj, J., Sutter, V. L., and Finegold, S. M.: Anaerobic pyogenic liver abscess. Ann Int Med 77:629, 1972.

vanSonnenberg, E., Ferrucci, J. T., Mueller, P. R., Wittenberg, J., and Simeone, J. F.: Percutaneous drainage of abscesses and fluid collections: Technique, results, and applications. Radiology 142:1, 1982.

149

SPLENIC ABSCESS

S. J. D. Brooks, M.D.

Splenic abscess results when a pyogenic infection in the splenic parenchyma causes inflammation and necrosis with or without cavitation.

INCIDENCE. Splenic abscess is not common, occurring in the preantibiotic era, in approximately 0.40 per cent of autopsies, and in the antibiotic era in .017 per cent. A major teaching institution would see one to three cases a year (Chulay and Lankerani 1976, Lawhorne and Zuidema 1976, Gadacz et al., 1974). A similar institution in Nigeria would average four cases per year (Kolawole and Bohrer 1973). Only 4 per cent of subphrenic abscesses arise in the spleen, and in a series of over 500 cases of intra-abdominal abscesses, none were in the spleen (Ochsner and Graves 1933, Altemeier et al., 1973).

Males outnumber females in a ratio of 5:3. It occurs at all ages and has the highest mortality in the seventh decade (Chun et al., 1980). Undiagnosed, and untreated it is always fatal. With correct treatment, the mortality is reduced to 7 per cent (Billings 1928, Wolfson 1944, Lawhorne and Zuidema 1976).

ETIOLOGY. Culture of pus from splenic abscesses has yielded an enormous variety of organisms. Splenic abscess formerly occurred more frequently in patients with malaria, relapsing fever, typhoid fever, and infective endocarditis, but has not been reported in malaria or relapsing fever in recent years, and only once lately in typhoid fever (Chun et al., 1980, Fonollosa et al., 1980).

The non-typhoidal salmonella are now of more etiologic importance. There is a particular association between abscesses due to these salmonella, and patients with a hemoglobinopathy (Kolawole and Bohrer 1973, Parrish and Sherman 1964). Isolated cases of splenic abscess due to these organisms have also been reported in patients with gastroenteritis, blunt trauma to the abdomen, and achlorhydria (Sharr et al., 1972, Rodan et al., 1981, Ralls et al., 1982, Brown et al., 1979, and Scott et al., 1977).

Infective endocarditis remains a common cause of splenic abscess despite the decline of rheumatic fever. This is due to intravenous drug abuse. The patients are nearly always infected by *Staphylococcus aureus*, but gram-negative organisms and anaerobes have also been isolated (Chulay and Lankerani 1976, Fry et al., 1978, Gangahar and Delaney 1981).

Streptococci, staphylococci, and gram negatives are the commonest organisms isolated in splenic abscess. Nearly 25 per cent of cases have sterile abscesses. Sixty per cent of blood cultures are positive for the causative organism (Chun et al., 1980). Many abscesses contain gas, with putrid but sterile pus. Such are the criteria for an anaerobic infection, but anaerobes are the etiologic agents in only 5.8 per cent of cases (Gorbach and Bartlett 1974, Chun et al., 1980). *Bacteroides spp.* and *Clostridial spp.* are most commonly isolated (Gadacz et al., 1974, Chulay and Lankerani 1976, Chun et al., 1980, Rosenblum 1974, Gangahar and Delaney 1981, Dylewski et al., 1979). Isolated instances of unusual organisms include *Brucella suis* (Spink 1964), *Candida pseudotropicalis* (Coopersmith et al., 1975), *Clostridium difficile* (Saginur et al., 1983), Nocardia (Chulay and Lankerani 1976), *Pseudomonas pseudomallei* (Levine et al., 1968), *Shigella flexneri* (Squires et al., 1981), and *Y. enterocolitica* (Rabson et al., 1972).

PATHOGENESIS. Both infarction and infection must exist before an abscess can result. The two can occur simultaneously, but usually infection occurs in an area of previous infarction. Infarction can be caused by blunt trauma to the splenic area. Enlarged spleens are more susceptible to trauma because they lack rib protection. They are also more likely to develop spontaneous subcapsular infarctions or hematomas (Kolawole and Bohrer 1973, Aleali et al., 1975). Splenic infarction occurs also in malaria, relapsing fever, infective endocarditis and hemoglobinopathies (HbSA, Hb-SC, and Hb-S/β-thalassemia). Infective endocarditis causes 12.1 per cent of cases and the incidence of spenic abscess in infective endocarditis is 2.4 per cent (Chun et al., 1980).

Apart from the heart, almost every organ system has been the source of the bacteremia responsible for a splenic abscess, and in one case the therapeutic use of gelfoam embolization resulted in a splenic abscess (Eron and Clark 1980). Local spread from infections or malignancies in contiguous organs may result in a splenic abscess, but this is unusual, and accounts for only 2.3 per cent of cases. (Chun et al., 1980, Ralls et al., 1982, Wagner et al., 1975). The mean splenic weight at removal is 655 g. Sixty per cent of removed spleens have solitary abscesses, and 40 per cent, multiple.

CLINICAL MANIFESTATIONS. The latent period between trauma or infection and the onset of symptoms can vary between days and weeks. Often the patient has forgotten the trauma or infection, but careful history taking should remind him (Chun et al., 1980). The systemic effects are invariably fever, and chills that only occur in about a quarter of febrile patients. Seventy per cent of patients have leukocytosis over 10,000/mm^3. Some patients may present as a fever of unknown origin if the abscess lies deep in the splenic substance and causes neither splenic enlargement nor capsular inflammation. Once capsular inflammation occurs, pain and tenderness appear in the left upper quadrant and the spleen becomes palpable in over 50 per cent of cases (Chun et al., 1980). When it impinges on the left hemidiaphragm, chest pain may occur, and in about 10 per cent there is left shoulder tip pain. A paralyzed hemidiaphragm and pleural effusion can develop on the left side. Extension of the spleen downwards causes a localized peritonitis, and displacement of surrounding organs. Untreated, the spleen may become matted to surrounding organs, obstruct the bowel, or rupture into the colon or peritoneal cavity (Podgorny 1971, Kennedy and Harvey 1961, Knauer and Abrams 1966, Vergne et al., 1975).

DIAGNOSIS. Computed tomography (CT), ultrasound, and radionuclide scans have brought new anatomical precision and accuracy to the diagnosis of this disease. In fact CT scan can be more reliable than visual examination at laparotomy (Moss et al., 1980).

The detection of splenic abscesses by CT is extremely accurate, and false normal CT scans are rare. An abscess appears as a circumscribed area of uniform low CT attenuation values, or as a fluid collection within the spleen. Gas presents as fine low attenuation bubbles or coalesces into fluid levels (Ferruci and vanSonnenberg 1981). Grey scale sonography is also highly accurate. Abscesses appear rounded, oval or ellipsoidal, and they have irregular, poorly defined anechoic masses of variable size. They have internal echogenicity, and decreased acoustic transmission. Gas causes dense echoes in the cavity with distal acoustic shadowing (Pawar et al., 1982, Ferruci and vanSonnenberg 1981).

Autologous leukocytes labeled with Indium III, can detect splenic abscess in over 90 per cent of cases. (Ferruci and vanSonnenberg 1981, Knochel et al., 1980). Critically ill patients and those with localizing signs should have CT scans and ultrasonography, because of the delays inherent in the use of radionuclide scans.

TREATMENT. Splenectomy, under antibiotic cover is the treatment of choice and usually lifesaving, although splenic abscess has been treated successfully with antibiotics (Dylewski et al., 1979). Percutaneous abscess drainage has also been reported (vanSonnenberg et al. 1982).

References

Aleali, S. H., Castro, O., Spencer, R. P., Finch, S. C.: Sideroblastic anemia with splenic abscess and fatal thromboemboli after splenectomy. Ann Intern Med 83:661, 1975.

Altemeier, W. A., Culbertson, W. R., Fullen, W. D., Shook, C. D.: Intra-abdominal abscesses. Am J Surg 125:70, 1973.

Beet, E. A.: Primary splenic abscess and sickle cell disease. East Afr Med J. 26:180, 1949.

Billings, A. E.: Abscess of the spleen. Ann Surg 88:416, 1928.

Brown, J. J., Sumner, T. E., Crowe, J. E., Shaffner, L. DeS.: Pre-operative diagnosis of splenic abscess by ultrasonography and radionuclide scanning. South Med J 72:5:575, 1979.

Chulay, J. D., Lankerani, M. R., Splenic Abscess. Report of ten cases and review of the literature. Am J Med 61:513, 1976.

Chun, C. H., Raff, M. J., Contreras, L., Varghese, R., Waterman, N., Daffner, R., Melo, J. C.: Splenic abscess. Medicine 59:50, 1980.

Coopersmith, A., Ritchey, A. K., Zinkham, W. H.: Fever of unknown origin and the value of gallium -67, and technetium 99M for defining abnormality of the spleen: a case report. The Johns Hopkins Med J 137:51, 1975.

Dylewski, J., Portnoy, J., Mendelson, J.: Antibiotic treatment of splenic abscess. Ann Intern Med 91:493, 1979.

Eron, L. J., Clark, L.: Gelfoam embolization complicated by splenic abscess. Virginia Medical 107:624, 1980.

Ferruci, J. T., Jr., vanSonnenberg, E.: Intra-abdominal abscess. JAMA 246:2728, 1981.

Fonollosa, V., Bosch, J. A., Garcia-Bragado F., Vilardell, M., Libenson, C., Tornos, J.: Hemolytic anemia, splenic abscess, and pleural effusion caused by S. typhi. J Inf Dis 142:6:945, 1980.

Fry, D. E., Richardson, J. D., Flint, L. M.: Occult splenic abscess: an unrecognized complication of heroin abuse. Surgery 84:650, 1978.

Gadacz, T., Way, L. W., Dunphy, J. E.: Changing clinical spectrum of splenic abscess. Am J Surg 128:182, 1974.

Gangahar, D. M., Delaney, M. M.: Intrasplenic abscess. Two case reports and review of the literature. The American Surgeon 47:488, 1981.

Gorbach, S. L., Bartlett, J. G.: Anaerobic infection. N Engl J Med 290:1177, 1974.

Kennedy, J. H., Harvey, C. A.: Ruptured splenic abscess—an unusual cause of acute abdominal disease. Report of a case. West J Surg Obstet, Gynecol 64:151, 1961.

Knauer, Q. F., Abrams, J. S.: Generalized peritonitis due to a ruptured splenic abscess. Am J Surg 112:923, 1966.
Knochel, J. Q., Koehler, P. R., Lee, T. G., Welch, D. M.: Diagnosis of abdominal abscesses with computed tomography, ultrasound and ^{111}In leukocyte scans. Radiology 137:425, 1980.
Kolawole, T. M., Bohrer, S. P.: Splenic abscess and the gene for hemoglobin S. Am J Roentgenol 119:175, 1973.
Lawhorne, T. W., Zuidema, G. D.: Splenic abscess. Surgery 79:686, 1976.
Levine, S., Wheland, T., Jr.: Melioidosis of the spleen. Am J Surg 115:849, 1968.
Moss, M. L., Kirschner, L. P.: Peereboom, G., Ferris, R. A.: CT demonstration of a splenic abscess not evident at surgery. AJR 135:159, 1980.
Ochsner, A., Graves, A. M.: Subphrenic abscess: An analysis of 3,372 collected and personal cases. Ann Surg 98:961, 1933.
Parrish, R. A., Sherman, H. C.: The surgical significance of splenic abscess. Am Surg 30:712, 1964.
Pawar, S., Kay, C. J., Gonzalez, R., Taylor, K. J. W., Rosenfield, A. T.: Sonography of splenic abscess. AJR 138:259, 1982.
Podgorny, G.: Splenic abscess causing obstruction of the large intestine. Am Surg 37:269, 1971.
Rabson, A. R., Koornhof, H. J., Notman, J., Maxwell, W. G.: Hepatosplenic abscesses due to *Yersinia enterocolitica*. Br Med J 4:341, 1972.
Ralls, P. W., Quinn, M. F., Colletti, P., Lapin, S. A., Halls, J.: Sonography of pyogenic splenic abscess. AJR 138:523, 1982.
Rodan, B. A., Max, R. J., Breiman, R. S., Rice, R. P.: Splenic abscess due to salmonella typhimurium bacteremia. Southern Medical Journal 74:382, 1981.
Rosenblum, A. C.: Cavitating splenic infarction. Am J Med 56:720, 1974.
Saginur, R., Fogel, R., Begin, L., Cohen, B., Mendelson, J.: Splenic abscess due to Cl. difficile. J Infect Dis 147:1105, 1983.
Scott, J. H. K., Thomas, H. W., Walters, R. O.: Acute splenic abscess due to *Salmonella chester*. Br Med J 1:688, 1977.
Sharr, M. M.: Splenic abscess due to *Salmonella agona*. Br Med J 1:546, 1972.
Spink, W. W.: Host-parasite relationship in human brucellosis with prolonged illness due to suppuration of the liver and spleen. Am J Med Sci 247:129, 1964.
Squires, R. H., Keating, J. P., Rosenblum, J. L., Askin, F., Ternberg, J. L.: Splenic abscess and hepatic dysfunction caused by *Shigella flexneri*. J of Ped 98:429, 1981.
vanSonnenberg, E., Ferruci, J. T., Mueller, P. R., Wittenberg, J., Simone, J. F., Malt, R. A.: Percutaneous radiographically guided catheter drainage of abdominal abscesses. JAMA 247:190, 1982.
Vergne, R., Selland, B., Gobel, F. L., Hall, W. H.: Rupture of the spleen in infective endocarditis. Arch Intern Med 135:1265, 1975.
Wagner, V. P., Smale, L. E., Lischke, J. H.: Amebic abscess of the liver and spleen in pregnancy and the puerperium. Obstet and Gynecol 45:562, 1975.
Walker, I. J.: Abscess of the spleen. N Engl J Med 203:1025, 1938.
Wolfson, I. N.: Abscess of the spleen. N Engl J Med 230:135, 1944.

150

GRANULOMATOUS HEPATITIS

STEVE KOHL, M.D.
HERBERT L. DUPONT, M.D.

Granulomatous hepatitis is the development of multiple granulomas in liver tissue. Granulomas are defined as "microscopic focal vascularized aggregation of histiocytes and hypertrophied fibroblasts that assume a round to oval shape" (Robbins, 1979).

PATHOGENESIS. Granuloma formation appears to be a normal response to certain indolent but persistent agents that are not readily degraded by phagocytic cells. Common etiologic agents include fungi, intracellular bacteria, mycobacteria, foreign bodies, and protozoa. It also appears to be a response of immune suppressed and immune deficient patients as in chronic granulomatous disease. Viral hepatitis is granulomatous in renal dialysis patients who are receiving immunosuppressant therapy, and *Listeria monocytogenes* elicits a granulomatous response in neonates and debilitated adults. Alteration of antigens or bacterial virulence can convert a stimulus that ordinarily produces a purulent response (such as that of live streptococci in mice) to one that produces a granulomatous response (live streptococci plus penicillin or heat-killed streptococci in mice). Antigen-antibody complexes can also induce granuloma formation.

The basic understanding of granuloma formation and classification has been advanced by animal experiments demonstrating that granulomas are a mononuclear cell (lymphocyte and macrophage) response to both inflammatory (agent-specific) and immunologic (host-specific) stimuli. An inflammatory granuloma is associated with a uniform, dose-dependent response that is independent of previous challenge. Granulomas generated by immunologic factors display an amnestic immunologic response when rechallenged with the sensitizing antigen, so that granuloma cells accumulate more rapidly (Warren, 1976). This is presumably due to previously sensitized memory lymphocytes (probably T cells) responding to antigens phagocytized by the liver macrophages (Kupffer cells). These lymphocytes begin the inflammatory cascade, recruiting other lymphocytes, monocytes, and macrophages to the site and orchestrating a complex combination of cellular and humoral responses that result in a granuloma formation with containment of the antigen. Identification of the various agents and mechanisms that cause an inflammatory and/or immunologic granulomatous response in man may eventually help facilitate their diagnosis and specific therapy.

In general, hepatic granulomas, though often numerous, have minor effects on liver function. These effects are usually manifested as mild obstructive signs (slight increase in bilirubin and serum transaminases and a greater elevation in serum alkaline phosphatase levels). There is often prolonged Bromsulphalein (BSP) retention, hypergammaglobulinemia, low serum albumin values, and elevated serum cholesterol levels. Occasionally, strategically located granulomas will produce striking abnormalities as a result of hepatic obstruction. A radionuclide liver scan in granulomatous hepatitis tends to reveal a patchy, mottled uptake or a normal liver. In one patient subjected to angiographic study there was a rich arterial supply and patchy patterns of increased vascularization on the arterial, parenchymal, and venous phases. This pattern is the same as that seen with metastatic lesions, regenerating nodular hyperplasia, and multiple small liver abscesses.

PATHOLOGY. A granuloma is a collection of mononuclear inflammatory cells (lymphocytes and macrophages) and epithelial cells (mononuclear inflammatory cells) usually arranged in an oval to round structure and often containing giant cells (formed by fusion of macrophages) and variable degrees of central necrosis. There may also be a minor infiltration of fibroblasts, plasma cells, eosinophils, and polymorphonuclear leukocytes. Active granulomas tend to contain more inflammatory cells, while older, more quiescent granulomas may be partially or entirely replaced by hyaline and calcified material, with or without a peripheral rim of mononuclear leukocytes. Despite the common notion that histologic variations have etiologic significance, there are few features that help identify the etiology. Caseous necrosis, classically linked to tuberculosis, is not diagnostic of the condition and can also be seen with tularemia, brucellosis, syphilis, fungal infection, Q fever, Wegener's granulomatosis, and chronic granulomatous disease of childhood. Although tuberculosis often produces less sharply defined granulomas with more inflammatory cells and necrosis, and sarcoidosis generally causes more circumscribed and compact masses of epithelial cells and giant cells without necrosis and surrounding inflammation, exceptions are frequently encountered. Other differences between the granulomatous reaction of tuberculosis and sarcoidosis have been suggested. The reticulum network tends to be damaged by tuberculosis, whereas in sarcoidosis it is generally well maintained. In one study, multiple granulomas were more typically associated with miliary tuberculosis (95 per cent) than with sarcoidosis (65 per cent) (Alexander and Galambos, 1973), although the opposite was found in another series (Hughes and Fox, 1972). Such generalities may influence a pathologist's opinion, yet the definitive etiologic diagnosis rests upon demonstration of the agent in the pathologic specimen, culture of the agent from the specimen, or ancillary clinical and laboratory data.

INCIDENCE. The incidence and etiology of granulomatous hepatitis depends on the patient population, geographic location, underlying disease state, reasons for pathologic examination of liver tissue (e.g., liver abnormalities, fever, incidental operative biopsy), and the method of tissue sampling. Granulomas have been identified in 0.7 to 9 per cent of more than 13,000 liver biopsies performed in published studies, with a mean of 4 per cent (Bunim et al., 1962; Guckian and Perry, 1966; Alexander and Galambos, 1973; Hughes and Fox, 1972; Klatskin and Yesner, 1950; Iverson et al., 1970; Wagoner et al., 1953; Pequignot et al., 1973; Bain et al., 1973; Mir-Madjlessi et al., 1973). In studies of patients with fever of undetermined origin, the diagnosis of granulomatous hepatitis was made in 2 to 11 per cent. Hepatic granulomas are found more often in cases of confirmed brucellosis or miliary tuberculosis. Results agree whether liver tissue is obtained through operative, autopsy, or needle biopsy procedures. The diffuse nature of the process is obvious when it is considered that a needle biopsy specimen represents approximately 1/50,000 of the liver (Klatskin and Yesner, 1950).

Tables 1 through 3 list the various etiologic agents and conditions associated with hepatic granulomas. Extrapulmonary tuberculosis and sarcoidosis are among the more common causes of granulomatous hepatitis. Other conditions such as brucellosis are almost invariably associated with hepatic granulomas.

Table 4 summarizes the relative incidence of etiologic agents from a review of ten published series containing 586 cases of granulomatous hepatitis (Bunim et al., 1962; Guckian and Perry, 1966; Alexander and Galambos, 1973; Hughes and Fox, 1972; Iverson et al., 1970; Wagoner et al., 1953; Pequignot et al., 1973; Bain et al., 1973; Mir-Madjlessi et al., 1973; Terplan, 1971). A search for recently

Table 1. INFECTIONS ASSOCIATED WITH GRANULOMATOUS HEPATITIS

Bacterial	**Viral**
Syphilis	Influenza
Tularemia	Viral hepatitis
Brucellosis	Cytomegalovirus disease
Meliodosis	Epstein-Barr virus infection
Listeriosis	
Tuberculosis	**Fungal**
Atypical mycobacterial disease	Histoplasmosis
Leprosy	Coccidioidomycosis
BCG infection	Aspergillosis
Granuloma inguinale infection	Cryptococcosis
Actinomycosis	Candidiasis
Nocardiosis	Blastomycosis
Typhoid fever	
Paratyphoid B	**Protozoan-Parasitic**
	Ascariasis
Rickettsia	Schistosomiasis
Q fever	Ancylostomiasis
Mediterranean fever	Amoebiasis
(*Rickettsia conorii*)	Strongyloidiasis
	Toxoplasmosis
Chlamydia	Tongue worm infection
Psittacosis	Visceral larval migrans
Lymphogranuloma venereum	Fascioliasis
infection	Capillariasis
	Malaria
	Giardiasis

Table 2. DRUGS AND TOXINS ASSOCIATED WITH GRANULOMATOUS HEPATITIS

Sulfonamides
Phenylbutazone
Allopurinol
Halothane
Methyldopa
Quinidine
Chlorpropamide
Penicillin
Hydralazine
Beryllium
Corn Starch
Copper
Talc
Tolbutamide
Quinine
Nitrofurantoin
Clofibrate
Procainamide
Carbamazepine
Isoniazid
Diazepam
Metahydrin
Metalozone
Phenytoin
Aspirin
Cephalexin
Procarbazine
Hydrochlorothiazide
Oxyphenbutazone
P-amino salicylic acid
Cromolyn sodium
Progesterone-estrogen contraceptives

Table 3. MISCELLANEOUS CONDITIONS ASSOCIATED WITH GRANULOMATOUS HEPATITIS

Cancer
Hodgkin's disease
Others
Immune Defects
Chronic granulomatous disease of childhood
Hypogammaglobulinemia
Liver Disease
Biliary cirrhosis
Chronic active hepatitis
Others
Sarcoid
Wegener's granulomatosis
Allergic granulomatosis
Inflammatory bowel disease
Whipple's disease
Collagen vascular disease
Systemic sclerosis
Lymphomatoid granulomatosis
Familial granulomatous arteritis
Giant cell arteritis
Polymyalgic rheumatica
Temporal arteritis
Celiac disease (after allergic granulomatosis)
Jejunoileal bypass surgery

discovered causes of granulomatous hepatitis not represented in these series, such as cytomegalovirus and certain drugs, will reduce the relative number of cases without diagnosis. Prospective studies have demonstrated that, with careful reevaluation, it is possible to increase the percentage of etiologic diagnoses (Guckian and Perry, 1968).

Table 4. ETIOLOGY OF 586 CASES OF GRANULOMATOUS HEPATITIS

Sarcoidosis	191 (34%)
Tuberculosis	173 (30%)
Hodgkin's disease	9
Viral hepatitis	8
Schistosomiasis	8
Histoplasmosis	8
Brucellosis	6
Syphilis	6
Berylliosis	3
Liver disease	
Cirrhosis	23
Fatty infiltration	13
First and second degree biliary cirrhosis	11
Hepatitis, nonviral	7
Unknown	102 (17%)

2 cases each: Lymphopathia venereum, infectious mononucleosis, cancer, erythema nodosum, fungal (unspecified)

1 case each: Q fever, visceral larval migrans, actinomycosis, systemic sclerosis, collagen vascular disease, blastomycosis, influenza B, viral (unspecified)

Bunim et al., 1962; Guckian and Perry, 1968; Alexander and Galambos, 1973; Hughes and Fox, 1972; Iverson et al., 1970; Wagoner et al., 1953; Pequignot et al., 1973; Bain et al., 1973; Mir-Madjlessi et al., 1973; Terplan, 1971.

ETIOLOGY AND CLINICAL MANIFESTATIONS

Infections

Tuberculosis. Infections are the most commonly diagnosed causes of granulomatous hepatitis, and tuberculosis is the most common infectious cause, accounting for nearly one third of all cases of granulomatous hepatitis (Table 4). The frequency of developing tuberculous hepatic granulomas is related directly to the extent and duration of the infection. In active pulmonary tuberculosis granulomas are found in 25 to 42 per cent of cases; in extrapulmonary nonmiliary disease they occur in 80 per cent; and in fatal, miliary, or chronic untreated tuberculosis granulomas are seen in nearly all cases (Alexander and Galambos, 1973; Frank and Raffensperger, 1965).

Patients with tuberculous granulomas of the liver are generally febrile, and 50 per cent have hepatomegaly. Liver function testing often reveals increased bilirubin, transaminase, alkaline phosphatase, and retention of BSP dye, particularly in miliary disease. Increased serum immunoglobulin levels are also common. Other than demonstrating the causative agent in a granuloma, the most helpful laboratory procedure is the tuberculin skin test. Most patients with tuberculosis, unless moribund, will respond to an intermediate or second strength PPD (purified protein derivative) skin test with Tween stabilized antigen, applied correctly and read at the appropriate time.

The characteristic granuloma of tuberculosis containing caseous necrosis is present in 15 to 50 per cent of cases showing a granulomatous reaction. As previously mentioned, granulomas of other causes may also show caseous necrosis, although the finding of caseation should lead to a suspicion of tuberculosis. Acid-fast bacilli are found in the liver with varying frequency in different series, although it is agreed that they are difficult to visualize. The frequency of positive acid-fast smears ranges from 0 to 45 per cent with the higher frequency seen among patients with miliary tuberculosis. The use of fluorescent-staining procedures may increase this low yield.

Culture of the bacillus from hepatic granulomas has been generally unrewarding except in miliary tuberculosis, where as many as 60 per cent of cultures may be positive (Alexander and Galambos, 1973). Other mycobacteria, including the leprosy bacilli in lepromatous leprosy, atypical mycobacteria (usually *M. avium-intracellulare*) in immunosuppressed patients, and bacille Calmette-Guérin (BCG) in patients receiving intralesional anticancer therapy, also cause granulomas.

The overall low incidence of positive cultures from lesions associated with mycobacteria supports the hypothesis that the granulomas are in large part hypersensitivity reactions to components of these organisms and not necessarily to the live bacillus.

The close association between mycobacterial infection and granulomatous hepatitis has led to the frequent empiric institution of antituberculous therapy in patients with granulomatous hepatitis when the diagnosis is not etiologically established. However, spontaneous remission of granulomatous hepatitis is common, making it difficult to ascribe etiologic significance to a satisfactory response to empiric tuberculosis therapy.

The presence of liver granulomas in a person with tuberculosis implies extrapulmonic mycobacterium infection, and the reader is referred to Chapter 120 for guidelines of specific therapy.

Syphilis. Syphilis involves the liver in 5 per cent of inadequately treated cases. Before 1941, approximately 5 in 1000 routine autopsies performed in the United States had evidence of syphilitic liver involvement. The granuloma (syphiloma) is found both in the second and third stages of disease. The granulomas often caseate and coalesce to form liver gummas, although at times no necrosis is found, and the histologic reaction is similar to that found in tuberculosis or sarcoid. Spirochetes have been found by careful darkfield examination of liver tissue, but diagnosis is most easily approached by serologic means. The finding of a positive serologic response for syphilis in a patient with hepatic granuloma is of course not diagnostic of syphilitic involvement of the liver, and the strength of the association relies on the incidence of positive serologic tests in the population from which the individual is drawn and exclusion of other causes of granulomatous liver reaction.

Brucellosis. Brucellosis, particularly that due to *Brucella abortus,* almost always involves the liver. *Br. suis* also may involve the liver. Granulomas are often found in the absence of hepatomegaly or altered liver function tests. The likelihood of finding granulomas in inactive cases is much lower. The histopathologic signs are non-specific and may include caseous necrosis. Diagnosis of brucellosis is made by culturing the causative organism from blood, marrow, or biopsy material or by a positive agglutination test with *Brucella* antigens in a significant titer (usually >1:100). Brucellosis of the liver rarely progresses to cirrhosis.

Tularemia. Although clinical liver manifestations are not common in tularemia, in one series 10 of 12 autopsy cases had hepatic lesions, and in another series of 21 cases, the majority had granulomas and caseous necrosis (Schiff, 1956). The agglutination test for tularemia is the most valuable for establishing the diagnosis. Cultivation of *Francisella tularensis* from tissues or blood is difficult and hazardous for laboratory technicians.

Listeriosis. *Listeria monocytogenes* infection occurs in immune-suppressed hosts, postpartum women, and neonates, as well as otherwise healthy people. Disseminated listeriosis in neonates can occur both prenatally and peripartum. The infant often has skin granulomas as well as granulomas in almost any organ, including the liver. The organism is easily cultured from the blood and granulomas. Mortality is high in the immunosuppressed patient or neonate with infection even though the organism is sensitive to readily available antimicrobials such as ampicillin and penicillin.

Viral Agents. Viral causes of liver granulomas are more difficult to verify. Although granulomatous hepatitis has been found in association with documented viral infection, the growth of virus from a granuloma has not been achieved. Infectious mononucleosis often involves the liver, with 85 per cent of affected individuals demonstrating altered liver enzymes. Focal round cell infiltrations occur but are not diagnostic of granulomatous hepatitis. One patient in each of two large series was felt to have liver granulomas associated with infectious mononucleosis.

Cytomegalovirus hepatitis resulted in a granulomatous reaction in three well-documented cases in two published series (Reller, 1973; Bonkowsky et al., 1975). In these cases no giant cells or viral inclusions were noted in the liver. Diagnosis was made by a fourfold or greater rise or fall in serologic titer and, in two patients, by concomitant isolation of cytomegalovirus from cervix or saliva. Influenza B virus infection has been associated with granulomatous hepatitis in one case (Klatskin and Yesner, 1950). Two series of small clusters of mononucleosis-like illness with granulomatous liver involvement involving five cases in Israel (Eliakim et al., 1968) and two cases in New York (Gelb et al., 1970) have been reported. Each series consisted of young to middle-aged people (16 to 52 years) with self-limited febrile illness, lymphocytosis, atypical lymphocytes seen on peripheral blood smear, and liver biopsies containing multiple granulomas without caseation or giant cells. In one of the series cytomegalovirus antibody titers were not obtained, and in both series heterophils were negative but Epstein-Barr virus antibody titers were not done.

Chronic active hepatitis has rarely been associated with granuloma formation, which may reflect a dysfunctional host response to persistent hepatitis B virus infection. During an outbreak of B-antigen–negative hepatitis in a renal dialysis unit, two patients showed changes of chronic persistent hepatitis on liver biopsy specimens and two had grade IV sclerosis, all with caseating granulomas present (Galbraith et al., 1975). The etiology of hepatitis that commonly occurs in patients undergoing renal hemodialysis is not always established and may be multifactoral. In a study of long-term dialysis patients, six of seven had mild focal hepatitis. One of these patients had severe involvement with noncaseating granuloma formation. Changes of viral hepatitis were not present (Bergman et al., 1972). Many of these patients had been treated with drugs that have been associated with hepatic granuloma formation, such as methyldopa, and many had had blood transfusions, increasing the risk of viral infections associated with granulomas. In addition, dialysis produces red cell sludging and offers opportunities for antigen challenge of patients who may be immunosuppressed for a variety of reasons.

Q Fever. The major rickettsial agent clearly associated with granulomatous hepatitis is *Coxiella burnetii*, the causative agent of Q fever. Common clinical manifestations of the disease are fever, severe headache, pneumonitis, and abnormal liver function. In one case, granulomas containing fluorescent antibody-positive organisms have been identified. The liver also was diffusely infiltrated with lymphocytes, polymorphonuclear leukocytes, eosinophils, plasma cells, and histiocytes (DuPont et al., 1971). In the same report, two volunteers experimentally infected with an aerosol challenge of *Coxiella burnetii* showed laboratory evidence of hepatitis 8 to 12 days after inoculation (during the late incubation period). Liver biopsy revealed foci of mononuclear cell inflammation and Councilman-like bodies, although rickettsiae were not seen.

Psittacosis. Psittacosis, an avian-acquired cause of interstitial chlamydial pneumonitis, has been associated with a hepatitic granulomatous response.

Fungal Agents. A wide variety of fungal diseases can cause granulomas of the liver (Table 1). Histoplasma is the most common fungal agent identified, and its incidence is related to geographic location. In a large series of patients with granulomatous hepatitis reported from the United States, histoplasmosis accounted for 12 per cent of the cases, the second most frequent diagnosis after sarcoid (Mir-Madjlessi et al., 1973). In this series, 80 per cent of the patients with histoplasmosis had fever while a third had hepatomegaly and/or splenomegaly. Laboratory and pathologic findings were nonspecific, with only 16 per cent having altered liver function tests. In a prospective evaluation of 26 patients with progressive disseminated histoplasmosis, 21 had liver abnormalities. Granulomas were present in five of eight undergoing liver biopsy, fungal cultures were positive in four, and fungi were visible in three culture-positive liver specimens (Fauci and Wolff, 1976). The diagnosis can be suspected by a positive serologic reaction (false-negative results are common) and can be confirmed only by direct visualization or by growth of the organism from liver or bone marrow. The skin test is of little clinical use and may confuse the serologic evaluation. Cryptococcosis can also produce a hepatitis, and encapsulated yeast may appear in the liver. The presence of fungus in liver signifies visceral dissemination and mandates careful search for other foci in the bone marrow, lung, or central nervous system. *Candida albicans* may be a cause of granulomatous hepatitis especially in patients with acute leukemia (Jones, 1980).

Parasitic Agents. Table 1 lists the many parasitic diseases that may elicit a granulomatous reaction. In one series of 214 cases reported from the United States, schistosomiasis accounted for eight (4 per cent) (Bunim et al., 1962). In Uganda, schistosomiasis is one of the most common causes of liver granuloma. Careful histopathologic examination of granulomas in certain cases may disclose eggs or migrating larvae such as those occurring in infection due to *Strongyloides stercoralis*. Trophozoites have been identified recently in the liver of a patient with acute granulomatous hepatitis due to *Toxoplasma gondii*. *Toxocara canis* and *T. cati*, which cause visceral larval migrans, may elicit a granulomatous reaction with eosinophilic infiltrates. In this situation, eosinophilia, high levels of isohemagglutinin antibody, and newly available serologic tests are diagnostically helpful.

Drugs. A variety of drugs have been associated with hepatic granuloma formation (Table 2). Recent drug associations have included allopurinol, methyldopa, and chlorpropamide as well as phenylbutazone, halothane, hydralazine, sulfonamides, quinine, nitrofurantion, clofibrate, procainamide, isoniazide, diazapam, carbamazepine, phenytoin, and others (Table 2). Quinidine is estimated to result in a hypersensitivity reaction in 6 per cent of individuals receiving it. In 32 patients (of 487) receiving quinidine who developed hypersensitivity reactions, 10 had clinical and biochemical evidence of hepatic abnormalities. Liver biopsy of four of these revealed granulomas upon rechallenge with quinidine (Geltner et al., 1976). In most instances, discontinuation of the offending drug has resulted in resolution of the clinical and histopathologic findings.

A recent review of 96 cases of granulomatous hepatitis (of 1500 liver biopsies, 6 per cent incidence) has implicated drugs as an etiology for 29 per cent (McMaster and Hennigan, 1981). These authors suggest that the early reaction in drug-induced granulomatous hepatitis is often (75 per cent of the time) characterized by an abnormal number of eosinophils (5 to 10 cells/granuloma) in noncaseating granulomas. Rechallenge studies were not performed on these patients and half the cases were classified as "probable" and the remainder "possible" drug-related. This highlights the difficulty of being certain that drug-related cases are truly representative of an etiologic situation (Table 2).

Chemical Agents. Table 2 enumerates the various chemicals that have been associated with liver granulomas. Many of these represent single case reports, and the patients may have had other underlying conditions, making it difficult to be sure of the association. Beryllium dust may result in an acute pneumonitis after only a brief exposure, but long-term exposure to beryllium oxide has been associated with diffuse hepatic granulomas that are histopathologically indistinguishable from sarcoid. Copper, particularly as Bordeaux mixture, which is copper sulfate neutralized with hydrated lime, has been associated with a syndrome of fever, pneumonitis, hypergammaglobulinemia, and lung or liver granulomas. This has occurred in vineyard sprayers using the copper solution for 3 to 15 years. Rubeanic acid stain has demonstrated the presence of copper in the liver and lungs of these individuals. The Kupffer cells often reveal yellow-brown copper-containing inclusions.

Sarcoidosis. Sarcoidosis and tuberculosis are the two most commonly diagnosed causes of granulomatous hepatitis. In more recent series from the United States and Europe, sarcoidosis is the leading cause, presumably because of the decreasing incidence of tuberculosis, especially the extrapulmonary form. In patients with liver granulomas from hospitals serving poor urban populations in the United States, however, the incidence of tuberculous liver involvement continues to exceed that of sarcoidosis. In our review of approximately 600 published cases of granulomatous hepatitis, sarcoidosis was the most common single diagnosis, accounting for approximately one third of all cases and 40 per cent of all diagnosed cases (Table 4). Two thirds of patients dying of sarcoid have liver lesions at postmortem examination. This figure agrees with the 75 to 85 per cent incidence of liver granulomas that are found when biopsies of the liver are made antemortem in patients with sarcoid (Bunim et al., 1962; Klatskin and Yesner, 1950; Wagoner et al., 1953; Frank and Raffensperger, 1965), although there is a selection factor here because liver biopsy is the primary method of diagnosis of the condition.

The clinical presentation of sarcoidosis with hepatic granuloma is not unlike that of other conditions causing granulomatous hepatitis. There is no sex predilection, and most patients are under the age of 50. From 13 to 50 per cent have fever, while 30 to 80 per cent or more have hepatomegaly. The associated findings of sarcoidosis—splenomegaly, weight loss, abnormal chest radiograph, cutaneous and ocular signs—are present with varying frequency, depending on how the patients reported are selected (that is, those referred to a sarcoid clinic versus those with fever of undetermined origin or those having a liver biopsy for a variety of reasons). Increases in alkaline phosphatase and BSP retention, and decreased prothrombin levels are found in half of the patients. The bilirubin level is less commonly elevated. The calcium, globulin, and eosinophil counts are often increased. The tuberculin test is usually negative in sarcoidosis, and the usefulness of the Kveim test remains highly controversial. In some hands Kveim antigen testing appears to have diagnostic value, but others find it negative in 80 per cent of patients diagnosed as having sarcoidosis (Israel and Goldstein, 1973). Whether these results depend on the antigen, the location of the series, multicausality of sarcoid, or other factors is unknown. The presence of serum angiotensin-converting enzyme may be helpful in establishing this diagnosis in selected cases.

The diagnosis of sarcoid is made by demonstrating granulomas in more than one organ and excluding other causes of granulomatous disease. The diagnosis at times may be made only after an extensive search for granulomas in the bone marrow, mediastinal or abdominal lymph nodes, spleen, and conjunctival tissue. The use of invasive procedures to establish the diagnosis is justified only in the patient in whom another diagnosis has not been made and who remains symptomatic with fever or liver abnormalities.

Steroids are the cornerstone of therapy for sarcoidosis. They are indicated in patients with unrelenting fever or progressive liver abnormalities. Although granulomas may be present for years, progression to fibrosis and cirrhosis occurs only rarely and does not appear to be related to type of treatment administered.

Neoplastic, Immune Disorder, and Liver Disease. Neoplastic diseases, in particular Hodgkin's disease, have been associated with granulomatous hepatitis. Liver biopsy obtained at staging laparotomy has shown granulomas in 5 per cent of patients with Hodgkin's disease. It is unclear if this represents a normal immunologic or inflammatory response to tumor products or whether it is the response of an immunologically abnormal host to an agent or agents that would ordinarily not elicit a granulomatous reaction. It is important to search carefully for infectious causes of granuloma formation in these patients, especially mycobacterial and fungal agents, in view of the high rate of infectious complications. The presence of Reed-Sternberg cells in liver granulomas indicates stage 4 Hodgkin's disease. Ovarian cancer and malignant melanoma have been associated rarely with a granulomatous reaction in the liver.

Several immune deficiency states have been associated with liver granuloma formation. Chronic granulomatous disease is a condition in which phagocytic leukocytes (polymorphonuclear leukocytes and monocyte-macrophages) can ingest certain organisms normally but fail to kill them. The basic biochemical defect appears to involve an inability by the host leukocyte to generate certain bactericidal chemicals (superoxide, hydrogen peroxide, and perhaps others). The condition is typically manifested as a sex-linked, or less commonly autosomal recessive-inherited, early onset (within the first 5 years of life) increase in susceptibility to infections. Although most commonly a pediatric disease, a milder form of this disease has been described in older individuals. The sites most often involved are the skin, lungs, liver, and lymph nodes. The common infecting organisms include *Staphylococcus aureus*, gram-negative bacilli, and fungi. The typical histologic picture is a granulomatous response with polymorphonuclear leukocyte infiltration. Bacteria that would cause abscess formation in a normal person produce granulomas instead, presumably because the leukocytes in chronic granulomatous disease cannot degrade or remove bacterial antigens. Diagnosis of chronic granulomatous disease is confirmed by assay of leukocyte function. Polymorphonuclear leukocytes from affected patients are unable to reduce nitro-blue tetrazolium dye, do not produce the oxygen burst or chemiluminescence that normally accompanies phagocytosis, and are unable to kill *S. aureus* in vitro.

Although hypogammaglobulinemia (a B cell defect) has been linked with granulomatous hepatitis, other concomitant defects of T cell function have not been defined in this syndrome. Collagen vascular diseases, vasculitides, and diseases of unknown etiology that are associated with autoimmune responses and immune alterations have been associated with granulomatous hepatitis (Table 3).

A variety of multisystem granulomatous diseases of unknown etiology, such as Wegener's granulomatosis, lymphomatoid granulomatosis (Fauci et al., 1982), and familial granulomatosis arteritis (Rotenstein et al., 1982) may manifest hepatic involvement. Recent therapeutic advances in the case of some of these syndromes utilizing cyclophosphamide and prednisone (Fauci et al., 1982) make their diagnosis increasingly important.

Granulomatous hepatitis, as well as the more common hepatic fatty metamorphosis, has been reported following jejunoileal bypass surgery performed for weight reduction. The etiology of granulomatous hepatitis in this setting is complex since these patients appear to have a higher incidence of acute tuberculosis. In the absence of infection, adsorption of bacterial antigens or toxins from the excluded segment of bowel has been hypothesized to cause hepatic granulomas. In uninfected patients, reanastomosis has been reported to reverse the granuloma formation (Kalat and Martin, 1981).

Primary liver abnormalities have been associated with granulomas. It is difficult to show clearly an association between granulomatous hepatic response and progressive liver fibrosis. It is evident that granulomatous hepatitis associated with a variety of causes can occasionally progress to cirrhosis (sarcoid, drugs, toxins). Also, when liver biopsy is performed on patients with cirrhosis, granulomatous reactions are encountered occasionally. Whether immune alterations that accompany cirrhosis predispose to granuloma formation when the host is challenged with various antigens, whether in cirrhotic patients an autoimmune phenomenon is initiated whereby the immune response is directed against liver tissue and leads to granuloma formation, or whether the occasional coexistence of cirrhosis and granulomatous reaction is merely a random phenomenon are unknown.

Biliary cirrhosis, in which there are characteristic lymphoid follicles, destructive lesions of small bile ducts, and antimitochondrial antibody, has been associated with granulomatous hepatitis. Biliary cirrhosis tends to be less of a diagnostic enigma owing to the characteristic histopathologic picture of the surrounding liver tissue. A series of patients recently reported with hepatic granulomas, antibodies to mitochondria, and pulmonary disease and granulomas have raised the question of a possible relation between primary biliary cirrhosis and sarcoidosis. Several of these cases had features of Sjogren's syndrome, celiac disease, and mixed connective tissue disease (Fagan et al., 1983)

Granulomatous Hepatitis of Unknown Etiology. The etiology of granulomatous hepatitis is often not identified. In most large studies, this group of patients is the second or third most common (after sarcoid and tuberculous liver disease). More intensive and thorough diagnostic evaluation has improved the frequency of establishing a diagnosis (Guckian and Perry, 1968). Serologic tests, biopsy of other tissues (peritoneal nodes, skin, bone marrow, spleen), review of tissue specimens by experts of some of the rarer granulomatous diseases (Wegener's, lymphomatoid granulomatosis), and judicious long-term observation have led to diagnoses that are not apparent on initial evaluation of the patient. The eventual diagnoses of these cases are similar to those of granulomatous hepatitis as a whole; sarcoid and tuberculosis are most common, followed by less commonly implicated infectious agents, malignancies, and hypersensitivity reactions.

Despite careful evaluation, however, in 10 to 40 per cent of cases no etiologic diagnosis is reached. In most series males outnumber females. The age range is usually older than that seen in the entire group of patients with liver granulomas. The clinical presentation is similar to that of cases of proven etiology, with common occurrence of high and prolonged fever, hepatomegaly, weight loss, and mildly elevated liver enzyme levels.

Associated laboratory abnormalities of undiagnosed granulomatous hepatitis often include increased erythrocyte sedimentation reaction and hypergammaglobulinemia. The histopathology is completely nonspecific and may include giant cells or caseous necrosis.

Although most of the available studies were published before certain infectious agents (cytomegalovirus, Epstein-Barr virus) and drugs were associated with granulomatous hepatitis, the chronicity of some of these cases (4 to 20 years in some series) would seem to exclude many of these causes (Terplan, 1971; Farrell and Powell, 1976; Simon and Wolff, 1973; Mir-Madjlessi et al., 1974). The granulomatous involvement of one organ system alone is not consistent with our current diagnostic criteria for sarcoidosis.

Management of these cases, after extensive evaluation, may include a trial of empiric therapy. Since the diagnosis of tuberculosis is often not excluded, the empiric use of antituberculous drugs is warranted in the patient with symptomatic or progressive disease. Response to antituberculous therapy may reflect an appropriate response in the patient with tuberculosis or it may be due to spontaneous remission of granulomatous hepatitis of unknown etiology. In addition, the use of certain antituberculous drugs such as streptomycin may affect other infections causing granulomatous hepatitis such as tularemia. If symptoms continue after two to four months' therapy with antituberculous medications in conjunction with attempts to exclude additional infectious diseases through appropriate serologic, histopathologic, and cultural studies, then corticosteroid therapy, which appears to be useful in controlling the symptoms if not the histopathology, is indicated. Antituberculous therapy should be continued in patients with positive skin tests for tuberculosis who are treated with corticosteroids. The prognosis of patients with this perplexing disease is good, and there is usually good to excellent response to empiric therapy as outlined above (Israel and Goldstein, 1973; Farrell and Powell, 1976; Neville et al., 1975; Simon and Wolff, 1973).

References

Alexander, J. F., and Galambos, J. T.: Granulomatous hepatitis. The usefulness of liver biopsy in the diagnosis of tuberculosis and sarcoidosis. Am J Gastroenterol 59:23, 1973.

Bain, B. J., Harris, O. D., and Quinn, R. L.: The contribution of percutaneous liver biopsy to the management of liver disease. Med J Aust 2:160, 1973.

Bergman, L. A., Thomas, W., Jr., Reddy, C. R., Ellison, M. R., Smith, E. C., and Dunae, G.: Nonviral hepatitis in patients maintained by long-term dialysis. Arch Intern Med 130:96, 1972.

Bonkowsky, H. L., Lee, R. V., and Klatskin, G.: Acute granulomatous hepatitis. Occurrence in cytomegalovirus mononucleosis. JAMA 233:1284, 1975.

Bunim, J. J., Kimberg, D. V., Thomas, L. B., VanScott, J., and Klatskin, G.: The syndrome of sarcoidosis, psoriasis and gout. Ann Intern Med 57:1018, 1962.

DuPont, H. L., Hornick, R. B., Levin, H. S., Rapoport, M. I., and Woodward, T. E.: Q fever hepatitis. Ann Intern Med 74:198, 1971.

Eliakim, M., Eisenberg, S., Levij, I. S., and Sacks, T. G.: Granulomatous hepatitis accompanying a self-limited febrile disease. Lancet 1:1348, 1968.

Fagan, E. A., Moore-Gillon, J. C., Turner-Warwick, M.: Multiorgan granulomas and mitochondrial antibodies. N Engl J Med 308:572, 1983.

Farrell, G. C., and Powell, L. W.: Chronic granulomatous hepatitis. Aust NZ J Med 6:474, 1976.

Fauci, A. S., and Wolff, S. M.: Granulomatous hepatitis. In Popper, H., and Schaffner, F. (eds.): Progress in Liver Disease, New York, Grune and Stratton, 1976.

Fauci, A. S., Haynes, B. F., Cost, J., Katz, P., and Wolff, S. M.: Lymphoid granulomatosis. Prospective clinical and therapeutic experience over 10 years. N Engl J Med 306:68, 1982.

Fitzgerald, M. X., Fitzgerald, O., and Towers, R. P.: Granulomatous hepatitis of obscure aetiology. Q J Med 150:371, 1971.

Frank, B. B., and Raffensperger, E. C.: Hepatic granulomata. Report of a case with jaundice improving on antituberculous therapy and review of the literature. Arch Intern Med 115:223, 1965.

Galbraith, R. M., Portmann, B., Eddleston, A. L., and Williams, R.: Chronic liver disease developing after outbreak of HBsAg-negative hepatitis in haemodialysis unit. Lancet 2:886, 1975.

Gelb, A. M., Brazenas, N., Sussman, H., and Wallach, R.: Acute granulomatous disease of the liver. Digest Dis 15:842, 1970.

Geltner, D., Chajek, T., Rubinger, D., and Levij, I. S.: Quinidine hypersensitivity and liver involvement. A survey of 32 patients. Gastroenterology 70:650, 1976.

Guckian, J. C., and Perry, J. E.: Granulomatous hepatitis. An analysis of 63 cases and review of the literature. Ann Intern Med 65:1081, 1966.

Guckian, J. C., and Perry, J. E.: Granulomatous hepatitis of unknown etiology. Am J Med 44:207, 1968.

Harrington, P. T., Gutierrez, J. J., Ramirez-Ronda, C. H., Quinones-Soto, R., Bermudez, R. H., and Chaffey, J.: Granulomatous hepatitis. Rev Infect Dis 4:638, 1982.

Hughes, M., and Fox, H.: A histological analysis of granulomatous hepatitis. J Clin Pathol 25:817, 1972.

Israel, H. L., and Goldstein, R. A.: Hepatic granulomatosis and sarcoidosis. Ann Intern Med 79:669, 1973.

Iverson, K., Christoffersen, P., and Poulsen, H.: Epithelioid cell granulomas in liver biopsies. Scand J Gastroenterol (Suppl) 7:61, 1970.

Jones, J. M.: Granulomatous hepatitis due to *Candida albicans* in patients with acute leukemia. Clin Res 28:736A, 1980.

Kalat, E. D., and Martin, D. B.: Granulomatous hepatitis associated with jejunoileal bypass surgery. JAMA 246:982, 1981.

Klatskin, G., and Yesner, R.: Hepatic manifestations of sarcoidosis and other granulomatous diseases. Yale J Biol Med 23:207, 1950.

McMaster, K. R., and Hennigan, G. R.: Drug induced granulomatous hepatitis. Lab Invest 44:61, 1981.

Mir-Madjlessi, S. H., Farmer, R. G., and Hawk, W. A.: Granulomatous hepatitis. A review of 50 cases. Am J Gastroenterol 60:122, 1973.

Mir-Madjlessi, S. H., Farmer, R. G., and Hawk, W. A.: Spectrum of hepatic manifestations of granulomatous hepatitis of unknown etiology. Am J Gastroenterol 62:221, 1974.

Neville, E., Piyasena, K. H. G., and Geraint James, D.: Granulomas of the liver. Postgrad Med J 51:361, 1975.

Pequignot, H., Cocheton, J., Christorofov, B., and Louvel, A.: Transparietal puncture biopsy of the liver. A review of 464 cases. Mater Med Pol 5:99, 1973.

Robbins, S. L.: Inflammation and repair. In Robbins, S. L., and Cotran, R. S. (eds.): Pathologic Basis of Disease. Philadelphia, W. B. Saunders Company, 1979, p. 55.

Rotenstein, D., Gibbas, D. L., Majmudar, B., Chastain, E. A.: Familial granulomatous arteritis with polyarthritis of juvenile onset. N Engl J Med 306:86, 1982.

Schiff, L.: Diseases of the Liver. Philadelphia, J. B. Lippincott Company, 1956.

Simon, H. B., and Wolff, S. M.: Granulomatous hepatitis and prolonged fever of unknown origin. A study of 13 patients. Medicine 52:1, 1973.

Terplan, M.: Hepatic granulomas of unknown cause presenting with fever. Am J Gastroenterol 55:43, 1971.

Wagoner, G. P., Anton, A. T., Gall, E. A., and Schiff, L.: Needle biopsy of the liver. VIII. Experiences with hepatic granulomas. Gastroenterology 25:487, 1953.

Warren, K. S.: A functional classification of granulomatous inflammation. Ann N Y Acad Sci 278:7, 1976.

151
FLUKE INFECTIONS

ELIZABETH BARRETT-CONNOR, M.D.

FASCIOLIASIS

Fascioliasis is a zoonosis caused by the liver fluke, *Fasciola hepatica*. Human infection occurs sporadically on a worldwide basis.

ETIOLOGY. Man is an accidental host. Fascioliasis is essentially a disease of sheep, goats, and cattle, in which it produces liver rot and therefore assumes economic importance. *F. hepatica* is enzootic in many wild animals, including rabbits and deer. Operculated eggs are passed in the feces of infected animals and hatch a ciliated miracidium into water. Larval development takes place in a fresh water snail, ultimately releasing cercaria that encyst on aquatic vegetation. When ingested by a suitable host, the parasites excyst and migrate through the intestinal wall into the peritoneal cavity. After penetrating the liver capsule, immature flukes migrate through the liver for several weeks and finally reach the bile ducts where they mature three months after infection and release eggs into the feces. Human infection is usually acquired by eating wild watercress grown in meadows frequented by sheep or other naturally infected herbivores. The use of casually gathered watercress to decorate food or drink has been followed by infection. Man can also be infected by chewing grasses containing metacercariae, and possibly by drinking contaminated water, since metacercariae can form on minute particles on surface water.

PATHOGENESIS AND PATHOLOGY. Migration of the immature flukes through the liver causes hepatitis, with parenchymal cell necrosis and an inflammatory and eosinophilic cellular response. Liver biopsy after recovery from this phase of illness shows no persistent hepatocellular pathology. The other characteristic finding is hyperplasia of the main bile duct with a thickened duct wall and an infolded endothelium surrounding an enlarged duct lumen. This process is probably essential for the establishment of the mature flukes, which are too large to be accommodated by unaltered bile ducts. Hyperplasia of the main bile duct occurs while immature *Fasciola* are still in the liver parenchyma, long before they enter the duct, and may be due to the stimulus of proline elaborated by the flukes (Isseroff et al., 1977). Experimentally, bile duct hyperplasia can be induced either by flukes maintained in the peritoneum without access to the liver, or by intraperitoneal proline.

CLINICAL MANIFESTATIONS. There are two phases of illness, the first caused by migration of young flukes through the liver, and a second caused by mature flukes in the biliary ducts. Infected patients may experience both phases, only the first phase, only the second phase, relapses of either phase, or may remain asymptomatic indefinitely.

Early symptoms due to transhepatic migration of flukes begin two to three months after ingestion of metacercariae; symptoms include intermittent fever, malaise, night sweats, weight loss, and pain in the right upper quadrant. Urticaria with dermatographia or persistent nonproductive cough may be the most prominent symptoms in some cases. Relapses of the acute phase may occur, possibly owing to flukes reentering the liver. This illness may last several weeks.

The adult flukes are established in the biliary tract three or four months after infection, where they may survive for over ten years and cause no symptoms. In some cases obstructive jaundice occurs months or years later. Most patients with *Fasciola* bile duct obstruction are diagnosed at surgery, when one or more large flukes are found obstructing the biliary tract. *F. hepatica* has also been recovered from many ectopic sites, including skin, brain, and lung.

GEOGRAPHIC VARIATIONS IN DISEASE. Most reported cases have originated in Latin America, particularly in Chile and Cuba, but the largest single outbreak occurred in France with 500 cases in 1956. *Fasciola gigantica*, closely related to *F. hepatica*, is a trematode infection of domestic stock, and occasionally man, in tropical and subtropical areas of Africa, Asia, Europe, Hawaii, and Russia.

In some parts of the mideast, notably Syria, Lebanon, and Armenia, raw sheep or goat liver is eaten. Flukes of *F. hepatica* become attached to the mucosa of the epiglottis or posterior pharynx and cause edema and suffocation. This condition is called halzoun.

DIAGNOSIS. Only a history of contact with a sheep-growing area and fondness for wild watercress offer clues to the diagnosis of the sporadic case. Eosinophilia, often exceeding 50 per cent, is common in the first phase, and liver function tests suggest hepatitis. During the first three months serologic tests are usually positive, but stools are negative for ova because the fluke is not yet mature in the biliary tract.

During the obstructive phase eosinophilia may persist, but is most often absent. A history of recent hepatitis may suggest the etiology of biliary tract disease to the astute clinician, but often hepatitis is denied or its significance is missed. Large operculate eggs, which must be differentiated from those of *F. buski*, are found in the stool of two-thirds of cases (Fig. 4, Chapter 86). Ova are not found in the stools at any time in nearly one-third of cases. Diagnosis in stool-negative cases can usually be made by demonstrating ova in duodenal aspirate or by serologic tests. False-positive diagnosis may be a problem in areas where raw liver is eaten and ingested *F. hepatica* are passed in the feces. This possibility can be excluded by examining the stool after several days on a liver-free diet.

On occasion, *F. gigantica* has induced an abscess or a tumor-like reaction in the liver, which can be seen as a low density, irregular calcification on abdominal roentgenogram. The appearance of this hepatic calcification is considered to be virtually diagnostic.

TREATMENT. No effective treatment is known for the migratory phase of illness. Symptomatic improvement may occur with chloroquine, emetine, or metronidazole therapy, leading to the mistaken diagnosis of amebic liver disease. Bithionol is the preferred treatment for preoperative or post-operative patients with ova in the stool. The recommended dose is 30 to 50 mg/kg on alternate days for 10 to 15 doses. Shorter course therapy with newer drugs, such as niclofolan, may be effective, but more data on toxicity and cure rates are needed.

PROPHYLAXIS. Avoiding watercress, unless known to be grown commercially under specific regulations, is the best way to prevent fascioliasis. Control measures aimed at reducing infection in domestic animals, including drainage of pastures and application of molluscicides, may be helpful.

OPISTHORCHIASIS

Opisthorchiasis is a common liver fluke infection of the dog, cat, fox, and pig. Although man is an incidental host, millions of people are infected. *Opisthorchis sinensis, Opisthorchis felineus,* and *Opisthorchis viverrini* are the major pathogens.

ETIOLOGY. In some endemic areas over 90 per cent of the population is infected. Infection rates increase with age. Man is infected by eating raw, pickled, or smoked fish containing encysted metacercariae. After ingestion the parasites excyst and attach to the duodenal wall. Subsequently they migrate through the ampulla of Vater into the biliary tree or, less often, up the pancreatic duct, and attach to the epithelial lining. The flukes mature in 1 month. Flukes do not multiply in man but may persist for many years, producing eggs that are passed in the feces. The life cycle requires two intermediate hosts. Ova released in feces are ingested by snails, which in time release cercaria. These infect freshwater fish, often of the carp family.

PATHOLOGY AND PATHOGENESIS. In the bile ducts adult flukes initially induce epithelial proliferation and adenomatous hyperplasia with the formation of new glands and goblet cells. Proliferation is gradually replaced by fibrosis around a dilated duct. These changes are irreversible. At autopsy, the dilated fibrosed ducts can be seen on the cut surface of the liver. The pancreatic duct, the only other structure affected by opisthorchiasis, may show hyperplasia, squamous metaplasia, or fibrosis. Ascending cholangitis, cholangiohepatitis, liver abscess, and pancreatitis are complications of obstruction and secondary infection. Intrahepatic gallstone formation is not unusual. Cirrhosis, at one time attributed to chronic liver fluke infection, is probably coincidental. Opisthorchiasis may increase the risk of cholangiocarcinoma. In Hong Kong, about 15 per cent of all primary liver cancers are cholangiocarcinomas attributed to opisthorchiasis. The majority of these are adenocarcinomas arising near the secondary bile ducts of the hepatic hilum. Animal studies suggest that nitrosamines derived from common popular foods are important factors in the development of carcinoma during opisthorchiasis (Schwartz, 1980).

CLINICAL MANIFESTATIONS. Prolonged exposure is required to achieve a heavy worm burden, so that flukes and disease attributed to them are not common in children. In general, the severity of liver fluke disease is proportional to the number of parasites, but there are patients with heavy infections (over 1000 flukes) who appear perfectly well, and others with relatively few flukes who suffer complications.

As with other intestinal parasites, most of those infected have no illness. Symptoms commonly attributed to moderate infection, such as low grade fever, anorexia, nausea, diarrhea, bloating, flatulence, and abdominal or back pain, have been equally common in uninfected controls. Right upper quadrant pain and weakness are more closely associated with the intensity of infection (Upatham et al., 1982). Some manifestations clearly reflect the effect of worms on bile or pancreatic duct function; these include hepatomegaly, jaundice, pyogenic cholangitis, liver abscess, and pancreatitis.

COMPLICATIONS AND SEQUELAE. Either opisthorchis ova or adults may form a nidus for gallstones. When worms obstruct the cystic or common bile duct, the enlarged gallbladder may simulate carcinoma of the pancreas. As noted above, cholangiocarcinoma of the liver is a late complication of opisthorchiasis.

The prognosis is uncertain. Patients may remain asymptomatic for years and then rather abruptly deteriorate and die of liver or pancreatic disease.

GEOGRAPHIC VARIATIONS. *Opisthorchis sinensis (Clonorchis sinensis)* is found in Indochina, Hong Kong, Japan, Korea, North Vietnam, and Taiwan. *Opisthorchis felineus* is found primarily in India, Vietnam, the Philippines, Korea, and Japan. *O. viverrini* is most common in northern Thailand, Laos, and West Malaysia. These flukes are morphologically and pathologically very similar, although *O. viverrini* may be less pathogenic than *O. sinensis*.

DIAGNOSIS. Opisthorchiasis should be suspected in a patient from an endemic area who presents with weakness, abdominal pain, jaundice, hepatomegaly, an enlarged gallbladder, or obscure liver disease (Hou and Pang, 1964). The peripheral white blood cell count may show eosinophilia, a polymorphonuclear leukocytosis, or be normal. Liver function tests are usually moderately deranged, even in patients who are completely asymptomatic. The diagnosis is made by identification of small operculate eggs (see Fig. 4 in Chapter 86) in unconcentrated feces. A direct smear should be positive in any patient with ten or more adult flukes, because the flukes are prolific egg producers. If stool examination is negative, diagnosis requires microscopic examination of a duodenal or bile duct aspirate. Serologic and intradermal tests can be used to confirm the diagnosis, but are rarely necessary and are not available in most areas.

Liver scan often shows hepatomegaly with diffusely poor uptake, a nonspecific finding. Intravenous cholangiography may show filling defects in the common bile duct and gall bladder. A percutaneous transhepatic cholangiogram showing multiple cystic ectasias of the intrahepatic bile ducts or mulberry-like dilatation is nearly pathognomonic of opisthorchiasis.

TREATMENT. Until recently, medical treatment has been unsatisfactory. Chloroquine, dehydroemetine, or bithionol usually suppress ova production, but do not cure the patient. Among the several recently introduced or investigational drugs, praziquantel (Merck-Bayer) is the most effective. The usual dose of 25 mg/kg two or three times a day for one or two days yields cure rates of 88 to 100 per cent. Toxicity is usually limited to transient diarrhea and epigastric pain. Dead or dying flukes are expelled with bile into the intestinal lumen, suggesting that surgery should rarely be necessary to relieve biliary obstruction (Bunnag and Harinasuta, 1980; Rim et al., 1980).

PROPHYLAXIS. Populations at risk should be taught about the route of infection and warned to avoid raw fish. Destruction of the intermediate snail host is an attractive idea but impractical.

FASCIOLOPSIASIS

Fasciolopsiasis is an intestinal infection of man and pigs caused by *Fasciolopsis buski*.

ETIOLOGY. *F. buski* normally lives in the small intestine of man and hogs. Large operculated eggs are excreted in the stool. The two intermediate hosts are freshwater snails and water plants. Water chestnuts, water lily shoots, water caltrops and other water plants may have hundreds of metacercariae on their outer coverings. Man becomes infected by placing one of these plants in the mouth either for eating, peeling, or holding during collection. Excysted metacercariae attach to the mucosa in the duodenum. Each fluke matures and releases eggs in one to three months. *F. buski* does not multiply in the intestine. In some endemic areas over two-thirds of the population is infected. Overt infection is most common in poor and malnourished children.

PATHOGENESIS AND PATHOLOGY. Very little has been written about the pathogenesis or pathology of *F. buski* infection. The large flukes apparently damage the mucosa of the intestine at the site of attachment, causing local ulceration, inflammation, and diarrhea. Abscess formation, hemorrhage from erosion of mucosal vessels, and local bowel obstruction have been described. Edema of the face and legs and ascites are usually attributed to an unidentified toxic metabolite of the parasite. Anemia and B12 deficiency are common.

CLINICAL MANIFESTATIONS. Most adults and approximately one-third of infected children are asymptomatic. The onset of illness coincides with the maturation of flukes in the intestine. Typically many flukes are present before symptoms attributable to *F. buski* occur: the usual worm burden of 10 to 20 flukes is probably of little clinical significance. At least 100 worms have been required to produce illness in an adult and in fatal cases 1000 to 3000 flukes may be recovered at autopsy. Many reported symptoms are nonspecific ones common in endemic areas, and, except in massive infections, are no more common in fasciolopsiasis than in uninfected controls. Typical symptoms attributed to *F. buski* infections are abdominal pain, often relieved by food and simulating peptic ulcer disease, intermittent nondysenteric diarrhea, flatus, excessive appetite, or anorexia.

COMPLICATIONS AND SEQUELAE. In heavily infected children, the disease may simulate protein-calorie malnutrition with massive edema, including facial edema and ascites, pallor, and hepatomegaly. Edema may occur because of competition by the flukes for limited nutrients in the malnourished, precipitating Kwashiorkor or may precede severe malnutrition or diarrhea. Heavily infected children often pass flukes per rectum and vomit flukes. Generally, the younger the patient, the larger the worm burden and the more inadequate the nutrition, the more severe the symptoms, and the greater the potential for a fatal outcome.

GEOGRAPHIC VARIATIONS. Fasciolopsiasis is found in rural parts of Central and South China, India, Bangladesh, Vietnam, Thailand, and Taiwan.

DIAGNOSIS. The clinical picture is not specific, unless the patient is passing worms, but is sufficiently characteristic to arouse suspicion in endemic areas (Plaut et al., 1969). Anemia, leukocytosis, and eosinophilia (5 to 30 per cent) are common. Diagnosis is based on finding the characteristic ova (Fig. 4, Chapter 86) in the stool.

TREATMENT. The traditional treatment has been hexylresorcinol (Crystoids anthelmintic). The dose is 0.4 g for patients less than seven years old and 1 g if older. Tetrachlorethylene, given in one dose of 0.12 cc/kg of body weight (maximum 5 cc dose), or niclosamide, two tablets as a single dose, are equally effective and now preferred. The latter is associated with fewer side effects (Suntharasamai et al., 1974).

PROPHYLAXIS. Prevention of *F. buski* infection would require public health education, improved sanitation, prohibition of swine access to areas where water plants are grown, and warning against consumption of raw water plants. Which, if any, of these measures are practical will depend on the endemic area under consideration.

HETEROPHYDIASIS

Heterophydiasis is infection caused by the *Heterophyidae* parasites of mammals and fish-eating birds. *Heterophyes heterophyes*, *Metagonimus yokogawai*, *Haplorchis yokogawai* and *H. pumilio* are the heterophyids most commonly recovered from man.

ETIOLOGY. The parasite life cycle requires both a fresh or brackish water snail and a fish, often of the mullet family, as intermediate hosts. Infection is acquired by the ingestion of uncooked fish. The adult parasite is found in the small intestine of man and a variety of fish-eating mammals and birds. Growth is rapid; mature ova are found in the stools less than two weeks after ingestion of metacercariae. Each fluke lives only about two months. In some areas the prevalence in young people exceeds 80 per cent.

PATHOLOGY AND PATHOGENESIS. The adult flukes are attached deep in the crypts of Lieberkühn of the small intestine. Infection may cause inflammation and increased mucous production, or there may be little tissue reaction. Ova or dying flukes in the bowel wall cause a granulomatous reaction. Rarely, ova embolize to distant sites, most notably the nervous system and heart. In some cases, eggs reach the mitral valve, eventually causing fibrosis and calcification.

CLINICAL MANIFESTATIONS. These parasites usually produce no symptoms unless present in large numbers. The most typical symptoms are abdominal pain simulating peptic ulcer disease or diarrhea (Sheir and El-Shabrawy, 1970). Diarrhea is usually nondysenteric, although bloody diarrhea has been reported. Diarrhea may persist for months.

COMPLICATIONS AND SEQUELAE. In the Philippines, heterophyid myocarditis is said to be an important cause of death. The clinical picture may be that of myocardial or valvular disease.

GEOGRAPHIC VARIATIONS. Human infection with *Heterophyes heterophyes* is found in Japan, China, the Philippines, Egypt, Israel, Greece, and Western India. A similar small fluke, *Metagonimus yokogawai*, is common in the Orient and is also found in the Balkans, Spain, Russia, and Israel.

DIAGNOSIS. Diagnosis is based on finding small operculated ova (Fig. 4, Chapter 86) in the feces. *Heterophyes* ova cannot be differentiated readily from *Metagonimus* ova, and both resemble those of *Opisthorchis*. Adult worms are not seen in the feces except after appropriate treatment.

TREATMENT. A 50 to 70 per cent cure rate can be achieved with the standard hookworm doses of tetrachlorethylene or bephenium hydroxynaphthoate, with the standard ascaris dose of piperazine, or with a three-day course of niclosamide. A single dose of piperazine, 50 mg/kg the evening preceding the first of two doses of niclosamide improves the cure rate.

PROPHYLAXIS. Eradication of heterophydiasis is precluded by the multiple reservoir hosts. Mollusciciding with present techniques also is not feasible. The only method of prevention is to avoid eating uncooked fish in endemic areas.

References

Bunnag, D., and Harinasuta, T.: Studies on the chemotherapy of human opisthorchiasis: I. Clinical trial of praziquantel. Southeast Asian J Trop Med Public Health 11:528, 1980.

Hammond, J. A.: Human infection with the liver fluke Fasciola gigantica. Trans Roy Soc Trop Med Hyg 68:253, 1974.

Hardman, E. W., Jones, R. L. H., and Davies, A. H.: Fascioliasis—a large outbreak. Br Med J 3:502, 1970.

Harinasuta, C. (ed.): Proceedings of the Fourth Southeast Asian Seminar on Parasitology and Tropical Medicine, Schistosomiasis and Other Snail-Transmitted Helminthiasis. Bangkok, Thai Watana Panich Press Co., Ltd., 1969.

Hou, P. C., and Pang, L. C. S.: Clonorchis sinensis infestation in man in Hong Kong. J Pathol Bacteriol 87:245, 1964.

Isseroff, H., Sawma, J. T., and Reino, D.: Fascioliasis: Role of proline in bile duct hyperplasia. Science 198:1157, 1977.

Koompirochana, C., Sonakul, D., Chinda, K., Stitnimankarn, T.: Opisthorchiasis: A clinicopathologic study of 154 autopsy cases. Southeast Asian J Trop Med Public Health 9:60, 1978.

Plaut, A. G., Kampanart-Sanyakorn, C., and Manning, G. S.: A clinical study of Fasciolopsis buski infection in Thailand. Trans R Soc Trop Med Hyg 63:470, 1969.

Rim, H. J., Lyu, K. S., Lee, J. S., and Joo, K. H.: Clinical evaluation of the therapeutic efficacy of Praziquantel against *Clonorchis sinensis* infection in man. Ann Trop Med Parasit 75:27, 1980.

Schwartz, D. A.: Helminths in the induction of cancer: *Opisthorchis viverrini, Clonorchis sinensis* and cholangio carcinoma. Trop Geogr Med 32:95, 1980.

Sheir, Z. M., and El-Shabrawy, Aboul-Enein M: Demographic, clinical and therapeutic appraisal of heterophydiasis. J Trop Med Hyg 73:148, 1970.

Suntharasamai, P., Bunnag, D., Tejavanij, S., Harinasuta, T., Migasena, S., Vutikes, S., and Chindanond, D.: Comparative clinical trials of niclosamide and tetrachlorethylene in the treatment of Fasciolopsis buski infection. Southeast Asian J Trop Med Public Health 5:556, 1974.

Upatham, E. S., Viyanant, V., Kurathong, S., Brockelman, Y., Menaruchi, A., Saowakontha, S., Intarakhao, C., Vajrasthira, S., and Warren, K. S.: Morbidity in relation to intensity of infection in *Opisthorchiasis viverrini:* study of a community in Khon Kaen, Thailand. Am J Trop Med Hyg 31:1156, 1982.

152
VISCERAL LEISHMANIASIS

ANTHONY D. M. BRYCESON, M.D.

Visceral leishmaniasis (kala-azar, ponos) is an infection with the viscerotropic species of parasites of the genus *Leishmania, L. donovani.* The disease is usually a zoonosis, transmitted by phlebotomine sandflies between wild or peridomestic animals. Man is infected when he interrupts the natural cycle, so that human disease is usually sporadic. Epidemics in which man is the only reservoir arise from time to time in the Indian subcontinent.

The disease is a severe chronic infection of the reticuloendothelial system, characterized by fever, chills, weight loss, splenomegaly, pancytopenia, malnutrition, immunosuppression, and a high natural mortality.

ETIOLOGY. *Leishmania* exist in two forms, one in the vertebrate host, including man, and the other in the sandfly and in artificial culture (Hommel, 1978). In the vertebrate host the parasite is in the amastigote (Leishman-Donovan body) stage, so called because it has no free flagellum. It is a round or oval body 2 to 3 μ across containing a nucleus and a smaller kinetoplast, which stain, respectively, red and purple with Geimsa, Wright's, or Leishman's stain, and stand out against the pale blue cytoplasm. *Leishmania* are strict intracellular parasites and are found in macrophages in which they multiply by binary fission. Heavily parasitized host cells rupture, and fresh cells are invaded. Sandflies become infected when they feed on an infected person or animal and take up parasites from blood or skin. In the sandfly the parasite is in the promastigote (leptomonad) stage, so called because of the anterior origin of its flagellum. Promastigotes are supple, highly motile, spindle-shaped organisms, 15 to 25 μ long and 1.5 to 3.5 μ broad. They are found in the hindgut or midgut of the sandfly, where they divide and migrate forward into the pharynx and buccal cavity, rendering the sandfly infective. The cycle of development in the sandfly takes about seven days. Once inoculated into man, the promastigotes rapidly penetrate macrophages, flagellum first, and transform into amastigotes.

Biochemical taxonomy of *Leishmania* (isoenzymes, DNA analysis) has proved a valuable adjunct to the traditional epidemiologic and serologic methods of species differentiation (World Health Organization, 1982).

It has been suggested that the zoonotic origin of *L. donovani* was among jackals in the steppes of Central Asia, where sporadic cases of visceral leishmaniasis are still seen among nomads and in settlers in the outskirts of rapidly expanding towns. From here the disease spread and developed three distinct epidemiologic patterns.

Visceral Leishmaniasis with a Canine Reservoir. This is the pattern in a belt that stretches from Portugal to Peking between latitudes 30 and 48 degrees North, the most important areas being the Mediterranean littoral, including North Africa, the shores of the Caspian Sea, central Soviet Asia, and northeast China. The main vectors are *Phlebotomus perniciosus* and *P. ariasi* in Western Europe, *P. major* in Eastern Europe, *P. papatasii* in the Middle East, and *P. chinensis* in China. In the Mediterranean and Chinese foci, the host-parasite relationship is relatively stable, and the disease is most common among children between one and four years of age. For this reason the parasite has also been designated *L. infantum,* although adults in areas into which the disease has newly been introduced or visitors of any age are highly susceptible. Domestic dogs and foxes are the reservoir. In West Africa, infected dogs have been found, but human cases are rare.

Portuguese and Spanish settlers possibly introduced *L. donovani* into the New World and initiated a zoonosis among foxes and dogs, although man may still be an occasional reservoir. The New World parasite has also been designated *L. chagasi.* The likely vector is *Lutzomyia longipalpis.* Visceral leishmaniasis is epidemic in northeast Brazil and sporadic in Amazonia, northern Argentina, and Paraguay. It extends up through Venezuela and Colombia as far as Guatemala and Mexico. It is a disease of towns and villages rather than of the forest. In Brazil male children are most commonly affected.

Visceral Leishmaniasis with Rodent Vector. This is the pattern in Africa south of the Sahara from Lake Chad in the west to Somalia in the east, sparing the highlands of Ethiopia. In the Sudan the zoonosis is between the Nile rat *(Arvicanthus niloticus)* and *P. orientalis* on the flood plains of the Nile and its tributaries. Visceral leishmaniasis is found among nomads who occupy temporary villages in riverine acacia woodland and migrant workers from adjoining countries.

In Kenya the disease is associated with termite hills where the vector *P. martini* rests and round which village men gather in the evenings. The reservoir has not been established, but is more likely to be in dogs or man than in rodents. The disease is usually sporadic, but epidemics have occurred. Males are affected four times as often as females, and the disease is most common in teenagers.

Visceral Leishmaniasis with a Human Reservoir. This is true epidemic kala-azar and is the pattern of the disease in northeast India, Bangladesh, Assam, and Burma. Classically, the disease spreads along the Brahmaputra valley every 20 years or so. Transmission is by the highly anthropophilic, domestic sandfly *P. argentipes.* Often, many cases are found to have originated from one house. The disease is commonest in young adults. Man is the only reservoir, and *P. argentipes* is readily infected from blood or from the lesions of post-kala-azar dermal leishmaniasis. The disease virtually disappeared over large areas as a result of DDT spraying for malaria control, but returned to Bihar in 1975, killing many thousands, and has spread into West Bengal.

Factors Affecting Transmission. Opportunities for contact with infected sandflies largely determine the pattern of disease in a given area. The pattern is modified by the level of immunity of the population or individual. An attack of visceral leishmaniasis confers lifelong immunity, which determines the periodicity of epidemics. Subclinical infections with *L. donovani* or possibly even lizard and rodent species of *Leishmania* may affect the pattern of spread in Africa.

PATHOGENESIS. Parasites inoculated by the infective sandfly are taken up by macrophages in which they multiply. The site of early multiplication may be in the skin or possibly in the viscera to which parasites have been carried by the blood stream.

Susceptibility and Resistance. Evidence from skin testing, serology, and liver biopsy suggests that subclinical cases outnumber clinical cases by about 30:1 during outbreaks of visceral leishmaniasis in the Mediterranean and in Africa. The situation in India is not known, but may be similar. Susceptibility of mice to *L. donovani* is genetically determined (Bradley, 1982), but genetic markers for human susceptibility have not yet been identified. Resistance to infection depends upon the development of specific cell-mediated immunity. When this response is efficient, the illness is mild or symptomless and pathology is limited to small self-healing tuberculoid granulomas in the liver, and possibly other organs. The leishmanin skin test becomes positive and antibodies appear transiently in the serum.

The Established Disease. Cell-mediated immunity fails to develop or is suppressed early in the infection and parasites spread through the blood stream to spleen, liver, bone marrow, lymph nodes, intestinal lymphatic tissue and submucosa and skin and multiply freely in macrophages or other reticuloendothelial cells. The small intestinal lesion may cause malabsorption and albumen loss. Enlargement of the spleen causes sequestration of erythrocytes, granulocytes, and platelets, all of whose half-lives are reduced. Increased plasma volume and immune lysis of erythrocytes due to complement activation also contribute to anemia. Cell-mediated immune responses to leishmanial antigens in vivo and in vitro are suppressed. They recover slowly after treatment in 75 per cent of patients. Cell-mediated responses to unrelated antigens and mitogens are also profoundly suppressed, but recover more rapidly after treatment (Ho et al., 1983). Leukopenia, and immunosuppression predispose to secondary infection. Reticuloendothelial bombardment leads to overproduction of globulin, especially IgG, little of which is specific antibody and none of which is protective. Some of it is autoantibody. Circulating immune complexes are found in high titer. They contain IgM and less frequently IgG and complement. It is possible that they contribute to anemia, nephritis, and amyloidosis. Bleeding, late in the disease, may be due to thrombocytopenia and clotting defects secondary to hepatocellular damage.

PATHOLOGY. Histologically the disease is characterized by massive proliferation of parasitized macrophages with little or no lymphocytic response (Winslow, 1971). The spleen is grossly enlarged, smooth, and firm, and the capsule is thick. The pulp is friable and infarcts are usual. There is massive hyperplasia of reticuloendothelial cells that are heavily parasitized. In the liver, Kupffer cells are hyperplastic and contain parasites. Occasionally, parenchymal cells are parasitized. In chronic untreated cases there may be parenchymal cell degeneration, which may be followed after several years by fibrosis and even cirrhosis with clinical and biochemical evidence of hepatic dysfunction.

The bone marrow is heavily infiltrated with parasitized

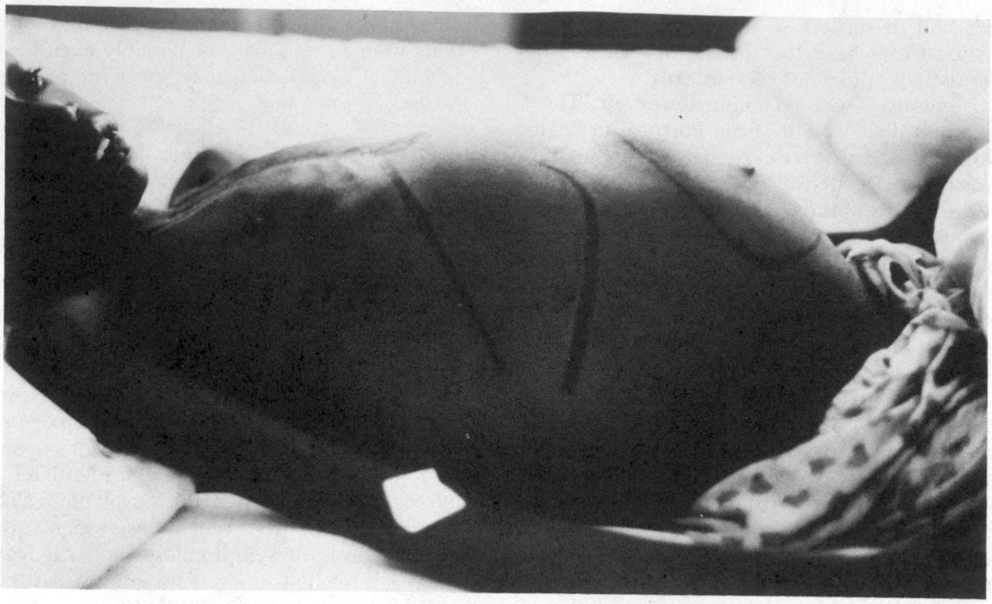

Figure 1. Gross hepatosplenomegaly and wasting in visceral leishmaniasis.

macrophages. Erythropoiesis and granulopoiesis are normal in the early stages of the disease, but may show maturation arrest. Later the marrow may be depressed. Lymph nodes and lymphoid tissue of the nasopharynx and gut are enlarged and contain many parasitized cells.

Immunoglobulin and complement may be deposited in the glomerular basement membrane, but in most cases neither protein nor cells are found in the urine. In fatal cases, hyaline thickening of the glomerular mesangium has been found. Amyloidosis may develop in chronic cases. The skin, although normal in appearance, contains many intracellular parasites. In post-kala-azar dermal leishmaniasis, there is variable infiltration with lymphocytes, histiocytes, and parasites.

CLINICAL MANIFESTATIONS. The incubation period is normally two to six months, but may be as short as ten days or as long as nine years. The onset is usually insidious, especially in indigenous peoples who may feel well and have a good appetite despite daily bouts of fever; however, in the poorly nourished with several underlying parasitic infections, the disease may progress rapidly. In Africa a primary cutaneous nodule may be noticed for a few months before there are any systemic symptoms. The earliest symptom is fever, usually gradual in onset and accompanied by sweats, often without preceding chills. Alternatively, the onset is sudden with high fever and chills. This is common in Americans and Europeans who have contracted the disease while visiting an endemic area. Associated with fever there may be dizziness, weakness, and weight loss. Other common early symptoms include cough, diarrhea, pain or discomfort in the left hypochondrium, and symptoms of complicating secondary infections.

The important physical findings are fever, splenomegaly, lymphadenopathy, malnutrition, and skin changes. At first fever is often inconstant, with apyrexial periods of several days or weeks. In over 80 per cent of cases, however, the fever eventually develops a characteristic pattern with twice daily elevations reaching 38 to 40° C, and may then undulate as in brucellosis. In the most acute cases, fever and toxemia may be the only signs. Splenic enlargement is not necessarily rapidly progressive, nor does the size of the spleen correlate with the duration of the disease. In many instances, however, it reaches the right iliac fossa (Fig. 1). It is firm and not tender, unless there has been a subcapsular infarct. The liver enlarges more slowly and becomes palpable in about 20 per cent of cases and is also firm and not tender. Generalized lymphadenopathy is common in patients from Mediterranean countries, Africa, or China. Appetite is usually good, and nutritional status is initially well maintained. Signs of hypoalbuminemia, however, develop. These include edema and loss of texture, curl, and color of hair. Later the patient becomes wasted. Various changes have been reported in the skin. Classically, there is hyperpigmentation of hands, feet, and abdomen. This may be missed in black Africans; in lighter-skinned Indians it looks gray or black (kala-azar means black sickness). In Africans warty eruptions or ulcers of the skin and oronasal lesions are occasionally seen (Abdalla et al., 1975).

COMPLICATIONS. As the disease progresses, anemia becomes clinically apparent. There may be bleeding from the nose or gums. In long-standing cases jaundice may develop. Finally, after a course that may run for a few months or for as long as five years, the patient becomes emaciated and exhausted. Intercurrent infections are the cause of death in 90 per cent of fatal cases. The most common are pneumonia, pulmonary tuberculosis, bacillary dysentery, amebic dysentery, pneumococcal otitis media and cancrum oris, and, in Africa, brucellosis. Massive gastrointestinal hemorrhage accounts for another 1 to 2 per cent.

Untreated, 75 to 90 per cent of patients with established disease die. Treated patients should recover. The mortality of late or severe disease in malnourished patients treated under difficult conditions can be over 25 per cent. Bad prognostic signs include extreme emaciation and toxemia, agranulocytosis, and the absence of the lymphocytosis, which usually appears during treatment.

SEQUELAE. A small, unknown proportion of recovered patients develop cirrhosis later. Another proportion may relapse. In the great majority, however, recovery, if it takes place, is complete, and the patient is immune against reinfection, probably for life. The role, or fate, of the 25 per cent who do not regain specific immune responsiveness is unknown.

Post-Kala-azar Dermal Leishmaniasis. About 20 per cent of Indian patients develop a rash one to two years after treatment or spontaneous recovery. The lesions develop slowly and may last for several, even 20, years. In Africa the rash develops in 2 per cent of cases, usually during treatment, and does not persist. It commonly starts as hypopigmented or erythematous macules on the face and sometimes on the arms, legs, and trunk. On the face, the rash gradually becomes papular (Fig. 2) or nodular, especially on the forehead, cheeks, and earlobes, and closely resembles lepromatous leprosy (Fig. 3). In 25 per cent of cases the lesions resolve spontaneously.

GEOGRAPHIC VARIATIONS IN DISEASE. Despite the extremely varied epidemiology of the disease, and despite the enormous opportunity for variation that the parasite is offered by continuous fly and animal passage, there is surprisingly little variation of the disease in man. Differences in age and sex patterns, due to endemicity, epidemicity, and opportunity for contact have been considered under Etiology.

In Africa, a primary leishmanioma has been described. In Europe and North Africa, self-healing skin lesions due to *L. donovani* have been reported. In the Sudan mucocutaneous lesions are seen, but it is not established whether they are due to *L. donovani* or to *L. major*. In Kenya lymphadenopathy may be the only sign of visceral disease. Spontaneous recovery is more common, up to 80 per cent, in Sudan than elsewhere.

Post-kala-azar dermal leishmaniasis is characteristic of Indian kala-azar, but rare elsewhere. For differences in response to treatment, see Treatment section.

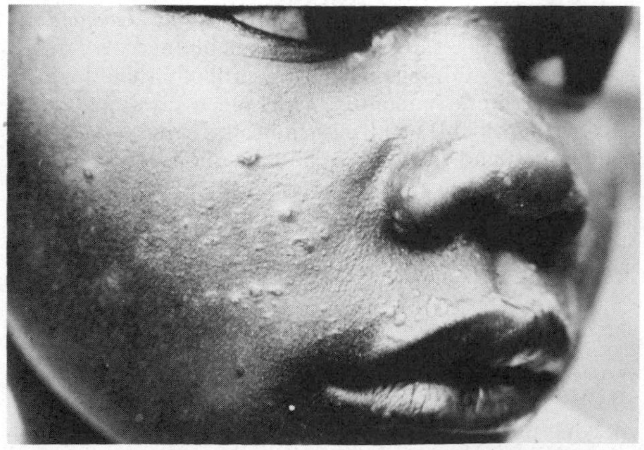

Figure 2. Papular rash of post kala-azar dermal leishmaniasis in a Kenyan child.

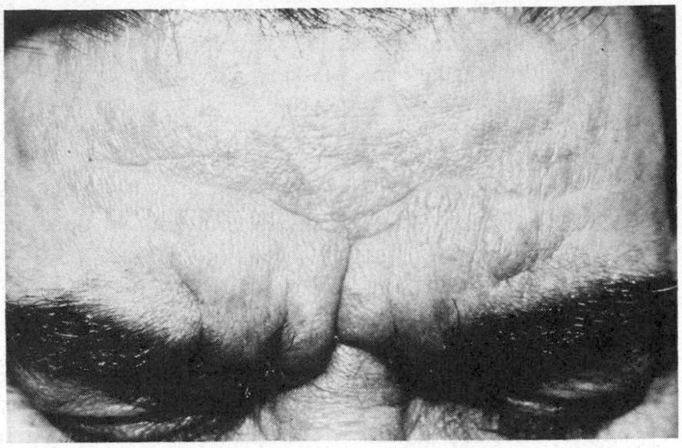

Figure 3. Nodular infiltration over the forehead in a European with post kala-azar dermal leishmaniasis of 15 years' duration, from India. (Courtesy of Dr. P. E. C. Manson-Bahr.)

DIAGNOSIS. The diagnosis must be suspected in any person living in, or having visited, an endemic area who has a prolonged fever. The diagnosis is likely in the presence of splenomegaly, granulocytopenia, anemia, hypoalbuminemia and hyperglobulinemia and is made by isolation of the parasite or by characteristic immunologic changes.

Isolation of Parasite. This is best done by needle aspiration of spleen, bone marrow, liver, or lymph nodes. Material obtained is:

1. Used to make a thin film on a glass microscope slide, stained, and examined under oil immersion for amastigotes, which must be distinguished from platelets. Parasitized macrophages usually rupture on smearing and free parasites must be looked for. Splenic aspiration is safe so long as the tip of the spleen is well below the costal margin, the prothrombin and bleeding times are normal and the platelet count is above 40,000/μl. A 1¼″ 21-gauge needle on a 5-ml syringe is passed through the skin at an angle of 45°, cranially. The plunger is withdrawn 1 ml to apply suction, and the needle is plunged into the spleen and withdrawn immediately. The trace of material obtained is adequate to set up cultures and make smears (Chulay and Bryceson, 1983). Organisms are seen in over 90 per cent of splenic aspirates and under 85 per cent from other tissues. Buffy coat preparations show parasites in over 90 per cent of cases in India, but in only about 1 per cent in Africa.
2. Inoculated onto suitable media such as NMN (Novy-MacNeal-Nicolle) medium overlaid with balanced salt solution, containing streptomycin and penicillin or Schneider's insect culture medium supplemented with fetal calf serum. Cultures are kept in the dark at 22 to 25° C (not at 37° C), and every three to four days a drop of fluid is examined wet for promastigotes. Culture improves parasitologic diagnosis in early cases, or if aspirates other than splenic are examined.
3. Inoculated intraperitoneally into hamsters, which are susceptible to a single amastigote. Although sensitive, this method is slow and seldom valuable.

Immunologic Tests. Anti-leishmanial antibodies can be demonstrated by indirect immunofluorescence of promastigotes in over 90 per cent of cases and by precipitation in gel or enzyme-linked immunosorbent assay in over 95 per cent (Ranque et al., 1975; Jahn and Diesfeld, 1983). Cross-reactions with *Trypanosoma cruzi* antibodies can be absorbed out. Complement fixation is positive in 65 per cent, but if the older antigen made from Kedrowsky's bacillus is used, reactions may be expected in some patients with mycobacterial disease. Serum obtained by eluting blood dried onto filter paper in the field can be used satisfactorily in all these techniques. The leishmanin test is negative in cases of active visceral leishmaniasis, but usually becomes positive after recovery (Pampiglione, 1975; Ho et al., 1983). It is most intense after one to two years, and slowly fades.

Other Laboratory Findings. Leukopenia is the most characteristic finding. The total count is below 2000 cells/mm^3 in 75 per cent of cases with absolute neutropenia and eosinopenia and relative lymphocytosis and monocytosis. Agranulocytosis occasionally develops. Anemia is slower in onset but becomes severe. It is normocytic and normochromic unless complicated by bleeding or deficiency states. There is often a mild reticulocytosis, and erythrocyte half-life is reduced. Thrombocytopenia is usual and progresses with the disease. Early on, tests of clotting are normal but later the prothrombin, partial thromboplastin, bleeding, and clotting times are prolonged. Total serum proteins are raised up to and over 10 g per 100 ml. This increase is due almost entirely to the IgG fraction of γ-globulin. On immunoelectrophoresis the IgG pattern is characteristically skewed. In some cases IgM is also slightly increased, but this is said to be transient and to revert rapidly to normal on treatment. In advanced cases serum albumin levels fall. Serum levels of liver enzymes are usually normal or nearly so. Plasma albumin is reduced to a mean 2.7 g/100 ml. There are no characteristic findings in the urine.

Differential Diagnosis. In Europeans, Americans, and others who are not immune, malaria must be excluded by examination of thick and thin blood films. In immunes, the presence of malarial parasites in the blood film does not exclude leishmaniasis. In many parts of the tropics where malaria and schistosomiasis are endemic, a palpable spleen is commonplace and is usually unrelated to a recent febrile illness. Diseases that can be confused with visceral leishmaniasis include aleukemic leukemia and lymphomas, tropical splenomegaly syndrome, cirrhosis of the liver with portal hypertension and hypersplenism, miliary tuberculosis, histoplasmosis, acute schistosomiasis, brucellosis, typhoid, and other septicemias, including bacterial endocarditis.

TREATMENT

Chemotherapy. Pentavalent antimonials are the drugs of choice. Two preparations are available. Sodium stibogluconate (pentostam, Stibanate, Dibanate, Stihek, Solyusurmin) contains 100 mg Sb/ml. Meglumine antimoniate (Glucantime) contains 85 mg Sb/ml. They are of equal potency, given in equivalent doses of Sb. The recommended dose is 10–20 mg Sb/kg of body weight daily by intramuscular or intravenous injection. Children require the higher dose. The maximum dose per injection is 850 mg Sb (8.5 ml sodium stibogluconate, 10 ml meglumine antimoniate). Treatment should be given for at least 21 consecutive days (World Health Organization, 1982b). Thirty days are necessary in Kenya. In India, the relapse rate has been reduced from 15 per cent to zero by extending treatment from 6 to 21 days. Interrupted treatment encourages relapse and the development of unresponsiveness to antimonials.

Over 90 per cent of the dose of pentavalent antimonial is excreted in 2 hours, in the urine. Side effects are cumulative but rare. They are nausea, vomiting, urticaria, bradycardia, and electrocardiographic changes. The response to antimonial treatment varies in kala-azar from different parts of the world. It is excellent in India and Brazil but less satisfactory in East Africa and the Mediterranean. Poor response may be due to inadequate dosage or duration of treatment. Relapsed patients are treated with 20 mg Sb/kg of body weight daily for 60 days. If antimony is unsuccessful, the choice then lies between two toxic drugs, pentamidine (isethionate or dimethanesulphonate: Lomidine) and amphotericin B (Fungizone). The dose of pentamidine is 4 mg/kg of body weight by intramuscular injection on alternate days for several weeks, or less frequently if side effects develop. If the drug is accidentally injected intravenously, the patient will collapse, but recovers quickly if the feet are raised. Cumulative side effects include fatigue, anorexia, nausea, abdominal pain and, in 2 per cent of cases, prolonged hypoglycemia. Ten per cent of patients develop diabetes, whose onset is not related to the duration of treatment. If this drug has to be used, a glucose tolerance test should be performed weekly. Amphotericin B is given by slow intravenous infusion in 5 per cent dextrose in a dose of 1 mg/kg of body weight on alternate days to a total of 2 g for a 50-kg adult. Side effects include rigors, thrombophlebitis, nausea, vomiting, fatigue, anemia, and uremia. This drug is more difficult to administer than pentamidine but is preferable.

Supportive Treatment. Bed rest, good nursing care, oral hygiene, an adequate fluid intake, and sufficient food are all desirable. Complicating infections must be sought and treated. Anemia responds as the patient recovers; but if severe, and especially if there is bleeding, blood transfusion should be given. Deficiencies of iron, folate, and other vitamins should be corrected.

Response to Treatment. The patient usually starts to feel better, and the fever to subside, within a week. The laboratory abnormalities start to improve in the second or third week. Lymphocytosis and reticulocytosis are good signs. No criterion of cure has been established. The patient should be seen at six weeks and six months, and in Africa at one year to detect 90 per cent of relapses. The spleen is measured and hemoglobin and serum albumin are estimated. A splenic aspirate is examined if relapse is suspected. At each visit blood is cultured for *Leishmania*, spleen size is measured, and hemoglobin and serum IgG are estimated. Complement-fixing antibody should not be detectable after six months. The spleen does not always become impalpable, and may indicate cirrhosis. Relapsed patients respond slowly to treatment and progress is monitored by splenic aspirates.

Post-Kala-azar Dermal Leishmaniasis. This usually responds to a 21-day course of pentavalent antimonial. If not, one of the other drugs may be used.

PROPHYLAXIS. On a mass scale the detailed epidemiology of the local disease must be known. This will permit reservoir control (destruction of stray dogs, early detection and treatment of cases) and vector control (insecticide spraying in the right places) to be carried out, and people may be able to avoid contact with infected flies. In some areas insecticide spraying against malarial mosquitoes reduced or eliminated kala-azar. Personal prophylaxis depends on wearing protective clothing in the evenings, the use of insect repellents, and sleeping under fine mesh netting.

References

Abdalla, R. E., El Hadi, A., Ahmed, M. A., and El Hassan, A. M.: Sudan mucosal leishmaniasis. Trans Roy Soc Trop Med Hyg 69:443, 1975.
Bradley, D. J.: Introduction and genetics of susceptibility to *Leishmania donovani*. Trans Roy Soc Trop Med Hyg 76:143, 1982.
Chance, M. L., Gardener, P. J., and Peters, W.: Biochemical taxonomy of *Leishmania* as an ecological test. Colloques Internationaux du C.N.R.S. No. 329, p. 53, 1977.
Chulay, J. D., and Bryceson, A. D. M.: Quantitation of amastigores of *Leishmania donovani* in smears of splenic aspirates from patients with visceral leishmaniasis. Am J Trop Med Hyg 32:475, 1983.
Ho, M., Koech, D. K., Iha, D. W., and Bryceson, A. D. M.: Immunosuppression in Kenyan visceral leishmaniasis. Clin Exp Immunol 32:475, 1983.
Hommel, M.: The genus *Leishmania:* biology of the parasites and clinical aspects. Bulletin de l'Institut Pasteur 76:5, 1978.
Jahn, A., and Diesfeld, H. J.: Evaluation of a visually read ELISA for serodiagnosis sero-epidemiological studies of Kala-azar in the Baringo District, Kenya. Trans Roy Soc Trop Med Hyg 77:451, 1983.
Pampiglione, S., Manson-Bahr, P. E. C., La Placa, M., Borgatti, M. A., and Musumeci, S.: Studies in Mediterranean leishmaniasis 3: The leishmanin test in kala-azar. Trans Roy Soc Trop Med Hyg 69:60, 1975.
Ranque, J., Quillici, M., Dunan, S., and Ranque, Ph.: Diagnostic immunologique de la leishmaniose viscerale (10 années d'expérience). Ann Soc Belge Méd Trop 55:579, 1975.
Winslow, D. J.: Visceral leishmaniasis. *In* Marcel-Rojas, R. A. (ed.): Pathology of Rickettsial and Helminthic Diseases. Baltimore, Williams and Wilkins Company, 1971, p. 86.
World Health Organization (a). Biochemical characterization of leishmania. Chance, M. L., and Walton, B. C. (Eds.). Geneva, WHO, 1982.
World Health Organization (b). Report of the informal meeting on the chemotherapy of visceral leishmaniasis. TDR/CHEMLEISH/VL/82.3. Geneva, 1982.

153
SYPHILITIC HEPATITIS

JÁNOS FEHÉR, M.D., D.SC.

Syphilitic hepatitis is an inflammatory disease of the liver that may develop either early or late in the course of syphilis and may occur in congenital syphilis and in lues congenita tarda.

ETIOLOGY. The pathogenic agent of syphilitic hepatitis is *Treponema pallidum*, a thin, delicate, spiral organism with 6 to 14 spirals and tapered ends, measuring 5 to 15 μm in total length and 0.2 to 0.3 μm in width. The depth and amplitude of the spirals is about 1 μm. In histologic preparations *T. pallidum* in barely stainable. It can be impregnated with silver because it reduces silver nitrate to metallic silver. In wet preparations it can be examined under the darkfield microscope. It also can be demonstrated by direct and indirect immunofluorescence (Al-Sammarrai, 1977) and by electronmicroscopic techniques (Ovcinnikov and Delektorskij, 1972). None of the pathogenic treponemes has yet been cultured in vitro. After drying in air and after oxidation, it perishes very quickly.

PATHOGENESIS AND PATHOLOGY. At the site of inoculation *T. pallidum* rapidly penetrates intact mucous membranes or abraded skin and enters the lymphatics and blood vessels within a few hours to produce systemic infection and metastatic foci long before the appearance of the primary lesion.

As a result of hematogenous dissemination, the treponemes may enter the liver and, in the early phase, may produce the characteristic early syphilitic hepatitis. In our syphilitic material we found early syphilitic hepatitis in about 10 per cent of early syphilitic patients. The liver is enlarged, and jaundice may occur (Fehér et al., 1975).

Early syphilitic hepatitis shows varying degrees of histologic abnormality. In the patients that show minimal changes, there is proliferation of sinus endothelial cells and Kupffer cells, together with many granulocytes, eosinophils, and lymphocytes in the sinusoids. The periportal region is swollen, and the walls of the arteries and portal vein branches are thickened and infiltrated with inflammatory cells. In these cases, the architecture of the liver is not altered, and there is no evidence of cholestasis. In more severe cases focal liver necrosis occurs. Only one or two liver cells may become necrotic in some cases, whereas necrosis is more extensive in others. In the necrotic areas, neutrophil and eosinophil granulocytes, lymphocytes, and mast cells are found, and the reticulin structure is destroyed (Fig. 1). In some areas of necrosis, fibroblasts and epithelioid cells are seen, as well as an acute inflammatory infiltrate. Necrotic foci are found in all parts of the lobules but are more common in the periportal region and around the central vein (Fig. 2). The necrotic inflammatory foci around the central vein appear to be characteristic of syphilitic hepatitis, as they were present in all of our patients with liver damage. The walls of the branches of the central vein are thickened with increased reticulin and collagen fibers. Glycogen content is markedly reduced in the necrotic areas and in their immediate neighborhood. In half of our cases, treponemes were demonstrated in liver biopsy material. They were found in the inflammatory necrotic foci, in the sinus endothelial cells, in the Disse spaces, and sometimes in the intrahepatic bile capillaries (Figs. 3 and 4).

After penicillin treatment, syphilitic hepatitis heals with accumulation of collagen in the walls of sinusoids and in the spaces between the liver cells.

CLINICAL MANIFESTATIONS. The *latent form* of syphilitic hepatitis can be detected only by liver function tests. It does not cause any clinical symptoms and develops after the primary infection.

Early syphilitic hepatitis occurs in the secondary stage of syphilis. The liver is enlarged, but there is no pain, and subicterus or icterus develops. Hepatitis often coincides with the appearance of luetic exanthems. It usually heals within a few weeks, but in some rare cases it undergoes yellow atrophy (Leonard, 1944).

Late luetic hepatitis is characterized by pain, fever, and

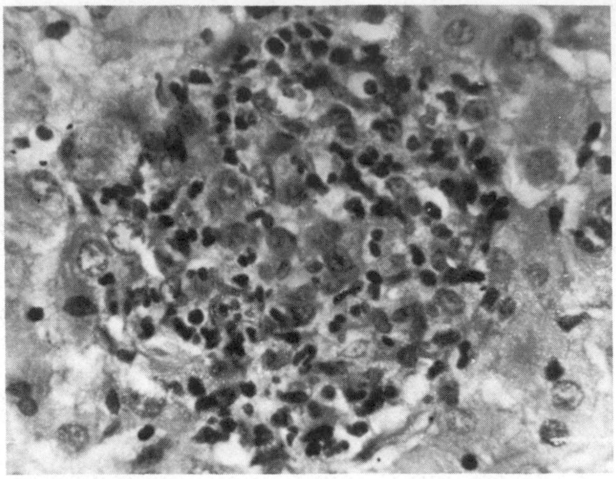

Figure 1. Light micrograph of liver tissue from patient with early syphilis, showing focal inflammatory reaction. (Hematoxylin and eosin, ×400.)

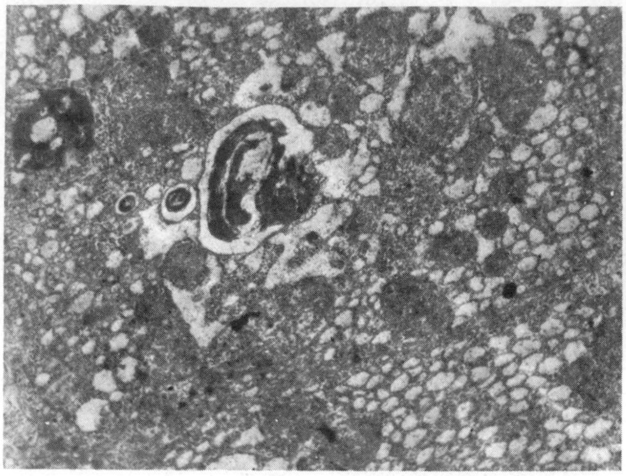

Figure 3. Electron micrograph of liver cell, showing tubularization of endoplasmic reticulum and intracellular treponema. (×9200.)

sometimes splenomegaly. The pain is colicky owing to tension of the liver capsule and to liver swelling. The fever is irregular and may be accompanied by chills. It is impossible to differentiate this interstitial form of hepatitis from luetic liver cirrhosis.

Some forms of *luetic liver cirrhosis* may arise from syphilitic hepatitis. We have observed the development of chronic aggressive hepatitis in certain cases of early syphilitic hepatitis. Luetic liver cirrhosis is thought to evolve from such chronic syphilitic liver lesions.

Hepatic gumma is the most frequent form of luetic liver disease. It is characterized by sudden sharp pain. The spleen is usually enlarged and irregular, and intermittent fever is a constant symptom. Without treatment, the patients become cachectic. The gummas are palpable as knots or lumps of various sizes, and occasionally liver tumor is suspected. Round masses are often palpable below the liver margin. Some patients present signs of cholangitis, while in others the symptoms are those of gallstones. The cicatrized contraction of gummas causes a lobular distortion of the liver known as *hepar lobatum.*

The *hepatitis of congenital lues* (brimstone liver) is not encountered in adults. Only its late form, the hepatomegaly of lues congenita tarda, occurs in adults.

COMPLICATIONS. With adequate penicillin therapy, the latent and early forms of syphilitic hepatitis usually heal completely. In some cases the picture of chronic aggressive hepatitis may develop and may progress to cirrhosis. Very rarely, acute hepatitis may undergo yellow atrophy. Cirrhosis, frequently in the company of hepatic gummas, may also develop from the hepatitis of late syphilis. Gummas in the portal region cause obstructive jaundice, and portal obstruction leads to the development of ascites.

Hepatitis B virus may be inoculated simultaneously with syphilis because the hepatitis B virus may be sexually transmitted (Papaevangelou et al., 1974).

GEOGRAPHIC VARIATIONS IN DISEASE. Syphilis and syphilitic hepatitis is endemic all over the world. There is no essential difference in the clinical symptoms and in the

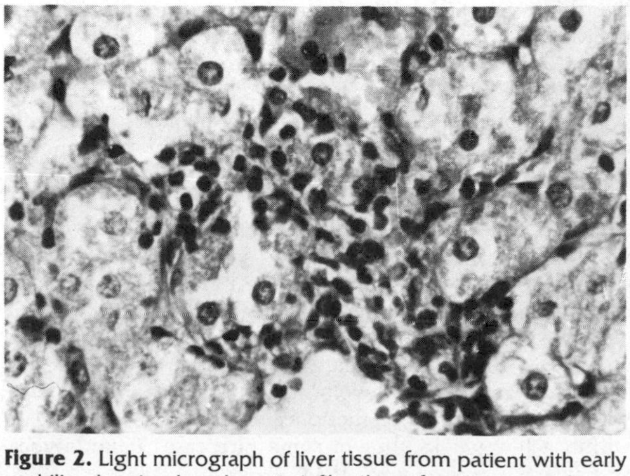

Figure 2. Light micrograph of liver tissue from patient with early syphilis, showing lymphocytic infiltration of region around vena centralis. (Hematoxylin and eosin, ×400.)

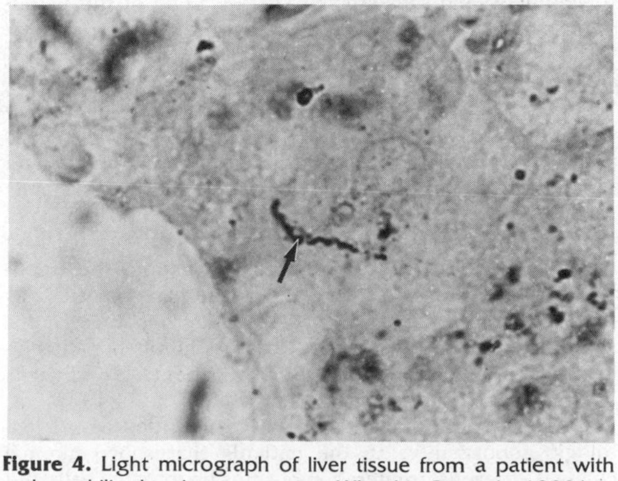

Figure 4. Light micrograph of liver tissue from a patient with early syphilis showing treponeme. Wharthin-Starry (×1000.)

course of the disease, unless it is associated with another infection or combined with malnutrition. More severe cases are found in less developed countries and in populations living under poor hygienic conditions.

DIAGNOSIS. The diagnosis of syphilis is based on serologic tests (VDRL, FABS, Kolmer) and on demonstration of treponemes in local lesions of the skin and mucous membranes. In syphilitic hepatitis, hepatomegaly and an increase in the serum bilirubin concentration are common. The SGOT and SGPT activity is increased, the prothrombin time and BSP value are abnormal, and serum protein levels are altered. Sometimes alkaline phosphatase activity is disproportionately higher than the serum bilirubin level (Keisler et al., 1982). The changes in serum immunoglobulins, especially IgG and IgM concentrations, resemble those found in viral hepatitis. The diagnosis can be established histologically by liver biopsy; treponemes can be demonstrated occasionally (Fehér et al., 1975). Renal involvement may occur concomitantly with the liver disorder.

TREATMENT. Syphilitic hepatitis should be differentiated from other forms of hepatitis. The specific therapy is penicillin treatment.

Patients with syphilitic hepatitis are treated with Procaine Penicillin G intramuscularly in doses of 1.0 million units daily for 15 consecutive days. This course of 15.0 million units is repeated after an interval of one month.

For patients allergic to penicillin, oral tetracycline hydrochloride may be given in a dose of 500 mg four times a day for 15 days. Erythromycin monostearate 500 mg every 6 hours for 15 days can be used if tetracycline is not tolerated. The tetracycline or the erythromycin therapy is repeated after a one-month interval. Cephaloridine or other cephalosporins have not been studied. Chloramphenicol should not be used because its efficacy is doubtful and the drug may be toxic.

Patients with early syphilitic hepatitis should be treated in the hospital. Bed rest is advised while the patient is symptomatic. The choice of diet should be left to the patient's discretion. A low fat, high carbohydrate diet is usually acceptable to a patient with anorexia, but does not alter the rate of recovery.

References

Al-Sammarrai, H. T., and Henderson, W. G.: Immunofluorescent staining of *Treponema pallidum* and *Treponema pertenue* in tissues fixed by formalin and embedded in paraffin wax. Br J Vener Dis 53:1, 1977.

Fehér, J., Somogyi, T., Timmer, M., and Józsa, L.: Early syphilitic hepatitis. Lancet 2:896, 1975.

Harrison, S. M.: Syphilis. In Conn, H. F. (ed.): Current Therapy. Philadelphia, W. B. Saunders Company, 1983, p. 568.

Keisler, D. S., Starke, W., Looney, D. J., and Mark, W. W.: Early syphilis with liver involvement. JAMA 247:1999, 1982.

Koff, R. S., and Gang, D. L.: Granulomatous hepatitis due to secondary syphilis. N Engl J Med 309:35, 1983.

Leonard, M. F.: Acute yellow atrophy of the liver in early syphilis: A case report with summary of the literature. Am J Med Sci 208:461, 1944.

Papaevangeolu, G., Trichopoulos, D., Papoutsakis, G., Kremastinou, T., and Pavlides, E.: Hepatitis B antigen in prostitutes. Br J Vener Dis 50:228, 1974.

Ovcinnikov, N. M., and Delektorskij, V. V.: Effect of crystalline penicillin and bicillin-1 on experimental syphilis in the rabbit. Electronmicroscopic study. Br J Vener Dis 48:327, 1972.

Sanford, J. P.: Leptospirosis. In Wintrope, M. M., et al. (eds.): Harrison's Principles of Internal Medicine. 7th ed. New York, McGraw-Hill Book Company, 1974, p. 887.

Sherlock, S.: Diseases of the Liver and Biliary System. 5th ed. Oxford, Blackwell Scientific Publications, 1975.

154

VIRAL HEPATITIS

SHALOM Z. HIRSCHMAN, M.D.

Viral hepatitis is a common infectious disease throughout the world. During the decade of 1966 to 1976 the case rate of viral hepatitis per 1000 population was at a low of 18.56 in 1966, reached a high of 33.64 in 1971, and declined to 26.46 in 1976. However, the case rate for hepatitis B virus infection has steadily increased from 1.79 in 1966 to 6.92 in 1976. The case rates for hepatitis A infection appeared to be declining during the six years from 1971 to 1976.

In Chapter 72, the properties of the hepatitis A and B viruses, including epidemiology and geographic distribution, were considered. In this chapter the pathogenesis, clinical manifestations, and untoward sequelae of infections with these viruses will be detailed.

HEPATITIS A

TRANSMISSION. The distribution of hepatitis A is worldwide, and disease is more prevalent in areas of poor hygiene and low socioeconomic standards (Murray, 1955). The infection appears to be spread by the fecal-oral route. Although sporadic cases of the disease develop from close person-to-person contact, many food- and water-borne epidemics have been reported (Dienstag et al., 1975). Occasionally, hepatitis A virus (HAV) infection is transmitted by parenteral injection. This route of infection may be more common in drug addicts. One of the most explosive water-borne outbreaks of hepatitis, presumed to be Type A, occurred in 1955 and 1956, when 29,000 people were infected within a six-week period in Delhi, India.

The incubation period of hepatitis A virus infection is usually about 30 days with a range of 15 to 50 days (Table 1). Hepatitis A antigen (HAAg) is found in the stool at least five days before the activities of transaminases in serum begin to increase and one to two weeks before the onset of clinical symptoms. The maximal fecal excretion of HAAg occurs at about the time of peak transaminase activity and then rapidly falls as jaundice ensues. The feces of patients with hepatitis A contain virus for about one to two weeks before, and about one week after, the appearance of jaundice. The total infectious period for the stool is about three weeks. When HAAg is no longer detectable in the stool, anti-HA is found in serum. The level of antibody rises quickly and remains elevated for at least ten years after recovery. The persistence of antibody may explain the long-lasting immunity of patients to reinfection with

Table 1. CLINICAL PRESENTATONS OF HEPATITIS A AND B

	Hepatitis A	Hepatitis B
Incubation period	15 to 50 days	40 to 180 days
Prodrome	Malaise, fever, gastroenteritis	Malaise, fever, urticaria, and arthritis
Onset	Acute	Gradual except in infancy
Clinical course	Usually mild with complete resolution in two to four weeks; fatal hepatic necrosis uncommon	Patient moderately ill; most recover; some develop chronic hepatitis; fatal hepatic necrosis uncommon
Chronic carrier	No	Yes
Chronic active hepatitis	No	Yes
Immunologic sequelae	None known	Glomerulonephritis, periarteritis nodosa

HAV. Recent serologic surveys have shown that only about 25 to 30 per cent of adults in the United States have anti-HA antibody. Where hepatitis A is endemic, 90 per cent of individuals acquire antibody by the age of 15. Thus, in underdeveloped areas, infection with HAV occurs mainly in the young.

CLINICAL PRESENTATION. Jaundice may be the first sign of hepatitis A virus infection, but most patients have symptoms for several days before jaundice becomes apparent. The most common prodromal symptoms are anorexia and malaise, often with abdominal discomfort and nausea. At times the abdominal pain may be acute and may suggest an acute abdomen. Although nausea is common, few patients vomit. Many patients also report losing their taste for cigarettes. Constipation may be as common as diarrhea. Patients in the pre-icteric stage also may complain of headaches and generalized myalgia. The headache is rarely severe but at times may suggest meningitis. The patient may have fever to 104° F and may even have chills. Rash, either papular, macular, or petechial, is uncommon. In general, children have much milder symptoms than adults. The prodromal or pre-icteric stage usually lasts less than one week, although some patients feel ill for as long as two weeks. The true nature of the illness becomes apparent with the onset of jaundice. Just before the jaundice, the patient usually notices dark urine and pale feces. As the jaundice appears, the patient becomes afebrile. The liver is often not enlarged but is usually tender. Hepatomegaly is often present in patients with severe illness unless massive necrosis develops, in which case the liver rapidly shrinks. Splenomegaly is present in less than 20 per cent of patients. The main symptom during the icteric phase is extreme fatigability. In milder cases, the patient feels well in a few days. However, many patients may feel tired and anorectic for one to two weeks. After two weeks, in most patients, the jaundice begins to recede and disappears by the end of the month. Some patients continue to complain of fatigability for many months after acute illness. In a few patients, especially women between 30 and 50 years of age, the jaundice may deepen and persist for two to three months before clearing. Pruritus may be a bothersome symptom, yet the patient remains relatively well. This type of illness, jaundice with cholestasis, always clears, although the duration of jaundice may be many weeks, especially in patients near puberty and in older individuals.

PATTERNS OF ILLNESS. The types of clinical illness caused by hepatitis A virus can be categorized as follows: anicteric hepatitis, icteric hepatitis, and fulminant hepatitis. Chronic hepatitis does not seem to occur. Many cases of hepatitis A are anicteric, and the patient may have very mild vague symptoms or none at all. Rarely, patients may suffer from a fulminant form of illness in which jaundice deepens rapidly, and the patient has frequent bouts of vomiting and rapidly falls into coma. Signs of hepatic failure are present. Such patients usually die within ten days of onset.

DIAGNOSIS. The activity of the aminotransferases in serum, aspartate aminotransferase or glutamic oxaloacetic transaminase (SGOT), and alanine aminotransferase or serum glutamic pyruvic transaminase (SGPT), begins to rise several days before clinical jaundice becomes apparent. The final peak level of transaminase activity found in serum is quite variable in patients with hepatitis. The activity of the transaminases usually peaks within one week and then begins to decline. As it declines, the activity of alkaline phosphatase is usually rising, reaching a peak several days to one week after the transaminase peak; gamma glutamyl transpeptidase activity is also elevated at this time. The bilirubin level rises as jaundice appears, preceded by bilirubinuria, and conjugated bilirubin predominates. Leukopenia is seen in the early stages of acute hepatitis, and atypical lymphocytes may be present in about 25 per cent of cases. Patients with fulminant hepatitis may have leukocytosis. The erythrocyte sedimentation rate (ESR) is often less than normal when jaundice appears. Elevation of the ESR later in illness may indicate persisting inflammatory changes in the liver. In most patients with acute hepatitis, the serum albumin and globulin remain normal. Prolongation of the prothrombin time and depletion of other clotting factors manufactured in the liver may be present during the acute phase of hepatitis. Hypoalbuminemia, acidosis, and hyperammonemia with encephalopathy are seen only in fulminant hepatitis.

Diagnosis and prognosis have been facilitated by needle biopsy. Pathologically, viral hepatitis is characterized by a combination of morphologic components that include (1) acute cytologic damage, (2) inflammation, and (3) hepatocellular necrosis (Schaffner, 1970). In acute hepatitis, single hepatocytes, or small groups of them, undergo necrosis that elicits both focal and portal inflammation (Fig. 1). The necrosis is located anywhere in the lobule but may be accentuated in the central zone. The inflammatory reaction consists of leukocytes, lymphocytes, and macrophages. The portal inflammation may vary from minimal to marked. The walls of the central veins are edematous and contain scattered macrophages and other inflammatory cells. Acidophilic or Councilman-like bodies are hepatocytes that have undergone coagulation necrosis (Fig. 2). Regeneration begins in the early stages of viral hepatitis

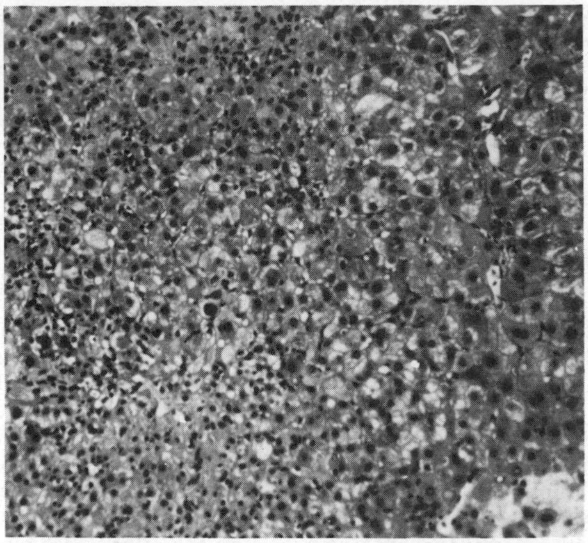

Figure 1. Liver biopsy specimen from patient with acute viral hepatitis showing diffuse spotty necrosis. Hematoxylin and eosin, ×40.

and is more prominent in the periportal region. Fulminant hepatitis causes massive necrosis of hepatocytes (Fig. 3).

All patients (except those few who die of massive necrosis) recover completely. However, in some patients the activity of the transaminases may be elevated for months. Liver biopsy of such patients may show minimal nonspecific inflammation or may be normal. Recent serologic evidence indicates that patients with hepatitis A do not develop chronic aggressive hepatitis. Aplastic anemia, usually fatal, may follow acute hepatitis on rare occasions.

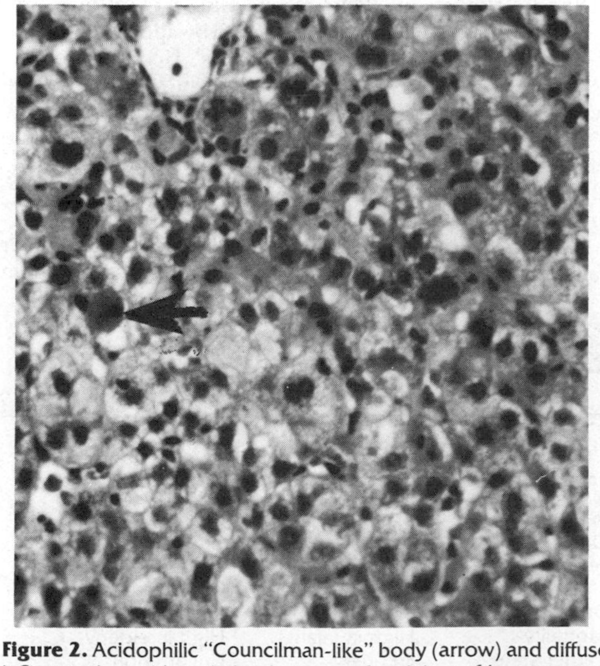

Figure 2. Acidophilic "Councilman-like" body (arrow) and diffuse inflammation with variation in size and staining of hepatocytes. A central vein in the center of the top edge shows inflammation in its walls (central phlebitis). Hematoxylin and eosin, × 100.

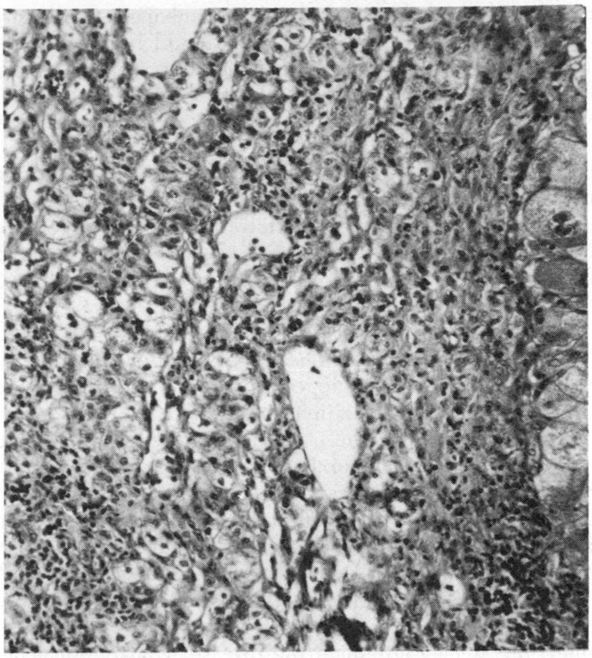

Figure 3. Early massive necrosis and beginning collapse in acute hepatitis. A row of surviving hepatocytes is seen at right border. Hematoxylin and eosin, × 100.

DIFFERENTIAL DIAGNOSIS OF ACUTE HEPATITIS. The differential diagnosis of acute hepatitis commonly focuses on infectious mononucleosis and cytomegalovirus infection. Infectious mononucleosis is usually accompanied by sore throat and lymphadenopathy; the heterophil agglutinins are positive by the second to fourth week of illness. Although the results of liver function tests are often mildly abnormal, jaundice is uncommon. Cytomegalovirus infection in adults usually involves the liver, but jaundice, when present, is mild; the diagnosis can be suggested by a fourfold rise in complement-fixing antibody. Leptospiral infection may also mimic acute hepatitis. The kidneys are often involved, and meningitis may be present. Serologic tests are most often used to establish a diagnosis. Yellow fever, the hemorrhagic fevers, and various other arbovirus infections must be considered in areas of endemicity. Parasitic diseases such as malaria, schistosomiasis, kala-azar, and clonorchiasis must also be considered in geographic areas of prevalence. Adverse reactions to drugs such as isoniazid, methyldopa, and chlorpromazine also cause acute and chronic hepatitis, which often cannot be separated from viral hepatitis.

TREATMENT. There is no specific treatment for hepatitis A virus infection. The patient's sense of well-being is the best guide for the amount of bed rest required; a simple guide is avoidance of fatigue. The patient in the acute stages of the illness usually does not feel like being up and around, and therefore should stay at reasonable rest. Simple exercises during convalescence may help restore a sense of well-being and forestall development of muscle weakness that accompanies protracted illness. In the early part of the illness, when anorexia is prominent, frequent small, light, and attractive feedings appear to be best tolerated. Intravenous fluid should be avoided if possible because overhydration and electrolyte imbalances are easily produced. A normal balanced diet should be prescribed. There is no rational basis for a low fat diet. Corticosteroids have no benefit in treatment of acute viral hepatitis and should be avoided. The treatment of acute fulminant hepatitis leaves much to be desired. A low protein diet, lactulose or neomycin, and bowel cleansing help reduce the intensity of encephalopathy. Exchange transfusions, parabiotic filtration, or in vitro filtration systems to remove toxic circulating substances are experimental and so far have been disappointing. A chronic carrier state for hepatitis A virus is not apparent.

PREVENTION OF HBA INFECTION. Patients should exercise good personal hygiene to prevent spread of disease to other patients and staff in hospital and to family members at home. In hospital, the usual enteric precautions should be used in handling materials from patients with acute viral hepatitis A. Good sanitation and high standards of hygiene among food handlers should help to prevent water-borne outbreaks. Many studies have substantiated the fact that gamma globulin offers good protection against hepatitis A (Krugman, 1976). It may be given to close contacts who are at special risk. Even if gamma globulin does not prevent infection, it may attenuate the disease. Conventional immune serum globulin (ISG) appears to be effective. Gamma globulin should be administered in doses of between 0.03 ml and 0.06 ml per pound of body weight. It is most effective if given during the first few days following contact with a patient with hepatitis A. Efforts to prepare an active vaccine against hepatitis A infection are hampered by lack of a tissue culture system for propagation of the virus.

HEPATITIS B

TRANSMISSION. Hepatitis B virus (HBV) infection is endemic throughout the world (Mosley, 1975). The virus can be transmitted from mother to child during delivery but rarely transplacentally. The rise in the use of blood transfusions has probably contributed to the increasing recognition of the disease in the western hemisphere. The increased use of donor blood in renal hemodialysis and in cardiovascular surgery also has increased the risk of transmission of HBV infection. Furthermore, the increase in drug addiction with intravenously used drugs such as heroin has led to the spread of HBV infection. Hepatitis B surface antigen (HBsAg) may also be found in the saliva and urine of infected patients, and there is much epidemiologic evidence for nonparenteral routes of transmission, especially from one sexual partner to the other. HBsAg has been detected in semen. HBV infection can be reactivated in patients who are treated with immunosuppressive agents.

CLINICAL PRESENTATION. The incubation period of HBV infection averages about 90 days, with a range of 40 to 180 days. Symptoms during the prodromal period that occur about one to three weeks before the appearance of jaundice are similar to those described for hepatitis A virus infection but are more gradual in onset. In addition, a symptom complex that includes urticarial skin eruption with arthritis has been described during the prodromal period of HBV infection. This prodrome seems to have an immunologic basis, and the complement levels in the synovial fluid of affected joints are low. Slowly increasing jaundice may be the first sign. Hepatitis B is considered to be a more severe disease than hepatitis A and causes more deaths. The greater severity is probably related to the older age of the patients and the frequent presence of some underlying disease. Patients may have anicteric disease, acute hepatitis with recovery, subacute fatal hepatitis, fulminant hepatitis, and chronic active or persistent hepatitis. The differences in clinical presentation of hepatitis A and hepatitis B are summarized in Table 1.

There are also several differences between HBV infection in adults and infection in children (Table 2). Hepatitis B in the neonatal period is rare and is usually transmitted from the mother during birth. However, the mortality rate is highest in infants, being 4 to 5/100,000 population under 1 year of age. Mortality drops greatly after 1 year of age and rises again slowly in later years, reaching a high level after age 60. In children, the onset of clinical symptoms is more abrupt, and the icteric phase is short. Gastrointestinal symptoms, particularly vomiting and abdominal pain, often with ketoacidosis, are usual; urticaria and arthritis are rare in children in contrast to adults. Immune complex phenomena such as glomerulonephritis and papular acrodermatitis are more common in children, while arthritis is more common in adults. Tender hepatomegaly with splenomegaly early in the course of disease is more frequent in children. Fever in children is high but brief, and is moderate but protracted in adults. The duration of hepatitis is usually short in children but is protracted in adults.

ANTIGENIC MARKERS OF HBV INFECTION. HBsAg usually appears in the serum several weeks after exposure before the onset of clinical symptoms and even before the activity of the transaminases in serum begin to rise (Krugman et al., 1974). Hepatitis B core antigen (HBcAg), DNA polymerase activity, and hepatitis Be antigen (HBeAg) usually appear when HBsAg is detected. In some patients, HBeAg, HBcAg, and DNA polymerase activity may precede the appearance of HBsAg. Anti-HBc appears in serum usually with the onset of acute illness (Hoofnagle et al., 1977). Anti-HBs usually appears during convalescence when circulating HBsAg has disappeared. Anti-HBe usually appears when anti-HBc is present. Anti-HBc may be the only viral marker detected during the "window period" after the disappearance of HBsAg but before the appearance of anti-HBs.

Abnormalities in the results of biochemical tests of liver function in HBV infection are similar to those found in

Table 2. COMPARISON OF HEPATITIS B INFECTION IN CHILDREN AND ADULTS

Clinical Presentation	Children	Adults
Susceptibility	High	Low
Peak incidence	Infants	Young adults
Onset	Acute	Gradual
Fever	High but brief	Moderate but protracted
Duration	Short	Often protracted
Mortality	High in infants	High in elderly
Carrier state	Frequent	Uncommon
Chronic hepatitis	Mainly infants	Mainly elderly

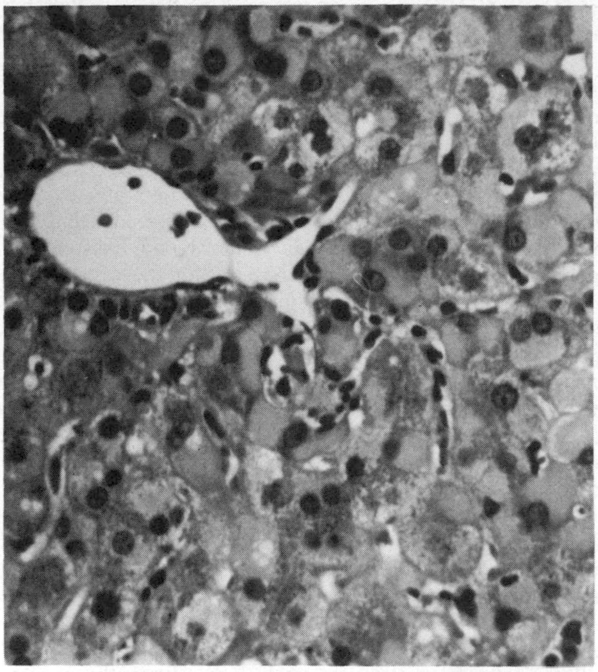

Figure 4. Ground glass hepatocytes near central vein on upper left in an HBsAg carrier. Hematoxylin and eosin, ×250.

hepatitis A infection. About 10 per cent of patients who have acute hepatitis B will become chronic carriers of HBsAg. The presence of HBeAg without anti-HBe, and the persistence of high levels of anti-HBc without anti-HBs are correlated with development of the carrier state. Hepatitis B surface antigenemia is found in approximately 0.1 to 0.4 per cent of apparently healthy volunteer blood donors in the United States. Anti-HBs is found in about 15 per cent of adults in the United States. The vast majority of these antibody-positive individuals had subclinical or anicteric hepatitis. The carrier state for HBsAg seems to develop more frequently in children after hepatitis B infection.

PATHOLOGY. Hepatocytes containing HBsAg can be recognized in liver biopsy specimens (Fig. 4). They are larger than normal, and the bulky cytoplasm has a smudged appearance similar to ground or frosted glass. These cells are usually present in small groups with no zonal predilection. Ground glass hepatocytes were first noted in asymptomatic carriers of HBsAg; they also have been seen in HBsAg-positive chronic hepatitis when diffuse liver cell injury is not severe. Electron microscopic studies have shown that HBsAg is associated with the endoplasmic reticulum of the cytoplasm of the hepatocyte. Naked core particles containing HBcAg are found in the nucleus of infected cells, especially in immunosuppressed individuals. Immunofluorescent studies have shown that anti-HBs attaches to particles in cytoplasm and anti-HBc attaches to particles in the cell nuclei of infected livers. Cytoplasmic HBsAg can also be detected by staining methods with paraffin sections. Due to the large antigenic load in hepatocytes and in serum of patients with hepatitis B virus infection, it has been hypothesized that the liver cell injury in this infection is caused by immunologic mechanisms.

Necrosis of hepatocytes in acute hepatitis B results in a focal scattered centrolobularly accentuated inflammatory response, portal inflammation, and endophlebitis of the central veins. In more severe cases, necrosis extends in a line from the portal tract to the central vein. This bridging necrosis often presages chronic hepatitis and cirrhosis (Fig. 5).

Most patients with hepatitis B virus infection survive the acute illness. Patients who become chronic carriers of HBsAg may be asymptomatic or symptomatic. Microscopic examinations of the liver in asymptomatic carriers of HBsAg may be normal or may show chronic portal hepatitis that is recognized clinically as chronic persistent hepatitis. In this entity, the inflammation that had extended from the parenchyma into the portal tracts in the acute state regresses until it is within the portal tracts, allowing the limiting plates of hepatocytes to restore themselves. This lesion will heal in most cases over a period of several years. However, progression to more serious disease does occur in a small percentage of patients. Some patients with HBV infection develop chronic periportal hepatitis known clini-

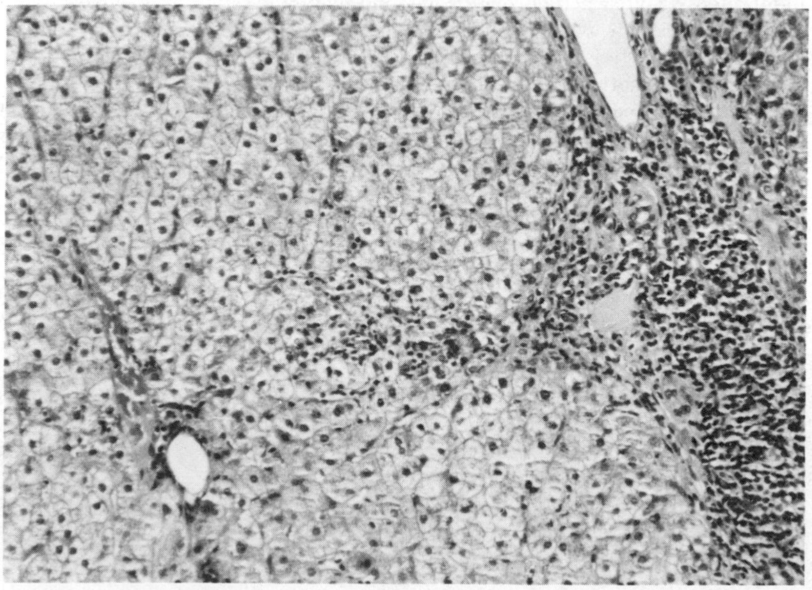

Figure 5. Beginning bridging necrosis in acute hepatitis from large portal tract on right to central area on left. Hematoxylin and eosin, ×40.

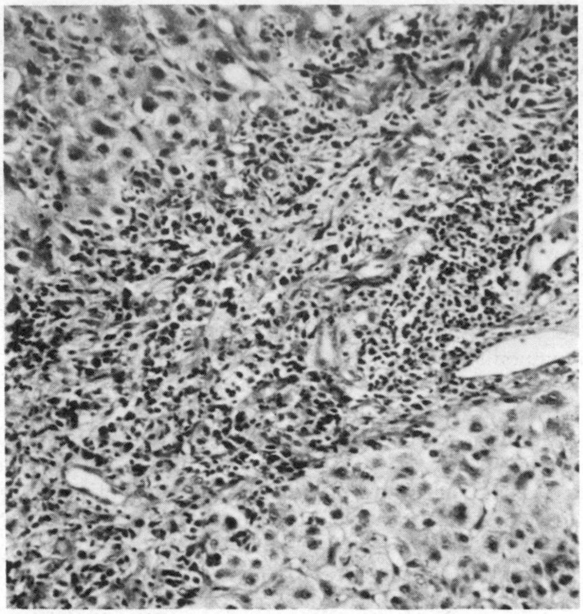

Figure 6. Large fibrotic and inflamed portal tract with piecemeal necrosis on upper left in patient with chronic active hepatitis. Hematoxylin and eosin, ×40.

cally as chronic aggressive or chronic active hepatitis. The portal and periportal inflammation in these patients does not subside, and the loss of hepatocytes in the limiting plates associated with inflammation and subsequent fibrosis is a process of piecemeal necrosis, the hallmark of chronic active hepatitis (Fig. 6). The bridging necrosis and collapse seen in acute hepatitis may persist or may develop anew from the chronic periportal hepatitis. Although this form of hepatitis may heal spontaneously in a minority of cases, it is more likely to progress to cirrhosis.

IMMUNOLOGIC SEQUELAE. HBV infection has several immunologic sequelae, the manifestations of which differ in children and adults. The lack of arthritis and urticaria in the early stages of the disease in children has already been mentioned. Papular acrodermatitis is found mainly in children in association with lymphadenitis and mild hepatitis. The skin disease is the major manifestation in these children, and virus antigen has been found in the skin. Papular acrodermatitis may be recurrent in young adults with persistent hepatitis B surface antigenemia. Glomerulonephritis, which is more common in children than in adults, results from the deposition of antigen-antibody complexes. Endocapillary proliferative, membrane proliferative, and membranous types of glomerulonephritis have been associated with hepatitis B infection. Aplastic anemia has been reported following hepatitis B infection in children and young adults. Periarteritis nodosa is another immunologic complication of HBV infection seen mainly in adults.

HEPATITIS B AND HEPATIC CANCER. There is a relationship among HBV infection, cirrhosis, and primary hepatocellular carcinoma in many areas of the world such as the Far East, where HBV is highly endemic and carriers of HBsAg are common. In these areas, primary hepatocellular carcinoma is one of the most common neoplasms. The exact role of HBV as an oncogenic agent in the liver has not yet been defined.

PREVENTION OF HBV INFECTION. The primary need is to eradicate the carrier state of hepatitis B. For the present, personal hygiene, control of drug abuse, and public education remain the mainstays of prevention. The most effective way of decreasing the incidence of hepatitis B virus infection in countries where the virus is spread mainly by blood transfusion is to test all donor blood by sensitive techniques such as radioimmunoassay for the presence of HBsAg. Such routine testing of all donors and all blood, combined with decreased use of commercial donors, has already lessened the incidence of hepatitis B following blood transfusion. Recent studies have shown that dentists with chronic hepatitis B surface antigenemia may spread disease to their patients. Hyperimmune globulin containing high titers of anti-HBs may be effective in reducing the incidence of hepatitis B infection in persons accidentally inoculated with infected blood, in patients and staff in renal dialysis units, and in spouses of patients with acute HBV infection. The protection is temporary, generally lasting from four to six months.

Vaccines prepared from purified HBsAg have been reported to be effective in protecting both people at risk and chimpanzees from infection with HBV. Recently, a commercially produced vaccine consisting of HBsAg purified from human serum has been approved. The vaccine is highly immunogenic; more than 90 per cent of healthy adults develop antibody after three 20-μg intramuscular doses are given. Injection of three 10-μg doses induces antibody in nearly all infants and children between the ages of three months and nine years. A well-designed trial of the vaccine showed it to be highly effective (Szmuness et al., 1980). Administration of hepatitis B immune globulin (HBIG) does not alter the anti-HBs response of adults who are given a simultaneous injection of vaccine. Side effects noted to date have been minor. Much work is being expended on the development of HBsAg protein subunit vaccines to preclude cross-reaction between vaccines containing purified HBsAg and normal human proteins and to produce vaccines by recombinant DNA techniques. Vaccination should be useful in groups at special risk of acquiring HBV infection. These include patients requiring repeated transfusions, patients and staff in renal dialysis units, staff in institutions for the mentally retarded, other health workers at risk of hepatitis B infection, homosexuals, drug addicts, and prostitutes, and persons in endemic areas (Hirschman, 1983).

Known antiviral chemotherapeutic agents are usually not helpful in the treatment of HBV infections (Dienstag and Isselbacher, 1981). The possible role of adenine arabinoside requires further study. However, preliminary studies have shown that injection of human interferon into patients with chronic HBsAg, including Dane particles and DNA polymerase activity, leads to a disappearance of the Dane particle and the surface antigenemia. Concomitantly, the patients did seem to have some symptomatic improvement, and liver function abnormalities returned to normal. Interferon is very expensive, the effect of its long-term administration in man is not known, and the studies were not randomized or controlled; thus, the ability of interferon to cure patients of hepatitis B virus infection remains to be established. Interferon has been combined with adenine

Table 3. CLINICAL PRESENTATIONS OF CHRONIC ACTIVE HEPATITIS

Clinical Presentation	Autoimmune	Associated with HBsAg
Sex	Mainly females	Mainly males
Age	Second and fifth decades	Infants and elderly; immunosuppressed patients
Increase in serum gammaglobulin	Marked	Moderate
Smooth muscle antibody	High	Low
LE cells	In 15 per cent	Absent
Corticosteroid therapy	Most respond	Few respond

arabinoside with beneficial effect in some patients. Larger controlled studies are still needed.

NON-A, NON-B HEPATITIS

Non-A, non-B hepatitis accounts for 50 per cent or more of post-transfusion hepatitis. The incubation period appears to be prolonged as in hepatitis B. Furthermore, the clinical presentation of non-A, non-B hepatitis, including chronic carriage of virus and risk of developing chronic active hepatitis, also resembles that of hepatitis B. There is no cross-antigenicity between HBV and the non-A, non-B viruses. However, no antigenic markers have been identified for the latter viruses. Non-A, non-B hepatitis is an infection that requires much epidemiologic and laboratory investigation (Hoofnagle et al., 1977).

CHRONIC ACTIVE HEPATITIS

Chronic active hepatitis is a chronic inflammatory disease of the liver, lasting at least six months without remission and appearing as a sequel to HBV infection or non-A, non-B hepatitis (Boyer, 1976). Chronic active hepatitis does not appear to be a sequel of hepatitis A virus infection. The onset of the disease is usually insidious with extreme fatigue. There may be fluctuating jaundice, anorexia with weight loss, intermittent fever, and amenorrhea. Examination of the patient shows spider nevi and hepatosplenomegaly. Late in the course of the disease, hepatic encephalopathy, edema, ascites, and bleeding from esophageal varices may develop.

The serum bilirubin level may or may not be increased, but the SGPT and SGOT activities are elevated often to more than five times normal, and there is polyclonal hypergammaglobulinemia. The same disease may occur, however, in congenital or acquired hypogammaglobulinemia. The serum alkaline phosphatase and gamma glutamyl transpeptidase values are also elevated. The prothrombin time may be increased.

Liver biopsy must be done to differentiate this condition from chronic persistent hepatitis and to delineate the extent of damage to the liver and of fibrosis. Microscopically, the liver shows lymphocytic and plasma cell infiltration of the portal areas with inflammation of the liver lobule, including erosion of the limiting plate or piecemeal necrosis, bridging necrosis, and fibrosis (Fig. 6). There is a wide spectrum in the clinical illness and presentation from mildly symptomatic to very ill patients; the clinical presentation often does not correlate with the pathology.

There are three major types of chronic active hepatitis—one associated with hepatitis B antigen, a non-B post-transfusion form, and an autoimmune or lupoid type (Table 3). The first affects mainly men 30 to 50 years old and is especially apt to develop in transfusion recipients, drug addicts, male homosexuals, immunosuppressed patients (such as renal dialysis patients), patients with malignancy, patients with organ transplants, and babies exposed to HBV. The autoimmune type affects mainly women (in a 3:1 ratio) in the second decade and may be associated with a variety of immunologic phenomena including positive LE cells, antinuclear factor, Coombs' positive hemolytic anemia, and particularly, smooth muscle antibody (Table 3).

Differential diagnosis includes granulomatous hepatitis, Wilson's disease, primary biliary cirrhosis, pericholangitis with inflammatory bowel disease, alcoholic liver disease, cytomegalovirus hepatitis, alpha 1-antitrypsin deficiency, and drug-related chronic hepatitis.

The mainstay of therapy is prednisone or prednisolone (Summerskill et al., 1975). Some patients require azathioprine in addition. Patients with non-B chronic active hepatitis respond better to therapy than those with HBsAg. Indeed, recent studies indicate that corticosteroid therapy may be detrimental in hepatitis B infection (Lam et al., 1981). In the individual patient, response to therapy must be weighed against the side effects of the corticosteroids.

References

Boyer, J. L.: Chronic hepatitis. A perspective on classification and determinants of prognosis. Gastroenterology 70:1161, 1976.

Dienstag, J. L., and Isselbacher, K. J.: Therapy for acute and chronic hepatitis. Arch Intern Med 141:1419, 1981.

Dienstag, J. L., Routenberg, J. A., Purcell, R. H., Hooper, R. R., and Harrison, W. O.: Foodhandler-associated outbreak of hepatitis A. Ann Intern Med 83:647, 1975.

Hirschman, S. Z.: The hepatitis B vaccine: current recommendations for use. Drug Therapy 8:21, 1983.

Hoofnagle, J. H., Gerety, R. J., and Barker, L. F.: Antibody to hepatitis B-virus core in man. Lancet 2:869, 1973.

Hoofnagle, J. H., Gerety, R. J., Tabor, J., Feinstone, S. M., Barker, L. F., and Purcell, R. H.: Transmission of non-A, non-B hepatitis. Ann Intern Med 87:14, 1977.

Krugman, S.: Effect of human immune serum globulin on infectivity of hepatitis A virus. J Infect Dis 134:70, 1976.

Krugman, S., Hoofnagle, J. H., Gerety, R. J., Kaplan, P. M., and Gerin, J. L.: Viral hepatitis type B. DNA polymerase activity and antibody to hepatitis B core antigen. N Engl J Med 290:1331, 1974.

Lam, K. C., Lai, C. L., Trepo, C., and Wu, P. C.: Deleterious effect of prednisolone in HBsAg-positive chronic active hepatitis. N Engl J Med 304:380, 1981.

Mosley, J. W.: Hepatitis types B and non-B. Epidemiologic background. JAMA 233:697, 1975.

Murray, R.: Viral hepatitis. Bull NY Acad Med 31:341, 1955.

Schaffner, F.: The structural basis of altered hepatic function in viral hepatitis. Am J Med 49:658, 1970.

Summerskill, W. H. J., Korman, M. G., Ammon, H. V., and Baggenstoss, A. H.: Prednisone for chronic active liver disease: dose titration, standard dose, and combination with azathioprine compared. Gut 16:876, 1975.

Szmuness, W., Stevens, C. E., Harley, E. J., Zang, E. A., Oleszko, W. R., William, D. C., Sadovsky, R., Morrison, J. M., and Kellner, A.: Hepatitis B vaccine: demonstration of efficacy in a controlled clinical trial in a high risk population in the United States. N Engl J Med 303:833, 1980.

155

YELLOW FEVER

FRANCISCO DE PAULA PINHEIRO, M.D.

Yellow fever is an acute viral illness characterized by jaundice, hemorrhage, and renal damage. It varies from a fulminant fatal disease to a mild febrile illness. Inapparent infections are frequent. The yellow fever virus is a member of the group B arboviruses, or *Flavivirus* genus of the family Togaviridae. The virus persists enzootically in forests of certain areas of Africa and South America through a cycle that is not yet fully understood and is transmitted to man by infected mosquitoes. In the past, yellow fever was also maintained in urban centers, where the agent was transmitted from man to man by the mosquito *Aedes aegypti*.

ETIOLOGY. In the older classification system (Casals, 1957), the yellow fever virus is a member of the group B arboviruses. It is now considered to be the type species of the genus *Flavivirus* of the Togaviridae family. The virus particles are spherical and possess a lipid-containing envelope and an icosahedral nucleocapsid. The virions contain an infectious single-stranded RNA genome. Electron microscopy of infected mouse brain and liver reveals that the virus particles exist in the cytoplasm of infected cells and that their diameter is about 38 nm, with a range of 33 to 43 nm (Bergold and Weibel, 1962). In the mouse brain, the particles are found only in the astrocytes, which are accumulated within the cisterna and ducts of the endoplasmic reticulum. The virus is labile in the absence of protein. It is more stable when suspended in phosphate buffer solution (pH 7.0) containing 10 per cent normal human serum, 10 per cent monkey serum, or 0.75 per cent bovine albumin. Virus infectivity can be preserved for one month in blood kept at 4° C and is destroyed by heating at 60° C for 10 minutes. The virus is inactivated by ether, sodium deoxycholate, and by common chemical disinfectants. It can be preserved for years in whole infected tissues or tissue suspensions at −60° C or in liquid nitrogen. Lyophilization, followed by cold storage, is the preferred method of preserving infectivity.

The virus possesses a hemagglutinin that is active against erythrocytes of several animal species, particularly those of the goose.

Yellow fever virus causes encephalitis and death in suckling mice after intracerebral, intraperitoneal, or subcutaneous inoculation. Many adult mice die when infected intracerebrally but usually not when infected by the other two routes. All primates are susceptible to infection, but mortality depends upon the species, route of inoculation, and strain of virus. Rhesus monkeys and other primates from India, as well as certain monkeys from South America, develop fatal infection. Wild strains are pantropic and affect a variety of the organs and tissues of rhesus monkeys but have a special predilection for the liver, kidneys, and heart. After serial passages in the mouse brain, the virus loses its affinity for monkey viscera and becomes markedly neurotropic. Some marsupials and a few rodents develop viremia without overt disease.

The agent has been propagated in several cell cultures of vertebrate origin such as primary chick embryo, BHK-21, Vero, HeLa, pig kidney, and others. It causes either plaque formation, cytopathic effect, or both. It also replicates and causes cytopathologic signs in the invertebrate cell line derived from *Aedes pseudoscutellaris*. Some strains of the virus multiply in the cell cultures of *Aedes albopictus*, but they do not produce cytopathologic signs (Varma et al., 1975/76).

PATHOGENESIS AND PATHOLOGY. The pathogenesis of yellow fever is not yet well understood. When rhesus monkeys are experimentally infected with small inocula, the virus cannot be detected for 24 hours (Strano et al., 1975). At the end of this period, Kupffer cells are found to contain intracytoplasmic areas of acidophilic degeneration. Between 24 and 48 hours after the infection, glycogen is reduced in the hepatocytes, and the titer of virus in the blood increases and peaks at about 96 hours postinfection. At 72 hours, many Kupffer cells are degenerating, and the alterations in hepatocytes are more evident. The glycogen gradually disappears, and fatty degeneration characterized by small and large droplets of fat both in the cytoplasm in the nucleus becomes apparent. Migration of chromatin to the nuclear membrane is followed by rupture of the membrane. Intranuclear eosinophilic bodies can also be recognized in the hepatic cells (Torres, 1928). Eosinophilic hyaline degeneration of the hepatocytes results in the formation of eosinophilic masses, known as Councilman bodies. Between 96 and 120 hours after the infection, the lesions are fully developed. Characteristically, the cells from the midzone of the hepatic lobule are more profoundly affected. At this site, the necrosis may become nearly confluent. Typically, the liver cords are discontinuously involved, so that living and necrotic cells are interspersed. The absence of significant inflammation is a cardinal feature.

The pathology in the liver of rhesus monkeys closely resembles that observed in the infected human liver. In human beings, midzone necrosis is also characteristic but may involve almost the entire lobule. Councilman bodies may be absent if death occurs after the tenth day of illness. Interestingly, the lesions in survivors are completely reversible. Classic histologic features of yellow fever are present only in the acute stage. During convalescence, the histologic picture resembles that of persistent, nonspecific hepatitis (Francis et al., 1972). Liver biopsy, however, is contraindicated in the acute phase of the illness.

The kidney, heart, and other organs of man may also be affected (Bugher, 1951). The tubular epithelium of the kidney undergoes changes varying from cloudy swelling and desquamation to simple necrosis. These changes are most severe in the convoluted tubules. The cells lining Bowman's capsule are also damaged, but the glomeruli are affected less than the tubules. Experimental findings suggest that acute tubular necrosis may result from prerenal hemodynamic alterations and azotemia, and thus be preventable (Monath et al., 1981).

Fatty degeneration of myocardial fibers is a uniform finding when the heart is involved. Lesions may occur in the sinoauricular node and the bundle of His. Involvement of the brain is minimal; perivascular hemorrhage is the most consistent finding. Significant necrosis of the cortical cells of the outer fascicular zone of the adrenals may occur.

CLINICAL MANIFESTATIONS, COMPLICATIONS, AND SEQUELAE. The incubation period varies from three to six days in naturally acquired yellow fever. It can be as long as ten days, however, in individuals accidentally exposed to infectious blood. Apparently the virus can penetrate either intact skin or areas of minor unnoticed abrasion.

The clinical course varies from benign febrile illness to the classic clinical picture of hepatic failure, albuminuria, hemorrhagic manifestations, coma, and death. During the 1960 to 1962 yellow fever outbreak in Ethiopia, a fulminating form of the disease was observed, characterized by high fever, severe headache, tachycardia, prostration, and death in two to three days (Sérié et al., 1968). Little or no hepatic or renal involvement was seen.

The following classification according to the severity of clinical disease has been suggested (Kerr, 1975): (1) Very mild. Patients experience only transient fever and headache that persists from a few hours to one or two days. (2) Mild. The fever and headache are more pronounced and may be accompanied by nausea, epistaxis, Faget's sign (see below), slight albuminuria, and subclinical elevations of bilirubin. The illness usually lasts from two to three days. Findings similar to these have been described among patients infected during outbreaks that occurred near Belem, Brazil (Causey and Maroja, 1959). Some of these patients also complained of epigastric pain, backache, general body pain, vertigo, vomiting, photophobia, and prolonged asthenia. Epistaxis was not observed. (3) Moderately severe. The fever is higher, the headache and backache are more severe, and the nausea and vomiting are more intense. Jaundice and albuminuria are usually present. Black vomitus, melena, or uterine hemorrhage may occur. The fever persists for about one week. (4) Malignant. All the classic signs and symptoms of the disease are present. Patients may die within three to four days.

Evolution of Severe Forms. Two periods can be recognized during the course of the moderately severe and malignant forms of the disease: the period of infection (viremia) and the period of intoxication.

The period of infection is characterized by the sudden onset of intense chills of short duration followed by fever of 39° to 40° C. There is severe headache, nausea, vomiting, generalized muscle pain, and backache. The face and sometimes the neck and upper part of the thorax are congested. The conjunctivae are suffused. The gums may be swollen and ooze blood on gentle pressure. Epistaxis is common. The patient is uncomfortable, anxious, and unable to sleep. By the second day, the appearance of a pulse-temperature dissociation begins: the temperature is high, and the pulse gradually slows down (Faget's sign). This viremic phase lasts about three days.

A remission follows that lasts from a few hours to two days. The general symptoms begin to diminish, the fever falls, and the headache decreases. After the remission, the period of intoxication is recognized by the appearance of hemorrhages, jaundice, and albuminuria. The fever rises, and the general symptoms reappear with great intensity.

Hemorrhagic manifestations are a major element of this stage. "Coffee-grounds" hematemesis from a small amount of swallowed blood and capillary hemorrhage into the stomach is followed by black vomitus, which is caused by massive hemorrhage into the stomach and the action of gastric juice on the blood. Melena, metrorrhagia, bleeding from the gums, and epistaxis also occur. Petechiae and ecchymoses of the skin are accompanied by bleeding from injection sites. Hematuria is rare. The jaundice is usually mild, although it may become pronounced if death is delayed.

Oliguria is common, but complete anuria is very rare. Albuminuria develops and increases rapidly. It is considered one of the most prominent findings in the disease, but it disappears in a few days in patients who recover. There is no hemoglobinuria. Hypotension occurs late in the course and may be accompanied by nonspecific abnormalities in the electrocardiogram. The liver and spleen are not palpable, but palpation of the epigastrium will elicit pain. Paroxysms of hiccoughing may occur, especially in severe cases.

Death occurs after one or two days of coma or suddenly after an attack of hematemesis. Death occurs most commonly between the sixth and eighth days of illness. The overall mortality rate among hospitalized patients may be as high as 40 to 50 per cent. Survivors exhibit long-lasting immunity.

Laboratory Findings. Leukopenia with a selective depression of polymorphonuclear cells occurs inconsistently. A moderate leukocytosis may be observed before death and during convalescence. The bilirubin level, especially the direct fraction, is increased. The serum glutamic pyruvic transaminase (SGPT) and serum glutamic oxaloacetic transaminase (SGOT) levels and the urea and creatinine concentrations in the blood are markedly increased in severe cases. Thrombocytopenia is also common in severe cases, with platelet counts as low as 30,000 per mm^3. The coagulation time and the prothrombin time are prolonged, and the levels of fibrinogen are reduced. Clot retraction may be poor. Coagulation factors II, V, and VII plus X, VIII, IX, X, and XIII may be depressed (Santos, 1973). The albumin concentration in the urine can reach 40 g per liter, but it is absent or shows only a moderate increase in mild cases. Casts may also be observed in the urine.

Differential Diagnosis. Mild cases of yellow fever cannot readily be distinguished from a number of other febrile conditions, including dengue, influenza, typhoid fever, and malaria. During the period of intoxication, this illness must be differentiated from infectious hepatitis, leptospirosis, malaria, Lassa fever, Bolivian hemorrhagic fever, the effects of certain chemical poisons, and other conditions that can cause jaundice and hemorrhage. A careful clinical history and the epidemiology, considered along with the laboratory findings, will help establish the diagnosis of yellow fever. The definitive diagnosis, however, can be established only by one of the following methods: virus isolation, serologic test, and/or liver histopathologic examination.

Complications that are not a part of the natural course of the disease are uncommon. Parotitis, usually unilateral, has been observed. In spite of marked renal and heart involvement in certain patients, survivors recover completely without sequelae.

GEOGRAPHIC VARIATIONS IN DISEASE. Yellow fever is currently maintained enzootically only in certain forested areas of South America and Africa. However, the virus has been historically endemic and even epidemic in several urban centers of the Americas, Africa, and Europe. Thus, two epidemiologic cycles of yellow fever can be recognized: urban and jungle. Each is quite distinct in the New World but less so in Africa.

Urban Cycle. This cycle is maintained by the transmission of virus from man to man by the bite of the mosquito *Aedes aegypti*. The mosquito can transmit the virus from 9 to 30 days after ingesting blood from a viremic patient and is thought to remain infected for life. Yellow fever transmitted by *Aedes aegypti* occurred in the past in many cities of South America, the Caribbean, the United States, and West Africa. It is also reported to have reached Spain, France, Italy, and England. The last case of urban yellow fever in the Americas was registered at Port-of-Spain in 1954 and in Africa at Sierra Leone, in 1975.

Jungle Yellow Fever. The two main foci of jungle yellow fever are considered to be the Amazon and Congo river basins. Although the maintenance of the virus in these regions is not fully understood, monkeys and certain mosquito species play an important role. In South America, mosquitoes of the genus *Haemagogus* e.g., *H. janthimomys (spegazzinii)* are the main vectors. These day-biting mosquitoes are found predominantly in the forest canopy, although they can be captured on the forest floor. They occasionally bite man inside houses located near forests. *Sabethes chloropterus* and *Haemagogus leucocelaenus* are considered to be secondary vectors of the virus in South and Central America. *Sabethes* species may be responsible for the persistence of the virus during dry periods in Central America from 1948 to 1957. Although monkeys are considered to be the main vertebrate hosts for the virus, it is thought that marsupials may also act as hosts in some areas. Experimentally, the three-toed sloth, *Bradypus tridactylus*, develops a heavy, persistent viremia but does not die (Johnson, 1978). There is no direct evidence, however, that *Bradypus* plays a role in the virus cycle.

In the rain forests of Africa, the mosquitoes of the *Aedes africanus* group are the main vectors among monkeys, but species of the *Aedes simpsoni* group may also transmit the virus. Both species can also infect man. The same species together with *Aedes luteocephalus* and *Aedes furcifer-taylori*, which are also antropophilic, play an essential role in transmission in savannah forests. In East African epidemics, *Aedes simpsoni*, *Aedes vittatus*, *Aedes metallicus*, and *Aedes taylori* have been implicated as vectors. The 1960 to 1962 epidemic of yellow fever in Ethiopia was basically rural in nature and was linked to villages harboring *Aedes simpsoni* (Sérié et al., 1968). In West Africa, yellow fever epidemics in rural environments have been associated with *Aedes luteocephalus*, *Aedes vittatus*, *Aedes taylori*, and *Aedes aegypti*, with possible mosquito transmission from man to man (Cordellier et al., 1977). Workers at the Institut Pasteur in Dakar have isolated three strains of yellow fever virus from *Aedes furcifer* males captured in Sénégal (Cornet et al., 1979). The tick *Amblyoma variegatum* can transmit the virus to its progeny, which can infect monkeys in experimental conditions.

In the enzootic areas of South America, the virus is believed to move in waves through populations of susceptible monkeys, with periodic invasions of other areas such as Central and Southern Brazil and northern Paraguay and Argentina (Kerr, 1975; Pinheiro et al., 1978). Northward migration of the virus to Central America was documented during 1948 to 1957. In West Africa, the virus spreads in similar wave-like movements (Cordellier et al., 1977). Nevertheless, the precise mechanism of virus persistence is unknown. Experimentally, transovarial transmission has been demonstrated in *Aedes aegypti* (Aitken et al., 1979) and in *Haemagogus equinus* (Dutary and LeDuc, 1980) and may play a role in viral persistence.

The number of cases of yellow fever reported to the World Health Organization during the period 1977-81 was 897 in the Americas and 889 in Africa. Cases reported from the Americas during this period occurred in Bolivia, Brazil, Colombia, Ecuador, Peru, Trinidad, and Venezuela. African reports came from Nigeria, Ghana, Cameroon, Gambia, and Senegal. The extensive Ethiopian epidemic of yellow fever in 1960 to 1962, in which there was an estimated morbidity of 100,000 and a mortality of 30,000, was especially severe (Sérié et al., 1968). Subsequently, smaller outbreaks have been recorded in both continents, including Brazil, Bolivia, Peru, Colombia, Trinidad, Venezuela, Nigeria, Upper Volta, Sierra Leone, Angola, Ghana, Gambia and Senegal.

DIAGNOSIS. Yellow fever is easy to diagnose when classic signs are present. The final diagnosis, however, depends upon laboratory methods, which are of particular importance for the recognition of modified cases of the illness. There are three laboratory procedures for the specific diagnosis of yellow fever: (1) Virus isolation. Blood must be drawn within the first three to four days of the infection. Although the virus has been isolated from blood stored for days or even weeks at 4° C, it should be kept at −50° C or below, if the inoculation cannot be performed on the day of collection. The virus has also been isolated from liver specimens collected from fatal cases. Serum, whole blood, or 10 per cent liver suspensions should be inoculated into infant white mice and tissue cultures. It is also desirable to inoculate an additional group of mice with a 1:10 dilution of serum or blood. When the mice sicken, the brain is harvested and used for virus identification by complement fixation or neutralization tests against yellow fever-specific antiserum. Vero and *Aedes pseudoscutellaris* cell lines are even more susceptible to the virus than mice (Varma et al., 1975/76). Monoclonal antibodies specific to yellow fever virus have now been developed and should be valuable for virus identification (Monath, T. P. et al., 1983). Virus growth can be detected in these cultures by the appearance of cytopathic effect. (2) Serologic tests. The first paired sera should be taken as soon as possible after the onset of illness and the second two to three weeks later. Sera should be tested by hemagglutination-inhibition, complement fixation, and neutralization procedures against yellow fever virus and other flaviviruses known to exist in the area where the case occurred. The convalescent serum should have an antibody titer to yellow fever antigen at least four times greater than the serum from the acute phase. Due to the antigenic cross-reactions between yellow fever and other group B arboviruses, it is sometimes difficult or even impossible to make a diagnosis by serologic tests. In patients who have experienced a previous *Flavivirus* infection of another type, antibody rises to a variety of *Flavivirus* antigens can be observed. However, IgM antibodies specific to yellow fever antigen can be found in such patients, although they may not be consistently present (Monath et al., 1981). (3) Histopathologic examination. This method depends upon the demonstration of Councilman bodies and the other characteristic lesions of yellow fever in liver sections. Liver specimens collected postmortem by direct incision of the abdominal wall or through a viscerotome should be preserved in 10 per cent formalin until examination. Immunofluorescence may be used for detection of YF virus antigen in liver sections.

TREATMENT. The treatment of yellow fever is symptomatic. Bed rest is important. The patient should be hospitalized under careful observation in order to avoid harm to the damaged liver. Oral fluids should be given in the form of salt solution for diarrhoeal diseases, sugared water, or citrus fruit juice. The fever must be controlled and pain may require analgesics. Salicylates (aspirin) should be avoided since they cause bleeding and acidosis. Tranquilizing drugs should be administered if the patient becomes agitated. Antiemetics should be used to control nausea and vomiting. Administration of intravenous fluids such as glucose in physiologic saline and electrolyte solutions are recommended to avoid dehydration and maintain the electrolyte balance. Blood transfusions may be required to replace blood loss by hemorrhage. Disseminated intravascular coagulation (Santos, 1973) may be improved by the intravenous use of 5000 units of heparin every six hours. This treatment, however, may not prevent death, indicating that other factors contribute to a fatal outcome. Dialysis should be performed when there is renal failure. The use of antibiotics is often necessary to combat secondary bacterial infections. New antiviral drugs such as ribavirin (1-β-D-ribofuranosyl-1,2,3, triazole-3-carboxamide) deserve evaluation through careful trials.

PROPHYLAXIS. Vaccination is essential for residents and visitors to endemic areas. Two attenuated strains of yellow fever virus are presently used for the protection of susceptible people. One is the 17D strain, derived from a wild strain passaged serially in tissue culture prepared from mouse and chick embryos and then grown in embryonated eggs. The other is the French neurotropic strain, which was attenuated by intracerebral passages in mice.

The 17D vaccine is the one most widely used, due to its safety and effectiveness. It has been given to more than 100 million persons with only a few serious complications. Complications attributed to 17D vaccine include 15 nonfatal cases of encephalitis in children under 1 year of age, all of whom recovered without sequelae, and a single fatal case in a 3-year-old child who developed encephalitis. Allergic reactions have also been observed and are probably due to the presence of egg protein in the vaccine. The vaccine is administered by subcutaneous inoculation with syringe or Ped-o-jet. Immunity develops within ten days and may last 18 years or more, although the International Regulations for travelers require booster shots every ten years. The vaccine is heat labile and must be carefully refrigerated. The commonly available 17D vaccine is contaminated with avian leukosis virus; however, a leukosis-free 17D vaccine produced in England is now available. The vaccine is not recommended for children less than 6 months of age.

The French neurotropic vaccine is also very effective, but serious neurologic complications have been associated with its use, especially in children less than 7 years old. It should be given only to those beyond this age. This vaccine is administered by cutaneous scarification. One advantage over the 17D vaccine is that it is much less heat labile.

Eradication of *Aedes aegypti* mosquitoes, the primary urban vector, is an important measure for control of yellow fever, especially in urban centers located near forests in which jungle yellow fever is present. Protective clothing can be worn, and insect repellents are useful.

References

Aitken, T. H. G., Tesh, R. B., Beaty, B. J., and Rosen, L.: Transovarial transmission of yellow fever virus by mosquitoes *(Aedes aegypti).* Am J Trop Med Hyg 28(1):119, 1979.

Bergold, G. H., and Weibel, J.: Demonstration of yellow fever virus with the electron microscope. Virology 17:554, 1962.

Bugher, J. C.: The pathology of yellow fever. In Strode, G. K. (ed.): Yellow Fever. New York, McGraw-Hill Book Company, 1951, p. 137.

Casals, J.: The arthropod-borne group of animal viruses. Trans NY Acad Sci Ser 2, 19:219, 1957.

Causey, O. R., and Maroja, O.: Isolation of yellow fever virus from man and mosquitoes in the Amazon region of Brazil. Am J Trop Med 8:368, 1959.

Cordellier, R., Germain, M., Hervy, J. P., and Mouchet, J.: Guide Pratique Pour Étude des Vecteurs de Fièvre Jaune en Afrique et Methodes de Lutte. Office de la Recherche Scientifique et Technique Outre-Mer, Documentations Techniques 33, 1977.

Cornet, M., Robin, Y., Heme, G., Adam, C., Renaudet, J., Valade, M., and Eyraud, M.: Une poussée épizootique de fièvre jaune selvatique au Sénégal Oriental. Isolement du virus de lots de moustiques adultes mâles et femelles. Médecine et Maladies Infectieuses, 9(2):63, 1979.

Dutary, B. E. and LeDuc, J. W.: Transovarial transmission of yellow fever virus by a sylvatic vector, *Haemagogus equinus. Trans Royal Soc Trop Med Hyg* 75:128, 1981.

Francis, T. L., Moore, D. L., Edington, G. M., and Smith, J. A.: A clinicopathological study of human yellow fever. Bull W H O 46:659, 1972.

Johnson, K. M.: Personal communication, 1978.

Kerr, J. A.: Yellow fever. In Tice: Practice of Medicine, Vol. 4. 1975.

Monath, T. P., Cropp, C. B., Muth, D. J., and Calisher, C. H.: Indirect fluorescent antibody test for the diagnosis of yellow fever. *Trans R Soc Trop Med Hyg* 75:282, 1981.

Monath, T. P., Brinker, K. R., Chandler, F. W., Kemp, G. E., and Cropp, C. B.: Pathophysiologic correlations in a rhesus monkey model of yellow fever with special observations on the acute necrosis of B cell areas of lymphoid tissues. *Am J Trop Med Hyg* 30:431, 1981.

Pinheiro, F. P., Travassos da Rosa, A. P. A., Moraes, M. A. P., Almeida Neto, J. C., Camargo, S., and Filgueiras, J. P.: An epidemic of yellow fever in Central Brazil 1972-1973. I. Epidemiological studies. Am J Trop Med Hyg 27:125, 1978.

Santos, F.: Dosagem dos fatores da coagulacão na febre amarela. Tese Faculdade de Medicina, Univ. Federal de Rio de Janeiro, 1973.

Sérié, C., Lindrec, A., Poirier, A., Andral, L., and Neri, P.: Études sur la fièvre jaune en Ethiopie. 1. Introduction. Symptomatologie clinique amarile. Bull W H O 38:835, 1968.

Sérié, C., Andral, L., Poirier, A., Lindrec, A., and Neri, P.: Études sur la fièvre jaune en Ethiopie. 6. Étude épidémiologique. Bull W H O 38:879, 1968.

Strano, A. J., Dooley, J. R., and Ishak, K. G.: Manual sobre la fiebre amarilla y su diagnostico diferencial histopatologico. Organizacion Pan Americana de la Salud Publicación Cientifica 299, 1975.

Torres, C. M.: Inclusions nucléaires acidophiles (dégénérescence exychromatique) dans le foie de *Macacus rhesus,* inoculé avec le virus brésilien de la fièvre jaune. C R Soc Biol 99:1344, 1928.

Varma, M. G. R., Pudney, M., Leake, C. J., and Peralta, P. H.: Isolation in a mosquito (*Aedes pseudoscutellaris*) cell line (Mos. 61) of yellow fever virus strains from original field material. Intervirology 6:50, 1975/76.

156

WHIPPLE'S DISEASE

STANLEY D. FREEDMAN, M.D.

In 1907, Dr. G. W. Whipple, a pathologist at Johns Hopkins University, described a fatal illness in a 36-year-old man who complained of arthralgias and arthritis for several years before developing cough, fever, weight loss, progressive debility and weakness, and malabsorption (Whipple, 1907). Pallor, wasting, a full abdomen, articular abnormalities, and lymphadenopathy were noted on physical examination. At autopsy, Whipple found enlarged mesenteric nodes, "foamy" mononuclear phagocytic cells especially in the lamina propria of the intestinal mucosa, and rod-shaped organisms in various tissues. The disease, in essence, remains well defined by Whipple's remarkable description.

ETIOLOGY. The foamy material in the macrophages of the lamina propria was shown to consist of periodic acid-Schiff (PAS)-positive particles by Black-Schaffer in 1949. This tinctorial identification of glycoproteins led to further speculation about the metabolic causes of the disease. Nine years later, Sieracki (1958) elaborated upon the morphologic appearance of these cytoplasmic particles, calling them "sickle-form particles" and the cells containing them "sickle-form particle-containing (SPC) cells." SPC cells were soon identified in tissues from all major organ systems and provided histologic confirmation of the systemic nature of Whipple's disease. These tinctorial reactions and morphologic characteristics were found to be present in Whipple's original case when reexamined by the PAS technique by Mendeloff; this histologic picture remains pathognomonic of the disease.

Electronmicroscopic studies suggested that the particles were bacillary bodies that had all the structural features of bacteria (Haubrich et al., 1960; Yardley and Hendrix, 1961; Chears and Ashworth, 1961). These rodlike organisms averaged 1.5 microns in length and 0.15 microns in width and had a three-component cell wall (Fig. 1 A and B). They divided by binary fission. The rods were both intra- and extracellular and disappeared with therapy. Bacterial cell walls remaining after treatment correlated with the PAS-positive material in the remaining macrophages. More recently, immunofluorescent studies of jejunal biopsy tissue demonstrated similar bacterial antigens in the macrophages of different patients and suggested that a single organism was responsible for the disease (Keren et al., 1976 and Kirkpatrick et al., 1978). Furthermore, there is strong morphologic data demonstrating the widespread nature of this infection, with involvement of different cell types and multiple organ systems. This information underscores the intracellular location of the bacilli, which is of considerable importance in immunologic, pathogenetic, and therapeutic discussions (Dobbins and Kawanishi, 1981).

This strong anatomic evidence for a bacterial etiology of Whipple's disease has not been confirmed by culture (Keren, 1981). Different organisms have been isolated and cell-wall deficient bacteria incriminated, but the identity of these rods is obscure, and Koch's postulates remain unfulfilled.

PATHOGENESIS AND PATHOLOGY

Pathogenesis. Disordered fat metabolism was first thought to explain the clinical and pathologic features, and numerous other theories have been proposed, but infection remains the most likely cause. In addition to the morphologic findings, the dramatic clinical response and the disappearance of the bacilli under electron microscopy after antibiotic therapy are compelling arguments in favor of a bacterial etiology.

The portal of entry is unknown, although the most likely route is oral. This is inferred from the demonstration of

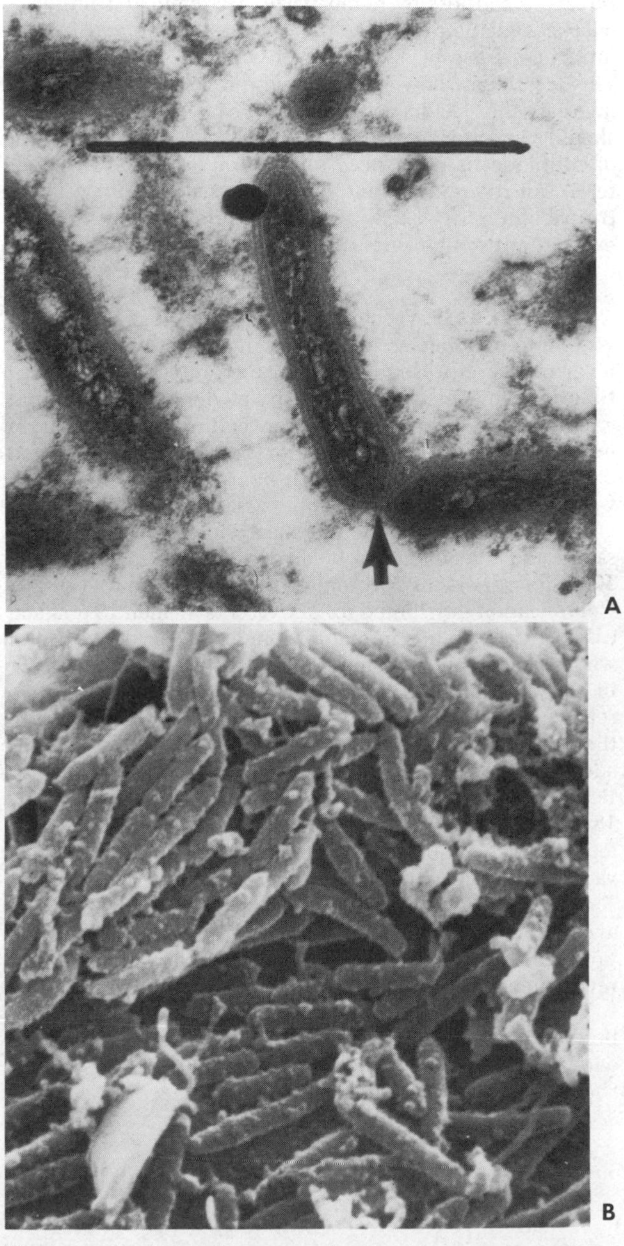

Figure 1. Electron microscopy showing the structure of the bacilliform bodies. (From Haubrich et al.: Gastroenterology 39:454, 1960.) Note 3 component cell wall in A and numerous bacilliform bodies with scanning electronmicroscope in B.

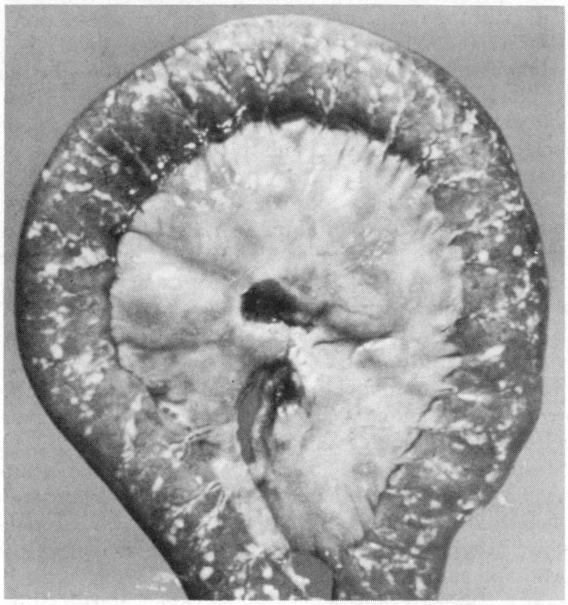

Figure 2. Appearance of large mesenteric nodes and fibrinous deposits in a case of Whipple's disease.

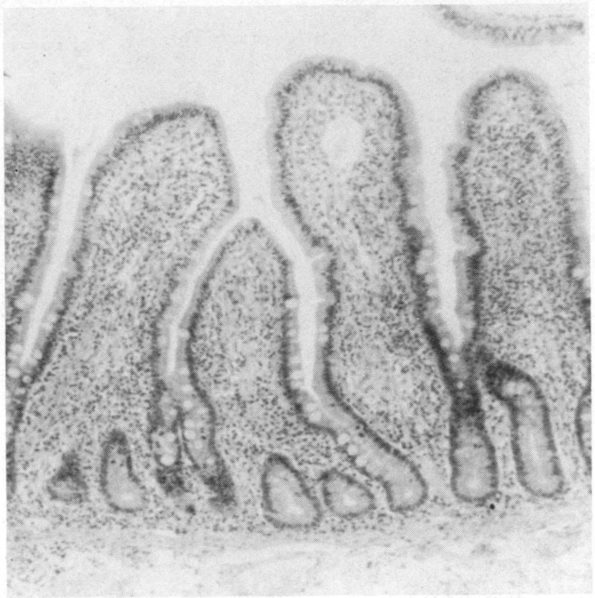

Figure 3. Small bowel morphology demonstrating enlarged, blunted villi.

more organisms in the upper portions of the gastrointestinal tract and a progressive decline as samples are obtained from the jejunum and ileum, and by the observation that the diagnostic morphologic abnormalities in the small intestine are almost universal, whether or not other tissues and organs are involved. Multiplication within the lamina propria and invasion of the absorptive cells and lymphatics with spread to the mesenteric nodes and beyond are the presumed mechanisms for subsequent hematogenous spread. The evidence for such dissemination is found in cases of Whipple's disease involving multiple systems.

Steatorrhea is caused mainly by functional and morphologic alterations of the absorptive cells, which are invaded by the bacillary structures. These cells revert to normal and the bacteria disappear soon after treatment, and coincident with this, fat absorption returns to normal. The dense infiltration of the lamina propria by the PAS-positive macrophages, the enlarged and abnormal mesenteric nodes, and the bacteria present in lysosomes within the lymphatic endothelium may impair lipid transport but are not thought to be a major cause of malabsorption.

The impressive predominance of Whipple's disease in middle-aged men, the chronicity and remittent nature of the illness, and the pathologic alterations all suggest that host factors play an important role in the expression of this disease, but these host factors are undefined. Some form of immunologic tolerance is thought to be present, but immunologic studies are inconclusive. Several investigators have demonstrated impaired cell-mediated immunity, mainly on the basis of altered delayed cutaneous hypersensitivity; however, these findings are inconsistent (Dobbins, 1981).

Pathology. The peritoneal and serosal surfaces of the bowel are covered with strands and nodular collections of soft, yellow-white, fibrinous material, and slight oozing occurs when the fibrinous adhesions are removed from the surface of the intestine. The small bowel wall can be thickened and irregular, particularly the proximal third. The colon is usually normal on gross inspection. Enlarged mesenteric nodes are striking (Fig. 2), and retroperitoneal adenopathy is present. Splenomegaly is frequent. Nodular excrescences on the ventricular surfaces of the brain, vegetations on the endothelial surfaces of the heart, pulmonary nodules, and pericarditis are some of the extraintestinal lesions described.

The small bowel villi are blunted and edematous (Fig. 3), and within these villi are large collections of foamy macrophages (Fig. 4). With the PAS stain, the sickle-form cytoplasmic particles (the bacilliform bodies) and the intra- and extracellular amorphous clumps of PAS-positive material appear as brilliant magenta (Fig. 5). These SPC cells, the hallmark of Whipple's disease, are most abundant in the lamina propria of the small bowel, but are also evident in the mesenteric nodes and have been demonstrated in most organs and tissues of the body. There may also be an increased number of plasma cells in the affected villi. Accumulations of neutral fat are seen in the intestinal mucosa and lymph nodes ("lipodystrophy"). Inflammation is minimal.

CLINICAL MANIFESTATIONS. Whipple's disease predominantly affects middle-aged white men, with manifestations usually appearing in the fourth and fifth decades. Exceptions to the usual picture continue to be reported, but the total number of such cases remains small.

Weight loss is almost universal and is sometimes extreme. Diarrhea occurs in over three fourths of the cases and can be watery stools or true steatorrhea. Abdominal pain is less frequent, usually epigastric. Articular manifestations provide the diagnostic clue and are present in at least 65 per cent of the cases (Maizel et al., 1970). The fascinating feature of the arthralgias is that they may precede the other manifestations by many years, frequently five to six. The arthralgia is migratory and involves multiple joints, with the ankles, knees, shoulders, and wrists most commonly involved. Arthritis can be dramatic and is an inflammatory, predominantly large-joint, asymmetric, monoarticular disease. Destructive arthritis is unusual.

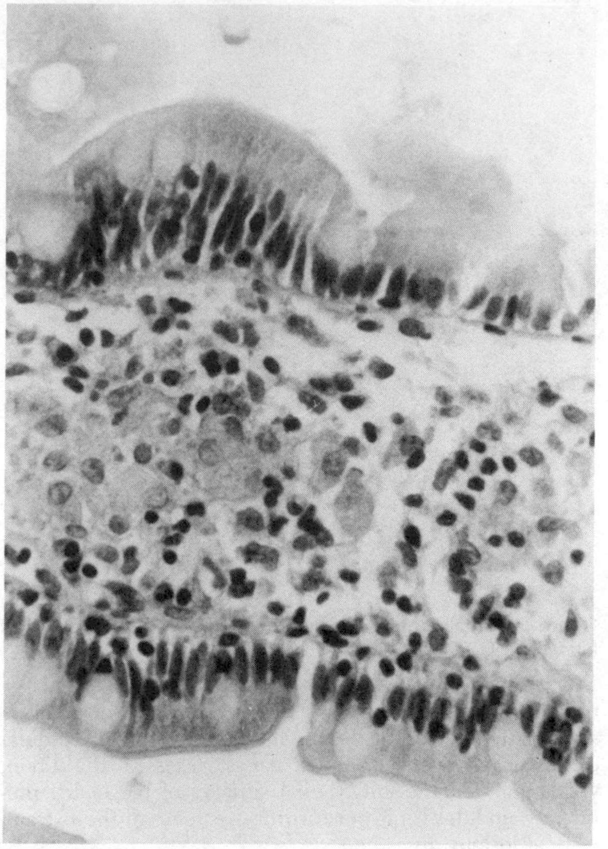

Figure 4. Foamy macrophages infiltrating the villi.

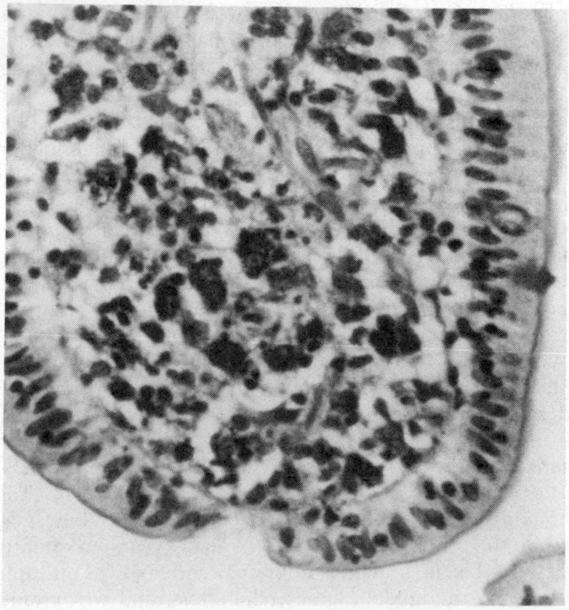

Figure 5. Note dark staining PAS-positive material, intra- and extracellular. Higher power necessary to identify SPC cells.

Axial arthropathy is uncommon, and the association of HLA-B27 and Whipple's disease is uncertain (Khan, 1982).

Abdominal distention and lymphadenopathy are the most common signs, occurring in over half of the cases. Hyperpigmentation, especially of the exposed skin, is frequently reported. Edema, glossitis, and splenomegaly are less often found.

Fever is present in approximately half of the patients reported and can be quite variable, ranging from low-grade pyrexia to intermittent fever with rigors. In fact, it is not uncommon for Whipple's disease to present as a "fever of unknown origin." Further, this illness should be added to the list of diseases associated with relapsing fever, as demonstrated in Figure 6.

There are a number of neurologic signs now reported, and the most common are dementia, myoclonus, supranuclear ophthalmoplegia, and ataxia (Knox et al., 1976). Brainstem and hypothalamopituitary dysfunction in association with a slowly progressive dementia is emerging as a diagnostic syndrome of central nervous system Whipple's disease (Halperin et al., 1982). Signs of valvular disease (aortic and mitral) related to endocarditis are noteworthy (Kraunz, 1969; Wright et al., 1978). Pleuropericarditis is part of the polyserositis, and manifestations of vasculitis have been described. Ocular inflammation is rare (Font et al., 1978).

Anemia is present in over 90 per cent of the patients and is most often attributed to impaired erythropoiesis due to chronic inflammation. Iron deficiency anemia associated with gastrointestinal blood loss has been documented. Megaloblastic anemia is rare. White blood counts are usually normal, but some eosinophilia occurs. Serum albumin is often reduced, and hypocalcemia occurs secondary to steatorrhea. Malabsorption is manifested by increased stool fat in most cases, impaired D-xylose absorption, and reduced serum carotene. The synovial fluid has an inflammatory character with high viscosity and protein and many leukocytes (predominantly mononuclear). There is roentgenographic evidence of sacroiliitis along with reports of HLA B27 positivity and circulating immune complexes. The cerebrospinal fluid is usually normal, but pleocytosis, elevated protein, and SPC cells have been found. Various gastrointestinal roentgenographic signs have been reported, but they are all nonspecific. Computerized scanning demonstrates the enlarged mesenteric and retroperitoneal lymph nodes and helps define central nervous system involvement (Ludwig et al., 1981).

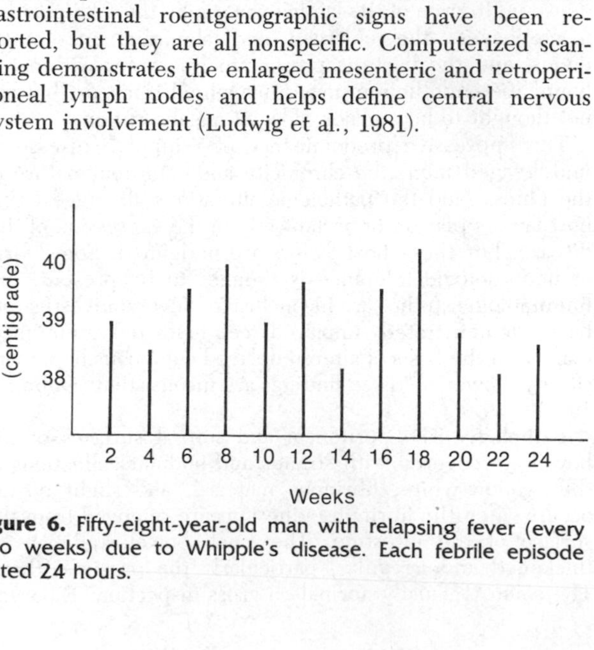

Figure 6. Fifty-eight-year-old man with relapsing fever (every two weeks) due to Whipple's disease. Each febrile episode lasted 24 hours.

COMPLICATIONS AND SEQUELAE. Whipple's disease is inexorably fatal if not treated. However, even with treatment, some neurologic manifestations may be permanent and even progressive (Feurle et al., 1979; Knox et al., 1976; Bayless and Knox, 1979; Schmitt, et al., 1981). Ocular changes may also persist. Stenotic and destructive valvular deformities require individualized study and management. Whipple's disease may preclude the use of tissue heart valves, since bacilliform bodies have been demonstrated in the porcine valve of a patient with Whipple's disease (Ratliff et al., 1984). The arthritides are nondeforming, and the vast majority of treated patients have a favorable outcome.

GEOGRAPHIC VARIATIONS IN DISEASE. Most cases are reported from the United States, Continental Europe, and England, and some from South America. Further, within the United States, there are areas (for example, the Southeast and upper Midwest) where the prevalence seems clearly higher. The reasons for this and for the other epidemiologic characteristics alluded to above remain unknown, but subtle ecologic factors related to the presumed causative agent may be responsible.

DIAGNOSIS. Recurring asymmetric arthralgias and inflammatory arthritis, involving large joints, in a white man over 35 years of age should suggest the diagnosis of Whipple's disease. The full-blown picture with weight loss and diarrhea is rather characteristic of this disorder. X-rays of the small bowel show mainly thickening of mucosal folds in the duodenum and proximal jejunum. In contrast to celiac sprue, there is little if any small intestinal dilatation, flocculation, or segmentation. Depending upon the predominant clinical features, however, the differential diagnosis frequently includes lymphoma, inflammatory bowel disease, connective tissue disorders, sarcoidosis, and a chronic infection such as tuberculosis (the main consideration in Whipple's original case).

Although the disease may be strongly suggested by a number of the clinical manifestations enumerated, the sine qua non for the diagnosis rests upon the demonstration of the foamy macrophages, which are PAS-positive and diastase-resistant, in the lamina propria of the enlarged and blunted villi. These macrophages have been found in the intestinal mucosa of patients whether or not gastrointestinal abnormalities were present. The necessary tissue can be obtained by peroral small bowel biopsy. Because of known irregular involvement, biopsies obtained endoscopically may increase the yield. The finding of PAS-positive material in cells from other sources, such as lymph nodes, cannot be considered pathognomonic of Whipple's disease. However, there is a disquieting report of a patient with presumed Whipple's disease who had negative small bowel biopsies and in whom the diagnosis was made by lymph node biopsy revealing PAS-positive cells, which on electron microscopy contained bacilliform bodies morphologically consistent with those seen in Whipple's disease (Mansbach et al., 1978). This raises important issues in our understanding of this disease. The same bacilliform bodies have been found from other extraintestinal sources, but rarely without bowel involvement.

THERAPY. It is only since the early 1960's that antibiotics were recognized as being curative (Maizel et al., 1970; Bayless, 1970). In fact, antibiotic treatment produces dramatic improvement in all signs and symptoms during the first few weeks. The optimum therapeutic program is not known. Mainly due to the increasing awareness of central nervous system (CNS) involvement, therapeutic recommendations are uncertain. One of the early suggestions was parenteral therapy with procaine penicillin G 1,200,000 units plus streptomycin 1 g daily for two weeks, followed with tetracycline 250 mg orally four times per day. It is not known if this regimen is preferable to tetracycline initially. Other oral drugs, including penicillin, ampicillin, and erythromycin all in a dose of 1 g per day, have been used successfully. Chloramphenicol and trimethoprim-sulfamethoxazole have also been used. It is clear that prolonged therapy is required, and the incidence of relapses is considerably less if such treatment is given for a full year. If relapses occur, indefinite therapy may be indicated, perhaps at reduced doses after remission is again achieved.

Poor response to tetracycline and progressive extraintestinal disease on this therapy is well reported. The recognition of progressing CNS disease while on tetracycline or oral penicillin has led some to suggest other forms of therapy with drugs that penetrate the CNS. This subject has been reviewed recently (Comer et al., 1983).

Whipple's disease involving the CNS is indeed a therapeutic challenge. In part, this may be due to the blood brain barrier and inadequate levels of antimicrobial agents in the CNS tissues. In such cases, it may be necessary to use over 12,000,000 units of penicillin IV per day and/or chloramphenicol to achieve a response; and then to rely on oral agents that do penetrate the CNS, such as trimethoprim-sulfamethoxazole, given indefinitely. Oral amoxacillin, erythromycin, and chloramphenicol have also been used in the treatment of CNS disease. The use of rifampin has not been reported, but its penetration into the CNS and into cells suggests that it may be of value in individuals unresponsive to other therapies. Yet, there are clearly other reasons for therapeutic failures in CNS disease such as multiply drug-resistant organisms and altered host responses.

Obviously, attention to nutritional needs, including vitamin and mineral replacement, and to the possible complications mentioned previously is mandatory. Corticosteroid therapy is no longer appropriate, but some have used it for short periods in severely ill cachectic patients. Further refinements in management await the identification of the still elusive rod-shaped organism.

References

Bayless, T. M.: Whipple's disease. Newer concepts of therapy. Adv Intern Med 16:171, 1970.

Bayless, T. M., and Knox, D. L.: Whipple's disease: A multisystem infection (editorial). N Engl J Med 300:920, 1979.

Black-Schaffer, B.: The tinctorial demonstration of a glycoprotein in Whipple's disease. Proc Soc Exp Biol Med 72:225, 1949.

Chears, W. C., and Ashworth, C. T.: Electronmicroscopic study of the intestinal mucosa in Whipple's disease. Gastroenterology 41:129, 1961.

Comer, G. M., Brandt, L. J., and Abissi, C. J.: Whipple's disease: a review. Am J Gastroenterol 78:107, 1983.

Dobbins, W. O.: Is there an immune deficit in Whipple's disease? Dig Dis and Sci 26:247, 1981.

Dobbins, W. O., and Kawanishi, H.: Bacillary characteristics in Whipple's disease: an electron microscopic study. Gastroenterol 80:1468, 1981.

Feurle, G. E., Volk, B., and Waldherr, R.: Cerebral Whipple's disease with negative jejunal histology. N Engl J Med 300:907, 1979.

Font Rao, N. A., Issareslu, S., and McEntee, W. J.: Ocular involvement in Whipple's disease. Arch Ophthalmol 96:1431, 1978.

Halperin, J. J., Landis, D., and Kleinman, G. M.: Whipple's disease of the nervous system. Neurol 32:612, 1982.
Haubrich, W. S., Watson, J. H. L., and Sieracki, J. C.: Unique morphologic features of Whipple's disease: A study by light and electronmicroscopy. Gastroenterology 39:454, 1960.
Keren, D. F.: Whipple's disease: a review emphasizing immunology and microbiology. CRC critical reviews in clinical laboratory sciences. May 1981.
Keren, D. F., Weisburger, W. R., Yardley, J. H., et al.: Whipple's disease: Demonstration by immunofluorescence of similar bacterial agents in macrophages from three cases. Johns Hopkins Med J 139:51, 1976.
Khan, M. A.: Axial arthropathy in Whipple's disease. J Rheumatol 9:928, 1982.
Kirkpatrick, P. M., Kent, S. P., Mihas, A., and Pritchett, P.: Whipple's disease: a case report with immunological studies. Gasteroenterol 75:297, 1978.
Knox, D. L., Bayless, T. M., and Pittman, F. E.: Neurologic disease in patients with treated Whipple's disease. Medicine 55:467, 1976.
Kraunz, R. F.: Whipple's disease with cardiac and renal abnormalities. Arch Intern Med 123:701, 1969.
Ludwig, B., Bohl, J., and Haferkamp, G.: Central nervous system involvement in Whipple's disease. Neuroradiology 21:289, 1981.
Maizel, H., Ruffin, J. M., and Dobbins, W. D.: Whipple's disease: A review of 19 patients from one hospital and a review of the literature since 1950. Medicine 49:175, 1970.
Mansbach, C. M., Shelburne, J. D., Stevens, R. D., and Dobbins, W. O.: Lymph-node bacilliform bodies resembling those of Whipple's disease in a patient without intestinal involvement. Ann Intern Med 89:64, 1978.
Ratliff, N. B., McMahon, J. T., Naab, T. J., Cosgrove, D. M.: Whipple's disease in the porcine leaflets of a Carpentier-Edwards prosthetic mitral valve. N Engl J Med 311:902, 1984.
Schmitt, B. P., Richardson, H., Smith, E. and Kaplan, R.: Encephalopathy complicating Whipple's disease. Ann Int Med 94:51, 1981.
Sieracki, J. C.: Whipple's disease—observation on systemic involvement. Arch Pathol 66:464, 1958.
Tauris, P., and Moesner, J.: Whipple's disease. Clinical and histopathologic changes during treatment with sulfamethoxazole-trimethoprim. Acta Med Scand 204:423, 1978.
Whipple, G. H.: A hitherto undescribed disease characterized anatomically by deposits of fat and fatty acids in the intestinal and mesenteric lymphatic tissues. Johns Hopkins Hospital Bull 18:382, 1907.
Wright, C. B., Hiratzka, L. F., Crossland, S., Isner, J., and Snow, J. A.: Insufficiency requiring valve replacement in Whipple's disease. Ann Thorac Surg 25:466, 1978.
Yardley, J. H., and Hendrix, T. R.: Combined electron and light microscopy in Whipple's disease. Demonstration of "bacillary bodies" in the intestine. Bull Johns Hopkins Hosp 109:80, 1961.

157
PERITONITIS

DENNIS L. KASPER, M.D.

Peritoneal infections involve the serous membrane that lines the abdominal cavity and covers most of the intraabdominal viscera. This membrane is divided into a parietal portion that lines the walls of the cavity and a visceral portion that encloses the intraperitoneal organs. In men, the peritoneal cavity is completely closed; in women it communicates with the environment through the genital viscera of the pelvis.

Two major inflammatory processes, peritonitis and abscesses, can affect the peritoneum. Peritonitis refers to nearly all inflammatory lesions of infectious etiology in which pus is not localized. Abscesses are localized collections of pus that can involve the abdominal viscera and either the intraperitoneal or retroperitoneal spaces.

ETIOLOGY. The most common causes of sterile peritonitis are blood, which causes chemical irritation and inflammation; bile from perforation or rupture of the biliary system; pancreatic enzymes, which are released into the peritoneum in acute hemorrhagic pancreatitis; carcinomatosis; and surgically introduced foreign materials, particularly talcum powder.

Bacteria are the most common cause of infectious peritonitis. These infections may be primary or secondary (Table 1). Primary bacterial peritonitis usually occurs in patients with altered susceptibility to infection. It is an acute or subacute infection caused by a single microbe that seeded the peritoneum either during a transient bacteremia or bacteremia from a distant site of infection.

In the past, children with the nephrotic syndrome developed primary peritonitis that was usually caused by *Streptococcus pneumoniae* or other species of *Streptococcus*, but this has subsequently become an unusual complication of nephrosis. Now, however, almost 10 per cent of patients with cirrhosis of the liver who also have portal hypertension and overt ascites develop spontaneous primary peritonitis for which there are multiple etiologic agents. *Escherichia coli* (36 per cent) and other enteric bacteria cause 60 per cent of these infections. The other enteric and gram-negative bacteria include *Pseudomonas*, *Proteus*, *Klebsiella*, *Bacteroides*, and *Salmonella* (Conn and Fessel, 1971). *S. pneumoniae* and other streptococci account for approximately 25 per cent of these infections.

Secondary peritonitis, which is more common than primary, is caused by: (1) lesions that damage the integrity of one of the viscera covered by the peritoneum, with leakage of microbes or irritants into the intraperitoneal or retroperitoneal space; (2) disruption of the peritoneum from outside the abdomen without actual penetration of the viscera; or (3) surgical contamination (Table 1). These lesions result in bacterial infection of the peritoneum with organisms that are usually part of the normal flora of the violated sites.

Mycobacterium tuberculosis is an important cause of chronic infectious peritonitis. In Osler's era, cirrhosis was thought to predispose to peritoneal tuberculosis. However, the validity of this observation depends upon the study population, and the relative risk for tuberculous peritonitis in cirrhosis is unknown. The prevalence of cirrhosis in patients with tuberculous peritonitis has varied from 0 of 32 patients in Iran to 20 of 47 patients at Boston City Hospital.

Peritoneal inflammation caused by fungi is distinctly uncommon, but *Candida albicans* can cause massive ascites by direct peritoneal involvement. Fungi have also caused secondary peritonitis after the organism has entered the peritoneum from intestinal leakage. Peritonitis occurs in 2 to 4 per cent of patients with disseminated histoplasmosis.

Parasitic infestations can lead to clinical peritoneal disease that can mimic tuberculosis or carcinomatosis. *Schistosoma mansoni* can cause granulomatous peritonitis without extraintestinal involvement. Enterobiasis has been reported to cause granulomatous peritonitis in women, apparently by retrograde migration through the genital

Table 1. ETIOLOGY OF BACTERIAL PERITONITIS

I. Primary peritonitis without disruption of the integrity of the gastrointestinal tract in:
  A. Nephrotics
  B. Cirrhosis
  C. Otherwise healthy young children occasionally
II. Secondary peritonitis
  A. Related to diseases and injuries of the gastrointestinal tract
    1. Appendicitis
    2. Diverticulitis
    3. Perforation due to malignant tumor
    4. Perforated peptic ulcer
    5. Devitalization of intestinal wall by circulatory impairment, volvulus, or intussusception
    6. Perforations caused by trauma such as gunshot or stab wounds
  B. Related to lesions of the biliary system and pancreas
    1. Suppurative cholecystitis
    2. Bile peritonitis
    3. Pancreatitis
  C. Related to lesions of the female genital tract
  D. Related to lesions of the male genitourinary tract, especially injuries or suppurating lesions of the bladder and, rarely, kidneys
  E. Postoperative
    1. Operative contamination of peritoneum
    2. Leaking anastomosis
    3. Retained foreign body
  F. Perforating wounds of abdominal wall only
III. *Mycobacterium tuberculosis*

tract. Amebiasis of the gastrointestinal tract, liver, or spleen can cause perforation of the involved viscera and secondary bacterial peritonitis. Ectopic *Paragonimus* cysts, as well as migratory *Ascaris*, may localize in the abdominal cavity and produce an acute abdomen. Mechanical irritation of the strobila and attachment of the scolex of intestinal tapeworms, especially *Taenia solium*, is a rare cause of intestinal perforation and secondary bacterial peritonitis. The hepatic cysts of *Echinococcus granulosus* can rupture into the abdominal cavity. Any of the migrating parasites may carry bacteria with them from the gastrointestinal tract and set up distant bacterial abscesses.

PATHOLOGY AND PATHOGENESIS. The inflammatory process in bacterial peritonitis is typical of other acute bacterial infections and consists primarily of an infiltration of neutrophils with a fibrinopurulent exudate. The membranes undergo sequential pathologic changes. Two to four hours after involvement, the membrane loses its gray, glistening quality and becomes dull. At this time, a small quantity of serous or slightly turbid fluid accumulates. Later, this fluid becomes creamy and suppurative and may either be confined by the omentum and viscera to a small area of the peritoneal cavity or become generalized. Rarely, the exudate resolves without residual fibrosis. Usually, the exudate eventually accumulates into well-loculated collections of pus called abscesses that may develop anywhere in the abdominal cavity, including the subhepatic and subdiaphragmatic spaces, the retroperitoneum, or within the viscera. The exudate may cause adhesions after the formation of abscesses.

The pathogenesis of primary peritonitis has not been well defined, but it is thought that ascites is an ideal culture medium for bacteria that reach the peritoneum by hematogenous spread. This is an attractive hypothesis to explain the development of peritonitis in cirrhotic patients with portal hypertension because their portal-systemic collaterals bypass the liver, a major bacterial filter.

It is probable that some cases of primary peritonitis originate from transmural migration of bacteria. The polymicrobic nature of some of these infections without evidence of a perforated bowel argues strongly for this mechanism of peritoneal contamination. Furthermore, ^{14}C-labeled *E. coli* have been shown to traverse the intact intestinal wall in dogs after hypertonic irrigations of the peritoneum (Schweinburg et al., 1950). For these reasons, it seems likely that the source of infection in some cirrhotics, and perhaps in a substantial number of patients receiving peritoneal dialysis, is transmural migration of intestinal bacteria.

The pathogenesis of secondary bacterial peritonitis, which has been well defined in the experimental animal, is dependent on the composition of the normal bowel flora. The largest populations of bacteria in the body reside in the lower tract where careful microbiological studies have revealed hundreds of bacterial species. Most of these bacteria are obligate anaerobes ($\sim 10^{11}$/gm), which outnumber aerobic bacteria ($\sim 10^{8}$/gm) 100- to 1000-fold. The stomach and upper small bowel support a rather sparse population ($<10^{5}$) of bacteria that are mainly washed down from the oropharynx. The lower ileum is a transitional area, with up to 10^{8} bacteria per ml. In the upper gastrointestinal tract, anaerobes and aerobes are equal in number. This quantitative anatomic distribution of bacteria in the gastrointestinal tract explains the fact that perforation of the upper intestine results in lower rates of infection and morbidity than colonic perforation. Careful bacteriology yields an average of five different species, often two aerobes and three anaerobes, from secondary intraabdominal infections due to colonic perforation. The prevalence of anaerobic microorganisms and the polymicrobial nature of these infections are characteristic of intraabdominal infection related to perforation of the lower gastrointestinal tract (Gorbach and Bartlett, 1974).

Careful bacteriologic studies have shown that certain species are predictably isolated from patients with intraabdominal infection. Of the aerobes, the gram-negative enteric bacilli are most common: these include *E. coli*, *Klebsiella*, *Proteus*, and *Pseudomonas*. Enterococci are the most common gram-positive aerobic bacteria. The major anaerobic isolates are *Bacteroides fragilis* (65 per cent of all cases), *Clostridium* species (60 per cent of cases), and anaerobic cocci (32 per cent). Studies using an animal model of intraabdominal sepsis have clarified the complex role of these bacteria in the pathogenesis of peritonitis and subsequent abscess formation (Weinstein et al., 1974). These studies, which employed an intraperitoneal implant of fecal contents in rats, showed a two-stage disease. During the first five days, there was acute peritonitis with free-flowing peritoneal exudate. The cumulative natural mortality rate during this stage was 43 per cent; this early stage was caused by aerobic gram-negative bacteria, particularly *E. coli*. The second stage, characterized by the formation of multiple intraabdominal abscesses in all survivors, was caused by anaerobic bacteria.

Abscess formation in the animal model usually required the synergistic interaction of an aerobe and an anaerobe. This requirement held unless the anaerobe was *Bacteroides fragilis*, which could induce abscesses without the synergistic help of an aerobe (*E. coli* or enterococci). *B. fragilis*, but not other *Bacteroides* species, contains a capsular polysaccharide, which is responsible for abscess formation (Zaleznik and Kasper, 1982).

Anaerobes are also more common in the vagina than aerobes and play a major role in secondary pelvic peritonitis and abscess after septic abortion, postoperative surgery on the reproductive tract, puerperal sepsis, and endometritis. Furthermore, *B. fragilis*, aerobic streptococci, and other enteric bacteria colonize the vagina in increased numbers postoperatively and after difficult deliveries (Gibbs et al., 1975). For these reasons, the microbiology of secondary peritonitis of pelvic origin is similar to that of intestinal origin, except for group B streptococci, *Corynebacterium (Haemophilus) vaginale*, and rarely gonococci, which are more common in pelvic infections. The prominence in these infections of *Bacteroides* species that are capable of degrading heparin (Gesner and Jenkin, 1961) may explain the tendency toward suppurative pelvic thrombophlebitis and septic pulmonary emboli.

The pathogenesis of tuberculous peritonitis is well understood. It is usually the result of reactivation of latent peritoneal foci that were established at the time of hematogenous spread from the primary pulmonary focus in patients who do not have active pulmonary tuberculosis. Tuberculous peritonitis can occur, however, at the time of hematogenous spread from active pulmonary or miliary tuberculosis.

CLINICAL MANIFESTATIONS. The clinical symptoms and onset of infectious peritonitis vary with the etiology, the precipitating event, and the population studied. The signs and symptoms may be deceptively absent in the very young, very old, or in patients on corticosteroids. Localizing signs may be absent in patients in shock. The presentation of patients with peritonitis may be acute, subacute, chronic, or insidious.

Of the more acute forms, primary spontaneous peritonitis usually occurs in patients with abnormal hepatic function and secondary ascites and jaundice. Portal-systemic collaterals are present in 80 per cent and azotemia in 55 per cent of patients. The symptoms or signs may be masked by hepatic failure; 35 per cent of patients have no peritoneal signs and 5 per cent are completely asymptomatic. Spontaneous primary peritonitis causes abdominal pain in 80 per cent and hypotension in 70 per cent; it is associated with hepatic encephalopathy in more than 70 per cent of cases. Sudden deterioration in the condition of a patient with cirrhosis should alert the physician to the possibility of bacterial peritonitis.

In patients with secondary peritonitis, the mode of onset varies with the precipitating event and may be acute or subacute. Abdominal pain and distention are usually prominent. Other findings include diffuse muscle spasm, absence of abdominal respiratory movement, abdominal tenderness, rebound tenderness, rigidity of the abdominal wall, and decreased or absent peristalsis. There may be tenderness or a mass on rectal or vaginal examination as well as fever, toxemia, or shock.

The onset of tuberculous peritonitis is insidious. More than 70 per cent of patients have had symptoms for more than four months before presentation. These signs are nonspecific, and the diagnosis of tuberculous peritonitis must be considered in any patient with ascites, fever, abdominal pain, anorexia, malaise, weakness, and weight loss. Abdominal pain, which is usually vague and dull, is reported by only 50 per cent of patients with tuberculous peritonitis. Some patients complain of vomiting, constipation, and diarrhea. Seventy-five per cent have ascites. Abdominal tenderness is reported by 65 per cent of patients. Despite classic descriptions, the "doughy" abdomen is rare. Twenty-five per cent of patients have hepatomegaly, and 20 per cent have an abdominal mass. More than half of these patients are thought to have evidence of tuberculosis elsewhere, particularly pleuropulmonary disease.

COMPLICATIONS AND SEQUELAE. The complications and sequelae of peritonitis can be divided into three general categories (Table 2). In the early phase of peritonitis, metabolic alterations place increased demands on the circulatory system. The amount of fluid lost into the peritoneal cavity may approach 50 per cent of the plasma volume. This fluid and electrolyte imbalance is complicated by ileus, which causes additional loss of fluid into the lumen of the bowel. There may be a large loss of potassium from the intracellular to the extracellular fluid with a shift of sodium into the intracellular compartment. The potassium loss may be masked by hemoconcentration and should be monitored by electrocardiography. Serum levels of glucocorticoids, aldosterone, and catecholamines are usually elevated. Elevation of catecholamines may contribute to peripheral vasoconstriction and decreased perfusion of vital organs, which can cause declining renal and cardiac function. The evolving ileus and progressive elevation of the diaphragm can interfere with ventilatory capacity and respiratory exchange.

Bacteremia with either aerobes (usually gram-negative rods) and/or anaerobes (most commonly *B. fragilis*) is common during the acute phase of peritonitis. All of these complications can contribute to the development of shock, which is associated with a high mortality rate, even in the face of appropriate therapy.

The major sequela of peritonitis is abscess formation. Intraperitoneal abscesses develop in one of two general patterns. The first is the result of diffuse peritonitis in which loculations of purulent material usually occur in anatomically dependent areas such as the pelvis, the kidney pouch, and the subphrenic or paracolic "gutter" areas. The second results from a localized focus of peritonitis related to some contiguous disease process such as pelvic inflammatory disease, in which the inflammatory response is rapid and effective enough to prevent diffuse peritonitis.

Adhesions may complicate either localized or generalized peritonitis and can cause intestinal, circulatory, or neural compression and obstruction. These are reported complications of tuberculous peritonitis as well. An additional

Table 2. COMPLICATIONS AND SEQUELAE OF PERITONITIS

I. Early acute phase
   A. Metabolic
      1. Fluid and electrolyte imbalance
      2. Hypokalemia
      3. Elevated glucocorticoids, aldosterone, catecholamines
      4. Vasoconstriction with decreased renal perfusion and cardiac action
   B. Respiratory embarrassment
   C. Bacteremia
   D. Shock
II. Abscesses
   A. Anatomically dependent areas
   B. Localized near the site of contamination
III. Adhesions

problem with tuberculous peritonitis is failure to make this difficult diagnosis early enough to prevent development of extensive disease of multiple organs. Local complications in the peritoneum have also been reported, including intestinal obstruction secondary to volvulus around tuberculous adhesions.

GEOGRAPHIC VARIATIONS IN DISEASE. Spontaneous primary and secondary bacterial peritonitis occur in all geographic areas and are caused by the same bacteria. Studies of human colonic flora have generally shown marked quantitative and qualitative similarities in bacterial species despite variations in race, diet, or geographic locale.

In the United States, tuberculous peritonitis is relatively uncommon, but is encountered in cities with large populations of individuals of lower socio-economic status who seem to be predisposed to the development of tuberculosis. This group includes the poorly nourished and debilitated as well as cirrhotic patients who are common on the wards of municipal hospitals. There is no age or sex predilection, but 80 to 90 per cent of people with this disease are black. The predisposition of blacks to tuberculosis is probably due to poverty and crowding, which also influence the relatively high rate of tuberculosis in developing countries. On a worldwide basis, tuberculosis is a widely distributed disease and peritonitis is a common manifestation.

Except for infections with *Candida,* which are part of the endogenous flora of patients all over the world, the rare fungal and parasitic infections of the peritoneum occur within the geographic distribution of the particular agent.

DIAGNOSIS. The differential diagnosis of peritonitis is extensive (Table 3). These etiologies can be grouped into intraabdominal inflammations (including septic and nonseptic conditions), metabolic processes, intrathoracic conditions, and infections that commonly cause the clinical picture of peritonitis.

Table 3. DIFFERENTIAL DIAGNOSIS OF PERITONITIS

I. Intraabdominal
  A. Septic, but contained within an organ (e.g., biliary)
    1. Primary
    2. Secondary
    3. Contained within an organ (e.g., cholecystitis)
  B. Nonseptic
    1. Intestinal obstruction
    2. Internal hemorrhage
    3. Pancreatitis
    4. Renal disease
II. Metabolic
  A. Porphyria
  B. Diabetic acidosis
  C. Plumbism
  D. Arachnidism
III. Intrathoracic
  A. Myocardial infarction
  B. Pleurisy
  C. Pneumonia
  D. Epidemic pleurodynia
IV. Infections with abdominal manifestations
  A. Tabetic crisis
  B. Malaria
  C. Typhoid fever
  D. Herpes zoster of the lower spinal roots
  E. Osteomyelitis
V. Others
  A. Periarteritis nodosa
  B. Retroperitoneal catastrophies
    1. Rupture of aneurysm
    2. Dissection of aorta
  C. Familial Mediterranean fever

The diagnosis of peritonitis can be additionally complex because of the great variation in the presenting signs and symptoms. Only careful evaluation of the patient, the clinical laboratory data, and the radiologic information can ensure an accurate diagnosis. First, careful attention must be paid to a history of antecedent illnesses, such as diverticulitis, duodenal ulcer, and pancreatitis, that would predispose to peritonitis from intraabdominal fecal contamination. The characteristics of the abdominal pain can help determine the etiology of the disease. The physician must determine its site of origin, the site of greatest intensity, and the radiation and character of the pain (Cope, 1963).

Most patients with bacterial peritonitis have fever and leukocytosis. The laboratory abnormalities are related to the involved viscera or the underlying etiology. Therefore, the physician must consider carefully the possible metabolic or intraabdominal nonseptic conditions that might mimic bacterial peritonitis. Urinalysis and measurement of blood sugar, bilirubin, amylase, alkaline phosphatase, serum ketones, or urinary porphyrins may be helpful, but all laboratory data must be assessed critically. For example, pyuria usually reflects pathology of the genitourinary tract but can be seen when adjacent viscera are inflamed as in diverticulitis or appendicitis. The serum amylase may be very high in acute pancreatitis, but modestly elevated levels can occur in peritonitis of many etiologies. Microbiologic studies are extremely important; in particular, aerobic and anaerobic cultures of the blood and peritoneal fluid are essential. Examination of the abdomen by x-ray may reveal displacement of the gastrointestinal tract or ureters, free air in the peritoneal cavity, encapsulated air or gas in an abscess, features of ileus or obstruction, evidence of peritoneal fluid, obliteration of the psoas shadows, calcification within the gallbladder or other organs, or restricted motion of the diaphragm (fluoroscopy). Chest x-ray may show unilateral elevation of the diaphragm and basilar atelectasis or pleural effusions and may help to differentiate peritonitis from an intrathoracic infection. Other radiologic procedures that can be of diagnostic value include radioisotopic scanning procedures for localization of abscesses, liver-lung scan (most useful for subdiaphragmatic abscesses) sonography, computerized tomographic scans, and abdominal arteriography.

Needle aspiration of the peritoneum can be diagnostic. Typical results of the laboratory examination of ascitic fluid from patients with bacterial and tuberculous peritonitis are outlined in Table 4. Peritoneal biopsy is also a valuable procedure and establishes the diagnosis in 50 to 60 per cent of patients with tuberculous peritonitis and in 25 to 40 per cent of cases of carcinoma.

The diagnosis of abscesses can be difficult. Persistence of fever and leukocytosis after abdominal surgery should be regarded as intraabdominal abscess until proved otherwise. Laboratory tests are of little aid in the diagnosis of intraperitoneal abscesses that do not involve organs, but roentgenologic examination can be very helpful for locating intraabdominal abscesses. In subdiaphragmatic abscess, the abnormalities are usually seen on chest x-ray; possible findings include pleural effusion; elevation and decreased mobility of the diaphragm; lower lobe infiltration or atelectasis; a unilateral widening of the angle between the chondral arch and the sternum; and obliteration of the costophrenic angle on lateral examination, all of which may

Table 4. TYPICAL LABORATORY CHARACTERISTICS OF THE PERITONEAL FLUID FROM PATIENTS WITH BACTERIAL PERITONITIS

	Bacterial Peritonitis	Tuberculous Peritonitis	Uninfected Cirrhotic Fluid
Specific gravity	↑	↑(↓[a])	↓(<1.012)
Protein	↑	↑(↓[a])	↓(<2.5 g per cent)
Cell count	↑	↑(↓[a])	↓(<250 WBC/mm³)
Differential	>50 per cent PMN	<30 per cent PMN	not helpful
Amylase	nl	nl	nl
Glucose	↓	↓	nl
Gram stain	+	–	–
Culture			
Culture			
Anaerobic	+	–	–
Aerobic	+	–	–
Tuberculous	–	+[b]	–
Fungi	–	–	–
Cytology	–	–	–
Lipid content	–	–	–

[a]Usually elevated, but can be normal or low in cirrhotic patients with tuberculous peritonitis.
[b]Greater yield if larger volumes are cultured.
↑, increase
↓, decrease
PMN, polymorphonuclear leukocytes
nl, normal

be mistaken for pneumonia postoperatively. Other important radiologic signs that may require contrast studies include gas-fluid levels (33 per cent positive in overpenetrated views) and displacement of the spleen, stomach (in the Trendelenburg position), colon, or left lobe of the liver. Combined liver-lung scan has been very helpful in the diagnosis of subdiaphragmatic abscess.

Abscesses elsewhere in the peritoneum or retroperitoneum may be more difficult to detect than subphrenic abscesses. Here again, an abscess may be demonstrable as a space-occupying lesion displacing loops of intestine or obliterating the intramuscular and subperitoneal fat layers of the adjacent abdominal wall. Perinephric abscesses usually present with fever, unilateral flank pain, abdominal pain, dysuria, and an abdominal or flank mass. Mild leukocytosis, normal or slightly elevated blood urea nitrogen, and pyuria are also common. Three fourths of the patients have abnormalities demonstrable by intravenous pyelogram; caliceal stretching and stones are common. Fifty per cent of these patients have abnormal chest x-rays with findings similar to those of subdiaphragmatic abscesses. Abscesses of the iliac fossa (psoas abscess) are also retroperitoneal and present with findings similar to those of perinephric abscesses, except that these patients may also have an unexplained limp, pain on walking, and pain on extension of the thigh. A history of a recent obstetric or gynecologic procedure, rectal and vaginal examination, positive smear or culture results from culdocentesis, and clinical or roentgenographic evidence of septic pulmonary emobli help to establish the diagnosis of pelvic peritonitis or abscess. Currently, the diagnosis of intraabdominal abscesses has been considerably improved by radioisotope scanning, ultrasound, and computerized tomographic scans.

TREATMENT. The general principles of therapy for peritonitis are: (1) improvement of vascular perfusion to correct fluid and electrolyte imbalances; (2) minimization of the effects of bacteria and their toxic components; (3) reduction of paralytic ileus; (4) elimination of the primary source of infection by excision, closure, or isolation; (5) drainage of the primarily infected site; and (6) treatment of local or distant complications (Finegold, 1977).

The initial treatment of peritonitis is supportive therapy in combination with appropriate antimicrobial agents. The choice of appropriate antimicrobials depends upon the sensitivity patterns of the microorganisms involved in the infectious process and the ability of an antibiotic to penetrate the peritoneum. Primary bacterial peritonitis is best treated with penicillin G if the causative agent is either *S. pneumoniae* or group A *Streptococcus*. If the etiologic agent is *E. coli*, an aminoglycoside is appropriate until the results of sensitivities are available.

Antimicrobial therapy of peritonitis secondary to a gastrointestinal or vaginal source should be directed at both aerobic and anaerobic gram-negative bacteria, particularly *B. fragilis*, because of the resistance of this organism to the penicillins. There are several commonly accepted alternative forms of therapy. The most widely accepted regimens are either clindamycin (25 to 35 mg/kg per day in four divided doses) or metronidazole (1500 to 2000 mg/day in three divided doses) and gentamicin (4 to 6 mg/kg per day in three divided doses). Clindamycin and metronidazole are active against anaerobes, including *B. fragilis*. Aminoglycosides (e.g., gentamicin, amikacin, tobramycin) are effective against the enteric aerobic bacteria. Recent data suggest that cefoxitin and some third generation cephalosporins are also effective against both the anaerobic and aerobic bacteria in peritonitis. Alternative regimens include either chloramphenicol (succinate derivative) in initial doses of 30 to 60 mg/kg per day, depending on the severity of the illness, or one of the cephalosporins mentioned above. These alternative antibiotics are active against *B. fragilis*, other anaerobes, and usually against the resident aerobic enteric gram-negative bacterial flora. Therapy of postoperative peritonitis should also include antibiotics that are active against penicillinase-producing staphylococci. Therefore, a penicillinase-resistant penicillin or a cephalosporin may be included. There is no substantial evidence that specific treatment for enterococci is necessary unless this organism is cultured from the blood. There is also no substantial evidence that intraperitoneal administration of antimicrobials is helpful; in fact, this form of treatment is not recommended. Infected peritoneal dialysates are an exception. In pelvic thrombophlebitis, heparin should be given in conjunction with antibiotics, and ligation of the inferior vena cava may be necessary in some patients with multiple episodes of septic pulmonary emboli.

Localized tuberculous peritonitis should be treated with two drug therapy, isoniazed and ethambutol. However, if the patient has miliary disease, as is frequently the case, isoniazied (300 mg/day) and rifampicin (600 mg/day) should be used.

In virtually all instances of secondary peritonitis or intraabdominal abscess, pus must be drained. Antibiotics may be useful in the early stages of abscess formation before the infection is walled off, and some patients can be treated with antimicrobials alone during this period if they can withstand a few days more of illness. Successful treatment with antibiotics may account for the reported cases of abscesses that resolved without drainage. In some patients with appendicitis, diverticulitis, or pancreatitis, a mass, frequently referred to as a phlegmon, is felt on examination of the infected area three to four days after the onset. In general, surgeons feel that this situation does not call for surgery because phlegmons resolve without intervention. Therefore, conservative therapy is advised in some forms of localized peritonitis, particularly appendiceal abscesses, diverticulitis, pancreatitis, or some cases of perforated peptic ulcers. However, surgical intervention is required in most cases of secondary peritonitis and abscesses. Recent evidence suggests that abscesses can be drained successfully by percutaneous needle aspiration under sonographic or computerized tomographic visualization. There is no justification for delaying incision and drainage in favor of antibiotic therapy in an extremely ill patient whose only chance for survival is surgical drainage. The overall mortality rate for this disease is extremely high, and early surgery is the only treatment that has been shown to reduce mortality.

PROPHYLAXIS. The only effective means of preventing peritoneal infections is early, appropriate attention to the primary conditions that cause the problem. Preventive measures for secondary peritonitis include early surgical intervention and appropriate antimicrobial chemoprophylaxis for cases in which there has been gross bacterial contamination of the peritoneal cavity. In such cases, appropriate antibiotics are effective in lowering the incidence of infectious complications. In the animal model of peritonitis discussed above, two agents used together had contrasting but important prophylactic effects. Gentamicin reduced mortality, but the survivors had abscesses. Clindamycin failed to reduce mortality rates significantly, but surviving animals did not have abscesses. When the combination of clindamycin and gentamicin was given, the salutary effects of the two drugs were additive. Similar results were obtained with some of the cephalosporins described above.

The short-term use (three doses on the first preoperative day) of oral preoperative neomycin (1 g) and erythromycin (1 g) combined with vigorous purgation has been shown to reduce the incidence of wound infections and other septic complications of elective operations on the colon and rectum (Clarke et al., 1977). Evidence is accumulating that prophylactic preoperative, intraoperative, and short-term postoperative cephalosporins and other antimicrobials may reduce the high incidence of infection after vaginal hysterectomy, radical surgery for gynecologic malignancy, and cesarean section after rupture of the membrane and labor.

References

Clarke, J. S., Conden, R. E., Bartlett, J. G., Gorbach, S. L., Nichols, R. L., and Ochi, S.: Preoperative oral antibiotics reduce septic complications of colon operations. Ann Surg 186:251, 1977.

Conn, H. O., and Fessel, M. J.: Spontaneous bacterial peritonitis in cirrhosis: Variations on a theme. Medicine 50:161, 1971.

Cope, F.: The Early Diagnosis of the Acute Abdomen, London, Oxford University Press, 1963, p. 196.

Finegold, S. M.: In Hoeprich, P. D. (ed): Peritonitis in Infectious Diseases, Hagerstown, Md., Harper and Row, 1977, p. 669.

Gesner, B. M., and Jenkin, C. R.: Production of heparinase by Bacteroides. J Bacteriol 81:595, 1961.

Gibbs, R. S., O'Dell, T. N., McGregor, R. R., et al: Puerperal endometritis: A prospective microbiologic study. Am J Obstet Gynecol 122:820, 1975.

Gorbach, S. L., and Bartlett, J. G.: Management of anaerobic infections. N Engl J Med 290:1177, 1237, 1289, 1974.

Schweinburg, F. B., Seligman, A. M., and Fine, J.: Transmural migration of intestinal bacteria: A study based on the use of radioactive *Escherichia coli.* N Engl J Med 242:747, 1950.

Weinstein, W. M., Onderdonk, A. B., Bartlett, J. G., and Gorbach, S. L.: Experimental intra-abdominal abscesses in rats: Development of an experimental model. Infect Immun 10:1250, 1974.

Zaleznik, D. F., and Kasper D. L.: The role of anaerobic bacteria in abscess formation. Ann Rev Med 1982; 33:217-29.

D. UROGENITAL INFECTIONS

158

URINARY TRACT INFECTION AND PYELONEPHRITIS

M. P. Glauser, M.D.

Urinary tract infections are among the most common human infections. They are responsible for considerable morbidity, and when associated with urinary obstruction or renal papillary damage lead to serious kidney damage.

DEFINITIONS. *Urinary tract infection* (UTI) is the presence of microorganisms in a properly collected specimen of urine (bacteriuria). UTI may be localized to any portion of the urinary tract and may be symptomatic or asymptomatic.

When present, the clinical presentation of UTI may be that either of *lower*, or of *upper* urinary tract symptoms.

Lower urinary tract symptoms are frequent urination, dysuria (difficult urination), odynuria (pain or burning while urinating), or suprapubic pain. Lower urinary tract symptoms most commonly result from vaginitis, cystitis, or the urethral syndrome. Acute *cystitis* defines those symptomatic patients having over 10^5 bacteria/ml upon culture of properly collected mid-stream urines, or any number of bacteria upon culture of urines collected directly from the bladder. The *acute urethral syndrome* refers to those symptomatic patients whose midstream urine culture grow less than 10^5 colonies/ml. Coliforms appear to cause most cases of either syndrome; the difference between both presentations is only in quantitative culture results.

Upper urinary tract symptoms are those of acute pyelonephritis.

Acute nonobstructive pyelonephritis, also referred to as acute pyelonephritis, is used *clinically* to describe the syndrome of acute illness with fever, flank pain, and tenderness combined with bacteriuria. Symptoms of lower urinary tract infection, such as frequency and dysuria, may coexist.

Acute suppurative pyelonephritis is acute inflammation, exudation, and suppuration due to bacterial infection of the kidney. This picture is seen when renal infection occurs during UTI in the presence of urinary tract abnormalities or underlying renal disease. It can lead to scar formation (chronic pyelonephritis).

Chronic pyelonephritis is the presence of scarring in the kidney parenchyma believed to be of infectious origin. Occasionally this may be extensive and severe enough to cause renal insufficiency. It probably occurs most often when children with urinary tract infection have severe vesico-ureteral reflux. Interstitial inflammation and scarring caused by infection is indistinguishable from renal inflammation of another origin (interstitial nephritis).

Interstitial nephritis is noninfectious renal interstitial inflammation and scarring from chronic obstruction, analgesic abuse, hyperuricemia, nephrosclerosis, diabetes, or sickle cell anemia.

ETIOLOGY. The vast majority of urinary tract infections are caused by Enterobacteriaceae originating from the gut. In ambulatory patients, the most common organism causing UTI is *Escherichia coli* (50 to 85 per cent of cases). This predominance is not as marked in patients who have hospital-acquired or repeated urinary tract infections treated with antibiotics, in whom *Proteus, Klebsiella, Pseudomonas*, and *S. faecalis* are frequently observed. Moreover, *Proteus* spp. may predominate in boys with UTI (Hallett et al., 1976). Brucellae and salmonellae may cause UTI, the latter especially in patients with associated urinary schistosomiasis (Hathout et al., 1966). Strict anaerobic bacteria are recovered from only 1 per cent of all cases of bacteriuria documented by suprapubic aspiration (Segura et al., 1972). Notwithstanding occasional anecdotal reports in immunocompromised patients, the role of "fastidious" slow-growing organisms, such as lactobacilli, microaerophilic streptococci, *Corynebacterium spp*, and *Gardnerella vaginalis*, in infections of the urinary tract and kidney is controversial (Maskell 1981).

Gram-positive cocci cause UTI less often than gram-negative bacteria. The frequency of coagulase-negative staphylococci *(S. saprophyticus)* is reported to be second only to *E. coli* as the cause of UTI in young women (Maskell, 1974; Stamm et al., 1980). *Staphylococcus aureus* found repeatedly in the urine may be the manifestation of renal microabscesses secondary to bacteremia, and a primary source of infection (e.g., endocarditis or osteomyelitis) should be sought.

Chlamydia trachomatis is a common cause of the urethral syndrome, in both sexes (Stamm et al., 1980). The roles of both *Mycoplasma hominis* and *Ureaplasma urealyticum* in urinary tract infections are much less well defined.

Candida albicans and other *Candida* spp may be found in diabetic women and in patients with indwelling catheters but usually represents harmless colonization. *Candida* found repeatedly in a properly collected urine specimen could originate from the kidney, a common site for metastatic infections during candidemia (Louria et al., 1962). Ascending *Candida* pyelonephritis is unusual (Tennant et al., 1968). Aspergillosis of the urinary tract is rare and occurs almost exclusively in patients with altered immunity (Flechner and McAninch, 1981). Cryptococcal pyelonephritis has been described in renal transplant patients (Hellman et al., 1981).

Viruses are frequently found in the urine during viral infections (Utz, 1974). Except for certain types of immune complex disease in which viruses could be deposited in the glomeruli, the role of viruses in kidney and urinary tract infections is poorly defined. Adenovirus Type 11 has been implicated in acute hemorrhagic cystitis in children (Numazaki et al., 1973). Cytomegalovirus and polyomavirus may cause persistent infections in transplanted kidneys, and have been implicated in acute rejection episodes (Fryd et al., 1980, Rosen et al., 1983).

PATHOGENESIS AND PATHOLOGY

Incidence. In the first week of life UTI appears to be mainly hematogenous and is more common in boys (Bergstrom et al., 1972). Thereafter, the incidence in girls rises almost linearly with increasing age, but boys are spared. UTI is found in about 1 per cent of school girls (Kunin et al., 1964) and reaches a peak of 10 to 12 per cent of women over 60 (Miall et al., 1962; Freedman et al., 1965). In men, on the other hand, infections are uncommon, with a prevalence of about 1 per cent at the age of 60 (Freedman et al., 1965). In certain areas endemic for urinary schistosomiasis, the prevalence in boys may be as high as 5 per cent (Laughlin et al., 1978).

Route of Infection and Host Defense Mechanisms. In nearly all patients, the microorganisms responsible for UTI originate from the intestinal aerobic gram-negative bacterial flora.

In women, the urethral meatus and the urethra normally harbor *Lactobacillus* spp, *S. epidermidis*, *Corynebacterium* spp, and anaerobes, but no aerobic gram-negative flora (Marrie et al., 1978). While urine does not seem to be inhibitory for enterobacteriaceae, it appears to possess some inhibitory activity against the indigenous urethral flora (Stamey and Mihara, 1980).

Enterobacteria are found in the vaginal vestibule of women who are about to develop UTI, sometimes just before the onset of bacteriuria (Stamey et al., 1971). Women resisting colonization possess vaginal antibodies against the fecal flora that are often lacking in women who become colonized (Stamey et al., 1978). Furthermore, vaginal cells from women with recurrent infections seem to attach *E. coli* more readily than cells from women who resist infection (Fowler and Stamey, 1977; Schaeffer et al., 1981). This may be mediated by attachment of bacteria to specific epithelial cell receptors, two of which have been well characterized so far. The first is a mannose-like receptor on the cell surface that binds to a mannose-specific substance on the surface of the bacterium (Ofek et al., 1977). This attachment may be prevented by specific competitive inhibition (Aronson et al., 1979), and possibly by the Tamm-Horsfall protein present in urinary slime (Orskov et al., 1980). Second, glycolipids of the globoseries, which are antigens of the P blood-group system, also seem to act as epithelial cell receptors. The P_1 blood-group phenotype seems to predispose to uncomplicated pyelonephritis (Lomberg et al., 1983), and glycolipid cell membrane analogues prevent experimental ascending UTI (Svanborg-Eden et al., 1982).

Whereas the vaginal vestibule is the reservoir for UTI in girls and women, there is evidence that in *boys* the preputial sac and possibly the urethra may play this role (Hallet et al., 1976). In *men* bacterial prostatitis, obstruction, and infection of the kidney are the major causes of UTI.

The short urethra of women favors the ascent of bacteria into the bladder. However, the antibacterial properties of prostatic fluid may also account for the increased resistance to UTI observed in men (Stamey et al., 1968). Mild trauma to the female urethra such as urethral milking (Bran et al., 1972) or sexual intercourse (Buckley et al., 1978) has been shown to increase the probability of finding bacteria in the bladder.

Incomplete emptying of the bladder with each voiding (congenital abnormalities, urethral strictures, cystocele, bladder diverticula, prostatic hypertrophy, neurologic disorders) favors UTI because it impedes the clearance of infected urine from the bladder lumen. The frequency of infection of retained urine may be increased in patients whose urine promotes growth of bacteria through factors such as high pH and favorable osmolality (Lees and Osborne, 1979). Furthermore, anatomic abnormalities and retention of urine may interfere with the natural bactericidal properties of the bladder mucosa and with the efficiency of phagocytosis. For these reasons, it may be particularly dangerous to carry vaginal and urethral microorganisms into the bladder with an instrument or indwelling catheter in patients with residual urine.

Urinary antibodies to the infecting microorganisms probably play a role in UTI. It has been observed that patients successfully treated for asymptomatic bacteriuria more often develop new symptomatic infections than do patients who have received no treatment at all (Asscher et al., 1969). This suggests that acquired antibodies might offer protection against the infecting strain and that treatment permits new virulent strains to infect the urinary tract. This observation is substantiated by the findings that specific urinary IgA antibodies prevent bacterial adherence to uroepithelial cells (Svanborg Edén and Svennerholm, 1978).

Bacterial Virulence. Several factors seem to play a role in the virulence of the *E. coli* strains that cause UTI. In symptomatic bacteriuric patients, the strains isolated from the urine are not necessarily the same as those isolated from a random sample of the fecal flora (Lindin-Janson et al., 1977). There is an increase in frequency and quantity of the K_1 capsular antigen on *E. coli* organisms cultured from patients with pyelonephritis (Kaijser, 1973), an observation also made in neonatal *E. coli* meningitis. The K_1 antigen appears to be related to increased tissue invasiveness and increased resistance to opsonization and phagocytosis.

Attachment of bacteria to epithelial cells appears to be an important mechanism of virulence in UTI. Bacterial adherence to human uroepithelial cells is increased in *E. coli* isolated from symptomatic bacteriuric patients and can be correlated with the presence of pili on their cell surfaces (Svanborg Edén and Hanson, 1978). It has been demonstrated experimentally that in ascending pyelonephritis pili are an important virulence factor and that antipili antibodies can protect against kidney infection (Silverblatt, 1974; Silverblatt and Cohen, 1979). At present two specific substances located on the pili seem to play a role in bacterial virulence. First, type I pili contain receptors for the epithelial cell surface mannose mentioned above. Second, mannose-independent pili are probably responsible for attachment to cell membrane glycolipids of the P blood-group system.

The need for attachment of bacteria to receptors on epithelial cells before inducing symptomatic UTI is controversial. Harder et al. (1982) have found that bacteria freshly voided from infected patients do not adhere well to epithelial cells, suggesting that bacterial factors promoting adherence might not be a virulence factor once bacteria have entered the urinary tract. Furthermore, receptors of the P blood-group do not correlate with recurrent pyelonephritis in patients with reflux, in contrast to the relationship mentioned above and found only in patients with *uncomplicated* pyelonephritis (Lomberg et al., 1983). These discordant findings might be reconciled by the hypothesis of Kunin (1982) that bacteria in the physiologically impaired urinary tract do not need special invasive properties. This hypothesis would fit very well with observations in experimental pyelonephritis, which show that almost any microorganism can cause pyelonephritis in the presence of obstruction (Glauser et al., 1985).

UTI in Patients with Indwelling Catheters. The risk of urinary infection in patients undergoing urethral catheterization is small in normal people but increases in hospitalized patients or in patients with urethrovesical abnormalities. In patients with long-term catheterization, infection is almost inevitable (Turck and Stamm, 1981). The routes of infection are mainly retrograde intraluminal bacterial spread in patients with "open" drainage systems, and retrograde extraluminal spread via the peri-urethral space in patients with "closed" drainage (Garibaldi et al., 1980). Despite all attempts at sterility when the catheter is inserted, regular cleaning of the meatal-catheter junction, closed drainage systems for collecting the urines, and regular antibiotic irrigations, infection rates increase steadily with the length of time the catheter is in place. Urethral catheter-associated infections are the most common hospital-acquired infections, cause considerable illness, and can be fatal. The most practical way to minimize this important problem is to use indwelling catheters only when absolutely necessary. When mandatory, the most important aspects of infection prevention are scrupulous aseptic technique in handling the catheter and cleansing the urethral meatal area.

Ascent of Infection to the Renal Pelvis and Parenchyma. Bacteria may ascend from the infected bladder to reach the kidney. There is no evidence of a lymphatic route of kidney infection. Hematogenous kidney infection occurs with *S. aureus*, *S. faecalis*, salmonellae and brucellae, fungi, *Mycobacterium tuberculosis*, and viruses. There is also experimental evidence that during severe reflux, *E. coli* may enter the bloodstream through pyelovenous communications and then recirculate to the kidney, producing pyelonephritis (Fierer et al., 1971). However, most infections spread to the kidney by way of the ureter and many factors predispose to it. A normal *vesicoureteral* valve probably prevents ascending infection. In children with vesicoureteral reflux, infected urine may reach the kidney freely. Furthermore, infection may cause vesicoureteral valve reflux (Kaveggia et al., 1966), and experimentally it has been shown to produce paralysis of ureteral peristalsis with subsequent dilatation. Reflux may not be necessary for bacteria to reach the renal pelvis because motile bacteria can ascend the ureter even against a descending flow (Braude, 1973).

Urinary tract obstruction occurring anywhere from the kidney to the urethral meatus predisposes not only to infection within the urinary tract but also to spread to the renal parenchyma. Calculi produce obstruction and act as a locus of infection where bacteria are protected from host defenses or antibacterial agents. Infection with urease-producing bacteria, such as *Proteus* spp or *Klebsiella*, results in alkaline urine, which favors the production of magnesium ammonium-phosphate stones. Thus, calculi may either be a cause or a result of urinary tract infections.

During pregnancy the incidence of UTI is not increased compared with nonpregnant women, but symptoms are more severe. The normal dilatation of the upper collecting system during pregnancy *increases the likelihood* that the infection will reach the kidney and produce the clinical syndrome of *acute pyelonephritis* (Norden and Kass, 1968).

Significance of Renal Involvement in Uncomplicated Urinary Tract Infections. Many methods for detecting kidney infection have been developed. These include measures of renal function (e.g., decreased urinary concentrating ability), increased serum antibody levels to the infecting organism, and increased leukocyte excretion (>20,000/ml) in the urine; culture of urine obtained by catheterization of the ureters; the bladder washout technique; and more recently, antibody coating of bacteria. It is generally believed that between 30 and 50 per cent of uncomplicated cases of UTI involve the kidney (Stamey et al., 1965; Fairley et al., 1971; Thomas et al., 1974).

The crucial question is: *what is the significance of kidney involvement during urinary tract infections in the absence of obstruction or underlying kidney disease?* Since population studies show that between 2 and 10 per cent of females have bacteriuria, and that between 20 and 50 per cent of women will contract UTI at some time during their lives, it is evidence that millions of people have kidney infections during their lifetime. If renal infection destroys kidney function, chronic pyelonephritis should be the leading cause of end-stage renal disease. Fortunately, this is not the case. Renal failure occurs in about 60 people per million population per year and is usually not of infectious origin. Among 173 dialysis candidates, Schechter and colleagues (1971) found that chronic pyelonephritis was the primary cause of end-stage renal failure in only 22 patients (13 per cent) and this condition was almost always associated with urinary tract abnormalities. Murray and Goldberg (1975) found that among 101 patients with end-stage interstitial nephritis, bacterial infection (present in 27 per cent) was found only in the presence of another preceding primary cause of renal damage. More recently, Huland and Bush (1982) in Germany described 42 patients with chronic pyelonephritis among 161 with end stage renal disease. All 42 had severe urinary tract abnormalities in addition to UTI. This epidemiologic evidence suggests that the bacteria reaching the kidney during uncomplicated UTI do not result in significant functional damage.

Acute Nonobstructive Pyelonephritis. This clinical symptom complex probably represents an acute infectious inflammatory episode occurring in the pelvis and/or the renal parenchyma. The evidence for parenchymal inflammation is the presence of white blood cell casts in the urine. However, very little is known about the pathologic features of this syndrome because the overwhelming majority of these patients recover and the kidneys are not examined histologically. Since multiple episodes of acute nonobstructive pyelonephritis do not seem to lead to kidney damage (Freedman and Andriole, 1974), the inflammation is probably not severe enough to cause irreversible necrosis.

Acute Suppurative Pyelonephritis and Papillary Necrosis. When kidney infection occurs in the presence of obstruction or renal disease such as chronic interstitial nephritis of various origins, susceptibility to renal damage increases considerably.

Much experimental as well as clinical evidence has shown that the papillae and the kidney medulla are especially susceptible to bacterial infection, particularly in the presence of obstruction (Freedman, 1979). Because antibacterial defenses are severely impaired in this hypertonic environment, the papillae and medulla have been called "an immunological desert" (Braude, 1973). Furthermore, the papilla and the medulla are susceptible to damage by analgesic drugs and probably to many other agents that are concentrated there during the process of excretion in the urine (chronic interstitial nephritis). The mechanism responsible for analgesic nephropathy seems to be mainly vascular insufficiency and secondary papillary and medullary ischemia (Freedman, 1979). When infection complicates obstruction or pre-existing papillary and medullary damage, it is so severe that the ensuing acute inflammation and suppuration cause permanent renal parenchymal damage (chronic pyelonephritis). *Papillary necrosis* may be precipitated and destroy a portion, if not all, of the kidney.

UTI in Childhood: Vesicoureteral Reflux, Intrarenal Reflux, and Renal Scarring. The greater part of progressive renal destruction due to infection probably occurs very early in life as a result of vesicoureteral reflux and infection. Most kidney scars develop before the age of 4 years. It has been demonstrated that the radiographic lesions called "chronic atrophic pyelonephritis" or "atrophic pyelonephritic scars" may be directly related to severe vesicoureteral reflux and intrarenal backflow of the urine (Hodson, 1969). In fact, the scars are most likely to develop at the very site where intrarenal reflux occurs (Rolleston et al., 1974). This clinical observation has been reproduced experimentally in piglets, in which intrarenal reflux has been shown to occur in those compound papillae whose papillary duct orifices cannot be occluded by a rise in the intracalyceal pressure (Ransley and Risdon, 1974). Furthermore, the renal scars develop in relation to refluxing papillae only when the urine is infected (Ransley and Risdon, 1978). In humans, because the scars occur very early in life and because reconstructive surgery in obstructive nephropathy should be performed before 1 year of age if renal function is to be preserved (Mayor et al., 1975), detecting reflux and infection in infancy may be a way of preventing chronic pyelonephritis. Prospective studies in girls have failed to show that persistent bacteriuria leads to scarring of the kidney if the kidneys were unscarred at the beginning of the follow-up period (Kincaid-Smith, 1983).

The Pathogenesis of Chronic Pyelonephritis. Chronic pyelonephritis may develop after acute infection of the kidney in the presence of obstruction or interstitial nephritis. More often it is the result of vesicoureteral reflux and infection early in childhood. When kidney scars are found in adults in the absence of complicating factors, the progression of lesions and the development of renal insufficiency does not seem to be related to urinary tract infection, but rather to hypertension or proteinuria (Arze et al., 1982). This suggests that continued kidney damage secondary to the presence of bacteria within the kidney parenchyma is of minor importance in the pathogenesis of chronic pyelonephritis.

Because chronic pyelonephritic kidneys are often sterile at autopsy, much experimental work has been performed in order to understand the pathogenesis of the disease. Mechanisms other than bacterial infection have been postulated. These include the persistence of bacterial protoplasts or of large amounts of bacterial antigens within the lesions and the existence of autoimmune mechanisms due to antigen-antibody complexes, immunity to Tamm-Horsfall protein, altered renal tissue antigenicity, or antibodies cross-reacting with common antigens shared by the infecting bacteria and renal tissue. A series of observations in both experimental animals and humans have suggested that chronic pyelonephritis results from kidney damage, scarring, and shrinkage secondary to suppuration and necrosis during acute complicated pyelonephritis and without persistent infection (Glauser et al., 1985).

CLINICAL MANIFESTATIONS. UTI may be asymptomatic. When symptomatic, the clinical manifestations of UTI are basically of two types: the symptoms of lower urinary tract infection (urethritis and cystitis) and the symptoms of upper urinary tract infection (acute nonobstructive pyelonephritis).

Urethritis and Cystitis

Patients with *urethritis* and/or bacterial cystitis complain of odynuria that is, pain or burning during urination, dysuria, i.e. difficulty urination, and urgency and frequency. *Cystitis* produces suprapubic pain, tenderness, and frequency due to diminished bladder capacity. In women, the symptoms of odynuria and frequency may also be due to vulvitis or vaginitis, both of which are usually accompanied by vaginal discharge. It has been suggested that when the complaint of pain or burning is felt to be inside the body ("internal" dysuria as opposed to "external" dysuria, in which pain or burning is felt to be in the labia) and when vaginal discharge is absent, there is a high probability that the cause is true urethritis due to UTI (Komaroff et al., 1978). Among women complaining of frequency and dysuria, between one-third and one-half do not have significant bacteriuria. These patients are regarded as having the *urethral syndrome*, the etiology of which seems to be either low numbers ($<10^5$/ml) of enterobacteria or *S. saprophyticus*, *C. trachomatis*, or, less often, *N. gonorrhoeae* in sexually active women. In a small portion of cases, the etiology is unknown (Stamm et al., 1980).

Fastidious anaerobic organisms from the vaginal flora may cause infection in some of these patients (Maskell et al., 1981). The study of Stamm et al. (1980) in young women with symptoms of dysuria and frequency has shown that the clinical presentation differed depending on the etiology of infection. Those women with bacteria recovered in bladder urine [whether in "significant" numbers ($\geq 10^5$/ml) or not ($<10^5$/ml)] more often had supra-pubic pain, a sudden onset of symptoms, a longer duration of illness, and a previous history of urinary tract symptoms during the preceding 2 years, than women with *C. trachomatis* infection. Furthermore, women with *C. trachomatis* infection used more oral contraceptives and more often had a new sex partner in the month before onset of symptoms.

Cystitis may be asymptomatic, or it may manifest itself, especially in older women, by malodorous urine or urinary incontinence. It is always difficult to be certain in the presence of cystitis symptoms that the infection is limited to the bladder, even in the absence of systemic symptoms such as fever. Their mere presence should alert the physician to possible renal infection and/or prostatitis or infection elsewhere in the body.

By far the most common cause of *cystitis* is the ascent of bacteria from the urethra in females. In males, it is almost always associated with prostatic or kidney infection. Rarely, cystitis may be due to urinary infections arising from contiguous infection from the bowel (diverticulitis, appendiceal abscess) or to viruses. *Acute cystitis* may occasionally develop without a demonstrable infectious agent, especially in men and boys (abacterial cystitis). *Chronic cystitis* may result if treatment of the acute phase has been insufficient or if incomplete voiding (residual urine) occurs. Chronic cystitis may be the manifestation of tuberculosis of the kidney and bladder, or it may be due to parasitic infections such as schistosomiasis or rarely, amebiasis or echinococcosis. *Interstitial cystitis* affects middle-aged women and is characterized by fibrosis of the bladder wall, thus decreasing the bladder capacity. Affected women present with a long history of progressive frequency and dysuria that mimics the urethral syndrome. Infection is rarely present, and the diagnosis is made by cystoscopy (Messing and Stamey, 1978). *Hemorrhagic cystitis* may follow radiation therapy of the bladder area or cyclophosphamide treatment.

Acute Nonobstructive Pyelonephritis ("Acute Pyelonephritis")

The syndrome of "acute pyelonephritis" is less frequently encountered as a manifestation of UTI than the symptoms of urethrocystitis. Acute pyelonephritis is predominantly a disease of young women. When it occurs in men, it is associated with a high incidence of obstruction (mainly prostatic hypertrophy), stones, or other urologic abnormalities. During pregnancy there is an increased likelihood of developing acute pyelonephritis from UTI.

The syndrome consists of flank pain, renal tenderness upon palpation, and fever and chills. It usually follows or is concomitant with symptoms of lower urinary tract infection. Nonspecific symptoms such as nausea, vomiting, diarrhea, or constipation may be confusing. Furthermore, flank pain and renal tenderness may be absent, or there may be a pain in the right upper abdominal quadrant that simulates acute cholecystitis. The symptoms of acute pyelonephritis may disappear spontaneously. Therefore, improvement of clinical symptoms does not indicate successful treatment once it has been started; improvement must be confirmed by sterility of subsequent urine cultures.

Next to bacteriuria, the key finding in confirming infectious inflammation of the kidney during acute pyelonephritis is leukocyte casts in fresh urine. Their absence should suggest a renal abscess or obstruction. Acute pyelonephritis is also accompanied by leukocytosis, and sometimes the infecting microorganism is recovered from the blood. Bacteremia should suggest the possibility of obstruction.

The prognosis for recovery from an episode of acute nonobstructive pyelonephritis is very good, and most patients respond rapidly to treatment.

COMPLICATIONS AND SEQUELAE

Gram-Negative Bacteremia. UTI is the main port of entry into the bloodstream by gram-negative rods and may be responsible for gram-negative septic shock and death (see Chapter 189). Bacteremia is especially likely to occur during UTI in patients who have underlying urologic or renal abnormalities. This is also true for patients who undergo urologic procedures because the instrument has to be introduced through the heavily colonized urethra and, in men, through an infected prostatic region. Metastatic infection secondary to urinary tract septicemia may localize in the spine, endocardium, or other parts of the body (Siroky et al., 1976).

Kidney Damage. Severe kidney damage has been described after acute pyelonephritis. In most cases, this is probably due to papillary necrosis in patients who had unrecognized or mild diabetes mellitus (Davidson and Talner, 1978) or other factors predisposing to interstitial nephritis.

The symptoms of acute infectious *papillary necrosis* are the same as those of acute pyelonephritis, but much more severe, and acute renal insufficiency follows if the process is bilateral. Death from intractable infection may also occur. In rare instances, papillary necrosis may evolve silently in the presence of UTI and may be identified later on pyelography. This is particularly likely to occur in diabetic patients.

End-stage chronic pyelonephritis, resulting from single or multiple bouts of exudative and suppurative infectious episodes, probably occurs in approximately 10 individuals per 1,000,000 population per year. It is doubtful if it ever occurs without concomitant urinary tract abnormality or underlying renal disease, either of which predisposes to progressive kidney damage (Schechter et al., 1971; Murray and Goldberg, 1975; Huland and Busch, 1982).

Renal and Perirenal Abscess, Emphysematous Pyelonephritis, and Xanthogranulomatous Pyelonephritis. Although renal and perirenal abscesses seem to have been caused in the past by the hematogenous spread of staphylococci (renal carbuncle), more recent series show that gram-negative rods predominate as the causative agents (Salvatierra et al., 1967; Thorley et al., 1974). A distinction has been proposed between the renal carbuncle, which is a blood-borne staphylococcal infection localized to the cortex of the kidney, and the gram-negative renal abscess, which originates in the renal medulla from urinary tract pathogens (Schiff et al., 1977). Most gram-negative bacterial *renal abscesses* are due to ascending UTI in association with obstruction, either in the kidney (renal calculi) or in the ureter. Less commonly, renal abscess is secondary to papillary necrosis, carcinoma, or infection of a renal cyst. Renal abscess may spread into the perinephric space, causing a *perinephric abscess.* Patients with renal and/or perirenal abscesses usually present with an insidious history of fever of two to three weeks' duration, flank and/or abdominal pain, leukocytosis, and, most often, pyuria. The long duration of the symptoms seems to distinguish these patients from those with acute nonobstructive pyelonephritis (Thorley et al., 1974). Furthermore, patients with renal and/or perirenal abscesses usually have an abnormal intravenous pyelogram (IVP) with an intrarenal mass, an altered renal silhouette, or a bulge in the renal outline. Perirenal abscess usually prevents movement of the affected kidney during deep inspiration and expiration (fixation of the kidney), a useful sign on IVP when abscesses are suspected. Ultrasound scans and computerized axial tomography may also be most helpful in this situation.

In diabetic patients, renal and perirenal suppuration and necrosis may be accompanied by the production of gas and may cause *emphysematous pyelonephritis* (Carris and Schmidt, 1977). This rare clinical picture is probably due to the bacterial fermentation of glucose by *E. coli* or other gram-negative enteric rods.

In some instances, mostly when obstruction is present, chronic renal infection and suppuration may evolve into *xanthogranulomatous pyelonephritis* (Goodman et al., 1979; Grainger et al., 1982). In this process, lipid-laden macrophages and epithelioid cells are found in the kidney and surrounding tissues. It occurs most frequently in middle-aged women, who present with nonspecific symptoms such as malaise and fatigue, fever and chills, flank pain, and recurrent episodes of UTI. In most cases there is pyuria, and IVP discloses an enlarged, nonfunctioning kidney, very often with calculi in the pelvis or ureter. The process is usually unilateral and may be localized to a part of the kidney, simulating a tumor. Cure is achieved by nephrectomy.

DIAGNOSIS

Collection of the Specimen. The diagnosis of UTI can be made only by finding bacteria in the urine. Because voided bladder urine may be contaminated by the resident microbiota of the urethra and vagina, urine collection must be performed with great care. In men, the glans penis must be cleansed with soap, water, and dried with sterile sponges. In women, while the labia are spread apart, careful washing of the urethral meatus must be performed from front to back with sponges soaked with soap. Disinfectants should not be used for cleaning because they may lower the bacterial count if they get into the urine sample. A specimen of "midstream" urine is then collected during forceful urination after the first 10 to 20 ml of urine have been voided ("urethral specimen"). When the patient cannot cooperate, catheterization or suprapubic aspiration may be necessary. The latter technique is safe and requires only a full bladder. After skin disinfection, a needle 10 to 12 cm long with a 0.9-mm diameter (3.5-inch, 20-gauge needle) affixed to a 20-ml syringe is inserted through the skin at the midline, about one-third of the distance from the symphysis pubis to the umbilicus, and directed toward the coccyx. Normal bladder urine is sterile, and microorganisms cultured from urine taken directly from the bladder should not be discarded as contaminants, even if present in low concentration. It is possible, however, that urine obtained by suprapubic aspiration may be contaminated by reversal of flow of urine which has already entered the urethra.

Because bacteria grow readily in urine, specimens that cannot be examined within one hour after collection should be kept refrigerated before being processed or discarded.

Quantitative Cultures. *Bacterial contamination* from the external genitalia usually results in less than 10^4 bacteria/ml of urine, provided the specimen has been properly collected and transported. However, it is not uncommon for even 10^5 bacteria/ml to be found in voided urine as a result of contamination, especially in elderly women (Moore-Smith, 1972). Two or more types of bacteria often indicate contamination. In *asymptomatic* patients, bacterial counts of 100,000 (10^5) or more per milliliter of clean-voided urine are usually found in true infections ("significant" bacteriuria). This large number of bacteria is partly due to bacterial multiplication in the bladder urine between urination.

The specimen of properly collected urine showing 10^5 bacteria makes a diagnosis of UTI 80 per cent likely; if two consecutive samples contain the same microorganism in concentrations of at least 10^5, there is a 95 per cent chance that true infection exists (Kass, 1957). In asymptomatic males, 10^5 bacteria recovered from a single clean-voided specimen of urine can be considered diagnostic of true UTI (Gleckman et al., 1979). In young *symptomatic* women, recent studies (Stamm, 1982) suggest that cultures should be examined for counts of coliform or *S. saprophyticus* starting at 10^2 bacteria/ml. Because pure cultures of the isolate obtained from midstream urine are not to be expected with such low numbers of bacteria (Stamey, 1965), Stamm's studies (1982) suggest that mixed cultures should not be disregarded. This is in contrast to the criterion of

10^5 colonies/ml when screening urine specimens from *asymptomatic* women.

Samples from the ureters, from the renal pelvis, or from renal urine may have few bacteria and yet indicate infection. Furthermore, lower bacterial counts may be found in patients who are undergoing diuresis, have indwelling catheters or ileal conduits, or receive inadequate antibacterial drugs. Therefore, any degree of bacteriuria should be evaluated in a patient with urinary tract symptoms. The *first morning specimen*, which should be examined whenever possible, may give more clear-cut results because it gives bacteria the opportunity to grow overnight in the bladder urine.

Quantitative cultures of urine are made by culturing a known amount of urine on a solid medium by either the pour-plate technique or the quantitative loop. The dip-slide method is simpler and probably dependable. Dip slides are plastic slides coated with culture media and are sold commercially so that quantitative cultures of urine are available in doctors' offices, and at the bedside at home or in the hospital.

Microscopic Examination. The fresh uncentrifuged urine may be looked at with or without gram staining (Barbin et al., 1978). When the bacteria count is around 10^5 or more, at least one bacterium per high-power field ($\times$ 1000) is likely to be seen, but specimens containing less than 10^4 organisms usually show no organisms in several fields. Pyuria (i.e., leukocytes in the urine) may also be found by microscopic examination of urine, but leukocytes in the urine of *asymptomatic* patients do not mean that UTI is present. Vaginal infection, prostatitis, urethritis, urinary stones, renal tuberculosis, glomerulitis, interstitial nephritis, and other diseases may produce white blood cells in the urine. Sterile urine samples with pyuria should be cultured for mycobacteria. In most *symptomatic* cases, leukocytes are present on microscopic examination of uncentrifuged urine. Women with lower UTI symptoms, whether caused by coliforms or by *C. trachomatis*, have $\geq$ 10/mm^3 leukocytes in centrifuged urine (Stamm 1980). Measurement of pyuria in symptomatic women may therefore be useful in diagnosis.

Red blood cells in the urine may result from UTI or other causes of inflammation, but red cell casts suggest glomerulitis. Microscopic or macroscopic hematuria (hemorrhagic cystitis) is often found in patients with coliform UTI but seems to be rare in *C. trachomatis* infections (Stamm, 1980).

Numerous squamous epithelial cells of vaginal origin indicate improper collection of the specimen and contamination. Squamous epithelial cells may also originate from the trigone; normally, this portion of the bladder is covered by a transitional epithelium, but inflammation may cause squamous metaplasia there, particularly in postmenopausal women.

Radiologic Evaluation. In women, an IVP should be performed only after repeated episodes of urinary infection that may be due to urinary tract abnormalities or stones. However, the vast majority of women with recurrent UTI do not present abnormalities (Fair et al., 1979). In men, urinary tract infections are relatively rare, so that IVP is warranted after the first infectious episode mainly to detect obstruction.

During acute nonobstructive pyelonephritis, the IVP is normal in most patients (Little et al., 1965). Severe involvement may cause enlargement of the kidney as well as a generalized or focal decrease in the nephrographic density, reflecting the patchy distribution of the pyelonephritic process. The ureter and pelvis often show dilatation resembling obstruction. This is due to inhibition of peristalsis by gram-negative bacilli (Harrison and Schaffer, 1979).

It seems reasonable to perform an IVP to rule out obstruction in patients presenting with symptoms of acute pyelonephritis that do not respond promptly to proper antibiotic treatment. Obstruction in the presence of acute pyelonephritis must be relieved.

Radiologic distinction between localized pyelonephritis and an abscess may be difficult. Evolution toward perirenal abscess may be indicated by disappearance of the renal outline and by fixation of the kidney (see Complications and Sequelae). Ultrasound examination and computerized axial tomography may help demonstrate pus in or around the kidney. The presence of gas indicates emphysematous pyelonephritis.

In the rare patient who presents late radiologic sequelae of acute nonobstructive pyelonephritis, wasting of the kidney parenchyma develops a few weeks after the acute episode, with deformities of the papillae and calyces (Davidson and Talner, 1978). This suggests that papillary necrosis may accompany the most severe forms of acute pyelonephritis.

TREATMENT

Asymptomatic Urinary Tract Infections. As already suggested in the *Pathogenesis* section, there is no real evidence of a need to treat asymptomatic urinary tract infections in nonpregnant women. On the other hand, asymptomatic UTI in preschool children with vesicoureteral reflux may need treatment because some of them are likely to develop kidney scarring and possibly renal failure. Similarly, patients with urinary tract obstruction or renal disease should be treated in order to prevent severe renal infection. Eradication of asymptomatic bacteriuria in a pregnant woman is mandatory because it will prevent acute pyelonephritis.

Symptomatic Urinary Infections. In symptomatic patients with infection, most antibacterial drugs that reach adequate urinary concentrations will clear the infection. The real questions—and the subject of controversy—are what dosage and for how long.

In an in vitro model simulating bladder conditions with periodic dilution and discharge, a heavy bacterial population is suppressed when exposed to a single dose of many antibacterial drugs (Greenwood and O'Grady, 1977). This experimental observation correlates with the clinical efficacy of a *single-dose treatment*, in patients with urinary infections localized to the bladder (Ronald et al., 1976; Fang et al., 1978; Fairley et al., 1978).

However, in patients with infection localized to the kidney, infection with the same bacteria (*relapse*) recurs frequently after single-dose treatment (Ronald et al. 1976). Even conventional therapy for 10 days may not prevent relapsing infection in half of the patients (Fang et al., 1978; Gargen et al., 1983). Nevertheless, since renal involvement during uncomplicated UTI is not an immediate threat to the patient, single-dose treatment is appropriate as initial therapy. If relapse does occur (usually during the days or first weeks following treatment), a more *prolonged course (10 to 15 days) of therapy* should be given. In fact, there are strong suggestions that 6 weeks of antimicrobial therapy might be needed to eradicate relapsing infections. This has been shown in women with infection originating from the upper urinary tract (Turck, 1978), in renal transplant pa-

Table 1. TREATMENT OF URINARY TRACT INFECTION

Infection	Treatment of Choice	Alternate
Lower urinary tract symptoms with >10 leukocytes/mm³ of urine		
Bacteria seen microscopically in uncentrifuged urines, microorganisms not yet identified.	A single dose of trimethoprim 160 mg—sulfamethoxazole 800 mg or amoxicillin 3 g	Sulfisoxasole 1.0 g two to four times daily for 5 to 8 days Ampicillin or amoxicillin 250 mg three to four times daily for 5 to 8 days Nalidixic acid 1.0 g four times daily Trimethoprim 200 mg twice daily for 5 to 8 days
No bacteria seen microscopically.	Doxycycline[2] 100 mg twice daily for 10 days	
Urethritis or cystitis symptoms, microorganism identified.	*E. coli* as above	As above
	P. mirabilis[1] Amoxicillin (or ampicillin) 250 mg three to four times daily for 5 to 8 days	Trimethoprim 160 mg* sulfamethoxazole 800 mg twice daily for 5 to 8 days or cephalexin 250 mg daily four times daily for 5 to 8 days
	K. pneumoniae[1] Trimethoprim 160 mg sulfamethoxazole 800 mg twice daily for 5 to 8 days	Cephalexin 250 mg three to four times daily for 5 to 8 days
	P. aeruginosa,[1] *E. aerogenes,*[1] *P. vulgaris*[1] Indanyl carbenillin 1.0 g or tetracycline 250 mg, four times daily for 5 to 8 days	Gentamicin or tobramycin 40 mg I.M. twice daily for 5 to 8 days
	S. fecalis Amoxicillin (or ampicillin) 250 mg three to four times daily for 5 to 8 days	Tetracycline[2] 250 mg orally four times daily for 5 to 8 days
	C. albicans Amphotericin B 50 mg in 1 liter for continuous irrigation of the bladder during 6 days (Wise et al., 1982)	
Upper Urinary Tract Symptoms		
Pyelonephritis, organism not known.	Amoxicillin (or ampicillin) 500 mg to 2.0 g four times daily I.V. (consider adding I.V. gentamicin or tobramycin 1.0 to 1.5 mg/kg three times daily) until evident clinical improvement Follow with amoxicillin (or ampicillin) 500 mg four times daily, for a minimum of 14 days	Amoxicillin or ampicillin 500 mg to 1.0 g orally four times daily for 10 to 14 days or trimethoprim 160 mg* sulfamethoxazole 800 mg orally or cefamandole or cefotaxime or moxalactam 1 g I.V. four times daily, until evident clinical improvement Follow with oral drug according to susceptibility testing; consider 6 weeks treatment
Pyelonephritis, microorganism identified.	*E. coli* As above	As above
	P. mirabilis[1] As above	As above, or cephalexin 500 mg four times daily for 14 days

Table continued on opposite page

Table 1. TREATMENT OF URINARY TRACT INFECTION (*Continued*)

Infection	Treatment of Choice	Alternate
	K. pneumoniae[1]	
	Cephamandole or cefotaxime or moxalactam 1 g I.V. four times daily (consider adding gentamicin or tobramycin 1.0 to 1.5 mg/kg three times daily) until evident clinical improvement Follow with cephalexin 500 mg to 1.0 g four times daily or trimethoprim 160 mg* sulfamethoxazole 800 mg twice daily for a total duration treatment of 14 days	Cephalexin 500 mg four times daily or trimethoprim 160 mg* sulfamethoxazole 800 mg orally twice daily for a minimum of 14 days
	P. aeruginosa[1], *P. vulgaris*[1], *E. aerogenes*[1]	
	Ticarcllin 5.0 g (or carbenicillin 10 g) I.V. three times daily (consider adding gentamicin[3] or tobramycin[3] 1.0 to 1.5 mg/kg three times daily) for 14 days	Piperacillin or azlocillin 5.0 g three times daily (consider adding amikacin 7.5 mg/kg I.M. or I.V. twice daily) for 14 days; consider following with indanylcarbenicillin 1.0 g or tetracycline 0.5 g orally four times daily for several weeks
	S. Fecalis	
	Amoxycillin (or ampicillin) 500 mg to 2.0 g I.V. four times daily plus gentamicin or tobramycin 1.0 to 1.5 mg/kg three times daily for 14 days	Vancomycin 1.0 g I.V. twice daily for 14 days or vancomycin 1.0 g I.V. twice daily plus gentamicin or tobramycin 1.0 to 1.5 mg/kg three times daily for a minimum of 14 days.
	B. suis	
	Tetracycline[2] 500 mg orally four times daily plus streptomycin 1.0 g I.M. daily, for two to four weeks	Tetracycline[2] 500 mg orally four times daily for two to four days or trimethoprim 160 mg* sulfamethoxazole 800 mg twice daily orally for 2 to 4 weeks
	C. albicans	
	Amphotericin B 20 to 50 mg I.V. every other day	Amphotericin B 20 to 30 mg I.V. every other day plus 5-fluorocytosine 30 to 40 mg/kg orally three to four times daily
	M. tuberculosis	
	Isoniazid 300 mg orally, plus ethambutol 1.0 g orally daily	Isoniazid 300 mg orally plus ethambutol 1.0 g orally plus rifampin 600 mg orally daily or streptomycin 1.0 g I.M. daily plus paraaminosalicylic acid 2.0 g orally every 6 hours

1. Because of inconstant sensitivity to antibiotics, susceptibility testing should be performed.
2. Tetracycline should be avoided in pregnant women, infants, and young children.
3. Gentamicin, tobramycin, and amikacin should *not* be mixed with ticarcillin or carbenicillin in the same solution. They must be injected separately.

*Trimethoprim-sulfamethoxazole.

tients with UTI (Rubin 1979) and in men with recurrent UTI (Gleckman 1979).

In addition to renal infection, relapse may be due to infection within a stone, or to prostatic hypertrophy or chronic bacterial prostatis. In selected patients, a relapse after single-dose therapy may warrant an IVP, since abnormal pyelograms are seen more frequently in relapsing patients treated with single-dose therapy (Fang et al., 1978; Fairley et al., 1978). However, the possible side effects and cost of IVP should be weighed against the good long-term prognosis of UTI.

In women, *reinfection* by new organisms is much more common than relapse. It usually occurs within one month of stopping treatment and increases in frequency with the passage of time.

Urine cultures performed 24 to 48 hours after starting or at the end of therapy should be sterile. The persistence of bacteria may represent inadequate dosage or, more likely, resistance to the drug.

Acute Pyelonephritis Syndrome, UTI in the Presence of Obstruction, and Renal Abscess. Acute pyelonephritis should be treated with drugs in dosages large enough to reach adequate concentrations in the renal parenchyma. There are several reasons why this attitude is justified. First, many patients are severely ill and when they are first seen, it is not known whether they have obstruction, deformity, or underlying renal disease that may precipitate bacteremia, renal abscess, or papillary necrosis. Experimentally, it has been shown that in acute suppurative pyelonephritis due to obstruction, the earlier treatment is initiated, the greater the protection against renal parenchymal destruction (Glauser et al., 1978). Furthermore, a combination of antibiotics that is synergistic in vitro against the infecting organism, such as a beta-lactam antibiotic with an aminoglycoside, has been experimentally shown in vivo to achieve sterility faster and more reliably than either drug alone (Glauser et al., 1979a). Since sterility must be achieved in order to prevent relapse in the presence of obstruction, a combination of synergistic antibiotics might be recommended whenever possible. In addition to surgical drainage, the same therapeutic considerations apply to the treatment of gram-negative renal and perirenal abscesses. Renal carbuncles (see Complications and Sequelae) have been successfully treated without drainage with long-term penicillinase-resistant penicillins (Schiff et al., 1977).

Choice of Drug. Most symptomatic patients with UTI can be treated with orally administered drugs such as a sulfonamide, a combination of sulfonamide and trimethoprim, ampicillin, or amoxycillin (see Table 1). Because of potentially fatal side effects, especially in older patients and women, the use of nitrofurantoin has been questioned (Holmberg et al., 1980). After microscopic examination for the presence of bacteria and enumeration of leukocytes in order to make a diagnosis of UTI likely, a dip-slide quantitative culture should be performed. Treatment then can be started without awaiting culture results. Symptomatic patients with pyuria and no bacteria visible microscopically (i.e., patients likely to have the acute urethral syndrome, due either to low count *E. coli* or *S. saprophyticus* or to *C. trachomatis* infections) may be successfully treated with doxycycline (Stamm, 1981).

Improvement of clinical symptoms does not correlate with successful treatment, since improvement frequently occurs in the absence of any treatment or in patients who receive ineffective treatment. If the culture performed 24 to 48 hours after starting therapy on ambulatory patients is sterile, the specimen cultured before treatment can be discarded without identification or antibiotic sensitivity tests. On the other hand, if there is any doubt about the efficacy of treatment, drug treatment should be adjusted according to sensitivity tests on the initial culture.

Patients with acute pyelonephritis should be treated with drugs that achieve serum and tissue bactericidal activity. Ampicillin or amoxicillin may be the drug of choice, but a cephalosporin may be necessary in some instances, depending upon the sensitivity tests, and the local epidemiologic situation. In Switzerland for instance, 18 per cent of *E. coli* strains isolated from the general population are resistant to ampicillin (Braun et al., 1981). A synergistic combination of a beta-lactam antibiotic with an aminoglycoside may be indicated if suppuration is suspected, especially in the presence of obstruction.

Specific treatment schedules are given in Table 1.

PROPHYLAXIS. Some patients are so disturbed or incapacitated by recurrent symptomatic episodes of UTI that prolonged therapy or prophylaxis may be necessary. Since these symptomatic episodes are often related to recent sexual activity, one dose of almost any oral antimicrobial, taken just after sexual intercourse, will prevent these episodes (Vosti et al., 1975).

Long-term prophylactic use of low-dose antimicrobial drugs reduces the frequency of recurrent symptomatic UTI in children, women, and men. Before such prophylaxis is started, however, the urine should be sterilized with an antimicrobial drug. Half a tablet of a combination of sulfamethoxazole-trimethoprim (200 mg and 20 mg, respectively), taken at bedtime (so that antibacterial activity will be maintained in the urine during the night) seems to be the best available drug, probably because it inhibits the enterobacteriaceae in the fecal flora and because trimethoprim concentrates in the vaginal secretions and prevents colonization of the periurethral area (Harding and Ronald, 1974; Stamey et al., 1977). In fact, half a tablet at bedtime three times a week seems to be just as effective as every day (Harding et al., 1979). Nitrofurantoin, 50 mg nightly, is also used with success but, at least in men, has not been shown to be as effective as the sulfamethoxazole-trimethoprim combination (Scherwin and Holm, 1977). A sulfonamide alone or methenamine-mandelate with acidification of the urine is probably less effective (Harding and Ronald, 1974; Vainrub and Muscher, 1977).

Because they accumulate and persist in the kidney parenchyma, from which they are slowly excreted, aminoglycoside antibiotics are promising prophylactic drugs. When used in low doses, they prevent experimental UTI and pyelonephritis, even in the presence of obstruction (Glauser et al., 1979b).

CONCLUSION. UTI occurs predominantly in females. Except in very young children with vesicourethral reflux, in pregnant women, and in the presence of obstruction or underlying renal disease, it is a self-limited disease with little risk of long-term damage to the patient Many drugs are available for treatment, but their cost and possible side effects should be weighed against the mildness of the disease. Very effective prophylaxis exists for patients with frequent recurrent symptomatic UTI.

References

Aronson, M., Medaliz, O., Schori, L. Mirelman, D., Sharon, N., and Ofek, I.: Prevention of colonization of the urinary tract of mice with *Escherichia coli* by blocking of bacterial adherence with methyl α-D-mannopyranoside. J Infect Dis 139:329, 1979.

Arze, R. S., Ramos, J. M., Owen, J. P., Morley, A. R., Elliott, R. W., Wilkinson, R., Ward, M. K., and Kerr, D. N. S.: The natural history of chronic pyelonephritis in the adult. Q J Med 204:396, 1982.

Asscher, A. W., Sussman, M., Waters, W. E., Evans, J. A. S., Campbell, H., Evans, K. T., and Williams, J. E.: Asymptomatic significant bacteriuria in the non-pregnant woman. II. Response to treatment and follow-up. Br Med J 1:804, 1969.

Barbin, G. K., Thorley, J. D., and Reinerz, J. A.: Simplified microscopy for rapid detection of significant bacteriuria in random urine specimens. J Clin Microbiol 7:286, 1978.

Bergstrom, T., Larsson, H., Lincoln, K., and Winberg, J.: Studies of urinary tract infections in infancy and childhood. XII. Eighty consecutive patients with neonatal infection. J Pediat 80:858, 1972.

Bran, J. L., Levison, M. E., and Kaye, D.: Entrance of bacteria into the female urinary bladder. N Engl J Med 286:626, 1972.

Braude, A. I.: Current concepts of pyelonephritis. Medicine 52:257, 1973.

Braun, R., Fitzi, K., Gutzwiller, F., Hohl, H. R., van der Linde, F., and Gelzer, J.: Resistenzhäufigkeit von *Escherichia coli* in der Schweiz. Schweiz med Wschr 111:1048, 1981.

Buckley, R. M., McGuckin, M., and MacGregor, R. R.: Urine bacterial counts after sexual intercourse. N Engl J Med 298:321, 1978.

Carris, C. K., and Schmidt, J. D.: Emphysematous pyelonephritis. J Urol 118:457, 1977.

Davidson, A. J., and Talner, L. B.: Late sequelae of adult-onset acute bacterial nephritis. Radiology 127:367, 1978.

Fair, W. R., McClennan, B. L., and Gilbert Jost, R.: Are excretory urograms necessary in evaluating women with urinary tract infection? J Urol 121:313, 1979.

Fairley, K. F., Whitworth, J. A., Kincaid-Smith, P., and Durman, O.: Single-dose therapy in management of urinary tract infection. Med J Aust 2:75, 1978.

Fang, L. S. T., Tolkoff-Rubin, N. E., and Rubin, R. H.: Efficacy of single-dose and conventional amoxicillin therapy in urinary-tract infection localized by the antibody-coated bacteria technic. N Engl J Med 298:413, 1978.

Fierer, J., Talner, L., and Braude, A. I.: Bacteremia in the pathogenesis of retrograde *E. coli* pyelonephritis in the rat. Am J Pathol 64:443, 1971.

Flechner, S. M., McAninch, J. W.: Aspergillosis of the urinary tract: ascending route of infection and evolving patterns of disease. J Urol 125:598, 1981.

Fowler, J. E., and Stamey, T. A.: Studies on introital colonization in women with recurrent urinary infections. VII. The role of bacterial adherence. J Urol 117:472, 1977.

Freedman, L. R., Phair, J. P., Seki, M., Hamilton, H. B., and Nefzger, M. D.: The epidemiology of urinary tract infections in Hiroshima. Yale J Biol Med 37:262, 1965.

Freedman, L. R.: Interstitial renal inflammation, including pyelonephritis and urinary tract infection. In Earley, L. E., and Gottschalk, C. W. (eds.): Strauss and Welt's Diseases of the Kidney. Boston, Little, Brown & Company, 1979, p. 817.

Freedman, L. R., and Andriole, V.: The long-term follow-up of women with urinary tract infections. Villareal, H. (ed.): Proceedings of the 5th International Congress of Nephrology, Mexico 1972, vol. 3. Basel, S. Karger, 1974, p. 230.

Fryd, D. S., Peterson, P. K., Ferguson, R. M., Simmons, R. L., Balfour, H. H., Jr., and Najarian, J. S.: Cytomegalovirus as a risk factor in renal transplantation. Transplantation 30:436, 1980.

Gargan, R. A., Brumfitt, W., and Hamilton-Miller, J. M. T.: Antibody-coated bacteria in urine: criterion for a positive test and its value in defining a higher risk of treatment failure. Lancet ii:704, 1983.

Garibaldi, R. A., Burke, J. P., Britt, M. R., Miller, W. A., and Smith, C. B.: Meatal colonization and catheter-associated bacteriuria. N Engl J Med 303:316, 1980.

Glauser, M. P., Lyons, J. M., and Braude, A. I.: Prevention of chronic experimental pyelonephritis by suppression of acute suppuration. J Clin Invest 61:403, 1978;

Glauser, M. P., Lyons, J. M., and Braude, A. I.: Synergism of ampicillin and gentamicin against obstructive pyelonephritis due to *Escherichia coli* in rats. J Infect Dis 139:133, 1979a.

Glauser, M. P., Lyons, J. M., and Braude, A. I.: Prevention of pyelonephritis due to *Escherichia coli* in rats with gentamicin stored in the kidney. J Infect Dis 139:172, 1979b.

Glauser, M. P., Ransley, P., and Bille, J.: Urinary tract infections, pyelonephritic scars, and chemotherapy. In Zak, O., and Sande, M. (eds.): Animal Models of infectious diseases. New York, Academic Press, in press, 1985.

Gleckman, R., Crowley, M., and Natsios, G. A.: Therapy of recurrent invasive urinary-tract infections of men. N Engl J Med 301:878, 1979.

Gleckman, R., Esposito, A., Crowley, M., and Natsios, G. A.: Reliability of a single urine culture in establishing diagnosis of asymptomatic bacteriuria in adult males. J Clin Microbiol 9:596, 1979.

Goodman, M., Curry, T., and Russel, T.: Xanthogranulomatous pyelonephritis: A local disease with systemic manifestations. Report of 23 patients and review of the literature. Medicine 58:171, 1979.

Grainger, R. G., Longstaff, A. J., and Larsons, M. A.: Xanthogranulomatous pyelonephritis: a reappraisal. Lancet i:1398, 1982.

Greenwood, D., and O'Grady, F.: Is your dosage really necessary? Antibiotic dosage in urinary infection. Br Med J 2:665, 1977.

Hallett, R. J., Pead, L., and Maskell, R.: Urinary infection in boys. A three-year prospective study. Lancet 2:1107, 1976.

Harber, M. J., Chick, S., Mackenzie, R., and Asscher, A. W.: Lack of adherence to epithelial cells by freshly isolated urinary pathogens. Lancet i:586, 1982.

Harding, G. K. M., and Ronald, A. R.: A controlled study of antimicrobial prophylaxis of recurrent urinary infection in women. N Engl J Med 291:597, 1974.

Harding, G. K. M., Buckwold, F. J., Marrie, T. J., Thompson, L., Light, R. B., and Ronald, A. R.: Prophylaxis of recurrent urinary tract infection in female patients: Efficacy of low-dose, thrice-weekly therapy with trimethoprim-sulfamethoxazole. JAMA 242:1975, 1979.

Harrison, R. B., and Schaffer, H. A.: The roentgenographic findings in acute pyelonephritis. JAMA 241:1718, 1979.

Hathout, S., Ghaffar, Y., Awny, A., and Hassan, K.: Relation between urinary schistosomiasis and chronic enteric carrier state among Egyptians. Am J Trop Med 15:156, 1966.

Hellman, R. N., Hinrichs, J., Sicard, G., Hoover, R., Golden P., and Hoffsten, P.: Cryptococcal pyelonephritis and disseminated cryptococcosis in a renal transplant recipient. Arch Intern Med 141:128, 1981.

Hodson, C. J.: The effects of disturbance of flow on the kidney. J Infect Dis 120:54, 1969.

Holmberg, L., Boman, G., Böttiger, L. E., Eriksson, B., Spross, R., and Wessling, A.: Adverse reactions to nitrofurantoin. Analysis of 921 reports. Am J Med 69:733, 1980.

Huland, H., and Busch, R.: Chronic pyelonephritis as a cause of end stage renal disease. J Urol 127:642, 1982.

Kaijser, B.: Immunology of *Escherichia coli:* K antigen and its relation to urinary-tract infection. J Infect Dis 127:670, 1973.

Kass, E. H.: Bacteriuria and the diagnosis of infections of the urinary tract. Arch Intern Med 100:709, 1957.

Kaveggia, L., King, L. R., Grana, L., and Idriss, F. S.: Pyelonephritis: A cause of vesicoureteral reflux? J Urol 95:158, 1966.

Kincaid-Smith, P.: Reflux nephropathy. Br Med J 286:2002, 1983.

Komaroff, A. L., Pass, T. M., McCue, J. D., Cohen, A. B., Hendricks, T. M., and Friedland, G.: Management strategies for urinary and vaginal infections. Arch Intern Med 138:1069, 1978.

Kunin, C. M., Deutscher, R., and Paquin, A., Jr.: Urinary tract infection in school children: an epidemiologic, clinical and laboratory study. Medicine 43:91, 1964.

Kunin, C. M.: Urinary tract infection: new information concerning pathogenesis and management. J Urol 128:1233, 1982.

Laughlin, L. W., Farid, Z., Mansour, N., Edman, D. C., and Higashi, G. I.: Bacteriuria in urinary schistosomiasis in Egypt. Am J Trop Med 27:916, 1978.

Lees, G. E., and Osborne, C. A.: Antibacterial properties of urine: A comparative review. J Am Anim Hosp Assoc 15:125, 1979.

Lindin-Janson, G., Hanson, L. A., Kaijser, B., Lincoln, K., Lindberg, U., Olling, S., and Wedel, H.: Comparison of *Escherichia coli* from bacteriuric patients with those from feces of healthy school children. J Infect Dis 136:346, 1977.

Little, P. J., McPherson, D. R., and de Wardener, H. E.: The appearance of the intravenous pyelogram during and after acute pyelonephritis. Lancet 1:1186, 1965.

Lomberg, H., Hanson, L. A., Jacobsson, B., Jodal, U., Leffler, H., and Svanborg Edén, C.: Correlation of P blood group, vesicoureteral reflux, and bacterial attachment in patients with recurrent pyelonephritis. N Engl J Med 308:1189, 1983.

Louria, D. B., Stiff, D. P., and Bennet, B.: Disseminated moniliasis in adults. Medicine 41:307, 1962.

Marrie, T. J., Harding, G. K. M., and Ronald, A. R.: Anaerobic and aerobic urethral flora in healthy females. J Clin Microbiol 8:67, 1978.

Maskell, R.: Importance of coagulase-negative staphylococci as pathogens in the urinary tract. Lancet 1:1155, 1974.

Maskell, R.: Should "fastidious" organisms alter our approach to the treatment of urinary symptoms? J Antimicrob Chemother 7:315, 1981.

Mayor, G., Genton, N., Torrado, A., and Guignard, J. P.: Renal function in obstructive nephropathy: long-term effect of reconstructive surgery. Pediatrics 56:740, 1975.
Meesing, E. M., and Stamey, T. A.: Interstitial cystitis: early diagnosis, pathology and treatment. Urology 12:381, 1978.
Miall, W. E., Kass, E. H., Ling, J., and Stuart, K. L.: Factors influencing arterial pressure in the general population in Jamaica. Br Med J 2:497, 1962.
Moore-Smith, B.: Bacteriuria in elderly women. Lancet ii:827, 1972.
Murray, T., and Goldberg, M.: Chronic interstitial nephritis: Etiologic factors. Ann Intern Med 82:453, 1975.
Norden, C. W., and Kass, E. H.: Bacteriuria of pregnancy—a critical appraisal. Annu Rev Med 19:431, 1968.
Numazaki, Y., Kumasaka, T., Yano, N., Yamanaka, M., Miyazawa, T., Takai, S., and Ishida, N.: Further study on acute hemorrhagic cystitis due to adenovirus type 11. N Engl J Med 289:344, 1973;
Ofek, I., Mirelman, D., and Sharon, N.: Adherence of *Escherichia coli* to human mucosal cells mediated by mannose receptors. Nature 265:623, 1977.
Orskov, I., Ferencz, A., and Orskov, F.: Tamm-Horsfall protein or uromucoid is the normal urinary slime that traps type I fimbriated *Escherichia coli*. Lancet i:887, 1980.
Ransley, P. G., and Risdon, R. A.: Renal papillae and intrarenal reflux in the pig. Lancet 2:1114, 1974.
Ransley, P. G., and Risdon, R. A.: Reflux and renal scarring. Br J Radiol Suppl 14, 1978.
Rolleston, G. L., Maling, T. M. J., and Hodson, C. J.: Intrarenal reflux and the scarred kidney. Arch Dis Childh 49:531, 1974.
Ronald, A. R., Boutros, P., and Mourtada, H.: Bacteriuria localization and response to single-dose therapy in women. JAMA 235:1854, 1976.
Rosen, S., Harmon, W., Krensky, A. M., Edelson, P. J., Padgett, B. L., Grinnell, B. W., Rubino, M. J., and Walker, D. L.: Tubulo-interstitial nephritis associated with polyomavirus (BK type) infection. N Engl J Med 308:1192, 1983.
Rubin, R. H., Fang, L. S. T., Cosimi, A. B., Herrin, J. I., Varga, P. A., Russel, P. S. and Tolkoff-Rubin, N. E.: Usefulness of the antibody coated bacteria assay in the management of urinary tract infection in the renal transplant patient. Transplantation 27:18, 1979.
Salvatierra, O., Buckley, W. B., and Morrow, J. W.: Perinephric abscess: a report of 71 cases. J Urol 98:296, 1967.
Savage, D. C. L., Adler, K., Howie, G., and Wilson, M. I.: Controlled trial of therapy in covert bacteriuria of childhood. Lancet 1:358, 1978.
Schaeffer, A. J., Jones, J. M., and Dunn, J. K.: Association of in vitro *Escherichia coli* adherence to vaginal and buccal epithelial cells with susceptibility of women to recurrent urinary-tract infections. N Engl J Med 304:1062, 1981.
Schechter, H., Leonard, C. D., and Scribner, B. H.: Chronic pyelonephritis as a cause of renal failure in dialysis candidates. JAMA 216:514, 1971.
Scherwin, J., and Holm, P.: Long-term treatment with sulfamethoxazole-trimethoprim (Bactrim) and nitrofurantoin in chronic urinary tract infections. A controlled clinical trial. Chemotherapy 23:282, 1977.
Schiff, M., Glickman, M., Weiss, R. M., Ahern, M. J., Touloukian, R. J., Lytton, B., and Andriole, V. T.: Antibiotic treatment of renal carbuncle. Ann Intern Med 87:305, 1977.
Segura, J. W., Kelalis, P. P., Martin, W. J., and Smith, L. H.: Anaerobic bacteria in the urinary tract. Mayo Clin Proc 47:30, 1972.
Silverblatt, F. J.: Host-parasite interaction in the rat renal pelvis. A possible role for pili in the pathogenesis of pyelonephritis. J Exp Med 140:1696, 1974.
Silverblatt, F. J., and Cohen, L. S.: Antipili antibody affords protection against experimental ascending pyelonephritis. J Clin Invest 64:333, 1979.
Siroky, M. B., Moylan, R. A., Austen, G., and Olsson, C. A.: Metastatic infection secondary to genitourinary tract sepsis. Am J Med 61:351, 1976.
Stamm, W. E., Wagner, K. F., Amsel, R., Alexander, E. R., Turck, M., Counts, G. W., and Holmes, K. K.: Causes of the acute urethral syndrome in women. N Engl J Med 303:409, 1980.
Stamm, W. E., Running K., McKevitt, M., Counts, G. W., Turck, M., and Holmes, K. K.: Treatment of the acute urethral syndrome. N Engl J Med 304:956, 1981.
Stamm, W. E., Counts, G. W., Running, K. R., Fihn, S., Turck, M., and Holmes, K. K.: Diagnosis of coliform infection in acutely dysuric women. N Engl J Med 307:463, 1982.
Stamey, T. A., Govan, D. E., and Palmer, J. M.: The localization and treatment of urinary tract infections: The role of bactericidal urine levels as opposed to serum levels. Medicine 44:1, 1965.
Stamey, T. A., Fair, W. R., Timothy, M. M., and Chung, H. K.: Antibacterial nature of prostatic fluid. Nature 218:444, 1968.
Stamey, T. A., Timothy, M., Millar, M., and Mihara, G.: Recurrent urinary infections in adult women. The role of introital enterobacteria. Calif Med 115:1, 1971.
Stamey, T. A., Condy, M., and Mihara, G.: Prophylactic efficacy of nitrofurantoin macrocrystals and trimethoprim-sulfamethoxazole in urinary infections. Biologic effects on the vaginal and rectal flora. N Engl J Med 296:780, 1977.
Stamey, T. A., Wehner, N., Mihara, G., and Condy, M.: The immunologic basis of recurrent bacteriuria: role of cervicovaginal antibody in enterobacterial colonization of the introital mucosa. Medicine 57:47, 1978.
Stamey, T. A., and Mihara, G.: Observations on the growth of urethral and vaginal bacteria in sterile urine. J Urol 124:461, 1980.
Svanborg Edén, C., Jodal, U., Hanson, L. A., Lindberg, U., and Akerlund, A. S.: Variable adherence to normal human urinary-tract epithelial cells of *Escherichia coli* strains associated with various forms of urinary-tract infection. Lancet 2:490, 1976.
Svanborg Edén, C., and Hanson, L. A.: *Escherichia coli* pili as possible mediators of attachment of human urinary tract epithelial cells. Infect Immun 21:229, 1978.
Svanborg Edén, C., and Svennerholm, A.-M.: Secretory immunoglobulin A and G antibodies prevent adhesion of *Escherichia coli* to human urinary tract epithelial cells. Infect Immun 22:790, 1978.
Svanborg Edén, C., Freter, R., Hagberg, L., Hull, R., Hull, R., Hull, S., Leffler, H., and Schoolnik, G.: Inhibition of experimental ascending urinary tract infection by an epithelial cell-surface receptor analogue. Nature 298:560, 1982.
Tennant, F. S., Remmers, A. R., and Perry, J. E.: Primary renal candidiasis. Associated perinephric abscess and passage of fungus balls in the urine. Arch Intern Med 122:435, 1968.
Thomas, V., Shelokov, A., and Forland, M.: Antibody-coated bacteria in the urine and the site of urinary-tract infection. N Engl J Med 290:588, 1974.
Thorley, J. D., Jones, S. R., and Sanford, J. P.: Perinephric abscess. Medicine 53:441, 1974.
Turck, M.: Importance of localization of urinary tract infection in women. In Kass, E. H., and Brumfitt, W. (eds.): Infections of the urinary tract. Proceedings of the third international symposium on pyelonephritis. The University of Chicago Press, 1978, p. 114.
Turck, M., and Stamm, W.: Nosocomial infection of the urinary tract. Am J Med 70:651, 1981.
Utz, J. P.: Viruria in man, an update. Prog Med Virol 17:77, 1974.
Vainrub, B., and Muscher, D. M.: Lack of effect of methenamine in suppression of, or prophylaxis against, chronic urinary infection. Antimicrob Agents Chemother 12:625, 1977.
Vosti, K. L.: Recurrent urinary tract infections. Prevention by prophylactic antibiotics after sexual intercourse. JAMA 231:934, 1975.
Williams, D. N., Lund, M. E., and Blazevic, D. J.: Significance of urinary isolates of coagulase-negative *Micrococcaceae*. J Clin Microb 3:556, 1976.
Wise, G. J., Kozinn, P. J., and Goldberg, P.: Amphotericin B as a urologic irrigant in the management of noninvasive candiduria. J Urol 128:82, 1982.

159

PROSTATITIS

WILLIAM R. FAIR, M.D.

The term prostatitis is often used to describe a symptom complex rather than a specific disease entity. Clinicians frequently make the diagnosis of prostatitis without objective evidence that the patient has an infected prostate. Furthermore, some patients who are said to have prostatitis have normal prostatic secretions, while the secretions of others reveal a marked inflammatory response. In an attempt to bring some order into the confusion surrounding the term prostatitis, a classification based on symptoms, urine and prostatic fluid cultures, and microscopic examination of the expressed prostatic secretion (EPS) appears to have decided advantages (Drach et al., 1978). In this classification, prostatitis is divided into four distinct categories. Although the specific symptoms of each entity are discussed in detail below, a general definition of each follows:

Acute Bacterial Prostatitis. Patients with acute bacterial infection of the prostate appear ill and have systemic symptoms and infected urine. Acute bacterial prostatitis is easily diagnosed. It should not present a diagnostic dilemma.

Chronic Bacterial Prostatitis. This diagnosis should be restricted to patients with chronic infections of the prostate proven to be caused by a specific microbial agent. Between episodes of urinary tract infection, *the patient is usually asymptomatic.* The EPS findings are variable. At times, the secretion may appear normal, but careful microscopic examination often reveals an increased number of leukocytes and fat-laden macrophages (oval fat bodies) and a decrease in or absence of the small, so-called lecithin bodies that are characteristically abundant in prostatic fluid.

Nonbacterial Prostatitis. This term is used when the diagnosis of bacterial prostatitis has been excluded by cultures but examination of the EPS reveals a consistent and prominent inflammatory reaction. Thus, the EPS findings are: (1) greater than 10 to 15 leukocytes per high-power microscopic field; (2) an increase in oval fat bodies (fat-laden macrophages, which are easily recognized as large cells partially or completely filled with doubly refractile lipid particles); and (3) a decrease in or total absence of "lecithin granules," the small particles characterized by Brownian movement that are abundant in the prostatic secretions of normal men.

Prostatodynia. Patients with prostatodynia, which simply means "prostatic pain," have the clinical symptoms of "prostatitis" (see below) but no objective evidence of prostatic inflammation. Microscopic examination of the EPS is entirely normal, and bacteriologic cultures are negative.

ETIOLOGY

Bacterial Prostatitis. The bacteria that cause both acute and chronic bacterial prostatitis are the same organisms responsible for most urinary infections, i.e., gram-negative aerobic enteric bacteria. *Escherichia coli, Pseudomonas, Klebsiella,* and *Proteus* are the most common. *Staphylococcus epidermidis* and *Streptococcus faecalis* (enterococci) are not uncommon but cause prostatitis less frequently than the gram-negative bacilli. The diagnosis of gram-positive bacterial prostatitis is more difficult because gram-positive organisms are part of the normal urethral flora of many men. Consequently, urine and EPS collections are frequently contaminated with these organisms, often in high colony counts. If the patient presents with symptoms suggesting prostatitis, and segmented cultures reveal gram-positive organisms in the EPS specimen, the clinician often assumes that a cause-and-effect relationship exists. Proof of this hypothesis is difficult unless bladder infections with the same organism (as is the case in gram-negative bacterial prostatitis) can be demonstrated. Some authorities feel gram-positive prostatitis is a common entity, however, and that urinary infection is uncommon only because most gram-positive organisms do not grow well in urine and cannot reach colony counts high enough to document a bladder infection (Drach, 1974).

Nonbacterial Prostatitis. The cause of nonbacterial prostatitis is unknown, although all of the following infectious agents have been suggested:

Anaerobic Bacteria. In a careful study of patients with nonbacterial prostatitis Meares (1973a) did not find one case of prostatitis due to anaerobic bacteria.

Viruses. There is no compelling evidence that viruses can cause prostatitis, although many cases of symptomatic prostatitis seem to develop following viral upper respiratory infections (Austen, 1966).

Parasites. *Trichomonas vaginalis* infection of the prostate is difficult to document since the prostatic secretions are readily contaminated if only the urethra is infected. However, I have successfully treated a few patients with *T. vaginalis* apparently localized to the prostate. As with urethral infestations, the sexual partner must be treated simultaneously to prevent rapid reinfection.

Fungi. Rare cases of fungal prostatic infection have been reported (Meares, 1975). These cases have all been secondary to generalized systemic infection.

Mycoplasma. T-strain mycoplasma (*Ureaplasma urealyticum*) have been shown to cause prostatitis in a few patients (Taylor-Robinson, 1977; Brunner et al., 1978). Although the precise incidence is unknown, *Ureaplasma* probably do not account for a significant number of cases. The fact that *Ureaplasma,* like bacteria, are part of the urethral flora of normal, asymptomatic men means that without the use of the segmented lower tract localization technique, it is difficult to establish a definite etiologic relationship.

Chlamydia. Recent reports have implicated *Chlamydia* as the cause of some cases of nonbacterial prostatitis (Bruce et al., 1979), but other investigators doubt, on the basis of the accumulated evidence to date, that chlamydia are a frequent cause of prostatitis (Mårdh et al., 1978).

Eosinophilic Granulomas. These have been found in the prostates of asthmatic patients and have been termed "allergic prostatitis" (Kelalis et al., 1964). Many cases of idiopathic granulomatous prostatitis have been reported (Schmidt, 1965). These appear unrelated to any infectious etiology.

Prostatodynia. The etiology of this condition is unknown, although a variety of causes, from neurogenic bladder dysfunction to a psychogenic disturbance, have been suggested.

DIAGNOSIS. The diagnosis of acute bacterial prostatitis is easily made from the clinical symptoms and the finding of infected urine. However, the diagnosis of chronic bacterial prostatitis as opposed to nonbacterial prostatitis and prostatodynia is more difficult. In the absence of a urinary tract infection, there are no characteristic symptoms that distinguish men with a chronic bacterial infection of the prostate from those in the latter two categories. The physical examination of the prostate is not particularly helpful. The oft-described "boggy prostate" is an extremely subjective description of the gland that varies from examiner to examiner. Pain on examination is also subjective and varies with the patient. Furthermore, prostatic biopsy is not an accurate way to confirm bacterial prostatitis. The problem encountered in making the diagnosis by histologic means is similar to that encountered in diagnosing pyelonephritis (the infection may be focal, in which case a single biopsy may completely miss the lesion, and a great many conditions other than bacterial infection produce an indistinguishable inflammatory reaction).

It is essential, however, that chronic bacterial prostatitis be excluded before the patient can be considered to have either nonbacterial prostatitis or prostatodynia. In summary, the diagnosis of chronic bacterial prostatitis can be made only by the obvious approach of culturing bacteria from the prostatic secretion.

It is difficult, however, to obtain a culture of prostatic secretion uncontaminated by urethral organisms. For this reason, the diagnosis of chronic bacterial prostatitis must be made by a technique that enables the physician to distinguish urethral from prostatic infection and minimizes the effect of urethral bacterial contamination. The excellent technique originally described by Meares and Stamey (1968) for localization of lower tract infection is the only way true bacterial prostatitis can be differentiated from urethral contamination. In this technique, clean-voided urines and expressed prostatic secretion are collected in such a way as to give four specimens: (1) the first-voided 10 ml (VB_1—the symbol for voided bladder No. 1); (2) the midstream aliquot (VB_2—the symbol for voided bladder No. 2); (3) the expressed prostatic secretion (EPS) obtained by prostatic massage; and (4) the first 10 ml of urine obtained immediately after prostatic massage (VB_3—the symbol for voided bladder No. 3).

Great care must be taken in the collection to minimize contamination. The patient must be well hydrated before the collections are attempted. In a circumcised man, no cleansing of the glans penis is necessary. Uncircumcised men should retract the foreskin fully and keep it retracted throughout the entire collection procedure. The glans is cleansed with a detergent soap, all soap removed with a rinse of sterile water, and the glans carefully dried with a sterile sponge. The first-voided 10 ml of urine (VB_1) is collected with a sterile culture tube held directly in front of the external meatus by the physician. As the patient continues to void, the physician removes the culture tube from the stream of urine. When the patient has voided approximately 200 ml, the second culture tube is inserted into the stream of urine for collection of the 10-ml midstream aliquot (VB_2). Immediately after collection of the second specimen, the patient is instructed to stop voiding and shake off any drops of urine at the urethral meatus. The patient then bends forward, keeping the foreskin retracted with one hand and holds a wide-mouth sterile container beneath the meatus with his other hand. As the physician massages the prostate, the drops of prostatic fluid fall directly into the specimen container. The collection is facilitated by intermittent gentle pressure from the examiner's thumb on the bulbar urethra. After the prostatic specimen is collected, the patient voids again. The first 10 ml of urine collected after prostatic massage is labeled VB_3 and is obtained in the same manner as the first-voided specimen. If the foreskin slips back over the meatus at any time during the procedure, it is important that the cleansing and drying be repeated in order to prevent bacterial contamination of the cultures. Gram-negative bacteria are plentiful beneath the foreskin and can easily contaminate the cultures. It is equally important to remove all of the detergent from the glans before collecting any cultures. Contamination of voided urine by even small quantities of the antibacterial detergent solution may invalidate the quantitative bacterial count.

The diagnosis of bacterial prostatitis or urethritis is made by comparing the quantitative colony count in the various specimens. If the bladder urine is sterile, comparison of the VB_1 and VB_3 bacterial counts localizes the infection to either the urethra or the prostate. When the VB_1 count exceeds that of the VB_3 by a factor of one log (a tenfold increase), the diagnosis is anterior urethritis. If the VB_3 count is substantially greater than the VB_1, the diagnosis is prostatitis. In acute bacterial prostatitis, the count in the prostatic secretion is much higher than the urethral count. The difference is usually smaller in chronic bacterial prostatitis. When the VB_1 and the VB_3 counts are approximately equal, the EPS culture is valuable for differentiating prostatitis from anterior urethritis.

If the bladder urine is infected with greater than 100,000 bacteria per milliliter, one cannot differentiate the focus of infection. In these cases, the patient is given an antibacterial drug to sterilize the urine. Either nitrofurantoin, 100 mg every 6 hours, or oral penicillin G, 250 mg every 6 hours, is satisfactory for this purpose. These agents sterilize the urine but have no effect on the bacterial count of the EPS specimen because they do not diffuse into the prostate. With the urine sterilized by one of these antibiotics that reach high levels in the urine, the localization procedure is repeated. The EPS and VB_3 cultures are streaked immediately on the agar plate to minimize contact of the prostatic fluid with the antibiotic-containing urine. When the urine is sterilized by antibiotics, even exceedingly low counts of bacteria in the EPS and VB_3 specimens establish the diagnosis of bacterial prostatitis. Actual counts obtained from a patient on antibiotics are illustrated in the following case history.

Clinical Case (Table 1). The following case illustrates the typical history, culture results, and course of a patient with recurrent episodes of bacterial prostatitis. His symptoms disappeared on antimicrobial therapy. When the antibiotic was stopped, the patient's urine became infected again, and his symptoms recurred. Despite treatment with a full therapeutic course of trimethoprim and sulfamethoxazole followed by long-term suppression with one nightly dose of the same drug, the *E. coli* persisted in the prostatic secretion.

L. N., a 59-year-old white man, first presented with low-grade fever, malaise, urgency, frequency, and dysuria on September 6, 1976. The spun urine sediment was loaded with white blood cells and motile bacilli, and a urine culture grew out greater than 100,000 *E. coli* per milliliter. The patient was given trimethoprim-sulfamethoxazole, 2 tablets twice a day, and quickly became asymptomatic. Although two urine cultures obtained while he was taking the drug were sterile, small numbers of *E. coli* were cultured from the prostatic fluid both times. The antibacterial agent was stopped after 24 days. He was asymptomatic for more than 1 month, but returned on November 1 with mild frequency and dysuria. Urine cultures again were positive for *E. coli*. He was treated with trimethoprim-sulfamethoxazole again, and his symptoms subsided. EPS cultures still grew a few *E. coli* while the patient was on the drug. When last seen, he was asymptomatic on a nightly dose of co-trimoxazole, but EPS cultures remained positive.

Thus, the diagnosis of chronic bacterial prostatitis is reserved for patients with recurrent urinary tract infection associated with bacteria in the prostatic secretions.

Patients with nonbacterial prostatitis have prostatic symptoms and a consistent, sterile inflammatory response in the prostatic secretions. If the patient has a history of urinary tract infection, lower tract bacterial localization studies, as described earlier, should be performed to ensure that the bacteria are not sequestered in the prostate and periodically seeding the urinary tract. However, the vast majority of patients with nonbacterial prostatitis do not have a history of even one episode of urinary tract infection. The diagnosis can be made from the characteristic symptoms and an inflammatory response in the expressed prostatic secretion; negative cultures confirm the diagnosis.

The diagnosis of prostatodynia is made by finding normal prostatic secretion in a patient with similar symptoms (but with no history of urinary tract infection) and sterile urine and prostatic secretion cultures.

CLINICAL MANIFESTATIONS

Acute Bacterial Prostatitis. Acute bacterial prostatitis is easily recognized. Typically the patient presents with sud-

Table 1. CHRONIC BACTERIAL PROSTATITIS
L.N., A 59-YEAR-OLD WHITE MAN

Date	Days on (+) or off (−) Drug	Colonies per ML				Organisms
		VB_1	VB_2	EPS	VB_3	
6 Sept 76	—	100,000	100,000	ND	ND	*E. coli*
13 Sept 76	+ 7 TMP-Sx ii b.i.d.	0	0	20	0	*E. coli*
27 Sept 76	+ 21 TMP-Sx	0	0	50	0	*E. coli*
4 Oct 76	− 4 TMP-Sx	100	0	20	200	*E. coli*
28 Oct 76	− 28 TMP-Sx	0	0	10,000	2,000	*E. coli*
1 Nov 76	− 32 TMP-Sx	100,000	0	ND	100,000	*E. coli*
8 Nov 76	+ 7 TMP-Sx ii b.i.d.	0	0	730	ND	*E. coli*
15 Nov 76	+ 14 TMP-Sx i nightly	0	0	10	0	*E. coli*
7 Jan 77	+ 67 TMP-Sx i nightly	0	0	30	0	*E. coli*
7 Feb 77	+ 98 TMP-Sx i nightly	0	0	70	10	*E. coli*

VB_1 = The first-voided 10 ml (void bladder No. 1)
VB_2 = Midstream specimen (void bladder No. 2)
EPS = Expressed prostatic secretion
VB_3 = Post-prostatic massage specimen (void bladder No. 3)
ND = Not done
TMP-Sx = Trimethoprim-sulfamethoxazole

den onset of fever, chills, and signs of a systemic illness. He usually has irritative voiding symptoms with prominent frequency and dysuria and may also complain of anorexia, malaise, perineal discomfort, arthralgias, and vague myalgias. The prostate is swollen, firm, indurated, warm to the touch, and exquisitely tender to palpation. Because of the risk of seeding bacteria into the bloodstream from an infected prostate, no attempt should be made to massage the prostate to obtain prostatic secretions. Only a very gentle diagnostic examination of the prostate should be done.

Classically, the urinalysis confirms the diagnosis of an acute urinary tract infection with bacteria and a large number of white cells in the spun urine sediment. Urine culture is invariably positive for bacteria.

Chronic Bacterial Prostatitis (CBP). The clinical presentation of the patient with chronic bacterial prostatitis is more subtle. The typical patient is a man with recurrent urinary tract infections. Frequently, the symptoms began during or after he had an indwelling catheter, but CBP may develop without prior catheterization. The unique feature of CBP is that most men have no specific symptoms until they develop symptoms of a bladder infection. These are most frequently dysuria, frequency, urgency, and nocturia, but fever and signs of systemic illness may herald the onset of the urinary tract infection, and the patient may appear to be quite ill. Although CBP may follow an episode of acute prostatitis in some patients, most men with CBP have no history of acute prostatitis.

The physical findings are variable. In long-standing bacterial prostatitis the prostate is usually small and may feel firm. Although the gland may be slightly tender during the symptomatic phase, pain on examination is not common. The term "boggy prostate" is often used as a synonym for prostatitis, but there is no typical consistency of the prostate in chronic bacterial prostatitis. The patients sometimes have prostatic calculi that can be palpated as firm areas in the gland, although most men with prostatic calculi never suffer with prostatitis.

When symptomatic, the patient invariably has pyuria, bacteriuria, and a positive urine culture. However, from a practical viewpoint, chronic bacterial prostatitis is the diagnosis of virtually every man with a history of recurrent urinary tract infections and an intravenous pyelogram that fails to reveal the source (such as stones or upper tract obstruction) for recurrent bacteriuria. The symptoms respond well to antimicrobials, and the patient is usually asymptomatic while he is taking the medication. However, at variable intervals after the antibiotics are stopped, the residual infection in the prostate seeds the bladder urine, and the symptoms recur.

The characteristics of the expressed prostatic secretion in chronic bacterial prostatitis are also variable. The secretion may be inflammatory and contain oval fat bodies on some occasions but, at other times, in the same person, it may be quite benign, particularly if the patient is on suppressive antimicrobials. In the latter situation, neither physical examination nor microscopic examination of the EPS gives any hint of persistent chronic bacterial infection. Cultures of the urine and EPS are mandatory in order to make the diagnosis.

Nonbacterial Prostatitis (NBP) and Prostatodynia. The symptoms of nonbacterial prostatitis and prostatodynia are indistinguishable. Generally, they consist of variable degrees of perineal aching; back pain; groin pain that occasionally radiates to the thigh, particularly its inner aspect; musculoskeletal soreness; and irritative voiding symptoms (frequency, urgency, and dysuria). The patients often refer to pain on ejaculation, although this is not always present. Urethral discharge is uncommon. A urethral discharge in a patient with these symptoms is much more likely to be caused by urethritis. There are no specific physical findings in nonbacterial prostatitis and prostatodynia. The term "boggy prostate," which is often used to describe the findings on rectal examination of these patients, is nonspecific. There is no characteristic consistency of the prostate in either of these conditions. Prostatic calculi can be found in these patients just as they can be in men with otherwise normal prostates. Thus, NBP and prostatodynia cannot be differentiated by symptoms or physical examination. The distinguishing features are many white blood cells, often in clumps or aggregates, an increase in the number of fat-laden macrophages (oval fat bodies), and a decrease in the number of lecithin bodies in the EPS of patients with nonbacterial prostatitis. In contrast, the EPS of patients with prostatodynia is perfectly normal. These unfortunate individuals simply have pelvic pain that may or may not emanate from the prostate, without any objective evidence of prostatic inflammation (Segura et al., 1979). Cultures of urine and prostatic secretion are sterile in both conditions.

PATHOGENESIS AND PATHOLOGY. The bacteria that infect the prostate probably reach the gland by ascending from the urethra. Although colonic bacteria are the most frequent cause of bacterial prostatitis, there is no strong evidence that the organisms spread to the prostate from the colon or by lymphatics from the rectum. Stamey (1972) has postulated that sexual intercourse may play a role in prostatic infection because the men develop transient urethral colonization with gram-negative bacteria if their sex partner's vagina is colonized with these bacilli.

The importance of the prostate in the genesis of urinary tract infections appears to be twofold. First, the antibacterial activity of the normal prostatic secretion is a significant defense mechanism against urinary infections, and is apparently related directly to the high concentration of zinc in the prostatic secretion (Fair and Stamey, 1969; Fair and Wehner, 1971; Fair et al., 1973). The prostatic secretion of some men with chronic bacterial prostatitis lacks this antibacterial activity (Fair et al., 1973). If this deficiency preceded the infection, it might have made these men more susceptible to prostatitis. Second, persistent bacteria in the prostate intermittently "seed" the bladder urine and cause most of the cases of recurrent bacteriuria in men. The failure of most antibacterials to diffuse into the gland and concentrate in its secretion accounts for the difficulty in eradicating organisms from the prostate. The gland thus serves as a reservoir of infection that often defies all attempts at cure.

Because of its diverse etiologies, there is no typical pathologic finding in patients with prostatitis. Acute bacterial prostatitis causes edema, capillary engorgement, a diffuse infiltration of neutrophils, and a few round cells. The infiltration of polymorphonuclear leukocytes is accompanied by profuse desquamation of epithelial cells and leukocytes into the tubular lumen. In severe cases, microabscesses may develop and completely break down prostatic tissue. As the process becomes more chronic, the neutrophils are replaced by plasma cells, lymphocytes, and monocytes, and the degree of fibrosis steadily increases.

There are no characteristic tissue changes noted in patients with nonbacterial prostatitis and prostatodynia. The tissue often appears normal.

COMPLICATIONS AND SEQUELAE. The complications of acute bacterial prostatitis are the same as those of any other severe urinary tract infection. Pyelonephritis is commonly seen if antibacterial treatment is delayed. If septicemia develops secondary to polynephritis, gram-negative shock and cardiovascular collapse may result. Recurrent bladder and upper tract infections are frequent complications of chronic bacterial prostatitis. Except for complications from secondary bacteriuria, chronic bacterial infection of the prostate does not appear to cause significant sequelae.

There is no documented evidence linking prostatitis to subsequent development of benign prostatic hypertrophy (BPH) or carcinoma of the prostate. True, documented chronic bacterial prostatitis is relatively uncommon, however. The possibility that the more frequent entities of nonbacterial prostatitis and prostatodynia might be associated with BPH and carcinoma of the prostate has not been carefully studied.

TREATMENT AND PROPHYLAXIS

Acute Bacterial Prostatitis. In contrast to chronic bacterial prostatitis, patients with acute bacterial prostatitis respond dramatically to antibacterials that do not diffuse into the normal prostate. It is thought that the intense acute inflammation increases the permeability of the prostatic membrane and permits drugs to penetrate the infected prostate. An antibiotic selected according to the results of in vitro sensitivity tests should be given in doses that achieve bactericidal concentrations in the serum. Most patients respond very rapidly if therapy is instituted immediately with trimethoprim-sulfamethoxazole (2 tablets twice daily), carbenicillin indanyl ester (382 mg, 2 capsules four times daily), ampicillin (250 mg four times daily), or one of the other penicillins or cephalosporins. Patients with pronounced systemic symptoms should be treated parenterally with the combination of gentamicin (5 mg/kg daily in three divided doses) or another aminoglycoside plus penicillin, ampicillin (4–8 g IV daily in four divided doses), or intravenous trimethoprim-sulfamethoxazole.

Systemic supportive measures such as bed rest, adequate hydration, analgesics, antipyretics, and stool softeners should also be used. Urethral instrumentation should *never* be considered. When the occasional instance of acute urinary retention occurs, suprapubic needle aspiration of the bladder is safer, more comfortable for the patient, and less likely to cause future complications than urethral catheterization.

Chronic Bacterial Prostatitis. The treatment of chronic bacterial prostatitis is unsatisfactory because most antimicrobials do not diffuse into the prostatic secretion of these patients (Winningham et al., 1968; Reeves and Gilchick, 1970; Stamey et al., 1970). In dogs, the most important factors influencing the diffusion of antimicrobials into the prostate are: (1) lipid solubility and (2) a favorable dissociation constant (pKa). An antibacterial with an alkaline pKa diffuses from serum into an acidic prostatic fluid and, by the mechanisms of "ion-trapping," concentrates in the secretion. In the presence of a highly alkaline secretion, however, the opposite occurs and the concentration in the prostatic fluid never approaches the serum levels. Trimethoprim (TMP) concentrates in the stimulated prostatic secretion of normal dogs and should be highly effective at eradicating chronic bacterial prostatitis. In clinical practice, however, cure remains a formidable task even when the organism is known to be sensitive to drugs that concentrate in uninfected canine prostatic fluid. Meares (1973b), Drach (1974b), and McGuire and Lytton (1976) found that only 30 per cent of patients treated with trimethoprim and sulfamethoxazole for CBP were cured after completion of therapy. These findings cast doubt on the applicability of the canine model to drug diffusion into the human prostate. The pH of normal canine prostatic fluid is approximately 6.4. Normal human prostatic fluid has a mean pH of 7.3, and it increases to 8.3 in the presence of CBP (Fair and Cordonnier, 1978). These observations probably explain the discrepancy between the experimental data and the clinical results.

No single drug is effective in the treatment of men with chronic bacterial prostatitis; despite the discouraging results of treatment with trimethoprim-sulfamethoxazole (TMP-Sx) in most series, it is still one of the orally effective drugs. An exception would be in patients with prostatitis due to *Pseudomonas aeruginosa*, an organism usually resistant to trimethoprim.

Carbenicillin indanyl ester appears to be at least equal to TMP-Sx in oral therapy of chronic prostatitis and is the agent of choice in most cases of *Pseudomonas* prostatitis. It is also valuable in chronic suppressive therapy as described below. Encouraging results with kanamycin suggest that this drug may be useful for sensitive organisms (Pfau and Sacks, 1976). Erythromycin (0.5 g four times daily) is the treatment of choice for gram-positive infections.

Transurethral resection of the prostate (TURP) is no better than treatment with antimicrobials. Only about one-third of patients subjected to TURP are permanently free of infection (Stamey, 1972). Moreover, the almost certain development of retrograde ejaculation and the possible risk of incontinence make most surgeons loath to perform TURP in young men unless the repeated infections cannot be controlled by medication.

Prevention of the symptoms of CBP is more successful than treatment. Men with CBP are asymptomatic between episodes of bladder bacteriuria, which can usually be prevented by a single nightly dose of an appropriate antimicrobial.

The drug chosen for chronic suppressive therapy should be one to which the organism in the prostatic secretion is sensitive. One nightly dose of TMP-Sx (½-1 tablet) or carbenicillin indanyl ester (1 capsule) will control symptomatic flare-ups of chronic bacterial prostatitis, just as low-dose therapy is effective prophylaxis of symptomatic urinary infections in females. Whether or not chronic suppressive therapy will eventually clear the organism from the prostatic secretion and cure the disease is under study.

While the prognosis of acute bacterial prostatitis is excellent, the prospect for cure of CBP is less favorable. However, prevention of bladder infection and control of symptoms in most patients with low-dose suppressive medication is easily accomplished.

Nonbacterial Prostatitis and Prostatodynia. Since the cause of these entities is unknown, no rational plan of therapy or prophylaxis can be formulated. Some patients respond symptomatically to empiric therapy with tetracycline or doxycycline. I believe one course of tetracycline (250 mg four times daily for 21 days), doxycycline (100 mg daily for 21 days), or minocycline (100 mg daily for 21 days) is warranted for nonbacterial prostatitis as empirical therapy for chlamydial or ureaplasma infection. If they give no relief, the patient should be informed that further antibiotic therapy is of no value. The expense and risk of side effects plus the lack of demonstrated efficacy make continued antibiotic administration inadvisable, and therapy should be symptomatic. On the theory that the prostate is "congested," some clinicians recommend periodic prostatic massages or more frequent ejaculations. The relief of pain is presumably the result of mechanical emptying or "drainage" of fluid from the engorged prostatic duct. Other patients seem to respond to anticholinergics, sedatives, muscle relaxants, or analgesics. Sitz baths are also often prescribed. Therapy with phenoxybenzamine has been reported to relieve the symptoms of prostatodynia (Drach, 1979). More recently, prazosin (1.0 mg one to two times daily) has largely replaced phenoxybenzamine in this regard.

Prophylactic recommendations have included prostatic massage, frequent sexual activity, sexual abstinence, vitamins, sunflower seeds, and oral zinc supplementation. To date, there are no data to support the value of any of these measures.

References

Austen, G., Jr.: The test of time. IX. Prostatitis: acute and chronic. Brit M Q 17:27, 1966.

Bruce, A. W., Willett, W. S., Chadwick, P., and O'Shaughnessy, M.: The role of Chlamydiae in genito-urinary disease. J Urol 126:625, 1981.

Brunner, H., Weidner, W., Krause, W., and Rothauge, C. F.: Zur Bedutung von Ureaplasma urealyticum bei unspezifischer prostatourethritis-quantitative Untersuchungen an 312 Patienten. Dtsch Med Wochenschr 103:465, 1978.

Drach, G. W.: Problems in diagnosis of bacterial prostatitis: Gram-negative, gram-positive, and mixed infections. J Urol 111:603, 1974a.

Drach, G. W.: Trimethoprim-sulfamethoxazole therapy of chronic bacterial prostatitis. J Urol 111:637, 1974b.

Drach, G. W.: Personal communication, 1979.

Drach, G. W., Meares, E. M., Jr., Fair, W. R., and Stamey, T. A.: Classification of benign diseases associated with prostatic pain: prostatitis or prostatodynia? (Letter to the Editor) J Urol 120:266, 1978.

Fair, W. R., and Cordonnier, J. J.: The pH of prostatic fluid: a reappraisal and therapeutic implications. J Urol 120:695, 1978.

Fair, W. R., Couch, J., and Wehner, N.: Purification and assay of the prostatic antibacterial factor (PAF). Biochem Med 8:329, 1973.

Fair, W. R., and Stamey, T. A.: Bactericidal properties of prostatic fluid. *In* Bacterial Infection of Male Genital System (Workshop), October 1967. Warrenton, Va., National Research Council, National Academy of Sciences, 1969.

Fair, W. R., and Wehner, N.: Further observations on the antibacterial nature of prostatic fluid. Infect Immun 3:494, 1971.

Kelalis, P. T., Harrison, E. G., Jr., and Greene, L. F.: Allergic granulomas of the prostate in asthmatics. JAMA 118:963, 1964.

Mårdh, P-A., Ripa, K. T., Colleen, S., Treharne, J. D., and Darougar, N. S.: The role of Chlamydia trichomatis in non-acute prostatitis. Br J Vener Dis 54:330, 1978.

McGuire, E. J., and Lytton, B.: Bacterial prostatitis—treatment with trimethoprim sulfamethoxazole. Urol 7:499, 1976.

Meares, E. M., Jr.: Bacterial prostatitis versus "prostatosis": a clinical and bacteriological study. JAMA 224:1372, 1973a.

Meares, E. M., Jr.: Observations on the activity of trimethoprimsulfamethoxazole in the prostate. J Infect Dis (Suppl):S679, 1973b.

Meares, E. M., Jr.: Prostatitis—a review. Urol Clin North Am 2:3, 1975.

Meares, E. M., Jr., and Stamey, T. A.: Bacteriologic localization patterns in bacterial prostatitis and urethritis. Invest Urol 5:492, 1968.

Pfau, A., and Sacks, T.: Chronic bacterial prostatitis: new therapeutic aspects. Brit J Urol 48:245, 1976.

Reeves, D. S., and Gilchick, M. B.: Secretion of the antibacterial substance trimethoprim in the prostatic fluid of dogs. J Urol 42:66, 1970.

Schmidt, J. D.: Non-specific granulomatous prostatitis: classification, review and report of cases. J Urol 94:607, 1965.

Segura, J. W., Opitz, J. L., and Greene, L. F.: Prostatosis, prostatitis or pelvic floor tension myalgia. J Urol 122:168, 1979.

Stamey, T. A.: Urinary Infections. Baltimore, Williams & Wilkins Co., 1972, p. 166.

Stamey, T. A., Meares, E. M., Jr., and Winningham, D. J.: Bacterial prostatitis and the diffusion of drugs into prostatic fluid. J Urol 103:187, 1970.

Taylor-Robinson, D.: Possible role of ureaplasmas in non-gonococcal urethritis. In Hobson, D., and Holmes, K. K. (eds.): Non-gonococcal Urethritis and Related Infections. Washington, D.C., American Society of Microbiology, 1977.

Winningham, D. J., Nemoy, N. J., and Stamey, T. A.: Diffusion of antibiotics from plasma into prostatic fluid. Nature 219:139, 1968.

160
NONVENEREAL INFECTIONS OF THE FEMALE GENITALIA

EDWARD BROOK ROTHERAM, JR., M.D.

Deep infections of the female genitalia not acquired or transmitted by sexual contact may be granulomatous (tuberculous) or pyogenic. Exogenous pyogenic infections are produced by single pathogens such as *Streptococcus pyogenes* or *Staphylococcus aureus*, microbes that are rarely recovered from normal vaginal and cervical secretions. When these specific infections occur after obstetric and gynecologic procedures, faults in aspetic technique should be suspected, especially if epidemic spread is observed. In endogenous pyogenic infections, the pus contains a mixture of poorly virulent aerobic and anaerobic bacteria that are frequently recovered from normal vaginal and cervical secretions. Most pyogenic infections occurring endemically within the hospital are endogenous.

PYOGENIC INFECTIONS

PATHOGENESIS AND PATHOLOGY. Nonvenereal pyogenic infections of the female genitalia originate in poorly oxygenated, poorly defended spaces or cavities containing material conducive to rapid bacterial growth. In abortal and postpartum sepsis, the uterine cavity contains dead fetal tissue. Before delivery, the amniotic space and its fluid are available for bacterial growth. Following obstetric and gynecologic surgery, collections of blood or lymph fulfill the criteria for bacterial growth admirably. A fallopian tube partially or totally occluded by inflammatory disease presents another nidus. Infection occurs when such spaces, regardless of their size, are inoculated with a specific pathogen. When large spaces are contaminated by vaginal and cervical secretions, certain members of the normal flora may proliferate. The strict anaerobes and the microaerophilic species of the normal flora usually become numerically dominant in these relatively avascular spaces. *Bacteroides*, *Peptostreptococcus*, and microaerophilic streptococcal species are often recovered in high concentrations when quantitative anaerobic cultural techniques are employed (Rotheram and Schick, 1969). Less frequently, other fastidious microbes such as *Actinomyces*, *Proprionibacterium*, *Clostridia* species, and even *Gardnerella vaginalis (Hemophilus vaginalis)* are recovered in large numbers. Certain facultative anaerobes such as *Escherichia coli*, *Proteus mirabilis*, *Staphylococcus epidermidis*, group B streptococci, and the enterococci are also frequently recovered. Although these facultative species are usually present in far smaller concentrations than the strict anaerobes, their importance in endogenous infections was overemphasized before the complete bacteriologic studies of the past 15 years because they grow so readily in air. Although they have now been placed in proper perspective, these facultative species, particularly the gram-negative bacilli, cannot be ignored. Not only may they occasionally dominate the pelvic infection but also produce shock when they enter the bloodstream.

Infection of a pelvic space may spread through lymphatic channels and produce cellulitis and abscesses of the broad ligaments and other retroperitoneal spaces of the pelvic floor. Infection can also extend from the uterine cavity into the fallopian tubes to produce tubal or tubo-ovarian abscesses. These may rupture and cause peritonitis and either local or remote intraperitoneal abscesses.

Many acute pyogenic infections of the female genitalia are accompanied by a bacteremia that reflects the local infection in that it is frequently anaerobic and polymicrobial. Hematogenous abscesses in distant organs show a similar flora. Septic thrombophlebitis explains the paradox of how a mixed infection in an avascular space gains ready access to the bloodstream. Since strict anaerobes induce thrombophlebitis more readily than facultative bacteria, *Escherichia coli* and the enterococci may often owe their access to the bloodstream to vascular lesions induced by the strict anaerobes. When confined to small tributaries, venous thrombosis may seal off the infection with spontaneous resolution of accompanying bacteremia. Conversely, thrombosis may extend to larger veins and produce a severe continuous septicemia.

CLINICAL MANIFESTATIONS

Septic Abortion (Postabortal Endometritis). Infection rarely complicates spontaneous abortion but frequently follows an induced incomplete abortion. Within two to five days of uterine instrumentation, the typical patient develops a shaking chill and high fever. An enlarged tender uterus discharges a foul-smelling mixture of blood and pus. Leukocytosis is expected. Bacteremia can be demonstrated in over 50 per cent of cases if the blood is cultured within 24 hours of the chill. Half of the positive blood cultures yield two or more bacterial species, and anaerobic and microaerophilic isolates outnumber facultative isolates 4 to 1. Bacterial species recovered in concentrations of more than 10^6 colonies/ml of uterine exudate show the same 4:1 ratio of fastidious to rapid-growing bacteria.

Despite early evidence of invasive infection, most patients recover promptly after evacuation of the uterus, a fact well known in the preantibiotic era. However, the complications of septic abortion, discussed separately below, are notoriously severe. The full spectrum of the disease ranges from death within hours of onset to a prolonged, debilitating illness.

The diagnosis of septic abortion is difficult only when local signs of infection develop with uncharacteristic indolence in a patient who falsely denies pregnancy and/or uterine instrumentation.

Puerperal Sepsis (Postpartum Endometritis). Chills and fever associated with a large tender uterus and profuse lochial flow begin abruptly two to five days after delivery, which may not have been difficult. Lacerations of the cervix or uterine wall obviously predispose to infection, but retained placental fragments are all that is needed to initiate endometritis. Before the use of aseptic technique, epidemics of puerperal sepsis with high mortality rates were reported from all countries where labor and delivery occurred in hospitals. These epidemics were undoubtedly caused by *Streptococcus pyogenes* transmitted from mother to mother by physicians' hands. This exogenous infection is characterized by the rapid development of intense pelvic cellulitis, and death can occur quickly from an overwhelming bacteremia (blood poisoning). This accelerated course is explained by the ability of *Streptococcus pyogenes* to spread rapidly through lymphatics despite the interposition of lymph nodes, which are ordinarily quite effective in limiting pyogenic infection. Sporadic cases of this specific exogenous infection still occur, although early treatment often results in a mild illness. *Staphylococcus aureus, Neisseria gonorrhea,* and even *Streptococcus pneumoniae* may also be recovered in puerperal cultures, but, as in septic abortion, the great majority of nonepidemic infections are caused by endogenous bacteria such as *E. coli* and anaerobes. The lower the virulence of the invading bacteria, the more important are local disturbances in tissue resistance. Hence, removal of retained tissues from the uterus is the cornerstone of treatment of endogenous infection. The complications of endogenous infection maintain puerperal sepsis as a leading cause of maternal death.

Subgluteal and Retropsoas Abscess. Although perivaginal tissues are remarkably resistant to infection, pudendal or paracervical block anesthesia during delivery can result in pelvic abscesses. Presumably a hematoma is induced and infected by the needle that must pass through the vagina. From this nidus, pus can dissect along the lumbosacral plexus superiorly to reach the retropsoas space and inferiorly to involve the subgluteal space posterior to the hip joint (Hibbard et al., 1972). Symptoms and signs of infection may develop insidiously after a normal delivery as the patient complains of increasingly severe pain and limitation of motion in the hip, with or without psoal spasm. Paraplegia, muscle destruction, bacteremic shock, and death have resulted from the failure to detect and drain these abscesses.

Chorioamnionitis. The chorioamniotic space is infected within 24 hours after rupture of the fetal membranes. When rupture is premature, 80 to 90 per cent of women go into spontaneous labor within this period of time. The longer the uterus remains unemptied, the greater the danger of infection to mother and child. Although some mothers may develop fever and bacteremia (with or without shock), others may show little or no evidence of infection while the fetus is suffering irreparable harm. Obviously, the temptation to delay delivery is greatest when the fetus is immature, but if amniocentesis confirms the suspicion of infection, nothing is gained by delay.

Postoperative Infections. Cesarean section must be considered a contaminated procedure if the fetal membranes have been ruptured for eight hours or longer. Nonelective hysterotomy yields an infection rate as high as 60 per cent when prophylactic antibiotics are not used. Fortunately many infections are endometrial or subcutaneous and respond promptly to intravenous antibiotics and drainage through the wound. A few involve the uterine wall, adnexa, intraperitoneal spaces, or bowel and may be fatal.

Abdominal and vaginal hysterectomies are also associated with a high incidence of infection with a broad range of morbidity (Ledger, 1969). Premenopausal women undergoing vaginal hysterectomy are at greatest risk: Hemostasis is difficult because their pelvic tissues are more vascular, ovulation exposes the ovarian stroma to infection, and preexisting salpingitis is more common. *Vaginal cuff abscess* is the most frequent and least serious infectious complication. Fever occurs early, usually within five days, symptoms are few, and drainage is followed by rapid recovery. The fever due to *pelvic cellulitis* tends to occur later in the postoperative period but still within the average hospital stay. Fever does not remit if an associated cuff abscess is drained. No other masses are felt, although the pelvis remains tender. The response to antibiotics is usually brisk.

Adnexal infection is often discovered after the patient has been discharged. The typical patient is readmitted with fever, lower abdominal pain, and a mass in the pelvis. Partial intestinal obstruction may be present. In *tubo-ovarian abscess,* tubal obstruction occurs when the ovary is caught up in an inflammatory reaction of the fimbria. Ultimately the ovary forms a tiny portion of an abscess within the tube. *Ovarian abscess* is quite distinct pathologically. Bacteria enter the ovary either through a ruptured follicle or by way of a surgical biopsy. The abscess develops within the ovarian tissue and spares the tubal structures. Although both types of abscesses may rupture, the ovarian abscess is particularly prone to this potentially fatal complication.

Nonspecific Pelvic Inflammatory Disease (Salpingo-oophoritis). Not all women who present with fever, lower abdominal pain, peritoneal irritation, cervical discharge, and adnexal masses have gonorrhea. When the syndrome is recurrent, recovery of the gonococcus in culture is unusual. The end stage of the recurrent disease is a fibrotic pelvis containing tubo-ovarian abscesses to which loops of small intestine may adhere. The abscesses typically contain a mixture of endogenous bacteria. In contrast to most of the infections already discussed, blood cultures are rarely positive.

The innate resistance of pelvic structures to endogenous bacteria suggests that this infection is superimposed upon a prior inflammatory process. Gonorrhea, puerperal endometritis, and adjacent abscesses of intestinal origin are long-recognized predisposing conditions. Intrauterine contraceptive devices also cause pelvic abscesses. Although milder than gonorrhea, acute salpingitis due to *Chlamydia trachomatis* might also lead to tubal infection with endogenous microbes.

COMPLICATIONS. Leakage or rupture of adnexal abscesses produces pelvic and generalized peritonitis, pelvic and remote intraperitoneal abscesses, mechanical intestinal obstruction, and adynamic ileus. Hemorrhage and/or acute bacteremias may produce hypovolemic and/or septic shock with a significant incidence of renal failure. Gram-negative bacteremias occurring in the peripartum period are likely to trigger disseminated intravascular coagulation. Indeed, human equivalents of the local and generalized Sanarelli-Shwartzman reactions occur complete with renal cortical necrosis. A rare complication of pregnancy, aptly termed the plasmapheresis syndrome, results from the body's failure to control yet another aspect of the inflammatory response: a global increase in capillary permeability rapidly leads to hypovolemia, hemoconcentration, and shock. Administration of salt and albumen results in more edema and damage to the brain and lungs.

Clostridial myonecrosis, uterine gangrene, and even tetanus can complicate the anaerobic infections. Clostridial septicemia (distinguished from bacteremia by intravascular hemolysis) originates in the postabortal and postpartum uterus. Suppurative thrombophlebitis in pelvic and ovarian veins produces fever, tachycardia, and multiple pulmonary emboli. Although this triad tends to respond slowly to treatment, proper antibiotic coverage prevents metastatic infection in the lungs, liver, brain, joints, and endocardium.

The youthful organs of most patients suffering these complications are valuable allies of the physician, who by skillful diagnosis and treatment can salvage most of these patients.

SEQUELAE. Sterility may follow any severe infection of the female genitalia. Pyogenic infections, however, do not cause the high incidence of sterility and ectopic pregnancy characteristic of tuberculosis. For example, most women who suffer recurrent salpingitis can carry out a successful pregnancy if one fallopian tube remains patent.

DIAGNOSIS. Diagnosis depends heavily upon a knowledge of the individual infectious entities, predisposing factors, and likely complications. Similarly, the pelvic examination is far more revealing if the mind as well as the fingers are exercised. Real-time gray-scale sector scanning ultrasonography has revolutionized the clinical evaluation of the pelvis. This technique can follow the development of an ovarian follicle. First detectable at a diameter of 8 millimeters, the follicle can be aspirated percutaneously when its diameter reaches 16 millimeters (Mantzavinos et al., 1983). Obviously ultrasound can detect and follow abscesses with similar precision. Abdominal laparoscopy requires general anesthesia but permits biopsy or aspiration of inflamed pelvic structures under direct vision. This technique has been used to investigate the etiology of acute salpingitis (Wolner-Hanssen et al., 1983).

Blood cultures are indicated not only before antibiotics are started but also when antibiotics do not appear to be working. Secretions for culture can be obtained on swabs from an operative wound, the cervical os, and the uterine cavity, but the swabs must not dry out before the culture is made. Hematomas and abscesses may be aspirated by both vaginal and abdominal routes. Culdocentesis and amniocentesis are now performed frequently with little morbidity. Secretions are sent to the laboratory in the syringe used for aspiration.

Regardless of the laboratory report, gross pus is rarely sterile and fetid pus is never free of strict anaerobes (Fig. 1). Smears often show an abundant variety of gram-positive and gram-negative bacteria. The aerobic culture identifies most exogenous pathogens. Those bacteria observed on Gram stain but missing in culture are usually fastidious anaerobes. For example, a light growth of enterococci cannot account for myriads of tiny, gram-positive cocci observed on the stain, nor can an abundant growth of *E. coli* explain the observation of many small encapsulated rods. Fortunately, *Bacteroides* and anaerobic streptococci are dependable in their sensitivity to various antibiotics, and patients can be successfully managed without optimal anaerobic bacteriology or sensitivity tests.

Clostridium perfringens may be recovered on culture in the absence of myonecrosis or septicemia. The diagnosis of these two complications must be based upon associated clinical manifestations if unnecessary surgery is to be avoided. Even at surgery, uterine gangrene may be a difficult diagnosis (Hawkins et al., 1975).

TREATMENT. Traditionally, treatment of pyogenic infections of the female genitalia has centered upon the evacuation or excision of infected cavities and associated abscesses. Delay in emptying an infected uterus is rarely justified. Surgical wounds are opened as soon as underlying pus is identified. An abscess pointing into the cul-de-sac is drained vaginally with little surgical morbidity. On the other hand, ultrasound and computed tomography have shown that many pelvic abscesses disappear under antibiotic therapy without surgical drainage. If a patient shows a prompt response to antibiotics, both clinically and by repeated imaging, surgical morbidity and loss of reproductive tissue can be avoided. The indications for percutaneous drainage of abscesses under ultrasonic guidance are being defined (vanSonnenberg et al., 1982). Physicians are increasingly ready to wait and see what course a pelvic infection will take before resorting to excisional surgery. Such conservatism must be tempered by the knowledge that an abscess high in the pelvis (such as an ovarian abscess) can rupture to produce a fatal peritonitis.

Most facultative and anaerobic bacterial species associated with endogenous pelvic infections are sensitive to

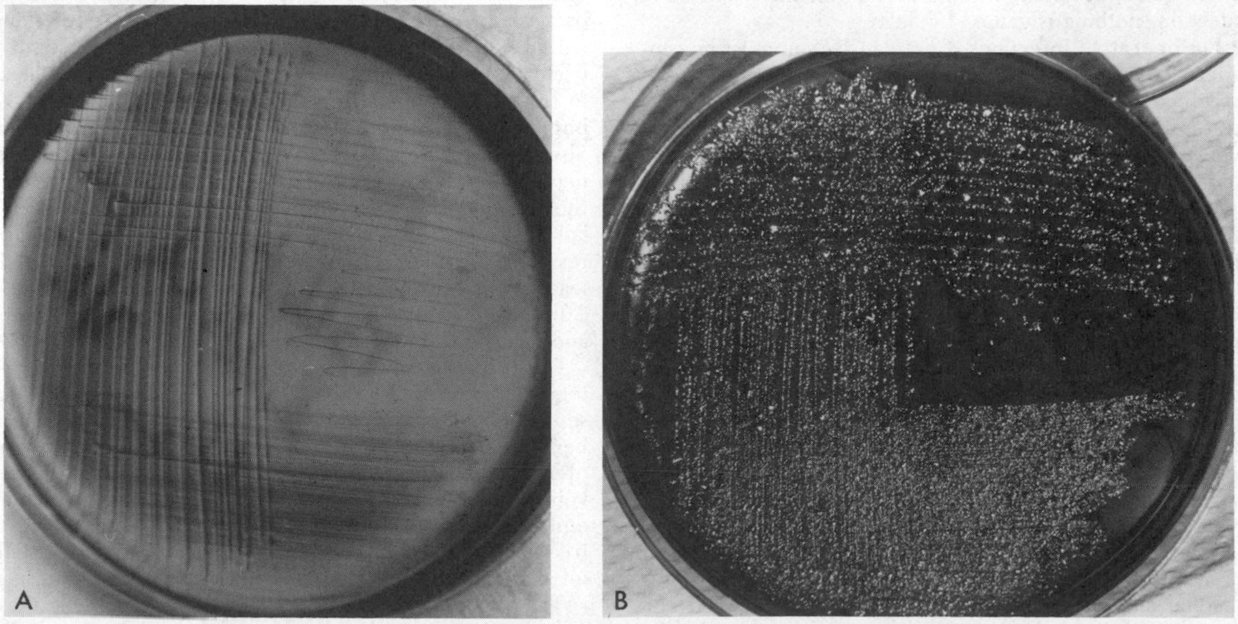

Figure 1. Both blood agar plates were inoculated with pus aspirated from a tubo ovarian abscess. *A*, This plate was incubated aerobically and remained sterile. The plate shown in *B* was incubated anaerobically and yielded six bacterial species, three of which were abundant.

Table 1. ANTIBIOTIC TREATMENT OF PYOGENIC INFECTIONS OF THE FEMALE GENITALIA

A. Severe infections with abscess formation in uterine wall, fallopian tubes, ovary, broad ligaments, peritoneum or cul-de-sac
   Penicillin G—3 million units every 3 hours, I.V.
   Clindamycin—600 mg every 6 hours, I.V.
   Gentamicin—2 mg/kg I.V. followed by 1.5 mg/kg I.V. every 8 hours in patients with normal renal function
   Notes:
   1. Metronidazole, 15 mg/kg I.V. followed by 7.5 mg/kg every 6 hours I.V. may be substituted for clindamycin.
   2. Length of I.V. therapy depends upon clinical and ultrasonographic response. Abscesses in the cul-de-sac are drained vaginally. Accessible simple abscesses can be drained percutaneously under ultrasonic guidance. Some patients will require excisional surgery.
   3. This regimen is classical "triple therapy" and remains the gold standard of treatment. The new beta-lactam antibiotics cannot substitute for clindamycin or metronidazole in the treatment of anaerobic infections which have progressed to deep abscess formation.

B. Moderately severe infections without deep abscess formation: postpartum and post-C-section endometritis, pelvic cellulitis, abscesses of abdominal wound or vaginal cuff
   Clindamycin and gentamicin—dosages as given in Section A or
   Cefoxitin—2 g every 6 hours I.V. or
   Cefotaxime or ceftizoxime—2 g every 6 hours I.V.
   Note:
   I.V. treatment is continued for at least 4 days and at least 48 hours after patient defervesces. Clindamycin, 450 mg four times daily by mouth, or tetracycline, 500 mg four times daily by mouth is continued after discharge from hospital to complete 14 days of therapy.

C. Moderately severe infections in which *N. gonorrhoeae* and *C. trachomatis* are suspected in addition to endogenous bacteria: acute pelvic inflammatory disease, postpartum endometritis and salpingitis
   Doxycycline—100 mg every 12 hours I.V. or
   Tetracycline—500 mg every 6 hours I.V. and
   Cefoxitin, cefotaxime or ceftizoxime—2 g every 6 hours I.V.
   Notes:
   1. I.V. treatment is continued for at least 4 days and at least 48 hours after patient defervesces. Doxycycline, 100 mg twice daily by mouth or tetracycline, 500 mg four times daily by mouth is continued after discharge from hospital to complete 14 days of therapy.
   2. These recommendations have evolved because *N. gonorrhoeae* may be resistant to penicillin and tetracycline, and gentamicin may not be effective in pus. *C. trachomatis* is resistant to beta-lactams, clindamycin, aminoglycosides and metronidazole but is dependably sensitive to the tetracyclines.

penicillin G. The two major exceptions are *Bacteroides fragilis* and *E. coli*. Before the complexity of endogenous infections was fully appreciated, the administration of penicillin in high doses permitted less destructive surgery or avoided surgery altogether (Franklin et al., 1973). To cover *B. fragilis*, tetracycline was added to penicillin. Tetracycline was replaced by clindamycin which is more potent in vitro, covers more strains of *B. fragilis*, inhibits *Staphylococcus aureus*, and produces little or no thrombophlebitis at the infusion site. An aminoglycoside (first streptomycin, then kanamycin and finally gentamicin) was added to cover *E. coli* to yield what became known as "triple therapy" (Section A, Table 1). Most recently metronidazole has emerged as an excellent drug against anaerobes, capable of deodorizing a foul pus discharge within 48 hours.

Triple therapy is not needed if deep infection has not progressed beyond the stage of cellulitis. Regimens of one or two drugs yield excellent cure rates in such circumstances (Section B, Table 1). It must be understood, however, that it is the prompt institution of antibiotics in high doses intravenously that has drastically reduced the morbidity of postpartum and postoperative infections (Sweet et al., 1983).

Dormant in the cervix throughout pregnancy, *Neisseria gonorrhoeae* and *Chlamydia trachomatis* can become invasive in the puerperium. This fact has led to the recommendations in Section C of Table 1.

Heparin appears to be a useful adjunct to antibiotics in the treatment of septic thrombophlebitis. Ligation of the inferior vena cava and left ovarian vein is required rarely today. Since pregnancy lowers reserves of folic acid, any myelopoietic stress, including infection, can produce a megaloblastic crisis with neutropenia and thrombocytopenia. All periparturient women who are seriously ill should receive folic acid to preserve the neutrophil response needed for control of infection.

PROPHYLAXIS. Although the vagina cannot be completely decontaminated, the number of resident bacteria can be reduced by the removal of excessive secretions through treatment of a specific vaginitis (due to *Trichomonas vaginalis* or *Candida albicans*) and by thorough mechanical cleansing before surgery. Conization of the cervix promotes bacterial multiplication, and hysterectomy should follow conization within 48 hours or be delayed several weeks to lower the risk of operative infection. To prevent exogenous infection, aseptic technique must be maintained even in the presence of gross contamination with vaginal flora. Hemostasis is a critical element of surgical technique for preventing infection. A biopsy of the ovary should never be made in a contaminated field such as that produced by culpotomy. Any patient at risk of an anaerobic infection should have had previous tetanus immunization.

A single antibiotic such as cephalothin given immediately before and for 24 hours after vaginal hysterectomy strikingly reduces postoperative infections in those (premenopausal) women at greatest risk (Mead, 1974). Apparently the presence of an antibiotic within the hematomas formed at surgery delays bacterial growth and often tips the early inflammatory battle in favor of the host.

GRANULOMATOUS INFECTIONS

Granulomatous infection would be synonymous with tuberculosis of the female genitalia if it were not for the rare infections with *Histoplasma capsulatum* and *Coccidioides immitis*. Tubercle bacilli reach the fallopian tubes hematogenously during the primary phase of pulmonary or intestinal tuberculosis. If infection is not arrested in one tube, it is rarely arrested in the other. Bacilli then spread upward to produce localized pelvic peritonitis in one half of patients and perioophoritis in one third. Downward spread produces endometritis in almost 60 per cent of cases, but the cervix and vagina are far more resistant. Coincidental renal tuberculosis occurs in less than 5 per cent of cases.

Systemic manifestations of chronic infection are often absent despite many years of involvement. Most patients without progressive pulmonary disease appear healthy, and fever is absent or low grade. However, 85 per cent of patients are nulliparous, and sterility is the chief complaint of 50 per cent. Mild pelvic pain and abnormal vaginal bleeding are the next most frequent complaints. The most common physical finding is an adnexal mass, which is often unilateral despite pathologic involvement of both tubes.

Local complications such as intestinal obstruction and fistula are rare. Generalized peritonitis and hematogenous dissemination develop only rarely from a genital focus. Thus, sterility reigns unchallenged as the major complication. Conception is more likely following treatment, but the risk of ectopic pregnancy is then increased.

If endometritis is present, diagnosis may be made by curettage performed near the end of the menstrual cycle. Endometrial tubercles are hard and contain few bacilli because the regular shedding of the endometrium allows no time for caseation to occur. Culture of the endometrial tissue is usually required for a definitive diagnosis. Peritoneal granulomas may be observed, and biopsies and cultures of them may be made by culdoscopy and peritoneoscopy. In geographic areas in which the disease is infrequently encountered, most cases are discovered unexpectedly at surgery.

Medical treatment is the same as for progressive pulmonary tuberculosis (Schaefer, 1967). Even large cold abscesses will resolve without surgical intervention, which may, however, be undertaken with little fear as long as medical treatment is begun postoperatively.

VULVOVAGINITIS

Vulvovaginitis is an abnormal increase in vaginal secretions with inflammation of the vaginal mucosa and adjacent vulvar skin. Purulent cervical discharge is a separate entity caused by *Neisseria gonorrhoeae, Chlamydia trachomatis,* nonspecific salpingo-oophoritis, an intrauterine contraceptive device, or erosive processes such as *Herpes simplex* and carcinoma.

At menarche, estrogen secretion causes glycogen to accumulate within a thickened vaginal squamous epithelium. The sparse but varied vaginal flora of childhood become dominated by *Lactobacillus* species that can use glycogen and lower the pH of the secretions to 5 or less. The vagina becomes resistant to pyogenic bacteria such as *Neisseria gonorrhoeae* and *Streptococcus pyogenes,* which cause vaginitis in childhood. *Trichomonas vaginalis* can proliferate in normal adult secretions. A significant proportion of women who acquire this motile protozoan through sexual intercourse promptly develop vaginitis that clears upon elimination of the trichomonads. *Candida albicans,* present in normal feces, has ready access to the vagina. Sexual transmission is not needed, and lowered resistance must play a large role in its ability to establish vaginal moniliasis. Pregnancy, oral contraceptives, cervical discharge, glycosuria, and oral antibiotics are believed to stimulate overgrowth of *C. albicans* through alterations in the volume, glycogen content, and pH of vaginal secretions and the suppression of competing fecal and vaginal bacteria. Vulvitis is partly a result of contact hypersensitivity to the parasite growing on epithelial cells.

Some women have increased vaginal secretions without abundant trichomonads or yeasts (nonspecific vaginitis). These secretions usually show some imbalance among "normal" vaginal microbes. *Gardnerella vaginalis (Hemophilus vaginalis), Ureaplasma urealyticum, Mycoplasma hominis,* and strictly anaerobic bacteria are often more numerous than *Lactobacilli* (as they may be in the specific forms of vaginitis). Although the pathogenesis of this mild illness is not understood, some investigators postulate a central role for *G. vaginalis* (Pheifer et al., 1978).

Classically, *T. vaginalis* produces a profuse, thin, greenish, malodorous discharge containing many granulocytes and so many motile trichomonads that microscopic examination of fresh wet secretions suffices for diagnosis. *C. albicans* causes a scantier, thicker exudate containing yeasts and granulocytes on wet mount or Gram stain. Epithelial cells scraped from inflamed vulvar skin show the fungus in its hyphal phase on Gram stain. Not infrequently, both agents of specific vaginitis occur simultaneously. Primary or recurrent *Herpes simplex* must be considered in the presence of vulvar vesicles or ulcers.

In nonspecific vaginitis, a scant discharge with a disagreeable odor but few granulocytes is present at the introitus. Vulvar irritation appears minimal, although the patient may complain of itching, burning, and dyspareunia. Diagnosis requires the exclusion of a purulent cervical discharge and the two specific agents.

T. vaginalis infection responds promptly to one oral dose of 2 g of metronidazole, which should not, however, be given during pregnancy (Dykers, 1975). To avoid reinfection, sexual partners should be treated simultaneously or they should use condoms for several months until trichomonads are eliminated spontaneously from the male urethra. *C. albicans* infection is treated by vaginal application of nystatin or miconazole daily for 14 days, and severe vulvitis responds promptly to topical corticosteroid cream. Initial results are good, but recurrence is common, even when predisposing factors are eliminated. Then, an attempt to reduce fecal yeast with oral nystatin seems reasonable (Miles et al., 1977).

With the possible exception of metronidazole, there is no evidence that any of the current therapies for nonspecific vaginitis is effective. Probably the less done the better, since local or systemic treatment may perpetuate a floral imbalance or produce inflammation itself.

References

Dykers, J. R.: Single dose metronidazole for trichomonal vaginitis. N Engl J Med 293:23, 1975.

Franklin, E. W., Hevron, J. E., and Thompson, J. D.: Management of the pelvic abscess. Clin Obstet Gynecol 16(2):66, 1973.

Hawkins, D. F., Sevitt, L. H., and Fairbrother, P. F.: Management of septic chemical abortion with renal failure. Use of a conservative regimen. N Engl J Med 292:722, 1975.

Hibbard, L. T., Snyder, E. N., and McVann, R. M.: Subgluteal and retropsoal infection in obstetrical practice. Obstet Gynecol 39:137, 1972.
Ledger, W. J.: Postoperative pelvic infections. Clin Obstet Gynecol 12(1):265, 1969.
Mantzavinos, T., Garcia, J. E., and Jones, H. W.: Ultrasound measurement of ovarian follicles stimulated by human gonadotropins for oocyte recovery and in vitro fertilization. Fertil Steril 40:461, 1983.
Mead, P. B.: Practical applications of antibiotics in prevention and treatment of pelvic infections. J Reprod Med 13:135, 1974.
Miles, M. R., Olsen, L., and Rogers, A.: Recurrent vaginal candidiasis. Importance of an intestinal reservoir. JAMA 238:1836, 1977.
Pheifer, T. A., Forsyth, P. S., Durfee, M. A., Pollock, H. M., and Holmes, K. K.: Nonspecific vaginitis. Role of *Haemophilus vaginalis* and treatment with metronidazole. N Engl J Med 298:1429, 1978.
Rotheram, E. B., and Schick, S. F.: Nonclostridial anaerobic bacteria in septic abortion. Am J Med 46:80, 1969.
Schaefer, G.: Diagnosis and treatment of female genital tuberculosis. Int Surg 48:240, 1967.
Sweet, R. L., Yonekura, M. L., Hill, G., Gibbs, R. S., and Eschenbach, D. A.: Appropriate use of antibiotics in serious obstetric and gynecologic infections. Am J Obstet Gynecol 146:719, 1983.
vanSonnenberg, E., Ferrucci, J. T., Mueller, P. R., Wittenberg, J., and Simeone, J. F.: Percutaneous drainage of abscesses and fluid collections: technique, results, and applications. Radiology 142:1, 1982.
Wolner-Hanssen, P., Mardh, P., Svensson, L., and Westrom, L.: Laparoscopy in women with chlamydial infection and pelvic pain: a comparison of patients with and without salpingitis. Obstet Gynecol 61:299, 1983.

161

GONOCOCCAL AND CHLAMYDIAL GENITAL INFECTIONS

J. Allen McCutchan, M.D.

Gonorrhea (from the Greek *gonos* [seed] and *rhoia* [a flow]) is a sexually transmitted infection of columnar and transitional epithelia by *Neisseria gonorrhoeae*. Genital infections (cervicitis in women and urethritis in men) may spread by ascending the genital tract or by invading the blood. The syndromes of gonococcal bacteremia are discussed in Chapter 192. Gonococci may directly infect extragenital mucous membranes such as the conjunctiva, pharynx, and rectum. Patients without symptoms may be colonized and can infect others.

Nongonococcal urethritis, a syndrome caused by several sexually transmitted agents, is usually less severe than gonorrhea. It may coexist with gonorrhea and make its appearance as postgonococcal urethritis after gonococci are eliminated by antibiotics. *Chlamydia trachomatis*, which appears to be the major cause of the syndrome, also infects the cervix and pelvic organs of women, the eyes of adults, and the eyes and lungs of neonates by way of the maternal cervix. *Ureaplasma urealyticum*, another candidate agent, is less clearly implicated.

ETIOLOGY

Gonorrhea. *Neisseria gonorrhoeae* is an aerobic, gram-negative diplococcus requiring enriched media and elevated levels of carbon dioxide for growth. Cytochrome oxidase distinguishes *Neisseria* from most Enterobacteriaceae. Pathogenic *Neisseria*, but not nonpathogens, produce an enzyme that cleaves one of the two subtypes of IgA (IgA_1) into Fab and Fc fragments. It is possible, but unproved, that inactivation of mucosal IgA is essential for virulence. Nongonococcal *Neisseria* organisms are frequently found in the pharynx and are rarely isolated from anogenital cultures but do not appear to produce local disease. A detailed discussion of the microbiology of the gonococcus is presented in Chapter 29.

The cell wall of the gonococcus is similar to that of other gram-negative bacteria. Several components of its outer membrane appear to contribute to virulence. Pili, which are found on fresh isolates, but are difficult to demonstrate in vivo, determine colonial morphology on agar and mediate attachment to mammalian cells. The lipopolysaccharide endotoxin can directly damage tissue and enhance the inflammatory response via interactions with cellular and humoral defenses. A capsule, thus far demonstrated only under special conditions in vitro, may be antiphagocytic, but its chemical or immunologic properties are unknown. Leukocyte association factor, a surface protein, enhances attachment of gonococci to polymorphonuclear leukocytes but not to other cells.

Strain-specific nutritional requirements for amino acids, purines, pyrimidines, and vitamins have been used to type gonococci (auxotyping). Dependence on arginine, hypoxanthine, and uracil or on proline characterizes many strains isolated from asymptomatic and bacteremic infections. These strains show a geographic distribution that parallels the incidence of these syndromes. This auxotype may identify a clone of unusual virulence and may help to account for the more frequent development of bacteremia in asymptomatic carriers.

Nongonococcal Urethritis. *Chlamydia trachomatis* is a strict intracellular bacterium (see Chapter 56). Certain serogroups cause lymphogranuloma venereum (see Chapter 164), and others cause nongonococcal urethritis (NGU). The evidence that *Chlamydia* causes NGU is as follows: (1) *Chlamydia* is more frequently isolated from men with NGU (30 to 60 per cent) than controls (about 5 per cent), (2) there is an acute antibody response in men with *Chlamydia*-positive NGU (Holmes et al., 1975), (3) *Chlamydia* causes urethritis in nonhuman primates, and finally, (4) when mixed gonococcal and chlamydial infections are treated with penicillin, *Chlamydia* organisms persist and are associated with a high incidence of postgonococcal urethritis (Bowie et al., 1977). When patients with NGU are treated with sulfisoxazole (active against *Chlamydia* but not *Ureaplasma*), response is common in *Chlamydia*-positive, *Ureaplasma*-negative cases, but is less frequent in *Ureaplasma*-positive, *Chlamydia*-negative cases. Aminocyclitols (active against *Ureaplasma* but not *Chlamydia*) cure *Ureaplasma*-positive, *Chlamydia*-negative cases but not *Chlamydia*-positive, *Ureaplasma*-negative cases. These studies suggest a role for both *Ureaplasma* and *Chlamydia* in NGU. The role of *Ureaplasma* remains controversial because it has not been possible to demonstrate an antibody response to infection and ureaplasmas are frequently found in men without urethritis. Intraurethral inoculation of ureaplasmas in two volunteers and several primates has produced urethritis. About 20 per cent of cases are negative for both organisms, do not respond well to antibiotics, and have not yielded a likely pathogen.

PATHOGENESIS

Gonorrhea. During transmission, gonococci are deposited with normal flora and genital secretions on the genital mucosa. To survive in the male urethra, they must avoid being washed out or killed by urine. In the cervix and vagina gonococci must survive hydrogen ion and other inhibitory products of the normal flora. The inhibitory effect of vaginal and urethral flora and of urine is well documented, and carriage of inhibitory lactobacilli in the endocervix has been correlated with resistance to gonorrhea (Saigh et al., 1978).

The susceptible columnar epithelium of the urethra, endocervix, or deeper genital tissues is invaded after gonococci penetrate the mucus and attach to epithelial cells. The major inflammatory response in gonorrhea occurs in the submucosa. Organisms apparently penetrate the intact mucosa before much inflammation begins, elicit an intense polymorphonuclear leukocyte response, and then destroy the overlying mucosa (Harkness, 1948). Experimental infection of the isolated human fallopian tube shows that gonococci adhere to specific appendages of the mucus-secreting epithelial cells of women, but not females of other species, are phagocytosed by these cells, and are then passed into the submucosa through and between them. They disrupt ciliary activity by means of a soluble toxin but do not attach to ciliated cells, and can severely damage tissues in the absence of an inflammatory response (Ward et al., 1974; McGee et al., 1978).

The mechanism by which gonococci ascend the genital tract is unknown. Their attachment to sperm is one potential mechanism of transport. Gonococcal endotoxin rapidly immobilizes cilia, thus preventing them from removing the gonococci from the fallopian tubes.

The intense submucosal inflammation in gonorrhea produces an exudate containing polymorphonuclear leukocytes (PMN) and gonococci. Some PMN have many gonococci in their cytoplasm either within individual phagosomes or, less commonly, as large clusters within a single phagosome. Most gonococci within PMN are rapidly killed, but some may escape destruction or even reproduce within the phagocytes (Veale et al., 1977). Acquired opsonizing antibody that increases phagocytosis of gonococci by human PMNs can be demonstrated in the sera of prostitutes (Bisno et al., 1975).

Despite the antibody response to gonococci, infection does not necessarily produce immunity. Treated patients can acquire the same strain from their untreated sexual partners. Women may develop partial immunity to upper genital tract infection with gonococci of the same principal outer membrane protein (protein I) serotype (Buchanan et al., 1980). Before antibiotic treatment became available, men with prolonged untreated infections commonly had multiple episodes of gonorrhea, presumably caused by different strains. Possible reasons for the ineffective immune response in patients with gonorrhea are treatment, antigenic variation among strains, and short-lived immunity. Furthermore, gonococci growing in vivo show a resistance to both phagocytosis and serum bactericidal activity that is not seen when the same strain is grown on agar (Penn et al., 1977).

Nongonococcal Urethritis. The pathogenesis of chlamydial infections has been extensively studied in the eye but not in the genital tract. The histopathology of experimental urethritis in nonhuman primates resembles that in human conjunctivitis and cervicitis. Follicular lesions in the eye and urethra contain intraepithelial inclusion bodies typical of *Chlamydia* and are composed of subepithelial collections of macrophages and lymphocytes. Human chlamydial urethritis has a similar follicular appearance, which is distinctly different from the deep mucosal erosions of gonorrhea. Local and systemic antibody responses occur, but their role in immunity is not clear. Recurrent infections are common in some men, others remain asymptomatic during prolonged carriage, and still others resist infection. The reasons for this variable response are not known.

CLINICAL SYNDROMES

Genital Infection in Men. Urethritis is the most common gonococcal infection in men, but less common than nongonococcal urethritis (NGU) in some groups. Gonococcal urethritis can be clinically distinguished from NGU in most cases (Jacobs and Kraus, 1975). After an incubation period of two to five days typical acute anterior gonococcal urethritis presents with severe dysuria, purulent discharge, and a positive gram stain of urethral pus (typical diplococci within polymorphonuclear leukocytes) (Fig. 1). In nongonococcal urethritis, dysuria is usually less severe and more chronic, discharge is mucoid and scant, and the exudate has no diplococci in the gram stain. The incubation period of nongonococcal urethritis is longer and more variable than that of gonorrhea (Fig. 2). Less common symptoms of either form of urethritis are frequency of urination, urgency, genital itching, inguinal adenitis, and fever. Age, marital status, sexual history, and history of gonorrhea or urethritis do not aid in separating these syndromes. In the United States and Britain, NGU is more common in whites than in blacks and in those of high socioeconomic status, but the reason for this difference is unknown.

Despite these differences in typical signs and symptoms, however, in certain patients NGU may be severely painful and purulent, and gonococci may colonize the urethra without producing symptoms. The importance of asymptomatic colonization of the male urethra by gonococci has only recently been appreciated (Handsfield et al., 1974). Asymptomatic men can transmit gonorrhea and may become symptomatic after prolonged carriage. For this reason, cultures of male contacts of infected women should be made (negative gram stain does not exclude asymptomatic colonization), and the men should be treated if the culture is positive or follow-up is not assured.

Gonococcal and nongonococcal urethritis may coexist. When gonorrhea is treated with drugs such as penicillin or spectinomycin that do not eliminate *Chlamydia*, about one third of patients develop recurrent urethritis two to three weeks later. Most cases of postgonococcal urethritis occur in men who harbor *Chlamydia* and respond to antichlamydial antibiotics. The cause of postgonococcal urethritis that is not associated with *Chlamydia* is unknown.

Untreated gonococcal anterior urethritis reaches a symptomatic peak in two to three weeks, but it may persist for months and relapse. Local extension to the posterior urethra, periurethral glands, prostate, seminal vesicles, and epididymis is common in patients with untreated disease but is rare in promptly treated cases. Complications of ascending infection include urethral stricture and sterility. The role of gonorrhea and the agents of nongonococcal urethritis in epididymitis and prostatitis is not clear. Cultures of epididymal aspirates from young men with acute epididymitis commonly grow *Chlamydia* and less frequently grow gonococci; those from older men grow coliform bacteria. Acute and chronic prostatitis is rarely associated with viable gonococci in prostatic secretions. Organisms that stain with fluorescent gonococcal antiserum but do not grow in culture are found in the prostatic

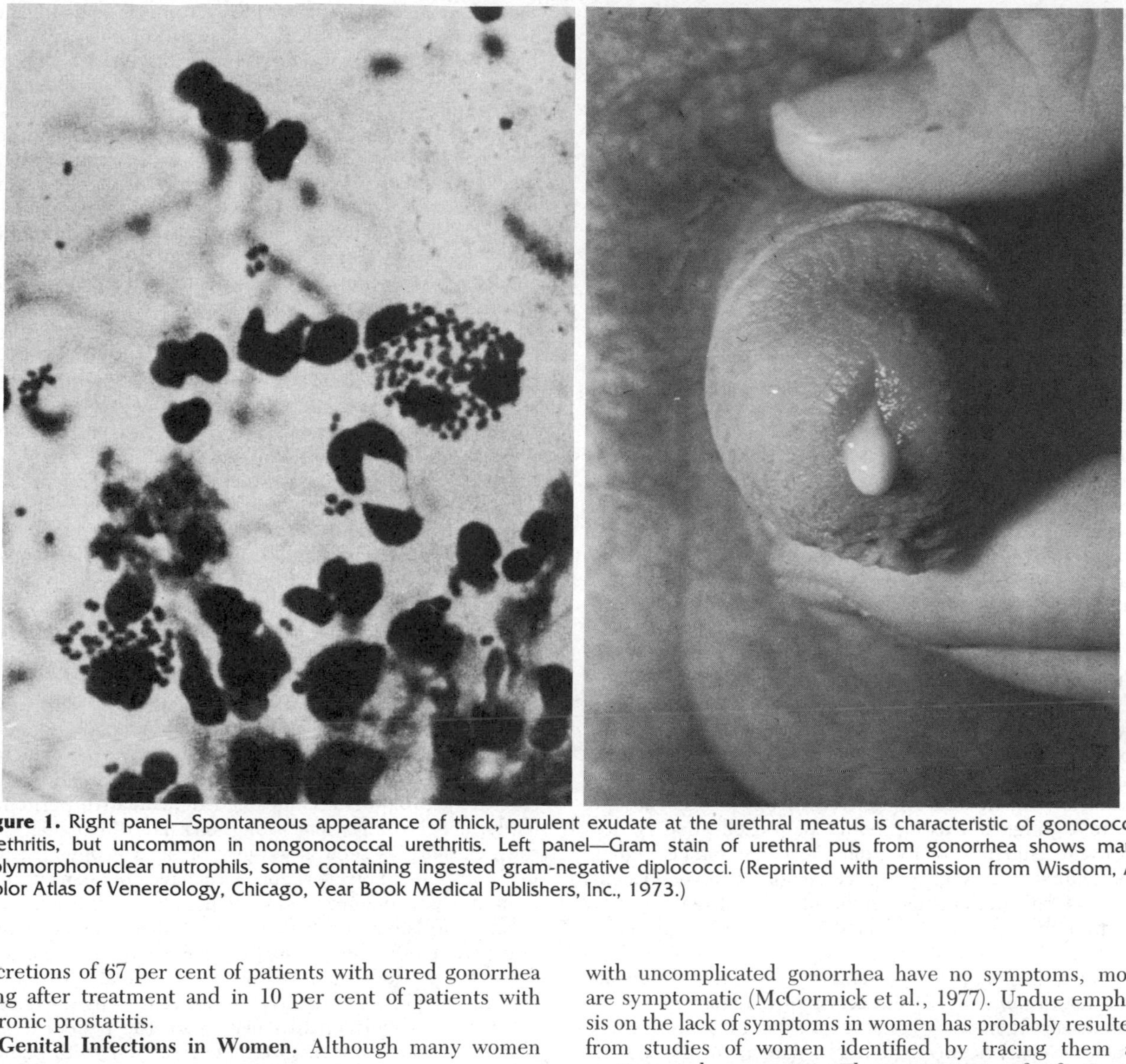

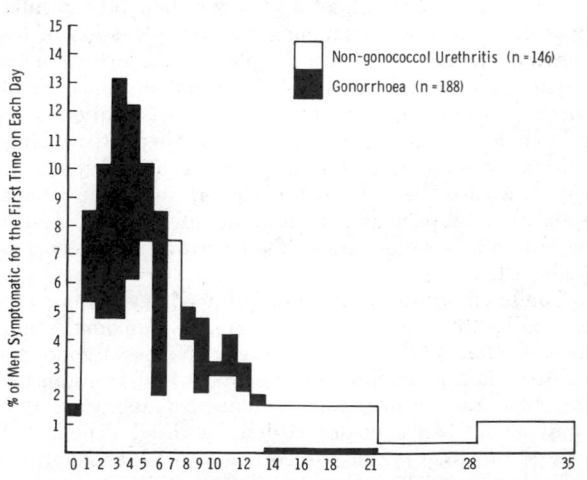

Figure 1. Right panel—Spontaneous appearance of thick, purulent exudate at the urethral meatus is characteristic of gonococcal urethritis, but uncommon in nongonococcal urethritis. Left panel—Gram stain of urethral pus from gonorrhea shows many polymorphonuclear nutrophils, some containing ingested gram-negative diplococci. (Reprinted with permission from Wisdom, A.: Color Atlas of Venereology, Chicago, Year Book Medical Publishers, Inc., 1973.)

secretions of 67 per cent of patients with cured gonorrhea long after treatment and in 10 per cent of patients with chronic prostatitis.

Genital Infections in Women. Although many women with uncomplicated gonorrhea have no symptoms, most are symptomatic (McCormick et al., 1977). Undue emphasis on the lack of symptoms in women has probably resulted from studies of women identified by tracing them as contacts or by screening. The primary site of infection is usually the endocervix with secondary infection or colonization of the urethra and rectum. Endocervical gonorrhea may produce increased or purulent vaginal secretions, menorrhagia, or intermenstrual bleeding. Urethritis gives rise to dysuria, urinary frequency, and urgency. Despite frequent colonization of the rectum, symptomatic proctitis is uncommon. Infection of the paraurethral (Skene's) glands simulates urethritis. Acute Bartholin's duct infection usually presents as a unilateral, exquisitely tender mass lateral to the introitus.

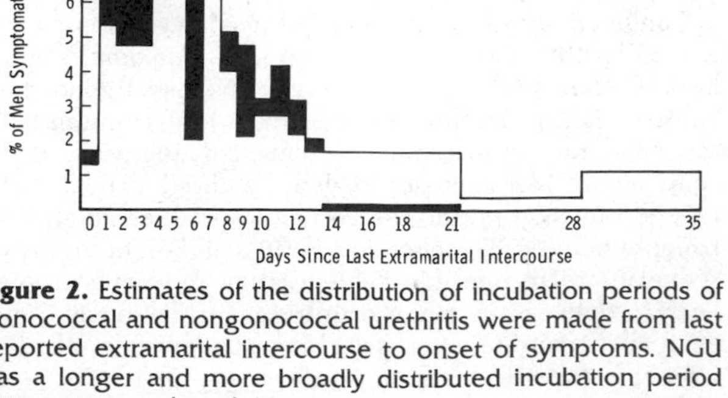

Figure 2. Estimates of the distribution of incubation periods of gonococcal and nongonococcal urethritis were made from last reported extramarital intercourse to onset of symptoms. NGU has a longer and more broadly distributed incubation period than gonococcal urethritis.

Gonococci ascend the genital tract in women to infect the fallopian tubes and pelvic peritoneum. This most common complication (10 to 20 per cent) of gonorrhea (often called pelvic inflammatory disease or salpingitis) occurs more frequently in women who have intrauterine devices or a history of prior attacks, but rarely occurs during pregnancy. Acute salpingitis usually begins with diffuse pelvic pain and tenderness, fever, malaise, and infrequently, vomiting. Tenderness may be lateralized and simulate appendicitis, ruptured ectopic pregnancy, or ovulation pain. Examination for pain on cervical movement and gram stain of urethral, endocervical, or rectal smears may help to confirm the diagnosis. Subacute salpingitis causes prolonged or recurrent attacks of pelvic pain and tenderness usually associated with episodic low-grade fever and menstrual disturbances. The intensity of pain and tenderness varies widely with time and among patients. Bilateral enlargement or thickening of the fallopian tubes is characteristic. Symptoms may simulate urinary tract, bowel, or lower back diseases. Chronic salpingitis is usually preceded by acute or subacute attacks but may appear de novo with sterility, ectopic pregnancy, or as asymptomatic thickening or abscess formation in the adnexal regions.

In any form of salpingitis, gonococci may not be recovered, and mixtures of anaerobic and aerobic vaginal flora may be found instead (Eschenback et al., 1975). The role of gonococci in cases of pelvic inflammatory disease from which other organisms are cultured is not clear. Experimental infection of human fallopian tubes by gonococci in vitro disrupts the function of the ciliated cells that maintain mucus flow toward the uterus. This damage to cilia could allow the normal vaginal flora to ascend and replace the gonococcus, which would explain why gonococci are most frequently cultured in acute salpingitis and diminish as symptoms continue (Lip and Burgoyne, 1966). Salpingitis causes sterility and ectopic pregnancy by obstructing the fallopian tubes. Sterility occurs in at least 20 per cent of women treated for salpingitis.

Of the agents of nongonococcal urethritis, *Chlamydia trachomatis* and *Herpes simplex* cause cervicitis and *Trichomonas* causes vaginitis. *Chlamydia trachomatis* of the NGU serotypes are commonly found in cervical cultures from asymptomatic women in developed countries. Their role in salpingitis is reinforced by a series of careful studies in which *Chlamydia* have been grown in one third of Swedish women undergoing laparoscopy for diagnosis of acute salpingitis. This technique allows collection of biopsies and exudate directly from the pelvic organs without contamination by vaginal or cervical flora. High or changing titers of IgG antibody or significant titers of IgM antibody support the claim that chlamydiae are involved in half of women with acute salpingitis (Ripa et al., 1980). Experimental infection by *Chlamydia* or *Mycoplasma hominis*, but not *Ureaplasma*, of the cervix or endometrium of the female grivet monkey resulted in salpingitis after several weeks, since *Chlamydia* required patency of the isthmus of the uterine tubes to ascend the genital tract. It would appear that they do not reach the fallopian tubes of women by hematogenous or lymphatic routes.

Proctitis. Sexually transmitted pathogens have been implicated in intestinal infections in homosexual men (Quinn et al., 1983). Most syndromes can be characterized clinically as enteritis (diarrhea, abdominal pain, nausea, flatulence, and normal sigmoidoscopic exam), proctocolitis (symptoms of enteritis associated with abnormal mucosa above 15 cm on sigmoidoscopy), or proctitis (constipation, anorectal pain or discharge, tenesmus, and abnormal mucosa limited to 15 cm from the rectum). While a variety of enteric pathogens (campylobacter, shigella, salmonella, giardia, and *Entamoeba histolytica*) probably descend the GI tract to cause enteritis and colitis, proctitis is caused by sexually transmitted organisms deposited directly on the rectal mucosa. In addition to the gonococcus and *Chlamydia*, *Herpes simplex* and *Treponema pallidum* frequently cause proctitis.

Gonococci infect the rectum during penoanal contact in women and male homosexuals or by secondary spread from the endocervix in women (Klein et al., 1977). The stratified squamous epithelium of the anus withstands invasion, but the columnar epithelium of the rectum becomes inflamed and friable. Mucopurulent or bloody discharge may occur, but most patients remain asymptomatic. Acute symptoms of proctitis (severe burning, tenesmus, or purulent discharge) are unusual (2 to 5 per cent) and even mild symptoms (itching, mucoid discharge, painful defecation, and constipation) are uncommon (< 10 per cent). Proctoscopic examination reveals mucosal pus in more than half of patients, rectal erythema and friability without ulcerations. *Chlamydia* are associated with two forms of proctitis. The lymphogranuloma venereum-associated serotypes of *Chlamydia trachomatis* cause acute, severe, ulcerative proctitis and granulomatous inflammation on biopsy. Non-LGV serotypes are found more frequently, but with milder signs and symptoms (Quinn et al., 1981; Bolan et al., 1982). Complications are rare in the postantibiotic era but include strictures, anal fistulas, and perianal abscesses.

Pharyngeal Gonorrhea. Gonococcal pharyngitis is primarily a disease of women and homosexual men who practice fellatio. Most carriers are asymptomatic, but pharyngitis, tonsillitis, and gingivitis have been ascribed to the gonococcus. Among patients with gonorrhea in other sites, about 20 per cent of homosexual men and 10 per cent of heterosexual women harbor gonococci in the pharynx. Gonococci disseminate in the blood more frequently from the pharynx than from other sites, but gonococci in the throat are rarely a source of transmission to sexual partners (Wiesner et al., 1973).

Perihepatitis (Fitz-Hugh-Curtis Syndrome). The association of acute, severe, pleuritic, right upper abdominal pain with salpingitis or cervical gonorrhea has led clinicians to formulate the concept of gonococcal perihepatitis. This clinical syndrome is accompanied by exudative peritonitis (early) and "violin string" adhesions (late) involving Glisson's capsule, as seen at surgery or laparoscopy. Despite many attempts, however, gonococci have not been cultured from the peritoneum. Association of the syndrome with chlamydial salpingitis has suggested that chlamydia may also play a role, but again they have not been cultured from the peritoneum (Wolner-Hansen et al., 1980). Although not proven by culture to be caused by gonococci, a diagnosis of perihepatitis may spare the patient an exploratory laparotomy and warrants treatment with penicillin. Perihepatitis simulates a variety of hepatic and biliary tract diseases with hepatomegaly, mild elevation of liver enzymes, leukocytosis, and elevated erythrocyte sedimentation rate (Litt and Cohn, 1978). Pleural effusions, hepatic friction rubs, and even transient nonvisualization of the gallbladder occur infrequently in perihepatitis. Clinical evidence of salpingitis is usually but not invariably present, and rare cases have been reported in men (see Chapter 180). Residual pain after medical therapy has been relieved by lysis of adhesions through the laparoscope (Reichert and Valle, 1976).

Conjunctivitis. Conjunctivitis in neonates is most often caused by the gonococcus but also by *Chlamydia*, staphylococci, *Hemophilus*, and *Moraxella*. Neonatal gonorrheal ophthalmia appears three to seven days postpartum, usually as a bilateral, profuse, and purulent conjunctivitis. If the conjunctival sac becomes sealed by dried exudate, the rapped pus may invade the cornea to produce keratitis or panophthalmitis (Thatcher and Pettit, 1971). These serious sequelae are responsible for legislation requiring prophylaxis at delivery in many countries. Instillation of 1 per cent silver nitrate after swabbing the eyes (method of Crede) is the safest and most effective prophylactic technique. Prophylactic local antibiotics or careful surveillance followed by specific diagnosis and treatment of the child and mother have also been successful. The latter method has the advantage of detecting gonorrhea in the mother but risks the vision of children who escape surveillance. The conjunctiva of children or adults can be infected by autoinoculation, sexual activity, laboratory accidents, or use of contaminated urine as a folk remedy for other forms of conjunctivitis. *Chlamydia trachomatis* causes conjunctivitis in both neonates and adults by spread from the genital areas.

Gonorrhea in Children. Aside from ophthalmia neonatorum, vulvovaginitis is the most common form of gonorrhea in prepubescent children (Barrett-Connor, 1973). Unlike the stratified squamous epithelium of the adult vagina, the immature vaginal and vulvar epithelium in girls is readily infected. Although fomites and nonsexual intimacy have been implicated, most cases result from sexual abuse by adult relatives. The medicolegal implications of this diagnosis require careful bacteriologic confirmation.

Painful inflammation and purulent or bloody discharge from the vulva and vagina are the most common symptoms, but associated urethritis, pelvic peritonitis, and proctitis also occur. Differential diagnosis includes thread worm (*Enterobius* or *Oxyuris*) infestations, shigellosis, or candidiasis. Boys and girls may also acquire the other syndromes of adult gonorrhea (Nelson et al., 1976). In all such cases other family members should be investigated for gonorrhea and child abuse.

DIAGNOSIS. Positive Gram stains show typical diplococci within polymorphonuclear leukocytes. Results of gram staining correlate well with cultures from men with urethritis but are often falsely negative in specimens from the endocervix and are of no value in rectal or pharyngeal disease. Fluorescent antibody staining finds rare organisms in joint fluids and skin lesions of patients with gonococcemia.

Culture of gonococci requires careful specimen collection and preservation during transport. Specimens should be collected on bacteriologic loops or nontoxic swabs because cotton, wood, wire, and other materials may contain inhibitors. Urethritis may be diagnosed by collecting urethral exudate or by culturing urinary sediment. When direct inoculation onto culture media is impossible, swabs should be placed in a transport medium appropriate to the time in transport and the environmental temperature. Cultivation and identification of *N. gonorrhoeae* require enriched and selective media. Because gonococci are inhibited by normal microbial flora, antibiotics should be incorporated into culture media. A combination of vancomycin (for gram-positive bacteria), colistin and trimethoprim (for gram-negative bacilli), and nysatin (for commensal fungi) have improved the yield from heavily contaminated areas such as the rectum, pharynx, and cervix. Because normal flora and nonpathogenic *Neisseria* organisms are suppressed on chocolate agar containing antibiotics (Thayer-Martin media), the growth there of characteristic small translucent colonies that are strongly oxidase-positive and composed of gram-negative diplococci allows presumptive diagosis of *N. gonorrhoeae*. The need to differentiate the gonococcus from nonpathogenic *Neisseria* strains or meningococci depends on the site cultured and the medicolegal and social consequences of the diagnosis. Other *Neisseria* organisms frequently live in the pharynx but are found only infrequently on other mucosal surfaces. Specific identification of the gonococcus can be made by saccharolytic reactions, commercially available staphylococcal coagglutination tests or by fluorescence with highly absorbed antiserum or monoclonal antibodies. The gonococcus produces acid from glucose only; and the meningococci does so from both glucose and maltose. Nonpathogenic *Neisseria* organisms have other saccharolytic patterns.

Diagnosis of nongonococcal urethritis can be made clinically but must be supported by negative cultures for gonococci and objective evidence of urethritis. Polymorphonuclear leukocytes in urethral discharge (>5/oil immersion field) or in sediment from the first 10 ml of overnight urine (>15/high-dry [×400] field) supports the diagnosis of urethritis. If there are no gram-negative diplococci on Gram stain and no signs or symptoms of prostatitis, a presumptive diagnosis of NGU can be made. Cultures for *Herpes*, *Chlamydia*, and *Ureaplasma* and cytology for chlamydial inclusion bodies may be useful but are not widely available. Examination of wet mounts for *Trichomonas* and *Candida* is unnecessary unless antibiotics fail.

EPIDEMIOLOGY AND GEOGRAPHIC VARIATION. Patients with gonorrhea are typically male, young, urban, and promiscuous. The male predominance (about 3:1) reflects the greater frequency of asymptomatic disease in women, so that fewer infected women are identified. When women are screened thoroughly and contacts are traced carefully, the ratio of men to women falls dramatically. The relative incidence is also affected by prostitution, which results in a small, highly promiscuous group of women transmitting gonorrhea to a larger group of men, and homosexuality, which allows transfer of infection between men. In the United States, gonorrhea shows a remarkably sharp peak in incidence among those 20 to 24 years old. The increase in cases during the current epidemic occurred in those under age 24. Women tend to contract gonorrhea at a younger age than men (e.g., modal age of 24 in men and 19 in women in Denmark). The higher incidence of gonorrhea reported in cities may reflect better reporting practices in large urban venereal disease clinics as well as real differences in rates. The effect of promiscuity is illustrated by the high rates of gonorrhea among female prostitutes and males with many sex partners.

Gonorrhea and other venereal diseases traditionally increase at times of social upheaval. The two world wars and the wars in Korea, Vietnam, and Bangladesh all resulted in epidemic peaks in those geographic regions. During the past 25 years a dramatic increase in gonorrhea has been reported from many countries throughout the world. This increase has leveled off or dropped slightly in most western countries since about 1975 (Fig. 3). There are two causes of this epidemic at a time of relative peace and prosperity: (1) changing sexual mores in the industrialized nations have allowed earlier, more frequent, and more promiscuous sexual activity in young adults, and (2) urbanization and economic immigration in the developing nations have separated people from their spouses and families.

At least two changes in the gonococcus may have contributed to the epidemic. One change is the increased resistance of gonococci to penicillin. This has resulted in increased failure rates with penicillin treatment. The second change is selection of strains that cause asympomatic disease in men (e.g., AHU auxotypes) by aggressive treatment programs. By remaining asymptomatic and thus untreated, these strains of gonococci continue to spread to female contacts of these colonized men.

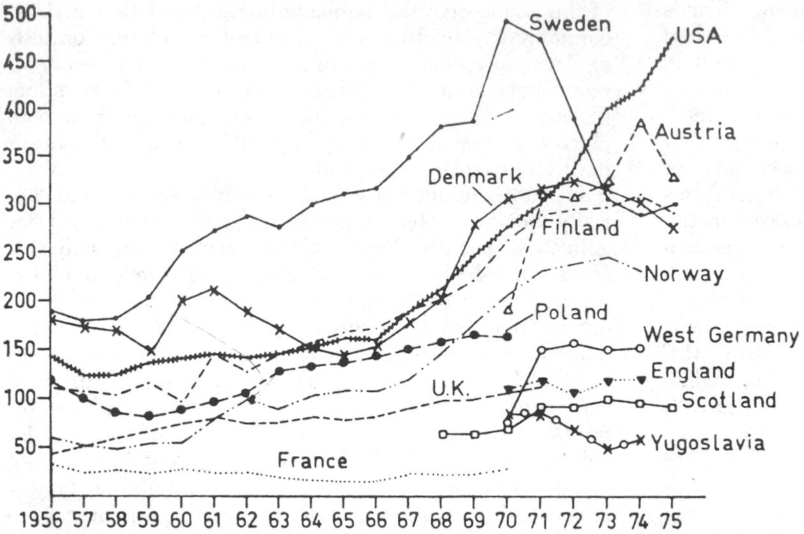

Figure 3. Incidence per 100,000 population of cases of gonorrhea reported to WHO by 12 European countries and the United States. Problems of reporting make it unlikely that these figures reflect the true incidence. Thus, they cannot be used as a basis for international comparisons but show the increasing incidence in many countries over the period from 1956 to 1975. Since the peaks in 1970 to 1975, incidence in many countries has leveled or declined. (Reprinted with permission—see Figure 2).

The incidence of various forms of gonorrhea, susceptibility to antibiotics, and patterns of spread vary geographically. Physicians must be aware of regional factors that could alter diagnosis and therapy. For example, isolates of gonococci from the western Pacific region are less likely to disseminate in the blood, are more resistant to penicillin by two different mechanisms, and are more often acquired from prostitutes than European or American strains (see Chapter 192 for further discussion). The spread of gonococci bearing plasmid-mediated penicillinase (PPNG = penicillin producing *N. gonorrhoeae*) as a marker can be traced to its geographic origin. After two different strains arose simultaneously in West Africa and Southeast Asia in 1976, the West African strain spread to Europe and the Southeast Asian strain spread to the United States. Despite aggressive attempts to control it, the Asian strain appears to be endemic at a low, but increasing, level in the United States and both strains have become endemic in western Europe. Furthermore, PPNG have increased in some areas of Europe, Asia, and Africa to levels (>5 per cent) at which penicillin can no longer be used with confidence. Spectinomycin-resistant PPNG are also being reported with increasing frequency. Thus, in the jet age strains acquiring drug resistance may spread rapidly throughout the world but have not replaced conventional strains.

Nongonococcal urethritis (NGU) and gonorrhea (GCU) are found in the same age group and both are frequently carried by asymptomatic female sex partners. Compared to GCU, NGU occurs in men of higher socioeconomic status, with fewer sexual partners, and in whites more frequently than blacks. In the United Stages NGU is as common as gonorrhea, and in England it is more common. Within the United States there appears to be marked geographic variation in ratios of NGU by region and type of population served by the reporting clinic. In England the number of reported cases of NGU has increased faster than GCU during the past two decades (Fig. 4). This greater increase in NGU than GCU may be an artifact of increased reporting of NGU because the ratio of NGU to GCU has remained constant in university-affiliated clinics in England, Sweden, and the United States (McCutchan, 1984).

THERAPY

Gonococcal Infections. Despite increasing resistance to penicillin over the past 20 years and the appearance of plasmid-coded penicillinase conferring high level resistance, penicillins remain the preferred therapy for most gonococcal infections (Table 1). In patients who are allergic to penicillins or harbor PPNG, tetracycline, spectinomycin, cefotaxime or cefoxitin are effective alternatives. Since gonococci are susceptible to many antibiotics, some regimens other than those listed may cure some infections but are not preferred because of efficacy, cost, and side effects.

It is important to consider the reliability of the patients, their history of drug intolerance, and the antibiotic susceptibility of the gonococcus in making a selection among the regimens recommended in Table 1. Tetracycline is cheap and lowers the rate of postgonococcal urethritis, but requires multiple doses and is contraindicated in children under 8 years old and in pregnant women. Doxycycline persists longer allowing for twice daily oral administration and potentially greater compliance, but is more expensive than tetracycline. Since spectinomycin is relatively expensive, it should be reserved for patients with penicillin allergy, treatment failure, or penicillinase-producing gon-

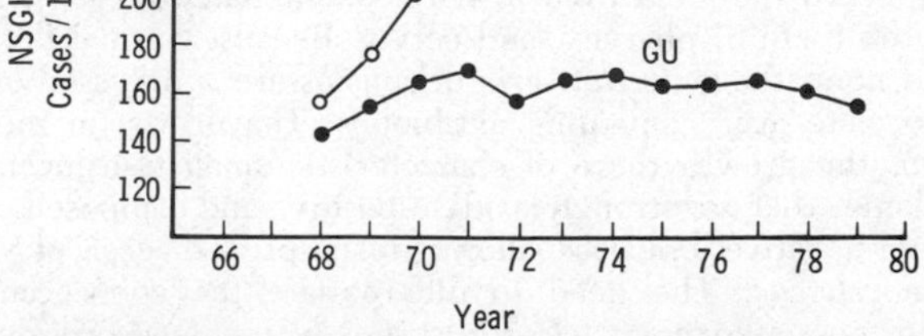

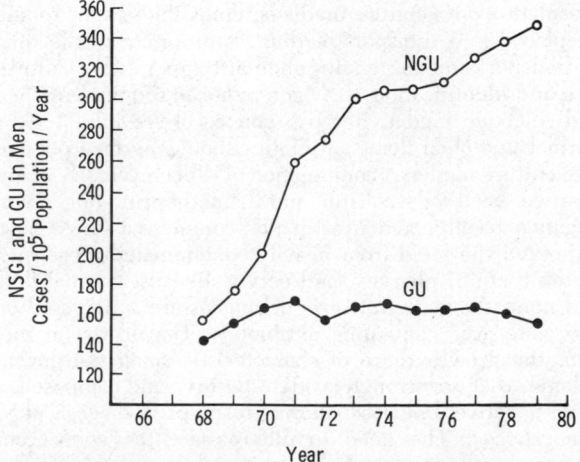

Figure 4. Reported incidence of gonococcal urethritis has been relatively stable in Great Britain during the period (1968 to 1979), during which time the reported incidence of nongonococcal urethritis doubled. Data from individual clinics suggest that most of the increase in NGU is the result of greater recognition rather than a true doubling in incidence.

Table 1. THERAPY OF GONOCOCCAL INFECTIONS

Uncomplicated Gonococcal Infections

Single Session, Intramuscular

A. Procaine penicillin G 4.8 million units (100,000 units/kg)[a] intramuscularly with probenecid 1.0 g orally
In patients allergic to penicillin, following treatment failure, or if gonococcus is penicillinase-producing (PPNG), use regimen B or C

B. Spectinomycin[b] 2 g (40 mg/kg) intramuscularly

C. Cefoxitin[b] 2 g intramuscularly with probenecid 1.0 g orally or cefotaxime 1 g intramuscularly without probenecid

Single Session, Oral

D. Ampicillin[b] 3.5 g (50 mg/kg)[a] or amoxicillin[b] 3.0 g (50 mg/kg)[a] either with probenecid 1.0 g orally

Multiple Dose, Oral

E. Tetracycline 0.5 g (10 mg/kg)[a] orally four times daily for 5 days or doxycycline 100 mg twice daily for 7 days (not to be used in pregnancy or in children less than 8 years of age)

Acute Salpingitis or Epididymitis

Oral

F. Tetracycline 0.5 g orally four times daily for 10 days or doxycycline 100 mg twice daily

G. Regimen A or D (above) initially followed by ampicillin or amoxicillin 0.5 g orally four times daily for 10 days

Intravenous

H. Cefoxitin 1 g intravenously four times daily plus doxycycline 100 mg intravenously two times daily for at least 4 days followed by regimen F

I. Clindamycin 600 mg every 6 hours plus gentamicin or tobramycin 2 mg/kg followed 1.5 mg/kg every 8 hours for at least 4 days followed by regimen F or G

J. Tetracycline 0.25 g intravenously four times daily (or doxycycline 100 mg every 12 hours) for at least 4 days followed by regimen F

K. Spectinomycin 2 g twice daily for 5 to 7 days

Conjunctivitis

Prophylaxis in Neonates

L. Tetracycline, erythromycin, or 1 per cent silver nitrate ophthalmic preparations in both eyes once immediately postpartum

Infants Born to Mothers with Gonorrhea

M. Aqueous penicillin G 50,000 units intramuscularly or intravenously once postpartum (treat as below if symptoms develop)

Neonatal Gonococcal Ophthalmia

N. Aqueous penicillin G 25,000 units/kg intravenously twice daily for 7 days plus saline irrigation of the eyes as needed to maintain drainage

Gonococcal Conjunctivitis (child or adult)

O. Aqueous penicillin G 100,000 units/kg/day intravenously in six to eight divided doses for 7 to 10 days plus irrigation and chloramphenicol (1 per cent ophthalmic) one drop every 5 to 30 minutes initially

[a]For children weighing less than 45 kg; larger children can receive adult doses.

[b]Not effective in gonococcal pharyngitis.

ococci (PPNG). Cefoxitin and cefotaxime are painful on intramuscular injection and expensive but, unlike most cephalosporins, are resistant to gonococcal penicillinase and therefore useful in treatment strains that are completely resistant to penicillins.

Most patients with gonococcal infections can be treated as outpatients. Patients with salpingitis who appear septicemic, have abscesses, are pregnant, fail to improve, or cannot be treated orally should be hospitalized. Gonococcal conjunctivitis requires hospitalization for intravenous antibiotics and saline lavage to maintain drainage. Patients with perihepatitis are usually hospitalized for observation to rule out more serious liver or biliary tract diseases. Patients with most other infections need no additional therapy, except for epididymitis, which may require scrotal suspension, sitz baths, analgesics, and occasionally bed rest.

The dose of penicillins and tetracyclines used to treat gonorrhea is also adequate for treatment of incubating syphilis, but a serologic test is necessary to exclude older disease that requires more prolonged treatment. All patients treated for gonorrhea should be recultured as a test of cure 7 to 14 days after treatment is completed, and women should be recultured six to eight weeks later. Culture of the rectum, the most likely site of failure in women, as well as the cervix is indicated at follow-up. Proctitis may need longer treatment (three to five days) with oral drugs if the first single-session treatment fails. Symptomatic pharyngitis should not be treated with a single dose of ampicillin, amoxicillin, or spectinomycin, but can be treated with nine tablets of sulfamethoxazole/trimethoprim once daily for five days, if patients are allergic to penicillin or harbor PPNG in the pharynx. Patients being treated with multiple dose regimens should be warned that they may remain infectious during treatment. Conjunctivitis is highly infectious and requires isolation during the first 24 hours of treatment, frequent irrigation of the eyes, and topical chloramphenicol or tetracycline as well as systemic penicillin.

Two complications of gonococcal therapy aside from drug allergy occasionally occur. Inadvertent intravenous injection of procaine penicillin G is followed by almost immediate development of transient neurologic and cardiorespiratory toxicity (procaine reaction). Patients with syphilis may experience the Herxheimer reaction (see Chapter 199) after receiving treatment for gonorrhea. Either of these reactions could simulate drug allergy and may produce severe symptoms.

Treatment of asymptomatic sexual contacts of patients with proven or suspected gonorrhea before culture results are known (epidemiologic treatment) is an accepted practice (Judson and Maltz, 1978). This practice is justified by the high likelihood of infection, opportunity for further transmission while awaiting diagnosis, and the inability or unwillingness of patients to return for follow-up. The decision to treat an exposed person should be based not only on the risk of infection as estimated from the nature of and time since last exposure, but also on the certainty of the diagnosis in the contact, the reliability of the patient in abstaining from additional exposures and returning for therapy, and the reliability of cultures. The following patients are usually considered for treatment because of high risk of infection (shown in parentheses): (1) female contacts of men with proven (two thirds) or suspected (one half) gonorrhea, (2) homosexual males with anal exposure to gonococcal urethritis (one half), (3) male contacts of women with suspected or proven gonorrhea (one third), and (4) neonates born to mothers with cervical gonorrhea.

Nongonococcal Urethritis. Tetracyclines give symptomatic relief in doses of 250 mg four times a day for two to three weeks and 500 mg four times a day for one week. Relapse and reinfection occur, and the latter can probably be reduced by simultaneous treatment of sexual partners. Doxycycline 100 mg twice a day for one to three weeks appears at least as good as tetracycline at 250 mg four times a day for the same period. Erythromycin 500 mg four times a day for 7 to 14 days can be used to treat pregnant contacts or men who cannot take tetracycline. Sulfonamides are active against *C. trachomatis*, and spectinomycin treats *U. urealyticum*, but neither is preferred for NGU or postgonococcal urethritis.

Undiagnosed Urethritis. Management of men with undiagnosed urethritis depends on Gram stain of urethral exudates. Positive Gram stains warrant treatment of the patients and their contacts for gonorrhea. Patients with negative or equivocal Gram stains should be treated for nongonococcal urethritis. Their sexual partners need culturing and epidemiologic treatment with the same regimen.

Recurrent Urethritis. Symptoms may recur after standard therapy for urethritis because of treatment failure, reinfection, dual infections, or incorrect diagnosis. Drug-resistant gonococci, failure to complete multiple dose regimens, and reinfection are important causes of recurrent gonococcal urethritis. Postgonococcal urethritis has been discussed in the section on clinical syndromes. If nongonococcal urethritis does not respond, treatment of both the patient and his sexual partner(s) with erythromycin 250 mg every six hours for seven days may be tried. If erythromycin fails to produce a response, prostatitis and other causes of urethritis (*Trichomonas*, condylomas, or urethral strictures or ulcers) should be searched for with smears and urethroscopy. If no other cause is found, a prolonged course of tetracycline (250 mg every six hours for 30 days) cures some patients.

PREVENTION. Gonorrhea can be prevented by condoms, postcoital antibiotics, or vaginal chemicals, contraceptives, and antibiotics. Because prophylactic antibiotics select for resistant strains, they are self-defeating if applied widely for an extended period, and therefore are not recommended. Most vaginal contraceptives and some intrauterine devices inhibit gonococci and some appear to prevent gonorrhea in women using them, but their impact on the spread of gonorrhea is unknown.

The recent epidemic occurred in several countries where aggressive programs of treatment and contact-tracing were already in operation. For this reason, this traditional approach to prevention needs revision. Immunization of the population at high risk remains attractive and candidate vaccines are being evaluated. Wide use of even a partially effective vaccine could dramatically reduce the high level of disease.

References

Barrett-Connor, E.: Gonorrhea. Curr Probl Pediatr 3, (11), 1973.

Bisno, A. L., Ofek, I., Beachy, E. H., and Curran, J. W.: Human immunity to *Neisseria gonorrhoeae:* Acquired serum opsonic antibodies. J Lab Clin Med 86:221, 1975.

Bolan, R. K., Sands, M., Schachter, J., Miner, R. C., Drew, W. L.: Lymphogranuloma venereum and acute ulcerative proctitis. Am J Med 72:703, 1982.

Bowie, W. R., Wang, S. P., Alexander, E. R., Floyd, J., Forsyth, P. S., Pollock, H. M., Lin, J. L., Buchanan, T. M., and Holmes, K. K.: Etiology of nongonococcal urethritis. J Clin Invest 59:735, 1977.

Buchanan, T. M., Eschenbach, D. A., Knapp, J. S., and Holmes, K. K.: Gonococcal salpingitis is less likely to recur with *Neisseria gonorrhoeae* of the same principal outer membrane antigenic type. Am J Obstet Gynec 138:978, 1980.

Eschenbach, D. A., Buchanan, T. M., Polloch, H. M., Forsyth, P. S., Alexander, E. R., Lin, J. S., Wang, S. P., Wentworth, B. B., McCormick, W. M., and Holmes, K. K.: Polymicrobial etiology of active pelvic inflammatory disease. N Engl J Med 293:166, 1975.

Handsfield, H. H., Lipman, T. O., Harnisch, J. P., Troncha, E., and Holmes, K. K.: Asymptomatic gonorrhea in men. N Engl J Med 290:117, 1974.

Harkness, A. H.: The pathology of gonorrhoeae. Br J Vener Dis 24:137, 1948.

Holmes, K. K., Handsfield, H. H., Wang, S. P., Wentworth, B. B., Turck, M., Anderson, J. B., and Alexander, E. R.: Etiology of non-gonococcal urethritis. N Engl J Med 292:1199, 1975.

Jacobs, N. F., and Kraus, S. J.: Gonococcal and non-gonococcal urethritis in man. Ann Intern Med 82:7, 1975.

Judson, F. M., and Maltz, A. B.: A rational basis for the epidemiological treatment of gonorrhea in a clinic for sexually transmitted diseases. Sex Trans Dis 5:89, 1978.

Klein, E. J., Fisher, L. S., Chow, A. W., and Guze, L. B.: Anorectal gonococcal infection. Ann Intern Med 86:340, 1977.

Lip, J., and Burgoyne, X.: Cervical and peritoneal bacterial flora associated with salpingitis. Obstet Gynecol 28:561, 1966.

Litt, I. F., and Cohen, M. I.: Perihepatitis associated with salpingitis in adolescents. JAMA 240:1253, 1978.

Mardh, P. A., Ripa, T., Svensson, L., and Weström, L.: *Chlamydia trachomatis* infection in patients with acute salpingitis. N Engl J Med 296:1377, 1977.

McCormick, W. M., Stumacher, R. J., Johnson, K., and Donner, D.: Clinical spectrum of gonococcal infection in women. Lancet 1:1182, 1977.

McCutchan, J. A.: The epidemiology of venereal urethritis. Rev Inf Dis 6:669, 1984.

McGee, Z. A., Melly, M. A., Gregg, G. R., Horn, R. G., Taylor-Robinson, D., Johnson, A. P., and McCutchan, J. A.: Virulence factors of gonococci: Studies using human fallopian tube organ cultures. In Brooks, G. F., et al. (eds.): Immunobiology of *Neisseria gonorrhea*. Washington, American Society for Microbiology, 1978, p. 258.

Nelson, J. D., Mohs, E., Dajani, A. S., and Plotkin, S. A.: Gonorrhea in preschool and school-aged children. JAMA 236:1359, 1976.

Penn, C. W., Veale, D. R., and Smith, H.: Selection from gonococci grown *in vitro* of a colony type with some virulence properties of organisms adapted *in vivo*. J Gen Microbiol 100:147, 1977.

Quinn, T. C., Stamm, W. E., Goodell, S. E., et al.: The polymicrobial origin of intestinal infections in homosexual men. N Engl J Med 309:576, 1983.

Reichert, J. A., and Valle, R. F.:Fitz-Hugh-Curtis syndrome. JAMA 236:266, 1976.

Ripa, K. T., Svenson, L., Treharne, J. D., Westom, L., and Mardh, P. A.: *Chlamydia trachomatis* infection in patients with laparoscopically verified acute salpingitis. Am J Obstet Gynec 138:960, 1980.

Saigh, J. H., Sanders, C. C., and Sanders, W. E.: Inhibition of *Neisseria gonorrhoeae* by aerobic and facultatively anaerobic components of the endocervical flora: Evidence for a protective effect against infection. Infect. Immun 19:704, 1978.

Taylor-Robinson, D., and McCormack, W. M.: The genital mycoplasmas. N Engl J Med 302:1003, 1980.

Thatcher, R. W., and Pettit, T. H.: Gonorrheal conjunctivitis. JAMA 215:1494, 1971.

Veale, D. R., Penn, C. W., and Smith, H.: The resistance of gonococci to killing by human phagocytes. In Skinner, F. A., et al. (eds.): Gonorrhea: Epidemiology and Pathogenesis. London, Academic Press, 1977, p. 97.

Ward, M. E., Watt, P. J., and Robertson, J. N.: The human fallopian tube: A laboratory model for gonococcal infection. J Infect Dis 129:650, 1974.

Weisner, P. J., Tronca, E., Bonin, P., Pederson, A. H. B., and Holmes, K. K.: Clinical spectrum of pharyngeal gonococcal infection. N Engl J Med 288:181, 1973

Wolner-Hansen, P., Westrom, L., and Mardh, P. A.: Perihepatitis and chlamydial salpingitis. Lancet 1:901, 1980.

162

SYPHILIS OF THE GENITAL TRACT

DANIEL M. MUSHER, M.D.

Syphilis is a venereally transmitted infection caused by *Treponema pallidum*. The biology of the infecting organism is reviewed in Chapter 53 and the pathogenesis and pathology of syphilitic infection is discussed in detail in Chapter 199.

CLINICAL MANIFESTATIONS. The earliest lesion of syphilis, the primary syphilitic chancre, appears after an incubation period of 2 to 3 weeks as a nontender papule that grows to 0.5 to 1 cm in size and promptly ulcerates leaving a clear, well-defined margin and a relatively clean, dull-red indurated base (Chapel, 1978). The progression from papule to ulcer is so rapid, and the lesion is so devoid of pain or tenderness that the papular stage is often overlooked by the patient, who presents for medical care with a chancre. Syphilitic chancres may occur anywhere in the genital or perineal areas (Fig. 1 and 2). In men, genital lesions most frequently involve the prepuce, coronal sulcus, and shaft of the penis, whereas in women the labia and fourchette are the most common sites. Multiple lesions are seen in one-quarter of cases. Because they cause no symptoms and tend to occur within a body orifice, primary syphilitic chancres in women are frequently not recognized; as a result, in most infected women the diagnosis of syphilis is made only in the secondary stage of the infection. The same is often true of homosexual men if the primary lesion occurs within the anus or rectum. Inguinal lymph nodes are enlarged in 80 per cent of patients with a genital chancre, two-thirds of whom have bilateral enlargement. The lymph nodes are tender in a relatively small proportion of cases. If untreated, chancres persist for 3 to 8 weeks. From a clinical point of view this means that lesions of secondary (disseminated) syphilis may appear while signs of the original chancre are still present.

Condyloma lata (Fig. 3) is a condition in which local spread of treponemes in a moist area causes formation of large whitish or grey plaques that exude serous material containing many infectious organisms. In the preantibiotic era condyloma lata often developed in the axilla or groin as a complication of secondary syphilis. Now the lesions usually occur in the perineal area as a result of local extension from an unrecognized chancre within the female genital tract or in the anus. Although condyloma lata may precede disseminated syphilis, it is generally regarded as part of secondary syphilis.

In its tertiary stages, syphilis can cause disease of the testis and epididymis, but, at the present time, this involvement must be exceedingly rare. Diffuse interstitial fibrosis may cause the testis to contract into a compact, hard mass that used to be called a billiard ball testis. Painful nodules of the spermatic cords and painless gummatous swelling of the epididymis or even a hydrocoele were seen when tertiary disease was more common.

DIAGNOSIS

Clinical Diagnosis. The diagnosis of syphilis should probably be considered in any patient who has any kind of a genital lesion. Chancroid (Hammond et al., 1980) is a venereal disease caused by *Haemophilus ducreyi* and characterized by one or more painful erosions that have an irregular margin and a nonindurated base. These lesions tend to occur in uncircumcised men who have social and domestic instability and extensive sexual contacts, features of epidemiologic interest but of no help in distinguishing chancroid from syphilis in an individual patient. Painful

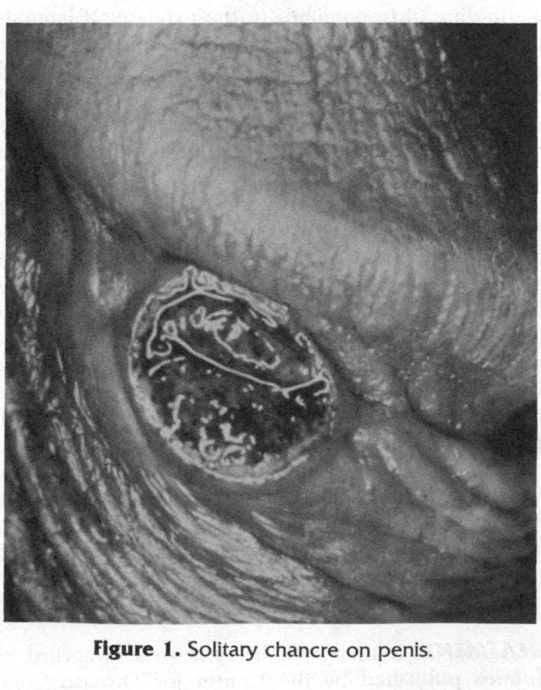

Figure 1. Solitary chancre on penis.

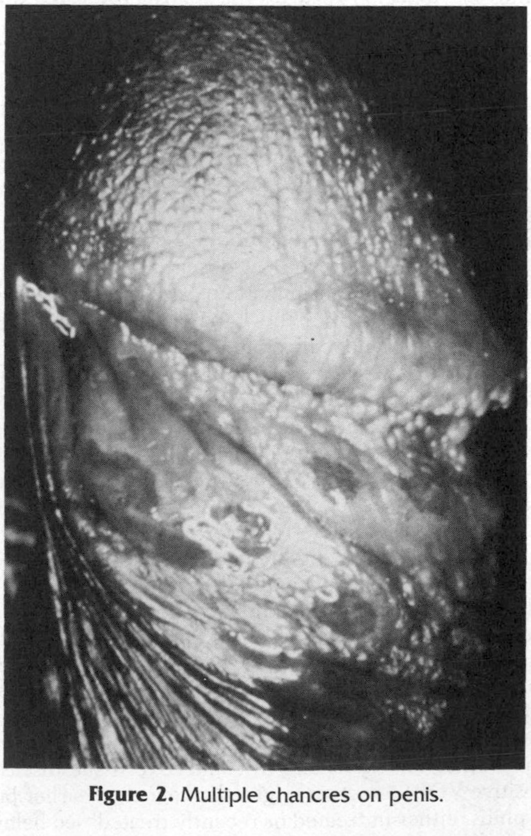

Figure 2. Multiple chancres on penis.

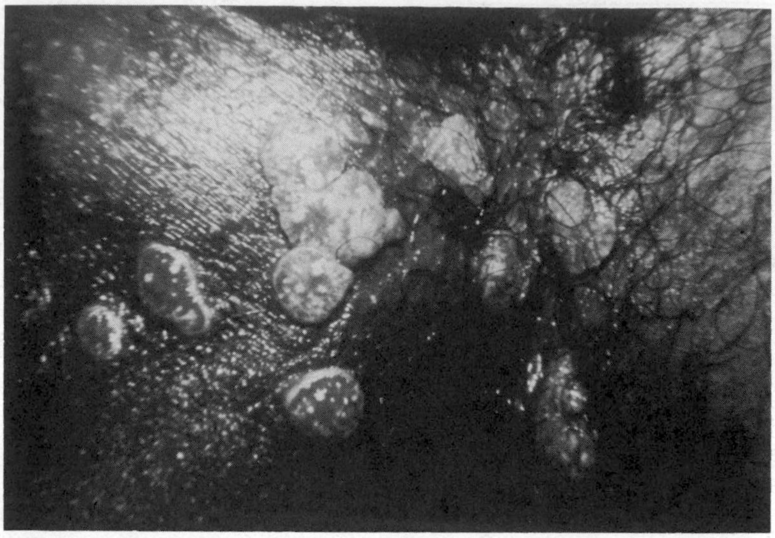

Figure 3. Condyloma lata in perineal area.

enlargement of inguinal lymph nodes is relatively common in chancroid and they sometimes ulcerate. Herpes simplex lesions of the genitalia are usually distinguishable from a syphilitic chancre by their size (1 to 4 mm), vesicular appearance, lack of induration, pain and history of recurring in the same area. Trauma during sexual intercourse or a fixed drug eruption may produce noninfectious penile lesions that resemble a chancre. Erosions on the cervix may be indistinguishable from syphilitic chancres. Reiter's syndrome may present with genital ulcers in the absence of conjunctivitis or arthritis, and the examiner may overlook oral lesions in Behcet's syndrome; genital lesions in these conditions are usually painful. Someone who has had syphilis may develop small, atypical chancres at the site of reinoculation of *T. pallidum* as a result of partial immunity. In prospective studies of patients who presented with a penile ulceration to a veneral disease clinic, an actual etiology (documented infection, history of trauma, etc.), was proven in no more than one-half of cases (Chapel et al., 1978); modern techniques that allow for culture of *H. ducreyi* may substantially increase the proportion of diagnosable lesions.

Laboratory Diagnosis. The etiology of a primary syphilitic chancre is best proven by observing treponemes on darkfield microscopic examination. The specimen should be obtained by abrading the base of the lesion without causing bleeding and collecting the serous exudate that accumulates in a capillary pipet. If necessary, one or two drops of a physiological saline solution can be placed on the base of the ulcer. False negatives occur with poor specimens and as a result of ointment having been applied to the lesion. False positives might result from the presence of nonpathogenic treponemes (a problem in evaluating oral lesions) or from artifact. With experience, the correct diagnosis is reached in the great majority of cases.

Serologic tests are distinctly less direct. Antibody to cardiolipin is detected by the VDRL (Veneral Disease Research Laboratory) test in 80 to 90 per cent of cases of primary syphilis (Moore, 1965; Chapel, 1978) and similar results are observed with the RPR (rapid plasma reagin) or its equivalent. The presence of this antibody signifies active treponemal infection, although positive titers under 1:8 are seen in other infections and in connective tissue diseases. A positive VDRL reaction might also reflect an earlier bout of syphilis, either untreated or recently treated (see below), and could be misleading if the lesion being evaluated were due to another cause.

Diagnosing primary syphilis by specific treponemal antibody tests is even more hazardous. The fluorescent treponemal antibody test (FTA-ABS) or more recently the *T. pallidum* hemagglutinating test (TPHA, MTPHA) are used to detect antibody to *T. pallidum*. These tests are positive in over 90 per cent of patients when they seek medical attention for primary syphilis and are highly specific for syphilitic infection. The problem is that they remain positive for life after an earlier case of syphilis, whereas the lesion under consideration at any given time may be due to another cause. Moreover, these serologic tests, which used to be done only at public health clinics and reference laboratories, are now being done routinely by private or individual hospital laboratories; false negatives and, especially, false positives are not uncommon. In summary, the clinical diagnosis of a primary syphilitic chancre is made most frequently and most reliably by the darkfield microscopic finding of treponemes in the exudate. If laboratory documentation is equivocal but the clinical appearance suggests a diagnosis of syphilis, most authorities urge that the patient be treated as if the diagnosis were proven. If a VDRL test obtained 2 to 4 weeks later shows a continued rise in titer the diagnosis would be supported, but the absence of such a rise does not exclude it.

Although in secondary syphilis of the skin it is more difficult to obtain a good specimen for darkfield examination, condylomatous lesions teem with infectious organisms. In addition, the VDRL is virtually always strongly positive (1:16 or greater). With the aforementioned decentralization of laboratory testing for syphilis it is necessary to caution the practitioner about the prozone phenomenon, in which a high titer of antibody leads to a test being read as negative if a full set of dilutions is not carried out. The VDRL and RPR should always be done with dilutions to avoid falsely negative results. If a diagnosis of condyloma lata or secondary syphilis seems certain on clinical grounds a negative serology should be questioned.

Tertiary syphilis with gummatous lesions causes a positive VDRL reaction, but biopsy and histologic examination is generally used for diagnosis.

TREATMENT. Genital syphilis is treated in accord with guidelines published by the Center for Disease Control (see Chapter 199). Primary or secondary syphilis is treated with a total of 2.4 million units of benzathine penicillin given on one occasion in two doses each of 1.2 million units. Tetracycline has been less extensively studied but is considered effective when 500 mg is given four times daily for 15 days. Erythromycin in the same dosage is probably efficacious, but incompletely studied. Syphilitic gummas (tertiary infection) should be treated with 2.4 million units of benzathine penicillin on three occasions one week apart after neurosyphilis has been excluded by lumbar puncture. Tetracycline or erythromycin in a dose of 500 mg four times daily for 30 days may be given if penicillin is absolutely contraindicated, but their efficacy is not well documented. Followup visits are recommended at 3, 6, and 12 months after treatment of primary or secondary syphilis to document a decline in VDRL titer; by the end of 12 months the VDRL is often negative although it may remain positive at a 1:2 dilution or less, especially in secondary infection. Special emphasis should be placed on followup visits when any drug regimen other than parenteral penicillin has been used.

References

Chapel T. A.: The variability of syphilitic chancres. Sex Trans Dis 5(2):68, 1978.

Chapel T., Brown W. J., Jeffries C., Stewart J. A.: The microbiological flora of penile ulcerations. J Infect Dis 137:50, 1978.

Hammond G. W., Slutchuk M., Scatliff J., Sherman E., Wilt J. C., Ronald A. R.: Epidemiologic, clinical, laboratory, and therapeutic features of an urban outbreak of chancroid in North America. Rev Infect Dis 2:867, 1980;

Moore, M. B. Jr., Knox J. M.: Sensitivity and specificity in syphilis serology. South Med J 48:963, 1965.

163

GENITAL HERPES

MICHAEL N. OXMAN, M.D.

Genital herpes (herpes genitalis) is an acute inflammatory herpes simplex virus (HSV) infection of the male or female genital tract. It may result from either a primary or a recurrent HSV infection. Primary genital herpes is a sexually transmitted exogenous infection that is usually caused by HSV Type 2 (HSV-2). Recurrent genital herpes almost always results from the reactivation of endogenous HSV-2, which is latent in sacral sensory ganglia. However, recurrent genital herpes may occasionally represent a sexually transmitted exogenous reinfection (Buchman et al., 1979).

Herpes genitalis in the female causes painful vesicles and ulcers of the vulva and vagina, and these may extend to the skin of the perineum, buttocks, and thighs. The cervix is also usually infected. In the male, painful vesicles and ulcers appear on the glans penis, prepuce and shaft of the penis, and sometimes extend to the scrotum and adjacent perineal areas. Bilateral inguinal lymphadenopathy is present in both sexes and, in primary infections, it is usually painful and accompanied by constitutional symptoms. The clinical manifestations of primary and recurrent herpes genitalis are similar, although primary episodes are usually more severe and slower to resolve. This is in marked contrast to oropharyngeal infections with HSV-1 (Chapter 105), in which primary and recurrent infections cause quite different syndromes (that is, acute herpetic gingivostomatitis vs herpes labialis).

ETIOLOGY. Genital herpes has been a recognized clinical entity for more than two centuries. It was described as a sexually transmitted disease as early as 1883, when Unna observed that it was a "vocational disease" of Hamburg prostitutes (Hutfield, 1966; Unna, 1883). In the 1920's, Lipschütz called attention to the transmission of "venereal herpes" by sexual contact and demonstrated that the viruses of "venereal herpes" and "herpes febrilis" (the fever blister) were biologically and antigenically different (Nahmias and Dowdle, 1968). However, the work of Lipschütz was ignored. Slavin and Gavett (1946) isolated HSV from lesions of the vulva, demonstrated that "herpetic vulvovaginitis" was a manifestation of primary HSV infection, and described the conjugal transmission of HSV from a husband with penile herpes to his wife. However, genital herpes was not really accepted as a sexually transmitted disease until the rediscovery of the two serotypes of HSV in the late 1960's and the development of assays to distinguish between them permitted the different epidemiology of HSV-1 and HSV-2 to be delineated (Nahmias and Dowdle, 1968).

HSV-1 and HSV-2 are very closely related members of the herpesvirus family, which includes three other human herpesviruses, varicella-zoster virus (VZV), cytomegalovirus (CMV) and Epstein-Barr virus (EBV). HSV-1 and HSV-2 are morphologically indistinguishable, share approximately 40 per cent of their DNA base sequences, have many antigens in common, and produce identical lesions in the skin and mucous membranes (Chapters 60 and 105). Although their similarities are much greater than their differences, HSV-1 and HSV-2 can be distinguished on the basis of certain antigenic, biologic, and biochemical differences (Table 1 in Chapter 105). Furthermore, they differ significantly in their clinical and epidemiologic behavior (Nahmias and Roizman, 1973; Nahmias and Josey, 1982). HSV-2 is transmitted sexually, or from a maternal genital infection to the newborn. It is the predominant cause of genital herpes, neonatal herpes, and herpetic infections of the skin below the waist. It is also associated epidemiologically with carcinoma of the cervix. HSV-1 is transmitted primarily by nonvenereal routes, usually involving contact with infected saliva. It is the principal cause of herpetic gingivostomatitis and pharyngotonsillitis, eczema herpeticum, skin infections above the waist, infections of the eye, and herpes simplex encephalitis. However, changing sexual practices and socioeconomic conditions are altering the epidemiology of HSV-1 and HSV-2; the proportion of cases of genital herpes caused by HSV-1 is increasing, presumably because of the increasing popularity of oral-genital sex and the growing number of adults who have escaped HSV-1 infection in childhood.

PATHOLOGY AND PATHOGENESIS. The pathology and pathogenesis of genital herpes appears to be analogous to the pathology and pathogenesis of oropharyngeal infections caused by HSV-1 (Chapter 105), and the skin and mucous membrane lesions of HSV-1 and HSV-2 are indistinguishable. HSV is introduced into the genital mucosa by genital or oral-genital sexual contact with a partner who has a symptomatic or asymptomatic genital or oropharyngeal HSV infection. It replicates in cells of the stratum spinosum, producing characteristic cytopathic effects that include cell swelling ("ballooning degeneration"), loss of intercellular bridges, the development of Cowdry Type A intranuclear inclusion bodies, and membrane changes that result in cell fusion with the formation of multinucleated giant cells. The infected cells are soon separated by intercellular edema which, together with inflammation and capillary dilatation in the underlying lamina propria, results in the formation of an erythematous papule. The infection and degeneration of additional epithelial cells and the continuing influx of edema fluid elevates the uninvolved stratum corneum to form a delicate, clear, intraepidermal vesicle that contains fibrin, degenerating epithelial cells, multinucleated giant cells, and large amounts of infectious virus. Inflammatory cells soon invade from below and the fluid becomes cloudy, transforming the vesicle into a pustule. Adjacent vesicles may coalesce to form small bullae. In moist areas, such as the cervix, vagina, and labial minora in women, and under the foreskin in uncircumcised men, the vesicles are macerated and quickly rupture, liberating infectious virus and leaving very tender, painful, shallow ulcers that are covered with a yellowish-gray exudate and surrounded by a narrow red areola. The virus liberated from ruptured vesicles spreads the infection locally to the cervix, vagina, vulva, and, often, to the surrounding skin. These may also be sites of initial infection or be infected by retrograde neural ("zosteriform") spread of HSV from infected sacral ganglia (Stanberry et al., 1982). During primary infections, there is significant involvement of regional lymph nodes and viremia. In the normal patient, local production of interferon, antibody formation, and various forms of cell-mediated immunity combine to localize the infection and eventually terminate virus multiplication. If these defenses are deficient, as they are in many immunosuppressed patients, primary (or recurrent) infection may result in viremic spread to the skin and visceral organs, or produce chronic progressive local lesions. Although we have not yet identified those host responses that are critical to the control of HSV infections, studies in animals and immunosuppressed patients indicate that cell-mediated responses are essential. Interestingly, antigens shared by HSV-1 and HSV-2 must be involved, for prior oropharyngeal infection with HSV-1 reduces the severity of initial episodes of herpes genitalis caused by HSV-2 (Nahmias et al., 1970; Rawls et al., 1971; Reeves et al., 1981; Corey et al., 1983a).

In primary genital herpes, even when it is asymptomatic, virus invades local sensory nerve endings, ascends within axons, and establishes a latent infection in sensory neurons within the corresponding sacral ganglia (Baringer, 1974). Despite the host's immunity, this latent infection persists for life and is periodically reactivated by various stimuli (for example, menses, sexual intercourse). The reactivated HSV then travels within axons from the neuronal soma to the genital skin or mucosa, where it replicates in epithelial cells and produces intraepidermal vesicles histologically indistinguishable from those observed during primary genital herpes. Preexisting humoral and cellular immunity normally limit this local virus replication, so that recurrent infections are generally less severe, more circumscribed, and of shorter duration than primary infections (Yen et al., 1965; Ng et al., 1970; Poste et al., 1972; Kaufman et al., 1973; Adams et al., 1976; Vontver et al., 1979).

CLINICAL MANIFESTATIONS. Genital HSV infections have usually been categorized as *primary* or *recurrent*, but this fails to reflect the true complexity of the situation. HSV-1 and HSV-2 have common antigenic determinants and can induce cross-reactive humorals and cellular immune responses. Consequently, infection with either serotype provides some protection against heterotypic infection, and this protection may be greater when both infections involve the same anatomic site. Previous infection with HSV-1 (presumably oropharyngeal in most cases) appears to protect against the acquisition of symptomatic genital HSV-1 infection, and to reduce the severity of initial genital HSV infections caused by HSV-2 (Reeves et al., 1981; Corey et al., 1983a). It is probable that previous HSV-1 infection also provides some protection against the acquisition of symptomatic genital HSV-2 infection and, likewise, that previous HSV-2 infection will reduce the incidence and severity of genital herpes caused by either HSV serotype. However, immunity to exogenous reinfection is not absolute, even at the same anatomic site; restriction endonuclease analysis of HSV isolates has demonstrated that symptomatic exogenous heterotypic (HSV-1) and homotypic (HSV-2) genital infections can occur in immunologically normal individuals with recurrent genital herpes caused by HSV-2 (Kit et al., 1983; Buchman et al., 1979). Finally, since even primary oropharyngeal and genital HSV infections are often asymptomatic, it is frequently impossible to ascertain the anatomic site of the previous HSV infection in patients with antibody to HSV who present with their first episode of symptomatic genital herpes. These considerations, which are especially important when one attempts to evaluate any form of treatment, have lead to the separation of initial or first episode symptomatic genital HSV infections into two categories: *primary* and *nonprimary*.

A *primary* genital HSV infection is one that occurs in a person with no previous HSV infection at any site, as evidenced by a lack of antibody to HSV-1 and HSV-2. A *nonprimary* first episode genital HSV infection is the first symptomatic genital HSV infection that occurs in a patient who already has antibody to HSV-1, HSV-2 or both. A *recurrent* genital HSV infection is one that occurs in a patient with a history of one or more previous episodes of symptomatic genital herpes. The average duration and severity of clinical disease is greater in *primary* than in *nonprimary* first episodes of genital herpes, and episodes of recurrent genital herpes are usually shorter and less severe than either primary or nonprimary first episode infections (Fig. 1). However, there is sufficient overlap so that these distinctions are often difficult to make clinically in any individual patient. Furthermore, the *nonprimary first episode* category is still very heterogeneous. It includes individuals previously infected with HSV-1, HSV-2 or both HSV serotypes, individuals with previous symptomatic and asymptomatic infections, and individuals previously infected at various anatomic sites (it even includes individuals with previous asymptomatic genital HSV infections). As more information is acquired (e.g., it is likely that a previous asymptomatic genital HSV-2 infection will provide

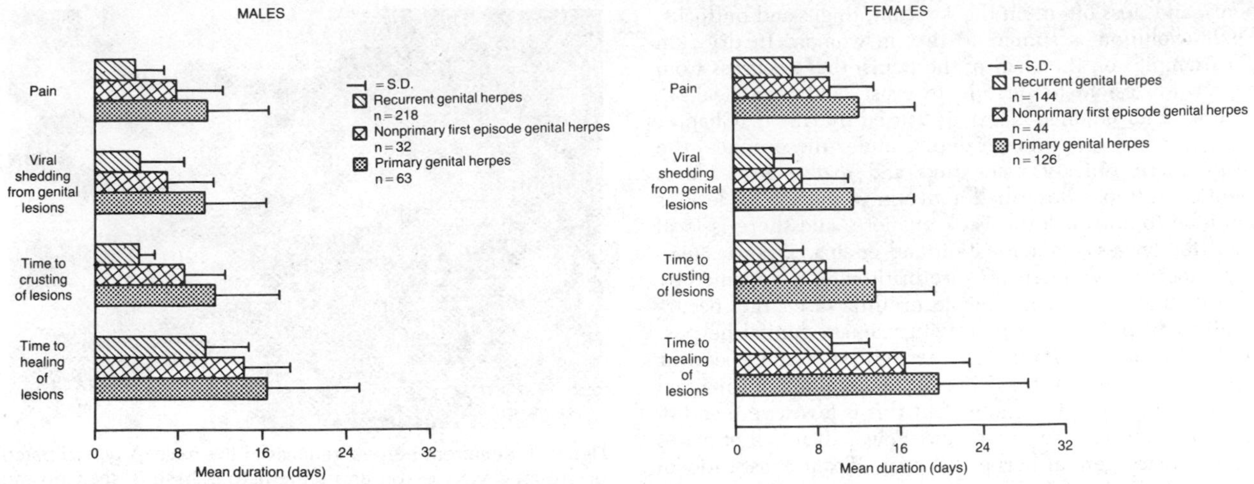

Figure 1. The duration of symptoms and signs of primary, nonprimary first episode, and recurrent genital herpes in men and women. SD = standard deviation (From Corey et al., 1983a, with permission.)

more protection against symptomatic genital infection with HSV-2 than a previous oropharyngeal HSV-1 infection) it may become appropriate to subdivide further this category of patients.

The incubation period following sexual contact is usually three to seven days, with a range of one day to more than two weeks (Poste et al., 1972; Kaufman et al., 1973; Brown et al., 1979; Corey et al., 1983a). Although many infections in both sexes are asymptomatic, primary genital herpes is more severe in women than in men. Women have a larger area of infection, more intense and prolonged local symptoms, more frequent constitutional symptoms, more extragenital lesions, and more complications (Corey et al., 1983a). Primary herpetic vulvovaginitis often begins with the appearance of herpetic vesicles, but this may be preceded by a short period of local burning, tenderness and erythema of the labia minora and vaginal introitus. Typical herpetic vesicles first appear on the external genitalia, usually involving the labia majora, labia minora, vaginal vestibule, and introitus. New lesions continue to appear bilaterally in the same areas and the eruption often spreads to the mons pubis, clitoris, urethral orifice and the perianal skin, buttocks, and thighs. In moist areas within the labial minora, vesicles quickly rupture, leaving shallow exquisitely tender ulcers covered with a yellowish-gray exudate and surrounded by a red areola (Fig. 2). In drier areas, such as the outer surface of the labia majora and the adjacent skin, vesicles may remain intact, evolve into pustules and then crust over several days. New lesions continue to appear for a week or more. They are often extensive and may coalesce, forming bullae and large areas of ulceration that resemble second-degree burn. The vaginal mucosa and vulva are inflamed and edematous. The cervix is almost always involved, and there is usually a profuse watery vaginal discharge. Examination most often reveals diffuse friability of the cervical epithelium, but sometimes there is extensive ulceration and, occasionally, severe necrotic cervicitis (Willcox, 1968). Most patients have severe vulvar pain, exquisite tenderness of affected tissues, and dysuria, which is sometimes severe enough to cause urinary retention. Bilateral painful inguinal and pelvic lymphadenopathy develops in most women with primary genital herpes, and most experience fever, headache, malaise, and myalgia. The local symptoms generally get worse during the first week, reach a peak between days 8 and 10, and then gradually subside. Constitutional symptoms usually peak within the first 3 or 4 days and disappear by the end of the first week. Even when severe, primary genital herpes is normally self-limited. Virus replication is maximal during the first 3 to 4 days and declines thereafter, although a few patients may shed virus for several weeks. Pain usually remits in 10 to 14 days, and healing occurs without residua in 2 to 5 weeks. Mucosal lesions heal without crusting. The cervix, which is involved in 90 per cent or more of women with symptomatic primary genital herpes, appears to be the source of virus that may be shed for weeks after visible lesions have healed and symptoms have disappeared (Nahmias et al., 1971; Adams et al., 1976; Ekwo et al., 1979; Adam et al., 1979).

In men, the lesions of primary genital herpes usually appear on the glans penis, the prepuce and the shaft of the

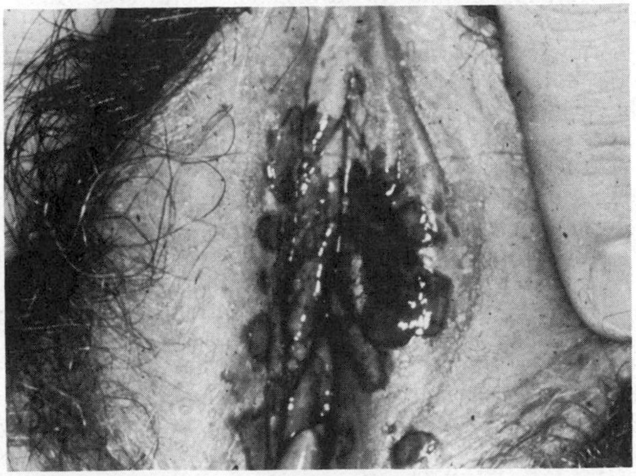

Figure 2. Herpes genitalis in the female. This young woman with primary herpetic vulvovaginitis has shallow, exquisitely tender ulcers on the inner surface of the labia majora, the labia minora, and the vaginal mucosa. The ulcers are covered with a yellowish-gray exudate and surrounded by a red areola. Further examination also reveals herpetic cervicitis.

penis, and, less often, on the scrotum, thighs and buttocks. Their evolution is similar to that in women. In dry skin (for example, on the shaft of the penis) they progress from papule to vesicle to pustule to crust, and then heal, as described for cutaneous lesions caused by HSV-1 (Chapter 105). In moist areas (for example, under the prepuce) the vesicles are quickly macerated and evolve into ulcers identical to those described above in women. New lesions continue to appear for a week or more, and there is local pain, tenderness, inflammation and edema. Dysuria, usually associated with herpetic urethritis and accompanied by a small amount of clear mucoid urethral discharge, occurs in 30 to 40 per cent of men with primary genital herpes. It is often more painful than the dysuria of gonococcal or nongonococcal urethritis. There is bilateral tender inguinal and pelvic lymphadenopathy, but this is less severe and of shorter duration than in women. Fewer than half of males with primary genital herpes have significant constitutional symptoms. Virus is present in large amounts during the first 3 to 5 days and it can usually be recovered for another week or more. Pain usually resolves during the second week, and healing occurs without scarring in 2 to 4 weeks.

The clinical manifestations and course of primary genital herpes caused by HSV-1 and HSV-2 are indistinguishable. However, the frequency of subsequent recurrences appears to be lower following primary genital HSV-1 infection (vide infra).

The clinical manifestations of nonprimary first episode genital herpes are similar to those of true primary genital herpes, but the disease is less severe and of shorter duration (Fig. 1). Women and men with nonprimary first episode genital herpes have fewer complications and less often develop constitutional symptoms or extragenital lesions; only about 65 per cent of women with nonprimary infections shed HSV from the cervix (Corey et al., 1983a).

Ninety per cent or more of individuals with symptomatic primary or nonprimary first episode genital herpes caused by HSV-2 will experience one or more episodes of symptomatic recurrent genital herpes during the subsequent year. The recurrences rate appears to be lower after primary genital herpes caused by HSV-1; it is about 0.1 episode per month, compared to 0.3 episode per month after primary genital HSV-2 infection (Corey et al., 1983a).

Recurrent genital herpes is usually less severe and of shorter duration than either primary or nonprimary first episode infection (Fig. 1). Although the same sites tend to be affected, there are fewer lesions, the area involved is more circumscribed, and the lesions are usually unilateral. Most patients have a prodrome of tenderness, pain, burning, tingling, or itching at the site of the impending eruption, beginning from a few hours to 1 or 2 days before the appearance of lesions. Some patients have a prodrome of ipsilateral sacral neuralgia, with pain in the leg, buttock, or genital area. The lesions of recurrent genital herpes begin as papules, but quickly develop into clusters of tiny vesicles on an erythematous base (Fig. 3). They often coalesce and evolve in the same manner as in primary genital herpes, but more rapidly. There are also fewer days of new lesion formation, and the total surface area involved is much smaller. The clinical manifestations of recurrent genital herpes are more severe in women than in men. In women, the lesions are almost always painful. They are most often located on the labia minora, labia majora, or perineum, but may also occur on the mons pubis, perianal skin, or buttocks; some women have linear ulcerations in the fourchette, which resemble inflammed excoriations (Brown et al., 1979; Guinan et al., 1981). Lymphadenopathy may be present, but fever and constitutional symptoms are uncommon, and only about a quarter of women with recurrent genital herpes have dysuria. Virus is present in much smaller amounts in recurrent than in primary herpetic lesions (mean peak titers of $\leq 10^3$ pfu per swab vs $\geq 10^5$ pfu per swab). Virus is shed for an average of 5 days, and its recovery after the seventh day is uncommon. Pain also disappears during the first week and the lesions generally heal within 8 to 10 days. The frequency of positive cervical cultures (about 10 per cent) is much lower during recurrent than during primary genital herpes. Furthermore, there are no visible cervical lesions, and the amount of virus present is at least 1000-fold less than the amount present during primary infections (Ekwo et al., 1979; Brown et al., 1979; Adam et al., 1980; Guinan et al., 1981). In men, recurrent genital herpes most often presents with one or more patches of grouped vesicles (Fig. 3) on the shaft of the penis, prepuce, or glans. Lesions begin as papules and, on dry skin, evolve into vesicles, pustules and crusts in the same manner as the lesions of herpes labialis. Under the prepuce, vesicles are quickly macerated, forming shallow painful ulcers. There may be mild inguinal lymphadenopathy, but constitutional symptoms are rare and urethritis is uncommon. Urethral cultures are positive for HSV in fewer than 5 per cent of males with recurrent genital herpes. The titer of virus is lower in recurrent than in primary lesions, and HSV can rarely be recovered after 4 or 5 days. Pain is present in about 60 per cent of males with recurrent genital herpes. It is usually mild and disappears with the virus. Lesions heal in 7 to 10 days.

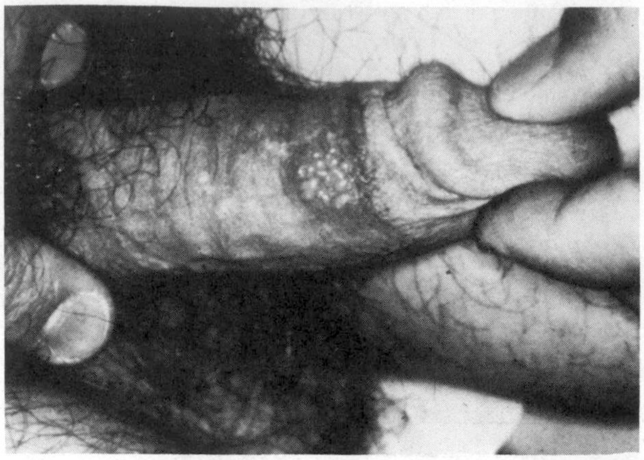

Figure 3. Recurrent herpes genitalis in the male. A typical patch of grouped vesicles on an erythematous base is seen on the shaft of the penis. (Courtesy of Dr. M. T. Jarratt.)

In approximately 5 per cent of patients, recurrent herpes genitalis may present with a single, large, shallow, minimally tender ulcer, up to 1 cm in diameter, which has a clean, granular base and sharply demarcated edges. This lesion, which has been called a herpetic chancre (Chang et al., 1974), may be mistaken for a syphilitic chancre. However, since both herpes genitalis and syphilis may coexist in the same patient (Chapel et al., 1979; Fiumara et al., 1980) laboratory diagnosis is essential.

Symptomatic genital HSV infections are only the tip of an iceberg. Examination of susceptible female contacts of males with genital herpes indicates that 50 per cent or more of primary genital HSV infections in women may be asymptomatic (Nahmias et al., 1969; Rawls et al.., 1971; Nahmias et al., 1971). Furthermore, only a minority of individuals with serologic evidence of prior HSV-2 infection give a history of symptomatic genital herpes. Asymptomatic recurrences of genital herpes are also extremely common, as evidenced by the frequent isolation of HSV from the cervix or vagina of asymptomatic women with a history of previous genital herpes (Ng et al., 1970; Poste et al., 1972; Adams et al., 1976; Bolognese et al., 1976; Ekwo et al., 1979; Adam et al., 1979 and 1980; Grossman et al., 1981; Guinan et al., 1981; Nahmias and Josey, 1982). Asymptomatic cervicovaginal shedding can be detected in 0.03 to 8 per cent of women, depending upon the patient population studied. For example, HSV was isolated from the cervix of 10 per cent of asymptomatic women with a history of genital herpes in the preceding 6 months (Adam et al., 1979). The frequency of reactivation and the duration of virus shedding may be increased during pregnancy (Nahmias et al., 1967; Ng et al., 1970; Nahmias et al., 1971). In one study of pregnant women, 35 per cent of whom were HSV antibody positive, HSV was isolated from the cervix in 0.65 per cent (Bolognese et al., 1976). Since only one culture was obtained per patient, this figure underestimates the prevalence of active HSV infection. HSV has been isolated from 0.7 to 4 per cent of genital cultures from asymptomatic pregnant women with a history of recurrent genital herpes, and asymptomatic shedding appears to be at least as common from the usual lesion site on the vulva as from the cervix (Scher et al., 1982; Vontuer et al., 1982; Harger et al., 1983; Wittek et al., 1984). The epidemiologic importance of asymptomatic genital HSV infection is underlined by the observation that the majority of the mothers of infants with neonatal herpes have had no signs or symptoms of genital herpes during pregnancy, and no history of prior symptomatic genital herpes (Whitley et al., 1980a; Boehm et al., 1981).

COMPLICATIONS AND SEQUELAE. Though often physically and mentally distressing, primary and recurrent genital herpes are self-limited and, in the normal host, almost always resolve spontaneously without complications or sequelae.

Those complications that do occur may be divided into three categories: (1) bacterial or fungal superinfection; (2) extragenital infection or aberrant behavior by the virus in an apparently normal person; and (3) HSV infections in compromised hosts.

Bacterial and fungal superinfections are surprisingly uncommon. Rarely, balanoposthitis occurs in an uncircumcised male from bacterial superinfection of herpetic ulcers on the prepuce, and *Candida* balanitis is seen occasionally. Ulcerative lesions in moist skin areas may also become superinfected, *Candida* vaginitis occasionally complicates herpetic vulvovaginitis, especially in patients with diabetes. These complications usually respond to local therapy and rarely require systemic antibiotics.

There are a number of examples of extragenital HSV-2 infections that may result from direct extension of the genital infection, autoinoculation, viremia, centrifugal neural ("zosteriform") spread from infected sacral ganglia, or exogenous extragenital infection (Hutfield, 1968). Herpetic urethritis usually occurs in association with primary genital herpes. Typical herpetic lesions may be visible near the urethral meatus or they may be intraurethral. There is usually severe burning pain on micturition, but minimal discharge. Typical intranuclear inclusion bodies and multinucleated giant cells may be demonstrated in urethral smears. The urethritis may recur, with or without recurrent genital lesions, and herpetic urethritis may be the only clinical manifestation of primary genital herpes. Herpetic cystitis has also been observed in patients with primary herpes genitalis and may account for some instances of dysuria and urinary retention (Person et al., 1973). In many cases, virus may reach the bladder by direct extension from the urethra, or by neural transmission from infected sacral ganglia (Stanberry et al., 1982). The occurrence of cystitis caused by HSV-1 in adults with oropharyngeal HSV infections suggests that the bladder may also be infected as a result of viremia.

Infection of the cervix occurs in almost every woman with symptomatic primary genital herpes, and probably causes much of the profuse watery vaginal discharge that usually begins shortly after the onset of the disease. In addition, the cervix appears to be the site of infection in many asymptomatic cases of genital herpes, which actually comprise the majority of genital HSV-2 infections. On occasion, the cervical infection may be extremely severe, producing necrotic cervicitis (Willcox, 1968). Symptoms include profuse vaginal discharge; dysuria; abdominal, pelvic, or genital pain; and constitutional symptoms. The cervix is extremely tender, bleeds easily, and exhibits extensive superficial necrosis with sloughing of necrotic epithelium. Healing occurs spontaneously in 2 to 3 weeks. One-half of the cases occur in the absence of other genital lesions. Rarely, extensive herpetic infection of the glans penis can produce necrotizing balanitis. Misdiagnosis and inappropriate therapy are common (Pertherer et al., 1979; Powers et al., 1982).

Anorectal herpes and herpetic proctitis may occur as complications of genital herpes in women, the virus spreading from the vulva to the perineum, anus, and anal canal directly, or by zosteriform spread from infected sacral ganglia. However, most cases occur as a result of anal intercourse, and the disease is seen most frequently in homosexual males. (Jacobs, 1976; Goodell et al., 1983). Typical herpetic lesions occur on the perianal skin and in the anal canal, where they frequently coalesce, producing an ulcerative cryptitis. Pain is severe, frequently radiating to the groin, buttocks, and thighs. There is often a serous rectal discharge and bilateral inguinal adenopathy, and constitutional symptoms are common. Pain in the anal canal usually results in reflex inhibition of defecation and sometimes tenesmus. Sacral ganglionitis and autonomic dysfunction frequently result in sacral neuralgia, urinary retention, and impotence (Oates and Greenhouse, 1979; Jacobs, 1976; Goodell et al., 1983). In spite of its severity, the disease is self-limited; the neurologic symptoms resolve and healing usually occurs without scarring in 2 to 4 weeks. Recurrent attacks of anal herpes are common after primary infection.

During primary genital herpes, contiguous spread, neural transmission from newly infected sacral ganglia, or autoinoculation frequently results in cutaneous lesions on the buttocks, thighs, or other areas of skin below the waist. When these lesions subsequently recur (typically in the absence of any genital lesions) they resemble herpes zoster and are often associated with a prodrome of deep neuralgic pain. However, frequent recurrence distinguishes this syndrome of "zosteriform herpes simplex" from true herpes zoster (Slavin and Ferguson, 1950). Autoinoculation of the finger during primary genital herpes may result in a herpetic whitlow which is indistinguishable from the whitlows that occur in hospital personnel as a result of contact with HSV-1 in saliva and respiratory secretions (Chapter 105). Most herpetic whitlows in adults (other than hospital personnel) occur in association with primary genital herpes and are caused by HSV-2 (Glogau et al., 1977). These troublesome lesions tend to recur.

The increasing popularity of oral-genital sexual practices is changing the epidemiology of HSV-1 and HSV-2 infections. HSV-1 is causing disease in territory formerly exclusively inhabited by HSV-2, and vice versa. Consequently, we are now finding that 10 to 50 per cent of genital herpes is caused by HSV-1, and that many cases of herpetic gingivostomatitis and pharyngotonsillitis in adults are caused by HSV-2. There is no detectable difference in these diseases when they are caused by HSV-1 or HSV-2, except that genital herpes caused by HSV-1 appears to have a lower recurrence rate than genital herpes caused by HSV-2. Herpetic pharyngotonsillitis, caused by HSV-1 or HSV-2, occurs in 10 to 20 per cent of patients with first episode genital herpes. Clinical manifestations range from mild erythema to severe exudative pharyngotonsillitis with pharyngeal obstruction (Tustin and Kaiser, 1979; Corey et al., 1983a), and the disease is frequently misdiagnosed as streptococcal pharyngitis. Symptomatic herpetic pharyngotonsillitis is usually a manifestation of primary HSV infection; it is rarely seen as a complication of recurrent or nonprimary first-episode genital herpes. When caused by HSV-2, it frequently occurs together with primary genital herpes, as result of oral-genital contact in conjunction with sexual intercourse (Kaufman and Rawls, 1972).

Severe disseminated HSV infections are common in immunosuppressed children and adults (see below). Yet, while viremia probably occurs during most primary HSV infections in normal hosts, it is seldom manifest clinically. Rarely, apparently healthy young adults with primary genital herpes develop disseminated infection. This generally involves the skin, rather than internal organs, and produces a disease that is virtually indistinguishable from varicella. The illness is self-limited and usually resolves in 12 to 15 days. However, skin lesions commonly recur at sites of primary cutaneous infection. Very rarely, genital herpes in an apparently normal adult may be complicated by fulminant HSV hepatitis, which is usually accompanied by disseminated intravascular coagulation and is almost always fatal (Whorton et al., 1983).

Neurons play a critical role in the pathogenesis of HSV infections, and thus it is not surprising that many complications involve the central and peripheral nervous system. An acute aseptic meningitis may occur in the course of primary genital herpes. HSV-2 can be isolated from the spinal fluid, but it is not clear whether the virus reaches the central nervous system by passage in sensory nerves or as a result of viremia. The meningitis usually follows a brief and benign course, although it may sometimes be associated with polyradiculitis or ascending myelitis (Chapter 180). Herpes simplex meningitis recurs in some patients in association with recurrent genital herpes. Recurrent genital herpes and recurrent zosteriform herpes involving the skin below the waist may be associated with severe local neuralgia, usually in a L5-S1 dermatome distribution. When the recurrent herpetic lesions and neuralgia involve the extremities, there may also be local edema and lymphangitis. The neuralgia may precede the eruption by several days and usually resolves along with the cutaneous lesions (Slavin and Ferguson, 1950; Layzer and Conant, 1974; Hinthorn et al., 1976). Although resolution is generally complete and multiple recurrences occur without any permanent residua, repeated attacks over a period of years may sometims result in chronic pain and permanent sensory and motor deficits. Primary genital or anal herpes is sometimes complicated by urinary retention, and this may be accompanied by neuralgic pain and blunting of sensation over the sacral dermatomes. Patients with this syndrome have hypotonic bladders and spinal fluid pleocytosis, indicating that the urinary retention reflects acute herpetic ganglionitis or lumbosacral radiculomyelitis (Caplan et al., 1977; Chang, 1979; Oates and Greenhouse, 1979). This complication of genital herpes normally resolves spontaneously without residua in 7 to 10 days; the only report of prolonged dysfunction was in a patient treated with corticosteroids (Craig and Nahmias, 1973).

Recurrent genital herpes may be associated with recurrent episodes of erythema multiforme or Stevens-Johnson syndrome. As is the case with HSV-1 (Chapter 105), this complication appears to be an allergic response to circulating HSV antigens or antigen-antibody complexes. The lesions are not the direct result of replications of HSV-2 in the skin or mucous membranes.

Compromised patients are at increased risk of severe, even fatal, HSV infections. Those at greatest risk appear to have abnormal cellular immunity, eczema, or burns. The risk to the compromised patient and the nature of the pathologic process appear to be the same with HSV-1 and HSV-2. Most reported infections in compromised patients have been with untyped HSV or with HSV-1, but this is mainly a matter of exposure and epidemiology. HSV-2 also causes many severe infections in patients with malignancies undergoing chemotherapy and in organ transplant recipients. Most of these result from local extension or systemic dissemination of herpes genitalis (Montgomerie et al., 1969; Logan et al., 1971; Muller et al., 1972; Sutton et al., 1974; Stone et al., 1977; Lopyan et al., 1977; Schneidman et al., 1979). Most episodes of genital herpes in these patients are recurrent infections, and they often evolve normally and resolve without complications. Sometimes, however, the local lesions do not resolve but slowly progress to form a deep, gradually enlarging ulcer with a sharp erythematous border and a necrotic base covered with purulent exudate; there are often satellite lesions in adjacent areas of skin. These chronic progressive herpetic ulcers are usually exquisitely tender. They contain large amounts of HSV and may persist for months. They occur most frequently in patients with severely depressed cellular immunity, and often heal spontaneously when cellular immunity improves upon induced remission of lymphoreticular malignancies or reduction in iatrogenic immunosuppression in organ allograph recipients. Male homosexuals with acquired immunodeficiency syndrome (AIDS) often have chronic progressive perianal herpetic ulcers (Siegal et al., 1981). In spite of their severity, these lesions are rarely associated with constitutional symptoms or hematogenous dissemination of HSV. Genital herpes sometimes disseminates in immunocompromised patients, producing widespread cutaneous lesions or fatal involvement of multiple visceral organs, especially the liver (Elliott et al., 1980; Taylor et al., 1981; Walker et al., 1981).

Disseminated HSV infections have been described in

otherwise normal women in their third trimester of pregnancy (Young et al., 1976; Hensleigh et al., 1979; Kobbermann et al., 1980). Some have been associated with primary oropharyngeal HSV-1 infections and others have followed primary or nonprimary first episodes of genital herpes caused by HSV-2. Fulminant HSV hepatitis with coagulopathy has been an almost constant feature and appears to be largely responsible for the high mortality observed. Other organs, including the brain, adrenal glands, pancreas, heart, and gastrointestinal tract have also been involved. The disease in these pregnant women resembles that observed in renal transplant recipients and other immunosuppressed patients (Taylor et al., 1981) and in the neonate (vide infra). HSV-specific cellular immunity is depressed during the third trimester of pregnancy (Kumar et al., 1984), and this may explain the susceptibility of pregnant women to disseminated HSV infections.

One of the most important complications of genital herpes occurs when infection in a pregnant woman is transmitted to her newborn infant (Hanshaw and Dudgeon, 1978; Whitley et al., 1980a; Nahmias et al., 1983; Oxman et al., 1983). The incidence of recognized neonatal HSV infection in the United States is estimated to be about one in 7500 deliveries, but it may vary from one in 3,000 to one in 30,000, depending upon the population studied, and may be increasing in parallel with the increasing prevalence of primary genital and nongenital HSV infections in young adults (Sullivan-Bolyai et al., 1983). In most cases, the infant appears to acquire infection perinatally during passage through the birth canal of a mother with genital herpes. Sometimes infection occurs *in utero*, as a result of maternal viremia or ascending infection from the cervix (Oxman et al., 1983); ascending infection can also be iatrogenic, introduced by a fetal monitor (Kaye and Dooling, 1981). A few infants with neonatal herpes (probably no more than 10 per cent) appear to acquire infection postpartum from the mother, other family members, or nursery personnel with nongenital HSV infections, or by nosocomial transmission from another infected infant (Light, 1979; Adams et al., 1981). Primary genital infection during the first trimester may, rarely, cause viremia and transplacental transmission of HSV-2 to the fetus. This is likely to cause fetal death and abortion but, occasionally, the infected fetus survives and is later born with multiple congenital anomalies (Florman et al., 1973; Hanshaw and Dudgeon, 1978). Only 30 per cent of mothers of infants with neonatal herpes have signs or symptoms of genital herpes at or around the time of delivery. While some of the other 70 per cent have a history of genital herpes or a sexual partner with a history of genital herpes, there are no discernible risk factors in fully half of the mothers of infants with neonatal herpes (Whitley et al., 1980a; Boehm et al., 1981). The risk of neonatal HSV infection after vaginal delivery in women with active genital herpes is not well defined, and is almost certainly affected by such factors as the nature (i.e., primary, nonprimary first episode, recurrent) and extent of the maternal genital infection, the newborn's level of passively acquired antibody to HSV (Yeager et al., 1980) and the degree to which normal barriers to HSV infection in the newborn (e.g., the skin) remain intact during delivery. The risk of neonatal infection has been estimated to be 10 per cent in infants delivered vaginally to mothers with symptomatic genital herpes after 32 weeks' gestation, and 40 per cent or more when active infection is present at term (Nahmias et al., 1971). However, these estimates were derived from a small series of patients selected primarily on the basis of cytologic or virologic evidence of HSV cervicitis. Since fewer than 10 per cent of women with symptomatic recurrent genital herpes have HSV cervicitis, and since Papanicolaou smears are usually negative in women with recurrent genital herpes, even when cervical cultures are positive for HSV (Guinan et al., 1981), these patients are certainly not representative of typical cases of recurrent genital herpes, and the estimates derived from them probably greatly exaggerate the risk of neonatal HSV infection. In fact, the risk of neonatal herpes is probably very much lower than 10 per cent in women with recurrent genital herpes, even when virus is present at term.

The initial clinical manifestations of neonatal herpes usually appear during the first or second week of life, but they may be present at birth or delayed until the infant is a month of age (Whitley et al., 1980a and 1983a; Nahmias et al., 1983). Many infants with neonatal herpes are born prematurely, usually between 30 and 37 weeks' gestation, and two-thirds of these develop complications of prematurity, principally respiratory distress syndrome, before the clinical onset of their HSV infection. In contrast, most term infants are discharged before their neonatal herpes becomes manifest. Skin lesions are present at onset in about 70 per cent, and develop sometimes during the course of the illness in 80 to 90 per cent of infected infants. They are usually vesicular or bullous, and may appear anywhere on the skin. The scalp is often involved, as are the sites of electrodes used for fetal monitoring. Visceral dissemination occurs in half of the infected infants, involving the liver, lungs, adrenal glands, brain and other organs. Initial manifestations in this group usually appear during the first week of life. They are relatively nonspecific, consisting of lethargy, fever or hypothermia, vomiting, and poor feeding. Jaundice, purpuric rash, apneic spells, respiratory distress and cyanosis may also appear. The clinical picture often resembles bacterial sepsis. Many of these infants have clinical evidence of central nervous system involvement, and seizures are common. The disease progresses rapidly, with the frequent development of pneumonia, shock, and disseminated intravascular coagulation. About 80 per cent of the infants with disseminated neonatal herpes die, usually in the second postpartum week, and most survivors have severe neurologic and ocular sequelae. The remaining infants with neonatal herpes have more localized infections, involving the skin, mouth, and eyes in various combinations, and extending to the central nervous system in over one-half. The infants with central nervous system involvement present with a clinical picture resembling bacterial meningitis, except that two thirds have herpetic skin lesions. Their symptoms begin later than those of infants with disseminated infection, usually during the second week of life. Approximately 40 per cent die and most of the survivors have severe neurologic and ocular sequelae. The small group of infected infants (approximately 20 per cent) in whom infection appears to remain localized to the skin, eyes, or mouth almost all survive, but 30 to 40 per cent develop significant neurologic or ocular sequelae. The overall mortality of untreated symptomatic neonatal herpes is 50 per cent. Asymptomatic neonatal HSV infections are uncommon. Earlier diagnosis, stimulated by the availability of experimental therapeutic protocols, has increased the proportion of infants recognized with localized infection of the skin, eye, or mouth. If untreated, most of these infections disseminate or spread to the central nervous system. Seventy-five to 85 per cent of neonatal HSV infections are caused by HSV-2. There is no apparent difference between the nature and severity of neonatal herpes in premature and full-term infants, in infants infected with HSV-1 and HSV-2, or in infants who acquire their infection during delivery and those infected postpartum. Yeager et al. (1980) has provided evidence that high levels of passively acquired maternal antibody to HSV-2 reduce the incidence and severity of infection in infants who are exposed to the virus during vaginal delivery, but this point is still controversial.

It has been suggested that HSV-2 may play a role in the etiology of carcinoma of the cervix (Rotkin, 1973; Rawls et al., 1977). This idea is based largely upon the capacity of HSV to induce cell transformation and the observation made in many seroepidemiologic studies that more patients with cervical carcinoma have antibody to HSV-2 than matched controls. In addition, several investigators have found HSV antigens and nucleic acid sequences in cervical carcinoma cells. However, epidemiologic studies indicate only that HSV-2 infection and carcinoma of the cervix are covariable, both linked to an early age of first coitus and multiple sexual consorts. Furthermore, HSV-2 is latent in sacral ganglia and is periodically reactivated, producing recurrent cervical infections that are generally asymptomatic. Thus, it would not be surprising, at least on occasion, to find evidence of HSV-2 in cervical tissues. Much work is still to be done to establish the exact relationship of HSV-2 infection to carcinoma of the cervix. Recently, more compelling data have been obtained implicating human papillomaviruses in the etiology of cervical carcinoma (Chapter 62).

GEOGRAPHIC VARIATION IN DISEASE AND EPIDEMIOLOGY. Although it differs from HSV-1 in its epidemiology, HSV-2 appears to be an almost equally successful and ubiquitous parasite of man (Chapter 105). Except for neonatal infections, which are rare, and which, because of their high mortality, contribute nothing to the survival of the virus in the human population, HSV-2 infections do not generally occur before puberty. Thereafter, the acquisition of HSV-2 infection is a function of sexual activity. The prevalence of antibody to the virus exceeds 70 per cent in prostitutes and is only 3 per cent in chaste women (Nahmias and Josey, 1982). In some populations genital herpes is now the most frequently occurring sexually transmitted disease and serologic data indicate that in the United States, 10 to 35 per cent of women of childbearing age have been infected with HSV-2. As in the case of HSV-1 (Fig. 3 in Chapter 105), latency and asymptomatic virus shedding play a critical role in maintaining HSV-2 in human populations.

Systematic virologic and cytologic surveys have revealed that more than one-half of all genital herpes infections in females are asymptomatic (Nahmias et al., 1969; Nahmias et al., 1971; Ng et al., 1970; Rawls et al., 1971; Dueñas et al., 1972; Poste et al., 1972; Whitley et al., 1980a; Nahmias et al., 1983). Primary HSV-2 infections are more often symptomatic than nonprimary first episode or recurrent infections. The overall rate of asymptomatic genital excretion of HSV in women varies from 0.03 per cent to 8 per cent, depending upon the population studied (Dueñas et al., 1972; Nahmias and Josey, 1982; Jeansson and Molin, 1970; Bolognese et al., 1976). The figure is highest in prostitutes and women attending venereal disease clinics, and lowest in private patients. Most of this virus shedding represents asymptomatic reactivation of latent endogenous HSV infection; virus is shed from the cervix and external genitalia. The rate of asymptomatic shedding of HSV from the cervix during pregnancy in women in the United States is 0.65 per cent (Bolognese et al., 1976); it is 2 to 4 per cent in pregnant women with a history of recurrent genital herpes (Scher et al., 1982; Harger et al., 1983; Wittek et al., 1984). In pregnant women with a history of recurrent genital herpes, but with no symptoms or detectable lesions, HSV is isolated more frequently from the external genitalia than from the cervix (Vontuer et al., 1982; Wittek et al., 1984).

The situation in males is less clear. In spite of the observation that males with a history of recurrent genital herpes may occasionally transmit infection to their sexual partner in the absence of symptoms or signs of active infection, virus is rarely isolated from semen or prostatic secretions. Deture et al. (1978) failed to isolate HSV from semen obtained during a symptom-free interval from 30 healthy males subject to recurrent genital herpes, and other workers have only rarely isolated HSV from the urethra in healthy, asymptomatic males. Jeansson and Molin (1974) reported the isolation of HSV from the urethra of 4.4 per cent of males and from the cervix of 5.2 per cent of females attending a Swedish venereal disease clinic. More than 25 per cent of the males and 30 per cent of the females who yielded virus were free of signs and symptoms of either genital herpes or gonorrhea. In contrast, no urethral isolates were obtained from 131 males attending a dermatology clinic. Longitudinal studies of individual patients demonstrated intermittent asymptomatic shedding by both males and females. More than 90 per cent of the isolates were HSV-2. Although the risk of infection is unknown when a susceptible individual has sexual intercourse with a partner asymptomatically shedding HSV-2, the rate of transmission during intercourse by symptomatic males is 75 to 80 per cent (Nahmias et al., 1969; Rawls et al., 1971).

DIAGNOSIS. The diagnosis of genital herpes is often clinically apparent, especially when there is a history of recurrent infections. In Europe and North America, HSV is now the most common cause of genital ulcers (Chapel et al. 1977; Catterall, 1981; Corey and Holmes, 1983), but there are a number of other diseases that can cause ulcerative genital lesions that may be confused with those of genital herpes. Moreover, the incidence of dual infections is higher than random (Hutfield, 1968; Young, 1972; Young et al., 1977; Fiumara et al., 1980; Chapel et al., 1979).

The methods for obtaining specimens for virus isolation, HSV antigen detection, and cytologic examination have already been described in detail (Chapter 105). The simplest and most rapid method of diagnosis is the examination of cells scraped from the base of a vesicle or ulcer (Tzanck smear) or scraped from the surface of the cervix or the vaginal mucosa (Papanicolaou smear) and stained by the Papanicolaou or Paragon Multiple stain technique as described in Chapter 105. Eosinophilic intranuclear inclusion bodies and multinucleated giant cells indicate HSV or VZV infection. Virus antigen detection and identification (e.g., by immunofluorescent or immunoenzyme staining) can give a rapid and specific diagnosis, if reagents are reliable. A punch biopsy taken at the edge of a lesion provides better tissue for cytologic and immunologic diagnosis. As with

HSV infections elsewhere, virus isolation is the most sensitive diagnostic technique. It is approximately twice as sensitive as cytology in genital herpes. Furthermore, it should be remembered that Papanicolaou smears of the cervix are usually negative during recurrent genital herpes, even when HSV can be isolated from the same specimen (Guinan et al., 1981). Specimens are more likely to yield virus if they are obtained from a vesicular lesions early in the course of the disease. This is especially true with recurrent infections. In pregnant women with a history of genital herpes (or with potential HSV exposure) it is recommended that the method of delivery be dictated by the presence or absence of HSV in the birth canal at the onset of labor (Nahmias et al., 1983; Oxman et al., 1983). However, this requires a rapid, sensitive and specific method for the detection of HSV or its components. Virus isolation is sufficiently sensitive and specific, but it is not widely available and does not yield results quickly enough. Furthermore, because virus shedding during episodes of recurrent genital herpes generally persists for less than 7 days (Harger et al., 1983; Wittek et al., 1984), asymptomatic shedding a week or more prior to delivery does not correlate with virus shedding at term (Harger et al., 1983; Wittek et al., 1984). Promising methods for the direct detection of HSV antigens and nucleic acids are being evaluated (Richman et al., 1984). Until they become available, management must still depend upon serial viral culture during the last weeks of pregnancy and careful physical examination at the onset of labor (vide infra).

The diseases to be considered in the differential diagnosis of herpes genitalis are syphilis, chancroid, lymphogranuloma venereum, donovanosis, vaccinia, herpes zoster, erythema multiforme, Behçet's syndrome, contact dermatitis, candidiasis, and impetigo (Corey and Holmes, 1983). Multinucleated giant cells and eosinophilic Cowdry Type A intranuclear inclusion bodies indicate the presence of either HSV or VZV; direct detection and identification of HSV antigens by immunologic methods, or virus isolation can give the specific diagnosis. However, patients are often simultaneously infected by more than one agent, and it is, therefore, important to rule out at least some of the other possibilities. Syphilis is the most important of these diseases (Chapel et al., 1977 and 1979; Fiumara et al., 1980). The chancre of syphilis may mimic the ulcerative lesions of genital herpes, although it tends to be more indurated, indolent, and painless. The mucous patches of secondary syphilis may also resemble the ulcerated lesions of genital herpes, but are usually accompanied by a generalized rash or other secondary manifestations. The diagnosis should be attempted by dark-field examination and serology. Serologic follow-up is essential. The ulcers of chancroid are soft and painful with ragged undermined margins, and there is prominent, painful, often fluctuant inguinal adenopathy. The demonstration of *Haemophilus ducreyi*, a small gram-negative rod, in smears of the ulcer or by culture, can help establish the diagnosis. The diagnosis of lymphogranuloma venereum and donovanosis are discussed in Chapter 164. Vaccinia, which should rarely be seen now that routine smallpox vaccination has been abandoned, can be differentiated from HSV and VZV infections by the presence of cytoplasmic inclusion bodies, and the absence of intranuclear inclusion bodies and multinucleated giant cells. The histopathology of erythema multiforme and Behçet's syndrome are very different from that of genital herpes, and both are accompanied by characteristic lesions outside of the genital area. However, erythema multiforme is induced in some patients by genital herpes, and the lesions may therefore coexist. Bacterial and candidal infections may be diagnosed by gram-stained smears and cultures.

Now that effective chemotherapy is available (vide infra) the diagnosis of neonatal herpes must be established early in the course of the disease. Because more than half of the infected infants are born to mothers without signs, symptoms, or a history of genital herpes, this will require a very high index of suspicion. Any skin lesion should be examined by Tzanck smear, one or more HSV antigen detection methods (e.g., immunoperoxidase staining), and viral culture. Lesions should be sought in the mouth, and the eyes should be examined for herpetic conjunctivitis. An infant with signs of sepsis or meningitis, but with negative bacterial cultures or a poor response to appropriate antibiotics, is suspect. Mouth, conjunctivae, urine, stool, blood, and cerebrospinal fluid should be cultured for HSV (Nahmias et al., 1983; Oxman et al., 1983) and the mother should be examined and cultured. Disseminated enterovirus infection can resemble neonatal herpes and, rarely, the two infections may coexist (Modlin, 1980; Boehm et al., 1981).

The serologic diagnosis of HSV infections is discussed in Chapter 105. Serologic assays are useful for confirming a diagnosis of primary HSV infection and for distinguishing between primary and nonprimary first episodes of HSV infection. However, because HSV-1 causes many cases of genital herpes and HSV-2 causes non-genital infections, type-specific serologic assays (when these are available) will not be able to rule in or rule out prior genital HSV infection. Recurrent genital herpes only rarely induces a significant increase in antibody titer to HSV. The antigenic cross-reactivity of HSV-1 and HSV-2 limits the usefulness of currently available serologic techniques (Rawls, 1979).

TREATMENT. Primary genital herpes is a self-limited disease which, in the normal person, resolves spontaneously without sequelae. However, it is followed by a latent HSV infection in sacral ganglia and, in most people, by repeated episodes of recurrent infection. While these, too, are ordinarily self-limited, they produce enough physical and psychological distress to cause most affected persons to seek some form of relief. The desire for relief from this recurrent affliction has been further stimulated by the recognition that genital herpes during pregnancy may cause serious infection of the fetus or newborn infant, and by the widely publicized epidemiologic association between HSV-2 infection and carcinoma of the cervix.

The topical application of a variety of agents designed to limit virus replication has been tried in patients with recurrent genital herpes. Each new regimen has been greeted with enthusiasm on the basis of anecdotal observations and uncontrolled trials, only to be proven ineffective when careful, double blind, placebo-controlled studies were carried out (Guinan, 1982; Corey and Holmes, 1983). Topical therapies that have proven to be ineffective for recurrent genital herpes include idoxouridine ointment, photodynamic inactivation with neutral red or proflavine and light, vidarabine (which is effective parenterally for HSV encephalitis and neonatal HSV infections), ether, surfactant, 2-deoxy-D-glucose, and adenine arabinoside monophosphate. In addition, L-lysine, BCG vaccine, levamisole, multiple smallpox vaccinations, and live and killed HSV vaccines have also proven to be ineffective.

To date, only one drug, acyclovir [9-(2-hydroxyethoxymethyl) guanine], has been proven effective for the treatment of genital herpes. Acyclovir is a guanosine analog that is selectively phosphorylated by HSV deoxypyrimidine kinase (thymidine kinase) and thus concentrated in HSV-infected cells. Cellular enzymes then convert the resulting acyclovir monophosphate to acyclovir triphosphate, which is a selective inhibitor of HSV DNA polymerase. In addition, any acyclovir triphosphate that is incorporated into DNA causes chain termination (Elion, 1982; McGuirt et al., 1984). As a consequence of these properties, acyclovir is a highly effective and nontoxic inhibitor of HSV replication in tissue culture and in animal models of HSV infection. Strains of HSV-1 are generally more sensitive to acyclovir than strains of HSV-2, but current dosages employed (vide infra) produce concentrations of acyclovir in serum and body fluids well in excess of those required to inhibit the replication of HSV-2 in vitro (Hirsch and Schooley, 1983; Corey and Holmes, 1983).

In considering chemotherapy of genital herpes, it is important ot recognize problems posed by the anatomy, pathophysiology, and natural history of genital HSV infections, and define therapeutic objectives. For example, the involvement of distant sites (e.g., the cervix, urethra, pharynx, and sacral ganglia) limits the potential efficacy of topical therapy applied to the external genitalia. The relatively short period of virus replication characteristic of recurrent genital herpes limits the potential clinical impact of any therapeutic agent that acts by inhibiting HSV multiplication. This is not the case when the period of virus replication is prolonged, as it is in primary genital herpes and in mucocutaneous HSV infections in immunocompromised patients. In primary or nonprimary first episode genital herpes, therapeutic objectives include: (1) to reduce the duration and severity of the genital infection itself; (2) to decrease the frequency and severity of complications, such as aseptic meningitis, urethritis, and infections at other extragenital sites; and (3) to prevent the development of latent neuronal infection, and thus prevent the subsequent development of recurrent genital herpes. In recurrent genital herpes, therapeutic objectives include: (1) to reduce the duration and severity of the recurrent episode itself; (2) to decrease the frequency and severity of complications; (3) to prevent subsequent recurrences, either by eradicating the latent neuronal infection or by preventing its subsequent reactivation; and (4) to decrease transmission of infection to other individuals.

A number of randomized placebo-controlled double-blind studies have demonstrated the therapeutic efficacy of intravenous, oral, and topical acyclovir in immunologically normal persons with first episode genital herpes. In patients with first episodes severe enough to warrant hospitalization, intravenous acyclovir (5 mg/kg every 8 hours for 5 days) begun within 7 days of onset, markedly reduced the subsequent duration of virus shedding (by more than 75 per cent), and of local and constitutional symptoms (by more than 50 per cent). Healing time was reduced by more than 50 per cent, and the development of new lesions and complications was prevented (Mindel et al., 1982; Corey et al., 1983b). Oral acyclovir (200 mg 5 times daily for 10 days) begun within 6 days of onset has also reduced virus shedding and new lesion formation (both by more than 70 per cent), shortened the duration of local and constitutional symptoms, and shortened the times to crusting and healing of lesions in patients with primary first episode genital herpes (Nilsen et al., 1982; Bryson et al., 1983; Mertz et al., 1984). In patients with nonprimary first episode genital herpes, oral acyclovir markedly reduced the duration of virus shedding, but did not have a significant effect upon the clinical course of the disease, presumably because of the late initiation of therapy relative to the shorter normal duration of nonprimary first episode disease (Mertz et al., 1984; Corey and Holmes, 1983). Topical acyclovir (5 per cent in polyethylene glycol ointment applied 4 times daily for 7 days) reduced the duration of virus shedding in patients with primary and nonprimary first episode genital herpes and shortened the clinical course of local disease in patients with primary infections. However, in contrast to oral and intravenous acyclovir, topical acyclovir did not decrease new lesion formation or reduce the duration of dysuria, vaginal discharge, or constitutional symptoms (Corey et al., 1982a and 1982b; Corey and Holmes, 1983). No form of therapy appears to prevent the establishment of neuronal latency, and in no group of treated patients has there been any reduction in the frequency or severity of subsequent recurrences.

In patients with recurrent genital herpes, oral acyclovir (200 mg 5 times daily for 5 days) begun within 48 hours of onset reduced the duration of virus shedding and new lesion formation, and modestly shortened the time to crusting and healing of lesions (Nilsen et al., 1982; Reichman et al., 1984). When therapy was initiated by patients at the onset of symptoms, the clinical effects of acyclovir were greater, but they were still far smaller than those observed in first episodes of genital herpes (Reichman et al., 1984). Trials of topical acyclovir (5 per cent in polyethylene glycol ointment 4 or 6 times daily for 5 days) begun within 48 hours of onset of recurrent genital herpes have demonstrated a small reduction in the duration of virus shedding, but no clinically significant effect on the course of disease (Corey et al., 1982a and 1982b; Reichman et al., 1983). Neither oral nor topical acyclovir treatment of recurrent genital herpes reduced the frequency or severity of subsequent recurrences.

A number of well-designed clinical trials have demonstrated that both oral and intravenous acyclovir are extremely effective for the treatment (and prophylaxis) of severe mucocutaneous HSV infections in immunocompromised patients (these are discussed in detail in Chapter 105). Although only a minority of the patients in these studies had genital herpes, their response to therapy was comparable to that of patients with oropharyngeal infections (Wade et al., 1982; Strauss et al., 1984). Excellent results have been obtained using oral dosages of 200 mg 4 or 5 times daily and intravenous dosages of 5 mg/kg every 12 hours, 5 mg/kg every 8 hours or 250 mg/m^2 of body surface area every 8 hours. No significant hematologic, renal or hepatic toxicity has been observed, although neurologic symptoms have been reported in several bone marrow transplant recipients treated with intravenous acyclovir (Wade and Meyers, 1983).

In the United States, intravenous acyclovir is approved for use in mucosal or cutaneous HSV infections in immunocompromised patients and for severe initial episodes of genital herpes in immunologically normal individuals. Acyclovir ointment (5 per cent acyclovir in a polyethylene glycol base) is approved for use in initial episodes of genital herpes in immunologically normal individuals and in mucocutaneous HSV infections in immunocompromised patients. Oral acyclovir represents a major advance in the treatment of genital herpes. When available, it will be the treatment of choice for primary and nonprimary first episode genital herpes, and will provide an alternative to intravenous acyclovir for such extragenital complications as herpetic whitlow, cutaneous dissemination, HSV meningitis, and sacral radiculopathy with urinary retention. Oral acyclovir also provides an alternative to intravenous acyclovir for the treatment of HSV infections in immunocompromised patients, especially when hospitalization is not otherwise required. Oral acyclovir may also be useful for selected patients with severe or prolonged recurrent genital herpes and for patients in whom recurrent genital herpes is associated with prolonged neuralgia or erythema multiforme. In these situations, patient-initiated therapy would permit acyclovir to be administered at the first sign of recurrent infection.

On the basis of the information discussed above, it is recommended that initial episodes of genital herpes in immunologically normal persons be treated by the application of acyclovir ointment to all external genital lesions 4 to 6 times daily for 7 to 10 days or until all lesions have entirely crusted. When available, oral acyclovir (200 mg 5 times daily for 10 days) should be used instead. Patients with severe initial infections should be treated with intravenous acyclovir (5 mg/kg or 250 mg/m^2 each 8 hours) for 5 to 7 days. Since significant complications, such as cutaneous dissemination, herpetic whitlow, HSV meningitis or sacral radiculopathy with urinary retention almost certainly involve HSV replication at extragenital sites, they should be treated systemically with intravenous acyclovir (5 mg/kg or 250 mg/m^2 each 8 hours) for 5 to 7 days. When available, oral acyclovir (200 mg 5 times daily for 7 to 10 days) can probably be substituted for intravenous acyclovir. Topical acyclovir is not recommended for recurrent genital herpes in immunocompetent individuals. When it is available, oral acyclovir (200 mg 5 times daily for 5 to 7 days) should be considered for selected patients with severe or prolonged recurrent genital herpes, and for patients in whom recurrent herpes is associated with prolonged neuralgia or erythema multiforme.

Primary and nonprimary first episode genital herpes in immunocompromised patients should be treated with intravenous acyclovir (5 mg/kg or 250 mg/m^2 each 8 hours) for 7 to 10 days, until involved sites are HSV culture negative, or until all lesions are entirely crusted. Recurrent genital herpes or mucocutaneous lesions at other sites in immunocompromised patients are rarely associated with early HSV dissemination and can often be successfully treated with topical acyclovir applied 4 to 6 times daily for 10 to 14 days, or until cultures are negative for HSV, or lesions have healed. If this is ineffective, or if there are any signs of dissemination or spread to extragenital sites, patients should be treated with intravenous acyclovir (5 mg/kg or 250 mg/m^2 each 8 hours) for 7 to 10 days, or until there is clinical and virologic resolution. When available, oral acyclovir (200 mg 5 times daily) can be substituted for intravenous acyclovir. In any immunocompromised patient with HSV infection, immunosuppressive therapy should be reduced, if possible.

Prophylactic administration of human interferon has decreased the frequency of reactivation of HSV-1 induced by surgical manipulation of the trigenimal ganglion (Pazin et al., 1979). Trials are underway to evaluate interferon for the treatment and prevention of genital herpes in normal and immunocompromised patients. However, unless interferon proves capable of preventing or abolishing latent neuronal HSV infection, bothersome side effects and the need for parenteral administration will limit its acceptance by most patients.

Detailed recommendations for the management of infants with neonatal herpes are available elsewhere (Nahmias et al., 1983; Oxman et al., 1983). Vidarabine (adenine arabinoside), administered intravenously at 15 mg/kg/day for 10 days, has reduced the mortality in infants with either disseminated or central nervous system HSV infection from 74 per cent in the placebo group to 38 per cent, and increased the proportion of survivors with normal psychomotor development at one year of life from 11 per cent in the placebo group to 29 per cent (Whitley et al., 1980b). In a second study (Whitley et al., 1983a), in which two dosage levels of Vidarabine (15 mg/kg/day and 30 mg/kg/day) were compared there was no significant differences in outcome in neonatal herpes. A collaborative study is underway comparing Vidarabine (30 mg/kg/day) with acyclovir (10 mg/kg every 8 hours) for 10 days in infants with neonatal herpes (Whitley et al., 1983b). Until the results of that study are available, infants with neonatal herpes should be treated with intravenous Vidarabine, 30 mg/kg/day administered over 12 hours for 10 days. It is clear from the clinical trials conducted to date that outcome is markedly improved if therapy is begun while disease is localized to the skin, mouth, or eye, i.e., before it disseminates to visceral organs or involves the central nervous system.

In the newborn, and perhaps also in HSV antibody negative immunosuppressed patients exposed to HSV-2 infection, the early administration of human HSV immune serum globulin containing high levels of antibody to HSV-2 should be considered.

PROPHYLAXIS. Primary and nonprimary first episode genital herpes can be prevented by avoiding exposure to the virus. Since males with symptomatic genital herpes appear to transmit infection to 75 per cent or more of susceptible consorts, males with prodromal symptoms or active genital herpes should refrain from sexual intercourse. Females with prodromal symptoms, symptomatic genital herpes, or visible but asymptomatic genital lesions should also refrain from sexual intercourse. Oral-genital contact can transmit infection in either direction. Thus, individuals with herpes labialis should refrain from oral-genital sexual activity. It should be recognized that asymptomatic virus shedding occurs between episodes of symptomatic genital herpes and herpes labialis. However, the concentration of virus and the duration of shedding are less during asymptomatic than symptomatic recurrences. Thus, the risk of transmission is lower. This risk can be further reduced by the use of condoms and spermicidal foams (which can inactivate extracellular HSV).

Because infants born by vaginal delivery to mothers with active genital herpes at term are at significant risk of developing neonatal herpes, it is generally advised that women with active genital herpes at term and intact membranes be delivered by Cesarean section (Kibrick, 1980; American Academy of Pediatrics, 1980; Nahmias et al., 1983; Oxman et al., 1983). It should be noted, however, that the efficacy of this procedure has never been proven. Because rupture of membranes facilitates ascending infection and may even be the result of herpetic chorioamnionitis (Oxman et al., 1983) many believe that if membranes have been ruptured for more than 4 hours, delivery by Cesarean section is probably not warranted. Others, noting that virus is shed from the cervix in only a minority of women with recurrent genital herpes, would deliver by Cesarean section whenever external genital lesions are present, irrespective of the duration of membrane rupture (Corey et al., 1983a). It is important to recognize the potential danger of manipulations that break or abrade fetal skin when there is a material history of recurrent genital herpes. Thus, such manipulations as vacuum extraction, the use of fetal scalp electrodes, and blood sampling should be avoided if possible. Infants delivered through an infected birth canal should probably be given large doses of immune serum globulin, preferably with a high titer of antibody to HSV-2. Although there is no evidence that passively administered antibody is protective, it reduces the mortality of primary HSV-2 infections in animals, and infants with high titers of transplacentally acquired antibody to HSV-2 appear to have a more favorable outcome than infants with low antibody titers (Yeager et al., 1980). Topical Vidarabine eye drops should also be administered, since the eye is one portal of entry for HSV.

The therapeutic and prophylactic efficacy of acyclovir in immunocompromised patients with HSV infections, and its capacity to prevent primary infection and the establishment of latency when given in advance of HSV inoculation in experimental animals (Field et al., 1979) suggest that acyclovir might be effective for the prophylaxis of genital herpes. In fact, studies to evaluate the capacity of oral acyclovir to prevent the development of primary genital herpes when administered after sexual exposure are underway, and consideration is being given to the use of acyclovir prophylaxis in infants delivered vaginally in the presence of active genital herpes. In addition, three recent double-blind placebo-controlled studies have demonstrated that daily prophylactic administration of oral acyclovir can markedly reduce the incidence and severity of recurrent genital herpes in immunocompetent persons with frequent recurrences (Douglas et al., 1984; Straus et al., 1984; Mindel et al., 1984). However, the effect of treatment was limited to the period of acyclovir administration, and there was no indication that neuronal latency was affected. In fact, acyclovir recipients frequently experienced typical prodromal symptoms, but these were rarely followed by the development of lesions. Moreover, after the treatment period, the median time to the first clinical recurrence was significantly shorter in recipients of acyclovir than in placebo recipients (Douglas et al., 1984) suggesting that the activity of some host factor(s) important in limiting the development of recurrences may have declined during the period of acyclovir prophylaxis. In regard to this, it has recently been observed that bone marrow transplant recipients with mucocutaneous HSV infections and normal patients with primary genital herpes treated with acyclovir (which was clinically highly effective) had diminished HSV-specific immune responses and earlier and more severe recurrences than placebo-treated controls (Wade et al., 1984; Ashley and Corey, 1984). In addition, Straus et al. (1984) isolated acyclovir resistant mutants of HSV from recurrent lesions which developed in patients receiving acyclovir. This is a worrisome finding, both with respect to the potential failure of longer-term prophylaxis, and because of the potential risk of transmission to susceptible sexual partners.

The use of oral acyclovir prophylaxis should be limited to selected seropositive patients undergoing finite periods of intensive immunosuppressive therapy (e.g., for organ allografts or cancer chemotherapy) and, perhaps, to a small number of immunocompetent patients with very frequent and severe recurrences of genital herpes. Prophylactic courses should be relatively brief because of the possibility of host cell DNA damage (most immunocompetent candidates will be of childbearing age) and the potential for emergence of resistant mutants of HSV. Furthermore, the failure of 4 months of effective prophylaxis to abolish HSV latency, and the rebound observed after cessation of therapy (Douglas et al., 1984; Straus et al., 1984) raises serious questions as to the advisability of long-term prophylaxis. The potential problems of the emergence of drug-resistant mutants of HSV and of alterations in host responses to HSV infection are discussed in Chapter 105.

The most effective method for the prevention of diseases caused by ubiquitous viruses is immunization. The reduced severity of initial genital infections with HSV-2 in individuals with prior HSV-1 infection, and the relative rarity and attenuated nature of exogenous HSV-2 infections in sexually active individuals with recurrent genital herpes caused by HSV-2, suggest that HSV vaccines can be expected to modify, if not prevent, primary HSV infections in susceptible immunocompetent individuals. It seems less likely that immunization will alter the natural history of recurrent herpes once latency has been established. A number of experimental HSV vaccines, including live attentuated and nucleic acid-free subunit vaccines, are currently being developed and evaluated. The subject of HSV vaccination is discussed in Chapter 105.

References

Adam, E., Dreesman, G. E., Kaufman, R. H., and Melnick, J. L.: Asymptomatic virus shedding after herpes genitalis. Am J Obstet Gynecol 137:827, 1980.

Adam, E., Kaufman, R. H., Mirkovic, R., and Melnick, J. L.: Persistence of virus shedding in asymptomatic women after recovery from herpes genitalis. Obstet Gynecol 54:171, 1979.

Adams, H. G., Renson, E. A., Alexander, E. R., Vontver, L. A., Remington, M. A., and Holmes, K. K.: Genital herpetic infection in men and women: Clinical course and effect of topical application of adenine arabinoside. J Infect Dis 133 Suppl.: A151, 1976.

Adams, G., Stover, B. H., Keenlyside, R. A., Hooton, T. M., Buchman, T. G., Roizman, B., and Stewart, J. A.: Nosocomial herpetic infections in a pediatric intensive care unit. Am J Epidemiol 113:126, 1981.

Ashley, R. L., and Corey L.: Effect of acyclovir treatment of primary genital herpes on the antibody response to herpes simplex virus. J Clin Invest 73:681, 1984.

American Academy of Pediatrics (Committee on Fetus and Newborn, Committee on Infectious Diseases): Perinatal herpes simplex virus infections. Pediatr 66:147, 1980.

Baringer, J. R.: Recovery of herpes simplex virus from human sacral ganglions. N Engl J Med 291:828, 1974.

Bolognese, R. J., Corson, S. L., Fuccillo, D. A., Traub, R., Moder, F., and Sever, J. L.: Herpesvirus hominis type II infections in asymptomatic pregnant women. Obstet Gynecol 48:507, 1976.

Buchman, T. G., Roizman, B., and Nahmias, A. J.: Demonstration of exogenous genital reinfection with herpes simplex virus type 2 by restriction endonuclease fingerprinting of viral DNA. J Infect Dis 140:295, 1979.

Boehm, F. H., Estes, W., Wright, P. F., and Growdon, J. F.: Maanagement of genital herpes simplex virus infection occurring during pregnancy. Am J Obstet Gynecol 141:735, 1981.

Brown, Z. A., Kern, E. R., Spruance, S. L., and Overall, J. C.: Clinical and virologic course of herpes simplex genitalis. West J Med 130:414, 1979.

Bryson, Y. J., Dillon, M., Lovett, M., Acuna, G., Taylor, S., Cherry, J. D., Johnson, B. L., Wiesmeier, E., Growdon, W., Creagh-Kirk, T., and Keeney, R.: Treatment of First episodes of genital herpes simplex virus infection with oral acyclovir. N Engl J Med 308:916, 1983.

Caplan, L. R., Kleeman, F. J., and Berg, S.: Urinary retention probably secondary to herpes genitalis. N Engl J Med 297:918, 1977.

Catterall, R. D.: Biological effects of sexual freedom. Lancet 1:315, 1981.

Chang, T. W., Fiumara, N. J., and Weinstein, L.: Genital herpes: Some clinical and laboratory observations. JAMA 229:544, 1974.

Chang, T-W.: Transient neurogenic bladder in genital herpes. J Infect 1:375, 1979.

Chapel, T. A., Jeffries, C. D., and Brown, W. J.: Simultaneous infection with treponema pallidum and herpes simplex virus. Cutis 24:191, 1979.

Chapel, T., Brown, W. J., Jeffries, C., and Stewart, J. A.: The microbiological flora of penile ulcerations. Sex Transm Dis 4:50, 1977.

Corey, L., and Holmes, K. K.: Genital herpes simplex virus infections: Current concepts in diagnosis, therapy, and prevention. Ann Intern Med 98:973, 1983.

Corey, L., Adams, H. G., Brown, Z.A., and Holmes, K. K.: Genital herpes simplex virus infections: Clinical manifestations, course, and complications. Ann Intern Med 98:958, 1983a.

Corey, L., Fife, K. H., Benedetti, J. K., Winter, C. A., Fahnlander, A., Connor, J. D., Hintz, M. A., and Holmes, K. K.: Intravenous acyclovir for the treatment of primary genital herpes. Ann Intern Med 98:914, 1983b.

Corey, L., Nahmias, A. J., Guinan, M. E., Benedetti, J. K., Critchlow, C. W., and Holmes, K. K.: A trial of topical acyclovir in genital herpes simplex virus infections. N Engl J Med 306:1313, 1982a.

Corey, L., Benedetti, J. K., Critchlow, C. W., Remington, M. R., Winter, C. A., Fahnlander, A. L., Smith, K., Salter, D. L., Keeney, R. E., Davis, L. G., Hintz, M. A., Connor, J. D., and Holmes, K. K.: Double-blind controlled trial of topical acyclovir in genital herpes simplex virus infections. Am J Med 73:326, 1982b.

Craig, C. P. and Nahmias, J.: Different patterns of neurologic involvement with herpes simplex virus type 1 and type 2 from the buffy coat of two adults with meningitis. J Infect Dis 127:365, 1973.

Deture, F. A., Drylie, D. M., Kaufman, H. E., and Centifano, Y. M.: Herpes virus type 2: Study of semen in male subjects with recurrent infections. J Urol 120:449, 1978.

Dueñas, A., Adam, E., Melnick, J. L., and Rawls, W. E.: Herpesvirus type 2 in a prostitute population. Am J Epidemiol 95:483, 1972.

Douglas, J. M., Critchlow, C., Benedetti, J., Mertz, G., Connor, J. D., Hintz, M. A., Fahnlander, A., Remington, M., Winter, C., and Corey, L.: A double-blind study of oral acyclovir for suppression of recurrences of genital herpes simplex virus infection. N Engl J Med 310:1551, 1984.

Ekwo, E., Wong, Y. W., and Myers, M.: Asymptomatic cervicovaginal shedding of herpes simplex virus. Am J Obstet Gynecol 134:102, 1979.

Elion, G. B.: Mechanism of action and selectivity of acyclovir. Am J Med 73(1A):7, 1982.

Elliott, W. C., Houghton, D. C., Bryant, R. E., Wicklund, R., Barry, J. M., and Bennett, W. M.: Herpes simplex type 1 hepatitis in renal transplantation. Arch Intern Med 140:1656, 1980.

Field, J. H., Bell, S. E., Elion, G. B., Nash, A. A., and Wildy, P.: Effect of acycloguanosine treatment on acute and latent herpes simplex infections in mice. Antimicrob Agents Chemother 15:554, 1979.

Fiumara, N. J., Schmidt-Ulrick, B., and Comite, H.: Primary herpes simplex and primay syphilis: A description of seven cases. Sex Transm Dis 7:130, 1980.

Florman, A. L., Gershon, A. A., Blackett, P. R., and Nahmias, A. J.: Intarauterine infection with herpes simplex virus: resultant congenital malformations. JAMA 225:129, 1973.

Glogau, R., Hanna, L., and Jawetz, E.:Herpetic whitlow as part of genital virus infection. J Infect Dis 136:689, 1977.

Goodell, S. E., Quinn, R. C., Mkrtichian, E., Schuffler, D., Holmes, K. K., and Corey, L.: Herpes simplex virus proctitis in homosexual men. Clinical, sigmoidoscopic, and histopathological features. N Engl J Med 308:868, 1983.

Grossman, J. H., Wallen, W. C., and Sever, J. L.: Management of genital herpes simplex virus infection during pregnancy. Obstet Gynecol 58:1, 1981.

Guinan, M. E.: Therapy for symptomatic genital herpes simplex virus infection: A review. Rev Infect Dis 4:S819, 1982.

Guinan, M. E., MacCalman, J., Kern, E. R., Overall, J. C., and Spruance, S. L.: The coure of untreated recurrent genital herpes simplex infection in 27 women. N Engl J Med 304:759, 1981.

Hanshaw, J. B., and Dudgeon, J. A.: Viral Diseases of the Fetus and Newborn. Vol 17 in series Major Problems in Clinical Pediatrics. Schaffer, A. J., and Markowitz, M. (eds.). Philadelphia, W. B. Saunders Co., 1978.

Harger, J. H., Pazin, G. J., Armstrong, J. A., Breinig, M. C., and Ho, M.: Characteristics and management of pregnancy in women with genital herpes simplex virus infections. Am J Obstet Gynecol 145:784, 1983.

Hensleigh, P. A., Glover, D. B., and Cannon, M.: Systemic herpesvirus hominis in pregnancy. J Reprod Med. 22:171, 1979.

Hinthorn, D. R., Baker, L. H., Romig, D. A., and Liu, C.: Recurrent conjugal neuralgia caused by herpesvirus hominis type 2. JAMA 236:587, 1976.

Hirsch, M. S., and Schooley, R. T.: Treatment of herpesvirus infections. N Engl J Med 309:963–970 and 309:1034, 1983.

Hutfield, D. C.: History of herpes genitalis. Br J Vener Dis 42:263, 1966.

Hutfield, D. C.: Herpes genitalis. Br J Vener Dis 44:241, 1968.

Jacobs, E.: Anal infections caused by herpes simplex virus. Dis. Colon Rectum 19:151, 1976.

Jeansson, S., and Molin, L.: Genital herpesvirus hominis infection: A venereal disease? Lancet 1:1064, 1970.

Jeansson, S., and Molin, L.: On the occurrence of genital herpes simplex virus infection. Clinical and virological findings and relation to gonorrhoea. Acta Dermatovener (Stockh) 54:479, 1974.

Kaufman, R. H., and Rawls, W. R.: Extragenital type 2 herpesvirus infection. Am J Obstet Gynecol 112:866, 1972.

Kaufman, R. H., Gardner, H. L., Rawls, W. E., Dixon, R. E., and Young, R. L.: Clinical features of herpes genitalis. Cancer Res 33:1446, 1973.

Kaye, E. M., and Dooling, E. C.: Neonatal herpes simplex meningoencephalitis associated with fetal monitor scalp electrodes. Neurol 31:1045, 1981.

Kibrick, S.: Herpes simplex infection at term: What to do with mother, newborn, and nursery personnel. JAMA 243:157, 1980.

Kit, S., Trkula, D., Qavi, H., Dreesman, G., Kennedy, R. C., Adler-Storthz, K., Kaufman, R., and Adam, E.: Sequential genital infections by herpes simplex viruses types 1 and 2: Restriction nuclease analyses of viruses from recurrent infections. Sex Transm Dis 10:67, 1983.

Kobbermann, T., Clark, L., and Griffin, W. T.: Maternal death secondary to disseminated herpesvirus hominis. Am J Obstet Gynecol 6:742, 1980.

Kumar, A., Madden, D. L., and Nankervis, G. A.: Humoral and cell-mediated immune responses to herpesvirus antigens during pregnancy—a longitudinal study. J Clin Immunol 4:12, 1984.

Layzer, R. B., and Conant, M. A.: Neuralgia in recurrent herpes simplex. Arch Neurol 31:233, 1974.

Light, I. J., and Linneman, C. C.: Neonatal herpes simplex infection following delivery by cesarean section. Obstet Gynecol 44:496, 1974.

Light, I. J.: Postnatal acquisition of herpes simplex virus by the newborn infant: A review of the literature. Pediatr 63:480, 1979.

Logan, W. S., Tindall, J. P., and Elson, M. L.: Chronic cutaneous herpes simplex, Arch Derm 103:606, 1971.

Lopyan, L., Young, A. W., and Menegus, M.: Generalized acute mucocutaneous herpes simplex type 2 with fatal outcome. Arch Derm 113:816, 1977.

McGuirt, P. V., Shaw, J. E., Elion, G. B., and Furman, P. A.: Identification of small DNA fragments synthesized in herpes simplex virus-infected cells in the presence of acyclovir. Antimicrob Agents Chemother 25:507, 1984.

Mertz, G. J., Critchlow, C. W., Benedetti, J., Reichman, R., Dolin, R., Connor, J., Redfield, D. C., Savoia, M. C., Richman, D. D., Tyrell, D. L., Mimedzinski, L., Portnoy, J., Keeney, R. E., and Corey, L.: Double-blind placebo-controlled trial of oral acyclovir in first episode genital herpes simplex virus infection. JAMA (in press).

Mindel, A., Adler, M. W., Sutherland, S., and Fiddian, A. P.: Intravenous acyclovir treatment for primary genital herpes. Lancet 1:697, 1982.

Mindel, A. Faherty, A., Hindley, D., Weller, I. V. D., Sutherland, S. and Fiddian, A. P.: Prophylactic oral acyclovir in recurrent genital herpes. Lancet 2:57, 1984.

Modlin, J. F.: Fetal echo II disease in premature neonates. Pediatr 66:775, 1980.

Montgomerie, J. Z., Becroft, D. M. O., Croxson, M. C., Doak, P. B., and North, J. D. K.: Herpes-simplex virus infection after renal transplantation. Lancet 2:867, 1969.

Muller, S.A., Herrmann, E. C., and Winkilmann, R. K.: Herpes simplex infections in hematologic malignancies. Am J Med 52:102, 1972.

Nahmias, A. J., and Dowdle, W. R.: Antigenic and biologic differences in herpesvirus hominis. Prog. Med Virol 10:110, 1968.

Nahmias, A. J., Dowdle, W. R., Naib, Z. M., Josey, W. E., McLone, D., and Domescik, G.: Genital infection with type 2 herpes virus hominis: A commonly occurring venereal disease. Br J Vener Dis 45:294, 1969.

Nahmias, A. J., Keyserling, H. L., and Kerrick, G. M: Herpes simplex in *Infectious Diseases of the Fetus and Newborn Infant* (eds. Remington, J. S., and Klein, J. O.) W. B. Saunders, Philadelphia, 1983, pp. 636–678.

Nahmias, A. J., and Josey, W. E.: Herpes simplex viruses 1 and 2 in *Viral Infections of Humans Epidemiology and Control* 2nd Ed. (ed. Evans, A. S.) Plenum Publishing Corp., New York, 1982, pp. 351–372.

Nahmias, A. J., Josey, W. E., Naib, Z. M.,Freeman, M. G., Fernandez, R. J., and Wheeler, J. H.: Perinatal risk associated with maternal genital herpes simplex virus infection. Am J Obstet Gynecol 110:825, 1971.

Nahmias, A. J., Josey, W. E., Naib, Z. M., Luce, C. F., and Duffey, A.: Antibodies to herpesvirus hominis types 1 and 2 in humans: I. Patients with genital herpetic infections. Am J. Epidemiol 91:539, 1970.

Nahmias, A. J., and Roizman, B.: Infection with herpes simplex viruses 1 and 2. N Engl J Med 289:667, 719, 781, 1973.

Ng, A. B. P., Reagan, J. W., and Yen, S. S. C.: Herpes genitalis: Clinical and cytopathologic experience with 256 patients. Obstet Gynecol 36:645, 1970.

Nilsen, A. R., Aasen, T., Halsos, A. M., Kinge, B. R.,Tjotta, E. A. L., Wikstrom, K., and Fiddian, A. P.: Efficacy of oral acyclovir in the treatment of initial and recurrent genital herpes. Lancet 2:571, 1982.

Oates, J. K., and Greenhouse, P. R. D. H.: Retention of urine in anogenital herpetic infection. Lancet 1:691, 1979.

Oxman, M. N., Richman, D. D., and Spector, S. A.: Management at delivery of mother and infant when herpes simplex, varicella-zoster, hepatitis or tuberculosis have occurred during pregnancy, in *Current Topics in Infectious Diseases,* Vol. IV. (Eds. Remington, J. S., and Swartz, M. N.) McGraw-Hill, Boston 224–280, 1983.

Pazin, G. J., Armstrong, J. A., Tai Lam, M.,Tarr, G. C., Jannetta, P. J., and Ho, M.: Prevention of reactivated herpes simplex infection by human leukocyte interferon after operation on the trigeminal root. N Engl J Med 301:225, 1979.

Person, D. A., Kaufman, R. H., Gardner, H. L., and Rawls, W. E.: Herpesvirus type 2 genitourinary tract infections. Am J Obstet Gynecol 116:993, 1973.

Pertherer, J. F., Smith, I. W., Robertson, D. H. H.: Necrotising balanitis due to a generalized primary infection with herpes simplex virus type 2. Br J Vener Dis 55:48, 1979.

Poste, G., Hawkins, D. F., and Thomlinson, J.: Herpesvirus hominis infection of the female genital tract. Obstet Gynecol 40:871, 1972.

Powers, R. D., Rein, M. F., and Hayden, F. G.: Nectrotizing balanitis due to herpes simplex type 1. JAMA 248:215, 1982.

Rawls, W. E.: Herpes simplex virus types 1 and 2 and herpesvirus simae. In Lennette, E. H., and Schmidt, N. J. (eds.): Diagnostic Procedures for Viral, Rickettsial and Chamydial Infections. Washington, D.C., American Public Health Association, p. 309, 1979.

Rawls, W. E., Bacchetti, S., and Graham, F. L.: Relation of herpes simplex viruses to human malignancies. In Arber, W., et al., (eds.): Current Topics in Microbiology and Immunology, Vol. 77. Berlin, Heidelberg, Springer Verlag, 1977.

Rawls, W. E., Gardner, H. L., Flanders, R. W., Lowry, S. P., Kaufman, R. H., and Melnick, J. L.: Genital herpes in two social groups. Amer J Obstet Gynec 110:682, 1971.

Reeves, W. C., Corey, L., Adams, H. G., Vontver, L. A., and Holmes, D. K.: Risk of recurrence after first episodes of genital herpes. N Engl J Med 305:315, 1981.

Reichman, R. C., Badger, G. J., Mertz, C. J., Corey, L., Richman, D. D., Connor, J. D., Oxman, M. N., Bryson, Y., Tyrell, L., Portnoy, J., Creagh-Kirk, T., Keeney, R. E., Ashikaga, T., Dolin, R.: Orally administered acyclovir in the therapy of recurrent herpes simplex genitalis: A controlled trial. JAMA 251:2103, 1984.

Reichman, R. C., Badger, G. J., Guinan, M. E., Nahmias, A. J., Keeney, R. E., Davis, L. G., Ashikaga, T., and Dolin, R.: Topically administered acyclovir in the treatment of recurrent herpes simplex genitalis: A controlled trial. J Infect Dis 147:336, 1983.

Richman, D. D., Cleveland, P. H., Redfield, D. C., Oxman, M. N., and Wahl, G. M.: Rapid viral diagnosis. J Infect Dis 149:298, 1984.

Rotkin, I. D.: A comparison review of key epidemiological studies in cervical cancer related to current search for transmissible agents. Cancer Res. 33:1353, 1973.

Scher, J., Bottone E., Desmond, E., and Simons, W.: The incidence and outcome of asymptomatic herpes simplex genitalis in an obstetric population. Am J Obstet Gynecol 144:906, 1982.

Schneidman, D. W., Barr, R. J., and Graham, J. H.: Chronic cutaneous herpes simplex. JAMA 241:592, 1979.

Siegal, F. P., Lopez, C., Hammer, G. S., Brown, A. E., Kornfeld, S. J., Gold, J., Hassett, J., Hirschman, S. Z., Cunningham-Rundles, C., Adelsberg, B. R., Parham, D. M., Siegal, M., Cunningham-Rundles, C., and Armstrong, D.: Severe acquired immunodeficiency in male homosexuals, manifested by chronic perianal ulcerative herpes simplex lesions. N Engl J Med 305:1039, 1981.

Slavin, H. B., and Ferguson, J. J.: Zoster-like eruptions caused by the virus of herpes simplex. Am J Med 8:456, 1950.

Slavin, H. B., and Gavett, E.: Primary Herpetic Vulvovaginitis. Proc Soc Exptl Biol Med 63:343, 1946.

Stanberry, L. R., Kern, E. R., Richards, J. T., Abbott, T. M., and Overall, J. C.: Genital herpes in guinea pigs: pathogenesis of the primary infection and description of recurrent disease. J Infect Dis 146:397–404, 1982.

Stone, W. J., Scowden, E. B., Spannuth, C. L., Lowry, S. P., and Alford, R. H.: Atypical herpesvirus hominis type 2 infection in uremic patients receiving immunosuppressive therapy. Am J Med 63:511, 1977.

Straus, S. T., Howard, H. E., Takiff, H. E., Seidlin, M., Bachrach, S., Lininger, L., DiGiovanna, J. J., Western, K. A., Smith, H. A., Lehrman, S. N., Creagh-Kirk, T., and Alling, D. W.: Suppression of frequently recurring genital herpes. A placebo-controlled double-blind trial of oral acyclovir. N Engl J Med 310:1546, 1984.

Strauss, S. E., Smith, H. A., Brickman, C., de Miranda, P., McLaren, C., and Keeney, R. E.: Acyclovir for chronic mucocutaneous herpes simplex virus infection in immunosuppressed patients. Ann Intern Med 96:270, 1982.

Sullivan-Bolyai, J., Hull, H. F., Wilson, C., and Corey, L.: Neonatal herpes simplex virus infection in King County, Washington. Increasing incidence and epidemiological correlates. JAMA 250:3059, 1983.

Sutton, A. L., Smithwick, E. M., Seligman, S. J., and Kim, D.-S.: Fatal disseminated herpesvirus hominis type 2 infection in an adult with associated thymic dysplasia. Am J Med 56:545, 1974.

Taylor, R. J., Saul, S. H., Dowling, J. N., Hakala, T. R., Peel, R. L., and Ho, M.: Primary disseminated herpes simplex infection with fulminant hepatitis following renal transplantation. Arch Intern Med 141:1519, 1981.

The Centers for Disease Control. Epidemiologic Notes and Reports: Genital herpes infection—United States, 1966–1979. *Morbidity and Mortality Weekly Report* 31:11, 1982.

Tustin, A. W., and Kaiser, A. B.: Life-threatening pharyngitis caused by herpes simplex virus, type 2. Sex Transm Dis 6:23, 1979.

Unna, P. G.: On herpes progenitalis, especially in women. J Cutan Vener Dis 1:321, 1883.

Vontver, L. A., Reeves, W. C., Rattray, M., Corey, L., Remington, M. A., Tolentino, E., Schweid, A., and Holmes, K. K.: Clinical course and diagnosis of genital herpes simplex virus infection and evaluation of topical surfactant therapy. Am J Obstet Gynecol 54:548, 1979.

Vontver, L. A., Hickok, D. E., Brown, Z., Reid, L., and Corey, L.: Recurrent genital herpes simplex virus infection in pregnancy: Infant outcome and frequency of asymnptomatic recurrences. Am J Obstet Gynecol 143:75, 1982.

Wade, J. C., Day, L. M., Crowley, J. J., and Meyers, J. D.: Recurrent infection with herpes simplex virus after marrow transplantation: Role of the specific immune response and acyclovir treatment. J Infect Dis 149:750, 1984.

Wade, J. C., and Meyers, J. D.: Neurologic symptoms associated with parenteral acyclovir treatment after marrow transplantation. Ann Intern Med 98:921, 1983.

Wade, J. C., Newton, B., McLaren, C., Flournoy, N., Keeney, R. E., and Meyers, J. E.: Intravenous acyclovir to treat mucocutaneous herpes simplex virus infection after marrow transplanation. Ann Int Med 96:265, 1982.

Walker, D. P., Longson, M., Lawler, W., Mallick, N. P., Davies, J. S., and Johnson, R. W. G.: Disseminated herpes simplex virus infection with hepatitis in an adult renal transplant recipient. J Clin Pathol 34:1044, 1981.

Whitley, R. J., Yeager, A., Kartus, P., Bryson, Y., Connor, J. D., Alford, C. A., Nahmias, A., and Soong, S-J.: Neonatal herpes simplex virus infection: Follow-up evaluation of vidarabine therapy. Pediatr 72:778, 1983a.

Whitley, R. J., and the NIAID Collaborative Antiviral Study Group: Interim summary of mortality in herpes simplex encephalitis and neonatal herpes simplex virus infections: vidarabine versus acyclovir. J Antimicrob Chemother 12:105, 1983b.

Whitley, R. J., Nahmias, A. J., Visintine, A. M., Fleming, C. L., and Alford, C. A.: The natural history of herpes simplex virus infection of mother and newborn. Pediatr 66:489, 1980a.

Whitley, R. J., Nahmias, A. J., Soong, S-J., Galasso, G. G., Fleming, C. L. and Alford, C. A.: Vidarabine therapy of neonatal herpes simplex virus infection. Pediatr 66:495, 1980b.

Whorton, C. M., Thomas, D. M., and Denham, S. W.: Fatal systemic herpes simplex virus type 2 infection in a healthy young woman. South Med J 76:81, 1983.

Willcox, R. R.: Necrotic cervicitis due to primary infection with virus of herpes simplex. Brit Med J 1:610, 1968.

Wittek, A. E., Yeager, A. S., Au, D. S., and Hensleigh, P. A.: Asymptomatic shedding of herpes simplex virus from the cervix and lesion site during pregnancy. Am J Dis Child 138:439, 1984.

Yeager, A. S., Arvin, A. M., Urbani, L. J., and Kemp III, J. A.: Relationship of antibody to outcome in neonatal herpes simplex virus infections. Infect Immun 29:532, 1980.

Yen, S. S. C., Reagan, J. W., and Rosenthal, M. S.: Herpes simplex infection in female genital tract. Obstet Gynecol 25:479, 1965.

Young, E. J., Vainrub, B., Musher, D. M., Kumpuris, A. G., Uribe, G., Gyorkey, P., Min, K-W., and Gyorkey, F.: Acute pharyngotonsillitis caused by herpesvirus type 2. JAMA 239:1885, 1978.

Young, E. J., Killam, A. P., and Greene, J. F.: Disseminated herpesvirus infection association with primary genital herpes in pregnancy. JAMA 235:2731, 1976.

Young, A. W.: Herpes genitalis. Med Clin North Am 56:1175, 1972.

Young, A. W., Tovell, H. M. M., and Sadri, K.: Erosions and ulcers of the vulva: Diagnosis, incidence and management. Obstet Gynecol 50:35, 1977.

164
LYMPHOGRANULOMA VENEREUM, CHANCROID, AND DONOVANOSIS

H. HUNTER HANDSFIELD, M.D.

LYMPHOGRANULOMA VENEREUM

Lymphogranuloma venereum (LGV) is a sexually transmitted infection caused by specific strains of *Chlamydia trachomatis*. It is characterized by a transient and often undiagnosed primary cutaneous or mucosal lesion, with subsequent regional lymphadenitis. Synonyms include lymphopathia venereum, lymphogranuloma inguinale, tropical bubo, climatic bubo, and others. Although it was recognized in the ninteenth century, Nicholas, Durand, and Favre provided the first definitive description in 1913.

ETIOLOGY. The chlamydiae are small bacteria that grow only within eukaryotic cells and require tissue culture for isolation. Two species are pathogenic for man: *C. psittaci*, the cause of psittacosis, and *C. trachomatis*, immunotype variants of which cause trachoma (primarily types A, B, Ba, and C), genital infections, and sporadic cases of inclusion conjunctivitis (primarily types D through K), and LGV (types L_1, L_2, and L_3). Compared with types A through K, the LGV strains of *C. trachomatis* cause greater cytopathic effect in tissue culture, are relatively resistant to neuraminidase, and, except for type L_3, are more lethal to mice after intracerebral inoculation.

EPIDEMIOLOGY AND GEOGRAPHIC VARIATION. LGV is worldwide in distribution, but is endemic in tropical climates and areas of economic deprivation. The greatest incidences are seen in Africa, Southeast Asia, and India, where LGV accounts for two to six per cent of diagnoses in sexually transmitted disease clinics. The disease is now uncommon in North America and Europe: only 235 cases were reported in the United States in 1982, although this figure probably reflects underdiagnosis and incomplete reporting. The influence of nonsexual socioeconomic factors is demonstrated by the decrease in incidence that has occurred in areas that have undergone economic improvement, such as the southeast United States.

The age distribution of LGV matches that of all sexually transmitted infections, with most cases in persons aged 15 to 40 years. The diagnosis is established 6 to 20 times more frequently in men, reflecting the greater incidence of minimal symptoms and perhaps asymptomatic carriage of *C. trachomatis* in women. In Europe and North America, LGV is seen predominantly in homosexual men. Active LGV is rarely documented in sex partners of infected patients, suggesting that asymptomatic carriage is common, and all partners should probably be treated routinely.

PATHOGENESIS AND PATHOLOGY. The histopathology of well-documented primary cutaneous lesions of LGV has not been described. In primary infection of the anorectal mucosa, crypt abscesses and multinucleated giant cells are seen, and the histologic picture is virtually identical to that of Crohn's disease (Quinn et al., 1981). Soon after the primary infection, probably within a few days, *C. trachomatis* is transported by the lymphatics to regional lymph nodes. At this time, a transient bacteremia may occur. Initially, the lymph node contains stellate microabscesses, with central granulocytes surrounded by palisading mononuclear inflammatory cells. The microabscesses later coalesce to form the classic fluctuant bubo. Several lymph nodes are usually infected simultaneously, becoming mutually adherent through an intense periadenitis. *C. trachomatis* may be isolated from the inflammatory exudate in 60 to 70 per cent of cases. Fixation to overlying skin is followed by spontaneous rupture and drainage. After a variable course that may include several cycles of partial healing, scarring, and recurrent drainage over months or years, chronic lymphatic obstruction may supervene, leading to the lymphedema, susceptibility to secondary infection, and tissue destruction that constitute the chronic sequelae of LGV.

Antibodies to *C. trachomatis* may be detected in the blood of persons with LGV by complement fixation, immunofluorescence, neutralization, and other techniques. Cell-mediated immunity also develops, as reflected in the Frei skin test and by species-specific lymphocyte transformation in vitro. Although these responses may be partially protective, reinfection is believed to occur in heavily endemic areas.

CLINICAL MANIFESTATIONS. The incubation period is four days to three weeks. The cutaneous primary lesion is usually described as an evanescent, painless 1 to 6 mm papule, vesicle, pustule, or ulcer, and is most commonly identified on the penis of men and the external genitalia, vaginal mucosa, or cervix in women. It is possible, however, that a cutaneous lesion often does not occur, and that chlamydial urethritis, cervicitis, or proctitis (with or without symptoms) are the primary lesions in some patients.

The location of the primary lesion in part determines the location of the subsequent lymphadenopathy, which develops after a latent period of a few days to several weeks. The lymphadenopathy usually involves the inguinal or femoral nodes, and is unilateral in approximately one-half to two-thirds of cases and bilateral in the remainder. Over one to four weeks, the nodes gradually become fluctuant and fixed to the overlying skin with erythema, warmth, and eventual rupture. Occasionally there is spontaneous regression without rupture. In 15 to 30 per cent of patients, both the femoral and inguinal nodes are involved; their separation by the inguinal ligament results in the pathognomonic "groove sign" (Fig. 1). The adenopathy initially causes little discomfort, but becomes increasingly painful and tender as the nodes enlarge and fluctuance and skin fixation progress.

Primary anorectal LGV is increasingly recognized, usually in homosexually active men (Quinn et al., 1981). This syndrome is manifested by symptoms and signs of severe proctocolitis, with tenesmus, diarrhea, bleeding, and abdominal cramps, often accompanied by fever, malaise, and weight loss. This now may be the most common form of LGV in the United States. Classical descriptions of LGV attributed the proctitis and its sequelae, such as perirectal abscess and rectal stricture, to involvement of perirectal lymph nodes following primary genital infection; however, the relative contributions of this mechanism and primary infection of the rectal mucosa are unknown.

In recent years, several cases of cervical, supraclavicular,

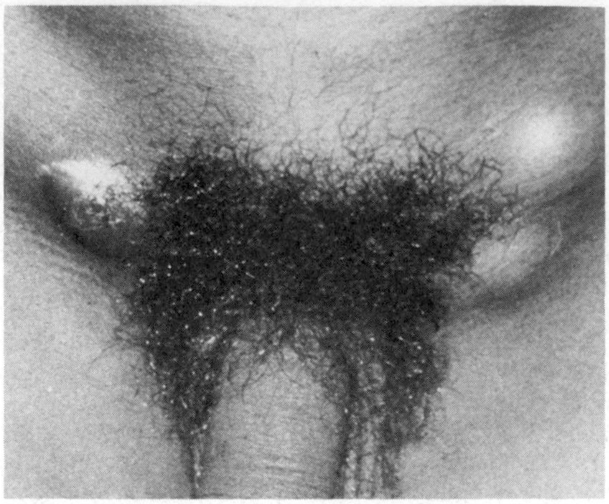

Figure 1. Inguinal and femoral lymphadenopathy and the "groove sign" in a case of lymphogranuloma venereum. (Reprinted with permission from Perine, P. L., and Osoba, A. O.: Lymphogranuloma venereum. *In* Holmes, K. K., et al. (eds.): Sexually Transmitted Diseases. New York, McGraw Hill, 1984.)

and mediastinal node involvement have been reported; all have been related to orogenital sexual practices.

Fever, chills, myalgia, headache, hyperglobulinemia with elevations of IgA, IgG, and IgM, leukocytosis, and elevation of the erythrocyte sedimentation rate are common. Less frequent are keratoconjunctivitis, meningoencephalitis, splenomegaly, erythema nodosum, erythema multiforme, polyarthritis, false-positive reagin tests for syphilis, circulating rheumatoid factor, and cryoglobulinemia.

COMPLICATIONS AND SEQUELAE. The majority of patients probably experience complete resolution, with or without antimicrobial therapy. Ten to 20 per cent of untreated patients, however, develop lymphatic obstruction with chronic lymphedema that may result in genital elephantiasis ("esthiomene" in women) and polypoid vulvar or perirectal masses of hypertrophied lymphoid tissue ("lymphorrhoids"). Chronic persistent chlamydial infection (often with bacterial super-infection) may result in draining inguinal sinuses, urethral fistulas and strictures, genital ulcerations, and rectal strictures.

DIAGNOSIS. The diagnosis of LGV commonly rests on clinical assessment and serologic testing. Isolation of an LGV strain of *C. trachomatis* or its identification by specific immunochemical methods is the only incontrovertible proof of the diagnosis, but the availability of laboratories with this capability varies widely. Identification of typical basophilic cytoplasmic inclusions by Giemsa staining of pus aspirated from a bubo is a highly specific but very insensitive test. The histopathology of the lymphadenitis is otherwise nonspecific, and biopsy or excision of involved lymph nodes usually is contraindicated on clinical grounds.

The complement-fixation (CF) test is the most widely available serologic test, and uses a heat-stable antigen common to all chlamydiae (Schachter et al., 1969). There is controversy regarding the definition of significant CF titers. In the United States, a titer of ≥ 1:64 has a sensitivity of about 70 to 80 per cent and probably is highly specific, especially when observed in conjunction with a fourfold rise or fall in titer. CF titers of 1:8 to 1:32 occur in 20 to 80 per cent of patrons of public venereal disease clinics in North America and Europe, and usually reflect past or present infection with non-LGV strains of *C. trachomatis*, rather than subclinical or previously treated LGV. The microimmunofluorescence test is more sensitive than the CF test and has the advantage of differentiation of strains of *C. trachomatis*, but requires laboratory facilities that are not available in the geographic areas with the highest incidences of LGV. A microimmunofluorescence titer of ≥ 1:1024 with specificity to an LGV strain of *C. trachomatis* or with broad reactivity to several serotypes is highly sensitive and specific for LGV.

The Frei test detects delayed hypersensitivity by using intradermal inoculation of material prepared from an LGV organism grown in chick embryo yolk sacs. In most investigators' hands, the Frei test is both insensitive and nonspecific, and is therefore of questionable diagnostic value (Schachter et al. 1969). Because of these problems, the antigen is no longer commercially available in the United States.

The differential diagnosis of LGV includes all causes of regional lymphadenopathy. Chancroid and granuloma inguinale are distinguished by the typical skin lesions and the usual absence of systemic symptoms. Anorectal LGV can be confused with ulcerative colitis, Crohn's disease, amebiasis, and other causes of proctocolitis and perirectal abscess. Because of the histopathologic similarities between LGV and Crohn's disease, rectal biopsy alone may not distinguish them, and tests for LGV are indicated for all sexually active persons with acute or chronic proctocolitis. Rectal stricture may be confused with carcinoma. Confusion with syphilis may occur because of occasional biologic false-positive reagin tests in patients with LGV.

TREATMENT. *C. trachomatis* is sensitive in vitro to the tetracyclines, the agents of choice. Tetracycline hydrochloride is given orally in a dose of 500 mg four times daily for at least two weeks. Effective alternatives include doxycycline (100 mg twice daily), erythromycin (500 mg four times daily), and the sulfonamides (e.g., sulfamethoxazole, 1.0 g twice daily), each given for at least two weeks. The lymphadenopathy resolves slowly, although systemic signs and symptoms subside promptly. Draining sinus tracts should be evaluated for bacterial superinfection and treated accordingly.

Fluctuant buboes should be aspirated with an 18-gauge needle as often as necessary to prevent rupture, taking care to enter the node through uninflamed skin in order to avoid establishing a sinus tract. Surgical incision or excision often leads to sinus formation and secondary infection, and is contraindicated.

PREVENTION. Condoms may provide some protection, but avoidance of sexual contact with infected individuals or carriers is the only sure means of prevention. An effective vaccine is not available and none is anticipated.

CHANCROID

Chancroid (soft chancre) is a sexually transmitted infection caused by *Haemophilus ducreyi*, and is characterized by painful genital ulceration and inguinal lymphadenitis, usually without systemic symptoms. Chancroid was differentiated from syphilis by Bassereau in 1852, and Ducrey described the causative bacillus in 1889.

ETIOLOGY. *H. ducreyi* is a small, facultatively anaerobic, nonmotile, gram-negative coccobacillus with fastidious nutritional requirements. In liquid media, and to a lesser extent in vivo, it tends to grow end-to-end in chains; two or more chains often lie in parallel. Using improved procedures for primary isolation and biochemical characterization, the inclusion of the Ducrey bacillus in the genus *Haemophilus* has recently been reconfirmed. Improved methodology has also established that other *Haemophilus* species and other genera morphologically indistinguishable from *H. ducreyi* commonly are isolated from genital ulcers or the normal genital tract. Their pathogenic roles, if any, are unknown.

EPIDEMIOLOGY AND GEOGRAPHIC VARIATION. Chancroid is transmitted almost exclusively by sexual contact. As is true for lymphogranuloma venereum and donovanosis, however, nonsexual socioeconomic factors have greatly influenced the frequency of chancroid in various populations, and the disease is now uncommon in Europe and North America, although it is not as rare as suggested by reported incidences. In the United States 1392 cases were reported in 1982. The greatest incidences occur in tropical and subtropical settings, where chancroid is among the most common sexually transmitted diseases, often with incidences severalfold greater than that of syphilis.

As for all sexually transmitted infections, most cases of chancroid occur in persons between 15 and 40 years of age. An asymptomatic carrier state in women has been postulated to explain the 80 to 90 per cent dominance of males in most published reports of chancroid, but bacteriologically confirmed asymptomatic carriage of *H. ducreyi* has been reported only rarely. Moreover, recent studies have shown male:female ratios between 1:1 and 3:1 and have documented genital ulcers in the majority of sexual contacts of patients with chancroid. The epidemiology of chancroid therefore requires further study using definitive bacteriologic techniques. Other sexually transmitted infections often are present simultaneously; syphilis was diagnosed in 7 per cent of U.S. military personnel who acquired chancroid in Korea, and 23 per cent of patients in a recent outbreak in Canada had concomitant gonorrhea (Hammond et al., 1980).

PATHOGENESIS AND PATHOLOGY. The primary lesion of chancroid begins as a small papule or vesicle that becomes pustular and ulcerates within two to three days. The ulcer may enlarge for several days or weeks. Three histologic zones have been described: a superficial zone of polymorphonuclear leukocytes, erythrocytes, bacteria, and necrotic debris; a central zone of edema and neovascularization; and a deep zone of macrophages, lymphocytes, and plasma cells. Central necrosis, spontaneous rupture, and drainage occur in the regional lymph nodes of many untreated patients. Fever, leukocytosis, and other signs of systemic illness are uncommon and suggest another diagnosis or superinfection; bacteremia and pathology distant from regional lymph nodes have not been described.

CLINICAL MANIFESTATIONS. The incubation period of one to five days is followed by the painful, nonindurated primary lesion, a round, irregular, or serpiginous ulcer of the external genitalia. In men, almost all lesions involve the penis, typically the glans, corona, or internal surface of the foreskin (Fig. 2); in women, lesions typically occur on the labia, fourchette, and in the perianal region. Individual lesions vary from 3 to 20 mm in diameter. The edges are undermined, the adjacent skin is inflamed, and the gray-white base bleeds readily when traumatized. Multiple primary lesions occur in up to half the cases, often in the form of "kissing" lesions caused by autoinoculation of normal skin in apposition to the initial lesion.

Regional lymphadenitis occurs in 30 to 50 per cent of cases, appears within a few days of onset of the primary lesion, and involves a single inguinal node unilaterally in about two-thirds of cases. Untreated, the involved node becomes fluctuant and ruptures spontaneously, followed by gradual healing.

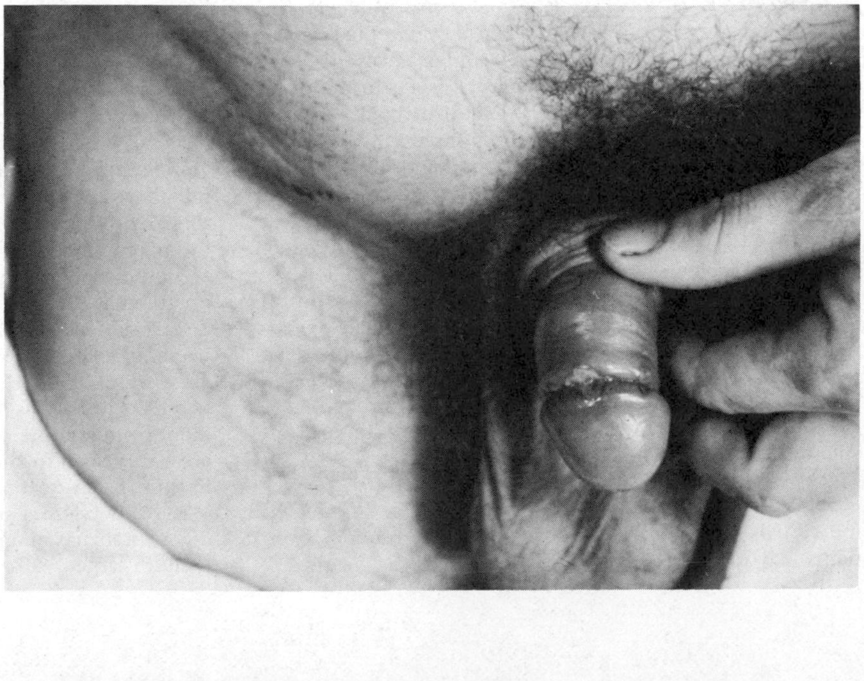

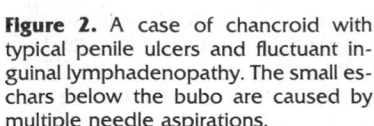

Figure 2. A case of chancroid with typical penile ulcers and fluctuant inguinal lymphadenopathy. The small eschars below the bubo are caused by multiple needle aspirations.

COMPLICATIONS AND SEQUELAE. "Phagedenic" chancroid, with large undermined ulcers that progress rapidly and cause extensive tissue destruction and scarring, is infrequent and probably results from secondary infection by a mixed aerobic and anaerobic flora. Uncomplicated chancroid usually heals spontaneously over several weeks or months, without significant scarring or lymphatic obstruction.

DIAGNOSIS. Although the clinical presentation of chancroid often is characteristic in areas of low prevalence, such as North America, most genital ulcers morphologically suggestive of chancroid are due to other causes, such as genital herpes virus infection. In all areas, isolation of *H. ducreyi* or its identification by specific immunochemical procedures is the only definitive means of diagnosis. Material from the undermined edge of an ulcer or pus aspirated from an infected lymph node should be inoculated onto chocolate agar containing 5 to 10 per cent fetal bovine serum, a defined supplement (e.g., IsoVitaleX), and 3 μg/ml vancomycin (Sottnek et al., 1980). Inoculated medium is incubated at 35-37°C in an atmosphere of 5 to 10 per cent CO_2 and increased humidity; these conditions are achieved in a candle-extinction jar that contains a small piece of saturated gauge or paper towel. Specific immunochemical tests for identification of the organism in infected material are under investigation and appear promising. Most authorities agree that microscopic examination of conventionally stained material obtained from genital ulcers is both insensitive and nonspecific. Serologic tests are under investigation but are not generally available.

In geographic areas where genital herpes virus infections are highly prevalent and chancroid is uncommon, cultures for both herpes simplex virus and *H. ducreyi* are indicated. Primary syphilis is distinguished by the nontender indurated chancre, but darkfield examination and syphilis serology are indicated in the evaluation of any genital ulceration. The systemic symptoms, more chronic course, and lymphadenopathy without prominent genital ulceration all help to distinguish LGV from chancroid. Traumatic or scabetic genital lesions may become secondarily infected and mimic chancroid, with or without regional lymphadenitis.

TREATMENT. *H. ducreyi* is usually susceptible to the sulfonamides, erythromycin, and the newer cephalosporin antibiotics. Most clinical isolates contain plasmids that encode for β-lactamase and are thus resistant to the penicillins. The regimens of choice for the treatment of chancroid are erythromycin, 500 mg orally three times daily for seven days, or the combination of trimethoprim and sulfamethoxazole (or sulfametrole), 160 mg and 800 mg, respectively, twice daily for five days. Preliminary studies suggest that several single-dose treatment regimens also are effective. These include oral sulfamethoxazole (or sulfametrole) plus trimethoprim, 3.2 g and 640 mg, respectively; intramuscular ceftriaxone, 250 mg; and intramuscular spectinomycin, 2.0 g. A 7 to 10 day course of a tetracycline may be effective, but is less reliable than the other regimens. Fluctuant lymph nodes should be aspirated through adjacent uninflamed skin as often as necessary to prevent spontaneous rupture.

PREVENTION. Avoidance of sexual contact with infected individuals is the only known means of prevention. Condoms may reduce the transmission rate.

DONOVANOSIS

Donovanosis (granuloma inguinale) is an infection caused by *Calymmatobacterium granulomatis*, and is characterized by indolent cutaneous or mucocutaneous ulceration, usually without systemic symptoms. Other synonyms include granuloma venereum, sclerosing granuloma, and granuloma donovani. The disease was recognized by McLeod in India in 1882, and Donovan described the characteristic intracellular bacterial inclusions in 1905.

ETIOLOGY. *C. granulomatis* is an encapsulated, bipolar-staining, short, nonmotile, fastidious gram-negative bacillus. It is antigenically related to *Klebsiella* species, and has been cultivated only in yolk sacs of embryonated chicken eggs and on media containing egg yolk. Its biochemical characteristics are unknown, and its antimicrobial susceptibilities have only been surmised on the basis of responses of patients to various drugs. The organism has been isolated from feces, and it is possible that a fecal reservoir plays an epidemiologic role in some populations.

EPIDEMIOLOGY AND GEOGRAPHIC VARIATION. Donovanosis is the rarest of all sexually transmitted infections in Europe and North America (17 cases were reported in the United States in 1982), but is an endemic problem in tropical and subtropical climates, especially among economically disadvantaged populations. Papua New Guinea (where donovanosis accounts for up to 50 per cent of genital ulcers), central Australia, and the Indian subcontinent apparently have the highest incidences.

The importance of sexual transmission of donovanosis has been debated, but most epidemiologic data and the weight of clinical experience indicate that sexual transmission is the rule (Lal and Nicholas, 1970). The age range reflects the frequency of sexual activity, with most cases occurring between ages 15 and 40. The reported male:female ratio varies from 2:1 to 10:1; in North America, many cases occur in homosexual men. Although most reports suggest that active disease is diagnosed in less than 20 per cent of sex partners of patients, a few studies have documented rates of 50 to 65 per cent. Donovanosis does not appear to be highly contagious, and sex partners have been reported free of infection despite several years of repeated intercourse with chronically infected patients.

PATHOGENESIS AND PATHOLOGY. The first identifiable lesion is an indurated papule that ulcerates over several days to weeks, with formation of pink-red hypertrophic granulation-like tissue with little or no purulent exudate or inflammation of the adjacent skin. There is extensive epithelial proliferation and acanthosis, and dense infiltration by macrophages and plasma cells, with variable numbers of polymorphonuclear leukocytes and lymphocytes; true granulomas do not form, the alternative names of the disease notwithstanding. The pathognomonic feature is the presence of large (25 to 90 μm) macrophages that contain large numbers of *C. granulomatis*, identified as Donovan bodies. These cells and the Donovan bodies are difficult to identify in routine paraffin-embedded tissue sections, but are easily seen in smears of scrapings or crushed tissue, or in thin (1 μm) sections of tissue embedded in plastic. With Wright or Giemsa staining, the organisms appear as blue-black bipolar-staining coccobacilli 1 to 2 μm in length, lying in large cytoplasmic vacuoles inside macrophages.

The ulcer may enlarge slowly for months or years, with extensive tissue destruction. Spontaneous resolution and healing may occur in some cases, but are often followed by later relapse. Bacteremia has not been documented, but metastatic systemic infection, manifested primarily by multifocal osteomyelitis, has been reported.

CLINICAL MANIFESTATIONS. The incubation period has been reported to vary between one week and six months, but probably averages two to four weeks. The primary cutaneous papule and subsequent ulcer are usually painless (Kuberski, 1980). In women and heterosexual men, over 90 per cent of lesions involve the external genitals, perianal skin, and the inguinal region. The anus and perianal skin are the usual sites in homosexual men. Almost any cutaneous or accessible mucous membrane site may be involved, and oral granuloma inguinale may follow orogenital sexual contact.

The ulcers have a characteristic appearance, with heaped-up pink or red granulation-like tissue; "kissing" lesions, due to local autoinoculation, are frequent. Extension, healing, and scarring may be observed simultaneously. Subcutaneous extension of induration and swelling into the inguinal region results in a "pseudobubo," which may subsequently break down into a typical ulcer. True lymph node involvement is uncommon. Fever, leukocytosis, and other signs of systemic illness are infrequent, and suggest secondary infection.

COMPLICATIONS AND SEQUELAE. When treated promptly, donovanosis is a benign disease with no known sequelae. However, extensive local tissue destruction may occur over months or years, resulting in autoamputation of external genitalia, local bone and deep soft tissue destruction, and sepsis and death due to bacterial superinfection. Systemic dissemination with focal osseous or visceral involvement is a rare complication. Squamous cell carcinoma has been reported to be a rare complication of chronic donovanosis, but the association is of uncertain significance, since the two diseases may share common risk factors such as poor hygiene and multiple sexual contacts.

DIAGNOSIS. The diagnosis is suspected on the basis of the clinical appearance of the lesions (Fig. 3) and is confirmed by identification of Donovan bodies after Wright or Giemsa staining of methanol-fixed smears of scrapings of a fresh ulcer or of crushed tissue obtained by biopsy. The appearance of the ulcers, the lack of suppuration of the pseudobuboes, and absence of systemic signs all serve to differentiate donovanosis from other causes of genital or perianal ulceration. Advanced disease may be mistaken for epidermoid carcinoma until histologic examination is complete. Isolation of *C. granulomatis* is not feasible, and there is no serologic test.

TREATMENT. Although few adequately controlled therapeutic trials have been reported, the combination of sulfamethoxazole and trimethoprim is considered the treatment of choice; the dose is 800 mg and 160 mg, respectively, given twice daily by mouth. Usually effective alternatives are tetracycline HC1 or chloramphenicol, each given orally in a dose of 500 mg four times daily. Erythromycin, ampicillin, and streptomycin have variable efficacies. In all cases, treatment is given for at least 10 to 14 days, or until healing is complete.

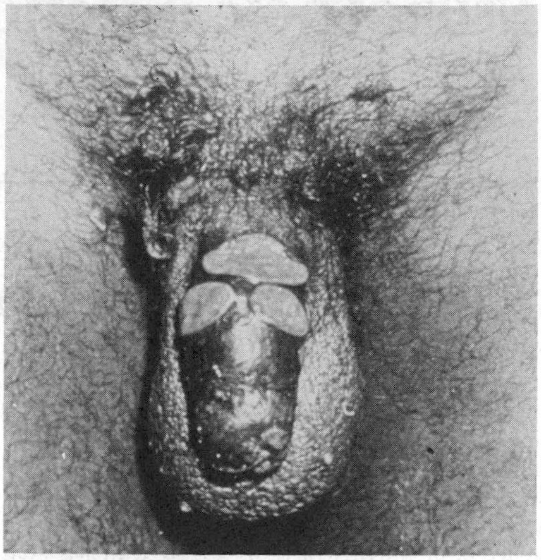

Figure 3. Multiple penile ulcerations in donovanosis. (Reprinted with permission from Sowmini, C. N.: Donovanosis. *In* Holmes, K. K., and Mårdh, P. A. (eds.): International Perspectives on Neglected Sexually Transmitted Diseases. Washington, D. C., Hemisphere/McGraw Hill, 1983.)

PREVENTION. As for all sexually transmitted infections, avoidance of sexual contact with infected individuals is the only sure means of prevention. There is no vaccine.

References

Current Treatments in the Control of Sexually Transmitted Diseases. Geneva, World Health Organization, 1984 (in press).

Hammond, G. W., Slutchuk, M., Scatliff, J., Sherman, E., Wilt, J. C., and Ronald, A. R.: Epidemiologic, clinical, laboratory, and therapeutic features of an urban outbreak of chancroid in North America. Rev Infect Dis 2:867, 1980.

Holmes, K. K., and Mårdh, P. A.: International Perspectives on Neglected Sexually Transmitted Diseases. Washington, D.C., Hemisphere/McGraw-Hill, 1983.

Kraus, S. J., Kaufman, H. W., Albritton, W. L., Thornsberry, C., and Biddle, J. W.: Chancroid therapy: a review of cases confirmed by culture. Rev Infect Dis 4 (suppl):S848, 1982.

Kuberski, T.: Granuloma inguinale (donovanosis). Sex Transm Dis 7:29, 1980.

Lal, S., and Nicholas, C.: Epidemiological and clinical features in 165 cases of granuloma inguinale. Br J Vener Dis 46:461, 1970.

Quinn, T. C., Goodell, S. E., Mkrtichian, E., Schuffler, M. D., Wang, S. P., Stamm, W. E., and Holmes, K. K.: *Chlamydia trachomatis* proctitis. N Engl J Med 305:195, 1981.

Schachter, J., Smith, D. E., Dawson, C. R., Anderson, W. R., Deller, J. J., Jr., Hoke, A. W., Smart, W. H., and Meyer, K. F.: Lymphogranuloma venereum. I. Comparison of the Frei test, complement fixation test, and isolation of the agent. J Infect Dis 120:372, 1969.

Sottnek, F. O., Biddle, J. W., Kraus, S. J., Weaver, R. E., and Stewart, J. A.: Isolation and Identification of *Haemophilus ducreyi* in a clinical study. J Clin Microbiol 12:170, 1980.

E. NEUROLOGIC INFECTIONS

165

PURULENT BACTERIAL MENINGITIS

THOMAS ALLAN HOFFMAN, M.D.

Purulent meningitis is an acute life-threatening illness caused by bacteria invading the meninges and eliciting a polymorphonuclear inflammatory reaction in cerebrospinal fluid (CSF). This disease occurs constantly in sporadic fashion throughout the world and in cyclic epidemics. The incidence of meningitis varies inversely with age. Age also affects the clinical expression of disease and the frequency with which different organisms cause meningitis. Prompt diagnosis and early treatment with specific antibiotics are essential steps in managing this condition. The case fatality rate continues to be an important concern, even though effective antimicrobial therapy is available. Neurologic sequelae occur in an appreciable number of surviving infants and children.

ETIOLOGY

Common Causative Agents. Three encapsulated organisms cause over 80 per cent of the cases of purulent meningitis. The most frequent cause is *Haemophilus influenzae,* a pleomorphic gram-negative rod that has a capsule composed of polyribitol phosphate. This polysaccharide is the specific antigen of type b strains of *H. influenzae* and is present in several other bacteria including those considered normal flora. Subclinical infection by these bacteria results in the formation of protective antibodies against *H. influenzae* type b in most individuals within the first five years of life. The attack rate of *H. influenzae* meningitis is highest among infants during the second six months of life. The age-related incidence of *H. influenzae* meningitis decreases with each succeeding year after one year and becomes almost negligible after childhood. Since the overall incidence of *H. influenzae* meningitis is apparently increasing in the antibiotic era, this organism has become an occasional cause of meningitis in adults. *Neisseria meningitidis* is the second most frequent cause of endemic purulent meningitis and is responsible for epidemics of meningitis. Pathogenic strains of this gram-negative diplococcus are, however, subdivided into at least four serologic groups based upon their capsular polysaccharides. The meningococcal polysaccharides of groups A, B, C, and Y organisms can induce the formation of group-specific antibodies. Asymptomatic nasopharyngeal infection by *N. meningitidis* is common and confers group-specific immunity. Immunity is also acquired by a complete cross-reaction between the group B meningococcal polysaccharide and the K1 capsule of *Escherichia coli.* The prevalence of protective antibodies against the various serogroups of *N. meningitidis* increases with age, and the age-related incidence of meningococcal meningitis declines during childhood. The disease occurs in adolescents and in adults at incidence rates that are substantially lower than those in children. *Streptococcus pneumoniae,* the other common cause of bacterial meningitis, and *N. meningitidis* are the principal causes of bacterial meningitis in people over ten years of age. All ages are susceptible to *S. pneumoniae* meningitis, since this gram-positive diplococcus has numerous capsular types that cause meningitis. However, 18 serotypes of *S. pneumoniae* cause 90 per cent of the disease (Gotschlich, 1978). Conditions that predispose to acquiring pneumococcal meningitis include sickle cell disease, splenectomy, alcoholism, and head trauma. Although most pneumococci are exquisitely susceptible to the bactericidal action of penicillin G, strains that have become either relatively resistant or highly resistant to this drug are known to cause meningitis. Relatively resistant strains are inhibited by penicillin at concentrations that are substantially higher than usual, but less than 1 μg/ml. These strains have been isolated from cases of prolonged and relapsing pneumococcal meningitis (Gartner and Michaels, 1979). An estimated 2 per cent of clinical isolates of *S. pneumoniae* meet these criteria for relative resistance to penicillin. An associated finding that allows these strains to be readily identified is resistance to oxacillin in disk susceptibility testing. Meningitis caused by pneumococci with higher degrees of resistance to penicillin (MICs above 1 μg/ml) is a very unusual occurrence, except in South Africa where this condition was first noted. Pneumococci that are highly resistant to penicillin are typically resistant to most other antibiotics, although they are usually susceptible to vancomycin. Isolates of *N. meningitidis* continue to be uniformly susceptible to penicillin. The penicillin derivative that has the most potent activity against *H. influenzae* is ampicillin; however, plasmid-mediated penicillinase activity has been noted in approximately 15 per cent of the strains causing meningitis. Chloramphenicol at levels that are clinically achievable in CSF is known to have bactericidal activity against the three organisms that commonly cause meningitis (Rahal and Simberkoff, 1974). In fact, the levels of chloramphenicol required for bactericidal activity against *H. influenzae* are equal or better than those of ampicillin.

The common causative agents of neonatal meningitis are *Streptococcus agalactica* (group B streptococci) and *E. coli.* These organisms are the most likely to colonize the newborn at birth. Approximately 80 per cent of the *E. coli* causing neonatal meningitis have a K1 capsular antigen, even though their somatic antigens differ. *S. agalactica* meningitis is commonly caused by strains with the serotype III capsule. Group B streptococci are uniformly susceptible to penicillin or ampicillin. Ampicillin also has activity against *E. coli;* however, approximately 20 per cent of strains causing neonatal meningitis are resistant to this drug.

Uncommon Causative Agents. A variety of organisms infrequently cause bacterial meningitis. *Listeria monocytogenes* is a gram-positive rod that accounts for approximately 2 per cent of the cases of bacterial meningitis. It is a well-recognized cause of meningitis in the neonate and in the elderly. This type of meningitis also occurs in adults with lymphoproliferative malignancies and in those, particularly transplant recipients, receiving immunosuppressive therapy (Nieman and Lorber, 1980). Alcoholism may also be a predisposing factor. Ampicillin is more bactericidal against *L. monocytogenes* than penicillin. Collectively, the enteric gram-negative bacilli and *Pseudomonas aeruginosa* constitute another important etiology of meningitis. These bacteria cause neonatal meningitis, meningitis occurring after neurosurgery or severe head trauma, and spontaneous forms of meningitis in adults. Neonatal meningitis may be caused by enteric organisms other than *E. coli*. Even gram-negative bacilli with low pathogenicity may produce overwhelming infection with central nervous system invasion in the neonate. For example, *Citrobacter* meningitis occurs almost exclusively in this age group and is frequently complicated by abscess formation in the brain (Levy and Saunders, 1981). Neonatal intensive care units may also experience outbreaks of meningitis caused by a gram-negative enteric organism with multiple antibiotic resistance. Purulent meningitis that occurs spontaneously in adults is only occasionally caused by gram-negative bacilli; however, these organisms are frequent causes of meningitis occurring after severe head injury or neurosurgical procedures (Berk and McCabe, 1980). Meningitis acquired in the hospital setting is likely to be caused by bacteria that are selected by prior antibiotic use. Antibiotic resistance is also frequently encountered in these circumstances. The gram-negative bacilli that are isolated from spontaneously occurring cases of meningitis have more predictable patterns of antibiotic susceptibility, but the range of causative organisms is extensive. Although *E. coli* is responsible for most cases, other *Enterobacteriaceae*, *Haemophilus* (other than type b), *Pseudomonas aeruginosa* and other nonfermentors may cause the spontaneous form of gram-negative bacillary meningitis. Included are *Pasteurella multocida*, a gram-negative bacillus that is susceptible to penicillin, and *Acinetobacter calcoaceticus*, a gram-negative coccobacillus that is resistant to penicillin, but in stained smears can be mistaken for a meningococcus. *Staphylococcus aureus* and *Streptococcus pyogenes* (Group A streptococci) are other pyogenic organisms that infrequently produce meningitis. *S. aureus* meningitis is an unusual metastatic complication of a suppurative process elsewhere in the body. Meningitis occurring in association with ventricular shunts used for the management of hydrocephalus may be caused by *Staphylococcus epidermidis*, but meningitis by either *S. aureus* or gram-negative bacilli is also associated with these shunts. Bacteremia by *S. pyogenes* infrequently results in bacterial meningitis (Murphy, 1983). Anaerobic bacteria can also cause meningitis, usually by spread from an adjacent focus of infection (Heerema, 1979).

PATHOGENESIS AND PATHOLOGY. Hematogenous spread from the upper respiratory tract is the principal route by which the common causative agents produce meningitis. The sequence of events has been examined in an experimental model of meningitis after intranasal inoculation of organisms (Moxon et al., 1974; Moxon and Ostrow, 1977). Although the size of the inoculum influences the occurrence of bacteremia, the intensity of the bacteremia varies inversely with age and has a direct relationship to the occurrence of meningitis. The severity of the bacteremia occurring within 24 hours after inoculation appears to be a primary determinant in the pathogenesis of meningitis. Invasion of organisms through the meningeal blood vessels apparently occurs in the large venous sinuses of the cranial dura. Organisms pass into the CSF through the delicate arachnoid membrane. CSF flows between this avascular membrane and the pia, another thin membrane that adheres to the surface of and carries the blood vessels to the brain. Diapedesis of polymorphonuclear (PMN) leukocytes occurs in the meningeal blood vessels, which become hyperemic and surrounded by purulent exudates. These inflammatory changes in the leptomeninges precede the appearance of inflammatory cells in the CSF. The inflammatory process increases progressively for 72 hours after the induction of meningitis (McAllister et al., 1975). Bacteria multiply in the CSF to levels that frequently exceed 10^5/ml, which is the concentration required for organisms to be visualized on Gram-stained smears (Feldman, 1977). As white blood cells (WBC) accumulate in the subarachnoid space, the CSF acquires a turbid appearance and the cortical areas of the brain become edematous. Occasionally, PMN leukocytes infiltrate the cortex, but the pia limits organisms from invading the brain tissue. These inflammatory changes cause increased intracranial pressure, which may eventually cause herniation. The extent to which inflammation progresses is the major determinant of the outcome (McAllister et al., 1975). Meningitis also affects the barrier that limits the entry of substances into the CSF from the blood. Inflammation of the meninges enhances the entry of solutes, serum proteins, and some antibiotics into the CSF from the blood. However, the transport of glucose into the CSF is decreased in bacterial meningitis.

Hematogenous spread from the gastrointestinal tract is the likely route by which *E. coli* causes meningitis in the neonate. The K1 capsular polysaccharide is a virulence factor that promotes systemic invasion and the subsequent development of meningitis by *E. coli* (Glode et al., 1977). The defense response of the neonate is limited and this is a particularly important reason for the occurrence of meningitis in this age. Premature rupture of the membranes and low birth weight increase the likelihood of meningitis during the neonatal period (Overall, 1970).

Bacterial meningitis may also result from contiguous spread of infection. Head trauma, even when seemingly minor, can disrupt the normal anatomic barriers and allow organisms in the nasopharynx to enter the meninges. Bacteria in foci of infection in the paranasal sinuses, mastoids, psoas muscles, or brain tissue may spread contiguously to invade the meninges.

CLINICAL MANIFESTATIONS. Bacterial meningitis in adults has a characteristic clinical pattern, although the progression of symptoms is somewhat variable. It is a febrile illness of short duration with the major symptoms being headache and stiff neck. Lethargy or drowsiness is frequent. Confusion, agitated delirium, and stupor are less frequent presenting findings; however, coma is an ominous prognostic sign. Most patients with bacterial meningitis are febrile, although the height of fever is variable. Pain and resistance to flexion of the neck are the characteristic findings on physical examination. Other signs of meningeal irritation can also be elicited. Kernig's sign is present when the leg cannot be extended more than 135 degrees on the thigh when flexed 90 degrees at the hip. Brudzinski's sign is present when flexion of the neck causes involuntary flexion of the thighs and legs. Focal neurologic signs are infrequent presenting findings. However, nuchal rigidity may not be elicited in comatose patients who may have signs of focal or diffuse neurologic impairment. Papilledema is not a presenting feature of bacterial meningitis and suggests the presence of an accompanying process (Swartz and Dodge, 1965). A frequent presenting sign in meningococcal meningitis is a petechial rash, which occurs rarely in other kinds of bacterial meningitis.

The clinical pattern of bacterial meningitis is often atypical in young children, since headache and nuchal rigidity are frequently absent. Irritability, especially with movement, is a common presenting manifestation of meningitis in a young child. Progression of the illness results in the development of lassitude and a more constant fever, often accompanied by abdominal discomfort. Projectile vomiting may occur. In addition, convulsions may signal the onset of meningitis in a young child.

Neonatal meningitis has an extremely varied and nonspecific clinical presentation. In a majority of cases, the disease begins within the first week of life and follows a fulminant course. If the onset is delayed until later in the neonatal period, the course tends to be more incremental. Nevertheless, any sudden change in the usual behavior of a neonate may be a sign of infection. Changes associated with meningitis include irritability, listlessness, convulsions, poor feeding, vomiting, and respiratory difficulty. Full-term infants with meningitis tend to be febrile, whereas low birth weight neonates may become hypothermic. Abdominal distention, jaundice and hypotension may occur. Bulging of the fontanelle due to increased intracranial pressure is a presenting sign that is found in less than half of the cases of neonatal meningitis.

Bacterial meningitis produces various changes in the CSF; however, their magnitude depends on the stage of disease in which the CSF is examined. The CSF pressure tends to be moderately elevated, but it may be markedly elevated in severely ill patients. Infected CSF appears turbid, and microscopic evaluation reveals a pleocytosis of PMN leukocytes. Although the number of white blood cells in infected CSF varies widely, counts range from 1000 to 10,000 WBC/mm^3 in the majority of cases. The concentration of proteins in CSF is increased in proportion to the concentration of white cells present. Reduction of the CSF glucose level to less than 40 per cent of the simultaneous blood glucose level is a feature that suggests bacterial meningitis. However, hypoglycorrhachia is found in only half of the patients with bacterial meningitis. These changes in the CSF reflect the intensity of the inflammatory process but have no prognostic significance.

COMPLICATIONS AND SEQUELAE. Several life-threatening complications may occur during the acute phase of bacterial meningitis. Marked cerebral edema, which may cause herniation of the temporal lobes or cerebellum, is manifested by coma, oculomotor nerve paralysis, and episodes of respiratory arrest. Coma may also result from diffuse cortical damage. This cortical lesion has a multifactorial etiology including increased intracranial pressure, cerebral vascular occlusions, hypoxia, and other toxic factors (Swartz and Dodge, 1965). Prolonged seizures that are either focal or generalized may also contribute to a fatal outcome. Death may also result from the systemic effects of an overwhelming bacteremia, as occurs in fulminant meningococcemia. Also, acute endocarditis may be a finding in fatal cases of pneumococcal meningitis.

Other acute complications of bacterial meningitis include seizures, cranial nerve impairment, focal cerebral deficits, and water retention due to inappropriate secretion of antidiuretic hormone (Kaplan and Feigin, 1978). Generalized brief seizures occur at some stage in approximately 20 per cent of patients with bacterial meningitis. The most frequent cranial nerve dysfunction is impaired ocular movement, which tends to be transient. Damage to the eighth cranial nerve complex, however, may persist. Focal cerebral necrosis resulting from cortical vein thrombosis is an infrequent complication of bacterial meningitis; focal cerebral signs tend to occur within the first few days of illness and often in association with seizures. Delayed thrombosis of the cortical veins is an unusual complication that results in the appearance of focal neurologic deficits after apparent clinical recovery. Another late complication is a subdural effusion that occurs in approximately 15 per cent of infants with bacterial meningitis. Blockade of the aqueduct by the inflammatory exudate causes a loculated infection in the ventricles that impairs the entry of antibiotics into this area. This condition has been termed ventriculitis and is a complication that occurs almost exclusively in infants.

The late sequelae of bacterial meningitis are deafness, mental deficits, and hydrocephalus. From 5 to 30 per cent of surviving infants and children have one or more of these sequelae (Swartz and Dodge, 1965; Feigin and Dodge, 1976).

GEOGRAPHIC VARIATION. Bacterial meningitis has a worldwide distribution; however, geographic location is a factor that affects the relative frequency with which the various pathogens cause meningitis. Epidemics of meningococcal disease occur at cyclic intervals in many parts of the world. Meningitis by some of the uncommon causative agents also shows geographic variation. For example, meningitis caused by *Salmonella* species tends to occur in underdeveloped countries where the sanitation is poor. Another consideration relates to the prevalence of antibiotic-resistant organisms in certain areas of the world. An example of this is ampicillin-resistant *H. influenzae* in the United States and elsewhere.

DIAGNOSIS. The organism is likely to be seen and recognized in a Gram-stained smear in over 70 per cent of the CSF specimens from which an agent is eventually cultured (Swartz and Dodge, 1965). Other rapid diagnostic tests involve the detection of specific capsular antigens by immunologic methods and endotoxin by the limulus assay. Although these newer tests have limitations, they may be used as an adjunct to the stained smear. A brisk pleocytosis by PMN leukocytes, hypoglycorrhachia, and an elevated protein concentration in CSF are characteristic of bacterial meningitis. The usual means for establishing the diagnosis of bacterial meningitis is culture of CSF. Blood cultures frequently yield the same organisms, but cultures of the nasopharynx are frequently misleading. Prior antibiotic therapy has been implicated as a reason for failure to isolate organisms from the CSF.

Recurrent episodes of bacterial meningitis that are commonly caused by *S. pneumoniae* suggest the presence of a skull defect and associated CSF rhinorrhea. Other causes of recurrent bacterial meningitis are parameningeal foci of infection, immunoglobulin disorders, and complement deficiencies.

Aseptic meningitis occasionally presents with a mild pleocytosis of predominantly PMN leukocytes and must be differentiated from bacterial meningitis. When aseptic meningitis presents in this manner, the proportion of PMN leukocytes in the CSF decreases markedly over the subsequent eight hours. Consequently, reexamination of the CSF after withholding antibiotic therapy for 8 to 12 hours is a useful means for distinguishing between these two syndromes (Feigin and Shackelford, 1973). The magnitude of the CSF pleocytosis and the predominance of PMN leukocytes in CSF aid in the rapid differentiation of bacterial meningitis from meningitis caused by other infectious agents except *Naegleria*. Bacterial endocarditis may produce a meningeal inflammatory reaction; however, the CSF is typically sterile in this condition. Meningeal reactions resembling bacterial meningitis also occur in neoplastic meningitis, chemical meningitis, sarcoidosis, and as a hypersensitivity reaction to drugs (e.g., sulfonamides). Parameningeal foci of infection including mastoiditis, sinusitis, brain abscess, subdural empyema, and epidural abscess typically have a mild pleocytosis in the CSF. Recurrent nonbacterial meningitis occurs in Behçet's syndrome, Mollaret's meningitis, and systemic lupus erythematosus.

TREATMENT. Specific antimicrobial therapy offers the most effective means for interrupting the progression of bacterial meningitis. This form of therapy is directed at reducing the number of viable organisms in the CSF and, thereby, allowing the inflammatory response in the meninges to subside. Control of the infection before the central nervous system is irreparably damaged permits the clinical manifestations to resolve without the occurrence of serious sequelae. Consequently, recognition of this disease process in its early stages is critical for the therapy to be effective. When the changes in the CSF are indicative of bacterial meningitis, it is imperative to begin antibiotic therapy promptly. Treatment of this disease appears to require the use of an antimicrobial agent that has bactericidal rather than just bacteriostatic activity against the causative organism (Cherubin et al., 1982). A prerequisite to successful therapy is the attainment of antimicrobial activity in the CSF (Sande, 1981). The blood-CSF barrier limits the entry of most antibiotics to the area of infection. Meningeal inflammation impairs the integrity of this barrier and permits parenterally administered penicillin antibiotics to enter the CSF in therapeutic concentrations. Most cephalosporins have proven unsuitable for the treatment of meningitis, because they are rapidly desacetylated to an inactive metabolite in the choroid plexus. The desacetyl derivate of cefotaxime, however, retains most of the activity of the parent compound. Moxalactam is apparently not metabolized by this mechanism. The efficacy of these two cephalosporin derivatives in the treatment of meningitis also depends upon the quantitative susceptibility of the causative organism. Cefotaxime and moxalactam have particularly excellent intrinsic activity against *Enterobacteriaceae*, including hospital strains that have acquired multiple antibiotic resistance. Both cephalosporins have proven efficacious in the treatment of meningitis caused by these organisms (Cherubin, 1982). These cephalosporins are not likely to be effective treatment of meningitis caused by *P. aeruginosa* or other organisms that are susceptible only at high levels of these drugs. Neither can they be recommended as a single drug for the treatment of neonatal meningitis, because they lack activity against *L. monocytogenes*. In patients who are allergic to penicillin, cefotaxime may represent an effective alternative therapy for meningitis caused by the three common agents. Chloramphenicol, which has excellent penetration into CSF, continues to be important in the therapy of meningitis and may be the preferred alternative therapy in penicillin-allergic patients. Vancomycin and co-trimaxazole also have enough penetration into CSF to be useful in treatment. Direct instillation of the aminoglycoside antibiotics is required to attain therapeutic levels in the CSF. Local injury at the site of instillation and uneven distribution throughout the CSF are limitations of this type of treatment, even though it represents a means for treating gram-negative bacillary meningitis.

Effective antimicrobial therapy exists for meningitis caused by most bacterial organisms (Table 1). The selection of an antimicrobial agent for initiating therapy of bacterial

Table 1. ANTIMICROBIAL TREATMENT OF BACTERIAL MENINGITIS

	Recommended Treatment Program			
Causative Organisms	***Antibiotic***	***Adult Dose***	***Pediatric Dose***[a]	***Route***[b]
S. pneumoniae, N. meningitidis, S. pyogenes, S. agalactica, P. multocida, and other penicillin-susceptible organisms	penicillin G	2×10^6 u every 2h	250,000 μ/kg/d	i.v.
H. influenzae (ampicillin-susceptible), *L. monocytogenes,* ampicillin-susceptible gram-negative bacilli	ampicillin	2.0 g every 4h	200 mg/kg/d	i.v.
H. influenzae (ampicillin-resistant), alternative therapy in penicillin-allergic patients	chloramphenicol	1.0 g every 6h	75 mg/kg/d	i.v. or p.o.
Enterobacteriaceae (ampicillin-resistant)	cefotaxime or moxalactam or	2.0 g every 4h	200 mg/kg/d	i.v.
	gentamicin	80 mg every 8h plus	7.5 mg/kg/d	i.v.
		5 mg once daily	2.5 mg once daily	i.t.
P. aeruginosa, A. calcoaceticus	piperacillin	3.0 g every 4h	300 mg/kg/d	i.v.
S. aureus (penicillin-resistant)	methicillin, nafcillin, or oxacillin	2.0 g every 4 h	150 to 200 mg/kg/d	i.v.
S. pneumoniae (penicillin-resistant)	vancomycin	0.5 g every 6h	50 mg/kg/d	i.v.

[a]Excludes neonates.
[b]Intravenously (i.v.), intrathecal (i.t.), orally (p.o.)

meningitis is influenced by a number of factors, including the likely etiologic agent and the clinical setting. Examination of the stained smear provides especially valuable information that aids in the choice of initial antibiotic therapy. Knowledge of the age-dependant frequency with which different organisms cause meningitis and of geographic considerations should also be taken into account. When bacterial meningitis occurs spontaneously in individuals over five years of age, penicillin is likely to be the most appropriate treatment. This drug is recommended for initiating treatment in adults with spontaneously occurring bacterial meningitis, when the stained smear examination of the CSF fails to reveal an organism. Chloramphenicol is recommended for initial treatment of children with bacterial meningitis in areas where ampicillin-resistant *H. influenzae* is known to exist. The American Academy of Pediatrics advises that both ampicillin and chloramphenicol be used for the initial treatment of bacterial meningitis in children. Neonates should not be treated with high doses of chloramphenicol because of the potential for producing the "gray baby" syndrome. Parenteral administration of ampicillin (infants $\leq$ 7 days: 100 mg/kg/d; $>$ 7 days: 200 mg/kg/d) and gentamicin (infants $\leq$ 7 days: 5.0 mg/kg/d; $>$ 7 days: 7.5 mg/kg/d) is advocated for initial treatment of neonatal meningitis. Intrathecal or intraventricular administration of an aminoglycoside does not have a beneficial effect upon the outcome of neonatal meningitis (McCrachen, 1980). The newer cephalosporins may prove useful in neonatal meningitis, especially against the gram-negative bacilli. Moxalactam or cefotaxime may also be selected for initial treatment of adults who acquired gram-negative bacillary meningitis in the hospital setting, unless *P. aeruginosa* is suspected. When gram-negative bacilli are recognized in stained smears of the CSF from adults with spontaneously occurring meningitis, piperacillin in combination with either intrathecal gentamicin or one of the newer cephalosporins is suggested as initial treatment. Antimicrobial therapy can be adjusted once the causative organism has been identified and its antimicrobial susceptibility determined. If cultures reveal a strain of *S. pneumoniae* that is relatively resistant to penicillin, it is advisable to complete the course of therapy with chloramphenicol. Since the penetration of antibiotics decreases as the meningeal inflammation subsides, large doses of these drugs must be given during the entire course of therapy. The duration of treatment for bacterial meningitis is usually 10 to 14 days.

Parenteral fluids should be carefully administered to avoid hyponatremia and water intoxication. Maintenance of adequate ventilation, prevention of aspiration, treatment of seizures with anticonvulsants, and reduction in fever constitute important supportive measures. Treatment of cerebral edema remains controversial. Corticosteroids have no beneficial effect on the outcome of purulent meningitis; repeated drainage of CSF has no therapeutic efficacy. Osmotic diuretics have been used successfully to reduce increased intracranial pressure, even though their administration may be associated with a late rebound effect.

Modern therapy allows many patients with bacterial meningitis to recover completely from an otherwise invariably fatal disease. Clinical improvement tends to be gradual and may not be appreciated during the first few days of treatment. Effective antimicrobial therapy for 48 h is expected to result in a clearance of visible organisms from stained smears of the CSF and an improvement in hypoglycorrhachia. Despite the availability of effective therapy, fatalities still occur. According to a 1978 survey of United States reported cases, the case fatality rates for meningitis caused by *H. influenzae, N. meningitidis,* and *S. pneumoniae* are 7, 14, and 28 per cent, respectively (Gold, 1983). Although the virulence of the causative organism may partially account for these differences, the severity of the disease at the time of presentation is the most important determinant of outcome. Pneumococcal meningitis is more likely to progress to coma by presentation than the other two types of meningitis (Underman et al. 1978). Other factors affecting prognosis include the age of the patient and underlying conditions. The mortality of *S. agalactica* meningitis is 22 per cent. The mortality of *L. monocytogenes* meningitis is 13 per cent in individuals without an underlying disease, but 30 per cent in renal transplant recipients and 60 per cent in those with malignancies (Nieman and Lorber, 1980). Gram-negative bacillary meningitis is also associated with a high mortality rate (Berk and McCabe, 1980).

The definitive treatment for recurrent bacterial meningitis associated with an anatomic defect is surgical correction.

PROPHYLAXIS. Prevention of bacterial meningitis by immunization is a desirable goal that is actively being pursued. A major problem is the limited immunogenicity of purified polysaccharide vaccines in children under 2 years of age, since this population is highly susceptible to bacterial meningitis (Gotschlich, 1978). A vaccine containing group A and group C meningococcal polysaccharides can be given to the population at risk when these serogroups of *N. meningitidis* cause epidemic meningitis. The polyvalent pneumococcal vaccine is indicated for children with sickle cell disease because of their high risk of pneumococcal meningitis.

Chemoprophylaxis of household contacts effectively reduces the secondary attack rate of meningococcal disease by interrupting the transmission of organisms to other susceptible family members. Chemoprophylaxis of meningococcal disease is described in Chapter 181. The prevention of secondary cases of *H. influenzae* disease by chemoprophylaxis is presently being studied, since the secondary attack rate in household contacts under 6 years of age is similar to that of meningococcal disease (Ward et al., 1979).

References

Berk, S. L., and McCabe, W. R.: Meningitis caused by gram-negative bacilli. Ann Intern Med 93:253, 1980.

Cherubin, C. E., Corrado, M. L., Nair, S. R., et al.: Treatment of gram-negative bacillary meningitis: Role of the new cephalosporin antibiotics. Rev Infect Dis 4:S453, 1982.

Feigin, R. D., and Dodge, P. R.: Bacterial meningitis: Newer concepts of pathophysiology and neurologic sequelae. Pediatr Clin North Am 23:541, 1976.

Feigin, R. D., and Schackelford, P. G.: Value of repeat lumbar puncture in differential diagnosis of meningitis. N Engl J Med 289:571, 1973.

Feldman, W. E.: Relation of concentrations of bacteria and bacterial antigen in cerebrospinal fluid to prognosis in patients with bacterial meningitis. New Engl J Med 296:433, 1977.

Gartner, J. C., and Michaels, R. H.: Meningitis from a pneumococcus moderately resistant to penicillin. JAMA 241:1707, 1979.

Glode, M. P., Sutton, A., Moxon, E. R., et al.: Pathogenesis of neonatal *Escherichia coli* meningitis: induction of bacteremia and meningitis in infant rats fed *E. coli* K1. Infect Immun 16:75, 1977.

Gold, R.: Bacterial meningitis—1982. Am J Med 75(suppl 1B):98, 1983.

Gotschlich, E. C.: Bacterial meningitis: The beginning of the end. Am J Med 65:719, 1978.
Heerema, M. S., Ein, M. E., Musher, D. M., et al.: Anaerobic bacterial meningitis. Am J Med 67:219, 1979.
Kaplan, S. L., and Feigin, R. D.: The syndrome of inappropriate secretion of antidiuretic hormone in children with bacterial meningitis. J Pediatr 92:758, 1978.
Levy, R. L., and Saunders, R. L.: *Citrobacter* meningitis and cerebral abscess in early infancy: cure by moxalactam. Neurology 31:1575, 1981.
McAllister, C. K., O'Donoghue, J. M., and Beaty, H. N.: Experimental pneumococcal meningitis: Characterization and quantitation of the inflammatory process. J Infect Dis 132:355, 1975.
McCracken, G. H., Mize, S. G., and Threlkeld, N.: Intraventricular gentamicin therapy in gram-negative bacillary meningitis of infancy. Report of the second neonatal meningitis cooperative study group. The Lancet, April 12:787, 1980.
Moxon, E. R., and Ostrow, P. T.: *Haemophilus influenzae* meningitis in infant rats: Role of bacteremia in pathogenesis of age-dependent inflammatory responses in cerebrospinal fluid. J Infect Dis 135:303, 1977.
Moxon, E. R., Smith, A. L., Averill, D. R., et al.: *Haemophilus influenzae* meningitis in infant rats after intranasal inoculation. J Infect Dis 129:154, 1974.
Murphy, D. J.: Group A streptococcal meningitis. Pediatrics 71:1, 1983.
Nieman, R. E., and Lorber, B.: Listeriosis in adults: a changing pattern. Report of eight cases and review of the literature, 1968–1978. Rev Infect Dis 2:207, 1980.
Overall, J. C.: Neonatal bacterial meningitis. J Ped 76:499, 1970.
Rahal, J. J., Jr., and Simberkoff, M. S.: Bactericidal and bacteriostatic action of chloramphenicol against meningeal pathogens. Antimicrob Agents Chemother 16:13, 1979.
Sande, M. A.: Antibiotic therapy of bacterial meningitis: Lessons we've learned. Am J Med 71:507, 1981.
Scheld, W. M., Park, T., Dacey, R. G., et al.: Clearance of bacteria from cerebrospinal fluid to blood in experimental meningitis. Infect Immun 24:102, 1979.
Spagnuolo, P. J., Ellner, J. J., Lerner, P. I., et al.: *Haemophilus influenzae* meningitis: the spectrum of disease in adults. Medicine 61:74, 1982.
Swartz, M. N., and Dodge, P. R.: Bacterial meningitis—a review of selected aspects. N Engl J Med 272:725, 779, 842, 898, 954, and 1003, 1965.
Underman, A. E., Overturf, G. D., and Leedom, J. M.: Bacterial meningitis—1978. Disease-a-Month 24:1, 1978.
Ward, J. I., Fraser, D. W., Baraff, L. J., et al.: *Haemophilus influenzae* meningitis: A national study of secondary spread in household contacts. N Engl J Med 301:122, 1979.

166

TUBERCULOUS MENINGITIS AND TUBERCULOMA OF THE BRAIN

Tuberculous Meningitis

GÉRARD DE CROUSAZ, M.D.

Tuberculous meningitis can occur at any age except in the newborn. It develops in tuberculosis in four particular settings:

1. As a complication of primary infection, with or without miliary spread. The younger the child is, the higher the risk is. In an unprotected population, the primary infection occurs before the age of 5 years in 75 per cent of children. Meningitis complicates 1 in 300 of such cases. It appears mainly within six months after contact and two months after conversion of the tuberculin test.

2. As a complication of end-stage chronic tuberculosis, predominantly of the lungs, with or without miliary spread. This affects mainly the elderly. The tuberculin test often becomes negative.

3. As a concurrent illness together with another localization of tuberculosis, mainly pulmonary or miliary. This affects older children and adults.

4. As an isolated form of tuberculosis. This condition overlaps the previous one because small lesions or even miliary spread found at necropsy are not detectable clinically. This type of meningitis constitutes about 20 per cent of adult cases.

Meningitis developing in each of these circumstances has many common features. It is fatal within one to eight weeks if untreated and carries a high risk of severe sequelae if treatment is delayed. The basal cisterns are principally affected by the exudate, which becomes granulomatous tissue. This can lead to three major complications: damage to cranial nerves, arteritis with cerebral infarction, and obstruction to cerebrospinal fluid (CSF) flow with hydrocephalus. The spinal cord and roots are likewise exposed to arteritis and compression.

The situations defined in paragraphs 1 and 2 above are by far the most common in those areas of the world in which tuberculosis still has a high prevalence, and meningitis affects mainly infants. These same conditions are practically extinct in the developed countries, in which meningitis can have a thousand-fold lower incidence and is nearly restricted to adults.

The patient's history, the clinical findings, and the pattern of CSF abnormalities together support the probability of diagnosis in the majority of cases. A specific therapy then has to be initiated without waiting for positive cultures, because a delay of three to six weeks would ruin the patient's chances of recovery.

ETIOLOGY. *Mycobacterium tuberculosis* infects the pia and arachnoid layers. The ratio of the human to bovine types differs in urban and rural areas. *Mycobacterium bovis* once caused up to 40 per cent of tuberculosis in children but is now absent in many countries in which bovine tuberculosis has been eradicated.

PATHOGENESIS AND PATHOLOGY. A hematogenous route is responsible for practically all cases of meningeal tuberculosis, but an intermediate cerebral lesion linking bacteremia to meningeal seeding is considered obligatory because injection of *M. tuberculosis* into the carotids or veins has repeatedly failed to produce meningitis in various animal species. Careful search of brains from patients dead after a short course of disease has revealed older tuberculous nodules, which are considered to be the link in 70 to 90 per cent of cases (Rich and McCordock, 1933). Bacteremia and the development of parenchymal nodules in the brain can be inapparent clinically or masked by some other manifestation of disease.

Release into the leptomeninges of bacilli and tuberculous antigens, hitherto enclosed within the parenchymal brain nodules, may occur early or after a latent period of months or years. A virulent or aggressive acute infection may be responsible for this release from recent lesions. In those nodules that were dormant for months or years, some disturbance in the patient's resistance is required. Corticosteroid therapy can activate a tuberculous meningitis, while other immunosuppressive drugs increase the risk of fungal meningitides (Stockstill and Kauffman, 1983). Recent measles (reported in 5 to 10 per cent of tuberculous meningitis complicating the primary infection), head trauma, sun exposure, and malnutrition are examples of conditions that cause release of tubercle bacilli from parenchymal brain nodules into the meninges (Illingworth, 1956; Lincoln et al., 1960; Tandon and Pathak, 1973).

Even though older nodules are often located on the convexity of the hemispheres, release of bacilli and antigens gives rise to an inflammation extending along the basal cisterns, the major route of CSF flow.

Direct spread from a site of tuberculous otitis, skull osteitis, or spondylitis is unusual.

The macroscopic appearance of meningeal tuberculosis varies from inconspicuous in acute cases to spectacular in patients whose death has been delayed by therapy. An exudate fills the basal cisterns, mainly interpeduncular and chiasmatic, extending laterally into the sylvian fissures and cisterna ambiens, downward along the prepontine, cisterna magna, and spinal spaces. Fibrocaseous transformation with eventual calcifications develops mainly in cases of long duration.

White tubercles, 1 to 3 mm in size, can be seen within the meningeal exudate on the convexity of the hemispheres (mainly around vessels of the sylvian fissure), on the ependyma and choroidal plexuses, and sometimes on the inner surface of the dura mater. On brain slices, many tubercles have a corticopial distribution, and a few lie deeper in the cortex.

Arteries embedded in the exudate may be occluded. Infarctions, occasionally hemorrhagic, are not uncommon in the basal nuclei and hypothalamus or in the corticosubcortical regions, mainly around the sylvian fissure and the inferior aspect of the frontal lobe. Brain edema is usual when death occurs early. Early hydrocephalus from ependymitis blocking the aqueduct is rare, but it is a common late finding due to atrophy.

Microscopically, lesions are initially exudative with a few tubercles. Tuberculous lesions of different ages are found throughout the evolution of the infection. Underlying parenchymal structures may be invaded, particularly along perforating vessels. Arteritis is more prominent than phlebitis. Many small vessels are occluded by thrombosis or a tuberculous granuloma; thrombosis occasionally occludes larger arteries.

Nonspecific features such as infarctions, areas of ischemic changes, and astrocytic proliferation may be found.

Spinal arteritis with infarction, cord or cauda equina compression from arachnoidal adhesions or granulomas, is found mainly in long protracted cases.

Besides the tuberculoma, some rare forms of neurotuberculosis deserve mention: tuberculous encephalopathy without meningitis; spinal meningitis around either an extradural tuberculous abscess with radiculopathy or a spinal cord tuberculoma; and localized meningitis "en plaque." These account for some 5 per cent of meningitides (Udani et al., 1971; Tandon and Pathak, 1973).

CLINICAL MANIFESTATIONS.* Most cases progress through three stages as defined by the British Medical Research Council (Streptomycin in Tuberculosis Trials Committee, 1948). The prognosis is correlated with the stage reached at the time treatment is initiated.

Stage 1 (early, prodromal): patients have mainly nonspecific symptoms, few or no signs of meningitis, are fully conscious, and have no neurologic defects.

Stage 2 (medium, intermediate): patients usually have signs of meningitis, minor or no neurologic defects, no marked change in the level of consciousness.

Stage 3 (advanced, late, paralytic): patients obviously are very ill, are deeply stuporous or comatose, or have gross pareses.

The prodromal stage lasts for two weeks to two to three months in 70 per cent of cases, excluding the extreme age groups, in which it is less often detected. Symptoms are nonspecific and misleading, except in cases with known tuberculosis of another organ, known contact, or documented tuberculin test conversion. In young children, a history of exposure to known contacts (mainly household) is nearly diagnostic. In older patients seen at a later stage, a history of this prodromal stage practically rules out a pyogenic or viral meningitis.

Apathy with bursts of irritability, nocturnal wakefulness, and minor headaches form a vague neurologic component. Pain may be localized in one ear or a paranasal sinus, and there is very often a coincident nonspecific upper respiratory infection. Anorexia, loss of weight, nausea and vomiting, abdominal pain (sometimes prominent), and constipation may erroneously point to some abdominal disorder. Myalgia and lumbosacral pain with radicular radiation in one or both lower limbs are frequent complaints in the adult. Transient or intermittent low-grade fever may add to the feeling that the patient has some "flu-like" disorder that fails to resolve.

The intermediate stage of meningitis develops over days or two to three weeks with no clear-cut separation from the prodrome; its onset is usually acute in infants and the elderly but in only 5 per cent of any other age groups (Taylor et al., 1955). Headaches and vomiting are the major complaints in 75 per cent of patients. Neck stiffness and the Kernig and Brudzinski signs are present in two thirds to three fourths of patients, though often inconspicuous; these signs are more often absent in the extreme age groups. Low to moderate fever (not above 39° C or 102° F) is the rule; isolated higher peaks are not unusual. Infants may have a persistent fever of 40° C (104° F) or more at this stage. An afebrile course is recorded in 3 to 5 per cent of pediatric and up to 10 per cent of adult series. At the other extreme, fever is reported as the presenting and only finding for days or weeks in about 10 per cent of cases.

*This description is based upon various large clinical series. Cases that are exclusively or mainly pediatric were found in Western (Illingworth, 1956; Lincoln et al., 1960), African (Freiman and Geefhuysen, 1970; Osuntokur et al., 1971), and Indian sources (Udani et al., 1971). In adults, the author's personal experience was consolidated with other large series (Lepper and Spies, 1963; Falk, 1965; Weiss and Flippin, 1965). More recent reports demonstrate diagnostic problems due to a decline in the frequency of the disease in Western countries (Meyers and Hirschman, 1974; Karandanis and Shulman, 1976; Haas et al., 1977; Crocco et al., 1980; Meyers, 1982; Roberts, 1981).

This stage may begin without fever in malnourished patients (Tandon and Pathak, 1973).

Apathy and irritability tend to evolve into confusion and lethargy. Psychotic behavior, and alcohol or drug withdrawal syndromes in chronic addicts, can mask the underlying disease. Intracranial hypertension is not impressive at this stage. Choroidal tubercles are found in less than 10 per cent of cases, more often in cases of concomitant miliary tuberculosis. The cranial nerves are involved in some 25 per cent of cases. An early sign that suggests the diagnosis consists of dilated pupils, reacting poorly or not at all to light, in fully awake patients without limitation of eye movements and with no ptosis (Fisher, 1974). External oculomotor paresis, usually incomplete and unilateral, affects mainly the third nerve, then the sixth and fourth nerves. Peripheral facial paresis is less common, and other cranial nerves are rarely affected. Focal or generalized convulsions are a presenting or early symptom in 10 to 15 per cent of children and in fewer adults. Transient or mild paresis can follow the seizure or occur alone in both groups.

The advanced stage is usually reached gradually, but at any age and especially in the extreme age groups, cases can suddenly become advanced with the onset of convulsions, coma, or hemiplegia. This accounts for some 10 per cent of patients with coma and/or gross paresis. A strokelike onset in adults, intracranial hypertension with focal cerebral signs, or poliomyelitis-like flaccid paralysis are some treacherous modes of onset.

Signs of meningeal irritation may disappear in a deep coma, but fever is persistent. Papilledema is seen in some 40 per cent of patients, and over one half have oculomotor or facial nerve involvement. Gross paralysis, mainly hemi-, tetra-, or paraplegia, is seen in up to 40 per cent of cases; these paralyses are reversible and may affect either side alternately. Abnormal movements, particularly ballismus, can occur. Other focal defects, such as aphasia or cerebellar signs, are detected only after improvement of stupor or coma. Over one half of the children have fits.

In the end-stage leading to death, there are decerebrate posture, disturbance in regulation of blood pressure and respiration, and hyperpyrexia followed by hypothermia.

Even successful therapy does not reverse the course of the disease immediately; on the contrary, an acute transient deterioration is actually frequent during the first week of treatment. Subsiding fever and clearing of consciousness occur mainly from the second to the fifth week in patients who are doing well. Some previously undetectable defects can appear, however, while new ones may develop.

Patients treated unsuccessfully or too late may survive in any degree of coma, mental deterioration, mono- to tetraparesis, blindness, or deafness. Later, death from intercurrent disease is frequent in these severely brain- or cord-damaged patients.

Relapses can occur when therapy is discontinued too early. Clear instructions on continuation of drugs must be given to the patient and to his family, and regular follow-up visits are important.

Many series originating from both developed and developing countries report a mortality rate of 5 to 20 per cent and full recovery in up to 60 to 70 per cent. It would seem realistic to expect a less optimistic prognosis, because most patients are not treated in specialized units. A mortality of one third to one half, with survivors distributed equally among those with moderate to severe sequelae and those with full recovery (or, at worst, mild sequelae) is probably closer to a worldwide situation. Unfavorable prognostic factors are a delay in treatment until a late stage, an age below 3 or over 40, the presence of associated diseases, and a very high initial CSF protein level (Lepper and Spies, 1963; Falk, 1965; Weiss and Flippin, 1965); either a basal or periventricular hypodensity on the cerebral CT scan is also a sign of poor prognosis (Bullock and Welchman, 1982).

COMPLICATIONS AND SEQUELAE. Two major complications can induce acute intracranial hypertension early in the course of the disease. Brain edema commonly aggravates the condition of critically ill patients in the first days of treatment. Great amounts of tuberculin released from the killed bacilli are thought to enhance abruptly this inflammatory swelling. Obstructive hydrocephalus due to ependymitis in the aqueduct, or cisternal exudate blocking the foramina of Magendie and Luschka, can cause tentorial herniation. CT scan is the safest procedure for differentiating these two complications.

Major neurologic complications that arise in Stages 2 and 3 have been described. The leptomeninges are occasionally superinfected by bacteria or fungi. Intracranial hemorrhages occasionally develop within infarcted areas. Both oversecretion and undersecretion of antidiuretic hormone are common in a mild form. Major extracranial complications are pyogenic infections (pneumonia, septicemia, urinary tract infection, infected bedsores) and gastric mucosal erosions with hemorrhage.

Complications can occur later as a result of progressive fibrosis; arachnoidal adhesions can block the pericerebral or spinal CSF flow even after the active phase is controlled by chemotherapy. Compressive-ischemic damage to the optic chiasm, hypothalamo-pituitary structures, spinal cord, or roots (especially of the cauda equina) can appear during convalescence. An increasing protein concentration in the lumbar CSF, with normal cells and glucose, is a warning sign of these spinal blocks. Focal or generalized epilepsy persists or appears in 10 per cent of survivors. Obesity, sexual precocity, Cushing's syndrome, and diabetes insipidus are occasional endocrine sequelae (Udani et al., 1971).

Drug-induced complications should be kept in mind. They were common when streptomycin was the only drug available (deafness, labyrinthine destruction, spinal dermoids or cholesteatomas from daily intrathecal injections). Neurologic side effects of the newer drugs include an occasional acute optic neuropathy (ethambutol) and cerebral dysfunction (cycloserine).

Sequelae range from mild to very severe. Intensive care reduces the mortality but increases the number of disabled survivors. A final assessment can be made only after one to two years, since many abnormalities in the active phase disappear, and a few others appear later.

The most disabled patients are often left with more than one of the following disorders: mental retardation or dementia, hemi- or paraplegia, epilepsy, cerebellar ataxia, blindness, deafness, or strabismus. Moderate sequelae include mild mental retardation, epilepsy, reduced vision, partial deafness, hemiparesis, and mild ataxia. Minor sequelae are more frequent if accurately sought and include some degree of behavioral or learning disorder, visual field defects, paresis of one oculomotor or facial nerve or of the lumbosacral roots, disturbance of micturition and hyperreflexia. Intracranial calcifications, mainly behind the optic chiasm, have been uncommon since isoniazid was introduced. Like diffuse or focal EEG abnormalities, they occur in survivors with or without clinical sequelae.

GEOGRAPHIC VARIATIONS. In developed countries, three factors account for the considerable decrease in incidence of the disease over the last century: improvement of overcrowded, substandard living conditions and personal hygiene; chemotherapy; and, to a lesser degree, public health programs.

Today, many developing countries have instituted public health programs; others have not. In those that have, the incidence of the disease has been rapidly reduced by 50 to 80 per cent or more, even without substantial changes in economic conditions. Mandatory BCG (bacille Calmette Guérin) inoculation in infancy and detection and treatment of pulmonary tuberculosis by mass chest roentgenography have thus proved their effectiveness here. The number of tuberculous meningitides per thousand hospital or pediatric admissions provides the only comparative figures. The highest incidence over the last 20 years has been recorded in South Asia, Africa, and South America and amounted to 10 to 50 cases per 1000 pediatric admissions. This incidence is no doubt similar to that in European and North American areas 80 years ago. Prophylactic measures have reduced this incidence to somewhere between 1 and 25 per 1000. However, tuberculous meningitis remains a major medical problem in developing countries, especially in children.

A steady decline of the disease has been reported in developed countries during the last three decades. In 1947, England and Wales reported about 2000 cases per year, accounting for 10 to 20 per cent of all bacterial meningitides; the annual rate fell to 56 from 1967 through 1971, or 3.9 per cent of all bacterial meningitides (Stevenson, 1973). Pediatric cases have virtually disappeared, and two thirds of cases occur in those aged 20 to 40 years, with a hint of a shift toward older age groups. Thus, 10 of 19 patients seen in 1966 through 1974 were over 40 years old (Haas et al., 1977); the mean age was 56 years in a series from Michigan during the years 1967 through 1981 (Stockstill and Kauffman, 1983).

An example of a very low incidence is that at the University Hospital in Lausanne, Switzerland, which serves an area without any economically depressed population group. The incidence was 0.019 per 1000 hospital admissions from 1972 through 1978, a three-fold decrease as compared with the previous decade. As a contrast, large indigent urban populations provide higher rates locally, especially if composed of immigrants. In Birmingham, England, during the period 1950 to 1960, the ratio of tuberculosis among Indians and Pakistanis versus the local British population was 20 to 1 (Springett, 1964). These findings were recently confirmed (Swarts et al., 1981). Immigrants from the Mediterranean area to Central Europe had a fairly high ratio of tuberculous meningitis. Rates nowadays should not exceed the 0.5 to 0.8 per 1000 hospital admissions recorded in 1959 in Cleveland, Ohio (Hinman, 1967).

DIAGNOSIS. Lumbar puncture is mandatory and urgent. It has to be repeated for diagnostic purposes if one or more of the classic abnormalities are lacking, which is more likely to occur in the early stages of the disease. Serial taps should, however, be avoided if the first one discloses a very high initial pressure (above 400 mm).

The CSF may be clear, opalescent, or turbid, and sometimes is xanthochromatic or slightly hemorrhagic.

CSF Cytology. The classic picture consists of 10 to 500 white blood cells per cmm, predominantly lymphocytic. Higher counts are seen in 10 to 15 per cent of cases, often concomitant with a predominantly polymorphonuclear reaction. On repeated diagnostic punctures within the first days, the marked variability of the total cell count with transient bursts of polymorphonuclears is, by itself, highly suggestive of the disease (Lepper and Spies, 1963). Erythrocytes in varying amounts are commonly found, presumably from traumatic tap.

Chemistry. Glucose concentration is below the normal range of 40 mg per 100 ml (or if blood levels are increased, below two fifths to one half of the blood glucose level) in 70 to 85 per cent of initial lumbar punctures. Repeated punctures in an early stage usually demonstrate the suggestive cross of the lowering glucose curve and the increasing protein curve, but this may not occur in adults. A low CSF glucose level should therefore not be required as a diagnostic criterion of tuberculous meningitis.

Protein levels are 60 to 200 mg per 100 ml in most initial samples. Initial values above 300 mg indicate a bad prognosis. Differential protein fractionation is useful if total levels are below 80 mg per 100 ml. Detectable IgM in the early phase of a lymphocytic meningitis without high protein levels argues against a viral infection (Smith et al., 1973). Intrathecal inflammation is more difficult to evaluate if total protein levels exceed 80 mg per 100 ml in the CSF, since above this level, any plasma globulins have free access to CSF.

Some elaborate diagnostic tests of the CSF are not yet widely used. The bromide partition test analyzes the ratio of serum to CSF bromide 48 hours after ingesting bromide. This ratio is below 1.9 in nearly all tuberculous and in a few pyogenic meningitides and is reported normal in all other neurologic diseases (Smith et al., 1955; Da Costa et al, 1977). CSF lactic acid is increased above 3.9 mEq/L in tuberculous meningitis but not in aseptic meningitis; it is also increased in cerebral anoxia and is therefore not discriminating (D'Souza et al., 1978). Measuring the titer of humoral antibodies to PPD tuberculin in CSF and serum appears to be highly specific and deserves a broader trial.

Bacteriology. If acid-fast bacilli are found on CSF smear, they are immediately diagnostic, but this painstaking procedure was positive in only 10 to 40 per cent of recent series (Barois, 1975; Haas et al., 1977; Stockstill and Kauffman, 1983). Older positive findings in up to 80 to 90 per cent required the centrifugation of 10 to 20 ml of lumbar CSF (Illingworth, 1956) or serial suboccipital punctures on the admission day.

Cultures are positive in 45 to 85 per cent of cases, depending on the amount of samples used and the laboratory's facilities (Haas et al., 1977; Karandanis and Shulman, 1976; Bertoye et al., 1970). Most Asian and African series attain bacteriologic proof in 10 to 15 per cent (Vejjajiva, 1974; Osuntokun et al., 1971). Initiation of treatment should by no means be delayed until the results of cultures are available, since this takes three to six weeks.

Guinea pig inoculation has the same rate of positive results, is more painstaking, and takes more time.

In the course of treatment, examination of CSF is advisable once a week for the first month, then every other week for two months, and later once a month. Usually the glucose level is the first parameter to improve, followed by cell count, and later by protein levels. Even in uncomplicated cases, it takes three to six months until CSF abnormalities disappear.

Neurodiagnostic Procedures. Electroencephalography, isotopic brain scan and cisternography, angiography, air encephalography are not diagnostic. The brain CT scan, usually normal in an early stage, often shows later a very suggestive picture: the basal cisterns are not detected on standard films but are strikingly enhanced after contrast injection. Further hypodensity of the periventricular and basal parenchyma worsens the prognosis (Bullock and Welchman, 1982). The CT scan can detect intracranial complications in the course of the disease: early edema or acute hydrocephalus, cerebral infarctions, and late atrophy (Newman et al., 1980).

Blood Studies. The peripheral neutrophil count does not exceed 10,000/cmm, and the total leukocyte count is usually not as high as in the pyogenic meningitides (Karandanis and Shulman, 1976). Hyponatremia is found on admission in 45 to 75 per cent of adults, a finding suggestive of meningeal tuberculosis if the CSF is not purulent and vomiting is not prominent. Hyponatremia is also common in *Herpes simplex* encephalitis. The blood glucose level is often above normal and must be taken into account in evaluating the CSF glucose level.

Intradermal Tuberculin Reaction (Mantoux). This test has a limited diagnostic value. It is reported negative in 3 to 15 per cent of tuberculous meningitides in European series (Barois, 1975), and up to 69 per cent in a recent series from the USA (Stockstill and Kauffman, 1983). African and Indian pediatric series reported a negative Mantoux test in 15 to 37 per cent of cases, possibly due to malnutrition and to the frequency of recent measles (Osuntokun et al., 1971; Da Costa et al., 1977). A positive test in infancy and documented positive conversions are highly informative, while a documented negative conversion suggests sarcoidosis or another disease capable of producing anergy.

Search for Other Localizations of Tuberculosis. This is imperative and is often more rewarding than CSF investigation. Direct examination and cultures of sputum, gastric washings, and urine should be performed before therapy is started.

Radiologic evidence of pulmonary tuberculosis is very frequent in meningitis following the primary infection: up to 90 per cent present the primary complex in various stages of evolution or a miliary spread. In older patients, the coincidence of meningitis with pulmonary lesions apparently dropped from around 70 per cent in the 1950s (Weiss and Flippin, 1961; Falk, 1965) to some 55 per cent in recent series (Haas et al., 1977; Stockstill and Kauffman, 1983), thus adding a further diagnostic problem where the disease is now rare. Meningeal tuberculosis is accompanied by lesions outside the chest in about 10 per cent of cases, and these lesions are mainly genitourinary. Tuberculous meningitis without evidence of tuberculosis elsewhere is found clinically in 20 to 30 per cent of adults and postmortem in 10 per cent (Falk, 1965).

Differential Diagnosis. Repeated lumbar taps, brain CT scan, a chest roentgenogram, and immunologic tests for infections other than tuberculosis are the most important procedures to exclude other causes.

Viral meningitis is either acute or the second part of a biphasic febrile disease and has no neurologic signs other than apathy, irritability, and some confusion. The CSF cell count can change from a predominance of polymorphonuclears to lymphocytes, but not the reverse; the CSF glucose is normal in 95 per cent of cases, and even when depressed, it becomes normal again when lymphocytes predominate (Karandanis and Shulman, 1976). The CSF protein level rarely exceeds 120 to 150 mg per 100 ml. All parameters usually improve on the next tap.

Subacute listeriosis with cerebral signs may be difficult to distinguish from tuberculous meningitis until the CSF culture is positive for *Listeria monocytogenes.* Partially treated bacterial meningitis rarely offers a confusing CSF picture (Mandal, 1976). Subarachnoid hemorrhage, in the absence of a history or in case of minimal leak, can resemble tuberculous meningitis. Hemosiderin-containing macrophages in the CSF may help in making the diagnosis.

In neurosyphilis, there may be cranial nerve signs and a CSF pattern like that in tuberculous meningitis, but a normal CSF glucose in syphilis and a positive serologic test for syphilis separate the two conditions. Sarcoid of the nervous system, with its depressed CSF glucose in two thirds of the cases (Gaines et al., 1970), can be indistinguishable from meningeal tuberculosis.

Leukemic meningitis occurs mainly in hematologic remission; the CSF glucose level and often the CSF protein level are within the normal range. Carcinomatous or sarcomatous meningitis can be easily confused with tuberculous meningitis because it may develop without a detectable primary tumor, tends to cause massive involvement of the cranial and spinal nerves and/or severe intracranial hypertension, and lowers the CSF glucose level while elevating the protein level. In all three conditions, the diagnosis depends on cytologic examination of the CSF.

Focal cerebral signs and/or intracranial hypertension with predominantly lymphocytic meningitis can be seen in any viral meningoencephalitis (particularly that due to *Herpes simplex* virus), bacterial brain abscess, fungal infection, parasitic disease, and intracranial venous thrombosis. Necrotic malignant tumors close to the pia or ependyma and benign intraventricular tumors can cause a "meningitis" with occasionally a low glucose level.

Focal neurologic or electroencephalographic findings pointing to temporal lobe disease may be helpful in recognizing herpes encephalitis. In cryptococcal meningitis there is seldom fever, an underlying immunosuppressive disease is often present, or immunosuppressive drugs are being given. The cryptococci are easily cultured in a week or less from the CSF and may be seen there in Gram stains. Cryptococcal antigen may be found in the CSF by immunologic tests. Brain abscesses can often be recognized because there is usually a chronic focus of infection in the ears, mastoid, sinuses, or lung from which the infection spreads to the brain. Cysticercosis of the brain can be a difficult diagnostic problem and may ultimately depend on cysticercal serology for diagnosis. Occasionally, the tell-tale subcutaneous cysticercal calcifications can be seen in roentgenograms of the chest or extremities, and a history of residence in an endemic area may be obtained. In Mexico, for example, cysticercosis is the main cause of epilepsy. The characteristic mass lesions of brain abscess and cysticercosis should be found by computerized axial tomography (CT) of the brain.

The fever with apathy and confusion of typhoid and brucellosis may be easily confused with that of meningeal tuberculosis, especially, if *Brucella* or typhoidal meningitis occurs. Both *S. typhosa* and *Brucella* sp. can be cultured from the blood without much trouble, and in brucellosis, the agglutinin test is invariably positive.

TREATMENT. A combination of several antituberculous drugs for several months, followed by one drug for a total of 18 to 24 months, is the usual therapy.

Isoniazid plus rifampin and ethambutol is one of the favorite combinations now. Isoniazid, 5 to 8 mg/kg in adults and 10 mg/kg in children, can be given in a single daily dose; 50 mg of pyridoxine daily is added to prevent neuropathy. As the single most effective drug, isoniazid is the one to continue for 18 to 24 months. Rifampin, 600 mg daily in adults (10 mg/kg if overweight or underweight) and 15 to 20 mg/kg in children, is given in one dose and for a period of five to six months. Ethambutol, 15 mg/kg in a single daily dose, should be given for three to six months. Feeding by nasogastric tube is often necessary for this combination. In case of intolerance to either drug, ethionamide, 15 to 30 mg/kg per day in children or 500 to 1000 mg in adults as a single dose (or para-aminosalicylic acid and streptomycin, as detailed below) can be substituted. Liver function tests must be made regularly.

The combination of streptomycin and isoniazid, with or without para-aminosalicylic acid, is still advocated in certain countries. Streptomycin, 40 mg/kg per day in children or 2 g daily in adults, is injected for three to four months; it can be reduced later. Isoniazid is recommended at an initial higher dose than in the previous regimen: 8 to 10 mg/kg in adults and 15 to 20 mg/kg in children. Control of renal function and of audiolabyrinthine function is necessary.

Corticosteroids are of debatable value but are widely used in practice. They should be restricted to those patients with early brain edema occurring spontaneously or after onset of treatment (dexamethasone, 4 to 10 mg I.V. every four hours for one or two days, tapered off over the next week). Corticosteroids do not prevent the fibrosis that results from organization of exudate in the subarachnoid spaces and produces cisternal or spinal blocks. Repeated intrathecal injections of hyaluronidase may reduce this late complication (Gourie-Devi and Satish, 1980).

Antiepileptic drugs are given if necessary. A possible interaction with antituberculous drugs should be kept in mind.

Nursing care in severely ill patients may require a nasogastric tube for feeding and drug intake, urinary catheter, pharyngeal aspiration, occasional tracheotomy, and assisted ventilation. Electrolytes must be monitored, and superinfections treated. Changes of posture are needed to prevent bed sores and ankylosis.

Surgical procedures consist mainly of ventricular shunt in case of obstructive hydrocephalus, which can be accurately determined by CT scan (Newman et al., 1980; Bullock and Welchman, 1982). A sudden blindness may occasionally justify a decompression of the optic chiasm.

PROPHYLAXIS. Pulmonary tuberculosis in one member of the household is the most common cause of tuberculous meningitis in infants and children. Isoniazid should be given in a daily dose of 10 mg/kg to all children under 5 years old who react to tuberculin. In the United States Public Health Service prophylaxis study of 275 children with positive tuberculin tests, there were no cases of meningeal tuberculosis among those given 4 to 6 mg/kg isoniazid daily for one year, whereas six cases of the disease occurred in the controls given a placebo instead of isoniazid. Mass BCG vaccination of the newborn has probably been the most effective step in dramatically reducing the disease in many developing countries. It confers a protection at best of about 80 per cent, so that a previous vaccination does not rule out the possibility that a case of meningitis is of tuberculous origin.

Tuberculomas of the Brain

Douglas D. Richman, M.D.

Tuberculomas of the brain are an uncommon extrapulmonary manifestation of tuberculosis. They are focal caseating granulomatous lesions within the substance of the brain that behave clinically as space-occupying lesions. Tuberculomas are important in the differential diagnosis of space-occupying lesions of the brain because they can be cured.

Tuberculomas of the brain are recognized predominantly in populations with a high incidence of tuberculosis, where they may comprise a large proportion of intracranial tumors (Dastur and Desai, 1965). They may occur at any age but are most frequent in children and young adults. However, in developed countries, where tuberculin reactivity has shifted largely to older persons, tuberculoma of the brain is also seen more at an older age (Anderson and Macmillan, 1975; Mayers et al., 1978).

The pathogenesis of brain tuberculomas can be deduced from Rich's studies of the pathogenesis of tuberculous meningitis (Rich, 1933 and 1951). He demonstrated that tuberculous meningitis was almost always associated with focal caseous lesions that were older than the meningitis and communicated with the meninges. The pathophysiology and the clinical picture of tuberculous meningitis are a consequence of the inflammatory response to the discharge of mycobacteria and their antigens into the cerebrospinal fluid from the local caseous lesion. Such local lesions far exceed in number the cases of meningitis because most do not rupture into the cerebrospinal fluid. A tuberculoma of the brain probably becomes evident clinically in the rare circumstance in which a caseous lesion of the brain grows without rupturing.

Tuberculomas of the brain are usually typical caseating granulomas containing variable microscopic calcification and surrounded by chronic and subacute inflammation. Tuberculomas may range in size from microscopic to those that extend throughout a whole lobe of the brain.

The failure of a tuberculoma to rupture results in a strikingly different clinical presentation from meningitis (Dastur and Desai, 1965; Anderson and Macmillan, 1975; Mayers et al., 1978; Loizou and Anderson, 1982; Harder et al., 1983). A tuberculoma may appear either abruptly with signs of a space-occupying lesion of the brain or as a slowly progressive intracranial tumor with symptoms lasting a year or longer. The patient may have seizures, focal neurologic signs, and, most frequently, signs and symptoms of elevated intracranial pressure such as headache, vomiting, visual disturbances, and papilledema. In the absence of extracranial tuberculosis, which is occasionally found, intracranial tuberculosis should be suspected from fever, a positive tuberculin test, an epidemiologic background of tuberculosis, or a past history of tuberculosis. There is nothing to distinguish the clinical manifestations of tuberculomas from other space-occupying lesions of the brain.

Tuberculomas may occur anywhere in the brain; however, they appear to have a slightly increased predilection for infratentorial structures, especially the cerebellum (Dastur and Desai, 1965). In the past, the diagnosis of a single lesion has been made as often as multiple lesions; however, with more sensitive and accessible radiographic techniques, including angiography and computerized tomography, multiple lesions are being recognized more frequently. This tendency to multiple lesions makes localization of a tuberculoma by neurologic examination less accurate than localization of a malignancy or another tumor.

The plain roentgenogram of the skull may show signs of increased intracranial pressure, such as increased convolutional markings, erosion of the dorsum sellae, or separation of the sutures in infants. Calcification in the lesion has been visualized only rarely by x-ray (Dastur and Desai, 1965; Anderson and Macmillan, 1975).

Radionuclide brain scans are often negative. Cerebral angiography has demonstrated displacement of vessels without the neovascularization seen with many malignancies. Computerized tomography is proving extremely valuable for the evaluation of tuberculomas of the brain (Whelan and Stern, 1981; Loizou and Anderson, 1982; Harder et al., 1983). They are of diminished or normal density without the administration of contrast medium, although calcification in older lesions may result in increased density. Following intravenous contrast medium, the lesions characteristically demonstrate either a uniform or ring-shaped enhancement. They resolve with antituberculous chemotherapy over a period of months.

Tuberculomas of the brain must be recognized early so that antituberculous drugs can be started before elevated intracranial pressure causes irreversible neurologic damage, such as blindness, or kills the patient. Most of the literature on this disease has been written by neurosurgeons who have treated patients for space-occupying lesions. With modern chemotherapy, surgery should be limited to biopsy or decompression; excision or drainage is not necessary except to relieve pressure and can cause complications (Harder et al., 1983). The role for excision becomes even more dubious now that multiple tuberculomas are being increasingly recognized. The response to chemotherapy is usually so prompt and clear-cut that a therapeutic trial has diagnostic value. Three hundred milligrams of isoniazid, along with 600 mg of rifampicin, daily in the adult probably constitute the best regimen currently available in view of their efficacy against *M. tuberculosis* and their ability to penetrate the brain. Although tuberculomas are too rare to allow a systematic evaluation of steroids, these drugs are probably indicated initially for a short period to diminish the inflammatory response. Steroids may preclude the need for surgical decompression, and a short course carries little risk in the presence of specific antituberculous chemotherapy (Harder et al., 1983). It must be remembered, however, that the nonspecific improvement with steroids will eliminate the diagnostic value of a therapeutic trial of antituberculous drugs.

References

Anderson, J. M., and Macmillan, J. J.: Intracranial tuberculoma—an increasing problem in Britain. J Neurol Neurosurg Psychiatry 38:194, 1975.

Balaparameswararao, M. S., and Dinakar, I.: Tuberculomas of the brain. Int Surg 57:216, 1972.

Barois, A.: Les méningites tuberculeuses. Rev Prat 25:633, 1975.

Bertoye, A., Garin, J. P., Vincent, P., Monier, P., Bertrand, J. L., Da Costa, H., Borker, A., and Loken, M.: Distribution of orally administered bromine-82 in tubercular meningitis: Concise communication. J Nucl Med 18:123, 1977.

Bullock, M. R. R., and Welchman, J. M.: Diagnostic and prognostic features of tuberculous meningitis on CT scanning. J Neurol Neurosurg Psychiat 45:1098, 1982.

Crocco, J. A.: Tuberculous meningitis in adults: clinical analysis. NY State J Med 80:1231, 1980.

Damergis, J. A., Leftwich, E. I., Curtin, J. A., and Witorsch, P.: Tuberculoma of the brain. JAMA 239:413, 1978.

Dastur, H. M., and Desai, A. D.: A comparative study of brain tuberculomas and gliomas based upon 107 case records of each. Brain 88:375, 1965.

D'Souza, E., Mandal, B. K., Hooper, J., and Parker, L.: Lactic-acid concentration in cerebrospinal fluid and differential diagnosis of meningitis. Lancet 2:579, 1978.

Falk, A.: Tuberculous meningitis in adults, with special reference to survival, neurologic residuals, and work status. Am Rev Resp Dis 91:823, 1965.

Fisher, C. M.: In Picard, E. H., and Richardson, E. P.: Seizures, hemiparesis and coma with cerebrospinal fluid pleiocytosis. N Engl J Med 290:1130, 1974.

Freiman, I., and Geefhuysen, J.: Evaluation of intrathecal therapy with streptomycin and hydrocortisone in tuberculous meningitis. J Pediatr 76:895, 1970.

Gaines, J. D., Eckman, P. B., and Remington, J. S.: Low CSF glucose level in sarcoidosis involving the central nervous system. Arch Intern Med 125:333, 1970.

Gourie-Devi, M., and Satish, P.: Hyaluronidase as an adjuvant in the treatment of cranial arachnoiditis (hydrocephalus and optochiasmatic arachnoiditis) complicating tuberculous meningitis. Acta Neurol Scand 62:368, 1980.

Haas, E. J., Madhavan, T., Quinn, E. L., Cox, F., Fisher, E., and Burch, K.: Tuberculous meningitis in an urban general hospital. Arch Intern Med 137:1518, 1977.

Harder, E., Al-Kawi, M. Z., and Carney, P.: Intracranial tuberculoma: Conservative management. Am J Med 74:570, 1983.

Hinman, A. R.: Tuberculous meningitis at Cleveland Metropolitan General Hospital 1959 to 1963. Am Rev Resp Dis 95:670, 1967.

Illingworth, R. S.: Miliary and meningeal tuberculosis. Difficulties in diagnosis. Lancet 2:646, 1956.

Karandanis, D., and Shulman, J. A.: Recent survey of infectious meningitis in adults: Review of laboratory findings in bacterial, tuberculous, and aseptic meningitis. South Med J 69:449, 1976.

Lepper, M. H., and Spies, H. W.: The present status of the treatment of tuberculosis of the central nervous system. Ann NY Acad Sci 106:106, 1963.

Lincoln, E. M., Sordillo, S. V. R., and Davies, P. A.: Tuberculous meningitis in children. A review of 167 untreated and 74 treated patients with special reference to early diagnosis. J Pediatr 57:807, 1960.

Loizou, L. A., and Anderson, M.: Intracranial tuberculomas: Correlation of computerized tomography with clinico-pathological findings. Q J Med 51:104, 1982.

Mandal, B. K.: The dilemma of partially treated bacterial meningitis. Scand J Infect Dis 8:185, 1976.

Mathew, N. T., Abraham, J., and Chandy, J.: Cerebral angiographic features in tuberculous meningitis. Neurology 20:1015, 1970.

Mayers, M. M., Kaufman, D. M., and Miller, M. H.: Recent cases of intracranial tuberculomas. Neurology 28:256, 1978.

Meyers, B. R., and Hirschman, S. Z.: Unusual presentations of tuberculous meningitis. Mount Sinai J Med 41:407, 1974.

Meyers, B. R.: Tuberculous meningitis. Med Clin North Am 66:755, 1982.

Newman, P. K., Cumming, W. J. K., and Foster, J. B.: Hydrocephalus and tuberculous meningitis in adults. J Neurol Neurosurg Psychiatry 43:1888, 1980.

Osuntokun, B. O., Adeuja, A. O. G., and Familusi, J. B.: Tuberculous meningitis in Nigerians. A study of 194 patients. Trop Geogr Med 23:225, 1971.

Rich, A. R.: The Pathogenesis of Tuberculosis, 2nd ed. Springfield, Ill. Charles C Thomas, 1951, pp. 882–894.

Rich, A. R., and McCordock, H. A.: The pathogenesis of tuberculous meningitis. Bull Johns Hopkins Hosp 52:5, 1933.

Roberts, F. J.: Problems in the diagnosis of tuberculous meningitis. Arch Neurol 38:319, 1981.

Smith, H., Bannister, B., and O'Shea, M. J.: Cerebrospinal-fluid immunoglobulins in meningitis. Lancet 2:591, 1973.
Smith, H. V., Taylor, L. M., and Hunter, G.: The blood-cerebrospinal fluid barrier in tuberculous meningitis and allied conditions. J Neurol Neurosurg Psychiatry 18:237, 1955.
Springett, V. H.: Tuberculosis in immigrants. An analysis of notification rates in Birmingham, 1960–62. Lancet 1:1091, 1964.
Stevenson, J.: Bacterial meningitis and tuberculous meningitis. Br Med J 2:411, 1973.
Stockstill, M. T., And Kauffman, C. A.: Comparison of cryptococcal and tuberculous meningitis. Arch Neurol 40:81, 1983.
Streptomycin in Tuberculosis Trials Committee, Medical Research Council: Streptomycin treatment of tuberculous meningitis. Lancet 1:582, 1948.
Swarts, S., Briggs, R. S., and Millac, P. A.: Tuberculous meningitis in Asian patients. Lancet 2:15, 1981.
Tandon, P. N., and Pathak, S. N.: Tuberculosis of the central nervous system. In Spillane, J. D. (ed.): Tropical Neurology. London, Oxford University Press, 1973, p. 37.
Taylor, K. B., Smith, H. V., and Vollum, R. L.: Tuberculous meningitis of acute onset. J Neurol Neurosurg Psychiatry 18:165, 1955.
Udani, P. M., Parekh, U. C., and Dastur, D. K.: Neurological and related syndromes in CNS tuberculosis. Clinical features and pathogenesis. J Neurol Sci 14:341, 1971.
Vejjajiva, A.: Neuro-tuberculosis. An unsolved problem. J Med Assoc Thai 57:89, 1974.
Weiss, W., and Flippin, H. F.: The prognosis of tuberculous meningitis in the isoniazid era. Am J Med Sci 242:423, 1961.
Weiss, W., and Flippin, H. F.: The changing incidence and prognosis of tuberculous meningitis. Am J Med Sci 250:80, 1965.
Whelan, M. A., and Stern, J.: Intracranial Tuberculoma. Radiology 138:75, 1981.

167
CRYPTOCOCCAL MENINGITIS

Gerald Medoff, M.D.

Cryptococcal meningitis is a chronic, subacute, or rarely, acute, central nervous system infection caused by the yeast *Cryptococcus neoformans*. It is the most familiar and most common manifestation of disease caused by this fungus and has the highest mortality.

ETIOLOGY. Cryptococcal meningitis is caused by one species, *Cryptococcus neoformans*, an encapsulated yeast-like fungus that is pathogenic for animals and man.

PATHOGENESIS AND PATHOLOGY. The presence of *C. neoformans* in bird droppings is well documented, and, at least in the case of human infection, epidemiologic data imply that the pigeon may be the chief vector of the disease. The organism is recovered in large numbers from pigeon feces and the debris of pigeon roosts in attics and old buildings. The recent discovery of the sexual (perfect) stage of *C. neoformans* and its phylogenetic relationships to various plant pathogens suggests that there may be other forms of this organism in nature that are important in the natural history of the disease (Kwon-chung, 1975).

Necropsy studies indicate that, with rare exceptions, cryptococci enter the body through the lungs by inhalation of the aerosolized infectious particles found in the dried pigeon droppings. The primary pulmonary focus is usually subclinical; if it is symptomatic, the infection usually resolves spontaneously. Cutaneous, skeletal, and visceral lesions may occur during hematogenous dissemination, but involvement of the central nervous system (CNS) with subacute or chronic meningoencephalitis is the most frequently diagnosed and most familiar form of the mycosis. The predilection of *C. neoformans* for the CNS has not been explained, but once dissemination to the CNS occurs, the infection is progressive and, in the absence of chemotherapy, fatal. The progressive nature of the infection in the CNS as compared with lung is unexplained but may be related to a less efficient cellular or phagocytic response or a deficiency of other factors important in an adequate host response to the cryptococci (Diamond et al., 1974; Henderson et al., 1982). In support of this concept, cryptococcal infection of the central nervous system is accompanied by minimal inflammatory reaction. Even in fatal cases of meningitis the gross appearance of the meninges and brain may be almost normal. Meningeal reaction is more pronounced at the base of the brain and in the dorsal area of the cerebellum, where thickening and opacity of the membrane may cause the meninges to adhere to the cortex. If the meningeal disease progresses to encephalitis, the brain may contain numerous cystic spaces. Characteristically, the subarachnoid space contains an adherent mucoid exudate with mononuclear cells and may present the picture of a pure histiocytic granuloma. Many microscopic fields may reveal no other inflammatory cells but a few lymphocytes.

In sections stained with hematoxylin and eosin, fungus cells appear as pale blue, often thin-walled, spherical or oval bodies either without visible internal structure or with a poorly defined, frequently eccentric pink cytoplasmic mass within the cells. The size of the fungi ranges from 3 to 10 μ. In the hematoxylin and eosin sections, there is frequently a clear halo separating the fungus wall from the cytoplasm of the phagocytic cell. When stained with mucicarmine, this clear zone is revealed as a pink capsule.

In active growing cryptococcal lesions, budding cells are found without difficulty. In old lesions or in lesions with a large amount of cellular reaction and few fungi, budding is difficult to demonstrate.

CLINICAL MANIFESTATIONS. Unlike the pulmonary infection, 50 per cent of patients with cryptococcal meningitis have an underlying disease such as lymphoma, other malignancies, diabetes, or other diseases that primarily affect the immune system or require therapy with immunosuppressive drugs.

Cryptococcal invasion of the central nervous system may produce signs and symptoms of meningitis, meningoencephalitis, or a space-occupying lesion. The clinical findings vary according to the location and extent of involvement of the fungus. The course is usually subacute or chronic and can vary from a few months to years, with periods of spontaneous remission followed by recurrence of progressive disease. A few patients have a fulminant downhill course that lasts from two days to three weeks. The usual course lasts weeks to months with progressive deterioration. Untreated, about 80 per cent of patients die within six months of the onset of infection.

The most frequent symptom is headache; other common

complaints include fever, weight loss, mental aberrations, nausea, and vomiting. On examination, obtundation or confusion, cranial nerve dysfunction, meningeal signs, and signs of increased intracranial pressure are found in varying degrees. Extraneural manifestations such as skin lesions, lymphadenitis, bone lesions, and other visceral involvement may occur in about 10 per cent of the cases of cryptococcal meningitis. The symptoms and physical findings in some patients may be very minimal, and many patients are afebrile and complain only of a slight headache. One must always suspect this disease in patients who are at high risk.

The cerebrospinal fluid formula usually provides the first clue to the diagnosis. The white cell count in the spinal fluid generally ranges between 40 and 400 per cubic millimeter with a predominance of lymphocytes. Early in the disease, however, polymorphonuclear leukocytes may be the major cell type. The glucose concentration is often, but not invariably, below 50 mg per 100 ml, or 50 per cent or less than a simultaneously obtained blood glucose value. The protein level is usually elevated, especially in the presence of hydrocephalus, and the CSF pressure may be normal or high. Thus, the cerebrospinal fluid abnormalities in this infection closely resemble those in tuberculous meningitis.

COMPLICATIONS AND SEQUELAE. Cryptococcal meningitis has a mortality of 100 per cent in untreated patients and 30 to 40 per cent in patients who are treated correctly. The mortality depends on age, underlying disease, and general physical status of the patient. Those who survive may suffer permanent damage to brain tissue as a result of the infection or may require placement of a ventricular shunt owing to hydrocephalus. Permanent deafness or dysfunction of any cranial nerve may also occur as a result of the infection.

GEOGRAPHIC VARIATION. Cryptococcal meningitis occurs sporadically and has a worldwide geographic distribution. It occurs more often than would be expected by chance in white males and in association with Hodgkin's disease, leukemia, lymphoma, diabetes mellitus, and in patients being treated with steroids or other immunosuppressive agents. However, 50 per cent of patients with the infection have no underlying disease and appear to be immunologically normal. Estimates of the incidence of cryptococcal meningitis range from 200 to 300 cases of meningitis per year in the United States, but this is probably a falsely low figure because the disease is not reportable. Of the four serotypes of *C. neoformans*, A is most commonly involved in meningitis. Types B and C are more common in southern California, and D may be more common in Europe (Bennett et al., 1977).

DIAGNOSIS. Routine laboratory studies of blood and urine are usually normal or have no diagnostic abnormalities. When a diagnosis of cryptococcal meningitis is suspected, the cerebrospinal fluid should be examined microscopically with the use of the India ink technique. This test is positive in 50 to 70 per cent of cases. The sensitivity of this test is increased by centrifuging several milliliters of CSF before mixing a drop of the sediment on a microscope slide with an equal volume of India ink reagent. Although typical cryptococci are easy to identify, artifacts can be mistaken for organisms by the inexperienced eye. Confirmation of positive results of this test by culture is obligatory.

The isolation of *C. neoformans* by culture is the best diagnostic test. Five to 10 ml of CSF should be centrifuged and the sediment inoculated on to fungal culture media without antibiotics. Incubation at 37° C should be aerobic. Ideally, three to five negative cultures should be obtained before the diagnosis is dismissed. Because cryptococci grow well on routine media such as chocolate agar plates, special fungal media are not an absolute necessity. The cultures will be positive in about 95 per cent of cases. Cultures of urine should be done and are positive in about a third of cases. Sputum and blood cultures may also be helpful, although the latter are usually positive only in fulminant disease. In some patients cerebrospinal fluid obtained by cisternal tap is positive when cultures obtained by lumbar puncture are negative.

The development of the latex agglutination test for the detection of cryptococcal antigen in CSF, blood, urine, or other body fluids has been a great advance in the diagnosis of cryptococcal meningitis (Gordon and Vedder, 1966). The polysaccharide antigen can be detected in the cerebrospinal fluid of patients with cryptococcal meningitis in about 94 per cent of cases. Tests for the demonstration of serum antibody to the cryptococcus have been somewhat less useful in diagnosis but may be more helpful in determining the responses of the patient to therapy. It is important to remember that patients with a positive rheumatoid factor may have a falsely positive result when blood is examined for cryptococcal antigen, and appropriate controls should be included for correct interpretation.

In a very small number of cases, all of the above tests are negative, and a positive diagnosis can then be made by culturing or seeing the organisms in a biopsy specimen taken from the central nervous system.

TREATMENT AND PROPHYLAXIS. Before the introduction of amphotericin B in 1957, cryptococcal meningitis was almost uniformly fatal. The intravenous administration of this drug has produced a cure rate of approximately 60 per cent (Diamond and Bennett, 1974). If treated daily, adults are usually given approximately 0.5 mg/kg of body weight, although doses as low as 0.3 mg/kg and as high as 1.0 mg/kg have been used. If the patient is to be treated every other day, twice as much is given per infusion. The duration of therapy has been guided by the rapidity with which the CSF findings become normal (including the antigen determination) and how well the patient does clinically. Generally, patients are treated for six to ten weeks with a total dosage of 1.5 to 3.0 g of amphotericin B (Bennett, 1974). Occasionally, the India ink test can remain positive for months to years even though cultures are negative. This finding is not an indication for continuation of therapy beyond the usually recommended dosages.

Because intravenously administered amphotericin B does not attain therapeutic concentrations in the CSF, the drug has been injected directly into the subarachnoid space. The value of this procedure is unknown. Probably intrathecal therapy should be reserved for patients who have not responded to an adequate course of systemic therapy or for those who have severe kidney disease and cannot tolerate systemic amphotericin B. If intrathecal treatment is to be used for longer than one or two weeks, it is preferable to administer the drug into a lateral cerebral ventricle through a subcutaneous siliconized rubber reservoir (Ommaya valve) rather than by lumbar or cisternal injection. Using this route, the drug is given two or three times weekly in graded doses up to a maintenance dose of about 0.5 mg per dose.

5-Fluorocytosine (5-FC) is an oral antifungal agent with good in vitro effect against *C. neoformans*. It readily penetrates the CSF, and toxic reactions are uncommon. Its use probably should be restricted in patients with compromised renal function. Unfortunately, at the dosage used (150 mg/kg/day), its therapeutic effect appears to be inferior to that obtained with amphotericin B (Bennett, 1974). In addition, drug resistance commonly occurs during therapy with 5-FC; this is not true for amphotericin B. For these reasons 5-FC alone is not recommended for use in cryptococcal meningitis.

Combination therapy of amphotericin B and 5-FC has shown in vitro (Medoff et al., 1972) and in vivo synergism (Block and Bennett, 1973) against *C. neoformans*. A controlled study in humans has shown that 0.3 mg/kg body weight of amphotericin B per day in combination with a daily dose of 150 mg/kg body weight of 5-FC may be the best treatment for cryptococcal meningitis (Bennett et al., 1979). The combined treatment is given for 6 weeks.

Other drugs such as ketoconazole and miconazole are under investigation to determine their therapeutic efficacy against cryptococcal meningitis. It is too early to tell whether these will prove to be an improvement over the existing regimens.

In addition to antifungal therapy, patients should be carefully monitored for complications of the infection such as seizures, inappropriate ADH, and hydrocephalus. If hydrocephalus occurs, a ventricular shunt may be necessary.

No prophylactic measures against *C. neoformans* infection are known at present.

References

Bennett, J. E.: Chemotherapy of systemic mycoses. N Engl J Med 290:30, 320, 1974.

Bennett, J. E., Kwon-chung, K. J., and Howard, D. H.: Epidemiologic differences among serotypes of *Cryptococcus neoformans*. Am J Epidemiol 105:582, 1977.

Bennett, J. E., Dismukes, W. E., Duma, R. J., et al.: A comparison of amphotericin B alone with flucytosine in the treatment of cryptococcal meningitis. N Engl J Med 301:126, 1979.

Block, E. R., and Bennett, J. E.: Combined effects of 5-fluorocytosine and amphotericin B in therapy of murine cryptococcosis. Proc Soc Exp Biol Med 142:476, 1973.

Diamond, R. D., and Bennett, J. E.: Prognostic factors in cryptococcal meningitis. Ann Intern Med 80:176, 1974.

Diamond, R. D., May, J. E., Kane, M. A., Frank, M. M., and Bennett, J. E.: The role of the classical and alternate complement pathways in host defenses against *Cryptococcus neoformans* infection. J Immunol 112:2260, 1974.

Gordon, M. A., and Vedder, D. K.: Serologic tests in diagnosis and prognosis of cryptococcosis. JAMA 197:961, 1966.

Henderson, D. K., Bennett, J. E., and Herber, M. A.: Long-lasting specific immunologic unresponsiveness associated with cryptococcal meningitis. J Clin Invest 69:1185, 1982.

Kwon-chung, K. J.: Description of a new genus Filobasidiella, the perfect state of *Cryptococcus neoformans*. Mycologia 67:1197, 1975.

Medoff, G., Kobayashi, G. S., Kwan, C. N., Schlessinger, D., and Venkov, P.: Potentiation of rifampicin and 5-fluorocytosine as antifungal antibiotics by amphotericin B. Proc Natl Acad Sci USA 69:196, 1972.

Spickard, A.: Diagnosis and treatment of cryptococcal disease. South Med J 66:26, 1973.

168
COCCIDIOIDAL MENINGITIS

DAVID A. STEVENS, M.D.

Coccidioidal meningitis is a granulomatous infection of the central nervous system (CNS) caused by *Coccidioides immitis*, a soil-associated fungus. This disease is the most severe and ominous complication of disseminated coccidioidomycosis because the mortality rate of untreated cases approaches 100 per cent. Dissemination occurs early after the primary pulmonary infection. The symptoms of meningitis usually appear within six months of primary coccidioidomycosis. Most primary infections are asymptomatic or undiagnosed, so that meningitis may be the first recognized manifestation of coccidioidomycosis (Kelly, 1980; Bouza et al., 1981). Less than 0.5 per cent of Caucasians with primary coccidioidomycosis develop disseminated disease.

ETIOLOGY. *C. immitis* is a dimorphic fungus that lives in the soil of the lower Sonoran life zone of the southwestern United States, Mexico, and South America. It is fully described in Chapter 77.

PATHOGENESIS AND PATHOLOGY. The fungus is inhaled into the lung and replicates there, stimulating cell-mediated immunity. If the host defenses fail to contain the infection, it may result in chronic pulmonary disease or hematogenous dissemination. The basilar meninges and sulci are the most common sites of metastatic CNS infection. Chronic meningitis may be complicated by hydrocephalus.

The basic tissue response to *C. immitis* is granulomatous, but focal areas of purulence occur, and fibrosis may develop in cases of long duration. Space-occupying lesions in the brain or spinal cord are rare. Intracranial or spinal epidural abscesses are usually secondary to an overlying osteomyelitis. The characteristic tissue form of the fungus, the spherule, can be found in the granulomas. Granulomatous cerebral arteritis can cause multiple areas of encephalomalacia. Granulomatous ependymitis may also be prominent.

CLINICAL MANIFESTATIONS AND DIAGNOSIS. The florid signs and symptoms of meningeal irritation that are common in bacterial meningitis are usually absent in coccidioidal disease. The most common symptom is headache. Fever, weakness, confusion, sluggishness, seizures, abnormal behavior, stiff neck, diplopia, ataxia, vomiting, and focal neurologic defects may occur. Coccidioidal skin lesions at the nasolabial fold are said to accompany meningeal disease frequently. Examination of the cerebrospinal fluid (CSF) reveals a pleocytosis that is usually mononuclear (eosinophils are sometimes seen), but polymorphonuclears may predominate early in the illness or during exacerbations. The CSF glucose level is decreased and the protein level is increased. Cisternal or lumbar CSF is a much better indicator of disease activity than ventricular fluid, which commonly has a higher glucose concentration, a lower protein concentration, lower antibody titers, and fewer cells. Cultures of the CSF are positive in less than one third of cases, and direct visualization of the organism is extremely rare. Complement-fixing (CF) antibody is present in the serum, but titers may not be high when meningitis is the only manifestation of coccidioidomycosis. When meningitis is associated with other forms of disseminated disease the CF titer is usually ≥1:32 in the serum. Most patients also have CF antibody to *C. immitis* in their CSF (70 per cent on the first examination). In those who do not and who also have low titers of antibody in the serum, it is difficult to establish the diagnosis. Repeated assays for antibody in the CSF must be performed. As the disease progresses, almost all patients develop antibody in the CSF. CF antibody can also be detected in the unconcentrated CSF in some patients with parameningeal lesions (e.g., epidural abscesses, bony lesions that abut the dura) but is not seen in other forms of coccidioidal disease without accompanying meningitis.

The diagnosis should be suspected in a patient with typical CSF findings and evidence of previous or concurrent coccidioidal disease anywhere in the body or appropriate exposure history. Other causes of meningitis should be excluded by appropriate cultures. The diagnosis of coccidioidal meningitis is confirmed either by detection of CF antibody in the CSF (in the absence of parameningeal disease) or by isolating the fungus from the CSF. It is important to make the diagnosis early because early treatment appears to correlate with a successful outcome.

The CF titers of the CSF parallel the course of the disease in the same way that serum CF titers follow the course of systemic infection (see Chapter 126). Rising titers indicate worsening disease, and falling titers indicate improvement. Patients who relapse after a response to therapy usually develop a pleocytosis or chemical abnormalities before the CSF antibody recurs.

TREATMENT AND COMPLICATIONS. Without treatment, about 90 per cent of patients die within one year. Untreated cases of chronic meningitis are rare but one reported case survived over 10 years. Intrathecal amphotericin B is the accepted treatment. Patients who have only meningitis are also treated with modest courses (0.5 to 1.0 g) of systemic amphotericin B. This practice is intended, at least in part, as prophylaxis against other occult foci of infection since intrathecal therapy is the essential treatment of meningitis. This situation differs from cryptococcal meningitis, which may be successfully treated by intravenous amphotericin B alone in some patients. If patients are known to have other foci of coccidioidal infection, the duration of systemic treatment should be altered to that usual for infection of that organ.

Intrathecal therapy can be administered by four routes: lumbar, cisternal, ventricular, and cervical. Corticosteroids (25 mg of hydrocortisone) may be administered simultaneously to reduce local reactions. It is advisable to begin therapy with low doses of amphotericin (0.01 to 0.025 mg) and increase the dose gradually as tolerated. Lumbar delivery is by barbotage or by suspension of the drug in hypertonic (10 per cent) glucose. With the patient on a table tilted head down, the hypertonic solution reaches the basilar area with minimal dilution. The maximum lumbar dose is usually about 0.5 mg, but the dose and frequency may need to be modified because of intolerance. Complications of lumbar therapy include local and radicular pain, headaches, paresthesias, nerve palsies that do not necessarily correspond to the level of injection, bladder dystonia, and impotence. The symptoms are usually transient. These problems have been attributed largely to amphotericin-induced arachnoiditis. However, amphotericin B can also cause neurotoxic myelopathy, probably on a vascular basis (Carnevale et al., 1980). Transient symptoms may precede more profound deficits. Cisternal therapy has the advantage of placing the drug closest to the site of maximum infection, the basilar meninges. Doses of 0.01 to 1.0 mg have been used; ≤0.25 mg in a ≤0.5 ml volume is most common. Complications of cisternal therapy are rare if the injections are given by a physician experienced in cisternal puncture. Headaches, nausea, vomiting, hypertension, bradycardia, arrhythmias, cranial palsies, dysequilibrium and gait problems, and rare instances of upper motor neuron impairment have occurred. These complications are caused by arachnoiditis, possibly by direct neurotoxicity, and by hemorrhage. Hemorrhage may cause meningismus, compression of the brain stem, and obstruction of the outflow of the fourth ventricle. Direct puncture of the brain, usually the medulla but occasionally the cerebellar tonsil or pons, causes immediate cough, vomiting, weakness, electric sensations, and respiratory difficulties. Ventricular therapy through an Ommaya reservoir places the drug distant from the usual principal site of infection but is necessary if the ventricles are infected. It is generally useless in the presence of a ventricular shunt because the drug is diverted out of the central nervous system unless the distal end of the tubing is placed in the cisterna magna. Some newer ventricular shunts have a valve permitting temporary occlusion by external pressure. The usual intraventricular dose is 0.01 to 0.5 mg. Mechanical problems often complicate this form of therapy, and the ventricular end of the catheter may cause damage. Bacterial superinfection is common. Experience with lateral cervical puncture is limited but this technique is reputedly safe and less troublesome than other methods if the physician is experienced. Obstruction by infection and/or fibrosis may prevent the movement of amphotericin B within the subarachnoid space no matter how the drug is administered. This complication may be detected by myelography, radioisotope flow studies, or computerized tomography.

There are no clear-cut guidelines for the frequency and duration of therapy. Recommendations for duration vary from three months after the CF antibody disappears from the CSF to treatment for life. Holeman had good results with a large, long-term series of patients treated with intrathecal amphotericin three times weekly for three months or until the cells in the CSF are $<10/mm^3$ (whichever is longer), then one to two times weekly for several months tapering to once every one to six weeks (Kelly, 1980). Whenever the cell count exceeds 10, the frequency is increased until the count falls below this level. If frank clinical relapse or marked abnormalities in the CSF recur, the patient is retreated like a new patient. Therapy is discontinued only after the CSF has been completely normal for at least a year on a once every six weeks treatment schedule. After treatment is discontinued, the CSF is examined every six weeks for at least one to two years. This is important because other studies have indicated that relapses occur most commonly one to two years after the end of a course of apparently successful therapy. We also have treated several patients by this regimen who appear to be cured more than 2 years after therapy was discontinued. Winn (1967) achieved comparable results with intrathecal amphotericin two times weekly until the CSF improved, then one to two times weekly until three months after the CF antibody disappeared from the CSF. He also examined the CSF intermittently for at least two years.

An imidazole, miconazole, offers a possible alternative to amphotericin. Some patients with disease unresponsive to amphotericin have responded to intravenous miconazole alone, intrathecal miconazole alone, or a combination of the two (Stevens, 1983). Doses of 20 mg intrathecally are well tolerated and produce CSF levels that exceed the minimal inhibitory concentration of *C. immitis* for 24 hours. Patients with meningeal disease of longer duration are less likely to respond, and relapses have occurred after short courses of therapy. The relative efficacy of miconazole and amphotericin B awaits comparative trials. The ability to treat meningitis by a systemic route of administration would represent a significant advance and is essential for patients with internal obstruction to the flow of CSF. Initial reports on an oral imidazole, ketoconazole, suggest patients with meningitis may respond to high (≥800 mg/day) doses (Craven et al., 1983).

Correct management of coccidioidal meningitis requires an awareness of the possibility of hydrocephalus and ventriculitis. Hydrocephalus is often the cause of deterioration in a patient whose CSF is unchanged or even improving on therapy. Patients with ventriculitis are refractory to therapy. Computerized tomography has replaced other methods in the detection of these complications. Shunting the flow of the CSF may prevent irreversible brain damage from hydrocephalus. Spread of infection from the distal end of the shunt is an unavoidable risk of this procedure. Concomitant intravenous therapy should be administered as long as ventricular cultures remain positive.

References

Bouza, E., Dreyer, J. S., Hewitt, W. L., et al.: Coccidioidal meningitis: An analysis of 31 cases and review of the literature. Medicine 60:139, 1981.

Carnevale, N. T., Galgiani, J. N., Stevens, D. A., et al.: Amphotericin B-induced myelopathy. Arch Int Med 140:1189, 1980.

Craven, P. C., Graybill, J. R., Jorgensen, J. H., et al.: High-dose ketoconazole for treatment of fungal infections of the central nervous system. Ann Intern Med 98:160, 1983.

Kelly, P. C. Coccidioidal meningitis. In Stevens, D. A. (ed.): Coccidioidomycosis: A Text. New York, Plenum Medical Book Co., 1980, pp. 163-193.

Stevens, D. A. An update on miconazole therapy for coccidioidomycosis. Drugs, 26:347, 1983.

Winn, W. A.: Coccidioidal meningitis: A follow-up report. In Ajello, L. (ed.): Coccidioidomycosis. Tucson, University of Arizona Press, 1967, pp. 55-61.

169

LYMPHOCYTIC CHORIOMENINGITIS

FRITZ LEHMANN-GRUBE, M.D.

Lymphocytic choriomeningitis is an illness of animals and man after infection with the lymphocytic choriomeningitis (LCM) virus. The symptomatology of the human disease ranges from a grippe-like syndrome to meningitis and encephalomyelitis. Lymphocytic choriomeningitis is a zoonosis; the principal reservoir in nature of LCM virus is the gray house mouse.

ETIOLOGY. The LCM virus was discovered independently and at about the same time on three occasions in the United States. Armstrong and Lillie (1934) encountered it when they passaged in monkeys "infectious materials" from a fatal case of the 1933 St. Louis epidemic of St. Louis encephalitis; Traub (1935) found albino mice from a laboratory colony to be infected; and Rivers and Scott (1935) isolated this agent from two cases of meningitis. The name was chosen to reflect the pathologic picture produced in monkeys and mice by intracerebral inoculation of the virus.

For a long time the LCM virus remained unclassified until other agents with similar properties were revealed, which led to the formation of a taxonomic group with the name arenoviruses (Rowe et al., 1970), later changed to arenaviruses (Matthews, 1982).

The LCM virus is released from the infected cell by a budding process in which the plasma membrane becomes the viral envelope. The infectious unit has a diameter of approximately 100 nm (Lehmann-Grube et al., 1983). The viral envelopes are covered with club-shaped projections that are approximately 10 nm long. In their otherwise unstructured interior, LCM virus particles contain one to several 20- to 25-nm electron-dense particles resembling cellular ribosomes (Dalton et al., 1968; Murphy and Whitfield, 1975). Their appearance is so characteristic for all the arenaviruses that they have formed the basis for the name *arenosus*, meaning sandy.

The genetic information of LCM virus resides in two classes of RNA called "L" and "S". They are of negative polarity and have molecular weights 2.1 and 1.1 $\times$ 10^6, respectively. Usually, virus preparations also contain cellular RNAs (Pedersen, 1979), but whether these are derived from the already mentioned ribosome-like granules seen with the electron microscope inside virions is not certain (Müller et al., 1983). Differences of biologic properties of strains of LCM virus were found to be reflected in differences of oligonucleotide patterns obtained by enzymatic digestion of their RNAs (Dutko and Oldstone, 1983).

Seven distinct virus polypeptides have so far been resolved, which we call, according to apparent molecular weight and glycosylation status, p200, gp85, p77, p63 ("NP"), gp60, gp44 ("GP-1"), and gp35 ("GP-2") (Buchmeier et al., 1980; Bruns et al., 1983b).

It is *a priori* likely and has been shown experimentally that many structural and nonstructural components of the LCM virus are immunogenic; three have been defined to some extent. One is gp44, which causes neutralizing antibody to be formed. It is situated on the surface of the virion and on infected cells. This antigen also fixes complement in the presence of the appropriate antibody, but the antigen titers are low (Bruns et al., 1983a). Cell-mediated immunity is induced by a structure that is expressed on cells and consists of two components, one being virus, the other a gene product of the major histocompatibility complex (Zinkernagel and Doherty, 1979). The third immunogen to be mentioned induces the formation of highly active complement-fixing antibody. It corresponds to the viral nucleoprotein (p63) and is not represented on either the virion or the infected cell, but a serologically indistinguishable substance is produced in large quantities in cells (Smadel et al., 1940; Gschwender et al., 1976). Besides the complement-fixation test, this antigen can be detected and measured by immunofluorescence procedures, double immunodiffusion tests, and radioimmunoassays.

PATHOGENESIS AND PATHOLOGY. The disease of the adult mouse infected with LCM virus is entirely immunopathologic in nature (Lehmann-Grube and Löhler, 1981). This well established fact has sometimes led to the assumption that in human lymphocytic choriomeningitis similar mechanisms are involved. There is nothing to indicate that the human illness has an allergic mechanism different from the immunopathologic component assumed to be associated with most viral diseases.

Human lymphocytic choriomeningitis is rarely fatal, and in the few cases with autopsy findings the etiology was not always convincingly revealed. In the case of Mitchell and Klotz (1942), in which the clinical diagnosis was LCM virus meningitis, the brain was swollen, thereby causing a cerebellar pressure cone. The arachnoid was markedly thickened and contained many lymphocytes and monocytes. With the severely altered vessels the inflammation extended into the Virchow-Robin spaces. There was little infiltration of the nervous tissue itself. Scheid et al. (1956b) described hemorrhagic necrotizing meningoencephalitis mainly involving the cortex. The central portions of the brain were less severely affected, showing predominantly perivascular infiltrations and glial proliferations. Capillary hemorrhages were also found in the cerebellar cortex, in the pontine nuclei, and in the nuclei of the cranial nerves with a pattern reminiscent of encephalitis caused by *Rickettsia prowazekii.* Death after meningoencephalitis was described by Warkel et al. (1973). In the brain there was marked meningeal perivascular inflammation, being most extensive in the sulci and over the brain stem and extending into dilated Virchow-Robin spaces. In the pons and medulla there were focal inflammatory nodules, and in the subcortical white matter of the cerebrum, pons, and cerebellum minimal to moderate signs of edema were observed. There was marked perivascular cuffing in the spinal cord and its coverings.

The infant that had died after transplacental infection (see below) and the three fatalities described by Armstrong are not included here because these cases were unusual and probably not representative of human lymphocytic choriomeningitis.

CLINICAL MANIFESTATIONS. When describing the symptomatology of human lymphocytic choriomeningitis, it is customary to disregard mode of infection and source of the virus. This approach does not appear permissible because the consequences of natural infections, accidental laboratory infections, and infections induced for therapeutic purposes (pyretotherapy) differ markedly. In particular, the history of the virus seems to have profound effects on the clinical picture in man. In the following, a subdivision will be made, and illnesses due to infection under natural conditions will be considered first.

Armstrong (1942) differentiated three major forms: the "grippal or non-nervous system," the "meningeal," and the "meningoencephalitic" types. This classification has been found useful (Scheid, 1957; Lehmann-Grube, 1971) and will be adhered to here. Inapparent infections with LCM virus seem to occur rather frequently.

The incubation period is 6 to 13 days or longer. The grippal type of lymphocytic choriomeningitis is characterized by malaise, fever, headache, myalgia, and may run a remittent course with two or three phases. The frequency of the grippal type is difficult to assess. Recent hamster-associated outbreaks indicate that it may be more common than previously assumed. Among 47 persons infected with LCM virus after contact with pet hamsters, Ackermann et al. (1972) in Germany observed the grippal type 16 times; under similar conditions Deibel et al. (1975) in New York made the diagnosis 34 times among a total of 60 cases.

The most frequent clinical manifestation of LCM virus infection is the syndrome designated by Wallgren (1925) as acute aseptic meningitis. I shall use the term LCM virus meningitis. Often preceded by a prodromic "grippe," the onset is acute with headache, fever, malaise, and muscular pain soon followed by stiff neck, vomiting, and Brudzinski's and Kernig's signs. The cerebrospinal fluid shows moderate to marked lymphocytic pleocytosis and moderate increase of protein. Hypoglycorrhachia is not a regular finding.

The distinction between meningitic and meningoencephalomyelitic types is not sharp. In meningoencephalomyelitis a multitude of symptoms and signs may be grouped in all possible combinations. Usually the course is mild and may consist solely of clouding of consciousness and fleeting organic signs of involvement of the central nervous system. Sometimes, however, the illness may be severe. Scheid et al. (1968) described in a young man a picture resembling von Economo's encephalitis lethargica. There are also cases with transverse myelitis (Werner and Wolf, 1972), and sometimes an organic type of psychosis develops lasting for a few days (Scheid and Jochheim, 1956).

The LCM virus has been incriminated in recurrent or chronic diseases, but in only a few patients was the etiology convincingly established (Treusch et al., 1943; Chesney et al., 1979). The case of encephalitis with unilateral orchitis and unilateral parotitis (Lewis and Utz, 1961) has remained a unique observation.

None of these syndromes is pathognomonic for lymphocytic choriomeningitis. Nor may the diagnosis be suspected from other nondescript symptoms associated with the disease, such as pharyngitis, sore throat, pain on moving the eyes, pleural pain, constipation or diarrhea, nausea and vomiting, skin rashes, swelling of lymph nodes, arthritis, coryza, and cough. The blood picture, too, is not very helpful. The erythrocyte sedimentation rate and leukocyte count are normal or slightly increased. Sometimes there is leukopenia.

The LCM virus may affect the unborn child if a pregnant mother becomes infected. Early in pregnancy, abortion seems to be the consequence (Ackermann et al., 1975; Biggar et al., 1975), but later the child may suffer malformations, especially hydrocephalus (Ackermann et al., 1974;

Sheinbergas, 1976; Chastel et al., 1978). In one case a pregnant woman fell ill with LCM virus meningitis and the newborn child died at the age of 12 days. LCM virus was recovered from its cerebrospinal fluid obtained one day before death (Komrower et al., 1955).

It has already been pointed out that lymphocytic choriomeningitis may exhibit unusual features if the infecting virus had been maintained under laboratory conditions. The most striking example is the three fatalities described by Armstrong (1942). Of these, two had been manufacturing distemper vaccine (presumably from cultivated dog tissues) and the third had assisted at their autopsy. There was cerebral edema but very little involvement of the meninges or choroid plexus. Rather, general damage to blood vessels was prominent. These unusually virulent isolates were shown to be LCM virus with specific antisera, but differed with respect to host range and pathologic changes they induced in experimentally infected animals. [Probably the two cases of lethal lymphocytic choriomeningitis described by Smadel et al. (1942) were among the three documented by Armstrong.]

Another case in point is H. L. W. described by Scheid et al. (1956a). This physician had worked experimentally with *Toxoplasma gondii*, employing monkeys, hamsters, and mice. He suffered from a severe illness with meningoencephalitis, myocarditis, and involvement of liver and kidneys, and for some time the prognosis was considered unfavorable. Laboratory mice were incriminated at first, but later found free of infection. Instead, the *Toxoplasma* strain with which the patient had been working, and which had been passaged for an unknown number of years in the peritoneal cavity of mice, turned out to be contaminated with LCM virus.

Of 30 persons who worked experimentally with Syrian hamsters in whom the LCM virus was unintentionally passaged together with an infected line of hamster fibrosarcoma, 10 had severe "grippe-like" illness with fever, headache, myalgias, anorexia, and chest pain. None had meningitis. During convalescence, unilateral orchitis developed in three of nine men. Arthralgias were invariably experienced, which, in two cases, progressed to frank arthritis of the hands (Baum et al., 1966).

Another unusual series of LCM virus infections involved personnel at a university medical center engaged in tumor research (Hinman et al., 1975; Vanzee et al., 1975). Again, the virus had come from transplantable tumors and had been passaged in Syrian hamsters from where it had spread to persons either handling them or working in the animal rooms. Of 48 infected individuals, only 21 had clinically apparent lymphocytic choriomeningitis. Fever, severe myalgias, headache, and chills were prominent. Two patients had LCM virus meningitis. Because leukopenia occurred in 10 of 11 patients and thrombocytopenia in eight of eight, Vanzee et al. (1975) suggested that these signs are characteristic for lymphocytic choriomeningitis. Although leukopenia has frequently been described in cases with unusual passage histories of the virus, the leukocyte counts are often normal when LCM virus comes directly from persistently infected house mice or from hamsters infected after a series of spontaneous transmissions from animal to animal. Death is an extremely rare outcome of LCM virus infection. The nine fatal cases with established etiology are listed in Table 1.

COMPLICATIONS AND SEQUELAE. Complications have not been described. Sequelae are uncommon even if the illness was initially severe. In a few patients paralyses or muscle weaknesses have remained, and in one person a "flu-like illness" was followed by lasting unilateral sensorineural deafness and labyrinth damage (Hirsch, 1976). The "severe sequelae" in one case of LCM virus encephalitis mentioned by Meyer et al. (1960) were not specified.

EPIDEMIOLOGY. It is often said that the LCM virus is distributed worldwide. Although this may be true, proof is available only for Europe (including western Russia) and North and South America (Lehmann-Grube, 1982).

When Rivers and Scott (1935) demonstrated an association between LCM virus and acute aseptic meningitis, it was thought that this syndrome was in fact a disease entity caused by the LCM virus, but it was soon realized that acute aseptic meningitis had numerous causes among which the LCM virus played but a minor role. It should be stressed that under natural conditions lymphocytic choriomeningitis is rare, as illustrated by the longitudinal study begun in 1941 by Rasmussen, continued by Adair and his colleagues, and concluded in 1958 by Meyer et al. (1960). In only 126 of 1568 patients (8 per cent) was the "acute infectious disease with CNS manifestations of apparent viral etiology" caused by the LCM virus.

The principal source of the LCM virus in nature is the gray house mouse (Armstrong, 1942) which may carry the virus lifelong in high concentrations in all its tissues. In mice the infection is perpetuated by vertical transmission. Carrier mice shed the virus with nasal secretions, saliva, and urine (Traub, 1939). Spread to other animals and man is accomplished either by direct contact, especially by a bite, or by contaminated fomites and possibly aerosols; vectors do not appear to play a role. Of the house mice, few are virus carriers and these are unevenly distributed among the mouse population (Lehmann-Grube, 1982).

As a rule, man is the last link of the infectious chain, and the same may be said about members of other species. There are, however, exceptions, of which the Syrian hamster (*Mesocricetus auratus*) is most noteworthy. This animal is easily infected by contact with carrier mice and produces large quantities of virus. Virus is shed for weeks and even months, predominantly with urine, thereby infecting other

Table 1. CASES OF FATAL LYMPHOCYTIC CHORIOMENINGITIS

Special Features	Author
1. Laboratory exposure to serially passed virus	Armstrong, 1942
2. Laboratory exposure to serially passed virus	Armstrong, 1942
3. Performed autopsies on case 1 or 2	Armstrong, 1942
4. LCM virus meningitis, 12-year-old child	Mitchell and Klotz, 1942
5. 12-day-old infant died of infection acquired transplacentally	Komrower et al., 1955
6. Bulbar paralysis	Adair et al., 1953
7. Landry-type ascending paralysis	Adair et al., 1953
8. Meningoencephalitis	Scheid et al., 1956b
9. Meningoencephalitis	Warkel et al., 1973

hamsters living in the same colony. Eventually, however, the virus is eliminated and, hence, infection of the hamster is not persistent in the way infection of a carrier mouse is (Skinner and Knight, 1979). Nonetheless, once a hamster colony is infested, it may remain so as long as susceptible young ones are born. Since LCM virus-infected hamsters are usually outwardly free of disease signs, they are not eliminated and, if sold, represent a hazard to their new owners.

Carrier mice and infected pet hamsters are the main sources of the LCM virus for man, and it is their distribution as well as frequency and intimacy of contact with people that determines the epidemiologic pattern of human infections. Cases have sometimes been observed sporadically over long periods of time in certain geographically confined rural areas. If looked for, carrier mice have invariably been found living in the same house as the diseased persons or in close proximity. If, on the other hand, the virus comes from freshly purchased hamsters, small or even large outbreaks are observed, mainly among city dwellers and often involving several members of a family.

DIAGNOSIS. No combination of symptoms or signs of human lymphocytic choriomeningitis is pathognomonic. Hence, confirmation of the etiology in a suspected case requires isolation of the agent and demonstration of a significant increase of specific antibodies. The virus may be detected during the acute stage in blood and cerebrospinal fluid that are inoculated into the brains of *adult* laboratory mice. A tentative diagnosis may be made if these animals exhibit characteristic neurologic disturbances five or more days after inoculation. Confirmation is obtained by protection tests employing LCM virus-immune mice that are challenged by intracerebral inoculation with the new agent.

For obscure reasons, the complement fixation test is often used for serologic diagnosis despite its severe limitations. In human infections LCM virus-specific complement-fixing antibody always remains in low concentration and sometimes is not detectable. Thus, false negative results are often obtained with this test. For diagnosis of a recent infection, antibody is most reliably determined by indirect immunofluorescent procedures and an infection of the more distant past is best verified by demonstrating neutralizing antibody with either mice or L cell cultures as assay hosts. Other methods have also been recommended, but they require experience and special facilities (Lehmann-Grube et al., 1979).

TREATMENT AND PROPHYLAXIS. Lymphocytic choriomeningitis is treated by supportive measures selected to meet the clinical requirements of each case. No specific antiviral drugs or vaccine for human use have been developed.

References*

Ackermann, R., Körver, G., Turss, R., Wönne, R., and Hochgesand, P.: Pränatale Infektion mit dem Virus der Lymphozytären Choriomeningitis. Bericht über zwei Fälle. Dtsch med Wschr 99:629, 1974.

Ackermann, R., Stammler, A., and Armbruster, B.: Isolierung von Virus der Lymphozytären Choriomeningitis aus Abrasionsmaterial nach Kontakt der Schwangeren mit einem Syrischen Goldhamster (Mesocricetus auratus). Infection 3:47, 1975.

*See Chapter 67 for References cited in text but not listed.

Ackermann, R., Stille, W., Blumenthal, W., Helm, E. B., Keller, K., and Baldus, O.: Syrische Goldhamster als Überträger von Lymphozytärer Choriomeningitis. Dtsch med Wschr 97:1725, 1972.

Adair, C. V., Gauld, R. L., and Smadel, J. E.: Aseptic meningitis, a disease of diverse etiology: clinical and etiologic studies on 854 cases. Ann Intern Med 39:675, 1953.

Armstrong, C.: Some recent research in the field of neurotropic viruses with especial reference to lymphocytic choriomeningitis and herpes simplex. Milit Surgeon, Wash 91:129, 1942.

Baum, S. G., Lewis, A. M., Rowe, W. P., and Huebner, R. J.: Epidemic nonmeningitic lymphocytic-choriomeningitis-virus infection. An outbreak in a population of laboratory personnel. N Engl J Med 274:934, 1966.

Biggar, R. J., Woodall, J. P., Walter, P. D., and Haughie, G. E.: Lymphocytic choriomeningitis outbreak associated with pet hamsters. Fifty-seven cases from New York state. JAMA 232:494, 1975.

Chastel, C., Bosshard, S., Le Goff, F., Quillien, M.-C., Gilly, R., and Aymard, M.: Infection transplacentaire par le virus de la chorioméningite lymphocytaire. Résultats d'une enquête sérologique retrospective en France. Nouv Presse Méd 7:1089, 1978.

Chesney, P. J., Katcher, M. L., Nelson, D. B., and Horowitz, S. D.: CSF eosinophilia and chronic lymphocytic choriomeningitis virus meningitis. J Pediat 94:750, 1979.

Dalton, A. J., Rowe, W. P., Smith, G. H., Wilsnack, R. E., and Pugh, W. E.: Morphological and cytochemical studies on lymphocytic choriomeningitis virus. J Virol 2:1465, 1968.

Deibel, R., Woodall, J. P., Decher, W. J., and Schryver, G. D.: Lymphocytic choriomeningitis virus in man. Serologic evidence of association with pet hamsters. JAMA 232:501, 1975.

Dutko, F. J., and Oldstone, M. B. A.: Genomic and biological variation among commonly used lymphocytic choriomeningitis virus strains. J Gen Virol 64:1689, 1983.

Hinman, A. R., Fraser, D. W., Douglas, R. G., Bowen, G. S., Kraus, A. L., Winkler, W. G., and Rhodes, W. W.: Outbreak of lymphocytic choriomeningitis virus infections in medical center personnel. Am J Epidem 101:103, 1975.

Hirsch, E.: Sensorineural deafness and labyrinth damage due to lymphocytic choriomeningitis. Report of a case. Arch Otolaryng 102:499, 1976.

Komrower, G. M., Williams, B. L., and Stones, P. B.: Lymphocytic choriomeningitis in the newborn. Probable transplacental infection. Lancet I: 697, 1955.

Lehmann-Grube, F.: Lymphocytic Choriomeningitis Virus. Virology Monographs Vol. 10. Vienna and New York, Springer-Verlag, 1971.

Lehmann-Grube, F., Kallay, M., Ibscher, B., and Schwartz, R.: Serologic diagnosis of human infections with lymphocytic choriomeningitis virus: comparative evaluation of seven methods. J Med Virol 4:125, 1979.

Lewis, J. M., and Utz, J. P.: Orchitis, parotitis and meningoencephalitis due to lymphocytic-choriomeningitis virus. N Engl J Med 265:776, 1961.

Meyer, H. M., Johnson, R. T., Crawford, I. P., Dascomb, H. E., and Rogers, N. G.: Central nervous system syndromes of "viral" etiology. A study of 713 cases. Am J Med 29:334, 1960.

Mitchell, C. A., and Klotz, M. O.: Lymphocytic choriomeningitis. Canad J Public Health 33:208, 1942.

Rivers, T. M., and Scott, T. F. M.: Meningitis in man caused by a filterable virus. Science 81:439, 1935.

Scheid, W.: Das Virus der lymphozytären Choriomeningitis und seine Bedeutung für die Neurologie. Fortschr Neurol Psychiatr 25:73, 1957.

Scheid, W., Ackermann, R., and Felgenhauer, K.: Lymphocytäre Choriomeningitis unter dem Bild der Encephalitis lethargica. Dtsch med Wschr 93:940, 1968.

Scheid, W., and Jochheim, K.-A.: Akute Encephalomyelitis und Virus der lymphocytären Choriomeningitis. Nervenarzt 27:385, 1956.

Scheid, W., Jochheim, K.-A., and Mohr, W.: Laboratoriumsinfektionen mit dem Virus der lymphocytären Choriomeningitis. Dtsch Arch klin Med 203:88, 1956a.

Scheid, W., Jochheim, K.-A., and Stammler, A.: Tödlicher Verlauf einer Infektion mit dem Virus der lymphocytären Choriomeningitis. Dtsch Zschr Nervenheilk 174:123, 1956b.

Sheinbergas, M. M.: Hydrocephalus due to prenatal infection with the lymphocytic choriomeningitis virus. Infection 4:185, 1976.

Traub, E.: A filterable virus recovered from white mice. Science 81:298, 1935.

Treusch, J. V., Milzer, A., and Levinson, S. O.: Recurrent lymphocytic choriomeningitis. Report of a case in which treatment was with pooled normal adult serum. Arch Intern Med 72:709, 1943.

Vanzee, B. E., Douglas, R. G., Betts, R. F., Bauman, A. W., Fraser, D. W., and Hinman, A. R.: Lymphocytic choriomeningitis in university hospital personnel. Clinical features. Am J Med 58:803, 1975.

Wallgren, A.: Une nouvelle maladie infectieuse du système nerveux central? (Méningite aseptique aiguë). Acta paediat 4:158, 1925.

Warkel, R. L., Rinaldi, C. F., Bancroft, W. H., Cardiff, R. D., Holmes, G. E., and Wilsnack, R. E.: Fatal acute meningoencephalitis due to lymphocytic choriomeningitis virus. Neurology 23:198, 1973.

Werner, W., and Wolf, G.: Akute Querschnittssyndrome bei lymphozytärer Choriomeningitis (LCM). Fortschr Neurol Psychiatr 40:662, 1972.

170

BACTERIAL BRAIN ABSCESS

HERBERT S. HEINEMAN, M.D.

A brain abscess, which is a focus of suppuration within the substance of the brain, is one of a group of intracranial suppurative diseases that includes extradural abscess, subdural abscess, and septic cortical thrombophlebitis.

ETIOLOGY. Nervous tissue appears to be highly resistant to bacterial invasion, in that bacteremia from any cause rarely results in infection of the brain. For example, in subacute endocarditis, where bacteremia may be sustained for weeks, damage to the brain is more likely to result from rupture of a mycotic aneurysm or cerebral infarction. Even the presence of highly virulent organisms in the subarachnoid space, as occurs in most cases of bacterial meningitis, almost never leads to infection of the brain. A brain abscess is most likely to occur in one of the following situations: (1) chronic cerebral anoxia, particularly when associated with a left-to-right intracardiac shunt; (2) chronic suppuration in the bone adjacent to the brain; (3) septic embolization from a chronic suppurative focus in another part of the body; and (4) direct implantation of bacteria by accidental or surgical trauma.

The role of chronic cerebral anoxia is best illustrated by the susceptibility of children with cyanotic congenital heart disease to brain abscess. In these patients, arterial hypoxemia complicated by polycythemia may result in cerebral infarction. Since brain abscess is a rare complication of cerebral infarction due to atherosclerosis, an additional etiologic factor in the children may be the bypassing of the pulmonary bacterial clearance mechanism.

The bacteriology of brain abscess has changed appreciably within the past 50 years. Hemolytic streptococci and pneumococci, leading pathogens in the past, are infrequently found nowadays, probably because the initial respiratory infections caused by them yield so readily to antibiotics. In other respects, the change is more apparent than real. Early descriptions of brain abscess referred to the frequent occurrence of "sterile" pus; from the remainder, hemolytic streptococci, pneumococci, staphylococci, and gram-negative enteric bacilli were recovered. In some cases, pus that yielded negative cultures showed an abundance of gram-positive cocci or gram-negative bacilli on microscopic examination. In the past two decades, the important role of endogenous anaerobic bacteria has been increasingly appreciated (Heineman and Braude, 1963; de Louvois, 1978; Ingham et al., 1978). The actual incidence of the various bacterial species recovered has varied from one report to another. For example, Heineman and Braude found anaerobic gram-positive cocci (streptococci) and gram-negative bacilli (*Bacteroides*) to be the most frequent; de Louvois and colleagues (1977), with equally meticulous attention to bacteriologic technique, noted a high incidence of capnophilic aerotolerant streptococci. In correlating bacteriology with localization (and portal of entry) of an abscess, de Louvois (1978) found that capnophilic streptococci (particularly *Streptococcus milleri*) were particularly associated with frontal lobe abscesses, while mixtures of anaerobic bacteria as well as aerobic enteric bacilli were typical of temporal lobe abscesses. Even allowing for these differences, the following generalizations appear to be justified: (1) hemolytic streptococci and pneumococci are now infrequent causes of intracranial suppurative disease; (2) staphylococci are associated with septicemia and penetrating trauma, including surgery, but are otherwise infrequently found; (3) *Haemophilus influenzae* is more or less limited to the age group showing high susceptibility to this organism (children from 2 to about 7 years), and aerobic enteric bacilli are limited to newborns and elderly debilitated patients; and (4) with the aforementioned exceptions, aerobic gram-negative bacilli are uncommonly found alone, and their importance, if any, is overshadowed by that of the mixture of anaerobes in whose company they occur.

Actinomyces israelii, *Nocardia asteroides*, and *Haemophilus aphrophilus* are occasionally implicated in brain abscess.

PATHOGENESIS AND PATHOLOGY. It is believed that infection with all but the most virulent bacteria (such as *Nocardia asteroides*) is preceded by damage to the nervous tissue. In the absence of trauma, the usual precipitating factor is infarction. In keeping with this concept, most abscesses originate at the junction of the gray and white matter, the least well perfused area of the brain. Septic embolization provides a mechanism for both infarction and infection. Its source may be distant, for example, the thorax or pelvis; in this case embolization occurs via the arterial blood, and the abscess may occur in any part of the brain but particularly in the distribution of the middle cerebral artery. More commonly, the source is a space in the skull from which sepsis travels via emissary veins to a nearby part of the brain: from the middle ear and mastoid, the temporal lobe and cerebellum are most commonly infected; from the frontal sinus, spread is typically to the frontal lobe.

As in other tissues, abscess formation is preceded by a stage of inflammation characterized by vascular congestion, edema, and infiltration with polymorphonuclear cells. This presuppurative stage, sometimes referred to as focal encephalitis or (when anatomically appropriate) cerebritis, is potentially reversible. The walling-off process begins at the end of the first week with a thin membrane. This is followed by the development of a fibrous capsule, thicker on the cortical than on the ventricular side, which matures after approximately three weeks from onset of infection. At this stage, the so-called acute abscess, the lesion is still surrounded by a varying zone of cerebral edema whose volume may be larger than that of the abscess itself. It is this edema that is largely responsible for persistent or progressive clinical manifestations leading to death or forced surgical intervention. In some cases, encapsulation is functionally complete, surrounding edema subsides spontaneously, and a chronic abscess may be tolerated for months or years with few or no symptoms.

Brain abscess almost never occurs as a consequence of bacterial meningitis. In the unusual cases where both coexist, they are believed to represent either concurrent infection or rupture of the abscess.

CLINICAL MANIFESTATIONS. Clinical manifestations of intracranial abscess reflect three separate processes: systemic reaction to infection, increased intracranial pressure, and damage or destruction of brain tissue. In addition, most patients will demonstrate a typical primary focus of infection.

Systemic manifestations, such as chills and fever, are most commonly associated with septicemia, acute sinusitis, or acute otitis. When the underlying process is indolent, the presence of a brain abscess may produce low-grade fever, but in some cases systemic reaction is totally absent.

Increased intracranial pressure almost always accompanies intracranial suppurative disease, contributes significantly to morbidity and mortality, and causes the commonest symptom, namely, headache. Nonspecific as headache is in infectious disease, and despite its more specific association with otitis and sinusitis, it has considerable value in the diagnosis of intracranial suppurative disease. This symptom is characterized by progressive severity, intractability, and occasional localization to the affected side of the head. In patients accustomed to headache because of their underlying infection, the change in character of this symptom coincident with intracranial spread should raise the suspicion of brain abscess. In advanced cases, vomiting may occur, consciousness may be clouded until coma supervenes, and funduscopic examination may reveal papilledema. Meningeal irritation is absent unless a subdural abscess is present or a brain abscess has ruptured, a complication that is frequently fatal.

Localizing neurologic signs reflect the particular site of the inflammatory process. For example, temporal lobe abscesses are characterized by expressive aphasia and a homonymous contralateral upper quadrant visual field defect; increased pressure may temporarily paralyze the ipsilateral third and sixth cranial nerves. In cerebellar abscesses, nystagmus with the fast component toward the lesion and ipsilateral incoordination and hypotonia occur; the ipsilateral sixth and seventh cranial nerves may be temporarily paralyzed by pressure. Parietal lobe abscesses may lead to contralateral hemisensory deficits. In frontal lobe abscesses, typical manifestations are impaired consciousness and contralateral motor deficits; however, lateralizing signs are frequently absent. Occipital lobe lesions may result in contralateral homonymous hemianopia.

Even focal neurologic dysfunction is as often due to inflammation or edema as to destruction of nervous tissue. Focal signs may even appear during antibiotic treatment and then regress as inflammation subsides (Heineman et al., 1971).

Although the clinical picture is dominated by the intracranial process, examination usually reveals evidence of suppuration elsewhere, for example, the middle ear.

The peripheral blood generally shows neutrophilic leukocytosis, but in subacute or chronic abscesses, the blood count may be normal.

COMPLICATIONS AND SEQUELAE. In a disease as severe as brain abscess, the chief complication is death, which until recently occurred in an average of about 40 per cent of patients. In one of the seeming paradoxes of modern medicine, reviews of several hundred cases of brain abscesses published during the first 30 years of the antibiotic era showed that this infectious disease, caused by bacteria susceptible to a wide range of antibiotics and treated by advanced surgical technique, carried no better a prognosis between 1962 and 1967 (Garfield, 1969) than it did between 1938 and 1951 (Jooma et al., 1951) or, for that matter, in 1893 (MacEwen, 1893). The logical conclusion was that irreversible damage had often occurred before any treatment was instituted, and that the chief obstacle to recovery was late diagnosis. With the availability of noninvasive radiologic techniques such as the technetium brain scan and computerized axial tomography (see section on Diagnosis), a more aggressive yet safer approach to early diagnosis is possible, and the pathologic process can be aborted much earlier, possibly without the need for surgery.

Death is often caused by intracranial hypertension leading to an uncinate or medullary pressure cone. In other cases, the abscess ruptures into a lateral ventricle, exciting a violent inflammatory response. Rupture through the cortex is comparatively infrequent, in keeping with the asymmetry of the abscess capsule (see Pathology section).

Among patients who survive, neurologic recovery on the whole is remarkably good. This discrepancy between severity of the acute illness and paucity of residual dysfunction can be explained by the relative roles of edema and suppuration in giving rise to clinical manifestations. If important motor, visual, or speech areas are actually destroyed, corresponding degrees of paresis, field defect, or speech impairment may result.

The most frequent sequela is focal epilepsy, which is presumably due to the inevitable scar that remains when an abscess is drained or excised. Several reviews have placed the frequency of this complication in the vicinity of 50 per cent. In the majority of affected survivors, seizures begin at some time during the first two years following surgery; in a small number, however, ten or more years may elapse.

DIAGNOSIS

Clinical. A high index of suspicion is necessary to diagnose intracranial suppurative disease at a stage when the prognosis is still favorable. The varied clinical manifestations have been described above. Since symptoms of intracranial hypertension or inflammation usually precede focal neurologic abnormalities by days or even weeks, close attention should be paid to such apparently nonspecific complaints as fever, headache, vomiting, visual disturbances, or drowsiness. When these symptoms occur in a patient with an appropriate portal of entry, a painstaking neurologic examination should be performed, with particular emphasis on visual fields, cognitive function, and coordination. Persistence of unaccustomed headache justifies a neuroradiologic investigation even when the physical examination of the nervous system discloses no abnormalities.

Radiologic. Routine skull radiographs are of limited value but are readily available. They may show a shift in a calcified pineal gland or, rarely, an air-fluid level in a gas-containing brain abscess. Films should be examined for clouding of the frontal sinuses and sclerosis of the mastoid bones, which support the presence of underlying suppurative disease in those areas.

An excellent screening technique for demonstrating a focal inflammatory process is the technetium-99m pertechnetate brain scan. However, although sensitive, it lacks discrimination, and the picture may be obscured by the underlying inflammatory process in the paranasal sinuses or mastoids or by blood in dilated dural venous sinuses.

The best combination of safety, sensitivity, and specificity is found in the computerized axial tomogram, or CAT scan. This scan has excellent localizing capability and, especially when used with a contrast medium, renders a picture that

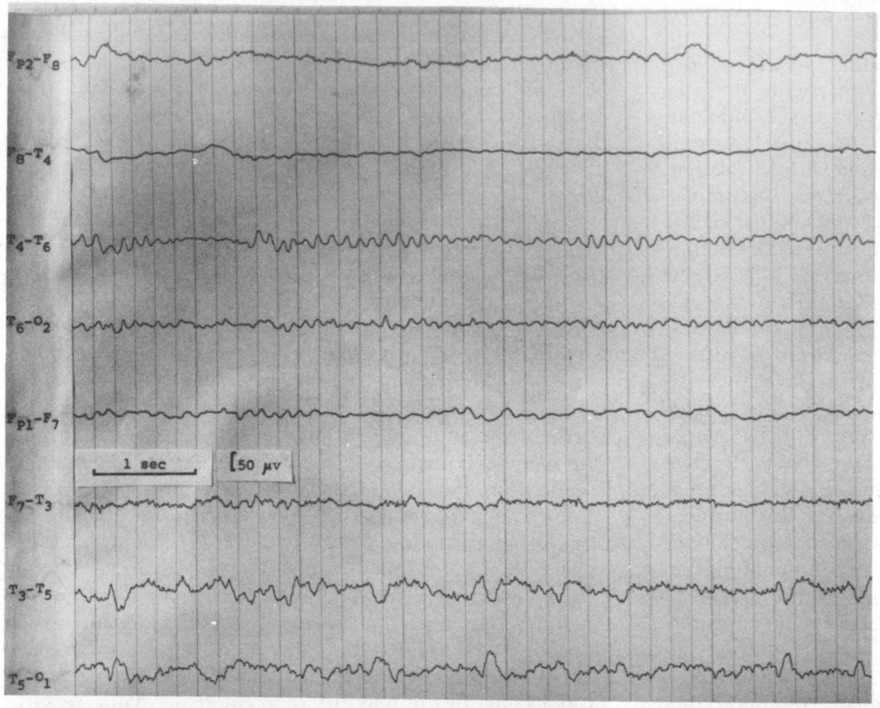

Figure 1. Demonstration of a left parieto-occipital abscess in a patient with congenital heart disease by four techniques. *A*, Electroencephalogram. Note high voltage slow waves in leads T_3–T_5 and T_5–O_1 (left) compared with normal alpha rhythm in leads T_4–T_6 and T_6–O_2 (right). *B* and *C*, Carotid arteriogram. Note straightened (stretched) branches of middle cerebral artery in *B* compared with normally tortuous branches in *C*. *D* and E, Technetium scan. "Hot spot" is visible in both lateral (*D*) and posterior (*E*) projections. *F*, CAT scan. "Doughnut" configuration, with central lucency surrounded by enhanced density, is typical of abscess.

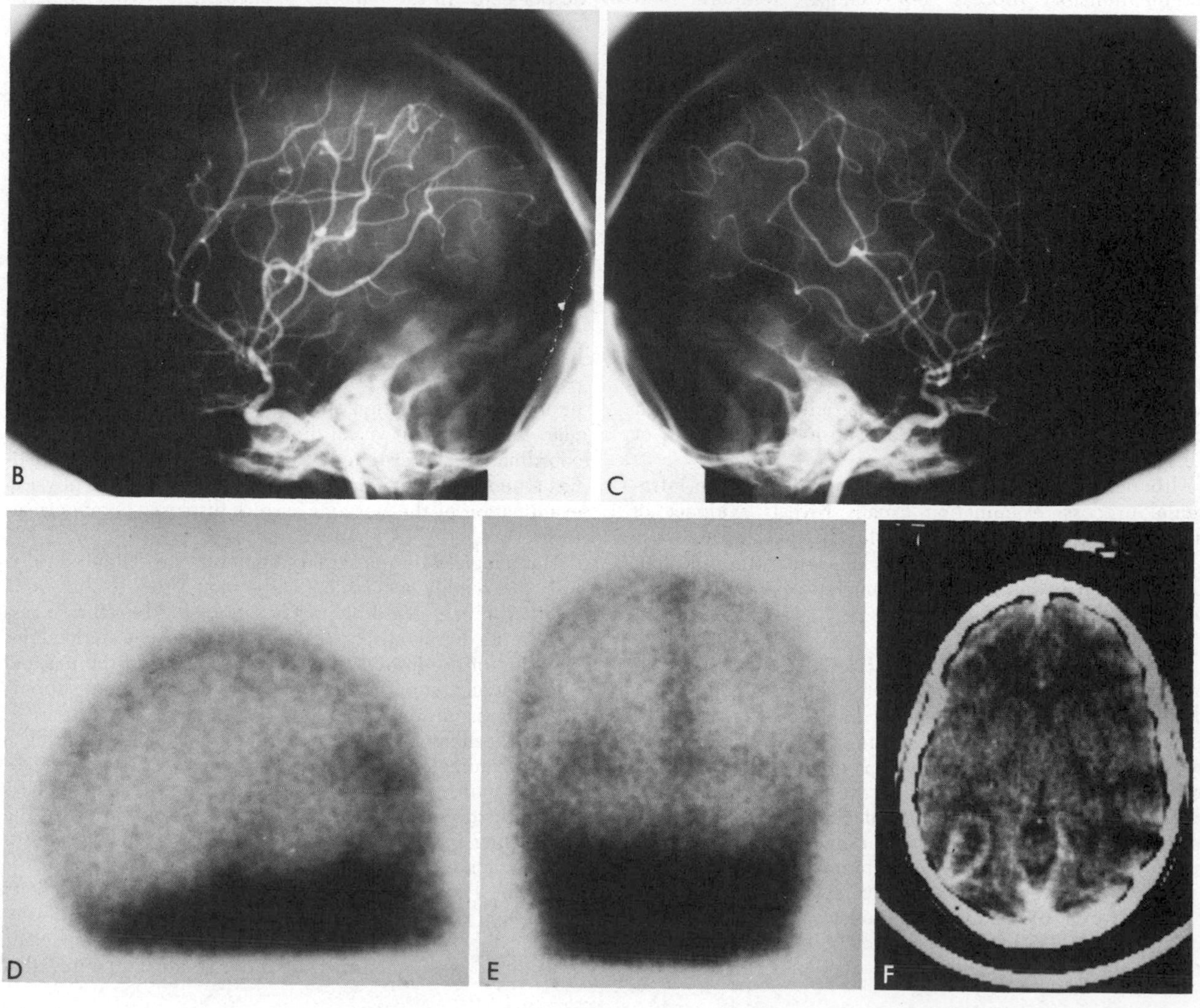

is quite characteristic of an abscess. When an abscess has not yet formed, that is, in the stage of focal encephalitis, this picture is less specific but its localization value is just as great. The CAT scan is useful not only for diagnosis, but also for monitoring progress during therapy (Rosenblum et al., 1978).

Arteriography, which is useful for demonstrating avascular mass lesions, and ventriculography, which shows lateral displacement of the ventricular system by a cerebral hemispheric mass or internal hydrocephalus due to an obstructing cerebellar mass, are invasive and hazardous. They have been largely replaced by the CAT scan.

Electroencephalography is useful for lateralizing a cerebral lesion, but the abnormalities are not specific for abscess. Posterior fossa (cerebellar) abscesses cannot be localized by this technique.

Figure 1 shows the appearance of a brain abscess by various techniques.

Lumbar puncture is contraindicated when a brain abscess is suspected (Garfield, 1969). As in the case of other asymmetrical space-occupying lesions associated with intracranial hypertension such as brain tumors, relief of pressure in the lumbar area may result in herniation of the brain through the tentorium cerebelli or the foramen magnum. Lethal compression of the hippocampal unci or the medulla oblongata may occur immediately or hours later. It should be emphasized that the slow withdrawal of a small amount of cerebrospinal fluid does not protect against this disastrous complication, as seepage continues through the punctured dura long after the needle has been withdrawn. In cases in which spinal fluid was examined, it showed at most a moderate mononuclear pleocytosis with normal glucose concentration; in other cases, no abnormalities were found. Therefore, this examination is not only dangerous but of little help.

Bacteriologic. Some of the bacteria most commonly found in brain abscesses are fastidious in their growth requirements and are killed by undue exposure to atmospheric oxygen. Pus should be submitted to the laboratory immediately upon withdrawal with instructions for prompt anaerobic as well as aerobic culture. Microscopic examination of a Gram-stained smear of the pus should be routine.

TREATMENT. In theory, treatment of intracranial suppurative disease is straightforward—drainage of pus and administration of antibiotics. In fact, acquired antibiotic resistance is not a serious problem and complications due to the surgical procedure itself are unusual. Yet despite these favorable conditions, the outcome still leaves much to be desired. As mentioned earlier, the chief reason for treatment failure appears to be delay in diagnosis, permitting the development of intolerable intracranial hypertension and, eventually, destruction of brain tissue. This situation can be remedied by clinical awareness and the ready use of safe and sensitive neuroradiologic tests.

The components of therapy are (1) timing and choice of neurosurgical procedure, (2) selection and dosage of antibiotic therapy, and (3) monitoring of the disease during recovery.

Surgery. There has been considerable debate on the relative merits of aspiration, drainage, and excision of the lesions (Jooma et al., 1951). Under ideal conditions of localization, as may be achieved with a technetium or CAT scan, aspiration and drainage have led to satisfactory results. However, reaccumulation of pus and failure to drain loculated daughter abscesses are potential dangers, and the patient's course must be closely followed by serial scans until the process is completely resolved. To avoid these problems, the prevalent opinion now is that excision is preferable, provided that the condition of the patient permits such surgery and the abscess is not in a vital area. Lesser procedures have been associated with slower convalescence and even relapse. Surgery is ideally performed when the abscess is well encapsulated, which may take three weeks or more to complete. A patient who survives that long without significant deterioration will probably withstand surgery well and recover. Unfortunately, progressive intracranial hypertension often demands surgical intervention at a time when both the poor clinical condition of the patient and the immaturity of the abscess militate against a successful outcome. As an ancillary measure, intracranial pressure can be temporarily lowered by an adrenocorticosteroid, for example, dexamethasone phosphate 4 mg parenterally every six hours. However, this treatment could interfere with the process of encapsulation.

The critical clinical indicator for assessing the urgency of operation is the patient's state of consciousness. More important than the development of new focal signs, progression from alertness to stupor or coma means that pressure must be relieved; the surgeon achieves this objective through the combined effects of craniotomy and removal of pus.

On the other hand, there is growing evidence that some cases of brain abscess can be successfully treated without surgery (Berg et al., 1978; Heineman et al., 1971; Rotheram and Kessler, 1979). The essential components of nonsurgical therapy appear to be (a) a stable state of consciousness, (b) aggressive use of rationally selected antibiotics, and (c) monitoring with repeated CAT scans.

Antibiotics. The contribution of antibiotics to surgical management so far has been disappointingly small, as judged by the overall lack of improvement in mortality since they were introduced. In part, this result is due to long-standing ignorance about the bacteriology of brain abscess and the pharmacokinetics of antibiotics in central nervous system infections, and in part to the inability to diagnose intracranial infection in a presuppurative stage when antibiotics are most effective.

It is almost axiomatic in the field of infectious diseases that antibiotics are selected on the basis of objective microbiologic data. When pus from a brain abscess is examined by appropriate microscopy, culture, and susceptibility tests, this requirement can be met. However, if the ideal time to treat such infection is before pus is formed, and the objective in fact is to avoid craniotomy altogether, then this crucial selection has to be made without the benefit of any direct examination. Unhappily, organisms cultured from the primary source, such as the middle ear cavity, or even from the blood may not accurately reflect the bacteriology of a brain abscess. On the other hand, published data (see Etiology section) indicate that certain bacterial species are characteristically found in abscesses of different origins. This justifies the general recommendation that brain abscesses originating from foci in the ear, sinus, chest, mouth, or pelvis receive treatment with 4 million units potassium penicillin G every 4 hours plus 1.0 g chloramphenicol succinate intravenously every 6 hours. Penicillin is particularly suitable because of overall lack of toxicity. Chloramphenicol has a broad antibacterial spectrum and penetrates well into the central nervous system.

First and second generation cephalosporins and aminoglycosides, as classes, are not as effective in central nervous system infections. The newer cephalosporins and related compounds, for example, moxalactam and cefotaxime, have been successfully used in gram-negative bacterial meningitis; their place in bacterial brain abscess has not yet been established.

A drug that shows promise of usefulness is metronidazole (Ingham et al., 1978). Because of its selective effectiveness against anaerobes, including *Bacteroides fragilis*, it should be considered for use in abscesses originating from the ear, sinus, or chest. However, it is ineffective against aerotolerant streptococci and, because the latter are especially common in frontal lobe infections (de Louvois, 1978), it should not be used alone. Doses of 400 to 600 mg intravenously every eight hours appear to be effective.

Sulfonamides are the drugs of choice for nocardial brain abscesses. Sulfadiazine can be given orally in a dose of 1 g every two hours. Trisulfapyrimidines have also been used successfully in this dosage.

Monitoring Recovery. There are no established criteria to determine the proper duration of therapy. The clinical course alone is unreliable as a guide, since patients may not fully recover or may suffer a relapse if antibiotics are discontinued too soon. If the abscess is surgically drained or excised, the cavity may be filled with a radiopaque material such as thorium dioxide or microbarium sulfate, which is taken up by the cells lining the cavity. This allows the progressive diminution of the lesion to be monitored by simple radiographs of the head. In cases managed without surgery, progress can be followed by the same techniques used in diagnosis, namely, technetium brain scans and computerized axial tomography. In the absence of objective indicators of healing, four to six weeks' therapy is recommended. In general, full doses should be administered parenterally for the entire duration of treatment; since subsidence of the inflammatory reaction reestablishes the normal blood-brain barrier, there is no reason for decreasing the dose or using a less reliable route of administration.

PROPHYLAXIS. Intracranial abscess is essentially a complication of extracranial disease; therefore, timely and effective treatment of the latter constitutes the best preventive measure. The relative decline in abscesses caused by hemolytic streptococci and pneumococci compared with earlier reports may be due in part to the ready susceptibility of these organisms to antibiotics, which are commonly given for acute otitis and sinusitis. Control of chronic infection in these sites, in which most intracranial abscesses in adults are found nowadays, is more difficult and often requires surgery. As an increasing variety of congenital cardiac anomalies yields to surgical correction, the incidence of brain abscess in these patients should diminish.

INTRACRANIAL SEPTIC THROMBOPHLEBITIS. Aseptic dural sinus or cortical vein thrombosis sometimes occurs as a late complication of bacterial meningitis. In these cases, thrombosis is secondary to a severe inflammatory process, perhaps aggravated by increased tissue pressure but not primarily a septic process. Septic thrombophlebitis, on the other hand, occurs by a mechanism similar to that involved in intracerebral suppuration, namely, direct spread of infection through the veins. The severity of this complication varies with the anatomic site. Among the more critical sites are the cavernous sinus and the superior sagittal sinus.

Cavernous Sinus Thrombosis. This sinus may be infected from the sphenoid or posterior ethmoid sinus or the mastoid. The most characteristic portal of entry, however, is the upper half of the face, with retrograde thrombosis or venous embolism via the facial, angular, and superior ophthalmic veins. Because cutaneous infections of the face are mostly caused by coagulase-positive staphylococci, these organisms are most commonly implicated in cavernous sinus thrombosis. The initial clinical manifestations of staphylococcal infection, such as rigors, fever, nausea, and lethargy, are predominantly constitutional. Peripheral leukocytosis is the rule, and the etiologic organisms can usually be cultured from the blood. In infections arising from a paranasal sinus or mastoid, the bacteria are those typically involved in infections in those areas and the systemic reaction may be less severe and acute. In either case, localizing signs due to venous obstruction soon evolve, making the diagnosis fairly easy. In typical cases, edema of the eyelids, forehead, and base of the nose is followed by chemosis and proptosis. Venous engorgement may be apparent on the forehead and in the retina. Compression of cranial nerves III to VI in the orbit or cavernous sinus results in pain and hyperesthesia and varying degrees of ophthalmoplegia and cycloplegia.

Although cavernous sinus thrombosis is basically a unilateral process, it may become bilateral if thrombosis extends through the intercavernous sinuses (circular sinus) to the opposite side. A rare complication in these cases is infarction or abscess of the pituitary, which is surrounded by the circular sinus.

Superior Sagittal (Longitudinal) Sinus Thrombosis. This is a relatively uncommon condition secondary to infection in a cavernous or lateral sinus, vertebral vein, or osteomyelitis of the calvaria. Clinical manifestations depend on the site of occlusion and involvement of tributary cortical veins. Posterior occlusion may lead to intracranial hypertension, engorgement of scalp veins, and edema of the forehead. Anterior occlusion of the sagittal sinus may be largely asymptomatic. However, if cortical veins are likewise occluded, the result may be varying degrees of cerebral infarction, with neurologic signs involving principally the legs, sometimes accompanied by focal seizures of first one and then the other side. The full-blown clinical picture is fairly easy to recognize.

Lateral Sinus Thrombosis. Involvement of the lateral sinus is usually secondary to infection in the middle ear. Although cerebral infarction is uncommon, increased intracranial pressure may result, especially if the right lateral sinus, which is usually the larger of the two, is involved. A diagnostic feature is edema and venous engorgement behind the ear of the affected side.

Treatment. The only useful form of therapy is the parenteral administration of large doses of antibiotics. Their selection is based on the known or suspected bacteriology of the initiating focus and the blood (see earlier section on Antibiotics).

CRANIAL EPIDURAL ABSCESS. There is normally no epidural (extradural) space, since the dura closely adheres to the inner table of the skull. A collection of pus creates an artificial epidural space by dissecting between the bone and the dura. This usually results by direct extension from osteomyelitis of the skull, which in turn is an extension of frontal sinusitis or mastoiditis or an infected wound. As long as the dura is not penetrated and no important venous channels are affected, the clinical manifestations are essentially those of the underlying osteomyelitis, with fever, local edema, pain, and tenderness. Neurologic findings may be totally absent, but there may be a low-grade mononuclear pleocytosis of the spinal fluid with all other values normal. Since the diagnosis is usually made at surgery, it can only be speculated that some cases may be aborted by antibiotic therapy directed at the underlying infection.

References

Berg, B., Franklin, G., Cuneo, R., Boldrey, E., and Strimling, B.: Nonsurgical cure of brain abscess: Early diagnosis and follow-up with computerized tomography. Ann Neurol 3:474, 1978.

de Louvois, J.: The bacteriology and chemotherapy of brain abscess. J Antimicrob Chemother 4:395, 1978.

de Louvois, J., Gortvai, P., and Hurley, R.: Bacteriology of abscesses of the central nervous system: A multicentre prospective study. Br Med J 2:981, 1977.

Garfield, J.: Management of supratentorial intracranial abscess: A review of 200 cases. Br Med J 2:7, 1969.

Heineman, H. S., and Braude, A. I.: Anaerobic infection of the brain: Observations on eighteen consecutive cases of brain abscess. Am J Med 35:682, 1963.

Heineman, H. S., Braude, A. I., and Osterholm, J. L.: Intracranial suppurative disease: Early presumptive diagnosis and successful treatment without surgery. JAMA 218:1542, 1971.

Ingham, H. R., Selkon, J. B., and Roxby, C. M.: The bacteriology and chemotherapy of otogenic cerebral abscesses. J Antimicrob Chemother 4 (Suppl C):63, 1978.

Jooma, O. V., Pennybacker, J. B., and Tutton, G. K.: Brain abscess: Aspiration, drainage, or excision. J Neurol Neurosurg Psych 14:308, 1951.

MacEwen, W.: Pyogenic and Infective Diseases of the Brain and Spinal Cord. Glasgow, J. Maclehose and Sons, 1893.

Rotheram, E. B., and Kessler, L. A.: Use of computerized tomography in nonsurgical management of brain abscess. Arch Neurol 32:25, 1979.

171

CEREBRAL MUCORMYCOSIS

ELIZABETH J. ZIEGLER, M.D.

Cerebral mucormycosis is a devastating condition in which fungi of the order Mucorales invade one or more structures within the cranial cavity of patients debilitated by acidosis or hematologic malignancy. These fungi spread through blood vessels to the brain either by direct extension from the nasopharynx or by embolization from a distant infection.

ETIOLOGY. The fungi causing cerebral mucormycosis are *Zygomycetes,* which belong to the large group of soil organisms known as *Phycomycetes.* In contrast to other pathogenic molds, they have nonseptate hyphae. The species or genera of *Zygomycetes* seen in brain sections are often not identified because they usually fail to grow from brain tissue, even when histologic sections show heavy infection. Almost all positive cultures have been identified as *Rhizopus, Mucor,* and *Absidia; Rhizopus oryzae* has been the most common species. *Cunninghamella, Mortierella,* and *Saksenaea* have been identified occasionally.

PATHOGENESIS AND PATHOLOGY. Cerebral mucormycosis can occur during generalized dissemination from the lung or gastrointestinal tract (Paltauf, 1885), as an isolated embolic episode (Mansucci et al., 1982) or in the classical rhinocerebral form by direct extension of infection from the nasopharynx (Gregory et al., 1943). All forms of the disease exhibit two common features in the pathogenesis: 1) metabolic and cellular abnormalities of the patient that permit spore germination at the body surface and uninhibited fungal growth in tissue and 2) the remarkable but poorly understood propensity of zygomycetes to invade and occlude blood vessels. Over half the cases are in uncontrolled diabetics (Blitzer et al., 1980), and the infection can be reproduced in ketotic alloxan-diabetic rabbits by nasal inoculation of spores (Bauer et al., 1955). Failure of experimental *Rhizopus* infection during hyperglycemia without acidosis and the development of cerebral mucormycosis in acidotic, normoglycemic babies after diarrhea (Hale, 1971) have focused attention on low pH as a critical predisposing factor. Phagocytes are important in the early response to invasion by Mucorales and are adversely affected by acidosis (Chapter 80; Bybee and Rogers, 1964). Acidosis may also stimulate fungal growth by inhibiting iron binding by transferrin so that more free iron is available to organisms in plasma (Artis et al., 1982). Neutropenia and congenital or acquired neutrophil dysfunction also increase the risk of mucormycosis (Chapter 80, Bruun et al., 1976, Meyer et al., 1972). Chronic sinusitis and trauma in the form of dental extraction or nasotracheal intubation may play a role. In addicts fungi directly injected into peripheral blood vessels may proliferate because occlusive thrombi cause local acidosis.

Inhaled spores first encounter the nasal turbinates, paranasal sinus mucosa or pulmonary alveoli. If allowed to germinate and form a nidus in tissue, the fungi quickly invade blood vessels, damage endothelium and produce infected clots, even in profound thrombocytopenia (Sims et al., 1976). Infection then proceeds by several mechanisms: 1) embolization of nearby or distant sites; 2) propagation of the clot antegrade and retrograde in both arteries and veins; 3) invasion of acidotic sterile infarcts by fungi in contiguous tissue; 4) progression of ischemic necrosis because edema from infarction and hemorrhage from ruptured mycotic aneurysms compress tissues and their blood vessels. Tissue damage by these means is rapid and irreversible. In many cases brain infection is well-established when the patient first complains of symptoms.

CLINICAL MANIFESTATIONS. Rhinocerebral mucormycosis commonly begins in the ethmoid, sphenoid or maxillary sinuses. The first symptoms are sinus tenderness, facial swelling, headache, retroorbital pain and fever. Fever may be low-grade. Occasional patients complain of nasal stuffiness or discharge, but many first seek medical attention because of double vision, sudden loss of vision, proptosis, ptosis or facial numbness (Fig. 1). These symptoms indicate that infection has spread through sinus walls or

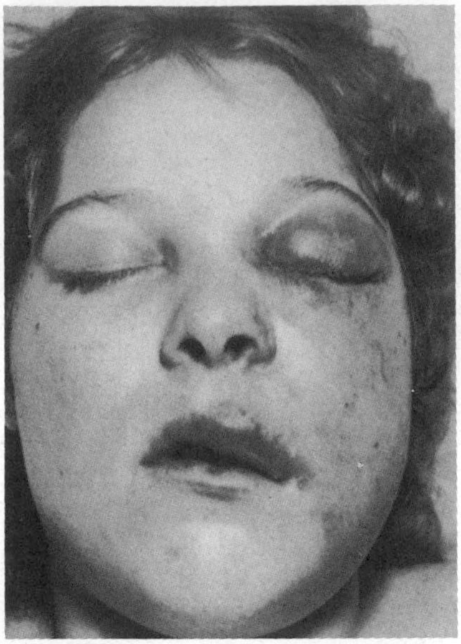

Figure 1. Rhinocerebral mucormycosis in a young diabetic woman with facial and orbital cellulitis, left ptosis, left facial weakness and blindness of the left eye. (From Kilpatrick, C. J., Speer, A. G., Tress, B. M. and King, J. O.: Med. J. Austr. *1*:308, 1983).

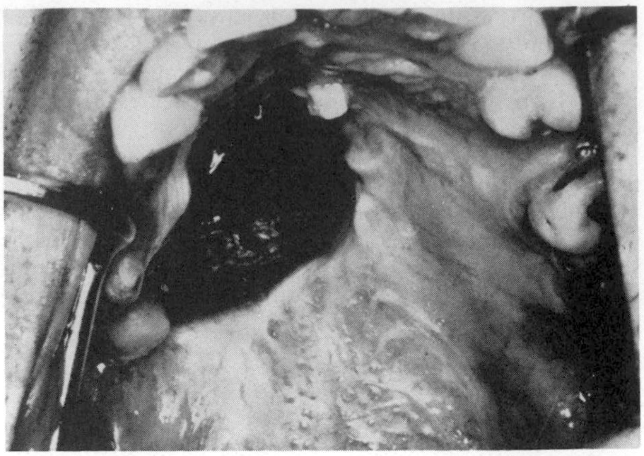

Figure 2. Ischemic necrosis of the palate in a middle-aged man with diabetic ketoacidosis, right-sided blindness and left hemiplegia. (From Yanagisawa, E., Friedman, S., Kundargi, R. S., and Smith, H. W.: Laryngoscope *87*:1319, 1977).

the nasolacrimal duct to the orbit and from the orbital apex into the cavernous sinus. Proptosis and ophthalmoplegia result from edema of extraocular muscles and compression of cranial nerves by the orbit. The fifth and seventh nerves are compressed in the thrombosed cavernous sinus (Pillsbury and Fischer, 1977). In a variant of this picture, palsies of cranial nerves V through XII occur without facial symptoms because a posterior nasopharyngeal ulcer penetrates the base of the brain without invasion of the nose or sinuses (Bahna et al., 1980). Extensive infection may evolve over one or two days in immunosuppressed patients or in diabetics as they recover from coma. Inspection of the nasal turbinates or palate frequently reveals ischemic lesions (Fig. 2). Biopsy of these lesions yields immediate diagnosis. The brain itself becomes infected either by direct extension to the frontal lobes, with edema and decreased mental status, or by carotid artery occlusion, with contralateral hemiplegia.

Occasionally, a diabetic has developed a chronic form of rhinocerebral mucormycosis with the sudden onset of some symptoms but slow evolution and prolonged survival (Ferstenfeld et al., 1977). The most likely explanation for the increased resistance of these patients is correction of ketoacidosis early in the course of infection.

The clinical picture of hematogenous cerebral mucormycosis depends upon the size and number of emboli. Addicts with endocarditis or peripheral artery thrombosis will first appear to have had a bland embolus but will worsen later as the fungus proliferates in the brain. Patients with leukemia and lymphoma who embolize from the lung are likely to have multiple lesions. If the emboli are small, the only symptoms may be fever, lethargy and confusion.

COMPLICATIONS AND SEQUELAE. The mortality rate of untreated cerebral mucormycosis is almost 90 per cent. Death is due to progressive infarction, ruptured mycotic aneurysm or brain herniation. In survivors, blindness, nerve damage and tissue necrosis are irreversible. Secondary, gram-negative meningitis has followed infection of the nasopharynx, antibiotic therapy, and surgical debridement.

DIAGNOSIS. The diagnosis of mucormycosis is made by visualizing broad, often fragmented, nonseptate hyphae in tissue (Fig. 3). Insistence on this criterion avoids the opposing pitfalls of false positive cultures due to environmental contamination and false negative cultures because Mucorales are difficult to isolate from tissue. Occasionally a rapid diagnosis can be made by swabbing the surface of a necrotic lesion. Negative smears should be immediately followed by biopsies. Tissue for biopsy often can be identified on sinus films or computed axial tomograms (CT) of the orbits and sinuses. Focal destruction of the walls of the bony sinuses or orbits, multiple lesions, irregular masses within sinuses and absence of air fluid levels suggest mucormycosis (Figs. 4 and 5). Conventional tomography is better than CT for detecting bone destruction but CT is superior for demonstrating orbital involvement (Centeno, 1981). These maneuvers are directed toward making a firm diagnosis before infection reaches the brain parenchyma. Brain infarction results in areas of decreased density on CT scan with or without rim enhancement. Cerebrospinal fluid findings are variable and influenced by proximity of infection to the meninges, duration of nervous system infection, and the patient's capacity to mount an exudative response to infarction.

The differential diagnosis of rhinocerebral mucormycosis is narrow. Aspergillus species can cause an almost identical syndrome, especially in immunosuppressed patients. Biopsy shows septate hyphae with acute angle branching. Cavernous sinus thrombosis from bacterial infection causes deep facial pain, orbital congestion, lid edema and ptosis, but proptosis is a late sign and visual loss is uncommon. Malignant external otitis due to *Pseudomonas aeruginosa* in diabetics is accompanied by cranial nerve palsies but obviously arises from the ear. *Pseudomonas* also can cause the necrotic lesions of ecthyma gangrenosum in the mouth and nose of neutropenics. Hematogenous cerebral mucormycosis can mimic bland embolic infarction, the cerebral form of disseminated aspergillosis, or embolization from

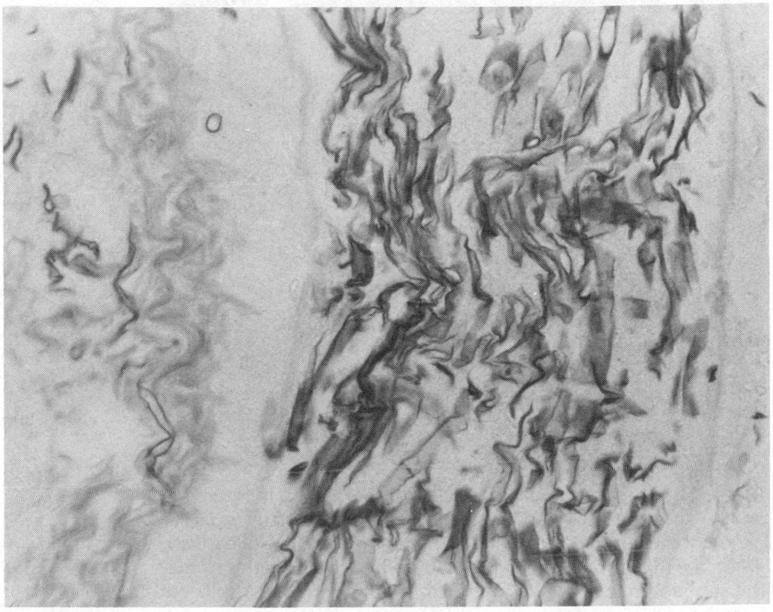

Figure 3. Biopsy of an ischemic mucormycotic palatal lesion from an adolescent leukemic. A longitudinal section of a blood vessel stained with methenamine silver shows obstruction of the lumen by broad ribbon-like nonseptate hyphae and early invasion of vessel wall.

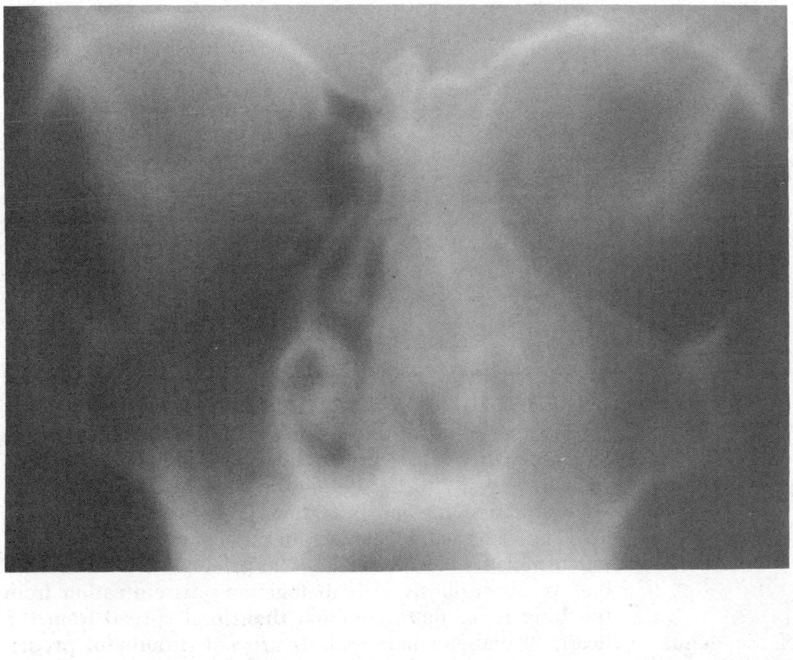

Figure 4. Sinus tomogram from the patient in Figure 3, showing opacification of the left maxillary, left ethmoid and right maxillary sinuses without air-fluid levels. Other films revealed destruction of the medial wall of the left maxillary sinus.

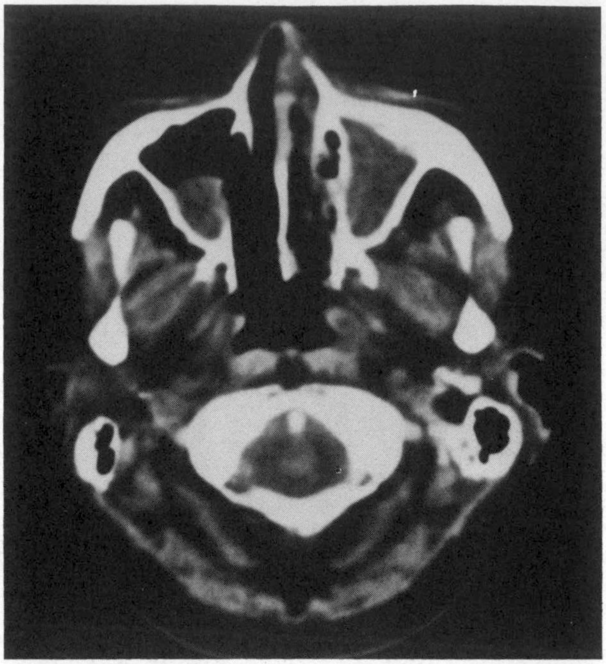

Figure 5. Computed axial tomogram of the patient in Figures 3 and 4, showing obliteration of the left ethmoid sinus, opacification of the left maxillary sinus, and a soft tissue density partially filling the right maxillary sinus. In another tomographic plane the superior medial portion of the right orbital rim was displaced laterally and eroded.

cardiac valves infected with Candida, Aspergillus, or bacteria.

TREATMENT. The four principles of treatment are early diagnosis, surgical debridement, amphotericin B and control of underlying disease. Often it is necessary to perform several debridement procedures guided by serial high resolution radiographic studies. The eye should not be removed from an infected orbit unless it has no remaining vision. Repair of tissues after radical debridement of the face, nose, and orbit will require extensive plastic surgery. Appropriate prosthetics have been helpful in acute and long-term management of palatal and orbital defects (Lapinski, 1979). The effect of amphotericin B alone on mortality has not been proven rigorously, but in combination with surgery it has lowered the death rate from rhinocerebral disease to about 30 per cent (Blitzer et al., 1980; Lehrer et al., 1980). No leukemics have survived. The drug should be given as aggressively as tolerated, up to 1.25 mg/kg/day. Total doses as high as 4 g have been suggested but cures are reported with much less.

References

Artis, W. M., Fountain, J. A., Delcher, H. K., and Jones, H. E.: A mechanism of susceptibility to mucormycosis in diabetic ketoacidosis: transferrin and iron availability. Diabetes 31: 1109, 1982.

Bahna, M. S., Ward, P. H., and Konrad, H. R.: Nasopharyngeal mucormycotic osteitis: a new syndrome characterized by initial presentation of multiple cranial nerve palsies. Otolaryngol Head Neck Surg 88: 146, 1980.

Bauer, H., Flanagan, J. F., and Sheldon, W. H.: Experimental cerebral mucormycosis in rabbits with alloxan diabetes. Yale J Biol Med 28: 29, 1955.

Blitzer, A., Lawson, W., Meyers, B. R., and Biller, H. F.: Patient survival factors in paranasal sinus mucormycosis. Laryngoscope 90: 635, 1980.

Bruun, J. N., Solberg, C. O., Hamre, E., Janssen, C. J. Jr., Thunold, S., and Eide, J.: Acute disseminated phycomycosis in a patient with impaired neutrophil granulocyte function. Acta Path Microbiol Scand C84: 93, 1976.

Bybee, J. D., and Rogers, D. E.: The phagocytic activity of polymorphonuclear leukocytes obtained from patients with diabetes mellitus. J Lab Clin Med 61: 1, 1964.

Centeno, R. S., Bentson, J. R., and Mancuso, A. A.: CT scanning in rhinocerebral mucormycosis and aspergillosis. Radiology 140: 383, 1981.

Ferstenfeld, J. E., Rose, H. D., Cohen, S. H., and Rytel, M. W.: Chronic rhinocerebral phycomycosis in association with diabetes. Postgrad Med J 53: 337, 1977.

Gregory, J. E., Golden, A., and Haymaker, W.: Mucormycosis of the central nervous system. Johns Hopkins Hosp Bull 73: 405, 1943.

Hale, L. M.: Orbital-cerebral phycomycosis. Arch Ophthal 86: 39, 1971.

Lapinski, M. V.: Phycomycosis: a case report combining surgical, therapeutic and dental management. Mt Sinai Med J 46: 205, 1979.

Lehrer, R. I., Howard, D. H., Sypherd, P. S., Edwards, J. E., Segal, G. P., and Winston, D. J.: Mucormycosis. Ann Int Med 93 (Pt I): 93, 1980.

Masucci, E. F., Fabara, J. A., Saini, N., and Kurtzke, J. F.: Cerebral mucormycosis (phycomycosis) in a heroin addict. Arch Neurol 39: 304, 1982.

Meyer, R. D., Rosen, P., and Armstrong, D.: Phycomycosis complicating leukemia and lymphoma. Ann Int Med 77: 871, 1972.

Paltauf, A.: Mycosis mucorina: ein Beitrag zur Kenntnis der menschlichen Fadenpilzerkrankungen. Virchow's Arch Pathol Anat Physiol 102: 543, 1885.

Pillsbury, H. C., and Fischer, N. D.: Rhinocerebral mucormycosis. Arch Otolaryngol 103: 600, 1977.

Sims, D. G., Scott, D. J., and Noble, T. C.: Multiple major cerebral artery thromboses with profound thrombocytopenia in acute leukaemia. Arch Dis Child 51: 74, 1976.

172

CEREBRAL ASPERGILLOSIS

Elizabeth J. Ziegler, M.D.

The brain becomes infected with fungi of the genus *Aspergillus* in the course of general dissemination from a pulmonary or intravascular source or occasionally by direct extension from paranasal sinus, orbit, or ear. Most cases occur in patients whose resistance has been impaired by corticosteroids, hematologic malignancy, or severe debility.

PATHOGENESIS AND PATHOLOGY. Like the *Zygomycetes,* aspergilli are ubiquitous in nature and bear spores that are easily inhaled. They also resemble *Mucorales* in their propensity to invade and occlude blood vessels with resultant ischemia and infarction. Thus, cerebral aspergillosis is remarkably similar in pathogenesis to cerebral mucormycosis (Chapter 171). The principal differences are that in aspergillosis 1) hematogenous dissemination from the lung is far more common than local spread from the head, 2) diabetes and acidosis are not prominent predisposing conditions, and 3) frank abscess formation is observed more frequently than in mucormycosis.

As in other forms of aspergillosis, *A. fumigatus* is the most frequent isolate from cerebral disease. However, other species can cause equally devastating infection.

Studies in mice have shown that macrophages prevent germination of aspergillus spores and that neutrophils kill mycelia. Cortisone, which interferes with macrophage function, and neutropenia destroy natural murine resistance against infection only when applied in combination (Schaffner, 1982). These defenses against dissemination of aspergillus also must be important in man. The only clinical series of any size are composed of patients with leukemia, lymphoma, high-dose immunosuppressive therapy (Young et al., 1970; Meyer et al., 1973; Fisher et al., 1981) or chronic granulomatous disease (Cohen et al., 1981). Analysis of these series of patients and the myriads of single case reports fails to identify a single predominant immune defect; this suggests that the pathogenesis of cerebral aspergillosis is complex and variable. The predisposition of patients with Cushing's syndrome (Walsh and Mendelsohn, 1981), however, highlights the importance of steroids.

Aside from the constant feature of vascular invasion, tissue reaction to infection is also varied. The pathological changes may include necrosis, frank abscesses, microabscesses, or granulomas. Lesions are often multiple. Small abscesses and granulomas are most frequent at the junction of the grey and white matter.

CLINICAL MANIFESTATIONS. Unfortunately, cerebral aspergillosis is recognized more frequently at autopsy than during life. Clinical manifestations correspond to the anatomic site of involvement. If lesions are large, seizures or localized neurologic findings are prominent. Multiple small lesions may cause only lethargy and confusion. Fever is usually present but may be blunted by corticosteroids. Mycotic aneurysms may be asymptomatic until rupture. Organisms proliferating in an ear or sinus may cause bleeding and often appear as a fungus ball on x-ray. *Aspergillus* may superinfect a pre-existing brain tumor (Beal et al., 1982) and give the clinical impression that the tumor has entered a new phase of rapid expansion. Occasionally, blindness is a manifestation of rather widespread cerebral dissemination (McCormick, 1975). Fungi introduced into the circulation during brain and cardiac surgery or during resection of a pulmonary aspergilloma may not become apparent in the brain until long afterwards. Chronic meningitis and ventriculitis occur in drug addicts, presumably from injecting a small inoculum of aspergilli along with intravenous heroin (Bryan et al., 1980; Morrow et al., 1983).

DIAGNOSIS. The only way to establish the diagnosis of cerebral aspergillosis is to see the characteristic septate hyphae in histologic sections of brain tissue (Chapter 79, Figure 4). Aspergillus grows well from brain, but false positive cultures may result from contamination during biopsy or handling of tissue. The brain is the most common extrapulmonary site of dissemination and most cases of cerebral disease have obvious pulmonary involvement. Nevertheless, pulmonary or cutaneous aspergillosis does not establish the diagnosis of cerebral aspergillosis, since immunosuppressed patients can suffer more than one opportunistic infection at a time. Even when the clinical condition of the patient precludes brain biopsy, empiric amphotericin B may be indicated because mucormycosis is the principal alternate diagnostic possibility. Blood and spinal fluid cultures are usually negative. The presence of specific serum precipitins is helpful, but most patients with disseminated disease do not make detectable antibody.

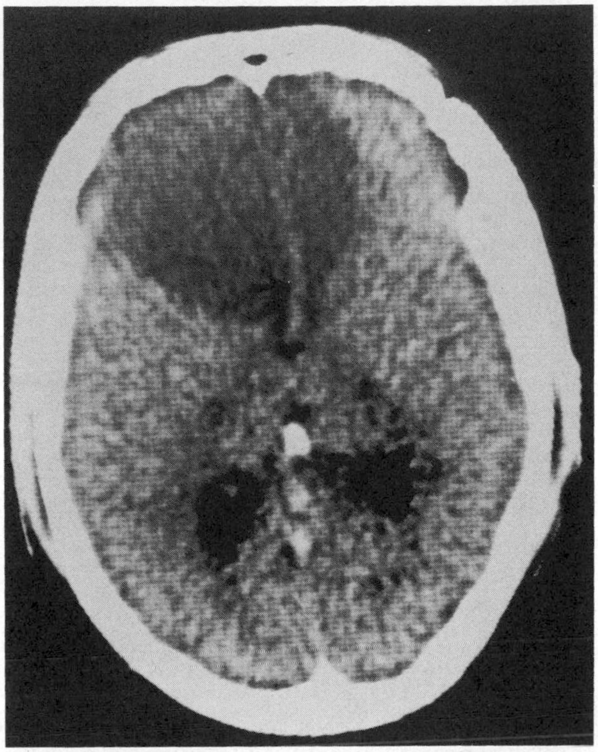

Figure 1. Computed axial tomogram of the head of a young leukemic man after administration of intravenous contrast material. The midline is displaced and there are bifrontal masses of decreased density without rim enhancement. (From Tubman, D. E., Yock, D. H., and Gold, L. H. A.: Invest. Radiol 17:525, 1982).

Radiographic techniques may be useful if lesions are large. Computed axial tomograms can be used to follow the course of treatment. Infarcts cause areas of decreased uptake (Fig. 1), whereas abscesses show rim enhancement with contrast. Arteriography may be necessary to find mycotic aneurysms.

TREATMENT. Amphotericin B is the mainstay of therapy. It is given in doses of 0.6 mg/kg/day intravenously and is coupled with vigorous debridement of all accessible dead tissue. To prevent dissemination or treat subclinical brain infection, amphotericin should also be used empirically and early in febrile cancer patients in whom an infectious agent has not yet been identified (Pizzo et al., 1980). Five-fluorocytosine has been effective when infection is limited to the meninges (Atkinson, 1973), but since confinement of infection to the meninges is difficult to determine with certainty, amphotericin B should also be given in most cases.

References

Atkinson, G. W., and Israel, H. L.: 5-Fluorocytosine treatment of meningeal and pulmonary aspergillosis. Am J Med 55: 496, 1973.

Beal, M. F., O'Carroll, C. P., Kleinman, G. M., and Grossman, R. I.: Aspergillosis of the nervous system. Neurology 32: 473, 1982.

Bryan, C. S., DiSalvo, A. F., Huffman, L. J., Kaplan, W., and Kaufman, L.: Communicating hydrocephalus caused by *Aspergillus flavus*. Southern Med J 73: 1641, 1980.

Cohen, M. S., Isturiz, R. E., Malech, H. L., Root, R. K., Wilfert, C. M., Gutman, L., and Buckley, R. H.: Fungal infection in chronic granulomatous disease. The importance of the phagocyte in defense against fungi. Am J Med 71: 59, 1981.

Fisher, B. D., Armstrong, D., Yu, B., and Gold, J. W. M.: Invasive aspergillosis. Progress in early diagnosis and treatment. Am J Med 71: 571, 1981.

McCormick, W. F., Schochet, S. S. Jr., Weaver, P. R., and McCrary, J. A. III.: Disseminated aspergillosis. *Aspergillus* endophthalmitis, optic nerve infarction, and carotid artery thrombosis. Arch Path 100: 353, 1975.

Meyer, R. D., Young, L. S., Armstrong, D., and Yu, B.: Aspergillosis complicating neoplastic disease. Am J Med 54: 6, 1973.

Morrow, R., Wong, B., Finkelstein, W. E., Sternberg, S. S., & Armstrong, D.: Aspergillosis of the cerebral ventricles in a heroin abuser. Case report and review of the literature. Arch Int Med 143: 161, 1983.

Pizzo, P. A., Robichaud, K. J., Simon, R., Siegel, B., and Manchester, B.: Empiric antifungal therapy for cancer patients with prolonged fever and granulocytopenia. Proc Am Soc Clin Oncol 21: 348, 1980.

Schaffner, A., Douglas, H., and Braude, A.: Selective protection against conidia by mononuclear and against mycelia by polymorphonuclear phagocytes in resistance to aspergillus. Observations on these two lines of defense in vivo and in vitro with human and mouse phagocytes. J Clin Invest 69: 617, 1982.

Walsh, T. J., and Mendelsohn, G.: Invasive aspergillosis complicating Cushing's syndrome. Arch Int Med 141: 1227, 1981.

Young, R. C., Bennett, J. E., Vogel, C. L., Carbone, P. P., and DeVita, V. T.: Aspergillosis. The spectrum of the disease in 98 patients. Medicine 49: 147, 1970.

173

CEREBRAL PHAEOMYCOSIS

ABRAHAM I. BRAUDE, M.D., PH.D.

In cerebral phaeomycosis, brain abscesses and, more rarely, meningitis are caused by cladosporia and other brown-pigmented soil fungi (Phaeo = brown).

ETIOLOGY. *Cladosporium bantianum* is the chief cause of cerebral phaeomycosis, having been isolated from over 20 cases of brain abscess. Occasional cases of cerebral phaeomycosis have been caused by species of *Curvularia (C. geniculata, C. lunata,* and *C. pallescens)* and *Drechslera hawaiiensis.*

PATHOGENESIS AND PATHOLOGY. *C. bantianum* is a neurotropic fungus that causes cerebral and cerebellar infections in animals as well as man (Binford et al., 1952; Critchlow et al., 1973). The portal of entry is unknown but inhalation or puncture wounds of the skin are likely. Immunosuppression has been a factor in cases due to *Cladosporium* and *D. hawaiiensis* (Symmons, 1969).

Those due to *C. bantianum* may be single or multiple encapsulated abscesses containing brown hyphae in the center. The hyphae are found in the thick neuroglial wall lying free or within foreign body giant cells. In the case due to *D. hawaiiensis,* a severe granulomatous and suppurative leptomeningitis was found at autopsy. Giant cells and hyphae were seen in areas of vasculitis (Fuste et al., 1973).

CLINICAL MANIFESTATIONS. The symptoms and findings in *C. bantianum* abscesses are those of a brain tumor and range from headache, seizures, and focal paralysis to coma. The protein and cell count of the cerebrospinal fluid are elevated as in other types of brain abscess.

In Curvularia infections, the cerebral lesions accompany disease in the chest or skin.

DIAGNOSIS. In *C. bantianum* infections computerized axial tomography will demonstrate one or more discrete abscesses. The organism has not been seen or cultured from the cerebrospinal fluid but careful search of the skin may disclose small lesions representing possible sites of primary infections from which *C. bantianum* could be seen or cultured from tissue removed by biopsy. After the lesion is excised, the fungus is recognized in the wall or center of the abscess by its brown pigmentation. Both hyphae and chains of yeast-like cells have been described in these lesions. *C. bantianum* is easy to isolate by culture and its ability to produce brain abscesses after inoculation into mice helps to establish its identity, although its morphology is distinctive (McGinnis and Borelli, 1981).

In the few cases with cerebral infections with *Curvularia,* lesions in the lung or skin may permit recognition by biopsy or sputum examination.

GEOGRAPHIC VARIATION. The dematiaceous fungi inhabit soil throughout the world and are saprophytes in decaying vegetation and lumber. Skin infections with these fungi occur mainly in the tropics and subtropics where they enter through puncture wounds of barefoot adults. The route of spread to the brain is not known; cerebral phaeomycosis might spread from puncture wounds, but very likely occurs after inhalation of the fungi. For this reason the disease can probably occur anywhere and is not limited to regions where shoes are seldom worn.

TREATMENT. Excision can sometimes cure the abscess but the tendency for these fungi to infect more than one cerebral focus warrants treatment with 5-fluorocytosine in conjunction with surgery for any type of cerebral phaeomycosis. The dose is 150 mg/kg/day. Amphotericin B, in doses of 0.4 mg/kg/day, should probably be used along with 5-fluorocytosine to prevent resistance of the fungi.

References

Binford, C. H. K., Thompson, R. K. and Gorham, M. E.: Mycotic brain abscess due to *Cladosporium trichoides,* a new species. Am J Clin Pathol 22:535, 1952.

Crichlow, D. K., Enrile, F. T., and Memon, M. Y.: Cerebellar abscess due to *Cladosporium trichoides* (bantianum). Am J Clin Pathol 60:416, 1973.

Fuste, F. J., Ajello, L., Threlkeld, R., et al.: *Drechslera hawaiiensis.* Causative agent of a fatal fungal meningoencephalitis. Sabouraudia 11:59, 1973.

Symmons, W.: A case of cerebral chromoblastomycosis (Cladosporiosis) occurring in Britain as a complication of polyarteritis treated with cortisone. Brain 83:37, 1960.

174

NEUROSYPHILIS

JOSHUA FIERER, M.D.

Neurosyphilis encompasses all the manifestations of syphilis consequent to the invasion of the central nervous system by *Treponema pallidum*. This includes symptomatic meningitis, which occurs during secondary syphilis, asymptomatic neurosyphilis, the various classical syndromes of tertiary syphilis including tabes dorsalis and general paresis, and several less distinctive manifestations of late infection. Because the neuropathology of tertiary syphilis involves the meninges, arteries, and the parenchyma of the cerebral cortex, the disease has many different manifestations that can resemble various neurological illnesses ranging from multiple sclerosis to strokes.

It has only been in the 20th century, since Wasserman devised the first serological test for syphilis, that there has been an objective way to diagnose the various forms of syphilis. Unfortunately, syphilis serology has not completely solved the problem of a working, clinical definition of neurosyphilis. Even with improved methods of measuring reaginic (non-treponemal) antibodies, and the development of serological tests for antibodies specific for *T. pallidum* (e.g. TPI, FTA-ABS), it is still not possible to distinguish between symptomatic neurosyphilis and latent syphilis complicated by other neurological illnesses.

PATHOLOGY AND PATHOGENESIS. All CNS infections take place within two years of the onset of primary syphilis (Hahn, 1961). *T. pallidum* invades the central nervous system in a small percentage of patients with primary syphilis and in about 25 per cent of cases of secondary syphilis, as judged by the prevalence of cerebrospinal fluid (CSF) pleocytosis and increased protein concentration (Hahn and Clark, 1946). Meningitis is the initial pathological lesion, persisting throughout the life of the patient and accounting for the pleocytosis that is characteristic of all stages of neurosyphilis. Untreated, a small percentage of infections may resolve spontaneously. The remainder stay asymptomatic for years. Eventually about half of those infected will develop signs and symptoms of neurosyphilis (Hahn and Clark). In addition to the meninges, the medium-sized arteries and the brain are affected, especially the parenchyma of the frontal and parietal lobes, which undergo cortical atrophy. The cerebral cortex of paretic patients shows widespread neural and axonal degeneration with such pronounced astrocytosis and gliosis that the brain gives the appearance of increased cellularity. Spirochetes can be found by using silver strains. Inflammation of the spinal dorsal roots, especially the lumbo-sacral roots, results in sensory neuropathy and secondary degeneration of the myelinated fibers that ascend the dorsal columns (Fig. 1).

Microscopic evidence of arteritis is common in all forms of neurosyphilis (Heubner's arteritis) (Fig. 2), but it is not known whether this is a specific syphilitic lesion or secondary to chronic meningitis, as occurs in other forms of granulomatous meningitis. The cerebral vascular lesion resembles syphilitic aortitis, so it may also be due to inflammation of the vasa vasorum. Discrete granulomatous reactions (gummas) can occur anywhere in the CNS but are extremely rare.

Since there are no animal models of tertiary syphilis, the pathogenesis of neurosyphilis is not known. It is not known why there is such a long-latent period between infection and symptoms, nor how the spirochete causes degeneration of neurons. Neither do we know how much of the neurologic damage is due to the spirochete and how much to the immune response of the patient.

CLINICAL MANIFESTATIONS

Meningitis. Symptomatic meningitis usually occurs during secondary syphilis but rarely may occur a few months later. Along with their rash, these patients have typical signs and symptoms of meningeal irritation. The CSF usually is moderately abnormal with an average of 500 lymphocyte per mm^3, increased protein, and a normal glucose. About 90 per cent of cases have a positive CSF VDRL, and the serum serology is positive in high titer in all cases (Merritt, 1935).

Optic neuritis may occur as a manifestation of secondary syphilis, with or without clinical meningitis (Weinstein et al., 1981). Typically, the peripheral optic nerve fibers are involved and there is concentric narrowing of the visual fields. This is due to inflammation of the perioptic meninges. The optic nerve appears swollen. Optic neuritis can also occur later in the course of infection as a manifestation of meningovascular syphilis.

Asymptomatic Neurosyphilis. By definition, patients have no signs or symptoms of a neurological or psychiatric disorder but have an abnormal CSF which contains 5 or more cells/mm^3, and an elevated concentration of protein. A variable percentage of patients have a positive CSF syphilis serology depending on whether the patient has been treated previously. About 75 per cent of patients have a positive serum VDRL, but the FTA-ABS is positive in 95 to 98 per cent of cases.

Patients with markedly abnormal CSF (pleocytosis, increased protein, and strongly positive serology) have 5 times the risk of developing symptomatic neurosyphilis than patients with weakly positive CSF, if untreated (Hahn and Clark, 1946).

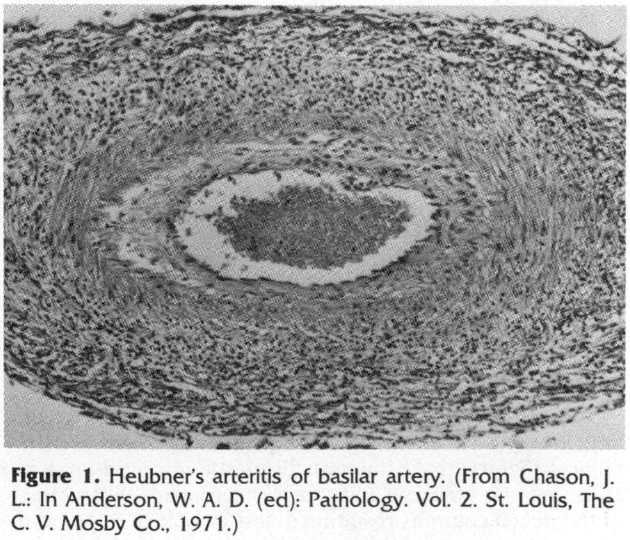

Figure 1. Heubner's arteritis of basilar artery. (From Chason, J. L.: In Anderson, W. A. D. (ed): Pathology. Vol. 2. St. Louis, The C. V. Mosby Co., 1971.)

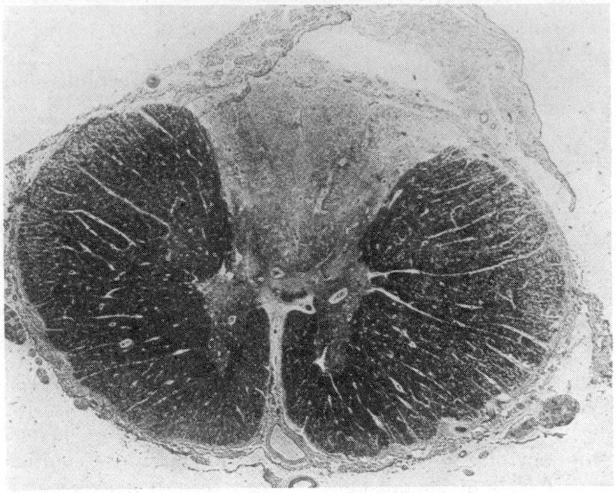

Figure 2. Tabes dorsalis with extreme sclerosis of the posterior columns. (From MacCallum, W. G.: A Textbook of Pathology. 6th ed. Philadelphia, W. B. Saunders Co., 1938.)

Meningovascular Syphilis. About 7 per cent of untreated patients with syphilis will develop one or more of the clinical forms of neurosyphilis (Gjestland, 1955). Meningovascular syphilis, which accounts for one third of those cases, usually appears earlier (5 to 15 years after infection) than other forms of neurosyphilis.

Generally speaking, the clinical manifestations of meningovascular syphilis are not uniquely characteristic of the disease so that correct diagnosis depends on serological tests and examination of the CSF. Patients may have symptoms due to vascular involvement or to chronic meningitis, or a combination of the two. Vasculitis (Fig. 2) can cause narrowing of large arteries with subsequent arterial thrombosis and strokes (Vatz et al., 1974). Either the brain or the spinal cord can be infarcted. Specific clinical manifestations reflect the anatomy of the vascular lesion and do not afford a clue to the infectious etiology. Therefore, syphilis should be considered in the differential diagnosis of all strokes in young people, and the CSF should be examined. Recovery from symptoms can be expected in most cases even without treatment, but there may be permanent sequelae.

Meningovascular syphilis may also be manifest as seizures, either grand mal or focal (Jacksonian), presumably due to irritation of the brain by meningitis. Meningitis may also damage cranial nerves at the base of the brain (3,6,7, and 8 most commonly) or produce communicating hydrocephalus with secondary increased intracranial pressure. None of these conditions are unique to syphilis. Some patients will have Argyll Robertson pupils. These are pinpoint (less than 4 mm in the dark), often irregular pupils that do not react to light but do maintain the reflex to accommodate. Visual acuity is maintained.

Parenchymatous Syphilis (General Paresis, Tabes Dorsalis and Taboparesis). These forms of syphilis always have their onset 10 or more years after infection and usually begin 15 to 20 years after primary disease (Gjestland).

The complete syndrome of tabes dorsalis is rarely seen any longer. An advanced case presents a characteristic clinical picture that is almost diagnostic of neurosyphilis. Inflammation of dorsal roots causes secondary destruction of the dorsal columns resulting in loss of joint position, and vibratory sensations. In advanced cases, deep-pain perception is also lost. Sensory complaints usually begin with lancinating (lightning) pains, especially in the legs, that can last from a few minutes to a few days. Hyperalgesia may accompany the pains. Activity does not precipitate them. Eventually the episodes decrease in frequency.

Ataxia is the next symptom to appear and is noted first at night or in the dark when there are no visual clues to aid in walking or balance. Eventually the patient develops a characteristic broad-based gait and lifts his feet high and slaps them down as he walks.

Paresthesias due to the sensory neuropathy, and atonic bladder and impotence due to involvement of sacral sympathetic ganglia are late manifestations. Abdominal crises occur in about 10 per cent of cases. They consist of acute episodes of pain and vomiting that can mimic surgical emergencies. Their pathogenesis is unknown.

The signs of tabes dorsalis are predictable from the neuropathology. Involved limbs have hypotonia but not muscle weakness. Deep tendon reflexes, especially at the ankle, are lost owing to damage to the afferent sensory nerves. Ataxia of the lower limbs gives rise to a positive Romberg test (imbalance with eyes closed but not with eyes open) and difficulty turning. Vibration sense in the feet and over the sacrum is lost early. The same early loss of position sense occurs in the toes. Diminished deep pain sensation can be demonstrated by squeezing the Achilles tendons or testicles. Loss of superficial sensation is much less regular and a typical peripheral (stocking) neuropathy is uncommon. Light touch may be lost in the Hitzig zones, i.e., the central face, around the nipples, on the ulnar borders of the arms, and the peroneal borders of the legs.

Many patients with tabes dorsalis will have ptosis and pupillary changes, including Argyll Robertson pupils. Optic atrophy, usually beginning in one eye, is found in about 15 per cent of untreated tabetics. Other cranial nerve palsies may also occur.

The earliest manifestation of general paresis is the gradual loss of higher cognitive functions. The patient is often unaware of his difficulties and may appear to be emotionally unstable and to have changed his personality. As the disease progresses, judgment becomes impaired and memory loss is great. The patient becomes easily confused and disoriented and may have poorly developed delusions, especially grandiose ones. Inevitably the dementia becomes worse and convulsions may develop. Rarely the disease will begin with convulsions and focal neurological deficits that remit after a short time. These symptoms may be due to concurrent vasculitis. Almost 80 per cent of paretics have an abnormal EEG, but the patterns are not diagnostic (Hooshmand, 1976). Computerized tomography may show cerebral atrophy with loss of both white and grey matters (Ganti, 1981).

Since nothing about the dementia of general paresis is unique to this disease, syphilis must be considered in the differential diagnosis of all dementias. If the patient has abnormal pupils, syphilis should be suspected strongly.

Taboparesis is the simultaneous involvement of the cord and the brain parenchyma. Usually general paresis develops first. Mixed presentations seem to be very common now (Hooshmand et al., 1971).

Other Syndromes. Gumma of the brain has always been a rare condition and is now almost unheard of (Perdrup et al., 1981). It presents as a single-mass lesion, and the correct diagnosis usually is made at surgery. Pachymeningitis hypertrophia is also a rare manifestation of neurosyphilis. The cervical spine is compressed by hypertrophic meninges, which causes symptoms and signs that mimic cervical spondylosis or a cord tumor.

Deafness is also a consequence of neurosyphilis, especially congenital infections. In congenital infections, late onset deafness is always associated with interstitial keratitis or Hutchinson's teeth (permanent incisors that are deformed to resemble screwdriver blades, sometimes with a notch on the cutting edge) (Fuimara and Lessell, 1970). In acquired syphilis, the onset of deafness may be either sudden or gradual. All varieties of conductive or sensineural hearing loss may result from infection, since all parts of the eighth nerve and its accessory organs can be affected. Acquired and congenital hearing loss is often accompanied by episodic vertigo that is almost indistinguishable from Meniere's disease. However, Meniere's disease is rare in children and usually is unilateral whereas syphilis is bilateral (Shulman, 1979). Hearing loss in acquired syphilis is usually due to meningovascular involvement and the CSF is abnormal in most cases (Rothenberg and Dancewicz, 1974).

COMPLICATIONS AND SEQUELAE. The different forms of neurosyphilis have different prognoses. General paresis is a progressive disease that is fatal, often within 5 years of diagnosis. Sometimes patients linger for years with progressive dementia and debility. In the late stages of this illness, the term paretic is apt (Adams and Victor, 1981). Tabes dorsalis is compatible with long life, even though the patients have residual disabilities. The sensory abnormalities can lead to progressive destruction of lower extremity joints (Charcot joints) that become deformed, swollen, and hyperextensible owing to lax ligaments. An atonic urinary bladder may develop chronic infection if catheter drainage is necessary. Blindness may be the consequence of optic atrophy, and deafness can occur as the result of eighth nerve involvement.

PROPHYLAXIS. Adequate treatment of secondary syphilis with penicillin results in a normal cerebrospinal fluid (CSF) in all cases (Fernando, 1965) and probably aborts neurosyphilis. Penicillin treatment of latent syphilis accompanied by asymptomatic neurosyphilis is also quite effective at clearing the CSF and at preventing the progression to symptomatic neurosyphilis. However, it is not effective in all cases (Hahn, 1961), so patients should have adequate follow-up. The CSF of treated patients should be examined six months after treatment to determine the adequacy of treatment. Patients with latent syphilis who have normal CSF are not at risk for developing neurosyphilis.

DIAGNOSIS. The diagnosis of neurosyphilis cannot be made with certainty on clinical grounds unless the patient has Argyll Robertson pupils. There are signs and symptoms associated with tabes dorsalis that are highly suggestive of neurosyphilis but not pathognomonic. Since neurosyphilis can be asymptomatic or can present with a myriad of signs and symptoms, all of which can be caused by other illnesses, the diagnosis of any given neurological disorder as syphilis can only be presumptive. The diagnosis ultimately rests on the interpretation of serological tests done on the serum and on examination of the CSF.

The serological tests for syphilis have been discussed in Chapters 53 and 199. Tests for reaginic antibody in the serum cannot be relied on to diagnose neurosyphilis, except for the CNS complications of secondary syphilis. Since reaginic antibody titers fall gradually with time after secondary syphilis, it is not surprising that some patients with late onset of neurosyphilis have negative serologies. This is especially true of patients with tabes dorsalis who may first be diagnosed 25 to 30 years after initial infection. It is also likely that early treatment, even if inadequate to eliminate the CNS infection, accelerates the rate of decline of reaginic antibody titers. It cannot be determined with certainty what percentage of patients with neurosyphilis have false negative serum serologies (reaginic antibody), but it is about 25 per cent. On the other hand, tests like the VDRL are not specific for syphilis. Other illnesses which may cause neurological symptoms, e.g., systemic lupus erythematosus, can produce false positive syphilis serologies.

Sensitive tests for antibodies that are specific for *T. pallidum* remain positive for a lifetime, even after treatment. Therefore, absence of antibody to *T. pallidum,* using a sensitive test such as the FTA-ABS or the hemagglutination test for syphilis, essentially excludes that diagnosis of neurosyphilis. A positive test, of course, does not establish the diagnosis of neurosyphilis since unrelated illness can affect people who have had syphilis.

If a patient has a clinical syndrome suggestive of neurosyphilis and a positive serum specific serology, the diagnosis of neurosyphilis should be considered. In order to increase the reliability of that diagnosis, the CSF should be examined. Since the pathology of neurosyphilis always involves the meninges, the CSF from patients with any clinical manifestation of neurosyphilis is abnormal. The findings are what one expects from a low-grade meningitis; the lymphocyte count is elevated (often between 5 and $50/mm^3$), the protein is modestly elevated, and the glucose is normal. The extent of these abnormalities varies somewhat in different forms of the infection. Cell counts and protein tend to be low in meningovascular syphilis and long-standing tabes dorsalis, and high in general paresis. All CSF should be tested for reaginic antibody because a positive CSF VDRL is indicative of neurosyphilis. Biologic false positives do not occur in the CSF.

Except for cases of "burned out" tabes dorsalis, it has been claimed that a normal CSF excludes the diagnosis of neurosyphilis (Adams and Victor). However, not all cases of neurosyphilis have positive VDRL. A rise in cell count immediately after therapy has been used as supportive evidence for the diagnosis of neurosyphilis, especially in cases with negative CSF serologies (Hooshmand et al., 1971). However, to be reliable the increase must be large enough so that it cannot be explained by random variation. In recent years, a number of clinicians have claimed that a normal CSF, including a negative VDRL, does not exclude the diagnosis of neurosyphilis (Hooshmand et al., 1971). They claim that if the serum FTA-ABS and the CSF FTA are positive, even in the absence of other CSF abnormalities, the patient has neurosyphilis. The benign nature of the CSF in these cases is explained by previous antibiotic therapy, which is presumed to have been sufficient to cure the meningitis but not the arterial or parenchymal infection. The validity of these diagnoses has not been established since there have not been any pathological studies on these cases. In addition, others have found that the CSF FTA is an unreliable test because of false positive results. The CSF FTA-ABS test is reliable and diagnostic of neurosyphilis (Sandra Larson, personal communication).

I think that current information supports the following conclusions about diagnosis. If patients have serum antibodies specific for *T. pallidum,* their neurological illnesses may be due to syphilis, and CSF should be examined. If the CSF shows increased numbers of lymphocytes, elevated protein, and a positive VDRL, a diagnosis of neurosyphilis is justified and the patient should be treated. In such a case, it is still possible that the patient has the coincidence of asymptomatic neurosyphilis and another cause for his symptom (Newman et al., 1980). If the CSF is abnormal but the CSF VDRL is negative, the patient may still have neurosyphilis. Other causes of aseptic meningitis must be excluded, but the patient should be treated for neurosyphilis. If the CSF is entirely normal, including a negative FTA-ABS, it is unlikely the patient has neurosyphilis.

TREATMENT. It is axiomatic that within the brain and spinal cord dead neurons do not rejuvenate. Therefore reflex abnormalities, pupillary abnormalities, ataxia in tabetic patients, and the dementia of general paresis, remain unaltered by treatment. We cannot expect penicillin to reverse cerebral atrophy. However, improvement can be expected in many signs and symptoms of meningovascular syphilis as they are often caused by inflammation, and adequate penicillin therapy can prevent or at least dramatically slow the progression of neurosyphilis. For instance, in a long-term study of paretic patients treated with penicillin, there were no deaths after 5 years and only 9 per cent of treated patients died of paresis within 10 years (Hahn, 1958).

Penicillin is the only antibiotic proven to be effective therapy for neurosyphilis. However, the amount of penicillin required is still controversial. Experimental and clinical observations have established the need for a minimal blood concentration of 0.03 units/ml of penicillin G, maintained for 7 to 10 days in order to treat early syphilis effectively. Later in syphilis, cure requires longer treatment rather than higher concentrations of penicillin (Rein, 1976). Prolonged blood levels are best achieved by using repository penicillin such as penicillin in oil with aluminum monostearate (PAM) or benzathine penicillin. Recommended regimens (Chapter 199) clear the spinal fluid of patients with secondary syphilis (Fernando, 1965) and prevent progression to neurosyphilis. In short-term follow up, 6 to 9 million units of penicillin G over 3 to 4 weeks was found to be satisfactory therapy for 90 per cent of patients with asymptomatic neurosyphilis. However, in paretic patients, Wilner and Brady (1968) found that 20 per cent had progression of their illness over 15 years of observation, even though they had previously received between 3 million and 30 million units of penicillin. The disease progressed even in patients whose CSF had reverted to normal after treatment. It should be emphasized, however, that the progression of the disease was much milder and slower than would have occurred in untreated patients. Subsequently, several authors have also reported individual examples of treatment failures in patients with symptomatic neurosyphilis despite the use of IM benzathine penicillin. Treponema have even been recovered from the CSF of treated patients (Tramont, 1976). After 2.4 million units of benzathine penicillin, CSF levels of penicillin are usually below 0.03 units/ml, which may explain the reported treatment failures (Mohr and Griffiths, 1976).

As a result of the uncertainty about the adequacy of previous recommendations, the United States Public Health Service and the WHO have revised their recommendations (Centers for Disease Control, 1982; Willcox, 1981). The WHO recommends a minimum of 20 daily injections of 600,000 units of aqueous procaine penicillin for treatment of neurosyphilis. The U.S.P.H.S. offers three alternative recommendations: A, aqueous procaine penicillin G, 2.4 million units IM plus probenecid 500 mg qid by mouth, both for 10 days, followed by benzathine penicillin G, 2.4 million units IM weekly for 3 doses; B, aqueous crystalline penicillin G, 12 to 24 million units IV per day in divided doses for 10 days followed by benzathine penicillin G, 2 to 4 million units IM weekly for 3 doses; or C, benzathine penicillin G, 2.4 million units IM weekly for 3 doses. This last choice is the same as their previous recommendation. Although there are no studies demonstrating that regimens A and B are more effective, both regimen C and the WHO recommended regimen have substantial failure rates and cannot be supported unless it is impossible to provide more intensive treatment.

There is no alternative antibiotic that can be given with confidence to patients with neurosyphilis. For patients who are allergic to penicillin, tetracycline 500 mg qid or minocycline 200 mg daily for 30 days may be used, but careful follow-up is necessary. If new signs or symptoms develop, it may be necessary to desensitize the patient to penicillin and then use either regimen A or B.

The *Jarisch-Herxheimer reaction* may occur within 3 to 12 hours after the first dose of penicillin, especially in patients with general paresis. The reaction consists of an increase in the temperature, intense headache, and a sudden deterioration in mental status, which may take the form of convulsions, stroke, or psychosis. The risk of such a reaction can be predicted somewhat by how abnormal the CSF is before therapy (Hahn, 1961). Although of unproven value, high-risk patients should receive 5 mg of prednisone qid for 3 days, beginning 1 to 2 days before penicillin is started.

Prednisone is also recommended as adjunct therapy for the treatment of nerve deafness due to congenital or acquired syphilis.

The clinical response to penicillin in tabes dorsalis is erratic. Lightning pains respond better to carbamazepine than to penicillin, and the former should be tried at 200 mg three or four times a day (Gimenez-Roldan, 1981). Patients with atonic bladders should be taught to empty their bladders mechanically so that catheter drainage is not needed.

References

Adams, R. D., and Victor, M.: Principles of Neurology. McGraw-Hill Book Co., New York, 1981, pp. 493–500.

Centers for Disease Control: Sexually transmitted diseases treatment guidelines. Morbid Mortal Wkly Rep. (Suppl.) 31:515, 1982.

Escobar, M. R., Dalton, H. P., and Allison, M. J.: Fluorescent antibody tests for syphilis using cerebrospinal fluid. American J of Clin Path 53:886, 1970.

Fernando, W. L.: Cerebrospinal fluid findings after treatment of early syphilis with penicillin. Br J Neur Dis 41:1168, 1965.

Fiumara, W. J., and Lessell, S.: Manifestations of late congenital syphilis. Arch Derm 102:78, 1970.

Ganti, B. R., Cohen, M., Sane, P., and Hilal, D. K.: Computed tomography of cerebral syphilis. J Comp Assist Tomography 5:345, 1981.

Gimenez-Roldan, S., and Martin, M.: Tabetic lightning pains: High dosage

intravenous penicillin versus carbamazepine therapy. Eur Neurol 20:424, 1981.
Gjestland, T.: The Oslo study of untreated syphilis. Acta Dermato-Venereologica: Supplement 34:12, 1955.
Hahn, R. D., Webster, B., Weickhardt, G., et al.: The results of treatment of 1,086 general paralytics, the majority of whom were followed for more than five years. J Chronic Dis 7:209, 1958.
Hahn, R. D.: Some remarks on the management of neurosyphilis. J Chronic Dis 13:1, 1961.
Hahn, R. D., and Clark, E. G.: Asymptomatic neurosyphilis: A review of the literature. Amer J of Syph, Gonorrhea, and Venereal Dis. 30:305, 1946.
Hooshmand, H., Escobar, M. R., and Kopf, S. W.: Neurosyphilis. A study of 241 patients. JAMA 219:726, 1971.
Hooshmand, H.: Seizure disorders associated with neurosyphilis. Dis Nerv Syst 37:133, 1976.
Jaffe, H. W., and Kabens, S. A.: Examination of cerebrospinal fluid in patients with syphilis. Rev Infect Dis 4 (Supplement 6), S842, 1982.
Luxon, L., Lees, A. J., and Greenwood, R. J.: Neurosyphilis today. Lancet 1:90, 1979.
Merritt, M. H., and Moore, M.: Acute syphilitic meningitis. Medicine 14:119, 1935.
Mohr, J. A., Griffiths, W., Jackson, R., et al.: Neurosyphilis and penicillin levels in cerebrospinal fluid. JAMA 236:2208, 1976.
Newman, P. E., Simon, D. B., Law, R. K., and Earnest, M. P.: Unusual causes of stroke in a young adult. Arch Int Med 140:1502, 1980.
Pedrup, A., Jorgensen, B. B., and Pedersen, N. S.: The profile of neurosyphilis in Denmark. Acta Dermato-Venereologica, Suppl 96:3, 1981.
Rein, M. F.: Biopharmacology of syphilotherapy. J Amer Ven Dis Assoc 3:109, 1976.
Rothenberg, R., and Dancewicz, E.: Significance of positive FTA-ABS test in Meniere's disease. JAMA 229:707, 1974.
Schulman, J. B.: Syphilis of the temporal bone. In Goodhill, V. (ed.). Ear Disease, Deafness, and Dizziness. Hagerstown, MD, Harper and Row, 1979, pp. 682–690.
Tramont, E. C.: Persistence of *Treponema pallidum* following penicillin G therapy. JAMA 236:2206, 1976.
Vatz, K. A., Scheibel, R. I., Keiffer, S. A., and Anjovi, K. A.: Neurosyphilis and diffuse cerebral angiography: A case report. Neurology 24:472, 1974.
Wienstein, J. M., Lexow, S. S., Ho, P., and Spickards, A.: Acute syphilitic optic neuritis. Arch Ophthalmol 99:1392, 1981.
Willcox, R. R.: Treatment of syphilis. Bull WHO 59:655, 1981.
Wilner, E., and Brody, J. A.: Prognosis of general paresis after treatment. Lancet 2:1370, 1968.

175

AMEBIC MENINGOENCEPHALITIS

LUBOR ČERVA, DR. SC.

The term amebic meningoencephalitis may designate any of three different diseases: (1) naegleriasis—primary amebic meningoencephalitis (PAME); (2) acanthamebiasis; or (3) amebiasis of the brain caused by *Entamoeba histolytica*.

NAEGLERIASIS

This is a primary type of acute purulent meningitis caused by the parasitic ameba *Naegleria fowleri*; it occurs mostly in young persons in robust health. Unless it is treated specifically, its outcome is generally fatal.

ETIOLOGY. The causative agent of PAME is the ameboflagellate *Naegleria fowleri*, which is free-living in either water or soil. Sessile amebic forms measure from 10 to 20 μm; mobile amebae produce wide eruptive lobopodia (Fig. 1); and their posterior ends may change into a specific supporting organ, the so-called uroid. They possess pulsating vacuoles and a single spherical nucleus with a characteristically big endosome. In a liquid environment, the amebae can transform into oval-shaped flagellates that are about 15 μm in length and have two flagella (Fig. 2). The transformation is reversible. The resting stages of the protozoan are spherical to discoid cysts, and they have a smooth surface measuring roughly 10 μm in diameter (Fig. 3). They are resistant to desiccation and to prolonged exposure to other nonphysiologic conditions.

PATHOGENESIS. In man the sole portal of entry of infection is the nasal mucosa and the olfactory nerve. Infection occurs after swimming and washing in infected

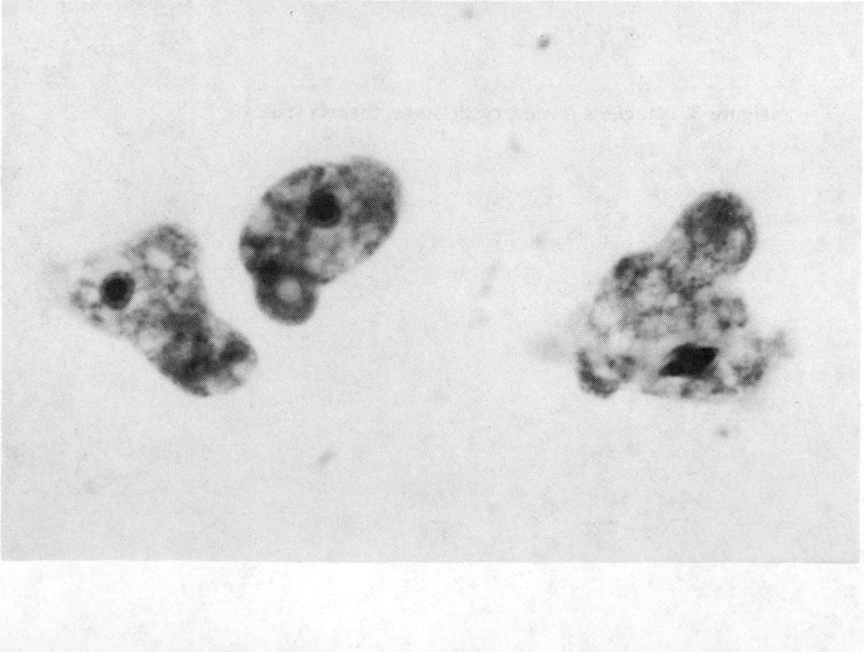

Figure 1. *Naegleria fowleri* in axenic culture. Note the typical rounded 1-obopodia, the structure of the nucleus, and the promitotic division of the nucleus in one of the amebae. Iron hematoxylin stain after Heidenhain. ×1300

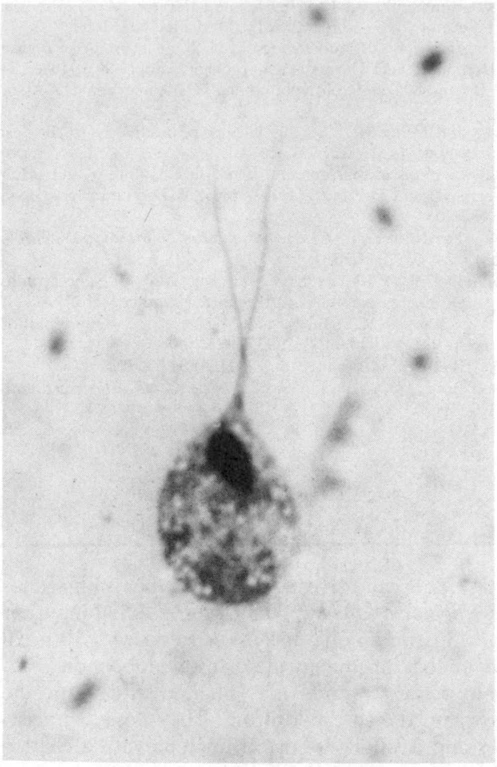

Figure 2. *Naegleria fowleri,* flagellate stage. Giemsa stain.

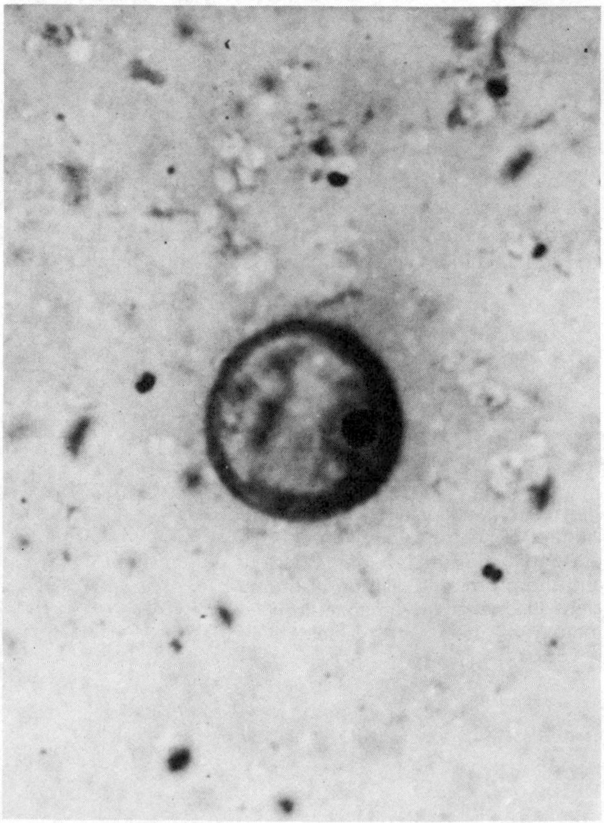

Figure 3. *Naegleria fowleri,* cystic stage. Giemsa stain.

water. For their critical stage of reproduction, pathogenic amebae need a water temperature over 20° C. Natural water reservoirs in the warm season, artificially heated water of swimming pools (Cerva et al., 1968), or warm industrial effluent, and occasionally warm mineral springs have been identified as the sources of the infectious agent. Amebae inhaled with water attach themselves to the nasal mucosa where they reproduce rapidly. They pass through the mucosa to the filaments of the olfactory nerve and along these to the base of the brain. They then spread actively in the brain or passively in the cerebrospinal fluid. From the meningeal spaces, they penetrate centripetally to the cortical and subcortical tissue of the brain and medulla.

PATHOLOGY. Brain edema varies from mild to moderate. The leptomeninges are infiltrated to a varying extent with a cellular exudate, which can be best observed at the base of the brain. Either one or both olfactory bulbs become necrotic and adhere to the cortex of the frontal lobes. The ventricular fluid is generally clear, and the chorioid plexus shows no gross changes. The cerebellum and the medulla are also the sites of edema and meningeal infiltration. Minute foci of softening or petechiae are present in areas of frank meningitis. Terminal changes in other organs (mainly in lungs) are not directly related to the amebic infection. Microscopically, the meninges of both the brain and the medulla are permeated with an infiltrate dominated by polymorphonuclears (PMNs). Among the PMNs, only solitary amebae can be identified, and these are frequently phagocytized. Masses of proliferating protozoans are present in the perivascular spaces of the cortical and subcortical layers of the brain (Fig. 4). These masses develop faster than the inflammatory cell reaction. The base, the frontal, and the temporal lobes tend to be affected most. Multiplication of amebae in the cerebellum is massive in the granular layer and destroys the ganglionic layer.

In histologic preparations, amebae measure 8 to 10 μ. They are spherical, and their nucleus, with its large endosome, is typical of the limax group (Fig. 5). In these preparations, no reliable generic and specific identification of amebae can be made on the basis of morphology. Cysts are not formed in the tissues.

CLINICAL FEATURES. The clinical picture of PAME is that of an acute purulent meningitis. It attacks mostly persons in robust health. The disease begins abruptly with headache and sometimes slight upper respiratory inflammation. It progresses rapidly with increasing headache, fever, and all the accompanying features of meningitis. Spasms of the face or extremities, mental disorders, parosmia (olfactory hallucinations), and other neurologic findings occur, depending on the location and extent of the cerebral lesions. Increasing intracranial pressure produces a deep coma and death.

The incubation period ranges from one to nine days (averaging five) after exposure to infected water. The disease lasts from one to seven days (averaging five).

COMPLICATIONS. Amebic infection of organs other than those of the CNS may occur, but this does not change the clinical picture.

GEOGRAPHIC DISTRIBUTION AND VARIATIONS. PAME has been reported in Australia (Fowler and Carter, 1965), Europe (Cerva et al., 1968), North America (Butt, 1966), New Zealand (Mandal et al., 1970), and Africa (Lawande et al., 1979). The clinical course is remarkably uniform in the various localities. The isolated causative agents are identical both morphologically and serologically.

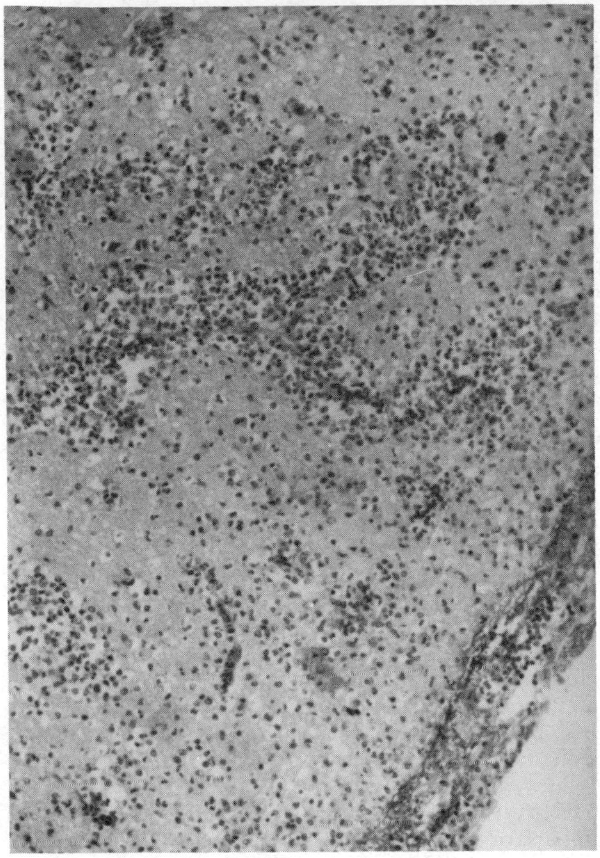

Figure 4. Naegleriasis in man. Heavily invaded cerebral subcortical tissue. Amebae are concentrated in perivascular spaces. Trichrome after Masson. × 200

DIAGNOSIS. The key to diagnosis is examination of *fresh* spinal fluid. PAME cannot be distinguished from other forms of purulent meningitis by clinical features or standard laboratory examinations of the cerebrospinal fluid (CSF). A specific diagnosis is made by finding naegleriae in *fresh* CSF either by microscopic examination or by culture. Motile amebae can be readily distinguished from other cellular elements in the purulent CSF. The CSF can be cultivated on both solid and liquid media or in tissue culture. Twenty-four hours at an incubation temperature of 37 to 42° C is the earliest possible time at which positive findings may be expected.

A specific examination for PAME should be made in any patient with purulent meningitis if the patient was in good health before the illness and has a history of swimming, if bacteriologic examination of the CSF is negative, and if the course of the disease has not been influenced by antibiotics or sulfonamides.

TREATMENT. The only drug that appears promising against *Naegleria fowleri* in vivo is amphotericin B in a dose of 1 mg/kg/day administered intravenously in a slow

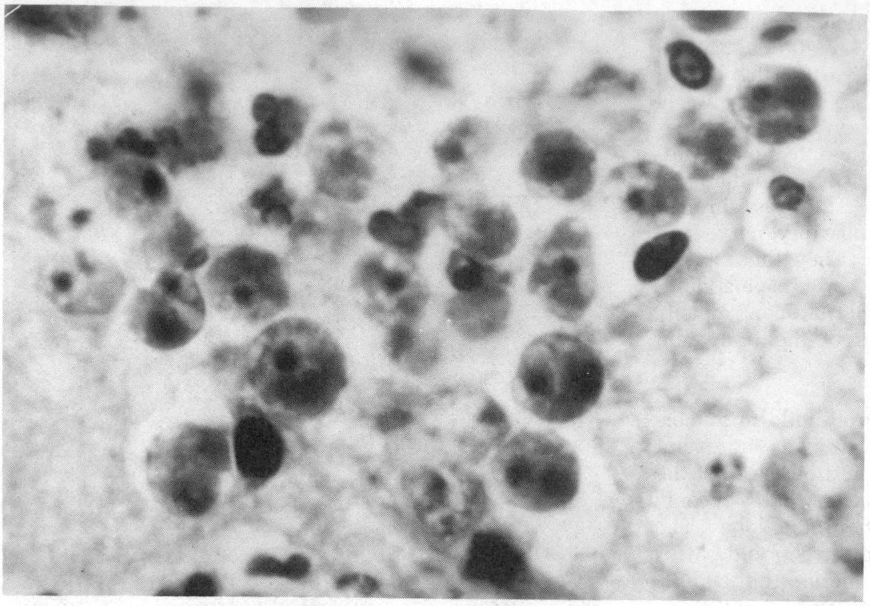

Figure 5. Detail of naegleriae in the cerebral tissue of man showing their typical morphology. Trichrome after Masson. ×1300

infusion or in combination with 0.7 mg amphotericin B intrathecally on alternate days. Only a few cases of successful treatment have been reported (Carter, 1972; Seidel et al., 1982).

PROPHYLAXIS. In endemic areas the only means of prophylaxis is to avoid swimming in water potentially contaminated with naegleriae.

ACANTHAMEBIASIS

Acanthamebiasis is a uniformly fatal acute or chronic protozoan infection of the brain, eye, lung, liver, kidney, pancreas, and skin of patients with underlying malnutrition, cirrhosis, chronic alcoholism, Hodgkin's disease, diabetes mellitus, immunosuppression due to therapy or disease, and other debilitating conditions. Meningoencephalitis is one of the most frequent forms of disease.

ETIOLOGY. Amebae of the genus *Acanthamoeba* (Hartmannella) have been seen but not isolated in culture, and the individual species have not been identified. This type of amebae live free in both water and soil. The living ameba is ovoid and measures from 20 to 50 μm (Fig. 6). The ameba moves by a slow flow of its plasma, which may form typical spiky acanthopodia. It has a pulsating vacuole and one nucleus. The latter is spherical with a large massive endosome. Amebic cysts measuring from 10 to 25 μm are covered with a thick multilayered membrane (Fig. 7). They are polygonal in shape and are most resistant to desiccation and other unfavorable physical influences.

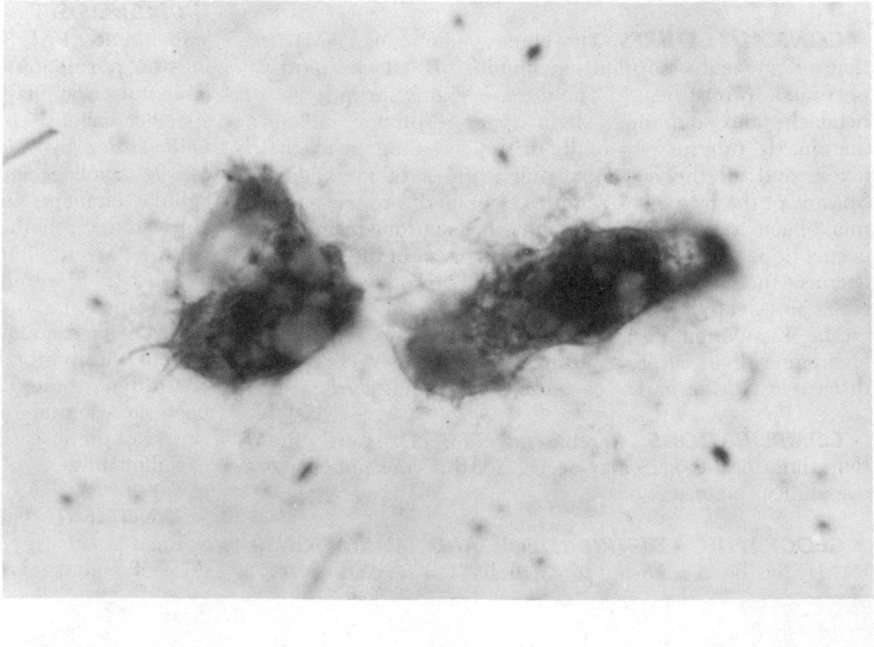

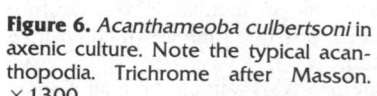

Figure 6. *Acanthameoba culbertsoni* in axenic culture. Note the typical acanthopodia. Trichrome after Masson. ×1300

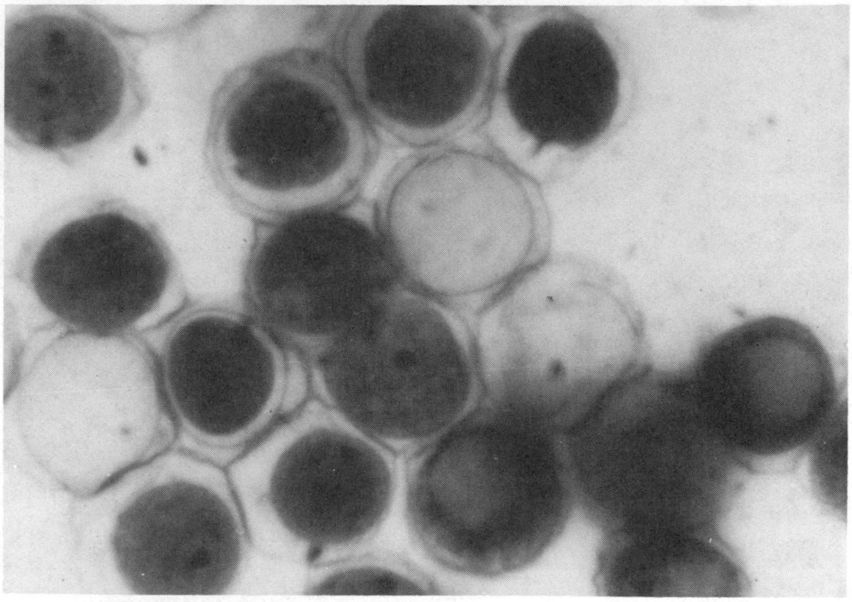

Figure 7. *Acanthamoeba culbertsoni,* cystic stages. Hematoxylin stain after Carazzi. ×1300

PATHOGENESIS. The portal of entry may be either the nasal mucosa (as with PAME) or an injury of the skin or eye. Sometimes the site of entry cannot be identified. The brain may be invaded either primarily via the nasal mucosa and the olfactory nerve (as with PAME) or secondarily by the hematogenous route. The clinical features are those of a fulminating meningoencephalitis (like PAME) or a chronic purulent meningitis, in which case the necrotic cerebral foci are smaller.

PATHOLOGY. In some cases the macroscopic picture is similar to that of PAME. In others, no cerebral edema and no other severe gross changes occur except necrotic foci that vary in size. Microscopic examination shows foci of necrotizing chronic granulomatous encephalitis in the cerebral cortex, cerebellar cortex, fornix, septal nuclei, thalamus, hypothalamus, pons, and midbrain. The lesions contain Langhans' giant cells. The individual lesions contain anywhere from solitary amebae to massive numbers in the perivascular spaces (Fig. 8), similar to *Naegleria* infection, but cellular reaction is better developed than in PAME. The size of the amebae in histologic preparations ranges from 10 to 50 μm; their nuclei are typical of the limax group (Fig. 9). An occasional characteristic polygonal cyst may be formed in the tissues.

CLINICAL FEATURES. Meningeal symptoms are usually preceded by headache and fever. The disease most often develops more slowly than PAME. Hemiparesis or ataxia follows frequently after the development of meningismus. Death occurs after a deep coma. The immediate cause of death is not necessarily central nervous system failure. If the focal lesions in the CNS are not extensive, the CSF may be clear. The number and type of cells have no relevance to the diagnosis; in some cases, lymphocytes predominate in the CSF. The incubation period may range

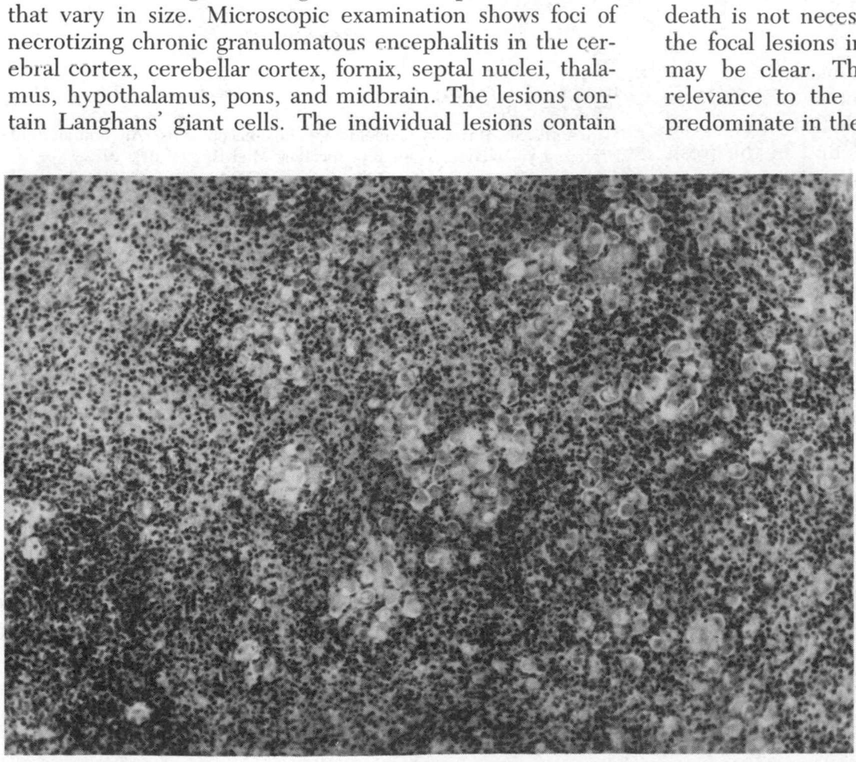

Figure 8. Experimental cerebral acanthamebiasis in guinea pig after intracerebral inoculation with *A. culbertsoni.* Perivascularly located amebae are surrounded by massive leukocytic infiltration. Trichrome after Masson. ×200

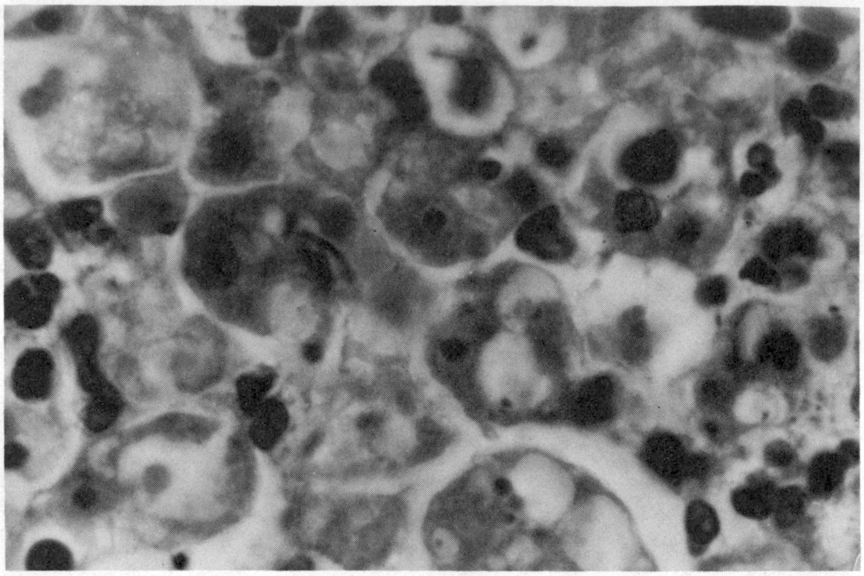

Figure 9. *Acanthamoeba culbertsoni* in cerebral tissue of an experimentally infected guinea pig (detail). Trichrome after Masson. ×1300

from roughly ten days to several months. The total duration of the disease from the first symptoms to death is three to seven weeks.

COMPLICATIONS. The incidence of focal lesions in other organs or generalized disease is frequent. The clinical picture is dominated by neurologic features. Acanthamebiasis may cause isolated keratoconjunctivitis and uveitis.

GEOGRAPHIC DISTRIBUTION. Cases of meningoencephalitis caused by acanthamebae have been reported from America, Africa, and Asia. However, the pattern of distribution of pathogenic amebae of the genus *Acanthamoeba* is cosmopolitan and so is the potential incidence of the infection.

DIAGNOSIS. Like PAME, acanthamebiasis cannot be distinguished by standard clinical or laboratory findings from an acute or chronic meningoencephalitis of bacterial origin. In some cases, no amebae are found in the fresh CSF. However, in the second week of the disease, it may be possible to obtain positive results from a serologic examination with antigens from several acanthamebic strains such as *A. culbertsoni, A. castellani, A. polyphaga* and *A. rhysodes*. The complement fixation, indirect hemagglutination, indirect fluorescent antibody, ELISA and immobilization tests are used for this purpose.

TREATMENT. Sulfonamides are of doubtful value, and other drugs with a satisfactory amebicidal effect in vitro do not enter the nervous tissue in high enough concentrations.

PROPHYLAXIS. Prophylaxis is unknown.

BRAIN AMEBIASIS CAUSED BY ENTAMOEBA HISTOLYTICA

This is a relatively infrequent form of extraintestinal amebiasis. It presents the picture of a brain abscess without marked meningeal features and no amebae in the cerebrospinal fluid. It is secondary to intestinal or hepatic disease and tends to produce multiple abscesses that vary in size (Lombardo et al., 1964). The treatment of choice is metronidazole because it combines strong antiamebic properties with good penetration of the drug into the brain. The dose is 500 mg intravenously every 6 hours.

References

Butt, C. G.: Primary amebic meningoencephalitis. New Engl J Med 274:1473, 1966.

Carter, R. F.: Primary amoebic meningo-encephalitis. An appraisal of present knowledge. Trans Roy Soc Trop Med Hyg 66:193, 1972.

Cěrva, L., Novak, K., and Culbertson, C. G.: An outbreak of acute, fatal amebic meningoencephalitis. Am J Epidemiol 88:436, 1968.

Fowler, M., and Carter, R. F.: Acute pyogenic meningitis probably due to Acanthamoeba sp.: a preliminary report. Br Med J 5464:740, 1965.

Lawande, R. V., John, I., Dobbs, R. H., and Egler, L. J.: A case of primary amebic meningoencephalitis in Zaria, Nigeria. Am J Clin Path 71:591, 1979.

Lombardo, L., Alonso, P., and Arroyo, L., et al.: Cerebral amebiases. Report of 17 cases. J Neurosurg 21:704, 1964.

Mandal, B. N., Gudex, D. J., Fitchett, M. R., Pullon, D. H. H., Malloch, J. A., David, C. M., and Apthorp, J.: Acute meningoencephalitis due to amoebae of the order Myxomycetale (slime mould). N Z Med J 71:16, 1970.

Seidel, J. S., Harmatz, P., Visvesvara, G. S., Cohen, A., Edwards, J., and Turner, J.: Successful treatment of primary amebic meningoencephalitis. New Engl J Med 306:346, 1982.

176
SPINAL EPIDURAL ABSCESS

ANN SULLIVAN BAKER, M.D.

Spinal epidural abscess is an uncommon disease; however, its importance stems not from its frequency but from its therapeutic implications. Effective treatment to prevent paraplegia requires early and accurate diagnosis of an often atypical and confusing group of symptoms and signs. Because the pace and evolution of the disease may be very rapid, it is important that the family practitioner, internist, and pediatrician recognize the features of the illness, make the diagnosis, and refer to the neurosurgeon for immediate treatment.

DEFINITION. Spinal epidural infections are purulent or granulomatous collections within the spinal epidural space. They lie over or encircle the spinal cord, roots, and nerves (Baker et al., 1975; Browder and Meyer, 1927; Dus, 1960). Infection is usually localized within three to four vertebral segments, although it may extend the length of the spinal canal. Spinal epidural abscesses are acute or chronic. The acute abscess has a rapid clinical course of less than two weeks. In chronic abscesses, more than two weeks elapse between back symptoms and surgical intervention, and granulation tissue rather than pus is found in the epidural space.

INCIDENCE. Spinal epidural abscess is less than one-twentieth as common as bacterial meningitis. Children and adults may be affected.

ETIOLOGY. *Staphylococcus aureus* is the organism most commonly isolated from epidural abscesses and accounts for 50 per cent of cases. Streptococci, including non-Group A species, composes the second major category. *Escherichia coli* and *Pseudomonas aeruginosa* have been isolated secondary to urinary tract or abdominal infections. Rarely, anaerobic or mixed organisms from dental or upper airway infections have been isolated from spinal epidural abscesses, in contrast to their much greater frequency as the cause of brain abscess. In a few patients, no organism has been found.

PATHOGENESIS. The most common focus for hematogenous spread to the epidural space is a skin infection, especially a furuncle. Dental and upper respiratory infections are frequent sources. Antecedent hematogenous vertebral osteomyelitis accounts for about 40 per cent of spinal epidural abscesses. A contiguous focus, such as a psoas abscess or sacral decubitus, may predispose to an epidural abscess. Congenital dermal sinuses may also be a source of infection.

In view of the frequency of transient bacteremic episodes, why do so few localize as spinal epidural abscesses? One possibility is that traumatic bleeding into the epidural space is often necessary to transmit the infection into this sequestered site, even some time after the injury. In one series, 13 of 38 patients (30 per cent) had a history of back trauma or back surgery.

ANATOMY. The clinical features and pathophysiology of spinal epidural abscess depend on certain key anatomic relationships. The epidural space contains fatty tissue and a rich, venous plexus (Fig. 1). Posteriorly, this space is relatively capacious, whereas anteriorly it narrows. The anterior spinal artery and central arteries supply most of the spinal cord. Indeed, occlusion of the anterior spinal artery or central arteries affects the anterior four fifths of the cord.

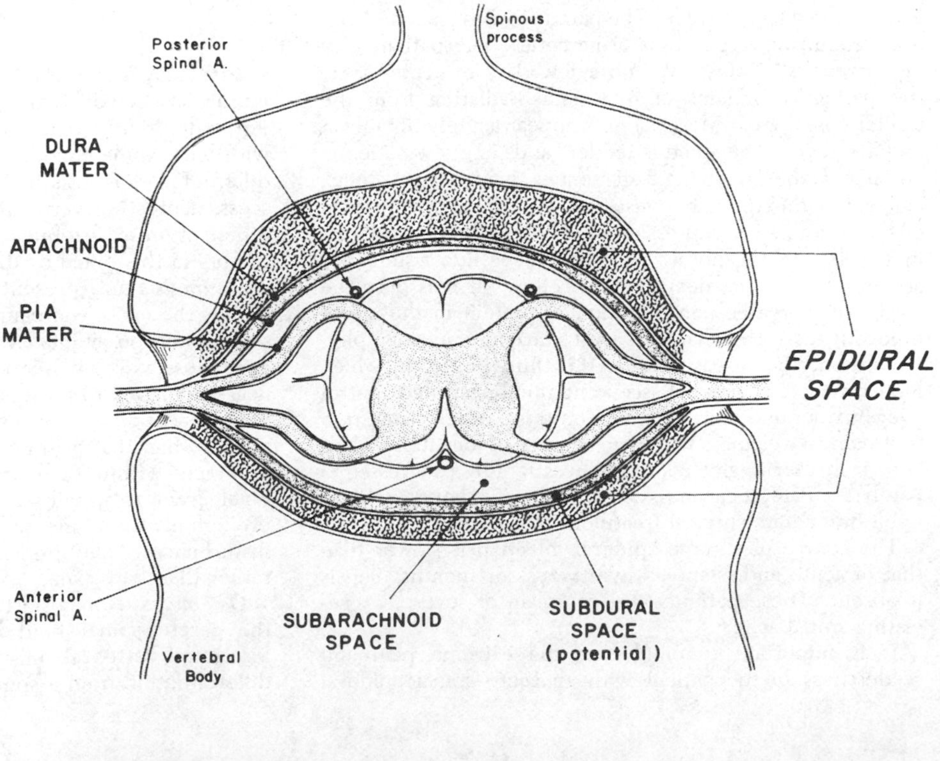

Figure 1. Anatomic relationship of epidural space. Note the larger capacity of the posterior space compared with the anterior space and the vulnerable positions of the spinal arteries.

The venous drainage of the spinal column consists of three communicating systems: (1) the internal or epidural plexus, (2) the intraosseous plexus, and (3) the external vertebral plexus. The internal network forms a meshwork around the dura, lining the adjacent bones, and connects with both the intraosseous and the external plexuses. The external plexus communicates freely with the vertebral and systemic circulations and with the intercostal, ascending lumbar, and lateral sacral veins, thus forming the well-known Batson's plexus (Batson, 1940).

PATHOLOGY. The average abscess extends over four to five vertebral segments. The primary site of involvement is, in order of frequency: thoracic, lumbar, or cervical. The posterior thoracic or lumbar extradural space of the spinal cord is the most common location for an epidural abscess. An anterior epidural abscess is almost always secondary to vertebral osteomyelitis.

The epidural space contains either pus in acute cases or granulation tissue in chronic cases without lesions in the spinal cord. In the more severe cases, examined postmortem, the spinal cord may become necrotic with early macrophage reaction in the disintegrating cord tissue, and many small arteries and veins in the subarachnoid space and spinal cord may be inflamed and thrombosed. The mechanism of the destructive changes in the spinal cord in cases of epidural abscess is not entirely clear. The lesions in the cord seem to be more extensive than can be accounted for by mechanical compression alone. Most probably, the rapidly growing infected inflammatory mass impairs the intrinsic circulation of the cord, perhaps by thrombosis. Thus, in addition to the serious effects of nerve root and cord compression from the epidural mass, there is the additional hazard of ischemic injury to the neural tissue.

CLINICAL MANIFESTATIONS. The clinical picture of an epidural abscess was classically described by Heusner (1948) as a progression from spinal ache to root pain to weakness and finally paralysis. The spinal ache starts at the level of the affected spine. The pain is usually excruciating, often requiring large doses of narcotics. The patient may be extremely restless. Within a few days in acute cases, the patient complains of root pains radiating from the tender spinal area. Most patients appear acutely ill; almost all have fever. The spine is tender, and, in a few patients, edema of the overlying soft tissues may occur. Reflex changes at this time are consistent with the anatomic level of the lesion, i.e., depression of the deep tendon reflexes in the legs if the abscess overlies the cauda equina, or accentuation of the deep tendon reflexes if it is over the cord. An increased concentration of protein in the spinal fluid suggests the diagnosis and warrants myelography. Untreated, the disease enters the third phase, in which motor weakness, gradual ascending numbness, and control over bladder and bowel is lost. There is a progression from root pain to weakness within an average of four to five days and, if further neglected, the illness rapidly progresses to paralysis. Paraplegia may occur within 24 hours, whereupon immediate surgical treatment is mandatory.

The course of chronic epidural infection is slower than that of acute and is spread over weeks or months. Sepsis is absent. These patients also complain of severe, excruciating spinal ache.

It is important to emphasize the extreme pain and restlessness in the patient with an acute spinal epidural abscess (Baker et al., 1975). The patients usually require large doses of narcotics. "Electric" pains or paresthesias (as described by Lhermitte) may be misinterpreted as hysterical (Liveson and Zimmer, 1972). Unfortunately, the patient with spinal epidural abscess is often labeled obstructive or malingering, and the psychiatrist may be consulted before the neurologist.

The mean peripheral white cell count is elevated in acute cases but is within normal limits in the chronic group. The cerebrospinal fluid (CSF) findings are typical of those of a parameningeal infection: the white cell count ranges from 0 to 1000 per mm^3; polymorphonuclear leukocytes and lymphocytes are present in roughly equal numbers; the protein level is markedly elevated with a mean value of about 500 mg per 1000 ml; and the glucose level is normal. Those patients with accompanying bacterial meningitis will have higher CSF white cell counts and may have low cerebrospinal fluid glucose values. If the spinal puncture needle enters the abscess, a very high white cell count is found.

Radiographs of the spine may reveal osteomyelitis in a significant number of patients. If spine films, including tomography, are negative, a CAT scan should be obtained. Myelograms show a partial, or most commonly, a complete block in most patients with spinal epidural abscess (Fig. 2).

COMPLICATIONS AND SEQUELAE. Because of the rapid progression of neurologic damage, failure to make an early diagnosis of spinal epidural abscess is often disastrous. Approximately 5 per cent of patients will have residual weakness, paralysis, or death.

The epidural abscess may extend into the vertebrae and cause osteomyelitis. This progression, however, is much less common than extension from vertebral osteomyelitis to an epidural abscess. Spread of the epidural abscess may also cause retroperitoneal psoas abscess, pleural effusion, or retropharyngeal abscess. Finally, the abscess may also spread through the vertebral system, erode through the subarachnoid space, and produce meningitis.

DIFFERENTIAL DIAGNOSIS. The diagnosis of spinal epidural abscess will be missed if this disease is not considered in the differential diagnosis of backache in a febrile patient with local spine tenderness. The major considerations in differential diagnosis are meningitis, spinal subdural abscess, acute transverse myelopathy, problems in the vertebral or intervertebral disk space, vascular lesions, and tumors in the spinal cord.

Meningitis may present with back pain, but headache is usually the major complaint. Local spine tenderness should suggest the possibility of an epidural process. *Spinal subdural abscess* is much less common but presents with signs nearly identical to those of an epidural abscess.

The onset of *acute transverse myelopathy* is usually more sudden than that of spinal epidural abscess, with paralysis occurring within 72 hours. Pain may be absent, and the myelogram is usually normal. *Infectious polyneuritis* is predominantly a motor disorder with minimal sensory disturbances. The initial symptom is usually weakness rather than back pain.

Osteomyelitis may start with back pain or root signs, but the cerebrospinal fluid analysis is normal. If there is associated vertebral collapse and spinal cord compression, differentiation from a spinal epidural abscess may be diffi-

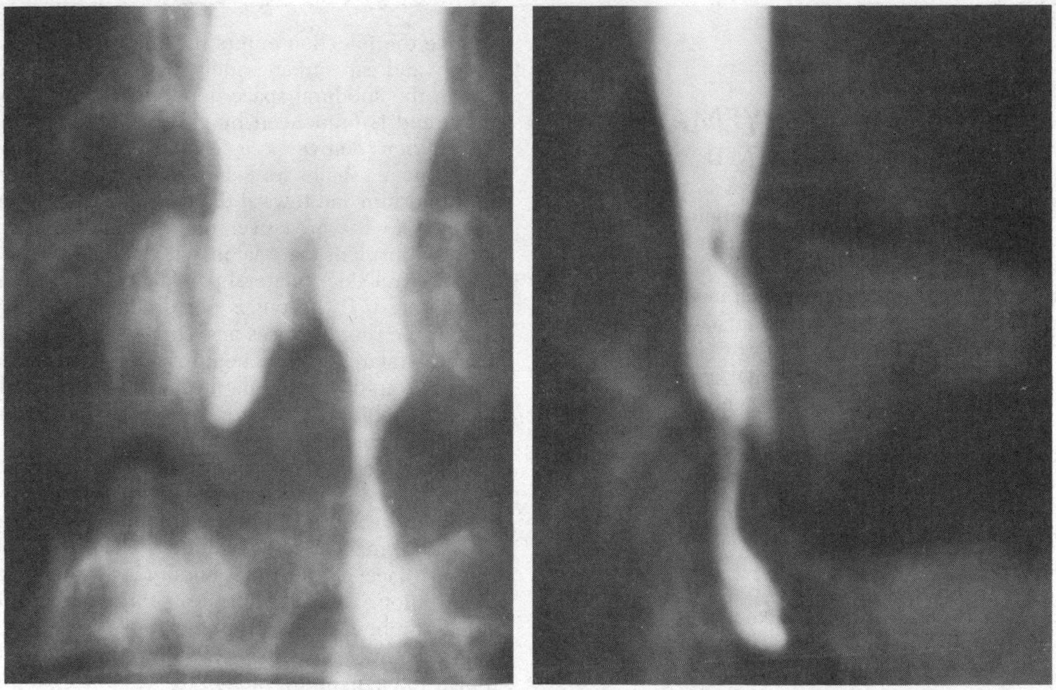

Figure 2. Myelogram of spinal epidural abscess showing complete block.

cult. *Extruded disks* may produce similar symptoms, but the cerebrospinal fluid is usually clear.

Most *vascular problems* such as an epidural hematoma or interruption of the vascular supply of the cord occur with sudden paralysis, often acute pain, and no fever. *Dissecting aortic aneurysm* often presents with severe stabbing pain and may be confused with epidural abscess.

Finally, *primary spinal tumors* may present in a manner similar to that of a chronic epidural abscess. This differentiation is difficult to make without a tissue biopsy of the epidural contents.

DIAGNOSIS AND TREATMENT. The patient with back pain, fever, and localized tenderness should have radiographs of the spine and a careful spinal puncture, with slow insertion of the needle and intermittent aspiration to ensure that epidural pus is detected. The risk of introducing infection from the epidural space is real, but is less a risk than not making the diagnosis of an epidural abscess. If involvement of the lumbar area is suspected, it is preferable to obtain the cerebrospinal fluid by lateral cervical puncture.

Signs of spinal cord or nerve root compression are an indication for myelography, preferably at the time of the spinal puncture. If a block or epidural mass is found on myelogram, laminectomy should be performed without delay, exposing the entire longitudinal extent of the abscess. If an acute abscess is found, the area is drained or packed open and subsequently closed secondarily. If the abscess is chronic and consists primarily of granulation tissue, the spinal cord should be fully decompressed and the wound closed.

When the primary abnormality is anterior, the extradural exposure should be done by removal of the pedicle or by a lateral or anterior approach. Blood cultures should be performed. The material obtained at operation should be immediately examined by Gram stain and cultured. Antibiotic treatment should be started during the operation or earlier. If there are no predisposing foci and no clues to the bacterial cause on examination of the Gram stained smear, a semisynthetic penicillin (nafcillin, oxacillin, or methicillin) in a dose of 2 g intravenously (I.V.) every four hours should be used initially. The combination of ampicillin (2.0 g I.V. every four hours) or carbenicillin (3.0 g I.V. every three hours) plus gentamicin (1 mg/kg I.V. every eight hours) is recommended in the setting of a known urinary tract focus. If penicillin allergy is present, a cephalosporin might be used in place of penicillin or semisynthetic penicillin.

Epidural abscess merits treatment with parenteral antibiotics for three to four weeks; concomitant vertebral osteomyelitis should be treated with antibiotics for six to eight weeks.

References

Baker, A. S., Ojemann, R. G., Swartz, M. N., and Richardson, E. P., Jr.: Spinal epidural abscess. N Engl J Med 293:463, 1975.

Batson, O. V.: The function of the vertebral veins and their role in the spread of metastases. Ann Surg 112:138, 1940.

Browder, J. R., and Meyer, R.: Infection of the spinal epidural space; an aspect of vertebral osteomyelitis. Am J Surg 37:4, 1927.

Dus, B.: Spinal peripachymeningitis (epidural abscess): Report of 8 cases. J Neurosurg 17:972, 1960.

Heusner, A. P.: Nontuberculous spinal epidural infections. N Engl J Med 239:845, 1948.

Liveson, J. A., and Zimmer, A. E.: A localizing symptom in thoracic myelopathy. A variation of Lhermitte's sign. Ann Intern Med 76:769, 1972.

177

SUBDURAL EMPYEMA

ANN SULLIVAN BAKER, M.D.

Subdural empyema is a purulent collection in the potential space between the dura and the arachnoid. The term subdural abscess has been applied to this condition, but a better term is subdural empyema, which indicates suppuration in a preformed space. More than half of the cases result from extension of infection from primary foci in the paranasal sinuses, especially the frontal sinuses; chronic otitis media and mastoiditis less commonly result in subdural empyema. Subdural empyema may also occur from direct introduction of infection through operative or traumatic wounds or, rarely, by arterial hematogenous dissemination. Finally, subdural empyema in infants may result from extension of bacterial meningitis (Jacobsen and Farmer, 1981).

INCIDENCE. Subdural empyema comprises about one-quarter of all localized intracranial bacterial infections. Mortality remains high, in the range of 20 to 40 per cent, because of errors in diagnosis, uncontrolled infection, and delayed surgical intervention.

ETIOLOGY. The organisms vary with the initiating process (Hitchcock and Andreadis, 1964; Swartz and Karchmer, 1974). Streptococci account for more than 50 per cent of the cases. The streptococci are frequently non-group A and often anaerobic. *Staphylococcus aureus* may account for as many as 30 per cent of the total isolates. Gram-negative bacteria, *E. coli, Proteus,* and *Pseudomonas,* cause approximately 20 per cent of the total cases. *Hemophilus influenzae* has been found in subdural empyema complicating *H. influenzae* meningitis in rare cases.

Anaerobic streptococci make up the largest portion of anaerobic bacteria isolated from subdural empyema, followed by *Bacteroidaceae* (Yoshikawa et al., 1975). This is not an unexpected finding, since the common predisposing factor to subdural empyema is paranasal sinus infection (Coonrod and Davis, 1972; Kubik and Adams, 1943; Kaufman et al., 1983), in which anaerobes are important pathogens (Frederick and Braude, 1974). Finally, unusual organisms or no organisms are found in 10 to 20 per cent of the cases.

PATHOGENESIS AND PATHOLOGY. The potential subdural space is unrestricted over and between the cerebral hemispheres but is restricted in the central basal region; hence most subdural empyemas are found either on the convexity (supratentorial region) or in the parafalx region. In cases of infection from a contiguous site, the empyema is usually located in the adjacent subdural spaces; for example, empyema following paranasal sinusitis is located primarily in the frontal subdural space. The spread in such cases occurs mainly via progressive thrombophlebitis of the mucosal veins, extending to the cerebral veins and to venous sinuses; less often, there is direct extension from bone or dura. Infection may also reach the subdural space by direct extension from osteomyelitis secondary to otogenic infection; the empyema may then be located in the adjacent temporal-parietal area.

Once the infection enters the subdural space, pus forms rapidly and can spread widely. The extension of the infection in the subdural space depends on the primary site of origin and is influenced by gravity and anatomic boundaries. When empyema is established following otogenic infection, it usually spreads posteriorly and medially over the tentorium and toward the falx. The empyema is usually confined to the area over one cerebral hemisphere, but because purulent material may spread under the falx to the contralateral side, bilateral parafalcine collections are often encountered. If the pus is not drained, the ensuing phlebitis of the dural sinuses and cortical veins causes areas of cerebral infarction and hemorrhage. Compression of the brain by rapidly accumulating pus and the cerebral injury due to phlebitis give rise to diffuse as well as focal neurologic abnormalities.

Subdural exudate generally covers a large part of one cerebral hemisphere and ranges in volume from a few milliliters to 200 ml. The arachnoid is cloudy and thrombosis of meningeal veins may be seen. The exudate on the inner surface of the dura undergoes variable degrees of organization. There is infiltration of the underlying pia with small numbers of neutrophilic leukocytes, lymphocytes, and mononuclear cells. The thrombi in cerebral veins appear to begin on the side of the vein nearest the subdural exudate. The superficial layers of the cerebral cortex then undergo ischemic necrosis.

CLINICAL MANIFESTATIONS. Subdural empyema is most often preceded by a flare-up of sinusitis or mastoiditis and symptoms of local pain with an increase in discharge from the nose or ear. Swelling, erythema, and local tenderness of the site overlying the primary infection may then become evident. In the early stages, pain or headache may be localized and moderate. As the illness progresses, the headache becomes generalized and severe. High fever, vomiting, and nuchal rigidity then develop. Focal or generalized seizures, hemiparesis, sensory deficits, visual field defects, and dysphasia may occur within several days. In dominant hemisphere collections, dysphasia is a frequent symptom, often appearing as a reluctance to talk and regarded by the inexperienced examiner as an expected accompaniment to the headache and systemic infection. Minimal weakness of one or more limbs progresses to complete paralysis. In some cases this is preceded by focal or generalized seizures. Papilledema may be seen. Seizures occur, owing partly to mass effect but also to the associated thrombophlebitis of cortical veins and infarction of cerebral tissue. Without treatment, progressive obtundation, coma, and death occur within 48 to 72 hours. Table 1 presents the relative frequency of symptoms and signs in 26 cases. Headache is present in every case in the early stages. The frequency of symptoms in patients with paranasal infections closely parallels that in otitic patients. Patients with pus on the convexity of the brain usually present with contralateral hemiplegia, often with focal seizures of face, arms, and legs. Sensory disturbances are less common, whereas in collections over the dominant hemisphere, aphasia is usual. The primary falcine collection begins with a lower limb monoplegia that rapidly progresses up the trunk to involve the arm but characteristically spares the face.

DIAGNOSIS. Sinusitis, fever, and focal neurologic signs and symptoms are major diagnostic clues in the diagnosis

Table 1. INCIDENCE OF DIFFERENT SYMPTOMS AND SIGNS

Symptoms and Signs	Paranasal (20 Cases) *At Onset*	Paranasal (20 Cases) *Established*	Otitic (6 Cases) *At Onset*	Otitic (6 Cases) *Established*
Evidence of systemic infection	19 (95%)	20 (100%)	5 (83%)	6 (100%)
Paralysis (usually hemiplegia)	13 (65%)	20 (100%)	4 (66%)	6 (100%)
Stiff neck and Kernigism	12 (60%)	18 (90%)	5 (83%)	6 (100%)
Disturbed consciousness	13 (65%)	16 (80%)	5 (83%)	6 (100%)
Headache	20 (100%)	15 (75%)	4 (66%)	4 (66%)
High intracranial pressure	8 (40%)	15 (75%)	2 (33%)	3 (50%)
Mental changes	10 (50%)	12 (60%)	3 (50%)	4 (66%)
Vomiting	10 (50%)	10 (50%)	4 (66%)	4 (66%)
Epilepsy	7 (35%)	9 (45%)	2 (33%)	3 (50%)
Visual field defects	1 (5%)	9 (45%)	2 (33%)	3 (50%)
Sensory changes	5 (25%)	8 (40%)	1 (17%)	4 (66%)
Aphasia (in left hemisphere involvement)	100%		80%	

From Hitchcock, E., and Andreadis, A.: J Neurol Neurosurg Psychiat 27:422, 1964.

of subdural empyema. A peripheral leukocytosis is often present. The cerebrospinal fluid (CSF) and white blood cell formula is variable—it may contain no cells, a few polymorphonuclear and/or mononuclear cells, or, most frequently, from 50 to 1000 white blood cells; usually there is an equal number of polymorphonuclear cells and mononuclear cells. The protein concentration is increased in the CSF (a range of 75 to 300 mg/100 ml) with a normal glucose level. Gram stain of the smear and cultures of the CSF are usually negative. The combination of focal signs, cells in the CSF, and a high protein concentration indicates a parameningeal focus. In general, the early performance of a lumbar puncture is important in the evaluation of patients with possible central nervous system infection. However, if papilledema or other signs of increased intracranial pressure are present, transtentorial herniation is apt to occur following lumbar puncture. This procedure should be omitted or postponed until after a mass lesion is excluded by CAT scan.

Skull films, with sinus or mastoid films, may confirm the existence of paranasal sinus or mastoid infection. These examinations and the selective use of conventional tomograms may demonstrate and delineate bony destruction from infection. Rarely, air fluid levels may be diagnostic of a subdural or epidural process. A shift of the calcified pineal may suggest an intracranial mass effect.

Computerized axial tomography, or CAT scan, is the single most useful procedure for making the diagnosis of subdural empyema (Joubert and Stephanov, 1977; Kaufman and Leeds, 1977). Typically, a low absorption mass is identified in an extracerebral location. A thin, moderately dense margin may be visualized after the injection of intravenous contrast material. The conventional axial CAT scan frequently shows the extent of the subdural mass, although coronal scans may help to define collections at the base of the brain or about the tentorium. Coexisting brain abscess, focal cerebritis, or infarction edema is detected as well. Bony involvement may also be documented by using special settings to visualize bone. The CAT scan may be negative if collections are small and may not distinguish a sterile collection from an empyema.

The radionuclide scan can also detect subdural empyema and associated brain abscess. It is less helpful in defining the exact anatomic location of the process, that is, in distinguishing a subdural collection from meningitis or infarction, and may miss small or parafalcine collections.

Cerebral angiography reliably demonstrates extracerebral collections and may be especially helpful for bilateral or small parafalcine lesions. Demonstration of irregular contours, spasm, small vessel occlusions, or venous obstruction in association with an extracerebral mass may suggest infection as the cause. Rarely, however, is the gain significant, and angiography should be avoided when possible because of its potential morbidity in the febrile, infected, neurologically impaired patient.

Differential Diagnosis. Subdural empyema may present the same symptoms and signs as brain abscess. The initial stage of cerebral abscess is often milder and more insidious in onset, and the course may be more protracted. The temperature is usually normal and the neck is rarely stiff except in the case of a complicating meningitis. Although the deterioration may be more acute in some cases of subdural empyema, the fact remains that making a clinical distinction from brain abscess may be quite difficult.

The clinical resemblance between subdural empyema and thrombophlebitis of the superior longitudinal sinus is close, and reference has already been made to their possible coexistence. Favoring the diagnosis of sinus thrombophlebitis are a septic temperature, bacteremia, absence of increased intracranial pressure or stiff neck, little or no pleocytosis, and bilateral signs such as focal convulsions or paralysis occurring first on one side of the body and then on the other.

Bacterial meningitis and subdural empyema may also present in a similar fashion, that is, with depressed sensorium, fever, and nuchal rigidity. However, sinusitis, especially frontal sinusitis, is an uncommon antecedent of bacterial meningitis. In addition, meningitis in adults, unlike subdural empyema, is usually not associated with focal seizures, hemiparesis, or papilledema. These findings suggest parenchymal brain involvement. Finally, slight pleocytosis, absence of organisms, a high protein concentration, and a normal glucose level in the spinal fluid are more suggestive of subdural empyema. Tuberculous, fungal (e.g., cryptococcal), and viral meningoencephalitis may all be confused with subdural empyema. Acid-fast smears and wet preparations of the spinal fluid, cultures for *Mycobacterium tuberculosis*, viruses, and fungi, and fungal or viral antibody titers of the cerebrospinal fluid and serum are helpful in the differential diagnosis of these entities.

COMPLICATIONS AND SEQUELAE. The mortality of subdural infections has decreased from 100 per cent to about 40 per cent since the introduction of antibiotics. A further decline in mortality has been prevented by persistent errors in diagnosis and by complications of the disease.

Frank meningitis seldom accompanies subdural empyema. Administration of antibiotics to patients with subdural empyema without concomitant drainage results in a chronic illness with a course resembling that of an intraparenchymal brain abscess.

Cortical venous or major dural sinus thrombophlebitis, cerebral abscess, or infarction or herniation may all complicate subdural empyema. At least one-half of the survivors from subdural empyema will have neurologic incapacities secondary to thrombosis of surface veins, dural sinuses, and areas of cerebral infarction.

TREATMENT. Subdural empyema is a life-threatening infection requiring prompt surgical drainage and intensive antimicrobial therapy. Both are crucial for a favorable outcome. Surgical management of the subdural empyema must provide for adequate drainage of all collections of purulent material. The simplest process is immediate drainage through enlarged multiple frontal burr holes. Craniotomy with contralateral placement of burr holes provides for full bilateral drainage, especially of loculated or viscous fluid, as well as for the proper exposure of parafalcine collections and cranial abscess formation. Surgical treatment of the accompanying sinusitis, frontal osteomyelitis, or mastoiditis is a secondary consideration and is usually postponed until the acute intracranial infection has subsided.

When the subdural contents are liquid, large amounts of purulent material are readily evacuated. In more chronic lesions, however, granulation tissue may be densely adherent to the underlying pia-arachnoid, making radical removal infeasible. Catheters may be left extending into each corner of the abscess cavity for drainage. At the time of surgery, purulent fluid should be obtained for a Gram-stained smear and aerobic and anaerobic cultures.

Antibiotic therapy should be instituted at the time of surgery or earlier. The initial choice of antibiotics should include penicillin, and, if recommended by the background of the case, an additional agent to cover gram-negative bacilli. Penicillin G, 20 million units/day in divided intravenous doses every four hours combined with chloramphenicol 50 mg/kg/day in divided doses every six hours, will be effective against most of the pathogens isolated from these infections. These antibiotics are also found in good concentrations in the cerebrospinal fluid. However, when infection follows surgery or a penetrating skull injury, a penicillinase-resistant penicillin should be substituted for penicillin G. Antibiotic therapy should be refined according to the background of the case, the Gram-stained smear of the pus obtained at surgery, and the results of cultures of this material. Antibiotics that do not penetrate cerebrospinal fluid, such as most cephalosporins and clindamycin, should be avoided. Although of unproven efficacy, bacitracin 500 to 2000 units/ml may be instilled into the subdural space at the time of surgery and for variable periods thereafter. Local therapy may also be beneficial when treatment requires that poorly diffusible aminoglycoside antibiotics be used. Administration of antibiotics should continue for at least three weeks after surgical drainage.

Since seizures are a frequent feature of subdural empyema, prophylactic use of anticonvulsants such as phenytoin seems reasonable. In addition, if signs of increased intracranial pressure are apparent, use of glucocorticosteroids such as dexamethasone should be considered to reduce inflammatory edema.

References

Coonrod, J. D., and Davis, P. E.: Subdural empyema. Am J Med 53:85, 1972.

Frederick, J., and Braude, A.: Anaerobic infection of the paranasal sinuses. N Engl J Med 290:135, 1974.

Hitchcock, E., and Andreadis, A.: Subdural empyema: A review of 29 cases. J Neurol Neurosurg Psychiatr 27:422, 1964.

Jacobsen, P. C., and Farmer, T. W.: Subdural empyema complicating meningitis in infants: Improved prognosis. Neurology (NY) 31:190, 1981.

Joubert, M. J., and Stephanov, S.: Computerized tomography and surgical treatment in intracranial suppuration. Report of 30 consecutive unselected cases of brain abscess and subdural empyema. J Neurosurg 48:73, 1977.

Kaufman, D. M., and Leeds, N. E.: Computed tomography (CT) in the diagnosis of intracranial abscesses. Brain abscess, subdural empyema and epidural empyema. Neurology 27:1069, 1977.

Kaufman, D. M., Miller, M. H., and Steigbigel, N. H.: Subdural empyema. Analysis of seventeen recent cases and review of the literature. Medicine 54:485, 1975.

Kaufman, D. M., Litman, N., and Miller, M. H.: Sinusitis: Induced subdural empyema. Neurology 33:123, 1983.

Kubik, R. S., and Adams, R. D.: Subdural empyema. Brain 66:18, 1943.

Swartz, M. N., and Karchmer, A. W.: Infections of the central nervous system. In Balows, A., et al. (eds.): Anaerobic Bacteria. Role of Disease. Springfield, Ill., Charles C Thomas, 1974.

Yoshikawa, T. T., Chow, A. W., and Guze, L. B.: Role of anaerobic bacteria in subdural empyema. Report of four cases and review of 327 cases from the English literature. Am J Med 58:99, 1975.

178

CEREBRAL ANGIOSTRONGYLIASIS

LEON ROSEN, M.D., DR. P. H.

Cerebral angiostrongyliasis results from the invasion of the human central nervous system by the rodent metastrongylid lungworm, *Angiostrongylus cantonensis* (Rosen et al., 1962).

ETIOLOGY. Both the male and female mature adult forms of *A. cantonensis* normally live within the pulmonary arteries of rodents (species of the genus *Rattus* and some related genera). In the course of their unusual life cycle, the parasites undergo an obligatory period of development within the central nervous system of the rodent before migrating to the pulmonary arteries. In man, however, development of the parasites almost always is arrested in the central nervous system, and the nematodes usually die there.

In the complete life cycle, eggs laid by fertilized females form emboli in the terminal branches of the pulmonary arteries and hatch there, and the resultant first-stage larvae enter the bronchial system. The larvae migrate up the trachea, pass into the alimentary canal, and are excreted in the feces. The parasites then must enter a molluscan intermediate host, usually a terrestrial or amphibious snail or slug. Two further stages of development occur in the mollusc, and the parasites then reach the third or infective larval stage. Development continues when infected molluscs are eaten by a rodent of the appropriate species. After liberation from molluscan tissue by digestive juices in the alimentary tract, third-stage larvae migrate to the brain and undergo two further stages of development within the parenchyma. The young adult nematodes then migrate to the surface of the brain and enter the venous system in order to reach their final destination, the pulmonary arteries. They attain full sexual maturity after they arrive in the arteries.

PATHOGENESIS AND PATHOLOGY. Man acquires cerebral angiostrongyliasis by accidental or intentional consumption of infected intermediate hosts (molluscs) or paratenic hosts (see below). Paratenic hosts become infected by consuming intermediate hosts. Infective larvae do not develop further in such hosts but remain viable. Although *A. cantonensis* does not develop completely in man, most ingested third-stage larvae apparently reach the human central nervous system, since disease has been observed in persons thought to have been exposed to relatively few larvae. (The parasite does not multiply in humans). The usual incubation period of the disease in man from the time of ingestion of infective larvae to the appearance of the first signs and symptoms is about 2 weeks (with a range of about 1 to 4 weeks).

Damage to the human host results from the development and movement of the living parasites (for example, to the anterior chamber of the eye), or, more commonly, from a granulomatous reaction to dead or dying parasites in the parenchyma of the central nervous system or the meninges. This inflammatory response, characterized by an abundance of eosinophilic leukocytes, gives rise to the eosinophilic pleocytosis characteristic of the disease. The degree of pathology usually is proportional to the number of parasites ingested, except in rare instances when parasites migrate to a critical area (such as the eye). Fatalities are rare, and most patients recover without sequelae. One episode of the disease does not confer immunity to subsequent exposure, and repeated episodes have been observed in individuals reexposed to infective larvae.

CLINICAL MANIFESTATIONS, COMPLICATIONS, AND SEQUELAE. The most common clinical expression of cerebral angiostrongyliasis is a meningitis characterized by headache, nausea and vomiting, moderate stiffness of the neck and/or back, paresthesias, and low-grade or no fever. Headache commonly is severe, intractable, and bitemporal in location, and is usually the symptom that brings the patient to a physician. Paresthesias are varied but commonly consist of exaggerated sensitivity to touch. They usually are unilateral and not limited to areas innervated by specific spinal segments or peripheral nerves. Unilateral facial paralysis of the lower motor neuron type occurs in about 5 per cent of patients. Other cranial nerves are affected more rarely. Fever is more common in children (Char and Rosen, 1967). Living young adult parasites have occasionally been observed in the eye. Characteristically, the disease is benign and self-limited with a case-mortality ratio of well under 1 per cent. However, severe permanent sequelae (such as blindness) and death may occur, presumably from infection with many parasites. Severe illness is characterized by somnolence or lethargy that may progress to unconsciousness. Paresthesias occasionally persist for years following mild disease.

GEOGRAPHIC VARIATIONS IN DISEASE. Although human disease caused by *A. cantonensis* generally is similar throughout the vast geographic area (see below) in which the parasite occurs, some variations in clinical manifestations are observed. These variations are believed to reflect the number of parasites that patients have ingested. In turn, this reflects differences in the epidemiology of the disease in various geographic areas and differences in the species of, and intensity of infection in, molluscan intermediate or paratenic hosts. For example, in Taiwan, where most human infection is acquired from heavily parasitized giant African snails (*Achatina fulica*), severe disease with permanent sequelae is fairly common (Yii, 1976). On the other hand, on South Pacific islands, where the disease most commonly is acquired from lightly infected paratenic hosts, serious sequelae or deaths are rare.

DIAGNOSIS. Cerebral angiostrongyliasis should be considered in evaluation of patients with severe headache and/or paresthesias who live in, or have recently visited, areas where *A. cantonensis* is known to occur. Until recently, the range of the parasite was believed to be limited by Madagascar in the west, the Hawaiian Islands in the east, Japan in the north, and Australia in the south. *A. cantonensis* has now been reported from Egypt (Yousif and Ibrahim, 1978) and Cuba (Aguiar et al., 1981) and disease presumed to be caused by it has been seen in the latter locality (Pascual et al., 1981). Since both the rodent vertebrate hosts and the molluscan intermediate hosts are commonly transported by human activity, it is probable that the geographic distribution of the parasite will continue to expand, both to new territory within the known geographic range and outside it. For example, neither rodent nor molluscan hosts of *A. cantonensis* occurred on Pacific islands before the arrival of humans. The parasite has been introduced on some of these islands but not on others.

The diagnosis of cerebral angiostrongyliasis usually can be made on clinical grounds alone in association with an epidemiologic history, provided one thinks of the possibility (Rosen et al., 1967). Most, but not all, cases have a characteristic pleocytosis consisting in large part of eosinophils. It is this characteristic that led to the designation of the disease as "eosinophilic meningitis" before its cause was discovered. Most patients have cerebrospinal fluid leukocyte counts of between 100 and 2000 cells/cm in conjunction with their symptoms, and characteristically 25 to 75 per cent of the leukocytes are eosinophils. In general, persons with the highest total cell counts have the highest percentages of eosinophils. Eosinophilia is observed also in the blood, but this finding is less useful because it is of lesser magnitude, more fleeting, and common in patients with other helmintic parasites.

Although living young adult *A. cantonensis* worms have been recovered from the eye and cerebrospinal fluid of patients, this is a rare occurrence. Despite considerable research, there is no satisfactory serologic or skin test that can diagnose the disease in man. Consequently, most cases can be diagnosed only on the basis of clinical, epidemiologic, and cerebrospinal fluid findings.

Infections with *A. cantonensis* often are not recognized because (1) patients are not sick enough to seek medical attention, (2) a spinal tap is not done because the meningitic nature of the illness is not recognized in the absence of fever, or (3) eosinophils in the cerebrospinal fluid are not detected because of failure to use suitable staining methods.

The finding of an eosinophilic pleocytosis does not, of course, establish the diagnosis of invasion of the central nervous system by *A. cantonensis.* Such a finding does, however, strongly suggest the invasion of the central nervous system by a helmintic parasite. Other than helmintic parasites, the only known causes of a significant eosinophilic pleocytosis are the intrathecal injection of various types of foreign proteins, rabies vaccination, the insertion of rubber tubing into the central nervous system in the course of neurosurgery, and coccidioidal meningitis. Helminths other than *A. cantonensis* that invade the central nervous system of man and that can give rise to an eosinophilic pleocytosis include the cysticercus of the pork tapeworm, *Taenia solium,* and the adult forms and eggs of the lung fluke, *Paragonimus westermani.* Both *T. solium* and *P. westermani* often give rise to signs and symptoms of space-occupying lesions and convulsions when the central nervous system is involved. *Gnathostoma spinigerum,* a nematode, can also invade the human central nervous system and cause an eosinophilic pleocytosis. Although larvae of *Trichinella spiralis* and *T. canis* can reach the central nervous system of humans, pleocytosis is uncommon and an eosinophilia pleocytosis has not been demonstrated.

It should be noted that sporadic cases of eosinophilic meningitis of unknown etiology have been described from many different parts of the world. Because of their geographic distribution, it is unlikely that many of these cases were caused by *A. cantonensis.* Thus, it is probable that there are as yet unknown etiologic agents that can give rise to a clinical picture indistinguishable from that of *A. cantonensis.*

TREATMENT. Once the diagnosis has been established, little can be done except to await recovery. Treatment is largely supportive and symptomatic. The diagnostic spinal tap often relieves headache. Aspirin and other analgesic agents are useful for fever and headache. In more severe cases, in which signs of cerebral edema may be prominent, corticosteroids or the osmotic brain-dehydrating agents such as urea or mannitol may be cautiously employed. Respiratory supportive measures, such as tracheostomy or artificial respiration, may be necessary if signs of brain stem compression appear. Recovery characteristically is slow but is usually complete.

Although thiabendazole, a broad spectrum anthelmintic, affects the development of *A. cantonensis* in rats, its use against the parasite in man has not been reported, and there is doubt as to the rationality of such use. It is suspected that most of the deleterious effects of *A. cantonensis* infection in humans are the result of reaction to dead or dying worms, and that not all parasites in a given patient die simultaneously. Consequently, if this view is correct, and if thiabendazole kills all the parasites at one time, treatment with the drug might do more harm than good.

PROPHYLAXIS. Human consumption of raw or incompletely cooked molluscs is sometimes deliberate (e.g., the consumption of chopped *Pila* species in Thailand) and sometimes accidental (e.g., the ingestion of small slugs on carelessly washed lettuce). Paratenic hosts of *A. cantonensis* include fish, amphibians, reptiles, crustaceans, and land planarians. The consumption of raw freshwater shrimp *(Macrobrachium lar)* or food containing extracts of these animals is an important source of human infection on some Pacific islands. Terrestrial or aquatic crabs have been suspected as sources of human infection in some instances. Thus, human infection with *A. cantonensis* is determined largely by cultural factors affecting types of foods consumed and the methods of their preparation. Sporadic cases occur, however, among individuals accidentally exposed to infected molluscs in the course of work or play (for example, contamination of hands in the course of gardening).

Since most species of terrestrial molluscs are susceptible to infection with *A. cantonensis,* their relative importance depends on their abundance near human habitations, their use as food, or their tendency to frequent vegetable gardens. The importance of the various paratenic hosts depends on the frequency with which they are infected and the degree to which they are used as human food in the raw or incompletely cooked state.

Perhaps the most important measure that can be used to control *A. cantonensis* infection in man is education about the nature and source of the disease. Individual measures depend on the way humans are infected in a given area and consist of avoiding the consumption of molluscs or paratenic hosts that may contain infective larvae (both freezing and cooking are effective in destroying larvae), the careful washing of green vegetation that is consumed raw, and careful washing of hands after working in areas likely to contain molluscs. Community-wide measures consist of the control of molluscs and land planarians in vegetable gardens, and perhaps the control of rodents in such areas. Attempts to control rodents and the molluscan intermediate hosts elsewhere appear almost futile at present.

Since *A. cantonensis* is disseminated by man and has yet to reach many geographic areas that appear to be suitable for its maintenance, it obviously is desirable to avoid the introduction of molluscs or rodents from endemic areas into such parasite-free areas.

References

Aguiar, P. H., Morera, P., and Pascual, J.: First record of *Angiostrongylus cantonensis* in Cuba. Am J Trop Med Hyg 30:963, 1981.

Alicata, J. E., and Jindrak, K.: Angiostrongylosis in the Pacific and Southeast Asia. Springfield, Ill., Charles C Thomas, Publisher, 1970.

Char, D. F. B., and Rosen, L.: Eosinophilic meningitis among children in Hawaii. J Pediatr 70:28, 1967.

Pascual, J. E., Bouli, R. P., and Aguiar, H.: Eosinophilic meningoencephalitis in Cuba, caused by *Angiostrongylus cantonensis.* Am J Trop Med Hyg 30:960, 1981.

Punyagupta, S., Bunnag, T., Juttijudata, P., and Rosen, L.: Eosinophilic meningitis in Thailand. Epidemiologic studies of 484 typical cases and the etiologic role of *Angiostrongylus cantonensis.* Am J Trop Med Hyg 19:950, 1970.

Punyagupta, S., Juttijudata, P., and Bunnag, T.: Eosinophilic meningitis in Thailand. Clinical studies of 484 typical cases probably caused by *Angiostrongylus cantonensis.* Am J Trop Med Hyg 24:921, 1975.

Rosen, L., Chappell, R., Laqueur, G. L., Wallace, G. D., and Weinstein, P. P.: Eosinophilic meningoencephalitis caused by a metastrongylid lungworm of rats. JAMA 179:620, 1962.

Rosen, L., Loison, G., Laigret, J., and Wallace, G. D.: Studies on eosinophilic meningitis. 3. Epidemiologic and clinical observations on Pacific islands and the possible etiologic role of *Angiostrongylus cantonensis.* Am J Epidemiol 85:17, 1967.

Yii, C.-Y.: Clinical observations on eosinophilic meningitis and meningoencephalitis caused by *Angiostrongylus cantonensis* on Taiwan. Am J Trop Med Hyg 25:233, 1976.

Yii, C.-Y., Chen, C.-Y., Chen, E.-R., Hsieh, H.-C., Shih, C.-C., Cross, J. H., and Rosen, L.: Epidemiologic studies of eosinophilic meningitis in southern Taiwan. Am J Trop Med Hyg 24:447, 1975.

Yousif, F. and Ibrahim, A.: The first record of *Angiostrongylus cantonensis* from Egypt. Z Parasitenkd 56:73, 1978.

179

RABIES

Bosko Postic, M.D.
Tadeusz J. Wiktor, D.V.M.

Rabies is a viral infection of the central nervous system affecting all warm-blooded animals including man. The disease is caused by rabies virus and is usually transmitted by saliva falling onto wounds inflicted by rabid animals. Overt disease, consisting of fever, excitation, convulsions, lacrimation, salivation, and dysphagia, is known as "furious rabies." The human disease is also known as hydrophobia. Another form of the disease is known as "dumb rabies." It is characterized by progressive lassitude, coma, and death. Human rabies is almost invariably fatal, except for an occasional documented survivor (Hattwick et al., 1972; Porras et al., 1976).

ETIOLOGY. Rabies virus belongs to a group of rhabdoviruses with a characteristic bullet-shaped form, dimensions of 75 × 180 nm, a ribonucleoprotein core, and a lipid envelope. Rhabdoviruses are inactivated by lipid solvents such as ether. They are described in greater detail in Chapter 69.

Rabies virus was isolated by Pasteur and coworkers in the 1880s. They discovered vaccination and introduced the widely used terms "street" and "fixed" strains. Fixed virus was produced in Pasteur's laboratory by repeated intracerebral passages of infected neural tissue in rabbits so that the incubation period became *fixed* at a shorter interval of five to ten days, whereas naturally circulating (street) strains produced encephalitis after a variable period of 15 to 30 days. Street strains have a wide host range and are infectious by peripheral inoculation. Transfer of infection in nature occurs by means of the virus in salivary glands. In contrast, fixed strains have diminished infectiousness when they are inoculated peripherally, and, as a rule, do not appear in the saliva of rabid animals. Fixed strains can serve for vaccine production because the original antigenicity appears to be maintained.

Previously, all strains of rabies virus, regardless of their geographic origin or the species of animal from which they were obtained, were considered to be antigenically indistinguishable. Presently, antigenic differences among strains of rabies virus can be readily demonstrated with monoclonal antibodies obtained by the fusion of mouse myeloma cells with cells derived from mice immunized with rabies virus. The analysis of many field virus isolates revealed a pattern of similar reactivity for strains of the same geographic origin (Wiktor et al., 1980).

PATHOGENESIS AND PATHOLOGY. After inoculation into experimental animals, the infectious virus can persist for four to six days close to the site of injection. The infection has been shown by immunofluorescence to start in striated muscle cells close to the site of inoculation. Amputation of the limb or cutting of the nerves proximal to inoculation prevents rabies in animals. The concept of neural spread of the virus is based on this observation. Viral replication has not been demonstrated in any of the peripheral nerve structures. After mouse foot pad inoculation, the virus moves probably passively via tissue interspaces within the nerve. More recent immunofluorescent studies suggest that the earliest replication in neural cells occurs in the dorsal root ganglia. Thereafter, the virus involves the adjacent cord segment.

After this initial invasion of the central nervous system, the virus disseminates in a rapid and selective manner: It attacks the neuronal cells of the brain stem, the hippocampus, the subcortical nuclei, the limbic cortex, and the Purkinje cells in the cerebellum. In the second phase, the virus spreads from the CNS through nerves to diverse organs such as the eye, salivary glands, tongue, skin, and heart. Replication takes place in these tissues. Certain cells, such as salivary glandular epithelium, efficiently support the production of rabies virions.

The histopathology of rabies consists of (1) encephalomyelitis and (2) inclusions known as Negri bodies.

This encephalomyelitis is characterized by neuronal changes and predominantly lymphocytic infiltration, both diffuse and perivascular. Negri bodies (Fig. 1) are intracytoplasmic inclusions in neurons. They are 2 to 10 μm in size and are found in the central pyramidal layer of Ammon's horn of the hippocampus, in the Purkinje cells of the cerebellum, and, less frequently, in the motor area of the cerebral cortex and medullary nuclei. Negri bodies consist of rabies virus ribonucleoprotein and are mostly acidophilic inclusions with central basophilic granules, which are demonstrable by the Seller's stain containing basic fuchsin and methylene blue. The reaction of these intracytoplasmic forms with rabies antibody, coupled to fluorescein dye or peroxidase, establishes the diagnosis of rabies histologically.

CLINICAL MANIFESTATIONS, COMPLICATIONS, AND SEQUELAE. The usual mode of infection for man is through a bite by a rabid animal. This does not necessarily lead to infection. In 1953, Iranian workers described an accident in which a rabid wolf bit 32 persons; rabies was contracted by 60 per cent of the victims sustaining head wounds and only 30 per cent of those with peripheral bites. Unlike most infectious diseases, subclinical rabies is not recognized in humans.

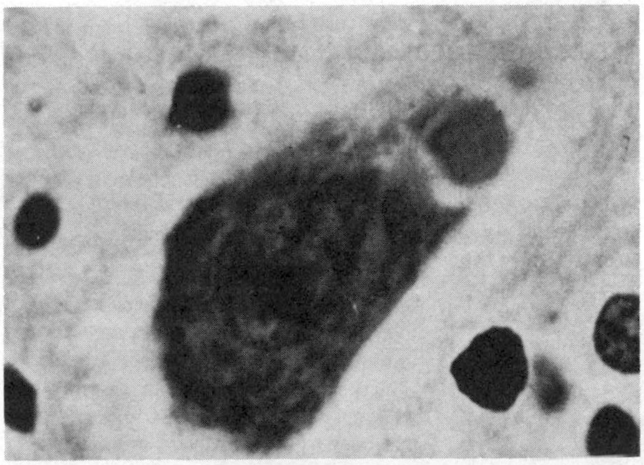

Figure 1. Purkinje cell with intracytoplasmic eosinophilic inclusion body (hematoxylin-eosin, paraffin embedded, × 600). (From Derakhshan, I: Arch Neurol 32:75, 1975.)

Bites are not the only mode of transmission. Scratches by rabid cats have produced rabies in humans, since transfer of virus from the saliva is easily accomplished. Only one human-to-human transmission through infective saliva has been recorded. Aerosol infection of man via the respiratory route has been observed also. In several instances rabies was transmitted to humans via transplanted corneas obtained post-mortem from donors in whom rabies infection was not recognized (Houff et al., 1970; Sureau et al., 1981).

The incubation period of human rabies is long. The median is 31 to 60 days. Approximately 15 per cent of victims develop rabies after three months, and only 1.2 per cent develop disease later than 1 year after exposure.

The clinical illness in man may be divided into five stages as seen in Figure 2 (Hattwick, 1974). During the incubation period, stage 1, there are generally no symptoms, and clinical illness begins with stage 2, the prodrome, consisting of malaise, anorexia, fatigue, headache, and fever. Pain or paresthesias at or close to the site of exposure are reported in 20 to 80 per cent of cases. After a prodromal period of from two to ten days, stage 3, the phase of acute neurologic symptoms, develops. The manifestations include hyperactivity, disorientation, hallucinations, seizures, bizarre behavior, and nuchal stiffness or paralysis. The hyperactivity is usually intermittent; periods of agitation, thrashing, or other bizarre behavior last a few minutes. They occur spontaneously or may be precipitated by tactile, auditory, visual, or other stimuli. Between these periods the patient is usually cooperative and able to communicate.

Hydrophobia or the fear of water results after attempts to drink or eat produce severe, painful spasms of the pharynx and larynx and precipitate hyperactivity. Subsequently, the mere sight of water may precipitate a similar episode. Many patients experience milder hydrophobia and are willing to drink, suffering pharyngeal spasms only upon contact of water with the oral or pharyngeal mucosa. Other abnormalities include muscle fasciculations, particularly near the site of exposure, hyperventilation, hypersalivation, and focal or generalized convulsions. Paralysis generally becomes the major problem unless the patient dies abruptly. In approximately 20 per cent of patients, paralysis dominates the clinical picture ("dumb rabies"). Paralysis may be generalized, asymmetrical with maximal involvement of the bitten extremity, or ascending as in the Landry Guillain-Barré syndrome. Paralytic rabies appears frequently after exposure to some strains of rabies virus, such as those from vampire bats.

During the acute neurologic phase, the patient's mental status gradually deteriorates over two to ten days, leading either to sudden fatal cardiac or respiratory arrest or to stage 4, the onset of coma lasting for hours or days, or rarely, months. The latter course has been seen in patients receiving modern cardiorespiratory supportive care. After a coma lasting from one to two weeks, the course has stabilized in several cases. In most, the patient died after prolonged support.

Recovery, stage 5, has been reported in two patients suffering from rabies, which was documented by exposures to rabid animals and elaborate serologic studies. In the first patient, a 6-year-old boy in the United States, and the second, a 45-year-old woman in Argentina, clinical recovery was complete or nearly complete within six months. No significant residual neurologic sequelae were observed after

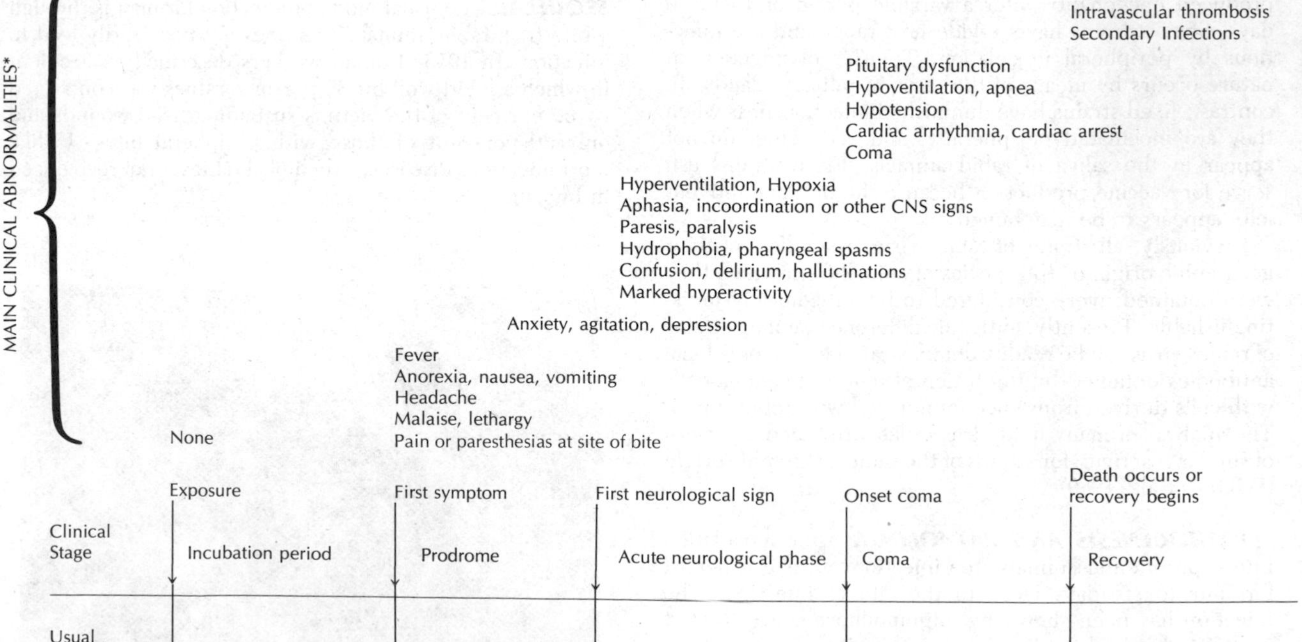

*All clinical abnormalities need not be present in each case

Figure 2. The natural history of clinical rabies in man, hypothetical composite case. (From Hattwick, M. A. W.: Human Rabies, Public Health Reports, 3:229, 1974.)

follow-up studies exceeding one year (Hattwick et al., 1972; Porras et al., 1972). In each surviving patient, the cerebrospinal fluid (CSF) contained a high level of antibody to rabies virus—approximately one third to one fourth of the serum titer. High CSF antibody is seen in viral encephalitis but not following vaccination. In neither survivor was rabies virus isolated.

GEOGRAPHIC VARIATION IN DISEASE. According to the report of the World Health Organization, only the following countries were considered to be free from rabies in 1981.

AFRICA

Djibouti
Lesotho
Mauritius

AMERICAS

Bahamas
Barbados
Jamaica
Netherlands Antilles

ASIA

Bahrain
Brunei
Japan
Malaysia—Sabah
Oman
Qatar
Singapore
United Arab Emirates

EUROPE

Bulgaria
Cyprus
Faroe Islands
Finland
Gibraltar
Iceland
Ireland
Malta
Netherlands
Portugal
Spain
Sweden
United Kingdom

OCEANIA

Australia
Fiji
Guam
New Caledonia
New Zealand
Papua New Guinea
Western Samoa

Cases in humans were reported from all continents except Australia and the Antarctic. About 700 deaths from rabies are reported to the World Health Organization annually, which is clearly an underestimate.

Rabies is a zoonosis with a vast natural reservoir in many animals. Global eradication is probably impossible. Wild animals, skunks and foxes particularly, emerged as important transmitters of the disease to man after 1960. In the United States, skunks are the most frequent rabid animals, accounting for approximately 50 per cent of animal cases reported in 1976. Skunks are also efficient transmitters, owing to the high content of virus in their saliva. Domestic animals, dogs, and cats have rarely transmitted disease in the United States since 1965 (Anderson et al., 1984); vaccination and the elimination of strays are to be credited for this reduced transmission. Raccoon rabies is enzootic in Florida and Georgia, but no case of rabies in man has resulted from this source. Approximately 1 per cent of bats are infected. Although they do not communicate the disease efficiently to terrestrial animals, several human cases have been traced to them.

DIFFERENTIAL DIAGNOSIS. Occasionally rabies is discovered at autopsy of persons dying of an unidentified encephalitis. This usually occurs in cases with an atypical onset—lack of prodromes, lack of hydrophobia, early coma, and early paralysis. Dramatic accidents can result from transplanting corneas from such patients (Plotkin and Koprowski, 1979).

On the other hand, local paresthesias at the site of the bite and hydrophobia are occasionally seen in persons who did not develop rabies. In cases of proven exposure to a rabid animal and a typical course, the differential diagnosis of rabies in man presents few problems.

Differentiation from other encephalitides may be more difficult. The enterovirus and arbovirus encephalitides commonly present diffuse alterations of the sensorium with no localizing signs and lack the characteristic waxing and waning course and hydrophobia. Cerebrospinal fluid in enteroviral and arboviral encephalitides, as well as in lymphocytic choriomeningitis, typically shows elevated leukocyte counts. In clinical rabies, CSF leukocyte counts may be normal or only slightly elevated. Herpes virus encephalitis may closely mimic clinical rabies, but brain scans often show focal herpetic lesions in contrast to the diffuse encephalitis of rabies. However, laboratory procedures may be necessary to distinguish these two infections.

LABORATORY DIAGNOSIS. This requires demonstration of specific inclusions (Negri bodies) in infected tissues, isolation and identification of the virus from brain tissue or saliva, and, in certain instances, special serologic tests.

Histopathologic Diagnosis. The diagnostic findings consist of acute encephalomyelitis and Negri bodies (Fig. 1) and the immunologic identification of the inclusion content as rabies virus ribonucleoprotein. Specific rabies antibody, conjugated with a fluorescent dye, is reacted with smears of frozen sections of brain tissue. The fluorescent antibody (FA) combines with antigen in the cytoplasm of the infected cells, and under the ultraviolet microscope, rabies virus ribonucleoprotein appears bright green against a dark background. Fluorescein-labeled monoclonal antibodies provide reagents with high purity and specificity. A panel of monoclonal antibodies directed against the nucleocapsid antigen of rabies and rabies-related viruses allows specific and rapid identification of rabies and Duvenhage, Mokola and Lagos bat virus antigens present in impression smears of brains. (Wiktor et al., 1980).

Several procedures have recently been introduced for the diagnosis of rabies in living patients (Bryceson et al., 1975). Since FA antigen can be present in the corneal epithelium during the incubation period, the "corneal test" was introduced with varying success. A positive test indicates rabies; a negative finding, however, does not rule it out. FA staining of scrapings from the oronasal mucosa and of frozen sections of skin biopsy specimens may also be used.

Isolation and Identification of Rabies Virus. For this purpose, young adult, weanling, or baby white mice are inoculated intracerebrally with a suspension of brain tissue. Newborn animals are most sensitive, permitting virus isolations that would otherwise be missed. Inoculated animals must be observed for sickness or death for at least four weeks. The incubation period in mice is from 9 to 18 days for street rabies virus but only 5 to 6 days for fixed strains. Rabies antigen can sometimes be detected by FA as early as the second day after inoculation in the brains of test mice. The virus must also be identified by the neutralization test. For this, antibody to rabies virus is mixed with infective brain tissue before it is inoculated into animals. In a positive test, the animals survive an otherwise lethal challenge. Neutralizing antibody in the serum or CSF of a victim can be evaluated in less than 24 hours by using the indirect FA method. Antibody conjugated to peroxidase can be used instead of fluorescein.

TREATMENT. Survival may be prolonged more than two weeks after the onset of symptoms in patients treated in intensive care units. Recovery from rabies has been reported in three patients, as described earlier. The first documented recovery from rabies in a patient was attributed to the anticipation and prompt treatment of hypoxemia and intracranial hypertension (through the insertion of an intraventricular catheter placed at the time of brain biopsy), as well as to the control of cardiac arrhythmia and seizures. Recovery from rabies may be obstructed by cardiac arrhythmias, cardiac arrest, pulmonary and systemic nosocomial infections, respiratory failure, and complications of neurosurgery following brain biopsy. Cardiac complications such as arrhythmia and congestive failure probably arise from the associated myocarditis or anoxia.

PROPHYLAXIS

Postexposure. This practice dates from Pasteur and is unique in the treatment of an infectious disease. Next to vaccine injections, known as the Pasteur treatment, two more measures are equally important and should be considered in each case. These are the local treatment of the wound and the administration of rabies-immune serum, or immunoglobulin.

After a bite, local treatment of the wound should be undertaken immediately. Experimental evidence indicates that washing with soap and water is very effective. The application of 40 to 70 per cent ethyl alcohol or an antiseptic such as benzyl ammonium chloride (Zephiran) should follow. The wound should not be sutured.

The epidemiologic circumstances of the bite must be examined before initiating immunoprophylaxis. Healthy dogs and cats are quarantined for ten days. If they show no signs of rabies, no treatment is offered to bitten persons. The risks of rabies from a vaccinated domestic animal is very small. Small rodents, mice, squirrels, and rats have not transmitted rabies to man in the United States and only very rarely elsewhere. Bites by wild animals, particularly bats and skunks, are an immediate indication for treatment with all measures available.

Animal brain samples should be secured whenever feasible. The physician should not wait for laboratory confirmation of rabies by FA to initiate treatment. The laboratory results should dictate the continuation or discontinuation of the prophylactic regimen described below.

The United States Public Health Service provided a postexposure guide, as shown in Table 1 (Centers for Disease Control, 1984). Most injuries sustained from animals suspected to be rabid call for both vaccine and serum therapy.

Until recently, duck embryo vaccine (DEV) and nervous tissue vaccine (NTV) were used. Both contain inactivated virus. The reputation for effectiveness of NTV is based on

Table 1. RABIES POSTEXPOSURE PROPHYLAXIS GUIDE—JULY 1984

The following recommendations are only a guide. In applying them, take into account the animal species involved, the circumstances of the bite or other exposure, the vaccination status of the animal, and presence of rabies in the region. Local or state public health officials should be consulted if questions arise about the need for rabies prophylaxis.

	Animal Species	Condition of Animal at Time of Attack	Treatment of Exposed Person*
Domestic	Dog and cat	Healthy and available for 10 days of observation	None, unless animal develops rabies†
		Rabid or suspected rabid	RIG‡ and HDCV
		Unknown (escaped)	Consult public health officials. If treatment is indicated, give RIG‡ and HDCV
Wild	Skunk, bat, fox, coyote, raccoon, bobcat, and other carnivores	Regard as rabid unless proven negative by laboratory tests§	RIG‡ and HDCV
Other	Livestock, rodents, and lagomorphs (rabbits and hares)	Consider individually. Local and state public health officials should be consulted on questions about the need for rabies prophylaxis. Bites of squirrels, hamsters, guinea pigs, gerbils, chipmunks, rats, mice, other rodents, rabbits, and hares almost never call for antirabies prophylaxis.	

**All bites and wounds should immediately be thoroughly cleansed with soap and water.* If antirabies treatment is indicated, both rabies immune globulin (RIG) and human diploid cell rabies vaccine (HDCV) should be given as soon as possible, *regardless* of the interval from exposure. Local reactions to vaccines are common and do not contraindicate continuing treatment. Discontinue vaccine if fluorescent antibody tests of the animal are negative.

†During the usual holding period of 10 days, begin treatment with RIG and HDCV at first sign of rabies in a dog or cat that has bitten someone. The symptomatic animal should be killed immediately and tested.

‡If RIG is not available, use antirabies serum, equine (ARS). Do not use more than the recommended dosage.

§The animal should be killed and tested as soon as possible. Holding for observation is not recommended.

From CDC, MMWR, July, 1984.

experience in countries with a high incidence of rabies such as India. Due to the relative frequency of postvaccinal neurologic complications with NTV and local reactions to DEV, which also showed poor immunogenicity, a new type of rabies vaccine was developed from virus grown on human diploid cell cultures (HDCV). As multiple doses of NTV or DEV occasionally fail to stimulate antibodies and protect from rabies, a combined treatment using anti-rabies serum in addition to vaccine was introduced. To overcome the possible interference by the passively administered antibodies (anti-rabies serum), to the induction of antibodies by vaccination, inoculations were increased: the full course consisted of 21 daily doses of NTV or DEV vaccine, followed by boosters on the 31st and 41st days.

If equine rabies anti-serum is used, the recommended dose is 40 international units per kilogram, and equal parts are instilled around the site of the bite and intramuscularly. Human rabies immunoglobulin (HRIG) is preferred because it produces fewer allergic reactions. The recommended dose is 20 international units per kilogram.

The effectiveness of serum plus vaccine treatment was established in a well-known trial in Iran in 1954 when a rabid wolf bit 18 persons. Rabies developed in three of the five victims receiving 21 injections of vaccine (NTV) alone, while only 1 of 13 persons receiving vaccine and serum succumbed to the disease.

Wiktor and Koprowski and their associates at the Wistar Institute in Philadelphia have developed a human diploid cell-derived rabies vaccine (HDCV), in which the virus was concentrated, purified, and inactivated by beta-propiolactone (Wiktor et al., 1964). After trials in volunteers established high immunogenicity and a low frequency of local reactions, the vaccine was used in a postexposure field trial in Iran. Forty-five persons bitten by rabid dogs and wolves were treated by Bahmanyar and co-workers (1976) with one dose of heterologous antiserum intramuscularly and only five doses of HDCV inoculated subcutaneously on days 0, 3, 7, 14, 30 with a booster on day 90. All patients survived. Case fatalities of no less than 35 per cent could have been expected had the victims not been treated. A fatality-free therapeutic trial of this magnitude has not been previously noted with other vaccines.

Table 2. RABIES IMMUNIZATION—JUNE 1984

I. PRE-EXPOSURE IMMUNIZATION. Pre-exposure immunization consists of three doses of HDCV, 1.0 ml, IM (i.e., deltoid area), one each on days 0, 7, and 28. (See text for details on use of 0.1 ml HDCV ID as an alternative dose/route.) Administration of routine booster doses of vaccine depends on exposure risk category as noted below. Pre-exposure immunization of immunosuppressed persons is not recommended.

Criteria for Pre-exposure Immunization

Risk Category	***Nature of Risk***	***Typical Populations***	***Pre-exposure Regimen***
Continuous	Virus present continuously, often in high concentrations. Aerosol, mucous membrane, bite, or nonbite exposure possible. Specific exposures may go unrecognized.	Rabies research lab workers.* Rabies biologics production workers.	Primary pre-exposure immunization course. Serologic tests every 6 months. Booster immunization when antibody titer falls below acceptable level.*
Frequent	Exposure usually episodic, with source recognized, but exposure may also be unrecognized. Aerosol, mucous membrane, bite, or nonbite exposure.	Rabies diagnostic lab workers,* spelunkers, veterinarians, and animal control and wildlife workers in rabies epizootic areas.	Primary pre-exposure immunization course. Booster immunization or serology every 2 years.†
Infrequent (greater than population-at-large)	Exposure nearly always episodic with source recognized. Mucous membrane, bite, or nonbite exposure.	Veterinarians and animal control and wildlife workers in areas of low rabies endemicity. Certain travelers to foreign rabies epizootic areas. Veterinary students.	Primary pre-exposure immunization course. No routine booster immunization or serologic testing.
Rare (population-at-large)	Exposure always episodic, mucous membrane, or bite with source recognized.	U.S. population-at-large, including individuals in rabies-epizootic areas.	No pre-exposure immunization.

II. POSTEXPOSURE IMMUNIZATION. All postexposure treatment should begin with immediate thorough cleansing of all wounds with soap and water.

Persons not previously immunized:	RIG, 20 I.U./kg body weight, one half infiltrated at bite site (if possible), remainder IM; 5 doses of HDCV, 1.0 ml IM (i.e., deltoid area), one each on days 0, 3, 7, 14 and 28.
Persons previously immunized‡:	Two doses of HDCV, 1.0 ml, IM (i.e., deltoid area), one each on days 0 and 3. RIG should not be administered.

*Judgment of relative risk and extra monitoring of immunization status of laboratory workers is the responsibility of the laboratory supervisor (see U.S. Department of Health and Human Service's *Biosafety in Microbiological and Biomedical Laboratories,* 1984).

†Pre-exposure booster immunization consists of one dose of HDCV, 1.0 ml/dose, IM (deltoid area). Acceptable antibody level is 1:5 titer (complete inhibition in RFFIT at 1:5 dilution). Boost if titer falls below 1:5.

‡Pre-exposure immunization with HDCV; prior postexposure prophylaxis with HDCV; or persons previously immunized with any other type of rabies vaccine *and* a documented history of positive antibody response to the prior vaccination.

From CDC, MMWR, June, 1984.

Experimental injection of hyperimmune serum alone after exposure usually delays the onset but does not prevent rabies. Antibodies probably neutralize the virus outside of the CNS during the early incubation period. Once the neurons are infected, antibodies are ineffective. The precise mechanism of protection produced by postexposure vaccination has not been fully defined. Both humoral and cellular immunity was induced by the inactivated rabies vaccines (Wiktor et al., 1977). In experimental animals, the HDCV induced interferon also (Wiktor et al., 1972). Thus antibody, cell immunity, and interferon may all contribute to protection.

HDCV is the only vaccine used in the USA and several European countries, and is the vaccine of choice whenever available and should be administered in conjunction with rabies immune globulin. Because of its high immunogenicity, only five 1-ml intramuscular doses of HDCV are required. The first injection should be given as soon as possible after exposure; additional dose should be given on days 3, 7, 14, and 28 totalling five injections. In many countries, however, NTV is still in use (CDC, 1980).

Pre-exposure Prophylaxis. This consists of three HDCV injections at weekly intervals, followed by a booster dose (Table 2). A successful prior vaccination, judged by seroconversion, allows a shorter course upon exposure to a suspected rabid animal: The first 1 ml intramuscular dose of HDCV should be given as soon as possible upon exposure and the second 3 days later. Persons working with rabies virus should be serologically tested every 6 months. In case of an inadequate (< 1:5) serum titer, a booster HDCV should be given (CDC, 1984).

Adverse reactions to HDCV include systemic allergic reactions ranging from hives to, rarely, anaphylactic shock. Transient fever and headache were noted also. The frequency of systemic allergic reactions was 11 per 10,000 vaccinees (CDC, 1984).

References

Anderson, L. J., Nicholson, K. G., Tauxe, R. V., and Winkler W. G.: Human rabies in the United States, 1960 to 1979: Epidemiology, diagnosis and prevention. Ann Int Med 100:728, 1984.

Bahmanyar, M., Fayaz, A., Nouri-Salehi, S., Mohammadi, M., and Koprowski, H.: Successful protection of humans exposed to rabies infection. JAMA 236:2751, 1976.

Bryceson, A. M. D., Grennwood, B. M., Warrell, D. A., Davidson, N., Pope, H. M., Lawrie, J. H., Barnes, H. J., Bailie, W. E., and Wilcox, G. E.: Demonstration during life of rabies antigen in humans. J Infect Dis 131:71, 1975.

Centers for Disease Control: Recommendations of the Public Health Service Advisory Committee on Immunization Practices: Rabies prevention. MMWR 33:July 20, 1984. Systemic allergic reactions following immunization with human diploid cell rabies vaccine. MMWR 33: April 13, 1984.

Derakhshan, I.: Is the Negri body specific for rabies? Arch Neurol 32:75, 1975.

Hattwick, M. A. W.: Human rabies. Public Health Rev 2:229, 1974.

Hattwick, M. A. W., Weis, T. T., Stechschulte, C. K., Baer, G. M., and Gregg, M. B.: Recovery from rabies. A case report. Ann Intern Med 76:931, 1972.

Houff, S. A., Burton, R. C., Wilson, W. T., Baer, G. M., Anderson, L. J., Winkler, W. G., Madden, D. L., and Sever, J. L.: Human-to-human transmission of rabies virus by corneal transplant. N Engl J Med 300:603, 1979.

Plotkin, S. A., Koprowski, H.: Phobia of Hydrophobia Justified. N Engl J Med 300:620, 1979.

Porras, C., Barboza, J. J., Fuenzaldia, Adaros, H. L., Oviedo de Diaz, A. M., and Furst, J.: Recovery from rabies in man. Ann Intern Med 85:44, 1976.

Sureau, P., Portnoi, D., Rollin, P., Lapresle, C., Chaouni-Berbich A.: Prevention de La Transmission Inter-humaine de Rage Après Greffe de Cornée, C. R. Acad Sc Paris, 293:689, 1981.

Wiktor, T. J., Doherty, P. C., and Koprowski, H.: In vitro evidence of cell-mediated immunity after exposure of mice to both live and inactivated rabies virus. Proc Natl Acad Sci USA 74:334, 1977.

Wiktor, T. J., Fernandes, N. V., and Koprowski, H.: Cultivation of rabies virus in human diploid cell strain WI38. J Immunol 93:353, 1964.

Wiktor, T. J., Postic, B., Ho, M., and Koprowski, H.: Role of interferon induction in the protective activity of rabies vaccines. J Infect Dis 126:408, 1972.

Wiktor, T. J., Flamand, A., Koprowski, H.: Use of monoclonal antibodies in diagnosis of rabies virus infection and differentiation of rabies and rabies-related viruses. J Virol Methods 1:33, 1980.

180

HERPES SIMPLEX ENCEPHALITIS AND MENINGITIS

MICHAEL N. OXMAN, M.D.

Symptomatic involvement of the central nervous system is a rare manifestation of herpes simplex virus (HSV) infection. It may take one of several forms depending, at least in part, upon the antigenic type of the HSV involved, the age and immunologic status of the host, and the route of infection.

Herpes simplex encephalitis is an acute necrotizing viral encephalitis that, beyond the neonatal period, is nearly always caused by HSV Type 1 (HSV-1). It has a higher mortality rate than most other forms of viral encephalitis and, although rare, appears to account for most cases of sporadically occurring acute necrotizing encephalitis in the Western World. In the neonate, herpes simplex encephalitis is usually caused by HSV Type 2 (HSV-2), which is acquired during passage through the birth canal of a mother with genital herpes. The encephalitis occurs most often as one component of a disseminated neonatal HSV infection. In the neonate, as in the adult, herpes simplex encephalitis carries a grave prognosis.

Herpes simplex meningitis is an acute aseptic meningitis that occurs mainly in young sexually active adults, frequently in association with genital herpes. It is generally caused by HSV-2, which may be isolated from the spinal fluid. In contrast to herpes simplex encephalitis, herpes simplex meningitis usually follows a brief and benign course, although it may sometimes be associated with polyradiculitis and, rarely, with ascending myelitis. In some patients, the meningitis may recur in association with recurrent episodes of genital or cutaneous herpes.

ETIOLOGY. Herpes simplex virus (HSV) is a member of the herpesvirus family, which includes three other human herpesviruses, varicella-zoster virus (VZV), cytomegalovirus (CMV), and Epstein-Barr virus (EBV). All of these herpesviruses are morphologically indistinguishable and share a number of properties, including a remarkable propensity for establishing latent infections that persist for the life of the host. In contrast to the other human herpesviruses, HSV has a wide host range. It can infect many experimental animals as well as a wide variety of cell cultures established *in vitro* from human and animal tissues. The cytopathic effect (CPE) of HSV in such cell cultures is characterized by the formation of acidophilic Cowdry Type A intranuclear inclusion bodies and multinucleated giant cells. These changes are indistinguishable from those produced by VZV.

There are two serotypes of HSV, HSV-1 and HSV-2, which have many common antigens, produce identical lesions in the skin, mucous membranes, central nervous system, and other organs, and produce identical CPE in cell cultures. Although their similarities are much greater than their differences, HSV-1 and HSV-2 can be distinguished unequivocally on the basis of certain antigenic, biological and biochemical differences (see Chapter 105). HSV-1 and HSV-2 also differ in their clinical and epidemiologic behavior (Nahmias and Josey, 1982). HSV-1 is transmitted primarily by contact with infected saliva and is the principal cause of herpetic gingivostomatitis and pharyngeotonsillitis, eczema herpeticum, skin infections above the waist, infections of the eye, and herpes simplex encephalitis beyond the neonatal period. HSV-2 is transmitted sexually or from a maternal genital infection to the newborn. It is the principal cause of genital herpes, neonatal herpes, skin infections below the waist, and herpes simplex meningitis. Changing sexual practices and socioeconomic conditions are altering the epidemiology of HSV-1 and HSV-2. An increasing proportion of genital HSV infections are being caused by HSV-1, and an increasing proportion of oropharyngeal HSV infections are being caused by HSV-2 (see Chapter 163). These epidemiologic changes may be expected, eventually, to alter the proportion of cases of herpes simplex encephalitis and meningitis caused by the two HSV serotypes.

Although HSV was isolated from the brains of several patients with encephalitis early in the century, its etiologic significance was not appreciated. Because of the ubiquity of HSV and its persistence as a latent infection in most adults, it was assumed that such isolations were merely coincidental (Drachman and Adams, 1962). It was not until 1941 that Smith, Lennette, and Reames established the etiologic role of HSV in acute necrotizing encephalitis. They isolated HSV from the brain of a 4-week-old infant with encephalitis and also demonstrated Cowdry Type A intranuclear inclusions characteristic of those produced by HSV in the cerebral lesions (Smith et al., 1941). Since then a number of reports, encompassing more than 500 cases of herpes simplex encephalitis, have described the clinical, pathologic, and epidemiologic features of the disease (Haymaker et al., 1958; Drachman and Adams, 1962; Leider et al., 1965; Rawls et al., 1966; Miller et al., 1966; Olson et al., 1967; Miller and Ross, 1968; Rappel et al., 1971; Illis and Gostling, 1972; Oxbury and MacCullum, 1973; Whitley et al., 1977 and 1982b). It is now clear that HSV is the most frequent cause of sporadically occurring acute necrotizing encephalitis in the Western World. When the virus isolated from the brain in adults and children beyond the neonatal period has been typed, it has almost always proven to be HSV-1. In herpes encephalitis in the neonate, the majority of virus isolates are HSV-2. However, herpes simplex encephalitis caused by HSV-1 and by HSV-2 are clinically and pathologically indistinguishable.

The association between benign aseptic meningitis and genital herpes was first reported by Ravaut and Darré in 1904 and has been reaffirmed in a number of later studies (Craig and Nahmias, 1973; Skoldenberg et al., 1975). While the number of reported isolates of HSV from the spinal fluid in cases of aseptic meningitis is small, the majority have been HSV-2, and serologic studies suggest that 1 to 5 per cent of all cases of aseptic meningitis are caused by this virus (Armstrong et al., 1943; Adair et al., 1953; Stalder et al., 1973; Skoldenberg et al., 1975; Wolontis and Jeansson, 1977).

PATHOLOGY AND PATHOGENESIS. In addition to the usual findings of viral encephalitis (that is, lymphocytic infiltration of the meninges; perivascular aggregates of lymphocytes, plasma cells, and histocytes in the cortex and subjacent white matter; and proliferation of microglia with formation of glial nodules), there are several distinctive features that serve to identify herpes simplex encephalitis (Haymaker et al., 1958; Drachman and Adams, 1962; Miller et al., 1966; Illis and Gostling, 1972; Esiri, 1982).

A. Severity of the process. Lesions are not uniform in their distribution or severity, but in each case the degree of necrosis is extremely severe in the regions of greatest involvement. There are focal areas of virtually total cortical necrosis with gross softening, destruction of architecture, hemorrhage, and extensive loss of neurons and glia.
B. Topography of the lesions. Although widespread involvement is usually present at autopsy, the distribution of lesions is asymmetric, and the pathologic process is generally further advanced in one hemisphere than in the other. The areas of greatest damage are in the temporal lobe, the orbital portion of the frontal lobe, and the structures forming the limbic system.
C. Inclusion bodies. Cowdry Type A intranuclear inclusion bodies are found in neurons, astrocytes, and oligodendrocytes (Fig. 1). These inclusions, the direct result of herpes simplex virus infection, are initially amphophilic and homogeneous. They fill the entire nucleus and displace the nucleolus to the periphery. The nuclear

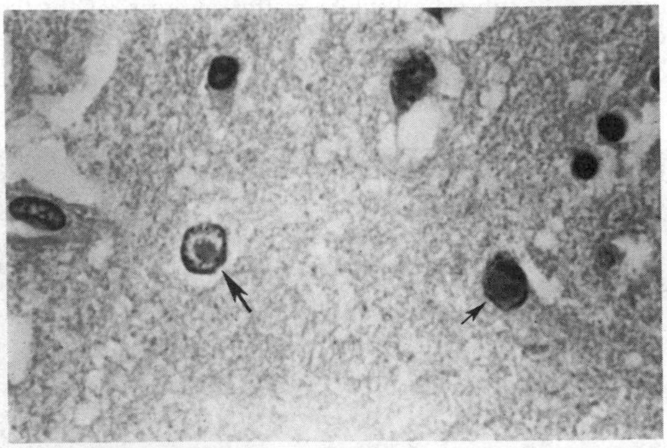

Figure 1. Temporal lobe biopsy from a patient with herpes simplex encephalitis stained with hematoxylin and eosin. An early amphophilic Cowdry type A intranuclear inclusion body (small arrow) fills the nucleus; displacing the nucleolus to the periphery. Margination of chromatin at the nuclear membrane is already apparent. A mature eosinophilic intranuclear inclusion body (large arrow) is surrounded by a clear zone or halo. The chromatin is distributed along the nuclear membrane. (Courtesy of Dr. R. Baringer.)

chromatin is distributed along the inner surface of the nuclear membrane. These early inclusions soon become condensed, granular, and eosinophilic, and they are then surrounded by a clear halo.

The nature and distribution of the lesions seen at autopsy are often so characteristic that the diagnosis is apparent on gross examination. In a typical case of rapidly fatal herpes simplex encephalitis (most deaths occur within 2 weeks of onset) examination of the brain reveals intense hemorrhagic necrosis of the inferior and medial parts of the temporal lobe, the insula, and the orbital portion of the frontal lobe, with distinct swelling and obvious softening of the brain. The cortical surface in these areas shows engorgement of small blood vessels and petechial hemorrhages (Fig. 2). When the brain is sectioned, the cortex in the areas of major involvement is found to be congested, soft, and swollen, and there is loss of the normal demarcation between cortex and white matter. The cortex is necrotic and friable, and it contains many small hemorrhagic foci (Fig. 3), which are also present in the underlying white matter. The meninges overlying these areas of intense cortical necrosis are opaque, but they appear normal in other areas. There is often evidence of extensive cerebral edema with uncal and cerebellar tonsillar herniation. Microscopic examination reveals hyperemia and perivascular infiltration by lymphocytes, plasma cells, and macrophages in the meninges overlying areas of obvious cortical pathology. In the underlying brain, the necrosis is primarily cortical, but the degree of destruction varies from place to place, even within regions of maximal involvement. In some places, the entire cortex is necrotic, with disintegration of nerve cells and glia and focal hemorrhage into the destroyed tissue. In other areas, there is glial proliferation and neuronophagia. The lesions are most pronounced beneath the pia in the upper cortical laminae. Small blood vessels are engorged and show endothelial cell hypertrophy. There are perivascular collections of lymphocytes, plasma cells and large mononuclear cells, and, in areas of severe cortical necrosis, perivascular hemorrhages. Necrotic foci may progress and coalesce, giving rise to areas of cavitation. Focal necrosis, hemorrhage, and pallor of myelin are seen in subcortical white matter in areas where the overlying cortex is severely affected, but there is no evidence of primary demyelination. Cowdry Type A intranuclear inclusion bodies (Fig. 1) are present in neurons, oligodendrocytes, and astrocytes.

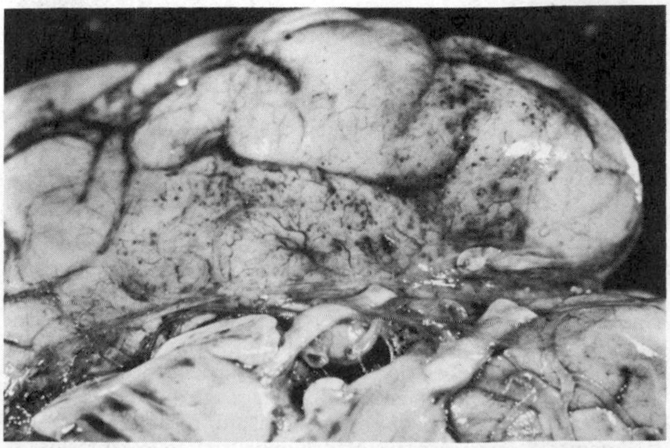

Figure 2. Medial aspect of the temporal lobe of a patient with herpes simplex encephalitis. Note the diffuse petechial eruption and the engorgement of small blood vessels (Courtesy of Dr. R. Baringer.)

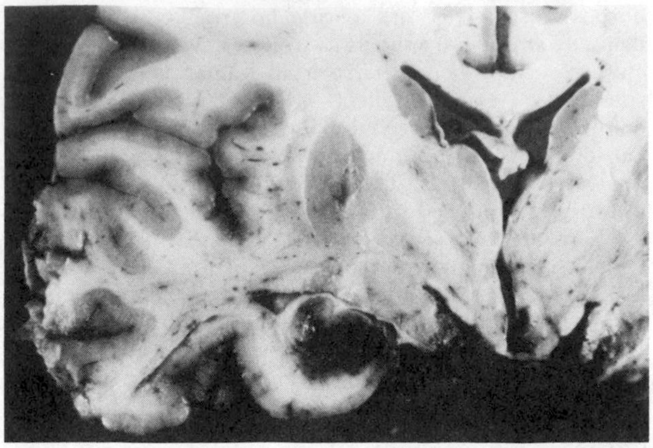

Figure 3. The brain of a patient with fatal herpes simplex encephalitis. Coronal section through the affected temporal lobe at the level of the thalamus showing hemorrhagic necrosis involving the hippocampus and adjacent cortical tissue, and focal areas of hemorrhage in the temporal lobe cortex. Congested vessels and small hemorrhages are also visible in the subjacent white matter.

Electron microscopic examination reveals viral nucleocapsids within the nuclei of infected neurons and glia. The nucleocapsids can be seen in clumps and also arrayed along the inner surface of the nuclear membrane (Fig. 4*A–C*). Occasionally, herpes simplex virus nucleocapsids can be seen budding through the inner lamella of the nuclear membrane in areas that are thickened by the addition of virus-specified glycoproteins (Fig. 4*D*). Complete enveloped virions can be seen in intercellular spaces and occasionally in the cytoplasm (Fig. 4*E*).

In neonatal herpes simplex encephalitis, the lesions are similar to those that are seen in older children and adults. However, they are generally more widely and uniformly distributed, without the characteristic orbitofrontal and temporal lobe localization described above.

In addition to their importance as diagnostic criteria, these unique pathologic features of herpes simplex encephalitis reflect its pathogenesis and provide the anatomic basis for the signs and symptoms of the disease. There are two major unanswered questions regarding the pathogenesis of herpes simplex encephalitis in children and adults: (1) What explains the unique anatomic distribution of infection in the brain, and (2) In view of the ubiquity of the virus and the high frequency of primary and recurrent HSV infections, why is herpes simplex encephalitis such a rare disease; its annual incidence is estimated to be only 1 to 2 cases per million persons (Nahmias and Josey, 1982; Skoldenberg et al., 1984).

Clinical and pathologic evidence indicates that in herpes simplex encephalitis in children and adults infection initially involves the orbitofrontal and temporal regions of one hemisphere and only later extends to contiguous areas and to the opposite hemisphere. This localization is not explained by the selective vulnerability of a specific subset of neurons. Unlike poliovirus, which essentially infects and destroys only motor neurons, HSV is unrestricted in its capacity to infect cells within the central nervous system. In involved regions of the brain, HSV inclusions and virions are seen in both neurons and glia over a contiguous anatomic area, as if the virus had spread locally from cell to cell. It has been suggested that the unique localization of infection in herpes simplex encephalitis may reflect the route of entry of HSV into the central nervous system. Thus, Johnson and Mims (1968) postulated that, during primary infection, HSV might infect the olfactory mucosa, enter the central nervous system via the olfactory nerve, and spread along olfactory pathways to the temporal lobe. While this explanation is consistent with the anatomy of the infection in many cases (Ojeda, 1980; Esiri, 1982) infection of the olfactory bulbs is not uniformally present in patients dying of herpes simplex encephalitis, and HSV is only rarely recovered from the nasopharynx early in the course of the disease. Even when HSV infection is observed in the olfactory tract, it is usually bilateral and may not reflect centripetal spread from the periphery to the temporal lobe. Instead, it may be the result of centrifugal spread of HSV from the infected brain to the olfactory bulb, a sequence of events similar to that responsible for the occurrence of HSV retinitis in patients with herpes simplex encephalitis (Cibis et al., 1978).

Herpes simplex encephalitis does not always represent primary infection with HSV-1. In 20 to 25 per cent of patients with herpes simplex encephalitis, there is a past history of recurrent herpes labialis, an incidence no different from that in the general population or in comparable patients with encephalitis not caused by HSV. In addition, serologic evidence of prior HSV-1 infection is found in the same proportion (about 30 per cent) of patients with herpes simplex encephalitis as comparable patients with encephalitis not caused by HSV (Nahmias et al., 1982; Whitley et al., 1982b). These observations indicate that the risk of herpes simplex encephalitis is neither greatly reduced nor greatly increased in people already infected with HSV-1—that is, in people for whom herpes simplex encephalitis would represent a recurrent infection.

It is now well established that during primary oropharyngeal HSV infections (which are usually asymptomatic) virus spreads centripetally to the trigeminal ganglia along branches of the trigeminal nerve and establishes latent infection in sensory neurons (Chapter 105). Episodes of recurrent herpes labialis or of asymptomatic oropharyngeal virus shedding result when this latent HSV in the trigeminal ganglion is activated and passes centrifugally down the axon to initiate infection in the skin or oropharyngeal mucosa. Between recurrences, the virus remains latent in sensory neurons in the ipsilateral trigeminal ganglion. Perhaps unfortunately, sensory fibers from the trigeminal ganglia also innervate basilar structures in the middle and anterior fossae, including the meninges over the areas of cortex most severely involved in herpes simplex encephalitis. These considerations have led Davis and Johnson (1979) to propose that herpes simplex encephalitis may result from the direct spread of HSV along nerve fibers from the trigeminal ganglion to the anterior and middle fossae. This would account for the orbitofrontal and temporal lobe localization, both in patients in whom the encephalitis is a manifestation of primary infection with HSV-1 and in patients with a prior history of recurrent herpes labialis, in whom encephalitis is almost certainly a recurrent infection. The recent demonstration that human superior cervical and vagus ganglia may also be latently infected with HSV-1 reveals another neural route by which this virus may reach the central nervous system (Warren et al., 1978). The trigeminal route would also explain the almost exclusive role of HSV-1 in herpes simplex encephalitis beyond the neonatal period. HSV-2 is at least as neuropathic as HSV-1, but it is very rarely isolated from patients with primary herpes stomatitis, herpes keratitis, recurrent herpes labialis, or recurrent herpetic lesions of the facial skin. Furthermore, only HSV-1 has been recovered from latently infected human trigeminal ganglia. Thus, in children and adults, HSV-2 does not ordinarily have access to the central nervous system by the trigeminal route. We can predict that, if sustained, the recent increase in the incidence of oropharyngeal infections caused by HSV-2 will eventually result in an increase in the frequency with which HSV-2 is isolated from cases of herpes simplex encephalitis in adults.

Attractive though it may be, the trigeminal route is not well supported by anatomic data (Ojeda, 1980; Esiri, 1982). Lesions produced by experimental infection via the trigeminal nerves are located in the brain stem, not the temporal lobes. Furthermore, in her detailed examination of the brains of 29 autopsied cases of herpes simplex encephalitis, Esiri (1982) did not find evidence of active HSV infection in the meninges at the base of the brain, in the trigeminal ganglia, or in the root entry zones of the trigeminal nerves. Moreover, while some patients with recurrent herpes labialis and herpes simplex encephalitis have an identical strain of HSV-1 isolated from their brain and lip lesion, others have quite different strains of HSV-1 isolated from the two sites (Whitley et al., 1982a). The most obvious explanation for this observation is that the trigeminal ganglion was not the source of the virus causing herpes simplex encephalitis in the latter patients. An alternative source of virus, other than exogenous infection, is the brain itself. Persistence of HSV and its DNA in sensory ganglia is well documented in humans and in animal models of HSV latency (Stevens, 1975; Wildy et al., 1982) but HSV DNA has also been detected in brain tissue from latently infected animals and humans (Sequiera et al., 1979; Cabrera et al., 1980; Fraser et al., 1981; Rock and Fraser, 1983). However, while infectious HSV can be recovered regularly from latently infected sensory ganglia by explantation and co-cultivation, recovery from brain tissue known to contain HSV DNA is uncommon (Cabrera et al., 1980; Rock and Fraser, 1983). This failure to recover infectious virus from brain tissue suggests that the HSV-cell interaction in brain may differ significantly from that in latently infected sensory neurons; this difference might explain the rarity of herpes simplex encephalitis versus herpes labialis.

Another potential explanation for the rarity of herpes simplex encephalitis is its causation by uniquely neurotropic strains of HSV, which constitute a very small minority of the strains of HSV causing human infections. However, the observations that all of the strains of HSV-1 isolated from temporal and geographic clusters of cases of herpes simplex encephalitis are different (Hammer et al., 1980; Landry et al., 1983) and that some isolates of HSV-1 from the brain are identical to those from the recurrent lesions of herpes labialis in the same patients (Whitley et al., 1982a) make this very unlikely.

Involvement of the central nervous system is recognized in 50 per cent or more of infants with neonatal HSV infection. In the majority, meningoencephalitis is but one component of a disseminated HSV infection in which there is extensive visceral involvement with viremic spread to the meninges and brain (Nahmias et al., 1983). Pathologic

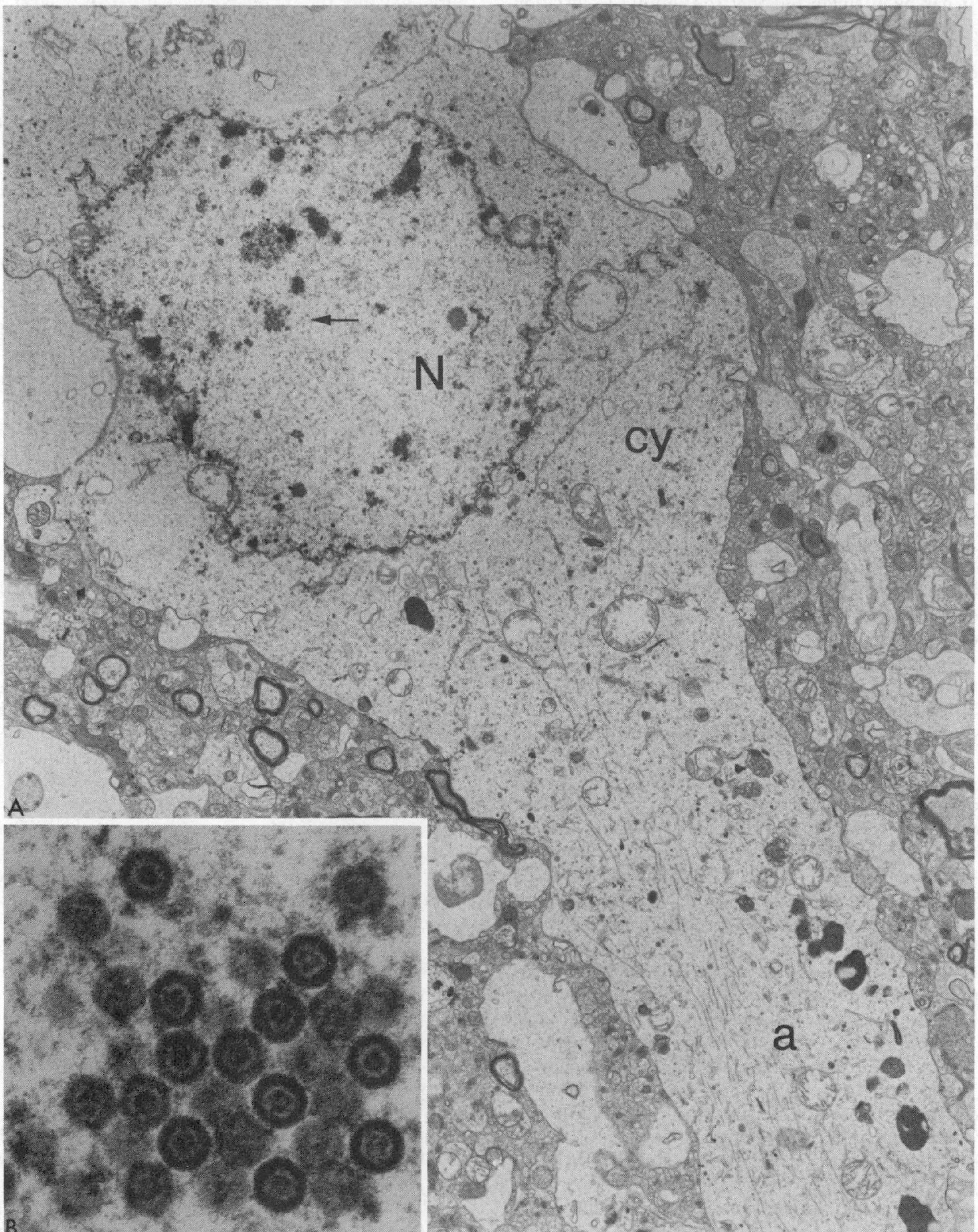

Figure 4. *Herpes simplex encephalitis.* (Courtesy of Dr. H. C. Powell and Mrs. M. A. Phillips.)

A, Electron micrograph of a herpes simplex virus-infected neuron from the brain of a patient with herpes simplex encephalitis. The cytoplasm and axon are indicated by (cy) and *(a),* respectively. The nucleus *(N)* contains small collections of herpes simplex virus nucleocapsids *(arrow).* Many other herpes simplex virus nucleocapsids are adjacent to the nuclear membrane and some are in the process of budding through its inner lamella in areas thickened by the addition of herpes simplex virus-specific glycoproteins. Magnification 7200×.

B, The herpes simplex virus nucleocapsids indicated by the arrow in *A* are shown at higher magnification (90,000×) in the set.

Illustration continued on opposite page

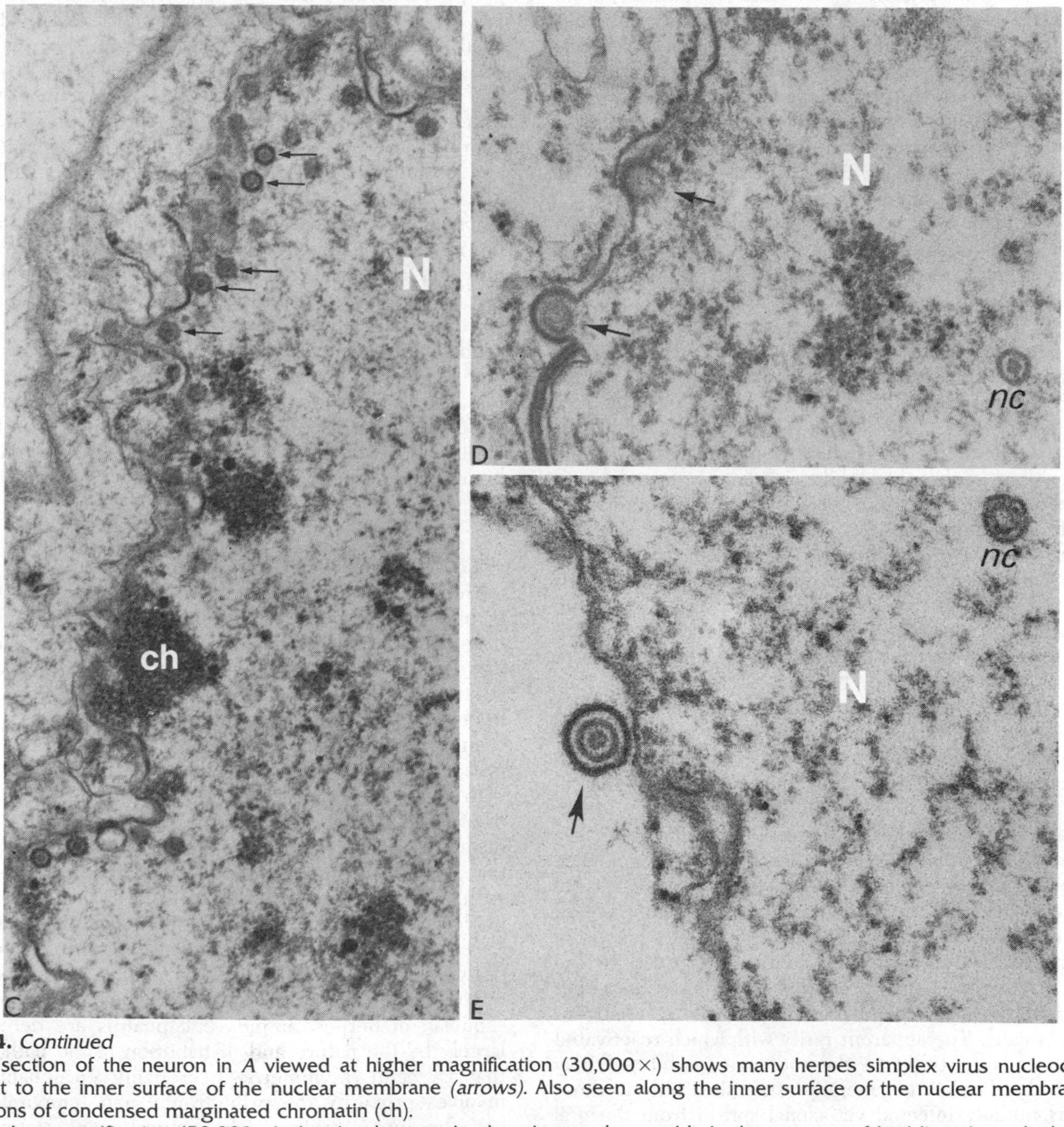

Figure 4. *Continued*

C, A section of the neuron in *A* viewed at higher magnification (30,000×) shows many herpes simplex virus nucleocapsids adjacent to the inner surface of the nuclear membrane *(arrows).* Also seen along the inner surface of the nuclear membrane are collections of condensed marginated chromatin (ch).

D, Higher magnification (50,000×) showing herpes simplex virus nucleocapsids in the process of budding through the inner lamella of the nuclear membrane in areas thickened by the addition of herpes simplex virus-specified glycoprotein *(arrows).* Nucleocapsids within the nucleus are indicated by (nc).

E, The process of budding completed, an enveloped (complete) herpes simplex virus particle *(arrow)* is seen in the cytoplasm adjacent to the nuclear membrane. Magnification 75,000×.

changes are similar to those observed in the adult, but in infants with disseminated infections there is generally no temporal lobe localization. Lesions are widely disseminated throughout the meninges and the entire brain, and virus can often be isolated from the spinal fluid. However, 30 to 40 per cent of infants with HSV infection involving the central nervous system have no evidence of disseminated disease. Almost all such infants also have herpetic lesions of the eye, mouth, or skin. Virus is less often isolated from the spinal fluid in infants with this localized central nervous system HSV infection, and several have had a more focal encephalitis, similar to that observed in older children and adults. Thus, although the pathogenesis of neonatal herpes simplex encephalitis usually involves the viremic spread of HSV to the central nervous system, there are some cases in which the virus may first infect the eye, mouth, or skin and then reach the brain by a neural route.

The virus in most cases of neonatal herpes simplex encephalitis is HSV-2. This reflects the importance of maternal genital herpes as the source of virus in neonatal infections, and the predominance of HSV-2 as the cause of genital herpes. There is no detectable difference in the pathogenesis, or in the nature, severity, or distribution of the pathology, in neonatal herpes simplex infections caused by HSV-1 and by HSV-2.

The risk of developing severe disease (and encephalitis) in the course of HSV infection is much greater in the neonate than in the older child or adult. In fact, beyond the neonatal period, most primary HSV infections are asymptomatic. Neonatal HSV infections, on the other hand, are almost always symptomatic. The majority result in viremia and visceral dissemination, more than half result in central nervous system involvement, and the overall mortality is greater than 60 per cent. The factors responsible for the increased pathogenicity of HSV in the neonate have yet to be identified, but it now appears that they include a deficit in one or more components of the cellular immune response to HSV antigens, as well as the inability of neonatal leukocytes to mediate antibody-dependent cellular cytotoxicity (ADCC), and the capacity of HSV to replicate in neonatal but not adult macrophages and peripheral blood leukocytes (Nahmias et al., 1983). We are even further from understanding what limits the incidence of herpes simplex encephalitis in adults, the majority of whom carry this potentially lethal virus as a lifelong tenant of their trigeminal ganglia. Reactivation of latent virus in the trigeminal ganglion, with centrifugal spread to the perioral skin, is certainly a common event, for at least one-quarter of the adult population is plagued by recurrent herpes labialis. The apparent rarity with which reactivated HSV spreads centrally to the meninges and brain may indicate that latency is generally established only in those neurons initially infected via axonal spread from the oral and perioral sites involved in primary infection, and that subsequent neuron-to-neuron spread within the trigeminal ganglion is uncommon.

It should be pointed out that neural and viremic spread from the ganglion are not mutually exclusive. The same immune deficit(s) that allow reactivated virus in the ganglion to replicate and spill over into the circulation may also favor spread via neural pathways.

Herpes simplex meningitis is usually associated with HSV-2. Because of its benign course, pathologic material has not been available from cases of uncomplicated herpes simplex meningitis. The disease afflicts mainly sexually active individuals between the ages of 15 and 35 years, and approximately one-half of the documented cases have occurred in temporal association with primary genital herpes. Herpes simplex meningitis has also been observed in association with herpetic pharyngotonsillitis and herpetic proctitis (Harford et al., 1975; Atia et al., 1982) and in children, in which case it is caused by HSV-1 (Sawanobori, et al., 1974). During the acute illness, HSV can frequently be isolated from the spinal fluid and sometimes from the peripheral blood (Stalder et al., 1973; Skoldenberg et al., 1975; Hevron, 1977; Craig and Nahmias, 1973; Morrison et al., 1979). The recovery of virus from the spinal fluid and blood has led Craig and Nahmias (1973) to propose that the route of central nervous system infection is viremic rather than neural. While this may be true in some cases, approximately one-third develop recurrent meningitis, usually accompanied by recurrent genital or perigenital herpes. These patients, as well as those in whom genital and cutaneous herpes is accompanied by radiculitis and ascending myelitis, suggest that the usual sequence of events is infection of dorsal root ganglia, followed by the direct spread of virus to the meninges and spinal cord, presumably via a neural pathway (Skoldenberg et al., 1975). This is probably the same sequence of events that leads to the motor paralysis that occasionally accompanies herpes zoster. The isolation of HSV-1 from the spinal fluid in cases of acute benign aseptic meningitis in children and adults indicates that both HSV types can cause the syndrome of benign herpes simplex meningitis.

CLINICAL MANIFESTATIONS

Herpes Simplex Encephalitis. The entire clinical spectrum of herpes simplex encephalitis in children and adults may not be known. It has been impossible to establish the diagnosis of herpes simplex encephalitis without demonstrating the virus or viral antigens in tissue obtained by brain biopsy or at autopsy (Johnson et al., 1968). However, brain biopsy has been reserved for patients whose clinical presentation is suggestive of the disease (that is, patients with evidence of an acute febrile encephalopathy with disordered mentation; focal cerebral signs; localization by diagnostic procedures such as electroencephalogram, brain scan, or arteriogram; and spinal fluid findings compatible with viral infection) (Whitley et al., 1977). Thus, milder, nonlocalized forms of herpes simplex encephalitis may go unrecognized. Nevertheless, analysis of recognized cases has yielded a reasonably coherent picture of the disease.

The mode of presentation, clinical manifestations, and sequelae of herpes simplex encephalitis are determined largely by the nature and distribution of the pathology—that is, acute asymmetric necrotizing encephalitis that involves primarily the orbitofrontal and temporal cortex and the limbic system. The clinical manifestations and course of the disease are quite variable, but most patients present with two recognizable groups of findings (Drachman and Adams, 1962):

1. Nonspecific changes that are seen in most forms of encephalitis. These include fever, headache, signs of meningeal irritation, nausea and vomiting, global confusion, generalized seizures, and an alteration of consciousness.

2. Changes referable to focal necrosis of the orbitofrontal and temporal cortex and the limbic system. These include anosmia, memory loss, peculiar behavior, defects of speech (especially expressive aphasia), hallucinations (particularly olfactory and gustatory hallucinations), and focal seizures.

More extensive involvement of the cerebral hemispheres is signaled by the appearance of reflex asymmetry, Babinski signs, focal (usually facial) paralysis, conjugate deviation of the eyes, ataxia, incontinence of stool and urine, hemiparesis, and coma. Cerebral edema contributes to these manifestations of herpes simplex encephalitis, and brain swelling often plays an important role in the outcome of the disease.

The most common early manifestations of herpes simplex encephalitis are fever, headache, and altered consciousness (Table 1). The onset of neurologic abnormalities is often dramatic; early appearance of delirium, hemiparesis and major motor seizures, and rapid progression to coma can make the presence of a severe encephalitic process immediately obvious. In many patients, the encephalitis progresses more slowly, with expressive aphasia, paresthesias, and mental changes preceding more severe neurologic abnormalities.

Another common and important mode of presentation of herpes simplex encephalitis is one in which the most striking initial symptoms are of a "psychological" nature (Drachman and Adams, 1962). There is usually a period of mild nonspecific illness lasting from one to several days and characterized by various combinations of headache, drowsiness, fever, malaise, fatigue, sore throat, rhinorrhea, photophobia, anorexia, nausea, vomiting, irritability, and abdominal pain. This is followed by the appearance of bizarre behavior characterized by disorientation, confusion, incoherent thought, memory disturbance, labile affect, and, often, sensory distortion and hallucinations. This bizarre behavior may be intermittent, alternating with periods of lethargy or sleep. The illness initially appears to be minor, and only the aberations of behavior call attention to its serious nature. The picture is often that of an acute psychosis or delirium tremens, and many patients with herpes simplex encephalitis are admitted for psychiatric care until the appearance of localizing neurologic signs, seizures, and coma alerts their physicians to the organic nature of the disease. This is tragic, for only early diagnosis and therapy offer hope of favorably altering the grim prognosis of this disease (Whitley et al., 1977 and 1981).

Fever is present initially in 90 per cent of patients and at some time during the course of the disease in almost every case. It ranges from 38 to 40.6° C (100 to 105° F) and is usually refractory to antipyretics. Headache is an early symptom in 70 to 80 per cent of patients. It is often severe and refractory to analgesics. Seizures, often focal, are also common. They occur early in 40 to 50 per cent, and at some time during the course of the disease in more than 80 per cent of patients. Other localizing neurologic signs, such as cranial nerve palsies, hemiparesis, and dysphasia, occur early in most patients and at some time during the course of the disease in nearly every case. The clinical picture often suggests a space-occupying lesion in the temporoparietal area, raising the possibility of an intracranial hemorrhage or cerebral abscess. Signs of meningeal irritation are uncommon early in the illness, but eventually develop in more than one-half of the patients. The optic fundi may show edema and swelling of the disk, and peripapillary retinal hemorrhages. This usually reflects cerebral edema, which frequently complicates the management of patients with herpes simplex encephalitis. In some cases, however, these abnormalities are a manifestation of herpes simplex optic neuritis and retinitis, which appear to be due to contiguous spread of infection from the brain (Minckler et al., 1976; Johnson and Wisotzkey, 1977; Cibis et al., 1978).

Although most patients with herpes simplex encephalitis present with fever, headache, alteration of consciousness, behavioral abnormalities, and localizing neurologic signs, Tucker et al. (1978) have recently described a patient with herpes simplex encephalitis whose initial illness was manifested solely as a seizure disorder. Because of the absence of fever, headache, and localizing neurologic signs until 7 days after hospital admission, the diagnosis was not made until late in the course of the disease. On rare occasions, perhaps reflecting an atypical route of entry of HSV into the central nervous system, the damage in herpes simplex encephalitis is concentrated in the brain stem. Such patients present with a brain stem encephalitis that bears little clinical resemblance to the usual case of herpes simplex encephalitis (Dayan et al., 1972).

Some cases of herpes simplex encephalitis are clearly primary infections with HSV-1, whereas others, occurring in patients with a history of recurrent herpes labialis and with antibody to HSV in their serum at the beginning of the illness, are almost certainly recurrent infections (Whitley et al., 1982a; Nahmias et al., 1982). Thus, it is surprising that typical herpetic lesions of the mouth, pharynx, perioral skin, or eyes are uncommon in the encephalitic patients. Furthermore, HSV is infrequently recovered from cultures of the oropharynx and has not been isolated from the blood, urine, or stool of otherwise healthy children and adults with herpes simplex encephalitis. In fact, the oropharyngeal isolation rate in patients with herpes simplex encephalitis (about 7 to 15 per cent) is no different from that in comparable patients without herpes simplex encephalitis (Nahmias et al., 1982).

The clinical course of herpes simplex encephalitis is variable, but the outlook in untreated patients is grim, with an overall mortality of 70 to 75 per cent (Whitley et al., 1981). The illness may fluctuate in intensity during the first several days, but thereafter it generally pursues an unremitting course with progression from lethargy to coma. Coma almost always indicates severe and irreversible brain damage, for almost all comatose patients die, and the rare survivor is left with severe neurologic sequelae. The average interval from onset of symptoms to coma is 6 to 7 days, with a range of 2 days to 2 weeks. The total duration of illness is often quite short, with more than three-quarters of the deaths occurring within the first 2 weeks. The average interval from onset to death is 10 to 12 days. If recovery occurs, it usually begins during the second or third week.

Results of routine laboratory tests are normal in most patients with herpes simplex encephalitis, unless it is complicated by respiratory infection or other intercurrent illness. Some patients have a moderate leukocytosis and a slightly elevated erythrocyte sedimentation rate. Hyponatremia and hyposmolality are often observed as a result of inappropriate secretion of antidiuretic hormone, but this can be seen in a wide variety of brain diseases.

The spinal fluid is usually abnormal from the outset, with pleocytosis and a moderately elevated protein. The spinal fluid pressure is frequently elevated, reflecting cerebral edema. However, 5 to 15 per cent of patients may have completely normal spinal fluid on the first examination and only subsequently show a rise in cell count and protein concentration. The cell count is variable, usually between 50 and 500 per mm^3, but with a range of 0 to 2500.

Table 1. FINDINGS IN PATIENTS ADMITTED FOR TREATMENT OF PRESUMED HERPES SIMPLEX ENCEPHALITIS WHO DID OR DID NOT PROVE TO HAVE THE DISEASE[a]

	% of Patients	
	Patients with Proven Herpes Simplex Encephalitis (n=113)[b]	***Patients Who Did Not Have Herpes Simplex Encephalitis (n=85)***[c]
Historical Findings		
Alteration in consciousness	97	98
CSF pleocytosis	97	87
Fever	90	78
Headache	81	77
Personality Change	71	68
Seizures	67	59
Vomiting	46	46
Hemiparesis	33	26
Memory loss	24	19
History of recurrent herpes	22	22
herpes labialis	16	14
genital herpes	2	2
cutaneous herpes simplex	5	6
Findings at Presentation		
Fever	92	81
Personality change	85	74
Dysarthria	76	67
Autonomic dysfunction	60	56
Ataxia	40	40
Hemiparesis	38	30
Seizures	38	47
focal	25	15
generalized	9	17
both	4	15
Cranial nerve defects	32	33
Visual field loss	14	12
Papilledema	14	11
Isolation of HSV from peripheral sites	15	11
Neurodiagnostic Assessment		
Focal EEG abnormality	81	59
Brain scan localization	50	14
CT scan localization	59	22
Localization by ≥ 1 test	82	63
Localization by ≥ 2 tests	48	18
Evidence of Intrathecal Production of Antibody to HSV[d]		
Day after Onset of Disease		
≤ 4	31	14
5	40	11
11–15	64	15
≥ 15	90	19
Examination of Brain Biopsy		
Histopathology		
Encephalitis	85	36
Encephalitis and intranuclear inclusion bodies	56	14
HSV Antigen by Immunofluorescence	70	9
Herpesvirus particles by EM	45	2[e]
≥ 1 test indicative of HSV infection	75	21
≥ 2 tests indicative of HSV infection	47	0
≥ 3 tests indicative of HSV infection	29	0

[a]Adapted from data in Whitley et al., 1982b and Nahmias et al., 1982.
[b]HSV isolated from brain tissue obtained by biopsy or at autopsy.
[c]HSV not isolated from brain tissue obtained by biopsy or at autopsy, and no other convincing evidence of herpes simplex encephalitis.
[d]Measured by passive hemagglutination and IgG-specific immunofluorescence assays. Intrathecal production of antibody is defined by a serum/CSF antibody ratio ≤20.
[e]Both of these patients had serologic evidence of EBV infection.

Lymphocytes or mononuclear cells generally predominate, but there are often 10 to 25 per cent polymorphonuclear leukocytes and, especially early in the disease, most or all of the cells may be polymorphonuclear leukocytes. The protein concentration is usually elevated to between 50 and 200 mg/dl and tends to increase during the course of the disease. The glucose concentration is usually normal on initial examination (5 per cent of patients have hypoglycorrhachia) but it may be depressed later in the presence of extensive cerebral necrosis. Erythrocytes are found in the spinal fluid initially in 40 per cent, and at some time in 70 to 80 per cent, of patients, reflecting the hemorrhagic nature of the cerebral lesions. Xanthochromia is sometimes observed. There is no clear relationship between the nature or magnitude of the spinal fluid abnormalities and the eventual outcome of the disease. HSV is rarely recovered from the spinal fluid in children and adults with herpes simplex encephalitis.

Most patients with proven herpes simplex encephalitis have shown temporal lobe localization on electroencephalogram, technetium brain scan, arteriogram, or computed tomography, singly or in combination. The changes observed are not pathognomonic of herpes simplex encephalitis (Table 1), but they do help to demonstrate the focal nature of the pathologic process and localize the area of greatest involvement for subsequent cerebral biopsy. Unfortunately, while one or more of these techniques eventually yields localizing findings in nearly every case, they often fail to do so on the first examination. The findings are nonspecific or normal in one-third of the patients during the first 5 days after the onset of neurologic signs and symptoms.

HSV infection in the newborn is often a disseminated visceral infection with severe involvement of the liver, adrenal glands, and many other organs (Nahmias et al., 1983). The brain is affected in more than one-half of the patients, but this may not be clinically apparent because of the severity of the disseminated visceral infection. The initial signs and symptoms of infection usually appear within the first week of life, but they may be present at birth or, rarely, appear as late as 4 weeks postpartum. The most common initial clinical manifestations are nonspecific, including lethargy, fever or hypothermia, vomiting, and poor feeding. Other early signs may include jaundice (with or without hepatomegaly), purpuric rash, apneic spells, respiratory distress, and cyanosis. The clinical picture resembles neonatal bacterial sepsis. Neurologic manifestations usually include generalized or focal seizures, increased intracranial pressure with a bulging fontanelle, cranial nerve palsies, opisthotonus, and flaccid or spastic paralysis. These signs and symptoms often progress to coma, decerebrate posturing, and continuous seizure activity that is difficult to control with anticonvulsants. The disease usually progresses rapidly, with death sometimes occurring within a few hours of the onset of symptoms. The mortality in untreated disseminated neonatal herpes, with or without encephalitis, is 70 to 80 per cent. The median interval from onset of symptoms to death is 7 days, and the median age at time of death is 2 weeks. In some patients with encephalitis, death results from the direct progression of neurologic symptoms. In others, the terminal events are respiratory failure or circulatory collapse with disseminated intravascular coagulation and bleeding from multiple sites. External herpetic lesions (that is, lesions of the skin, eyes, or oral cavity) are present at the onset of the disease in 70 per cent of the patients. They appear at some time during the course of the disease in 90 per cent of the infants with disseminated neonatal herpes.

Approximately 40 per cent of neonates with herpes simplex encephalitis have no evidence of disseminated disease. The onset of symptoms in this group is later (average, 11 days) than in infants with disseminated disease. In over one-half of these patients, the disease begins with the development of herpetic skin lesions, oropharyngeal lesions, or HSV infection of the eye, with subsequent development of signs and symptoms of encephalitis. In the remainder, the earliest manifestations of infection are lethargy, irritability, tremors, and focal or generalized seizures, but most of these patients also develop visible lesions of the skin, mouth, or eyes at some time during the disease. These are probably the sites of initial infection from which virus then spreads to the central nervous system, perhaps by neural routes. Progression of neurologic signs and symptoms eventually leads to death in about 40 per cent of these patients, and most survivors are left with severe neurologic sequelae.

The spinal fluid is abnormal in both forms of neonatal herpes simplex encephalitis, but not invariably so on the first examination. There is usually a mononuclear pleocytosis with 50 to 200 cells per mm^3, and the cell count seldom exceeds 400 per mm^3. Polymorphonuclear leukocytes occasionally predominate, and erythrocytes are frequently present. The protein concentration is usually elevated and, in the presence of extensive cerebral necrosis, may sometimes exceed 1000 mg/dl. The glucose concentration is usually normal, but it may be depressed, and a low spinal fluid glucose concentration may sometimes reflect hypoglycemia. The spinal fluid is not discernibly different in the two forms of neonatal herpes simplex encephalitis except for the presence of virus. HSV is more often isolated from the spinal fluid of infants in whom encephalitis is associated with disseminated infection. In the disseminated infection, HSV can also be isolated from lesions of the skin, from the eyes, throat, nasopharynx, blood, sputum, urine, and feces, and from multiple organs at autopsy. In infants with localized central nervous system infection, virus can be isolated from the peripheral lesions that are usually present in the skin, mouth, or eyes. When peripheral lesions are absent, brain biopsy is required to establish the diagnosis.

In some infants with localized central nervous system infection, electroencephalogram, brain scan, and computerized axial tomography may provide evidence of temporal lobe localization, as observed in older children and adults. This is in contrast to the diffuse bilateral involvement that characterizes the encephalitis that occurs in the course of disseminated neonatal HSV infections.

Herpes Simplex Meningitis. Herpes simplex meningitis is an acute, generally benign, lymphocytic meningitis that occurs primarily in otherwise normal young adults, often in temporal association with genital or perigenital HSV infections (Terni et al., 1971; Craig and Nahmias, 1973; Skoldenberg et al., 1975; Hevron, 1977). It usually starts abruptly with headache, fever, photophobia, nausea and vomiting, myalgias, and nuchal rigidity. There are no seizures, focal neurologic signs, or behavioral disturbances. In most cases, the disease follows a brief, benign course, and symptoms disappear in about a week without residua. An occasional patient may develop radiculitis or ascending myelitis, with neurologic symptoms, such as dysesthesia and paresthesia, which persist for months. Approximately one-half of the documented cases of herpes simplex meningitis have occurred in the company of genital herpes, usually following the onset of the genital lesions by 5 to 10 days. Clinical and serologic data indicate that most of the episodes of genital herpes that are associated with herpes simplex meningitis are primary infections with HSV-2.

There is spinal fluid pleocytosis, with from 25 to 2500 cells per mm^3. Most patients have cell counts between 100 and 500 per mm^3, but one-quarter exceed 500 per mm^3. Generally, 75 to 100 per cent of the cells are mononuclear, but polymorphonuclear leukocytes may predominate early in the illness. The protein is moderately elevated, to greater than 100 mg/dl in one-half of the patients, but rarely exceeding 250 mg/dl. The glucose concentration is abnormally low in about 20 per cent of samples. Virus, usually HSV-2, can be isolated from the spinal fluid early in the disease. Abnormalities of spinal fluid often resolve slowly, and lymphocytic pleocytosis may persist for several weeks after clinical recovery.

Recurrences of benign aseptic meningitis are reported in 25 to 30 per cent of the patients, usually in association with episodes of recurrent genital or cutaneous herpes. Such recurrences are usually milder than the initial episode.

COMPLICATIONS AND SEQUELAE. In children and adults, herpes simplex encephalitis is entirely a disease of the central nervous system, and most of its complications and sequelae are the direct result of neuronal destruction by HSV. Complications outside the central nervous system are typical of those in any severely ill, unconscious patient with seizures. They include anoxic episodes, aspiration, pulmonary and urinary tract infections, fluid and electrolyte imbalance, cardiovascular problems, pulmonary embolus, stress ulcer, and bed sores. Inappropriate secretion of antidiuretic hormone and diabetes insipidus have also been observed.

The hemorrhagic necrosis produced by the virus also results in cerebral edema, leading to extensive brain swelling and increased intracranial pressure. This major and almost universal complication is an important cause of death in the acute phase of the disease. By increasing the extent of cerebral necrosis, the cerebral edema also contributes to the frequency and severity of sequelae in survivors.

The development of optic neuritis and retinitis, with unequivocal evidence of HSV infection of the retina, choroid, and optic nerve, has been observed in adults with herpes simplex encephalitis (Minckler et al., 1976; Johnson and Wisotzkey, 1977; Cibis et al., 1978). The pallor and edema of the optic disk and the retinal hemorrhages may be misinterpreted clinically as papilledema, and thus this complication may frequently be overlooked.

Reports of recurrent herpes simplex encephalitis are extremely rare and have not been documented by isolation of virus from the brain or spinal fluid. However, a number of patients with well documented herpes simplex encephalitis have been observed to relapse after an apparently successful course of antiviral chemotherapy. This has occurred in patients treated with vidarabine, acyclovir, and cytosine arabinoside (which is not an effective therapeutic agent in herpes simplex encephalitis). Typically, antiviral therapy of the initial episode resulted in dramatic improvement, but after 2 to 10 weeks, the symptoms and signs of encephalitis returned and there was progressive neurologic deterioration in spite of retreatment. Repeat brain biopsy at the time of clinical relapse has generally revealed an inflammatory infiltrate consisting of lymphocytes, macrophages and plasma cells, perivascular cuffing with lymphocytes and mononuclear cells, widespread gliosis and perivascular hemorrhages, but no intranuclear inclusion bodies, herpesvirus particles or HSV antigens. In one patient, a pattern of cell-mediated demyelination was observed, which resembled that seen in postinfectious encephalomyelitis (Koenig et al., 1979). Thus it appears that postinfectious encephalomyelitis, an acute, presumably autoimmune, demyelinating disease most frequently observed following virus infection or vaccination, may occur as a complication of herpes simplex encephalitis. However, demyelination was not observed in the other cases reported (Whitley et al., 1981; Abramson et al., 1984) and HSV-1 was isolated from brain tissue obtained by biopsy during the relapse in two patients (Dix et al., 1983; Davis and McLaren, 1983). It must be remembered that even in acute herpes simplex encephalitis, it can be very difficult to demonstrate HSV in the brain more than two weeks after onset (Olson et al., 1967). In this regard, it is noteworthy that both of the above-mentioned isolates of HSV-1 were obtained by inoculating susceptible cell cultures with finely minced fragments of brain, and that HSV CPE was not observed until more than 2 weeks after inoculation. Although this may suggest that the virus recovered was latent in the brain tissue, the difficulty in recovering HSV seems more likely related to the presence of large amounts of antibody to HSV in the biopsied tissue. Immunologic responses are undoubtedly important in producing the pathology observed in patients who relapse after therapy. However, the failure to detect HSV in brain biopsies from some of these patients does not exclude the possibility that the pathologic process is directly related to the continued replication of HSV.

It has often been suggested that subacute or chronic herpes simplex encephalitis might be responsible for some cases of psychosis (Wilson, 1976; Koehler and Guth, 1979), but the presence of HSV in the brain in such patients has rarely been documented. When it has (Rhodes et al., 1984) it may simply represent the occurrence of herpes simplex encephalitis in a psychotic patient, or the predominance of "psychological" symptoms in an otherwise unremarkable case of the disease (Oommen et al., 1982). However, the case of a 9-year-old boy with recurrent episodes of organic psychosis, each of which occurred in association with an episode of recurrent herpes labialis, suggests that self-limited recurrences of herpes simplex encephalitis may occur (Shearer and Finch, 1964). This interesting possibility, which has been observed in animal models of herpes simplex encephalitis, has yet to be documented adequately in humans. The case reported is reminiscent of the association of recurrent HSV-2 meningitis with episodes of recurrent herpes genitalis.

The sequelae observed in patients surviving herpes simplex encephalitis reflect the severe cortical damage sustained by the temporal lobes and adjacent structures. They include memory loss, anosmia, ageusia, dysphasia, alexia and other agnosias, confusion, personality changes, hemiparesis, ataxia, autonomic nervous system dysfunction, seizures, and chorioretinitis. In some patients, memory loss, confabulation, and personality change result in a picture that closely resembles Korsakoff's psychosis.

When neonatal herpes simplex encephalitis occurs during disseminated infection, the complications are primarily the result of viremia with extensive involvement of the liver, adrenal glands, lungs, and other organs and tissues throughout the body. Mortality exceeds 70 per cent, and death often results directly from virus infection and necrosis of vital organs. Severe complications include cerebral edema, status epilepticus, hypoglycemia, acidosis, pneumonitis, disseminated intravascular coagulation with hemorrhage and shock, and bacterial or fungal superinfection. More than one-half of the survivors have significant sequelae attributable to central nervous system damage. Infants with herpes simplex encephalitis without disseminated infection have a lower acute mortality, about 40 per cent. However, at least 75 per cent of the survivors have severe sequelae. The neurologic sequelae of neonatal herpes simplex encephalitis include microcephaly, multicystic encephalomalacia, porencephalic cysts, hydrocephaly, seizures, motor deficits, and varying degrees of psychomotor retardation. Ocular sequelae include corneal scarring, cataracts, chorioretinitis, and blindness. Some of these sequelae may not be recognized for months or years and may even develop following vidarabine therapy in infants whose disease remained limited to the skin, eyes, or mouth (Whitley et al., 1983b; Nahmias et al., 1983).

In contrast to herpes simplex encephalitis, herpes simplex meningitis is usually benign and self-limited, without significant complications and residua. However, an occasional patient may suffer a protracted illness with signs and symptoms of ascending myelitis or radiculitis (Hunt and Comer, 1955; Klastersky et al., 1972), and 25 to 30 per cent have recurrent episodes of aseptic meningitis, often in association with recurrences of genital or cutaneous herpes. Increased intracranial pressure and papilledema have been reported in one patient with recurrent herpes meningitis, with isolation of HSV-2 from the spinal fluid (Stalder et al., 1973).

As with HSV infections at other sites, the course of HSV infections of the central nervous system may be particularly severe and atypical in immunosuppressed patients, especially patients with defects in cellular immunity. Such severe and atypical infections have included fatal HSV-2 meningoencephalitis in renal transplant recipients (Linnemann et al., 1976); HSV-2 encephalitis in patients with cerebral metastases (Manz et al., 1979); and slowly progressive herpes simplex encephalitis without inflammatory changes or hemorrhagic necrosis in a patient with Hodgkin's disease (Price et al., 1973).

GEOGRAPHIC VARIATION IN DISEASE AND EPIDEMIOLOGY. Herpes simplex viruses are distributed worldwide without evidence of differing racial or sexual susceptibility. While many experimental animals can be infected, humans are the only known reservoir of natural infection. The principal mode of transmission is through direct contact with infected secretions, and there are no known animal vectors. HSV-1 is transmitted primarily by contact with oral secretions and HSV-2 by contact with genital secretions.

Following primary infection, these viruses establish latent infections that persist for life. Latently infected persons are a stable reservoir of virus, and this explains why HSV infections are endemic everywhere, even in small, totally isolated populations in which the pool of susceptibles is too small to maintain the continuous circulation of such epidemic diseases as measles (Black, 1975). Primary and recurrent infections with both HSV types can be symptomatic or asymptomatic, and transmission can occur from either.

Age-related patterns of infection differ for HSV-1 and HSV-2. Antibodies to HSV-1 rise rapidly during childhood, and, by puberty, nearly everyone in lower socioeconomic groups has been infected. Infection rates are inversely related to socioeconomic status. The incidence of infection is lower in higher socioeconomic groups, in which antibody prevalence in young adults is only 30 to 50 per cent. The major period of HSV-2 infection follows puberty, transmission being directly related to sexual activity.

Infection of neurons plays a crucial role in HSV latency, but symptomatic infection of the central nervous system is extremely uncommon. Herpes simplex encephalitis (beyond the neonatal period) is a rare manifestation of primary and recurrent HSV-1 infection. Nevertheless, it is the most common sporadic form of encephalitis in the United States, where it accounts for approximately 10 per cent of all reported cases of encephalitis of determined etiology. It also appears to be the most frequently identified form of severe sporadic encephalitis in the United Kingdom and Western Europe. The incidence is estimated to be 1 to 2 cases per million population per year and may well be substantially higher (Nahmias and Josey, 1982). Herpes simplex encephalitis occurs sporadically throughout the year in all parts of the world and in patients of both sexes and all ages, reflecting the ubiquity of HSV infection. It is caused almost exclusively by HSV-1. Approximately 10 per cent of the cases occur in the first year of life but, thereafter, the age-specific attack rate appears to be relatively constant. There is no seasonal variation in its occurrence, as there is with central nervous system infections caused by togaviruses and enteroviruses, and there is no temporal association with epidemic diseases such as measles, mumps, or varicella.

Neonatal herpes simplex encephalitis is a manifestation of neonatal HSV infection, which is worldwide and sporadic. There is no discernible seasonal variation, and infection appears to be distributed about equally between males and females. The incidence of recognized neonatal HSV infections in the United States has been estimated to be about 1 in 7500 deliveries (Nahmias et al., 1983) but it is probably somewhat lower. In the majority of cases, infection is acquired perinatally from the birth canal of a mother with genital herpes. In some cases, infection may occur in utero, as a result either of maternal viremia or of ascending infection from the cervix. Rarely, infection may be acquired postnatally from the mother, other family members, or nursery personnel with symptomatic or asymptomatic HSV infections, or by nosocomial spread from another infected infant. Most infections are caused by HSV-2, but there is no discernible difference in the nature or severity of the disease caused by HSV-1 and HSV-2. Neonatal HSV infection is more common in premature infants, who comprise 40 to 50 per cent of reported cases. While this may reflect increased susceptibility to HSV, the outcome appears to be as poor in full-term infants as in premature infants. A more likely explanation is a higher frequency of premature deliveries in women with severe genital herpes, perhaps associated with ascending HSV infection and herpetic chorioamnionitis (Chapter 163).

Herpes simplex meningitis is also worldwide in distribution. Some cases, caused by HSV-1, have been reported in children. However, herpes simplex meningitis is primarily a disease of sexually active young adults, 15 to 35 years of age. In this age group, it is usually caused by HSV-2. Serologic and virologic data from Sweden and the United States indicate that herpes simplex meningitis accounts for about 1 to 5 per cent of all cases of "aseptic" meningitis. In addition to its well recognized association with genital herpes, herpes simplex meningitis has also been observed in association with HSV pharyngotonsillitis and proctitis. Changing sexual practices and socioeconomic conditions are altering the epidemiology of HSV-1 and HSV-2 infections. As a consequence, we are likely to see an increase in the proportion of cases of herpes simplex meningitis caused by HSV-1.

DIAGNOSIS. Although herpes simplex encephalitis is a relatively uncommon disease, it is unique among the viral encephalitides in its susceptibility to specific antiviral therapy. It is also an extraordinarily severe disease, usually characterized by extensive and rapidly progressive cerebral necrosis. Even the most effective antiviral drug will not restore life to dead neurons, and thus it is not surprising that antiviral therapy has proved futile once the disease has progressed to the point at which the patient is comatose. In a recent study, mortality in comatose patients exceeded 60 per cent in spite of therapy with vidarabine, and virtually all of the survivors were severely debilitated (Whitley et al., 1977, 1981 and 1983a). Since the mean interval from onset of symptoms to coma is only 6 to 7 days, there is an enormous premium on early diagnosis. Unfortunately, herpes simplex encephalitis is difficult to diagnose, especially early in the disease, because its occurrence is sporadic and its manifestations protean. Many other pathologic processes mimic herpes simplex encephalitis.

The problem is well illustrated by the results of a recent multicenter collaborative study (Whitley et al., 1981). The clinical criteria for entry—"evidence of an acute, febrile encephalopathy with disordered mentation, focal cerebral signs, localization by diagnostic procedures (electroencephalogram, arteriogram, or brain scan, singly or in combination), and cerebrospinal-fluid findings compatible with viral infection"—were so stringent that more than 25 per cent of the patients with herpes simplex encephalitis were already comatose when admitted to the study. Nevertheless, brain biopsy demonstrated herpes simplex encephalitis in only 54 per cent of the patients entered into the study. In approximately one-half of the remaining 46 per cent, brain biopsy yielded other specific diagnoses, many of which required other forms of therapy. These included brain abscess, toxoplasmosis, tuberculosis, cryptococcal infection, rickettsial infection, leptospiral meningitis, cerebrovascular disease, metastatic tumor, toxic encephalopathy, Epstein-Barr virus infection, and more than one dozen cases of meningoencephalitis caused by RNA viruses (which are not inhibited by vidarabine). Biopsies in the remaining patients showed histologic changes suggesting viral meningoencephalitis caused by agents other than HSV. Ten per cent of the patients who did not have herpes simplex encephalitis had nonviral central nervous system infections for which effective specific therapy is presently available. It is already clear that as the clinical criteria are being relaxed in order to start treatment earlier in the course of herpes simplex encephalitis, an even higher proportion of nonherpetic patients are being included. These considerations emphasize the need to establish firmly the etiology before accepting the diagnosis of herpes simplex encephalitis. Unfortunately, the only means of establishing the diagnosis of herpes simplex encephalitis is the demonstration of HSV or HSV antigens in brain tissue obtained by biopsy or at autopsy (Johnson et al., 1968; Boston Interhospital Virus Study Group, 1975; Whitley et al., 1981 and 1982b). The morbidity and mortality that will result from the failure to diagnose promptly and treat other treatable diseases far exceeds the morbidity of brain biopsy (Whitley et al., 1981; Morawetz et al., 1983).

Signs and symptoms referable to the orbitofrontal and temporal cortex and the limbic system, especially peculiar behavior, anosmia, dysphasia, memory loss, olfactory, gustatory or auditory hallucinations, and focal seizures can provide the earliest evidence of serious disease and of localization.

Routine laboratory tests are of no value in diagnosing herpes simplex encephalitis. Examination of the spinal fluid is helpful only in providing data consistent with a viral infection or in identifying bacterial, parasitic, or fungal infections. The cell count is quite variable but usually ranges from 50 to 500 per mm^3. Lymphocytes and mononuclear cells generally predominate but there are often 10 to 25 per cent polymorphonuclear leukocytes. The protein concentration is usually elevated, and the glucose concentration is usually normal on initial examination. The spinal fluid pressure is often elevated and erythrocytes are frequently present, reflecting the hemorrhagic nature of the cerebral lesions. However, 5 to 15 per cent of patients with herpes simplex encephalitis may have normal spinal fluid on the first examination, and others have a cellular response consisting predominantly of polymorphonuclear leukocytes early in the disease. The spinal fluid examination cannot rule out many alternative diagnoses, such as bacterial cerebritis, cerebral abscess, tumor, central nervous system manifestations of bacterial endocarditis, postinfectious encephalomyelitis, cerebral hemorrhage or infarction, tuberculous or fungal meningitis, or meningoencephalitis caused by other viruses (Whitley et al., 1981).

Unfortunately, herpes simplex virus is rarely (i.e., fewer than 5 per cent of cases) isolated from the spinal fluid in children and adults with herpes simplex encephalitis. Attempts have been made to detect HSV antigens in the spinal fluid in the hope of circumventing the need for brain biopsy to establish the diagnosis. Immunofluorescent staining of leukocytes in spinal fluid to detect HSV antigens has not given positive results in most cases (Nahmias et al., 1982). The use of sensitive assays to detect HSV antigens or nucleic acids in spinal fluid is currently being evaluated, but at present, brain biopsy remains the only reliable method for early diagnosis.

Serologic tests are of no value in the *early* diagnosis of herpes simplex encephalitis because of the necessity for convalescent specimens and because an increase in antibody titer, even from undetectable levels, may simply reflect the reactivation of latent HSV unrelated to the encephalitic process (Johnson et al., 1968). Furthermore, many cases of herpes simplex encephalitis represent recurrent rather than primary infection, further complicating the interpretation of serologic data. However, the presence or appearance of IgM antibody to HSV in newborns provides reliable evidence of neonatal HSV infection.

Intrathecal synthesis of antibody to HSV can be detected in patients with herpes simplex encephalitis soon after onset by sensitive assays (Skoldenberg et al., 1981). An altered serum/CSF antibody ratio (e.g., <20) has been considered indicative of local antibody production (MacCallum et al., 1974, Levine et al., 1978), but alterations in the blood: brain barrier must be taken into account, ideally, by simultaneously measuring the serum/CSF ratio of antibody to another virus not likely to infect the central nervous system (e.g., rubella). Documentation of intrathecal synthesis of antibody to HSV can provide retrospective evidence of herpes simplex encephalitis, but the specificity of this diagnostic test is only about 80 per cent (Nahmias et al., 1982). Furthermore, the delay in the appearance of intrathecal antibody makes it unlikely that this approach will yield an early diagnosis.

The electroencephalogram is almost always abnormal, and often localizes the area of maximum involvement. The typical pattern is one of widespread arrhythmic slow wave activity, sometimes with unilateral or regional predominance, and the appearance of periodic sharp waves or spike-and-wave complexes ("periodic lateralized epileptiform discharges" or "PLEDS") over one or both temporal lobes. These changes are not always present, nor are they pathognomonic of herpes simplex encephalitis. They may occur in cerebral infarcts, increased intracranial pressure, various inflammatory conditions, and encephalitis caused by other viruses. Nevertheless, they may aid in distinguishing herpes simplex encephalitis from other processes and help determine the best site for cerebral biopsy (Illis and Taylor, 1972).

Cerebral arteriography and technetium brain scan reveal a temporal lobe mass, with abnormal uptake of isotope in most cases, but the changes are not specific, and they are often absent early in the course of the disease (Table 1). Computed tomography (CT) reveals an area of diminished attenuation in the medial portion of the temporal lobe with extension into the insular area in most patients. Mass effect and streaky enhancement on contrast administration are also seen (Davis et al., 1978; Enzmann et al., 1978; Zimmerman et al., 1980). Unfortunately, these changes are often not seen within the first 5 days of illness. Nevertheless, in most patients, CT scan has obviated the need for angiography.

Definitive diagnosis of herpes simplex encephalitis requires cerebral biopsy. The biopsy should be performed early in order to start specific therapy as soon as possible, and tissue should be obtained from an area of obvious pathology. The medial and inferior surfaces of the temporal lobe are so regularly involved that if any doubt exists as to the site of maximum pathology, these areas should be selected. Biopsied tissue should be divided under sterile conditions into pieces for histopathologic examination, electronmicroscopy, routine bacterial and fungal cultures, and virus isolation. Care should be taken so that each sample includes cortex. In addition, impression smears should be made and fixed in chilled acetone for immunofluorescent or immunoperoxidase staining (Flewett, 1973). The tissue for histopathologic examination should be fixed in Bouin's or another acid fixative to best demonstrate intranuclear inclusions. The tissue for viral culture should be carried to the virology laboratory in ice-cold transport medium, finely minced (or dispersed with trypsin or collagenase), washed several times with tissue culture medium, and inoculated into tissue cultures of primary human embryonic kidney, diploid human lung or skin fibroblasts, primary guinea pig embryo, or primary rabbit kidney cells. The inoculation of viable brain cells, rather than a clarified suspension of homogenized brain, increases the chances of isolating small amounts of virus, especially if there is antibody to HSV present in the biopsied tissue. Typical HSV CPE is usually apparent within 48 hours, and more than 90 per cent of positive biopsies are recognized as such within 3 days of inoculation. However, tissue obtained from a minimally involved area of brain or taken more than 2 weeks after onset of disease may contain very little virus and large amounts of antibody. Under these circumstances, the appearance of HSV CPE in tissue culture has been delayed for as long as 21 days (Johnson et al., 1972). These cultures should be held for a minimum of 3 weeks and, in situations in which the diagnosis remains obscure, blind passaged once before being discarded. Isolation of HSV represents the most sensitive and reliable means of establishing the diagnosis of herpes simplex encephalitis. The incidence of culture-negative biopsies in cases in which virus is subsequently isolated at autopsy is very low (in the neighborhood of 1 to 3 per cent). Immunofluorescent or immunoperoxidase staining provides a rapid means of establishing the diagnosis. Unfortunately, the results are positive in only 70 per cent of culture-positive biopsies (Table 1), because the technique fails to detect HSV antigens in biopsies with a low concentration of virus (Cho and Feng, 1978). False-positive fluorescent antibody staining appears with a frequency of at least 5 per cent. It has been reported in cases of tuberculosis, cryptococcal meningitis, brain abscess, and St. Louis encephalitis. The use of HSV-specific monoclonal antibodies may improve the specificity of fluorescent antibody staining, but it is unlikely to improve its sensitivity. The identification of Cowdry Type A intranuclear inclusion bodies and the electronmicroscopic detection of herpesvirus particles (Figs. 1 and 4) are both less sensitive and less specific diagnostic techniques (Table 1). Similar inclusion bodies can be produced by VZV, measles virus, and the human papovaviruses responsible for progressive multifocal leukoencephalopathy; the virions of all of the herpesviruses are morphologically indistinguishable. Furthermore, at least one-third of biopsy specimens that are positive by culture and fluorescent antibody staining do not contain detectable inclusion bodies or virions. It should be emphasized that the likelihood of isolating virus from the brain in herpes simplex encephalitis is greatly reduced when tissue is obtained more than 2 weeks after the onset of symptoms (Olson et al., 1967). Although virus is rarely isolated from the lumbar spinal fluid, ventricular fluid is frequently culture-positive (Flewett, 1973). However, this may simply reflect the passage of the needle used to obtain ventricular fluid through infected brain.

The differential diagnosis of herpes simplex encephalitis encompasses most viral and many nonviral diseases of the central nervous system. It includes encephalitis produced by other viruses, particularly togaviruses and mumps virus; postinfectious encephalomyelitis; bacterial, rickettsial, fungal, and parasitic infections; toxic encephalopathy (for example, lead poisoning); cerebrovascular disorders; and tumors. Although other viruses are less likely to produce focal disease in the temporal lobe, the clinical distinction between herpes simplex encephalitis and other forms of viral encephalitis rests primarily on epidemiologic data and is never secure. Virus isolation and serologic data are required to establish the etiologic diagnosis. The possibility of postinfectious encephalomyelitis is raised by a history of antecedent viral illness, such as measles or varicella, or recent vaccination. Toxic encephalopathy may be suggested by a history of ingestion or exposure, and the diagnosis is supported by detection of the toxic substance in the blood, urine, or other body fluid. A thorough examination of the spinal fluid usually distinguishes fungal, parasitic, or bacterial meningitis from herpes simplex encephalitis. In these non-viral infections, the spinal fluid glucose concentration is consistently depressed. The detection of organisms on microscopic examination and culture, or of specific microbial antigens or antibodies (for example, cryptococcal antigen or antibody to *Coccidioides immitis*) by immunologic assay, often gives a rapid and definitive diagnosis. Cerebral infarction, subarachnoid hemorrhage, subdural hematoma, subdural empyema, epidural abscess, and brain tumors may also be confused with herpes simplex encephalitis (Whitley et al., 1981). Examination of the spinal fluid is rarely helpful, but technetium brain scan, arteriography, and, especially, CT scan help to distinguish these disorders from herpes simplex encephalitis. Cerebral abscess presents a difficult differential diagnosis because fever, headache, obtundation, seizures, and other focal neurologic signs are frequent. The spinal fluid findings are not distinctive, and, while personality changes and isolated disorders of memory are more common in herpes simplex encephalitis, they may occur in brain abscess as well. The electroencephalogram and CT scan may suggest one or the other diagnosis, but none of the noninvasive diagnostic procedures is reliable enough to obviate the need for diagnostic brain biopsy. The necessity for brain biopsy to establish the diagnosis of herpes simplex encephalitis is clearly demonstrated by the fact that nearly one-half of the patients with the clinical diagnosis of herpes simplex encephalitis who have undergone brain biopsy have proved to have some other disease (Whitley et al., 1981).

In the neonate, as in the adult, the key to the early diagnosis of herpes simplex encephalitis is a high index of suspicion. The presence of skin lesions, oral ulcers, or keratoconjunctivitis greatly facilitates the diagnosis of neonatal HSV infection, and such lesions should be carefully sought at birth and frequently thereafter in any infant who is unwell. The skin lesions may initially be maculopapular and only later become vesicular. They are often on the presenting part, especially the scalp. Enlarged epithelial cells and multinucleated giant cells containing acidophilic Cowdry Type A intranuclear inclusion bodies distinguish the lesions of herpes simplex from all others except varicella-zoster, which can usually be dismissed on epidemiologic grounds. These cells can be seen in Tzanck smears (Chapter 105). A punch biopsy provides more reliable material for histopathologic examination, especially in atypical or prevesicular lesions. Tzanck smears should also be made from the base of oral ulcers and from conjunctival scrapings in infants with keratoconjunctivitis. Because more than one-half of maternal genital infections associated with neonatal herpes are clinically inapparent, cells for histopathologic examination should also be obtained from the mother's cervix, even in the absence of genital lesions. All of these materials should be carefully examined for HSV antigens by immunofluorescent or immunoperoxidase staining, or with some other technique to detect HSV antigens or nucleic acids (Chapter 105). This often gives a rapid and specific diagnosis. They may also be examined for herpes virus particles by electron microscopy. Cells scraped from all visible lesions should be immediately inoculated into appropriate tissue cultures (Chapter 105) in order to isolate the virus.

Unfortunately, visible stigmata of HSV infection may be absent at the outset of neonatal herpes. However, virus can usually be isolated from the spinal fluid, throat, nasopharynx, sputum, blood, urine, and feces. It should be sought in any infant with the clinical picture of neonatal sepsis or meningitis in whom the bacteriologic diagnosis is not rapidly established. In the absence of herpetic skin lesions, neonatal herpes may be indistinguishable from disseminated neonatal enterovirus infections; in fact, the two may occasionally coexist in the same infant.

The presence or appearance of IgM antibodies to HSV provides reliable evidence of neonatal infection. Unfortunately, the progression of the disease is usually so rapid that antibody is rarely present soon enough to aid in early diagnosis.

Herpes simplex meningitis is indistinguishable from the benign aseptic meningitis caused by a number of other viruses. The diagnosis should be suspected when aseptic meningitis develops in association with genital or cutaneous herpes. Isolation of HSV from the blood and serologic evidence of primary HSV infection are highly suggestive, but the diagnosis is firmly established only by the isolation of HSV from the spinal fluid.

TREATMENT. General supportive measures directed at the care of the comatose patient with seizures are extremely important. The airway must often be maintained by intubation or tracheostomy, and mechanical ventilation may be required. Frequent turning and careful skin care are essential to avoid decubitus ulcers. There must also be careful attention to the bowel, bladder, eyes, and tracheal toilet, and to the maintenance of body temperature, fluid and electrolyte balance, and blood glucose levels. Seizures may be controlled with diphenylhydantoin or phenobarbital, and diazepam may help in status epilepticus. The respiratory tract, urinary tract, skin, and intravenous sites are common loci of nosocomial infections. Such infections should be carefully sought, vigorously treated, and avoided by meticulous nursing care.

Cerebral edema with brain swelling and tentorial herniation are lethal in many cases of herpes simplex encephalitis. Large doses of corticosteroids are frequently given for this complication, but the effectiveness of this form of therapy has not been substantiated, and the possibility that it may lower resistance to HSV infection has not been adequately evaluated. Osmotic diuretics, such as glycerol, may also help to control cerebral edema. An alternative approach, extensive decompressive craniotomy, has been extremely useful in selected patients (Illis and Gostling, 1972).

The development of agents capable of inhibiting the replication of HSV in tissue cultures has provided a means for the effective specific treatment of herpes simplex encephalitis. Most of these antiviral agents are nucleoside analogs that interfere with the synthesis of HSV DNA. Unfortunately, they may also interfere with host-cell DNA synthesis and thus be toxic when administered systemically. Among the typical manifestations of such toxicity are myelosuppression and immunosuppression leading to uncontrolled bleeding and infection. Evaluation of the efficacy of antiviral agents in humans with herpes simplex encephalitis has been difficult because of the frequent failure to establish clearly the diagnosis in treated patients. The mortality in cases diagnosed clinically as herpes simplex encephalitis but negative for HSV on brain biopsy is much lower than that in untreated biopsy-proven cases (Whitley et al., 1977) so that the inclusion of biopsy-negative patients in a treatment group results in lower mortality, regardless of the efficacy of the treatment. Variations in the stage of the disease at start of therapy, uncertainties as to the natural history of the disease in untreated patients, and difficulty in distinguishing between complications of the disease itself and complications reflecting drug toxicity have contributed to the problem. To date, four nucleoside analogs have been evaluated for the therapy of herpes simplex encephalitis in humans. In the process, we have come to the painful realization that the evaluation of such therapeutic modalities can be accomplished only by means of double-blind, placebo-controlled studies in proven cases of the disease.

5-iodo-2′-deoxyuridine (idoxuridine), a thymidine analog that is effective when applied topically for the treatment of HSV keratitis, was the first antiviral drug used to treat herpes simplex encephalitis. Despite early optimism based upon case reports and uncontrolled trials, a double-blind, placebo-controlled study demonstrated lack of efficacy and unacceptable myelosuppressive toxicity (Boston Interhospital Virus Study Group, 1975). Similarly, case reports and uncontrolled trials of another pyrimidine analog, 1-B-D-arabinofuranosyl cytosine (cytosine arabinoside, cytarabine or ara-C) were thought by some to indicate efficacy until a recently completed placebo-controlled study carried out in the United Kingdom demonstrated a mortality in excess of 70 per cent in both the treated and placebo groups (Whitley et al., 1981). Another nucleoside analog, 9-B-D arabinofuranosyl adenine (adenine arabinoside, vidarabine, or ara-A), has yielded more promising results. In a double-blind, placebo-controlled study in biopsy-proven cases of herpes simplex encephalitis, vidarabine (15 mg/kg/day intravenously for 10 days) reduced the mortality, measured at 30 days, from 70 per cent to 28 per cent. The proportion of patients who survived without debilitating neurologic sequelae was increased from 20 per cent to 40 per cent. Later fatalities among patients with severe sequelae brought the mortality to 90 per cent in the placebo group and 40 per cent in the treated group at 120 days (Whitley et al., 1977). Although the number of patients in the study was small, comparable results have since been obtained in a larger group of biopsy-proven cases, all of whom were treated with this dose of vidarabine. The importance of early initiation of antiviral therapy was also clearly demonstrated. Patients who were lethargic when therapy was initiated had a 78 per cent survival rate, and 53 per cent returned to normal function. In contrast, patients who were comatose when treatment began had a 33 per cent survival rate, and only 8 per cent returned to normal function (Whitley et al., 1981). In a similar double-blind, placebo-controlled study, vidarabine (15 mg/kg/day intravenously for 10 days) reduced the mortality in newborns with disseminated HSV infection and localized herpes simplex encephalitis from 74 per cent to 38 per cent. The proportion of infants who survived without significant sequelae was also increased from 11 to 29 per cent (Whitley et al., 1980a). As in the case of herpes simplex encephalitis in children and adults, infants treated early (before dissemination) had a much lower mortality and fewer sequelae than infants treated when HSV had already disseminated to vital organs.

These results are encouraging, but the mortality in treated patients is still excessive and the quality of life is poor in many survivors. Vidarabine, though somewhat more active in inhibiting HSV than cellular DNA synthesis, still interferes with host-cell DNA replication and, at higher doses, produces myelosuppression and other toxic manifestations in vivo (Hirsch and Schooley, 1983). Moreover, vidarabine is relatively insoluble in aqueous solutions, and the large volume of intravenous fluid required to administer the drug frequently exacerbates cerebral edema.

The first of a new generation of truly selective inhibitors of HSV replication is now being compared to vidarabine in children and adults with herpes simplex encephalitis and in infants with neonatal HSV infections (Whitley et al., 1983a). This drug, 9-(2-hydroxyethoxymethyl) guanine (acycloguanosine or acyclovir) is selectively phosphorylated by the HSV-specified deoxypyrimidine kinase, but is a poor substrate for cellular thymidine kinases. As a result, the concentration of acyclovir monophosphate in HSV-infected cells is 30 to 100 times greater than that in uninfected cells. Cellular enzymes convert acyclovir monophosphate to acyclovir triphosphate, which is a selective inhibitor of HSV DNA polymerase. In addition, any acyclovir incorporated into DNA causes chain termination. Acyclovir is a highly effective and nontoxic inhibitor of HSV replication in tissue culture and in animal models of HSV infection. At therapeutic concentrations, it has no observable effects on hematopoietic precursor cells or on the immune system (Hirsch and Schooley, 1983).

Adults with herpes simplex encephalitis have been treated for 10 days with intravenous vidarabine (15 mg/kg/day over 12 hours) or acyclovir (10 mg/kg each 8 hours) in randomized double-blind collaborative trials in the United States and Europe. The results of one such trial carried out in Sweden (Skoldenberg et al., 1984) and the preliminary results of a larger study carried out in the United States demonstrated the superiority of acyclovir. The mortality in the patients treated with acyclovir was less than half that in the vidarabine recipients, and the incidence of significant sequelae in survivors was also much lower in the acyclovir recipients. On the basis of these results, it is recommended that patients with herpes simplex encephalitis be treated with intravenous acyclovir, 10 mg/kg each 8 hours for 10 days. Brain biopsy should also be carried out in these patients to rule out other treatable diseases. Infants with neonatal HSV infections are being treated for 10 days with intravenous vidarabine (30 mg/kg/day over 12 hours) or acyclovir (10 mg/kg each 8 hours) in a similar randomized double-blind collaborative trial, but this study has not yet been completed. Many additional compounds designed to interfere selectively with HSV-specific functions are under development and should soon be ready for testing in patients.

Because of the likelihood that relapses of herpes simplex encephalitis involve active replication of HSV in the brain, patients should be promptly re-evaluated and re-biopsied. They should then be retreated with acyclovir, unless there is evidence for the presence of acyclovir resistant HSV. Every attempt should be made to recover virus from the biopsy and test its sensitivity to vidarabine and acyclovir (and to any newer antiviral drugs that may become available) in parallel with the initial virus isolate. If corticosteroids are administered, the patient should also receive antiviral chemotherapy.

Interferons are natural antiviral glycoproteins produced by cells in response to virus infection. They are an important component of our natural resistance to infection by many viruses, including HSV. When given before infection or early in infection, interferons can inhibit the replication of HSV in tissue culture and in animals without apparent toxicity. In humans, interferon has been effective against herpes simplex keratitis, and, administered perioperatively, has reduced the frequency of reactivation of latent

HSV infection after surgical manipulation of the trigeminal nerve root (Pazin et al., 1979). The most likely use of interferon is in combination with an antiviral chemotherapeutic agent such as vidarabine or acyclovir. In a recent uncontrolled trial of human leukocyte interferon plus vidarabine in patients with herpes simplex encephalitis, no therapeutic effect was discernable and toxicity was greater than that expected with either agent alone (Koskiniemi et al., 1982).

In the newborn, the early administration of human HSV immune globulin containing high levels of antibody to HSV-2, as well as the use of hyperthermia, needs to be evaluated, especially in combination with antiviral agents.

Herpes simplex meningitis is usually a benign and self-limited disease. Nevertheless, when oral acyclovir is available, its use in herpes simplex meningitis should be considered, especially if there is any compromise in host immunity. Complications, such as ascending myelitis, should be treated with intravenous acyclovir (5 mg/kg or 250 mg/m^2 each 8 hours) for 7 to 10 days.

PROPHYLAXIS. Herpes simplex encephalitis beyond the neonatal period is a rare complication of both primary and recurrent HSV-1 infections. Because we do not understand its pathogenesis and, in particular, what causes on rare occasions this otherwise temperate virus to produce a highly fatal encephalitis, we are far from developing any specific prophylactic measures. Nevertheless, it seems likely that prophylactic measures effective against primary and recurrent HSV-1 infections in general will also reduce the frequency of herpes simplex encephalitis. Such measures would include anything that could reduce the incidence of primary infection, interfere with the establishment of latent infections of sensory neurons, or prevent the reactivation and spread of latent virus. Because primary and recurrent HSV infections in general, and herpes simplex encephalitis in particular, are sporadic in occurrence and afflict individuals of all ages, prevention will require lifelong prophylaxis. The only practical means of achieving lifelong prophylaxis of viral infections is active immunization. The development and evaluation of HSV vaccines is discussed in Chapter 105. Even when HSV vaccines are available, their effect on herpes simplex encephalitis is likely to be difficult to measure because of the rarity of the disease.

In the newborn, herpes simplex encephalitis is always a manifestation of primary infection, which is usually acquired from a mother with genital herpes. Most infections are acquired during passage through the infected birth canal or result from an ascending infection after rupture of the membranes. Thus, cesarean section has been recommended prior to rupture of the membranes when clinically apparent genital herpes is present at term (Chapter 163). However, the majority of the infants with neonatal herpes are born to mothers without clinically apparent genital herpes. Consequently, when there is a history of genital herpes in either parent, it is generally recommended that the mother's cervix, labia and vaginal secretions be cultured at least weekly during the last 2 months of gestation, even in the absence of symptoms of genital infection, and that the infant be delivered by cesarean section if virus is present at term. However, the frequency with which infants with neonatal herpes are born to mothers with no history of genital herpes and no known exposure to HSV, as well as the poor correlation between virus shedding a week or more before delivery and virus shedding at term, limits the efficacy of this approach. The management of the mother and infant in this situation is discussed in Chapter 163 and elsewhere (Oxman et al., 1983; Nahmias et al., 1983). Infants exposed to HSV during delivery should probably be given large doses of immune serum globulin, preferably from a lot with a high titer of antibody to HSV-2. Although there is no evidence that passively administered antibody is protective, infants with high titers of transplacentally acquired antibody to HSV-2 have a more favorable outcome than infants with low antibody titers (Yeager et al., 1980). The topical application of idoxuridine or adenine arabinoside drops to the eyes, which are sometimes the portal of entry of virus, should also be considered. These recommendations are based upon limited epidemiologic data, and their efficacy is unproven.

Herpes simplex meningitis is generally a benign and self-limited infection. There is no known specific prophylaxis, except the avoidance of genital HSV infection, with which it is often associated.

References

Abramson, J. S., Roach, E. S., and Levy, H. B.: Postinfectious encephalopathy after treatment of herpes simplex encephalitis with acyclovir. Pediatr Infect Dis 3:146, 1984.

Adair, C. V., Gauld, R. L., and Smadel, J. E.: Aseptic meningitis, a disease of diverse etiology: Clinical and etiology studies on 854 cases. Ann Intern Med 29:675, 1953.

Armstrong, C.: Herpes simplex virus recovered from the spinal fluid of a suspected case of lymphocytic choriomeningitis. Public Health Rep 58:16, 1943.

Atia, W. A., Ratnatunga, C. S., Greenfield, C., and Dawson, S.: Aseptic meningitis and herpes simplex proctitis. Br J Vener Dis 58:52, 1982.

Black, F. L.: Infectious diseases in primitive societies. Science 187:515, 1975.

Boston Interhospital Virus Study Group and the NIAID Sponsored Cooperative Antiviral Clinical Study. Failure of high dose 5-iodo-2′-deoxyuridine (IDU) in the therapy of herpes simplex virus encephalitis: Evidence of unacceptable toxicity. N Engl J Med 292:599, 1975.

Cabrera, C. V., Wohlenberg, C., Openshaw, H., Rey-Mendez, M., Puga, A., and Notkins, A. L.: Herpes simplex virus DNA sequences in the CNS of latently infected mice. Nature 288:288, 1980.

Cho, C. T., and Feng, K. K.: Sensitivity of the virus isolation and immunofluorescent staining methods in diagnosis of infections with herpes simplex virus. J Infect Dis 138:536, 1978.

Cibis, G. W., Flynn, J. T., and Davis, E. B.: Herpes simplex retinitis. Arch Ophthalmol 96:299, 1978.

Craig, C. P., and Nahmias, A. J.: Different patterns of neurologic involvement with herpes simplex virus types 1 and 2: Isolation of herpes simplex virus type 2 from the buffy coat of two adults with meningitis. J Infect Dis 127:365, 1973.

Davis, J. M., Davis, K. R., Kleinman, G. M., Kirchner, H. W., and Taveras, J. M.: Computed tomography of herpes simplex encephalitis with clinicopathological correlation. Radiology 129:409, 1978.

Davis, L. E., and Johnson, R. T.: An explanation for the localization of herpes simplex encephalitis: Ann Neurol 5:2, 1979.

Davis, L. E. and McLaren, L. C.: Relapsing herpes simplex encephalitis following antiviral therapy. Ann Neurol 13:192, 1983.

Dayan, A. D., Gooddy, W., Harrison, M. J. G., and Rudge, P.: Brain stem encephalitis caused by *Herpesvirus hominis*. Br Med J 4:405, 1972.

Dix, R. D., Baringer, J. R., Panitch, H. S., Rosenberg, S. H., Hagedorn, J., and Whaley, J.: Recurrent herpes simplex encephalitis: Recovery of virus after Ara-A treatment. Ann Neurol 13:196, 1983.

Drachman, D. A., and Adams, R. D.: Herpes simplex and acute inclusion-body encephalitis. Arch Neurol 7:61, 1962.

Enzmann, D. R., Ranson, B., Norman, D., and Talberth, E.: Computed tomography of herpes simplex encephalitis. Radiology 129:419, 1978.

Esiri, M. M.: Herpes simplex encephalitis. An immunohistological study of the distribution viral antigen within the brain. J Neurol Sci 54:209, 1982.

Flewett, T. H.: The rapid diagnosis of herpes encephalitis. Postgrad Med J 49:398, 1973.

Fraser, N. W., Lawrence, W. C., Wroblewski, Z., Gilden, D. H., and

Koprowski, E.: Herpes simplex type 1 DNA in human brain tissue. Proc Natl Acad Sci U.S.A. 78:6461, 1981.

Hammer, S. M., Buchman, T. G., D'Angelo, L. J., Karchmer, A. W., Roizman, B., Hirsch, M. S.: Temporal cluster of herpes simplex encephalitis: investigation by restriction endonuclease cleavage of viral DNA. J Infect Dis 141:436, 1980.

Harford, C. G., Wellinghoff, W., and Weinstein, R. A.: Isolation of herpes simplex virus from the cerebrospinal fluid in viral meningitis. Neurol 25:198, 1975.

Haymaker, W., Smith, M. G., van Bogaert, L., and de Chenar, C.: Pathology of viral disease in man characterized by nuclear inclusions, with emphasis on herpes simplex and subacute inclusion encephalitis. In Fields, W. S., and Blattner, R. J. (eds.): Viral Encephalitis. Springfield, Charles C Thomas, p. 95, 1958.

Hevron, J. E., Jr.: Herpes simplex virus type 2 meningitis. Obstet Gynecol 49:622, 1977.

Hirsch, M. S., and Schooley, R. T.: Treatment of herpesvirus infections. New Engl J Med 390:963 and 309:1034, 1983.

Hunt, B. P. and Comer, E. O'B.: Herpetic meningo-encephalitis accompanying cutaneous herpes simplex. Am J Med 19:814, 1955.

Illis, L. S., and Gostling, J. V. T.: Herpes Simplex Encephalitis. Scientechnica Ltd., Bristol, 1972.

Illis, L. S., and Taylor, F. M.: The electroencephalogram in herpes-simplex encephalitis. Lancet 1:718, 1972.

Johnson, B. L., and Wisotzkey, H. M.: Neuroretinitis associated with herpes simplex encephalitis in an adult. Am J. Ophthalmol 83:481, 1977.

Johnson, K. P., Rosenthal, M. S., and Lerner, D. I.: Herpes simplex encephalitis. The course in five virologically proven cases. Arch Neurol 27:103, 1972.

Johnson, R. T., and Mims, C. A.: Pathogenesis of viral infections of the nervous system. N Engl J Med 278:23, 84, 1968.

Johnson, R. T., Olson, L. C., and Buescher, E. L.: Herpes simplex virus infections of the nervous system. Problems in laboratory diagnosis. Arch Neurol 18:260, 1968.

Juel-Jensen, B. E., and MacCallum, F. O.: Herpes Simplex, Varicella and Zoster, Clinical Manifestations and Treatment. Philadelphia, J. B. Lippincott Co., 1972.

Klastersky, J., Cappel, R., Snoeck, J. M., Flament, J., and Thiry, L.: Ascending myelitis in association with herpes-simplex virus. N Engl J Med 287:182, 1972.

Koehler, K. and Guth, W.: The mimicking of mania in "benign" herpes simplex encephalitis. Biol Psychiarty 14:405, 1979.

Koenig, H., Rabinowitz, S. G., Day, E., and Miller, V.: Post-infectious encephalomyelitis after successful treatment of herpes simplex encephalitis with adenine arabinoside. N Engl J Med 300:1089, 1979.

Koskiniemi, M. L., Vaheri, A., Valtonen, S., Haltia, M., Kaste, M., Manninen, V., Salonen, E. M., Icen, A., Cantell, K. and Study Group. Trial with human leucocyte interferon and vidarabine in herpes simplex virus encephalitis: Diagnostic and therapeutic problems. Acta Med Scan (Suppl) 668:150, 1982.

Landry, M. L., Berkovits, N., Summers, W. P., Booss, J., Hsiung, G. D., and Summers, W. C.: Herpes simplex encephalitis: Analysis of a cluster of cases by restriction endonuclease mapping of virus isolates. Neurology 33:831, 1983.

Leider, W., Magoffin, R. L., Lennette, E. H., and Leonards, L. N. R.: Herpes-simplex-virus encephalitis. Its possible association with reactivated latent infection. N Engl J Med 273:341, 1965.

Levine, D. P., Lauter, C. B., and Lerner, M.: Simultaneous serum and CSF antibodies in herpes simplex virus encephalitis. J Am Med Assn 240:356, 1978.

Linnemann, C. C., Jr., First, M. R., Alvira, M. M., Alexander, J. W., and Schiff, G. M.: Herpesvirus hominis type 2 meningoencephalitis following renal transplantation. Am J Med 61:703, 1976.

MacCallum, F. O., Chinn, I. J., and Gostling, J. V. T.: Antibodies to herpes-simplex virus in the cerebrospinal fluid of patients with herpetic encephalitis. J Med Microbiol 7:325, 1974.

Manz, H. J., Phillips, T. M., and McCullough, D. C.: Herpes simplex type 2 encephalitis concurrent with known cerebral metastases. Acta Neuropathol (Berl.) 47:237, 1979.

Meyer, H. M., Jr., Johnson, R. T., Crawford, I. P., Dascomb, H. E., and Rogers, N. G.: Central nervous system syndromes of "viral" etiology: a study of 713 cases. Am J Med 29:334, 1960.

Miller, J. D., and Ross, C. A. C.: Encephalitis, a four year survey. Lancet 1:1121, 1968.

Miller, J. K., Hesser, F., and Tompkins, V. N.: Herpes simplex encephalitis, a report of 20 cases. Ann Int Med 64:92, 1966.

Minckler, D. L., McLean, E. B., Shaw, C. M., and Hendrickson, A.: Herpesvirus hominis encephalitis and retinitis. Arch Ophthalmol 94:89, 1976.

Morawetz, R. B., Whitley, R. J., and Murphy, D. M.: Experience with brain biopsy for suspected herpes encephalitis: A review of forty consecutive cases. Neurosurgery 12:654, 1983.

Morrison, R. E., Shatsky, S. A., Holmes, G. E., Top, F. H., and Martins, A. N.: Herpes simplex virus type 1 from a patient with radiculoneuropathy. JAMA 241:393, 1979.

Nahmias, A. J. and Josey, W. E.: Herpes simplex viruses 1 and 2 in *Viral Infections of Humans: Epidemiology and Control* 2nd Ed. (ed. Evans, A. S.) Plenum Publishing Corp, New York, 1982, pp. 351–372.

Nahmias, A. J., Whitley, R. J., Visintine, A. N., Takei, Y., Alford, C. A., Jr., and the Collaborative Antiviral Study Group. Herpes simplex virus encephalitis: Laboratory evaluations and their diagnostic significance. J Infect Dis 145:829, 1982.

Nahmias, A. J., Keyserling, H. L., and Kerrick, G. M.: Herpes simplex in *Infectious Diseases of the Fetus and Newborn Infant* (eds. Remington, J. S. and Klein, J. O.) W. B. Saunders, Philadelphia, 1983, pp. 636–678.

Ojeda, V. J.: Fatal herpes simplex encephalitis with demonstration of virus in the olfactory pathway. Pathology 12:429, 1980.

Olson, L. C., Buescher, E. L., Artenstein, M. S., and Parkman, P. D.: Herpes virus infections of the human central nervous system. N Engl J Med 277:1271, 1967.

Oommen, K. J., Johnson, P. C., and Ray, C. G.: Herpes simplex type 2 virus encephalitis presenting as psychosis. Am J Med 73:445, 1982.

Oxbury, J. M., and MacCallum, F. O.: Herpes simplex virus encephalitis: clinical features and residual damage. Postgrad Med J 49:387, 1973.

Oxman, M. N., Richman, D. D., and Spector, S. A.: Management at delivery of mother and infant when herpes simplex, varicella-zoster, hepatitis or tuberculosis have occurred during pregnancy. *In* Current Topics in Infectious Diseases. Vol. IV (Eds. Remington, J. S., and Swartz, M. N.). New York, McGraw-Hill, 1983, 224–280.

Pazin, G. J., Armstrong, J. A., Tai Lam, M., Tarr, G. C., Jannetta, P. J., and Ho, M.: Prevention of reactivated herpes simplex infection by human leukocyte interferon after operation on the trigeminal root. N Engl J Med 301:225, 1979.

Price, R., Chernik, N. L., Horta-Barbosa, L., and Posner, J. B.: Herpes simplex encephalitis in an anergic patient. Am J Med 54:222, 1973.

Rappel, M., Dubois-Dalcq, M., Sprecher, S., Thiry, L., Lowenthal, A., Pelc, S., and Thys, J. P.: Diagnosis and treatment of herpes encephalitis, a multidisciplinary approach. J Neurol Sci 12:443, 1971.

Ravaut, P., and Darré, M.: Les réactions nerveuses au cors de herpes génitaux. Ann Dermatol Syphiligr (Paris) 5:481, 1904.

Rawls, W. E., Dyck, P. J., Klass, D. W., Greer, H. D., and Hermann, E. C., Jr.: Encephalitis associated with herpes simplex virus. Ann. Intern Med 64:104, 1966.

Rhodes, R. H., Novak, R., Beattie, J. F., West, H. M., and Whetsell, W. O., Jr.: Immunoperoxidase demonstration of herpes simplex virus type 1 in the brain of a psychotic patient without history of encephalitis. Clin Neuropathol 3:59, 1984.

Rock, D. L. and Fraser, N. W.: Detection of HSV-1 genome in central nervous system of latently infected mice. Nature 302:523, 1983.

Sawanobori, S., Onishi, S., Matsuyama, S., and Irie, H.: HSV-1 and acute aseptic meningitis. Lancet 1:756, 1974.

Sequiera, L. W., Carrasco, L. H., Curry, A., Jennings, L. C., Lord, M. A., and Sutton, R. N. P.: Detection of herpes-simplex viral genome in brain tissue. Lancet 2:609, 1979.

Shearer, M. L., and Finch, S. M.: Periodic organic psychosis associated with recurrent herpes simplex. N Engl J Med 271:494, 1964.

Skoldenberg, B., Alestig, K., Burman, L., Forkman, A., Lovgren, K., Norrby, R., Stiernstedt, G., Forsgren, M., Bergstrom, T., Dahlqvist, E., Fryden, A., Norlin, K., Olding-Stenkvist, E., Uhnoo, I., and De Vahl, K.: Acyclovir versus vidarabine in herpes simplex encephalitis. Randomised multicentre study in consecutive Swedish patients. Lancet 2:707, 1984.

Skoldenberg, B., Jeansson, S., and Wolontis, S.: Herpes simplex virus type 2 and acute aseptic meningitis. Clinical features of cases with isolation of herpes simplex virus from cerebrospinal fluids. Scand J Infect Dis 7:227, 1975.

Skoldenberg, B., Kalimo, K., Carlstrom, A., Forsgren, M., and Halonen, P.: Herpes simplex encephalitis: A serological follow-up study. Synthesis of herpes simplex virus immunoglobulin M, A, and G antibodies and development of oligoclonal immunoglobulin G in the central nervous systems. Acta Neurol Scan 63:273, 1981.

Smith, M. G., Lennette, E. H., and Reames, H. R.: Isolation of the virus of herpes simplex and the demonstration of intranuclear inclusions in a case of acute encephalitis. Am J Pathol 17:55, 1941.

Stalder, H., Oxman, M. N., Dawson, D. M., and Levin, M. J.: Herpes simplex meningitis: isolation of herpes simplex virus type 2 from cerebrospinal fluid. N Engl J Med 289:1296, 1973.

Stevens, J. G.: Latent herpes simplex virus and the nervous system. Curr Top Microbiol Immunol 70:31, 1975.

Terni, M., Caccialanza, P., Cassai, E., and Kieff, E.: Aseptic meningitis in association with herpes progenitalis. N Engl J Med 285:503, 1971.

Tucker, B. A., Doekel, R. C., Jr., Whitley, R. J., and Dismukes, W. E.: Herpes simplex virus encephalitis: an atypical presentation. South Med J 71:1431, 1978.

Warren, K. G., Brown, S. M., Wroblewska, Z., Gilden, D., Koprowski, H., and Subak-Sharpe, J.: Isolation of latent herpes simplex virus from

the superior cervical and vagus ganglions of human beings. N Engl J Med 298:1068, 1978.
Whitley, R. J., Soong, S-J., Dolin, R., Galasso, G. J., Ch'ien, L. I., Alford, C. A., and the Collaborative Study Group. Adenine arabinoside therapy of biopsy-proved herpes simplex encephalitis. N Engl J Med 297:289, 1977.
Whitley, R. J., Nahmias, A. J., Soong, S-J., Galasso, G. J., Fleming, C. L., and Alford, C. A.: Vidarabine therapy of neonatal herpes simplex virus infection. Pediatr 66:495, 1980a.
Whitley, R. J., Nahmias, A. J., Visintine, A. M., Fleming, C. L., and Alford, C. A.: The natural history of herpes simplex virus infection of mother and newborn. Pediatr 66:489, 1980b.
Whitley, R. J., Soong, S-J., Hirsch, M. S., Karchmer, A. W., Dolin, R., Galasso, G. J., Dunnick, J. K., Alford, C. A., and the NIAID Collaborative Antiviral Study Group. Herpes simplex encephalitis: Vidarabine therapy and diagnostic problems. N Engl J Med 304:313, 1981.
Whitley, R. J., Lakeman, A. D., Nahmias, A. J., and Roizman, B.: DNA restriction-enzyme analysis of herpes simplex virus isolates obtained from patients with encephalitis. N Engl J Med 307:1060, 1982a.
Whitley, R. J., Soong, S-J., Linneman, C., Liu, C., Pazin, G., Alford, C. A., and the NIAID Collaborative Antiviral Study Group. Herpes simplex encephalitis: Clinical assessment. JAMA 247:317, 1982b.
Whitley, R. J. and the NIAID Collaborative Antiviral Study Group.: Interim summary of mortality in herpes simplex encephalitis and neonatal herpes simplex virus infections: vidarabine versus acyclovir. J Antimicrob Chem 12 (Suppl B):105, 1983a.
Whitley, R. J., Yeager, A., Kartus, P., Bryson, Y., Connor, J. D., Alford, C. A., Nahmias, A. J., and Soong, S-J.: Neonatal herpes simplex virus infection: Follow-up evaluation of vidarabine therapy. Pediatr 72:778, 1983b.
Wildy, P., Field, H. J., and Nash, A. A.: Classical herpes latency revisited. in *Virus Persistence Symposium 33.* (eds, Mahy, B. W. J., Minson, A. C. and Darby G. K.), Society for General Microbiology Ltd Cambridge University Press, 1982, pp. 133–167.
Wilson, L. G.: Viral encephalopathy mimicking functional psychosis. Am J Psychiatry 133:165, 1976.
Wolontis, S., and Jeansson, S.: Correlation of herpes simplex virus types 1 and 2 with clinical features of infection. J Infect Dis 135:28, 1977.
Yeager, A. S., Arvin, A. M., Urbani, L. J., and Kemp, III, J. A.: Relationship of antibody to outcome in neonatal herpes simplex infections. Infect Immun 29:532, 1980.
Zimmerman, R. D., Russell, E. J., Leeds, N. E., and Kaufman, D.: CT in the early diagnosis of herpes simplex encephalitis. Am J Radiol 134:61, 1980.

181

HERPESVIRUS SIMIAE (B VIRUS) ENCEPHALITIS

JOSHUA FIERER, M.D.

Herpesvirus simiae (B virus) encephalitis is a rare disease characterized by diffuse inflammation of the central nervous system consequent to infection with *H. simiae.*

ETIOLOGY. This sporadic infection occurs in people who have had occupational exposure to monkeys or their tissues. B virus infection occurs naturally in Old World monkeys, principally *Macaca mulatta.* In the primate, *H. simiae* causes a benign, self-limited, superficial infection of the oral mucosa similar to *Herpesvirus hominis* infections in humans (Keeble et al., 1958). Apparently healthy monkeys may have latent infections and their saliva may contain virus. Although B virus is genetically distinct from human herpesviruses, it shares at least one common antigen (Norrild et al., 1978) and there is cross neutralization of *H. simplex* by antiserum raised to *H. simiae* (Plummer, 1964).

PATHOGENESIS AND PATHOLOGY. Infection is acquired from infected monkeys or their tissues. Many cases, but not all, are initiated by a monkey bite, by minor trauma inflicted by a monkey, or by puncture wounds with objects that were contaminated with monkey tissue. Since an aerosol of the virus can infect experimental animals, it is possible that those patients without a history of direct trauma were infected by airborne virus (Benda and Cerva, 1969). The virus is quite neurotropic in humans. It presumably spreads along neural routes from the point of inoculation to the spinal cord and then cephalad within the central nervous system. There may also be hematogenous spread to the brain. In one patient there was circumstantial evidence that encephalitis followed reactivation of a latent infection of the trigeminal nerve (Fierer et al., 1973).

The specific pathologic changes produced by B virus are limited to regional lymph nodes and the central nervous system. Lymph nodes draining a site of inoculation may be hemorrhagic and show focal necrosis. Within the central nervous system, the pons and medulla are always involved with a lymphocytic infiltrate, glial proliferation, and edema. In some cases there is necrosis and death of neurons. Giant cells are not seen, and the microscopic appearance of the brain is not specific for B virus infection. In some patients there is a prominent myelitis of the cervical and thoracic cord that is not limited to specific tracts. Diffuse cortical encephalitis is a feature of some cases. Virus has been isolated from all affected areas of the central nervous system and from lymph nodes distal to the site of inoculation but never from blood, cerebrospinal fluid, or other organs (Davidson and Hummeler, 1960).

CLINICAL MANIFESTATIONS. A vesicular rash may develop at the site of inoculation within two or three days of the inciting injury. This is followed by lymphangitis and regional lymphadenopathy. Within three days to five weeks fever and symptoms of central nervous system infection develop. The disease may present either as ascending myelitis with flaccid motor paralysis and bladder paresis or as a diffuse encephalitis without localizing signs. Brain stem dysfunction is often prominent, with diplopia, dysphagia, and respiratory paralysis in most patients (Davidson and Hummeler, 1960). Hemorrhagic chorioretinitis has been reported in one case and one patient had a corneal ulcer associated with a zosteriform rash in the distribution of the ophthalmic branch of the V nerve (Fierer et al., 1973; Roth and Purcell, 1977).

COMPLICATIONS AND SEQUELAE. In clinically apparent infections, death results in most cases. The few people who survive are left with residual neurologic damage of varying severity.

GEOGRAPHIC VARIATIONS. About half the reported cases were from the United States. The rest occurred in Canada and Great Britain. This distribution probably reflects the number of individuals with occupational exposure to monkeys and their tissues.

DIAGNOSIS. The diagnosis should be suspected in any patient who develops encephalitis or encephalomyelitis and who has had direct contact with monkeys or with monkey tissue. A definite premortem diagnosis can only be established by isolating the virus but this is rarely done because the virus cannot be recovered from secretions, CSF, or the blood, although it has been recovered from vesicular skin lesions. Premortem diagnosis usually depends on demonstrating a rise in antibody during the course of the disease. Infection with *H. simiae* stimulates neutralizing antibody for both *H. simplex* and *H. simiae* but *H. simplex* infections in humans do not stimulate neutralizing antibody to *H. simiae*. Viral neutralizing assays should be done only in research laboratories that have facilities to protect laboratory workers from B virus infection.

TREATMENT. There is no proven specific treatment. Corticosteroids and cytosine arabinoside have been used, but there is no evidence that they were beneficial. Acyclovir is the most effective anti-*H. simiae* drug in vitro and has been used successfully to treat experimental infections in rabbits (Boulter et al., 1980). However, treatment had to be continued for 14 days. A dose of 10 mg/kg three times/day is recommended with attention to maintaining hydration.

PROPHYLAXIS. Everyone who works with monkeys and their tissues should be aware of the potential danger of the infection and use protective clothing. Monkeys with active infections should be placed in quarantine (Perkins and Hartley, 1966). A killed virus vaccine has been developed but is not produced commercially (Hull et al., 1962). Antibody to *H. hominis* is not protective and antibody to *H. simiae* is not effective if raised in a heterologous species. It is suggested that a person who is injured by a monkey with active stomatitis should receive a therapeutic course of acyclovir.

References

Benda, R., and Cerva, L.: Course of air-borne infection caused by B virus *(Herpesvirus simiae)*. J Hyg Epidemiol Microbiol Immunol 13:307, 1969.

Boulter, E. A., Thornton, B., Bauer, D. J., and Bye, A.: Successful treatment of experimental B virus *(Herpesvirus simiae)* infection with acyclovir. Br Med J 280:681, 1980.

Davidson, W. L., and Hummeler, K.: B virus infection in man. NY Acad Sci Ann 85:970, 1960.

Fierer, J., Bazeley, P., and Braude, A. I.: Herpes B virus encephalomyelitis presenting as ophthalmic zoster. Ann Intern Med 79:225, 1973.

Hull, R. M., Peck, F. B., Jr., Ward, T. G., and Nash, J. C.: Immunization against B virus infection. II. Further laboratory and clinical studies with an experimental vaccine. Am J Hyg 76:239, 1962.

Keeble, S. A., Christofinis, G. J., and Wood, W.: Natural virus-B infection in rhesus monkeys. J Pathol Bacteriol 76:189, 1958.

Norrild, B., Ludwig, H., and Rott, R.: Identification of a common antigen of Herpes simplex virus, Bovine herpes mammillitis virus, and B virus. J Virol 25:712, 1978.

Perkins, F. T., and Hartley, E. G.: Precautions against B virus infections. Br Med J 1:899, 1966.

Plummer, G.: Serological comparison of the herpes viruses. Br J Exp Pathol 45:135, 1964.

Roth, A. M., and Purcell, T. W.: Ocular findings associated with encephalomyelitis caused by *Herpesvirus simiae*. Am J Ophthalmol 84:345, 1977.

182

CENTRAL NERVOUS SYSTEM INFECTIONS CAUSED BY TOGAVIRIDAE AND RELATED AGENTS

MONTO HO, M.D.

GENERAL ASPECTS OF TOGAVIRIDAE

Viral encephalitis and meningoencephalitis may be either *epidemic* (and endemic) or *sporadic* (Dickerson et al., 1952). Sporadic cases occur irrespective of time, season, and place. One example is herpes simplex encephalitis (Chapter 180), which occurs in any population at any time and place. Epidemic encephalitis occurs at particular times of the year and in particular places. The reason is that the implicated viruses are maintained in well-defined biologic reservoirs and are transmitted to man by specific biologic vectors.

Togaviridae and related agents are the most important causes of epidemic encephalitis. Almost every large geographic region in the world has its own particular agent of this type. Every physician should be familiar with the arthropod-borne encephalitides peculiar to his own region.

General comments about the epidemiologic and clinical aspects of this group of viruses will be given here and will not be repeated for each agent and disease. More basic virologic material is covered in Chapter 66. There are over 350 viruses that are transmitted by arthropods or cause febrile illnesses in man and animals. In man, these range from inapparent infection to febrile diseases with or without rashes, hemorrhagic shock syndromes, and infections of the central nervous system (Theiler and Downs, 1973). The important agents causing encephalitis and infection of the central nervous system are listed in Table 1 and will be discussed here. There are subgroups of Togaviridae as well as additional virus groups such as Arenaviridae (South American hemorrhagic fevers, Lassa fever, Rift Valley fever) and Orbiviridae (Colorado tick fever), which cause infections not usually involving the central nervous system. These are discussed elsewhere.

One important newly discovered agent of hemorrhagic fever is the cause of epidemic (Korean) hemorrhagic fever (Lee et al., 1978). It belongs to the Bunyamwera group, which includes the California encephalitis virus, and it is also arthropod-borne. It causes a series of illnesses ranging from hemorrhagic fever in China, Korea, and northern Eurasia to nephropathia epidemica in Finland. Encephalitis may be a part of the picture, but tubular nephropathy is a common denominator. West Nile fever (flavivirus) and the *Phlebotomus* fever group also cause febrile syndromes and also only occasionally they involve the central nervous system. These agents are included in Table 1 but are not separately discussed in the text.

Table 1. TOGAVIRUSES AND RELATED AGENTS CAUSING ENCEPHALITIS

Virus Family	Genus	Representative Species Infecting Man	Vector	Disease	Geographic Distribution
Togaviridae	Alphavirus	Eastern equine encephalitis (EEE) virus	Mosquito	Encephalitis	Eastern U.S., Canada, Brazil
		Western equine encephalitis (WEE) virus	Mosquito	Encephalitis	Western U.S.
		Venezuelan equine encephalitis (VEE) virus	Mosquito	Encephalitis	Northern Latin America, Southern U.S.
Togaviridae	Flavivirus	St. Louis encephalitis virus	Mosquito	Encephalitis	United States
		Japanese encephalitis virus	Mosquito	Encephalitis	Japan, China, Korea, Southeast Asia
		Tick-borne virus group (Russian spring-summer encephalitis, Powassan encephalitis, Louping ill). Nine viruses	Tick	Encephalitis, meningoencephalitis, hemorrhagic fever	European Russia, Siberia, Central Europe; Canada, U.S. (Powassan); United Kingdom (Louping ill)
		Murray Valley encephalitis virus	Mosquito	Encephalitis	Australia, New Guinea
		West Nile virus	Mosquito	Usually a febrile rash disease, occasionally meningoencephalitis	Israel, Egypt
Bunyaviridae	Bunyamwera	Bunyamwera and 13 other viruses	Mosquito	Fever, headache	Africa, India, South America
		California group	Mosquito	Meningitis, encephalitis	United States
		Epidemic (Korean) hemorrhagic fever	? Flea	Hemorrhagic fever, renal failure, encephalopathy	Far East, Northern Eurasia
Phlebotomus fever group (ungrouped)		Three species	Phlebotomus (sandfly)	Usually a three-day febrile illness; may be associated with aseptic meningitis	Italy, Egypt

Many, but not all, of these agents are transmitted by arthropods, and the term arbovirus is no longer de rigueur. Nevertheless, almost all the viruses in the group that causes encephalitis and meningoencephalitis are arthropod borne. According to the new terminology, which is based on the physicochemical rather than the epidemiologic properties of these agents, most of them belong to the Togaviridae (Table 1). Some important exceptions, such as California viruses, belong to the Bunyaviridae. They are distinct from the Togaviridae because their proteins are arranged in helical symmetry. Unlike the Togaviridae, the complement fixation test is more specific for these viruses than the hemagglutination inhibition test.

EPIDEMIOLOGY. The fact that the most important epidemic encephalitides and meningoencephalitides are transmitted by arthropods (usually mosquitoes or ticks) has profound clinical as well as public health implications. Concepts of diagnosis and prevention of these infections are largely based on the peculiar epidemiology of these viruses. For example, if a suspected case occurs during a season or in a climate or region that cannot support the presence of responsible vectors, one can safely exclude the diagnosis of this type of encephalitis. There are several basic patterns of transmission of these agents. In the most important pattern, the vector transmits the infection from the animal reservoir to man but not from man to man. The reservoirs for the viruses are usually lower vertebrates such as fowl, rodents, and pigs. Hence, these encephalitides are "zoonoses," and man is an accidental host who does not serve as a source of infection. All the major arthropod-borne encephalitides, such as eastern equine encephalomyelitis (EEE), western equine encephalomyelitis (WEE), St. Louis, Venezuelan, Japanese, California, and the tick-borne encephalitides belong to this pattern. The isolation of the patient is usually unnecessary in these diseases with the exception of Venezuelan encephalitis and Russian spring-summer encephalitis. In another pattern of transmission, the mosquito transmits the infection from man to man. This is the pattern of yellow fever and dengue, which are discussed elsewhere. Finally, some of these related viruses are transmitted directly from man to man without a vector and cause certain exotic hemorrhagic fevers such as Lassa fever and Marburg disease, but no important virus causing epidemic encephalitis is transmitted in this pattern.

CLINICAL MANIFESTATIONS. The patient with arthropod-borne encephalitis usually presents with signs of infection and inflammation of the central nervous system. There is fever, headache, and disturbed consciousness, ranging from lethargy to stupor and coma. Convulsions, paralysis, involuntary movements, and other localizing signs may be present. There may also be signs of meningitis.

The onset and progression of each disease varies considerably with each virus, and even with particular localities and epidemics. In general, however, the infection is of sudden onset, runs an acute or subacute course, and is strikingly different from slow infections of the central nervous system (see Chapter 183). No chronic infection from arthropod-borne encephalitic viruses has been described in man.

DIAGNOSIS. Diagnosis of arthropod-borne encephalitides is not difficult during an epidemic. In isolated cases, clinical acumen and epidemiologic awareness is required. Every physician should know what is "going around." This requires communication with the local health authorities and subscription to their bulletins. In the United States, all physicians dealing with communicable diseases should subscribe to the Morbidity and Mortality Weekly Reports, available from the Centers for Disease Control (CDC), Atlanta, Georgia. The precise diagnosis of these infections requires laboratory proof.

DIFFERENTIAL DIAGNOSIS. Arthropod-borne encephalitides usually have a more acute onset than herpes encephalitis. They also appear more suddenly and have a shorter duration than encephalitides associated with tuberculosis, cryptococcosis, other fungal infections, or brain abscess. Fever is a dependable sign, and its absence is rare in arthropod-borne encephalitides. In contrast, fever may be absent in cryptococcosis, brain abscess, para- and postinfectious encephalitis, and encephalopathy due to connective tissue diseases such as disseminated lupus erythematosus or cancer.

It may not be possible to distinguish clinically between arthropod-borne encephalitis and meningoencephalitis and encephalitis due to mumps and enteroviruses. Para- and postinfectious meningoencephalitis may also be difficult to rule out. Epidemiologic and laboratory aid is essential.

In viral meningoencephalitides, the cerebrospinal fluid is usually clear and colorless. There is a moderate number of cells, usually less than 1000, over 70 per cent of which are lymphocytes. In early taps there may be a predominantly neutrophilic response. The protein concentration is only moderately elevated (<100 mg/dl) and the glucose level not at all.

LABORATORY DIAGNOSIS. Laboratory diagnosis of diseases caused by Togaviridae and related agents is based on a serologic rise of specific antibody titer or isolation of the causative agent from the patient. The main source of viral isolation is blood. Since viremia in man lasts only a short time, the virus is frequently not isolated from the blood. But when it is, a specific diagnosis may be made. The virus is even more rarely isolated from the cerebrospinal fluid. By and large, the suckling mouse is more satisfactory and more sensitive than cell cultures for isolation of these viruses. The number of viruses involved is so large that not even well-equipped laboratories or specialized centers have the reagents and sera necessary to identify all of them. Unknown isolates should be sent to the CDC in the United States or to national public health authorities in other countries for identification or confirmation. Through these agencies, the specimen may be referred to a regional laboratory for arboviruses or to an international reference center for arboviruses designated by the World Health Organization.

The most important laboratory method in diagnosis is serologic examination. Occasionally a diagnosis is made by the height of the antibody titer, but usually it is better to demonstrate a rise of titers in paired sera because almost all togaviruses can produce infection without disease, and a large segment of the population in an endemic area may already have antibodies to a particular virus without having had disease from it. The time to collect the first serum specimen is when the diagnosis is suspected. The titer in an acute phase blood specimen is then compared with the titer of a "convalescent" specimen obtained weeks after the first one.

The main serologic tests are the complement fixation, hemagglutination inhibition, and neutralization tests. The complement fixation test is the most widely used. Antibodies that fix complement are frequently of brief duration and hence are particularly significant when they are found in acute infections. Occasionally they appear too late to be useful. The hemagglutination inhibition test in togavirology is more group-specific and less type-specific, which is the reverse of the situation in the Bunyamwera group (California viruses), influenza, and other myxoviruses. Hemagglutination-inhibiting antibodies usually appear earlier than complement-fixing and neutralizing antibodies and disappear more rapidly than neutralizing antibodies.

TREATMENT AND CONTROL. There is no specific treatment for togavirus infections. Interferon and ribavirin are under consideration. Supportive care, however, is essential, since even patients with serious encephalitis recover. Rehabilitative care is essential for patients with residual neurologic defects.

The only widely used and well-proven human vaccine in the togavirus field is the live attenuated yellow fever vaccine, the Theiler 17-D chick embryo tissue culture strain. Formalin-inactivated mouse brain vaccine against Japanese encephalitis has been used extensively in Japan and to a lesser extent by the American armed forces. Several attenuated live vaccines are undergoing study in Japan.

There are no accepted human vaccines against the arthropod-borne encephalitides in the United States. The amount of infection and morbidity is insufficient for widespread immunization programs. Vector and reservoir control is more important, although it is by no means simply achieved.

EASTERN EQUINE ENCEPHALOMYELITIS (EEE)

EEE is caused by an alphavirus. This frequently fatal encephalitis of children and the elderly was first described on the eastern seaboard of the United States in 1938.

EPIDEMIOLOGY. In endemic areas more than 50 per cent of birds tested may have antibodies. This suggests a natural cycle in which birds and mosquitoes are essential links. Horses and humans are probably dead ends in the infection cycle. In most epidemics, epizootics among horses and occasionally pheasants precede human illness. Inapparent infection in man is less common in this disease than in other togavirus infections.

PATHOLOGY. Extensive necrosis may involve large areas of the midbrain. Neuronal damage and neuronophagia occur, with a predominance of neutrophils in infiltrates as an outstanding feature.

CLINICAL MANIFESTATIONS. The severity of EEE encephalitis is notable in almost all epidemics. Cases are concentrated in the 0 to 14 and over 55 age groups.

The onset of encephalitis is abrupt in young children. In older patients there may be a longer prodromal period of malaise, headache, and nausea before drowsiness, confusion, stiff neck, or convulsions supervene. The temperature rises sharply. Nonpitting edema of the face and distal parts of the limb has frequently been described in infants during the second and third days of illness. Leukocytosis is common. CSF is under increased pressure, with 200 to 2000 cells/mm^3. Neutrophils may comprise over 50 per cent of the cells and may persist to the second week of illness before mononuclear cells predominate. Infants who survive the acute illness almost always have neurologic sequelae.

WESTERN EQUINE ENCEPHALOMYELITIS (WEE)

WEE is caused by an alphavirus endemic in wildlife and in horses. Human disease was first described in 1938. It is generally less severe than EEE.

EPIDEMIOLOGY. The WEE virus is found in wildlife in the United States, Canada, Brazil, British Guiana, and Argentina. Human disease caused by this virus has been described only in the United States, Canada, and Brazil. The virus is found in practically all sections of the United States but most frequently in the western states and western Canada. An important endemic area is the Central Valley of California. The principal vector in this area is *Culex tarsalis*, which also transmits St. Louis encephalitis.

PATHOLOGY. Damage to the brain and spinal cord may be extensive in small children. In severe cases, the pathologic signs are similar to those of EEE.

CLINICAL MANIFESTATIONS. The disease is more common and more severe in children. About 20 to 30 per cent of all cases occur in infants under 1 year. Fever and drowsiness are common. Convulsions occur in 90 per cent of infected infants and in 40 per cent of children between 1 and 4 years old, but rarely in adults. In all age groups remission is sudden. Even those with convulsions or in coma may recover in five to ten days. The illness ends in less severe cases in three to five days. The overall mortality is 2 to 3 per cent.

Permanent sequelae are rare in adults but are more frequent in younger children. More than half of afflicted infants less than a month old are left with recurring convulsions or motor or behavioral disorders requiring institutionalization. Inapparent infections far outnumber clinical illness, probably in the range of 60 to 1 in young children and 1000 to 1 in adults. The spinal fluid and other laboratory findings are similar to those in St. Louis encephalitis.

VENEZUELAN EQUINE ENCEPHALOMYELITIS (VEE)

The alphavirus that causes VEE is transmitted sporadically to man, producing a mild encephalomyelitis during epizootics afflicting horses in Venezuela, Central America, and southwestern United States.

EPIDEMIOLOGY. The virus passes through a sylvan cycle of mosquitoes and wild rodents such as cotton rats. Many mammals and birds compose the reservoir for the virus and develop antibodies to it, but the important amplifying host for man is the horse. Viremia in horses persists for only a few days, but this is sufficient to infect mosquitoes that can then transmit the virus to man. Usually a large number of infected horses is necessary to reach an infective threshold for human disease.

CLINICAL MANIFESTATIONS. The disease in man is not usually fatal. Children account for about half of the cases, but any age group may be affected. Usually more males than females are attacked. Clinical diagnosis is based on seizures or any three of the following features: severe drowsiness, agitation, confusion, disorientation, hallucinations, and ataxia. There may be only a short febrile illness with sudden onset of malaise, chills, fever, nausea, vomiting, headache, muscle and bone aches, and fever lasting one to four days. Convalescence with marked asthenia may last up to three weeks.

ST. LOUIS ENCEPHALITIS (SLE)

St. Louis encephalitis is the most important epidemic encephalitis in the United States in terms of number and severity of cases. It was first recognized in 1933, when an epidemic of 1100 cases with 221 deaths occurred in the St. Louis area (Kinsella and Brown, 1934).

EPIDEMIOLOGY. St. Louis encephalitis occurs in three distinct regions in the United States, each with distinct types of mosquito vectors. The vectors explain why this disease may occur in either rural or urban areas. In the west, principally in irrigated rural and suburban areas, the vector is the same as that for WEE, i.e., *Culex tarsalis*. In the midwestern and occasionally eastern states such as the urban area of St. Louis, Kansas City, Houston, and Dallas, the vector is the *Culex pipeinsquinquefasciatus* complex. In Florida, the vector is *Culex nigripalpus*, which is a semitropical mosquito prevalent in both rural and urban areas.

CLINICAL MANIFESTATIONS. SLE shows a striking and unique increase of incidence with age. Children are spared, and the elderly are preferentially afflicted. The case-fatality ratio (deaths among cases) also increases with age, and most of the deaths occur among the elderly. The incubation period is 9 to 14 days.

The typical case starts abruptly with fever, headache, nuchal rigidity, nausea, vomiting, and usually somnolence, tremors, and difficulty in speaking. As a rule, the disease reaches its height within the first 24 to 48 hours of illness. Many patients show disorientation, inability to remember earlier events, slurred speech, lethargy, insomnia, and occasionally delirium, but rarely deep coma. In children, convulsions may occur. Objective findings of stiff neck and positive Kernig signs are common. The fever is highest in the first two or three days of infection and returns to normal after seven to ten days. Rarely, it persists up to a month or six weeks. Urinary frequency, dysuria, hyponatremia, and inappropriate secretion of antidiuretic hormone may occur. The white cell count varies between 12,000 and 20,000. The spinal fluid is clear and under moderate pressure. The average cell count is between 50 and 250 cells/mm^3, rarely rising to 500 or 1000. In the first count one-third or even one-half of the white cells may be neutrophils. Later mononuclear cells predominate.

In mild or abortive cases the chief symptoms are fever, moderate headache, and perhaps mild systemic manifestations. Occasionally there is suspicion of a rigid neck and slight tremors. Spinal fluid reveals mononuclear cells. Symptoms of clouded consciousness, apathy, and, in some cases, night-prowling and senile dementia may follow the acute disease for weeks or months. Permanent sequelae are uncommon.

PATHOLOGY. The basic lesions are perivascular round cell cuffing, hemorrhages, and neuronal damage. They predominate in the thalamus and substantia nigra. The cerbral cortex, cerebellum, and in particular the Purkinje cells may also be affected.

JAPANESE ENCEPHALITIS

Japanese encephalitis is caused by a flavivirus that produces serious epidemics that affect more people in larger areas of the world than any other togavirus. The disease was distinguished from von Economo's (A) type encephalitis in 1924.

EPIDEMIOLOGY. Like other togaviruses, Japanese encephalitis virus is maintained in extrahuman reservoirs such as wild and domestic birds that develop sustained viremia. Man is an incidental host and plays no role in its transmissions. The disease has a seasonal incidence, although in tropical regions where mosquitoes are active throughout the year, it can occur in any season. In addition to Japan, it occurs in eastern Siberia, China, Korea, Taiwan, Southeast Asia, and India. The most important vector is a rural mosquito, *Culex tritaeniorhynchus,* which prefers to bite large domestic animals but also feeds on birds and man. In Japan this virus probably overwinters in hibernating adult female mosquitoes.

CLINICAL MANIFESTATIONS. Japanese encephalitis occurs more frequently in children than in adults. There is another peak of incidence in patients over 60 years old. In general, the disease is more severe and has a longer course, slower convalescence, higher incidence of sequelae, and higher case-fatality rate than St. Louis encephalitis. Mortality, which varies greatly from epidemic to epidemic, ranges from 10 to 40 per cent.

Encephalitis usually takes two to four days before it becomes full-blown. The presenting symptoms are headache, fever, shaking chills, nuchal rigidity, vomiting, and nausea. Several distinguishing characteristics of the encephalitis may be noted (Dickerson et al., 1952). Altered sensorium is characterized by retardation or a flattened affect. There is no anxiety or apprehension. Patients may present a mask-like facies reminiscent of Parkinsonism. The speech is thick and slow, and there are frequently coarse ocular tremors. There is an unusually severe symmetrical neurogenic paresis, which is not specifically localizing and lacks sensory abnormalities. Frequently the deep tendon reflexes are increased. The patients are extremely ill. They may be bedridden for two weeks and convalesce for four weeks. There may be long-term mental and psychiatric residual effects, with intellectual impairment, confusion, psychosis, and delusions.

The CSF is uniformly abnormal and frequently may not return to normal for seven weeks. Pleocytosis may reach 1000 cells/mm^3. Blood leukocytosis is common, with a predominance of neutrophils. The erythrocyte sedimentation rate is elevated.

PATHOLOGY. There is vascular congestion in the meninges and brain, with widespread perivascular lymphocyte infiltration and cuffing. Neuronal degeneration, neuronophagia, microglial proliferation, and petechial hemorrhages are common. The cerebral cortex and frequently the thalamus and substantia nigra are particularly involved.

DIAGNOSIS. The specific complement fixation test is frequently unsatisfactory if only one specimen is obtained, because no titer rise may be obtained until more than five weeks after onset. Multiple hemagglutination inhibition and neutralization tests should be done to observe a diagnostic rise in titer.

MURRAY VALLEY ENCEPHALITIS

The responsible flavivirus is antigenically related to Japanese encephalitis virus. It is enzootic in birds and mosquitoes in northern tropical Australia and New Guinea. Infection in man occurs only in these two areas. A high proportion of human infections is inapparent with an estimated ratio of inapparent to apparent infections of between 500 to 1000:1. The highest attack rate occurs in children, in whom the case-fatality rate and the incidence of serious sequelae are both higher than in older patients. Despite high infection rates, epidemics are relatively infrequent, and the population at risk is not large.

The clinical features and pathologic findings at autopsy resemble those seen in encephalitis caused by other viruses transmitted by arthropods.

TICK-BORNE ENCEPHALITIDES

An indefinite number of flaviviruses are transmitted by ticks and cause encephalitis. Two clinical forms are identified, a severe form occurring primarily in the Soviet Far East (Russian spring-summer encephalitis), and a milder form occurring in Central Europe (diphasic meningoencephalitis) (Henner and Hanzal, 1963).

EPIDEMIOLOGY. Probably small wild rodents are the reservoir of these viruses, which accounts for the stationary endemicity of the disease. The larvae and nymphs of ticks grow only in field mice, whereas the adult forms feed on larger mammals. Humans are an incidental host for the virus when they are exposed to ticks in rural wooded areas. An unusual method of acquiring the infection is by consumption of raw milk from cows or sheep, which become infected by infected ticks. Of all togaviruses this one shares with the virus of VEE the distinction of creating the greatest hazard for laboratory workers. The virus may also cause infection by the respiratory route.

CLINICAL MANIFESTATIONS. The Far Eastern or more severe form of the disease has an incubation period of 8 to 14 days. There is violent onset of headache, fever, nausea, vomiting, hyperesthesia, and photophobia. Nuchal rigidity, weakness, and drowsiness follow rapidly. At the height of illness, delirium or coma, convulsions, pareses, or paralysis may develop. Severe disease is characterized by involvement of the bulbar centers and the cervical cord. Ascending paralysis or hemiparesis may result. The more benign course is essentially that of aseptic meningitis. In the nonfatal case, fever lasts five to eight days. Convalescence may be prolonged for months. Residual paralysis typically involves the arms and shoulder girdle. The case-fatality rate is estimated to be 20 to 30 per cent, death occurring within one to seven days. Infection is more severe in children than in adults.

The Central European form is more benign and often runs a diphasic course. The first phase is a period of viremia characterized by a febrile influenza-like illness that lasts for two to seven days. The liver may be tender, and liver function tests are abnormal, but the CSF is normal. Leukopenia is characteristic. This phase is followed by an asymptomatic period of 8 to 15 days. The second phase is characterized by signs and symptoms of meningoencephalitis—that is, fever, severe headache, nuchal rigidity, nausea, and vomiting. The temperature rises rapidly to 40° C or more. There may be diplopia, blurring of vision, slowed mentation, mental confusion, and delirium. Coma is rare. Most patients recover completely. The case-fatality ranges from 0.5 to about 5 per cent depending on the locality of outbreaks. Patients have a more severe form of disease in newly endemic areas such as Austria, and are less ill in Czechoslovakia, Western U.S.S.R., and Eastern Europe. Convalescence may be prolonged, with tremors and psychic or emotional disturbances. Permanent disability is uncommon.

Louping ill, a rare cause of tick-borne flavivirus encephalitis in the British Isles, produces a benign diphasic illness resembling the Central European form of tick-borne encephalitis.

POWASSAN VIRUS ENCEPHALITIS

Powassan virus was isolated in 1958 from a human case of fatal encephalitis and is distantly related to the tick-borne encephalitis virus group. Antibodies to this virus have been found in wild mammals and, very infrequently, in humans in Ontario and New York State. The evidence indicates that man was not infected by this virus in the past, but his inroads into wild habitats may cause human infections in the future.

CALIFORNIA ENCEPHALITIS

The California virus group, now under the Bunyaviridae, was first isolated from mosquitoes in California in 1943. It was shown to cause encephalitis in man in 1952. Since then it has become the most frequently reported cause of arthropod-borne meningoencephalitis in the United States. Most patients recover.

EPIDEMIOLOGY. The reservoir of infection is probably rodents, such as squirrels, cotton rats, and rabbits. Birds are not important in transmission of this virus. The constant and relatively immobile sylvatic reservoir may account for the constancy of infection rates in many parts of the United States. The infection is transmitted accidentally from this reservoir to man by a large variety of *Aedes* mosquitoes in rural areas. The virus is endemic in California and the Midwest, including Wisconsin and Ohio. Human infection was apparently absent before 1950.

CLINICAL MANIFESTATIONS. This virus group causes a significant amount of inapparent infection. For example, in Kern County in the Central Valley in California, 39 per cent of rural residents were inapparently infected as demonstrated by the presence of antibodies. Encephalitis does not occur in infants but is frequent in young children. Adults may develop only meningitis.

There may be prodromal fever, headache, nausea, vomiting, and abdominal pain lasting one to four days. As in other types of encephalitides, headache, stiff neck, sensorial disturbance, and convulsions are common. The peripheral blood count is usually elevated with predominance of the neutrophils. Lymphocytosis is usually seen in the cerebrospinal fluid.

Residual neurologic defects such as recurrent seizures, depressed intellectual function, and abnormal EEG have been described. Usually the patient recovers completely, and mortality is very low.

References

Dickerson, R. B., Newton, J. R., and Hansen, J. E.: Diagnosis and immediate prognosis of Japanese B encephalitis. Am J Med 12:277, 1952.

Hammon, W. McD., and Ho, M.: Viral encephalitis. Disease-a-Month, February, 1973.

Henner, K., and Hanzal, F.: Les encéphalites européennes à tiques. Rev Neurolog 108:697, 1963.

Kinsella, R. A., and Brown, G. O.: Clinical features of epidemic (St. Louis) encephalitis. JAMA 103:462, 1934.

Lee, H. W., Lee, P. W., and Johnson, K. M.: Isolation of the etiologic agent of Korean hemorrhagic fever. J Infect Dis 137:298, 1978.

Theiler, M., and Downs, W. G.: The Arthropod-Borne Viruses of Vertebrates. New Haven, Yale University Press, 1973.

183
SLOW INFECTIONS

Ashley T. Haase, M.D.

Sigurdsson first introduced the term "slow infections" to capture the novel time scale of a group of chronic transmissible diseases of Icelandic sheep (Sigurdsson, 1954). The characteristics of slow infections are as follows: 1) a long preclinical phase, generally months to years, from exposure to the infectious agent to appearance of symptoms; 2) a protracted clinical course; 3) pathologic manifestations frequently confined to a single organ system, most often the central nervous system (CNS). The medical importance of slow infections became evident with the discovery by Gajdusek that degenerative diseases of man, like kuru and Creutzfeldt-Jakob disease (CJD), were transmissible diseases with incubation periods exceeding one year.

DIVERSITY OF ETIOLOGIC AGENTS OF SLOW INFECTIONS. Diseases that fulfill Sigurdsson's criteria for slow infections are caused by viruses from most major taxonomic

Table 1. TAXONOMY OF AGENTS OF SLOW INFECTIONS

A. Slow Infections of Man Caused by Viruses

Classification	*Virus*	*Disease*
RNA Viruses		
Paramyxovirus	Measles variant	Subacute sclerosing panencephalitis (SSPE)
Rhabdovirus	Rabies	Rabies
DNA Viruses		
Papovavirus	JC, SV40	Progressive multifocal leukoencephalopathy (PML)
Parvovirus	Hepatitis A,B	Hepatitis, arteritis

B. Slow Infections of Animals Caused by Viruses

Classification	*Virus*	*Disease*	*Host*
RNA Viruses			
Retrovirus	Visna	Meningoencephalitis	Sheep
	Maedi	Pneumonitis	Sheep
	Progressive pneumonia (PPV)	Pneumonitis	Sheep
	Equine infectious anemia (EIA)	Hemolytic anemia, arteritis	Horse
	Gardner agent	Lower motor neuron	Feral Mouse
	Xenotropic C Type	Hemolytic anemia, SLE-like	NZB Mouse
Arena Virus	Lymphocytic choriomeningitis (LCM)	Meningitis glomerulonephritis	Mouse
Paramyxovirus	Canine distemper	Encephalitis	Dog
Togavirus	Lactate dehydrogenase (LDV)	Elevated LDH; mild nephritis	Mouse
Picornavirus	Theiler's agent	Demyelination	Mouse
DNA Viruses			
Parvovirus	Aleutian disease (ADV)	Arteritis, anemia, nephritis	Mink
Papovavirus	SV40	Progressive multifocal leukoencephalopathy	Monkey

classes (Table 1), and by agents designated unconventional (Table 2A), because they are filterable, replicate, and transmit disease like viruses, but have other properties (Table 2B) quite unlike conventional viruses (Gajdusek 1977; Prusiner 1982). Particularly important is the unusual resistance of these agents to commonly employed disinfectants; effective methods for inactivation are listed in Table 2C. Slow infections frequently are called slow virus infec-

Table 2. UNCONVENTIONAL AGENTS OF SLOW INFECTIONS

A. Slow Infections Caused by Unconventional Agents

In Man	*In Animals*
Creutzfeldt-Jakob Disease (CJD)	Scrapie in sheep, goats
Kuru	Transmissible mink encephalopathy

B. Unusual Properties of Unconventional Agents

1. Resistance to physical, chemical treatments: Not wholly inactivated by boiling, sonication; resistant to UV irradiation, proteases, nucleases, formaldehyde, B propiolactone.
2. Genome: Small target size to UV irradiation, equivalent to molecular weight of about 100,000 or less; atypical action spectrum-inactivation 237 nm greater than 254 nm.
3. Virus particles: No virus particles evident in electron micrographs of tissues with 10^8 infectious units/g. Although abnormal fibrils have been observed in scrapie brain preparations (Mertz, et al. 1981).
4. Host response: No inflammatory reaction; antigenicity questionable, as humoral or cellular immunity not demonstrable, disease unaltered in immunosuppressed animals; interferon not induced, no response to exogenously administered interferon.
5. Replication in tissue culture: Replication to low titers in explanted fragments of brain; no cytopathic effect; no interference with growth of conventional viruses.

C. Inactivation of Unconventional Agents

Autoclaving (121°C; 20 psi; 30 minutes)
Hypochlorite (Clorox NaOCl 0.5–5.0 percent) iodine disinfectants
Lipid solvents: Ether, acetone, chloroform, chloroform-butanol, 2 chlorethanol, strong detergents, 6 M urea
Carbohydrate active reagents: 0.1 M periodate

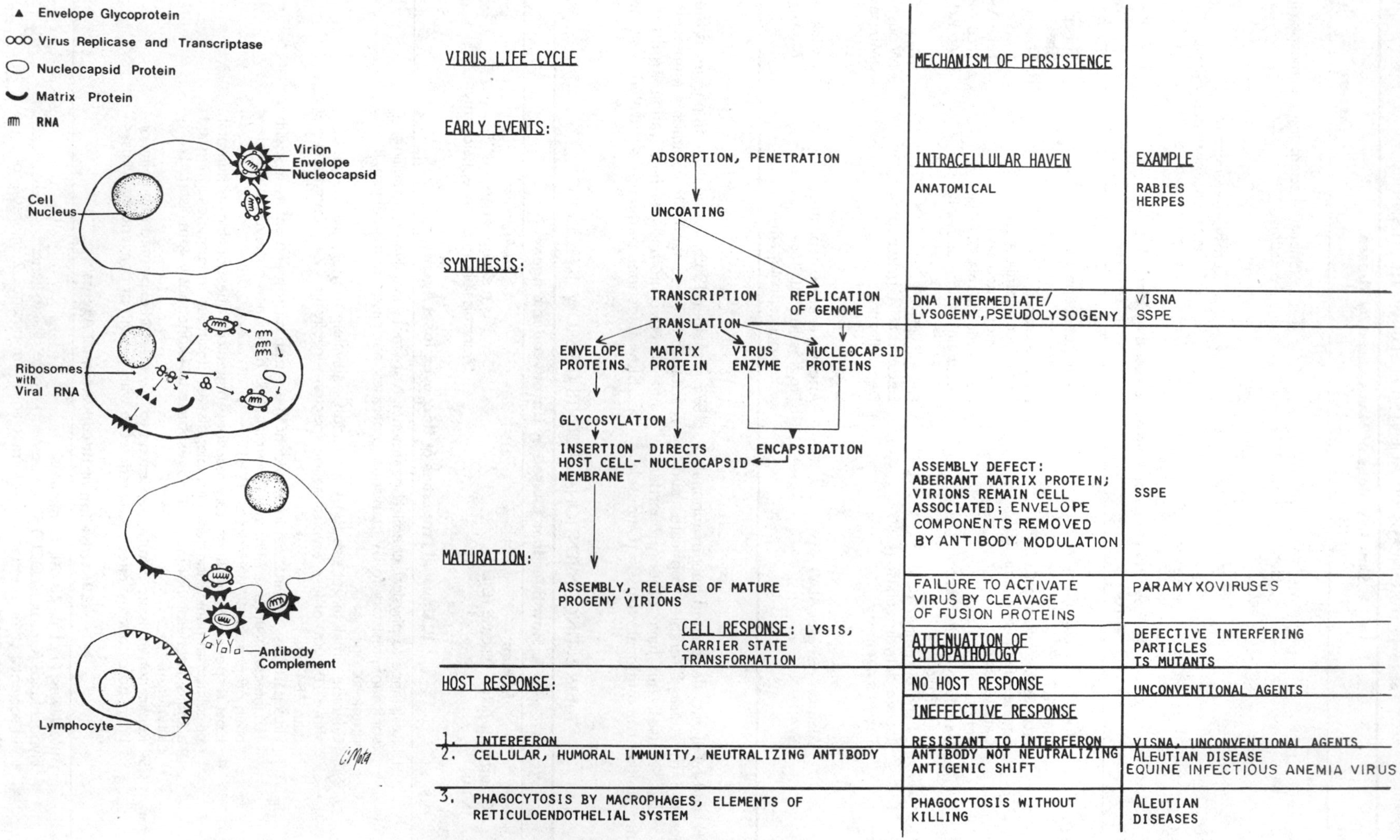

Figure 1. Mechanisms of Virus Persistence: A generalized virus life cycle and the attendant effects on the cell and host response is presented schematically in the left half of the diagram; explanations proposed for persistence are tabulated in the right half.

tions because they are caused by viruses or viral-like agents with one exception, Johne's disease of sheep caused by mycobacteria. However, except for the unconventional agents the pace of viral replication is not inherently slow in animals or tissue culture. Rather, only the appearance of symptoms from cumulative pathology is slow.

PATHOLOGY. In many slow infections the pathologic alterations are confined largely to the CNS; in immunopathologic syndromes to be described any organ system may be involved. The tissue lesions in the CNS are described as demyelinating, inflammatory, or spongioform. Unconventional agents produce a degenerative lesion giving tissue sections a spongy appearance at the light microscopic level. This is due to vacuolation primarily in neurons and neuropil. Hypertrophy and proliferation of astrocytes are also characteristic of spongioform encephalopathies. Visna and subacute sclerosing panencephalitis (SSPE) are prototypes of inflammatory encephalitides in which lymphocytes and plasma cells infiltrate the CNS, often arrayed as cuffs around blood vessels, or collected discretely in foci (microglial nodules). Sclerosing refers to the relative firmness of the end-stage lesion vis a vis normal neural tissue. Destruction of neurons in inflammatory foci may lead secondarily to demyelination. In progressive multifocal leukoencephalopathy (PML), demyelination is primary, that is, axis cylinders are relatively preserved. Demyelination in this situation is a direct consequence of destruction of oligodendrocytes, the cells that furnish myelin sheaths in the CNS. PML is thus almost exclusively a disease of white matter (leukoencephalopathy).

PATHOGENESIS. Persistence of virus in the face of host defense mechanisms, and the evolution of disease over a period often of years are two aspects of slow infections that require explanation and continue to inspire investigative efforts in this area.

Mechanisms of Persistence. Mechanisms for virus persistence can be considered in a logical framework of the virus life cycle, the fate of the infected cell, and the host response to virus infection (Fig. 1). In acute infections viruses invade cells and subvert them to production of a new crop of virions. The cells often die and virus spreads until host defenses are mobilized to limit infection. Evidently in persistent infections virus host cell interactions must be different; the destructive effects of virus growth must be mitigated in order to provide for survival of the host beyond the initial phase of infection, and host defenses must not eliminate the infecting agent. A virus may escape elimination because 1) it remains inside the cell, where humoral and cellular immunity are powerless; 2) host defense mechanisms are not evoked; and 3) defense mechanisms are ineffective. Generally several mechanisms play a part in persistence. Herpetic infections, visna, and SSPE illustrate the first stratagem. Herpes virus travels to and from the nervous system in axoplasm. In visna a DNA intermediate or provirus conserves viral genetic information inside the cell, but, analogous to lysogeny, this information is not expressed. Consequently the infected cells are not detected and destroyed by immune surveillance (Haase et al., 1977). In SSPE the synthesis and expression of the viral genome also is reduced (Haase et al., 1981). Moreover, the causative variant of measles virus is entrapped in the cell because the protein required for virus assembly (matrix protein) is abnormal in structure, stability, or amount (Hall and Choppin, 1981; Roux and Waldvogel, 1982). Residual virion envelope components are then stripped from the cell membrane by antibody modulation so that the cell is refractory to immune lysis (Joseph and Oldstone, 1975), and persistently infected (Rommohon et al., 1981).

Unconventional agents exemplify immunologically silent infections in which host defenses are not engaged. In other slow infections virus persists because the host response is ineffective. Aleutian disease is representative of a group of immune complex diseases in which antibody is produced and combines with virus without neutralizing infectivity. Humoral immunity may be ineffective too, at least temporarily, if antigenic variants arise that are not neutralized by antibody to the strain of virus-initiating infection. Such is the case in equine infections anemia (Kono et al., 1973). Antigenic variants have been described in visna (Gudnadottir, 1974; Narayan et al., 1977), but it seems unlikely that they play an essential role either in persistence or the evolution of neurological disease (Thormar et al., 1983; Lutley et al., 1983). Other reasons for the failure of host defense mechanisms include phagocytosis of virus by cellular elements of the reticuloendothelial system without killing, and resistance to interferon.

Persistent infections imply moderation in the severity of viral cytopathology; otherwise susceptible cells would be consumed, or the host would succumb to acute infection. Defective interfering particles have been invoked to explain initiation of persistent infections because they diminish cytopathology. These particles have lost a portion of the genome of standard virus and can replicate only in a dual infection where standard virus supplies the missing genetic information (Huang, 1973). Such a co-infection is a competitive situation that sharply reduces the production of standard virus. Whether defective particles play a role in human infections is unknown. Their participation in the chronic infections of tissue culture cells is more securely supported by available evidence, and co-infection with defective particles prolongs some experimental infections of animals by days. Viral temperature-sensitive (ts) mutants also reduce growth of standard virions and lessen cytopathology. They arise later in persistent infections of tissue culture cells, and may play a role in the maintenance of persistent infections (Preble and Youngner, 1975).

Slowness and Mechanisms of Disease. Slowness refers to the tempo of development of discernible pathology and this in turn is a reflection of the kinetics of replication and spread of the causative agents and the mechanisms involved in tissue damage. The rate of replication of unconventional agents in the nervous system is inherently slow, and this is also true in visna, SSPE, and equine infectious anemia where virus gene expression is restricted, or the spread of virus is intermittent. In other instances the virus may replicate at a relatively rapid rate, but the disease evolves slowly because the immunopathological mechanisms involved in tissue damage become manifest over a protracted period. The pathological mechanisms in slow diseases summarized in Table 3 fall into two classes. Some viruses that cause persistent infections directly impair differentiated functions of their host cells, or kill the specialized host cell with consequences cited in the table. In many instances, however, it is the host's immune response to infection that is responsible for pathological alterations, e.g., through innocent bystander damage in sites of inflammation where immune cells are attacking infected cells; or by deposition of virus-antibody immune complexes in glomeruli and the walls of blood vessels. Recent work also points to the

Table 3. MECHANISMS OF DISEASE*

Direct Mechanisms	Examples
1. Cell Dysfunction.	Rabies virus impairs binding of acetylcholine to neurons (Tsiang, 1982).
	Lymphocytic choriomeningitis (LCM) virus persistently infects cells in the anterior lobe of the pituitary and causes runting in infected mice (Oldstone et al., 1982).
2. Cell Death.	In PML and coronavirus infections virus induced lysis of oligodendroglial cells causes demyelination.
Indirect Immunopathological Mechanisms	**Examples**
1. Immune attack is directed toward viral antigens borne on the infected cells.	Cytolytic T cells mediate neurological disease in LCM infected mice (Cole, et al., 1972), and a behavioral disease in rats caused by Borna virus (Narayan et al., 1983.)
2. Immune attack is directed toward shared determinants on viral and host antigens: molecular mimicry.	Antibodies to proteins of measles virus and herpes simplex virus types cross react with human intermediate filaments (Fujinami et al., 1983).
	Autoantibodies to neurofilaments are found in patients with spongioform encephalopathies (Sotelo et al., 1980).
3. Infection elicits autoantibody.	Mice infected with reovirus type 1 develop an autoimmune polyendocrinopathy (Haspel et al., 1983).
4. Deposition of immune complexes causes inflammation and destruction of tissue.	Aleutian disease (Porter et al., 1969).

*Modified from Conference Report on Detection of Viral Genes and Their Products in Chronic Neurological Diseases. Ann. Neurol. 15:119, 1984.

possibility of autoimmune disease provoked by infection, either through shared antigenic determinants, or through some other as yet unknown autosensitization process.

CLINICAL DESCRIPTION AND DIAGNOSIS OF SLOW INFECTIONS IN MAN

Unconventional Agents Causing Spongioform Encephalopathies

Kuru. Kuru is a neurologic affliction at one time epidemic among the peoples of the Fore cultural and linguistic group inhabiting the remote mountainous regions of New Guinea. Kuru means trembling or shivering, a name derived from the most prominent symptoms, tremors of the head, trunk, and extremities. These symptoms disappear with sleep. The tremors and unsteadiness in gait are manifestations of cerebellar involvement; the symmetric cerebellar ataxia and motor dysfunction are progressively incapacitating. Flaccid paralysis, abnormalities of extraocular movements, incontinence, mental changes, and emaciation precede death three to nine months from the onset of symptoms. Patients are afebrile, there are no inflammatory cells or increase in the protein in cerebral spinal fluid (CSF), and the pathologic changes are degenerative ones, most evident in cerebellum and pons. An infectious basis for kuru was discounted initially on these grounds, until Hadlow pointed out the remarkable similarities in the pathology of the slow infection of sheep (scrapie) and kuru in man. This stimulated renewed efforts to transmit kuru to animals, and ultimately led to the demonstration that homogenates of kuru brain would elicit a similar clinical pathologic picture in chimpanzees 13 to 18 months after inoculation.

Natural infections probably were transmitted by autoinoculation of the kuru agent into breaks in skin and mucous membranes occurring during preparation and consumption of the dead in a mourning rite. Since usually only adult women and young children of either sex were involved in this ritual, most cases of kuru occurred in these groups. The practice of cannibalism has been discontinued with a marked decline in the overall number of cases of kuru and the disappearance of kuru in children born since cannibalism ceased (Gajdusek, 1977).

Creutzfeldt-Jakob Disease and other Transmissible Dementias. Success in transmitting kuru to experimental animals prompted a search for other degenerative conditions that might represent slow infections. The striking similarities in the pathology of kuru and CJD made the latter a prime candidate, and in 1966 Gajdusek and his collaborators reported transmission of CJD to chimpanzees. Dementias other than CJD are also transmissible in some cases that include familial Alzheimer's disease, supranuclear palsy, and sporadic presenile dementia in a variety of clinical contexts.

CJD is a rare presenile dementia of worldwide distribution most prevalent between the ages of 40 and 65. The combination of dementia progressing noticeably from week to week, myoclonus, and an abnormal electroencephalogram with a pattern of overall suppression on which paroxysmal bursts of high voltage slow waves are superimposed, suggest the diagnosis antemortem. Pneumoencephalogram and CT scan may disclose dilated ventricles consistent with diffuse cortical atrophy. The disease pursues a relentless downhill course with death 3 to 16 months from the onset of symptoms.

The origins and transmission of CJD are enigmatic. In about 10 per cent of cases there is a familial pattern suggesting transmission as an autosomal dominant. Clustering of disease in Jewish immigrants of Libyan origin, whose religious practices involve consumption of uncooked sheep brain, has provoked speculation that CJD may have arisen by transmission of scrapie to man. Inadvertent human transmission of CJD by corneal transplantation, and by improperly sterilized electroencephalographic electrodes has been reported.

Conventional Agents

Progressive Multifocal Leukoencephalopathy. PML is a neurologic condition usually of immunologically compromised patients in which the protean symptomatology reflects the distribution of multiple foci of demyelination. Cerebral cortical involvement is most frequent with confusion, disorientation, personality change, poor memory, speech and visual disturbances, weakness, and paralysis. Dysarthria and abnormalities of sensation are common. The electroencephalogram is abnormal but not diagnostic, and although not always useful in detecting early lesions CT scans can be used to follow the progression of late lesions.

Eosinophilic or basophilic intranuclear inclusion bodies in enlarged oligodendroglia at the periphery of demyelinated foci first suggested viruses as the cause of PML. Subsequently, electron micrographs demonstrated viral particles with the morphologic characteristics of papovaviruses in the inclusion bodies, and the causative agent was isolated in cultures of glial cells. In most cases PML is caused by a new member of the papovavirus group, designated JC virus (Padgett et al., 1976); two reported cases of PML appear to have been caused by SV40 virus. This virus also causes a PML-like condition in macaque monkeys. Another human papovavirus, the BK agent, has been isolated from the urine of patients undergoing renal transplantation. Although BK virus may be an adventitous agent in most situations, it also has been associated with interstitial nephritis (Rosen et al., 1983). Serologic surveys indicate that JC and BK viruses are acquired early in life by a large proportion of populations (see Chapter 62).

Most cases of PML occur in patients with some underlying disorder that impairs host defenses, most recently in patients with AIDS (Miller et al., 1982). Presumably the impaired defenses in these patients provide an opportunity for JC virus to replicate to high titer in CNS, either by reactivation, by spread from an extraneural site, or by newly acquired infection. These explanations reconcile the ubiquitous nature of the virus with the rarity of PML (one to two cases per million in the United States).

Subacute Sclerosing Panencephalitis (Dawson's Inclusion Body Encephalitis). SSPE is a rare disease of children and young adults between the ages of 4 and 20 years. Disease most often occurs in males from rural areas infected with measles before age 2. The initial phase is characterized by insidiously progressive deterioration of intellectual function and by behavioral changes. School performance declines and affected children are forgetful and temperamental In the second phase these changes are more marked and are associated with myoclonic movements of the head, trunk, or extremities repeated at intervals of 10 to 60 seconds. The electroencephalogram is abnormal with a pattern of periodic synchronous bursts of high voltage slow and sharp waves on a background of generalized suppression. Inflammatory lesions of the optic nerve may lead to chorioretinitis, papilledema, and pigmentary retinopathy. The terminal phase is one of profound dementia, decorticate spasticity, blindness, and hypothalamic dysfunction. Death occurs by infection or vasomotor collapse one to three years from the onset of symptoms.

Inflammatory changes in SSPE and eosinophilic intranuclear inclusion bodies pointed to a viral etiology, a suspicion heightened by finding tubular structures resembling paramyxovirus nucleocapsids in the inclusions, and by the very high titers of antibody to measles virus consistently demonstrated in the serum and CSF of these patients (Johnson et al., 1974). Later a variant of measles virus was isolated. Antigens of the measles variant can be demonstrated by immunofluorescence in cells in inflammatory foci. These foci also contain plasma cells that produce antibody to the virus; consequently the levels of IgG in CSF are elevated, and, on electrophoresis, specific bands appear (oligoclonal pattern) that can be absorbed with viral antigens.

Progressive Rubella Encephalitis. Progressive motor and mental deterioration in the second decade of life has been recognized recently in patients chronically infected with rubella virus (Townsend et al., 1975). Other abnormalities include ataxia, myoclonus, elevated protein and IgG, and increased cells in the CSF. Inflammatory changes with moderate loss of neurons and cerebellar atrophy were found postmortem in addition to the calcification and deposition of basophilic granular material in the walls of blood vessels and in perivascular spaces that occur in rubella. Rubella virus was isolated in one case.

TREATMENT AND PREVENTION. No specific therapy is available currently for most slow infections. Antiviral drugs such as IudR, Ara-A, Ara-C, and amantidine, immunopotentiation (γ-globulin, adjuvants, transfer factor), immunosuppression, and steroids have been used without objectively arresting disease. The incidence of SSPE has declined markedly after widespread vaccination against measles. Special care must be exercised with demented patients with known or suspected spongioform encephalopathy. Corneas should not be transplanted from these patients, and the measures delineated in Table 2C should be employed to sterilize equipment or to disinfect CSF and pathologic specimens.

PROSPECTUS. Slow infections will continue to be the focus of major research efforts because of the possibility that far more prevalent chronic degenerative diseases of man may be attributed to viral infection. The demonstration of viral antigens in Paget's disease (Mills et al., 1981) and measles and herpes virus genes in the brains of patients with multiple sclerosis as well as normal controls (Haase et al., 1981; Fraser et al., 1981) continue to support the possibility of virus involvement in chronic diseases, but there is no conclusive evidence that this is the case.

References

Andrewes, C. H.: The troubles of a virus. J Gen Microbiol 40:140, 1965.

Cole, G. A., Nathanson, N., and Prendergast, R. A.: Requirement for Θ-bearing cells in lymphocytic choriomeningitis virus-induced central nervous system disease. Nature 238:335, 1972.

Fraser, N. W., Lawrence, W. C., Wroblewska, A., Bilden, D. H., and Koprowski, H.: Herpes simplex type 1 DNA in human brain tissue. Proc Natl Acad Sci USA 78:6461, 1981.

Fujinami, R. S., Oldstone, M. B. A., Wroblewska, Z., Frankel, M. E., and Koprowski, H.: Molecular mimicry in virus infection: Crossreaction of measles virus phosphoprotein or of herpes simplex virus protein with human intermediate filaments. Proc Natl Acad Sci USA 80:2346, 1983.

Gajdusek, D. C.: Unconventional viruses and the origin and disappearance of kuru. Science 197:943, 1977.

Gudnadottir, M.: Visna-maedi in sheep. Prog in Med Virol 18:336, 1974.

Haase, A. T., Stowring, L., Narayan, O., Griffin, D., and Price, D.: Slow persistent infection caused by visna virus: Role of host restriction. Science 195:171, 1977.

Haase, A. T., Swoveland, P., Stowring, L., Ventura, P., Johnson, K. P., Norrby, E., and Gibbs, Jr., C. J.: Measles virus genome in infections of the central nervous system. J Infect Dis 144:154, 1981.

Haase, A. T., Ventura, P., Gibbs, Jr., C. J., and Tourtellotte, W. W.: Measles virus nucleotide sequences: Detection by hybridization in situ. Science 212:672, 1981.

Hall, W. W., and Choppin, P. W.: Measles-virus proteins in the brain tissue of patients with subacute sclerosing panencephalitis: Absence of the M protein. N Engl J Med 304:1154, 1981.

Haspel, M. V., Onodera, T., Prabhakar, B. S., Horita, M., Suzuki, H., and Notkins, A. L.: Virus-induced autoimmunity: Monoclonal antibodies that react with endocrine tissues. Science 220:304, 1983.

Huang, A. S.: Defective interfering viruses. Ann Rev Microbiol 27:101, 1973.

Johnson, K. P., Byington, D. P., and Gaddis, L.: Subacute sclerosing panencephalitis. Adv Neurol 6:77, 1974.

Joseph, B. S., and Oldstone, M. B. A.: Immunologic injury in measles virus infection. II. Suppression of immune injury through antigenic modulation. J Exp Med 142:864, 1975.

Kono, Y., Kobayashi, K., and Fukunaga, Y.: Antigenic drift of equine infectious anemia virus in chronically infected horses. Arch ges Virusforsch 41:1, 1973.

Lutley, R., Petursson, G., Palsson, P. A., Georgsson, G., Klein, A., and Nathanson, N.: Antigenic drift in visna: Virus variation during long-term infection of Icelandic sheep. J Gen Virol 64:1433, 1983.

Mertz, P. A., Somerville, R. A., Wisniewski, H. M., and Iqbal, K.: Abnormal fibrils from scrapie-infected brain. Acta Neuropathol (Berl) 54:63, 1981.

Miller, J. F., Barrett, R. E., Britton, C. B., Tapper, M. L., Bahr, G. S., Bruno, P. J., Marquardt, M. D., Hays, A. P., Mcmurtry, J. G., Weissman, J. B., and Bruno, M. S.: Progressive multifocal leukoencephalopathy in a male homosexual with T-cell immune deficiency. New Eng J of Med 307:1436, 1982.

Mills, B. G., Singer, F. R., Weiner, L. P., and Holst, P. A.: Immunohistological demonstration of respiratory syncytial virus antigens in Paget disease of bone. Proc Natl Acad Sci USA, 78:1209, 1981.

Narayan, O., Herzog, S., Frese, K., Scheefers, H., and Rott, R.: Behavioral disease in rats caused by immunopathological responses to persistent Borna virus in the brain. Science 220:1401, 1983.

Narayan, O., Griffin, D. E., and Chase, J.: Antigenic shift of visna virus in persistently infected sheep. Science 197:376, 1977.

Oldstone, M. B. A., Sinha, Y. H., Blount, P., Tishon, A., Rodriguez, M., von Wedel, R., and Lampert, P. W.: Virus-induced alterations in homeostasis: Alterations in differentiated functions of infected cells in vivo. Science 218:1125, 1982.

Padgett, B. L., Walker, D. L., ZuRhein, G. M., Hodach, A. E., and Chou, S. M.: Jc papovavirus in progressive multifocal leukoencephalopathy. J Infect Dis 133:686, 1976.

Porter, D. D., Larsen, A. T., and Porter, H. B.: The pathogenesis of aleutian disease of mink. I. *In vivo* replication and the host antibody response to viral antigen. J Exp Med 130:575, 1969.

Preble, O. T., and Youngner, J. S.: Temperature-sensitive viruses and the etiology of chronic and inapparent infections. J Infect Dis 131:467, 1975.

Prusiner, S. B.: Novel proteinaceous infectious particles cause scrapie. Science 216:136, 1982.

Rammohan, K. W., McFarland, H. F., and McFarlin D. E.: Induction of subacture murine measles encephalitis by monoclonal antibody to virus haemagglutinin. Nature 290:588, 1981.

Rosen, S., Harmon, W., Krensky, A. M., Edelson, P. J., Padgett, B. L., Grinnell, B. W., Rubino, M. J., and Walker, D. L.: Tubulo-interstitial nephritis associated with polyomavirus (BK type) infection. N Engl J Med 308:1192, 1983.

Roux, L., and Waldvogel, F. A.: Instability of the viral M protein in BHK-21 cells persistently infected with sendai virus. Cell 28:293, 1982.

Sigurdsson, B.: Rida, a chronic encephalitis of sheep—with general remarks on infection which develop slowly and some of their special characteristics. British Vet J: Series of special university lectures, University of London, March, 1954.

Sotelo, J., Gibbs, Jr., C. J., and Gajdusek, D. C.: Autoantibodies against axonal neurofilaments in patients with kuru and Creutzfeldt-Jakob disease. Science 210:190, 1980.

Thormar, H., Barshatzky, M. R., Arnesen, K., and Kozlowski, P. B.: The emergence of antigenic variants is a rare event in long-term visna virus infection *in vivo*. J Gen Virol 64:1427, 1983.

Townsend, J. J., Baringer, J. R., Wolinsky, J. S., Malamud, N., Mednick. J. P., Panitch, J. S., Scott, R. A. T., Oshira, L. S., and Cremer, M. E.: Progressive rubella panencephalitis—late onset after congenital rubella. N Engl J Med 292:990, 1975.

Tsiang, H.: Neuronal function impairment in rabies-infected rat brain. J Gen Virol 61:277, 1982.

184

REYE'S SYNDROME

DORIS A. TRAUNER, M.S., M.D.

Reye's syndrome is an acute encephalopathy of childhood associated with diffuse fatty infiltration of the viscera. Before 1963 this disorder was frequently diagnosed as "acute toxic encephalopathy of unknown etiology." The full clinicopathologic syndrome was described by Reye and his co-workers in Australia in 1963, and numerous reports of this same disease from many parts of the world have since been published. The disease appears to be confined primarily to children, with most cases reported in patients 7 weeks to 22 years of age. It occurs with equal frequency in males and females. Recently, several cases have been reported in adults.

ETIOLOGY AND PATHOGENESIS. The cause of Reye's syndrome is unknown. Numerous viruses have been associated with the prodromal illness. The most common are influenza B, A1 and A2, and varicella. Other viruses implicated in reported cases include herpes simplex, rubella, rubeola, poliovirus type I, adenovirus type III, echovirus, coxsackievirus types A, A1, B1, and B4, parainfluenza, and Epstein-Barr virus. Although a viral prodrome is present in almost all cases of Reye's syndrome, there is no evidence that the virus itself causes the encephalopathy.

There are several hypotheses regarding the cause of this disorder. Various potential toxins, including salicylates and phenothiazines, have been thought to play a possible causal role. Several case-control studies have documented that salicylate use is more common in children who develop Reye's syndrome than in their peers with a similar prodromal illness (Waldman et al., 1982). The American Academy of Pediatrics recommends that children with flu-like symptoms or varicella not be given aspirin-containing compounds because of the possible relationship between salicylate use and subsequent development of Reye's syndrome. The suggestion that a virus-toxin interaction may produce Reye's syndrome also has some foundation experimentally. Toxins such as insecticides and 4-pentenoic acid (an analogue of hypoglycin A) can produce an encephalopathy associated with fatty accumulation in the viscera of rats with viral infections.

Two disorders similar to Reye's syndrome are caused by exogenous toxins. Jamaican vomiting sickness is characterized by vomiting, coma, and seizures. It affects children in Jamaica and is caused by ingestion of unripe Ackee fruit, which contains the toxin hypoglycin A. Udorn encephalopathy, described from Thailand, is an acute encephalopathy of childhood that is identical to Reye's syndrome clinically and biochemically. This disorder is produced by ingestion of aflatoxin, a plant toxin present in some foods.

Patients with Reye's syndrome have elevated concentrations of serum short-chain fatty acids. These have been implicated as possible endogenous toxins. If short-chain fatty acids are injected into laboratory animals, an encephalopathy develops that has clinical and pathologic features identical to those of Reye's syndrome. Ammonia has also been considered as an endogenous toxin, but the levels of hyperammonemia seen in children with Reye's syndrome are generally lower than those required to produce coma in experimental animals. Short-chain fatty acids potentiate the effects of ammonia on the central nervous system in experimental animals, and it is possible that the presence of both toxins simultaneously may produce the encephalopathy of Reye's syndrome.

Finally, it has been suggested that some genetic factor may be involved. In a few instances Reye's syndrome has occurred in two or more family members. The presence of an inborn error of urea cycle metabolism would account for the hyperammonemia, lethargy, and coma. The activity of the mitochondrial urea cycle enzymes ornithine transcarbamylase and carbamyl phosphate synthetase have been decreased in liver biopsy specimens of patients during the acute phase of the disease. It is unlikely that this decreased activity represents an inborn metabolic error, since Reye's syndrome is not a recurrent disease and survivors exhibit no further evidence of metabolic derangements; rather, these enzyme abnormalities probably reflect mitochondrial injury during the acute illness.

PATHOLOGY. Pathologic changes are found in liver, kidney, heart, pancreas, lungs, thymus, and brain. The liver may be enlarged and is usually yellow. Histologic examination reveals diffuse accumulation of small fatty droplets within the cytoplasm of hepatocytes (Fig. 1). There is no evidence of extensive necrosis of liver cells. Histochemical stains for succinic dehydrogenase demonstrate decreased enzyme activity. Ultrastructural changes include mitochondrial swelling with distortion of cristae, dilatation of the cisternae of the rough endoplasmic reticulum, proliferation of the smooth endoplasmic reticulum, and fat droplets within the cytoplasm of hepatocytes. The glycogen content is reduced in the liver. These abnormalities disappear after the patient recovers.

The kidneys may also appear swollen and pale. Fatty infiltration is present in the proximal tubules and loops of Henle. In the heart, myocardial tissue contains fat droplets, and fibers may be swollen and vacuolated. The pancreas also contains an accumulation of fat droplets. Nonspecific intranuclear inclusions may be seen on ultrastructural examination. Histiocytes and alveolar lining cells of the lungs may also contain fat droplets.

The brain is grossly edematous and heavier, and the cortical surface is flattened. Cerebellar tonsillar or temporal lobe herniation may be present. The cerebral ventricles are smaller than normal. Microscopic examination of the brain reveals evidence of cellular and interstitial edema. No specific pathologic abnormalities are seen. There is no accumulation of fat. Anoxia may cause necrosis of cortical neurons, loss of cerebellar Purkinje cells, and reactive astrocytes.

CLINICAL MANIFESTATIONS. Reye's syndrome in infants and children over 1 year of age is a biphasic illness with the features shown in Table 1. The first phase, or prodrome, is a viral illness, usually an upper respiratory infection or flu-like syndrome. This prodrome may be mild. As the child recovers from the viral illness, he begins to vomit repeatedly, and over a period of hours becomes delirious and agitated, then comatose. Generalized or focal seizures are common. Marked hyperventilation occurs with a mixed respiratory alkalosis and metabolic acidosis. Tachycardia may persist until improvement begins. Fever may be high even though no infection can be found. The liver is enlarged in the great majority of cases.

The encephalopathy varies in severity. In a recent study of children who had vomiting and elevated serum transaminases after a viral illness, 74 per cent had liver biopsies that were diagnostic of Reye's syndrome. All children had minimal neurologic symptoms and were classified as Stage I. The conclusion reached was that mild Reye's syndrome may be much more common than was previously believed (Lichtenstein et al., 1983).

Table 1. CLINICAL FEATURES OF REYE'S SYNDROME

Prodromal viral illness
Vomiting
Lethargy, delirium, coma
Hyperventilation
Seizures
Enlarged liver

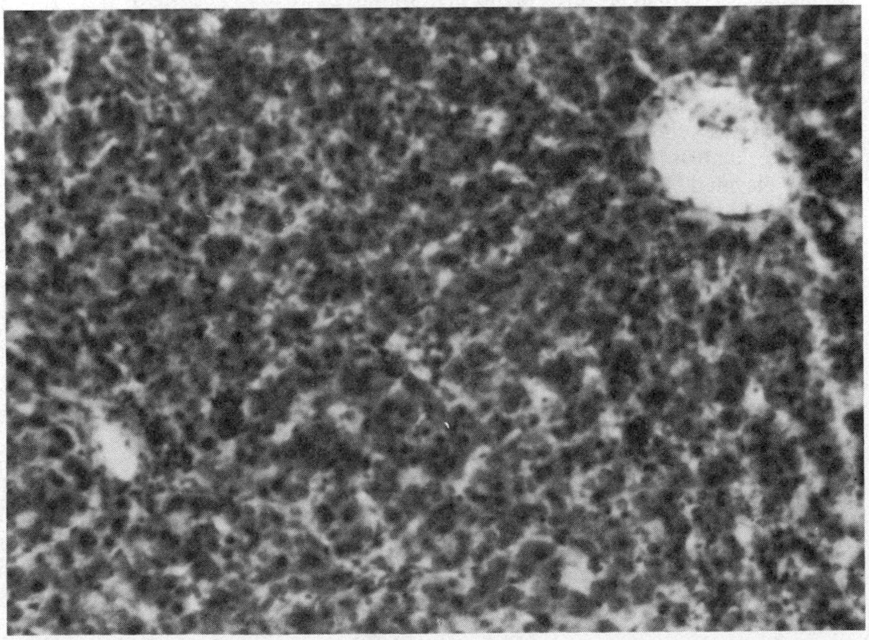

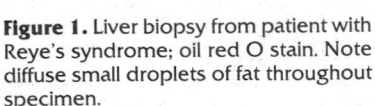

Figure 1. Liver biopsy from patient with Reye's syndrome; oil red O stain. Note diffuse small droplets of fat throughout specimen.

Several methods of staging coma in Reye's syndrome have been suggested. One commonly used set of criteria is that of Lovejoy and colleagues (1974), which consists of five stages.

Stage 1: vomiting and lethargy.
Stage 2: disorientation, delirium, combativeness; hyperventilation, hyperactive deep tendon reflexes, inappropriate responses to noxious stimuli.
Stage 3: coma, hyperventilation, decorticate rigidity, preservation of pupillary reflexes.
Stage 4: deepening coma, decerebrate rigidity, loss of oculocephalic reflexes, dilated pupils unresponsive to light, dysconjugate eye movements in response to caloric stimulation.
Stage 5: seizures, loss of deep tendon reflexes, respiratory arrest, flaccidity.

As the coma deepens, the central nervous system dysfunction progresses in a rostral-caudal direction down the brain stem. In the final stage the brain stem stops functioning.

The clinical picture of Reye's syndrome in infants under 1 year of age differs somewhat from that in older children. Vomiting is less prominent. Respiratory abnormalities occur early and consist of marked hyperventilation and at times intermittent apnea. Seizures are common and may occur in the early encephalopathic stage. Infants tend to be limp and hypotonic with loss of primitive reflexes such as the Moro and tonic neck reflexes. The course is fulminant and the mortality and morbidity are high.

LABORATORY ABNORMALITIES. Numerous biochemical abnormalities are present in patients with Reye's syndrome (Table 2). Abnormalities in liver function are distinctive. The prothrombin time is prolonged, and the serum glutamic oxaloacetic transaminase (SGOT), serum glutamic pyruvic transaminase (SGPT), and lactic dehydrogenase (LDH) concentrations are elevated. Yet the bilirubin concentration is typically normal. Serum creatine phosphokinase (CPK) levels are also elevated. Hyperammonemia is present in virtually all patients early in the disease, but ammonia levels may return to normal within 24 to 48 hours.

Hypoglycemia is found in only 40 per cent of patients and is not a reliable diagnostic criterion. It is more common in children under 4 years of age. Arterial blood gas determinations may show a metabolic acidosis, respiratory alkalosis, or a mixture of both. Blood urea nitrogen is usually mildly elevated. Rarely, a significant azotemia is present, and transient anuria may occur. Although clinical evidence of pancreatitis is usually lacking, the serum amylase level may be elevated. Except for low glucose concentrations, the cerebrospinal fluid is normal.

Table 2. LABORATORY ABNORMALITIES IN REYE'S SYNDROME

Hyperammonemia
Hypoglycemia
Hypoglycorrachia
Abnormal liver function tests
Prolonged prothrombin time
Metabolic acidosis
Respiratory alkalosis
Hyperaminoacidemia
Short-chain fatty acidemia
Lactic acidemia

Certain serum amino acids (alanine, glutamine, lysine, α-amino *n*-butyrate) have been abnormally elevated. Lactic acidosis may occur. Elevated serum concentrations of the short-chain fatty acids propionate, butyrate, isobutyrate, valerate, isovalerate, and octanoate have also been found in patients with Reye's syndrome.

DIAGNOSIS. No single abnormality is pathognomonic for Reye's syndrome. Recognition of the disease is based on several criteria. The biphasic clinical course—an antecedent viral illness followed by repeated vomiting and progressing rapidly to lethargy and coma—is characteristic. This course, coupled with abnormal liver function tests, normal bilirubin levels, and a negative toxicology screen for toxins such as salicylates, leads to a diagnosis of Reye's syndrome. In doubtful or atypical cases, a biopsy of liver tissue may show diffuse accumulation of small fatty droplets.

A differential diagnosis should consider acute hepatitis, salicylate poisoning, other toxins (aflatoxin ingestion in Thailand, unripe Ackee fruit ingestion in Jamaica), encephalitis, severe hypoglycemia, and inborn errors of urea cycle and organic acid metabolism.

TREATMENT. Since the cause of Reye's syndrome is unknown, treatment is empirical. Therapy is aimed at stabilizing the patient's clinical status and correcting metabolic abnormalities.

Several procedures have been suggested to clear possible toxins from the body. Exchange blood transfusion and peritoneal dialysis have both been employed. Recent studies have found no additional benefit to the patients from these modes of therapy. A comprehensive treatment plan of intensive supportive care has been successful in many patients. This plan consists of the following steps:

1. Control respiration by nasotracheal intubation and mechanical ventilation.
2. Monitor blood pressure and central venous pressure with arterial and CVP lines.
3. Use neomycin enemas as necessary to decrease serum ammonia concentrations.
4. Administer vitamin K, 5 mg, intramuscularly or intravenously to help correct clotting abnormalities. Fresh frozen plasma can be given as well.
5. Monitor serum electrolytes, osmolality, glucose concentrations, prothrombin time, and blood urea nitrogen frequently.
6. Administer intravenous fluids consisting of 20 per cent glucose with appropriate electrolyte solutions.
7. Administer insulin, 1 unit per 5 g of glucose, every four hours intravenously. Blood glucose should be maintained at between 150 and 200 mg per 100 ml and insulin dosage altered as required to accomplish this. (Both hypertonic glucose and insulin help decrease serum accumulation of short-chain fatty acids.)
8. Place the child on cooling blanket or sponge him frequently to keep temperature down to 37° C.
9. An intracranial pressure monitor should be inserted (in either the epidural or the intraventricular space) to monitor intracranial pressure continuously. Pressure should be kept below 20 mm of mercury. Control of

intracranial pressure may be accomplished by the following methods:

a. Controlled hyperventilation to a pCO_2 of 25 mm mercury.
b. Intravenous mannitol 1/4 to 1/2 g per dose repeated as often as necessary. Serum osmolality should be kept below 320 to ensure continued efficacy of mannitol therapy and to decrease the incidence of complications.
c. Paralysis of the patient with pancuronium bromide after mechanical ventilation has been instituted.

These measures should be continued until the patient begins to awaken from the coma.

PROGNOSIS. Prognosis has become more favorable over the past several years. In Reye's original case reports (1963) there was an 80 per cent mortality. In subsequent years mortality has dropped, and with the treatment outlined above the mortality is less than 40 per cent.

Some survivors of Reye's syndrome are left with permanent neurologic sequelae, including seizure disorders, mental retardation, and spasticity. However, many patients survive with no neurologic deficits. Since the encephalopathy is metabolic rather than structural in origin, early recognition and aggressive therapy, with particular attention to control of intracranial pressure, can result in complete recovery with return to normal function for many children with Reye's syndrome.

EPIDEMIOLOGY. Reye's syndrome occurs sporadically and in "epidemics." The epidemic cases are geographically and temporally associated with outbreaks of influenza B infection. Sporadic cases have been reported from all parts of the world. There appears to be no clear racial or geographic predilection, although in the United States the vast majority of reported cases occur in Caucasians. With the exception of cases following influenza B infections, there is no seasonal predilection.

References

Huttenlocher, P. R., and Trauner, D. A.: Reye's syndrome. In Vinken, P. J., and Bruyn, G. W. (eds.): Handbook of Clinical Neurology. Vol. 29. Amsterdam, North-Holland Publishing Company, 1977.

Lichtenstein, P. K., Heubi, J. E., Daugherty, C. C., et al: Grade I Reye's syndrome: A frequent cause of vomiting and liver dysfunction after varicella and upper-respiratory-tract infection. N Engl J Med 309:133, 1983.

Lovejoy, F. H., Smith, A. L., Bresnan, J. J., Wood, J. N., Victor, D. J., and Adams, P. C.: Clinical staging in Reye's syndrome. Am J Dis Child 128:36, 1974.

Pollack, J. D. (ed.): Reye's Syndrome, New York, Grune & Stratton, 1975.

Reye, R. D. K., Morgan, G., and Baral, J.: Encephalopathy with fatty degeneration of the viscera. Lancet 2:749, 1963.

Trauner, D. A.: Treatment of Reye's syndrome. Ann Neurol 6:1, 1980.

Trauner, D. A., Brown, R. A., Ganz, E., and Huttenlocher, P. R.: Treatment of elevated intracranial pressure in Reye's syndrome. Ann Neurol 4:275, 1978.

Waldman, R. J., Hall, W. N., McGee, H., et al: Aspirin as a risk factor in Reye's syndrome. JAMA 247:3089, 1982.

185
POLIOMYELITIS

ALBERT B. SABIN, M.D.

Poliomyelitis (infantile paralysis, acute anterior poliomyelitis, poliomyélite, Kinderlähmung, Heine-Medin disease) is a clinical-pathologic syndrome caused by enteroviruses. It is characterized by an acute febrile illness, which, in its paralytic form, presents within one or more days after onset varying degrees of usually asymmetric, flaccid paralysis of various striated muscles and sometimes also respiratory and vasomotor disturbances. The paralysis is caused by primary neuronal damage accompanied by cellular infiltration mainly in the spinal cord and medulla.

HISTORY. Poliomyelitis is a worldwide infectious disease of human beings that probably dates back to earliest evolutionary times. The characteristic muscular atrophy and deformities resulting from paralysis of various muscles in early life has permitted identification of the disease from drawings made thousands of years ago. Poliomyelitis became a clinical entity in the 19th century after epidemics occurred in several countries. Rissler's (1888) description of the specific neuronal damage and inflammatory reaction in the central nervous system (CNS) established poliomyelitis as a neuropathologic entity. The experimental transmission of the disease to monkeys by Landsteiner and Popper (1909) and the subsequent work of Flexner and Lewis (1909) established the viral nature of the disease. The studies of Sabin and Ward (1941a) on fatal cases of human poliomyelitis proved that the human disease, in contrast to some artificial experimental models in monkeys, is predominantly an infection of the alimentary tract and of certain portions of the CNS. A collaborative effort of many investigators demonstrated that polioviruses belong to only three distinct serologic types (Committee on Typing, 1951). The work of Enders, Weller, and Robbins (1949) initiated the tissue culture era that revolutionized all further studies on poliomyelitis. Tissue cultures provided (1) simple in vitro procedures for the isolation, identification, and typing of the polioviruses and for determination of antibodies (Robbins et al., 1951); (2) new information on the nature and epidemiology of the disease including the fact that other viruses (Coxsackie and ECHO) can cause most cases of so-called nonparalytic poliomyelitis and occasionally persistent paralytic and fatal poliomyelitis; (3) the possibility of demonstrating that polioviruses of different neurovirulence exist in nature and that polioviruses with different capacities for multiplication in the nervous system, alimentary tract, and other extraneural tissues can be artificially selected in the laboratory (Sabin, 1956; 1965a); and (4) the basis for the development of both the killed (Salk) and live, attenuated, orally administered (Sabin) poliovirus vaccines. In many parts of the world, where the oral vaccine has been used on a mass scale, the paralytic disease caused by the polioviruses has almost completely disappeared (Sabin, 1965a; 1977), and the naturally occurring polioviruses have been replaced by the attenuated vaccine strains that are excreted by millions of vaccinated children and their nonimmune contacts.

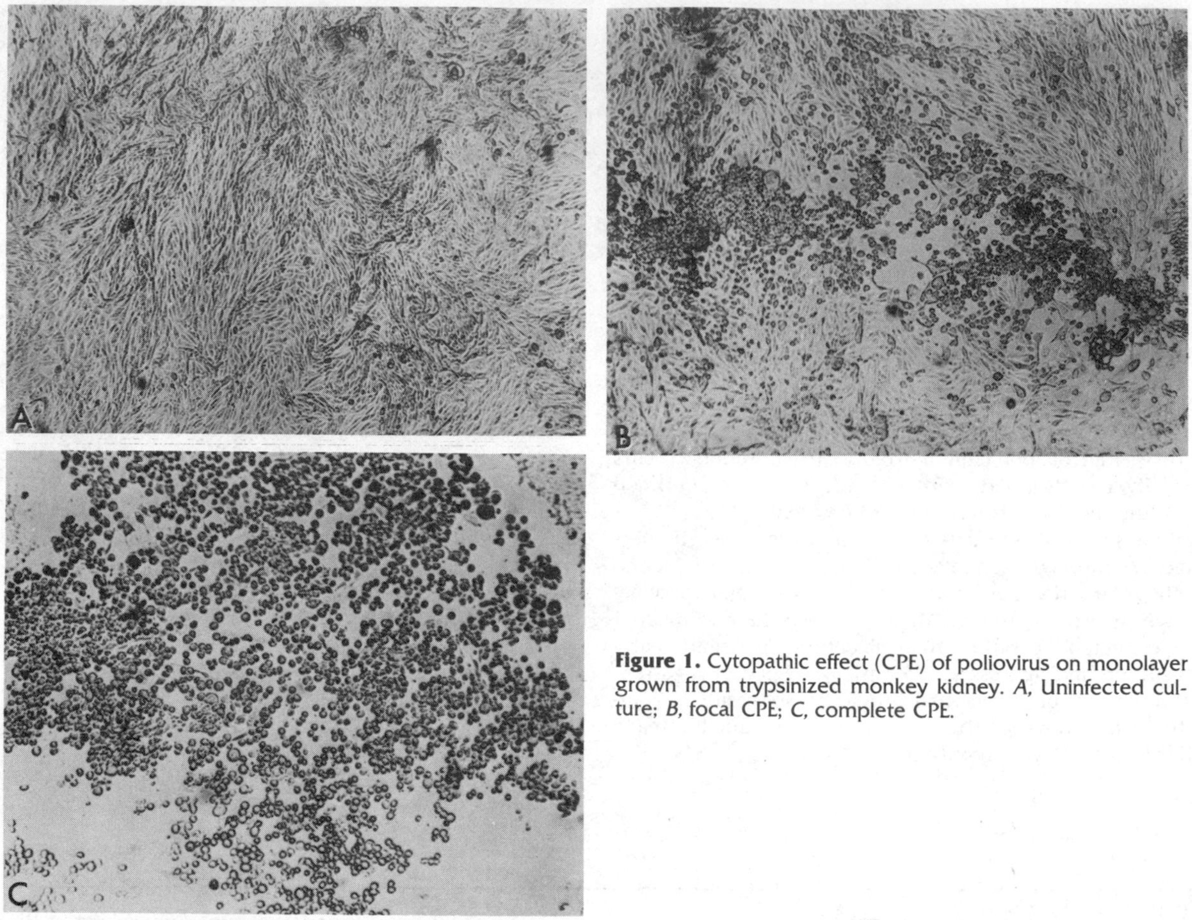

Figure 1. Cytopathic effect (CPE) of poliovirus on monolayer grown from trypsinized monkey kidney. *A*, Uninfected culture; *B*, focal CPE; *C*, complete CPE.

ETIOLOGY. Poliomyelitis is caused by enteroviruses, a group that consists of the polioviruses, the Coxsackie A and B viruses, and the ECHO viruses. These RNA viruses have a size of 15 to 30 nm (mμ), are resistant to ether, chloroform, bile, and detergents, and are stable at pH 3. Some naturally occurring strains of these viruses can produce in intrathalamically inoculated monkeys paralytic disease that is associated with the characteristically located neuronal damage and inflammatory response. All naturally occurring polioviruses, ECHO viruses, Coxsackie B viruses, and some Coxsackie A viruses multiply with production of a characteristic cytopathic effect (CPE) in monkey kidney monolayer cultures (Fig. 1). Inhibition of this CPE by appropriate sera establishes their identity and serologic type. These viruses also multiply and produce CPE in various normal and malignant human cell cultures. Naturally occurring polioviruses neither multiply nor produce CPE in monolayer cultures of nonprimate tissues. Continuous serial passages in the nervous system of monkeys can select polioviruses that multiply in vitro in the nervous but not in the non-nervous tissues of human embryos (Sabin and Olitsky, 1936) and those that do not produce CPE in monkey kidney cultures (Sabin, 1954).

Although all three serotypes of poliovirus sooner or later infect almost all human beings, about 85 per cent of the persistent paralytic cases and most of the epidemics over the years have been caused by type 1 polioviruses. In the prevaccine era, the polioviruses caused only a small proportion of "abortive" or "nonparalytic" poliomyelitis and probably about 99 per cent of the *persistent* paralytic cases. Paralytic poliomyelitis, occasionally severe and permanent, has been reportedly caused by Coxsackieviruses A7, A9, and B2 to B5 (Dalldorf and Melnick, 1965) and ECHO viruses types 1, 2, 4, 6, 7, 9, 11, 16, 18, and 30 (Melnick, 1965; Sabin et al., 1961 [for persistent ECHO 6 virus paralysis]). ECHO viruses types 2, 11 (Steigman, 1958; Steigman and Lipton, 1960), and 6 (Francis and Ceballos, 1959), and Coxsackievirus A7 (Grist, 1962) have been etiologically implicated in fatal cases of paralytic poliomyelitis.

Persistent lower motor neuron paralysis has recently been found to be caused by enterovirus types 70 and 71. The virus of acute hemorrhagic conjunctivitis (EV 70) has been found in Africa, Asia, Europe, and Oceania (Kono, 1975) and was first isolated in North America from Asian refugees in 1980. With rare exceptions, the EV 70 paralytic disease occurred in 20 to 50 year old persons in association with epidemics of acute hemorrhagic conjunctivitis (Kono et al., 1977; Hung and Kono, 1979). Enterovirus 71 epidemics with persistent and also fatal lower motor neuron paralytic disease occurred in Bulgaria in 1975 and in Hungary in 1978. Enterovirus 71 paralytic disease occurred predominantly in very young children (Sabin, 1981; Melnick, 1984).

Viral studies on 497 patients with a clinical diagnosis of paralytic poliomyelitis in 1955 to 1957 incriminated polioviruses in only 57 per cent (more often in unvaccinated than in vaccinated paralytic patients), Coxsackie and ECHO viruses in 8 per cent, mumps virus in 3 per cent, herpes simplex virus in 1 per cent, mixed infections in 1 per cent, and *no evidence of viral infection in 30 per cent* (Lennette et al., 1959). In a subsequent study (Lennette et al., 1962) on 69 patients with a clinical diagnosis of poliomyelitis, 30 per cent again yielded negative results, 13 per cent had evidence of concurrent infection with Coxsackie B or ECHO viruses, 1 per cent had mumps virus, and only 52 per cent had polioviruses. Poliovirus infection was demonstrated in 75 per cent of 35 unvaccinated paralyzed patients in this group and in only 18 per cent of 17 who had received three doses of Salk vaccine, which indicated that the proportion of other causes of clinically diagnosed paralytic poliomyelitis became relatively higher as vaccination diminished the role of the polioviruses. The clinical diagnosis of paralytic poliomyelitis, even in good hospitals, is not always made on the strict criteria that would increase the probability that the disease is the result of the neuropathologic changes of poliomyelitis (Sabin, 1981). Thus, Ramos-Alvarez (1967) isolated polioviruses from 91 per cent of 105 children under 2 years of age whose clinically diagnosed paralytic poliomyelitis was associated with fever, but from none of 74 children aged 1 to 12 years when the paralytic disease was afebrile.

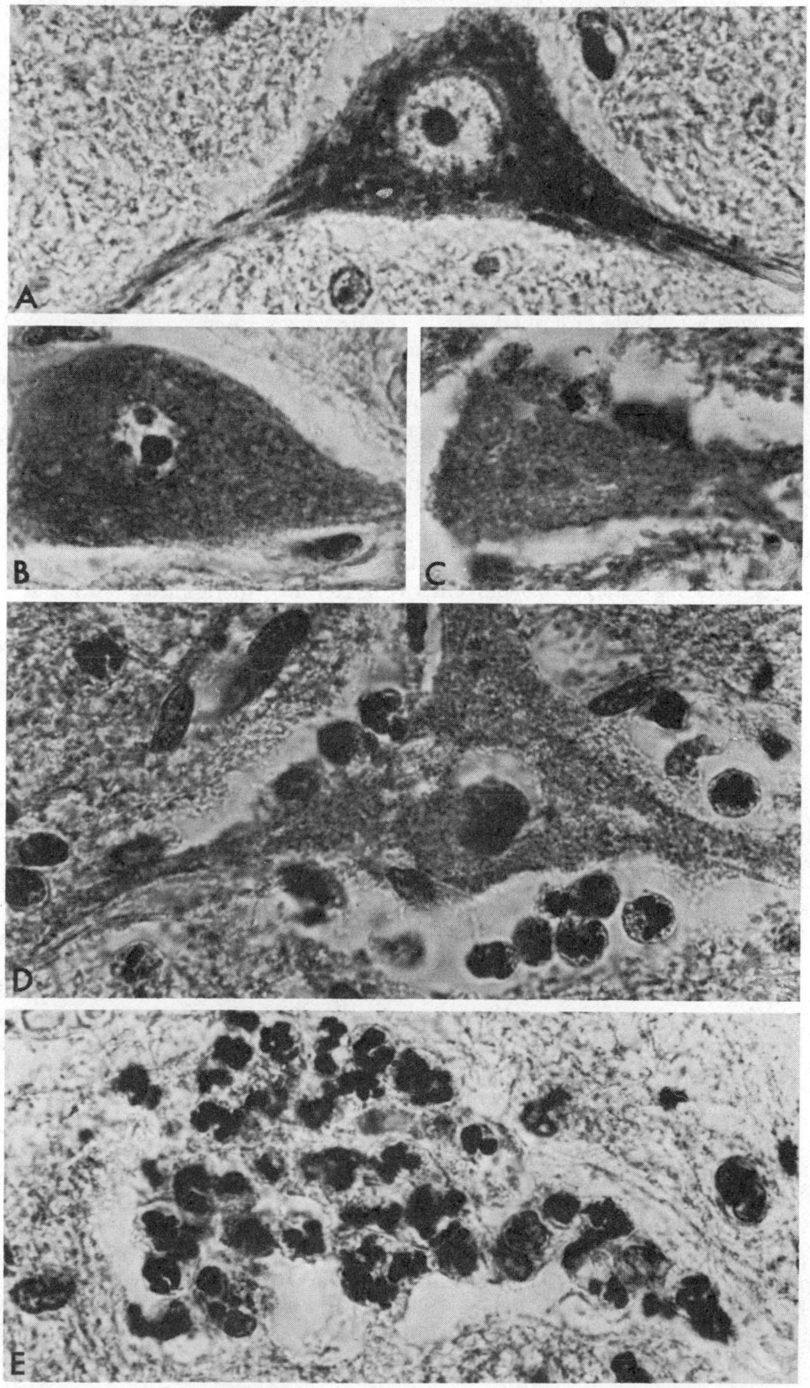

Figure 2. Successive stages in destruction of an anterior horn cell of monkeys experimentally infected by nasal route with virulent poliovirus. *A,* normal appearance about three days before onset of paralysis; *B,* diffuse chromatolysis and three acidophilic, intranuclear inclusions grouped around the darker and larger nucleolus, found almost exclusively in monkeys sacrificed one day before onset of paralysis; *C,* complete acidophilic necrosis; *D,* polymorphonuclear leukocytes invading necrotic neuron; *E,* neuronophagia by polymorphonuclear leukocytes seen during the first day of paralysis. (From Sabin, A. B., and Ward, R.: J. Exp Med 73:757, 1941.)

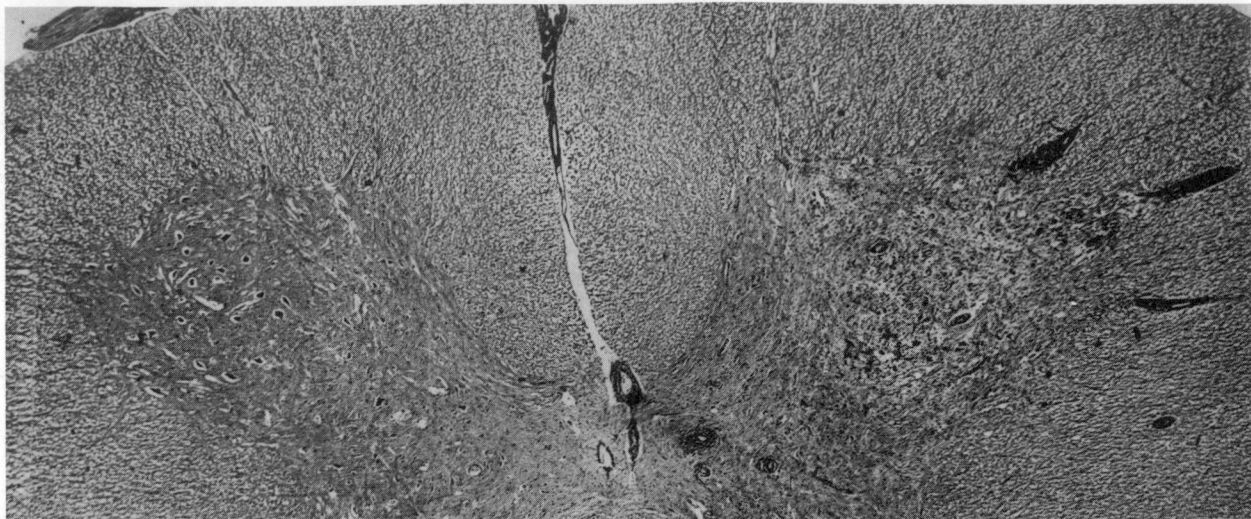

Figure 3. Anterior horn of monkey with nonparalytic poliomyelitis. Note normal architecture on left and necrosis with inflammatory reaction and perivascular infiltration on right. (From Sabin, A. B., and Ward, R.: J. Exp Med 73:757, 1941.)

PATHOLOGY. Significant virus-induced morphologic changes have been described only in the nervous system, where neuronal damage is primary and inflammatory reaction secondary. The fate of an anterior horn neuron attacked by virulent poliovirus is shown in Figure 2. The location, extent, and persistence of paralysis depend on the location and number of neurons so affected. Since any one muscle fibril is innervated by motoneurons from several levels of the spinal cord, even extensive destruction of anterior horn cells limited to one level of the spinal cord can occur in nonparalytic infections as was found in monkeys with nonparalytic poliomyelitis (Fig. 3). In experimental nonparalytic and transitory paralytic poliomyelitis in monkeys (Sabin and Ward, 1941a), one finds not only complete destruction of some neurons, resulting in neuronophagia, but also partial degenerative changes of chromatolysis and acidophilic-intranuclear inclusions from which the cells may recover (Fig. 4). The inflammatory cells in the meninges represent an overflow from the interstitial and perivascular infiltration that follows neuronal damage. The familiar spasm of the neck and back, along with other so-called signs of "meningeal irritation" actually are early manifestations of neuronal damage.

In human poliomyelitis, the extent of involvement of the spinal motoneurons observed postmortem depends on the neural pathways that first brought the virus to the CNS and on the duration of paralysis before death occurs. Figure 5A shows an essentially normal anterior horn of the lumbar cord of a patient who died within 24 hours after onset of palatal and pharyngeal paralysis. An anterior horn from the lumbar cord of a patient with bulbar poliomyelitis of somewhat longer duration shows only a few foci of neuronophagia and perivascular infiltration in the midst of a majority of intact neurons (Fig. 5B). In patients who die within a few days after onset of paralysis in the extremities the motoneurons in the lumbar cord are completely destroyed (Fig. 6). The relative distribution of neuronal lesions in the spinal cord and medulla in bulbar and spinal poliomyelitis is shown in Figure 7. Dorsal root ganglions show neuronophagia and interstitial infiltration (Fig. 8). In cynomolgus monkeys, experimentally infected by the oral route, poliovirus was demonstrated in the regional ganglia of the alimentary tract when no virus was found in the CNS (Verlinde et al., 1955).

The medulla has neuronal lesions in the nuclei of various cranial nerves, in the vestibular nuclei, and in the reticular formation. The cerebellum has neuronal lesions in the roof nuclei and vermis but not in the hemispheres. The midbrain has lesions in the periaqueductal gray matter, tectum, and tegmentum. Neuronal lesions are also present in the thalamus, hypothalamus, globus pallidus, and motor cortex, especially in area 4 of Brodmann. This localization differentiates the pathology of poliomyelitis from the more diffuse lesions seen in human encephalitis produced by a variety of different viruses.

PATHOGENESIS. The pathogenesis of the disease in human beings is determined by (1) the extent of viral multiplication at the portal of entry in the alimentary tract; (2) the extent (if any) of multiplication in other extraneural tissues after the virus finds its way into the bloodstream from the lymph nodes draining the initial sites of viral multiplication; (3) the neurovirulence of the invading virus, which determines its capacity to invade the sensory neurons supplying the extraneural sites of viral multiplication and then to multiply in them sufficiently to spread to the motoneurons; and finally, (4) capacity of the virus that reaches the initial motoneurons to multiply in them enough to progress to and destroy the numerous motoneurons required to produce clinical paralysis.

The experimental studies on chimpanzees and cynomolgus monkeys that develop paralysis following ingestion of appropriate strains of polioviruses have been helpful in indicating potential pathogenic mechanisms but not in showing precisely what happens in man, because the relative susceptibility of the upper and lower alimentary tracts and nervous system has been found to be quantitatively different in monkeys, chimpanzees, and humans (Sabin, 1956). The source of virus spread among humans must be the feces of infected persons because virus multiplying in the oropharynx is not found in the mouth, gums, or anterior third of the tongue. Moreover, the predominant

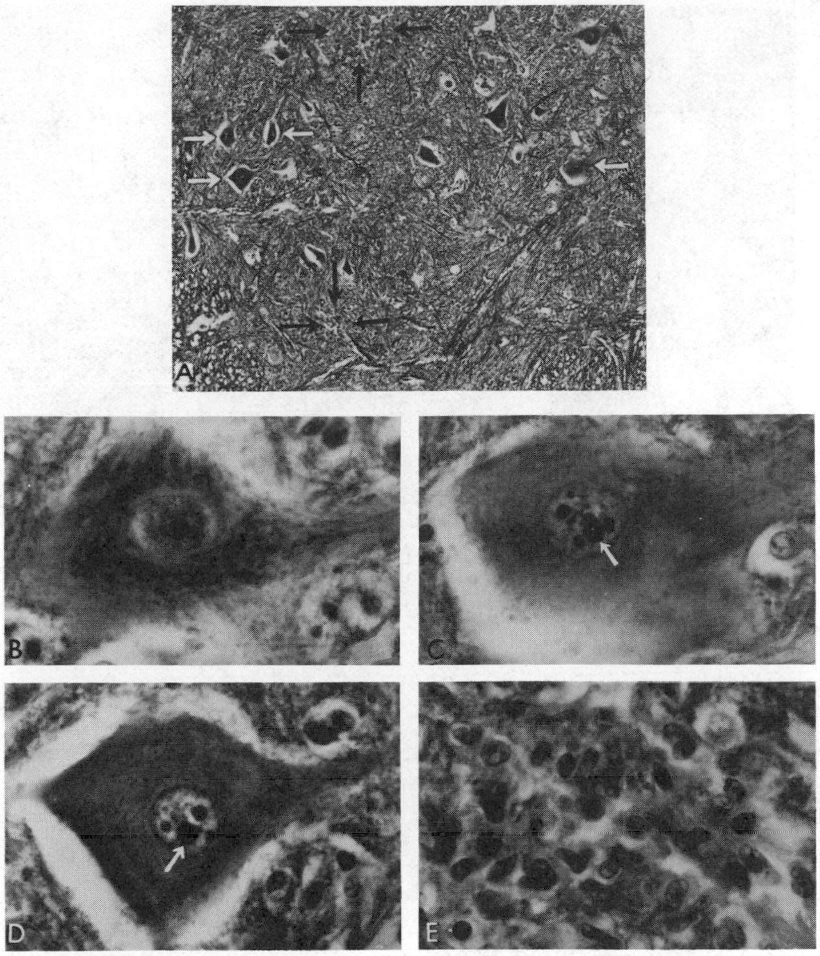

Figure 4. *A,* Anterior horn in spinal cord of monkey killed two days after spontaneous recovery from paralysis of lower extremities; black arrows point to foci of glial neuronophagia shown enlarged in *E* and white arrows point to neurons with diffuse chromatolysis and acidophilic intranuclear inclusions shown enlarged in *C* and *D* with arrows pointing to basophilic nucleoli; *B,* one of only two almost normal neurons in *A.* (From Sabin, A. B., and Ward, R.: J. Exp Med 73:757, 1941.)

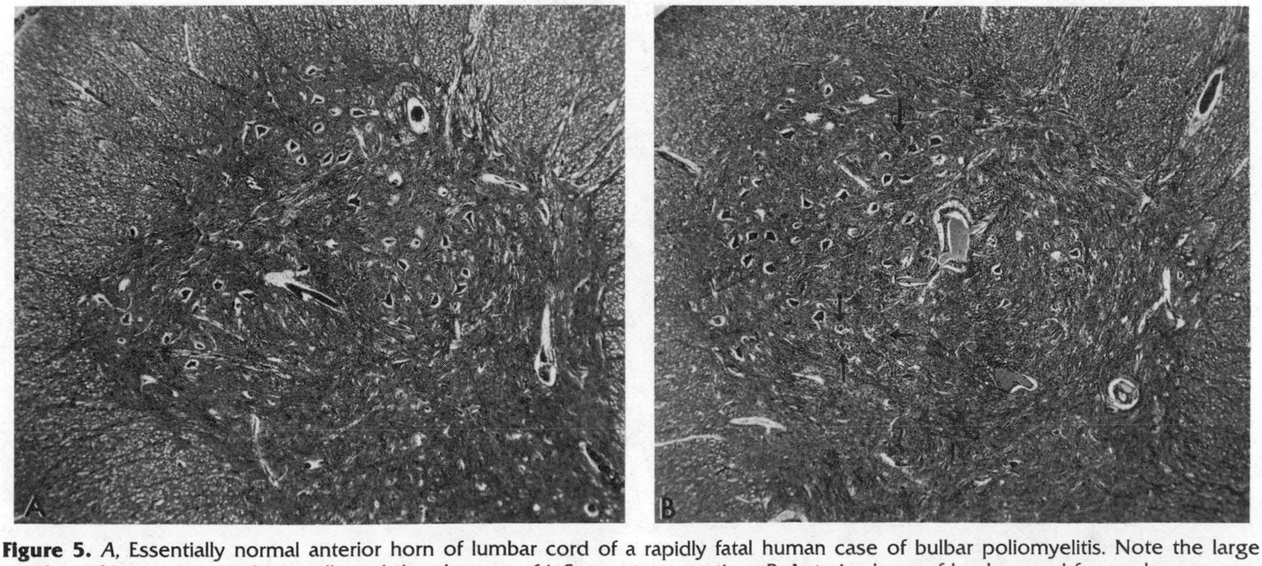

Figure 5. *A,* Essentially normal anterior horn of lumbar cord of a rapidly fatal human case of bulbar poliomyelitis. Note the large number of intact anterior horn cells and the absence of inflammatory reaction. *B,* Anterior horn of lumbar cord from a human case of bulbar poliomyelitis. Note foci of neuronophagia (arrows) and perivascular infiltration in the midst of many normal neurons. (From Sabin, A. B.: JAMA 120:506, 1942.)

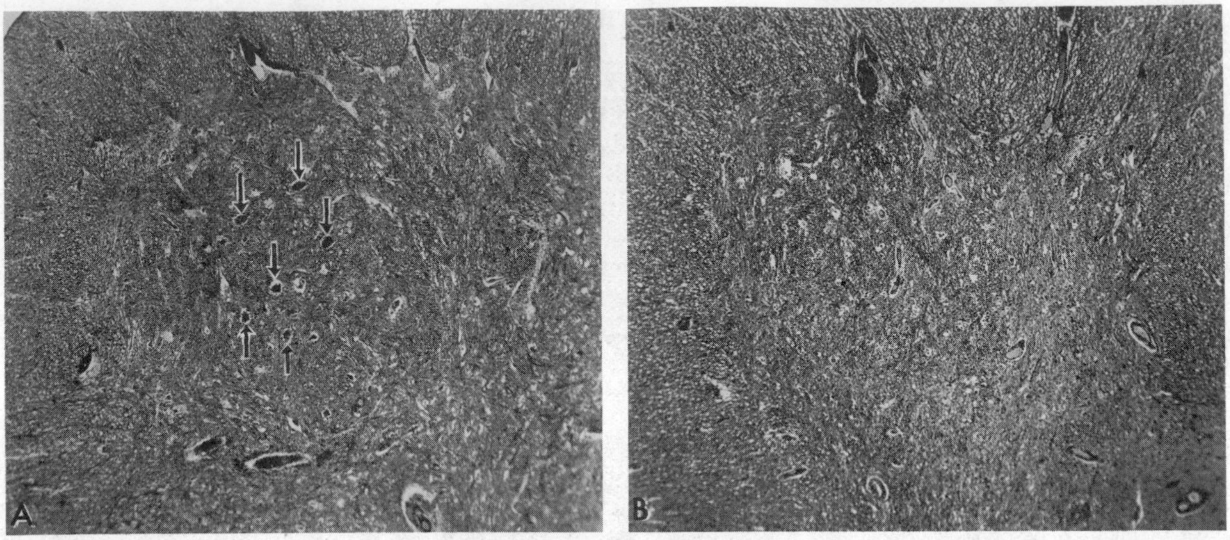

Figure 6. *A,* Anterior horn of lumbar cord from a human case of initial spinal paralysis. Note destruction of all anterior horn cells and few remaining foci of neuronophagia (arrows). *B,* Anterior horn of lumbar cord from a human case of initial spinal paralysis of somewhat longer duration than that in *A.* Note complete disappearance of all neurons. (From Sabin, A. B.: JAMA 120:506, 1942.)

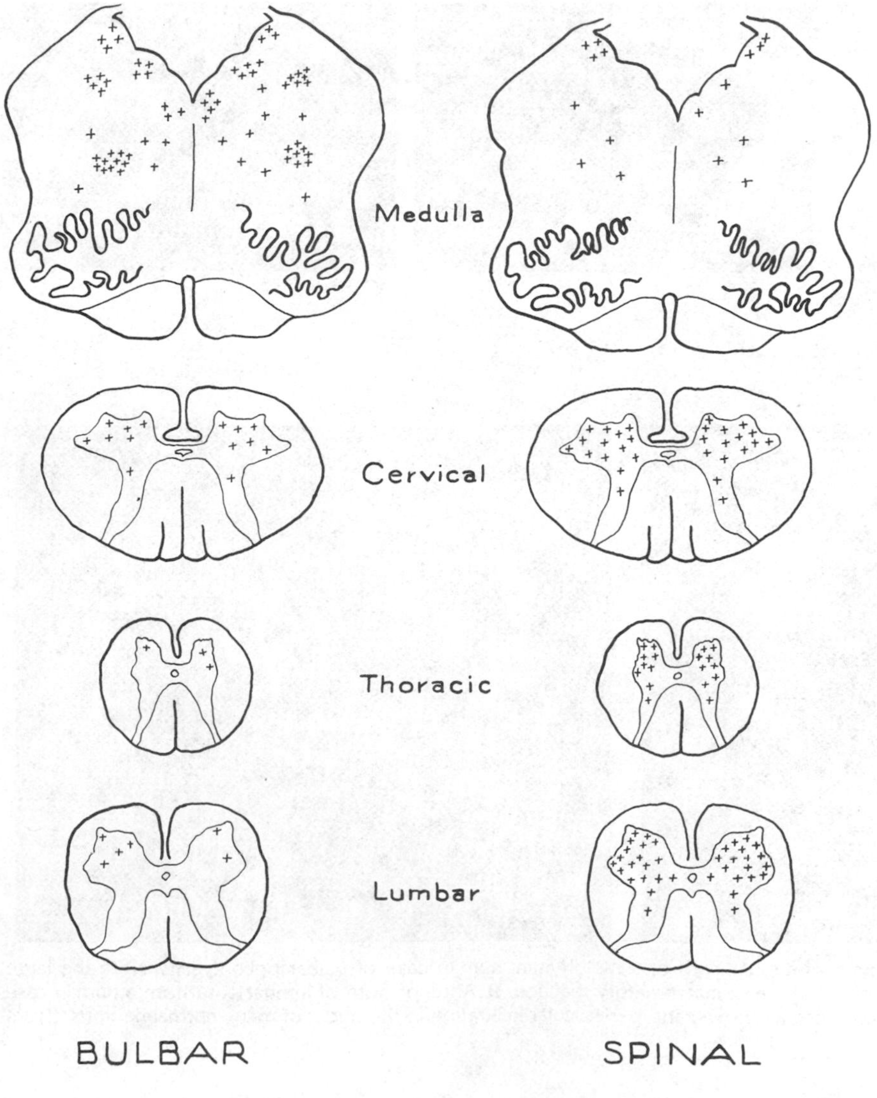

Figure 7. Distribution of neuronal lesions in primary bulbar and primary spinal human poliomyelitis. (From Sabin, A. B.: JAMA 120:506, 1942.)

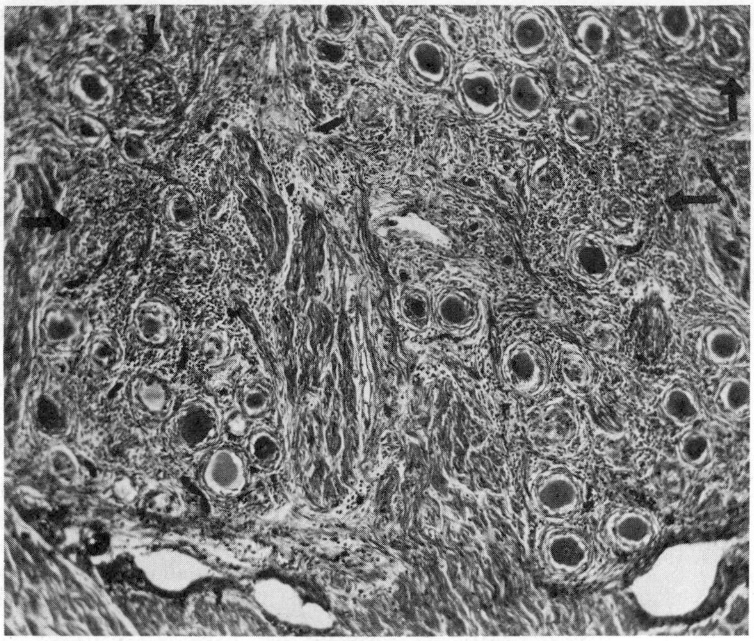

Figure 8. Spinal dorsal root ganglion in human poliomyelitis. Note destruction of some neurons, focal neuronophagia, and interstitial cellular infiltration. (From Sabin, A. B.: JAMA 120:506, 1942.)

dissemination of the viruses during hot weather in countries with high standards of sanitation and hygiene in temperate climates is in accord with fecal-borne rather than with pharyngeal transmission.

Figure 9 shows a schema of the possible pathogenesis of human poliomyelitis (Sabin, 1956). The virus enters by way of the mouth on contaminated fingers or food and not by aspirated droplets. When the amount of ingested virus is less than 100,000 to one million tissue culture infective doses—and only under exceptional circumstances can it be assumed to be as much or more—it is usually swallowed without multiplication in the oropharynx. After passing through the stomach, the virus attaches itself to the superficial epithelium of the intestinal mucosa, and multiplication occurs within 24 hours. The virus is shed in the lumen and spreads from one superficial group of cells to another until

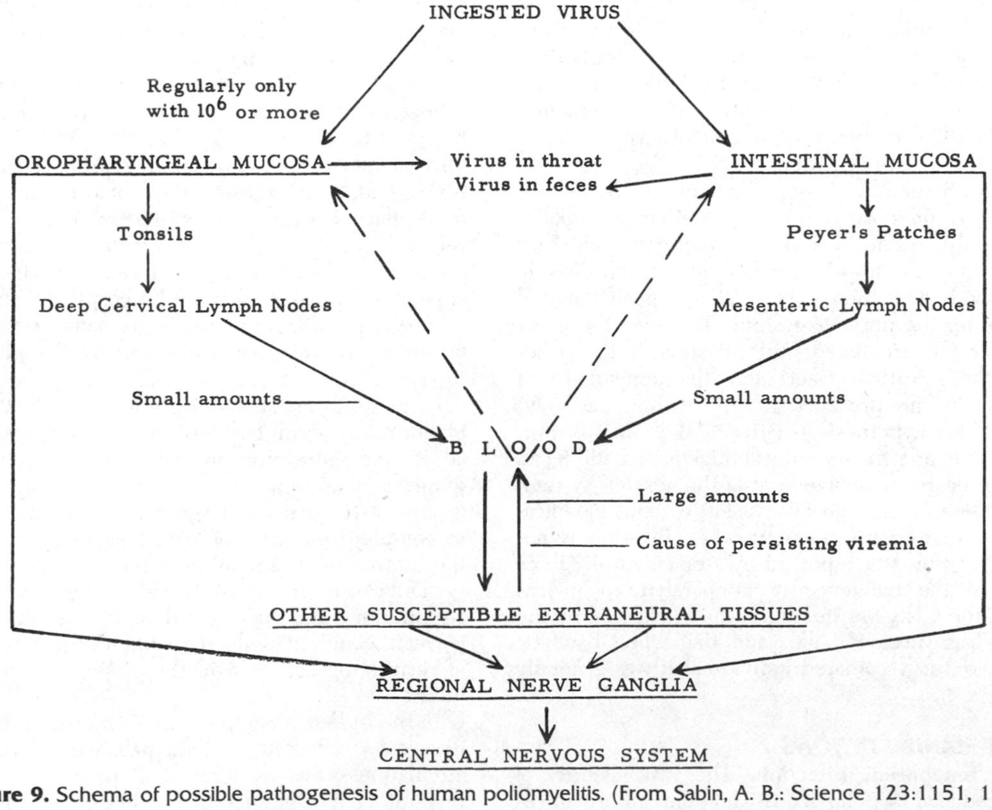

Figure 9. Schema of possible pathogenesis of human poliomyelitis. (From Sabin, A. B.: Science 123:1151, 1956.)

local resistance halts further propagation, which may not happen for many weeks after initial infection and development of antibody. From the intestinal mucosa, virus is absorbed into the regional lymph nodes, from which small amounts may escape into the bloodstream before early local antibody formation. The appearance of larger amounts of virus in the bloodstream must depend on the capacity of a particular strain of virus to multiply in other extraneural tissues, because extensive multiplication of certain attenuated strains in the intestinal tract of human beings is not usually associated with detectable viremia, and intramuscular injection of as much as one million tissue culture infective doses of such a strain produces neither viremia, intestinal infection, nor antibody formation. However, with the usual paralytogenic strains, larger amounts of virus appear in the blood early after infection (Horstmann et al., 1954; Bodian and Paffenberger, 1954). Secondary spread to the oropharyngeal mucosa accounts for the high frequency of recovery of virus from the throat of patients with clinical signs of systemic illness. From various sites of multiplication in the alimentary tract and other extraneural tissues, the virus is assumed to invade the corresponding sensory peripheral ganglia. If the amount of virus is large enough and the strain sufficiently neurotropic, enough multiplication occurs in the first group of sensory neurons to permit spread by axonal pathways to the corresponding area of the CNS. This course of events would account for the hyperesthesias, paresthesias, and pain so often noted especially in adults before onset of paralysis, and for the different localizations of paralysis depending on the parts of the spinal cord or medulla that are invaded. After invasion of the CNS, the virus also progresses across synaptic junctions and insulated axonal pathways; the extent of progression and the number of neurons affected is influenced by the neurovirulence of the virus. According to this interpretation of the available data and observed phenomena, placentally transmitted or killed virus vaccine-induced antibody, which does not prevent multiplication in the superficial cells of the intestinal mucosa, could prevent or limit secondary spread to other extraneural tissues and thereby reduce the amount of virus available for invasion of the sensory ganglia.

According to Bodian's view of pathogenesis (1955), which is based largely on observations in chimpanzees, polioviruses multiply in the lymphatic structures and other extraneuronal tissues, invade the nervous system directly from the blood, and then spread along specific neural pathways within the nervous system. This hypothesis explains neither the prolonged multiplication of the polioviruses in the intestinal tract after the appearance of antibody nor in the presence of pre-existing antibody. Moreover, if this hypothesis is correct, the effect of pre-existing antibody on primary natural infection should be all or none with regard to involvement of the nervous system, that is, complete prevention of invasion without modification of the extent of involvement when invasion is not prevented. Yet the data reported by Francis et al. (1955) indicated that the incidence of nonparalytic poliovirus infections of the CNS was not significantly affected by the killed poliovirus vaccine (Salk), and that when paralytic disease occurred in vaccinated individuals it was generally milder.

CLINICAL MANIFESTATIONS

Clinically Inapparent Infection. The vast majority of infections produced by polioviruses and other enteroviruses are clinically inapparent or unrecognized. Differences in virulence (i.e., tissue affinities) of naturally occurring viruses and other factors such as amount of virus ingested, interference by other enteroviruses, or infections modified by placentally transmitted or breast milk-ingested antibodies, are probably responsible for the very high incidence of inapparent infections.

"Minor Illness." So-called minor illness is characterized by fever, sore throat, headache, nausea and vomiting, anorexia, and abdominal pain lasting a few hours to a few days. Enteroviruses generally, as well as other viruses, can cause the same type of illness. These symptoms are usually not associated with spinal fluid pleocytosis and are not a consequence of involvement of the CNS.

Nonparalytic or "Major Illness." This illness includes the various manifestations of the "minor illness," often in more severe form, plus pain and stiffness of the neck, back, and legs (demonstrable by the tripod sign when sitting up, and by the kiss the knee, Kernig's, and Brudzinski's signs). These signs, as well as occasional hyperesthesias and paresthesias, indicate involvement of neurons before appearance of paralysis. The cerebrospinal fluid (CSF) during this period shows an increased number of leukocytes (usually between 15 and 500 cells per cubic mm) with a predominance of polymorphonuclear cells early and of lymphocytes later. The protein concentration is normal or slightly elevated at first and increases later as the leukocytes disappear. Glucose level is normal. This syndrome, also called "aseptic meningitis," can be caused by many enteroviruses as well as by other viruses. Most cases of what was reported as nonparalytic poliomyelitis before the early 1950s were not caused by polioviruses.

Paralytic Poliomyelitis. The paralytic disease, fulfilling the clinical criteria for a diagnosis of poliomyelitis, is occasionally preceded by the "minor illness" and usually by the "major illness." Excruciating muscle pain and spasm may precede or accompany onset of paralysis of the extremities. Localized hyperesthesia, fasciculation of muscle groups, loss or diminution of cremasteric and abdominal reflexes, and hyperactivity of the deep tendon reflexes may be indicators of pending paralysis. Paralysis may develop fully in one or two days or increasing weakness may be present for two or three days before the appearance of frank, flaccid paralysis associated with loss of deep tendon reflexes, which usually does not progress further after the temperature has returned to normal. The paralytic disease appears in spinal, bulbar, or bulbospinal form.

In the *spinal form* there can be asymmetric involvement of any of the muscles innervated by the motoneurons in the spinal cord—that is, legs, abdomen, back, intercostals, diaphragm, arms, shoulder girdle, or neck. Paralysis of the bladder may accompany paralysis of the legs, especially in adults and more often in males, but is usually transitory. Paralysis may remain localized in certain large muscle groups of the arms and legs but occasionally can progress to complete paralysis of both legs and arms. Paralysis of the intercostal and diaphragmatic muscles is life-threatening and causes great anxiety and restlessness in the patient. Respirations are shallow and rapid but regular, the voice is weak, cough is ineffective, and all the accessory muscles of respiration are used in the struggle to get air into the lungs.

In the *bulbar form* the muscles innervated by the cranial nerves are affected, and disturbances of respiration and circulation occur as a result of neuronal damage in the respiratory and vasomotor centers of the medulla. Weak-

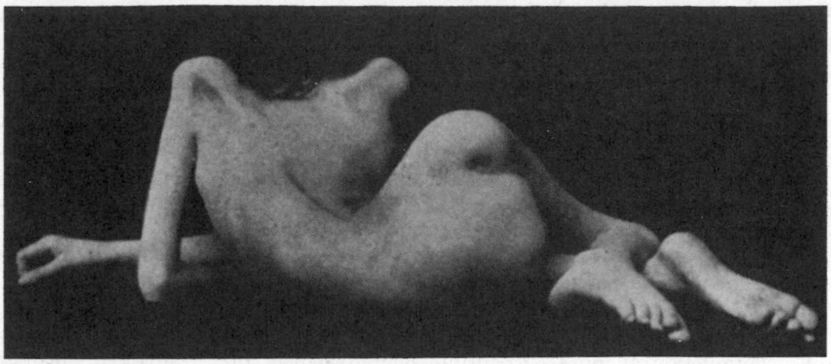

Figure 10. Severe, untreated infantile paralysis of nine years' duration. Extensive scoliosis, contraction of both hips and both knees, double knock-knee, severe equinus of one foot, and paralysis of one arm. (From Lovett, R. W.: The Treatment of Infantile Paralysis. Philadelphia, Blakiston's Son and Company, 1916.)

ness or paralysis of the soft palate, pharynx, and vocal cords, resulting from damage in the vagal nuclei, causes difficulty in swallowing, accumulation of pharyngeal secretions, regurgitation through the nose, nasal voice, hoarseness, and occasionally laryngeal stridor. Peripheral facial paralysis, and less often ocular palsies, pupillary disturbances, and paralysis of the tongue and masticator muscles are also seen. Involvement of the eleventh cranial motoneurons manifests itself by weakness or paralysis of the trapezius and sternocleidomastoid muscles. Involvement of the respiratory center neurons gives rise to the most serious manifestation of bulbar poliomyelitis, that is, respiratory failure resulting from irregularities in rhythm, depth, and rate. Shallow respirations with irregular periods of apnea of varying duration and Cheyne-Stokes respiration lead to acid-base imbalance, confusion, delirium, and coma. Circulatory disturbances due to involvement of the vasomotor center are indicated by a flushed, dusky facies with cherry-red lips progressing to mottled cyanosis, a pulse of 150 to 200 per minute that may be irregular and difficult to palpate, and a fluctuating blood pressure with a small pulse pressure.

The *bulbospinal form* may either begin with bulbar manifestations and descend to produce spinal manifestations, or cause ascending paralysis.

In the 90 to 95 per cent of patients who survive the most severe forms of the disease, the further course of the paralytic disease is in most instances stationary for a period of days or weeks after the temperature returns to normal. Improvement may then occur during the subsequent year or two. Atrophy of paralyzed muscles appears within less than eight weeks. When extensive paralysis occurs early in life, growth of paralyzed extremities is arrested, and severe deformities result from involvement of the back, chest, and shoulder muscles (Figs. 10 and 11).

COMPLICATIONS. In patients with disturbances of deglutition and respiration, the airways become obstructed, and pulmonary atelectasis or pneumonia may be fatal. Long immobilization of extensively paralyzed patients may lead to decalcification of bones with high concentrations of calcium in the blood and urine and formation of kidney stones.

GEOGRAPHIC VARIATION IN DISEASE. Fecal-borne microbial agents, including the polioviruses and other enteroviruses, are maximally disseminated during hot weather. Accordingly, the summer and early autumn months were the peak months for the occurrence of endemic and epidemic paralytic poliomyelitis in countries with temperate climates before the disease was controlled by vaccination. In tropical and subtropical countries, dissemination of these viruses and the resulting disease occur throughout the year. In countries with poor sanitation and hygiene, which predominate in the tropical and subtropical regions of the world, dissemination of these viruses is constant and is so extensive that most children become infected very early in life. Whatever paralytic disease occurs under these conditions is truly infantile paralysis because most cases occur in children under 2 years of age. In tropical and subtropical communities, paralysis was until recently believed to be uncommon, incomplete persistent paralysis often goes unrecognized until children begin to walk, and epidemics were rare. However, large epidemics have occurred in Africa and elsewhere when such popula-

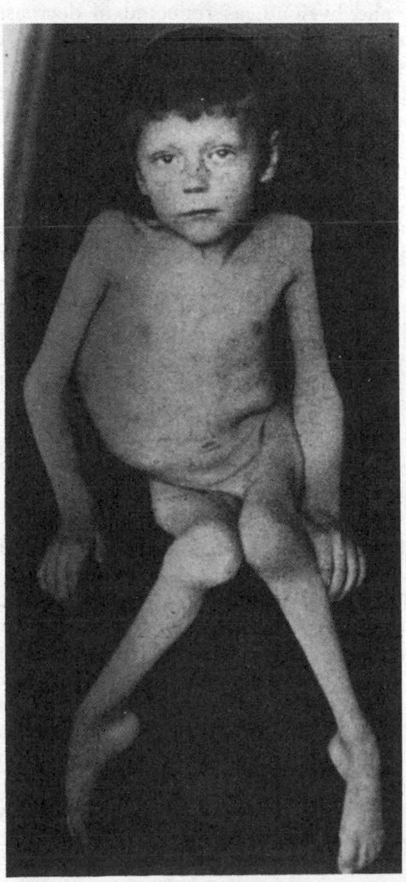

Figure 11. Extensive paralysis and deformity in untreated infantile paralysis. (From Römer, P. H.: Epidemic Infantile Paralysis (English translation). New York, Prentice, 1913.)

tion groups have left their villages and congregated in large numbers in very crowded conditions to work in large development projects. Most of the paralytic cases in these epidemics still occur in children under 2 years of age, indicating that the older children had acquired immunity from inapparent infections in their small communities.

Increasing numbers of older children and adults began to have paralytic poliomyelitis in countries with temperate climates when improved sanitation and hygiene, better housing with less crowding, and higher living standards for ever larger numbers of people diminished the dissemination of all enteroviruses and postponed the age at which immunity was naturally acquired. The same factors led to the accumulation of more susceptible people, which, together with increased opportunities for the spread of highly neurovirulent polioviruses provided by increasing mobility of populations, led to the emergence of large-scale summer epidemics at different times in different countries.

A study that I carried out in Brazil in 1980 showed that small epidemics, affecting children predominantly under three years, also occur with considerable frequency in tropical and subtropical areas. In Brazil, such epidemics often begin in September-December of one year and continue until March-May of the following year, lasting four to eight months instead of four to eight weeks, the usual duration of epidemics in temperate climates in the prevaccine era (Sabin, 1981).

The old dogma that paralytic poliomyelitis is rare in tropical, economically underdeveloped countries until there is a marked improvement in the standard of living, sanitation, and hygiene, as reflected in decreasing infant mortality rates, has been found to be a fallacy, especially by surveys for residual paralysis in school-age children in Africa, Asia, and Latin America. These "lameness" surveys have shown that the number of officially reported cases is but a small and varying fraction of the actual number that can be estimated to have occurred (Sabin, 1980). Even in the absence of recognized epidemics, the estimated average annual incidence of paralytic poliomyelitis in rural and urban tropical regions has been found to be as high or higher than the average of 135 paralytic cases per annum per million total population in the USA during the five years in the pre-poliovaccine era (Sabin, 1981). The lameness surveys in Ghana, Burma, the Philippines, Indonesia, Thailand, Malawi, Ivory Coast (summarized by Sabin, 1981) and Brazil (Sabin and Silva, 1983) yielded estimates of 123 to 589 paralytic cases for the average annual incidence per million total population in regions with limited or no vaccination programs (see also Bernier, 1984).

DIAGNOSIS. A clinical diagnosis of paralytic poliomyelitis is based on a history of an acute febrile illness, associated signs and symptoms of "aseptic meningitis," and appearance during the febrile period of asymmetric, flaccid, lower motor neuron type of muscle paralysis accompanied by loss of deep tendon reflexes. The paralysis usually fails to progress significantly after defervescence. Pleocytosis of the spinal fluid during the first week after onset of paralysis is essential for establishing the diagnosis of poliomyelitis, because noninflammatory lower motor neuron paralytic syndromes without pleocytosis resemble poliomyelitis but are pathologically distinct. In postmortem studies on 57 Mexican children with acute lower motor neuron paralytic disease, Ramos-Alvarez et al. (1969) found the neuropathologic changes of poliomyelitis in only 32. Among the remaining 25 without inflammatory changes in the CNS, 10 exhibited the neuropathologic changes of polyradiculitis and 15 presented hitherto unrecognized neuropathologic syndromes. Eight showed widespread and extensive "cytoplasmic neuronopathy" and 7 showed "nuclear neuronopathy." Although 7 of 9 patients with polyradiculitis showed albumino-cytologic dissociation during the first week after onset of paralysis, only 1 of the 14 patients with the other noninflammatory neuropathologic syndromes tested during the first week after onset of paralysis had a slightly elevated concentration of CSF protein. From a differential diagnosis point of view, it is noteworthy that in 23 of the 25 patients with noninflammatory paralytic syndromes, there was no fever at onset of paralysis and none exhibited nuchal or spinal rigidity. It is also noteworthy that virologic tests on the spinal cords of 17 of the patients with the noninflammatory lower motor neuron paralytic syndromes were negative, but in one of these patients (a 2-year-old child with nuclear neuronopathy who died three days after onset of paralysis), type 1 poliovirus was recovered in repeated tests from suspensions of colon, jejunum, ileum, and mesenteric lymph nodes. This important finding, as well as the presence of enteroviruses in the stools of seven other paralytic patients who showed no neuropathologic evidence of poliomyelitis, emphasizes the fact that mere isolation of a poliovirus or other enterovirus from the intestinal tract does not by itself prove an etiologic role of the virus in the paralytic condition. The statement in some textbooks (Bodian and Horstmann, 1965; Krugman et al., 1977) that the CSF may remain normal in a small proportion, or 10 per cent, of poliomyelitis cases even in the presence of severe paralysis, is not supported by acceptable evidence. The recently recognized infantile infectious botulism syndrome (Berg, 1977; Arnon et al., 1977), characterized by constipation, general weakness, paralysis of neck muscles, and dysfunction of various cranial nerves, can be confused with bulbar poliomyelitis but has no pleocytosis and usually no fever. Bell's palsy and a predominantly motor neuritis in older persons, occasionally misdiagnosed as poliomyelitis, are also without pleocytosis. A critical evaluation of the available data indicates that a diagnosis of poliomyelitis should not be made in patients without pleocytosis during the *first week* after onset of paralysis, especially when there is neither fever nor nuchal or spinal rigidity at the first appearance of paralysis.

Paralytic conditions associated with pleocytosis that occasionally are confused with paralytic poliomyelitis include transverse myelitis and postinfectious myelitis when the lesions are located predominantly in the gray matter. Encephalomyelitis caused by arboviruses, mumps, or herpesvirus have in atypical forms occasionally erroneously been diagnosed as bulbar poliomyelitis (Sabin, 1981).

A valid clinical-pathologic diagnosis of poliomyelitis does not establish the etiologic diagnosis per se. However, as discussed previously under Etiology, *concurrent* infection with *naturally occurring* polioviruses (established by isolation of virus from the stools or throat and by a rising titer of antibody *shortly after onset* of paralysis) may in the prevaccine era have been responsible for about 99 per cent of all the *correctly* diagnosed cases of *persistent* poliomyelitic paralysis. Incrimination of enteroviruses in the etiology of poliomyelitic paralysis must depend not only on isolation of the virus and evidence of *concurrent* infection by antibody tests but also on the demonstration that wild polioviruses have not caused infection at the time of the clinical manifestations. In countries where paralytic poliomyelitis has become exceedingly rare following extensive use of oral poliovirus vaccine, the mere demonstration of concurrent infection with a poliovirus vaccine strain does not establish it as the etiologic agent of the paralytic condition; the mere failure to isolate other potentially neurovirulent enteroviruses from the intestinal tract shortly after onset of paralysis does not exclude the demonstrated possibility that it may have been there prior to onset of clinical illness and subsequently been replaced by poliovirus vaccine strains (Sabin, 1963; 1969; 1980; 1981).

TREATMENT. During the acute paralytic phase of the disease, treatment should relieve pain and discomfort and deal with spinal or medullary respiratory failure or airway obstruction from aspirated fluids. If facilities are inadequate for proper home care or for prompt transfer to a hospital during an emergency, the patient should be hospitalized as soon as possible after onset of paralysis. Complete rest in a hard bed with a footboard is essential. Changes in posture are helpful for relief of discomfort and essential when the respiratory muscles are weak. Pain and muscle spasm can be relieved by judiciously applied hot packs for 20-minute periods several times a day. Aspirin and codeine relieve headache and generalized pain and discomfort. Sedatives that depress respiration should be avoided. Catheterization should be avoided for urinary retention that may respond to parasympathomimetics. Constipation and abdominal distention may be relieved by small doses of neostigmine. Voluntary movements of partly paralyzed extremities and passive movements of extensively paralyzed extremities should be started as soon as pain disappears.

Swallowing problems need special care. Mechanical suction and postural drainage should be used to prevent secretions from blocking the airway. Tracheostomy should be performed when these measures prove to be inadequate, or when paralysis of the vocal cords, ineffective cough, and laryngeal stridor result in life-threatening respiratory embarrassment—preferably before bouts of choking and cyanosis begin. Respiratory failure of medullary origin should not be treated in a tank respirator in the absence of tracheostomy or when throat secretions cannot be adequately removed. Humidified oxygen (40 to 60 per cent and in emergencies 100 per cent for brief periods) can be given through the tracheostomy tube. A cuffed tracheostomy tube may be used for positive pressure respiration when artificial respiration is required.

Respiratory embarrassment resulting from paralysis of intercostal muscles and the diaphragm, without bulbar involvement, is best treated in a tank respirator during the acute progressive phase of paralysis as soon as the vital capacity falls to less than 50 per cent. When no tank respirator is available, Thompson's method of artificial respiration (1935) can be life-saving in patients with rapidly progressing paralysis. It consists of "lifting the pelvis of a subject in the prone position and allowing it to fall back to the floor" (Fig. 12) six to ten times per minute. This procedure, combined with the Schafer prone pressure method after the patient is lowered to the floor, produces a large respiratory exchange. When possible, weaning from the tank respirator should begin as soon as paralysis stops progressing. Pulmonary atelectasis, a frequent complication of respiratory failure, may require bronchoscopic aspiration. Pulmonary infection is not prevented by prophylactic antibiotics, but when it occurs it requires antibiotics for treatment.

A

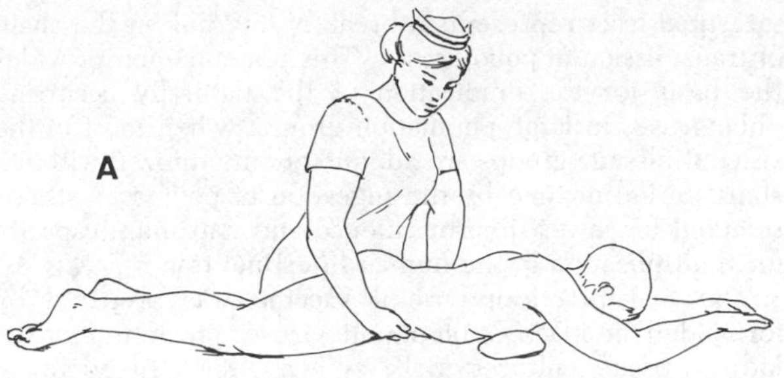

Position of patient.

B

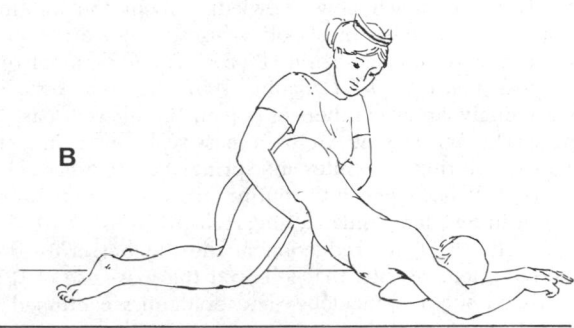

Procedure by operator.

Figure 12. Emergency artificial respiration for spinal respiratory paralysis when tank respirator is not available. *A,* Patient is in prone position on a hard surface. A folded coat or small pillow is placed beneath the clavicles and upper part of chest. *B,* Operator, kneeling or seated on a low chair, puts one hand beneath each anterior superior spine and lifts the pelvis off the ground until the back arches and the abdomen sags down. The patient is then slowly lowered to the original position. At this point the chest may be compressed by pushing downward and forward over the lower ribs to obtain additional air exchange. (From Thompson, T. C.: JAMA 104:307, 1935.)

Proper physiotherapy and orthopedic intervention, when indicated after the acute phase of paralysis is over, can help to achieve the maximum possible return of muscle function and prevent the tragic crippling deformities shown in Figures 10 and 11.

PROPHYLAXIS. Natural infection with polioviruses, even in the absence of reinfection (Paul et al., 1951), provides lifelong immunity that is associated with neutralizing antibodies in the blood and partial or complete resistance of the intestinal tract to reinfection (Sabin, 1957; 1965a). Resistance of the intestinal tract has been found in some individuals in the absence of demonstrable neutralizing antibodies both after natural infection and after experimental infection of volunteers with attenuated strains. Placentally transmitted antibody does not confer intestinal resistance to poliovirus infection. The incomplete intestinal resistance in some persons with antibody acquired after natural infection or after ingestion of attenuated strains is characterized by brief periods of limited viral multiplication that usually are insufficient for transmission. This limited intestinal reinfection in persons with infection-acquired immunity usually induces complete resistance to subsequent infection even by very large doses. Each resistant intestinal tract represents a break of one link in the chain of transmission of polioviruses. This phenomenon provides the basis for the eradication of the naturally occurring polioviruses in large population groups, when most of the susceptible age groups are adequately immunized within a short period of time by the ingestion of poliovirus strains selected for lowest neurovirulence and maximum capacity for multiplication in the human intestinal tract.

The first practically useful vaccine was prepared by formaldehyde inactivation of polioviruses grown in monkey kidney tissue cultures (Salk et al., 1954). In adequate dosage the inactiviated poliovirus vaccine (IPV) produces neutralizing antibodies that can protect against paralytic poliomyelitis caused by the polioviruses (Francis et al., 1955). The development of an acceptable live, attenuated vaccine for oral administration (OPV) depended on the acquisition of much new knowledge about the multiple properties and behavior of polioviruses in monkeys, chimpanzees, and humans (Sabin, 1965a). The OPV in current use was ready in 1957 (Sabin, 1957) for field tests on increasingly larger numbers of persons in different parts of the world, and routine use on a mass scale began in many countries during the winter and spring of 1960. Since about 1965, OPV has come into routine use all over the world except in Sweden, Finland, and Holland.

Despite extensive reduction in the number of cases of paralytic poliomyelitis that followed the mass use of IPV, increased summer incidence and epidemics continued to occur. Because IPV has no effect on multiplication of virus in the intestinal tract, polioviruses continued to circulate in communities where IPV had been used on a large scale, and paralysis continued to occur in significant numbers among those who remained unvaccinated, or received an insufficient number of doses, or lost their vaccine-acquired immunity. Approximately 20 to 30 per cent of the paralytic cases during epidemics had received three or more doses of IPV. The antibody response to IPV is particularly poor and transitory (especially for types 1 and 3) in children and older persons who have never had natural infections with any of the three types of poliovirus. Surveys of young children who had received multiple doses of Salk vaccine in the United States and South Africa showed that about 50 per cent had no neutralizing antibodies for the important type 1 virus, and about 60 per cent had none for type 3 virus, reflecting partly a poor initial response and partly a higher loss of acquired antibody within one year. During the first five years after mass use of IPV, epidemics occurred in the United States, Canada, Australia, Finland, Hungary, Israel, Japan, and other countries. In 1959 and 1960, Finland had epidemics of a magnitude comparable to those of the prevaccine years of 1949 and 1950, despite the use of IPV on an increasingly larger scale since 1956. In 1959, four years after extensive use of IPV, the United States had 6289 reported cases of paralytic poliomyelitis, of which 5472 had residual paralysis two months after onset. In 1961, seven years after extensive use of IPV, Denmark had an epidemic of 148 paralytic cases caused by type 1 poliovirus, which on a population basis is comparable to the number of paralytic cases in the United States in 1959.

OPV has the following properties not possessed by IPV that are of special importance for a rapid elimination of the paralytic disease (Sabin, 1962):

1. Immunity can be produced quickly—within about a week—after ingestion of a single dose of any one of the three types of vaccine. Thus, when type 1 monovalent vaccine is given first, protection is quickly obtained against the most important cause of paralytic poliomyelitis. Protection against the other two types is subsequently quickly achieved when they are given separately at a suitable interval or together in a single dose. During the winter and spring months in temperate climates when the incidence of infection by enteric viruses is low, this procedure has yielded an antibody response of 100 per cent or close to it for all three types (when low antibody titers are included) in the United States, Britain, Switzerland, Czechoslovakia, and Yugoslavia.

2. Extensive multiplication of the vaccine strains in the intestinal tract produces local resistance to reinfection that is independent of antibody in the blood.

3. Some unvaccinated persons, both children and adults, become immune by contact with young vaccinated children. During extensive community-wide programs, the incidence of such immunization has been especially high.

4. Intestinal resistance in a *large proportion of the child population*, the most important spreaders of polioviruses, leads to a break in the chain of transmission of the naturally occurring polioviruses of varying neurovirulence, which results in the elimination of the paralytic disease from the unvaccinated as well as the vaccinated persons in a community.

5. The fact that OPV begins to multiply in the intestinal tract within 24 hours after ingestion, creating the potential for immediate interference with subsequently ingested virulent polioviruses, combined with the early immunogenic effect of monovalent vaccine and the simplicity of mass administration, makes possible the rapid termination of epidemics.

The main disadvantages of OPV result from interference by enteric viruses that may be multiplying in the intestinal tract when the vaccine is ingested or when the three types of polioviruses are competing with one another after ingestion of a dose of trivalent vaccine. The types 2 and 3 vaccine strains have the advantage because they multiply more rapidly and extensively than type 1. In tropical and subtropical regions, where enteric viruses including naturally occurring polioviruses are widely disseminated throughout the year, mass administration of OPV within a period of a day or two has been shown to curtail temporarily the dissemination of the other enteric viruses as a result of a massive dissemination of the vaccine strains. Moreover, the *annual* administration of two doses of OPV, each given in a mass campaign on a single day with an interval of two months, to all children under 3 or 4 years of age, can keep a subtropical country free of paralytic poliomyelitis (Sabin, 1977; 1980; 1981; 1982). In temperate climates, where after initial mass campaigns with monovalent vaccines for all susceptible age groups, trivalent OPV is now used for routine immunization of children during the first year of life, multiple trivalent doses have proved to be as effective as the separately administered monovalent vaccines.

The rapidity with which a properly executed mass campaign with OPV can alter the incidence of paralytic poliomyelitis in a country with a large population and considerable variations in climate and social conditions is exemplified by the events in Italy with a population of 51 million during 1962 to 1966 (Fig. 13). By May 1965, the three monovalent doses and one trivalent dose had been given to 80 to 90 per cent of the children under 6 years of age in most of the northern provinces and to only about 50

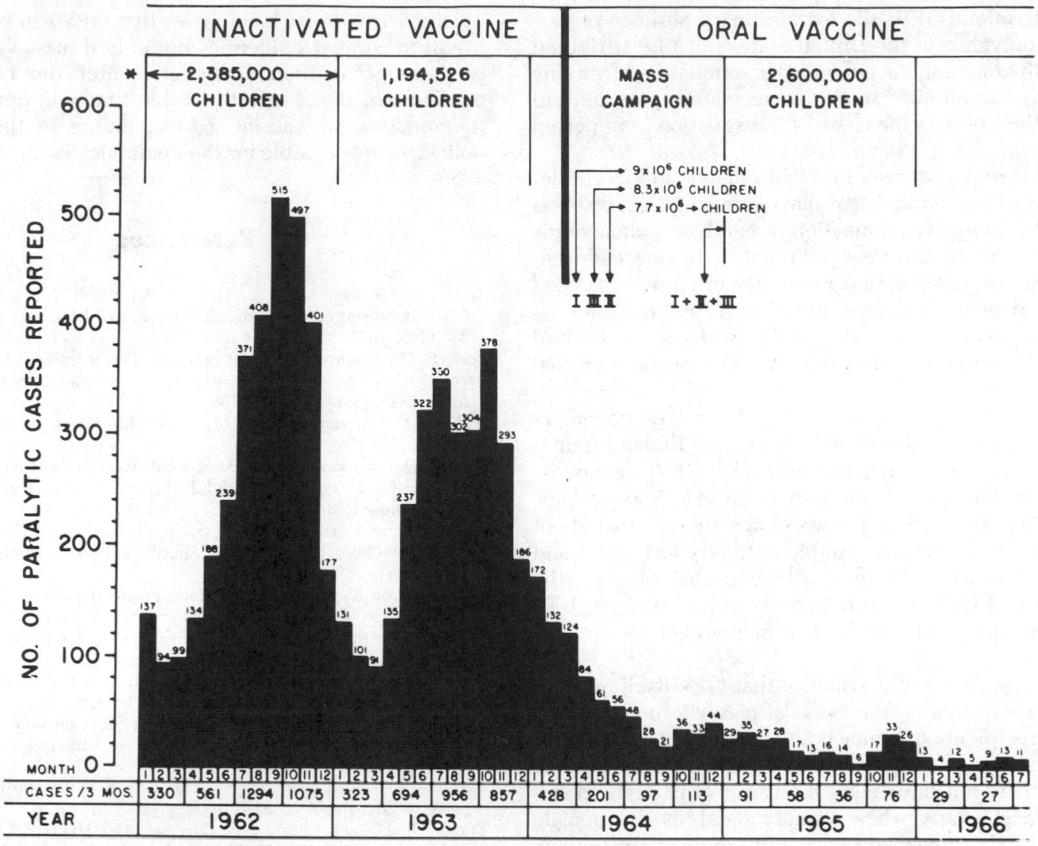

* FROM 1958 TO 1961 INACTIVATED VACCINE WAS GIVEN TO 9,349,846 CHILDREN.

Figure 13. Paralytic poliomyelitis in Italy from 1962–1966. (From Sabin, A. B.: Washington, D. C., PAHO Sc Pub No. 147, 1967.)

to 60 per cent in most of the southern provinces. More extensive vaccination was then carried out in the southern provinces, and 80 to 90 per cent of the new generations of children have continued to be vaccinated each year. According to Volpi et al. (1976), "only four cases of paralytic disease, which were not conclusively defined as poliomyelitis, were reported in 1975." In Rome in 1974 and 1975 nearly 100 per cent of all age groups had antibody for each of the three types of poliovirus (Volpi et al., 1976).

Table 1 summarizes what happened in the United States, where OPV was introduced in stages, and the mass campaigns, which covered only about 50 per cent of the total population, were followed by the routine use of trivalent vaccine for immunization of children during the first year of life (Sabin, 1981). No other country of comparable size has achieved as good a record in the complete or almost complete elimination of paralytic poliomyelitis caused by polioviruses, particularly in view of the large immigration from Mexico where paralytic polioviruses are still prevalent. The very few indigenous cases of paralytic poliomyelitis that still occur in the United States are of doubtful clinical diagnosis and are sometimes based on isolation of harmless OPV strains from the stools. Even so, it is remarkable that during the entire eight-year period of 1969 to 1976 inclusive, 18 states and the District of Columbia, with a total population of about 36 million (1970 census), did not report a single case, while the Mexican border states of California and Texas, with a combined 1970 population of a little over 31 million, reported 52 cases (6.5 per annum), some of which were probably real poliomyelitis of poliovirus etiology and some clinically or etiologically something else. This is an incredible record, since on the basis of data presented earlier under Etiology one would expect a small number of cases of persistent paralytic poliomyelitis caused by enteroviruses other than polioviruses to occur each year. Since in the 1- to 4-year-old age group about 34 per cent of white children (82 per cent of the total population in this age group) and about 60 per cent of children of other races have had less than three

Table 1. PARALYTIC POLIOMYELITIS REPORTED IN UNITED STATES, 1951 TO 1983

Period	Vaccine Used	Cases/100 million/year
1951–55	None	13,500*
1956–60	IPV† only	2,600
1961–65	IPV + OPV‡	240§
1973–78	OPV only	4§
1980–83	OPV only	4§

*Number of reported as paralytic plus percentage of unspecified cases estimated to be paralytic (see Sabin, A. B.: Rev Infect Dis 3:543, 1981).

†IPV = inactivated polio vaccine.

‡OPV = oral polio vaccine.

§Includes imported and clinically and etiologically questionable cases.

Reproduced from Sabin, A. B.: J Infect Dis, March 1985 (in press).

doses of trivalent OPV, the extraordinary absence of paralytic poliomyelitis in the United States must be attributed partly to the ongoing documented dissemination of vaccine strains that immunize some unvaccinated persons and partly to the break in the chain of transmission of imported virulent polioviruses (Sabin, 1981).

A 1976 serologic survey on 3022 persons in Czechoslovakia, where the initial OPV mass campaign in 1960 was followed by complete elimination of paralytic poliomyelitis and ongoing immunization was limited to the new children, showed almost 100 per cent immunity in all persons aged 2 years and over, indicating persistence of antibodies for at least 14 years without booster doses of vaccine beyond the first 18 months of life (Dr. V. Skovranek, personal communication).

The complete absence since 1965 of paralytic poliomyelitis and apparently also of polioviruses in Finland (population 4.7 million), which has used only IPV, cannot be explained on the basis of immunity because a 1966 serologic survey of children under 3 years of age showed that about 60 per cent had no demonstrable antibody for type 1 and type 3 polioviruses. There is a high probability that the massive use of OPV in the remainder of Europe from 1960 to 1964 has protected Finland from invasion by virulent polioviruses.

There is no acceptable evidence that OPV itself may be, even in rare instances, the cause of paralytic poliomyelitis in either recipients or contacts. Nor is there any evidence that IPV as it was prepared in the United States in 1959 and 1960 may not have been the cause of paralytic poliomyelitis (particularly when primary paralysis occasionally occurred in the inoculated extremity) (Sabin, 1963; 1969; 1977; 1978).

The strategy of initial mass vaccination of all susceptible age groups with OPV followed by ongoing vaccinations of infants concurrently with other routine immunizations has worked very well in many "developed" countries, but for a variety of reasons has been only partly effective in "developing" countries (Sabin, 1967; 1977; 1980). Mass administration of OPV *each* year to *all* children under 36 or 48 months of age, without reference to previous vaccination history, on each of two days separated by an interval of at least two months, can produce optimum results in developing countries in tropical and subtropical regions. There are valid reasons for proposing that the annual two-dose schedule should consist of 300,000 $TCID_{50}$ (50 per cent tissue culture infective doses) of only type 1 for the first dose, and of trivalent vaccine (300,000 $TCID_{50}$ of each of the three types) for the second dose (Sabin, 1977; 1980). Cuba initiated such a program in 1962 and has reported no indigenous paralytic poliomyelitis since then. Brazil rapidly brought poliomyelitis under control by well-organized, national campaigns of vaccination of almost all children under 5 years of age that have been carried out with great success annually since 1980. Mexico began annual campaigns in 1981 using only type 1 vaccine for the first of the two annual doses (Sabin, 1982). In 1983, the Dominican Republic demonstrated the possibility of vaccinating all children under 3 years of age in their own homes by thousands of nonprofessional community volunteers (Sabin, 1984; 1985).

It is difficult to set up arbitrary rules regarding the stage at which an economically developing country, with many health problems and limited health facilities, should undertake an ongoing program of vaccination against poliomyelitis. It is in such countries that OPV can be especially useful to combat epidemics but only if mass vaccination is carried out as soon as possible after the onset of the epidemic in the shortest possible time and optimally with the monovalent vaccine corresponding to the particular poliovirus responsible for the epidemic (Sabin, 1965b; 1967; 1980).

References

Arnon, S. S., Midura, T. F., Clay, S. A., Wood, R. M., and Chin, J.: Infant botulism; epidemiological, clinical, and laboratory aspects. JAMA 237:1946, 1977.

Berg, B. O.: Syndrome of infant botulism. Pediatrics 59:321, 1977.

Bernier, R. H.: Some observations on poliomyelitis lameness surveys. Rev Infect Dis 6 (Suppl 2):S371, 1984.

Bodian, D.: Emerging concept of poliomyelitis infection. Science 122:105, 1955.

Bodian, D., and Horstmann, D. M.: Polioviruses. In Horsfall, F. L., Jr., and Tamm, I. (eds.): Viral and Rickettsial Infections of Man, 4th ed. Philadelphia, J. B. Lippincott Company, 1965, p. 449.

Bodian, D., and Paffenberger, R. S., Jr.: Poliomyelitis infection in households; frequency of viremia and specific antibody response. Am J Hyg 60:83, 1954.

Committee on Typing of the National Foundation for Infantile Paralysis: Immunologic classification of poliomyelitis viruses. I. A cooperative program for the typing of one hundred strains. Am J Hyg 54:191, 1951.

Dalldorf, G., and Melnick, J. L.: Coxsackie viruses. In Horsfall, F. L., Jr., and Tamm, I. (eds.): Viral and Rickettsial Infections of Man, 4th ed. Philadelphia, J. B. Lippincott Company, 1965, p. 492.

Enders, J. F., Weller, T. H., and Robbins, F. C.: Cultivation of the Lansing strain of poliomyelitis virus in cultures of various human embryonic tissues. Science 109:85, 1949.

Flexner, S., and Lewis, P. A.: The nature of the virus of epidemic poliomyelitis. JAMA 53:2095, 1909.

Francis, R. D., and Ceballos, R.: Viremia in ECHO type 6 infection. Proc Soc Exp Biol Med 101:479, 1959.

Francis, T., Jr., Korns, R. F., Voight, R. B., Boisen, M., Hemphill, F. M., Napier, J. A., and Tolchinsky, E.: An evaluation of the 1954 poliomyelitis vaccine trials. Am J Public Health 45:Suppl 5, 1955.

Grist, N. R.: Type A7 Coxsackie (type 4 poliomyelitis) virus infection in Scotland. J Hyg London 60:323, 1962.

Horstmann, D. M., McCollum, R. W., and Mascola, A. D.: Viremia in human poliomyelitis. J Exp Med 99:355, 1954.

Hung, T. P., and Kono, R.: Neurological complications of acute haemorrhagic conjunctivitis (A polio-like syndrome in adults). In Vinken, P. J., and Bruyn, G. W. (eds.): Handbook of Clinical Neurology; Neurological Manifestations of Systemic Diseases, Part I (Klawans, H. L. ed.), Amsterdam, North-Holland Publishing Company, 1979, p. 595.

Kono, R.: Apollo 11 disease or acute hemorrhagic conjunctivitis: a pandemic of a new enterovirus infection of the eyes. Am J Epidemiol 101:383, 1975.

Kono, R. Miyamura, K., Tajiri, E., Sasagawa, A., Phuapradit, P., Roongwithu, N., Vejjajiva, A., Jayavasu, C., Thongcharoen, P., Wasi, C., and Rodprassert, P.: Virological and serological studies of neurological complications of acute hemorrhagic conjunctivitis in Thailand. J. Infect Dis 135:706, 1977.

Krugman, S., Ward, R., and Katz, S. L.: Infectious Diseases in Children, 6th ed. S. Louis, C. V. Mosby Company, 1977, p. 41.

Landsteiner, K., and Popper, E.: Übertragung der Poliomyelitis acuta auf Affen. Zschr Immunitätsforsch Orig 2:377, 1909.

Lennette, E. H., Magoffin, R. L., Schmidt, N. J., and Hollister, A. C., Jr.: Viral disease of the central nervous system; influence of poliomyelitis vaccination on etiology. JAMA 171:1456, 1959.

Lennette, E., Magoffin, R. L., and Knouf, E. G.: Viral central nervous system disease: An etiologic study conducted at the Los Angeles County General Hospital. JAMA 179:687, 1962.

Melnick, J. L.: Echoviruses. In Horsfall, F. L., Jr., and Tamm, I. (eds.): Viral and Rickettsial Infections of Man, 4th ed. Philadelphia, J. B. Lippincott Company, 1965, pp. 528–529.

Melnick, J. L.: Enterovirus type 71 infections: A varied clinical pattern sometimes mimicking paralytic poliomyelitis. Rev Infect Dis 6 (Suppl 2):S387, 1984.

Paul, J. R., Riordan, J. T., and Melnick, J. L.: Antibodies to three different antigenic types of poliomyelitis virus in sera from North Alaskan eskimos. Am J Hyg 54:275, 1951.

Ramos-Alverez, M.: Discussion. In Vaccines Against Viral and Rickettsial Diseases of Man. Pan American Health Organization Sc Pub No. 147, Washington, 1967, p. 235.

Ramos-Alvarez, M., Bessudo, L., and Sabin, A. B.: Paralytic syndromes associated with noninflammatory cytoplasmic or nuclear neuronopathy; acute paralytic disease in Mexican children, neuropathologically distinguishable from Landry-Guillain-Barré syndrome. JAMA 207:1481, 1969.
Rissler, J.: Zur Kenntniss der Veränderungen des Nervensystems bei Poliomyelitis anterior acuta. Nord Med Ark 20:1, 1888.
Robbins, F. C., Enders, J. F., Weller, T. H., and Florentino, G. L.: Studies on the cultivation of poliomyelitis viruses in tissue culture. V. The direct isolation and serologic identification of virus strains in tissue culture from patients with nonparalytic and paralytic poliomyelitis. Am J Hyg 54:286, 1951.
Sabin, A. B.: Pathology and pathogenesis of human poliomyelitis. JAMA 120:506, 1942.
Sabin, A. B.: Nonctyopathogenic variants of poliomyelitis viruses and resistance to superinfection in tissue culture. Science 120:357, 1954.
Sabin, A. B.: Pathogenesis of poliomyelitis—reappraisal in the light of new data. Science 123:1151, 1956.
Sabin, A. B.: Properties and behavior of orally administered attenuated poliovirus vaccine. JAMA 164:1216, 1957.
Sabin, A. B.: Oral poliovirus vaccine; recent results and recommendations for optimum use. Roy Soc Hlth J 82:51, 1962.
Sabin, A. B.: Is there an exceedingly small risk associated with oral poliovirus vaccine? JAMA 183:268, 1963.
Sabin, A. B.: Oral poliovirus vaccine—history of its development and prospects for eradication of poliomyelitis. JAMA 194:872, 1965a.
Sabin, A. B.: Immunization against poliomyelitis with particular reference to the tropics. Industry Trop Health 5:74, 1965b.
Sabin, A. B.: Poliomyelitis; accomplishments of live virus vaccine. In Vaccines Against Viral and Rickettsial Diseases of Man. Pan American Health Organization Sc Pub No. 147, Washington, 1967, p. 171.
Sabin, A. B.: Vaccine-associated poliomyelitis cases. Bull WHO 40:947, 1969.
Sabin, A. B.: Oral poliomyelitis vaccine: Achievements and and problems in worldwide use. Bull Internat Pediatr Assn 2:6, 1977.
Sabin, A. B.: Poliomyelitis vaccination; evaluation and direction of continuing application. Am J Pathol 70(Supplement):136, 1978.
Sabin, A. B.: Vaccination against poliomyelitis in economically underdeveloped countries. Bull WHO, 58:141, 1980.
Sabin, A. B.: Paralytic poliomyelitis: old dogmas and new perspectives. Rev Infect Dis 3:543, 1981.
Sabin, A. B.: Vaccine control of poliomyelitis in the 1980s. Yale J Biol Med 55:383, 1982.
Sabin, A. B.: Strategies for elimination of poliomyelitis in different parts of the world with oral poliovirus vaccine. Rev Infect Dis 6(Suppl 2):S391, 1984.
Sabin, A. B.: Oral poliovirus vaccine: History of its development and use and current challenge to eliminate poliomyelitis from the world. J Infect Dis, March 1985 (in press).
Sabin, A. B., and Olitsky, P. K.: Cultivation of poliomyelitis virus in vitro in human embryonic nervous tissue. Proc Soc Exp Biol Med 34:357, 1936.
Sabin, A. B., and Silva, E.: Residual paralytic poliomyelitis in a tropical region of Brazil, 1969–1977: Prevalence surveys in different age groups as indicators of changing incidence. Am J Epidemiol 117:193, 1983.
Sabin, A. B., and Ward, R.: Nature of non-paralytic and transitory paralytic poliomyelitis in rhesus monkeys inoculated with human virus. J Exp Med 73:757, 1941a.
Sabin, A. B., and Ward, R.: The natural history of poliomyelitis. I. Distribution of virus in nervous and nonnervous tissues. J Exp Med 73:771, 1941b.
Sabin, A. B., Michaels, R. H., Spiegland, I., Pelon, W., Rhim, J. S., and Wehr, R. E.: Community-wide use of oral poliovirus vaccine; effectiveness of the Cincinnati program. Am J Dis Child 101:546, 1961.
Salk, J. E., Krech, U., Youngner, J. S., Bennett, B. L., Lewis, L. J., and Bazeley, P. L.: Formaldehyde treatment and safety testing of experimental poliomyelitis vaccines. Am J Public Health 44:563, 1954.
Steigman, A. J.: Poliomyelitic properties of certain non-polio viruses: Enteroviruses and Heine-Medin disease. J Mt Sinai Hosp 25:391, 1958.
Steigman, A. J., and Lipton, M. M.: Fatal bulbospinal paralytic poliomyelitis due to ECHO 11 virus. JAMA 174:178, 1960.
Thompson, T. C.: A method of artificial respiration especially useful for the paralyzed patient. JAMA 104:307, 1935.
Verlinde, J. D., Kret, A., and Wyler, R.: The distribution of poliomyelitis virus in cynomolgus monkeys following oral administration, tonsillectomy, and intramuscular injection of diphtheria toxoid. Arch Ges Virusforsch 6:175, 1955.
Volpi, A., Ragona, G., Biondi, W., Rocchi, G., and Archetti, I.: Seroimmunity to polioviruses in an urban population of Italy. Bull WHO 54:3518, 1976.

186

ENTEROVIRAL INFECTIONS OTHER THAN POLIOMYELITIS

REISAKU KONO, M.D., M.P.H.

Enteroviral infections of the central nervous system other than poliomyelitis take three clinical forms: aseptic meningitis, encephalitis (meningoencephalitis), and poliolike paresis or paralysis. Aseptic meningitis is predominantly a syndrome of infants and children who have signs and symptoms of meningitis and a benign prognosis. Wallgren (1925) established the concept of "aseptic meningitis" without knowledge of the viral etiology of the disease, and later Goldfield (1957) proposed the name "lymphocytic meningitis" for the same syndrome. When lymphocytic choriomeningitis (LCM) virus was isolated from such cases, the cause seemed to have been discovered, but later it became clear that LCM virus was infrequent, and other viruses were more important as etiologic agents. Accordingly, the term "viral meningitis" has been widely used to identify this disease complex, which is most often due to enteroviruses. The term "aseptic meningitis" applies not only to cases due to viruses but also to meningeal infections caused by *Chlamydia*, *Leptospira*, fungi, and some bacteria. There are also certain noninfectious causes (Krugman and Ward, 1973). Aseptic meningitis is a more suitable clinical term than viral meningitis because the viral etiology cannot be recognized at the bedside and requires laboratory confirmation.

The encephalitis or meningoencephalitis that I refer to in this chapter is regarded as an advanced state of aseptic meningitis; meningitic inflammatory reactions spread to the central nervous system via the blood vessels but do not severely affect the parenchyma. Although encephalitic symptoms such as disturbed consciousness and convulsions occur with meningitis, they tend to be transient, and the prognosis is usually benign.

Sabin (1981) claimed that paralytic poliomyelitis should be regarded as a syndrome caused not only by the three types of poliovirus but probably also by 19 other enteroviruses, and that it is unnecessary to call the disease due to nonpolio enteroviruses "poliolike paresis or paralysis." However, it is generally considered that the term poliomyelitis has become so closely associated with the disease caused by human polioviruses 1–3 that it would be confusing to apply it to similar conditions caused by other enteroviruses. Therefore, the Council for International Organization of Medical Science and World Health Organization (1983) assigned to it the designation "enteroviral encephalomyelitis" and, if the causative organism is identified, a specific name is described by the use of the words "due to" in the usual manner; example: encephalomyelitis due to human coxsackievirus A7 in the International Nomenclature of Diseases. The word "paralytic" should precede "encephalomyelitis" when appropriate.

ETIOLOGY. The enteroviruses other than poliovirus that are involved are: coxsackievirus A1 through A22 and A24; coxsackievirus B1 through B6; echovirus Types 1 through 9, 11 through 27, and 29 through 33; and enterovirus Types 68 through 72. They share some common properties with poliovirus in that the virions are ether-resistant, have cubic symmetry, and have diameters of about 20 to 30 nm and densities of 1.34 g/ml in CsCl. Their RNA genomes are single-stranded and have molecular weights of 2 to 2.8 $\times$ 10^6 daltons. The enteroviruses do not have as strong a neurovirulence as do poliovirus infections of primates, although the AB IV variant of coxsackievirus A7 (Voroshilova and Chumakov, 1959) and enterovirus 70 (Kono et al., 1973) and 71 (Hashimoto et al., 1978) display a weak but definite neurovirulence. Greater acid stability and lower buoyant density in CsCl are the main characteristics distinguishing the enteroviruses from the rhinoviruses, which are also picornaviridae but cause the common cold and are not neurotropic.

Coxsackieviruses were first distinguished from echoviruses by their pathogenicity for suckling mice, but the pathogenicity for mice was later found to vary from virus strain to strain. For example, some strains of coxsackievirus B1 through B6, A7, A9, and A16 can grow in monkey kidney cell cultures and are harmless to mice, whereas some strains of echovirus 9 are pathogenic to suckling mice. Because of this variability, a subclassification of coxsackieviruses or echoviruses is no longer applied to new enteroviruses, and they are simply numbered as enterovirus 68, 69, 70, 71, and so forth (Melnick et al., 1974).

It is clear from the following statistical data that enteroviruses play an important role in neurologic infections. In the grand total of 23,824 viral infections of the central nervous system reported to the World Health Organization (WHO) during three years (1974 through 1976), 10,370 cases (43.5 per cent) were ascribed to enteroviruses other than poliovirus, followed in frequency by 5152 cases (21.6 per cent) of mumps virus infection (World Health Organization, 1974, 1975, 1976).

According to the aseptic meningitis surveillance summary covering the period 1969 through 1971 by the Center for Disease Control (CDC), nonpolio enteroviruses were the most prevalent cause of aseptic meningitis each year, comprising over 80 per cent of the identified etiologic agents (Center for Disease Control, 1969 to 1971 and 1971 to 1975). However, among the pathogens causing encephalitis, enteroviruses played a relatively minor role; they represented only 6.2 per cent of the total known causative agents of viral encephalitis in the CDC surveillance reports (Center for Disease Control, 1973). Table 1 summarizes the etiologic relationships among enterovirus types and clinical manifestations from past reports. Table 2 shows the reported numbers of enterovirus infections that appeared in the WHO yearly virus reports during the ten years from 1971 to 1980 (World Health Organization, 1971 through 1980). The large number of isolations of coxsackievirus A9 seems to reflect simply that coxsackievirus A9 can be easily isolated by tissue culture methods while other coxsackie A viruses require cumbersome inoculations into suckling mice; hence, fewer attempts were made to isolate other coxsackie A viruses. In spite of the small number of isolations of coxsackie A viruses, coxsackieviruses A1 and A4 have been isolated relatively frequently from patients with paralysis, although their real etiologic relationship with the disease is still uncertain.

As indicated by their generic name, enteroviruses are transient inhabitants of the human alimentary tract; hence, they are apt to be recovered from throat secretions and stools. Enteroviruses isolated from feces may or may not have an etiologic role in paralytic or other diseases that occur sporadically, since enteroviruses are often coincidentally carried in the alimentary tract of children. An isolate from nervous tissue or cerebrospinal fluid (CSF) has more etiologic significance. Although they possess the properties of enteroviruses, most strains of enterovirus 70 cannot grow in the alimentary tract but do multiply in the human conjunctiva. They are normally isolated from eye swabs but rarely from the throat or feces.

PATHOGENESIS AND PATHOLOGY. Infections with enteroviruses show themselves through either subclinical or apparent illness, and about half of them occur in the central nervous system (World Health Organization, 1974, 1975, and 1976). The primary sites of infection with enteroviruses, other than enterovirus 70 and 72 (hepatitis A virus) are the pharynx and intestine. In this alimentary phase, there are often no apparent signs or symptoms of infection, although sometimes there is a slight fever and a respiratory or intestinal disorder. On the other hand, the primary site of enterovirus 70 infection is the eyes, and this results in a high incidence of acute hemorrhagic conjunctivitis (AHC) (Kono and Uchida, 1977). The virus spreads from the primary site of infection to local lymph nodes, and then a transient viremia carries it to the central organs. From these, a secondary viremia probably ensues, eventually reaching the central nervous system. It was reported that viremia was proved in five of nine blood specimens taken within five days after the onset of echovirus 4 meningitis (Ishii et al., 1968). Most enteroviruses probably infect the choroid membrane at this stage and then invade the

Table 1. ENTEROVIRUS TYPES AND CLINICAL SYNDROMES

Aseptic meningitis	CA	1, 2, 3, 4, 5, 6, 7, 8, 9, 10, 11, 14, 16 17, 18, 22, 24.
	CB	1, 2, 3, 4, 5, 6.
	E	1, 2, 3, 4, 5, 6, 7, 9, 11, 12, 13, 14, 15, 16, 17, 18, 19, 20, 21, 22, 23, 25, 30, 31, 32, 33.
	EV	71.
Poli-like motor paralysis	CA	1, 4, 7, 9, 10, 14.
	CB	1, 2, 3, 4, 5.
	E	1, 2, 4, 6, 7. 9, 11, 14, 16, 18, 22, 30.
	EV	70, 71.
Encephalitis or meningoencephalitis	CA	2, 5, 6, 7. 9.
	CB	1, 2, 3, 4, 5.
	E	2, 3, 4, 6, 7, 9, 11, 14, 16, 18, 19, 33.
	EV	71.

CA, coxsackievirus A Types 1, 2, etc.
CB, coxsackievirus B Types 1, 2, etc.
E, echovirus Types 1, 2, etc.
EV 70, EV 71, enterovirus Types 70 and 71.
Lines under the figure represent the types reported in outbreak.

Table 2. MAJOR ENTEROVIRUS TYPES THAT AFFECT THE CENTRAL NERVOUS SYSTEM

Virus Types	Total CNS Disease No.	Total CNS Disease %	Polio-Like Paralysis No.	Polio-Like Paralysis %
Coxsackie A				
Total	2201	100.0	167	100.0
CA 1	47	2.1	29	20.3
CA 4	65	3.0	16	9.6
CA 7	77	3.5	2	1.2
CA 9	1517	68.9	27	18.9
CA 16	61	2.8	3	1.8
Coxsackie B				
Total	6197	100.0	180	100.0
CB 1	419	6.9	23	12.8
CB 2	1105	18.1	26	14.4
CB 3	1247	20.4	36	20.0
CB 4	1247	20.4	40	22.2
CB 5	2201	32.7	47	26.1
Echoviruses				
Total	19718	100.0	236	100.0
E 4	1124	5.8	3	1.3
E 6	1520	7.8	22	10.0
E 7	891	4.6	17	7.7
E 9	2202	11.3	25	11.4
E 11	3062	15.5	34	15.5
E 19	2122	10.9	10	4.5
E 30	4880	22.2	19	8.6
Enterovirus*				
Total	82	100.0	2	100.0
EV 71	82	100.0	2	100.0

Compiled from WHO Yearly Virus Reports, 1971–1980.
*From 1975–1980.
Total numbers and percentages include all the enterovirus types, from which major ones are selected. Therefore, summations of number of each type shown here do not reach to 100 per cent.

leptomeninges and ependyma, causing aseptic meningitis. Such enteroviruses are isolated from the CSF at a high rate but have little neurovirulence. On the other hand, some strains of coxsackievirus A7 enterovirus 70 and 71 like poliovirus, seem to have a special affinity for the motor neurons, which they destroy, causing paralysis (Horstmann and Manuelidis, 1958; Voroshilova and Chumakov, 1959; Kono et al., 1973; Hashimoto et al., 1978). This neurovirulence is weaker than that of wild-type poliovirus. A diffuse meningoencephalitis may follow aseptic meningitis, but it is transitory and benign. Generally speaking, the pathogenesis and pathology of enteroviral infections of the central nervous system are not clearly understood because there have been few autopsied cases, and no suitable studies have been made in animal models.

Factors like physical and/or mental strain may precipitate the central nervous system disease. In the polio-like motor paralysis due to enterovirus 70, intramuscular injection of a drug seemed to provoke paralysis of the injected limb (Phuapradit et al., 1976).

Persistent CNS infections with enterovirus have attracted increasing attention. Wilfert et al. (1977) reported five cases with agammaglobulinemia and persistent echovirus infection of CNS, from whose CSF echovirus 30, 19, 9 and 33 were recovered for periods varying from two months to three years. However, they had few signs of acute CNS disease and three of them had a dermatomyositis-like syndrome. These data suggest that B cell function is essential to eradicate CNS infection with enterovirus.

CLINICAL MANIFESTATIONS. Acute aseptic meningitis can begin abruptly with fever, headache, and signs of meningeal irritation, or it can occur diphasically with prodromal symptoms and then meningitis. The prodromal symptoms are usually fever, anorexia, malaise, and sore throat, which, after a remission for a few days, are followed by meningitis and a second temperature rise. It is likely that the alimentary phase of infection is subclinical in the former case and symptomatic in the latter.

When the central nervous system is attacked, body temperature rises, headache intensifies, and nausea and vomiting follow. During this stage, older children and adults often complain of nuchal pain, backache, or lumbago. Nuchal rigidity is often found, Kernig's and Brudzinski's signs are positive, and patellar and other deep tendon reflexes are exaggerated. However, nuchal rigidity is not so prominent as in bacterial meningitis; especially in infections of young infants, it is often absent or obscure. At the height of illness, various grades of disturbances of consciousness from somnolence to coma may appear, but convulsions are rather exceptional. Convulsions are considered to be the result of a diffuse meningoencephalomyelitis.

Often aseptic meningitis due to some enteroviruses (echoviruses 4, 6, 9, and 16 and coxsackieviruses A9 and A16) is accompanied by skin rash, and hence may be designated as meningitis exanthematica. Maculopapules, 2 to 4 mm in diameter, appear on the trunk and face most abundantly at the onset or during the second phase. The rash is sometimes scarlatina-like, vesicular, or, rarely, petechial. An enanthem may be seen on the tonsils and buccal mucosa. Meningitis is accompanied by a high incidence of rash, especially with echovirus 9 infections; in the Milwaukee epidemic of 1957, most such rashes occurred in infants under 3 years old; 44 per cent were between 5 and 15 years; and 6 per cent were above 15 years (Sabin et al., 1958). I have observed skin rash in only 11 per cent of the cases of echovirus 4 meningitis in Niigata, Japan, in 1964 (Ishii et al., 1968), which suggests that the incidence of skin rash is lower in aseptic meningitis due to enteroviruses other than echovirus 9.

Aseptic meningitis due to coxsackie B viruses is often accompanied by myalgia and is called meningitis myalgica. Coxsackie B viruses tend to cause aseptic meningitis in infants and epidemic myalgia or epidemic pleurodynia in adults. If the two clinical conditions happen to manifest themselves at the same time, a coxsackie B virus etiology is suggested, although the final diagnosis cannot be made without laboratory confirmation.

One of the newer enteroviruses, enterovirus 71, was isolated from patients with the hand, foot, and mouth disease syndrome complicated by aseptic meningitis in Japan (Hagiwara et al., 1978); Sweden (Blomberg et al., 1974); and Australia (Kennett et al., 1974). Hand, foot, and mouth disease has been known to result from coxsackievirus A16 infections but has seldom led to neurologic complications. In the United States, it was reported that enterovirus 71 was isolated from the brain of a patient with encephalitis (Schmidt et al., 1974). The most severe outbreak of enterovirus 71 occurred in 1975 in Bulgaria: about 700 children were suffering from meningoencephalitis, of whom 21 per cent developed polio-like paralysis and 44 died (Melnick et al., 1979). Therefore, enterovirus 71 appears to be more neurovirulent than many other enteroviruses (Hashimoto et al., 1978).

Cerebellar and other ataxias have been observed during the course of proven infections by coxsackievirus A and B; echovirus 6 and 9 (McAllister et al., 1959); and enterovirus 71 (Ishimaru et al., 1974), but the actual etiologic relationship between ataxia and these enteroviruses is unsolved.

Associations between Guillain-Barré syndrome and some enteroviruses have been reported but are unconfirmed (Gear, 1961 to 1962). In these cases, late examinations of CSF in patients with enteroviral meningitis may seemingly give a picture of protein increase without pleocytosis and thus lead to a misdiagnosis of Guillain-Barré syndrome. Mild paresis or paralysis may appear during the course of enterovirus infections other than poliovirus, but it occurs sporadically, and the recovery is usually complete. However, three exceptions have been recorded in the past during outbreaks of polio-like motor paralysis caused by the AB IV variant of coxsackievirus A7 (Voroshilova and Chumakov, 1959), enterovirus 70 (Kono et al., 1977; Hung and Kono, 1979; Wadia et al., 1983) and enterovirus 71 (Melnick et al., 1979).

COMPLICATIONS AND SEQUELAE. Enteroviral meningitis or meningoencephalitis is usually benign and resolves within two weeks. However, neonatal infections with enteroviruses, particularly with coxsackieviruses B1 through B5, require special attention (Kibrick, 1964) because they tend to be generalized diseases (encephalohepatomyocarditis) with a high fatality rate. Kibrick (1961) examined 54 newborns with disease caused by coxsackie B viruses; 45 of them had generalized infections, in which the major illness was myocarditis; one fourth of them had meningoencephalitis; and only 12 survived. The onset was abrupt and the clinical course was rapid, terminating in collapse and death within a few days. Tachycardia, tachypnea, and cyanosis were common; and cardiomegaly, hepatomegaly, and systolic murmurs were present, accompanied by electrocardiographic changes. Autopsies revealed that the patients had myocarditis (100 per cent), meningoencephalitis (76 per cent), hepatitis (43 per cent), pancreatitis (41 per cent), and adrenal cortical involvement (16 per cent). Many such illnesses are the result of infections of the mother just prior to birth (Kibrick and Benirschke, 1958), but others are transmitted by nursery personnel (Gear, 1958). Other enteroviruses are occasionally reported to cause fatal infections of newborn children, but their etiologic significance has not always been clear.

Children who experience enteroviral central nervous system diseases during their first year of life may have neurologic sequelae and lowered intelligence in later life. Sells et al. (1975) carried out a controlled follow-up study of 19 children 2½ to 8 years of age who had been hospitalized with enterovirus infection 17 to 67 months before. Three children (16 per cent) had definite neurologic impairment, 5 (26 per cent) had possible impairment, and 11 (58 per cent) were free of detectable abnormalities. Children whose illness occurred during the first year of life were found to have significantly smaller mean head circumferences, lower IQs and depressed language and speech skills. Farmer et al. (1975) reported that two of three infants who were noted to be irritable or twitching in association with coxsackie B5 meningoencephalitis in the neonatal period developed spasticity, and their intelligence was below the mean for the group six years after the onset.

Since the motor paralysis due to enterovirus 70 is a newly discovered disease and has several unique clinical features, some important clinicoepidemiologic points are described here (Kono et al., 1977; Hung and Kono, 1979). The neurologic disease usually appears two to five weeks or more after the onset of acute hemorrhagic conjunctivitis (AHC) (Fig. 1). Consequently, the relationship between conjunctivitis and the neurologic disorders is often overlooked by physicians as well as by the patients themselves. The patients sustain a systemic illness (i.e., pyrexia, general malaise, headache, nuchal pain, dizziness, and vomiting) one to three days before the onset of the neurologic symptoms. The most frequent initial symptoms are radicular pains in the muscles and limbs and aching in the lower back. Flaccid paresis or paralysis usually follows, occurring in one or more limbs, being asymmetrical and more severe in the lower limbs than in the upper, and often more proximal than distal. Tendon reflexes are abolished or diminished in the affected muscles. Cranial nerve involvement (e.g., difficulty in swallowing and facial palsy) is noted in some patients; in these cases, the interval between conjunctivitis and paralysis seems to be shorter than that found in patients with paralysis of the limbs (Fig. 1). A preponderance of male patients is usually observed. Unlike poliomyelitis, the highest incidence is found in patients who are 20 to 40 years old (Fig. 1). Pleocytosis of the CSF is found in the first three weeks from onset of neurologic symptoms, and the total protein level is raised from the second week of illness up to seven weeks or later in the CSF. Death from the disease has not been confirmed, although there was one suspicious case in Taiwan. Permanent incapacitation due to paralysis and muscular

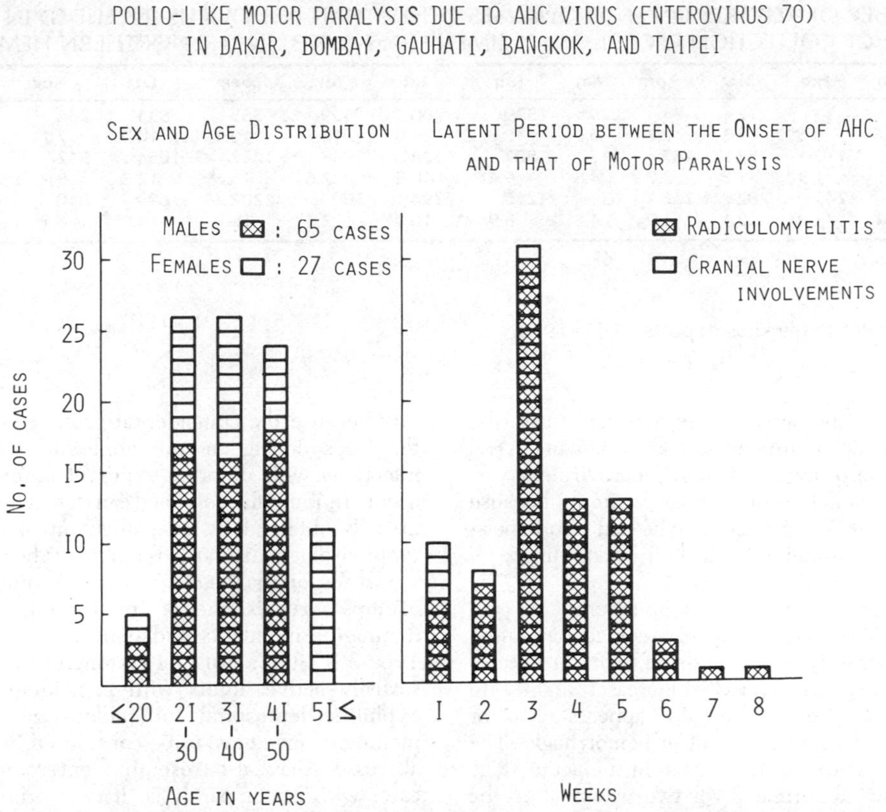

Figure 1.

atrophy in the affected proximal muscles of the limbs is observed in roughly one fourth of the patients.

EPIDEMIOLOGIC FEATURES AND GEOGRAPHIC VARIATION IN DISEASE. Enteroviruses have a worldwide distribution, but their spread is influenced by climatic conditions; they are prevalent in summer and early fall in the temperate zone and throughout the year in the tropics. Table 3 shows that the peak incidence of coxsackie A virus infection was found in July and those of coxsackie B and echoviruses occurred in August in the temperate zone of the northern hemisphere. The epidemics that occurred seemed to increase only the total number of cases, without displacing or distorting the seasonal pattern. All epidemics occurred in the season in which maximum enterovirus activity would be expected to occur in a normal, nonepidemic year.

Enterovirus infections were consistently reported more frequently in males than in females. The male to female ratio ranged from 1.33 to 1.54 in the enterovirus surveillance report, 1971 through 1975, of the Center for Disease Control (1977), but it was sometimes over 2.0.

In the temperate zone, one particular type of enterovirus becomes prevalent within a particular time and space. When that occurs, the population lacks immunity against that particular enterovirus type. An epidemic of enteroviral meningitis and meningoencephalitis represents an epiphenomenon in that setting. Therefore, an enormous number of patients with summer grippe or other minor illnesses and healthy virus carriers are usually seen along with the patients with neurologic diseases during an epidemic.

In the tropical countries, several types of enteroviruses often circulate at the same time. Therefore, the local population experiences infections with many types of enteroviruses in early life. However, there is no evidence indicating that the neurologic diseases are more prevalent in the tropics than in the temperate zone.

When new types of variants of enteroviruses appear in a country, they spread from area to area. Because of a lack of immunity, all ages are affected in a pandemic fashion. For instance, enterovirus 70 appeared in West Africa in 1969 and within a few years spread to other parts of Africa, Europe, and Asia. In 1981 the second pandemic of AHC appeared for the first time in South America, having reached Central America, the Caribbean Islands, and the southeastern United States (Center for Disease Control, 1981). Africa (Desmyter et al., 1981) and India (World Health Organization, 1982a) were revisited by the outbreaks. In the next year the disease spread to the South Pacific Islands (World Health Organization, 1982).

Outbreaks of polio-like motor paralysis due to the AB IV variant of coxsackievirus A7 were recorded in the 1950's in Karanganda and the U.S.S.R. (Voroshilova and Chumakov, 1959) and in the 1960's in Scotland (Grist, 1962), while paralytic outbreaks of enterovirus 70 occurred in Senegal (1970), India (1971), Thailand (1974), and China (Taiwan) (1971 through 1977) (Hung and Kono, 1979). In the 1981 pandemic of AHC, Wadia et al., (1983) observed 70 cases with AHC and neurologic complication in Bombay, India, and presumed that more than 1000 cases should have been found in India as a whole. It is likely that similar cases following AHC might have occurred but went unrecognized

Table 3. NUMBER OF REPORTS ON ENTEROVIRUSES OTHER THAN POLIOVIRUS INCLUDED IN THE STUDY BY MONTH OF COLLECTION RECEIPT OF SPECIMEN (1967–1973) IN THE NORTHERN HEMISPHERE

Virus Type		Jan	Feb	Mar	Apr	May	Jun	Jul	Aug	Sep	Oct	Nov	Dec	Total
CA	No.	81	53	72	74	229	529	700	559	365	333	236	108	3339
	%	2.4	1.6	2.2	2.2	6.9	15.8	21.0	16.7	10.9	10.0	7.1	3.2	100.0
CB	No.	128	113	152	187	417	807	1624	1948	1427	1054	512	247	8616
	%	1.5	1.3	1.8	2.2	4.8	9.4	18.8	22.6	16.6	12.2	5.9	2.8	100.0
E	No.	289	249	282	261	651	1210	2294	3007	2202	1899	840	374	13555
	%	2.1	1.8	2.1	1.9	4.8	8.9	16.9	22.1	16.2	14.0	6.1	2.8	100.0

CA, coxsackievirus A.
CB, coxsackievirus B.
E, echovirus.
Compiled from WHO Yearly Virus Reports, 1967–1973.

in other countries. At the present time, it is hard to ascribe the occurrence of the neurologic disease following AHC either to the local appearance of more neurovirulent variants or to the accumulation of such cases simply because of the enormous number of patients who had also experienced hemorrhagic conjunctivitis in their backgrounds.

DIAGNOSIS. Recognition of the aseptic meningitis syndrome is usually not difficult. Signs of meningeal irritation should prompt laboratory examination of CSF. In enterovirus infections, the pressure of CSF increases slightly (to 200 to 300 mm of water). The CSF appears clear or somewhat cloudy but never purulent or hemorrhagic. The protein content tends to remain normal in the acute stage but increases to an abnormal level two weeks after the onset of infection. The sugar content does not decrease as it does in cryptococcal meningitis, tuberculous meningitis, and other bacterial meningitides. In contrast to the pattern of elevated protein concentration, the pleocytosis (30 to 4000 cells, average 150 cells) tends to be confined to the acute rather than to the late stage. The pleocytosis usually consists of lymphocytes, but sometimes polymorphonuclear leukocytes also appear in the early stage of illness. The pleocytosis usually returns to normal within a few weeks after the onset of meningitis.

Etiologic diagnosis can be achieved by virus isolation and/or serologic reactions. However, the materials and methods used for virus isolation differ depending on what virus is sought. For isolation of enteroviruses from patients, CSF, throat swabs, and feces are the specimens of choice, and they should be sent in a frozen state (−70°C) to the virus laboratory for inoculation into human cell cultures of fetal kidney or lung and primary monkey kidney. They should also be inoculated into suckling mice. Many types of enteroviruses are readily recovered from the CSF (echoviruses 4 and 6 and coxsackie B viruses, for example), but some types (e.g., enterovirus 70 [Kono et al., 1977] and 71 [Kennett et al., 1974]) are not. A virus isolation from CSF taken during the early stage of illness (within three to five days after the onset) renders a positive diagnosis of viral etiology. In the early stage of aseptic meningitis, the virus isolation rate from CSF was reported to be as high as 87.5 per cent and 73.0 per cent in echovirus 4 (Ishii et al., 1968) and 18 (Wilfert et al., 1975) in meningitis, respectively. If an enterovirus has been isolated from only a throat swab or feces, a diagnosis should not be made unless serologic confirmation is possible with paired sera from the same patient, and/or epidemiologic considerations indicate that the patient has encountered the same virus type during an outbreak. Serologic confirmation is necessary because the coincidental presence of enteroviruses in the feces during an unrelated illness is frequent. Dual infections with different types of enteroviruses may also occur. Immunofluorescence can detect enterovirus antigens in cells obtained by centrifugation of CSF and makes a rapid virologic diagnosis possible (Taber et al., 1973).

Viruses other than enteroviruses must be considered. Mumps virus is one of the common causes of aseptic meningitis in infants and children; herpes simplex virus Type 2 is often a cause of meningitis of the neonate and of sexually active adults with coincidental genital herpes. Syphilitic, leptospiral, tuberculous, cysticercal, and fungal meningitis may have to be considered in some cases. Brain abscesses may also resemble enteroviral meningitis. In cases with motor paralysis, it is of primary importance to exclude poliovirus by virus isolation and serologic methods.

TREATMENT AND PROPHYLAXIS. There is no specific therapy for enteroviral neurologic diseases. However, the clinician often faces the problem of antimicrobial treatment of patients with encephalitis and/or meningitis, since it is usually very difficult to eliminate a bacterial etiology solely on clinical grounds during the early phases of illness. Antimicrobial treatment may be started in such cases of uncertain diagnosis and be discontinued if the CSF cultures prove to be sterile. Other treatments are symptomatic. In case of polio-like motor paralysis, physiotherapy must be given as soon as the aching of limbs and muscle pains subside and the progression of motor paralysis stops. Immunization with vaccines and prophylaxis with gamma globulin are impractical. The avoidance of possible precipitating or aggravating factors that could lead to encephalomeningitis and motor paralysis (such as intramuscular drug administration and undue physical exertion) must be emphasized to patients with enteroviral infections.

As already described, enteroviruses are present in throat secretions for about two weeks and in stools for several weeks or more. Infection spreads most often by the fecal-oral route among playmates in summer. Therefore, while it is theoretically possible to prevent infection with nonpolio enteroviruses by cutting the chain of infection, it is difficult in practice because there are many healthy virus carriers, and the environment is easily contaminated by the virus during the epidemic. Avoidance of contact with patients exhibiting acute febrile illness, especially those with a rash, is advisable for very young children. Newborns acquire infection vertically from their infected mothers or horizontally from medical personnel carrying the virus and/or contaminated utensils in the nursery. Since neonatal infections tend to be more severe, strict precautions must be taken to prevent cross-infections. Members of the institutional staffs responsible for caring for infants should be tested for carriage of enteroviruses.

Since enteroviruses cannot withstand temperatures of over 50°C, either boiling or autoclaving or dry heat sterilization is an effective method for killing them. Sodium hypochlorite is generally used as a disinfectant for enteroviruses.

As already mentioned, enterovirus 70 is present in eye discharges for a few days after the onset of AHC. Accordingly, it is most often transmitted on the contaminated hands of patients and medical personnel or by other vehicles, particularly ophthalmologic instruments. Since it is highly communicable, contaminated utensils should not be used by healthy persons unless they are sterilized or carefully disinfected in the household. In eye clinics, AHC patients must be treated separately from non-AHC patients. The disinfection of hands of ophthalmologists and nurses and of ophthalmologic instruments is of primary importance in the prevention of institutional outbreaks.

References

Blomberg, J., Lycke, E., Ahlfors, K., Johnsson, T., Wolontis, S., and von Zeipel, G.: New enterovirus type associated with epidemic of aseptic meningitis and/or hand, foot, and mouth disease. Lancet 2:112, 1974.

Center for Disease Control, Neurotropic Viral Diseases Surveillance: Annual encephalitis summaries. In Krugman, S., and Ward, W.: Infectious Diseases of Children and Adults. 5th ed. St. Louis, C. V. Mosby Company, 1973, p. 26.

Center for Disease Control, Neurotropic Viral Diseases Surveillance: Aseptic meningitis annual summaries 1969–1971. Atlanta, U.S. Public Health Service, Center for Disease Control, 1970, 1972, 1973.

Center for Disease Control, Neurotropic Viral Diseases Surveillance: Enterovirus summary 1971–1975. Atlanta, U.S. Public Health Service, Center for Disease Control, 1977.

Center for Disease Control: Acute hemorrhagic conjunctivitis-Latin America. Morbidity Mortality Weekly Rep. 30: 450, 1981; Acute hemorrhagic conjunctivitis-Key West, Florida. ibid. 30:463, 1981; Acute hemorrhagic conjunctivitis-Panama and Belize. ibid. 30:497, 1981; Acute hemorrhagic conjunctivitis-Florida and North Carolina. ibid. 30:501, 1981.

Council for International Organizations of Medical Science and the World Health Organization.: International Nomenclature of Diseases. Vol. II Infectious Diseases, Part 3: Viral diseases 1st Ed., p. 64, CIOMS, Geneva, 1983.

Desmyter, J., Colaert, J., Maertens, K., and Muyembe, T.: Enterovirus 70 haemorrhagic conjunctivitis in Zaïre, 1981 versus 1972 [letter] Lancet 2:1054, 1981.

Farmer, K., MacArthur, B. A., and Clay, M. M.: A follow-up study of 15 cases of neonatal meningoencephalitis due to coxsackie virus B5. J Pediatr 87:568, 1975.

Gear, J. H. S.: Coxsackie virus infection in South Africa. Yale J Biol Med 34:289, 1961–1962.

Gear, J. H. S.: Coxsackievirus infections of the newborn. Progr Med Virol 1:106, 1958.

Grist, N. R.: Type A-7 coxsackie (type 4 poliomyelitis) virus infection in Scotland. J Hyg 60:323, 1962.

Goldfield, M.: Viral meningitis. Am J Med Sci 234:91, 1957.

Hagiwara, A., Tagaya, I., and Yoneyama, T.: Epidemic of hand, foot, and mouth disease associated with enterovirus 71 infection. Intervirology 9:60, 1978.

Hashimoto, A., Hagiwara, A., and Kodama, H.: Neurovirulence in cynomolgus monkeys of enterovirus 71 isolated from a patient with hand, foot and mouth disease. Arch Virol 56:257, 1978.

Horstmann, D. M., and Manuelidis, E. E.: Russian coxsackie A-7 virus (AB IV strain)—neuropathogenicity and comparison with poliomyelitis. J Immunol 81:32, 1958.

Hung, T.-P., and Kono, R.: Neurologic complications of acute hemorrhagic conjunctivitis—A polio-like syndrome in adult. In Vinken, P. J., and Bruyn, G. W. (eds.): Handbook of Clinical Neurology. Vol. 38, Amsterdam, North-Holland Publishing Company 1979, p. 595.

Ishii, K., Matsunaga, Y., Onishi, E., and Kono, R.: Epidemiological and virological studies of echovirus type 4 meningitis in Japan, 1964. Jap J Med Sci Biol 21:11, 1968.

Ishimaru, K., Ishiki, M., and Yamaoka, K.: Aseptic meningitis accompanied by hand-foot-mouth disease and ataxia. Igaku-no-ayumi 89:108, 1974 (in Japanese).

Kennett, M. L., Birch, C. J., Lewis, F. A., Yung, A. P., Locarnini, S. A., and Gust, I. D.: Enterovirus type 71 infection in Melbourne. Bull WHO 51:609, 1974.

Kibrick, S.: Viral infections of the fetus and newborn. In Perspectives in Virology, Vol. 2. Minneapolis, Burgess Publishing Company, 1961, p. 140.

Kibrick, S.: Current status of coxsackie and echo viruses in human disease. Progr Med Virol 6:27, 1964.

Kibrick, S., and Benirschke, K.: Generalized disease (severe encephalohepatomyocarditis) occurring in the newborn period due to infection with coxsackievirus group B. Pediatrics 22:857, 1958.

Kono, R., Miyamura, K., Tajiri, E., Sasagawa, A., Phuapradit, P., Roongwithu, N., Vajjajiva, A., Jayavasu, C., Thongcharoen, C., Wasi, C., and Roodprassert, P.: Virological and serological studies of neurological complications of acute hemorrhagic conjunctivitis in Thailand. J Infect Dis 133:706, 1977.

Kono, R., and Uchida, Y.: Acute hemorrhagic conjunctivitis. Ophthalmol Dig 39:14, 1977.

Kono, R., Uchida, N., Sasagawa, A., Akao, Y., Kodama, H., Mukoyama, J., and Fujiwara, T.: Neurovirulence of acute-hemorrhagic-conjunctivitis virus in monkeys. Lancet 1:61, 1973.

Krugman, S., and Ward, W.: Infectious Diseases of Children and Adults. 5th ed. St. Louis, C. V. Mosby Company, 1973.

McAllister, R. M., Hummeler, K., and Coriell, L. L.: Acute cerebellar ataxia: Report of a case with isolation of type 9 echovirus from the cerebrospinal fluid. N Engl J Med 261:1159, 1959.

Melnick, J. L., Tagaya, I., and Von Magnus, H.: Enterovirus 69, 70 and 71. Intervirology 4:369, 1974.

Melnick, J. L., Schmidt, N. J., Mirkovic, R. R., Chumakov, M. P., Lavrova, I. K., and Voroshilova, M. K.: Identification of Bulgarian strain 258 of enterovirus 71. Intervirology 12:297, 1979.

Phuapradit, P., Roongwithu, U., Linsukon, P., Boongird, P., and Vejjajiva, A.: Radiculomyelitis complicating acute hemorrhagic conjunctivitis: A clinical study. J Neurol Sci 27:117, 1976.

Sabin, A. B.: Paralytic poliomyelitis: old dogmas and new perspectives. Rev Inf Dis 3:543, 1981.

Sabin, A. B., Krumbiegel, E. R., and Wigand, R.: Echo 9 virus disease: Virologically controlled clinical and epidemiological observations during 1957 epidemic in Milwaukee with notes on concurrent similar diseases and associated coxsackie and other echo viruses. J Dis Child 96:197, 1958.

Schmidt, N. J., Lennette, E. H., and Ho, H. H.: An apparently new enterovirus isolated from patients with disease of the central nervous system. J Infect Dis 129:304, 1974.

Sells, C. J., Carpenter, R. L., and Ray, C. G.: Sequelae of central nervous system enterovirus infections. N Engl J Med 293:1, 1975.

Taber, L. H., Mirkovic, M. R., Adam, V., Ellis, S. S., Yow, M. D., and Melnick, J. L.: Rapid diagnosis of enterovirus meningitis by immunofluorescent staining of CSF leukocytes. Intervirology 1:127, 1973.

Voroshilova, M. K., and Chumakov, M. P.: Poliomyelitis-like properties of AB IV coxsackie A-7 group of viruses. Progr Med Virol 2:106, 1959.

Wadia, N. H., Katrak, S. M., Mirsa, V. P., Wadia, P. N., Miyamura, K., Hashimoto, K., Ogino, T., Hikiji, T., and Kono, R.: Polio-like motor paralysis associated with acute hemorrhagic conjunctivitis in an outbreak in 1981 in Bombay, India: Clinical and serological studies. J Inf Dis 147:660, 1983.

Wallgren, A.: Une nouvelle maladie infecteuse du system nerveux central. Acta Paediat 4:158, 1925.

Wilfert, C. M., Lauer, B. A., Cohen, M., Costenbader, M. L., and Myers, E.: An epidemic of echovirus 18 meningitis. J Infect Dis 131:75, 1975.

World Health Organization, Virus Disease Unit: WHO Yearly Virus Report. Geneva, World Health Organization, 1971 VIR/72.10; 1972 VIR/73. 12; 1973 VIR/74. 18; 1974 VIR/75. 18; 1975 VIR/77. 3; 1976 VIR/78. 4; 1977 VIR/78. 9; 1978 VIR/79. 5; 1979 VIR/81. 3; 1980 VIR/82. 3.

World Health Organization. Acute Haemorrhagic conjunctivitis. Weekly Epidemiological Record. 57:111, 1982.

World Health Organization: Acute haemorrhagic conjunctivitis, India. Weekly Epidemiological Record. 57:161, 1982a.

187

TETANUS

RICARDO VERONESI, M.D.
ROBERTO FOCACCIA, M.D.

Tetanus (lockjaw) is a disease of humans and some warm-blood animals, caused by a potent neurotropic exotoxin released by the tetanus bacilli. Rigidity and spasms of the skeletal musculature are the most important clinical features of the disease.

ETIOLOGY. The etiological agent of tetanus is an anaerobic spore-bearing gram-positive rod called *Clostridium tetani*. The vegetative forms of the tetanus bacilli release potent toxins (tetanospasmin and tetanolysin) that can be lethal for many susceptible animals and man. Depending on its H antigen the strains of *C. tetani* can be differentiated into nine H-serovars (Bytchenko, 1981). There is variation in the prevalence of different serovars in different parts of the world. Tetanus bacilli are encountered in most of the surface of earth, mostly in tropical and sub-tropical areas. It is isolated very frequently from the soil and feces of man and animals, mainly herbivores. Bacilli can survive unfavorable environmental conditions due to their ability to sporulate. There is an established correlation between the amount of soil contamination and morbidity rates of tetanus. The production of toxin by bacilli is mediated by a large plasmid whose presence differentiates toxigenic from nontoxigenic strains (Laird et al., 1981). Tetanus toxin can be degraded by action of trypsin or papain into different fragments (α, β-1, β-2, and γ) each of which has been incriminated as responsible for different symptoms of the disease. Beta fragments may cause asphyxia, cardiac arrest, and general exhaustion in laboratory animals, without causing any muscle spasms or hypertonicity (Bizzini, 1981). Tetanolysin, another component of the tetanus toxin, causes intravascular hemolysis, pulmonary edema, and cardiovascular disturbances when injected intravenously in rabbits (Bizzini, 1975).

PATHOGENESIS AND PATHOLOGY. The tetanus toxin released from the tetanus bacilli at the portal of entry binds to the gangliosides of the nerve cell membrane, and then enters the axons to be transported retrograd (intra and peri-axonal transport) through the ventral roots of the peripheral nerves to the ventral horns of the spinal cord (or the motor nuclei of the cranial nerves). The targets of the neurotropic toxin (tetanospasmin) are the presynaptic terminal endings on the motoneurones in the ventral horns, where it acts by preventing the release of inhibitory transmitters (Kryzhanovsky, 1981). Also, the release of acetylcholine is impaired and this chemical mediator accumulates substantially in the damaged synapses. Besides the disturbance of inhibition, there is the formation of a generator of pathologically enhanced excitation which results in enhanced propagation of high-frequency impulses to the periphery (Kryzhanovsky, 1981). These physiological alterations are responsible for the muscle spasms and rigidity of striated muscles that are characteristic of tetanus. The inhibitory control of sympathetic neurons is also impaired by the toxin so that the patient presents the "sympathetic overactivity syndrome" characterized by hyperhydrosis, hyperthermia, tachycardia, arrhythmias, labile hypertension, increased respiratory secretions, and gastrointestinal hemorrhages. These symptoms appear in the most severe cases of tetanus and have been correlated with the levels of catecholamines in the blood. Visible pathologic changes in tetanus are usually minimal and nonspecific. The central nervous system usually shows swelling of the motor ganglion cells of the spinal cord and medulla, associated with nuclear swelling and chromatolysis. Vertebral fractures due to mechanical compression of the vertebral bodies (usually dorsal vertebrae) are very common (Veronesi, 1960).

Portals of Entry. Tetanus has been differentiated into accidental, neonatal, gynecological, obstetrical, otogenic, and surgical. In about 20 per cent of all cases the portal of entry remains unrecognized (Veronesi, 1960); these cases are probably due to small skin abrasions or G.I. ulcerations, injections with contaminated needles or infected dental decays. In adult cases the most common portals of entry are wounds on the lower limbs, most frequently the feet. The tetanus bacilli usually penetrate through a breach in the skin or mucosa resulting in suppuration, spore germination, and release of tetanus toxin. Burns and bites or scratches by animals are also common tetanus-prone injuries. The presence of foreign bodies in the wound constitutes an important predisposing factor. In the primitive communities of the world, the most frequent portal of entry is the umbilical stump. Uterine injuries by contaminated objects inserted for the purpose of abortion are common causes of tetanus in such communities.

The period between the injury and the first symptoms is the *incubation period*. The shorter the incubation period, the worse the prognosis; an incubation period of less than one week is usually followed by severe tetanus. The time elapsed between the first symptoms and the first muscular spasm is called a "period of progression." Periods of progression shorter than 48 hours are usually a prediction of severe forms of tetanus (Armitage, 1978; Veronesi, 1960).

CLINICAL MANIFESTATIONS. Tetanus is characterized by generalized hypertonia (generalized tetanus) or, less frequently, localized hypertonia (usually cephalic) of the striated musculature, and is frequently accompanied by clonic paroxysmal muscular spasms. Trismus (lockjaw) is usually the first symptom of the disease. Throughout the illness the patient is conscious and mentally clear. As the disease progresses, muscular rigidity increases and causes stiff neck, opisthotonus (see Chapter 5, Fig. 1) or less frequently orthotonus, dysphagia, rigidity of the abdominal wall, and rigidity of the lower limbs. Rigidity of the facial muscles causes "risus sardonicus" and gives the false impression that the patient is smiling. Dorsal kyphosis and dorsolumbar lordosis are the result of stiffness of the paravertebral musculature. Paroxysmal tonic spasms usually appear a few hours after onset of trismus. Paroxysms can be precipitated by the slightest stimuli such as noise, swallowing, a draft of air, or even the touching of the patient when he is sleeping. Such spasms are usually of short duration but very painful. In the more severe forms, the spasms are very frequent and persistent enough to interfere with breathing. When the spasms of the respiratory and laryngeal musculature last a long time, the patient becomes cyanotic, and death may result if he is not immediately relaxed. Frequently in the more severe forms of tetanus symptoms of sympathetic overactivity appears. High fever is a bad prognostic sign.

Neonatal Tetanus. Neonatal tetanus is practically a synonym for *umbilical tetanus*, since at this age the portal of entry is, with rare exception, the umbilical stump. Usually the incubation period is one week. The first symptom is usually difficulty in sucking either the breast or the bottle. The clinical picture progresses rapidly and does not differ greatly from that described for adult tetanus. The permanent rigidity of the striated musculature brings about a posture that strongly suggest the diagnosis of tetanus. The main symptoms of neonatal tetanus are: trismus, opisthotonos (rigidity of paravertebral musculature), hyperflexion of the upper limbs bringing the hands close to the thorax, hyperextension of the lower limbs, complete flexion of the fingers of hands and feet, and contracted facial musculature (closed eyes, forehead wrinkled, half-opened mouth and lips contracted). Usually the muscular spasms are very intense and frequent. Spasms of the respiratory muscles are accompanied by apnea and cyanosis and can be fatal unless muscle-relaxing drugs are injected immediately. Manifestations of sympathetic overactivity may also occur. High fever is either due to the severity of the disease itself or, more frequently, due to secondary bacterial superinfections, usually bronchopneumonia.

COURSE AND PROGNOSIS. These correlate closely with the severity of the disease, the age of the patient, superimposed infections, hospital facilities availability, and previous state of health. The fatality rate is highest in newborns and in the elderly. The fatality rates in generalized tetanus range from 10 to 60 per cent. Local tetanus is mild and has a fatality rate of around 1 per cent. The full course of the disease takes about 2 to 4 weeks. When the patient survives, complete recovery is usually observed without sequelae. After the acute stage, patients usually experience some muscular rigidity for 1 to 2 months, which improves with physiotherapy. Great loss of weight and mild anemia often follow severe tetanus. Except for the newborn, most patients have fractures of the vertebral bodies (Veronesi, 1960).

COMPLICATIONS AND SEQUELAE. Respiratory complications are frequent in tetanus. Because of spasms of the respiratory muscles there is difficulty expelling secretions that accumulate in the bronchial tree. Bronchitis, bronchiolitis, bronchopneumonia, atelectasis, and diaphragmatic paralysis (Focaccia et al., 1980) are common complications that bring on respiratory failure. Over sedation or an obstructed tracheostomy may also contribute to respiratory failure. Aspiration pneumonia is frequent in neonatal tetanus because liquids are regurgitated during muscle spasms.

Transitory electrocardiographic alterations are frequently observed. In severe cases of tetanus marked cardiovascular changes occur, (tachycardia, arrythmias, cardiac failure, labile hypertension, and shock). These signs, added to profuse sweating, hyperthermia, and intense diaphoresis, are described as the "sympathetic overactivity syndrome" (Kerr et al., 1968).

Other less frequent complications are septicemia, bed sores, thromboembolism, G.I. hemorrhages, urinary infections, acute renal failure, dehydration, and metabolic acidosis. In neonatal tetanus, herniations of the abdominal wall may appear or become accentuated.

GEOGRAPHIC VARIATIONS IN DISEASE. The incidence of tetanus varies in different areas of the world, in accordance with the following: 1) conditions that affect the density of *C. tetani* in the soil, such as presence of organic substances, its pH and moisture, environmental temperature, and presence of herbivorous animals (mainly equines and bovines); 2) the frequency of tetanus-prone wounds, which is influenced by cultural and socio-economic standards of living, frequency of tetanus-prone wounds, abortion practices, medical attendance during pregnancy and delivery, and medical care for wounded people, and 3) the immune status of the population. More recently it was demonstrated in Brazil and in India that naturally acquired tetanus antibodies affect the prevalence and severity of the disease and, influence the response to tetanus toxoid (Veronesi et al., 1983). In well developed countries, where tetanus is mainly confined to the aged, fatality rates may be higher than in developing countries where tetanus hits mainly younger people. In African countries, where septic abortion is frequent tetanus is very severe and highly lethal. Neonatal tetanus is the most prevalent form of tetanus in developing countries, and responsible for 60 to 70 per cent of the total number of cases. In well developed countries, tetanus is most often a consequence of drug addiction (Furste, 1981).

DIAGNOSIS. Since there are no routine laboratory tests for specific diagnosis, this is based mainly on data provided by the patient's history, epidemiologic, and clinical data. Epidemiological data are mainly concerned with tetanus-prone wounds and the prevalence of the disease in the community. The most common tetanus-prone wounds are: umbilical stumps (for neonatal tetanus), burns, non-medical abortions, gun shot injuries, dirty wounds that contain foreign materials (earth, wood, glass, cat-gut, etc.), and necrotic tissues.

Specific laboratory diagnosis is based mainly in the inoculation of the debrided suspected tissues in the hind leg of mice or guinea pigs where the first local symptoms of tetanus may appear as early as 12 hours thereafter. Fluorescent labeled antitoxin may also be used for detection of *C. tetani* in tissues or dressings. Differential diagnosis should include the following diseases that share symptoms with tetanus: Bell's palsy and trigeminal neuritis, tetany, rabies, meningitis, and temporomandibular arthralgia. Bell's palsy and trigeminal neuritis are not accompanied by trismus, dysphagia, or nuchal rigidity that are seen in tetanus. Meningitis does not cause trismus and usually results in disturbances of consciousness, which is not characteristic of tetanus. The CSF is abnormal in meningitis but not in tetanus. Tetany causes spasm of the limbs in extension (Trousseau sign) and is usually due to low blood levels of calcium. Rabies in its early stages may simulate cephalic tetanus (dysphagia, dyspnea) but the disease progresses more rapidly to death. Rabies causes paralysis instead of the muscular hypertonicity seen in tetanus. Temporomandibular arthralgia (as seen with serum sickness) improves and may disappear with the use of corticosteroids whereas trismus due to tetanus is unaffected by such therapeutics.

TREATMENT. The treatment of tetanus includes: 1) specific therapy; 2) control of muscle spasms; 3) supportive measures. All patients suspected of having tetanus should be admitted to the hospital and treated in an intensive care unit. Patients must be protected against bright light, high environment temperature, and noise. During the acute stage of the disease patients must remain under the close supervision of nursing and medical personnel.

Specific Treatment. Serum therapy includes the following drugs:

a) *Heterologous tetanus antitoxin* (20,000 to 100,000 I.U.), when given by the intramuscular route is not curative because the antitoxin cannot displace the toxin that has already bound to nervous tissues. Antitoxin acts only to neutralize the circulating toxin and the newly formed toxin being produced in the portal of entry (Rey et al., 1981). The administration of 250 to 500 I.U. of heterologous antitoxin by the intrathecal route (cisternal) may reduce the fatality rates, which suggests that the antitoxin may reach the CNS when injected by such route. Corticosteroids intravenously may diminish the meningeal reactions to the drug injected intrathecally.

b) *Human tetanus immune globulin* (HTIG) should be administered intramuscularly (500 to 10,000 I.U.) or intrathecally (500 to 1,000 I.U.). There is no evidence that it is more effective than the heterologous antitoxin; the main advantages of its use is avoidance of allergic reactions and longer duration of adequate blood levels. We observed a statistically significant reduction in the fatality rates when the drug was administered as a single dose of 1,000 I.U. intrathecally, combined with 10,000 I.U. intravenously (Veronesi et al., 1980).

c) *Treatment of the wound*: the portal of entry should be debrided and thoroughly cleansed after infiltrating the wound with tetanus antitoxin. All necrotic tissues and foreign bodies should be carefully removed.

d) *Antibiotic therapy:* penicillin, 12 million U/day, has been recommended for its effectiveness against the vegetative forms of the *C. tetani*. Specific antibiotics are indicated for treatment of complicating infections.

Control of Spasms. It is of vital importance to avoid tetanic spasms and its most important consequence laryngeal spasms, which can produce apnea. Treatment often requires the continuous intravenous infusion of sedatives and muscle-relaxing drugs. Various drugs have been used, but benzodiazepines are preferred, especially diazepam in doses up to 7 mg/kg/day. Whenever necessary, add other sedative drugs such as chlorpromazine (up to 25 mg/kg/dose) or chloral hydrate (0.5 g/dose). Chloral hydrate is excellent for treatment of newborns and infants in developing countries. When the spasms are not controlled with such drugs, curarization and artificial ventilation may be necessary.

SUPPORTIVE MEASURES. Oral feeding is avoided during the acute spasmodic stage, hydration is maintained by continuous intravenous infusion. Urine output is maintained with a catheter in the bladder. Patients must be monitored for respiratory complications. Uncontrolled apneic spasms require tracheostomy to allow easier aspiration of pharyngeal and tracheal secretions in order to maintain a patent airway. The control and prevention of respiratory complications requires periodic chest roentgenograms. Cardiovascular disturbances secondary to sympathetic overactivity may be controlled by adrenergic blocking drugs, such as propanolol (up to 10 mg/dose).

PROPHYLAXIS. Human tetanus is prevented by: active immunization with tetanus absorbed toxoid, passive immunization with tetanus antitoxin (homologous or heterologous), antibiotics, wound debridement, perinatal maternal assistance, and prevention of injuries.

Active immunization with adsorbed tetanus toxoid is the safest prophylactic procedure, and also the most effective; it is innocuous and cheap compared to other preventive measures. However, most inhabitants of developing countries are denied immunization and more than one million people die with tetanus every year in the world. A crucial human experiment that established the effectiveness of tetanus toxoid was the prevention of tetanus made during the Second World War. Greater purity, potency, and efficacy of tetanus toxoid allow shorter schedules of immunization (2 or even 1 dose). This has been achieved through better detoxification of the toxin and more effective adjuvants. Primary immunization is best achieved with 2 shots of regular tetanus toxoid (10 to 20 Lf) injected intramuscularly at 1 to 2 month intervals, and a reinforcing dose given 6 to 12 months later. Protective blood levels of antitoxin (0.01 I.U/ml) are maintained for 5 to 10 years after immunization and during this period of time only one booster dose is required for protection against tetanus. All injured persons with a tetanus-prone wound should receive one shot of adsorbed tetanus toxoid intramuscularly at the time of injury unless they have received a booster injection or has completed the basic immunization within the last 12 months. For those previously vaccinated the toxoid works as a booster, but for those not previously vaccinated it serves as the first immunizing dose and should be accompanied by passive immunization (see below).

Pregnant women living in areas of high prevalence of tetanus should be vaccinated in order to protect the newborn against neonatal tetanus. Three shots of toxoid should be injected intramuscularly at one month intervals, the last dose given one month in advance of the delivery. For tetanus-prone wounds seen in emergency medical services, tetanus toxoid should be injected as a booster only in previously vaccinated people, within 10 years of vaccination. Beyond that period passive immunization should accompany active immunization. *Untoward reactions* to tetanus toxoid are unusual and limited to local erythema, edema, nodules, or pain. Very exceptionally, arthralgia, urticaria, edema of eyelids, nephrosis, or, even, anaphylactic shock can occur.

Passive Immunization. Either equine or human tetanus immune globulin may be used to prevent tetanus in those who were never vaccinated against tetanus. Tetanus immune globulin is indicated in cases of tetanus-prone wounds, i.e., dirty wounds with necrotic tissues, foreign bodies, and pus. The dosage of heterologous (equine) antitoxin ranges from 5 to 10,000 I.U., independent of age and weight. Skin or ocular tests for hypersensitivity are mandatory before injecting heterologous antitoxin. Heterologous antitoxin affords antitetanus protection for up to 10 days. The dosage of homologous antitoxin ranges between 500 and 1,000 I.U. and protection is maintained for 3 to 4 weeks.

Combined active-passive immunization is advised for those who were never vaccinated against tetanus, and who need optimal protection after injury. In developing countries where tetanus is a major public health problem, mass tetanus immunization is advised, mainly for children and people at high risk. Tetanus-diphtheria and pertussis is the preferable combination of antigens for infants; after six years of age the adult-type of diphtheria toxoid is advised.

Antibiotics and surgical debridement of damaged tissues

contribute to the effectiveness of prophylaxis. Antibiotics should be maintained for 3 to 5 days. For better results, antibiotics should be started within the first six hours after injury (Veronesi, 1981).

Surgical Prophylaxis. Surgical debridement and removal of the damaged tissues may eliminate the anaerobic local conditions required for the germination of the tetanus spores. In areas of developing countries where people cannot afford professional medical assistance, primary health care delivered by laymen may be very effective in preventing tetanus.

References

Armitage, P., and Clifford, R.: Prognosis in tetanus: use of data from therapeutic trials. J Infect Dis 138 (1): 1, 1978.

Bizzini, B.: Toxines-Toxinogénèse. In Proceedings of the Fourth International Conference on Tetanus. Lyon (France), Lips, 1975, p. 119.

Bizzini, B.: Structure-function relationship of tetanus toxin. In Proceedings of the Sixth International Conference on Tetanus. Fondation Marcel Merieux. Lyon (France), 1981, p. 1.

Bytchenko, B.: Microbiology of tetanus. In Veronesi, R. (ed.): Tetanus—Important New Concepts. Amsterdam-Oxford-Princeton, Excerpta Medica, 1981, p. 28.

Focaccia, R., Veronesi, R., Magalhães, A. E. A., Mazza, C. C., Feldman, C., and Hutzler, R. U.: Paralisia diafragmática no tétano. Relato de 37 casos. Rev Bras Clin Terap 9(5): 321, 1980.

Furste, W.: Tetanus. In Braude, A. I. (ed.): Medical Microbiology and Infectious Diseases. Philadelphia. W. B. Saunders Company, 1981, p. 1373.

Kerr, J. H., Corbert, J. L., Prys-Roberts, C., Crampton-Smith, A., and Spalding, J. M. K.: Involvement of the sympathetic nervous system in tetanus, studies on 82 cases. Lancet 2:236, 1968.

Kryzhanovsky, G. N.: Tetanus pathophysiology. In Veronesi, R. (ed.): Tetanus—Important New Concepts. Amsterdam-Oxford-Princeton, Excerpta Medica, 1981, p. 109.

Laird, W. J., Aaronson, W., Habig, W. H., Hardegree, M. C., and Silver, R. P.: Genetics of the virulence plasmids of *Clostridium tetani*. In Proceedings of the Sixth International Conference on Tetanus. Fondation Marcel Merieux. Lyon (France), 1981, p. 9.

Rey, M., Diop-Mar, I., and Robert, D.: Treatment of tetanus. In Veronesi, R. (ed.): Tetanus—Important New Concepts, Excerpta Medica, Amsterdam-Oxford-Princeton, 1981, p. 207.

Veronesi, R.: Contribuicão para o estudo clínico e experimental do tétano. Thesis. Faculty of Medicine, University of São Paulo, Brazil, 1960.

Veronesi, R., Bizzini, B., Hutzler, R. U., Focaccia, R., Mazza, C. C., and Feldman, C.: Eficácia do tratamento do tétano com antitoxina tetânica por via raquiana e/ou venosa: estudo de 101 casos, com pesquisa sobre a permanência da gamaglobulina humana - F(ab)^2 - no líquor e no sangue. Rev Bras Clin Terap 9(5):301, 1980.

Veronesi, R., and Focaccia, R.: Tetanus—The clinical picture. In Veronesi, R. (ed.): Tetanus-Important New Concepts, Excerpta Medica, Amsterdam-Oxford-Princeton, 1981, p. 183.

Veronesi, R.: Tetanus—Prophylaxis. In Veronesi, R. (ed.): Tetanus-Important New Concepts. Excerpta Medica, Amsterdam-Oxford-Princeton, 1981, p. 238.

Veronesi, R., Bizzini, B., Focaccia, R., Coscina, A. L., Mazza, C. C., Focaccia, M. T., Carraro, F., and Honningman, M. N.: Naturally acquired antibodies to tetanus toxin in humans and animals from the Galapagos Islands. J Infect Dis 147 (2):308, 1983.

188
LEPROSY

ROBERT R. JACOBSON, M.D., PH.D.

Leprosy (Hansen's disease) is a chronic infection primarily affecting the skin, peripheral nerves, eyes, and mucous membranes. It has been known for over 2000 years and afflicts more than 12,000,000 people worldwide. The etiologic agent is a bacterium (*Mycobacterium leprae*) that has never definitely been cultured in artificial media, although it will grow in the mouse footpad and produce disseminated disease in the armadillo. There is much about the disease we do not understand, but we can manage nearly all patients satisfactorily without removing them from their normal position in society.

PATHOGENESIS AND PATHOLOGY. There are several theories regarding transmission. The oldest holds that bacilli are shed from the skin of a patient and pass through the skin of a new host. Recently it has been argued that respiratory spread is more probable. The upper respiratory tract in a patient with active disseminated (lepromatous) disease is heavily infected, and with each cough or sneeze huge numbers of bacilli are blown out. When inhaled by a susceptible host, these bacilli presumably grow in the upper respiratory tract and disseminate therefrom via the bloodstream. A third theory suggests that insect vectors might occasionally transmit leprosy (Navayanane, et al., 1977) and another that since *M. leprae* may occur in nature, as among some wild armadillos, transmission from them to humans could occur. Because no definitive studies have been done in humans, opinions vary, but the theory that transmission is respiratory seems to be favored now.

However it is transmitted, leprosy seems to be very contagious as measured by lymphocyte transformation to *M. leprae* antigens in exposed persons (Godal, 1974), yet the incidence of the disease in most areas remains very low, presumably because the overwhelming majority of people are not susceptible. Data suggest that susceptible persons have a defective cell-mediated immune (CMI) response toward *M. leprae*. Thus, when a normal person is exposed, the invading bacilli are engulfed by macrophages and destroyed, and no outward sign of infection develops. Although the macrophages in a person with the specific CMI defect ingest the bacilli, they do not fully recognize them as pathogens and allow them to multiply and disseminate to a variable degree. The source of the defective immune response to *M. leprae* is unknown. The evidence for a genetic origin is inconclusive. It is specific for *M. leprae*, since the CMI response to other pathogens is normal in patients with leprosy.

Leprologists often describe the different forms of leprosy as separate disease entities. This distinction is important clinically but tends to obscure the fact that these are different manifestations of the same disease. Since its presentation in a given patient is related to the degree of immune deficit present, any description should integrate the clinical and immunologic aspects. It is for this reason that the classification of Ridley and Jopling has gained relatively widespread acceptance (Ridley and Jopling, 1966). Figure 1 illustrates the five-part Ridley-Jopling classification. As noted, almost everyone (> 95 per cent) can apparently resist a routine exposure to this infection.

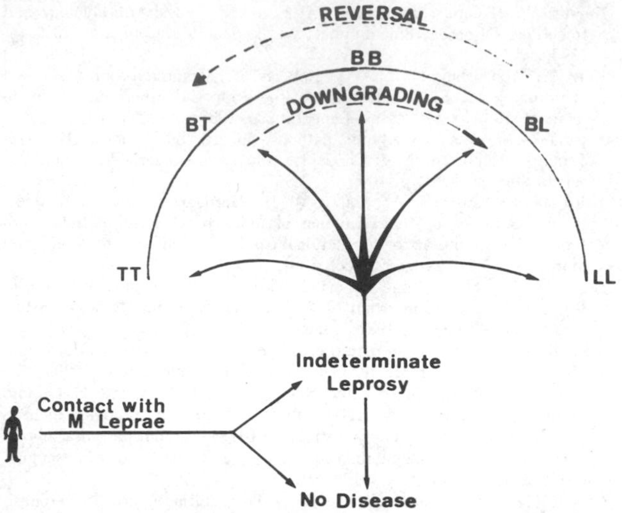

Figure 1. The Ridley-Jopling classification of leprosy.

The remainder develop indeterminate leprosy. Unless it heals spontaneously or is treated the disease will progress to one of the three common clinical types. Those with the greatest resistance keep the infection localized and develop tuberculoid disease (TT), while those with the least resistance develop generalized or lepromatous disease (LL). Between these two extremes is a broad zone (BT, BB, and BL), which is usually referred to as borderline (dimorphous) leprosy. The disease in a patient at either pole (TT or LL) tends to be stable, but in the broad borderline portion of the spectrum relatively wide shifts in disease type can occur. Without treatment there is a tendency for immunity to diminish with a consequent shift toward lepromatous disease. With effective chemotherapy, on the other hand, the tendency is to shift in the other direction toward tuberculoid disease with an enhanced immune response. These shifts may be accompanied by reactive episodes, referred to as downgrading (rare) or reversal reactions, respectively. Thus, although an infection may start out as BT, extensive disease may develop (downgrading), and it may be classified upon diagnosis as BB or beyond. With treatment, on the other hand, the patient's immunity and clinical course may improve (reversal), and the disease moves toward BT again. Although these immunologic shifts are seldom demonstrated histologically, they explain the course of the disease.

Biopsy sections in patients with indeterminate leprosy will usually show minimal nonspecific chronic inflammation of the upper dermis consisting of round cells around nerves, blood vessels, and glands. These may be mistaken for a chronic nonspecific dermatitis unless leprosy is suspected and an acid-fast stain is done to demonstrate bacilli, particularly in the dermal nerves, which may have an associated infiltrate. The mycobacteria may be difficult to find because of their small numbers.

Tuberculoid leprosy is characterized by epithelioid cell granulomas containing occasional giant cells and surrounded by lymphocytes (Fig. 2). The infiltrate extends up to the epidermis and sometimes invades the basal epithelium. Nerve involvement is pathognomonic of leprosy, and in tuberculoid disease, nerve bundles are invaded and destroyed, often to the point of being unidentifiable. Bacilli are most likely to be found in the nerves but only with extreme difficulty.

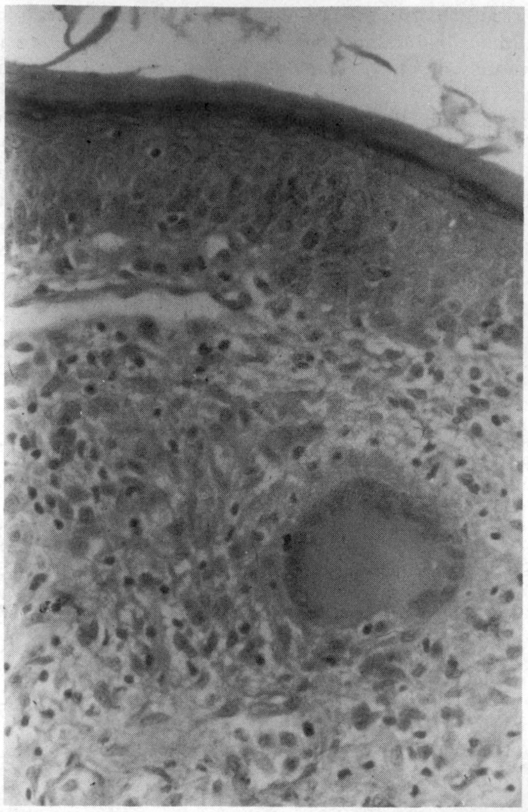

Figure 2. Tuberculoid leprosy granuloma, consisting mainly of epithelioid cells, some lymphocytes, and a giant cell. It extends up to the epidermis.

The cutaneous infiltrate in lepromatous leprosy initially consists of macrophages that proliferate around dermal appendages, nerves, and blood vessels. This infiltrate gradually increases and may eventually replace much of the dermis, always, however, separated from the epidermis by a clear zone (Fig. 3). *M. leprae* organisms are found in macrophages, and their numbers steadily increase, gradually replacing the cytoplasm, which becomes vacuolated with accumulated lipid forming foam cells. Although the infiltrate is apparent around the nerves, intraneural invasion by macrophages is seldom significant until late in advanced cases. Numerous bacilli may be seen within the nerves, however, particularly within Schwann cells. Edema and pressure from these cells filled with bacilli probably account for the gradual diminution of neural function seen in lepromatous leprosy. The gradual loss of nerve function is to be contrasted with the rapid destruction of nerves by the intense cellular infiltrates of tuberculoid leprosy and many borderline cases.

The lesions of borderline leprosy present a very mixed picture. In general, in BT leprosy the infiltrate is composed of lymphocytes, epithelioid, and giant cells as in TT disease. A clear zone may be found; however, nerves tend to be more readily identifiable, and acid-fast bacilli (AFB) are easier to find. As the disease moves toward BL, the infiltrate is composed mostly of macrophages, the clear zone becomes more prominent, bacilli steadily increase in numbers, and the infiltration of nerves becomes mostly perineural rather than intraneural. Lymphocytes are plentiful but nearly disappear as the LL end of the spectrum is reached.

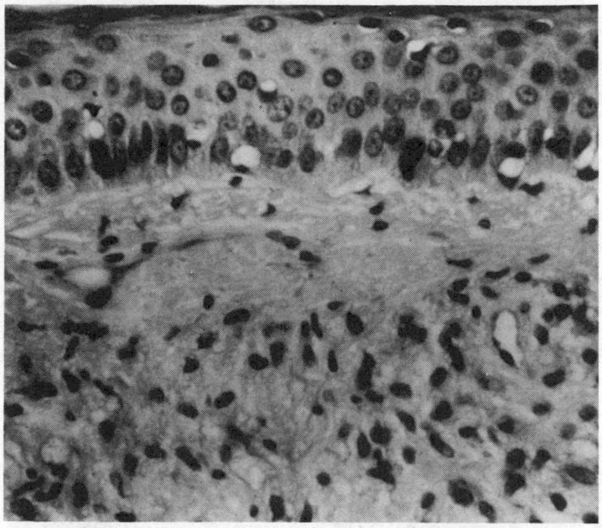

Figure 3. Lepromatous leprosy with infiltrate consisting of macrophages, many having foamy cytoplasms. It is separated from the epidermis by a clear zone (zone of Grenz).

CLINICAL MANIFESTATIONS AND DIAGNOSIS. A diagnosis of leprosy should always be considered in a patient with skin lesions and sensory loss. The ideal examination would include routine laboratory studies, a G-6-PD screening test plus skin scrapings, a biopsy, examination of the eyes, a test of motor strength in the hands and feet, palpation of peripheral nerves, a sensory examination, inspection of the skin to determine the extent and type of lesions, and, in certain instances, a lepromin test.

Smears are taken by scraping the edge of small skin slits and smearing the material obtained on a microscopic slide. Since the bacillus grows best in cooler regions of the body, we routinely scrape the earlobes, elbows, and knees in addition to select lesions in newly diagnosed borderline and lepromatous patients.

A biopsy specimen should be taken entirely from within the margin of the chosen lesion. Separate sections of it are then stained for routine histopathology and AFB. The skin scrapings are also stained for AFB, and the numbers of bacilli in biopsy sections and scrapings are counted by using a semilogarithmic scale called the bacteriologic index (BI). (See Figure 4.) Typically, the BI on scrapings and biopsy will be 0 to 1+ in indeterminate and tuberculoid disease, 1 to 4+ in borderline disease, and 4 to 6+ in lepromatous cases. The morphologic index (MI) is also determined. This is the percentage of bacilli that appears normal in size, shape, and uniformity of staining (1 to 5 per cent in a typical newly diagnosed case). The figure is correlated to some extent with viability in that, when the MI becomes 0, the bacilli cannot be routinely grown in the mouse footpad, and the disease is no longer considered communicable.

BI	
0	NO BACILLI IN 100 OIF*
1+	1-10 BACILLI PER 100 OIF
2+	1-10 BACILLI PER 10 OIF
3+	1-10 BACILLI PER OIF
4+	10-100 BACILLI PER OIF
5+	100-1000 BACILLI PER OIF
6+	OVER 1000 BACILLI PER OIF
	(*OIL IMMERSION FIELDS)

Figure 4. The bacteriologic index (BI).

The eyes are tested for lagophthalmus, visual acuity, circumcorneal hyperemia, tear production, corneal sensation, pupillary shape, and response to light.

Motor strength should be examined in the face, hands, and feet. The face is inspected for seventh nerve paralysis. In the hand, complete ulnar nerve paralysis will result in a partial claw-hand deformity, flattening of the hypothenar eminence and thenar web space, and wasting of the interosseous muscles. Lesser involvement will cause only weakness in the ulnar innervated muscles. The median nerve may be affected but only with or after the ulnar nerve. This combined paralysis leads to the classic complete claw-hand deformity. The radial nerve may be involved rarely, producing a wrist-drop. In the lower extremities claw-toe (posterior tibial nerve) and foot-drop (common peroneal nerve) deformities may be seen. The ulnar, median, superficial radial cutaneous, great auricular, and common peroneal nerves should be palpated for evidence of enlargement and/or tenderness.

Sensory loss will involve light touch, pain, and temperature. In general, in tuberculoid leprosy sensory loss will be confined to the lesion or lesions and in borderline disease it may be found in and around the lesions or in the lepromatous pattern—i.e., in the distal extremities—or any combination in between. Sensory loss in the lepromatous case may advance to nearly total body anesthesia, sparing only the warmer regions such as the axillae, groin, and midline of the back. The ability to sweat is lost in insensitive areas owing to damage to autonomic fibers and destruction of sweat glands, and this often leads to severe dryness.

The lepromin test is a useful measure of immune status toward *M. leprae*, but it is not a diagnostic test. The Mitsuda-type lepromin contains 160×10^6 heat-killed *M. leprae* per ml, and 0.1 ml of this suspension is injected intradermally. A positive result consists of a tuberculin-like response (Fernandez reaction) at 48 hours and/or a nodular, occasionally ulcerated response (Mitsuda reaction) at 21 days. The test is invariably positive in TT and BT cases, negative in BL and LL cases, and may be positive or negative in indeterminate, BB cases, and the general population depending upon their ability to generate a delayed hypersensitivity response to *M. laprae*.

The skin manifestations of leprosy are remarkably varied, sometimes resembling those seen in many other skin diseases. In the section that follows the usual manifestations of the various types are described, but variations occur.

Indeterminate Leprosy. This usually presents as a hypopigmented macule that may have slight erythema. It appears most commonly on the face, extremities, or buttocks, and more than one lesion may be present. Sensation is usually normal or only mildly diminished. The lesion appears insignificant and is most often detected during contact examinations or leprosy case-finding surveys. Diagnosis can be confirmed only by biopsy.

Tuberculoid Leprosy. There is usually only one or at most a very few lesions with well-defined margins that vary in size from a few to 30 or more centimeters. They are hypopigmented and may be purely macular, macular with an irregularly or uniformly raised edge, or occasionally plaque-like (Fig. 5). The surface is usually scaly and sen-

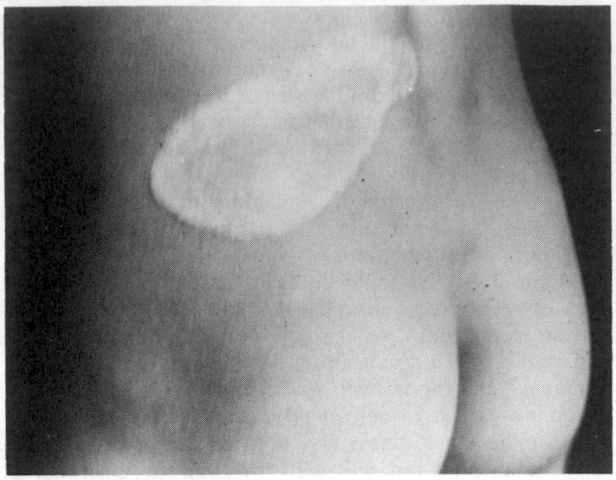

Figure 5. Tuberculoid leprosy (TT). A large solitary lesion with a sharply demarcated raised margin and a scaly hypopigmented surface.

sation is absent. Only cutaneous or peripheral nerves in the area are usually enlarged and tender.

Lepromatous Leprosy. This form of disease is usually generalized at the time of diagnosis, but occasionally patients are seen so early that only a few lesions are present. It may present in several different ways. Disseminated faint erythematous macules with vague margins may occur; if allowed to progress, they tend to increase in number, enlarge, coalesce, and become plaque-like. Second, this disease may present with generalized papular and nodular lesions, and third, it may present as diffuse disease with no distinct lesions, although the skin may have a slight generalized erythema and a somewhat glossy appearance. Here as in all lepromatous cases, complete or partial loss of eyebrows and eyelashes (lateral portions) and diminished body hair may be seen. Where the infiltration becomes more pronounced, as on the face, corrugation may develop, leading to the classic leonine facies (Fig. 6). Finally, a mixed picture may occur. Another variation, referred to as the histoid variety, is most commonly seen in relapsed cases and presents as multiple, firm, waxy nodules. Other findings in lepromatous cases include the following:

1. There may be varying degrees of motor loss.
2. Heavy infiltration of the upper respiratory tract may cause nasal stuffiness, epistaxis, and voice changes. The nasal lesions may destroy the cartilage and bone, produce a septal perforation, and then result in collapse of the nose.
3. Small lepromatous nodules may be seen in the conjunctiva, sclera, and episclera, particularly at the corneal-scleral junction, and there may be beading of the corneal nerves. Lagophthalmos from facial nerve paralysis may cause exposure keratitis.
4. In theory, *M. leprae* organisms may be found anywhere in the body outside of the central nervous system, but only the following areas are of interest or significance clinically:
   a. A granulomatous infiltrate and multiple bacilli may be found in the liver, spleen, lymph nodes, and testes. No alteration of function is usually seen except in the testes, which may be destroyed or atrophied by the process. Gynecomastia often accompanies testicular atrophy, but a direct causal relationship has not been established.
   b. The small bones of the hands and feet occasionally contain lepromatous granulomas that may appear cystic on radiographs.
   c. *M. leprae* bacteremia is common.
5. A false-positive serologic result (VDRL) is frequently observed. The FTA will be negative, however.

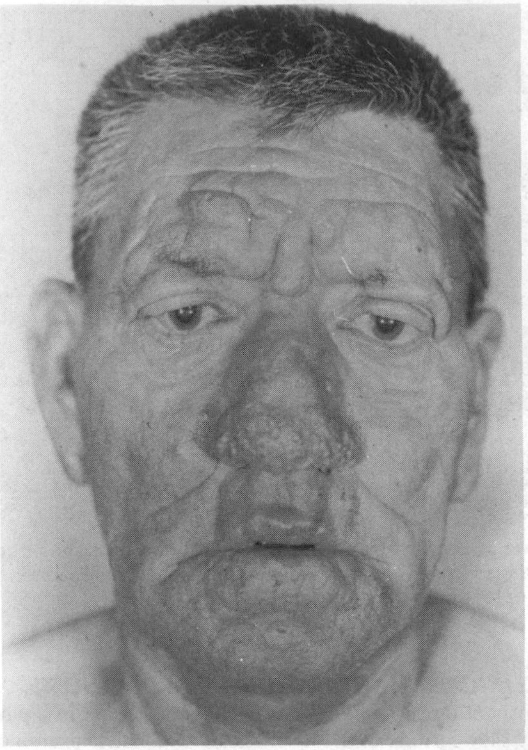

Figure 6. Lepromatous leprosy (LL). An early leonine facies with diffuse infiltration, particularly of the nose. Note the loss of eyelashes and lateral eyebrows.

Borderline Leprosy. Borderline disease occupies most of the leprosy spectrum from localized disease with large lesions on one end to generalized disease with small lesions on the other, with all possible gradations and mixtures between. In BT disease the lesions vary in size but tend to be large. They may be macules, plaques, or annular (Fig. 7) with diminished sensation in and around many of them and sometimes small satellite lesions nearby. BB disease shows a similar picture but has more (although smaller) lesions, a higher BI, and a mixed tuberculoid-lepromatous sensory picture (Fig. 8). At the BL region, we usually find extensive disease with small lesions, a high BI, and a mostly lepromatous-type sensory loss (Fig. 9). Some borderline lesions may have indented or depressed hypopigmented centers, giving them a "punched out" appearance. Nerve involvement tends to be extensive and severe in borderline cases, and paralysis is frequent, particularly with reactive episodes. In some geographic areas, particularly India, cases are occasionally seen in which the disease in fact appears to involve only the nerves, and these are referred to as polyneuritic or pure neuritic leprosy.

TREATMENT. Successful treatment requires patient education and rehabilitation as well as antibacterial therapy.

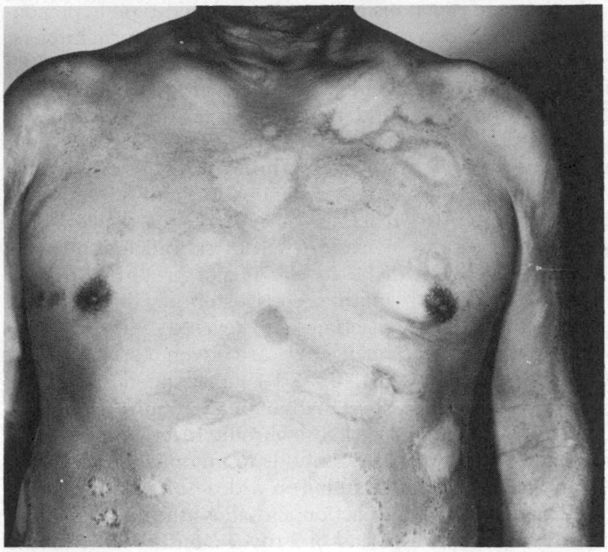

Figure 7. Borderline tuberculoid leprosy (BT). Multiple, scaly hypopigmented lesions with sharp raised margins and a bacteriologic index of 0 to 1+.

The patient must understand his disease, the reasons for his treatment (to help him *and* prevent transmission of the infection), and the fact that he may temporarily feel worse (reactions) with treatment. The importance of never interrupting medications must be emphasized if the development of sulfone-resistant disease is to be minimized.

Dapsone (DDS), clofazimine (Lamprene, B663), rifampin and ethionamide are the major drugs available for the treatment of leprosy. Rifampin is strongly bactericidal, ethionamide intermediate, and dapsone and clofazimine weakly bactericidal against *M. laprae*.

The normal adult dose of dapsone is 100 mg daily. Hemolysis, its most common side effect, is usually mild except in occasional patients with a G6PD deficiency. Mild gastrointestinal complaints occur but rarely necessitate interrupting therapy. Agranulocytosis, the dapsone syndrome, peripheral neuropathies, and hepatitis are rare but serious complications of dapsone therapy. Other sulfones include DADDS (Hansolar), which is not recommended because it produces very low blood levels of dapsone, and sulfoxone sodium (Diasone) an enteric coated preparation given in a dose of 330 mg daily.

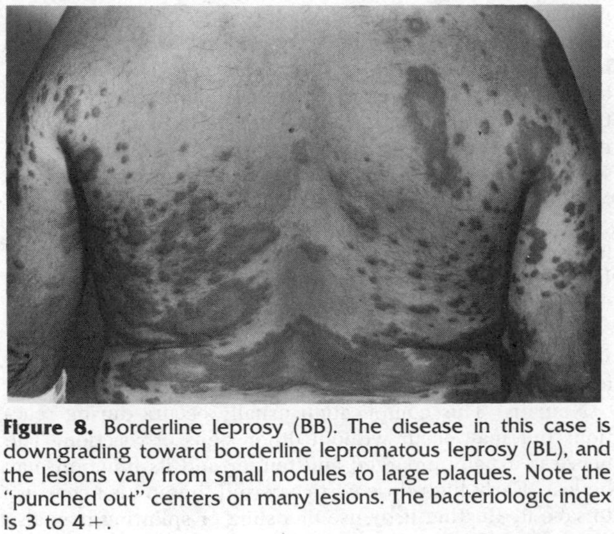

Figure 8. Borderline leprosy (BB). The disease in this case is downgrading toward borderline lepromatous leprosy (BL), and the lesions vary from small nodules to large plaques. Note the "punched out" centers on many lesions. The bacteriologic index is 3 to 4+.

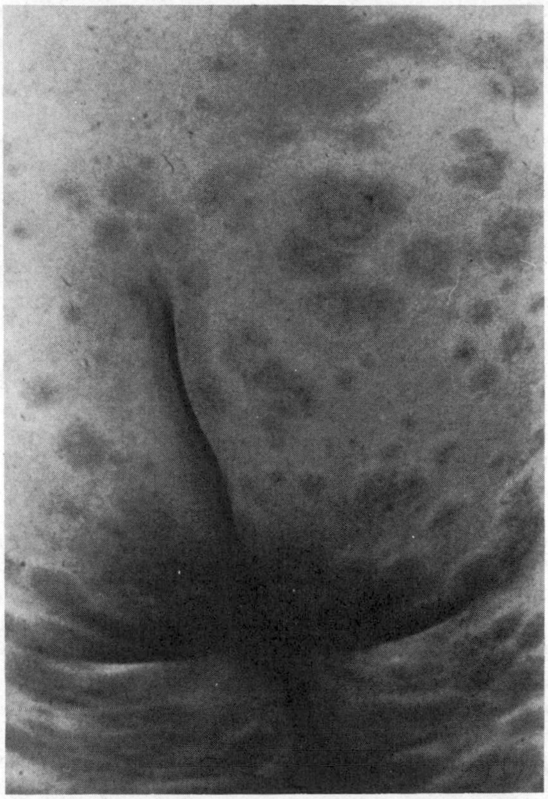

Figure 9. Borderline lepromatous leprosy (BL). Multiple small plaques, papules, and nodules symmetrically distributed. The bacteriologic index is 4 to 5+.

Clofazimine is commonly used in a dose of 50 to 100 mg daily. Higher doses are anti-inflammatory and useful for the management of reactions. Side effects include skin pigmentation, gastrointestinal complaints and diminished sweating and tearing. The pigmentation is uneven, occurs in essentially all cases and varies from reddish-tan to black. It diminishes as the disease approaches negativity and eventually clears completely if the drug is discontinued. Clofazimine accumulates in the wall of the small bowel, particularly on doses over 100 mg daily and this may produce pain, nausea, vomiting, diarrhea, and decreased motility with obstructive symptoms. Decreasing the dose or temporarily discontinuing the drug usually eliminates the problem.

The usual adult dose of rifampin is 600 mg daily, but as little as 600 mg once monthly has demonstrable activity. Its major side effect is hepatotoxicity, but thrombocytopenia, a flu-like syndrome, and other toxic effects are occasionally seen. Ethionamide and the similar prothionamide are usually used in a dose of 250 to 500 mg daily. Gastrointestinal complaints are common and hepatotoxicity occurs in about 5 per cent of cases. When used in combination with rifampin, hepatotoxicity is more common and severe, necessitating discontinuance of the drug in 10 to 20 per cent of cases.

Three factors complicate leprosy chemotherapy: drug resistance, persistent viable bacilli, and the length of treatment required. Dapsone monotherapy was the standard approach to treatment for nearly 3 decades. It was frequently taken irregularly or in low doses, however, favoring the development of secondary dapsone resistance after prolonged therapy. Resistance can be confirmed by mouse footpad drug sensitivity testing or a monitored clinical trial of dapsone. In the last decade primary dapsone resistant cases have been found but many of these display only low levels of resistance in mouse footpad testing and may still respond to full dose dapsone therapy. Strains of *M. leprae* resistant to clofazimine, rifampin or ethionamide have also been isolated from patients taking these drugs as monotherapy.

Persistent viable *M. leprae* have been isolated from patients receiving the various anti-leprosy drugs either alone or in combination drug regimens. Whether their existence necessitates life-time therapy in patients with BL and LL disease is uncertain. Satisfactory initial results have been obtained in trials where treatment was discontinued after either long-term dapsone monotherapy or short-term combination drug therapy with regimens containing rifampin. Thus combination drug therapy should avoid development of drug resistance and may shorten the treatment period, but for now leprosy chemotherapy remains in a state of flux and only the results of long-term trials will resolve these questions.

Dapsone 100 mg daily plus rifampin 600 mg daily is recommended for all adult BB, BL, and LL cases. This is continued for at least 2 years, followed by dapsone monotherapy until 10 years beyond inactivity in BB cases and for life in BL and LL cases. Indeterminate, TT and BT cases can be treated with dapsone monotherapy, but rifampin is often combined with it for the first 6 months. Treatment is continued 3 years beyond inactivity in indeterminate and TT cases and 5 years in BT cases. Inactivity is defined as at least 1 year of negative (BI = 0) skin scrapings and biopsies with no clinical evidence of activity such as reactions. Typically this requires 1 to 2 years in indeterminate and TT cases, 2 to 6 years in BT and BB cases and 5-10 years in BL and LL cases. Sulfone resistant cases can be treated with clofazimine plus either rifampin or ethionamide for at least 2 years, followed by clofazimine monotherapy. Those who will not accept clofazimine because of the pigmentation can be given rifampin plus ethionamide, but this combination is relatively hepatotoxic. A WHO Study Group (1982) has recommended that indeterminate, TT, and BT cases be given daily dapsone plus rifampin 600 mg once monthly for 6 months with all therapy then discontinued. BB, BL and LL cases would receive daily dapsone and clofazimine plus 300 mg of clofazimine with 600 mg of rifampin once monthly for at least 2 years and preferably to bacterial negativity with therapy then discontinued. These regimens remain unproven, but may be effective and if so could avoid problems associated with drug resistance and the maintenance of patients on chemotherapy for prolonged periods of time.

Attempts to correct the specific CMI defect in leprosy patients such as through administration of transfer factor (Hastings, 1977) or vaccinotherapy with a mixture of killed *M. leprae* and BCG (Convit et al., 1982) have shown promise, but remain experimental.

COMPLICATIONS AND SEQUELAE

Reactions. Reactions occur in about 50 per cent of leprosy patients and probably produce most of the deformities in this disease. There are basically two types:

1. *Reversal reactions* represent a delayed-type hypersensitivity response to *M. leprae* antigens. As the term implies, a change or "reversal" has apparently occurred in the individual's responsiveness to these antigens. They may occur in borderline and tuberculoid cases, usually those receiving treatment. The clinical findings are fever, neuritis, edema and erythema of preexisting lesions (which may ulcerate), new lesions, adenopathy, and a high white blood count. Any reaction that carries a danger of a significant motor or sensory deficit or skin ulceration must be treated daily with 60 to 100 mg of prednisone or an equivalent dose of another corticosteroid. Steroids will usually control the reaction and reverse nerve damage within 24 to 48 hours if they are given early enough. Patients with a low BI (0 to 1+) may need only brief therapy, but multibacillary patients may require months or even years of treatment. These chronic reactions should be managed by alternate day steroids to minimize side effects. As an alternative, clofazimine in a dose of 200 to 300 mg daily may control the reaction and allow the steroids to be discontinued over a period of 2 to 12 months. Care should be taken to avoid small bowel toxicity, however. Therapy should be continued without interruption, since stopping it has no immediate effect on the reaction.

2. *Erythema nodosum leprosum* (ENL) usually occurs and is more severe in BL and LL cases under treatment but may occur in untreated patients. It seems to be the result of Arthus reactions (immune complex deposition in vessels) at multiple sites. Erythematous, often painful, nodules develop in large crops within a matter of hours. Less commonly, the lesions may be pustular, necrotic, erythema multiforme-like, or hemorrhagic. All but the mildest episodes are febrile. Neuritis, malaise, arthralgias, leukocytosis, iridocyclitis, lymphadenitis, periostitis (particularly pretibial), orchitis, and nephritis may also occur. The nephritis may be an immune complex type, and a nephrotic syndrome may occur. Stress may bring on an episode, but the precipitating cause is usually unknown. Therapy is continued and the reaction is suppressed by thalidomide, the treatment of choice, in a dose of 100 mg four times daily. This dose usually controls the reaction within 48 hours, and it can then be tapered to a maintenance level of about 100 mg daily, which may have to be continued for years in some cases. If acute neuritis is present, corticosteroids should be used. Although very effective, their prolonged use for the treatment of ENL itself often results in serious steroid side effects even if they are given on alternate days. Thus, in fertile women in whom thalidomide is contraindicated because of its teratogenicity and in cases where thalidomide is not effective or available, clofazimine should be used as in reversal reactions. Antimonials and chloroquine are also effective in some cases, but thalidomide and clofazimine are preferred. Mild cases of ENL may require only aspirin and rest.

In Mexico and some other areas patients with diffuse lepromatous leprosy may develop a reaction called the Lucio phenomenon. Many punched-out skin ulcers develop, and patients may occasionally die of septic complications. High doses of corticosteroids usually control the Lucio phenomenon, but they may need to be continued for years.

Neuritis. This complication usually occurs during reactions but may occur without other signs of reaction. The nerve is usually enlarged and tender and its function may be lost. Early high-dose corticosteroid therapy is necessary to save it. Resting it by use of a sling or splinting may also help. Surgical intervention, e.g., neurolysis or drainage of the nerve abscesses as sometimes seen in tuberculoid cases, is occasionally necessary.

Eye Problems. Iridocyclitis is heralded by photophobia and blurring of vision. It is a medical emergency! Corticosteroid and atropine eye drops should be started at once to avoid permanent damage. Glaucoma may eventually occur in these cases. Lagophthalmos and decreased lacrimation are treated with a tear substitute to avoid development of an exposure keratitis.

Injuries. Most patients have varying degrees of permanent sensory and/or motor impairment. They must be taught to use their eyes as a substitute for other sensations and to rely on protective measures such as gloves and special footwear. When injuries occur, they must be protected from trauma while healing occurs, e.g., by resting a foot with a plantar ulcer or by using a total skin-contact walking cast. Repeated trauma and infection may lead to absorption of bones in hands and feet. Proper management of these problems is essential for the success of any leprosy control program, or the patient may feel that treatment has failed and abandon it.

Orchitis. This may accompany a reactive episode or occur independently. A short tapered course of corticosteroids will usually control the problem, but sterility may ultimately result.

Renal Disease. Renal amyloidosis or glomerulonephritis is a complication of long-standing active leprosy or a chronic reaction. The patients usually progress to renal failure unless the underlying process is controlled.

GEOGRAPHIC VARIATIONS IN DISEASE. Leprosy today is mostly a disease of tropical and semitropical areas and occurs mainly in the underdeveloped nations. The incidence of the disease varies markedly between countries and within a given country, and in the proportions of indeterminate, tuberculoid, borderline, and lepromatous cases. The reasons for this variation are unknown.

CONTROL AND PROPHYLAXIS. First, the prevalence and incidence rates should be determined for each type of leprosy and case-detection surveys should be repeated at regular intervals. Outpatient treatment and close follow-up should be provided for all cases, and programs for health education should be established. Household contacts of lepromatous patients are at greatest risk, but most new cases will be detected outside the household. Serodiagnostic tests for leprosy now being developed may greatly aid control efforts (Melsom, 1983).

The value of prophylaxis remains uncertain, and it can never be used as a substitute for active case-finding programs. Trials of BCG vaccination have shown marked variation in the degree of protection afforded. One can conclude only that BCG might be useful in areas with a high prevalence rate for tuberculoid leprosy. A specific antileprosy vaccine is under development but is many years away from regular use. Chemoprophylaxis with dapsone is plagued by administrative and medical uncertainties. For this reason, WHO does not recommend it for large-scale control programs. Nonetheless, many workers feel that it is indicated for household contacts.

References

Convit, J., Aranzaau, N., Ulrich, M., Pinardi, M. E., Reyes, O., and Alvarado, J.: Immunotherapy with a mixture of *Mycobacterium leprae* and BCG in different forms of leprosy and in Mitsuda-negative contacts. Int J Lepr 50:415, 1982.

Godal, T.: Growing points in leprosy research. 3. Immunological detection of sub-clinical infection in leprosy. Lepr Rev 45:22, 1974.

Hastings, R. C.: Transfer factor as a probe of the immune defect in lepromatous leprosy. Int J Lepr 45:281, 1977.

Melsom, R.: Serodiagnosis of leprosy: the past, the present, and some prospects for the future. Int J Lepr 51:235, 1983.

Navayanane, E. S., Kirchheimer, W. B., and Bedi, M. B. S.: Transfer of leprosy bacilli from patients to mouse footpads by *Aedes aegypti*. Lepr India 48:181, 1977.

Ridley, D. S., and Jopling, W. H.: Classification of leprosy according to immunity. A five-group system. Int J Lepr 34:255, 1966.

World Health Organization Study Group: Chemotherapy of leprosy for control programmes. WHO Technical Report Series No. 675. Geneva, World Health Organization, 1982.

F. INTRAVASCULAR AND DISSEMINATED INFECTIONS

189
GRAM-NEGATIVE BACTEREMIA

William R. McCabe, M.D.

Gram-negative bacilli have assumed the paramount role in producing nosocomial infections over the past few decades. Although these organisms have become increasingly prevalent causes of hospital-acquired pulmonary, wound, and urinary tract infections, bacteremia caused by Enterobacteriaceae and Pseudomonadaceae provides the most definitive and striking example of the increasing frequency of gram-negative bacillary infections. Bacteremia caused by coliform bacilli was originally recognized shortly after the turn of the century but was considered a clinical rarity until the 1950's. Since this time, however, a progressive increase, as great as 20-fold in some hospitals, in the frequency of gram-negative bacteremia has been documented by McCabe and Jackson, 1962a; Dupont and Spink, 1969: McCabe, 1974; Young et al., 1977. The frequency of occurrence of gram-negative bacteremia currently exceeds a rate of 1 per 100 hospital admissions in many major medical centers in the United States. Estimates of the frequency of gram-negative bacteremia in the United States range from 71,000 to 300,000 episodes annually.

Table 1. ETIOLOGIC AGENTS IN GRAM-NEGATIVE BACTERIA

Etiologic Agent	Relative Frequency (Per Cent)
E. coli	35
Klebsiella-Enterobacter-Serratia sp.	27
(*Klebsiella*, 16%; *Enterobacter*, 9%; *Serratia*, 2%)	
P. aeruginosa	12
Proteus sp	11
Bacteroides sp	8
Other gram-negative bacilla	7
(*Acinetobacter, Alcaligenes, Hafnia, Providencia, Achromobacter, Flavobacter*, etc.)	

More than one species of gram-negative bacilli or gram-negative bacilli and gram-positive cocci are isolated from blood cultures from approximately 16 per cent of patients with gram-negative bacteremia.

DEFINITION. The term *bacteremia* indicates the presence of bacteria in the blood and, although the diagnosis may be suspected on clinical grounds, it can be confirmed only by culture of the blood. The term *septicemia* is often used interchangeably and implies the occurrence of "toxemia" and other ill-defined clinical manifestations in addition to bacteremia. Since clinical features may vary considerably depending on the duration of infection and other factors, the diagnosis of septicemia is largely dependent on subjective interpretation. Bacteremia is a more precise term that is preferable for clinical use. In some instances, bacteremia may be transient and associated with minimal clinical symptoms, but most patients with gram-negative bacteremia are acutely and severely ill.

ETIOLOGY. Although almost all gram-negative bacteria may produce bacteremia, the term *gram-negative bacteremia* is usually reserved for bacteremias produced by members of the families Enterobacteriaceae and Pseudomonadaceae. Bacteremias caused by other gram-negative bacteria (such as meningococci, gonococci, *Brucella, Salmonella typhosa,* and *Hemophilus influenzae*) may be associated with similar clinical manifestations but are usually considered as discrete clinical entities rather than under the general term of gram-negative bacteremia.

The most frequent causative agents of gram-negative bacteremia observed in 612 patients in a Boston hospital are shown in Table 1, with *Escherichia coli* accounting for slightly more than one third of cases, and *Klebsiella pneumoniae, Pseudomonas aeruginosa,* and species of *Proteus* and *Bacteroides* following in this order. A variety of other genera of gram-negative bacilli, such as *Serratia, Acinetobacter, Providencis,* and *Flavobacter,* also are responsible for occasional instances of bacteremia, but the total number of cases caused by these less frequent species constitutes only about 10 per cent of cases of bacteremia. Mixed or polymicrobic bacteremias, in which more than one species of gram-negative bacilli or cocci and gram-negative bacilli are isolated, occur in approximately 15 per cent of cases.

Some variation in the relative frequency of etiologic agents may occur in individual hospitals. A higher incidence of bacteremia with *Bacteroides* and other anaerobic gram-negative bacilli would be anticipated in hospitals with a large volume of abdominal and gynecologic surgery or large numbers of patients with abdominal trauma. Similarly, a higher proportion of bacteremias from *P. aeruginosa* occurs in hospitals with large numbers of patients with burns or hematologic malignancies. Outbreaks of nosocomial bacteremias caused by gentamicin-resistant *K. pneumoniae, P. aeruginosa, P. rettgeri,* and *Serratia marcescens* have also been reported in a number of hospitals.

Other factors (such as site of local infection or source of bacteremia, prior antibiotic therapy, and whether the infection is nosocomial or community-acquired) also may determine the most likely etiologic agent of bacteremia. Table 2 lists the most frequent sites of origin of gram-negative bacteremia, factors predisposing to bacteremia, and the species most often causing bacteremia originating from these sites. Generally, bacteria that comprise the major constituents of the bacterial flora of the gastrointestinal tract are the most frequent causes of bacteremia originating from the genitourinary, gastrointestinal, or female genital tract. *E. coli* is the most frequent etiologic agent in bacteremia originating from the genitourinary tract, with *Klebsiella* and *Enterobacter, Proteus,* and *Pseudomonas* being much less frequent and tending to occur only in patients with obstruction, repeated urinary infections, or protracted indwelling catheterization. Anaerobic bacilli, such as *Bacteroides,* are more frequent as the etiologic agent when the bowel or the female genital tract is the source of bacteremia.

In contrast, when bacteremia originates from unidentifiable sites, from tracheostomies or the use of ventilatory equipment, intravascular foreign bodies, or the skin, a different group of gram-negative bacilli is more prevalent. Bacteria such as *P. aeruginosa, Acinetobacter,* and *Serratia,* which are often found in dust, water, or on the human skin, become relatively more frequent.

PATHOGENESIS AND PATHOLOGY. Gram-negative bacilli usually enter the blood from extravascular foci but also may originate from intravascular foci such as intravascular catheters, septic thrombophlebitis, or, more rarely, bacterial endarteritis, endocarditis, mycotic aneurysms, or infected vascular grafts. The latter types of infection usually result from localization from prior bacteremic episodes or from direct invasion of large blood vessels from areas of adjacent infection. Most often, gram-negative bacilli gain access to the blood from extravascular septic foci by passage through the lymphatics or by direct invasion of small blood vessels within a local area of infection.

Factors involved in the increasing incidence of gram-negative bacteremia are more a reflection of the population affected and changing medical practices than of the virulence of gram-negative bacilli. Several factors appear to be implicated in the continuing increase in frequency of bacteremia:

Bacterial Characteristics. Despite the relatively limited capacity to produce invasive infection, other properties of gram-negative bacilli make them ideal for the production of opportunistic infections. Gram-negative bacilli are ubiquitous in their distribution. Some are major components of the fecal flora, others occur as normal inhabitants of the skin, and gram-negative bacilli are also found in large numbers within the hospital environment. In addition, gram-negative bacilli are relatively resistant to moisture, drying, and some disinfectants; and some are able to persist and multiply in water. Equally important is the proclivity among gram-negative bacilli for the development of anti-

Table 2. FACTORS INFLUENCING ETIOLOGIC AGENTS IN BACTEREMIA

Site of Origin	Precipitating Events	Most Frequent Etiologic Agents
Genitourinary tract	Indwelling catheters Instrumentation Obstruction	*E. coli* *Klebsiella-Enterobacter-Serratia* *Proteus* sp *P. aeruginosa*
Gastrointestinal tract Bowel	Obstruction Perforation Abscesses Neoplasia Diverticula	*Bacteroides* sp *E. coli* *Klebsiella-Enterobacter-Serratia* *Salmonella*
Biliary tract	Cholangitis Obstruction (stones) Surgical procedures	*E. coli* *Klebsiella-Enterobacter-Serratia*
Reproductive system	Abortion Instrumentation Postpartum	*Bacteroides* sp *E. coli*
Vascular system	Venous cutdowns Intravenous catheters Intracardiac pacemakers Surgical procedures	*P. aeruginosa* *Acinetobacter* sp *Serratia* *Erwinia* *E. cloacae*
Skin	Leukemia Agranulocytosis Immunosuppressive and cancer chemotherapeutic agents	*P. aeruginosa* *Acinetobacter* sp *Serratia*
Respiratory tract	Tracheostomy Mechanical ventilatory assistance	*P. aeruginosa* *Klebsiella-Enterobacter-Serratia* *Acinetobacter* sp *E. coli*
	Aspiration	*E. coli* *Bacteroides* sp *Klebsiella-Enterobacter-Serratia*

biotic resistance, which is much greater than that observed with gram-positive bacteria. Resistance is mediated by self-replicating, extrachromosomal genetic material termed *plasmids*. These plasmids are composed of two components: the resistance transfer factor (RTF), which is responsible for the transfer of resistance from one bacterium to another, is linked to resistance determinants (RD), which provide the genetic information required to enable recipient bacteria to perform the biochemical changes responsible for antibiotic resistance (Chapter 21). Transfer of RTF and RD occurs between bacteria of the same and different species. Although exposure to antibiotics per se does not induce antibiotic resistance, it does provide a selective reproductive advantage to bacteria that are resistant and enhances the development of a resistant hospital flora. For this reason, the frequency of antibiotic resistance among bacteria within a hospital tends to reflect the intensity of antibiotic usage.

Susceptible Population. Striking changes in the characteristics of hospitalized patients have occurred over the past few decades. There has been a progressive increase in age of hospitalized patients and an increasing proportion of the hospital population is composed of patients with abnormal defense mechanisms who are most susceptible to infections with opportunistic pathogens such as gram-negative bacilli. The demonstration that the severity of the host's underlying disease is the major determinant of the outcome of gram-negative bacteremia further emphasizes the importance of the susceptible host in the pathogenesis of bacteremia (McCabe and Jackson, 1962a and b).

Circumvention or Alteration of Host Defenses. Many procedures in hospitals, such as intravenous and bladder catheters and ventilatory assistance equipment, allow a direct means by which gram-negative bacilli may be introduced or gain access to body sites that are normally protected against bacterial ingress by host defense mechanisms. Increased likelihood of infection may result from prolonged operative procedures required by newer, more complex surgical techniques. In addition, commonly used therapeutic measures such as corticosteroids, cytotoxic agents, and irradiation therapy deleteriously affect host defense mechanisms and greatly enhance susceptibility to infection.

Thus, the modern hospital provides the optimal conditions for the occurrence of opportunistic infections (Myerowitz et al., 1971). The extensive use of antimicrobial agents results in the selection of a hospital flora composed largely of antibiotic-resistant gram-negative bacilli, while the patient population represents a concentration of patients most susceptible to infections with relatively avirulent microorganisms such as gram-negative bacilli. In addition, many therapeutic agents and procedures either deleteriously affect host defense mechanisms or provide mechanisms that circumvent normal defense mechanisms and allow access of bacteria into normally protected body sites. This combination of circumstances affords a ready explanation of the progressively increasing frequency of gram-negative bacillary infections.

The clinical features of bacteremia caused by various species of gram-negative bacteria are virtually identical regardless of the etiologic agent. In addition, intravenous administration of killed gram-negative bacteria or purified endotoxin extracted from the cell walls of gram-negative bacteria produces manifestations similar to those observed in bacteremia. This has led to the assumption that endotoxin, which is present in all gram-negative bacteria, is released during the course of infection and is the primary pathogenetic mechanism in bacteremia (Young et al., 1977). Despite the attractiveness of this concept, the actual role of endotoxin in the pathogenesis of the manifestations of gram-negative bacteremia is not clearly defined. Other studies have suggested that endotoxin per se may play a negligible role in the pathogenesis of the manifestations of certain bacteremias (McCabe, 1975).

A variety of substances (histamine, 5-hydroxytryptamine, glucocorticoids, lysosomal enzymes, epinephrine, norepinephrine, β endorphin, and prostaglandins and related compounds) have also been proposed as mediators of many of the clinical features observed in gram-negative bacteremia, but their actual importance in clinical infections has yet to be documented. More recent laboratory and clinical studies have indicated that concomitant activation of the coagulation, fibrinolytic, and complement systems, depicted in Figure 1, may be important in the development of the hemodynamic and hemostatic changes sometimes observed in gram-negative bacteremia. Gram-negative bacilli or their endotoxins can activate Hageman factor (Factor XII). This is followed by activation of the intrinsic clotting system and also the fibrinolytic system as a result of the conversion of plasminogen to plasmin. Concomitant activation of the coagulation and the fibrinolytic systems provides the circumstances required for the development of disseminated intravascular coagulation or consumptive coagulopathy occasionally seen in gram-negative bacteremia. The magnitude of activation of the complement system, primarily via the properdin C3-C9 pathway, has been shown to parallel the severity of bacteremia. Similarly, conversion of kallikreinogen ultimately to bradykinin, which increases vascular permeability and produces vascular dilatation, has been demonstrated to occur in gram-negative bacteremia. Thus, intravascular coagulation, fibrinolysis, and shock may result from activation of Hageman factor. These interrelated changes in the coagulation, fibrinolytic, complement, and kinin systems as a result of contact with gram-negative bacilli or their products have been documented to occur in bacteremia and may be responsible for the pathophysiologic changes observed.

CLINICAL MANIFESTATIONS. The diagnosis of bacteremia can be established with certainty only by isolation of

Activation of Humoral Mediators by Gram-negative Bacteria

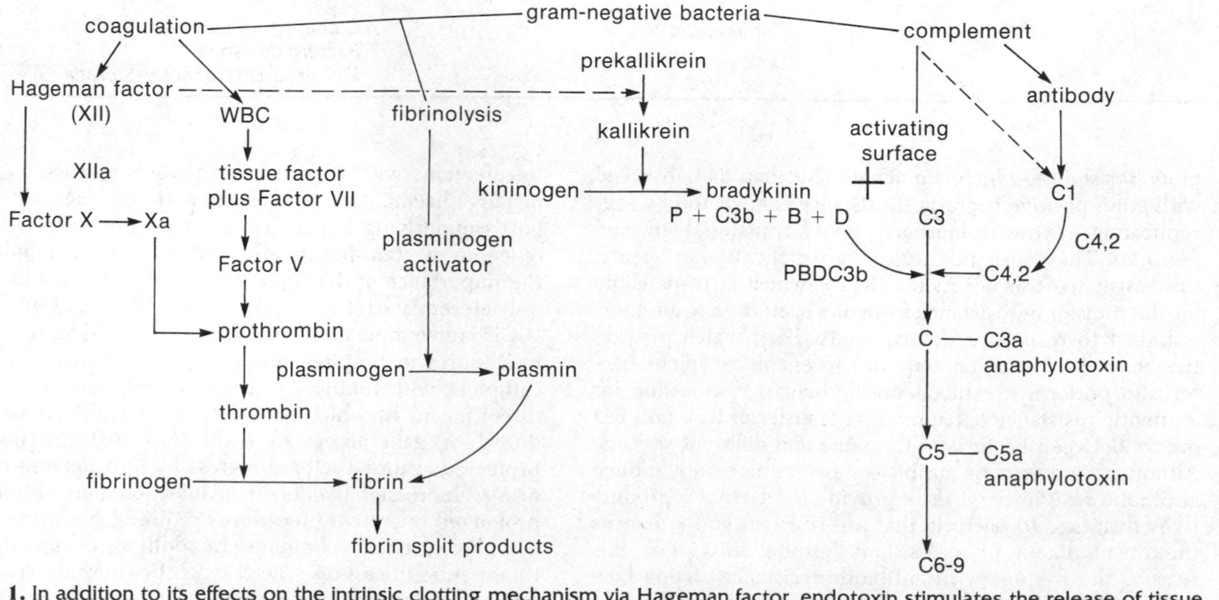

Figure 1. In addition to its effects on the intrinsic clotting mechanism via Hageman factor, endotoxin stimulates the release of tissue factor from phagocytic leukocytes (WBC) and thereby activates the extrinsic clotting pathway. Both PMN and monocytes have been implicated as sources of procoagulant activity. In addition, macrophages are stimulated by endotoxin to release plasminogen activator. The complement system, as well as the clotting system, can also be activated as a result of gram-negative bacteremia, and there is evidence that the magnitude of activation parallels the severity of the bacteremia. Complement activation can be reproduced in vitro and in vivo by endotoxin. It appears that both the classic and the alternative complement pathways can be activated by endotoxin and by gram-negative bacteremia. Activation of complement generates the anaphylatoxins C3a and C5a, which increase vascular permeability. In addition, C3d is generated and causes the initial leukopenia that is characteristic of gram-negative bacteremia. Thus, activation of proenzymes by the bacteria or their endotoxins may cause intravascular coagulation, fibrinolysis, complement activation, and even shock.

the infecting organism from cultures of the blood. The rapid course and high fatality rate of bacteremia, however, often require the formulation of clinical diagnosis and initiation of treatment before the results of blood culture are known. Although there may be considerable case-to-case variation in the severity of the disease, the clinical signs of bacteremia produced by individual species of gram-negative bacilli are virtually identical. Thus, the clinical manifestations do not readily allow identification of the etiologic agent. In the typical case, shaking chills, high fever, prostration, and occasionally nausea and vomiting develop within one to two hours after manipulation, insertion, or removal of a bladder catheter or manipulation of an area of focal infection. Shock, or hypotension, usually appears within two to eight hours after the initial manifestations of bacteremia. Regrettably, however, this typical sequence of events occurs in only 30 to 40 per cent of patients with gram-negative bacteremia, and the clinical manifestations are more subtle in the majority of patients. Table 3 lists some of the clinical manifestations that may be observed in gram-negative bacteremia. Fever is almost universal at the onset but may be minimal in uremics, the elderly, and patients receiving corticosteroids. The development of fever after genitourinary and gastrointestinal procedures, in patients with bladder or venous catheters, and in patients with leukemia or hematologic disorders, especially if associated with granulocytopenia, may be the only manifestation of bacteremia. Despite considerable variation in the magnitude of fever, higher fevers tend to occur in bacteremias caused by gram-negative bacilli than in those caused by gram-positive bacteria. Very rarely, hypothermia may be the presenting feature of bacteremia.

Hyperpnea, tachypnea, and respiratory alkalosis, in the absence of pulmonary abnormalities, may be the mode of presentation of bacteremia. Similarly, bacteremia may present as hypotension, anuria or oliguria, or acidosis without apparent cause. Clinical manifestations of bacteremia tend to be less flagrant in the elderly, and confusion, delirium or agitation, or stupor may be the initial symptom. Thrombocytopenia of mild to moderate degree occurs in approximately 60 per cent of patients and may suggest the diagnosis of bacteremia. In patients in whom bacteremia results from extension of previously localized pulmonary, genitourinary, and gastrointestinal infections, manifestations of the local infection may obscure those of bacteremia. As a result, bacteremia should always be considered a likely possibility in patients with severe pulmonary, genitourinary, and gastrointestinal infections.

Although it is generally not possible to identify the specific etiologic agent of bacteremia on the basis of clinical findings, there is one manifestation that may allow clinical identification of the specific etiologic agent. The appearance of tender, indurated, or ulcerative lesions with black, necrotic centers, ecthyma gangrenosum, or erythematous vesicles filled with cloudy fluid is almost diagnostic of bacteremia with *P. aeruginosa*, although there have been isolated reports of similar lesions in *Citrobacter* and *Aeromonas* bacteremia.

The above-described features, except for ecthyma gangrenosum, are not specific, but they should alert the physician to the possibility of bacteremia. Their occurrence should stimulate prompt collection of blood cultures and other appropriate specimens for culture and Gram stain.

DIAGNOSIS AND TREATMENT. Optimal treatment of gram-negative bacteremia is based on (1) early recognition of bacteremia and its source; (2) identification of the etiologic agent and determination of its antimicrobial susceptibility; (3) administration of adequate doses of an appropriate antibiotic parenterally; (4) correction of obstructive lesions, drainage of purulent accumulations, or removal of foreign bodies; and (5) prevention or treatment of complications.

Once the etiologic agent has been identified and its antimicrobial susceptibility determined, the treatment of bacteremia is not difficult. This is different from the usual clinical situation, however, when the physician is presented with an ill, febrile patient suspected of having bacteremia but in whom the etiologic agent and its antibiotic susceptibility are unknown. In these circumstances, two to three blood cultures should be obtained at intervals of no less than ten minutes. Appropriate specimens should also be collected from any possible site of infection, e.g., urine, sputum, purulent exudates, and intravenous catheters, for immediate Gram stain and culture. Total and differential leukocyte counts, urinalysis, and x-ray of the chest should also be included in the evaluation of patients with suspected bacteremia. Prior culture and sensitivity results that may have been obtained also may provide clues for the initiation of therapy.

Identification of the source of bacteremia can assist in estimation of the most likely etiologic agent and selection of appropriate antibiotic therapy. Those bacterial species that produce infections most often in specific organs or body sites also are the species most often found in bacteremias originating from infections at these sites. Table 2

Table 3. CLINICAL FEATURES SUGGESTIVE OF GRAM-NEGATIVE BACTEREMIA

Chills, fever and hypotension	
Fever alone (particularly in patients with malignancies, hematologic, urinary tract, or gastrointestinal disorders, and following instrumentation or insertion of urinary or intravenous catheters)	
Hyperpnea, tachypnea, and respiratory alkalosis	} Without apparent cause
Oliguria and anuria	
Hypotension	
Thrombocytopenia	
Change in mentation (agitation, confusion, stupor)	
Acidosis	
Hypothermia	
Evidence of urinary tract infection	
Evidence of pulmonary infection (associated with ventilatory assistance)	
Ecthyma gangrenosum	

lists the bacterial species most often isolated from blood cultures in instances of bacteremia originating from various organs. It is important to recognize that anaerobic bacteria, such as *Bacteroides* sp, are frequent causes of bacteremia originating from the gastrointestinal and female genital tracts since the antibiotic sensitivity of anaerobes varies markedly from that of aerobic gram-negative bacilli. Overall, *E. coli* is the most frequent cause of gram-negative bacteremia and is especially likely to be found in bacteremias originating from the urinary, gastrointestinal, and female reproductive systems. *Pseudomonas* is relatively more frequent in bacteremias occurring in leukemics and in patients with thermal injuries, and in infections secondary to intravascular catheters and tracheostomies.

Initial antibiotic therapy is selected on the basis of the most likely etiologic agent and its antimicrobial sensitivity pattern. Estimation of susceptibility to various antimicrobial agents should include consideration of whether the infection was hospital-acquired and a knowledge of the sensitivity patterns of bacteria indigenous to individual hospitals, since there may be considerable variation in antibiotic susceptibility patterns of gram-negative bacilli from hospital to hospital. In general, an agent is usually selected for initial therapy of suspected gram-negative bacteremia that provides the broadest spectrum of activity against the most likely causative gram-negative bacilli. Gentamicin, 1.5 mg/kg body weight every eight hours; tobramycin, 1.5 mg/kg body weight every eight hours; and amikacin, 5 mg/kg body weight every eight hours are the antimicrobials most frequently used for initial therapy of suspected gram-negative bacteremia in most centers because of the frequency of resistance to other antibiotics. The much broader spectrum of activity of newer cephalosporin and penicillin derivatives (cefaperazone, cefotaxime, ceftizoxime, moxalactam, azlocillin, mezlocillin, piperacillin) against gram-negative bacilli than their precursors suggests that they might serve for initial therapy of suspected gram-negative bacteremia. The lack of comparative trials and the relatively limited clinical experience to date with these newer agents in bacteremia make it uncertain whether they should supplant the aminoglycosides as agents of choice for initial therapy, however. After receipt of culture and antibiotic sensitivity results, it is preferable to change to a less toxic effective agent whenever possible. Clindamycin, metronidazole, or chloramphenicol is usually administered simultaneously with one of the aminoglycosides when the concomitant presence of anaerobic gram-negative bacilli is suspected. Combined therapy with one of the above aminoglycosides and a cephalosporin or anti-Pseudomonas penicillin has been proposed, but such combinations do not materially increase the spectrum of activity against aerobic gram-negative bacilli over that of the aminoglycosides, and the clinical value and predictability of synergistic effects of these agents has not been convincingly demonstrated. In addition, the use of such combinations may enhance toxicity and the likelihood of superinfection. Antibiotic treatment is continued until the patient has been afebrile for at least three to five days, and the ultimate duration is usually determined by the time required for optimal treatment of the primary infection.

Drainage of abscesses, correction of obstruction, and removal of infected intravenous or bladder catheters also constitute an important aspect of the management of bacteremia.

COMPLICATIONS AND SEQUELAE. Shock is the most frequent and serious complication of gram-negative bacteremia. It occurs in approximately 40 per cent of such patients. Characteristically, hypotension tends to appear within six to eight hours after the first manifestations of bacteremia. Diminution in peripheral resistance, normal venous pressure, and variable alterations in cardiac output are the characteristic hemodynamic findings in shock associated with gram-negative bacteremia. Steps involved in the treatment of shock consist of (1) administration of an appropriate antimicrobial agent; (2) monitoring of central venous pressure (CVP) or wedged pulmonary capillary pressure (PWP); (3) expansion of intravascular fluid volume; (4) monitoring of arterial pressure, mental status, and urinary output; and (5) administration of vasoactive agents.

After initial evaluation has been completed and an adequate airway has been ensured, plasma volume deficits and anemia should be corrected immediately using CVP or PWP to assess the adequacy of volume replacement. Because the major functional defect in bacteremic shock is the result of diminished peripheral resistance not compensated by an adequate increase in cardiac output, attempts are made to expand plasma volume and increase cardiac output in order to provide an adequate perfusion volume. Expansion of plasma volume requires monitoring of CVP or PWP. Changes in CVP or PWP in response to volume expansion provide better indices of the adequacy of volume expansion and fluid overload than absolute values. Initially, saline, plasma, or blood is administered rapidly, then more slowly with frequent measurement of CVP or PWP until the arterial blood pressure rises. If the CVP rises to 110 to 120 mm of water or the PWP rises to 18 to 20 mm of mercury and persists at this level or continues to rise, volume expansion is discontinued. Repetitive measurement of urinary output and mental status provide an assessment of perfusion of vital organs in addition to information obtained from arterial blood pressure measurements.

If blood pressure is not restored by fluid replacement, vasoactive amines should be used. Disagreement exists over the relative merits of various agents in shock. Dopamine, which has recently been used frequently in patients with bacteremic shock, should be started in a dose of 1 to 10 μg/kg/min because this amount dilates renal vessels and increases urine output. At higher doses (10 to 50 μg/kg/min), it stimulates alpha reactors so that arterial pressure rises due to peripheral vasoconstriction. Isoproterenol should be used if there is no response to dopamine and is given in a dose of 1 to 2 μg/kg/min. It stimulates myocardial contractility and heart rate and causes vasodilatation, but renal blood flow is unchanged and arrhythmias are frequent. Older patients especially must be watched closely for supraventricular tachycardias. Norepinephrine is the agent of last resort. It produces severe peripheral vasoconstriction and thrombosis that may cause irreversible ischemic injury to the extremities. Nevertheless, it may restore blood pressure when other treatment fails. Its dose is 0.05/μg/kg. The alpha adrenergic blocking agent phentolamine has also been used in dosages of 0.1 to 2 mg over a 20-minute period with reported good results. There is even more controversy over the value of corticosteroid therapy in bacteremic shock. Early controlled studies failed to demonstrate any beneficial effects of doses of steroids equivalent to 300 mg of hydrocortisone per day but, more recently, doses of 30 mg/kg of body weight of methylprednisolone were reported to be of benefit in the treatment of bacteremic shock (Schumer, 1976). Other recent studies demonstrated greater fatality rates in patients with bacteremic shock treated with large doses of steroids than in similar patients not receiving steroids (Kreger et al., 1980).

Anuria, oliguria, and retention of urea nitrogen may complicate shock. If correction of hypotension does not induce increased urine output, osmotic diuresis with 12.5 to 25 g of mannitol, given intravenously, may be attempted. Failure to obtain diuresis necessitates modification of antibiotic dosage and initiation of measures such as hemodialysis for management of renal failure.

Respiratory alkalosis often occurs early in the course of bacteremia but metabolic acidosis usually supervenes in severe shock and may require correction with bicarbonate. Pulmonary changes, termed *shock lung*, also may result from bacteremic shock and are manifested by roentgenographic evidence of diffuse opacification of the lung and severe hypoxemia, which is relatively refractory to oxygen administration.

Disseminated intravascular coagulation with thrombocytopenia, fibrinogenopenia, decreased levels of clotting Factors II, V, and VIII, and the presence of circulating fibrin split products may occur in 5 to 10 per cent of patients with bacteremia. Its occurrence is limited almost exclusively to patients with shock, and correction of the hypotension is usually associated with improvement of coagulation abnormalities. Heparin has been used in the treatment of disseminated intravascular coagulation with equivocal results.

PREVENTION. Prevention is much more effective than treatment of gram-negative bacteremia. Care in the use of the most frequent sources of bacteremia (intravenous catheters, urinary catheters, and ventilatory equipment) can materially reduce the frequency of bacteremia. The use of these devices should be limited to instances in which they are absolutely necessary. If the use of an intravenous catheter is mandatory, it should be inserted under scrupulously sterile conditions and removed within 48 to 72 hours. Similarly, care should be exercised to ensure that bladder catheters are also inserted under sterile conditions and that closed drainage systems, which prevent contamination between the drainage tube and the collection bottle, are used. Continuous irrigation with antibiotic solutions is not of value if closed drainage systems are carefully maintained. Equipment used for ventilatory assistance and therapy should be gas-sterilized before use, and reservoir nebulizers and humidifiers removed daily and cleaned with 0.25 per cent acetic acid. Additional control measures should include insistence on strict aseptic precautions for the care of wounds, tube drainage systems, catheters, and tracheostomies, prevention of decubiti, and limitation of prophylactic antibiotics. Diligent application of techniques for infection control can materially reduce the incidence of nosocomial bacteremia and effect reductions in the costs of medical care by shortening the duration of hospitalization for many patients.

References

DuPont, H. L., and Spink, W. W.: Infections due to gram-negative organisms. An analysis of 860 patients with bacteremia at the University of Minnesota Medical Center, 1958-1966. Medicine 48:307, 1969.

Kreger, B. E., Craven, D. E., Carling, P. C., and McCabe, W. R.: Gram-negative bacteremia. III. Reassessment of etiology, epidemiology, and ecology in 612 patients. Am J Med 68:332, 1980.

Kreger, B. E., Craven, D. E., and McCabe, W. R.: Gram-negative bacteremia. IV. Re-evaluation of clinical features and treatment in 612 patients. Am J Med 68:344, 1980.

McCabe, W. R.: Gram-negative bacteremia. Adv Intern Med 19:135, 1974.

McCabe, W. R.: Antibiotics and endotoxic shock. Bull NY Acad Med 51:1084, 1975.

McCabe, W. R., and Jackson, G. G.: Gram-negative bacteremia. I. Etiology and ecology. Arch Intern Med 110:847, 1962a.

McCabe, W. R., and Jackson, G. G.: Gram-nagative bacteremia. II. Clinical, laboratory, and therapeutic observations. Arch Intern Med 110:856, 1962b.

Myerowitz, R. L., Medeiros, A. A., and O'Brien, T. F.: Recent experience with bacillemia due to gram-negative organisms. J Infect Dis 124:239, 1971.

Schumer, W.: Steroids in the treatment of clinical septic shock. Ann Surg 184:333, 1976.

Young, L. S., Martin, W. J., Meyer, R. D., Weinstein, R. J., and Anderson, E. T.: Gram-negative rod bacteremia: Microbiologic, immunologic and therapeutic considerations. Ann. Intern. Med. 86:456, 1977.

190
STAPHYLOCOCCAL BACTEREMIA

MARIA C. SAVOIA, M.D.
STEPHEN I. MORSE, M.D.

Coagulase-positive staphylococci are among the most common human pathogens. Manifestations of infection with these important bacteria range from trivial skin infections to overwhelming septicemia. In the preantibiotic era, patients with *Staphylococcus aureus* bacteremia were often young, healthy people with an obvious source of infection that predisposed to invasion of the blood stream. Most developed metastatic abscesses, and mortality was exceptionally high (82 per cent) (Skinner and Keefer, 1941). *S. aureus* is still a common cause of both community and hospital acquired bacteremia, with many deaths despite antibiotics.

Coagulase-negative staphylococci, the most common bacteria isolated from blood cultures, are often not fully identified in clinical microbiology laboratories and are commonly called *Staphylococcus epidermidis.* Although the vast majority are contaminants or are of no clinical importance, (Zierdt, 1983), significant coagulase-negative staphylococcal bacteremia can occur in patients with prosthetic valves, cerebrospinal fluid shunts, indwelling intravenous catheters, or profound granulocytopenia (Wade et al., 1982).

ETIOLOGY AND PATHOGENESIS. *S. aureus* can often be cultured from clothing, bedding, and floors. Ten to 40 per cent of healthy people carry *S. aureus* in moist skin areas and the anterior nares. Carriage rates are even higher in drug addicts (Tuazon and Sheagren, 1975), insulin-dependent diabetics (Tuazon et al., 1975), and hemodialysis patients (Kirmani et al., 1978). These individuals are often infected with the phage type that they carry, and there is some evidence that the incidence of staphylococcal disease may be higher in chronic *S. aureus* carriers (Sewell et al., 1982).

Intact skin and mucous membranes are a major defense against invasion by staphylococci. Once these barriers are breached, bloodstream dissemination of staphylococci can arise from any site, most commonly from a clinically apparent primary infection in the skin and soft tissues, (20 to 50 per cent), operative wounds (13 to 20 per cent), intravenous catheters or vascular access devices (7 to 22 per cent), bone and joints (1 to 15 per cent), and lungs (1 to 12 per cent). In large series, 20 to 40 per cent of patients with *S. aureus* bacteremia have no identifiable primary focus of infection. Some of these patients are drug addicts, who probably injected the bacteria. In others, bacteremia may have developed from trivial skin infection or colonized areas after mild or even unrecognized trauma.

Staphylococci probably disseminate from localized abscesses into the bloodstream by invading blood vessels and producing septic thrombi, or by traveling up the lymphatics through incompetent lymph nodes into the general circulation. Although *S. aureus* produces a number of toxins and enzymes that might promote bloodstream invasion, none has been proven to be of primary importance in the development of bacteremia. Strains isolated from the blood are no more virulent for experimental animals than other strains.

About 80 per cent of patients with staphylococcal bacteremia have serious associated medical conditions (Musher and McKenzie, 1977). Among the factors that appear to predispose to staphylococcal bacteremia are uncontrolled diabetes mellitus, renal insufficiency requiring hemodialysis, extensive surgery, malignancies, malnutrition, corticosteroids, granulocytopenia, liver disease, and immunosuppressive drugs. All decrease local or systemic defense mechanisms, and also predispose to other infections.

Metastatic foci of infection are very common in the absence of a primary focus of infection (Nolan and Beaty, 1976), but also occur in 15 to 30 per cent of patients with identifiable portals of entry. The most common sites are the lungs, bone and joints, soft tissue, and kidney. Extravascular lesions, such as osteomyelitis, may be the only manifestations of transient staphylococcal bacteremia. These lesions can, in turn, cause continuing bacteremia.

Coagulase negative staphylococci are part of the normal skin flora. They lack most of the pathogenic properties of *S. aureus*. Bacteremia occurs most commonly when organisms are allowed direct access to the bloodstream via intravenous devices (Wade et al., 1982; Winston et al., 1983). Foreign material, such as a prosthetic heart valves or cerebrospinal fluid shunts, commonly predisposes to bacteremia.

PATHOLOGY. The pathologic findings in staphylococcal bacteremia are those of the metastatic or primary abscesses which have the same basic histopathologic findings regardless of site. The hallmark of the abscess is a central core of liquefaction necrosis containing dead polymorphonuclear leukocytes, other cells, and bacteria, surrounded by a zone of fibrin in which viable organisms and newly recruited granulocytes are found. In *S. aureus* endocarditis, destructive lesions of the valve leaflet and ring are serious complications. Although abscesses may completely replace an organ, as with renal abscesses, or affect such vital sites as the brain, meninges, and myocardium, the immediate cause of death cannot always be determined in overwhelming staphylococcal sepsis.

CLINICAL MANIFESTATIONS AND LABORATORY FINDINGS. *S. aureus* bacteremia from any source may be a fulminating disease beginning suddenly with high fever, chills, and tachycardia, and rapidly progressing to death within 24 to 48 hours. More often, however, the disease progresses more slowly. There are no specific symptoms of staphylococcal bacteremia, although shock is less frequent than with gram-negative septicemia. Most patients with *S. aureus* bacteremia have fever and look acutely ill and confused. They often have specific symptoms referable to areas of primary infection or secondary involvement. Occasionally *S. aureus* endocarditis may present as a subacute febrile illness. Mild musculoskeletal symptoms or headache may be the only complaint.

Anemia and polymorphonuclear leukocytosis with many immature granulocytes ("shift to the left") are characteristic. Leukocyte counts may be normal or depressed in severe infections, but the proportion of immature neutrophils is still greatly elevated. The sedimentation rate is often increased. Thrombocytopenia and hypocomplementemia may occur (O'Connor et al., 1978). Proteinuria and microscopic hematuria are usually secondary to immune complex disease rather than septic emboli and patients may be azotemic.

Bacteremia due to *S. epidermidis* is usually more indolent. Hypotension is rare. In bacteremia secondary to infection of intravascular catheters, local inflammation is common, but fever may be the only indication of infection in patients with prosthetic valve endocarditis or infected CSF shunts. Mucositis and other alimentary tract disturbances may be present and serve as portals of entry in granulocytopenic patients who become colonized with antibiotic resistant *S. epidermidis*.

COMPLICATIONS AND SEQUELAE

Endocarditis. The most serious complication of staphylococcal bacteremia is endocarditis. Although *S. aureus* endocarditis in experimental animals can only be established in the presence of a valvular abnormality (Garrison and Freedman, 1970), human endocarditis often occurs on previously normal valves. However, abnormal valves also predispose to endocarditis. In early published series composed of a large percentage of patients with underlying valvular heart disease, *S. aureus* bacteremia was associated with endocarditis in greater than 60% of patients (Wilson and Hamburger, 1957). *S. aureus* and *S. epidermidis* are both common causes of prosthetic valve endocarditis, which is associated with high mortality (63 to 74 per cent), especially in the early post-operative period (Masur and Johnson, 1980).

Patients with *S. aureus* endocarditis may have classic presentations with new pathologic or changing murmurs, splenomegaly, hematuria, multiple metastatic abscesses, and evidence of peripheral emboli (see Chapter 213). Although a murmur is often absent in tricuspid endocarditis, it is easy to make this diagnosis in the setting of intravenous drug abuse, fever, pulmonary infiltrates and positive blood cultures. However, it is difficult to distinguish some bacteremic syndromes from endocarditis. Hemodialysis access site infections and septic venous thrombophlebitis may mimic right–sided endocarditis, and the presence of left-sided endocarditis is a matter of expert clinical judgement in many bacteremic patients.

Osteomyelitis. Osteomyelitis is a common complication of staphylococcal bacteremia. Hematogenous osteomyelitis is primarily a disease of children under 12 years of age. The source of the bacteria is not found in over half of patients, and only about 50 per cent are bacteremic when bone symptoms begin. Trauma is thought to cause transient dissemination from the skin. S. *aureus* has a predilection for the diaphyseal ends of the femur and tibia. Usually, only one bone is involved. In adults, the subchondral vertebral end plates are another common site of hematogenous staphylococcal osteomyelitis. The presenting symptoms of osteomyelitis are almost always pain and swelling of overlying soft tissue, either from secondary inflammation or extension of infection. Radiographic evidence of bone disease may not appear for two weeks or more after the onset of symptoms but may be found earlier by radionuclide scanning. In patients with endocarditis or complicated bacteremia, bone scans may disclose areas of unsuspected osteomyelitis (Musher and McKenzie, 1977).

Septic Arthritis. S. *aureus* is a common cause of pyogenic arthritis in children and adults. In adults, infection often occurs in previously abnormal joints, such as those affected by rheumatoid arthritis or osteoarthritis. In drug addicts, the sternoclavicular or sacroiliac joints may be involved. Staphylococci can be seen in smears and isolated from aspirated joint fluid.

Pulmonary Abscesses. Multiple lung abscesses can arise hematogenously, particularly during endocarditis of the tricuspid valve. Lung abscesses may be the only evidence of right-sided endocarditis, since tricuspid infections are often silent. Scanning techniques will often demonstrate lesions before chest X-rays. The usual radiographic findings are multiple, small (<3 cm), peripheral lung densities that cavitate and coalesce, and may develop after antibiotics are begun. They may either be silent clinically or produce fever and pulmonary symptoms for several weeks. Empyema is a rare complication.

Kidney Lesions. Septic emboli to the kidneys may cause cortical and perinephric abscesses or pyelonephritis that can be demonstrated by radiographic and scanning techniques. Proteinuria, hematuria and hypocomplementemia may accompany the rapidly progressive noninfectious lesions of immune complex glomerulonephritis. Renal insufficiency usually improves quickly with antibiotic therapy. Indolent immune complex nephritis is a particular complication of prolonged S. *epidermidis* bacteremia and may lead to nephrotic syndrome in children with infections of ventriculo-atrial shunts.

Skin and Soft Tissue Lesions. A spectrum of lesions ranging from petechiae on the digits and distal extremities to metastatic cutaneous abscesses may be found in staphylococcemia. Although some of these lesions may be immunologic (Davis et al., 1978), others represent septic embolization, and aspirates reveal neutrophils and staphylococci (Musher and McKenzie, 1977).

Over 95 per cent of reported cases of pyomyositis are caused by S. *aureus*. Although blood cultures are usually sterile when symptoms appear, pyomyositis is probably hematogenous in origin. Abscesses are usually deep within striated muscle and involvement of overlying tissues does not occur for several weeks. Uncommon in temperate zones, pyomyositis may be responsible for 1 to 2 per cent of surgical admissions to hospitals in some tropical areas ("tropical" pyomyositis, Chapter 220).

Central Nervous System Lesions. The relatively uncommon lesions of meningitis, brain abscess, cerebral infarct, and mycotic aneurysm are more frequent during endocarditis than simple bacteremia and have a poor prognosis. More commonly, bacteremic patients present with a sterile CSF and altered mental status without focal findings. The combination of pleocytosis and a sterile CSF usually represents multiple cerebral microabscesses.

Disseminated Intravascular Coagulation (DIC). DIC occurs much less often in staphylococcal bacteremia than in gram-negative bacteremia. Hemorrhagic skin lesions, thrombocytopenia, clotting abnormalities, and increased plasma levels of fibrin split products all occur. DIC can occasionally be severe enough to mimic meningococcemia.

DIAGNOSIS. Bacteremia is often unsuspected and overlooked in patients who have severe underlying disorders because the basic disease may mask infection. Although it is difficult to diagnose staphylococcal bacteremia on clinical grounds alone, certain clinical settings warrant a high index of suspicion. Staphylococcal bacteremia should be considered as the possible etiology of any newly acquired fever in a hospitalized patient with an intravenous cannula. S. *aureus* is the most common cause of bacteremia and endocarditis in drug addicts and S. *epidermidis* is the most common cause of prosthetic valve endocarditis (Karchmer et al., 1983). Skin or skeletal foci in a patient with symptoms of bacteremia may point to disseminated staphylococcal infection. As previously noted, however, staphylococcal bacteremia may occur without an overt focus of infection. Clinical observations, radionuclide scanning and x-ray procedures may reveal metastatic lesions.

Specific diagnosis can be made only by isolation of the bacteria from the blood, but accessible lesions should be aspirated and cultured because the presence of staphylococci in the primary or secondary lesions suggests the diagnosis and affects treatment and prognosis. Staphylococci are usually detectable in cultures within 24 to 48 hours. In heavy infections stained specimens of the buffy coat of peripheral blood sometimes reveal staphylococci within neutrophils.

Since both coagulase-positive and coagulase-negative staphylococci are part of the normal skin flora, specimens must be obtained with sterile techniques. Although 90 per cent of bloodstream isolates of coagulase negative staphylococci are contaminants, the likelihood of clinical significance increases with increasing numbers of positive blood cultures, and these isolates should not be dismissed in patients with prosthetic devices or profound granulocytopenia.

S. *aureus* is usually easily identified. Since a rare S. *aureus* strain may be coagulase negative (Smith and Farkas-Hemsley, 1969), infection in the absence of a foreign body should not be ascribed to S. *epidermidis* without testing for lysostaphin susceptibility, DNAse activity, bacteriophage sensitivity and/or protein A determination.

The frequency of endocarditis in S. *aureus* bacteremia is controversial. Differentiation of endocarditis from bacteremia is not always simple, but certain clinical parameters are more useful than others. Bacteremia with endocarditis is classically persistent and "high grade" (30 to 100 organisms/ml blood) (Beeson et al., 1945). Unfortunately, however, bacteremia may also be persistent in patients with large abscesses or infected intravenous devices (Musher and McKenzie, 1977). S. *aureus* bacteriuria also occurs with equal frequency in bacteremia with and without endocarditis (Lee et al., 1978). Although complicated staphylococcal infections without endocarditis may rarely be accompanied by immune complex glomerulonephritis, its presence strongly suggests valvular involvement. Detection of cardiac vegetations by echocardiography is specific but not sensitive (Mintz and Kotler, 1980).

With no obvious portal of entry at the time of clinical presentation, the likelihood of *S. aureus* endocarditis increases, so that 60 to 70 per cent of such patients have prominent clinical features of endocarditis or vegetations at surgery or autopsy. These bacteremias often arise in the community rather than the hospital and frequently cause metastatic abscesses (Nolan and Beatty, 1976; Iannini and Crossley, 1976; Mirimanoff and Glauser, 1982).

The reported frequency of endocarditis in patients with a primary focus of infection ranges from 0% to 38 per cent (Ianinni and Crossley, 1976; Mirimanoff and Glauser, 1982). When bacteremia is acquired in the hospital, if the portal of entry is easy to identify (usually an infected intravenous catheter) and promptly treated with the right antibiotics, the risk of endocarditis is low.

THERAPY. The suspicion of staphylococcal bacteremia demands prompt intravenous administration of bactericidal antibiotics in high doses after cultures have been obtained. Since most strains of *S. aureus* are resistant to penicillin, treatment should start with a semisynthetic penicillin (oxacillin, nafcillin, methicillin) or a cephalosporin with good anti-staphylococcal activity (cephalothin or cefazolin) (see Table 1). Drug sensitivities should include the minimal inhibitory concentration (MIC), the minimal bactericidal concentration (MBC), and a test for beta-lactamase production. If the strain is penicillin sensitive (i.e., MIC < 0.1 mg/ml) and does not produce beta-lactamase, penicillin G should be given. Most authorities recommend continued treatment of penicillinase-producing *S. aureus* bacteremia with a semisynthetic penicillin. Nafcillin, oxacillin, and methicillin appear to be equally effective. When given in high doses for prolonged ($>$ 2 weeks) periods, the incidence of side effects may be higher with methicillin, but fever, eosinophilia and granulocytopenia may occur with any of these agents. Renal and hepatic abnormalities that occasionally occur with methicillin and oxacillin therapy are reversible. Although ototoxic at high serum levels, vancomycin offers significant advantages in the treatment of staphylococcal bacteremia in patients undergoing chronic hemodialysis, since it can be administered as a single, weekly, intravenous dose (Barcenas et al., 1976).

Table 1. PARENTERAL DOSES OF ANTIMICROBIAL DRUGS IN STAPHYLOCOCCAL BACTEREMIA IN ADULTS

A. Patients not allergic to penicillins:
 1. Initial therapy
  Oxacillin, 8–12 grams per day in divided doses every 4 hours
  or
  Nafcillin, 8–12 grams per day in divided doses every 4 hours
  or
  Methicillin, 12–16 grams per day in divided doses every 4–6 hours
 2. Definitive therapy
  a. Penicillin-sensitive staphylococcus
   Change to penicillin G, 12×10^6 units per day in divided doses every 4 hours
  b. Penicillin-resistant staphylococcus
   Continue initial therapy

B. Patients allergic to penicillin but not to cephalosporins:
 1. Initial and definitive therapy (if organism sensitive)
  Cephalothin, 12–16 grams per day given in divided doses every 4–6 hours; *or* Cefazolin 3–4 grams per day in divided doses every 6–8 hours

C. Patients allergic to both penicillin and cephalosporins *or* organisms resistant to penicillin G, semisynthetic penicillins and cephalosporins:
  Vancomycin 2 grams per day in divided doses every 6 hours

The role of the cephalosporins (and in particular, cefazolin) in the treatment of serious *S. aureus* infections is more controversial. Cefazolin therapy costs less than treatment with other agents, and it is particularly useful when venous access is difficult, since intramuscular administration produces high blood levels. Whether first generation cephalosporins and semisynthetic penicillins are equally effective is a matter of debate. This controversy revolves around one major issue. In animal models of *S. aureus* endocarditis, valvular vegetations may contain 10^8 to 10^9 bacteria per gram of tissue (Sande and Johnson, 1975), and, *in vitro*, with large ($> 10^7$ organisms/ml) inocula, the first generation cephalosporins are more susceptible to β-lactamase inactivation than the semisynthetic penicillins (Sabath et al., 1975). However, cephalothin and cefazolin have been used successfully in the treatment of bacteremia with and without endocarditis (Carrizosa et al., 1978). Anecdotal case reports of treatment failures with these and other agents should be interpreted cautiously, since treatment failures have occurred with all the major antistaphylococcal antibiotics. Because of poor penetration, cephalothin and cefazolin should not be used in the treatment of central nervous system infections. Although the third generation cephalosporins achieve high cerebrospinal fluid levels, these agents, in general, have reduced antistaphylococcal activity. In complicated bacteremias and endocarditis, once a therapeutic regimen has been established, the results of standardized serum bactericidal titers (Reller, 1981) may be useful in guiding subsequent therapy.

Soon after the introduction of methicillin, virulent *S. aureus* strains appeared in Europe that were resistant by a nonpenicillinase mechanism to all penicillins. Infections with these organisms have become increasingly important worldwide. Individual cocci in a resistant culture may show wide quantitative differences in resistance and growth characteristics, making standard disk susceptibility testing unreliable. This phenomenon has been termed "staphylococcal heteroresistance" (Hewitt et al., 1969). Methicillin-resistant *S. aureus* are usually resistant to multiple antibiotics. Vancomycin is the only antibiotic that is effective against all methicillin-resistant *S. aureus* isolated to date (Watanakunakorn, 1982) and is the drug of choice in this situation.

In 1977, Sabath and colleagues described another kind of resistance of *S. aureus* to cell-wall-active antibiotics, termed tolerance because of similarities to the tolerant pneumococci described by Tomasz (1970). Tolerance is defined as a dissociation between bacterial inhibition (MIC) and bacterial killing (MBC) in vitro. Tolerant bacteria are inhibited but not killed after 24 hours of incubation with the antibiotic. In many instances, however, tolerance merely represents slower killing, since 99.9 per cent killing is achieved with longer incubations. In addition, multiple variables in the assay procedures profoundly affect the expression of tolerance (Sabath and Mokhbat, 1983). This lack of standardization complicates interpretation of the literature. It appears, however, that tolerance after 24 hours of incubation is a fairly common phenomenon and that the percentage of tolerant bacteria in clinical isolates varies widely (Bradley et al., 1978). In the rabbit model of endocarditis, tolerance does not affect the outcome of treatment (Goldman and Petersdorf, 1979). In patients, retrospective reports have suggested that tolerance may be associated with a less favorable course or outcome (Sabath et al., 1977; Denny et al., 1979; Rajashekaraiah et al., 1980). In general, however, *in vitro* tolerance of *S. aureus* to an antibiotic does not correlate with the clinical response to treatment with that drug (Thompson, 1982). Although the clinical significance of tolerance is unproven, a change of antibiotics on the basis of *in vitro* tolerance may be warranted in patients whose response to treatment is poor when other causes for poor response cannot be found.

Therapy of *S. aureus* endocarditis should continue for four to six weeks, depending on the patient's clinical course. Not all patients with staphylococcal bacteremia require prolonged treatment. When patients without underlying valvular disease are treated promptly for uncomplicated, intravenous catheter-associated bacteremia, two weeks of intravenous antibiotics appear to be enough (Ianinni and Crossley, 1976; Nolan and Beatty, 1976). Most patients, however, have neither clearcut endocarditis nor simple catheter-associated bacteremia, and the length of their treatment is more difficult to decide. A number of serologic tests have been proposed to distinguish those patients requiring long duration of therapy from those who do not (Wheat et al., 1979). Some of these are based on the observation that patients with clinically obvious endocarditis or deep seated *S. aureus* infection (with the exception of osteomyelitis) (Mackowiak and Smith, 1978), develop antibodies to ribitol teichoic acid, a component of the *S. aureus* cell wall, within two weeks after symptoms begin (Tuazon and Sheagren, 1976; Wheat et al., 1979). The value of these tests in determining length of treatment, however, is not settled (Kaplan et al., 1981). At present, serologic tests appear to be of limited usefulness and tend to confirm the clinically obvious.

Although most patients with intravenous catheter-associated bacteremia will be cured by 2 weeks of treatment, reduction in the length of therapy should be considered only after careful clinical observation because patients who develop complications often do so after therapy has begun. In special circumstances, intravenous antibiotic therapy at home (Stiver et al., 1982) or intravenous followed by high dose oral therapy (Carney et al., 1982) may avoid prolonged hospitalization, but such innovations should be approached cautiously.

Despite appropriate antibiotic therapy, some patients with serious *S. aureus* infections respond slowly. In endocarditis, fever and positive blood cultures may last over a week on an antibiotic regimen that will ultimately be curative. Because the addition of an aminoglycoside to a semisynthetic penicillin kills more rapidly both *in vitro* (Licht, 1979) and in animal models (Sande and Johnson, 1975), some have proposed combination antibiotic therapy of *S. aureus* endocarditis. They reason that earlier sterilization of vegetations might reduce valvular damage and infectious sequelae. Several published studies, however, suggest that the addition of an aminoglycoside has no beneficial effect on eventual outcome (Abrams et al., 1979; Watanakunakorn and Baird, 1977), although fever and bacteremia may resolve more quickly in some patients. Any potential benefits must, however, be weighed against the additional risk of the renal and auditory toxicity of aminoglycosides.

Antibiotics play a major role in the successful treatment of *S. aureus* bacteremia, but local adjunctive therapy is often equally important. Intravenous catheters must be removed and atrioventricular shunts and valve prostheses may also have to be removed or replaced. Abscesses should be incised and drained and deep-seated lesions may need surgical treatment after antibiotics have been started. Treatment fails if bacteria are in a locus where antimicrobials cannot act, if serum levels of antibiotic are too low, or if drug therapy is too brief. *S. aureus* rarely loses its sensitivity to antimicrobial drugs during therapy but repeat cultures of patients with persistent signs of infection may reveal an unrecognized mixed infection or superinfection.

The vast majority of coagulase-negative staphylococcal infections are acquired in the hospital and caused by bacteria resistant to multiple drugs (Archer, 1978). Vancomycin appears to be the best single drug in the treatment of these drug resistant organisms (Wade et al., 1982; Karchmer et al., 1983). Much of the concern over methicillin resistance in *S. aureus* applies to coagulase negative staphylococci as well; disk diffusion methods of susceptibility testing may not be reliable.

A short course of treatment with a semisynthetic penicillin (if the organism is sensitive) or vancomycin, coupled with catheter removal, is sufficient for most patients with catheter-associated *S. epidermidis* bacteremia. The results of treatment of more serious infections, such as prosthetic valve endocarditis or cerebrospinal fluid shunt infections, are surprisingly poor. Removal of the device is usually necessary (Karchmer et al., 1983; Schoenbaum et al., 1975). Prosthetic valve endocarditis in the early postoperative period is often associated with tissue invasion or valve destruction (Karchmer et al., 1983) and is frequently fatal (Masur and Johnson, 1980). Combination therapy with semisynthetic penicillins or vancomycin plus rifampin and/or an aminoglycosides appears to be beneficial (Gombert et al., 1981; Sande and Scheld, 1980).

PROPHYLAXIS. Prevention of staphylococcal disease is exceedingly difficult because the organisms are part of the normal flora of the skin and mucous membranes. Normal individuals are resistant to serious staphylococcal infections although minor disease, particularly of the skin, is common. Simple preventative measures can, however, reduce the incidence of nosocomial staphylococcal infection. Personnel with open, draining lesions should be excluded from contact with highly susceptible patients. Intravenous access sites should be observed daily, and peripheral intravenous catheters should be changed every 48 to 72 hours. Education of hospital personnel about their role in the propagation of nosocomial infections and the institution of control measures in outbreaks of methicillin resistant *S. aureus* or *S. aureus* of the same phage type may decrease rates of hospital acquired infection.

References

Abrams, B., Sklaver, A., Hoffman, T., and Greenman, R.: Single or combination therapy of staphylococcal endocarditis in intravenous drug abusers. Ann Intern Med 90:789, 1979.

Archer, G. L.: Antimicrobial susceptibility and selection of resistance among Staphylococcus epidermidis isolates recovered from patients with infections of indwelling foreign devices. Antimicrob Agents Chemother 14:353, 1978.

Barcenas, C. G., Fuller, T. J., Elms, J., Cohen, R., and White, M. G.: Staphylococcal sepsis in patients on chronic hemodialysis regimens. Arch Intern Med 137:1131, 1976.

Beeson, P. B., Brannon, E. S. and Warren, J. V.: Observations on the sites of bacteria from the blood in patients with bacterial endocarditis. J Exp Med 81:9, 1945.

Bradley, J. J., Mayhall, C. G., and Dalton, H. P.: Incidence and characteristics of antibiotic-tolerant strains of Staphylococcus aureus. Antimicrob Agents Chemother 13:1052, 1978.

Carney, D. N., Fossieck, B. E., Jr., Parker, R. H., and Minna, J. D.: Bacteremia due to Staphylococcus aureus in patients with cancer: Report on 45 cases in adults and review of the literature. Rev Infect Dis 4:1, 1982.

Carrizosa, J., Santoro, J., and Kaye, D.: Treatment of experimental Staphylococcus aureus endocarditis: Comparison of cephalothin, cefazolin, and methicillin. Antimicrob Agents Chemother 13:74, 1978.

Christensen, G. D., Bisno, A. L., Parisi, J. T., McLaughlin, B., Hester, M. G., and Luther, R. W.: Nosocomial septicemia due to multiple antibiotic-resistant Staphylococcus epidermidis. Ann Intern Med 96:1, 1982.

Cooper, G., and Platt, R.: Staphylococcus aureus bacteremia in diabetic patients. Amer J Med 74:658, 1982.

Davis, J. A., Weisman, M. H., and Dail, D. H.: Vascular disease in infective endocarditis; Report of immune-mediated events in skin and brain. Arch Intern Med 138:480, 1978.

Denny, A. E., Peterson, L. R., Gerdine, D. N. and Hall, W. H.: Serious staphylococcal infections with strains tolerant to bactericidal antibiotics. Arch Intern Med 139:1026, 1979.

Garrison, P. K., and Freedman, L. R.: Experimental endocarditis. I. Staphylococcal endocarditis in rabbits resulting from the placement of a polyethylene catheter in the right side of the heart. Yale J Biol Med 42:394, 1970.

Goldman, P. L., and Petersdorf, R. G.: Significance of methicillin tolerance in experimental staphylococcal endocarditis. Antimicrob Agents Chemother 15:802, 1979.

Gombert, M. E., Landesman, S. H., Corrado, M. L., Stein, S. C., Melvin, E. T., and Cummings, M.: Vancomycin and rifampin therapy for Staphylococcus epidermidis meningitis associated with CSF shunts. J Neurosurg 55:633, 1981.

Hewitt, J. H., Coe, A. W., and Parker, M. T.: The detection of methicillin resistance in Staphylococcus aureus. J Med Microbiol 2:443, 1969.

Iannini, P. B., and Crossley, K.: Therapy of Staphylococcus aureus bacteremia associated with a removable focus of infection. Ann Intern Med 84:558, 1976.

Kaplan, J. E., Palmer, D. L., and Tung, K. S. K.: Teichoic acid antibody and circulating immune complexes in the management of Staphylococcus aureus bacteremia. Amer J Med 70:769, 1981.

Karchmer, A. W., Archer, G. L., and Dismukes, W. E.: Staphylococcus epidermidis causing prosthetic valve endocarditis: Microbiologic and clinical observations as guides to therapy. Ann Intern Med 98:447, 1983.

Kirmani, N., Tuazon, C. U., Murray, H. W., Parrish, A. E., and Sheagren, J. N.: Staphylococcus aureus carriage rate of patients receiving long term hemodialyses. Arch Intern Med 138:1657, 1978.

Lee, B. K., Crossley, K., and Gerding, D. N.: The association between Staphylococcus aureus bacteremia and bacteriuria. Amer J Med 65:303, 1978.

Licht, J. H.: Penicillinase-resistant penicillin/gentamicin synergism. Effect in patients with Staphylococcus aureus bacteremia. Arch Intern Med 139:1094, 1979.

Mackowiak, P. A., and Smith, J. W.: Teichoic acid antibodies in chronic staphylococcal osteomyelitis. Ann Intern Med 89:494, 1978.

Masur, H., and Johnson, W. D., Jr.: Prosthetic valve endocarditis. J Thorac Cardiovasc Surg 80:31, 1980.

Mintz, G. S. and Kotler, M. N.: Clinical value and limitations of echocardiography. Its use in the study of patients with infectious endocarditis. Arch Intern Med 140:1022, 1980.

Mirimanoff, R. W., and Glauser, M. P.: Endocarditis during Staphylococcus aureus septicemia in a population of non-drug addicts. Arch Intern Med 142:1311, 1982.

Musher, D. M. and McKenzie, S. O.: Infections due to Staphylococcus aureus. Medicine 56:383, 1977.

Nolan, C. M., and Beaty, H. N.: Staphylococcus aureus bacteremia. Current clinical patterns. Amer J Med 60:495, 1976.

O'Connor, D. T., Weisman, M. H., and Fierer, J.: Activation of the alternate complement pathway in Staph. aureus infective endocarditis and its relationship to thrombocytopenia, coagulation abnormalities, and acute glomerulonephritis. Clin Exp Immunol 34:179, 1978.

Rajashekaraiah, K. R., Rice, T., Rao, V. S., Marsh, D., Ramakrishna, B., and Kallick, C. A.: Clinical significance of tolerant strains of Staphylococcus aureus in patients with endocarditis. Ann Intern Med 93:796, 1980.

Reller, L. B.: Laboratory procedures in the management of infective endocarditis. In Bisno, A. L. (ed.): Treatment of Infectious Endocarditis N.Y., Grune and Stratton, 1981, p. 235.

Sabath, L. D., Garner, C., Wilcox, C., Finland, M.: Effect of inoculum and of beta-lactamase on the anti-staphylococcal activity of thirteen penicillins and cephalosporins. Antimicrob Agents Chemother 8:344, 1975.

Sabath, L. D., and Mokhbat, J. E.: What is the clinical significance of tolerance to β-lactam antibiotics? In Remington, J. S., and Swartz, (eds.) Current Clinical Topics in Infectious Diseases Vol. 4 New York, McGraw-Hill, Inc., 1983, p. 358.

Sabath, L. D., Wheeler, N., Laverdiere, M., Blazevic, D., and Wilkinson, B. J.: A new type of penicillin resistance of Staphylococcus aureus. Lancet 1:443, 1977.

Sande, M. A., and Johnson, M. L.: Antimicrobial therapy of experimental endocarditis caused by Staphylococcus aureus. J Infect Dis 131(4):367, 1975.

Sande, M. A., and Scheld, W. M.: Combination antibiotic therapy of bacterial endocarditis. Ann Intern Med 92:390, 1980.

Schoenbaum, S. C., Gardner, P., and Shilleto, J.: Infections of cerebrospinal fluid shunts: epidemiology, clinical manifestations and therapy. J Infect Dis 131:543, 1975.

Sewell, C. M., Clarridge, J., Lacke, C., Weinman, E. J., and Young, E. J.: Staphylococcal nasal carriage and subsequent infection in peritoneal dialysis patients. JAMA 248:1493, 1982.

Skinner, D., and Keefer, C. S.: Significance of bacteremia caused by Staphylococcus aureus. A study of one hundred and twenty-two cases and a review of the literature concerned with experimental infection in animals. Arch Intern Med 68:851, 1941.

Smith, H. B. H., Farkas-Hemsley, H.: The relationship of pathogenic coagulase-negative staphylococci to Staphylococcus aureus. Can J Microbiol 15:879, 1969.

Stiver, H. G., Trosky, S. K., Cote, D. D., and Oruck, J. L.: Self-administration of intravenous antibiotics: an efficient, cost-effective home care program. CMA J 127:207, 1982.

Thompson, R. L.: Staphylococcal infective endocarditis. Mayo Clin Proc 57:106, 1982.

Tomasz, A., Albino, A., and Zanati, E.: Multiple antibiotic resistance in a bacterium with suppressed autolytic system. Nature 227:138, 1970.

Tuazon, C. U., Perez, A., Kishaba, T., and Sheagren, J. N.: Staphylococcus aureus among insulin-injecting diabetic patients. JAMA 231:1272, 1975.

Tuazon, C. U., and Sheagren, J. N.: Staphylococcal endocarditis in parenteral drug abusers: source of the organism. Ann Intern Med 82:788, 1975.

Tuazon, C. U., and Sheagren, J. N.: Teichoic acid antibodies in the diagnosis of serious infections with Staphylococcus aureus. Ann Intern Med 84:543, 1976.

Wade, J. C., Schimpff, S. C., Newman, K. A., and Wiernik, P. H.: Staphylococcus epidermidis: an increasing cause of infection in patients with granulocytopenia. Ann Intern Med 97:503, 1982.

Watanakunakorn, C.: Treatment of infections due to methicillin-resistant Staphylococcus aureus. Ann Intern Med 97:376, 1982.

Watanakunakorn, C., and Baird, I. M.: Prognostic factors in Staphylococcus aureus endocarditis and results of therapy with a penicillin and gentamicin. Amer J Med Sci 273:133, 1977.

Weinstein, M. P., Reller, L. B., Murphy, J. R., and Lichtenstein, K. A.: The clinical significance of positive blood cultures: a comprehensive analysis of 500 episodes of bacteremia and fungemia in adults. I. Laboratory and epidemiologic observations. Rev Infect Dis 5:35, 1983.

Wheat, L. J., Luft, F. C., Tabbarah, Z., Kohler, R. B., and White, A.: Serologic diagnosis of access device-related staphylococcal bacteremia. Amer J Med 67:603, 1979.

Williams, R. E. O.: Healthy carriage of Staphylococcus aureus: its prevalence and importance. Bacteriol Rev 27:56, 1963.

Wilson, R., and Hamburger, M.: Fifteen years' experience with staphylococcus septicemia in a large city hospital. Amer J Med 22:437, March, 1957.

Winston, D. J., Dudnick, D. V., Chapin, M., Ho, W. G., Gale, R. P., and Martin, W. J.: Coagulase-negative staphylococcal bacteremia in patients receiving immunosuppressive therapy. Arch Intern Med 143:32, 1983.

Zierdt, C. H.: Evidence for transient Staphylococcus epidermidis bacteremia in patients and in healthy humans. J Clin Microbiol 17:628, 1983.

191

TYPHOID FEVER

GERALD T. KEUSCH, M.D.

Typhoid fever, which is caused by a motile, gram-negative bacillus, *Salmonella typhi*, is an acute febrile illness that was originally named for its clinical resemblance to typhus (the word typhoid means typhus-like). The names for both diseases were derived from the Greek word *typhos*, which means smoke in both a literal and a metaphoric sense, because the diseases were thought to have their origin in miasmic vapors and to cause mental clouding with high fever. Typhoid and typhus were clinically distinct, however, being designated "putrid-malignant" and "slow nervous" fevers, respectively. In fact, in all aspects of etiology, pathogenesis, and pathology, they are entirely distinct, but "typhoid" is still the accepted term for infection with *S. typhi*.

Actually, the clinical syndrome of typhoid fever can be caused by other salmonellae, including *S. enteritidis* bioserotype paratyphi A (*S. paratyphi* A), *S. enteritidis* serotype paratyphi B (*S. schottmuelleri* or *S. paratyphi* B), and on rare occasions even by *S. enteritidis* serotype typhimurium (*S. typhimurium*). Thus, some have advocated calling these various diseases "enteric fevers" because of the consistent involvement of Peyer's patches in the intestine by infecting organisms. Although this term is useful to indicate a family of infections with similar clinical manifestations, involvement of the enteric tract is not the essential feature of the disease. Rather, invasion of, and multiplication within, the mononuclear phagocytic cells in the liver, spleen, lymph nodes, and Peyer's patches by these infecting organisms is the hallmark of this syndrome.

ETIOLOGY

Microbiology. Microbiologic identification of *S. typhi* is simple because its biochemical reactions are different from those of all of the more than 2200 distinct salmonellae currently known. Salmonellae belong to the family Enterobacteriaceae (Chapter 31) because they all ferment glucose, reduce nitrate to nitrite, and synthesize peritrichous flagella when motile.

Biochemical features of importance in distinguishing *S. typhi* and *S. enteritidis* bioserotype paratyphi A and paratyphi B are shown in Table 1. *S. typhi*, a lactose and sucrose nonfermenting bacterium, produces a characteristic pattern that initially resembles *Shigella* more than *Salmonella*. It is anaerogenic (does not produce gas from glucose) and usually produces a trace of hydrogen sulfide (H_2S), which, in conjunction with motility and its inability to utilize citrate (Simmons') and to decarboxylate ornithine, is sufficient for a presumptive identification of *S. typhi*. Confirmation is easily obtained by serologic testing of agglutination patterns with commercially available antisera (Table 2).

Identification of *S. enteritidis* bioserotype paratyphi A may be confusing at first glance because, unlike nearly all other salmonellae, it does not produce H_2S (10 per cent of strains produce trace amounts but only after several days in culture). Initial biochemical screening may therefore suggest identification as a *Shigella*, *Alkalescens dispar*, *Citrobacter freundii* (H_2S negative variety), *Enterobacter hafnia*, or even *Yersinia enterocolitica*. Use of pooled *Salmonella* O-antigen grouping sera can quickly establish the correct genus and, in conjunction with the biochemical data and flagellar antigen typing, the species as well.

S. enteritidis serotype paratyphi B resembles biochemically the majority of the remaining salmonellae. Because its somatic antigens are also identical to those of *S. enteritidis* serotype typhimurium, the single most common *Salmonella* species isolated from humans, further characterization is required for specific identification. Serologic detection of flagellar antigens is essential in making this distinction.

Serology. Salmonellae possess many different antigens. Detection of some of these antigens by agglutination with antisera is the basis for serologic classification and identification. Specific antisera are used to determine the particular kind of envelope (K), somatic (O), or flagellar (H) antigens that are present. The resulting antigenic formula is the fingerprint that helps to identify specific strains.

Envelope antigens are the most exterior of the three antigenic types; they form a capsule on the surface of the organism. In fact, colonies of *S. enteritidis* serotype paratyphi B, when left at room temperature for a few days, may form a distinctive raised moist rim composed of K polysaccharide, the so-called "slime wall." The most important K antigen, however, is the highly polymerized acidic polysaccharide, the Vi factor, found in *S. typhi*, *S. enteritidis* serotype paratyphi C, and in *Citrobacter*. Vi antigens cover the somatic O antigens of these bacteria and render the strains inagglutinable in anti-O serum. Vi was originally discovered in this fashion by Felix and Pitt, who also showed that Vi-positive strains of *S. typhi* were more virulent for mice (hence the designation Vi). Experimental studies in human volunteers have documented a similar role of Vi in man, although the mechanism is not clear. Vi

Table 1. BIOCHEMICAL DIFFERENCES BETWEEN *S. typhi* and *S. enteritidis*

		S. Enteritidis	
	S. Typhi	***Bioserotype paratyphi A***	***Serotype parathyphi B***
Acid from glucose	+	+	+
Gas from glucose	−	+ (trace)	+
H_2S production	+(trace) (5% −)	− (10% late+)	+
Citrate utilization	−	− (25% late +)	+
Lysine decarboxylase	+	−	+
Ornithine decarboxylase	−	+	+

Table 2. ANTIGENIC FORMULAE OF CERTAIN SALMONELLAE

Organism	O Antigen Group	O Antigens	H Antigens	K Antigens
S. enteritidis				
bioserotype paratyphi A	A	1, 2, 12	a	—
serotype paratyphi B	B	1, 4, 5, 12	b:1, 2	—
serotype typhimurium B	B	1, 4, 5, 12	i:1, 2	—
bioserotype paratyphi C	C	6, 7	c:1, 5	Vi
S. typhi	D	9, 12	d	Vi

also determines phage susceptibility but is most useful in the laboratory for rapid identification of *S. typhi* by a slide agglutination test against Vi antisera. Fresh isolates of *S. typhi* that are Vi-positive are usually poorly motile and are thus not flocculated by antiflageller antisera. Because of blocking by the Vi antigen, they are not agglutinated by anti-O sera either. However, they may be quickly identified by agglutination with anti-Vi. Boiling a suspension of these organisms in physiologic saline for 20 minutes removes the Vi (and reaction with anti-Vi) and permits agglutination with anti-O serum for confirmation of the identification of *Salmonella*.

O antigens are heat-stable oligosaccharides composed of repeating units of specific sequences of simple and amino sugars at the terminal end of the lipopolysaccharide of the bacterial cell wall. Several different O antigens (designated by Arabic numerals) are usually present in each individual organism. Salmonellae with identical major O antigens are grouped together in serogroups (A, B, C, etc.), although some minor O antigens occur in more than one serogroup (Table 2). *S. typhi* is one of many organisms in group D, while *S. enteritidis* bioserotype paratyphi A is in group A, and *S. enteritidis* serotype paratyphi B is in group B. Pooled grouping antisera are commercially available for use in slide agglutination tests. A serologic distinction among the many organisms that group together in the same serogroup is made on the basis of Vi and flagellar antigens.

H antigens are flagellar proteins. In contrast to O antigens, tests for the presence of flagellar antigens are usually made in broth cultures because the organisms must be actively motile for the antigens to be detectable. Many *Salmonella* strains possess both specific and nonspecific H determinants; the latter result in significant cross-agglutination between strains. These antigens are now designated phase 1 (specific) and phase 2 (nonspecific) antigens; they are denoted by lower case Roman letters and Arabic numbers, respectively. Thus, *S. enteritidis* serotype paratyphi B expresses b antigen in phase 1 and antigens 1, 2 in phase 2 (Table 2). A fresh isolate is likely to express only one H antigen phase. In order to test for antigens of the variant phase, it is usually necessary to select colonies expressing such antigens. This is generally accomplished by the use of a phase reversal medium, a semisolid agar containing antibody to the expressed H phase. The antiserum immobilizes colonies with the homologous antigen but permits motility of organisms expressing the other phase. These organisms may then be selected for testing.

EPIDEMIOLOGY. *S. typhi*, *S. enteritidis* bioserotype paratyphi A, and serotype paratyphi B infect only humans. Christie (1980) suggests that this evolution and adaptation to the human environment constitute an "epidemiologic rut" because every case of typhoid fever may ultimately be traced back to a human carrier. There are limited possibilities for transmission of infection. Theoretically, this situation should facilitate efforts to mount an epidemiologic attack on the organisms because the transmission routes should be easily followed.

However, this is not necessarily the case. First, while patients may excrete many viable organisms in the feces, urine, vomitus, and respiratory secretions, and although the stools of chronic carriers usually contain more than one million *S. typhi* organisms per gram, direct person-to-person transmission is rare. In addition to the human source, a vehicle is required. Second, while most infections are food-borne or water-borne, there are a multitude of secondary pathways and vehicles. For example, shellfish such as mussels, living in waters contaminated with sewage, may become highly infectious although the water itself is not. This occurs because the mussel picks up and filters out the microbial content of over 10 gallons of water per day. This marked concentration of the inoculum in the creature creates a highly infectious meal for a human. The chain of causative events in this situation involves a carrier who sheds organisms into inadequately processed sewage, which is discharged into waters inhabited by edible shellfish. It is apparently safer to swim in such polluted water than it is to eat its shellfish. Third, *S. typhi* can persist for weeks in water, ice, or even dust or dried sewage. If such organisms reach a suitable vehicle, they can multiply to an infectious dose and complete the epidemiologic life cycle by reinfecting a human subject. It is not unusual to be unable to isolate *S. typhi* from the contaminated water source when clinical cases develop, because the responsible contamination occurred two or more weeks before. Nevertheless, in the classic epidemiologic investigation of a waterborne outbreak of typhoid fever, the disease is traced backward along waterways and septic systems to the chronic carrier.

The incidence of typhoid fever will therefore be determined by the prevalence of human carriers, the adequacy of environmental sanitation, and the purity of the water supply. In industrialized nations, technical improvements in handling wastes and water have contributed to a steady decline in typhoid fever, while mass production and distribution of food, which is often poorly stored and handled, have led to an explosive increase in all other forms of salmonellosis. This is perhaps the clearest example of the limited epidemiologic potential of the Salmonellae adapted to humans and the unlimited potential of the nonadapted strains. In developing countries with poor sanitation and primitive water systems, typhoid fever remains a common endemic illness.

PATHOGENESIS. Experimental studies in volunteers infected with *S. typhi* and in mice infected with *S. enteritidis* serotype enteriditis or typhimurium ("mouse typhoid") have shed considerable light on the pathogenesis of typhoid fever. Oral administration of the virulent Quailes strain of *S. typhi* has shown that the intestine, not the pharynx, is the portal of entry. Organisms must be swallowed in order to initiate disease; gargling and expectoration of large inocula failed to cause typhoid. About 50 per cent of adults are infected after ingestion of 10^7 organisms of the Quailes strain, whereas 28 per cent and 95 per cent of humans are infected by 10^5 or 10^9 organisms, respectively. Doses below 10^5 do not cause disease. Limited comparisons with other Vi-positive strains have shown a similar degree of virulence. Vi-negative strains are less virulent.

Ingested organisms must traverse the stomach to reach the small bowel. Gastric acid appears to affect *S. typhi* less than *V. cholerae, E. coli,* and other salmonellae. Viable *S. typhi* organisms can be isolated from gastric secretions for at least 30 minutes after ingestion. Organisms reaching the proximal small intestine rapidly penetrate the mucosa and begin the process of systemic invasion and frank clinical illness. Biopsy of the proximal small intestine of humans during the incubation period of typhoid, before bacteremia occurs, shows focal inflammation and suggests that this is the site of penetration. Electron micrographs of the small bowel of animals during experimental salmonellosis have demonstrated a remarkable sequence in which the epithelial cell brush border seems to melt away in advance of the penetrating organisms but is quickly restored after invasion is complete.

In monkeys, invading *S. typhi* organisms remain briefly in the regional mesenteric nodes before spreading to the liver and spleen. In the mouse, however, transient bacteremia occurs within 20 seconds of ingestion, and bacteria reach the liver and spleen shortly thereafter. *S. typhi* is rapidly taken up by mononuclear phagocytes in the liver and spleen, but instead of being quickly killed by these phagocytes, the organism multiplies intracellularly. It is precisely this characteristic of *S. typhi* that determines the nature of the illness it produces. After this period of intracellular multiplication (corresponding to the incubation period), organisms escape into the bloodstream, cause a second bacteremia, which is now sustained, and usher in the febrile symptomatic phase of the disease. In experimental animals the duration of the symptom-free interval varies inversely with the size of the inoculum. Establishment of bacteremia seems to require a set number of viable intracellular organisms; the smaller the inoculum, the longer it takes to reach this critical mass of bacteria.

Bacteremia also leads directly to two critical events in typhoid fever—invasion of the gallbladder and the Peyer's patches of the bowel. Infection of either site leads to positive stool cultures, and invasion of the gallbladder may lead to long-term carriage of the organism. When the inflammatory response of either tissue is severe, necrosis may occur, presenting clinically as necrotizing cholecystitis or hemorrhage and/or perforation of the bowel.

The role of endotoxin in the pathogenesis of typhoid fever is unclear. Although the systemic symptoms (including chills, fever, headache, myalgia, anorexia, nausea, leukopenia, and thrombocytopenia) produced by intravenous injection of *S. typhi* endotoxin resemble those of the actual disease, subjects rendered unresponsive (tolerant) to these effects of *S. typhi* endotoxin nevertheless develop typical typhoid symptoms during experimental infection. It is possible that the intracellular location of the typhoid bacillus stimulates the release of endogenous mediators directly from leukocytes and macrophages, relegating endotoxin to an unessential role.

The histopathology of typhoid is directly related to the proliferation of large mononuclear cells. This infiltration is most pronounced in the Peyer's patches of the terminal ileum but is also prominent in the liver, spleen, and mesenteric lymph nodes. Focal hepatic necrosis and cloudy swelling of hepatic cells are responsible for abnormalities of liver function during typhoid fever.

Much of our understanding of host defenses against *S. typhi* has been derived from investigations of an experimental model of typhoid fever in mice produced by mouse-passaged strains of *S. typhimurium* or *enteritidis*. Although humoral antibody reduces the number of organisms in the blood of infected mice, bacterial multiplication in tissues such as the liver and spleen is unaffected. The systemic bacterial population is reduced and the infection controlled only when the intracellular bacterial activity of macrophages is activated. Circulating specific antibody appears to contribute little to the cell-mediated immune response responsible for this critical intracellular bactericidal process. Mouse typhoid, and by extrapolation human typhoid as well, has therefore been classified as a facultative intracellular infection in which the causative organism can multiply freely within nonimmune macrophages (Hornick et al., 1970). These pathogens are rapidly killed, however, by macrophages that have been activated by lymphokines from specifically sensitized T lymphocytes, which develop early in infection.

The ability of different strains of *S. typhimurium* to survive within normal mouse peritoneal macrophages varies with the intrinsic virulence of the organism. As a consequence, the need for the development of specific cellular immunity varies as well. Furthermore, experimental studies do not exclude a role for humoral factors in the host defense response, in the form of either free antibody or cytophilic antibody on lymphocyte or macrophage membranes. Passive immunization of normal mice with isolated B, but not T, lymphocytes sensitized to *S. typhimurium* reduces the tissue multiplication of bacteria and enhances survival. This mechanism is probably distinct from the partial protection offered by circulating anti-Vi or O antibody in the vaccinated person, a protection that is most likely due to serum bactericidal activity during the initial transient bacteremia before the organism is sequestered inside macrophages.

Recent studies also provide evidence for a cell-mediated immune response in acute human typhoid fever, including lymphocyte proliferative responses and lymphokine responses to *S. typhi* antigens in vitro (Rajagopalan et al., 1982). These responses are reduced in complicated compared to uncomplicated cases, and correlate with a marked decrease in the ratio of helper to suppressor T lymphocytes.

CLINICAL MANIFESTATIONS, COMPLICATIONS, AND SEQUELAE. The incubation period of typhoid fever is generally one to two weeks, but it varies inversely with the size of the inoculum, and may be as short as three days or as long as two months. Classically, clinical disease is ushered in with fever as the phase of sustained bacteremia begins. The peak temperatures typically increase in stepwise fashion over three to four days to 104 to 105° F. Nonspecific symptoms, including anorexia, malaise, lethargy, myalgia, and continuous dull frontal headache, accompany the fever. In the past, patients have been noted to have constipation rather than diarrhea, nonproductive cough with evidence of bronchitis, and a relative bradycardia for the height of the fever response. More recent observations suggest that diarrhea is in fact more commonly observed, that cough is present in only 10 to 15 per cent of patients, and that relative bradycardia is observed in fewer than 25 per cent of cases (Samantry et al., 1977; Gulati et al., 1968). Moreover, the step-wise pattern of temperature elevation is no longer common either, and sustained or intermittent fevers often occur from the outset. A few patients may be afebrile.

Although some patients experience spontaneous remission of illness in one week or less, high sustained fevers characteristically occur during the second and third weeks. The patient looks acutely ill and has prominent facial flushing, dry skin, dilated pupils, and an asthenic, dulled, and detached appearance. Frank prostration or, particularly in children, delirium may occur at this stage. This distinctive appearance is often referred to as "toxic," although the participation of a toxin in its genesis has not been shown. Clinical symptoms usually abate within four weeks, but may last much longer. During the second week, vague abdominal discomfort with diffuse lower quadrant tenderness and distension may be experienced. At times the examiner can readily palpate loops of bowel filled with air and fluid. The liver and spleen are enlarged in about one third of these patients. Thus, the traditional clues to diagnosis, including the step-wise rise in fever, the relative bradycardia, and splenomegaly, may be absent. The value of splenomegaly in the diagnosis must be further discounted in regions of the world in which endemic malaria is a common cause of splenic enlargement. Rose spots, which are transient blanching rose-colored papules that often occur in the second week of fever in the periumbilical region, are not specific for typhoid fever but are very suggestive of it. Many observers feel that the presence of herpes labialis rules out the diagnosis of typhoid fever.

In perhaps 15 per cent of adults and 30 per cent or more of children, the onset of disease does not fit the above description. In some, the mildness of the clinical presentation is misleading, and the correct diagnosis is made only by subsequent isolation of the organism. In others, symptoms affecting the central nervous system (convulsions, meningismus, altered sensorium) or the lungs (cough, bronchitis, pneumonia), or an acute condition of the abdomen suggest focal rather than systemic disease. Isolation of *S. typhi* comes as a surprise, but this should not be the case, for a bewildering array of clinical syndromes has been reported as either the principal or an accompanying feature of typhoid. These include a number of other complications of the nervous system (encephalitis or encephalomyelitis; myelitis with spastic paraplegia; peripheral or cranial neuritis, especially involving the eighth nerve; meningitis; and Guillain-Barré syndrome), psychiatric presentations (including acute psychoses, mania, catatonia, or depression), acute myocarditis, hepatitis (possibly related to deposition of immune complexes (Dan et al., 1982), necrotizing cholangitis, immune-complex nephritis, hemolytic-uremic syndrome, and osteomyelitis or septic arthritis.

Typhoid fever has been associated traditionally with two late complications: significant intestinal hemorrhage and frank perforation. These problems occur secondary to bacterial invasion of the Peyer's patches, which in turn may lead to necrosis, ulceration, and erosion of blood vessels. Although the lesions are usually restricted to the superficial mucosa, they may extend to the serosa and cause perforation, which always occurs on the antimesenteric border of the bowel. These complications occur in 2 to 3 per cent of patients, most often in the third week of illness. Many more, perhaps 20 per cent, have minor intestinal blood loss. In developing countries, an acute bowel catastrophe may be the event that brings the patient to medical attention. Typhoid perforation is clinically manifested by a sudden drop in temperature, a rise in the pulse, and rapid development of the signs of peritonitis, with pain, tenderness, rebound, and rigidity, most often in the right lower quadrant. Seventy-five per cent of perforations occur within 40 cm of the ileocecal valve and 90 per cent within 60 cm. In about one fifth of patients operated on more than 24 hours after perforation, focal abscesses will be found in the subphrenic or subhepatic spaces or in the pelvis. Perforation and massive hemorrhage are important causes of the reported mortality rate of about 10 per cent in untreated infection.

Relapse is common and usually occurs one to three weeks after therapy is discontinued. The signs and symptoms are similar to the first episode, but usually milder and respond promptly to antimicrobials.

GEOGRAPHIC VARIATIONS. The clinical presentation of typhoid has changed considerably throughout the world in the past three decades because of several factors related to host, agent, and environment. These changes have tended to sharpen rather than lessen the geographic variations in disease patterns. Thus, age, underlying illness, nutritional state, and R factor-mediated antimicrobial resistance of the organisms have caused differences in the severity of the disease, while water supply, environmental sanitation, and the degree of environmental contamination have contributed to differences in the prevalence of typhoid (Levine et al., 1982).

In industrial countries, the incidence of typhoid has steadily declined, so that most cases are now imported by young adult travelers to endemic regions (dubbed holiday typhoid in England). Complications (except for relapse) are unusual. Indeed, the sole clinical presentation can be that of fever of undetermined origin. The emergence of chloramphenicol-resistant *S. typhi* has led to occasional cases of severe "old-time" disease, but this is a limited phenomenon at present.

In contrast, in the developing nations intestinal perforation still occurs in as many as 10 to 20 per cent of patients hospitalized with typhoid fever. Because of the long delay before obtaining medical care, these patients are usually gravely ill when they present with high fever, profound toxemia, delirium, stupor, or even frank coma. High mortality rates (over 50 per cent) are observed in these patients, even with prompt institution of appropriate antimicrobial therapy (Hoffman et al., 1983). Hypothermia and cardiovascular collapse may accompany signs of an acute abdomen. The death rate from this complication remained high in the mid-1970s, with a mortality rate of 70 to 80 per cent regardless of surgery.

In Africa, Indonesia, and some parts of India, central nervous system and psychiatric symptoms are prominent (Scragg et al., 1969). These include acute confusional, delirious, or psychotic states; nuchal rigidity; cog-wheel extrapyramidal rigidity of extremities; incontinence; and motor seizures. Patients may occasionally be admitted to psychiatric units with a diagnosis of catatonic schizophrenia; however, the finding of fever usually leads to more appropriate medical care. Examination of the cerebrospinal fluid is invariably negative in these patients.

In these endemic regions of the world, there is a higher

relative incidence of typhoid fever in children, including infants in the first two years of life, a rarity elsewhere. Although childhood typhoid in the affluent nations is typically a mild disease, it is severe in the tropics, with a high incidence of pulmonary, central nervous system, and intestinal complications (Duggan and Beyer, 1975). Because the omentum may be short or relatively immobile in this age group, extensive peritoneal soiling and early abscess formation is not uncommon. This is often worsened by delay in bringing patients to the hospital. A few specific geographic clinical associations have also been made. These are (1) a syndrome of prolonged, intermittent fever and bacteremia, persisting for as long as two years in patients with *Schistosoma mansoni* infection. It has been suggested but not proved that salmonellae infecting the gut of the worm may be the source of recurrent bacteremia, although altered blood flow due to intrahepatic fibrosis may also alter mononuclear cell function. (2) Chronic urinary tract carriage of organisms, which may be a source of sporadic or epidemic infection in patients with *Schistosoma haematobium* infection. These individuals experience intermittent bacteremia and fever. (3) Intrahepatic (as opposed to gallbladder) carriage among Chinese suffering from concomitant *Clonorchis sinensis* infection. This is associated with a spectrum of clinical manifestations ranging from asymptomatic excretion of S. *typhi* in the stool to recurrent cholangitis. In these patients, the sex ratio of carriers is close to 1:1 instead of the usual predominance of women, which is probably related to the sex distribution of cholelithiasis.

DIAGNOSIS. More than 90 per cent of untreated patients will have a positive blood culture during the first week of illness. Unfortunately, the incidence of isolations drops to 40 per cent in the face of antecedent antimicrobial therapy. However, cultures of the bone marrow are still positive 90 per cent of the time, even after a few doses of antibiotics. The yield of positive blood cultures slowly diminishes with time, but there is a concomitant rise in stool (85 per cent) and urine (25 per cent) isolates in the third and fourth weeks because of invasion of Peyer's patches and the kidneys. More recent studies (Wicks et al., 1974; Gilman et al., 1975) suggest a much lower incidence of positive stool and urine cultures, especially in the treated patient. Cultures from the center of rose spots are positive in two thirds of patients. Fecal excretion ceases by three months in 90 per cent of patients, but about 3 per cent may go on to become long-term fecal carriers (more than one year). These chronic enteric carriers may excrete S. *typhi* for life, and they are the usual source for new cases. Adults more frequently than children, and women more frequently than men, become chronic carriers, probably because of the relative incidence of gallstones in these groups (Levine et al., 1982).

Serologic diagnosis depends upon antibody rises to O and H antigens, detected by agglutination reactions (Widal test). Antibody to O antigens in group D develops during the first week of illness, peaks at three to four weeks, and declines after nine months to one year. A rising titer (greater than fourfold) is suggestive of acute infection but of course may be produced by any group D salmonella sharing the 9, 12 somatic antigens with S. *typhi.* Prior immunization with typhoid-paratyphoid vaccine may also result in an anamnestic antibody response of group D titers due to infection with many other salmonellae and other enteric bacteria. Additional specificity can be ascribed to the O antibody response if there is also a rise in titer of antibody to the d flagellar antigen of S. *typhi.* These antibodies rise in titer after the first week and peak in four to six weeks. However, titers remain high for years, whether stimulated by infection or vaccine, and a single determination of a high titer of flagellar antibody cannot be considered diagnostic of recent infection. The effect of vaccine may be particularly vexing, because patients often cannot remember their immunization history. It has been suggested that a distinctive and unusual H antigen be included in the vaccine to facilitate identification of vaccine-induced titers, but this has not been done. For all these reasons, a single high Widal titer or even rising titers are even less specific than most serologic tests. A recent study (Abraham et al., 1981) reported O and or H titers ≥ 1:160 in 86 per cent of bacteriologically proven cases of typhoid in contrast to 4-8 per cent in healthy or nontyphoid patients, respectively.

Diseases that are most commonly confused with typhoid clinically include nontyphoidal salmonellosis, brucellosis, tularemia, shigellosis, tuberculosis, malaria, Rocky Mountain spotted fever, murine typhus, or even lymphoproliferative or collagen-vascular diseases. All of these diseases can present with similar high sustained fevers, splenomegaly, and, in some instances, rashes that can be confused with rose spots. Appropriate cultures will usually establish the correct diagnosis, but other laboratory tests are also useful. The white blood count is normal or reduced, but a pronounced left shift in the differential is common. The serum transaminases are often elevated without other evidence of liver disease. Anemia and occult blood in the feces are common during the third and fourth weeks of the disease, even in patients without frank perforation.

THERAPY. Effective antimicrobial therapy has reduced the mortality rate to 1 per cent or less in recent reported series. At the same time, the incidence of relapse, which usually occurs one to three weeks after antibiotics are discontinued, has doubled to about 15 to 20 per cent. Although recrudescent illness may be severe or complicated, it is usually less severe than the original illness and responds promptly to therapy. Second and even third relapses have been reported.

Since 1948, chloramphenicol has been the chemotherapeutic standard against which the efficacy of other drugs has been measured. Typhoid fever is one of the classic infections in which in vitro sensitivity does not predict in vivo efficacy, although drugs ineffective in vitro will surely be clinically ineffective. For chloramphenicol sensitive strains, no other agent has been found to produce a superior clinical response. Except for concern about effects on the bone marrow, chloramphenicol would be the clear-cut agent of choice. Other drugs that are nearly as effective, such as ampicillin, amoxicillin, or trimethoprim-sulfamethoxazole, are less toxic and may be chosen for the initial therapy of patients who are not severely ill. Chloramphenicol should be given orally in a dose of 60 mg/kg/day in four divided doses. Many alternate regimens have been suggested in an attempt to reduce the relapse rate, but none seem superior. One reasonable program is to continue therapy until the temperature becomes normal (usually four to eight days), then lower the oral dose to 30 mg/kg/day and treat the patient for two additional weeks. Chloramphenicol may be given intravenously in the same fashion. Because it is not absorbed well from muscle, chloramphenicol should not be given intramuscularly. Bleeding or perforation may occur during therapy, even in afebrile patients. Treatment with chloramphenicol does not prevent the carrier state.

Intravenous ampicillin (100 mg/kg/day) or oral amoxicillin (100 mg/kg/day) is also effective. However, both forms of ampicillin and especially amoxicillin are considerably more expensive than chloramphenicol. Ampicillin or amoxicillin is the drug of choice for chloramphenicol-resistant strains of *S. typhi*.

S. typhi may also be resistant to ampicillin and amoxicillin. In the typhoid outbreak in Mexico in 1972, strains resistant to these drugs and to chloramphenicol were recovered (Overturf et al., 1973). The recommended treatment for these organisms, as well as for patients who are unable to take penicillins or chloramphenicol because of allergy or toxicity, is 320 mg of trimethoprim in combination with 1600 mg of sulfamethoxazole divided into two daily doses or half the amount in children under 12 years (Butler et al., 1982).

In a recent report (Hoffman et al., 1984) the mortality in severe typhoid fever (delirium, coma, or shock) fell from 56 per cent in controls given chloramphenicol plus placebo to 10 per cent in those treated with high dose dexamethasone (3 mg/kg intravenously followed by 1 mg/kg every 6 hours for 2 days).

Hemorrhage is generally managed by conservative supportive measures, including transfusions. Occasionally, bowel resection has been employed for massive or recurrent bleeding, but this can be difficult because there are usually multiple bleeding sites in a friable bowel.

Results of surgical repair of perforations have improved with modern fluid and electrolyte replacement. Early recognition and aggressive correction of hypovolemic shock permit successful simple operative repairs, without the need for wedge excision or resection and anastomosis (Kim et al., 1975). Mortality rates are considerably reduced when the diagnosis is made quickly and the surgery performed rapidly, but may remain unacceptably high (50 per cent) when patients first present to the hospital because of perforation (Chouhan and Pande, 1982).

Treatment of the chronic carrier state has always been a problem, particularly in gallbladder carriers with stones. In vitro experiments demonstrate the ease with which *S. typhi* can move to the interior of a gallstone and the difficulty of killing these protected organisms, even by immersing the infected stone in a very high concentration of a bactericidal antibiotic. Approximately 3 per cent of appropriately treated typhoid patients become chronic carriers. In the absence of cholelithiasis, most of these subjects will be cured by a course of oral ampicillin or amoxicillin, 100 mg/kg/day, plus probenecid, 30 mg/kg/day, or trimethoprim-sulfamethoxazole, 2 tablets twice daily for three months (Johnson et al., 1973). In the presence of cholelithiasis, the likelihood of cure with antimicrobials alone is much reduced, and cholecystectomy and antimicrobials may be needed. Nevertheless, an adequate course of one or both antimicrobials should be tried before a decision for surgical intervention is made. Known chronic enteric carriers should, of course, be urged to maintain strict standards of hygiene and particularly to wash their hands thoroughly after defecation. They should not work as food handlers.

Chronic urinary carriers of *S. typhi* are often infected with *Schistosoma haematobium* or *Schistosoma mansoni* at the same time. The best results are obtained when the schistosomiasis is treated first, the current drug of choice being praziquantel. Excellent results have been reported recently when antischistosomal treatment is followed by 250 mg of amoxicillin every six hours for four weeks.

IMMUNIZATION. Current vaccines consist of killed bacterial suspensions, prepared for subcutaneous inoculation, of either *S. typhi* alone (monovalent) or *S. typhi* in combination with *S. enteritidis* bioserotype paratyphi A and serotype paratyphi B (TAB). Recent studies have confirmed the original observations of Almford Wright at the turn of the century that such vaccines afford protection, at least for the *S. typhi* component (Warren and Hornick, 1979). Because the efficacy of the TAB vaccine for the nontyphi strains is unverified and the risk of adverse side reactions such as severe local inflammatory responses is increased with TAB vaccine, monovalent *S. typhi* vaccine is the preferred vaccine. This preparation does not induce cell-mediated immunity, but stimulates the production of serum antibody to Vi, O, and H antigens. Human trials show no correlation between anti-Vi or anti-O responses and protection, but a number of studies suggest an association between anti-H antibodies and resistance. It is likely that serum antibody would assist host defenses during the initial bacteremia, before the invasion of mononuclear phagocytes, by reducing the number of organisms capable of intracellular multiplication. The mechanism of action of the antibody is unknown. Anti-H antibodies stop motility of the microorganisms, but the importance of this effect is uncertain.

Human studies have documented three key points about killed vaccines (Warren and Hornick, 1979). (1) Immunity can be overcome by increasing the bacterial inoculum. This is probably important when the route of transmission is considered because food-borne inocula may be considerably greater than water-borne inocula. (2) The method of vaccine preparation is important. Acetone-killed and preserved vaccine is more effective than the classic heat-killed, phenol-preserved vaccine. (3) Two doses are better than one; both increase the degree and duration of protection. The recommended routes and schedules for immunization are arbitrary and are based on tradition rather than data. From the field trial experiences, however, a reasonable primary schedule would include two 0.5 ml subcutaneous injections of acetone-inactivated vaccine given four weeks apart. In endemic regions, boosters should probably be given every three years. While the acetone vaccine is intended for subcutaneous (or intramuscular) inoculation, the phenol vaccine can be administered intradermally by Jet injection. However, the primary injection should be given by syringe because it is difficult to guarantee delivery of the required dose by Jet injector. The Jet method is suitable for revaccination (booster doses).

Because of new concepts of mucosal immunity, recent studies have been directed towards production of an oral vaccine in order to promote local resistance in the small intestine, the initial site of infection. There is now little doubt about the increased efficacy of live attenuated compared to dead virulent oral vaccines. Live vaccines are more likely to activate mucosal and cell-mediated immune responses, but dead vaccines are safer because they preclude the possibility of reversion to virulence. The few human studies of killed oral vaccine have been disappointing. Because the critical protective antigen is undefined, these failures may represent specific faults of the vaccines rather than the general method. On the other hand, oral vaccination with a live mutant, which synthesizes incomplete O antigen because it lacks UDP-glucose-4-epimerase, is very effective (Warren and Hornick, 1979). When grown in excess exogenous galactose, this mutant synthesizes complete O side chains but eventually lyses. In a recent large field trial with three years of observation (Wahdan et al., 1982) oral immunization with this TY21a vaccine strain demonstrated impressive protection (attack rate, confirmed cases, of 2/100,000 compared to 49/100,000 per year in placebo immunized controls). Lyophilized vaccine was reconstituted in 20-30 ml of sweetened phosphate buffer and three doses were administered on alternate days immediately after ingestion of 1 g of sodium bicarbonate as a chewable tablet. A more recent trial of an enteric coated formulation given once or twice without bicarbonate has been disappointing and further trials are underway to determine the best form of vaccine and dose schedule.

References

Abraham, G., Teklu, B., Gedebu, M., Selassie, G. H., Azene, G.: Diagnostic value of the Widal test. Trop Geogr Med 33:329, 1981.

Butler, T., Rumans, L., Arnold, K.: Response of typhoid fever caused by chloramphenicol-susceptible and chloramphenicol-resistant strains of *Salmonella typhi* to treatment with trimethoprim-sulfamethoxazole. Rev Infect Dis 4:551, 1982.

Chouhan, M. K., Pande, S. K.: Typhoid enteric perforation. Br J Surg 69:173, 1982.

Christie, A. N.: Typhoid and paratyphoid fevers. In Infectious Diseases: Epidemiology and Clinical Practice. London, E & S Livingstone, Ltd. 1980, pp. 47–102.

Dan, M., Bar-Meir, S., Jedwab, M., Shibolet, S.: Typhoid hepatitis with immunoglobulins and complement deposits in bile canaliculi. Arch Int Med 142:148, 1982.

Duggan, M. D., and Beyer, L.: Enteric fever in young Yoruba children. Arch Dis Childh 50:67, 1975.

Gilman, R. H., Terminel, M., Levine, M. M., Hernandez-Mendoza, P., and Hornick, R. B.: Relative efficacy of blood, urine, rectal swabs, bone marrow and Rose spot cultures for recognition of *Salmonella typhi* in typhoid fever. Lancet 1:1211, 1975.

Gulati, P. D., Saxena, S. N., Gupta, P. S., and Chuttani, H. K.: Changing pattern of typhoid fever. Am J Med 45:544, 1968.

Hoffman, S. L., Punjabi, N. H., Kemala, S., Moechtar, A., Pulungsih, S., Rivai, A., Rockhill, R., Woodward, T. E., Loedin, A. A.: Reduction of mortality in chloramphenicol treated severe typhoid fever with high dose dexamethasone. N Engl J Med 310:82, 1984.

Hornick, R. B., Greisman, S. E., Woodward, T. E., DuPont, H. L., Dawkins, A. T., and Snyder, M. J.: Typhoid fever: Pathogenesis and immunologic control. New Engl J Med 283:686, 739, 1970.

Johnson, W. D., Jr., Hook, E. W., Lindsey, E., and Kaye, D.: Treatment of chronic typhoid carriers with ampicillin. Antimicrob Ag Chemother 3:439, 1973.

Kim, J. P., Oh, S. K., and Jarrett, F.: Management of ileal perforation due to typhoid fever. Ann Surg 181:88, 1975.

Levine, M. M., Black, R. E., Lanata, C.: Precise estimation of the numbers of chronic carriers of *Salmonella typhi* in Santiago, Chile, an endemic area. J Infect Dis 146:724, 1982.

Overturf, G., Martin, K. I., and Mathies, A. W., Jr.: Antibiotic resistance in typhoid fever. New Engl J Med 289:463, 1973.

Rajagopalan, P., Kumar, R., Malaviya, N.: Immunological studies in typhoid fever. II. Cell mediated immune responses and lymphocyte subpopulations in patients with typhoid fever. Clin Exp Immunol 47:269, 1982.

Samantry, S. K., Johnson, S. C., and Chakrabarti, A. K.: Enteric fever: An analysis of 500 cases. Practitioner 218:400, 1977.

Scragg, J., Rubridge, C., and Wallace, H. L.: Typhoid fever in African and Indian children in Durban. Arch Dis Childh 44:18, 1969.

Wahdan, M. H., Serie, C., Cerisier, Y., Sallam, S., Germanier, R.: a controlled field trial of live *Salmonella typhi* strain Ty 21a oral vaccine against typhoid: Three-year results. J Infect Dis 145:292, 1982.

Warren, J. W., and Hornick, R. B.: Immunization against typhoid fever. Annu Rev Med 30:457, 1979.

Wicks, A. C. B., Cruickshank, J. G., and Musewe, N.: Observations on the diagnosis of typhoid fever. S Afr Med J 68:1368, 1974.

192

GONOCOCCEMIA

J. ALLEN McCUTCHAN, M.D.

Gonococci infecting the genitalia, pharynx, or rectum may invade the blood to produce a variety of syndromes collectively called disseminated gonococcal infection (DGI). Patients with DGI usually have no symptoms of gonorrhea because DGI complicates asymptomatic infection. Arthritis-dermatitis, the most common form of DGI, is characterized by fever and chills, typical skin lesions, and arthralgias or transient arthritis. Gonococcal septic arthritis, a less common form of DGI, is a typical, culture-positive, purulent arthritis with minimal systemic symptoms and negative blood cultures. Metastatic infection of the heart (endocarditis or pericarditis) or the meninges is rare. In contrast to meningococci, gonococci in the blood do not produce shock or disseminated intravascular coagulation and thus rarely kill patients.

ETIOLOGY. *Neisseria gonorrhoeae* and gonococcal infections without gonococcemia are discussed in Chapters 29 and 161. Gonococci from cases of DGI are usually resistant to killing by serum, very sensitive to penicillin, nutritionally fastidious, and slow growing. These traits (DGI biotype), which help to explain some features of disseminated gonococcal infections, occur less frequently in gonococci that cause genital infections.

Almost all DGI isolates resist killing by antibody and complement in normal human sera (Schoolnik et al., 1976). Gonococci causing the arthritis-dermatitis syndrome are more likely to be resistant to normal human sera and the patient's convalescent serum than those that cause septic arthritis (OBrien et al., 1983). This resistance results from the binding of a natural IgG antibody that blocks killing by bactericidal IgM antibody (McCutchan et al., 1978). Resistant gonococci avidly bind the blocking antibody to their surfaces, but sensitive strains do not. The mechanism by which blocking antibodies protect serum-resistant gonococci is not completely understood. The entire membrane attack complex (a structure composed of terminal complement components that can create a lethal transmembrane channel) is deposited on the surface of serum-resistant gonococci, but fails to kill the bacteria (Harriman et al., 1982; Joiner et al., 1983). A transmembrane protein, or porin, found in most DGI stains may be the target for the IgG blocking antibody (Hilderrandt et al., 1978; Rice et al., 1982). Since many gonococci that cause only local infections also resist killing by serum but do not invade the blood, serum resistance is necessary but not sufficient for dissemination.

Gonococci that cause DGI usually are extremely sensitive to penicillin (minimum inhibitory concentration less than 0.06 μg/ml) (Weisner et al., 1973). In contrast, gonococci causing local infection have become increasingly resistant (see Chapter 161). Most disseminated gonococci cannot synthesize certain nutrients made by most local strains. By adding these growth factors (e.g., proline, arginine, hypoxanthine, or uracil) to nutritionally deficient media, the pattern of growth requirements (auxotype) of gonococci can be determined. Gonococci requiring either proline or the triad of arginine, hypoxanthine, and uracil (AHU), or both are isolated much more commonly from disseminated disease than from local disease. The proportion of various auxotypes varies both geographically and over time. For example, in the northwestern United States, AHU-negative strains cause about 90 per cent of DGI. In the southeastern United States, about 25 per cent of DGI strains are AHU-negative and 50 per cent are proline-negative. Since the mucosal infections in patients with DGI are usually asymptomatic, it is significant that AHU-negative gonococci also cause most cases of asymptomatic urethritis (Crawford et al., 1977). Because they cause no symptoms, nutritionally dependent gonococci escape treatment and, by persisting, increase their chances of invading the blood. Careful examination of these traits (serum resistance, penicillin susceptibility, and auxotype) suggests that they are not genetically linked (Eisenstein et al., 1977). Each trait probably promotes dissemination independently. Identical gonococci are isolated from mucosal and disseminated sites in patients with DGI and from their contacts. Thus, it appears that only those patients initially infected with strains capable of invading the blood are at risk for DGI.

DGI strains are more difficult to grow, their colonies are smaller, and they are more sensitive to undefined, methanol-soluble toxins in agar. These properties may be related to their nutritional dependence and help to account for the difficulty encountered in cultivating gonococci from some patients with clinically typical DGI.

PATHOGENESIS AND PATHOLOGY. Although certain characteristics of gonococci determine their potential for dissemination, the sporadic pattern of DGI suggests that the response by the patient is more important than virulence in determining who gets DGI. If the virulence of certain strains were the key factor, epidemics of DGI would be common. Paired cases and a "microepidemic" have been reported, but infected partners of patients with DGI rarely develop disseminated infection. Two groups of patients appear to be at increased risk for gonococcemia: women during the menses and pregnancy and patients with genetic deficiency of the terminal components of complement. Alterations in levels of sex hormones may explain the increased frequency of dissemination at the menses and during pregnancy. In addition, mucin and hemoglobin, which flood the endocervix at the menses, may increase gonococcal invasiveness. When gonococci are injected into the peritoneal cavities of mice, they multiply, invade the blood, and kill the animals only if mucin and hemoglobin are added (Corbeil et al., 1978). Neisserial bacteremias recur in patients with congenital deficiency of one of the terminal components of complement (Table 1). Since these components (C6 through C8) mediate lysis of gonococci but not opsonization or chemotaxis, gonococci are phagocytosed but not killed in their sera. Patients with deficiency of the final component of complement, C9, do not appear to be at risk of disseminated neisserial infections. This is explained by the fact that the ability of sera from C9-deficient persons to kill gonococci is nearly normal (Harriman et al., 1981). The striking association of complement deficiency with recurrent DGI emphasizes the importance of complement-mediated bacteriolysis in protection against DGI. However, since most patients with DGI have normal levels of hemolytic complement, complement deficiency explains only a minority of cases of DGI.

Table 1. ASSOCIATION OF NEISSERIAL BACTEREMIAS AND DEFICIENCY OF THE TERMINAL COMPONENTS OF COMPLEMENT

	Type of Neisserial Infection		
Deficient C Component	***DGI***[a]	***MI***[b]	***Total Neisserial Infections***
C6	2/6[c]	5/6	6/6
C7	1/11	4/11	5/11
C8	2/8	1/8	3/8
Total	5/25	10/25	14/25

[a]DGI, Disseminated gonococcal infection.
[b]MI, Meningococcal infection (implies bacteremia).
[c]No. of infections/no. of complement-deficient patients at risk. Data from Petersen et al., 1979.

Susceptibility to gonococcemia, unlike that to meningococcemia, is not predictable except in these rare patients with complement deficiency. Patients with either type of neisserial bacteremia (gonococcal or meningococcal) lack complement-mediated serum bactericidal activity against their infecting strain. Patients whose serum does not kill their colonizing meningococcal strain are at high risk for meningococcemia in epidemics (Goldschneider et al., 1969). This susceptibility apparently results from inexperience with the infecting strain and can be corrected by immunization with meningococcal vaccine, which enhances bactericidal activity. Patients fail to kill DGI strains because blocking antibody protects the strains from bactericidal antibody. Since these blocking antibodies are present in most people, sera from few normal persons kill DGI strains. Because most carriers of gonococci do not develop DGI, something other than serum bactericidal activity must protect them from gonococcemia.

Two stages of DGI are postulated (Keiser et al., 1968). In the bacteremic (arthritis-dermatitis) stage, gonococci can be cultured from the blood and skin but not from the joints. In the septic joint stage, the blood is sterile but gonococci are found in one or a few infected joints. In one study, patients presenting with arthritis-dermatitis had had symptoms for an average of three days, and patients with septic joints for eight days. In another large prospective study, patients with both syndromes reported symptoms for four days before seeking care. Not all patients with septic joints have antecedent polyarthritis or dermatitis, and some patients have features of both syndromes. It appears that bacteremia produces polyarthritis early and that septic arthritis develops only after bacteremia is over, but this interpretation is controversial.

Joint fluid from patients with polyarthritis is sterile despite positive blood cultures. The polyarthritis resembles that seen in acute immune complex diseases (i.e., serum sickness or the prodrome of hepatitis B). Circulating immune complexes are found in most DGI patients and are associated with joint disease and a history of previous gonococcal infection but not skin rash (Walker et al., 1978). A possible interpretation is that the initial polyarthritis results from immune complex disease that favors localization of circulating gonococci in joints. Since most people have natural antibodies to gonococci, the formation of immune complexes may not require an antibody response to the infection.

In gonococcal dermatitis skin biopsy shows collections of neutrophils and monocytes around small arteries in the dermis. Lysis of white cells around arterioles produces leukocytoblastic angiitis, which is often associated with allergic diseases (Seifert et al., 1974). Gonococci grow from only a minority of lesions but are frequently seen after immunofluorescent antibody staining (Barr and Danielsson, 1971). Thus, circulating gonococci seem to localize in dermal arterioles and evoke an immune cellular response.

In acute septic arthritis, the synovial membranes are invaded by an intense cellular infiltrate of polymorphonuclear leukocytes, lymphocytes, macrophages, and neutrophils. A lymphocytic perivascular infiltrate develops in the deeper synovium, and gonococci can be seen in the tissues. The synovium is destroyed and replaced by granulation tissue, and the underlying cartilage may be invaded and destroyed.

Untreated patients dying of gonococcal endocarditis in the pre-antibiotic era resembled patients with other forms of subacute endocarditis (Williams, 1938). Similar valves (aortic, mitral, pulmonary, tricuspid) were involved and similar complications (nephritis, myocarditis, splenitis, arterial emboli) were found postmortem. Most patients died of cardiac or renal failure.

A striking but unexplained feature of DGI is the inverse relationship between the degree of local inflammation and dissemination: most patients with DGI have asymptomatic local infection, and those with pelvic inflammatory disease seldom develop DGI. Thus, vigorous local inflammation may prevent dissemination. As discussed in the previous section, the nutritional fastidiousness and consequent slow growth of DGI strains may explain why they elicit little local inflammation.

CLINICAL COURSE AND COMPLICATIONS. DGI causes clinical syndromes ranging from low-grade fever or dermatitis alone to severe metastatic infection of joints, heart, or meninges. Bacteremia is usually a complication of asymptomatic local infection, especially of the pharynx; less frequently it arises from symptomatic genital infections and rarely occurs with pelvic inflammatory disease. Dissemination occurs more frequently during the first week of the menstrual cycle or during pregnancy and perhaps most frequently after genital trauma. Most patients have an acute febrile illness with polyarthritis of the hands, knees, wrists, ankles, or feet. When polyarthritis accompanies the characteristic dermatitis in a sexually active young person, the diagnosis of disseminated gonococcal infection can be made at the bedside.

Uncomplicated Gonococcemia (Arthritis-Dermatitis Syndrome). The cardinal symptoms of gonococcemia are fever, chills, malaise, polyarthritis, and dermatitis. Any or all of these symptoms may be absent. In addition to arthritis and dermatitis, asymptomatic myocarditis (transient electrocardiographic changes) and hepatitis (elevated liver enzymes) can be found in about half the patients (Holmes et al., 1971). Polyarthritis occurs in about 90 per cent of patients with gonococcemia and has a migratory or additive pattern, small effusions, and less than 20,000 white cells per mm^3 in sterile joint fluids (Handsfield, 1975). The knee is most commonly affected, followed by the wrists, hands, ankles, feet, elbows, and shoulders (Fig. 1). Arthralgia, often without arthritis, is usually the first symptom and is succeeded by fever, chills, malaise, and frank arthritis. Periarticular inflammation, especially tenosynovitis, is frequent. Dermatitis is present in 50 to 70 per cent of patients. Lesions start as small red papules on an erythematous base and may evolve through vesicular, pustular, hemorrhagic, and occasionally bullous or necrotic stages. These skin lesions usually are tender and number between 2 and 10 per patient. They are found on the hands and feet (including the palms and soles) or near the joints but spare the head, trunk, and mucous membranes. Lesions may be in various stages of development. They evolve over one to three days, are arrested by therapy, and heal quickly (three to seven days) and completely unless they are necrotic.

Septic Arthritis. Patients with gonococcal septic arthritis complain of severe pain in one or two joints with only minimal systemic symptoms. They often report antecedent fever, malaise, polyarthritis, or dermatitis that resolved without treatment. On average their symptoms have been present longer than those of patients with uncomplicated gonococcemia. Septic arthritis involves the same joints, especially the knees, wrists, and ankles, as gonococcal

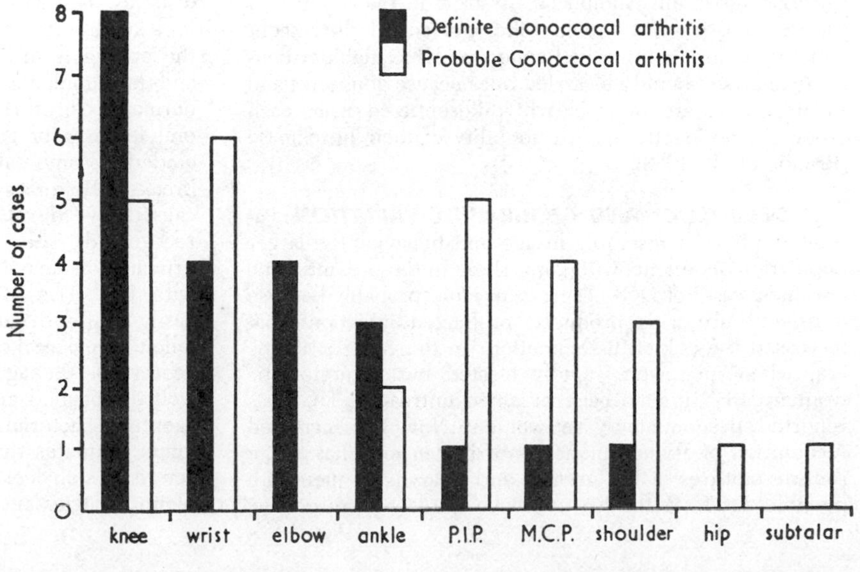

Figure 1. Frequency of involvement of various joints in gonococcemia.

polyarthritis. Joint fluid is usually purulent with more than 20,000 leukocytes per mm^3 and more than 75 per cent polymorphonuclear leukocytes. Gonococci can be grown from the joint in about half the cases and can be seen by Gram stain or fluorescent antibody staining in some of the sterile fluids. Untreated arthritis progressively destroys the joint and leads to periarticular fibrosis and adhesions between articular cartilages (Keefer and Spink, 1937). Response to treatment is slower in patients with septic arthritis than in those with polyarthritis, but residual joint dysfunction is unusual by six months after treatment.

Endocarditis. *Neisseria gonorrhoeae* was an important cause of endocarditis in the pre-antibiotic era, accounting for 20 to 25 per cent in several series (Jones, 1950; Williams, 1938), but it is rare in developed countries today. Gonococci usually infect normal cardiac valves, involve the right heart about one third of the time, and create large vegetations that frequently embolize (Thayer, 1922). The course of untreated gonococcal endocarditis is intermediate in length and severity between the subacute disease cause by *Streptococcus viridans* and the acute disease caused by the pneumococcus and *Staphylococcus aureus*. Fever, chills, arthritis, skin lesions, cardiac murmurs, mild hepatitis, and markedly elevated sedimentation rates and white blood counts are characteristic. Only a new pathologic cardiac murmur or embolus clearly differentiates endocarditis from benign gonococcemia, but sustained gonococcemia, anemia, nephritis, or a very high erythrocyte sedimentation rate at presentation (>100) should suggest endocarditis. Complications include arterial emboli, myocarditis, pericarditis, nephritis with renal failure, and valvular destruction with cardiac failure. Before the antibiotic era only a few untreated patients survived. Antibiotic therapy has cured most of the recently reported cases.

Gonococcal Meningitis. In contrast to the frequency of meningeal infection with meningococci, gonococcal meningitis is rare. Of 16 cases collected by Holmes et al. (1971), six had skin lesions, nine had arthritis, three of six had positive blood cultures, and only three of nine untreated patients died. All treated cases survived. Cerebrospinal fluids show the typical polymorphonuclear pleocytosis and low glucose levels typical of bacterial meningitis. Because only one saccharolytic reaction differentiates meningococci from gonococci, *Neisseria* organisms isolated from cerebrospinal fluid (CSF) should not agglutinate in meningococcal capsular antiserum, should fail to grow in the absence of carbon dioxide, and should bind gonococcal fluorescent antibody before being called gonococci. If available, isoenzyme analysis should be carried out because gonococci and meningococci are most clearly differentiated from each other by the electrophoretic mobility of their hexokinase (Braude et al., 1983).

EPIDEMIOLOGY AND GEOGRAPHIC VARIATION. Patients with DGI resemble in age and behavior the larger population of patients with gonorrhea. In the pre-antibiotic era, most cases of DGI occurred in men, probably because untreated urethritis produced prolonged infections that increased the risk of dissemination. In the early antibiotic era, when men were rapidly treated but asymptomatic women carrying gonococci remained untreated, DGI was reported predominantly in women. Now the increased recognition of asymptomatic gonorrhea in men has led to routine cultures of the urethra and pharynx in men with possible DGI. With this approach a recent prospective study found that DGI occurred in nearly equal numbers of men and women (Handsfield et al., 1976). Thus, the sex distribution and the frequency of dissemination probably depend on the number of patients carrying gonococci that can invade the blood.

The emergence in some areas of the world of the DGI biotype (auxotrophic, penicillin-sensitive, and serum-resistant gonococci) may have increased both asymptomatic disease in men and DGI in both sexes. DGI appears to have increased during the past 20 years along with uncomplicated gonorrhea. Rates of dissemination as high as 1 to 3 per cent have been calculated, but marked geographic variations occur. In the western Pacific area, where the DGI biotype is rare (Knapp and Holmes, 1975), DGI is also rare despite high rates of gonorrhea in some populations. Penicillinase-producing *Neisseria gonorrhoeae* are found predominantly in the western Pacific, are probably not of the DGI biotype, and only rarely cause DGI.

DIAGNOSIS. DGI is diagnosed clinically from combinations of dermatitis, arthritis, and other symptoms of gonorrhea or a history of recent unusual sexual exposures. Symptomatic gonorrhea occurs in only a minority of patients with DGI, but it is a helpful sign when present. Polyarthritis and typical dermatitis in a sexually active young adult is nearly diagnostic of DGI. On the west coast of the United States, where DGI is common, gonococci cause over half the hospital admissions for acute arthritis in adults under 30 years of age. Gonococcal dermatitis is often so characteristic in location and appearance that a presumptive diagnosis can be made even in the absence of arthritis.

When gonococcemia is suspected, cultures of blood, the genitalia, pharynx, and rectum should be taken (see Chapter 161). Standard blood culture media incubated aerobically are suitable for isolation of gonococci from blood. Positive cultures are most frequently obtained from genital sites, but occasionally only the pharynx or rectum yields the gonococcus. Joint fluid, if obtained, should always be cultured and is frequently positive if many (>80,000 per mm^3) polymorphonuclear leukocytes are present. Immunofluorescent stains frequently detect gonococci in skin lesions and buffy coats of blood even when cultures of these sites are negative.

Gonococcemia must be distinguished from several similar diseases. Polyarthritis, dermatitis, and fever occur in Reiter's syndrome, acute rheumatic fever, meningococcemia, the prodrome of hepatitis B, and various other infections and immunologic diseases. Reiter's syndrome (arthritis, dermatitis, urethritis, and conjunctivitis) can simulate several features of gonococcemia and was unknowingly included in some early reviews of gonococcal arthritis. Outbreaks of Reiter's syndrome following epidemics of diarrhea caused by *Shigella*, *Salmonella*, or *Yersinia* are easily recognized. The endemic (or venereal) form, occurring primarily in sexually active, often promiscuous young men with the HLA-B27 histocompatibility antigen, is more easily confused with DGI. Although Reiter's disease may follow gonococcal or nongonococcal urethritis, neither gonococci nor the agents of nongonococcal urethritis are as well established antecedents of Reiter's syndrome as the agents of bacterial diarrheas. The distribution of involved joints simulates that of gonococcal arthritis, but the characteristic skin lesions of Reiter's syndrome (keratodermia blennorrhagica and balanitis circinata) differ from those of gonococcemia. In addition, Reiter's syndrome does not respond to antibiotics and often relapses. Skin lesions of acute rheumatic fever are uncommon, do not resemble gonococcal dermatitis, and progress despite antibiotics. Meningococcemia frequently produces petechiae and only rarely causes lesions that are indistinguishable from gonococcal dermatitis. The prodromes of hepatitis B, serum sickness, and other immune complex diseases produce polyarthritis, but their skin lesions (petechiae, urticaria, and erythemas) are easily differentiated from gonococcal dermatitis.

TREATMENT. Because gonococci are usually very sensitive to penicillin G, ampicillin, and amoxicillin, these are the antibiotics of choice (Thompson, 1979). Seven-day courses of oral erythromycin or tetracycline are also effective. Experience with parenteral cephem antibiotics is limited, but they should be effective in penicillin-allergic patients who are unable to take oral agents. DGI caused by penicillinase-producing gonococci is rare but should respond to cefoxitin or spectinomycin.

Table 2 lists acceptable regimens for treating various syndromes of gonococcemia. Penicillin regimens are preferred unless penicillin allergy or penicillinase-producing gonococci are involved. Although some physicians treat patients with septic arthritis for 10 to 14 days, three days of intravenous high-dose penicillin therapy (Blankenship, 1974) or seven days of oral ampicillin and amoxicillin (Handsfield et al., 1976) have been uniformly successful. Septic arthritis does not require surgical drainage (except perhaps in the hip), and intra-articular injections of antibiotics are contraindicated. Joint immobilization, repeated aspiration of purulent joint fluid, and anti-inflammatory agents may be used, but their efficacy has not been studied. Gonococcal endocarditis should be treated with three to four weeks of parenteral penicillin because experience with shorter regimens and other drugs is not available. Because of poor penetration into the CSF, high doses of penicillin G or chloramphenicol (in penicillin-allergic patients) are recommended for meningitis.

Table 2. TREATMENT OF DISSEMINATED GONOCOCCAL INFECTIONS

Uncomplicated Gonococcemia and Septic Arthritis

Intravenous

1. Penicillin G, 10 million (10^7) units daily in four divided doses (2.5 mU) every six hours for three days; in neonates or children use 100,000 (10^5) u/kg/day for three to seven days
2. Cefoxitin, 8.0 g daily in four divided doses (2.0 g every six hours) for seven days
3. Cefazolin, 3.0 g daily in three divided doses (1.0 g every eight hours) for seven days

Intramuscular

1. Spectinomycin, 2 g intramuscularly every 12 hours for three days
2. Procaine penicillin G, 1.2 million units daily (600,000 units every 12 hours) for seven days

Oral

1. Ampicillin or amoxicillin, 0.5 g every six hours for seven days after either ampicillin, 3.5 g plus probenecid, 1.0 g or amoxicillin, 3.0 g
2. Tetracycline or erythromycin, 0.5 g every six hours for seven days

Gonococcal Endocarditis (Intravenous)

1. Penicillin G, 8 million units daily intravenously (1.0 million units every three hours) for three weeks
2. Cefoxitin, 8 g daily intravenously (1.0 g every three hours) for three weeks

Gonococcal Meningitis (Intravenous)

1. Penicillin G, 4 million units daily intravenously (2 g every two hours) for ten days
2. Chloramphenicol, 8 g daily intravenously (1 g every three hours) for ten days

References

Barr, J., and Danielsson, D.: Septic gonococcal dermatitis. Br Med J 1:482, 1971.

Blankenship, R. M., Holmes, R. K., and Sanford, J. P.: Treatment of disseminated gonococcal infection. N Engl J Med 290:267, 1974.

Braude, A. I., McCutchan, J. A., Ison, C., and Sargeaunt, P.: Differentiation of Neisseriaceae by isoenzyme electrophoresis. J Inf Dis 147:247, 1983.

Corbeil, L. B., Wunderlich, A. C., McCutchan, J. A., and Braude, A. I.: In Brooks, G. F. (ed): Immunobiology of *Neisseria gonorrhoeae*. Washington, D.C., American Society for Microbiology, 1978, p. 318.

Crawford, G., Knapp, J. S., Hale, J., and Holmes, K. K.: Asymptomatic gonorrhea in men: Caused by gonococci with unique nutritional requirements. Science 196:1352, 1977.

Eisenstein, B., Lee, T. J., and Sparling, P. F.: Penicillin sensitivity and serum resistance are independent attributes of strains of *Neisseria gonorrhoeae* causing disseminated gonococcal infection. Infect Immun 15:834, 1977.

Goldschneider, I., Gotschlich, E. C., and Artenstein, M. S.: Human immunity to the meningococcus. I. The role of humoral antibodies. J Exp Med 129:1307, 1969.

Handsfield, H. H.: Disseminated gonococcal infection. Clin Obstet Gynecol 18:131, 1975.

Handsfield, H. H., Weisner, P. J., and Holmes, K. K.: Treatment of the gonococcal arthritis-dermatitis syndrome. Ann Intern Med 84:661, 1976.

Harriman, G. R., Esser, A. F., Podack, E. R., Wunderlich, A. W., Braude, A. I., et al.: The role of C9 in complement-mediated killing of *Neisseria*. J Immunol 127:2386, 1981.

Harriman, G. R., Podack, E. R., Braude A. I., Crobeil, L. C., Esser, A. F., et al.: Activation of complement by serum-resistant *Neisseria gonorrhoeae*. J Exp Med 156:1235, 1982.

Hildebrandt, J. F., Mayer, L. W., Wong, S. P., and Buchanan, T. M.: *Neisseria gonorrhoeae* acquire a new principal outer membrane protein when transformed to resistance to serum bactericidal activity. Infect Immun 20:267, 1978.

Holmes, K. K., Counts, G. W., and Beaty, H. N.: Disseminated gonococcal infection. Ann Intern Med 74:979, 1971.

Jones, M.: Subacute bacterial endocarditis of non-streptococcic etiology. Am Heart J 40:106, 1950.

Joiner, K. A., Warren, K. A., Brown, E. J., Swanson, J., and Frank, M. M.: Studies on the mechanism of bacterial resistance to complement mediated killing. IV. C56-9 forms high molecular weight complexes with bacterial outer membrane constituents on serum resistant, but not on serum sensitive *Neisseria gonorrhoeae*. J Immunol 131:1443, 1983.

Keefer, C. S., and Spink, W. W.: Gonococcic arthritis: Pathogenesis, mechanism of recovery and treatment. JAMA 109:1448, 1937.

Keiser, H., Ruben, F. L., Wolinsky, E., and Kushner, I.: Clinical forms of gonococcal arthritis. N Engl J Med 279:233, 1968.

Knapp, J. S., and Holmes, K. K.: Disseminated gonococcal infection caused by *Neisseria gonorrhoeae* with unique nutritional requirements. J Infect Dis 132:204, 1975.

McCutchan, J. A., Katzenstein, D., Norquist, D., Chikami, G., Wunderlich, A., and Braude, A. I.: Role of blocking antibody in disseminated gonococcal infection. J Immunol 121:1884, 1978.

O'Brien, J. P., Goldenberg, D. L., and Rice, P. A.: Disseminated gonococcal infection: a prospective analysis of 49 patients and a review of pathophysiology and immune mechanisms. Medicine 62:395, 1983.

Payne, S. M., Holmes, K. K., and Finkelstein, R. A.: Role of iron in disseminated gonococcal infections. Infect Immun 20:573, 1978.

Partain, J. O., Cathcart, E. S., and Cohen, A. S.: Arthritis associated with gonorrhea. Ann Rheum Dis 27:156, 1968.

Petersen, B. H., Lee, I. J., Synderman, R., and Brooks, G. F.: *Neisseria meningitidis* and *Neisseria gonorrhoeae* bacteremia associated with C6, C7, and C8 deficiency. Ann Intern Med 90:917, 1979.

Rice, P. A., and Kasper, D. L.: Characterization of serum resistance of gonococci that disseminate: the role of blocking antibody and outer membrane protein. J Clin Invest 70:152, 1982.

Seifert, M. H., Warin, A. P., and Miller, A.: Articular and cutaneous manifestations of gonorrhea. Ann Rheum Dis 33:140, 1974.

Schoolnik, G. K., Buchanan, T. M., and Holmes, K. K.: Gonococci causing disseminated gonococcal infection are resistant to the bactericidal action of normal human serum. J Clin Invest 58:1163, 1976.
Thayer, W. S.: On the cardiac complications of gonorrhea. Bull Johns Hopkins Hosp 33:361, 1922.
Thompson, S. E.: Treatment of disseminated gonococcal infections. Sex Transmitted Dis 6:181, 1979.
Walker, L. C., Ahlin, T. D., Tung, K. S. K., and Williams, R. C.: Circulating immune complexes and disseminated gonorrheal infection. Ann Intern Med 88:28, 1978.
Weisner, P. J., Handsfield, H. H., and Holmes, K. K.: Low antibiotic resistance of gonococci causing disseminated infection. N Engl J Med 288:1221, 1973.
Williams, R. H.: Gonococcic endocarditis. Arch Intern Med 61:26, 1938.

193
MENINGOCOCCEMIA

THOMAS ALLAN HOFFMAN, M.D.

Invasion of the bloodstream by *Neisseria meningitidis* causes a spectrum of disease ranging from a benign transient bacteremia to an overwhelming infection that is rapidly fatal. Meningitis commonly intervenes during the course of meningococcemia. Meningococcal disease occurs sporadically or in episodic epidemics throughout the world. The incidence of meningococcal disease is highest in children from six months to one year of age and then declines. Meningococcal disease is a relatively common affliction of military recruits.

ETIOLOGY. *N. meningitidis* is a gram-negative diplococcus, commonly named the meningococcus. It grows well on solid media supplemented with blood and incubated in a moist CO_2-enriched atmosphere, and in liquid media used to culture blood aerobically. After 24 hours it should be subcultured onto blood agar or chocolate agar because turbidity may be difficult to recognize. Oxidase and catalase are biochemical markers for preliminary identification and sugar fermentations for final identification of the species. *N. meningitidis* ferments glucose and maltose, but not sucrose or lactose. Agglutination reactions with immune serum subdivide the species into serogroups A, B, C, W 135, X, Y, and Z, depending upon a group-specific capsular polysaccharide antigen. The group A meningococcal polysaccharide consists mainly of acetylated mannosamine phosphate whereas the group C polysaccharide is a polymer of acetylated sialic acid (Goldschneider et al., 1969). Sialic acid is also found in the group B polysaccharide, but it is antigenically distinct from that in group C polysaccharide (Goldschneider et al., 1969). Most strains causing meningococcal disease have the polysaccharide antigen of groups A, B, or C. Group Y and group W 135 meningococci cause disease more commonly than groups X and Z, which are rarely associated with disease. Meningococcal strains that lack these group-specific antigens are thought to be nonpathogenic.

The cell wall of pathogenic meningococci contains a toxic lipopolysaccharide or endotoxin. Meningococcal endotoxin appears to be chemically identical to endotoxin of enteric bacilli, but meningococcal endotoxin has greater potency for inducing the dermal Shwartzman reaction than enteric endotoxin (Davis and Arnold, 1974). Since the dermal Shwartzman reaction is the experimental equivalent of meningococcal purpura, endotoxin appears to be the cause of certain meningococcal lesions (Sotto et al., 1976).

Meningococci are susceptible to several antimicrobial agents. The activity of penicillin G against these organisms is greater than that of other penicillins or cephalothin. Minimal inhibitory concentrations of penicillin G usually range between 0.02 and 0.2 μg/ml. Chloramphenicol, rifampin, erythromycin, and tetracyclines are also active against meningococci. Meningococci have appeared that are resistant to 0.01 mg of sulfadiazine per milliliter. Meningococci are not susceptible to vancomycin, polymyxin, or achievable serum levels of aminoglycoside antibiotics.

PATHOGENESIS AND PATHOLOGY. The human nasopharynx is the only known reservoir of meningococcal infection. Meningococci are spread from person to person by airborne droplets of infected nasopharyngeal secretions. Organisms attach to mucosal surfaces where droplets deposit. Concomitant viral respiratory infection, particularly infection by influenza viruses, appears to enhance the spread of meningococcal infection and the likelihood of nasopharyngeal carriage after exposure to meningococci. Meningococcal infection of the nasopharynx produces few symptoms and is usually subclinical. Asymptomatic nasopharyngeal carriage of meningococci is transient and resolves within several weeks. In a few individuals the infection invades the circulation, causing either transient bacteremia, metastatic infection that most commonly involves the meninges, or a fulminant, overwhelming systemic infection with circulatory collapse. Many of the manifestations of this fulminant form of meningococcemia can be reproduced experimentally by meningococcal endotoxin. This substance can cause hypotension, margination of circulating leukocytes, aggregation of platelets, and disseminated intravascular clotting (Davis and Arnold, 1974; Mellins et al., 1972).

The fundamental pathologic change in meningococcemia is widespread vascular injury characterized by endothelial necrosis, intraluminal thrombosis, and perivascular hemorrhage (Sotto et al., 1976; Mellins et al., 1972). Organisms in blood invade through damaged vessels in the skin and elicit a perivascular infiltration of neutrophils. Skin lesions usually contain numerous meningococci undergoing phagocytosis by neutrophils. Occlusive thrombi composed of platelets, red blood cells, and fibrin are most prominent in vessels deep in the dermis and suggest a local Shwartzman reaction (Sotto et al., 1976). Immunologic factors probably contribute to vascular injury, since the walls of damaged vessels usually contain deposits of immunoglobulins, complement, and meningococcal antigen (Sotto et al., 1976). Serous surfaces and other organs have the same vascular injury (Mellins et al., 1972), although bacteria are difficult to find in tissues other than the skin.

Patients who die of meningococcemia develop thrombosis and hemorrhage in the skin, mucous membranes, serosal surfaces, adrenal sinusoids, and renal glomeruli (Wolf and Birbara, 1968). Adrenal hemorrhage is rarely extensive. Thrombosis of the glomerular capillaries may cause renal cortical necrosis, the chief characteristic of the generalized Shwartzman reaction, which can be induced experimentally by meningococcal endotoxin (Davis and Arnold, 1974). In the lung, thrombi containing numerous leukocytes are occasionally seen, and extensive intra-alveolar hemorrhage can occur. Myocarditis has been frequent in adults with fatal meningococcal infections (Hoffman and Edwards, 1972; Wolf and Birbara, 1968).

Susceptibility to meningococcal disease has been correlated with the absence of bactericidal antibody against pathogenic meningococci (Goldschneider et al., 1969). Bactericidal activity is mediated by IgG antibodies that have specificity for the meningococcal polysaccharides; however, activation of the complement system is required for expression of this activity. Asymptomatic carriage of meningococci in the nasopharynx induces a humoral antibody response and most individuals acquire immunity to meningococcal disease by age 20. Passively transferred maternal antibody provides temporary protection to infants for the first six months. Colonization with nonpathogenic meningococci seems to induce cross-reacting, protective antibodies. An episode of meningococcal disease confers group-specific immunity, but a second episode may be caused by another meningococcal serogroup. Complement deficiencies may allow repeated episodes of severe meningococcal infection.

CLINICAL MANIFESTATIONS. The clinical pattern of meningococcemia is varied (Hoffman and Edwards, 1972; Wolf and Birbara, 1968). The mildest form is a transient bacteremic illness that begins insidiously with fever and malaise. Petechial skin lesions do not appear in this form and the symptoms resolve spontaneously within one to two days. It is learned, subsequently, that blood cultures obtained during the febrile episode are growing *N. meningitidis*.

Acute meningococcemia is more serious. After a few days of upper respiratory prodromal symptoms, the temperature rises abruptly, often after a chill. Malaise, weakness, myalgias, headache, nausea, vomiting, and arthralgias are frequent presenting symptoms. The most characteristic manifestation of meningococcemia is the skin rash, which is essential for its recognition (Wolf and Birbara, 1968). Petechiae are the most common type of skin lesion and they may be sparsely distributed over the body. Ill-defined pink macules have sometimes been noted. Maculopapular lesions also occur and are sometimes large plaque-like lesions with a central petechia. The skin lesions of meningococcemia tend to occur in crops, and on any part of the body, although the face is usually spared and involvement of the palms and soles is less common. Petechiae are occasionally present on the conjunctiva and mucous membranes. The skin rash may advance from a few ill-defined lesions to a widespread eruption within a few hours. Patients with acute meningococcemia usually present with moderate fever (average 39.5° C) and marked leukocytosis (average 19,000/mm^3). Signs of shock are not present. Coagulation is normal except for elevated fibrinogen (Hoffman and Edwards, 1972). Other acute phase reactants, such as the serum complement, may be elevated.

Fulminant meningococcemia is the most serious form of meningococcal disease because of the high mortality rate. This form, which is also called the Waterhouse-Friderichsen syndrome, occurs in approximately 5 to 15 per cent of the cases of meningococcal disease (Hoffman and Edwards, 1972). It begins abruptly with sudden high fever, chills, myalgias, weakness, nausea, vomiting, and headache. Apprehension, restlessness, and frequently delirium occur within the next few hours. The rash appears suddenly and is widespread, purpuric, and ecchymotic. Hemorrhages appear on the buccal mucosa and conjunctiva. Less frequently, this form presents as purpura fulminans and, rarely, no skin lesions are recognized. Typically, no signs of meningitis are present. Cyanosis, hypotension, and profound shock eventually appear. Patients with the fulminant form of meningococcemia usually present with a high fever (average of 40.6° C) and either a normal WBC count or leukopenia. The blood pressure is lowered and shock may be present. Thrombocytopenia and other changes of disseminated intravascular clotting are also present (Hoffman and Edwards, 1972). These changes include a lowered prothrombin time, an increased partial thromboplastin time, a lowered fibrinogen level, and circulating levels of fibrin split products. The cell count, glucose, and protein in the cerebrospinal fluid are usually normal even though meningococci can frequently be cultured from it. The serum complement may be lowered. Pulmonary insufficiency develops within a few hours and many patients die despite appropriate antibiotic therapy and intensive care. Patients with fatal forms of fulminant meningococcemia are likely to succumb within 24 hours of being hospitalized.

Chronic meningococcemia is a rare form of meningococcal disease. This is an intermittent bacteremic illness that lasts for at least one week and as long as several months. The fever tends to be intermittent with afebrile periods ranging from two to ten days, during which the patient seems well. As the disease progresses the temperature rises daily and the fever may be continuous. Eventually, a skin eruption appears during the febrile episodes. The skin lesions are usually maculopapular, but may be hemorrhagic or pustular. Leukocytosis is noted during the febrile episodes but coagulation studies are usually normal.

COMPLICATIONS AND SEQUELAE. The most frequent complication of meningococcemia is meningitis. This complication is present in approximately half the patients with meningococcal disease. Other metastatic meningococcal infections are arthritis and, rarely, pericarditis (Hoffman and Edwards, 1972; Wolf and Birbara, 1968). Although joint involvement in meningococcal disease may be that of a septic arthritis, it frequently appears as an effusion after several days of antibiotic treatment. Meningococcal infection is associated with reactivation of herpes labialis.

In fulminant meningococcemia many complications are related to the circulatory changes of overwhelming infection. Acute renal failure can necessitate dialysis. Occlusion of pulmonary vessels and pulmonary hemorrhage may produce respiratory insufficiency. Acute adrenal failure has also been described, but infrequently. Cardiac insufficiency is frequent in fatal cases of meningococcemia.

GEOGRAPHIC VARIATIONS. Meningococcemia occurs sporadically in all inhabited areas of the world. The prevalence of meningococcal disease is highest in the spring. Meningococci have also caused massive outbreaks. Large-scale outbreaks of meningococcal disease have spread at cyclic intervals through Central African countries north of the equator. The recent outbreaks in Africa have been caused by group A meningococci. An outbreak of unusually massive proportions began in São Paulo, Brazil, during 1971. The predominant serogroup during the initial years of this epidemic was group C meningococci, but group A organisms became prevalent during the later years. The last extensive outbreak of meningococcal disease in the United States occurred during World War II when group A organisms were the prevalent serogroup. This serogroup has been subsequently replaced by group B and then by group C meningococci. Although sulfonamide-resistant meningococci were initially identified in the United States, they have subsequently been recovered in several parts of the world.

DIAGNOSIS. Recovery of *N. meningitidis* from cultures of the blood or petechiae is the usual means for establishing the diagnosis of meningococcemia. Positive blood cultures may not be obtained until late in the course of chronic meningococcemia. Detection of group-specific meningococcal antigen in serum offers a new and rapid means of diagnosis (Hoffman and Edwards, 1972). Studies with group-specific immune sera in counterimmunoelectrophoresis have shown that serum from patients with fulminant meningococcemia contains detectable levels of the polysaccharide antigen. The concentration of antigen in serum is likely to be related to the intensity of the bacteremia and to have prognostic significance (Hoffman and Edwards, 1972).

Meningococcal disease must be differentiated from Rocky Mountain spotted fever, bacterial endocarditis, hemorrhagic fevers due to arboviruses, enteroviral infection with exanthem, thrombotic thrombocytopenic purpura, and anaphylactoid purpura. The skin lesions of disseminated gonococcemia can usually be distinguished from those of meningococcemia.

TREATMENT. Specific antimicrobial therapy should be instituted promptly when the clinical features are suggestive of meningococcemia. The preferred drug for the treatment of meningococcal disease is penicillin G, and it should be given intravenously (Wolf and Birbara, 1968). Patients suspected of having meningococcemia should receive a high dosage of penicillin G for the initial 48 hours of therapy, since meningitis is a likely complication. Recommended initial therapy in adults with meningococcemia is one to two million units of penicillin G given by intermittent intravenous infusions every two hours; a dosage of 250,000 units/kg of body weight can be given daily in divided doses to pediatric patients. Most patients with uncomplicated meningococcemia defervesce within the first 24 hours of antibiotic therapy. Antibiotic therapy for uncomplicated meningococcemia need be given for only 4 to 5 days after defervescence occurs, and the dosage needed to complete the course of therapy in adults can be reduced to 600,000 units of procaine penicillin G given every 12 hours intramuscularly. Alternate therapy in penicillin-allergic patients is chloramphenicol, which is given in a dosage of 75 mg/kg/day intravenously until defervescence occurs, and then 50 mg/kg/day orally to complete a seven- to ten-day course of therapy.

Patients with fulminant meningococcemia may require supportive therapy to maintain perfusion to vital organs (Wolf and Birbara, 1968). Electrolyte-containing fluids should be administered aggressively in a critical care setting where cardiovascular monitoring is available. Rapid digitalization is indicated when evidence of cardiac insufficiency is present. A single intravenous infusion of either 30 mg of methylprednisolone per kilogram or 3 mg of dexamethazone per kilogram may be beneficial for profound hypotension that is unresponsive to other supportive measures. One additional dose can be administered four hours later if no response has occurred. A continuous infusion of dopamine or another ionotropic agent may also be needed for the management of shock. Anticoagulant therapy in fulminant meningococcemia remains controversial although it is generally accepted that heparin therapy does not improve survival in this condition.

PROPHYLAXIS. Meningococcal disease can be prevented by vaccination with group-specific meningococcal polysaccharides and by chemoprophylaxis (Artenstein, 1975). Purified polysaccharides of group A and group C meningococci have been used to stimulate group-specific humoral bactericidal antibodies. Vaccination with these polysaccharide antigens appears to be a highly effective means of preventing disease caused by these serogroups of meningococci. A single dose of vaccine, however, does not protect younger children, especially those under two years of age. Nevertheless, use of the vaccines is indicated for the population at risk whenever an outbreak caused by group A or group C meningococci becomes evident. Vaccination with the meningococcal polysaccharides has also been used effectively in military recruit populations to control disease caused by group A and group C organisms (Artenstein, 1975). Efforts to obtain a satisfactory vaccine for group B meningococcal disease have been unsuccessful.

Household contacts of patients with meningococcal disease are an identifiable population in which the risk of acquiring illness is definable (Artenstein, 1975). The secondary attack rate is inversely proportional to age and estimated to be approximately 10 per cent in household contacts between the ages of one and four years. Meningococcal infection is postulated to be introduced commonly into families by asymptomatic adults and then spread through one or more household contacts to reach the younger family members. Person-to-person transmission can be interrupted by chemoprophylaxis, which eradicates the asymptomatic nasopharyngeal carrier state. Sulfonamides, rifampin, and minocycline are the only drugs that have been shown to eradicate meningococci from the nasopharynx. Meningococcal isolates that are susceptible to 0.01 mg of sulfadiazime per milliliter can be eradicated by a two-day course of sulfadiazine given to adults in a dosage of 2 g per day. The dosage of sulfadiazine for children from 1 to 12 years of age is 1 g per day; children under 1 year are given 500 mg per day. Where the prevalent strains are sulfadiazine-resistant, rifampin is commonly used for meningococcal prophylaxis of household contacts. A two-day course of rifampin at doses of 600 mg every 12 hours for adults and 20 mg per kg per day for children is recommended. The rapid emergence of rifampin-resistant meningococci precludes the use of this drug in large populations; the high incidence of side effects has limited the wide acceptance of minocycline. Many experts believe that chemoprophylaxis of sulfadiazine-resistant meningococci by either of these agents is less preferable than close observation of household contacts for signs of disease (Artenstein, 1975).

References

Artenstein, M. S.: Prophylaxis of meningococcal disease. JAMA 231:1035, 1975.

Davis, C. E., and Arnold, K.: Role of meningococcal endotoxin in meningococcal purpura. J Exp Med 140:159, 1974.

Goldschneider, I., Gotschlich, E. C., and Artenstein, M. S.: Human immunity to the meningococcus: The role of humoral antibodies. J Exp Med 129:1307, 1969.

Greenwood, B. M., Oduloju, A. J., and Ade-Serrano, M. A.: Cellular immunity in patients with meningococcal disease and in vaccinated subjects. Clin Exp Immunol 38:9, 1979.
Griffiss, J. M., and Bertram, M. A.: Immunoepidemiology of meningococcal disease in military recruits. II. Blocking of serum bactericidal activity by circulating IgA early in the course of invasive disease. J Infect Dis 136:733, 1977.
Hoffman, T. A., and Edwards, E. A.: Group-specific polysaccharide antigen and humoral antibody response in disease due to Neisseria meningititis. J Infect Dis 126:636, 1972.
Lee, T. J., Snyderman, R., Patterson, J., et al: *Neisseria meningitidis* bacteremia in association with deficiency of the sixth component of complement. Infect Immun 24:656, 1979.
Mellins, R. B., Levine, O. R., Wigger, H. J., et al.: Experimental meningococcemia. J Appl Physiol 32:309, 1972.
Sotto, M. N., Langer, B., Hoshino-Shimizu, S., et al.: Pathogenesis of cutaneous lesions in acute meningococcemia in humans. J Infect Dis 133:506, 1976.
Wolf, R. E., and Birbara, C. A.,: Meningococcal infections at an army training center. Am J Med 44:243, 1968.

194
LISTERIOSIS

ANDREAS SCHAFFNER, M.D.

Listeria monocytogenes causes 3 major, distinct infectious syndromes: 1) meningoencephalitis, the most common manifestation of listeriosis; 2) intrauterine infection of the fetus resulting in abortion, stillbirth, or neonatal listeriosis; and 3) septicemia, which usually occurs in immunocompromised individuals or newborns. Endocarditis, lymphadenitis, skin pustules, ocular infections, and isolated abscesses of parenchymatous organs and soft tissue are rare manifestations of listeriosis.

ETIOLOGY. Listeriosis is caused by *L. monocytogenes*, a hemolytic, gram-positive, nonsporulating, motile bacillus. Because its morphology varies, it can easily be confused with either streptococci or corynebacteria unless careful attention is given to the appropriate microbiological tests (See Chapter 26). The possibility of *L. monocytogenes* must always be considered when a hemolytic, gram-positive coccobacillus is isolated from tissue, blood, cerebrospinal fluid, or any other body fluid.

PATHOGENESIS AND PATHOLOGY. Evidence is accumulating that the gastro-intestinal tract is frequently the portal of entry in adult patients with listeriosis. The major evidence includes the following observations: 1) *L. monocytogenes* is often isolated from the fecal flora; 2) like *Salmonella*, it can penetrate intestinal epithelial cells of experimental animals, multiply intracellularly, and reach subepithelial structures (Racz et al., 1972); 3) enteric symptoms are recognized early in the course of infection in an increasing number of patients; and 4) epidemiologic data suggest that food-borne transmission is responsible for some case clusters of listeriosis (Schlech et al., 1983).

Early neonatal listeriosis is usually a consequence of transplacental infection as evidenced by the high frequency of maternal infection and bacteremia and infectious placental foci (Gray and Killinger, 1966).

Symptomatic illness usually occurs at the extremes of life or in individuals with underlying conditions affecting their immune system (Table 1). As many as 25 to 30 per cent of patients with meningoencephalitis are young (<50 years), healthy people without recognized immune defects (Nieman and Lorber, 1981); Bouvet et al., 1982). In these patients infection of the CNS arises from low-grade septicemia, which is probably more prevalent than generally suspected. Once the organism penetrates the blood brain barrier, it is protected from host defense mechanisms that control the disease in other organs. Listeriosis of the pregnant woman is similar. The woman usually experiences a transient, "flu-like" illness that is recognized as listeriosis only because of its devastating effects on the fetus.

Because serology is not reliable, the incidence of subclinical and mild infections with *L. monocytogenes* is unknown. In a few instances, bacteremia has been documented in benign, self-limited febrile episodes of healthy, non-pregnant individuals.

In laboratory animals *L. monocytogenes* is an intracellular pathogen that survives and multiplies inside "resting" macrophages. The infection is controlled only after immune activation of the mononuclear phagocyte by lymphokines (see Chapter 26). There is no proof that listeriosis in humans is an intracellular infection and the microorganism is readily killed *in vitro* by human PMN's and blood monocytes (Felice et al., 1980). Furthermore, the low incidence of clinical disease compared to the high carrier rate and the

Table 1. CONDITIONS PREDISPOSING TO LISTERIOSIS. UNDERLYING DISORDERS IN 148 PATIENTS WITH LISTERIC MENINGITIS (102) AND SEPTICEMIA (40)*

Underlying Condition	Patients (% Mortality)
TOTAL MALIGNANCY	26% (40%)
.....Malignant Lymphoma	..13%
.....Leukemia	...9%
.....Carcinoma	...4%
TOTAL IMMUNOSUPPRESSION**	31% (24%)
.....Renal transplant	..23%
.....Other indication	...8%
TOTAL OTHER	19% (15%)
.....Alcoholism	...6%
.....Cirrhosis, hemochromatosis	...3%
.....Pregnancy***	...4% (0%)
.....Miscellaneous	...6%
NONE****	24% (11%)

*Data from the English language literature from 1968—1978, modified from Nieman and Lorber, 1980.
**Most immunosuppressive regimens included corticosteroids.
***All pregnant patients had bacteremia without CNS involvement.
****In patients with no underlying illness, meningitis was the most common form of listeriosis (31 of 36) and was responsible for most of the deaths.

ability of immunocompetent people to limit the infection to a short-lived, benign febrile disease suggest that people have strong natural resistance to *Listeria*. The nature of these defense mechanisms is unknown.

Analysis of the incidence of severe listeriosis among different groups of immunocompromised individuals (Table 1) suggests that cell-mediated immunity is also important for control of listeriosis in humans, because patients with renal transplants and malignant lymphomas have the highest predisposing conditions. On the other hand, most of these patients are treated with corticosteroids (Nieman and Lorber, 1980). In the experimental mouse, corticosteroids inhibit the early nonspecific resistance provided by macrophages, rather than acquired cell-mediated immunity (Schaffner et al., 1983).

In the meninges *Listeria* usually produces a granulocytic infiltration that cannot be distinguished from other purulent infections. In a minority of cases, the reaction is predominantly mononuclear and often reflects an underlying defect of the granulocytic defense system. The pathologic changes in the brain may consist of purulent cerebritis, necrotic encephalitis, or frank abscesses (Larsson and Linell, 1979). Septicemic listeriosis is frequently accompanied by small granulomas, consisting chiefly of macrophages and small foci of necrosis, scattered throughout many organs. Abscesses also occur and are most common in the liver (Yu et al., 1982). *Granulomatosis infantiseptica* is the name given to a distinct syndrome in early congenital listeriosis characterized by disseminated granulomas, necrosis, and abscesses of multiple internal organs.

CLINICAL MANIFESTATIONS

Meningoencephalitis in the Adult. Meningitis is the most frequent form of listeriosis in humans and *L. monocytogenes* is one of the leading causes of CNS infection in immunocompromised individuals, (Nieman and Lorber, 1980). In New York City from 1972 to 1979 it was the fifth most commonly reported cause of meningitis in adolescents and adults (Cherubin et al., 1981). Listeric meningitis usually presents as an acute febrile illness that cannot be differentiated clinically from other purulent meningitides. Nuchal rigidity in 80 per cent, a disturbance of consciousness ranging from confusion to coma in 60 per cent and seizures in 25 per cent of patients direct attention to the CNS. Tremors, cerebellar ataxia, or fasciculations are reported in over 10 per cent (Nieman and Lorber, 1980). In a few patients the manifestations are more subtle with a subacute course, low-grade fever and personality changes as the only discrete signs of CNS infection. CSF findings vary. The cell count usually ranges from 50 to several thousand cells per mm^3 with a predominance of PMN's in 75 per cent of the cases, but pleocytosis may be minimal or absent in patients with underlying conditions affecting mobilization of phagocytes. Protein concentrations are usually elevated to 200 mg/dl or more but may be normal. Less than half of the CSF glucose levels are below 40 mg/dl. CSF lactate is usually elevated. Gram stains of CSF are often negative. In a large review of case reports, examination of gram stains revealed no microorganisms in 59 per cent, gram-positive bacilli or coccobacilli in 33 per cent, and gram-positive diplococci in 8 per cent of patients (Nieman and Lorber, 1980).

Localizing neurologic findings such as motor disturbances and aphasia suggest encephalitis or brain abscess. Ten to 15 per cent of patients develop CNS listeriosis without meningitis (normal cell count or modest pleocytosis and negative culture of CSF) and present with hemiparesis, cranial nerve pareses, aphasia, or other focal neurologic signs with fever and positive blood cultures (Nieman and Lorber, 1980).

Septicemia in the Adult. Immunocompromised adults with *Listeria* septicemia usually present with severe illness, high fever, and prostration. There is usually no feature to distinguish listeremia from other causes of septicemia. Symptoms are nonspecific and include fatigue, malaise, nausea, and vomiting. Abdominal pain and diarrhea are not uncommon. Hypotension and disseminated intravascular coagulation may suggest gram-negative bacteremia. In some instances extensive seeding of the liver with abscesses causes the manifestations of acute hepatitis with massive elevation of transaminases (Yu et al., 1982).

Listeremia in pregnant women is usually a benign self-limited "flu-like" illness. Mild forms have also been observed in alcoholics and non-pregnant immunocompetent people. Nevertheless, all patients with septicemia should be treated. Seeding of the CNS should be suspected and a lumbar puncture performed in suspicious cases.

Neonatal Listeriosis. Neonatal listeriosis resembles group B streptococcal disease in that there are two forms, according to the age of the infant at onset. "Early-onset disease" is septicemia that occurs within the first few hours of life. "Late-onset disease" is meningitis that usually presents after 3 days of life (Ahlfors et al., 1977; Halliday and Hirata, 1979).

In "early-onset disease," infection originates *in utero*, the mother frequently reports a significant febrile illness before delivery, the baby is born prematurely, and *L. monocytogenes* can often be isolated from the mother's cervix, lochia, or blood. Prolonged rupture of the membranes is not a feature of neonatal listeriosis. Meconium staining of the amniotic fluid is common and fetal distress is recognized in about 50 per cent of cases. Presenting signs occur within the first hours of life and include respiratory distress, bilateral pneumonia, hepatosplenomegaly, rash, leukopenia, and thrombocytopenia. Diagnosis depends on cultures of blood, urine, gastric and tracheal aspirates, amniotic fluid, and meconium. Gram stain of the gastric aspirate is helpful when gram-positive coccobacilli are present. The CSF is usually culturally negative but the cell count may be elevated (Halliday and Hirata, 1979).

The meningitis of "late-onset disease," which makes up about one-third to one-fourth of all cases of neonatal listeriosis, commonly reflects infection during the birth process or in the postnatal period. Pregnancy, labor, and delivery are generally unremarkable. Meconium staining and birth asphyxia are not features of the disease and babies are frequently term (Larsson, 1979). Three to 15 days, or occasionally longer, after birth, the infant presents with fever, irritability and poor feeding. CSF cultures are always positive for *L. monocytogenes* but blood cultures are frequently negative. The finding that serotype 4b predominates in "late-onset disease" (Albritton et al., 1976) has not yet been confirmed (Larsson, 1979).

Rare Forms of Listeriosis. *L. monocytogenes* is a rare cause of endocarditis and has been reported to infect normal as well as injured and prosthetic valves (Nieman and Lorber, 1980). The clinical presentation is typical of subacute endocarditis. Other rare manifestations of listeriosis include endophthalmitis, peritonitis, pleurisy, osteomyelitis, lymphadenitis, skin lesions, conjunctivitis, cholecystitis, and abscesses of the spleen, liver, and soft tissues (Gray and Killinger, 1966; Nieman and Lorber, 1980). Pustular skin lesions have been observed in veterinarians after contact with infected placentas. Purulent keratoconjunctivitis has been reported in laboratory and poultry plant workers after accidentally splashing infectious material into their conjunctivae. The first such incident revealed the potential of pathogenic *Listeria* to penetrate the intact conjunctiva and cornea and led to the use of experimental keratoconjunctivitis in rabbits for identification of *L. monocytogenes* (Anton, 1934). *L. monocytogenes* does not cause monocytosis or a syndrome simulating infectious mononucleosis in human beings (Gray and Killinger, 1966).

COMPLICATIONS AND PROGNOSIS. Respiratory insufficiency is an important complication in the neonate, often necessitating aggressive ventilatory support. In spite of prompt treatment, neonatal "early-onset disease" causes high mortality and a high incidence of neurologic sequelae including retardation, focal deficits, hydrocephalus, and seizures. The prognosis of "late-onset disease" is considerably better. Most infants recover completely if therapy is promptly instituted (Visintine et al., 1977). In adults, the prognosis depends on the underlying condition (Table 1). Septicemia without CNS involvement carries a lower mortality rate (11 per cent) than meningoencephalitis (30 per cent). Adolescents and young adults without severe underlying disease usually recover uneventfully from meningitis (Cherubin et al., 1981; Larsson et al., 1978), but half of all surviving adults suffer neurologic sequelae, including cranial nerve and major limb palsies, mental deficits, and aphasia (Bouvet et al., 1982).

Unconfirmed studies suggest the possibility that *L. monocytogenes* might be responsible for some cases of "habitual" abortion (Gray and Killinger, 1966).

GEOGRAPHIC VARIATIONS. The three important clinical forms of listeriosis have been reported from all continents, as expected from the worldwide distribution of the organism. Differences in the incidence, age distribution, and relative frequency of the various syndromes appear to reflect the characteristics of the population studied and the awareness of listeriosis rather than true geographic variation. The yearly incidence of listeriosis fluctuates considerably for unknown reasons (Larsson, 1979) and complicates the interpretation of comparative studies.

DIAGNOSIS. Diagnosis of listeriosis depends on culture. In septicemia and meningitis the organism is often recoverable within 24 hours on routine media. Sufficient amounts (at least 1 ml) of CSF should be cultured because bacterial counts may be low in meningitis. If early neonatal listeriosis is suspected, fetal blood, meconium, and gastric and tracheal aspirates should be cultured. Cultures of the maternal cervix and the placenta may provide additional information. Listeremia should be considered in pregnant women with unexplained fever because early treatment of listeremia has a beneficial effect on the outcome of the pregnancy or neonatal infection (Zervoudakis and Cederqvist, 1977).

Identification of the organism is simple if the possibility is considered (see Chapter 26). The chief danger is that isolates may be discarded as a "diphtheroid contaminant" because the possibility of *Listeria* is not considered.

Serological diagnosis of listeriosis by demonstration of anti-listeric antibodies is not helpful because antibody responses do not occur until late in the disease (Larsson et al., 1978), are erratic in the immunocompromised, and are not very specific because of cross-reactions with antigens of other gram-positive bacteria (Gray and Killinger, 1966).

THERAPY. *L. monocytogenes* is inhibited by achievable concentrations of many antimicrobial agents but killing often requires much higher concentrations (see Chapter 26). Therefore, it is usually necessary to treat patients for prolonged periods. Relapses of meningoencephalitis in immunocompromised patients (Watson et al., 1978) and of meningitis in newborns (Halliday and Hirata, 1979) have been documented after antibiotic therapy of less than 3 weeks. Because CNS involvement is frequent and not always recognized clinically (Larsson et al., 1978), the ability of the drug to penetrate the CSF should be considered. Clinical experience is most extensive with penicillin G and ampicillin. Based on *in vitro* data and limited clinical studies, ampicillin may be preferable, but treatment failures have been reported with both drugs. The usual dose for meningoencephalitis, encephalitis, septicemia, and endocarditis is 240,000 to 320,000 units of penicillin G/kg/day or 250-350 mg/kg/day of ampicillin divided into 4 to 6 equal doses. Therapy should always be continued for at least 3 weeks with longer regimens in patients with endocarditis and all immunocompromised patients, especially with CNS infection. On the basis of *in vitro* synergism of gentamicin with ampicillin or penicillin and a superior effect of the combinations compared to ampicillin alone in a rabbit model of meningitis, therapy with two drugs has been proposed (Scheld et al., 1979). For severe listeriosis a combination of ampicillin or penicillin with gentamicin in a dose of 5 to 6 mg/kg/day in 3 equally divided doses may be considered but there are no clinical data in patients to support combined therapy that is certainly more toxic. Because gentamicin penetrates the CSF poorly, intrathecal gentamicin has been advocated for combination therapy in patients with listeria meningoencephalitis (Cherubin et al., 1981).

Penicillin allergy greatly complicates treatment because clinical experience with alternative drugs is limited. Erythromycin, tetracycline, and chloramphenicol have all been used successfully but the limited data do not permit a definite choice. Erythromycin appears to be an adequate substitute for patients with septicemia. Although chloramphenicol has been used frequently in adults with meningoencephalitis, a recent retrospective study suggests that it is significantly less effective than ampicillin (Cherubin et al., 1981). Trimethoprim is very active against *Listeria in vitro* (MIC < 0.5 μg/ml) with little disparity between the minimal inhibitory and minimal bactericidal concentrations (Tuazon et al., 1982). Because trimethoprim and sulfonamides also penetrate into the CSF very well and have been used in combination successfully in a few patients (Larsson et al., 1978), they are a promising alternative in patients allergic to penicillin. It is also possible that oral trimethoprim or trimethoprim-sulfonamide might be used to shorten hospitalization solely for the purpose of parenteral therapy with penicillin.

PROPHYLAXIS. Control of listeriosis in animals does not affect the incidence of human disease (Kampelmacher and Van Norle Jansen, 1980) nor the frequency of isolation from environmental sources (Dijkstra, 1982). Transmission by milk from infected cows can be prevented by avoiding raw milk. An epidemic of human listeriosis has recently been attributed to contamination of vegetables by manure from a herd infected by *Listeria*. Neither untreated manure (Schlech et al., 1983) nor raw sewage from sewage plants (Watkins and Sleath, 1981) should be used on crops designated for human use. No vaccine is available.

References

Ahlfors, C. E., Goetzman, B. W., Halsted, C. C., et al.: Neonatal listeriosis. Am J Dis Child 131:405, 1977.

Albritton, W. L., Wiggins, G. L., and Feeley, J. C.: Neonatal listeriosis: distribution of serotypes in relation to age at onset of disease. J Pediatr 88:481, 1976.

Anton, W.: Kritisch experimenteller Beitrag zur Biologie des *Bakterium monocytogenes*. Zentr Bakteriol Parasitol Abt I Orig 131:89, 1934.

Bouvet, E., Suter, F., Gibert, C. et al.: Severe meningitis due to *Listeria Monocytogenes*. A review of 40 cases. Scand J Infect Dis 14:267, 1982.

Cherubin, C. E., Marr, J. S., Sierra, M. F., and Becker, S.: Listeria and gram-negative bacillary meningitis in New York City, 1972–79. Frequent causes of meningitis in adults. Am J Med 71:199, 1981.

Dijkstra, R. G.: The occurrence of *Listeria monocytogenes* in surface water of canals and lakes, in ditches of one big polder and in the effluents and canals of a sewage treatment plant. Zbl Bakt Hyg I Abt Orig B 176:202, 1982.

Felice, G. A., Beaman, B. L., Krick, J. A., and Remington, J.: Effects of human neutrophils and monocytes on *Nocardia asteroides:* failure of killing despite occurrence of the oxidative metabolic burst. J Infect Dis 142:432, 1980.

Gray, M. L., and Killinger, A. H.: *Listeria monocytogenes* and listeric infections. Bacteriol Rev 30:309, 1966.

Halliday, H. L., and Hirata, T.: Perinatal listeriosis—a review of twelve patients. Am J Obstet Gynecol 133:405, 1979.

Kampelmacher, E. H., and Van Noorle Jansen, L. M.: Listeriosis in humans and animals in the Netherlands (1958–77). Zbl Bakt Hyg I Abt Orig A 246:211, 1980.

Larsson, S., Cronberg, S., and Winblad, S.: Clinical aspects of 64 cases of juvenile and adult listeriosis in Sweden. Acta Med Scand 204:503, 1978.

Larsson, S.: Epidemiology of listeriosis in Sweden 1958–74. Scand J Infect Dis 11:47, 1979.

Larsson, S., and Linell, F.: Correlations between clinical and postmortem findings in listeriosis. Scand J Infect Dis 11:55, 1979.

Nieman, R. E., and Lorber, B.: Listeriosis in adults: a changing pattern. Report of eight cases and review of the literature, 1968–78. Rev Infect Dis 2:207, 1980.

Racz, P., Tenner, K., and Mero, E.: Experimental listeria enteritis. 1. An electron microscopic study of the epithelial phase in experimental listeria infection. Lab Invest 26:694, 1972.

Schaffner, A., Douglas, H., and Davis, C. E.: Models of T cell deficiency in listeriosis: The effects of cortisone and cyclosporin A on normal and nude BALB/c mice. J Immunol 131:450, 1983.

Scheld, W. M., Fletcher, D. D., Fink, F. N., and Sande, M. A.: Response to therapy in an experimental rabbit model of meningitis due to *Listeria monocytogenes*. J. Infect Dis 140:287, 1979.

Schlech, W. F., Lavigne, P. M., Bortolini, R. A., et al.: Epidemic listeriosis—evidence for transmission by food. New Engl J Med: 308:203, 1983.

Tuazon, C. U., Shamuddin, D., and Miller, H.: Antibiotic susceptibility and synergy of clinical isolates of *Listeria monocytogenes*. Antimicrob Agents Chemother 21:525, 1982.

Visintine, A. M., Oleske, J. M., Nalimias, A. J.: *Listeria monocytogenes* infection in infants and children. Am J Dis Child 131:393, 1977.

Watkins, J., and Sleath, K. P.: Isolation and enumeration of *Listeria monocytogenes* from sewage, sewage sludge and river water. J Appl Bacteriol 50:1, 1981.

Watson, G. W., Fuller, T. J., Elms, J., and Kluge, R. M.: *Listeria cerebritis*: relapse of infection in renal transplant patients. Arch Intern Med 138:83, 1978.

Yu, V. L., Miller, W. P., Wing, E. J., et al: Disseminated listeriosis presenting as acute hepatitis. Case reports and review of hepatic involvement in listeriosis. Am J Med 73:773, 1982.

Zervoudakis, A. L., and Cederqvist, L. L.: Effects of *Listeria monocytogenes* septicemia during pregnancy on the offspring. Am J Obstet Gynecol 129:465, 1977.

195

BACTEROIDES SEPTICEMIA

DONALD L. BORNSTEIN, M.D.

The obligately anaerobic gram-negative bacilli of clinical importance, the *Bacteroides*, make up the major portion of the normal microflora of the lower intestinal tract and are prevalent in the oropharynx, in the female genital tract, and on certain areas of the skin. Disease, surgery, or trauma involving these colonized sites is often complicated by opportunistic infection with *Bacteroides*, usually in combination with other resident anaerobic or aerobic microorganisms. Many species of the two important genera, *Bacteroides* and *Fusobacterium*, can cause suppurative infections and bacteremia, but the pre-eminent pathogen and the organism most frequently isolated from purulent sites and from the blood is *B. fragilis*. *Bacteroides* septicemia usually follows the development of a suppurative and necrotizing process that has originated from and around the gastrointestinal or the female genital tract. Advanced cases may be associated with marked leukocytosis, septic thrombophlebitis, jaundice, metastatic infection, obtundation, and refractory shock. Because *B. fragilis* is generally resistant to penicillin, cephalosporins, and aminoglycosides, infection with this organism should be seriously considered when febrile illness develops or persists despite use of these antibiotics after abdominal or pelvic surgery or in other appropriate clinical settings.

ETIOLOGY. The Family *Bacteroidaceae* comprises three genera: the genus *Bacteroides*, with over twenty species; the genus *Fusobacterium*, with fourteen species; and the genus *Leptotrichia*, with one species. In a two-year study at the Mayo Clinic, *Bacteroides* organisms were recovered from 19 per cent of all clinical specimens that contained bacteria (Martin, 1974). Bacteremia due to *Bacteroides* has increased in incidence from 1 to 2 per cent of all positive blood cultures between 1955 and 1965 to 6 to 12 per cent in more recent studies (Wilson et al., 1972; Chow and Guze, 1974). Over 60 per cent of strains of *Bacteroides* isolated from all clinical specimens and over 80 per cent of strains isolated from the blood are of the *B. fragilis* group.

The distribution of species of *Fusobacterium* and *Bacteroides* varies throughout the body, and this fact is reflected in the patterns of infection associated with the different species. In the oropharynx, Fusobacteria (*F. necrophorum*, *F. nucleatum*, *F. varium*, *F. mortiferum*), *B. oralis*, *B. corrodens*, and *B. melaninogenicus* are common, while *B. fragilis* is rare. In the distal ileum and colon and on the perineum, the *B. fragilis* group predominates, but *B. melaninogenicus* and *F. necrophorum* are also commonly present. In the healthy female genital tract, other Bacteroides species are more prevalent, but *B. fragilis* is the most commonly isolated species from pelvic abscesses. *B. fragilis* rarely causes infections that arise above the diaphragm, although septic embolization and metastatic infection to the lungs or to the brain can occur. Chronic sinusitis, chronic otitis media, and mastoiditis are occasionally caused by *B. fragilis*. Conversely, *Bacteroides* infection originating from an abdominal or pelvic source, a wound, or a decubitus ulcer should be considered to be due to *B. fragilis* until proved otherwise.

The distribution of *Bacteroides* organisms recovered from clinical specimens by species and site was reviewed by Martin (1974). Of 4433 clinical isolates of *Bacteroides*, 56 per cent were of the *B. fragilis* group, 25 per cent were *B. melaninogenicus*, 13 per cent were other *Bacteroides*, 4 per cent were *F. nucleatum*, and 1 per cent were other fusobacteria. *B. fragilis* was recovered from 13 per cent of 134 sputum specimens containing *Bacteroides* organisms, 65 per cent of specimens from abdominal wounds, and 87 per cent of 326 positive blood cultures for *Bacteroides*. These figures indicate the rarity of *B. fragilis* in the lung, its prevalence in abdominal sites, and its greater virulence as indicated by a disproportionate presence in the blood.

Until 1976, five subspecies were recognized within the species *B. fragilis:* s.s. *fragilis*, s.s. *thetaiotamicron*, ss. *distasonis*, s.s. *vulgatus*, and s.s. *ovatus*. Subsequently, each has been raised to full species rank on the basis of DNA homology (Cato and Johnson, 1976). Most clinical studies begun before 1977 have not distinguished among the five species, and the term *B. fragilis* used in earlier reports refers to what is now described as the *B. fragilis* group. This group shares a common habitat, many common cultural characteristics, and a common special pattern of antibiotic susceptibility. The potential virulence varies considerably, however, among these five species, from the highly pathogenic *B. fragilis* to the essentially nonpathogenic *B. ovatus*. Of the five species of the *B. fragilis* group, *B. fragilis* is the most prevalent in clinical specimens, while the other species are more prevalent in the normal bowel flora. About 70 to 80 per cent of clinical isolates described as *B. fragilis* in the recent past were truly *B. fragilis*, 10 to 20 per cent were *B. thetaiotamicron*, and 5 to 10 per cent were *B. vulgatus* or *B. distasonis* (Polk and Kasper, 1977).

PATHOGENESIS AND PATHOLOGY. *Bacteroides* organisms are opportunistic pathogens without primary invasive ability, and a breach of local anatomic defenses is usually required to initiate infection. However, the intense colonization of the lower bowel—over 10^9 organism per gram of stool (100 to 1000 times the number of *Escherichia coli*)—and the consequent colonization of adjacent skin surfaces and, in 50 to 70 per cent of women, of the female genital tract, pose a constant threat of infection. The oropharynx also carries a large number of other *Bacteroides* species as part of its complex microflora. Ulcerating or necrotizing inflammatory or malignant disease, trauma, or surgery involving heavily colonized skin or mucosal surfaces is the usual means of introducing *Bacteroides*, along with other indigenous flora, into normally sterile deeper tissues. Since *Bacteroides* organisms are obligate anaerobes, the presence of any necrotic tissue, foreign material, impaired blood flow, anoxia or acidosis, or aerobic bacterial growth, which reduces the redox potential (Eh) in the tissues, provides a potent stimulus for rapid bacterial growth.

Bacteremia may be initiated directly by minor injury to a colonized mucous membrane, but most *Bacteroides* sepsis involves an established local suppurative infection. The major sources of *Bacteroides* septicemia have been the gastrointestinal tract (50 to 65 per cent of cases), the female genital tract (20 to 30 per cent), decubiti and other wounds (10 to 15 per cent), the respiratory tract (2 to 5 per cent), and the oropharynx (1 to 3 per cent).

The predisposing event involving the gastrointestinal tract has been disease (appendicitis, diverticulitis, acute pancreatitis, intestinal obstruction, vascular disease, malignancy, inflammatory bowel disease, perforated ulcer, other surgical problems), trauma (gunshot wounds), or surgery that has caused a spill of bowel contents into the peritoneum. The disease that follows depends on the magnitude of the spill, the prior health of the patient, and the subsequent medical and surgical management. A large leak can lead to frank peritonitis and gram-negative sepsis within 2 to 24 hours owing to rapidly growing facultative enteric bacilli. *Bacteroides* infection may first become apparent after the acute problem has been corrected, from 5 to 20 days after the initiating event. An experimental animal model of the events that follow fecal contamination of the peritoneum has shown a similar biphasic illness: an early acute peritonitis and bacteremia after one to two days due to *E. coli* or *Klebsiella*, followed in all survivors by intra-abdominal abscess formation after a week or so due to *B. fragilis* (Weinstein et al., 1974).

Bacteroides septicemia originating in the female genital tract is usually secondary to septic abortion, to amnionitis and puerperal complications, to cesarean section, or to vaginal hysterectomies (Ledger et al., 1975). Less common but more serious septicemia can be seen in older women with more extensive gynecologic surgery or radiation therapy for malignant disease.

Surgical or traumatic wounds of the back, hips, buttocks, or thighs, and decubitus ulcers are often heavily soiled with fecal flora. This is an exceedingly serious problem in paraplegics and other immobile or bedridden patients. It is further intensified by diabetes mellitus, peripheral vascular disease, obesity, and fecal incontinence (Galpin et al., 1976).

Neither the lung nor the oropharynx is a common portal of entry of *Bacteroides* sepsis today. In the pre-antibiotic era, however, over 30 per cent of cases developed from the oropharynx. A severe pharyngitis with suppurative complications, which dissected into the neck and mediastinum, and which caused septic thrombophlebitis of the jugular vein, was a common presentation. This was associated with heavy persistent bacteremic seeding and serious metastatic infection of lungs, joints, and meninges (Gunn, 1956). The oral *Bacteroides* and Fusobacteria are generally sensitive to common antimicrobial agents, and antibiotics abort most of these infections in their early stages today. The remaining infections of the mouth and lung are secondary to local tissue injury and to aspiration.

Surgery of the bowel can be complicated by intraoperative spills, by anastomotic leaks or fistulae, and by abdominal wound infections. When penicillins, cephalosporins, or aminoglycoside antibiotics are administered, or when oral neomycin or nonabsorbable sulfonamides are given for "preparation" of the bowel before colon surgery, significant changes occur in the microbial ecology of the bowel. These drugs suppress enteric bacteria and many of the antibiotic-sensitive anaerobes and allow the more pathogenic and drug-resistant *B. fragilis* to proliferate, increasing the risk of postoperative or other opportunistic infection. The addition of erythromycin base to oral neomycin reduces the overgrowth of *B. fragilis*, and this regimen appears to be somewhat safer in regard to opportunistic infection (Nichols et al., 1973).

In 1976, Kasper and co-workers demonstrated an important virulence factor in *B. fragilis*. Electron micrography of various species of *Bacteroides* stained with ruthenium red revealed a capsular structure on fresh isolates of *B. fragilis* that was not seen in any other species. Specific capsular antibody was prepared and immunofluorescence studies demonstrated capsules on *B. fragilis* strains but on no other *Bacteroides*. Isolates of *B. thetaiotamicron*, *B. distasonis*, *B. vulgatus*, and *B. ovatus* showed no evidence of capsules by ruthenium red and no capsules by immunofluorescence (Kasper et al., 1977). Two capsular types are now recognized and the chemical structure of these complex polysaccharides has been analyzed (Kasper et al., 1983). Subsequently, an analogous specific capsular material has been demonstrated on a subspecies of *B. melaninogenicus*, ss. *asaccharolyticus*, which has now been assigned full species status as *B. asaccharolyticus*. It appears to be more pathogenic than other isolates of *B. melaninogenicus* and may have accounted for many of the serious *B. melaninogenicus* infections (Mansheim et al., 1978). *B. thetaiotamicron*, *B. distasonis*, and *F. necrophorum* exhibit significant pathogenicity in some cases, and it is conceivable that some isolates of these species will eventually be shown to possess a capsule.

The capsular material of *B. fragilis* has been shown to be antiphagocytic and to be highly leukotactic for polymorphonuclear leukocytes. Killed *B. fragilis* or partially purified capsular material placed in the peritoneal cavity of a rat can elicit a massive accumulation of polymorphonuclear cells and abscess formation. This may explain, in part, the markedly purulent nature of the host response to *B. fragilis* infections, which is more like a pyogenic infection than a coliform infection.

Active immunization of rats or mice with purified capsular polysaccharide leads to protection against abscess formation after intraperitoneal infection with *B. fragilis*. This protection is not transferable with immune serum to normal rats or mice; splenic cell transfer to syngeneic mice is protective, however. The cell that appears to be responsible for transferring resistance to abscess formation is a T lymphocyte with surface markers typical of a suppressor cell (Lyt $1\text{-}2^{+}$) (Shapiro et al., 1983). Elucidation of the mechanisms involved should provide new insights into a currently unrecognized host defense system.

Other factors that may be involved in the pathogenicity of *B. fragilis* include proteolytic and collagenolytic enzymes, heparinase, which may promote septic thrombophlebitis and interfere with anticoagulant therapy, and the presence of a unique lipopolysaccharide (LPS). The LPS of the genus *Bacteroides*, unlike that of the classical endotoxins, lacks 2 keto-3-deoxyoctonate and L-glyceromannoheptose residues, and is devoid of the hypotensive, toxic, and lethal properties of typical LPS. Intravenous infusion of *B. fragilis* does not cause the refractory hypotension in rabbits that is seen after infusions of E. coli. Shock does occur in *Bacteroides* sepsis, but it may be unrelated to endotoxin, since it generally occurs later in the course of the illness, as is seen in continuing sepsis due to gram-positive pathogens.

Chromosomal beta-lactamase activity is present in the whole *B. fragilis* group, although it is not the only mechanism of penicillin or cephalosporin resistance. Recently, plasmids bearing R factors for clindamycin and for chloramphenicol have been described. Such plasmids, may introduce other factors that enhance bacterial virulence and their role in the pathogenesis of *Bacteroides* infections requires further careful study.

CLINICAL PICTURE. *Bacteroides* septicemia typically appears as a prostrating and toxemic febrile illness that develops over several days in a patient hospitalized for other medical problems or recovering from recent abdominal or gynecologic surgery. A more acute onset may be seen in young women following septic abortion or puerperal complications. In contrast to gram-negative rod bacteremia, *Bacteroides* sepsis rarely originates from the urinary tract and is relatively uncommon in severely immunocompromised patients (acute leukemics, transplant recipients). The clinical picture is usually less precipitous in onset and is more protracted than typical gram-negative bacteremia.

Most nonobstetrical patients are over 40 years of age, have had recent surgery or a biopsy, and have been on antibiotics or have received oral neomycin or other agents in preparation for bowel surgery. Common clinical features are a brisk peripheral leukocytosis, sometimes exceeding 40,000 white blood cells per mm^3, spiking fevers and repeated chills, persistence of bacteremia over several days, and, usually, some signs and symptoms of the initial infection in the abdomen, the pelvis, or an infected wound. In other patients persistent low-grade fever and malaise may be the only findings.

Jaundice (12 to 29 per cent), septic thrombophlebitis (5 to 44 per cent), septic embolization to the lungs, liver, or brain (23 to 29 per cent), and septic shock (25 to 35 per cent) can be seen in far-advanced cases and constitute a classic but uncommon syndrome of *Bacteroides* septicemia. Most cases will not present with these findings.

The bacteremia and the toxemia of *Bacteroides* sepsis can persist intermittently or continuously for up to several weeks despite the use of appropriate antibiotics unless all suppurative lesions are identified and are drained effectively. Bacteremia that persists after effective drainage often indicates bacterial invasion of veins in the infected area. Septic thrombophlebitis is more common following pelvic infection or surgery. Venous cords may be palpated or clinical evidence of venous obstruction may be noted in some cases. Septic emboli to the liver and, and more often, to the lungs may be the first evidence of venous infection. Antibiotics and heparin therapy can usually correct the phlebitis, but venous ligation is still required in some cases.

Metastatic infection can develop into more extensive and life-threatening problems than the original suppurative lesion. Large or multiple liver abscesses or extensive pleuropulmonary suppuration can become the source of persistent bacteremia and further metastatic infection to the brain, to joints, to other serosal surfaces, and to the heart valves.

About 3 to 8 per cent of patients with *Bacteroides* bacteremia have only transient bacteremia—a brief fever elevation without significant toxemia. They do not have an established local infection and they recover without specific therapy. Another significant portion of cases (10 to 25 per cent) are polymicrobial; anaerobic streptococci, facultative streptococci, and enterobacteria are common associated organisms. These cases are usually associated with less morbidity and mortality than pure *B. fragilis* septicemia.

Oropharyngeal sepsis due to *F. necrophorum* or oral strains of *Bacteroides*, although rare, still occurs and diagnosis is usually seriously delayed or missed. Seidenfeld et al. (1982) describe 5 recent cases complicated by septic thrombophlebitis of the internal jugular vein. The clinical presentations suggested acute bacterial endocarditis because of the hectic course and the rapid development and progression of cavitating lung nodules and septic arthritis in young adults. The pharyngeal findings were not very impressive or were resolving in several of the cases. Tenderness and swelling along the sternocleidomastoid muscle can be an important clue. The slow growth of these organisms in blood culture can delay their recognition for 4 to 7 days or longer.

COMPLICATIONS. The major hazards of *Bacteroides* septicemia are serious metastatic infection, septic thrombophlebitis, septic shock and its consequences, and, rarely, bacterial endocarditis. Metastatic complications include lung, liver, spleen, myocardial and brain abscesses, empyema, meningitis, and septic arthritis. Local complications (extension, obstruction, and necrosis) at the initial site of infection can themselves be life-threatening.

The diagnosis of endocarditis due to *Bacteroides* is difficult to establish unless there is clear-cut peripheral embolization or unequivocal evidence of new valve injury, because persistent bacteremia is often due to undrained abscesses or septic thrombophlebitis. Finegold (1977) reviewed 56 case reports of *Bacteroides* endocarditis. Most cases were in older persons without predisposing valvular abnormalities; over 50 per cent of these patients died. About one half of cases were due to *B. fragilis* and originated mainly from the abdomen, pelvis, or perineum. The other cases were of dental, pharyngeal, and pulmonary origin and involved *B. melaninogenicus*, *B. oralis*, and fusobacteria. The validity of the diagnosis of endocarditis in many of the patients who recover on antibiotic therapy is open to question. The need for effective bactericidal therapy to cure *Bacteroides* endocarditis was underlined by Nastro and Finegold (1973), who recommend the use of intravenous metronidazole for this disease.

DIAGNOSIS. When fever and toxemia develop or progress in a patient with puerperal or postabortal complications, gynecologic or intra-abdominal problems, chronic decubiti, or after recent abdominal or pelvic surgery, one must strongly suspect either enterobacterial or *Bacteroides* sepsis. If blood cultures are still sterile after 48 hours of incubation, *Bacteroides* septicemia is more likely, since it often takes three to seven days, and occasionally longer, for these slower growing organisms to be recognized. If the febrile illness developed or progressed despite antimicrobial therapy with a cephalosporin and an aminoglycoside, the diagnosis of *Bacteroides* sepsis is strongly supported.

Surgical wounds, decubitus ulcers, or other accessible sites that could be the source of bacteremia should be examined and swabbed for smears and anaerobic and aerobic cultures. The presence of foul-smelling exudate and of small or pleomorphic gram-negative rods on gram-stained smears should heighten suspicion. In over 70 per cent of patients, however, the seeding site is not accessible to direct culture. It must be localized by other means in order to identify the origin of the bacteremia and to render proper treatment. Thorough physical examination, including repeat rectal and pelvic examinations, plain and barium contrast x-ray films, and liver function tests, will often identify the site of a septic focus. A pocket of gas in an extra-intestinal site or in the soft tissues may indicate the source of the sepsis. Liver-spleen scans, gallium scans, sonography, and computer-assisted axial tomography are of great value in localizing intra-abdominal and hepatic abscesses and other masses or suppurative lesions that cannot be observed by routine x-rays. They are invaluable adjuncts in finding the source of *Bacteroides* septicemia.

Diagnosis rests on recovery of the agent in blood cultures, and success here relates directly to the use of proper media and bacteriologic methods. Although most *Bacteroides* are not very stringent anaerobes and need only moderate reduction in the redox potential (Eh) for growth, acceptable recovery rates require enriched anaerobic media. Some strains of *B. melaninogenicus* require media enriched with hemin and menadione and some *Bacteroides*, seen on initial gram-stains, are not recoverable with commonly used bacteriologic media.

In polymicrobial bacteremia (about 10 to 25 per cent of all *Bacteroides* bacteremia) it is possible to overlook the slower growing *Bacteroides* if an enteric gram-negative rod is present. The coexisting *Bacteroides* will be detected only if the laboratory routinely subcultures all turbid blood culture bottles to two blood agar plates, one of which is cultured under anaerobic conditions. Unfortunately, this is not a routine for many laboratories. *Bacteroides* bacteremia may be recognized belatedly in such cases, after therapy aimed at the aerobic isolate has cleared this organism but allowed the *Bacteroides* to persist. Such belated recognition adds significantly to the morbidity and mortality of *Bacteroides* infection. Fluorescein-conjugated antisera to capsular antigens of *B. fragilis* and *B. asaccharolyticus* allow rapid recognition of pathogenic *Bacteroides* organisms in wound exudates and more rapid speciation in the laboratory, speeding diagnosis and delivery of appropriate antimicrobial therapy.

As a general rule, *B. fragilis*, when present in a mixed aerobic-anaerobic infection, is the most important pathogen, and the infection will not be cured without specific and effective therapy against this organism. One exception is in idiopathic lung abscess. In this condition *B. fragilis* has been isolated from 15 to 20 per cent of cases as part of a mixed flora, but therapy with penicillin, which is normally ineffective against this organism, has been very successful.

GEOGRAPHIC CONSIDERATIONS. The extent of colonization of the bowel by the various species of *Bacteroides* and of fusobacteria does vary in different parts of the world, primarily because of dietary differences. Significant colonization with the major pathogenic species of *Bacteroides* is universal, however. The incidence of illness caused by these endogenous organisms varies in relation to the extent of obstetric infections, abdominal and pelvic surgery, and malignancy. When hospital facilities are more limited and when less extensive surgery is carried out, infection rates will appear lower. However, more fatal cases will develop in the home and will not be recognized as due to *Bacteroides*.

TREATMENT. Because abscesses and other local suppurative lesions are the usual sources of *Bacteroides* septi-

Table 1. ANTIMICROBIAL SUSCEPTIBILITY OF BACTEROIDES AND FUSOBACTERIA[a]

Antimicrobial Agent	Concentration (μg/ml)	B. Fragilis Group	B. Melaningogenicus	Bacteroides Species	Fusobacterium Species
Penicillin G	2	0	++−+++	+	++−+++
	8	0−±	+++	++	+++
Cephalothin	8	0	++	+	++−+++
Gentamicin	4	0	0−+	0	0
Polymyxin	4–8	0	0−±	0−±	++
Tetracycline	1–2	±−+	++	±−+	+++
Erythromycin	1–2	±	+++	++	0−+
Chloramphenicol	8	++−+++	+++	+++	+++
Clindamycin	4	+++	+++	+++	+++
Metronidazole	8	+++	+++	++−+++	+++
Carbenicillin	64	++	+++	+++	+++
Cefoxitin	16	++	+++	++−+++	+++

[a]Per cent susceptible at concentration tested: +++, over 95%; ++, over 75%; +, over 50%; ±, over 25%; 0, less than 25%. Data from Finegold (1977), Martin (1972), and other sources.

cemia, antimicrobial therapy must be supplemented with effective surgery in many cases. Abscesses must be drained, necrotic tissues excised, decubitus ulcers debrided, obstructed bowel or viscera relieved, and infected veins that do not respond to heparin must be ligated. Sites of metastatic infection may also require surgical drainage to terminate bacteremia. Patients who succumb to *Bacteroides* septicemia usually have collections of undrained pus at autopsy (Lawrence et al., 1977).

There are important differences in antimicrobial susceptibility among the *Bacteroides.* Most fusobacteria and many *Bacteroides* species *(B. oralis, B. melaninogenicus)* have been highly susceptible to penicillin G and, to a lesser extent, to the other penicillins and cephalosporins (Table 1). An increasing number of isolates of *B. melaninogenicus* that produce a beta-lactamase (primarily a penicillinase) is being reported. This is a cause for concern and requires careful observation. *B. fragilis,* however, and the related strains of the *B. fragilis* group, are intrinsically resistant to penicillins and cephalosporins, to all aminoglycosides, and to polymyxins. In 50 to 70 per cent of cases they are also resistant to tetracyclines. Fortunately over 95 per cent of isolates of the *B. fragilis* group are susceptible to clindamycin, metronidazole and chloramphenicol and 85 to 90 per cent are susceptible to cefoxitin or moxalactam. Newer drugs under development, which appear to be highly effective, include *N*-formimidoyl thienamycin, tinidazole, and some of the newer quinoline derivatives.

Clindamycin is effective against *B. fragilis*, the other Bacteroides, and Fusobacteria. Intravenous doses of 600 mg q6 hours or 900 mg q8 hours in adults produce mean peak blood levels exceeding the MIC_{90} by three- to five-fold. These levels are bactericidal for over 60 per cent of strains. Once reported to cause antibiotic-associated colitis (AAC) due to *C. difficile* overgrowth in upwards of 10 per cent of cases, the overall rate is clearly below 1 per cent. Most of these cases can be averted by discontinuing clindamycin promptly if the patient develops diarrhea that persists over 48 hours or is associated with abdominal cramps. Should it develop, *C. difficile* colitis can be treated with oral vancomycin, 125 mg po qid.

Plasmid-borne high level resistance to clindamycin and to macrolides has been recognized. Such isolates are rare in the U.S. although there are clusters of cases in certain hospitals and cities. The problem is more widespread in Spain and France (Linares et al., 1983). Resistance to clindamycin has been transferred to sensitive recipient strains in the laboratory by strains that lack plasmids but that have sequences homologous to the R factor DNA integrated into their chromosomal DNA (Guiney et al., 1983). Despite this and other novel aspects of transfer of clindamycin and of tetracycline resistance, 98 per cent of *B. fragilis* isolates in most U.S. hospitals are still susceptible to clindamycin (Tally et al., 1981).

Metronidazole is an effective bactericidal drug for most obligate anaerobes but does not inhibit microaerophilic or aerobic organisms that frequently accompany *Bacteroides* infections. Like chloramphenicol and unlike clindamycin it diffuses very well into the central nervous system and the cerebrospinal fluid, which makes it a drug of choice for *B. fragilis* infections of the CNS. Most *Bacteroides* infections of the CNS, however, are caused by the penicillin-sensitive species resident in the oropharynx. Metronidazole is administered I.V. as an initial loading dose of 15 mg/kg followed by 7.5 mg/kg q6 hours. Oral metronidazole can be substituted to complete a course of therapy after a good clinical response has been obtained (Bergan, 1982).

Chloramphenicol has been associated with more treatment failures than would be anticipated from its in vitro sensitivity, probably because it lacks bactericidal activity and possibly because it can be inactivated within abscesses. The usual adult dose is 1 g I.V. q6 hours. Plasmid R factors that acetylate the drug have been recognized but are rare. Resistance mechanisms to metronidazole and chloramphenicol have recently been reviewed by Britz (1981).

The *B. fragilis* group shares a chromosomal constitutive beta-lactamase, which is primarily a cephalosporinase that inactivates penicillins and most cephalosporins. Cefoxitin resists inactivation by these beta-lactamases by virtue of its 7 α-methoxy group and can inhibit 70 to 80 per cent of strains at 16 μg/ml and 85 to 95 per cent of strains at 32 μg/ml. Because 2-g doses are required to achieve peak blood levels of 32 μg/ml at 1 hour after infusion, and because of its relatively short half-life, an effective regimen is 2 g I.V. every 4 hours (12 g/day). Moxalactam has a similar degree of beta-lactamase resistance and in vitro activity but has occasional failures in vitro that are not well explained. Further successful experience against *B. fragilis* infections is required before it replaces cefoxitin as the alternative drug to clindamycin or metronidazole. Other members of the *B. fragilis* group appear to be less susceptible than *B. fragilis* to these cephalosporins.

Table 2. INHIBITORY INDEX (I. I.) OF ANTIMICROBIAL AGENTS ACTIVE AGAINST B. FRAGILIS

Antimicrobial Agent	Parenteral Dose	Achievable Serum Concentrations[a] (μg/ml)	MIC for 95% of Strains	I. I. (Serum Concentration/MIC 95)
Clindamycin	600 mg every six hrs	8–10	3	3.0
Chloramphenicol	1000 mg every six hrs	12–16	12	1.2
Metronidazole	750 mg every eight hrs	16–24	8	2.5
Carbenicillin	5000 mg every four hrs	125	128	1.0
Cefoxitin	2000 mg every four hrs	30	32	0.8

[a]Serum concentration one hour after IV infusion or IM injection.

Carbenicillin, ticarcillin, and the newer acylureidopenicillins have been recommended for *B. fragilis* infections. However, because their activity is low, because very large doses are required, and because they lack a record of clinical success in established *B. fragilis* sepsis, these are not first line drugs. The relative blood concentrations and MIC_{95} for these antibiotics are summarized in Table 2.

For infections with *Fusobacteria* and with oropharyngeal strains of *Bacteroides*, penicillin G (12 to 36 million units/day I.V.) has been the drug of choice. In penicillin-allergic patients, either clindamycin, metronidazole, chloramphenicol, cefoxitin, or another parenteral cephalosporin is an effective alternative. There is growing concern about beta-lactamase production by oropharyngeal *Bacteroides* (especially *B. melaninogenicus)*, which has been found in 5 to 10% of isolates overall and, in some reports, in excess of 50% of strains (Brown and Waati, 1980). If a poor clinical response is seen to I.V. penicillin, another effective agent should be substituted promptly. In vitro susceptibility testing for anaerobes is not routinely offered by most hospital laboratories, but if increasing drug resistance continues, it may become necessary for effective management of *Bacteroides* sepsis.

The in vitro susceptibility patterns of the five species of the *B. fragilis* group are very similar. *B. distasonis* is somewhat more susceptible to penicillins and *B. thetaiotamicron* is slightly more resistant to clindamycin (Jones and Fuchs, 1976).

Because of some increasing resistance to all the effective agents (Sutter et al., 1979), unnecessary use of these drugs must be discouraged and appropriate infection control measures must be taken when plasmid-borne resistance is detected to prevent the spread of resistant *B. fragilis* strains. Although the prophylactic use of antibiotics active against *B. fragilis* in surgery must be carefully considered, early surgical use in conditions in which an actual spill of bowel contents has occurred would appear to be clinically indicated (Thadepalli et al., 1973).

Bacteroides septicemia has a poor prognosis, despite the availability of effective antimicrobial drugs. In large collected series 25 to 45 per cent of patients have died. Important prognostic factors are age, site of infection, underlying disease, choice of antibiotic, adequacy of drainage, and especially, promptness of recognition and treatment.

Bacteroides bacteremia arising from an obstetrical infection is, by contrast, a very mild illness. In 184 cases reviewed by Chow and Guze (1974) there was only one fatality (0.6 per cent), as compared with a mortality rate of 35 to 45 per cent for nonobstetrical cases. Infection is rare in childhood, but young adults can develop serious septicemia from decubiti (in paraplegics), trauma, surgery, or appendiceal disease. Mortality is higher in the nonobstetrical group for older patients, in postsurgical cases, in bedridden patients, and in the presence of advanced diabetes, arteriosclerosis, liver or kidney disease, and malignant disease. Inadequate surgical drainage, inappropriate antibacterial therapy, and the development of septic shock are associated with a poorer prognosis. Deferring surgery to allow an extended period of antimicrobial therapy is generally unwise. Surgical drainage should be carried out as soon as the need is recognized, even if the patient appears acutely ill. When effective drainage is not possible (as in patients with multiple abdominal fistulae or severe eroding decubiti), survival rates are poor.

PREVENTION. Neither active or passive immunization against *Bacteroides* infection is available. It is conceivable that protective anticapsular antibody or cell-mediated immunity can be elicited in man and that there may be a role for active immunization in selected high-risk settings in the future.

Antimicrobial prophylaxis of postoperative infection after bowel or uterine surgery is widely practiced. If the regimen does not include an agent effective against *B. fragilis*, overgrowth of *Bacteroides* in the gut and an increased risk of *Bacteroides* infection can be anticipated. Although the inclusion of clindamycin, metronidazole, chloramphenicol, or cefoxitin might reduce the incidence or delay the onset of *Bacteroides* infections, the risk/benefit ratio must be considered. The risks include: drug toxicity (hypersensitive, idiosyncratic, and other adverse reactions) altered normal flora (colonization with resistant organisms, superinfection, pseudomembranous enterocolitis); and the epidemiologic consequences (selection of R factor plasmid-bearing organisms and eventual selection of drug-resistant *B. fragilis* strains). Prophylaxis should be brief, brisk, and be based on sound indications.

The best preventive measures against bacteroides sepsis are early recognition and effective treatment of localized *Bacteroides* infections.

References

Bergan, T.: The pharmacokinetics of metronidazole. In First United States Metronidazole Conference. Finegold, S. M., George, W. L., and Rolfe, R. D. (eds.): Biomedical Information Corp, New York, 1982, pp. 83–112.

Britz, M. L.: Resistance to chloramphenicol and metronidazole in anaerobic bacteria. J Antimicrob Chemother 8 (Suppl. D): 49, 1981.

Brown, W. J., and Waatti, P. E.: Susceptibility of clinically isolated anaerobic bacteria by an agar-dilution technique. Antimicrob Agents Chemother 17:629, 1980.

Cato, E. P., and Johnson, J. L.: Reinstatement of species rank for *Bacteroides fragilis, B. ovatus, B. distasonis, B. thetaiotamicron* and *B. vulgatus.* Int J Syst Bacteriol 26:230, 1976.

Chow, A. W., and Guze, L. B.: Bacteroidaceae bacteremia: Clinical experience with 112 patients. Medicine 53:93, 1974.
Finegold, S. M.: Anaerobic Bacteria in Human Disease. New York, Academic Press, 1977.
Finegold, S. M., Bartlett, J. G., Chow, A. W., Flora, D. J., Gorbach, S. L., Harder, E. J., and Tally, F. P.: Management of anaerobic infections. Ann Intern Med 83:375, 1975.
Galpin, J. E., Chow, A. W., Bayer, A. S., and Guze, L. B.: Sepsis associated with decubitus ulcers. Am J Med 61:346, 1976.
Guiney, D. G., Jr., Hasegawa, P., Stalker, D., and Davis, C. E.: Genetic analysis of clindamycin resistance in *Bacteroides* species. J Infec Dis 147:551, 1983.
Gunn, A. A.: Bacteroides septicemia. J R Coll Surg Edinb 2:41, 1956.
Holdeman, L. V., Cato, E. P., and Moore, W. E. C.: Anaerobic Laboratory Manual. 4th ed. Blacksburg, Va., Virginia Poytechnic Institute and State University, 1977.
Jones, R. N., and Fuchs, P. C.: Identification and antimicrobial susceptibility of 250 *Bacteroides fragilis* subspecies tested by broth microdilution methods. Antimicrob Agents Chemother 9:719, 1976.
Kasper, D. L., Hayes, M. E., Reinap, B. G., Craft, F. O., Onderdonk, A. B., and Polk, B. F.: Isolation and identification of encapsulated strains of *Bacteroides fragilis*. J Infect Dis 136:75, 1977.
Kasper, D. L., Weintraub, A., Lindberg, A. A., and Lonngren, J.: Capsular polysaccharide from two *Bacteroides fragilis* strains: chemical and immunochemical characterization. J Bacteriol 153:991, 1983.
Lawrence, P. F., Tietgen, J. W., Gingrich, S., and King, T. E.: Bacteroides bacteremia. Ann Surg 186:559, 1977.
Ledger, W. J., Norman, M., Gee, C. L., and Lewis, W. P.: Bacteremia on an obstetric-gynecologic service. Am J Obstet Gynecol 121:205, 1975.
Linares, J., Perez, J. L. and Martin, R.: Susceptibility studies on the *B. fragilis* group resistant to clindamycin. J Antimicrob Chemother 12:253, 1983.
Mansheim, B. J., Solstad, C. A., and Kasper, D. L.: Identification of a subspecies-specific capsular antigen from *Bacteroides melaninogenicus*, subspecies *asaccharolyticus* by immunofluorescence and electron microscopy. J Infect Dis 136:736, 1978.
Martin, W. J.: Isolation and identification of anaerobic bacteria in the clinical laboratory. Mayo Clin Proc 49:300, 1974.
Nastro, L. J., and Finegold, S. M.: Endocarditis due to anaerobic gram-negative bacilli. Am J Med 54:82, 1973.
Nichols, R. L., Broido, P., Condon, R. E., Gorbach, S. L., and Nyhus, L. M.: Effect of pre-operative neomycin-erythromycin intestinal preparation on the incidence of infectious complications following colon surgery. Ann Surg 178:453, 1973.
Polk, B. F., and Kasper, D. L.: *Bacteroides fragilis* subspecies in clinical isolates. Ann Intern Med 86:569, 1977.
Seidenfeld, S. M., Sutker, W. L., and Luby, J. P.: *Fusobacterium necrophorum* septicemia following oropharyngeal infection. JAMA 248, 1982.
Shapiro, M. E., Onderdonk, A. B., Kasper, D. L., and Finberg, R. W.: Cellular immunity to *Bacteroides fragilis* capsular polysaccharide. J Exp Med 154:1188, 1982.
Sutter, V. L., Vargo, V. L., and Finegold, S. M.: Wadsworth Anaerobic Bacteriology Manual. 2nd ed. Los Angeles, Extension Division, University of California at Los Angeles, 1975.
Sutter, V. L., Kirby, B., and Finegold, S. M.: In-vitro activity of cefoxitin and parenterally administered cephalosporins against anaerobic bacteria. Rev Infect Dis 1:128, 1979.
Tally, F. P., Sosa, A., Jacobus, M. V., and Malamy, M. H.: Clindamycin resistance in *Bacteroides fragilis*. J Antimicrob Chemother 8 (Suppl D): 43, 1981.
Thadepalli, H., Gorbach, S. L., Broido, P. W., Norsen, J., and Nyhus, L. M.: Abdominal trauma, anaerobes and antibiotics. Surg Gynecol Obstet 137:270, 1973.
Weinstein, W. M., Onderdonk, A. B., Bartlett, J. G., and Gorbach, S. L.: Experimental intraabdominal abscesses in rats: Quantitative bacteriology of infected animals. Infect Immun 10:1250, 1974.
Wilson, W. R., Martin, W. J., Wilkowske, C. J., et al.: Anaerobic bacteremia. Mayo Clin Proc 47:639, 1972.

196
CLOSTRIDIAL SEPTICEMIA
DONALD L. BORNSTEIN, M.D.

Clostridial septicemia is a rare, highly lethal illness due to heavy bacteremic seeding with pathogenic clostridia originating primarily from the uterus, colon, or biliary tract. The characteristic clinical presentation, as seen following septic abortion, is that of high fever, extensive intravascular hemolysis due to circulating clostridial alpha toxin (lecithinase C), hypotension, and acute renal tubular necrosis. Fatal sepsis can occur without significant hemolysis. Episodes of transient clostridial bacteremia are much more common than septicemia and do not necessarily carry a serious prognosis. Clostridial myonecrosis (gas gangrene) may give rise to transient bacteremia but is very rarely associated with septicemia and hemolysis. In rare cases, protracted clostridial septicemia may induce "metastatic" or "spontaneous" gas gangrene. Clostridial bacteremia can also occur agonally or in the last hours of life, especially in patients with impaired resistance or intestinal ulceration, and may produce striking postmortem changes of crepitus and gas-filled cysts in many organs.

ETIOLOGY. Although many of the 60-odd species of *Clostridium* can colonize humans and cause local infections and a transient bacteremia, only a few are significant pathogens. *Clostridium perfringens*, the major pathogen, causes over 90 per cent of cases of septicemia as well as most of cases of transient bacteremia. *C. septicum*, which may be relatively more common in patients with malignant disease, and, very rarely, *C. sordelli*, or *C. novyi* account for the other cases. Clostridia are recovered from 1 to 2.5 per cent of all positive blood cultures. The large majority of isolations represent transient bacteremia; the septicemic cases are rare. In about 30 to 40 per cent of positive cultures, clostridia are mixed with other aerobes and/or anaerobes (Martin, 1974; Gorbach and Thadepalli, 1975).

A site of origin can be identified in less than half of the patients; an intestinal, biliary, or gynecologic origin is assumed for the others. Transient bacteremias due to nonpathogenic species, for example, *C. ramosum, C. tertium, C. difficile,* and *C. bifermentans,* arise from the same sites and from secondarily infected necrotic processes. Bacteremia with these organisms, usually benign, can produce shock or lethal illness in newborns or in severely compromised patients (Alpern and Dowell, 1971).

PATHOGENESIS AND PATHOLOGY. The pathogenesis of clostridial septicemia involves colonization of a site with pathogenic clostridia, a local environment that promotes rapid growth of clostridia, and local factors that help to introduce organisms into the bloodstream.

The vast intestinal reservoirs of pathogenic and nonpathogenic clostridia are concentrated in the large intestine, but colonization of the small intestine can occur and is favored by disordered or reverse peristalsis, antibiotic use (including some nonabsorbable drugs), and surgery, especially gastrojejunostomy or bypass jejunoileostomy.

The biliary tract is sterile in health but becomes susceptible to colonization with enteric bacteria via portal venous blood as a result of disease, surgery, or obstruction. Clostridia have been recovered in pure or mixed culture in 5 to 27 per cent of infected cases (Fukunaga, 1973). Pneumocholecystitis (or emphysematous cholecystitis), an unusual condition in which gas can be seen in the wall or the lumen of the gallbladder, is caused by clostridia in 25 to 30 per cent of cases.

The perineal area and the skin of the thighs and abdomen and, to a lesser extent, the hands, other skin areas, and the oropharynx are contaminated with clostridia as a consequence of the heavy intestinal carriage of this organism. Clostridia also colonize the genital tract of 4 to 9 per cent of healthy women. Carriage increases in complicated pregnancy or after surgical intervention and reaches rates of 18 to 27 per cent following septic abortion.

Clostridia, like other obligate anaerobes, can proliferate in tissues only when the oxidation-reduction potential (Eh) falls or when, at any level of Eh, the pH is reduced. Rapid growth of clostridia is promoted by foreign material, lactic acid accumulation due to tissue anoxia, arterial injury or compression of vessels by edema, and above all, the presence of necrotic tissue (Oakley, 1954). While *C. perfringens* requires anaerobiosis for growth, its pathogenicity is enhanced by its ability to survive for considerable periods of time at atmospheric oxygen tensions. Even exposure to oxygen at three atmospheres pressure for several hours does not kill this hardy organism (Fredette, 1965).

Most cases of clostridial septicemia originate from the genital tract of women; a few occur after complicated term delivery, cesarean section, gynecologic surgery, or, very rarely, from infected necrotic tumors (leiomyomas or malignant lesions), but the vast majority of cases follow septic abortion. In septic abortion a foreign body (catheter, wire, slippery elm stalk) or a solution (soap, phenolics, quinine) is introduced through the cervix. In this process clostridia from the perineum or the vagina or occasionally from the foreign object itself can be introduced into the uterus, where there are usually residual necrotic fetal and placental tissues and traumatized areas of endometrium that favor the rapid heavy growth of clostridia. In addition, the pregnant uterus is a highly vascular organ and any infected retained placental tissue is intimately apposed to vascular beds, a feature that is responsible for the early intense and persistent septicemia that can follow. Fortunately, only a small fraction of cases of septic abortion are followed by serious bacteremic illness. The conditions required to permit clostridial sepsis occur in only about 0.2 to 1.5 per cent of all women hospitalized after septic abortion, which is fortunate in view of the poor salvage rate in this disease. This catastrophic illness has almost disappeared in the United States since abortion has been legalized.

Dissemination of clostridia into the blood from the gastrointestinal tract is favored by ulcerative processes of the small or large intestine (bleeding peptic ulcer in a patient with a gastrojejunostomy, enteritis necroticans); intestinal obstruction; necrotic or infiltrating malignancy; abdominal catastrophe (perforation, diverticulitis, ruptured appendix, acute pancreatitis); or recent bowel surgery. Anaerobic cellulitis, decubitus ulcers, and ischiorectal abscesses have also caused septicemia. A special group at high risk for clostridial septicemia are patients with hematologic or other malignant disease, especially carcinoma of the colon. Primary or metastatic disease, and cytotoxic or radiation therapy can cause intestinal ulceration that allows clostridia ready access to the bloodstream. Clostridial septicemia can originate from acute cholecystitis (especially emphysematous or gangrenous cases) or surgery (operative cholangiography, common duct exploration, or cholecystectomy).

Many of the features of clostridial sepsis are due to exotoxins. Alpha toxin, the important hemolytic toxin of *C. perfringens*, is an enzyme, lecithinase C, which cleaves phosphorylcholine from lecithin to leave an insoluble diglyceride. It also acts similarly on sphingomyelin. Both phospholipids are vital structural components of the surface membranes and of mitochondrial and lysosomal membranes of mammalian cells.

Alpha toxin has the most obvious effects on erythrocytes. It causes cell fragmentation, loss of volume, and formation of osmotically fragile and morphologically distinctive microspherocytes. The ensuing hemolysis releases free hemoglobin intravascularly in amounts that rapidly overload clearance by haptoglobin and the reticuloendothelial system. Injury to endothelial cells and platelets induces the disseminated intravascular coagulation (DIC) that is seen in the most severe cases. Alpha toxin can also damage muscle and is responsible for the severe muscle tenderness seen in advanced clostridial sepsis.

The contribution of the other toxins of *C. perfringens* is not clear, although some may play an important role (see Chapters 49 and 253). *C. septicum* lacks lecithinase C and the lethal septicemia that it can produce is not accompanied by significant hemolysis. Septic shock is common in clostridial sepsis and occurs within the first 12 to 24 hours of illness, a pattern that is unusual for bacteremia caused by other gram-positive organisms. This may be due to the intensity of the bacteremic seeding or may be a reflection of the toxicity of *C. perfringens* for leukocytes and other tissues. Clostridial sepsis is frequently so intense that organisms can be demonstrated on smears of the buffy coat or peripheral blood (Brooks, 1973).

The combination of massive hemolysis, sudden high fever, and hypotension causes the characteristic renal lesion of acute tubular necrosis with hemoglobinuria and subsequent oliguria or anuria. Intravenous infusion of hemoglobin solutions does not cause acute renal failure in normal man or animals, but rapid intravascular hemolysis, especially in combination with the circulatory changes of an acute febrile illness or impending shock, will produce this lesion.

At autopsy there is evidence of intravascular hemolysis such as pink discoloration of blood vessels, bronzing of the skin, icterus, hemoglobin casts in renal tubules, and erythropoiesis in the marrow. Lesions may be found at the site of origin in the uterus, gastrointestinal tract, biliary tree, or skin. Changes compatible with acute renal tubular necrosis may also be present.

Welch in 1892 described masses of clostridia and gas-filled bubbles and cysts in many tissues (liver, heart, muscle, and others) and recognized that they represented the effects of continued postmortem proliferation of clostridia with accompanying gas production in the tissues. Too often these postmortem changes have been erroneously described as "gas gangrene" of the liver or of other viscera and have been misinterpreted as antemortem events. On occasion, however, patients with severely depressed resistance (advanced malignancy, acute leukemia, immunosuppression) have such overwhelming septicemia that they may develop multiple foci of metastatic gas infection during life (Boggs et al., 1958; Cabrera et al., 1965).

CLINICAL MANIFESTATIONS. Clostridial sepsis, fever, and chills usually begin 24 to 72 hours after attempted abortion and are associated first with malaise, headache, severe myalgias, crampy or sharp abdominal pain, nausea, vomiting, and occasionally diarrhea. A foul bloody or brown vaginal discharge is noted. Within a matter of hours symptoms may increase dramatically with the development of oliguria, hypotension, and jaundice. Dark mahogany urine due to hemoglobinuria may be noticed. A characteristic bronzing of the skin can occur within several hours of the onset of hemolysis. On admission to the hospital patients are often gravely ill, jaundiced, and hypotensive. They are characteristically apprehensive, mentally alert although hypotensive, tachypneic, and often display tachycardia out of proportion to the temperature elevation. The skin may be cold and mottled and the sclerae icteric. Pelvic examination reveals red-brown, foul cervical drainage, sometimes with gas bubbles. Laceration marks around the cervix or perforation of the cervical segment may be detected. The uterus is slightly enlarged and tender, but if infection involves the myometrium or has spread to the adnexa, extreme tenderness, guarding, and an adnexal mass may be detected (Mahn and Dantuono, 1955; MacLennan, 1962).

Laboratory studies show a neutrophilic leukocytosis with leukocyte counts of 15,000 to 50,000 per mm^3, normal or pink to port-wine colored plasma, with plasma hemoglobin concentrations as high as 8000 mg/100 ml. Anemia is proportional to the degree of hemolysis; hematocrits may be as low as 10 per cent. The platelet count may be moderately or significantly reduced, either as an isolated finding or as part of an unfolding pattern of disseminated intravascular coagulation. Microspherocytes and deformed erythrocytes may be seen on the peripheral smear. Under observation, oliguria or anuria, increasingly refractory hypotension, and, in severe cases, hemorrhagic phenomena and bruising, as well as the laboratory stigmata of disseminated intravascular coagulation, may develop.

Clostridial septicemia arising from the biliary or gastrointestinal tract usually presents as an acute and serious febrile illness with chills and fevers but often with no other specific or localizing findings. Intravascular hemolysis is observed in less than 30 per cent of cases. Biliary or gastrointestinal symptoms may be the only clues to the etiology of the apparent bacteremic episode, and the underlying infections would be presumed to be due to gram-negative bacilli until blood culture results are reported.

Patients with malignant disease, especially those receiving treatment with radiation or cytotoxic agents, can rapidly develop fatal clostridial sepsis from a minor gastrointestinal focus or surgical trauma. They have fever, tachypnea, hypotension, abdominal pain or tenderness, nausea, vomiting, and coma. Crepitus may develop in the flanks or over a recent incision, and the temperature and pulse rate may become dissociated. Significant hemolysis is recognized in only 20 to 30 per cent of cases. In studies from oncologic hospitals, a striking feature was the lethality of this syndrome and the rapidity of death. Half the deaths occur less than 12 hours after onset of symptoms, and almost all occur within 24 hours (Wynne and Armstrong, 1972). Physicians should consider clostridial sepsis in any patient with advanced malignancy who develops abdominal pain or tenderness and fever, and an effective drug for clostridia should be part of any empirical antibiotic therapy, pending the results of blood cultures. Early appropriate antimicrobial therapy can be life-saving (Koransky, 1979).

The milder transient bacteremias, which are significantly more common than the septicemic cases, can arise in any hospitalized patient but are most common when there is a predisposing lesion or impaired resistance (cirrhosis, neutropenia, prior antibiotic therapy, immunosuppression). These illnesses have few distinctive clinical features. Blood cultures reveal either *C. perfringens* or nonpathogenic clostridia, and, with or without antibiotics, the fever usually disappears within 24 to 48 hours. Although usually self-limited, clostridial bacteremia is associated with a mortality rate of 20 to 40 per cent overall, which is due primarily to the serious underlying diseases that permit entry of clostridia into the blood. This mortality demonstrates the gravity, if not the severity, of this illness. Persistent or polymicrobial bacteremia may carry an even poorer prognosis (Pietrafitta and Deckers, 1982; Ramsay, 1949; Bornstein et al., 1964; Rathbun, 1968).

The syndrome of life-threatening *C. septicum* septicemia in association with carcinoma of the cecum or hematologic malignancy deserves special mention. This organism is not commonly isolated from normal fecal samples and comprises less than 5 per cent of all clinical isolates of clostridia. However, in recent reports, 76 of 98 patients with *C. septicum* bacteremia had an underlying malignant disease, 28 of which were carcinoma of the cecum or ascending colon and 38 acute leukemia, lymphoma, or other hematologic malignancy. Others had neutropenia, ischemic bowel, or other malignancy. Autopsy findings in 24 patients without bowel malignancy implicated the terminal ileum, the cecum and the ascending colon as the site of entry in 18 cases. Since *C. septicum* bacteremia is uncommon in other types of immunocompromised patients, these highly associated diseases must establish unique local conditions favoring heavy growth of *C. septicum* in the cecum. (Koransky et al., 1979).

COMPLICATIONS AND SEQUELAE. The major complications of clostridial septicemia are refractory shock, disseminated intravascular coagulation, and, if significant hemolysis occurs, acute tubular necrosis with oliguric renal failure. Metastatic myonecrosis is a very rare but dramatic complication most often associated with carcinoma of the cecum or acute leukemia (Chapter 253).

GEOGRAPHIC VARIATIONS IN DISEASE. *C. perfringens* is present as a major component of human intestinal flora through the world. Hygienic practices vary considerably, however, and much higher carriage rates on the skin, in the oropharynx, and in the female genital tract may be expected in areas with poor sanitary facilities.

Geographic differences in rates of clostridial septicemia are probably related primarily to the level of obstetrical care and to variations in the incidence of septic abortion. With poor sanitation and home deliveries a greater incidence of puerperal clostridial infection may be anticipated. In countries where abortion is legal and freely available, cases of postabortal clostridial sepsis are rare. In countries where religious beliefs interdict rational policies on abortion or where sterile surgical facilities are not available, this preventable disease is still far too prevalent. Socioeconomic factors within a society also play a role in clostridial sepsis. In 1963, before legal abortions were freely available in the United States, postabortal septicemia accounted for 45 per cent of all puerperal mortality in New York and for 80 per cent of the puerperal mortality in black and Puerto Rican women, reflecting a greater incidence of abortion among those of poor socioeconomic status and the dangers of illegal abortion.

DIAGNOSIS. Although overt hemolysis, telltale gas shadows, or crepitus can provide clues to clostridial sepsis, they are often absent. In such a case Gram-stained smears,

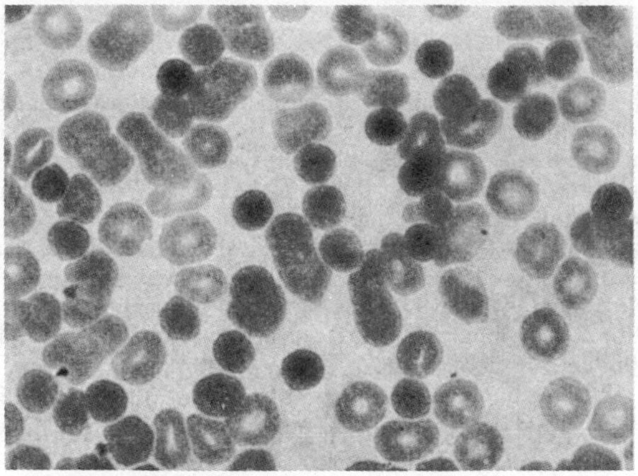

Figure 1. Peripheral blood smear (×715) of a patient with frank hemolysis secondary to clostridial septicemia. Numerous microspherocytes are present. (From Bennett, J. M., and Healey, P. J. M.: N Engl J Med 268:1070, 1963.)

timely cultures and a high index of suspicion are required for early diagnosis.

A Gram-stained smear of peripheral blood or buffy coat may demonstrate clostridia in cases with very heavy bacteremia, as can be seen when there is overt hemolysis and severely impaired resistance.

Gram-stained smears of cervical drainage, of wound drainage, or of aspiration from crepitant wounds should be examined promptly. In post-abortal cases the absence of plump gram-positive rods militates against clostridial infection: their presence is supportive but may represent only vaginal carriage of *C. perfringens* or of a nonpathogenic species. A constellation of findings on Gram stains of cervical swabs that is highly associated with clostridial sepsis was described by Butler (1942): many plump gram-positive rods with a heavy capsule (by Muir stain) associated with no more than a few ragged polymorphonuclear leukocytes (PMNs). The presence of many PMNs, active phagocytosis, or the absence of capsule augured against clostridial sepsis. If the gram-positive rods contain spores, they are not *C. perfringens*, which forms no spores in human tissues. They may represent *C. septicum* or *C. novyi*, but statistically they are more likely to represent one of the numerous nonpathogenic species.

Wright-stained blood films may show a distinctive pattern of microspherocytosis—small dense erythrocytes that have been injured by alpha toxin and are soon to lyse (Fig. 1) (Hadley and Ekroth, 1954; Bennett and Healey, 1964). Several cases have been first diagnosed when this striking abnormality was recognized in the clinical laboratory (Willis, 1969). Serial observation of serum samples for evidence of hemolysis and of urine samples for hemoglobinuria, and serial examination for new physical findings may help establish the diagnosis early. If overt hemolysis develops during observation, the diagnosis is established.

An abdominal x-ray may detect gas in the uterus, uterine wall, or free in the pelvis (Fig. 2), or gas may be found in the gallbladder or biliary tree (Fig. 3).

Cultural techniques for isolating and identifying clostridia are described in Chapter 49. Positive blood cultures will be the only evidence for clostridial bacteremia and sepsis in many cases.

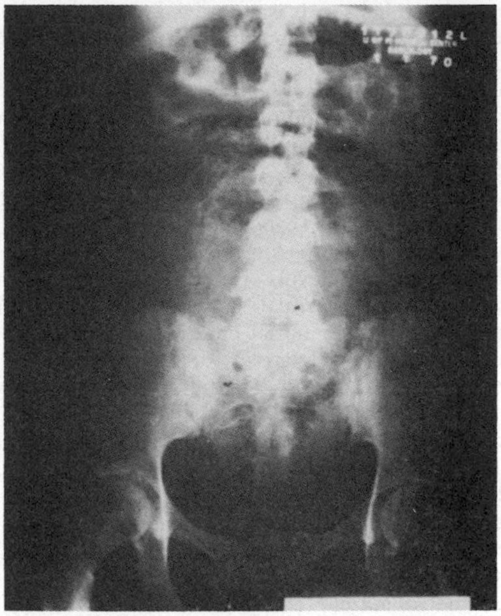

Figure 2. Clostridial infection of the uterus. Gas bubbles can be seen in the myometrium. (From Eaton, C. J., and Peterson, E. P.: Am J Obstet Gynecol 109:1162, 1971.)

TREATMENT. Clostridial septicemia carries a very poor prognosis, with a mortality of 25 to 75 per cent despite treatment. The results reflect patient delay in seeking help (especially among postabortal cases), delays in diagnosis in the more unusual cases, and the serious underlying disease that may have caused the bacteremia.

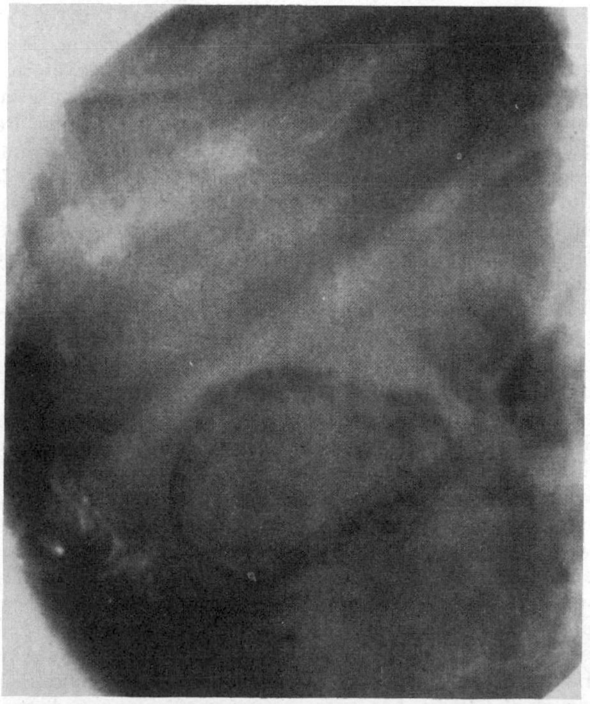

Figure 3. Emphysematous cholecystitis. (Courtesy of Alfred Berne, M.D.)

Once clostridial sepsis is suspected or proved, the treatment of choice is 3 million units penicillin G every three hours intravenously (I.V.). If the patient is allergic to penicillin, parenteral cephalosporins (cefazolin 1 g every six hours I.V.), cephalothin, cephapirin, or cefamandole 2 g every 4 hours I.V.), clindamycin (600 mg every six hours I.V.), chloramphenicol (1 g every six hours I.V.), or vancomycin (0.5 g every six hours I.V.) are effective alternatives. Aminoglycosides and polymyxins are ineffective. Tetracycline resistance is too prevalent to rely on this drug, and blood and tissue levels of erythromycin are inadequate for treatment of clostridial sepsis. Antibiotics should be begun promptly after initial cultures have been obtained in suspected cases.

Since coliforms and other enterics are even more common causes of sepsis of uterine, biliary, or intestinal origin than are clostridia, and since mixed infections can occur, an aminoglycoside, in full I.V. doses, should be added pending results of the initial cultures and adjusted for renal function. If the clinical situation suggests that *Bacteroides* may be involved, then intravenous clindamycin 600 mg every six hours, chloramphenicol succinate 1 g every six hours, metronidazole 500 mg I.V. every six hours or cefoxitin 2 g I.V. every 4 hours should be part of the initial therapy.

Antitoxin should be used to prevent further hemolysis and tissue injury by circulating alpha toxin. Because equine antitoxin can induce serum sickness, it should be used in the absence of hemolysis only when the diagnosis of postabortal clostridial sepsis is strongly suggested. It is most effective if given before gross hemolysis has occurred. A recommended dose is 40,000 units (four vials) of monospecific anti-*C. perfringens* alpha toxin initially followed by 20,000 to 40,000 units every six hours until hemolysis is controlled. It can be given intramuscularly or by I.V. drip; the latter may be more effective in acute hemolysis, the former may be safer. Local instillation into the uterus has been advocated but not carefully studied.

When clostridial sepsis follows septic abortion, it is generally necessary to empty or to remove the uterus. There is considerable controversy about the proper surgical approach in different stages of this disease. If clostridia are demonstrated in Gram stains of cervical smears, the first decision is whether there is evidence of bacteremia. If there is no hemolysis and only moderate fever and illness, fluids and antibiotics are administered, and any retained fetal and placental tissues are removed by aspiration or by curettage. If the patient is seriously ill or if there is hemolysis, antitoxin, antibiotics, and fluids are administered and a surgical approach is chosen and carried out. If gas is found in the wall of the uterus or free in the pelvis by x-ray or sonogram, and if there is uterine or adnexal tenderness, a total abdominal hysterectomy is indicated. The decision to remove tubes and ovaries is best made after direct observation during surgery. The most controversial situation arises from the uncertainty of whether the infection has penetrated into the myometrium in a woman who is clearly ill and has hemolysis. Some would opt for curettage if such patients want to remain fertile; others would choose early hysterectomy for all patients. The best plan for these cases is uncertain but involves important personal choices for the woman as well as the physician. Hyperbaric oxygen, which is recommended by some (Perrin et al., 1970), has only limited use in serious disease and is fraught with complications (Smith et al., 1971). It does not appear to be an important alternative.

If oliguria ensues, an effective means of dealing with the problems of hyperkalemia, fluid balance, and azotemia is required. If massive hemolysis and shock occur early in the illness, a protracted period of renal shutdown can be anticipated, and if facilities are available for hemodialysis, an AV shunt should be placed. Such a shunt allows, in addition, a convenient route for exchange transfusions, which have been recommended by some early in the course to remove toxic products of hemolysis and residual circulating toxins. This therapy may be lifesaving in cases of disseminated intravascular coagulation and may reduce the extent of hemoglobinuric renal injury (Rubenberg et al., 1967; Strum et al., 1968).

Hypotension carries a very grave prognosis in this disease. It is best treated as other cases of septic shock (Chapter 92) by prompt correction of hypovolemia, anemia, lactic acidemia and hypoxia, by early surgical intervention to remove or drain the source of sepsis, and by appropriate antibiotic and, if indicated, antitoxin administration. Rapid and precise hemodynamic and biochemical monitoring to guide proper fluid, blood, bicarbonate, and electrolyte replacement, as well as the need for and use of pressor drugs and ventilatory support, can be lifesaving at this stage.

PROPHYLAXIS. Clostridial sepsis is a rare disease, and specific indications for immunoprophylaxis are few. There is no effective toxoid or vaccine for active immunization in humans.

Chemoprophylaxis with parenteral penicillin does appear warranted during and after cholecystectomy or common duct exploration in elderly patients and when acute pathologic changes or intramural or intraluminal gas are encountered at surgery. Intraoperative Gram stains of bile have been urged as a guide to the choice of prophylactic antibiotics (Keighley et al., 1977).

An important general preventive measure is the removal of the need for women to seek illegal and unsterile abortions by providing birth control education and assistance and safe surgical facilities for those who require abortions. Upgrading sanitary facilities generally will reduce puerperal and post-traumatic clostridial infections.

References

Alpern, R. J., and Dowell, V. R., Jr.: Clostridium septicum infections and malignancy. JAMA 209:385, 1969.

Alpern, R. J., and Dowell, V. R., Jr.: Non-histotoxic clostridial bacteremia. Am J Clin Pathol 55:717, 1971.

Bennett, J. M., and Healey, P. J. M.: Spherocytic hemolytic anemia and acute cholecystitis caused by *Clostridium welchii*. N Engl J Med 268:1070, 1963.

Boggs, D. R., Frei, E., and Thomas, L. B.: Clostridial gas gangrene and septicemia in patients with leukemia. N Engl J Med 295:1255, 1958.

Bornstein, D. L., Weinberg, A. N., Swartz, M. N., and Kunz, L. J.: Anaerobic infections: Review of current experience. Medicine 43:207, 1964.

Brooks, G. F.: Early diagnosis of bacteremia by examination of buffy coat. Arch Intern Med 132:673, 1973.

Butler, H. M.: The examination of cervical smears as a means of rapid diagnosis in severe *C. welchii* infection following abortion. J Pathol Bacteriol 54:39, 1942.

Cabrera, A., Tsukada, Y., and Pickren, J. W.: Clostridial gas gangrene and septicemia in malignant disease. Cancer 18:800, 1965.

Fredette, V.: Effect of hyperbaric oxygen on anaerobic bacteria and toxins. Ann NY Acad Sci 117:700, 1965.

Fukunaga, F. H.: Gallbladder bacteriology, histology, and gallstones. Arch Surg 106:169, 1973.

Gorbach, S. L., and Thadepalli, H.: Isolation of *Clostridium* in human infections: Evaluation of 114 cases. J Infect Dis Suppl 13:S81, 1975.

Hadley, G. G., and Ekroth, R. D.: Spherocytosis as a manifestation of postabortal *C. welchii* infection. Am J Obstet Gynecol 67:691, 1954.
Keighley, M. R. B., McLeish, A. R., Bishop, H. M., et al: Identification of the presence and type of biliary microflora by immediate gram stains. Surgery 81:469, 1977.
Koransky, J. R., Stargel, M. D., and Dowell, V. R. Jr.: Clostridium septicum Bacteremia. Its clinical significance. Am J Med 66:63, 1979.
MacLennan, J. D.: The histotoxic clostridial infections of man. Bacteriol Rev 26:177, 1962.
Mahn, E., and Dantuono, L. M.: Postabortal septicotoxemia due to *Clostridium welchii*. Am J Obstet Gynecol 70:604, 1955.
Martin, W. J.: Isolation and identification of anaerobic bacteria in the clinical laboratory. Mayo Clin Proc 49:300, 1974.
Oakley, C. L.: Gas gangrene. Br Med Bull 10:52, 1954.
Perrin, L. E., Ostergard, D. R., and Mishell, D. R.: The use of hyperbaric oxygen in the treatment of clostridial septicemia complicating septic abortion. Am J Obstet Gynecol 106:666, 1970.
Pietrafitta, J. J., and Deckers, P. J.: Significance of clostridial bacteremia. Am J Surg 143:519, 1982.
Ramsay, A. M.: The significance of *Clostridium welchii* in the cervical swab and blood stains in postpartum and postabortion sepsis. J Obstet Gynecol Br Commonw 56:247, 1949.
Rathbun, H. K.: Clostridial bacteremia without hemolysis. Arch Intern Med 122:496, 1968.
Rubenberg, M. L., Baker, L. R. I., McBride, J. A., Sevitt, L. H., and Brain, M. C.: Intravascular coagulation in a case of *Clostridium perfringens* septicemia: Treatment by exchange transfusion. Br Med J 4:271, 1967.
Smith, J. W., Southern, P. M., Jr., and Lehmann, J. D.: Bacteremia in septic abortion: Complications and treatment. Obstet Gynecol 35:704, 1970.
Smith, L. P., McLean, A. P., and Maughan, G. B.: *Clostridium welchii* septicotoxemia. A review and report of three cases. Am J Obstet Gynecol 110:135, 1971.
Strum, W. B., Cade, J. R., Shires, D. L., and deQuesada, A.: Postabortal septicemia due to *C. welchii*. Treatment with exchange transfusion. Arch Intern Med 122:73, 1968.
Welch, W. H., and Nuttall, G. H. F.: A gas-producing bacillus *(Bacillus aerogenes capsulatus)* capable of rapid development in the blood vessels after death. Bull Johns Hopkins Hosp 3:81, 1892.
Willis, A. T.: Clostridia of wound infection. London, Butterworths, 1969.
Wynne, J. W., and Armstrong, D.: Clostridial septicemia. Cancer 29:215, 1972.

197
BRUCELLOSIS

WESLEY W. SPINK, M.D.

DEFINITION. Brucellosis is an infectious disease caused by bacteria in the genus *Brucella*. The disease is transmitted to humans, directly or indirectly, from the natural animal reservoirs of sheep, goats, cattle, swine, and reindeer. Acute brucellosis can simulate many other infections. Chronic brucellosis with fever, weakness, and complaints of vague origin usually has demonstrable localizing manifestations. It is unusual for chronic disease to follow acute brucellosis if properly treated.

Brucellosis has probably existed for centuries in the Mediterranean areas, causing an illness known as Mediterranean fever, Malta fever, Gibraltar fever, Neapolitan fever, Cyprus fever, and undulant fever. David Bruce first isolated brucellae from patients in Malta in 1887. Hughes described the human disease definitively in 1897. Thereafter reservoirs of the disease were traced to domestic animals (Spink, 1956).

ETIOLOGY. Three classic species of *Brucella* cause human disease, originating from their own animal reservoirs: *Brucella melitensis* from sheep and goats, *Brucella abortus* from cattle, and *Brucella suis* from swine. Because of certain biochemical or metabolic differences, each of the species is divided into subtypes. *Br. melitensis* has three, *Br. abortus* nine, and *Br. suis* three. *Br. suis*, Subtype II, called *Brucella rangiferi tarandi*, is found in the reindeer of Alaska and Siberia and is a cause of human illness. The species *Br. canis* causes epidemic disease in dogs but has caused only a few human cases. Recognition of the species causing human illness is important epidemiologically in the control of animal reservoirs of the disease. *Br. abortus*, Strain 19, a live vaccine widely used for immunizing cattle, has caused human illness through accidental self-inoculation by veterinarians. There is no evidence that Strain 19 is transmitted from vaccinated animals to humans, either directly or indirectly.

GEOGRAPHICAL DISTRIBUTION. The species of *Brucella* causing illness depends upon the species present in the natural reservoir of animals. Brucellosis afflicts dairy cattle in most parts of the world (Stableforth, 1959). In the United States for many years the predominant cause has been *Br. abortus*, because cattle, especially dairy herds, harbor the organisms. Range cattle in the United States and elsewhere in the world are uncommon reservoirs of brucellosis. Foci of infections due to *Br. suis* appear in workers in abattoirs where infected swine are slaughtered. *Br. melitensis* in sheep and goats is a minor problem in the United States, occurring in the southwestern part of the country. Most cases of brucellosis in the United States involve men between the ages of 20 and 50 years, principally abattoir employees, farmers, and veterinarians. Children rarely have the disease because milk is pasteurized.

In many areas, *Br. melitensis* is the predominant cause of disease because sheep and goats are infected. These areas include Mexico, Central and South America, France and southeastern Europe, countries bordering on the Mediterranean, and parts of Africa, southern Russia, Iran, and India.

Human cases originating from infected swine occur in the United States, Germany, Austria, Bulgaria, and Russia. *Br. suis* Type 4 (*rangiferi tarandus*) parasitizes reindeer in Siberia and Alaska, where it is a common, and the only, cause of human brucellosis. *Br. suis* Type 2, found in the hare and swine of Denmark and southeastern Europe, is not a cause of human disease.

There are other, less commonly distributed animal reservoirs of brucellosis that cause human disease, such as camels (*Br. melitensis*), yaks in Mongolia (*Br. abortus*), bison, elk, and moose (*Br. abortus*).

For a worldwide comprehensive review of the incidence of brucellosis up to 1980 in humans and in animals consult the WHO Guide (Elberg, 1981).

PATHOGENESIS AND PATHOLOGY. The portals of entry for *Brucella* are minute abrasions of the skin, oropharynx, and conjunctivae. Entering the blood stream, the organisms localize preferentially in tissues having an abundance of reticuloendothelial cells such as lymph nodes, liver, spleen, and bone marrow, although the kidneys, central and peripheral nervous systems, testes, and bone are also involved (Spink, 1956). The circulating polymorphonuclear leukocytes are the first line of defense against *Brucella*, but the macrophages in the blood and tissues are the major cells that ingest and destroy the bacteria. The tissue reaction in brucellosis is primarily granulomatous. It consists of epithelioid cells, giant cells, and an infiltrate of lymphocytes and plasma cells. The lesions simulate those of sarcoidosis. Almost simultaneously with the formation of granulomas, *Brucella* disappears from the tissues.

Occasionally, however, the focal lesion becomes necrotic, and caseation appears similar to that of tuberculosis. This occurs particularly with the suppurating lesions caused by *Br. suis*, but also occasionally with *Br. melitensis* or *Br. abortus*.

Toward the second week after invasion by *Brucella*, the tissues develop hypersensitivity to *Brucella* antigens, and circulating antibodies appear. The *Brucella* hypersensitivity very likely contributes to the systemic reaction of the patient, much like the patient with tuberculosis and his reaction to tuberculin.

CLINICAL MANIFESTATIONS. The incubation period of the disease is from one to three weeks. Brucellosis is usually an acute febrile disease with chills, sweats, headache, aches and pains, and weakness like that occurring in influenza. There are usually few or no localizing findings except lymphadenopathy and a palpable spleen and liver. With rest and supportive treatment, most patients recover within three to six months, and even earlier with tetracycline therapy. Although much has been written about a condition known as "chronic brucellosis" in which symptoms endure for years, the number of proved cases having a continued illness after 12 months is relatively small. This is particularly true of patients who have received adequate therapy. Relapses are uncommon in treated patients. Treated individuals who have illness after one year usually have a demonstrable suppurative localization, especially of the bone or joints.

COMPLICATIONS. The most common complication involves the bones and joints. Spondylitis involving an intervertebral area of the lumbar spine, which can be associated with a sciatic distribution of severe pain, is the most frequent manifestation. The larger joints, such as the hip joint, may have localized suppuration. Brucellosis does not cause chronic polyarthritis of the smaller joints.

During the acute phase, peripheral neuritis may occur and gradually subside. Meningitis is an uncommon complication. Localization in the kidneys causes chronic pyuria, as in tuberculosis. Orchitis, usually unilateral, mimics mumps, but sterility does not follow. Suppurative endocarditis is a rare complication, and pulmonary lesions rarely occur. Brucellosis does not cause human abortions any more frequently than other bacterial infections.

Brucellosis, like typhoid fever, does cause mental depression, especially if convalesence is prolonged. This can result in a state of chronic neurasthenia after recovery from the disease. Patients must be reassured that lingering fatigue and weakness do not imply that they have chronic brucellosis, a diagnosis that must be applied cautiously. Unless severe inflammatory complications have occurred, brucellosis does not result in sequelae.

DIAGNOSIS. Brucellosis simulates many other febrile diseases such as infectious mononucleosis, typhoid fever, malaria, and influenza. Because the infection is an occupational disease, knowledge of exposure to potentially infected animals is a distinct aid in differential diagnosis. Likewise, the ingestion of unpasteurized milk or *fresh* milk products, such as cheese, from a questionable source is helpful. Enlarged peripheral lymph nodes and a palpable spleen are consistent with the disease.

A definitive diagnosis is dependent upon laboratory data (Alton et al., 1975). A characteristic finding in the peripheral blood is an increase in lymphocytes, which have at times a morphology like that in infectious mononucleosis. The total leukocyte count may be normal, elevated, or reduced. The erythrocyte sedimentation rate is of no aid, since it may be accelerated or normal.

The most reliable procedure for screening suspected cases of brucellosis is the tube-dilution saline agglutination test in which a reliable Brucella antigen is used. The test has minor limitations as far as specificity is concerned. Cross-agglutination occurs with *Vibrio cholera, Francisella tularensis*, and *Yersinia enterocolitica* when the test is done with the sera of patients who have had these diseases or received vaccines containing these organisms. The antigen-serum mixtures should be incubated for 48 hours at 37° C and then examined. Titers of 1:100 and above are significant, although individuals who have had the disease months and years previously may have titers of 1:100 and below, and occasionally higher. "Blocking antibodies" may interfere with a clear-cut reading in the lower dilutions, where little or no agglutination may occur, and prevent complete agglutinations in the higher dilutions. When such blocking is present, centrifuging the mixtures at 3000 rpm may reveal further clumping. The presence of blocking antibody can also be detected by incubating the suspect serum with a known serum of high antibody content. Dilutions of the serum mixture are then incubated with antigen, and if blocking is present, the titer will be lower than that in the untreated serum.

Although agglutinins are rarely absent in patients with active disease, especially in those with blood cultures that reveal *Brucella* organisms, the interpretation of agglutinin titers of 1:100 or less is often difficult when the cultures remain sterile. The *Brucella* agglutinin in active disease is IgG antibody, whereas in those who have recovered from the disease it is IgM. The type of antibody present in the serum may be differentiated by adding 2-mercaptoethanol to the antigen-antibody mixtures. Under these circumstances, IgM is degraded, and no agglutination occurs.

The complement fixation, Coombs' antiglobulin, and fluorescent antibody tests add nothing to the ordinary agglutination test in routine clinical diagnosis.

Blood cultures should be made for every suspected case of brucellosis before therapy is attempted. We prefer two cultures, each performed one day apart. In the Castaneda technique, blood is introduced into rectangular bottles of 120 ml capacity. Trypticase soy broth or tryptose broth is the culture medium, and agar composed of the same basic medium is layered along a flat side of the bottle. Ten per cent of the air is displaced with carbon dioxide. After the blood is mixed with the broth, the mixture is spread over the agar, and then the bottle is placed in the incubator at 37° C. The agar layer is examined daily for at least 21 days for evidence of bacterial colonies, which usually appear within a week. Cerebrospinal fluid, urine, and tissues minced with sterile saline solution can be cultured in the same manner.

The *Brucella* skin test is specific for the disease, and,

like the tuberculin reaction, a positive test indicates past or recent exposure to the disease. Because skin reactivity may endure for years after recovery from disease, it is of little value in diagnosis. Skin testing is useful in epidemiologic studies for determining the degree of exposure to brucellosis in a population.

TREATMENT. The physician should convey the diagnosis of brucellosis to the patient only if definitive diagnostic laboratory data support this conclusion, since popular and medical literature portray a disease leading to a life of chronic and disabling illness. Furthermore, the physician should reassure the patient that health will be restored after proper antibiotic therapy.

During the acute phase of the illness, rest is paramount. Supportive treatment should include sedation and analgesics, such as salicylates. Tetracycline should be administered orally with an initial dose of 1.0 g, followed by a second dose in four hours, and then 0.5 g four times daily for 21 days. In severe cases, 1.0 g of streptomycin daily can be given simultaneously intramuscularly for ten days. Occasional relapses may occur within one to three months for which a similar course of tetracycline should be given, with or without streptomycin. There is no advantage in giving repeated courses of therapy to any patient, particularly in those with *presumed* chronic brucellosis.

Patients with severe brucellosis accompanied by fever, marked toxicity, and anorexia can obtain marked relief from an adrenal steroid such as prednisone in an oral dose of 20 mg two to three times a day for up to five days.

Brucella vaccines are not recommended for "desensitization" of patients with chronic disease.

Patients who recover from brucellosis become immune to the disease. Reinfection can result in a milder febrile illness, that responds readily to tetracycline for a week or ten days, according to the foregoing schedule.

PROPHYLAXIS. The control of human brucellosis depends upon the eradication of brucellosis in animal reservoirs. Although prophylatic vaccines for humans have been proposed in certain areas in the world, there is no general acceptance of such procedures.

References

Alton, G. G., Jones, L. M., and Pietz, D. E.: Laboratory Techniques in Brucellosis. 2nd ed. Geneva, World Health Organization, 1975.

Elberg, S. S. (ed.): A guide to Diagnosis, Treatment, and Prevention of Human Brucellosis, Document VPH/81.31, 1983.

Spink, W. W.: The Nature of Brucellosis. Minneapolis, University of Minnesota Press, 1956.

Stableforth, A. W.: Brucellosis. *In* Stableforth, A. W., and Galloway, I. A. (eds): Infectious Diseases of Animals. Vol. I. Diseases Due to Bacteria. New York, Academic Press, 1959, Chapter 3.

198

BARTONELLOSIS

M. Cuadra, M.D.

Bartonellosis is a human infection caused by *Bartonella bacilliformis*, a bacterium that has an affinity for vascular endothelial and red blood cells. Transmitted by certain species of *Phlebotomus*, it is confined to certain Andean valleys in Peru, Ecuador, and Colombia. The disease occurs in two stages: the first, named Oroya fever or Carrión's disease, is characterized by an acute febrile hemolytic anemia; the second stage, verruga peruana, is characterized by the appearance of hemangioma-like nodules on the skin.

ETIOLOGY. After a short period of confusion (Strong et al., 1913), it has been firmly established that both Oroya fever and verruga peruana are caused by the same organism, *B. bacilliformis* (Noguchi, 1927a, b; Pinkerton and Weinman, 1937–38; Strong, 1945), and that the conditions represent two stages of the same disease. The experiment of Carrión, who was voluntarily inoculated with the exudate from a verruga nodule and succumbed to Oroya fever, represents one of the most solid supports for the etiologic unity of both entities. The taxonomic position of *B. bacilliformis* (Moulder, 1974) is still unsettled.

PATHOGENESIS AND PATHOLOGY. In the stage of Oroya fever or Carrión's disease only two types of host cells are parasitized—vascular endothelial cells and red blood cells. In the stage of verruga peruana the organisms are found only in the verruga nodules; no *Bartonella* organisms can be seen in erythrocytes, although blood cultures frequently are positive. In the "verrucoma," abundant organisms are found within the cytoplasm of endothelial cells lining the vessels (angioblasts) in both human nodules (Mayer et al., 1913; Mackehenie and Weiss, 1926; Weiss, 1932; Weinman and Pinkerton, 1937; Alzamora Castro, 1945; Urteaga and Calderón, 1965) and in nodules experimentally induced in monkeys (Mayer et al., 1913; Noguchi, 1926a,b; Noguchi and Battistini, 1926; Mackehenie and Weiss, 1926; Marquez de Cunha and Muniz, 1928; Kikuth, 1931; Weinman and Pinkerton, 1937). By electron microscopy, both intracellular (Takano, 1970) and extracellular organisms (Recavarren and Lumbreras, 1972) have been found. This discrepancy remains to be clarified. These findings are consistent with the ability of *Bartonella* to grow intra- and extracellularly in tissue cultures (Pinkerton and Weinman, 1937).

Oroya Fever Stage. Neither the cycle of *B. bacilliformis* within the *Phlebotomus* nor the mechanism of penetration of the agent into or through the skin is known. Scratching of the *Phlebotomus* bite may favor penetration. From the skin (first station) the *Bartonella* organisms travel to the regional lymph nodes (second station). From there the infection enters the bloodstream and then the vascular endothelium (third station). Endothelial cells fully loaded with microorganisms have, in fact, been found by a number of authors (Strong and Tyzzer, 1915; Aldana, 1929; Pinkerton and Weinman, 1937–38; Alzamora Castro, 1940; Urteaga, 1948). The presence of *Bartonella* organisms in the blood causes symptoms (fever) if the organisms exceed a certain concentration. The time elapsing from the first station (skin) to the third one (blood) is approximately three weeks. This is the *incubation period*.

After infecting the endothelial cells, the parasites can

involve nearly all the red blood cells of the host. It appears that when infected endothelial cells burst (Aldana, 1929, 1947), the released organisms enter the blood directly and penetrate the red blood cells. The propensity of *Bartonella* to attach to red blood cells has, in fact, been demonstrated in vitro (Cuadra, 1978). The possibility of transmission of *Bartonella* organisms from erythrocyte to erythrocyte appears to be unlikely (although intracellular organisms are viable since multiplication can be observed under the microscope in broth cultures of blood from patients with Oroya fever) because the organisms are intracellular (Cuadra and Takano, 1969) and no rupture of parasitized erythrocytes occurs within the bloodstream.

B. bacilliformis appears in the erythrocytes of Oroya fever patients in two discrete forms: as rods (so-called bacillary forms) and as coccoid forms. The pathogenic significance of the two forms has been deduced from correlating them with the course of the fever (Cuadra, 1957). Bacillary *Bartonella* is an active or vegetative form, since its presence is always associated with fever, while the coccoid *Bartonella* is an inactive (stationary) form incapable of generating fever. In typical cases of Oroya fever, within the first or second day of the disease the patient has high fever and only a very low number of rods in the peripheral blood. During subsequent days, the fever continues while the bacillary forms increase geometrically in number until they parasitize nearly 100 per cent of red blood cells by the end of the first week. At this time the coccoid forms begin to appear in increasing numbers. By about the end of the second week, rods and coccoid forms reach approximately equal numbers. During the resolution of the fever by lysis (about the third week), coccoid forms increasingly predominate in number over the rods. Finally, during convalescence, rods have disappeared and the patient is afebrile, but coccoid forms parasitize nearly 100 per cent of red blood cells (see Fig. 1, Chapter 55). If the patient relapses in the convalescent period, fever reappears and bacillary forms are again found in the erythrocytes (Cuadra, 1957). The coccoid forms seem to originate from the rods by multisegmentation; rosary-like (intermediate) forms are seen frequently. A similar transformation occurs in vitro on blood agar cultures.

The anemia caused by *B. bacilliformis* is hemolytic in nature inasmuch as the lifespan of parasitized erythrocytes is notably shortened (Reynafarge and Ramos, 1961). The serum indirect bilirubin (Guzman Barrón, 1926; Hurtado et al., 1938), urobilin, and stercobilin concentrations (Urteaga, 1948), and iron stores in the spleen, liver, and lymph glands are notably increased (Strong and Tyzzer, 1915; Weiss, 1933; Urteaga, 1948). In addition, erythromyeloid hyperplasia of the bone marrow occurs (Carvallo, 1911; Hurtado et al., 1938; Urteaga, 1948), and reticulocytes in the peripheral blood are increased. *Bartonella* does not directly destroy the erythrocyte it parasitizes because intravascular hemolysis, which characteristically occurs in hemobartonellosis, never occurs in Oroya fever despite the high rate of parasitism and the significantly increased mechanical fragility of the parasitized erythrocytes (Reynafarge and Ramos, 1961). Red blood cell ghosts were found in smears of peripheral blood from Oroya fever patients and rat hemobartonellosis, slightly increased in the former and strongly in the latter (Cuadra, 1957). Neither hemagglutinins nor hemolysins are present in serum (Guzman Barrón, 1926), and the Coombs' test is negative (Reynafarge and Ramos, 1961). The finding in histologic sections of spleen, liver, and lymph nodes of large quantities of macrophages overloaded with erythrocytes (Strong, 1915; Aldana, 1929; Weiss, 1932; Urteaga, 1948) is evidence that the anemia occurs as a consequence of erythrophagocytosis (Aldana, 1929). The fact that the severity of the anemia is proportional to the degree of erythrocytic parasitism (Gonzalez Oechea, 1932; Cuadra, 1970) indicates that only parasitized erythrocytes are phagocytized. Such selective phagocytosis implies that the macrophages can recognize parasitized erythrocytes. Since *Bartonella* is an intracellular organism, it is not understood how this recognition occurs. It is suggested that *Bartonella* organisms release some antigen that coats the erythrocyte and renders it subject to antibody-mediated phagocytosis. The rapidity with which the anemia occurs (there is a decrease of approximately 200 to 400 thousand circulating red cells per mm^3 per day) is also consistent with antibody-mediated phagocytosis in which the estranged erythrocytes are removed. The anemia tends to be normocytic and normochromic during the stage of red blood cell destruction.

Hypersplenism exists in Oroya fever and may contribute to the anemia. It is evidenced by the hematologic changes that occur during the febrile period compared with those of the convalescent period. During the febrile period, in which bacillary forms of *Bartonella* are present, relative leukopenia and thrombocytopenia, and at times thrombocytopenic purpura (Ricketts, 1942) occur. When fever disappears and the convalescent period, in which only coccoid forms of *Bartonella* are present, commences, leukocytosis (at times a leukemoid reaction) and thrombocytosis occur. Large lymphocytes (40 to 60 per cent) with wide ameboid and basophilic cytoplasm are usually found. Reticulocytes also increase abruptly (10 to 30 per cent or more), and there is anisocytosis and polychromatophilia. The anemia in this stage of hematologic regeneration tends to be macrocytic and hypochromic.

In pure cases of Oroya fever there is an extraordinary hyperplasia of the reticuloendothelial system in the spleen, the lymph nodes, the liver, and the bone marrow. The hyperplasia serves to increase the removal of parasitized erythrocytes and to consolidate the immunity against *Bartonella*. Zonal necrosis of the liver around the central veins of the lobules has been reported to occur in Oroya fever (Strong, 1915). Since this has been reproduced in monkeys in which neither severe anemia nor salmonellosis occurred (Noguchi, 1927a,b,c), and since *Bartonella* does not invade the hepatocytes, the necrosis is probably caused by a *Bartonella* toxin circulating in the blood. However, there is no significant increase of serum transaminase in typical Oroya fever. Anoxemia and secondary *Salmonella* septicemia kill patients without producing gross pathologic lesions.

Verruga Peruana Stage. Histologically, the verruga nodule is a dense network of blood vessels lying in a matrix or interstitium of edematous connective tissue within which lymphatic vessels, angioblasts, histiocytes, and leukocytes are associated with fibroblasts (Rocha Lima, 1913; Mackehenie, 1938; Hercelles, 1935). The relative amount of these components varies with the age and developmental stages of the nodules. Thus, according to Mackehenie (1938), early nodules are rich in histiocytes, mature ones in blood vessels and angioblasts, and old nodules in fibroblasts. The angioblasts derive from the endothelium of the vessels. They proliferate outward, forming buds of variable size

(Rocha Lima, 1913). The new capillaries probably develop from the buds as a result of canalization of a lumen into which blood then flows (McCutcheon, 1948). According to the type of predominant tissue or cells, the verruga nodule may resemble a hemangioma or a fibrosarcoma. Most nodules show few leukocytes; occasionally lymphocytes or granulocytes may be present in appreciable numbers. In this latter case a secondary infection should be considered. In hematoxylin–eosin-stained sections of nodules the organisms are not visible. Sections should be fixed in Regaud's solution and stained with Giemsa's stain to demonstrate organisms (Noguchi, 1927a; Pinkerton and Weinman, 1937–38). *B. bacilliformis* is doubtless present within the verruga tissue, but its precise localization, whether intracellular (Takano, 1970) or extracellular (Recavarren and Lumbreras, 1972), and the cells involved are unknown. When the nodules are full-grown, outgrowths of fibroblasts are obtained (Cuadra, 1966). The identity of the inclusion-like bodies found within cells, which presumably are densely packed *Bartonella* organisms, must be elucidated by electronmicroscopy.

CLINICAL MANIFESTATIONS

Oroya Fever or Carrión's Disease. The cardinal manifestations of Oroya fever (Carrión's disease) are fever, anemia, and enlargement of the spleen, lymph nodes, and liver. Fever represents the best indicator of disease activity and in most cases lasts as long as two to three weeks. It is irregular or remittent in type and considerable sweating occurs with it. Its onset may occur suddenly or be preceded by prodromal symptoms and it terminates usually by lysis. No chronic Oroya fever has been reported. The temperature reaches 39 to 40° C and is accompanied by intense toxemic manifestations (headache, malaise, pains in the bones and large joints). Anemia develops so rapidly that in a week an intense pallor of the skin and mucous membranes of the mouth and conjunctivae occurs. The pallor is accompanied by slight jaundice. The resulting anoxemia may be reflected in clouding of consciousness, apathy, rapid pulse, and a great tendency to circulatory collapse. The enlargement of the lymph nodes (cervical, axillary, epitrochlear, inguinal) is painless and less than that in infectious mononucleosis. The spleen is less enlarged than in typhoid fever or brucellosis. The enlargement of the liver is moderate and is more marked in young people than in adults. After the fever stops, patients feel well in spite of the profound anemia, and complete recovery occurs in three to four weeks. In some patients slight edema of the face and feet and effusion in serous cavities may occur during the first week of convalescence. This is probably due to protein deficiency (Merino, 1939). In severe forms of Oroya fever death is caused by both toxemia and anemia or by any intercurrent infection, of which salmonellosis is the most common (Cuadra, 1956).

In addition to the pattern of Oroya fever described above, in which there is a high rate of parasitism, there are cases with a very low parasitism rate throughout the course of the disease (paucibacillary form of Oroya fever) (Figs. 1

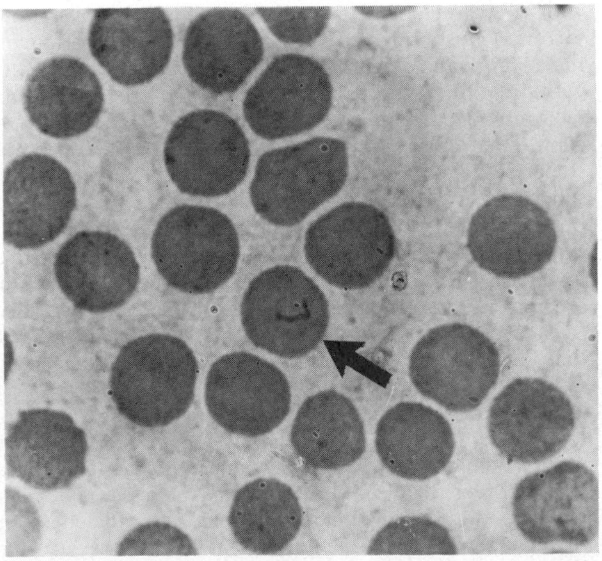

Figure 1. Blood film of a patient suffering from a paucibacillary form of Oroya fever. A very low parasitism rate, illustrated by the photograph in which only one red blood cell (arrow) appears parasitized by a bacillary *Bartonella*, was observed throughout the course (27 days) of the disease. No antibiotics were used and the verruga peruana stage occurred 55 days after spontaneous remission of the fever.

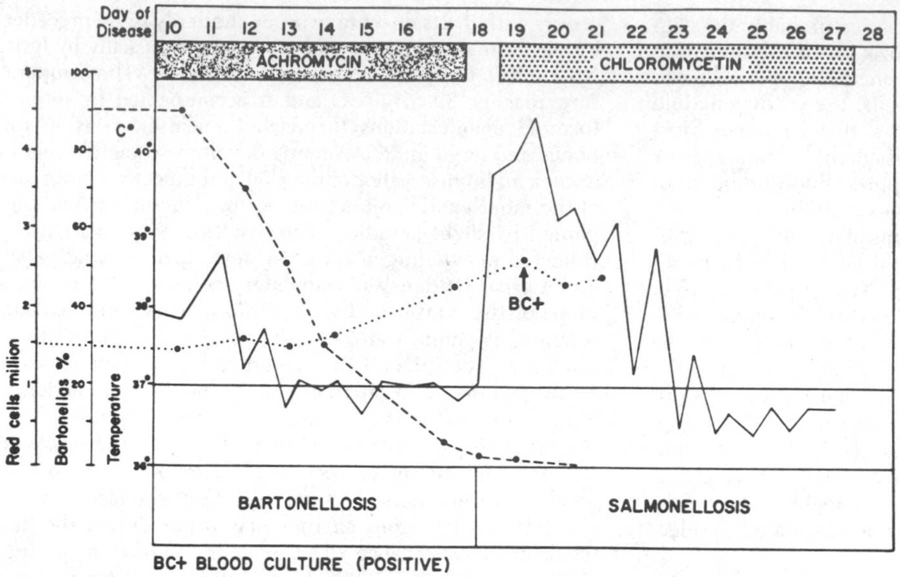

Figure 2. Salmonella bacteremia in the convalescent stage of Oroya fever *(S. typhimurium)*. Typical response to chloramphenicol occurred with recovery of patient.

and 5). In these cases there is at most a slight anemia (Gonzalez Oechea, 1932; Cuadra, 1970). The fever may last as long as the ordinary type or only one to three days. Between these extremes there is a range of intermediate forms. Milder forms of Oroya fever may go untreated and be followed later by the verruga peruana stage.

COMPLICATIONS AND SEQUELAE. Approximately 40 per cent of cases of Oroya fever are complicated by septicemia caused by *Salmonella* species (Tamayo, 1907; Ribeyro, 1932; Ricketts, 1948; Aldana, 1949; Cuadra, 1954; 1956), of which S. *typhimurium* is the most frequent (Colichón and Cuadra, 1954). This complication occurs during the course of Oroya fever, or, more frequently, in the period of convalescence (Fig. 2). High temperature with wide oscillations, sweating, rapid pulse, malaise, and extreme prostration are the main manifestations. Before the advent of chloramphenicol, 90 per cent of patients died within the first week (Cuadra, 1954; 1956). In contrast, the mortality of uncomplicated Oroya fever is as low as 5 per cent. The pathogenesis of the complication is not understood. Septicemia occurs in individuals who previously had solid immunity to *Salmonella*. The blockade of the macrophages by phagocytized red blood cells probably facilitates the invasion of the blood by salmonellae from the intestinal lumen or mesenteric lymph nodes. The fact that the secondary infection is not caused by agents other than *Salmonella* (e.g., *Staphylococcus, Streptococcus*) suggests that bartonellosis selectively suppresses anti-*Salmonella* immunity.

Verruga Peruana. One or more weeks, sometimes months, after the termination of Oroya fever, verruga peruana appear on the body as hemangiomatous nodules. The nodules may be localized in the skin (cutaneous verruga), in the subcutaneous tissue (subcutaneous verruga), in the mucous membranes (mucous verruga), or in internal organs such as muscles, bones, or viscera (Odriozola, 1898; Rebagliati, 1940). Blood capillaries, in any location, are the only structures for which *Bartonella* shows affinity, and infection of the capillaries induces the verrucoma. The most frequent localization is apparently the skin. Perhaps because of the benignity of the disease, reports of internal verruga are scarce.

The eruption is pleomorphic (Fig. 3) as it occurs in successive episodes over a period of one to three, rarely up to six, months. It is usually preceded or accompanied by fever that varies in intensity and duration. Pains in the joints of the extremities (verrucous rheumatism), especially the knees, are very frequent and can immobilize the patient. A typical cutaneous nodule is as large as a pea, bright red in color, soft in consistency and smooth and shiny (its surface does not belong to the nodule itself but is the surface of the original skin, distended and made extremely thin by the growing nodule). A nodule is fragile and bleeds easily. On the mucous membranes nodules tend to be pedunculated. The nodules vary in size from about 1 to 2 mm in diameter (Fig. 3) up to several cm (Fig. 4). Two types are recognized: the miliary and the nodular. In the miliary type the nodules, measuring 1 to 2 mm in diameter, are distributed on the face and extremities and vary from a few to innumerable. Usually there is a heavy concentration on the legs. The eruption begins as pruritic petechiae or as small conical papules with a minute vesicle or keratinous thickening at their apex (Cuadra, 1962). The new verruga nodules emerge at the petechiae or at the base of the vesicles or the keratinous thickening and appear as red dots that grow in a few days to become a miliary lesion. The nodules may behave in one of two ways: either growth stops and they remain as miliary nodules until they degenerate and crust (which occurs within a few weeks), or the growth continues and produces the nodular type of eruption. The size of the nodules may vary to a large extent from pea-sized (small nodular verruga) to giant tumors (Figs. 3 and 4). Figure 4 shows one of the largest reported in the literature (Ricketts, 1942). Between these two extremes there is a range of middle-sized nodules; however, the small and middle-sized nodules are much more frequent than the large or giant tumors. The large verruga nodules are also called "verruga mular" because of their resemblance to certain skin tumors (probably of viral etiology) that affect mules in verrucous endemic areas. The density of the nodular eruption is in general lower than that of the miliary type; the larger the nodules the lower their density. The lifespan of the nodular type is much longer (up to six months (Odriozola, 1898) than that of the miliary type (weeks). Miliary and nodular verruga can

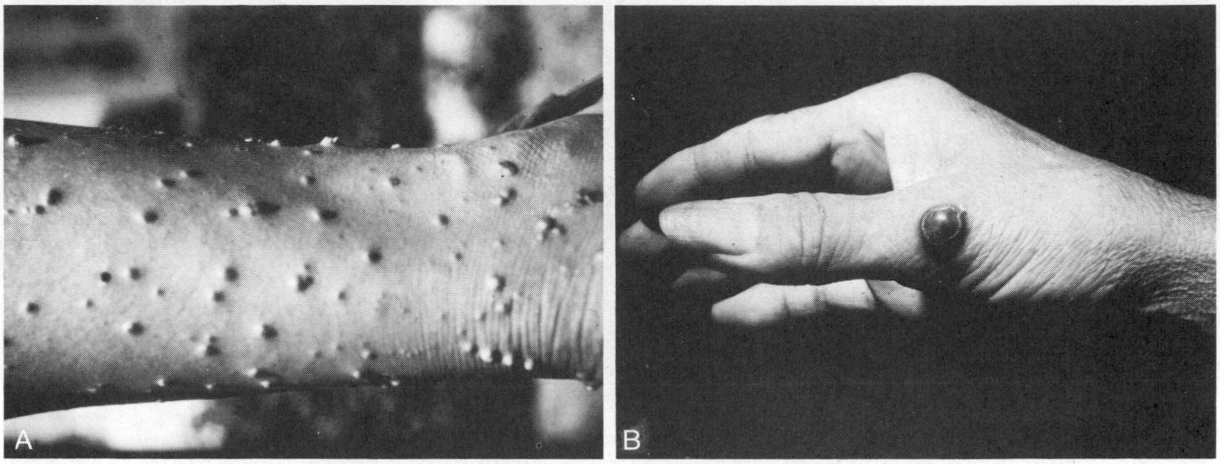

Figure 3. Verruga peruana. The lesions vary greatly in size. *A,* The smallest, verrugas of miliary type, are early lesions. The larger, verrugas of nodular type, are old lesions. *B,* A large solitary, nodular verruga with the histological character of a hemangioma.

coexist in the same individual; this fact also contributes to the pleomorphism of the eruption (Fig. 3).

Nodules localized in the subcutis tissue (subcutaneous verruga) are usually scarce and appear preferentially on the extremities. Some of these nodules are detectable only by palpation, others make a prominence above the skin or, when the growth is excessive, the skin covering them becomes distended and extremely thin.

In the internal organs (muscles, lungs, serous membranes, spleen, gastrointestinal tract, or meninges) only miliary or small nodular types have been reported. However, in the interstitium of the muscles larger nodules can be found (Odriozola, 1898).

Although verruga peruana usually occurs as a stage that follows Oroya fever, there are some important variations. (1) Eruption occuring as a primary condition—that is, cases not preceded by Oroya fever—after an incubation period of less than 40 days (Odriozola, 1898; Rebagliati, 1940). When verruga is experimentally induced in humans and monkeys, the eruption occurs mostly as a primary condition at the points of inoculation (exceptionally at a distance) after about two to three weeks of incubation. The existence of mild forms of Oroya fever (see above) and even of infection without disease suggests that "primary eruptions" are secondary to subclinical forms of Oroya fever. On the other hand, *Bartonella* inoculated by *Phlebotomus* should also be able to induce verruga nodules directly at the point of inoculation. (2) The eruption can occur precociously, that is, during the course of Oroya fever (Odriozola, 1898). (3) The usual sequence may be reversed so that the eruption precedes Oroya fever (Odriozola, 1898). (4) A second attack (relapse) of Oroya fever can follow the eruption ("retrocession") (Odriozola, 1898). (5) Some individuals can suffer periodically throughout their lives from attacks of verruga peruana (chronic verruga peruana).

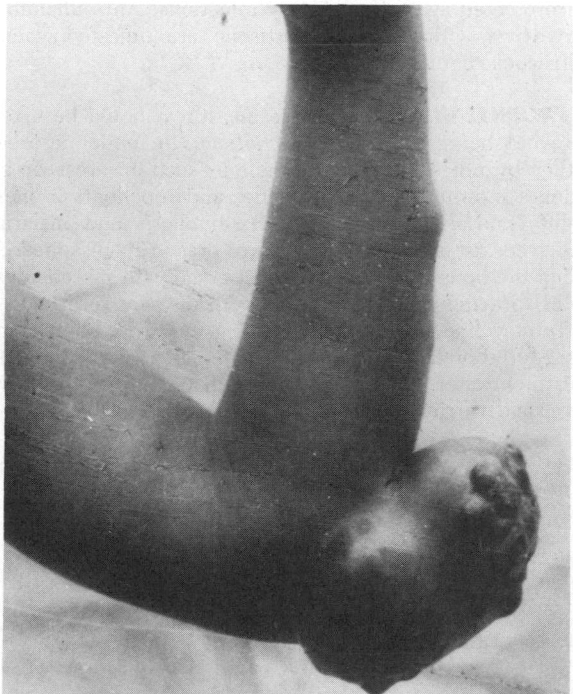

Figure 4. Verruga peruana. A giant verrucoma. Case reported by Ricketts (1942).

Variations 2, 3, and 4, which were reported at a time when neither *Bartonella* nor secondary infections caused by *Salmonella* were known, remain to be confirmed.

COMPLICATIONS AND SEQUELAE. Hemorrhage is the most important complication. The nodules, though appearing fragile, do not have a tendency to bleed spontaneously; bleeding is provoked by mechanical injury. Only the bleeding from nodules localized on mucous membranes (nose, larynx, trachea, bronchi, gastrointestinal tract), which are fortunately rare, may be serious. On the other hand, nodules localized on the respiratory tract, especially the larynx, may provoke serious respiratory difficulty.

Other complications, such as secondary infection or ulceration of the nodules, are infrequent.

The crusts, which are the final stage of the nodules, drop off without leaving a scar, except those that may be infected secondarily.

GEOGRAPHIC VARIATIONS IN DISEASE. In some endemic areas of Peru, for example, Callejón de Huaylas, verruga peruana without Oroya fever occurs much more frequently than the eruption preceded by anemia. In other areas, such as the Rimac valley, the reverse is true.

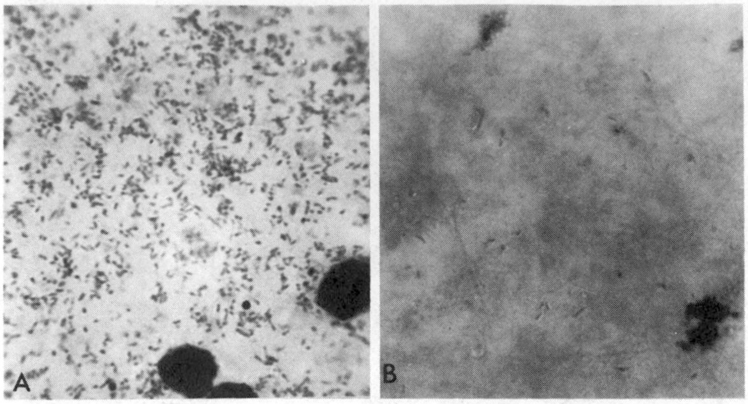

Figure 5. Thick film preparations. *A,* From a patient with a high rate of parasitism involving nearly 100 per cent of red blood cells, the usual occurrence in Oroya fever. *B,* From a patient with a paucibacillary form of Oroya fever. Scarcely 15 organisms appear in the field.

DIAGNOSIS. Fever and anemia, or fever alone, suggests Oroya fever if the patient has visited an endemic area within the preceding three weeks. Abundant *Bartonella* organisms can be found on conventional blood smears (Fig. 1 in Chapter 55). In the paucibacillary form of the disease, finding the infectious agent may be difficult. Oroya fever can be excluded in those cases only after exhaustive examinations of the blood, including thick film preparations (Fig. 5). A blood culture should be made to confirm or exclude Oroya fever and, above all, to diagnose salmonellosis.

The diagnosis of verruga peruana is suggested by the presence of the characteristic verruga nodules after residence in an endemic area. Culture and histopathology of the nodule can clarify the diagnosis in difficult cases.

TREATMENT AND PROPHYLAXIS. Although *B. bacilliformis* is highly susceptible to many antibiotics, chloramphenicol is the antibiotic of choice because of its effectiveness against both *Bartonella* and the frequently associated *Salmonella* (Cuadra, 1956). All severely ill patients should be considered as potentially infected with *Salmonella.* Therefore, the laboratory diagnosis of bartonellosis should be established as rapidly as possible in order to initiate treatment.

Chloramphenicol is administered orally to adults at an initial dose of 1 g followed by 0.5 g every six hours. In uncomplicated cases the temperature should drop abruptly within the first 24 hours (Cuadra, 1957). After the temperature is normal, treatment should be continued for five days more. In some patients a relapse may occur, usually within the first week after the termination of therapy. The relapse responds favorably to a second course of chloramphenicol (Cuadra, 1957). If there is concomitant salmonellosis, the temperature drops by lysis in three to five days. After the temperature is normal the therapy should be continued for five days more at a dose of 0.5 g every six hours. Salmonellosis occurring during the period of convalescence from Oroya fever should be treated similarly.

Blood transfusion is indicated only for patients with profound anemia. Patients who are convalescent from Oroya fever (anemia without fever) when first seen should still be treated with chloramphenicol to prevent salmonellosis and to prevent a verrucous eruption. *No verruga stage occurs in patients with Oroya fever who have been treated with antibiotics.* At most there is a pruriginous papulovesicular or papulokeratinous eruption, which vanishes within one to two weeks and is considered to be an abortive form of verruga peruana (Cuadra, 1962).

The effectiveness of antibiotics against verruga peruana is doubtful, since a dramatic response has never been observed. Since *Bartonella* is a highly susceptible organism, both in patients with Oroya fever (Larrea, 1958) and in vitro (Wigand, 1952), perhaps the organisms within the verruga nodule are killed by antibiotic therapy but the tumor is still able to continue its normal evolution, or perhaps the intracellular localization of *Bartonella* within the verrucoma can protect the organism against antibiotics.

Care should be taken to avoid mechanical injury of the nodules. Hemorrhage should be stopped by compression of the bleeding nodule. Surgical extirpation, which should be as complete as possible, or cauterization may be indicated if the tumors are in a dangerous location (larynx, conjunctivae). Antibiotics are especially indicated if the nodules become secondarily infected (Biffi and Carbajal, 1904), an unusual complication. Ulcerated nodules should be protected against secondary infections. Anti-inflammatory drugs, with or without cortisone, are indicated against verrucous rheumatism.

PROPHYLAXIS. All available measures should be taken to avoid being bitten by *Phlebotomus* in endemic areas either by not spending the night in such an areas or by using a mosquito net, insecticide, and repellents if overnight exposure is necessary. Bartonellosis and malaria, which coexist in many areas of Peru, practically disappeared when the houses were regularly sprayed with insecticides. After spraying was discontinued both diseases returned.

Tetracycline in low doses (0.25 g every 12 hours), administered orally while in an endemic area or as a five-day treatment after leaving the area, will prevent both Oroya fever and verruga peruana. No vaccine is available.

References

Aldana, L.: Bacteriologia de la enfermedad de Carrión. Cron Med Lima 46:237, 1929.

Aldana, L.: Estados biológicos de la *Bartonella* en la enfermedad de Carrión. Rev Sanid Polic Lima 7:391, 1947.

Aldana, L. A.: Contribución al estudio de la complicación salmonelósica en la enfermedad de Carrión. Rev Sanid Polic Lima 9:9, 1949.

Alzamora Castro, V.: Enfermedad de Carrión: Ensayo de etiopatogenia. Anal Fac Cien Med Lima 23:1, 1940.

Alzamora Castro, V.: Contrbución al estudio de la bartonellosis humana o enfermedad de Carrión. Gac Med Lima 2:78, 1945.

Biffi, U., and Carbajal, G.: Sobre un caso de enfermedad de Carrión con verrucomas supurados. Cron Med Lima 21:379, 1904.
Carvallo, C.: La médula osea en la enfermedad de Carrión. Cron Med Lima 28:135, 1911.
Colichón, H., and Cuadra, M.: La salmonellosis en la verruga peruana. Rev Med Per Lima 25:30, 1954.
Cuadra, M.: La complicación salmonelósica en la bartonelosis aguda (anemia de Carrión). Rev Med Per Lima 25:3, 1954.
Cuadra, M.: Salmonellosis complication in human bartonellosis. Tex Rep Biol Med 14:97, 1956.
Cuadra, M.: Tratamiento con cloranfenicol de casos de bartoelosis aguda (enfermedad de Carrión) en periodo de inicio. Anal Fac Med Lima 40:747, 1957.
Cuadra, M.: Mecanismo de destrucción de los eritrocitos. La hemólisis intravascular. Anal Fac Med Lima 40:872, 1957.
Cuadra, M.: Erupción verrucosa frustra en pacientes tratados con antibióticos. Anal Fac Med Lima 45:302, 1962.
Cuadra, M.: Bartonellosis. Cultivo del tejido del verrucoma. Anal Fac Med Lima 40:646, 1966.
Cuadra, M., and Takano, J.: The relationship of *Bartonella bacilliformis* to the red blood cell as revealed by electron microscopy. Blood 33:708, 1969.
Cuadra, M.: Fiebre bartonellósica aguda con parasitismo escaso y anemia subclínica. Anal Progr Acad Med Lima 53:87, 1970.
Cuadra, M.: The ability of *Bartonella bacilliformis* growing in culture to attach to red blood cells. Abstract 12, International Congress of Microbiology, Munich, 1978, p. 178.
Guzman Barrón, A.: La reacción de Van den Bergh, hemoaglutininas y hemolisinas en la enfermedad de Carrión. Cron Med Lima 48:753, 1926.
Gonzalez Oechea, M.: Algunas consideraciones sobre la fiebre grave de Carrión y la infección verrucosa aguda poco anemizante. Rev Med Per Lima 46:407, 1932.
Hercelles, O.: Estudio de la *Bartonella* en los órganos y tejidos, y deducciones que de él se sacan sobre el proceso anátomoclínico de la enfermedad. Rev Med Per Lima 7:235, 1935.
Hurtado, A., Pons, J., and Merino, C.: La anemia de la enfermedad de Carrión. Anal Fac Med Lima 21:25, 1938.
Kikuth, W.: Experimentelle Untersuchungen über Oroyafieber und Verruga Peruana. Z Immunforsch 73:1, 1931.
Larrea, P.: Los antiobióticos en la bartonelemia humana. Arch Per Pat Clin Lima 12:1, 1958.
Mackehenie, D., and Weiss, P.: Contribución al estudio de la verruga peruana. Gac Med Per Lima 4:51, 1926.
Mackehenie, D.: Estudio del noduloma verrucoso. Ref Med Lima 24:50, 1938.
Mayer, M., Rocha Lima, H., and Werner, H.: Untersuchungen über Verruga peruviana. Muench Med Wschr 60:739, 1913.
McCutcheon, M.: Inflamation. In Anderson, W. A. D.: Pathology. St. Louis, C. V. Mosby Company, 1948.
Marquez da Cunha, A., and Muniz, J.: Pesquisas sobre la verruga peruana. Mem Inst O Cruz 21:161, 1928.
Merino, C.: Las seroproteinas en la enfermedad de Carrión. Thesis (medicine). Lima, Faculty of Medicine of the San Marcos University, 1939.
Moulder, J. W.: The rickettsias. In Bergey's Manual of Determinative Bacteriology. 8th ed. Baltimore, The Williams & Wilkins Company, 1974, p. 882.
Noguchi, H., and Battistini, T.: Etiology of Oroya fever. I. Cultivation of *Bartonella bacilliformis*. J Exp Med 43:851, 1926a.
Noguchi, H.: Etiology of Oroya fever. III. The behavior of *Bartonella bacilliformis* in *Macacus rhesus*. J Exp Med 44:697, 1926b.
Noguchi, H.: Etiology of Oroya fever. IV. The effect of inoculation of anthropoid apes with *Bartonella bacilliformis*. J Exp Med 44:715, 1926c.
Noguchi, H.: The etiology of verruga peruana. J Exp Med 45:175, 1927a.
Noguchi, H.: Etiology of Oroya fever. VIII. Experiments on cross-immunity between Oroya fever and verruga peruana. J Exp Med 45:781, 1927b.
Noguchi, H.: Etiology of Oroya fever. VI. Pathological changes observed in animals experimentally infected with *Bartonella bacilliformis*. The distribution of the parasites in the tissues. J Exp Med 45:437, 1927c.
Odriozola, M.: La Maladie de Carrión ou la Verruga Péruvienne. Paris, 1898.
Pinkerton, H., and Weinman, D.: Carrión's disease. I. Behavior of the etiological agent within cells growing or surviving in vitro. Proc Soc Exp Biol Med 37:587, 1937.
Pinkerton, H., and Weinman, D.: Carrión disease. II. Comparative morphology of the etiological agent in Oroya fever and verruga peruana. Proc Soc Exp Biol Med 37:591, 1937-38.
Rebagliati, R. Verruga Peruana (Enfermedad de Carrión). Lima, Imprenta Torres Aguirre, 1940.
Recavarren, S., and Lumbreras, H.: Pathogenesis of the verruga of Carrión's disease. Am J Pathol 66:461, 1972.
Reynafarge, C., and Ramos, J.: The hemolytic anemia of human bartonellosis. Blood 17:562, 1961.
Ribeyro, R.: Verruga peruana y paratifico beta. Cron Med Lima 49:361, 1932.
Ricketts, G.: Contribución al estudio clinico de la enfermedad de Carrión. Thesis (medicine). Lima, 1942.
Ricketts, G.: Intercurrent infections of Carrión's disease observed in Peru. Am J Trop Med 28:437, 1948.
Rocha Lima, H.: Zur Histologie der Verruga peruviana. Verh Dtsch Pathol Ges 16:409, 1913.
Strong, R. P., Tyzzer, E. E., Brues, C. T., Sellard, A. B., and Gastiaburu, J. C.: Verruga peruviana, Oroya fever and uta, JAMA 61:1713, 1913.
Strong, R. P., and Tyzzer, E. E.: Pathology of Oroya fever. JAMA 64:965, 1915.
Strong, R. P.: Verruga peruana and Oroya fever. In Stitt's Diagnosis, Prevention and Treatment of Tropical Diseases. Philadelphia, The Blakiston Company, 1945, p. 997.
Takano, J.: Enfermedad de Carrión (Bartonellosis humana). Estudio morfológico de la fase hemática y del periodo eruptivo con el microscopio electrónico. Thesis (Medicine). Lima, Faculty of Medicine of the San Marcos University, 1970.
Tamayo, M. O.: Un ensayo de clasificación de los tifosimiles de la Verruga peruana. Cron Med Lima 14:21, 1907.
Urteaga, O.: Histopatogenia de la anemia en la Verruga peruana. Arch Per Pat Clin Lima 2:355, 1948.
Urteaga, O., and Calderón, J.: Ciclo biológico de reproducción de la *Bartonella bacilliformis* en los tejidos de pacientes de Verruga peruana o enfermedad de Carrión. Arch Per Pat Clin Lima 19:1, 1965.
Weinman, D., and Pinkerton, H.: Carrión's disease. III. Experimental production in animals. Proc Soc Exp Biol Med 37:594, 1937.
Weiss, P.: Contribución al estudio de la verruga peruana o enfermedad de Carrión. Rev Med Per Lima 4:5, 58, 1932.
Weiss, P.: Contribución al estudio de la verruga peruana. Rev Med Lat Am Buenos Aires 18:214, 1933.
Wigand, R.: Neue Untersuchungen über *Bartonella bacilliformis*. 2. Verhalten gegenüber Sulfonamide und Antibiotica in vitro. Z Tropenmed Parasitol 3:453, 1952.

199

SYPHILIS

DANIEL M. MUSHER, M.D.

DEFINITION. Syphilis is a venereal infection caused by *Treponema pallidum*. The ulcer that arises within 3 weeks at the initial site of treponemal inoculation is called a chancre. Verifying the presence of a syphilitic chancre establishes the diagnosis of *primary* syphilis. Clinically unrecognized dissemination of treponemes from this primary site results in systemic symptoms and widespread cutaneous lesions that appear 3 to 6 weeks after the development of the chancre and are the major presenting symptoms in *secondary syphilis*. Disseminated skin lesions do not resemble chancres, because by the time of their appearance some degree of protective immunity has developed. Although involvement of skin and mucous membranes usually predominates in secondary syphilis, the lymph nodes, bones, joints, eyes, central nervous system, and kidneys may also be involved. Without treatment, the lesions of secondary syphilis resolve spontaneously, but only after a period of 1 to 3 months has transpired. During the first year without signs of disease, termed *early latent syphilis*, a relapse to active, secondary syphilis occurs in up to 20 per cent of patients. Primary, secondary, and early latent syphilis together comprise early syphilis. After 1 year of latency, relapses no longer occur and late latent syphilis is said to be present. The diagnosis of late latent syphilis is also made as a matter of public health policy in an asymptomatic person who has serologic evidence of infection, whose cerebrospinal fluid is normal, and who has not received definitive treatment for syphilis. *Tertiary syphilis* becomes clinically apparent after months or years of latency in one-third or more of those who do not receive treatment for early syphilis. Tertiary syphilis is often divided into: (1) "benign" infection, in which the disease is limited to granulomatous involvement of skin, bones, cartilage, soft tissue, and viscera; (2) cardiovascular syphilis in which the ascending aorta is involved; and (3) neurosyphilis, which has a remarkably broad range of neurologic and psychiatric manifestations. *Congenital syphilis* is acquired by the fetus when *T. pallidum* crosses the placenta. *Endemic syphilis* or bejel, a nonvenereally acquired infection caused by *T. pallidum*, occurs in the Middle East, Africa, and rarely in Eastern Europe. The early age of acquisition of bejel by nonvenereal routes, together with malnutrition and primitive living conditions, is probably responsible for the different clinical manifestations of endemic and sporadic syphilis, although some differences in the pathogenicity of the causative organisms have been demonstrated in laboratory animals.

ETIOLOGY. *T. pallidum*, a highly motile, helical organism in the order Spirochetales, is discussed in depth in Chapter 53. *T. pallidum* is a natural pathogen only for man, although infection has been produced experimentally in primates and a few laboratory animals. With the rare exception of laboratory accidents (including transfusion of blood), all cases are acquired by direct contact among human beings.

PATHOGENESIS AND PATHOLOGY. *T. pallidum* enters the body after intimate, usually sexual, contact presumably through tiny breaks in squamous or mucous epthelium. As with other infections, some organisms lodge in the dermis immediately after inoculation, while others escape to draining lymph nodes. During the ensuing weeks, treponemes proliferate locally in the dermis and continue to escape into the bloodstream; this spirochetemia sets the stage for disseminated and perhaps for late forms of syphilis, as is discussed below. After a 14- to 21-day incubation period, a painless papule appears at the site of inoculation; within a few days, it ulcerates, producing a syphilitic chancre. Histologic examination of the papule reveals a relatively acellular central area rich in mucopolysaccharides, surrounded by an infiltrate consisting of degranulated polymorphonuclear leukocytes and lymphocytes. As the lesion evolves, plasma cells and macrophages come to predominate at the periphery. Endothelial proliferation and perivascular infiltration by lymphocytes and plasma cells are characteristically present. Syphilitic chancres heal spontaneously within 3 to 6 weeks. The mechanism for healing is obscure; some kind of local immunity perhaps related to local activation of macrophages appears to be largely responsible since disseminated (secondary) lesions appear and progress while the primary lesion is regressing. These disseminated lesions result from spirochetemia that has occurred during the incubation period or, more likely, result from the chancre itself. Three or more weeks elapse between deposition of *T. pallidum* in the dermis and emergence to secondary lesions. The curious progression of infection despite the presence of specific antitreponemal antibody and other immunologic aspects of the infection are discussed elsewhere in this textbook and reviewed in depth in other sources. (Schell and Musher, 1983). The tendency of syphilis to produce skin lesions may reflect the preference of *T. pallidum* for cooler areas; in experimental animals, disseminated skin lesions appear only in areas that have been shaved. Although primary lesions ulcerate, secondary lesions do not, presumably because some degree of systemic immunity has already developed. Despite this difference, the histology of disseminated lesions is similar to that of syphilitic chancres.

Late syphilitic lesions, called gummas, have a granulomatous appearance, often with epithelioid and giant cells, although only infrequently are palisading cells seen at the periphery; central necrosis is often present without frank caseation. Their pathogenesis is not fully understood; they arise in areas that are not the most frequently involved ones in disseminated syphilis, and the presence of treponemes has not been consistently demonstrated.

CLINICAL MANIFESTATIONS

Primary Syphilis. Most clinical lesions in heterosexual men occur on the penis (Fig. 1) and in women on the labia, fourchette, and cervix, although lesions frequently occur elsewhere on the genitalia, in the mouth, and in other

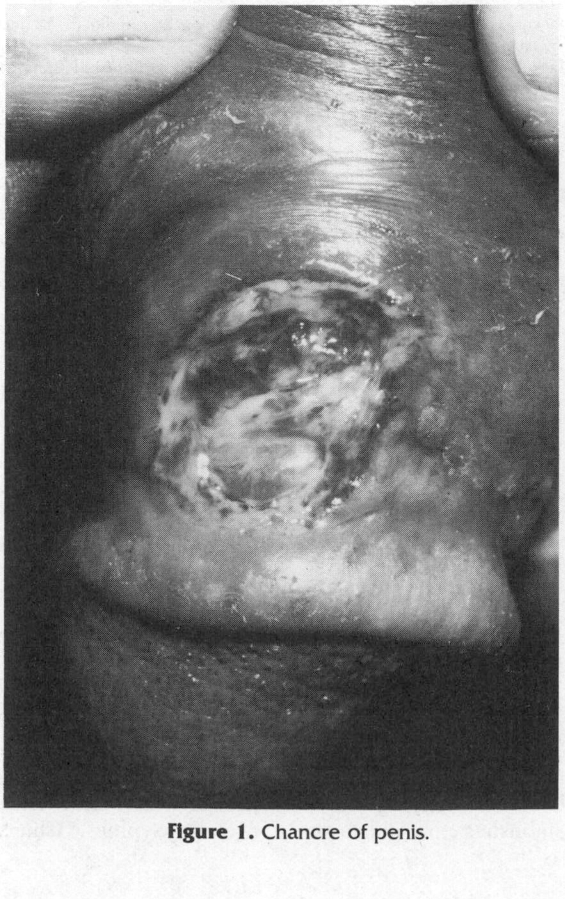

Figure 1. Chancre of penis.

erogenous zones (genital lesions of syphilis are also discussed in Chapter 162). Examination at the time a lesion first appears usually reveals one or more painless papules, 0.5 to 1 cm in diameter. Within a few days, these papules ulcerate, producing syphilitic chancres that are usually round but may be elongated, depending on their relation to tissue lines. Although solitary lesions were once said to be characteristic, multiple lesions are seen almost as frequently (Chapel, 1978). Lymph nodes that drain the infected area are enlarged in 80 per cent of cases. Because the chancre is painless and occurs in women inside the labia or on the cervix, primary syphilis is easily overlooked; as a result, the diagnosis of syphilis is frequently not made until the secondary stage is reached. The same is true of homosexual or bisexual men whose primary lesion may be an asymptomatic anal or rectal chancre. Alternatively, chancres in the anus in homosexual or bisexual men may cause irritation, pain on defecation, and/or blood-streaking of the feces.

Secondary Syphilis. This disseminated disease involves many organ systems and causes a wide variety of symptoms and physical findings (Chapel, 1980). Dermatologic manifestations are virtually always present, although they can be overlooked by incomplete physical examination, or ignored because the diagnosis of syphilis is not entertained and/or because they may be attributed to one of a great variety of other dermatologic conditions. The initial lesion is an evanescent, diffuse macular eruption that may involve the trunk or occur everywhere except the face, hands, and feet. This eruption is usually not recognized, especially in dark-skinned individuals. Within a few days well demarcated papules 0.5 to 2 cm in size appear, occurring symmetrically nearly everywhere on the body including palms and soles, but often sparing the face (Fig. 2). The lesions may be smooth, follicular, or scaly in texture and dusky red or brownish in color. Vesicles occur only very rarely, although vesicular-pustular lesions may well have been the rule centuries ago when syphilis was called the great pox, and lesions on the palms tend to have a pustular appearance even today. Leukoderma rarely occurs. Mucosal lesions, either in the form of superficial erosions or grayish plaques are not uncommon. Circular "annular" lesions may appear on the face in dark-skinned individuals. Hypo- or hyperpigmentation may be seen. Patchy alopecia results from syphilitic involvement of hair follicles. Condylomata, large plaque-like vegetative lesions, occur in warm, moist areas such as the perineum or groin and represent a confluent area of syphilitic infection that results from local spread of *T. pallidum*, either from primary or secondary lesions.

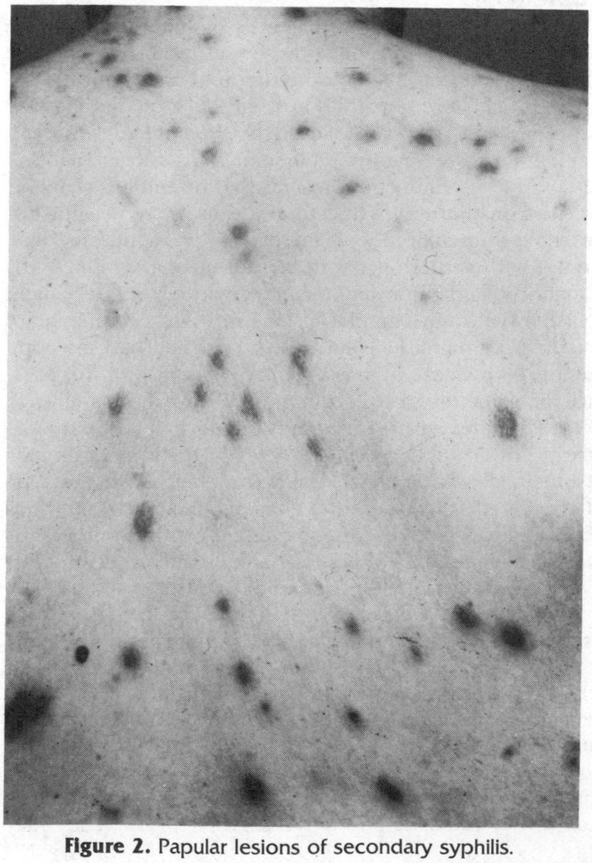

Figure 2. Papular lesions of secondary syphilis.

The physician must not forget that disseminated or secondary syphilis is a systemic disease. Pruritis, sore throat, headache, muscle aches, fever, and malaise occur, although less frequently now than in the preantibiotic era (Table 1). Symmetric nontender lymphadenopathy is present in one or more areas in 85 per cent of patients and may be generalized. Periostitis, which is usually asymptomatic, may be found in one-third of cases by bone scan; the skull, tibia, sternum, and ribs are most frequently involved. Radiographs show osteolytic areas without sclerosis (Dismukes et al., 1976). Arthritis, more frequently of large joints, occurs, with a synovial effusion that may contain large numbers of white blood cells equally divided between polymorphonuclelar leukocytes and lymphocytes; Chesney showed that 3 of 10 such fluids contained infective *T. pallidum*. Low-grade abnormalities of liver function may be present in up to 10 per cent of patients with disseminated syphilis (Feher et al., 1975); histologic examination shows focal inflammatory changes, but true granulomas have not been observed. Iritis, anterior uveitis, and meningitis also occur in secondary syphilis. Glomerulitis with a nephrotic syndrome may result from glomerular deposition of immune complexes that contain treponemal antigen and antibody (Baughn et al., 1983). Rarely, hematuria may be a prominent finding.

Late Syphilis. Clinical manifestations of tertiary syphilis develop in untreated syphilitic patients after a highly

Table 1. SYMPTOMS REPORTED BY PATIENTS WITH SECONDARY SYPHILIS IN TWO STUDIES, ONE OF WHICH WAS PROSPECTIVE (CHAPEL, 1980)

	No. (%) of Patients	
Symptom	***Chapel (1980) n= 105***	***Stokes et al., (1945) n= 178***
Sore throat	16 (15.2%)	53 (29.8%)
Malaise	No data	42 (23.6%)
Headache	9 (8.6%)	24 (13.5%)
Weight loss	2 (1.9%)	18 (10.1%)
Fever	5 (4.8%)	14 (7.9%)
Meningismus	3 (2.8%)	8 (4.5%)
Musculoskeletal aches	6 (5.7%)	14 (7.9%)
Iritis	0	3 (1.7%)
Hoarseness	0	2 (1.1%)
Hair loss	3 (2.9%)	No data
Pruritus	44 (41.9%)	No data

variable time period that is dependent, in large measure, upon how carefully an examination is made to detect them; usually more than 1 year of latency elapses before late syphilis is detectable. Thus, the incidence of late or tertiary syphilis varies greatly with how the diagnosis is established. Of a large group of patients who were observed with untreated syphilis for many years, late benign syphilis became clinically apparent in 15 per cent, and cardiovascular syphilis in 10 to 25 per cent (Clark et al., 1964). However, a substantially higher percentage of patients may develop cardiovascular syphilis, and some cardiovascular abnormalities attributable to syphilis have been said to be present at autopsy in up to 80 per cent of affected subjects (Kampmeier, 1964; Heggtveit, 1964). Benign late syphilis is a term used when nonvital structures such as skin, soft tissue, bones, and cartilage or certain parenchymal organs such as the liver or testes are involved. In recent years it has become exceedingly unusual to diagnose a case of benign late syphilis.

Benign late syphilis most commonly involves the skin and subcutaneous tissues; lesions usually occur singly, although asymmetric involvement of a few areas may occur simultaneously. The face, neck, and extremities are most commonly affected. Indurated, nodular ulcerated lesions that describe an arc of an irregular full circle are characteristic. Peripheral hyperpigmentation is seen and there is often central scarring. These lesions may be indolent or aggressive; frequently tissue destruction with ulceration results, producing small nodular ulcers that may progress to large confluent ulcerated areas (Olansky, 1964). If untreated, these may persist for several years.

Late syphilis of the bone most commonly affects tibia, fibula, clavicle, and skull, although any bone or multiple areas may be involved (Kampmeier, 1964). The symptoms of pain and swelling, which are nearly always present, are consistent with the periosteal location of the granulomatous reaction. Roentgenograms reveal periosteal thickening that may be accompanied by erosion and/or an osteoblastic response of the underlying bone. Syphilis of the tibia or fibula with ulceration of overlying soft tissue often causes symptoms and signs suggestive of chronic venous stasis. Destruction of cartilage plays an important part in determining the clinical appearance of the lesions. Subperiosteal gummas of the nose and hard palate cause perforation and eventually destroy the involved structures. Gummas of the joints are frequently found in the company of syphilitic osteomyelitis as painless swellings of the knee or sternoclavicular joints. Gummas of the joint may take the form of single tumors or diffuse synovitis, which causes thickening of the synovium, extensive effusion, and destruction of the cartilage; in the case of the knee this sequence results in a nonfunctional joint. Gummas of the joint must be distinguished from Charcot's joint, in which neurotropic disturbances due to tabes dorsalis causes painless destruction of cartilage and adjacent bones.

Visceral gummas occur mainly in the liver and testes. Hepatic involvement includes solitary gummas that present as a hepatic mass, multiple large gummas with subsequent scarring (hepar lobatum), or widespread small gummas that produce a picture resembling Laennec's cirrhosis. Syphilis of the testis causes diffuse interstitial fibrosis with contraction of the testis into a round, hard mass. Nodules of the spermatic cords and epididymis or a hydrocele may also be present. Syphilis of the stomach may imitate peptic ulcer or carcinoma of the stomach. Gummatous infiltration rarely occurs in the rectum.

Neurosyphilis, which eventually appeared in 7% of patients with untreated syphilis, is discussed in Chapter 174. Syphilitic involvement of the vasa vasorum of the aorta with resulting medial necrosis of the aorta produces a spectrum of disease under the general category of syphilitic aortitis. The majority of patients are asymptomatic. Clinical syndromes that used to be observed relatively frequently and still occur occasionally include aortic insufficiency, left ventricular hypertrophy, congestive heart failure, and aneurysm of the ascending aorta, sometimes with erosion into the bones of the thorax (Kampmeier, 1964; Heggtveit, 1964; Grabau et al., 1976). Involvement of the coronary artery ostia occasionally causes symptoms of ischemic heart disease. Syphilis of the aorta is recognized radiographically by calcifications in the ascending aorta or by an aneurysm of the ascending aorta with or without erosion of adjacent bones. At autopsy, the proximal aorta has a shaggy appearance and the aortic valve is dilated. Microscopic examination shows the presence of patchy destruction of the media and obliterating endarteritis of the vasa vasorum with plasma cell infiltration. Syphilitic aneurysm may occur years after active disease of the aorta has subsided, probably resulting from continued mechanical stress in an already damaged vital area. This hypothesis is consistent with the finding that the VDRL reaction is negative in one-third of patients at the time that syphilitic disease of the aorta is diagnosed. An interesting but unexplained observation is that syphilitic disease of the aorta does not appear in patients who contracted their infection before adolescence.

DIAGNOSIS

Clinical Diagnosis. The diagnosis of syphilis should be considered in any patient with genital lesions. A chancre due to *T. pallidum* needs to be differentiated from the so-called soft chancre, a painful erosion 1 to 2 cm in diameter with a necrotic exudate caused by *Hemophilus ducreyi.* Trauma during sexual intercourse or a fixed drug eruption may produce noninfectious lesions that resemble a chancre. Erosions on the cervix due to any cause may be indistinguishable from syphilitic chancres. Reiter's syndrome may present with genital ulcers in the absence of conjunctivitis or arthritis, and the examiner may overlook oral lesions in Behcet's syndrome; genital lesions in these conditions are usually quite painful. A person who has had past infection may develop small, atypical chancres because of the presence of some degree of immunity. The lesions due to Herpes simplex virus are usually small, painful, and vesicular; a history of recurring vesicles in the same area may be obtained. A variety of lesions in the mouth must be differentiated from syphilitic chancre, including aphthous ulcers and cancer of the lip or tongue. Syphilis of the anus may cause symptoms of hemorrhoidal irritation or proctitis or may be confused with carcinoma (Drusin et al., 1977).

Secondary syphilis of the skin may be confused with diseases that produce widespread, symmetric skin lesions. These include acute exanthems of any kind (except vesicular), pityriasis rosea, psoriasis, erythema multiforme, and drug eruptions. The association of diffuse lymphadenopathy and splenomegaly may also raise the possibility of infectious mononucleosis or lymphoma. Late (tertiary) lesions of the skin need to differentiated from other chronic infections such as tuberculosis, blastomycosis, or leprosy. They may simulate the lesions of discoid lupus erythematosus, especially when they occur on the face. Sarcoidosis, basal cell carcinoma, or cutaneous involvement by lymphoma may cause confusion. Ulcers from stasis or factitious causes must also be differentiated.

Late syphilis of the bone may be confused with osteogenic sarcoma or osteomyelitis, whether pyogenic or mycobacterial. Disfiguring late syphilitic lesions of the nasal septum, palate, or pharynx may simulate leprosy, carcinoma, Wegener's (midline) granuloma, and related conditions or autoimmune vasculitides such as systemic lupus erythematosus. Although syphilitic aortic insufficiency must be differentiated from that due to other causes, an aneurysm of the ascending aorta is relatively specific in suggesting the diagnosis of syphilis.

Laboratory Diagnosis. In early syphilis, the use of darkfield microscopy to detect *T. pallidum* in exudate obtained directly from suspicious lesions remains the most direct, immediate, and specific way of establishing the diagnosis of syphilis. This examination is positive in most chancres, although bacterial superinfection and/or prior local use of ointments may obscure the treponemes. Darkfield microscopy in secondary lesions is less rewarding, especially if the examiner is not skilled in exposing the base of the ulcer while maintaining a blood-free field before aspirating material for examination. Gram stains of exudates are not helpful because the narrow width of the causative organism precludes visualization by light microscopy and cultures cannot be used since *T. pallidum* has not yet been cultivated successfully in vitro.

The presence of antibodies to cardiolipin has been used widely since the time of Wassermann to diagnose syphilis. These antibodies are detected in reference or city and state health laboratories by the VDRL (Venereal Disease Research Laboratory) test or, increasingly, in hospital and office practices with the RPR (rapid plasma reagin) test or a modification thereof, which gives nearly identical results. Results are reported with dilutions (titers) so that the degree of reactivity can be determined. Some laboratories may take shortcuts and not carry out a full set of dilutions, in which case the prozone phenomenon may lead to a falsely negative result. The VDRL is reactive in about 80 per cent of patients at the time that they seek medical attention for primary syphilis. After treatment, it nearly always reverts to negative over a period of 12 months (Fiumara, 1977). It is worthwhile to document this reversion in order to avoid problems relating to diagnosis of reinfection at a later date. Secondary syphilis is always characterized by a reactive VDRL, usually in a high titer (1:16 or greater). With treatment, the VDRL usually becomes negative, although low-grade reactivity may persist (serofast state). In the absence of treatment, the VDRL slowly returns to normal and is, in fact, negative in nearly half of patients with late syphilis. It should be stressed, however, that active late benign syphilis with periostitis or gumma is virtually always associated with a positive serologic reaction. One-third of patients with syphilitic aortitis have a negative VDRL; in some of these individuals, the aorta may have been damaged during active infection, but the resulting weakness may lead to aneurysm formation long after the infection and/or immunologic reaction has subsided. The VDRL may be reactive, generally in a low dilution (less than 1:8), in nonsyphilitic patients who have infections due to viruses (especially infectious mononucleosis and hepatitis), mycoplasma or protozoa. A positive VDRL is also seen in the absence of syphilis in heroin addicts and elderly subjects, and also in patients with cirrhosis, malignancy (especially if associated with production of excess globulin), or autoimmune disease. VDRL reactivity in these conditions has acquired the unfortunate designation "biologic false-positive" to indicate that it does not connote infection due to *T. pallidum*; this term is best avoided.

Specific antibodies to *T. pallidum* are detected by using the FTA-ABS or the TPHA tests. FTA-ABS stands for Fluorescent Treponemal Antibody, following absorption with *T. phagedenis* (*T. reiteri*) to eliminate nonspecific group antibodies that crossreact with other treponemes. TPHA stands for *T. pallidum* hemagglutinating antibody; MTHPA is a micro-method that is also automated. Because of ease in performing and interpreting the hemagglutination test it has largely replaced the FTA-ABS. However, as carried out in individual hospital laboratories, these tests are not as reliable as they used to be when only health department laboratories did them, and questionable results should lead to restudy by such a reference laboratory. About 90 per cent of patients with a primary syphilitic chancre have a positive FTA-ABS and TPHA by the time they come to medical attention (Duncan et al., 1974). All patients with disseminated and late infection have positive reactions. These tests are highly specific as well as being extremely sensitive. A few disease states such as systemic lupus erythematosus, polyarteritis, and related conditions are said to cause a falsely positive FTA-ABS, but the sophisticated observer can often detect a distinctive beaded pattern in these reactions. The FTA-ABS usually remains positive for life; the TPHA probably does, as well, although declining levels have been detected and the test has not been available for long enough to be certain. As a result, despite their exquisite sensitivity and specificity, these tests may *not* be helpful diagnostically in evaluating an individual patient who might have had syphilis in the past except to *exclude* a diagnosis of secondary or late syphilis if the results are negative.

TREATMENT. Syphilis is generally treated in accord with recommendations of the United States Public Health Service with little, if any attempt to tailor the therapy to individual cases. This treatment generally succeeds in arresting the infection; the question of ultimate cure will be discussed below. Early syphilis (primary or secondary) is treated with a single injection of 2.4 million units of benzathine penicillin or with daily injection of 600,000 units of procaine penicillin for 8 days. Patients with early syphilis who are allergic to penicillin should receive tetracyline 500 mg four times daily for 15 days. Erythromycin is a third choice and is considered less reliable. Early latent syphilis (defined as the unusual situation in which an asymptomatic individual has had untreated primary or secondary syphilis within the past year or has a positive VDRL that was known to have been negative 1 year ago) is treated in the same fashion. Patients who have a positive VDRL and FTA-ABS that is of indeterminate age or in whom syphilis occurred more than 1 year ago and was treated inadequately are considered, albeit somewhat arbitrarily, to have late latent syphilis. A lumbar puncture should be done in such cases to exclude asymptomatic neurosyphilis. If the cerebrospinal fluid is entirely normal, three doses of benzathine penicillin, 2.4 million units 1 week apart, are currently recommended. If cerebrospinal fluid abnormalities suggest a diagnosis of neurosyphilis, or if this diagnosis is made clinically in the absence of such abnormalities, 10 daily injections of 1.2 million units procaine penicillin, or even larger doses of aqueous penicillin, intravenously, are recommended. The need to do a lumbar puncture has received some emphasis since neurosyphilis has failed to respond to benzathine penicillin in a few cases.

Late benign syphilis usually responds promptly to treatment with procaine penicillin G; 600,000 units should be given each day for 10 days. Symptoms resulting from granulomas of skin, bone, or viscera rapidly disappear, as do the lesions themselves; obviously, cartilaginous stuctures that have already been destroyed do not regenerate. Three doses of benzathine penicillin, 2.4 million units at weekly intervals, are thought to give equivalent results. Tetracycline, 2 g daily for 30 days, is prescribed for patients who cannot take penicillin and appears to be effective, although this has not been as well studied as penicillin therapy. Cardiovascular syphilis should be treated similarly. Patients with symptomatic aortic insufficiency should be evaluated for valve replacement (Grabau et al., 1976).

Several investigators have presented evidence that *T. pallidum* persist in the central nervous system, the aqueous humor, and lymph nodes despite recommended doses of penicillin (Dunlop, 1972; Tramont, 1976). Much of this evidence is thought to represent artifactual finding of treponeme-like structures in darkfield examination of tissues, although infective organisms have been found in some instances. It is not clear that persistence of treponemes is associated with increased morbidity or that the therapeutic recommendations need to be changed.

A complication of therapy for syphilis is the Jarisch-Herxheimer reaction, the development of fever, malaise, and other constitutional symptoms that reach a peak of 39.5° C within 6 to 8 hours of treatment and last up to 24 hours, sometimes associated with increased prominence of skin lesions. This reaction occurs in some patients with primary syphilis, and in three-quarters of those with secondary syphilis. The mechanism is unclear; release of treponemal endotoxin is not responsible, and increased levels of circulating antigen-antibody complexes have not been demonstrated consistently, although release of other pyrogenic substances from *T. pallidum* is probably responsible (Young et al., 1982).

Congenital Syphilis

Congenital syphilis is acquired by transplacental passage of *T. pallidum* from an infected pregnant woman to the fetus. Infection is said not to occur until after the fourth month of pregnancy and not be common until after the sixth month (Dippell, 1944) when atrophy of the Langhans cell layer permits passage of the treponemes. One study has used light microscopy to show structures resembling *T. pallidum* in aborted fetuses in the ninth to tenth weeks (Harter and Benirschke, 1976). Hager (1978) has hypothesized that treponemes may regularly be present in the fetus early in pregnancy, but that the search for characteristic syphilitic lesions has been unsuccessful because of the immunologic immaturity of the fetus. Since the fetus acquires infection directly by the hematogenous route, it is not surprising that widespread, disseminated disease occurs.

A stillbirth may result, or the infant may be born with a variety of signs and symptoms of disseminated syphilis (Ingall and Musher, 1983). Generally, the disease appears in the second to sixth weeks of life. The first symptom is usually snuffles; this resembles a head cold, with a purulent nasal discharge, resulting from involvement of the nasal mucous membranes. Skin lesions and mucous patches then appear in the mouth, lips, nose, pharynx, and anogenital region. The infant may also have fever. Enlargement of the spleen and liver, often accompanied by jaundice, and hematologic abnormalities are present in nearly all affected infants, and lymph nodes are enlarged in more than one-half. Meningitis is present in up to 60 per cent of infected infants although usually it is clinically inapparent. Chorioretinitis also occurs. Radiologic and histologic findings of periostitis and osteochondritis can be found in nearly all patients. In the absence of treatment, wasting culminates in marasmus and death. This set of symptoms and signs is rapidly reversed by treatment (Ingall and Musher, 1983).

Late manifestations of congenital syphilis are those that appear after 2 years of age. They are divided into two kinds. (1) "Stigmata" become apparent as structures such as teeth and long bones develop, but actually result from damage to these tissues during intrauterine infection. Examples include abnormalities of the upper incisors ("Hutchinson tooth"), osteochondritis of the tibia causing "saber shin," and sternoclavicular involvement with resulting deformity. These changes are prevented completely by treatment before the third month of life. (2) Other late manifestations resemble, by analogy, the lesions of late (tertiary) syphilis in the adult in that continued signs of active disease are present in involved tissues, although the pathogenesis is obscure. These include lesions of the eye (keratitis and uveitis) and skin, eighth cranial nerve damage with deafness, gummas of nasal and facial bones, periostitis, and central nervous system disease.

Adequate treatment of the infected pregnant woman prevents congenital syphilis. Infants with active infection should be separated, for the purposes of treatment, into those with normal and those with abnormal cerebrospinal fluid (CSF). If the CSF is normal, definitive therapy is 50,000 units benzathine penicillin per kilogram body weight on a single day. In cases in which abnormalities of the CSF suggest that the central nervous system is thought to be involved procaine penicillin G, 50,000 units/kg, should be given daily for 10 days. Antibiotics other than penicillin are not currently recommended for the treatment of congenital syphilis.

References

Baughn, R. E., Adams, C., Musher, D. M.: Circulating immune complexes in experimental and human syphilis. Infect Immun 42:585, 1983.

Chapel, T. A.: The variability of syphilitic chancres. Sex Transm Dis 5:68, 1978.

Chapel, T. A.: The signs and symptoms of secondary syphilis. Sex Trans Dis 7(4):161, 1980.

Clark, E. G., Danbolt, N., Chapel, T. A.: The Oslo study of the natural course of untreated syphilis. An epidemiologic investigation based on a restudy of the Boeck-Bruusgaard material. Med Clin North Amer 48:613, 1964.

Dippell, A. L.: The relationship of congenital syphilis to abortion and miscarriage, and the mechanism of intrauterine protection. Am J Obstet Gynecol 47:369, 1944.

Dismukes, W. E., Delgado, D. G., Mallernee, S. V., and Myers, T. C.: Destructive bone disease in early syphilis. JAMA 236:2646, 1976.

Drusin, L. M., Singer, C., Valenti, A. J., and Armstrong, D.: Infectious syphilis mimicking neoplastic disease. Arch Intern Med 137:156, 1977.

Duncan, W. C., Knox, J. M., and Wende, R. D.: The FTA-ABS test in dark-field-positive primary syphilis. JAMA 228:859, 1974.
Dunlop, E. M. C.: Persistence of treponemes after treatment. Brit Med J 2:577, 1972.
Feher, J., Somogyi, T., Timmer, M., and Jozsa, L.: Early syphilitic hepatitis. Lancet 2:896, 1975.
Fiumara, N. J.: The treatment of seropositive primary syphilis—an evaluation of 196 patients. Sex Transm Dis 4:92, 1977.
Fulford, K. W. M., Johnson, N., Loveday, C., Storey, J., and Tedder, R. S.: Changes in intra-vascular complement and anti-treponemal antibody titres preceding the Jarisch-Herxheimer reaction in secondary syphilis. Clin Exp Immunol 24:483, 1976.
Grabau, W., Emanuel, R., Ross, D., Parker, J., and Hedge, M.: Syphilitic aortic regurgitation. An appraisal of surgical treatment. Brit J Vener Dis 52:366, 1976.
Harter, C. A., and Benirschke, K.: Fetal syphilis in the first trimester. Am J Obstet Gynecol 124:705, 1976.
Hager, W. D.: Transplacental transmission of spirochetes in congenital syphilis: a new perspective. Sex Transm Dis 5:122, 1978.
Heggtveit, H. A.: Syphilitic aortitis. A clinicopathologic autopsy study of 100 cases, 1950 to 1960. Circulation 29:346, 1964.
Ingall, D., and Musher, D. M.: Syphilis. In Remington, J. S., and Klein, J. O. (eds): Infectious Diseases of the Fetus and Newborn Infant, Second Edition, Philadelphia, W. B. Saunders Co., 1983, pp. 335-374.
Kampmeier, R. H.: The late manifestations of syphilis: skeletal, visceral, and cardiovascular. Med Clin North Amer 48:667, 1964.
Olansky, S.: Late benign syphilis (gumma). Med Clin North Amer 48:653, 1964.
Schell, R. F., and Musher, D. M. (eds): Pathogenesis and Immunology of Treponemal Infection. New York, Marcel Dekker, 1983.
Stokes, J. H., Bearman, H., Ingraham, N. R.: Modern Clinical Syphilology. W. B. Saunders, Philadelphia, 1945.
Tramont, E. C.: Persistence of *Treponema pallidum* following penicillin G therapy. Report of two cases. JAMA 236:2206, 1976.
Young, E. J., Weingarten, N., Baughn, R. E., Duncan, W. C.: Studies on the pathogenesis of the Jarisch-Herxheimer reaction: development of an animal model and evidence against a role for classical endotoxin. J Infect Dis 146:606, 1982.

200

EPIDEMIC (LOUSE-BORNE) TYPHUS

R. Brezina, M.D.

Epidemic typhus is an acute infectious disease that is caused by *Rickettsia prowazekii* and transmitted from man to man by the human body louse, *Pediculus humanus corporis*. It is characterized clinically by a high fever, severe encephalitis, and a generalized macular or papular rash. The overall case fatality of untreated patients ranges from 8 to 40 per cent. Fever lasting for 14 to 18 days subsides by lysis. Antibiotic therapy shortens the disease dramatically and substantially reduces its lethality. Clinical recovery from typhus is accompanied by development of solid immunity to reinfection, but a few rickettsiae may persist in the tissues. Relapse of disease caused by these persisting organisms may occur decades after the primary infection (Brill-Zinsser disease).

Epidemic typhus is the only rickettsial disease that has the potential for explosive epidemics in man. In the past, outbreaks of epidemic typhus have been associated with major historical events such as wars, famines, and large migrations of populations. It still represents a serious public health problem in some countries (Tarizzo, 1978). In 1975, 10,548 cases of epidemic typhus with 146 deaths were reported to the World Health Organization. Its highest prevalence is in the developing countries of Africa (Rwanda, Burundi, Ethiopia, Uganda, Zaire) and, to a lesser extent, of Latin America (Peru, Bolivia, Ecuador, Mexico) and Asia (Afghanistan). This geographic distribution is related to the high level of louse infestation caused by low socioeconomic standards, lack of education, and climate. The high incidence of primary cases creates a reservoir of possible cases of Brill-Zinsser disease. These cases can serve as the source for future outbreaks of epidemic typhus if the population is infested with lice. Furthermore, individuals who had typhus during World War II and now live in countries without a focus of primary epidemic typhus may develop Brill-Zinsser disease.

ETIOLOGY. *Rickettsia prowazekii* is antigenically similar to *Rickettsia typhi* and *Rickettsia canada*. Under natural conditions, it multiplies in the epithelium of the louse gut. Lice succumb to this infection within one to four weeks. *R. prowazekii* is excreted in the feces of infected lice four to five days after infection and may remain infectious, depending on the environmental temperature, for up to six months. Feces of infected lice infect human beings when driven into the skin by the process of scratching. Transmission is accomplished mainly by *Pediculus humanus corporis* (the body louse), but *Pediculus humanus capitis* (the head louse) may also be a vector. Lice can be infected experimentally via the rectum. Fleas are also susceptible to experimental infection. The existence of an extrahuman reservoir was demonstrated by Bozeman et al. (1975, 1977) who recovered several strains of *R. prowazekii* from flying squirrels (*Glaucomys volans volans*) in Virginia and Florida. The agent was also detected in fleas and lice (possible natural vectors) removed from these animals (Bozeman et al., 1978; Sonenshine et al., 1978). Human infections in the eastern United States were described by McDade et al. (1980) and Duma et al. (1981).

R. prowazekii forms short rods 0.3 to 0.7 μm by 0.8 to 2.0 μm. It multiplies well in the yolk sac of chick embryos, in chick embryo cell culture, and in established lines such as mouse lymphoblasts, mouse L cells, or monkey kidney cells. The growth is restricted to the cytoplasm of the cells. The organism is unstable outside of the cells but remains viable for several years at -70° C. It contains a hemolysin and toxin that kills mice within 24 hours after intravenous administration. Both the toxin and the hemolytin are firmly bound to viable rickettsiae.

The two major antigenic components of *R. prowazekii* are a heat-stable, soluble, group-specific antigen and a heat-labile, species-specific antigen. The group antigen, released in the aqueous phase after ether treatment, is identical to that of *R. typhi*. The species-specific antigen, which remains after thorough washing of *R. prowazekii*, distinguishes *R. prowazekii* from *R. typhi*. Recently major species-specific protein antigens of *R. prowazekii* and *R. typhi* were prepared and identified by rocket immunoelectrophoresis (Dash, 1981; et al., 1981). The common polysaccharide antigen shared with *Proteus vulgaris* strain OX 19 explains the agglutinability of the sera of acute epidemic typhus patients in the Weil-Felix reaction. Sera of patients with Brill-Zinsser disease are Weil-Felix negative. The guanine plus cytosine (G + C) content of *R. prowazekii* DNA is approximately 30 moles per cent.

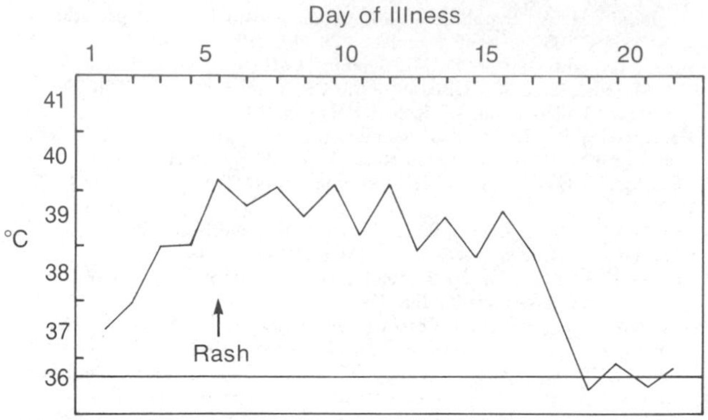

Figure 1. The temperature curve in an epidemic typhus patient untreated with antibiotics.

The guinea pig is highly susceptible to infection and is commonly used for primary isolation. The highest titers of rickettsiae are in the brain and spleen. Mice are killed by the toxin of *R. prowazekii.* The cotton rat, *Sigmodon hispidus*, is as susceptible to infection as the chick embryo. Although mice are not susceptible to intraperitoneal infection, *R. prowazekii* can be adapted to growth in the mouse lung after serial intranasal passage.

PATHOGENSIS AND PATHOLOGY. Infection is established by forcing infected louse feces into the skin by scratching. In rare instances, infection may be acquired by pulmonary inhalation or conjunctival absorption of airborne suspensions of the organisms. Rickettsiae may circulate in the blood well before the onset of clinical disease. During rickettsemia, organisms penetrate the endothelium of small vessels, principally those of the skin, brain, heart, and kidneys. Rickettsial growth results in cell destruction, endovasculitis, thrombosis, and hemorrhage. So-called Fraenkel's nodules consisting of accumulations of polymorphonuclear leukocytes, macrophages, and lymphoid cells are located perivascularly. In addition to the vascular lesions of the skin, necropsy reveals interstitial pneumonitis and mononuclear infiltration of the myocardium. Panencephalitis may dominate the clinical picture of epidemic typhus. Histologically, the encephalitis is also perivascular. Experimentally, the toxin of *R. prowazekii* seems to cause some of the histopathology by increasing capillary permeability, resulting in the loss of plasma and hemoconcentration. Toxic vascular damage may lead to intravascular coagulation and peripheral vascular collapse, which is the principal cause of death.

CLINICAL MANIFESTATIONS. The incubation period of epidemic typhus ranges from 5 to 23 days, with an average of 11 days. Usually, clinical illness begins abruptly with chills, fever, malaise, headache, weakness, backache, and generalized myalgia. Vomiting and vertigo are infrequent at the onset of the disease. During the first two or three days the temperature fluctuates from normal to 39° C, and afterwards remains at 39° to 40° C, until death or recovery of the patient (Fig. 1). Conjunctivitis with photophobia, orbital pain aggravated by pressure or ocular movement, and flushing of the face and the neck are common. Headache increases in severity and may be either generalized or most severe in the frontal region. Coughing and vomiting increase. Constipation or, less commonly, diarrhea may occur.

The appearance of a characteristic, generalized eruption, usually between the fifth and ninth days, is accompanied by progressive central nervous system (CNS) involvement. The rash, which is first apparent on the lateral chest, spreads first to the abdomen and during the next one to two days to the entire body, except the face, palms, and soles (Fig. 2). At first the skin lesions are separate macules or maculopapules about the size of a pinhead or a lentil (2 to 4 mm in diameter) that blanch on pressure. Later on they fail to blanch, become purpuric, and form groups but do not become confluent. In some instances, there may be a transient marbled appearance of the skin before the onset of the rash. The exanthem is usually visible for 10 to 12 days, at which time it begins to change to a brown color. Desquamation occurs during convalescence.

At the end of the first week meningoencephalitis begins to dominate the clinical picture. Manifestations include psychosis, meningismus, Kernig's and Brudzinski's signs, and hyperesthesia. The second and third weeks of illness are the critical period.

Dysphagia, inability to eat and drink without assistance, and prostration develop during this stage. Stupor or coma may be interrupted by episodes of delirium and violence, which tend to subside into apathy. Catalepsy, muscle stiffness, aphasia, and hemianopsia signify diffuse brain damage. Extrapyramidal symptoms include tremor, choreiform movements, and myoclonus. Splenomegaly, cough and tachypnea, and myocarditis complete the picture of the critical period of illness. Tachycardia, hypotension, and gangrene of the toes, feet, tips of fingers, ear lobes, nose, penis, scrotum, or vulva may occur in severe cases.

Albuminuria, microhematuria, and casts are common.

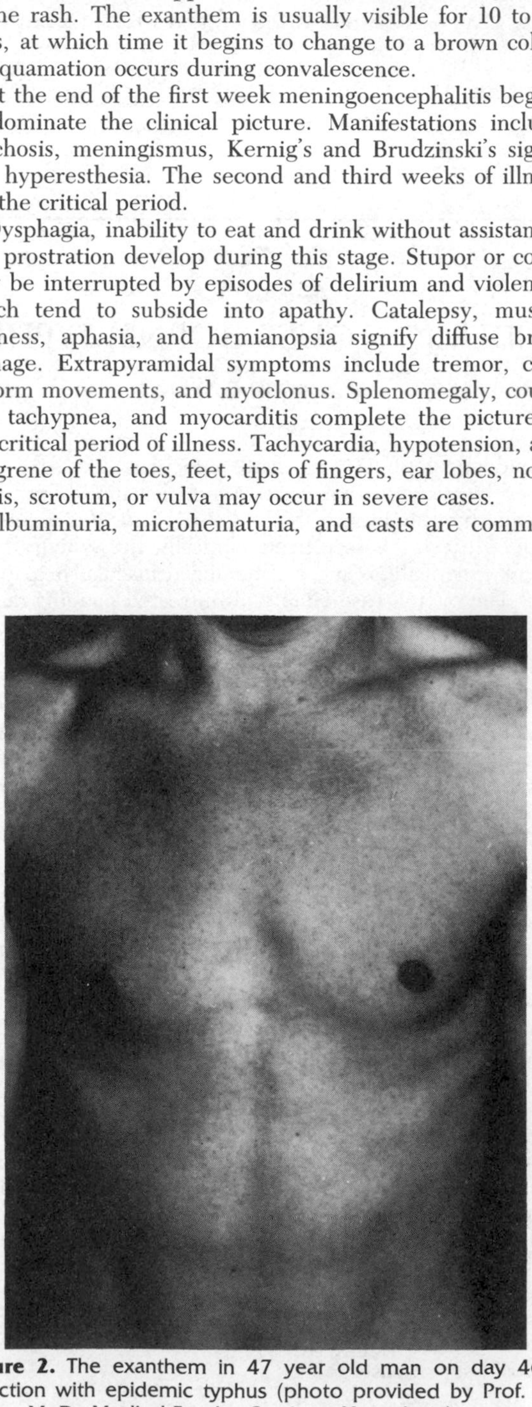

Figure 2. The exanthem in 47 year old man on day 46 of infection with epidemic typhus (photo provided by Prof. J. A. Gaon, M. D., Medical Faculty, Sarajevo, Yugoslavia).

Oliguria and azotemia are signs of fulminating, preterminal disease.

The white blood count is normal or low in the first week of illness and slightly elevated later on. The decrease in red blood cell count is accompanied by a corresponding reduction of hemoglobin. Toward the end of the first week, the serum albumin is reduced and the serum globulin increased. Increased protein and pleocytosis may be found in the spinal fluid.

In fatal cases, the terminal period is characterized by uremia, stupor, and coma. Death from epidemic typhus is caused by peripheral vascular collapse or by complications such as pneumonia. If a patient recovers, the fever generally subsides by rapid lysis in the third week of the illness. Recovery from severe encephalitis is not so rapid and the patient may be irritable or apathetic for a prolonged period. Full strength and normal mental and physical activity are regained in two or three months.

COMPLICATIONS AND SEQUELAE. Pneumonia is one of the most important complications of epidemic typhus. Bronchopneumonia during the first week is usually of rickettsial origin. About 10 per cent of patients develop bacterial pneumonia in the third or fourth week of the disease. It may be accompanied by leukocytosis, pleuritis, and empyema. Purulent tonsillitis, otitis, parotitis, and pharyngitis are the other common bacterial complications. Thrombosis, thrombophlebitis, and gangrene are caused by the classic vascular lesions of epidemic typhus.

Serious sequelae are rare, despite extensive involvement of the central nervous system, myocardium, and kidneys during the acute stage. The most important sequelae are disturbances of the central nervous system, including deformation and enlargement of the third ventricle (Mohr et al., 1972), personality changes, impairment of mental function, epilepsy, and disorders of the cranial nerves and extrapyramidal system.

Brill-Zinsser Disease

Brill-Zinsser disease is recurrent epidemic typhus that appears from 4 to 50 years after the primary attack. Its clinical features are the same as those of classic epidemic typhus but with lower intensity, shorter duration, infrequent complications, and only an exceptional fatality (Fig. 3). Rickettsemia is shorter and rashes are infrequent. Although recrudescence is known to be caused by rickettsiae that persist in lymph nodes, the factors that precipitate Brill-Zinsser disease are unknown. Intercurrent diseases such as paratyphoid fever, common cold, influenza, bacillary dysentery, sunstroke, and leptospirosis preceded Brill-Zinsser disease in a recent study in East Slovakia (Mittermayer, 1978).

Cases of Brill-Zinsser disease are important from the standpoint of epidemic typhus control because they represent a potential reservoir of epidemic typhus in louse-infested populations. Brill-Zinsser disease can occur in any country with European immigrants who developed the primary attack during World War II or shortly afterwards. Otherwise, the geographic distribution of Brill-Zinsser disease is associated with the distribution of typhus epidemics in the past. Brill-Zinsser disease is not of public health significance in countries where lice are uncommon.

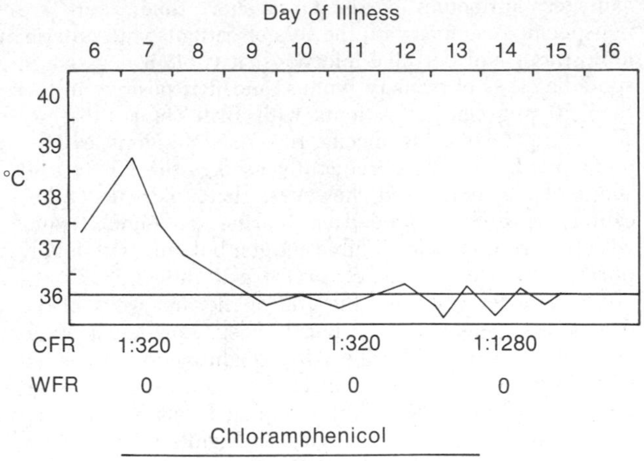

Figure 3. The temperature curve and antibody response in a patient suffering from Brill-Zinsser disease (with permission of Prof. J. A. Gaon, M.D., Medical Faculty, Sarajevo, Yugoslavia).

GEOGRAPHIC VARIATIONS IN DISEASE. There are no known geographic variations in antigenic properties or virulence of wild strains of *R. prowazekii*. Variations in the severity of disease depend more on the quality of care provided to the patient. Because of improvement in care during World War II, the mortality dropped below 8 per cent. Under peaceful conditions, the mortality in treated sporadic cases may be less than 1 per cent.

DIAGNOSIS. The clinical diagnosis is not difficult during epidemics or in areas with a high prevalence of epidemic typhus. It is based on the typical rash, unremitting high fever, headache, and other signs of CNS involvement. In contrast, the clinical diagnosis of Brill-Zinsser disease is difficult and depends on a careful history. The differential diagnosis of epidemic typhus includes other rickettsioses, relapsing fever, smallpox, malaria, measles, and yellow fever.

The definitive diagnosis is made in the laboratory either by isolation of *R. prowazekii* or by a rising, specific serologic tests.

Isolation. *R. prowazekii* can be isolated during rickettsemia by inoculating a suspension of clotted blood intraperitoneally into guinea pigs or the yolk sac of the chick embryo. Several blind passages may be necessary to isolate *R. prowazekii* in the yolk sac. Guinea pigs develop a mild febrile disease after an incubation period that varies directly with the number of rickettsiae in the inoculum. Rickettsiae can be harvested from the guinea pig brain or spleen by inoculation into yolk sacs. As early as the end of the first week after intraperitoneal inoculation, guinea pigs develop specific antibodies detectable by complement fixation (CF) or agglutination tests. Rickettsiae in the patient's blood can also be demonstrated by xenodiagnosis, in which clean, hungry lice are allowed to feed on the patient. After three to four days rickettsiae are detected in the louse gut by immunofluorescence or by injection and isolation in laboratory animals.

Serology. An increase in the titer of antibodies to *R. prowazekii* in paired, acute, and convalescent sera can be sought by several techniques. The Weil-Felix reaction for agglutinins against *Proteus vulgaris* OX 19, which starts to be positive from the fifth to eighth day, has many disadvantages: antibodies persist for a short time, there are nonspecific reactions with the sera of patients with enteric, leptospiral, and borrelial infections, it is often negative in sporadic cases of primary typhus, and it is positive in less than 20 per cent of patients with Brill-Zinsser disease. Therefore, tests using specific rickettsial antigens are recommended. The most frequently used is the CF test. It should be remembered, however, that epidemic typhus cannot be differentiated from murine (endemic) typhus with the group-specific soluble antigen but only with highly purified, species-specific *R. prowazekii* antigen. CF antibodies are detectable by the end of the first week of the disease and peak about the fourth week. Low levels of CF antibody may persist for life. Microagglutination of washed suspensions of purified rickettsiae is as sensitive as the CF test (Fiset et al., 1969). Passive hemagglutination of sheep or human O group erythrocytes or agglutination of latex particles (Hechemy et al., 1981) sensitized with boiled, alkaline-treated rickettsiae is positive only through early convalescence and does not differentiate epidemic from murine typhus. An indirect microimmunofluorescence test (Philip et al., 1976), which determines the class of antibody made by the patient, is said to differentiate primary epidemic typhus from Brill-Zinsser disease (Ormsbee et al., 1977). Since patients with early epidemic typhus make predominantly IgM antibodies and those with Brill-Zinsser disease make IgG, differentiation by heating sera or treatment with mercaptoethanol (Ormsbee et al., 1977) is also possible.

In all these serologic tests, the possibility of cross-reactivity, not only with the typhus group rickettsiae but also with the spotted fever group (Ormsbee et al., 1977) should be taken into consideration. The specificity of serologic tests may differ in individual situations; for example, the sera of patients convalescent from epidemic typhus usually reacts with *R. canada* (see Chapter 54) in the CF and immunofluorescence tests, but only slightly or not at all in the microagglutination reaction (Urvölgyi, 1978). Recently the ELISA proved to be a highly sensitive and reliable test for detection of the human serological response to typhus antigens (Halle and Dash, 1980).

TREATMENT. Chloramphenicol and tetracycline are the only effective specific treatments for epidemic typhus. The first dose, depending on the weight of the patient, is 2 to 3 g, followed by 1 to 2 g/day, in four divided doses. Although patients become afebrile within two to three days, the antibiotic should be continued for several days after the temperature becomes normal to avoid relapses. Doxycycline, an antibiotic from the tetracycline series that persists in the blood and tissues for prolonged periods, has been effective in a single 100- to 200-mg dose (Wisseman, 1973; Huys et al., 1973). Antibiotics dramatically shorten the duration of the disease and reduce lethality practically to zero. Because they are rickettsiostatic but not rickettsiocidal, they do not affect rickettsial persistence and the possibility of recrudescent typhus.

Symptomatic therapy is aimed at relief of headache and delirium, maintenance of fluid balance, and circulatory support. Oral hygiene, skin care, and maintenance of bowel function are also important in severely ill patients.

PROPHYLAXIS. Epidemic typhus can be prevented either by control of lice with insecticides or by human vaccination.

Depending on the circumstances, one or more of the following vector control techniques may be used effectively; (1) delousing of all contacts of a typhus patient; (2) delousing of small focal populations; and (3) mass delousing. Ultimately, effective louse control depends upon education and improvement of the standard of living in developing countries.

Resistance of lice to commonly used insecticides of the DDT, lindane, and malathion groups has been demonstrated in various areas. Resistance is usually related to the use of specific insecticides as agricultural pesticides over long periods. Other insecticides found effective against body lice are 2 per cent temephos, 5 per cent carbaryl, 1 per cent propoxur and the synthetic pyrethroid, permethrin (1 per cent powder). The use of juvenile hormones as insecticides is experimental.

Typhus fever vaccines have been used widely and extensively, but only limited information on the effectiveness of the standard formalin inactivated vaccine is available. Furthermore, commercially produced killed vaccines are not tested and standardized properly. A killed yolk-sac vaccine, used extensively during World War II, either prevented disease or greatly reduced its severity. An attenuated strain of *R. prowazekii* (Madrid E strain) has been tested experimentally by many investigators. A single dose of this live vaccine prevents disease under epidemic conditions and changes the antibody profile of a population enough to break the transmission cycle (Wisseman, 1978). The most important question at this time about the usefulness of the E strain as a vaccine is whether the attenuation is stable. Some experimental data by Soviet and Slovak investigators suggest that under appropriate selective conditions the E strain can revert to virulence. Despite this fact, live E vaccine could be administered to a population that was at very high risk of an epidemic (Wisseman, 1978).

References

Bozeman, F. M., Masiello, S. A., Williams, M. S., and Elisberg, B. L.: Epidemic typhus rickettsiae isolated from flying squirrels. Nature (London) 255:545, 1975.

Bozeman, F. M., Williams, M. S., Stocks, N. I., Chadwick, D. P., Elisberg, B. L., Sonenshine, D. E., and Lauer, D. M.: Ecologic studies on epidemic typhus infection in the southern squirrel. In Kazar, J (ed): Proceedings of the Second International Symposium on Rickettsiae and Rickettsial Diseases. Bratislava, Veda, Publishing House of Slovak Academy of Sciences, 1978.

Dash, G. A.: Isolation of species-specific protein antigens of *Rickettsia typhi* and *Rickettsia prowazekii* for immunodiagnosis and immunoprophylaxis. J Clin Microbiol 14:333, 1981.

Duma, R. J., Sonenshine, D. E., Bozeman, F. M., Veazey, J. M., Elisberg, B. L., Chadwick, D. P., Stocks, N. I., McGill, T. M., Miller, G. B., MacCormack, J. N.: Epidemic typhus in the United States associated with flying squirrels. J Am Med Ass 245:2318, 1981.

Fiset, P., Ormsbee, R. A., Silberman, R., Peacock, M., and Spielman, S. H.: A microagglutination technique for detection and measurement of ricksettsial antibodies. Acta Virol 13:60, 1969.

Halle, S., Dash, G. A.: Use of a microplate enzyme-linked immunosorbent assay in a retrospective serological analysis of a laboratory population at risk to infection with typhus group rickettsiae. J Clin Microbiol 12:343, 1980.

Hechemy, K. E., Osterman, J. V., Eiseman, C. S., Elliot, L. B., Sasowski, S. J.: Detection of typhus antibodies by latex agglutination. J Clin Microbiol 13:214, 1981.

Huys, J., Kayhigi, J., Freyens, P., and Vanden Berge, G.: Single-dose treatment of epidemic typhus with doxycycline. Chemotherapy 18:314, 1973.

McDade, J. E., Shepard, C. C., Redus, M. A., Newhouse, V. F., Smith, V. F.: Evidence of R. prowazekii infections in the United States. Am J Trop Med Hyg 29:227, 1980.

Mittermayer, T.: Intercurrent diseases as possible provocative factors of Brill-Zinsser disease. In Kázar, J., Ormsbee, R. A., and Tarasevich, I. V. (eds.): Rickettsiae and Rickettsial Diseases. Bratislava, Veda, Publishing House of Slovak Academy of Sciences, 1978, p. 465.
Mohr, W. Weyer, F., and Asshauer, E.: Klassisches Fleckfieber. In Gsell, O., and Mohr, W. (eds.): Infektionskrankheiten. Bd. IV. Berlin, Springer-Verlag, 1972, p. 23.
Ormsbee, R.A., Peacock, M., Philip, R., Casper, E., Plorde, J., Gabre-Kindan, T., and Wright, L.: Serologic diagnosis of epidemic typhus. Am J Epidemiol 105:261, 1977.
Philip, R. M., Caster, E. A., and Ormsbee, R. A.: Microimmunofluorescence test for the serological study of Rocky Mountain spotted fever and typhus. J Clin Microbiol 3:51, 1976.
Sonenshine, D. E., Bozeman, F. M., Williams, M. S., Masiello, S. A., Chadwick, D. P., Stocks, N. I., Lauer, D. M., and Elisberg, B. L.: Epizootology of epidemic typhus (Rickettsia prowazeki) in flying squirrels. Am J Trop Med Hyg 27:339, 1978.
Tarizzo, M. L.: Public health significance of rickettsial diseases. In Kázar, J., Ormsbee, R. A., and Tarasevich, I. V. (eds.): Rickettsiae and Rickettsial Diseases. Bratislava, Veda, Publishing House of Slovak Academy of Sciences, 1978, p. 539.
Urvölgyi, J.: New achievements in serological diagnosis of rickettsial diseases. In Kázar, J., Ormsbee, R. A., and Tarasevich, I. V. (eds.): Rickettsiae and Rickettsial Diseases. Bratislava, Veda, Publishing House of Slovak Academy of Sciences, 1978, p. 361.
Wisseman, C., Jr.: Concepts of typhus control and factors influencing choice of methods. In Proceedings of the Symposium on the control of lice and louse-borne diseases, Washington, D.C., 4–6December 1972. Washington, D.C., Pan American Health Organization, 1973, p. 267.
Wisseman, C., Jr.: Prevention and control of rickettsial diseases, with emphasis on immunoprophylaxis. In Kázar, J., Ormsbee, R. A., and Tarasevich, I. V. (eds.): Rickettsiae and Rickettsial Diseases. Bratislava, Veda, Publishing House of Slovak Academy of Sciences, 1978, p. 553.

201

ENDEMIC (MURINE) TYPHUS

R. BREZINA, M.D.

Endemic flea-borne (murine) typhus is an acute febrile disease caused by *Rickettsia typhi*, which is transmitted to man by the rat flea (*Xenopsylla cheopis*). The reservoir of this zoonosis is rats and mice. Man is an accidental victim who breaks the usual rat-flea-rat cycle. Clinically, endemic typhus resembles a mild form of epidemic typhus (Chapter 200). The mortality is negligible, and late recrudescence (Brill-Zinsser disease) is unknown. Infection stimulates solid immunity, not only to endemic, but also to epidemic typhus.

ETIOLOGY. *R. typhi* belongs to the typhus group (biotype) of rickettsia (see Chapter 54). This group also includes *R. prowazekii* (epidemic typhus) and *R. canada*, a recently described rickettsia that has not yet been definitely associated with human disease. *R. typhi* is very closely related to *R. prowazekii*. They share a common, thermostable, soluble antigen and another common antigen with *Proteus vulgaris* OX19. They can be separated in complement fixation tests by antisera against a species-specific, cell-associated antigen obtained by repeated washing of the rickettsiae. They can also be differentiated by cross challenges of vaccinated guinea pigs or by mouse toxin neutralization tests. Recently Dash et al. (1981) found that the two typhus agents can be differentiated in rocket immunoelectrophoresis by using species-specific protein antigens solubilized by French pressure cell extraction or sonication of rickettsiae purified in a Renografin density gradient. The guanine plus cystosine content of the DNA in *R. typhi* is approximately 30 moles per cent, similar to that of *R. prowazekii*. *R. typhi* is slightly more sensitive to environmental effects than *R. prowazekii*, but it can persist in flea feces for two weeks at normal humidity and room temperature, and for four months at 4° C. It grows well in the yolk sac of the chick embryo. *R. typhi* is more virulent for the guinea pig than *R. prowazekii*. In addition to fever, it causes scrotal erythema and swelling. Adhesions develop between the testes and the tunica vaginalis so that the testes cannot be pushed up into the abdomen (Neill-Mooser reaction). The mesothelial cells of the tunica vaginalis are packed with masses of rickettsiae (Mooser's cells). White rats and mice are also highly susceptible to intraperitoneal infection and develop peritonitis with abundant rickettsiae in the peritoneal exudate. Mice die between the third and eighth days. White rats survive the infection, but *R. typhi* may persist in their brains for as long as 380 days.

The rat flea, *Xenopsylla cheopis*, is the classic vector for the transmission of the organisms from rat to rat and from rat to man. It contracts *R. typhi* by feeding on an acutely infected rat. Rickettsiae multiply in the epithelium of the gut and are shed in the feces of the flea throughout its life. Man can be infected by scratching and driving infected feces into the skin, by inhalation, by conjunctival absorption of airborne rickettsiae, or by ingestion of contaminated food. *R typhi* multiplies in the human flea (*Pulex irritans*), the human body louse (*Pediculus humanis corporis*), and the rat louse (*Polyplax spinulosa*). *Xenopsylla brasiliensis* is thought to be a vector of *R. typhi* in Kenya. In the United States, infected cat fleas (*Ctenocephalides felis*) have been found. In Java, *R. typhi* was isolated from a trombiculid mite, and in India from a tick (*Boophilus annulatus*).

Rats (*Rattus norvegicus* and *Rattus rattus*) are the primary reservoir of the organism. Mice can also be infected, but they are not as important a reservoir as rats. The small mammalian hosts and vectors may vary from one locality to another.

PATHOGENESIS AND PATHOLOGY. The pathogenesis and pathology of endemic typhus is identical to that of epidemic typhus (Chapter 200). Rickettsemia occurs during the febrile phase of infection, and rickettsiae penetrate and multiply in the endothelium of small vessels, causing vascular damage and necrosis. The pathologic findings in experimentally infected laboratory animals and in the brains of human beings at postmortem are identical to those of epidemic typhus. It is difficult to explain the mild clinical course of endemic typhus, since the pathogenesis and pathology of the diseases are so similar. Some investigators feel that the toxin of *R. prowazekii* is more potent than that of *R. typhi*.

CLINICAL MANIFESTATIONS, COMPLICATIONS, AND SEQUELAE. The incubation period of endemic typhus varies from 4 to 15 days. The onset is sudden, but the course of the illness is more gradual than in epidemic typhus. Fever rises by steps; it may drop to normal and rise again to 40.0° C. Later in the illness, it is still remittent and varies from 38.5 to 40.0° C. In about half the cases, the rash appears first on the abdomen and spreads to the chest, back, and upper extremities. Small papules and macules are replaced later by poorly delineated roseolae. Compared with epidemic typhus, the rash is shorter in duration, skin lesions are less numerous, and petechiae are very uncommon.

Conjunctivitis may occur early in the disease. Headache and arthralgia persist throughout the course. Involvement of the central nervous system, myocardium, kidneys, and liver are less frequent and substantially less severe. The white and red blood cell counts are normal. The sedimentation rate and the concentration of serum proteins are increased.

Fever terminates by lysis after 9 to 14 days. Complications, such as thrombosis, thrombophlebitis, gangrene, azotemia, and bronchopneumonia, are infrequent. Mortality in untreated patients is about 2 per cent. Recovery is prompt without sequelae and is followed by solid immunity to *R. typhi* and cross-immunity to epidemic typhus. Clinical relapses have occurred in patients treated with a short course of antibiotics early in the disease (Wisseman et al., 1962). Spontaneous late relapse (Brill-Zinsser disease) has not been described in murine typhus.

GEOGRAPHIC VAIRATIONS. The disease has wide distribution over the world, and its importance as a human disease is probably grossly underestimated. Serosurveys of human and rat populations in tropical and subtropical urban centers suggest that this disease occurs more frequently than recognized.

DIAGNOSIS. Endemic (murine) typhus cannot be clinically distinguished from epidemic typhus. It can also be confused with spotted fevers (Chapters 203 and 204) that occur in the same geographic areas. In endemic typhus the rash appears first on the body and spreads to the extremities; in spotted fevers the reverse is true, and the rash tends to become petechial and hemorrhagic. The incidence of the diseases in a particular area, exposure to rats, the presence of lice and the absence of the typical primary lesions of the spotted fevers may help to establish the diagnosis of endemic typhus. Viral exanthems and drug eruptions must be ruled out.

The definitive diagnosis can be made only in the laboratory by isolation of the agent or specific serologic changes. *R. typhi* can be isolated by inoculating the patient's blood into the peritoneal cavity of guinea pigs or white rats. Infected animals develop fever and scrotal swelling. Rickettsiae are easily discernible in the cells of the tunica vaginalis stained by the Giemsa, Macchiavello, or Gimenez methods. Similarly, after intraperitoneal inoculation of mice, abundant *R. typhi* can be detected in stained preparations from the peritoneal exudate. It is also possible to isolate *R. typhi* by inoculating infected blood into the chick embryo yolk sac.

Cross-reactive antibodies against *Proteus vulgaris* OX 19 (the Weil-Felix reaction) develop by the fourth day of the disease with a peak around the tenth day, but there are substantially lower antibody levels than in epidemic typhus. The complement fixation test and microagglutination reaction (Fiset et al., 1969) are the serologic methods of choice, however. The common soluble antigen shared with *R. prowazekii* makes it impossible to distinguish endemic typhus from epidemic typhus by the complement fixation test, but extensively washed rickettsial suspensions possess species-specificity in the microagglutination reaction. Endemic typhus can also be differentiated from epidemic typhus by the mouse-toxin neutralization test. As with *R. prowazekii* (Chapter 200) antibodies to *R. typhi* can be detected by the immunofluorescence test in either its macro- or micromodification (Goldwasser et al., 1959; Philip et al., 1976; Ormsbee et al., 1977). Serologic diagnosis is difficult in patients who have been vaccinated against epidemic typhus. The relative antibody titers against *R. prowazekii* and *R. typhi* may or may not be helpful. The microagglutination test with washed suspensions of *R. typhi* may be definitive if the titer rises.

TREATMENT. Treatment of endemic (murine) typhus is the same as that of epidemic typhus. Treatment with a tetracycline should be continued for at least ten days after the onset of symptoms and for 48 hours after the patient becomes afebrile in order to prevent relapses. A single dose of 200 mg of doxycycline may also be effective against endemic typhus.

PROPHYLAXIS. Since commensal rats and their ectoparasites are the main reservoirs and vectors of endemic typhus, prophylaxis should be directed at their elimination or control. To avoid temporary increases in human cases, rodent control measures (poisoning) should be delayed until the flea population has been reduced. The most suitable preparation for the elimination of fleas is 10 per cent DDT. Because of its residual effect, this insecticide needs to be used only once a year.

Vaccines prepared from killed *R. typhi* probably do not protect against *R. prowazekii.* Because of the mild course of endemic typhus and its rapid response to antibiotic therapy, vaccination against endemic typhus only is not necessary.

References

Dash, G. A., Samms, J. R., and Williams, J. C.: Partial purification and characterization of the major species-specific protein antigens of *Rickettsia typhi* and *Rickettsia prowazekii* identified by rocket immunoeleletrophoresis. Infection and Immunity, 31:276, 1981.

Fiset, P., Ormsbee, R. A., Silberman, R., Peacock, M., and Spielman, S. H.: A microagglutination technique for detection and measurement of rickettsial antibodies. Acta Virol 13:60, 1969.

Goldwasser, R. A., Shepard, C. C., Jordan, M. E., and Fox, F. P.: The specificity of antibody response in typhus fever. Its alteration during murine typhus infection as a result of previous exposure to epidemic typhus antigen. J Immunol 83:491, 1959.

Ormsbee, R. A., Peacock, M., Philip, R., Casper, E., Plorde, J., Gabre-Kindan, T., and Wright, L.: Serologic diagnosis of epidemic typhus. Am J Epidemiol 105:261, 1977.

Philip, R. N., Casper, E. A., and Ormsbee, R. A.: Microimmunofluorescence test for the serological study of Rocky Mountain spotted fever and typhus. J Clin Microbiol 3:51, 1976.

Wisseman, C. L., Jr., Wood, W. H., Jr., Noriega, A. R., Jordan, M. E., and Rill, D. J.: Antibodies and clinical relapse of murine typhus fever following early chemotherapy. Ann Intern Med 57:743, 1962.

202
SCRUB TYPHUS

GARRISON RAPMUND, M.D.

DEFINITION. Scrub typhus (Tsutsugamushi disease, mite-borne typhus, chigger-borne rickettsiosis) is characterized by a primary cutaneous lesion or eschar, fever, and rash. It is caused by *Rickettsia tsutsugamushi*, which is transmitted to man by certain larval trombiculid mites called chiggers. The disease occurs throughout Asia and the western Pacific region, reflecting the distribution of vector chiggers. Death can occur, but many infections are mild or inapparent. The immunologic heterogeneity of scrub typhus rickettsiae may explain reinfection.

HISTORY. The disease first appeared in Western medical literature in 1879 but was known earlier in Chinese and Japanese writings. Long after 1879 the only known foci of disease were along rivers in three prefectures of northwestern Honshu Island, Japan. Disease occurred in farmers who entered low-lying grasslands to plant crops after the spring floods had subsided, hence the early name Japanese flood fever. The red larval mite called akamushi (red mite) was plentiful and was assumed to be the vector of disease. In 1920 Hayashi isolated from patients an organism that he called *tsutsugamushi*, meaning noxious mite, but this was probably not the disease agent. Nagayo and coworkers in 1930 isolated a rickettsia-like agent from patients and called it *Rickettsia orientalis*, the name still commonly used in Japan. Ogata shortly thereafter isolated a similar organism from patients. He called the agent *Rickettsia tsutsugamushi*, which has become the name commonly used outside Japan (Blake et al., 1945).

Scrub typhus was first recognized outside Japan in Formosa by Hatori in 1915 in persons who collected camphor in forests. At about the same time it was recognized in northern Sumatra by Schuffner, in Malaya by Dowden, in northern Queensland by Breinl and co-workers, and in Indochina by Lagrange. In the early 1920s in Malaya, Fletcher, Lesslar, and Lewthwaite distinguished shop typhus in town dwellers from rural typhus in plantation workers. Rural typhus was similar to tsutsugamushi disease in Japan but milder. Rural typhus patients developed agglutinins to the OX-K strain of *Proteus* but not to the X-19 strain, which was agglutinated by sera from patients with shop typhus. Rural typhus occurred in laborers and European planters who worked in terrain covered with mixed grass and low shrub vegetation, loosely referred to as scrub, hence the name scrub typhus. Scrub typhus has become the predominant name in Western literature, while in Japan it remains tsutsugamushi disease. Cross-immunity experiments in animals have proved that rural typhus in Malaya and the disease in Sumatra and Japan are caused by the same organism (Blake et al., 1945).

The role of the red mite *Leptotrombidium akamushi* as a vector was established after *R. tsutsugamushi* was isolated from this mite. Its prevalence in hyperendemic foci corresponds to the incidence of disease; it transmits the disease to a monkey by feeding; its ability to infect man has been confirmed; and its principal natural host, the field vole, *Microtus montebelli*, has been shown to be infected with *R. tsutsugamushi*. The life cycle of *L. akamushi* has been established and shows that only the larval stage feeds on vertebrates. Other larval mites have been found to be vectors in other countries. *L. deliense* has been incriminated over most of tropical Asia and Australia (Audy, 1961). *L. fletcheri* was the vector mite encountered in New Guinea during World War II and it also transmits disease in Malaysia. *L. pallida* and *L. scutellare* are prevalent in Japan in the winter, in contrast to the summer prevalence of *L. akamushi* (Tamiya, 1962). In Malaysia other vectors occur, for example, *L. arenicola*, near sandy beaches (Upham et al., 1971). One recognized and several other proposed species are possible vectors in far eastern Siberia (Shubin et al., 1970). Thus, an array of mites, mostly of the same genus and having many characteristics in common, are vectors of scrub typhus to man, but ecologic differences such as seasonal occurrence and habitats determine the local epidemiology.

During World War II, an estimated 40,000 combatants contracted scrub typhus (Audy, 1961). Penicillin was soon found to be ineffective (Sayen et al., 1946), but in 1948 Smadel and co-workers demonstrated the value of chloramphenicol in these patients (Smadel et al., 1949). Vaccines composed of killed rickettsiae developed in Britain and the United States failed to protect against all strains of the organism.

Confronted with the failure of killed vaccines and lacking a genuinely nonpathogenic strain of *R. tsutsugamushi*, Smadel and co-workers examined live rickettsiae as a vaccine, ameliorating the consequent disease with chloramphenicol (Smadel et al., 1952). From these studies in volunteers in Malaya, it was observed that immunity to challenge with the vaccine strain Karp was complete more than one year later, but challenge with a different strain, Gilliam, resulted in disease as early as four months postvaccination. Thus, the immunologic heterogeneity of rickettsial strains, documented in the laboratory (Rights et al., 1948), was confirmed in humans.

ETIOLOGY. *Rickettsia tsutsugamushi* is a small, gram-negative microorganism that multiples intracellularly and does not grow on cell-free media. Its cell wall is composed of five layers as seen by electronmicroscopy and consists of protein, lipid, polysaccharides, and muramic and diaminopimelic acids, typical of gram-negative bacteria. The microorganism is pleomorphic but generally occurs as short rods measuring about 2.0 by 0.5 μm, visible by light microscopy. The organism is stained with basic fuchsin dyes such as those in the Giemsa and Machiavello stains. It does not possess a true capsule, but the cell is surrounded by an amorphous layer that contains soluble antigen. *R. tsutsugamushi* is immunologically heterogeneous, and classification of strains is incomplete. Nevertheless, three strains, Karp, Gilliam, and Kato, have been adopted as reference strains and have received wide use, especially in the immunofluorescence procedure for the diagnosis of human disease.

PATHOGENESIS AND PATHOLOGY. The fundamental abnormality in scrub typhus is a disseminated focal perivasculitis with endothelial damage. Various organs develop interstitial edema, endothelial swelling in capillaries and small vessels, and infiltration of lymphocytes and large macrophages. Perivascular tissues and adventitia of vessels are widely involved, but arteritis, thrombosis, and gangrene, which are common in other rickettsial infections, are rare. The necrotizing arteritis of epidemic typhus and spotted fever is not seen in scrub typhus. Small platelet thrombi along with enlarged and hyperchromatic endothelial cells in capillaries, venules, and veins occur in the skin. Perivascular infiltration consists of lymphocytes, plasma cells, and macrophages, which need not correspond in location to the endothelial changes. Focal infiltrates are seen as an interstitial myocarditis, with myocardial fibers intact. Major coronary arteries are fully patent.

Interstitial pneumonitis and acute necrotizing bronchiolitis are seen, with only minimal changes in blood vessels, but areas of bronchopneumonia may be present. A mononuclear cell meningitis is almost always found; in half the cases of one series, meningitis occurred without brain involvement. The brain lesion consists of proliferating oligodendroglial cells and a few lymphocytes, plasma cells, and macrophages, all collected around capillaries, whose walls are disrupted and contain enlarged and hyperchromatic endothelial cells. Although these lesions are like those described in epidemic typhus, they are much less frequent in tsutsugamushi disease and are confined chiefly to the pons and medulla. Various authors report rickettsia-like organisms in lesions of skin vessels, heart, lung, and brain, but human tissue has not been examined by modern methods for specific identification of whole organisms or their antigens. Rickettsiae and rickettsial antigen are widely distributed in tissues of infected mice (Kundin et al., 1964).

Knowledge of pathophysiology is limited because severe disease in man has not been available for study since the advent of antibiotics. Abnormal pulmonary, myocardial, renal, and neurologic function may be caused by local reaction to the presence and multiplication of rickettsiae. The endothelial lesions presumably increase vascular permeability, but there are no published studies of peripheral vascular function similar to those for spotted fever, which showed increased permeability, thrombosis, and vascular occlusion before rickettsiae could be demonstrated. Schramek and co-workers report isolation of a lipopolysaccharide with endotoxin properties from *R. tsutsugamushi* (Schramek et al., 1976). Since cell wall constituents of *R. tsutsugamushi* and other rickettsiae closely resemble those of gram-negative bacteria (Perkins and Allison, 1963), and since endotoxin-like activity has been isolated from cell walls of *R. mooseri* (Wood and Wisseman, 1967), the isolation of endotoxin from *R. tsutsugamushi* would not be surprising and might provide one mechanism for the peripheral circulatory collapse seen in rapidly fatal cases. Hemorrhagic manifestations of disease described formerly were probably associated with disseminated intravascular coagulation (DIC). DIC has been well documented (Ognibene et al., 1971; Suzuki et al., 1981). The basis for DIC is the widespread endothelial damage caused by rickettsial multiplication in endothelial cells. In the laboratory mouse, effects attributed to a rickettsial toxin have been described (Kitaoka and Tanaka, 1973). Suspensions of live rickettsiae inoculated intravenously kill mice within one hour. Very high titers of rickettsiae are required, and the relationship of this phenomenon in mice to disease in man is uncertain.

CLINICAL MANIFESTATIONS. The incubation period is usually 8 to 10 days with extremes of 6 to 19 days. Onset is usually abrupt and is sometimes precisely timed by patients. The initial symptom is severe frontal and occipital headache followed within hours by fever to 39° C with shaking chills. Most patients also complain of general malaise, severe backache, and profuse sweating. Some have anorexia, and a few report nausea and vomiting.

Fever is remitting, rising to 40° C and higher by the fourth or fifth day. The pulse rate generally remains under 100 for a relative bradycardia during the first week of fever. In the second week, fever continues to peak near 40° C with daily remissions until it falls by lysis, around the fourteenth day. In severe cases, fever lasts for up to three weeks. Blood pressure may fall below 100 mm Hg systolic at the peak of illness but returns to normal with defervescence.

A primary lesion, or eschar, develops at the site of chigger feeding and is pathognomonic. A small papule forms within hours after the chigger has completed its painless feeding of 48 to 72 hours duration. When special attention is paid to attached chiggers, slight burning or itching at the feeding site is sometimes recalled but is ordinarily overlooked (Kitaoka et al., 1974). The papule develops into a pustule that loses its top to become a shallow ulcer about 5 mm in diameter, surrounded by a flat red margin. The base of the ulcer usually becomes yellowish-gray, lacks exudate, and is painless by the time symptoms begin (Fig. 1). Before the end of the first week of disease, a black scab covers the ulcer (Fig. 2), which slowly regresses, leaving at most a point scar. First episodes of tsutsugamushi disease do not always cause an eschar, and proven second infections usually produce no eschars, presumably because of partial immunity (Morris, 1965). As many as six eschars may appear simultaneously, and two are not unusual in persons exposed in hyperendemic areas. Eschars occur on every part of the body, predominating in the genital and inguinal areas, axilla, lower trunk, and neck. Eschars are frequently overlooked by patients, especially when they are located posteriorly. A number of studies have shown that the skin must be thoroughly examined if all eschars are to be found and that their absence does not rule out tsutsugamushi disease. In certain series, 20 to 50 per cent of proven cases did not have

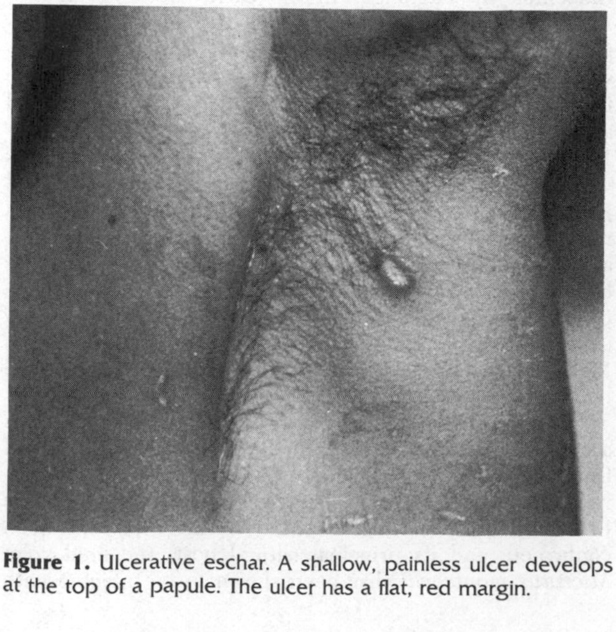

Figure 1. Ulcerative eschar. A shallow, painless ulcer develops at the top of a papule. The ulcer has a flat, red margin.

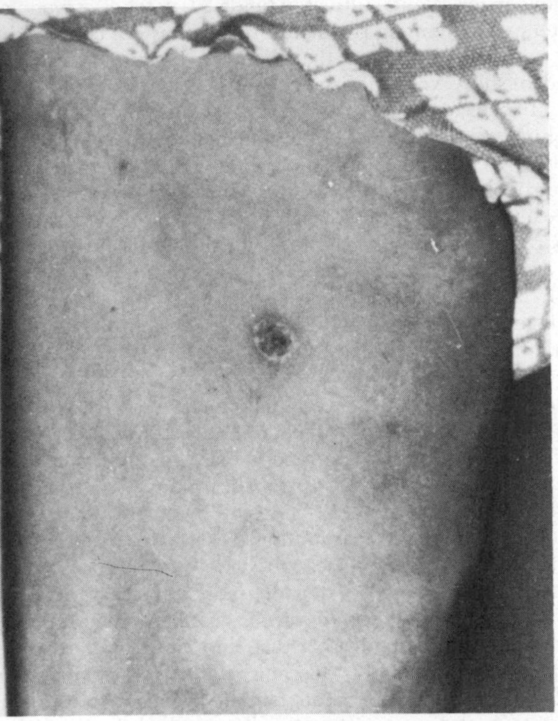

Figure 2. Crusted eschar.

eschars (Berman and Kundin, 1973; Sheehy et al., 1973; Yosano, 1953).

Lymph nodes draining the eschar are invariably enlarged and tender during the first week of disease. Generalized lymph node enlargement is also common but abates during the second week. Conjunctival hyperemia is very typical at first and about 25 per cent of cases also exhibit pharyngeal hyperemia.

Pink, maculopapular skin lesions about 0.5 cm in diameter are present from the third to ninth day in 40 to 60 per cent of cases (Fig. 3). The rash usually begins on the face, chest, and abdomen and extends to the anterior aspects of the extremities, but it may involve all parts of the body, including the palms and soles. The buccal mucosa is occasionally involved. The rash is difficult to see in darker-skinned persons and may be present for only a few hours. It is not pruritic, never confluent, and almost never hemorrhagic. Purpuric lesions are described in isolated cases, but petechiae have not been reported. Subconjunctival hemorrhage and epistaxis, the principal hemorrhagic phenomena, are most common in severe disease.

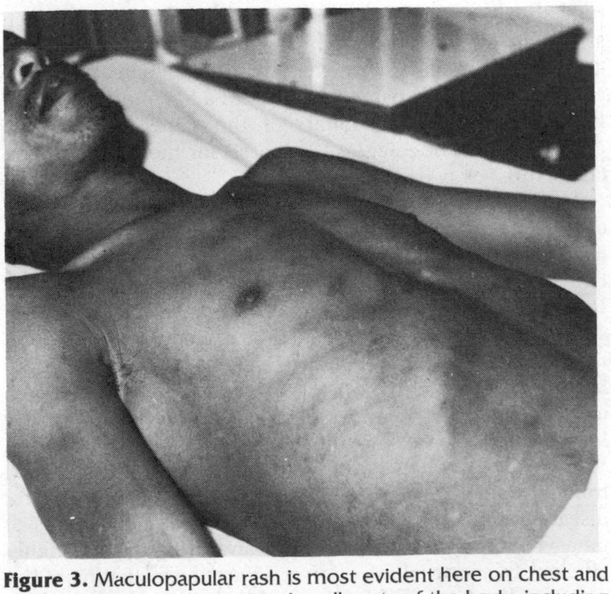

Figure 3. Maculopapular rash is most evident here on chest and upper abdomen but may involve all parts of the body, including palms and soles.

Bronchitis, with moderate to severe cough, is very common. Rickettsial interstitial pneumonia is common, but physical findings are usually limited to rhonchi and occasional basilar crepitant rales. Signs of bronchopneumonia are not found. Dyspnea and cyanosis seldom occur except in fatal cases, and bacterial superinfection is rare. Although myocarditis is common at autopsy, clinical abnormalities of the heart are usually minimal. The usual findings are progressive cardiac enlargement, an apical systolic murmur, and a transient gallop rhythm, with normal central venous pressure. Electrocardiographic findings include extrasystoles, variable degrees of AV block, shifts in electrical axis, and variable T-wave changes (Ognibene et al., 1971). The spleen and liver are palpable 1 to 3 cm below the costal margins in 25 to 50 per cent of cases by the beginning of the second week.

Renal involvement is usually minor except in severely ill patients, who may develop massive albuminuria and cylindruria, oliguria, pitting peripheral edema, and, rarely, ascites.

Meningeal involvement, as evidenced by pain and tenderness in the neck muscles and some resistance to flexion, was present in 13 per cent of one large series of patients (Sayen et al., 1946), but severe nuchal rigidity was rare. In most patients lumbar puncture revealed an elevated cerebrospinal fluid pressure, 15 cells or less with a predominance of mononuclear cells and a protein concentration of 68 to 156 mg per 100 ml. Signs of generalized cerebral involvement ranged from hyperesthesias (5 per cent) and transient mental confusion (22 per cent) to delirium (13 per cent), severe persistent restlessness (13 per cent), convulsions (6 per cent), and coma (7 per cent). Focal neurologic signs such as dysarthria, dysphagia, paraplegia, and urinary retention were less frequent. The majority of patients complained of tinnitus and deafness during the second and third weeks.

R. tsutsugamushi is now known to be a frequent cause of fever without rash or eschar. At one hospital in peninsular Malaysia, scrub typhus was diagnosed in 23 per cent of cases admitted for fever (Brown et al., 1976). It was also a major cause of febrile illness among American servicemen in Vietnam (Berman et al., 1973).

In the pre-antibiotic era patients usually defervesced by lysis near the end of the second week of disease. More recently, the same fever pattern has been observed in patients who were not treated because the diagnosis of scrub typhus was made only retrospectively by positive serologic tests (Berman and Kundin, 1973).

A recent clinical study of Taiwanese soldiers by Bourgeois et al. (1982) confirmed earlier experimental work (Morris, 1965) that suggested the possibility of reinfections with scrub typhus. Reinfected patients may be either completely asymptomatic or develop mild disease. Primary infections occur in younger patients and are accompanied by a higher incidence of rash, conjunctivitis, and relapse. Generalized lymphadenopathy is more common in reinfections. Reinfection with heterologous serotypes may occur within 2 months of the primary infection, but it is likely that immunity to the homologous strain persists for 1 to 3 years. Although primary infections can be differentiated from reinfections by the nature of the antibody response (See Diagnosis section), Bourgeois et al. (1982) showed that reinfected patients also developed higher ratios of activated lymphocytes during acute infection and early convalescence.

COMPLICATIONS AND SEQUELAE. Death usually occurs between the tenth and fourteenth days of disease. Nothing in the early clinical picture points to a severe or fatal course, which usually results from progressive pneumonia and circulatory collapse, sometimes associated with an encephalitis that is manifest by delirium and coma. Convulsions, cyanosis that is resistant to oxygen therapy, and pulmonary edema are usual terminal events. In the preantibiotic era mortality rates in hospitalized patients ranged from less than 1 per cent to 60 per cent (Audy, 1961). Elsom and co-workers (Elsom et al., 1961) found no permanent sequelae in 524 untreated persons 11 or more years after recovery from severe disease contracted in the China-Burma-India region. Although rickettsiae persist for many months in lymph nodes and perhaps in other tissues after recovery, even in patients treated with antibiotics, clinical relapse some years after initial infection like that seen in epidemic typhus has never been recognized.

GEOGRAPHIC VARIATIONS AND EPIDEMIOLOGY. In November, 1950, a nonfatal noncommunicable exanthematous febrile illness resembling tsutsugamushi disease was observed on Hachijo Island (Yosana, 1953), one of a chain of islands stretching south from Toyko Bay for several hundred miles. Unlike tsutsugamushi, it occurred in the colder months and affected many small children and women, as well as agricultural laborers. The disease prevalence matched the seasonal occurrence of the chigger *L. scutellare*, which attacks man. *R. tsutsugamushi* was isolated both from patients with so-called winter disease and from *L. scutellare* larvae. Investigation of the main Japanese islands (Tamiya, 1962) disclosed febrile disease caused by *R. tsutsugamushi* in eight widely separated prefectures, and *R. tsutsugamushi* was isolated from small mammals trapped in almost every prefecture in Japan and from several zoophilic species of chiggers not known to parasitize man. The vectors of human disease were recovered from birds, and more recent observations of *L. scutellare* in peninsular Malaysia at elevations above 5000 feet suggest that vector chiggers are dispersed over great distances by migratory birds. Widespread mild and inapparent infection with *R. tsutsugamushi* occurs in Malaysia (Brown et al., 1976) just as it does in Japan.

The cardinal epidemiologic feature of scrub typhus is its highly focal nature, with outbreaks traceable to common sites of exposure. The principal determinant of epidemiology is the vector chigger, which requires a vertebrate on which to feed as a larva and a favorable microenvironment within and on the surface of the ground to complete its life cycle. Other requirements are poorly defined but are met by a variety of ecologic habitats, including: (1) grassy banks of water-courses; (2) grassland covered with kunai or lallang grass (*Imperata cylindrica*); (3) uncultivated agricultural land that has been allowed to overgrow, or marginal land between forest and cultivated fields; (4) patches of woodland interspersed among populated rural areas; (5) certain kinds of volcanic soil such as that found in Japan near Mt. Fugi and offshore volcanic islands; (6) hedgerows composed of coral rock, as in the Pescadores Islands; (7) shaded areas behind sandy beaches in peninsular Malaysia; (8) abandoned vegetable plots and other marginal land within metropolitan areas such as Bombay, and Djakarta; and (9) pockets of ecologic disturbance within the forest in which aboriginal people practice shifting slash-and-burn methods of agriculture.

In all these circumstances, the natural hosts of vector chiggers, chiefly small rodents of the genus *Rattus*, are plentiful. Larger animals, wild and domestic fowl, and even domestic cattle may also act as vector hosts. Chiggers attach to the host for several days and feed on tissue fluids rather than blood. After feeding, the larvae drop to the soil, where they develop through several additional stages into free-living adults. After fertilization by acquiring spermatophores deposited in the soil by males, one female adult can produce many hundreds of larval offspring. The entire life cycle requires about 60 to 90 days in the laboratory but may be shorter under ideal natural conditions. Chiggers, which require a ground surface microenvironment of favorable moisture and air temperature, disappear during drought, flooding, and extremes of heat and cold. Thus, in the temperate climate of Japan, scrub typhus is a seasonal disease occurring when and where the climate is favorable for a particular vector. The risk of contracting scrub typhus in the summer is greatest along certain watercourses when the temperature exceeds 20° C, which favors the prevalence of *L. akamushi*. In the winter the risk is associated with certain volcanic soil and nonriverine areas when the temperature falls to 10 to 18° C, favoring *L. scutellare* and *L. pallida*. In tropic and subtropic areas, the principal vector is *L. deliense*. When the tropic climate is moist throughout the year, as in Malaysia, there is little monthly fluctuation in the number of cases, whereas in tropic areas with sharp wet and dry seasons, as in India, disease is usually confined to the wet season (Traub and Wisseman, 1974).

Chiggers are barely visible to the naked eye as red or reddish-white spots moving across a black background such as boots. Within typical habitats, the distribution of chiggers on the ground is uneven, with collections or foci of chiggers on certain patches of ground a few meters square. By contrast, nearby habitats of the same type can be entirely devoid of chiggers. The basis for these distribution characteristics is unknown.

The risk of disease is determined both by the distribution of vector chiggers and the presence of rickettsiae in the chigger population. It has been estimated that only one or two per cent of chiggers are infected (Kitaoka et al., 1974). Rapmund and co-workers showed, however, that all offspring of an infected adult female may be infected (Rapmund et al., 1969). Since adult chiggers are thought to have a limited range of movement, highly infectious, concentrated foci of chiggers may occur, with an attendant high risk of disease for humans exposed to them. During World War II, when military personnel moved on a broad front through terrain typical for scrub typhus vectors, disease was often limited to certain very small groups of men (Philip et al., 1946; Sayers and Hill, 1948). Highly efficient transovarial infection is a partial explanation of the very focal nature of the disease. Dohany and co-workers have recently developed an immunofluorescence procedure by which unfed chiggers collected from the ground can be speciated and examined for the presence of scrub typhus rickettsiae (Dohany et al., 1978). This provides a much needed tool for the assessment of the relative infectiousness of chigger foci. The phenomenon of highly efficient transovarial transmission of rickettsiae suggests that the reservoir of *R. tsutsugamushi* in nature is the chigger itself.

All age groups and both sexes acquire scrub typhus. The ecologic circumstances of an area determine whether scrub typhus affects chiefly agricultural workers, individuals around the immediate environs of the home, or children and young adults who become infected on vacant land used for playing fields.

R. tsutsugamushi has been recovered from chiggers that are not known to feed on humans (Kitaoka et al., 1973), from tropic forest animals remote from humans (Muul et al., 1977), and from animals and chiggers in sparsely populated mountainous and subarctic terrain (Traub and Wisseman, 1974), suggesting that sylvan reservoirs of rickettsiae exist in nature. It was Audy's evolutionary view of scrub typhus that a preexisting sylvan, chigger-borne rickettsiosis has been extended and amplified by human encroachment on and alteration of primary forest, leading to creation of hyperendemic foci of vectors to which humans are exposed (Audy, 1961). A full analysis of the ecology of scrub typhus has been published by Traub and Wisseman (Traub and Wisseman, 1974). The evolutionary view is important because humans continue to alter the land, eliminating some hyperendemic foci but creating new ones elsewhere. The disease epidemiology is not static. Physicians must be alert for the appearance of new foci of scrub typhus—for example, in the vicinity of rural land settlement schemes located where forest has recently been cleared.

The current geographic distribution of scrub typhus encompasses Asia and contiguous islands of the western Pacific region, including the island continent of Australia. Known extreme limits of vector chiggers are the Maldive and Chagos Archipelagos in the Indian Ocean (Audy, 1961), the New Hebrides Islands east of New Guinea (Audy, 1961), the Tadzhik SSR in the Soviet Union adjacent to Afghanistan (Kulagin et al., 1968), and the islands of Shikotan and Kunashir in the Kuril Island chain near Japan (Somov et al., 1976). In countries or regions within this broad geographic zone in which the disease has not been reported, its eventual recognition can be anticipated. There is serologic evidence of *R. tsutsugamushi* infection in rodents in eastern Iran, but human disease has not been reported there (Hamidi et al., 1974). Scrub typhus antibody and skin-test reactivity have been reported from Ruanda in central Africa (Giroud and Jadin, 1951). *R. tsutsugamushi* has not been isolated in Africa, however, Until that is accomplished, the specificity of these reactions must be questioned.

DIAGNOSIS. If no eschar or rash is present, the differential diagnosis includes most etiologies contributing to fever of unknown origin syndrome, especially malaria, typhoid fever, infectious mononucleosis, leptospirosis, dengue, and other arbovirus infections. Concurrent malaria and scrub typhus are seen (Berman and Kundin, 1973). Scrub typhus must be considered in malaria patients who have persistent fever after adequate treatment, especially in southeast Asia, where such a response may be viewed as a drug-resistant falciparum infection. Ulcerative eschars in the genital area and tender regional lymph nodes may be mistaken for veneral disease (Levy, 1959).

Laboratory findings are not distinctive. Leukocyte counts may be normal. When abnormal, there is usually a leukopenia of 2000 to 4000 cells per mm^3 during the first week of disease with a predominance of polymorphonuclear cells and a leukocytosis of up to 25,000 cells per ml^3 during the second week with a predominance of small lymphocytes. Red blood cell count and hematocrit are usually normal. Total platelet count may be as low as 10,000 per mm^3, but the frequency and mechanism of thrombocytopenia are unknown. Urinalysis may be normal at first, but in the more severe cases it usually shows moderate albuminuria, elevated specific gravity, occasional red and white blood cells, and granular casts. Nitrogen retention may occur. The serum chloride concentration is low and total protein levels are usually normal. In one series of 41 patients (Berman and Kundin, 1973), serum glutamic oxalacetic transaminase (SGOT) levels were highly variable and were not correlated with rash, severity of fever, or hepatomegaly. Hypofibrinogenemia, increased levels of circulating fibrin-split products, and general consumption of clotting factors, which are typical of disseminated intravascular coagulation (DIC), have been described (Ognibene et al., 1971; and Suzuki et al., 1981).

Laboratory diagnosis is achieved by isolation of rickettsiae and by demonstration of specific antibody in convalescent serum. Intraperitoneal inoculation of white laboratory mice with whole blood or blood clot collected from untreated febrile patients should yield *R. tsutsugamushi*. Identification of rickettsiae requires at a minimum several weeks and often several months. Chloramphenicol or tetracycline rapidly eliminates rickettsemia, but mouse inoculation up to 24 hours after initiation of antibiotics occasionally yields rickettsiae. When mouse inoculation is delayed, the blood clot should be stored at or below $-60°$ C.

Serologic diagnosis must contend with the immunologic heterogeneity of scrub typhus rickettsial strains. Bozeman and Elisberg (1963) developed an indirect immunofluorescent procedure using three strains—Karp, Gilliam, and Kato—isolated from human infections in New Guinea, Burma, and Japan, respectively. Because suspensions of whole rickettsiae are used as an antigen that is not available commercially, the test is usually performed in reference laboratories. The antigen is stable when dried on microscope slides stored frozen so that the procedure can be performed wherever fluorescent microscopy is available. Sera from some patients react with only one strain, others with two or all three. Patients with typical clinical courses, or from whom rickettsiae have been isolated, almost always produce antibody against one of these strains. One exception is 18 of 27 strains of *R. tsutsugamushi* isolated from febrile patients in Queensland, Australia, that were immunologically distinct from these three reference strains but were similar to isolates from small animals in Thailand (Shirai et al., 1982). Other rickettsial strains that are immunologically distinct from these reference strains have also been isolated from nature. The extent to which these other strains cause human disease is unknown. Shishido prepared purified complement-fixing antigens from Karp, Gilliam, and Kato strains that have been used widely in Japan (Shishido, 1962). Antibody can usually be detected by immunofluorescence on about the eighth or ninth day of disease, and by complement fixation on about the fourteenth day. During primary infection IgM appears within 8 days of the onset of illness and rises rapidly; IgM does not appear until about day 12 and rises more slowly (Bourgeois et al., 1982). The IgM response is more specific for the infecting strain. During reinfection, on the other hand, IgG is detectable by day 6, while the appearance and persistence of IgM is variable. Antibody can be detected for years by CF test, but IF antibody disappears more rapidly after a single infection. More recently, ELISA (Crum et al., 1980) and the indirect immunoperoxidase (Yamamoto and Minamishima, 1982) techniques have been applied successfully to serodiagnosis. Collection of blood specimens on filter paper for easy storage and shipment has been described by Gan and co-workers (Gan et al., 1972).

The Weil-Felix *Proteus* agglutination test has been widely used for nearly 50 years. The agglutination reaction is based on possession of common antigens by *R. tsutsugamushi* and *Proteus mirabilis* OX-K strain. Agglutinins are found as early as the ninth day of disease. Low titers of agglutinins (less than 1:100) occur in some normal individuals. Therefore, a diagnosis can be made only upon demonstration of a four-fold or greater increase in agglutinins or a high titer in a single convalescent serum specimen. However, not all scrub typhus infections stimulate these agglutinins. Indeed, in some reported case series, fewer than 25 per cent of the patients developed them. OX-K agglutinins also occur in other diseases: leptospirosis (Carley et al., 1955), rat-bite fever (Lewthwaite, 1940), and relapsing fever (Zarafonetis et al., 1946). Thus, the Weil-Felix test is unreliable and with the increasing availability of other specific serologic procedures should not be relied upon.

TREATMENT. Scrub typhus responds rapidly to antibiotics. In adults, oral tetracycline, 2.0 g per day in divided doses, clears all manifestations of disease in 36 to 48 hours. Children should be given 20 to 40 mg per kg per day in four divided doses. Chloramphenicol was the original drug of choice (Smadel et al., 1949), but it has been supplanted by tetracycline, which is less toxic and produces a faster response (Sheehy et al., 1973). Because all effective drugs are rickettsiostatic, treatment should be continued until about the fourteenth day, when the immune response is well developed. Clinical relapse with rickettsemia occurs within four to five days if treatment is stopped earlier, especially if it was begun in the first week of disease. Humoral antibody, which may be detected as early as the ninth day, does not prevent relapse. Cell-mediated immunity seems to be the principal mechanism of acquired resistance in experimentally infected mice and probably plays a role in humans as well (Sheehy et al., 1973 and Bourgeois et al., 1982). Peripheral vascular collapse should be managed as septic shock. DIC should subside quickly with antibiotic therapy. Only in instances of severe hemorrhagic diathesis should heparin therapy be necessary. Single-dose treatment of scrub typhus with 200 mg of doxycycline, a long-acting tetracycline, has been successful in Malaysia in more than 30 patients without relapse, but treatment was almost always begun on or after the seventh day of disease (Brown et al., 1978). This simplified approach must be evaluated further before it can be recommended for use earlier in disease.

PROPHYLAXIS. No vaccine against scrub typhus is available. The immunologic heterogeneity of *R. tsutsugamushi* has proved to be an insurmountable obstacle thus far, but the limited number of immunologically distinct strains causing human disease in certain areas (Brown et al., 1976; Kitaoka et al., 1974) provides some encouragement that a vaccine may be developed eventually.

Individuals can be protected by two other means, however. Diethyltoluamide (DEET), a highly effective mite repellent suitable for skin and clothing, is sold commercially. The most effective formulation includes 50 per cent active material. Its disadvantages are that it washes off easily and has organic solvent properties that affect certain plastics used in personal and household articles. The second approach is chemoprophylaxis. Smadel first demonstrated that chloramphenicol in oral doses of 3.0 to 4.0 g every four to seven days for four weeks or longer protects persons from disease while they are taking the drug and after its discontinuance (Smadel et al., 1950). The long-acting tetracycline, doxycycline, usually prevents clinical scrub typhus in endemic areas when given orally 200 mg once weekly (Olson et al., 1980; Twartz et al., 1982). Mild disease requiring treatment occasionally occurs among individuals on this regimen, and mild self-limited symptoms may occur 10 to 14 days after the last dose of doxycycline. More frequent doxycycline may eliminate these problems. Chemoprophylaxis should be reserved for persons who must enter known hyperendemic areas of disease for short periods.

Direct control of chiggers is also possible. The residual chlorinated hydrocarbon insecticide, dieldrin, sprayed over a hyperendemic focus of disease, eradicated vector chiggers for up to two years with one application (Traub and Dowling, 1961). Concern for the environmental impact of residual insecticides has limited the use of this highly effective chemical. In the United States, a nonresidual organophosphate, chlorpyrifos, has controlled the American chigger *Eutrombicula alfreddugesi* for four weeks with one application (Mount et al., 1978). Since this chigger is similar to scrub typhus vector chiggers, the use of chlorpyrifos should be tested against vectors in Asia. Dohany has described a systemic acaracide, dimethoate, which is effective against American chiggers. Dimethoate, an organophosphate, is placed in food for vertebrate hosts, which transfer it to chiggers during feedings (Dohany et al., 1977). One field trial in the Pescadores Islands was not successful (Trooper, 1979). Since the mite is apparently both the vector and the reservoir of the disease, elimination of rats does not reduce the risk of disease and, in the short term, may increase it by substituting humans as the only available chigger host (Audy, 1961).

References

Audy, J. R., The ecology of scrub typhus. In May, J. M. (ed.): Studies in Disease Ecology. New York, Hafner Publishing Company, 1961.

Berman S. J., and Kundin, W. D.: Scrub typhus in South Vietnam. A study of 87 cases. Ann Intern Med 79:26, 1973.

Berman, S. J., Irving, G. A., Kundin, W. D., Gunning, J., and Watten, R. H.: Epidemiology of the acute fevers of unknown origin in South Vietnam: Effect of laboratory support upon clinical diagnosis. Am J Trop Med Hyg 22:796, 1973.

Blake, F. G., Maxcy, K. F., Sadusk, J. F., Jr., Kohls, G. M. and Bell, E. J.: Studies on tsutsugamushi disease (scrub typhus, mite-borne typhus) in New Guinea and adjacent islands. Am J Hyg 41:243, 1945.

Bourgeois, A. L., Olson, J. G., Fang, R. C. V., Huang, J., Wang, C. L., Chow, L., Bechthold, D., Dennis, D. T., Coolbaugh, J. C., and Weiss, E.: Humoral and cellular responses in scrub typhus patients reflecting primary infection and reinfection with *Rickettsia tsutsugamuchi.* Am J Trop Med Hyg 31:532, 1982.

Bozeman, F. M., and Elisberg, B. L.: Serological diagnosis of scrub typhus by indirect immunofluorescence. Proc Soc Exp Biol Med 112:568, 1963.

Brown, G. W., Robinson, D. M., Huxsoll, D. L, Ng, T. S., Lim, K. J., and Sannasey, G.: Scrub typhus: A common cause of illness in indigenous populations. Trans R Soc Trop Med Hyg 70:444, 1976.

Brown, G. W., Saunders, J. P., Singh, S., Huxsoll, D. L., and Shirai, A.: Single dose doxycycline therapy for scrub typhus. Trans R Soc Trop Med Hyg 72:412, 1978.

Carley, J. G., Doherty, R. L., Derrick, E. M., Pope, J. M., Emanuel, M. L., and Ross, C. J.: The investigation of fever in North Queensland by mouse inoculation, with particular reference to scrub typhus. Austral Ann Med 4:91, 1955.

Crum, J. W., Hanchaley, S., and Eamsila, C.: New paper enzyme-linked immunosorbent technique compared with microimmunofluorescence for detection of human serum antibodies to *Rickettsia tsutsugamushi.* J Clin Microbiol 11:584, 1980.

Dohany, A. L., Cromroy, H. L., and Cole, M. M.: Laboratory tests of dimethoate for systemic control of chiggers (Acarina: Trombiculidae), populations on rodents. J Med Ent 14:79, 1977.

Dohany, A. L., Shirai, A., Robinson, D. M., Ram, S., and Huxsoll, D. L.: Identification and antigenic typing of *Rickettsia tsutsugamushi* in naturally infected chiggers by direct immunofluorescence. Am J Trop Med Hyg 27:1261, 1978.

Elsom, K. A., Beebe, G. W., Sayen, J. J., Scheie, H. G., Cannon, G. D., and Wood, F. C.: Scrub typhus: A follow-up study. Ann Intern Med 55:784, 1961.

Gan, E., Cadigan, F. C., Jr., and Walker, J. S.: Filter paper collection of blood for use in a screening and diagnostic test for scrub typhus using the IFAT. Trans R Soc Trop Med Hyg 66:588, 1972.

Giroud, P., and Jadin, J.: Presence des anticorps vis-a-vis de *Rickettsia orientalis* chez les indigenes et des asiatiques vivant au Ruanda-Urindi (Congo Belge). Bull Soc Pathol Exot 44:50, 1951.

Hamidi, A. N., Saadatezadeh, H., Tarasevich, I. V., Arata, A. A., and Farbangazad, A.: A serological study of rickettsial infections in Iranian small mammals. Bull Soc Pathol Exot 67:607, 1974.

Kitaoka, M., and Tanaka, Y.: Rickettsial toxin and its specificity in three prototype strains, Karp, Gilliam and Kato, of *Rickettsia orientalis.* Acta Virol 17:426, 1973.

Kitaoka, M., Asanuma, K., Okubo, K., Tanegugh, H., Tsubo, M., and Hattor, K.: Seasonal occurrence of trombiculid mites species and *Leptotrombidium kawamurai* (Acarina, Trombiculidae) as a carrier of *Rickettsia orientalis* in the Noporro area, Hokkaido, Japan. J Hyg Epidemiol Microbiol Immunol 17:478, 1973.

Kitaoka, M., Asanuma, K., and Otsuji, J.: Transmission of *Rickettsia orientalis* to man by *Leptotrombidium akamushi* at a scrub typhus endemic area in Akita Prefecture, Japan, Am J Trop Med Hyg 23:993, 1974.

Kulagin, S. M., Taresevich, I. V., Kudryashova, N. I., Plotnikova, L. F.: The investigations of scrub typhus in the USSR. J Hyg Epidemiol Microbiol Immunol 12:257, 1968.

Kundin, W. D., Liu, C., Harmon, P., and Rodina, P.: Pathogenesis of scrub typhus infection (*Rickettsia tsutsugamushi*), as studied by immunofluorescence. J Immunol 93:772, 1964.

Levy, B.: Scrub typhus in the differential diagnosis of veneral disease. J R Army Med Corps 105:125, 1959.

Lewthwaite, R.: Agglutination of *Proteus* in rat-bite fever. Lancet 1:390, 1940.

Morris, J. A.: Early development in monkeys of cutaneous resistance to reinfection with *Rickettsia tsutsugamushi.* Proc Soc Exp Biol Med 119:736, 1965.

Mount, G. A., Grothaus, R. H., Reed, J. T., and Baldwin, K. F.: Area control of chigger mites with granules and concentrated sprays of chlorypyrifos. J Econ Entomol 71:27, 1978.

Muul, I., Lim, B. L., and Walker, J. S.: Scrub typhus infection in rats in four habitats in peninsular Malaysia. Trans R Soc Trop Med Hyg 71:493, 1977.

Ognibene, A. J., O'Leary, D. S., Czarnecki, S. W., Flannery, E. P., and Grove, R. B.: Myocarditis and disseminated intravascular coagulation in scrub typhus. Am J Med Sci 262:233, 1971.

Olson, J. G., Bourgeois, A. L., Fang, R. C. Y., Coolbaugh, J. C., and Dennis, D. T.: Prevention of scrub typhus. Prophylactic administration of doxycycline in a randomized double blind trial. Am J Trop Med Hyg 29:989, 1980.

Perkins, H. R., and Allison, A. C.: Cell-wall constituents of rickettsiae and psittacosis-lymphogranuloma organisms. J Gen Microbiol 30:469, 1963.

Philip, C. B., Woodward, T. E., and Sullivan, R. R.: Tsutsugamushi disease (scrub or mite-borne typhus) in the Philippine Islands during American reoccupation in 1944–45. Am J Trop Med 26:229, 1946.

Rapmund, G., Upham, R. W., Jr., Kundin, W. D., Manikumaran, C., and Chan, T. C.: Transovarial development of scrub typhus rickettsiae in a colony of vector mites. Tran R Soc Trop Med Hyg 63:251, 1969.

Rights, F. L., Smadel, J. E., and Jackson, E. B.: Studies on scrub typhus (tsutsugamushi disease). III. Heterogeneity of strains of *R. tsutsugamushi* as demonstrated by cross vaccination studies. J Exp Med 87:339, 1948.

Sayen, J. J., Pond, H. S., Forrester, J. S., and Wood, F. C.: Scrub typhus in Assam and Burma. A clinical study of 616 cases. Medicine 25:155, 1946.

Sayers, M. H. P., and Hill, I. G. W.: The occurrence and identification of the typhus group of fevers in South East Asia Command. J R Army Med Corps 90:6, 1948.

Schramek, S., Brezina, R., and Tarasevich, I. V.: Isolation of a lipopolysaccharide antigen from *Rickettsia* species. Acta Virol 20:270, 1976.

Sheehy, T. W., Hazlett, D., and Turk, R. E.: Scrub typhus. A comparison of chloramphenicol and tetracycline in its treatment. Arch Intern Med 132:77, 1973.

Shirai, A., Campbell, R. W., Gan, E., Chan, T. C., and Huxsoll, D. L.: Serologic analysis of *Rickettsia tsutsugamushi* isolates from North Queensland. Aust J Exp Biol Med Sci 60:203, 1982.

Shishido, A.: Identification and serologic classification of the causative agent of scrub typhus in Japan. Jap J Med Sci Biol 15:308, 1962.

Shubin, F. N., Natsky, K. V., and Somov, G. P.: Concerning the vector of tsutsugamushi fever in the Far East. Zh Mikrobiol Epidemiol Immunobiol 47:112, 1970.

Smadel, J. E., Woodward, T. E., Ley, H. L., Jr., and Lewthwaite, R.: Chloramphenicol (Chloromycetin) in the treatment of tsutsugamushi disease (scrub typhus). J Clin Invest 28:1196, 1949.

Smadel, J. E., Traub, R., Frick, L. P., Diercks, F. H., and Bailey, C. A.: Chloramphenicol (Chloromycetin) in the chemoprophylaxis of scrub typhus (tsutsugamushi disease). Suppression of overt disease by prophylactic regimens of four-week duration. Am J Hyg 51:216, 1950.

Smadel, J. E., Ley, H. L., Jr., Diercks, F. H., Paterson, P. Y., Wisseman, C. L., Jr., and Traub, R.: Immunization against scrub typhus. Duration of immunity in volunteers following combined living vaccine and chemoprophylaxis. Am J Trop Med Hyg 1:87, 1952.

Somov, G. P., Shubin, F. N., Gopachenko, I. M., and Kononova, D. G.: Tsutsugamushi fever in the Kuril Islands. Zh Mikrobiol Epidemiol Immunobiol 53:69, 1976.

Suzuki, T., et al.: Four cases of tsutsugamushi disease (scrub typhus) complicated with disseminated intravascular coagulation. Kansenshogaku Zasshi 55:642, 1981.

Tamiya, T.: Recent Advances in Studies of Tsutsugamushi Disease in Japan. Tokyo, Medical Culture, Inc., 1962.

Traub, R., and Dowling, M. A. C.: The duration of efficacy of the insecticide Dieldrin against the chigger vectors of scrub typhus in Malaya, J Econ Entomol 54:654, 1961.

Traub, R., and Wisseman, C. L., Jr.: The ecology of chigger-borne rickettsiosis (scrub typhus). J Med Entomol 11:237, 1974.

Trooper, J. M.: Field evaluation of dimethoate as a systemic for the control of chigger mites in the Pescadores Islands of Taiwan. Southeast Asian J Trop Med Public Health 10:62, 1979.

Twartz, J. C., Shirai, A., Selvaraju, G., Saunders, J. P., Huxsoll, D. L., and Groves, M. G.: Doxycycline prophylaxis for human scrub typhus. J Inf Dis 146:811, 1982.

Upham, R. W., Jr., Hubert, A. A., Phang, O. W., Yusof bin Mat, and Rapmund, G.: Distribution of *Leptotrobidium (Leptobrombidium) arenicola* (Acarina: Trombiculidae) on the ground in West Malaysia. J Med Entomol 8:401, 1971.

Wood, W. H., Jr., and Wisseman, C. L., Jr.: Studies of *Rickettsia mooseri* cell walls. II. Immunologic properties, J Immunol 98:1224, 1967.

Yamamoto, S., and Minamishima, Y.: Serodiagnosis of tsutsugamushi fever (scrub typhus) by the indirect immunoperoxidase technique. J Clin Microbiol 15:1128, 1982.

Yosana, H.: Studies on Shichito Fever: Winter Scrub Typhus of Izu Shichito Islands, Japan. Tokyo, Health Bureau, Tokyo Metropolitan Office, 1953.

Zarafonetis, C. J. D., Ingraham, H. S., and Berry, J. F.: Weil-Felix and typhus complement fixation tests in relapsing fever, with special reference to B. *Proteus* OX-K agglutination. J Immunol 52:189, 1946.

203

ROCKY MOUNTAIN SPOTTED FEVER

Alan L. Bisno, M.D.

Rocky Mountain spotted fever is an acute infectious disease caused by a rickettsial agent, transmitted to man by several species of infected ticks, and characterized by fever, skin rash, myalgias, intense headache, and prostration.

ETIOLOGY. The causative agent, *Rickettsia rickettsii*, is an obligate intracellular parasite belonging to the spotted fever group of rickettsiae. It shares a common antigen with other members of this group but may be differentiated from them serologically by means of a species-specific antigen. The organism measures approximately 1 μ by 0.2 to 0.3 μ and may be visualized under the light microscope in sections of infected tissues stained by the Gimenez, Giemsa, or Macchiavello methods. In such specimens, *R. rickettsii* often appears in pairs and surrounded by a halo, as if encapsulated.

EPIDEMIOLOGY. The disease is limited to North and South America. It was first described during the late nineteenth century in the western United States. Its initial recognition in the mountainous areas of Montana and Idaho led to the name Rocky Mountain spotted fever. This appellation is now a misnomer, however, since in the United States the disease is much more prevalent along the Atlantic seaboard and in the southeastern states than in the Rockies. Rocky Mountain spotted fever has also been described in Canada, Mexico, Brazil, Panama, and Colombia.

Between 1906 and 1910, Howard Taylor Ricketts proved that ticks transmit the disease, described the appearance of the causative organism in human and animal tissues, and demonstrated that ticks can transmit the rickettsiae from generation to generation transovarially.

Several species of ticks transmit Rocky Mountain spotted fever. In the western United States, the wood tick, *Dermacentor andersoni*, is the principal vector, whereas east of the Mississippi River most cases are initiated by the bite of the American dog tick, *Dermacentor variabilis*. A third species, *Amblyomma americanum*, the Lone Star tick, is responsible for some cases in the southwestern United States. *Haemaphysalis leporispalustris*, the rabbit tick, is also a natural carrier of the disease but has not been definitely implicated in spread to man. *Amblyomma cajennense* transmits the disease in Brazil, Colombia, and Mexico. This tick, which parasitizes a number of wild and domestic animals and fowl, also avidly parasitizes man. It is a possible vector in the United States, where its range is limited to southern Texas and Florida.

Ticks become infected either transovarially or by feeding on infected animals. Once infected, they can harbor the rickettsiae throughout their lifetime. Thus, the tick serves as both a vector and a reservoir of Rocky Mountain spotted fever. Infection of man is an incidental event unnecessary for the persistence of *R. rickettsii* in nature. Although Rocky Mountain spotted fever is generally transmitted by tick bite, tick feces are also infectious; accidental self-inoculation, as by scratching, may cause illness. Aerosol transmission has occurred among laboratory personnel involved in rickettsial research.

Epidemiologic features of this disease are those that might be predicted from its known method of transmission. In temperate climates almost all cases occur during the warmer months of the year; approximately 60 per cent of cases occur in males and nearly 90 per cent in individuals less than 30 years of age (Hattwick et al., 1976). Cases do occur in winter on rare occasions. Clusters of cases involving families or extended family groups are well documented.

PATHOGENESIS AND PATHOLOGY. Rocky Mountain spotted fever is characterized by rickettsial invasion of small blood vessels throughout the body. The process first involves capillary endothelial cells, where the organisms multiply rapidly and cause endothelial cell swelling, proliferation, and degeneration. Subsequently the lesions extend to veins and arterioles (Fig. 1). The pathologic process in arterioles involves the entire vascular wall, with necrosis of smooth muscle cells of the media as well as mononuclear and plasma cell infiltration of the adventitia (Fig. 2). The end result of this intense infectious vasculitis is diffuse thrombosis and microinfarction, particularly involving skin, subcutaneous tissue, and the central nervous system. Necrosis of arteriolar walls leads to rupture with local areas of hemorrhage. In the brain, in addition to vascular proliferative, necrotic, and thrombotic changes, foci of cerebral astroglial proliferation (so-called "glial nodules") may be seen (Fig. 3).

The exact cause of the toxic, febrile state in Rocky Mountain spotted fever is unknown. Although products of host tissue destruction are undoubtedly involved, the rickettsial agent itself can produce both a toxin and a hemolysin, which are specifically neutralized by immune sera and which may play a role in the pathogenesis of the disease.

CLINICAL MANIFESTATIONS. Approximately three-quarters of patients give a history of tick bite or tick exposure. The incubation period ranges from two days to two weeks, averaging seven days. The onset is frequently abrupt, consisting of severe headache, chills, fever in excess of 102° F, generalized myalgias involving especially the back and legs, anorexia, malaise, and prostration. Additional symptoms may include nausea, vomiting, upper abdominal pain, photophobia, and arthralgias. This nondescript toxic, febrile illness resembles other acute infectious processes, and specific diagnosis at this stage is extremely difficult.

The characteristic rash appears between the second and sixth day of illness (average, fourth day). It usually appears first as an erythematous macular eruption involving the wrists, ankles, palms, soles, and forearms (Fig. 4). The rash rapidly becomes maculopapular and spreads centripetally to involve the proximal extremities and trunk (Fig. 5). After three to four days the lesions become petechial (Fig. 6) and, in more severe cases, may coalesce to form ecchymoses. Although the above description presents the usual features of the rash, exceptions do occur. The rash may at times begin on the trunk rather than the distal extremities. On rare occasions, the appearance of the rash may be delayed until the ninth day of illness or later,

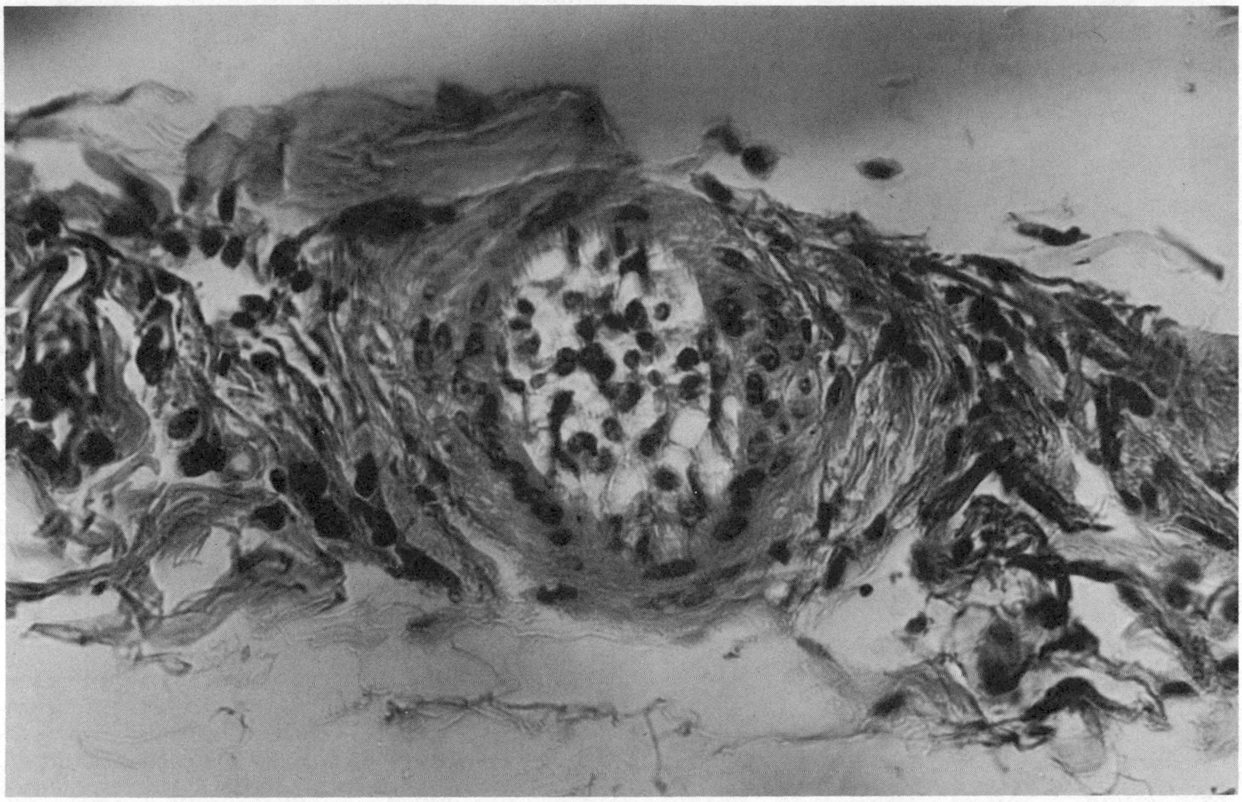

Figure 1. Cutaneous arteriole, demonstrating endothelial damage and mononuclear infiltration of vessel wall (hematoxylin-eosin, ×400). (From Archives of Internal Medicine, Sept. 1973, 132:40. Copyright 1973, American Medical Association.)

making specific diagnosis extremely difficult. Very rarely, the rash may be absent (Westerman, 1982). More frequently a mild or transient rash may be overlooked, especially in black patients.

When diagnosed and treated early, the course of the disease may be relatively mild. More severe cases, however, are characterized by profound alterations in the neurologic, hematologic, cardiovascular, and metabolic status of the patient. Neurologic abnormalities are an extremely prominent feature of the clinical illness. In addition to intense headache, these may include nuchal rigidity, delirium, stupor, coma, or grand mal seizures. Lumbar puncture may be normal or may show a mild pleocytosis and increase in protein concentration. Cerebrospinal fluid sugar concentration remains normal.

Approximately one-half of patients admitted to the hospital with severe forms of Rocky Mountain spotted fever exhibit thrombocytopenia. This finding is presumably due to margination of platelets at sites of vascular inflammation. In patients with fulminant infections, the diffuse intravascular coagulation that characterizes this disease gives rise to consumptive coagulopathy, manifested by hypofibrinogenemia, elevated levels of fibrin degradation products, depletion of circulating clotting factors, and severe hemorrhagic diathesis. Such a sequence of events is associated with a poor prognosis.

Another consequence of the diffuse vascular damage in Rocky Mountain spotted fever is increased capillary permeability, with loss of plasma and erythrocytes from the capillary bed into the interstitial space. Severely ill patients exhibit hypovolemia, hypoproteinemia, and edema (Fig. 7). The loss of blood volume may be severe enough to cause hypotension, oliguria, azotemia, and circulatory collapse. Marked hyponatremia is frequent in seriously ill patients. Antidiuretic hormone (ADH) levels may be elevated relative to plasma osmolality in certain of these hyponatremic patients (Kaplowitz and Robertson, 1983). It is not always clear, however, whether this is due to inappropriate secretion of ADH or whether it is a result of nonosmotic stimuli such as decreased intravascular volume and systemic hypotension.

Although nonspecific electrocardiographic abnormalities may occur, clinically significant cardiovascular dysfunction is more frequently secondary to circulatory collapse or to iatrogenic fluid overload during therapy. Nonproductive cough may be present, as well as localized pneumonitis. Pulmonary consolidation is uncommon. Modest hepatic and splenic enlargement frequently occur, but jaundice is unusual.

DIAGNOSIS. Since rickettsiae cannot be cultivated upon artificial media, diagnosis of Rocky Mountain spotted fever by culture of blood or tissue specimens is beyond the capability of most routine clinical laboratories. Moreover, attempts at isolation of the organism by inoculation of tissue culture, guinea pigs, or embryonated eggs may be hazardous to technical personnel in laboratories inexperienced in these procedures. Diagnostic serologic tests are available (see below), but these usually do not become positive until late in the course of the disease. Therefore, the disease

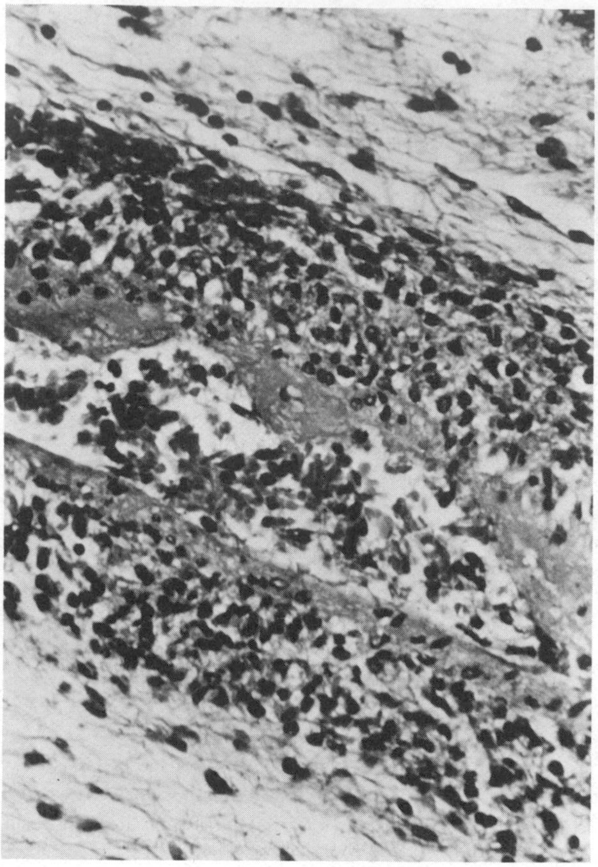

Figure 2. Tangential section of an arteriole from seminal vesicle in a fatal case of Rocky Mountain spotted fever. The endothelium is denuded, and there is fibrin deposition along the vessel lining. Intense cellular infiltration involves all layers of the vessel (hematoxylin-eosin, ×400). (Courtesy of W. Manford Gooch, M.D.)

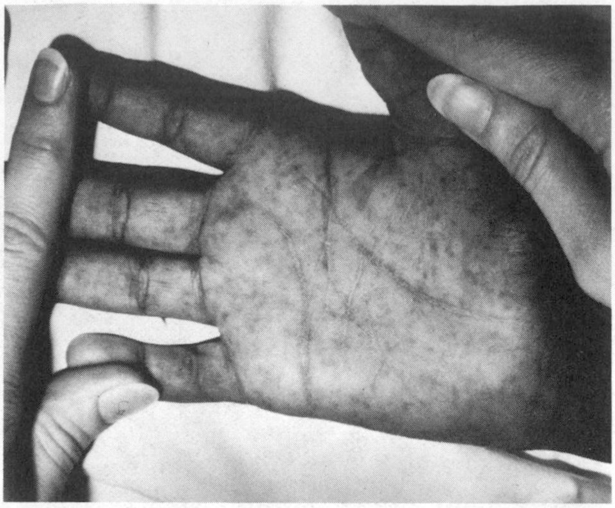

Figure 4. Palmar rash in patient with Rocky Mountain spotted fever. (From Archives of Internal Medicine, Sept. 1973, 132:40. Copyright 1973, American Medical Association.)

must be suspected and appropriate therapy instituted on clinical grounds alone. The diagnosis of Rocky Mountain spotted fever should be strongly entertained in patients living or visiting in endemic areas who present during the warmer months of the year with an illness characterized by fever, headache, and maculopapular or petechial rash. The diagnosis is particularly likely if there is a history of tick bite or intimate exposure to ticks, but lack of such a history by no means excludes the diagnosis. In more severely ill subjects, the presence of thrombocytopenia or hyponatremia is highly suggestive of Rocky Mountain spotted fever. Total leukocyte counts are variable but are

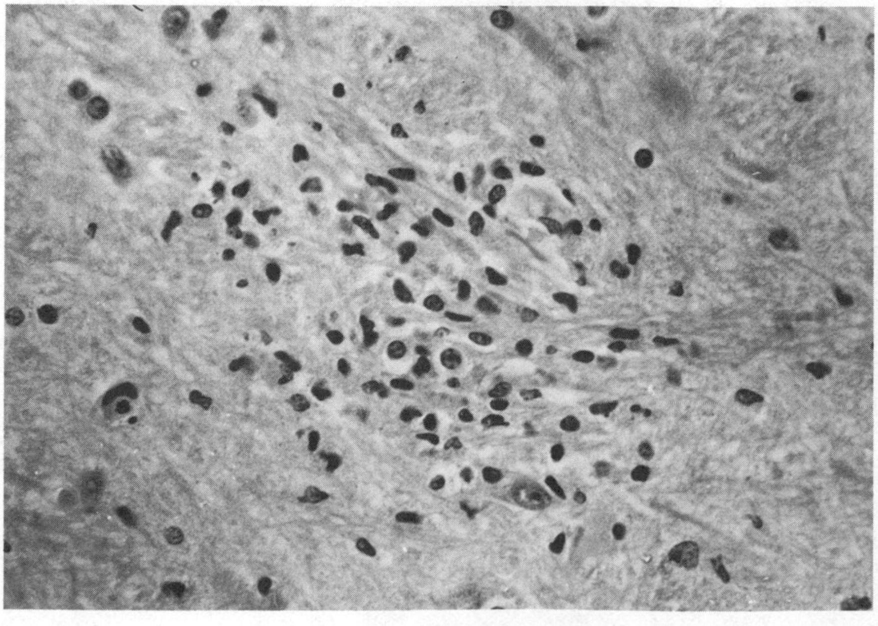

Figure 3. Focus of cerebral astroglial proliferation ("glial nodule") in a fatal case of Rocky Mountain spotted fever (hematoxylin-eosin, ×400). (From Archives of Internal Medicine, Sept. 1973, 132:40. Copyright 1973, American Medical Association.)

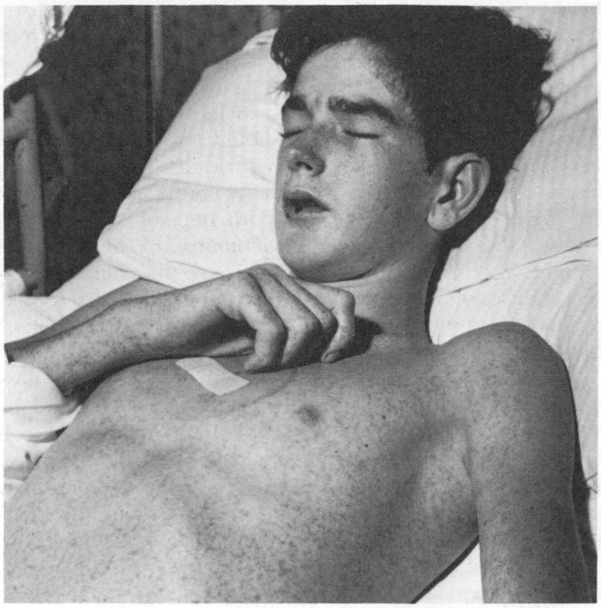

Figure 5. Appearance of generalized rash on tenth hospital day. Bleeding about the mouth was related to mild consumptive coagulopathy. (From Archives of Internal Medicine, Sept. 1973, 132:40. Copyright 1973, American Medical Association.)

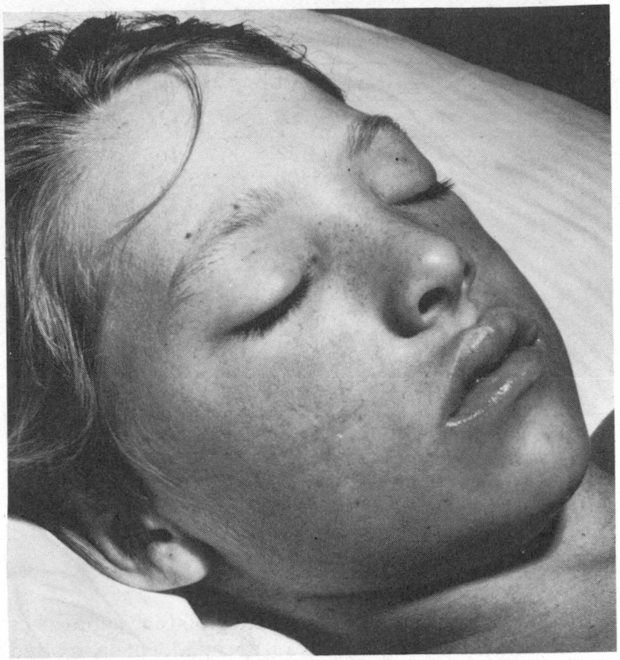

Figure 7. Periorbital and facial edema in a child with Rocky Mountain spotted fever.

usually within normal limits. Anemia and a shift to the left in the differential leukocyte count are frequently present.

The differential diagnosis is a broad one, involving a variety of febrile rash illnesses. In the early rash stage, the disease is frequently misdiagnosed as measles, although measles does not usually occur during the summer. The petechial rash and neurologic abnormalities may lead to the diagnosis of meningococcal meningitis. Time lost during consequent administration of penicillin or its congeners,

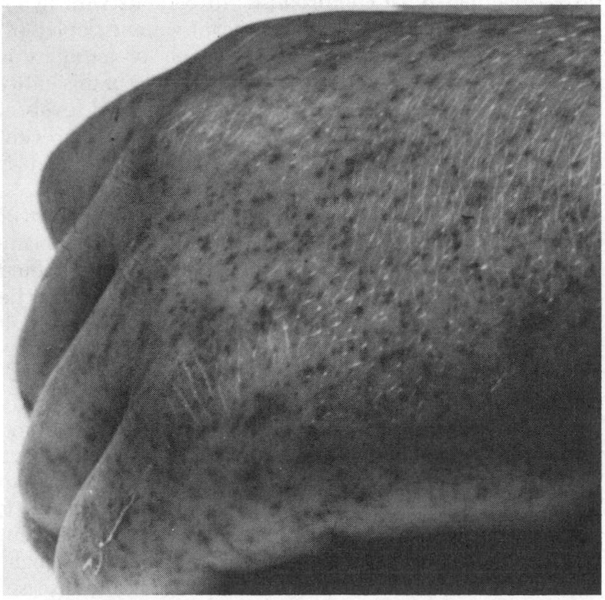

Figure 6. Close-up view of the hand illustrates petechial nature of the rash. (From Archives of Internal Medicine, Sept. 1973, 132:40. Copyright 1973, American Medical Association.)

which are ineffective against *R. rickettsii*, may have disastrous results. Additional diseases to be differentiated include other rickettsioses (murine and epidemic typhus and, to a lesser extent, rickettsialpox), infectious mononucleosis, typhoid fever, rat bite fever, atypical measles, leptospirosis, exanthematous enteroviral infections, toxic shock syndrome, mucocutaneous lymph node syndrome, and various acute vasculitides of noninfectious origin.

Two types of serologic tests are generally available. The Weil-Felix agglutination reaction depends upon a fortuitous cross-antigenicity between *R. rickettsii* and certain strains of *Proteus*, namely OX-2 and OX-19. *Proteus* OX-K agglutinins are of no value in diagnosis of Rocky Mountain spotted fever. The complement-fixation test is performed with purified rickettsial antigens. In either agglutination or complement-fixation tests a four-fold or greater rise of serum antibody titers between acute and convalescent phases of illness is considered diagnostic. If only a single convalescent serum sample is available, Weil-Felix titers of 1:320 or greater and complement-fixation titers of 1:16 or greater, when accompanied by a compatible clinical picture, confirm the diagnosis. Other serologic tests, such as microagglutination, indirect immunofluorescence, indirect hemagglutination, and latex agglutination, are being used with success in certain laboratories. Regardless of the test used, serum antibody titers do not ordinarily achieve diagnostic levels until the second or third week of illness (Table 1).

Investigators have demonstrated rickettsiae by immunofluorescence technique in biopsies of skin lesions taken from patients within the first few days of their illnesses (Woodward et al., 1976). In other studies, peripheral blood monocytes from monkeys experimentally infected with *R. rickettsii* have been maintained in in vitro tissue cultures on glass coverslips. In such preparations it has been possible to visualize rickettsiae within monocytes within three to five days after specimen collection. Both the skin biopsy

Table 1. TIME OF DEVELOPMENT OF ELEVATED WEIL-FELIX AND COMPLEMENT FIXATION (CF) TITERS*

	Days after Onset of Symptoms			
Test	***1–7***	***8–14***	***15–21***	***>22***
OX-2	1/9 (11%)†	11/33 (33%)	5/10 (50%)	5/6 (83%)
OX-19	0/14 (0%)	16/40 (40%)	11/15 (73%)	4/5 (80%)
OX-K	0/10 (0%)	0/19 (0%)	0/9 (0%)	0/1 (0%)
CF	1/4 (25%)	7/17 (41%)	3/4 (75%)	8/8 (100%)

*Weil-Felix titers of 1:320 or greater and complement fixation titers of 1:16 or greater were considered elevated.

†No. positive/No. tested (per cent positive).

(From Torres, J. et al. Archives of Internal Medicine, 132:40. Copyright 1973, American Medical Association.)

and monocyte culture techniques are promising approaches to earlier laboratory diagnosis of Rocky Mountain spotted fever.

TREATMENT. Specific antimicrobial therapy is the cornerstone of management of the patient with Rocky Mountain spotted fever. It has cut the case-fatality ratio from 20 per cent to the current figure of approximately 5 per cent. Both tetracycline and chloramphenicol are effective, and apparently equally so.

Because of the potentially serious hematologic side effects of chloramphenicol therapy, tetracycline is preferred in the usual case. Before the antibiotic era, para-aminobenzoic acid was used with good results, but this drug is no longer employed. Penicillin, cephalosporins, or aminoglycosides are of no known value. Sulfonamides may actually have a deleterious effect and should be avoided.

Insofar as is known, the various tetracycline preparations are essentially equivalent in treatment, although adequate data are lacking for some of the newer preparations. Doxycycline has been reported by various investigators to be effective in prophylaxis of scrub typhus and in treatment of scrub typhus and epidemic typhus. In vitro, one strain of *R. rickettsii* has been shown to be susceptible to doxycycline. The drug has been used with apparent success to treat induced cases of Rocky Mountain spotted fever in volunteers.

Tetracycline may be administered in a total dosage of 25 to 40 mg/kg body weight per day, given in equally divided doses every six hours by mouth. (Some authorities also favor an initial loading dose of 25 mg/kg.) Since the majority of patients with Rocky Mountain spotted fever are children, the hazard of dental problems in tetracycline-treated subjects in the first decade of life must be kept in mind. The risk associated with a single course of therapy, however, is small and must be balanced against the risk of serious side effects from the alternative drug, chloramphenicol. Tetracycline is relatively contraindicated in patients with compromised renal function. If administered to patients with renal insufficiency, it should be used in decreased dosage. The half-life of doxycycline, however, is not significantly prolonged in patients with renal insufficiency. Tetracyclines have been associated with severe and even fatal hepatotoxic reactions. Significant toxicity has usually been associated with high dose intravenous therapy in patients with severe pyogenic infections. Most, but not all, instances have occurred in women in the last trimester of pregnancy. Thus, intravenous tetracycline should not be administered in doses greater than 2 g per day to adults (proportionately less in children) and should probably not be used in women late in pregnancy (to prevent both hepatotoxicity in the mother and abnormal tooth development in the fetus). In patients requiring intravenous therapy, the choice of tetracycline vs. chloramphenicol must be individualized, taking into account the patient's clinical status and the potential adverse effects of each drug.

Chloramphenicol should be administered in a total dosage of 50 mg/kg of body weight per day, divided into four equal doses to be given every six hours. The drug is well absorbed from the gastrointestinal tract but may be given by the intravenous route if necessary. Chloramphenicol is inactivated primarily by liver enzymes and should be given in decreased dosage to patients with hepatic insufficiency. The principal side-effects are dose-related, reversible marrow depression and very rare instances of non-dose related, usually irreversible, aplastic anemia.

If treatment is initiated early in the disease, the patient usually becomes afebrile in three or four days. Relapses are uncommon unless treatment is begun within the first two days of illness.

Supportive care is particularly critical in severely ill patients. Loss of fluid, electrolytes, and protein from the intravascular space may bring on hypotension, circulatory collapse, oliguria, and azotemia. Therefore, monitoring of central venous pressure and replacement of volume are crucial features of management. Fluid therapy should include judicious replacement of electrolytes but also may require colloid-containing solutions such as plasma or albumin. When anemia is severe, whole blood transfusions may be required. Care must be taken, however, to avoid fluid overload and precipitation of pulmonary edema in these patients, some of whom may, in addition, have myocardial and renal compromise. In patients with hyponatremia without evidence of significant volume depletion, the diagnosis of inappropriate secretion of antidiuretic hormone should be entertained, since therapy of this entity requires fluid restriction. Subjects with impaired levels of consciousness require meticulous nursing care to prevent decubitus ulcers or aspiration. A high protein diet is ordinarily indicated in patients able to eat.

Adrenal corticosteroids decrease the toxicity and fever of Rocky Mountain spotted fever. In view of the many problems associated with their use, these agents should ordinarily be avoided. If prescribed at all, they should be given in pharmacologic doses only to the most severely ill patients and their use limited to a few days.

PREVENTION. The most effective measures involve prevention of tick exposure by avoiding tick-infested areas and by keeping household pets tick-free. Wearing protective clothing (long-sleeved garments, trousers tucked into lace-up boots) is often impractical in hot weather when risk is the greatest. Impregnation of clothing with tick repellent may be a useful measure when risk of tick-exposure is high.

For persons at increased risk of contracting the disease, such as recreational campers in areas endemic for Rocky Mountain spotted fever, one of the most practical and effective preventive measures is careful examination of all individuals at least twice daily. Care should be taken to avoid crushing attached ticks while removing them and to avoid scratching the area of the bite, since infective tick juices or feces may be inoculated. After removal of the tick, the area of attachment should be washed with soap and water or treated with a disinfectant. There is no evidence that antibiotic treatment of infected individuals during the incubation period will prevent the disease.

A Rocky Mountain spotted fever vaccine, previously available commercially and recommended for certain high-risk groups, has been withdrawn from the market because of lack of evidence of efficacy.

References

Hattwick, M. A. W., O'Brien, R. J., and Hanson, B. F.: Rocky Mountain spotted fever: epidemiology of an increasing problem. Ann Intern Med 84:732, 1976.

Kaplowitz, L. G., and Robertson, G. L.: Hyponatremia in Rocky Mountain spotted fever: role of antidiuretic hormone. Ann Intern Med 98:334, 1983.

Torres, J., Humphreys, E., and Bisno, A. L.: Rocky Mountain spotted fever in the mid-South. Arch Intern Med 132:340, 1973.

Westerman, E. L.: Rocky Mountain spotless fever: a dilemma for the clinician. Arch Intern Med 142:1106, 1982.

Woodward, T. E., Pedersen, C. E., Jr., Oster, C. N., Bagley, L. R., Romberger, J., and Snyder, M. J.: Prompt confirmation of Rocky Mountain spotted fever: identification of rickettsiae in skin tissues. J Infect Dis 134:297, 1976.

204

OTHER RICKETTSIAL SPOTTED FEVERS

R. Brezina, M.D.

FIÈVRE BOUTONNEUSE

Fièvre boutonneuse (South African tick bite fever, Kenya tick typhus, Indian tick typhus) is a mild or moderately severe, acute febrile disease caused by *Rickettsia conorii.* It is characterized by a primary lesion (tâche noire) at the site of tick attachment, a maculopapular exanthem, headache, photophobia, arthralgia, and diffuse myalgia. Fièvre boutonneuse is widely distributed along the Mediterranean and the Black and Caspian Sea littorals (Spain, France, Italy, Greece, Rumania, Bulgaria, Turkey, Israel, U.S.S.R., Morocco, Algeria, Libya, and Egypt). Kenya tick typhus and South African tick bite fever, which occur in the bush areas of West, Central, and East Africa and in all parts of the Union of South Africa (Gear, 1954), and Indian tick typhus are apparently variants of the same disease. Rickettsial strains identical to *R. conorii* have also been isolated in Pakistan, Thailand, and Malaysia.

ETIOLOGY. Rickettsiae of the spotted fever group are divided into several antigenic subgroups (see Chapter 54). *R. parkeri,* which causes disease only in guinea pigs, and *R. conorii* make up subgroup B of the spotted fever group (Lackman et al., 1965). They cross-react in toxin-neutralization tests in mice and in complement fixation tests with the soluble, group-specific antigen. They can be distinguished by complement fixation tests performed with the cell-associated antigen derived from repeated washing of *R. conorii.* This CF test against mouse antibodies differentiates *R. conorii* from all other rickettsiae of the spotted fever group. *R. conorii* can also be separated from *R. rickettsii* (Rocky Mountain spotted fever) and *R. siberica* (North Asian tick typhus) by toxin-neutralization tests in mice.

Except for lower virulence for the guinea pig, the morphologic and biologic properties of *R. conorii* are similar to those of *R. rickettsii* (Chapter 54). *R. conorii* causes fever and scrotal swelling in guinea pigs but not scrotal necrosis and death. Intravenous injections of mice with heavy suspensions of viable *R. conorii* cause acute toxic deaths. Strains of *R. conorii* collected in the Mediterranean region, Kenya, South Africa, and India are antigenically indistinguishable. *R. conorii* grows relatively well in the chick embryo yolk sac. Rickettsiae are found in both the cytoplasm and the nucleus of infected cells. *R. conorii* elicits cross-reactive antibody to *Proteus* OX-2 and OX-19 antigens. The guanine plus cytosine (G + C) content of the DNA in *R. conorii* is approximately 32.5 moles per cent.

The most important vector and arthropod host of *R. conorii* in the Mediterranean, Caspian, and Black Sea regions and in parts of the Indian subcontinent is the dog tick, *Rhipicephalus sanguineus.* In Europe, other species of the genera *Ixodes* and *Dermacentor* can probably be vectors. In Africa, *R. conorii* has been isolated from *Haemaphysalis leachi, R. sanguineus, Amblyomma hebraeum, R. appendiculatus, R. evertsi, Hyalomma aegyptium,* and *R. simus. H. leachi* and *R. simus* are the most important vectors. All stages of *H. leachi,* a dog tick, are infective. Transovarial transmission provides a permanent reservoir of *R. conorii.* In Malaysia, *R. conorii* was isolated from *Ixodes granulatus* and *Haemaphysalis* species. *R. conorii* has been isolated from rats and mice in South Africa, Kenya, and Malaysia (Marchette, 1965), where they may be important reservoirs. The reservoir animals of Indian tick typhus are unknown.

PATHOGENESIS AND PATHOLOGY. Because fatal human cases of fièvre boutonneuse are unknown, the pathologic changes have been studied in experimentally infected guinea pigs. Rickettsemia occurs during the early febrile period, after the rickettsiae invade the body through the tick bite. Secondary invasion of the endothelium of capillaries, arterioles, and venules leads to thrombosis and formation of perivascular nodules. There is less necrosis of these small vessels than in Rocky Mountain spotted fever.

CLINICAL MANIFESTATIONS. The incubation period of fièvre boutonneuse varies from three to 15 days. The onset is usually abrupt with chills and fever to 39 to 40° C, conjunctivitis, myalgia, and arthralgia. Disturbances of the sensorium may occur in more severe cases. The rash, which usually appears between the second and fifth days of fever, consists of pink, lentil-sized maculopapules (Fig.

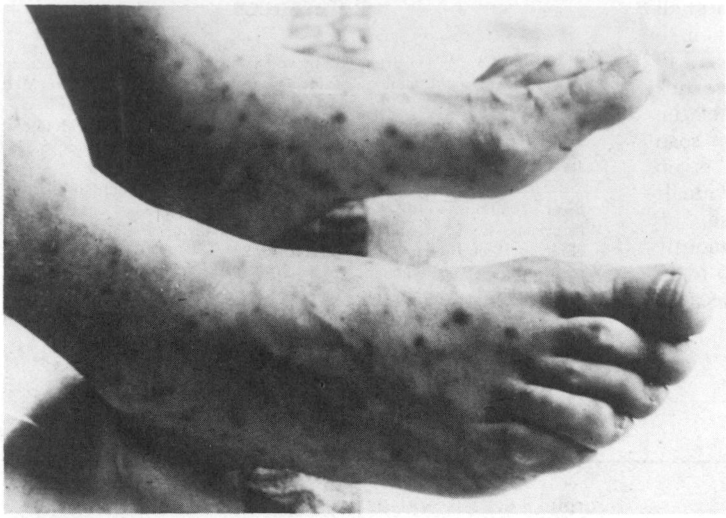

Figure 1. The maculopapular rash on the lower extremities of a patient with fièvre boutonneuse (photo kindly provided by Prof. V. Scaffidi, M.D., University of Palermo, Italy).

1). The rash is noted first on the extremities and rapidly spreads to the trunk, scalp, face, palms, and soles. Exanthems were present in 100 per cent of 73 cases reported from Sicily (Romano, 1977). Fever, often remittent, continues for approximately 10 to 20 days, the rash for 5 to 10 days. The primary lesion (tâche noire, Fig. 2), which ranges from the size of a pinhead to that of a lentil, ulcerates and forms a brown to black eschar. It is usually accompanied by regional lymphadenopathy. Splenomegaly, hepatomegaly, transitory proteinuria and hematuria, bronchitis, ECG abnormalities (T-wave changes, bundle branch block), and signs of meningeal irritation may occur. Bradycardia and hypotension are unusual.

COMPLICATIONS AND SEQUELAE. Complications are extremely rare. In the group of 73 patients with fièvre boutonneuse reported from Sicily, complications included microhematuria and albuminuria, bronchopneumonia and bronchitis, myocarditis, hypotension, and meningismus (Ferrarini et al., 1977).

There are no permanent sequelae. Insomnia and irritability may occur during convalescence. Recovery is accompanied by the development of solid immunity.

GEOGRAPHIC VARIATIONS. Fièvre boutonneuse, African tick bite fever, Kenya tick typhus, and Indian tick typhus are thought to represent geographic variations of one disease caused by the same agent. The rickettsiae isolated from patients with each of these diseases are morphologically and antigenically indistinguishable from type strains of *R. conorii.* The vectors and the virulence of *R. conorii* (see etiology) strains may differ depending on the geographic areas from which they were collected. Strains of *R. conorii* with extremely low virulence have been isolated in Malaysia (Marchette, 1965).

DIAGNOSIS. A primary, and typical exanthem and contact with tick-infected dogs in an endemic area strongly suggest the diagnosis. Dogs, however, do not appear to be a necessary link between ticks and man. Other exanthematous diseases, including rickettsial infections, are difficult to exclude clinically, especially when the primary lesion is absent in abortive cases of fièvre boutonneuse.

The guinea pig is the animal of choice for primary isolation. A few days after intraperitoneal inoculation of infected blood, guinea pigs develop fever and scrotal swelling without necrosis. *R. conorii* can also be isolated by

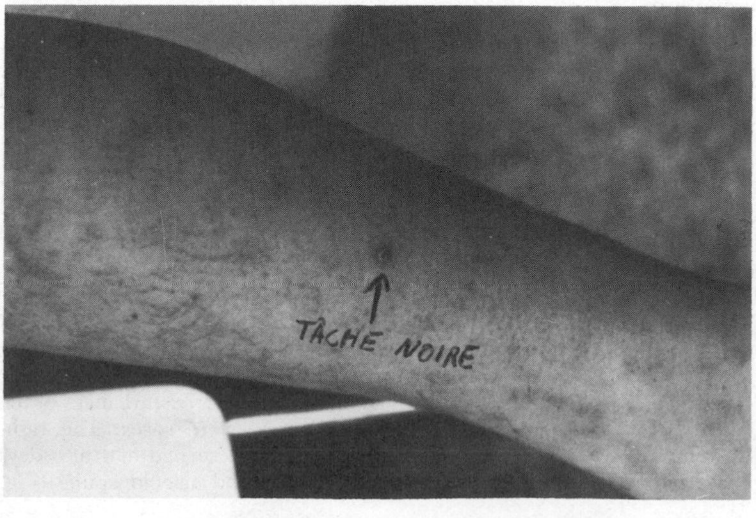

Figure 2. The primary lesion (tâche noire) in a patient with fièvre boutonneuse (photo kindly supplied by Prof. O. Restivo, M.D., Department of Infectious Diseases, Caltanissetta, Italy).

inoculation of blood, infected guinea pig tissue, or tick suspensions into the chick embryo yolk sac.

Serologic diagnosis is based on the examination of sera by complement fixation tests against the soluble group-specific antigen or, more specifically, against the highly purified species-specific cell-associated antigen. The species-specific antigen differentiates *R. conorii* from all other rickettsial species of the spotted fever group. So does the microimmunofluorescence test (Philip et al., 1976), which makes it possible to establish the exact diagnosis as early as the fourth to eighth day of the disease by examination of skin lesions as described for Rocky Mountain spotted fever (Woodward et al., 1976). The Weil-Felix reactions do not distinguish fièvre boutonneuse from most other rickettsial infections.

TREATMENT. As with other rickettsioses, chloramphenicol and the tetracyclines are the drugs of choice. Patients generally become afebrile within two to three days of the institution of one to two grams per day of either antibiotic. Treatment should be continued for four to seven days after the temperature returns to normal.

PROPHYLAXIS. Fièvre boutonneuse is usually a sporadic disease of low incidence and low mortality. Under these circumstances, the only practical control measures are tick repellents and removal of ticks before attachment. Detachment or any handling of infected ticks should be done carefully to avoid contamination of the skin and environment with highly infectious tick juices.

ASIAN TICK-BORNE TYPHUS

Asian tick-borne typhus is an acute febrile infection, caused by *Rickettsia siberica*. It is characterized by the sudden onset of headache, myalgias, a maculopapular (or, less frequently, a petechial) exanthem, chills, and fever. The fever is usually remittent and lasts from 6 to 17 days, depending on the severity of the disease. It occurs not only in Siberia, the Far East, Central Asia, Armenia, Azerbaijan, Mongolia, and Pakistan, but also in the European part of the U.S.S.R., especially in the Tula region and the Bashkir A.S.S.R.

ETIOLOGY. *R. siberica* belongs to subgroup A of the spotted fever group along with *R. rickettsii*, the cause of Rocky Mountain spotted fever (Lackman et al., 1965). The close antigenic relationship of these two species was first proved by mouse toxin-neutralization tests with immune guinea pig sera (Bell and Stoenner, 1960). This test, in combination with a complement fixation system using washed *R. siberica* and immune guinea pig sera or soluble antigen and immune mouse sera, differentiates *R. siberica* from other species of the spotted fever group. The morphologic and biologic properties of *R. siberica*, including its occurrence both in the cytoplasm and in the nucleus of infected cells, are similar to those of the other species of the spotted fever group. The experimentally infected guinea pig develops fever, splenomegaly, and scrotal swelling. *R. siberica* grows relatively well in the chick embryo yolk sac and kills most embryos within four to five days. It proliferates in guinea pig kidney and chick embryo cell cultures, as well as in various established cell lines.

R. siberica has been isolated from many species of ixodid ticks (*Dermacentor sylvarum, D. marginatus, D. pictus, D. nuttallii, Haemaphysalis concinna, H. japonica, H. punctata, Hyalomma marginatum, Ixodes persulcatus*), from several species of gamasid ticks, and from chiggers (*Trombicula autumnalis* and *T. zachvatkini*). It multiplies in the salivary glands, testes, and ovaries. Except for *H. concinna*, transstadial and transovarial transmission occurs in all tick vectors. Therefore, ticks are not only vectors but also the primary reservoir. Adult ticks parasitize larger wild and domestic animals; larvae and nymphs feed on small wild animals and birds. The peak incidence of human cases occurs in April to May and corresponds to the highest activity of adult ticks. Many domestic and wild animals that are hosts of ticks have been shown to harbor *R. siberica* and have been implicated as possible reservoirs (Tarasevich et al., 1977).

PATHOGENESIS AND PATHOLOGY. Following the tick bite, rickettsemia occurs and an eschar (tâche noire) develops at the site. It resembles a cigarette burn or a black button-like lesion with a central dark necrotic area and a surrounding reddish areola. This local lesion is accompanied by regional lymphadenitis and is probably the primary site of rickettsial propagation, as Woodward et al. (1976) demonstrated in Rocky Mountain spotted fever.

The pathologic lesions in fatal cases resemble those of Rocky Mountain spotted fever and other rickettsioses. Damage to the endothelium of capillaries, small arteries, and veins leads to thrombosis and formation of reactive perivascular nodules.

CLINICAL MANIFESTATIONS. The incubation period of about five to seven days is followed by sudden fever, headache, myalgia, and conjunctivitis. The fever may reach 40° C or more and may persist for seven to ten days. It is usually remittent and ends by lysis. Soviet authors distinguish subclinical, mild, and severe forms of the disease. In addition to the primary lesion and fever, the most distinct clinical sign is a pink to red maculopapular eruption, which infrequently becomes petechial or hemorrhagic. It appears on about the third to fourth febrile day on the extremities and rapidly spreads over the entire body, including the scalp, face, palms, and soles. The exanthem persists during the febrile period.

There are no characteristic changes in the white blood cell count. The sedimentation rate is slightly elevated. Splenomegaly and hepatomegaly may occur with little disturbance of function. Involvement of the central nervous system or the cardiovascular system is unusual.

COMPLICATIONS AND SEQUELAE. Complications are uncommon, but pneumonia, myocarditis, nephritis, and meningitis have been reported. Convalescence may be prolonged, but no serious or permanent sequelae occur. In contrast to Rocky Mountain spotted fever, relapses have not been observed. Recovery from the disease is accompanied by development of solid immunity to reinfection with *R. siberica* and to infections caused by other rickettsiae of the spotted fever group.

DIAGNOSIS. The clinical diagnosis is based on the presence of the primary lesion, regional lymphadenitis, fever, and the maculopapular rash in a patient exposed to ticks in an endemic area. Other rickettsial infections and viral exanthems must be excluded, especially if there is no primary eschar.

The definitive diagnosis can be established only in the

laboratory. Intraperitoneal inoculation of infected blood into male guinea pigs causes fever and scrotal swelling with a serofibrinous exudate in the tunica vaginalis. Surviving guinea pigs develop specific antibody that can be demonstrated by the CF test with washed *R. siberica* antigen.

By the end of the first week, the Weil-Felix reaction is positive with *Proteus* OX-2 and later *Proteus* OX-K antigen. Complement-fixing antibody is detectable by the tenth day. To distinguish Asian tick-borne typhus from other spotted fevers, highly purified washed corpuscular antigen must be used in the complement fixation or microagglutination tests. Microimmunofluorescence will also distinguish these organisms (Philip et al., 1976).

TREATMENT. Chloramphenicol and the tetracyclines are equally effective. Patients generally become afebrile after two to three days of treatment with 2 g per day of either antibiotic.

PROPHYLAXIS. Control measures are aimed at avoiding tick bites by using repellents, by wearing clothing that interferes with attachment, and by prompt removal of attached ticks. Vaccines of purified killed suspensions of *R. siberica* and ether-treated *R. siberica* have been used. Kekcheeva (1963) recommended a so-called chemovaccine of the live *R. siberica* suspension attenuated by the addition of tetracycline.

QUEENSLAND TICK TYPHUS

Queensland tick typhus is an acute febrile exanthematous disease caused by *Rickettsia australis*, one of the spotted fever rickettsiae. It was first recognized at Atherton in North Queensland (Andrew et al., 1946; Brody, 1946), and its etiology was established by demonstration of rickettsiae in smears from the peritoneal fluid of mice inoculated with blood from the infected patient (Andrew et al., 1946). The primary lesion or eschar is a common feature of the disease, whether it occurs in North or South Queensland.

ETIOLOGY. *R. australis* and *R. akari* (the cause of rickettsialpox) (see Chapter 205) belong to subgroup C of the spotted fever rickettsiae (Lackman et al., 1965). *R. australis* shares the common soluble antigen of this group. It can be differentiated from the others by complement fixation with washed corpuscular antigens, by cross-challenge of immunized guinea pigs, and by toxin-neutralization tests in mice (Bell and Stoenner, 1950; Bozeman et al., 1960). It can be best distinguished from *R. akari* by complement fixation tests with immune mouse sera. The morphologic and biologic properties of *R. australis* are similar to those of the other spotted fever rickettsiae, except that acute mouse toxicity has not been demonstrated. Although guinea pigs and adult mice are susceptible to intraperitoneal inoculation with *R. australis*, the best results are achieved with weaned or newborn mice.

The Australian ticks *Ixodes holocyclus* and *I. tasmani* are the major vectors of *R. australis* (Campbell and Domrow, 1978). Epidemiologic evidence implicates these ticks as reservoirs as well. Specific complement-fixing antibodies and evidence of active infection have been found in several species of marsupials and wild rodents, including bandicoots, opossums, kangaroos, and mice (Cock and Campbell, 1965, cited by Campbell and Domrow, 1978).

PATHOGENESIS AND PATHOLOGY. The pathogenesis and pathology of Queensland tick typhus are similar to those of the other species of the spotted fever group of rickettsiae.

CLINICAL MANIFESTATIONS. The incubation period varies from seven to ten days after the tick bite. A primary eschar is common but is not always easily found. Regional lymph nodes are enlarged and tender. The disease is not fatal and is characterized by a mild course with headache, malaise, and a maculopapular rash on the face, scalp, trunk, palms, and soles. Complications and sequelae are infrequent.

DIAGNOSIS. A primary lesion, rash, and fever in someone exposed to ticks in the endemic area provide strong clinical evidence of the diagnosis. Scrub typhus (Chapter 202) is the only other exanthematous rickettsial infection that occurs in Australia. The macular rash of scrub typhus begins on the trunk and spreads later to the upper and lower extremities. The reverse is usually true in Queensland tick typhus.

The laboratory diagnosis is established by the isolation of *R. australis* from suckling or weaned mice and guinea pigs injected intraperitoneally with the blood of the patient. *R. australis* does not cause acute toxicity in the mouse.

The Weil-Felix reactions are positive with *Proteus* OX-19 and OX-2 antigens. The complement fixation reaction is positive with the soluble antigens of the spotted fever group but specific when washed suspensions of *R. australis* are used as the antigen. It can also be differentiated from other members of the spotted fever group by cross-challenge of immune guinea pigs and by toxin-neutralization tests in mice.

TREATMENT. Two grams per day of either tetracycline or chloramphenicol are effective.

PROPHYLAXIS. The control measures are aimed at preventing tick bites. No effective vaccine is available.

References

Andrew, R., Bonnin, J. M., and Williams, S.: Tick typhus in North Queensland. Med J Aust 2:253, 1946.

Bell, E. J., and Stoenner, H. G.: Immunologic relationships among the spotted fever group of rickettsias determined by toxin neutralization test in mice with convalescent animal serum. J Immunol 84:171, 1960.

Bozeman, F. L., Humphries, J. W., Campbell, J. M., and O'Hara, P. L.: Laboratory studies of the spotted fever group of rickettsiae. In Symposium on the Spotted Fever Group of Rickettsiae. Med Sci Pub No. 7, Walter Reed Army Institute of Research. Washington, D.C., U.S. Government Printing Office, 1960, pp. 7–11.

Brody, J.: A case of tick typhus in North Queensland. Med J Aust 1:511, 1946.

Campbell, R. W., and Domrow, R.: Rickettsioses in Australia: Ecology of *Rickettsia tsutsugamushi* and *Rickettsia australis*. In Kazár, J., Ormsbee, R. A., and Tarasevich, I. V. (eds.): Rickettsiae and Rickettsial Diseases. Bratislava, Veda, Publishing House of Slovak Academy of Sciences, 1978, p. 505.

Ferrarini, E., Distefano, G., and Barca, S.: Esperienze cliniche su una casistica di rickettsiosi dermotifose. Minerva med Siciliana 68:2369, 1977.

Gear, J.: The rickettsial diseases of Southern Africa. A review of recent studies. J Clin Sci 5:158, 1954.

Kekcheeva, N. (1963) cited in Zdrodovskij, P. F., and Golinevich, H. M.: La rickettsiose à tiques d'Asie. Bull WHO 35:105, 1966.

Lackman, D. B., Bell, J. E., Stoenner, H. G., and Pickens, E. G.: The Rocky Mountain spotted fever group of Rickettsias. Hlth Lab Sci 2:135, 1965.

Marchette, N. J.: Rickettsioses—tick typhus, Q fever, urban typhus in Malaya. J Med Entomol 2(4):339, 1965.

Philip, R. N., Casper, E. A., and Ormsbee, R. A.: Microimmunofluorescence test for the serological study of Rocky Mountain spotted fever and typhus. J Clin Microbiol 3:51, 1976.

Romano, A.: Osservazioni su 73 casi di febbre bottonosa verificatisi nella Provincia di Trapani nel decenio 1966–1975. Minerva med Siciliana 68:2365, 1977.

Tarasevich, I. V., Panfilova, S. S., and Fetisova, N. F.: Ecological geography of rickettsioses of tick spotted fever group (in Russian). In Lebedev, A. D. (ed.): Medicinskaja geografia, Vol. 8. Moskva, Viniti, 1977, pp. 7–103.

Woodward, T. E., Pedersen, C. F., Oster, C. N., Bagley, L. R., Romberger, J., and Snyder, M. J.: Prompt confirmation of Rocky Mountain spotted fever: Identification of rickettsiae in skin tissues. J Infect Dis 134:297, 1976.

205

RICKETTSIALPOX

GARRISON RAPMUND, M.D.

DEFINITION AND ETIOLOGY. Rickettsialpox is a febrile disease distinguishable by the presence of a primary cutaneous lesion, or eschar, and a papulovesicular eruption. The disease is caused by *Rickettsia akari*, a member of the spotted fever group of rickettsiae and is transmitted to man by the bite of a blood-sucking mite, *Allodermanyssus sanguineus*, an ectoparasite of the house mouse (Huebner et al., 1946; Huebner, Jellison, and Pomerantz, 1946). The disease was first described by Greenberg (1947) in 1946 in New York City and shortly thereafter in the Soviet Union by Drobinskii (1962). The incidence has declined sharply in the last 20 years, but recent case reports (Wong et al., 1979; Brettman et al., 1981) prove that the disease has not disappeared. More likely, rickettsialpox is being overlooked by physicians, which is unfortunate because the disease can be severe, although nonfatal, and specific therapy is available.

CLINICAL MANIFESTATIONS. After an incubation period of 10 to 24 days, patients have sudden onset of fever, chills, headache, and malaise. A rash follows, usually within one to four days, consisting of red maculopapules 2 to 10 mm in size and ranging in number from a few scattered lesions to a diffuse rash over most of the body, including the mucous membranes. Involvement of the palms and soles is rare. Two to three days later vesicles form at the apices of the papules, and then crust and fall off, leaving pigmented areas but no scars. The rash persists for three to eight days and is not pruritic. Patients are not infectious for others. The fever is remittent with peaks ranging from 38.5° to 40.5° C, falling to normal after about seven days. Headache is usually frontal and can be severe. The primary cutaneous lesion can be located anywhere, developing at the site of the mite feeding. By the time a rash develops, the lesion is either ulcerated or crusted with a black top. Patients are unaware of the mite feeding and usually overlook the developing lesion as well. In up to 10 per cent of patients the primary lesion is not evident. The disease abates spontaneously in 10 to 14 days, without sequelae. Occasionally the clinical course of disease can be so mild that patients remain ambulatory. A leukopenia of 2500 to 5000 cells per cubic millimeter is seen in the acute phase, lymphocytes predominating, sometimes with large vacuolated mononuclear cells also present. Heterophil antibody is absent.

GEOGRAPHIC VARIATIONS IN DISEASE. Rickettsialpox is an urban domiciliary disease. In the first recognized epidemic in New York City in 1946 (Greenberg et al., 1947), the disease affected middle income families living in multistoried apartment blocks. American cases were contracted infrequently in single family dwellings or at work. Disease was always associated with places having large house-mouse populations and heavy infestations of the rodent mite *A. sanguineus*. The circumstance favoring mouse proliferation was incomplete incineration of garbage in basement incinerators, which also provided warmth needed for mite proliferation. In the years after 1946 several hundred cases were reported annually in New York City and isolated outbreaks occurred in other northeastern American cities. In 1949 Drobinskii (1962) described a "vesicular rickettsiosis" in urban populations in the Donetz Basin of the Ukraine that closely resembled the disease in America. Subsequently the disease agent, called by Russian workers *Dermacentroxenus murinus* (Zdrodovskii et al., 1960), was shown to be serologically identical to *R. akari* isolated in New York City. Rickettsialpox was reported clinically in the 1950s from equatorial Africa (Central African Republic) by LeGac and coworkers (1953) and from southern Africa by Gear (1954). By 1963 disease incidence was reported to be much reduced, ascribed to improved rodent control (Lackman, 1963). Since then, sporadic cases have been recorded in New York City (Wong et al., 1979); none elsewhere. Recently, Brettman and coworkers (1981) described an outbreak of five cases in one apartment building in New York City.

Evidence suggests that *R. akari* exists in nature apart from man. The rickettsia has been isolated from a single specimen of wild-caught reed vole in Korea (Jackson et al., 1957). The rickettsia is passed transovarially in *A. sanguineus* mites; so this mite as well as its rodent host may serve as a natural reservoir. *A. sanguineus* has been recovered in diverse locations around the world since its first description in Egypt in 1914. Finally, the ubiquitous tropical rat mite, *Liponyssus bacoti*, is capable experimentally of transmitting *R. akari* to mice by feeding and of passing *R. akari* transovarially to its progeny but it is not an efficient vector (Philip and Hughes, 1948). However, a thorough investigation of the natural ecology of *R. akari* has not been undertaken. Physicians should consider rickettsialpox in any patient with a vesicular eruption.

DIAGNOSIS. The clinical differential diagnosis must take into account varicella, typhoid fever, infectious mononucleosis, other spotted fever rickettsial infections such as fièvre boutonneuse and murine typhus. A specific laboratory diagnosis is possible by isolation of *R. akari* from acute phase blood inoculated into laboratory mice or guinea pigs and from the fourteenth day on by detection of complement-fixing antibody in convalescent serum using washed *R. akari* organisms as antigen. More commonly, spotted fever group antigens are used to detect antibody in the CF and IF procedures, the latter being more sensitive. Agglutinins to *Proteus* OX-19, OX-2, or OX-K strains are not present at significant dilutions of serum (>1:100). Since *Proteus* agglutinins to strains OX-19 and/or OX-2 are usually present at these serum dilutions in other spotted fever infections, their absence serves to differentiate rickettsialpox from other members of the spotted fever group of diseases, especially when a vesicular eruption is absent.

TREATMENT. Tetracycline, 250 mg every six hours, produces rapid clinical response within 48 hours.

References

Brettman, L. R., Lewin, S., Holzman, S., Goldman, W. D., Marr, J. S., Kechijian, P., and Schinella, R.: Rickettsialpox: report of an outbreak and a contemporary review. Medicine 60:363, 1981.

Drobinskii, I. R.: Gamazov'y rikketsioz. Klinika I diagnostika. Kishinev: Akademiya Naul Moldarskoi SSR, 1962.

Gear, J.: The rickettsial diseases in Southern Africa. A review of recent studies. South African J Clin Sci 5:158, 1954.

Greenberg, J., Pelliteri, O. J., and Jellison, W. L.: Rickettsialpox—a newly recognized rickettsial disease. III. Epidemiology. Am J Pub Hlth 37:860, 1947.

Huebner, R. J., Jellison, W. L., and Pomerantz, C.: Rickettsialpox—a newly reocgnized rickettsial disease. IV. Isolation of a rickettsia apparently identical with the causative agent of rickettsialpox from *Allodermanyssus sanguineus*, a rodent mite. Public Health Rep 61:1677, 1946.

Huebner, R. J., Stamps, P., and Armstrong, C.: Rickettsialpox—a newly recognized rickettsial disease. I. Isolation of the etiological agent. Public Health Rep 61:1605, 1946.

Jackson, E. B., Danauskas, J. X., Coale, M. C., and Smadel, J. E.: Recovery of *Rickettsia akari* from the Korean vole *Microtus fortis pelliceus*. Am J Hyg 66:301, 1957.

Lackman, D. B.: A review of information on rickettsialpox in the United States. Clin Ped 2:296, 1963.

Le Gac, P.: Research on rickettsial pox in Oubangui-Chari. West African Med J 2(n.s.):42, 1953.

Philip, C. B., and Hughes, L. E.: The tropical rat mite *Liponyssus bacoti* as an experimental vector of rickettsialpox. Am J Trop Med 28:697, 1948.

Rose, H. M.: The clinical manifestations and laboratory diagnosis of rickettsialpox. Ann Int Med 31:871, 1949.

Wong, B., Singer, C., Armstrong, D., and Millian, S. J.: Rickettsialpox. Case report and epidemiologic review. JAMA 242:1998, 1979.

Zdrodovskii, P. F., and Golinevich, H. M.: The rickettsial diseases. New York, Pergamon Press, 1960, p. 340.

206

TRENCH FEVER

GARRISON RAPMUND, M.D.

DEFINITION AND ETIOLOGY. Trench fever is a louse-borne febrile disease that is indistinguishable clinically from many other infections. It was first widely recognized during World War I in Europe when epidemics occurred in military personnel engaged in trench warfare. In Europe the disease is also called Wolhynian fever after a district in Poland where epidemic disease occurred. The causative agent, *Rochalimaea quintana*, originally considered a *Rickettsia*, is distinguished from rickettsiae by its ability to grow extracellularly on bacteriologic media and in the lumen of the louse gut. One form of the disease consists of recurrent febrile episodes with intervening afebrile periods of roughly five days, hence the specific name quintana. The disease has many other patterns including a single three- to four-day fever, continuous fever for several months, and relapsing fever at irregular intervals for many months (Byam, 1919; Strong, 1918).

CLINICAL MANIFESTATIONS. Like epidemic typhus, the disease is transmitted to man through infected louse feces. Patients inoculate themselves by scratching skin contaminated with louse feces. The incubation period is 9 to 25 days. At onset, patients experience severe headache, usually postorbital, profuse sweating, pain in the lower back that extends to both legs by the second or third day, neck pain simulating meningitis, and fever of 38.5 to 40° C. Mild sore throat occurs without catarrhal rhinitis or bronchitis. Muscle and bone pain, especially in the tibiae, is very typical. Abdominal pain simulating appendicitis occurs. A macular rash of discrete spots 1 centimeter or less in diameter occurs on the anterior chest and abdomen, rarely elsewhere, on the second and third days and lasts at the most for several days. The most striking physical finding is an enlarged spleen, which is often found on the first day and persists throughout the clinical course. A mild leukocytosis may accompany the acute phase (Hurst, 1942; Mohr, 1956; Zdrodovskii and Golinevich, 1960).

The disease always remits completely without specific therapy. Occasionally convalescence is protracted, and *Rochalimaea* organisms may circulate in the blood for many months in asymptomatic convalescent patients (Vinson et al., 1969). Relapse after a year or more of good health has also been described (Mohr and Weyer, 1964).

GEOGRAPHIC VARIATIONS. The distribution of the disease has never been accurately established. Specific antibody has been found in persons in Europe (Weyer et al., 1962), and in Tunisia, Burundi, Ethiopia, Mexico, and Bolivia (Meyers and Wisseman, 1973; Vinson, 1973), but broad-scale seroepidemiologic studies have not been undertaken. The only known reservoir of *Rochalimaea* is man. This agent does not pass transovarially in the louse, *Pediculus humanis* (Weyer, 1962), which parasitizes only man. There is evidence that movement of infected persons can introduce the disease to new areas, as in Greece and Iraq in World War I (Hurst, 1942). Infected human lice have been found in Mexico City (Varela, 1969) but no naturally occurring disease has been reported in the western hemisphere. Weiss and co-workers (1978) reported that a microorganism isolated by Baker (1946) in 1943 from voles *(Microtus pennsylvanicus)* captured in Grosse Isle, Quebec, Canada was very similar to *R. quintana*. Grosse Isle was a quarantine station in the St. Lawrence River where in 1847 thousands of immigrants died of epidemic typhus and were buried. As Weiss and his colleagues point out, thorough study of voles and other small rodents elsewhere has failed to recover this agent. This finding may represent an unusual isolated extension of an *R. quintana*–like organism from man to voles. Myers and coworkers (1979) have concluded that the two agents, though similar, can be distinguished serologically and the Baker vole agent may be classified separately within the genus (Weiss, 1982).

Weiss and Dasch (1982) have proposed the name *Rochalimaea vinsonii* for Baker's vole agent.

DIAGNOSIS. Formerly, the diagnosis could be confirmed only by allowing rickettsia-free lice to feed on patients and identifying the organism growing extracellularly in the louse intestinal lumen (xenodiagnosis). Now the organism can be cultured on specially prepared blood agar (Varela et al., 1969), and specific antibody can be detected by a variety of serologic procedures including complement fixation (Weyer et al., 1962), passive hemagglutination (Cooper et al., 1976), and enzyme immunoassay (Hollingdale et al., 1978). Antibodies appear within several weeks of the onset of disease and persist in some cases for years. Studies of volunteers during World War I show that persons are susceptible to reinfection and disease within three to six months of the initial attack, but an assessment of immunity to trench fever by current methods has not been reported (Byam, 1919; Strong, 1918). Trench fever may be particularly difficult to distinguish clinically from malaria, influenza, and relapsing fever caused by *Borrelia recurrentis*.

TREATMENT AND PROPHYLAXIS. Rapid clinical response to treatment with tetracycline and chloramphenicol has been reported (Mohr and Weyer, 1964). The disease can be controlled by measures that curtail louse infestation and decontaminate lousy clothing. Dry louse feces remain infectious for many months.

Although it has not been reported in recent years, cases of trench fever surely must continue to occur in louse-infested populations. Recent advances in laboratory diagnosis should improve the chances of recognizing endemic disease.

References

Baker, J. A.: A rickettsial infection in Canadian voles. J Exp Med 84:37, 1946.

Byam, W.: Trench Fever. London, Oxford University Press, 1919.

Cooper, M. D., Hollingdale, M. R., Vinson, J. W., and Costa, J.: A passive hemagglutination test for the diagnosis of trench fever. J Infect Dis 134:605, 1976.

Hollingdale, M. R., Herrmann, J. E., and Vinson, J. W.: Enzyme immunoassay of antibody to *Rochalimaea quintana:* Diagnosis of trench fever and serologic cross-reactions among other rickettsiae. J Infect Dis 137:578, 1978.

Hurst, A.: Trench fever. Br Med J 2:318, 1942.

Meyers, W. F., and Wisseman, C. L., Jr.: Louse-borne diseases worldwide: Trench fever. Serologic studies of trench fever employing a microagglutination procedure. In Proceedings of the International Symposium on the Control of Lice and Louse-borne Diseases. Publication No. 263. Washington, D.C. Pan American Health Organization, 1973, pp. 79–81.

Myers, W. F., Wisseman, C. L., Fiset, P., Oaks, E. V., and Smith, J. F.: Taxonomic relationship of vole agent to *Rochalimaea quintana*. Infect Immun 26:976, 1979.

Mohr, W.: Das Wolhynische Fieber. Med Wochenschr 10:220, 1956.

Mohr, W., and Weyer, F.: Spätrückfälle bei wolhynischem Fieber. Dtsch Med Wochenschr 89:244, 1964.

Strong, R. P. (ed.): Trench Fever. Report of Commission Medical Research Committee, American Red Cross. London, Oxford University Press, 1918.

Varela, G.: Nuevas rickettsias encountradas en la Republica Mexicana, fiebre Q y fiebre de las trincheras. Ga Med Mexico 85:275, 1955.

Varela, G., Vinson, J. W., and Molina-Pasquel, C.: Trench fever. II. Propagation of *Rickettsia quintana* on cell-free medium from the blood of two patients. Am J Trop Med Hyg 18:708, 1969.

Vinson, J. W., Varela, G., and Molina-Pasquel, C.: Trench fever. III. Induction of clinical disease in volunteers inoculated with *Rickettsia quintana* propagated on blood agar. Am J Trop Med Hyg 18:713, 1969.

Vinson, J. W.: Louse-borne diseases worldwide: Trench fever. Geographic distribution of trench fever. Proceedings of the International Symposium on the Control of Lice and Louse-borne Diseases. Publication No. 263. Washington, D.C., Pan American Health Organization, 1973, pp. 76–78.

Weiss, E.: The biology of Rickettsiae. Ann Rev Microbiol 36:345, 1982.

Weiss, E., and Dasch, G. A.: *Rochalimaea vinsonii*, sp. nov., the Canadian vole agent. Int J Syst Bacteriol 32:305, 1982.

Weiss, E., Dasch, G. A., Woodman, D. R., and Williams, J. C.: Vole agent identified as a strain of the trench fever rickettsia, *Rochalimaea quintana*. Infect Immun 19:1013, 1978.

Weyer, F.: Experimente zur Frage der transovarienen Übertragung von Rickettsien. Z Tropenmed Parasitol 13:409, 1962.

Weyer, F., Vinson, J. W., Mannweiler, E., and Mohr, W.: Serologische Untersuchungen bei wolhynischem Fieber. Z Tropenmed Parasitol 23:187, 1962.

Zdrodovskii, P. F., and Golinevich, H. M.: The Rickettsial Diseases. London, Pergamon Press, 1960, pp. 431–440.

207

CHRONIC Q FEVER

WALTER P. G. TURÇK, M.B., F.R.C.P., F.R.C.P. (EDIN.)

Chronic Q fever is a chronic disease caused by persistent infection with *Coxiella burnetii* and characterized by prolonged illness, continuous or recurrent fever, and the development of sinister complications within the cardiovascular system. In most cases there are chronic hepatitis and thrombocytopenia. In contrast to the negligible mortality of acute disease (see Chapter 116) even in the absence of antibiotic therapy, untreated chronic Q fever with cardiovascular complications is invariably fatal. Although in most reports endocarditis is the dominant feature, the term chronic Q fever is preferred to Q fever endocarditis to encompass the whole spectrum of disease—from the simple prolonged fever extending over weeks and months in which there is minor hepatic involvement, to the insidious but grossly destructive endocarditis accompanied by granulomatous hepatitis or even cirrhosis.

ETIOLOGY. The disease is caused by *C. burnetii*, a species of bacteria belonging to the family Rickettsiaceae. *C. burnetii* is named after H. R. Cox, who was a codiscoverer of the agent of Q fever in the United States after its discovery in Australia, and F. M. Burnet, the Australian who first isolated the organism. It is a short rod that grows only intracellularly in vacuoles outside the nucleus. In contrast to other rickettsiae, *C. burnetii* is resistant to drying and relatively high temperatures. It can be cultured in chick embryos and cell cultures and readily infects guinea pigs, rabbits, hamsters, and mice.

PATHOGENESIS AND PATHOLOGY. The ability of *C. burnetii* to cause persistent and latent infection, to become embedded within and directly destroy heart valves, and to induce immune-complex phenomena seem to be the main factors contributing to the pathogenesis of chronic Q fever.

C. burnetii may persist in various hosts for as long as

526 days after infection, and it can be isolated from the placenta of animals infected up to 92 days before conception. In the pregnant guinea pig *C. burnetii* exists in the spleen throughout gestation, but in the placenta only in early and late pregnancy. Experimentally, both in domestic ruminants and in humans, the infective agent, after causing an initial mild or inapparent infection, remains latent until parturition, when large numbers may be found in placentae and birth fluids, in feces and urine, and later in milk. In human infection the urine may remain infective for four months. *C. burnetii* may be recovered from the placentae of women two to three years after their initial Q fever infection, and also in subsequent pregnancies. The rickettsemia of acute Q fever usually lasts no more than 15 days, but rare instances of rickettsemia persisting for more than 12 months have been recorded (Robson and Shimmin, 1959).

Although high titers of complement-fixing antibodies to phase I and phase II antigens of *C. burnetii* may be found in chronic Q fever, the role of these antibodies in its pathogenesis is not entirely clear. Phase II complement-fixing antibody develops relatively early but persists in some patients for more than ten years after the initial infection, suggesting persistence of rickettsiae. Phase 1 complement-fixing antibody, which is also a neutralizing antibody, develops late in acute Q fever, if at all, but correlates then with prolonged incapacity in the older patient and a complicated illness.

Marmion (1959) has suggested that absence of phase I antibody in the early stages may allow seeding of *C. burnetii* throughout the body. Later, after phase I antibody has appeared, *C. burnetii* may be limited to an intracellular location where it cannot be reached by antibody. Antibody may thereby contribute to latency. However, the duration of the latent state is possibly related to the physiologic and metabolic state of the cell rather than to the level of antibody of the host. Experimentally, reactivation of latent infection has been provoked by x-rays and multiple cortisone injections (Sidwell et al., 1964). The factors that cause the rickettsiae to reappear in large numbers in the placenta at parturition are unknown.

The impression gained from accounts of the clinical picture is that chronic Q fever arises most readily when acute Q fever is superimposed upon another disease such as chronic rheumatic valvulitis or alcoholic liver disease. However, apart from the frequent demonstration of evidence of pre-existing heart disease, it has not been possible to substantiate this theory pathologically. Although in some cases the underlying cardiac lesion does not appear to play a significant role clinically, such patients who have come to autopsy, or whose heart valves have been replaced, have invariably shown evidence of Q fever endocarditis. Accompanying lesions such as hepatitis or glomerulonephritis may contribute materially to the disability of the patient even to the extent of overshadowing any due to endocarditis.

Q fever endocarditis affects the aortic valve more frequently than the mitral valve. In some patients, both valves may be affected. The aortic valve lesion may be superimposed upon chronic rheumatic valvulitis, but congenital bicuspid aortic valves are commonly found, and in rare instances subaortic stenosis and syphilitic aortitis have been the underlying lesions. In many cases the macroscopic picture has been that of a florid and destructive endocarditis. Large vegetations, either firm and granular or friable and fungating, arise from the valve cusps. The cusps are frequently ulcerated or perforated and a sinus of Valsalva may be ruptured. False aneurysms of the aortic wall may develop behind the aortic valve cusps, and may extend into the intraventricular septum and ventricular wall. The valve cusps are often fused and may be heavily calcified. On occasion the picture is less dramatic, with tiny vegetations similar to those found on the cusps of an affected valve in acute exacerbation of rheumatic valvular disease. Fibrosis and adhesions may extend from the mitral valve to the tips of the papillary muscles.

The vegetations are composed of fibrinoid material embedded in and fused with the collagen of the valve and overlaid with thrombus. There is an infiltrate of large mononuclear cells and neutrophils. At the bases of the infected cusps there may be ingrowth of large reticulum cells, and swelling and proliferation of endothelial cells lining the valve leaflets may be present. Microcolonies of rickettsiae with tinctorial characteristics of *C. burnetii* may be found within degenerating infected cells in the center of the vegetations or scattered extracellularly owing to breakdown of the cells.

A similarly destructive picture may be seen in the tissues around a valve prosthesis, in a homograft valve, or in a porcine bioprosthesis when chronic Q fever develops as a complication of open heart surgery.

Cardiovascular involvement is not restricted to heart valves. Coronary, carotid, and renal arteritis and abdominal aortitis have been described. Vasculitis may also involve the venous system, causing thrombophlebitis, deep venous thrombosis, and pulmonary embolism and infarction. Q fever infection in a large ventricular aneurysm has been described (Willey et al., 1979).

Myocarditis is not uncommon. Numerous small foci of necrotic and swollen muscle fibers are distributed throughout the myocardium, resembling lesions seen in acute rickettsial fevers such as typhus. Evidence of ischemic heart disease has been found at autopsy in some instances, but this has been either accompanied by more florid structural damage in or around the valve or associated with coronary arteritis. Pericardial effusions may occur, but chronic pericarditis is rare.

Multiple large emboli frequently lodge in the iliac arteries as saddle emboli or in the popliteal arteries where mycotic aneurysms may develop. Splenic, renal, femoral, radial, and cerebral emboli are regular features of the disease. Emboli may arise from infected abdominal aortic dacron grafts (Ellis et al., 1983).

The liver is almost invariably involved in Q fever endocarditis. From liver biopsy and postmortem studies there is clear evidence that the histologic changes in Q fever hepatitis (see Chapter 116) can persist and progress, although they are variable and nonspecific (Turck et al., 1976). The most consistent feature of the chronic lesion is an infiltration of the portal tracts with lymphocytes and occasional plasma cells. A few cases have patchy parenchymal necrosis, parenchymal granulomata, and prominence of sinusoidal Küpffer cells. Periportal or diffuse fatty change is not uncommon. These appearances may persist for more than a year and may progress to portal tract fibrosis and cirrhosis. Although rickettsiae have never been seen in histologic sections of liver in chronic Q fever, the organism has been isolated from hepatic tissue.

In the kidneys of patients with endocarditis, renal infarcts secondary to embolization or arteritis are common. Hematuria occurs infrequently, but proteinuria is always present and may be heavy. A diffuse glomerulonephritis, similar to that found in the secondary immunologic disease that may accompany subacute bacterial endocarditis, has been seen in some patients at autopsy. Renal biopsy specimens show either hypercellularity of the glomeruli, capsular adhesions and diffuse mesangial thickening, or glomerulosclerosis. In such cases, electron microscopy may show granular deposits on glomerular basement membranes and fusion of the foot processes of the epithelial cells, and immunofluorescence studies show granular distribution of immunoglobulins and C3 in the glomeruli. Serum complement is reduced (Dathan and Heyworth, 1975).

Acute tubular necrosis occurred in one fatal case, and rickettsia-like organisms were noted in the tubular epithelium in another case with mild membranous glomerulonephritis.

Although *C. burnetii* has been frequently isolated from splenic tissue, the morphology of the spleen is usually unremarkable, apart from occasional splenic infarction and microscopic evidence of hypertrophy and hyperplasia of the endothelial cells of the sinuses. Massive splenomegaly with splenic sinus congestion may occur (Spring and Hampson, 1982). No *Coxiella* organism has ever been found in lymph nodes, in contrast to observations in persistent infections with rickettsiae of epidemic typhus, Rocky Mountain spotted fever, and scrub typhus.

Peripheral pulmonary infarction, interstitial pneumonitis, or pleural effusions occur occasionally.

In most cases the IgG and IgM are elevated. In some instances the elevation of IgM is the dominant feature, but in other cases normal or low levels of IgM have been recorded. The variability of IgM levels probably reflects a nonspecific reaction rather than a response to continuous intravascular antigenic stimulation by *C. burnetii* (Kazár et al., 1977). Even when IgM is elevated, the most specific Q fever antibodies may be found in the IgG fraction.

Thrombocytopenia is common, but the cause is not clear. Marrow examination shows no reduction in numbers of megakaryocytes nor abnormal megakaryocyte morphology. The combination of thrombocytopenia, persistent liver disease, glomerulonephritis with deposition of immunoglobulins and complement on glomerular basement membranes, and a coupled rise of IgG and IgM with reduction of complement in the serum strongly suggests that immune complex formation and deposition occurs.

C. burneti may be isolated by guinea pig inoculation from blood or unfixed tissue from heart valve, spleen, kidney, or embolus. Infectivity titrations of organ suspensions may indicate the primary focus.

CLINICAL FEATURES. The peak age-group of patients with Q fever endocarditis is approximately 20 years lower than that of patients with other causes of infective endocarditis. The onset is insidious. Persistent or recurrent fever is often the only symptom, although it may be accompanied by sweats and rigors. Its commencement may date from an illness strongly suggestive of acute Q fever, but an asymptomatic interval of weeks, months, or even years may be recognized. A few patients with endocarditis remain afebrile but present with angina and progressive dyspnea. There may be a history of previous medical treatment for rheumatic or congenital heart disease, previous valve surgery, alcoholic liver disease, diabetes, pneumoconiosis, lymphoma, or other conditions associated with impaired immune mechanisms.

On physical examination those patients without endocarditis have few signs apart from hepatomegaly, splenomegaly, and, occasionally, a petechial rash.

Patients with endocarditis have signs of the underlying cardiac disease, which may include finger clubbing, splenomegaly, murmurs, embolic phenomena, and anemia. In such cases hepatomegaly and petechial rashes are particularly common, but jaundice and ascites are infrequent.

Patients whose illness is complicated by hepatitis, myocarditis, or pericarditis may have signs and symptoms of the complication in addition to the persistent fever.

Occasionally, patients present with signs of chronic active hepatitis without any clinical evidence of active infective endocarditis. Episodes of deep venous thrombosis and pulmonary embolism may occur at any time in the illness.

Chronic Q fever, even without endocarditis, may cause osteomyelitis, and the premature birth of an infected fetus (Ellis et al., 1983).

Very rarely chronic Q fever may be silent and cryptic, detected only on incidental serologic testing (Willey et al., 1979).

COMPLICATIONS AND SEQUELAE. Arterial embolism is common, particularly in the cerebral and popliteal arteries, but all major arteries may be affected. Arteritis may involve coronary arteries with myocardial ischemia and infarction, or carotid and cerebral arteries with secondary cerebral ischemia or hemorrhage.

Pulmonary embolism, occasionally massive and fatal, may follow deep venous thrombosis.

Progression from hepatitis to cirrhosis, ascites, and fatal hepatic failure has been recorded.

Hematuria is less frequent than in subacute bacterial endocarditis. Rarely, there may be heavy proteinuria, or even a frank nephrotic syndrome due to an immune complex glomerulonephritis that may terminate in renal failure (Dathan and Heyworth, 1975). Neuropsychiatric complications are rare, but two patients displayed fatalistic personality change and paranoid psychosis respectively.

Without treatment, Q fever endocarditis is invariably fatal. Death may be due to pulmonary embolism, intractable cardiac failure arising from destruction of the valve, or chronic myocarditis.

GEOGRAPHIC VARIATIONS IN DISEASE. Chronic Q fever under the age of 30 is exceedingly rare. The male preponderance may be extreme. In Australia, Q fever endocarditis appears to be exclusively a disease of males.

Despite the worldwide prevalence of Q fever, the geographic distribution of chronic Q fever appears to be far more restricted. Over three quarters of the cases reported have occurred in the British Isles, and another tenth in Australia. A few cases have occurred in France, Switzerland, Spain, Portugal, Greece, Yugoslavia, and South Africa, but, interestingly, no reports have emerged from Italy, where so much Q fever occurred during World War II. In the United States, where persistent fever and protracted illness have been well recognized, Q fever endocarditis has been reported very infrequently. No cases have been reported from South America, East Africa, Russia, the Indian subcontinent, or Far East Asia.

Failure to recognize chronic Q fever probably accounts for this geographic imbalance. Experience in the British Isles and Australia in recent years indicates that increasing awareness of the disease has been accompanied by an apparent increase in incidence (Turck et al., 1976; Wilson et al., 1976).

DIAGNOSIS. The diagnosis should be considered whenever a patient with clinical evidence of infective endocarditis presents with hepatomegaly, biochemical evidence of liver involvement, thrombocytopenia, and negative bacterial blood cultures. Endocarditis due to fungal or exotic bacterial infection may have to be excluded. The diagnosis of chronic Q fever should also be suspected in any patient with fever of unknown origin, persistent hepatitis, myocarditis, pericarditis, or osteomyelitis, particularly when the patient is discovered to have the appropriate epidemiologic background, as outlined in Chapter 116.

Confirmation of the diagnosis is obtained serologically by means of the complement fixation test using phase I and phase II antigens of *C. burnetii.* In view of the chronicity of the infection, a single estimation usually suffices, the height of the antibody titer being more important than a rising titer. Both phase I and phase II antibody are elevated, the latter usually being slightly higher than the former. In patients with clinical evidence of endocarditis, a titer of complement-fixing antibody to phase I greater than 1:200 is strongly suggestive of chronic Q fever. Titers of phase I antibody greater than 1:200 in patients without clinical evidence of endocarditis indicate probable cryptic infection. When phase I antibody is detected in patients with valvular heart disease but at titers below this figure, the diagnosis should not be rejected, even if the abnormal heart valve is considered to be free of infective endocarditis, since such results may represent chronic Q fever in evolution. In those circumstances attempts should be made to isolate the organism from the blood by guinea pig inoculation. If signs or symptoms in such patients are mild or absent, repeat testing for phase I antibody should be performed after an interval of one month. Titers that do not fall confirm chronic infection. Since high titers of complement-fixing antibody frequently exist in Q fever endocarditis, prozone phenomena may cause the unwary to record false negative results. Positive sera are often anticomplementary, probably because of circulating immune complexes.

Guinea pig inoculation of embolus or valve tissue obtained at operation may establish the diagnosis where it was unsuspected previously.

TREATMENT. Tetracycline is the mainstay of antibiotic therapy in chronic Q fever, but recent clinical reports suggest that in Q fever endocarditis, lincomycin, 2 g per day, in combination with tetracycline, 1 g per day, may be even more effective in eradicating the infection. Co-trimoxazole has been used with variable results, but experience with this drug combination is limited. Rifampicin, which is more potent than tetracycline in vitro, may also prove effective (Kimbrough et al., 1979). In view of the indolent and destructive nature of the disease, even those patients with low titers of antibody to phase I complement-fixing antigen who may have chronic Q fever in evolution should receive the full antibiotic regimen. Antibiotic therapy should be maintained for at least 12 months and withdrawn only in the presence of clinical, biochemical, and serologic evidence suggesting quiescence of the disease.

Valve replacement should be reserved for those patients requiring it for hemodynamic reasons. Antibiotic therapy should be continued postoperatively for at least one year. Continued careful monitoring of patients after antibiotic withdrawal is mandatory.

PROPHYLAXIS. Acute Q fever should be suspected and treated adequately. In all elderly patients and in patients with underlying disease who have illness characterized by prolonged fever, pneumonitis, or hepatitis, it is particularly vital that tetracycline not be discontinued prematurely.

Patients with valvular heart disease should be advised not to pursue occupations where the risk of Q fever is high, nor to spend their vacations in areas where Q fever is endemic, nor to drink raw milk. If a satisfactory vaccine becomes readily available, such patients should be immunized, bearing in mind that live vaccines are not suitable for this purpose.

Experimental evidence suggests that it is important to be alert to the possibility of reactivation of latent disease by x-ray or corticosteroid therapy in patients who are known to have had Q fever.

References

Dathan, J. R. E., and Heyworth, M. F.: Glomerulonephritis associated with *Coxiella burnetii* endocarditis. Br Med J 1:376, 1975.

Ellis, M. E., Smith, C. C., and Moffat, M. A. J.: Chronic or fatal Q fever infection; a review of 16 patients seen in North-East Scotland (1967–80). Q J Med 52:54, 1983.

Kazár, J., Schramek, S., and Brezina, R.: Analysis of serum immunoglobulins in a patient with chronic Q fever and endocarditis. Bratisl Lek Listy 67:109, 1977.

Kimbrough, R. C., Ormsby, R. A., Peacock, M., Rogers, W. R., Bennetts, R. W., Roof, J., Krause, A., and Gardner, C.: Q fever endocarditis in the United States. Ann Intern Med 91:400, 1979.

Marmion, B. P.: Latency and rickettsial infections. Proc 6th International Congress of Tropical Medicine and Malaria, Lisbon, Sept, 1958. 5:711, 1959.

Robson, A. O., and Shimmin, C. D. G. L.: Chronic Q fever. I. Clinical aspects of a patient with endocarditis. Br Med J 2:980, 1959.

Sidwell, R. W., Thorpe, B. D., and Gebhardt, L. P.: Studies of latent Q fever infections. II. Effects of multiple cortisone injections. Am J Hyg 79:320, 1964.

Spring, W. J. C., and Hampson, J.: Chronic Q fever endocarditis causing massive splenomegaly and hypersplenism. Br M J 2:1244, 1982.

Turck, W. P. G., Howitt, G., Turnberg, L. A., Fox, H., Longson, M., Matthews, M. B., and Das Gupta, R.: Chronic Q fever. Q J Med 45:193, 1976.

Willey, R. F., Matthews, M. B., Peutherer, J. F., and Marmion, B. P.: Chronic cryptic Q fever infection of the heart. Lancet 2:270, 1979.

Wilson, H. G., Neilson, G. H., Galea, E. G., Stafford, G., and O'Brien, M. F.: Q fever endocarditis in Queensland. Circulation 53:680, 1976.

208
MALARIA

DAVID FRANCIS CLYDE, M.D., PH.D.

Malaria is a disease characterized by fever, anemia, and splenomegaly, and is often attended by dangerous complications. It results from infection of hepatic parenchymal cells and erythrocytes by sporozoa of the genus *Plasmodium.* Four species may infect humans: *Plasmodium falciparum* produces malignant tertian, subtertian, or falciparum malaria; *Plasmodium vivax* produces benign tertian or vivax malaria; *Plasmodium ovale* produces benign tertian or ovale malaria; *Plasmodium malariae* produces benign quartan or malariae malaria.

These parasites are carried by female *Anopheles* mosquitoes. Their development in the mosquito is sexual (sporogony), and in the human asexual (schizogony) (see Chapter 84). A few cases of malaria occur through congenital transmission, blood transfusion, or shared syringes in drug users.

ETIOLOGY, DISTRIBUTION, AND GEOGRAPHIC VARIATIONS. Because malaria transmission is dependent on the presence of *Anopheles* mosquitoes, it occurs primarily in rural areas. The degree of endemicity is determined by several factors, the principal ones being: (1) *the reservoir*—the prevalence of infection in the community; (2) *the vector*—the abundance of *Anopheles* mosquitoes and their species suitability as hosts for the parasite; and (3) *the victim*—the presence of a susceptible human population.

Malaria is distributed mainly between latitudes 45° north and 40° south (Fig. 1). The most common type, caused by *P. vivax,* occurs also in temperate regions, whereas *P. falciparum* is largely confined to the tropics. *P. malariae* is considerably rarer and has a focal distribution. *P. ovale,* rather than *P. vivax,* is the benign relapsing type of malaria in West Africa, but it is found less frequently in other parts of Africa and is rare elsewhere. It has this distribution because *P. vivax* (but not *P. ovale*) requires Duffy blood group receptors on erythrocytes in order to penetrate the erythrocyte membrane, and these receptors are lacking in many Africans, particularly West Africans.

In the cooler parts of endemic areas, vivax malaria is first to appear each spring, while *P. falciparum* and *P. malariae* infections appear later in the summer. In tropical countries, all species of *Plasmodium* may occur in the humid lowlands, particularly at the peak periods of *Anopheles* mosquito breeding at the beginning and end of the rainy season. In the highlands *P. falciparum* disappears, although *P. vivax* may persist at altitudes higher than 2500 meters. In the individual untreated patient, falciparum infections (when not fatal) persist for up to one year, vivax up to five years, and malariae much longer.

The distribution and prevalence of the different kinds of malaria are modified by various human genetic traits. Glucose-6-phosphate dehydrogenase, essential to parasite metabolism, may be deficient in the erythrocytes of certain people, and these erythrocytes are from 2 to 80 times as resistant to invasion by *P. falciparum* as are normal erythrocytes. Various hemoglobinopathies, particularly the presence of Hb S, also result in premature death of intraerythrocytic *P. falciparum.* The geographic distribution of people having these traits—in Africa, the eastern Mediterranean, and parts of Asia, and their descendants elsewhere—is such that it has been assumed that possession of the trait confers a selective advantage against malaria.

This advantage permits patients to survive and enhances their ability to develop immunity to malaria. At the same time, they remain infective to the mosquito and thus maintain transmission. People who are relatively asymptomatic, because of enhanced partial immunity or in the intervals between paroxysms, are usually ambulatory, remain at their rural homes, and thus constitute reservoirs of infection to the mosquito. The stage of the parasite infective to the mosquito, the circulating gametocyte, appears early in the vivax or malariae attack, but does not appear for some 10 days after the first falciparum paroxysm and even then is not immediately infective—an important epidemiologic factor.

PATHOGENESIS AND PATHOLOGY. The exoerythrocytic stage of the malaria parasite in the liver is not pathogenic nor does a local inflammatory reaction occur. Pathology is associated with the erythrocytic phase, in which many red blood cells, both infected and uninfected, are destroyed.

In vivax/ovale and malariae infections destruction of erythrocytes is limited, in the former to a maximum of 2 per cent because reticulocytes are preferentially invaded, and in malariae because only older erythrocytes are invaded and each schizogonic cycle is lengthy. In contrast, the hemolysis in falciparum infections, which involve erythrocytes of all ages, may be so extensive that hemoglobinuria results.

Many erythrocytes are sequestered by the reticuloendothelial system, particularly in the spleen, where parasitized cells are either phagocytosed by macrophages or hemolyzed. Destruction of circulating and sequestered erythrocytes, parasitized as well as unparasitized, quickly produces a severe anemia. This is accompanied by thrombocytopenia. The principal site of platelet destruction is the spleen. Infected erythrocytes and free merozoites are also phagocytosed in the circulation; monocytes, which show an absolute increase in numbers, play a major role, despite an overall leukopenia. Monocytes, polymorphonuclear leukocytes, and visceral reticuloendothelial cells remove hemozoin from the circulation. This malarial pigment colors the organs, particularly the spleen, liver, and brain, slate-gray or black.

The spleen may be enlarged and slate-colored, weighing 1000 grams or more after protracted infections. The reticuloendothelial elements are markedly hyperplastic, and the cells contain malarial pigment in brown blocks or small black masses. In acute malaria the spleen is congested and soft with a distended capsule, and is susceptible to spontaneous or traumatic rupture. Thrombosis and areas of infarction occur in the arterioles, while the pulp may be hemorrhagic. The follicles are reduced in size and rarely contain phagocytosed pigment. In chronic malaria, fibrosis of trabeculae is prominent and the organ becomes hard and shrunken.

The liver may be enlarged and discolored owing to black pigmentation of the endothelial and Küpffer cells. Hepatic parenchymal cells do not take up this malarial pigment but, as with the spleen pulp, may contain dark yellow hemosiderin and show vacuolization and cloudy swelling. Small necrotic foci may occur in the portal areas and in the central zones of the liver lobules.

The brain may be similarly discolored. Particularly in severe falciparum malaria, the cerebral capillaries are engorged with, and may be plugged by, masses of parasitized erythrocytes (Fig. 2). Areas of necrosis ringed by hemorrhages develop around the thrombosed vessels in the subcortical white matter, the pons, medulla, and cerebellum, but not in the gray matter (Young, 1976).

Because the basic pathologic process is generalized and includes anemia, disseminated intravascular coagulation, tissue anoxia, and necrosis, other organs are damaged, particularly in falciparum infections. Symptoms resembling those of acute toxic, focal, or interstitial myocarditis and pneumonitis may occur. In chronic malariae infections of African children especially, a nephrotic syndrome with excretion of large amounts of albumin and massive edema has been observed. Severe falciparum infections may produce glomerulonephritis with nitrogen retention and uremia. This is characteristically associated with the hemoglobinuria of blackwater fever. Gastrointestinal lesions may simulate appendicitis. In the placentas of infected women, erythrocytes in the intervillous spaces (maternal portions) but not in the chorionic villi (fetal portion) are parasitized.

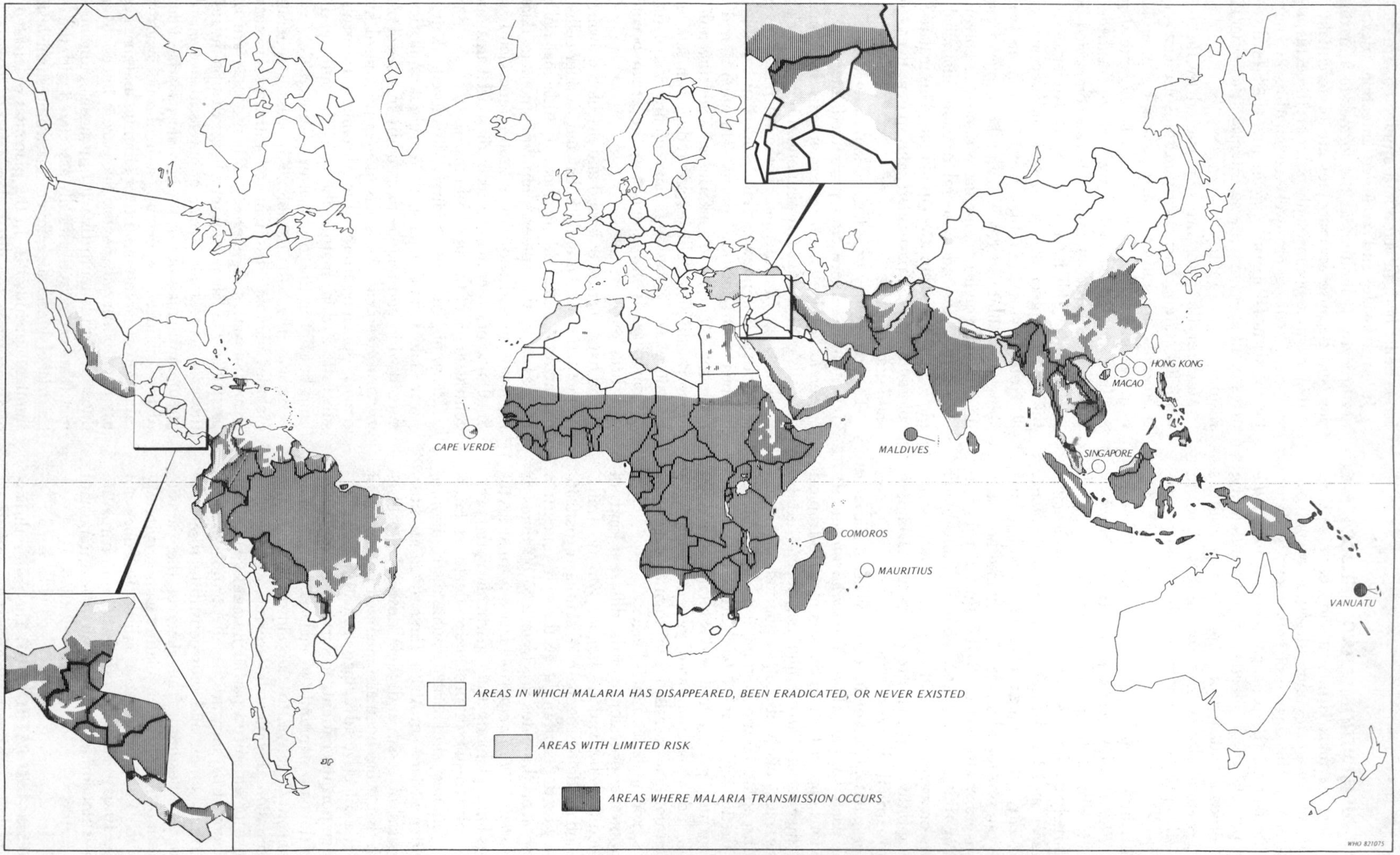

Figure 1. Distribution of malaria in 1983 (Courtesy of the World Health Organization).

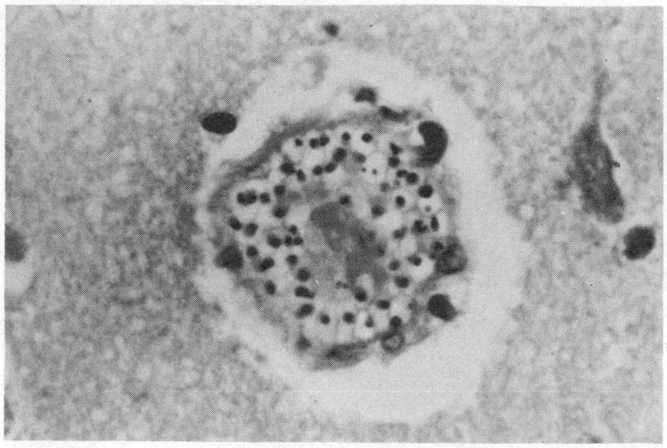

Figure 2. Blood vessel in brain largely blocked by parasitized erythrocytes adherent to endothelium and to each other. A granule of pigment marks each parasitized red cell. (Courtesy of G. W. Hunter, III. In Hunter, G. W., et al.: Tropical Medicine. 5th ed. Philadelphia, W. B. Saunders Company, 1976.)

Congenital malaria may be transmitted to the fetus by a nonimmune infected woman. Although this is a rare event in regions where mothers have acquired a considerable degree of immunity, the birth weight of such infected babies is often subnormal.

Biochemical abnormalities are prominent during the acute attack. Plasma proteins are reduced, the albumin-globulin ratio is reversed, and the serum potassium and euglobulin levels are increased. Cholesterol, lecithin, and glucose concentrations increase during the febrile paroxysms. Disturbance of the glycogenetic function of the liver results in a decrease in levulose and galactose tolerance. Bilirubin appears in the plasma in quantities that parallel the intensity of the infection.

Acquired immunity greatly modifies these pathologic processes. Malaria infections produce partial immunity that is species-specific and to some extent strain-specific; an attack of falciparum malaria, for example, does not decrease the severity of a vivax infection but confers tolerance to the existing infection and to new falciparum infections. Such tolerance, manifested by reduced severity of symptoms, wanes rapidly in parallel with antibody decay after the infection is cured. Agglutinins, precipitins, complement-fixing and fluorescent antibodies appear. Soon after parasites become patent, immunoglobulins M, A, and G increase in parallel with the rising parasite density. After the parasitemia peaks, IgM and IgA levels decline; but IgG may remain elevated for many months or years. Long-persisting IgG fluorescent antibodies are a valuable epidemiologic indication of past infection. Peaked elevations of IgM indicate infection within the past three months.

Transplacental passage of IgG from a malarious mother provides the neonate with protection that diminishes in strength over about 12 weeks. The breast milk of infected women also contains protective IgG, and is additionally protective because of its deficiency in the para-aminobenzoic acid essential to plasmodial metabolism.

The antigens stimulating production of the IgG-related antibodies are complex and are not only species-specific but, for the erythrocytic cycle, largely stage-specific. In humans, inoculation by irradiated biting mosquitoes of live falciparum and vivax sporozoites has resulted in "sporozoite neutralizing antibody" that provides solid immunity against further sporozoite inocula of each species for up to six months (Clyde et al., 1973). Furthermore, "merozoite inhibitory" and "gametocyte-sterilizing" antibodies have been demonstrated in animal models. Although vaccines against human malaria are not yet available, their production is increasingly promised through the use of hybridoma and genetic engineering technology.

CLINICAL MANIFESTATIONS. The clinical triad characteristic of malaria consists of periodic fever, splenomegaly, and anemia. The periodicity of the fever is related to maturation of erythrocytic schizonts and their synchronous release into the plasma as the red cells are ruptured (Fig. 3). Parasite pigment in the circulation is thought to cause leukocytes to release endogenous pyrogen into the serum, which, together with prostaglandins, stimulates hypothalamic temperature sensors. Splenomegaly and to a lesser extent hepatomegaly reflect the great increase in reticuloendothelial cells, which are phagocytic for merozoites, pigment, erythrocyte remnants, whole parasitized erythrocytes, and sometimes unparasitized erythrocytes. Anemia results from the cyclical destruction of parasitized erythrocytes and concomitant lysis of large numbers of uninfected erythrocytes. Consequently, it is normocytic and normochromic.

The *intrinsic incubation period* (the interval between the infecting bite and elevation of temperature to 37.8° C) in falciparum malaria is 11 to 14 days, in vivax 11 to 15 days, in ovale 14 to 26 days, and in malariae 21 to 28 days. It is usually a day or two longer than the appearance of parasites in the erythrocytes, which indicates the end of the *prepatent period*. In the temperate climates of northern Europe and Asia, vivax infections may incubate for nine months or longer, and ovale malaria has been known to behave similarly. Before the onset of the first paroxysm of fever, prodromal symptoms of malaise, headache, anorexia, and a slightly elevated temperature may occur.

Thereafter, clinical malaria may develop into one of two types. The more serious, produced by *P. falciparum*, may be fatal, owing to (1) the capacity of this parasite to enter both reticulocytes and mature erythrocytes, develop rapidly, and thus build up high levels of parasitemia, and (2) the tendency of infected erythrocytes to agglutinate and adhere to vascular endothelium, plugging capillaries and producing thrombosis with local anoxia and ischemia in many organs, most dangerously the brain.

Falciparum malaria may develop insidiously, with various nonspecific symptoms including gradually increasing pyrexia, headache, and gastrointestinal disturbances. Or it may have an abrupt onset of the paroxysmal type popularly associated with malaria—initial sensations of chilliness, often with marked shivering, followed by a prolonged hot stage, terminating in sweating and a fall in temperature with temporary relief of the symptoms of intense throbbing headache, nausea, and vomiting. When it occurs, the periodicity of fever is around 36 hours, but the fever can continue for 24 hours or more without relief of symptoms. The spleen becomes palpable and painful. Prostration is a marked feature of the acute attack in a nonimmune patient. Mental confusion warns of the extremely dangerous complication of cerebral malaria that may develop rapidly.

Vivax, ovale, and malariae infections, although less life-threatening, are also accompanied by marked symptoms. The fever at first may be sustained or irregular in periodicity owing to the presence of two or more groups of

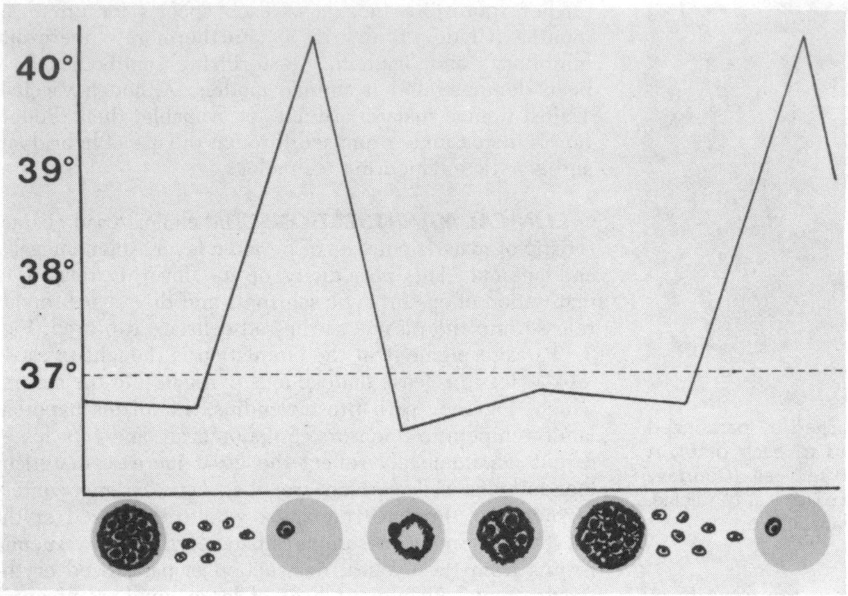

Figure 3. Relationship between periodicity of fever and rupture of malaria parasites from erythrocytes.

parasites maturing on alternate days. Soon, however, one group begins to dominate and the characteristic periodicity of fever is established. In vivax and ovale infections the intervals are 40 to 50 hours, and in malariae they are 72 hours. The onset is more abrupt in vivax than in ovale and malariae, which tend to run a milder course. The paroxysm commences with a rigor, during which the temperature rises rapidly to peaks as high as 41° C, although the patient feels chilly or cold. Nausea and vomiting are prominent, and the pulse is rapid and weak. Within an hour a sensation of heat develops, accompanied by severe headache and continual nausea and vomiting. The skin is dry. This stage is followed by profuse sweating lasting two to three hours, during which the temperature and pulse rate subside. The paroxysm usually lasts 10 to 12 hours and is accompanied by a moderate leukocytosis, but in the relatively asymptomatic intervals between paroxysms, leukopenia with monocytosis prevails.

The primary untreated attack of *P. malariae* terminates spontaneously in three weeks to six months. Thereafter, latent infections with a few circulating parasites may persist and set up recrudescent attacks for as long as 40 years. Such latent infection is also sufficient to establish the disease in another person receiving that blood by transfusion.

The primary attack of falciparum malaria in a nonimmune patient is short and severe. If untreated and not fatal, it subsides within three weeks. Recrudescences of latent blood stages may occur for a year.

Mixed infections, usually consisting of *P. falciparum* and *P. vivax,* may occur. *P. falciparum* initiates the clinical symptoms. Only when it has run its course do the vivax symptoms become manifest. Similarly, *P. vivax* predominates over *P. malariae* in mixed infections.

COMPLICATIONS AND SEQUELAE. Complications of malaria attacks may be life-threatening. Unless the attack is cured quickly, anemia is an increasingly severe problem, and dehydration and electrolyte disturbances develop. The acutely enlarged spleen may rupture spontaneously or by trauma in vivax infections. Nephrosis with marked albuminuria may occur in chronic malariae infections.

Falciparum infections are much more liable than the others to produce serious complications. Although plugging of capillaries by infected erythrocytes occurs throughout the body, one of the organ systems is usually most affected. When this is the brain, *cerebral malaria* develops, either gradually with increasing headache, confusion, and psychotic manifestations lapsing into delirium and coma, or suddenly with abrupt rise in temperature sustained at high levels, convulsive seizures (particularly in children), and coma. Cerebral edema develops, and the cerebrospinal fluid pressure may increase. The condition can be fatal within a few hours.

Other complications of falciparum infections include the following. (1) *Bilious remittent fever,* in which the liver is the main organ affected, is characterized by continuous vomiting (sometimes of coffee-ground vomitus from gastric hemorrhage), epigastric and liver tenderness, and marked jaundice. (2) *Algid malaria,* in which the adrenal gland fails and the gastrointestinal tract is extensively involved, leads to shock, prostration, syncope, and circulatory collapse. The temperature may not be elevated. Diarrhea, sometimes bloody, is often present. (3) *Acute renal failure* due to tubular necrosis is characterized clinically by prolonged oliguria leading to anuria. (4) *Blackwater fever,* with hemoglobinuria due to massive sudden hemolysis, is believed to be triggered by hypersensitivity to drugs including quinine. (5) *Pneumonic malaria,* a rare complication, is accompanied by pulmonary edema.

Recurrent attacks generally follow inadequate treatment. The untreated primary attack of vivax malaria may persist for two months; toward the end of that time the paroxysms diminish and then cease, but in at least 50 per cent of the cases relapses develop from latent exoerythrocytic stages in the liver within a few weeks to a year or more later. Untreated relapses may continue for as long as five years at a steadily decreasing intensity. The untreated primary ovale attack tends to subside spontaneously within three weeks; relapses occur infrequently and then rarely persist longer than one year.

DIAGNOSIS. The diagnosis of malaria depends on identification of parasites in blood smears. Morphology and species differentiation are described in Chapter 84. The thick blood film, in which a dried drop of defibrinated blood is dehemoglobinized before staining with Giemsa stain buffered to pH 7.0 to 7.2, is superior to the usual methyl alcohol-fixed thin film because low densities of parasitemia may be detected. A minimum of 100 oil immersion fields should be examined in the thin film. Leukocytes containing malarial pigment may be seen. Leukopenia and monocytosis are usual. In the rare cases in which parasitemia is not detected in thick films taken morning and afternoon for three consecutive days but clinical indications persist, sternal puncture and examination of the stained marrow smear may reveal the parasites.

Immunodiagnosis has limited clinical usefulness but positive indirect hemagglutination (IHA) and indirect fluorescent antibody (IFA) tests are valuable for epidemiologic surveys and, with the complement fixation test, for screening potential blood donors. Wassermann and Kahn reactions are often positive in malaria.

Malaria must be differentiated from other systemic infectious diseases, particularly typhoid fever, brucellosis, miliary tuberculosis, diverticulitis, and abscesses of the liver, kidney, or pelvis. Tropical diseases such as visceral leishmaniasis, extra intestinal amebiasis, and relapsing fever may resemble malaria. In temperate zone countries, a patient who is comatose from cerebral malaria poses a particularly difficult and critical diagnostic problem if no history of recent tropical sojourn is available. Because cerebral malaria may be so quickly fatal, it must be considered in any unconscious or semiconscious patient who has an undiagnosed fever, and appropriate blood microscopy undertaken without delay.

TREATMENT. The specific chemotherapy of malaria is directed at (1) prompt abatement of the acute clinical attack and its complications by rapid elimination of asexual erythrocytic parasites (using blood schizonticidal drugs), (2) prevention of relapses of vivax or ovale malaria by destruction of their latent exoerythrocytic stages in the liver (using tissue schizonticidal drugs), (3) prevention of the initial attack by suppression of parasites entering the blood from the liver (using suppressive prophylactic drugs) or by destroying them when they first enter the body (using casual prophylactic drugs—still largely theoretical), and (4) prevention of transmission of malaria via the mosquito by interference with gametogony (gametocyticidal and sporonticidal drugs).

Abatement of the Attack. Blood schizonticidal drugs generally used in the treatment of the acute attack of malaria include quinine, and the 4-aminoquinolines chloroquine, hydroxychloroquine, and amodiaquine. Except for falciparum malaria originating in areas of known resistance to the 4-aminoquinolines, chloroquine is the drug of choice. Symptoms are generally relieved within 24 hours, and parasites are cleared from the blood by about 60 hours, although *P. malariae* may persist for several days. Infections produced by strains of *P. falciparum* sensitive to these drugs will be cured, but gametocytes of this species are not damaged, although those of the other species will disappear rapidly.

Dosage. The initial dose of chloroquine per kilogram of body weight is 10 mg of the base (equivalent to 17 mg of chloroquine sulfate or diphosphate). This is followed by three doses of 5 mg (base) per kg, at 6, 24, and 48 hours after the initial dose. Hydroxychloroquine sulfate may be used similarly. Alternatively, amodiaquine 10 mg (base) per kg (equivalent to 13 mg of amodiaquine dihydrochloride) may be used on the first day, then 7 mg (base) per kg daily on the second and third days.

In severe illness with vomiting, parenteral treatment may be necessary. Chloroquine hydrochloride may be given intramuscularly in doses of 5 mg (base) per kg, injected every six hours until treatment by mouth is resumed. Alternatively, and particularly if cerebral malaria threatens, quinine dihydrochloride may be given intravenously in a dose of 10 mg/kg in normal saline diluted to 1 mg/ml, administered very slowly at a flow rate of 1 mg per minute. This should be repeated every 9 hours (in adults) or 12 hours (in children) until oral treatment is feasible. Because of the hazard of circulatory collapse from rapid or excessive intravenous administration of quinine, pulse and blood pressure must be monitored frequently. Parenteral treatment should not be continued longer than two days: if parasitemia does not diminish, the parasites are drug resistant (see below).

Complications of malaria occur most commonly in falciparum infections. In the treatment of cerebral malaria, quinine given intravenously as described above may be lifesaving. In patients with renal failure, fluid management is necessary, drug dosage, particularly of quinine, should be reduced, and peritoneal or hemodialysis may be necessary if the plasma urea concentration nears 200 mg per 100 ml. On the other hand, acute dehydration requires fluid replacement. Symptoms such as convulsions, shock, and hyperpyrexia should be managed according to general principles. Anemia should be treated with iron or, if severe, by blood transfusion.

Pregnancy is not a contraindication to administration of these antimalarials, since malaria itself constitutes a much greater hazard.

The side effects of treatment may be difficult to distinguish from the symptoms of the disease. Vomiting is sometimes brought on by the intensely bitter taste of the 4-aminoquinolines and quinine. Children are given coated tablets or syrup preparations, and a tasteless base preparation of amodiaquine is available. Side effects of the 4-aminoquinolines include headache and pruritus, and more rarely an eruption resembling lichen planus, depigmentation of the hair, discoloration of the nails, visual disturbances, and (after higher doses of chloroquine than are used in malaria) retinal damage. Quinine produces cinchonism, early signs of which have been used as an indication of effective dosage and include giddiness, tinnitus, and transitory deafness. Permanent deafness, amblyopia, and blindness have occurred in patients who were overdosed or had an idiosyncratic reaction to quinine. When quinine is given intravenously too rapidly, circulatory collapse and death may occur owing to cardiac depression and vasodilatation. Patients with renal failure should receive no more than half the usual doses.

Resistance to 4-aminoquinolines is apparent when appropriate treatment does not reduce parasitemia and relieve symptoms in 24 hours. Falciparum malaria in much of South America and Panama and in Southeast Asia from the Solomon Islands, New Guinea, and the Philippines west to eastern India is resistant to these drugs, and such resistance is beginning to appear in East Africa. Oral treatment with quinine sulfate must be instituted immediately in the following regimen:

Adults:	650 mg every 8 hours
6 to 12 years:	325 mg every 8 hours
3 to 6 years:	160 mg every 6 hours
1 to 3 years:	80 mg every 4 hours
Less than 1 year:	80 mg every 6 hours

This treatment should continue for 14 days. While some strains of *P. falciparum* may be eliminated by shorter courses, others may recrudesce after the full 14 days of treatment. Additional drugs must then be given with the quinine. One combination consists of sulfadiazine 500 mg every six hours for five days (adult dosage) with pyrimethamine 25 mg every 12 hours for three days (folinic acid 10 mg/kg is also given daily to counteract hematologic toxicity of pyrimethamine).

Alternative methods for treating drug-resistant falciparum malaria include the above quinine schedule for 3 rather than 14 days with a full dose of a tetracycline for seven days; or, when quinine is not used, a combination of trimethoprim with a long-acting sulfonamide for three days; or a single dose of sulfadoxine 1.5 g with pyrimethamine 75 mg. A newly developed 4-quinolinemethanol compound, mefloquine, has proved effective in adults when given in a 1.5 g single dose.

Consideration must be given to the potentially dangerous side effects of long-acting sulfonamides, particularly the development of erythema multiforme, and to the question of inducing bacterial resistance by indiscriminate use of drugs such as the sulfonamides, trimethoprim, and tetracycline.

Severe or complicated cases are treated by intravenous administration of quinine as described above.

Malaria in partially immune patients may be treated with lower doses of schizonticides.

Prevention of Vivax and Ovale Relapses. Destruction of the latent exoerythrocytic stages of *P. vivax* and *P. ovale* in the liver is achieved by administering the 8-aminoquinoline drug primaquine. Patients treated for acute attacks of vivax or ovale malaria with blood schizonticides should also receive primaquine diphosphate 0.45 mg/kg body weight (containing 0.25 mg/kg of base primaquine) each day for 14 consecutive days; for adults, this amounts to 15 mg (base) daily. The course of primaquine may commence concurrently with the blood schizonticide but, if vomiting is a problem, it can be delayed for two or three days until the patient is stabilized. In pregnancy, use of primaquine should be delayed until after the first trimester. Some strains of *P. vivax*, notably the Chesson of New Guinea (now being found more widely in Southeast Asia), may require twice the daily dosage.

Side effects of treatment consist of hemolytic reactions to primaquine in individuals whose erythrocytes are deficient in glucose-6-phosphate dehydrogenase (G-6-PD). These reactions tend to be severe in some Mediterranean Caucasians and Southeast Asians and milder in some Africans. Acute intravascular hemolysis occurring in these individuals is self-limited because only the older erythrocytes are affected. Because the larger dosage regimen used in Chesson-type vivax malaria may bring on hemolytic reactions, G-6-PD-deficient patients infected with this type should be given no more than the 0.25 mg (base) per kg course, to be repeated should relapse take place later. Alternatively, primaquine may be given once a week for eight weeks, in the amount of 0.75 mg (base) per kg each dose. The drug should be discontinued in patients developing hemolytic anemia or methemoglobinemia manifested by marked cyanosis (Bruce-Chwatt et al., 1981).

Prevention by Suppression of Parasitemia. Chemoprophylaxis of malaria is effective only if a drug to which the local parasites are susceptible is taken regularly.

Chloroquine is the most widely used suppressive drug, and is taken by mouth once each week in the amount of 5 mg (base) per kg body weight, which, for an adult, is 300 mg base. Amodiaquine or hydroxychloroquine may be used in the equivalent dosage. All may be taken in suitably divided doses at shorter intervals (e.g., daily) or, in the case of partially immune patients, at intervals of two weeks without increasing the quantity. People who visit malarious areas should continue the treatment for six weeks after the last possible exposure. During or following visits to areas of high vivax transmission, primaquine may be taken in addition to the 4-aminoquinolines.

Pyrimethamine, in a once-weekly dosage of 25 mg (for those aged 10 years or more), 12.5 mg (ages 4 to 10), or 6.25 mg (children under 4 years), or proguanil (chlorguanide) in a daily dosage of 100 mg for adults (proportional for children) may be used alone, but resistance by *P. falciparum* may develop rapidly, requiring either the addition of chloroquine to the regimen or a change to that drug.

Resistance to 4-aminoquinolines, notably chloroquine, by *P. falciparum* in Southeast Asia and South America is often accompanied by resistance to pyrimethamine and proguanil. Because these multi-drug-resistant parasites may be suppressed by sulfones and sulfonamides, which are ineffective against *P. vivax* and *P. malariae*, and because pyrimethamine, proguanil, and the 4-aminoquinolines remain effective against *P. vivax* and *P. malariae*, combinations of drugs are used for prophylaxis in these regions. These combinations include chloroquine (weekly or daily) with (adult doses listed) dapsone 25 mg (daily), proguanil 100 mg with dapsone 25 mg (daily), chloroquine with sulfadoxine 500 mg (weekly), chloroquine with primaquine 45 mg (base) (weekly), or, most commonly, pyrimethamine 25 mg with sulfadoxine 500 mg (weekly). Dapsone has produced agranulocytosis.

Prevention of Transmission. For epidemiologic purposes, the nonpathogenic circulating gametocytes of *P. falciparum* may be destroyed or their development in the mosquito inhibited by primaquine or (provided the parasites are not resistant) by proguanil or pyrimethamine. Gametocytes of the other species are eliminated during routine treatment of the acute attack by chloroquine, quinine, and so forth. Primaquine as a single dose in the amount of 0.75 mg (base; adult dose listed) is the most effective gametocyticide and sporonticide.

PROPHYLAXIS. Attainment of the goal of worldwide malaria eradication through destruction of *Anopheles* mosquitoes by spraying houses with residually acting insecticides has proved more elusive than was expected when the World Health Organization sponsored the campaign in 1956. Although nearly 40 per cent of people at risk have been freed of the threat of malaria, a resurgence of the disease is again threatening the health and economic well-being of entire populations in South and Central America, Southeast Asia, the Indian subcontinent, and equatorial Africa. The disease is also being imported increasingly to countries in the temperate zones. One factor has been the development of resistance to insecticides by mosquitoes. More significant factors include adverse international economic trends and the expense of unexpectedly protracted eradication campaigns. Strengthening of these campaigns by mass chemoprophylaxis has been partly counteracted by the spread since 1960 of parasites resistant to chloroquine.

In these circumstances, control of malaria must revert to a variety of measures directed against the vector and the parasite, including mosquito source reduction by water management; larvicidal, and biologic control methods; continuation on a selective basis of the attack on adult mosquitoes by use of residually acting insecticides and space sprays; separation of people from the night-feeding mosquitoes by use of house screening and bed nets; and reduction of the parasite reservoir in humans by use of chemoprophylaxis and sporonticidal drugs (Bruce-Chwatt, 1980).

References

Bruce-Chwatt, L. J.: Essential Malariology. London, William Heinemann Medical Books Ltd, 1980.

Bruce-Chwatt, L. J., Black, R. H., Canfield, C. J., Clyde, D. F., Peters, W., and Wernsdorfer, W. H.: Chemotherapy of Malaria. Geneva, World Health Organisation, 1981.

Clyde, D. F., Most, H., McCarthy, V. C., and Vanderberg, J. P.: Immunization of man against sporozoite-induced falciparum malaria. Am J Med Sci 266:169, 1973.

Young, M. D.: Malaria. In Hunter, G. W., Swartzwelder, J. C., and Clyde, D. F. (eds.): Tropical Medicine. 5th ed. Philadelphia, W. B. Saunders Company, 1976.

209

BABESIOSIS

Michael G. Groves, D.V.M., Ph.D.
Charles E. Davis, M.D.

Babesiosis is a tick-borne protozoan disease that affects primarily wild and domestic animals. It is a major veterinary medical problem in many areas of the world. Until recently, human disease was considered a medical curiosity limited exclusively to splenectomized individuals. Since 1970, however, interest in human babesiosis has been stimulated by several case reports of people uncompromised by splenectomy and by the isolation of *Babesia* from the blood of asymptomatic individuals. Most of the recognized infections of intact individuals have occurred on five neighboring islands off the northeastern shore of the United States.

ETIOLOGY. *Babesia* are small, malaria-like protozoan parasites of red blood cells (RBC). Although they are closely related to plasmodia, the *Babesia* are placed in a different class, because they are small, nonpigmented, and pyriform (see Chapter 16). For many years, *Babesia* were called *Piroplasma* because of their shape, and the disease is still sometimes referred to as piroplasmosis.

Since Babes first observed *Babesia* in the red blood cells of Romanian cattle in 1888, more than 70 species have been identified in animals. Table 1 summarizes the host and geographic distribution of some of the more common species. For many years, the various species were thought to be quite host-specific. Although most *Babesia* species do display at least a limited host preference, a few, like *B. divergens,* which infects cattle, rodents, and splenectomized primates, cause infections across both species and generic boundaries.

Babesia do not necessarily retain their typical morphology in aberrant hosts. Nevertheless, the species of the host and the intraerythrocytic morphology of the parasite are the principal taxonomic criteria by which the organisms are identified. Understandably, definitive identification of the *Babesia* species that occasionally spill over from animal transmission cycles to infect man may be difficult. However, three species have been identified with some degree of certainty: *B. bovis* and *B. divergens,* which normally infect cattle, and *B. microti,* which usually infects rodents. Bovine *Babesia* (*B. divergens* and *bovis*) have caused most of the infections of splenectomized human beings, while *B. microti* is responsible for the clinical infections of intact individuals observed in the United States.

The vectors of *Babesia* are several species of hard ticks in the family *Ixodidae.* The principal vector of *B. microti* in the United States is *Ixodes dammini.* This tick was probably imported in the 1930s when a large number of wild deer were shipped from the northcentral United States to Nantucket Island in the northeast to replenish hunting stock (Spielman et al., 1979). In 1893, Smith and Kilborne proved the tick transmission of *B. bigemina* in cattle and thereby created a unique historic niche for *Babesia* as the first pathogenic protozoan proven to be transmitted to mammals by an arthropod. Within the tick, *Babesia* proceed through a developmental cycle that results in a generalized infection. Infections acquired by an immature stage are generally transmitted by the next stage in the tick life cycle (transstadial transmission). *Babesia* can also pass from an infected female to her offspring, producing infective larvae that have never taken a blood meal (transovarial transmission).

Ixodes are three-host ticks; that is, the larva, nymph, and adult seek a new host (of the same or different species) for a blood meal. *I. dammini* feeds primarily on the white-

Table 1. PRINCIPAL *BABESIA* OF DOMESTIC AND WILD ANIMALS

Parasite	Usual Host	Distribution
B. bigemina	Cattle	Europe, Africa, Australia, South America
B. bovis	Cattle	Europe, Africa, Asia, East Indies
B. divergens	Cattle	Northern Europe, United Kingdom
B. ovis	Sheep and goats	Southern Europe, Middle East, U.S.S.R., Southeast Asia, Africa
B. motasi	Sheep and goats	Same as *B. ovis*
B. equi	Horse	Tropical and subtropical areas of the world
B. caballi	Horse	Same as *B. equi*
B. trautmani	Swine	Southern Europe, U.S.S.R., Central and South Africa
B. canis	Dog	Tropical and subtropical areas of the world
B. microti	Rodents	North America and Europe

footed deer mouse (larvae and nymphs) and deer (adults). Although all stages will feed on man, only the nymphs appear to be capable of transmitting *B. microti.*

Details of the life cycle of *Babesia* are not completely known. In contrast to plasmodia, the development of *Babesia* in the mammalian host occurs exclusively within the RBC. After invading the RBC, new trophozoites are apparently formed by budding. Budding produces pairs and tetrads, but the organisms remain as ring and oval forms. They do not develop into schizonts. Instead, parasites are released into the bloodstream to infect new RBCs when the infected cell ruptures.

Ring forms are occasionally seen extracellularly, especially in very heavy infections. *Babesia* are not pigmented because they completely metabolize hemoglobin. This absence of the brownish, hemoglobin-derived pigment (hemozoin) is an important differential point between *Babesia* and *Plasmodium falciparum.* When stained by the Giemsa technique, the cytoplasm of *Babesia* is blue, but it contains a compact mass of red chromatin. Only a small percentage of the erythrocytic forms survive after ingestion by ticks. This has given rise to speculation that some intraerythrocytic developmental change occurs in a small number of the parasites to make them infectious for the tick. Various babesial forms observed in the gut contents of ticks are thought to be sexual stages that presumably unite to form the zygote. The zygote, then, undergoes a succession of multiple fission divisions in the gut cells of the tick. The numerous vermicules that are formed by these divisions invade other tissues and multiply. When the ovary is involved, the infection is transmitted to the guts of developing larval offspring. A final division in the salivary gland or in lymph cells produces infective *Babesia* that closely resemble the trophozoites found in the mammalian host.

PATHOGENESIS AND PATHOLOGY. The pathophysiology of babesiosis has been studied primarily in animals and has been found to vary greatly depending on the host and the species or strain of parasite. The disease is often quite mild. The one consistent finding throughout all infections is the invasion and destruction of RBC's by the parasites. The ability of at least some *Babesia* to penetrate erythrocytes depends on an intact alternative complement pathway through C3 (Jack and Ward, 1980). C3b is a critical determinant in the interaction between *Babesia* and red cells, and C3b receptors, either on the red cell or the parasite, are necessary for penetration of the erythrocyte by *Babesia* (Jack and Ward, 1980a). In any event, hypocomplementemia and transient glomerulonephritis occur in experimental babesiosis (Annable and Ward, 1974) and circulating immune complexes have been demonstrated in people with *B. microti* infections (Gombert et al., 1982).

Electron microscopy of RBC penetration by *B. microti* (Rudzinska, et al., 1976) showed that the merozoite first touches its anterior end to the RBC and then quickly becomes attached to it. The RBC membrane invaginates and forms a vacuole that disappears as the red cell membrane disintegrates. Thus, when the process is complete, the organism lies free in the cytoplasm separated from the RBC only by the babesial membrane.

Lysis of erythrocytes is responsible for many of the most severe manifestations of babesiosis. Hemolytic anemia, bilirubinemia, hemoglobinemia, hemoglobinuria, and renal failure with hemoglobinuric nephrosis occur in fatal cases.

Wright and Mahoney (1974) ascribe the early dramatic findings of hypotension, vascular congestion, and anoxia that occur in bovine babesiosis to the release of kallikreins. The role of pharmacologic mediators in human disease is unknown.

Splenomegaly is a uniform finding in babesiosis of animals and occurs in many human infections. The spleen may be two to five times its normal size with soft, dark red pulp and prominent lymphoid follicles. In some infections, large numbers of parasitized RBCs line the walls of the capillaries and small blood vessels. These "sticky cells" cause sludging of the blood and capillary occlusion that can result in ischemia and necrosis of the affected organ. The brain is frequently affected in animal babesiosis. In the liver, stasis of blood in hepatic sinusoids leads to swelling, cellular degeneration, and necrosis, especially around the central veins. The enlarged liver and other organs are bile-stained. Erythrophagocytosis in the spleen and liver is common. Proliferation of hematopoietic tissue in the bone marrow, spleen, and liver is extensive.

After recovery from the initial illness, animals continue to carry the parasite at low levels for months and even years. *B. microti* parasitemias have been documented in people for up to one year after infection (Wittner et al., 1982). The persistence of the parasites may be explained by antigenic variation. Like the African trypanosomes (Chapter 210), *Babesia* may be capable of eluding the immune response by altering their surface antigens (Mahoney, 1977). These chronic infections appear to be important in maintaining the humoral and cellular defense mechanisms. If the parasitemia is eliminated, either spontaneously or by successful chemotherapy, the host becomes susceptible to reinfection.

Splenic function is extremely important in the maintenance of resistance to babesiosis. Many *Babesia* species do not infect secondary hosts unless they have been splenectomized. Furthermore, the spleen restricts the degree of parasitemia and therefore the severity of the disease. Of the 11 cases of acute babesiosis reported in splenectomized people, five have been fatal (Garnham, 1980; Jacoby et al., 1980; Scholten et al., 1968; Teutsch et al., 1980). In contrast, only one fatal case has been recorded in the over 50 clinical cases of *B. microti* infections in intact individuals (Marcus et al., 1982). Furthermore, the results of serologic surveys indicate that milder subclinical infections are most common in intact individuals (Filstein et al., 1980; Osorno et al., 1976; Ruebush et al., 1977). Removal of the spleen from chronically infected animals increases the parasitemia and may precipitate a fatal infection. Cellular immunity is probably also an important factor in restricting parasitemia. Hamsters given antilymphocyte serum before infection with *B. microti* develop dramatic, fulminating disease.

CLINICAL MANIFESTATIONS. The severity and the clinical manifestations of acute human babesiosis depend upon the presence of a spleen. Seven of the 11 reported *Babesia* infections of splenectomized people were fulminating, and five ended fatally within a week. Fever, chills, anemia, vomiting, hemoglobinuria, and jaundice are the most common findings. Renal failure, hypotension, and coma may occur in fatal cases. Two of the six nonfatal infections were mild like those of intact individuals. A probable twelfth case of babesiosis in a splenectomized subject was diagnosed serologically two years after the original illness (Grunwaldt, 1977). The individual lived in the area of the United States where infections with *B. microti* are endemic, had a history of a tick bite two weeks before the symptoms started, and recovered spontaneously.

To date, only *B. microti* has caused overt disease in persons with spleens, and these infections have been restricted to the northeastern United States. The disease is typically nonfatal, with a gradual onset and a protracted recovery. Clinically, it is characterized principally by fever, fatigue, myalgia, and anemia. Splenomegaly, nausea, chills, and sweating occur less commonly. The severe manifestations of hemoglobinemia do not occur (Ruebush et al., 1977).

The laboratory manifestations in splenectomized and intact individuals vary chiefly in magnitude. The major changes are secondary to hemolysis and abnormal liver function. Anemia, decreased hemoglobin concentration, elevated erythrocyte sedimentation rate, reticulocytosis, and elevated serum glutamic oxaloacetic transaminase and lactic dehydrogenase are consistent findings. Proteinuria, elevated bilirubin, thromboytopenia and a modest leukopenia may also occur. Splenectomized individuals may develop azotemia, thrombocytopenia, and hypocomplementemia.

The mild or subclinical form of babesiosis has been studied extensively in North America. Thirty-eight of 101 people in an enzootic area of animal babesiosis in rural Mexico reacted positively to an indirect hemagglutination test, and *Babesia*, probably of rodent origin, was isolated in splenectomized hamsters from three asymptomatic carriers (Osorno et al., 1976). In the same study, 29 individuals living in Mexico City were all negative for antibody. In a similar survey on Nantucket Island, the *B. microti* endemic area of the United States, 10 of 133 sera from asymptomatic individuals with a recent history of fever or tick bite were positive by a fluorescent antibody test (Ruebush et al., 1977). This survey also found evidence of undiagnosed infections in unselected patients undergoing routine diagnostic tests. Eleven of 577 specimens were seropositive for *Babesia*. *B. microti* was isolated in splenectomized hamsters from the blood of one seropositive patient nine weeks after discharge from the hospital, and rare *Babesia* organisms were seen in thin blood smears of another seropositive individual. In still another study, seven of 102 sera collected on Shelter Island, New York, had antibody to *Babesia* (Filstein et al., 1980).

COMPLICATIONS AND SEQUELAE. The development of a chronic low-level parasitemia following acute disease has been discussed above (see section on *Pathogenesis and Pathology*). No long-term side effects have been attributed to these parasitemias in either animals or man, although patients frequently complain of fatigue for four to eight weeks following the disappearance of parasites from routine blood smears. Patients who have recovered from babesiosis must be considered carriers and should not be used as blood donors. At least three cases of transfusion-induced babesiosis have been documented (Marcus et al., 1982). If splenectomy of a possible *Babesia* carrier is required, the patient should be closely observed, and peripheral blood smears should be carefully monitored for signs of an acute exacerbation.

GEOGRAPHIC VARIATIONS IN DISEASE. *Babesia* species, like their tick vectors, are distributed throughout most of the tropical and temperate areas of the world. However, animal babesiosis is more prevalent in tropical and subtropical zones due to the longer tick seasons. Paradoxically, acute human babesiosis has only been diagnosed in temperate, nonmalarious areas. Clinical disease may be suppressed in malarious areas either by antimalarial antibody that cross-reacts with *Babesia* (Chisholm et al., 1978) or by prophylactic antimalarial drugs, an unlikely possibility because antimalarial compounds are not very effective against *Babesia*. It seems more likely that babesiosis is overlooked in these areas, because it is misdiagnosed as malaria. This diagnostic error is common even in temperate climates. Because the disease is self-limited in normal individuals, any treatment may appear to be effective. Fatal babesiosis in splenectomized persons could certainly mimic fulminating drug-resistant malaria, since the resistance of these individuals to *Plasmodium* would also be severely compromised.

By far the largest concentration of reported human babesiosis cases has occurred in a small area of the northeastern United States. Most affected persons were 48 years of age or older, possessed a spleen, and contracted the infection on one of five coastal islands. The age distribution of acute infections is interesting. It seems unlikely that older individuals were exposed more frequently to the vectors or that they all had some form of splenic dysfunction. Babesiosis in young animals is often asymptomatic.

The causative agent in the northeastern United States has been identified as *B. microti*. Because this parasite is widely distributed throughout North America and Europe but seems to produce disease only in this location, it has been suggested that a more virulent strain of the organism has emerged on these islands. A number of other factors (such as an abundant *B. microti* reservoir in the form of the white-footed mouse; a vector tick, *I. dammini*, which feeds both on mouse and man; and an intimate tick–man contact on islands that are popular summer vacation areas) have certainly contributed to the establishment of this endemic focus of disease. At least one case contracted on the mainland close to Nantucket Island has been reported (Teutsch et al., 1980).

DIAGNOSIS. The diagnosis of acute disease depends upon the demonstration of *Babesia* in peripheral blood smears stained with either Wright's or Giemsa's stain. The parasites may be pyriform, round, ameboid, rod- or ring-shaped (Fig. 1), and are frequently mistaken for *Plasmodium*. Pairs and tetrads ("maltese-cross" forms) are common. *Babesia* differ from plasmodia in that they do not produce hemozoin pigment in the RBC and do not develop into schizonts or gametocytes.

The diagnosis of chronic babesiosis is more difficult because parasites are scarce in the peripheral blood. Serodiagnosis by the indirect fluorescent antibody, complement fixation, capillary tube agglutination, or indirect hemagglutination tests is sensitive and reliable in malaria-free areas. The immunofluorescent test is especially useful. Infected individuals develop very high titers that drop to 1:64 or less within 8 to 12 months (Chisholm et al., 1978). Thus, a titer greater than 1:64 usually indicates active or recent infection. However, because many *Babesia* antigens cross-react with those of *Plasmodium*, serology is of limited value in areas endemic for malaria. The presence of parasites in chronic infections is usually detectable only by subinoculating large quantities of blood into a susceptible animal (usually splenectomized). Asymptomatic infections of animals have been detected by administering corticosteroids and monitoring blood smears for an exacerbation of the parasitemia.

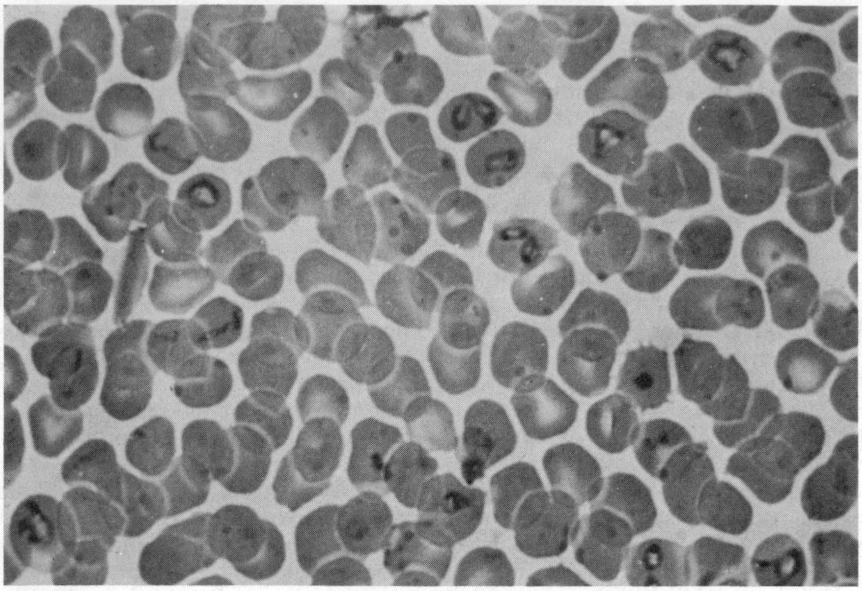

Figure 1. *Babesia microti* in hamster red blood cells. The parasites were isolated from the blood of a person with acute babesiosis. Photomicrograph courtesy of Dr. Miodrag Ristic, University of Illinois.

TREATMENT. Although the antimalarial drug, chloroquine, has been the most common chemotherapeutic agent used in the treatment of human babesiosis, clinical and laboratory findings do not support its use. Patients treated with the drug fail to eliminate their parasitemias, and the drug is ineffective against experimental *B. microti* and *B. rodhaini* infections in rodents (Miller et al., 1978). Pentamidine has also proved ineffective in the treatment of human babesiosis despite its successful use against *Pneumocystis* infections (Chapter 130) and African trypanosomiasis.

Another aromatic diamidine, diminazene aceturate (Berenil), may be more useful. Both pentamidine and Berenil are effective in the treatment of animal babesiosis and have been used in humans for the treatment of other parasitic diseases. However, they were only partially successful against experimental *B. microti* infections of hamsters (Miller et al., 1978). One patient with human *B. microti* infection has been treated with an unstated dose of diminazene and cleared his parasitemia but developed Guillain-Barré syndrome (Ruebush, 1978). Since diminazene can cause central nervous system toxicity in dogs, it is possible that this complication was caused by the drug. On the other hand, some patients with African trypanosomiasis have been treated with I.M. (intramuscular) diminazene, 5 mg/kg for three doses on alternate days, without serious side effects (Temu, 1975).

Until more information is available, it is probably prudent to give only symptomatic treatment to intact individuals with babesiosis since all but one 79-year old patient have recovered (Marcus et al., 1982). Patients who are asplenic or otherwise compromised and develop fulminating disease should probably be treated with one of the diamidines. These drugs should be used with caution, however, because of their intrinsic toxicity and because some animals treated with these drugs for experimental babesiosis died despite an impressive reduction in their parasitemia (Miller et al., 1978). Exchange transfusions have been used successfully in splenectomized patients with life-threatening disease (Gombert et al., 1982).

PROPHYLAXIS. Prevention of naturally occurring human babesiosis would depend on: (1) reduction of ticks below disease maintenance levels, (2) removal of susceptible reservoir animals, or (3) isolation of humans from vector ticks. The rare incidence of this disease and our limited knowledge of the control of wildlife babesiosis make institution of any of these measures difficult or impractical. Blood donors in endemic areas should be questioned about tick bites, but the screening of blood for parasites is impractical.

References

Annable, C. R., and Ward, P. A.: Immunopathology of the renal complications of babesiosis. J Immunol 112:1, 1974.

Babés, V.: Sur l'hémoglobinurie bactérienne du boeuf. C R Acad Sci (Paris) 107:692, 1888.

Chisholm, E. S., Ruebush, T. K. II, Sulzer, A. J., and Healy, G. R.: *Babesia microti* infection in man: Evaluation of an indirect immunofluorescent antibody test. Am J Trop Med Hyg 27:14, 1978.

Filstein, M. R., Benach, J. L., White, D. J., Brody, B. A., Goldman, W. D., Bakel, C. W., and Schwartz, R. S.: Serosurvey for human babesiosis in New York. J Infect Dis 141:5/8, 1980.

Garnham, P. C. C.: Human babesiosis: European aspects. Trans R Soc Trop Med Hyg 74:153, 1980.

Gombert, M. E., Goldstein, E. J. C., Benach, J. L., Tenenbaum, M. J., Grunwaldt, E., Kaplan, M. H., Eveland, L. K.: Human Babesiosis. Clinical and therapeutic considerations. JAMA 248:3005, 1982.

Grunwaldt, E.: Babesiosis on Shelter Island. NY State J Med 77:1320, 1977.

Jack, R. M. and Ward, P. A.: The role *in vivo* of C3 and the C3b receptor in babesial infection in the rat. J Immunol 124:1574, 1980.

Jack, R. M. and Ward, P. A.: *Babesia rodhaini* interactions with complement: relationship to parasitic entry into red cells. J Immunol 124:1566, 1980.

Jacoby, G. A., Hunt, J. V., Kosinski, K. S., Demirjian. Z. N., Huggins, C., Etkind, P., Marcus, L. C., and Spielman, A.: Treatment of transfusion-transmitted babesiosis by exchange transfusion. N Engl J Med 303:1098, 1980.

Mahoney, D. F.: Babesiosis of domestic animals. In Kreier, J. P. (ed.): Parasitic Protozoa. Vol IV. New York, Academic Press, 1977, pp. 1–52.

Marcus, L. C., Valigorski, J. M., Fanning, W. L., Joseph, T., and Glick, B.: A case report of transfusion babesiosis. JAMA 248:465, 1982.

Miller, L. H., Neva, F. A., and Gill, F.: Failure of chloroquine in human babesiosis (*Babesia microti*). Case report and chemotherapeutic trials in hamsters. Ann Intern Med 88:200, 1978.

Osorno, M., Vega, C., Ristic, M., Roble, C., and Ibarra, S.: Isolation of *Babesia sp.* from asymptomatic human beings. Vet Parasitol 2:111, 1976.

Ruebush, T. K. II: Human babesiosis in the United States. Ann Intern Med 88:263, 1978.

Ruebush, T. K. II, Cassady, P. B., Marsh, H. J., Lisker, S. A., Voorhees,

D. B., Mahoney, E. B., and Healy, G. R.: Human babesiosis on Nantucket Island. Clinical features. Ann Intern Med 86:6, 1977.
Ruebush, T. K. II, Juranek, D. D., Chisholm, E. S., Snow, P. C., Healy, G. R., and Sulzer, A. J.: Human babesiosis on Shelter Island. Evidence for self-limited and subclinical infections. N Engl J Med 297:825, 1977.
Rudzinska, M. A., Trager, W., Lewengrub, S. J., and Gubert, E.: An electron microscopic study of *Babesia microti* invading erythrocytes. Cell Tissue Res 169:323, 1976.
Scholten, R. G., Braff, E. H., Healey, G., and Gleason, N.: A case of babesiosis in man in the United States. Am J Trop Med Hyg 17:810, 1968.
Smith, T., and Kilbourne, F. L.: Investigation into the nature, causation, and prevention of Texas or south cattle fever. Washington D.C., U.S. Department of Agriculture Bur Anim Ind Bull 1:1, 1893.
Spielman, A., Carlton, C. M., Piesman, J., and Carlton, M. D.: Human babesiosis on Nantucket Island, U.S.A.: Description of the vector *Ixodes dammini*, N. sp. (*Acarina Ixodidea*). J Med Entomol 15:218, 1979.
Temu, S. E.: Summary of cases of human early trypanosomiasis treated with Berenil at E.A.T.R.O. Trans R Soc Trop Med Hyg 69:277, 1975.
Teutsch, S. M., Etkind, P., Burwell, E. L., Sato, K., Dana, M. M., Fleishman, P. R., and Juranek, D. D.: Babesiosis in post-splenectomy host. Am J Trop Med Hyg 29:738, 1980.
Wittmer, M., Rowin, K. S., Fanowitz, H. B., Hobbs, J. F., Saltzman, S., Wentz, B., Hirach, R., Chisholm, E., and Healy, G. R.: Successful chemotherapy of transfusion babesiosis. Ann Intern Med 96:601, 1982.
Wright, I. G., and Mahoney, D. F.: The activation of plasma kallikrein in acute *Babesia argentina* infections of splenectomized calves. Z Parasitenkd 43:271, 1974.

210

TRYPANOSOMIASIS

W. H. R. Lumsden, D.Sc., M.D., F.R.C.P.E., F.R.S.E.

Trypanosomiasis of man is surpassed only by malaria as an infection that inhibits the development of tropical lands. There are two distinct forms of trypanosomiasis, American trypanosomiasis or Chagas' disease and African trypanosomiasis or sleeping sickness. Both are transmitted by blood-sucking insects, infect other vertebrates in addition to man, and occur mainly in rural environments. But they differ in the mechanisms of their transmission and are caused by different species of trypanosomes. *Trypanosoma cruzi*, the agent that causes Chagas' disease, belongs to the section Stercoraria of *Trypanosoma*. Stercoraria are transmitted, as the name indicates, via the feces of blood-sucking insects. *Trypanosoma brucei*, the agent of African sleeping sickness, belongs to the section Salivaria, which are transmitted via the bite or saliva of the vector (Hoare, 1972). Because the geographic distributions differ and because of linguistic barriers between investigators, the two diseases have been studied independently and will be described separately in this chapter. Nevertheless, there are many general similarities between their clinical course, pathology, and epidemiology, and instructive comparisons may be drawn.

AMERICAN TRYPANOSOMIASIS—CHAGAS' DISEASE

Chagas' disease is caused by infection with *Trypanosoma (Schizotrypanum) cruzi*, which is transmitted by blood-sucking bugs (Hemiptera). The disease occurs in Central America, Panama, Guatemala, and Costa Rica, and in all the states of South America as far south as central Argentina. It has been estimated that 30 million people are at risk of infection and 7 million infected. There are probably more cases of cardiac disease in the world due to Chagas' disease than to any other cause.

ETIOLOGY AND TRANSMISSION. *Trypanosoma cruzi* exists in two morphologic forms in the vertebrate (Fig. 1). Amastigotes are rounded, nonmotile, aflagellate forms, about 3 μm in diameter that multiply by binary fission inside the cells of many different tissues of the body but particularly in muscle cells. Amastigotes multiply until nearly all the cytoplasm of the cell is consumed, resulting in a mass of amastigotes surrounded by the remains of the cell membrane. This structure is called a pseudocyst. When the pseudocyst ruptures, the amastigotes transform into trypomastigotes—motile forms about 15 to 20 μm long with a flagellum and undulating membrane. These nonmultiplying forms serve two purposes: to disseminate the infection from cell to cell and to initiate infection in the vector. The insects are nocturnally active blood-sucking bugs of the family Reduviidae, sub-family Triatominae (*Triatoma, Rhodnius*, and *Panstrongylus* spp, Chapter 18). In the midgut of these bugs the ingested trypomastigotes transform into epimastigotes—motile, multiplying forms with a flagellum and a short undulating membrane. These proliferate in the lumen of the midgut and eventually invade the hindgut. In the rectum trypomastigotes are formed again; these are the infective forms. The bugs defecate when they feed, and trypomastigotes in the feces enter the body of a new vertebrate through the bite, skin abrasions, or the intact mucous membranes.

In addition to man, a wide variety of wild and domestic animals have been found infected with *T. cruzi*-like organisms. These animals may be important reservoirs of infection. *T. cruzi* has been isolated from wild mammals and triatomes in the southern and southwestern United States, but the human disease is virtually nonexistent there because man does not live in close association with either the vector or these mammalian reservoirs. It is difficult to judge the magnitude of the threat of thc nonhuman reservoirs in endemic areas because many of these organisms may well be transmitted exclusively among wild animals and not impinge upon man at all. Methods for the infraspecific characterization of *T. cruzi* by means of isoenzyme patterns are now giving information on this point. In one case it was clear that the *T. cruzi* organisms circulating in the domestic environment in man, cats, dogs, rodents, and *Panstrongylus megistus* were different from those found in sylvatic mammals and bugs. Thus, the most common epidemiologic picture is probably transmission to man in the house by domiciliated bugs sheltered in crevices of mud-and-wattle walls or palm-leaf roofs, with only an occasional introduction of trypanosomes from sylvatic environments. Transmission by blood transfusion has also become an important hazard.

PATHOLOGY AND PATHOGENESIS. At the site of inoculation (chagoma), *T. cruzi* multiplies mainly in macrophages. When systemic dissemination occurs, *T. cruzi* multiplies in cells of many different tissues. There is a predilection for nerve cells and muscle cells, particularly of the heart and the gut. The pathological effects of the acute stage seem to be due mainly to direct damage to these cells by multiplication of the organisms.

Later, in the chronic phase, when circulating and intracellular organisms are very few, the mechanisms of pathology are more controversial. In addition to direct damage to muscle tissue, destruction of the autonomic nerve-ganglion cells that control function seems to be important. One school of thought holds that the onset of symptoms is determined by the proportion of these cells damaged during the acute stage combined with the rate of further natural loss of cells by senescence (Köberle, 1968). Others consider the damage to be the result of a continuing, progressive, immunologically mediated process. This mechanism has received support from clinical studies that show widespread inflammation of the heart in the absence of parasites and from experimental studies that show similar lesions in mice injected with extracts of *T. cruzi*.

In its reproductive stages, *T. cruzi* evades the immune response by living within the cytoplasm of the cells of the host. In this location the amastigotes provoke little host reaction. The immunologic response to the breakdown products of the parasitized cells may be greater than that to the organisms themselves. However, there is a humoral response to the circulating trypomastigotes. This antibody is the basis of the complement fixation test. There is no evidence of the antigenic variability that is characteristic of the African trypanosomes.

The immunologic mechanisms that reduce the number of organisms to low levels after the acute phase of the infection are poorly understood, but cell-mediated mechanisms are likely to be operative because immune macrophages can kill *T. cruzi* and delayed hypersensitivity skin reactions to soluble antigens of *T. cruzi* become positive (WHO, 1974).

A severe inflammatory reaction characterized by lymphangitis, edema, and infiltration of polymorphonuclears, lymphocytes, and monocytes is responsible for the appearance of the chagoma. Muscle cells that have become packed with amastigotes are called pseudocysts. These rupture and release toxic products and the developing trypomastigotes, provoking the early inflammatory response consisting primarily of neutrophils, followed by lymphocytes, plasma cells, and histiocytes. In chronic disease, these lesions become granulomatous with pseudotubercles and giant cells in affected muscles. Adjacent cells degenerate. Lesions in the central nervous system (CNS) consist of lymphocytic perivascular cuffing, focal endarteritis, neuronal degeneration, and leptomeningitis. The focal nature of the vascular and neuroglial lesions may produce glial nodules scattered throughout the brain.

CLINICAL MANIFESTATIONS. Three stages of Chagas' disease can be recognized: the primary lesion, the acute stage, and the chronic stage. The primary lesion marks the site of entry of the organism into the body and appears after an incubation period of one to two weeks. It is not invariably present. When infection occurs through a skin abrasion, the primary lesion is an inflamed swelling of the skin, some 10 cm in diameter, called a chagoma. If the portal of entry is the conjunctiva, a common route, the primary lesion is a unilateral, bipalpebral edema of the conjunctiva (Romaña's sign).

When the acute stage of the disease is recognized, it follows the appearance of the primary lesion by 7 to 14 days and lasts about 30 days. It is characterized by pyrexia, headache, facial and generalized edema, and signs of heart damage. The acute stage occurs mostly in children and is believed to cause a mortality of about 5 per cent. Meningoencephalitis or heart failure is the usual cause of death. The acute stage is usually not recognized, however. When it does occur, it often resolves with little or no immediate damage. After this stage, the infection becomes latent, and the individual may remain healthy and asymptomatic for the rest of his life.

The infection is probably rarely eliminated, however, and an unknown proportion of cases enters the so-called chronic phase. This stage is characterized by disturbances of the function of the hollow organs, particularly the heart, esophagus, and colon. The cardiac changes include myocardial insufficiency, cardiomegaly, disturbances of atrioventricular conduction, and the Adams-Stokes syndrome. Disturbances of peristalsis in the esophagus and colon lead to distention of these organs (megaesophagus and megacolon). Food may accumulate in the lower esophagus, and the patient may be able to transfer it to the stomach only by a jolt, such as that produced by jumping off a chair to the floor. Huge quantities of feces may accumulate in the colon. Megacolon and megaesophagus occur because of invasion and destruction of cells of the autonomic ganglia.

Sudden death on exertion is a common terminal event in chronic Chagas' disease. Many macabre anecdotes illustrate the frequency of this type of death. One of the most impressive is that football teams from affected communities may carry a large number of reserves to replace the losses occasioned by the rigor of the game! The late effects of Chagas' disease appear mainly in the third to fifth decades of life. They are of great social significance because they tend to occur when the family responsibilities of the subject are at their most demanding.

DIAGNOSIS. A distinction should be made between protozoologic and serologic diagnosis because each gives fundamentally different information. Protozoologic diagnosis, which depends on the actual demonstration of the organism, proves that the patient is still infected. It has two implications: the pathologic process is continuing and the patient is still a source of infection to vector insects. Serologic positivity is evidence only of past infection with either *T. cruzi* or some other antigenically similar agent. False positive and negative results are not infrequent.

Protozoologic Diagnosis. This procedure is usually straightforward during the acute phase of the disease. The organisms are multiplying actively and amastigotes are plentiful in tissue cells. Consequently, trypomastigotes are also plentiful in the peripheral blood. Trypomastigotes can be detected in the peripheral blood by examination of thin or thick films stained with Romanowsky stain. Later, however, organisms become very scarce and can be demonstrated only by the use of multiplicative methods. *T. cruzi* is comparatively easy to cultivate on simple blood-agar slants and these may be used. However, the most sensitive method is generally believed to be xenodiagnosis, the process of allowing laboratory-bred, uninfected bugs to feed on the patient and examining the gut of these bugs subsequently for the presence of *T. cruzi* epimastigotes or trypomastigotes. The method, although sensitive, has obvious shortcomings: it is distasteful to patients, it is slow (since infection may not be detectable in bugs for as long as 90 days), and it is dangerous to the personnel who perform it.

Trypanosoma (Herpetosoma) rangeli, a nonpathogenic

organism that occurs in man in Guatemala and El Salvador in Central America and in Colombia, Venezuela, and Chile in South America, is readily distinguished from *T. cruzi* in the peripheral blood. It is much longer—up to 36 μm long—and its kinetoplast is much smaller than that of *T. cruzi*. It also is transmitted by triatomid bugs.

Serologic Diagnosis. Complement fixation, introduced in the 1930's, demonstrated the wide distribution and high prevalence of antibodies to *T. cruzi* in South America and established it as an important cause of disease. It is still the most widely used test, although there have been problems with variability of the antigen that is derived from *T. cruzi* cultures (Lumsden, 1973; WHO, 1974). Some of the more modern tests for recognition of humoral antibody, such as immunofluorescence (IF) and enzyme-linked immunosorbent assay (ELISA), are coming into use (PAHO, 1975).

GEOGRAPHIC VARIATIONS. Because the disease is chronic and occurs mainly in rural communities that are often largely illiterate and deficient in health records, it is difficult to document the anecdotal geographic variations in the disease. However, the acute stage of the disease is more frequently recognized in western Argentina than elsewhere and the "mega" conditions occur most commonly in southern Brazil.

TREATMENT. The disease is feared out of proportion to the chance of infection because it is widely accepted in South America that there is no really effective chemotherapy against it. The most active drug available so far is a nitrofurazone compound, nifurtimox (Bayer 2502 or Lampit) (Lumsden, 1972). It appears to be effective against circulating trypomastigotes but less so against the intracellular amastigotes.

An experimental imidazole (R07-1051, *N*-benzyl-2-nitro-1-imidazolacetamide) may be useful against circulating and intracellular *T. cruzi* (Lugones et al., 1974). There is good evidence that it may cure acute Chagas' disease and a possibility that it may also be effective against chronic disease.

PROPHYLAXIS AND CONTROL. Control measures are limited to those that reduce contact between the vectors and man. Measures to improve housing and to use materials that do not provide shelter for the bugs are obvious but are often precluded economically. The disease is one of poverty-stricken rural communities. When housing cannot be improved, spraying with the insecticide benzene hexachloride (BHC) is widely used.

AFRICAN TRYPANOSOMIASIS—SLEEPING SICKNESS

Sleeping sickness is caused by infection with *Trypanosoma (Trypanozoon) brucei*, which is transmitted by blood-sucking tsetse flies (Muscidae: *Glossina)*. The disease occurs widely in sub-Saharan Africa from Senegal in the west to Ethiopia in the east and as far south as Zambia and Rhodesia. It is not coextensive with the distribution of the vector tsetse flies. Instead, it occurs focally within that distribution, depending on the habits and customs of the people and the ecologic characteristics of the local flies and wild animals (Ford, 1971).

ETIOLOGY AND TRANSMISSION. *T. brucei* exists in the vertebrate in only one morphologic form, the trypomastigote (Fig. 1). The trypomastigote is pleomorphic, however, and may occur as "long slender," 23 to 30 μm in length with a long flagellum, or "short stumpy" forms, 17 to 22 μm in length. The short stumpy forms have no, or only a very short, free flagellum. The long slender trypomastigote is the reproductive form in the vertebrate. The function of the short stumpy form is more controversial, but it is generally believed that it has altered respiratory metabolism that permits it to survive in the gut of *Glossina* and infect this vector insect.

T. brucei is divided into three subspecies on the basis of differences in host susceptibility and in the characteristics of the diseases they cause (Mulligan, 1970). All are identical morphologically. *T.b. brucei* is by definition noninfectious for man but infects a wide variety of domestic and wild artiodactyls, including cattle, waterbuck, bushbuck, and buffalo. The other two species infect man as well as lower animals. *T.b. gambiense* causes a slowly developing disease (Gambian disease) with an incubation period that may last many months and a course that may permit the patient to survive for many years. *T.b. rhodesiense* is also infectious for man, but it is associated with a rapidly progressive disease (Rhodesian disease) that has a short incubation period and usually kills the patient within a few months. These are the classic courses of the two diseases, but evidence is accumulating that there may be a significant number of subclinical cases.

All three subspecies of *T. brucei* are transmitted by the bite of tsetse flies (*Glossina* spp), which typically inhabit woodland or forest. Short stumpy trypomastigotes from the circulation of an infected patient are ingested in the blood meal of the fly and multiply first as trypomastigotes in the midgut of the fly. Later, infection extends to the salivary glands and after about 15 days, metacyclic, mammal-infective forms develop (Mulligan, 1970). These are trypomastigotes clothed in a glycoprotein outer coat, which equips them for survival in the mammalian host. These forms are injected into a mammal during the next blood meal of the fly. It was formerly thought that the entire development of the trypanosome in the fly took place in the lumina of the gut and in the salivary glands, but recent evidence indicates that organisms may alternatively pass through the intestinal wall and the hemocoele to reach the salivary glands.

The patterns of transmission and maintenance of *T.b. rhodesiense* and *T.b. gambiense* differ. In the rapidly progressive Rhodesian disease, infected humans cannot provide a continuous source of infection in nature because they are soon removed from the scene by treatment, hospitalization, or death. Thus, this type of disease is a true zoonosis; humans are infected by flies that acquired their infection from wild animals. Intrahuman cycles of transmission are unimportant. A preponderance of males is infected because it is mainly men who go hunting, fishing, or honey-gathering (or, as tourists, go game-watching) and expose themselves to attack by flies that usually feed only on wild animals.

In the more slowly progressive Gambian disease, humans are available to provide long-term sources of infection for flies, and purely intrahuman cycles of transmission are more frequent. Thus, in the classic epidemiology of West African sleeping sickness a small population of flies is concentrated in a riverine forest by the prevailing aridity of the surrounding terrain and feeds repetitively on the

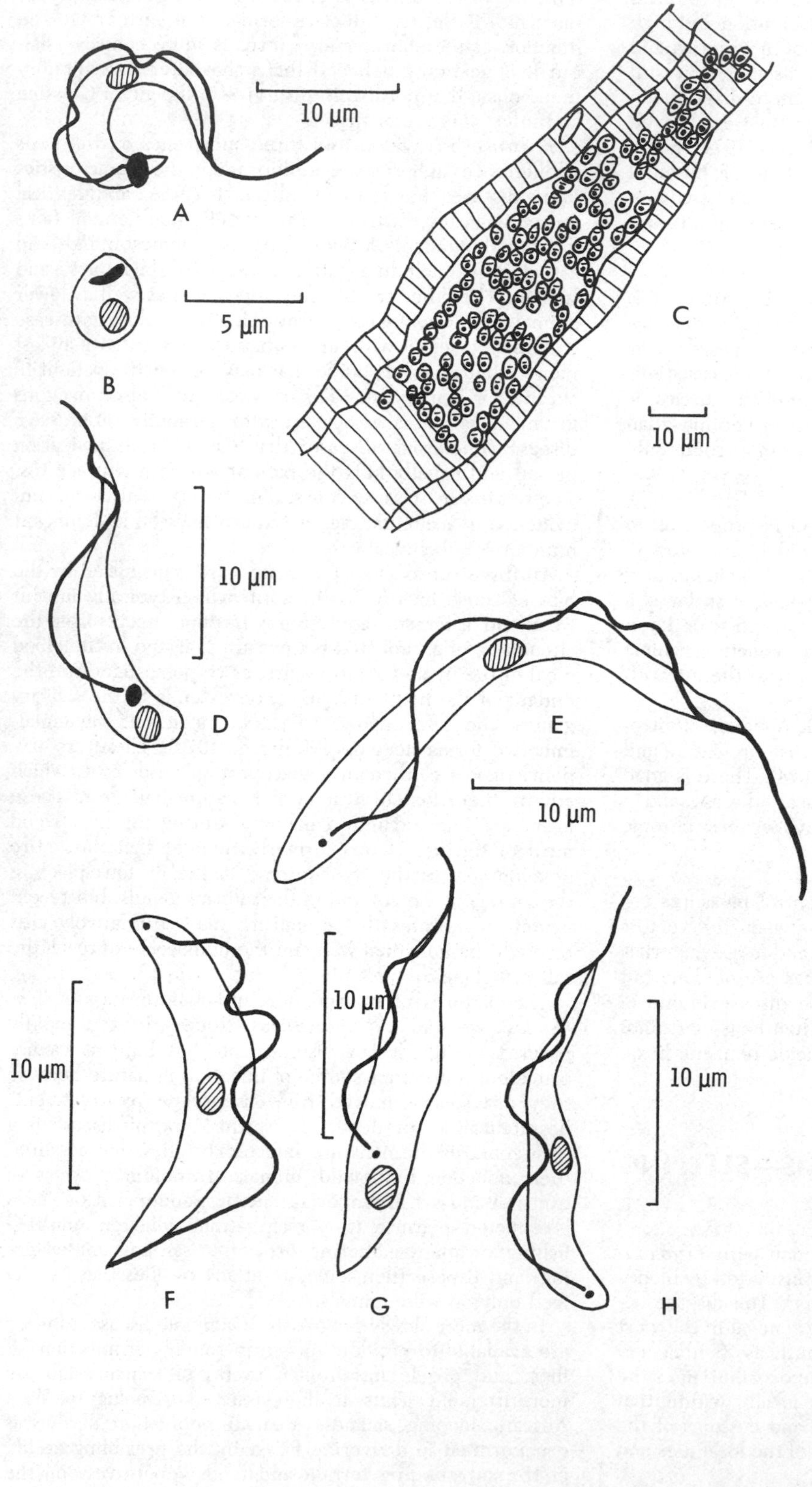

Figure 1. *Trypanosoma cruzi: A,* Trypomastigote from mammalian blood; *B,* amastigote from mammalian cell; *C,* pseudocyst packed with amastigotes in mammalian muscle; *D,* epimastigotes from midgut of bug vector. *Trypanosoma brucei: E,* Long slender form from mammalian blood; *F,* short stumpy form from mammalian blood; *G,* epimastigote form from salivary gland of *Glossina; H,* metacyclic trypomastigote from salivary gland of *Glossina.*

people coming to the river bed to collect water. Women and children are infected most often because they visit the river bed more frequently.

PATHOLOGY AND PATHOGENESIS. *T. brucei* differs from *T. cruzi* in the behavior it adopts to evade the immune response of the host. Instead of sheltering within cells, the organisms alter their external antigens about every five or six days. Thus, the infection consists of a series of waves of parasitemia, each differing antigenically from those that preceded it and from those that will follow. This antigenic change occurs in the "outer coat," a glycoprotein layer outside the plasmalemma that is the true boundary of the cell. The antigenic repertoire of a single trypanosome may include 100 to 1000 different variable surface glycoproteins (VSGs). This number is reached by a form of genetic rearrangement that may involve the synthesis of duplicate copies of genes. In some strains, only the duplicate (expression-linked copy) can express new VSGs. The new VSG becomes dominant when antibody selects against trypanosomes carrying the preceding glycoprotein coat (reviewed by Englund et al., 1982). The antigens of *T. brucei* can, therefore, be divided into two classes: the variable antigens contributed by this outer coat and the stable antigens—internal run-of-the-mill cell constituents such as enzymes and structural proteins.

The multiplicity and rapid succession of variable antigens bombards the immune response like a succession of infections by different organisms and induces a profuse production of IgM antibody, the antibody that is stimulated by new particulate antigens. The towering IgM levels produced both in serum and in cerebrospinal fluid (CSF) are characteristic of salivarian trypanosomiasis, are exploited for diagnostic purposes, and may be responsible for many of the manifestations of the disease. This profuse production of antibody causes hyperplasia of the reticuloendothelial system, particularly the lymph nodes and the spleen. The small lymphocytes in the germinal centers are replaced by macrophages and plasma cells. The patient eventually becomes immunosuppressed, and the lymph nodes become atrophic and fibrotic.

The high levels of IgM and antigen-antibody complexes are thought to cause many of the pathologic manifestations of trypanosomiasis. The markedly elevated erythrocyte sedimentation rate is caused by the high immunoglobulin levels. Antigen-antibody complexes are thought by some investigators to contribute directly to the pathology of trypanosomiasis by immune injury to the blood vessels and by stimulating the production of "kinins" and other mediators, which are elevated during salivarian trypanosomiasis (Boreham, 1968). Glomerulonephritis occurs during the course of the disease and has been taken as evidence of the importance of immune complex disease.

Immune complexes and mediators have also been blamed for the destruction of red blood cells and platelets that often occurs during the course of salivarian trypanosomiasis. There is also evidence, however, that parasite metabolites or even protein toxins may be responsible for destruction of these formed elements of the blood (Davis et al., 1974; Tizard et al., 1978). Immunosuppression precedes the late atrophy of the germinal centers and may also be caused by massive antigenic stimulation and immune complexes.

Cardiac dilatation and hypertrophy is usually caused by myocarditis but may also be associated with valvulitis, pancarditis, pericarditis, or lesions of the conduction system. Interstitial hemorrhage and interstitial and perivascular mononuclear infiltration are characteristic.

The most attention, however, has been devoted to the late-stage changes in the CNS, which include diffuse meningoencephalitis, swelling of the brain, and dura-arachnoid adhesions. The membranes are "felted" on to the surface of the brain and there is infiltration by lymphocytes. The infiltration of lymphoid cells into the brain via the Virchow-Robin space surrounding the blood vessels is particularly striking. This layer of perivascular cuffing around the vessels is sometimes 20 to 30 cells thick and separates them from the brain substance. Morula or Mott cells, lymphoid cells containing a large mulberry-like eosinophilic mass, are found in these "cuffs," in the brain substance, and in the lymph nodes. These are thought to be IgM-secretory plasma cells that have failed to externalize their secretion. They are very characteristic although not pathognomonic of sleeping sickness.

The immediate cause of the cerebral damage in sleeping sickness is still uncertain, but it seems likely that the neural damage is mediated by immunologic reactions that take place around the blood vessels and invade the brain substance.

CLINICAL MANIFESTATIONS. As in Chagas' disease, three stages can be recognized: the primary lesion, the early stage, and the late stage. The primary lesion, called the trypanosome chancre, develops at the site of the infected tsetse bite after a period of two to three weeks. It is an indurated, inflamed area about 10 cm in diameter that resolves in a week or two to an area of shiny desquamation. It seems to be more often recognized in the rapidly progressive Rhodesian disease than in the Gambian disease. Local multiplication of trypanosomes in the chancre is followed in the early stage by dissemination of the organisms, which multiply as trypomastigotes in the blood and interstitial fluids of most tissues. This early stage is characterized by fever, debilitation, anemia, and cardiac signs, including tachycardia and right bundle branch block. The fever tends to be intermittent, with weekly peaks that correspond to the waves of parasitemia. Each of these waves is different antigenically from those that precede or succeed it. By this phenomenon of antigenic variation, the trypanosome avoids the effects of humoral antibody.

During this early stage, the organism is multiplying not only in the blood but also in the tissue fluids, particularly the lymphatics. The distribution of lymphadenopathy varies but is particularly prominent in the nodes of the posterior cervical triangle. This finding, called Winterbottom's sign, was well known to the 18th-century slavers and used by them to exclude individuals with sleeping sickness from their shipments. Localized edema of the face and other tissues is common. Caucasians may develop a fugitive, erythematous circinate rash, mainly on the trunk and shoulders. Disseminated intravascular coagulation (Barrett-Connor et al., 1973) or thrombocytopenia (Robins-Browne et al., 1975) may occur during this stage.

There is no clear distinction or period of latency between this early stage and the late stage of the disease. Although there is often invasion of the CNS very early in the disease, the late stage can be defined clinically by the onset of symptoms of interference with mental function, headache, irritability, insomnia, and changes in mood. These progress to the more obvious signs of tremors of the hands, muscle fasciculations (particularly of the tongue), muscular rigidity, indistinct speech, difficulty in walking, and, finally, somnolence gradually deepening to coma and loss of sphincter control. Death is usually due to bronchopneumonia or other intercurrent infections.

The foregoing is a short summary of the main characteristics of a very variable and protean disease. Both types, Gambian and Rhodesian, are fundamentally similar and differ primarily in the speed of their progression. In Gambian disease the onset may be mild and unnoticed, so that the first signs are those of mental damage and somnolence. The typical duration of disease is about three years to death. In Rhodesian disease, the onset is almost invariably acute, but it may be followed by a relatively asymptomatic and afebrile period until the disease resumes its progress and leads to death six to nine months after onset. In general, the disease is more acute in Europeans than in Africans, but its manifestations are quite variable in both groups.

DIAGNOSIS

Protozoologic Diagnosis. The problems of establishing the diagnosis of *T. brucei* infections are similar to those of *T. cruzi* infections. The recognition of organisms in the early stage is simple because the concentrations in the blood are high. They are readily recognized in wet blood films or in thin or thick blood films or in aspirates of chancres or lymph nodes stained with Romanowsky stains. In the later stages of the disease, organisms are scanty, so concentrative or multiplicative methods must be used. For blood, double centrifugation, that is, a first centrifugation just sufficient to deposit the erythrocytes followed by a second centrifugation of the supernatant and examination of the pellet, is often successful. There are other more sensitive methods of concentration. Blood samples taken in microhematocrit tubes are centrifuged and examined microscopically, preferably directly in the tube. The trypanosomes are concentrated in the plasma immediately above the buffy layer. The anion exchange/centrifugation method is more sensitive and has been miniaturized and streamlined for field use (Lumsden et al., 1981). The blood is diluted with buffers of suitable osmolarity and pH and passed through anion-exchange columns. Blood cells are adsorbed to the anion exchanger; trypanosomes pass through unimpeded and can be found in the eluate on direct microscopic examination after centrifugation. Anion exchange/filtration may also be used. In this technique, the eluate from the column is passed through a millipore filter, which then is fixed, stained, and searched for trypanosomes under the microscope. But this is less immediate and more time-consuming than the anion-exchange/centrifugation method. Examination of the CSF is also important. Increases in the cell count above 5 cells/mm^3 and a protein content above 40 mg/100 ml, or the presence of trypanosomes indicate that the infection has entered the late stage and changes the choice of antitrypanosomal drugs.

As a multiplicative method, blood, lymph node aspirate, or CSF should be inoculated into laboratory rodents. This is effective for Rhodesian infections but less so for Gambian, which typically produces only very low parasitemias that may be difficult to recognize. Other more susceptible hosts for *T.b. gambiense* are inconvenient and expensive.

Serologic Diagnosis. The antigenic variability of *T. brucei* has impeded the development of serologic diagnostic tests, but CF, immunofluorescent, and ELISA tests for antibody to stable antigens are becoming available (Lumsden, 1972). The simple, nonspecific estimation of serum IgM by radial immunodiffusion is also useful. High concentrations in the serum of an individual exposed to an endemic area should stimulate an intensive search for trypanosomes and trypanosomal antibody.

GEOGRAPHIC VARIATIONS. The more slowly progressive Gambian disease is characteristic of the western and northern part of the distribution from Senegal on the African west coast through west and central Africa as far as the Sudan and Uganda. The rapidly progressive Rhodesian disease is characteristic of eastern Africa from Ethiopia and eastern Uganda south to Zambia and Rhodesia. These distinctions, however, are not hard and fast; for example, virulent infections have been reported from eastern Nigeria and mild infections from Malawi.

TREATMENT. In contrast to the situation in Chagas' disease, effective curative and prophylactic chemotherapy is available for African trypanosomiasis. Successful treatment depends, however, on early recognition of the disease and the use of drugs appropriate for the stage of infection. The important distinction is between the early stage of the disease, when CNS invasion is absent or minimal, and the late-stage disease, when CNS involvement is well established. Successful treatment of late disease depends on the use of drugs that cross the blood-brain barrier. Patients with CNS symptoms, abnormal cerebrospinal fluid, or trypanosomes in the spinal fluid should be treated as late disease. Because the nervous system is invaded early in Rhodesian trypanosomiasis, patients who have been infected longer than four weeks should be treated as if they had late disease.

Intravenous suramin sodium, 1 g on days 1, 3, 7, and 14, is the treatment of choice for early infections. A test dose of 100 mg should be given and the patient carefully monitored for a few hours before the remainder of the first dose is given because some patients experience shock and collapse after intravenous suramin. Common toxic reactions include rashes and renal damage. Suramin should be discontinued if proteinuria or marked changes in the urine sediment occur. Pentamidine is a good alternative for early disease in a daily dose of 3 mg base per kg intramuscularly for ten days. When CNS invasion is established or suspected, melarsoprol must be used, often after a preliminary course of suramin, which clears the parasitemia and improves the general condition of the patient so that he can withstand the toxic effects of melarsoprol (Melarsen-oxide/BAL; Mel B). Melarsoprol should be administered cautiously intravenously at 48-hour intervals. In one recommended schedule, 1.5, 2.0, and 2.2 mg/kg are given the first week; one week later 2.5, 3.0 and 3.6 mg/kg are administered, and after another week a final course of three injections of 3.6 mg/kg is given. Patients should be watched closely for signs of arsenic poisoning such as encephalopathy, exfoliative dermatitis, or enteritis.

CONTROL AND PREVENTION. Prevention of infection with Rhodesian trypanosomes is primarily a matter of personal protection against tsetse bites; no general attack against the tsetse is feasible because of the huge areas of country involved. Prevention of Gambian disease can be accomplished by measures against the vector including clearing of the forest and the use of insecticides because the infested forest areas are usually circumscribed. Prophylactic chemotherapy with pentamidine has also been widely employed against *T.b. gambiense*, but the success of this method is dependent on well-organized survey teams and regular surveillance of the infected areas. The usual prophylactic dose of pentamidine isethionate is 250 mg intramuscularly every six months. It is better, however, to permit the short-incubation, acute Rhodesian disease to declare itself and treat the patient early. The problem with chemoprophylactic campaigns is the possibility of suppression of the disease so that it is only recognized in the late stages, when radical cure is more difficult to accomplish.

References

Barrett-Connor, E., Ugoretz, R. J., and Braude, A. I.: Disseminated intravascular coagulation in trypanosomiasis. Arch Intern Med 131:574, 1973.

Boreham, P. F. L.: Immune reactions and kinin formation in chronic trypanosomiasis. Br J Pharmacol Chemother 32:493, 1968.

Davis, C. E., Robbins, R. S., Weller, R. D., and Braude, A. I.: Thrombocytopenia in experimental trypanosomiasis. J Clin Invest 53:1359, 1974.

Englund, P. T., Hadjuk, S. L., and Marini, J. C.: The molecular biology of trypanosomes. Ann Rev Biochem 51:695, 1982.

Ford, J.: The Role of the Trypanosomes in African Ecology. Oxford, Clarendon Press, 1971.

Hoare, C. A.: The Trypanosomes of Mammals. Oxford, Blackwell Scientific Publications, 1972.

Köberle, F.: Chagas' disease and Chagas' syndrome: The pathology of American trypanosomiasis. In Dawes, B. (ed.): Advances in Parasitology. Vol. 6. London, Academic Press, 1968.

Lugones, H., Rabinovich, B., Cerisola, J. A., Ledesma, O., and Barclay, C.: Preliminary results of the anti-*T. cruzi* activity of RO7-1051 in man. In Proceedings of the Third International Congress of Parasitology 3:1297, 1974.

Lumsden, W. H. R.: Trypanosomiasis. Br Med Bull 28:34, 1972.

Lumsden, W. H. R.: Demonstration of antibodies to protozoa. In Weir, D. M. (ed.): Handbook of Experimental Immunology. 2nd ed. Oxford, Blackwell Scientific Publications, 1973.

Lumsden, W. H. R., Kimber, C. D., Dukes, P., Haller, L., Stanghellini, A., and Duvallet, G.: Field diagnosis of sleeping sickness in the Ivory Coast. 1. Comparison of the miniature anion–exchange/centrifugation technique with other protozoological methods. Trans R Soc Trop Med Hyg 75:242, 1981.

Mulligan, H. W. (ed.): The African Trypanosomiases, London, George Allen and Unwin, 1970.

Pan American Health Organization: New Approaches in American Trypanosomiasis. Washington, D.C., Pan American Health Organization, 1975.

Robins-Browne, R. M., Schneider, J., and Metz, J.: Thrombocytopenia in trypanosomiasis. Am J Trop Med Hyg 24:226, 1975.

Tizard, I., Nielson, K. H., Seed, J. R., and Hall, J. E.: Biologically active products from African trypanosomes. Microbiol Rev 42:661, 1978.

World Health Organization: Immunology of Chagas' disease. Bull WHO 50:459, 1974.

211 BANCROFTIAN AND MALAYAN FILARIASIS

ABRAHAM I. BRAUDE, M.D., PH.D.

Bancroftian and Malayan filariasis are infections that are transmitted by mosquitoes and located in the lymphatics. Adult worms can cause lymphatic inflammation or obstruction and release microfilariae that enter the peripheral blood at night. Bancroftian filariasis occurs throughout the tropics and subtropics, including Central Africa, North Africa along the Mediterranean, Southeast Asia, the Philippines, Indonesia, China, Korea, Japan, Polynesia, the West Indies, Venezuela, Brazil, and Colombia. Malayan filariasis is much less extensive, but foci are found in India and Southeast Asia, including Burma, Malaysia, Vietnam, Borneo, and Indonesia. Manson proved that mosquitoes suck the filarial larvae from the blood of patients and thus demonstrated for the first time that arthropods can be a vector of a parasitic infection. Manson, however, had the mistaken notion that *Filariae* are released into water from dying mosquitoes, and transmitted to humans who drink the infected water. Bancroft demolished this thesis and proposed, correctly, that "young filariae may gain entrance to the human host whilst mosquitos bearing them are in the act of biting" (Chernin, 1983).

ETIOLOGY. Bancroftian filariasis is caused by *Wuchereria bancrofti*. The adults are white, thread-like worms with tapering ends. The males can measure 1.5 inches and the females twice as long. The two exist intertwined in human lymphatic vessels and lymph nodes, in which they mate, and the female gives birth to minute eel-like embryos, the microfilariae. These remain coiled within the egg shell when first developed but later elongate and retain the shell as a thin delicate sheath. The microfilaria is a diminutive worm with graceful sweeping curves and a pointed tail. In blood smears, the sheathed larva measures 245 to 295 microns. It has rudimentary organs, no alimentary canal, and numerous nuclei except in the rear end of the tail. This absence of terminal nuclei is used to differentiate it from *Brugia malayi*, whose tail is swollen at the tip with two nuclei. The larvae of bancroftian filariasis were proved to be the cause of this disease by the Brazilian physician, Wucherer, who found them in the urine of patients with chyluria and whose name has become identified with the parasite. Further development of *W. bancrofti* takes place in the mosquito after the larvae are ingested with a blood meal obtained by biting an infected person at night during the periodic entry of microfilariae into the circulation. The larva loses its sheath in the stomach of the mosquito, leaves the alimentary canal, and migrates to the breast muscles, in which it changes its shape and structure within ten days to become infective for man. In maturing to the infectious third stage, the microfilaria grows to 1.5 to 2.0 mm and becomes filiform. Then, it goes to the head of the mosquito and down into the proboscis. When the mosquito bites a warm, moist skin, the larvae creep out and penetrate through the mosquito bite. The infectious larvae then migrate to lymph nodes and lymph vessels, in which they mature, sexually mate, and produce embryos in about one year after the bite.

The adult worms do not multiply in people, nor do the larvae multiply in mosquitoes, so that the extent and severity of human infection depend on the total number of bites each person receives from an infected vector. In addition, the filariae are not highly infective for human beings because many larvae fail to penetrate the skin after a mosquito bite or cannot reach the lymphatics if they do penetrate. Others are injured by the immune response in the lymphatics, so that microfilariae never enter the blood for further transmission. This situation was common in American troops in the South Pacific in World War II, when soldiers frequently had inguinal lymphadenitis and lymphangitis of the spermatic cord but rarely had microfilariae in the blood. Because of these obstacles to infection, an enormous number of bites is required to maintain the disease in a community; perhaps as many as 15,000 infective bites per person are needed to ensure transmission (Hairston and DeMerllon, 1968).

The filaria belonging to the genus *B. malayi* are smaller than *W. bancrofti*. Male adult forms of *B. malayi* measure only 0.5 to 1.0 and the females 1.5 to 2.2 inches in length. The sheathed larvae are also smaller than those of *W. bancrofti*; the microfilariae of *B. malayi* have a length of only 175 to 230 microns. The life cycles of the two species of filaria are the same, but the mosquito vectors are somewhat different. The important vectors of bancroftian filariasis are *Culex*, *Anopheles* and *Aedes* mosquitoes, whereas Malayan filariasis is transmitted primarily by members of the genera *Mansonia* and *Anopheles*. Both forms of filariasis exhibit nocturnal periodicity, a condition in which the number of microfilariae in the peripheral blood increases at night and decreases during the day. As a result, both forms of disease are transmitted by mosquitoes that bite at night when there are more than 15 microfilariae per drop of blood, the minimum number that can infect mosquitoes. An exception to this periodicity in bancroftian filariasis is seen under two circumstances: (1) If the infected person changes his sleeping habits and stays awake at night, the microfilariae increase in the peripheral blood during the day. This change in periodicity occurs about a week after daytime sleeping begins. (2) In the Polynesian islands (Samoa, Fiji, Tonga, and Cook islands) the microfilariae are found in the blood at all times but increase after noon and decrease after sunset. This is known as the subperiodic form of filariasis, and the filaria involved is regarded by some (Manson-Bahr and Muggleton, 1952) as a separate variety or species, to be designated *Wuchereria pacifica*. Most authorities feel this distinction is not justified because, under close scrutiny, the two forms appear to be identical, except that the adult worms in most periodic cases are slightly longer.

PATHOGENESIS AND PATHOLOGY. The adult worms cause lymphatic inflammation and obstruction in the scrotum, spermatic cords, epididymis, testis, arms, legs, abdomen, and retroperitoneal area. Lymphangitis and lymphadenitis are thought to be allergic reactions to worm secretions or antigens liberated from dead filariae periodically so that the attacks of chills and fever are recurrent. Obstruction probably results from the lymphangitis and secondary fibrosis rather than from simple mechanical blockade by the worm. Lymph varices are among the early signs of lymphatic obstruction, and if they rupture, lymph (chyle) is released into the peritoneum, kidney, bladder, scrotum, or bowel. Chyluria and chylous ascites are manifestations of this phenomenon. Obstruction of the smaller subcutaneous lymphatic vessels produces lymphedema of the scrotum, vulva, legs, arms, and breast. As lymphedema gives way to subcutaneous fibrosis and hyperkeratosis, the skin takes on the character of elephant hide and becomes thick, hard, and dry from loss of sweat glands.

In contrast to the adult worms, microfilariae contribute little to the pathology of the disease. In fact, there is a negative correlation between lymphatic obstruction and positive blood smears for microfilariae. There may be 20,000 microfilariae per milliliter of blood from people with no symptoms, and negative blood smears in patients with elephantiasis. This is probably because the adults have died before lymphatic injury becomes severe enough to produce clinical disturbances. A positive correlation exists, however, between clinical severity and the development of rapid infection with many worms. Thus, foreigners residing in endemic areas seldom show symptoms for 10 to 15 years, whereas American troops in the South Pacific developed lymphangitis, lymphadenitis, and swelling of the genitalia or arms in about nine months (Huntington et al., 1944). The difference can probably be explained by the speed and intensity of infection. Europeans and Americans living in the tropics under peacetime conditions can protect themselves well enough from night-biting mosquitoes to avoid heavy infections. The troops in the South Pacific, on the other hand, were heavily exposed to the day-biting mosquitoes *(Aëdes scutellaris polynesiensis)* near native villages, and received bites from more infected mosquitoes in a few weeks than foreigners residing in other endemic regions would get in years. Individual variation in sensitization to worm antigens probably explains why, among persons with equal exposure to infection, some develop lymphangitis and lymphedema, and some do not. A definite association exists between certain immune phenomena and clinical manifestations of filariasis. For example, the titer of IgG antibodies against surface antigens of microfilariae, the prevalence of immune complexes, and the degree of in vitro lymphocyte reactivity is higher in patients with hydrocoeles or elephantiasis than in those with acute filarial adenitis and lymphangitis. Similarly, there is evidence the tropical eosinophilia is a form of occult filariasis that results from excessive hypersensitivity to the microfilaria, which ordinarily cause lymphatic disease alone (Piessens, 1981; Ottesen et al., 1979). Biopsies showing acute lymphangitis with no adult worms in sight are consistent with the idea that inflammatory lesions are the result of allergy to worm antigens carried along the lymph channels rather than a nonspecific reaction to the intact worm.

The tissue reaction in lymph nodes and lymph vessels is an infiltration of histiocytes, lymphocytes, and eosinophils, along with hyperplasia of the lymphatic endothelium. The lymphatic wall becomes thickened and edematous so that its lumen narrows and dilatation occurs beyond it. Within the dilatations of the lymph vessels and nodes lie the tightly coiled adult worms. Later, small granulomas appear in the lymph nodes. When the active inflammation is replaced by fibrosis, sclerotic lymph channels become permanently obstructed. The granulomatous tissues are eventually absorbed, and the scar sometimes calcifies around dead worms. The obstructed lymph channels develop varices; in some areas, they become obliterated, fibrous strands.

The location of elephantiasis depends on which lymph nodes are obstructed. Obstruction of the para-aortic nodes blocks drainage of lymph from the tunica vaginalis, epididymis, and spermatic cord so that hydrocele develops (Jordan, 1955) without edema of the scrotal skin, which drains into the superficial inguinal glands. In patients with elephantiasis of the leg, the obstruction is in the inguinal or iliac group of nodes.

CLINICAL MANIFESTATIONS. After an incubation period of about one year, the acute stage begins with frequent attacks of fever to 104° F, lymphangitis, and lymphadenitis. The lymphangitis usually occurs on the legs, hands, and scrotum, where it produces tenderness and red streaks or cord-like swellings that extend peripherally from the infected swollen lymph nodes in the groin, axilla, or epitrochlear region. In the early attacks, the pain and swelling of the scrotum, spermatic cord, testis, or limb may be only mild and transient, but later the lymphedema becomes more marked and persistent. Abdominal lymphangitis may produce a clinical picture suggesting an acute abdomen if there is pain, or unexplained fever if painless. The fever and chills last for several days and then stop suddenly with profuse sweating. The clinical picture during acute attacks varies with the population and their location. In American troops exposed to the nonperiodic strain of *W. bancrofti* in the South Pacific islands, for example, the attacks of lymphangitis were often accompanied by headache, backache, fatigue, nausea, and mental depression, but fever was unusual. Lymphangitis of the spermatic cord and orchitis were the most common clinical signs in these soldiers.

After a couple of years of recurring attacks, permanent edema sets in and most often causes swelling of the legs, scrotum, and penis. Lymphatic obstruction causes subcutaneous lymph varices. These soft, lobular, elastic structures develop in the groin or axilla. Numerous varices also develop within the scrotum and on its surface, a condition known as "lymph scrotum." It has a characteristic velvety feel and produces a steady ooze from the skin after surface blebs rupture. If the thoracic duct is obstructed, the urinary lymphatics may rupture into the bladder and produce chyluria. The chyluria tends to be transient, lasting usually for only a few days at a time but sometimes for months. The incidence of chyluria varies considerably from one geographic zone to another. Rupture of lymphatics in the peritoneal or pleural spaces can produce chylous ascites or chylothorax.

Hydrocele is probably the most common sign of long-standing bancroftian filariasis. The significance of this finding as a sign of filariasis tends to be ignored in areas of low endemicity and exaggerated in highly endemic areas. It may affect as many as 40 per cent of the male population (Nelson, 1979).

Filariasis caused by *Brugia malayi* usually produces a more acute clinical picture than bancroftian filariasis. Elephantiasis of the limbs is common, but the genitalia and bladder are usually spared.

COMPLICATIONS AND SEQUELAE. Although patients with filariasis have a morbid fear of developing elephantiasis, especially of the genitalia, this complication occurs in only a small percentage of cases. Elephantiasis most often affects the legs but can occur in any part of the body, including the arms, breast, scrotum, and vulva (Fig. 1). The mistaken belief that elephantiasis is an inevitable consequence of bancroftian filariasis has caused much unnecessary mental anguish and neurotic problems, which can thus be serious sequelae of the disease.

Elephantiasis is further complicated by attacks of inflammation in the swollen part. These may be due to filariasis itself or to secondary bacterial infection.

Elephantiasis appears to be a function of high rates of microfilarial infection. In areas with microfilarial rates over 10 per cent, elephantiasis is one of the most common complications. In areas with lower rates, hydrocele and chyluria predominate (Edeson, 1972).

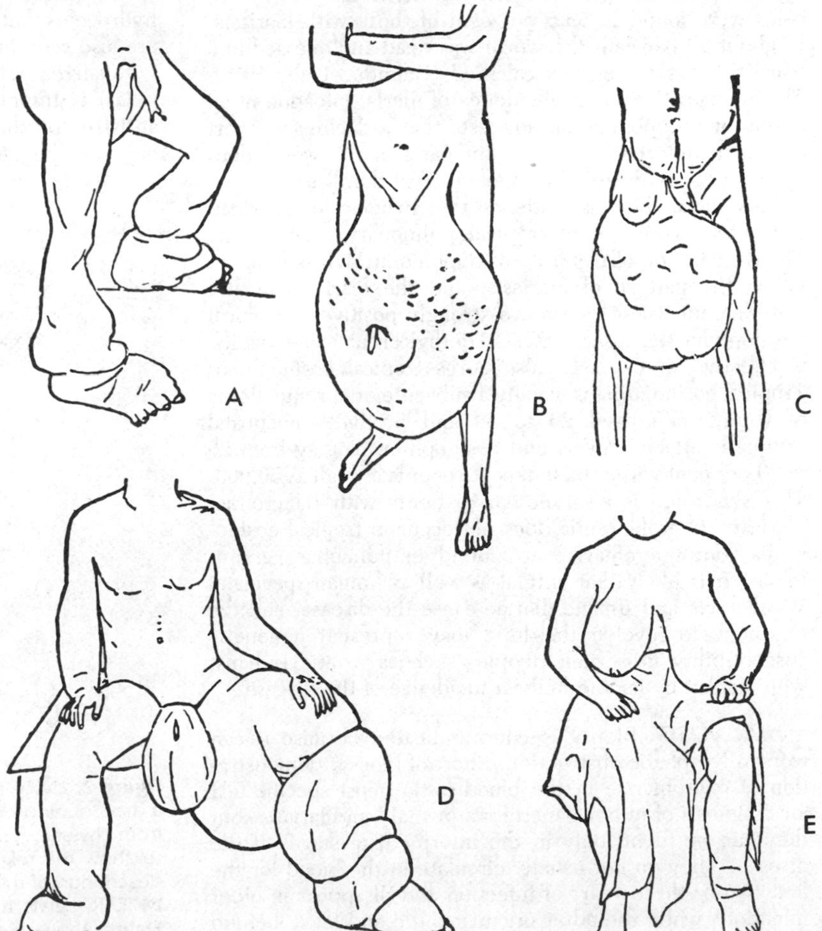

Figure 1. Extreme cases of elephantiasis sketched by A. C. Chandler from photographs. *A*, Legs and feet. *B*, Scrotum. *C*, Varicele of inguinal lymph node. *D*, Scrotum and legs. *E*, Breasts. (Chandler, A. C.: Introduction to Parasitology. New York, John Wiley and Sons, 1955.)

GEOGRAPHIC VARIATIONS IN DISEASE. Chyluria has been the most important and frequent clinical manifestation of bancroftian filariasis in the temperate zone countries such as Japan. In 111 cases of filariasis reported in 1961 from Ehime, Japan, 103 (92.8 per cent) had chyluria, but only four had hydrocele, and another four had elephantiasis. Among 3407 cases of filariasis in Sri Lanka, on the other hand, only two had chyluria and 2983 (87.5 per cent) had elephantiasis (Sasa, 1976).

Another interesting symptom reported from Sri Lanka is chest pain. Among students at the University of Ceylon, this was the second most common symptom (after headache) in early bancroftian filariasis. The pain was usually precordial, retrosternal, or infraclavicular and worse at night. It was also recurrent and severe enough to suggest a myocardial infarction (Wijetunge, 1967).

The periodicity of *W. bancrofti* infection also follows geographic patterns. The periodic form, in which the microfilariae enter the blood at night, occurs in the tropics throughout the world, whereas the nonperiodic diurnal form occurs in Polynesia. *B. malayi*, which is limited to Asia, produces a somewhat different clinical picture than *W. bancrofti*. Infections by *B. malayi* tend to have a shorter incubation period, to involve the upper limbs more frequently, and to be free of genital or urinary disease.

In Puerto Rico, serial observations over 40 years show a tendency toward a declining incidence of microfilaremia and the emergence of a persistent subclinical form of bancroftian filariasis. In a study of intrascrotal organs in 330 autopsies, 23.9 per cent had filarial worms, and hydroceles were found in 59.5 per cent of those with filariasis. In about 90 per cent the worm was dead and encased in a scar that was sometimes calcified (Galindo et al., 1962). This unexpectedly high incidence of filarial infection in an asymptomatic population suggests that a decline in overt clinical manifestations in certain parts of the world does not necessarily mean a disappearance of the disease.

In Malaya, there is evidence that Brugian filariasis can cause the syndrome of tropical pulmonary eosinophilia. The distribution of tropical eosinophilia in Malaya tends to follow the pattern of filariasis, and the filarial skin and complement fixation tests are strongly positive in tropical eosinophilia (Janssens, 1974). Diethylcarbamazine, which is effective in filariasis, also cures tropical eosinophilia. Tropical eosinophilia is usually a subacute or chronic illness of young men aged 20 to 30 and produces nocturnal asthmatic attacks, fever, and eosinophilia ranging from 20 to 90 per cent with total leukocyte counts as high as 50,000. This syndrome is also seen in patients with Bancroftian filariasis. Microfilaremia does not occur in tropical eosinophilia, but microfilariae are found in pulmonary granulomas. It is likely that animal as well as human species of *Wuchereria* and *Brugia* filariae cause the disease, and the tendency to involve the lung may represent a genetic susceptibility in certain people, such as Asiatic Indians, who display by far the highest incidence of the disease.

DIAGNOSIS. Biopsy is contraindicated because it can worsen lymphatic obstruction. Short of biopsy, demonstration of microfilariae in the blood is the most specific test for diagnosis of either bancroftian or malayan filariasis, but they can be found only in the intermediate stages of the disease. They do not usually circulate in the blood for the first two or three years of infection and disappear in older infections when the adult organisms die and leave behind lymphatic pathology, the "tombstones of their obstructive existence." If parasitemia is heavy, the microfilariae can be demonstrated easily in Giemsa-stained smears of blood taken between 10 P.M. and 2 A.M. In a wet preparation of the blood under a coverslip, the microfilaria is seen in constant motion, coiling and uncoiling itself increasingly and lashing the blood corpuscles in all directions (Lewis, 1872) (Fig. 2). If parasitemia is light, the blood should be passed through a membrane filter with a 5 μm pore, so that the microfilariae (but not the blood cells) are collected on the membrane, where they can be stained. In the Pacific areas where the nonperiodic strains prevail, blood should be examined in the early afternoon. The nocturnal forms of microfilariae can be driven from lung capillaries into the circulation in the daytime by giving 100 mg of diethylcarbamazine orally and making smears one hour later. This technique is risky, however, for patients who may have onchocerciasis and loa loa infections because it may cause severe allergic reaction when the worms are killed (Nelson, 1979; WHO report, 1974).

In the early stages before blood smears are positive, the clinical signs are usually typical enough to make the diagnosis. In an endemic area, recurrent attacks of "elephantoid" fever with lymphadenitis and lymphangitis of a limb, scrotum, or spermatic cord are almost diagnostic. The attack starts with a chill; the fever comes down in three to five days; the lymphatics are swollen and tender; and the overlying skin is inflamed. The diagnosis is more difficult if there is only recurrent fever without lymphangitis. When abscesses form in the lymph node or lymphatic vessels, the diagnosis can be made by finding remnants of dead filarial worms in the pus. Microfilariae can be found in fluid from hydroceles that result from rupture of a lymph vessel. They are also seen in chylous urine.

Recurrent streptococcal lymphangitis (relapsing erysipelas) is important in differential diagnosis. The titer of antistreptolysin O is characteristically elevated, and a trial of penicillin abruptly terminates the fever and prevents

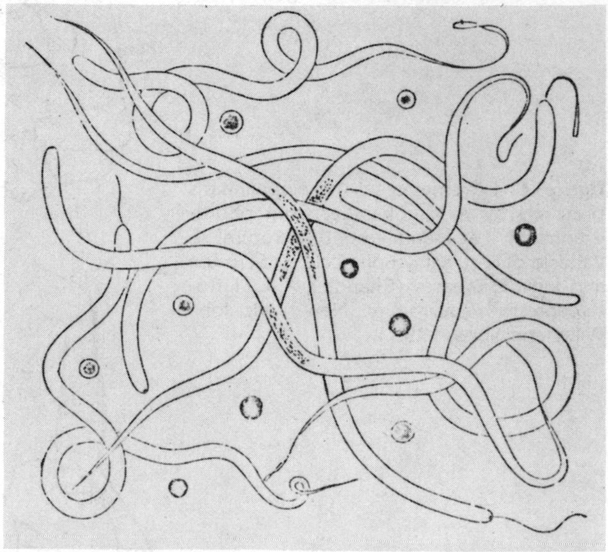

Figure 2. Living microfilariae observed by T. R. Lewis (1872) in a drop of blood from the finger of a European woman suffering from chyluria. A few red blood corpuscles have been introduced to show the relative size of the microfilariae. This was the first description of microfilariae in the blood. (From a woodcut made by T. R. Lewis to show a composite picture of several fields. Eighth Annual Report of the Public Health Commissioner with the Government of India. Calcutta Office of Superintendent of Gov. Prints, 1872, p. 243.)

future attacks of streptococcal lymphangitis. Unfortunately, streptococci are difficult to isolate from the bullae that are characteristic of this condition, and cultures of biopsies of the deep lymphatics may be needed to find the organism. In sporotrichosis, there is thickening of the lymphatics, but there is no fever and no local erythema or pain. Although the fungus cannot be seen in smears of the pus, the diagnosis is easily made by culture of *Sporothrix schenckii.*

Hereditary lymphedema (Milroy's disease) can be difficult to distinguish from filariasis. The familial history and the involvement of both legs are helpful since elephantiasis tends to be unilateral. Lymphangiography is useful in the early stages of filarial elephantiasis when the lymphatic vessels are dilated and tortuous because the lymphatics are hypoplastic in Milroy's disease. In advanced elephantiasis, the lymphatics atrophy, and lymphangiography loses its differential value.

The occurrence of nonfilarial elephantiasis must be kept in mind in the highlands of East Africa where there is no filariasis because the altitude is too great for mosquitoes to live. People cultivating the red clays of Africa develop nonfilarial elephantiasis of the legs secondary to the absorption of aluminosilicate and silicon from the soil through the skin of the feet. Irritation of the different lymphatics by particles of these substances causes fibrosis and obstructive lymphopathy (Price and Henderson, 1979).

Many patients with filariasis have eosinophilia, but this sign is too nonspecific to be of much help in diagnosis. There are no serologic tests of value because it has not been possible to obtain enough antigen of *W. bancrofti.* The reason for this problem is that there is no susceptible laboratory animal in which to propagate the worm.

TREATMENT. Both bancroftian and Malayan filariasis can be cured with diethylcarbamazine (Hetrazan), which kills both adult worms and microfilariae. Treatment is usually started with a small oral dose of 0.25 mg/kg and then gradually increased to 6 mg/kg per day. A total dose of 72 mg/kg is then given in divided doses at daily or weekly intervals as best tolerated (WHO Report, 1974). Schedules vary from 6 mg/kg once daily to 3 mg/kg three times daily. The schedule is less important than the total dose in achieving a high cure rate. Febrile reactions occur after the first dose and are especially severe in infections by *B. malayi,* which is much more susceptible to diethylcarbamazine. In addition to fever, patients complain of headache, nausea, and painful swellings of the lymph nodes and lymph vessels early in the course of treatment. In some patients, filarial abscess may occur along the lymphatics during treatment as a result of an allergic reaction to the dead worm. If care is taken to start treatment with small doses and to increase them slowly, severe symptoms can be avoided. These allergic reactions result from the release of antigens upon disintegration of killed microfilariae or adult worms. The reactions respond to Phenergan in doses of 10 mg. Phenergan is also useful with aspirin in controlling attacks of filarial lymphangitis in patients who are not under treatment with diethylcarbamazine. After diethylcarbamazine therapy, the microfilariae disappear from the blood in a period ranging from several days to a few weeks, but relapses can occur. For this reason, blood smears should be reexamined, and another course of treatment should be given if microfilariae are still present.

Although radical cure of infection with chemotherapy can eliminate the febrile attacks, the acute lymphangitis, and early lymphedema, it does little to improve the stigmata of chronic filariasis such as elephantiasis, chronic hydrocele, chyluria, or draining sinuses. Instead, it is necessary to resort to nonspecific treatment for these problems. Hydroceles and scrotal elephantiasis can be corrected by surgery, but precautions must be taken to protect the spermatic cord and testes during the operation. Excisional treatment of elephantiasis of the limbs, on the other hand, is often unsatisfactory, and this condition should be treated conservatively with pressure bandages and elevation of the swollen part during bed rest. The swelling in elephantiasis of the leg, for example, diminishes considerably in a week if the foot of the bed is raised as much as possible. If an elastic stocking is applied before the patient leaves the bed, recurrent swelling and discomfort is minimized. The patient can then be mobilized and even undertake useful work. Prednisone, in doses of 40 mg per day, helps to soften the tissues and reduce the swelling if it is given for a few weeks before the elastic bandage is applied.

Chyluria should be treated with diethylcarbamazine to eliminate the obstructing worms. In chyluric patients, such treatment does not produce the side effects otherwise found during treatment of filariasis. It is difficult to evaluate chemotherapy, however, because chyluria undergoes frequent remissions and exacerbations. Since eating fat provokes chyluria, fatty foods are restricted. Some success has been achieved by repeated injection of 25 per cent sodium iodide or 3 per cent silver nitrate into the renal pelvis through retrograde catheters. A cure rate of 51.5 per cent has been reported in Japan with this treatment (Sasa, 1976). In very severe cases, chyluria has been radically cured by surgical removal of collateral lymph vessels that empty into the renal pelvis.

PROPHYLAXIS. Mass chemotherapy has been used against the parasite, and insecticides against the mosquitoes, but each approach has met with difficulties. When diethylcarbamazine is used for treatment of whole populations in endemic areas, it meets resistance because of the febrile reactions in carriers of filariasis. Yet it is worth pursuing despite the missed doses from febrile reactions and the problems in getting the drug to many people because microfilariasis rates can be reduced greatly by mass treatment and then retreatment of positive carriers (Edeson, 1972). The microfilariasis rates were reduced in this way from 26.0 per cent to 0.7 per cent in Malaysia, and an 82 per cent cure rate was obtained in the Ryuka islands by giving one course of treatment to known microfilaria carriers.

Prevention of filariasis through mosquito control has met two serious obstacles. One of these is the resistance acquired by *Culex fatigans* to insecticides. This mosquito is the chief vector of bancroftian filariasis in many parts of the world and is almost impossible to control because population growth has overwhelmed the attempts in large cities to provide sanitation and disposal of waste waters. The problem with Malayan filariasis is even worse because the subperiodic (diurnal) type in Malaya and Indonesia has a reservoir in monkeys and is transmitted in the forests by mosquitoes that bite rubber plantation workers in the daytime (Nelson, 1979).

References

Chandler, A. C.: Introduction to Parasitology. New York, John Wiley and Sons, 1955, p. 469.

Chernin, E.: Sir Patrick Manson's studies on the transmission and biology of filariasis. Rev Infect Dis 5:148, 1983.

Edeson, J.: Filariasis. Br Med Bull 28:60, 1972.
Galindo, L., von Lichtenberg, F., and Boldizon, C.: Bancroftian filariasis in Puerto Rico: Infection pattern and tissue lesions. Am J Trop Med Hyg 11:739, 1962.
Hairston, N., and DeMerllon, B.: On the inefficiency of transmission of *Wuchereria bancrofti* from mosquito to human host. Bull WHO 38:935, 1968.
Huntington, R., Fogel, R., Eichold, A., and Dickson, J.: Filariasis among American troops in a South Pacific Island. Yale J Biol Med 16:529, 1944.
Janssens, P.: Filariasis. In Woodruff, A. W. (ed): Medicine in the Tropics. Edinburgh, Churchill Livingstone, 1974, p. 244.
Jordan, R.: Notes on elephantiasis and hydrocoele due to *Wuchereria bancrofti*. J Trop Med Hyg 58:113, 1955.
Lewis, T. R.: On a *Haematozoan* inhabiting human blood, its relation to chyluria and other diseases. Eighth annual report of the Public Health Commissioner with the Government of India. Calcutta Office of Superintendent of Government Prints, 1872, p. 243.
Manson-Bahr, P., and Muggleton, W.: Further research on filariasis in Fiji. Trans R Soc Trop Med Hyg 46:301, 1952.
Nelson, G.: Current concepts in parasitology: Filariasis. N Engl J Med 300:1136, 1979.
Ottesen, E., Neva, F., Paranjape, R., Tripathy, S., Thiruvengadam, K., and Beaven, M.: Specific allergic sensitization to filarial antigens in tropical eosinophilia syndrome. Lancet 1:1158, 1979.
Piessens, W.: Lymphatic filariasis in humans: an immunologic maze. Ann Int Med 95:778, 1981.
Price, E., and Henderson, W.: Silica and silicates in femoral lymph nodes of bare-footed people in Ethiopia with special reference to elephantiasis of the lower limbs. Trans R Soc Trop Med Hyg 73:640, 1979.
Sasa, M.: Human filariasis. Baltimore, University Park Press, 1976.
Wijetunge, H.: Clinical manifestations of early Bancroftian filariasis. A study of 212 cases of microfilariaemia. J Trop Med Hyg 70:90, 1967.
World Health Organization Expert Committee on Filariasis: Third report. WHO Tech Rep Ser 542:1, 1974.

212
FUNGEMIA

JOHN E. EDWARDS, JR., M.D.

Fungemia denotes fungi in the circulating venous or arterial blood.

ETIOLOGY. *Candida* is by far the most frequent fungus isolated from the blood. Candidemia has become a major problem in centers in which critically ill patients are managed. The emergence of this problem over the past three decades is a result of new therapeutic modalities; candidemia and candidiasis are, for the most part, iatrogenic conditions.

Although *Candida albicans* is the most frequent species of *Candida* found in blood and was once thought to be the only pathogenic species of the genus *Candida*, it is now clear that several *Candida* species can cause disseminated candidiasis. These species include *C. tropicalis*, *C. pseudotropicalis*, *C. guilliermondii*, *C. stellatoidea*, *C. krusei*, *C. glabrata*, and *C. parapsilosis*. A blood isolate of any of these species has the same significance as isolation of *C. albicans*. In recent years, *C. tropicalis* isolates have been increasing in frequency compared to the other *Candida* species, particularly from immunocompromised patients.

Cryptococcus, *Histoplasma*, *Rhodotorula*, *Geotrichum*, and *Trichosporon* and *Cladosporium* are only rarely recovered from blood (Sheehy et al., 1976; Winston et al., 1977). In unusual instances of fungal endocarditis, *Aspergillus*, *Paecilomyces*, *Hormodendrum*, and *Curvularia* also have been recovered from blood (Hartford, 1974). Despite the fact that aspergillosis is the second most common cause of disseminated mycosis in the compromised patient, and widespread hematogenous seeding undoubtedly occurs, aspergilli are almost never cultured from blood. Since aspergilli are common laboratory contaminants, it is difficult to know whether a positive blood culture actually represents an *Aspergillus* fungemia. In one series, 20 per cent of patients with cryptococcal meningitis had positive blood cultures (Butler et al., 1964). *Rhodotorula* organisms have been recovered from blood occasionally, but in four cases of *Rhodotorula* fungemia, no disseminated fungal disease was present (Louria et al., 1967). One case of *Rhodotorula* septicemia has been associated with the picture of endotoxic shock. Patients with histoplasmosis may have positive blood cultures and the organism may be seen in peripheral smears.

PATHOLOGY AND PATHOGENESIS. *Candida* fungemia occurs more frequently in the following clinical settings: (1) intravenous hyperalimentation, (2) intravenous polyethylene catheters, (3) immunosuppressive drug therapy, (4) postoperative complications, (5) cancer, and (6) multiple antibiotic therapy. Burn patients, heroin addicts, and patients receiving prosthetic cardiac valves are at special risk for developing candidemia and/or endocarditis.

Disseminated candidiasis and candidemia probably originate from the gastrointestinal tract. Two important observations substantiate that hypothesis. (1) An investigator drank a suspension of *C. albicans* and became candidemic and candiduric afterward. This heroic experiment is almost irrefutable evidence that the gastrointestinal route can be a source for dissemination (Krause et al., 1969). (2) H. H. Stone (Stone et al., 1974) injected suspensions of *Candida* into various levels of canine and primate gastrointestinal tracts and found that the yeasts crossed the gastrointestinal tract and entered the bloodstream. To determine whether the yeasts gained entrance into the blood from colonized wounds, he injected *Candida* into canine muscles, fat, and granulating pouches and found no candidemia. In patients who have been treated with multiple antibiotics, *Candida* probably overgrow the gastrointestinal tract because the resident bacteria are suppressed. This risk is compounded after abdominal surgery because the gastrointestinal trauma may facilitate entry of organisms through injured mucosa or open vessels. The pathogenesis of candidemia after hyperalimentation is not fully understood. Since high glucose concentrations promote the growth of yeasts, it is theoretically possible for hyperglycemia to foster growth of organisms that enter the bloodstream from the gastrointestinal tract or skin. Another possibility is that the foreign body (hyperalimentation catheter) may provide a site for the localization and multiplication of circulating yeasts that come from the gastrointestinal tract. Catheters acquire vegetations that are sites of prolific growth after localization on the catheter.

CLINICAL MANIFESTATIONS. If contamination is excluded, growth of fungi in blood cultures can represent fungemia with or without underlying disseminated mycosis of various organs. Clinical recognition of the complications that result from the fungemia are of utmost importance, not only for diagnosing the fungemia but also for determining its significance. Unfortunately, with the exception of blood cultures, there are practically no laboratory tools to assist in detection of fungemia.

There are several peripheral manifestations that suggest candidemia. Candidal endophthalmitis is one of the more easily recognizable. The lesions begin in the chorioretina, extend into the vitreous, and are covered by an overlying vitreous haze (Fig. 1). The chorioretinal-vitreal reaction has the appearance of a cottonball, off-white in color. Both experimental and clinical evidence suggest that when candidal eye lesions are present, there is a high likelihood that other organs are involved as well (Edwards et al., 1974). Although the evidence is incomplete, it appears that many patients with candidemia have ocular lesions. Therefore, patients must have thorough serial ocular examinations, preferably with an indirect ophthalmoscope. By far the most common species cultured from *Candida* endophthalmitis has been *C. albicans*. Experimental evidence suggests that other species may have less predilection for the eye. Because of the frequency, importance, and significance of these lesions, any patient who is predisposed to candidemia should have a thorough baseline ocular examination and regular evaluations for hematogenous *Candida* endophthalmitis.

Macronodular skin lesions are another peripheral sign of candidemia and disseminated candidiasis (Bodey and Luna, 1974). The lesions are 0.5 to 1.0 cm in diameter and pink to red in color. Either single or multiple lesions may occur (see Chapter 225). Occasionally they have a hemorrhagic base. *Candida* organisms have been found more often in biopsy sections than by culture of the lesion. Finding the lesion and demonstrating the causative organism may not increase the frequency of diagnosis of disseminated candidiasis but may reduce the time required, because blood cultures may become positive only after several days (often after the patient has died).

Hematogenous *Candida* osteomyelitis and arthritis may also be clues to candidemia and underlying disseminated candidiasis. Candida osteomyelitis may affect the spine (intervertebral disks and adjacent vertebrae), wrist, femur, neck, costochondral junction, scapula, and proximal humerus. Diagnosis is made by biopsy (usually percutaneous); blood cultures are generally negative. *Candida* arthritis usually follows direct hematogenous infection but can also develop after extension from an adjacent area of hematogenous osteomyelitis or from direct inoculation into the joint.

In addition to these "peripheral manifestations," visceral infection should be sought in the patient who is predisposed to candidemia and disseminated candidiasis. Frank myocarditis, which occurs in about half of the patients with disseminated candidiasis, may cause chest pains, congestive heart failure, or cardiac arrhythmias. Diffuse candidal brain involvement may first produce obtundation, and later focal neurologic findings or frank meningitis. Hematogenous pyelonephritis occurs, renal function may fail rapidly, and *Candida* may be found in the urine. The shock syndrome that has been described might be related to the endotoxin-like substance in its cell wall.

The clinical manifestations of *C. glabrata* septicemia are less well defined than those of *Candida* septicemia, primarily because the experience has been much smaller. A review of 10 cases (Pankey and Dalaviso, 1973) indicated that rapid elevation of temperatures was characteristic. In this series, hypotension was not seen; in other series, an endotoxic shock-like picture has been described (Valdivieso

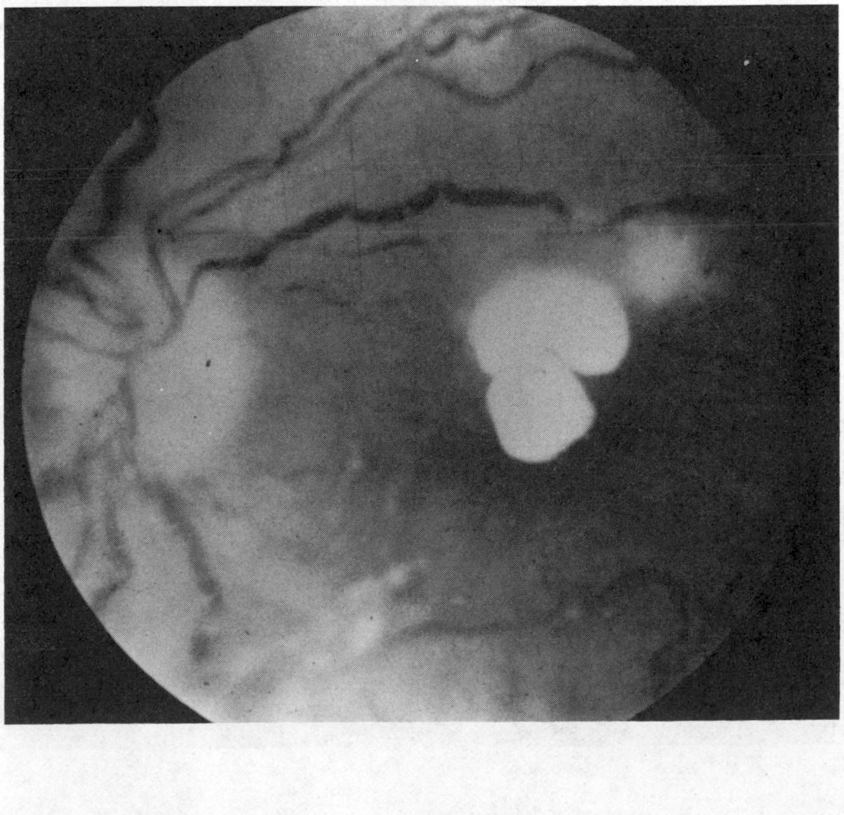

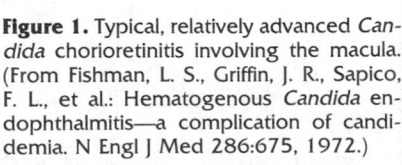

Figure 1. Typical, relatively advanced *Candida* chorioretinitis involving the macula. (From Fishman, L. S., Griffin, J. R., Sapico, F. L., et al.: Hematogenous *Candida* endophthalmitis—a complication of candidemia. N Engl J Med 286:675, 1972.)

et al., 1976). Since this organism is distributed to multiple organs during hematogenous infection one would expect the focal manifestations observed in candidemia, but there are only a few reports of such findings. Several comprehensive reviews of *C. glabrata* septicemia fail to mention involvement of the eye, skin, bone, or joint. Instead, *C. glabrata* produces disseminated disease in the lung and kidney and in the mucosa of the gastrointestinal and genitourinary tracts, uterus, and fallopian tubes.

Blood cultures are frequently positive in acute disseminated histoplasmosis but only rarely positive in the chronic disseminated form (Goodwin et al., 1980). Indirect evidence suggests that many, if not all, cases of primary pulmonary histoplasmosis disseminate hematogenously. Culture of both blood and bone marrow may assist in the diagnosis of disseminated histoplasmosis.

Clinically detectable *Aspergillus* fungemia is so rare that it is impossible to derive a meaningful account of the clinical manifestations of the fungemic period.

Recovery of cryptococcus from blood is not common. Fungemia has occurred in 15 to 18 per cent of patients with cryptococcal meningitis (Perfect et al., 1983) and has accounted for only 5 per cent of fungal isolates in a large population of immunocompromised patients. Patients with cryptococcal septicemia have tended either to be seriously ill or to be treated with steroids. Their prognosis has been very poor.

Reviews of blastomycosis, sporotrichosis, mucormycosis, and coccidioidomycosis reveal positive blood cultures only rarely. Widespread organ involvement and subcutaneous nodules (which are consistent with hematogenous spread rather than direct inoculation) suggest that these fungi disseminate hematogenously.

DIAGNOSIS. The diagnosis of fungemia is made by blood culture. Admitting air into the routine blood culture bottles improves the rate of recovery of candida. The time required to detect growth of *Candida* may be reduced by placing an aliquot of blood directly onto agar or into the Castaneda bottle, which contains a layer of agar on the side. Blood cultures for fungi should be held for at least 21 days to allow the slower growing organisms to become visible. A lysis of polymorphonuclear leukocytes may facilitate recovery of intracellular *Candida*. Promising results for increasing recovery of fungi from blood have been obtained recently with a cell lysis centrifugation system (Freeman et al., 1984). Experiments in dogs suggest that right atrial or arterial cultures may give a higher yield than peripheral venous cultures. Gas-liquid chromatography of the serum for mannose is being evaluated in *Candida* septicemia for rapid diagnosis. Radioimmunoassay techniques for the detection of *Candida* and *Aspergillus* antigen in serum are also under study. Preliminary data suggests that bacteria may obscure the recovery of fungi in polymicrobial septicemia and, in selected patients, it may be necessary to suppress bacterial growth in cultures (Hockey et al., 1982).

In addition to culturing blood for fungi, a peripheral smear may help identify fungemia due to *Candida*, *Geotrichia*, and *Histoplasma*. Figure 2 shows candida in peripheral blood.

High or rising precipitin titers for *Candida* antigens in selected patients may help confirm the presence of disseminated candidiasis. However, the incidence of false-negative titers is high, especially in the terminally ill or severely immunocompromised patient, so that the value of the test is limited.

Because of the low rate of positive blood cultures, the diagnosis of a fungemia is often made only after complications of the disseminated form of the disease become evident.

TREATMENT AND PROPHYLAXIS. The treatment for fungemias other than those caused by *Candida* is described in each chapter for the specific disseminated mycosis, because the fungemia is a manifestation of the disseminated infection.

In some patients with *Candida* septicemia, removal of the catheter is followed by clearance of *Candida* organisms from the blood, with no identifiable sequelae. However, in the severely immunocompromised patient (Young et al., 1974) or the complicated postsurgical patient, it is dangerous to assume that a catheter-associated fungemia is either "benign" or a contaminant. A recent study (Weinstein et al., 1983) of 500 bacteremias and fungemias has shown that the vast majority of fungemias represent true infection. Some patients in whom the fungemia clears after removal

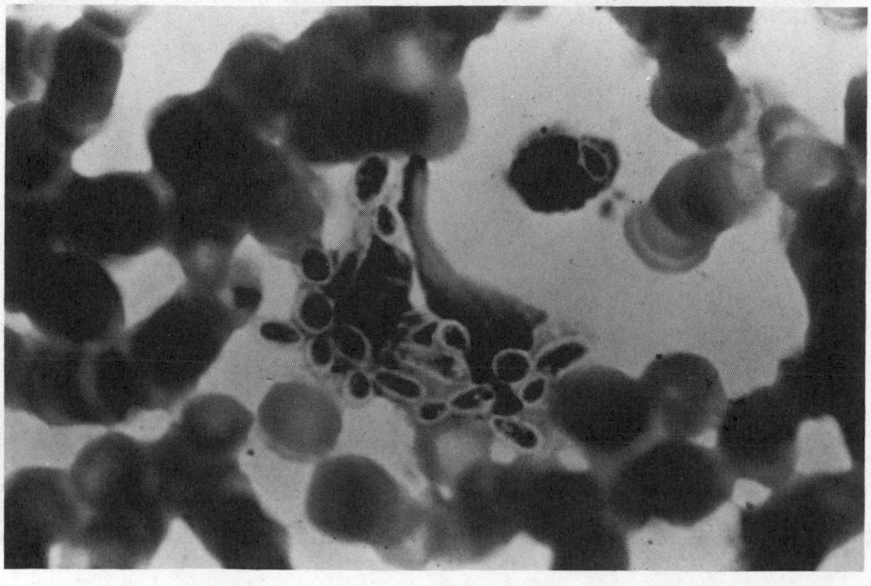

Figure 2. *Candida* in a peripheral blood smear. (Courtesy of Dr. Jack S. Remington.)

Table 1. MANAGEMENT OF CANDIDEMIA ASSOCIATED WITH INTRAVENOUS CATHETERS

Axiom: Patients with catheter-associated candidemia may have disseminated candidiasis despite resolution of the candidemia.

Plan:
1. Remove catheter.
2. If patient has inexplicable worsening course: Treat
3. If patient has stable course:
   a. Eliminate predisposing factors
   b. Complete evaluation:
      (1) Physical examination: eyes, blood smear, skin, bone, muscle, auscultation, neurologic
      Other studies: EKG, EMG, spinal tap (if indicated), muscle biopsy (if clinical myositis is present)
      (2) Serologic tests: Candida precipitins, antigen
      (3) Repeat blood cultures

If result is positive, treat; if negative, continue observation with extreme caution.

of the catheter may have disseminated disease despite negative follow-up blood cultures. With any patient who has candidemia, whether or not it is associated with an indwelling polyethylene catheter, a thorough examination should be performed to detect both peripheral and deep organ involvement, and serial blood cultures should be obtained. If the titers of *Candida* precipitins exceed 1:8 by counterimmunoelectrophoresis or if they are rising, dissemination rather than benign candidemia is more likely. However, since some patients, especially those who are terminally ill, may not be able to mount an antibody response during dissemination, a negative titer is of limited value. If the patient's course is inexplicably worsening, antifungal therapy should be initiated while a decision regarding the significance of the fungemia is made. An algorithm for the management of candidemia is diagrammed in Table 1.

Once the decision to treat has been made, several options are available. Because most *Candida* strains are highly susceptible to amphotericin B, this drug is the mainstay of therapy for candidemia and disseminated candidiasis. If the patient is deteriorating rapidly, the addition of 5-fluorocytosine (5-FC) to the regimen may help to achieve therapeutic antifungal levels sooner than the use of amphotericin B alone. In addition, the two drugs are synergistic for many *Candida* strains. The organism should be tested for susceptibility to 5-FC and to the synergistic action of 5-FC with amphotericin B. Many isolates of *Candida* are completely resistant to 5-FC on initial isolation, and others become resistant during therapy. The length of therapy and the total amount of medication necessary to treat disseminated candidiasis are unknown. A reasonable approach is to treat the patient with 0.5 mg/kg amphotericin B intravenously daily until the patient is stable (usually total dose is approximately 1.0 g).

If the course is fulminant, 150 mg/kg of 5-FC can be added and the amphotericin B can be advanced at 12-hour intervals until 0.7 to 1.0 mg/kg doses are reached. When the patient is stable, both drugs will require reduction (amphotericin B to approximately 0.5 mg/kg/day and 5-FC to 100 mg/kg/day or less) because of the hematologic toxicity of the combined agents. One or both drugs can be given until substantial clinical improvement is evident and then withheld as the patient is watched cautiously for recurrent signs of infection.

Minimizing the use of broad spectrum antibiotics, hyperalimentation catheters and fluids, steroids, and antineoplastic therapy will reduce the incidence of candidemia and perhaps septicemia. Prophylactic oral nystatin may be useful in burn patients and postsurgical patients. However, its usefulness in the severely immunocompromised patient is not clear. Flushing intravenous lines with small quantities of amphotericin B has been attempted, but the value of that technique has not been established.

References

Bodey, G. P., and Luna, M.: Skin lesions associated with disseminated candidiasis. JAMA 229:1466, 1974.

Butler, W. T., Alling, D. W., Spickard, A., and Utz, J. P.: Diagnostic and prognostic value of clinical and laboratory findings in cryptococcal meningitis. N Engl J Med 270:59, 1964.

Edwards, J. E., Jr., Foos, R. Y., Montgomerie, J. Z., Shaw, V., and Guze, L. B.: Ocular manifestations of Candida septicemia: Review of seventy-six cases of hematogenous Candida endophthalmitis. Medicine 53:47, 1974.

Fishman, L. S., Griffin, J. R., Sapico, F. L., et al: Hematogenous Candida endophthalmitis—a complication of candidemia. N Engl J Med 286:675, 1972.

Freeman, D., Bille, J., Edson, R. S., Roberts, G. D.: Clinical evaluation of the lysis-centrifugation blood culture system for the detection of fungemia and comparison with a conventional broth blood culture system. J Clin Microbiol 19:126, 1984.

Goodwin, R. A., Shapiro, J. L., Thurman, G. H., Thurman, S. S., Des Prez, R. M.: Disseminated histoplasmosis: clinical and pathologic correlations. Medicine 59:1, 1980.

Hartford, C. G.: Postoperative fungal endocarditis. Fungemia, embolism, and therapy. Arch Intern Med 134:116, 1974.

Hockey, L. J., Fujita, N. K., Gibson, T. R., Rotrosen, D., Montgomerie, J. Z., Edwards, J. E., Jr.: Detection of fungemia obscured by concomitant bacteria: in vitro and in vivo studies. J Clin Microbiol 16:1080, 1982.

Krause, W., Matheis, H., and Wulf, K.: Fungemia and funguria after oral administration of Candida albicans. Lancet 1:598, 1969.

Louria, D. B., Blevins, A., Armstrong, D., Burdich, R., and Lieberman, P.: Fungemia caused by "nonpathogenic" yeasts. Arch Intern Med 119:247, 1967.

Pankey, G. A., and Dalaviso, J. R.: Fungemia caused by Torulopsis glabrata. Medicine 52:395, 1973.

Perfect, J. R., Durack, D. T., Gallis, H. A.: Cryptococcemia. Medicine 62:98, 1983.

Sheehy, T. W., Honeycutt, B. K., and Spencer, J. T.: *Geotrichum* septicemia. JAMA 235:1035, 1976.

Stone, H. H., Kolb, L. D., Currie, C. A., Geheber, C. E., and Cuzzell, J. Z.: Candida sepsis: pathogenesis and principles of treatment. Ann Surg 179:697, 1974.

Valdivieso, M., Luna, M., Bodey, G. P., Rodriguez, V., and Groschel, D.: Fungemia due to *Torulopsis glabrata* in the compromised host. Cancer 38:1750, 1976.

Weinstein, M. P., Reller, L. B., Murphy, J. R., Lichtenstein, R. S.: The clinical significance of positive blood cultures: a comprehensive analysis of 500 episodes of bacteremia and fungemia in adults. I. Laboratory and epidemiologic observations. Rev Inf Dis 5:35, 1983.

Winston, D. J., Balsley, G. E., Rhodes, J., and Linne, S. R.: Disseminated *Trichosporon capitatum* infection in an immunosuppressed host. Arch Intern Med 137:1192, 1977.

Young, R. C., Bennett, J. E., Geelhoed, G. W., and Levine, A. S.: Fungemia with compromised host resistance. Ann Intern Med 80:605, 1974.

213

INFECTIVE ENDOCARDITIS AND OTHER INTRAVASCULAR INFECTIONS

LAWRENCE R. FREEDMAN, M.D.

Intravascular infection is established when circulating microorganisms colonize platelet-fibrin vegetations covering altered vascular endothelium. Intravascular infection within the heart is referred to as infective endocarditis (IE). These infections occur in all parts of the world and affect approximately 60 per 1,000,000 persons per year.

There are few other examples in medicine in which simple and inexpensive diagnostic methods are sufficient to indicate the presence of a lethal disease that can be cured with antibiotics. Nevertheless, despite the technical simplicity of diagnosis, many patients die or suffer the consequences of serious arterial embolization or heart valve damage because of a long delay in establishing the diagnosis or because the diagnosis is not thought of at all. Part of the reason for this delay is that the clinical picture is nonspecific and does not conform to the "classic textbook description" derived from observation of patients with long-established disease in the preantibiotic era.

Prevention of IE with antibiotics is theoretically possible in about 25 per cent of persons in whom the infection develops. However, patients at risk are often unaware of the need for antibiotic prophylaxis in the face of procedures known to induce bacteremia, and physicians and dentists often do not prescribe prophylactic measures despite having facts available that should have warranted their doing so.

Clearly, merely having the information and the means available to prevent, diagnose, and treat potentially fatal illness does not ensure that the disease will be prevented, diagnosed, or treated correctly. In addition, several dramatic technical advances in medicine (chronic hemodialysis, cardiac surgery) have created a new population of patients who are at special risk for developing IE. It is no wonder that there is considerable interest in intravascular infections in the clinic and in the laboratory.

DEFINITION. Infective endocarditis is a microbial infection of a platelet-fibrin vegetation located on the endothelial surface of the heart. Similar infections occur less frequently within the vascular system outside the heart: mycotic aneurysms, infections of aortic prosthetic grafts, infections of patent ductus arteriosus and coarctation of the aorta, and septic thrombophlebitis. The principles of pathogenesis, prevention, and treatment are similar for all of these infections.

It has been customary in the past to divide patients with infective endocarditis into categories of acute (malignant) and subacute (lenta) endocarditis. The differences of clinical course and infecting microorganisms (subacute, predominantly alpha-hemolytic streptococci; acute, staphylococci, pneumococci, gonococci), although statistically valid, overlap sufficiently to argue against continuing the distinction. The lethal complications of infection, aortic valve perforation or cerebral embolization, are frequent and may occur with any type of infection. It is therefore incumbent upon the physician to establish the diagnosis and begin treatment as soon as possible. The decision to begin treatment in the absence of definite proof of the diagnosis is not an easy one and will, of course, be influenced by the clinical state of the patient.

PATHOGENESIS. The development of any intravascular infection depends upon the presence of a lesion of the vascular endothelium susceptible to infection, and the arrival at that lesion of sufficient organisms capable of establishing infection. Experimental studies have shown that the endothelial injury susceptible to infection may be so small as to escape detection. When endothelial damage was produced in rabbits by the mere placement of a plastic catheter within the heart chambers, the intravenous inoculation of only 10^3 streptococci (viridans group) or staphylococci (*aureus* species) was enough to produce infection in 25 per cent of animals. (Larger inocula produce infection regularly under these circumstances.) Vegetations in the rabbit are more susceptible to infection with *Staphylococcus aureus* than with streptococci, and still less susceptible to infection with *Escherichia coli.* Although it is not clear how many factors influence the ability of bacteria to colonize such vegetations, one of them seems to be increased stickiness of those gram-positive cocci that produce dextran. Infections in the left side of the heart of rabbits achieve higher microbial populations than infections of the right heart and have a more severe "clinical" course; right heart infections are rarely fatal and often have an evolution leading to spontaneous sterilization (without antibiotics). In rabbits infection is much more difficult to establish in the vena cava or aorta than in the left heart (Freedman, 1982).

All of these experimental phenomena have their counterparts in human disease. In man, vegetations (or areas of endothelial damage) susceptible to infection are found in the following conditions: rheumatic heart (valvular) disease, congenital heart disease (except for atrial septal defect, which rarely becomes infected), mitral valve prolapse (a forme fruste of Marfan's syndrome?), Marfan's syndrome, idiopathic hypertrophic subaortic stenosis, patent ductus arteriosus, coarctation of the aorta, peripheral arteriovenous fistulas (either on the fistula or in the heart), indwelling intravenous or intra-arterial plastic catheters or intracardiac pacemakers, prosthetic valve surgery, placement of prosthetic aortic grafts, and myocardial infarction.

Sterile valvular vegetations are frequent at autopsy in patients with cancer and in patients who had disseminated intravascular coagulation during life. These vegetations probably result from generalized hypercoagulability or valve damage by circulating immune complexes. In addition, unknown mechanisms induce susceptibility of heart valves to infection by chronic hemodialysis and intravenous drug usage.

It is often difficult to identify the source of bacteremia that initiates the infection because the number of bacteria required to induce infection may be too small to detect, since the first symptoms of IE may be too vague and insidious to pinpoint the onset of infection, and because there are so many causes of bacteremia that it is difficult to be certain of the relation between a particular bacteremia-producing event and the onset of infection.

Bacteremia often occurs after any procedure that breaks the normal mucosal or epithelial barrier. Bacteremia can occur after almost any dental treatment. It is more frequent with gingival disease and results from procedures as non-traumatic as tooth-brushing, gingival irrigation, nasotracheal suctioning, and chewing hard candy. In the gastrointestinal tract, bacteremia is provoked by liver biopsy, gastroscopy, sigmoidoscopy, and barium enema. In the genitourinary tract, bacteremia has been documented during normal delivery, cesarian section, normal menstruation, and uterine dilatation and curettage. Urinary tract instrumentation and prostatectomy produce bacteremia. The risk is higher with established urinary tract infections. Virtually any procedure that involves cannulation of veins, arteries, or the heart can give rise to bacteremia. Particularly dangerous is total parenteral nutrition, from which 27 per cent of patients developed bacteremia in one series. Bacteremia can also arise from any local infection, especially if manipulated or incised, and from any severe infection in patients with impaired defense mechanisms. In many patients with infective endocarditis, no source of bacteremia is apparent.

Infective endocarditis is thought to develop frequently on normal heart valves. It is often not possible, however, to rule out tiny underlying endocardial lesions; even at autopsy, the reason for the development of an impressive vegetation may not be apparent. Nevertheless, there is general agreement (and considerable clinical and experimental evidence to support the view) that *infective endocarditis begins when circulating microorganisms colonize sterile vegetations covering a damaged endothelium.* In the laboratory, normal endocardium is resistant to infection.

The platelet-fibrin vegetation, once colonized by bacteria, grows quickly by the further deposition of platelets and fibrin, thus rapidly isolating the bacteria from the few polymorphonuclear leukocytes that might arrive from the vessels in the heart valve or from the circulation. *This "protection" of bacteria from phagocytic cells* is one of the most important features of the infection and creates, in fact, an infection in a *zone of localized agranulocytosis.* This phenomenon explains why cure of these infections requires prolonged administration of bactericidal antibiotics. Intensive antibiotic therapy may also be needed for the old bacterial colonies at the base of infected vegetations that metabolize at a much slower rate than those on the surface. Thus, even bactericidal antibiotics that depend on active bacterial cell-wall synthesis for their activity are less effective in sterilizing these deep colonies than in sterilizing rapidly growing bacteria (Durack and Beeson, 1978).

At first, the vegetation remains fairly constant in size because of a balance between growth, resorption, and fragmentation. New surface growth of the vegetation is due to the continued deposition of circulating bacteria. Growth of the vegetation due to its continual reseeding is compensated for by resorption at its base or fragmentation and embolization. One of the hallmarks of these infections is *constant bacteremia* with little variation in the number of circulating bacteria over long periods of time.

There are four mechanisms by which these infections affect the patient:

1. *Constant bacteremia* produces fever, loss of appetite, anemia, splenomegaly, and metastatic infection.
2. *Local invasion* can produce disturbances of cardiac conduction, myocardial infarction, valve ring abscesses and pericarditis, mycotic aneurysm of the sinus of Valsalva, and valve perforation.
3. *Peripheral embolization* of fragments of infected vegetation are responsible for mycotic aneurysm formation and septic infarction of any organ. Most commonly, these emboli involve the brain, spleen, kidneys, bone, and myocardium. Abscesses in these organs may be a source of reinfection of the vegetation and consequent treatment failure. Emboli from mycotic vegetations are larger than in bacterial endocarditis and occlude major vessels.
4. *Circulating immune complexes* are another distinctive feature of infective endocarditis (see Chapter 89). Aside from patients with salmonellosis, brucellosis, leprosy, and quartan malaria, it is unusual to find viable microorganisms in the bloodstream simultaneously with their specific antibody, yet this is the rule in infective endocarditis. The simultaneous presence of antigen (bacteria) and antibody leads to the formation of circulating immune complexes. In other infections the presence of antibody and the availability of polymorphonuclear leukocytes effectively block the shedding of bacteria into the blood. In infective endocarditis this mechanism is ineffective.

Circulating immune complexes probably cause petechiae, Osler and Janeway lesions, arthritis, and, most important, glomerulonephritis. Immune complexes may be detected as cryoprecipitates and stimulate antibody formation against globulins (rheumatoid factor).

EPIDEMIOLOGY AND BACTERIOLOGY. The frequency of infective endocarditis and the types of bacteria isolated depend on the population under study. For example, in Western Europe and North America, streptococci (excluding group A) and staphylococci account for about 90 per cent of the infecting microorganisms. In Nigeria, on the other hand, streptococci are rarely recovered from patients with infective endocarditis.

In narcotic addicts with endocarditis, infections with certain organisms tend to cluster in different cities in the United States. *Staphylococcus aureus* is prevalent in some areas, enterococci or *Serratia marscesens* in others, and *Pseudomonas aeruginosa* in others. The explanation for this is not clear, since specific microorganisms are not found in the drugs or equipment used for injections in specific geographic locations. In addicts with *S. aureus* infections, skin and mucous membranes were often colonized with the infecting bacteria, thus suggesting that they spread to the heart from the carrier sites.

Although streptococci and staphylococci are the most common causes, almost any bacteria can infect a susceptible intravascular site including, rarely, tubercle bacilli, meningococci, *Brucella* spp., and rickettsiae. *Candida albicans* and *Aspergillus* spp. have produced such infections, but viruses and cell-wall-defective bacteria have not been proved to cause infective endocarditis in man. *Candida* endocarditis occurs mainly in drug addicts and recipients of prosthetic heart valves. *Candida albicans* and *Candida parapsilosis* are the main species of *Candida* involved in endocarditis and also always require underlying valve injury to cause infection of the heart. For this reason, nearly all cases of *Candida* endocarditis in addicts affect the mitral or aortic valves, in contrast to staphylococci, which often attack the right side of the heart.

Extracardiac intravascular infections are frequently caused by bacteriologic contamination during surgery or accidental trauma. *Salmonella* spp. is among the most common bacteria recovered from spontaneous infections of abdominal aortic aneurysms. The explanation for this peculiar predilection is not known, since *Salmonella* very rarely causes infective endocarditis.

Recovery of more than one bacterial species from the blood of patients with infective endocarditis, although unusual, is being reported with increasing frequency. The antibiotic sensitivities of bacteria recovered in these "double infections" may differ considerably, thus complicating the choice of antibiotics and the evaluation of bactericidal drug activity in the serum.

When *Streptococcus bovis* causes IE, colonic disease, frequently carcinoma, is often present. Gastrointestinal cancer must be sought in any patient from whose blood *S. bovis* is recovered, even when no symptoms of bowel disease are present.

PROPHYLAXIS. Although it would appear to be a simple matter to prevent infective endocarditis, the problem is complex (Everett and Hirschmann, 1977; Kaplan et al., 1977; Sipes et al., 1977; Sternon, 1975). If one starts with those patients given a diagnosis of endocarditis, about 50 per cent are unaware of any cardiac abnormality or predisposing condition, and about 50 per cent (probably more) have no evident source of bacteremia. Thus, with our present understanding of the disease, it would be possible to prevent only about 25 per cent of identified cases.

Many patients in apparent good health have "innocuous" heart murmurs—should they be protected? In a recent study of "normal" young women, between 6 and 28 per cent were considered to have mitral valve prolapse, regarded by some authorities as the underlying lesion in one-third of patients with infective endocarditis and mitral valve insufficiency.

Another problem is to decide against which organisms to direct antibiotic prophylaxis. For example, it is customary to cover high risk of infection by staphylococci after open heart surgery with prophylactic penicillins that are resistant to β-lactamase. The only studies of the efficacy of this prophylaxis found no difference between treated and nontreated patients except for infections in the treated group that were resistant to the antibiotics administered.

Finally, there is no evidence in man that prophylactic antibiotics work, even for reasonably well-defined procedures involving dental manipulations. The low frequency of infection and the ethical impossiblity of withholding antibiotics from susceptible patients prevent investigation of the problem.

Nevertheless, despite these difficulties and unknown factors, there is general agreement that prophylactic antibiotics should be given to patients subjected to procedures described below. The patients are those with a history of infective endocarditis, valvular heart disease, prosthetic valves or aortic grafts, coarctation of the aorta, patent ductus arteriosus, and, prolapse of the mitral valve accompanied by the murmur of mitral regurgitation.

It is astonishing how often patients with known heart disease are not aware of the risk of developing infective endocarditis and of the recommendations for prophylactic antibiotics. It is equally astonishing how infrequently dentists ask their patients about a history of heart disease. Some patients who have developed endocarditis of prosthetic heart valves after dental extraction believed that their heart surgery eliminated the risk of endocarditis. This problem was not discussed by their physicians and they were not told, at least for a while, that the risk of endocarditis is probably greater than before operation and that the risk will always remain.

The following procedures increase the risk of endocarditis:

1. *Oropharyngeal procedures,* such as dental extraction, dental prophylaxis, oral surgery, and rigid-tube bronchoscopy. The frequency of bacteremia varies after these procedures, but it is generally detected in 30 to 80 per cent of patients. The bacteria recovered from the blood are those resident in the mouth, especially various streptococci.
2. *Urologic procedures,* such as instrumentation or catheterization of the urethra and prostatectomy. The frequency of bacteremia varies between about 10 and 80 per cent of patients, the higher rates being seen with established urinary infections. The urinary tract is considered to be the portal of entry in about 50 per cent of patients with group D streptococcus endocarditis.
3. *Gastrointestinal procedures,* such as sigmoidoscopy, upper GI tract endoscopy, barium enema, colonoscopy, and liver biopsy. About 10 per cent of patients undergoing these examinations develop bacteremia. The bacteria in the blood may be any of those in the normal bowel flora. After barium enema and sigmoidoscopy, blood cultures often reveal enterococci.
4. *Gynecologic procedures,* such as normal pregnancy, uterine dilation and curettage, and cesarian section. The frequency of bacteremia in these patients is reported to be low. Nevertheless, obstetric and gynecologic procedures are believed to be the source of group D streptococcal endocarditis in about 20 per cent of patients. The problem of defining the indications for antibiotic prophylaxis is well illustrated by considering the procedure of insertion of an intra-uterine device. Although no bacteremia was detected in one group of 84 patients, in others with infective endocarditis it is highly probable that insertion of an IUD was the source of infection.

The choice of antibiotics will depend on the probability that certain bacteria will cause bacteremia after a given procedure. The dose of antibiotics has not been established by studies in man. There are two clues that past recommendations are inadequate. One such clue is the failure of prophylaxis in a number of patients and another is the failure of recommended doses for man to prevent infective endocarditis in rabbits. The problem is complicated, and the recommendations of the American Heart Association for antibiotic prophylaxis in the prevention of infective endocarditis have recently been revised (Table 1).

The basic prophylaxis for dental procedures and surgery of the upper respiratory tract is either penicillin or penicillin plus streptomycin. Parenteral antibiotics are preferred. Regimen A or B is recommended for patients with congenital, rheumatic, or other acquired heart disease. Regimen C is recommended in these instances for patients allergic to penicillin. Regimen B is recommended for patients with prosthetic heart valves, and for these patients Regimen D in the case of allergy to penicillin. These recommendations are intended to prevent infection with non-group A streptococci. For instrumentation and surgery of the genitourinary or gastrointestinal tract, at which time enterococcus bacteremia might be provoked, the recommendation is to administer penicillin plus gentamicin or streptomycin, or ampicillin plus gentamicin or streptomycin. For patients allergic to penicillin, vancomycin plus streptomycin is recommended. In view of the frequent finding of streptomycin resistance in enterococci recovered in the United States, it would seem preferable to use

Table 1. PROPHYLAXIS OF INFECTIVE ENDOCARDITIS*
(Risk of Infection with non-group A streptococci from the upper respiratory tract)

Drug	Time of Administration	Preparation†	Dose
A. Penicillin (parenteral-oral)	Before procedure 30 min to 1 hr	ACPG + PPG	1,000,000 units I.M. 600,000 units I.M.
	After procedure every 6 hr for 8 doses	PV	500 mg orally
OR:			
Penicillin (oral)	Before procedure 30 min to 1 hr	PV	2.0 g orally
	After procedure every 6 hr for 8 doses	PV	500 mg orally
B. Penicillin + Streptomycin	Before procedure 30 min to 1 hr	ACPG + PPG + streptomycin	1,000,000 units I.M. 600,000 units I.M. 1.0 g I.M.
	After procedure every 6 hr for 8 doses	PV	500 mg orally
C. Patients Allergic to Penicillin (parenteral-oral)	During procedure over 30 min to 1 hr	vancomycin	1.0 g I.V. (start 30 min to 1 hr before procedure)
	After procedure every 6 hr for 8 doses	erythromycin	500 mg orally
D. Patients Allergic to Penicillin (oral)	1 ½–2 hr before procedure	erythromycin	1.0 g orally
	After procedure every 6 hr for 8 doses	erythromycin	500 mg orally

*For details concerning these recommendations and for children's dosages, see Kaplan, E. L., et al.: A. H. A. Committee Report: Prevention of bacterial endocarditis. Circulation 56:139A, 1977.

†ACPG—aqueous crystalline penicillin G; PV — penicillin V (phenoxymethyl penicillin); PPG — procaine penicillin G.

vancomycin or vancomycin and gentamicin to prevent enterococcal endocarditis. These antibiotics have been shown to be most effective in preventing streptomycin-resistant enterococcal endocarditis in animals (Guze et al., 1983).

The recommendations in the United Kingdom differ from those in the United States, principally in recommending amoxicillin rather than penicillin and in advising a single dose of 3.0 g of amoxicillin one hour before dental procedures in the hope of increasing compliance (Report of a Working Party of the British Society for Antimicrobial Chemotherapy. 1982).

CLINICAL FINDINGS. Infective endocarditis may produce symptoms related to any organ, with or without fever, and with or without evidence of heart disease. Symptoms range from vague complaints of poor health to those of an acute illness of the central nervous system. Many patients are referred to the hospital for possible intestinal cancer, arthritis, or back pain. The nonspecific symptoms in these patients are the reason why the interval between the onset of symptoms and the diagnosis is usually several weeks and often many months.

The clinical findings are related to bacteremia (fever, weight loss, anemia, splenomegaly), local invasion by the infection (valve perforation, congestive heart failure, cardiac arrhythmias), peripheral emboli (symptoms of embolization, infarction, abscess formation, and mycotic aneurysm), and circulating immune complexes (skin lesions, arthritis, glomerulonephritis) (Kaye, 1976; Sternon, 1975; Weinstein and Schlesinger, 1974).

Patients usually have fever and a heart murmur, but other signs of infective endocarditis may be absent. Fever may be slight or absent in 5 to 15 per cent of patients. Similarly, there may be no heart murmur (about 15 per cent of patients). But absence of both fever and heart murmur is exceedingly rare. A changing quality of systolic heart murmurs is unusual and to be expected only in exceptional cases. Even when present this finding is often difficult to interpret.

The murmur of aortic insufficiency is easily recognized, and may be an ominous prognostic sign. Clubbing of the fingers, Osler's nodes, retinal "Roth spots" (Fig. 1), and Janeway lesions (Table 2) are unusual today. Migrating polyarthritis and osteomyelitis are seen occasionally.

The laboratory findings are seldom helpful (except for blood cultures). There may be an anemia without reticulocytosis, an elevated titer of rheumatoid factor, decreased levels of complement, circulating immune complexes, and cryoglobulinemia. There may be laboratory findings associated with infarctions or abscess in any organ and, of course, the findings in the blood (azotemia) and urine (hematuria, red cell casts, proteinuria) typical of glomerulonephritis. In addition, patients may develop the clinical syndrome of disseminated intravascular coagulation.

DIAGNOSIS. *The diagnosis of infective endocarditis depends on the culturing of bacteria from the blood.* It is

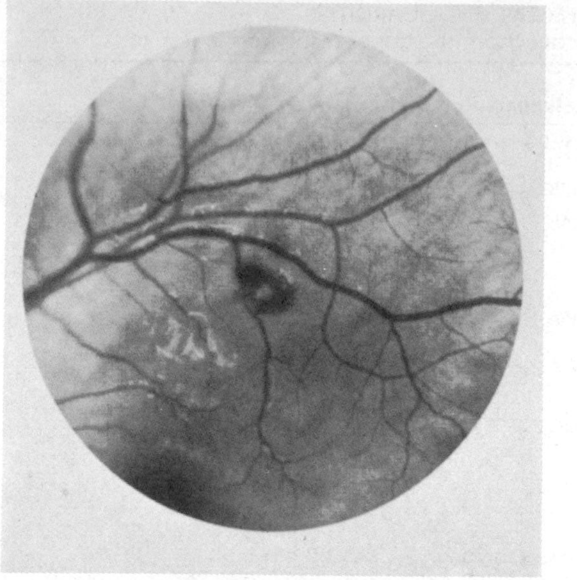

Figure 1. Roth spot (hemorrhage with white center) in a patient with subacute bacterial endocarditis. (From Cogan: Ophthalmic Manifestations of Systemic Vascular Disease, W. B. Saunders Co., 1974.)

necessary to obtain cultures aerobically and anaerobically. *Bacteria may be cultured from the blood in this infection in the absence of fever.* Since there is insignificant filtration of bacteria in the peripheral circulation, there is no advantage in obtaining cultures from arterial blood—venous blood is satisfactory. Occasionally, special culture techniques are necessary to cultivate fungi or mycobacteria and microorganisms with peculiar nutritional requirements. In endocarditis due to *Coxiella burnetii* (Q fever), serologic evidence of infection is essential for diagnosis (see Chapter 207).

Because of the constancy of the bacteremia in infective endocarditis, three to five blood culture pairs (aerobic and anaerobic) are sufficient to establish the diagnosis in about 90 per cent of patients who will ever have a positive blood culture. Occasionally, it takes several days, and rarely, weeks, for the microorganisms to be detectable in blood cultures.

A certain number of patients have infective endocarditis detected at autopsy in whom it was not possible to culture microorganisms from the blood during life. This may be due to several phenomena:

1. Prior administration of antibiotics. The administration of even small quantities of antibiotics may suppress bacterial growth (without sterilization of the lesion) in the vegetation for prolonged periods. We have followed a patient whose daily blood cultures were sterile for 12 days after the administration of a few doxycycline tablets. Blood cultures became consistently positive from the thirteenth day onward. The practice of treating febrile illnesses with antibiotics without undertaking bacteriologic studies to establish the nature of the infection is generally to be condemned.
2. Infection with peculiar microorganisms whose growth needs are not satisfied by "routine" culture media. Examples are tubercle bacilli, *Coxiella burnetii*, and vitamin B_6-dependent streptococci.
3. The biology of the infection. Infections on the right side of the heart are occasionally accompanied by negative blood cultures. Blood cultures in patients with infections of the abdominal aorta are negative about 50 per cent of the time. Experiments in rabbits show that the density of bacterial populations in these locations is lower than in vegetations in the left side of the heart. This could explain the negative blood cultures in these clinical circumstances.
4. Rarely, infective endocarditis is seen at autopsy for which none of the above explanations for negative blood cultures is applicable.

Echocardiography may provide evidence of vegetations on heart valves. Vegetations do not necessarily indicate infection, since nonbacterial thrombotic endocarditis, found frequently in patients with cancer, may produce a clinical picture very similar to that of infective endocarditis, but with negative blood cultures. A negative echocardiogram does not rule out vegetations.

Heart antibodies occur with infective endocarditis, but it is not yet clear how useful these will be in diagnosis.

Radioactive scanning of the heart after administration of technetium-99-labeled pyrophosphate or after injection of radioactive-labeled antibodies to the infecting organism has been useful in the laboratory, but has not yet been applied to human infections.

DIFFERENTIAL DIAGNOSIS. Infective endocarditis may mimic a wide variety of disorders and may be superimposed on underlying unrelated disease. The clinical features of infective endocarditis may not be distinguishable from those of nonbacterial thrombotic endocarditis (often seen in patients with cancer), atrial myxoma, or endothelial tumors. The presence of circulating immune complexes, cryoglobulinemia, rheumatoid factor, hypocomplementemia, and arteritis in skin biopsy has led to the mistaken diagnosis of collagen-vascular disease and treatment of patients with endocarditis with adrenocortical steroids.

Any febrile patient with clinical evidence of glomerulo-

Table 2. COMPARISON OF SMALL FOCAL LESIONS CHARACTERISTIC OF ENDOCARDITIS

Lesion	Location	Appearance
Osler node	Pads of fingers and toes, thenar or hypothenar eminence, soles	Raised, *tender,* discolored (bluish, pink, or red), pea sized. Last several hours to several days
Janeway lesion	Palms or soles	Small area of erythema or hemorrhage, sometimes raised but *never* painful
Roth's spots (Fig. 1)	Retina	Round hemorrhage with white center near disk

nephritis should be suspected of having endocarditis. In the aged the diagnosis may be exceptionally difficult, and some authors have gone so far as to recommend culturing the blood of any elderly person who doesn't feel well.

A difficult problem arises in the interpretation of positive blood cultures without other signs of infective endocarditis. In these instances it is necessary to try to determine the source of the bacteremia. Even when a peripheral source for bacteremia is evident, it is possible that the peripheral infection is secondary to endocarditis.

TREATMENT. The principles of antibiotic treatment in infective endocarditis are determined by two important features of the pathologic lesion: (1) the ineffective participation of polymorphonuclear leukocytes and (2) the decreased metabolic activity of bacteria located at the base of infected vegetations.

The vegetation of infective endocarditis can be considered a zone of "localized agranulocytosis," so that bactericidal antibiotics are needed to sterilize the lesions. Treatment of infective endocarditis with bacteriostatic antibiotics may suppress clinical signs and symptoms, but signs of infection invariably reappear when antibiotics are discontinued. In view of the lowered metabolic activity of bacteria buried in vegetations and in view of the dependence of penicillin upon bacterial cell-wall synthesis, it is not surprising that even bactericidal antibiotics must be administered for long periods.

Benzyl penicillin is the mainstay of treatment for streptococcal endocarditis and a β-lactamase–resistant penicillin for staphylococcal endocarditis. Drugs for the treatment of less common infections are selected according to in vitro antibiotic sensitivities.

It is not a simple matter to know when to start antibiotic treatment if the causative organism has not been isolated from the blood. If the clinical diagnosis is clear, therapy can be started immediately after obtaining three to five blood cultures. If the patient has already received antibiotics and the clinical diagnosis is uncertain, it may be advisable to wait up to several weeks in an effort to identify the causative microorganism. These are decisions that require judgment; the risk of blind treatment without an established diagnosis or sensitivities of the organism must be weighed against the risk of sudden cerebral embolism or valve perforation.

It is relatively easy to judge response to treatment when there is prompt disappearance of fever, reduction in size of the spleen, cessation of new skin petechiae, and increase in general well-being. On the other hand, low-grade fever (often due to drug hypersensitivity) commonly persists throughout treatment. It is important, therefore, to examine indirect indices of the effectiveness of treatment: reticulocyte response in anemic patients, decrease in titer of rheumatoid factor, and decrease in circulating immune complexes. Unfortunately, none of these changes is conclusive evidence of response, nor is absence of change a conclusive argument for lack of response. As a rough guide to effective antibiotic treatment, it is common practice to adjust antibiotics so as to achieve a peak bactericidal effect in vitro with a dilution of serum of at least ¼ to ⅛. This is easily achieved with infections by viridans streptococci and bacteriologic cure is the rule. Experimental studies have substantiated this relation in viridans streptococcal infections. In staphylococcal infections, however, it is frequently impossible to achieve in vitro evidence of satisfactory bactericidal levels in the serum and yet such patients may also be cured bacteriologically. Despite experimental evidence suggesting the usefulness of serum bactericidal levels as a guide to proper therapy, conclusive proof is lacking of their value in man.

Some infections do not respond to antibiotics despite in vitro effectiveness as measured by sensitivity testing. For example, the treatment of endocarditis due to *Candida* and other fungi is unsatisfactory, and fungal infections on prosthetic valves are usually impossible to sterilize without removal of the valve (Duma, 1977). It may be necessary to observe patients for several years after the treatment of fungal endocarditis to be certain that the infection has been eradicated. *Candida* endocarditis should be treated postoperatively with 8.0 g 5-fluorocytosine orally, daily, and 40 mg amphotericin B every other day. The 5-fluorocytosine should be continued for six weeks and the amphotericin B for a total dose of 1200 mg.

In contrast to the uncertainty regarding the effectiveness of antibiotics in the prophylaxis of infective endocarditis, there is no question regarding their effectiveness in treatment of the established infection. Choice of antibiotic depends, obviously, on the bacteria or fungi recovered from the bloodstream. The relapse rate in this disease can be related inversely to the duration of treatment with effective antibiotics.

Many reports appear in the literature on the successful use of antibiotics for short periods of time in small numbers of patients. These reports are useful in indicating which antibiotics can work, but they do not tell us how regularly they work. For example, overall the relapse rate after a two-week penicillin-streptomycin treatment of penicillin-sensitive ($\leq$ 0.1 μg/ml-MIC) viridans streptococcus infections is between 6 and 10 per cent. After four weeks of treatment no relapses are reported. Clearly, two weeks of this treatment program can work, but four weeks works better. The life-threatening consequences of this infection are such that antibiotics should be administered so as to reduce to a minimum (zero, if possible) the rate of relapse. Recent analyses of patients treated with penicillin-streptomycin indicate that two weeks of treatment of infection due to sensitive streptococci is sufficient provided that infection was of short duration (symptoms less than three months) and that subjects with prosthetic valve endocarditis, mycotic aneurysm, cerebritis, shock, and abnormal renal function were excluded. This two-week therapy is also contraindicated in patients infected with nutritionally-dependent streptococci. (Bisno, 1981; Wilson et al. 1982).

Antibiotics should be administered parenterally. There are reports of the successful use of oral antibiotics in patients with infective endocarditis, but the uncertainities of intestinal absorption of large quantities of antibiotics would seem to introduce a dangerous element of uncertainty in the treatment of a lethal disease. If long-term intravenous or intramuscular therapy cannot be pursued, oral treatment can be substituted, with frequent monitoring of serum bactericidal activity.

A major cause of death in infective endocarditis is congestive heart failure due to aortic valve perforation. We do not know whether treatment that sterilizes a valve more rapidly is more likely to prevent dangerous local complications. Nevertheless, it is logical to assume that the most rapid sterilization of valves is one of the goals of therapy. For this reason, treatment programs have been adjusted recently to take into consideration experimental data in rabbit endocarditis that show that for penicillin-sensitive streptococcal and staphylococcal infections, the addition to a penicillin of an aminoglycoside that is synergistic in vitro significantly speeds the sterilization of the valve. There is evidence that infections with bacteria tolerant to antibiotics (MBC ≥16 × MIC) were associated with a less favorable outcome in man and animals. The combination of penicillin and streptomycin is synergistic even against tolerant strains of bacteria.

The following recommendations take into consideration data derived from experimental studies.

Penicillin-sensitive viridans streptococci (MIC ≤0.1 μg/ml): pencillin, 10 to 20 million units I.V.; or 1.6 million units (procaine penicillin G) I.M. every six hours for four weeks, plus streptomycin, 0.5 I.M. every 12 hours for two weeks. Two weeks of penicillin-streptomycin appear to be satisfactory in patients with uncomplicated infection of short duration (see above).

Other viridans streptococci (MIC ≥0.1 μg/ml) or *enterococci*: penicillin, 20 million units I.V. for six weeks, plus streptomycin, 1.0 g I.M. every 12 hours (or 0.5 g every six hours) for two weeks, then 0.5 g I.M. every 12 hours (or 0.25 g every six hours) for four weeks.

In the case of vestibular or auditory impairment, streptomycin may be discontinued after four weeks for the treatment of penicillin-resistant streptococci. Cephalosporins should not be used for the treatment of penicillin-resistant streptococci, since clinical results have been unsatisfactory.

In view of the frequent finding of streptomycin resistance (>2000μg/milliliter) in as many as 50 per cent of enterococci isolated from the blood stream it is recommended that therapy be started with gentamicin 3mg/kg IV or IM in 3 equally divided doses per 24 hours until sensitivity to streptomycin is tested. Ampicillin, 12 g per day I.V. continuously or 2.0 g I.V. q4h, may be substituted for penicillin.

Staphylococci sensitive to penicillin (MIC <0.1 *μg/ml):* as for penicillin-sensitive streptococci, but with administration of 20 million units of penicillin and continuing treatment for six weeks.

Other staphylococci (penicillinase producers): methicillin, oxacillin, or nafcillin 2 g every four hours I.V. for six weeks plus gentamicin, 3 to 5 mg/kg I.M. daily in three divided doses every eight hours for one week.

There is disagreement whether aminoglycosides are necessary for penicillin-sensitive streptococcal or staphylococcal infection and many authorities do not recommend their use. However, studies in animals and man demonstrating more rapid sterilization of infection with the addition of gentamicin, argue for the use of combined therapy (Korzeniowski et al., 1982). In the case of penicillin allergy, it is possible to substitute vancomycin, 0.5 g I.V. every six hours. Some authors believe cephalothin or cefazolin should be given to patients with penicillin allergy because they feel these cephalosporins are as effective in staphylococcal endocarditis as β-lactamase–resistant semisynthetic penicillins. It is difficult to evaluate the relative effectiveness of different antibiotics in staphylococcal endocarditis, since comparative clinical studies have not been done. In addition, many patients with staphylococcal endocarditis reported in the literature had right heart infection due to intravenous narcotic usage; the likelihood is that infections in the right heart are easier to sterilize than those in the left heart. It may thus not be possible to translate the results of treatment of right heart infections to infections of the left heart.

In circumstances where streptomycin or gentamicin is recommended, it is reasonable to substitute tobramycin or amikacin according to in vitro sensitivity tests. Antibiotic dosages should be adjusted to avoid toxic blood levels and still obtain peak serum bactericidal concentrations of ⅛.

Methicillin-resistant staphylococci (aureus or epidermidis) require therapy with vancomycin and gentamicin and perhaps a third drug, rifampin. These infections are difficult to treat and data are not yet available to permit definition of an optimal drug regimen.

The treatment of endocarditis due to other microorganisms is determined by the antibiotic sensitivities demonstrated in vitro. As a general rule, it is desirable to combine an aminoglycoside with a penicillin (or cephalosporin). In *Pseudomonas* endocarditis, carbenicillin is given in a dose of 2.5 g I.V. every two hours with gentamicin, 100 mg I.V. every six hours. Some authors recommend the use of ticarcillin, 3.0 g I.V. every 4 hours with tobramycin 8 mg/kg/day I.V. in 3 divided doses. This is combined with prompt surgical removal of the valve when infection is on the left side of the heart. On the right side, surgery is undertaken if the blood culture remains positive after two weeks of therapy or if infection recurs after the completion of six weeks of therapy (Reyes, Lerner, 1983). When antibiotic treatment must be initiated in the absence of a bacteriologic diagnosis, the regimen chosen is that for treatment of either enterococcal or penicillin-resistant staphylococcal infection.

Anticoagulants have no place in the treatment of infective endocarditis. On the other hand, there is no contraindication to their use for other reasons in patients receiving proper antibiotic treatment for infective endocarditis. Patients with prosthetic heart valves receiving long-term anticoagulant treatment may experience difficulties in the regulation of their anticoagulants as an initial sign of the presence of infective endocarditis. It is generally felt that the risk of discontinuing anticoagulants in these patients exceeds that of continuing them during antibiotic treatment.

Whereas in the preantibiotic era virtually all patients died of infection, today it is exceptional not to be able to sterilize intravascular vegetations. Mortality, on the other hand, remains between 0 to 5 per cent and 30 to 40 per cent depending on the patient population under study. Factors of obvious importance to the outcome of treatment include age, associated disease, alcoholism, drug addiction, severity and nature of underlying heart disease, and embolic complications. Although there is variation from one series to another, valve perforation (and resulting congestive heart failure) and neurologic complications are among the most serious.

Valve perforation with resultant congestive heart failure is usually an indication for surgical replacement of the damaged valve with a prosthesis. This complication may occur as late as one week after the institution of antibiotic therapy and has been noted in about 25 per cent of patients with streptococcal endocarditis. Surgery is lifesaving in such patients, and is successful even when carried out within hours of starting antibiotic therapy. It is desirable, however, to delay surgery as long as possible in order to achieve maximal antibiotic effectiveness before exposing the prosthetic valve to possible infection.

In patients with prosthetic heart valves who develop infective endocarditis, it is usually but not always necessary to replace the valve in order to eliminate the infection.

Antibiotics without surgery are often successful in patients who acquire endocarditis many months or years after insertion of a prosthetic valve, and whose infection is caused by a drug-sensitive organism. Mortality is considerable when such infections require surgery. In some patients, osteomyelitis or splenic abscess may serve as a source of reinfection of heart valves after antibiotic therapy is completed.

In rare patients with severe renal insufficiency due to immune complex glomerulonephritis renal function does not improve despite sterilization of the intravascular infection. Immune complexes have been found to persist in the circulation of these patients, an indication for their removal by plasmapheresis.

If the patient cannot withstand heart surgery, he can be treated effectively with continuous suppressive drug therapy given orally or even intramuscularly. Dicloxacillin, for example, can be given in doses of 1.0 g three times daily for suppression of staphylococcal bacteremia in patients with inoperable endocarditis.

References

Bisno, A. L.: Treatment of Infective Endocarditis. New York, Grune and Stratton, 1981.

Duma, R. J.: Infections of Prosthetic Heart Valves and Vascular Grafts. Baltimore, University Park Press, 1977.

Durack, D. T., and Beeson, P. B.: Pathogenesis of Infective Endocarditis. In Rahimtoola, S. H. (ed.): Infective Endocarditis. New York, Grune and Stratton, 1978.

Everett, E. D., and Hirschmann, J. V.: Transient bacteremia and endocarditis prophylaxis—a review. Medicine 56:61, 1977.

Freedman, L. R.: Infective Endocarditis and Other Intravascular Infections. New York, Plenum, 1982.

Guze, P. A., Kalmanson, G. M., Freedman, L. R., Ishida, K., and Guze, L. B.: Antibiotic prophylaxis against streptomycin-resistant and -susceptible *Streptococcus faecalis* endocarditis in rabbits. Antimicrob Agents Chemo 22:514, 1983.

Kaplan, E. L., Anthony, B. F., Bisno, A., Durack, D., Houser, H., Millard, H. D., Sanford, J., Shulman, S. T., Stillerman, M., Taranta, A., and Wenger, N.: A.H.A. Committee Report: Prevention of bacterial endocarditis. Circulation 56:139A, 1977.

Kaye, D.: Infective Endocarditis. Baltimore, University Park Press, 1976.

Korzeniowski, O., Sande, M. A. and The National Endocarditis Study Group. Combination antimicrobial therapy for *Staphylococcus aureus* endocarditis in patients addicted to parenteral drugs and nonaddicts. Ann Int Med 97:496, 1982.

Report of a Working Party of the British Society for Antimicrobial Chemotherapy: The antibiotic prophylaxis of infective endocarditis. Lancet 2:1323, 1982.

Reyes, M. P., and Lerner, A. M.: Current problems in the treatment of infective endocarditis due to *Pseudomonas aeruginosa*. Rev Inf Dis 5:314, 1983.

Sipes, J. M., Thompson, R. L., and Hook, E. W.: Prophylaxis of infective endocarditis: A reevaluation. Ann Rev Med 28:371, 1977.

Sternon, J.: Les endocardites bactériennes de l'adulte. Clinique, anatomie pathologique, thérapeutique et prophylaxie. Paris, Masson et Cie, 1975.

Weinstein, L., and Schlesinger, J. M.: Pathoanatomic, pathophysiologic and clinical correlations in endocarditis. N Engl J Med 291:832, 1974.

Wilson, W. R., Giuliani, E. R. and Geraci, J. E.: Treatment of penicillin-sensitive streptococcal infective endocarditis. Mayo Clin Proc 57:95, 1982.

214

MYOCARDITIS AND PERICARDITIS

A. Martin Lerner, M.D.

Infections and inflammation within the myocardium, endocardium, or pericardium are always a potential threat to life that may develop during systemic infections or as a primary focus of infection. The major infectious causes of myopericardial dysfunction in the United States are enteroviruses, certain pyogenic bacteria, *Mycobacterium tuberculosis*, and a few fungi.

ETIOLOGIC AGENTS

Enterovirus. Enteroviruses, pyogenic bacteria, *Mycobacterium tuberculosis*, and fungi (*Candida, Aspergillus*) are the most important infectious causes of myopericarditis, but the heart and pericardium may also be involved in many systemic infections (Table 1) (Fowler and Monitsas, 1973). Available data, however, indicate that enteroviruses are the dominant cause of so called idiopathic myopericarditis. Because of difficulties inherent in diagnosing enteroviral infections, the incidence of enteroviral infections is probably greatly underestimated. Over a 6-year period, Grist and Bell at the Regional Virus Laboratory (Ruchill Hospital, Glasgow, Scotland) examined sera from 385 patients with suspected heart disease (Grist and Bell, 1974). On the basis of their studies of type-specific neutralizing antibodies, they suggested that coxsackieviruses belonging to Group B accounted for at least half of the cases of acute myocarditis and an additional one-third of the cases of acute nonbacterial pericarditis. These cases occurred throughout the year, but fewest cases were found in the first quarter, and most in the second and third quarters of the year. This incidence corresponds to the seasonal distribution of enterovirus infections. Serologic results inferred that (compared with coxsackieviruses) influenza viruses, adenoviruses, *Chlamydia*, Q fever, and *Mycoplasma pneumoniae* contributed few cases.

In order to sharpen the criteria for the diagnosis of enteroviral myopericarditis, we have proposed the following scheme for evaluating diagnostic criteria (Lerner et al., 1975).

1. High-Order Associations (H).
   A. Virus is isolated from the myocardium, endocardium, or pericardial fluid; or
   B. Type-specific virus is localized in the myocardium, endocardium, or pericardium at sites of pathologic change by methods of immunofluorescence or peroxidase-labeled antibody. These studies may be possible only at autopsy. Specimens must be properly taken and stored (−50°C), but cannot be placed in formalin.

   H-order associations are strengthened if virus isolated from the myocardium produces similar heart disease in an experimental model (for example, mouse).
2. Moderate-Order Associations (M): (moderate probability of a true positive diagnosis):
   A. Virus is isolated from pharynx or feces, and a fourfold rise in type-specific neutralizing, hemagglutinating-inhibiting, or complement-fixing antibodies is demonstrated; or

Table 1. INFECTIOUS CAUSES OF MYOPERICARDITIS

Viruses
Adenoviruses
Cytomegalovirus
Enteroviruses (coxsackieviruses, Groups A and B, echoviruses, polioviruses)
Epstein-Barr virus
Hepatitis A virus
Herpes simplex viruses, Type 1 and Type 2
Influenza viruses A and B
Lymphocytic choriomeningitis virus
Mumps virus
Rubella virus
Vaccinia virus
Varicella-zoster virus

Bacteria
Actinomyces israelii
Corynebacterium diphtheriae
Neisseria gonorrhoeae
Neisseria meningitidis
Pasteurella (Francisella) tularensis
Pseudomonas pseudomallei
Staphylococcus aureus
Streptococcus pneumoniae
Streptococcus pyogenes
Various aerobic gram-negative bacilli
Bacteroides and *Peptostreptococci*

Mycobacteria
Mycobacterium chelonei
Mycobacterium tuberculosis

Fungi
Aspergillus sp.
Blastomyces dermatitidis
Candida sp.
Coccidioides immitis
Cryptococcus neoformans
Histoplasma capsulatum
Nocardia asteroides
Sporothrix schenckii

Parasites
Echinococcus granulosus
Entamoeba histolytica
Plasmodium sp.
Schistosoma sp.
Toxoplasma gondii
Treponema pallidum
Trichinella spiralis
Trypanosoma cruzi

Rickettsia
Rickettsia burnetii
Rickettsia mooseri
Rickettsia rickettsii

Other
Chlamydia psittaci
Mycoplasma pneumoniae

B. Virus is isolated from pharynx or feces, and a concomitant titer in serum of 1/32 or greater of type-specific immunoglobulin M (IgM) (mercaptoethanol-sensitive) neutralizing or hemagglutinating-inhibiting antibodies is demonstrated.

The evidence used to establish a moderate-order association (M) can attain a higher order of probability (H) if significant numbers of appropriate controls do not show the findings of 2A or 2B.

3. Low-Order Associations (L).
   A. Virus is isolated from pharynx or feces; or
   B. A fourfold rise in type-specific neutralizing, hemagglutinating-inhibiting, or complement-fixing antibodies is demonstrated; or
   C. A single serum shows a titer of 1/32 or greater of type-specific IgM (mercaptoethanol-sensitive) neutralizing or hemagglutinating-inhibiting antibodies.

A low-order association (L) can attain a higher (M) order of probability if significant numbers of appropriate controls do not show the findings of 3A, 3B, or 3C. For instance, a CF titer $>1/32$ is more suggestive of a recent infection if <5 per cent age-matched controls have titers $\geq 1/32$.

Only high-order associations can be accepted as firm evidence for a viral infection as the etiology of myopericarditis.

High-order associations with acute myocardiopathies have been established in man for coxsackieviruses Group A, Types 4 and 16; coxsackieviruses Group B, Types 1, 2, 3, 4, 5, and 6; and echoviruses, Types 9, 11, and 22 (Table 2). Lower degrees of evidence are available for coxsackieviruses Group A, Types 1, 2, 5, 8, and 9; and echoviruses, Types 1, 4, 6, 7, 14, 16, 19, 25, and 30. Therefore, we conclude that coxsackieviruses belonging to Group B (Types 1 through 6) are established causes of virus myocardiopathy. There are also data implicating certain coxsackieviruses belonging to Group A and some echoviruses (Table 2). Coxsackieviruses may cause 23 per cent of acute virus myocardiopathies (Bell and Grist, 1968). No estimate of the proportion of cases due to echoviruses is available (Bell and Grist, 1970).

A characteristic postvaccinial myopericarditis has been observed 10 to 14 days after primary smallpox vaccination. Severe local reactions have occurred, but generalized vaccinia is not accompanied by heart disease. When congestive heart failure ensues, it responds dramatically to corticosteroids, digoxin, and diuretics without sequelae (Matthews and Griffith, 1974).

Bacteria. Significant changes in the incidence of several bacterial pathogens in purulent pericarditis were shown in an 86-year review of autopsy experience with 200 patients at the Johns Hopkins Medical institutions by Klacsmann, Bulkley, and Hutchins (Klacsmann et al., 1977). They studied 145 patients with purulent pericarditis at Johns Hopkins from 1889 through 1943 (Group 1) and compared them with 56 patients admitted since 1943 (Group 2). The median age of patients in Group 1 was 22 years, but it was 49 years in the later period. Whereas 80 per cent of the cases formerly were caused by aerobic, gram-positive cocci (*Streptococcus pneumoniae, Staphylococcus aureus, Streptococcus pyogenes*), these organisms accounted for 44 per cent of the cases since 1943. On the other hand, gram-negative bacilli (*E. coli, Proteus* sp., and *Pseudomonas aeruginosa, Salmonella* sp., *Shigella* sp., *Neisseria meningitidis*) were 39 per cent in Group 2, but only 5 per cent in Group 1. This remarkable increase in the occurrence of gram-negative bacilli in Group 2 was due to more infections with *E. coli, Proteus,* and *Pseudomonas.*

Mycobacteria. The number and percentage of cases of tuberculous pericarditis varies with the prevalence of tu-

Table 2. COXSACKIEVIRUSES OR ECHOVIRUSES ASSOCIATED WITH ACUTE PHASE OF VIRUS MYOCARDIOPATHY

Enterovirus		Order of Association*
Coxsackieviruses A		
Types	1	L, M
	2	L, M
	4	H
	5	L, M
	8	L, M
	9	L, M
	16	H
Coxsackieviruses B		
Types	1	H
through	6	
Echoviruses		
Types	1	L, M
	4	L, M
	6	L, M
	7	L, M
	9	H
	11	H
	14	L, M
	16	L, M
	19	L, M
	22	H
	25	L, M
	30	L, M

*L = low; M = moderate; H = high.

berculosis in the region. There are rare postoperative infections of the pericardium and mediastinum due to rapid growing mycobacteria—for example, *M. chelonei.*

Fungi. *Candida* and *Aspergillus* pericarditis occur in immunocompromised patients receiving cancer chemotherapy (Franklin et al., 1976). *Histoplasma capsulatum* uncommonly causes pericarditis either as an isolated infection or as part of disseminated disease.

PATHOGENESIS AND PATHOLOGY. The anatomy of the pericardium has an influence on both the pathogenesis of infection and the physiologic consequences of infection. The parietal pericardium separates the heart and proximal segments of the main vessels (aorta, pulmonary artery and veins, superior and inferior vena cava) from surrounding mediastinal tissues. A central tendon fuses the diaphragm with the pericardium. Laterally, *the parietal pericardium* is separated by pleura from the external surface of the lungs. On each side, a phrenic nerve passes vertically between the membranes of pleura and pericardium. The *visceral pericardium* is continuous with interstitial tissues of the myocardium. The pericardial sac normally contains 15 to 20 ml of clear fluid (Hipona and Paredes, 1976).

A fine capillary endomyocardial lymphatic system arises in the endocardium and interstitial areas of the myocardium and condenses into collecting channels subjacent to myocardial fibers. Lymphatic channels coalesce to form tertiary lymphatic vessels, or lymphatic trunks, which again join at the epicardium in a septal lymphatic system. The subepicardial tissues, therefore, have a diffuse lymphatic network.

Lymph flows from endocardial and interstitial myocardium to epicardial lymphatics, and, finally, to tracheobronchial lymph nodes in the mediastinal collecting system. The parietal pericardium has no lymphatics (Kline, 1969; Miller, 1970; Cohen, 1976; Drinker and Field, 1931).

Pathologic Physiology of Pericardial Effusion. Blockade of lymphatics in the mediastinum *plus* epicardium causes pericardial effusion. Impedance of venous drainage from the heart at the coronary sinus facilitates formation of pericardial effusion. Isolated mediastinal lymphatic obstruction causes pleural effusion but not pericardial effusion.

Pathologic Anatomy

Virus Pericarditis. Usually, both pericardium and myocardium are simultaneously affected (myopericarditis). Clinically, there may be predominantly myocarditis or pericarditis. The acute process may be benign with a mixed inflammatory response limited to interstitial areas of the heart and indistinguishable from acute rheumatic fever with carditis (Fig. 1). In benign myopericarditis, muscle-cell necrosis is minimal and recovery is anatomically and physiologically complete. An intervening ventricular arrhythmia can lead to death, but this is unusual. Virulent infections have varying degrees of interstitial myocarditis and myocardial cellular necrosis. Lesions heal with permanent scar and sometimes with myocardial calcification. Virus-induced myocardial necrosis is indistinguishable from that of myocardial infarction secondary to coronary atherosclerosis and thrombosis (Woods et al., 1975). Of course, in virus myocarditis, coronary arteries and veins are patent, and vasculitis is absent. Coronary atherosclerosis does not prevent, however, supervening virus myocarditis.

The special tropism of enteroviruses for the human heart is virus-specific, genetically determined by the histocompatibility type of the host, and age-specific. These viruses

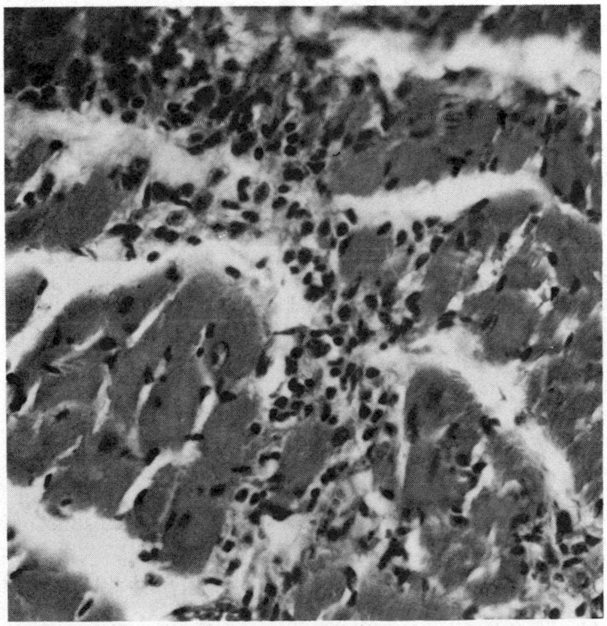

Figure 1. Benign coxsackievirus A9 myocarditis (acute infectious phase of myocardiopathy). With this virus strain, complete healing occurs without sequelae; there is no late noninfectious phase. Myocarditis was induced by coxsackievirus A9, strain 711, in 8-month-old Swiss mice by intraperitoneal inoculation of $10^5 TCD_{50}$. An area of moderate focal inflammation was seen after 9 days. (Reprinted from Progress in Medical Virology, by permission.)

attach as the result of specific interaction between outer capsid viral protein and enterovirus receptors on cell membranes. The subunit structure of the outer protein capsid (capsomeres) determines species, tissue, and age specificities for infection, as well as antigenicity. Enterovirus receptors on cell membranes are present in limited number (1 to 10 × 10^4 per cell). Coxsackievirus B all share the same receptor, but this is distinct from the poliovirus receptor. Adenoviruses Types 2 and 5 also share the coxsackievirus B receptor (Lonberg-Holm et al., 1976).

Infections with enteroviruses are common. By adult life, most people in the United States have neutralizing antibodies to many of the viruses. Contagium spreads from person to person by the fecal-oral route. (Transplacental spread of coxsackievirus and echoviruses also occurs.) Spread to the heart is presumably hematogenous and occurs at about 5 per cent of all symptomatic coxsackievirus infections.

Once myopericarditis is established, it may progress to death (especially in newborns), or it may be self-limited, or relapsing. There is both clinical and experimental evidence to suggest that the inflammatory reaction is due to an immunopathologic process (Wilson et al., 1969). During the early stages of the infection in the mouse model of myopericarditis, viruses are shed from the cell surface through vacuoles that fuse with the plasma membrane. Virus is discharged from infected cells as they lyse. Later in the process, myonecrosis results from the activity of cytotoxic T-lymphocytes. B-lymphocytes and macrophages do not play an important role (Lerner, 1969; Wong et al., 1977).

There is evidence that stress, such as forced swimming, enhances viral virulence, especially with coxsackievirus B3. The myocardium transforms into a wholly necrotic, inflamed, calcified mass (Fig. 2). This is accompanied by increased replication of the virus (Gatmaitan et al., 1970). The mechanism of this reaction to stress is unknown, but interferon production is delayed. Exercise is also a potent immunosuppressive agent (Reyes and Lerner, 1976). Adrenal corticoids also exacerbate infection, and stress may act through that mechanism. Additional adverse influences on experimental myocarditis include genetic susceptibility of mice, pregnancy, male sex, and undernutrition (Grodums, 1972). Whether these factors contribute to human infection is not known. A composite view of the varied effects and mechanisms of virus infection of the heart may be summarized as follows. A benign coxsackievirus myopericarditis produces interstitial inflammation affecting the endomyocardial lymphatic network. When lymphatic obstruction occurs, pericardial effusion results. Myocyte necrosis does not occur in this animal model of disease and when lymphatic obstruction is relieved, pericarditis resolves, (e.g., coxsackievirus A9, adult Swiss mice). Healing is usually complete without any residue (Fig. 1, Lerner and Shaka, 1962), Kinetic curves of this multiplication of virus in the cardiac interstitium correlate directly with the inflammatory exudate. On the other hand, a similar productive infection with coxsackievirus B1 (or B4) in 24–28 hour-old Swiss mice induces focal transmural myocardial necrosis. If death does not ensue, survivors show ventricular aneurysms (Fig. 3) (Khatib, R., et al., 1982).

Finally, infection of 14 day old Swiss mice with coxsackievirus B2 (or B3) results in diffuse myocyte necrosis which is mediated by thymocyte-derived lymphocytes. A dilated type of cardiomyopathy is the end-point here, with atrial hypertrophy, thrombi, and myocardial fiber disintegration and replacement by fibrous scar. Pathologic changes concentrate in the left ventricle interventricular septum and atrioventricular junction (Fig. 4) (Reyes, M. P., et al., 1981; Reyes, M. P., et al., 1984).

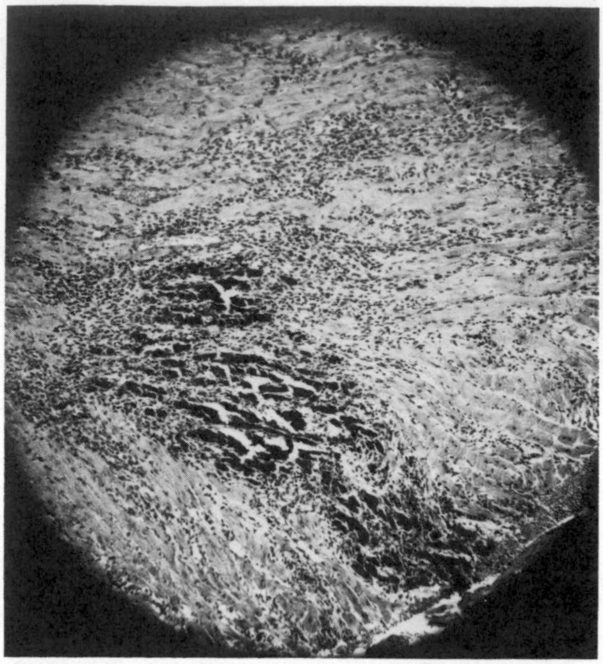

Figure 2. Effect of swimming on pathologic findings in acute coxsackievirus B3 myocardiopathy. The extensively involved myocardium of a 27-day-old mouse on the thirteenth day after infection is shown (HE × 90). (Reprinted from Progress in Medical Virology, by permission.)

Pyogenic Pericarditis. Acute purulent pericarditis induces a thickened (8 to 12 mm) pericardium usually containing 500 to 2000 ml of viscid fibrinous or frankly yellow purulent exudate and granulation tissue under varying degrees of tension. The left lower lung may be adherent

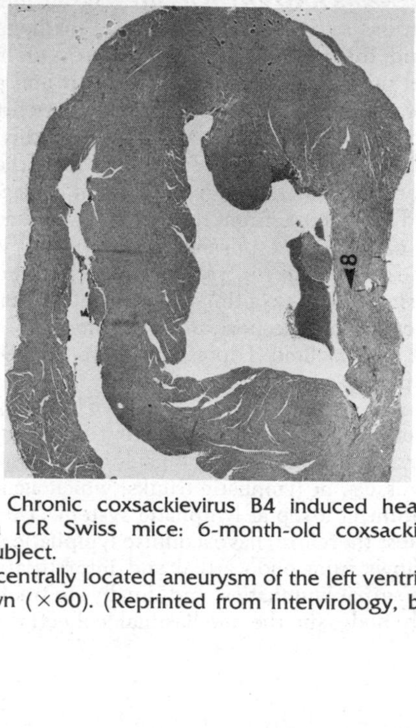

Figure 3. Chronic coxsackievirus B4 induced heart muscle disease in ICR Swiss mice: 6-month-old coxsackievirus B4 infected subject.

A large centrally located aneurysm of the left ventricle (arrow 8) is shown (×60). (Reprinted from Intervirology, by permission).

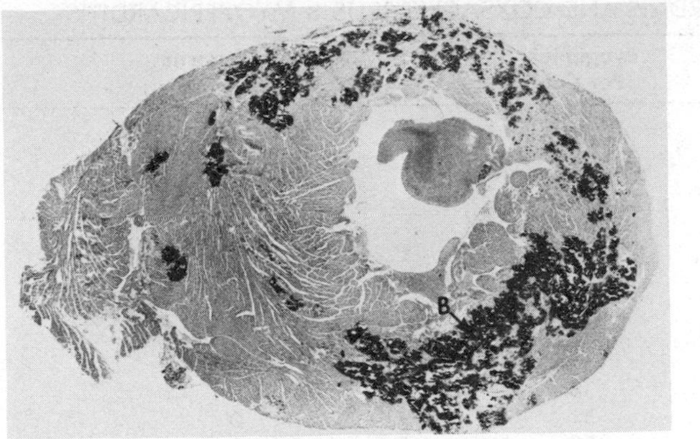

Infection +, exercize +, NS

Figure 4. A cross-section of the dilated cardiomyopathic heart of a Swiss mouse earlier infected with coxsackievirus B3 augmented by exercise. The black areas (arrow) show calcification of sites of myocyte necrosis anal drop-out. Pathologic changes are concentrated in the left ventricular wall.

to the thoracic wall. Pericardium is often adherent to myocardium and covered with "cottage-cheese-like" material. On the other hand, there may be a fibrinous granulomatous pericarditis and no free fluid (Liedtke et al., 1976; Cameron, 1975; Das and Ray, 1976).

Bacteria. Most adult patients who develop pyogenic pericarditis today have chronic underlying conditions or diseases (for example, recent thoracic surgery, chronic renal failure, carcinoma, myocardial infarctions, diabetes mellitus, myeloproliferative disorders, or sickle cell anemia) (Liedtke et al., 1976). In contrast to the preantibiotic era, primary infectious diseases in patients without underlying diseases account for only 22 per cent of the cases of purulent pericarditis since 1943 at the Johns Hopkins Medical Institutions. Pneumonia, meningitis, otitis media, subacute bacterial endocarditis, skin infections, and endometritis are primary infections that can spread to the pericardium. Extension of infection from the lung to the pericardium is now less common (20 per cent of cases versus 64 per cent before 1943), but perforating injury to the chest wall (for example, surgery, trauma) as a cause of pericarditis increased to 24 per cent from 4 per cent. Rupture of myocardial abscess, embolization from acute endocarditis, and extension from a subdiaphragmatic suppurative lesion are other routes of infection. Some patients with meningococcemia develop pericarditis 4 to 16 days after treatment begins. The exudate is sterile, and symptoms respond to anti-inflammatory drugs. This condition is believed to represent a hypersensitivity response to bacterial antigens (Morse et al., 1971).

Fungus Myopericarditis. These systemic infections often complicate cancer chemotherapy. The heart as well as the kidneys, gastrointestinal tract, lungs, brain, liver, and thyroid are often simultaneously affected. Opportunistic *Candida* and *Aspergillus* species are the most frequent. Myocardial abscesses are uniformly present. Palpable 3 to 15 mm white-yellow nodules with or without hyperemic borders distribute themselves randomly through both ventricles. Fibrinous pericarditis may also occur.

If histologic secretions are stained with periodic acid-Schiff or silver-methenamine stains, microcolonies of fungi can be seen in the pericardial and myocardial abscesses. Depending upon the patient's underlying disease, the inflammatory response varies from none to marked acute suppuration. Microcolonies may also infiltrate between myocardial fibers. Myocardial fibers can show coagulative necrosis. Coronary vessels occasionally are invaded by hyphae, but valves remain free (Franklin et al., 1976).

CLINICAL MANIFESTATIONS (Table 3). Regardless of the infectious agent, the symptoms and signs of myopericarditis are similar, except that bacterial disease is generally more dramatic than viral. In cases ascribed by Sainani, Dekate, and Rao to coxsackieviruses B, Types 2, 3, 4, or 5; dyspnea (16 of 19 patients); pain in the chest (15 of 19 patients); and malaise and fever (12 of 19 patients) were common, but cough, myalgia, arthralgia, preceding upper respiratory infections, nausea, vomiting, or diarrhea occurred in only a minority (Sainani et al., 1975).

All patients with pyogenic pericarditis have toxic signs and become acutely ill with anorexia, fever, chills, and chest pain. Physical findings also help differentiate pyogenic pericarditis from virus myopericarditis. Raised jugular venous pulsations (16 of 16 patients); adynamic pericardiums with impalpable apical pulses (16 of 16 patients); muffled heart sounds (15 of 16 patients); hepatomegaly (15 of 16 patients); paradoxic pulses (14 of 16 patients); and cardiac tamponade (14 of 16 patients) are the striking physical findings of pyogenic pericarditis (Klacsmann et al., 1977). Pleural effusions (9 of 16 patients), ascites (5 of 16 patients), and pitting edema (4 of 16 patients) are also more common in purulent pericarditis. None of these signs are common in coxsackievirus, Group B myopericarditis.

Pericardial friction rubs are heard to the left of the midsternal border while the patient is sitting up, leaning forward, and not breathing. The rubs are accentuated during inspiration or expiration and may be mono-, di- or tri-phasic, corresponding to atrial or ventricular systole or early ventricular diastole. At phonocardiogram, systolic murmurs or clicks may be detected. Pericardial or pleuropericardial friction rubs are often palpable (Spodick, 1971).

The heart may not be enlarged in patients with cardiac disability that results from virus cardiomyopathies. Further, there may be no pericardial rub, arrhythmia, congestive heart failure, questionable ischemic myocardial pain, or congestive heart failure. However, systolic time intervals may be prolonged, indicating myocardial dysfunction. The latter tests, along with the usual observations (clinical findings, EKG, chest x-ray, phonocardiogram, echocardiogram), should be used to follow convalescent patients (Weissler, 1974). Cardiac catheterization may be needed to confirm pulmonary embolization or restrictive/constrictive cardiomyopathies before decisions are made to perform pericardial drainage or decortication.

DIAGNOSIS

Microbiologic Diagnosis. In human enterovirus infections, virus often multiplies in the heart when the same virus is no longer recoverable from pharynx or feces, the initial sites of infection. When acute myocardiopathy is discovered, antibody titers may already have risen. On the other hand, if a chronic myocardiopathy has been induced, replicating virus may not even be present in the heart at the time of clinical presentation. The etiologic diagnosis of virus myocardiopathy is difficult.

Criteria for the diagnosis of enterovirus myopericarditis have been outlined (see *Etiologic Agents*). Rhesus-kidney

Table 3. CLINICAL FINDINGS IN PYOGENIC PERICARDITIS AND COXSACKIEVIRUS B MYOPERICARDITIS

	Pyogenic*† (Per Cent)	Coxsackiervirus B* (Per Cent)
SYMPTOMS/SIGNS		
Acutely ill (toxic, fever, dyspnea)	100*†	58
Raised jugular venous pulse	100	21
Enlarged cardiac dullness	100	74
Adynamic pericardium	100	11
Muffled heart sounds	94	11
Hepatomegaly	94	21
Paradoxic pulse	88	11
Cardiac tamponade	88	0
Pleural effusion	56	5
Pericardial friction rub	38	26
Ascites	31	0
Pitting edema	25	5
Apical systolic murmur	10	68
LABORATORY		
Polymorphonuclear leukocytosis	100	74
Enlarged cardiac silhouette	100	74
Abnormal EKG (low voltage; ↓ ST, ↑ ST segments)	100	100
Arrhythmia	rare	common
Pericardiocentesis with isolation of bacterium or virus from fluid	100*	rare
Pericardial fluid	exudate	usually exudate

*Estimates of occurrence of symptoms/signs are made from the following references: Klacsmann et al., 1977, and Sainani et al., 1975.

†Isolation of etiologic organism is routine prior to therapy. This is possible in only about 40% of cases of tuberculous pericarditis.

cultures and intraperitoneal inoculation of suckling mice are best for isolation of enteroviruses from throat, rectal swabs, blood, or pericardial fluid. Enteroviruses are rarely recovered from pericardial fluid. Pyogenic pericarditis is proved by isolation of the causative bacteria at pericardiocentesis or from blood cultures. Tubercle bacilli are isolated from pericardial fluid in about 40 per cent of cases. Gram, acid-fast, and methenamine silver stains of pericardial exudates must be examined.

Serologic Diagnosis. Within 3 days after onset of a virus myocardiopathy, IgM neutralizing antibodies are often found in sera, but, when bloods are taken several weeks later, fourfold rises in titers are often not demonstrable. IgM antibodies normally disappear from sera about 39 days later. Considerable cross-reacting IgM neutralizing antibody occurs among the coxsackievirus B serotypes. Schmidt, Magoffin, and Lenette demonstrated IgM antibody to Group B coxsackieviruses in 27 per cent of 148 patients with pericarditis, 25 per cent of 92 patients with myocarditis, and 8 per cent of 259 controls taken from age- and place-matched patients with pneumonia (Schmidt et al., 1973). The data were not diagnostic in the individual patient. These are M-order associations.

Chances for demonstrating significant increases in neutralizing antibodies to enteroviruses are greatly reduced if the titer in the acute-phase serum is 1/32 or greater. Neutralizing-antibody responses are highly type-specific in primary or initial infections with any of the five immunotypes of Group B coxsackievirus. However, in subsequent infections heterotypic responses occur with increasing frequency, and presumably arise from a booster effect of the current infecting virus on the level of antibodies to other enteroviruses with which the individual has previously been infected. Titers of heterotypic antibody frequently exceed those of homotypic antibody. Neutralizing antibodies to Group B coxsackievirus, Types 1 through 5, are frequently found at titers of 1/64 to 1/512 in patients without other evidence of current coxsackievirus infections. The prevalence of neutralizing antibody at these high residual titers precludes diagnosis on the basis of elevated neutralizing antibody in the absence of a fourfold or greater increase in titer. The finding of IgM antibodies is a reliable indicator of recent infection but does not preclude heterotypic reactions that may be of greater magnitude. However, even in initial infections with coxsackievirus, complement-fixing antibodies are invariably 7S immunoglobulins. Antibodies to heart muscle, γ-globulins bound to the myocardium, decreases in serum complement, and biologic false-positive serologic tests for syphilis have occasionally been found in patients with idiopathic myocardiopathies.

Other Laboratory Findings. Electrocardiograms in purulent and coxsackievirus B myopericarditis show low voltage and ST segment elevation and/or depression. On the other hand, left ventricular hypertrophy, systolic murmurs, and arrhythmias (sinus bradycardia, atrial fibrillation, complete heart block, and low voltage) are more frequent in viral myopericarditis. Leukocytosis, an enlarged cardiac silhouette, and an elevated erythrocyte sedimentation rate are frequent in both acute pyogenic and virus pericarditis.

Radiography. (Echocardiogram, Isotopic Scan, Angiocardiogram, Pericardiocentesis with Contrast Material).

A sonolucent space on echocardiograph (ultrasound) separating the ventricular wall motions from nonmoving pericardial echo indicates pericardial effusion. Echocardiograms validate the presence of significant pericardial effusion, but a negative examination does not exclude significant effusion. In fact, a pericardiocentesis has relieved severe cardiac tamponade after an echocardiogram failed to reveal a diagnostic sonolucent space.

Intravenous radioisotope (technetium-99 bound to serum

albumin or technetium-99 per technetate) outlines the intracardiac blood pool, and this is compared with the cardiac silhouette at chest x-ray. At angiocardiography, the distance between the endocardial surface of a cardiac chamber and its adjacent pericardial/pleural lung surface is determined.

At pericardiocentesis, contrast material may be injected directly into the pericardial sac.

Pericardiocentesis. Pericardiocentesis has the risk of hemopericardium and cardiac tamponade. This procedure is safer when done by a cardiothoracic surgeon in the operating room with electrocardiographic monitoring. Advice about inoculations for culture/stains of pericardial fluids should be obtained from physicians with special competence in infectious diseases.

Fenoglio et al. (1983) and Mason et al. (1980) have used endomyocardial biopsies for the diagnosis and treatment of recurring episodes of myopericarditis. If mononuclear inflammatory cells are seen in the sections, azathioprine or corticosteroids have been employed, but their value is unknown.

COMPLICATIONS. The possible courses that enteroviral myopericarditis may take are diagramed in Figure 5. This scheme is based on clinical observations and data obtained from experimental murine infections. The coxsackievirus B3 infections can produce permanent myocardial injury in mice (Wilson et al., 1969) that may progress to cardiomyopathy. The mild, focal infection produced by coxsackievirus A9 (Fig. 1) does not progress to congestive failure.

Roberts and Ferrans described idiopathic cardiomyopathies as (1) dilated and (2) hypertrophic (Roberts and Ferrans, 1975). In hypertrophic cases, the ventricular septum is often thicker than the free ventricular wall. There is indirect (low-order) serologic evidence that both forms may result from enteroviral infection. Some cases of myocarditis may affect the subendocardium (for example, mumps), resulting in endocardial fibroelastosis (St. Geme, Jr., et al., 1966). Recent observations suggest that myocardial infarction in patients with normal coronary arteries may be due to coxsackievirus infection (Desa'neto et al,. 1980).

The prognosis in purulent bacterial pericarditis is good if the specific etiologic diagnosis is made early and proper therapy instituted. At follow-up several months after treatment ended, only 3 of 16 patients had died, and those that recovered had no residua (Klacsmann et al., 1977).

Tuberculous pericarditis can progress to fibrosis and calcification. This process causes constrictive pericarditis, and ultimately myocardial failure.

TREATMENT

Purulent Pericarditis. Purulent pericarditis is a medical and surgical emergency because of the tendency for cardiac tamponade and shock to develop rapidly. Pericardial drainage by pericardiostomy is rarely sufficient (Das and Ray, 1976). Decortication is usually necessary in order to drain adequately the otherwise closed space and to prevent the development of adhesive pericarditis and later constriction. Antibacterial therapy for 4 to 6 weeks (Table 4) is necessary. Local instillation of antibiotics into the pericardial sac is not indicated.

Tuberculous Pericarditis. This complication of tuberculosis is treated with the same antituberculous agents that are used to treat pulmonary infection. However, adrenal corticosteroids are also indicated and should be given promptly. They promote the reabsorption of the effusion and reduce the risk of constrictive pericarditis (Rooney et al., 1970). If the diagnosis is not made until constrictive pericarditis has already developed, then surgical excision

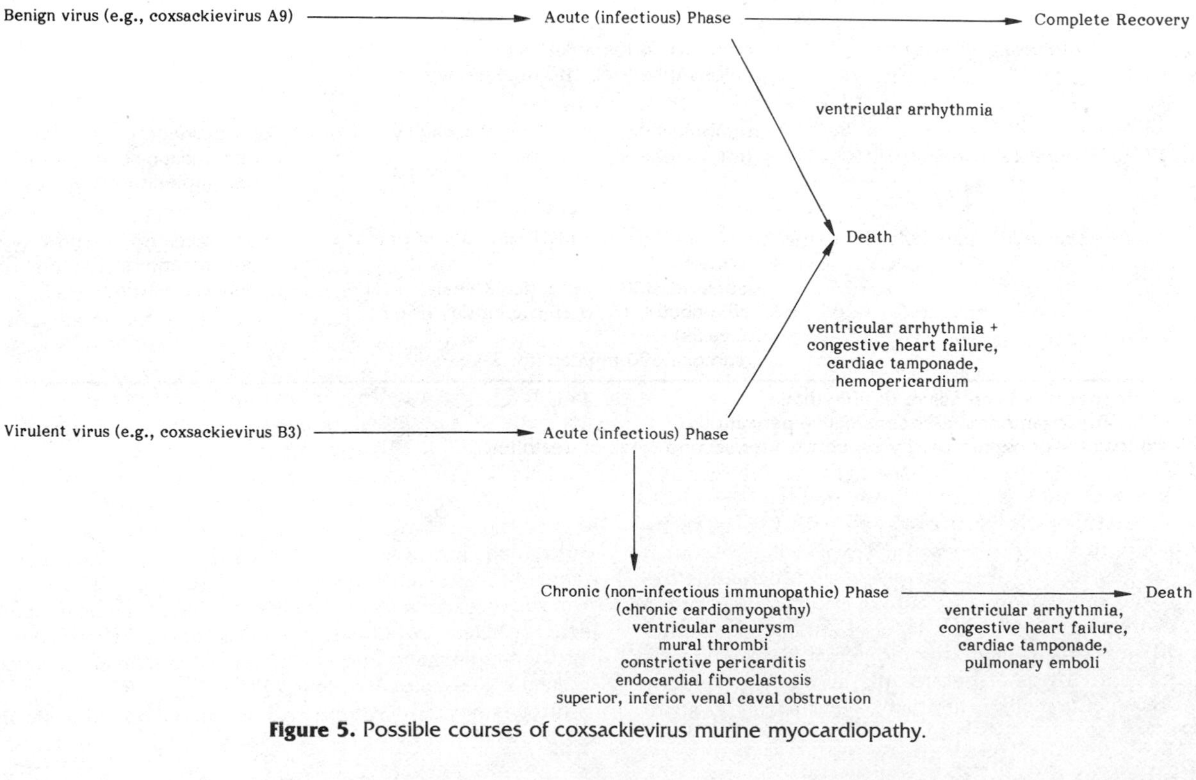

Figure 5. Possible courses of coxsackievirus murine myocardiopathy.

Table 4. TREATMENT OF ENTEROVIRUS MYOPERICARDITIS AND PURULENT PERICARDITIS

Etiologic Agent(s)	**Treatment**	
	Medical	***Surgical***
Enterovirus myopericarditis	Acute phase (first 14 days of disease). Avoid: corticosteroids, anti-coagulants, exercise, alcohol.	Pericardiocentesis†
	Use: digitalis, diuretics, antiarrhythmic agents.*	Pericardiocentesis† or pericardiectomy†
	Chronic phase (after 14 days of disease). Corticosteroids (see text); otherwise as for acute phase	
Purulent pericarditis		
Gram-positive cocci		
Staphylococcus aureus *Streptococcus pneumoniae* *Streptococcus pyogenes*	Penicillin G: 30,000,000 u/day, I.V. (for 4 to 6 weeks) or Methicillin, 1.5 g I.V., q 4 h (for 4 to 6 weeks) for resistant staphylococci	Tube drainage†/ decortication†/ pericardiectomy†
Gram-negative bacilli *Esch. coli, Proteus, Enterobacter, Pseudomonas*	Two appropriate antibiotics: carbenicillin, 20 to 30 g/day, I.V. (for 4 to 6 weeks) gentamicin, 3 to 5 mg/kg/day, I.V. in 3 divided doses‡ (for at least 2 weeks) amikacin, 15 mg/kg/day, I.V. in 2 divided doses (for at least 2 weeks). cephalothin, 1.5 g q 4 h I.V. (for 4 to 6 weeks) ampicillin, 1.5 g q 4 h, I.V. (for 4 to 6 weeks)	Tube drainage†/ decortication†/ pericardiectomy†/
Hemophilus influenza b	ampicillin, 400 mg/kg/day chloramphenicol, 100 mg/kg/day	
Fungi *(Aspergillus, Candida)*	Amphotericin B, 20 to 45 mg/kg/day I.V. (for 10 weeks)	Tube drainage†/ decortication†/ pericardiectomy†
Mycobacterium tuberculosis	Corticosteroids (see text) plus two of the following: isoniazid, 300 mg/day (for 2 years) ethambutol, 15 to 25 mg/kg/day (for 2 years) rifampin, 600 mg/day (for 2 years)	Tube drainage†/ decortication†/ pericardiectomy†

*Use for congestive heart failure or arrhythmia.
†Use for cardiac tamponade/or constrictive pericarditis.
‡Watch for oto- or nephrotoxicity especially after second week of treatment.

of the fibrotic pericardium is required. Pericardiectomy may actually precipitate left ventricular failure in patients who have had long-standing pericardial constriction.

Enterovirus Pericarditis. No specific therapy is available. Once the diagnosis is suspected, patients are treated exactly as they would be with myocardial necrosis due to coronary atheromatous disease. Those without evidence of muscle necrosis should rest for about 30 days; others with destruction of muscle should rest for 3 months or more. Arrhythmias, congestive failure, angina-like pain, and cardiomegaly are all poor prognostic signs. Alcohol, strenuous exercise, and reserpine should be avoided during convalescence.

Adrenal corticosteroids are avoided during the acute infectious phase (about the first 14 days), but, if the disease lasts longer, patients should receive adrenal steroids. After an initial dose of 20 mg prednisone four times a day, the amount is decreased by 25 per cent weekly until the lowest effective dose is reached. At times, patients with congestive heart failure that is refractory to digitalis and diuretics respond dramatically to prednisone.

Fungal Pericarditis. Intravenous amphotericin B is given for 4 to 6 weeks in *Candida* or *Aspergillus* myocarditis (Table 4).

Parasitic Pericarditis. American trypanosomiasis (Chagas' disease), trichinosis, toxoplasmosis, amebiasis, and echinococcosis are systemic parasitic diseases sometimes producing myopericarditis (Turner, 1975). Treatment is that of the systemic disease. Echinococcal cysts of the heart must be carefully removed surgically to avoid anaphylaxis and allergic phenomena resulting from dissemination of cysts to other organs, or their rupture into the pericardial cavity (Heyat et al., 1971).

References

Bell, E. J., and Grist, N. R.: Coxsackievirus infections in patients with acute cardiac disease and chest pain. Scott Med J 13:47, 1968.

Bell, E. J., and Grist, N. R.: Echoviruses, carditis, and acute pleurodynia. Lancet 1:326, 1970.

Cameron, E. W. J.: Surgical management of staphylococcal pericarditis. Thorax 30:678, 1975.

Cohen, J. L.: Neoplastic pericarditis. In Spodick, D. (ed): Pericardial Diseases. Philadelphia, F. A. Davis Co., 1976, p. 257.

Das, P. B., and Ray, D.: Surgical management of pyogenic pericarditis. International Surgery 61:483, 1976.

Desa'neto, A., Bullington, J. D., Bullington, R. H., Desser, K. B., and Benchimol, A.: Coxsackie B5 heart disease (Demonstration of inferolateral wall myocardial necrosis). Am J Med 68:295, 1980.

Drinker, C. K., and Field, M. E.: Absorption from pericardial cavity. J Exp Med 53:143, 1931.

Fenoglio, J. J., Ursel, P., Kellog, C. F., Dursin, R. E., and Weis, M. B.: Diagnosis and classification of myocarditis by endomyocardial biopsy. N Engl J Med 308:12, 1983.

Fowler, N. O., and Monitsas, G. T.: Infectious pericarditis. Prog Cardiovasc Dis 16:323, 1973.

Franklin, W. G., Simon, A. B., and Sodeman, T. M.: Candida myocarditis without valvulitis. Am J Cardiol 38:924, 1976.

Gatmaitan, B. G., Chason, J. L., and Lerner, A. M.: Augmentation of the virulence of murine coxsackievirus B-3 myocardiopathy by exercise. J Exp Med 131:1121, 1970.

Grist, N. R., and Bell, E. J.: A six-year study of coxsackievirus B infections in heart disease. J Hyg 73:165, 1974.

Grodums, E. I.: The effect of reserpine upon experimental coxsackievirus B-3 infection in mice. Can J Microbiol 18:577, 1972.

Heyat, J., Mokhtari, H., Hajaliloo, J., and Shakibi, J. G.: Surgical treatment of echinococcal cyst of the heart. Report of a case and review of the world literature. J Thorac Cardiovasc Surg 61:755, 1971.

Hipona, F. A., and Paredes, S.: The radiology of pericardial disease. In Spodick, D. (ed): Pericardial Diseases. Philadelphia, F. A. Davis Co., 1976, p. 91.

Khatib, R., Chason, J. L., Silberberg, B. K., and Lerner, A. M.: Age-dependent pathogenicity of group B coxsackieviruses in Swiss-Webster mice: Infectivity for myocardium and pancreas. J Infect Dis 14 (3):343, 1980.

Khatib, R., Chason, J. L., and Lerner, A. M.: A mouse model of transmural myocardial necrosis due to coxsackievirus B4: Observations over 12 months. Intervirology 18:197, 1982.

Klacsmann, P. G., Bulkley, B. H., and Hutchins, G. M.: The changed spectrum of purulent pericarditis. An 86-year autopsy experience in 200 patients. Am J Med 63:666, 1977.

Kline, I. K.: Lymphatic pathways in the heart. Arch Path 88:638, 1969.

Lerner, A. M.: Coxsackievirus myocardiopathy. J Infect Dis 120:496, 1969.

Lerner, A. M., and Shaka, J. A.: Coxsackie A9 myocarditis in adult mice. Proc Soc Exper Bio and Med 111:804, 1962.

Lerner, A. M., Wilson, F. M., and Reyes, M. P.: Enteroviruses and the heart (with special emphasis on the probable role of coxsackieviruses, group B types 1-5). II. Observations in humans. Mod Concepts Cardiovasc Dis 44:11, 1975.

Liedtke, A. J., DeJoseph, R. L., and Zelis, R.: Echocardiographic observations in inflammatory pericarditis. Ann Intern Med 84:573, 1976.

Lonberg-Holm, K., Crowell, R. L., and Philipson, L.: Unrelated animal viruses share receptors. Nature 259:679, 1976.

Mason, J. W., Billingham, M. E., and Ircci, D. R.: Treatment of acute inflammatory myocarditis assisted by endomyocardial biopsy. Am J Cardiol 45:1037, 1980.

Matthews, A. W., and Griffiths, I. D.: Postvaccinial pericarditis and myocarditis. Br Heart J 36:1043, 1974.

Miller, A. J.: Some observations concerning pericardial effusions and their relationship to the venous and lymphatic circulation of the heart. Lymphology 3:76, 1970.

Morse, J. R., Onetsky, M. T., and Hudson, J. A.: Pericarditis as a complication of meningococcal meningitis. Ann Intern Med 74:212, 1971.

Reyes, M. P., Ho, K. L., Smith, F., and Lerner, A. M.: A mouse model of dilated-type cardiomyopathy due to coxsackievirus B3. J Infect Dis 144:232, 1981.

Reyes, M. P., and Lerner, A. M.: Interferon and neutralizing antibody in sera of exercised mice with coxsackie B-3 myocarditis. Proc Soc Exp Biol Med 151:333, 1976.

Reyes, M. P., Smith, F. E., and Lerner, A. M.: An enterovirus-induced murine model of an acute dilated-type cardiomyopathy. Intervirology (in press, 1984).

Roberts, W. C., and Ferrans, V. J.: Pathologic anatomy of the cardiomyopathies. Idiopathic dilated and hypertrophic types, infiltrative types, and endomyocardial disease with and without eosinophilia. Human Path 6:287, 1975.

Rooney, J. J., Crocco, J. A., and Lyons, H. A.: Tuberculous pericarditis. Ann Intern Med 72:73, 1970.

Sainani, G. S., Dekate, M. P., and Rao, C. P.: Heart disease caused by coxsackievirus B infection. Br Heart J 37:819, 1975.

Schmidt, N. J., Magoffin, R. L., and Lennette, E. H.: Association of group B coxsackieviruses with cases of pericarditis, myocarditis, or pleurodynia by demonstration of immunoglobulin M antibody. Infect Immun 8:341, 1973.

Spodick, D. H.: Acoustic phenomena in pericardial disease. Am Heart J 81:114, 1971.

St Geme, Jr., J. W., Noren, G. R., and Adams, Jr., P.: Proposed embryopathic relation between mumps virus and primary endocardial fibroelastosis. N Engl J Med 275:339, 1966.

Turner, J. A.: Parasitic causes of pericarditis. West J Med 122:307, 1975.

Weissler, A. M.: Noninvasive cardiology. Clinical cardiology monographs. New York, Grune & Stratton, 1974.

Wilson, F. M., Miranda, Q. R., Chason, J. L., and Lerner, A. M.: Residual pathologic changes following murine coxsackie A and B myocarditis. Am J Path 55:253, 1969.

Wong, C. Y., Woodruff, J. J., and Woodruff, J. F.: Generation of cytotoxic T lymphocytes during coxsackievirus B-3 infection. II. Characterization of effector cells and demonstration of cytotoxicity against viral-infected myofibers. J Immunol 118:1165, 1977.

Wood, J. D., Nimmo, M. J., and Mackay-Scollay, E. M.: Acute transmural myocardial infarction associated with active coxsackievirus B infection. Am Heart J 89:283, 1975.

215

KAWASAKI SYNDROME (THE MUCOCUTANEOUS LYMPH NODE SYNDROME)

MARIAN E. MELISH, M.D.

Kawasaki syndrome or the mucocutaneous lymph node syndrome (MCLS, MLNS) is an acute, febrile, exanthematous childhood illness of unknown etiology. It was first recognized in Japan by Dr. Tomisaku Kawasaki in 1967 (Kawasaki, 1967; Kawasaki et al., 1974). Since its first description, more than 25,000 cases have been reported to the national research committee from all over Japan.

The disease was recognized independently in Hawaii by Melish, Hicks, and Larson, who encountered 12 cases between 1971 and 1974 (Melish et al., 1974, 1976, 1979). Without knowledge of the Japanese experience, these American workers independently identified the same diagnostic criteria. Since 1974, Kawasaki syndrome has been recognized worldwide in children of all racial and ethnic groups, but the highest prevalence has been reported among Japanese children in Japan and Hawaii (Melish et al., 1979).

ETIOLOGY. The etiology of Kawasaki syndrome is unknown. No bacterial or viral agent has been isolated consistently; reports of a rickettsial etiology have not been confirmed. Nevertheless, Kawasaki syndrome is suspected to have a microbial component because the sudden onset of a febrile, largely self-limited, exanthematous disease strongly resembles an infectious disease. A pronounced tendency for time-space clusters of cases also favors an infectious etiology.

CLINICAL MANIFESTATIONS, COMPLICATIONS, AND SEQUELAE. The diagnosis of Kawasaki syndrome is based on strict adherence to clinical criteria and exclusion of other clinically similar diseases. The principal diagnostic criteria are listed in Table 1. To fit the diagnosis of Kawasaki syndrome, the patient should meet five of the six criteria. In practice, most patients have all of the first five criteria, whereas the sixth, lymphadenopathy, is seen in 70 per cent of cases or less.

Table 1. PRINCIPAL DIAGNOSTIC CRITERIA

1. Fever, persisting for greater than 5 days (mean 11 days), usually > 39°C
2. Conjunctival injection without purulent exudate or corneal involvement
3. Changes in the mouth consisting of:
   (a) Erythema, fissuring, and crusting of the lips
   (b) Diffuse oropharyngeal erythema
   (c) "Strawberry" tongue
4. Changes in the peripheral extremities consisting of:
   (a) Induration and swelling of hands and feet during acute febrile stage
   (b) Erythema of palms and soles during acute febrile stage
   (c) Desquamation of finger and toetips approximately two weeks after onset of fever progressing to extensive peeling of palms and soles
   (d) Transverse grooves across fingernails two to three months after onset
5. Erythematous rash of morbilliform, multiforme, urticarial, or scarlatiniform character
6. Enlarged lymph node mass measuring greater than 1.5 cm in diameter, usually unilateral in the cervical region.

The clinical course of the illness is best described as triphasic with an acute febrile phase, a subacute phase, and a convalescent phase. Fever is generally the first sign of illness and is followed within one to three days by discrete vascular injection of bulbar conjunctivae, changes in the mouth, hands, and feet, an erythematous rash, and lymphadenopathy. The most distinctive features of the syndrome are moderate, often painful, swelling and firm induration of the hands and feet. The skin is so tightly stretched and shiny that it resembles acute scleroderma with fusiform swelling of the fingers. The palms and soles take on a diffuse, deep red-purple color during the acute stage. The erythematous rash is diffuse and may be morbilliform, urticarial, polymorphous, or scarlatiniform, but not vesicular, bullous, or petechial. The associated features of aseptic meningitis, diarrhea, and hepatic dysfunction may occur during the acute phase. Children are moderately to severely ill, extremely irritable, and anorectic throughout this acute period.

After a mean of 11 days (range 6 to 35) the fever, rash, and lymphadenopathy subside, and the subacute phase begins. This stage is characterized by persistent anorexia, irritability, conjunctival injection, thrombocytosis, and desquamation of the palms and soles. The convalescent phase lasts from the time all signs of illness have disappeared until the sedimentation rate has returned to normal, usually six to eight weeks after onset.

The associated features of Kawasaki syndrome (Table 2) attest to the multisystem involvement of the disease. Pyuria/urethritis is seen in over two thirds of cases during the acute phase. Aseptic meningitis associated with irritability, lethargy, meningismus, or semicoma complicates the acute stage of about one fourth of patients. The cerebrospinal fluid (CSF) contains 25 to 100 white cells that are predominantly lymphocytes; the glucose and protein levels are normal. About one fourth of patients have diarrhea and abdominal pain. In approximately 10 per cent there is obstructive jaundice with mild elevations of the liver enzymes. Both American and Japanese patients have developed acute gallbladder hydrops late in the acute period. This complication is manifested by a right upper quadrant abdominal mass, which resolves spontaneously in two to three weeks. It can be monitored by repeated ultrasound examinations.

Table 2. ASSOCIATED FEATURES IN ORDER OF FREQUENCY

Pyuria and urethritis
Arthralgia and arthritis
Aseptic meningitis
Pericardial effusion
Diarrhea
Abdominal pain
Myocardopathy
Obstructive jaundice
Hydrops of gallbladder
Acute mitral insufficiency
Myocardial infarction

The most serious and important complications of Kawasaki syndrome are arthritis and cardiac involvement. Frank arthritis with erythema, warmth, edema, and effusion occurs in nearly 40 per cent of patients. Two patterns are observed. In one third of those with arthritis, multiple joints (>24) are involved, including both the large weight-bearing joints (knees, ankles, and hips) and the smaller joints (wrists and interphalangeal joints). Polyarticular involvement usually begins in the first week of illness. Oligoarticular involvement (two thirds of patients with arthritis) usually begins in the second and third weeks of illness. Large weight-bearing joints are involved. Joint fluid aspirate reveals a highly cellular fluid (frequently over 100,000 per mm^3) with a polymorphonuclear predominance. Immune complexes can be demonstrated in the joint fluid. Arthritis is entirely self-limited with an average duration of 2 weeks, but it may persist for several months.

Kawasaki syndrome was originally described as benign mucocutaneous lymph node syndrome because it was primarily a self-limited, febrile illness. By 1970 however, it had become obvious that 2 to 3 per cent of patients died suddenly, usually in the third to sixth week after onset with coronary aneurysms, acute coronary artery thrombosis, or massive myocardial infarction. It is now known that cardiac involvement ranges from relatively minor problems, gallop rhythm, first-degree heart block, minor arrhythmias, and pericardial effusions, to inflammatory myocarditis with congestive heart failure, mitral valve dysfunction, coronary aneurysm, and coronary thrombosis.

Cardiac complications are the only ones that may lead to death or permanent disability. Clinical cardiac disease with evidence of pericardial effusion, congestive heart failure, and/or mitral valve disease with insufficiency occurs in 10 to 15 per cent of patients. Overt cardiac complications may occur at any time during the first 4 weeks of illness. Nonfatal myocardial infarction is less frequent than a fatal outcome but may occur at any time from the second week to many years after onset. Biplanar electrocardiograms or coronary angiography of unselected patients demonstrate coronary artery dilatation or aneurysm in 15 to 25 per cent in the fourth week of illness. Coronary aneurysms are more common in younger infants, males, and patients with more severe clinical illness or congestive heart failure, but there are no clinical or laboratory features that reliably predict the presence of aneurysms. The natural history of coronary aneurysms has been studied by repeat angiography or echocardiography in both Japan and the United States. One half to two thirds of aneurysms regress with restoration of normal caliber of the arterial lumen within 12 to 18 months. Abnormalities (aneurysms and/or areas of stenosis or irregular arterial wall) persist in one third. The mechanism of regression is either massive intimal hypertrophy or thrombosis, recanalization, and organization. Late complications of myocardial infarction, angina pectoris, and coronary insufficiency occur almost exclusively in the group that have developed aneurysms by 4 weeks.

Laboratory abnormalities in Kawasaki syndrome are generally nonspecific and nondiagnostic. The white blood cell count is greater than 20,000 with a left shift in more than half the patients during the acute febrile phase. The sedimentation rate and C-reactive protein are uniformly elevated in the acute stage and gradually subside to normal six to ten weeks after the onset of fever. Unlike the white blood count, the platelet count is normal during the acute stage but rises after the tenth day to levels of 600,000 to 1.8 million by the fifteenth to twenty-fifth day of illness. Elevation of platelet count during this period is a universal feature of the disease. The period of the elevated platelet count is the period of greatest risk of coronary thrombosis. The SGOT and SGPT levels may also be modestly elevated. The SGOT, creatine phosphokinase and lactic dehydrogenase may be elevated in patients with myocarditis or myocardial infarction.

IgG, IgA, and IgM are normal early in the disease, but increase from weeks 2 to 5, and fall during convalescence. IgE may be normal or modestly to moderately elevated during weeks 2 to 5 (Kusakawa and Heiner, 1976). None of these tests has any diagnostic value. Complement levels are normal, antinuclear antibodies are absent, and rheumatoid factor is negative.

PATHOGENESIS AND PATHOLOGY. The pathologic changes of Kawasaki syndrome are better understood than the etiology. The cardinal pathologic feature is multisystem arteritis of the medium-sized muscular arteries. In fatal cases the most profound changes occur in the coronary arteries, with scattered and variable involvement of other blood vessels. The cardiac pathology varies with the stage of illness. The main changes in the few patients who have died during the first ten days of illness were pancarditis and acute perivasculitis of the coronary arteries and aorta. Intimal hypertrophy with edema, acute inflammatory infiltration, and fragmentation of the internal elastic lamina occurred during this period, but aneurysmal dilation was unusual, and the coronary arteries were patent. An inflammatory infiltrate was also noted in the AV conduction system of these patients. The cause of death was presumed to be cardiac arrythmia.

The most typical pathologic changes are seen in the hearts of children who die from day 15 to day 50, when more than 70 per cent of deaths occur. These patients have severe panvasculitis of the coronary arteries with coronary aneurysms. The immediate cause of death is either coronary thrombosis or rupture of the coronary aneurysm. Massive myocardial infarction may occur. Pericarditis, myocarditis, and endocarditis are less pronounced than in the early deaths, and some fatal cases have had a variable degree of extracardiac vasculitis (Fujiwara and Hamashima, 1978). The extraparenchymal portion of the musculoelastic arteries such as the mesenteric, adrenal, splenic, renal, and genital arteries is most frequently involved. Extracoronary aneurysms are rare but do occur, especially in the axillary and mesenteric arteries.

The pathologic features of fatal Kawasaki syndrome are indistinguishable from those of what had been known as infantile periarteritis nodosa (IPN) (Landing and Larson, 1976). IPN was a rare pathologic entity diagnosed only at autopsy. The clinical course of these patients was similar to that of patients with Kawasaki syndrome. Therefore, the Kawasaki syndrome appears to be the clinical expression of an illness that, in its most severe form (the 2 per cent who die), has the pathologic features of IPN. It is likely that similar but less severe vascular changes are present in the vessels of all children with the disease. Although the names are confusingly similar, IPN differs considerably from adult or classic periarteritis not only in the ages affected but also in the vessels involved (Landing and Larson, 1976).

Late deaths that occur from more than 50 days to years after the clinical illness are characterized by coronary scarring, aneurysms with recanalization, and old myocardial infarction with fibrosis. Active inflammation of vessels is not a feature of the late deaths, but the cardiac and vascular pathologic changes appear to be caused by the vasculitis of the acute episode. A few children with a history of Kawasaki syndrome who died from trauma or malignancy had intimal abnormalities with chronic thickening, disrupted internal elastic lamina, and other focal abnormalities of the coronary arteries.

Circulating immune complexes can be detected in the blood of 30 to 60 per cent of patients during the first 5 weeks of illness. Complement levels remain normal or are even elevated, and immune complexes are not deposited in skin and other tissues. The role of immune complexes in the pathogenesis of vascular lesions is uncertain. They may merely represent acute immunologic stimulation.

EPIDEMIOLOGY AND GEOGRAPHIC VARIATIONS IN DISEASE. Kawasaki syndrome is overwhelmingly a disease of young children. In Japan and in our series in Hawaii, the incidence peaks at 1 year of age with almost equal numbers affected in the first and second years of life. Eighty per cent of patients are less than 4 years of age, and the age-specific incidence declines steadily to age 8. Very few cases occur after 10 years of age. In Japan and Honolulu, males predominate by over 1.5:1 (Kawasaki et al., 1974; Melish et al., 1976; Landing and Larson, 1976). The epidemiology has been carefully studied in Japan, where the MCLS research committee of the Ministry of Health and Welfare has conducted seven nationwide surveys involving more than 47,000 patients. There were no clear geographic or urban-rural differences in the incidence of the disease in children aged 0 to 4 years. The reported yearly incidence has increased steadily since the survey began. There were no dramatic seasonal differences. Nearly all cases were sporadic with no evidence of secondary cases in the school, home, or neighborhood. In a small case-control study, affected children showed few important differences from neighborhood controls except that they were more likely to have had common colds and "viral" infections, or allergic rhinitis, at some time before the development of Kawasaki syndrome. Diet, general health, and environment were unremarkable and equivalent to that of controls (Yanigawa et al., 1983).

Community-wide outbreaks of disease with sharply increased incidence were first recognized in the United States, Japan, and Korea in the late 1970's. Outbreaks have been reported from several United States cities and two large nationwide outbreaks occurred in Japan in 1979 and 1982. In Hawaii, where active surveillance has been maintained for over a decade, outbreaks were seen in 1978, 1981, and 1983. In both Japan and Hawaii, years after epidemics have had an unusually low incidence of disease. Despite community-wide epidemics, neither person-to-person spread nor attendance at common events has been demonstrated.

Since its first description in the English language, Kawasaki syndrome has been reported worldwide among children of all racial groups. Outside of Japan, the highest incidence of disease has been reported from Hawaii. Clusters of cases have been encountered in the continental United States; scattered cases have been reported from other areas of the world. Among 280 cases in Hawaii, children of Japanese ancestry were markedly overrepresented compared with their proportion of the population; Caucasian children were markedly underrepresented. Chinese, Polynesian, and Filipino children and children of mixed race appeared to have an intermediate incidence (Melish et al., 1979). National surveillance data obtained by the Centers for Disease Control confirm that the incidence is highest in Orientals, intermediate in Blacks and Hispanics, and lowest in Caucasians (Bell et al., 1983). Nevertheless, in communities where Caucasians are numerically dominant, many Caucasian cases will be encountered.

Because this disease appears to be most prevalent in Japan and among Japanese children in Hawaii, a unique genetic susceptibility is suspected. HLA typing of cases compared with controls has given conflicting results. No single HLA antigen has been common to all cases. A report from Japan showing a modest excess in frequency of HLA antigen BW 22 subtype J_2 differs from the negative findings of three other studies.

DIAGNOSIS. The diagnosis of Kawasaki syndrome is entirely a clinical one based on firm adherence to the clinical criteria and exclusion of other possible causes. For example, leptospirosis and infection with streptococci and other bacteria should be ruled out by cultures and serology. Patients should meet five of the six principal diagnostic criteria (Table 1). The clinical course should also be typical. If hand and foot desquamation and thrombocytosis do not occur within 12 to 20 days after the onset of fever, the diagnosis of Kawasaki syndrome should be seriously questioned.

TREATMENT. Effective therapy for Kawasaki syndrome awaits discovery of its etiology and pathogenesis. The present treatment is supportive and consists of a careful program of repeated clinical and laboratory evaluations designed to detect and manage arthritis and serious cardiac and vascular abnormalities.

Since vasculitis is the major pathologic change, aspirin is an attractive therapeutic agent because it is anti-inflammatory and inhibits platelet aggregation. We have found that aspirin administered in standard anti-inflammatory doses of 80 to 100 mg/kg/day shortens the mean duration of fever. Approximately two thirds of patients become afebrile within two days of starting aspirin therapy; the remaining third remains febrile for several days (Melish et al., 1979). Once fever has been controlled or the platelet count has started to rise, the aspirin dose should be reduced to 5 to 10 mg/kg/day and continued for the additional six to eight weeks that the sedimentation rate remains elevated. This lower dose of aspirin should suppress platelet aggregation and inhibit formation of thromboxane A_2 with minimal suppression of prostacycline.

Corticosteroids have been used in the United States and Japan. Two recent controlled studies demonstrate that corticosteroids given orally on a daily basis are contraindicated because they were associated with an increased frequency of aneurysms in patients studied by routine aortography or echocardiography (Kato et al., 1979; Kusakawa, S., presented at Fuji Conference on Kawasaki Disease, Fuji, Japan, Oct. 29, 1983.) Corticosteroids may also increase the platelet count without decreasing platelet adhesiveness. For these reasons, corticosteroids are specifically contraindicated in Kawasaki syndrome.

Hospitalization during the acute febrile stage facilitates diagnostic testing, but patients can be managed as outpatients if they are seen frequently. Blood, urine, throat, and stool cultures must be obtained to exclude a treatable bacterial disease. Streptococcal infection should also be excluded by serial antistreptococcal antibody titers. If available, leptospiral cultures and serology should be obtained. Chest radiograph and EKG should be performed to monitor cardiac function. Careful follow-up with repeated physical examinations is mandatory to detect arthritis and cardiac disease, which may appear after the acute symptoms have cleared.

If cardiac decompensation occurs, the patient should be hospitalized for digitalization monitoring and anti-arrythmia therapy, if indicated. Biplanar echocardiography is a useful noninvasive method of detecting and evaluating aneurysms at the origin of the coronary arteries (Yoshida et al., 1979). In the early stage of the disease through the first 2 months after onset, echocardiography is nearly as sensitive as angiography for the detection of aneurysms. Later (2 months to several years after onset), angiography may be needed for patients with aneurysms to detect stenosis or peripheral coronary vessel disease, which may develop many months to years after the acute episode.

PROGNOSIS. In Japan approximately one per cent of children with Kawasaki syndrome die in the subacute or early convalescent phase. Ten to 20 per cent develop coronary aneurysms detectable by routine angiography or echocardiography. Resolution of angiographic abnormalities over a 1 year follow-up period has been noted in a third of those with aneurysms (Kato et al., 1981). Resolution does not indicate that the coronary vessels have returned to normal. Regression of the size of aneurysms results from either intimal hypertrophy or thrombosis, recanalization and organization (Kato, 1981). Stenosis is a frequent sequel and may cause angina pectoris, myocardial insufficiency, and infarction months to years after the acute episode. Kawasaki syndrome is self-limited in the overwhelming majority of patients. If cardiac damage is not detected by careful follow-up through the convalescent period, it is not likely to pose major clinical problems in the next three to five years. However, because some degree of coronary vasculitis may be present in all patients, long-term follow-up studies of complicated and uncomplicated cases are necessary to determine whether they may be susceptible to premature coronary atherosclerosis.

References

Bell, D. M., Morens, D. M., Holman, R. C., Hurwitz, E. S., and Hunter, M. K.: Kawasaki Syndrome in the United States 1976–1980. Am J Dis Child 137:211, 1983.

Fujiwara, H., and Hamashima, Y.: Pathology of the heart in Kawasaki disease, Pediatrics 61:100, 1978.

Kato, H., Ishinose, E., Yoshioka, F., Takachi, T., Matsunaga, S., Suzuki, K., and Rikitake, N.: Fate of coronary aneurysms in Kawasaki disease: Serial coronary angiography and long-term follow-up study. Am J Card 49:1758, 1982.

Kato, H., Koike, S., and Yokoyama, T.: Kawasaki disease: Effect of treatment on coronary artery involvement. Pediatrics 63:175, 1979.

Kato, H., Koike, S., Yamamoto, M., Ito, Y., and Yano, E.: Coronary aneurysms in infants and young children with acute febrile mucocutaneous lymph node syndrome. J Pediatr 86:892, 1975.

Kawasaki, T.: Acute febrile mucocutaneous syndrome with lymphoid involvement with specific desquamation of the fingers and toes. Jap J Allergy 16:178, 1967.

Kawasaki, T., Kosaki, F., Okawa, S., Shigematsu, I., and Yanagawa, H.: A new infantile febrile mucocutaneous lymph node syndrome (MLNS) prevailing in Japan. Pediatrics 54(3):271, 1974.

Kusakawa, S., and Heiner, D.: Elevated levels of immunoglobulin E in the acute febrile mucocutaneous lymph node syndrome. Pediat Res 10:108, 1976.

Landing, B. H., and Larson, E. J.: Are infantile periarteritis nodosa with coronary artery involvement and fatal mucocutaneous lymph node syndrome the same? Comparison of 20 patients from North America with patients from Hawaii and Japan. Pediatrics 59:651, 1976.

Melish, M. E., Hicks, R. M., and Dean, A. G.: Kawasaki syndrome in Hawaii (abstract). Pediat Res 13:451, 1979.

Melish, M. E., Hicks, R. M., and Larson, E. J.: Mucocutaneous lymph node syndrome in the United States (abstract). Pediat Res 8:427, 1974.

Melish, M. E., Hicks, R. M., and Larson, E. J.: Mucocutaneous lymph node syndrome in the United States. Am J Dis Child 130:599, 1976.

Yoshida, H., Funabashi, T., Nakaya, S., and Taniguchi, N.: Mucocutaneous lymph node syndrome: A cross-sectional echocardiographic diagnosis of coronary aneurysms. Am J Dis Child 133:1244, 1979.

216

DENGUE AND OTHER HEMORRHAGIC FEVERS

ABRAHAM I. BRAUDE, M.D., PH.D.

AMORN LEELARASAMEE, M.D.

The hemorrhagic fevers are a collection of diverse epidemic virus infections transmitted by arthropod bites or contact with rodents. They are severe, life-threatening illnesses with fever, thrombocytopenia, hemorrhages, shock, and neurologic disturbances.

ETIOLOGY. The viruses known to cause the hemorrhagic fever syndrome are shown in Table 1. They belong mainly to the families Togaviridae and Arenaviridae. The viruses causing dengue, Kyasanur forest disease, Omsk hemorrhagic fever, and yellow fever belong to the genus *Flavivirus* in the togavirus family; and Junin, Lassa, Muchupo, and Pichinde viruses are arenaviruses. The virus of Crimean hemorrhagic fevers is classified as a Bunyavirus (Viral Hemorrhagic Fever, 1983). The virus of hemorrhagic fever with renal syndrome closely resembles members of the bunyaviruses, especially with respect to its tripartite, single-stranded RNA genome (Schmaljohn et al., 1983).

Marburg and Ebola viruses have striking similarities in size, shape, and ultrastructure that they share with no other viruses. For this reason, they are considered the first representatives of a new group. Their superficial similarity to rabies virus does not warrant their classification as a rhabdovirus. The togaviruses are described in Chapter 66, the arenaviruses in Chapter 67, the bunyaviruses in Chapter 8, and Marburg-Ebola viruses in Chapter 71.

The viruses spread by arthropods are also placed in a category known as the *Arbovirus group*. This grouping, based on transmission, is considered useful, even though nearly all members are characterized well enough by modern methods to be classified according to the taxonomic scheme in Chapter 8. Two groups of arthropods are responsible for transmission: ticks and mosquitoes (Table 1). The mosquito *Aedes aegypti* is the main vector of dengue, yellow fever, and chikungunya fever, although other species of *Aedes* have been shown occasionally to carry dengue

Table 1. VIRAL CLASSIFICATION OF HEMORRHAGIC FEVERS

Virus (Family:Genus)		Disease	Vector
Togaviridae:	*Flavivirus*	Dengue	*Aedes aegypti* (and other mosquitoes)
		Kysasanur forest disease	*Haemaphysalis* (ticks)
		Omsk hemorrhagic fever	*Dermacentor* (ticks)
		Yellow fever	*Aedes aegypti*
Togaviridae:	*Alphavirus*	Chikungunya fever	*Aedes aetypti*
Bunyaviridae:	Possible member Crimean hemorrhagic fever Congo virus	Crimean hemorrhagic fever	*Hyalomma marginatum* (ticks)
	Probable member, Hantaan virus	Hemorrhagic fever with renal syndrome	*Apodemus agrarius coreae*
Arenaviridae:	*Arenavirus*		
	Junin virus	Argentine hemorrhagic fever	*Calomys* laucha*
	Lassa virus	Lassa fever	*Mastomys natalensis*
	Machupo virus	Bolivian hemorrhagic fever	*Calomys callosus*
Marburg-Ebola group:			
	Marburg virus	Marburg virus disease	Unknown
	Ebola virus	Ebola virus disease	Unknown

*The species *Calomys* comprises wild mice and *Mastomys* house rats.

and yellow fever viruses. Because *A. aegypti* is a domestic mosquito, it spreads disease in urban areas. The cycles for transmission of dengue and chikungunya viruses appear to involve only human beings and mosquitoes. Yellow fever virus, on the other hand, is transmitted from monkey to monkey, from monkey to person, and from person to person. Lassa, Ebola, Marburg, and Crimean-Congo hemorrhagic fevers can also be transmitted from person to person.

PATHOGENESIS AND PATHOLOGY. Not every patient infected with the hemorrhagic fever viruses develops the hemorrhagic fever syndrome. On the contrary, benign febrile illnesses may be the only clinical evidence of infection, and the reason why other patients develop increased vascular permeability and come down with lethal hemorrhages and shock is largely a mystery. This question has been studied most extensively in dengue, a disease in which a child with an apparently benign fever may suddenly develop severe abdominal pain, intestinal bleeding, and shock. There appear to be three factors in the pathogenesis of dengue hemorrhagic shock. One of these is the existence of four serotypes of dengue virus. The second is the presence on these four serotypes of cross-reacting antigenic determinants that give no lasting protection against heterologous serotypes. The third is a previous dengue infection. Infection with the first serotype sensitizes the child to produce a secondary type of immune response to infection with the second serotype, so that IgG is generated. This IgG is believed to bind but not neutralize the heterologous serotype of dengue virus. There is evidence that such ineffectual neutralization by bound antibody not only enhances the growth of virus but also produces damage by immune complexes composed of IgG and viral antigen (Sobel et al., 1975; Theofilopoulos et al., 1976). Growth enhancement would occur when virus antibody complexes are attached to human monocytes by their Fc receptors so that entry into the cell is facilitated. Damage from immune complexes has been attributed to complement activation (Russel, 1971). During the shock stage of dengue infections, blood levels of complement components Clq, C3, C4, C5–C8, and C3 proactivator were depressed (Bokish et al., 1973), and there were low levels of blood-clotting Factor XII (Hageman factor) and activation of intravascular clotting. From these data, a hypothesis has been formulated that proposes that massive viral synthesis produces excess viral antigen for complexing with IgG, that the complexes activate complement to provide C3A and C5A, and that these complement-cleavage products increase capillary permeability by their anaphylatoxin activity (i.e., release of histamine and other mediators from mast cells). The immune complexes can also produce intravascular coagulation, a prominent finding in some cases at autopsy.

The malignant form of dengue has appeared mainly since the end of World War II and can be traced to an increased movement of people between rural and urban areas so that the chance for exposure to a new serotype is increased. There is no reason to believe that reinfection is important in the pathogenesis of the other hemorrhagic fevers, however, because the syndromes have been seen in accidental laboratory infections acquired thousands of miles from endemic areas. Although it is possible that immune complexes could develop in the nondengue hemorrhagic fevers as a result of antibody formation during their incubation and prodromal periods, there is no evidence of such complexes.

Biopsies of nonfatal, uncomplicated cases and autopsies both show findings consistent with a vascular injury in dengue. In skin biopsies of volunteers with benign illnesses, there were endothelial swelling, perivascular edema, and infiltration of mononuclear cells in or around small blood vessels (Sabin, 1952). The outstanding findings in fatal cases were edema, petechial hemorrhages in all tissues including the heart, some blood in the intestines and stomach, and fluid in the serous cavities. In other words, the most common finding was that resulting from diffuse, general capillary oozing of fluid and cells (Hammon et al., 1960).

Experimental infection of guinea pigs with Junin virus produces a disease that resembles human Argentine hemorrhagic fever (AHF). In this model, both clotting and complement systems are activated at the same time, with complement activation occurring through the classic pathway as would occur with immune complexes. Complement activation occurs in human cases of AHF also, with total serum-complement activity reduced to 68 per cent of control values in severe or moderate cases during the early acute stage. Complement-fixing antibodies, however, do not appear until 12 to 17 days, when clinical recovery begins. Moreover, the profile of change in the complement components is not that of complement activation by immune complexes, and there has been no binding of C3 or immunoglobulins in glomeruli or other vessels in fatal cases. In addition, there has been no histologic evidence that disseminated intravascular coagulation (DIC) contributes to the lesions (deBracco et al., 1978). For these reasons, it is believed that neither immune complexes nor DIC are involved in the pathogenesis of human AHF.

The role of interferon in the pathogenesis of certain manifestations of AHF has also been investigated. Very high titers of circulating endogenous interferon are present during the most active stage of the disease and fall when the infection is controlled with immune plasma. Since exogenous interferon causes many adverse effects like those of AHF, it has been suggested that interferon contributes to their development in that disease. For example, fever, granulocytopenia, lymphocytopenia, malaise, and hair loss are observed in AHF and are prominent effects of exgenous interferon (Levis et al., 1984).

The autopsy findings in other forms of viral hemorrhagic fever disclose little that would help in determining the pathogenesis of bleeding. Lassa fever resembles dengue hemorrhagic fever in its tendency for severe edema as well as hemorrhage throughout all tissues. The occurrence of severe edema with the bleeding indicates that increased capillary permeability from diffuse vascular injury is the basic disturbance, and that it results from infection of the capillary endothelium, from the action of pharmacologic mediators, such as histamine, or from both. In other hemorrhagic fevers, edema is less prominent or absent so that focal vascular injury and coagulation disturbances are the likely defects. In human infections due to Marburg, Ebola, Junin, Lassa, and yellow fever viruses, there are hepatic lesions that might help to explain the hemorrhagic disorder. In yellow fever, for example, the prothrombin time is characteristically prolonged, indicating a disturbance in hepatic synthesis of prothrombin and the other clotting factors measured by the prothrombin screening test. In general, however, the pathogenesis of bleeding in the viral hemorrhagic fevers needs further study.

CLINICAL MANIFESTATIONS, DIAGNOSIS, AND TREATMENT. Separate chapters are devoted to yellow fever (Chapter 155), Lassa fever (Chapter 218), Marburg virus disease (Chapter 266), and Ebola virus disease (Chapter 267). This discussion takes up mainly the other viral hemorrhagic fevers listed in Table 1.

DENGUE

Dengue may start as an explosive urban epidemic in the rainy season and affect many people. It may also attack tourists or other travelers who visit endemic areas. Epidemics of dengue were known in the Caribbean countries and United States of America in the early 19th century, shifted westward to Texas between 1885 and 1920, and back to the southeastern United States between 1920 and 1950. Each of the American epidemics was preceded by an Asian outbreak, and both probably spread from Africa, the original home of *Aedes aegypti*, through slave traffic (Ehrenkranz et al., 1971). In recent years, an outbreak of dengue Type 4 infection began in French Polynesia (Tahiti and Moorea) in early 1979 after never before appearing outside Southeast Asia. A few years earlier, a dengue epidemic due to Types 1, 2, and 3 broke out in the Caribbean and represented the first time that Type 1 virus had been isolated in the Western Hemisphere. The number of cases of dengue imported into the United States has increased lately because of increased epidemic activity in the tropics. At least two patients who came into the United States with imported dengue also had hemorrhagic manifestations. One of these had been exposed in Puerto Rico and the other in India (Annual Summary, 1982).

After an incubation period of five to eight days, the nonfatal, uncomplicated form of dengue starts abruptly with severe generalized aches, excruciating muscle pains, severe headache, pain behind the eyes, and fever to 104° F. Fever lasts three to six days. After two to three days the fever may rapidly subside but reappears again at a lower peak than the first. The two separated peaks give the fever curve an appearance of a saddleback. A transient punctate rash may appear on the knees and elbows early in the illness, and a morbilliform or scarlatiniform rash develops between the third and fifth days on the trunk. From there, it spreads to the face and extremities and may desquamate. Generalized lymphadenopathy is usually present, especially in children, and leukopenia is prominent. During convalescence, the patient is often exhausted for weeks.

Dengue hemorrhagic fever is almost exclusively Asiatic now, although many cases of dengue, shown serologically to be due to Type 1 virus, were hemorrhagic in epidemics that broke out in Durban in 1927 and Athens in 1928 (Theiler et al., 1960). Dengue viruses were first isolated in 1956 from hemorrhagic fever patients by Hammon in Manila. The patients were children between the ages of 6 months and 16 years (median 5 to 9 years) who had extensive petechiae, ecchymoses, nose bleeds, melena, and shock. Thrombocytopenia as low as 10,000 and a prolonged bleeding time were the most prominent laboratory abnormalities (Hammon, 1973). The severe myalgias of classic dengue were usually not present. Hemorrhages started on the third and fourth days of fever (Fig. 1) when leukopenia was replaced by leukocytosis in about one third of patients. Part of the leukocytosis may have resulted from hemoconcentration. Fluid loss from the vessels into the tissues raised the hematocrit over 50 per cent during shock. The fatality rate in the Manila outbreak was 10 per cent and has been 4 to 12 per cent in other epidemics. Dengue viruses belonging to Types 2, 3, and 4 were isolated from the specimens of blood and serum, and from mosquitoes.

Subsequent epidemics of hemorrhagic fever have occurred repeatedly in Bangkok and also in Singapore, South Vietnam, and Calcutta. In each of these, as well as in rare sporadic cases recently described in Curaçao and Jamaica, the clinical pattern has been substantially the same as that described by Hammon (van Der Sar, 1979; Fraser et al., 1978). The World Health Organization has formulated a classification of dengue hemorrhagic fever into four clinical grades of severity (WHO, 1975):

Grade I: Fever, constitutional symptoms, and positive tourniquet test.
Grade II: Grade I plus spontaneous bleeding into skin, gums, gastrointestinal tract, and elsewhere.
Grade III: Grade II plus circulatory failure and agitation.
Grade IV: Profound shock; blood pressure unobtainable.

In all stages, there is thrombocytopenia and hemoconcen-

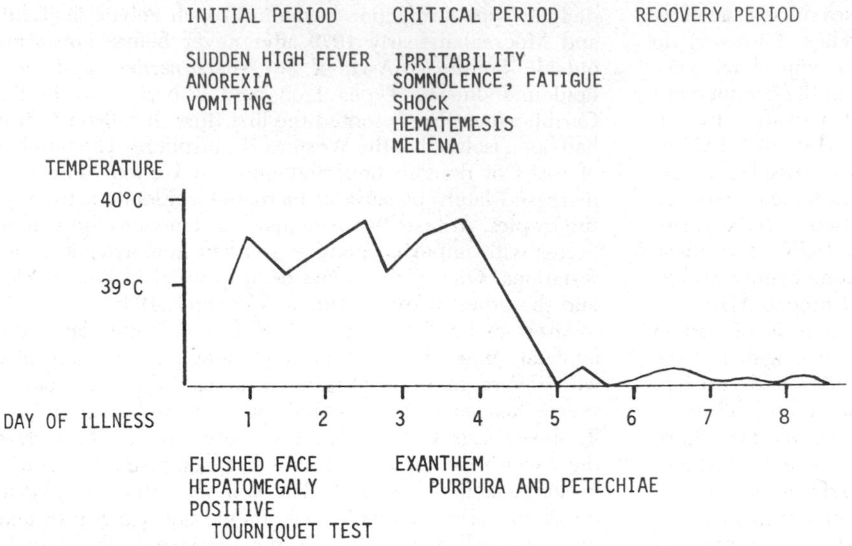

Figure 1. Febrile response and clinical course in dengue hemorrhagic fever. (Courtesy Prasert Thongcharoen, M.D.)

tration. Grades III and IV are also called the *dengue shock syndrome.*

DIAGNOSIS. Dengue hemorrhagic fever is easy to recognize during an outbreak of dengue in Bangkok and other known epidemic areas of Asia. An elevated hematocrit ≥40, low platelet counts (<100,000/mm^2) and a scarcity of platelets in the peripheral blood smear are usually suggestive of the disease. In the rare child who comes down with the illness when visiting an endemic area, the diagnosis can be confirmed by measuring hemagglutination-inhibition (HI) and complement-fixation (CF) antibodies to dengue Subtypes 1, 2, 3, and 4. The HI antibodies rise early in the illness, and recent dengue infection is indicated by a rise in HI titer of at least four-fold. In first infections, there is usually a type-specific rise to one virus with lower rises to other types. In second or third infections, a secondary type of response occurs, which shows an increase of antibody reacting broadly to all dengue serotypes and to other flaviviruses but to higher titer (>1:640) against one of the dengue types. Virus isolation can be made by inoculation of .015 ml of serum intracerebrally in 1- to 4-day-old Swiss mice or baby hamsters. Monolayer cell cultures are inoculated with 0.1 ml and observed for cytopathogenic changes. A variety of cell lines are used, including chick embryo, hamster kidney, Vero, HeLa, BHK-21, and others. Dengue virus can also be isolated from peripheral blood leukocytes, even after high levels of serum antibody appear (Scott et al., 1980). Presumed isolates can be sent to WHO regional reference centers for identification.

The disease closely resembles fulminant meningococcal purpura, and the distinction may not be possible until the blood culture is positive for the meningococcus one or two days after it is drawn.

TREATMENT. Treatment depends on the stage of the disease (Fig. 1). Patients who are beginning to show signs of hypovolemia, such as orthostatic hypotension but no bleeding, are given intravenously 5 per cent dextrose in normal saline until these signs are corrected and the hematocrit stabilized. This treatment cannot be overemphasized because it is perhaps the only way to prevent further deterioration in those who present with nausea and vomiting. At Children's Hospital in Bangkok, the mortality rate of dengue hemorrhagic fever has been decreasing significantly since prompt intravenous fluid therapy has been emphasized and started upon hospitalization. The mortality rate now is about 0.3 per cent and S. Nimmammilya anticipates that the mortality rate should be zero if early hospitalization and intravenous fluid are instituted in every case. Relative hypovolemia on the 2nd and 3rd day of illness seems to accelerate the deterioration of the disease and results in the grave situation seen on the 5th day of illness. It is imperative to avoid aspirin for relief of fever or headache because of the drug's adverse effect on bleeding. The relatives of the patient should be alerted to the possible need for blood donation.

If there is hemorrhage, a falling hematocrit, shock, and thrombocytopenia, the patient should receive whole blood and platelet transfusions. An aluminum hydroxide antacid suspension is taken orally for gastric bleeding. Additional fluids are given intravenously in the form of 5 per cent dextrose in saline, and, if this does not correct hypotension, the patient should receive plasma or plasma expanders other than dextran. Dextran carries the risk of causing platelet dysfunction and further bleeding. Adrenal steroids, norepinephrine, epinephrine, dopamine, or other sympathicoamines appear to be contraindicated.

PROPHYLAXIS. The prevention of dengue depends on control of *A. aegypti*. This has been accomplished in urban areas in which yellow fever was prevalent in the western hemisphere and has also provided freedom from dengue when epidemics of dengue swept through neighboring Caribbean islands. In contrast to yellow fever, for which an effective vaccine is available, vaccination against dengue carries the theoretical risk of sensitizing the person so that hemorrhagic fever would be more likely to occur (Ehrenkranz et al., 1971). Although attenuated experimental live vaccines appear to give protection, the need for vaccines against all four types and the risk of sensitization have probably discouraged the development of a vaccine.

CHIKUNGUNYA FEVER

Chikungunya fever resembles dengue in its transmission by *A. aegypti*, its benign clinical syndrome, its ability to cause hemorrhagic fever, and its prominence in Southeast Asia and Africa.

Like dengue, the usual picture of chikungunya fever is "break-bone fever." After an incubation period of 3 to 12 days, there is a sudden onset of high fever with muscle and joint pains that are so severe that the patient literally folds up and becomes immobile. The fever may go away any time during the first week and reappear one to three days later at a lower level. This febrile relapse is accompanied in three fourths of cases by a maculopapular pruritic rash on the trunk and limbs. In addition to these dengue-like features, there is a leukopenia of 4000 to 5000. In contrast to dengue, retroorbital pain does not occur, and headache is mild. The main sequelae are crippling joint pains that may return periodically over the next four months.

Much more rarely, chikungunya virus can cause hemorrhagic fever. An outbreak of chikungunya hemorrhagic fever occurred along with dengue hemorrhagic fever in Bangkok in 1962. Nearly 90 per cent of those involved in these epidemics were children under 10 years old. They had a fever up to 104° F, vomiting, abdominal pain, and a positive tourniquet test. Purpura occurred in three fourths of the patients. The overall mortality in the combined epidemic was about 10 per cent, but there is evidence that chikungunya hemorrhagic fever was milder (Dasaneyavaja et al., 1963). Chikungunya hemorrhagic fever has also occurred in Calcutta, Madras, and Vellore, India, but not in Africa. Thus, Asiatic children appear to be uniquely susceptible to hemorrhagic fever by chikungunya as well as dengue viruses. These outbreaks have been distinguished from dengue hemorrhagic fever by isolation in suckling mice of chikungunya virus from the blood of patients during the first five days of illness.

KYASANUR FOREST DISEASE

Kyasanur forest disease (KFD) was discovered in 1957 following the death of wild monkeys and human beings in Mysore State in India (Work, 1958). It is transmitted by several species of hard ticks belonging to the genus *Haemaphysalis*, and the reservoir consists of small rodents such as voles and forest rats. Rhesus and Langur monkeys are also infected but, like man, are not part of the natural chain.

The illness occurs about four to eight days after exposure to ticks in the forest with a sudden onset of headache, fever, severe prostration, severe pains in the lower back and extremities, and insomnia. The fever has a biphasic course like that described in dengue and chikungunya fever. The phases are separated by an afebrile period of 10 to 20 days, with the second fever lasting 2 to 10 days. During the second phase, there may be evidence of meningoencephalitis, such as severe headache, vertigo, tremors, and mental changes (Webb and Rao, 1961).

There is no skin eruption, but after three or four days there is bleeding from the gums as well as epistaxis, hemoptysis, hematemesis, and melena. Death results from blood loss, intrapulmonary hemorrhage, and shock in the second week. Bronchopneumonia is also present in some cases. The mortality among virologically proven cases in the 1957 outbreak in India was about 5 per cent.

The chief laboratory findings are a severe leukopenia of 2000 or less and thrombocytopenia. In those cases with signs of meningoencephalitis, the cerebrospinal fluid may have an increase in protein and mononuclear cells, ranging from 5 to 70 per mm^3. Autopsies have shown massive hemorrhage into the gastrointestinal tract, hemorrhage into the lungs, pneumonia, and occasional focal areas of necrosis in the liver. Erythrophagocytosis is prominent in the spleen and liver. No encephalitis has been found.

Patients are treated with enough fluids to restore hydration, blood pressure, and urinary output; and plasma is given to those who do not respond to normal intravenous saline. Those who recover may have prolonged muscle weakness, but there are no permanent sequelae.

Virologic diagnosis is made by isolation of KFD virus from serum during the long period of viremia. The virus multiplies readily in suckling or 3-week-old mice after intracerebral, subcutaneous, or intraperitoneal inoculation. It will also multiply in various tissue culture cell lines, where it may produce no cytopathogenic effect but can be recognized by the hemadsorption phenomenon. The virus is easily identified by complement fixation or neutralization with specific antiserum. Serologic diagnosis is made by complement fixation or hemagglutination-inhibition tests with blood samples taken during the acute and convalescent stages of the disease.

There is no vaccine for the disease, and prophylaxis depends entirely on preventing tick bites. To some extent, this can be done by applying repellents, such as dimethyl phthalate, and by wearing protective clothing. Persons in endemic forest areas should make a careful search for ticks and remove them from the skin.

OMSK HEMORRHAGIC FEVER

This infection resembles Kyasanur forest disease very closely in its clinical manifestations (Gajdusek, 1953). Both are due to togaviruses belonging to *Flavivirus* group B and are transmitted by ticks. Omsk hemorrhagic fever occurs in Omsk and Novosibirsk in western Siberia, and possibly Bukovina in northern Romania. It has its reservoir in water voles and the Asiatic ground squirrels (or susliks). Human infections occur from bites of the tick *Dermacentor* or after contact with muskrats killed by fur trappers. The muskrats, which are not part of the primary cycle, are infected by bites from ticks infected with the virus acquired from voles or susliks. Treatment of Omsk hemorrhagic fever is the same as that of other hemorrhagic fevers. The mortality is less than 3 per cent and the incidence of disease has dropped since the epidemics in 1945 through 1948. A formalin-inactivated mouse brain vaccine is reported to be effective in lowering the incidence of disease. Prophylaxis involves mainly wearing protective gloves when handling carcasses of muskrats.

CRIMEAN HEMORRHAGIC FEVER

ETIOLOGY. Infection of human beings with the virus of Crimean hemorrhagic fever (CHF) occurs during spring and summer from the bites of infected ticks in Central Asia and the Crimea. This hemorrhagic fever virus is antigenically identical to a virus, designated Congo virus, which was isolated from cattle, goats, febrile patients, and *Hyalomma* ticks in equatorial Africa and Pakistan. Even though hemorrhagic fever due to this virus has not been described in equatorial Africa, the agent of the disease is now referred to as Crimean-Congo hemorrhagic fever virus (or CHF-Congo virus). It is classified as a Bunyavirus. Its natural reservoir is wild and domesticated mammals such as sheep, cattle, goats, and hares.

CLINICAL MANIFESTATIONS. About four to eight days after a tick bite, patients become acutely ill with fever to 104° F, diffuse myalgia, flushing of the face and neck, conjunctival infection, and severe hemorrhages. As in the other hemorrhagic fevers, bleeding begins on about the fourth day with petechiae, ecchymoses, melena, and hematemesis. There are also nosebleeds and bleeding from the gums. The liver is enlarged in half the patients, and the spleen in a few. The mortality rate in man reaches 50 per cent from hemorrhage, shock, and neurologic complications. As many as 20 per cent of patients have evidence of meningoencephalitis with stiff neck, mental changes, and coma. During the prolonged convalescence, there may be postinfectious neuritis.

DIAGNOSIS. The clinical pattern of hemorrhagic fever with neurologic disease is easily recognized as that of the CHF syndrome in Central Asia. If it should occur in Africa, however, it would need to be distinguished from other African hemorrhagic fevers by virus isolation. CHF-Congo virus can be isolated from blood by inoculation of serum into newborn mice. Diagnosis is also made serologically by complement fixation, indirect-hemagglutination, or indirect fluorescent antibody tests. Other laboratory findings are severe leukopenia to 1000 per mm^3, severe thrombocytopenia, proteinuria, and hematuria.

The epidemiologic history is also helpful in diagnosis because the disease is spread by ticks in regions where cattle are raised. Milkmaids are infected by the ticks on teats of dairy cows, and cowhands by ticks in the cow pastures. Thus, in contrast to dengue, CHF is a rural disease.

TREATMENT. Blood transfusion is needed to combat the blood loss and shock. Platelet transfusions, avoidance of aspirin, and use of plasma or plasma expanders other than dextran are important measures for preventing more severe bleeding. The value of immune plasma is uncertain.

PROPHYLAXIS. There is no vaccine. The most practical method for preventing the disease has been education of milkers and cowhands in the risks of tick infestation, so that they can take steps to avoid these vectors. Since the infection can also spread to hospital personnel, strict isolation is required to protect those involved in the care of the patient. Infection is thought to be transmitted from person to person by infected blood, rather than by the airborne route (Suleiman et al., 1980). The mortality rate jumps from 15 per cent among sporadic cases to 70 per cent in hospital outbreaks (Al-Tikriti et al., 1981).

ARGENTINE HEMORRHAGIC FEVER

ETIOLOGY. Argentine hemorrhagic fever, caused by Junin virus (Chapter 67) is an epidemic disease primarily of young rural men working in the rich agricultural region of Argentina known as the humid pampa. Epidemics involving 300 to 1000 cases occur every year.

The disease is transmitted in the urine of rodents of the genus *Calomys* that develop immune tolerance to Junin virus so that they have steady viremia. The immune tolerance is explained by acquisition of infection within the first week after birth and the failure of an antibody response to develop against the virus. A chronic infection of the salivary glands and kidney results in constant excretion in saliva and urine. Other weanling rodents can develop neutralizing antibody that terminates the viremia but not the kidney infection, so that infected urine persists. When corn is harvested in the pampa, the harvest workers are exposed to the infected urine of *Calomys* rodents and come down with hemorrhagic fever.

CLINICAL MANIFESTATIONS. After an incubation period of 8 to 14 days, the patients become ill with malaise, fever, hemorrhages, leukopenia, and thrombocytopenia. The onset of the symptoms is relatively gradual and slow when compared with the abrupt onset of other hemorrhagic fevers (Arribalzaga, 1955). Patients complain of headache, generalized myalgia, nausea, and vomiting. The face is flushed, the conjunctivae inflamed, and the eyelids swollen. An enanthem occurs in the mouth and eyes, and a light exanthem also develops. Neither the spleen nor liver are enlarged, and the chest x-ray is negative. About 50 per cent of patients are troubled with loss of equilibrium. There may also be tremors of the tongue and limbs. Most patients develop hypotension and signs of hemoconcentration before shock becomes definite. Hemorrhages begin on the fifth day when the gums bleed and petechiae appear on the axillae and chest. In severe cases, there are widespread hemorrhages from mucous membranes, epistaxis, hematemesis, hematuria, and melena. Death occurs from hemorrhage, shock, secondary bacterial infection, and renal failure. Those who recover become afebrile in about eight days and improve quickly after a profuse diuresis. Some patients relapse four to six weeks after the onset of symptoms, with fever and cerebellar signs that subside within a few days.

DIAGNOSIS. Junin virus is recovered from the blood during the first week by inoculation of guinea pigs or newborn mice. Guinea pigs die in about two weeks from a hemorrhagic disease resembling human AHF. The hemorrhages occur on the skin, intestine, adrenals, and mesenteric lymph nodes. The antibody response is generally too slow to help in diagnosis of the acute illness, but complement fixation and neutralization tests on serial samples of serum make a retrospective diagnosis. The virus must be handled in specialized laboratories, because fatal infections have occurred in laboratory workers.

Other laboratory findings are severe leukopenia (lasting about a week), severe thrombocytopenia, azotemia, pronounced proteinuria, and a fall in serum albumin.

TREATMENT. Patients must be monitored closely for the first signs of hypotension and hemoconcentration so that intravenous saline or plasma can be started before frank shock appears. The treatment outlined for dengue hemorrhagic fever also applies for AHF. The observation that recovery occurs when antibody appears in the blood suggests that convalescent serum may have a place in treatment or even prophylaxis (deBracco et al., 1978). This idea was examined in a double-blind study in which patients received intravenously 500 ml of either convalescent plasma with antibodies against Junin virus or normal plasma obtained from donors without a history of AHF (Maiztegui et al., 1979). The mortality fell from 16.5 per cent in 97 patients given nonimmune plasma to 1.1 per cent in 91 who were given convalescent immune plasma ($P<0.01$). Ten patients treated with immune plasma developed late neurologic complications, which were generally benign and self-limiting. The association between treatment with immune plasma and a late neurologic relapse suggests either that the neurologic disease has an immunologic mechanism or that immune plasma prevented death in those who had infection of the central nervous system but could not prevent late neurologic complications. No other form of treatment has proved so effective as immune plasma in reducing the mortality of AHF.

The mortality is about 10 to 15 per cent. Those who recover have no sequelae, although convalescence may be long.

BOLIVIAN HEMORRHAGIC FEVER

The etiologic agent, epidemiology, and clinical features of Bolivian hemorrhagic fever (BHF) are closely related to those of Argentine hemorrhagic fever (AHF). Machupo virus is antigenically and morphologically similar to Junin virus and is transmitted to man from *Calomys callosus* by the same processes.

The disease first came to serious attention between 1959 and 1962 when it occurred near San Joaquin, Bolivia. It produced a similar clinical picture to that of AHF: fever to 104° F, severe myalgias, intention tremors of the hands and tongue, melena, hematemesis, petechiae of the skin and pharynx, hypotension, leukopenia, and proteinuria. Death usually occurred after seven to ten days from severe hypotension and shock. There were 650 cases and 115 deaths in a population of 2500. (This attack rate and severity was so great that people fled their homes in terror.) The epidemic was finally terminated by eradication of *Calomys* from the vicinity of San Joaquin. The high population of *Calomys* had been attributed to attrition in the population of cats from fatal poisoning with DDT that had been heavily sprayed for malaria control. The situation is similar to that in West Africa, where Lassa fever broke out when control of the house rat enabled *Calomys* to infest human dwellings.

In recent years the disease has been found to spread among people by direct contact. In an outbreak in 1971 of 20 cases in Cochabamba, Bolivia, all patients had been exposed to a 20-year-old nursing student who later died of the disease (Mercado et al., 1971).

HEMORRHAGIC FEVER WITH RENAL SYNDROME (HFRS) (KOREAN HEMORRHAGIC FEVER)

Korean hemorrhagic fever (KHF) is the name given to an epidemic form of hemorrhagic fever with renal involvement. This disease first generated interest when it broke out among United Nations troops in 1951, but similar diseases had been reported in Manchuria in 1942, the Soviet Union in 1950, Scandinavia in 1951, Eastern Europe in 1962, Japan in 1964, and in Belgium in 1978. In Korea the disease was acquired by farmers and soldiers stationed in rural areas from the excreta of a wild rodent, *Apodemus agrarius coreae*. The disease has remained endemic near the demilitarized zone between North and South Korea. The related hemorrhagic fever in Scandinavia and Finland, known as nephropathia epidemica, is transmitted by the bank vole *Clethrionomys glareolus*. Outbreaks have been traced to laboratory rats in Japan, Korea, and Belgium (Desmyter et al., 1983; Umenai et al., 1979; Lee and Johnson, 1982) and to wild rats in Korea and China. Studies on the antigenic relationship between these apodemus-borne and rat-borne hemorrhagic fever viruses indicate that the two are related but not identical.

ETIOLOGY. Earlier studies by Japanese and Russian investigators indicated that the causative agent was viral because the disease could be transmitted to volunteers by injecting blood or urine from febrile patients, and the agent was filterable (Brummer-Korvenkontio et al., 1980). In 1978, Lee propagated the agent serially in adult *A. agrarius* and demonstrated specific immunofluorescent reactions when lung tissues of the rodents reacted with sera from patients convalescing from Korean hemorrhagic fever. The agent could not be cultivated then in continuous cell cultures of African green monkey kidney, dog embryo, porcine kidney, human embryo lung (W1–38), mink kidney, or Chinese hamster lung; nor in primary cell cultures prepared from rhesus monkey kidney, duck and chicken embryo, rat liver, and human embryonic liver. No infections could be established in suckling white mice, weaned mice, hamsters, guinea pigs, rats, or rabbits. Antisera to Lassa, Machupo, Marburg, and Ebola viruses gave no fluorescence when reacted with infected *A. agrarius* lung tissues, but raised titers of antibody to the agent of KHF were found by the fluorescent antibody method in Finnish patients with nephropathia epidemica (NE) (Lee and Lee, 1979). Thus, the agents of KHF and NE appeared to be closely related.

In 1981, G. R. French and associates reported on the propagation of the prototype virus of hemorrhagic fever with renal syndrome in a pulmonary alveolar epithelial cell line of human origin (French et al., 1981). Subsequent adaptation of this strain, designated Hantaan virus, to Vero cells permitted sufficient yield of the agent to characterize it and to show that it has properties similar to some members of the virus family Bunyaviridae (Schmaljohn et al., 1983). The most compelling evidence in support of its classification among Bunyaviridae is the demonstration that it contains three separate species of nucleic acid. The Bunyaviridae are the only group of animal viruses known to possess a tripartite single-stranded RNA genome.

PATHOGENESIS AND PATHOLOGY. In addition to shock, acute renal failure and pulmonary edema kill the patient. In early deaths, retroperitoneal edema is marked but not in deaths that occur later. There are hemorrhages from distended small vessels in the right atrium, anterior pituitary, adrenal medulla, and especially the renal medulla, where intense vascular congestion separates the tubules that undergo focal necrosis, resembling that seen in lower nephron nephrosis (Lukes, 1954). The necrosis may be limited to the tubules or involve the pyramids. The shock is oligemic and secondary to the loss of plasma into the tissues. There is reduced cardiac output and increased peripheral resistance.

CLINICAL MANIFESTATIONS. The disease occurs in three phases: invasion, toxic, and convalescent (Powell, 1953). The invasion stage starts suddenly, and the symptoms are those of any acute febrile illness. After an incubation period of 10 to 30 days, the illness begins with chilliness or chills, high fever reaching 104 to 106° F by the third day, severe myalgias, and frontal headaches. Photophobia and pain on moving the eyes are especially prominent and last into the second stage. Some patients complain of sore throat, dry cough, or diarrhea, but these are mild and transient. The main physical findings are a flush of the face and neck, giving a characteristic "sunburned" appearance, a relative bradycardia, generalized lymph node enlargement with no tenderness, normal heart and lungs, negative neurologic examination, and only occasional splenomegaly. The temperature falls rapidly to subnormal levels on the third to sixth day, along with a drop of blood pressure to near shock levels.

The toxic stage starts about the fourth day with defervescence. Thus, the disappearance of fever is not a hopeful sign as it is in most infections because it indicates the start of a more severe illness. The patients feel worse and develop a sense of desperation; prostration increases, and extreme restlessness develops. Hematemesis, hemoptysis, and melena begin, abdominal pain increases, and thirst becomes intense but cannot be satisfied because of intense vomiting. Renal failure with oliguria or anuria sets in between the fourth and ninth days. Disorientation, delirium, coma, and convulsive seizures develop in the severest cases. The systolic blood pressure drops to 80 mm Hg, and shock may become irreversible. Ocular hemorrhages vary from conjunctival petechiae to the typical "red eyes" of severe episcleral bleeding. Severe petechiae also occur in the soft palate, pharynx, axillae, chest, scapulas, and arms. Almost all patients have some evidence of uremia. Periorbital, severe conjunctival, facial, and pulmonary edema are features of the uremic phase. The heart is usually normal, but a few deaths have occurred from myocardial failure and ventricular fibrillation. Abdominal tenderness is usually severe and raises the question of an acute surgical problem.

The convalescent stage starts about ten days to two weeks after onset of illness. The symptoms usually disappear suddenly. Immediately after the oliguria subsides, marked polyuria begins with daily urine outputs of 4 to 10 liters and marked thirst. This diuretic phase may last as long as two to three months.

LABORATORY DIAGNOSIS. Heavy proteinuria begins about the fourth day of illness when oliguria occurs. During the polyuric phase the specific gravity of the urine is below 1.010 and remains low for up to three months. Creatinine levels of 5 to 6 mg per 100 ml are common during the uremic phase. A polymorphonuclear leukocytosis of 20,000 to 40,000 is uniformly present in the toxic stage and can reach 100,000 in patients with a myeloid type of leukemoid reaction. Atypical lymphocytes are also common, reaching 5 to 25 per cent. Thrombocytopenia is present between the fourth and tenth days, when platelets fall to 20,000 or less, but the prothrombin time and other clotting factors are normal. The hematocrit depends on the balance between the loss of blood and water into the circulation. Loss of plasma can raise the hematocrit to 70 per cent in shock.

Specific diagnosis is made by demonstrating rising antibody titers to the KHF agent in lung tissues of *Apodemus agrarius jejudoici* by the indirect fluorescent antibody techniques of Lee et al. (1978). A rise in titer in serial samples must be obtained because antibodies from a past infection can still be present ten years later. It may also be possible to make a specific diagnosis by complement fixation, viral neutralization, and other serologic tests now that the virus has been propagated in tissue culture.

TREATMENT. Fluids must be kept at the minimum requirements needed to replace what is lost in the urine, feces, vomitus, sweat, and evaporation during fever. This can be determined by measuring output and weighing the patient. If the overpowering thirst is allowed to determine water intake, the patient becomes overloaded with fluid and suffers pulmonary edema. When vomiting is severe, 10 per cent glucose in water should be given intravenously in minimal quantities and saline should be avoided. Mild hypotension is treated by placing the patient in the Trendelenburg position and bandaging the extremities. When the hematocrit reaches high levels (55 to 60 per cent) in more advanced shock, the patient should receive plasma or salt-free human albumin. Pressors such as 1-norepinephrine are ineffective. The treatment of severe renal failure is probably best accomplished by early and frequent dialysis. Either peritoneal or extracorporeal hemodialysis may be used. Frequent dialysis cuts down on the need for strict water restriction, makes fluid balance easier to manage, and helps avoid serious problems with hyperkalemia and other electrolyte disturbances. If dialysis cannot be done, the hyperkalemia should be treated with intravenous glucose and insulin and calcium chloride to protect against the cardiotoxic effects of potassium. Enemas of potassium-binding resins (such as Kayexelate, a sodium cycle resin), given two to four times daily, can prevent dangerous levels of potassium, but rectal impaction is a risk when these are given to severely dehydrated patients. Sodium bicarbonate may be needed to keep the plasma bicarbonate above 15 mEq per liter.

During the diuretic phase of convalescence, fluid intake must be carefully maintained to prevent dehydration and shock. For this reason, the patient should be kept in the hospital until the urine is concentrated to 1.020.

The mortality rate depends on the quality of the care. In early reports, before the pathophysiology and treatment were understood, one third of the patients died in some outbreaks, and the overall death rate was 15 per cent. Troops in Korea receiving better treatment had a mortality of about 6 per cent, and no deaths have occurred in specialized centers for treating hemorrhagic fever.

The main sequela is persistent disturbance in renal tubular function, which occurs in only a few patients. This may last for many years without causing serious disability.

References

Al-Tikriti, S., Al-Ani, F., Jurgi, F., et al.: Congo/Crimean hemorrhagic fever in Iraq. Bull WHO 59:85, 1981.

Annual Summary, 1982, Morbidity and Mortality Weekly Report. Dengue-confirmed imported cases and distribution of Aedes aegypti mosquitos in the United States, 1982. Morbidity and Mortality Weekly Report 31:113, 1983.

Arribalzaga, R.: Una nueva enfermedad epidémica a german desconocido: Hipertermia nefrotóxica, leukopenica y enantemática. Dia Méd 27:1204, 1955.

Bokish, V., Franklin, H., Russel, P., Dixon, F., and Müller-Eberhard, H.: The potential pathogenic role of complement in dengue hemorrhagic shock syndrome. J Immunol 102:412, 1973.

Brummer-Korvenkontio, M., Vaheri, A., Hori, T., H. von Bonsdorff, C., Vuorimies, J., Manni, T., Penttinen, K., Oker-Blom, N., and Lĕhdevirta, J.: Nephropathia epidemica: Detection of antigen in bank voles and serologic diagnosis of human infection. J Infect Dis 141:131, 1980.

Dasaneyavaja, A., Robin, Y., and Yenbutia, D.: Laboratory observations related to prognosis in Thai hemorrhagic fever. J Trop Med Hyg 66:35, 1963.

Desmyter, J., Johnson, K. M., Deckers, C., LeDuc, J., Brasseur, F., and van Ypersele de Strihou, C.: Laboratory rat-associated outbreak of haemorrhagic fever with renal syndrome due to Hantaan-like virus in Belgium. Lancet 2, 1445, 1983.

deBracco, M., Rimoldi, M., Cossio, P., Rabinovich, A., Maiztegui, J., Carballal, G., and Arana, R.: Argentine hemorrhagic fever. N Engl J Med 299:216, 1978.

Ehrenkranz, N. J., Ventura, A., Cuadrado, R., Pond, W., and Porter, J.: Pandemic dengue in Caribbean countries and the southern United States—past, present, and potential problems. N Engl J Med 285:1460, 1971.

Fraser, H., Wilson, W., Thomas, E., and Sissons, J.: Dengue shock syndrome in Jamaica. Br Med J 1:893, 1978.

French, G. R., Foulke, R. S., Brand, O., Eddy, G., Lee, H. W., and Lee P. W.: Korean hemorrhagic fever: propagation of the etiologic agent in a cell line of human origin. Science 211:1046, 1981.

Gajdusek, D.: Acute infectious hemorrhagic fevers and mycotoxicoses in the Union of Soviet Socialist Republics. Medical Science Publications no. 2. Washington, Army Medical Service Graduate School, 1953, pp. 19–35.

Hammon, W.: Dengue hemorrhagic fever. Do we know its cause? Am J Trop Med Hyg 22:82, 1973.

Hammon, W., Rudnick, A., Sather, G., Rogers, K., and Morse, L.: New hemorrhagic fevers of children in the Philippines and Thailand. Trans. Assoc Am Physicians 73:140, 1960.

Lee, H., and Lee, P.: Etiological relation between Korean haemorrhagic fever and nephropathia epidemica. Lancet 1:186, 1979.

Lee, H., Lee, P., and Johnson, K.: Isolation of the etiologic agent of Korean hemorrhagic fever. J Infect Dis 137:298, 1978.

Lee, H., and Johnson, K.: Laboratory-acquired infections with Hantaan virus, the etiologic agent of Korean hemorrhagic fever. J Infect Dis 146:645, 1982.

Levis, S., Saavedra, Ceccohi, C., Falcoff, E., Feiullade, D., Enria, D., Maztegui, J., and Falcoff, R.: Interferon in Argentine hemorrhagic fever. J Infect Dis 149:428, 1984.

Lukes, R.: The pathology of 39 fatal cases of epidemic hemorrhagic fever. Am J Med 16:639, 1954.

Maiztegui, J., Fernandez, N., and Damilano, A.: Efficacy of immune plasma in treatment of Argentine haemorrhagic fever and association between treatment and a late neurological syndrome. Lancet 2:1216, 1979.

Mercado, R., Valverde, L., Webb, P., Peters, C., and Johnson, K.: Hemorrhagic fever. Bolivia Morbid Mortal Weekly Rep May 1, 1971, p. 162.

Powell, G.: Clinical manifestations of epidemic hemorrhagic fever. JAMA 151:1261, 1953.

Russel, P.: Immunopathologic mechanism in the dengue shock syndrome. In Amos, B. (ed.): Progress in Immunology. New York, Academic Press, 1971, pp. 831–838.

Sabin, A.: Research on dengue during World War II. Am J Trop Med Hyg 1:30, 1952.

Schmaljohn, C., Hasty, S., Harrison, S., and Darrymple, J.: Characterization of Hantaan virions, the prototype virus of hemorrhagic fever with renal syndrome. J Inf Dis 148:1005, 1983.

Scott, R., Nisalak, A., Cheaumudon, U., Seridhoranakul, S., and Nimmannityia, S.: Isolation of dengue virus from peripheral blood leukocytes of patients with hemorrhagic fever. J Infect Dis 141:1, 1980.

Sobel, A., Bodusch, V., and Müller-Eberhard, H.: C1q deviation test for the detection of immune complexes, aggregates of IgG, and bacterial products in human sera. J Exp Med 142:139, 1975.

Sugiyama, K., Matsuura, Y., Morita, C., Morikawa, S., Komatsu, T., Shiga, S., Akao, Y., and Kitamura, T.: Determination by immune adherence HA of the antigenic relationship between Rattus and Apodemus-borne viruses causing hemorrhagic fever with renal syndrome. J Infect Dis 149:472, 1984.

Suleiman, M., Muscat-Baron, J., Harries, J., et al.: Congo/Crimean haemorrhagic fever in Dubai: an outbreak at the Rashid Hospital. Lancet 2:939, 1980.

Theiler, M., Casals, J., and Moutousses, C.: Etiology of the 1927–1928 epidemic of dengue in Greece. Proc Soc Exp Biol Med 103:244, 1960.

Theofilopoulos, A., Wilson, C., and Dixon, F.: The Raji cell radioimmune assay for detecting immune complexes in human sera. J Clin Investig 57:169, 1976.

Umenai, T., Lee, H., Lee, P., et al.: Korean haemorrhagic fever in staff in an animal laboratory. Lancet 1:1314, 1979.

van Der Sar, A.: An outbreak of dengue hemorrhagic fever in Curaçao. Trop Geogr Med 25:119, 1979.

Viral hemorrhagic fever: initial management of suspected and confirmed cases. MMWR Supplement 32:275, 1983.

Webb, H., and Rao, R. L.: Kyasanur forest disease: A general clinical study in which some cases with neurological complications were observed. Trans R Soc Trop Med Hyg 55:284, 1961.

Work, T.: Russian spring-summer virus in India. Kyasanur forest disease. Progr Med Virol 1:248, 1958.

World Health Organization: Technical guides for diagnosis, treatment, surveillance, prevention and control of Dengue hemorrhagic fever. Geneva, 1975.

217

INFECTIOUS MONONUCLEOSIS DUE TO EPSTEIN-BARR VIRUS AND CYTOMEGALOVIRUS

M. Colin Jordan, M.D.

Infectious mononucleosis is characterized by the intense proliferation of lymphoid cells in the spleen, lymph nodes, and peripheral blood. The clinical signs and symptoms of the disease result primarily from this cellular proliferation, and the presence of atypical lymphocytes for several weeks in the peripheral blood is pathognomonic of the illness (Hoaglund, 1967). Recent studies have indicated that infectious mononucleosis is caused by two herpesviruses, the Epstein-Barr virus (EBV) and cytomegalovirus (CMV). When caused by EBV, infectious mononucleosis is accompanied in most cases by heterophile antibody (Evans et al., 1968). On the other hand, CMV mononucleosis is a "heterophile-negative" form of the disease (Klemola and Kaariainen, 1965.).

ETIOLOGY. EBV, a herpesvirus, was first discovered by electron microscopic studies of Burkitt's African lymphoma. Since then, the virus has been associated with three other clinical entities: infectious mononucleosis, nasopharyngeal carcinoma, and a diffuse polyclonal B-cell lymphoma seen primarily in young boys (Robinson et al., 1980). EBV is unusual in that it cannot be propagated in standard tissue culture. The virus replicates partially, however, in human B lymphocytes in vitro, which causes indefinite proliferation of the infected cells ("immortalization"). Each infected cell contains many copies of the viral DNA genome, which persists as an extrachromosomal element (Robinson and Smith, 1981). During infectious mononucleosis, EBV is shed in the respiratory secretions. This appears to result from lytic virus replication in the salivary glands or in pharyngeal epithelium.

Another herpesvirus, CMV, causes a syndrome which meets the hematologic criteria for a diagnosis of infectious mononucleosis (Klemola and Kaariainen, 1965). The pathogenesis of this disease is not as well defined as that caused by EBV. CMV does not immortalize lymphocytes in vitro. As with EBV, however, CMV is shed for prolonged periods in the respiratory secretions and also in the urine. CMV can be readily cultivated in human diploid cell cultures, although two to four weeks may be required to detect the virus (Jordan et al., 1973).

EPIDEMIOLOGY. Infections with EBV are extremely common throughout the world; most are subclinical. The incidence of infection is especially high in lower socioeconomic groups and under crowded living conditions. A few studies have indicated that EBV may cause nonspecific respiratory illnesses in young children. Most of the clinically apparent illness, however, occurs in the form of infectious mononucleosis among adolescents and young adults. Because of the high frequency of subclinical EBV infections among children in lower socioeconomic groups, infectious mononucleosis is largely a disease of middle-income to upper-income groups who are exposed to the virus for the first time in adolescence or young adulthood. Patients with Burkitt lymphoma in Africa and anaplastic nasopharyngeal carcinoma in the Orient have a high prevalence of EBV antibody and also extraordinarily high antibody titers. EBV DNA is present in these tumors in large amounts as well. In the normal population, most EBV infections are probably transmitted by close contact with people shedding the virus in respiratory secretions. Intimate or close contact (i.e., kissing) is probably necessary.

The epidemiology of CMV infection is similar to that of EBV. Early studies documented that CMV is a leading cause of in utero infection. Classic cytomegalic inclusion disease of the newborn may result when the mother acquires her primary CMV infection during pregnancy. Subclinical in utero infection with CMV is more common, occurring in approximately 2 per cent of all pregnancies. Asymptomatic infection with active viral replication is common among children in day care centers (urine and saliva), pregnant women (cervicovaginal secretions), postpartum women (breast milk), homosexual men (urine and semen), and immunocompromised patients (urine and saliva). Transmission of CMV infection probably results from contact with asymptomatic shedders, primarily children. Other vehicles of transmission include breast milk, cervicovaginal secretions during parturition, organ transplants (kidney and heart), blood and granulocyte transfusions, and possibly sexual contact. The "posttransfusion" or "postperfusion" syndrome can be caused by either CMV or EBV in transfused blood, although CMV infection is much more common in this setting.

As with other herpesviruses, EBV and CMV establish lifelong latent infection in their host. Latent EBV infection is established in B lymphocytes, whereas the cellular site(s) of CMV latency are not yet known definitively. Either virus may be activated as a result of immunosuppression from underlying disease or from superimposed chemotherapy. Activation of latent CMV in immune-deficient patients may result in serious disseminated infection, often causing life-threatening interstitial pneumonitis.

The highest frequency of infectious mononucleosis is seen among college students and military personnel. The vast majority of these infections, which are heterophile-antibody positive, are caused by EBV. Recently, however, EBV-mononucleosis has been described in the elderly (Horwitz et al., 1983). Mononucleosis due to CMV is always heterophile-antibody negative and tends to occur in a somewhat older age group (mid- to late-twenties) than EBV infection. Of heterophile-negative cases, about two thirds are caused by CMV. Most of the remaining cases are caused by EBV. Thus, EBV can cause infectious mononucleosis with or without a positive heterophile-antibody test, although the vast majority are heterophile-positive (Jordan, 1975). A syndrome mimicking infectious mononucleosis in all respects is also caused by *Toxoplasma gondii*. The heterophile test in these cases is negative. Finally, dual infections with EBV or CMV are occasionally seen during infectious mononucleosis as determined by specific antibody studies. Most likely, these infections result from activation of one latent virus as a consequence of acute primary infection with the other.

PATHOGENESIS. Presumably, initial viral infection takes place in epithelium of the pharynx or salivary glands. Subsequently, EBV disseminates to virtually all lymphoid tissues in the body including the spleen. In the peripheral blood, B lymphocytes are infected with the virus and are induced to proliferate. However, the classic atypical lymphocytes or "Downey" cells are T lymphocytes that have been mobilized, presumably in an attempt to eliminate EBV-infected B cells, which now have altered membrane antigens. Thus, the peripheral blood cells that are the hallmark of infectious mononucleosis are not themselves infected. "Suppressor" T lymphocytes predominate early in the illness, causing anergy and immune suppression. Later, helper "T cells" proliferate and are associated with eventual recovery from the infection.

Another characteristic feature of mononucleosis is disordered immune regulation involving B lymphocytes. Infection of these cells with EBV eventually results in secretion of a variety of polyclonal antibodies, including the heterophile agglutinin, which is a macroglobulin. Other such antibodies include cryoglobulins, cold agglutinins, red blood cell hemolysins with anti-i specificity, false-positive serologic tests for syphilis, and rheumatoid factor.

The pathogenesis of CMV mononucleosis is less well understood. In general, the degree of lymphoproliferation is less intense than in EBV mononucleosis. In CMV disease, virus can be recovered from the peripheral blood and is associated with polymorphonuclear leukocytes or monocytes. The lymphocytes do not appear to be infected. Except for the heterophile antibody, CMV causes disordered production of diverse antibodies as seen in EBV infection.

CLINICAL MANIFESTATIONS. The characteristic clinical features of mononucleosis in its classic form include fever, tonsillopharyngitis, diffuse lymphadenopathy, and splenomegaly (Hoaglund, 1967). Other less specific manifestations include chills, anorexia, headache, abdominal pain, arthralgias, and inspiratory pain involving the costal margins. It is important to realize, however, that in many cases a number of the classic symptoms may be lacking. This is especially true in the "typhoidal" form of the disease in which pharyngitis and lymphadenopathy may be minimal or absent altogether. In other instances, the tonsillopharyngeal involvement may be so prominent that a diagnosis of streptococcal pharyngitis is made without an appreciation of the systemic nature of the illness. Profound fatigue and malaise are the presenting complaints in some patients.

The most common physical findings include fever, pharyngitis with or without exudate, palatal petechiae, cervical lymphadenopathy, and splenomegaly. On occasion, tonsillopharyngeal involvement and exudation may be so intense as to cause airway obstruction and severe dysphagia. Other signs include axillary and epitrochlear lymphadenopathy, hepatomegaly, a variety of skin rashes (maculopapular, urticarial, petechial or erythema multiforme-like), icterus, and periorbital edema.

The liver is virtually always involved in either EBV or CMV mononucleosis. In fact, the presence of completely normal liver function tests would make the diagnosis of mononucleosis highly unlikely. Histologically, nonspecific hepatitis is usually present, although granulomatous changes have been documented in few instances. In laboratory studies, the hepatic involvement is most frequently manifested by elevations of SGOT and SGPT, usually in the range of two to four times the normal values. The alkaline phosphatase concentrations are characteristically normal but may be elevated in granulomatous hepatitis. Slight elevations of the serum bilirubin are common, although frank jaundice is seen in only 5 per cent of cases. The hepatitis usually resolves simultaneously with the other clinical manifestations of mononucleosis.

Although there is considerable overlap in terms of clinical manifestations, CMV mononucleosis is characterized by less intense tonsillopharyngeal involvement and lymphadenopathy. Pharyngeal exudate is particularly uncommon. Similar presentations are also seen with EBV-induced disease, however. When mononucleosis occurs in older patients (ages 40 to 70), it frequently occurs in this "typhoidal" form (Horwitz et al., 1983).

COMPLICATIONS. Although convalescence may be protracted, the majority of patients with mononucleosis recover completely. However, there are several complications which, although uncommon, may cause difficulties in diagnosis and management. Because of intense congestion and subcapsular hemorrhage, splenic rupture may occur spontaneously, from minor trauma or as a result of injudicious exercise. Hematologic complications include hemolytic anemia and profound thrombocytopenia in 0.5 to 4.0 per cent of cases. The latter may be associated with serious hemorrhagic complications, including splenic rupture. Although nonspecific ST-T wave abnormalities are frequently detected by electrocardiography, frank pericarditis is rare.

Neurologic complications occur in approximately 1 per cent of cases of infectious mononucleosis, particularly in association with EBV infection. Such involvement may actually dominate the clinical picture at the time of initial presentation. Diffuse or focal encephalitis, sometimes primarily involving the cerebellum, may be seen. Varying degrees of aseptic meningitis are often present as well. The spinal fluid is usually typical of that found in other forms of viral meningoencephalitis, including a mononuclear pleocytosis with normal glucose values. Although meningoencephalitis is the most common cause of death in infectious mononucleosis, complete recovery ensues in approximately 90 per cent of patients. Other neurological findings of infectious mononucleosis include transverse myelitis, cranial nerve palsies (including Bell's palsy), optic neuritis, retrobulbar neuritis, and mononeuritis multiplex. Recently, the Guillain-Barré syndrome has been reported repeatedly in association with EBV or CMV infection. At the present time, these two viruses appear to be the most common known infectious cause of this syndrome.

A peculiar propensity for the development of maculopapular rashes in patients with mononucleosis who have been given ampicillin has been described repeatedly. It may occur in either EBV or CMV mononucleosis. In one series, 19 of 20 patients with EBV mononucleosis developed a rash during or immediately after administration of the antibiotic. When these patients are rechallenged with ampicillin after recovery from mononucleosis, the rash does not develop, indicating that specific allergy is not the cause.

DIAGNOSIS. Diagnosis of classic heterophile-positive mononucleosis is usually not difficult provided the physician considers the possibility. The characteristic clinical findings, the atypical lymphocytosis, and the positive test for heterophile agglutinin are usually present. However, the diagnosis may be missed for a variety of reasons. The tonsillopharyngeal involvement may suggest streptococcal pharyngitis if the systemic nature of the illness is not appreciated. In some patients, the heterophile test may be negative initially, only to become positive 3 to 4 weeks later. In others, the initial hematologic response may be characterized by a proliferation of polymorphonuclear leukocytes. However, even in these patients, the lymphocytes present may be atypical in type. The diagnosis is also frequently missed in patients without prominent tonsillopharyngeal involvement, splenomegaly, or lymphadenopathy ("typhoidal" presentation). Such patients may be subjected to expensive and potentially hazardous diagnostic tests. Finally, the characteristic findings of infectious mononucleosis may be overshadowed by complicating features such as hemolytic anemia, thrombocytopenia with hemorrhage, jaundice, splenic rupture, and neurologic manifestations.

The detection of serum heterophile antibody has been used for many years in the diagnosis of infectious mononucleosis and is a hallmark of EBV-induced disease. The heterophile antibody is a polyclonal macroglobulin that does not appear to be directed toward any of the known EBV antigens. Presumably, synthesis of this macroglobulin reflects the disordered regulation of B cell function previously noted. In the clinical laboratory, the heterophile agglutinin is sought after removal of the Forssman antibody (which is present in normal serum) by adsorption with guinea pig kidney. If heterophile antibody is present, the serum will then agglutinate sheep red blood cells at a dilution of 1:28 or greater. In many laboratories, sheep red cells have been replaced by beef or horse red cells because of greater sensitivity and because differential adsorption with guinea pig kidney is not necessary. More recently, commercially available slide kits have become widely used for demonstration of heterophile antibody. These tests are generally quite specific, and they are slightly more sensitive than the traditional tube-dilution studies.

More than 85 per cent of cases are associated with a positive heterophile test (Davidsohn and Lee, 1962). Diagnostic tests using horse red blood cells appear more sensitive than those employing sheep or beef red cells. The currently available diagnostic slide or spot tests are as sensitive as the traditional tube-dilution studies. False-positive tests are quite rare. It should be remembered, however, that the characteristic hematologic abnormalities must be present for a definitive diagnosis of infectious mononucleosis. All cases with a positive heterophile test are caused by EBV. Virus-specific serologic studies are not necessary in these cases.

Approximately 15 per cent of cases meeting the hematologic criteria for infectious mononucleosis are persistently heterophile-negative. Of these, two thirds are caused by CMV with the remaining one third due to EBV. Why the heterophile antibody does not develop in these cases due to EBV is not known. A previous bout of EBV mononucleosis does not protect against CMV mononucleosis or vice-versa.

In heterophile-negative mononucleosis or in cases with atypical features, further evaluation in terms of etiology may be indicated. This is especially true of pregnant women with heterophile-negative disease because of the possibility of in utero infection of the fetus with CMV or toxoplasma. In CMV mononucleosis, the diagnosis may be made by demonstration of a four-fold or greater rise in CMV antibody titers. It is usually difficult to demonstrate a seroconversion against CMV because antibodies are usually present by the time the patient seeks medical attention. Virus can be recovered from several sites in patients with CMV mononucleosis, including urine, saliva, and cervicovaginal secretions. Since CMV shedding in urine and saliva is protracted, it may be possible to make a presumptive diagnosis retrospectively in some cases.

In heterophile-negative mononucleosis due to EBV, a thorough evaluation of the patient's serologic response is required for viral diagnosis. The presence of IgM antibodies against EBV is virtually diagnostic of acute infection. The immunofluorescence test for IgM is difficult to perform, however. Antibody against the EBV viral capsid antigen (VCA) develops in all cases but the test is rarely useful in diagnosis because the titers are usually in the same range as seen in individuals with previous EBV infection. If the development of antibody against EB nuclear antigen (EBNA) can be demonstrated in paired sera, it is virtually diagnostic of acute infection. This antibody remains present for years after initial infection. Antibodies against the diffuse component of the EBV early antigen (anti-D EA antibody) are present transiently in the sera of 70 per cent of patients with mononucleosis. The lack of anti-VCA antibody in the serum, especially when the patient has been ill for two weeks or longer, essentially rules out a diagnosis of EBV mononucleosis.

DIFFERENTIAL DIAGNOSIS. Occasionally, infection with *Toxoplasma gondii* can closely mimic infectious mononucleosis. Fever, pharyngitis, lymphadenopathy, hepatosplenomegaly, and skin rash may be present. The proliferation of atypical lymphocytes is less intense and shorter in duration than that seen in infectious mononucleosis. Other causes of atypical lymphocytosis include hepatitis A, scrub typhus, blood transfusions, and drug reactions (diphenylhydantoin, para-aminosalicylic acid, allopininol, hydralazine, methyldopa). Acute infectious lymphocytosis, Hodgkin's disease, lymphoma, and angioimmunoblastic lymphadenopathy may present with some of the manifestations of mononucleosis.

MANAGEMENT. The vast majority of patients with infectious mononucleosis recover completely, although the convalescent phase may be protracted in some. Relapses of low-grade fever, generalized malaise, and fatigue are not uncommon, especially after injudicious exercise. The recurrence of symptoms is not associated with reappearance of laboratory abnormalities. Adequate rest and nutrition are important in the recovery process. Aspirin should not be used as an analgesic because subcapsular splenic hemorrhage may result. When the airway or swallowing mechanisms are severely compromised as a result of tonsillopharyngeal involvement, a short course of corticosteroids is indicated. Prednisone 40 mg/day for five days is usually sufficient. Parenteral steroid therapy may be necessary in some patients who cannot swallow tablets. Other indications for corticosteroids include severe hemolytic anemia or thrombocytopenia, and possibly, encephalitis or aseptic meningitis. Steroids are probably not indicated for the Guillain-Barré syndrome. Nonspecific symptoms such as protracted fatigue and malaise are not indications for corticosteroids. Currently, there are no antiviral compounds that have been shown to enhance recovery from either EBV or CMV mononucleosis.

References

Davidsohn, E., and Lee, C.: The laboratory in diagnosis of infectious mononucleosis (with additional notes on epidemiology, etiology, and pathogenesis). Med Clin N Am 46:225, 1962.

Evans, A. S., Niederman, J. C., and McCollum, F.: Seroepidemiologic studies of infectious mononucleosis with EB virus. N Engl J Med 279:1123, 1968.

Hoaglund, R. J.: Infectious Mononucleosis. New York, Grune & Stratton, 1967.

Horwitz, C. A., Henle, W., Henle, G., Schapiro, R., Borken, S., and Bundtzen, R.: Infectious mononucleosis in patients aged 40 to 72 years: report of 27 cases, including three without heterophile-antibody responses. Medicine (Balt) 62:256, 1983.

Jordan, M. C., Rousseau, W. E., Stewart, J. A., Noble, G. R., and Chin, T. D. Y.: Spontaneous cytomegalovirus mononucleosis. Clinical and laboratory observations in nine cases. Ann Intern Med 79:153, 1973.

Jordan, M. C.: Nomenclature for the mononucleosis syndrome. JAMA 234:45, 1975.

Klemola, E., and Kaariainen, L.: Cytomegalovirus as a possible cause of a disease resembling infectious mononucleosis. Br Med J 2:1099, 1965.

Robinson, J. E., Brown, N., Andiman, W., Halliday, K., Kranke, U., Robert, M. F., Anderson-Anvret, M., Horstmann, D., and Miller, G.: Diffuse polyclonal B-cell lymphoma during primary infection with Epstein-Barr virus. N Engl J Med 302:1293, 1980.

Robinson, J., and Smith, D.: Infection of human B-lymphocytes with high multiplicities of Epstein-Barr virus: Kinetics of EBNA expression, cellular DNA synthesis, and mitosis. Virology 109:336, 1981.

218

LASSA FEVER

Abraham I. Braude, M.D., Ph.D.

Lassa fever is a severe infection caused by an arenavirus. The disease is named for Lassa, a lonely herdsmen's village in the northern Nigerian Sudan where the first outbreak was recognized in 1969. The virus is spread to man from its reservoir, a multimammate rat, and from one person to another in households and hospitals. The outstanding symptoms are fever, prostration, severe pharyngitis, vomiting, abdominal pain, and dyspnea. Serous effusions, facial edema, generalized hemorrhages, and fatal shock occur later. The mortality rate is between 30 and 50 per cent.

ETIOLOGY. The Lassa fever virus is one of the arenaviruses pathogenic for man; the others cause lymphocytic choriomeningitis, Argentine hemorrhagic fever, and Bolivian hemorrhagic fever. The term arenavirus is taken from the Latin word *arenosus*, which means sandy and refers to the characteristic granules seen by electron microscopy in infected cells (Rowe et al., 1970). Like other arenaviruses, Lassa virus is released from infected cells by budding and has an envelope formed from the plasma membrane. Its nucleic acid is single-stranded RNA (Chapter 67).

The apparent recent emergence of the disease suggests the possibility that Lassa virus is a virulent mutant of lymphocytic choriomeningitis virus or some nonpathogenic arenavirus.

PATHOGENESIS AND PATHOLOGY. Man is infected through contact with *Mastomys natalensis*, a multimammate rat widespread in Africa. Lassa virus was recovered from tissues of *Mastomys* captured in houses occupied by Lassa fever patients during the 1972 epidemic in Sierra Leone. Ironically, the more vicious *Rattus rattus* seems to protect communities from Lassa fever by competing for food and space and thus driving away *Mastomys* and its Lassa virus. The rodents have easy access to the open African dwellings to which they are attracted by grains and food that are stored without protection. *Mastomys* sheds virus in the urine for long periods of time and spreads the infection to human beings by crawling over the beams and rafters of huts or houses and urinating on the sleeping inhabitants, their personal articles, and their food. The routes of entry are thus surmised to be inhalation of virus, direct contact with infected urine, or eating contaminated food. The prominence of sore throat and abdominal pain early in the illness would fit with a gastrointestinal or inhalational route of infection. Spread from patient to medical personnel takes place after direct contact, exposure to respiratory droplets, and accidental cuts from needles or scalpels. Airborne dissemination is the best way to explain infections in hospital visitors or patients who had no direct contact with hospitalized cases of Lassa fever and who developed prominent respiratory symptoms. Infection in households is probably transmitted by eating contaminated food or drinking infected water. Lassa virus has been recovered from the throat two to three weeks after symptoms began, and from the urine four to five weeks thereafter. Viremia is heavy enough to explain the spread of infection by sharp instruments. There are records of infection that occurred after sticking a finger with a needle being used for intravenous injection of fluid. One death from Lassa fever was the result of a cut received while performing an autopsy. Thus Lassa virus differs from other arenaviruses in the ease with which it spreads from person to person.

Whether the portal of entry is the throat, gastrointestinal tract, or lung, a persistent viremia develops that carries the Lassa virus to all organs, apparently damaging capillaries everywhere so that water and blood is lost into the tissues, producing edema and hemorrhages. Thrombocytopenia and other coagulation disturbances contribute to these hemorrhages, which have been noted in the skin, intestine, myocardium, and kidney. A distinctive lesion has been found throughout the liver where the virus has been seen by electron microscopy. Individual hepatocytes, or groups of hepatocytes, undergo eosinophilic necrosis with no accompanying inflammatory exudate, inclusions, or fatty changes. Unusual lesions also occur in the spleen where the malpighian bodies have been found depleted of lymphocytes and surrounded by an eosinophilic zone of coagulation necrosis. Focal pneumonitis has also been present (Edington and White, 1972; Frame et al., 1970).

CLINICAL MANIFESTATIONS. Symptoms usually start gradually after an incubation period of 7 to 17 days. An exact incubation period was calculated in the case of a pathologist who cut her finger on January 25, 1970 with a scalpel while freeing the ribs of a dead patient with Lassa fever in Jos, Nigeria. Ten days later, on February 3, the pathologist had a severe chill, felt severe muscle pains, and became very tired. The next day her temperature was over 102° F, and her throat became so sore she could hardly swallow. On February 11 she complained of greatly increased malaise, her skin became flushed, and petechiae began to appear. Her course thereafter was steadily downhill. Blood oozed from anywhere an injection had been made, oliguria set in, and she became hypothermic to 94.6°. Her white count, which had been low, suddenly jumped to over 37,000, a puzzling feature noted in other Lassa cases. She went into shock and her respirations became labored, but she remained conscious until her death on February 18, 15 days after the illness began (Fuller, 1974).

The features of this case are typical of the severe form of Lassa fever with its fatality rate of 41 per cent in Africans to 64 per cent in whites (Frame et al., 1970; Monath, 1975). In milder cases the mortality rate is only 8 per cent (Monath et al., 1974). In most patients the onset is more insidious than that described in the pathologist, possibly because she gave herself a massive inoculum of Lassa virus from a fatal case. The symptoms of chills, fever, and muscle aches are regularly seen at the beginning, but they are usually not bad enough to see a doctor until four to nine days after they start. Sometimes there is improvement on the second and third days before the progressive illness sets in. Sore throat is usually present after the third day and may become so severe that swallowing is impossible. In about half the patients, pains are also noticed in the head, chest, and abdomen. Headache is mild but persistent and either frontal or generalized. The abdominal pain may be localized over the liver, or diffuse and colicky, with frequent loose stools. Chest pain tends to occur along the costal margins or under the sternum and is made worse by a frequent nonproductive cough (Monath, 1974).

The severe sore throat is accompanied by an exudative pharyngitis and tonsillitis. The yellowish or white exudate may coalesce to form a pseudomembrane. Aphthous ulcers with a yellow center and bright red rim may occur singly or in clusters on the back of the throat, buccal mucosa, and palate. The cervical and submaxillary lymph nodes are enlarged and often tender. Axillary lymphadenopathy is also present.

Signs of capillary leakage, such as facial edema, pleural effusion, and ecchymoses occur in the more severe cases. The pleural effusion, which is a clear serous fluid, is accompanied by dyspnea. Rales are more common than edema or serous effusions, last only a few days, and are not accompanied by signs of heart failure. It is also of interest that the edema does not tend to be dependent. The blood pressure is low (systolic under 90 mm Hg) during the acute stage, but shock occurs only in fatal cases.

COMPLICATIONS AND SEQUELAE. Abortion and hearing loss are the only two complications of Lassa fever. Women with severe Lassa fever often abort within four days of admission (Fabiyi, 1975), and others may deliver a dead fetus during convalescence. The death rate from Lassa fever in pregnant women is twice that in nonpregnant women (Monath, 1975).

About half the patients have symptoms referable to the eighth nerve, and a few continue to have trouble hearing after recovery from the acute illness. Ataxia may also be a problem in convalescence (Fuller, 1974).

GEOGRAPHIC VARIATIONS IN DISEASE. There are no clinical differences in the Lassa fever syndrome seen in Nigeria, Sierra Leone, and Liberia, the three epidemic areas of the disease.

DIAGNOSIS. The disease should be suspected in anyone living in, or coming from, Nigeria, Sierra Leone, or Liberia and who becomes ill with fever, prostration, severe ulcerative pharyngitis, cervical adenopathy, rales, cough, and abdominal pain. Leukopenia and proteinuria are also useful diagnostic points, and a history of employment in a hospital in these epidemic regions is important. The pharyngitis is perhaps the distinctive feature of the illness because no other tropical infection is characterized by this combination of a severe sore throat with severe febrile prostration. It resembles infectious mononucleosis, but mononucleosis is seldom seen in the tropics. Streptococcal sore throat and diphtheria would be important diagnostic considerations if there were no facilities for bacteriologic diagnosis, but otherwise the distinction is easy to make. Dengue hemorrhagic fever and yellow fever are tropical diseases with severe prostration and bleeding, but the rash of dengue and the jaundice of yellow fever are not seen in Lassa fever.

The specific diagnosis of Lassa fever can be made by serologic tests and virus isolation. Lassa virus can be rapidly isolated from the throat, blood, and urine in Vero cells and other tissue culture cell lines, and by mouse inoculation. Such isolation should be attempted, however, only in laboratories equipped with iron-clad safety precautions against laboratory infection with this lethal virus (such as the Maximum Security Laboratory at the Center for Disease Control [CDC]). Lassa virus can be isolated from the blood, throat, and urine for at least two weeks and rarely more than three. Hence, quarantine for three weeks is probably long enough.

Serologic diagnosis is made by complement fixation, neutralization, and indirect immunofluorescence. Complement-fixing antibody does not appear until two weeks after onset of infection, and antigenic differences in strains from different outbreaks have been noted that could give negative results in proven infections if a nonreacting strain is used for complement fixation. Thus, sera from Lassa fever patients in Nigeria did not fix complement in the presence of strains from Liberia and Sierra Leone (Monath, 1975). Such antigenic differences have not been encountered with the indirect immunofluorescence test. For this reason, and also because it has been positive with sera as early as seven days after onset of infection, it is probably the diagnostic test of choice in Lassa fever. The test must also be done in high-security laboratories because live virus is used to prepare the antigenic substrates to which the human sera are applied. The reaction between human serum and Lassa virus is detected on slides with fluorescein isothiocyanate-conjugated antihuman immunoglobulin.

TREATMENT. Transfusions of immune plasma have been given to Lassa fever patients who recovered, but their number is too small to draw conclusions about the value of such immunotherapy. In monkeys infected with Lassa fever virus, treatment with convalescent immune human plasma dramatically terminated viremia and lowered mortality, especially when used against homologous strains (Jahrling and Peters, 1984). One patient died after such treatment, possibly because renal failure was precipitated by the plasma (White, 1972). Otherwise, treatment is supportive and should be directed at relieving the sore throat, removing pleural fluid when such effusions compromise breathing, treating the bleeding disorder with transfusions of platelets, and replacing blood lost by hemorrhage. Dialysis may be of value for patients with renal failure. Ribavarin, an antiviral drug used successfully against Lassa virus infections in monkeys, may help in treating patients with Lassa fever (Jahrling et al., 1980). It has been suggested that effective treatment of human Lassa fever may require both plasma and ribavarin.

PREVENTION. Current epidemiologic information would suggest that prevention of Lassa fever will require rodent control, isolation of patients, and personal precautions by hospital personnel or laboratory workers who must deal with infected excreta, blood specimens, or tissues. *Mastomys natalensis* are the rodents that must be controlled, since the virus has been found in no other animal reservoir. Unfortunately the crowded living conditions, poor sanitation, open houses, and unprotected food storage that encourage this rodent in epidemic areas are too widespread and too difficult to change. A more realistic approach is to prevent spread in the hospital where the source of nosocomial outbreaks is a patient admitted with an unexplained fever. A high index of suspicion should prevail in West Africa in epidemic areas so that the index case can be spotted and isolated. Surgeons, nurses, pathologists, and laboratory technicians are among those at greatest risk and should be most alert to the danger of infection from cases of unexplained fever with sore throat who might have the Lassa syndrome. Although food and water are vehicles for transmission, the danger of this route of transmission from the index cases is minimized in African hospitals by the practice of feeding patients with food brought by their relatives. Isolation of index cases should be carried out in a way that would not allow airborne dissemination. In addition, linens, bedpans, and other utensils must be carefully handled and sterilized because the virus is shed in excreta for at least two weeks.

Travelers who arrive from West Africa with pharyngitis and fever should be hospitalized in strict isolation. Throat swabs and urine and blood samples should be collected for shipment to a diagnostic center by a physician wearing a mask and protective clothing. High-risk contacts known to have had intimate contact, including face-to-face conversation, should be identified and kept under close surveillance if the diagnosis is confirmed. It should be kept in mind that Lassa fever is not highly communicable outside the home or hospital. At least five patients have traveled aboard commercial airplanes, but no secondary cases have been found among airline passengers (Editorial note, 1978). There is no vaccine, but convalescent plasma has protected monkeys and might be beneficial for prophylaxis in exposed humans (Jahrling and Peters, 1984).

References

Edington, G., and White, H.: The pathology of Lassa fever. Trans R Soc Trop Med Hyg 19:670, 1970.

Fabiyi, A.: In discussion of paper by Monath, T., 1975.

Frame, J., Baldwin, J., Gocke, D., and Troup, J.: Lassa fever, a new virus disease of man from West Africa. I. Clinical description and pathological findings. Am J Trop Med Hyg 19:670, 1970.

Fuller, J. G.: Fever! The Hunt for a New Killer Virus. New York, Ballantine Books, 1974, pp. 183–205.

Jahrling, P., Hesse, R., Eddy, G., Johnson, K., Callis, R., and Stephen, E.: Lassa virus infections of rhesus monkeys: pathogenesis and treatment with ribavarin. J Infect Dis 141:580, 1980.

Jahrling, P., and Peters, C.: Passive antibody therapy of Lassa fever in cynomolgus monkeys: Importance of neutralizing antibody and Lassa virus strain. Infect and Immun 44:528, 1984.

Monath, T. P.: Lassa fever: Review of epidemiology and epizootiology. WHO Bull 52:577, 1975.

Monath, T., Maher, M., Casals, J., Kissling, R., and Cacciapuoti, A.: Lassa fever in the Eastern Province of Sierra Leone, 1970–1972. II. Clinical observation and virologic studies on selected hospital cases. Am J Trop Med Hyg 23:1140, 1974.

Rowe, W., Murphy, F., Bergold, G., Lasak, J., Hotchin, J., Johnson, K., Lehman-Grube, F., Mims, C., Traub, E., and Webb, P.: Arenaviruses: Proposed name for a newly defined virus group. J Virol 5:651, 1970.

U.S. Public Health Service, Center for Disease Control: Editorial note: Suspected Lassa fever—Washington, D.C. Morbid Mortal Weekly Rep May 26, 1978, p. 182.

White, H.: Clinical findings in 23 cases of Lassa fever hospitalized in Jos, Nigeria. Trans R Soc Trop Med Hyg 66:390, 1972.

G. DERMAL INFECTIONS, EXANTHEMS, AND INFESTATIONS

219

IMPETIGO

MARIAN E. MELISH, M.D.

ETIOLOGY. There are two clinically and bacteriologically distinct superficial skin infections that are commonly called "impetigo." These two basic forms are: (1) the thick crusted variety that is primarily of streptococcal origin, and (2) the bullous form that is caused exclusively by coagulase-positive staphylococci. Either or both may be referred to as impetigo. In the United States, however, the term impetigo generally refers to the thick crusted variety and "bullous impetigo" to the staphylococcal form.

Bacterial culture of typical crusted impetigo lesions generally yields either group A β-hemolytic streptococci or a mixed flora of group A streptococci and coagulase-positive staphylococci. Several lines of evidence indicate that the streptococcus is the primary etiologic agent and the staphylococcus merely a secondary invader or "fellow traveler."

1. Streptococci are frequently isolated in pure culture from typical thick crusted lesions, whereas staphylococci are almost never encountered alone.

2. Sequential cultures of typical lesions show the same strain of streptococci as permanent residents, whereas staphylococci of varying types are only intermittently present.

3. Early lesions are often purely streptococcal; later cultures yield mixed flora. An increasing yield of staphylococci as the lesion ages suggests that staphylococci are secondary invaders.

4. Treatment of patients with antibiotics active against streptococci, but not staphylococci, gives as good a cure rate as treatment directed against both organisms (Dajani et al., 1972; Dillon, 1970).

A number of different M types (see Chapter 24) are associated with impetigo, particularly those of higher numbers; for example, M-33, M-49 (Red Lake), and M-52 to M-61. Many strains cannot be typed by antibody to known M types and are identified by antisera to their T antigens (Chapter 24).

Only strains of *S. aureus* that produce epidermolytic toxin (see Chapter 5) cause bullous impetigo. Pustular folliculitis (Chapter 220) is the superficial dermatitis commonly caused by nontoxigenic strains of staphylococci.

IMPETIGO (STREPTOCOCCAL PYODERMA)

PATHOGENESIS AND PATHOLOGY. Direct inoculation of group A hemolytic streptococci into superficial abrasions or compromised areas of skin is the usual route of infection. The most common skin conditions predisposing to impetigo are insect bites, maceration (by sweat or rhinorrhea), atopic dermatitis, and eczema. Biopsy of lesions is not needed for diagnosis and is rarely indicated. The typical pathology is

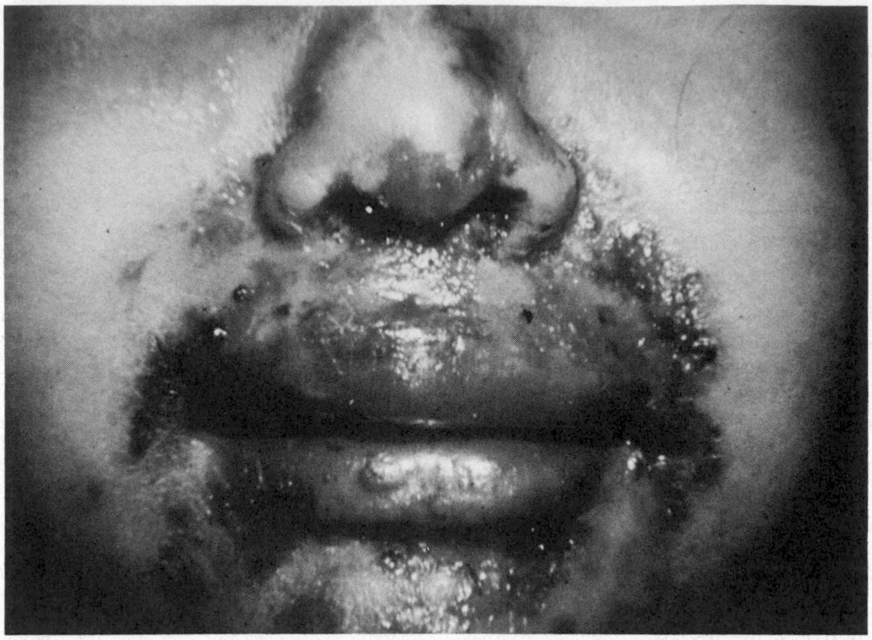

Figure 1. Common impetigo. Extensive thick crusted lesions are present around the nose and mouth of this preschool child. The lesion is a dark yellow-brown crust composed of dried cloudy serous exudate. This lesion is predominantly streptococcal.

restricted to the epidermis and is characterized by subcorneal inflammatory infiltrate containing bacteria, polymorphonuclear leukocytes, and scattered areas of liquefactive degeneration. There may be a perivascular cellular infiltrate within the dermis.

CLINICAL MANIFESTATIONS. This thick crusted superficial skin infection is exceedingly common, especially in children. It is sufficiently distinctive to be diagnosed and treated on clinical grounds alone (Fig. 1). The typical lesion begins as an erythematous papule or an erythematous zone surrounding an abrasion or insect bite. Small vesicles may appear transiently, but these are rarely appreciated because the lesion rapidly evolves to the crusted form. The usual lesion varies in size from a few millimeters to 1 to 2 cm and consists of a central crusted plaque surrounded by a discrete erythematous margin. The crust is thick, raised, and of an amber or dirty honey color. Lesions are generally not purulent; when the crust is removed, a cloudy amber fluid issues from the moist erythematous base. With time, lesions may become extensive and coalescent, particularly on the scalp. Systemic signs are unusual even in patients with extensive impetigo; the appearance of fever and pain generally heralds development of significant cellulitis. For this reason, there is frequent delay in seeking medical attention; several series of children in the United States demonstrated a two to three week period of lesions before patient presentation. This delay is even more likely in tropical areas or medically underserved regions where sores are frequently considered a normal attribute of childhood. Lesions are only moderately tender to touch. Exposed areas such as the face and extremities are most often involved. Regional adenitis is common.

COMPLICATIONS AND SEQUELAE. Impetigo is usually indolent and may remain stable for considerable periods. Many lesions heal spontaneously, particularly in people with good personal hygiene, but the infection may spread from the dermis and cause deeper suppurative disease, including cellulitis, lymphadenitis, and bacteremia. Neglected lesions may also form chronic ulcers with erosion through the dermis.

The most important complication of streptococcal impetigo, however, is acute poststreptococcal glomerulonephritis. The pathogenesis of this complication is similar to that described for experimental immune-complex disease with glomerular deposition of IgG, complement, and fibrin.

GEOGRAPHIC VARIATIONS IN DISEASE. Climate dramatically affects the prevalence of impetigo. It occurs during warm humid seasons in temperate areas but year around in tropical areas. It is strikingly less common in arid climates. Warm humid weather apparently enhances the establishment of impetigo by providing maximum opportunities for inoculation sites (insect bites and abrasions on uncovered limbs) and for bacterial multiplication.

Impetigo is generally endemic but may spread in epidemic fashion among people who are in close contact such as families, schools, military camps, and athletic teams.

DIAGNOSIS AND TREATMENT. The diagnosis of impetigo can usually be made clinically. Cultures of the lesions are not necessary unless the presentation is atypical or the response to therapy is poor. Serum antibodies to the enzymes of group A streptococci are most often measured as an aid to establishing the diagnosis of poststreptococcal glomerulonephritis. The antibody response to streptolysin O after impetigo is often poor, but antibodies are uniformly produced to hyaluronidase and DNAse B.

Multiple studies have demonstrated the superiority of systemic antibiotic therapy over local measures such as scrubbing, soaking, or topical antibiotics. One dose of intramuscular benzathine penicillin (600,000 units for patients weighing less than 60 pounds, 1.2 million units for patients weighing more than 60 pounds) or a 10-day course of oral penicillin, erythromycin, or lincomycin are of equal efficacy and superior to local therapy. Systemic antibiotic therapy is important for all but the most trivial lesions to prevent deeper suppurative disease and bacteremia. Antibiotic therapy will not prevent acute poststreptococcal nephritis, at least in part because so much antigenic exposure has already occurred during the delay between first appearance of the lesion and therapy (Anthony et al., 1967; Dillon, 1968).

PROPHYLAXIS. Prevention of impetigo depends on good general hygiene, bathing of insect bites and abrasions, and recognition of early lesions. Scrubbing and application of antibiotic ointment to incipient lesions will prevent extensive disease.

BULLOUS IMPETIGO

PATHOGENESIS AND PATHOLOGY. Staphylococci from the focus of infection within the epidermis produce epidermolytic toxin that separates the granular cells of the superficial epidermis to form the characteristic thin-roofed bullae with a cleavage plane high in the epidermis at the granular cell layer just below the stratum corneum (Fig. 2). Staphylococci and polymorphonuclear leukocytes are seen within the bullae. Epidermolytic toxin can be demonstrated within bullae fluid. Biopsy is diagnostic but is rarely needed unless extensive lesions suggest another diagnosis.

CLINICAL MANIFESTATIONS, COMPLICATIONS, AND SEQUELAE. Bullous impetigo presents a completely different clinical picture from the thick crusted appearance of the streptococcal disease. It can be recognized by the superficial thin-walled, flaccid bullae ranging from 0.5 to 3 cm in diameter that erupt on otherwise normal-appearing skin (Fig. 3). Only a small ring of erythema surrounds the bullae. They may be grouped or coalescent. The fluid within the bulla is generally thin and varies from slightly cloudy to frankly purulent. Bullae rupture easily and spontaneously, revealing a moist, circular erythematous plaque (Fig. 4). Soon after rupture a thin, varnish-like crust forms over the surface of this plaque. Bullous impetigo is usually localized to a few lesions or a few areas of the body; however, widely disseminated disease may result when the skin has been macerated or soaked. Coagulase-positive staphylococci that produce the epidermolytic toxin are recovered from the bullae.

If neglected or untreated, bullous impetigo may spread to large areas of skin. Disseminated staphylococcal septicemia may also occur. Although antitoxin to epidermolytic toxin develops after an episode of bullous impetigo, the disease can develop and progress despite serum antibody (Melish et al., 1978).

DIAGNOSIS. Bullous impetigo occurs both in endemic and epidemic patterns. In neonates, the disease has been seen frequently in association with common nursery epidemics of staphylococcal disease. Among older children and adults, disease is generally sporadic and relatively uncommon compared to streptococcal impetigo. The lesions of bullous impetigo are generally correctly identified when present in small groups in a single area. Single lesions may be mistaken for thermal burns. Extensive, coalescent lesions are likely to be confused with generalized bullous dermatoses such as dermatitis herpetiformis, pemphigus and bullous erythema multiforme (Stevens-Johnson syndrome). A firm diagnosis can be made by aspirating intact bullae and demonstrating staphylococci and polymorphonuclear leukocytes within the fluid. Skin biopsy is definitive and occasionally necessary (Dillon, 1968; Melish and Glasgow, 1978).

TREATMENT. Systemic antistaphylococcal antibiotics, usually given by the oral route, eradicate the infection. Infections may progress rapidly if untreated, particularly in neonates and individuals with pre-existing skin disease.

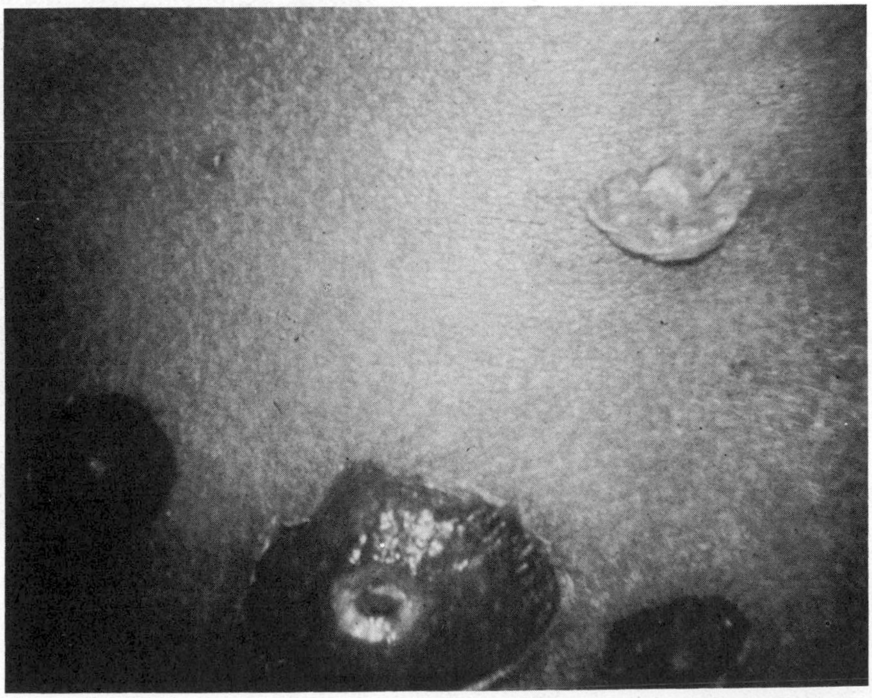

Figure 2. Bulla in bullous impetigo. The lesion is composed of a cavity containing leukocytes. Staphylococci and epidermolytic toxin. The cleavage plane is located at the granular cell layer.

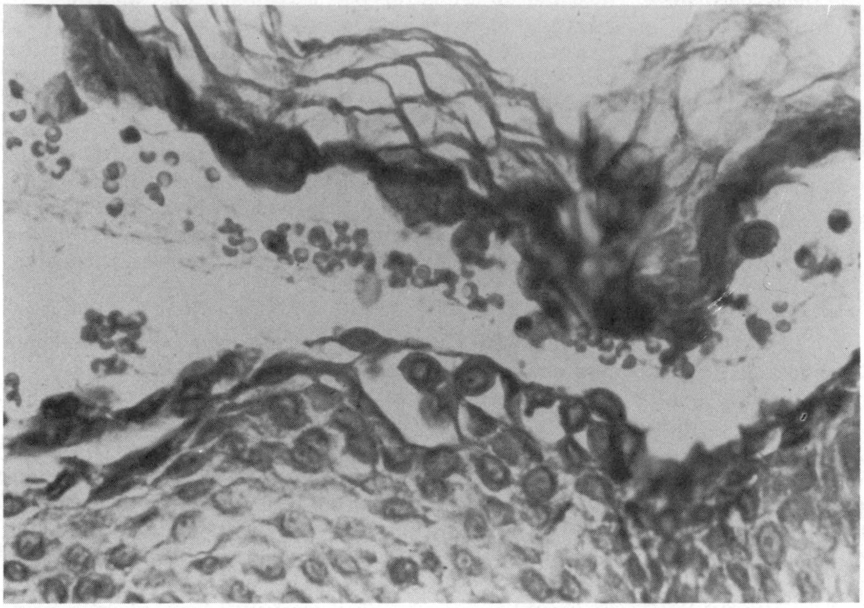

Figure 3. Bullous impetigo. In contrast to common impetigo, bullous impetigo is composed of superficial bullae that rupture spontaneously, revealing a moist surface that may dry to a thin collodion-like veneer.

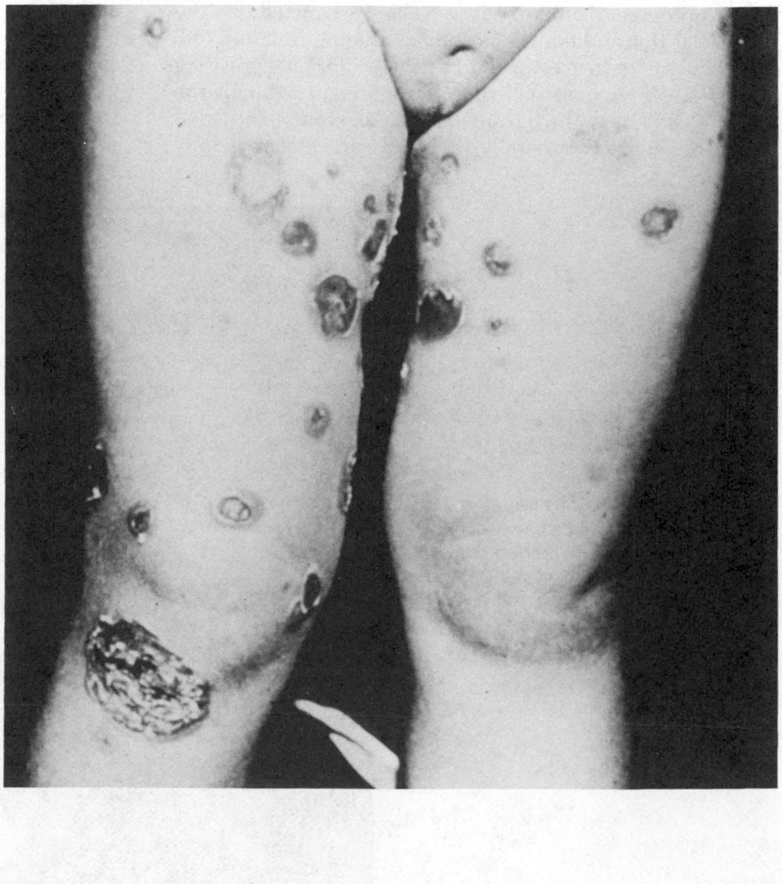

Figure 4. Bullous impetigo.

Staphylococci that produce epidermolytic toxin are overwhelmingly penicillin-resistant, at least in North America and Europe, and should be treated either with β-lactamase-resistant penicillins, cephalosporins, erythromycin, or lincomycin.

References

Anthony, F. B., Perlman, L. V., and Wannamaker, L. W.: Skin infections and acute nephritis in American Indian children. Pediatrics 39:263, 1967.

Dajani, A. S., Ferrieri, P., and Wannamaker, L. W.: Natural history of impetigo. II. Etiologic agents and bacterial interactions. J Clin Invest 51:2863, 1972.

Dillon, H. C.: Impetigo contagiosa: Suppurative and non-suppurative complications. Am J Dis Child 115:530, 1968.

Dillon, H. C.: The treatment of streptococcal skin infections. J Pediatr 76:676, 1970.

Melish, M. E., and Glasgow, L. A.: The staphylococcal scalded skin syndrome: The expanded clinical syndrome. J Pediatr 78:958, 1971.

Melish, M. E., Stuckey, M., and Sprouse, S.: Development of antibody to staphylococcal epidermolytic toxin (ET). Clin Res 26:188A, 1978.

220

PYOGENIC SKIN INFECTIONS

MARIAN E. MELISH, M.D.

Most of the infections considered in this chapter are more extensive and involve deeper tissue planes than superficial impetigo.

Only bacterial skin infections that elicit a pyogenic response and are not usually a manifestation of a specific systemic disease are included. Thus, cutaneous anthrax, erysipeloid, actinomycotic mycetoma, and swimming pool granuloma (*Mycobacterium marinum*) are not considered. Although *Staphylococcus aureus* and group A β-hemolytic streptococci are the most common causes of pyogenic skin infections, a rich array of other bacteria may be involved in certain environmental and clinical situations. These clinical settings and the clinical manifestations are sometimes specific enough to permit the institution of appropriate treatment while awaiting the results of smears and cultures.

FOLLICULITIS, FURUNCULOSIS, AND CARBUNCLES

This group of infections all arise in hair follicles, form abscesses with central purulence, and are generally caused by coagulase-positive staphylococci (*S. aureus*). The lesions differ in extent. *Folliculitis* is limited to small abscesses involving single hair follicles with only a small amount of surrounding tissue reaction. *Furuncles* develop in hair follicles but become larger and deeper inflammatory nodules surrounded by a wide zone of intense tissue reaction. *Carbuncles,* which are composed of several interconnecting furuncles or abscesses, are much wider and deeper.

ETIOLOGY. Coagulase-positive staphylococci cause the overwhelming majority of these infections. Rarely, other organisms may cause the same lesions in immunocompromised patients or in persons who have experienced unusual environmental exposure. For example, *Pseudomonas aeruginosa* can cause folliculitis after the use of heavily contaminated hot tubs or whirlpools. These lesions occur only on immersed areas of the body and resolve spontaneously if use of the tubs is discontinued.

PATHOGENESIS AND PATHOLOGY. Lesions are limited to hair-bearing areas and are most common in the axillae, perineum, extremities, neck, and around the breast. They appear to arise de novo without preexisting foci. Poor personal hygiene, occlusion and maceration of the skin, and warm, moist, tropical climates appear to be powerful predisposing factors to the development of these lesions. Nevertheless, trouble may occur in persons with meticulous hygiene. Environmental exposure to virulent staphylococci has also been the source of widespread outbreaks of folliculitis and furunculosis in normal newborn nurseries. In addition to infants, adolescents, young adults, and diabetics are more susceptible to these infections. Experimentally, folliculitis can be induced regularly in laboratory animals and in man when coagulase-positive staphylococci are applied to mildly traumatized or occluded skin. Infection cannot be induced in normal, unmanipulated skin, even with extremely large inocula. In either experimental or natural infections, a thick-walled abscess eventually becomes established in the hair follicle. Lesions have a purulent necrotic center that may rupture spontaneously. Although most are well contained by the surrounding inflammatory reaction, infection may spread to adjacent tissues and cause a diffuse cellulitis or metastasize hematogenously.

DIAGNOSIS AND MANAGEMENT. The diagnosis can be made by inspection (Fig. 1) and confirmed by gram stain. If the lesions or history are atypical or if organisms other than *Staphylococcus aureus* are seen in the gram stain, cultures must be obtained.

Early lesions may be treated with warm soaks to encourage spontaneous drainage. Larger, localized lesions must be incised and drained. Patients with an extensive carbuncle or a furuncle associated with cellulitis may also require an oral antistaphylococcal antibiotic, such as dicloxacillin or cephalexin (0.5 g four times a day for seven to ten days). Penicillinase-negative *S. aureus* should be treated with 1.0 g of penicillin V four times a day. Patients must be cautioned that draining lesions are a hazard to others and should not be allowed to work as food handlers or have contact with hospitalized patients. After adequate drainage, the erythema and edema subside, but a dense scar frequently follows all but the most trivial lesions.

COMPLICATIONS AND SEQUELAE. Local or metastatic spread of infection, the most serious complication, can usually be avoided by prompt drainage. If the patient is

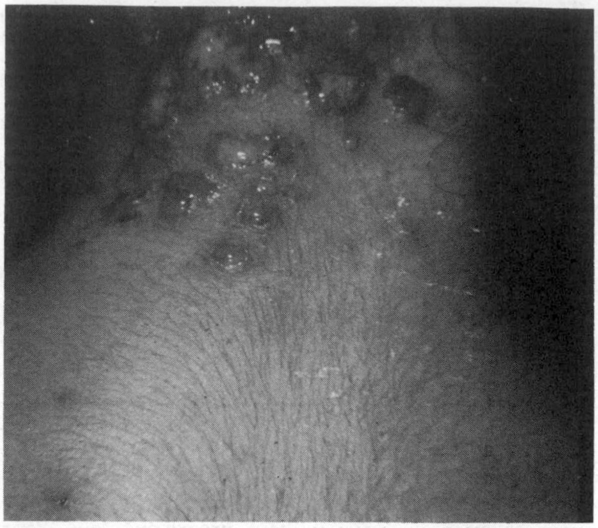

Figure 1. Superficial staphylococcal furunculosis. All stages in the development of superficial staphylococcal skin abscess are depicted here from early folliculitis to multiple nodular furuncles to a small carbuncle made up of interconnecting furuncles.

already febrile and systemically ill when first evaluated, blood and the lesion should be cultured and metastatic foci should be sought in the heart, bones, joints, brain, muscles, and endocardium.

PROPHYLAXIS. Certain patients predisposed to recurrent infections should have careful physical examinations, with particular attention to underlying disease, nutritional status, personal hygiene, and any potential breaks in the skin barrier. Chronic dermatoses such as eczema, icthyosis, or seborrhea may be predisposing factors and should be treated. A meticulous regimen of personal hygiene and antibiotic ointment for use on all minor wounds and early lesions should be prescribed. No other regimens are of proven value. Staphylococcal vaccines have been widely used but have never been adequately evaluated.

WOUND INFECTIONS

When the protective barrier of the skin is breached by traumatic or surgical invasion, infection may be introduced and develop in the skin and adjacent tissues. The ubiquitous, coagulase-positive staphylococcus and group A streptococcus are most often responsible for wound infections. However, a variety of other organisms may be introduced under specific environmental conditions. These organisms require specific consideration. (Those responsible for infections from animal bites are discussed in Chapter 256.)

HUMAN BITE WOUND INFECTIONS. Human bites frequently result in rapidly progressive destructive infections of soft tissues, tendons, joints, and bones. The hand is commonly infected after tooth lacerations to the fist or full mouth bites to the hand or fingers. Signs of infection develop rapidly within 24 hours of injury. Bite wound infections are nearly always polymicrobial. Normal mouth flora, particularly anaerobic streptococci, oral spirochetes, staphylococci, aerobic streptococci, and mouth aerobes, are involved. The pus is malodorous because of the presence of anaerobic bacteria. Bite wounds should be carefully inspected and irrigated, and devitalized tissue should be debrided. The wounds should not be sutured primarily, because adequate drainage is very important. Penicillinase-resistant penicillins or cephalosporins directed at staphylococci and mouth bacteria may be given even before signs of infection appear, because the fully developed infection is so destructive.

Patients who present with an established infection after a human bite frequently require radical débridement, deep wound culture, and high-dose systemic antibiotics directed at the organisms isolated from the deep wound culture (Shields et al., 1975).

SOIL-CONTAMINATED WOUNDS. The gram-negative enteric bacilli and the clostridia responsible for gas gangrene and tetanus are prominent in soil-contaminated wounds. The wound must be completely explored for foreign material, debrided adequately, and irrigated. Primary closure should be avoided. Clostridial cellulitis and myonecrosis (gas gangrene) can be prevented only by making the local environment unsatisfactory for the growth of clostridia by removal of foreign material and dead tissue and ensuring that oxygen can enter the wound.

An established wound infection should be surgically inspected for its full extent and any foreign material removed. Bullae, tissue crepitation, and/or gas in tissue on x-ray suggests clostridial infection. Deep wound culture and gram stain should be made. If the gram stain shows gram-positive rods and there is clinical evidence of clostridial cellulitis, extensive surgical débridement with multiple incisions into the involved tissue must be made. Large intravenous doses of penicillin (200,000 units/kg) should be given. Necrotic muscle containing gram-positive rods and gas in the tissue establish the diagnosis of gas gangrene and constitute a medical emergency. Amputation or extensive débridement and hyperbaric oxygen treatment should be instituted immediately (see Chapter 253).

Wound infections that are not obviously clostridial should be managed in a similar way. Deep wound culture and gram stain should be taken at the time of débridement. A penicillinase-resistant penicillin plus an aminoglycoside should be given for all significant infections, pending the results of cultures and sensitivities. If the primary gram stain suggests the presence of *Bacteroides*, clindamycin can be substituted for the semisynthetic penicillin until the cultures are completed.

WATER-CONTAMINATED WOUNDS. Organisms found in stagnant fresh water, particularly *Aeromonas hydrophila*, pseudomonads, and coliforms, may infect wounds that are sustained in fresh water. *Aeromonas* causes a particularly rapid progressive necrotizing infection. Wounds sustained in salt water may be contaminated with *Vibrio parahemolyticus* and other noncholera vibrios. Deep culture, adequate surgical exploration and exposure, and careful follow-up are especially important measures in the management of traumatic wounds sustained under unusual circumstances because unusual bacteria may be encountered.

SURGICAL WOUNDS. Surgical wound infections are caused primarily by coagulase-positive staphylococci and group A streptococci. Occasionally, the anaerobic and aerobic enteric flora infect abdominal incisions after surgery for peritonitis or gross fecal contamination.

The condition of the wound plays a major role in its resistance to infection. The presence of a hematoma, necrotic tissue, diminished blood flow, and foreign bodies all decrease innate local resistance. The type of suture material is also important; braided silk sutures are more likely to form a nidus of infection than monofilament nylon or wire.

The nature of the infecting organism dictates the clinical manifestations. Group A β-hemolytic streptococci, which cause surgical infections far less commonly than coagulase-positive staphylococci, present the most immediate and serious problem. Within one to two days after the operation, the patient may develop high fever, leukocytosis, tachycardia, and even vascular collapse. Erysipelas may develop around the wound. Often, however, the wound appears normal, but large numbers of streptococci are seen in the deep wound aspirate. Because streptococcal postoperative wound infections may cause fulminant disease, a high degree of suspicion, careful wound evaluation, and deep cultures are essential measures in the management of patients who develop fever soon after surgery. Penicillin at a dose of 100,000 units/kg/day should be started intravenously. If the gram stain shows gram-positive cocci that are not clearly differentiated from staphylococci, methicillin, or oxacillin should be used instead of penicillin at doses of 200 mg/kg/day.

Staphylococci and enteric bacilli usually cause a less dramatic illness. Early signs of infection are insidious and begin four to six days after surgery with wound tenderness, low-grade fever, and mild systemic signs, such as lethargy and anorexia. The wound may look normal, but careful inspection and removal of sutures may reveal infection deep within the wound. Gram stain of the exudate distinguishes between staphylococci and enterics, which are the usual causes of this common, more indolent presentation. The wound should be opened to allow drainage and to determine the extent of involvement. Antibiotics are given to prevent dissemination of the infection but are less important than surgical drainage. Staphylococcal infections should be treated with an antistaphylococcal penicillin. Gram-negative infections of abdominal wounds, are likely to be caused by *Bacteroides fragilis*. In this case, therapy with chloramphenicol, clindamycin, or metronidazole is required. An aminoglycoside is preferred for aerobic enteric flora.

ERYSIPELAS

Erysipelas is a specific form of superficial cellulitis that involves the dermis and uppermost subcutaneous tissue. It is caused exclusively by group A β-hemolytic streptococci that pack and obstruct the superficial lymphatics beneath the involved skin. Erysipelas has a characteristic appearance consisting of a rapidly enlarging, deeply erythematous plaque with a sharply demarcated, raised border. The involved area is indurated, tender, and may have a "peau d'orange" appearance (Fig. 2). Large tension bullae may develop within the erythematous zone because the lymphatics are obstructed by streptococci.

Group A streptococci may be recovered either from the advancing margin or from the central primary wound, if present, but a punch biopsy from the center of the erysipeloid lesion is the most reliable way to obtain the organism for gram stain and culture. The portal of entry may be a surgical wound or an excoriated insect bite but is most frequently inapparent. Erysipelas may occur on any area of the body; we have seen it most frequently as a circumferential, rapidly progressive lesion on the extremities, but it is also common on the face or with surgical wounds.

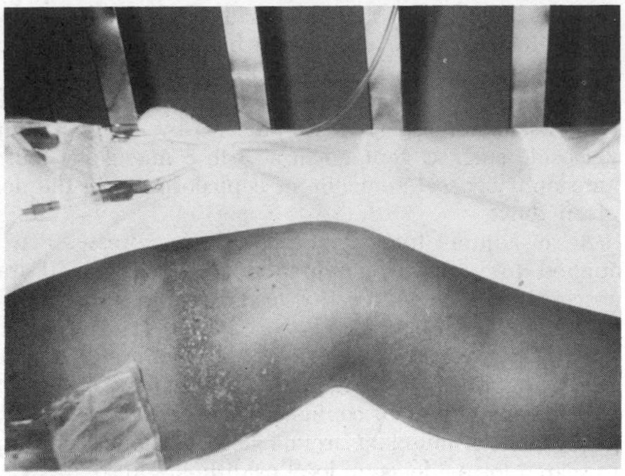

Figure 2. Erysipelas. This form of superficial streptococcal cellulitis presents with a sharply demarcated, slightly elevated, tender erythroderma, here forming a band around the thigh and calf of a child. Small bullae are seen at the uppermost extent of the lesions.

Patients with erysipelas are frequently febrile and toxic. Because of the characteristic rapid progression, we initiate therapy with 600,000 units of procaine penicillin twice daily for the first 24 to 48 hours followed by 500 mg of penicillin V four times each day for 10 days.

CELLULITIS

Cellulitis refers to infections that involve primarily the subcutaneous tissues with some secondary involvement of the dermis. Clinically, cellulitis is manifest as an area of edema, erythema, warmth, and tenderness. Because the area of involvement is primarily in the subcutaneous tissue, the lateral margins of the infection appear indistinct, and the edema and erythema merge into the surrounding area.

A wide variety of organisms may cause cellulitis, particularly after trauma or in immunocompromised patients, but group A streptococci and *Staphylococcus aureus* are by far the most common. In children under 5 years, *Haemophilus influenzae* Type b is a frequent cause of cellulitis, especially on the face.

Staphylococcal and streptococcal cellulitis may have identical clinical appearances. Both are associated with cutaneous trauma and tend to be more frequent on the extremities. Aspiration of the central and lateral margins of the cellulitis or a punch biopsy of the central area should be done for culture. Blood cultures may also be positive. Therapy should be started before the culture results are known and should include an antistaphylococcal agent, unless gram stain of the aspiration or punch biopsy clearly shows streptococci. Streptococcal cellulitis should be treated with penicillin by the same routes and doses listed above for erysipelas. Cefazolin (1.0 g I.M. four times daily for two days) followed by cephalexin (500 mg orally four times daily for ten days) is good treatment for staphylococci and satisfactory for streptococci until the culture results are known. Gram-negative bacilli and fungi may also cause cellulitis in the immunocompromised patient. For these patients, every effort should be made to obtain the etiologic agent, including the use of skin biopsy. Empiric therapy for cellulitis in the immunocompromised should include coverage for *Pseudomonas aeruginosa*, gram-negative enterics, staphylococci, and streptococci by using an aminoglycoside such as gentamicin at 3 to 5 mg/kg/day plus an antistaphylococcal penicillin or cephalosporin in the doses given above.

As an adjunct to antibiotics, warm compresses may be applied to promote suppuration and drainage. If frank abscesses occur within the lesion, surgical drainage is indicated.

The prognosis of cellulitis in the normal host is excellent after antibiotics are begun. Cellulitis may disseminate hematogenously or to contiguous underlying foci, such as bone, joint, or muscle. Careful follow-up should be planned to search for evidence of local or distant spread.

TROPICAL PYOMYOSITIS

Tropical pyomyositis is an acute staphylococcal infection of skeletal muscle that occurs spontaneously in the absence of other known foci of infection. Myositis secondary to hematogenous spread from a distant focus or to local spread from a contiguous site of infection in the bone or overlying soft tissue is excluded from this definition. Patients with tropical pyomyositis rarely develop septicemia, and hematogenous spread to other organs is distinctly unusual. Isolated staphylococcal pyomyositis may account for as many as 4 per cent of hospital admissions in the tropics (Levin et al., 1971; Horn and Master, 1968), but it is very rare in temperate climates.

PATHOGENESIS AND CLINICAL MANIFESTATIONS. The pathogenesis of tropical pyomyositis is unknown. Attempts to explain its high prevalence in the tropics have been unsuccessful. There is no convincing evidence that any tropical disease or parasite is responsible either for damaging the affected muscle or seeding it with staphylococci. A history of recent trauma can be elicited from about 20 per cent of patients, and it seems likely that at least some of the cases develop from seeding a traumatized muscle during a transient, asymptomatic bacteremia.

The muscles of the leg and trunk are most commonly affected. The typical patient presents with fever, leukocytosis, and a history of a few days of localized muscle pain and tenderness. A firm swelling may be present over the affected muscle, but local heat and erythema are absent until the infection breaks through the muscle into the overlying tissue. One or more muscles may be affected (Horn and Master, 1968; Shepard, 1983).

DIAGNOSIS AND TREATMENT. The diagnosis of tropical myositis is established by cultivating *S. aureus* from aspiration or surgical drainage of an infected muscle in a patient with negative blood cultures and no other detectable focus of infection (Levin et al., 1971). If blood cultures are positive, the patient should be carefully evaluated for the presence of endocarditis or other foci of infection in the bone or joints. *Streptococcus pneumoniae* and group A streptococci have been isolated from rare cases of isolated pyomyositis.

The cornerstone of treatment is surgical drainage of all muscle abscesses. A penicillinase-resistant penicillin should be administered intravenously in doses of 100 to 200 mg/kg/day until the cultures and sensitivities are completed. Penicillinase-negative *S. aureus* and the rare isolates of streptococci should be treated with similar doses of I.V. penicillin G. If the patient becomes afebrile promptly, and there is no evidence of endocarditis or osteomyelitis, antibiotics can be discontinued after the abscess has resolved.

References

Horn, C. V., and Master, S.: Pyomyositis tropicans in Uganda. E Afr Med J 35:463, 1968.

Levin, M. J., Gardner, P., and Waldvogel, F. A.: "Tropical" pyomyositis: An unusual infection due to *Staphylococcus aureus*. N Engl J Med 284:196, 1971.

Shephard, J. J.: Tropical myositis: Is it an entity and what is its cause? Lancet, 1240, 1983.

Shields, C., Patzakis, M. S., Myers, M. H., and Harvey, J. P., Jr.: Hand infections secondary to human bites. J Trauma 15:235, 1975.

221

THE STAPHYLOCOCCAL SCALDED SKIN SYNDROME

MARIAN E. MELISH, M.D.

Staphylococcus aureus is associated with a spectrum of dermatologic diseases that range from localized bullae to diffuse exfoliative disease with systemic toxemia. These conditions are caused by an epidermolytic toxin that is produced only by *S. aureus*. In the localized form of the disease, called bullous impetigo, the toxin is produced in a focus of infected skin, remains at that site, and produces localized bullae. By contrast, in the other two forms of the scalded skin syndrome, the toxin is produced at a site that may be distant from the skin, is disseminated hematogenously, and produces widespread skin disease at sites distant from the focus of infection. The two generalized forms of the scalded skin syndrome are associated with systemic toxemia and present clinically as either an acute generalized exfoliative disease or an acute scarlatiniform eruption.

These toxin-mediated diseases have been called a bewildering variety of names. The diffuse exfoliative form of the disease has been known as Ritter's disease and pemphigus neonatorum when it occurs in neonates, and as Lyell's disease and toxic epidermal necrolysis when it occurs in children and adults. We refer to the entire spectrum of dermatologic diseases caused by the epidermolytic toxin as the staphylococcal scalded skin syndrome (SSSS) and to the clinical varieties as the diffuse exfoliative form of SSSS, the scarlatiniform variety of SSSS, and bullous impetigo. SSSS may be a cumbersome term, but it is encompassing, descriptive, and etiologic rather than eponymic. Lyell has recently suggested that these conditions would be more appropriately called the Staphylococcal Epidermolytic Toxin Syndrome.

PATHOGENESIS AND PATHOLOGY. The skin changes are caused by a soluble protein exotoxin, epidermolytic toxin, that is elaborated in vitro and in vivo by *S. aureus*, primarily but not exclusively those belonging to phage group II. Epidermolytic toxin can be detected in the blood during the early stages of the exfoliative diseases (Melish et al., 1972). At least two separate antigenic forms of the toxin, referred to as epidermolytic toxins A and B, have been isolated in the United States and in Japan (Kondo et al., 1975). Both have molecular weights of about 25,500, but they differ in other physical properties. Toxin A is sometimes called the stable toxin because it is resistant to boiling. Toxin B is referred to as labile toxin because it is inactivated at 60° F. Toxin A is chromosomally determined, but toxin B may be extrachromosomally mediated because it can be eliminated by DNA intercalating agents (Warren et al., 1974). Between 70 and 90 per cent of toxin-positive *S. aureus* produce A, up to 30 per cent produce A and B, but only 15 per cent produce toxin B only (Melish et al., 1979).

The toxin causes the separation of granular cells within the epidermis (Fig. 1). Intact cells lose their attachments to each other, and a cleavage plane develops just below the stratum corneum. There is no inflammatory response. Antitoxic antibody develops after infection and appears to be protective against the hematogenous dissemination of toxin that is responsible for the generalized manifestations of the scalded skin syndrome. Antitoxic antibody does not prevent local production and action of the toxin. Bullous impetigo and secondary infections of other skin lesions such as bullous varicella may occur and progress despite the presence of antitoxic antibody.

The generalized forms of the scalded skin syndrome occur almost exclusively in children less than 5 years old. There are only twelve reports of staphylococcal toxic epidermal necrolysis in adults, and all have been immunocompromised or have had renal failure. This age-related susceptibility to generalized disease has been explained by a survey of antibody prevalence in people of different ages. In the United States, more than three-quarters of the population over 10 years of age but only one-quarter of children less than 2 years old have antibody to epidermolytic toxin A. Antitoxic antibody develops early in life, probably from minor, inapparent infections with toxin-producing staphylococci (Melish et al., 1979). Although bullous impetigo occurs in the presence of antibody to epidermolytic toxin, immunity even to the diffuse forms of the disease is unusual because humoral immunity to other staphylococcal extracellular products or toxins does not prevent staphylococcal infections.

CLINICAL MANIFESTATIONS

Bullous Impetigo. The lesion is a superficial, localized bulla arising on areas of apparently normal skin (also see Chapter 219). The bullae are flaccid and contain clear, pale to dark yellow fluid. They usually appear on moist or opposing surfaces of the skin, such as the diaper area, the neck, and the axilla, and are easily denuded by slight trauma. The lesions are superficial and heal without scarring or systemic illness. Nikolsky's sign, in which the outer layer of the skin is easily rubbed off by slight friction, is not present, and there is no exfoliation beyond the local lesion.

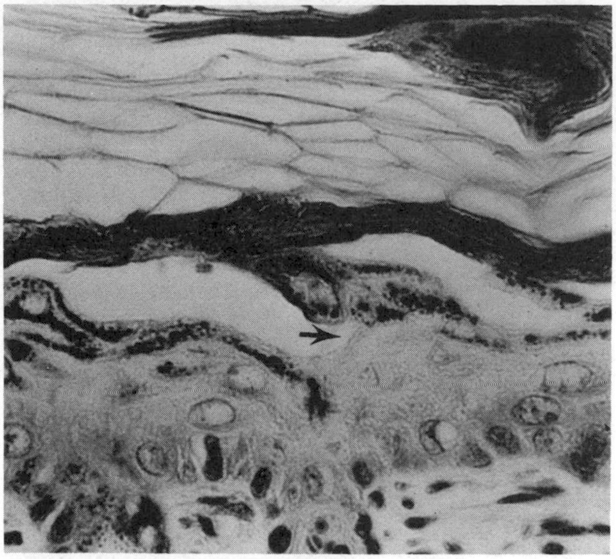

Figure 1. Site of action of epidermolytic toxin. In this early lesion, a cleavage plane is developing at the granular cell layer high in the epidermis.

Bullous varicella is a variant of localized SSSS that usually occurs two to five days after the onset of the skin lesions of chickenpox. Variable numbers of the varicella lesions become secondarily infected with staphylococci. Small crops of bullae may develop around each secondarily infected vesicle. After the bullae become denuded, the clinical appearance of denuded skin surrounding crusted varicella lesions is very characteristic.

Diffuse Exfoliative Disease. This illness generally begins with the sudden appearance of a diffuse scarlatiniform erythroderma. This rash is tender to the touch and has a rough sandpaper-like texture. In the early stages, it is indistinguishable from the rash of streptococcal scarlet fever except for its tenderness. Within one to three days, generalized bullae appear in the skin, the Nikolsky sign becomes positive, and the epidermis separates and peels off in large sheets, revealing a moist, red surface beneath (Figs. 2 and 3). Areas of exfoliation generally involve most of the body surface but are occasionally limited to smaller areas. Bullae in this disease are quite transient, and diffuse erythroderma with large areas of exfoliation may be all that is seen when the patient presents. Cultures of aspirates from intact bullae are generally sterile, but a focus of staphylococcal infection is found at a distant site. This focus is often trivial, such as conjunctivitis or throat colonization, but serious infections like bacteremia, omphalitis, osteomyelitis, endocarditis, or major wound infections also occur. The patient is usually febrile, irritable, and in pain. Small infants may develop serious problems with dehydration and temperature regulation secondary to evaporative losses. Within 24 hours, the exposed exfoliative areas dry with a thin, shiny, varnish-like crust. Cracks and fissures develop spontaneously in the skin surrounding the eyes and mouth. Secondary desquamation of large, thick flakes of skin follows during the next five to seven days. Within 14 days from the onset, the skin has healed without scarring.

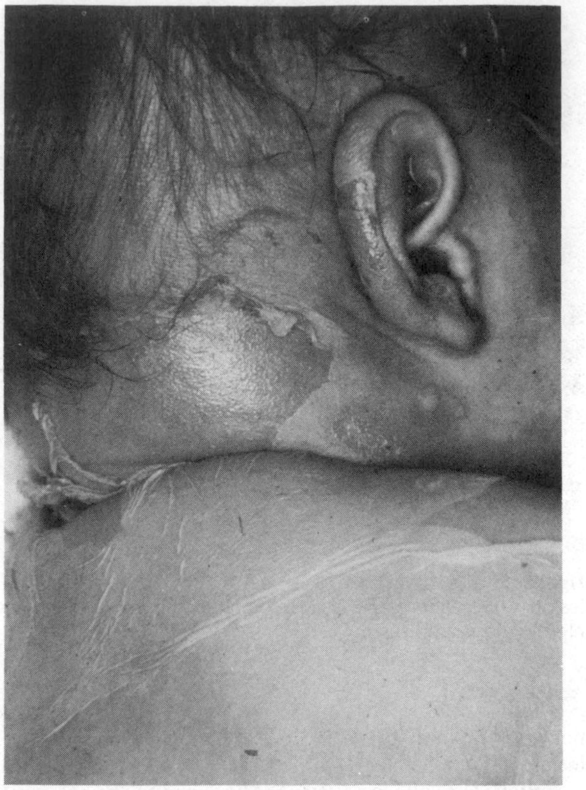

Figure 2

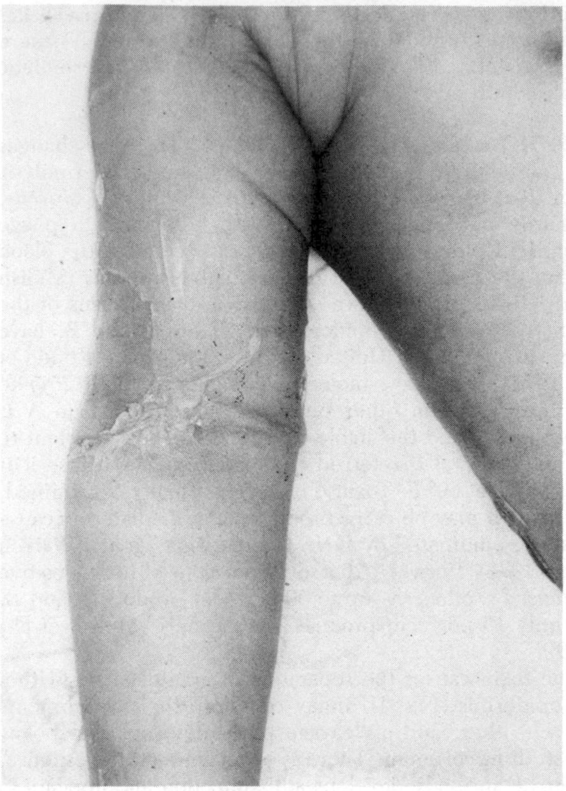

Figure 3

Figures 2 and 3. Generalized staphylococcal scalded skin syndrome (toxic epidermal necrolysis). Extensive superficial skin separation is seen in this child who had generalized tender erythroderma with increased erythema in skin creases, transient flaccid bullae, and extensive denudation of skin, revealing a moist, red surface that rapidly dried. In this child, staphylococcal epidermolytic toxin was disseminated from a focus of infection in the eye. (Photographed by Mitsuo Tottori, M.D.)

Staphylococcal Scarlatiniform Eruption. Children with this form of the staphylococcal scalded skin syndrome develop a generalized erythroderma that is usually associated with fever. The skin has a roughened sandpaper-like texture with increased erythema in skin creases similar to the rose-red, transverse Pastia's lines in the skin over the fold of the elbow in patients with scarlet fever. The appearance of the skin in these early stages can be indistinguishable from streptococcal scarlet fever. Patients with Toxic Shock Syndrome (TSS) may also present with generalized erythroderma and a severe acute illness characterized by high fever, myositis, gastroenteritis, hypotension, and renal impairment. Both streptococcal scarlet fever and TSS can be differentiated from the scarlatiniform variant of SSSS in which the skin is tender to the touch and there is no palatal enanthem or strawberry tongue. The resolution of the rash differs from both scarlet fever and TSS. Within one to four days of the onset, cracks and fissures develop about the eyes and mouth. Thick flakes appear and the entire skin surface undergoes desquamation within ten days of onset. This pattern of desquamation differs from the fine, branny flaking that begins on the fingers ten days or longer after the onset of streptococcal scarlet fever.

The staphylococcal scarlatiniform eruption and diffuse exfoliative SSSS are identical during the initial stage of generalized erythroderma and the final stage of secondary desquamation, but the intermediate stages of bullae formation and generalized exfoliation do not occur in the scarlatiniform disease.

DIAGNOSIS. The clinical presentation of diffuse exfoliative disease or toxic epidermal necrolysis may be identical whether it is caused by staphylococcal epidermolytic toxin or is of the idiopathic variety. The idiopathic type of toxic epidermal necrolysis has been associated with hypersensitivity reactions to drugs, viral infections, and graft-versus-host reactions. It is far rarer than the staphylococcal disease and usually occurs in adults. Despite the clinical similarity, the idiopathic variety has a completely different histologic appearance. In the idiopathic variety, the inflammatory response is intense, the epidermis is necrotic, and a cleavage plane develops either at the level of the dermal-epidermal junction or within the upper dermis. In the staphylococcal variety, the cleavage plane develops just below the cornified layer, and there is no inflammatory reaction within the epidermis (Fig. 1). A simple punch skin biopsy can make this differentiation. Even simpler, one can obtain a frozen section of bulla roof or freshly exfoliative skin (Fig. 4). If only cornified cells with one epidermal cell layer are seen, the process is toxin-mediated. The full epidermis is present in the idiopathic variety. Many clinicians are satisfied with a diagnosis in children of staphylococcal toxic epidermal necrolysis based upon the typical clinical appearance plus identification of a focus of staphylococcal infection. If the clinical appearance and biopsy suggest staphylococcal disease, a search must be made for the infective focus. Blood, wounds, eye exudates, and the throat should be cultured. Osteomyelitis, septic arthritis, or other occult foci should be sought if the source of

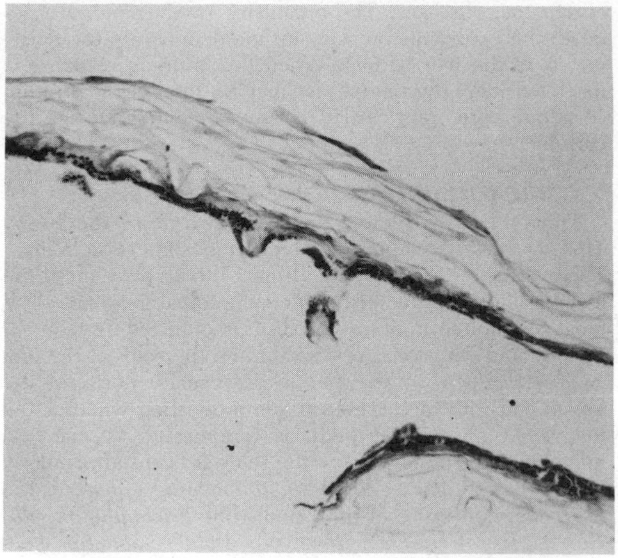

Figure 4. Rapid diagnosis of SSSS. Firm diagnosis of SSSS can be made by skin biopsy or by examination of an excised bulla roof, as seen here. Only the stratum corneum and uppermost granular cell layer are present, indicating SSSS. A deeper cleavage plane is seen in idiopathic toxic epidermal necrolysis, Stevens-Johnson syndrome, and other bullous exfoliative diseases.

infection is not obvious. Because the skin disease is toxin-mediated, its severity is not necessarily related to the severity of the infection; the focus is often trivial, and purulent conjunctivitis is the most common infection in our experience. The importance of making the correct etiologic diagnosis is to ensure effective therapy. An antistaphylococcal antibiotic aimed at eradicating the focus of staphylococcal infection is indicated for staphylococcal disease. Corticosteroids are contraindicated because they have no beneficial effect on toxin-mediated skin changes and may enhance the infection. On the other hand, the idiopathic variety is primarily an inflammatory condition, and corticosteroids are indicated.

TREATMENT. In severe cases with considerable loss of skin surface, we prefer to hospitalize patients and administer intravenous antistaphylococcal antibiotics, usually methicillin at 200,000 mg per kg per day or another penicillinase-resistant penicillin in high doses. Almost all phage group II *S. aureus* produce penicillinase. Weight, urine output, and temperature are closely monitored. Small children may be dehydrated or hypothermic because of the evaporation of fluid from denuded skin. The patient is nursed on clean linen and handled as little as possible. We do not apply topical therapy or dressings of any kind. Once the focus of infection has been identified, therapy should be continued as indicated for the basic condition. If the infection is minor, intravenous therapy is discontinued in three to five days when the skin begins to heal, and oral therapy is given for a total treatment course of 10 days. Staphylococcal scarlatiniform rash may be treated at home with oral antistaphylococcal therapy, providing that the focus of infection is minor. When the skin disease is limited, the nature of the underlying infection should dictate the route, duration, and intensity of therapy. Bullous impetigo and bullous varicella should also be treated with oral antistaphylococcal drugs. Local therapy should be avoided because of the dangers of skin maceration and sensitization to topical antimicrobials.

The prognosis for recovery from the skin disease is excellent once the underlying infection is controlled. The skin heals without scarring within 14 days of the institution of antibiotic therapy. The mortality is low (5 per cent even in infants) provided that prompt therapy and proper supportive care are given during the acute phase. Mortality from the idiopathic disease in adults is much higher and may be over 50 per cent.

References

Kondo I., Sakurai, S., and Sarai, Y.: Two serotypes of exfoliation (epidermolytic toxin) and their distribution in staphylococcal strains isolated from patients with scalded skin syndrome. J Clin Microbiol 1:397, 1975.

Melish, M. E., Glasgow, L. A., and Turner, M. D.: The staphylococcal scalded skin syndrome: Isolation of a new exfoliative toxin. J Infect Dis 1255:129, 1972.

Melish, M. E., Sprouse, S., and Stuckey, M.: Development of antibody to staphylococcal epidermolytic toxin (abst.). Clin Res 78:188A, 1979.

Warren, R., Rogolsky, M., Wiley, B. B., and Glasgow, L. A.: Effect of ethidium bromide on elimination of exfoliative toxin and bacteriocin production in *Staphylococcus aureus*. J Bacteriol 118:980, 1974.

222

DERMATOPHYTOSIS

RICHARD B. STOUGHTON, M.D.

The dermatophytoses are the superficial fungus infections of the skin. The fungi are confined to the dead stratum corneum, hair, and nails. These organisms are nourished by keratin and can survive only in the keratin structures. Dermatophytosis is classified broadly into tinea versicolor, tinea nigra, tinea capitis, tinea cruris, tinea corporis, tinea pedis, and onychomycosis.

ETIOLOGY. Sabouraud (1910) discovered the relationship between certain skin fungi and specific diseases. Emmons (1934) classified these pathogenic fungi into three main genera: *Trichophyton*, *Microsporum*, and *Epidermophyton*. Each of the many species in these genera may produce clinical variations. At least 35 species have been identified in superficial skin infections (Ajello, 1968).

PATHOGENESIS AND PATHOLOGY. The organisms of dermatophytosis live in balance with the functional changes in the stratum corneum, hair, and nails. These constantly growing structures shed at the surface (stratum corneum), at the ends (nails), or at the base (hair). The infection can maintain itself only if the fungi invade at a rate equal to the rate of sloughing (stratum corneum), extension (nail), or growing out (hair). Thus, there is a dynamic, perpetual battle between the invading force of the organism and the counterflow of the biologic river in which it has to survive. There are factors in serum and in live epidermal cells that kill the dermatophytic fungus. Thus, when the organism invades beyond the stratum corneum into the nucleated epidermis the host factors rapidly destroy the invading organism. Again we see the precarious balance that the organism must maintain to survive. If it invades too fast it will provoke a lethal response; if it invades too slowly it will be ejected.

The first contact of the organism with its host is in the top layer of the stratum corneum. This lipid film contains a variety of chemical agents derived from sweat, sebaceous glands, and the keratinization process. Sebaceous glands contribute triglycerides that are hydrolyzed by surface bacteria to fatty acids. Many of these fatty acids are potent inhibitors of dermatophytes that limit their invasion of the cutaneous surface. The soles of the feet have no sebaceous glands and this may account for the high incidence of dermatophyte infection of this area. It is rare, for instance, to see a fungus infection of the sole extend onto the dorsum of the foot, where sebaceous glands are present.

Tinea capitis caused by *Microsporum audouini* is limited essentially to prepuberty. The disease is cured spontaneously at puberty and practically never starts in adults. The enormous increase of sebaceous glands at puberty probably explains spontaneous regression of *M. audouini* tinea capitis at puberty and its absence in adults. During the 1940s *M. audouini* tinea capitis was epidemic but has been relatively uncommon since. The episodic nature of tinea capitis epidemics is unexplained.

The immunologic state is important in determining the type of infection. In subjects infected for the first time with *Trichophyton rubrum* mild erythema and scaling develop slowly and gradually spread peripherally. As delayed skin tests to the trichophyton antigen become reactive, the clinical course becomes more intense and rapid. Some patients who cannot develop delayed hypersensitivity to the organism usually have enhanced immediate-type hypersensitivity and tend to be atopic. In them, tinea pedis is chronic, scaling, and noninflammatory. The studies of Ray et al., (1976) have implicated the complement system and chemotaxis in the resistance to *Candida albicans* infections. Typical pustules can be created in newborn mice by applying *C. albicans* to the skin under occlusion. Polymorphonuclear leukocytes densely infiltrate the epidermis (pustule) and *C. albicans* is walled off in the epidermis with *no* invasion of the lower layers of the skin. In mice deficient in the fifth component of complement (C5) this experiment evoked a minimal response of polys (lack of the chemotactic agent C5a) and *C. albicans* invades the deep skin and subcutaneous tissues. *C. albicans* infections (moniliasis) are common in diabetes mellitus, a disease with defective chemotaxis.

Dermatophytes live only in the stratum corneum, hair, or nails, where their hyphae or spores can be identified with special stains—for example, periodic acid-Schiff.

Lymphocyte invasion of the corium, particularly in the upper layer, is evidence of an active immunologic response to dermatophytes. Along with this early invasion of lymphocytes, the cytoplasm of the nucleated epidermal cells breaks down and spaces between the cells widen. This epidermal response, known as spongiosis, is also seen in eczematous diseases. The organisms rarely penetrate beneath the epidermis but may invade deeply into the horny matrix of the hair or nail. When the immune response is inactive, many dermatophytes may be seen in the stratum corneum with very little, if any, inflammation in the corium.

CLINICAL MANIFESTATIONS

Tinea Pedis (Athlete's Foot, Ringworm of the Feet). This is probably the most common fungus infection in man. The organism can be isolated from 25 to 40 per cent of the feet of normal adults whether symptomatic or not. The most common form of tinea pedis is manifested by redness, scaling, and occasional vesiculation on the soles of the feet and particularly in the toe webs, usually between the fourth and fifth toes. There is some question whether the toe web type of tinea pedis is complicated by bacterial infection, but the lesions on the soles are caused primarily by the dermatophyte. *Trichophyton mentagrophytes* is the most common cause of tinea pedis but *Trichophyton rubrum* is also frequently involved. *Epidermophyton floccosum* is not usually found in this infection. These three organisms account for over 95 per cent of fungus infections of the soles.

Minimal scaling is common but seldom bothers anyone enough to send him to the doctor. The physician is consulted usually because of intense pruritus or very noticeable scaling or vesiculation. Acute episodes build up to maximum severity in 7 to 16 days and spontaneously subside over two to three weeks. It is common in individuals wearing unventilated shoes in moist, warm climates. In societies where shoes are rarely used, this type of acute tinea pedis is rare. The more acute vesicular type of tinea pedis most often occurs in patients with a positive delayed skin test to trichophyton antigen. Those having a negative delayed test to *Trichophyton* but a positive immediate test usually show a chronic scaling, erythematous type of tinea pedis, frequently caused by *T. rubrum.* This latter type of tinea pedis is difficult to eradicate and seldom undergoes spontaneous remission.

The clinical picture is highly suggestive of a fungus infection but proof resides in demonstrating hyphae in the stratum corneum. This can be done by treating scales from the lesion by the potassium hydroxide technique, which is the most reliable for identifying dermatophytic infection (see below). Culture is positive in only about 50 per cent of active infections. Cultural identification of the organism is not necessary for diagnosis of tinea pedis.

Tinea Manus (Ringworm of the Hands). Tinea manus is relatively rare. The usual cause is *T. rubrum* and the infection is almost always associated with the chronic dry scaling type of *T. rubrum* tinea pedis.

In general, chronic scaling of the hands is not a fungus infection and is more likely an eczematous reaction of contact dermatitis, neurodermatitis, or atopic dermatitis.

Tinea Cruris (Jock Itch). This occurs mainly in the moist, warm inguinal areas and more often in males than females. There is a sharp strongly erythematous, scaling border. The area behind the advancing margin has less erythema but as many scales. The inflammatory margin is the most characteristic feature of this disease. The fungi most often associated with this infection are: *E. floccosum, T. rubrum,* and *T. mentagrophytes.*

Tinea Corporis (Tinea Circinata, Tinea Glabrosa). Superficial fungus infections outside the hands, feet, groin, and scalp are much more common in hot, humid climates than in the cool northern latitudes. The lesions are usually circinate, have an active spreading erythematous inflammatory border, and heal behind the advancing border. The term "ringworm" is probably derived from this lesion. They frequently regress without treatment. In patients with diabetes or lymphoma these lesions may become enormous and cover most of the body.

The classic annular lesion of tinea circinata may be caused by a variety of dermatophytes, but most commonly in the United States by *Microsporum audouini, Microsporum canis*, and *T. mentagrophytes*.

Occasionally no clearing occurs behind the border and a large plaque of eczematous vesicular lesions develops. This more inflammatory ringworm can be caused by an endothrix, *Trichophyton* or *M. canis*. In severe inflammatory ringworm, known as kerion, there are large vesicles, extensive edema, and pustulation. Kerion is self-curing because the intense inflammatory response sterilizes the lesion. Self-sterilization also makes it difficult to demonstrate the organism.

Majocchi's granuloma is a variant of more inflammatory ringworm that involves hair follicles, mainly in the lower extremities and usually is caused by deep infection of the skin with *T. rubrum*. It is treated with griseofulvin.

Tinea Capitis (Ringworm of the Scalp). Inflammation of the scalp can be induced by many species of dermatophytes in the genera *Microsporum* and *Trichophyton*. Severity depends on the organism.

Most cases of tinea capitis in the United States are caused by *Microsporum audouini*. It causes epidemics and during the 1940s was severe in the United States, but occurs only sporadically now in children and practically never in adults. The infection is easily transmitted from child to child and is difficult to control during epidemics. Broken hairs are the first obvious sign of the disease, and cause partial alopecia of the scalp. Scaling and mild erythema around the broken hairs in tinea capitis help to distinguish it from alopecia areata, trichotillomania, and other causes of hair loss.

Onychomycosis. Fungus infections of the toenails are very common, are more frequent in men, and are unusual before puberty. Other cutaneous disease may give nail changes that can resemble fungus infections of the nail. Probably less than half of distorting afflictions of the nail are caused by fungi; the most common are *T. rubrum*, and *T. mentagrophytes*. *Epidermophyton* and *Microsporum* rarely infect nails. In Asia, *T. violaceum* commonly infects fingernails.

Onychomycosis is not common in societies where footwear is not used. Shoes may account for the much higher incidence of fungus infections of toenails than fingernails.

Onychomycosis ordinarily is not a severe disease but one of cosmetic importance to women but not men. Women are distressed by infection of the toenails, particularly if they wear open toed shoes. Both men and women are upset by fungus infection of the fingernails. Onychomycosis of the fingernails is most often caused by *T. rubrum*. It is rare for *T. rubrum* to infect the hand or fingernail and spare the feet and toenails. The big toenail is most often infected by a fungus, but all other nails can be. Usually one or two nails are involved and the others are spared. Secondary bacterial infection is rare in severe onychomycosis. The nail may become severely disfigured and impinge upon footwear so that it has to be cut down or filed.

Tinea Versicolor. This superficial fungus infection of the skin is easy to diagnose. It causes discolored, slightly hyperpigmented spots or plaques on the chest and back. These lesions have a slight scale and gentle trauma with the fingernail will expose a branny-type scaling within the lesion. The disease is most common in young adults but may occur at any age. It is much more common in hot humid areas. It tends to recur but is usually not contagious to others even after intimate contact.

Tinea Nigra. This disease is characterized by black discolorations resembling stains of silver nitrate and usually on the palms or sides of the fingers. It is more common in South America than in the United States. The cause is *Cladosporium wernecki*.

COMPLICATIONS AND SEQUELAE. Most dermatophyte infections are mild, self-limited, and reversible with little or no permanent change in the invaded tissue. The repair process causes no permanent damage.

Severe tinea capitis, tinea barbae, or trichophyton granuloma are rare causes of scarring. Some fungi are more likely to cause permanent damage, but severe inflammation may destroy or scar the skin, even when the infection is caused by a benign organism such as *T. rubrum*.

Secondary infection with pathogenic bacteria is unusual but when it occurs is generally caused by *Staphylococcus aureus* or of Group A streptococci. Secondary streptococcal skin infection rarely can lead to acute glomeronephritis.

GEOGRAPHIC VARIATIONS. The incidence of clinical types and etiologic fungi of dermatophyte infection varies in different parts of the world.

In India, tinea pedis is less frequent than in the United States, where it is the commonest dermatophyte infection, probably because occlusive shoes are worn by almost everybody. *Epidermophyton* is a rare cause of dermatophytosis in India but common in the United States. The same is true for *T. mentagrophytes*, a common cause of tinea pedis in the United States.

Tinea capitis seems to be caused by different organisms in different parts of the world. *T. tonsurans* is a common offender in Mexico and *T. violaceum* is common in India.

Tinea versicolor is a common problem in tropical areas and relatively rare in cold, dry climates.

DIAGNOSIS. To substantiate the clinical impression two laboratory methods are useful.

The first is the KOH preparation, in which 10 per cent potassium hydroxide solution is used to digest the scales on a glass slide under a cover slip. After heating over a mild flame just to the point of boiling, the slide is examined under 40 × magnification with subdued lighting. The hyphae of the fungus show up as clearly outlined, branched filaments, which are easily distinguished from the outlines of the skin cells. It is best to learn this technique from one with experience before attempting it by yourself.

The other method is to culture the skin scales on Sabouraud's medium. Dermatophytes take 7 to 14 days to grow at room temperature. Usually, the organism can be classified by its gross and microscopic characteristics. Often a KOH preparation will be positive and the culture negative.

Tinea pedis can mimic other diseases. Dyshidrosis, a variant of atopic eczema and neurodermatitis, can give a similar clinical picture. Dyshidrosis is usually bilateral and tinea pedis is not. Dyshidrosis tends to be more intensely pruritic and is frequently associated with lesions of neurodermatitis or atopic dermatitis elsewhere. The lesions of dyshidrosis will rarely contain hyphae. Contact dermatitis can mimic dermatophytosis of the feet. The most common cause of contact dermatitis of the feet is allergy to something in the shoes. Patch tests to elements in the shoes will show such allergy. Occasionally psoriasis can mimic tinea pedis but lesions of psoriasis elsewhere on the skin and nails distinguish it from a fungus infection.

The organism in tinea cruris or corporis is best identified by scraping horny material from the inflamed, advancing margin, and making a KOH preparation. The hyphae can then be demonstrated under the microscope. Again, the KOH preparation is more reliable than culture.

In tinea capitis the fungi can easily be seen in the hair on KOH preparations. Greenish fluorescence of the hair under black light is characteristic of tinea capitis due to *Microsporum,* including *M. canis, M. ferrugineum,* and *M. distortum.* Other types of tinea capitis do not fluoresce. Cultures help distinguish these fungi.

Onychomycosis is diagnosed by KOH preparation or culture. It is best to scrape away superficial debris and use the scales beneath for examination. Many nonpathogenic fungi are saprophytic on human toenails and rarely cause disruption of the nail. Nail distortion can occur with many other dermatoses such as psoriasis, eczema, and lichen planus so it is important not to ascribe the nail disease to a saprophyte that is cultured.

In tinea versicolor the hyphae and spores are sometimes called "spaghetti and meatballs." The stratum corneum is invaded by thick masses of these hyphae and spores and they are easy to see on the KOH preparation. They are difficult to culture and standard culture media are of no value in identification of the organism.

In tinea nigra a KOH preparation will disclose the dark green segmented hyphae and the organism is fairly easy to culture on standard media. This disease is occasionally misdiagnosed as junctional nevus or melanoma and unnecessary surgery is performed.

TREATMENT. The only systemic drug for dermatophytoses is griseofulvin. It is particularly useful in resistant cases of tinea pedis, tinea manus, onychomycosis, and tinea cruris, and is the only treatment for tinea capitis. Griseofulvin should be used with discretion, however, because tinea pedis, tinea manus, onychomycosis, and tinea cruris tend to recur soon after discontinuing the drug even though it takes up to 12 to 18 months to clear onychomycosis and up to two to three months to clear tinea pedis or tinea manus. Tinea capitis responds rapidly and completely.

The dosage is 500 mg/day of micronized griseofulvin. The crystals of griseofulvin are ground to a minute size (micronized) to facilitate gastrointestinal absorption. Griseofulvin sometimes causes headaches but very few other complaints. Although it can cause porphyria and liver tumors in animals it has been relatively safe in patients for the past 20 years.

Most dermatophytic infections are treated first with topical fungistatic or fungicidal agents. One of the oldest is precipitated sulfur 2 to 5 per cent in a cream or ointment. Newer agents have a wider spectrum of activity against yeasts and bacteria. Because some tinea infections are complicated by bacterial infection and some are mimicked by bacterial and yeast infections, these newer agents are usually preferred. Miconazole, clotrimazole, and ciclopirox are the most widely used among these broad spectrum agents. Tolnaftate is also widely used but its spectrum is confined to dermatophytes and it is inactive against most yeasts and bacteria.

These antifungal drugs are supplied in 1 per cent concentration in liquid or cream vehicles. Generally, the liquid preparations are more active and better tolerated by the patient. They are applied as a thin layer twice a day to the affected area. Occasionally allergic drug reactions occur. Length of treatment varies greatly. Tinea corporis or tinea cruris usually responds well in two weeks or less. In tinea pedis or tinea manus treatment is often prolonged indefinitely and usually without a cure.

Tinea pedis or tinea manus is treated topically with a potent antifungal agent such as tolnaftate, ciclopirox, miconazole, or clotrimazole in lotions or creams. In tinea pedis the thick, horny layer on the soles prevents penetration of antifungal drugs to fungi in the depths of the stratum corneum. Most patients improve with topical therapy but the infection is likely to reappear from external reinfection. The answer may be a combination of topical therapy and oral griseofulvin. The most difficult tinea pedis to treat has chronic, scaling nonvesicular lesions over large areas of both soles. Topical antifungal agents offer little in this disease. During oral griseofulvin therapy most of these infections subside but recur soon after griseofulvin is stopped. In some cases the fungus becomes resistant to griseofulvin.

The usual course of tinea cruris infection is for spontaneous flares, which frequently subside without treatment but do respond rapidly to topical tolnaftate, miconazole, clotrimazole or ciclopirox. In about 10 per cent of subjects the infection is persistent and resistant, and topical agents help but do not eradicate the disease. Only rarely is oral griseofulvin necessary.

Some forms of tinea capitis tend to be more inflammatory than those caused by *M. audouini* and rarely give rise to large boggy draining lesions of the kerion type. Although usually self-healing the severe inflammatory types of tinea capitis are treated with griseofulvin. Tinea barbae, an inflammation of the beard caused by a zoophilic fungus, is easily controlled with oral griseofulvin.

Topical antifungal agents are of little, if any, value in onychomycosis because they do not penetrate to the fungus in the nail bed and nail plate. Over 50 per cent of toenail infections subside after oral griseofulvin. The faster growing fingernails respond in six months, whereas the toenails need treatment for one year. When griseofulvin is stopped the nail infection almost invariably returns. Griseofulvin cannot be taken indefinitely and topical antifungals prevent reinfection of the fingernails after griseofulvin is stopped. Removal of the nail is generally ineffective because the new nail becomes reinfected despite prophylactic topical antifungals.

Tinea versicolor responds readily to precipitated sulfur or selenium sulfide. Tolnaftate, miconazole, clotrimazole, and ciclopirox also seem to be effective. If treatment is applied once a day in a thin layer, the fungi will not be detectable after two to three weeks. If treatment is stopped then the disease will often recur, but application of one of these fungicides once or twice a week will prevent recurrence. Discoloration will remain up to six months after fungi have been cleared.

PROPHYLAXIS. Since almost all attempts to clear the environment of dermatophytes have failed exposure of the population to dermatophytes seems inevitable. Nevertheless, tinea pedis would be rare if no one wore shoes. In most societies this is impractical, but people who suffer from resistant severe tinea pedis may get considerable relief by wearing open shoes or sandals. There is little gain in forbidding people with scaly feet from entering locker rooms or swimming pool areas. About 25 per cent of people without scaly feet carry dermatophytes on their feet and about 50 per cent of those with scaly feet do not have tinea pedis. In any event, it is host resistance that determines susceptibility rather than the size or frequency of the inoculum.

Occasionally an infected pet (cat or dog) will pass on tinea corporis to a group of children. Elimination of the infection of the pet will prevent spread of the disease. The same holds for infection of farmers by animal carriers.

Eliminating local moisture can help tinea cruris. Loose underclothes, drying powders, and air conditioned rooms are helpful but usually not curative or fully effective in prophylaxis.

Epidemic tinea capitis (*M. audouini*) is spread by direct or intermediate contacts. Yet extreme measures of isolation and protection of children during the USA epidemic in the 1940s seemed to help little in preventing spread.

Topical antifungal drugs seem to prevent recurrent dermatophytosis, especially stubborn infections due to tinea pedis, onychomycosis, or tinea cruris that had required oral griseofulvin.

References

Ajello, L.: A taxonomic review of the dermatophytes and related species. Sabouraudia 6:147, 1968.

Conant, N. F., Smith, D. T., Baker, R. D., et al.: Manual of Clinical Mycology. 3rd ed. Philadelphia, W. B. Saunders Company, 1971.

Emmons, E. W.: Dermatophytes. Natural grouping based on the form of the spores and accessory organs. Arch Derm Syph 30:337, 1934.

Hildick-Smith, G., Blank, H., and Sarkany, I.: Fungus Diseases and Their Treatment. Boston, Little, Brown & Company, 1964.

Ray, T. L., Baker, D., and Weupper, K.: Experimental cutaneous candidiasis. Role of stratum corneum. J Invest Dermatol 66:278, 1976.

Sabourand, R.: Les Teignes. Paris, Masson et Cie, 1910.

223

SPOROTRICHOSIS

ABRAHAM I. BRAUDE, M.D., PH.D.

Sporotrichosis is a chronic infection due to the soil fungus *Sporothrix schenckii*. In most cases suppurating nodules form along the lymphatics of the skin and subcutaneous tissues. Hematogenous dissemination also occurs rarely and pulmonary infection is occasionally produced by inhaled fungi.

ETIOLOGY. The fungus *S. schenckii* is dimorphic on Sabouraud's agar. At room temperature its growth is mycelial, but in the tissues it takes the form of tiny cigar-shaped, gram-positive yeast cells. These yeast cells are seen abundantly in experimental lesions but are rarely found in infected lesions of patients. The yeast stage can develop in culture if the organism is incubated under CO_2 at 37° C on blood agar containing cystine.

PATHOGENESIS AND PATHOLOGY. The fungus lives as a saprophyte on vegetation and penetrates the hands or feet when the skin is broken. Many cases have followed injury by thorns or wood splinters. Sporotrichosis is primarily an occupational disease in people working with plants. Sphagnum moss is an important source of infection.

From 7 to 40 weeks after penetrating the skin the fungus produces at the incubation site a reddish-purple necrotic nodule, the sporotrichotic chancre. This lesion has marked hyperkeratosis and intradermal microabscesses that rupture into the dermis. The most distinctive feature is a suppurative granuloma that contains polymorphonuclears in the center of a zone of histiocytes and giant cells. The entire lesion is surrounded by lymphocytes and plasma cells (Lurie, 1963). Occasionally the lesion at the inoculation site remains confined to the skin or epidermis without lymphatic involvement and has been called fixed cutaneous sporotrichosis. In the vast majority of cases the fungus spreads from the chancre up the extremities and evokes nodular lesions along the thickened lymphatics. It seems that tolerance for higher temperatures is essential for lymphatic spread beyond the cooler superficial tissues at the inoculation site. Thus, conidia of strains isolated from fixed cutaneous lesions without lymphangitis cannot grow at 37° C even though they multiply at 35° C. Conidia from isolates recovered from lymphangitic or disseminated infections multiply at both 35° and 37° C (Kwon-Chung, 1979). Microscopically, the nodules along the lymphatics are also granulomas with abscesses in their center. Sometimes asteroid bodies can be found scattered irregularly in the pus (Splendore, 1908). These bodies are spherical structures measuring 5 to 10 μ in diameter and resemble spores. When stained by the periodic acid-Schiff method, the wall seems to have a double contour. This round structure is surrounded by eosinophilic material arranged in the form of a star. Similar radial formation of eosinophilic material has been found around schistosome ova (Hoeppli, 1932), microfilaria, and *Entomophthora coronata*, the cause of African nasal phycomycosis. Known as the Splendore-Hoeppli phenomenon, it is thought to result from an antigen-antibody reaction.

Primary infections of the extremities almost never become disseminated through the bloodstream. In the rare case of disseminated infection the portal of entry is thought to be the gastrointestinal tract, and lesions predominate in the skin, bones, muscles, and joints. Occasionally the liver, testicles, eye, and lung may also be involved. Sporotrichosis of the central nervous system is the most unusual form of disseminated infection and produces a granulomatous basilar meningitis. The rarity of any form of disseminated infection can be appreciated from the fact that in South Africa, where 3300 cases of sporotrichosis had been seen by 1963, only five were disseminated (Lurie, 1963). More recently, sporotrichosis has shown a tendency to be an opportunistic infection that disseminates in compromised patients with such disorders as Hodgkin's disease, multiple myeloma, leukemia, diabetes, nephrosis, and especially alcoholism (Lynch et al., 1970). The disseminated lesions have the same granulomatous appearance as those described in primary lymphocutaneous infection. In some disseminated lesions abundant yeast forms have been visible.

CLINICAL MANIFESTATIONS

Primary Cutaneous Sporotrichosis. The primary lesion is usually found on the hands or fingers but can appear on any exposed part of the body, including the face (Pepper and Rippon, 1980). It starts as a small red papule and progresses to a pustular nodule of firm, rubbery consistency. An ulcer forms on the pustule, exudes pus on pressure, and is frequently surrounded by tiny papules. Later the lesion may be covered by a hard scab. In about 20 per cent of cases, there is no extension of disease along the lymphatics. This is especially likely to be the case in endemic areas where repeated exposure to the fungus is thought to sensitize or immunize the patient so that infection is confined to the area of inoculation. In these infections, known as the fixed cutaneous form, the lesions may also be verrucous, papillomatous, acneiform, or nonulcerative papules.

In most patients, however, the infection begins to spread along the lymphatics in about a week after the primary lesion appears. A chain of hard, red discrete lumps extends up the arm or leg to the axilla or groin, and the intervening lymphatics become red and thickened. The epitrochlear lymph node frequently enlarges, but the axillary or inguinal glands usually do not. The disproportion between symptoms and findings is striking; there is no pain, fever, or other constitutional symptoms. Older nodules may rupture to produce fistulas or ulcers, but these remain relatively indolent.

Disseminated Sporotrichosis. There are two forms of disseminated infection. In one, the patient has multiple, scattered, dusky red skin nodules. These may begin anywhere, with one nodule and then multiple nodules appearing on the trunk, face, scalp, arms, and legs. Most of these patients also have lesions in the bones or joints and may complain of migratory arthritis, with joint swellings and effusion. This form of arthritis in sporotrichosis is especially easy to confuse with rheumatoid arthritis (Molstad and Strom, 1978). A few patients develop metastatic deep-seated abscesses of the muscles, including the trapezius, biceps, gastrocnemius, and triceps (Lurie, 1963). Lymphangitis is not a characteristic feature of disseminated disease, but lymphadenopathy is found in some cases. Meningitis and brain infection are exceedingly unusual. Metastatic lung nodules and mucosal lesions are also rare. Sporotrichosis of mucous membranes may occur in the nasopharynx, mouth, or larynx and may produce ulcers, soft scars, and suppurating nodules with regional lymphadenopathy. Sporotrichosis of bone in these patients usually causes local swelling over the area of bone destruction. Warmth and tenderness may also be present. Sinuses drain from the bone through the skin, and adjacent joints become infected by contiguous spread. The bones of the arms, legs, wrists, ankles, hands, and feet are most often infected. In contrast to the classic lymphocutaneous infection, this form of disseminated sporotrichosis may be accompanied by mild fever (<39° C), anorexia, and weight loss.

The other form of disseminated sporotrichosis has only one metastatic focus that involves primarily a joint but sometimes the eye, genitourinary tract, or bone. Because any one of these occurs with no contiguous skin lesion and without direct trauma into the infected site, each is presumed to be infected by hematogenous spread.

Primary Pulmonary Sporotrichosis. In primary pulmonary sporotrichosis the patient usually has slight respiratory symptoms, if any, until the disease becomes well advanced. A number of cases have been identified when routine x-ray examinations disclosed an upper lobe infiltrate or cavity. These infiltrates resemble those of tuberculosis (Fig. 1), and patients are often given antituberculous drugs even though tubercle bacilli are never seen or cultured. When symptoms occur, a mild or moderate cough is noted at first, and a small amount of sputum may be produced. Chest pain, fever, chills, night sweats, and hemoptysis are not the rule when the disease is first recognized, and there are no skin nodules or other signs of disseminated infection. Later, however, fever, hemoptysis (Fig. 1), and respiratory insufficiency may become prominent.

Traumatic Synovitis. Penetrating injury of a joint or tendon sheath may cause synovitis. It has been suggested that these infections tend to occur in alcoholics because the fungus can penetrate deeper than in the ordinary patient, whose coordination and sensitivity to pain are not affected during gardening. Traumatic synovitis tends to involve the wrist, which becomes swollen, painful, and red (Kedes et al., 1964; DeHaven et al., 1972; Marrocco et al., 1975). The diagnosis is usually missed and the patient treated unsuccessfully with antituberculous drugs and synovectomy. A diagnosis of chronic granulomatous synovitis

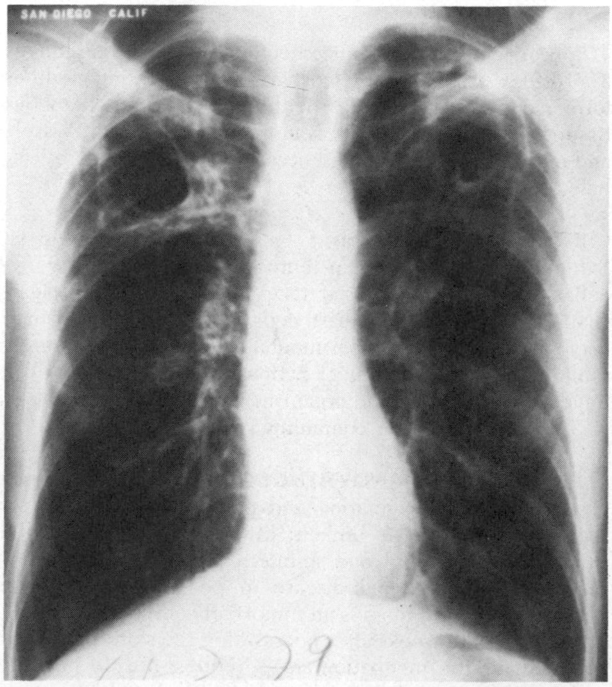

Figure 1. Pulmonary sporotrichosis with bilateral apical cavities resembling tuberculosis. Patient was treated unsuccessfully for tuberculosis despite negative smears and cultures of sputa for mycobacteria. Diagnosis of sporotrichosis was made by repeated culture of Sporothrix schenckii from sputum. Chief clinical problem had been ten years of marked hemoptysis that did not abate with treatment of sporotrichosis and required therapeutic embolization of the bleeding vessel.

is made from the infected synovium, but no etiology can be found by the pathologist because the fungus cannot be seen microscopically, and routine cultures for bacteria are negative. Cases are on record in which multiple surgical procedures were done over a period of seven years without a correct diagnosis.

Ocular Sporotrichosis. The fungus has a predilection for the conjunctiva and eyelids but may infect any part of the eye, either exogenously or endogenously (Francois, 1972). It is a special hazard to laboratory workers who handle the fungus. Primary sporotrichosis of the eyelid starts as a hard inflammatory nodule that involves the overlying skin and underlying conjunctiva. Primary sporotrichosis of the conjunctiva produces small, hard, yellow nodules, usually on the inner surface of the lids but also on the bulbar conjunctiva. Both conjunctival and palpebral nodules become abscesses that discharge pus and are accompanied by enlarged preauricular lymph nodes. The cornea is resistant to spread of infection from the conjunctiva, and sportrichotic ulcers are rare. Intraocular sporotrichosis is relatively common and may be caused by traumatic inoculation or metastatic spread during hematogenous dissemination. Several cases of intraocular sporotrichosis have followed cataract surgery. The first lesion is usually a nodular iritis.

Central Nervous System Sporotrichosis. Both meningitis and brain abscess have occurred but are exceedingly rare. One of the reported infections started two years after a myelogram was done for a herniated intervertebral disk and was probably a form of inoculation sporotrichosis. The patient complained of occipital headache and dizziness for a year (Shoemaker et al., 1957). He also lost weight, became confused, and deteriorated neurologically until his death. Another case occurred in a 58-year-old farmer who also suffered from confusion, weakness, ataxia, weight loss, and impaired vestibular function (Klein et al., 1966). He responded to treatment with amphotericin B. In a third case no neurologic symptoms were noted during the course of disseminated sporotrichosis, but suppurative granulomas were scattered throughout the cerebral cortex at postmortem examination (Collins, 1947).

Genitourinary Sporotrichosis. Metastatic lesions can develop in the epididymis, testis, and kidney. Pyonephrosis has been reported in a patient with stones in the renal pelvis.

COMPLICATIONS. These depend on the site of infection. Secondary bacterial infection of open lesions may spread to produce septicemia. Pulmonary sporotrichosis can be complicated by pulmonary insufficiency and severe chronic hemoptysis. If hilar adenopathy occurs in pulmonary sporotrichosis, it may be so great that it causes bronchial obstruction. Pulmonary infections can disseminate hematogenously or by swallowing heavily infected sputum; a case of perirectal abscess has been attributed to swallowed fungi (Khan et al., 1975). Sporotrichotic osteomyelitis of the tibia has been complicated by pathologic fracture.

GEOGRAPHIC VARIATIONS IN DISEASE. The common denominator of sporotrichosis throughout the world is occupational exposure during agricultural work and gardening. In certain areas, however, special forms of exposure have been noted. For example, in a huge epidemic in South Africa, nearly 3000 cases occurred in gold miners who were infected by exposure of skin abrasions to *S. schenckii* growing as a saprophyte on timbers supporting the mine. In the United States, several epidemics of cutaneous sporotrichosis have been traced to sphagnum moss contaminated with the fungus (Powell et al., 1978). In Mexico, where sporotrichosis is the most common fungus infection, the pattern of disease varies with age, sex, and occupation. Thus, women get lesions on their fingers from weaving baskets of grass, children on the face from scratches of branches, and men on the fingers and wrists from collecting grasses or on the legs from thorns (Rippon, 1974). Steady exposure to spores in endemic areas of Mexico is thought to produce immunity and sensitization to antigens of *S. schenckii* so that infections remain localized to the inoculation site and take on the character of verrucous, acneiform, plaque-like, papular, or crusted weeping lesions that behave more like allergic reactions than infections. Patients in endemic areas develop strong intradermal allergic reactions to sporotrichin, an antigen of *S. schenckii.*

The nutritional status of the population is probably another important factor in determining the incidence and severity of sporotrichosis. The declining frequency in France has been attributed to improved nutrition, whereas the high frequency in the poor areas of Latin America can be correlated there with poor diets. Nutritional disturbances would also account for the increased prevalence of sporotrichosis in alcoholics, and its tendency to become disseminated in patients with an underlying illness. Thus sporotrichosis appears to be an opportunistic infection, and its geographic or clinical pattern can be explained to some extent on this premise. It is not surprising that the highest incidence of sporotrichosis is in poor areas of southern Brazil and the central highlands of Mexico, and that it is practically nonexistent in Germany (Travassos and Lloyd, 1980).

DIAGNOSIS

Lymphocutaneous Sporotrichosis. The fungus cannot be seen upon microscopic examination of biopsied material or pus in most cases. Cultural isolation is always successful, however, if pus is taken from an unbroken nodule or ulcer and inoculated into Sabouraud's agar at room temperature. The growth at first has the soft creamy character of bacterial colonies and later develops a wrinkled dark-brown appearance without the cotton-like filament of most molds. Microscopically, typical clusters of pear-shaped spores are found at the tips of tiny conidiophores arising from the tangled mass of delicate branched mycelia. If the mold or pus is inoculated intraperitoneally into mice or rats, numerous yeast forms will be seen in lesions of the peritoneal cavity or testicle, where they take the form of gram-positive, cigar-shaped rods within polymorphonuclear leukocytes.

Recovery of the organism is so reliable that sporotrichosis can be recognized in a week or two and thus differentiated from other chronic infections of the subcutaneous tissues such as tularemia, blastomycosis, coccidioidomycosis, syphilis, and mycobacterial infections. The lymphangitic ("sporotrichoid") forms of *Mycobacterium marinum* and *Mycobacterium kansasii* infections cannot be distinguished from sporotrichosis clinically, but skin injuries in an aquarium or swimming pool point to *M. marinum.*

Disseminated Cutaneous Sporotrichosis. In contrast to the lymphocutaneous type, subcutaneous nodules are scattered all over the body, and no primary lesion is found. As the scattered nodules grow, they soften and form a central depression with hard peripheries. Although they may run their course without ulcerating, when perforation does occur, the indolent ulcers are indistinguishable from those in the localized form of the disease. Pus aspirated from the unbroken disseminated nodules may have numerous cigar-shaped, gram-positive yeast forms of *S. schenckii,* so that this less typical clinical variety of sporotrichosis can be more easily identified in the laboratory. The combination of bone or joint lesions with such skin lesions should always suggest the possibility of sporotrichosis, especially in alcoholics or immunosuppressed patients.

Extracutaneous Sporotrichosis. Sporotrichosis of joints is difficult to differentiate from rheumatoid arthritis, because both diseases may be multiarticular, chronic, and relapsing; the joint fluids both have high neutrophil counts; the chronic inflammatory response in synovial biopsies looks the same in both diseases; the fungus is not usually seen in the tissues in sporotrichosis; and in both diseases subcutaneous nodules may occur. In addition, rheumatoid arthritis and articular sporotrichosis respond somewhat to rest, heat, salicylates, and intra-articular steroids. The diagnosis of sporotrichosis can be suspected if a synovial fistula to the skin develops and if the small joints of the foot are affected. Culture of the synovial biopsy will always be positive.

In osseous sporotrichosis the lesion is osteolytic, and x-ray examination shows destruction of bone without reactive osteoblastic change (Gladstone and Littman, 1971). About two thirds of patients have distant skin lesions from which the fungus can be cultured, if not seen in direct examination. Nearly 80 per cent have signs of joint involvement, and over 40 per cent have draining sinuses from which positive cultures can be made.

In pulmonary or meningeal sporotrichosis differential diagnosis centers first around tuberculosis. In pulmonary sporotrichosis the fungus grows heavily from the sputum, and sputum culture on Sabouraud's medium is imperative in any patient with upper-lobe cavities whose sputum has no acid-fast bacilli in smears. This test will also help exclude histoplasmosis, which can be endemic in the same regions as sporotrichosis and is another important cause of upper-lung cavitation with negative acid-fast smears in the sputum.

Limited experience in the rare cases of meningeal sporotrichosis indicates that *S. schenckii* can also be readily grown from the spinal fluid. In addition to clinical signs of a chronic basilar meningitis, meningeal sporotrichosis produces cerebrospinal fluid changes like those of tuberculosis—i.e., low sugar levels, moderate lymphocytosis, and elevated protein levels.

TREATMENT. The common lymphangitic form of sporotrichosis is almost invariably and dramatically cured by saturated potassium iodide (de Beurmann and Gougerot, 1907; Auld and Beardmore, 1979; Powell et al., 1978). This should be given orally in starting doses of 10 drops three times daily after meals and gradually increased to the point of maximum tolerance. Treatment should be continued for a month after lesions disappear. Additional local therapy may be required for cutaneous ulcers, which should be painted with tincture of iodine. It may also be necessary to excise epidermal lesions, because these may not subside with oral iodides. Systemic sporotrichosis is resistant to iodides but often responds well to intravenous treatment with amphotericin B, given in a total dose of 1.5 to 2.0 g over a period of six to eight weeks. There is some evidence that intravenous miconazole may be of value in patients who do not respond to amphotericin B because of drug resistance, clinical resistance, or drug intolerance (Rohwedder and Archer, 1976). Miconazole is given in a dose of 800 to 1000 mg three times daily through a central venous catheter to avoid phlebitis. The chief side effects of miconazole are itching and water retention due to inappropriate secretion of antidiuretic hormone. Antipruritic drugs and water restriction can control these problems. More studies will be needed to determine the value if any of ketoconazole in sporotrichosis.

Heat treatment has been advocated for skin lesions in patients who cannot tolerate iodides or amphotericin B. An attempt is made to kill the fungus in the lesions by raising the temperature of the infected area above 39° C for an hour or more four times daily. This can be done with hot packs or an electric heating pad. Surgical resection is required for pulmonary cavities that do not respond to amphotericin B or iodides (Jung et al., 1979a).

PROPHYLAXIS. Sporotrichosis can be prevented when epidemic sources are identified. For example, in a recent epidemic traced to sphagnum moss, the incriminated moss was buried in order to control the outbreak (Powell et al., 1978). Other lots of sphagnum moss are stored indoors, the storage buildings are scrubbed monthly with a disinfectant, and the moss is cultured regularly for *S. schenckii.* The massive epidemic in South African gold mines was controlled by disinfecting the timber where *S. schenckii* was growing as a saprophyte. Laboratory infections can be prevented by reasonable precautions among technicians, who should be made aware of the risk of autoinoculation, especially of the eyelids. For the most part, however, the simple precautions needed to prevent infection in agriculture workers are difficult to enforce because they cannot afford the clothing needed to protect their hands, legs, and feet.

References

Auld, J., and Beardmore, G.: Sporotrichosis in Queensland: a review of 137 cases at the Royal Brisbane hospital. Aust J Dermatol 20:14, 1979.

Collins, W.: Disseminated ulcerating sporotrichosis with widespread visceral involvement: Report of a case. Arch Derm Syph (Chicago) 56:523, 1947.

de Beurmann, L., and Gougerot, H.: Les Sporotrichses, Paris, Felix Alcan, 1912.

DeHaven, K., Wilde, A., and O'Duffy, J.: Sporotrichosis arthritis and tenosynovitis. J Bone Joint Surg 54A:874, 1972.

Francois, J.: Sporotrichosis. In, Francois, J.: Oculomycoses. Springfield, Ill., Charles C Thomas, 1972, p. 375.

Gladstone, J., and Littman, M.: Osseous sporotrichosis. Am J Med 51:121, 1971.

Hoeppli, R.: Histologic observation in experimental schistosomiasis Japonica. Chinese Med J 43:1179, 1932.

Jung, J., Almond, C., et al.: Role of surgery in the management of pulmonary sporotrichosis. J Thor Cardiovasc Surg 77:234, 1979.

Kedes, L., Siemienski, J., and Braude, A.: The syndrome of the alcoholic rose gardener Sporotrichosis of the radial tendon sheath. Ann Intern Med 61:1139, 1964.

Khan, F., Guarneri, J., and Sierra, M.: Primary pulmonary sporotrichosis complicated by perirectal abscess. Am Rev Resp Dis 112:119, 1975.

Klein, R., Ivens, M., Seabury, S., and Dascomb, H.: Meningitis due to *Sporotrichum schenckii.* Arch Intern Med 118:145, 1966.

Kwon-Chung, K. J.: Comparison of isolates of *Sporothrix schenkii* obtained from fixed cutaneous lesions with isolates from other types of lesions. J Inf Dis 139:424, 1979.

Lurie, H.: Histopathology of sporotrichosis. Arch Pathol 75:421, 1963.

Lynch, P., Voorhees, I., and Harrell, E.: Systemic sporotrichosis. Ann Intern Med 73:23, 1970.
Marrocco, G., Tihen, W., Goodnough, C., and Johnson, R.: Granulomatous synovitis and osteitis caused by *Sporothrix schenckii*. Am J Clin Pathol 64:345, 1975.
Molstad, B., and Strom, R.: Multiarticular sporotrichosis. JAMA 240:556, 1978.
Pepper, M., and Rippon, J.: Sporotrichosis presenting as facial cellulitis. JAMA 242:2327, 1980.
Powell, K., Taylor, A., Phillips, B., Blakey, D., Campbell, G., Kaufman, L., and Kaplan, W.: Cutaneous sporotrichosis in forestry workers. JAMA 240:232, 1978.
Rippon, J.: Sporotrichosis. In Medical Mycology. Philadelphia, W. B. Saunders Company, 1974, p. 250.
Rohwedder, J., and Archer, G.: Pulmonary sporotrichosis: Treatment with miconazole. Am Rev Resp Dis 114:403, 1976.
Shoemaker, E., Bennett, H., Fields, W., Whitcomb, F., and Halpert, B.: Leptomeningitis due to *Sporotrichum schenckii*. Arch Pathol 64:222, 1957.
Splendore, A.: Sobre acultura d'uma nova especie de cogumello pathogenico. Rev Soc Sci S Paulo 3:62, 1908.
Travassos, L., and Lloyd, K.: *Sporothrix schenckii* and related species of Ceratocystis. Microbiol Rev 44:683, 1980.

224

CHROMOBLASTOMYCOSIS

ALBERTO THOMAZ LONDERO, M.D.

Chromoblastomycosis is a chronic indolent granulomatous infection, usually confined to the skin, caused by several dematiaceous fungi, which develop in the tissue as round, dark-brown bodies and multiply by equatorial splitting.

ETIOLOGY. Five closely related dematiaceous fungi are the etiologic agents of chromoblastomycosis. The most important are: *Cladosporium carrionii, Fonsecaea pedrosoi, Fonsecaea compacta,* and *Phialophora verrucosa. Rhinocladiella aquaspersa* has also caused a few cases of chromoblastomycosis. The most common agent is *F. pedrosoi.*

EPIDEMIOLOGY. The mycosis primarily affects rural adults, usually between 30 and 50 years of age. The infection is rare in children, even in highly endemic areas, and is more frequent among men than women. All races seem to be susceptible to the infection, and its prevalence is closely related to the social and economic habits of the people.

PATHOGENESIS AND PATHOLOGY. The agents of chromoblastomycosis are soil-inhabiting fungi, but they have been isolated more frequently from wood than from soil itself (Gezuele et al., 1972). *F. pedrosoi* and *P. verrucosa* have been recovered from rotting wood, wood pulp, and plant debris. *C. carrionii* has been isolated from fence posts in Australia, and Salonen and Ruokola (1969) recovered *P. verrucosa* from the wooden furniture and floor of rustic saunas in Finland.

The fungus enters the skin through an abrasion or trauma caused by decaying wood. Inadequate nutrition, immunologic deficiency, and poor general health seem to play a role in allowing the infection to evolve.

The lesions appear at the site of the trauma and remain circumscribed for some time. After months, the lesions spread slowly to adjacent areas through the superficial lymphatics, extending after many years over large areas of the body. Some lesions may heal and form scars. Metastatic lesions, located some distance from uninvolved areas, may be caused by autoinoculation and either by lymphatic or, more rarely, by hematogenous spread. There is no known transmission from person to person.

The chromoblastomycotic lesions, usually confined to the skin, are sharply limited. Histologic section under low-power microscopic observation shows hyperkeratosis, pseudoepitheliomatous hyperplasia, papillomatosis, and microabscesses. A granulomatous infiltrate of the upper and lower dermis is also seen. The pleomorphic infiltrate, composed of lymphocytes, plasma cells, some eosinophils, and multinulceated giant cells, of either the Langhans or the foreign-body type, surrounds the tuberculoid granulomata and the microabscesses. Dermal tuberculoid granulomas are formed by clusters of epithelioid cells. Microabscesses consist of masses of polymorphonuclear leukocytes surrounded by histiocytes or epidermal cells. Usually there is slight fibrosis. Fungal elements may be seen within granulomata, microabscesses, and giant cells. They are described under *Diagnosis*.

Secondary bacterial invasion, with or without ulceration, may obscure the histologic picture of chronic inflammation by evoking a pyogenic reaction.

CLINICAL MANIFESTATIONS. In chromoblastomycosis, cutaneous lesions are nearly always unilateral and situated on an exposed part of the body. They occur on the lower limbs, upper limbs, face, and trunk, in that order of frequency.

Bopp (1959) classified the lesions in two types: (1) nodular or tumoral and (2) smooth or vegetating plaque-like lesions. The plaque-like lesions may be subdivided into tuberculoid, syphiloid, psoriasiform, and mycetoma-like subtypes. The noncharacteristic early lesions are still another type.

The noncharacteristic early lesions have been described as either a pink scaly papule, a nodule that ulcerates, a subcutaneous abscess, a ringworm-like lesion, a superficial ulceration with a slightly verrucoid basis, or an erythematous violaceous pustule. A nodule or a papule has been reported to be the starting lesion in experimental inoculations in man.

Nodular or tumoral lesions are characteristic of the mycosis, but usually they are seen in the distal part of the lower limbs. At first a hemispheric, soft or fibrous, glistening pink to violaceous, small nodule is seen. After months or perhaps years, other nodules appear in adjacent areas or ascend irregularly along the limbs, covering large areas (Fig. 1). As the lesions progress, the nodules became raised, up to 1 or 2 cm above the skin, and are sometimes pedunculated. Their surface may be smooth or verrucoid. These crops of nodules are hard and dry, but, when pressed, a caseous or purulent secretion emerges. Some nodules may ulcerate, and from the ulceration many tumoral lobulated masses arise, resembling the florets of the cauliflower. At the proximal part of the limb these nodular

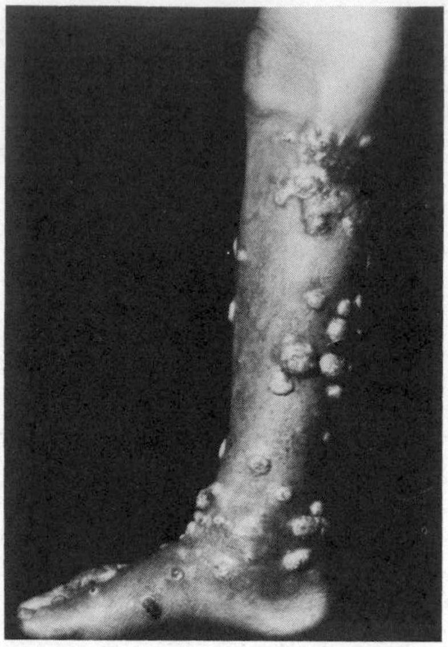

Figure 1. Nodular or tumoral form of chromoblastomycosis. (Courtesy of Dr. C. Bopp, Brazil.)

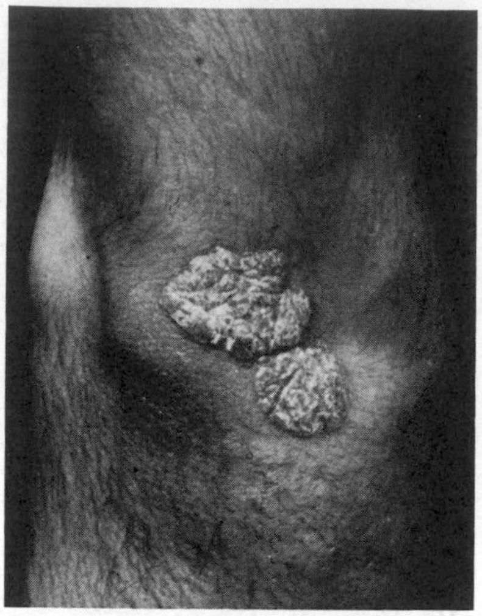

Figure 2. psoriasiform subtype of the plaque-like form of chromoblastomycosis.

overgrowths usually are isolated and moderately elevated from the skin, presenting a violaceous surface that is sometimes covered by dirty, grayish crusts.

Plaque-like lesions are seen almost exclusively on the upper limbs, face, and trunk. These lesions result from the eccentric progress of the small initial infiltrated area. After months or perhaps years, they became round or oval lesions, elevated up to 1 to 5 mm above the skin, measuring 5 to 10 cm in diameter, sometimes greater. These lesions are formed of packed papillomatous vegetations, either denuded and pink colored or covered by horny, grayish crusts. Pus or caseous material may be obtained by pressing, and when the crusts are picked up the surface bleeds easily. Sometimes the plaque-like lesions extend over a large area of the body. In those cases the surface becomes smooth and glistening, pink or violaceous, and covered by grayish crusts.

The plaque can heal spontaneously in the center or on a segment of the border of the lesion. If the remaining lesion is semilunar, elevated, and heavily infiltrated, it is considered to be of the tuberculoid subtype. If the atrophic cicatricial area is bordered by an infiltrated and ulcerated serpiginous or arciform lesion that progresses centrifugally, it is called the syphiloid subtype. On the other hand, if the area has some slightly infiltrated plaques, whose surface is a conglomerate of closed minute papillae covered by micaceous adherent scales, it is called the psoriasiform subtype (Fig. 2). The mycetomatoid subtype is a heavily infiltrated plaque with scattered mammillated elevations containing apertures at their apex, through which pus may drain.

Primary lesions on the mucous membranes of the nose, eye, larynx, and vulva are rare. Disseminated hematogenous lesions of the skin or internal organs, especially the brain, are also unusual. Lymphatic spread may cause lymphangitis and regional lymphadenopathy.

COMPLICATIONS AND SEQUELAE. The most frequent complication is elephantiasis of the extremities. It is caused by lymphatic blockade from extensive fibrosis in the deeper tissues. Another complication is secondary bacterial infection producing ulcerations that are sometimes extensive. Scars take the form of smooth, atrophic areas of glistening skin and result from spontaneous partial healing of the lesions, or from treatment.

DIAGNOSIS. Diagnosis of chromoblastomycosis can only be established by demonstrating the infective agent in the lesion.

Clinical Diagnosis. Chromoblastomycosis may be suspected in advanced cases, especially in patients presenting the tumoral form. The early lesions must be differentiated from bacterial infections and the initial lesions of the other subcutaneous mycoses. The circumscribed tumoral, plaque-like, and mixed types of the mycosis must be differentiated from similar lesions seen in other mycoses (e.g., lobomycosis, sporotrichosis, blastomycosis, tropical mossy foot, yaws, syphilis, tuberculosis, lupus erythematosus, lupus vulgaris, leishmaniasis, and psoriasis).

Laboratory Diagnosis. Mycologic diagnosis is very simple and inexpensive. A little drop of pus or caseous material, obtained by squeezing the lesions or puncturing a small abscess, should be placed on a slide with 10 per cent potassium hydroxide and examined under a coverglass. Crusts should be removed and mounted in the same way. *All the agents of chromoblastomycosis present identical forms in tissue or pus.* They appear as single or clustered round, dark-brown, thick-walled bodies, 8 to 12 μm in diameter, some of them dividing by splitting (Fig. 3). In the epithelial crusts the fungal elements are seen occasionally as brown septate-branching hyphae, 2 to 5 μm in width, germinating from muriform bodies. The diagnosis may also be made by histologic examination and culture of biopsied tissue.

Cultures of crusts, pus, exudate, and biopsied tissue should be placed on Mycosel or Sabouraud's dextrose agar, in tubes or plates, and incubated at 25 to 30° C (see Chapter 81).

GEOGRAPHIC VARIATIONS. With the exception of the frigid polar regions, chromoblastomycosis has been reported from every continent in the world, but its geographic distribution is not uniform. In the New World

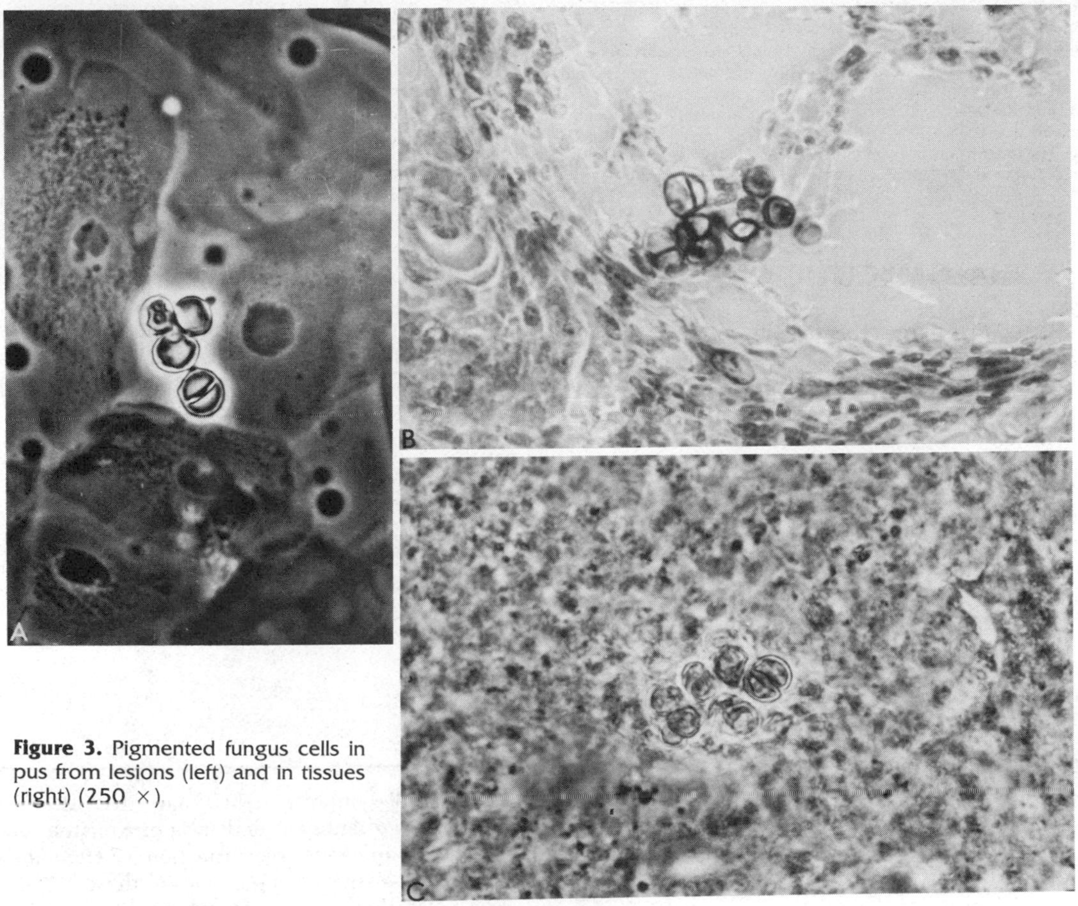

Figure 3. Pigmented fungus cells in pus from lesions (left) and in tissues (right) (250 ×).

almost all cases have been reported in a belt limited by 30° N and 30° S. In this zone there are highly endemic circumscribed areas, such as Costa Rica and the Dominican Republic. In Europe most cases have been seen in countries above 45° N, with the greatest number appearing in Finland. In Africa the endemic zone is below the equator, with a highly endemic area in the Malagasy Republic. In Asia, with the exception of Japan, the mycosis has not been frequently reported. In Australasia almost all cases have been reported in Australia.

Throughout the world, *F. pedrosoi* is the agent most commonly isolated from chromoblastomycosis. It prevails in humid areas with more than 2000 mm annual rainfall. *C. carrionii*, the agent isolated next most frequently, infects patients in regions with less than 600 mm annual rainfall (Mexico, Venezuela, South Africa, Malagasy Republic, and Australia). *P. verrucosa*, less frequently found as an agent of chromoblastomycosis, generally occurs in patients living in the temperate regions of the New World, and sporadically in patients from Africa and Asia. *F. compactum* has been isolated sporadically from patients in the New World, Europe, and Asia. *R. aquaspersa* is an occasional cause of the infection in Mexico, Costa Rica, and Brazil.

TREATMENT. In the early small lesions the most suitable treatment is local heat administered as a water bath or infrared rays (Conti-Diaz et al., 1969). Heat treatment can be combined with perilesional infiltration of amphotericin B. The drug is infiltrated weekly for three months in a concentration of 40 mg/5 ml of 2 per cent procaine solution (Costello et al., 1959).

Patients with nonextensive lesions, especially those caused by *C. carrionii*, can be treated with 5-fluorocytosine in a dose of 100 mg/kg body weight daily, in three daily doses for 8 to 12 weeks. Treatment may be stopped three weeks after the first negative culture. An alternative is thiabendazole in a dose of 25 mg/kg body weight daily, for 6 to 22 months (Bayles, 1971).

Advanced cases may be treated with a combination of 1 g of thiabendazole and 4 g of 5-fluorocytosine daily, in three daily doses for 6 to 8 months (Solano, 1983).

PROPHYLAXIS. The exposed parts of the body, especially the distal parts of the limbs, must be covered during work in the fields or with wood.

References

Bayles, M. A. H.: Chromomycosis. Treatment with thiabendazole. Arch Derm 104:476, 1971.

Bopp, C.: Cromoblastomicose. Contribuição ao estudo de alguns de seus aspectos. Thesis. Porto Alegre, Livraria Globo, 1959.

Conti-Diaz, I. A., Vignale, R. A., and Pereira, M. E. P.: Cromoblastomicosis tratada con termoterapia local. Med Cut ILA 3:383, 1969.

Costello, M. J., DeFeo, C. P., Jr., and Littman, M. L.: Chromoblastomycosis treated with local infiltration of amphotericin B solution. Arch Derm 79:184, 1959.

Gezuele, E., Mackinnon, J. E., and Conti-Diaz, I. A.: The frequent isolation of *Phialophora verrucosa* and *Phialophora pedrosoi* from natural sources. Sabouraudia 10:266, 1972.

Ridey, M. F.: The saprophytic occurrence of fungi causing chromoblastomycosis. In: Recent Advances in Botany. Univ. Toronto Press, Toronto, 1961, p. 312.

Salonen, A. and Ruokola, A. L.: Mycoflora of the Finnish "sauna." Mycopathologia 38:327, 1969.

Solano, E.: Tratamiento de la cromomicosis con thiabendazole y 5-fluorocytosine. X Congr Ibero Latino Amer, Rio de Janeiro, April, 1983.

PHAEOMYCOTIC CYSTS

Phaemycotic cysts are subcutaneous or intramuscular lesions caused by certain dematiaceous (pigmented) fungi. The fungus *Exophiala jeanselmei* is the commonest cause; other agents isolated from these lesions are other species of *Exophiala* or *Phialophora* and *Wangiella dermatiditis*. These organisms can be seen within the cysts as brown pigmented hyphae, or in pus extruded from ruptured cysts. The fungi are introduced by puncture wounds beneath the skin where they produce slowly developing granulomatous masses that gradually soften in the center. The granulomatous portion, which contains sheets of epitheloid and giant cells, has a fibrous capsule and central foci of microabscesses (Binford and Dooley, 1976). They appear as single or multiple superficial cysts on the legs or arms; if near a joint they may resemble a synovial cyst. Although most cysts occur in healthy persons, the size and character of the local lesion is influenced by debility and underlying disease. A very large subcutaneous phaeomycotic cyst over most of the thigh developed in a diabetic who introduced *W. dermatiditis* with an insulin injection (Rippon, 1982).

The cysts are easily cured by surgical excision because they are not attached to the skin and are easily shelled out. Simple aspiration is unsatisfactory and may cause sinus tracts. If the cyst ruptures during excision, 5-fluorocytosine should be given to prevent recurrence and spread of infection. A dose of 100 mg/kg/day by mouth should be given for 5 days. If recurrence develops this treatment must be continued until the lesion resolves.

References

Binford, C., and Dooley, J. R.: Phaeomycotic cysts. *In*: Binford, C. and Connor, D., Pathology of Tropical and Extraordinary Diseases, Armed Forces Institute of Pathology, Washington, D.C. 1976, p. 589.

Rippon, J. W.: Medical Mycology: The Pathogenic Fungi and Pathogenic Actinomycetes. 2nd ed. Philadelphia, W. B. Saunders Company, 1982.

225

MONILIASIS OF THE SKIN

J. E. Edwards, Jr., M.D.

CHRONIC MUCOCUTANEOUS CANDIDIASIS

DEFINITION. This term applies to a heterogeneous group of refractory *Candida* infections of the skin, mucous membranes, hair, and nails that persist and recur in spite of therapy. These infections generally occur in patients with specific immunologic abnormalities; however, as many as one-third may have no definable immune abnormality.

ETIOLOGY. Cellular immunity, [usually thymus-derived lymphocytes (T cells)] is abnormal (see section on Pathogenesis and Pathology) in most patients with chronic mucocutaneous candidiasis. In some forms, genetic factors are obvious from familial trends. Several mechanisms, all speculative, have been considered responsible for failure of cellular immunity: (1) failure of antigen recognition by the T-cell, (2) failure of T-cell mediator production (macrophage inhibition factor [MIF]), (3) abnormality in the inflammatory cell itself (defective monocyte chemotaxis), (4) inhibition of T-cell function by a population of suppressor cells, (5) abnormal thymic function, and (6) immune tolerance for a specific antigen shared by *Candida* organisms.

PATHOGENESIS AND PATHOLOGY. T-cell dysfunction is evident from the following observations (Stiehm, 1977): in approximately half of patients there is cutaneous anergy to *Candida* antigen, in 80 per cent there is diminished synthesis of lymphocyte MIF (in vitro) after stimulation with *Candida* antigen, and in approximately one-third of patients lymphocyte transformation by *Candida* antigen is depressed. Various combinations of these T-cell abnormalities exist. Some patients, whose lymphocytes undergo transformation, do not synthesize MIF, but virtually all patients with negative transformation lack MIF production. Diminished MIF production is closely correlated with cutaneous anergy. However, the number of T cells, the lymphocyte proliferative responses to phytohemagglutinins, and the allogenic cells are usually normal. The quantity of B lymphocytes and serum immunoglobulins is also normal.

Certain patients with chronic mucocutaneous candidiasis have had additional immunologic abnormalities, such as cutaneous anergy to other delayed hypersensitivity skin-test antigens (e.g., streptokinase-streptodornase, tetanus toxoid, and mumps). Their lymphocyte transformation to PHA and other mitogens and their monocyte chemotaxis may be defective. In addition, anti-*Candida* antibody may be absent from salivary IgA immunoglobulins. Various degrees of thymic aplasia are also observed.

Generally, the earlier the onset of chronic mucocutaneous candidiasis, the more severe the immune abnormalities. Some patients with early onset disease and severe immune abnormalities have had negative skin tests to all common antigens, including *Candida*, and cannot be sensitized to dinitrochlorobenzene.

In the resultant infection of the mucous membranes, skin, and nails, chronic inflammation with plasma cells and lymphocytes is associated with hyperkeratosis and parakeratosis in the epidermis. Deep penetration into the dermis is rare. Giant cells and fungi may be seen in the epidermis. Candidal granuloma, the most severe cutaneous form, is characterized by pronounced papillomatosis, hyperkeratosis, and dense infiltrate in the dermis of lymphoid cells, neutrophils, plasma cells, and multinucleated giant cells. The infiltrate may extend to the subcutis. Organisms have been found only in the stratum corneum.

CLINICAL MANIFESTATIONS. Most forms of chronic mucocutaneous candidiasis begin in infancy or within the first two decades. Rarely, the onset may be after age 30. Thrush is usually the first sign of the disease, followed by nail infection and then by cutaneous moniliasis. The spectrum of severity ranges from chronic involvement of a single nail to disfigurement by the worst form of infection, candidal granuloma (Fig. 1).

Endocrine disorders are associated with chronic mucocutaneous candidiasis in half the patients. These are hypoparathyroidism, Addison's disease, hypothyroidism, and diabetes. Pernicious anemia, ovarian insufficiency, chronic active hepatitis, hepatic cirrhosis, alopecia, depigmentation, cheilosis, blepharitis, keratoconjunctivitis, corneal ulcers, iron deficiency anemia, chronic pulmonary disease, malabsorption, hemolytic anemia, and thymoma, autoantibodies to melanin producing cells, vitiligo, and dental dysplasia have also accompanied the disease.

Stiehm has proposed the working classification of these disorders outlined in Table 1. In addition, this form of candidiasis has been described in patients with thymic dysplasia and agammaglobulinemia (Swiss type agammaglobulinemia), and thymic dysplasia without agammaglobulinemia (Nezelof-Allibone syndrome).

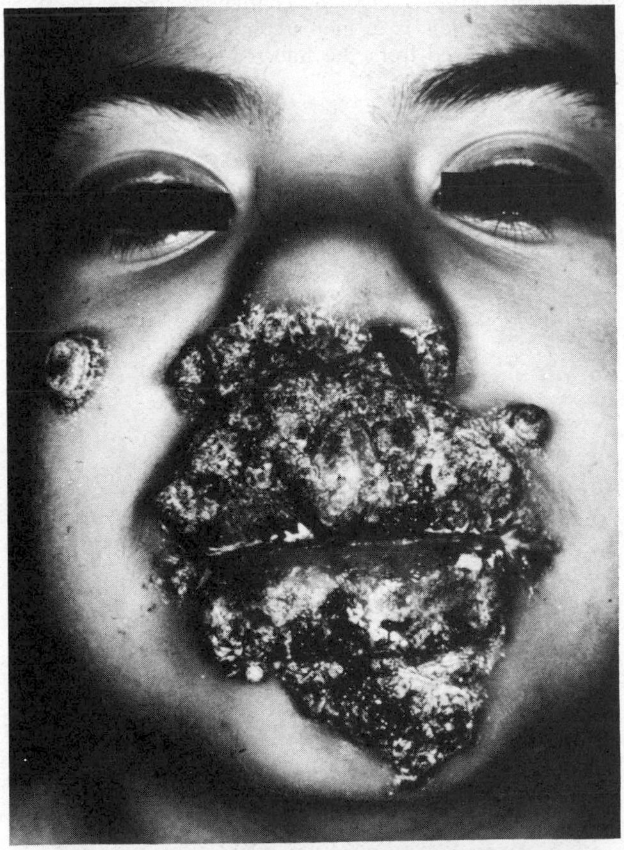

Figure 1. Severe disfiguration from *Candida* granuloma involving the perioral area. (Courtesy of Dr. Victor Newcomer.)

Table 1.

	Severity of Candidiasis	Endocrinopathy	Inheritance
I. Early onset chronic mucocutaneous candidiasis	Moderate to severe	Common	Sporadic
Subtype candidal granuloma	Severe	Common	Sporadic
II. Late onset CMC	Mild	Rare	Sporadic
III. Familial CMC	Mild to moderate	Rare	Autosomal recessive
IV. Juvenile familial polyendocrinopathy with candidiasis (candida-endocrinopathy syndrome)	Mild to moderate	Always	Autosomal recessive

From Stiehm, E. R.: Chronic mucocutaneous candidiasis. Clinical perspectives, pp. 96–99. In Edwards, J. E., Jr. (moderator): Severe candida infections. Clinical perspective, immune defense mechanisms, and current concepts of therapy. Ann Intern Med 89:91–106, 1978.

COMPLICATIONS AND SEQUELAE. If cutaneous involvement and the immunodeficiencies are severe enough, the condition may be fatal, usually as a result of disseminated bacterial infection. Surprisingly, disseminated candidiasis has been a rare complication of chronic mucocutaneous candidiasis. Squamous carcinoma of the mouth and esophageal carcinoma may develop at the site of chronic candidal inflammation. Inflammation may cause loss of hair and nail, and scarring. In addition to direct complications of candidal infection, these patients may develop thymomas and sequelae related to their endocrine disorders.

DIAGNOSIS. Diagnosis of chronic mucocutaneous candidiasis is based on finding refractory candidal infections and the characteristic immunologic abnormalities, genetic background, and endocrinopathies. Proof of chronic candidiasis is established by biopsy and by demonstration of the typical histopathologic signs. Classification of the disease type requires skin testing with the appropriate antigens, evaluation of in vitro lymphocyte function, and assessment of immunoglobulin status. The endocrinopathy must also be identified.

TREATMENT AND PROPHYLAXIS. Efforts to correct immune deficiencies with transfer factor, levamisole (a synthetic anthelmintic agent capable of T-cell activation), and thymus extracts (thymosin fraction 5 or fetal thymus) are experimental and their effects are doubtful. Amphotericin B has been the mainstay of treatment, given in a dose of 0.5 mg/kg intravenously every other day for two to four weeks, depending on the clinical response. However, impressive and long lasting remissions have been obtained with ketoconazole, which may become the drug of choice (Petersen et al.) 1980. 5-Fluorocytosine (5-FC) in a dose of 100 mg/kg can be given alone or in conjunction with amphotericin B. 5-FC is taken in divided doses every six hours orally and should be continued as long as clinical improvement occurs. These drugs are repeated as tolerated for relapses. Topical preparations of these and other antifungal drugs may also be of value. Amphotericin B is applied in 2 per cent concentration as a lotion and 5-FC as a 1 per cent solution. Miconazole nitrate ointment (2 per

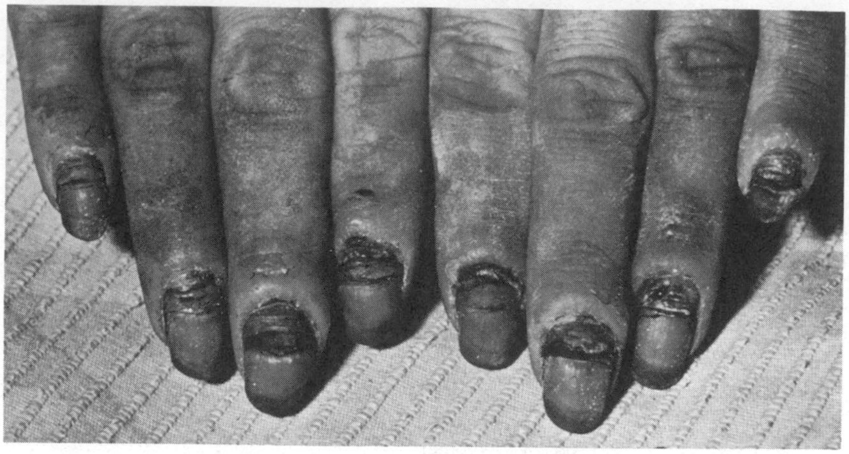

Figure 2. *Candida* paronychia. (Courtesy of Dr. Victor Newcomer.)

cent) or Mycostatin ointment can be applied twice daily to the skin lesions in place of amphotericin B or 5-FC.

OTHER CUTANEOUS CANDIDAL INFECTIONS

CANDIDA INTERTRIGO. This common disease affects any skin surfaces that are in close enough approximation to provide a warm moist environment. The crural folds, interdigital areas of hands and feet, submammary area, submaxillary area, gluteal folds, and ear folds are examples. The first lesions are vesicopustules that enlarge, rupture, macerate the skin, and produce fissures. The lesions have a scalloped border rimmed by a white necrotic epidermis with the appearance of overhanging scales. The base of the lesion is erythematous, and satellite flaccid vesicopustules or white colloid macules often appear on adjacent skin. These may coalesce and extend the area of involvement. Although *Candida* may be cultured from an intertriginous area of inflammation, one should not conclude that *Candida* is the cause without proof by biopsy of cutaneous invasion by *Candida* organisms. Even without biopsy, however, a presumptive diagnosis is enough to undertake a therapeutic trial.

In addition to intertrigo, candidiasis of the skin may take on a miliary appearance from the erythematous macules or vesicopustules resembling miliaria rubra or a drug eruption (Kozin and Taschdgian, 1977).

CANDIDAL PARONYCHIA. This is an inflammatory reaction around the nail attributed to candidal infection. The exact role that *Candida* organisms play in this reaction is not clear, however, since many skin bacteria, in addition to *Candida*, are usually cultured from the infected area. The importance of *Candida* as the primary pathogen has been challenged.

Because frequent immersion of the hands in water is highly correlated with this condition, there is a high incidence of it in dishwashers and laundry workers. Young children may develop a candidal paronychia as a complication of thumbsucking. Diabetics have a higher incidence of paronychia than do those who are not diabetics.

The clinical appearance of a paronychia is that of a relatively well localized periungual inflammation that becomes warm, glistening, and tense. It may extend under the nail and gradually destroy the nail plate so that the nail develops secondary thickening, ridging, and discoloration (Fig. 2). Pain varies from severe to mild or may even be absent. The histologic changes include acanthosis and parakeratosis in the presence of chronic inflammatory infiltration. Candidal hyphae are seen penetrating the stratum corneum. The specific diagnosis is made by Gram stain, potassium hydroxide preparation, or culture showing predominantly *Candida* organisms. Major complications are loss of the nail and/or cellulitis of the finger.

CUTANEOUS GENITAL CANDIDIASIS. This condition may be a direct extension of candidal vaginitis or may occur in intertriginous areas of the perineum. In addition to the vulvar skin, the urethral orifice and urethral mucosa may be involved. As the infection progresses, the vulva becomes very red and the skin erodes. The process may spread onto the perineum and contiguous areas (Fig. 3).

Genital candidiasis in men is thought to be a venereal infection acquired from the infected vagina. The process

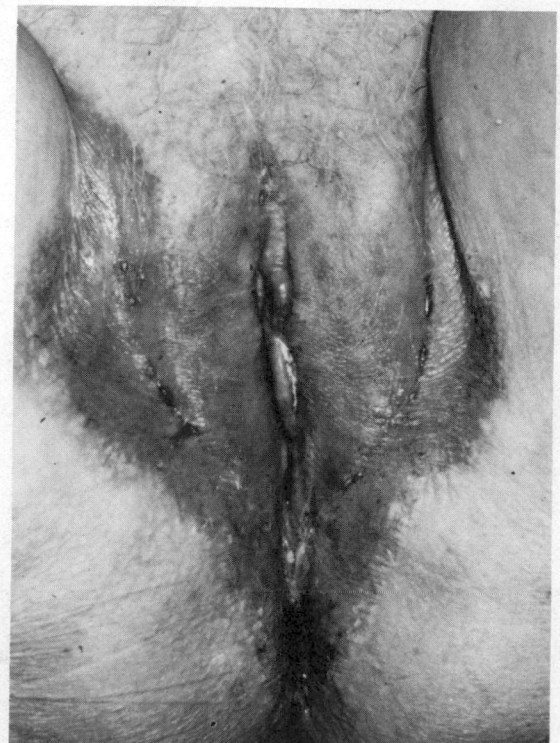

Figure 3. Severe vulvar and intercrural Candida intertrigo. (Courtesy of Dr. Victor Newcomer.)

begins on the penis as vesicles that evolve into painful, itchy, burning patches resembling thrush. It can spread to the thighs, gluteal folds, buttocks, and scrotum.

PERIANAL CANDIDIASIS. *Candida* may be one of the numerous micro-organisms associated with pruritus ani, either alone or in combination. *Candida* has been implicated as the predominant cause in some cases, resulting in erythema that progresses to maceration and generally intense pruritus, especially at night (Fig. 4). It can spread to the anal canal and cause frank proctitis.

GENERALIZED CUTANEOUS CANDIDIASIS. This is an unusual form of cutaneous candidiasis seen primarily in infants. It causes a widespread eruption that is particularly severe in the genitocrural folds, anal region, axillae, hands, and feet. The process begins as vesicles or vesicopustules that rupture and leave a denuded surface. Eventually it spreads peripherally, and large confluent areas develop (Fig. 5). Paronychia occur and the mucocutaneous area may be involved. This condition may simulate acrodermatitis enteropathica, seborrheic dermatitis, psoriasis, contact dermatitis, and pityriasis rubra pilaris.

MACRONODULAR CUTANEOUS LESIONS OF DISSEMINATED CANDIDIASIS. These are lesions of disseminated candidiasis in which multiple blood cultures are positive (Bodey and Luna, 1974). They are pink to red lesions 0.5 to 1.0 cm in diameter and occur either as single lesions or scattered over the entire body (Fig. 6). Occasionally, they have a hemorrhagic base. Organisms have been demonstrated most frequently on histologic sections of punch biopsy.

CANDIDAL DIAPER RASH. *Candida* is a very common cause of diaper rash in infants. The initial perianal localization suggests that the gastrointestinal tract is the site of origin. Spread to the diaper area occurs rapidly and is facilitated by cutaneous maceration from wet diapers. Scaly macules and vesicles characterize the rash, which is very uncomfortable because of itching and burning (Fig. 7). Diagnosis is made by scraping the involved area (simple swabbing is inadequate) and demonstrating the organisms on potassium hydroxide preparation or culture.

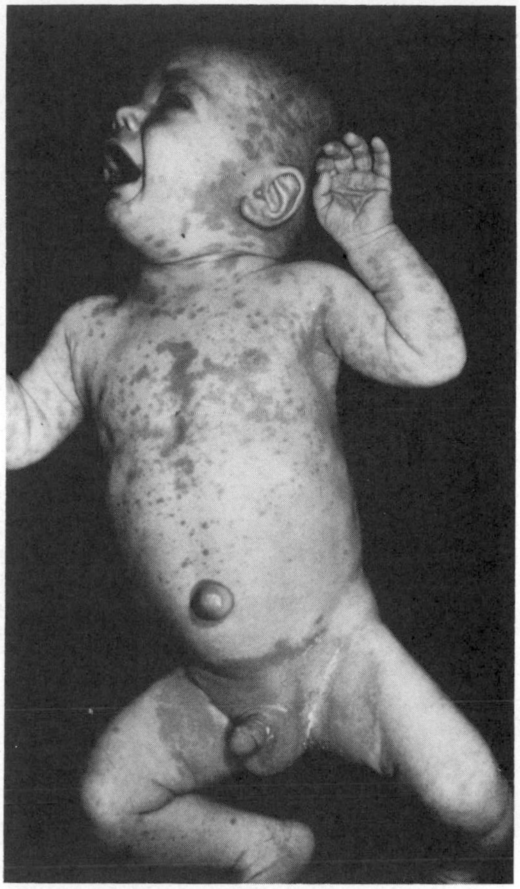

Figure 5. Generalized cutaneous candidiasis that began in the diaper distribution in this patient. (Courtesy of Dr. Victor Newcomer.)

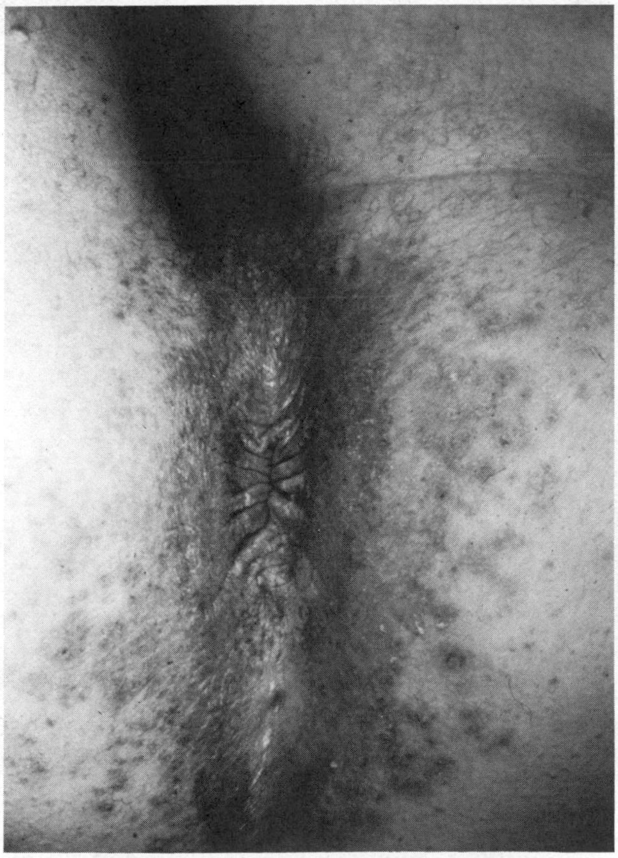

Figure 4. Perinal candidiasis. (Courtesy of Dr. Victor Newcomer.)

ADDITIONAL FORMS OF CUTANEOUS CANDIDIASIS. Candida may cause onychomycosis with extensive nail plate involvement, but this is usually associated with paronychia. Erosia interdigitalis blastomycetica is a term applied to a form of candidal infection that occurs between the fingers (Fig. 8) or between the toes and extends onto the sides of the digits. It causes a red base, maceration, and pain. Candidal folliculitis may also occur (Fig. 9). Ecythma gangrenosum-like lesions due to *Candida* have been reported (Fine et al., 1981) as well as subcutaneous *Candida* abscesses in an operative site (Feldman et al., 1980).

TREATMENT AND PROPHYLAXIS. Successful treatment of all forms of mucocutaneous candidiasis requires the elimination of local irritation and moisture. The hands must be spared excessive immersion in dish water, thumb-sucking must stop, moist skin should be dried, and diapers should be changed more frequently. Powders or creams can reduce skin moisture, especially in intertriginous areas. Vaginal, oral, or gastrointestinal candidiasis must be treated

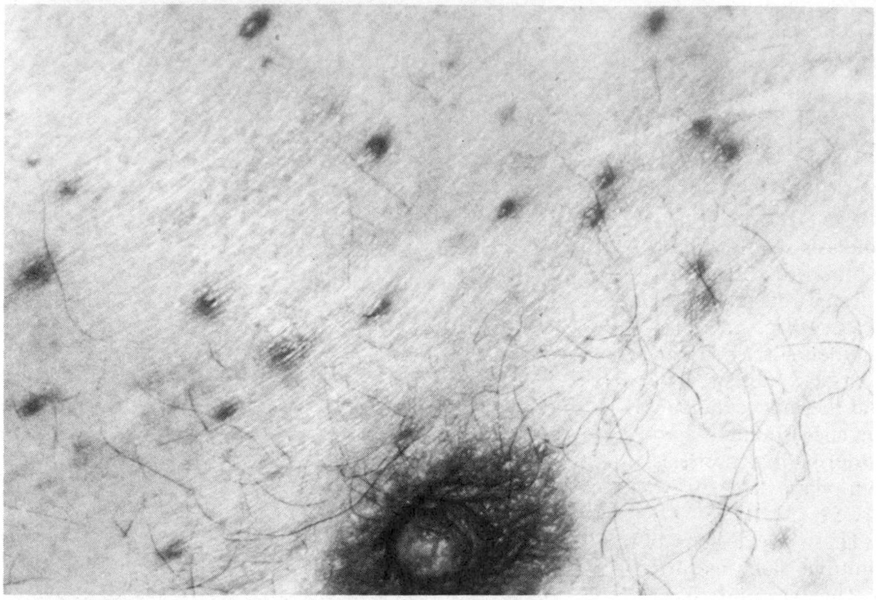

Figure 6. Typical macronodular lesions of disseminated candidiasis. (Courtesy of Dr. Gerald P. Bodey.)

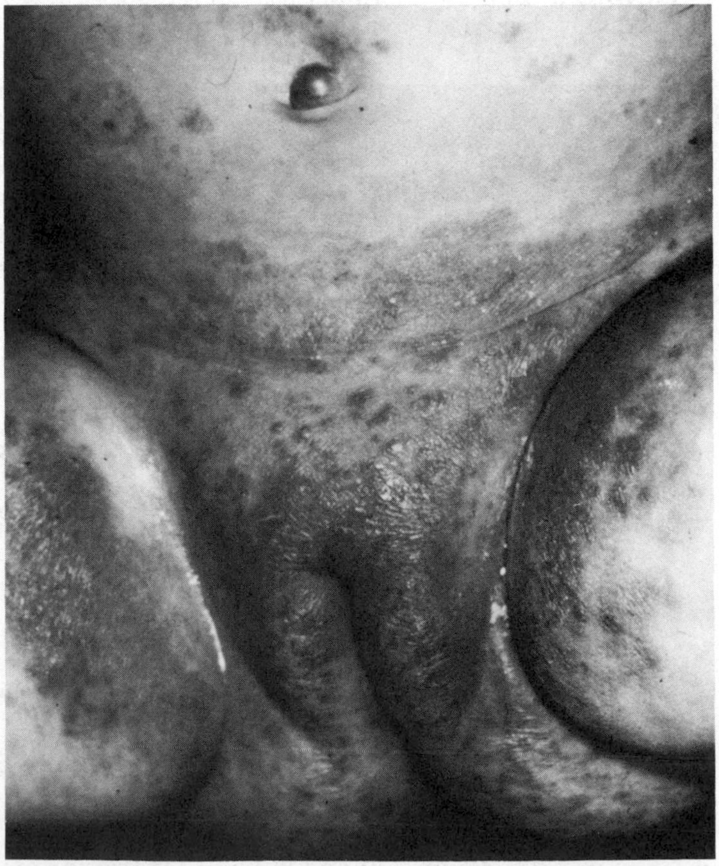

Figure 7. Typical *Candida* diaper rash. (Courtesy of Dr. Victor Newcomer.)

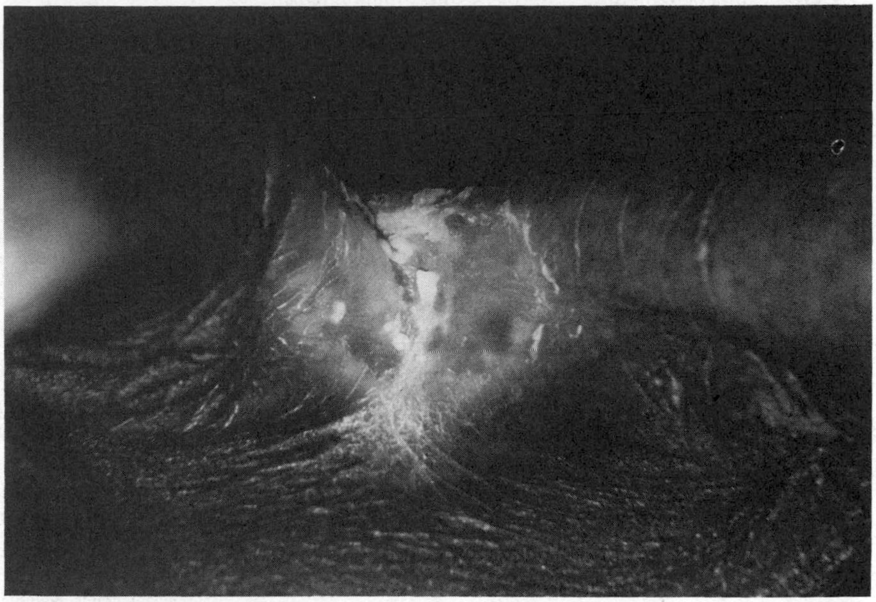

Figure 8. Erosio interdigitalis blastomycetica. (Courtesy of Dr. Arnold Gurevitch.)

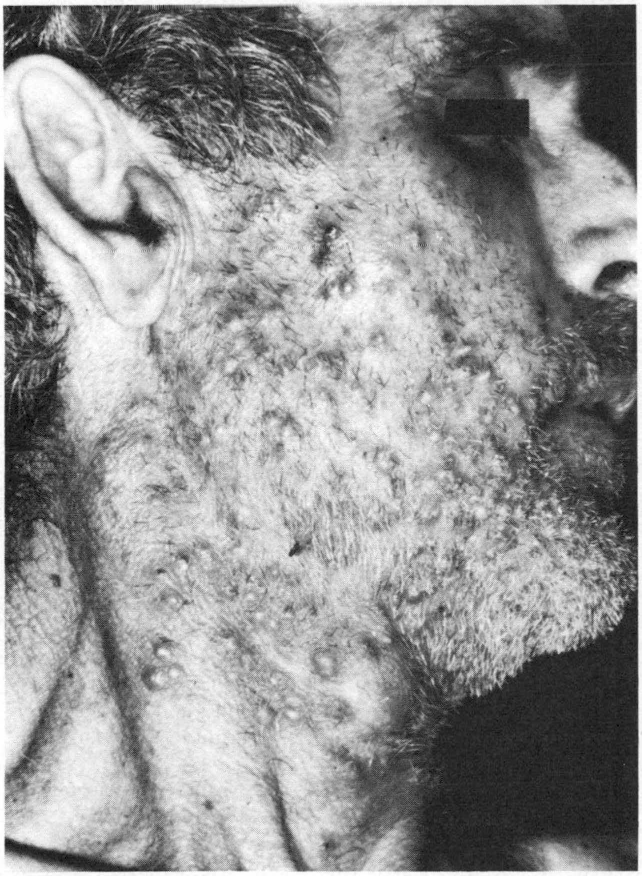

Figure 9. Severe *Candida* folliculitis. (Courtesy of Dr. Victor Newcomer.)

if it is the source of cutaneous disease (such as vulvar disease).

Chronic mucocutaneous candidiasis and cutaneous candidiasis not associated with T-cell defects are usually treated with either nystatin or amphotericin B topical preparations. Amphotericin B 3 per cent in vanishing cream base or 100,000 units of nystatin in the same base can be used with equal efficacy. On the other hand, calamine lotion is relatively ineffective by comparison (Stritzler, 1966). For candidal paronychia, either the 3 per cent amphotericin B or resorcin (3 per cent in 70 per cent isopropyl alcohol) lotions can be followed by application of a cream containing 3 per cent iodochlorhydroxyquin. Candidal diaper rash has been treated successfully with nystatin powder or cream in combination with a corticosteroid such as Mycolog cream (Squibb). Other successful compounds include amphotericin cream or lotion, Castellani paint, 1 per cent gentian violet applied once daily, or chlordantoin lotion (Sporostecin [Ortho]). The agents used for diaper rash are generally successful for pruritus ani as well.

Newer antifungal agents—miconazole, sulconazole, (Tanenbaum et al., 1983) and clotrimazole—are undergoing trial for their efficacy in controlling mucocutaneous candidiasis (Cullen, 1977; Keczkes et al., 1975). Intial studies are encouraging; however, further evaluation of their advantages over existing agents is necessary. In severe cases oral ketoconazole may be warranted but the risk of hepatic toxicity must be clarified.

Finally, correction of iron deficiency has been associated with rapid improvement of clinical manifestations in some patients with chronic mucocutaneous candidiasis. It has been postulated that iron deficiency contributes to an immune deficiency against *Candida* (Higgs and Wells, 1972).

References

Bodey, G. P., and Luna, M.: Skin lesions associated with disseminated candidiasis. JAMA 229:1466, 1974.

Cullen, S. I.: Cutaneous candidiasis: Treatment with miconazole nitrate. Cutis 19:126, 1977.

De Villez, R. L., Lewis, C. W.: Candidiasis seminar. Cutis 19:69, 1977.

Feldman, W. E., et al.: Skin abscesses caused by Candida albicans: Unusual presentation of *C. albicans* disease. J Clin Microbiol, July 12(1):44, 1980.

Fine, J. D., Miller, J. A., Harrist, T. J., et al.: Cutaneous lesions in disseminated candidiasis mimicking ecthyma gangrenosum. Am J Med 70:1133, 1981.

Hay, R. J.: Management of chronic mucocutaneous candidosis. Clin Exp Dermatol 6:515–519, 1981.

Higgs, J. M., and Wells, R. S.: Mucocutaneous candidiasis. Br J Dermatol 86, Supplement 8:88, 1972.

Jorizzo, J. L.: Chronic mucocutaneous candidiasis. An Update. Arch Dermatol 118:963, 1982.

Keczkes, K., Leighton, I., and Good, C. S.: Topical treatment of dermatophytoses and candidoses. Practitioner 214:412, 1975.

Kozinn, P. J., and Taschdgian, C. L.: Candidiasis (unit 17–16). In Dennis, D. J., Dobson, R. L., and McGuire, J. (eds): Clinical Dermatology, Hagerstown, Harper and Row, 1977.

Petersen, E. A., Alling, D. W., Kirkpatrick, C. H.: Treatment of chronic mucocutaneous candidiasis with ketoconazole. A controlled clinical trial. Ann Intern Med 93:791, 1980.

Stiehm, E. R.: Chronic mucocutaneous candidiasis. Clinical aspects, pp. 96–99. In Edwards, J. E., Jr. (moderator): Severe candida infections: Clinical perspectives, immune defense mechanisms, and current concepts in therapy. Ann Intern Med 89:91–106, 1978.

Tanenbaum, L., Anderson, C., Rosenberg, M., Darr, A.: A new treatment for cutaneous candidiasis: Sulconazole nitrate cream 1%. International J Dermatol 22:318, 1983.

226
LOBOMYCOSIS

JOSÉ LISBÔA MIRANDA, M.D.

Lobomycosis (keloidal blastomycosis, Jorge Lôbo's disease, Lôbo's mycosis) is an autonomous, chronic fungus infection that produces lesions only in the skin. Its etiologic agent has probably not yet been cultured. The disease has been found in humans living in the torrid zone of the Americas and in dolphins from the waters of the Florida and Surinam coasts.

The epidemiology and pathogenesis of the disease are still unclear, since it is difficult to reproduce experimentally in animals. Immunologic studies have been inconclusive, and there is no effective treatment for this infection. Diagnosis can be easily made because its clinical and histopathologic features are characteristic and the parasites are very abundant in the lesion.

DEFINITION. Lobomycosis is a chronic skin infection characterized chiefly by slow-growing, keloid-like tumors caused by a fungus that abounds in the tissues as round, thick-walled cells. It excites a massive proliferation of histiocytes and giant cells in the dermis.

ETIOLOGY. The causative agent of lobomycosis has not been cultured, and whatever fungi that have been isolated and reported should be considered as contaminants. Several names were proposed for the fungus, but it is best to call it *Loboa loboi*. Using this name discourages the use of names based on cultures of contaminants. There is no reason for classifying the fungus in the genus *Paracoccidioides*.

HISTORY. The disease was first described in a preliminary report in 1930 by Jorge Lôbo, who published further studies of the case in 1931 and 1933. The patient had keloidal skin lesions without lymphatic or visceral involvement. Lôbo gave an accurate account of the main histopathologic features and of the morphology of the parasite in tissues. He could not reproduce the infection in guinea pigs, rats, or Rhesus monkeys but claimed to have obtained cultures of the fungus on Sabouraud's glucose agar. Intradermal and complement fixation tests for *Paracoccidioides brasiliensis* were negative in his patient, and he concluded that he had found a new form of blastomycosis caused by a new fungus.

The cultures first obtained by Lôbo were probably contaminants, since a fungus like the one originally described has never again been isolated from other patients with the disease. Furthermore, the original strain appears to have been lost and a colony of *P. brasiliensis* mislabeled with its name (Carneiro, 1952; Da Fonseca Filho, 1955).

EPIDEMIOLOGY. Lobomycosis has a limited geographic distribution. With only one exception, all human cases of the disease have lived in tropical rain forests and bush country of South and Central America, chiefly the Amazon basin. Most patients have been reported from Brazil, but the infection has been found also in French Guiana, Surinam, Venezuela, Colombia, Panama, Costa Rica and Peru. In North America there is a registered case in Mexico (Zavala-Velazques and Perez, 1978).

The disease is not as rare as first thought, and increasing numbers of reports have appeared during the last 20 years. There are published references to 199 patients (Baruzzi et al., 1979), but many other cases are unreported and it is now considered a relatively frequent fungus infection in Amazon State (Brazil).

This mycosis does not appear to have a racial preference. Most cases reported were in mulattos because they predominate in the area where the disease occurs. However, it has been found also in 50 Brazilian Indians of the Caiabi tribe (Baruzzi et al., 1967; Baruzzi et al., 1979), in 13 Negroes from Surinam (Wiersema and Niemel, 1965), and in a white Portuguese male living in Amazon State, Brazil (Lacaz et al., 1955).

Most patients are men who have worked on rubber plantations or in other agricultural occupations. The infection has been found in females very rarely.

It is difficult to determine the age at the time of acquisition of the disease because most patients seek medical care many years, even decades, after the first lesions are apparent. The age at diagnosis varies between 20 and 83 years old.

The lesions are found commonly on exposed skin, particularly ear lobes and legs (Fig. 1*A*, *B*, *E*). Many patients state that the lesions appeared at sites of previous injuries, including snake and insect bites. There are no data suggesting that this mycosis is contagious from person to person.

Natural infection of animals was not known until recently. A first reported case of lobomycosis in a bottle-nosed dolphin (*Tursiops truncatus*) on the west coast of Florida in 1971 (Migaki et al., 1971) was followed by findings in another infected dolphin (*Sotalia guianensis*) in the estuary of the Surinam river (De Vries and Laarman, 1973), in one on the east coast of Florida, and still another captured in the Gulf of Mexico (Caldwell et al., 1975).

The ecology of the parasite is unknown. The fact that the fungus cannot be grown from tissue obtained from humans or naturally infected dolphins and that most attempts to reproduce the disease experimentally in animals have not been successful suggest the existence of an obligatory natural host of the parasite. However, there is no proof to substantiate this theory.

CLINICAL MANIFESTATIONS. Lobomycosis is a chronic disease of the skin without systemic involvement. Cases are known in which the infection has persisted for several decades without impairment of the general health of the patient.

The characteristic lesion is a very slow-growing keloid-like tumor surrounded by apparently normal skin (Fig. 1*C*). In addition, one can sometimes see papules, verrucoid, nodular lesions, or infiltrated plaques.

The isolated keloid-like lesion is freely movable and usually has a smooth, shiny surface with telangiectases. Old lesions may become scaly or verrucous and occasionally ulcerate or become pedunculated. Large lobulated tumors may be produced by confluence of several growing nodules (Fig. 1*E*). The lesions may remain confined to one area, growing in diameter or showing new nodules in the surrounding skin, or they may be scattered to several different regions of the body.

Symptoms are negligible, and only a few patients complain of slight pruritus. As a rule regional lymph nodes are not involved, but occasionally they become enlarged.

A somewhat different clinical appearance is seen in infected Brazilian Indians (Fig. 1*D*). They present, besides the characteristic keloid-like tumors, papules and infiltrated plaques like those seen in tuberculoid leprosy. In its classic form the lesions of lobomycosis have no tendency to heal spontaneously, but in the Brazilian Indians one can see hypertrophic scarring and wrinkled atrophic skin following a natural involution of the nodules.

PATHOLOGY AND PATHOGENESIS. The histopathologic picture is characteristic and diagnostic. The lesions are located in the dermis, but the epidermis shows some changes.

The epidermis frequently is atrophic and may be stretched, with disappearance of the rete pegs (Fig. 2*A*) owing to pressure from the diffuse dermal lesion. When ulceration occurs, the borders show acanthosis or pseudoepitheliomatous hyperplasia. In old scaly lesions there is hyperkeratosis and focal parakeratosis.

The whole dermis is obliterated by a massive infiltrate consisting mainly of histiocytes and giant cells (Fig. 2*B*,*D*). The parasites abound in the affected area, and because many organisms seem to be empty cells, the skin sections have a sieve-like appearance (Fig. 2*C*). A narrow band of normal connective tissue is frequently present in the subpapillary dermis (Fig. 2*A*), but sometimes the lesions reach the epidermis and even destroy its basal layer. In the same way, the dermal infiltrate may occasionally extend downward into the upper hypodermis. Giant cells are more numerous in the center of the lesions, while at the borders the histiocytes predominate in such a way as to give an appearance of cultured cells (Fialho, 1938). The histiocytes are large with foamy cytoplasm and eccentric nuclei. The giant cells vary in size and disposition of nuclei and contain many parasites and sometimes asteroid bodies (Fig. 2*D*). Small foci of lymphocytes and plasma cells may be found at the periphery of the histiocytic proliferation. Collagen fibers are seen dividing the entire lesion into lobules. In old lesions there is an increase of these collagen fibers. There is no necrosis in the affected tissues.

A striking feature in the tissue sections of lobomycosis is the great abundance of parasites (Fig. 3*A*). They are seen in long chains (Fig. 3*A*), in rosettes (Fig. 3*D*), or isolated (Fig. 3*A*). The author (Miranda, 1972a) found the maximum diameter to be 15.2μ, the minimum 6.0μ, and the average 9.6μ. Organisms of apparently small diameter may be only segments of cells (Wiersema and Niemel, 1965). The relative uniformity in size of the yeasts distinguishes them from the yeast cells of *P. brasiliensis*. Many of the organisms appear as empty cells; some are deformed; some have a homogeneous cytoplasmic mass that may be shrunk at the center of the cell, while in others the cytoplasm is seen as irregular masses or dust-like material. The wall of the fungus is 1μ in thickness, and the parasite has no capsule. Both wall and cytoplasm are PAS-positive. In PAS- or silver-stained specimens some cells show the walls with

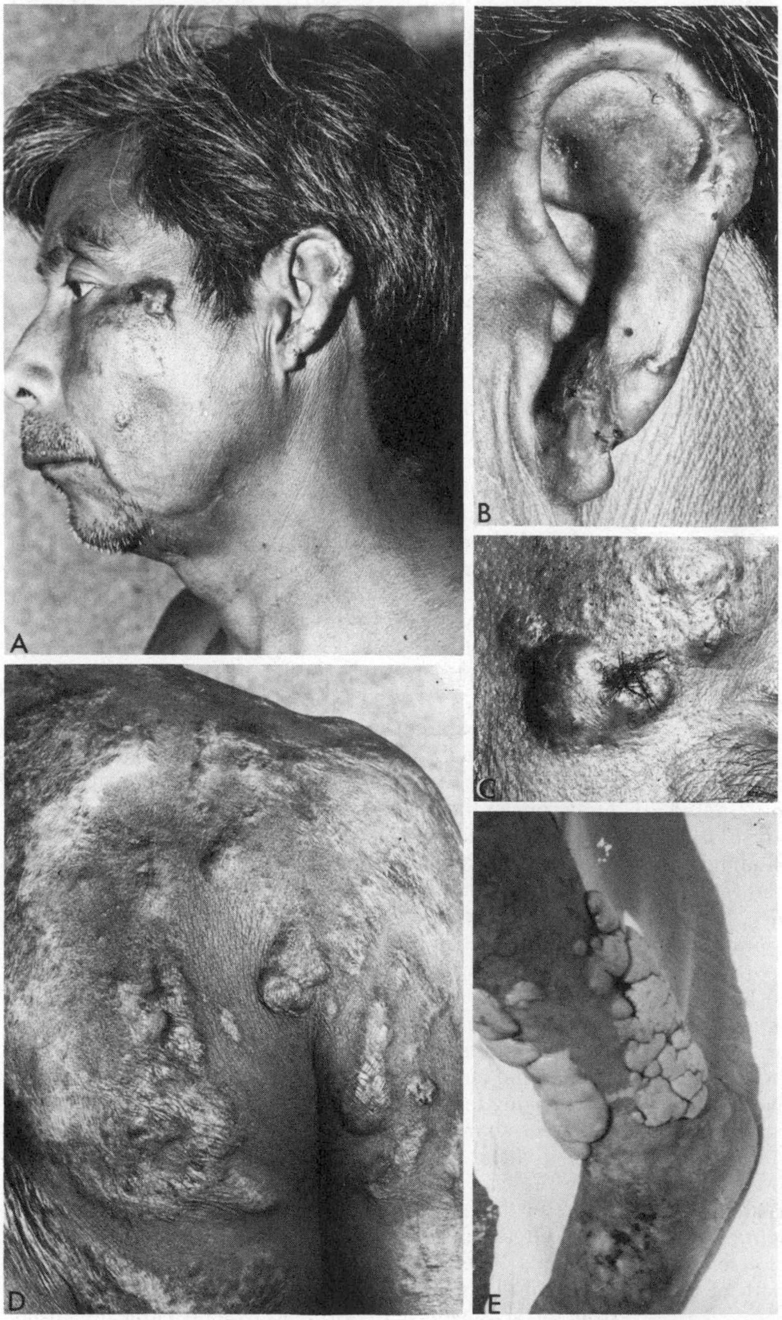

Figure 1. Lobomycosis. A, Cutaneous lesions on zygomatic area and ear. *B,* Close-up of the ear showing nodular lesions on helix and ear lobe. Note traumatic erosion on ear lobe. *C,* Close-up of zygomatic arch showing keloid-like lesions surrounded by apparently normal skin. The stitches were done to repair the biopsy area. *D,* Keloid-like tumors, infiltrated plaques, hypertrophic scarring and wrinkled atrophic skin are shown in a Brazilian Indian. *E,* Lobulated tumors resulting from confluence of growing nodules.

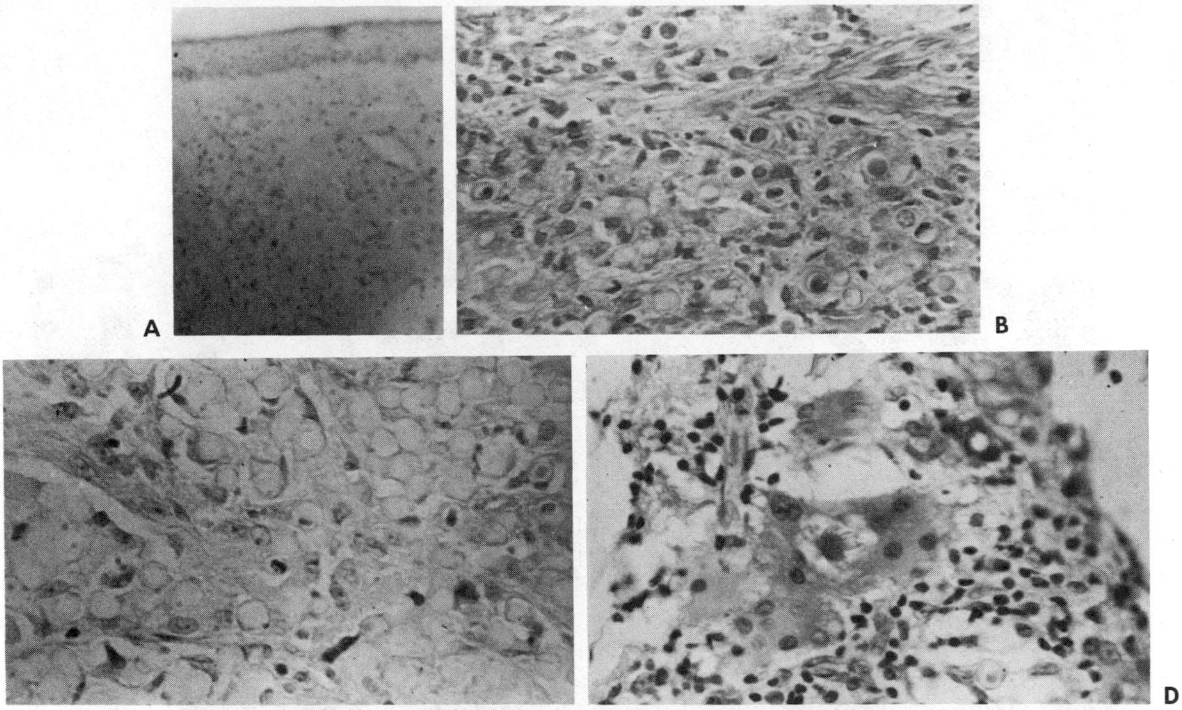

Figure 2. Lobomycosis. A, Stretched epidermis with disappearance of rete pegs. Subpapillary dermis with narrow band of normal connective tissue (H & E, × 120). *B,* Proliferation of histiocytes and numerous parasites (PAS, × 480). *C,* Abundant fungi seen as empty cells, giving a sieve-like appearance (H & E, × 480). *D,* Asteroid body in a giant cell (PAS, × 480).

radiating spines (Fig. 4*B*). Scanning electron microscopy (Abreu and Miranda, 1972; Miranda, 1972b) seems to corroborate the impression that the radiations are part of the parasite's wall and not a host-tissue reaction. Those observations revealed a thick three-layer wall whose outermost layer was made of irregular overlapping scales (Fig. 4*C, D*).

The fungus apparently reproduces by single, double, and rarely by three or more gemmations (Fig. 3*C*). Cryptosporulation with numerous small buds around the mother cell, such as that observed in *P. brasiliensis,* is not seen in lobomycosis. Buds have a tendency to remain permanently attached to the cell from which they originate, which explains the long chains of parasites. Because the parasites may have multiple buddings, those chains sometimes are branched (Fig. 3*B*). It is estimated that 90 per cent of the organisms found in the lesions are strung together (Wiersema and Niemel, 1965). The walls of the parasites continue from one cell to another as short, narrow, bridge-like structures. This connection may be severed by pressure and a bud scar shows at the site of the fracture (Fig. 3*G*).

Following the several stages of budding, the yeast-like cell first appears pear-shaped (Fig. 3*E*), then exhibits a finger-like projection with a nodular end (Fig. 3*F*) that widens to become knob-like (Fig. 3*E*), finally growing up to form a new cell. At the beginning, the cytoplasm of both cells is continuous (Fig. 4*A*), but later communication is interrupted.

The pathogenesis of lobomycosis is still unclear. The infection probably follows direct implantation of the fungus into the skin. This is in accordance with the belief of many patients that the first lesions appeared at the site of a previous injury. It also explains why most sufferers show the disease on exposed skin areas. The occurrence of lesions at scattered regions of the body might suggest hematogenous spread of the organism, but autoinoculation is more likely to be the cause. This autoinoculation would also explain the appearance of new satellite nodules around the original one.

Some authors (Leite, 1954; Teixeira, 1962; Wiersema and Niemel, 1965) have tried to reconstruct the pathogenesis of the infection from the pathologic findings. They postulate that the large size of the parasites, their rigid wall, and their disposition to chains of cells do not permit hematogenous or lymphatic dissemination. The proliferating histiocytes and giant cells of the host and the causative agent of the disease do not seem to harm each other. There is no sign in the lesions of digested parasites or tissue necrosis. The fungi are apparently not killed.

Most attempts to infect animals by inoculation of material from humans have failed. The few successful attempts did not clarify our understanding of the disease. Material from dolphins' lesions have been passed through three generation of mice inoculated in their footpads (Chandler et al., 1980). A few successful experimental infections were obtained with difficulty in hamsters (Guimaraes, 1964; Sampaio and Dias, 1970; Wiersema and Niemel, 1965), rats (Azulay et al., 1970), tortoises (Sampaio et al., 1971), and an armadillo (Sampaio and Dias, 1977). In the armadillo the lesion developed more rapidly than in natural human infection and the microscopic aspect showed areas of liquefactive necrosis similar to those observed in natural infection of dolphin (Caldwell et al., 1975).

DIAGNOSIS. Clinical diagnosis is based on the finding of slow-growing nodules resembling keloids on agricultural workers who live or have lived in the torrid zone of the Americas. Brazilian Indians with the disease present with

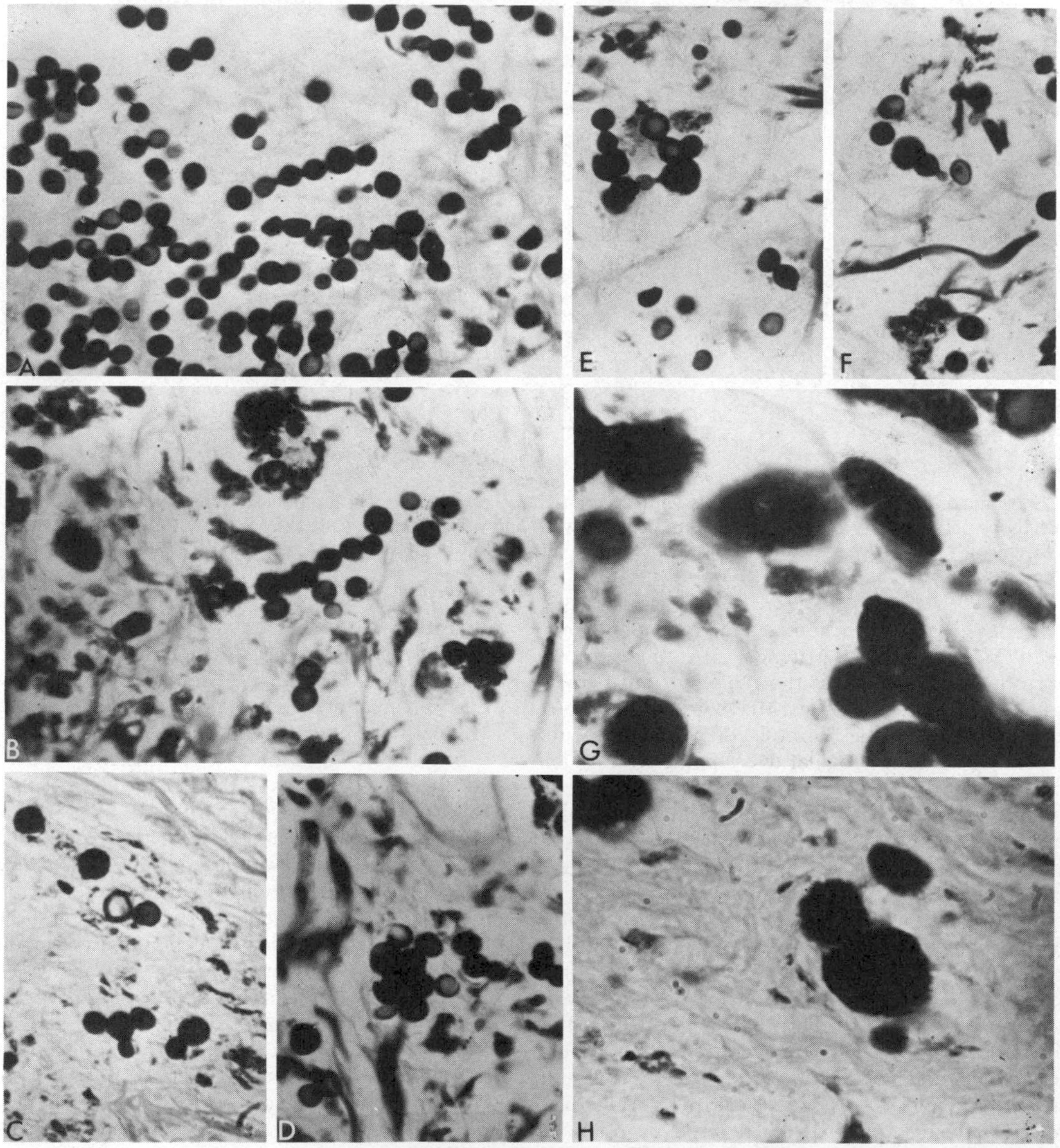

Figure 3. Lobomycosis. A, Abundance of parasites with little variation in size. Fungi are isolated or arranged in chains. Narrow tubes connect the cells (methenamine silver, × 480). *B,* Branched chain of parasites (methenamine silver, × 480). *C,* Cell showing three buds (Grocott, × 480). *D,* Fungi arranged in rosette (methenamine silver, × 480). *E,* First stage of budding: pear-shaped cell at lower right quadrant. At center is a further stage of reproduction: the knob-like aspect of the bud (methenamine silver, × 480). *F,* Early stage of budding: finger-like projection with nodular ending (methenamine silver, × 480). *G,* Bud scar where connecting tube was severed (methenamine silver, × 1200). *H,* Parasite's wall with radiating spines (Grocott, × 1200).

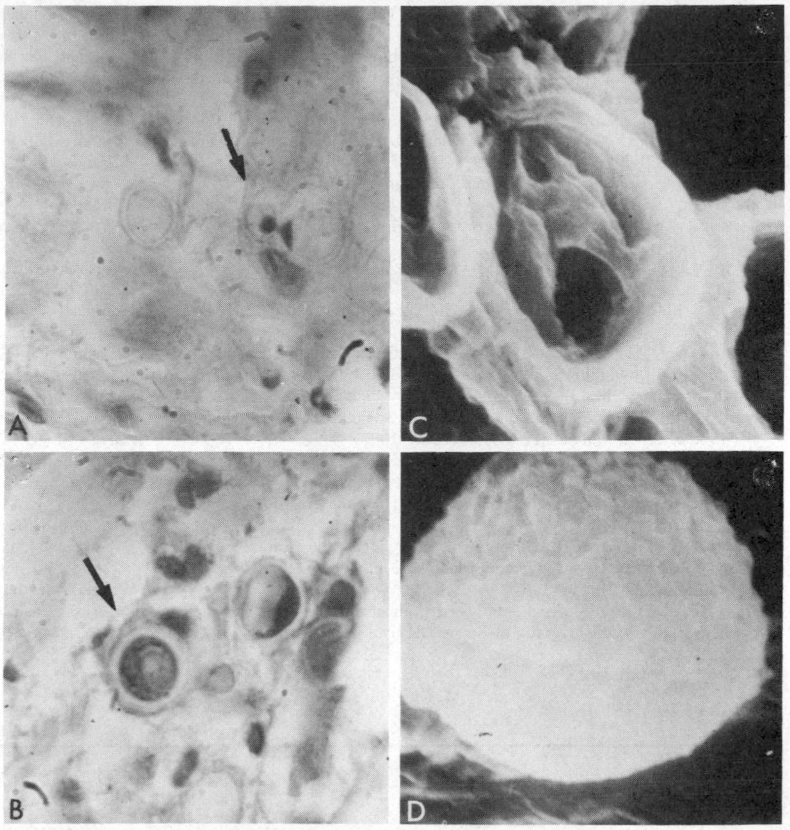

Figure 4. Lobomycosis. *A,* The arrow points to budding cell showing continuity of its cytoplasm with that of the mother cell (PAS, × 1200). *B,* Fungus wall with radiating spines (PAS, × 1200). *C,* Thick three-layered wall of the parasite (scanning electron microscopy, × 5000). *D,* Parasite's wall with irregular overlapping scales (scanning electron microsopy, × 5000).

infiltrated plaques, hypertrophic scars, and atrophic wrinkled lesions, as well as the typical keloids. True keloids, leprosy, and xanthomatoses should be considered in the differential diagnosis. Old verrucous lobomycosis lesions may resemble chromomycosis, tuberculosis verrucosa cutis, or chronic pyogenic infection.

The diagnosis is confirmed by direct mycologic and histopathologic examinations. For the direct mycologic examination, the material obtained through scarification of a lesion or from a biopsied nodule is digested in 10 per cent potassium hydroxide. The parasites appear as numerous yeast-like cells with thick refractile walls. Often they are arranged in chains, but isolated cells are also frequently seen. Most organisms show single or double budding, rarely three or more gemmulations. Each cell is attached to the next by a short and narrow tubular structure. The fungi have little variation in size, averaging 9 to 10μ in diameter. The histopathologic picture is typical, showing a dense dermal infiltrate with intense proliferation of histiocytes, the presence of giant cells, and a great abundance of parasites. The fungus does not have cryptosporulation (numerous small buds) like *P. brasiliensis,* its buds are not connected to the mother cell by a broad base as in *Blastomyces dermatitidis,* and it has no capsule like *Cryptococcus neoformans.* Transmission electron microscopy demonstrates that the parasite is multinucleated (Furtado et al., 1967).

The fungus cannot be cultivated *in vitro.* Serology and skin tests do not contribute to the diagnosis. Complement fixation test with the polysaccharide antigen of *P. brasiliensis* and paracoccidioidin skin test are negative or weakly positive (Lacaz et al., 1955; Fonseca and Lacaz, 1971). Immunofluorescence studies (Silva et al., 1968) showed that *Loboa loboi* is more closely related antigenically to some strains of *P. brasiliensis* than to others. It also has antigens in common with the yeast forms of *Histoplasma capsulatum, B. dermatitidis, Candida albicans,* and the mycelial form of *Coccidioides immitis.* However, labeled serum globulins from three patients with lobomycosis did not stain cells of *L. loboi* from tissues and yeast-like cells of *P. brasiliensis.*

COMPLICATIONS, SEQUELAE, AND PROGNOSIS. The only frequent complications observed are traumatic ulceration and secondary bacterial infection of ulcerated lesions. Lesions may increase in size until they cover extensive areas and produce incapacitating deformities.

The prognosis is good as far as general health is concerned, but the lesions persist without self-healing.

TREATMENT. Wide surgical excision of the lesion is the only effective treatment, but recurrences are frequent.

References

Abreu, W. M., and Miranda, J. L.: Microscopia electrônica scanning: Agente da micose de Jorge Lôbo. An Bras Dermat 47:115, 1972.

Azulay, R. D., Carneiro, J. A., and Andrade, L. C.: Blastomicose de Jorge Lôbo. Contribuiçao ao estudo da etiologia, inoculação experimental, immunologia e patologia da doença. An Bras Derm Sif 45:47, 1970.

Baruzzi, R. G., D'Andretta, C., Jr., Carvalhal, S., Ramos, O. L., and Pontes, P. L.: Ocorrência de blastomicose queloideana entre índios Caiabí. Rev Inst Med Trop S Paulo 9:135, 1967.

Baruzzi, R. G., Lacaz, C. S., and Souza, F. A. A.: Historia natural da doença de Jorge Lôbo. Ocorrência entre os índios Caiabí (Brasil Central). Rev Inst Med Trop São Paulo 21:302, 1979.

Caldwell, D. K., Caldwell, M. C., Woodard, J. C., Ajello, L., Kaplan, W., and McClure, H. M.: Lobomycosis as a disease of the Atlantic bottle-

nosed dolphin (*Tursiops truncatus* Montagu, 1821). Am J Trop Med Hyg 24:105, 1975.
Carneiro, L. S.: Contribuiçao ao Estudo Microbiológico do Agente Etiológico da Doença de Jorge Lôbo. Thesis, University of Recife. Recife, Imprensa Industrial, 1952.
Chandler, F. W., Kaplan, W., and Ajello, L.: Color Atlas and Text of Histopathology of Mycotic Diseases. Chicago, Year Book Medical Publishers, Inc., 1980, p. 73.
Da Fonseca Filho, O.: Deep skin and pulmonary mycosis in Brazil. In Sternberg, T. H., and Newcomer, V. D. (eds.): Therapy of Fungus Diseases. An International Symposium. Boston, Little Brown & Company, 1955, p. 56.
De Vries, G. A., and Laarman, J. J.: A case of Lôbo's disease in the dolphin *Sotalia guianensis*. Aquatic Mammals 1:26, 1973.
Fialho, A.: Blastomicose do tipo "Jorge Lôbo" Hospital (Rio de J) 14:903, 1938.
Fonseca, O. J. M., and Lacaz, C. S.: Estudo das culturas isoladas de blastomicose queilodiforme (doença Jorge Lôbo). Denominação ao seu agente etiológico. Rev Inst Med Trop S Paulo 13:225, 1971.
Furtado, J. S., Brito, T., and Freymuller, E.: Structure and reproduction of *Paracoccidioides loboi*. Mycologia 59:286, 1967.
Guimarães, F. N.: Inoculações em hamsters da blastomicose sulamericana (doençã de Lutz), da blastomicose queloidiforme (doença de Lôbo), e da blastomicose dos índios do Tapajós-Xingú. Hospital (Rio de J) 66:581, 1964.
Lacaz, C. S., Sterman, L., Monteiro, E. V. L., and Pinto, D. O.: Blastomicose queloideana. Comentários sobre novo caso. Rev Hosp Clín Fac Med S Paulo 10:254, 1955.
Leite, J. M.: Doença de Jorge Lôbo. (Contribuiçao ao seu Estudo Anátomopatológico). Thesis, University of Recife. Revista da Veterinaria, 1954.
Lôbo, J.: Nova espécie de blastomicose. Brasil Méd 44:1327, 1930.
Lôbo, J.: Um caso de blastomicose produzido por uma espécie nova, encontrada em Recife. Rev Med Pernambuco 1:763, 1931.
Lôbo, J.: Contribuiçao ao estudo das blastomicoses. An Bras Derm Sif 8:43, 1933.
Migaki, G., Valerio, M. G., Irvine, B., and Garner, F. M.: Lôbo's disease in an Atlantic bottle-nosed dolphin. J Am Vet Med Assoc 159:578, 1971.
Miranda, J. L.: Lôbo's mycosis. In Marshall, J. (ed.): Essays on Tropical Dermatology. Vol. 2. Amsterdam, Excerpta Medica 1972a, p. 356.
Miranda, J. L.: Lobomicose (blastomicose queilodiforme, micose de Jorge Lôbo, morbus Jorge Lôbo). An Bras Dermat 47:273, 1972b.
Sampaio, M. M., and Dias, L. B.: Experimental infection of Jorge Lôbo's disease in the cheek pouch of the golden hamster *(Mesocricetus auratus)*. Rev Inst Med Trop S Paulo 12:115, 1970.
Sampaio, M. M., Dias, L. B., and Scaff, L.: Bizarre forms of the etiologic agent in experimental Jorge Lôbo's disease in tortoises. Rev Inst Med Trop S Paulo 13:191, 1971.
Sampaio, M. M., and Dias, L. B.: The armadillo *Euphractus sexcintus* as a suitable animal for experimental studies of Jorge Lôbo's disease. Rev Inst Med Trop São Paulo 19:215, 1977.
Silva, M. E., Kaplan, W., and Miranda, J. L.: Antigenic relationship between *Paracoccidioides loboi* and other pathogenic fungi determined by immunofluorescence. Mycopathologia (Den Haag) 36:97, 1968.
Teixeira, G. A.: Doença de Jorge Lôbo. Aspectos microscópicos. Hospital (Rio de J) 62:813, 1962.
Wiersema, J. P., and Niemel, P. L. A.: Lôbo's disease in Surinam patients. Trop Geogr Med 17:89, 1965.
Zavala-Velazques, J., and Perez, A. R.: Enfermedad de Lôbo (Lobomicosis). Primer caso mexicano. Dermatologia (Mex.) 22:5, 1978.

227

MYCOBACTERIAL INFECTIONS OF THE SKIN

WAYNE M. MEYERS, M.D., PH.D.

In 1882 Robert Koch identified *Mycobacterium tuberculosis* as the cause of tuberculosis. Thus, by priority this bacillus became the "typical" mycobacterium. Other mycobacteria, however, were soon observed that differed from *M. tuberculosis,* and these became known as "atypical" mycobacteria. In 1954 Timpe and Runyon first classified atypical mycobacteria into four groups on the basis of their growth characteristics. This system, known as the Runyon Classification (Table 1), has undergone so many modifications that it has been more or less abandoned in favor of a new system that recognizes ten species or species complexes of mycobacteria pathogenic for man: *M. leprae, M. tuberculosis* complex, *M. ulcerans, M. marinum, M. kansasii, M. szulgai, M. simiae, M. avium-scrofulaceum-intracellulare* complex, *M. xenopi,* and *M. fortuitum* complex. All of these mycobacteria except *M. simiae* and *M. xenopi* cause diseases of the skin. The optimal growth temperature of 43° C makes *M. xenopi* an unlikely pathogen of the skin. *M. leprae,* the cause of leprosy, is discussed in Chapter 188.

M. TUBERCULOSIS INFECTION

DEFINITION AND ETIOLOGY. *M. tuberculosis* is the predominant cause of cutaneous tuberculosis, but *M. bovis,* sometimes called *M. tuberculosis* (var. *bovis*), also infects the skin. Cutaneous tuberculosis is classified as follows:

1. *Primary inoculation tuberculosis.* Infection starts in the skin.
2. *Reinfection tuberculosis.* The skin becomes infected in a patient sensitized by co-existing or previous tuberculosis.
3. *Tuberculids.* Some authorities believe that tuberculids are local hyperergic reactions to mycobacteria or their antigens that are spread hematogenously to the skin from foci of active tuberculosis. Others, however, consider tuberculids a misnomer for a phenomenon that is unrelated to tuberculosis. The skepticism about tuberculids as an entity may be explained in part by their rarity in countries with relatively little active tuberculosis (Iden et al. 1978). The various forms of tuberculids are: erythema induratum, lichen scrofulosorum, papulonecrotic tuberculid, and lupus

Table 1. CLASSIFICATION OF THE ATYPICAL MYCOBACTERIA THAT CAUSE LESIONS OF SKIN IN MAN (RUNYON SYSTEM)

Group	Pigment Production in Culture	Growth Rate	Species Identified
I	Photochromogens[a]	Slow	*M. kansasii* *M. marinum*
II	Scotochromogens[b]	Slow	*M. scrofulaceum* *M. szulgai*
III	Nonphoto-chromogens[c]	Slow	*M. avium* *M. intracellulare* (Battey)
IV	Variable	Rapid	*M. fortuitum* *M. chelonei*

[a]Pigment produced only on exposure to light.
[b]Pigment produced in dark or light.
[c]Nonpigmented.
Note: *M. ulcerans* has not been classified in the Runyon system.

miliaris disseminatus faciei. Tuberculids will not be discussed further in this chapter.

EPIDEMIOLOGY. With the marked reduction of pulmonary tuberculosis in many countries, cutaneous tuberculosis has become rare. Tuberculosis of the skin is more common in colder humid climates and is uncommon in tropical Africa, even though pulmonary tuberculosis is highly prevalent there. For example, in Kenya, Verhagen et al. (1968) found only 14 patients with cutaneous tuberculosis among 3168 patients with skin disease.

PATHOGENESIS AND PATHOLOGY

Primary Tuberculosis

Primary Inoculation Tuberculosis. In patients who have not been sensitized to *M. tuberculosis*, the inoculation of tubercle bacilli into the skin produces a local lesion and enlargement of regional lymph nodes. This is *primary inoculation tuberculosis* and is analogous to the Ghon complex. Within two weeks after inoculation into the skin there is an infiltration of polymorphonuclear leukocytes, necrosis, and ulceration. In approximately six weeks this acute reaction is replaced by epithelioid cells and giant cells. Tubercles may develop in the later stages, but caseation is not a constant feature. Acid-fast bacilli are abundant in early lesions but gradually decrease and become rare as granulomas develop.

Generalized Miliary Tuberculosis of the Skin. In anergic patients with fulminating tuberculosis of other organs there may be hematogenous spread to the skin. In the dermis there is a perivascular infiltration of polymorphonuclear leukocytes and lymphocytes. Acid-fast bacilli are easily demonstrated in vessels and surrounding tissues. Tuberculoid granulomas develop in older lesions.

Reinfection Tuberculosis. Patients who are sensitized to *M. tuberculosis*, either by previous infection or by coexisting tuberculosis, usually develop local delayed-type hypersensitivity reactions when reinfected by *M. tuberculosis*. Histopathologic changes in the common variants of these lesions are as follows:

Lupus Vulgaris. In the dermis there are admixtures of epithelioid cells, giant cells, lymphocytes, and plasma cells (Fig. 1). There often are tuberculoid granulomas with only slight necrosis or none. Acid-fast bacilli are rare. Squamous cell carcinomas may develop at the borders of the lesion.

Tuberculosis Verrucosa Cutis. In the upper dermis there are marked hyperkeratosis and parakeratosis with abscesses containing polymorphonuclear leukocytes (Fig. 2). Pseudoepitheliomatous hyperplasia may be marked. There may be tuberculoid granulomas with slight to moderate necrosis. Acid-fast bacilli are uncommon but are more numerous than in lupus vulgaris.

Scrofuloderma A tract of necrosis extends through the dermis and ulcerates the epidermis (Fig. 3). Tuberculoid

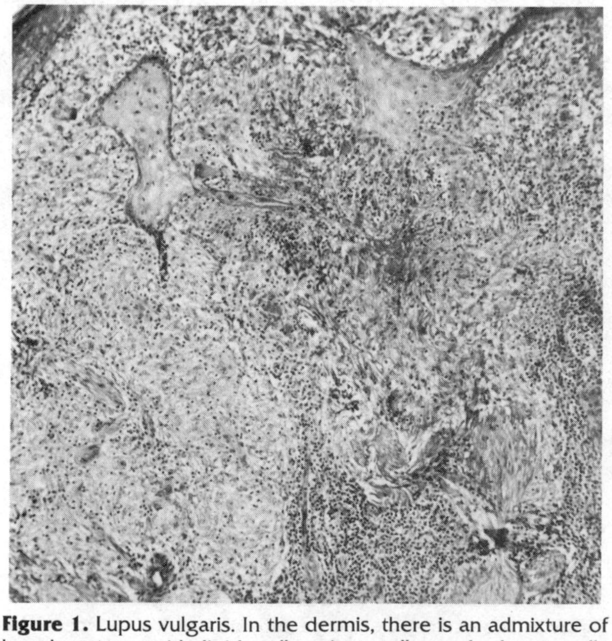

Figure 1. Lupus vulgaris. In the dermis, there is an admixture of lymphocytes, epithelioid cells, giant cells, and plasma cells without caseation necrosis. × 40, AFIP 57-9803.

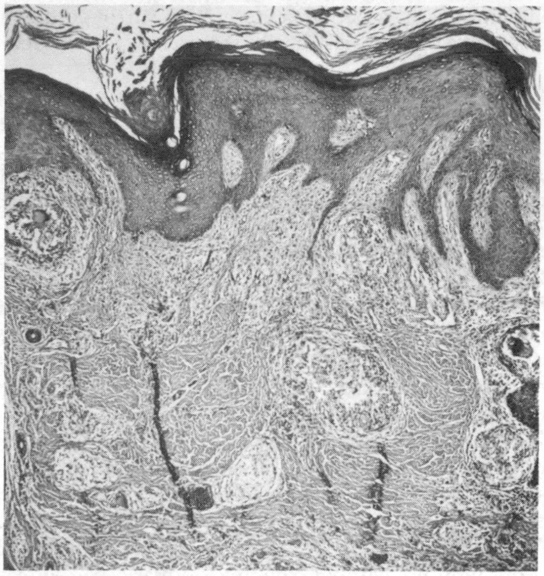

Figure 2. Tuberculosis verrucosa cutis showing hyperkeratosis and acanthosis. There are several granulomas in the dermis. × 40, AFIP 58-4939.

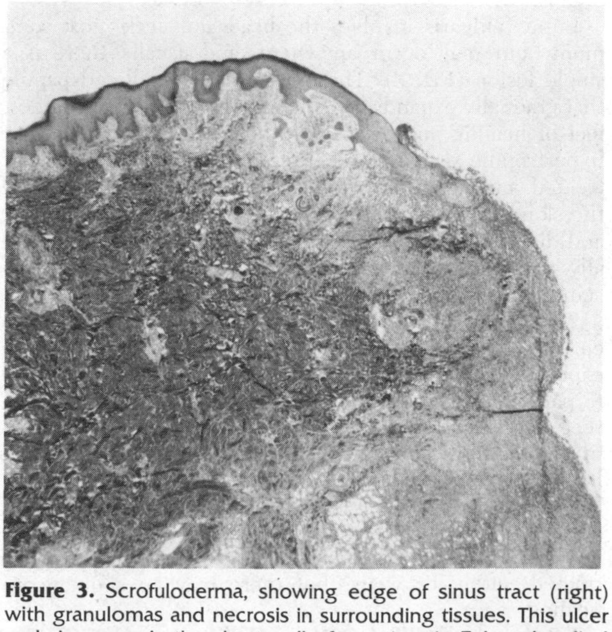

Figure 3. Scrofuloderma, showing edge of sinus tract (right) with granulomas and necrosis in surrounding tissues. This ulcer and sinus was in the chest wall of a patient in Zaire who died of pulmonary tuberculosis. The sinus communicated with the diseased lung. × 18, AFIP 78-729.

granulomas with caseation necrosis often surround the ulcer and sinus tract. Acid-fast bacilli are usually readily demonstrable.

Tuberculosis Cutis Orificialis. The mucous membrane is ulcerated with acute inflammatory cells in the ulcer base and a mixture of acute and chronic inflammation beneath the base. In long-standing lesions there may be tuberculoid granulomas with caseation. Acid-fast bacilli are abundant.

CLINICAL MANIFESTATIONS

Primary Tuberculosis

Primary Inoculation Tuberculosis. Approximately 0.15 per cent of all primary tuberculosis occurs in the skin. Infants and those whose occupations bring them in contact with tuberculosis are at risk, for example, "prosector's paronychia" in those who perform autopsies (Goette et al., 1978). Lesions appear as papules or crusted ulcers about two weeks after infection. These ulcers, or "tuberculous chancres," gradually enlarge to up to 5 cm in diameter. Often, about one month after infection, there is regional painful lymphadenopathy. Most infections subside after several months without therapy. Miliary dissemination from the skin is rare. A serious form of primary tuberculosis has been reported in subjects who have undergone circumcision by circumcisers with active tuberculosis.

Generalized Miliary Tuberculosis of the Skin. This rare complication of tuberculosis is usually seen in infants. There are widely disseminated small erythematous macules, papules, or vesicles in the skin. Prognosis is poor.

Reinfection Tuberculosis

Lupus Vulgaris. Lupus vulgaris is the most common form of cutaneous tuberculosis and is more frequent in women. Peak incidences occur at ages 20 years and 50 years. Horwitz (1960) studied 3902 patients with lupus vulgaris in Denmark and found that one-third of them eventually developed pulmonary tuberculosis, one-third had pulmonary tuberculosis before the onset of lupus vulgaris, and one-third had onset of pulmonary tuberculosis and lupus vulgaris simultaneously. Three-quarters of all patients with lupus vulgaris had tuberculosis of other organs.

Lupus vulgaris involves the head and neck most commonly but may occur anywhere, and usually there is a single lesion (Fig. 4). There is an early small red papule that gradually expands peripherally. As the lesion enlarges, foci of healing and active growth occur with atrophic or hypertrophic scarring and ulceration. This process, if not treated, may continue for decades and cover large areas of the skin. Loss of function of vital structures (e.g., eyelids) and disfigurement are serious sequelae. Skin cancers, usually squamous cell carcinomas, are not uncommon in long-standing lesions.

Tuberculosis Verrucosa Cutis. Tuberculosis verrucosa cutis is a disease of adults. Lesions are most frequent on exposed parts of the body (e.g., hands). Individuals exposed to patients or cadavers with tuberculosis are at risk. "Prosector's" and "anatomist's" wart are synonyms for lesions in those who perform autopsies. Lesions begin as papules, become hyperkeratotic, and resemble verrucae vulgaris. These "warts" gradually expand peripherally to form verrucose, reddish-brown, irregular patches (Fig. 5). Regional lymphadenopathy is usually absent. The course is protracted, often for years, but there may be spontaneous healing.

Scrofuloderma (Tuberculosis Colliquativa Cutis). Scrofuloderma is an extension of tuberculosis into the skin from

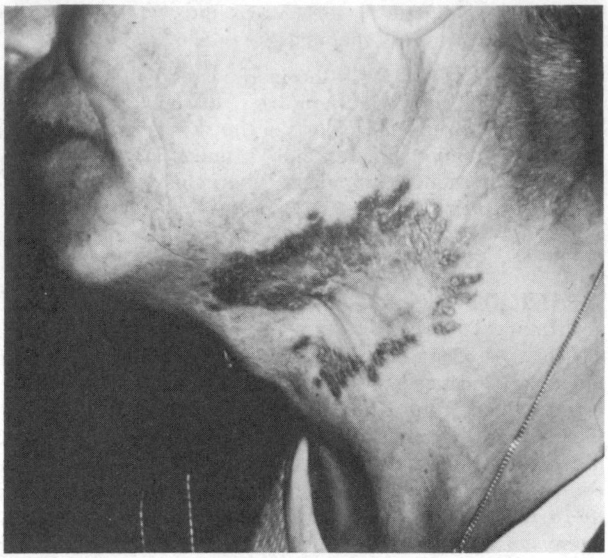

Figure 4. Lupus vulgaris. Lesion began in the central scarred area and in 40 to 50 years enlarged to its present size. AFIP 75-15588. (Photograph by Dr. B. Rasaiah).

underlying structures such as lymph nodes, bone, or lung. A subcutaneous swelling progresses into cold abscesses, multiple ulcers, and sinus tracts. Lesions on the neck are common, especially in children, and develop from mycobacterial cervical lymphadenitis (Fig. 6). Lincoln and Gilbert (1972), in 340 patients throughout the world with culturally proven nontuberculous mycobacterial cervical lymphadenitis, found that 208 were caused by scotochromogens, 108 were caused by organisms in the *M. avium-intracellulare* complex, 21 were in Runyon group I (probably *M. kansasii*), and three were rapid growers. *M. scrofulaceum* is the most frequently identified scotochromogen. *M. bovis* is a well-known cause of scrofuloderma. The course is protracted but eventually heals with residual keloidal scars.

Tuberculosis Cutis Orificialis. Tuberculosis cutis orifici-

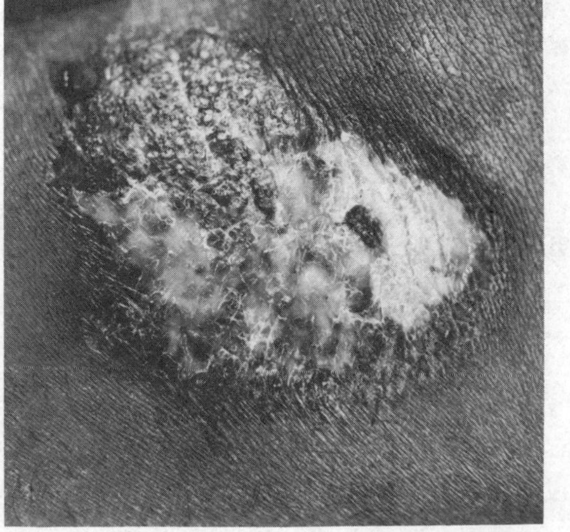

Figure 5. Tuberculosis verrucosa cutis on leg. The surface of the lesion is hyperkeratotic and verrucose. AFIP 53-1664.

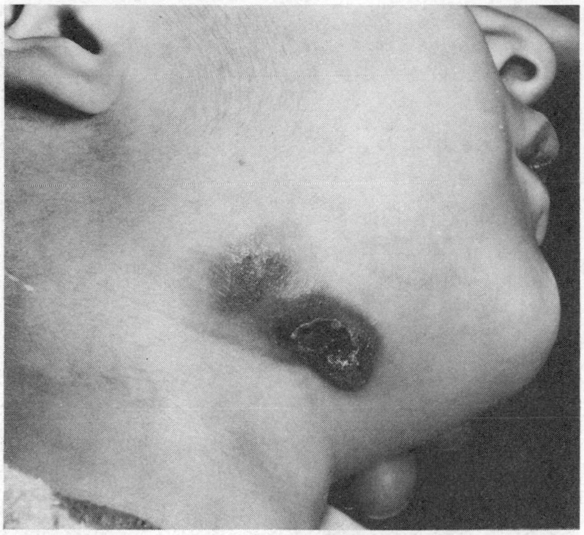

Figure 6. Scrofuloderma in a child. There is cervical lymphadenitis with a communicating sinus tract and ulcer. AFIP 53-11701.

alis arises by autoinoculation of mucous membranes from internal tuberculosis and is rare where there are effective tuberculosis control programs. There are shallow crusted ulcers in or around the mouth, anus, or vulva. Although the lesions regress with effective chemotherapy, involvement of orifices often portends a poor prognosis.

TREATMENT. All patients with cutaneous tuberculosis should be studied to determine if there are other foci of tuberculosis. Tuberculosis of the skin usually responds rapidly to chemotherapy. The drugs commonly used for internal tuberculosis are effective. Combined therapy with isoniazid (300 mg orally) and streptomycin (1 to 2 g daily IM) is commonly employed, but isoniazid alone is effective in many cases. The duration of chemotherapy is variable. Some believe that isoniazid therapy should be continued for up to three years and streptomycin for two months. Rifampicin (daily oral doses of 600 mg), ethambutol (15 to 25 mg/kg daily), and 0.5 gr. cycloserine may be used in patients infected with mycobacteria that are resistant to isoniazid or streptomycin. Calciferol (vitamin D_2) and radiotherapy are not recommended.

Small lesions of lupus vulgaris and tuberculosis verrucosa cutis may be excised if there is no fever or evidence of spread to lymph nodes. Tuberculostatic drug therapy should precede surgical intervention for cutaneous tuberculosis.

In a series of 21 patients with cervicofacial nontuberculous mycobacteriosis, Olson (1981) found that excisional surgery or curettage alone or combined with drug therapy gave equally excellent results. If applicable, curettage was preferred.

DIAGNOSIS. Identification of mycobacteria requires cultivation. In primary tuberculosis acid-fast organisms may be seen in Ziehl-Neelsen-stained smears or by fluorescent microscopy of auramine-rhodamine-stained smears. Histopathologic evaluation of biopsy specimens is often diagnostic. Cutaneous reactions to tuberculin or PPD must be correlated with other diagnostic findings; a positive reaction is never diagnostic by itself.

MYCOBACTERIUM ULCERANS INFECTION (BURULI ULCER)

DEFINITION AND ETIOLOGY. *M. ulcerans* is a slow-growing organism that infects the skin and subcutaneous tissues of man, giving rise to indolent ulcers with undermined edges. *M. ulcerans* grows optimally on routine mycobacterial media at 32° C and elaborates a cytotoxin (Hockmeyer et al., 1978) that causes necrosis of skin and subcutaneous tissue. Growth in culture is usually inhibited at temperatures above 35° C, but a rare strain will grow at 37° C. Large undermined ulcers, almost certainly caused by *M. ulcerans*, were first described by Cook in Uganda in 1897 (Connor and Lunn, 1966), but *M. ulcerans* was not identified until 1948 in Australia (MacCallum et al., 1948).

EPIDEMIOLOGY. All major endemic foci are located in swampy terrain of tropical or subtropical countries. The largest known foci are in Uganda (Barker, 1972) and Zaire (Meyers et al. 1974a). The source of *M. ulcerans* in nature is unknown. Infection probably begins when *M. ulcerans* is introduced into the skin by minor trauma or by hypodermic needle (Meyers et al. 1974c), presumably from the contaminated surface of the skin. Spread from patient to patient is rare. Persons of all age groups are infected, but the highest frequency of infection occurs in the second and third decades.

PATHOGENESIS AND PATHOLOGY. *M. ulcerans* organisms elaborate a toxin that causes necrosis of the dermis, panniculus, and deep fascia (Krieg et al., 1974) (Figs. 7 and 8). Early lesions are closed, but the necrosis spreads to the overlying dermis and epidermis, and in two to three months produces an ulcer with undermined borders and a necrotic base. Microscopically, there is contiguous coagulation necrosis of the deep dermis and panniculus with destruction of all tissue including nerves, appendages, and vessels. There is interstitial edema without conspicuous inflammatory cells. Extracellular clumps and masses of acid-fast bacilli are found in the necrotic areas, especially in the ulcer bed (Figs. 8 and 9). Necrosis may spread to the deep fascia and muscle, and rarely to bone. In the healing phase there is a granulomatous response and eventual scarring.

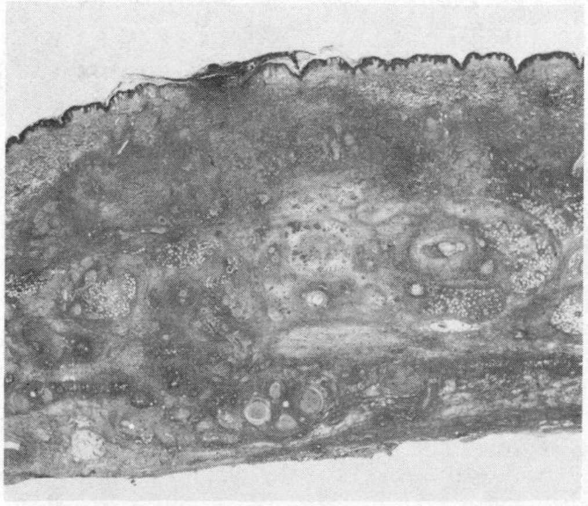

Figure 7. *Mycobacterium ulcerans* infection, preulcerative lesion. This section, through the center of the lesion, shows massive coagulation necrosis in the lower dermis and subcutaneous tissue. × 4, AFIP 65-1411.

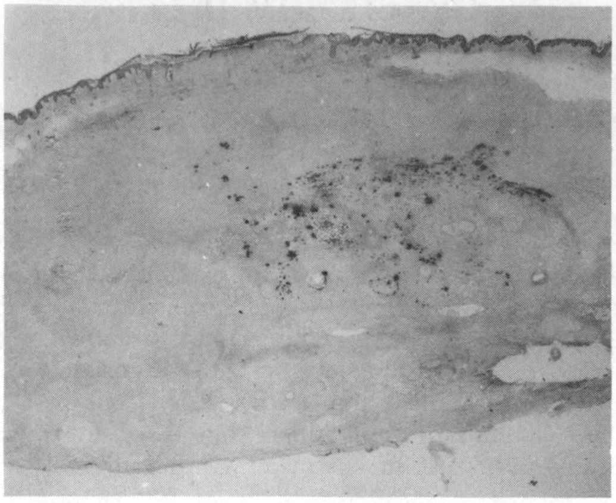

Figure 8. *Mycobacterium ulcerans* infection. This is a parallel section of the lesion in Figure 10 stained by the Ziehl-Neelsen method. There are many clumps of acid-fast bacilli in the necrotic area. × 4, AFIP 65-1413.

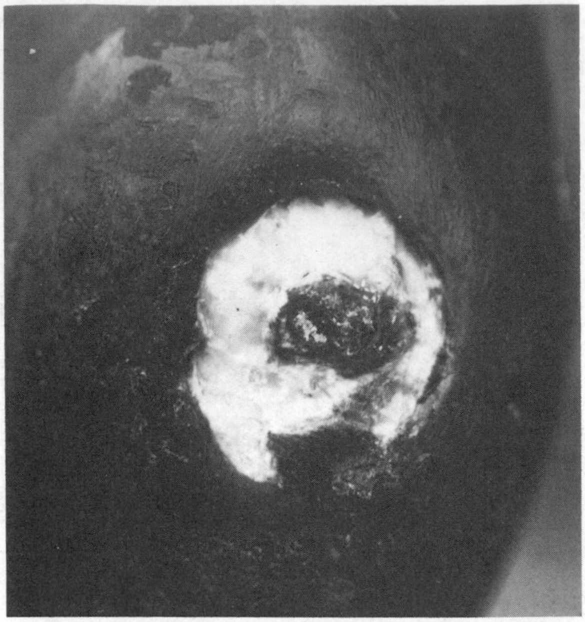

Figure 10. *Mycobacterium ulcerans* infection in the deltoid area of a Zairian boy. Lesion developed at the site of a hypodermic injection. The border of the ulcer was undermined and there is a necrotic slough in the base. AFIP 76-11034-5.

CLINICAL MANIFESTATIONS. The first sign is a firm, painless, nontender, movable nodule 1 to 2 cm in diameter in the subcutaneous tissue. Within one to two months the nodule becomes fluctuant, spreads peripherally, and ulcerates. The border of the ulcer is undermined up to 15 cm or more, and the adjacent skin is edematous (Fig. 10). Even with large ulcers, there is usually no regional lymphadenopathy or systemic symptoms. Ulcers may remain small and heal within a few months without treatment, or spread rapidly, undermining the skin of large areas, even an entire leg, thigh, or arm. Occasionally, important structures such as an eye are lost (Fig. 11). Lesions tend to heal spontaneously in months or years, but without therapy contraction deformities and lymphedema may result (Fig. 12).

TREATMENT. Early pre-ulcerative nodules are excised and closed primarily. Ulcers are widely excised and skin is grafted. Continuous heating at 40° C (e.g., by a heated water jacket) will promote healing without wide excision, but this must be used cautiously when vital structures are threatened (Meyers et al., 1974b). Amputation of limbs is rarely necessary and should be done only as a last resort. Rifampin promotes healing of pre-ulcerative nodules or small ulcers but has not been adequately evaluated. Other antimicrobial agents are ineffective. Physical therapy must be instituted early when there is danger of contraction deformities.

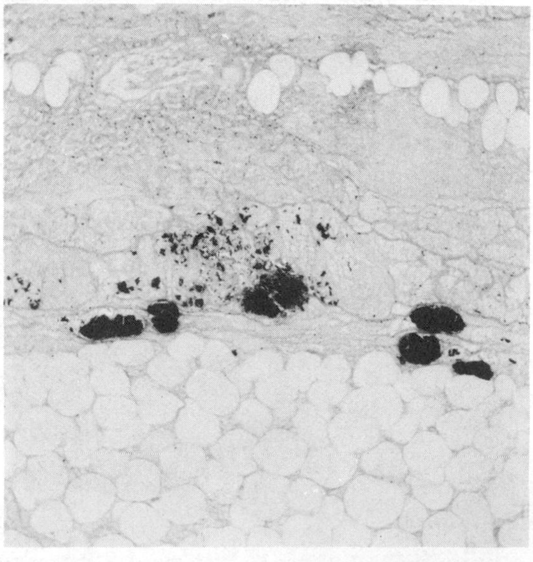

Figure 9. *Mycobacterium ulcerans* infection showing large numbers of acid-fast bacilli in the subcutaneous area of the edge of an ulcer. The surrounding tissue is nonviable and there are many "ghosts" of fat cells. Ziehl-Neelsen stain. × 80, AFIP 65-5851.

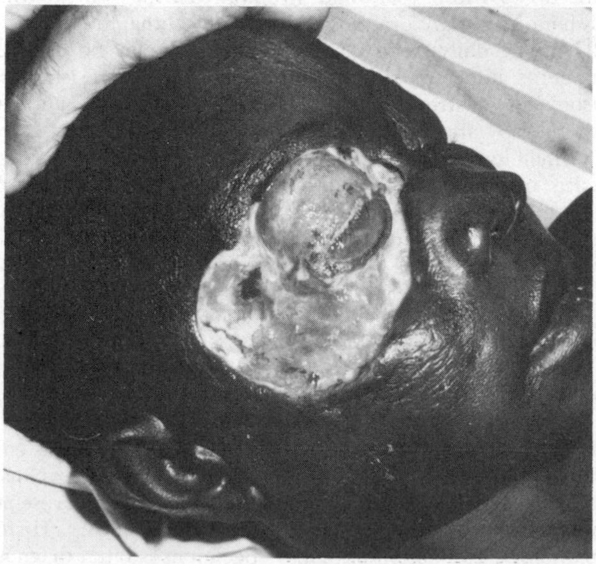

Figure 11. *Mycobacterium ulcerans* infection in a Zairian woman. The eye was lost because of damage to the eyelids. AFIP 76-11034-6.

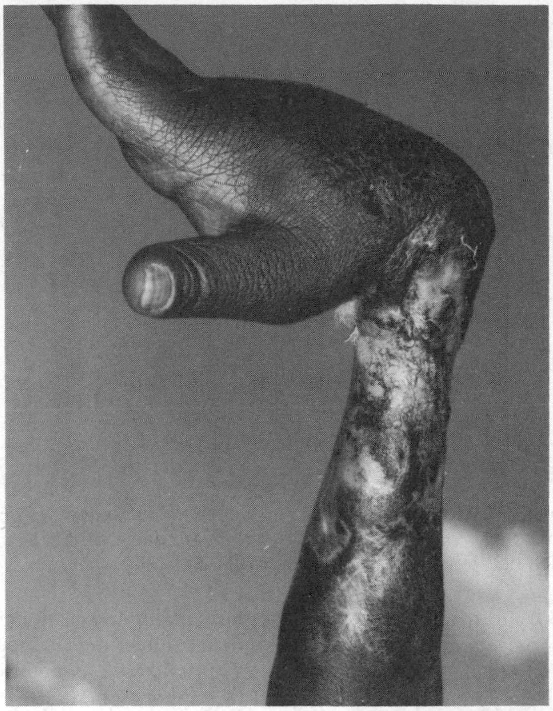

Figure 12. *Mycobacterium ulcerans* infection of forearm and wrist. Lesion is healed but the scar has caused a contraction deformity with subluxation at the wrist. AFIP 65-2982-1. (Photographed by Dr. D. H. Connor).

DIAGNOSIS. Smears from the necrotic base of ulcers, stained by the Ziehl-Neelsen technique, often reveal clumps of acid-fast bacilli. Biopsy specimens of the necrotic base and undermined periphery of the ulcer usually reveal necrosis of the dermis and subcutaneous tissue and acid-fast bacilli and establish the diagnosis. Culture of *M. ulcerans* from exudates or biopsy specimens is successful in 50 to 75 per cent of active lesions, but visible growth often requires six to eight weeks. Skin tests are of no diagnostic value.

PROPHYLAXIS. There is no effective prophylaxis, but vaccination with BCG may give short-lived protection (Uganda Buruli group, 1969).

MYCOBACTERIUM MARINUM INFECTION

DEFINITION AND ETIOLOGY. Aronson (1926) first identified *M. marinum* in marine fish in an aquarium in Philadelphia. Linell and Norden (1954) isolated this mycobacterium from patients who developed granulomas of the skin after swimming in a pool in Sweden; hence infections by *M. marinum* are commonly called "swimming pool granulomas." *M. marinum* grows within two weeks at 30 to 32° C on mycobacterial media, but growth is inhibited at 37° C. *M. balnei* is a synonym for *M. marinum*.

EPIDEMIOLOGY. *M. marinum* infections have been reported from Australia, Belgium, England, Germany, Israel, Japan, Sweden, and the United States (including Hawaii), and the organism is presumed to be ubiquitous. Most patients have been in contaminated swimming pools. Philpott et al. (1963), for example, described 290 patients who had been in a single swimming pool in Colorado. Occasionally a hobbyist who keeps tropical fish, or people who work or swim in bayous, rivers, or coastal or brackish water are infected (Miller and Toon, 1973; Zeligman, 1972). Sometimes the patient has not been exposed to any known source of *M. marinum*. The organism is introduced into the skin at sites of trauma, and there is no evidence of man-to-man transmission. In nature, water-dwelling animals can become infected from water contaminated with *M. marinum* and in turn shed *M. marinum* into the water. The "water flea," Daphnia, can serve as a host. Because of cross-reactivity with other mycobacterial antigens, epidemiologic studies based on skin testing are not valid.

PATHOGENESIS AND PATHOLOGY. Incubation periods are often difficult to establish in natural infections, but usually last from one to six weeks. A laboratory infection is reported that became clinically apparent ten days after an accident, and *M. marinum* was cultured at 15 days (Chappler et al., 1977). The low temperature growth requirement limits infections to the skin, usually to the focus of inoculation. The disease, however, may spread along the lymphatics and may resemble sporotrichosis (Dickey, 1968). Spread may be enhanced by local infiltration with corticosteroids (Aaronson and Park, 1974). In early lesions a mixture of lymphocytes, histiocytes, and polymorphonuclear leukocytes infiltrates the dermis (Fig. 13). In older lesions there are tuberculoid granulomas that may show caseation necrosis (Fig. 14). Acid-fast rods with crossbands that are wider and longer than *M. tuberculosis*, although scarce, are often seen in the granulomas. In immunosuppressed patients *M. marinum* may mimic undermined lesions caused by *M. ulcerans*.

CLINICAL MANIFESTATIONS. The earliest sign is usually a mildly tender erythema at the inoculation site. This erythema develops into a papule that gradually enlarges into an erythematous or violaceous nodule that occasionally

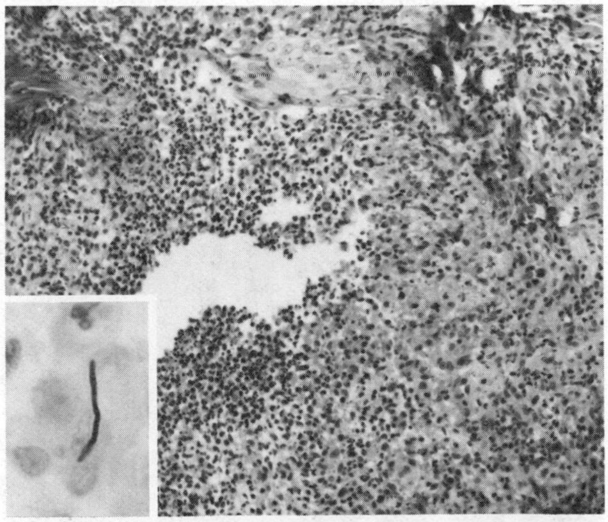

Figure 13. *Mycobacterium marinum* infection, "swimming pool granulomas," showing a mixed inflammatory reaction in dermis. × 100, AFIP 73-3053. *Inset:* A single *M. marinum* in area of inflammation. Ziehl-Neelsen, × 1190, AFIP 73-3054. These sections are from the lesions shown in Figure 13.

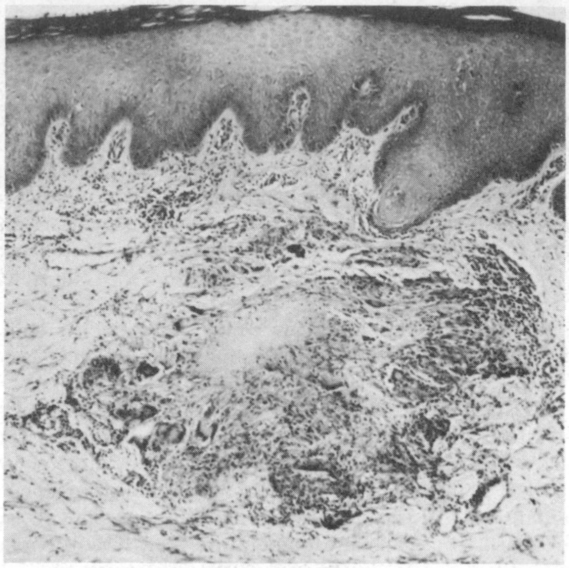

Figure 14. *Mycobacterium marinum* infection, "swimming pool granulomas," showing granuloma with necrosis in dermis. × 40, AFIP 69-9675.

ulcerates and discharges pus (Fig. 15). Older lesions may become verrucose (Fig. 16). Because bony prominences are prone to trauma, the hands, elbows, and knees are sites of predilection (Philpott et al., 1963), and the bursae of the elbows and knees are sometimes invaded. Sporotrichoid *M. marinum* infections are uncommon and rarely patients may have widely disseminated lesions in the skin (King et al., 1983). Spontaneous cure is the rule, usually requiring three months to three years for complete resolution, but infections have persisted 4 to 17 years.

TREATMENT. Most lesions are self-healing. Because of the protracted course of the disease, many patients demand therapy. The following drugs have been used orally with some success; tetracycline, 1 to 2 g daily (Kim, 1974; Izumi et al., 1977); minocycline, 200 mg daily (Hanke et al.,

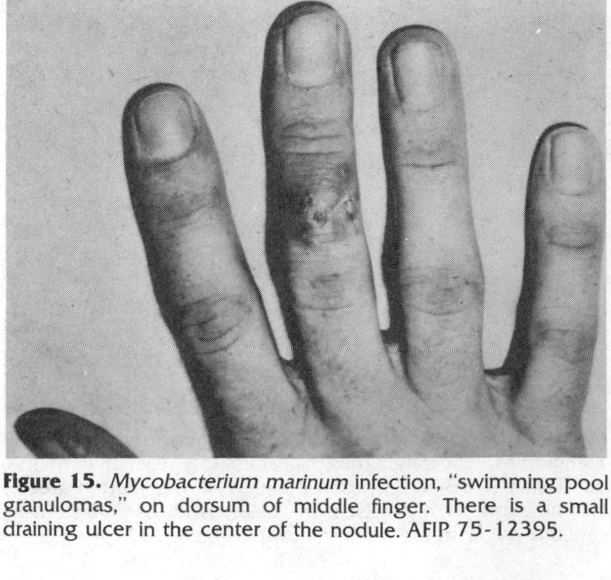

Figure 15. *Mycobacterium marinum* infection, "swimming pool granulomas," on dorsum of middle finger. There is a small draining ulcer in the center of the nodule. AFIP 75-12395.

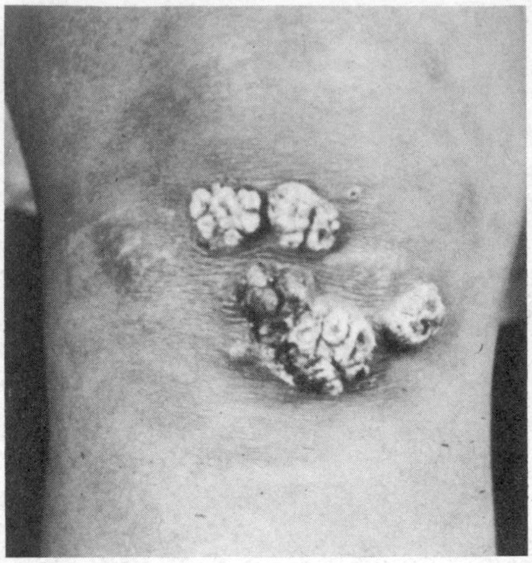

Figure 16. *Mycobacterium marinum* infection, "swimming pool granuloma," on knee showing verrucose nature of this lesion, which had persisted for 6 years. AFIP 75-12396.

1980) and trimethoprim, 60 mg, plus sulfamethoxazole, 800 mg, twice daily. Antituberculosis drugs, including rifampin, streptomycin, isoniazid, and ethambutol, have been tried with varying success. Local heat therapy may be beneficial (Sutherland et al., 1980). When possible, surgical excision or curettage and electrodesiccation have been recommended as the treatments of choice.

DIAGNOSIS. Diagnosis requires cultivation of *M. marinum* from the lesion because histopathologic changes are not specific. Positive skin tests, even with antigens prepared from *M. marinum,* are not diagnostic owing to strong cross-reactions with other mycobacteria (Judson and Feldman, 1974).

PROPHYLAXIS. Adequate maintenance of swimming pools (Philpott et al., 1963) interrupts epidemics; however, sporadic cases cannot be prevented except by avoiding potentially contaminated sources such as home aquariums.

MYCOBACTERIUM KANSASII INFECTION

DEFINITION AND ETIOLOGY. Typical *M. kansasii* strains grow at 37° C and are photochromogens, but there are nonchromogenic and scotochromogenic strains that are otherwise identical. *M. kansasii* commonly infects the lungs, but only approximately 12 patients with skin lesions have been reported. *M. kansasii* infections protect against *M. tuberculosis* infections in the guinea pig and hence are more closely related to *M. tuberculosis* than any other mycobacterium except BCG (Palmer and Long, 1966). Consequently, cross-reactions to skin-test antigens of *M. kansasii* and *M. tuberculosis* are common.

EPIDEMIOLOGY. In nature, *M. kansasii* is found most frequently in tap water but occasionally also in cows and swine. *M. kansasii* infections are worldwide in distribution, and in the United States occur most frequently in the Midwest and Southwest. Among 1185 consecutive patients admitted to a Denver, Colorado, hospital during the period 1960 to 1964, 4.2 per cent had atypical mycobacteriosis, and 60 per cent of these were infected by *M. kansasii*

(Fischer et al., 1968). Pulmonary infections are acquired by inhalation and are probably transmissible. The mode of primary infections of the skin is not known but may be by inoculation.

PATHOGENESIS AND PATHOLOGY. The length of the incubation period of primary cutaneous lesions is not known. One infection occurred approximately one year after a local injury. Histopathologic changes in pulmonary and systemic lesions are similar to those caused by *M. tuberculosis* (i.e., granulomas with caseation). Acid-fast bacilli are few and difficult to find in smears and tissue sections.

Lesions of the skin that have spread from primary infections elsewhere have often been seen in immunosuppressed patients. These lesions show a variable acute and chronic inflammatory response that is sometimes pyogenic. Acid-fast organisms may be numerous. No systemic spread has been reported from primary lesions of the skin.

CLINICAL MANIFESTATIONS. Primary lesions of the skin may present as single nodules or as sporotrichoid spread. Some nodular lesions are preceded by erythematous tender swellings. In patients with sporotrichoid spread the lesions appear on the hand and extend to the forearm but do not involve the lymph nodes. Chronic infections may last as long as 22 years. Four patients with disseminated *M. kansasii* have been reported; they had erythema induratum, abscesses, cellulitis, and ulcers of the skin (Fraser et al., 1975; Hirsh and Saffold, 1976).

TREATMENT. Treatment with antibiotics or by chemotherapy should be based on sensitivity studies on cultured organisms. Primary lesions have healed after four months of combined therapy with isoniazid, para-aminosalicylic acid, and streptomycin. Rosen (1983) obtained a favorable response with rifampin, ethambutol, and kanamycin in combination. One immunosuppressed patient with disseminated disease responded to specific transfer factor (Hirsh and Saffold, 1976).

DIAGNOSIS. Diagnosis requires the cultivation of *M. kansasii* from biopsy specimens or exudates. Skin reactions to mycobacterial antigens are not specific.

PROPHYLAXIS. No prophylactic measures are known.

INFECTIONS CAUSED BY THE "RAPID-GROWING" MYCOBACTERIA

DEFINITION AND ETIOLOGY. These bacteria grow within five days (usually in 48 hours) on routine laboratory media at 32 to 37° C. Nomenclature of the "rapid-growers" is imprecise: Some employ the term "*M. fortuitum* complex" for all members of this group, whereas others (e.g., Inman et al., 1969) separate *M. fortuitum* from *M. chelonei* because of their antigenic and biochemical differences. Stanford et al. (1972) concluded that *M. abscessus*, *M. runyonii*, and *M. borstelense* are synonymous with *M. chelonei*.

EPIDEMIOLOGY. These ubiquitous organisms are common saprophytes in soil and water. *M. fortuitum* and *M. chelonei* have been reported from nearly all continents. Cruz (1938) first identified *M. fortuitum* as the cause of an injection abscess in the arm of a patient in Brazil. Penetrating wounds of the skin, including surgical wounds and hypodermic injections, may introduce the organism (Hand and Sanford, 1970). In local epidemics of "injection abscesses" the injected medication may be contaminated (Inman et al., 1969). Although these organisms may cause disease in amphibians, rodents, and other animals, there are no epidemiologic data linking disease in man to these sources.

PATHOGENESIS AND PATHOLOGY. The incubation period is ordinarily two to seven months. The early histopathologic changes have not been described. The earliest lesion presented for medical examination is a fluctuant abscess that may form one or more sinuses that discharge pus. In closed lesions the predominant feature is liquefactive necrosis with an intense polymorphonuclear leukocytic infiltrate into the dermis and subcutaneous tissue. In chronic lesions there is fibrosis of the abscess wall or sinus tract. Epithelioid cell granulomas with suppuration and caseation have been described (Moore and Frerichs, 1953). Acid-fast bacilli are present, but are often scarce and are most consistently seen in well-defined spherical vacuoles in the dermis (Fig. 17). This appears to be a unique histopathologic feature of *M. chelonei* infections. Most lesions of the skin and subcutaneous tissue remain localized. There may be regional lymphadenopathy. Systemic spread is rare, but immunosuppression may cause multiple skin lesions and dissemination (Graybill et al., 1974). Pulmonary infections are common, but there is no evidence that pulmonary disease has arisen from skin infections.

CLINICAL MANIFESTATIONS. Mild local inflammation develops within a few days at the site of an injection or injury. These changes are minor, and the physician often does not see the patient until there is a subcutaneous nodule, fluctuation, or ulceration. Lesions are painless and are frequently on the buttocks and deltoid areas (usual sites of injections), and range from 1 cm in diameter to those that cover the entire buttock (Fig. 18). Larger lesions may

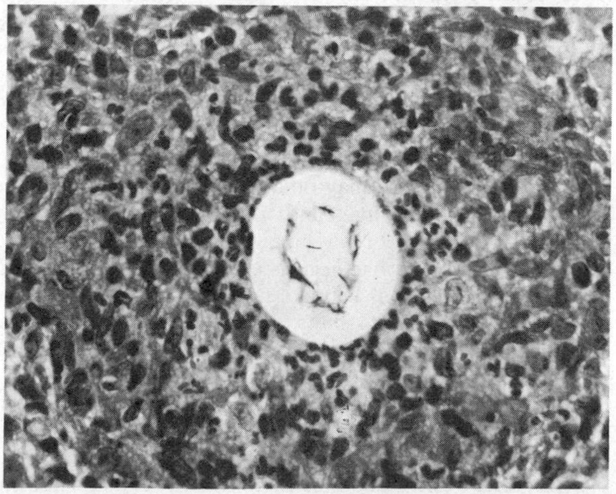

Figure 17. Skin of patient with *M. chelonei* infection. In the dermis there is a spherical vacuole surrounded by mixed suppurative and granulomatous reaction. This vacuole contains acid-fast bacilli in a delicate matrix. Ziehl-Neelsen, × 630, AFIP 81-13871.

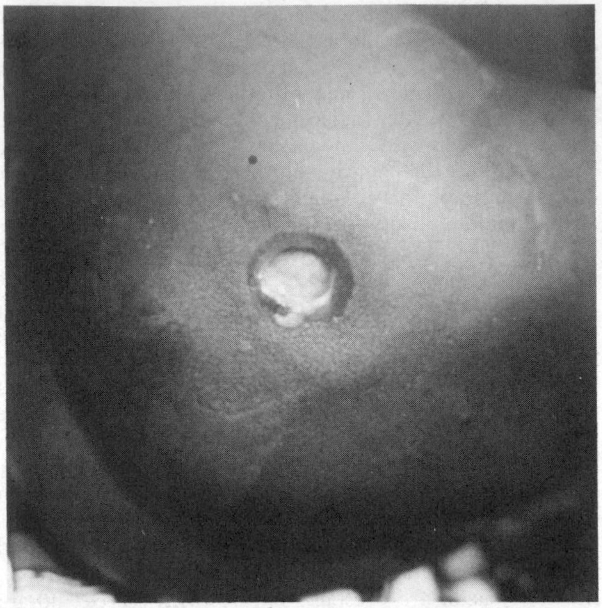

Figure 18. Injection ulcer caused by *M. fortuitum* in buttock of Zairian infant. Infant had received a hypodermic injection at this site approximately 2 months previously. AFIP 78-3306.

have multiple sinuses. Regional lymph nodes may be enlarged and tender. Healing requires several months to over two years.

TREATMENT. Incision and drainage is adequate therapy for most abscesses. Repeated incisions may be necessary to maintain drainage. If practicable, sinuses may be excised. On the mistaken clinical diagnosis of a pre-ulcerative *M. ulcerans* infection, the author excised an abscess on the deltoid area that was caused by *M. chelonei*. The skin was closed primarily and the wound healed without recurrence. *M. fortuitum* and *M. chelonei* are frequently resistant to antibiotics and chemotherapy; however, Dalovisio et al. (1981) found amikacin and doxycycline, alone or in combination, effective in 9 of 10 patients. Nevertheless, sensitivity tests should be performed, and if the organism proves to be sensitive, specific therapy should be given. Drug therapy, like incision and drainage, requires prolonged treatment.

DIAGNOSIS. There may be a history of trauma, but the incubation period is long and many patients forget they have had injections or an injury. Diagnosis depends on identifying the mycobacteria in exudates or biopsy specimens. In closed lesions exudate may be obtained by needle aspiration. If acid-fast stains are not routinely done on exudates, the diagnosis may be missed, and the bacteria misidentified as "diphtheroids" on gram stains. Because the organisms grow rapidly on simple media, the diagnosis can be made within a few days.

PROPHYLAXIS. Infections acquired by hypodermic injections are preventable by ensuring sterility and practicing antisepsis of the skin (Vandepitte et al., 1969). Many infections acquired in hospitals and clinics could be prevented by asepsis in wound care.

MISCELLANEOUS AND UNCOMMON MYCOBACTERIAL INFECTIONS OF THE SKIN, SCOTOCHROMOGENIC MYCOBACTERIA AND THE M. AVIUM-SCROFULACEUM-INTRACELLULARE COMPLEX

This is a composite of mycobacteria. Their nomenclature and interrelationships, involving both Runyon groups II and III organisms, present problems in identification. The most common pathogenic scotochromogen is *M. scrofulaceum (M. marianum)*, found in soil and water and sometimes cultured as a contaminant in secretions and tissues from humans. Primary *M. scrofulaceum* infections of the skin are rarely reported with positive identification of the etiologic agent. *M. scrofulaceum* is a common cause of cervical lymphadenitis and scrofuloderma in children (Lincoln and Gilbert, 1972). Dustin et al. (1980) noted a fatal infection by *M. scrofulaceum* in an immunosuppressed boy with severe involvement of the skin and reviewed the literature on all six previously reported patients. One patient on corticosteroid therapy developed multiple cutaneous nodules, cellulitis, and ulcers caused by the scotochromogen *M. szulgai* (Sybert et al., 1977).

Organisms of the *M. avium-intracellulare* complex rarely cause primary skin lesions. An ulcer of the foot caused by a "Runyon group III" organism occurred in a patient who claimed to have had a minor abrasion at the site about one month before the lesion appeared (Schmidt et al., 1972). This patient responded to combined isoniazid, cycloserine, and streptomycin therapy.

Skin Lesions Caused by Unidentified Mycobacteria. A group of 29 patients in the period 1957 to 1971 from north central United States and Canada developed indurated erythematous papules, primarily of the extremities, and regional lymphadenitis (Feldman and Hershfield, 1974).

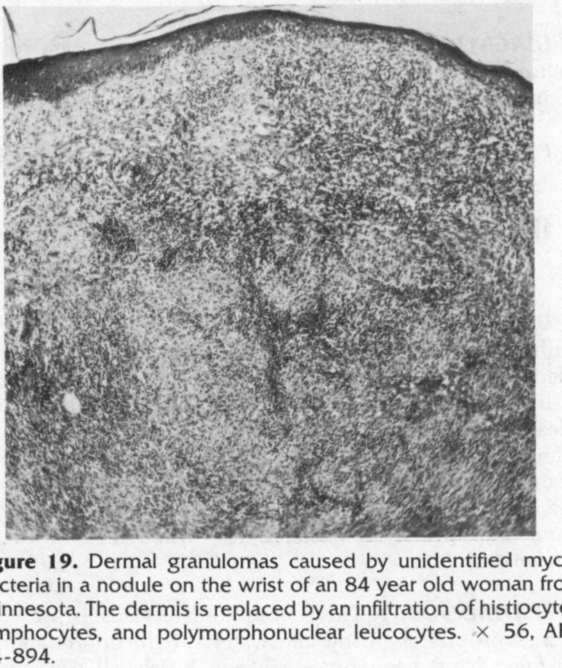

Figure 19. Dermal granulomas caused by unidentified mycobacteria in a nodule on the wrist of an 84 year old woman from Minnesota. The dermis is replaced by an infiltration of histiocytes, lymphocytes, and polymorphonuclear leucocytes. × 56, AFIP 74-894.

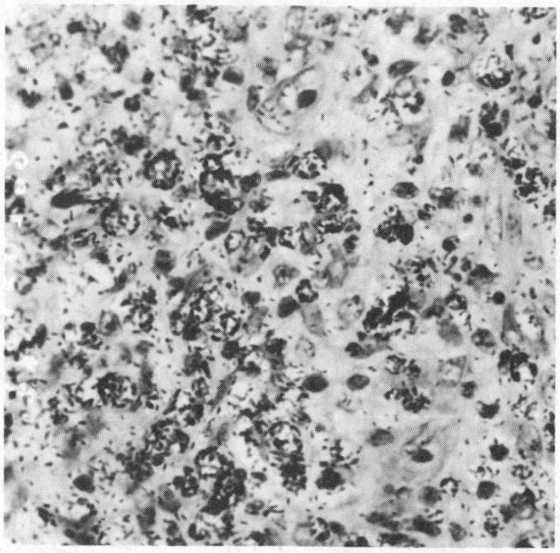

Figure 20. Higher magnification of lesion of Figure 19 showing masses of acid-fast bacilli in infiltration. This area is undergoing necrosis. × 485, AFIP 74-896.

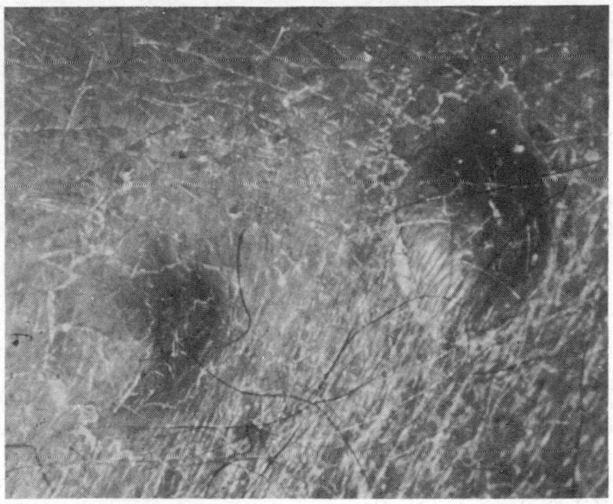

Figure 21. Two of many similar nodules in the skin of a 51 year old man under immunosuppressive therapy following an organ transplant. Nodules were caused by an unidentified mycobacterium. AFIP 75-1220-1.

The lesions ulcerated and were found to contain numerous intracellular and extracellular acid-fast bacilli in exudates and histopathologic sections. The organisms could not be cultured (Figs. 19 and 20). The mycobacterium causing these infections has not been identified, but it was not *M. leprae* as originally suspected.

Atypical Mycobacterial Infections and Immune Deficiency. Patients with cutaneous lesions who have diseases that are associated with immunosuppressed states, or who have had known immunologic deficiencies, must be monitored for atypical mycobacterial infections. Conversely, any dissemination of atypical mycobacterial infections should alert the physician to the possibility of an underlying immune deficiency or neoplastic disease (Dibella et al., 1977 and Dalovisio et al., 1981). Patients with hairy cell leukemia appear to be unusually predisposed to disseminated *M. kansasii* and *M. intracellulare* infections (Weinstein et al., 1981). The acquired immune deficiency syndrome (AIDS) is commonly associated with disseminated *M. avium-intracellulare* infections (Zakowski et al., 1982 and Reichert et al., 1983). Disseminated *M. avium-intracellulare* may first be manifested as a panniculitis (Sanderson et al., 1982). Mechanisms for the unusual susceptibility of immunosuppressed patients to atypical mycobacterial infections have not been delineated, but helper T-lymphocyte deficiency may predispose patients to dissemination (Bultmann et al., 1982). Several cutaneous mycobacterial infections reminiscent of those reported by Feldman and Hershfield (1974) have occurred in immunosuppressed patients and have been studied at the Armed Forces Institute of Pathology. The acid-fast bacilli in these lesions have not been identified (Figs. 21 and 22).

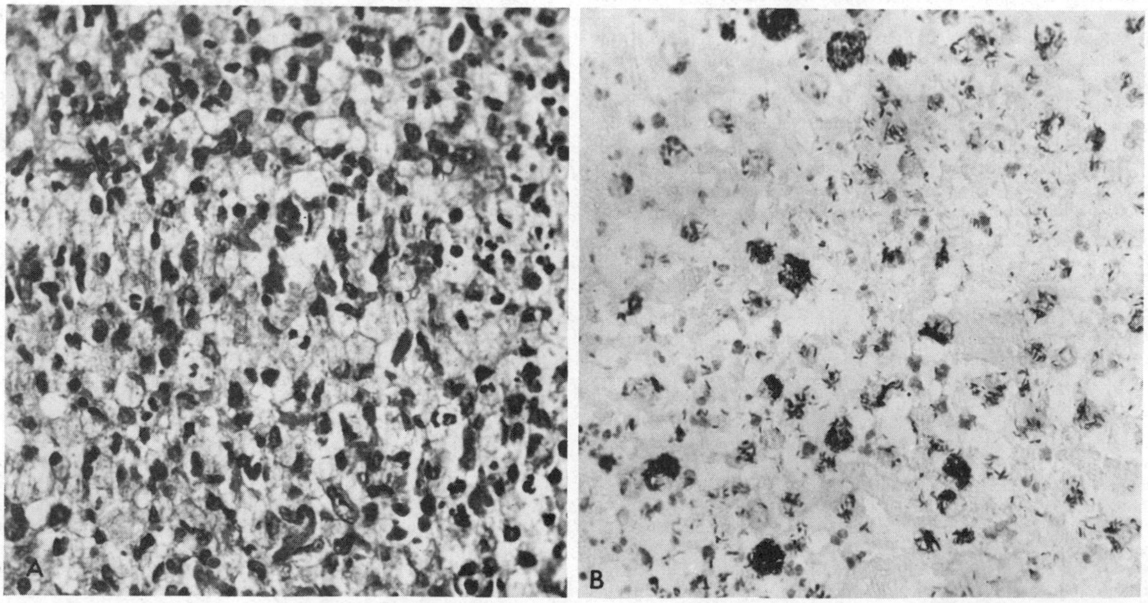

Figure 22. *A*, Histiocytic infiltration of dermis in lesion shown in Figure 21. × 440, AFIP 74-889. *B*, Parallel section stained by Ziehl-Neelsen method and showing clumps of acid-fast bacilli in histiocytes. × 440, AFIP 74-890.

Complications of Vaccination with the Bacillus of Calmette-Guerin (BCG). Occasionally, vaccination with BCG (a viable attenuated strain of *M. bovis*), which is given to prevent tuberculosis or to treat cancer, results in progressive disease. Local lupus vulgaris-like lesions with or without regional lymphadenopathy may develop. Immunosuppressed patients can develop fatal systemic infections (Aungst, 1975). Most progressive infections by BCG respond to isoniazid therapy.

References

Aaronson, C. M., and Park, C. H.: Sporotrichoid infection due to *Mycobacterium marinum:* Lesion exacerbated by corticosteroid infiltration. South Med J 67:117, 1974.

Aronson, J. D.: Spontaneous tuberculosis in salt water fish. J Infect Dis 39:315, 1926.

Aungst, C. W., Sokal, J. E., and Jager, B. V.: Complications of BCG vaccination in neoplastic diseases. Ann Intern Med 82:666, 1975.

Bailey, R. K., Wyles, S., Dingley, M., Hesse, F., and Kent, G. W.: The isolation of high catalase *Mycobacterium kansasii* from tap water. Notes. Am Rev Resp Dis 101:430, 1970.

Barker, D. J. P.: Epidemiology of *Mycobacterium ulcerans* infection. Trans R Soc Trop Med Hyg 67:43, 1973.

Bultmann, B. D., Flad, H. D., Kaiserling, E., Muller-Hermelink, H. K., Kratzsch, G., Galle, J., Schachenmayr, W., Heimpel, H., Wigger, H. J., and Haferkamp, O.: Disseminated mycobacterial histiocytosis due to *M. fortuitum* associated with helper T-lymphocyte immune deficiency. Virchow's Arch. Pathol Anat 395:217, 1982.

Chappler, R. R., Hoke, A. W., and Borchardt, K. A.: Primary inoculation with *Mycobacterium marinum.* Letter. Arch Dermatol 113:380, 1977.

Connor, D. H., and Lunn, F.: Buruli ulceration. A clinicopathologic study of 38 Ugandans with *Mycobacterium ulcerans* ulceration. Arch Pathol 81:183, 1966.

Cruz, J. C.: *Mycobacterium fortuitum,* um novo bacilo acido-resistente patogenico para o homem. Acta Med Rio de Janeiro 1:297, 1938.

Dalovisio, J. R., Pankey, G. A., Wallace, R. J., and Jones, D. B.: Clinical usefulness of amikacin and doxycycline in the treatment of infection due to *Mycobacterium fortuitum* and *Mycobacterium chelonei.* Rev Infect Dis 3:1068, 1981.

Dibella, N. J., Buchanan, B. D., and Koontz, C. H.: Disseminated atypical tuberculosis antedating the clinical onset of neoplasia. Cancer 40:1276, 1977.

Dickey, R. F.: Sporotrichoid mycobacteriosis caused by *M. marinum (balnei).* Arch Dermatol 98:385, 1968.

Dustin, P., Demol, P., Derks-Jacobvitz, D., Cremer, N., and Vis, H.: Generalized fatal chronic infection by *Mycobacterium scrofulaceum* with severe amyloidosis in a child. Path Res Pract 168:237, 1980.

Feldman, R. A., and Hershfield, E.: Mycobacterial skin infections by an unidentified species: A report of 29 patients. Ann Intern Med 80:445, 1974.

Fischer, D. A., Lester, W., and Schaefer, W. B.: Infections with atypical mycobacteria. Five years' experience at the National Jewish Hospital. Am Rev Resp Dis 98:29, 1968.

Fraser, D. W., Buxton, A. E., Naji, A., Barker, C. F., Rudnick, M., and Weinstein, A. J.: Disseminated *Mycobacterium kansasii* infection presenting as cellulitis in a recipient of a renal homograft. Am Rev Resp Dis 112:125, 1975.

Goette, D. K., Jacobson, K. W., and Doty, R. D.: Primary inoculation tuberculosis of the skin. Prosector's paronychia. Arch Dermatol 114:567, 1978.

Graybill, J. R., Silva, J., Fraser, D. W., Lordon, R., and Rogers, E.: Disseminated mycobacteriosis due to *Mycobacterium abscessus* in two recipients of renal homografts. Am Rev Resp Dis 109:4, 1974.

Hand, W. L., and Sanford, J. P.: *Mycobacterium fortuitum*—a human pathogen. Ann Intern Med 73:971, 1970.

Hanke, C. W., Bergfeld, W. F., and Shear, H.: Sporotrichoid *Mycobacterium marinum* infection treated with minocycline hydrochloride. Cleve Clin Q 47:339, 1980.

Heineman, H. S., Spitzer, S., and Pianphongsant, T.: Fish tank granuloma. A hobby hazard. Arch Intern Med 130:121, 1972.

Hirsh, F. S., and Saffold, O. E.: *Mycobacterium kansasii* infection with dermatologic manifestations. Arch Dermatol 112:706, 1976.

Hockmeyer, W. T., Krieg, R. E., Reich, M., and Johnson, R. D.: Further characterization of *Mycobacterium ulcerans* toxin. Infect Immun 21:124, 1978.

Horwitz, O.: Lupus vulgaris cutis in Denmark 1895-1954: Its relation to the epidemiology of other forms of tuberculosis. Epidemiology and course of the tuberculous infection based on 3902 cases from the Finsen Institute, Copenhagen. Acta Tuberc Scand (Suppl) 49:1, 1960.

Iden, D. L., Rogers, R. S., and Schroeter, A. L.: Papulonecrotic tuberculid secondary to *Mycobacterium bovis.* Arch Dermatol 114:564, 1978.

Inman, P. M., Beck, A., Brown, A. E., and Stanford, J. L.: Outbreak of injection abscesses due to *Mycobacterium abscessus.* Arch Dermatol 100:141, 1969.

Izumi, A. K., Hanke, W., and Higaki, M.: *Mycobacterium marinum* infections treated with tetracycline. Arch Dermatol 113:1067, 1977.

Judson, F. N., and Feldman, R. A.: Mycobacterial skin tests in humans 12 years after infection with *Mycobacterium marinum.* Am Rev Resp Dis 109:544, 1974.

Kim, R.: Tetracycline therapy for atypical mycobacterial granuloma. Letter. Arch Dermatol 110:299, 1974.

King, A. J., Fairley, J. A., and Rasmussen, J. E.: Disseminated cutaneous *Mycobacterium marinum* infection. Arch Dermatol 119:268, 1983.

Koch, R.: Die Aetiologie der Tuberkulose. Berl Klin Wochnschr 19:221, 1882.

Krieg, R. E., Hockmeyer, W. T., and Connor, D. H.: Toxin of *Mycobacterium ulcerans.* Production and effects on guinea pig skin. Arch Dermatol 110:783, 1974.

Lincoln, E. M., and Gilbert, L. A.: Disease in children due to mycobacteria other than *Mycobacterium tuberculosis.* Am Rev Resp Dis 105:683, 1972.

Linell, F., and Norden, A.: *Mycobacterium balnei.* A new acid-fast bacillus occurring in swimming pools and capable of producing skin lesions in humans. Acta Tuberc Scand (Suppl) 33:1, 1954.

MacCallum, P., Tolhurst, J. C., Buckle, G., and Sissons, H. A.: A new mycobacterial infection in man. J. Pathol Bacteriol 60:93, 1948.

Meyers, W. M., Connor, D. H., McCullough, B., Bourland, J., Morris, R., and Proos, L.: Distribution of *Mycobacterium ulcerans* infections in Zaire, including the report of new foci. Ann Soc Belg Med Trop 54:147, 1974a.

Meyers, W. M., Shelly, W. M., and Connor, D. H.: Heat treatment of *Mycobacterium ulcerans* infections without surgical excision. Am J Trop Med Hyg 23:924, 1974b.

Meyers, W. M., Shelly, W. M., Connor, D. H., and Meyers, E. K.: Human *Mycobacterium ulcerans* infection developing at sites of trauma to skin. Am J Trop Med Hyg 23:919, 1974c.

Miller, W. C., and Toon, R.: *Mycobacterium marinum* in gulf fishermen. Arch Environ Health 27:8, 1973.

Moore, M., and Frerichs, J. B.: An unusual acid-fast infection of the knee with subcutaneous, abscess-like lesions of the gluteal region. Report of a case with a study of the organism, *Mycobacterium abscessus* n. sp. J Invest Dermatol 20:133, 1953.

Olson, N. R.: Nontuberculous mycobacterial infections of the face and neck—Practical considerations. The Laryngoscope 91:1714, 1981.

Palmer, C. E., and Long, M. W.: Effects of infection with atypical mycobacteria on BCG vaccination and tuberculosis. Am Rev Resp Dis 94:553, 1966.

Philpott, J. A., Woodburne, A. R., Philpott, O. S., Schaefer, W. B., and Mollohan, C. S.: Swimming pool granuloma. A study of 290 cases. Arch Dermatol 88:158, 1963.

Reichert, C. M., O'Leary, T. J., Levens, D. L., Simrell, C. R., and Macher, A. M.: Autopsy pathology in the acquired immune deficiency syndrome. Am J Pathol 112:357, 1983.

Rosen, T.: Cutaneous *Mycobacterium kansasii* infection presenting as cellulitis. Cutis 31:87, 1983.

Sanderson, T. L., Moskowitz, L., Hensley, G. T., Cleary, T. J., and Penneys, N.: Disseminated *Mycobacterium avium-intracellulare* infection appearing as a panniculitis. Arch Pathol Lab Med 106:112, 1982.

Schmidt, J. D., Yeager, H., Jr., Smieth, E. B., and Raleigh, J. W.: Cutaneous infection due to a Runyon Group III atypical mycobacterium. Am Rev Resp Dis 106:469, 1972.

Stanford, J. L., Pattyn, S. R., Portaels, F., and Gunthorpe, W. J.: Studies on *Mycobacterium chelonei.* J Med Microbiol 5:177, 1972.

Sutherland, G. E., Lauwasser, M., McNeely, D. J., and Shands, J. W.: Heat treatment for certain chronic granulomatous skin infections. South Med J 73:1564, 1980.

Sybert, A., Tsou, E., and Garagusi, V. R.: Cutaneous infection due to *Mycobacterium szulgai.* Am Rev Resp Dis 115:695, 1977.

Timpe, A., and Runyon, E. H.: Relationship of "atypical" acid-fast bacilli to human disease: Preliminary report. J Lab Clin Med 44:202, 1954.

Uganda Buruli Group: B.C.G. vaccination against *Mycobacterium ulcerans* infection (Buruli ulcer). First results of a trial in Uganda. Lancet 1:111, 1969.

Vandepitte, J., Desmyter, J., and Gatti, F.: Mycobacteria, skins, needles. Lancet 2:691, 1969.

Verhagen, A. R., Koten, J. W., Chaddah, V. K., and Patel, R. I.: Skin

diseases in Kenya. A clinical and histopathological study of 3168 patients. Arch Dermatol 98:577, 1968.
Weinstein, R. A., Golomb, H. M., Grumet, G., Gelmann, E., and Schechter, G. P.: Hairy cell leukemia: Association with disseminated atypical mycobacterial infection. Cancer 48:380, 1981.
Zakowski, P., Fligiel, S., Berlin, G. W., and Johnson, L.: Disseminated *Mycobacterium avium-intracellulare* infection in homosexual men dying of acquired immunodeficiency. JAMA 248:2980, 1982.
Zeligman, I.: *Mycobacterium marinum* granuloma. A disease acquired in the tributaries of Chesapeake Bay. Arch Dermatol 106:26, 1972.

228

YAWS, PINTA, AND BEJEL

PETER M. MOODIE, M.D., B.S., D.T.M. & H.

Yaws, pinta, and bejel are endemic nonvenereal treponemal infections of humans (treponematoses). They share many clinical, pathologic, and immunologic features with venereal syphilis, and the causative treponemes are morphologically identical to each other and to *Treponema pallidum* (Chapter 53).

The endemic treponematoses are characterized by a superficial primary lesion at the site of inoculation and secondary, blood-borne, satellite lesions that are usually superficial. Destructive granulomas of skin, subcutaneous tissues, bones, and joints are tertiary manifestations of yaws and bejel, and pigmented tertiary skin changes of pinta.

Yaws, pinta, and bejel constitute a clinical and pathologic spectrum of diseases in which bejel most resembles venereal syphilis, pinta least resembles venereal syphilis, and yaws occupies an intermediate position. Differentiation of the treponematoses, including venereal syphilis (Chapter 162), is based on clinical, epidemiologic, and geographic considerations and may be difficult in the individual case.

Yaws (frambesia, pian, buba, bouba, parangi) is a disease of the humid tropics throughout the world. *Pinta* (carate, mal del pinto, tian, lota, azul) is confined to parts of Latin America and the Caribbean. *Bejel* (or endemic syphilis) occurs in cooler, drier climates in all regions of the world except the Americas, under a variety of local names—for example, bejel or balash in the Middle East, dichuchwa in Botswana, irkintja in Central Australia, njovera in Rhodesia, siti in Gambia, and skerlievo in Bosnia.

Once widespread throughout the rural tropics and subtropics (Fig. 1), the endemic treponematoses were greatly reduced in incidence or eradicated locally by mass treatment campaigns with penicillin. However, they still occur in remote rural communities with poor hygiene, and their sequelae may be encountered in areas where the endemic infection has been eradicated.

ETIOLOGY. The treponemes cannot be cultured on artificial media or otherwise distinguished from each other in the laboratory but have been given the following specific names: *Treponema pertenue* (yaws), *Treponema carateum* (pinta), and *Treponema pallidum* (bejel, endemic syphilis). Sometimes the agent of bejel is referred to as *T. pallidum II* or *T. pallidum endemicum* to distinguish it from *T. pallidum* of venereal syphilis.

There is a continuing controversy about the origins and interrelationships of the treponematoses. Hackett (1963) believes that they have all evolved from pinta over about 15,000 years into distinct treponemal species with relatively fixed disease-producing characteristics. Hudson (1958) holds that they all derived from a yaws-like disease in Africa about 100,000 years ago and that the organisms are no more than intraspecific strains of *T. pallidum.* Willcox (1974) considers the evolution of treponemal diseases to be continuing through the natural selection of strains suited to local conditions and modes of transmission. Turner and Hollander (1957) have demonstrated characteristic, but not particularly consistent, differences in the lesions produced by inoculating and passing the treponemes of syphilis, yaws, and bejel in laboratory hamsters and rabbits. Pinta treponemes did not produce lesions and could not be passed in these animals, but Kuhn et al. (1968) have produced typical pinta lesions in inoculated chimpanzees.

The reservoir of yaws, pinta, and bejel is humans. Yaws may have an additional animal reservoir of unknown significance in human disease, in West African cynocephalic baboons (Hardy, 1976). In endemic areas, the incidence of yaws is highest in children, who therefore form the main reservoir. The main reservoir of pinta is older children and young adults.

PATHOGENESIS AND PATHOLOGY

Source. The sources of the infectious agents of yaws, pinta, and bejel are cases with active primary or secondary lesions, which are usually on the skin in yaws and pinta and in the mouth or on the lips in bejel.

Because treponemes are fragile and are very easily killed by drying, they are short-lived in the external environment. They survive best in serum or living cellular material, and the diseases are usually acquired by direct contact of the abraded or minimally injured epithelium with an exudative lesion. Pinta lesions are not normally exudative but are characteristically pruritic. Scratching the lesions causes oozing of infectious serum.

Indirect Transmission. Indirect transmission of bejel may occur through shared eating and drinking utensils, toothpicks, and tobacco pipes, as well as by kissing or biting. Biting insects may play a part in the mechanical transmission of pinta, and sucking flies in the transmission of yaws and bejel. The fingers of children may also transfer infection. Child-to-mother transmission of yaws and bejel is not uncommon. Indirect skin-to-skin spread by way of floors, furniture, clothing, bedding, or the ground underfoot is unlikely unless the time interval between contamination and inoculation is very brief.

Venereal transmission is rare because of the rarity of genital lesions in adults. Congenital transmission does not occur.

Susceptibility and Immunity. Susceptibility is general. More than 80 per cent of adults in highly endemic areas may show serologic evidence of past infection. Susceptibility is altered by acquired immunity, but in a variable and unpredictable manner. Cross-immunity occurs between each of the endemic treponematoses (particularly yaws and bejel) and between the endemic treponematoses and venereal syphilis but is not complete and may be overcome

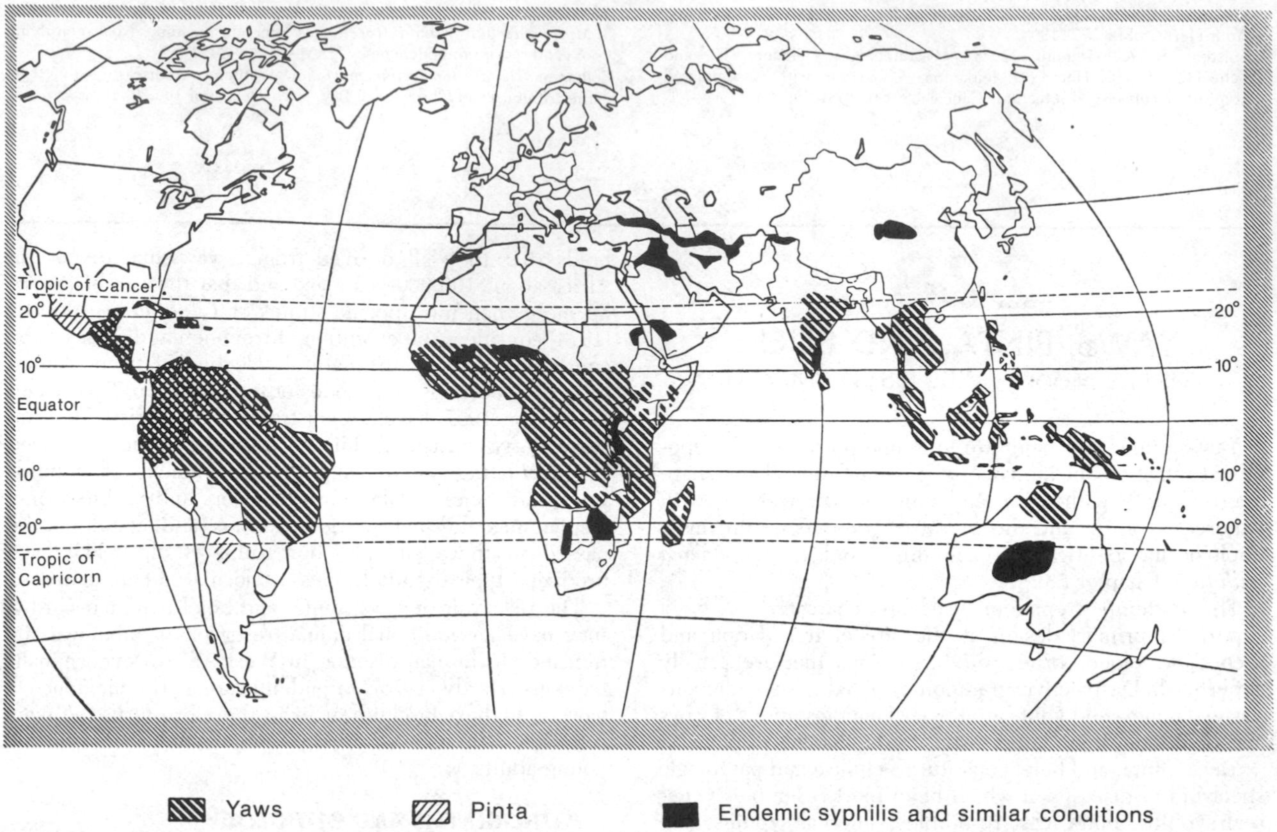

Figure 1. Geographical distribution of the endemic treponematoses about 1950, at the beginning of the WHO-supported mass eradication campaign. (Modified from World Health Organization: International Work in Endemic Treponematoses and Venereal Infections 1948–1963. Geneva, World Health Organization, 1965.)

by a large inoculum of treponemes. Immunity to homologous strains of treponemes is stronger and develops more rapidly but is also incomplete.

Incubation Period. In most cases the time from inoculation to the appearance of the primary lesion varies from a few weeks to a few months. The results of animal studies suggest that the incubation period is directly related to the size of the infecting dose, which may be as small as a single organism.

Pathology of Primary Infection. As in venereal syphilis, the basic pathologic processes in the endemic treponematoses may be grouped into three characteristic but often overlapping stages. The primary stage includes the relatively slow development of an inflammatory reaction at the inoculation site. During this stage, organisms multiply in the primary lesion, spread to the regional lymph nodes and the blood, and are disseminated throughout the body. Histopathologically, early edema of the corium is followed by infiltration with lymphocytes, plasma cells, and polymorphonuclear leukocytes associated with micro-abscesses. Unless it is secondarily infected, the primary lesion heals slowly with minimal scarring.

Pathology of Secondary Lesions. Yaws and bejel, but not pinta, may pass through a latent phase before the appearance of secondary lesions. The usual sites of secondary lesions are the skin in pinta, the skin and subperiosteum in yaws, and the skin, subperiosteum, and mucous membranes in bejel. The secondary lesions usually contain numerous treponemes but show a greater and more accelerated tissue reaction than primary lesions. They develop and heal faster than the primary lesions in yaws and bejel and induce pronounced hyperplasia (of epithelium or periosteum) and marked perivascular, round-cell cuffing. Allergic reactions of the syphilide ("ide") type may also occur, particularly in bejel and yaws. These lesions contain very few treponemes and are probably not infectious.

Pathology of the Tertiary Stage. Tertiary lesions are usually grossly destructive (gummas of skin, subcutaneous tissues, or bone in yaws and bejel) or grossly hyperplastic (hyperkeratosis or hyperostosis in yaws and bejel; hyperkeratosis and hyperpigmentation in pinta). Bone lesions commonly show a mixture of hyperplastic and destructive processes. Superficial gummas commonly ulcerate. The histopathology features necrosis, epithelioid and giant-cell aggregation, capillary obstruction, and fibrous tissue scarring. Surface scars are usually depigmented.

The histopathologic aspects of the three stages may be viewed as the result of three grades of immunologic response to treponemes: (1) slowly developing cell-mediated immunity and relatively ineffective humoral immunity in the primary stage; (2) fairly effective cell-mediated and humoral immunity in the secondary stage; and (3) a late, cell-mediated local hypersensitivity reaction to a few surviving treponemes in the tertiary stage.

CLINICAL MANIFESTATIONS. The following descriptions emphasize the typical clinical features of the various stages of the endemic treponematoses. Atypical lesions are common in the individual case, and the stages may overlap. Very few clinical manifestations are unique to a particular treponemal disease, including venereal syphilis. With the probable exception of Bosnian endemic syphilis (now eradicated), the endemic treponematoses do not attack the central nervous system, the eye, the cardiovascular system, or the abdominal viscera (Turner, 1959).

Primary Infection. The primary papilloma of yaws ("mother yaw") usually occurs on the lower leg, face, or arm in children and may also occur on the breast or hip of nonimmune women nursing infected children. The lesion begins as a papule, without prodromal or general symptoms, and evolves slowly and relatively painlessly into a raised pseudogranulomatous lesion as large as 8 cm in diameter. It appears to be bursting through the skin, and oozes serum or becomes covered with a thin, tough scab. Untreated, it may take 6 to 12 months to heal and usually leaves a faint, slightly pitted circular scar. It is usually accompanied by moderate, nontender regional lymphadenopathy.

The primary oral lesion of bejel is seldom noticed. On the lips, nipple, or elsewhere on the skin it is similar to an extragenital chancre of venereal syphilis.

The primary lesion of pinta is an itchy red papule, usually on the exposed skin of the dorsum of the foot or hand. It occurs rarely on the trunk. It spreads slowly and becomes more raised and scaly but never ulcerates unless it is scratched or injured. Regional lymph nodes may enlarge. The primary lesion usually persists for years, overlapping with the secondary manifestations and eventually becoming indistinguishable from them.

Secondary Manifestations. In yaws, multiple secondary lesions may appear either before the primary lesion heals or up to several years later. Their appearance is accompanied by fever, malaise, bone and joint pains, and headache. The skin lesions vary in appearance from large, oozing or crusted papillomas that resemble the typical primary lesion (Fig. 2) to small, scattered or diffuse papular lesions like syphilides. Hyperplastic subperiosteal changes with or without small foci of rarefaction may be visible in x-rays, particularly of the anterior cortex of the tibia, the ulna, and the small bones of the hands and feet. Scaly or papillomatous lesions of the soles and palms are not uncommon. General lymphadenopathy is common. The lesions heal in a few months, usually without permanent structural change or scarring.

In pinta, pruritic, erythematous macules or papules erupt 5 to 12 months after the first appearance of the primary lesion. They are usually widespread and are accompanied by generalized lymphadenopathy. The lesions persist without intervening latency, but they often appear in crops that later coalesce into irregular patterns. Plantar and palmar hyperkeratoses have been reported only in Cuban pinta. Pigmentation in various colors appears as the lesions enter the tertiary stage.

In bejel, secondary manifestations include macular and papular rashes (syphilides), condylomatous papillomas in the skin folds, "split papules" at the corners of the mouth, oral mucous patches, laryngitis and pharyngitis, periostitis, and generalized lymphadenopathy. Scaly lesions of the palms and soles may also appear. Relapses, especially of the "-ide" lesions, may alternate with periods of latency over several years. Bone pain is common in some populations.

Tertiary Manifestations. Tertiary yaws and bejel cause nodular or ulcerative necrosis (gummas of skin and subcutaneous tissue); gummas and subperiosteal thickening of the long bones, and plantar hyperkeratosis (Fig. 3). Nasopalatal destructive lesions (gangosa), destruction of joints (particularly the interphalangeal joints in yaws), and mobile soft tissue nodules near the joints (juxta-articular nodes) occur in both diseases, but are more common in yaws. Healed ulcerative lesions leave thin depigmented scars (Hackett, 1957; Hackett and Loewenthal, 1960).

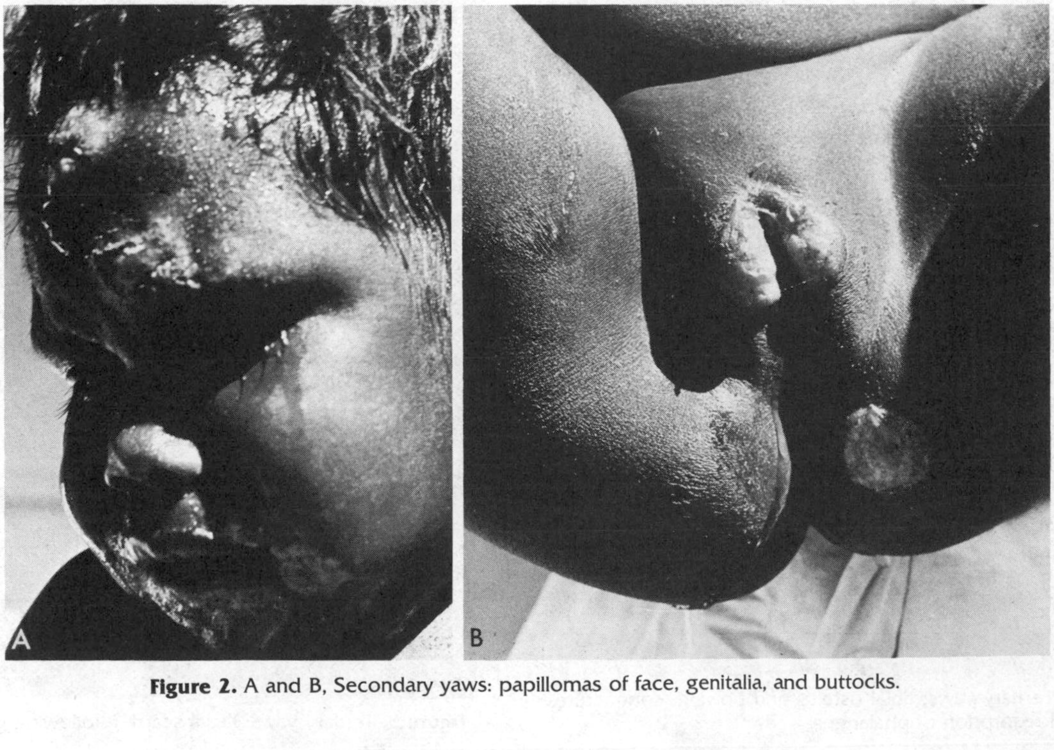

Figure 2. A and B, Secondary yaws: papillomas of face, genitalia, and buttocks.

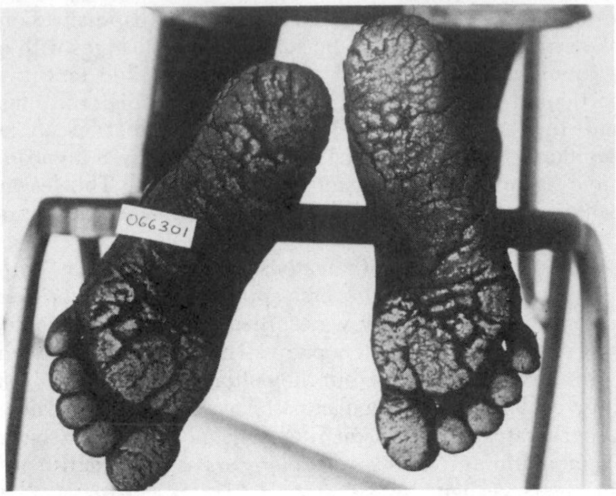

Figure 3. Tertiary yaws: plantar hyperkeratosis.

Tertiary pinta lesions are generally limited to dyspigmented patches (gray, black, bluish, purplish, red, coppery), which may heal spontaneously or become depigmented (leukodermic) in the center before they heal as atrophic white patches. Aortitis has been reported in some cases of Cuban pinta.

The progress of untreated treponemal diseases through the three stages is not inevitable. Primary lesions may be so insignificant that they are never noticed, and spontaneous cure during one of the periods of latency before the onset of tertiary manifestations is the rule rather than the exception in yaws and bejel.

COMPLICATIONS AND SEQUELAE. Complications and sequelae are uncommon in the primary and secondary stages. Joint effusions may occur in yaws and bejel. Respiratory obstruction and dysphagia have been reported in bejel due to extensive laryngeal or pharyngeal involvement during the secondary stage (Hudson, 1958). Plantar hyperkeratosis or papillomas in secondary yaws and bejel may become ulcerated and make walking painful and difficult. The minor subperiosteal changes in secondary yaws and bejel and the very rare massive periostitis of the nasal processes of the maxillae (goundou) are mainly of cosmetic importance.

Functional handicaps may follow secondarily infected skin lesions that ulcerate and cause deep scarring and contractures. Polydactylitis in childhood yaws may be temporarily disabling.

Destructive tertiary lesions of bone and subcutaneous and submucous tissues in yaws and bejel are responsible for nearly all the serious permanent sequelae in the endemic treponematoses. Spontaneous fractures may occur and heal imperfectly. Gross bony deformities, particularly of the tibia and ulna; destruction or partial resorption of the phalanges, metacarpals, metatarsals, and tarsal bones (Fig. 4); palatal perforation; pharyngeal stenosis; and scar-tissue contractures of joints, tendons, and fascia may be severely disabling. Gangosa, a massive and grossly mutilating gummatous destruction of the nose, mouth, nasal septum, palate, and pharynx is a late complication of yaws and occasionally of bejel (Fig. 5).

The sequelae of pinta are patches of permanently depigmented, atrophic areas of skin. Similar sequelae may occur in yaws and bejel (Fig. 6).

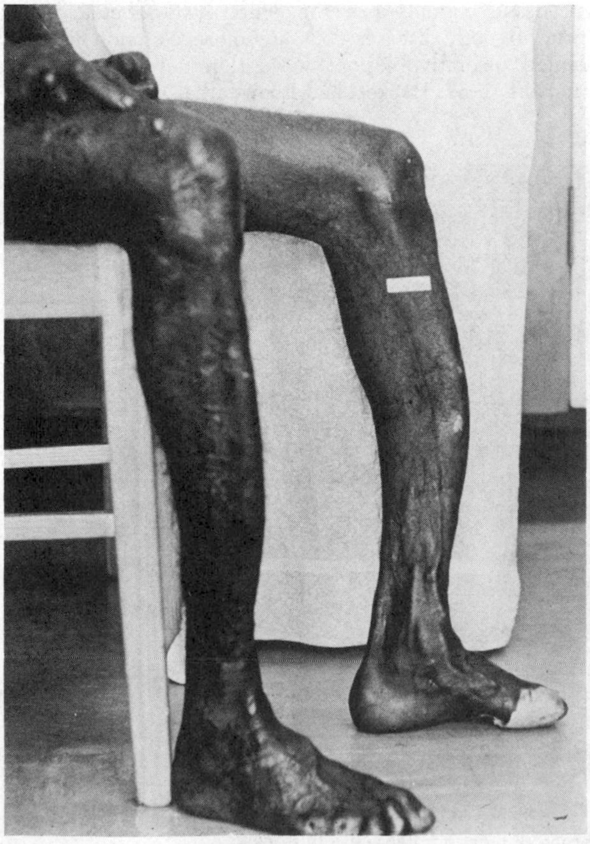

Figure 4. Tertiary yaws: tibial osteitis and bowing; contractures and partial resorption of phalanges.

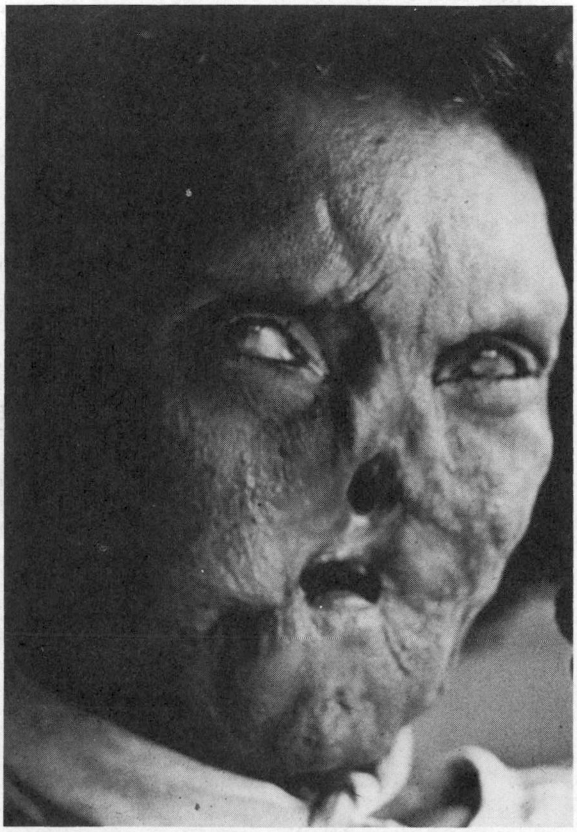

Figure 5. Tertiary yaws: facial scarring following gangosa.

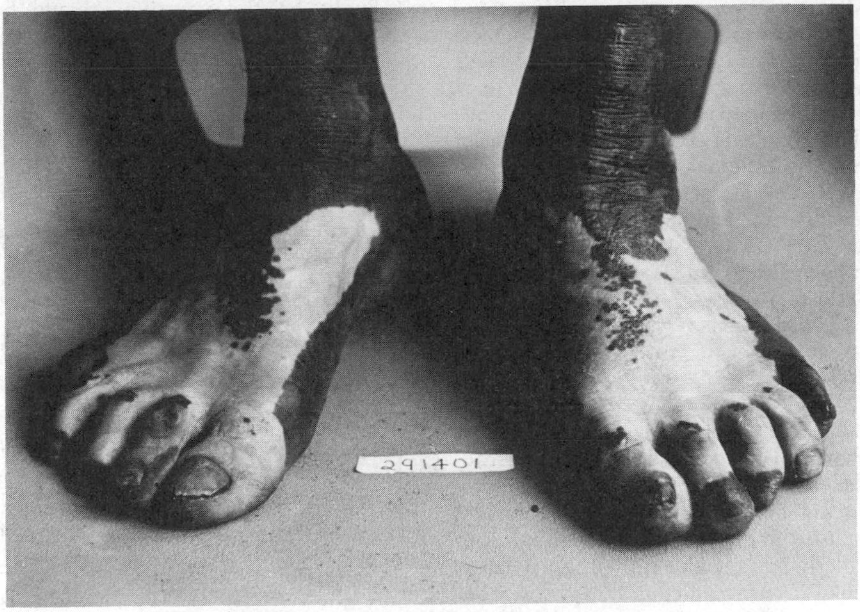

Figure 6. Tertiary yaws: symmetrical depigmentation of feet.

GEOGRAPHIC VARIATIONS. Variations in the clinical features of the endemic treponematoses appear to be related more to climate, clothing, behavior, and life style than to geography or race in the usual sense. These factors may act to select strains, but they certainly also influence the age of onset and the site and type of primary (and possibly secondary and tertiary) lesions. Because all treponemes are highly sensitive to penicillin, the tetracyclines, erythromycin, chloramphenicol, and other antibiotics, local variations in the extent and frequency of general exposure to these antibiotics (for any kind of infection) is another potent factor that influences the pattern of clinical treponemal disease. The "incidental" cure of many treponemal infections at an early stage in their evolution decreases the rate of transmission as well as the incidence of late disease and complications. There is no evidence anywhere in the world of development of resistance by treponemes to antibiotics.

The geographic variation of greatest significance is the restriction of pinta to the Americas, where today it is a disease of remote jungle Amerindian communities in Mexico, Venezuela, Colombia, Peru, and Ecuador, and probably in parts of Argentina, Chile, Dominican Republic and Haiti (Willcox, 1976).

DIAGNOSIS. The firm diagnosis of one of the nonvenereal treponematoses depends on establishing two or more of the following: (1) a history of exposure to the disease; (2) appropriate clinical or radiologic findings; (3) the presence of typical treponemes; and (4) treponemal seroreactivity. The diagnosis is most difficult to establish in patients with early primary lesions, atypical secondary lesions, and latent disease discovered by routine serologic screening.

In all suspected cases, a history of contact with other cases or residence in an endemic area should be pursued. In possible secondary, latent, and tertiary disease, a history of earlier lesions should be sought and a search made for a primary scar and minor abnormalities of bone and skin. In adult latent or tertiary disease, evidence of neurologic and cardiovascular syphilis should be specifically excluded before making the diagnosis of endemic treponematosis.

An essential step in early primary infection is darkfield microscopy of fresh exudate or a saline suspension of material swabbed or scraped from the lesion. This can confirm the presence of treponemes before serologic tests become positive, but it is also important in later primary and secondary stages. If darkfield microscopy is unsuccessful, immunofluorescent staining of scrapings or biopsy material may confirm the presence of treponemes. Treponemes are rarely found in "-ide" lesions, but may be found in lymph node aspirates in the secondary stage.

All the serologic tests for venereal syphilis become positive after three to four weeks in yaws and bejel, and during the secondary rash in pinta. Nonspecific reactions such as the Cardiolipin Wassermann reaction (CWR), Venereal Disease Research Laboratory (VDRL) test, rapid plasma reagin (RPR) test, and the Reiter protein complement fixation (RPCF) test may be converted to false positivity by other tropical diseases, and should be confirmed by treponeme-specific tests such as the fluorescent treponemal antibody-absorption (FTA-ABS) test, the *Treponema pallidum* hemagglutination (TPHA) test, or the *Treponema pallidum* immobilization (TPI) test. Quantitative versions of the serologic tests are helpful in evaluating current or recent disease activity and the evidence for spontaneous or therapeutic cure.

Venereal syphilis is generally increasing in incidence in areas where endemic treponematosis has been reduced, and the two diseases may coexist in the same community. In these areas, a specific diagnosis of one or the other may be impossible without a detailed and accurate history.

TREATMENT. Penicillin is the antibiotic of choice unless it is contraindicated by allergy. Primary and secondary stages of yaws and bejel and all stages of pinta respond rapidly to a single intramuscular injection of long-acting penicillin. The recommended adult dose is 1.2 mega units of procaine penicillin G in oil with 2 per cent aluminum monostearate (PAM), or 1.2 mega units of benzathine penicillin. Infected children and adult household contacts should receive 0.6 mega units, and child contacts 0.3 mega units. Standard four- to five-day courses of tetracycline or erythromycin may be substituted. Because recent evidence suggests that a single dose of long-acting penicillin may not cure all patients, active cases should be treated, registered, re-examined in 2 years, and retreated.

Late latent and tertiary yaws and bejel should be treated in the same way as late venereal syphilis; for example, PAM or benzathine penicillin 0.6 mega units twice weekly or daily for 15 to 20 doses.

Local treatment of early lesions is usually unnecessary. Reconstructive surgery may be indicated in late tertiary yaws and bejel with deformities.

PROPHYLAXIS. Individual prophylaxis depends entirely on attention to personal hygiene and appropriate precautions when in contact with early cases. Community prophylaxis is important and depends on general improvement of living conditions, case finding, and treatment of cases and contacts (particularly household contacts). Early latent cases of yaws and bejel may exceed clinical cases by ratios of 5:1 or more. For this reason, community protection cannot be achieved by clinical case finding alone.

Public health authorities should be notified of cases diagnosed in hospitals and clinics even in areas where it is not a statutory requirement.

References

Hackett, C. J.: An International Nomenclature of Yaws Lesions. Monograph Series No. 36. Geneva, World Health Organization, 1957.

Hackett, C. J.: On the origin of the human treponematoses. Bull WHO 29:7, 1963.

Hackett, C. J., and Loewenthal, L. J. A.: Differential Diagnosis of Yaws. Monograph Series No. 45. Geneva, World Health Organization, 1960.

Hardy, P. H.: Pathogenic treponemes. In Johnson, R. C. (ed.): The Biology of the Parasitic Spirochetes. New York, Academic Press, 1976, p. 107.

Hudson, E. H.: Non-Venereal Syphilis: A Sociological and Medical Study of Bejel. London, E. & S. Livingstone Ltd., 1958.

Kuhn, U. S. G., Varela, G., Chandler, F. W., and Bsuna, C. G.: Experimental pinta in the chimpanzee. JAMA 206:829, 1968.

Turner, L. H.: Notes on the Treponematoses with an Illustrated Account of Yaws. Bulletin No. 9, Institute for Medical Research, Federation of Malaya. Kuala Lumpur, Government Press, 1959.

Turner, T. B., and Hollander, D. H.: The Biology of the Treponematoses. Monograph Series No. 35. Geneva, World Health Organization, 1957.

Willcox, R. R.: Changing patterns of treponemal disease. Br J Vener Dis 50:169, 1974.

Willcox, R. R.: The epidemiology of the spirochetoses: A worldwide view. In Johnson, R. C. (ed.): The Biology of the Parasitic Spirochetes. New York, Academic Press, 1976, p. 133.

229

LOAIASIS

B. A. Southgate, M.B., B.S., F.F.C.M.

Loaiasis is the state of infection with the filarial nematode *Loa loa*. This infection is confined to the equatorial rain forest regions of West and Central Africa, particularly cleared areas on the edge of natural forests where trees such as rubber have been planted. One exception is the focus situated in moist savanna in the southwest of Sudan.

The principal countries affected by loaiasis are Zaire, Cameroon, Nigeria, Angola, Gabon, Congo (Brazzaville), Central African-Republic, Chad, and Sudan. Autochthonous cases have been reported from Equatorial Guinea, Sierra Leone, Guinea, Ghana, Benin, Ruanda, Burundi, and Senegal, but infection in these countries is very rare and some reports require confirmation. In East Africa the infection is rare, but cases have been reported from Uganda, Ethiopia, Zambia, and Malawi.

ETIOLOGY. The causative agent of loaiasis, *L. loa* is transmitted to man by the bites of large tabanid flies of the genus *Chrysops*. (See Chap. 18, Fig. 7). The most important species are *C. silacea* and *C. dimidiata*, but all species of *Chrysops* can transmit *L. loa*. *C. zahrai* and *C. distinctipennis* may be locally important vectors, and *C. langi*, *C. centurionis*, and *C. longicornis* are under study as possible vectors.

L. loa is closely related to a number of other sibling species of the same genus that infect nonhuman primates, particularly baboons, mandrills, vervet monkeys, and gorillas in endemic regions. Although human infections are occasionally acquired from other primates, it seems certain that human loaiasis is primarily an anthroponosis, and an animal reservoir of infection can be ignored in considering etiology and control.

The life cycle in the fly begins when it bites an infected person and ingests microfilariae with its blood meal. The microfilariae penetrate the stomach wall and migrate through the body cavity to the thoracic muscles. There they develop in 10 to 12 days into infective larvae, which migrate onto the human skin and enter it through the bite of the fly. After maturing to adults, the female worms produce eggs containing embryos that uncoil to become microfilariae. The eggshell persists, however, to produce a "sheathed" microfilaria that enters the blood circulation diurnally.

PATHOGENESIS AND PATHOLOGY. All three phases of the life cycle of *L. loa* that occur in the human body can be involved in the pathogenesis of loaiasis. These are the third stage larvae introduced by the bite, the adults in the subcutaneous tissue, and the microfilariae in the blood. The most serious and sometimes fatal lesions result either from the immune response to the parasite or specific drug treatment.

A characteristic wheal frequently appears at the site of an infected *Chrysops* bite if infective third-stage larvae from the vector reach the subcutaneous tissues. This wheal is particularly pronounced in previously infected subjects and may progress to a small induration lasting for several days in heavily infected individuals. The lesion, which results from both immediate and delayed hypersensitivity, indicates the presence of circulating IgE or reaginic antibody and a well-developed, cell-mediated immune response to the infective larvae of *L. loa*.

The most common and widely studied lesions of loaiasis

are associated with subcutaneous and transocular migrations of the sexually mature adult worms. These evoke transient episodes of local inflammation and edema. The swellings usually range from 2 to 20 cm in diameter, but occasionally involve a whole limb, most often the arm. The pathogenesis of these reactions is uncertain. Some workers hold that they are a response to mechanical damage of the tissues by the rapid (at least 1 cm/minute) movement of the large adult worms. Others postulate that they result from immunologic lysis of many microfilariae shortly after they are produced by the migrating adult female. Histologic sections usually contain adult worms, surrounded by an edematous reaction containing polymorphonuclear neutrophils and eosinophils, plasma cells, and macrophages. If a dead adult worm is seen the reaction tends to be lymphocytic, producing a granuloma and later a fibrous nodule.

The third main element in the pathogenesis of loaiasis is the interaction between the embryo worms or microfilariae and either circulating antimicrofilarial IgG antibodies or the specific therapeutic drug diethylcarbamazine citrate. The most important organs in which these reactions occur are the kidneys and brain. Renal damage is evident from proteinuria, microfilariae in the urine, and occasionally the nephrotic syndrome. Proteinuria is often provoked or made worse by diethylcarbamazine. Two theories have been proposed to explain the glomerular lesions: penetration of and mechanical damage by circulating microfilariae, and precipitation of antigen-antibody complexes on the glomerular endothelium.

A more severe and sometimes fatal aspect of loaiasis is the production of meningoencephalitis by the administration (often unsupervised self-administration) of diethylcarbamazine to patients with high-density microfilaremia. The syndrome does occur rarely without drug therapy, probably due to specific immune responses. Diethylcarbamazine causes massive invasion of the cerebrospinal fluid by microfilariae when it is administered to heavily infected persons. Cerebral hypoxia and coma result from capillary obstruction by masses of moribund or dead microfilariae. Two distinct pathologic features are seen in fatal cases: an acute and diffuse edema of the brain with many occluded capillaries, and localized, partially necrotic granulomas containing much microfilarial debris. These chronic granulomas appear to be long-standing reactions around dying microfilariae, and their presence in the brain may determine whether diethylcarbamazine administration will precipitate acute meningoencephalitis. Some workers have attributed the cerebral lesions in loaiasis to a Jarisch-Herxheimer type reaction caused by the liberation of enormous quantities of specific neurotropic somatic toxins from microfilariae by diethylcarbamazine. The histologic evidence, however, indicates that such a mechanism could only be secondary in importance to cerebral hypoxia and edema resulting from capillary blockade. A frequent complication of meningoencephalitis in loaiasis is retinal hemorrhage and exudates probably secondary to raised intracranial venous pressure. Retinal lesions occur most often in individuals with pre-existing retinopathy of another cause.

A report from Nigeria implicates *L. loa* as the etiologic agent of a form of endomyocardial fibrosis associated with eosinophilia, fever, skin irritation, and transient localized subcutaneous swellings, particularly of the face. This report clearly needs further investigation.

CLINICAL MANIFESTATIONS. The hypersensitivity reactions associated with the entry of infective *L. loa* larvae into the body after *Chrysops* bites can cause intense itching and irritation. Scratching this painful site causes secondary pyoderma.

Between 6 and 12 months after entry into the body, worms attain sexual maturity and start their migrations through the connective tissues. The pathologic reactions to these migrations, which are mainly subcutaneous, give rise to the most common clinical effect of loaiasis, the so-called Calabar swelling. This is a firm area of edema, usually painless but sometimes showing signs of acute inflammation and becoming hot, tender, and painful. The swellings are often accompanied by pruritus and fever and, if they occur near a joint, can cause limitation of movement. Calabar swellings are most frequent on the hands and arms, but patients complain most vigorously when they occur on the face, particularly the bridge of the nose. They can, however, occur on any part of the body. Swelling is usually transient, lasting a few days or rarely a few weeks, and has often been graphically described as a "hen's egg" or "wasp sting" swelling. Less commonly, worm migrations produce fugitive swelling of a complete limb, usually the arm.

Transocular migration of adult worms is common and the worms are easily seen migrating across the conjunctiva, causing painful conjunctivitis and lacrimation.

At any stage of loaiasis, subcutaneous or deep abscesses may occur, usually in areas of inflammation surrounding a dead adult worm.

Proteinuria is common in loaiasis, and a nephrotic syndrome occurs occasionally. Both may be precipitated or exacerbated by diethylcarbamazine therapy.

Meningoencephalitis appears as a severe and progressive headache leading rapidly to coma. It is most common in heavily infected adults and is usually provoked by diethylcarbamazine treatment. However, it must be stressed that a history of drug treatment may be impossible to obtain, since the drug is widely sold by retail stores in endemic areas. Furthermore diethylcarbamazine causes the visible expulsion of intestinal roundworms in feces, and patients may not connect taking "worm" medicine with questions about self-treatment for Calabar swellings or pruritus. Retinal hemorrhage is always a grave prognostic sign in cerebral loaiasis. Even after recovery, there is usually complete or partial blindness.

COMPLICATIONS AND SEQUELAE. The main complications and sequelae of long-standing loaiasis are lichenification of the skin in areas where multiple Calabar swellings have occurred. Abscesses, meningoencephalitis, and renal complications have been described above.

GEOGRAPHIC VARIATIONS IN DISEASE. The only geographic variations recorded in the clinical picture of loaiasis relate to the local intensities of transmission, and hence to the numbers of live adult worms and microfilariae in the body at any given time. The frequency of clinical manifestations, their severity, and the frequency of complications are directly correlated with worm burdens. No evidence has yet been presented of geographic strain variation in the pathogenicity of *L. loa*.

DIAGNOSIS. The typical history of loaiasis is diagnostic, given the fugitive swellings with or without pain and fever,

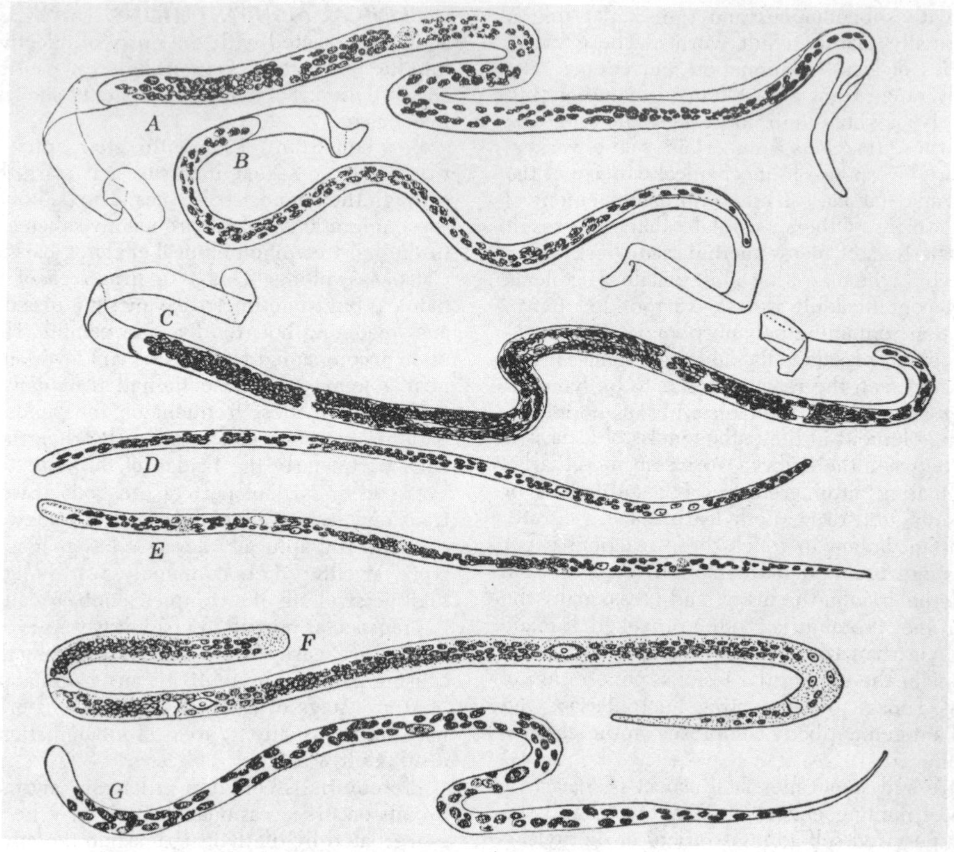

Figure 1. Various species of microfilariae drawn to scale.
A, Wuchereria bancrofti; sheathed, no nuclei in tip of tail, 270 × 8.5 μ.
B, Brugia malayi; sheathed, 2 nuclei in tail, 200 × 6 μ.
C, Loa loa; sheathed, nuclei to tip of tail, 275 × 7 μ.
D, Tetrapetalonema perstans; no sheath, tail blunt with nuclei to tip, 200 to 4.5 μ.
E, Mansonella ozzardi; no sheath, pointed tail without nuclei at tip, 205 × 5 μ.
F, Onchocerca volvulus; no sheath, no nuclei in end of tail, 320 × 7.5 μ.
G, Dirofilaria immitis; no sheath, sharp tail without nuclei in end, 300 × 6 μ.

and the occasional dramatic migration of an adult worm across the eye. Worms in the conjunctiva or under the skin can be easily removed under local anesthesia and identified by a parasitologist. The adults resemble pieces of surgical catgut, females measuring 20 to 70 mm and males 20 to 35 mm. The cuticle has numerous little dewdrop-like warts along the lateral lines of the body, which distinguishes *Loa* from other filariae.

A definitive diagnosis of loaiasis can be made only by recovery and identification of the adult worms or the typical sheathed microfilariae in peripheral blood. (See Fig. 1). However, many patients with loaiasis are amicrofilaremic, either because they have unisexual infections or because infection with both sexes is too sparse for mating. Further, a vigorous immune response appears to render a few heavily infected persons amicrofilaremic. Conversely, many persons with microfilaremia may have no signs or symptoms of clinical loaiasis.

Since the microfilariae of *L. loa* are diurnally periodic, blood samples for examination should be taken as close as possible to 12 noon. Microfilariae must be counted as well as identified in blood samples of known volume in order to plan treatment schedules for the individual patient and to assess the effectiveness of control measures in community surveys. Depending on the desired degree of sensitivity, blood sample sizes are usually 20 mm³, 100 mm³, 1 ml, or 10 ml. The first two sample volumes are usually obtained by stylet puncture of skin to produce capillary blood from the finger, thumb, heel, or earlobe. Volumes of 1 ml or 10 ml require venipuncture. Three main methods for processing the blood are available: smearing, fixing, and staining on a glass microscope slide; hemolysis and counting in a counting-chamber; or concentration and filtration through a Millipore or Nuclepore membrane. Details of the techniques can be found in textbooks of medical helminthology such as Muller (1975).

Hypereosinophilia of 60 to 90 per cent (20,000 to 50,000 per mm³) is common in loaiasis and as confirmatory evidence in diagnosis. Serodiagnosis and skin testing are under intensive research but are too nonspecific to help the practitioner.

TREATMENT. The drug of choice in loaiasis is diethylcarbamazine. In different dosages, it is effective against all the life-cycle stages of *L. loa* that occur in humans—adult worms, microfilariae, and infective larvae. Diethylcarbamazine has no effect on *L. loa* in vitro. In vivo, it is an extremely effective microfilaricide in small doses, apparently inducing an opsonin-like effect which sensitizes microfilariae to destruction by phagocytes, primarily the Kupffer cells. In larger doses it kills adult worms more slowly, apparently by inducing them to migrate to the dermis, where they are killed by a foreign body type of reaction.

Dosage schedules in loaiasis should be planned according to circulating microfilarial densities. Dosages refer to oral administration of diethylcarbamazine citrate, and are planned to bring about radical cure in adults.

1. For amicrofilaremic patients:
   Day 1, 50 mg in one dose
   Day 2, 100 mg in one dose
   Day 3, 200 mg in divided doses every 12 hours
   Day 4, 400 mg in divided doses every 12 hours
   Day 5 to day 26, 600 mg in divided doses three times daily
2. For microfilaremic patients with less than 30 microfilariae per mm³ blood:
   Day 1, 6.25 mg
   Day 2, 12.5 mg
   Day 3, 25 mg — in one dose each day
   Day 4, 50 mg
   Day 5, 100 mg
   Day 6, 200 mg in divided doses every 12 hours
   Day 7, 400 mg in divided doses every 12 hours
   Day 8 to day 29, 600 mg in divided doses three times daily
3. For microfilaremic patients with more than 30 microfilariae per mm³ blood:
   As in (2) above, with the addition of oral prednisone 20 mg daily for the first seven days of treatment.

The adult doses given above are suitable for a 70-kg patient; doses for children should be reduced proportionally. All treated patients should be given a follow-up blood examination after six months, and further treatment if necessary.

Individual inflammatory lesions of loaiasis should be treated by the application of cold compresses and antihistamine creams to the affected area to relieve itching and pain. Visible adult worms in the eye or the skin should be removed under local anesthesia by passing a curved bayonet-edged surgical needle under them and gently extracting them by traction through a small incision, controlled by a mounted needle.

PROPHYLAXIS. Personal prophylaxis against *L. loa* can be achieved by taking 200 mg of diethylcarbamazine citrate twice daily for three consecutive days once a month. Less specific measures are the use of insect repellents such as dimethylphthalate when in areas where *Chrysops* is present, and the careful screening of houses against insects.

Community prophylaxis by environmental and insecticidal control of *Chrysops* breeding sites has been tried, but measures have not been developed that are practical and cheap.

References

Fain, A: Les problemes actuels de la loase. Bull WHO 56:155, 1978.
Muller, R.: Worms and Disease. London, William Heinemann Medical Books Ltd., 1975, p. 142.
Sasa, M.: Human Filariasis. Baltimore, University Park Press, 1976, p. 122.

230
DRACUNCULIASIS
D. W. Belcher, M.D.

Dracunculiasis is an acquired parasitic infection of subcutaneous and connective tissues caused by a large nematode, *Dracunculus medinensis*. Because of its unique clinical presentation—a long, string-like worm protruding from a shallow skin ulcer—it has been recognized since ancient times. Local names like guinea worm (Africa) and Medina worm (Middle East and Nile valley) reflect its endemic distribution. In these areas and in India and in Pakistan it is a major health problem because it incapacitates many farmers (Belcher et al., 1975a).

ETIOLOGY AND LIFE CYCLE. Man becomes infected when he drinks unfiltered water containing *Cyclops* infected with *D. medinensis* larvae. After the *Cyclops* are digested by gastric secretions, larvae are freed and penetrate the intestinal wall. In about six weeks they migrate to subcutaneous tissues, where they mature into worms. Males die after fertilizing the female, a few months after entering the human host. Males are absorbed or encysted in experimental animals, while the fertilized female burrows deeper into connective tissue until its uterus becomes distended with an estimated three million embryos. About eight months after entering the human host, the gravid female worm begins to migrate back to subcutaneous tissue, usually in the person's legs. Ten to 14 months after infection, the female emerges through the skin to release larvae into the water. The stage is now set for a new cycle. Larvae are released into water through the prolapsed uterus over a two- to four-week period before the worm dies. Repeated contact with water produces vigorous contraction of the uterus which expels the embryos.

D. medinensis is an obligate parasite that alternates between man, the definitive host, and its intermediate arthropod host. In 1870 Fedchenko discovered that a freshwater crustacean, *Cyclops* (water flea), contained *D. medinensis* larvae. He suggested that infected *Cyclops* were the source of guinea worm disease. His report is the first that showed that an arthropod could serve as the intermediate host for an agent of human disease. Since *Dracunuculus* larvae possess no boring apparatus, only large predatory *Cyclops* strains that can ingest larvae become infected. These include *C. leukarti* (West Africa, Middle East, India) and *C. hyalinus* (West Africa, India). Endemic areas are sharply demarcated tropical locations because disease transmission is dependent upon an appropriate *Cyclops* species and a water temperature above 20° C. Warm water is necessary for larvae inside the Cyclops host to develop into the infective third stage in about two weeks.

Since *Cyclops* organisms propagate best in stagnant surface water, communities that are dependent on ponds, cisterns (Iran), and step-down wells (India) for drinking water have the greatest risk of infection. Water becomes contaminated when patients with guinea worm infections wade in to obtain water or bathe their ulcers to relieve pain.

D. medinensis is the only member of the Dracunculidae family that is known to infect man. A related nematode, *D. insignis,* infects North American mammals such as the raccoon and fox, but not man. Although *D. medinensis* infections of dogs, cats, monkeys, and several domesticated animals are known, no definite reservoir host has been demonstrated.

EPIDEMIOLOGY AND GEOGRAPHIC VARIATIONS. The actual number of cases per year is unknown because official statistics grossly underestimate the extent of the problem. Dracunculiasis is not a notifiable disease in endemic areas. Because most patients are from rural areas, they are likely to have poor access to clinics and to prefer traditional treatment methods. Thirty years ago, an estimated 48 million persons were infected annually in areas with long dry seasons and ponds, cisterns, or step-down wells as water sources.

West Africa, Ethiopia, the Nile valley, Saudi Arabia, Iran and the Middle East, and Pakistan and India are endemic areas because water supplies are poor, an appropriate *Cyclops* species is present, and the water temperature is above 20° C. (Fig. 1). Previous foci in the West Indies and northeastern South America are no longer active because of improved economic conditions and better water supplies (Reddy et al., 1969).

Peak attack rates occur in men aged 16 to 44 years, probably because of their heavy seasonal farming activities and increased consumption of contaminated water. Females are infected as often as males in communities that use a common source of water. Infants and toddlers are rarely infected because they are breast-fed.

The source of water in tropical areas varies with the season. During a rainy season lasting two or three months, ponds fill and overflow as small streams. Villagers collect roof water in barrels and water pots. As the dry season progresses, these sources are expended and shallow surface ponds are used. Near the end of the dry season, the volume of pond water becomes low, so that the density of *Cyclops* is increased. Experimental evidence shows that infected *Cyclops* organisms lie near the bottom, where low pond volume may increase the likelihood of their being scooped up with drinking water (Muller, 1970a). Seasonal rains interrupt the transmission of dracunculiasis because the increased water volume and turbidity reduce the density of *Cyclops.* In areas where wells and cisterns are used, *Cyclops* tend to persist in larger numbers and transmission periods are longer.

Agricultural activities in the tropics have clear seasonal patterns. Land-clearing and planting are done at the end of the dry season, just before the rains. This peak farming period coincides with the major transmission period of dracunculiasis. When the patent worm emerges about one year later, ulcers located on the feet or ankles and secondary bacterial infections can incapacitate the farmer at this critical time. In southern Ghana three out of four adult farmers are affected in some villages. The impact of this painful and disabling illness on communities where it recurs year after year is difficult to measure. Adults lying around with guinea worm ulcers and swollen legs explain the ill-kept and listless atmosphere of some of these villages (Kale, 1977a).

Some people who use larvae-contaminated water do not develop dracunculiasis, but little is known about factors that influence individual host resistance. The effect of gastric acidity on the infectivity of ingested larvae is controversial. However, gastric emptying time is clearly an important factor. Experimental animals that have rapid passage of infected cyclops through the stomach are more readily infected (Muller, 1970b). This observation suggests that gastric contents interfere with the infectivity of larvae. The fact that previously infected adults acquire fewer patent worms suggests that acquired immunity limits infection.

PATHOGENESIS AND CLINICAL MANIFESTATIONS. The infected patient is asymptomatic for about one year, the prepatency period. Shortly before emerging, the female worm migrates to a subcutaneous location where she lies in a fibrous tunnel. Localized skin changes develop over the anterior end, apparently caused by the premature release of larvae into subcutaneous tissue. Localized swelling, accompanied by intense burning or itching, is followed within a few days by the formation of a blister made up of granulation tissue, fibrin, and a sterile yellow fluid containing eosinophils and larvae. Within a week the blister ruptures, leaving a shallow, 1- to 2-cm erosion. In its center is a tiny hole through which a portion of the uterus may protrude. Such ulcerations are not disabling unless they are numerous, located near a joint, or secondarily infected (Price and Child, 1971).

The vast majority of patients have one to three patent worms. Only 10 per cent develop four or more lesions. One third of skin lesions are on the foot and ankle and one

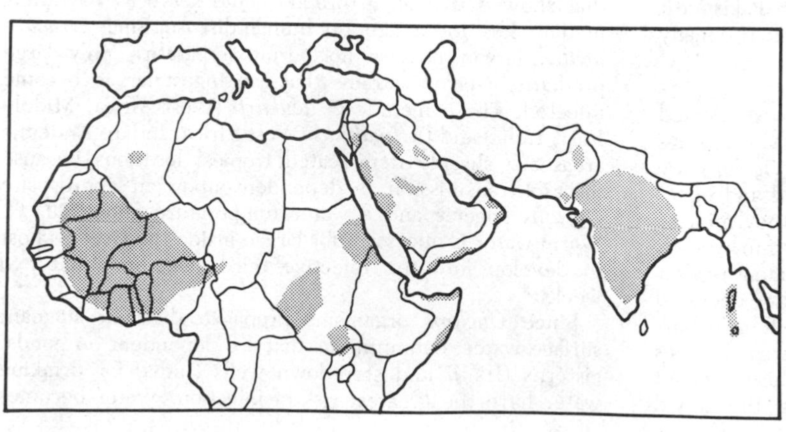

Figure 1. Geographic distribution of dracunculiasis.

half are on the leg. The rest occur on the trunk and arms and, rarely, on the head and neck. One to three days before the appearance of skin lesions, about one third of patients develop prodromal symptoms including fever, generalized urticaria, dizziness, vomiting, diarrhea, and occasionally dyspnea.

A small number of gravid females do not reach the surface of the skin and produce deep, sterile abscesses causing swollen extremities. Cryptic infection by nonemergent worms is often confused with bacterial pyomyositis of the extremities (Davey, 1971). Clinical differentiation between these two conditions is usually possible because pyomyositis is characterized by fever, induration with marked tenderness, and occasionally scaling of the overlying skin. In contrast, the abscesses of dracunculiasis are much less tender, and patients are generally afebrile. There is often an associated eosinophilia attributed to release of larvae into tissue. Other parasitic skin conditions caused by nonhuman hookworm or the Tumbu fly can be differentiated because they are smaller in size and occur in a wider range of anatomic locations.

COMPLICATIONS AND SEQUELAE. Nonemergent female worms sometimes invade other organs. Infrequent extracutaneous manifestations of dracunculiasis include genitourinary symptoms, retroplacental bleeding, pericarditis, pulmonary scarring, ophthalmic disease, and paraplegia secondary to extradural spinal cord involvement. The underlying etiology should be suspected if a calcified worm is detected on radiography or if the patient comes from an endemic area. More commonly, the unexpected diagnosis is established at surgery or by examination of the histologic sections.

Periarticular tissue and even joint spaces are invaded occasionally. The resulting pain and immobility cause knee and ankle contractures, which leave patients crippled and unable to work. Bony ankylosis is rare.

Prolonged incapacitation may occur secondary to cellulitis and abscess formation. Ulcers of the leg are frequently secondarily infected because patients continue to farm, make unsuccessful attempts to extract a worm, or apply local herb poultices. Colonization with *Streptococcus*, *Staphylococcus*, or coliforms produces a local cellulitis or a spreading infection along the subcutaneous worm track. These may be the "fiery serpents" described by Moses during the exodus through the Sinai peninsula in Numbers 21. Other complications include bacterial abscesses, septic arthritis, and large, persistent ulcerations. These painful conditions prevent normal activity for months. Numerous cases of fatal tetanus originating in guinea worm ulcerations have been reported from West Africa.

DIAGNOSIS. In endemic areas dracunculiasis can be diagnosed on clinical grounds. The diagnosis is usually obvious when the slender, string-like uterus protrudes from the ulcer or if the long serpentine configuration of the subcutaneous worm can be seen or palpated. Microscopic examination of ulcer fluid to identify larvae is rarely used. Fluorescent antibody tests are positive six months or more before the worm emerges, but this technique is feasible only in a research setting. Eosinophilia of about 15 per cent may be helpful in diagnosis. Nonemergent, calcified worms in atypical locations are occasionally an incidental finding on radiographs.

TREATMENT. Four drugs are currently used to treat dracunculiasis. Niridazole was the first agent tested, but frequent side-effects have shifted the interest of clinicians to metronidazole (Kulkarni and Nagalotimath, 1975), thiabendazole, and mebendazole (Kale, 1977b). Published results of trials are difficult to interpret because different criteria of efficacy are used, control groups are infrequent, and many patients drop out of studies. Furthermore, study patients often had lighter worm loads than nonparticipating patients, so that they were able to walk to clinics where the research was being conducted. Drug treatment was less effective in patients with recently emerged worms than in those with lesions of longer duration. Since patent worms only live two to four weeks anyway, it is not clear that the drugs are useful (Belcher, 1975b).

Experimental animal work suggests that niridazole, metronidazole, and thiabendazole provide symptomatic relief and make patent worms easier to extract (Muller, 1970b). These effects are apparently related to a nonspecific anti-inflammatory action (Muller, 1971b). No direct toxicity or interference with guinea worm metabolism has been demonstrated (Muller, 1971a).

None of these drugs affect either the latent larvae or the pre-emergent worm. For weeks after a completed drug course, viable adult worms continue to emerge in patients with heavy infections. Diethylcarbamazine, which is used in filariasis, destroys latent *Dracunculus* larvae but has no effect on the adults. It is not recommended for mass chemotherapy in latent asymptomatic cases.

Since drug treatment reduces pain and swelling within a few days, treatment of individual patients with currently available drugs (Table 1) should be considered. Cost may preclude widespread application in developing countries. Repeated courses are necessary for symptomatic relief as new worms emerge.

Because well-designed comparative drug trials are unavailable, the drug of choice is unclear; however, the shorter course required for thiabendazole should promote better compliance by patients with instructions. After chemotherapy, some physicians use local anesthesia and make multiple incisions along the worm track to remove the entire female.

In isolated areas, the use of traditional therapy will continue. The protruding worm is tied to a piece of wood and a few centimeters are extracted each day for two to three weeks. Frequent moistening of the ulcer facilitates removal, because water produces uterine contraction, expulsion of larvae, and reduced worm resistance to traction. Patients are advised to elevate the affected limb, cleanse the wound, and apply clean dressings. Secondary bacterial complications are treated with oral penicillin (400,000 units three times daily for adults) for 5 to 7 days.

Table 1. DRUGS USED IN TREATMENT OF DRACUNCULIASIS

Drug	Schedule	Duration
Thiabendazole	25 mg/kg twice a day	2 days
Metronidazole[a]	500 mg three times a day	7 days
Mebendazole	400 mg twice a day	7 days
Niridazole	25 mg/kg in divided doses	7 days

[a]25 mg/kg in children (maximum 500 mg/day); generally not used in pregnant women.

PROPHYLAXIS AND CONTROL. There appears to be little likelihood for some years that piped water or bore wells can be afforded in most rural communities where dracunculiasis is prevalent, although this is the most direct approach to interrupting transmission. Since the epidemiology and seasonality of dracunculiasis are well understood, several methods to achieve control can be considered (Workshop, 1982).

Because man is the definitive host, eradication of the infection in patients would be one means of controlling dracunculiasis. Unfortunately, no drug will suppress latent human infection. Even if effective anthelmintics were available, residents in endemic areas generally have poor access to regular medical services. Furthermore, patients have depended on traditional treatment for years. There may be a long time lag before modern clinical care is sought, particularly when patients are too ill to walk.

Another approach is to educate residents of endemic areas to avoid water contaminated by patients suffering from dracunculiasis, but there are numerous obstacles to such education. Residents often have supernatural explanations for the appearance of dracunculiasis in some individuals or communities while others are spared. The long incubation period of about one year also makes it difficult to explain the transmission cycle to local inhabitants in an effort to modify their behavior. The construction of walls that prevent wading in water reservoirs and platforms that are combined with a device to lower a utensil into the pond have helped to end the transmission cycle.

Control methods can also be directed at the intermediate host. Because cyclops are macroscopic crustaceans, they can be removed from water by filtering through a cloth. Thirsty farmers working in fields some distance from a village rarely take time to filter nearby pond water. Boiling is also effective, but few households will regularly boil all their drinking water if wood and other fuels are scarce.

Biologic and chemical approaches have suppressed *Cyclops* populations during the transmission season. Large year-round ponds might be successfully stocked with *Cyclops*-consuming fish, but transient seasonal rural ponds are best managed by periodic application of chemical compounds (Muller, 1971b). Several compounds have been field tested. In Iran widespread chlorination of cisterns has met with marked success (Sahba et al., 1973). In India, however, the taste of chlorinated water was poorly accepted. DDT is also effective but affects other life forms and is not recommended in water used for drinking purposes.

Abate (temephos, tetramethyl thiophenylene-phosphorothioate), an organophosphorus insecticide originally developed for control of mosquitoes, is one of the more successful anti-*Cyclops* chemicals (Lyons, 1973). Abate in a sand granule form at one part per million suppresses *Cyclops* for six weeks. In areas where ponds are associated with short transmission periods, Abate could be applied near the end of the dry season in two courses at a four-week interval. Repeated cycles of Abate would be required to suppress *Cyclops* effectively in areas where water sources are associated with longer transmission periods.

References

Belcher, D. W., Wurapa, F. K., Ward, W. B., and Lourie, I. M.: Guinea worm in southern Ghana: Its epidemiology and impact on agricultural productivity. Am J Trop Med Hyg 24:243, 1975a.

Belcher, D. W., Wurapa, F. K., and Ward, W. B.: Failure of thiabendazole and metronidazole in the treatment and suppression of guinea worm disease. Am J Trop Med Hyg 24:444, 1975b.

Davey, W. W.: Guinea worm disease versus pyomyositis. In Companion to Surgery in Africa. Edinburgh, E. & S. Livingstone, 1971, p. 100.

Kale, O. O.: The clinico-epidemiologic profile of guinea worm in the Ibaden district of Nigeria. Am J Trop Med Hyg 26:208, 1977a.

Kale, O. O.: Clinical evaluation of drugs for dracontiasis. Tropical Doctor 7:15, 1977b.

Kulkarni, D. R., and Nagalotimath, S. J.: Guinea worms and metronidazole. Trans R Soc Trop Med Hyg 69:169, 1975.

Lyons, G. R.: The control of guinea worm with Abate: A trial in a village in northern Ghana. Bull WHO 49:215, 1973.

Muller, R.: Laboratory experiments in the control of cyclops transmitting guinea worm. Bull WHO 42:563, 1970a.

Muller, R.: Pathology and chemotherapy of dracunculiasis infection in rhesus monkeys. Trans R Soc Trop Med Hyg 64:24, 1970b.

Muller, R.: The possible mode of action of some chemotherapeutic agents in guinea worm disease. Trans R Soc Trop Med Hyg 63:843, 1971a.

Muller, R.: Dracunculus and dracunculiasis. In Dawes, B. (ed.): Advances in Parasitology. New York, Academic Press, 1971b, p. 73.

Price, D. L., and Child, P. L.: Dracontiasis (dracunculiasis, dracunculosis, medina worm, guinea worm). In Marcial-Rojas, R. A. (ed.): Pathology of Protozoal and Helminthic Diseases with Clinical Correlation. Baltimore, The Williams & Wilkins Company, 1971, p. 852.

Reddy, C. R. R. M., Narasaiah, I. L., and Parvathi, G.: Epidemiological studies on guinea worm infection. Bull WHO 40:521, 1969.

Sahba, G. H., Afraa, F., Fardin, A., and Ardalan, A.: Studies in dracontiasis in Iran. Am J Trop Med Hyg 22:343, 1973.

Workshop, June 16–19, 1982 Washington, D.C. Opportunities for control of dracunculiasis. National Academy Press, 1983. BOSTIC, National Academy of Sciences, 2101 Constitution Avenue, Washington, D.C. 20418.

231

CUTANEOUS ONCHOCERCIASIS

HORACIO FIGUEROA MARROQUIN

Cutaneous onchocerciasis is the term applied to certain dermal changes in man caused by an infestation with *Onchocerca volvulus*.

The first recorded observation of the skin lesions produced by *O. volvulus* dates back to 1875, when O'Neill discovered microfilariae in patients with craw-craw, a condition identified with filaric scabies. In 1893 Leuckart reported filariae in tumors excised from natives of Ghana by German missionaries. He named the parasite *Filaria volvulus*. In 1910 Raillet and Henry classified it in the genus *Onchocerca* as *Onchocerca volvulus*.

For many years the parasite was regarded as a curiosity that could infect man with no untoward effects. Robles in Guatemala discovered, after excising many nodules, that infestation with *O. volvulus* resulted in blindness (Robles, 1919). This news was received with skepticism, and it was not until 17 years later in 1932 that Hissette observed ocular lesions in the Belgian Congo similar to those found by Robles and Pacheco Luna in Guatemala.

ETIOLOGY. The etiologic agent of onchocerciasis is *Onchocerca volvulus*, a nematode of the superfamily Filarioidea, genus *Onchocerca*, species *volvulus*. It is a white

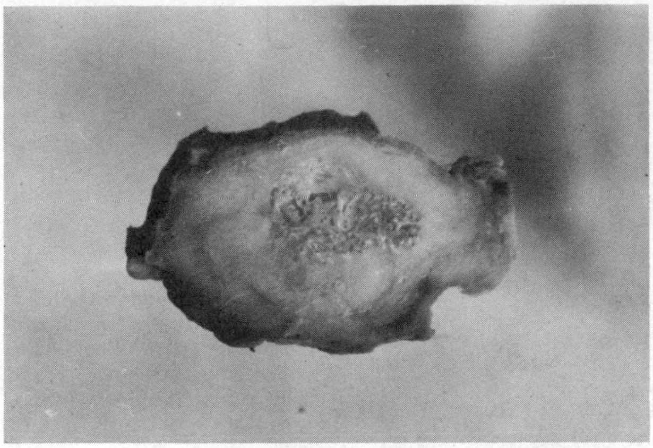

Figure 1. Section of a nodule showing the two main portions: the central part, or stroma, and the peripheral fibrous capsule.

thread-like worm measuring up to 50 cm in length and 0.45 mm in width. Uteri filled with mature microfilariae are prominent in sections of the midbody of the gravid worm. It is transmitted from man to man by several species of Simuliidae. The main vectors are *S. damnosum* in Africa, *S. ochraceum* in Mexico and Guatemala, and *S. metallicum* in Venezuela. These insects are known as buffalo gnats or black flies. (See photograph in Chapter 18). These black flies develop in fast streams and rivers.

PATHOGENESIS AND PATHOLOGY. The larvae of O. volvulus are introduced into the human skin by the proboscis of the fly and develop into the adult parasite there. A bleeding point may appear after the fly bite. Adult parasites live in nodules or onchocercomas. The nodules are either superficial or deeply embedded in the tissues. The parasites also live free in the tissues with no inflammatory reaction. In Africa most of the nodules are located from the waist down, whereas those in the Americas usually appear from the waist up.

Two regions are observed in sections of nodules (Fig. 1) —a central region or stroma where the thread-like adult worms are found, and a peripheral section formed by fibrous tissue. The female liberates her embryos around the nodule, from which site they migrate to the skin and eyes (Figueroa, 1972). Enormous numbers of microfilariae reach the skin and produce the various skin lesions described below. The microfilariae live in the outer dermis where they are ingested by the fly. In the fly they pass from the gut to the muscles, and become infective larvae there after several molts.

Although several theories have been advanced to explain the symptoms produced by *O. volvulus*, most authorities favor the idea of an immunologic reaction to substances liberated by the disintegration of microfilariae. Immune complexes develop about vessels that induce injurious Arthus-type reactions in the eye or testis, causing blindness or infertility (see Chapter 85). In contrast to the serious lesions caused by the microfilariae, those caused by adult worms are trivial and amount to little more than the nodule shown in Figure 1.

There are no specific pathologic findings. The most frequent are hyperkeratosis, acanthosis, papillomatosis, and perivascular inflammation.

CLINICAL MANIFESTATIONS. Regardless of geographic location, nodules, eye lesions, and dermatitis are uniformly present. This triad is found in Africa, Mexico, Central America, and South America, but with some geographic differences. There are striking differences between African and American onchocerciasis. Lymphatic symptoms, elephantiasis, and hanging groin are never seen in Mexico and Guatemala, whereas "erysipela de la costa" (coast erysipelas) and "mal morado" (purple disease) are never observed in Africa.

Skin Lesions. The findings usually include pruritus, erythema, papules, scab-like eruptions, pigmentation, depigmentation, and lichenification, all intermingled in the different lesions. The types of lesions vary according to the geographic location.

GEOGRAPHIC VARIATIONS

Yemen and Asia. The typical form of onchocercal dermatitis found in Yemen is "sowda" (Fig. 2). The name is taken from its main characteristic, a black pigmentation of the skin (*sowda* is Arabic for black). It is usually observed in one or both of the lower limbs. Intense pruritus, papules, thickening and roughness of the skin, and hypertrophy of the inguinal glands are present (Anderson and Fuglsang, 1900). It is very unusual to find microfilariae in a skin biopsy specimen unless it is taken deep enough (Fig. 3). The Mazzotti test (see below) is positive.

Africa. Pruritus is one of the main symptoms but is not unique to the African disease. It can be mild or acute, localized or generalized, continuous or intermittent, and it sometimes disappears spontaneously.

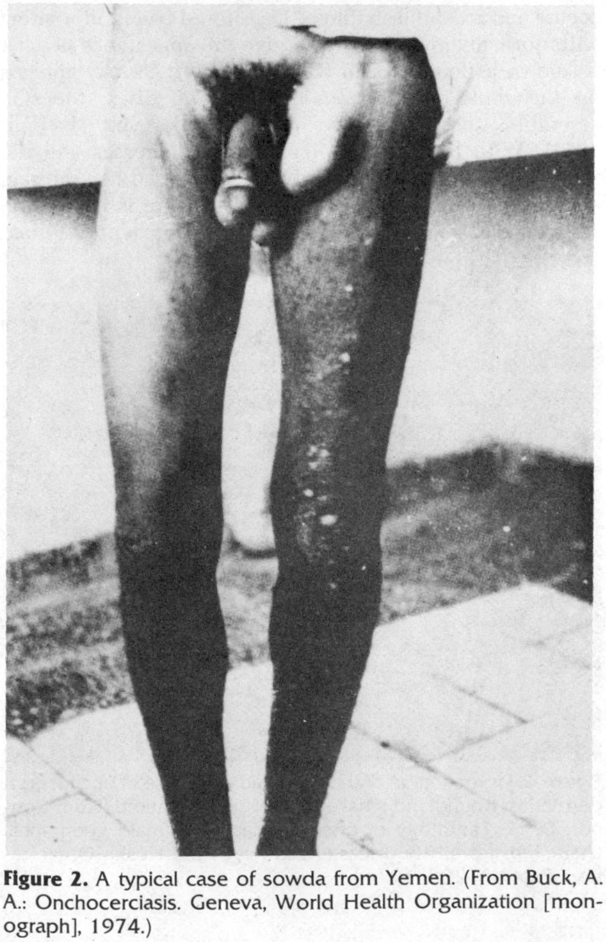

Figure 2. A typical case of sowda from Yemen. (From Buck, A. A.: Onchocerciasis. Geneva, World Health Organization [monograph], 1974.)

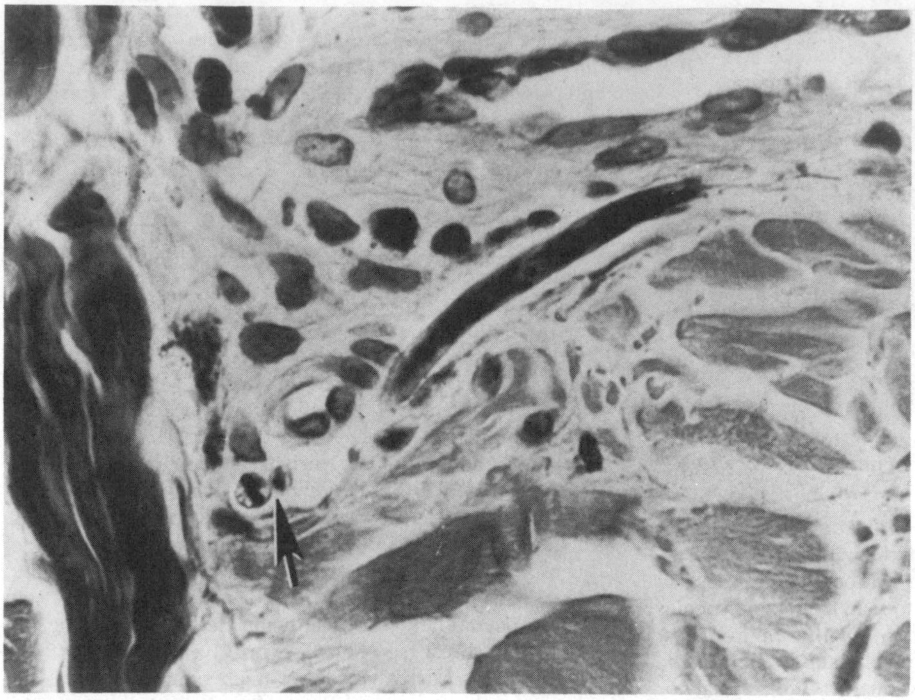

Figure 3. Microfilaria in the mid-dermis in a case of sowda (Giemsa stain). (From Buck, A. A.: Onchocerciasis. Geneva, World Health Organization [monograph], 1974.)

Round pigmented spots (Fig. 4) result from hyperkeratosis, increased pigmentation of the basal epidermis, and perivascular inflammation (Fig. 5). Depigmentation also occurs and resembles vitiligo. Discolored bands alternating with normally pigmented skin give the appearance of what is known as leopard skin (Buck, 1974). It usually appears on the shins (Fig. 6). In long-standing cases, the skin resembles that of various animals (Reber and Hoeppli, 1964). With lizard skin, pigmentation increases and the skin becomes scaly and geometrically squared like the skin of an alligator (Fig. 7). Histologically, there is hyperkeratosis, separation of the corneous stratum, perivascular infiltration, and atrophy of the epidermis (Fig. 8). When the lesions are very old, atrophy of the papillary body, which histologically looks like the skin of an old man, ensues. Because of its shiny and scaly appearance it is known as xeroderma ichthyosiformes, or fish skin (see Fig. 20). When the skin atrophies completely it loses its elasticity and resembles crushed tissue or crushed paper. There are fewer dermal papillae and almost complete disappearance of elastic fibers (Fig. 9) but no hyperkeratosis.

In African onchocerciasis lymphatic obstruction causes "hanging groin" (Fig. 10). The skin atrophies, becomes flaccid, and hangs like a bag containing lymph nodes (Buck, 1974) (Fig. 11).

Central America and Mexico. Onchocerciasis in Mexico

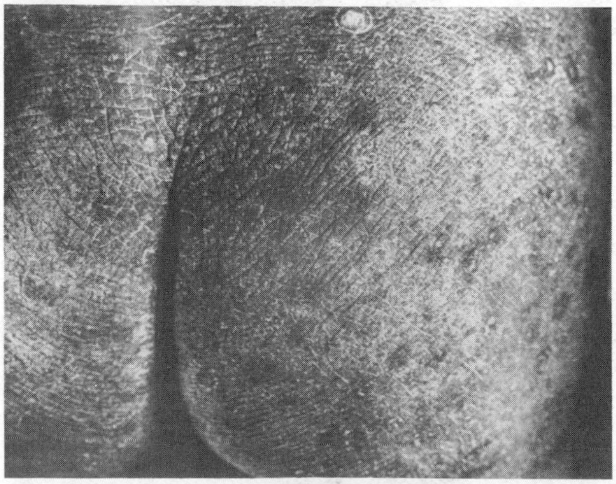

Figure 4. Pigmentation of the skin in an early case of onchocercal dermatitis. Round and small spots of pigmentation. (From Connor, D. H.: Pathology of onchocerciasis and main geographic characteristics of the disease. Geneva, World Health Organization, Pub. No. 298, 1974.)

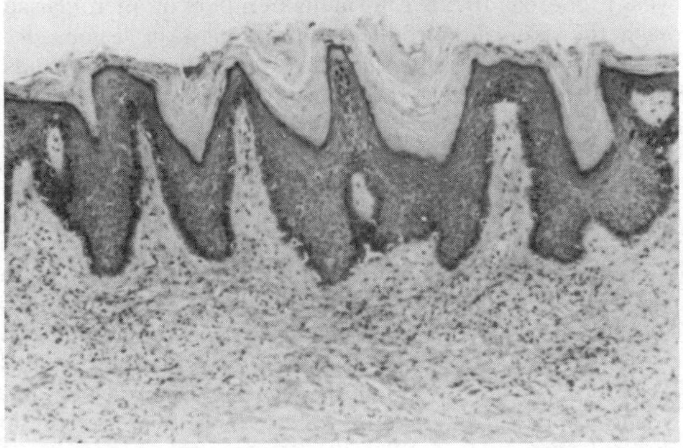

Figure 5. Slight acanthosis, elongation of the rete ridges, pigmentation of the basal layer and inflammatory cell infiltrates (hematoxylin-eosin). (From Connor, D. H.: Pathology of onchocerciasis and main geographic characteristics of the disease. Geneva, World Health Organization, Pub. No. 298, 1974.)

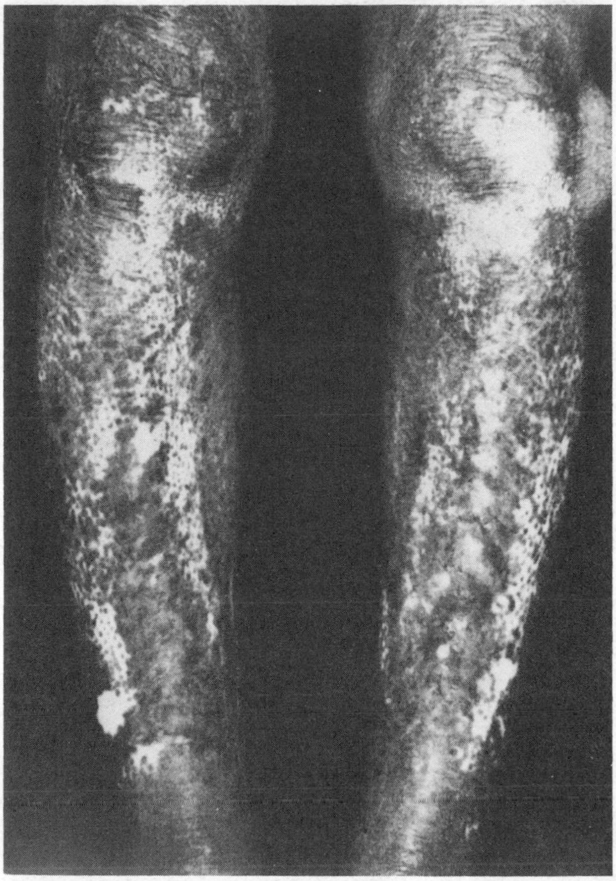

Figure 6. A case of "leopard skin." Depigmentation is more common at the shins. (From Buck, A. A.: Onchocerciasis. Geneva, World Health Organization [monograph], 1974.)

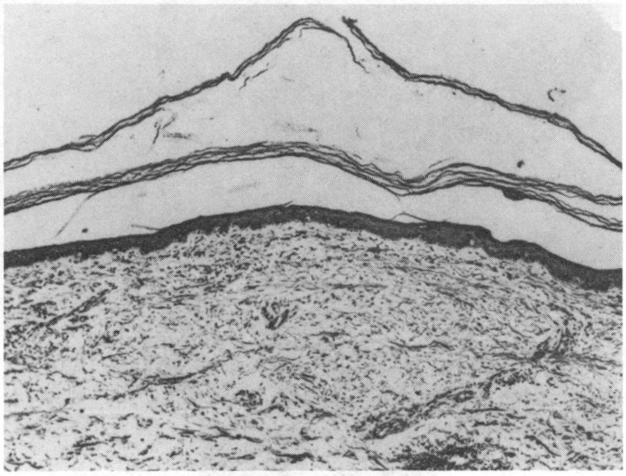

Figure 8. "Lizard skin." Separation of the keratin, atrophy of the epidermis, and chronic inflammation of the dermis. (From Connor, D. H.: Pathology of onchocerciasis and main geographic characteristics of the disease. Geneva, World Health Organization, Pub. No. 298, 1974.)

and Guatemala is known as Robles' disease. The most typical form is erysipela de la costa (coast erysipelas), so-called for its resemblance to streptococcal erysipelas. First the skin becomes tense, smooth, and shiny, and acquires a red pigmentation. Then it becomes edematous, and when the face is affected, the lips, nose, ears, and eyelids become swollen and intensely pruritic (Fig. 12). In chronic disease the skin loses elasticity, atrophies, becomes wrinkled, and causes a leonine face (Fig. 13).

Sometimes the color of erysipelas is replaced by a blue cast to the skin, called mal morado in Mexico (Salazar Mallen, 1962).

In Mexico and Guatemala almost all the skin manifestations are seen, but with differences from the African disease. Hyperpigmentation, especially of the face and

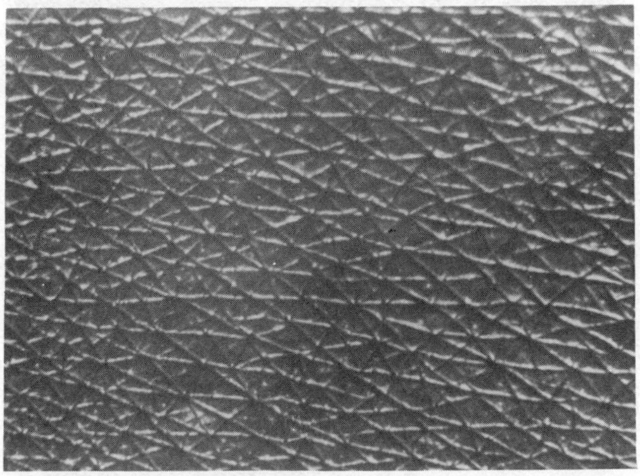

Figure 7. "Lizard skin." Increased pigmentation. Skin alterations in onchocercal dermatitis. (From Reber, W. W., and Hoeppli, R.: The relationship between macroscopic skin alterations, histological changes and microfilaria in one hundred Liberians with onchocercal dermatitis. Z Tropenmed Parasitol 15(2), July 1964.)

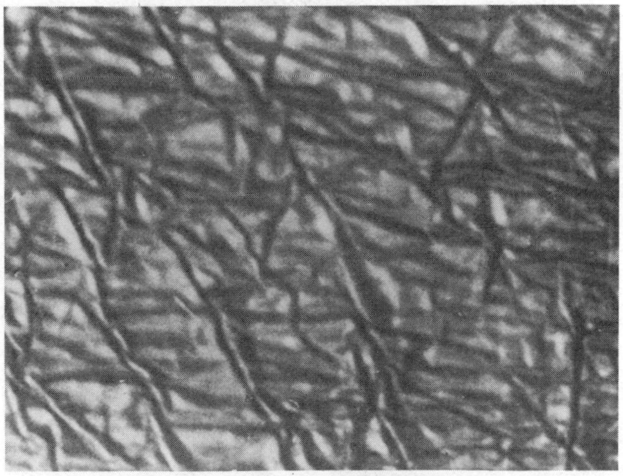

Figure 9. Crushed tissue or crushed paper appearance of xeroderma ichthyosiformes. The skin is thin and pale and loses its elasticity and luster. (From Reber, W. W., and Hoeppli, R.: The relationship between macroscopic skin alterations, histological changes and microfilaria in one hundred Liberians with onchocercal dermatitis. Z Tropenmed Parasitol 15(2), July 1964.)

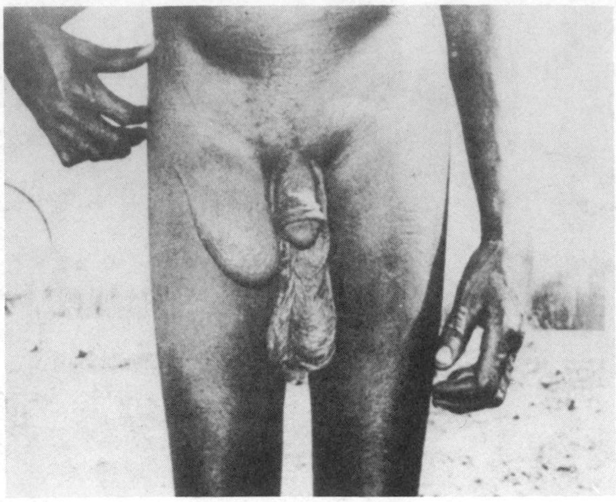

Figure 10. Unilateral hanging groin. The inguinal glands are enlarged. (From Buck, A. A.: Onchocerciasis. Geneva, World Health Organization [monograph], 1974.)

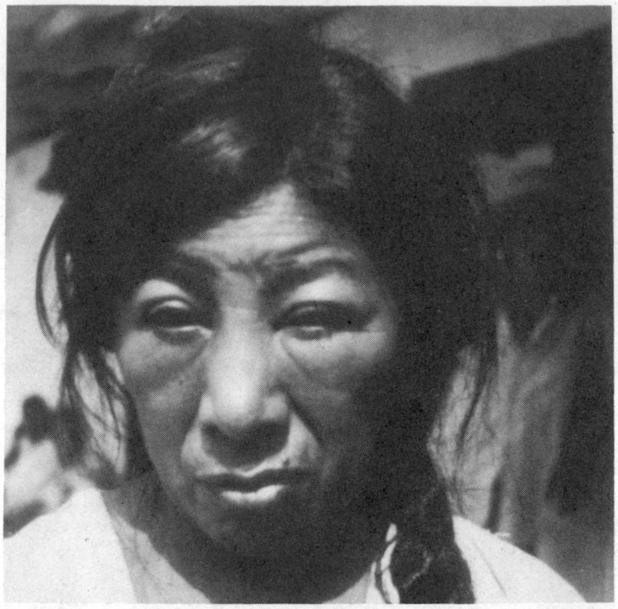

Figure 12. Erisipela de la costa.

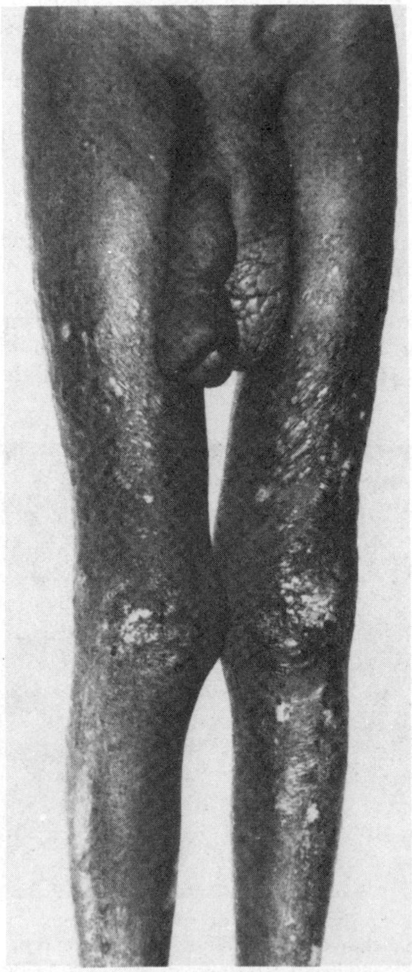

Figure 11. Elephantoid changes of the penis, the scrotum, and the thigh. (From Buck, A. A.: Onchocerciasis. Geneva, World Health Organization [monograph], 1974.)

chest, occurs but not very intensely. Depigmentation is also present, not as leopard skin but rather as small or medium sized spots. Onchocercotic scabies is frequent and is accompanied by pruritus, itching lesions, and papules that sometimes resemble craw-craw (Fig. 14).

One type of onchocercotic dermatitis that appears commonly on the ears, chest, and arms resembles the keratinization observed in vitamin A deficiency. The skin becomes dry, and pin-point papules appear as a result of obstruction of the pilosebaceous ducts (Fig. 15).

Lichenification is also common in the form of thick folds

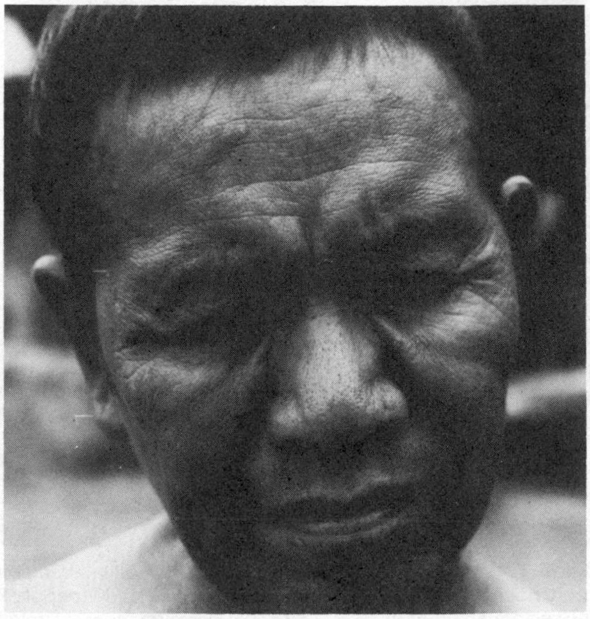

Figure 13. "Leonine facies" in a case of severe, chronic onchocercal dermatitis.

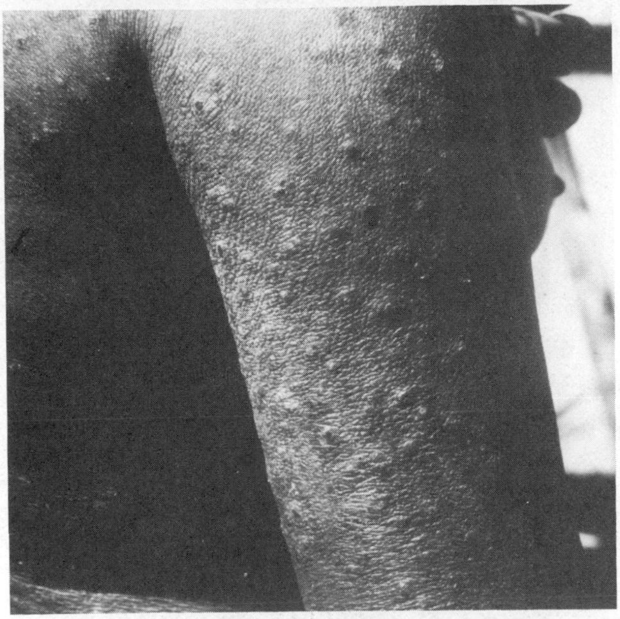

Figure 14. Scabies-like onchocercal dermatitis in a very old and severe case.

on the anterior surface of the arm (Fig. 16); the skin becomes very thick and dry.

Pseudosowda is a new kind of dermatitis that resembles sowda in that it is also black; however, it lacks some of the characteristics of true sowda (Fig. 17).

All the skin lesions mentioned are almost always bilateral. Biopsy specimens taken from the lesions are usually positive for microfilariae.

South America. South American onchocerciasis is found in Venezuela, Colombia, Ecuador, and Brazil. The skin lesions there resemble those observed in Africa more than those found in Mexico and Guatemala. Pruritus and scabies-like onchodermatitis as well as atrophy and hypertrophy of the skin occur. More acute manifestations have been found in a geographic focus of onchocerciasis recently discovered by Rassi and his colleagues (1977) in the Amazonian Federal Territory. As in Africa, there are conditions that closely resemble hanging groin (Fig. 18). Skin depigmentation appears as white small spots covering the entire body, in some cases giving the patient a mottled appearance (Fig. 19). Xeroderma ichthyosiformes or fish skin (Fig. 20) and acute atrophy of the skin (Fig. 21) also have been observed. Erythematous dermatitis, like that in erysipela de la costa, is present.

Microfilariae can invade any part of the eye and cause conjunctivitis, keratitis, iridocyclitis, chorioretinitis, and optic atrophy. In endemic areas of West Africa, onchocerciasis causes blindness in nearly half of the men over 40 years of age.

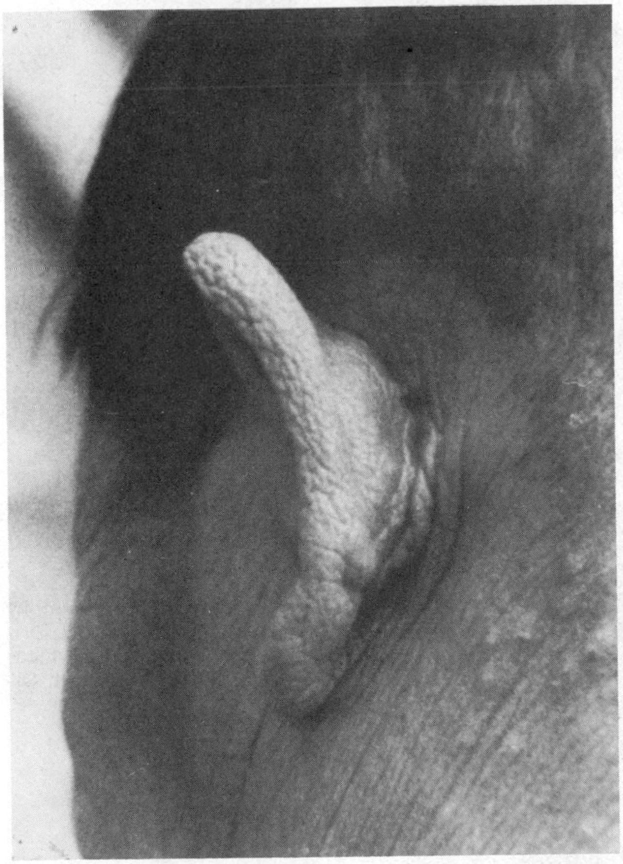

Figure 15. Pinpoint papules caused by plugging of the pilosebaceous follicles. The ear is frequently enlarged and displaced from its normal position.

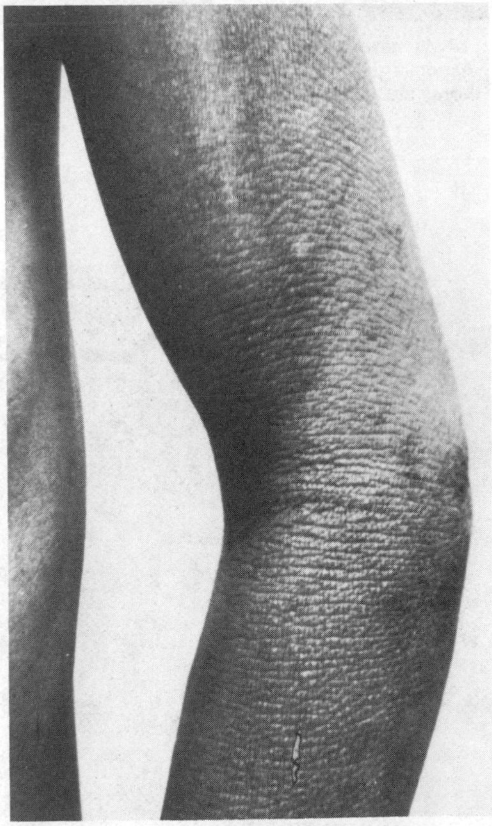

Figure 16. Lichenification in a severe case of onchocercal dematitis. Transverse and prominent folds of the skin appear.

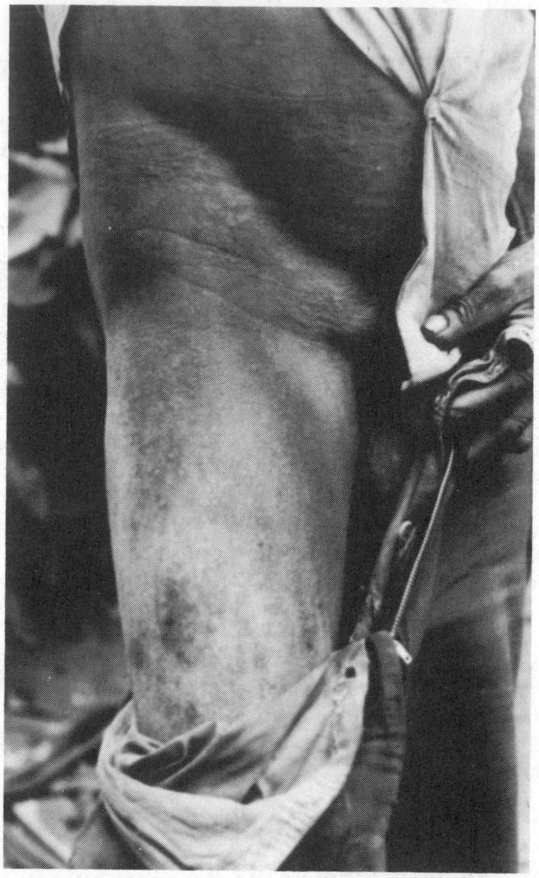

Figure 17. A case of pseudosowda. The inguinal nodes are somewhat enlarged. The black coloration of the skin is also seen in the thorax and arms.

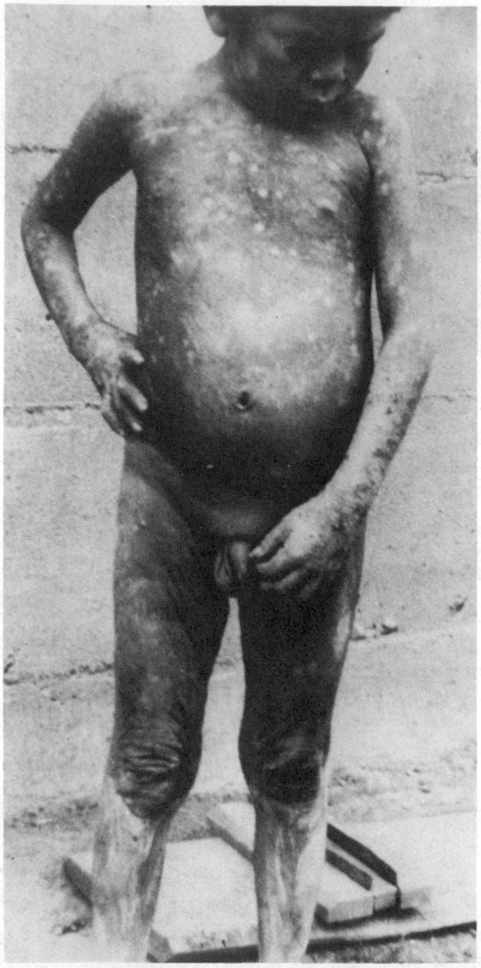

Figure 19. Generalized depigmentation. Small white spots covering almost the entire body (mottled depigmentation). (From Rassi, E., et al.: Discovery of a new onchocerciasis focus in Venezuela. Bull Pan Am Health Organ 11(1):41, 1977.)

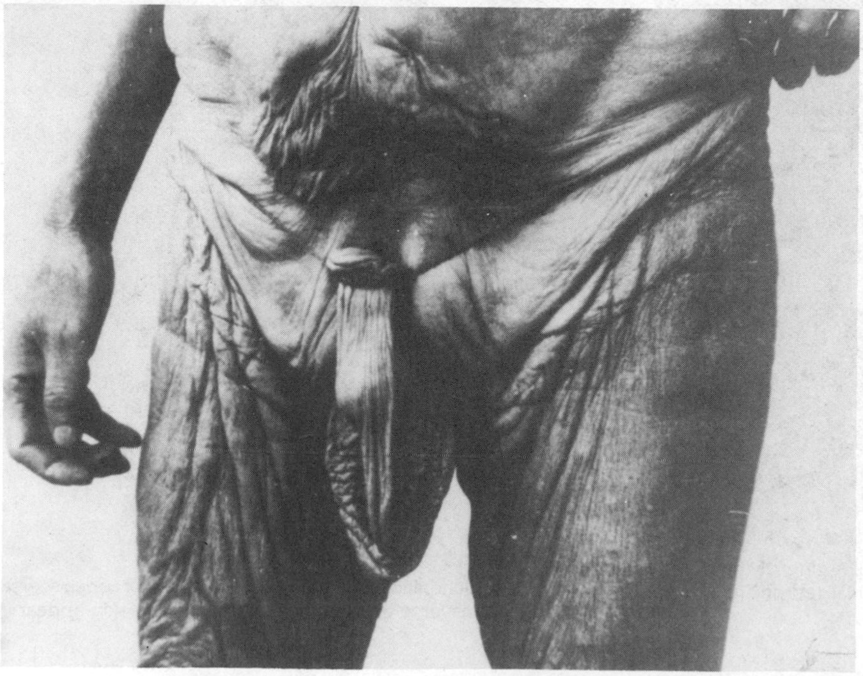

Figure 18. Hanging groin and atrophy of the skin. (From Rassi, E., et al.: Discovery of a new onchocerciasis focus in Venezuela. Bull Pan Am Health Organ 11(1):41, 1977.)

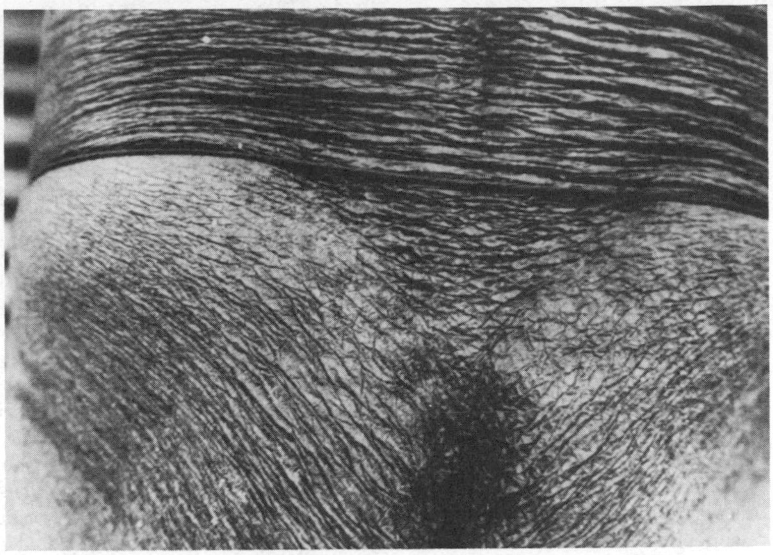

Figure 20. Fish skin (xeroderma ichthyosiformes). There is atrophy of the skin. (From Rassi, E., et al.: Discovery of a new onchocerciasis focus in Venezuela. Bull Pan Am Health Organ 11(1):41, 1977.)

Keratitis may be punctate or sclerosing. The punctate lesions are small inflammatory opacities about 0.5 mm in diameter. They develop around dead microfilariae and are located mainly at the periphery of the cornea. For this reason, visual impairment is not a serious problem. Sclerosing keratitis is a consequence of heavy microfilarial infection. Hundreds of these parasites can invade the corneal stroma and produce chronic inflammation, vascularization, and scarring that extends inward from the periphery until the pupil is covered and vision is lost. Blindness from sclerosing keratitis is common in West Africa and Central America. Sclerosing keratitis and severe iridocyclitis are often joint manifestations of the heavy invasion of the anterior part of the eye by microfilariae. The iris may adhere to the cornea, posterior synechiae may develop, and the pupil may become distorted or occluded.

In chorioretinitis the choroid and retina undergo patchy atrophy and scarring. The lesions are at first small and focal but spread over most of the posterior pole, causing chorioretinal degeneration, hyperpigmentation, and optic atrophy. Throughout all this, the macula tends to be spared and central vision may be preserved (Rodger, 1960; Paul and Zimmerman, 1970).

DIAGNOSIS. Diagnosis is easy when the triad of nodules, eye lesions, and skin changes is found. However, there are persons with the disease in whom none of these signs are observed. In such cases, microfilariae can sometimes be found in the anterior chamber of the eye.

Skin Biopsy. A skin site is selected where experience in a given geographic region has demonstrated that microfilariae are more likely to be found. The suprascapular or

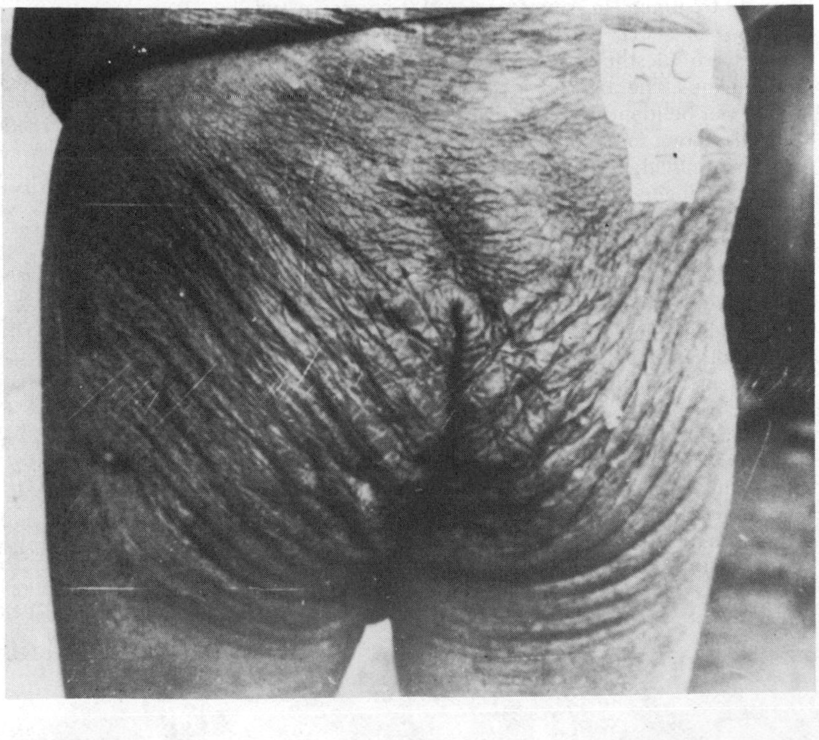

Figure 21. Complete atrophy of the skin. (From Rassi, E., et al.: Discovery of a new onchocerciasis focus in Venezuela. Bull Pan Am Health Organ 11(1):41, 1977.)

deltoid region, iliac crest, and malleolus (Yemen) are common sites. A skin fold is pinched to avoid bleeding and snipped with a razor blade. The excised skin snip is placed in a drop of water or saline on a microscope slide, and 30 minutes later the microfilariae are counted under the microscope. For maximum accuracy a biopsy may be taken from three of the sites mentioned. Another procedure is to raise a thin portion of the skin with a needle and cut it at the base with a razor blade, or use a corneal scleral punch of 2.3 to 3 mm bite.

In countries where there are other microfilariae (*Dipetalonema streptocerca* in Africa and *Mansonella ozzardi* in the Americas) besides *O. volvulus* that may be infecting the skin, it is necessary to differentiate them. The length and location of the cephalic and caudal nuclei are different in stained preparations.

When no microfilariae show up in the biopsy it is necessary to resort to the Mazzotti test.

Mazzotti Test. The test consists of an oral dose of one or two 50 mg tablets of diethylcarbamazine. Patients with onchocerciasis develop severe local symptoms in 30 minutes to a few hours after ingesting the drug. The symptoms include localized or generalized pruritus and papular erythema, eye congestion, and edema of the limbs or face. Less frequently, painful axillary or inguinal adenopathy, fever, and headache are observed. In infected patients who have never been exposed to the drug, a positive reaction is almost universal; if the drug has been taken previously, the test may be negative (Figueroa and Garcia, 1972).

PROGNOSIS. In patients with chronic and massive infestations, prognosis is not good because the disease can lead to complete blindness. Widespread dissemination of microfilariae may cause several systemic reactions.

TREATMENT. Treatment can be surgical or chemotherapeutic and must be individualized according to the severity of the lesions and general state of the patient. Treatment must be initiated before lesions become irreversible.

Surgical Treatment: Nodulectomy. This is the most common treatment in Americans, and it has decreased the incidence of ocular and cutaneous invasion. All palpable nodules are anesthetized with 2 per cent Novocain with epinephrine. The overlying skin is dissected until the nodule can be identified by its white color or by palpation. With dissecting forceps and curved scissors the lips of the incision are widened in order to isolate and excise the nodule. A finger is inserted into the cavity to ensure that the entire nodule has been removed, and then the incision is closed with one or two sutures. All this should be done with aseptic and antiseptic precautions.

If there are deep nodules or free filariae the treatment is only palliative; if not, recovery is excellent.

Chemotherapy. The drugs in common use are diethylcarbamazine, which kills microfilariae, and suramin (Germanine, Antripol, Moranil), which kills adult parasites and microfilariae.

Diethylcarbamazine. Reaction to this drug, which can be violent, calls for caution in undernourished or heavily infested patients. After two or three days the reaction subsides and the patient can continue taking the drug without any problem. To minimize the reaction, Antistin (100 mg) or Betamethasone (1 mg three times a day) may be administered during the first three or four days of treatment.

Diethylcarbamazine can be given in several dosages. An average dose is from 6 to 10 mg/kg of body weight per day (up to 600 mg per day), in three divided doses at meal times. Other schedules give 2 mg/kg body weight, three times daily for two to three weeks (Mazzotti, 1962) or 100 mg twice daily for 15 days.

Treatment of acute infections starts with lower doses that are gradually increased. Periodic treatment is palliative and not without risk.

Suramin. This is a synthetic drug derived from urea. A 10 per cent solution of the white powder is given intravenously. In patients weighing 60 kg or more, the usual dose is 1 g weekly for six or seven weeks. In patients weighing less than 60 kg, the first dose is 0.01 g/kg, and the six remaining doses are each 0.02 g/kg (Rivas, 1965). Treatment is stopped if significant proteinuria develops. Before starting treatment, the patient can be challenged with 0.1 g of the drug to determine sensitivity.

The drug kills adult parasites and microfilariae. It can cause serious toxic reaction to the patient, including edema and renal injury, and is contraindicated in patients with kidney disease. It can also cause severe exfoliative dermatitis, urticaria, and hyperkeratosis in the palms and soles. It is not recommended for mass treatment, and its use has been discontinued after several deaths in trials carried out in Africa and Guatemala (Aguilar et al., 1955). But in Venezuela, where it is still being used, 2432 cases were reported to have been treated in 1974 with no deaths.

References

Aguilar, G., Barrera, M., et al.: Proyecto piloto de una campaña de tratamiento médico de la oncocercosis, basado en la admínistración de suramina sódica (U.S.P. XIII). Bol Of Sanit Panama, 38(2), Feb. 1955.

Anderson, J., and Fuglsang, H.: Clinical aspects of onchocerciases in Uganda and Yemen Arab Republic compared with rain forest and savanna focus in Cameroon. World Health Organization-ONCHO Series No. 102. Mimeographed.

Buck, A. A.: Onchocerciasis. Symptomatology, Pathology, Diagnosis. Geneva, World Health Organization [monograph], 1974.

Castro, F.: Histological findings in some onchocercal dermatitis. Unpublished data. Pathol Laboratory, General Hospital, Guatemala.

Figueroa Marroquin, H.: Enfermedad de Robles. ¿Como salen las microfilarias del oncocercoma? Rev Invest Salud Publica 32:9, 1972.

Figueroa Marroquin, H., and Garcia, G. C.: Especificidad de la reacción de Mazzotti en el diagnóstico de la enfermedad de Robles. Rev Semana Médica Centroamérica Panamá 29(240), January 12, 1972.

Hissette, J.: Mémoire sur l'onchocerca volvulus "Leuckart," et ses manifestations oculaires au Congo Belge. Ann Soc Belge Med Trop 12(4), Dec. 1932.

Mazzotti, L.: Tratamiento de la oncocercosis. Rev Salud Publica Mexico. Epoca 5., 4(6), Nov.–Dec. 1962.

O'Neill, J.: On the presence of a filaria in craw craw. Lancet, Feb. 20, 1875.

Paul, E., and Zimmerman, L.: Some observations on the ocular pathology of onchocerciasis. Human Pathology 1:581, 1970.

Rassi, E., et al.: Discovery of a new onchocerciasis focus in Venezuela. Bull Pan Am Health Organ 11(1):41, 1977.

Reber, W. W., and Hoeppli, R.: The relationship between macroscopic skin alterations, histological changes and microfilaria in one hundred Liberians with onchocercal dermatitis. Z Tropenmed Parasitol 15(2):153, 1964.

Rendon, A., Tito, B.: La "oncocercosis," enfermedad desconocida aparece en el pais. Diaro "Universal," Section 2, Ecuador, August 30, 1980.

Rivas, A., et al.: La oncocercosis en Venezuela. Acta Med Venezol (Suppl 1), Dec. 1965.

Robles, R.: Onchocercose humaine au Guatemala produisant la cécité et "l'erysipele du littoral" (erysipela de la costa). Bull Soc Pathol Exot Paris 7, July 1919.

Rodger, F. C.: The pathogenesis and pathology of ocular onchocerciasis. Am J Opthalmol 49:104, 327, 560, 1960.

Salazar Mallen, M.: Los síntomas cutáneos de la oncocercosis. Rev Salud Publica Mexico, Epoca 5., 4(6), Nov.–Dec., 1962.

232
CUTANEOUS LARVA MIGRANS (CREEPING ERUPTION)

CHARLES E. DAVIS, M.D.

DEFINITION. Cutaneous larva migrans and creeping eruption are synonyms for the prolonged migration of dog and cat hookworm larvae in the skin of man. Because they have penetrated the skin of an "abnormal" host, these parasites cannot complete their life cycle. Instead, they wander for weeks or months in the epidermis and leave a pruritic, elevated, erythematous trail along the path of their migration. By contrast, reactions at the site of skin penetration by *Necator americanus*, *Ancylostoma duodenale* (human hookworms), and *Strongyloides stercoralis* are only a macule or papule without migration and are called "ground itch."

ETIOLOGY. By far the most common cause of cutaneous larva migrans is *Ancylostoma braziliense*, the hookworm of dogs and cats (Beaver, 1956). In 1926, Kirby-Smith et al. identified larval nematodes in skin biopsies of people in Florida with creeping eruption. Experiments on human volunteers by these investigators (White and Dove, 1928 and 1929) with third-stage infective filariform larvae of *A. braziliense* reproduced the disease that was seen in thousands of people in the southeastern United States. Many similar trials (Dove, 1932; Maplestone, 1933) with *A. caninum*, the dog hookworm, established that it could also cause creeping eruption but usually penetrated the skin less readily and migrated for less than 2 weeks. Other experiments and observations (Fulleborn, 1926a; Mayhew, 1947) established that *Uncinaria stenocephala*, the European dog hookworm, and the cattle hookworm *(Bunostomum phlebotomum)* could occasionally cause cutaneous larva migrans that was also of shorter duration than typical creeping eruption caused by *A. braziliense*.

Experiments with *Ancylostoma duodenale*, *Necator americanus*, and *Strongyloides stercoralis* (Beaver, 1945; Fulleborn, 1930; Fulleborn, 1926) indicated that these natural parasites of people cause creeping eruption rarely and only in sensitized individuals, either during or recently after intestinal infection.

The development and life cycle of the hookworms of dogs and cats is the same as the human hookworm (see Nemathelminthes, Chapter 85). After ova are passed in the feces, rhabditiform larvae hatch within 24 hours under ideal conditions in moist, sandy soil in subtropical or tropical zones. After feeding on bacteria and organic debris, the larvae molt twice, grow, and become slender, nonfeeding, infectious filariform larvae. These larvae stand upright on pieces of dirt or other organic material and wait for a warm-blooded host. They penetrate the skin on contact and reach the circulation of the normal host by migration to capillary beds. They remain localized in the skin of "abnormal" hosts and die after a few weeks to months.

A. braziliense, the usual cause of typical cutaneous larva migrans, is distributed most heavily in the southeastern and southern United States, the coastal regions of Mexico, Central America, and the tropical and subtropical coastal areas of South America and Africa. It also occurs in India, Southeast Asia, the Philippines, Taiwan, and Hong Kong. Because moist and warm sandy soil, loam, or humus favors development of the larvae, typical high risk areas include swimming beaches, sand piles, and crawl spaces under houses where dogs and cats defecate.

PATHOGENESIS AND PATHOLOGY. Penetration of the skin appears to be mechanical but is probably aided by collagenases. The adherence of caked earth or sand to the skin probably also adds purchase to the slender, filariform larvae that usually penetrate through a hair follicle. A small papule or macule may develop at the site of invasion. After 2 to 3 days, the larvae begin to migrate in the stratum germinativum with the corium as a floor and the stratum granulosum as a roof (Fig. 1). Local infiltration of eosinophilic and lymphocytic leukocytes and the movements of the larvae cause intense pruritis. Secondary bacterial infection from inoculation of bacteria by scratching may induce surrounding cellulitis and polymorphonuclear infiltration. It is likely that penetration into the dermal capillary beds or hypodermal lymphatics of the usual host is aided by enzymes that are ineffective against the dermal structures of the human being in whom the migration seems aimless and serpentine.

Since human hookworms and *S. stercoralis* cause creeping eruption primarily in sensitized individuals, it would seem that they are temporarily confined to the skin of these individuals by immune reactions.

There have been scattered reports of human intestinal infections with adult *A. braziliense*. Many of these probably represent infections with distinct but closely related species. It is possible, however, that *A. braziliense* may rarely complete its life cycle in the human being because transient pulmonary infiltrations, eosinophilia, and cough (Loeffler's syndrome) have been reported in conjunction with cutaneous larva migrans (Wright and Gold, 1946). The mere demonstration of hookworm ova in the stools of patients with cutaneous larva migrans must be interpreted with caution, however, because the ova of many hookworms are identical.

CLINICAL MANIFESTATIONS. Lesions may be single or multiple and occur most often on the hands, feet, and

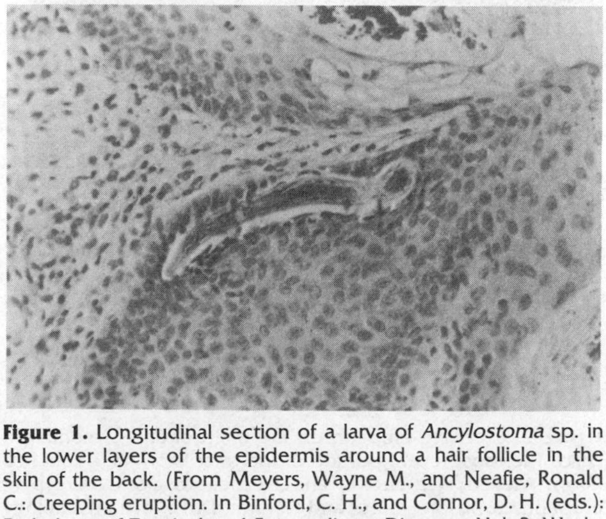

Figure 1. Longitudinal section of a larva of *Ancylostoma* sp. in the lower layers of the epidermis around a hair follicle in the skin of the back. (From Meyers, Wayne M., and Neafie, Ronald C.: Creeping eruption. In Binford, C. H., and Connor, D. H. (eds.): Pathology of Tropical and Extraordinary Diseases, Vol. 2. Washington, D.C., Armed Forces Institute of Pathology, 1976.)

buttocks of sunbathers and on the hands, shoulders, and torso of plumbers, pipefitters, and others who work under buildings and crawlspaces of houses where dogs and cats defecate. A sensation of tingling or itching at the time of penetration may be recalled by the patient. A pruritic, red papule forms within a few hours to a day after penetration. Migration begins 2 to 3 days later and causes a conspicuous, elevated, serpiginous, erythematous, intensely pruritic tunnel that marks the trail of the migrating larva. The larva, which may migrate at a rate of 1 to 2 cm per day, lies just in advance of the conspicuous portion of its trail. The unoccupied portion of the burrow dries and becomes crusted within a few days, but the larva of *A. braziliense* continues its migration for up to 1 year, circling on its own trail and producing a serpentine design (Fig. 2). The path is so serpentine that the larva usually lies only a few centimeters from the site of penetration even after months of migration. The local pruritis is enough to bring on prominent insomnia and anorexia.

Symptoms from the migration of *A. caninum, Unicinaria stenocaphala*, and *Bunostomum phlebotomum* (see *Etiology*) are indistinguishable, but the worm usually dies and the symptoms disappear within 2 weeks instead of several months. The human hookworms and *S. stercoralis* usually cause only "ground itch," a localized pruritic macule or papule at the site of penetration, but they occasionally migrate in the skin of sensitized victims for a few days or weeks. *S. stercoralis* also causes a rare form of creeping eruption called *larva currens* that is unique in two of its clinical characteristics (Fulleborn, 1926a; Caplan, 1949). First, the migration is perianal because it occurs by autoinoculation of filariform larvae that mature at the anus.

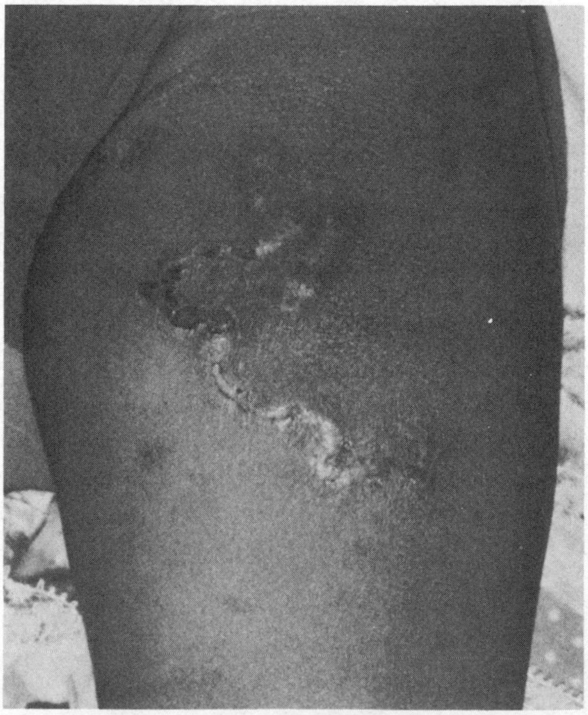

Figure 2. Creeping eruption on the thigh of an 11-month-old child. The most recent portion of the tract is on the upper left. (From Meyers, Wayne M., and Neafie, Ronald C.: Creeping eruption. In Binford, C. H., and Connor, D. H. (eds.): Pathology of Tropical and Extraordinary Diseases, Vol. 2. Washington, D.C., Armed Forces Institute of Pathology, 1976.)

Second, the migration is incredibly rapid. Instead of the rate of 1 to 2 cm per day that is characteristic of *A. braziliense* larvae, the perianal migration of *S. stercoralis* may advance at a rate of 10 cm in the first 2.5 hours. Obvious migration does not continue after 1 or 2 days; fleeting burrows at distant sites and urticarial wheals replace the typical picture of larva migrans and underscore the hypersensitive nature of this syndrome.

Cutaneous larva migrans causes only a low-grade eosinophilia and no other laboratory abnormalities.

COMPLICATIONS AND SEQUELAE. Secondary infections from autoinoculation of bacteria by scratching are common and are usually manifest by cellulitis. In the rare instances of Loeffler's syndrome, there are cough, transient pulmonary infiltrates, and eosinophilia to 50 per cent.

GEOGRAPHIC VARIATIONS IN DISEASE. There are no known geographic variations in cutaneous larva migrans, but *A. caninum* occurs as far north as New York City (Dormand and Van Ostrand, 1958) and Montreal (Choquette and Gelinas, 1950) in the Western Hemisphere. Since its northern distribution probably exceeds that of *A. braziliense*, it is likely that cutaneous larva migrans in temperate and northern climates is milder and of shorter duration than that in subtropical and tropical climates.

DIAGNOSIS. The diagnosis of cutaneous larva migrans can almost always be made clinically. The patient should recall exposure of the affected part of the body to the earth and often remembers a tingling or itching sensation that occurred within a few hours of exposure. Even without a typical history, the characteristics of the lesions are pathognomonic. Only lesions caused by *Gnathostoma spinigerum* and bot flies are easily confused with cutaneous larva migrans caused by hookworm larvae.

G. spinigerum, a natural parasite of the intestine of dogs, cats, and other carnivores, requires two waterborne intermediate hosts (microscopic crustaceans and either a fish, frog, or snake). Man becomes infected by eating the incompletely cooked flesh of the fish, frog, or snake. The larvae migrate and cause visceral larval migrans in man that may involve the lungs, meninges, and eyes. The cutaneous form may be indistinguishable clinically from creeping eruption caused by hookworm larvae except that it commonly causes nodules and abscesses that do not occur in creeping eruption. Gnathostomasis is endemic in Israel, the Indian subcontinent, Southeast Asia, and the Far East.

Larvae of the bot flies of horses (*Gasterophilus* spp.) and cattle (*Hypoderma* spp.) may also migrate superficially and be indistinguishable from true creeping eruption, but they frequently migrate into deeper tissue temporarily, leaving gaps in their trail. This condition should be considered in patients with creeping eruption who also have heavy exposure to livestock.

All larvae that migrate in the skin lie just in advance of their burrow and may be removed, examined, and identified by a skin biopsy of this area. This procedure is seldom necessary, however, because *A. braziliense* and the larvae of other hookworms cause the vast majority of creeping eruption.

TREATMENT. The traditional treatment is freezing the area around the leading edge of the tunnel with ethyl chloride spray or carbon dioxide snow. Because this treatment does not always provide permanent relief and is impractical if there are multiple lesions, treatment with local and oral anthelmintics is becoming more popular. Thiabendazole, 25 mg per kg orally twice daily for 2 days, has been used most commonly. A suspension of thiabendazole (500 mg per 5 ml) may be applied to the leading area in addition to, or instead of, oral therapy. Oral mebendazole at 1 to 2 mg per kg may be equally effective, and an ointment made up of mebendazole tablets and tetracaine (for the pruritis) cured four patients with typical creeping eruption (Winter and Fripp, 1978). Topical application of 50 per cent thiabendazole paste, an oral veterinary preparation, has been effective (Bardach, 1980).

PROPHYLAXIS. Dogs and cats should be prohibited from public beaches, and people should avoid contact with beaches on which these animals are permitted. Sandboxes in which children play should be covered to protect them from dogs and cats. Workmen who come into contact with the soil under buildings and crawl spaces under houses should wear protective clothing. Finally, dogs and cats should be dewormed periodically.

References

Bardach, H.: Topically applied thiabendazole in the treatment of creeping eruptions (cutaneous helminthiasis). Wien Med Wochenschr 130:761, 1980.

Beaver, P.: Immunity to *Necator americanus* infection. J Parasitol 31 (Suppl.):18, 1945.

Beaver, Paul C.: Parasitological Reviews. Larva migrans. Exp Parasitol V:587, 1956.

Caplan, J. P.: Creeping eruption and intestinal strongyloidiasis. Br Med J 1:396, 1949.

Choquette, L. P. E., Gelinas, L. de G.: The incidence of intestinal nematodes and protozoa in dogs of the Montreal area. Can J Comp Med 24:33, 1950.

Dormand, D. W., and Van Ostrand, J. R.: A survey of *Toxocara canis* and *Toxocara cati* in the New York City area. NY State J Med 58 (Part 2):2793, 1958.

Dove, W.: Further studies on *Ancylostoma braziliense* and the etiology of creeping eruption. Am J Hyg 15:664, 1932.

Fulleborn, F.: Hautquaddeln und "Autoinfection" bis Strongyloid estragern. Arch. Schiffs- U. Tropen-Hyg 30:721, 1926a.

Fulleborn, F.: Experimental erzeugte "Creeping eruption." Dermatol Wochschr 83:1474, 1926b.

Fulleborn, F.: Über die durch die larvae von *Ancylostoma caninum* verursachten Hauterscheinungen. Giorn Clin Med Festschr Prof Gabbi Part 1:37, 1930.

Kirby-Smith, J., Dove, W., and White, G.: Creeping eruption. Arch Dermatol Syphilol 13:137, 1926.

Maplestone, P. A.: Creeping eruption caused by hookworm larvae. Indian Med Gaz 68:251, 1933.

Mayhew, R. L.: Creeping eruption caused by the larvae of the cattle hookworm *Bunostomum phelobotomum*. Proc Soc Exp Biol Med 66:12, 1947.

White, G., and Dove, W.: The causation of creeping eruption. JAMA 90:1701, 1928.

White, G., and Dove, W.: A dermatitis caused by larvae of *Ancylostoma caninum*. Arch Dermatol Syphilol 20:191, 1929.

Winter, P. A. D., and Fripp, P. J.: Treatment of cutaneous larva migrans (Sandworm disease). S Afr Med J 52:556, 1978.

Wright, D. O., and Gold, E. M.: Löffler's syndrome associated with creeping eruption. Arch Intern Med 78:303, 1946.

233

CUTANEOUS AMEBIASIS

FRANCISCO BIAGI, M.D.

Cutaneous amebiasis is an ulcer of the skin that sometimes extends to the contiguous mucous membranes. It can occur as a complication of intestinal or hepatic amebiasis or as a primary infection with exogenous trophozoites of *Entamoeba histolytica*. It is sporadically seen in geographic areas where amebiasis is severe and common. Cutaneous amebiasis should always be included in the differential diagnosis of skin lesions in endemic areas because it is often fatal if untreated but is easy to diagnose and responds promptly to treatment.

PATHOGENESIS AND CLINICAL MANIFESTATIONS. The source of the trophozoites of *E. histolytica* and their pathway to the skin determine the location of amebic skin lesions.

1. When the skin is invaded by trophozoites from fistulae or surgery on intestinal amebiasis, the lesions are located on the perineum or the anterior abdominal wall (Fig. 1).
2. Trophozoites from spontaneous or surgical drainage of a liver abscess are located on the skin over the abdominal wall or the base of the right hemithorax. These lesions sometimes communicate with the lungs.
3. Trophozoites may be directly implanted from the exterior:
   a. Genital lesions may develop in infants with acute intestinal amebiasis because infected feces are held in contact with the skin by diapers (Fig. 2). This type of cutaneous amebiasis is more common in girls.
   b. Penile lesions may occur after rectal intercourse (Fig. 3).
   c. Rarely, cutaneous amebiasis may occur on the nose or face (Fig. 4) after implantation of trophozoites by contaminated fingers or hands. These lesions may occur in patients with no other evidence of amebiasis.

The basic pathologic process is lysis of the tissues with formation of ulcers. The inflammatory response is minimal. *E. histolytica* produces several enzymes that may be capable of degrading skin.

The ulcers are painful, bleed easily, and grow rapidly. The edges are well-defined, thick, and dark red. Small early lesions resemble cutaneous leishmaniasis. These ulcers may become very large and destroy the skin, mucous membranes, and subcutaneous tissues. Muscles are usually not invaded. The process may destroy the external genitalia. If untreated, the lesions may spread from the perineum, abdomen, thorax, or face, and become so large that the patient dies (Fig. 5).

DIAGNOSIS. The diagnosis is confirmed by demonstrating trophozoites in a fresh microscopic preparation of a

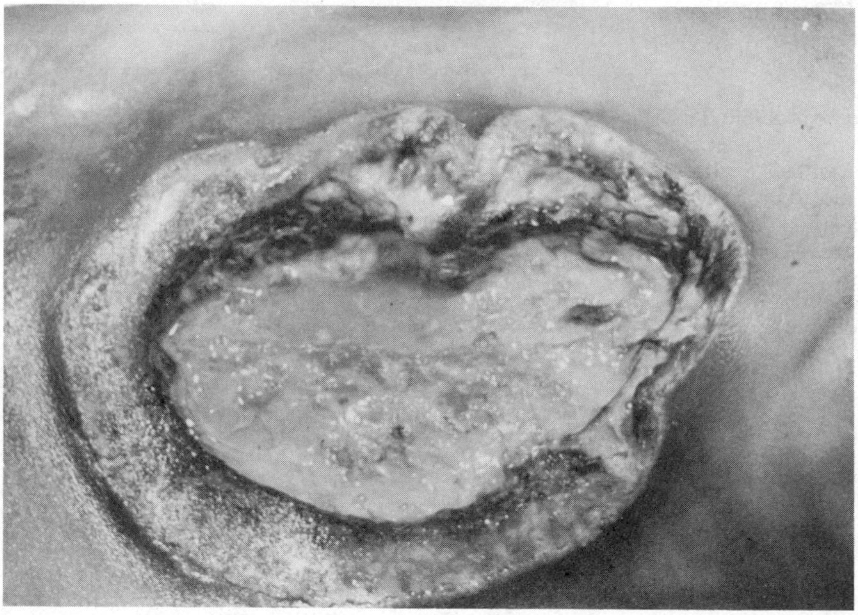

Figure 1. Cutaneous amebiasis of the abdomen after surgery for unsuspected amebic appendicitis.

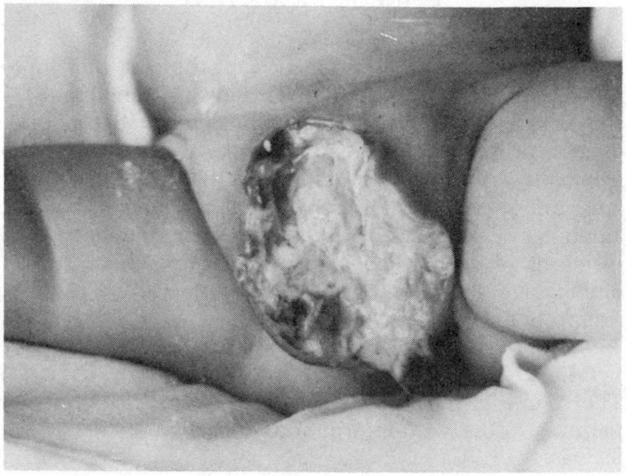

Figure 2. Infant with acute intestinal amebiasis and genital amebiasis secondary to reinvasion of trophozoites.

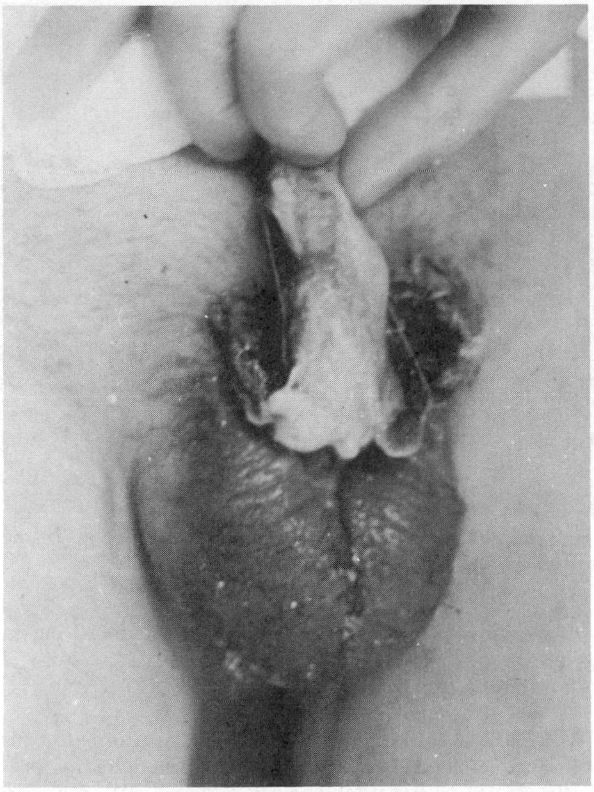

Figure 3. Cutaneous amebiasis of the penis.

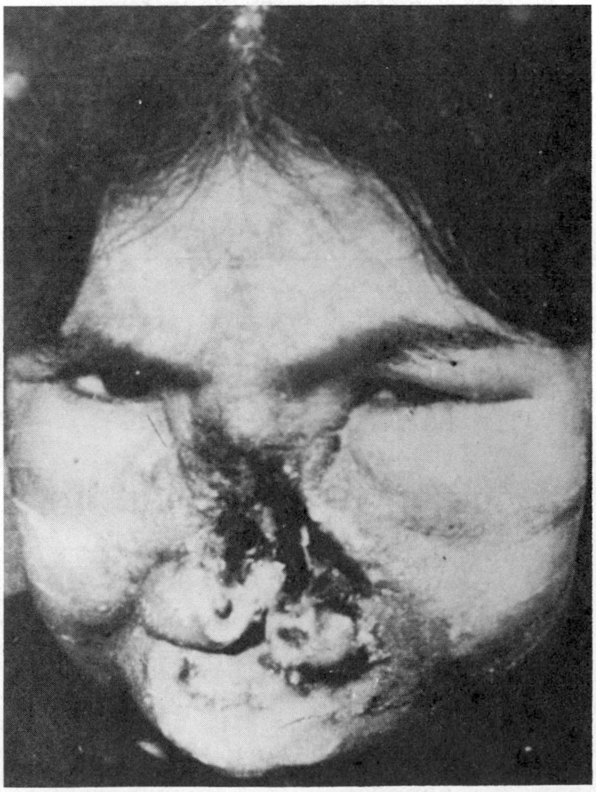

Figure 4. Cutaneous amebiasis of the face.

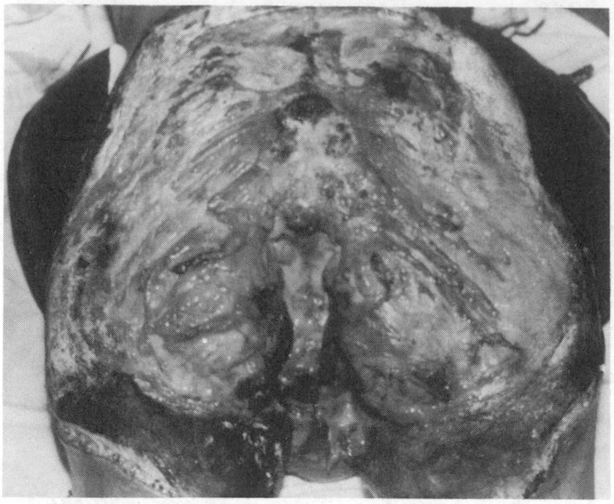

Figure 5. Fatal cutaneous amebiasis of the perineal and gluteal regions.

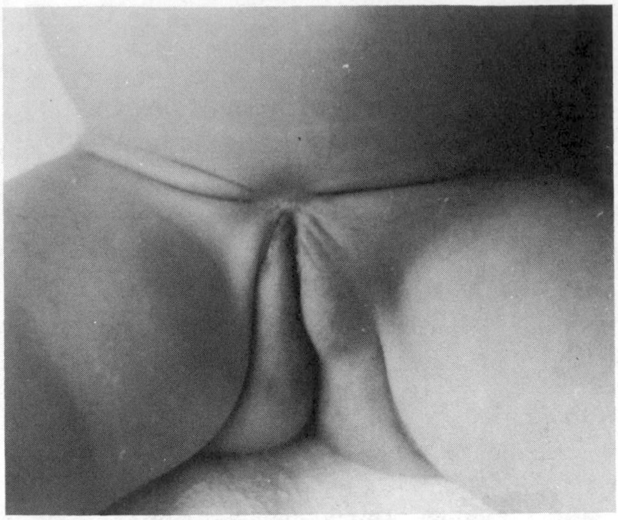

Figure 6. Healed cutaneous amebiasis after emetine. (Same case as Fig. 2)

scraping from the edge of the ulcer. The smears can be stained with iron hematoxylin to bring out details of the internal structure and permit more precise identification. Trophozoites can also be shown on histologic sections of skin biopsies stained with iron hematoxylin or hematoxylin and eosin. The amebae may also be cultivated in one of the standard media from a scraping or biopsy of the edge of the ulcer. Serologies for amebiasis are usually positive.

TREATMENT. Emetine or dehydroemetine is very effective (1 mg/kg of body weight daily for ten days) (Fig. 6). Metronidazole and nimorazole are also very effective (20 to 40 mg/kg of body weight daily for ten days), and other nitroimidazoles may be equally effective. Granulation of the skin is rapid and clean and produces good healing with little fibrosis. This prompt, complete healing may occur because of the minimal inflammatory reaction provoked by amebae. Reconstructive surgery is usually not necessary. If the lesions have grown too large (more than 20 cm in diameter), however, the patient usually dies in spite of appropriate therapy.

PROPHYLAXIS. In addition to general measures to control or avoid amebiasis, a few specific principles for prevention of cutaneous amebiasis can be listed: (1) Amebiasis should be treated early, preferably during the carrier state; (2) infants with diarrhea should be cleaned and changed frequently; and (3) surgery of amebic bowel lesions or liver abscesses should be done under cover of emetine or a nitroimidazole.

References

Biagi, F.: Amibiasis cutánea. Prensa Med Mex 30(5–6):155, 1965.

Meleney, F. L., and Meleney, H. E.: Gangrene of the buttocks, perineum and scrotum due to *Entamoeba histolytica*. Arch Surg 30:980, 1953.

234

CUTANEOUS AND MUCOCUTANEOUS LEISHMANIASIS (ORIENTAL SORE, ESPUNDIA)

ANTHONY D.M. BRYCESON, M.D., F.R.C.P.E.

Cutaneous leishmaniasis is an infection with one of the cutaneous species of parasites of the genus *Leishmania* (see Table 1). It is usually a zoonosis transmitted by phlebotomine sandflies between wild or peridomestic animals, especially rodents or carnivores. Man is infected when he interrupts the natural cycle. Human infection is characterized by one or several chronic sores that usually heal spontaneously. In parts of South and Central America, severe mutilating metastatic lesions of the mouth and nose are seen.

ETIOLOGY AND EPIDEMIOLOGY. The morphology and biology of *Leishmania* are described in Chapter 84 (Hommel, 1978).

In the Old World the innumerable names of this disease (Delhi or Baghdad boil, Biskra button, Aleppo evil, bouton de Crete, little sister) testify to its scope and familiarity throughout the Mediterranean basin, the Near and Middle East, and parts of India. At least six epidemiologic situations are recognized.

"Rural" leishmaniasis throughout these areas is caused by *L. major*. The disease is a zoonosis among the desert gerbils (*Rhomobomys opimus*, *Psammomys obesus*, *Meriones* spp.) and is transmitted to man by *Phlebotomus papatasii*. When village settlements are close to gerbil colonies, 100 per cent of the population may become

Table 1. EPIDEMIOLOGY OF CUTANEOUS LEISHMANIASIS

Parasite	Vector to Man	Reservoir	Geography	Human Disease
		OLD WORLD		
L. tropica	*Phlebotomus sergenti*	Man, dog	Middle East, Mediterranean	"Urban" sores and leishmaniasis recidivans
L. major	*Phlebotomus papatasi,* etc.	Rodents, esp. *Rhombomys, Meriones*	Middle East, India, Pakistan, Central Asia, North Africa	"Rural" sores
L. major	*Phlebotomus duboscqi*	*Arvicanthus,* etc.	West Africa, Sudan	"Rural" sores
L. aethiopica	*Phlebotomus longipes, pedifer*	Hyraxes	Ethiopian and Kenyan highlands	Simple sores and diffuse cutaneous leishmaniasis
L. donovani	*Phlebotomus ariasi,* etc.	Dogs	Southern Europe, North Africa	Simple sores
Unnamed	*Phlebotomus rossi*	?	Namibia	Simple sores
		NEW WORLD		
L. mexicana mexicana	*Lutzomyia olmeca*	Numerous forest rodents	Yucatan, Belize, Guatemala	"Chicle ulcer," "bay sore" in forest workers; diffuse cutaneous leishmaniasis
L. mexicana amazonensis	*Lutzomyia flaviscutellata*	Numerous rodents, esp. *Proechimys,* marsupials, fox	All South American forests; ? = *L. pifanoi,* Venezuela	Rare, single skin lesions; diffuse cutaneous leishmaniasis
L. brasiliensis brasiliensis	*Psychodopygus wellcomei, Lutzomyia* spp.	Several forest rodents	All South American forests, Costa Rica, Belize	Single or few large, persistent, destructive skin ulcers; oronasal metastases common: "espundia"
L. brasiliensis guyanensis	*Lutzomyia umbratilis*	Sloth *(Choloepus didactylus),* anteaters	Guyanas, Surinam, into Brazil and Venezuela	"Forest yaws," "pian-bois," ?oronasal metastases
L. brasiliensis panamensis	*Lutzomyia trapidoi, Psychodopygus, panamensis,* etc.	Sloths, esp. *Choloepus hoffmanni,* procyonids, monkeys	Panama, Costa Rica, Colombia	Skin ulcers, ?oronasal metastases
L. brasiliensis peruviana	*Lutzomyia verrucarum, Lutzomyia peruensis*	Dogs	Peru, west slopes of Andes to 3000 meters, Argentinian highlands	"Uta;" single or few skin lesions, healing in one year

infected, usually in early childhood, but there may be periodic epidemics. Travelers, hunters, and soldiers also get the disease. In "urban" leishmaniasis, the parasite *L. minor* is adapted to dogs and to man, either of which can act as a reservoir. *P. sergenti* is the main vector. This disease was formerly the scourge of Middle Eastern cities. Every adult inhabitant bore the scars, and few visitors were spared. Iso-enzyme typing of human isolates has shown that *L. donovani* may also cause self-healing sores, without visceral disease, in patients living in certain parts of the Mediterranean basin.

In Africa two distinct zoonoses exist. In the sub-Saharan savanna belt of West Africa, extending as far east as Sudan, the situation is "rural." *L. major* is the parasite. Human cases are uncommon and sporadic. Rodents, especially the Nile rat, *Arvicanthus niloticus,* and *Tatera* spp., are the reservoir and *P. duboscqi* the vector. In Ethiopia and Kenya the disease is caused by *L. aethiopica* and is confined to the highlands, where the reservoir is the rock hyrax (*Procavia*). The vector, *P. longipes,* or *P. pedifer,* bites villagers at night in their houses. A few isolated cases of cutaneous leishmaniasis have been reported in Central Africa, and there is a focus in Namibia. The epidemiology is unknown.

In the New World, cutaneous leishmaniasis is endemic in Central and South America as far south as the Parana Estuary in the east and the Peruvian Andes in the west, and the border of Mexico with Texas to the north. In this extensive and varied terrain many different zoonoses exist, each associated with its own reservoirs and vector and a particular pattern of human disease (Lainson, 1983). Two groups of parasites are distinguished, those of *L. mexicana* and of *L. brasiliensis. L. mexicana,* which grows easily in NNN medium and in the hamster, is responsible for most of the cutaneous leishmaniasis in Mexico, and a little in Central and South America. Rates of infection among forest rodents may be as high as 20 per cent, but the vector is not attracted to man, so human infection is rare except in Mexican chicle collectors who are exposed to intense contact with infective sandflies at the time of maximum transmission. *L. brasiliensis,* which grows poorly in NNN medium and in the hamster and has a distinctive phase of development in the hind gut of the sandfly, is responsible for most of the disease in South America, including mucocutaneous leishmaniasis. All the vectors of *L. brasiliensis* are highly anthropophilic and will bite man viciously by night or day, so that the rate of infection among those who enter the forest is high. In Panama the natural sloth-sandfly cycle takes place in the treetops rather than on the forest floor, but the vector rests on the lower parts of tree trunks, from which it is attracted to man.

Cutaneous leishmaniasis presents a formidable obstacle to the development of the Central and South American forests. This is particularly true in Brazil, where new settlers and workers in the forest, become infected and run the risk of developing mutilating oronasal metastatic lesions.

In the Peruvian Andes and Argentinian highlands the parasite *L. b. peruviana* has adapted to the high, dry climate and sparse vegetation. The dog is the reservoir, and transmission is domiciliary.

Epidemiologic data are summarized in the table.

PATHOGENESIS. The patterns of disease in man are partly determined by the parasite and partly by man's response to the parasite (Bryceson, 1975; Ridley, 1979). Dermatotropic species of *Leishmania* are sensitive to temperatures above 35° C and will grow only on the exposed, cooler areas of skin. Some species are more immunogenic and allergenic than others. *Leishmania* organisms may eventually destroy the macrophages in which they multiply but do not otherwise damage their host directly. Resistance to *Leishmania* depends on the development of specific cell-mediated immunity. The capacity of individuals to mount such a response varies, and consequently cutaneous leishmaniasis presents a spectrum of disease similar to that seen in leprosy. At one end of the spectrum is diffuse cutaneous leishmaniasis, characterized by an abundance of parasites, absence of lymphocytes in lesions, dermal insensitivity to injection of leishmanin (a suspension of promastigotes), and poor prognosis. At the other end are the self-healing sores, characterized by relatively scanty parasites, marked lymphocytic infiltration, and leishmanin sensitivity. Accompanying cell-mediated immunity is delayed hypersensitivity to numerous parasite antigens, which seems to cause the destructive pathology of leishmanial ulcers, which in turn seems to be an essential step toward healing, unlike the situation in leprosy. In the chronic conditions of mucocutaneous leishmaniasis and leishmaniasis recidivans the normal balance between immunity and hypersensitivity has been lost, so that healing is prevented.

PATHOLOGY. At the site of inoculation there is a massive infiltration of monocytes and histiocytes, which take up the parasites and support their growth. The lesion then becomes surrounded by or mixed with lymphocytes and a few plasma cells. Macrophages develop into epithelioid cells, foci of necrosis appear, the overlying dermis ulcerates, and parasites diminish. Later, tubercles composed of loosely packed cells may develop. The epidermis shows hyperkeratosis, acanthosis, pseudo-epitheliomatous hyperplasia, intraepidermal necrosis, and ulceration. Healing is accompanied by fibrosis.

In diffuse cutaneous leishmaniasis, cell-mediated immunity fails to develop, and the disease spreads to other parts of the skin (Petersen et al., 1982). Histologic study shows masses of heavily parasitized macrophages with little or no lymphocytic infiltration or epidermal change.

In leishmaniasis recidivans, failure to heal is associated with extreme chronicity, a tuberculoid histology with epithelioid giant cells but no caseation, and scanty or undetectable parasites.

Metastatic lesions of *L. brasiliensis* arise in the mucosa of the nose and mouth and show at first a typical leishmanial granuloma with numerous parasites. The parasites later become scanty, and can be seen also in cells in cartilage, which is rapidly invaded and destroyed. There is vasculitis with edema, necrosis, and fibrosis.

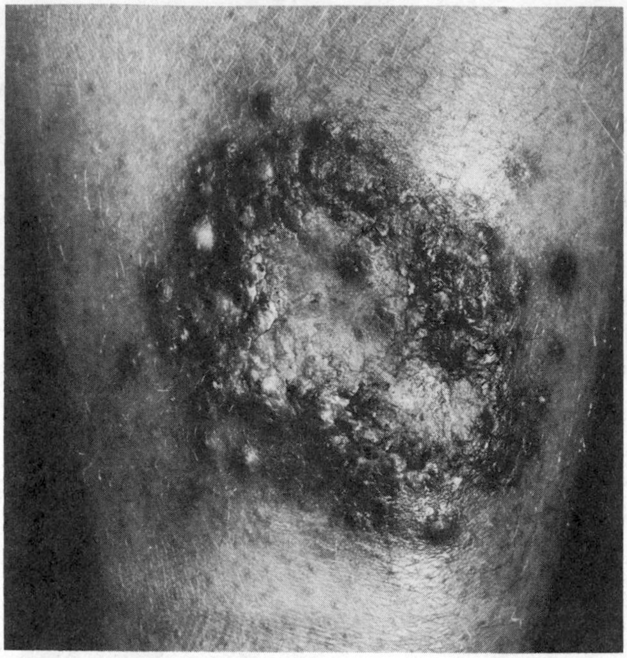

Figure 1. Oriental sore from the Middle East, showing the classic appearance of cutaneous leishmaniasis: elevated lesion with central crusting, satellite papules, and little peripheral inflammation. (Courtesy of St. John's Hospital for Diseases of the Skin, London.)

CLINICAL MANIFESTATIONS. The earliest lesion is a small erythematous papule, appearing two to eight weeks after the sandfly bite. It may itch slightly. The prototype is the "urban" sore, caused by *L. tropica* which grows slowly into a nodule 1 to 2 cm across, and after a period of weeks or months forms a central crust overlying a shallow ulcer with an elevated margin (Fig. 1). The edge of the lesion is characteristically studded with small satellite papules. The sore usually remains in this state for a few more months and then heals gradually, leaving a depressed, mottled scar. The whole process takes from three months to two years. The most common site is the face, followed by the arms and legs. Soles, palms, axillae, and scalp are usually spared. There may be one or several sores.

COMPLICATIONS AND SEQUELAE. Healing is usually followed by lifelong immunity. Second infections are seen in only about 2 in 1000 cases of oriental sore, usually in older patients or in those taking corticosteroid drugs. Immunity is usually species-specific, but *L. major* protects against *L. tropica.* About 1 per cent of patients with urban sores develop leishmaniasis recidivans (lupoid leishmaniasis) (Fig. 2). In this condition the ulcer fails to heal completely. It either spreads peripherally from the central scar or heals and recrudesces at the edge of the scar. The lesion lasts for many years and resembles cutaneous tuberculosis. This complication is less common with *L. major* and *L. aethiopica* and is not seen in the New World.

Diffuse cutaneous leishmaniasis develops in the rare patient without specific cellular immunity. This complica-

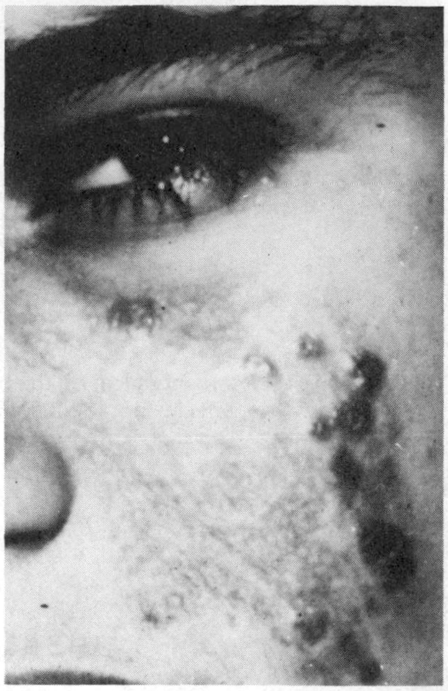

Figure 2. Leishmaniasis recidivans from Baghdad. Nodules persist in the edge of a scarred healed sore. (Courtesy of Professor G. F. Rhahim.)

tion is associated with only three species of parasite (see next section).

GEOGRAPHIC VARIATIONS. The diverse epidemiology of cutaneous leishmaniasis is associated with many different clinical patterns. Some of these patterns are distinct, while others are themselves a spectrum of disease that merges into other patterns.

There are many variants of the typical pattern of the Old World oriental sore. "Rural" sores, caused by *L. major*, are commonly multiple, rapid in evolution, more florid, heal in 3 to 5 months and produce more scarring. West African sores, usually found on the limbs, are often multiple and extremely crusty. Ethiopian lesions are solitary, facial, milder, and slower in evolution, often lasting several years before healing with little or no ulceration. Primary lesions affecting the mucocutaneous border of the nose are common in Ethiopia and are extremely chronic and disfiguring.

Ethiopia and Kenya are the only Old World countries where diffuse cutaneous leishmaniasis is found. It is a rare condition, occurring in perhaps 1 in 3,000 cases of leishmaniasis due to *L. aethiopica*. The primary nodule does not ulcerate. After a period of months or years it spreads locally, and the disease is disseminated to other parts of the skin, notably the face and the extensor surfaces of the limbs. These infiltrative and nodular lesions may resemble lepromatous leprosy (Fig. 3) and do not heal spontaneously. The viscera are not involved, and the patient feels well.

In the New World, many sores conform to the Old World prototype, especially "uta" due to *L. b. peruviana* and the majority of lesions due to *L. m. mexicana*, the "chicle ulcer" or "bay sore" (Fig. 4) of forest workers in Yucatan and Central America that is commonly seen on the face and heals in less than six months. *L. m. mexicana* lesions are, however, especially common on the pinna, where they may last for many years, slowly destroying the cartilage (Fig. 5). Human infections with *L. m. amazonensis* are rare, but up to 30 per cent cause diffuse cutaneous leishmaniasis. There is a focus of diffuse cutaneous leishmaniasis in the Dominican Republic, due to an unnamed parasite. The validity of *L. m. pifanoi*, *L. m. garnhami*, and *L. m. venezuelensis*, as distinct agents of cutaneous leishmaniasis, is not yet fully established.

Primary lesions of *L. b. brasiliensis* are often frankly and deeply ulcerative. They occur most commonly on the limbs, are often multiple, and heal spontaneously. American Indians commonly develop transient mild infections, so that by the age of 40 almost all are sensitive to leishmanin. They rarely develop mucocutaneous lesions. Lesions due to *L. b. guyanensis*, known as "forest yaws" or "pian bois,"

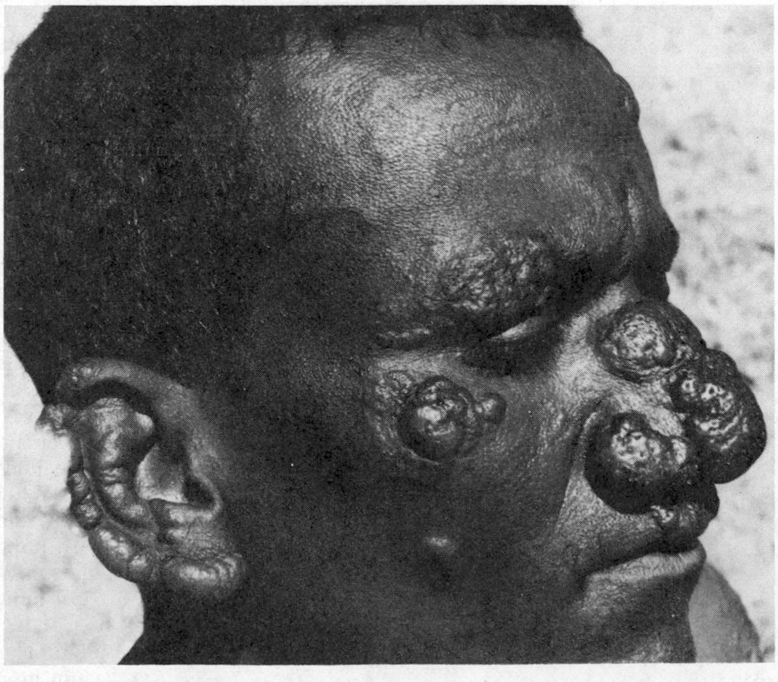

Figure 3. Diffuse cutaneous leishmaniasis caused by *L. aethiopica* in an Ethiopian. Note the resemblance with post–kala-azar dermal leishmaniasis and lepromatous leprosy. (Courtesy of Dr. A. Bryceson and Trans. R Soc Trop Med Hyg.)

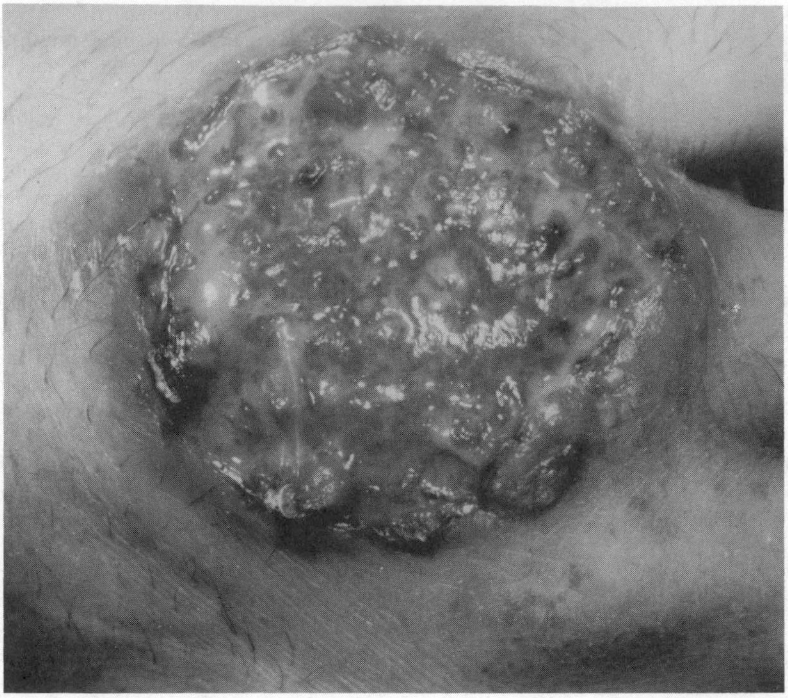

Figure 4. Leishmanial ulcer on the back of hand. From Belize; species not identified.

and *L. b. panamensis* have a tendency to produce nodular or cord-like lesions in the draining lymphatic vessels.

American Mucocutaneous Leishmaniasis. Primary lesions of *L. b. brasiliensis* are followed after a period ranging from a few days to 25 years by metastatic lesions of the nose or mouth, most commonly on the mucocutaneous borders, but sometimes on the palate or larynx and rarely on the conjunctiva or external genitalia (Marsden and Nonata, 1975). Nasal obstruction is the most common early symptom. These lesions may arise many years after the primary lesion has healed. At first there is crusting or polyp formation, and then ulceration and perforation of the septum. Alternatively, large protruding granulomas of the nose and lips develop (Fig. 6). The lesion heals slowly, if at all, after many years. Scarring may constrict the nose or mouth, producing gross deformity and making eating difficult. Secondary sepsis is common and increases the patient's debility. The prevalence of this complication, sometimes called espundia (Portuguese for sponge), varies from 2 per cent in Panama, where few cases of the disease are due to *L. b. brasiliensis*, to 80 per cent in Paraguay, where most cases of the disease are due to this agent. The complication is usually prevented by adequate chemotherapy of the primary lesion.

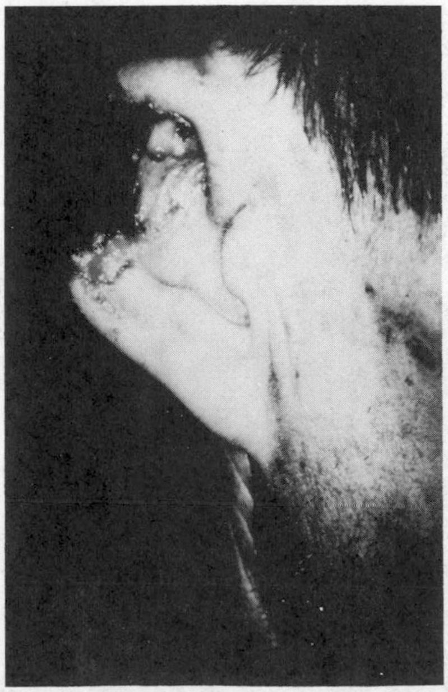

Figure 5. Chronic destructive lesion caused by *L. mexicana mexicana* on the pinna of a Mexican chiclero. (Courtesy Dr. J. E. Ash.)

Diffuse cutaneous leishmaniasis has been described in Venezuela, northern Brazil, Mexico, and Texas. Its clinical features are the same as in Ethiopia.

DIAGNOSIS. Leishmaniasis must be suspected as the cause of any chronic nodule or ulcer in a person who lives in or has recently visited an endemic area. Typical sores can be diagnosed on sight. Diagnosis is confirmed by finding parasites in stained slit-skin smears taken from a nonulcerated part of the lesion (Fig. 7). The slit must reach the dermis; the smears must contain tissue juice, not blood or pus. If this technique is unsuccessful, the crust should be removed, the ulcer cleaned of all debris, and smears made of tissue scraped from the base of the ulcer. These methods are simpler and more likely to show parasites than histology. In lesions of leishmaniasis recidivans and in mucocutaneous lesions, parasites are scanty, and culture of tissue juice or biopsy tissue may be necessary (Chapter 152). Whenever possible, parasites should be isolated in culture and identified by iso-enzyme typing. This is especially important in areas where *L. b. brasiliensis* or *L. donovani* occur.

Leishmanin (Montenegro) Test. Leishmanin is a suspension of 10^6 promastigotes in 1 ml of 0.5 per cent phenol-saline. The test is performed by injecting 0.1 ml of leishmanin intradermally into the volar surface of the forearm.

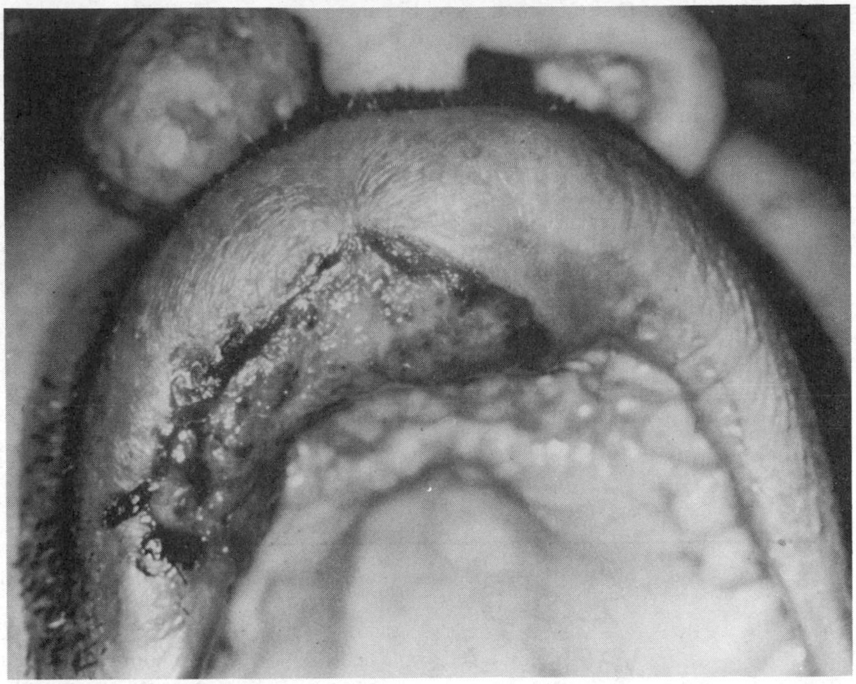

Figure 6. Mucocutaneous leishmaniasis caused by *L. braziliensis.* There is granulomatous infiltration of the palate, ulceration of the lip, and a polypoid lesion in the right nostril. (Courtesy of Professor A. Pons.)

A palpable nodule, 5 mm or more in diameter after 48 to 72 hours, is considered positive. The test is an index of delayed hypersensitivity but not necessarily of immunity to *Leishmania*. It is not species-specific. It is used to map out the extent of past infection in a community and may help in the diagnosis of individual patients.

The leishmanin test becomes positive as the lesion ulcerates and is of diagnostic value in patients who do not live in endemic areas; it also may help to distinguish lupoid leishmaniasis from cutaneous tuberculosis, late syphilis, blastomycosis, histoplasmosis, and other fungal granulomas that may be histologically similar.

Antibodies may be detected by indirect immunofluorescence in over 90 per cent of patients with American mucocutaneous leishmaniasis, and in a smaller proportion of patients with simple sores from the New World (Walton et al., 1972). Serologic tests have not generally been found helpful in the diagnosis of cutaneous leishmaniasis in the Old World.

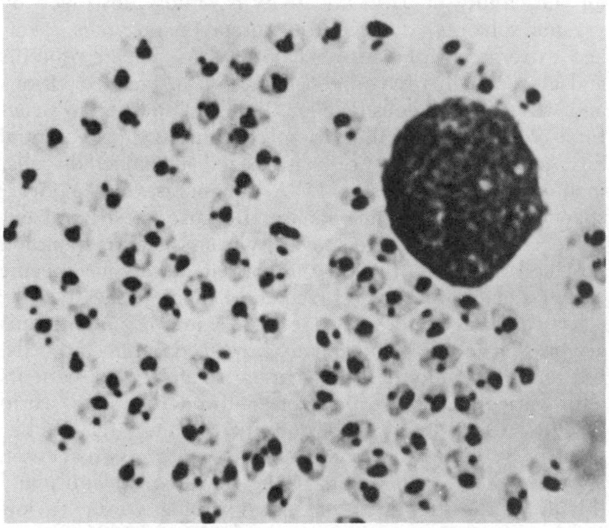

Figure 7. Macrophage containing numerous amastigotes of *Leishmania* in a smear from the tail of *Oryzomys capito*, a rodent reservoir of *L. mexicana amazonensis.* A similar appearance is seen in slit skin smears from human cutaneous lesions or marrow aspiration smears in visceral leishmaniasis. (Courtesy of Dr. R. Lainson, Dr. J. Shaw, and Trans R Soc Trop Med Hyg.)

TREATMENT. Treatment is unsatisfactory (World Health Organization, 1983). In most parts of the world lesions heal spontaneously, and the systemic use of toxic drugs is seldom justified. Any patient with a lesion that could be due to *L. brasiliensis* should be thoroughly treated with systemic pentavalent antimony as described in Chapter 152.

Local Treatment. Success has been claimed for local infiltration with 15 per cent mepacrine, or 0.3 to 0.8 ml sodium stibogluconate. The local application of heat, whereby the lesion is held at 40 to 43° C for several hours daily, is usually successful. Cryotherapy has also been used successfully (Bassiouny et al., 1982).

Leishmaniasis recidivans heals poorly and may require intralesional injections of corticosteroids combined with a course of antimony, or curettage and skin grafting.

Systemic Treatment. Most cases respond to a course of pentavalent antimony, which is usually not toxic and should be given until the lesion is nearly healed (see Chapter 152). *L. brasiliensis* lesions are treated until they are well healed. Failure to respond is usually due to inadequate dosage or duration of treatment. Established American mucocutaneous lesions often fail to respond to antimony or relapse after its use. Amphotericin B is then the drug of choice (see Chapter 152). Diffuse cutaneous leishmaniasis responds initially to antimony in South America but is resistant in Ethiopia. Amphotericin B- or pentamidine may then be tried. Treatment must be given for several months without interruption, but frequent relapses are the rule.

PROPHYLAXIS. Detailed epidemiologic knowledge has permitted attacks on the reservoir of this disease in Central Asia and in Middle Eastern cities, where demolition of mud buildings and antimalarial spraying have reduced the number of sandflies. Destruction of gerbil burrows removes the reservoir. Immunization with live, virulent organisms is practiced on a mass scale in Russia and in the Middle East.

Prevention in South America is difficult. Intensity of transmission in the forest and lack of detailed epidemiologic information make mass prophylaxis a hopeless approach at the moment. People who are obliged to enter the forest should try to apply insect repellents every few hours and sleep under a fine mesh netting, even though these procedures are uncomfortable and inconvenient, and wear long sleeved shirts and trousers.

References

Bassiouny, A., Meshad, M. El., Talaat, M., Kutty, K., and Metawa, B.: Cryosurgery in cutaneous leishmaniasis. Br J Derm 107:467, 1982.

Bryceson, A. D. M.: Mechanisms of disease in leishmaniasis. In Taylor, A., and Muller, R. (eds.): Pathogenic Processes in Parasitic Infections. Oxford, Blackwell Scientific Publications, 1975, p. 85.

Hommel, M.: The genus *Leishmania*: biology of the parasite and clinical aspects. Bull Inst Pasteur 76:5, 1978.

Lainson, R.: The American leishmaniases: some observations on their ecology and epidemiology. Trans R Soc Trop Med Hyg 77:569, 1983.

Marsden, P. D., and Nonata, R. R.: Mucocutaneous leishmaniasis: A review of clinical aspects. Rev Soc Bras Med Trop 9:309, 1975.

Petersen, E. A., Neva, F. A., Oster, C. N., and Diaz, H. B.: Specific inhibition of lymphocyte-proliferation responses by adherent suppressor cells in diffuse cutaneous leishmaniasis. N Engl J Med 306:387, 1982.

Ridley, D. S.: The pathogenesis of cutaneous leishmaniasis. Trans R Soc Trop Med Hyg 73:150, 1979.

Walton, B. C., Brooks, W. H., and Aronja, I.: Serodiagnosis of American leishmaniasis by indirect fluorescent antibody test. Am J Trop Med Hyg 21:296, 1972.

World Health Organization: Report of the workshop on chemotherapy of Old World Cutaneous Leishmaniasis. TDR/LEISH/CL-JER/83.3 Geneva, 1983.

235

VARICELLA

MICHAEL N. OXMAN, M.D.

Varicella (chickenpox) and herpes zoster (shingles, zoster) are distinct clinical entities which are both caused by the same virus, varicella-zoster virus (VZV), a member of the herpesvirus family. The differences between these two diseases result from differences in the host and in the circumstances of infection, and not from differences in the etiologic agent.

Varicella, an acute, highly contagious exanthematous disease that occurs most often in childhood, is the result of primary exogenous infection of a susceptible individual. It is characterized by a short or absent prodromal period and a generalized pruritic rash consisting of successive crops of lesions that progress rapidly from macules and papules to vesicles, pustules, and crusts. In normal children, systemic symptoms are usually mild, and serious complications are extremely rare. In adults and in immunologically compromised individuals of any age, varicella is more likely to be associated with an extensive eruption, high fever, severe constitutional symptoms, pneumonia, and other life-threatening complications.

ETIOLOGY. Heberden (1767) is credited with first differentiating varicella from smallpox, the former being a benign pruritic eruption without residua and the latter being a serious disease causing disfigurement and death. However, more than a century later such authorities as Osler (1892) deemed it necessary to emphasize that the two diseases were indeed etiologically distinct. The name "chickenpox" is probably derived from the Old English *gican*, to itch (Scott-Wilson, 1978). Steiner in 1875 transmitted the disease to volunteers by the inoculation of vesicle fluid from patients with varicella. Tyzzer described the histopathology of the skin lesions of varicella in 1906 and called attention to the characteristic multinucleated giant cells and intranuclear inclusion bodies. However, it was not until 1952 that Weller and Stoddard succeeded in isolating and propagating the virus from varicella vesicle fluid in vitro.

VZV is a member of the herpesvirus family. Other members pathogenic for humans include herpes simplex virus type 1 (HSV-1) and type 2 (HSV-2), cytomegalovirus (CMV), and the Epstein-Barr virus (EBV) of infectious mononucleosis (Roizman et al., 1981). All of these herpesviruses are morphologically indistinguishable and share a number of properties, including a remarkable propensity for establishing latent infections that persist for the life of the host. VZV consists of an icosahedral capsid 100 nm in diameter that encloses the viral genome, a linear molecule of double-stranded DNA with a molecular weight of about 90 million daltons. The capsid is composed of 162 protein subunits (capsomers), which resemble elongated hexagonal or pentagonal prisms with an axial hole (Fig. 1B). The nucleocapsid is surrounded by one or two additional layers of protein and, finally, by a loose lipoprotein envelope derived from the nuclear membrane of the host cell and containing radially oriented viral glycoproteins on its surface (Fig. 1A). The complete virion is roughly spherical with a diameter of 150 to 200 nm (Almeida et al., 1962). Only enveloped virions are infectious, and this accounts for the lability of VZV; infectivity is rapidly destroyed by organic solvents, detergents, proteolytic enzymes, heat, and extremes of pH. More than 40 virus-specific proteins and glycoproteins have been identified in purified virions and VZV-infected cells (Weller, 1983). In addition to structural components of the virion, certain enzymes essential for virus replication are synthesized in infected cells, including a virus-specific DNA polymerase and a virus-specific deoxypyrimidine kinase. Because these viral enzymes differ in substrate specificity from the corresponding host cell enzymes, they are important targets for specific antiviral chemotherapy (Hirsch and Schooley, 1983).

There is only one VZV serotype. A number of antigens are present in the virion and are produced in infected cells, but these are identical in viruses isolated from patients with varicella and herpes zoster throughout the world (Weller, 1979; Taylor-Robinson and Caunt, 1972; Weller et al., 1958). However, some VZV antigens cross-react with antigens of other members of the herpesvirus family and this limits the usefulness of certain serologic tests (Taylor-Robinson and Caunt, 1972; Weller, 1979 and 1982; Shiraki et al., 1982).

The DNA of VZV is a double-stranded linear molecule composed of a long unique region and a short unique region flanked by inverted repeat sequences. VZV DNA

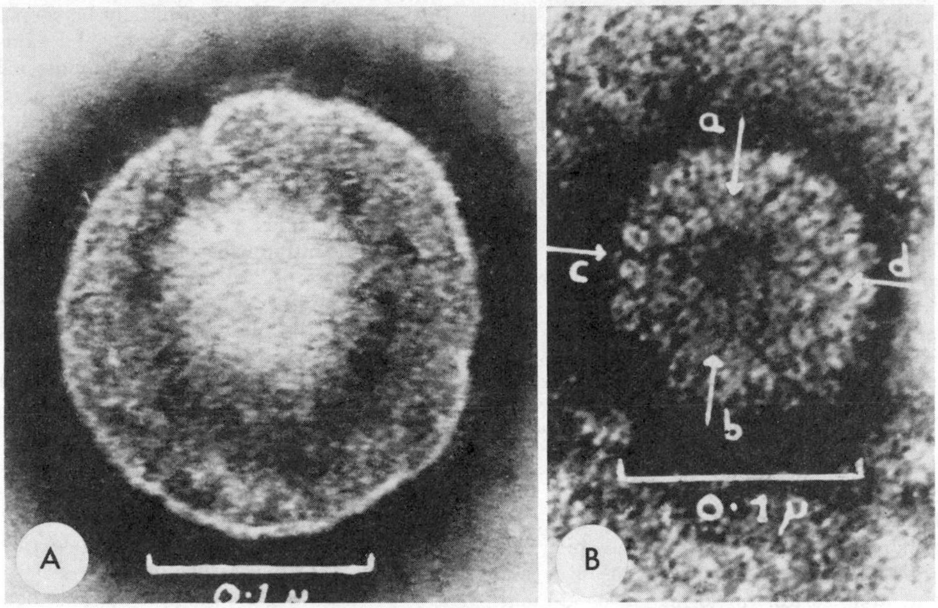

Figure 1. Varicella-zoster virus stained with phosphotungstic acid. *A,* Intact particle showing envelope with radially oriented glycoproteins on its surface. *B,* Rupture of the envelope reveals the nucleocapsid within. (From Almeida, J. D., Howatson, A. F., and Williams, M. G.: Virology 16:353, 1962.)

extracted from purified virions or infected cells is a mixture of two isomers that differ by inversion of the short unique region; the biological significance of this phenomenon is unknown (Straus et al., 1981; Ecker and Hyman, 1982; Gilden et al., 1982). The DNA of viruses isolated from cases of varicella and herpes zoster throughout the world is basically similar, but minor variations in nucleotide sequence give the genomes of different clinical isolates of VZV slightly different restriction endonuclease cleavage patterns (i.e., each isolate has a unique pattern or "fingerprint"). More substantial differences distinguish the OKA live attenuated VZV vaccine (vide infra) from wild-type VZV isolates, and there is little resemblance between the restriction endonuclease cleavage pattern of VZV and those of the other human herpesviruses (HSV-1, HSV-2, CMV, and EBV). These differences are useful epidemiologically, in that isolates from common source outbreaks will have identical restriction endonuclease cleavage patterns, and when illness occurs in vaccinees or their contacts the responsible agent, vaccine virus or wild-type VZV, can be determined (Ecker and Hyman, 1981; Martin et al., 1982; Hyman, 1983; Weller, 1983; Hayakawa et al., 1984).

VZV can be isolated and progated in vitro in monolayer cultures of a variety of human (and certain simian) cells (Taylor-Robinson and Caunt, 1972; Weller, 1979 and 1983). The cytopathic effect in such cell cultures is characterized by the formation of acidophilic intranuclear inclusion bodies and multinucleated giant cells similar to those seen in the cutaneous lesions of the disease. These changes are indistinguishable from those produced by herpes simplex virus. Herpes simplex virus is released into the medium by initially infected cells and rapidly spreads to infect the remaining cells in the culture, whereas the cytopathic effect of VZV remains focal. This is because infectious VZV remains cell-associated and is not released into the medium by the initially infected cells; infection proceeds from cell to cell only by direct contact, and the initial foci of infection gradually enlarge. Serial passage of VZV in tissue culture requires the transfer of infected cells.

Studies of the molecular biology and pathogenesis of VZV infection have been hampered by difficulty in obtaining adequate quantities of cell-free virus and by the absence of suitable animal models. Some progress has been made in preparing cell-free virus, and the application of molecular cloning procedures has facilitated the physical mapping of the VZV genome (Straus et al., 1982). VZV has now been isolated and propagated in guinea pig cells, and a guinea pig model of VZV infection and transmission has been established (Myers et al., 1980; Weller, 1983).

PATHOGENESIS AND PATHOLOGY. Our concept of the pathogenesis of varicella is based primarily on circumstantial evidence, analogy with experimental models of other exanthematous diseases (Fenner, 1948), and postmortem examination of fatal cases. The virus probably enters through the mucosa of the upper respiratory tract and oropharynx. Initial multiplication there results in dissemination of small amounts of virus via the blood and lymphatics (the primary viremia) to the reticuloendothelial system, which is probably the major site of virus replication during the remainder of the incubation period. The incubating infection is partially contained by nonspecific defenses (e.g., interferon and nonspecific killer [NK] cell activity) and developing immune responses. In most individuals, virus replication eventually overwhelms these defenses so that at about two weeks after infection a much larger viremia (the secondary viremia) occurs (Feldman and Epp, 1979). This causes fever and malaise and disseminates virus throughout the body, especially to the skin and mucous membranes, where foci of infection are initiated by the infection of capillary endothelial cells (Tyzzer, 1906; Bruusgaard, 1932; Cheatham et al., 1956; Johnson, 1940; Eisenbud, 1952). The appearance of lesions in successive crops probably reflects a cyclic viremia which, in the normal host, is terminated by specific humoral and cellular immunity after about three days. Virus in the blood is cell-associated; it probably circulates and replicates in monocytes (Myers, 1979; Arbeit et al., 1982). Abnormal electroencephalograms and elevated serum levels of hepatocellular enzymes in the acute stage of uncomplicated varicella (Gibbs et al., 1959; Pitel et al., 1980; Myers, 1982; Ey et al., 1981) suggest the regular occurrence of asymptomatic viremic infection of many organs, including the CNS. These visceral infections are normally terminated by host defense mechanisms before they become symptomatic. When host defenses are deficient (e.g., in patients receiving cancer chemotherapy), these visceral infections are not suppressed and are responsible for most of the varicella-associated mortality observed (Cheatham et al., 1956; Feldman et al., 1975).

Pneumonia and most other complications of varicella reflect a failure to limit virus replication and dissemination (Gold, 1966; Feldman and Epp, 1976; Myers, 1979). Their frequency in newborns and in patients with congenital, acquired, or iatrogenic immunodeficiencies is almost certainly due, in large part, to depressed cellular immunity. The reason for the greater severity of varicella in normal adults than in children, however, is unknown.

The characteristic changes in infected cells, which can be observed in tissue culture as well as in vivo, are "ballooning degeneration" with the formation of intranuclear inclusion bodies and multinucleated giant cells (Taylor-Robinson and Caunt, 1972). Individual infected cells become greatly enlarged with pale vacuolated cytoplasm. The nuclei exhibit margination of chromatin and contain inclusion bodies. Early in the course of the infection, the inclusion bodies may be homogeneous and moderately basophilic, and they often fill the nucleus. However, they rapidly evolve into sharply demarcated acidophilic inclusion bodies that are separated from the deeply basophilic ring of marginated chromatin at the nuclear membrane by a clear zone or halo. Multinucleated giant cells are formed primarily by the fusion of adjacent infected cells (Johnson, 1940). Cell fusion, which is mediated by viral glycoproteins that appear on cell membranes early in the VZV replication cycle, facilitates cell-to-cell spread of infection, even in the presence of antibody capable of neutralizing extracellular virus. Neither multinucleated giant cells nor intranuclear inclusions are found in the vesicular lesions caused by poxviruses (smallpox, vaccinia) or enteroviruses (echoviruses, coxsackieviruses).

The initial event in the formation of the cutaneous lesions of varicella is probably infection of capillary endothelial cells in the papillary dermis, with subsequent spread of virus to epithelial cells in the epidermis, hair follicles, and sebaceous glands (Tyzzer, 1906; Bruusgaard, 1932; Lipschutz, 1921; Johnson, 1940; Taylor-Robinson and Caunt, 1972; Cheatham et al., 1956; Olding-Stenkvist and Grandien, 1976). In early papular lesions, the epithelium is slightly elevated owing to swelling of the infected epithelial cells and to edema and vascular congestion in the underlying dermis. In the superficial dermis, capillary endothelial cells are swollen, and their nuclei frequently contain intranuclear inclusions. Similar inclusions may be seen in the nuclei of fibroblasts in the surrounding connective tissue, which is edematous and infiltrated sparsely by mononuclear cells. Superficial lymphatics are dilated, and cells lining these structures are also swollen and may contain intranuclear inclusions. In the epidermis, the cells initially involved are those of the germinal layer and the deeper portion of the stratum spinosum. These cells show ballooning degeneration with loss of intercellular bridges, and they soon become separated by intercellular edema (acantholysis). A few small multinucleated giant cells, containing three to eight nuclei, can usually be seen at the base and periphery of these early epithelial lesions. The papular lesions rapidly evolve into intraepidermal vesicles as a result of infection and degeneration of more epithelial cells and the influx of edema fluid, which elevates the uninvolved stratum corneum to form a delicate clear vesicle (Fig. 2A). At this stage, the vesicle fluid contains fibrin, degenerating and "ballooned" epithelial cells, and abundant cell-free infectious VZV. Multinucleated giant cells with eosinophilic intranuclear inclusions are readily found in the walls and base of the vesicle (Fig. 2B). Polymorphonuclear leukocytes and a smaller number of macrophages then invade from the underlying dermis, and the vesicle fluid becomes cloudy; this transforms the vesicle into a pustule. The fluid is subsequently absorbed, with the formation of a flat adherent crust that is eventually detached by the regrowth of subjacent epithelial cells. The lesion can evolve from papule to early crusting in 8 to 12 hours. Lesions of uncomplicated varicella usually heal without scarring. Lesions in mucous membranes develop in the same way, but the thin roof of the vesicle breaks down quickly, producing a shallow ulcer that heals rapidly.

In fatal varicella, focal lesions have been found in the mucous membranes of the respiratory, gastrointestinal, and genitourinary tracts, in the serosa of the pleural and peritoneal cavities, and in the parenchyma of virtually every organ, the lungs being the most frequent site of severe involvement (Taylor-Robinson and Caunt, 1972; Krugman et al., 1977; Cheatham et al., 1956; Christie, 1980; Johnson, 1940; Waring et al., 1942; Eisenbud, 1952). There is widespread vascular damage, with characteristic acidophilic intranuclear inclusions in the endothelial cells lining small blood vessels and lymphatics; capillaries within individual lesions are often destroyed, with thrombosis and hemorrhage. In varicella pneumonia, the pleura are studded with hemorrhagic nodules, and the lungs show widely disseminated interstitial pneumonia with numerous foci of hemorrhagic necrosis. Alveoli are filled with red cells, fibrin, inclusion-bearing mononuclear cells, and occasional multinucleated giant cells. Hyalin membranes are frequently seen. Typical acidophilic inclusions are also seen within hyperplastic alveolar septal cells, swollen capillary endothelial cells, fibroblasts, and bronchiolar and tracheobronchial epithelial cells. Similar areas of vascular damage and focal necrosis are found in the liver, spleen, and other organs. In some cases, characteristic intranuclear inclusions may be nearly or totally absent, in spite of unmistakable clinical and pathologic evidence of extensive VZV infection and the isolation of VZV from the liver, lungs, brain, and other tissues (Waring et al., 1942; Rotter and Collins, 1961; Sander et al., 1970; author's unpublished observations).

There is now increasing evidence that (except for Reye's syndrome) the central nervous system (CNS) complications of varicella may be caused by direct VZV infection of the CNS (vide infra), rather than autoimmune demyelination, as previously thought by many observers (Griffith et al., 1970; McKendall and Klawans, 1978).

CLINICAL MANIFESTATIONS

Prodrome. In young children prodromal symptoms are infrequent and the illness usually begins, after an incubation period of 14 or 15 days, with the rash. The rash may be accompanied by low-grade fever and malaise. In older children and adults the rash is often preceded by two to three days of fever, chills, malaise, headache, anorexia, severe backache, and, in some patients, sore throat and

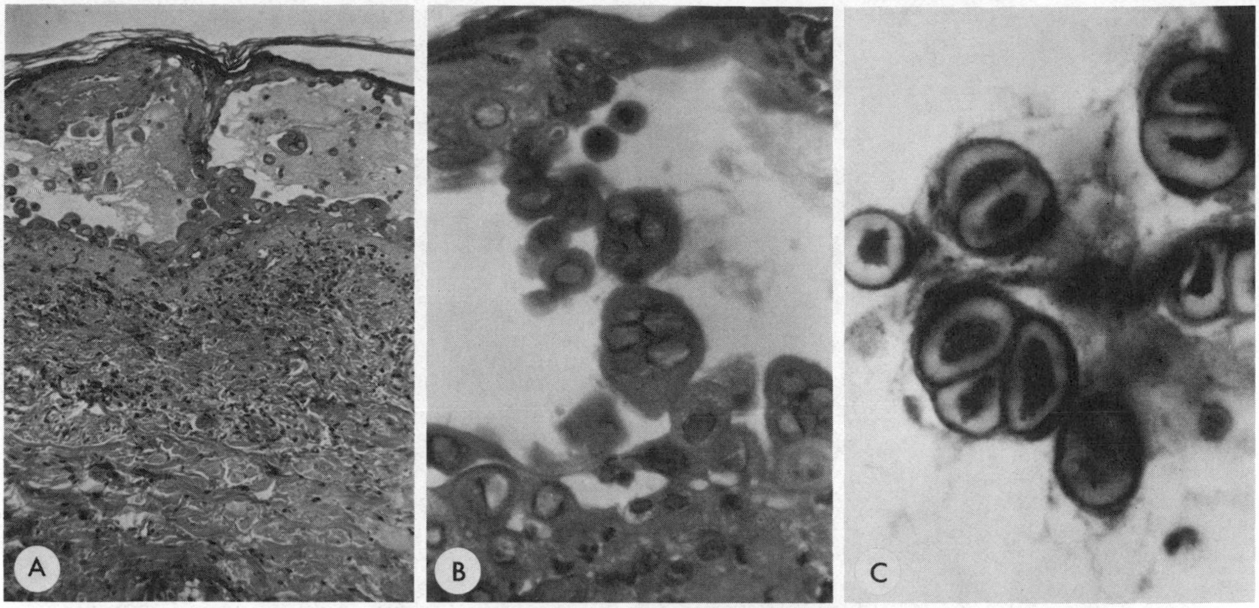

Figure 2. Varicella, early vesicle. *A,* Intraepidermal vesicle. Infected epithelial cells show acantholysis, "ballooning degeneration," intranuclear inclusions, and multinucleated giant cell formation. Underlying dermis shows edema and mononuclear cell infiltration (hematoxylin-eosin stain × 200). (Courtesy of Dr. R. J. Barr). *B,* Multinucleated giant cells in the walls and base of the vesicle (hematoxylin-eosin stain × 800). (Courtesy of Dr. R. J. Barr.) *C,* Tzanck smear from the base of the vesicle, showing multinucleated giant cells with intranuclear inclusion bodies (hematoxylin-eosin stain. × 2000).

dry cough. A fleeting scarlatiniform rash may occur occasionally just before or coincident with the vesicular eruption.

Rash. The rash begins on the face and scalp, and spreads rapidly to the trunk with relative sparing of the extremities. New lesions appear in successive crops, but their distribution remains central. The rash tends to be more profuse in hollows and protected parts of the body than on prominent and exposed parts. Thus it is denser in the hollow of the small of the back and the furrow between the shoulder blades than on the scapulae and buttocks, and more profuse on the medial than on the lateral aspects of the limbs. It is not uncommon to have a few lesions on the palms and soles. Vesicles often appear earlier and in larger numbers in areas of inflammation, such as diaper rash, sunburn, or eczema.

The most striking feature of the lesions of varicella is their rapid progression from rose-colored macules to papules to vesicles to pustules to crusts. The entire transition may take only 8 to 12 hours. The typical superficial, thin-walled vesicle of varicella looks like a drop of water lying on the skin. It is usually 2 to 3 mm in diameter and elliptical; its long axis is parallel to the folds of the skin (Fig. 3A) and it is surrounded by an irregular area of erythema, which gives the lesions the appearance of a "dewdrop on a rose petal" (Wesselhoeft, 1944). The vesicle fluid soon becomes cloudy with the influx of inflammatory cells, and the lesion begins to dry. Drying begins in the center, first producing an umbilicated pustule and then a crust. Crusts fall off in one to three weeks, depending upon the depth of the skin involvement, leaving shallow pink depressions that gradually disappear. Scarring is rare in uncomplicated varicella.

Vesicles also develop in the mouth, occurring most commonly over the palate. Mucosal vesicles rupture so rapidly that the vesicular stage may be missed. Instead, one sees shallow ulcers 2 to 3 mm in diameter. Vesicles may also appear on other mucous membranes, including those of the nose, pharynx, larynx, trachea, gastrointestinal tract, urinary tract, and vagina, as well as on the conjunctivae.

A distinctive feature of varicella is the simultaneous presence, in any one area of the skin, of lesions in all stages of evolution (Fig. 3B). This is due to the rapid development of individual lesions and the appearance of successive crops involving the same anatomic areas. In the typical case, three crops of lesions appear over a three-day period, but there are wide variations, ranging from a single crop of a few scattered lesions to a series of five or more crops developing over a period of one week with innumerable lesions over the entire body. In general, the mildest cases are seen most frequently in infants, and the most severe in adults. Inapparent infections occur but are rare (Ross, 1962).

Fever usually persists as long as new lesions continue to appear, and its height is generally proportional to the severity of the rash. In typical cases it rarely exceeds 102° F; it may be absent in mild cases and rise to 105° F in severe cases with extensive rash. Prolonged fever or recurrence of fever after defervescence may be associated with secondary bacterial infection or other complications. Headache, malaise, myalgia, and anorexia accompany the fever and are more severe in older children and adults. However, the most distressing symptom is usually pruritus, which is present throughout the vesicular stage.

COMPLICATIONS AND SEQUELAE. In the normal child varicella is a benign disease rarely attended by serious complications. The most frequent complication is staphylococcal or streptococcal infection of skin lesions, which may produce impetigo, furuncles, cellulitis, erysipelas, and, rarely, gangrene. These local infections often lead to

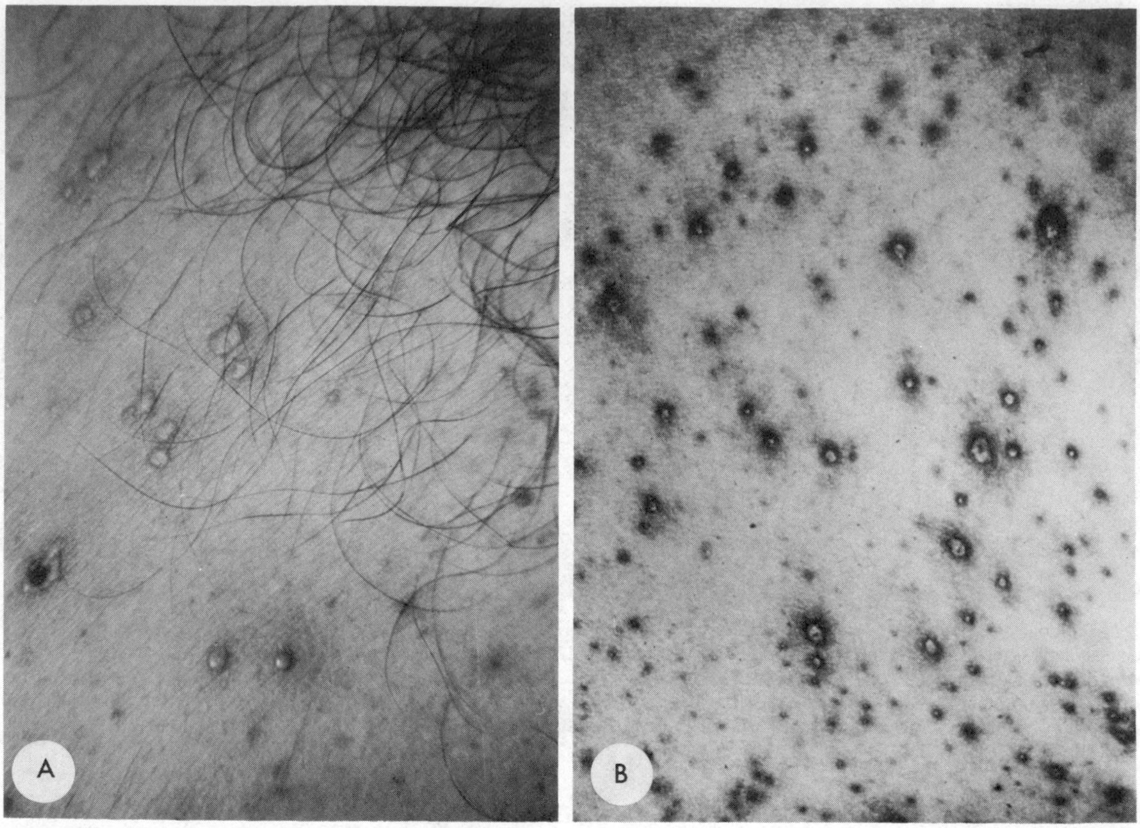

Figure 3. Varicella. A, Superficial, thin-walled, elliptical vesicles with their long axis parallel to the skin folds. B, Lesions in all stages of evolution.

scarring and, very rarely, to septicemia with metastatic infection of other organs (Bullowa and Wishik, 1935; Krugman et al., 1977; Smith et al., 1976; Fleischer et al., 1981). Bullous lesions may be produced when vesicles are infected with staphylococci that elaborate exfoliative toxin (Melish, 1973). Secondary bacterial pneumonia is rare, occurs mainly in children under seven years of age, and responds to antibiotics, as do otitis media and suppurative meningitis (Bullowa and Wishik, 1935; Weinstein and Meade, 1956; Singer, 1979). In contrast to the normal host, bacterial superinfection is frequent and life-threatening in leukopenic patients, especially children with leukemia.

Other complications, which result directly from the replication and dissemination of VZV, account for the increased morbidity and mortality of varicella in adults, in newborns, and in immunocompromised patients of any age (Krugman et al., 1977; Weinstein and Meade, 1956; Juel-Jensen and MacCallum, 1972; Gold and Nankervis, 1973; Triebwasser et al., 1967; Cheatham et al., 1956; Boughton, 1966a; Feldman et al., 1975; Haggerty and Eley, 1956; Gershon et al., 1972).

Varicella is generally more severe in adults. Fever and constitutional symptoms are more prominent and prolonged. The rash is more profuse and complications more frequent. Primary varicella pneumonia is the major complication of adult varicella. It is rarely observed in normal children; adults account for more than 90 per cent of reported cases (Bullowa and Wishik, 1935; Krugman et al., 1977; Weinstein and Meade, 1956; Triebwasser et al., 1967).

The incidence of primary varicella pneumonia depends upon the population of patients studied and the diagnostic criteria employed. Roentgenographic evidence of pneumonia was found in 16 per cent of healthy male military recruits with varicella, but clinical signs of pneumonia were present in only 4 per cent (Weber and Pellecchia, 1965). The incidence and severity are substantially higher in older patients and in the subset of adults with varicella who are admitted to hospitals (Weinstein and Meade, 1956; Triebwasser et al., 1967). Pneumonia generally appears one to six days after the onset of rash, and the degree of pulmonary involvement correlates best with the severity of the cutaneous eruption; oropharyngeal mucosal lesions are usually extensive. Some patients are asymptomatic, but others develop cough, dyspnea, tachypnea, high fever, pleuritic chest pain, cyanosis, and hemoptysis. The severity of the symptoms is usually out of proportion to the physical findings in the chest, but the roentgenogram typically reveals diffuse nodular or miliary densities throughout both lung fields, often peribronchial in distribution, with a tendency to concentrate in the perihilar regions and at the bases. Roentgenographic abnormalities disappear more slowly than do the symptoms of pneumonia, and occassionally the pulmonary lesions calcify and persist for years (Krugman et al., 1977; Gold and Nankervis, 1973; Triebwasser et al., 1967; Mackay and Cairney, 1960). The mortality in adults with varicella pneumonia has been estimated to be between 10 and 30 per cent, but it is probably closer to 10 per cent if immunocompromised patients are excluded (Krugman et al., 1977; Boughton; 1966a; Sargent et al., 1967; Triebwasser et al., 1967). It is clear from postmortem examination of fatal cases that the pneumonia is only one manifestation of widespread hematogenous dissemination, with evidence of varicella infection in virtually every organ examined (Triebwasser et al., 1967; Sargent et al., 1967; Waring et al., 1942).

It is unclear whether either the incidence or the severity of varicella pneumonia is greater when varicella occurs during pregnancy than when it occurs in the normal nonpregnant adult (Oxman et al., 1983; Young and Gershon, 1983). The fetus may sometimes die as a consequence of premature labor or maternal death in severe varicella pneumonia, but varicella during pregnancy has not increased the background level of fetal morbidity, mortality, or congenital malformations (Oxman et al., 1983; Young and Gershon, 1983). Nevertheless, varicella during pregnancy may result in intrauterine (congenital) VZV infection.

When congenital VZV infection occurs early in gestation, the spectrum of disease ranges from severe congenital malformations to asymptomatic neuronal latency. A characteristic syndrome of developmental abnormalities (including hypoplasia of an extremity, cicatricial skin scarring, cortical atrophy, ocular abnormalities, and low birth weight) has been observed in infants born to women who had varicella between the seventh and twentieth weeks of gestation (Williamson, 1975; Oxman et al., 1983; Young and Gershon, 1983). This is a rare occurrence, with fewer than 30 cases reported worldwide. However, maternal varicella at any stage of pregnancy can cause a fetal infection that resolves before parturition without obvious sequelae. These infants are born without visible evidence of infection, but frequently develop herpes zoster at an early age without any history of previous varicella (Brunell and Kotchmar, 1981; Oxman et al., 1983; Young and Gershon, 1983).

Congenital varicella (i.e., varicella occurring within 10 days of birth) appears to be more serious than varicella in infants infected postnatally, and the severity varies markedly depending upon the proximity of maternal disease to delivery. When an infant acquires VZV infection in utero but is born before the transplacental passage of sufficient maternal antibody to modify the infection during its incubation period (i.e., when the rash of varicella occurs in the mother less than five days before or within two days after delivery, or begins in an infant between five and ten days of age), the result is often severe disseminated varicella, and the mortality is about 30 per cent. When the onset of rash in the mother is 5 days or more before delivery (onset of rash in the infant at 0 to 4 days of age) sufficient maternal antibody has crossed the placenta to modify the infection, and all such infected infants can be expected to survive. These observations imply that immature perinatal defenses cannot restrain VZV replication and dissemination (Oxman et al., 1983; Young and Gershon, 1983).

The morbidity and mortality of varicella are markedly increased in immunocompromised patients, including patients with leukemia and other malignancies who are receiving corticosteroids, chemotherapeutic agents, or radiotherapy at the time of infection; patients receiving corticosteroids for diseases such as nephrotic syndrome and rheumatic fever; and patients with congenital immunologic deficiencies (Cheatham et al., 1956; Finkel, 1971; Feldman et al., 1975; Haggerty and Eley, 1956; Gershon et al., 1972; Scheinman and Stamler, 1969; Lux et al., 1970; Hattori et al., 1976; Feldhoff et al., 1981; Whitley et al., 1982a and b). These patients have a more extensive rash and a longer period of new vesicle formation, as well as frequent involvement of the lungs, liver, central nervous system and other organs, in association with prolonged high-level viremia (Feldman and Epp, 1976; Myers, 1979). In one series, 19 of 60 children with leukemia who were receiving chemotherapy at the time of infection had visceral dissemination, and four died (Feldman et al., 1975). There was varicella pneumonia in all four fatal cases and fulminant encephalitis in two. Varicella hepatitis was also frequently present, but was not fatal in the absence of pneumonia. Disseminated varicella occurred more frequently in children with absolute lymphopenia (less than 500 lymphocytes per cubic millimeter). Immunosuppressed and corticosteroid-treated patients may also develop hemorrhagic complications of varicella that range in severity from mild febrile purpura to severe and often fatal purpura fulminans and "malignant varicella with purpura" (Smith, 1967; Juel-Jensen and MacCallum, 1972; Feusner et al., 1979; Christie, 1980; Charkes, 1961; Yeager and Zinkham, 1980). The etiology of these hemorrhagic complications is complex and probably not the same in every case. In some, thrombocytopenia may be associated with the underlying disease, its therapy, the direct effect of VZV infection on the bone marrow, or immune-mediated platelet destruction (Espinoza and Kuhn, 1974; Feusner et al., 1979). In others, particularly those with malignant varicella and purpura fulminans, the primary factor may be infection of vascular endothelial cells, with endothelial damage initiating disseminated intravascular coagulation and thrombotic purpura.

Central nervous systems complications of varicella, which occur in fewer than 1 in 1000 cases, include several distinct syndromes (McKendall and Klawans, 1978): (1) Reye's syndrome, (2) acute cerebellar ataxia, (3) encephalitis or meningoencephalitis, (4) acute ascending or transverse myelitis, and (5) Guillain-Barré syndrome. Varicella-associated Reye's syndrome (acute encephalopathy with fatty degeneration of the viscera) occurring 2 to 7 days after the appearance of the rash is not discernibly different from Reye's syndrome associated with influenza A, influenza B, or other viral infections. Although its pathogenesis is not understood, there is no inflammatory response in the CNS, and pathologic and virologic studies have essentially ruled out direct virus infection of the liver or brain. Instead, Reye's syndrome may be caused by some circulating toxin, perhaps a component of the virus or a substance elaborated by virus-infected cells (Ladisch et al., 1979). From 15 to 40 per cent of all cases of Reye's syndrome occur in association with varicella (Center for Disease Control, 1980; Lichtenstein et al., 1983), and the mortality may be as high as 40 per cent (Fleisher et al., 1981). Reexamination of older reports of the CNS complications of varicella suggests that many of the cases described as "varicella encephalitis" in immunologically normal children were probably Reye's syndrome. Furthermore, Reye's syndrome appears to account for most of the fatalities in normal children that were attributed to varicella encephalitis. Two recent series (Takashima and Becker, 1979; Fleisher et al., 1981) support this conclusion. In Takashima and Becker's review of 32 fatal cases of varicella in children, all 12 that occurred in otherwise normal children had clinical and pathologic findings compatible with Reye's syndrome. Of the remaining 20, 18 occurred in children with underlying diseases (12 of whom were receiving corticosteroids) and 2 were cases of neonatal varicella. Although typical inclusions were demonstrated in the brains of only 2, all 20 of these children had evidence of widespread VZV dissemination with inclusions in many internal organs. In a series of 96 patients hospitalized with varicella (Fleisher et al., 1981), there were 17 cases of Reye's syndrome in 81 immunologically normal children, and these accounted for 7 of the 10 fatalities recorded. Another of the deaths occurred in an infant who developed varicella 7 days after delivery; CNS involvement in this case was part of a widely disseminated VZV infection.

Varicella-associated Guillain-Barré syndrome is extremely rare, and many of the cases reported are almost certainly examples of varicella myelitis. Apart from the temporal association in the few cases recorded, there is no evidence directly implicating VZV in the pathogenesis of Guillain-Barré syndrome.

In acute cerebellar ataxia the onset of neurologic symptoms has ranged from 11 days before to 20 days after the appearance of the rash. Recovery without sequelae is the rule, and no pathologic data are available. However, its occurrence as early as 11 days before the onset of rash, i.e., during the primary viremia (Goldston et al., 1963) and the detection of VZV antigens in the cerebrospinal fluid (CSF) of two patients with this complication (Peters et al., 1978) suggest that acute cerebellar ataxia may reflect direct invasion of the CNS, presumably as a consequence of viremia and infection of vascular endothelial cells.

The pathogenesis of varicella encephalitis (meningoencephalitis) and myelitis remains obscure. Although many observers favor a post-infectious (autoimmune) demyelinating process like that observed in measles encephalomyelitis (Johnson et al., 1984), there is increasing evidence that these complications of varicella result from direct VZV infection of the CNS. The therapeutic implications of this distinction are obvious (vide infra). Many cases of varicella meningoencephalitis and myelitis (and most cases that have come to postmortem examination) have occurred in patients with prolonged high-grade viremia and infection of many organs in addition to the skin and mucous membranes—a setting in which direct infection of the CNS is to be expected (Waring et al., 1942; Appelbaum et al., 1953; Boughton, 1966b; Feldman et al., 1975; Myers, 1979; Takashima and Becker, 1979). Furthermore, whereas characteristic intranuclear inclusions in the CNS have been reported in only a few cases (Nicolaides, 1957; Takashima and Becker, 1979), many others have shown pathologic features more consistent with direct VZV infection than with post-infectious (autoimmune) encephalomyelitis (Griffith, 1970). These have included perivascular infiltrates in the cortex and brain stem, scattered foci of necrosis, often hemorrhagic and often associated with endothelial swelling and injury to vessel walls, and inflammatory infiltration of the leptomeninges. Moreover, because isolation of VZV from skin vesicles after more than 4 days of rash is uncommon (Gold, 1966) and because characteristic intranuclear inclusions are not always observed in infected tissues, the failure to isolate VZV or demonstrate inclusions is not compelling evidence against direct CNS infection. Finally, the infectious nature of varicella encephalitis and myelitis is further supported by the recent demonstration of antibody to VZV (presumably locally produced within the CNS) in the CSF of patients with varicella encephalitis and transverse myelitis, and by the direct isolation of VZV from the CSF of a patient with varicella encephalitis (Gershon et al., 1980).

Other rare complications of varicella include myocarditis, glomerulonephritis, orchitis, appendicitis, pancreatitis, arthritis, optic neuritis, keratitis, and iritis. The pathogenesis of these complications has not been delineated, but direct parenchymal infection or vasculitis induced by endothelial VZV infection appears to be responsible in many instances.

Although chemical evidence of mild hepatitis is common in uncomplicated varicella (Pitel et al., 1980; Myers, 1982; Ey et al., 1981), clinical hepatitis is rare, except as a complication of progressive varicella.

GEOGRAPHIC VARIATION IN DISEASE AND EPIDEMIOLOGY. Varicella occurs worldwide, and there is no evidence of differing racial or sexual susceptibility. Humans are the only known reservoir of infection, and arthropod vectors play no apparent role in transmission. Varicella is endemic in metropolitan communities in temperate climates, with a regularly recurring prevalence in winter and spring, and periodic epidemics when susceptibles accumulate. In urban areas of the United States, 90 per cent of cases occur in children under 10 and fewer than 5 per cent in individuals over 15 years old (Gordon, 1962, Weller, 1982 and 1983). In semitropical and tropical countries, infection is delayed, and varicella is seen more often in adults. In a survey of parturient women in New York City, only 4.5 per cent of those born in the United States lacked antibody to VZV, whereas 16 per cent of those from Latin America were seronegative (Gershon et al., 1976). The proportion of susceptible adults is even higher in areas of Asia, Africa, and the Middle East (Weller, 1982 and 1983). This becomes an important consideration in delivering health care to immigrant populations and in controlling nosocomial varicella in hospitals with patients and staff from these areas.

Despite the lability of the virus, varicella is highly contagious. Attack rates of 87 per cent among susceptible siblings in households and nearly 70 per cent among susceptible patients on hospital wards have been reported (Gordon, 1962; Ross, 1962). Most cases of varicella are clinically apparent, although the exanthem may be so sparse and transient that it is unnoticed. A typical patient is probably infectious for one to two days (rarely, three to four days) before the exanthem appears, and for four or five days thereafter—i.e., until the last crop of vesicles has crusted (Evans, 1940). The immunocompromised patient, who may experience successive crops of lesions for one week or more, is infectious for a longer period. The average incubation period of varicella is 14 or 15 days, with a range of 10 to 23 days (Gordon, 1962; Ross, 1962). The incubation period is often prolonged in patients who develop varicella after passive immunization with zoster-immune globulin (ZIG) or plasma (ZIP) (Gershon et al., 1974; Balfour et al., 1977; Orenstein et al., 1981). Varicella is thought to be acquired and transmitted mainly via the respiratory tract by airborne droplets (Leclair et al., 1980; Gustafson et al., 1982), but also by direct contact and, less frequently, by indirect contact. Unlike smallpox, varicella crusts are not infectious, and the duration of infectivity of droplets containing the labile VZV must be relatively limited. The mechanism by which VZV is shed is unclear. Viremia occurs during the prodromal stage, when varicella can be transmitted to the fetus in utero and by blood transfusion from a donor incubating the infection. Lesions are not confined to the skin, but occur also in the respiratory, genitourinary, and gastrointestinal tracts. Though infectiousness is thought to depend largely upon virus shed from the upper respiratory tract, VZV has only rarely been isolated from pharyngeal secretions, whereas it can regularly be recovered from vesicle fluid (Weller, 1982 and 1983).

IMMUNE RESPONSES AND VIRUS-HOST INTERACTION. Antibodies to VZV can be measured by a variety of techniques that vary in their sensitivity and specificity

(Gershon, 1980; Weller, 1983; Cradock-Watson, et al., 1979; Arvin and Koropchak, 1980; Shanley et al., 1982; Kamiya et al., 1982; Shiraki et al., 1982; Iltis et al., 1982; Wittek et al., 1983; Schmidt and Gallo, 1984; Weigle and Grose, 1984). Sensitive assays show that IgG, IgM, and IgA antibodies to VZV appear within 2 to 5 days after the onset of clinical varicella and reach maximum titers during the second or third week. Thereafter, IgG antibodies decline slowly and persist at low levels for life. IgM and IgA antibodies decline more rapidly and are generally undetectable a year after infection, although IgA antibodies may persist at low levels in some individuals.

Cell-mediated immunity (CMI) to VZV also develops during the course of varicella and persists for many years (Jordan and Merigan, 1974; Zaia et al., 1978). The assays most frequently employed measure the capacity of peripheral blood leukocytes to synthesize DNA and proliferate in vitro in response to VZV antigens (Zaia et al., 1978; Kumagai et al., 1980). CMI to VZV has also been demonstrated by other techniques (Gershon, 1980; Weller, 1983) including a skin test that correlates well with the results of antibody assays and efficiently identifies susceptible individuals (Kamiya et al., 1977; Asano et al., 1981).

The relative importance of humoral and cellular immunity in recovery from varicella is not clear. The disease is not particularly severe in children with agammaglobulinemia (Good and Zak, 1956), and there is no obvious correlation between the endogenous antibody response and the severity of varicella (Gold, 1966; Feldman et al., 1975; Brunell et al., 1975). Cellular immune responses, and perhaps interferon, appear more important in limiting the extent and duration of VZV infection, and it is patients with defects in CMI who suffer severe and life-threatening varicella (Feldman et al., 1975; Armstrong et al., 1970; Stevens et al., 1975; Ruckdeschel et al., 1977; Patel et al., 1979; Gershon and Steinberg, 1979). However, passive immunization of these immunocompromised patients with antibody to VZV can protect them from severe or fatal varicella (Gershon et al., 1974; Orenstein et al., 1981; Zaia et al., 1983). Control of primary VZV infection must involve a number of host defenses; augmenting one (e.g., by administering antibody to VZV) may compensate for deficiencies in another.

The nature of immunity to varicella (i.e., to exogenous reinfection) is another important question. One attack of varicella confers lasting immunity in immunologically normal individuals. Although this statement is validated by vast quantities of clinical and epidemiologic data, it requires some qualification. Immunity to VZV is exceedingly complex; for example, whereas varicella may immunize against a second attack of varicella, it does not prevent herpes zoster, a disease caused by the same virus. Serum antibody to VZV is an important factor in immunity to exogenous reinfection. People with detectable serum antibody do not usually become ill after exogenous exposure, whereas those devoid of serum antibody to VZV develop varicella (Gershon and Krugman, 1975; Zaia and Oxman, 1977). Moreover, passive immunization can prevent varicella in susceptible immunocompetent individuals exposed to exogenous VZV (Ross, 1962; Brunell et al., 1969; Gershon et al., 1974). However, the development and application of sensitive assays for humoral and cell-mediated immunity to VZV has revealed the dynamic nature of the VZV-host interaction. Subclinical reinfection, evidenced by a boost in the titer of IgG antibody to VZV, by the reappearance of IgM and IgA antibodies, and by an increase in the in vitro lymphoproliferative response to VZV antigens, is a frequent occurrence in normal immune individuals following household exposure to varicella (Brunell et al., 1975; Iltis et al., 1982; Arvin et al., 1983). This implies limited replication of VZV, at least at the portal of entry. Repeated exposures of this sort may help adults to maintain a high level of immunity to VZV (Hope-Simpson, 1965). Furthermore, infants with transplacentally acquired maternal antibody regularly develop mild varicella after exposure (Baba and Yabuuchi, 1982), as do immunocompromised children who are passively immunized with varicella-zoster immune globulin (VZIG) (Zaia et al., 1983). It would thus appear that the presence of antibody to VZV in a normal host, with or without the VZV-specific cellular immune responses induced by previous varicella, will prevent the development of disease but not the local replication of exogenous VZV at the portal of entry. The failure of the same antibody preparations to prevent disease in immunosuppressed patients implies the need for some nonspecific, presumably cellular, component(s) that may interact with antibody—perhaps cells capable of mediating antibody-dependent cytotoxicity.

It also appears that persons who develop modified varicella (e.g., because they are infected as infants in the presence of transplacentally acquired maternal antibody) may be susceptible to exogenous reinfection and clinical varicella (Weller, 1983; Gershon et al., 1984a). In this regard, Baba et al., (1982) observed that among institutionalized infants developing varicella after exposure, those with preexisting maternal antibody who had mild (modified) varicella developed relatively low levels of antibody and VZV skin test reactivity during convalescence. Finally, although immunologically normal recipients of live attenuated VZV vaccines (vide infra) have had a greatly reduced incidence of varicella after subsequent exposures, a few have developed mild varicella in spite of having vaccine-induced antibody to VZV (Arbeter et al., 1984; Gershon et al., 1984b).

Taken together, these observations suggest that antibody alone will not guarantee total immunity to varicella unless it is the result of a previous unmodified natural infection.

DIAGNOSIS. Varicella can usually be recognized by the character and evolution of the rash, particularly when there is a history of exposure within the preceding two to three weeks (Wesselhoeft, 1944; Krugman et al., 1977; Christie, 1980). Characteristic diagnostic features include (1) a papulovesicular eruption accompanied by fever and mild constitutional symptoms; (2) crops of lesions with a predominantly central distribution including the scalp; (3) rapid evolution from macules to papules to delicate thin-walled vesicles to pustules and, finally, to crusts; (4) the presence of lesions in all stages of development in any one anatomic area throughout the acute disease; and (5) lesions in the oral mucous membranes.

Disseminated herpes simplex may occasionally resemble varicella, especially in the neonate, in immunosuppressed patients, and in patients with eczema. However, the distribution of lesions is rarely typical of varicella, and there may be an obvious concentration of lesions at the site of the primary or recurrent infection (e.g., the mouth or external genitalia). Marked toxicity and encephalitis are more common in neonatal herpes simplex than in neonatal varicella. However, the histopathology of lesions caused by HSV and VZV is indistinguishable. Thus differentiation of the two requires virus isolation or the detection and identification of viral antigens or nucleic acids in the lesions.

Severe varicella, especially in immunosuppressed patients, may resemble smallpox or generalized vaccinia. Conversely, mild variola, especially when modified by vaccination, may be indistinguishable from varicella. Generalized vaccinia, especially in patients with immunologic defects or eczema, may also be confused with varicella. Since the distinction between varicella and these poxvirus infections cannot be made with certainty on clinical grounds, prompt laboratory diagnosis is required. However, the eradication of smallpox and the consequent cessation of smallpox vaccination should eliminate this diagnostic problem.

Other diseases that may be confused with varicella include impetigo, the vesicular exanthems of coxsackievirus and echovirus infections (e.g., hand-foot-mouth syndrome), rickettsialpox, insect bites, papular urticaria, scabies, contact dermatitis, dermatitis herpetiformis, drug eruptions, secondary syphilis, and erythema multiforme. The character, distribution, and evolution of the lesions, together with a careful epidemiologic history, usually differentiate these diseases from varicella (Krugman et al., 1977). When any doubt exists, the clinical impression should receive laboratory confirmation.

Multinucleated giant cells and epithelial cells containing acidophilic intranuclear inclusion bodies distinguish the cutaneous lesions produced by VZV from all others except herpes simplex (see Fig. 2). These cells can be demonstrated in Tzanck smears; material is scraped from the base of an early vesicle and stained with hematoxylin-eosin, Giemsa, Papanicolaou, or Paragon multiple stain (Blank et al., 1951; Barr et al., 1977) (see Fig. 2C). Every physician should use this simple procedure for the evaluation of any patient with a vesicular eruption. Punch biopsies provide more reliable material for histologic examination and also facilitate diagnosis in the prevesicular stage. Sputum from patients with varicella pneumonia may contain desquamated respiratory epithelial cells with acidophilic intranuclear inclusions, but such cells are also found in patients with measles pneumonia. The identification of herpesvirus particles in vesicle fluid or biopsy material by electronmicroscopy provides another diagnostic technique. However, neither electronmicroscopy nor Tzanck smears can distinguish VZV from HSV infections.

The distinction between VZV and HSV, as well as the definitive diagnosis of VZV infection, can be made by isolating VZV from fresh vesicle fluid inoculated into suitable tissue cultures (Weller, 1979; Levin et al., 1984) or by the direct identification of virus antigens or nucleic acids in material from skin lesions or infected tissues (Weller, 1979; Richman et al., 1984). Viral antigens can be demonstrated by using countercurrent immunoelectrophoresis (Frey and Steinberg, 1981). Direct fluorescent antibody staining of cellular material from fresh vesicles or prevesicular lesions is a rapid and specific method of diagnosis, and it can identify individual infected cells and structures (Esiri and Tomlinson, 1972; Aoyama et al., 1974; Weller, 1979; Olding-Stenkvist and Grandien, 1976; Schmidt et al., 1980). Enzyme immunoassay provides another rapid and sensitive method for antigen detection (Cleveland et al., 1982; Richman et al., 1984). Monoclonal antibodies can improve the specificity of these techniques, but it is always important to examine aliquots of each specimen with antisera to VZV, HSV-1, HSV-2, and control antigen in parallel, together with positive and negative virus-infected tissue controls. Nucleic acid hybridization with radiolabeled or biotinylated probes can detect viral nucleic acids in clinical specimens (Richman et al., 1984) and offers another sensitive, specific means for rapid diagnosis.

Serologic tests allow a retrospective diagnosis by comparing acute and convalescent sera, and can be used to identify susceptible candidates for isolation or prophylaxis. The complement fixation (CF) test has two disadvantages (Weller, 1979; Schmidt, 1980): (1) a rise in CF titer to VZV or HSV is not diagnostic if antibody to both viruses increases, because infection by either virus can induce a heterologous anamnestic response, and (2) CF antibody drops within months after varicella infection and may reach undetectable levels. Thus, many adults who are immune to varicella may be CF antibody-negative. Consequently, the CF test is not useful for distinguishing between immune and susceptible adults. In addition to virus neutralization and indirect immunofluorescence assays, a number of new and more sensitive techniques can measure humoral responses to VZV (Weller, 1983). These include an immunofluorescence assay for antibody to VZV-induced membrane antigens (FAMA) (Williams et al., 1974; Zaia and Oxman, 1977) that distinguishes immune from susceptible adults; an immune adherence hemagglutination assay (IAHA), which is slightly less sensitive than the FAMA assay (Kalter et al., 1977); a rapid ^{125}I-staphylococcal protein A radioimmunoassay, which is more sensitive and easier to perform than the FAMA assay (Richman et al., 1981); enzyme-linked immunosorbent assays (ELISA), which are comparable to the FAMA assay in their ability to distinguish immune from susceptible adults, but which are more sensitive and simpler to perform (Iltis et al., 1982; Shanley et al., 1982); and a solid-phase radioimmunoassay (RIA) for measuring VZV-specific IgG, IgM, and IgA responses (Arvin and Koropchak, 1980). Of these, the ELISA appears most promising. In addition, measurement of the in vitro proliferative response of peripheral blood lymphocytes to VZV antigens (Zaia et al., 1978; Arvin et al., 1983) correlates well with immunity, as measured by FAMA, RIA, and ELISA, and a VZV skin test has been widely and successfully used in Japan to distinguish between immune and susceptible individuals (Kamiya et al., 1977; Asano et al., 1981; Steele et al., 1982). With all of these assays, adequate controls are required to deal with the problem of heterotypic responses to infections by other herpesviruses (Schmidt and Gallo, 1984).

TREATMENT. In normal children, varicella is generally benign and self-limited. Cool compresses or calamine lotion locally and antihistamines orally may help control the intense pruritus of the rash. Tepid baths with baking soda (¼ cup per tub of water) may also relieve itching. Creams or lotions containing corticosteroids and occlusive ointments should not be used. Antipyretics are rarely indicated, and it has been recommended that salicylates be avoided because of their possible association with Reye's syndrome (Fulginiti et al., 1982). Fingernails should be kept short and clean to minimize secondary skin infections and scarring that may result from scratching.

Complications are most frequently due to bacterial superinfection. Bacterial infections of local lesions are treated with warm soaks. Systemic antimicrobial drugs are indicated for bacterial cellulitis, otitis media, sepsis, bacterial meningitis, osteomyelitis, septic arthritis, and bacterial pneumonia. The prominence of *Staphylococcus aureus* and group A β-hemolytic *Streptococcus* as causes of these complications should be recognized, but therapy should be guided by the results of gram-stained smears and cultures. Antibiotics are useless in varicella pneumonia unless there is bacterial superinfection.

Reye's syndrome must be considered when a child with otherwise uncomplicated varicella develops lethargy, persistent vomiting, and confusion. Early diagnosis, with supportive care and aggressive control of increased intracranial pressure and hypoglycemia, should reduce the mortality and morbidity of this mysterious complication.

The most common neurologic complication of varicella in normal children is cerebellar ataxia, which is usually self-limited. However, recent evidence that it may involve VZV infection of the CNS (vide supra) warrants consideration of antiviral chemotherapy. Varicella encephalitis, meningoencephalitis and myelitis are very rare complications in normal children. However, evidence that they may also involve VZV infection of the CNS, rather than a postinfectious autoimmune mechanism (vide supra), make it reasonable to treat them with an antiviral agent.

Varicella pneumonia is rare in normal children, but more common in adults. Although it usually responds to supportive measures, including positive-pressure ventilation, antiviral chemotherapy should be used early to inhibit VZV replication. Antibiotics are indicated only when bacterial superinfection develops. There is no evidence that corticosteroids are beneficial, and their use is not recommended.

Hemorrhagic complications should be treated on the basis of the results of coagulation studies and bone marrow examination. It is always important to rule out bacterial sepsis. Because of the possible involvement of VZV-induced endothelial damage in purpura fulminans, especially if this complication occurs when new vesicles are continuing to appear, antiviral therapy should probably be administered in such situations.

In contrast to varicella in normal children, varicella in immunocompromised children and adults may be severe and life-threatening. Thus every effort should be made to prevent its occurrence (see *PROPHYLAXIS*). When this fails, antiviral therapy should be initiated as early in the illness as possible, and certainly before any clinical evidence of disseminated disease. Patients at risk include those with leukemia, lymphoproliferative disorders, metastastic malignancies, and congenital or acquired immunodeficiency diseases, as well as newborns and patients receiving cytotoxic drugs, corticosteroids, radiotherapy or antithymocyte globulin because of organ allografts, nephrotic syndrome, collagen-vascular diseases, and so on. The risk is low in patients receiving low-dose alternate-day steroid therapy, but is substantial in those receiving higher doses (e.g., 1–2 mg/kg/day of prednisone). If possible, cancer chemotherapy should be temporarily interrupted; however, treatment of malignancy should take precedence during induction therapy or therapy for disease in relapse. When treatment is stopped, it should be resumed 21 days after exposure or 7 days after complete crusting of all lesions. Steroids should be tapered during the incubation period and cytotoxic therapy stopped if possible. However, patients who have received prolonged courses of corticosteriods should continue to receive replacement therapy.

Two antiviral chemotherapeutic agents are effective in VZV infections (Hirsch and Schooley, 1983). Vidarabine (9-β-D-arabinofuranosyladenine, adenine arabinoside, Vira-A), a purine nucleoside analog, is phosphorylated by cellular kinases to the triphosphate, which appears to act as a competitive inhibitor of DNA polymerases. Its capacity to inhibit selectively the replication of HSV and VZV in vitro and in vivo has been attributed to the greater effect of vidarabine triphosphate on viral than cellular DNA polymerases (Schwartz et al., 1976; Whitley and Alford, 1981). In a placebo-controlled therapeutic trial in immunosuppressed patients with varicella, intravenous vidarabine (10 mg/kg/day for 5 days) decreased new vesicle formation, mean daily vesicle counts, and the duration of fever. Of greater import, vidarabine reduced the incidence of life-threatening visceral dissemination from 53 per cent in the placebo group to 5 per cent, with minimal evidence of drug toxicity (Whitley et al., 1982a). The capacity of vidarabine to inhibit VZV replication and dissemination in immunosuppressed patients has been further demonstrated with the same dose and treatment schedule in immunocompromised patients with herpes zoster (Whitley et al., 1982b). Treatment begun within 72 hours of onset of the initial dermatomal lesions reduced cutaneous dissemination from 24 to 8 per cent and visceral dissemination from 19 to 5 per cent. Treatment also accelerated the disappearance of infectious virus from cutaneous lesions. In spite of its efficacy, vidarabine has drawbacks (Hirsch and Schooley, 1983; Whitley and Alford, 1981). It is not a selective inhibitor of virus replication (vidarabine triphosphate also inhibits cellular DNA polymerases) and thus it is potentially cytotoxic. It is also mutagenic and teratogenic in some experimental models. Finally, its low solubility requires that it be administered in large volumes of fluid.

Acyclovir [9-(2-hydroxyethoxymethyl) guanine, acycloguanosine] is the first of a new generation of truly selective inhibitors of herpesvirus replication (Elion, 1982). The drug, a guanosine analog, is selectively phosphorylated by HSV and VZV deoxypyrimidine kinases (it is a poor substrate for cellular thymidine kinase). As a result, the concentration of acyclovir monophosphate in infected cells is 30 to 100 times greater than that in uninfected cells. Cellular enzymes convert acyclovir monophosphate to acyclovir triphosphate, which is a selective inhibitor of HSV and VZV DNA polymerases (Elion, 1982). In addition, any drug that is incorporated into DNA causes chain termination. Acyclovir, at therapeutic concentrations, is remarkably nontoxic, with no observed effects on hematopoietic precusor cells or the immune system (Hirsch and Schooley, 1983). Most studies of mutagenicity and teratogenicity in model systems have been negative. Acyclovir has been tested in a small placebo-controlled therapeutic study in immunosuppressed patients with varicella (Prober et al., 1982). Acyclovir (500 mg/m^2 intravenously every 8 hours for 7 days) reduced the incidence of pneumonitis from 45 per cent (5/11) in the placebo group to 0 per cent (0/7) with no evidence of toxicity. In a placebo-controlled study in immunocompromised patients with herpes zoster, intravenous acyclovir at this dose inhibited cutaneous and visceral dissemination of VZV, with no evidence of toxicity (Balfour et al., 1983). These results, as well as experience gained in open protocols (Serota et al., 1982; Balfour, 1984), suggest that acyclovir is at least as effective as vidarabine in patients with VZV infections but is free of vidarabine's toxicity and problems of fluid overload (Hirsch and Schooley, 1983). However, randomized controlled studies directly comparing vidarabine and acyclovir in patients with VZV infections have only recently been initiated.

All studies indicate that to be effective, antiviral therapy must be initiated early in the disease before the occurrence of significant visceral dissemination. The recommended dose of acyclovir is 500 mg/m^2 every 8 hours intravenously for 7 days; vidarabine is administered in a dose of 15 mg/kg/day in a 12-hour intravenous infusion for 5 to 7 days. The doses of both drugs are reduced in patients with renal insufficiency. Pending the results of comparative studies, I prefer to use acyclovir in these patients because of its ease of administration and lower toxicity.

Interferon has also been evaluated in randomized placebo-controlled treatment studies of varicella in children with cancer (Arvin et al., 1982). Parenteral administration of human interferon alpha (3.5×10^5 units/kg/day for 2 days, then 1.75×10^5 units/kg/day for 3 days) shortened the period of new lesion formation and reduced the incidence of fatal and life-threatening dissemination from 29 per cent in the placebo group to 9 per cent. Though reasonably well tolerated in these studies, interferons appear to be somewhat more toxic than acyclovir or vidarabine (Hirsch and Schooley, 1983).

Oral formulations of acyclovir are being tested in patients with VZV infections (Novelli et al., 1984), and a number of promising new selective antiviral chemotherapeutic agents are beginning to be evaluated in clinical trials (Hirsch and Schooley, 1983). Systemic cytosine arabinoside (Ara-C) or iododeoxyuridine (IdR) should *not* be used in patients with varicella or its complications because both drugs are too toxic and are likely to adversely affect the outcome, especially in immunosuppressed patients.

PROPHYLAXIS. Varicella is almost always a benign disease in normal children. Since infection results in life-long immunity, its acquisition in childhood eliminates the problem of varicella in the adult. Consequently, no preventive measures are recommended for a normal child who has been exposed to varicella.

On the other hand, varicella is potentially fatal in susceptible patients undergoing immunosuppressive therapy, patients with an immunosuppressive malignancy such as Hodgkin's disease, susceptible newborn infants, and even normal adults. Thus it is desirable to prevent or modify varicella in these high-risk individuals. Potential approaches include passive immunization, active immunization, chemoprophylaxis, and prevention of exposure.

Passive immunization with large doses (0.6 to 1.2 ml/kg) of standard human immune serum globulin (ISG) administered within three days of exposure was shown to attenuate but not prevent varicella in normal children (Ross, 1962). Passive immunization with zoster immune globulin (ZIG), prepared from the plasma of donors recovering from herpes zoster and containing a high titer of antibody to VZV, prevented varicella in susceptible normal children when administered within three days of exposure (Brunell et al., 1969) and modified the disease in immunosuppressed children (Gershon et al., 1974; Orenstein et al., 1981). One third of the immunosuppressed recipients developed subclinical infection, and the disease was mild in most of the others. Similarly, zoster immune plasma (ZIP) obtained from otherwise healthy individuals during convalescence from varicella or herpes zoster has been shown to modify or prevent varicella in susceptible high-risk children when it is administered within five days of exposure (Geiser et al., 1975; Balfour et al., 1977; Balfour and Groth, 1979). In contrast to the favorable outcome in these passively immunized, high-risk children is the 32 per cent mortality reported in a group of 106 leukemic children with unmodified varicella (Hattori et al., 1976). In order to overcome the relative shortage of zoster convalescent plasma and ZIG for the growing population of immunosuppressed patients, Zaia et al. (1978) screened outdated blood from blood banks and used those units with high levels of antibody to VZV to prepare batches of immune globulin (varicella-zoster immune globulin, VZIG) with antibody levels equivalent to those in ZIG. In a randomized double-blind trial of their capacity to protect immunosuppressed children from severe varicella, ZIG and VZIG were comparable (Zaia et al., 1983). Clinical infection occurred in 44 per cent of VZIG recipients and 37 per cent of ZIG recipients, with no significant difference in severity in the two groups. Subclinical infections occurred in 16 per cent of VZIG and 31 per cent of ZIG recipients. It was also observed that 28 per cent of patients with a negative history of previous varicella, but with FAMA antibody to VZV detectable in preimmunization serum, developed mild clinical illness. This suggests that in patients receiving blood and blood products, low levels of antibody to VZV do not indicate immunity in patients without a history of varicella or herpes zoster. Thus such patients remain at risk of serious infection. When exposed to VZV they should receive passive immunization and require isolation procedures to prevent nosocomial varicella. Note that the incubation period is prolonged in ZIG, ZIP, and VZIG recipients who develop clinical disease.

VZIG has now been licensed for use by the FDA and can be bought from a number of regional distribution centers (Centers for Disease Control, 1984). The following is a list of criteria recommended for VZIG use:

1. One of the following illnesses or conditions: A. Leukemia or lymphoma. B. Congenital or acquired immunodeficiency. C. Bone marrow transplant recipient *regardless of pretransplantation history of varicella or herpes zoster.* D. Under immunosuppressive treatment (including corticosteroid treatment). E. Newborn of mother who had onset of varicella within 5 days before delivery or within 48 hours after delivery. F. Premature infant, <28 weeks gestation or ≤ 1000 grams regardless of maternal history of varicella or herpes zoster. G. Premature infant, ≥ 28 weeks gestation, whose mother lacks a history of varicella or herpes zoster. H. Any infant ≤ 14 days of age whose mother lacks a history of varicella or herpes zoster. I. Susceptible pregnant or nonpregnant adult.*
2. One of the following types of exposure to person or persons with varicella or herpes zoster: A. Continuous household contact. B. Playmate contact (generally >1 hour play indoors). C. Hospital contact (in same 2-bed to 4-bed room *or* adjacent beds in a large ward *or* prolonged face-to-face contact with an infectious staff member or patient. D. Intrauterine contact (newborn of mother with onset of varicella 5 days or less before delivery or within 48 hours after delivery).
3. Negative or unknown history of varicella or herpes zoster (except bone marrow transplant recipients).
4. Time elapsed after exposure is such that VZIG can be administered within 96 hours of exposure.

New serologic tests (vide supra), which permit the rapid identification of susceptible individuals, and the increased availability of VZIG, now make it possible to identify and

*Immunologically normal adults with no history of varicella or herpes zoster are generally considered immune unless serologic testing shows that they lack serum antibody to VZV.

passively immunize *susceptible* pregnant and nonpregnant adults with recognized exposure to varicella.

Unfortunately, protection afforded by VZIG is transient, whereas most susceptible people will experience repeated exposures to VZV. Furthermore, exposure to VZV is often unrecognized, and thus large numbers of immunocompromised patients will continue to develop unmodified varicella in spite of the availability of VZIG. Continuous prophylaxis by administration of VZIG on a monthly or bimonthly schedule is impractical; what is needed is a safe means of inducing long-lasting immunity to VZV in immunocompromised patients and susceptible adults.

A decade ago Dr. M. Takahashi and his colleagues announced the development of a live attenuated VZV vaccine (OKA strain) prepared from a clinical (varicella vesicle fluid) isolate of VZV by serial passage in human and guinea pig cell cultures (Takahashi et al., 1974). Despite concerns about its degree of attenuation, capacity to induce latent infections, and safety in immunocompromised patients, it has been extensively evaluated in Japan and, more recently, in the United States (Gershon, 1980; Brunell et al., 1982; Asano et al., 1982 and 1983; Gershon, 1983; Arbeter et al., 1984; Hayakawa et al., 1984; Gershon et al., 1984b). Administered to normal children and adults, it induces a mild papular or papulovesicular rash and slight fever in a small minority. Antibody to VZV, VZV-specific lymphoproliferative responses, and VZV-specific skin test reactivity are induced in almost all normal recipients and are generally long-lasting. Virus is almost never isolated from the rash in normal recipients, and there is no apparent transmission to contacts. However, in contrast to natural varicella, a few of these immunized normal persons have developed very mild varicella on subsequent exposure to VZV; the virus isolated from such patients is wild-type VZV. Herpes zoster has developed in less than 0.3 per cent of normal recipients of the vaccine. Interestingly, the vaccine can prevent varicella in normal children if administered within the first 3 days after exposure. When children with leukemia in remission and off chemotherapy are vaccinated, fewer than 10 per cent develop a papular or papulovesicular rash, and most develop antibody and CMI to VZV. When children on chemotherapy have it stopped for one week before and one week after vaccination, up to 40 per cent develop rash. When the rash is vesicular, vaccine virus can be isolated and transmitted to susceptible normal siblings (who develop mild varicella). However, when vaccinated leukemic children are exposed to VZV, most are protected and only about 10 to 20 per cent develop clinical varicella, which is generally mild. Leukemic vaccinees do develop herpes zoster (caused by the vaccine virus) at a rate comparable to that in similar patients with a history of natural varicella. In summary, the OKA VZV vaccine can be safely administered to susceptible immunosuppressed children, who are then markedly protected from the morbidity and mortality that would otherwise result from subsequent exposures to varicella. However, even in normal individuals, the immunity induced by the vaccine is not as solid or as durable as that induced by wild-type VZV. Furthermore, vaccine virus can be transmitted from vaccinated patients to susceptible normal contacts, who develop varicella, and it appears that a single passage in humans may result in increased virulence. Although many questions remain, the attenuated OKA VZV vaccine represents a tremendous advance in our ability to cope with the problem of varicella in immunocompromised patients. While a safe and effective VZV vaccine will be very useful for immunosuppressed patients and susceptible adults, questions of long-term safety and efficacy are still likely to preclude its use in normal children (Brunell, 1977).

Chemoprophylaxis has not been developed for VZV. Exposure of susceptible patients to VZV warrants reduction in the dosage of corticosteroids to physiologic levels and elimination or reduction of immunosuppressive drugs until the varicella has resolved or until it is clear that they have escaped infection. Such patients should receive VZIG immediately after exposure.

No attempts need to be made to prevent exposure of susceptible normal children; patients with varicella need only be kept at home until all vesicles have crusted (Weller, 1982; Krugman et al., 1977). On the other hand, rigid isolation should be enforced to prevent infection of susceptible immunosuppressed patients and newborn infants. Contact with patients with varicella and herpes zoster, and with persons who may be incubating varicella, must be avoided. Hospital personnel without a clear history of varicella or herpes zoster should be tested for antibody to VZV. Hospitals should develop and implement clear procedures to prevent nosocomial varicella (Weller 1982; Krugman et al., 1977; Leclair et al., 1980, Myers et al., 1982). If such exposure occurs or is suspected, VZIG prophylaxis is warranted.

References

Almeida, J. D., Howatson, A. F., and Williams, M. G.: Morphology of varicella (chickenpox) virus. Virology 16:353, 1962.

Aoyama, Y., Kurata, T., Kurata, K., Hondo, R., and Ogiwara, H.: Demonstration of viral antigens in herpes simplex and varicella-zoster infection. Recent Adv RES Res 14:90, 1974.

Appelbaum, E., Rachelson, M. H., and Dolgopol, V. B.: Varicella encephalitis. Am J Med 15:223, 1953.

Arbeit, R. D., Zaia, J. A., Valerio, M. A., and Levin, M. J.: Infection of human peripheral blood mononuclear cells by varicella-zoster virus. Intervirology 18:56, 1982.

Arbeter, A. M., Starr, S. E., Preblud, S. R., Ihara, T., Paciorek, P. M., Miller, D. S., Zelson, C. M., Proctor, E. A., and Plotkin, S. A.: Varicella vaccine trials in healthy children. Am J Dis Child 138:434, 1984.

Armstrong, R. W., Gurwith, M. J., Waddell, D., and Merigan, T. C.: Cutaneous interferon production in patients with Hodgkin's disease and other cancers infected with varicella or vaccinia. N Engl J Med 283:1182, 1970.

Arvin, A. M., and Koropchak, C. M.: Immunoglobulins M and G to varicella-zoster virus measured by solid-phase radioimmunoassay: antibody responses to varicella and herpes zoster infections. J Clin Microbiol 12:367, 1980.

Arvin, A. M., Koropchak, C. M., and Wittek, A. E.: Immunology evidence of reinfection with varicella-zoster virus. J Infect Dis 148:200, 1983.

Arvin, A. M., Kushner, J. H., Feldman, S., Baehner, R. L., Hammond, D., and Merigan, T. C.: Human leukocyte interferon for the treatment of varicella in children with cancer. N Engl J Med 306:761, 1982.

Asano, Y., Albrecht, P., Vujcic, L. K., Quinnan, G. V., Kawakami, K., and Takahashi, M.: Five-year follow-up study of recipients of live varicella vaccine using enhanced neutralization and fluorescent antibody membrane antigen assays. Pediatr 72:291, 1983.

Asano, Y., Hirose, S., Iwayama, S., Miyata, T., Yazaki, T., and Takahashi, M.: Protective effect of immediate inoculation of a live varicella vaccine in household contacts in relation to the viral dose and interval between exposure and vaccination. Biken J 25:43, 1982.

Asano, Y., Shiraki, K., Takahashi, M., Nagai, H., Ozaki, T., and Yazaki, T.: Soluble skin test antigen of varicella-zoster virus prepared from the fluid of infected cultures. J Infect Dis 143:684, 1981.

Baba, K., Yabuuchi, H., Takahashi, M. and Ogra, P. L.: Immunologic and epidemiologic aspects of varicella infection acquired during infancy and early childhood. J Pediatr 100:881, 1982.

Balfour, H. H., Jr.: Intravenous acyclovir therapy for varicella in immunocompromised children. J Pediatr 104:134, 1984.

Balfour, H. H., Jr., Bean, B., Laskin, O. L., Ambinder, R. F., Meyers, J. D., Wade, J. C., Zaia, J. A., Aeppli, D., Kirk, L. E., Segreti, A. C., and Keeney, R. E.: Acyclovir halts progression of herpes zoster in immunocompromised patients. N Engl J Med 308:1448, 1983.

Balfour, H. H., and Groth, K. E.: Zoster immune plasma prophylaxis of varicella: a follow-up report. J Pediatr 94:743, 1979.

Balfour, H. H., Jr., Groth, K. E., McCullough, J., Kallis, J. M., Marker, S. C., Nesbit, M. E., Simmons, R. L., and Najarian, J. S.: Prevention or modification of varicella using zoster immune plasma. Am J Dis Child 131:693, 1977.

Barr, R. J., Herten, R. J., and Graham, J. H.: Rapid method for tzanck preparations. JAMA 237:1119, 1977.

Blank, H., Burgoon, C. F., Baldridge, G. D., McCarthy, P. L., and Urbach, F.: Cytologic smears in diagnosis of herpes simplex, herpes zoster, and varicella. JAMA 146:1410, 1951.

Boughton, C. R.: Varicella-zoster in Sydney: I. Varicella and its complications. Med J Aust 53:392, 1966a.

Boughton, C. R.: Varicella-zoster in Sydney: II. Neurological complications of varicella. Med J Aust 53:444, 1966b.

Brunell, P. A.: Protection against varicella. Pediatrics 59:1, 1977.

Brunell, P. A., Geiser, C., Shehab, Z., and Waugh, J. E.: Administration of live varicella vaccine to children with leukaemia. Lancet 1069, 1982.

Brunell, P. A., Gershon, A. A., Uduman, S. A., and Steinberg, S.: Varicella-zoster immunoglobulins during varicella, latency, and zoster. J Infect Dis 132:49, 1975.

Brunell, P. A., and Kotchmar, G. S.: Zoster in infancy: Failure to maintain virus latency following intrauterine infection. J Pediatr 98:71, 1981.

Brunell, P. A., Ross, A., Miller, L. H., and Kuo, B.: Prevention of varicella by zoster immune globulin. N Engl J Med 280:1191, 1969.

Bruusgaard, E.: The mutual relation between zoster and varicella. Br J Dermatol 44:1, 1932.

Bullowa, J. G. M., and Wishik, S. M.: Complications of varicella. I. Their occurrence among 2,534 patients. Am J Dis Child 49:923, 1935.

Center for Disease Control. Epidemiologic notes and reports: Follow-up on Reye syndrome—United States. Morbidity and Mortality Weekly Report 29:1, 1980.

Centers for Disease Control. Varicella-zoster immune globulin for the prevention of chickenpox. Ann Intern Med 100:859, 1984.

Charkes, N. D.: Purpuric chickenpox: Report of a case, review of the literature, and classification by clinical features. Ann Intern Med 54:745, 1961.

Cheatham, W. J., Weller, T. H., Dolan, T. F., and Dower, J. C.: Varicella: Report of two fatal cases with necropsy, virus isolation, and serologic studies. Am J Pathol 32:1015, 1956.

Christie, A. B.: Chickenpox; herpes zoster. In *Infectious Diseases: Epidemiology and Clinical Practice*. 3rd ed. Edinburgh, Churchill Livingstone, 1980, pp. 262–277; 278–287.

Cleveland, P. H., Richman, D. D., Redfield, D. C., Disharoon, D. R., Binder, P. S., and Oxman, M. N.: An enzyme immunofiltration technique for the rapid diagnosis of herpes simplex virus eye infections. J Clin Microbiol 16:676, 1982.

Cradock-Watson, J. E., Ridehalgh, M. K. S., and Bourne, M. S.: Specific immunoglobulin responses after varicella and herpes zoster. J Hyg Camb 82:319, 1979.

Ecker, J. R., and Hyman, R. W.: Varicella-zoster virus vaccine DNA differs from the parental virus DNA. J Virol 40:314, 1981.

Ecker, J. R., and Hyman, R. W.: Varicella zoster virus DNA exists as two isomers. Proc Natl Acad Sci 79:156, 1982.

Eisenbud, M.: Chickenpox with visceral involvement. Am J Med 12:740, 1952.

Elion, G. B.: Mechanism of action and selectivity of acyclovir. Am J Med 73(1A):7, 1982.

Esiri, M. M., and Tomlinson, A. H.: Herpes zoster: Demonstration of virus in trigeminal nerve and ganglion by immunofluorescence and electron microscopy. J Neurol Sci 15:35, 1972.

Espinoza, C., and Kuhn, C.: Viral infection of megakaryocytes in varicella with purpura. Am J Clin Pathol 61:203, 1974.

Evans, P.: An epidemic of chickenpox. Lancet 2:339, 1940.

Ey, J. L., Smith, S. M., and Fulginiti, V. A.: Varicella hepatitis without neurologic symptoms or findings. Pediatrics 67:285, 1981.

Feldhoff, C. M., Balfour, H. H., and Najarian, J. S.: Varicella in children with renal transplants. J Pediatr 98:25, 1981.

Feldman, S., and Epp, E.: Isolation of varicella-zoster virus from blood. J Pediatr 88:265, 1976.

Feldman, S., and Epp, E.: Detection of viremia during incubation of varicella. J Pediatr 94:746, 1979.

Feldman, S., Hughes, W. T., and Daniel, C. B.: Varicella in children with cancer: Seventy-seven cases. Pediatrics 56:388, 1975.

Fenner, F.: The pathogenesis of the acute exanthems: An interpretation based on experimental investigations with mousepox (infectious ectromelia of mice). Lancet 2:915, 1948.

Feusner, J. H., Slichter, S. J., and Harker, L. A.: Mechanisms of thrombocytopenia in varicella. Am J Hematol 7:255, 1979.

Finkel, K. C.: Mortality from varicella in children receiving adrenocorticosteroids and adrenocorticotropin. Pediatrics 28:436, 1971.

Fleisher, G., Henry, W., McSorley, M., Arbeter, A., and Plotkin, S.: Life-threatening complications of varicella. Am J Dis Child, 135:896, 1981.

Frey, H. M., and Steinberg, S. P.: Rapid diagnosis of varicella-zoster virus infections by countercurrent immunoelectrophoresis. J Infect Dis 143:274, 1981.

Fulginiti, V. A., Brunell, P. A., Cherry, J. D., Ector, W. L., Gershon, A. A., Gotoff, S. P., Hughes, W. T., Jr., Mortimer, E. A., Jr., and Peter, G.: Special Report: Aspirin and Reye syndrome. Pediatrics 69:810, 1982.

Gershon, A. A.: Live attenuated varicella-zoster vaccine. Rev Infect Dis 2:393, 1980.

Gershon, A. A.: Varicella vaccine. Isr J Med Sci 19:1024, 1983,

Gershon, A. A., Brunell, P. A., Doyle, E. F., and Clapps, A. A.: Steroid therapy and varicella. J Pediatr 81:1034, 1972.

Gershon, A. A., and Krugman, S.: Seroepidemiologic survey of varicella: Value of specific fluorescent antibody test. Pediatrics 56:1005, 1975.

Gershon, A. A., Raker, R., Steinberg, S., Topf-Olstein, B., and Drusin, L. M.: Antibody to varicella-zoster virus in parturient women and their offspring during the first year of life. Pediatrics 58:692, 1976.

Gershon, A. A., and Steinberg, S. P.: Cellular and humoral immune responses to varicella-zoster virus in immunocompromised patients during and after varicella-zoster infections. Infect Immun 25:170, 1979.

Gershon, A. A., Steinberg, S., and Brunell, P. A.: Zoster immune globulin, a further assessment. N Engl J Med 290:243, 1974.

Gershon, A. A., Steinberg, S. P. and Gelb, L.: Live attenuated varicella vaccine: Efficiency for children with leukemia in remission. JAMA 1984a, in press.

Gershon, A. A., Steinberg, S. P., Gelb, L., and The National Institute of Allergy and Infectious Diseases Collaborative Varicella Vaccine Study Group. Clinical Reinfection with varicella-zoster virus. J Infect Dis 149:137, 1984b.

Gershon, A. A., Steinberg, S., Greenberg, S., and Taber, L.: Varicella-zoster-associated encephalitis: Detection of specific antibody in cerebrospinal fluid. J Clin Microb 12:764, 1980.

Gibbs, F. A., Gibbs, E. L., Carpenter, P. R., and Spies, H. W.: Electroencephalographic abnormality in "uncomplicated" childhood diseases. JAMA 171:1050, 1959.

Gilden, D. H., Shtram, Y., Friedmann, A., Wellish, M., Devlin, M., Fraser, N., and Becker, Y.: The internal organization of the varicella-zoster virus genome. J Gen Virol 60:371, 1982.

Goffinet, D. R., Glatstein, E. J., and Merigan, T. C.: Herpes zoster-varicella infections and lymphoma. Ann Intern Med 76:235, 1972.

Gold, E.: Serologic and virus-isolation studies of patients with varicella or herpes-zoster infection. N Engl J Med 274:181, 1966.

Gold, E., and Nankervis, G. A.: Varicella-zoster viruses. In Kaplan, A. S. (ed.): The Herpesviruses. New York, Academic Press, 1973, pp. 327-351.

Goldston, A. S., Millichap, J. G., and Miller, R. H.: Cerebellar ataxis with preeruptive varicella. Am J Dis Child 106:197, 1963.

Good, R. A., and Zak, S. J.: Disturbances in gamma globulin synthesis as "experiments of nature." Pediatrics 18:109, 1956.

Gordon, J. E.: Chickenpox: An epidemiological review. Am J Med Sci 244:362, 1962.

Griffith, J. F., Salam, M. V., and Adams, R. D.: The nervous system diseases associated with varicella. Acta Neurol Scand 46:279, 1970.

Gustafson, T. L., Lavely, G. B., Brawner, E. R., Jr., Hutcheson, R. H., Jr., Wright, P. F., and Schaffner, W.: An outbreak of airborne nosocomial varicella. Pediatrics 70:550, 1982.

Haggerty, R. J., and Eley, R. C.: Varicella and cortisone. Pediatrics 18:160, 1956.

Hattori, A., Ihara, T., Iwasa, T., Kamiya, H., Sakurai, M., Izawa, T., and Takahashi, M.: Use of live varicella vaccine in children with acute leukaemia or other malignancies. Lancet 2:210, 1976.

Hayakawa, Y., Torigoe, S., Shiraki, K., Yamanishi, K., and Takahashi, M.: Biologic and biophysical markers of a live varicella vaccine strain (Oka): Identification of clinical isolates from vaccine recipients. J Infect Dis 149:956, 1984.

Hirsch, M. S., and Schooley, R. T.: Treatment of herpesvirus infections. N Engl J Med 309:963 and 309:1034, 1983.

Hope-Simpson, R. E.: The nature of herpes zoster: A long-term study and a new hypothesis. Proc R Soc Med 58:9, 1965.

Hyman, R. W.: Molecular biology of varicella-zoster virus. In Roizman, B. (ed.): The Herpesviruses. New York, Plenum, 1983, pp. 115–134.

Iltis, J. P., Castellano, G. A., Gerber, P., Le, C., Vujcic, L. B., and Quinnan, G. V., Jr.: Comparison of the Raji cell line fluorescent antibody to membrane antigen test and the enzyme-linked immunosorbent assay for determination of immunity to varicella-zoster virus. J Clin Microbiol 16:878, 1982.

Johnson, H. N.: Visceral lesions associated with varicella. Arch Pathol 30:292, 1940.

Johnson, R., and Milbourne, P. E.: Central nervous system manifestations of chickenpox. Can Med Assoc J 102:831, 1970.

Johnson, R. T., Griffin, D. E., Hirsch, R. L., Wolinsky, J. S., Roedenbeck, S., de Soriano, I. L., and Vaisberg, A.: Measles encephalomyelitis—clinical and immunologic studies. N Engl J Med 310:137, 1984.

Jordan, G. W., and Merigan, T. C.: Cell-mediated immunity to varicella-zoster virus: in vitro lymphocyte responses. J Infect Dis 130:495, 1974.

Juel-Jensen, B. E., and MacCallum, F. O.: Herpes Simplex Varicella and Zoster. Philadelphia, J. B. Lippincott Company, 1972.

Kalter, Z. G., Steinberg, S., and Gershon, A. A.: Immune adherence hemagglutination: Further observations on demonstration of antibody to varicella-zoster virus. J Infect Dis 135:1010, 1977.

Kamiya, H., Ihara, T., Hattori, S., Iwasa, T., Sakurai, M., Izawa, T., Yamada, A., and Takahashi, M.: Diagnostic skin test reaction with varicella virus antigen and clinical application of the test. J Infect Dis 6:784, 1977.

Kamiya, H., Starr, S. E., Arbeter, A. M., and Plotkin, S. A.: Antibody-dependent cell-mediated cytotoxicity against varicella-zoster virus-infected targets. Infect Immun 38:554, 1982.

Krugman, S., Ward, R., and Katz, S. L.: Varicella-zoster infections. In Infectious Diseases of Children. 6th ed. St. Louis, C. V. Mosby Company, 1977, pp. 451-471.

Kumagai, T., Chiba, Y., Wataya, Y., Hanazono, H., Chiba, S., and Nakao, T.: Development and characteristics of the cellular immune response to infection with varicella-zoster virus. J Infect Dis 141:7, 1980.

Ladisch, S., Lovejoy, F. H., Hierholzer, J. C., Oxman, M. N., Strieder, D., Vawter, G. F., Finer, N., and Moore, M.: Extrapulmonary manifestations of adenovirus type 7 pneumonia simulating Reye syndrome and the possible role of an adenovirus toxin. J Pediatr 95:348, 1979.

Leclair, J. M., Zaia, J. A., Levin, M. J., Congdon, R. G., and Goldmann, D. A.: Airborne transmission of chickenpox in a hospital. N Engl J Med 302:450, 1980.

Levin, M. J., Leventhal, S., and Masters, H. A.: Factors influencing quantitative isolation of varicella-zoster virus. J Clin Microbiol 19:880, 1984.

Lichtenstein, P. K., Heubi, J. E., Daugherty, C. C., Farrell, M. K., Sokol, R. J., Rothbaum, R. J., Suchy, F. J., and Balistreri, W. F.: Grade I Reye's syndrome. A frequent cause of vomiting and liver dysfunction after varicella and upper-respiratory-tract infection. N Engl J Med 309:133, 1983.

Lipschutz, B.: Untersuchungen über die Ätiologie der Krankheiten der Herpesgruppe (Herpes zoster, Herpes genitalis, Herpes febrilis). Arch Dermatol 136:428, 1921.

Lux, S. E., Johnston, R. B., Jr., August, C. S., Say, B., Penchaszadeh, V. B., Rosen, F. S., and McKusick, V. A.: Chronic neutropenia and abnormal cellular immunity in cartilage-hair hypoplasia. N Engl J Med 282:231, 1970.

Mackay, J. B., and Cairney, P.: Pulmonary calcification following varicella. N Z Med J 59:453, 1960.

Martin, J. H., Dohner, D. E., Wellinghoff, W. J., and Gelb, L. D.: Restriction endonuclease analysis of varicella-zoster vaccine virus and wild-type DNAs. J Med Virol 9:69, 1982.

McCormick, W. F., Rodnitzky, R. L., Schochet, S. S., Jr., and McKee, A. P.: Varicella-zoster encephalomyelitis. Arch Neurol 21:559, 1969.

McKendall, R. R., and Klawans, H. L.: Nervous system complications of varicella-zoster virus. In Vinken, P. J. and Bruyn, G. W. (eds.): Handbook of Clinical Neurology. vol. 34. Amsterdam, North Holland Publishing Co., 1978, pp. 161–183.

Melish, M. E.: Bullous varicella: Its association with the staphylococcal scalded skin syndrome. J Pediatr 83:1019, 1973.

Meyers, J. D.: Congenital varicella in term infants: risk reconsidered. J Infect Dis 129:215, 1974.

Myers, M. G.: Viremia caused by varicella-zoster virus; association with malignant progressive varicella. J Infect Dis 140:229, 1979.

Myers, M. G.: Hepatic cellular injury during varicella. Arch Dis Child 57:317, 1982.

Myers, M. G., Duer, H. L., and Hausler, C. K.: Experimental infection of guinea pigs with varicella-zoster virus. J Infect Dis 142:414, 1980.

Myers, M. G., Rasley, D. A., and Hierholzer, W. J.: Hospital infection control for varicella zoster virus infection. Pediatrics 70:199, 1982.

Nicholaides, N. J.: Fatal systemic varicella. A report of 3 cases. Med J Aust 2:88, 1957.

Novelli, V. M., Marshall, W. C., Yeo, J., and McKendrick, G. D.: Acyclovir administered perorally in immunocompromised children with varicella-zoster infections. J Infect Dis 149:478, 1984.

Olding-Stenkvist, E., and Grandien, M.: Early diagnosis of virus-caused vesicular rashes by immunofluorescence on skin biopsies. Scand J Infect Dis 8:27, 1976.

Orenstein, W. A., Heymann, D. L., Ellis, R. J., Rosenberg, R. L., Nakano, J., Halsey, N. A., Overturf, G. D., Hayden, G. F., and Witte, J. J.: Prophylaxis of varicella in high-risk children: Dose-response effect of zoster immune globulin. J Pediatr 98:368, 1981.

Osler, W.: The Principles and Practice of Medicine. New York, D. Appleton and Company, 1892, p. 65.

Oxman, M. N., Richman, D. D., and Spector, A. A.: Management at delivery of mother and infant when herpes simplex, varicella-zoster, hepatitis or tuberculosis have occurred during pregnancy. In Remington, J. S., and Swartz, M. N. (eds.): Current Topics in Infectious Diseases. vol. 4. Boston, McGraw-Hill, 1983, pp. 224–280.

Patel, P. A., Yoonessi, S., O'Malley, J., Freeman, A., Gershon, A., and Ogra, P. L.: Cell-mediated immunity to varicella-zoster virus infection in subjects with lymphoma or leukemia. J Pediatr 94:223, 1979.

Peters, A. C. B., Versteeg, J., Lindeman, J., and Bots, G. T. A. M.: Varicella and acute cerebellar ataxia. Arch Neurol 35:769, 1978.

Pitel, P. A., McCormick, K. L., Fitzgerald, E., and Orson, J. M.: Subclinical hepatic changes in varicella infection. Pediatrics 65:631, 1980.

Prober, C. G., Kirk, L. E., and Keeney, R. E.: Acyclovir therapy of chickenpox in immunosuppressed children—a collaborative study. J Pediatr 101:622, 1982.

Richman, D. D., Cleveland, P. H., Oxman, M. N., and Zaia, J. A.: A rapid ^{125}I-staphylococcal protein A radioimmunoassay for antibody to varicella-zoster virus. J Infect Dis. 1981, in press.

Richman, D. D., Cleveland, P. H., Redfield, D. C., Oxman, M. N., and Wahl, G. M.: Rapid viral diagnosis. J Infect Dis 149:298, 1984.

Roizman, B., Carmichael, L. E., Deinhardt, F., de-The, G., Nahmias, A. J., Plowright, W., Rapp, F., Sheldrick, P., Takahashi, M., and Wolf, K. Herpesviridae. Definition, provisional nomenclature, and taxonomy. Intervirology 16:201, 1981.

Ross, A. H.: Modification of chicken pox in family contacts by administration of gamma globulin. N Engl J Med 267:369, 1962.

Rotter, R. and Collins, J. D.: Fatal disseminated varicella in adults; report of a case and review of the literature. Wis Med J 60:325–332, 1961.

Ruckdeschel, J. C., Schimpff, S. C., Smyth, A. C., and Mardiney, M. R.: Herpes zoster and impaired cell-associated immunity to the varicella-zoster virus in patients with Hodgkin's disease. Am J Med 62:77–85, 1977.

Sander, J., Serck-Hanssen, A., and Ulstrup, J. C.: Fatal varicella pneumonia. Scand J Infect Dis 2:231–234, 1970.

Sargent, E. N., Carson, M. J., and Reilly, E. D.: Varicella pneumonia. A report of 20 cases, with postmortem examination in six. Calif Med 107:141, 1967.

Scheinman, J. I., and Stamler, F. W.: Cyclophosphamide and fatal varicella. J Pediatr 74:117, 1969.

Schimpff, S., Serpick, A., Stoler, B., Rumack, B., Mellin, H., Joseph, J. M., and Block, J.: Varicella-zoster infection in patients with cancer. Ann Intern Med 76:241, 1972.

Schmidt, N. J.: Varicella-zoster virus. In Lennette, E. H., Balows, A. Hausler, W. J., Jr., and Truant, J. P. (eds.): Manual of Clinical Microbiology, Third Edition. Washington, American Society for Microbiology, 1980, pp. 798–806.

Schmidt, N. J., and Gallo, D.: Class-specific antibody responses to early and late antigens of varicella and herpes simplex viruses. J Med Virol 13:1, 1984.

Schmidt, N. J., and Gallo, D.: Class-specific antibody responses to early and late antigens of varicella and herpes simplex viruses. J Med Virol 13:1, 1984.

Schmidt, N. J., Gallo, D., Devlin, V., Woodie, J. D., and Emmons, R. W.: Direct immunofluorescence staining for detection of herpes simplex and varicella-zoster virus antigens in vesicular lesions and certain tissue specimens. J Clin Microbiol 12:651, 1980.

Schwartz, P. M., Shipman, C., and Drach, J. C.: Antiviral activity of arabinosyladenine and arabinosylhypoxanthine in herpes simplex virus-infected db cells. Selective inhibition of viral deoxyribonucleic acid synthesis in the presence of adenosine deaminase inhibitor. Antimicrob Agents Chemother 10:64, 1976.

Scott-Wilson, J. H.: Why "chicken" Pox? Lancet I:1152, 1978.

Serota, F. T., Starr, S. E., Bryan, C., Koch, P. A., Plotkin, S. A., and August, C. S.: Acyclovir treatment of herpes zoster infections. JAMA 247:2132, 1982.

Shanley, J., Myers, M., Edmond, B., and Steel, R.: Enzyme-linked immunosorbent assay for detection of antibody to varicella-zoster virus. J Clin Microbiol 15:208, 1982.

Shiraki, K., Okuno, T., Yamanishi, K., and Takahashi, M.: Polypeptides of varicella-zoster virus (VZV) and immunological relationship of VZV and herpes simplex virus (HSV). J Gen Virol 61:255, 1982.

Singer, J.: Postvaricella suppurative meningitis. Case reports and review of the literature. Am J Dis Child 133:934, 1979.

Smith, H.: Purpura fulminans complicating varicella: Recovery with low molecular weight dextran and steroids. Med J Aust 2:685, 1967.

Smith, E. W. P., Garson, A., Boyleston, J. A., Katz, S. L., and Wilfert, C. M.: Varicella gangrenosa due to group A-hemolytic streptococcus. Pediatrics 57:306, 1976.

Sokal, J. E., and Firat, D.: Varicella-zoster infection in Hodgkin's disease. Am J Med 39:452, 1965.

Steele, R. W., Coleman, M. A., Fiser, M., and Bradsher, R. W.: Varicella zoster in hospital personnel: skin test reactivity to monitor susceptibility. Pediatrics 70:604, 1982.

Steiner: Zur Inokulation der Varicellen. Wien Med Wochenschr 25:306, 1875.

Stevens, D. A., Ferrington, R. A., Jordan, G. W., and Merigan, T. C.: Cellular events in zoster vesicles: Relation to clinical course and immune parameters. J Infect Dis 131:509, 1975.

Straus, S. E., Aulakh, H. A., Ruyecnan, W. T., Hay, J., Casey, T. A.,

Vande Woude, G. F., and Hay, J.: Molecular cloning and physical mapping of varicella-zoster virus DNA. Proc Natl Acad Sci 79:993–997, 1982.
Takahashi, M., Otsuka, T., Okuno, Y., Asano, Y., Yazaki, T., and Isomura, S.: Live vaccine used to prevent the spread of varicella in children in hospital. Lancet 2:1288–1290, 1974.
Takashima, S., and Becker, L. E.: Neuropathology of fatal varicella. Arch Pathol Lab Med 103:209, 1979.
Taylor-Robinson, D., and Caunt, A. E.: Varicella Virus. Vienna, Springer-Verlag, 1972.
Triebwasser, J. H., Harris, R. E., Bryant, R. E., and Rhoades, E. R.: Varicella pneumonia in adults. Medicine 46:409, 1967.
Tyzzer, E. E.: The histology of the skin lesions in varicella. Philipp J Sci 1:349, 1906.
Uduman, S. A., Gershon, A. A., and Brunell, P. A.: Rapid diagnosis of varicella-zoster infections by agar-gel diffusion. J Infect Dis 126:193, 1972.
Underwood, E. A.: The neurological complications of varicella; a clinical and epidemiological study. Brit J Child Dis 32:83, 1935.
Waring, J. J., Neubuerger, K., and Geever, E. F.: Severe forms of chickenpox in adults. Arch Int Med 69:384, 1942.
Weber, D. M., and Pellecchia, J. A.: Varicella pneumonia: Study of prevalence in adult men. JAMA 192:527, 1965.
Weigle, K. A., and Grose, C.: Molecular dissection of the humoral immune response to individual varicella-zoster viral proteins during chickenpox, quiescence, reinfection, and reactivation. J Infect Dis 149:741, 1984.
Weinstein, L., and Meade, R. H.: Respiratory manifestations of chickenpox. Arch Intern Med 98:91, 1956.
Weller, T. H.: Varicella and Herpes Zoster. *In* Lennette, E. H., and Schmidt, N. J. (eds.): Diagnostic Procedures for Viral, Rickettsial and Chlamydial Infections, Fifth Edition. Washington, American Public Health Association, 1979, pp. 375–398.
Weller, T. H.: Varicella-herpes zoster virus. In Evans, A. S. (ed.): Viral Infections of Humans. New York, Plenum, 1982, pp. 569–595.
Weller, T. H.: Varicella and herpes zoster. Changing concepts of the natural history, control, and importance of a not-so-benign virus. N Engl J Med 309:1362 and 309:1434, 1983.
Weller, T. H., and Stoddard, M. B.: Intranuclear inclusion bodies in cultures of human tissue inoculated with varicella vesicle fluid. J Immunol 68:311, 1952.
Weller, T. H., and Witton, H. M.: The etiologic agents of varicella and herpes zoster: Serologic studies with the viruses as propagated *in vitro* J Exp Med 108:869, 1958.
Weller, T. H., Witton, H. M., and Bell, E. J.: The etiologic agents of varicella and herpes zoster: Isolation, propagation, and cultural characteristics *in vitro*. J Exp Med 108:843, 1958.
Wesselhoeft, C.: The differential diagnosis of chicken pox and smallpox. N Engl J Med 230:15, 1944.
Whitley, R. J., and Alford, D. C.: Parenteral antiviral chemotherapy of human herpesviruses. In Nahmias, A. J., Dowdle, W. R., and Schinazi, R. F. (eds.): The Human Herpesviruses: An Interdisciplinary Perspective. New York, Elsevier, 1981, pp. 478–490.
Whitley, R., Hilty, M., Haynes, R., et al.: Vidarabine therapy of varicella in immunosuppressed patients. J Pediatr 101:125, 1982a.
Whitley, R. J., Soong, S., Dolin, R., Betts, R., Linnemann, C., Jr., Alford, C. A., Jr., and The NIAID Collaborative Antiviral Study Group: Early vidarabine therapy to control the complications of herpes zoster in immunosuppressed patients. N Engl J Med 307:971, 1982b.
Williams, V., Gerson, A., and Brunell, P. A.: Serologic response to varicella-zoster membrane antigens measured by indirect immunofluorescence. J Infect Dis 130:669, 1974.
Williamson, A. P.: The varicella-zoster virus in the etiology of severe congenital defects. Clin Pediatr 14:553, 1975.
Wittek, A. E., Arvin, A. M., and Koropchak, C. M.: Serum immunoglobulin A antibody to varicella-zoster virus in subjects with primary varicella and herpes zoster infections and in immune subjects. J Clin Microbiol 18:1146, 1983.
Yeager, A. M., and Zinkham, W. H.: Varicella-associated thrombocytopenia: Clues to the etiology of childhood idiopathic thrombocytopenic purpura. Johns Hopkins Med J 146:270, 1980.
Young, N. A., and Gershon, A. A.: Chickenpox, measles and mumps. In (eds. Remington, J. S., and Klein, J. O.) *Infectious Diseases of the Fetus and Newborn Infant* Philadelphia, W. B. Saunders, 1983, pp. 375–449.
Zaia, J. A., Leary, P. L., and Levin, M. J.: Specificity of the blastogenic response of human mononuclear cells to herpesvirus antigens. Infect Immun 20:646, 1978.
Zaia, J. A., Levin, M. J., Preblud, S. R., Leszczynski, J., Wright, G. G., Ellis, R. J., Curtis, A. C., Valerio, M. A., and LeGore, J.: Evaluation of varicella-zoster immune globulin: Protection of immunosuppressed children after exposure to varicella. J Infect Dis 147:737, 1983.
Zaia, J. A., Levin, M. J., Wright, G. G., and Grady, G. F.: A practical method for preparation of varicella-zoster immune globulin. J Infect Dis 137:601, 1978.
Zaia, J. A., and Oxman, M. N.: Antibody to varicella-zoster virus-induced membrane antigen: Immunofluorescence assay using monodisperse glutaraldehyde-fixed target cells. J Infect Dis 136:519, 1977.

236

HERPES ZOSTER

MICHAEL N. OXMAN, M.D.

Herpes zoster (shingles, zoster) is a localized disease that occurs most frequently in elderly and immunocompromised people and is characterized by unilateral radicular pain and a vesicular eruption that is limited to the dermatome innervated by a single spinal or cranial sensory ganglion. It is caused by varicella-zoster virus (VZV), the same virus that causes varicella. In contrast to varicella, which follows primary exogenous VZV infection, herpes zoster appears to represent reactivation of an endogenous infection that has persisted in latent form after an earlier attack of varicella.

ETIOLOGY. The relationship of herpes zoster to varicella was first noted by von Bokay in 1888, who observed that susceptible children acquired varicella after contact with individuals with herpes zoster (von Bokey, 1909; Bruusgaard, 1932). Lipschutz (1921) noted that the skin lesions of herpes zoster were histologically identical to those of varicella.

Kundratitz (in 1922) and Bruusgaard (in 1925) inoculated children with zoster vesicle fluid and demonstrated that the same agent caused both diseases (Bruusgaard, 1932). Some developed varicella-like lesions at the site of inoculation; others developed, in addition, generalized varicella. Uninoculated children in contact with affected recipients developed typical varicella after a normal incubation period and transmitted the disease to other contacts. Children who had previously had varicella developed no disease when inoculated with herpes zoster vesicle fluid or when exposed to children who had developed varicella after such inoculation. Vesicles from the site of inoculation and in the generalized exanthem were histologically identical to those of ordinary varicella and herpes zoster. In early studies, antigens from vesicles and crusts of varicella and herpes zoster were shown to react equally well in complement fixation tests with convalescent sera from patients with either disease (Taylor-Robinson and Caunt, 1972; Weller 1982). Final proof of their common cause was provided when Weller and his colleagues found that the viruses recovered from patients with varicella and herpes zoster were identical (Weller and Coons, 1954; Weller, 1983). The properties of the virus are described in the previous chapter on varicella (Chapter 235).

PATHOGENESIS AND PATHOLOGY. The neurologic implications of the segmental distribution of the lesions of herpes zoster were recognized as long ago as 1831 by

Richard Bright, and the inflammatory changes in the corresponding sensory ganglion and spinal nerve were first described by von Barensprung in 1862. The definitive work is that of Head and Campbell (1900), who correlated postmortem examinations of 21 persons with herpes zoster with the clinical observations on 450 individuals with the disease. They described acute lymphocytic inflammation, focal hemorrhage, and neuronal destruction in sensory ganglia, the degeneration of sensory nerve fibers linking the affected neurons peripherally to the involved skin and centrally to the spinal cord and brain, and the later fibrosis of severely involved ganglia and nerves. They also mapped the area of skin (dermatome) innervated by each of the sensory ganglia. Their findings have been repeatedly confirmed (Stern 1937; Denny-Brown et al., 1944; Muller and Winkelmann, 1969; Esiri and Tomlinson, 1972; Bastian et al., 1974; Aoyama et al., 1974); some of these later studies used electronmicroscopy and fluorescent antibody staining to demonstrate virus and viral antigen within neurons and satellite cells in the sensory ganglia, and within peripheral sensory nerves early in the disease. Together, these observations indicate that in herpes zoster, active infection of sensory neurons precedes involvement of the skin.

Although the histopathology of the skin lesions of herpes zoster and varicella is the same, herpes zoster is accompanied by acute inflammation of the corresponding sensory nerve and ganglion. The ganglion shows intense lymphocytic infiltration, necrosis of nerve cells and fibers, endothelial proliferation and lymphocytic cuffing of small vessels, focal hemorrhage, and inflammation of the ganglion sheath (Head and Campbell, 1900; Denny-Brown et al., 1944). Satellite cells and neurons contain characteristic acidophilic intranuclear inclusions, virus particles visible by electronmicroscopy, and VZV antigens demonstrable by immunofluorescence (Esiri and Tomlinson, 1972; Ghatak and Zimmerman, 1973; Bastian et al., 1974; Aoyama et al., 1974; Juel-Jensen and MacCallum, 1972). Some neuronal degeneration and lymphocytic infiltration is also generally present in adjacent ganglia on the same side. The peripheral nerve shows diffuse lymphocytic infiltration and focal hemorrhage, with axonal degeneration and demyelination of sensory fibers; virus particles and VZV antigens are present in Schwann and perineural cells. These inflammatory and degenerative changes can be traced distally to branches innervating the affected skin (Muller and Winkelmann, 1969). The inflammatory reaction in the ganglion also extends proximally to the posterior nerve root and into the adjacent region of the cord or brain stem, producing a localized segmental poliomyelitis. This segmental myelitis is predominantly unilateral and involves the posterior horns more than the anterior ones. There is degeneration of nerve fibers in the posterior columns and inflammatory changes in the gray matter of the posterior and anterior horns, with perivenous lymphocytic infiltration, scattered neuronal necrosis, and neuronophagia. These changes may extend two or more segments from the one corresponding to the cutaneous eruption. A mild lymphocytic leptomeningitis is generally present and is most intense over the involved segments and nerve roots. Marked inflammation and degeneration of the anterior nerve root within the meninges and in the portion contiguous to the involved sensory ganglion can produce a true motor radiculitis (Denny-Brown et al., 1944) and, when extensive, results in fibrosis of the ganglion and nerve (Head and Campbell, 1900). These observations, as well as the isolation of VZV from the sensory ganglion (Aoyama et al., 1974; Bastian et al., 1974; Shibuta et al., 1974), cerebrospinal fluid (Gold and Robbins, 1958; Feldman et al., 1973; O'Donnell et al., 1981; Andiman et al., 1982) and central nervous system tissue (McCormick et al., 1969; Hogan and Krigman, 1973; Horton et al., 1981) indicate that the pathologic changes in herpes zoster are the direct result of VZV infection. These pathologic changes account for the segmental nervous system complications that are frequently observed in patients with herpes zoster, e.g., neuralgic pain, anesthesia, dysesthesia, and lower motor neuron paresis (McKendall and Klawans, 1978).

Herpes zoster is occasionally complicated by meningoencephalitis or myelitis, in which central nervous system involvement is not restricted to segments corresponding to the involved dermatone (McKendall and Klawans, 1978). The pathologic findings in herpes zoster meningoencephalitis vary from focal mononuclear cell infiltration of the leptomeninges (Norris et al., 1970; Juel-Jensen and MacCallum, 1972) to acute necrotizing encephalitis with perivenous encephalomalacia, myelin and axonal degeneration, macrophage infiltration, and typical intranuclear inclusions and virus particles in oligodendrocytes, neurons, and astrocytes. The presence of VZV in the involved brain tissue has been documented by virus isolation or immunoperoxidase staining in at least three of these patients (McCormick et al., 1969; Horten et al., 1981). Herpes zoster myelitis is rarely fatal, but in two patients who died of pulmonary embolism 12 days and 12 weeks, respectively, after the onset of herpes zoster, autopsy revealed extensive inflammatory necrosis of the spinal cord, which was maximal at the level of the dermatomal rash and extended above and below in a continuous but irregular pattern that did not correspond to any vascular topography (Rose et al., 1964; Hogan and Krigman, 1973). In areas of most recent extension where necrosis was less complete, intranuclear inclusion bodies were present in glial nuclei (Hogan and Krigman, 1973). VZV has also been isolated from the cerebrospinal fluid (CSF) of a number of patients with herpes zoster memingoencephalitis and myelitis (Gershon et al., 1980; O'Donnell et al., 1981; Andiman et al., 1982; Jemsek et al., 1983). In herpes zoster myelitis, it seems clear that VZV reaches the spinal cord by direct extension from the infected dorsal root ganglion. The pathogenesis of herpes zoster encephalitis (or meningoencephalitis) is more obscure. The presence of perivascular mononuclear cell infiltrates and demyelination, and the lack of direct evidence of VZV infection in autopsied cases, caused many observers to favor a post-infectious (autoimmune) encephalomyelitis (McKendall and Klawans, 1978) like that observed in measles encephalomyelitis (Johnson et al., 1984). However, there is now much evidence that most or all of the CNS complications of herpes zoster result directly from VZV infection of the tissues involved, and that the demyelination observed in herpes zoster encephalitis can be accounted for by VZV infection of oligodendrocytes (Horten et al., 1981). The frequent occurrence of herpes zoster encephalitis or meningoencephalitis in association with disseminated herpes zoster suggests that virus often reaches the brain as a result of viremia (McKendall and Klawans, 1978; Jemsek et al., 1983). However, it may also reach the brain along neural routes, especially when meningoencephalitis occurs in association with herpes zoster of cranial dermatomes (Horten et al., 1981; Jemsek et al., 1983).

The contralateral hemiplegia that sometimes develops in patients with ophthalmic herpes zoster appears to be caused by segmental granulomatous angiitis involving ipsilateral cerebral arteries (Rosenblum and Hadfield, 1972; Hilt et al., 1983; Bourdette et al., 1983). The temporal association with herpes zoster and the electronmicroscopic observation of herpesvirus-like particles in the walls of involved vessels and in adjacent glial cells (Reyes et al., 1976; Linnemann and Alvira, 1980; Doyle et al., 1983) suggest that the angiitis is due to VZV infection of arterial walls. The virus may reach the vessels by direct spread from the trigeminal ganglion or along branches of the ophthalmic nerve that supply the meninges and most of the intracranial arteries that have been involved.

Lesions of the skin, lungs, and other organs in fatal cases of disseminated herpes zoster are identical to those observed in fatal cases of varicella (Cheatham, 1953; Merselis et al., 1964). They result from the viremic spread of VZV in both diseases (Cheatham, 1953; Feldman et al., 1977; Myers, 1979).

The pathogenesis of herpes zoster is not fully understood but clinical, epidemiologic, and pathologic data, as well as analogy with recurrent herpes simplex virus infections (Stevens, 1975; Chapter 105), support the following model (Hope-Simpson, 1965). During varicella, VZV passes from skin and mucosal lesions into the contiguous endings of sensory nerves and travels centripetally up the sensory fibers to the sensory ganglia. In the ganglia, a latent infection is established in sensory neurons, and the virus then persists silently and harmlessly; it is no longer infectious and does not multiply, but it retains the capacity to revert to full infectiousness. Herpes zoster occurs most frequently in dermatomes in which the rash of varicella achieves the greatest density (Hope-Simpson, 1965; Stern, 1937), and this is probably because, during varicella, larger amounts of virus are transmitted to the corresponding ganglia, and latent infections are established in more sensory neurons. If reactivation occurs at random, zoster should occur most frequently in areas of skin innervated by ganglia with the most latently infected neurons. Two recent reports support the hypothesis that VZV is latent in sensory neurons. Gilden et al. (1983) detected small amounts of VZV DNA in trigeminal ganglia from 4 of 10 persons who died without clinical evidence of active VZV infection. Hyman et al. (1983), employing in situ hybridization with a cloned VZV DNA probe, detected VZV-specific RNA in neurons in trigeminal ganglia from 3 of 5 persons who died without evidence of active VZV infection. Only 0.08 to 0.3 per cent of the neurons in positive ganglia contained detectable VZV-specific RNA.

Although the latent virus in the ganglia retains its potential for full infectivity, reversions are sporadic and infrequent. The mechanisms involved in the reactivation of latent VZV are unclear, but a number of conditions have been associated with the occurrence and localization of herpes zoster. These include immunouppression in Hodgkin's disease and other malignancies; administration of immunosuppressive drugs and corticosteroids; irradiation of the spinal column; tumor involvement of the cord, dorsal root ganglion, or adjacent structures; local trauma; surgical manipulation of the spine; heavy metal poisoning or therapy; and frontal sinusitis, as a precipitant of ophthalmic zoster (Head and Campbell, 1900; Shanbrom et al., 1960; Hope-Simpson, 1965; Juel-Jensen and MacCallum, 1972; Schimpff et al., 1972; Feldman et al., 1973; Reboul et al., 1978).

Even when latent virus is reactivated, usually nothing perceptible happens. The minute dose of infectious virus that results is immediately neutralized by circulating antibody or destroyed by cellular immune responses before it can infect other cells and multiply enough to cause perceptible damage. The small quantity of viral antigen released into the bloodstream during such "contained reversions" stimulates host immune responses (Hope-Simpson, 1965; Luby et al., 1977; Weigle and Grose, 1984), and this raises the level of host resistance (Fig. 1). A similar boost in the level of host resistance frequently follows contact with a patient with varicella (Fig. 1), reflecting subclinical exogenous reinfection (Gershon et al., 1982; Iltis et al., 1982; Arvin et al., 1983). When host resistance falls to a level at which reactivated virus can no longer be contained, reversion is "successful." Virus multiplies and spreads within

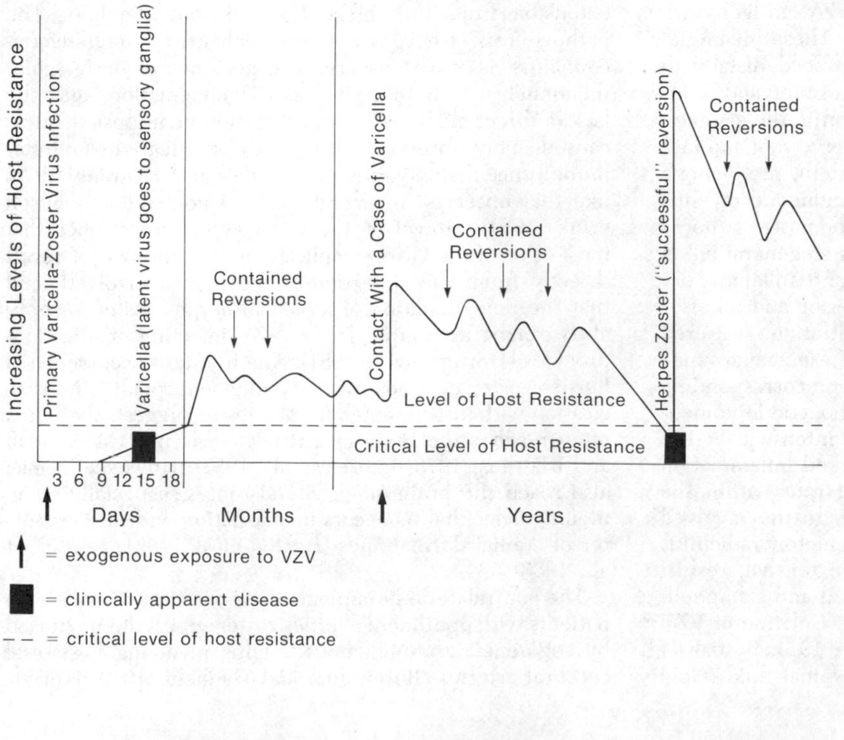

Figure 1. Pathogenesis of herpes zoster. (Modified from Hope-Simpson, R. E.: Proc R Soc Med 58:9, 1965.)

the ganglion, causing neuronal necrosis and intense inflammation, and this is usually accompanied by severe neuralgia. Infectious VZV then spreads antidromically down the sensory nerve, causing intense neuritis, and is released around the nerve endings, where it produces the characteristic cluster of zoster vesicles. The frequent occurence of neuralgia several days before the rash appears and the presence of degenerative changes in cutaneous nerve fibrils on the first day of the eruption (Muller and Winkelmann, 1969) provide additional evidence that infection in the sensory ganglion precedes involvement of the skin. Spread of the ganglionic infection proximally along the posterior nerve root results in local leptomeningitis, spinal fluid pleocytosis, and segmental myelitis. Infection of motor neurons in the anterior horn and inflammation of the anterior nerve root occasionally cause local palsies, and extension of infection within the central nervous system may cause ascending myelitis or meningoencephalitis, rare complications of herpes zoster (Dolin et al., 1978; McKendall and Klawans, 1978).

During each successful reversion, hematogenous dissemination of virus from the ganglion often produces aberrant vesicles at a distance from the primary dermatome, even in uncomplicated herpes zoster (Oberg and Svedmyr, 1969), and stimulates an anamnestic immune response that terminates or may even prevent the cutaneous lesions. Sometimes this results in radicular pain without eruption *(zoster sine herpete)*, but with a coincident rise in antibody to VZV. The occurrence of this syndrome has now been well documented (Juel-Jensen and MacCallum, 1972; Easton, 1970; Luby et al., 1977), as have completely asymptomatic rises in antibody to VZV that presumably reflect "contained reversions" (Luby et al., 1977; Gershon et al., 1982; Arvin et al., 1983). If the anamnestic immune response is delayed or deficient, as it appears to be in many immunosuppressed patients, the duration and severity of the local infection are increased, and the hematogenous dissemination of VZV is more prolonged and extensive (Feldman et al., 1977; Gallagher and Merigan, 1979; Mazur et al., 1979).

Hope-Simpson considered the level of antibody to be the critical determinant of the host's capacity to contain VZV reversions (Hope-Simpson, 1965). However, it now appears that cellular immunity is more important in resistance to recurrent VZV infections (Miller and Brunell, 1970; Schimpff et al., 1972; Feldman et al., 1973; Pollard et al., 1982; Arvin et al., 1980; Meyers et al., 1980).

A selective decline in cellular immune responses to VZV has been documented in elderly individuals (Miller, 1980; Berger et al., 1981; Burke et al., 1982), and this may explain the increased incidence and severity of herpes zoster observed in older people.

CLINICAL MANIFESTATIONS

Prodrome. The first symptom of herpes zoster is usually pain and paresthesia in the involved dermatome. This generally precedes the eruption by several days and varies from superficial itching, tingling, or burning to severe, deep pain. It may be constant or intermittent, and it is often accompanied by tenderness and hyperesthesia of the skin in the involved dermatome. The pre-eruptive pain of herpes zoster may simulate pleurisy, myocardial infarction, duodenal ulcer, cholecystitis, biliary or renal colic, appendicitis, prolapsed intervertebral disk, or early glaucoma, and it may thus lead to serious misdiagnosis. Regional lymphadenopathy and a dermatomal pattern of cutaneous sensory changes may be useful diagnostic clues. Constitutional symptoms, including headache, malaise and fever, occur in about 5 per cent of patients, mostly in children, and may precede the rash by one or two days (Burgoon et al., 1957; Rogers and Tindall, 1972; Juel-Jensen and MacCallum, 1972).

A few patients experience acute segmental neuralgia without ever developing a cutaneous eruption, a syndrome called *zoster sine herpete* (Juel-Jensen and MacCallum, 1972; Lewis, 1958; Easton, 1970). Although zoster sine herpete may explain some cases of trigeminal neuralgia, most patients with this syndrome do not have serologic evidence of herpes zoster. Similarly, while facial palsy frequently complicates cephalic herpes zoster, VZV infection does not appear to be responsible for most cases of "idiopathic" facial (Bell's) palsy (Adour, 1982).

Rash. The most distinctive feature of herpes zoster is the localization of the rash, which is nearly always unilateral, does not cross the midline, and is usually limited to the area of skin innervated by a single sensory ganglion (Fig. 2). Individual sensory ganglia are not attacked at random; herpes zoster occurs with greatest frequency where the rash of varicella is most abundant (Hope-Simpson, 1965; Stern, 1937). The areas supplied by the trigeminal nerve, particularly the ophthalmic division, and the trunk from T3 to L2 are most frequently affected; the thoracic region alone accounts for more than one-half of reported cases, and lesions rarely occur below the elbows or knees (Head and Campbell, 1900; Hope-Simpson, 1965; Burgoon et al., 1957; Juel-Jensen and MacCallum, 1972; Ragozzino et al., 1982a). Regional lymphadenopathy occurs in most cases, and the spinal fluid frequently shows a mild pleocytosis, predominantly lymphocytic, and an elevated protein content. Although individual lesions of herpes zoster and varicella are usually indistinguishable, those of herpes zoster tend to evolve more slowly and often consist of closely grouped vesicles on an erythematous base rather than the discrete, randomly distributed vesicles of varicella. The lesions begin as erythematous maculopapules that often first appear where superficial branches of the affected sensory nerve are given off—e.g., the posterior primary division and the lateral and anterior branches of the anterior primary division of the spinal nerves (Head and Campbell, 1900; Stern, 1937). Vesicles form within 12 to 24 hours and become pustules by the third day. These dry up and crust in seven to ten days. Crusts generally persist for two to three weeks. In normal individuals, new lesions continue to appear for one to four days (occasionally for as long as seven days), and virus may be recovered from lesions for as long as a week after the appearance of the rash. The rash is most severe and lasts longest in older individuals and is mildest in children (Burgoon et al., 1957; de Moragas and Kierland, 1957; Brown, 1976; Juel-Jensen and MacCallum, 1972). Segmental pain, a prominent feature of herpes zoster in older individuals, generally remits as the crusts fall off. Pain is seldom a significant symptom of herpes zoster in children (Winkelman and Perry, 1959; Brunell et al., 1968).

From 10 to 15 per cent of reported cases of herpes zoster involve the ophthalmic division of the trigeminal nerve. The rash of ophthalmic zoster may extend from the level of the eye to the vertex of the skull, but it does not cross the midline of the forehead. When only the supratrochlear and supraorbital branches are involved, the eye is usually spared. Involvement of the nasociliary branch, as evidenced by a herpetic rash on the tip and side of the nose (Fig. 3), occurs in one-third or more of patients and is usually accompanied by conjunctivitis and occasionally by keratitis,

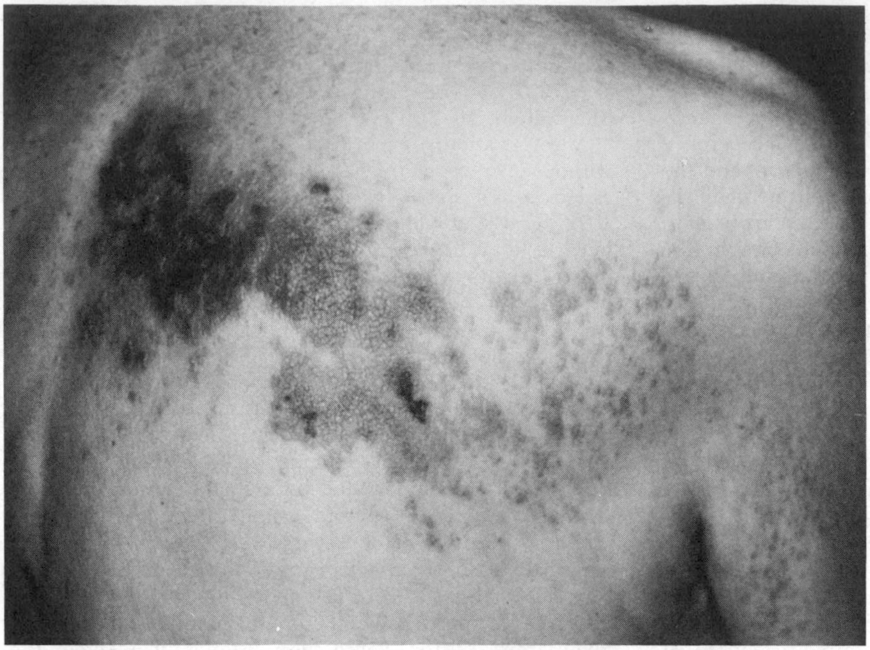

Figure 2. Herpes zoster in the right second thoracic dermatome involving primarily skin innervated by the posterior primary division and by the posterior branch of the lateral cutaneous nerve (Courtesy Dr. D. A. Lopez).

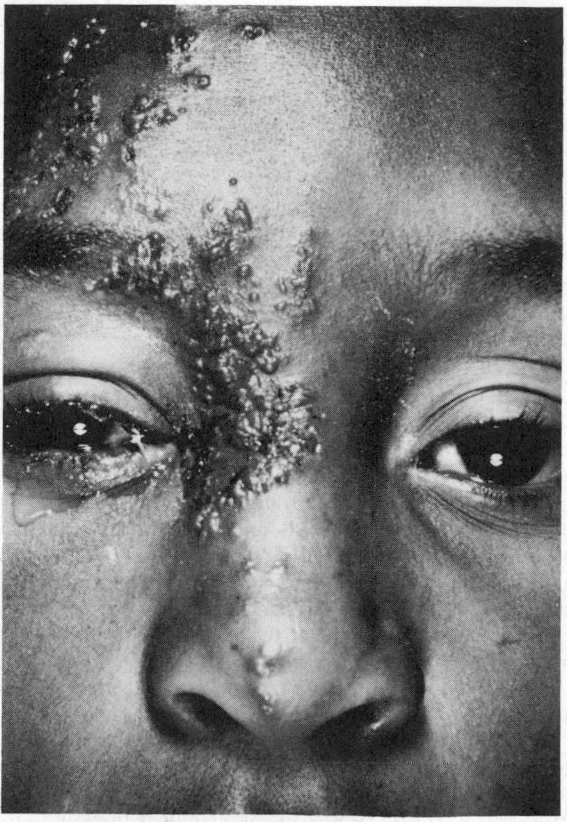

Figure 3. Herpes zoster of the ophthalmic division of the fifth cranial nerve. Involvement of the nasociliary branch results in lesions on the tip and side of the nose and unilateral conjunctivitis. (Courtesy of Dr. D. A. Lopez.)

scleritis, iridocyclitis, extraocular muscle palsies, ptosis, and mydriasis. Thus, when ophthalmic zoster involves the side of the nose, careful attention must be given to the condition of the eye. VZV is not, however, as pathogenic for the eye as herpes simplex virus (HSV).

Herpes zoster affecting the second and third divisions of the trigeminal nerve and other cranial nerves is uncommon, but when it occurs, it may produce symptoms and lesions in the mouth, ears, pharynx, or larynx (Denny-Brown et al., 1944; Eisenberg, 1978; Clark, 1979). The so-called Ramsay Hunt syndrome, which consists of facial palsy in combination with herpes zoster of the external ear or tympanic membrane, with or without tinnitus, vertigo, and deafness, results from involvement of the facial and auditory nerves (Denny-Brown et al., 1944).

Complications. Postherpetic neuralgia (pain persisting after all crusts have fallen off) occurs in 10 to 15 percent of patients with herpes zoster (Hope-Simpson, 1975; Ragozzino et al., 1982a). It is uncommon in patients under 40 years of age, but occurs in more than one third of patients 60 years old or older, especially those with ophthalmic zoster (Burgoon et al., 1957; de Moragas and Kierland, 1957; Juel-Jensen and MacCallum, 1972; Hope-Simpson, 1975). Anesthesia in the involved dermatome is another common sequela, and is particularly troublesome when it occurs in the area innervated by the ophthalmic nerve (Juel-Jensen and MacCallum, 1972; Pavan-Langston, 1983; Womack and Liesegang, 1983). Postherpetic neuralgia is refractory to treatment but usually remits spontaneously in one to six months.

When the rash is particularly severe, there may be superficial gangrene wih delayed healing and subsequent scarring. As in varicella, secondary bacterial infection may also delay healing and cause scarring.

Ophthalmic zoster has a relatively high complication rate, especially when involvement of the nasociliary branches provides VZV with direct access to intraocular structures (Ragozzino et al., 1982a; Womack and Liesegang, 1983; Pavan-Langston, 1983). The eye is involved in 20 to 70 per cent, depending upon the population of patients. Complications include cicatricial lid retraction, paralytic ptosis, acute epithelial keratitis, scleritis, uveitis, secondary glaucoma, oculomotor palsies, chorioretinitis, and optic neuritis. Corneal sensation is almost always impaired, and when the impairment is severe it may lead to neurotrophic keratitis and chronic ulceration. Rarely, secondary bacterial infection may result in panophthalmitis requiring enucleation. Granulomatous cerebral angiitis with contralateral hemiplegia (vide supra) was observed in 4 of 86 patients with ophthalmic zoster seen at the Mayo Clinic between 1975 and 1980 (Womack and Liesegang, 1983).

Most other complications of herpes zoster appear to be associated with spread of virus from the involved ganglion, either via the bloodstream or by direct neural extension. When patients with herpes zoster are carefully examined, 17 to 35 per cent are found to have at least a few vesicles in areas remote from the involved dermatome; this is due presumably to hematogenous dissemination of virus from the affected ganglion, nerve, or skin (Oberg and Svedmyr, 1969; Juel-Jensen and MacCallum, 1972). The disseminated lesions usually appear within a week of onset of the segmental eruption and, if few in number, are easily overlooked. More extensive dissemination, producing a varicella-like eruption (generalized herpes zoster), occurs in 2 to 10 per cent of unselected patients with localized zoster, most of whom have immunologic defects due to underlying malignancy (particularly lymphomas) or immunouppressive therapy (Burgoon et al., 1957; de Moragas and Kierland, 1957; Oberg and Svedmyr, 1969; Rogers and Tindall, 1972; Merselis et al., 1964).

On rare occasions, most often in children, infection disseminates widely from a small, painless area of zoster (Rogers and Tindall, 1972), so that the zoster is unnoticed and the disseminated eruption is mistaken for varicella. This probably explains some reports of second attacks of varicella, as well as some cases of "atypical generalized zoster" (a disseminated varicella-like eruption without an accompanying dermatomal rash in a person with a history of varicella) reported in immunocompromised patients (Schimpff et al., 1972) . However, symptomatic reinfections do occur, especially in immunocompromised patients and in people whose initial infection was modified by passively acquired antibody to VZV (Weller, 1983; Gershon et al., 1984). Such symptomatic reinfections, which may have a prolonged incubation period, probably explain many of the cases of "atypical generalized zoster" observed in immunocompromised and apparently normal patients (Schimpff et al., 1972; Patterson et al., 1980).

Motor paralysis is reported in 1 to 5 per cent of patients with herpes zoster; it results from spread of infection from the sensory ganglion to adjacent parts of the nervous system (Head and Campbell, 1900; Denny-Brown et al., 1944; Juel-Jensen and MacCallum, 1972; Grant and Rowe, 1961; Thomas and Howard, 1972). When zoster involves the cranial nerves or the extremities, the incidence of motor involvement is 10 to 20 per cent; mild motor deficits are often missed in thoracolumbar zoster (McKendall and Klawans, 1978). Paralysis usually begins within two weeks of the onset of the rash and almost always involves muscle groups with innervation that is contiguous with that of the affected dermatome; oculomotor and facial palsies are seen with cephalic zoster, unilateral diaphragmatic paralysis with homolateral cervical zoster, paralysis of the trunk and limbs with zoster involving corresponding dermatomes, and dysfunction of the bladder and anus with sacral zoster (Head and Campbell, 1900; Kendall, 1957; Brostoff, 1966; Juel-Jensen and MacCallum, 1972; Thomas and Howard 1972; Izumi and Edwards, 1973; Jellinek and Tulloch, 1976). Rare cases in which the involved myotome and dermatome are widely separated may represent the result of more extensive myelitis (Rose et al., 1964; Thomas and Howard, 1972). Total or functional recovery occurs in most cases.

Posterior nerve roots contain sensory fibers originating in the viscera as well as the skin, which explains the occasional occurrence of visceral lesions in patients with herpes zoster. The affected viscera usually have innervation corresponding to the infected dermatome. Thus, vesicular lesions in the gastric mucosa have been observed in patients with thoracic herpes zoster (Wissloff et al., 1979), and herpes zoster hemicystitis has frequently been observed in association with sacral herpes zoster (Gibbon, 1956; Richmond, 1974).

Although a lymphocytic pleocytosis, with or without an increase in protein in the CSF, is a regular feature of uncomplicated herpes zoster, the incidence of acute symptomatic meningoencephalitis and myelitis is low (0.2 to 0.5 per cent). When these complications do occur, their onset usually follows that of herpes zoster by 7 to 10 days, but it may precede the rash by a week or more, or follow it by up to 2 months (Appelbaum et al., 1962; McKendall and Klawans, 1978; Jemsek et al., 1983). Clinical manifestations include fever, altered sensorium (frequently with delirium and hallucinations), headache, meningismus, and cranial or extracranial nerve palsies, often at a cord level corresponding to the rash. There is a lymphocytic CSF pleocytosis, which usually ranges from 10 to 500 cells/mm^3, a moderate elevation in protein concentration, and a normal glucose concentration. However, the cell count occasionally exceeds 1000/mm^2, there may be 30 to 40 per cent neutrophils, and the sugar concentration may be low. The incidence of meningoencephalitis appears to be increased in cranial zoster and in immunocompromised patients, and most cases occur in association with VZV dissemination (Dolin et al., 1978; Jemsek et al., 1983). Most patients recover and return to their pre-encephalitis cognitive status, but many are left with postherpetic neuralgia, chronic ophthalmologic infections, and motor palsies. In herpes zoster meningoencephalitis and myelitis, virus appears to reach the CNS by the hematogenous route in the course of disseminated herpes zoster, or by direct extension from the involved sensory ganglion (McCormick et al., 1969; McKendall and Klawans, 1978; Jemsek et al., 1983).

Another complication of herpes zoster, which is being recognized with increasing frequency, is granulomatous angiitis of cerebral arteries, which is responsible for a syndrome of ophthalmic zoster and delayed contralateral hemiplegia (Bourdette et al., 1983; Hilt et al. 1983). This complication, which may present as an isolated cerebral infarction, multiple cerebral infarctions, stroke-in-evolution or transient ischemic attacks, usually occurs weeks to months after ophthalmic zoster (average interval about 8 weeks). The clinical manifestations are similar to hypertensive strokes and the delayed onset may obscure the relationship to herpes zoster. Thus, the syndrome is probably underdiagnosed. Cerebral arteriograms almost always reveal segmental narrowing or occlusion of cerebral arteries ipsilateral to the ophthalmic zoster. Although multiple strokes may occur for several weeks, later recurrences are rare and the disease appears to be self-limited. The mortality in reported cases is about 15 per cent.

Herpes Zoster in the Immunosuppressed Host. Certain types of malignancy, especially Hodgkin's disease and lymphocytic leukemia, and the administration of immunosuppressive therapy (e.g., radiation, antimetabolites, antilymphocyte serum, and corticosteroids) to patients with malignancies and nonmalignant diseases markedly increase the incidence and severity of herpes zoster (Schimpff et al., 1972; Goffinet et al., 1972; Feldman et al., 1973; Reboul et al., 1978). In fact, serious complications of herpes zoster occur almost exclusively in such immunosuppressed patients. From 20 to 50 per cent of patients with Hodgkin's disease develop herpes zoster, with the highest incidence in patients with far advanced disease and those receiving radiation and combination chemotherapy (Schimpff et al., 1972; Goffinet et al., 1972; Feldman et al., 1973; Reboul et al., 1978). The severity of the disease is also increased; necrosis of skin and scarring are relatively common, as is postherpetic neuralgia; and the incidence of cutaneous dissemination is 25 to 50 per cent. Approximately 10 per cent of patients with disseminated cutaneous lesions develop widespread, frequently fatal visceral involvement, particularly of the lungs, liver, and brain (Cheatham, 1953; McCormick et al., 1969; Merselis et al., 1964). The incidence of herpes zoster is also markedly increased in immunosuppressed kidney, heart, and bone marrow transplant recipients (Luby et al., 1977; Rifkin, 1966; Pollard et al., 1982; Atkinson et al., 1980) and patients with AIDS (Chapter 273).

A syndrome resembling progressive multifocal leukoencephaly (PML) has recently been reported following herpes zoster in two immunocompromised patients with cancer (Horten et al., 1981). Both patients exhibited steadily progressive, asymmetric, multifocal neurologic deficits, including impaired mental function and focal seizures, and died after several months. At autopsy, there were multifocal lesions, primarily at the gray-white cortical junction, with demyelination, necrosis, and eosinophilic Cowdry type A intranuclear inclusion bodies in oligodendrocytes, neurons, and astrocytes. Herpesvirus-like particles and VZV antigens were detected in these cells. A remarkable feature of these two cases was the long interval (9 to 20 months) between their episode of herpes zoster and the onset of neurologic symptoms. This, as well as the long interval between ophthalmic zoster and the onset of symptoms in patients with granulomatous angiitis, suggests that in addition to latent infections, VZV can produce prolonged "smoldering" subclinical infections, especially in patients lacking the normal defenses that eliminate virus-infected cells and prevent cell-to-cell spread of VZV infection.

The cellular rather than the humoral response to VZV appears to determine the response of these patients to herpes zoster (Miller and Brunell, 1970; Feldman et al., 1973; Pollard et al., 1982; Gold, 1966; Brunell et al., 1975; Armstrong et al., 1970; Stevens et al., 1975; Gallagher and Merigan, 1979; Arvin et al., 1980; Meyers et al., 1980). Lymphocyte blastogenesis and interferon production after exposure to VZV antigens, both of which are indicators of cellular immunity, appear to correlate well with resistance to VZV replication and dissemination.

EPIDEMIOLOGY. Herpes zoster occurs sporadically throughout the year without seasonal prevalence and affects both sexes and all races with equal frequency. As expected wih a disease that reflects the reactivation of latent endogenous infection, the occurrence of herpes zoster is independent of the prevalence of varicella, and there is no convincing evidence that zoster can be acquired by contact with persons with varicella or herpes zoster (Hope-Simpson, 1965; Seiler, 1949; Burgoon et al., 1957; Hope-Simpson, 1975). Rather, the incidence of herpes zoster is determined by factors that influence the host-parasite relationship. One of these is age. The rate of occurrence is in the range of 1.3 to 5 per 1000 persons per year, and although the disease may be seen in any age group, including children, more than two thirds of reported cases occur in individuals over 50 years of age, and less than 10 per cent of cases occur in persons under the age of 20 years (Gordon, 1962; Hope-Simpson, 1965; Seiler, 1949; Burgoon et al., 1957; de Moragas and Kierland, 1957; Miller and Brunell, 1970; Rogers and Tindal, 1972; Ragozzino et al., 1982a). Hope-Simpson's tabulation of data from 192 cases occurring over a 16-year period in a population of 3500 individuals showed that the annual incidence per 1000 rises from 0.74 in children under 10 years of age to a plateau of approximately 2.5 between ages 20 and 50, and thereafter increases to reach a level of over 10 in octogenarians. The incidence of zoster among those who have already had an attack appears to be at least as high as that of first attacks in individuals of comparable age. Second attacks comprise 4 to 5 per cent of reported series, and third attacks are not unheard of (Ragozzino et al., 1982a). Hope-Simpson estimated that if a cohort of 1000 people were to live to be 85 years old, half would have had an attack of zoster and ten would have had two attacks. However, multiple episodes of zoster-like disease, especially in the same anatomic location, are far more likely to be recurrent zosteriform herpes simplex virus infections. The incidence of herpes zoster in immunosuppressed patients is increased by 20- to 100-fold, and the severity of the disease is also increased. The increased incidence and severity of herpes zoster in older individuals, as well as in individuals of any age who are immunosuppressed, is correlated with a deficient cell-mediated immune response to VZV antigens (Miller, 1980; Patel et al., 1979; Pollard et al., 1982; Arvin et al., 1980; Meyers et al., 1980).

Herpes zoster is rare during the first few years of life. When it occurs in infants, there is usually no history of postnatal varicella, but there is almost always a history of maternal varicella during gestation (Brunnell and Kotchmar, 1981). Presumably, primary VZV infection and the establishment of neuronal latency occurred in utero.

Patients with herpes zoster are infectious. Virus can be isolated from vesicles in uncomplicated herpes zoster for up to seven days after the appearance of the rash and for much longer periods in immunocompromised individuals. However, herpes zoster is less contagious than varicella; the infection rate in susceptible household contacts appears to be only about one-third that of varicella (Gordon, 1962; Bruusgaard, 1932; Hope-Simpson, 1965; Seiler, 1949).

The increased incidence of herpes zoster in immunocompromised patients with cancer has led many to assume that patients presenting with herpes zoster have an increased prevalence or an increased subsequent incidence of malignancy. Consequently, many apparently normal patients with herpes zoster are subjected to aggressive and expensive workups for occult cancer. However, a recent prospective population-based study of 590 patients with herpes zoster demonstrated that the incidence of cancer during the first year and the first 5 years after the diagnosis of herpes zoster is the same as the incidence of cancer in the general populations (Ragozzino et al., 1982b).

DIAGNOSIS. In the pre-eruptive stage, herpes zoster is easily confused with other causes of pain such as pleurisy, myocardial infarction, cholecystitis, appendicitis, renal colic, or collapsed intervertebral disk. Sometimes the early appearance of regional lymphadenopathy and localized cutaneous sensory abnormalities provide a clue to the diagnosis. When the eruption appears, the diagnosis is almost always obvious.

Zosteriform herpes simplex eruptions are often impossible to distinguish from herpes zoster on clinical grounds or by the complement fixation test. Multiple recurrences at the same site are common in herpes simplex but exceedingly rare in herpes zoster. Virus isolation or the identification of VZV (or herpes simplex virus) antigens and nucleic acids in material obtained from the lesions is the only reliable means of differential diagnosis (see Chapters 105 and 235 for details).

Contact dermatitis, burns, vaccinia autoinoculation, and localized bacterial skin infections may resemble herpes zoster, but a careful history and examination of the lesions (including a Tzanck smear with the identification of multinucleated giant cells and intranuclear inclusion bodies) eliminates any confusion.

Most immunocompetent patients with herpes zoster show an anamnestic increase in humoral and cell-mediated immunity to VZV (Gershon et al., 1982; Arvin et al., 1983; Weigle and Grose, 1984), but this often fails to occur in immunocompromised patients. Antibody to VZV appears in the CSF of most patients wiht herpes zoster meningoencephalitis, presumably as a result of intrathecal synthesis (Gershon et al., 1980). As in the case of herpes simplex encephalitis (Chapter 180) this may provide a useful means for retrospective diagnosis.

TREATMENT. The major goals of therapy in patients with herpes zoster are to (1) limit the extent, duration, and severity of disease in the primary dermatome; (2) prevent disease elsewhere; and (3) prevent postherpetic neuralgia. Since pathology in the primary dermatome, as well as that responsible for the visceral and central nervous system complications of herpes zoster, appear to require replication of VZV, the first two goals can be achieved by limiting VZV replication and spread. If immunity is intact, herpes zoster is usually self-limited and rarely spreads outside of the initially involved dermatome. In contrast, immunocompromised individuals, particularly those with deficiencies in cell-mediated immunity, have more severe and prolonged local disease and a much higher incidence of visceral and central nervous system complications. Obviously, it is these patients who have the most to gain from effective antiviral therapy.

The pathogenesis of postherpetic neuralgia is obscure, as is the reason why this complication develops almost exclusively in persons over 50 years of age. Both cytolysis by the virus and inflammation cause tissue injury. Postinflammatory scarring of neural structures may be important in the pathogenesis of postherpetic neuralgia, and this possibility has provided the rationale for the use of corticosteroids to prevent this complication (vide infra).

Nucleoside analogs capable of inhibiting VZV replication have been administered parenterally in attempts to control the multiplication and dissemination of VZV in immunocompromised patients with herpes zoster. Cytosine arabinoside (Ara-C) and iododeoxyuridine (IUdR) have proven ineffective and toxic when administered systemically. Two other nucleoside analogs, vidarabine (9-β-D-arabinofuranosyladenine, adenine arabinoside) and acyclovir (9-[2-hydroxyethoxymethyl] guanine, acycloguanosine) have proven effective for the treatment of VZV infections (Wong and Hirsch, 1984). Their mechanisms of action are discussed in Chapters 105 and 235. The efficacy of vidarabine in immunocompromised patients with acute herpes zoster was established in a double-blind placebo-controlled crossover study (Whitley et al., 1976) and, more recently, in a randomized double-blind placebo-controlled study (Whitley et al., 1982). When administered within 72 hours of the onset of rash, vidarabine (10 mg/kg intravenously over 12 hours each day for 5 days) shortened the period of new vesicle formation, accelerated healing, and reduced the spread of the rash over the primary dermatome. Vidarabine also reduced the incidence of cutaneous dissemination from 24 per cent in placebo recipients to 8 per cent, and the incidence of visceral or central nervous system complications from 19 per cent to 5 per cent. Patients with lymphoproliferative malignancies and those older than 38 years of age had the greatest risk of complications and thus benefited most from therapy. Vidarabine did not reduce the incidence of postherpetic neuralgia (45 per cent in patients older than 38 years of age) but appeared to reduce its duration, and to reduce the duration of acute pain. Vidarabine toxicity, consisting mainly of nausea, vomiting, subclinical abnomalities in liver enzymes, jitteriness, and hallucinations, was self-limited and did not necessitate cessation of therapy. Analysis of placebo recipients revealed that concomitant administration of corticosteroids did not reduce the frequency of postherpetic neuralgia, but did delay healing and prolong new vesicle formation.

Acyclovir, a more selective and less toxic inhibitor of VZV replication, is also effective in patients with herpes zoster. A randomized double-blind placebo-controlled study in 94 immunocompromised patients with acute herpes zoster demonstrated that acyclovir (500 mg/m^2 intravenously each 8 hours for 7 days) halted progression of herpes zoster, both in patients with localized disease and in patients with cutaneous dissemination before treatment (Balfour et al., 1983). Acyclovir accelerated the rate of clearance of virus from vesicles and reduced the incidence of visceral or progressive cutaneous dissemination from 26 per cent in placebo recipients to 4 per cent. Pain subsided faster in acyclovir recipients, and fewer reported postherpetic neuralgia, but these differences were not statistically significant. No acyclovir toxicity was observed.

Three small double-blind placebo-controlled trials have examined the effect of acyclovir (5 mg/kg or 500 mg/m^2 intravenously 3 times daily for 5 days) on acute herpes zoster in immunocompetent adults (Peterslund et al., 1981; Bean et al., 1982; McGill et al., 1983). Acyclovir shortened the period of virus shedding and of new vesicle formation, accelerated healing, and shortened the duration of pain during the acute phase of the disease. However, there was no effect upon the incidence of postherpetic neuralgia. The greatest effect of acyclovir treatment was observed in patients older than 67 years of age and those with fever (i.e., patient in whom the disease is more severe and prolonged without therapy) and in patients treated early (Peterslund et al., 1981). No toxicity was observed in acyclovir recipients.

These results, as well as experience gained in open protocols and in treating varicella (Chapter 235) suggest that acyclovir is at least as effective as vidarabine in patients with VZV infections, but is free of vidarabine's toxicity and problems of fluid overload (Hirsh and Schooley, 1983). Randomized double-blind studies directly comparing the two drugs in patients with VZV infections are now in progress. Human trials are also under way to assess the efficacy and toxicity of several other promising nucleoside derivatives that resemble acylovir in their mechanism of action (Wong and Hirsch, 1984).

The efficacy of human leukocyte interferon (interferon alpha) has also been evaluated in a series of randomized placebo-controlled studies in immunocompromised patients with localized herpes zoster (Merigan et al., 1978 and 1981). Patients receiving 1.7 or 5.1×10^5 units/kg/day intramuscularly for 7 or more days, beginning within 72 hours of the onset of rash, showed a reduction in new vesicle formation, cutaneous and visceral dissemination, visceral and central nervous system complications, and postherpetic neuralgia. A two-day course of therapy at the higher interferon dose reduced the incidence of cutaneous dissemination and may also have reduced the duration and severity of postherpetic neuralgia, but it did not alter the progression of disease in the primary dermatome. Although reasonably well tolerated in these trials, interferon appears to be somewhat more toxic than vidarabine (Hirsch and Schooley, 1983).

Immunocompromised patients with herpes zoster who have a deficient or delayed antibody response to VZV have an increased incidence of severe disease and dissemination (Rifkind, 1966; Miller and Brunell, 1970; Mazur et al., 1979). This led Stevens and Merigan (1980) to conduct a double-blind controlled therapeutic trial of zoster immune globulin (ZIG) in immunocompromised patients with herpes zoster. Despite a much higher titer of antibody to VZV, ZIG did not appear superior to the normal immune serum globulin (ISG) control in preventing dissemination or diminishing postherpetic neuralgia.

It is clear that in immunocompromised patients, parenterally administered acyclovir, vidarabine, or interferon can shorten the course of acute herpes zoster and markedly reduce the incidence of serious complications. However, parenteral antiviral therapy has only a small effect upon the course of herpes zoster in immunocompetent individuals (because normal host defenses alone are effective in limiting VZV replication and spread) and does not appear to alter the incidence or severity of postherpetic neuralgia, which is the major cause of morbidity in immunologically normal patients with herpes zoster. Thus, while antiviral therapy might well prevent complications such as motor paresis and meningoencephalitis, the potential benefits for most immunologically normal individuals do not appear to outweigh the expense and inconvenience of hospitalization for intravenous therapy. What is needed is an effective outpatient regimen, and progress is being made in this direction; studies are under way to determine the therapeutic potential of intramuscularly administered interferon alpha and of orally administered acyclovir in immunologically normal individuals with herpes zoster. Oral acyclovir has already been proven effective in patients with genital herpes (Chapter 163), but treatment of VZV, which is less sensitive to acyclovir than HSV, will require larger doses than those used to treat genital herpes. Oral administration of acyclovir (400 mg 5 times daily for 10 days) to 10 immunocompromised children with varicella or herpes zoster has been reported to produce serum levels higher than that required to inhibit VZV replication in vitro (Novelli et al., 1984). All 10 children recovered without complications and there was no evidence of drug toxicity.

In view of the early and extensive involvement of the sensory ganglion and nerve, and the importance of contiguous rather than viremic spread in the genesis of central nervous system complications of herpes zoster in immunocompetent individuals, it seems unlikely that topical therapy applied to the skin will reduce the incidence or severity of most complications of herpes zoster (including postherpetic neuralgia) in immunologically normal persons. Moreover, while many forms of topical therapy have been advocated, few have been subjected to well-controlled clinical evaluation. An exception is iododeoxyuridine (IUdR) in dimethylsulfoxide (DMSO). Well-controlled studies have demonstrated that topical application of 5 to 40 per cent IUdR in 100 per cent DMSO, beginning early in the course of uncomplicated herpes zoster, shortens the vesicular phase and accelerates healing, and may also reduce the duration of pain (Juel-Jensen and MacCallum, 1972; Wildenhoff et al., 1979). However, these effects are small, the treatment protocol is inconvenient, and IUdR is not effective in more convenient ointment formulations. The IUdR-DMSO preparation is not licensed for use in the United States, and the cost and potential long-term toxicity of such high concentrations of drug and solvent should discourage its use elsewhere. The use of other forms of topical therapy, including topical and intralesional corticosteroids, should be avoided until their safety and efficacy are demonstrated by means of well-designed double-blind placebo-controlled clinical trials.

During the acute phase of herpes zoster, analgesics and the application of cool compresses, calamine lotion, cornstarch, or baking soda may help to alleviate local symptoms and hasten the drying of vesicular lesions. Occlusive ointments should be avoided, and creams or lotions containing corticosteroids should not be used. After the acute phase, a bland ointment or olive oil dressings may help to soften and separate adherent crusts. Bacterial superinfection of local lesions is uncommon and should be treated with warm soaks; bacterial cellulitis requires systemic antibiotic therapy.

The possibility that postherpetic neuralgia may be caused by inflammation, necrosis, and subsequent scarring of the sensory ganglion and continguous neural structures has provided the rationale for the use of corticosteroids during the acute phase of herpes zoster in an attempt to prevent this complication. However, the host defenses that cause tissue injury appear to be identical to those that terminate dermatomal VZV infection and prevent dissemination, and patients who develop herpes zoster while being treated with corticosteroids have an increased risk of dissemination and visceral complications. Nevertheless, two small controlled trials have suggested that the oral administration of 48 mg of triamcinolone or 40 mg of prednisolone per day, beginning during the early eruptive phase of the disease, may reduce the duration of postherpetic neuralgia in otherwise healthy patients over 60 years of age (Eaglestein, 1970; Keczkes and Basheer, 1980). No complications of corticosteroid therapy were observed in either study. In view of the possibility that such large doses of corticosteroid may induce VZV dissemination, and the reported failure of corticosteroid therapy to reduce the incidence of postherpetic neuralgia in immunocompromised patients treated with vidarabine (Whitley et al., 1982), these results should be confirmed by means of a larger double-blind placebo-controlled trial before this form of therapy is accepted for general use. If the capacity of corticosteroid to reduce the incidence and severity of postherpetic neuralgia can be confirmed, any associated increase in VZV replication and dissemination might be prevented by the simultaneous administration of an antiviral agent. However, a recent trial of acyclovir and corticosteroid in patients with herpes zoster kerato-uveitis (McGill et al., 1983) does not support this assumption. Topical acyclovir was found to control herpes zoster kerato-uveitis without recurrences, whereas recurrence of disease was common after corticosteroid therapy. When corticosteroids were used in combination with acyclovir, patients suffered the same problems (slow resolution and high recurrence rates) as they did when corticosteroids were used alone. The NIAID Collaborative Antiviral Study Group has initiated a double-blind randomized study in which immunocompetent persons > 50 years of age with herpes zoster will be treated orally with prednisone, acyclovir, prednisone plus acyclovir, or placebo. This trial should resolve the questions of the safety and efficacy of corticosteroid therapy and, in addition, determine the therapeutic potential of oral acyclovir alone and in combination with corticosteroid.

Postherpetic neuralgia, once established, is often refractory to therapy. Fortunately, it resolves spontaneously in most patients; within 3 months in about 50 per cent and within a year in 75 per cent or more. Nevertheless, a number of patients are left with persistent, often disabling, pain. Conventional analgesics should be tried, but they often fail, as do narcotics, which also carry a risk of addiction. A wide range of therapies have been advocated, including epidural injection of local anesthetic and corticosteroid, acupuncture, biofeedback, subcutaneous injections of triamcinolone, and systemic administration of a variety of compounds, but most have not been validated by controlled trials. Though of unproven benefit, an initial trial of cutaneous stimulation, either by frequent rubbing with a dry towel or with a cutaneous electrical stimulator, is advocated by many experts (Price, 1982). This should be continued for several weeks before being abandoned. The typical dull persistent aching pain of postherpetic neuralgia will often respond to tricyclic antidepressants (Price, 1982). In a controlled trial, amitriptyline provided excellent pain relief in about two thirds of patients with postherpetic neuralgia. Carbamazepine may also be effective, especially for the lancinating pain that develops in some patients (Price, 1982).

The eye is involved in 20 to 70 per cent of patients with ophthalmic zoster, and the advice of an ophthalmologist should be sought in treating these patients. Therapy of ocular VZV infections is controversial. Mydriatics are used to prevent synechiae, and topical corticosteroids are frequently recommended for keratitis and uveitis, although their efficacy is unproven (Paven-Langston, 1983). Topical antiviral drugs (IUdR, vidarabine, trifluorothymidine) are also frequently recommended and should be included whenever corticosteroids are used. A recent study indicates that topical acyclovir alone is superior to corticosteroid or to the combination of acyclovir and corticosteroid in patients with herpes zoster kerato-uveitis (McGill and Chapman, 1983).

The following recommendations reflect the author's views and current state of knowledge. Progress in antiviral therapy is rapid, and these recommendations are certain to be altered by the results of studies now under way.

Herpes zoster in immunologically normal persons less than 50 years of age is generally benign and self-limited and is very rarely complicated by postherpetic neuralgia. Thus antiviral therapy is not recommended and the use of corticosteroids, even if it is proven effective in preventing postherpetic neuralgia, is not warranted.

In immunologically normal older persons (> 50 years of age) the major complication of herpes zoster is postherpetic neuralgia, which can be expected to develop in 20 per cent or more of these patients. Until a regimen of antiviral drug, corticosteroid, or both is clearly demonstrated to reduce the incidence or severity of this complication, neither is recommended for routine use. However, the high incidence of ocular and CNS complications observed in patients with ophthalmic zoster, including the syndrome of delayed contralateral hemiplegia (Ragozzino et al., 1982a; Womack and Liesegang, 1983; Bourdette et al., 1983) warrants consideration of antiviral therapy. The cost and inconvenience of intravenous therapy would almost certainly be justified if there were unequivocal evidence that the early initiation of antiviral therapy prevented the development of these complications. Until such evidence is available, therapeutic decisions should be made on a case-by-case basis, recognizing that the frequency and severity of complications increases with age. When a safe and effective oral regimen is available, its use will probably be warranted in all patients with herpes zoster who are more than 50 years of age.

Immunocompetent patients of any age who develop significant cutaneous dissemination (e.g., 20 or more vesicles at a distance from the primary dermatome) should be carefully evaluated and those with evidence of visceral or CNS involvement should receive antiviral therapy. Pending the availability of the results of comparative studies, the author prefers to use acyclovir (500 mg/m^2 or 10 mg/kg intravenously every 8 hours for 5 days) because of its ease of administration and lower toxicity.

In immunocompromised patients of any age with herpes zoster, the major objective is to prevent local, visceral, and CNS complications, which are the direct consequence of VZV replication and spread. Accordingly, such patients are prime candidates for antiviral therapy. The only significant deterrant is the cost and inconvenience of intravenous administration. The development of safe and effective oral regimens will make it practical to treat most or all of these patients early in the course of their disease, when infection is localized to the primary dermatome. Early initiation of therapy is important because of the close temporal proximity of the onset of cutaneous dissemination to the onset of visceral and CNS complications; one would rather not wait for the occurrence of cutaneous dissemination to initiate antiviral therapy. Until an effective outpatient regimen is available, it would seem reasonable to treat herpes zoster in more severely immunocompromised patients (e.g., those with lymphoproliferative malignancies, advanced Hodgkin's disease, and organ allografts) with intravenous acyclovir (500 mg/m^2 or 10 mg/kg each 8 hours for 7 days). Older patients with lesser degrees of immunosuppression, and all immunocompromised patients with ophthalmic zoster should probably also be treated. Treatment should be continued for 7 days or more, or until there is no longer evidence of VZV replication. Untreated immunocompromised patients who develop cutaneous dissemination or evidence of visceral or CNS involvement should be treated with intravenous acyclovir at this dosage for 7 to 10 days or until there is no longer evidence of VZV replication. Patients with CNS involvement should probably be treated longer, and their physician should be alert for relapse.

Both acyclovir and vidarabine require dose reduction in patients with renal insufficiency. Furthermore, the widespread use of antiviral drugs in patients with VZV infections will pose two potential problems: (1) the emergence of drug-resistant mutants and (2) an alteration in host immune responses that could increase the frequency and severity of recurrent infections. The mechanisms of action of vidarabine, acyclovir, and other antiviral drugs appear to be similar for HSV and VZV, and drug-resistant mutants of VZV exist in nature. Efforts will have to be made to prevent the abuse of antiviral drugs, and surveillance carried out to detect the emergence of drug-resistant mutants in treated patients. It is now clear, as originally proposed by Hope-Simpson (1965), that resistance to clinically apparent recurrent VZV infections is maintained by antigenic stimulation provided by subclinical exogenous and endogenous reinfections (see Fig. 1). By inhibiting VZV replication, early antiviral therapy might reduce the "booster" effect of herpes zoster and thus increase the incidence and severity of subsequent recurrences.

PROPHYLAXIS. Herpes zoster is a sporadic disease that results from reactivation of latent endogenous VZV, rather than from exogenous infection. Thus, attempts at prophylaxis must be aimed at preventing the reactivation of endogenous VZV or inhibiting its subsequent replication and spread. It appears that natural resistance to herpes zoster is maintained by periodic antigenic stimulation, which results from subclinical episodes of exogenous reinfection and endogenous reactivation (see Fig. 1). The increased incidence and severity of herpes zoster observed in elderly persons appears to be associated with depressd immunity to VZV, primarily depressed cell-mediated immunity. Depressed cell-mediated immunity also appears to be responsible for the increased incidence and severity of herpes zoster in immunocompromised patients. Accordingly, one approach to the prevention of herpes zoster is the stimulation of immunity to VZV in elderly and other high risk individuals. The development of live attenuated VZV vaccines (Chapter 235) provides an opportunity to test this approach to prophylaxis in immunologically normal elderly individuals. (The use of live attenuated vaccines is generally to be avoided in immuncompromised individuals, although the current VZV vaccines have proven to be relatively safe and effective in immunocompromised children with leukemia and other malignancies [Chapter 235].) Berger et al. (1984) have recently administered attenuated VZV vaccine to 33 elderly adults with a history of varicella and antibody VZV, but with a negative in vitro lymphoproliferative response to VZV antigen (stimulation index < 3). Seventeen (52 per cent) of the vaccine recipients subsequently developed a positive lymphoproliferative response to VZV antigen (stimulation index > 5), and an additional 11 (33 per cent) became weakly positive (stimulation index of 3 to 5). It remains to be seen whether immunization of such elderly individuals will also result in a reduction in the incidence and severity of herpes zoster. Experimental vaccines consisting of purified VZV envelope glycoproteins and free of VZV DNA will provide another means of stimulating immunity that is more suitable for use in immunocompromised patients.

References

Adour, K. K.: Current Concepts in Neurology: Diagnosis and management of facial paralysis. N Engl J Med 307(6):348, 1982.

Andiman, W. A., White-Greenwald, M., and Tinghitella, T.: Zoster encephalitis. Isolation of virus and measurement of varicella-zoster-specific antibodies in cerebrospinal fluid. Am J Med 73:769, 1982.

Aoyama, Y., Kurata, T., Kurata, K., Hondo, R., and Ogiware, H.: Demonstration of viral antigens in herpes simplex and varicella-zoster infection. Recent Adv RES Res 14:90, 1974.

Applebaum, E., Kreps, S. I., and Sunshine, A.: Herpes zoster encephalitis. Am J Med 32:25, 1962.

Armstrong, R. W., Gurwith, M. J., Waddell, D., and Merigan, T. C.: Cutaneous interferon production in patients with Hodgkin's disease and other cancers infected with varicella or vaccinia. N Engl J Med 283:1182, 1970.

Arvin, A. M., and Koropchak, C. M.: Immuoglobulins M and G to varicella-zoster virus measured by solid-phase radioimmunoassay: antibody response to varicella and herpes zoster infections. J Clin Microbiol 12:367, 1980.

Arvin, A. M., Koropchak, C. M., and Wittek, A. E.: Immunologic evidence of reinfection with varicella-zoster virus. J Infect Dis 148:200, 1983.

Arvin, A. M., Pollard, R. B., Rasmussen, L. E., and Merigan, T. C.: Cellular and humoral immunity in the pathogenesis of recurrent herpes viral infections in patients with lymphoma. J Clin Invest 65:869, 1980.

Atkinson, K., Meyers, J. D., Storb, R., Prentice, R. L., and Thomas, E. D.: Varicella-zoster virus infection after marrow transplantation for aplastic anemia or leukemia. Transplantation 29:47, 1980.

Balfour, H. H., Jr., Bean, B., Laskin, O. L., Ambinder, R. F., Meyers, J. D., Wade, J. C., Zaia, J. A., Aeppli, D., Kirk, L. E., Segretti, A. C., and Keeney, R. E.: Acyclovir halts progression of herpes zoster in immunocompromised patients. N Engl J Med 308:1448, 1983.

Bastian, F. O., Rabson, A. S., Yee, C. L., and Tralka, T. S.: Herpesvirus varicellae: Isolated from human dorsal root ganglia. Arch Pathol 97:331, 1974.

Bean, B., Braun, C., and Balfour, H. H., Jr.: Acyclovir therapy for acute herpes zoster. Lancet II:118, 1982.

Berger, R., Florent, G., and Just, M.: Decrease of the lymphoproliferative response to varicella-zoster virus antigen in the aged. Infect Immun 32(1):24, 1981.

Berger, R., Luescher, D., and Just, M.: Enhancement of varicella-zoster-specific immune responses in the elderly by boosting with varicella vaccine. J Infect Dis 149:647, 1984.

Bourdette, D. N., Rosenberg, N. L., and Yatsu, F. M.: Herpes zoster ophthalmicus and delayed ipsilateral cerebral infarction. Neurology 33:1428, 1983.

Bright, R.: Reports of Medical Cases, London: Longmans, Ltd. 1831, vol. 2, p. 383.

Brostoff, J.: Diaphragmatic paralysis after herpes zoster. Br Med J 2:1571, 1966.

Brown, G. R.: Herpes zoster: Correlation of age, sex, distribution, neuralgia, and associated disorders. South Med J 59:576, 1976.

Brunell, P. A., and Kotchmar, G. S.: Zoster in infancy: Failure to maintain virus latency following intrauterine infection. J Pediatr 98:71, 1981.

Brunell, P. A., Gershon, A. A., Uduman, S. A., and Steinberg, S.: Varicella-zoster immunoglobulins during varicella, latency, and zoster. J Infect Dis 132:49, 1975.

Brunell, P. A., Miller, L. H., and Lovejoy, F.: Zoster in children. Am J Dis Child 115:432, 1968.

Bruusgaard, E.: The mutual relation between zoster and varicella. Br J Dermatol 44:1, 1932.

Burgoon, C. F., Burgoon, J. S., and Baldridge, G. D.: The natural history of herpes zoster. JAMA 164:265, 1957.

Burke, B. L., Steele, R. W., Beard, O. W., Wood, J. S., Cain, T. D., and Marmer, D. J.: Immune response to varicella-zoster in the aged. Arch Intern Med 142:291, 1982.

a central ulcer on their arm, hand, or eyelid. The lesions may take as long as two months to heal.

In lambs the infection produces pustules on the lips, mouth, vulva, and cornea. The virus can be recovered on the chorioallantoic membrane of chick embryos where it produces very small pocks. It can be recognized under the electron microscope in scrapings from the lesions. It is antigenically related to vaccinia virus.

References

Bauer, D. J., St. Vincent, L., Kempe, C. H., and Downie, A. W.: Prophylactic treatment of smallpox contacts with N-methyl isatin beta thiosemicarbazone. Lancet 2:494, 1963.

Behbehani, A. M.: The smallpox story: Life and death of an old disease. Microbiol Rev 47:455, 1983.

Curshmann, H. In Ziemssen: Cyclopedia of the Practice of Medicine. Vol. 2. London, Samson Low, Martson Low, Searle, 1875. (Cited by Dixon, C. W.: 1962).

Dixon, C. W.: Smallpox. London, J. & A. Churchill Limited, 1962.

Downie, A. W., Meiklejohn, G., St. Vincent, L., Rao, A. R., Sundarababu, B. V., and Kempe, C. H.: The recovery of smallpox virus from patients and their environment in a smallpox hospital. Bull WHO 33:615, 1965.

Kempe, C. H., Bowles, C., Meiklejohn, G., Berge, T. O., St. Vincent, L., Sundarababu, B. V., Govindarajan, S., Ratnakannan, N. R., Downie, A. W., and Murray, V. R.: The use of vaccinia hyperimmune gammaglobulin in the prophylaxis of smallpox. Bull WHO 25:41, 1961.

Kempe, C. H., Dekking, F., St. Vincent, L., Rao, A. R., and Downie, A. W.: Conjunctivitis and subclinical infection in smallpox. J Hyg (Camb) 67:631, 1969.

McKenzie, P. J., Githens, J. H., Harwood, M. E., Roberts, J. R., Bao, A. R., and Kempe, C. H.: Hemorrhagic smallpox—Specific bleeding and coagulation studies. Bull WHO 33:773, 1966.

Meiklejohn, G., Kempe, C. H., Downie, A. W., Berge, T. O., St. Vincent, L., and Rao, A. R.: Air sampling to recover variola virus in the environment of a smallpox hospital. Bull WHO 25:63, 1961.

Ramachandra Rao, A., McFedzean, J. A., and Kamalakshi, S.: An isothiazole thiosemicarbazone in the treatment of variola major in man. Lancet 1:1072, 1966a.

Ramachandra Rao, A., McKendric, G. D. W., Velayudhan, L., and Kamalakshi, S.: Assessment of an isothiazole thiosemicarbazone in the prophylaxis of contacts of Variola major. Lancet 1:1072, 1966b.

Rao, A. R.: Smallpox. Bombay, Kothari Book Depot, 1972.

Rao, A. R., Jacobs, E. S., Kamalakshi, S., Appaswasmy, M. S., and Bradbury: Epidemiological studies of smallpox–A study of intrafamilial transmission in a series of 254 infected families. Ind J Med Res 56:1826, 1968.

Rao, A. R., Jacobs, E. S., Kamalakshi, S., et al.: Chemoprophylaxis and chemotherapy in variola major. Part 1. An assessment of CG662 and Marboran in prophylaxis of contacts of variola major. Ind J Med Res 57:477, 1969a.

Rao, A. R., Jacobs, E. S., Kamalakshi, S., et al.: Chemoprophylaxis and chemotherapy in variola major. Part 2. Therapeutic assessment of CG662 and Marboran in treatment of variola major in man. Ind J Med Res 57:484, 1969b.

Rao, A. R., McFedzean, J. A., and Squires, S.: The laboratory and clinical assessment of an isothiazole thiosemicarbazone (M&B 7714) against pox-viruses. Ann NY Acad Sci 130:118, 1965.

Rao, A. R., Savithri Sukumar, M., Kamalakshi, S., Paramasivam, T. V., Parasuram, A. R., and Shantha, M.: Experimental Variola in monkeys. Part 1. Studies on the disease-enhancing property of cortisone in smallpox. Ind J Med Res 56:1855, 1968b.

Roberts, J. F., Coffee, G., Creel, S. M., Gall, A., Githens, J. H., Rao, A. R., Sundarababu, B. V., and Kempe, C. H. Hemorrhagic smallpox. 1. Preliminary hematologic studies. Bull WHO 35:607, 1965.

World Health Organization: Report of WHO Expert Committee on Smallpox Eradication. Technical Report Series No. 493. Geneva, World Health Organization, 1972.

238

MEASLES

GILBERT M. SCHIFF, M.D.

Measles (rubeola) is a highly contagious viral disease of childhood that is recognized by a typical prodrome of fever, conjunctivitis, coryza, cough, and enanthem followed by a generalized maculopapular eruption. Complications are common, and some are of a serious nature. Measles has occurred in all countries since antiquity. Because the measles virus has been cultivated in tissue culture, it has been possible to develop reliable diagnostic laboratory tests and effective vaccines. Widespread vaccination has altered the familiar epidemiologic patterns of the disease and has reduced the incidence. However, measles is still prevalent in lesser developed countries.

ETIOLOGY. The measles virus is a member of the paramyxovirus group and is closely related to canine distemper and rinderpest viruses. On examination by the electronmicroscope, the virus appears as a circular structure 1200 to 1500 Å in diameter with an outer lipoprotein envelope 100 to 200 Å in width and containing short spike-like projections. The envelope surrounds an inner core of elongated nucleocapsid consisting of spirally arranged protein units dispersed around an RNA nucleic acid. The envelope contains hemagglutination and complement-fixation antigens, and the nucleocapsid contains a complement-fixation antigen. The virus is stable at lower temperatures but relatively unstable at room and body temperature.

Measles virus requires the entire virion to produce infection. Infection produces two types of giant cells in the body. One type consists of large, multinucleated lymphoid giant cells, which are present in lymphoid tissues and occasionally contain inclusion bodies. The second type is the syncytial epithelial giant cell found in the upper and lower respiratory tract. These cells may contain 40 or more nuclei and inclusion bodies in the nucleus and cytoplasm and may be readily found in nasal secretions.

Infection with measles virus results in the development of neutralizing, hemagglutination-inhibiting, and complement-fixing antibodies. The neutralizing and hemagglutination-inhibiting antibodies generally parallel each other and first appear within a few days after onset of the rash. They reach peak titers two to four weeks later and persist for many years (probably for life). The complement-fixing antibodies appear and peak somewhat later, and disappear after 6 to 12 months or more. The primary antibody response to measles infection is characterized by the production of both IgM and IgG immunoglobulins, with disappearance of IgM after 21 days.

Measles infection stimulates the development of cellular immunity. Patients incapable of responding with humoral immunity have nonetheless been protected against subsequent measles virus challenge.

PATHOGENESIS AND PATHOLOGY. Measles virus enters the body via the upper respiratory tract (or possibly by the conjunctival sac), multiplies locally, and soon spreads to the regional lymphoid tissues. Following a primary viremia, the virus disseminates and multiplies throughout the reticuloendothelial system. A secondary viremia then takes place and seeds the respiratory tract and conjunctival sac. Ultimately the virus localizes in the skin and/or other organs. Replication of the virus in leukocytes aids in dissemination.

The lesions of measles are generalized throughout the body, and multinucleated giant cells are found widely in hypoplastic lymphoid organs. The epithelial cells of the upper respiratory tract and bronchi may lose their cilia and their ability to secrete mucus and contain intranuclear and cytoplasmic inclusions. Koplik's spots are inflamed, submucosal glands, in which the endothelium of the inflamed vessels proliferates and becomes necrotic. The cutaneous lesions are caused by a serous perivascular exudate into the epidermis and by vacuolization and necrosis of the epithelial cells, which eventually form vesicles. Both Koplik's spots and skin lesions have foci of syncytial giant cells. The lesions in measles encephalitis are described under Complications.

CLINICAL MANIFESTATIONS. Measles is a seven- to ten-day illness. Following an incubation period of 8 to 12 days, there are two to four days of prodromal symptoms and then an eruptive phase. The prodromal period begins with malaise and fever, followed within 24 hours by a copious coryza, a dry brassy cough, and conjunctivitis. These symptoms become progressively more severe until the sixth day, when there is rapid improvement. The temperature varies from 101 to 105° F during the early rash stage, and falls rather quickly to normal about the third day of the rash. The conjunctivitis is frequently associated with photophobia. The cough may persist in a mild form for one or two weeks. Small bluish-white spots on a red areolar base (Koplik's spots) appear in the buccal mucosa opposite the molars two days before the onset of the rash. They rapidly spread over the entire oral mucous membrane during the next few days. Examination of the blood during the prodromal period shows a leukopenia.

The eruption begins behind the ears and on the forehead, and then spreads onto the face and neck within 24 hours. Soon afterward, the eruption spreads to the chest and downward over the trunk and extremities; the soles and palms are spared. The rash is initially maculopapular, light pink, and discrete. Later, it becomes deeper red and may remain discrete or coalesce. By the fifth day, the color has become brownish, and the lesions eventually become desquamative. At the height of the illness, usually two days after the appearance of the rash, the child appears miserable. He is covered with a maculopapular rash, has a high fever, malaise, copious nasal discharge, a distressful cough, swollen and inflamed eyes, photophobia, and Koplik's spots on the buccal mucosa. However, there is usually a relatively uneventful, short convalescence.

Modified measles occurs in infants who have residual maternal antibody and in children who have been given immune globulin early in the incubation period. The incubation period is prolonged, the prodromal symptoms are diminished or absent, Koplik's spots are few in number or absent, and the eruption is mild and discrete. Hemorrhagic measles is a rare severe form featuring a sudden rise in temperature to 105 to 106° F; convulsions, delirium, stupor, and coma; and marked respiratory distress. There is hemorrhage into the cutaneous lesions and mucous membranes. The outcome is usually fatal.

"Atypical measles" is a newer syndrome that occurs in children who have previously been immunized with inactivated (and in some cases live, attenuated) measles vaccine (Fulginiti et al., 1967). There is high fever, interstitial pneumonitis, edema of the extremities, myalgia, and prostration. An atypical rash occurs that may be urticarial, vesicular, petechial, or maculopapular. The rash tends to be located primarily on the extremities and appears on the palms and soles. Atypical measles frequently resembles the exanthem of Rocky Mountain spotted fever.

COMPLICATIONS. Complications of measles are common. They can be caused by the virus or secondary bacterial invasion, or both. Sudden appearance of leukocytosis is indicative of a bacterial complication. The most common complication is otitis media. This is generally caused by secondary invasion by beta-hemolytic streptococci, pneumococci, or *Haemophilus influenzae.* Bacterial invasion of the lower respiratory tract causes the next most frequent complication. There may be bronchiolitis (in infants), bronchopneumonia, or lobar pneumonia. The bacteria involved are beta-hemolytic streptococci, pneumococci, or staphylococci. Giant cell pneumonias occur in patients with immunologic deficiencies. The pulmonary complications account for more than 90 per cent of measles-related deaths.

Upper respiratory tract complications include laryngotracheitis or obstructive laryngitis. These are caused by extension of the usual respiratory tract inflammation found in measles and may result in a need for tracheostomy.

Acute encephalitis occurs in approximately 0.1 per cent of measles cases. The encephalitis varies in severity from mild to fulminant. Usually it appears suddenly during the eruptive stage, but can precede the rash. The fever returns, and there may be headache, confusion, convulsions, and coma as a result of cerebral edema, hemorrhages, cellular infiltration, and perivascular demyelination. Paresis of the limbs or bladder indicates myelitis. The cerebrospinal fluid is characterized by a pleocytosis in which lymphocytes are predominant, protein level is elevated, and glucose concentration is normal. Although measles virus has been recovered from the brain tissue of patients, some feel that the encephalitis is caused by activation of a second latent virus or by an allergic phenomenon. The mortality rate is 15 per cent; 25 per cent have significant residual neurologic deficiencies, and 60 per cent recover fully.

An uncommon complication is the development of subacute sclerosing panencephalitis (SSPE) (Wechsler and Meisner, 1982). This is a progressive deteriorating neurologic disease with a fatal outcome. Pathologically, there is perivascular lymphocytic and plasma cell infiltration, astrocyte hypertrophy, neuroglial proliferation, and demyelination in the brain. Measles-like virus has been recovered from the brain tissue of patients with SSPE. These patients also exhibit very high titers of measles antibody in the cerebrospinal fluid and serum. The disease begins insidiously several months to years (average five years) after the child has had clinical measles. There are also documented cases in which the child's only *known* experience with measles virus was the receipt of attenuated measles vaccine. However, in none of these vaccine-associated cases were studies done before vaccination to rule out previous subclinical measles. Subtle disturbances in mental and emotional activity occur at the onset. The child's memory may begin to fail, and his performance may decline at school. Nightmares, crying spells, and involuntary movements or "spasms" become prominent. Coordination becomes poor, seizures develop, and ataxia appears. The electroencephalogram exhibits a characteristic suppression-burst pattern. There may be temporary remissions, but a general downhill course ensues, ending in death 6 to 12 months later.

There are several theories concerning the pathogenic mechanisms involved (see Chapter 183). Most believe that the measles virus becomes latent in the brain, and some unknown mechanism later reactivates the latent virus. Such a triggering event may involve a second virus (McDonald, 1977). Others advocate the concept of a hypersensitivity mechanism, pointing out the simultaneous presence of virus and high levels of specific antibody (Termeislen, 1973).

There has been much consternation that the inoculation of an attenuated measles virus vaccine might create a favorable circumstance for the development of the chronic carrier state of the virus in the brain with a predisposition to subsequent SSPE. This fear is apparently unfounded. The widespread use of further attenuated measles vaccines to prevent active measles could conceivably decrease or eliminate cases of SSPE.

GEOGRAPHIC CONSIDERATIONS. Measles is found all over the world. In most areas it is endemic, with epidemics occurring every six to seven years. In island populations, however, the epidemiology is much different in that the disease is not endemic, and explosive outbreaks occur when the virus is reintroduced (Panum, 1940). The epidemiology of measles is changing in countries practicing widespread immunization of the young. In these countries, outbreaks of measles are occurring in older adolescents and young adults rather than in elementary school–age children (Werner et al., 1977).

The severity of measles varies around the world. It is more severe in children in underdeveloped countries and in island populations, where more adults become ill.

DIAGNOSIS. In cases of typical measles, the clinical diagnosis is reliable. The observation of Koplik's spots strengthens the diagnosis. The difficulty comes in cases of modified or atypical measles. In such circumstances laboratory diagnosis is required for confirmation. Laboratory diagnosis may be accomplished by isolation of the measles virus in tissue culture systems or through documentation of a significant (four-fold or greater) rise in antibody titer in acute and convalescent blood specimens. A serologic diagnosis is preferred because of the relative difficulty in growing the virus from clinical specimens. Nasopharyngeal secretions taken during the acute period of the illness are the best source for isolation of the virus. Measles virus grows in human and simian renal cells and in human amnion cells. A typical cytopathic effect is found in cell cultures featuring the formation of syncytia or multinucleated giant cells, with intranuclear and intracytoplasmic inclusion bodies. The hemagglutination-inhibition antibody test is the most practical serologic test.

The diseases most likely to be confused with measles are rubella, scarlet fever, erythema infectiosum, exanthem subitum, Rocky Mountain spotted fever, enteroviral infections, and drug eruptions. Laboratory tests are available for the diagnosis of rubella, scarlet fever, Rocky Mountain spotted fever, and enteroviral infections.

In rubella the prodromal period is unremarkable. The rash is discrete, spreads quickly, and disappears by 72 hours without desquamation. Posterior auricular and/or occipital adenopathy is quite prominent. In adults, there may be joint symptoms that mimic rheumatoid arthritis.

In scarlet fever, the rash occurs within 12 hours of the prodromal period of high fever, vomiting, and sore throat. The rash is erythematous with punctiform eruption and blanches on pressure. It first appears on the flexural surfaces of the extremities and rapidly becomes generalized. A characteristic circumoral pallor is present. The characteristic "strawberry tongue" and a membranous tonsillitis help in making the diagnosis. Group A hemolytic streptococci are cultured from the nasopharynx, and there is usually a rise in the titer of antistreptolysin O.

Erythema infectiosum (fifth disease) has a characteristic rash without any prodromal symptoms. There is first a "slapped cheek" appearance. Then a secondary generalized discrete maculopapular rash that may be pruritic and remains for five days or more appears; it resembles a "chicken-wire" effect as it fades. Finally, there is a variable period lasting for weeks in which the eruption recurs after stimulation of the skin with sunlight or hot baths. Lymphadenopathy and low-grade fever may be present but are frequently absent. The disease tends to occur in explosive classroom epidemics. Occasionally adults become involved and may develop transient arthralgia or arthritis. Although it is believed to be of viral etiology, no specific viral agent has been recovered from patients with erythema infectiosum.

Exanthem subitum is a disease of infants characterized by several days of high fever, irritability, and a discrete maculopapular rash of 48 hours. The fever abates dramatically when the eruption occurs. No etiologic agent has been discovered.

Rocky Mountain spotted fever (RMSF) is frequently confused with typical measles but is most likely to be mistaken for atypical measles. In RMSF, there is a three- to four-day prodrome of fever, chills, headache, and malaise followed by a maculopapular and petechial eruption with a centrifugal distribution including the palms and soles. A history of tick bite or discovery of a tick on the child's body suggests the diagnosis. The scalp should be searched as a likely place for ticks. Laboratory tests include recovery of rickettsial organisms from the ticks and complement-fixation antibody assay. A Giemsa stain of skin biopsy may disclose coccobacilli in the endothelial cells.

Many of the enteroviruses can cause a rubella-like rash. Frequently, there are other signs of enteroviral infection such as aseptic meningitis, pleurodynia, and herpangina. These infections tend to occur in the summer in the northern hemisphere and can be identified by recovery of the viruses from stools, spinal fluid, or throat cultures and by specific serologic tests.

Occasionally a drug eruption will mimic the rash of measles. Differential diagnosis is based on lack of prodromal symptoms and a history of drug administration.

TREATMENT. There is no specific treatment for measles. Symptomatic treatment and supportive therapy include bed rest, hydration, eye washes, dim lighting, antipyretics, and non-narcotic cough medications. Antibiotics are indicated when secondary bacterial invasion occurs. Routine prophylactic antibiotics are to be discouraged except in high-risk children with chronic illnesses such as heart disease, cystic fibrosis, tuberculosis, and immunopathologic deficiencies. Adrenal corticosteroids have not been of proven benefit in the treatment of measles encephalitis.

Antiviral agents have been empirically given to patients

with SSPE. Amantadine, 5-iodo-2-deoxyuridine, and cytosine arabinoside have not stopped the downhill course significantly. Isoprinosine has given some favorable indications of effectiveness in early noncontrolled trials. Various forms of interferon are being evaluated.

PREVENTION. It is desirable to prevent or modify measles infection in children under 5 years of age, in chronically ill patients, and in patients who are immunosuppressed. Immune human globulin serum (gamma globulin) in a dose of 0.25 ml/kg body weight administered within 48 hours of exposure will prevent measles infection. Measles may be modified by a dose of 0.05 ml/kg body weight of immunoglobulin given within six days of exposure. The advantages of modifying measles are that a milder disease occurs and natural immunity develops. However, in order to ensure the development of immunity, patients given immune globulin should be immunized no sooner than six weeks after the administration of immune globulin or after 15 months of age unless there is a contraindication for the vaccine.

Highly effective, safe vaccines are available for measles (Proceedings 1962; Rauh and Schmidt, 1965). In the 1960s both inactivated and attenuated live measles vaccines were developed. The inactivated vaccines required a series of primary inoculations, and subsequent boosters were required to maintain vaccine-induced immunity. Because the attenuated live vaccine had a high rate of side effects when given alone, measles immune globulin was recommended for simultaneous administration. In 1965, further attenuated live measles vaccines were developed that had an acceptable rate of side-effects and produced long-standing immunity after one subcutaneous inoculation.

Measles vaccines have dramatically lowered the incidence of measles (Hinman et al., 1983). A resurgence of measles in the United States in 1970 to 1971 (cases occurring among previously immunized children) was attributed to improper use of the vaccines (Linneman et al., 1972). Vaccination may fail in patients under 1 year of age when maternal antibody may still be present, when too much measles immune globulin is used, or when vaccine is stored improperly. The resurgence of measles cases brought up the consideration of routine "booster" immunization. It appears unnecessary, but a final decision awaits continued surveillance of vaccinees.

Further attenuated vaccine is recommended for routine use at 15 months of age. There were more vaccine failures in children who were vaccinated before 15 months of age, probably because of maternal antibody (Yeager et al., 1977). The measles vaccine may be given alone or in combination with other viral vaccines. Revaccination is recommended in children who received inactivated measles vaccine or measles immune globulin to prevent measles. Exposed adults may be vaccinated if they have no history of measles. Vaccination is contraindicated in children with altered immune status due to underlying disease and/or therapy, and in pregnancy.

Aerosolized measles vaccines appear encouraging in early studies aimed at more effective vaccination in lesser developed countries (Sabin et al., 1983).

References

Fulginiti, V. A., Eller, J. J., Downie, A. W., and Kempe, C. H.: Altered reactivity to measles virus. JAMA 202:1075, 1967.

Hinman, A. R., Kirby, C. D., Eddens, D. L., et al: Elimination of indigenous measles from the United States. Rev Infect Dis 5:538, 1983.

Linneman, C. C., Jr., Rotte, T. C., Schiff, G. M., and Youtsey, J. L.: A seroepidemiologic study of a measles epidemic in a highly immunized population. Am J Epidemiol 95:238, 1972.

McDonald, R.: SSPE (subacute sclerosing panencephalitis). Clin Pediatr 16:124, 1977.

Panum, P. L.: Observations Made During the Epidemic of Measles on the Faroe Islands in the Year 1846. Berkeley, Delta Omega Society, 1940.

Proceedings of the International Conference on Measles Immunization. Am J Dis Child 103:211, 1962.

Rauh, L. W., and Schmidt, R.: Measles immunization with killed virus vaccine. Am J Dis Child 109:232, 1965.

Sabin, A. B., Arechiga, A. F., Fernandex de Castro, J., et al.: Successful immunization of children with and without maternal antibody by aerosolized measles vaccine. 1. Different results with undiluted human diploid cell and chick embryo fibroblast vaccines. JAMA 249:2651, 1983.

Termeislen, V.: SSPE and measles virus: Current state of our knowledge. Neuropädiatric 4:347, 1973.

Wechsler, S. L. and Meisner, H. C.: Measles and SSPE viruses: Similarities and differences. Prog Med Virol (Ed., J. Melnick), 28:65, 1982, Karger, Basel.

Werner, L. B., Corwin, R. M., Nieburg, P. F., and Feldman, H. A.: A measles outbreak among adolescents. J Pediatr 90:17, 1977.

Yeager, A. S., Davis, J. H., Ross, L. A., and Harvey, B.: Measles immunization: Successes and failures. JAMA 237:347, 1977.

239
RUBELLA

Gilbert M. Schiff, M.D.

Rubella is a childhood disease highlighted by a three-day generalized maculopapular rash, posterior auricular and/or occipital lymphadenopathy, and low-grade fever. The disease is endemic throughout the world and occurs in periodic epidemics. Rubella is not considered as contagious as measles or chickenpox, requiring relatively close exposure for transmission. Adults with rubella tend to develop arthralgia or arthritis.

The disease has serious implications when it occurs in a pregnant woman. The rubella virus can create an intrauterine infection and cause fetal death, spontaneous abortion, or a variety of congenital anomalies. For this reason, it is desirable to prevent rubella.

The isolation of the etiologic agent in 1962 in tissue culture was followed by the development of diagnostic laboratory tests and live, attenuated vaccines (Parkman et al., 1962; Weller and Neva, 1962; Schiff and Sever, 1966). A severe, widespread epidemic in 1964–65 provided many cases of acquired and congenital rubella for study, and the availability of the newly developed diagnostic tools permitted great advancement in our knowledge of the disease. Widespread application of rubella vaccines has reduced the incidence of rubella (and congenital rubella), has changed its epidemiology, and provides a basis for effective control.

ETIOLOGIC AGENT. The rubella virus is an RNA virus classified in the togavirus group. The 60-nm viral particles are made up of a 150s nucleocapsid with single-stranded RNA and a surrounding lipid-containing envelope. Three proteins have been detected: two glycoproteins and a capsid protein. The virus hemagglutinates at low temperatures only.

The virus is stable for years at −70° C, for short periods at −20° C, and is thermolabile at room and body temperature. It can be inactivated by radiation, chemicals (chloroform, formalin, or beta-propriolactone), and low pH (<6.5) or high pH (>8.1).

Rubella virus can be grown in many tissue culture cell lines. In some cell lines (RK_{13}, SIRC) there is a direct cytopathic effect, while in others (primary African green kidney, Vero) the virus is detected only by interference with a superinfecting enterovirus. Some workers feel that the interference method is the most sensitive for recovering rubella virus from clinical specimens.

Experimental rubella infections have been produced in subhuman primates and rodents. These animals do not develop clinical signs of illness. Intrauterine infection has been reported in rabbits, mice, and ferrets. Specific antisera can best be made in African green monkeys and ferrets.

Rubella infection generates specific antibodies that can be measured by a variety of tests. Neutralizing and hemagglutination-inhibition antibodies parallel each other and are a reliable index of immunity. These antibodies first appear at the time of clinical symptoms and reach a peak two to four weeks later. They remain for long periods of time, if not for life. Complement-fixation antibodies develop a week or two after the onset of symptoms, peak two to four weeks later, and disappear six months to two years later.

There are conflicting reports on the effect of rubella infection on cell-mediated immunity.

CLINICAL MANIFESTATIONS. Subclinical infection with rubella virus occurs at least as often as clinical infection. The incubation period varies from 12 to 21 days. There is little prodromal symptomatology. Illness begins with the appearance of posterior auricular, occipital, and/or cervical lymphadenopathy that is usually nontender. Within a day or two a maculopapular rash begins on the face and rapidly spreads downward over the rest of the body, sparing the palms and soles. The discrete rash turns into an erythematous blush and disappears without desquamation by the third to fourth day. The rash is usually nonpruritic. A low-grade fever may accompany the eruptive period. Lymphadenopathy may persist for a week or so. Some children have a mild to moderate sore throat. Early in the illness there may be a leukopenia, but later the white cell count is within normal limits or may be slightly elevated.

In adults constitutional symptoms are usually more severe and adenopathy less so. Adults frequently (25 per cent) develop arthralgia and/or arthritis. The joint manifestations usually appear when the rash is disappearing but may occur earlier, or may occur without the rash. The arthritis resembles acute rheumatoid arthritis and may persist for weeks. Joint involvement is 10 to 25 times more common in women than men, and occurs in about 1 per cent of children.

The virus may be found in the nasopharynx for a week to ten days before the onset of rubella and for up to two weeks afterward. The peak period of viral shedding in the nasopharynx occurs during the eruptive phase. Viremia and viruria have been detected from six days after exposure to virus until soon after the appearance of the rash (Schiff et al., 1969).

COMPLICATIONS. Except for arthralgia and arthritis, complications from rubella are very uncommon. There have been reports of thrombocytopenic purpura and encephalitis with coma, post-encephalitic sequelae, and death.

A fatal degenerative neurologic disease very similar to subacute sclerosing panencephalitis (SSPE) has been found in several patients with congenital rubella (Weil, 1975). The patients were all in their second decade. They presented with signs like those in SSPE, and had very high rubella antibody titers in cerebrospinal fluid and serum. Rubella-like virus has been recovered from the brain tissue of one of these patients. There were thousands of patients born with congenital rubella in 1964–65 who are now in their second decade, but an epidemic of rubella-associated SSPE has not materialized.

GEOGRAPHIC VARIATIONS. Rubella is distributed worldwide and is endemic in most locations. Epidemics occur every seven to ten years. Island populations may be spared outbreaks for longer periods but often experience explosive epidemics that affect those born since the previous outbreak.

Although there appears to be only one serologic type of rubella virus, there is some evidence that the virus varies in its teratogenic potential in different locations (Cockburn, 1969). Thus, in Japan, the incidence of teratogenic effect of the virus is much less than it is elsewhere.

DIAGNOSIS. There are many viral infections that can produce a symptom complex similar to that of rubella. These infections are caused by viruses that do not appear to have teratogenic potential. Also, rubella may produce an atypical clinical picture or be subclinical. *A clinical diagnosis of rubella is unreliable and requires laboratory confirmation.* This is especially true in pregnant women. The two reliable methods of making a laboratory diagnosis of rubella are isolation of the virus and serologic test. Virus may be recovered from the nasopharynx for up to two weeks after appearance of the rash. The isolation of the virus requires tissue culture systems and may take a week to ten days. The most sensitive method for isolation of the virus is the enteroviral interference technique. A more practical method of laboratory diagnosis is the demonstration of a four-fold or greater rise in hemagglutination-inhibition antibody in paired specimens taken at the time of clinical illness and two to three weeks later. When the first specimen is collected a week or two after onset of symptoms, the complement-fixation antibody test may be used. Detection of specific IgM antibody in an acute phase serum specimen may also be used for diagnosis of acute rubella.

Blood counts and urinalysis are not useful in the diagnosis of acute rubella.

For the determination of immune status to rubella, the hemagglutination-inhibition antibody assay has been the standard. This antibody is a good index of immunity and persists after natural infection. The complement-fixation antibody disappears within a year or two after natural infection and is therefore not a valuable assay for the determination of immune status. The enzyme-linked immunosorbent assay, latex-agglutination, and radioimmune assay appear to be more sensitive but their specificity is not established (Sever and Cleghorn, 1982).

CONGENITAL RUBELLA

Although rubella had been recognized as an entity for many years previously, it was in 1941 that Gregg first noted the teratogenic potential of the disease (Gregg, 1942). Since then much information has been compiled concerning congenital rubella. Intrauterine infection with rubella virus often results in a child with one or more birth abnormalities, although the infection may be entirely subclinical. In the newborn with congenital rubella infection, rubella virus multiplies in the nasopharynx, urine, cerebrospinal fluid, and many internal organs. Circulating antibody is present at the same time. Virus is shed for months to years, whereas the antibody level persists for years and then may disappear. During the first few weeks of life there is both IgM and IgG; later only IgG persists.

The viremia in the mother leads to infection restricted to the placenta, or it involves many fetal tissues. The viral infection in the fetus causes degenerative and inflammatory reactions with intravascular thrombosis. Fewer parenchymal cells are found in infected organs. The timing of the initial fetal infection determines the type of teratogenic effects. Chronic infection may produce continuous damage throughout gestation and early life of the infant.

Fetal infection during the first trimester of pregnancy appears to be most critical. The generally accepted rates for subsequent anomalies are 50 per cent, 20 per cent, and 4 per cent if maternal rubella occurs in the first, second, or third month of pregnancy, respectively. Inapparent maternal infection can produce anomalies. The incidence of stillbirths and spontaneous abortion caused by maternal infection may reach 75 per cent.

The clinical manifestations of congenital rubella are varied. Some may be life-threatening, some may result in handicaps that require institutional care, and some are only temporary. The major abnormalities are patent ductus arteriosus, pulmonary and aortic stenosis, coarctation of the aorta, and atrial and/or ventricular septal defects; ocular lesions such as unilateral or bilateral cataracts, glaucoma, and chorioretinitis; deafness, unilateral or bilateral, partial or complete; microcephaly; and mental retardation and generalized growth retardation. There may be acute, self-limited lesions such as thrombocytopenic purpura, anemia, hepatitis, interstitial pneumonitis, myocarditis, encephalitis, and radiolucencies of the long bones.

The diagnosis of congenital rubella is easily made by isolation of the virus from the nasopharynx and/or documentation of elevated IgM antibodies in the first few weeks of life. The newborn with congenital rubella is literally pouring out virus in the nasopharynx. Since most congenital rubella cases may be subclinical, laboratory diagnosis becomes essential. The differential diagnosis includes cytomegalovirus disease, toxoplasmosis, and syphilis. Laboratory tests are available for each of these.

Many of the abnormalities can be corrected by surgery or may respond to medical therapy. Early intervention in hearing and speech deficiencies is critical for proper social adjustments. Amantadine, an antiviral drug, is effective against rubella virus in vitro (Maassab and Cockran, 1964) but was disappointing in a few cases of congenital rubella in children. At best, amantadine temporarily decreased viral shedding.

TREATMENT. There is no specific treatment for rubella, and the disease is seldom severe enough to require even supportive treatment. The arthalgia/arthritis is treated with analgesics. Corticosteroids are not indicated.

Encephalitis requires supportive therapy; corticosteroids have been administered, but their effectiveness has not been determined. Patients with thrombocytopenic purpura often require corticosteroids and platelet transfusions.

Amantadine, which has activity against rubella virus, in vitro, has not been used in clinical cases of acquired rubella.

PREVENTION. Administration of immune globulin has been reported to prevent or modify rubella infection. However, the value of immune globulin for the exposed pregnant woman is controversial. The controversy is the result of several variables that can confuse the interpretation of clinical trials if they are not well controlled: immune status of the recipient, accurate diagnosis of rubella infection, variation in dose of immune globulin, variation in rubella antibody titer of immune globulin, and variation in the time of administration of immune globulin in relation to time of exposure. The important goal in administering immune globulin to a susceptible pregnant woman is prevention of viremia. Experimental human challenge studies have shown that viremia is first detected on day 6 after intranasal administration of rubella virus. In practice it is difficult to pinpoint the time of exposure. It must be taken into consideration that a person with clinical symptoms of rubella has been contagious for a week or so before the onset of symptoms. A series of human experimental rubella challenge studies indicated that a specifically prepared, high-titered (2048) immune globulin prevented clinical symptoms and signs and viremia when rubella virus was given 24 hours later, but viremia occurred when commercially available immune globulin (titer 64–256) was used (Schiff, 1969).

The hazard of administering immune globulin to the exposed susceptible pregnant woman is that it might convert a clinical disease into a subclinical infection without preventing the viremia. Therefore, it is imperative, if immune globulin is administered, that pre-administration and follow-up antibody titers be assayed to determine if subclinical infection has occurred. This would be important if termination of pregnancy were to be considered for rubella infection. Certainly, in cases in which termination of pregnancy is not permissible under any circumstances, immune globulin should be administered to the exposed woman as the one positive measure that might be helpful. Twenty milliliters of immune globulin is the recommended dose.

Several effective, safe, live attenuated rubella vaccines have been developed (Buynak et al., 1969; Musser and Hilrabeck, 1969; Huggelen et al., 1969). These vaccines are more than 95 per cent effective in stimulating protective levels of antibody. The vaccines cause few side effects in children, and are not transmitted to susceptible contacts. The duration of vaccine-induced immunity can be determined only by continuous monitoring of vaccinees, but studies to date reveal persistence of immunity in more than 90 per cent for at least seven to nine years (Schiff et al., 1974, Herrmann et al., 1982).

In women, the vaccines are equally effective but produce more side effects, including parethesias and/or temporary joint manifestations, which may mimic rheumatoid arthritis. The vaccines should not be given to women who are pregnant or become pregnant within two months of vaccination on the theoretical grounds that the vaccines may be teratogenic. Vaccine strain viruses can cross the placenta, but there has been no proof that they are teratogenic. The vaccines can be given to women of childbearing age if the following recommendations are heeded: (1) the woman has been tested and shown to lack rubella hemagglutination (HI) antibody, (2) pregnancy has been ruled out, (3) the woman will not get pregnant for eight weeks after vaccination, and (4) postvaccination blood test is performed to confirm the development of antibody.

In the United States, rubella vaccination is part of the well-baby routine care. The vaccine may be given singly or in combination with other vaccines at 15 months of age or older. The goal is to create a "herd immunity" and thus indirectly protect pregnant women. After 13 years of administering rubella vaccines to well babies and pre-pubertal children, there has been a dramatic reduction in cases of acquired and congenital rubella, but outbreaks of cases have occurred among nonvaccinated teenagers and young adults (Centers for Disease Control, 1983). Thus an effective herd immunity has not been achieved. The danger of rubella vaccination at an early age is that it may not induce lifelong immunity or that vaccine-induced immunity will wane in the childbearing age.

In England, the rubella vaccination program provides for vaccination of girls at puberty. The overall effect of this program has not been determined.

An effective rubella control program should not rely on vaccination alone. Equally important are identification of susceptible women of childbearing age by antibody testing so that careful vaccination or intelligent management may be instituted if exposure occurs during pregnancy, and use of laboratory tests to diagnose the infection properly.

References

Buynak, E. B., Larson, V. M., McAleer, W. Y., Mascoli, C. C., and Hilleman, M. R.: Preparation and testing of duck embryo cell culture rubella vaccine. Am J Dis Child 118:347, 1969.

Centers for Disease Control. Rubella and Congenital Rubella—United States, 1980–1983. MMWR 32:505, 1983.

Cockburn, W. C.: World aspects of the epidemiology of rubella. Am J Dis Child 118:112, 1969.

Gregg, N. M.: Congenital cataract following German measles in the mother. Trans Ophthalmol Soc Aust 3:35, 1942.

Herrmann, K. L., Halstead, S. B., and Wiebenga, N. H.: Rubella antibody persistence after immunization. JAMA 247:193, 1982.

Huggelen, C., Sigel, M. M., Zygraich, N., Peetermans, B. S., Colinet, G., Leyton, R., Raupp, W. G., Pinto, C. A., Garg, S. G., Boyle, J. J., and Haff, R. F.: Safety testing of rubella virus vaccine (Cendehill strain): Preparation in primary rabbit kidney cells. Am J Dis Child 118:362, 1969.

Maassab, H. F., and Cockran, K. W.: Rubella virus. Inhibition in vitro by amantadine hydrochloride. Lancet 287:1443, 1964.

Musser, S. J., and Hilrabeck, L. Y.: Production of rubella virus vaccine: live, attenuated in canine renal cell cultures. Am J Dis Child 118:362, 1969.

Parkman, P. O., Buercher, E. L., and Artenitein, M. S.: Recovery of rubella virus from army recruits. Proc Soc Exp Biol Med 111:225, 1962.

Schiff, G. M.: Titered lots of immune globulin (IG): Efficacy in the prevention of rubella. Am J Dis Child 118:322, 1969.

Schiff, G. M., Donath, R., and Rotte, T.: Experimental rubella clinical and laboratory features of infection. Am J Dis Child 118:269, 1969.

Schiff, G. M., Rauh, J. R., Linnemann, C. C., Jr., Shea, F., Rotte, T. C., and Trimble, S.: Rubella vaccinees in a public school system. A 4½ year follow-up. Am J Dis Child 128:180, 1974.

Schiff, G. M., and Sever, J. F.: Rubella. Recent laboratory and clinical advances. Progr Med Virol 8:30, 1966.

Sever, J. L., and Cleghorn, C.: Rubella diagnostic tests, what is a specific result. Postgrad Med 71:73, 1982.

Weil, M. F., Itabashi, H. H., Cremer, N. E., Oshiro, L. S., Lennette, E., H., and Carnay, F.: Chronic progressive panencephalitis due to rubella virus simulating subacute sclerosing panencephalitis. N Engl J Med 292:994, 1975.

Weller, T. H., and Neva, F. A.: Propagation in tissue culture of cytopathic agents from patients with rubella-like illness. Proc Soc Exp Biol Med 111:215, 1962.

240

WARTS

SEPPO PYRHÖNEN, M.D.

ETIOLOGY. Human warts are induced by human papilloma viruses (HPV), a subgroup of the papovavirides (see Chapter 62). They are stable, cubical, icosahedral viruses with a diameter of 52 to 55 nm; occasionally tubular forms are observed. The viral capsid is composed of 72 capsomer units. The genome of HPV is a covalently closed, circular, double-stranded DNA with a molecular weight of about 5×10^6. The heterogeneity of the HPV genome is currently well established. More than 30 different subtypes of HPV have been recognized, and additional microheterogeneity of genomes within the viruses of a single wart has been demonstrated. The structural proteins of the various subtypes also differ. Different protein patterns and serologic groups corresponding to genetic subtypes have been demonstrated. The total number of different proteins varies among the groups, but the exact numbers are still unknown. In many respects the human papilloma viruses so far identified are still far from being fully characterized, and additional subtypes are currently to be detected.

PATHOGENESIS. Warts are generally regarded as a simple hyperplasia rather than a true neoplasm. In the normal epidermis, cell division is limited to the basal layer of cells. In warts, mitotic figures are seen in cells of higher layers. Proliferation of keratinocytes and elongation of rete pegs accompany the development of protruding papilloma topped by extensive hyperkeratosis.

Warts are transmitted either by autoinoculations from one site of the body to another or from one person to another, both directly by contact with wart tissue and indirectly by contact with contaminated objects. The incubation period after experimental inoculation averages about four months but varies from a few weeks up to two years (Rowson and Mahy, 1967). Microtrauma and pressure probably aid in skin penetration by the virus. Accordingly, the most common sites for lesions are the palmar and plantar areas. Hyperhidrosis and certain hormonal states (puberty, pregnancy) may predispose the patient to infection. After infection, latent virus may become manifest during immunosuppression or immunodeficiency.

The number of viral particles in wart tissue seems to be highly variable. Viruses are abundant in plantar warts, particularly within a year after their appearance (Shirodaria and Matthews, 1975). By contrast, genital warts contain remarkably fewer detectable viruses. Virus particles cannot be found in the proliferating cells of the wart; they first appear within the nucleoli of the cells in the stratum spinosum. In the stratum granulosum, nucleoli disappear and may be replaced by virus particles. Virus aggregates can be seen in the stratum corneum. Thus, virus maturation seems to be linked to cell differentiation.

It has been suggested that warts are made up of proliferating epidermal cells that arise from a single clone of infected cells (Murray et al., 1971). Another possible mechanism of origin is infection and subsequent transformation of adjacent cells into wart tumor cells. This type of multicellular origin has been suggested for genital warts (Friedman and Fialkow, 1976).

Warts are self-limiting tumors. Their natural lifespan varies from a few months to decades but averages about two years. Cell-mediated immunity (Morison, 1974; Ivanyi and Morison, 1976) and specific antibodies, particularly of the IgG class (Pyrhönen and Johansson, 1975), probably limit growth, produce spontaneous resolution, and prevent reinfection.

PATHOLOGY. Warts are local accumulations of hyperplastic epithelial cells. The basement membrane remains intact and the basal cells appear normal. Hyperplasia (acanthosis) occurs in the stratum spinosum. The keratinization pattern differs from normal skin. Parakeratosis in cells of the stratum corneum and thickening (hyperkeratosis) of this layer and the underlying stratum granulosum are characteristic. Certain features predominate in warts on different skin sites. Hyperkeratosis is marked in plantar and common warts. Plane warts show acanthosis but little papillomatosis or hyperkeratosis. Acanthosis and papillomatosis without hyperkeratosis are the typical histopathologic forms of warts on thin skin and genital warts of the vagina and cervix. Two types of intranuclear inclusions occur in warts. Eosinophilic and basophilic inclusions first appear in the nuclei of cells in the stratum spinosum and increase in size in the overlying, more superficial layers. The basophilic inclusions are viral in origin. The eosinophilic inclusions are caused by abnormal keratinization of wart tissue. One of the most characteristic histologic features of genital warts is the koilocytic atypia. The koilocytic cells have a prominent perinuclear clearing or "halo" that fails to stain with eosin or periodic acid–Shiff (PAS). Dyskeratotic, bi- or multinucleate cells are also observed in these lesions. (Syrjänen, 1980).

Histopathologic findings during spontaneous regression of plane and common warts differ. In plane warts, a dense mononuclear cell infiltration of the upper dermis and epidermis occurs first and is replaced by spongiosis and necrotic eosinophilic cells (Tagami et al., 1977). During regression of common warts, there is no infiltration of mononuclear cells. Instead, blood vessels are occluded with thrombi (Matthews and Shirodaria, 1973). The epidermis retains the typical structure of common warts.

CLINICAL MANIFESTATIONS. Skin warts are the most common disease caused by HPV. The appearance of warts varies remarkably depending on the site and the duration of the tumor. The *common wart* (verruca vulgaris), a round papillomatous tumor with a horny surface, is most often located on the dorsal aspects of the hands and fingers. Larger and older lesions develop a verrucous surface with clefts. These warts are usually 1 to 10 mm in size, but they may form lesions 2 cm or more in diameter. Warts located on areas of soft skin like the eyelids, face, neck, and nasolabial area have slender finger-like projections, 2 to 10 mm long on a narrow base, and are called *filiform warts.* Flat and smooth warts, *plane warts* or verruca plana, are found primarily on the face and dorsal aspects of the hands but also occur on the extensor surfaces of the arms and legs. They are flat-topped, round, slightly raised, 2- to 6-mm lesions with a granular surface. Plantar, palmar, and subungual warts do not project but lie deep in the epidermis. The most typical of these are the so-called *plantar warts,* which may be of several different types: a single wart, multiple warts containing small satellite warts around a central primary lesion, or a mosaic wart, which is a thick coalescence of smaller warts with extensive involvement of the sole of the foot (Fig. 1). Warts may cover a large area of the skin, particularly on the head and neck region. This disease is called *epidermodysplasia verruciformis.*

Another group of HPV tumors is *genital* or *venereal warts* (condyloma acuminata). Transmission is mainly venereal (Oriel, 1971). In males the lesions are usually located on the glans penis and prepuce but also occur in the urethra and occasionally in the bladder and ureters. In females the lesions are most frequent on the external genitals and perianal area but also occur frequently in the vagina and on the cervix. The warts often have a cauliflower-like appearance, but the virus may affect the cervical and vaginal epithelium without producing typical papillary condylomatous lesions (Purola and Savia, 1977). At least three different manifestations of human wart virus infections in the uterine cervix have been discovered: the papillomatous, the flat, and the inverted type of lesions. All have the typical histologic features induced by HPV. Genital warts may occur in male homosexuals around the anus. They are usually small, discrete tumors but may be giant condylomata, which can cause obstruction.

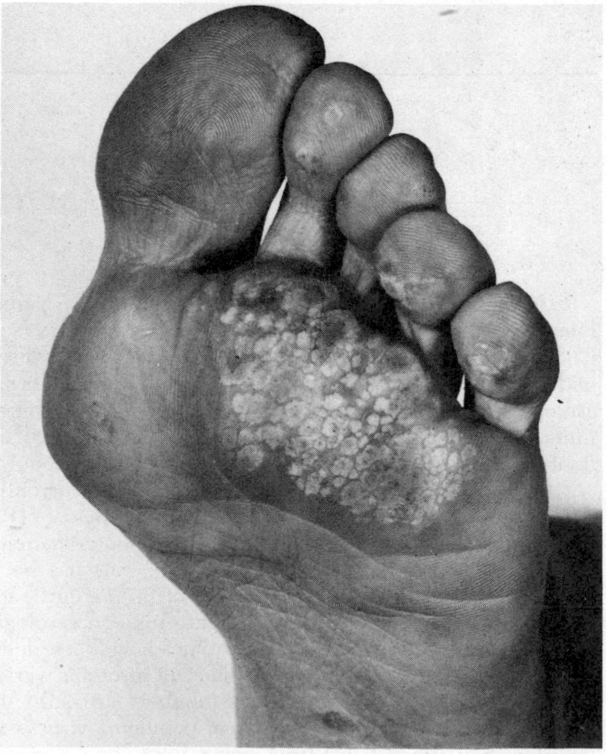

Figure 1. Typical mosaic type of plantar wart with extensive involvement of the sole.

Papillomatous tumors sometimes occur in the larynx. At least some of these *laryngeal papillomas* are induced by HPV, particularly in children. Infection may be acquired from vaginal condylomata during delivery (Cook, 1973).

Different clinical types of warts are preferentially associated with some types of HPVs. Typical plantar warts have been associated with HPV-1, multiple common warts mainly with HPV-2, and multiple flat warts with HPV-3. Different subtypes like 6, 11, and 16 have been identified in genital lesions, and laryngeal papillomas seem to be associated preferentially with types 6 and 11. Multiple subtypes like 3, 5, 8, 10, and 12 and many of the remaining poorly characterized subtypes have been isolated from epidermodysplastic lesions. Some of these patients seem to be infected by several HPV types.

COMPLICATIONS AND SEQUELAE. The vast majority of warts are benign tumors; malignant transformation is rare. A simple cutaneous wart almost never becomes malignant, but the lesions in about 20 per cent of patients with epidermodysplasia verruciformis undergo malignant changes (zur Hausen, 1977). These tumors can spread to other tissues and even produce destruction of the underlying bone. Malignant conversion seems to depend on the virus type, e.g., HPV-5 is associated with malignant forms, whereas HPV-3 is found in benign lesions.

Malignant transformations of condylomata have also been reported (zur Hausen, 1977), and the distinction between verrucous carcinoma and benign condyloma may be difficult. Exceptional extension of growth may lead to a giant condyloma called Buschke-Loewenstein's tumor. Clinically, they appear to be malignant, but the tumor is usually found to be benign histologically. Women with typical genital condylomata frequently have premalignant dysplasia of the vaginal and cervical epithelium (Purola and Savia, 1977; zur Hausen, 1977). Several types of evidence indicate that HPV might be one of the most important causal agents in cervical carcinomas (Syrjänen, 1980; zur Hausen, 1982; Zoler, 1983). The most severe epithelial atypia are often associated with the flat and inverted condylomas. Part of these lesions may undergo change into cervical neoplasias or their precursors (dysplasia and in situ carcinomas).

Juvenile laryngeal papillomas may also sometimes be transformed into malignant tumors, particularly if the papillomas were treated by x-rays.

After appropriate therapy or spontaneous recovery, cutaneous warts usually leave no detectable sequelae. Plantar warts may cause painful scars that interfere with normal walking for a long time. Periungual warts may scar the nail matrix and cause permanent deformity. Plane warts can cause spotty hyperpigmentation, especially in dark-skinned people. Certain warts, especially in soft and moist skin, may develop into large masses with secondary bacterial infection and ulceration.

GEOGRAPHIC VARIATIONS IN DISEASE. Warts are common diseases with a worldwide distribution. The highest incidence is during childhood and adolescence. Most people have had some kind of wart by the age of 20. The incidence is probably similar throughout Europe and the United States, but warts are much less common in most tropical regions (Rook et al., 1972).

DIAGNOSIS. There is usually no doubt about the clinical diagnosis of viral warts. However, a few other lesions can simulate these common warts. Simple calluses and corns, especially on the sole of the foot, are probably confused most often with warts. The correct diagnosis can be verified by removing the thick covering of horny cells. In warts, the infected central area has a white surface in which the capillary loops are seen as bleeding points or as thrombosed black dots. In contrast, calluses have a smooth, normal epidermis under the horny layer. Molluscum contagiosum (Chapter 242) may also mimic warts. The surface of these small, pearly tumors is smooth except for a central umbilicus from which infected cell debris can be extruded. Seborrheic warts and squamous cell papillomas or keratoacanthomas can also simulate viral warts but are seen mainly in older people. The discrete horny papules of punctate keratoderma that develop during childhood or early adult life can sometimes mimic plantar warts. The differential diagnosis also includes intradermal foreign bodies (e.g., glass and splinters), neurofibroma, and painful scars. The definitive diagnosis can be established by histologic examination of tissue. This is most important in cases of venereal warts, when malignancy must be excluded. Gynecologic condylomata also can be identified by vaginal and cervical cytologic examinations (Purola and Savia, 1977).

TREATMENT AND PROPHYLAXIS. Therapy that might lead to permanent scarring or other sequelae should be avoided because most warts will involute spontaneously within two years. Warts that are painful, subject to trauma and infection, or cosmetically objectionable should be treated. Sometimes treatment is indicated to prevent further dissemination. The type of therapy should be determined by the type and location of the wart and the response to treatment. The treatment may include destructive therapy such as electrocoagulation, curettage, cryotherapy, or superficial radiotherapy, but less destructive treatment should be favored, especially for plantar warts, to avoid scarring. Daily application of one of the following agents often leads to the resolution of plantar as well as other types of warts: 10 to 20 per cent glutaraldehyde solution, 15 to 20 per cent lactic and salicylic acid in flexible collodion, or 20 to 40 per cent salicylic acid ointment or plaster. The combination of one of these agents with curettage often gives good results. Cantharidin, 0.7 per cent solution in acetone collodion 1:1, is especially effective against common warts, particularly in the periungual area. Genital warts are usually treated by a weekly application of 20 per cent podophyllin in tincture of benzoin or in alcohol. The surrounding normal skin should be covered with a protective ointment. Podophyllin should never be used for pregnant women. The therapy of recurrent warts has included application of topical antiviral agents like iododeoxyuridine (IDU), topical antitumor agents such as 5-fluorouracil and bleomycin, and immunotherapy with dinitrochlorobenzene (DNCB), smallpox vaccination, or autogenous wart vaccines. Some of these agents may be helpful but their efficacy is unproved. Interferon therapy has also been observed to be effective in recurrent laryngeal papillomas as well as in skin and genital warts.

Because of the lack of a vaccine and the ubiquitous nature of HPV, there is no effective prophylaxis for common warts. Genital warts can be prevented by avoiding infected sexual contacts. Avoiding common bathing and swimming pools may prevent some exposure to HPV, but other sources of infection are widespread throughout the environment.

References

Cook, T. A.: Maternal condyloma linked to lesions in babies. JAMA 224:1475, 1973.
Fletcher, S.: Histopathology of papilloma virus infection of the cervix uteri: the history, taxonomy, nomenclature and reporting of koilocytic dysplasias. J Clin Pathol 36:616, 1983.
Friedman, J. M., and Fialkow, P. J.: Viral "tumorigenesis" in man: Cell markers in condylomata acuminata. Int J Cancer 17:57, 1976.
Ivanyi, L., and Morison, W. L.: In vitro lymphocyte stimulation by wart antigen in man. Br J Dermatol 94:523, 1976.
Matthews, R. S., and Shirodaria, P. V.: Study of regressing warts by immunofluorescence. Lancet 1:689, 1973.
Morison, W. L.: In vitro assay of cell-mediated immunity to human wart antigen. Br J Dermatol 90:531, 1974.
Murray, R. F., Hobbs, J., and Payne, B.: Possible clonal origin of common warts (verruca vulgaris). Nature 232:51, 1971.
Oriel, J. D.: Natural history of genital warts. Br J Vener Dis 47:1, 1971.
Purola, E., and Savia, E.: Cytology of gynecologic condyloma acuminatum. Acta Cytol 21:26, 1977.
Pyrhönen, S., and Johansson, E.: Regression of warts. An immunological study. Lancet 1:592, 1975.
Rook, A., Wilkinson, D. S., and Ebling, F. J. G.: Textbook of Dermatology. Vol. I, 2nd ed. Oxford, Blackwell Scientific Publications, 1972, p. 550.
Rowson, K. E. K., and Mahy, B. W. J.: Human papova (wart) virus. Bact Rev 31:110, 1967.
Shirodaria, P. V., and Matthews, R. S.: An immunofluorescence study of warts. Clin Exp Immunol 21:329, 1975.
Syrjänen, K. J.: Condylomatous epithelial changes in the uterine cervix and their relationship to cervical carcinogenesis. Int J Gynaecol Obstet 17:415, 1980.
Tagami, H., Takigawa, M., Ogino, A., Imamura, S., and Ofugi, S.: Spontaneous regression of plane warts after inflammation. Arch Dermatol 113:1209, 1977.
Zoler, M. L.: Human papilloma virus linked to cervical (and other) cancers. JAMA 249:2997, 1983.
zur Hausen, H.: Human genital cancer: synergism between two virus infections or synergism between a virus infection and initiating event? Lancet 2:1370, 1982.
zur Hausen, H.: Human papillomaviruses and their possible role in squamous cell carcinomas. Curr Top Microbiol Immunol 78:1, 1977.

241

HAND-FOOT-MOUTH DISEASE

DAVID I. MINKOFF, M.D.
JAMES D. CONNOR, M.D.

Hand-foot-mouth disease is a mild exanthematous infection of children due to coxsackieviruses A. Its name comes from a characteristic vesicular eruption of the hands, feet, and mouth and must not be confused with foot and mouth disease of cattle.

ETIOLOGY. Since the isolation of coxsackieviruses in 1947 by Dalldorf and Sickles (1948) and subsequent recognition of two distinct biologic groups, A and B, recurring clinical patterns of disease caused by specific coxsackievirus serotypes have been recognized. One such epidemic was investigated by Robinson, Doane, and Rhoades in 1957. It was linked with coxsackievirus A16 and was characterized by vesiculo-ulcerative lesions of the oropharynx and exanthems on the hands and feet. Alsop subsequently reported an epidemic in Birmingham, England, in 1960 and gave the name hand-foot-mouth disease to the syndrome he observed. Many epidemics have been reported since then with similar clinical characteristics and demonstration of coxsackievirus A16 as the etiologic agent of hand-foot-mouth syndrome. Clinical cases associated with coxsackieviruses A5 and A10 have also been described.

PATHOLOGY. The characteristic histologic change is a subepidermal vesicle with a mixed inflammatory exudate of lymphocytes, monocytes, and polymorphonuclear leukocytes. The overlying dermis shows extensive acantholysis with reticular degeneration. Intracytoplasmic inclusions have been seen. There are no multinucleated giant cells on Tzanck preparations from active vesicles.

CLINICAL MANIFESTATIONS. The illness is typically mild without obvious prodromal signs and seldom lasts over a week. In one outbreak, the disease was so mild that only 2 per cent of the patients had fever. However, the same virus may cause aseptic meningitis, paralysis, a life-threatening systemic disease resembling measles, myocarditis, and death.

The incubation period is usually three to five days. Mild fever, sore mouth, and refusal to eat are the most common presenting symptoms (Richardson and Leibovitz, 1965). The oral lesions begin as small red macules and then form vesicles on an erythematous base in the pharynx, soft palate, buccal mucosa, gingivae, and tongue. The vesicles are 1 to 3 mm in diameter but may coalesce to form bullae. Some vesicles may ulcerate while others absorb without breaking the mucous membrane. Those that break down form shallow ulcers 1 to 2 cm across in the oropharynx, with yellowish gray bases and hyperemic margins. These are often so painful that children refuse to eat. The exanthem is maculopapular and often evolves to vesicles containing clear watery fluid. The vesicles measure 0.5 to 1 cm in diameter and have a narrow rim of erythema around the base of the lesion. They usually appear on the back of the hands and the lateral margins of the feet; less often they are found on the palms, soles, and between the fingers and toes. The number varies from as few as 2 or 3 to 30 to 40. They are non-pruritic, rarely painful, and usually absorbed in three to four days without scarring. The buttocks are sometimes involved, and scattered single vesicles may appear over the proximal extremities, penis, ear lobes, and face. During the acute illness there may also be malaise, anorexia, abdominal pain, diarrhea, cough, coryza, chest pain, and headache.

The disease is most common in preschool children from birth to age 4. There is no sex predilection. The incidence of infection is difficult to determine because most cases are too mild to need the patient seeing a doctor. In epidemics, the high attack rate of the virus can be demonstrated because clinical illness develops in more than half of the contacts in affected households. In epidemics, up to 44 per cent of asymptomatic contacts without a past history of hand-foot-mouth disease have evidence of infection as demonstrated by stool culture and/or neutralizing antibody titer rises.

DIAGNOSIS. The diagnosis is usually made when vesicular ulcerative stomatitis occurs along with exanthems of the hands and feet during a mild febrile illness. The leukocyte count ranges from 3750 to 16,200, occasionally with an atypical lymphocytosis. If coxsackievirus A16 is cultured or neutralizing antibody rises fourfold or more, the diagnosis is established. Inoculation of stool (not a rectal swab) into tissue culture and suckling mice produces a viral isolation rate of 75 to 80 per cent in most series. Twenty-five to 50 per cent of throat swabs and vesicle fluid cultures from patients contain coxsackievirus.

Since a high neutralizing antibody titer is sometimes present in "acute phase" serum two to seven days after onset of symptoms, the antibody titer may not rise in convalescent serum.

The distribution of vesicular lesions in herpes simplex stomatitis may be similar to those of hand-foot-mouth infection but herpes infection often involves the perioral structures and may cause high fever and cervical and submandibular lymphadenopathy, all of which are unusual with hand-foot-mouth disease. Herpangina, caused by another coxsackie A virus, most frequently involves the anterior fauces, tonsillar pillars, soft palate, and uvula, and is not commonly associated with lingual, buccal mucosal, or gingival lesions. Erythema multiforme may involve the mouth and skin, but typical target or iris lesions are the rule, and its association with other underlying viral infections and drug ingestions is well known. Aphthous stomatitis causes no fever or systemic signs or symptoms and is confined to the anterior mouth. It is not known to be caused by a specific viral agent and has a tendency to recur in certain individuals, occasionally after trigger stimuli.

GEOGRAPHIC VARIATIONS. Although first reported in Canada, outbreaks have occurred in areas of the world as widely separated as South Africa (Gear, 1962), Australia, Japan (Togaya and Tachibana, 1975), and the United States (Adler et al., 1970). The Japanese outbreaks have been the most extensive, involving thousands of cases.

TREATMENT. There is no specific drug therapy.

References

Adler, J. L., Mostow, S. R., Mellin, H., et al.: Epidemiologic investigation of Hand-Foot-Mouth disease. Am J Dis Child 120:309, 1970.

Dalldorf, G., and Sickles, G.: An unidentified, filterable agent isolated from the feces of children with paralysis. Science 108:61, 1948.

Gear, J.: Coxsackie virus infections in Southern Africa. Yale J Biol Med 34:289, 1962.

Richardson, H. B., and Leibovitz, A.: "Hand-Foot-Mouth disease" in children. J Pediatr 67:6, 1965.

Robinson, C. R., Doane, F. W., and Rhoades, A. J.: Report of an outbreak of febrile illness with pharyngeal lesions and exanthem: Toronto, summer, 1957. Isolation of group A Coxsackie virus. Can Med Assoc J: 79(8):1958.

Togaya, I., and Tachibana, K.: Epidemic of hand, foot, and mouth disease in Japan 1972–1973: Difference in epidemiologic and virologic features from the previous one. Jpn J Med Sci Biol 28:231, 1975.

242
MOLLUSCUM CONTAGIOSUM

ROY POSTLETHWAITE, B.SC., M.D.

Molluscum contagiosum is a benign epidermal tumor of characteristic appearance. It occurs only in human beings and is caused by a poxvirus (Postlethwaite, 1970).

ETIOLOGY. An unclassified member of the pox group, molluscum contagiosum virus (Fig. 1) is distinct from the parapoxviruses and resembles vaccinia virus in size (300 × 240 nm) and shape and in its linear, duplex DNA genome with a molecular weight of 118×10^6 (Parr et al., 1977). It differs from vaccinia in some structural details (Peters and Küper, 1970), in G + C (guanine plus cytosine) content and base sequence of its DNA, and in some properties of its DNA-dependent RNA polymerase (Shand et al., 1976). Virion DNA from different patients shows genetic and structural heterogeneity and structural polypeptides also differ amongst isolates (Oda et al., 1982). Homologous sera react weakly with viral antigen in complement fixation, precipitation, immunofluorescence, and neutralization tests. There is no cross-reactivity with vaccinia, cowpox, mousepox, rabbitpox, or fowlpox antigens. Molluscum virus fails to reactivate other poxviruses and has not consistently been grown in serial passage outside man. An etiologic relationship to similar rare lesions in chimpanzees, macropod marsupials and horses has not been established.

PATHOGENESIS AND PATHOLOGY. An ordered array of proliferating epidermal cells extends as pear-shaped lobules into the dermis (Lever and Schaumburg-Lever, 1975), compressing papillae but not breaching the basement membrane (Fig. 2). The surrounding epidermis is undermined and stretched over the projecting tumor, and a central pore appears over the degenerating apical portions, which are rich in molluscum inclusion bodies. Virus growth is confined to the epidermis (Epstein and Fukuyama, 1973; Vreeswijk et al., 1976) and is associated with extensive development of gap junctions, increased turnover of basal cells, and adjacent stromal proliferation. The phagosomes of these basal cells contain virions but do not fuse with lysosomes (Vreeswijk et al., 1977). Released viral cores cluster alongside the Golgi apparatus, centrioles, and spindle fibers of cells in early mitosis where second-stage uncoating may occur. Nuclear DNA synthesis declines as the viral DNA begins to replicate in the cytoplasm of the infected prickle cell layer and tiny eosinophilic inclusions appear. Granular masses of viroplasm are enveloped in membranes, forming immature and then mature virions. These pack the developing inclusions, which, as the cells migrate synchronously to the surface, reach up to 30 μm in diameter and displace the nuclear remnants (Fig. 3). Infected cells reach the horny layer by 7 days and are shed by 9 to 15, the glassy molluscum bodies now being basophilic and Feulgen positive, possibly due to capsid damage with exposure of viral DNA (Kwittken, 1980). We still need to elucidate the precise relationship of infection to cell division, whether virus is transmitted between cells, and the mechanisms of initiation and maintenance of infection.

Molluscum virus does not grow reproducibly in cell cultures. Even without propagation, however, it is cytotoxic and induces interference, interferon, and a transient "transformed" phenotype (Barbanti-Brodano et al., 1974) in cell cultures. Along with the lack of reactivating capacity, these

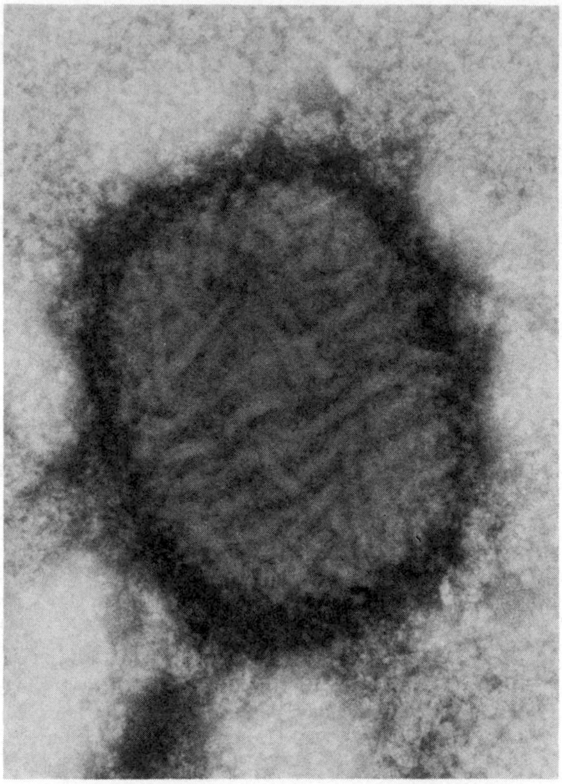

Figure 1. Molluscum contagiosum virion negatively stained with ammonium molybdate. ×210,000. (Courtesy Dr. D. W. Gregory.)

properties are consistent with the behavior of a mutant, defective, or partially inactivated virus, which achieves partial genome expression but is unable to synthesize uncoating protein except in human skin in situ (La Placa et al., 1967; McFadden et al., 1979). In cell cultures, indeed, ingested virions are either destroyed in phagolysosomes like heated vaccinia virus or, after first-stage uncoating, remain as cytoplasmic cores that fail to become fully uncoated (Prose et al., 1969). Anecdotal reports suggest that some viral properties are relatively heat-labile, and in vitro growth has been reported at 30° C but not at 37° C. An unconfirmed report of virus growth in cell cultures suggested a novel mechanism of DNA replication (Francis and Bradford, 1976) because of the surprising failure of base analogues and of rifampicin and methisazone to inhibit viral replication.

Although viral antigen is present in all lesions, the cellular response is usually slight and antibody may not be detectable. However, inflammatory reactions, cellular infiltration around regressing lesions, tuberculin-type responses after experimental inoculation, and the predominance of IgG antibody in most patients (Shirodaria and Matthews, 1977), sometimes only after treatment, all suggest that specific sensitization occurs when viral antigens reach subepidermal tissues. Sera from 60 per cent of patients have IgM anticellular antibodies (Shirodaria et al., 1979). The relationship of these responses to immunity, regression, recurrence, and the age distribution of the disease is unknown.

CLINICAL MANIFESTATIONS. The incubation period of experimental infection ranges from 14 to 50 days and, in the natural infection, extends to 6 months. Up to 20 or more discrete pearly papules about 2 to 7 mm in diameter appear singly or in groups on the face, neck, trunk (Fig. 4), and limbs. They are rare on the palms, soles, and mucous membranes. A cheesy white core may be expressed from the central pore. Children of more than 1 year are most commonly affected, but the reported age range extends from 6 weeks to 72 years. Lesions may itch and autoinoculation is common. Outbreaks suggesting direct or indirect contagion are recorded in wrestlers, in children's homes, and in association with tattooing, swimming pools, and beauty parlors. However, most cases are sporadic, experimental infection is frequently unsuccessful, and the precise mode of transmission is unknown. Venereal infections, with genital lesions and an appropriate contact his-

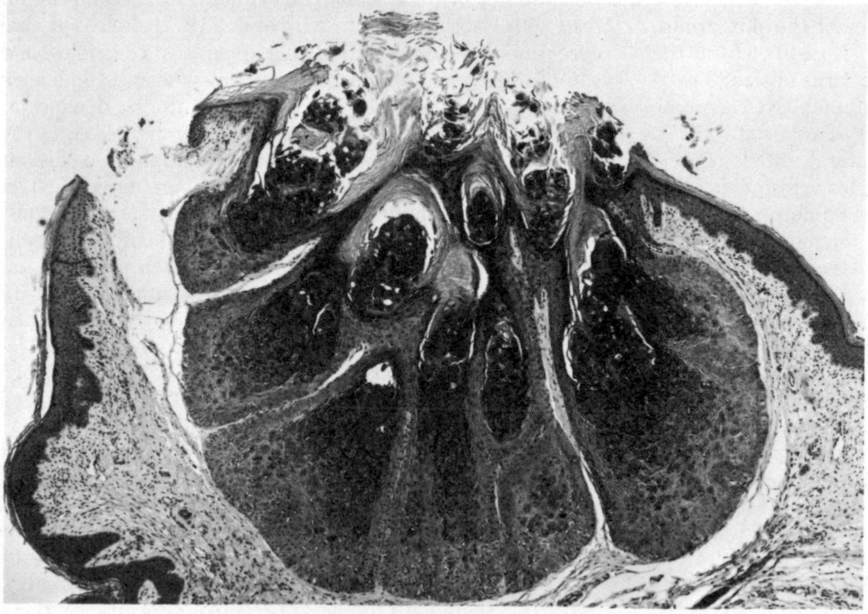

Figure 2. Molluscum contagiosum. Section through entire lesion. Hematoxylin and eosin stain. ×37. (Courtesy Dr. S. W. B. Ewen.)

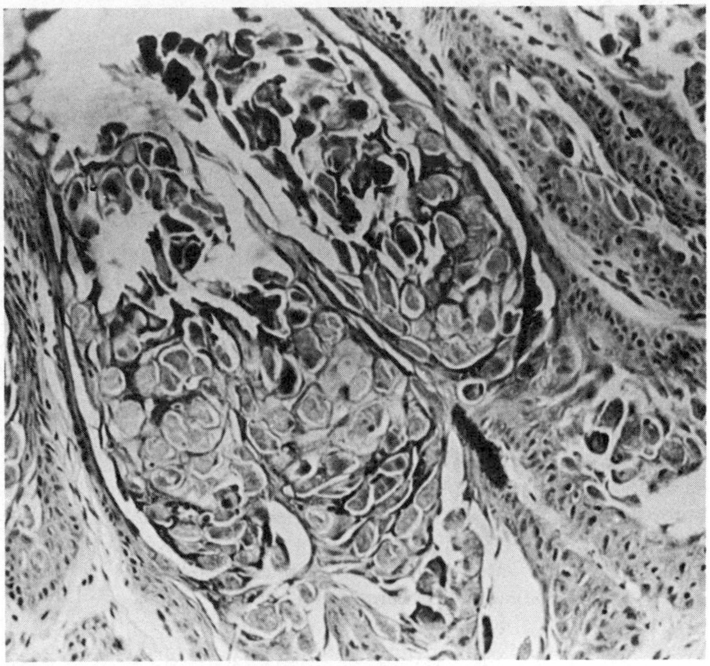

Figure 3. Molluscum contagiosum. Section through apical part of lesion showing molluscum bodies. Phloxine-tartrazine stain. ×160. (From Postlethwaite, R., Watt, J. A., Hawley, T. G., Simpson, I., and Adam, H.: Features of molluscum contagiosum in the northeast of Scotland and in Fijian village settlements. Journal of Hygiene, Cambridge 65:281, 1967.)

tory, are recognized with increasing frequency in young adults (Lynch, 1972; Wilkin, 1977). Both indigenous and imported infections have been reported. A specific diagnosis in the sexual partner is more usually inferred than proved. Lesions regress spontaneously or after trauma or bacterial infection; new ones appear intermittently during a total course of six months to four years. The presence of antibody and skin hypersensitivity in patients without lesions may imply inapparent, unrecognized, or unreported infection.

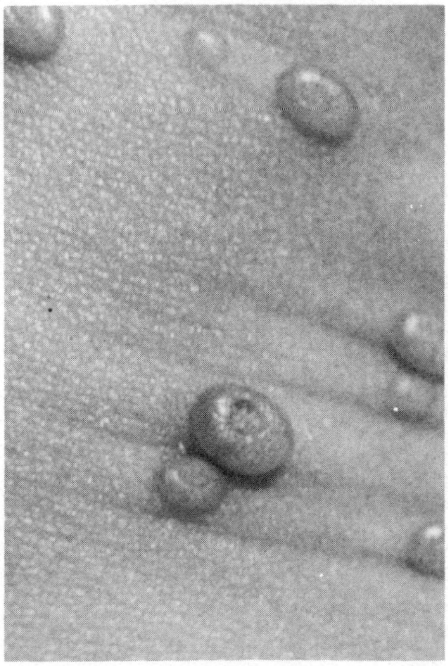

Figure 4. Molluscum contagiosum lesions. ×2½. (Courtesy Dr. R. F. Menzies.)

COMPLICATIONS AND SEQUELAE. Minor bleeding after trauma, secondary bacterial infection, and perilesional depigmentation may occur. Conjunctivitis may complicate eyelid lesions. An eczematous reaction occurs in 10 per cent of patients after a month or more and may represent a nonspecific or an immunologic response to the extension of products of the lesions into the dermis. The claim that treatment of preexisting eczema with topical steroids predisposes to molluscum contagiosum is disputed. Subjects treated with immunosuppressive drugs (Rosenberg and Yusk, 1970), and those with atopic dermatitis, AIDS, or lymphoid malignancy sometimes develop several hundred lesions within a few days. This phenomenon also occurs rarely in apparently normal patients. Extensive chronic infection in a patient with atopic dermatitis was attributed to impaired cellular immunity (Pauly et al., 1978). New lesions may appear two months or more after apparent cure.

GEOGRAPHICAL VARIATIONS IN DISEASE. Regional variations in prevalence and in age and lesion distribution (Rook et al., 1979; Noble, 1983) of this worldwide condition may reflect local patterns of hygiene, social custom, nutrition, and climate. However, sampling differences also contribute to such prevalence variations as 0.1 per cent in Scottish dermatology outpatients, 4.5 per cent of an entire Fijian village settlement, and 22 per cent of children under 10 in villages in New Guinea (Sturt et al., 1971). A remarkable outbreak in Maasai pastoralists in Kenya coincided with a period of relief feeding following famine, suggesting activation of a previously quiescent infection (Murray et al., 1980). Household spread is rare in Aberdeen, Scotland, but common in Fiji. The peak age incidence is 10 to 12 years in Aberdeen outpatients, predominantly in boys attending public swimming baths; 2 to 3 years in the Pacific Islands, with both sexes equally affected; and 1 to 4 years in the Congo. Infrequent infection among adults in countries with widespread infection in early childhood may reflect persisting specific immunity, which, combined with the long incubation period, may also contribute to the low prevalence during the first year of life.

DIAGNOSIS. Diagnostic difficulties (Molluscum contagiosum, 1968) arise with giant, isolated, miliary, and confluent lesions, and those in unusual locations such as the soles of the feet and the glans penis. Secondarily infected lesions simulate furuncles or folliculitis, and eyelid lesions may resemble chalazions or sebaceous cysts. Some mistaken diagnoses include (Mehregan, 1961) epithelioma, basal cell carcinoma, keratoacanthoma, and verruca vulgaris. The presence of multiple lesions or freezing with ethyl chloride to accentuate the central dimple may help establish the diagnosis.

Molluscum bodies are readily recognized by microscopic examination of expressed core material, either unstained or stained by the Giemsa or Papanicolaou techniques. Virions may be detected by Morosow's stain or by electron microscopy (Fig. 1). Biopsies may be examined histologically (Fig. 2) or by immunofluorescence and electronmicroscopy for viral antigen and viral particles, respectively. Molluscum virus cannot be directly isolated from lesions in standard tissue culture lines, but three different types have been recognized by restriction endonuclease analysis of viral DNA (Parr et al., 1977). Antibodies may be demonstrated by gel diffusion and immunofluorescence techniques.

TREATMENT. Since lesions resolve spontaneously, treatment for cosmetic reasons or to prevent spread should aim at painless destruction, without other damage or residual scarring. Removal of the core with fine forceps or curette, when tolerated, produces rapid resolution. Other physical treatments, transiently painful, include puncture with a toothpick dipped in liquor iodi fortis or freezing with liquid nitrogen. Treatment by chemicals, such as trichloroacetic acid or 20 per cent podophyllin in 95 per cent ethanol is prolonged and may produce unpleasant burns. By contrast, twice daily application of 0.05 per cent tretinoin (vitamin A acid) cream (Papa and Berger, 1976) is effective and painless, and the antikeratolytic "salactol" (16.7 per cent each of lactic and salicylic acids in flexible collodion) prevents spread. Skin emollients relieve associated dermatitis, which, as with conjunctivitis, disappears following lesion removal. Methisazone, an antiviral agent for other poxviruses, is not effective. Follow-up examinations for four months are necessary to treat previously undetected lesions.

PROPHYLAXIS. There is no specific prophylaxis. General measures include successful treatment of patients and their exclusion from, for instance, communal swimming pools until cured. The general principles of epidemiology and hygiene should be applied to common source outbreaks. Patients with genital lesions should be examined for other sexually transmitted diseases and followed up by contact-tracing and health education. Similarly, patients with other sexually transmitted infections should be examined for coexistent molluscum contagiosum.

References

Barbanti-Brodano, G., Mannini-Palenzona, A., Varoli, O., Portolani, M., and La Placa, M.: Abortive infection and transformation of human embryonic fibroblasts by molluscum contagiosum virus. J Gen Virol 24:237, 1974.

Epstein, W. L., and Fukuyama, K.: Maturation of molluscum contagiosum virus (MCV) in vivo: Quantitative electron microscopic autoradiography. J Invest Dermatol 60:73, 1973.

Francis, R. D., and Bradford, H. B., Jr.: Some biological and physical properties of molluscum contagiosum virus propagated in cell culture. J Virol 19:382, 1976.

Kwittken, J.: Molluscum contagiosum: some new histologic observations. Mount Sinai J Med 47:583, 1980.

La Placa, M., Portolani, M., Mannini-Palenzona, A., Barbanti-Brodano, G., and Bernardini, A.: Further studies on the mechanism of the cytopathic changes produced by the molluscum contagiosum virus into human amnion cell cultures. G Microbiol 15:205, 1967.

Lever, W. F., and Schaumburg-Lever, G.: Histopathology of the Skin. 5th ed. Philadelphia and Toronto, J. B. Lippincott Company, 1975.

Lynch, P. J.: Molluscum contagiosum venereum. Clin Obst Gynecol 15:966, 1972.

McFadden, G., Pace, W. E., Purres, J., and Dales. S.: Biogenesis of poxviruses: transitory expression of molluscum contagiosum early functions. Virology 94:297, 1979.

Mehregan, A. H.: Molluscum contagiosum—a clinicopathologic study. Arch Dermatol 84:123, 1961.

Molluscum contagiosum. Br Med J 1:459, 1968.

Murray, M. J., Murray, A. B., Murray, N. J., Murray, M. B., and Murray, C. J.: Molluscum contagiosum and herpes simplex in Maasai pastoralists; refeeding activation of virus infection following famine. Trans Roy Soc Trop Med Hyg 74:371, 1980.

Noble, W. C.: Microbial Skin Disease; its Epidemiology. London, E. Arnold, 1983.

Oda, H., Ohyama, Y., Sameshima, T., and Hirakawa, K.: Structural polypeptides of molluscum contagiosum virus: their variability in various isolates and location within the virion. J Med Virol 9:19, 1982.

Papa, C. M., and Berger, R. S.: Venereal herpes-like molluscum contagiosum: Treatment with tretinoin. Cutis 18:537, 1976.

Parr, R. P., Burnett, J. W., and Garon, C. F.: Structural characterization of the molluscum contagiosum virus genome. Virology 81:247, 1977.

Pauly, C. R., Artis, W. M., and Jones, H. E.: Atopic dermatitis, impaired cellular immunity, and molluscum contagiosum. Arch Dermatol 114:391, 1978.

Peters, D., and Küper, H.: The nucleoid structure of molluscum contagiosum virus during maturation. Arch Ges Virusforsch 31:137, 1970.

Postlethwaite, R.: Molluscum contagiosum—a review. Arch Environ Health 21:432, 1970.

Prose, P. H., Friedman-Kien, A. E., and Vilček, J.: Molluscum contagiosum virus in adult human skin cultures: An electron microscopic study. Am J Pathol 55:349, 1969.

Rook, A., Wilkinson, D. S., and Ebling, F. J. G. (eds.): Textbook of Dermatology. 3rd ed. Oxford, Blackwell Scientific Publications, 1979.

Rosenberg, E. W., and Yusk, J. W.: Molluscum contagiosum. Eruption following treatment with prednisone and methotrexate. Arch Dermatol 101:439, 1970.

Shand, J. H., Gibson, P., Gregory, D. W., Cooper, R. J., Keir, H. M., and Postlethwaite, R.: Molluscum contagiosum—a defective poxvirus? J Gen Virol 33:281, 1976.

Shirodaria, P. V., and Matthews, R. S.: Observations on the antibody responses in molluscum contagiosum. Br J Dermatol 96:29, 1977.

Shirodaria, P. V., Matthews, R. S., and Samuel, M.: Virus-specific and anti-cellular antibodies in molluscum contagiosum. Br J Dermatol 101:133, 1979.

Sturt, R. J., Muller, K. H., and Francis, G. D.: Molluscum contagiosum in villages of the West Sepik district of New Guinea. Med J Aust 2:751, 1971.

Vreeswijk, J., Leene, W., and Kalsbeek, G. L.: Early interactions of the virus molluscum contagiosum with its host cell. Virus-induced alterations in the basal and suprabasal layers of the epidermis. J Ultrastruct Res 54:37, 1976.

Vreeswijk, J., Leene, W., and Kalsbeek, G. L.: Early host cell-molluscum contagiosum virus interactions. II. Viral interactions with the basal epidermal cells. J Invest Dermatol 69:249, 1977.

Wilkin, J. K.: Molluscum contagiosum venereum in a women's outpatient clinic: A venereally transmitted disease. Am J Obstet Gynecol 128:531, 1977.

243
MYIASIS

ALEXANDER W. PIERCE, JR., M.D.

The order Diptera includes all insects with only one pair of functional wings—flies, gnats, and mosquitoes. Diptera undergo complex metamorphosis and transform from ovum to larva to pupa to the adult insect (imago). Parasitic disease of man and other vertebrates caused by larvae of Diptera (maggots) is termed myiasis.

The typical larva is a cylindrical, headless, legless, segmented, white or gray maggot. The length ranges from 2 to 30 millimeters. The anterior end may be prominently tapered. Larvae respire through two posterior respiratory spiracles that are frequently mistaken for eyes. The morphology of different species and, on occasion, developmental stages of the same species may vary markedly.

A newly hatched larva is termed the first instar. After a period of feeding and growth, the larva molts and discloses a second instar. The number of repetitions of this process varies with the species, but there are usually three developmental stages or instars. The skin of the final instar does not shed but hardens into a dark, protective shell that encloses a nonfeeding semiquiescent pupa. Pupation of all the Diptera that produce myiasis occurs in the soil. Weeks to months later, varying both with the species and the climatic conditions, an adult fly emerges from the pupal case. Most adult females are oviparous, but a few give birth to live larvae.

Obligate parasites feed and develop in nature only in living tissue. They may be host-specific. Incidental parasitism is the invasion of an unusual host by an obligate parasite. The symptoms of the incidental host may differ from those of the usual host because the parasite may fail to complete normal growth and development or may behave in an unusual manner. Facultative parasites feed and develop in dead and decaying organic matter under most circumstances but occasionally infect a living organism. A temporary parasite lives free of its host during part of its existence.

Accidental parasitism refers to infection resulting from the unknowing transfer of an infectious parasite from a previous location. Accidental myiasis is usually the result of the ingestion of food on which oviposition has occurred.

ETIOLOGY. Dipterous species that cause human myiasis may be divided into four groups: (1) obligate myiasis-producing Diptera for which man is a favored host, (2) obligate myiasis-producing Diptera for which man is an incidental host, (3) facultative myiasis-producing Diptera, and (4) accidental myiasis-producing Diptera. Diptera that cause facultative and accidental myiasis are traditionally differentiated, although many species are classified in both groups.

The Diptera listed in Table 1 are obligate parasites for which man may be the host.

The primary screwworm (*Cochliomyia hominivorax*), the Old World screwworm (*Chrysomyia bezziana*), and the larvae of *Wohlfahrtia magnifica* are the most virulent dipterous larvae. The human botfly (*Dermatobia hominis*) and the tumbu fly (*Cordylobia anthropophaga*) account for the majority of human disease caused by Dipterous larvae that are obligatory parasites. Attacks by the Congo floor maggot (*Auchmeromyia luteola*) are not considered true myiasis by many authorities. Man is, however, the only known host for this temporary parasite.

Obligate parasites that may incidentally infect man are listed in Table 2.

Larvae of the *Gasterophilus* spp are gastrointestinal parasites of horses. Cattle and deer are the usual hosts for larvae of the *Hypoderma* species. Larvae of the sheep botfly, *Oestrus ovis*, infect the nasal passages and paranasal sinuses of sheep and goats. *Rhinoestrus purpureus* larvae cause similar infections of horses. *Wohlfahrtia opaca* and *W. vigil* are probably a single species. *W. opaca vigil* larvae usually infect mink and fox pups. The antelope is the primary host for larvae of *C. rodhaini*. Larvae of *Cuterebra* spp infect rodents and lagomorphs.

More than 150 dipterous species have been implicated in facultative myiasis of man. Among the most common are the larvae of *Phormia* spp, *Phoenicia* spp, *Sarcophaga* spp, *Calliphora* sp, and the common house fly, *Musca domestica*. Rarely, deliberate inoculation of a necrotic wound with larvae of a facultative dipterous species has been used to facilitate wound débridement.

Over 50 dipterous species have been reported to cause accidental human gastrointestinal myiasis. The most frequently reported species are the cheese skipper (*Piophila casei*), the rat-tailed maggot (*Eristalis tenax*), and *M. domestica*.

Specific identification of dipterous larvae requires entomologic expertise. Differentiation of the obligate parasites

Table 1. HUMAN OBLIGATORY MYIASIS

Geographic Distribution	Genus/Species	Anatomic Localization
North America and South America	*Cochliomyia hominivorax* (primary screwworm)	Aural, ophthalmic, genitourinary, nasopharyngeal, integumentary
Africa, Asia and Indonesia	*Chrysomyia bezziana* (Old World screwworm)	Aural, ophthalmic, genitourinary, nasopharyngeal, integumentary
Asia, Africa and Europe	*Wohlfahrtia magnifica*	Aural, ophthalmic, genitourinary, nasopharyngeal, integumentary
Central America and South America	*Dermatobia hominis* (human botfly)	Integumentary
Africa	*Cordylobia anthropophaga* (tumbu fly)	Integumentary
Africa	*Auchmeromyia luteola* (Congo floor maggot)	Bloodsucking

Table 2. HUMAN INCIDENTAL MYIASIS

Geographic Distribution	Genus/Species	Anatomic Localization
Worldwide	*Gasterophilus nasalis*	Integumentary
	Gasterophilus intestinalis	Integumentary
	Gasterophilus hemorrhoidalis	Integumentary
Africa	*Cordylobia rodhaini*	Integumentary
North America	*Wohlfahrtia opaca*	Integumentary
	Wohlfahrtia vigil	
Europe, Asia and North America	*Hypoderma lineatum*	Integumentary, ophthalmic
	Hypoderma bovis	
Europe	*Hypoderma diana*	Integumentary, ophthalmic
North America	*Cuterebra buccata*	Integumentary, nasopharyngeal
Europe, Asia, Africa, and Australia	*Oestrus ovis*	Ophthalmic, nasopharyngeal
Europe, Asia, and Africa	*Rhinoestrus purpureus*	Ophthalmic, nasopharyngeal

C. hominivorax and *C. bezziana* from their respective facultative counterparts, *C. macelleria* and *C. megacephala*, has been particularly difficult. Species identification of the first larval instar is not always possible.

PATHOGENESIS AND PATHOLOGY. Screwworm flies oviposit up to several hundred eggs next to minor integumentary lesions such as scratches, insect bites, or abrasions. The ova are glued to adjacent intact skin. Upon hatching, the first instar of the primary screwworm (*C. hominivorax*) enters the break in the integument and actively invades, digests, and liquefies normal tissue. The first larval instar of the Old World screwworm (*C. bezziana*) remains superficial, but the second instar is invasive. The growth rate of these biophagous larvae is remarkable. The primary screwworm increases in size 15-fold in eight days. It is believed that previously infected wounds attract gravid females of the species for further oviposition.

Wohlfahrtia magnifica is larviparous. Larviposition of the 100 to 200 first larval instars is adjacent to minor integumentary lesions of a mammalian host. The first instar is invasive and biophagous.

The human botfly (*D. hominis*) oviposits 15 to 25 ova on the ventral surface of a captured, but unharmed, insect vector, usually a mosquito. The egg hatches in 5 to 15 days, and the first larval instar abandons the chorion while the vector is in contact with a mammalian host. The larva does not penetrate intact skin but may penetrate even minimal lesions such as the bite of the mosquito vector. Once established in the subcutaneous tissue, the larvae do not migrate but live singly in furuncular lesions. Their lifespan averages five to ten weeks but may last up to three months.

The tumbu fly (*C. anthropophaga*) oviposits several hundred ova in the soil, usually in sand contaminated by urine or feces. Oviposition occurs only in shaded places. Larvae hatch in one to three days and remain viable awaiting a host for one to two weeks. When the soil is disturbed, the larvae extend themselves upward from the soil and wave actively, seeking a host. After attachment, the larva penetrates intact skin. These maggots also dwell singly in subcutaneous furuncular lesions. The usual three instars are passed in eight to ten days, whereupon the larva leaves the wound and returns to the soil for pupation.

Gravid *A. luteola* flies oviposit on dry soil or sand in shaded areas, usually in the crevices of huts. The larvae, the Congo floor maggots, live in crevices and emerge at night to attach to a human host by means of powerful mouth hooks. The maggot sucks blood for 15 to 20 minutes, then detaches and returns to its hiding place, returning to the host the following evening. Sleep disturbances with heavy infestations are the sole symptoms caused by this sanguinivorous, temporary parasite. Moreover, it is not known to be the vector for any other infectious agent.

Dipterous species whose larvae fail to grow and develop as incidental parasites in man include *Gasterophilus* spp, *O. ovis*, *R. purpureus*, and probably the *Cuterebra* species. *Gasterophilus* species, *O. ovis*, and *R. purpureus* larvae fail to develop beyond the first instar in man. *Hypoderma* spp may achieve normal larval development in humans, but the extended subcutaneous wandering of the parasite is not comparable to the highly directed migration that occurs in the preferred bovine host. Human infection by *W. opaca vigil*, *C. rodhaini*, and the *Cuterebra* spp. is rare.

Oviposition on a living host by Diptera species that are facultative parasites is generally on diseased, frequently necrotic, exposed, and neglected tissues. Similarly, a fetid discharge from a body orifice, such as the ear, urethra, or vagina, or the external accumulation of body excrement perianally in a neglected and debilitated elderly individual may invite oviposition by facultative Diptera species.

CLINICAL MANIFESTATIONS. Symptoms and signs of myiasis are related to the infected organ or tissue. Classifications of myiasis based on organ system involvement are more useful clinically than those based on the identity of the infecting parasite. The most commonly involved organ is the skin. Integumentary myiasis may be either furuncular or a creeping eruption.

Furuncular myiasis is characterized by one or more erythematous nodules, each with one or more ulcers (Fig. 1). Visualization of single or multiple motile larvae is diagnostic and easily achieved by careful inspection. There is usually a serous or purulent discharge from the ulcer. The discharge may be stained with blood or larval feces. A single large furuncle with several ulcers and containing numerous larvae is characteristic of infections by the screwworms or larvae of *W. magnifica*. Infection by tumbu fly larvae is manifested by multiple furuncles, each with a single maggot. One to three furuncles of long duration, each with a single maggot, are characteristic of *D. hominis* infection. *Wohlfahrtia opaca vigil* infections usually present with 5 to 15 pustulofuruncular lesions of 1 to 5 mm on the neck, upper trunk, or arms of an infant. Each furuncle contains one to four larvae.

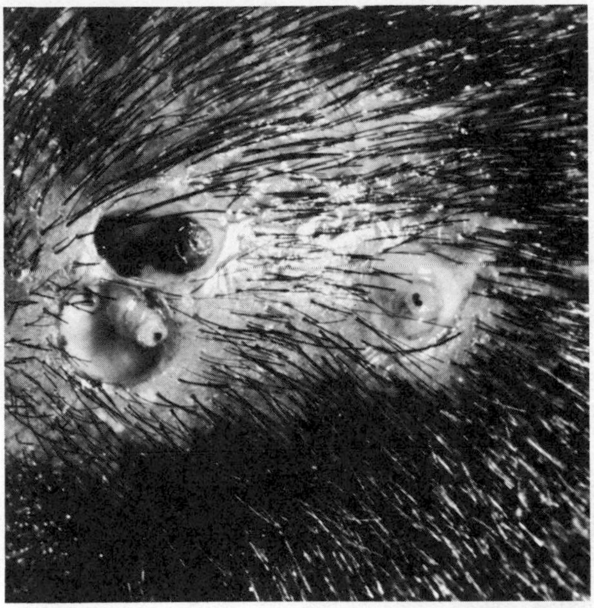

Figure 1. Furuncular myiasis of the scalp. The parasite is *Cochliomyia hominivorax.*

In man, infection by larvae of *Gasterophilus* spp produces a creeping eruption. The lesions are visible, palpable, serpiginous, intradermal tracts. The larva is found distal to the more prominent end of the tract. The lesion will be single and pruritic. By contrast, the lesions of cutaneous larva migrans due to the dog and cat hookworm, *Ancylostoma braziliense,* are multiple and on skin surfaces that have been in contact with the soil.

Larvae of *Hypoderma* spp produce furuncular myiasis in cattle and deer after extensive migration through tissue. The furuncles in cattle are known as warbles. In man, the maggot migrates in the subcutaneous tissue over extensive distances, frequently disappearing and re-emerging at a distant site. The general direction of the larval migration is cephalad. The subcutaneous tracts are not sharply demarcated. They may be tender at the site of the most recent migration and become increasingly tender and inflamed as furuncles form. Several furuncles at several sites may form and resolve before the definitive surface furuncle with ulcer formation develops. The definitive warble is usually on the shoulder, neck, or head and may be associated with diffuse edema.

Nasopharyngeal myiasis may be fatal. Infection usually occurs in debilitated patients with antecedent nasopharyngeal disease. The screwworms and the larvae of *W. magnifica* produce extensive tissue destruction that may involve the paranasal sinuses. The palate or nasal septum may be perforated. There may be extension into the eye or through the calvarium into the central nervous system. Manifestations include a malodorous, serosanguineous, or purulent nasal discharge, nasal obstruction, pain, and the sensation of "something moving." Less destructive nasopharyngeal lesions are produced by the incidental parasites *O. ovis* and *R. purpureus.*

These same maggots, *O. ovis* (the sheep botfly) and *R. purpureus* (the equine head maggot), may be found in ophthalmomyiasis. External ophthalmic involvement with conjunctivitis is usual, but the first larval instar has been found in both the anterior and posterior chambers of the eye in association with uveitis. *Cuterebra* species may also be found in either the anterior or posterior chamber and may produce multiple linear and arcuate subretinal tracts. These tracts are believed to be diagnostic by virtue of their extent, size, and circuity even in the absence of a visible larva. Rarely, the larva of *Hypoderma* spp migrates into the orbit and produces extensive ocular damage.

Aural myiasis usually occurs in the presence of preexisting diseases of the external ear. *Phoenicia* species have been recovered from the external ear, however, in the absence of known antecedent pathology. Pain and noise are the major manifestations of myiasis of the external auditory canal. The larva of *Hypoderma* spp may produce extensive middle ear damage in the course of its wandering. The screwworms and *W. magnifica* may invade the middle ear directly or extend into the middle ear from the paranasal sinuses.

Symptoms of urinary myiasis may include abdominal pain, dysuria, frequency, urgency, gross hematuria, priapism, and spontaneous ejaculation. The ejaculate may contain larvae. Urethral obstruction may occur. There is usually antecedent urogenital disease. It is hypothesized that oviposition occurs at the urethral meatus, and the first larval instar migrates into the posterior urethra or bladder. The larvae are usually facultative parasites, and these infections generally remit spontaneously when the maggots are passed.

Larvae of facultative Diptera organisms may be found in excrement, leading to confusion about their origin. Oviposition in excrement after its passage is far more common than infection of the gastrointestinal tract. Most ova deposited in food do not survive passage through the gastrointestinal tract. Classification of this benign infestation as myiasis is controversial. It has therefore been called pseudomyiasis. Symptoms attributed to enteric myiasis include malaise, pallor, abdominal pain, diarrhea, hematochezia, vomiting, and anorexia.

COMPLICATIONS AND SEQUELAE. Most infections by dipterous larvae result in uncomplicated cutaneous myiasis. "Ver du Cayor," furuncular myiasis due to tumbu fly larvae, may leave persistent, pigmented scars. *Hypoderma* species may invade the spinal canal with resulting paresis. Inflammation, edema, and suppuration may be manifestations of the larval infection and do not necessarily require antimicrobial therapy. Rarely, isolated granulomatous lesions of viscera have been attributed to dipterous larvae. A larva of *Gasterophilus* sp has been found in a pulmonary coin lesion, and a *Hypoderma* sp has been demonstrated in a hepatic granuloma.

GEOGRAPHIC VARIATIONS. Although myiasis due to certain dipterous larvae is endemic to specific geographic regions, and case clusters of human myiasis may be seen in association with epizootics in domestic animals, human myiasis is usually seen as isolated cases. The geographic distribution of the Diptera species for which myiasis is obligatory is shown in Tables 1 and 2. Case importation has been repeatedly documented, however. Instances of infection by both *D. hominis* and *C. anthropophaga* have been documented on the North American continent. Climatic conditions have a major influence on pupation, and many species such as the primary screwworm will not maintain sustained colonization outside a subtropical climate.

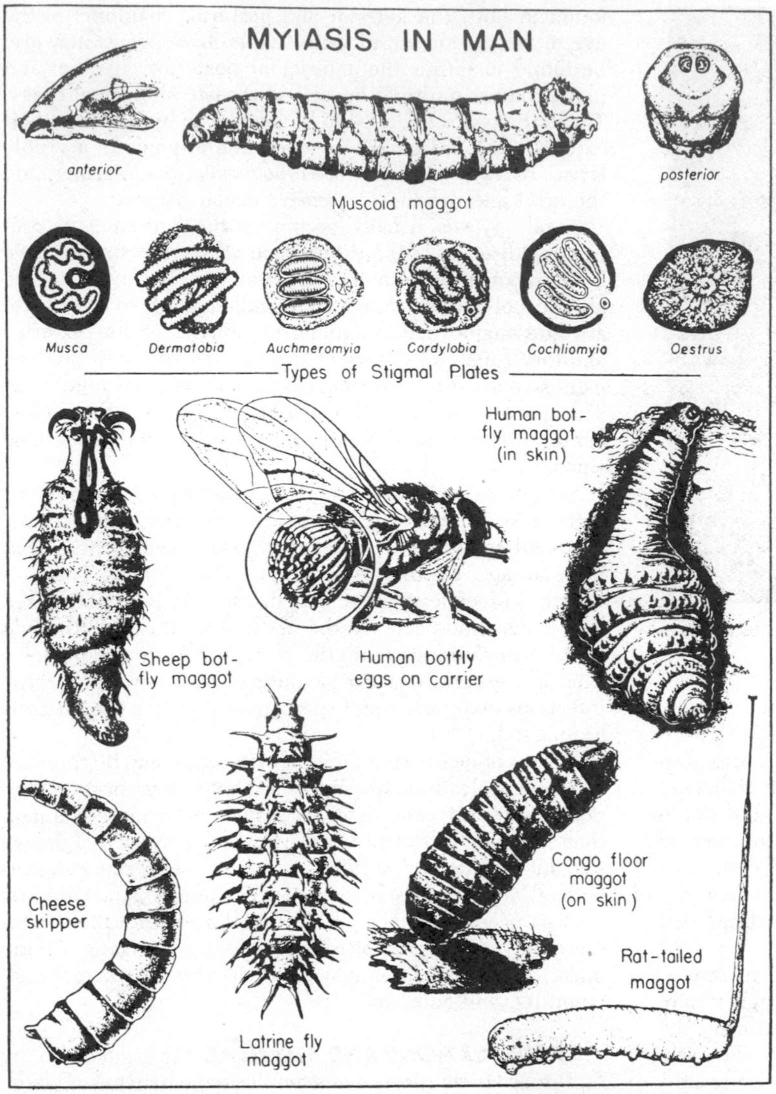

Figure 2. Agents of human myiasis. (From Newson, H. D.: Order Diptera. *In* Hunter, G. W., Swartzwelder, J. C., and Clyder, D. F. (eds.): *Tropical Medicine.* 5th Ed. Philadelphia, W. B. Saunders Company, 1976.)

DIAGNOSIS. Diagnosis requires the demonstration of dipterous larvae in tissue or wounds. Preservation of maggots for entomologic identification is important and can be achieved by placing specimens in a solution of 70 to 80 per cent alcohol. If an antiseptic has been applied to the wound, the specimens should be rinsed in saline before suspension in alcohol. Figure 2 illustrates some of the maggots that are common causes of human myiasis. Saprophytic species may be reared on blood agar plates at 30° C, but obligate dipterous larvae require specialized rearing techniques. In the United States, an entomologic identification service is provided by the Department of Agriculture, Animal and Plant Health Inspection Service, Post Office Box 969, Mission, Texas 78572.

TREATMENT. Removal of the maggots is curative. This is usually easily accomplished by saline irrigation and extraction with forceps. Large furuncles with multiple larvae produced by obligate parasites such as the screwworms or larvae of *W. magnifica* may require surgical enlargement of an ulcer under local anesthesia to achieve complete removal of all the maggots. The local application of oils, paraffin, chloroform, or ether to interfere with larval respiration will produce increased larval activity and migration to the surface. Extensive surgical débridement may be required for nasopharyngeal myiasis. Antimicrobial therapy should be employed for culturally documented secondary bacterial infections.

PROPHYLAXIS. Good personal and environmental hygiene is the most effective prophylaxis. These measures include appropriate disposal of human and animal excreta and screening of homes and public buildings. Endemic or epidemic outbreaks may require spraying with chlorinated hydrocarbons to control the adult fly and veterinary care for domestic animals. Prompt, appropriate therapy for pyoderma or pediculosis capitis will eliminate potential sites of oviposition.

The Screwworm Eradication Program of the United States Department of Agriculture has resulted in eradication of the primary screwworm from the southern United States. The last self-sustaining colonies in the continental United States were eliminated by 1966. This eradication program consists of aerial release of irradiated pupae from which infertile flies emerge. Because the female *C. hominivorax* mates but once, the reproductive cycle is interrupted. A barrier aerial release zone is maintained along the border of the United States with Mexico. A new barrier zone is being established across the Tehuantepec isthmus in southern Mexico. Eradication of the primary screwworm from northern Mexico is now under way.

References

James, M. T.: The Flies That Cause Myiasis in Man. U.S. Department of Agriculture, Miscellaneous Publication No. 631. Washington, D.C., U.S. Government Printing Office, 1948.

Harwood, R. F., and James, M. T.: Entomology in Human and Animal Health. 7th ed. New York, Macmillan Publishing Co., Inc., 1979.

Newsom, H. D.: Order Diptera. In Hunter, Swartzwelder, and Clyde (eds.): Tropical Medicine. 5th ed. Philadelphia, W. B. Saunders Company, 1976.

Zumpt, F.: Myiasis in Man and Animals of the Old World. London, Butterworths, 1965.

H. OCULAR INFECTIONS

244

OCULAR BACTERIAL INFECTIONS

PERRY S. BINDER, M.D., F.A.C.S.

INTRODUCTION

The hallmark of an ocular infection is a red eye. The location of the erythema usually occurs near the infected structure. For instance, the eyelid margins are red in cases of blepharitis; the conjunctiva are injected in bacterial and viral conjunctivitis; and the deep blood vessels adjacent to the cornea and sclera are dilated (ciliary flush) in cases of iritis. Erythema of all ocular structures suggests a severe infection of the entire globe and orbit, such as panophthalmitis (abscess of the globe). The presence of edema, in addition to erythema, suggests severe or advanced infection or inflammation. An ocular discharge is not normal, and its character indicates the type of disease that caused it. For example, the discharge is watery in allergies, serosanguineous in severe viral conjunctivitis, and purulent in bacterial infections.

The first symptoms of an ocular infection are a mild sensation of a foreign body, tearing, and sensitivity to sunlight. More advanced infection causes pain and decreased vision. The sensation of a foreign body is common in patients with any type of mild conjunctivitis, and any source of irritation to the fifth nerve reflexly stimulates the lacrimal gland and causes tearing.

Sensitivity to light is usually produced by a corneal abnormality, or an intraocular inflammation or infection that affects the pigmented tissues of the eye. Decreased vision is a very serious sign of advanced infection and is usually associated with an opacity in the path of light from the cornea to the retina, such as a corneal abscess or severe intraocular inflammation that clouds the vitreous.

A careful history is important in the evaluation of a patient with a red eye. Factors that predispose to infection include recent or previous trauma, previous infections, contacts with family members or friends who have acute red eyes, diabetes mellitus, malnutrition, and diseases or drugs that diminish cell-mediated immunity. The use of ocular medications and their frequency of administration must be determined because they can produce toxic and/or allergic changes. Unlabeled bottles with red tops contain medications that dilate the pupil; green-topped bottles contain medications that constrict the pupil. Milky white drops are usually glucocorticoids, and clear drops in clear bottles are usually anesthetics.

The examination of the patient with a red eye must be done carefully in order to avoid contaminating the physician's hands and instruments. Because ocular viral infections are highly contagious, it is important to clean carefully any instruments that may have come in contact with an infected eye before examining another patient. It is best not to touch a patient who you suspect has viral conjunctivitis.

The routine administration of antibiotics, topical glucocorticoids, or topical anesthetics to every patient with a red eye is inappropriate because this treatment does not help the patient and may make his condition worse. For example, steroids aggravate a herpes simplex infection of the cornea, and anesthetics, which are toxic to the cornea, can produce severe sloughing of the entire epithelium, subsequent scarring, and neovascularization. The administration of antibiotics before obtaining cultures of a corneal abscess may hinder later efforts to determine the cause of infection by temporarily suppressing growth.

Most patients with *redness*, a *sudden* change in *vision*, or ocular *pain* (RSVP) should be examined immediately and referred to an ophthalmologist (an M.D.) for evaluation. Referral to an optometrist (a doctor of optometry, who is not an M.D.) who is untrained in the diagnosis and therapy of ocular disease, only delays accurate diagnosis and appropriate therapy.

ORBITAL CELLULITIS

ETIOLOGY AND PATHOGENESIS. Orbital cellulitis is an acute inflammation of the orbital tissues that may threaten the patient's vision or even his life if it is not diagnosed and treated immediately. It may be produced by spread of an infection from either nearby structures or distant foci. In children, ethmoiditis is a common focus of spread to the orbit. In adults, infections of the other sinuses are equally

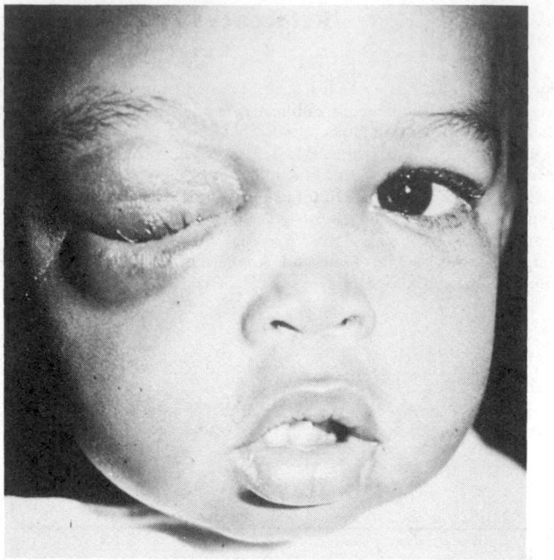

Figure 1. *Haemophilus influenzae* orbital cellulitis in a 2-year-old. The eyelid edema is sharply demarcated by the orbital septum in the upper and lower eyelids.

common foci. Sinus infections spread to the orbit by causing thrombophlebitis of the communicating veins between the orbit and sinuses.

Hemophilus influenzae is the most common cause of orbital cellulitis in children less than 5 years of age. *Staphylococcus aureus*, group A streptococci, and pneumococci are the predominant organisms in adults and also occur in children. When the infection spreads from chronic sinusitis, anaerobic bacteria may be prominent (Frederick and Braude, 1974). Almost any microorganism may be introduced by penetrating trauma or during surgery.

CLINICAL MANIFESTATIONS. The clinical presentation depends upon the location of the infection in the orbit. The infected area displaces the globe in the opposite direction (proptosis). For instance, a superior abscess produces a downward displacement of the globe.

The patient may or may not be systemically ill. There is usually orbital pain and eyelid erythema with edema of the upper lid (Fig. 1). The eye usually protrudes (proptosis), and the lids are usually swollen shut with a discharge that may or may not be purulent. Early in the disease, the cornea and conjunctiva are uninvolved. As the proptosis progresses, however, the cornea can become exposed, ulcerated and perforated, which may lead to panophthalmitis. If the apex of the orbit is affected, the optic nerve and cranial nerves III through VI may be infected. This complication causes optic neuritis with decreased vision and an afferent pupillary defect with decreased extraocular muscle movements (progressive ophthalmoplegia). The extraocular muscle movements become restricted slowly, but with advanced disease, there are no extraocular muscle movements. The pupil becomes fixed and dilated only if the cavernous sinus is involved. Compression and/or infiltration of the optic nerve produces optic neuritis and decreased vision.

The pocket of purulent material may either point or produce fluctuance. When the pus is confined to the episcleral space, there is less eyelid swelling and more conjunctival involvement at the site of the extraocular muscle insertions near the junction of the cornea and sclera (limbus). This causes severe pain when the patient attempts to move the eye.

Some bacteria cause these signs and symptoms over a slower time course. Tuberculous or syphilitic periostitis and granulomas may produce swelling and a hard mass behind the globe either unilaterally or bilaterally. Erythema and pain may or may not be prominent, and most of these patients may be thought to have an orbital tumor. Opportunistic organisms can infect the orbit from a simple external lesion and slowly produce a large external orbital mass before they produce the typical signs and symptoms of acute orbital cellulitis (Fig. 2).

DIAGNOSIS AND THERAPY. It is easy to make a diagnosis when a patient presents with a rapid onset of lid and orbital swelling with erythema of the eyelid, proptosis of the globe, pain in the eye and orbit, and decreased vision. The presence of a pointing abscess or a fluctuant mass in a systemically ill patient is further evidence of orbital infection. The extent of the infection is determined by examining the retina and by measuring the patient's visual acuity, pupillary reaction, corneal sensation, and extraocular muscle movements. Sinus x-rays may confirm disease of an adjacent sinus, and ultrasound can be used to define the extent of the abscess within the orbit.

Blood cultures are usually positive in children with orbital cellulitis caused by *H. influenzae*, but are frequently negative in children and adults when staphylococci, streptococci, pneumococci, or anaerobes have spread from the paranasal sinuses. Since there is usually no external drainage from the orbital infection, and it is usually undesirable to aspirate the orbital abscess, therapy is often directed at the most likely organism. If there is clinical or radiologic evidence of sinusitis, sinus aspiration usually yields the responsible organism. In the absence of definitive bacteriology, children less than 5 years of age are usually treated with I.V. ampicillin at 200 mg per kg per day or chloramphenicol (50 mg per kg per day). A specific antistaphylococcal antibiotic may be added to this regimen. Since *Staphylococcus aureus* is the most common cause of orbital

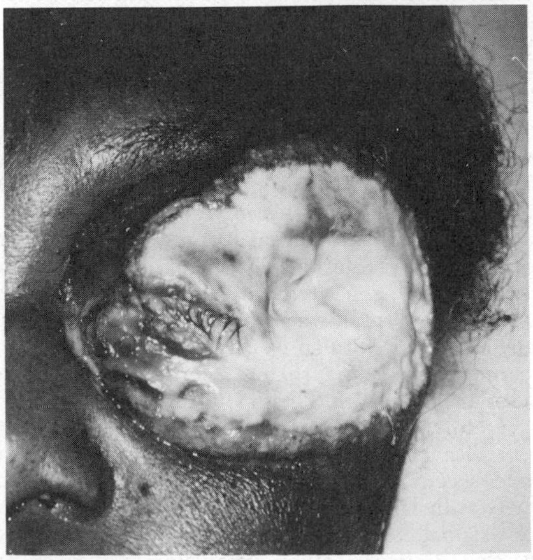

Figure 2. *Pseudomonas* orbital abscesses in a diabetic following a minor injury to the skin of the left upper eyelid.

cellulitis in older children and adults, they are usually treated with a penicillinase-resistant penicillin at 200 mg per kg per day. This treatment is also adequate for pneumococci and group A streptococci.

Surgical decompression of the orbit is necessary only in cases of optic nerve compression and/or progressive exposure of the cornea. Topical hotpacks and daily evaluation of the visual acuity and extraocular muscle movements are important adjuncts to the systemic antibiotics. With appropriate therapy, the signs and symptoms abate rapidly, and the patients are left without sequelae (Gombos, 1973; Trevor-Roper, 1974).

INFECTION OF THE EYELIDS AND OCULAR ADNEXAE (LACRIMAL GLAND, LACRIMAL DUCTS AND LACRIMAL SAC)

DEFINITION AND CLINICAL MANIFESTATIONS. Infection of the eyelids and adnexae produces redness and swelling of the involved structure(s) and ultimate compromise of the particular function (for example, interference with tearing when the tear ducts or lacrimal sac is occluded). Chronic infection produces permanent changes in the structures and may cause permanent loss of function.

The sty, or hordeolum, is an acute staphylococcal abscess of the oil-secreting glands of the eyelids. It may occur on the inner lid (internal hordeolum) when the meibomian glands are involved and on the outer surface of the lid (external hordeolum—Fig. 3) when the glands of Zeiss and Moll are infected. The patient develops acute localized swelling of the lid with pain and erythema. In time, the abscess may point through the skin of the lid. The conjunctiva and remainder of the eye are usually uninvolved. Extension of the infection into the entire eyelid produces a lid abscess (Fig. 4).

A chalazion is a sterile granulomatous inflammation of the meibomian glands. It may or may not follow a hordeolum, but many patients with chalazia have a history of previous episodes of acute inflammation. The lesion develops slowly, and patients may only notice a "lump" in their eyelids. Chalazia seldom subside spontaneously. If chalazia become large enough to induce abnormal curvatures in the cornea, they can cause visual symptoms.

Chronic low-grade infection of the oil-secreting glands by *Staphylococcus aureus* and/or *Staphylococcus epidermidis* (blepharitis) is another common disease of the eyelid. This infection produces a vascularized and erythematous lid margin with scale formation, loss of lashes, production of white lashes, misdirection of lashes, and deposits around the base of the eyelashes (collarettes—Fig. 5). Staphylococcal exotoxins erode the superficial corneal epithelium, and the bacteria metabolize the oil to nonesterified free fatty acids, which destabilize the tear film and add to the disruption of the corneal epithelium. These patients may develop a punctate pattern of erosions on the inferior cornea, ulceration of the cornea at the junction of the cornea and sclera (limbus), or other acute inflammatory lesions of the cornea with neovascularization (phlyctenulosis) (Smolin and Okumoto, 1977).

The corneal debris seen at the base of the lashes may also consist of greasy scales from coexistent seborrheic dermatitis. The conjunctiva is often mildly injected. Staphylococcal blepharitis is common in patients with atopic dermatitis and in the immunologically suppressed. A previous history of hordeola and chalazia is common. The destruction of the tear film produces a dry, gritty feeling, and the patients may sometimes complain of a foreign body

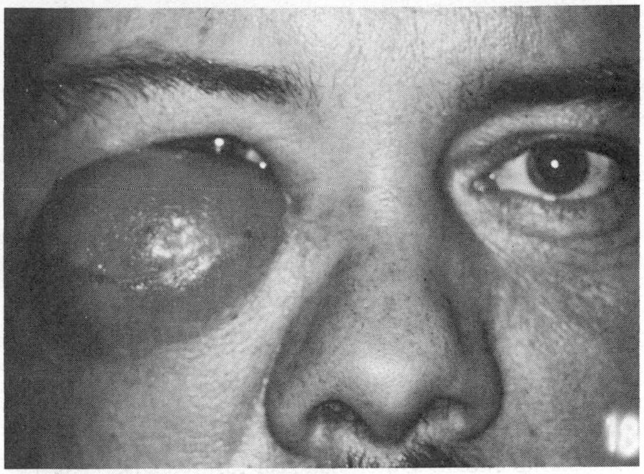

Figure 4. Pneumococcal eyelid abscess following repair of a blow-out fracture. The infection is limited by the orbital septum. The old incision was reopened, and a drain was placed in the wound after removal of 15 ml of pus.

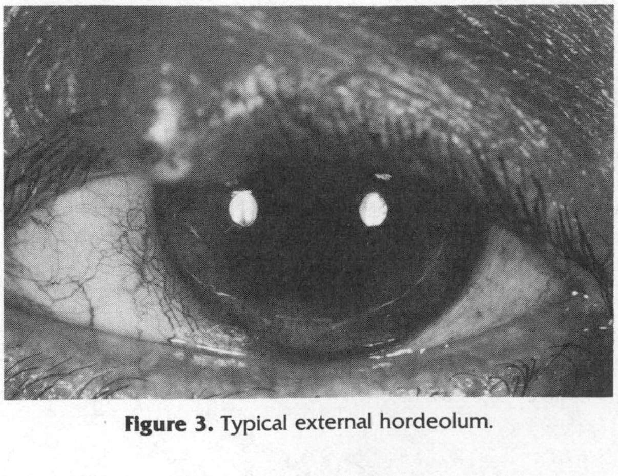

Figure 3. Typical external hordeolum.

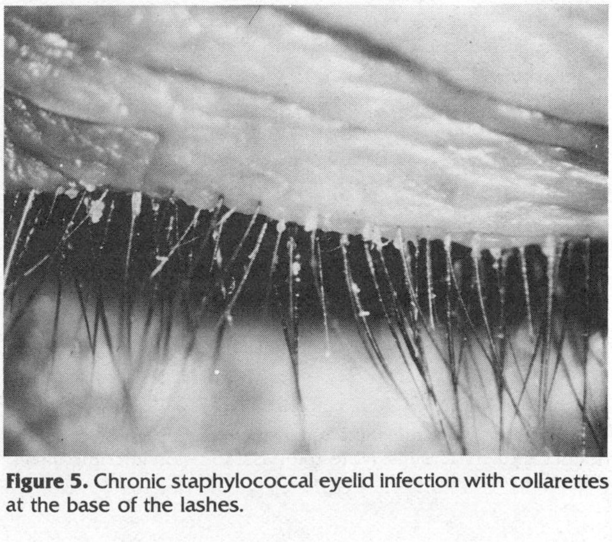

Figure 5. Chronic staphylococcal eyelid infection with collarettes at the base of the lashes.

in the eye. Scarring of the eyelids may cause the lashes to rub on the cornea and produce corneal scarring. These patients may complain of photophobia from the abnormalities in their corneal epithelium. Other common presenting complaints include burning, itching, and red eyelid margins. Chronic, untreated blepharitis may cause inferior corneal scarring and loss of vision. When the area of erythema is fixed in the corners of the eye and spares the central lids (angular blepharitis), either staphylococci or *Moraxella* may be responsible for the infection.

Infection of the lacrimal ducts (canaliculitis) usually produces a unilateral red eye. There is localized redness and swelling in the area in which the duct opens into the eyelid (punctum), and granular material can usually be expressed from the duct. If the infection is untreated, purulent conjunctivitis may result. Fungi or *Actinomyces* usually cause this infection. Other bacteria rarely cause canaliculitis.

Dacryoadenitis is a rare unilateral infection of the lacrimal gland that occurs in children as a complication of mumps, measles, or influenza and in adults as a complication of gonococcal bacteremia. Other purulent infections of the lacrimal gland may follow penetrating injuries to the eyelid. Patients develop pain, swelling, and redness in the upper outer quadrant of the orbit in which the lacrimal gland is located.

When the duct from the lacrimal sac becomes occluded, usually near its opening into the nose, stagnation in the sac promotes infection. Most cases are unilateral. Patients complain of tearing (from lacrimal duct obstruction), redness, swelling, and tenderness over the area of the tear sac that is adjacent to the nose below the junction of the upper and lower lids (Fig. 6).

Pressure over the sac usually expresses purulent material from the ducts. The most common offending organisms are *Staphylococcus aureus*, *Streptococcus pneumoniae*, or *Hemophilus influenzae*, although almost any organism may infect the sac. In severe cases, the abscess may point through the skin or a fistula may develop. In contrast to canaliculitis, concomitant unilateral conjunctivitis is uncommon.

DIAGNOSIS AND TREATMENT. All of these infections of the eyelid and ocular adnexae are treated as localized abscesses. The infected area is drained by massage or surgery; heat is applied; and topical or systemic antibiotics are given.

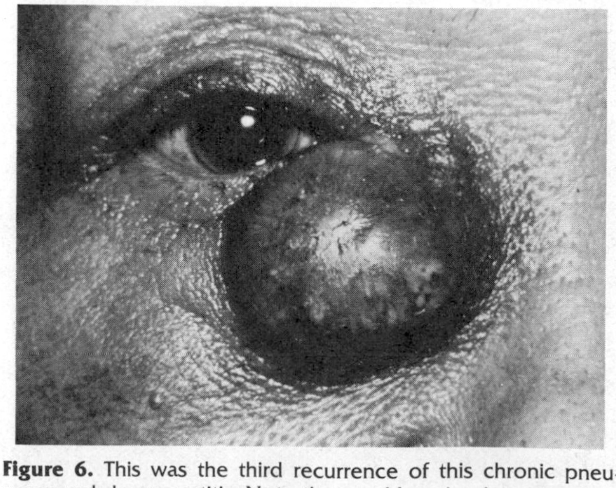

Figure 6. This was the third recurrence of this chronic pneumococcal dacryocystitis. Note the nasal location in comparison with the eyelid abscess in Figure 4.

Topical heat and instillation of antibiotic drops (10 per cent sulfacetamide or 0.5 per cent chloromycetin) for a minimum of six times a day is recommended for acute hordeolum. If the lesion points, incision and drainage promote rapid healing. Chalazia do not respond to this treatment, and excision is recommended for cosmetic purposes.

Treatment of staphylococcal blepharitis is designed to decrease the number of organisms, promote healing of the corneal epithelium, and restabilize the tear film. Patients are instructed to "scrub" the eyelid margins at the base of the lashes daily with a cotton-tipped applicator moistened in dilute baby shampoo. This treatment promotes drainage from the stagnant oil glands and cleans the lid margin. Topical antibiotic drops (10 per cent sulfacetamide or tetracycline) should be instilled at a minimum of six to eight times per day initially, and antibiotic ointments (erythromycin or bacitracin) should be applied to the base of the lashes four times a day with a cotton-tipped applicator. Artificial tears should be applied frequently to smooth out the tear film.

In severe, recurrent cases, oral dicloxacillin (500 mg four times daily) may be added to the treatment schedule, but the major cause of treatment failure is noncompliance with or incorrect use of the eyelid scrubs.

Cultures of hordeola and blepharitis are usually not necessary because the diagnosis is obvious, and they are always caused by *S. aureus*. If a culture is taken, a broth-moistened, cotton-tipped applicator should be rubbed gently to and fro across the base of the lashes after the lids have been compressed between two applicators to express material from the meibomian glands.

Infection of the lacrimal ducts is controlled by removal of the organism by expression, irrigation of the ducts with an antibiotic (Gantrisin), application of topical heat, and frequent instillation of topical antibiotics (sulfacetamide or chloromycetin). If *Actinomyces* is isolated, tetracycline (500 mg orally every eight hours until two weeks after clinical cure) may be necessary but does not replace irrigation to keep the canaliculi patent.

Infections of the lacrimal sac (dacryocystitis) cannot be cured until the obstruction in the nasal lacrimal duct is relieved. If the duct fails to open by repeated digital pressure on the lacrimal sac, the nasal lacrimal system should be probed. Infection of the sac is treated with topical and systemic antibiotics chosen on the basis of cultures and sensitivities, irrigation with antibiotics, and hot packs. Pointing lesions should be incised and drained. If the nasal lacrimal duct cannot be unobstructed, a new opening into the nose is produced surgically (dacryocystorhinostomy). The site of obstruction in chronic recurrent cases can be determined clinically by staining the tear film with fluorescein or radiographically by injecting radiopaque dyes into the lacrimal duct system (dacryocystography). Applying a radioactive tracer to the tear film and following its path is another technique that has been used to locate obstruction.

Purulent dacryoadenitis is treated with heat and topical and systemic antibiotics chosen according to the cultures of the red eye or penetrating wound. Diagnostic biopsy of the chronically infected, swollen lacrimal gland is seldom necessary.

CONJUNCTIVITIS

ETIOLOGY. The normal conjunctival flora consists of *S. epidermidis*, *S. aureus*, diphtheroids, some gram-negative rods, a few other aerobic organisms (Locatcher-Khorazo and Seegal, 1972), and two major anaerobes (*Propionibacterium acnes* and *Peptostreptococcus* species) (Perkins et al., 1975). The conjunctival sac is difficult to sterilize because of easy contamination from the eyelid margins. Positive cultures can be obtained from 80 to 95 per cent of normal eyes when a cotton swab moistened in a broth medium is rubbed gently back and forth across the conjunctival sac without contamination from the eyelid margins. Fungi can be cultured from 2 to 22 per cent of normal patients, and viruses from 1 per cent of conjunctival cultures (Table 1).

Most ophthalmologists have regarded "conjunctivitis" as a mild, self-limited disease and until recently have felt that the etiology of conjunctivitis could be established by clinical signs and symptoms supported by Gram and Giemsa smears of the conjunctiva and cultures of the conjunctival sac. Unfortunately, the same aerobic organisms are found in cultures of the normal and infected conjunctival sac. There is no increase in aerobic bacteria during bacterial conjunctivitis (Leibowitz et al., 1976). However, there is some new evidence that anaerobic organisms may play a role in the etiology of conjunctivitis (Perkins et al., 1975).

CLINICAL MANIFESTATIONS AND DIAGNOSIS. A patient with conjunctivitis has a red eye. Conjunctivitis is an extremely common disease and may present unilaterally or bilaterally. The patient may awaken with matter on the lid margins, and the lids may be "stuck together." The conjunctiva is injected in all areas but is usually not as severely injected adjacent to the junction between the cornea and sclera (limbus). The conjunctiva on the surface of the eyelids (palpebral conjunctiva) and on the surface of the eyeball (bulbar conjunctiva) is usually affected. The application of one drop of 2.5 per cent phenylephrine usually clears this infection temporarily, whereas a red eye caused by glaucoma or iritis is unaffected by this agent.

Tearing is a nonspecific response to inflammation and is not diagnostic. The discharge in conjunctivitis ranges from minimal and serous to profuse and purulent. This profuse, purulent discharge is diagnostic only in *Neisseria* infections (*Neisseria gonorrhoeae* or *Neisseria meningitidis*), where it is extremely thick and appears to pour out between the eyelids (Fig. 7). Purulent conjunctivitis in a newborn child can be caused by *Neisseria*, almost any other bacterium, chemicals such as silver nitrate, and *Chlamydia* (inclusion blenorrhea). A purulent discharge in a newborn should be considered to be gonorrhea until proved otherwise because this organism can produce blindness in a very short time. In most cases of bacterial conjunctivitis, however, the discharge can be of any type. It may also vary in severity and change in quality during the course of the disease from serous to purulent.

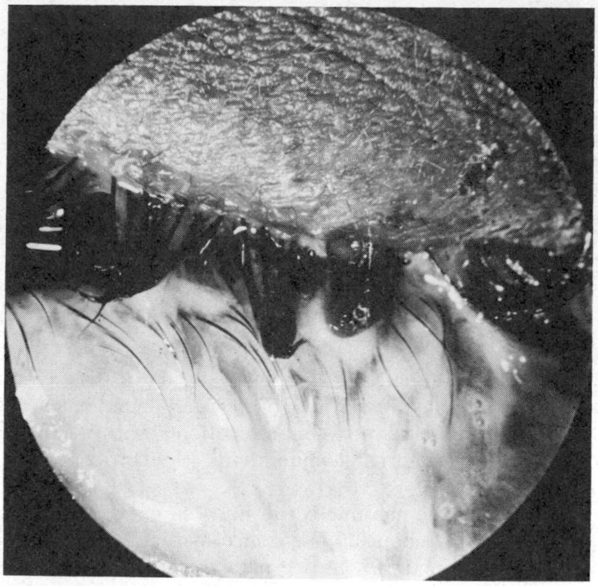

Figure 7. Purulent gonococcal conjunctivitis. The pus is so profuse that it will return within minutes of irrigation.

Table 1. NORMAL CONJUNCTIVAL FLORA

Aerobic Bacteria	Anaerobic Bacteria
Staphylococcus epidermidis	*Propionibacterium acnes*
Staphylococcus aureus	*Peptostreptococcus* species
Corynebacterium species	*Lactobacillus* species
Micrococcus species	*Clostridium* species
Streptococcus species	*Eubacterium* species
Gram-negative rods	
Streptococcus pneumoniae	**Fungi**
Bacillus species	*Candida* species
	Aspergillus species
Viruses	*Rhodotorula* species
Adenoviruses	

The presence of conjunctival membranes (not mucus), which can be removed and peeled off the conjunctival surface, suggests a diagnosis of diphtheria. Immediate therapy is indicated because this organism can penetrate the intact epithelium and produce blindness within hours (Chandler and Milam, 1978).

A palpable preauricular node is most commonly found in viral infections but occasionally occurs in bacterial disease. Its presence during purulent conjunctivitis suggests severe infections such as tularemia, glanders, and granulomatous diseases. Most cases of bacterial conjunctivitis do not cause systemic symptoms or affect the peripheral white count.

Patients complain of mild discomfort or a feeling of "something in the eye." They are usually comfortable, and few are sensitive to the sunlight or a flashlight. The visual acuity and intraocular pressures are normal. Patients complain of itching and burning, but ocular itching is more commonly associated with allergy. The presence of blood beneath the conjunctiva is rare in bacterial conjunctivitis. It is more commonly associated with severe viral conjunctivitis, especially adenovirus infection. The bacterial causes of subconjunctival hemorrhage are the pneumococcus, *Hemophilus*, or Koch-Weeks bacillus (*"H. aegyptius"*). Eyelid disease such as blepharitis or disease of the lacrimal ducts can produce a concomitant conjunctivitis and should be sought in patients with unilateral conjunctivitis.

The diagnosis of a bacterial conjunctivitis can be made clinically in the presence of the appropriate signs and symptoms (Table 2). A Giemsa smear of the conjunctival sac shows a predominance of polymorphonuclear leukocytes in only about 50 per cent of patients with a clinical diagnosis

Table 2. SIGNS AND SYMPTOMS OF BACTERIAL CONJUNCTIVITIS

Signs	Symptoms
Preauricular node	Burning
Purulent discharge	Itching
Matted eyelashes	Pain
Conjunctival injection	Foreign body sensation
Eyelid disease	Photophobia
Subconjunctival hemorrhage	Tearing

of bacterial conjunctivitis (Leibowitz et al., 1976a). Gram stains are even less rewarding; bacteria are found in smears from only about 12 per cent of patients with a clinical diagnosis of bacterial conjunctivitis (Leibowitz et al., 1976a).

Cultures of the conjunctiva in injected eyes also have a poor yield; only about 30 per cent of patients with clinical bacterial conjunctivitis harbor pathogenic organisms, and more than 50 per cent of patients with a clinical diagnosis of viral conjunctivitis harbor the same organisms (Leibowitz et al., 1976a). These results, coupled with the expense of the diagnostic tests, have discouraged their use in the routine diagnosis of conjunctivitis. The poor correlation between the clinical and laboratory diagnoses of bacterial (and viral) conjunctivitis should make us less dogmatic about the clinical manifestations that we have considered to be specific for a given type of conjunctivitis.

THERAPY. The time-honored treatment of conjunctivitis has been the instillation of topical antibiotic drops four times a day. The reason this regimen was chosen is not clear because there is good evidence that this frequency of medication does nothing to the normal conjunctival flora (Binder et al., 1975; Binder and Worthen, 1976; Leibowitz et al., 1976b). In fact, it is almost impossible to sterilize the conjunctival sac under ideal conditions, and the normal flora return after topical therapy is discontinued.

While it is clear that this regimen of antibiotic drops decreases the signs and symptoms of conjunctivitis when compared with placebo artificial tears, it is not clear why topical steroids or a steroid in combination with an antibiotic are even better at decreasing the signs and symptoms of conjunctivitis (Leibowitz et al., 1976b). In spite of these findings, steroids should never be used in the routine treatment of "conjunctivitis" because they predispose patients to cataracts and glaucoma and potentiate infections of the cornea with herpes simplex virus.

The recommended treatment of conjunctivitis (bacterial or viral) is the application of topical antibiotic drops at least six times a day because four times per day has no effect on the conjunctival flora (Binder et al., 1975; Binder and Worthen, 1976). The application of a hot pack over the closed eyelids after the use of eye drops makes the patient more comfortable but usually does not affect the course of the disease. An antibiotic that is not allergenic or toxic is the best choice, and most ophthalmologists recommend chloramphenicol or sulfacetamide as the drug of first choice. Neomycin-containing drops are highly allergenic, and like other aminoglycosides such as gentamicin are toxic to the epithelium of the cornea when used frequently.

The drops are continued for about 48 hours after signs and symptoms are gone. If a patient has not improved after 48 hours and has been using the drops appropriately, it is possible there is an underlying problem such as infection of the lacrimal system, the eyelid, or the cornea. Alternatively, the original diagnosis of conjunctivitis may have been incorrect, and the patient may have iritis or glaucoma. The most likely cause of conjunctivitis persisting beyond 48 hours of proper therapy is an adenovirus infection that may last two to three weeks. In case of doubt, it is best to refer the patient to an ophthalmologist.

Gonococcal conjunctivitis must be treated immediately. All patients should be hospitalized, and the purulent drainage cultured on Thayer-Martin media and chocolate agar. Topical penicillin G drops, prepared by diluting the parenteral preparation to 10,000 units per ml, should be instilled hourly. Hourly 30 per cent sulfacetamide may be substituted. Systemic penicillin (see Chapter 161), topical atropine, and very frequent irrigation of the eyes are also mandatory.

BACTERIAL CORNEAL ULCERS

ETIOLOGY. The normal eye has very effective defenses against infection. The eyelids and lashes prevent foreign debris from striking the eye. The lashes wash the tears across the cornea and cleanse the eyes. Tears also contain secretory immunoglobulins and lysozymes that help prevent infection. The corneal epithelium and the underlying strong band of collagenous tissue (Bowman's layer) act as strong barriers to infection and injury by foreign bodies. The eye becomes susceptible to infection only when these defense mechanisms are altered.

Most bacterial ulcers occur after trauma to the cornea disrupts the epithelium. A mild injury such as a fingernail scratch or a glancing blow from a tree branch or a moderately severe injury such as a foreign body can disrupt the epithelium of the cornea, which permits bacterial colonization. In most instances of mild trauma, the eye heals without complications, but this type of mild trauma may proceed to frank abscess formation in a few cases.

In the presence of predisposing factors such as concomitant eyelid infection (blepharitis or dacryocystitis), decreased corneal sensation due to a fifth nerve lesion (neurotrophic keratitis), or decreased tear film (keratoconjunctivitis sicca), even very mild trauma can produce ulceration.

Contaminated ocular solutions, contaminated makeup (Wilson and Ahern, 1977), or contaminated soft or hard contact lenses also promote the progression of an ulcerative process (Krachmer and Purcell, 1978). Topical anesthetics or steroids severely increase the risk of infection and should not be prescribed. Only those organisms capable of epithelial colonization and penetration can produce spontaneous infections (*Neisseria gonorrhoeae*, *Corynebacterium diphtheria*, and Koch-Weeks bacillus).

PATHOGENESIS, CLINICAL MANIFESTATIONS, AND DIAGNOSIS. Once the organisms penetrate the corneal stroma, they can proliferate freely. They may spread either into superficial areas or into the deep stroma. In the past, ophthalmologists attempted to identify the infecting organism by the morphology of the corneal abscess and the location of the abscess. It is true that some bacteria such as the pneumococcus and *Pseudomonas* produce fairly typical ulcerations, but the accepted and superior practice is to scrape and culture the abscesses in order to obtain a definitive diagnosis. Too much emphasis has been placed on the clinical morphology of the abscess.

All corneal ulcer cases must be cultured, and most should be admitted to the hospital. Neurotrophic keratitis, herpes simplex keratitis, and corneal transplant rejections can present with findings similar to bacterial corneal abscesses. It is very important to make the correct diagnosis because these diseases require different therapy.

Injury to the cornea causes the sensation of a foreign body because the corneal nerves are exposed. An interruption of the normally smooth optical surface also produces a dispersion of light rays with the production of glare and photosensitivity. Any infection in the cornea is usually associated with pain and internal ocular inflammation (iritis). An inflamed iris and ciliary body produce severe pain when they are moved, as occurs when light is shined into the eye. Increased opacity in the corneal stroma also decreases vision. In summary, patients with corneal ulcers experience pain, the sensation of a foreign body, photophobia, and decreased vision.

The hallmark of bacterial corneal ulceration is pus. The stroma, which is normally crystal clear, becomes opaque and the surface irregular. An overlying epithelial defect is almost always present. The underlying stroma becomes soft and mushy and is often discolored to a white, yellow, or brown color (Fig. 8). The stromal abscess may be single or interconnected with other smaller abscesses. The ulcer is usually located near the center of the cornea. A similar abscess in the periphery of the cornea is usually associated with a specific organism such as *Staphylococcus aureus*, *Hemophilus aegyptius*, or *Moraxella lacunata*, but cultures and scrapings must always be performed.

Bacterial ulceration produces pus on the surface of the cornea, the conjunctiva, and the lid margins, which causes matted eyelashes (Fig. 9). As the corneal abscess enlarges, the cornea swells and becomes opaque in areas adjacent to the ulcerative process, and folds are produced in the back layer of the cornea (Descemet's membrane) that appear as white lines.

Increased ocular inflammation produces pus in the anterior chamber (hypopyon), which appears as a yellow to white layer in the inferior part of the anterior chamber (Fig. 10). This severe intraocular inflammation causes constriction of the pupil (miosis), which fails to dilate even in a dark room. With advanced infection, the lens may become opaque (cataract), the entire eye may become infected, or the cornea may perforate. The conjunctiva is always severely injected and is usually edematous. The lids are red and may be swollen. All of these signs depend on the duration of the infection, the pathogenicity of the organism, previous antibiotic therapy, and predisposing factors such as topical steroid therapy.

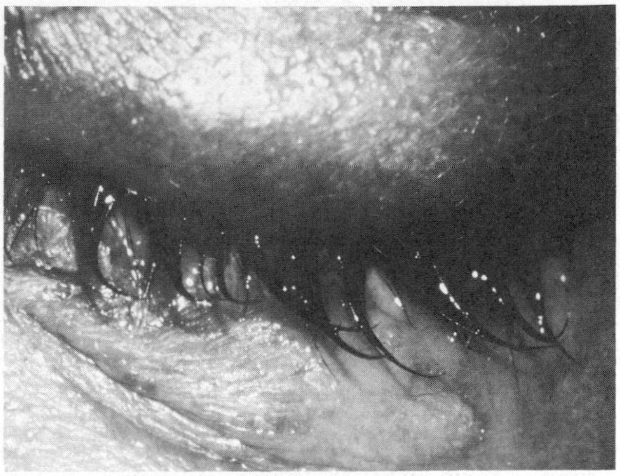

Figure 9. Matted eyelashes in a case of a bacterial corneal ulceration.

A history of a foreign body injury with the associated signs and symptoms described above is usually indicative of bacterial ulceration, but patients with viral corneal ulceration, neurotrophic keratitis, or recent corneal transplantation may have similar clinical findings. In order to establish a specific diagnosis, all corneal ulcers must be carefully examined and cultured.

Because very few organisms can be obtained by scraping the cornea, it is important to make smears for Gram, Giemsa, potassium hydroxide, and acid-fast stains and to plate the cultures directly from the spatula that is used to scrape the cornea (Jones, 1980). Because this procedure is technically difficult and because the area of tissue to be scraped is small, the procedure is usually performed under magnification with a slit-lamp microscope by an ophthalmologist. Diagnostic paracentesis of the anterior chamber

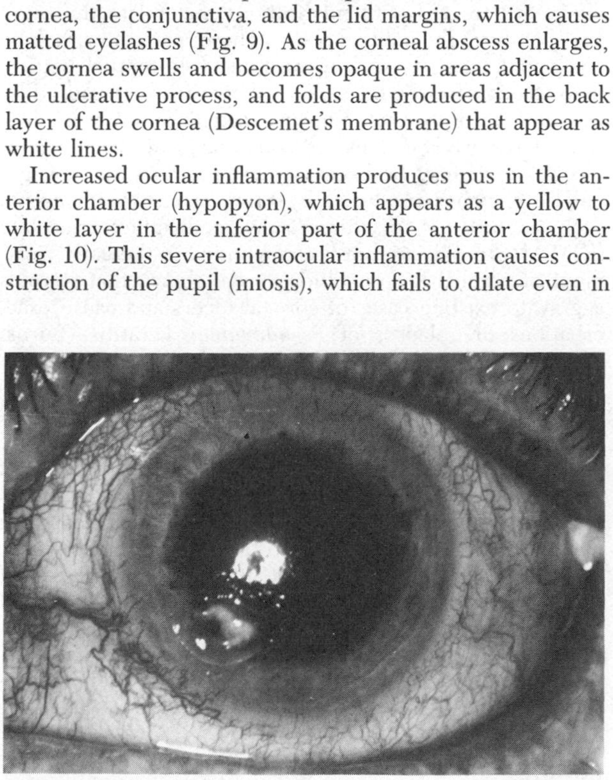

Figure 8. *Staphylococcus aureus* corneal ulcer in a 65-year-old man with rheumatoid arthritis and mildly dry eyes. The patient had been treated with topical steroids for two months before the infection.

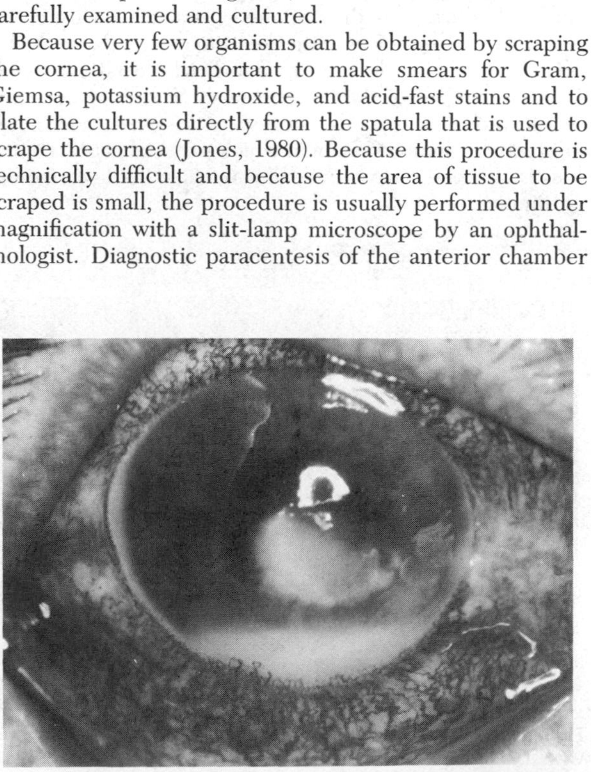

Figure 10. This *Moraxella lacunata* ulcer occurred one week after a "scratch" to the eye of a 45-year-old chronic alcoholic.

is necessary only in severely advanced cases with deep stromal abscesses.

The most common bacteria cultured from bacterial corneal ulcers are *S. pneumonia*, *S. aureus*, *Pseudomonas*, and *Moraxella*, but almost every bacterium has been isolated from corneal ulcerations. More and more so-called nonpathogens have been isolated as opportunists from eyes of patients with decreased cell-mediated immunity or after treatment with corticosteroids.

TREATMENT. Bacterial corneal ulcers may be treated topically with frequent instillation of antibiotic drops and systemic or periocular injections of antibiotics. The antibiotic is selected on the basis of the Gram stain and modified according to the results of the cultures. When no organisms are seen in the Gram stain, one must assume that the ulcer is caused by a penicillin-resistant staphylococcus or *Pseudomonas aeruginosa* until proved otherwise (Jones, 1980). This decision is based on the fact that more than 50 per cent of *S. aureus* isolated from corneal ulcers produce penicillinase and that *Pseudomonas* ulcers are so virulent that they can perforate a cornea in one day if not treated promptly and appropriately.

The topical treatment of choice for Pseudomonas is 0.3 per cent gentamicin drops. *Staphylococcus aureus* infections may be treated with chloramphenicol (1.0 g orally every six hours) or with 200 mg per kg per day I.V. of a penicillinase-resistant penicillin. *Pseudomonas aeruginosa* ulcers can be treated with 2.5 g of carbenicillin I.V. every two hours. The dose and circumstances under which subtenon's gentamicin is given are described below.

Topical antibiotic drops should be applied hourly around the clock until the signs and symptoms abate and should be continued a minimum of six times a day for at least seven to ten days after the corneal ulcer completely resolves. If therapy is discontinued prematurely, especially for *Pseudomonas* ulcers, the keratitis may relapse or become exacerbate. In cases of superficial ulceration, topical therapy may be all that is necessary. In very severe cases of ulceration, it may be necessary to use a continuous antibiotic irrigation system in which a special plastic contact lens is attached to an intravenous infusion bottle containing antibiotics.

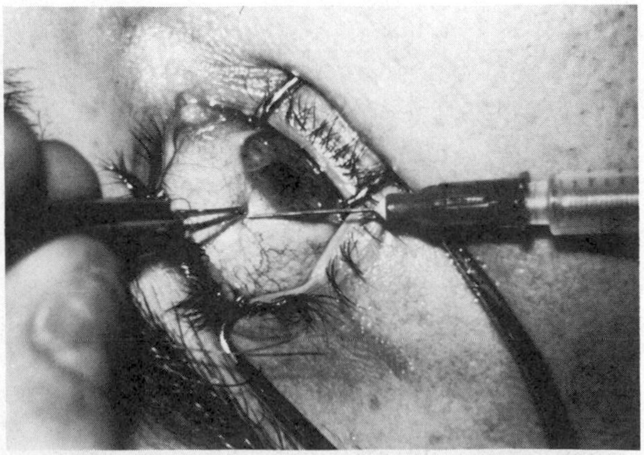

Figure 11. Example of a subconjunctival injection of antibiotics with a 25-gauge needle and topical cocaine anesthesia. About 1½ ml of antibiotic can be injected at one time.

Periocular injections of antibiotics are also used in modern therapy. These injections are made underneath the conjunctiva or under the deep fibrofatty capsule that surrounds the globe (Tenon's capsule). Most ophthalmologists prefer a subtenon's injection with a 25-gauge needle (Fig. 11) under topical anesthesia, although there is some evidence that higher aqueous levels of antibiotics may be obtained by subconjunctival injection (Patterson, 1973). It is clear that periocular injection provides higher levels of antibiotics in the ocular tissue and fluid than those obtained with intravenous or intramuscular injection (Baum, 1977). Recommended dosages of subconjunctival and subtenon's injections have been published and are presently in use (Jones, 1980; Baum, 1977). Gentamicin (60 mg by subtenon's injection or 20 mg by subconjunctival injection) is effective treatment for staphylococcal and *Pseudomonas* corneal ulcers.

The periocular injection is repeated daily until the signs of infection decrease. The frequency of repeated injections is limited primarily by discomfort to the patient and by the condition of the periocular tissues. Since this mode of therapy produces measurable blood levels of antibiotics, renal function should be evaluated during repeated therapy with nephrotoxic drugs.

Intravenous and intramuscular routes of therapy were in vogue until periocular injections were used. Systemic therapy provides acceptable ocular fluid levels of antibiotics in inflamed eyes but not as high as those obtained with periocular injection (Baum, 1977). Intraocular injections are not performed in the routine treatment of most bacterial corneal ulcers, but may be the therapy of choice for endophthalmitis (Peyman, 1977).

In addition to antibiotic therapy, patients with corneal ulcers are treated with medications that dilate the pupil and paralyze the ciliary body. These parasympatholytic (cycloplegic) agents such as atropine (red-topped bottles) help to decrease the discomfort of ciliary spasm caused by iritis and help prevent glaucoma secondary to fibrin adhesion of the iris and lens. In some cases of *Pseudomonas* ulceration, it may be necessary to neutralize the collagenolytic enzymes produced by this organism with agents such as 0.01 M disodium ethylenediaminetetraacetate (EDTA). Steroids are not recommended in the early treatment of corneal ulcers. Studies have shown that steroids aggravate existing cases of corneal ulcers and cause exacerbations or relapses of *Pseudomonas* keratitis (Burns, 1969).

The following parameters should be specifically measured in patients with bacterial corneal ulcers before beginning antibacterial therapy and daily during the entire course of treatment: best obtainable visual acuity, size of corneal abscess, size of corneal epithelial defect, height of a hypopyon, and pupillary diameter. Measurements are made with a light beam ruler on the slit-lamp microscope. All of the findings decrease as the infection improves except the pupil size, which becomes larger (assuming the patient is being treated with daily cycloplegic agents). The medications are tapered as the signs and symptoms improve. Any underlying disease or abnormality is treated concurrently. Medications are continued for several days after the abscess has resolved.

Some patients recover good visual acuity, but most are left with a corneal opacity which may interfere with vision. When the opacity is severe, a corneal transplant (Fig. 12) and a cataract extraction are required. Any underlying

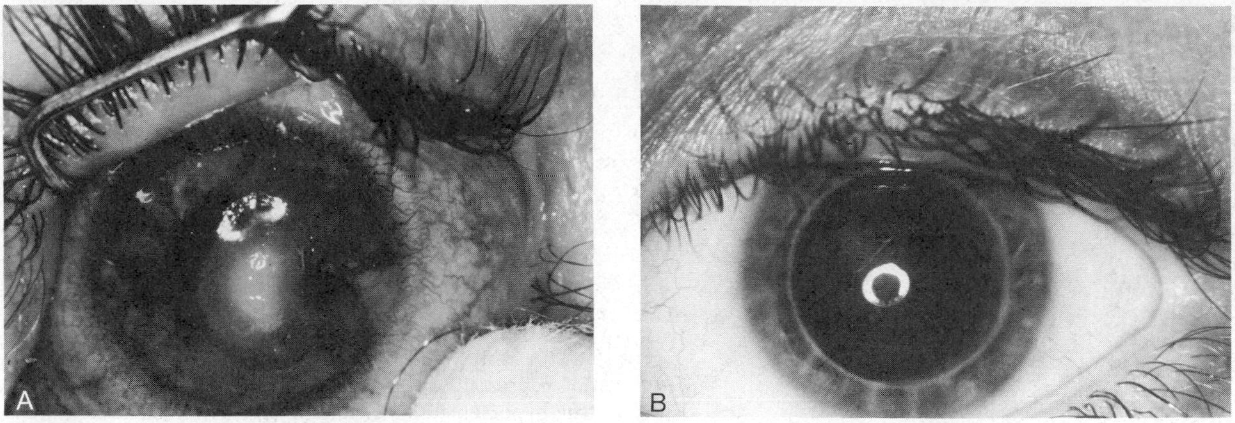

Figure 12. *A,* Six-year-old boy with an allergic conjunctivitis which was treated with steroids. He developed a *Staphylococcus aureus* infection and required general anesthesia for a subconjunctival injection of antibiotics (11/18/76). *B,* This patient underwent a corneal transplant in December, 1976, because of corneal scarring and finger counting vision. His vision with glasses after surgery is 20/30 (5/2/80).

disease process or predisposing factor should be eliminated and the patient instructed to return if inflammation recurs after treatment is discontinued.

References

Baum, J. L.: Antibiotic administration in the treatment of bacterial endophthalmitis. I. Periocular injections. Surv Ophthalmol 21:332, 1977.
Binder, P. S., Abel, R. A., Jr., and Kaufman, H. E.: The effect of chronic administration of a topical antibiotic on the conjunctival flora. Ann Ophthalmol 7:1429, 1975.
Binder, P. S., and Worthen, D. M.: A continuous-wear hydrophilic lens. Prophylactic topical antibiotics. Arch Ophthalmol 94:2109, 1976.
Burns, R. P.: *Pseudomonas aeruginosa* keratitis: Mixed infections of the eye. Am J Ophthalmol 67:257, 1969.
Chandler, J. W., and Milam, D. F.: Diphtheria corneal ulcers. Arch Ophthalmol 96:53, 1978.
Frederick, J., and Braude, A. I.: Anaerobic infections of the paranasal sinuses. N Engl J Med 290:1177, 1974.
Gombos, G. M.: Handbook of Ophthalmologic Emergencies. Medical Examination Publishing Company, Inc., 1973, p. 55.
Jones, D. B.: Strategy for the initial management of suspected microbial keratitis. In Symposium on Medical and Surgical Diseases of the Cornea. C. V. Mosby Co. St. Louis, Mo. 1980, p. 86.
Krachmer, J. H., and Purcell, J. J., Jr.: Bacterial corneal ulcers in cosmetic soft contact lens wearers. Arch Ophthalmol 96:57, 1978.
Leibowitz, H. M., Pratt, M. V., Flagstad, I. J., Berrospi, A. R., and Kundsin, R.: Human conjunctivitis. I. Diagnostic evaluation. Arch Ophthalmol 94:1747, 1976a.
Leibowitz, H. M., Pratt, M. V., Flagstad, I. J., Berrospi, A. R., and Kundsin, R.: Human conjunctivitis. II. Treatment. Arch Ophthalmol 94:1752, 1976b.
Locatcher-Khorazo, D., and Seegal, B. C.: The bacterial flora of the healthy eye. In Microbiology of the Eye. St. Louis, C. V. Mosby Company, 1972, p. 13.
Patterson, C. A.: Intraocular penetration of C^{14}-labelled penicillin after subtenons or subconjunctival injection. Ann Ophthalmol 5:17, 1973.
Perkins, R. E., Kundsin, R. B., Pratt, M. V., Abrahamsen, I., and Leibowitz, H. M.: Bacteriology of normal and infected conjunctiva. J Clin Microbiol 1:147, 1975.
Peyman, G. A.: Antibiotic administration in the treatment of bacterial endophthalmitis. II. Intravitreal injections. Surv Ophthalmol 21:331, 1977.
Smolin, G., and Okumoto, M.: Staphylococcal blepharitis. Arch Ophthalmol 95:812, 1977.
Trevor-Roper, P. D.: Diseases of the Orbit. Int Ophthalmol Clin 14:323, 1974.
Wilson, L. A., and Ahern, D. G.: Pseudomonas-induced corneal ulcers associated with contaminated eye mascaras. Am J Ophthalmol 84:112, 1977.

245

VIRAL KERATOCONJUNCTIVITIS

HERBERT E. KAUFMAN, M.D.

HERPES SIMPLEX

In the United States and Europe, herpes simplex infection is the most common corneal infection and the most important ocular virus disease from the point of view of morbidity and mortality. Its importance stems not only from the frequency of initial attacks, but from its likelihood of recurrences with progressive scarring and morbidity, and also from the fact that this is one of the few virus diseases that may be successfully treated with chemotherapeutic agents.

CLINICAL MANIFESTATIONS

Primary Herpes Simplex. Primary herpes simplex most commonly occurs between the ages of six months and five years (Duke-Elder, 1965). In its classic form it involves not only the eyes but also areas of skin, most commonly the face. In children with eczema, the primary infection with herpes simplex can be an acute disseminated infection with a generalized rash (Kaposi's varicelliform eruption) as well as necrotic lesions of the liver and other organs, and encephalitis. The mortality in this type of infection may be as high as 50 per cent. Most commonly, primary herpes simplex is associated with blisters over the face and lips, and sometimes lesions elsewhere on the body. With this there may be an acute keratoconjunctivitis, and sometimes an involvement of the cornea, with preauricular lymphadenopathy and fever. It is clear, however, that the most common type of ocular infection with herpes simplex is the so-called recurrent, or secondary, herpes simplex, which

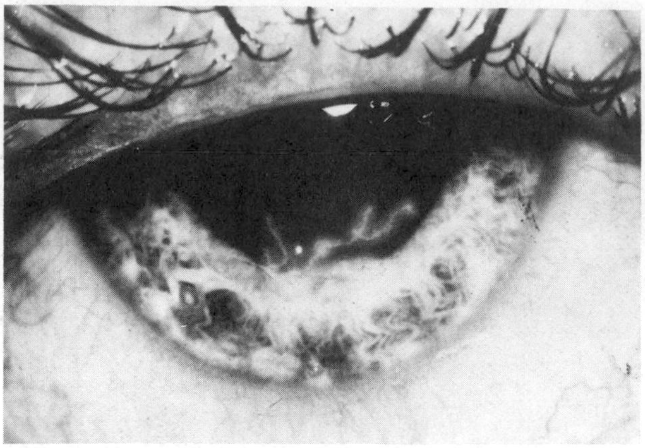

Figure 1. Typical dendritic lesion caused by herpes simplex infection of the superficial cornea. Stained with fluorescein.

develops in the presence of circulating antibodies even though there may be no history of previous infection.

Dendritic Keratitis. As virus infection begins in the cornea, small punctate epithelial spots or tiny vacuoles may appear in the corneal epithelium. As the disease progresses, these rapidly coalesce to form the familiar, branching dendritic figure (Fig. 1). Although corneal sensation may be lost early in infection with herpes simplex, in our experience this has not been an invariable sign of herpes simplex infection.

The symptomatology of herpetic infection varies widely in patients of different age groups. In older adults this disease tends to be relatively asymptomatic, in that the eye is not red and pain is not severe. In children and even in young adults, this is not the case. In children, herpes simplex is one of the most common causes of the red, sore, painful eye. In a young child, a red eye with pain and photophobia and the absence of obvious conjunctivitis should suggest herpes simplex infection until proved otherwise. Especially in infants and young children, the morphology of the corneal infection loses its dendritic character and large areas of the cornea appear to be involved by ulceration and vascularization in a process whose etiology frequently is not apparent until virus cultures are done. The reason for this apparent pleomorphism may be that infants come to an ophthalmologist only later in the course of the disease. Pleomorphism is a common clinical finding.

In the early dendritic ulcer, and in the dendritic ulcer with some stromal involvement beneath it, multiplying virus is generally present in the cornea. When virus cultures are done on such patients, most are positive, and virus multiplication appears responsible for the tissue damage. If corticosteroids are used inadvertently on dendritic ulcers, the ulcers usually extend and invade the stroma, and the cornea may perforate. The typical adult with epithelial herpes simplex complains only of a foreign body sensation and may have little redness and reaction around the eye. The physician should be especially alert to the patient who complains of a foreign body sensation of the cornea without a clear history of having been struck in the eye by a foreign body. The patient, for example, who awakens with a foreign body sensation would be most likely to have some primary corneal disease rather than a true foreign body injury, since any epithelial damage is felt as a foreign body injury.

Stromal Herpes. The original epithelial defect, if left untreated, may progress to a much larger map-like lesion and may invade the stroma. The involvement of the corneal stroma seems to take three clinically different forms which are treated differently:

1. Stromal ulceration may occur with direct invasion of the stroma and is facilitated by the inadvertent administration of corticosteroids.

2. In the absence of ulceration, however, virus may also directly invade the stroma, causing a cheesy white infiltrate with iritis that is difficult to treat.

3. A third type of stromal involvement probably does not represent direct viral invasion but may represent a true hypersensitivity reaction. This hypersensitivity disease can be mimicked by injecting sensitized animals with dead herpes antigen and is seen in infected animals who have previously been sensitized to the virus. It consists primarily of a round patch of corneal edema (disciform edema) and, like many types of hypersensitivity reaction, responds rapidly to very small doses of topical corticosteroids (Fig. 2).

Stromal herpes may also be accompanied by severe iritis, which may persist for long periods of time and usually is amenable to corticosteroid treatment with coverage by an antiviral agent. Herpetic retinitis has been seen in a few neonatal cases of disseminated herpes but is rare.

Recurrent Herpes Simplex. In the eye, recurrent herpes simplex causes much greater morbidity than on the lips and elsewhere. The progressive scarring of the cornea makes it one of our most serious clinical problems. The chance for recurrence after a first attack of herpes is almost 25 per cent within two years. After two or more attacks the chances are approximately 43 per cent of a recurrence within two years.

Patients with recurrent herpes, as well as some who remain asymptomatic, intermittently shed virus in the tears and in the saliva for months or even years. It appears that the virus is harbored in a latent state in the trigeminal ganglia and that recurrences are triggered by the virus traveling along the nerves to the end organ, i.e., the cornea, where the disease process is manifested.

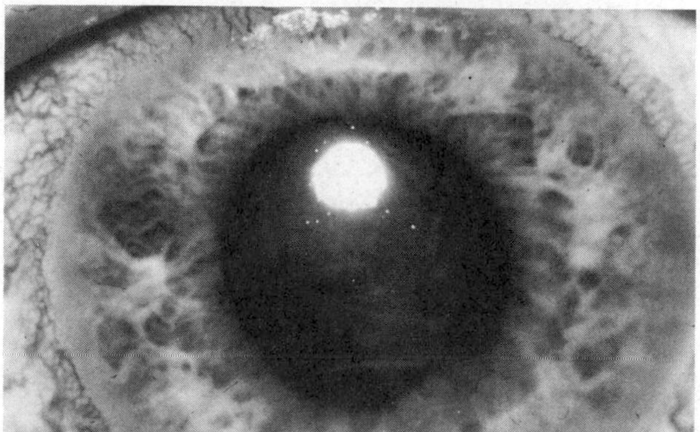

Figure 2. Patch of corneal edema with folds in Descemet's membrane caused by hypersensitivity to herpesvirus.

The precise mechanisms by which recurrences occur are uncertain, but most patients with recurrent herpes have high stable levels of neutralizing antibody in their blood before their recurrences. Similarly, no definite correlation with local IgA secretory antibody has been found, although we have found that such antibody to herpesvirus is produced in the eye.

Current studies indicate that within a single herpesvirus type, such as HSV type 1, there are individual strains or isolates that have unique biological properties. Some of these strains produce minimal conjunctivitis with virtually no ocular disease, whereas other strains produce moderate to severe disease, or even corneal necrosis and death. This relationship between strain and disease characteristics appears to be independent of inoculum size, and occurs in immunocompetent animals; therefore, virulence seems to be an inherent genetic property of the virus strain. It also appears that stromal disease is determined not entirely by the immune reactivity of the patient, but at least in part by the production of specific types and amounts of glycoproteins by individual herpesvirus strains. Furthermore, there is some experimental evidence that early infection with a relatively avirulent strain and subsequent colonization of the trigeminal ganglia prevents later ganglionic colonization even by a more virulent strain after superinfection. Other evidence indicates that all the cervical ganglia of a person are colonized by only one virus strain. Also, sequential isolates from patients with recurrent herpes simplex seem to be identifiable as a single herpesvirus strain by DNA fingerprinting. All of this implies that an individual is infected early in life by a particular strain of herpes simplex, and that this strain colonizes the ganglia and determines the character of both the initial episode of herpetic disease and the kind of recurrent disease that will follow. The history of the patient with herpes is, therefore, primarily determined by the initial infecting strain and the characteristics of the disease it produces.

THERAPY OF HERPES SIMPLEX. Two basic groups of herpes simplex virus are known to infect man, type 1 and type 2. Type 1 is generally responsible for recurrent disease of the eye, lips, and face, whereas type 2 is associated primarily with genital infections, has a reservoir in the male genitourinary tract, and may occasionally cause keratitis in infants. Most therapeutic studies have been done with type 1 virus, which seems slightly more susceptible to chemotherapy than type 2.

IDU (idoxuridine; Stoxil) was the first antiviral drug proven in controlled studies to be effective in the treatment of corneal herpes. Later, adenine arabinoside (vidarabine; Vira-A) and trifluridine (trifluorothymidine; Viroptic) were approved for use in corneal herpetic disease. Of these three drugs, trifluridine is clearly the agent of choice; with this antiviral, 97 per cent of dendritic ulcers are healed within two weeks. Trifluidine also has the advantage of being a clear drop that does not blur vision, as the ointment-based drugs do. Therefore, compliance is improved, and effectiveness is increased. Trifluridine can be applied as often as 5 to 10 times a day with no apparent toxic effects.

Trifluidine is effective against epithelial herpes because it inhibits the multiplying virus; however, this drug has no apparent effect on stromal herpes, such as disciform edema, which is a corneal hypersensitivity reaction and becomes manifest after the virus is gone from the corneal tissue. Corticosteroids suppress pain and reduce edema, but can reactivate and worsen local herpetic infections. Clinical studies indicate that the addition of an antiviral, such as trifluridine, greatly increases the safety of corticosteroid therapy; however, even in conjunction with antivirals, corticosteroids should be used carefully and in minimal quantities.

IDU, adenine arabinoside, and trifluridine are relatively nonselective DNA inhibitors that can be incorporated into normal cellular DNA to some extent, but are therapeutically effective at concentrations with reasonably low toxicities. Recently, a new class of drugs has been developed that is nontoxic by virtue of its mechanism of action. Such drugs include acyclovir (acycloguanosine, Zovirax), which is not yet approved for use in the treatment of ocular herpes, and BVDU (bromovinyl deoxyuridine, E-5-(2 bromvinyl-2′-deoxyuridine), FIAC (arabinosyl cytosine, 2′-fluoro-5-iodo-ara-C), and FMAU (2′-fluoro-5-methyl-ara-U), which are still in the experimental or investigational stages. These compounds are phosphorylated, and therefore, activated only by virus-specific thymidine kinase, and not by the thymidine kinase of normal cells. Therefore, they inhibit replication only in virus-infected cells, and have no toxic effects on normal corneal cells. However, viruses can become resistant to these drugs by dropping out or modifying their thymidine kinase, or by altering their DNA polymerase. The emergence of virus resistance to this class of drugs remains a potential problem, the exact importance of which is unclear now. Nevertheless, acyclovir has already been approved for the topical treatment of primary genital herpes infection, and the oral and systemic use of these agents may hold great promise for future antiviral chemotherapy.

Interferon is available in large quantities and relatively inexpensively as a result of new techniques, such as plasmapheresis and stimulation of leukocytes, tissue-culture of fibroblasts and other cells, and other types of genetic engineering. Yet, the role of interferon in antiviral therapy is still not clear. It may be that interferon is not useful alone, but may potentiate the effects of other drugs and reduce the tendency toward the development of resistance. In addition, chronic administration of interferon may have some role in preventing recurrences of herpes.

In some recurrent ulcers, the problem is not direct reinvasion by herpesvirus giving a new dendritic lesion, but rather an erosion of the epithelium. In these erosions, the epithelium does not attach well to its basement membrane because of previous basement membrane damage, and is peeled off by the motion of the lids. This recurrent-erosion type of ulcer is not caused by multiplying virus, does not have the irregular dendritic projections of its margins, and must be recognized and treated by patching and other techniques that favor epithelial healing rather than by frequent administration of antiviral compounds that do not help in the absence of multiplying virus.

ADENOVIRUS INFECTION

Infection due to adenovirus is fairly common in the United States and can be more serious than many physicians realize. Many syndromes are presently associated with adenovirus infection. For example, types 1, 2, and 5 can cause a febrile disease in young children, and this can be accompanied by gastrointestinal symptoms. Types 3, 4, and 7 cause pharyngoconjunctival fever or an acute respiratory disease. Types 2, 3, 4, 5, 6, 7, 8, and 9, as well as others, can be associated with a simple conjunctivitis. Most

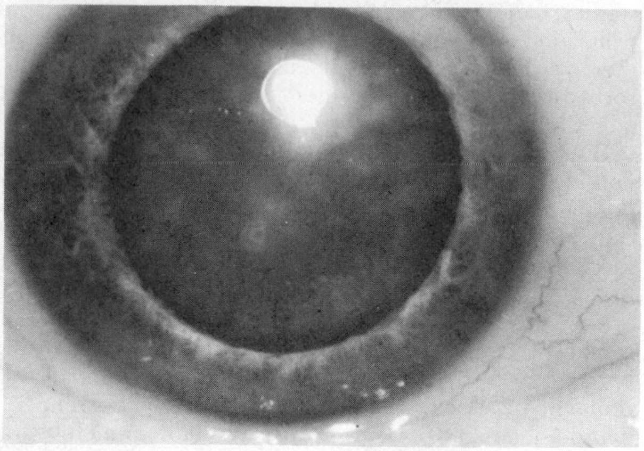

Figure 3. Subepithelial infiltrates of the cornea caused by adenovirus.

of the epidemic keratoconjunctivitis, however, appears due to type 8, although cases caused by types 3, 7, 19, and 22 have also been reported. All of these types, except the avian adenoviruses, share a specific complement-fixing antigen and produce generally similar cytopathogenic changes in tissue culture.

OCULAR MANIFESTATIONS OF ADENOVIRUS INFECTION. A simple, mild follicular conjunctivitis is associated with many types of adenovirus infection. Often, this is unilateral, and associated with pharyngitis, lymphadenopathy (usually either preauricular or submaxillary), and severe gastrointestinal symptoms, coryza, or even meningismus. Similarly, conjunctivitis due to adenovirus is sometimes acquired through swimming pool contacts, without either apparent systemic manifestations or enlargement of the preauricular or submaxillary nodes. In most cases the conjunctivitis is mild, but in epidemic keratoconjunctivitis it can be severe and disabling (Duke-Elder, 1965; and Kaufman, 1964).

Epidemic keratoconjunctivitis (EKC) is most commonly caused by adenovirus type 8, and is rarely associated with systemic symptoms of fever, nausea, vomiting, and adenopathy. The conjunctivitis is sometimes mild, but may be so severe as to cause petechiae and bleeding into the conjunctiva and even pseudomembrane formation. EKC tends to be bilateral, although unilateral cases sometimes occur. It is common for one eye to be more severely involved than the other. During the acute phase of adenovirus infection, symptoms may be severe. Pain, redness of the eye, and severe photophobia often are present and, on some occasions, the symptoms are so severe that patients are too uncomfortable to read; some even require hospitalization. The keratitis of this disease usually begins within two weeks after the onset of symptoms of conjunctivitis but may be more delayed. In the initial phases it is common to see subepithelial corneal infiltrates that are small, round translucent infiltrates varying widely in their distribution and number (Fig. 3). During the initial formation of the subepithelial infiltrates, tiny pits in the epithelium, which stain with fluorescein, sometimes occur over the infiltrates. The *acute* phase of EKC usually lasts from four to six weeks. After this time, however, although symptoms of conjunctivitis and epithelial pits may disappear, the subepithelial infiltrates may persist for years.

The presently available antiviral agents have not been shown to be effective in adenovirus infection, but, occasionally, if the disease is severe and there is significant iritis, corticosteroids may give some symptomatic benefit. In addition, corticosteroids seem temporarily to make the subepithelial infiltrates smaller and may be of limited use when these infiltrates are central and reduce vision.

The most important fact about EKC is that it is frequently spread by the general physician or ophthalmologist through unwashed hands or unsterile tonometers.

VACCINIA

Now that smallpox vaccination is no longer a part of the routine immunization schedule in the United States, vaccinia keratitis is extremely rare. However, when it occurs, it greatly resembles herpes simplex keratitis in its clinical manifestations and its good response to trifluridine therapy.

VARICELLA-ZOSTER

Primary infection of the eye in patients with chickenpox can occur with lid lesions, a red elevated "pock" on the conjunctiva, or direct infection of the cornea with scarring of the corneal stroma. This is relatively uncommon.

Involvement of the first division of the fifth nerve, however, is much more likely to involve the eye, since the cornea is innervated by the nasociliary branch of the first division of the trigeminal nerve. This branch innervates both the eye and the tip of the nose and when the tip of the nose is involved with herpetic vesicles, eye involvement is relatively common and should be suspected (Fig. 4).

The eye is involved as a severe iridocyclitis that lasts for months or even years. In zoster the cornea may be denervated and the eye dry. It is common to see serious corneal disease. It may be treated with cycloplegics and mydriatics to dilate the pupil and prevent the formation of iris adhesions; corticosteroid therapy may be necessary. In addition to the iritis, primary involvement of the cornea may cause corneal ulcers (dendritic ulcers) and, less commonly, dense white corneal scarring. In addition, optic neuritis, ophthalmoplegia, and pupillary paralysis have all been observed after herpes zoster, and ocular motor paralyses should be recognized as a rare but definite part of this syndrome.

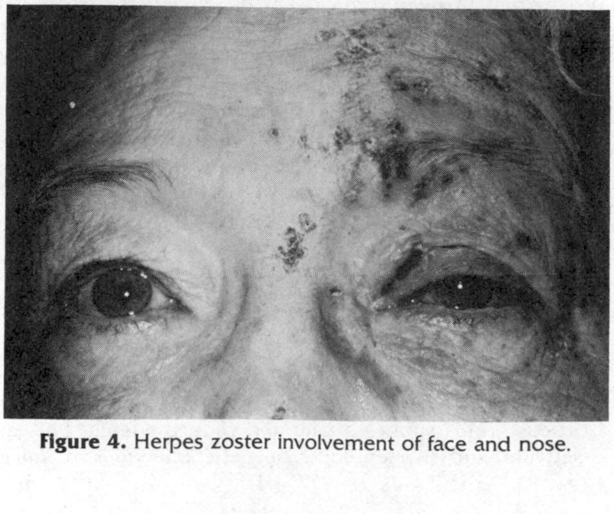

Figure 4. Herpes zoster involvement of face and nose.

The treatment of ophthalmic zoster with specific antivirals is in its infancy, but systemic adenine arabinoside or acyclovir may prove to be useful. In England, high concentrations of IDU in dimethylsulfoxide are used topically on the skin with apparent good success.

ACUTE (EPIDEMIC) HEMORRHAGIC CONJUNCTIVITIS

This disease appears in tropical countries, usually in the warm, moist seasons. Most cases are caused by Enterovirus 70 (See Chapter 186). Its secondary attack rate is high, and hundreds of thousands of cases can be involved. Typically, a severe conjunctivitis with hemorrhages in the conjunctiva is seen, with little corneal involvement except for some stippling. The disease usually clears spontaneously within a week, although in rare cases (1 in 10,000) neurological involvement resembling poliomyelitis may occur. Because of the high attack rate, there can be considerable disability. A recent study indicates that human leukocyte interferon does not alter the course of the disease in the individual patient, but can prevent the transmission of this disease to contacts, and thus stop an epidemic.

OTHER VIRUSES

Virtually all the exanthems can produce a mild conjunctivitis and even keratitis with punctate stippling of the cornea. The condition in which this is most common is measles, where the keratitis and mild iritis may make it desirable to reduce the light level for the patient's comfort. In North America and Europe, severe corneal disease from these infections is rare and the ocular irritation is generally transient, but in parts of Africa, measles can produce severe corneal scarring and blindness.

On occasions, systemic infection with a variety of viruses can also produce an iritis and a disturbance of the pigment epithelium of the eye as well as optic neuritis. Although the frequency and importance of viral uveitis are uncertain, viruses may be an important cause of nonspecific iridocyclitis. Placoid pigmentary epitheliopathy, a transient depigmenting choroiditis that does not cause permanent visual loss, occurs after viral upper respiratory infections.

References

Duke-Elder, S.: System of Ophthalmology. Vol. 8, p. 310. St. Louis, C. V. Mosby Co., 1965.
Kaufman, H. E.: Viral diseases. Int Ophthalmol Clin, 4:267, 1964.

246
OCULAR FUNGAL AND PARASITIC INFECTIONS

PERRY S. BINDER, M.D., F.A.C.S.

OCULAR FUNGAL INFECTIONS

Orbital Fungal Infections

ETIOLOGY. The most common causes of orbital fungal infections are the *Phycomycetes (Mucor* and *Rhizopus),* but almost any fungus can cause primary or secondary infections of the orbit (See Chapters 80, 103, and 171). These infections can be secondary to trauma (with or without retained foreign material), to immune suppression, and, most commonly, to spread from infected paranasal sinuses. There are also a few reports of spontaneous orbital infections in normal people without apparent antecedent sinus involvement (Schwartz et al., 1977).

CLINICAL MANIFESTATIONS. Most cases of cerebrorhinoorbital phycomycosis (CROP) occur in diabetics. Diabetics in good control may suddenly develop facial pain, sinusitis, and/or rhinitis, and become obtunded within hours. Alternatively, a diabetic who has just recovered from ketoacidosis may suddenly develop the same rapid progression of symptoms. Infected wounds or spontaneous infections of the skin about the orbit can also spread into the orbit. Acidosis in infancy, leukemia, and lymphomas also predispose patients to CROP.

The early orbital manifestations of CROP are similar to bacterial infections of the orbit and include a lid droop (ptosis), injection and edema of the lids and conjunctiva (chemosis), and proptosis. As the infection progresses, the lids become more involved and may become gangrenous. Because the *Phycomycetes* have a predilection for invasion of blood vessels, ischemic necrosis and infarction of all structures in the orbit and nose may occur. The extent of involvement can be more easily outlined when the necrotic areas are cleaned with hydrogen peroxide.

Involvement of the cranial nerves as they enter the orbital apex may produce extraocular muscle palsies, convulsions, hemiplegia, hemianesthesia, and death. This infection causes bilateral disease rarely and only after one side is severely affected. The patients are febrile, systemically ill, and have a peripheral leukocytosis.

DIAGNOSIS AND TREATMENT. A diabetic who develops facial pain, sinusitis, and rhinitis with neurologic signs and symptoms fits easily into the diagnosis of CROP. Roentgenograms of the sinuses are usually abnormal and may show an air-fluid level. Portions of the palate and nose may be ischemic or necrotic. The best way to make the diagnosis is by examination of wet mounts, smears, histologic sections, and cultures of biopsies from the orbit, sinuses, or skin. Histologic examination of biopsy specimens demonstrates the organisms (nonseptate hyphae in the case of *Phycomycetes*), vascular thrombosis, coagulative necrosis, and gangrene.

Treatment includes the surgical removal of foreign bodies and necrotic tissue, control of the underlying disease process, and systemic antifungal therapy. Amphotericin B (0.7 to 1.0 mg/kg/day I.V.) is the treatment of choice for the phycomycoses. CROP causes a severe illness in immunosuppressed patients and has a mortality rate as high as 68 per cent (Schwartz et al., 1977).

Fungal Infections of the Eyelids and Ocular Adnexa

Fungal infections of the eyelids are rare. They usually cause rashes, ulcers, granulomas, nodules, or verrucous lesions on the lid margin and surrounding skin. The diagnosis is made by scraping the lesion onto a glass slide, treating the scrapings on the slide with potassium hydroxide to eliminate the keratin, and examining the slide microscopically for mycelial elements. Another portion of the scrapings may be cultured for fungi. Treatment is by topical application of antifungal agents. The subject of fungal eyelid infections has been well reviewed recently (Ostler et al., 1978).

Fungal infection of the lacrimal system is much more common and is usually associated with a stone in the lacrimal sac (dacryolith) or an obstructed lacrimal drainage system (canaliculitis). *Candida albicans* is the most common organism associated with dacryoliths, but many other fungi and bacteria may be involved (Wolter, 1977). Canaliculitis is usually caused by bacteria. *Actinomyces* is the most common, but fusobacteria have also been reported (Weinberg et al., 1977).

Patients complain of unilateral tearing, conjunctivitis, or discharge. The eyelid or skin overlying the nasal lacrimal sac or canalicular system may be injected (Fig. 1), and solid lesions may be outlined when radiopaque dyes are injected into the canalicular system. In canaliculitis, firm concretions can be seen at the opening of the puncta. The dacryolith or canalicular obstruction should be removed and cultured and the canalicular system irrigated with penicillin diluted to 10,000 units per ml. Topical sulfacetamide drops should be used for treatment of *Actinomyces* and *Fusobacterium* canaliculitis. After removal of dacryoliths, *C. albicans* and other fungi should be treated with topical antifungal agents as described for fungal infections of the cornea.

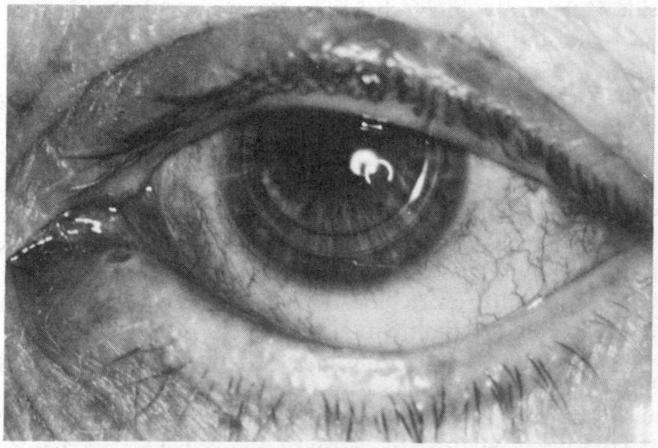

Figure 1. *Actinomyces* canaliculitis. The punctum is swollen and the adjacent eyelid and conjunctiva are infected. (Eye infections with this branching, filamentous bacterium have traditionally been included with fungal eye infections.)

Conjunctival Fungal Infection

ETIOLOGY. Some fungi are normal inhabitants of the conjunctival sac and may be cultured from 2 to 20 per cent of normal eyes. After treatment of nonspecific inflammation with topical antibiotics or corticosteroids, fungi may be cultured from a much higher percentage. Most are nonpathogens and rarely produce ocular disease except in the immunodeficient or after severe ocular trauma.

DIAGNOSIS AND CLINICAL MANIFESTATIONS. Most fungal infections of the conjunctiva occur in a setting of chronic conjunctivitis that has not responded to antibiotic therapy, but in the early stages they can resemble almost any "conjunctivitis." Fungi can produce deep purulent lesions with ulcerating nodules, granulomatous lesions surrounding ulcers, pseudomembranes, or large polypoid growths. Follicular conjunctivitis with a palpable preauricular node is a rare manifestation of fungal infection. Skin lesions are usually present. Fungal infections should be considered in all cases of chronic conjunctivitis with or without concomitant skin disease that have not responded to standard therapy and in any conjunctivitis in a compromised host. The clinical manifestations of the most common causes of fungal conjunctivitis are listed in Table 1. The organisms may be identified by examination of conjunctival scrapings with potassium hydroxide, by biopsy of the conjunctiva, and by cultures of the scrapings and biopsies on standard fungal media.

TREATMENT. Predisposing factors, such as infection of the lacrimal system and chronic antibiotic and/or corticosteroid therapy, must be eliminated or discontinued. Eyelid lesions may be treated with the standard topical antifungal agents that are used to treat skin disease. Topical diluted amphotericin B, natamycin (pimaricin), or miconazole may also be used in the same doses used for fungal infections of the cornea. Surgical excision of large conjunctival lesions with cautery may accelerate healing. Systemic amphotericin B or oral 5-fluorocytosine may be useful in specific cases. Scarring usually follows resolution of the lesions and may cause the eye lashes to rub on the cornea (trichiasis).

Table 1. CLINICAL MANIFESTATIONS OF FUNGAL CONJUNCTIVITIS[a]

Sporothrix schenckii
Ulcerating nodules, purulent discharge, lymphadenopathy
Blastomyces
Ulcer surrounded by granuloma, lymphadenopathy
Coccidioides immitis
Nodules, peripheral corneal vascularization
Rhinosporidiosis
Unilateral pink polypoid growths resembling granulomas; pus may be expressed from center of growth
Candida albicans
Pseudomembranous conjunctivitis
Ringworm fungi
Diffuse conjunctivitis

[a]After Ostler, H. B., et al.: J Cont Ed Ophthalmol, Feb., 1978, p. 3.

Fungal Corneal Infections

ETIOLOGY. The normal cornea is rarely infected by fungi, but damage to the normal protective mechanisms permits fungal invasion. Patients who are predisposed to fungal corneal ulceration include those who have received topical corticosteroid therapy, immunosuppressed patients, and those with antecedent or concurrent bacterial ulceration or herpes simplex keratitis.

CLINICAL MANIFESTATIONS. Most patients have a history of antecedent ocular trauma, especially trauma due to plant material or to accidents that occur during outdoor activity. Many have received topical antibiotics or steroids before the diagnosis of fungal keratitis is made, but a significant proportion have not had antecedent trauma or therapy (Forster and Rebell, 1975a).

The patient complains of pain, photophobia, tearing, and decreased vision. The conjunctiva is injected, and the eyelids are swollen. The corneal abscess may be accompanied by a hypopyon (Fig. 2). Mycelial fungi (molds) tend to produce a gray-white elevated lesion with a stromal abscess whose edges are "feathery." Satellite lesions are common. Lesions that are caused by yeasts are more yellow-white and tend to be single and focal. They resemble bacterial ulcers (Fig. 3). Occasionally, white blood cells adhere to the posterior surface of the stromal lesion in solid plaques (Fig. 2). An accurate clinical diagnosis cannot be made on the basis of the morphology of the lesion alone. The differential diagnosis includes chronic herpes simplex stromal keratitis and bacterial stromal abscess.

DIAGNOSIS. A fungal ulcer should be suspected in any patient who presents with a stromal corneal abscess and a history of foreign body trauma from plant material, a history of a chronic corneal ulcer that has not responded to standard therapy, or a history of antecedent treatment with corticosteroids. Fungal ulcers are also common in the immunosuppressed or after cerebrovascular accidents that cause chronic corneal exposure.

The lesion is cultured in the same fashion as bacterial ulcers (Chapter 244) with a platinum spatula under microscopic control. Glass slides are prepared for a potassium hydroxide mount, Gram stain, Giemsa stain, acid-fast stain, and special stains for fungi such as the Gridley, periodic acid–Schiff (PAS), or Gomori methenamine silver (GMS) stain. These stains supplement each other and increase the percentage of positive diagnoses (Polack, 1973). The scrapings are also directly streaked onto media appropriate for bacterial and fungal culture (Forster and Rebell, 1975a). If the index of suspicion is high and no organisms are seen on the slides, a biopsy of the edge of the lesion may reveal the fungi. It is rarely necessary to perform an anterior chamber paracentesis. The organisms most frequently cultured from keratomycoses are listed in Table 2.

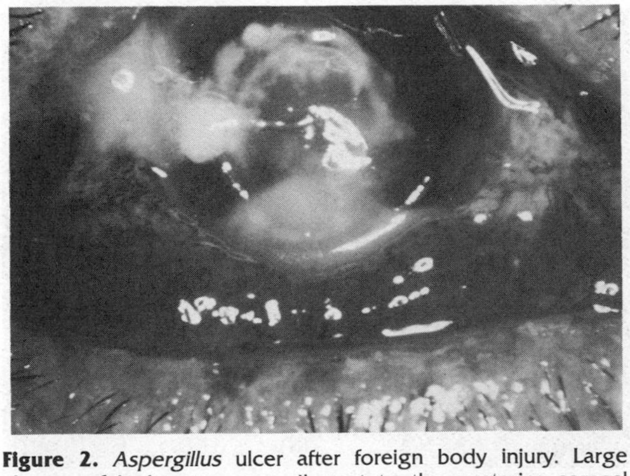

Figure 2. *Aspergillus* ulcer after foreign body injury. Large clumps of leukocytes are adherent to the posterior corneal surface (plaques) above the ulcer. A fluffy hypopyon can be seen below.

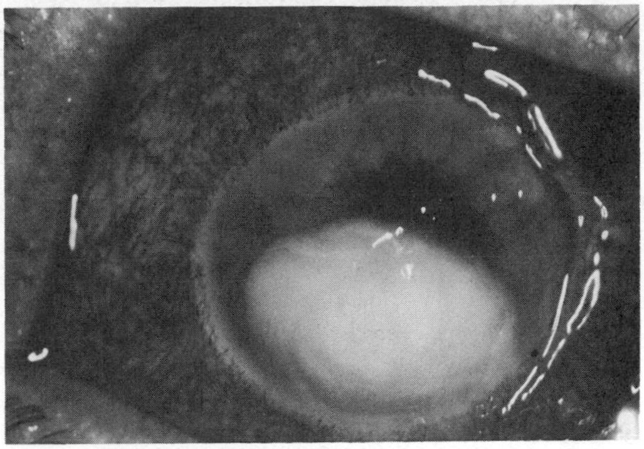

Figure 3. *Candida* ulcer in a chronic diabetic. Only a small corneal abscess can be seen because of the very large hypopyon filling most of the anterior chamber.

TREATMENT. The necrotic cornea is usually removed at the time of diagnostic scraping. The lesions are then treated with topical antifungal agents. The topical application of one of the polyene antibiotics such as amphotericin B or natamycin (pimaricin) either directly to the ulcer (amphotericin B or natamycin) or subconjunctivally (amphotericin B) is standard therapy. Topical and oral therapy with 5-fluorocytosine is effective against *Candida*, *Cryptococcus*, and some strains of *Aspergillus* and *Penicillium* (Table 3). Newer agents with a broader antifungal spectrum that are less toxic to the eye include clotrimazole and miconazole. Amphotericin B or natamycin should be used until the responsible organism is identified (Table 3). Concomitant cycloplegics and antibiotics should also be given.

If the infection fails to respond to medical therapy, it is necessary to excise the superficial cornea and cover the infected cornea with conjunctiva (conjunctival flap). After the eye heals, a corneal transplant should be done. An

Table 2. CAUSES OF KERATOMYCOSIS

Common	Rare
Fusarium	Tetraploa
Cephalosporium	Curvularia
Candida	Phialophora
Aspergillus	Nocardia[a]
Pencillium	

[a]This filamentous, branching bacterium is included because the disease is similar to that caused by fungi.

Table 3. MEDICAL THERAPY FOR KERATOMYCOSIS

Amphotericin B	
Topical	
	0.01 to 2.5 mg/ml, every 2 to 3 hours
Subconjunctival	
	0.15 to 2.0 mg as necessary
Natamycin	
	50 mg/ml topically every 1 to 2 hours
5-Fluorocytosine	
Topical	
	10 to 15 mg/ml, every 1 to 2 hours
Oral	
	50 to 150 mg/kg/day in 4 divided doses
Miconazole	
Topical	
	5 to 10 mg/ml every 1 to 2 hours
Ketoconazole	
Oral	
	200 mg daily

emergency corneal transplant is only necessary for acute perforations in order to halt the disease process (Forster and Rebell, 1975b). Fungal ulcers rarely progress to endophthalmitis.

Intraocular Fungal Infections

ETIOLOGY. Fungi can be introduced into the interior of the eye through a corneal ulceration, by intraocular trauma with retained intraocular plant material, cataract surgery, or from metastatic spread (Fig. 4). The infection usually presents as a fulminant endophthalmitis. It should be treated with topical, subconjunctival, systemic, and intravitreous antifungal agents and by surgical removal of the foreign body and the infected vitreous (vitrectomy) (Snip and Michaels, 1976). Rarely, the fungal infection presents as retinal and vitreal inflammation (Fig. 5) instead of a fulminating infection. The diagnosis and management of fungal endophthalmitis are discussed in Chapter 248.

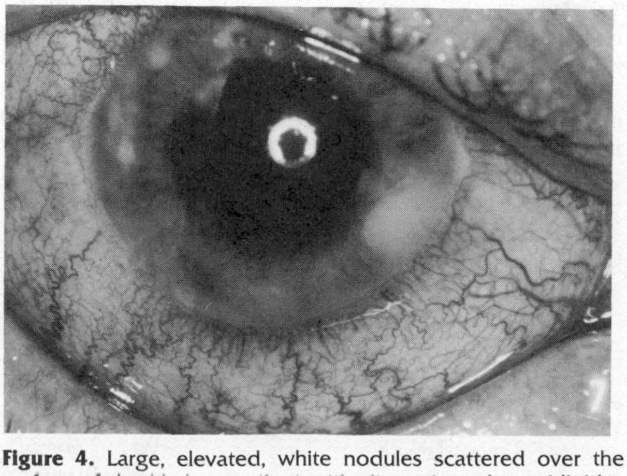

Figure 4. Large, elevated, white nodules scattered over the surface of the iris in a patient with disseminated coccidioidomycosis.

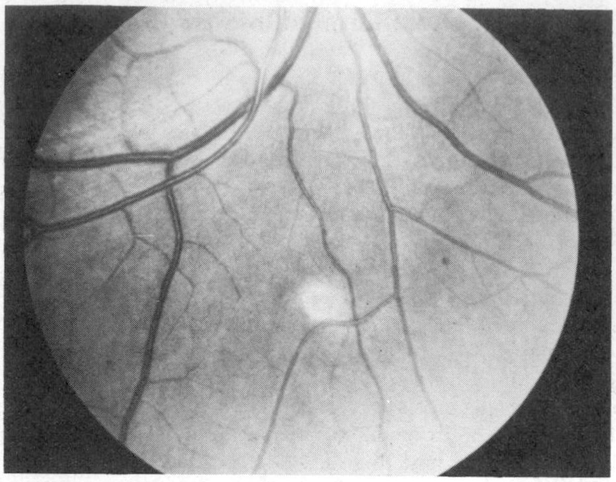

Figure 5. Isolated, focal, yellow-white retinal abscess in a patient with disseminated coccidioidomycosis.

OCULAR PARASITIC INFECTIONS

Orbital Parasitic Infections

Parasitic orbital infections are rare. Trichinosis, cysticercosis, echinococcosis, and onchocerciasis produce granulomatous infections and mild irritation until the organisms die, when they produce a severe inflammatory reaction. Trichina cysts within the extraocular muscles cause pain on eye movement, extraocular muscle paralysis, and edema of the conjunctiva and eyelids that resemble Chagas' disease (Romaña's sign). All of these organisms tend to invade the globe more frequently than the orbit.

Parasitic Infections of the Eyelids and Ocular Adnexa

The two most common parasites that affect the eyelids are lice (Fig. 6) and mites. The specific organisms include *Pediculus humanis* var. *capitis,* the head louse; *Pediculus*

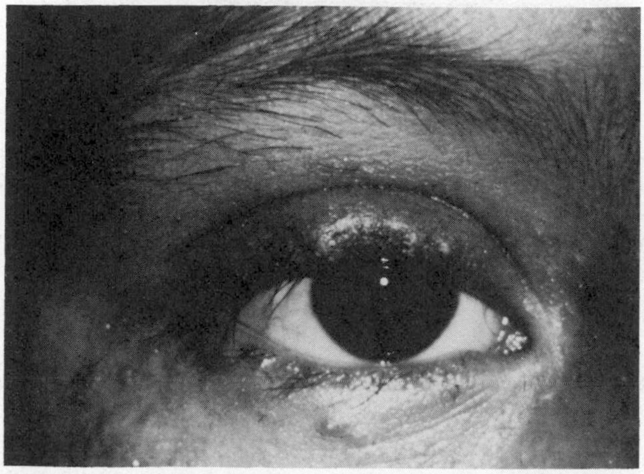

Figure 6. Tinea capitis infection of the eyelid. Note loss of lashes above, scarred and irregular lid margin, and depigmentation.

Table 4. CAUSES OF PARASITIC INFECTIONS OF THE EYELIDS[a]

Pediculus humanis	*Demodex folliculorum*
Leishmaniasis	*Enterobius vermicularis*
Loa loa	*Ascaris lumbricoides*
Ancylostoma duodenale	*Necator americanus*
Trichinella spiralis	Schistosoma
Flukes	Sparganum
Echinococcus	Cysticercus

[a]After Ostler, H. B., et al.: J Cont Ed Ophthalmol, Feb, 1978, p. 3.

humanis var. *corporis*, the body louse; *Phthirus pubis*, the crab louse; and *Demodex folliculorum*, the common mite of hair follicles and sebaceous glands (Table 4).

Phthirus pubis produces complaints similar to those of staphylococcal blepharitis. High magnification examination of the base of the eyelashes may reveal the transparent organism (Fig. 7) or the nits. The nits should be removed and the eyelid margins treated by smothering the organisms with ointment and directly killing them with 0.25 per cent physostigmine (eserine ointment) or careful application of 1 per cent gamma benzene hexachloride (Kwell). The pubic area should also be treated with Kwell.

Demodex folliculorum is a common contaminant of the hair follicle (Coston, 1967). Slit-lamp examination of the base of the eyelashes reveals a fine or waxy brownish debris. If the lashes are pulled out and examined microscopically, the mite may be seen attached to the base. Itching is the main symptom. *Demodex* may also carry staphylococci into the hair follicle. The treatment is to maintain good eyelid hygiene and to kill the mites by applying camphor, acetone, or ether to the lid margin with a cotton-tipped applicator (using care to avoid the cornea) or by topical application of 10 per cent sulfacetamide ointment (Ostler et al., 1978).

Other parasites that infect the eyelids produce chronic lid infections that may present as nodules, depigmented areas (Fig. 6), hyperkeratosis, edema, loss of lashes, or erythema (Table 4). After the organisms are removed and identified microscopically, the affected area is treated topically as described above.

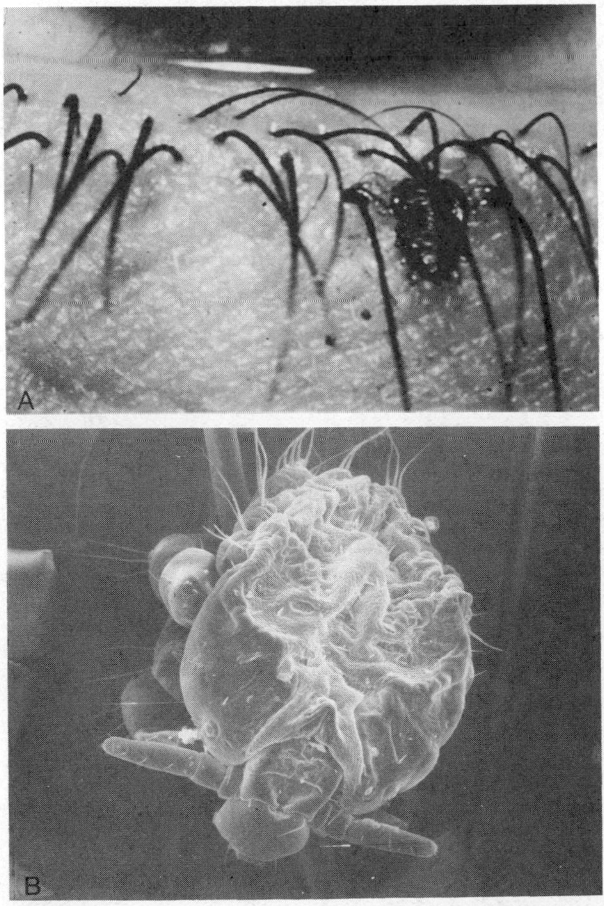

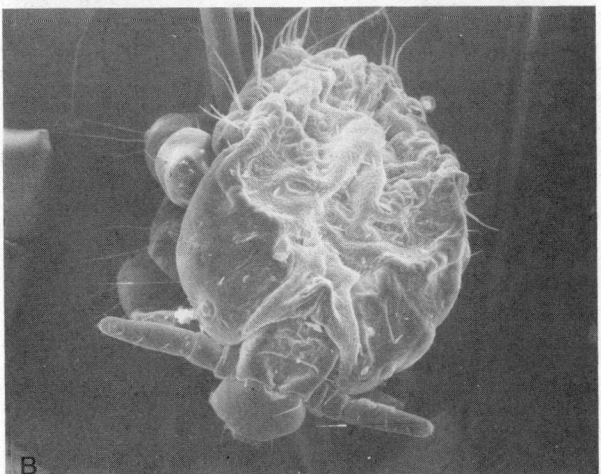

Figure 7. *A, Phthirus pubis* on eyelid margin. The patient complained of itching and redness. *B*, Scanning electron micrograph of *Pediculus humanis* removed from the base of an eyelash. × 128.

Conjunctival Parasitic Infections

Parasitic conjunctival disease is very rare in the United States but common in areas where the parasites listed in Table 4 and 5 are endemic. The ease of jet travel, however, has increased the number of patients with parasitic conjunctivitis in nonendemic areas. Therefore, the possibility of a parasitic infection should be considered in any patient who presents with conjunctivitis following a trip into an endemic area. Unfortunately, the manifestations of some parasitic infections occur months to years after exposure (Duke-Elder, 1965).

CLINICAL MANIFESTATIONS AND DIAGNOSIS. Tearing, photophobia, itching, erythema, chemosis, and mass lesions of the conjunctiva are common to all parasitic infections of the conjunctivae. Concomitant disease of the eyelids and periorbital skin is frequent. A history of recent exposure to an endemic area is helpful. The organism may be directly visualized in the conjunctiva or in a biopsy of a conjunctival mass. Eosinophils are prominent in Giemsa smears of conjunctival scrapings. Corneal lesions may be present. Many patients also have symptoms and signs of systemic infection with the parasite. Some of the clinical presentations are listed in Table 5.

TREATMENT. If an organism is either visible or thought to be alive and near the surface of the eye, the topical application of 4 to 10 per cent cocaine paralyzes the organism (Hennessy et al., 1977) so that it can be removed with a blunt forceps. Topical physostigmine ointment (eserine) can also be used for this purpose and to smother the organism. Deep burrowing or encysted parasites must be excised surgically. Patients are also treated systemically with the appropriate antiparasitic drug. The eye is carefully monitored for the acute ocular inflammation that occurs when the organisms die, and topical corticosteroids and cycloplegic agents such as atropine are given to control this inflammatory response. The number of eosinophils in serial conjunctival Giemsa smears decreases as the disease is controlled.

Parasitic Corneal Infections

Corneal infections usually spread from the conjunctivae. The etiology cannot be established by the type and appearance of the corneal lesions alone (Table 5). The organ-

Table 5. CLINICAL MANIFESTATIONS OF CONJUNCTIVAL AND CORNEAL PARASITIC INFECTION[a]

Protozoa	
Leishmaniasis	Ulcerating granuloma, gelatinous avascular nodules, peripheral corneal vascularization, corneal abscess
Nemathelminthes	
Loa loa	Visible movement under conjunctiva, irregular symptoms
Onchocerciasis	Chronic conjunctivitis, diffuse edema and erythema, conjunctival pigmentation, conjunctival nodules, peripheral corneal vascularization, fluffy (temporary) or discrete superficial (permanent) corneal opacities
Platyhelminthes	
Schistosomiasis	Conjunctival tumors
Echinococcosis	Conjunctival cyst
Cysticercosis	Conjunctival cyst
Arthropods	
Ocular myiasis	Irregular foreign body sensation, maggot visible in conjunctiva, marginal corneal ulcers, subconjunctival mass

[a]After Ostler, H. B., et al.: J Cont Ed Ophthalmol, Feb., 1978.

ism can only rarely be visualized in the corneal stroma. The diagnosis frequently must be established by obtaining the organism from the cornea or from other organs. Treatment is directed toward decreasing the corneal inflammation and eliminating the organism systemically.

Intraocular Parasitic Infections

ETIOLOGY. Most intraocular parasitic infections are produced by organisms that enter the globe hematogenously or directly from adjacent orbital or conjunctival infections. Living parasites usually do not cause intraocular inflammation but may produce cataracts, lens dislocation, vitreous hemorrhage, or retinal detachment. When the organism dies, it elicits severe inflammation that usually destroys the eye in spite of appropriate therapy. (See also Chapters 229 (Loaisis), 231 (Onchocerciasis), 243 (Myiasis), and 264 (Visceral Larva Migrans).)

Table 6. CHARACTERISTICS OF INTRAOCULAR PARASITIC INFECTION[a]

Protozoa	
Leishmaniasis	Endophthalmitis following corneal perforation
Nemathelminthes	
Loa loa	Free floating in vitreous
Onchocerciasis	Choroiditis, iritis, "retinal degeneration" with pigment dispersion
Platyhelminthes	
Echinococcosis	Vitreous cysts
Cysticercosis	Chorioretinal scars, vitreous cysts
Coenurosis	Vitreous cysts
Arthropods	
Oculomyiasis	Subretinal scars ("tracks"), endophthalmitis
Visceral larva migrans	Subretinal granulomas, endophthalmitis

[a]After Ostler, H. B., et al.: J Cont Ed Ophthalmol, Feb., 1978.

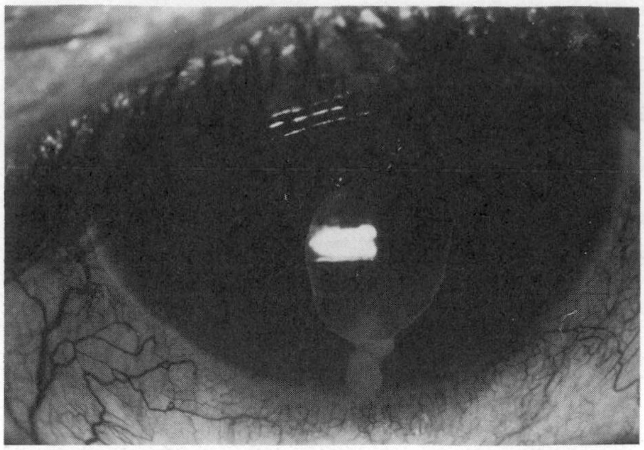

Figure 8. Free-floating cyst (*Cysticercus*) in anterior chamber.

CLINICAL MANIFESTATIONS AND DIAGNOSIS. Patients often have no ocular complaints when only the posterior segment is involved. The first symptoms may be severe and may include inflammation, bleeding, cataracts, retinal scars, and/or detachment. If the symptoms suggest infection of the anterior part of the eye, the vitreous and retina should be examined (Table 6).

A history of exposure to insect vectors or unsanitary eating conditions in an endemic area adds further to the suspicion of a parasitic infection. The visual acuity is usually unaffected by early infection. Even if only minimal inflammation can be detected, examination may reveal floating cysts in the vitreous, tracks under the retina (Gass and Louis, 1976), or chorioretinal scars; or the organism may be seen (rarely) with an ophthalmoscope or at the slit lamp (Fig. 8) (Fitzgerald and Ruben, 1974). The parasites tend to avoid the light and make visualization by the ophthalmoscope difficult.

When isolated intraocular parasitic infections occur, the specific serologic tests are negative.

TREATMENT. The parasite must be removed alive without disturbing the intraocular structures. This type of operation is technically difficult but must be attempted because dead parasites produce such severe inflammation that blindness may result (Hutton et al., 1976). Successful treatment without surgery has been reported but is rare (Fitzgerald and Ruben, 1974). Cycloplegics and periocular corticosteroids are essential adjuncts to surgery.

References

Coston, T.: *Demodex folliculorum* blepharitis. Trans Am Ophthalmol Soc 65:361, 1967.

Duke-Elder, S.: System of Ophthalmology. VIII. Diseases of the Outer Eye. Part I. Parasitic Infections of the Conjunctiva. London, Henry Kimpton, 1965a, p. 398.

Fitzgerald, C. R., and Ruben, M. L.: Intraocular parasite destroyed by photocoagulation. Arch Ophthalmol 91:162, 1974.

Forster, R. K., and Rebell, G.: The diagnosis and management of keratomycoses. I. Cause and diagnosis. Arch Ophthalmol 93:975, 1975a.

Forster, R. K., and Rebell, G.: The diagnosis and management of kerato-

mycoses. II. Medical and surgical management. Arch Ophthalmol 93:1134, 1975b.
Gass, J. D. M., and Louis, R. A.: Subretinal tracts in ophthalmomyiasis. Arch Ophthalmol 94:1500, 1976.
Hennessy, D. J., Sherrill, J. W., and Binder, P. S.: External ophthalmomyiasis caused by *Estrus ovis*. Am J Ophthalmol 84:802, 1977.
Hutton, W. L., Vaiser, A., and Snyder, W. B.: Pars plana vitrectomy for removal of intravitreous *Cysticercus*. Am J Ophthalmol 81:571, 1976.
Ostler, H. B., Thygeson, P., and Okumoto, M.: Infectious diseases of the eye. J Cont Ed Ophthalmol, Feb 1978, p. 3.
Polack, F. M.: Diagnosis and treatment of keratomycosis. Int Ophthalmol Clin 13:75, 1973.
Schwartz, J. N., Donnelly, E. H., and Klintworth, G. K.: Ocular and orbital phycomycosis. Surv Ophthalmol 22:3, 1977.
Smith, T. W., and Burton, T. C.: The retinal manifestations of Rocky Mountain spotted fever. Am J Ophthalmol 84:259, 1977.
Snip, R. C., and Michaels, R. G.: Pars plana vitrectomy in the management of indigenous *Candida* endophthalmitis. Am J Ophthalmol 82:699, 1976.
Weinberg, R. J., Sartoris, M. J., Buerger, G. F., Jr., and Novak, J. F.: *Fusobacterium* in presumed Actinomyces canaliculitis. Am J Ophthalmol 84:371, 1977.
Wolter, J. R.: *Pityrosporum* species associated with dacryoliths in obstructive dacryocystitis. Am J Ophthalmol 84:806, 1977.

247
OCULAR CHLAMYDIAL AND RICKETTSIAL INFECTIONS

PERRY S. BINDER, M.D., F.A.C.S.

Chlamydial and Rickettsial Infections of the Eyelids and Ocular Adnexa

These infections are always associated with active conjunctivitis (Ostler et al., 1978). Rickettsiae and Chlamydiae are sensitive to tetracycline, and the eyelid and conjunctival lesions clear simultaneously during topical and systemic therapy.

Conjunctival Rickettsial Infections

Rickettsiae may infect the eye as part of the generalized rickettsial illness. They have a predilection for vascular endothelium and may produce angiitis with necrosis and thrombosis of conjunctival and intraocular vessels. Rickettsial conjunctivitis is characterized by subconjunctival hemorrhage, erythema, and edema. The organisms may be cultured from conjunctival scrapings. Topical and systemic tetracycline or chloramphenicol is the treatment of choice.

Intraocular Rickettsial Infections

The manifestations of intraocular rickettsial infections include venous engorgement, retinal edema, papilledema, cytoid bodies, retinal hemorrhages, arteriolar branch occlusions, and severe inflammation (Smith and Burton, 1977). Although these findings are not diagnostic, they suggest rickettsial infection in a patient with an acute febrile exanthematous illness. Systemic tetracycline, as given for the generalized illness, is the only treatment necessary.

Conjunctival Chlamydial Diseases

TRACHOMA

ETIOLOGY. *Chlamydia* is divided into two species or groups, *C. psittaci* and *C. trachomatis*. *C. psittaci* causes ornithosis or psittacosis. Trachoma, inclusion conjunctivitis, and lymphogranuloma venereum (LGV) are caused by *C. trachomatis*. Unlike those of *C. psittaci*, the intracellular inclusion bodies of this species contain glycogen that stains with iodine. All chlamydial organisms show a common lipopolysaccharide group antigen, but they can be separated by other type-specific cell-wall antigens. The subgroup of *C. trachomatis* that causes trachoma and inclusion conjunctivitis (TRIC agents) can be divided into nine antigenic types (A through I) by microimmunofluorescence. Types A, B, and C cause trachoma in hyperendemic areas (Afro-Oriental), where poor social conditions and poor hygiene favor eye-to-eye transmission. Inclusion conjunctivitis (occidental trachoma or paratrachoma), which is caused by Types D through I, is spread from the genital areas to the eyes. The agents of lymphogranuloma venereum can be divided into three separate antigenic types.

The history of trachoma and the discovery of its etiology are outlined by Duke-Elder (Duke-Elder, 1965b).

DIAGNOSIS. Trachoma is the major cause of preventable blindness in the world. The organism infects the conjunctiva and produces hypertrophy of the lymphoid follicles underneath the upper eyelid and nonspecific inflammation of the remaining conjunctiva. When untreated, this process causes scarring of the conjunctiva (Fig. 1), dry eyes, and inturning of the scarred upper eyelid margin (entropion) so that the lashes continuously rub the cornea (trichiasis). Corneal infection and scarring (Fig. 2) eventually result in blindness.

Certain characteristic lesions (Table 1) strongly suggest the diagnosis. An ingrowth of blood vessels from the superior junction of the cornea and sclera (limbus) into the clear corneal stroma (corneal pannus) and an overlying

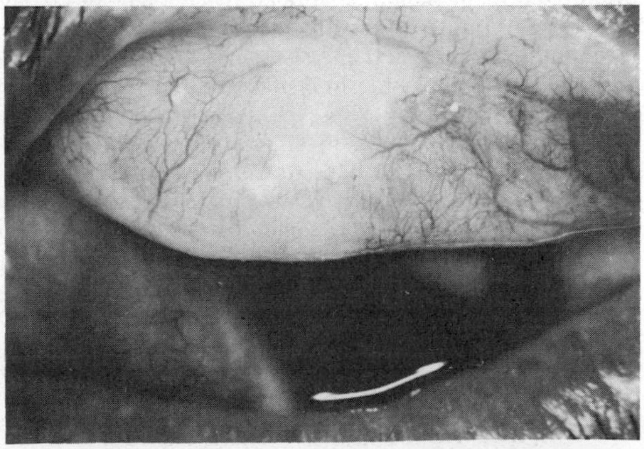

Figure 1. Severe conjunctival scarring on the everted upper eyelid in a patient with end-stage trachoma.

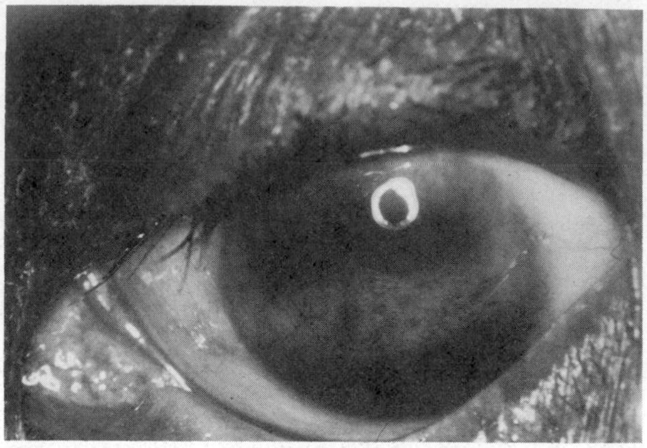

Figure 2. Diffuse corneal scarring of the superior and central cornea in a patient with advanced trachoma.

disturbance of the corneal epithelium (punctate keratitis) are particularly characteristic of trachoma (Table 1). The diagnosis is established by the clinical presentation and the demonstration of the organism in smears or cultures. Blunt scrapings of the superficial conjunctiva under topical anesthesia with a platinum spatula should be stained by the Giemsa technique and examined microscopically. If intracytoplasmic inclusion bodies are found, a definitive diagnosis can be made. Special fluorescent-labeled monoclonal antibody stains are as sensitive and specific as tissue culture. The types of white blood cells in the scrapings help to stage the disease. Polymorphonuclear leukocytes and lymphocytes are prominent in acute disease, whereas monocytes and lymphoblasts are predominant in the chronic stage. The conjunctival scrapings may be cultured in HeLa cells or McCoy cells treated with iododeoxyuridine or cyclohexamide, in which they cause typical iodine-positive, intracytoplasmic inclusions. The microimmunofluorescence test measures type-specific antibodies in serum and tears and greatly facilitates diagnosis (see Table 3, Chapter 56 for relative sensitivity of diagnostic tests).

TREATMENT. Hyperendemic trachoma is difficult to treat because of continuous reexposure. Treatment must include improvement of hand and facial hygiene to prevent reinfection by eye-to-eye and hand-to-eye contact. The treatment of choice is topical and systemic tetracycline. Tetracycline ointment should be applied twice a day for 60 days or on an intermittent schedule of five days each month for six months. Oral tetracycline (1 gram each day for three to six weeks), vibramycin (3 to 5 mg/kg initially, followed by 2 to 5 mg/kg for three to six weeks), or sulfonamides (2 to 4 gm per day for three to six weeks provide effective systemic therapy. Most patients respond within 12 to 17 weeks after starting therapy (Dawson, 1973; Yoneda et al., 1975). All members of the same social group should be treated to eliminate repeated transmission of the infection. The anatomic ocular complications must be treated to prevent or arrest corneal scarring. Surgical correction of the lids, the use of artificial tears, and corneal transplantation may all be necessary.

Table 1. CLINICAL FINDINGS IN TRACHOMA

Eyelids:	Papillae, follicles, scarring, trichiasis
Limbus:	Follicles, Herbert's pits, scars
Cornea:	Pannus, keratitis, scars

PARATRACHOMA (ENDEMIC, OCCIDENTAL PARATRACHOMA)

ETIOLOGY. Paratrachoma is a sexually transmitted infection caused by *Chlamydia trachomatis* of Types D through I. It is transmitted by genital secretions either to the genital area or to the eyes. The clinical presentation depends on the age of the contact and the portal of entry. Neonates develop inclusion blennorrhea (TRIC ophthalmia neonatorum), and adults develop either inclusion conjunctivitis or genital infection (TRIC urethritis, cervicitis, proctitis).

INCLUSION BLENNORRHEA (TRIC OPHTHALMIA NEONATORUM). Newborns are exposed to *Chlamydia* during passage through the infected birth canal. After 5 to 12 days, the infant develops a severe mucopurulent discharge from one or both eyes, with swelling and redness of the lids and diffuse conjunctival injection. Unlike the adult with inclusion conjunctivitis whose conjunctiva reacts by producing lymphoid follicles, the newborn does not produce follicles until 3 months of age. Giemsa stains of the conjunctival scrapings reveal diagnostic intracellular inclusions in 50 to 90 per cent of the cases (Yoneda et al., 1975), a much higher yield than in adults with inclusion conjunctivitis. Conjunctival cultures of the infant and cervical cultures of the mother are also usually positive.

The infants are treated with topical tetracycline or sulfa ointment at least six times per day for five to six weeks, and both parents are treated for chronic inclusion conjunctivitis. The ocular complications are usually mild and include minimal conjunctival scarring and some neovascularization of the superior cornea, but a rare patient may develop considerable scarring (Markham et al., 1977).

ADULT INCLUSION CONJUNCTIVITIS (OCULOGENITAL INCLUSION CONJUNCTIVITIS). *C. trachomatis* causes asymptomatic, nonspecific urethritis in men and chronic cervicitis with or without vaginal discharge in women. The infection is transferred to the eye by the hands or by direct transfer from the genitals to the eye. The incubation period varies from 4 to 12 days (Dawson, 1973). The disease presents in sexually active adults, usually 18 to 30 years of age, as acute (or chronic) unilateral or bilateral conjunctivitis with a palpable preauricular node, conjunctival lymphoid follicles, and mild mucopurulent discharge. Fever and respiratory symptoms are absent. Lymphoid follicles are most prominent in the lower conjunctiva but can spread to the entire conjunctiva. Conjunctival infection is moderate. The patient complains of tearing, a mild foreign body sensation, and lid fullness. The corneal epithelium becomes involved in the second week. Sequelae include scarring, opacities, and, rarely, iritis.

The patients are treated with systemic tetracycline or sulfa in the same doses prescribed for trachoma but only for three weeks. Topical ointments may also be used if the response to therapy is unsatisfactory. All sexual consorts must be treated to prevent reinfection. If untreated, the disease becomes chronic and produces corneal scarring.

References

Dawson, C.: Therapy of diseases caused by *Chlamydia* organisms. Int Ophthalmol Clin 13:93, 1973.

Duke-Elder, S.: System of Ophthalmology. VIII. Diseases of the Outer Eye. Part I. Trachoma. London, Henry Kimpton, 1965b, p. 258.

Markham, R. H. C., Richmond, S. J., Walshaw, N. W. D., and Easty, D. L.: Severe persistent inclusion conjunctivitis in a young child. Am J Ophthalmol 83:414, 1977.
Ostler, H. B., Thygeson, P., and Okumoto, M.: Infectious diseases of the eye. J Cont Ed Ophthalmol, Feb 1978, p. 3.
Yoneda, C., Dawson, C. R., Daghfous, T., Hoshiwara, I., Jones, P., Messadi, M., and Schachter, J.: Cytology as a guide to the presence of chlamydial inclusions in Giemsa-stained conjunctival smears in severe endemic trachoma. Br J Ophthalmol 59:116, 1975.

248

ENDOPHTHALMITIS

BURT R. MEYERS, M.D.

Endophthalmitis is an inflammation of the interior of the eye that may involve the vitreous body and/or the anterior chamber. The inflammatory process may spread to the uvea or the retina. If all the tunics are involved, the process is called panophthalmitis. Endophthalmitis may be caused by infection, blood, retained lens material, trauma, or neoplasm. It may be classified according to the anatomic location of the inflammation (anterior or posterior), the type of infectious agent (bacterial or fungal), or the route of entry of the infectious agent (endogenous or exogenous). Infection acquired during trauma, ophthalmic surgery, or by direct extension from adjacent tissues is called exogenous. Endophthalmitis acquired by hematogenous, lymphatic, or neural pathways is classified as endogenous.

Bacteria and fungi, including strains of questionable pathogenicity for other tissues, are the most common causes of endophthalmitis. Parasites and viruses cause occasional infections of the globe, but rickettsial and chlamydial infections are extremely uncommon.

ETIOLOGY AND PATHOGENESIS

Exogenous Endophthalmitis. The bacteria and fungi that make up the normal flora of the conjunctivae are the most common causes of endophthalmitis acquired at the time of trauma or surgery. Infants usually acquire an aerobic flora similar to the aerobic vaginal flora of the mother. *Staphylococcus epidermidis*, streptococci, *Escherichia coli*, and *Staphylococcus aureus* have been isolated at birth and persist through the fifth day even after topical penicillin or silver nitrate therapy. Cultures of more than 10,000 healthy conjunctivae have shown that *S. epidermidis* is the most common isolate, followed by *S. aureus* and diphtheroids. Other gram-positive bacteria and Enterobacteriaceae are isolated less frequently (Locatcher-Khorazo and Gutierrez, 1972). This pattern of normal flora is independent of age, season, and sex. There is no significant geographic variation in the conjunctival flora. The cultural results from many different countries are strikingly similar (Locatcher-Khorazo and Seegal, 1972). Obligate anaerobes are rarely isolated from normal conjunctivae. In the United States, fungi have been recovered much less frequently than bacteria from healthy eyes; 1.5 per cent of the age group from 10 to 18 years were positive compared with 4.4 per cent of adults (Locatcher-Khorazo and Seegal, 1972). Comparative reports of the incidence of fungi recovered from healthy eyes range from 2.5 per cent in the U.S.S.R. (Ovsepian and Osipian, 1965) to 52 per cent in Spain (Vasquez de Parga and Pereira, 1965). Over 80 species of fungi belonging to 50 genera have been isolated from the conjunctivae, but *Aspergillus* species are by far the most common. The bacterial flora of the eyelid margins and the conjunctival sac are the same, but fungi are more common on the lid margin. Urban dwellers have a lower incidence of fungal isolates than those in rural settings. The instillation of topical steroids and antibiotics, a warm, moist climate, an agricultural environment, and advanced age increase the number of fungal isolates from the conjunctivae. The local microbial flora is probably prevented from causing infections by local protective mechanisms such as lid closure, mechanical washing by the tears, and the lysozyme and IgA in the tears.

Endophthalmitis following surgery or trauma is usually caused by the introduction into the interior of the eye of one of these members of the normal conjunctival flora. The commonest cause of endophthalmitis after surgery, most often a cataract extraction, is staphylococci. *S. epidermidis* may now be a more common isolate than *S. aureus* (Puliafito et al., 1982). Gram-negative bacteria including Enterobacteriaceae and *Pseudomonas* spp have become more prominent since the advent of preoperative topical antibiotics. These bacteria are associated with a poor visual outcome. The most common causes of fungal endophthalmitis after surgery or trauma are *Candida* spp, *Aspergillus* spp, *Fusarium*, *Penicillium*, *Cephalosporium*, *Alternaria*, and *Allescheria boydii (Monosporium apiospermum)*. Abrasions and ulcers from contact lenses have also been the portal of entry for fungal endophthalmitis.

The interior of the eye can also be infected by direct extension of orbital cellulitis or sinusitis, but the globe is remarkably resistant to invasion unless the natural defenses are breached by surgery or trauma. *S. aureus* is the most common microbe that extends into the globe from the orbit or sinuses, but the Phycomycetes (*Rhizopus* and *Mucor)* and *Aspergillus* have a predilection to invade local blood vessels and can also extend through facial planes into the globe.

Endogenous Ophthalmitis. Endogenous endophthalmitis usually occurs from seeding of the globe during hematogenous infection. When the infection is localized, the vessels of the choroid and ciliary body are often involved. The first intraocular focus is often in the choroid and retina, with direct extension into the vitreous body. The retina may become necrotic, especially with fungal infections. *Candida* spreads through the intraocular tissues, whereas Phycomycetes invade the vascular supply and cause thrombosis of the retinal artery. Abscesses of the vitreous body and choroid and uveitis are frequent complications. Granulomatous chorioretinitis also occurs. Endogenous endophthalmitis can be caused by *Aspergillus*, *Cryptococcus neoformans*, *Blastomyces dermatitidis*, and *Sporothrix schenckii*, but *Candida* spp (usually *C. albicans*) are the most common causes of endogenous fungal endophthalmitis (Meyers et al., 1973). Metastatic endophthalmitis from bacteremia due to *S. aureus*, pneumococci, meningococci, *Streptococcus pyogenes*, *E. coli*, *Klebsiella*, and *Pseudo-*

monas spp has also been reported. Endophthalmitis may follow puerperal sepsis, pneumococcal pneumonia, endocarditis, and meningitis.

Endophthalmitis complicates 0.3 to 6 per cent of cases of meningococcemia. The tubercle bacillus and *Treponema pallidum* may also involve the globe secondary to hematogenous spread. *T. pallidum* has been found in the anterior chamber many years after the initial diagnosis of primary syphilis.

The prominence of *Candida* as a cause of endophthalmitis parallels the increasing incidence of candidemia. The rising number of patients with underlying malignancies, mainline drug addiction, intravenous or intra-arterial catheters, indwelling urinary catheters, and parenteral hyperalimentation increases the incidence of candidemia and secondary endophthalmitis. Periocular devices such as encircling bands placed around the eye at the time of surgery for retinal detachment can become contaminated and cause orbital and intraocular infection. Disseminated aspergillosis is a significant cause of endophthalmitis and death in leukemia patients. Unfortunately, the diagnosis is frequently made at necropsy.

Toxocara and *Toxoplasma* are the most common causes of parasitic intraocular infections. *Toxoplasma* usually causes posterior uveitis and is discussed in Chapter 262. Intraocular infection with *Toxocara* is discussed in Chapter 264, and viral ocular infections are discussed in Chapter 245.

CLINICAL MANIFESTATIONS. Endophthalmitis may present as an acute fulminating infection or as a more prolonged, subacute disease. In a patient who has either bacteremia or fungemia the development of eye symptoms of even the mildest degree should alert one to the possibility of ophthalmic infection. Complaints of eye irritation, pain, photophobia, blurred vision, or loss of vision are most common. Redness, hyperemia, and edema of the conjunctiva are early findings. Chemosis of the lids and proptosis follow.

Ophthalmic examination may reveal decreased vision with scotomas. Yellow-white opaque lesions may be seen on the retina and appear to be growing into the vitreous (Fig. 1). The iris may be involved and on slit-lamp examination a flare and cells are noted in the anterior chamber. The vitreous body may also appear hazy. In fungal endophthalmitis the retinal lesions may be fluffy with indistinct borders and look like cotton-wool spots.

If the disease is secondary to local extension from the nasal sinuses there are usually complaints of facial pain and headache; tenderness over the maxillary or frontal sinus will usually be elicited. Radiographs of the sinuses may reveal distortion of the normal architecture, bony erosion, and fluid. CAT (computerized axial tomography) scans will more clearly delineate involvement of the orbit and surrounding structures.

Patients are usually febrile with a leukocytosis and a left shift. Endophthalmitis may be the first manifestation of meningococcemia or occur concomitantly with bacterial pneumonia. In this event blood cultures should be performed before therapy is initiated.

The subacute form of this disease may occur 6 to 12 weeks after trauma, eye surgery, or fungemia. Endophthalmitis secondary to intravenous drug abuse usually has a subacute presentation. These patients may have no history of chills or fever and present with only minor eye complaints of blurring, redness, or irritation. An eye complaint in an addict warrants a thorough ophthalmoscopic examination.

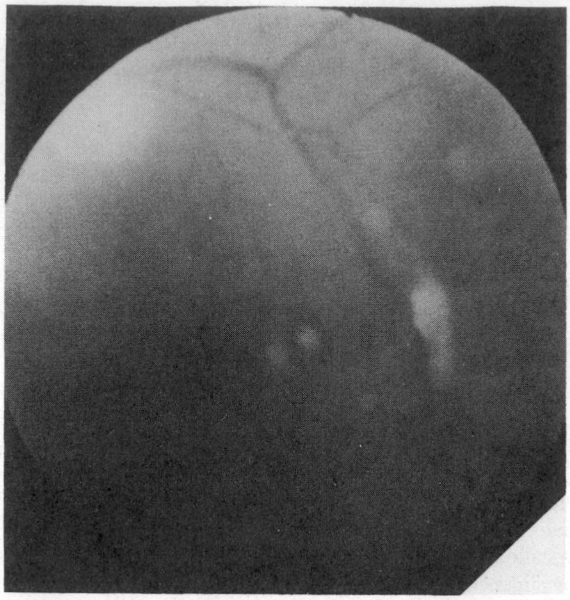

Figure 1.

In subacute endophthalmitis blood cultures are usually negative, and the peripheral white count is normal. Aspiration of the vitreous body for smear and culture may establish the etiology. Paracentesis of the anterior chamber is positive less frequently. In one study in which 78/140 eyes had a positive diagnostic aspiration, 27 eyes had a vitreous culture that was positive, while the anterior chamber was sterile (Forster et al., 1980). The presence of either white blood cells or bacteria in the gram stain of aspirated fluid suggests a suppurative infection. Fluids should be cultured for fungi and aerobically and anaerobically for bacteria. Serologic determinations for *Candida* precipitins and agglutinins have not been of value. The hemagglutination test for *Toxocara* may be reactive, but cross-reactions with gastrointestinal nematode infections have limited its usefulness.

Noninfectious endophthalmitis secondary to metastatic bronchogenic carcinoma, melanoma, and primary reticulum cell sarcoma causes similar symptoms and signs. Behçet's syndrome usually involves the uvea but can cause endophthalmitis. Asteroid hyalitis (inflammation of the vitreous body with star-shaped inclusions) may produce endogenous opacities, but these are of no clinical importance. Endophthalmitis phakoanaphylactica, a sterile, postoperative inflammatory process, must be considered after cataract surgery. Phacolytic glaucoma, a condition in which lens protein leaks through the intact lens capsule, may cause severe sterile inflammation and glaucoma.

GEOGRAPHIC VARIATIONS. Postoperative bacterial and fungal endophthalmitis and endogenous *Candida* endophthalmitis associated with hospitalization, radical surgery for neoplasms, and indwelling lines are diseases of medical progress and occur more frequently in industrialized countries. *Toxocara* and *Toxoplasma* eye infections have been reported most frequently from the United States but depend on exposure to cats (*Toxocara cati* and *Toxoplasma*) or dogs (*Toxocara canis*) and probably occur worldwide. Except for *Candida, Aspergillus,* and *Cryptococcus,* the fungi that cause endogenous endophthalmitis are restricted in their distribution. *Coccidioides* occurs in the arid southwest region of the United States, Mexico, and Argentina; *Blastomyces dermatitidis* (North American blastomycosis) in the southeastern United States, Canada, and Africa; and *Histoplasma capsulatum* primarily in the Mississippi and Ohio river valleys of the United States but also in Central and South America. The bacteria that cause endophthalmitis and the fungi that cause exogenous endophthalmitis are ubiquitous. As noted in the *Etiology and Pathogenesis* section, the conjunctivae of people from rural environments and moist, warm climates are more frequently colonized with fungi, but there is no clear-cut evidence that exogenous fungal endophthalmitis is more common in these populations.

TREATMENT AND SEQUELAE. Bacterial infections of the globe are usually very destructive. Early therapy is mandatory in order to avoid enucleation and save vision (Peyman and Sanders, 1975). Since the etiology of most cases is not known when therapy is started, it is necessary to give broad-spectrum antibiotic coverage for both gram-positive and gram-negative bacteria. For example, the antibiotic regimen must cover beta-lactamase—producing *S. aureus* and *Pseudomonas aeruginosa* since these are common causes of this condition. Furthermore, the route of administration and the pharmacology of the antibiotics must be carefully considered because most antibiotics do not penetrate into the eye very well. It is believed that antibiotics diffuse from the blood into the aqueous and that inflammation increases diffusion. Lipophilic compounds like chloramphenicol achieve higher intraocular levels than the penicillins, cephalosporins, or aminoglycosides. Protein-binding decreases penetration, so antibiotics like methicillin, cephaloridine, and gentamicin with a relatively high percentage of free drug should be selected. Therapeutic concentrations of trimethoprim-sulfamethoxazole have been detected in the anterior chamber, but the levels in the vitreous are unknown. Many antibiotics reach reasonable levels in the aqueous after systemic administration, but penetration into the vitreous is usually very poor. These observations and the high frequency of treatment failures have prompted the use of periocular injections to increase antibiotic penetration into the globe. Based on these considerations, therapy could be started with cephalothin or methicillin 2 g I.V. every four hours. The drug should be given as a pulse because the high serum levels diffuse into the eye against a gradient more effectively. Gentamicin sulfate should also be given parenterally in a dose of 5 mg/kg daily in three divided doses. Topical and periocular administration (by an ophthalmologist) of gentamicin is also recommended. Some authorities believe that intraocular antibiotics should be administered; however, complications are increased with this procedure, and the benefits are not certain. Infections secondary to *S. epidermidis* that are treated rapidly within 24 hours may respond to antibiotics alone (O'Day et al., 1982). Infections due to either gram-negative bacilli or fungi are more virulent in nature and may require more aggressive therapy. In many open uncontrolled trials intra-ocular antibiotics are administered often in conjunction with a therapeutic vitrectomy. Vitrectomy will remove infected material and membranes but could lead to detachment of the retina and ciliary body. These procedures are reserved for the opthalmologist (Baum et al., 1982). When blood or intraocular culture reports are available and antibiotic sensitivities known, more specific therapy should be given. Therapeutic efficacy is not increased by multiple drugs, and continued use of combinations may increase toxicity and superinfection. The optimal duration of therapy is unknown, but parenteral antibiotics should probably be given for four to six weeks.

Inflammation can destroy vision and cause cataracts, retinal detachment, and glaucoma. Topical and periocular administration of corticosteroids reduce inflammation of the retina and choroid in an animal model, and clinical studies have suggested that their use with antibiotics has been of value in preserving vision. Intravitreal administration of corticosteroids is also considered an experimental procedure.

Coexisting infections such as meningitis, pneumonia, or endocarditis must be treated effectively. Débridement of wounds and removal of foreign bodies, indwelling lines, and urinary catheters is necessary to prevent further hematogenous seeding. If contiguous structures such as the sinuses are involved, they should be drained immediately.

Studies of the comparative efficacy of different treatment regimens are not available, since only case reports have been presented in the literature. When antimicrobial therapy fails, enucleation or evisceration is necessary. Data derived from clinical studies of postoperative endophthalmitis revealed that 66 per cent of patients were blinded by inflammatory destruction or enucleation. Additional patients were left with almost useless vision.

Subacute endophthalmitis is more difficult to diagnose. If blood cultures are negative and there is either a history or a strong suspicion of prior fungemia, the vitreous should be aspirated. Even if the cultures are negative, therapy with amphotericin B should be started if there is a definite history of previous candidemia.

Data on the intraocular penetration of antifungal drugs in humans are also scanty (Leopold, 1973). Amphotericin B penetrates into the inflamed rabbit eye, but the intraocular levels of this compound and of 5-fluorocytosine in man have been measured only rarely. 5-Fluorocytosine has been used to treat only a few patients with endophthalmitis, and its efficacy is unknown. Data are also unavailable on miconazole, a newer antifungal agent.

Amphotericin B is the drug of choice for proven or suspected fungal endophthalmitis. A total of 1 to 2 g should be given intravenously over a four-to six-week period, although regression of lesions has been observed with less. The earliest response to therapy is decreased inflammation and clearing of the vitreous haze; regression of vitreous inflammation may take longer. Visual acuity will improve if the patient is responding to antifungal therapy.

The combination of 5-fluorocytosine (150 mg/kg/day) with nontoxic doses of amphotericin B (0.3 to 0.4 mg/kg/day) to prevent 5-fluorocytosine resistance has been used successfully in a few cases of postsurgical candidal endophthalmitis (Jones, 1978), but this regimen should probably not be used routinely until more information on the intraocular concentrations of 5-fluorocytosine is available.

Débridement, surgical drainage, and removal of all intraocular and intravascular devices should prevent further hematologic seeding. Periocular corticosteroids and vitrectomy are recommended by some clinicians. Intraorbital injections of corticosteroids and amphotericin B have been attempted, but the efficacy and safety of these agents by this route are unclear.

Tuberculosis of the eye, a rare condition, usually presents as choroiditis with whitish tubercles on the retinal surface, but tuberculous endophthalmitis has also been reported. Standard systemic antituberculous therapy should be administered and other sites of infection thoroughly sought.

Intraocular syphilis is treated with 15 daily intramuscular injections of 600,000 units of procaine penicillin.

PROPHYLAXIS. Preoperative antibiotics have been recommended to prevent postoperative endophthalmitis. Most studies compare different drug regimens, and comparative data without antibiotics are unavailable. Improvement of surgical techniques may have lowered the rate of infection. Postoperative infections often occur in spurts, which suggests that the source of these infections may be contaminated instruments or eye solutions. Elective surgery should never be performed in the presence of eye, lid, or adjacent infections of the face. Trauma to the eye should be attended to at once by an ophthalmologist. The incidence of candidemia can be lowered by avoiding the use of unnecessary antibiotics, and by removal or frequent replacement of intravascular lines and Foley catheters. The eyes of candidemic patients should be examined even in the absence of symptoms. If lesions are seen or suspected, antifungal therapy should be instituted promptly after appropriate cultures are obtained.

References

Baum, J., Peymon, G. A., Barza, M.: Intravitreal administration of antibiotics in the treatment of bacterial endophthalmitis III Consensus. Survey of Opthalmol: 26:204, 1982.

Forster, R. K., Abbott, R. L., Glender, H.: Management of infectious endophthalmitis. Opthalmology 87:313, 1980.

Jones, D. B.: Therapy of postsurgical fungal endophthalmitis. Ophthalmology 85:357, 1978.

Leopold, I. H. (ed.): Symposium on Ocular Therapy. Vol. 6. St. Louis, C. V. Mosby Company, 1973.

Locatcher-Khorazo, D., and Gutierrez, E.: Unpublished data quoted in Locatcher-Khorazo, D., and Seegal, B. C.: Microbiology of the Eye. St. Louis, C. V. Mosby Company, 1972, p. 15.

Locatcher-Khorazo, D., and Seegal, B. C.: Microbiology of the Eye. St. Louis, C. V. Mosby Company, 1972.

Meyers, B. R., Lieberman, T. W., and Ferry, A. P.: Candida endophthalmitis complicating candidemia. Ann Intern Med 79:647, 1973.

O'Day, D. M., Jones, D. B., Patrinely, J., and Elliot, J. H.: Staphylococcus epidermidis endopthalmitis: Visual outcome following noninvasive therapy. Opthalmology 89:354, 1982.

Ovsepian, T. L., and Osipian, L. L.: Mycologic flora of the conjunctival sac. Zh Eksp Klin Med 5:78, 1965.

Peyman, G. A., and Sanders, D. R.: Advances in Uveal Surgery, Vitreous Surgery and the Treatment of Endophthalmitis. New York, Appleton Century Crofts-Prentice Hall, 1975.

Puliafito, C. A., Baker, A. S., Haaf, J., and Foster, C. S.: Infectious endopthalmitis. Review of thirty-six cases. Opthalmology 89:921, 1982.

Vasquez de Parga, A. S., and Pereiro, M.: Flora micotica de la conjunctiva. Arch Soc Oftal Hisp Am 25:168, 1965.

I. MUSCULOSKELETAL INFECTIONS

249
BACTERIAL ARTHRITIS

PATRICK J. KELLY, M.D.
ROBERT H. FITZGERALD, JR., M.D.

This entity is also known as infectious arthritis, septic arthritis, suppurative arthritis, and pyoarthrosis. Granulomatous infections such as those caused by *Mycobacterium, Brucella,* and fungi are discussed in other chapters.

ETIOLOGY

Adults. *Staphylococcus aureus* causes three fourths of all joint infections (Kelly, 1977). Beta-hemolytic streptococci (nearly all group A), *Streptococcus pneumoniae,* and *Neisseria gonorrhoeae* are the only other bacteria that cause a sizable number of infections. All gram-negative bacilli together account for 10 to 20 per cent of infections. Bacterial arthritis due to obligate anaerobic bacteria is infrequent (Ziment et al., 1969). Many different anaerobic organisms, often in mixed culture, have been isolated from joints. Most mixed anaerobic infections are due to the contiguous spread of infection from adjacent soft tissue infections. *Haemophilus influenzae* arthritis is rare in adults (Krauss et al., 1974).

Children. The principal organisms isolated from infected joints in children are *S. aureus* and *H. influenzae* type B. They occur with approximately equal frequency in children between 6 months and 5 years of age. In older children, *S. aureus* predominates. Group A hemolytic streptococci and the pneumococci are isolated less frequently. Gram-negative bacilli such as *Pseudomonas aeruginosa* are much less common causes of arthritis except as complications of direct puncture wounds of metatarsophalangeal joints.

Nearly all cases of bacterial arthritis are due to hematogenous spread of bacteria to the joint. The bacteria evoke hyperemia and edema of the synovial membrane, which becomes infiltrated with leukocytes. Small vessels may rupture and cause microscopic hemorrhages. Fluid accumulates in the joint space and probably interferes with normal nutrition of the cartilage. The most devastating aspect of bacterial arthritis is the inflammatory damage to articular cartilage. The leukocytes in the joint release lysosomal enzymes that can digest cartilage and seem to destroy tissue. Since bacterial antigens, especially endotoxin, are themselves chemotactic, inflammation may persist after viable bacteria are killed (Braude et al., 1963; Curtiss and Klein, 1963; Dingle, 1973). The proteolytic enzymes produced by bacteria may also help destroy the joint. Inflammation can denude the joint of cartilage, but it rarely leads to spontaneous ankylosis in the adult. If the articular plate is penetrated by the infection, frank osteomyelitis can result. Pannus may form if the infection is not promptly controlled.

Predisposing Conditions. The principal predisposing factor is infection outside the joint. However, bacterial arthritis can occur following a bacteremia without any other apparent focus of infection. The knee, hip, and shoulder are most often affected. There is often no explanation for localization of infection in a particular joint, but previously damaged joints, especially those with rheumatoid arthritis, seem particularly vulnerable. (Hypocomplementemia may also increase the susceptibility of rheumatoid joints [Hunder and McDuffie, 1973]). Bacterial arthritis is also associated with diseases and treatment in which immune mechanisms are impaired, such as malignancy, diabetes mellitus, and sickle cell anemia. Patients with sickle cell anemia are especially prone to *Salmonella* infections, probably because of decreased splenic function as well as iron overload. High local concentrations of injected corticosteroids may also predispose to joint infection and may account for the increase in the incidence of shoulder joint infections that has been observed in the last ten years (Chartier et al., 1959; Kelly, 1977). Heroin addicts are peculiarly disposed to infections of axial skeletal joints with *P. aeruginosa* and *Serratia marcescens.* There is no explanation for the unusual distribution of these infections or for their unusual etiology (Kido et al., 1973).

Patients who develop gonococcal arthritis may be predisposed to disseminated infection by a deficiency of serum bactericidal activity (McCutchan et al., 1978). The strains that cause disseminated infections are often auxotrophs and differ from strains of *N. gonorrhoeae* that are limited to mucosal surfaces (see Chapter 192). Patients with congenital absence of one of the terminal complement components (C6 through C8) are uniquely predisposed to disseminated neisserial infections (Lee et al., 1978).

Infections of prosthetic arthroplasties are initiated either at the time of surgery or any time afterward by the hematogenous route. Operative sepsis, when due to organisms of low virulence, may not become apparent for several weeks. The prosthetic joint apparently remains susceptible to hematogenous infection indefinitely. These late infections often originate from urinary tract infections. Residual synovium, the pseudocapsule, or the bone in which the prosthesis is anchored may be infected (Wilson et al., 1975).

CLINICAL MANIFESTATIONS

Adults. The infection usually starts abruptly with fever, pain, and swelling of the affected joints. Rarely, multiple joints may be affected simultaneously. Gonococcal infections involve small joints more commonly than do staphylococcal infections. Gonococcal arthritis is classified into two clinical categories: disseminated gonococcal arthritis (DGA) and gonococcal arthritis (GCA). The first is associated with bacteremia and its manifestations: fever, chills, characteristic skin lesions, and multiple joint involvement (See Chapter 192). The latter (GCA) presents as a "septic joint." Masi and Eisenstein (1981) consider this classification an oversimplification and view the disease as a continuum. The infected joint is characteristically warm, painful, tender, and swollen with joint fluid. Movement of the joint, either active or passive, produces pain. Occasionally, these signs of joint infection are less dramatic so that the diagnosis is delayed. Infected rheumatoid joints are often mistaken for an exacerbation of the rheumatoid process. Other noninfectious conditions, such as gout and Reiter's syndrome, may mimic infection. Patients with gonococcal arthritis may or may not have clinical evidence of genital infection or pharyngitis.

The most direct avenue to diagnosis of bacterial arthritis is aspiration of joint fluid. Infected fluids are usually yellow, turbid, and have a friable mucin clot. The white blood cell count is 10,000 to 100,000 and most of the cells are granulocytes. The protein content is elevated and the glucose concentration is almost always less than half the serum value. Gram stains are often positive except in gonococcal infections. A specific etiologic diagnosis is made by culturing the joint fluid. Blood cultures should also be obtained because in many cases *Neisseria meningitidis* and *N. gonorrhoeae* cannot be recovered from joint fluid cultures but can be grown from blood cultures. All joint fluids should be cultured on chocolate agar under CO_2 for *Neisseria* and on blood agar for *H. influenzae.*

Most patients with septic arthritis have leukocytosis and elevated erythrocyte sedimentation rates, an exception being patients with acute gonococcal infections. X-rays show only enlargement of the joint space and soft tissue swelling due to edema of periarticular structures. After several weeks of infection, rarefaction of subchondral bone develops along with narrowing of the joint space because of destruction of the articular cartilage.

Infections of prosthetic joints may cause characteristic signs and symptoms of inflammation, especially those infections that begin in the immediate postoperative period. There is usually drainage (sometimes bloody), which contains the responsible bacteria; blood cultures may also be positive. Delayed infections often occur without producing any signs of inflammation, and pain is the only symptom. Radiographic evidence of a loose prosthesis and an elevated erythrocyte sedimentation rate may be the only clues preoperatively that there is an infection. The diagnosis is made by surgical exploration, biopsy, and culture (Fitzgerald et al., 1977).

Children. Bacterial arthritis in children presents with more characteristic symptoms and signs than does acute hematogenous osteomyelitis. Bacterial arthritis must be distinguished from rheumatic fever and rheumatoid arthritis. The most difficult distinction to make is that between benign, self-limited, sterile inflammation of the hip and bacterial arthritis of the hip. In bacterial infections, the patient is younger, the temperature and erythrocyte sedimentation rate are elevated, polyarticular involvement is more likely, and cell counts of joint fluid are higher. In the final analysis, only a positive culture or isolation of the organism from a focus in another system or from the blood may give the final answer (Molteni, 1978).

DIFFERENTIAL DIAGNOSIS. Suppurative bacterial arthritis must be distinguished from arthritis caused by mycobacteria, *Brucella* organisms, syphilis, *Streptobacillus moniliformis*, *Salmonella* organisms, fungi, and viruses. Arthritis can be caused by any of the 3 species of *Brucella* and usually has an acute onset with purulent joint fluid. Like pyogenic arthritis, *Brucella* arthritis attacks the large joints, especially the hips, ankles, and sacroiliac joints and cannot be distinguished on clinical grounds from acute pyogenic arthritis. *Brucella* organisms can be cultured from the joint fluid and blood, and serum agglutinins usually reach a titer of 1:320 or more. Mycobacterial (usually *M. tuberculosis* but sometimes *M. kansasii* or *M. intracellu-*

lare) arthritis is milder than pyogenic arthritis and may last for months or years without recognition. It is often confused with rheumatoid arthritis. Only about 50 per cent of patients with skeletal tuberculosis have active concomitant pulmonary tuberculosis, and there is often a history of antecedent local trauma to the affected joint, or of steroid injections. The mild clinical manifestations are attributed to the fact that the joint inflammation from caseating granulomas is milder than that with acute suppuration. Next to the spine, tuberculous arthritis attacks chiefly the hips or knees. The warm, swollen soft tissues around these joints have a peculiar doughy consistency and are not usually red. A surprising feature is the cell count of the joint fluid: there are usually over 10,000 cells/mm^3 and the majority are often polymorphonuclears. Acid-fast smears are positive in only 30 per cent but cultures of the fluid or synovial biopsy tissue yield the tubercle bacillus in over 80 per cent of cases. Biopsies of the synovium show granulomas in over 90 per cent.

Septic arthritis due to *Salmonella, E. coli,* and other enteric bacilli is an acute pyogenic infection but occurs mainly in sickle cell disease, systemic lupus erythematosus, chronic rheumatoid arthritis, and other debilitating diseases. These infections tend to be monoarticular and usually in the knee. Arthritis due to *E. coli* is often accompanied by *E. coli* cystitis or pyelonephritis. Because of the underlying problems, these gram-negative bacillus infections show a poor response to treatment. *Pseudomonas aeruginosa* has become the most important nonenteric gram-negative bacillus causing arthritis. It is especially prominent as a cause of monoarticular infection in heroin addicts, in whom it has a predilection for the sternoclavicular and sacroiliac joints.

Three other bacterial infections must also be kept in mind in the differential diagnosis of septic arthritis. *Streptobacillus moniliformis*, the cause of rat bite fever, produces a very painful migratory polyarthritis in 50 per cent of cases, and tends to involve large joints. Syphilis produces migratory polyarthralgia due to periostitis in the secondary stage, Clutton's joints in older children (8 to 16 years), and Charcot joints in tabes dorsalis. The painless bilateral hydroarthrosis of Clutton's joints, and the noninflammatory neuropathic joint of Charcot's disease are easy to distinguish from acute bacterial arthritis. The third bacterial infection to be considered is septic bursitis. This is a disease of the olecranon (80 per cent) and prepatellar bursae, and is sometimes confused with infection of the elbow or knee joints themselves. It is not, however, associated with septic arthritis and is recognized by the characteristic swelling of the bursa, by a history of trauma or sustained pressure, and by examination of bursa fluid, which is purulent and usually infected with staphylococci.

Bacterial arthritis must also be differentiated from acute viral arthritis due to rubella, mumps, hepatitis B, and certain togaviruses. Before its eradication, smallpox was also a cause of infectious arthritis. Most of these tend to be polyarticular and can cause severe pain. Rubella arthritis is a common problem in adolescents and adults. It usually starts when the rash is fading and it involves both large and small joints. Because of its migratory polyarticular nature, it tends to resemble rheumatic fever or rheumatoid arthritis more than septic arthritis. Although massive effusions can occur in large joints, much more commonly fusiform swellings develop in the fingers. All manifestations usually go away in 5 to 10 days. Mumps arthritis is also polyarticular and migrates to large and small joints, but is rare. Varicella is another rare cause of arthritis; it can produce pain and a monoarticular effusion in the knee without erythema. The synovial fluid has a few thousand lymphocytes. The polyarthritis of hepatitis B virus infection occurs in the preicteric stage, is usually a symmetric disease of distal joints, but may affect large joints as well. Patients with hepatitis may seem to have various forms of acute arthritis, only to have the diagnosis clarified when jaundice appears. The two togaviruses that cause prominent joint symptoms are both alphaviruses: Chikungunya fever virus and Ross River virus. Chikungunya fever is a disease of Southeast Asia and Africa in which joint pain is so severe that the patient literally folds up from the immobilizing discomfort. The crippling joint pains may return periodically over the next four months. The occurrence of a maculopapular rash and the leukopenia help differentiate this disease from pyogenic infections. In addition, joint swelling and redness is not common. Ross River virus also causes an illness with febrile rash and is endemic in Australia, but has recently caused a large outbreak in Fiji, where a number of American tourists became infected. The disease in Australia, known as epidemic polyarthritis is characterized by mild joint pains and is transmitted by bites of *Aedes vigilax* and *Culex annulirostris.*

Any of the deep fungus infections can produce arthritis by extension from adjacent areas of osteomyelitis. This form of secondary fungal arthritis is most common in mycetomas, and easily recognized by the characteristic antecedent infection of the bone and soft tissues (Chapter 252). Occasionally, however, the agents of mycetoma, such as *Petriellidium boydii*, can be inoculated directly into the joint and cause primary arthritis, especially of the knee. Coccidioidomycosis and sporotrichosis are much more important causes of fungal arthritis and need to be distinguished from bacterial arthritis. Primary pulmonary coccidioidomycosis can be accompanied by a transient arthritis in which the joints are painful, tender, swollen, and red. The fungus is not present in the joint and the arthritis disappears. In about 33 per cent of cases of chronic dissemination, *Coccidioides immitis* invades the joints, usually the ankle, but the knee, elbow, wrist, shoulder, and hand are also infected in the order of frequency listed, and often more than one at a time. The infection starts as an acute arthritis with swelling and redness but later causes a chronic monoarticular arthritis. This may occur without evidence of coccidioidomycosis elsewhere, usually involves the knee, and no adjacent bone involvement is seen on x-ray examination. *Coccidioides immitis* is readily cultured from joint fluid, synovial biopsy tissue, or drainage from articular sinuses. In sporotrichosis, arthritis can be secondary either to hematogenous dissemination or trauma. The hematogenous form of arthritis can be one of several sites of disseminated infection with migratory joint swellings and effusions, or it may be the only metastatic focus. Traumatic synovitis results from penetrating injury of a joint or tendon sheath and tends to occur in alcoholic gardeners because the fungus can penetrate deeper when pain is blunted by inebriation. It tends to involve the wrist, which becomes swollen, painful, and tender. Unless the synovium is biopsied and cultured with *Sporothrix* in mind, the diagnosis is usually missed and the patient mistakenly treated for tuberculosis after granulomas are seen in the joint tissue. *Candida* arthritis can also be hematogenous or traumatic. Hematogenous infection sometimes spreads to two or more joints and affects the knee, hip, and elbow in that order of frequency. Traumatic candidal arthritis is a complication of steroid injection. In contrast to other fungal infections, candidal arthritis is not granulomatous, and causes a polymorphonuclear exudate in acute infections. The yeast is seen and grown with ease in the joint fluid.

COMPLICATIONS AND SEQUELAE

Adults. Although bacterial arthritis is not a common disease, death attributable to this disorder has occurred in as many as 15 per cent of proven cases (Kelly, 1977). Spread to bone and ligaments around the joint can lead to a markedly unstable joint and necessitate external support or a surgical arthrodesis after infection is controlled. In adults, spontaneous bony ankylosis is not common. Because of loss of bone or poor positioning during the healing period, flexion contractures, inequality of limb length, and a painful joint may result. Persistent drainage may occur, especially if there is secondary osteomyelitis.

Children. Delay in diagnosis and therefore delay in treatment are the most important factors adversely affecting prognosis. One study of 49 patients indicated that 31 per cent were functionally impaired as the result of their infections (Howard et al., 1976). Bacterial arthritis of the hip may have serious sequelae such as discrepancies in limb length, persistent pain, and limitation of hip motion. These complications may require arthrodesis of the hip, epiphysiodesis to correct leg length, or an osteotomy to correct deformity. The hip and shoulder joints are especially prone to late sequelae because the ends of the bone are within the joint space. With accumulation of pus, increased pressure compromises the blood supply, and necrosis of the femoral or humoral head can occur. The destruction of joints seems to be equally likely with *S. aureus* and *H. influenzae* infections.

GEOGRAPHIC VARIATIONS. Geographic variation in the occurrence of bacterial arthritis is not striking if granulomatous infections are excluded. Large series with late follow-up are now available from North America (Morrey et al., 1975; Howard et al., 1976; Newman, 1976; Nade, 1977), Australia, and England, and no major differences in pattern are evident.

TREATMENT

Adults. It is necessary to identify the specific microorganism responsible for the infection and determine its susceptibility to antibacterials. If the diagnosis is established early, antibacterial treatment alone may cure the patient. Most antibiotics are transported into the synovial fluid, and concentrations are approximately equal to serum levels (Nelson, 1971; Parker and Schmid, 1971; Marsh et al., 1974). There is no reason to inject antibiotics directly into the joint space. Pneumococci and beta-hemolytic streptococci should be treated with penicillin G in a dose of 1 million units intravenously (I.V.) every 6 hours for 1 week. There are no convincing data to guide one in deciding how long the patient with *S. aureus* arthritis should receive antibiotics. However, it appears to us that a month of parenteral antibacterials is a helpful, albeit an arbitrary guide. Penicillin-sensitive (penicillinase-negative) staphylococci should be treated with 2 million units I.V. every 4 hours. Joint infections due to penicillinase-producing staphylococci require nafcillin or oxacillin in doses of 1.5 g I.V. every 3 hours; or cefazolin in a dose of 1.0 g I.V. every 8 hours in adults. Uncomplicated gonococcal arthritis can be cured with seven to ten days of either oral ampicillin, 2 g/day, or tetracycline, 2 g/day. More acutely ill patients should be treated with intravenous penicillin G in a dose of 10 million units/day for three days or until improvement occurs. Treatment is then continued with ampicillin for a total of ten days' combined therapy. Treatment of arthritis due to gram-negative bacilli depends on the results of sensitivity tests. In general, arthritis due to *P. aeruginosa* can be treated with gentamicin or tobramycin (80 mg I.V. every 8 hours) in combination with either ticarcillin, azlocillin, or mezlocillin (2.0 g every 3 hours I.V.).

There is controversy regarding removal of infected joint fluid. Experiments in animal models support a hypothesis that infected joint fluid interferes with metabolism of cartilage (Curtiss and Klein, 1965) and that its removal diminishes this damage (Daniel et al., 1975). On this basis surgeons favor removal of infected joint fluid. Easily accessible joints such as the knee, ankle, and shoulder can be aspirated by needle and syringe. If the fluid thickens or if the joint is one that is not easily aspirated—for example, the hip or sacroiliac joint—it may be necessary to open the joint and remove infected material by suction-irrigation. However, some cautionary notes must be made: (1) Addition of antibacterials to the irrigant may not only be unnecessary but can be harmful because potentially toxic antibacterials can be absorbed by synovial tissues and the antibacterial may be damaging to articular cartilage. (2) Suction-irrigation may allow entry of secondary invaders and cause superinfection, especially if kept in place beyond three to four days. Some authorities believe that periodic distention of the joint prevents adhesions.

Open drainage has been advocated recently (Ballard et al., 1975), as it was after World War I (Willems, 1919). Establishing open drainage may be necessary if purulent material tends to loculate in the recesses of the joint. This method may be useful in post-traumatic joint infections, which represent a different category of patients from those with hematogenous septic arthritis.

In the adult, the following brief outline suggests the management of bacterial arthritis when the diagnosis and institution of treatment have been delayed and one is faced with a surgical as well as a medical problem.

1. Débridement and arthrodesis are recommended for the knee, ankle, elbow, wrist, and subtalar joints. Compression by means of the Hoffman apparatus is useful.
2. For the hip, joint resection should be done, followed by skeletal traction and gradual ambulation with an ischial weight-bearing brace for three months.
3. For the glenohumeral, sternoclavicular, and acromioclavicular joints, débridement of the joint and immobilization in a sling are recommended. The treatment of infected prosthetic joints is often difficult. Most acute infections should be treated by removal of the prosthesis, surgical débridement, and four weeks of parenteral antibiotics, chosen according to the in vitro susceptibility of the pathogen. In some cases, if the components are not loose and there is no x-ray evidence of osteomyelitis, it may be possible to suppress the infection without removing the prosthesis. Once the infection has been brought under control, these patients should receive oral antibiotics indefinitely. Some patients with infections due to bacteria of low virulence, for example, *Staphylococcus epidermidis*, can be treated by removal of the prosthesis, débridement,

and antibiotics with reinsertion of a new prosthesis in six months (Wilson, 1978).

Children. It appears that bacterial arthritis of the hip in the child is best treated by immediate open surgical drainage. This statement may be controversial, but long-term follow-up studies suggest that the majority of bad results from bacterial arthritis occur after hip infections. In one series, 50 per cent of the late results were unsatisfactory. In the other joints that are more accessible to needle aspiration, daily needle aspiration may be adequate; if not, open drainage is preferable to no drainage. Management of late sequelae are discussed above.

In summary, early diagnosis, identification of the causative organism, and proper choice of antibacterial agent, plus removal of infected joint material, are the essential steps in the treatment of infections of the joint. Early diagnosis is all too often not established, and when first seen, some patients have irreparably injured joints. Once invasion of bone has occurred and ligamentous structures have been damaged, it seems likely that stability, mobility, and freedom from pain will have been lost.

References

Ballard, A., Burkhalter, W. E., Mayfield, G. W., Dehne, E., and Brown, P. W.: The functional treatment of pyogenic arthritis of the adult knee. J Bone Joint Surg [Am] 57:1119, 1975.

Braude, A. I., Jones, J. L., and Douglas, H.: The behavior of *Escherichia coli* endotoxin (somatic antigen) during infectious arthritis. J Immunol 90:297, 1963.

Chartier, Y., Martin, W. J., and Kelly, P. J.: Bacterial arthritis: Experiences in the treatment of 77 patients. Ann Intern Med 50:1462, 1959.

Curtiss, P. H., Jr., and Klein, L.: Destruction of articular cartilage in septic arthritis. I. In vitro studies. J Bone Joint Surg [Am] 45:797, 1963.

Curtiss, P. H., Jr., and Klein, L.: Destruction of articular cartilage in septic arthritis. II. In vivo studies. J Bone Joint Surg [Am] 47:1595, 1965.

Daniel, D., Akeson, W., and Amiel, D.: The effect of joint lavage in preventing cartilage destruction in an experimentally produced *Staphylococcus aureus* joint infection (abstract). J Bone Joint Surg [Am] 57:583, 1975.

Dingle, J. T.: The role of lysosomal enzymes in skeletal tissues. J Bone Joint Surg [Br] 55:87, 1973.

Fitzgerald, R. H., Nolan, D. R., Ilstrup, D. M., Van Scoy, R. E., Washington, J. A. II, and Coventry, M. B.: Deep wound sepsis following total hip arthroplasty. J Bone Joint Surg 59:847, 1977.

Howard, J. B., Highgenboten, C. L., and Nelson, J. D.: Residual effects of septic arthritis in infancy and childhood. JAMA 236:932, 1976.

Hunder, G. G., and McDuffie, F. C.: Hypocomplementemia in rheumatoid arthritis. Am J Med 54:461, 1973.

Kelly, P. J.: Infections of bones and joints in adult patients. Instructional Course Lectures 26:3, 1977.

Kido, D., Bryan, D., and Halpern, M.: Hematogenous osteomyelitis in drug addicts. Am J Roentgenol Rad Ther Nucl Med 118:356, 1973.

Krauss, D. S., Aronson, M. D., Gump, D. W., and Newcombe, D. S.: *Hemophilus influenzae* septic arthritis: A mimicker of gonococcal arthritis. Arthritis Rheum 17:267, 1974.

Lee, T. J., Utsinger, P. D., Snyderman, R., Yount, W. J., and Sparling, P. F.: Familial deficiency of the seventh component of complement associated with recurrent bacteremic infections due to *Neisseria*. J Infect Dis 138:359, 1978.

Marsh, D. C., Jr., Matthew, E. B., and Persellin, R. H.: Transport of gentamicin into synovial fluid. JAMA 228:607, 1974.

Masi, A. T., and Eisenstein, B. I.: Disseminated gonococcal infection (DGI) and gonococcal arthritis (GCA). II. Clinical manifestations, diagnosis, complications, treatment, and prevention. Semin Arthritis Rheum 10:173, 1981.

McCutchan, J. A., Katzenstein, D., Norquist, D., Chikami, G., Wunderlich, A., and Braude, A. I.: Role of blocking antibody in disseminated gonococcal infection. J Immunol 121:1884, 1978.

Molteni, R. A.: The differential diagnosis of benign and septic joint disease in children: Clinical, radiologic, laboratory, and joint fluid analysis, based on 37 children with septic arthritis and 97 with benign aseptic arthritis. Clin Pediatr 17:19, 1978.

Morrey, B. F., Bianco, A. J., Jr., and Rhodes, K. H.: Septic arthritis in children. Orthoped Clin North Am 6:923, 1975.

Nade, S.: Choice of antibiotics in management of acute osteomyelitis and acute septic arthritis in children. Arch Dis Child 52:679, 1977.

Nelson, J. D.: Antibiotic concentrations in septic joint effusions. N Engl J Med 284:349, 1971.

Newman, J. H.: Review of septic arthritis throughout the antibiotic era. Ann Rheum Dis 35:198, 1976.

Parker, R. H., and Schmid, F. R.: Antibacterial activity of synovial fluid during therapy of septic arthritis. Arthritis Rheum 14:96, 1971.

Willems, C.: Treatment of purulent arthritis by wide arthrotomy followed by immediate active mobilization. Surg Gynecol Obstet 28:546, 1919.

Wilson, M. R., Fitzgerald, R. H., Jr., and Coventry, M. B.: Reconstruction (delayed) by total hip arthroplasty after resection arthroplasty for infection. Proc Sci Meet Hip Soc 6:149, 1978.

Wilson, P. D., Jr., Salvati, E. A., and Blumenfeld, E. L.: The problem of infection in total prosthetic arthroplasty of the hip. Surg Clin North Am 55:1431, 1975.

Ziment, I., Davis, A., and Finegold, S. M.: Joint infection by anaerobic bacteria: A case report and review of the literature. Arthritis Rheum 12:627, 1969.

250

BACTERIAL OSTEOMYELITIS

ROBERT H. FITZGERALD, JR., M.D.

PATRICK J. KELLY, M.D.

Although osteomyelitis refers to an inflammation of the marrow (myelitis) of bone *(osteo)*, the term is generally understood to signify an infection of either the cortical or the medullary portion of a bone. Pyogenic or bacterial osteomyelitis can be subdivided into hematogenous and secondary forms of osteomyelitis; the latter includes osteomyelitis from a contiguous focus of infection and post-traumatic and postoperative osteomyelitis. The selection of treatment requires further subdivision into acute and chronic stages according to the clinical signs and symptoms and the pathologic changes.

PATHOGENESIS AND PATHOLOGY. The exact pathophysiologic changes in hematogenous osteomyelitis are incompletely understood. Although the initial pathologic changes may occur in various anatomic locations, the relatively high frequency of involvement of the metaphyses suggests that this site is vulnerable to infection. The vascular anatomy of the metaphysis (end arteries, capillary loops, and venous sinusoids) creates the necessary environment for the propagation of infective emboli (Trueta, 1959). Hobo (1921) demonstrated that the afferent capillary has no phagocytes and that in the efferent venous sinusoid, phagocytosis by leukocytes and endothelial cells is ineffective.

The infective embolus probably enters through the nutrient artery and lodges in the metaphyseal end artery–venous sinusoid. The local nidus of sepsis creates arterial occlusion. Both the host's humoral and cellular responses and the toxins released by the invading bacteria combine to produce tissue necrosis. The resulting debris, exudate, and acidosis increase the local pressure, which further compromises the circulation and promotes more necrosis. When defense mechanisms fail to eradicate the bacteria, an abscess (Brodie's abscess) surrounded by a fibrous membrane and a wall of dense bone may occur (Fig. 1). The infection may then become quiescent only to undergo recrudescence. Frequently, the bacteria are destroyed, and serous fluid or fibrous tissue fills the cavity. More frequently, the necrosis and increased pressure spread the infection through the paths of least resistance: the haversian and Volkmann canals and the intramedullary space. As the process continues, the pus forms a subperiosteal abscess and deprives the cortex of its periosteal blood supply. If the endosteal blood supply is occluded simultaneously, the entire cortex can become necrotic and sequestrated (Fig. 2). New periosteal bone is formed, and this creates an involucrum about the necrotic bone (the sequestrum). A reactive synovitis frequently occurs in adjacent joints. Healing with resolution of the infection may occur at any stage, by natural recovery or through the influence of antimicrobial agents.

Hematogenous osteomyelitis in adults is uncommon and usually affects the axial skeleton of patients in the fifth and sixth decades of life. An underlying debilitating condition such as diabetes mellitus is frequently noted. Most commonly, the thoracolumbar segments of the spinal column are involved. An antecedent infection of the pelvic organs or instrumentation of the urogenital tract is frequently associated with vertebral osteomyelitis and is considered to create a bacteremia, with retrograde seeding of the vertebral body through the interconnecting plexus of valveless veins, as described by Batson (1957). Arterial seeding through posterior spinal arteries into the nutrient artery is also believed to occur, and this is undoubtedly the route of infection in drug addicts (Wiley and Trueta, 1959). The vertebrae have capillary arcades and venous sinusoids adjacent to the vertebral end plate, reminiscent of the metaphysis of a long bone in a growing child. The intervertebral disk space becomes involved only after the end plate has been destroyed by the infection.

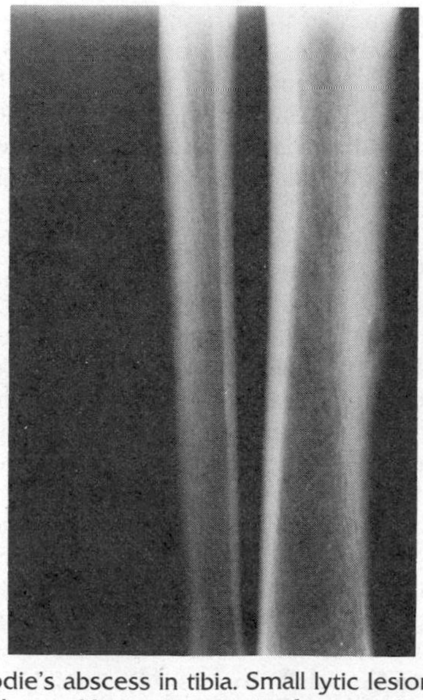

Figure 1. Brodie's abscess in tibia. Small lytic lesion surrounded by sclerotic bone. Note attempt to form a sinus tract, with erosion of sclerotic bone.

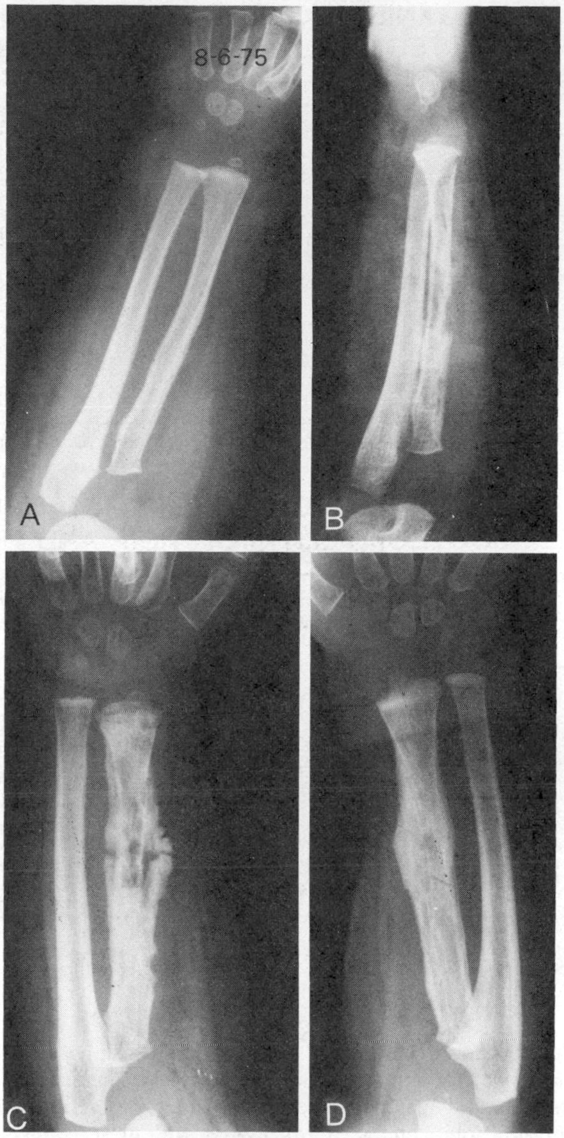

Figure 2. Acute osteomyelitis of radius and ulna in a child. *A,* Soft tissue changes can be seen within the first week after onset of symptoms. *B,* Lytic destruction of osseous architecture is seen in the third week. *C,* Elevation of periosteum with new periosteal bone formation has resulted in sequestration of entire radius. *D,* Healing of osteomyelitic process is well demonstrated.

ETIOLOGY

Hematogenous Causes. *Staphylococcus aureus* causes 80 to 90 per cent of hematogenous bone infections in children (Morrey and Peterson, 1975). Group A beta hemolytic streptococci are seen most frequently in children under 3 years. Gram-negative bacteria, other than *Haemophilus influenza*, are encountered very infrequently in children, except for those with sickle cell anemia who are susceptible to infection with *Salmonella enteritidis*.

Adults with acute vertebral osteomyelitis are also most often infected with *S. aureus*. Enteric gram-negative bacilli such as *Escherichia coli* also cause vertebral osteomyelitis, especially when the infection originates in the urinary tract. In drug addicts *Pseudomonas aeruginosa*, *Serratia marcescens*, or *S. aureus* often causes osteomyelitis.

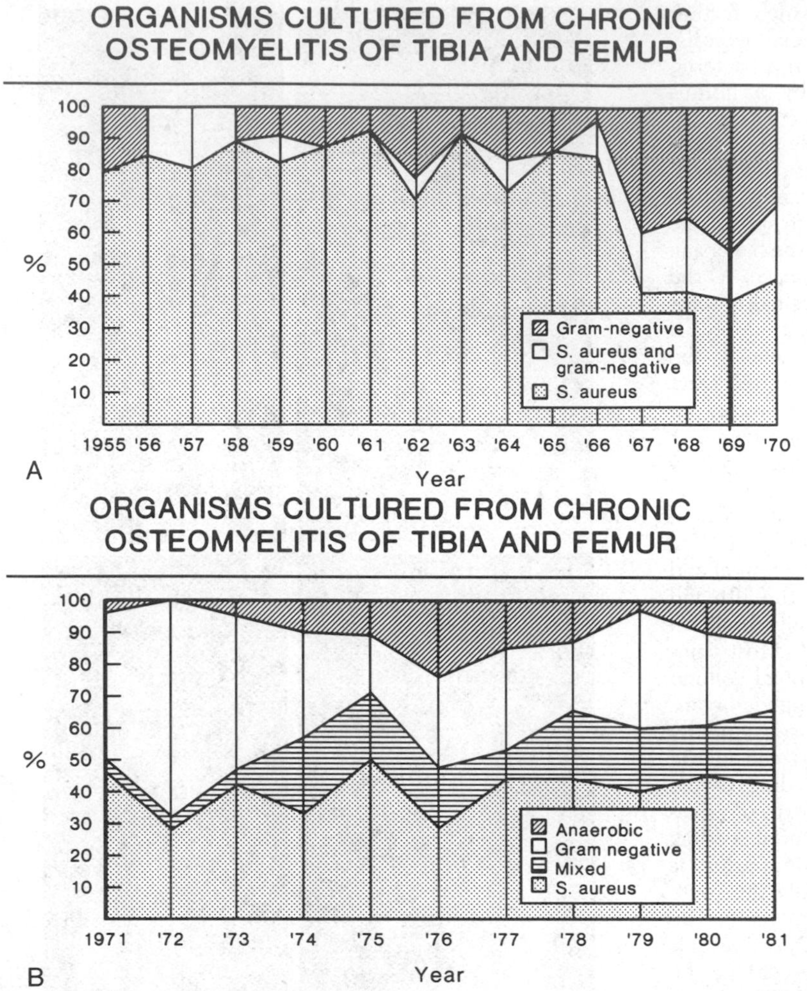

Figure 3. Isolates recovered from tissue cultures obtained at débridement in patients with chronic osteomyelitis.

Contiguous Focus. Bone infections that originate from contiguous soft tissue infections can have various bacterial etiologies and may even be due to mixtures of bacteria from multiple genera. *S. aureus* is the most common etiology, but various gram-negative bacteria can cause osteomyelitis in this clinical setting (Fierer et al., 1979). Identification of the etiologic agent can be difficult in these cases because many have received an antibiotic for their soft tissue infection, which prevents the growth of the primary pathogen but allows the superficial overgrowth of antibiotic-resistant, colonizing bacteria in the wound. A specific syndrome of osteomyelitis due to *P. aeruginosa* has been recognized in patients who sustain a puncture wound of the foot.

Post-traumatic and Postoperative Causes. Whereas *S. aureus* is the cause of hematogenous osteomyelitis in the vast majority of patients, contamination of traumatic wounds with soil and water results in infections due to a diverse group of microorganisms. Gram-negative bacilli, in particular *Pseudomonas aeruginosa,* have been isolated in more than half the patients, and even fungi are occasionally isolated in post-traumatic osteomyelitis. When anaerobic bacteria are isolated, it is usually as part of a mixed culture containing facultative anaerobes.

The microbiologic findings in chronic hematogenous osteomyelitis are different from those in post-traumatic and postoperative osteomyelitis. Gram-positive bacteria, especially *S. aureus,* are isolated in patients with postoperative and chronic hematogenous osteomyelitis. Gram-negative bacilli predominate in post-traumatic osteomyelitis. The increasing frequency of post-traumatic osteomyelitis is reflected in our overall experience with the microbiologic findings in chronic osteomyelitis (Fig. 3). *S. aureus,* formerly the causal organism in 80 per cent of patients with chronic osteomyelitis, is still most frequently isolated, but gram-negative bacilli and anaerobes are cultured with increasing frequency.

CLINICAL MANIFESTATIONS

Hematogenous. Acute hematogenous osteomyelitis is primarily a disease of children between the ages of 3 and 15 years. The abrupt onset of pain of increasing severity, frequently after minor trauma, and fever are the cardinal symptoms. Irritability, lethargy, and dehydration are usually present as well. The principal signs are tenderness, erythema, and swelling. The joints of the involved extremity are held in flexion, and the enveloping muscles are in spasm. Unless done gently, passive motion in the adjacent joints is resisted. Fluctuation is not found until the abscess cavity has ruptured through the periosteum. Pseudoparalysis is frequent. Leukocytosis, with counts as high as $30{,}000/mm^3$, and a shift to the left usually occur. An elevated erythrocyte sedimentation rate is characteristic. Although roentgenographic examination in the acute phase demonstrates a normal osseous pattern, careful inspection frequently identifies alteration of the soft tissues. A localized destructive process surrounded by a zone of decalcification in the metaphysis is observed 10 to 14 days after the onset of the disease (Fig. 4). Subsequently, the periosteal shadow at the same level is elevated, and periosteal calcification may occur. In the untreated patient, the periosteum may be elevated in a circumferential fashion, creating an involucrum of the entire bone. Eventually, the trabeculae of the metaphysis are eroded, giving a moth-eaten appearance (Fig. 4B).

Before definitive roentgenographic changes of the osseous structure are seen, a technetium-99 scan frequently demonstrates the area of involvement. The earliest detectable change may be a decrease in uptake of the isotope in the metaphysis. Increased uptake occurs a few days later. Because the isotope is normally concentrated in the metaphysis, it may be difficult to distinguish changes due to infection, and a normal scan does not exclude the diagnosis within the first five days of infection.

Hematogenous osteomyelitis has a predilection for the metaphyseal region of a long tubular bone. The distal femoral and the proximal and distal tibial metaphyses are the most frequent sites of involvement. Infection of the proximal femoral metaphysis is intracapsular and frequently is associated with septic arthritis of the hip. The humerus, fibula, radius, and ulna are involved less frequently. The pelvis is infected but only uncommonly. In the child with spinal involvement, the arterial blood supply to the disk space results in disk space infections rather than vertebral osteomyelitis, as seen in the adult.

A subacute form of the disease is occasionally encountered in a child who has received inadequate antimicrobial therapy. This illness has few systemic symptoms and a persistence of regional physical findings. Although the leukocyte count may have returned to normal as the result of incomplete therapy, the erythrocyte sedimentation rate remains elevated. Roentgenographic changes usually are seen.

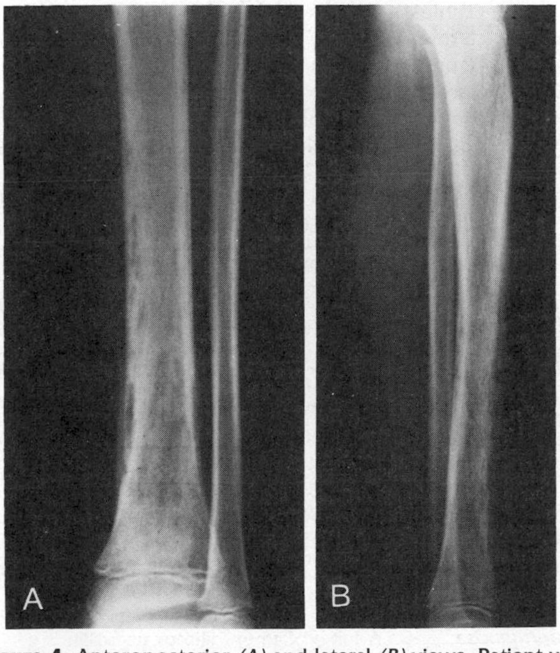

Figure 4. Anteroposterior *(A)* and lateral *(B)* views. Patient with osteomyelitis of distal tibial metaphysis. Periosteal elevation and localized lytic destruction with surrounding zone of decalcification are well illustrated.

Although the patient with acute vertebral hematogenous osteomyelitis may have severe back pain and systemic signs of acute sepsis, the clinical signs and symptoms are frequently insidious, with little systemic reaction. Localized pain to the area of involvement is the most characteristic symptom. There is usually severe paraspinal spasm and splinting to prevent spinal motion. Palpation and percussion over the afflicted area precipitate exquisite pain.

There is frequently a normal or slightly elevated leukocyte count. Elevation of the erythrocyte sedimentation rate is the most frequent abnormal laboratory finding. During acute systemic disease, the causal organism may be identified with cultures of blood and tissue obtained by needle biopsy of the vertebral body. In the subacute and chronic phases of the disease, the causal organism is difficult to isolate. As with other types of acute osteomyelitis, roentgenographic findings are normal for the first 10 to 14 days. The earliest changes include narrowing of the disk space and demineralization of the end plate. Erosion of the vertebral body and end plate follows. Loss of vertebral height frequently occurs. During the early phase, a technetium-99 scan can be helpful in identifying the level involved.

Blood cultures are positive in approximately two thirds of patients with acute osteomyelitis. In the remaining third, the diagnosis is made by aspiration of a contiguous abscess or needle biopsy of the subperiosteal space or metaphysis. If needle aspiration yields only sterile blood, it may be necessary to repeat the procedure if the patient has not responded to empiric therapy. Open biopsy of the affected vertebrae may be necessary to establish the diagnosis in adults.

Osteomyelitis from a Contiguous Focus of Infection. Osteomyelitis secondary to exogenous contamination or spread from a contiguous focus of infection that has been incompletely treated is being seen with increasing frequency (Fitzgerald et al., 1975). This form of osteomyelitis usually occurs after a puncture wound to the foot but also after an inadequately treated soft tissue abscess or septic arthritis. The patients usually have received incomplete antimicrobial therapy, which changed their clinical picture. They are frequently afebrile but have a limp or a painful extremity with regional muscular spasm. The sedimentation rate is usually elevated.

Because most of these patients are seen late in the infection, characteristic roentgenographic changes are present. Surgical débridement is invariably necessary. A retained foreign body is common after puncture wounds. When a foreign body is not encountered, the central focus involves a cartilaginous surface (articular, epiphyseal, apophyseal, or some combination of these).

With the improved diagnostic techniques and treatment of acute hematogenous osteomyelitis, the incidence of chronic hematogenous osteomyelitis has decreased and should continue to do so. The most common sites of involvement (the femur, tibia, and humerus) reflect the high incidence of osteomyelitis in these sites in children. The femur and tibia constitute almost 80 per cent of the long bones involved. Disease of the soft tissues about the involved bone can vary considerably. Contracted scar with little healthy tissue is noted in patients who have had repeated surgery or chronic drainage.

Laboratory tests are rarely of value in patients with

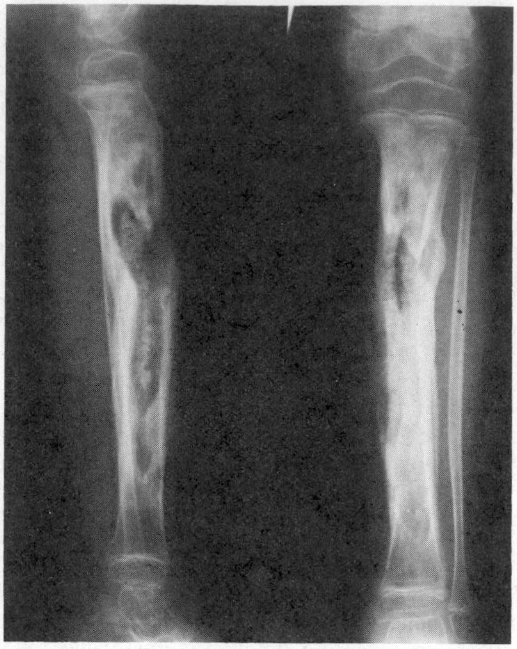

Figure 5. Chronic osteomyelitis of tibia, with sequestrum in intramedullary canal.

chronic osteomyelitis. Roentgenographic examination of the involved extremity demonstrates deformity with a mixture of lucent and sclerotic changes. Although sequestrum may be noted on routine roentgenograms, tomography may be needed to visualize the sclerotic changes (Fig. 5).

Post-traumatic and Postoperative Osteomyelitis. The neurovascular and other soft tissue injuries associated with fractures and dislocations of the musculoskeletal system increase the risk of infection in patients with severe traumatic injuries. The areas of involvement reflect the high incidence of traumatic injuries to the tibia and femur and, to a lesser extent, the bones of the upper extremity. Concomitant nonunion of fractures in as many as one third of the patients with post-traumatic osteomyelitis was noted by Fitzgerald and Kelly (1980).

Although comparisons are difficult, the prognosis in patients with either post-traumatic or postoperative osteomyelitis is similar to that in patients with chronic hematogenous osteomyelitis. Successful eradication of the infection is most frequent in the upper extremity, followed by the femur and tibia. Infection recurs more often in patients with a concomitant nonunion than in those with a united but infected fracture. Gram-negative bacilli are often isolated in pure or mixed culture in recurrent infections.

The incidence of osteomyelitis and postoperative wound infection after musculoskeletal surgery is unknown. The incidence of postoperative wound sepsis has been reported to vary from 1.0 to 7.4 per cent (Howard, 1964; Patzakis et al., 1974). However, most major institutions have reported an incidence of deep wound infection of 1 to 2 per cent after musculoskeletal surgery (Fitzgerald, 1979), the infection rate varying with the type of surgery. Elective procedures without the implantation of foreign bodies and procedures performed on children have a low infection rate (0.5 per cent) (Patzakis et al., 1974). In surgery after fractures and dislocations, especially with an open injury, the infection rate is usually 1 to 2 per cent. Procedures for implantation of a foreign body, especially the newer ones involving implantation of a total joint arthroplasty, have an infection rate of approximately 1 per cent (Fitzgerald et al., 1977).

Osteomyelitis frequently develops from infections after surgery that involves a foreign body: a plate, screws, a rod, or a total joint arthroplasty (Burri, 1975). Most infections are due to gram-positive bacteria acquired in the operating rooms. In recent years, anaerobic isolates have been identified in almost 25 per cent of such infections (Fitzgerald et al., 1977).

The prognosis is poor when infection occurs after the implantation of the foreign body. In general, the infection does not respond to treatment until the foreign body is removed. When infection occurs after open reduction and internal fixation of an acute fracture, débridement of the wound is done, leaving the foreign bodies in situ until first-stage osseous healing occurs if the device provides stability to the fracture. If the fracture is unstable, the internal fixation device should be removed, and an external fixation device or cast is used for immobilization until the fracture is healed. When an infection develops after an open fracture or fracture-dislocation, gram-negative bacilli predominate.

TREATMENT OF OSTEOMYELITIS

Acute Hematogenous Osteomyelitis. This is often a life threatening disease in children because of the associated staphylococcal bacteremia. Early treatment with antibiotics often obviates the need for surgery (Morrey and Peterson, 1975). If bony destruction is present on the initial radiograph or if there is soft tissue fluctuance indicating abscess formation, surgical débridement is necessary to prevent bone necrosis. Blood cultures should be obtained and abscesses aspirated before starting antibiotics. Since most infections are caused by *S. aureus* organisms that produce penicillinase, therapy should be started with a penicillinase-resistant beta lactam antibiotic. If a penicillin-sensitive strain of *S. aureus* is isolated, penicillin G is the treatment of choice (Table 1). Parenteral therapy should be continued for three to four weeks (Waldvogel et al., 1970). However, cooperative patients may be treated with parenteral therapy until they are afebrile for three days and then oral drugs in high doses for a total of four weeks of therapy (Bryson et al., 1979). The high doses of dicloxacillin and cephalexin

Table 1. ANTIBIOTICS USED IN THE TREATMENT OF OSTEOMYELITIS

Organism	Age	Antibiotics
S. aureus (beta-lactamase producing)	Adult	Oxacillin 3 g every six hours or cefazolin 1 g every six hours
	Child	Oxacillin 200 mg/kg/day or cefazolin 60 mg/kg/day
S. aureus (beta-lactamase negative)	Adult	Penicillin G 2 mega units every four hours or cefazolin 1 g every six hours
	Child	Penicillin G 0.5 mega units/kg or cefazolin 60 mg/kg/day
H. influenzae and	Child	Ampicillin 100 mg/kg or chloramphenicol 100 mg/kg
S. enteritidis	Adult	Ampicillin 2 g every six hours or co-trimoxazole 2 tabs twice daily
P. aeruginosa	Adult	Carbenicillin or ticarcillin 3 g every two hours plus gentamicin 1.5 mg/kg every eight hours

used in these studies are rarely tolerated by children, and comparable studies of oral therapy have not been done in adults.

When *H. influenzae* is the causal organism, antibiotic susceptibility studies are mandatory. In the past, isolates have been universally susceptible to ampicillin. However, in recent years, laboratory and clinical experience has unfortunately documented resistance to ampicillin and cefamandole. Chloramphenicol, with its effective bactericidal activity and favorable pharmacokinetic properties, remains an alternative agent. Moxalactam, a third generation cephalosporin, is highly active against *H. influenzae* and does not carry the serious toxic side effects of chloramphenicol (Marks, 1981).

Treatment of vertebral osteomyelitis in adults varies with the clinical condition of the patient. Immobilization of the spinal column relieves pain and promotes new bone formation, fusion of the involved disk space, and healing of the infection (Fig. 5). Antibiotics are administered intravenously until the patient is afebrile and has no systemic symptoms. Oral therapy can be continued for a total of four weeks if the pathogen is susceptible to orally absorbed antibiotics.

Chronic Osteomyelitis. In chronic hematogenous and post-traumatic osteomyelitis, it is essential to excise infected granulation tissue, including the dead and infected bone. Saucerization of the infected cavities of bone by unroofing procedures is frequently necessary. Once all the infected and dead tissues have been excised, the dead space can be eradicated at a subsequent operation. When the femur or humerus is involved, there is frequently sufficient healthy soft tissue to permit delayed primary or secondary closure over an irrigation-suction system. A myocutaneous flap or a muscle pedicle and split-thickness skin graft can be used to obliterate the dead space when the tibia, ulna, or radius is involved (Ger, 1977). Alternatively, the wound can be packed open, and, when a healthy granulating bed has been achieved, a split-thickness skin graft can be applied. Papineau (1973) has had good results with the application of cancellous bone grafts in the cavity with secondary split-thickness skin graft. In the distal forearm and hand, abdominal and thoracic pedicle flaps have been used with success. The use of the free-flap or composite free-tissue transfer can offer dramatic results if successful, but they are demanding techniques with the potential for complications (Taylor and Daniel, 1973; Serafin et al., 1980).

When osteomyelitis is associated with a nonunion of a fracture, control of the infection has first priority. In the past, the nonunion has been treated with a bone graft or internal fixation only after eradication of the infection and healing of soft tissue have occurred. However, with the advent of rigid external fixation devices, the fracture can be rigidly stabilized while the infection is being treated. Frequently, union occurs, thus obviating the need for subsequent internal fixation and bone grafting. Once the infectious process has been controlled, it is also possible to insert small divided cancellous bone grafts if the cavity has a good clean base of granulation tissue.

Results of susceptibility studies are considered in the selection of specific antimicrobial therapy in the adult with chronic osteomyelitis. The polymicrobic nature of post-traumatic osteomyelitis frequently warrants more than one antibiotic. Parenteral therapy for four weeks is essential for eradication of infection (Dich et al., 1975). If secondary bacterial invasion occurs with the isolation of nosocomial organisms from the irrigation-suction tubes or wound drainage, they should be treated with specific antimicrobial therapy. When the causal organism(s) is susceptible to an oral agent, it should be administered for 8 to 12 weeks following completion of parenteral therapy.

The recovery of a mixed flora consisting of gram-negative and gram-positive isolates from specimens of deep tissue can be difficult to evaluate. If necessary, multiple antimicrobial agents should be administered in order to treat all of the isolates, including anaerobes. If untreated, anaerobes are often isolated from the bone when infection recurs. The presence of mixed aerobic-anaerobic flora in an osteomyelitic lesion carries a poorer prognosis than a pure anaerobic or aerobic flora (Hall et al., 1983).

When second-stage surgical débridements are performed, additional specimens should be analyzed to ensure that the bacteria remain susceptible to the antibiotic drug used. Frequently, a gram-negative bacillus that is initially susceptible to the antimicrobial administered develops resistance, necessitating change of the treatment.

Irrigation-suction tubes are valuable in the management of the dead space that remains after saucerization of an osteomyelitic cavity (Kelly et al., 1970). In the past, such irrigation systems were empirically used for three weeks. Contamination of an irrigation-suction system with secondary gram-negative bacillary organisms is common after the reversal of the system if clotting or leakage occurs. Reversal of the system can lead to nosocomial colonization of the wound. Irrigation-suction tubes continue to be used in the management of osteomyelitis, but specimens of ingress and egress tubes for culture should be obtained every third day. The irrigation-suction system should be discontinued after five days, or after the first negative culture is obtained. The irrigation-suction tubes are rarely needed beyond ten days.

Creation of healthy tissue, both osseous and soft, with a good blood supply is the fundamental principle on which the treatment of osteomyelitis is based. Failure to remove inadequate fixation devices or to stabilize a nonunion by internal or external means can contribute to recurrent infection.

COMPLICATIONS OF CHRONIC OSTEOMYELITIS.

Three major complications of chronic osteomyelitis are seen: recurrent infection, malignant change, and amyloidosis. Recurrent infection is seen in 15 to 20 per cent of patients with chronic osteomyelitis and is usually associated with inadequate antimicrobial therapy, inadequate surgical treatment, or both (West, Kelly, and Martin, 1970).

Malignant change in association with chronic osteomyelitis can be carcinomatous or sarcomatous (Baitz and Kyle, 1964; Fitzgerald et al., 1976). Either tumor can occur as a consequence of post-traumatic or hematogenous osteomyelitis. Both types of malignant change probably result from a long-standing reparative process: either hyperplastic reparative epithelium or stimulated reticuloendothelial elements become neoplastic. Squamous cell carcinoma occurs in 0.2 to 1.7 per cent of patients with osteomyelitis (Sedlin and Fleming, 1963). The incidence in patients with wounds that drain for 20 to 30 years appears to be higher. Fitzgerald et al. (1976) reported that 19 of the 23 patients with squamous cell carcinoma complicating chronic osteomyelitis had post-traumatic osteomyelitis. All of the patients had long-standing osteomyelitis, ranging in duration from 18 to 72 years (mean, 42 years).

The clinical features of squamous carcinoma include a

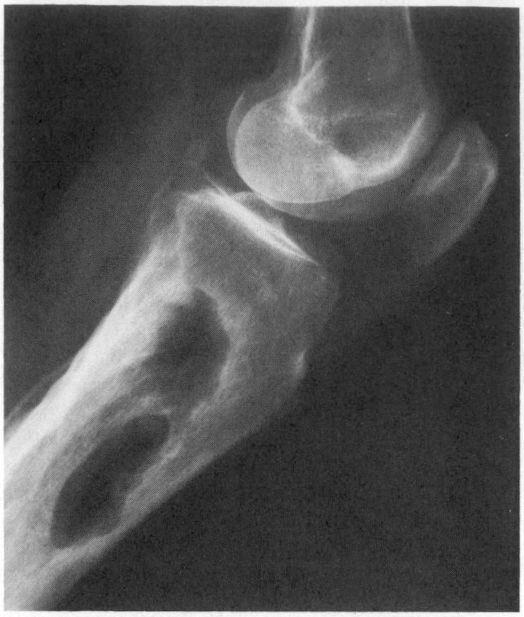

Figure 6. Squamous cell carcinoma in chronic osteomyelitis of tibia. Findings are indistinguishable from those of chronic osteomyelitis without carcinomatous change.

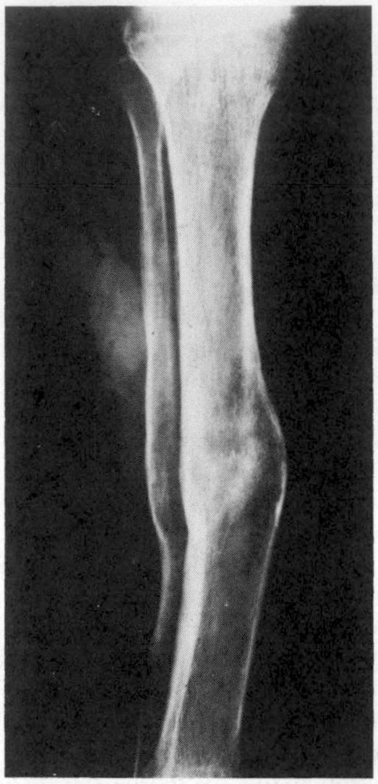

Figure 7. Squamous cell carcinoma in chronic osteomyelitis of tibia. Large soft tissue defect located posteriorly with a fungating soft tissue mass is demonstrated. It is highly suggestive of malignant change.

draining sinus that spontaneously develops a foul odor, increased pain, and increased drainage that is often bloody. An enlarging mass or a pathologic fracture may occur. Males predominate in a ratio of 10 to 1. Because osteomyelitis is tolerated longer in the lower extremity than in the upper, the femur and tibia are the most frequent sites of involvement.

Routine laboratory tests, including the sedimentation rate and leukocyte count, are of limited diagnostic value. A routine roentgenogram of the chest should be performed to evaluate the possibility of pulmonary metastasis. Osseous roentgenograms usually demonstrate lytic and sclerotic changes indistinguishable from chronic osteomyelitis (Fig. 6). However, a severely destructive lesion clearly different from the usual osteomyelitic process can be seen in some cases (Fig. 7).

Histologically, low-grade (Broders' classification), malignant-appearing squamous epithelium invading bone is seen. With ablative surgery (which is the treatment of choice), the prognosis for patients with carcinomatous degeneration is good. Only 2 of 21 patients who received aggressive surgical treatment reported by Fitzgerald et al. (1976) had metastatic disease and died secondary to the malignancy. Regional lymphadenopathy is usually inflammatory. Regional lymphadenectomy need not be performed unless lymphadenopathy persists longer than three months after ablative surgery.

Sarcomatous change in chronic osteomyelitis is much less common (Baitz and Kyle, 1964). Approximately 20 acceptable examples have been documented in the literature. Liposarcoma, myeloma, reticulum cell sarcoma, polymorphic sarcoma, myxofibrosarcoma, synovial sarcoma, and unclassified sarcomas have been reported. Pathologic fracture or a growing mass is the most common variety. Biopsy makes the histologic diagnosis. The prognosis for patients with sarcomatous degeneration is similar to that of patients with sarcomas without osteomyelitis.

The association of amyloidosis with long-standing osteomyelitis and tuberculosis was recognized years ago. Modern drug therapy has significantly limited this complication of osteomyelitis (Dahlin, 1949; Sherman, 1949; Cohen, 1967). Secondary amyloidosis is seen with equal frequency in patients with chronic hematogenous and post-traumatic osteomyelitis. In general, chronic or recurring osteomyelitis will have been present for 20 years or more before amyloidosis becomes evident. Most patients in whom secondary amyloidosis develops secondary to chronic osteomyelitis have osteomyelitis of the lower extremity.

Hepatosplenomegaly, a common finding in primary amyloidosis, is noted infrequently. Occasionally, peripheral edema of the involved extremity is seen. Laboratory evaluation of renal function is helpful in identifying the patient who has secondary amyloidosis. The serum creatinine and blood urea nitrogen levels are elevated. Proteinuria is seen on urinalysis. Renal biopsies are necessary to confirm the diagnosis. Hypertension is present in a minority of the patients with secondary amyloidosis. Improvement can be achieved by eradication of the infection. It is hoped that the improved prognosis for patients with osteomyelitis will make this complication of historic interest.

References

Baitz, T., and Kyle, R. A.: Solitary myeloma in chronic osteomyelitis. Report of case. Arch Intern Med 113:872, 1964.

Batson, O. V.: The vertebral vein system. Am J Roentgenol 78:195, 1957.

Bryson, Y. J., Connor, J. D., LeClerc, M., and Giammona, S. T.: High-dose oral dicloxacillin treatment of acute staphylococcal osteomyelitis in children. J Pediatr 94:673, 1979.

Burri, C.: Post-traumatic Osteomyelitis. Bern, Hans Huber Medical Publishers, 1975.

Cohen, A. S.: Amyloidosis. N Engl J Med 277:522, 574; 628, 1967.
Dahlin, D. C.: Secondary amyloidosis. Ann Intern Med 31:105, 1949.
Dich, V. Q., Nelson, J. D., and Haltalin, K. C.: Osteomyelitis in infants and children: A review of 163 cases. Am J Dis Child 129:1273, 1975.
Fierer, J., Daniel, D., and Davis, C.: The fetid foot: Lower extremity infections in patients with diabetes mellitus. Rev Infect Dis 1:210, 1979.
Fitzgerald, R. H., Jr.: Laboratory diagnosis of postoperative sepsis of the musculoskeletal system. Orthrop Clin North Am 10:361, 1979.
Fitzgerald, R. H., Jr., Brewer, N. S., and Dahlin, D. C.: Squamous-cell carcinoma complicating chronic osteomyelitis. J Bone Joint Surg [Am] 58:1146, 1976.
Fitzgerald, R. H., Jr., and Kelly, P. J.: Recurrent sepsis, malignant change, and sarcoidosis following post-traumatic osteomyelitis. In Hierholzer, G., and Lob, G. (eds.): Posttraumatic Osteomyelitis. New York, Springer Verlag, 1980.
Fitzgerald, R. H., Jr., Landells, D. G., and Cowan, J. D. E.: Osteomyelitis in children: Comparison of hematogenous and secondary osteomyelitis. Can Med Assoc J 112:166, 1975.
Fitzgerald, R. H., Jr., Nolan, D. R., Ilstrup, D. M., Van Scoy, R. E., Washington, J. A., II, and Coventry, M. B.: Deep wound sepsis following total hip arthroplasty. J Bone Joint Surg [Am] 59:847, 1977.
Ger, R.: Muscle transposition for treatment and prevention of chronic post-traumatic osteomyelitis of the tibia. J Bone Joint Surg [Am] 59:784, 1977.
Hall, B. B., Fitzgerald, R. H., Jr., and Rosenblatt, J. E.: Anaerobic osteomyelitis. J Bone Joint Surg [Am] 65:30, 1983.
Hobo, T.: Zur Pathogenese der akuten haematogenen Osteomyelitis, mit Berücksichtigung der Vitalfärbungslehre. Acta Sch Med Univ Imp Kioto 4:1, 1921.
Howard, J. M. (Chairman): Postoperative wound infections: The influence of ultraviolet irradiation of the operating room and of various other factors. Ann Surg 160 Suppl:1, 1964.
Kelly, P. J., Martin, W. J., and Coventry, M. B.: Chronic osteomyelitis. II. Treatment with closed irrigation and suction. JAMA 213:1843, 1970.
Marks, M. I.: Antibiotic therapy of serious Hemophilus infections—a continuing problem. J Pediatr 98:910, 1981.
Morrey, B. F., and Peterson, H. A.: Hematogenous pyogenic osteomyelitis in children. Orthoped Clin North Am 6:935, 1975.
Papineau, L.-J.: L'excision-greffe avec fermeture retardée délibérée dans l'ostéomyélite chronique. Nouv Presse Med 2:2753, 1973.
Patzakis, M. J., Harvey, J. P., Jr., and Ivler, D.: The role of antibiotics in the management of open fractures. J Bone Joint Surg [Am] 56:532, 1974.
Sedlin, E. D., and Fleming, J. L.: Epidermoid carcinoma arising in chronic osteomyelitic foci. J Bone Joint Surg [Am] 45:827, 1963.
Serafin, D., Sabatier, R. E., Morril, R. L., and Georgiade, N. G.: Reconstruction of the lower extremity with vascularized composite tissue: Improved tissue survival and specific indications. Plast Reconstr Surg 66:230, 1980.
Sherman, M. S.: Acute and chronic osteomyelitis. Surg. Clin North Am 29:117, 1949.
Taylor, G. I., and Daniel, R. K.: The free flap: Composite tissue transfer by vascular anastomosis. Aust NZ J Surg 43:1, 1973.
Trueta, J.: The three types of acute haematogenous osteomyelitis: A clinical and vascular study. J Bone Joint Surg [Br] 41:671, 1959.
Waldvogel, F. A., Medoff, G., and Swartz, M. N.: Osteomyelitis: A review of clinical features, therapeutic considerations, and unusual aspects. N Engl J Med 282:198; 260; 316, 1970.
West, W. F., Kelly, P. J., and Martin, W. J.: Chronic osteomyelitis. I. Fractures affecting the results of treatment in 186 patients. JAMA 213:1837, 1970.
Wiley, A. M., and Trueta, J.: The vascular anatomy of the spine and its relationship to pyogenic vertebral osteomyelitis. J Bone Joint Surg [Br] 41:796, 1959.

251

VERTEBRAL OSTEOMYELITIS

FRANCISCO L. SAPICO, M.D.
JOHN Z. MONTGOMERIE, M.D.

PYOGENIC VERTEBRAL OSTEOMYELITIS

Vertebral osteomyelitis is an infection of the axial, or vertebral, part of the skeletal system, arising by hematogenous or contiguous spread from adjacent soft tissue infection such as pressure sores. Vertebral osteomyelitis is the most common form of hematogenous bone infection in adults.

ETIOLOGY. *Staphylococcus aureus* accounts for more than 50 per cent of the bacteria responsible for hematogenous pyogenic vertebral osteomyelitis in the general population. Gram-negative aerobic bacilli have been isolated in 30 per cent of cases, with *E. coli*, *Proteus sp.*, and *Pseudomonas aeruginosa* being the most common pathogens, especially in association with preceding urinary tract infections. In contrast, among intravenous drug users, *Pseudomonas sp.* is most frequently isolated, with *S. aureus* second in frequency (Table 1). Other gram-negative bacilli, such as *Serratia sp.*, *Klebsiella sp.*, and *Enterobacter sp.*, as well as yeasts such as *Candida sp.* are also occasionally isolated from drug users. Hematogenous vertebral osteomyelitis is almost always monomicrobial, and polymicrobial infections are primarily secondary to contiguous spread from an infected pressure sore. In contrast to the frequent isolation in vertebral infections associated with a contiguous pressure sore, anaerobes are distinctly uncommon in hematogenous vertebral osteomyelitis.

The lumbar vertebrae are involved in about one-half of the cases of hematogenous vertebral osteomyelitis, followed by the thoracic and the cervical segments. Although occasionally affected along with adjacent L5 disease, the sacral

Table 1. DIFFERENCES IN CLINICAL FEATURES OF PYOGENIC VERTEBRAL OSTEOMYELITIS IN INTRAVENOUS DRUG ABUSERS AND IN THE GENERAL POPULATION*

	Drug Abusers	General Population	p Value (Chi Square Analysis)
Age group most frequently affected	Young adults	Elderly	
Male to female ratio	6:1	2:1	
Duration of symptoms > 3 months (%)	19	50	< 0.001
Involvement of cervical vertebrae (%)	27	7	< 0.001
Fever on presentation (%)	43	52	< 0.005
"Normal" admission plain spine films (%)	22	2	< 0.05
Most commonly isolated microorganism	*P. aeruginosa*	*S. aureus*	
Permanent neurologic sequelae (%)	0	6	0.07

*Data derived from Sapico, F. L., and Montgomerie, J. Z., 1979, and Sapico, F. L., and Montgomerie, J. Z., 1980.

vertebrae are frequently involved in contiguous spread from an adjacent infected pressure sore. In intravenous drug abusers, however, the most common site next to the lumbar segment is the cervical region, and thoracic involvement is much less common (Table 1).

PATHOGENESIS AND PATHOLOGY. The observation that adjacent vertebral end plates are very often involved simultaneously is consistent with arterial spread via the posterior spinal arteries. During embryogenesis, one sclerotome contributes to the formation of the two adjacent segments of the vertebral bodies as well as the intervening disk. The blood supply established during embryogenesis is therefore carried throughout life.

A complex network of intercommunicating paravertebral veins known as Batson's plexus has been considered a possible route of spread from communicating pelvic veins, especially when the postulated source of infection is the urinary tract. However, the infrequency of involvement of more than two vertebrae at a time and of "skip lesions" (presence of normal vertebrae in between affected ones) makes this route less likely than the arterial.

Lysosomal activity brought on by leukocytic infiltration is believed to cause destruction of bony trabeculae, penetration of the subchondral plate, and involvement of the intervertebral disc. Adjacent vertebral bony involvement is felt to be present even in cases where only disk-space narrowing is evident on plain x-rays. "Ballooning" of the intervertebral disk space may be associated with erosion of the vertebral bodies. Sequestration, although uncommon, may occur in advanced cases. Involvement of the posterior elements of the vertebrae is also uncommon, although neural arch involvement may be seen in advanced cases.

More than one-third of patients have no obvious demonstrable source of infection. Demonstrable or putative sources of infection in the remainder include the urinary tract (especially in the elderly), soft tissues, teeth, respiratory tract, intravenous foci, spinal surgery, endocarditis, and intravenous drug abuse.

CLINICAL MANIFESTATIONS. Pyogenic vertebral osteomyelitis is uncommon in children under 10 years. The so called "diskitis" of children is usually a benign disease of uncertain etiology and is considered a separate entity of nonbacterial origin. There is an increased frequency from 10 to 19 years of age, but the distinct majority of cases occurs after 50 years of age. Males outnumber females two to one. Diabetics appear to have an increased predilection for the disease.

Back or neck pain with or without stiffness is the most common presenting complaint, and is seen in at least 90 per cent of cases. About one-half of patients may have indolent symptomatology lasting for at least three months before presentation. A shorter duration of symptoms, however, is curiously seen in intravenous drug abusers (Table 1). Approximately 15 per cent of all patients may present primarily with atypical symptoms, such as occipital, arm, chest, abdominal, or leg pains. Patients with cervical osteomyelitis may complain primarily of sore throat and/or dysphagia. These complaints may overshadow any coexistent back pain, and are felt to be secondary to inflammatory irritation of nerve roots resulting in referred pain. Only slightly more than one-half of the patients are febrile. About 17 per cent of patients have variable degrees of neurologic deficits on presentation and limitation of back motion and/or a positive straight-leg raising sign are seen in 15 per cent.

Among the routine laboratory studies performed on admission, leukocytosis is seen in less than one-half of the cases, and the ESR is elevated in more than 90 per cent.

COMPLICATIONS AND SEQUELAE. Permanent neurologic deficits have been seen in about 6 per cent of patients overall, and less than 5 per cent die from the disease. These figures, however, include patients managed during the early years of antibiotic availability, and the adequacy of antibiotic therapy in some cases is questionable. Paraplegia usually results from extension and abscess formation in the epidural space. In these cases the diagnosis has been made too late. Paresis of an extremity as well as causalgia have been reported in a few patients. Permanent neurologic deficits and development of epidural or paravertebral abscesses appear to be significantly more common in diabetics. However, complications seem to be distinctly unusual in intravenous drug abusers (Table 1). Meningitis is a rarely observed complication. Large subcutaneous and intramuscular abscesses have been observed in patients with pre-existent sensory deficits, such as in spinal cord injury (Figure 1).

DIAGNOSIS. Erosive irregularities of the vertebral end plates with or without disk space narrowing is detectable

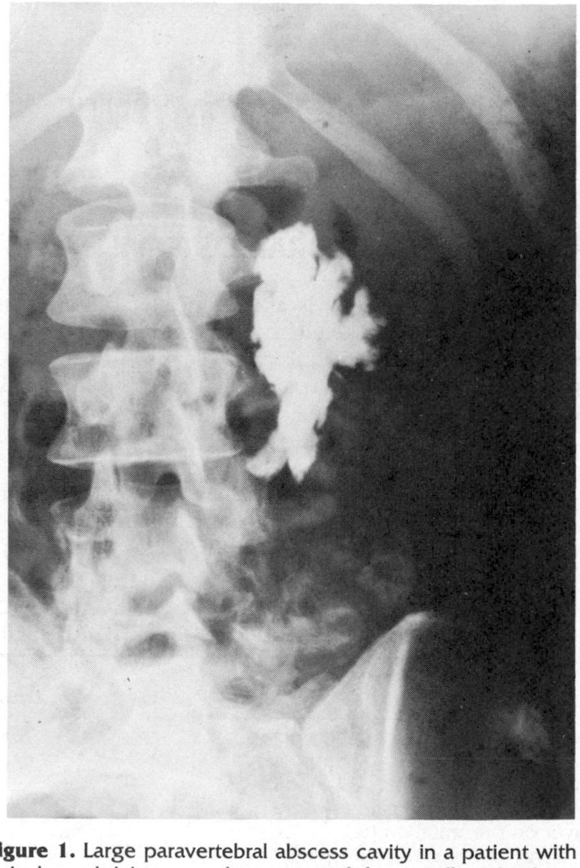

Figure 1. Large paravertebral abscess cavity in a patient with a spinal cord injury, as demonstrated by needle injection of contrast material. Note marked destructive changes of L4 and L5 vertebrae.

in 95 per cent of cases or more from plain antero-posterior and lateral spine films. Plain films, however, may appear normal in as much as 20 per cent of intravenous drug abusers on initial presentation (Table 1). Tomograms, technetium bone and gallium scans, however, should demonstrate the abnormalities in these cases.

Bulging of the psoas margins on plain x-ray films does not always mean that a psoas abscess is present, since it is also produced by inflammatory edema and chronic granulation tissue. Ultrasonography and, better yet, computerized axial tomography, appear very promising tests for these purposes. Any uncertainty may be resolved by needle aspiration.

In view of the wide spectrum of microorganisms capable of producing osteomyelitis, microbiologic diagnosis is of utmost importance. In most instances this can be carried out by needle biopsy and aspiration with the Craig needle under fluoroscopic, tomographic, or ultrasonic guidance. Failure is frequently followed by success on a second try. Otherwise open biopsy may be necessary.

The indolence and chronicity of some cases of pyogenic vertebral osteomyelitis may frequently make it difficult to distinguish from the chronic granulomatous processes such as tuberculous and fungal osteomyelitis. The ESR is more often in the normal range in tuberculous or brucella vertebral osteomyelitis than in the pyogenic variety. Concomitant reparative (i.e., sclerotic) and destructive changes on x-ray, although more common in tuberculosis, brucellosis, and actinomycosis, may also be seen in pyogenic vertebral osteomyelitis. Actinomycotic disease may have a "sieve-like" or honeycombed appearance on x-ray, produced by alternating areas of osteolysis and sclerosis. Disk space involvement and collapse are uncommon in actinomycosis and coccidioidomycosis. Coccidioidal vertebral osteomyelitis has a tendency to present with "skip" lesions and to involve the posterior elements of the vertebrae and ribs. A proclivity for rib involvement has also been described in blastomycosis. Metastatic neoplasms and multiple myeloma characteristically spare the disk space.

TREATMENT. Antimicrobial therapy has to be tailored to the microbiologic etiology of the disease as determined by needle biopsy or aspiration of the infected site, or by blood culture. Parenteral therapy should be given for a minimum of four weeks because shorter courses have failed. Single-antibiotic therapy with a semisynthetic penicillin appears adequate for *S. aureus* infections. Double-antibiotic therapy with an aminoglycoside plus an antipseudomonal penicillin has often been used for *P. aeruginosa* infections. Oral therapy after parenteral therapy has not been adequately evaluated and at present its use cannot be justified.

X-ray improvement may be quite slow despite proper therapy, and deterioration with increased demineralization may often be seen 3 to 4 weeks after starting antibiotics. Bony fusions may not be detectable for at least one year in some patients. A state of fibrous immobilization, however, may serve a similar function in the absence of complete arthrodesis. The ESR should drop to two-thirds of the pretherapy value by the end of four weeks of antibiotics. Longer courses may be indicated in patients who do not show this improvement in the ESR value.

Bed rest is an adequate method of immobilization in the vast majority of cases. If significant spinal stability exists, body jackets or braces may be used. Total body casts are seldom indicated.

SURGICAL MANAGEMENT. Epidural abscess requires immediate surgical decompression. In rare instances with longstanding extensive disease, the infected vertebra may be sequestered. Paravertebral abscesses have to be evacuated. Large subcutaneous or abdominal abscesses, which have been seen in patients with sensory loss, require drainage.

In the past, many surgeons performed debridement of the infected vertebra at the time of diagnosis or 3 or 4 weeks after starting antibiotics. One reason for this, (as mentioned earlier) was deterioration on x-ray after starting therapy. Demineralization of the bone may occur after starting therapy, but if other findings (i.e., pain, fever, and ESR) are improving, this does not necessarily indicate that the disease is progressing and surgical intervention is not indicated.

PROPHYLAXIS. Theoretically, prevention of bacteremia or its prompt treatment may decrease the frequency of vertebral osteomyelitis but this has not been demonstrated. In this respect we have been surprised that this disease is seldom associated with infective endocarditis.

TUBERCULOUS SPONDYLITIS

ETIOLOGY. Tuberculous spondylitis tuberculosis of the spine, the most common form of skeletal tuberculosis, is caused by *Mycobacterium tuberculosis*. It is predominantly a disease of children in developing nations and of the elderly in industrialized nations.

PATHOGENSIS AND CLINICAL MANIFESTATIONS. In contrast to its pyogenic counterpart, the lower thoracic and thoraco-lumbar segments are the most commonly involved. Collapse, gibbus formation, and paravertebral abscess formation are more common in tuberculosis as compared to pyogenic disease. Cold psoas abscess can track down within the muscle or muscle sheath and drain into the hip, the gluteal area, the groin, or the thigh. Most patients do not present with concomitant active pulmonary disease, and the radiological appearance of the vertebral lesion may be indistinguishable from pyogenic disease. The tuberculin skin test is characteristically positive. Vertebral instability or an epidural abscess or granuloma may result in paraplegia. Other causes of neurologic deficits are direct involvement of the spinal cord from contiguous spread, localized arachnoiditis, and thrombosis of a spinal artery. The progression of neurologic deficits tends to be more indolent than in pyogenic disease. The ESR may be normal in most patients with tuberculous vertebral osteomyelitis. Definitive diagnosis can be reached by needle biopsy or by open biopsy with subsequent histological examination and culture.

TREATMENT. The routine use of surgical anterior fusion in the management of spinal tuberculosis has been advocated, but is controversial. Conservative therapy without surgery is recommended by some authorities. If no improvement is noted after four to six weeks of triple antituberculous therapy, if there are severe neurologic deficits on admission, or if progressive neurological deterioration continues despite adequate chemotherapy, surgical decompression and stabilization surgery is indicated. Before the advent of rifampin, triple therapy with isoniazid, ethambutol, and paraminosalicylic acid had been advocated for a minimum of 18 months. Since infected bone has a paucity of tubercle bacilli, 300 mg isoniazid and 600 mg rifampin daily may be just as efficacious.

References

Gorse, G. J., Pais, M. J., Kusske, J. A., and Cesario, T. C.: Tuberculous spondylitis: A report of six cases and a review of the literature. Med 62:178, 1983.

Malik, G. M., Sapico, F. L., and Montgomerie, J. Z.: Severe vertebral osteomyelitis in patients with spinal cord injury. Arch Int Med 142:807, 1982.

Musher, D. M., Thorteinsson, S. B., Minuth, J. N., and Luchi, R. J.: Vertebral osteomyelitis: Still a diagnostic pitfall. Arch Int Med 136:105, 1976.

Sapico, F. L., and Montgomerie, J. Z.: Pyogenic vertebral osteomyelitis: Report of nine cases and review of the literature. Rev Inf Dis 1:754, 1979.

Sapico, F. L., and Montgomerie, J. Z.: Vertebral osteomyelitis in intravenous drug abusers: Report of three cases and review of the literature. Rev Inf Dis 2:196, 1980.

Waldvogel, F. A., Medoff, G., and Swartz, M. N.: Osteomyelitis: A review of clinical features, therapeutic considerations and unusual aspects. N Engl J Med 282:198, 260, 316, 1970.

Waldvogel, F. A., and Vasey, H.: Osteomyelitis: The past decade. N Engl J Med 303:360, 1980.

252

MYCETOMA

TARALAKSHMI V. VENUGOPAL, M.D.
PANKAJALAKSHMI V. VENUGOPAL, M.D.

Mycetoma is a chronic, suppurative, granulomatous disease of the subcutaneous tissues and bones. It is characterized by localized swellings with multiple sinuses discharging granules or grains that are the microcolonies of the causal agents.

ETIOLOGY. The etiologic agents of this clinical entity range from bacteria (actinomycotic mycetoma) to fungi (eumycotic or maduromycotic mycetoma). They exist free in nature as soil saprophytes or plant pathogens and enter the tissues through abrasion or implantation.

Actinomycotic mycetoma is caused by aerobic species of the actinomycetes group, belonging to the genera *Nocardia, Streptomyces,* and *Actinomadura* (Table 1). Eumycotic mycetoma is associated with a variety of fungi (Table 2); the most common are *Madurella mycetomii, Pseudallescheria boydii,* and *Acremonium* species (*Cephalosporium* species).

PATHOGENESIS AND PATHOLOGY. Mycetoma generally affects those parts of the body surface that come into contact with the soil. The agents from the soil are introduced into the tissues through traumatic or imperceptible abrasions of the skin. Acute suppurative inflammation burrows and spreads through the soft tissues and bones until sinuses communicate with the skin surface and discharge granules or microcolonies of the organism.

The size, shape, color, and texture of the granules vary with the infecting agent. Actinomycotic mycetomas have granules composed of filamentous mycelium of bacterial width and without chlamydospores. In eumycotic mycetoma, the granules consist of broad septate hyphae with well-defined walls and chlamydospores.

The histologic appearance of the granules in tissue sections is characteristic for most of the species of organisms (Figs. 1 through 5). The initial response of the host tissue to all agents of mycetoma is acute suppuration. This pyogenic reaction persists in actinomycotic mycetoma, whereas the true fungi evoke a foreign body response with the formation of granulomata with epithelioid hyperplasia and multinucleated giant cells.

CLINICAL MANIFESTATIONS. The exact incubation period of mycetoma is not known, but may vary from a few days to several months. The disease may develop at any age, with the maximal incidence between 21 and 40. Men are affected five times as often as women. The most common location of the infection is on the foot, although no site is exempt from mycetoma.

The condition often begins as a small, painless subcutaneous nodule at the site of previous injury, which then

Table 1. COMMON CAUSAL AGENTS OF ACTINOMYCOTIC MYCETOMA

Agent	Grain: Color	Grain: Approximate Diameter (mm)	Geographic Distribution	Rainfall (mm/year)
Actinomycetes:				
Nocardia asteroides	White	0.5	Ubiquitous	1000–2000
Nocardia brasiliensis	White	0.2	Mexico, South America, Africa, India	500–1500
Nocardia caviae	White	0.5	Ubiquitous	—
Actinomadura madurae	White to yellow	2	Africa, India, North and South America, Europe	250–500
Actinomadura pelletierii	Red to pink	1	Africa, India, North and South America	500–800
Streptomyces somaliensis	White to yellow	1	Africa, North and South America, Arabian peninsula, Israel, India	50–250

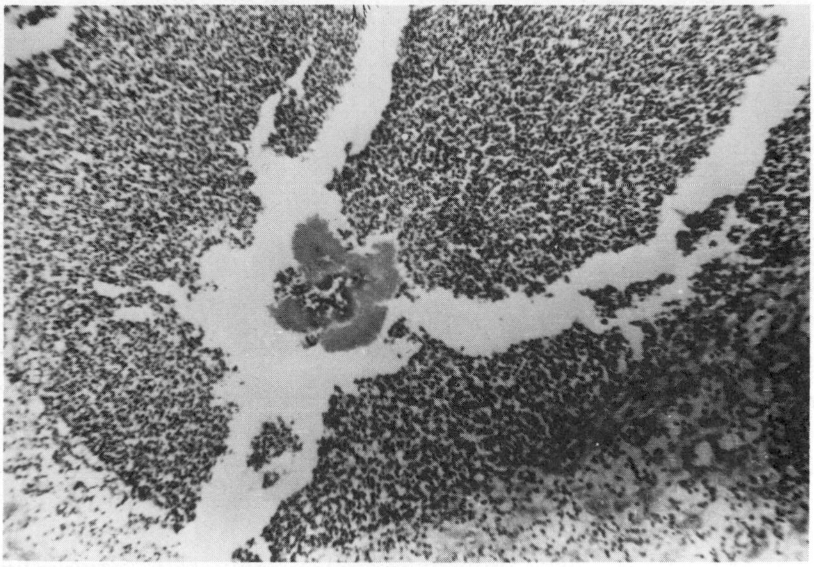

Figure 1. Small granule of *N. asteroides* surrounded by inflammatory cells. Hematoxylin and eosin stain. (×100)

Table 2. COMMON CAUSAL AGENTS OF EUMYCOTIC MYCETOMA

Agent	Grain: Color	Grain: Approximate Diameter (mm)	Geographic Distribution	Rainfall (mm/year)
Fungi				
Madurella mycetomii	Black to brown	1	Africa, India, Indonesia, North and South America, Europe	250–500
Madurella grisea	Black to brown	1	North and South America, Africa, India	—
Leptosphaeria senegalensis	Black	1	Senegal, Chad, Mauritania, India	250–500
Pyrenochaeta romeroi	Black	1	Mexico, South America, Africa, India	—
Phialophora jeanselmei	Brown to black	1	North America, Martinique, Congo, Europe	—
Pseudallescheria boydii	White to pale yellow	1	North and South America, Europe, Africa, India	1000–2000
Acremonium species	White to yellow or black	1	North and South America, Africa, Europe, India, Japan, Thailand, Malaysia	—
Neotestudina rosatti	Yellow	1	Somali, Senegal	—

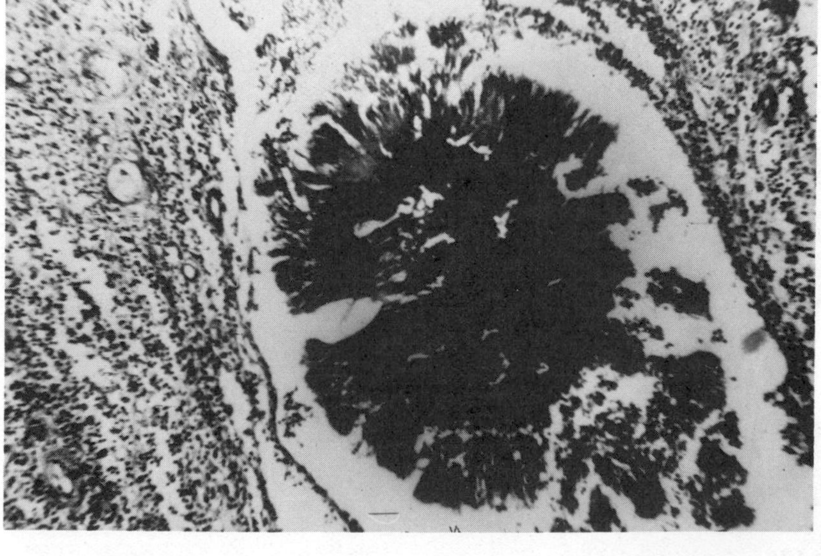

Figure 2. Large granule of *A. madurae* in subcutaneous tissue with characteristic fringe at the periphery. Hematoxylin and eosin stain. (× 100)

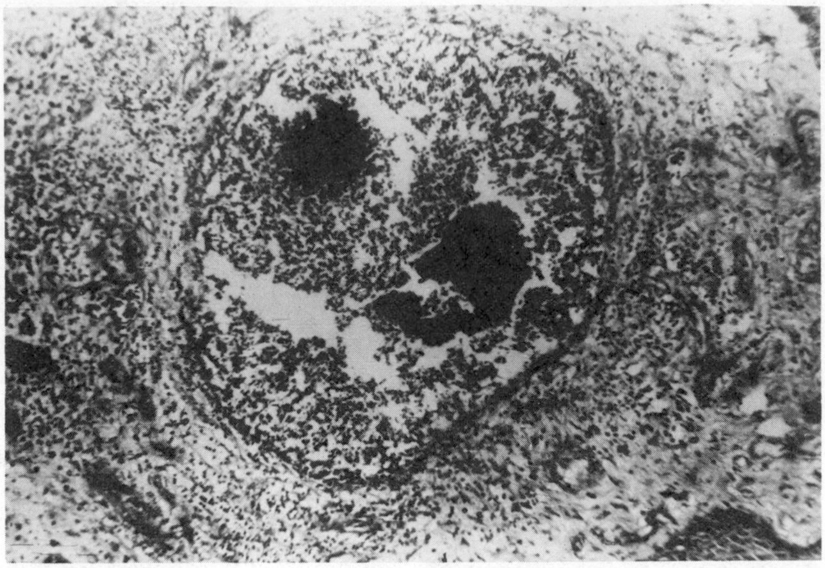

Figure 3. Granules of *A. pelletierii* with densely staining homogeneous matrix. Hematoxylin and eosin stain. (×100)

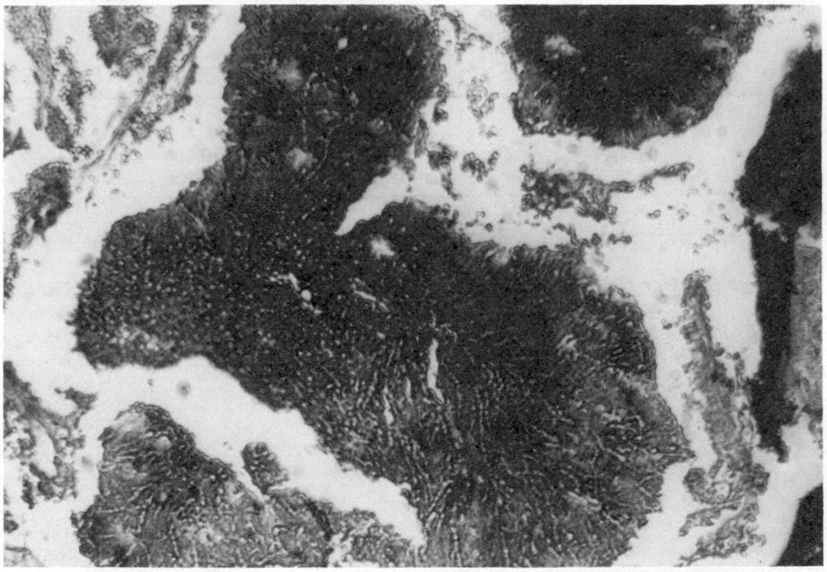

Figure 4. Granules of *M. mycetomii* with hyphae embedded in interstitial cement. Hematoxylin and eosin stain. (×100)

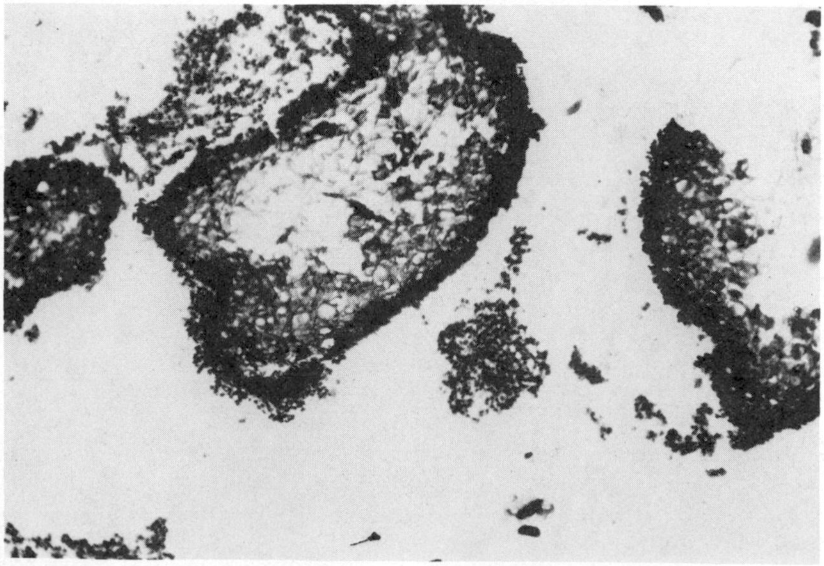

Figure 5. Granules of *L. senegalensis* with large vesicles. Hematoxylin and eosin stain. (×100)

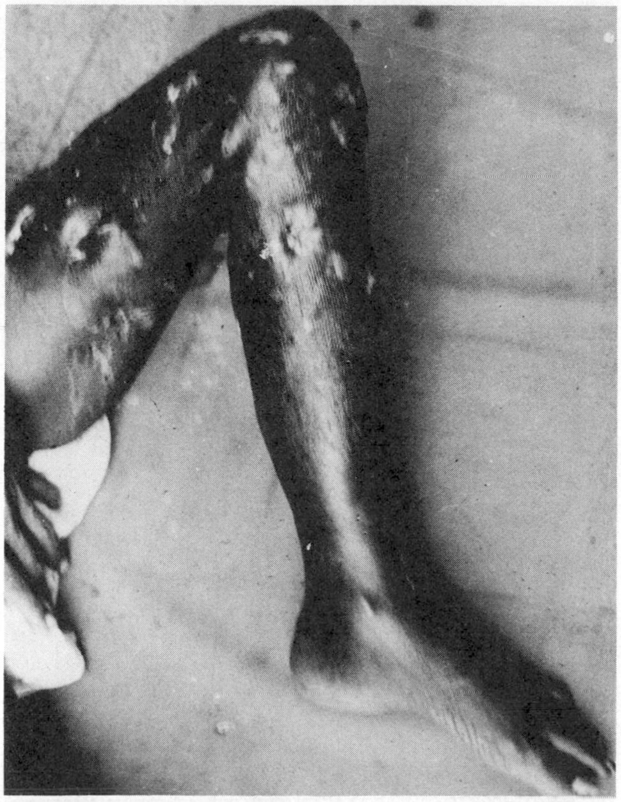

Figure 6. Mycetoma of the thigh and leg caused by *N. brasiliensis.*

softens, forming a sinus that discharges pus. Gradually, multiple nodules develop, ulcerate, and drain through sinus tracts (Figs. 6 and 7). The tracts may remain open for months, or heal only to open again in other areas (Fig. 6). The discharge may be serosanguineous, seropurulent, or purulent, and often contains the characteristic granules (Fig. 7), which can be white, yellow, cream, pink, red, brown, or black, depending on the etiologic agent. As the disease progresses, the surrounding tissue becomes swollen and deformed by fibrous tissue reaction and multiple sinus formation (Fig. 8). Pain is not a serious complaint when only the soft tissues are invaded. However, the condition can be very painful if there is involvement of bone or secondary bacterial infection. Often the disease exists for a number of years before the patient seeks medical advice. The general health is not affected, although the disease may incapacitate the patient.

COMPLICATIONS AND SEQUELAE. Mycetoma usually remains localized, extending slowly by direct contiguity along fascial planes and invading the subcutaneous tissue, fat, ligaments, muscles, and bones but sparing the tendons until very late. Although penetration of the bone is an important feature of mycetoma, the degree and extent of bone involvement varies with the species of infecting agent, the site of the lesion, the stage of development, and the intensity of infection. The osseous lesions (periostitis and round cavities of various sizes) may evolve slowly, as with localized foci of *M. mycetomii*, or be highly invasive and destructive, as with *Actinomadura pelletierii* (Cockshott, 1968).

Destruction of the joint ligaments and articular surfaces results in ankylosis.

When the infection occurs in the head, neck, chest, or buttocks, visceral invasion by contiguity is not rare. Hematogenous spread is very rare, whereas lymphatic spread of mycetoma agents to regional lymph nodes with consequent enlargement have been reported (Koshi et al., 1972; Symmers, 1978). This is most commonly found in *Nocardia* and *Streptomyces* infections in which encapsulation is rare (Hassan and Mahgoub, 1972). Secondary bacterial infection may result in large open ulcers. Extensive fibrosis in the tissue may cause elephantiasis.

GEOGRAPHIC VARIATIONS IN DISEASE. Although mycetoma has been reported from all over the world, it is more common in tropic and subtropic regions in which few people wear shoes. The species responsible for mycetoma varies from country to country, and the etiologic agents that are common in one region are rarely reported from another (Tables 1 and 2).

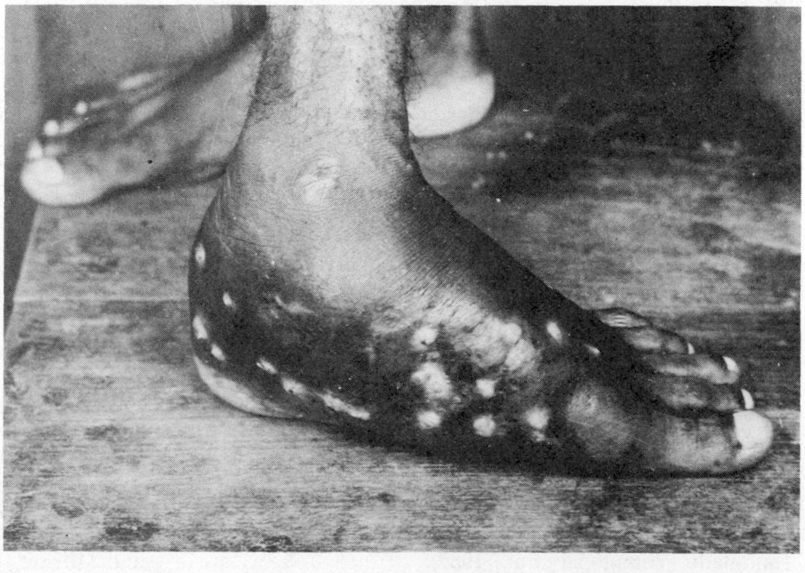

Figure 7. Mycetoma caused by *M. mycetomii* with sinuses discharging black granules.

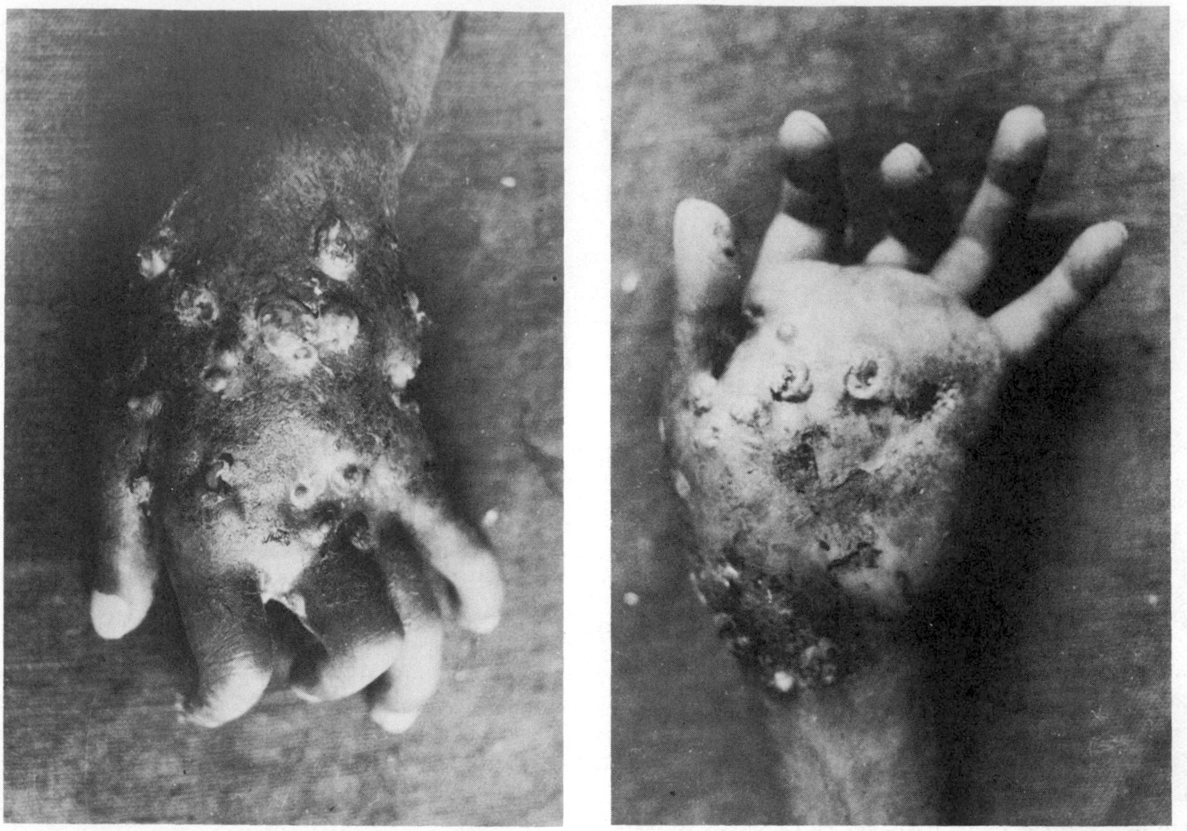
A B

Figure 8. *A* and *B*, Mycetoma of the hand caused by *M. mycetomii. A*, Dorsal aspect. *B*, Palmar aspect.

Climate exerts some influence on the prevalence of the disease and distribution of the causative agents. *M. mycetomii* and *Streptomyces somaliensis* are found in dry arid regions with sandy soils and thorny vegetation, where the rainfall ranges from 50 to 500 mm per year (Vanbreuseghem, 1967). Mycetoma caused by *M. mycetomii* is common in Africa, but the organism has been found in several regions of the world. In Sudan 70 per cent of all recorded cases are caused by *M. mycetomii* (Mahgoub, 1968), and this is the major cause of black grain mycetoma in India, which is responsible for most of the cases encountered in the dry arid regions of the North (Mohapatra and Bhargava, 1967; Andleigh, 1957; Harbans Singh, 1976).

S. somaliensis has been reported mainly from Africa, including Sudan, Somalia, Senegal, Ethiopia, Nigeria, Republic of South Africa, and Tanzania, and in the Western Hemisphere from Brazil and Mexico. In Sudan it accounts for 20 per cent of mycetoma cases (Mahgoub, 1968). Three to 10 per cent of mycetomas in India are due to *S. somaliensis*, which is more common in the southern region of the country (Grueber and Kumar, 1970). One-third of the reported cases in India are from Tamilnadu (Venugopal et al., 1982).

A. pelletierii infection is especially prevalent in relatively humid areas that have a rainfall of 500 to 800 mm or more per year (Rey, 1961). This agent has been reported mainly from African and Latin American countries. The infection is rarely seen in northern India as single cases (Bedi et al., 1978; Talwar Sehgal, 1979; Joshi et al., 1980), and most of the cases reported from the southern region were from Tamilnadu (Venugopal et al., 1982).

Nocardia is more commonly seen in wet forest countries, and small grain mycetoma due to *Nocardia brasiliensis* is prevalent in Mexico, Central and South America, and Africa. *Nocardia* species, once considered rare in Asia, were found to be present in a considerable percentage of cases in India (Venugopal et al., 1977).

Leptosphaeria senegalensis infection, which is native to Africa (seen in Senegal and Chad only), has also been encountered in a significant number of cases from southern India (Klokke et al., 1968; Reddy et al., 1972; Venugopal et al., 1980).

Actinomadura madurae as a causative agent of mycetoma has mainly been reported from North and South America, Africa, and Asia. It is the predominant pathogen in India, along with *M. mycetomii.*

Only a few sporadic cases of mycetoma have been recorded in Europe, Canada, and the United States, and in the last two areas, *Pseudallescheria boydii* has been the most common agent.

Although certain agents of mycetoma show some geographic and ecologic prevalence, most of them have been found all over the world, and it is quite probable that they are ubiquitous, awaiting the proper circumstances for expression.

The factors that determine the susceptibility of humans to mycetoma are unknown. Wounds, personal hygiene, nutrition, general health of the patient, and virulence of the causative agent may all play a role. Sensitization of the body by repeated infections may be a prerequisite to the development of mycetoma in a given individual (Mahgoub and Murray, 1973).

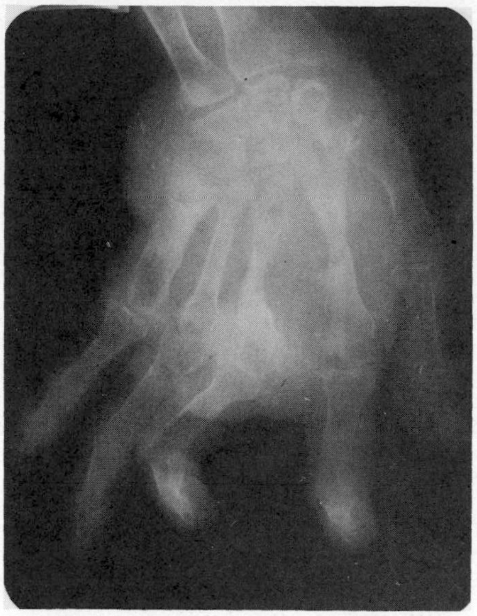

Figure 9. Mycetoma. X-ray of hand showing osteolytic lesions due to *M. mycetomii.*

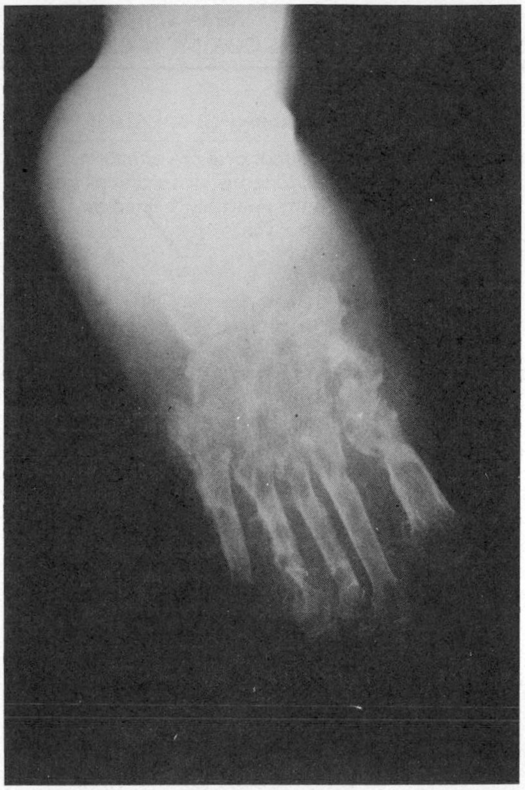

Figure 10. Mycetoma. X-ray of foot showing osteosclerotic and osteolytic lesions due to *A. madurae.*

DIAGNOSIS

Clinical Diagnosis. A fully developed mycetoma can be easily diagnosed by the pathognomonic triad of swelling, sinuses, and grains in the discharge. Diagnosis may be very difficult in the early stages, especially when the lesion is located at an unusual site.

Radiologic Diagnosis. The radiologic manifestations of mycetoma are late sequelae and are of no help in early diagnosis. However, certain radiologic features help to distinguish different types of mycetoma. In eumycotic mycetoma the lesion takes the form of single or multiple, punched-out lytic areas with well-defined walls and little sign of bone reaction, owing to localized masses of grains that gradually replace the osseous tissue and marrow with absence of sequestration (Fig. 9). In actinomycotic mycetoma, both osteolytic and osteosclerotic changes are present at the same time (Fig. 10). The affected bone thickens as fresh lamellae are deposited beneath the active periosteum (Mahgoub, 1968). The size and number of cavities in the bone may give a clue to the identity of the causal agent (Destombes et al., 1958; Delahaye et al., 1962). A few large single cavities generally suggest *M. mycetomii* infection; large multiple cavities with limited destruction suggest *A. madurae;* and a large number of small cavities with extensive fuzzy destruction of bones are probably caused by *A. pelletierii* or *S. somaliensis*. Extensive bone destruction without cavities is generally suggestive of *N. asteroides* (Desai et al., 1970).

LABORATORY DIAGNOSIS

Direct Examination. The pus, serosanguineous fluid that either drains from or is aspirated from unopened lesions, scraping of sinuses, or biopsy material should be examined for granules. The granules should be washed in sterile saline and examined microscopically in a drop of 10 per cent potassium hydroxide. Actinomyotic granules are further stained by Gram's and Kinyoun's acid-fast methods after crushing. The actinomycotic granules are tangled masses of delicate branching gram-positive filaments, 0.5 to 1 μ in diameter, which may break up into bacillary and coccoid forms. *Nocardia* species are partially acid-fast, whereas *Actinomadura* and *Streptomyces* organisms are not. Eumycotic granules contain wide septate hyphae with hyphal swellings and chlamydospores.

Culture. A deep biopsy is ideal for culture, because it is free from external contamination. Granules from open lesions should be washed repeatedly with sterile saline, inoculated onto Sabouraud's dextrose agar slants with and without chloramphenicol (0.05 mg/ml), and incubated at both 26° C and 37° C. The characteristics of the common agents are given in Tables 3 and 4.

Histopathology. Histologic sections of the biopsy material stained by hematoxylin and eosin are examined for the presence of characteristic granules within the abscess cavities. If no granule is seen, deeper sections should be examined. Mere histologic examination of the biopsy material not only establishes the diagnosis of the disease but also allows specific identification of the causal agent in 94 per cent of mycetomas (Klokke et al., 1968). However, histologic examination has its limitations, and it should always be supplemented by culture.

Sections of actinomycotic mycetoma are further stained by Brown and Brenn's modification of Gram's and Kinyoun's acid-fast methods, and eumycotic mycetomas are stained by Bauer chromic acid–Schiff and Gomori Grocott's methenamine silver stains. A detailed morphologic study of the organism in the granule should be made for establishing the identity of different species.

Table 3. HISTOLOGIC AND CULTURAL CHARACTERISTICS OF COMMON CAUSAL AGENTS OF ACTINOMYCOTIC MYCETOMA

Organism	Histology (H & E Stain)	Culture	
		Macroscopic	*Microscopic*
N. asteroides	Small; round, oval or vermiform; homogeneous loose clumps of filaments; partially stained by hematoxylin	Fast-growing, glabrous, chalky; folded or wrinkled, white to orange-pink; no enzymatic activity	Delicate branched filaments fragmenting into bacillary and coccoid forms; gram-positive, partially acid-fast
N. brasiliensis	Same as above	Fast-growing, small, heaped, wrinkled or folded, yellow to orange; enzymatically active	Same as above
N. caviae	*Same as above*	*Resembles N. asteroides;* differentiated by special tests	Same as above
A. madurae	Large; round or lobulated; center eosinophilic, amorphous; dense basophilic mantle peripherally surrounded by an eosinophilic fringe; clubs	Slow-growing, glabrous or waxy; wrinkled and folded, white to cream-color colonies; adherent to the medium; enzymatically active	Delicate branched nonfragmenting filaments and arthrospores; gram-positive, not acid-fast
A. pelletierii	Small; round or irregular with denticulate edge: homogeneous matrix staining deeply with hematoxylin; no clubs	Very slow growing; small, glabrous, waxy, wrinkled or irregularly folded, pink to coral-red colonies	Delicate branched nonfragmenting filaments; gram-positive, not acid-fast
S. somaliensis	Variable size; round or oval with smooth borders; center amorphous and lightly stained; no clubs	Fast-growing, glabrous, folded or wrinkled, cream to brown in color	Delicate branched nonfragmenting filaments and arthrospores; gram-positive, not acid-fast

Immunologic Diagnosis. Although precipitins, agglutinins, and complement-fixing antibodies have been demonstrated, immunologic diagnosis of mycetoma is of only academic value because no standard antigen was available until recently. However, this method is gaining importance as a highly useful diagnostic procedure, especially in the very early stages of the disease, during which the granules are not found. In addition, serology can be of value in distinguishing between the pathogenic and saprophytic status of an agent isolated in culture, in suggesting the identity of the species involved, and in monitoring therapy (Peloux and Quilici, 1979).

Demonstration of precipitins by immunodiffusion has been useful in identifying the causal agents of mycetoma (Mahgoub, 1964; Murray and Mahgoub, 1968). Counterimmunoelectrophoresis is more sensitive than immunodiffusion for the diagnosis of early cases of mycetoma (Gumaa and Mahgoub, 1975). Enzyme-linked immunosorbent assays appear to be sensitive tests for the detection of antibodies in mycetoma infections, especially in epidemiological work. The specificity of reactions, however, was more variable and cross-reactions were observed because of close relationship between the causal agents (Mc Laren et al., 1978).

Mycetoma patients seem to be deficient in cell-mediated immunity as measured by the tuberculin test, dinitrochlorobenzene reaction, and lymphocyte transformation test (Mahgoub et al., 1977). Type 4 skin reactions, produced to purified protein antigens, are of some value in actinomycotic mycetoma, but eumycotic mycetoma patients failed to react (Murray and Moghraby, 1964).

TREATMENT. Unlike eumycotic mycetoma, actinomycotic mycetoma responds to chemotherapy. Treatment should be continued for several months after clinical cure to prevent a relapse. Surgical procedures such as exploration and drainage of sinus tracts, debridement of diseased tissue, and removal of bone cysts assist greatly in healing. Favorable responses have been reported with drug therapy alone in actinomycotic mycetoma even when there are extensive long-standing lesions involving the bone and lymphatics (Mahgoub, 1976).

The treatment of choice for nocardial mycetoma is a sulfonamide or its derivatives. The most common drug used is sulfadiazine, and the dose varies from 3 to 8 g per day. Dapsone (diaminodiphenylsulfone), long-acting sulfonamides, and a combination of sulfamethoxazole and trimethoprim are reported to be useful (Latapi, 1963; Lavalle, 1966; Vanbreuseghem, 1967; Mahgoub and Murray, 1973). Treatment is usually very effective in these cases because the small nocardial granules offer less resistance to drug penetration (Mariat et al., 1977).

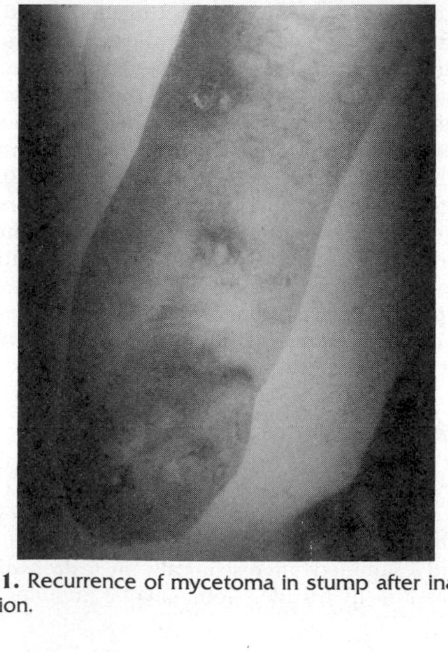

Figure 11. Recurrence of mycetoma in stump after inadequate amputation.

Table 4. HISTOLOGIC AND CULTURAL CHARACTERISTICS OF CAUSAL AGENTS OF EUMYCOTIC MYCETOMA

		Culture	
Organism	**Histology (H & E Stain)**	***Macroscopic***	***Microscopic***
M. mycetomii	Large, dark brown, lobulated; compact type with even distribution of brownish cement intersected by a network of hyphae; vesicular type with peripheral localization of brown cement around hyaline hyphae and chlamydospores; brown pigment particles in hyphal cells	Slow-growing, cottony to membranous, flat or folded, white, yellowish brown or brown with diffusible pigment; growth better at 37° C	Branched septate hyphae with chains of chlamydospores; black sclerotia; rare phialides and conidia
M. grisea	Small, oval or lobed; hollow center with loose hyaline hyphae; dark colored periphery with dense network of hyphae and chlamydospores embedded in brown cement; brown granules of intracellular pigment absent	Slow-growing, leathery, folded, black colonies with gray mycelium; red diffusible pigment	Fine septate hyphae and larger moniliform hyphae with chains of chlamydospores; sterile pycnidia.
L. senegalensis	Small, irregular, tubular or hollow; central core of hyaline hyphae; periphery dense with black hyphae and large vesicular cells imbedded in black cement	Fast-growing, gray-brown colony with black reverse, rare diffusible rose pigment	Dark brown or black perithecia; septate ascospores
P. romeroi	Small, tubular, central network of hyphae with thick band of chlamydospores in the periphery; dark swollen cells in the outer edge surrounded by an eosinophilic zone	Rapid-growing, dark gray, floccose; white periphery; black pigment in reverse	Brownish black pycnidia; elliptical conidia
P. jeanselmei	Small, vermiform, crescent-shaped; hollow center; hyphae and chlamydospores brown; cement absent	Slow-growing, leathery, black and moist; later velvety, reverse black	Toruloid yeast cells; moniliform cells; long unbranched phialides
P. boydii	Large; round or lobulated; broad septate hyaline hyphae with numerous, swollen hyphal cells (< 20 μ)	Rapid-growing, white, cottony, or fluffy; later grayish white, reverse gray to black	Hyaline hyphae, ovoid to pyriform conidia borne singly or in groups; dark brown perithecia; evanescent asci and ascospores
Acremonium spp	Small, irregular; hyaline hyphae with numerous swollen cells (> 12 μ) surrounded by an eosinophilic zone	Slow-growing, white, glabrous colony; later downy, diffusible violet	Hyaline hyphae; curved septate conidia in mucoid clusters at the tips of conidiophores
N. rosatii	Small, polyhedral; center basophilic with vesicles and few hyphae; periphery with narrow septate hyphae imbedded in cement	Slow-growing, dark, flat or wrinkled colonies with light gray aerial mycelia; reverse dark brown	Black perithecia; kidney-shaped ascospores

In mycetomas caused by *A. madurae*, *A. pelletierii*, and *S. somaliensis*, streptomycin has been used most successfully (Abbot, 1956; Lynch, 1964). Combinations of dapsone with streptomycin or sulfamethoxazole-trimethoprim with streptomycin are the most effective treatments. Streptomycin 1 g daily for one month and then on alternate days with either dapsone 100 mg twice daily or 800 mg sulfamethoxazole plus 160 mg trimethoprim twice daily should be used initially in all cases. Treatment requires 4 to 24 months, averaging 9 months, and relapse is uncommon. Hematological monitoring is essential because of bone marrow depression. Chemotherapy is less successful in *S. somaliensis* mycetomas (Mahgoub, 1976).

Until recently, there had been no specific therapy for eumycotic mycetoma, and the prognosis was poor. Complete surgical excision of the early lesions may prevent spread. There have only been a few isolated instances of improvement following the use of a variety of agents from griseofulvin to amphotericin B. In vitro studies have shown that dapsone causes inhibition of growth of *M. grisea*, *A. madurae*, *S. somaliensis*, and *N. brasiliensis* (Mackinnon et al., 1958). A preliminary course of broad spectrum antibiotics combined with a prolonged course of dapsone in a dosage of 100 mg twice daily, together with immobilization of the affected part, has been effective in the treatment of mycetomas caused by fungi as well as actinomycetes (Cockshott, 1957; Cockshott and Rankin, 1960).

Although miconazole and ketoconazole are inhibitory in vitro against many pathogenic fungi (Van Cutsem and Theinpont, 1972; Van Cutsem, 1983), their effectiveness in cases of mycetoma is equivocal. Miconazole therapy has been reported to be effective with no sign of recurrence after surgery in a case of mycetoma due to *Acremonium* species (Hay, 1979). Excellent results have been obtained with ketoconazole in 3 cases of mycetoma, 2 due to *P. boydii* and 1 due to a dematiaceous fungus (Droubet and Dupont, 1983). But treatment with ketoconazole was to little avail in most patients with mycetoma. However, some improvement has been reported in infections due to *P. boydii* (Symoens et al., 1980; Hay, 1983). In advanced cases, amputation is necessary and it should be well above the seat of the disease. Unless the entire lesion is removed, it is likely to recur in the stump (Fig. 11).

PROPHYLAXIS. Prevention is not possible, but the disease is likely to disappear with better standards of living. Since trauma, often inflicted by a thorn, is generally found to be the basis of mycetoma, shoes would be a practical control measure.

References

Abbott, P.: Mycetoma in the Sudan. Trans R Soc Trop Med Hyg 50:11, 1956.
Andleigh, H. S.: Etiology of maduromycosis in India. Mycopath Mycol Appl 8:138, 1957.
Bedi, T. R., Kaur, S., and Kumar, B.: Red grain mycetoma of the scalp, (A. pelletieri). A case report from India. Mycopathologia 63:127, 1978.
Cockshott, W. P.: The therapy of mycetoma. W Afr Med J 6:101, 1957.
Cockshott, W. P.: Radiological patterns of the deep mycoses. In Wolstenholme, G. E. W., and Porter, R. (eds): Systemic Mycoses. London, J. & A Churchill Ltd., 1968, p. 113.
Cockshott, W. P., and Rankin, A. M.: Medical treatment of mycetoma. Lancet 2:1112, 1960.
Delahaye, R. P., Destombes, P., and Moutounet, J.: Les aspects radiologiques des mycétomes. Ann Radiol (Paris) 5:817, 1962.
Desai, S. C., Pardanani, D. S., Sreedevi, N., and Mehta, R. S.: Studies on mycetoma. Indian J Surg 32:427, 1970.
Destombes, P., Andre, M., Segretain, G., Mariat, F., Camain, R., and Nazimoff, O.: Contribution a etude des mycétomes en Afrique francaise. Bull Soc Pathol Exot 51:815, 1958.
Drouhet, E., and Dupont, B.: Laboratory and clinical assessment of ketoconazole in deep seated mycoses. Am J Med 74:30, 1983.
Grueber, H. L. E., and Kumar, T. M.: Mycetoma caused by *Streptomyces somaliensis* in North India. Sabouraudia 8:108, 1970.
Gumaa, S. A., and Mahgoub, E. S.: Counterimmunoelectrophoresis in the diagnosis of mycetoma and its sensitivity as compared to immunodiffusion. Sabouraudia 13:309, 1975.
Hassan, E. A. M., and Mahgoub, E. S.: Lymph node involvement in mycetoma. Trans R Soc Trop Med Hyg 66:165, 1972.
Hay, R. J.: Mycoses imported from the West Indies. A report of three cases. Postgrad Med J 55:603, 1979.
Hay, R. J.: Ketoconazole in the treatment of fungal infection: Clinical and laboratory studies. Am J Med 74:16, 1983.
Joshi, K. R., Malthur, D. R., Sharma, K., and Chawla, S. N.: Mycetoma caused by *Streptomyces pelletierii* in India (case report). Indian J. Dermatol Venereol Lepr 46:123, 1980.
Klokke, A. H., Swamidasan, S., Anguli, R., and Verghese, A.: The causal agents of mycetoma in South India. Trans R Soc Trop Med Hyg 62:509, 1968.
Koshi, G., Victor, N., and Chacko, J.: Causal agents in mycetoma of the foot in Southern India. Sabouraudia 10:14, 1972.
Latapi, F.: Das Mycetom; in Handbuch der Haut und Geschlechtskrankheiten. Springer, Berlin, 1963.
Lavalle, P.: Clinica Y terapeutica de los micetomas. Dermat Intern 5:117, 1966.
Lynch, J. B.: Mycetoma in the Sudan. Ann R Coll Surg Engl 35:319, 1964.
Mackinnon, J. E., Artagaveytia-Allende, R. C., Gracia-Zorron, N.: The inhibitory effect of chemotherapeutic agents on the growth of the causal organisms of exogenous mycetomas and Nocardiosis. Trans R Soc Trop Med Hyg 58:78, 1958.
Mahgoub, E. S.: The value of gel diffusions in the diagnosis of mycetoma. Trans R Soc Trop Med Hyg 58:560, 1964.
Mahgoub, E. S.: Clinical aspects. In Wolstenholme, G. E. W., and Porter, R. (eds.) Systemic Mycoses. London, J. & A. Churchill Ltd. 1968, p 125.
Mahgoub, E. S.: Medical management of mycetoma. Bull WHO 54:303, 1976.
Mahgoub, E. S., Gumaa, S. A., and Hassan, E. A. M.: Immunological status of mycetoma patients. Bull Soc Pathol Exot 70:48, 1977.
Mahgoub, E. S., and Murray, I. G.: Mycetoma. London, William Heinemann Medical Books Ltd., 1973.
Mariat, F., Destombes, P., and Segretain, G.: The mycetomas: Clinical features, pathology, etiology and epidemiology. Contrib Microbiol Immunol 4:1, 1977.
McLaren, M. L., Mahgoub, E. S., and Georgakopoulos, E.: Preliminary investigation on the use of the enzyme-linked immunosorbent assay (ELISA) in the serodiagnosis of mycetoma. Sabouraudia 16:225, 1978.
Mohapatra, L. N., and Bhargava, S.: Mycetoma. Indian J Ortho 1:172, 1967.
Murray, I. G., and Mahgoub, E. S.: Further studies on the diagnosis of mycetoma by double diffusion in agar. Sabouraudia 6:106, 1968.
Murray, I. G., and Moghraby, I. M. E.: The value of skin tests in distinguishing between maduromycetoma and actinomycetoma. Trans R Soc Trop Med Hyg 58:557, 1964.
Peloux, Y., and Quilici, M.: Les agents des mycétomes: étude bactériologique et parasitologique. Med Trop 39:9, 1979.
Reddy, C. R. R. M., Sundareshwar, B., Pattabhi Rama Rao, A., and Reddy, S. S.: Mycetoma: Histopathological diagnosis of causal agents in 50 cases. Indian J Med Sci 26:733, 1972.
Rey, M.: Les mycetomes dans ouest africain. Paris, R. Foulon et Cie, 1961.
Singh, H.: Black grain perianal mycetoma. Indian J Surg 38:530, 1976.
Symmers, W. St. C.: The lymphoreticular system—Lymphadenitis caused by actinomycetes and true fungi. In Symmers, W. St. C. (ed.): Systemic Pathology. Edinburgh, Churchill Livingstone, 1978, p.616.
Symoens, J., Moens, M., Dom, J., Scheijgrond, H., Dony, J., Schuermans, V., Legendre, R., and Finestine, N.: An evaluation of two years of clinical experience with ketoconazole. Rev Infect Dis 2:674, 1980.
Vanbreuseghem, R.: Early diagnosis, treatment and epidemiology of mycetoma. Rev Med Vet Mycol 6:49, 1967.
Van Cutsem, J.: The antifungal activity of ketoconazole. Am J Med 74:9, 1983.
Van Cutsem, J. M., and Thienpont, D.: Miconazole, a broad spectrum antimycotic agent with antibacterial activity. Chemotherapy 17:392, 1972.
Venugopal, T. V., Venugopal, P. V., Paramasivan, C. N., Shetty, B. M. V., and Subramanian, S.: Mycetomas in Madras. Sabouraudia 15:17, 1977.
Venugopal, T. V., Venugopal, P. V., Kamalakannan, R., Annamalai, R., Shetty, B. M. V., Subramanian, S., and Shanmugasundaram, T. K.: Mycetomas caused by *Streptomyces pelletierii* in Madras, India. Arch Derm 114:204, 1978.
Venugopal, T. V., Venugopal, P. V., and Pandurangan, C. N.: *Leptosphaeria senegalensis* causing mycetoma pedis in Madras (case report). Indian J Dermatol Venereol Lepr 46:364, 1980.
Venugopal, T. V., Venugopal, P. V., and Arumugam, S.: *Streptomyces somaliensis* causing mycetomas in South India. Indian J Dermatol Venereol Lepr 48:35, 1982.

253
CLOSTRIDIAL MYONECROSIS

DONALD L. BORNSTEIN, M.D.

Clostridial myonecrosis (gas gangrene) is a rapidly progressive, highly toxemic, and life-threatening illness caused by the invasion of previously healthy skeletal muscle by pathogenic clostridia. Most cases occur following serious injuries or surgical procedures. The involved muscle and the overlying soft tissues undergo necrosis and autolysis with little inflammatory cell reaction (myonecrosis). Severe toxemia with tachycardia, hypotension, and mental changes accompanies this process.

ETIOLOGY. Over 60 species of *Clostridium* can be isolated from man and his environment, but only six seem able to induce myonecrosis: *C. perfringens (C. welchii), C. septicum, C. novyi (C. oedematiens), C. sordelli (C. bifermentans),* and, very rarely, *C. histolyticum* and *C. fallax.* Of these, *C. perfringens,* Type A, is by far the most important pathogen, accounting for 90 to 95 per cent of cases of myonecrosis. *C. septicum* and *C. novyi*, Type A, cause the balance of cases of civilian gas gangrene. More than one pathogenic species of clostridia may be isolated from a wound.

C. perfringens is prominent among the normal bowel microflora in man and is typically 10 to 100 times more prevalent than *Escherichia coli* in fecal specimens. Clostridia can be found on the skin, especially over the buttocks, thighs, and perineum, and less frequently in the vagina and in the diseased biliary tract. Our environment is heavily contaminated with clostridia, which can be found on clothing, in the air of operating rooms, in water, on food, in dust, and in soil. The ability of clostridia to form spores allows them to persist in the environment under adverse conditions.

PATHOGENESIS AND PATHOLOGY. The virulence of pathogenic clostridia is a consequence of their potent exotoxins and their ability to grow rapidly under favorable growth conditions. There is apparently no difference in the virulence of strains of *C. perfringens* that are isolated from cases of gas gangrene and strains that are commensals. Isolates from normal bowel flora and from fatal cases of myonecrosis are not distinguishable in toxin production or in animal virulence tests. Rather, myonecrosis occurs because damaged tissue presents this common enteric organism with an unusual opportunity to proliferate and thereby brings out the full latent toxigenic and invasive characteristics of the species.

Pathogenic clostridia are obligate anaerobes and cannot proliferate unless the oxidation-reduction or redox potential (Eh) of their microenvironment is reduced well below the +120 mv potential of well-oxygenated human tissues. They are not killed in atmospheric concentrations of oxygen but they will not multiply in such conditions. Lacerated, crushed, or dead tissues have redox potentials as low as −150 to −250 mv and provide excellent growth conditions.

With impaired blood flow in tissue, anaerobic glycolysis occurs, lactic acid accumulates, and pH falls. A fall in pH creates new opportunities for clostridia to grow. *C. perfringens*, which could not grow at redox potentials above +60 mv at pH 7.4, was able to grow at an Eh of +160 mv when the pH was reduced to 6.4 (Oakley, 1954).

Like other anaerobic infections, most infections with *C. perfringens* are endogenous. Exogenous infection is more likely only in cases of major trauma in which gross contamination with soil, water, or foreign material has occurred.

Wounds at highest risk for developing gas gangrene are those produced by high velocity missiles, severe compound fractures, and badly contaminated crush injuries. In all of these, muscle is lacerated, circulation and local perfusion are badly compromised, clothing, dirt, and foreign material are buried deep within a wound, and pH and Eh fall. Clostridia from the skin, clothing, or external sources are often introduced along with other bacteria. The longer this dangerous situation persists before effective surgical care is initiated, the greater the risk of gas gangrene (Langley and Winkelstein, 1945).

The major toxin of *C. perfringens* is the alpha toxin, a lecithinase C, which has lethal, hemolytic, and necrotizing effects. This toxin can cause massive hemolysis by its action on the cell membranes of erythrocytes, as in clostridial septicemia (Chapter 196) or after intravenous administration to experimental animals. When injected intramuscularly, however, hemolysis is not significant, perhaps because the toxin is fixed at the injection site where it damages tissue and increases vascular permeability. Alpha toxin is believed to initiate the injury to myofibril membranes that triggers the invasion of previously normal muscle.

The severe toxemia observed in gas gangrene, however, is not due to alpha toxin itself, because alpha toxin is not usually detected in the circulation, gross hemolysis is not seen, and specific antitoxin does not reduce the toxemia. Excision of all affected muscle or, in some cases perhaps, hyperbaric oxygen therapy, can reverse the toxemia. Products of clostridial-infected muscle, as yet uncharacterized, appear to be responsible for toxemia.

The role of the other toxins in the genesis of clostridial myonecrosis is obscure, except for their potent leukocidal activity, which eliminates phagocytosis and facilitates invasion by the organism (Smith, 1979). The major toxin of *C. novyi* is also a lecithinase C, but the major toxin of *C. septicum*, which produces an equally severe myonecrosis, has no lecithinase activity.

The important pathologic change in myonecrosis is a progressive destruction of muscle. The process disrupts the

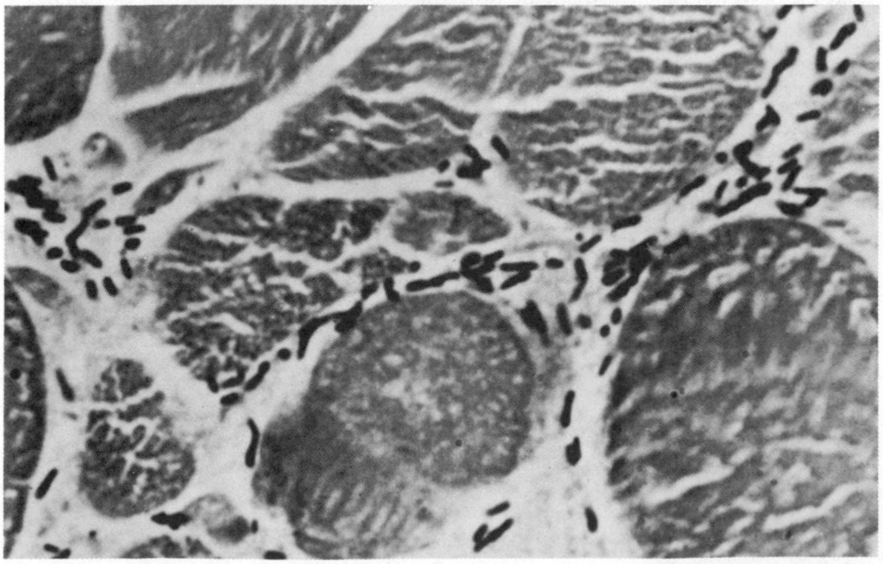

Figure 1. Pathologic changes in muscle in clostridial myonecrosis (×400). Necrotic muscle fibers are separated by gas and edema fluid. Many clostridia are present with minimal inflammatory response. (From Boyd, N. A., Walter, P. D., and Thomson, R. O.: J Med Microbiol 5:459, 1972.)

sarcolemma and fragments the muscle fibers, but the myofibrils are preserved. There is gas and edema between the muscle fibers, some loss of reticulin and collagen, and karyolysis. There is no vascular congestion, no marked fibrin deposition, and no neutrophilic exudate (Robb-Smith, 1945) (Fig. 1). Electronmicrographs suggest a primary attack on the lecithin in the cell membranes of muscle where small membrane gaps can be observed (Strunk et al., 1967).

With the exception of uterine infections (Chapter 196), serious clostridial wound infection is confined to skeletal muscle. Necrosis of the overlying connective tissue and skin in clostridial infection is a secondary phenomenon. There is no evidence that clostridia can cause a primary destructive or invasive infection of skin or soft tissues, a fundamental distinction that has been obscured in some recent reviews.

Localized infections with clostridia can occur almost anywhere if organisms are introduced into a normally sterile area such as the pleural space, peritoneum, subarachnoid space, a joint, the brain, the eye, or the gallbladder. Although local tissue injury, edema, gas formation, and purulence or abscess formation may ensue, and although bacteremia may on rare occasions develop from such a site without muscle infection, these are rarely progressive, toxemic, or life-threatening infections, and they respond to antibiotic therapy and simple drainage procedures (Bornstein et al., 1964).

CLINICAL MANIFESTATIONS. Sixty to 70 per cent of civilian gas gangrene follows trauma, usually a major injury that breaks the skin, crushes tissue, introduces dirt and foreign materials, compromises the vascular supply, and in most cases badly fractures one or more long bones. The thigh and/or hip are involved in most cases. Motorcycle or other traffic accidents, falls, crushing by industrial or farm machinery, gunshot wounds, and penetrating injuries are the most common precipitating events. The common features in these cases are ill-advised, early internal fixation of contaminated open fractures, primary wound closure, inadequate débridement, unrelieved tension in fascial compartments, or application of tight casts (Fig. 2).

Twenty to 30 per cent of cases follow clean surgical procedures. Biliary surgery with common duct exploration (Fig. 3), bowel surgery, orthopedic procedures on the hip or femur, amputation, or attempted vascular repair for arterial insufficiency of the leg are the most common offenders.

The remaining 10 to 15 per cent of cases occur after intramuscular injections, minor trauma or superficial lesions in patients with impaired circulation, and in immunosuppressed patients. There are also cases of "spontaneous" and "metastatic" gas gangrene. Intragluteal injection of epinephrine is the most common cause of post-injection gas gangrene. Epinephrine should never be injected in the buttocks because it constricts blood flow and can introduce clostridial spores into ischemic tissue. Ischemic or neuropathic ulcers and decubitus ulcers have served as other points of entry. Neutropenia, immunosuppression, advanced Hodgkin's disease, and acute leukemia all predispose to clostridial myonecrosis. In such patients minor trauma such as an infiltrated venipuncture site can usher in atypical, rapidly advancing, and usually fatal myonecrosis. "Spontaneous" or "idiopathic" gas gangrene involves a previously uninjured site. Occult bowel leakage (diverticulitis, necrotic malignancy, fistulae) that drains down along the iliopsoas sheath can sometimes initiate myonecrosis in the upper thigh or buttock. "Metastatic" gas gangrene develops in muscle groups that have been seeded by heavy clostridial bacteremia, usually originating from a carcinoma or an ulcerated lesion of the bowel. *C. septicum* has been involved in many of the reported cases (Chapter 196). Very rarely in advanced myonecrosis a metastatic patch of disease will develop at a new and distant site presumably because of blood-borne spread.

The first symptom of myonecrosis in most cases is the development of heaviness or pain in the affected area beginning 6 to 120 hours (usually 24 to 48 hours) after injury. The pain is unrelenting and increases in degree and in extent. The painful area is not red and inflamed but appears cool, pale, and swollen, often with tense, white, shiny skin. Crepitus is not prominent because it is obscured by the increasing edema, which is most severe in infections caused by *C. novyi*. The area becomes swollen and tense, and a dark, thin, serous fluid drains from existing wounds. A blotchy bronze or brown discoloration and thin-walled blebs filled with dark fluid containing clostridia but few white cells develop in the affected skin. These changes progress to patches of frank necrosis in the initial sites of

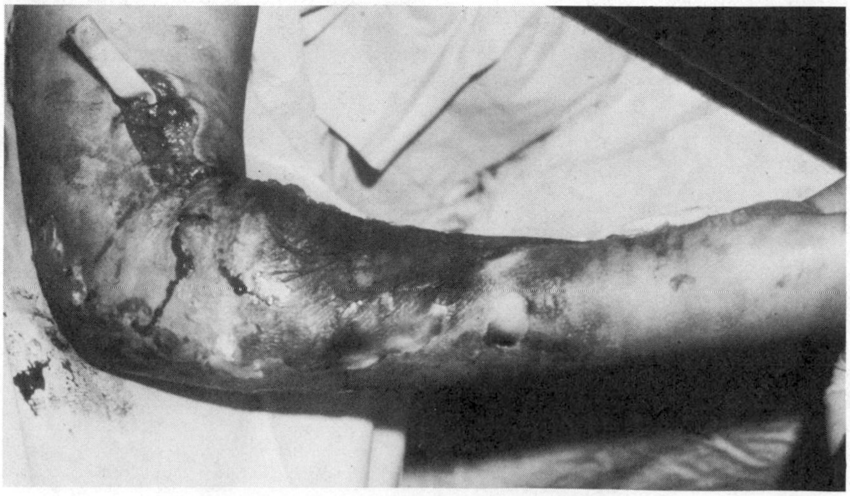

Figure 2. Gas gangrene of the forearm following an open fracture of the proximal ulna resulting from a fall. When the cast was opened because of severe pain, discoloration, serous discharge, bleb formation, and frank necrosis of the skin were apparent. Amputation above the elbow was required.

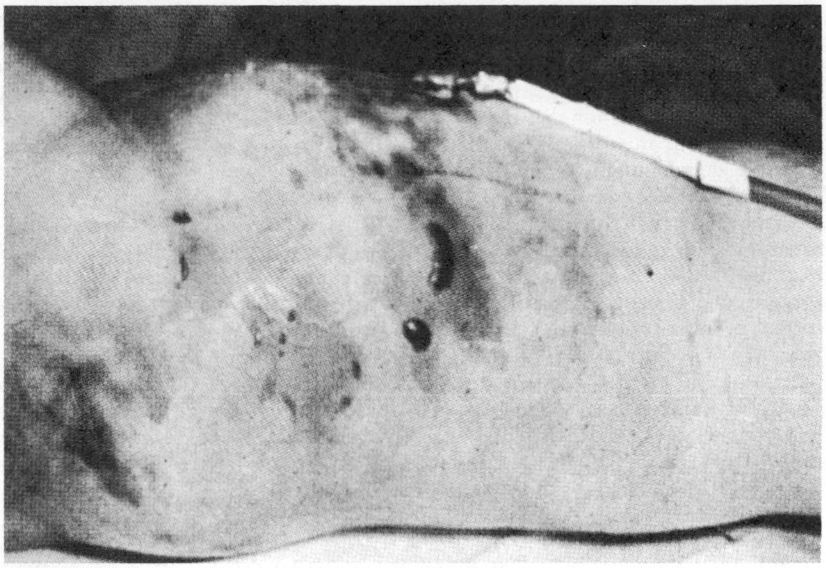

Figure 3. Gas gangrene of the abdominal wall following gallbladder surgery. The patient survived after extensive resection of necrotic muscle and soft tissue. (From Bornstein, D. L. et al.: Medicine 43:207, 1964. Courtesy of The Williams & Wilkins Company.)

involvement, while pain, edema, and discoloration advance to involve new areas.

With the onset of pain and edema, a marked systemic reaction appears, with myalgias, tachycardia, sweating, and restlessness that are disproportionate to the local changes and to the low-grade fever. Within several hours a rapidly advancing toxemic state with prostration, hypotension, and either agitation or signs of obtundation appears. Most patients are febrile, some with rigors and high fever; a few are hypothermic. Without prompt and effective therapy, refractory septic shock, circulatory failure, central nervous system depression, and death soon follow (MacLennan, 1962; Altemeier and Fullen, 1971).

COMPLICATIONS AND SEQUELAE. The major complication in survivors of myonecrosis is loss of a limb by amputation or weakness caused by extensive removal of necrotic muscle. Defects in the abdominal wall from myonecrosis may be of such magnitude that extensive and prolonged plastic surgery may be needed before the patient can resume a normal life (Phillips et al., 1974).

GEOGRAPHIC VARIATIONS. Although the content of clostridia in soils varies geographically, the major reservoir of pathogenic clostridia is the human intestinal tract. The most important geographic factor in the incidence of myonecrosis is the level of hygiene and the availability of medical facilities at which effective primary surgical care of contaminated open fractures, crush injuries, and penetrating wounds can be carried out. Local customs such as the use of contaminated soil or other natural materials as poultices for traumatic wounds may introduce infection.

DIAGNOSIS. Early recognition and prompt therapy are vital to minimize tissue destruction and to prevent death. Definitive diagnosis in early cases can be made only by surgical examination of muscle in the affected area. Persistent pain in a high-risk surgical or traumatic wound should always be evaluated. Casts should be split, sutured wounds opened, and dressings taken down to evaluate the state of the wound and to obtain smears and cultures.

If local edema or early skin discoloration is found, or if the patient appears unduly toxemic, confused, or hypotensive, prompt muscle exploration is required. The finding of clostridia on gram-stained smears of wound exudate with only a few neutrophils supports the diagnosis of gas gangrene. Once gas gangrene is considered, exploration should not be deferred. A two-hour delay may cost a patient a limb that could otherwise have been saved. First priority for operating room use must be granted for this emergency (Altemeier and Fullen, 1971). Crepitus in a wound in the absence of local pain or systemic signs also requires limited surgical exploration of the underlying muscle, but is a lesser emergency.

The first changes in involved muscle are pallor, edema, loss of tone, and poor contractility when pinched. With further involvement an unhealthy brick red color appears that progresses to a brown or gray "cooked meat" appearance. The excised muscle does not bleed freely and soon becomes necrotic with green-black discoloration, liquefaction, and gas bubbles. The extent of myonecrosis must be determined surgically because it is usually greater than the skin changes might indicate.

Gram-stained smears from the gangrenous muscle reveal plump gram-positive rods (with no spores if *C. perfringens*) and very few leukocytes. The rare cases of anaerobic streptococcal myositis, which can mimic early stages of clostridial myonecrosis, are clearly distinguished by large numbers of streptococci and heavy neutrophilic infiltration (Chapter 254). Wound and blood cultures are obtained to confirm the diagnosis, to speciate the clostridia, to determine the extent of other bacterial contamination, and to rule out any associated bacteremia. *C. perfringens* bacteremia can be detected in 5 to 10 per cent of patients with advanced myonecrosis. The bacteremia is rarely heavy and is only occasionally associated with significant in vivo hemolysis caused by circulating alpha toxin, although significant anemia and some degree of hyperbilirubinemia are commonly seen in myonecrosis due to other mechanisms than hemolysis.

If muscle is not involved, surgical examination can identify and help correct other infections, such as necrotizing fasciitis or crepitant or noncrepitant cellulitis. In civilian practice, many crepitant infections are not caused by clostridia but rather by facultatively anaerobic gram-negative bacilli, or nonclostridial obligate anaerobes. Gram stains will give clues to the etiologic agents and will guide the initial antimicrobial therapy. Culture of *C. perfringens* from a wound does not make the diagnosis of myonecrosis because it may represent simple contamination, anaerobic cellulitis (a gas infection that spreads along superficial fascial plains without muscle involvement and that is treated by limited débridement), or a localized ("Welch") abscess (Wilson, 1960).

X-ray films can sometimes differentiate the feathery or fern-like pattern of gas within muscle bundles that generally signifies myonecrosis from the linear patterns or rounded or irregular pockets of gas in subcutaneous tissues due to other crepitant processes (Fig. 4). Because these x-ray findings may be late in developing, surgical exploration should not be delayed in their absence. Crepitus in tissues and extraluminal gas shadows on X-ray should not be equated with clostridial myonecrosis. A logical diagnostic approach to gas-forming processes is required, which begins with gram-stains, proper anaerobic and aerobic cultures of exudates and blood, and clinical evaluation of the patient. (Chapter 254; Bornstein, 1964).

There are no other specific tests for the early detection of myonecrosis. Leukocytosis, anemia, elevated transaminase, and slight hyperbilirubinemia are common. An increase in the blood of myoglobin and muscle enzymes (creatine phosphokinase, aldolase, LDH isozymes) is not helpful because they are also elevated by the trauma or surgery that preceded the development of myonecrosis. Laboratory studies of fluid and electrolyte balance, renal function, hepatic function, and the blood picture are required for proper management of this disease and its complications.

Without muscle examination it may not be possible to distinguish between clostridial myonecrosis and a variety of other crepitant or necrotizing infections of the skin and soft tissues, especially clostridial anaerobic cellulitis, which can be managed by simple débridement of necrotic tissue in the wound and antimicrobial therapy. Necrotizing fasciitis—a mixed infection with hemolytic streptococci, staphylococci, or gram-negative bacilli—and synergistic necrotizing cellulitis due to aerobic gram-negative rods plus peptostreptococci or *Bacteroides* are likely to be the most confusing because they cause local pain, discoloration and necrosis of the skin, and marked systemic reactions (Ledingham and Tehrani, 1975; Chapter 254). Necrotizing fascitis of the perineum is frequently misdiagnosed as gas gangrene (Finegold, 1977).

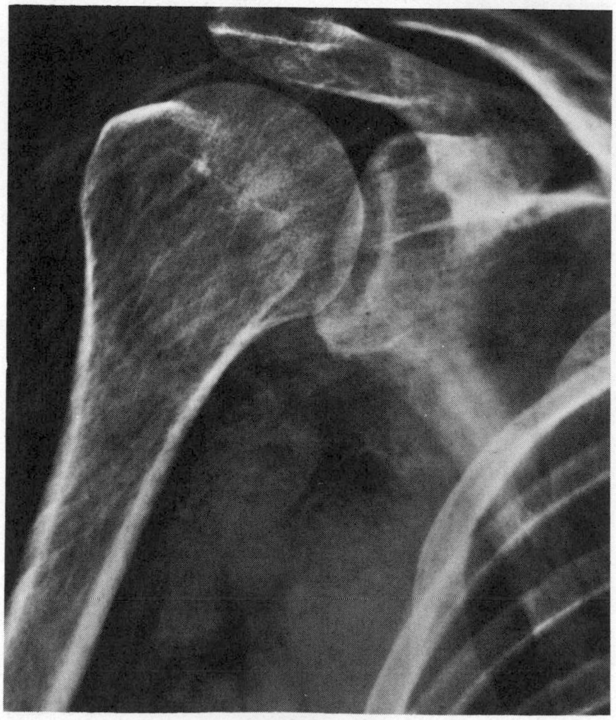

Figure 4. Regular linear pattern of gas within muscle bundles in "spontaneous" clostridial myonecrosis of the shoulder in a young man with advanced Hodgkin's disease.

TREATMENT. Complete excision of diseased muscle has been the only effective treatment for gas gangrene in the past. It has been repeatedly observed that when affected muscle was overlooked or could not be removed, the disease progressed despite antibiotics or antitoxin.

Myonecrosis in an extremity may involve only a few muscle bundles if it is detected at an early stage. If these are excised a functional limb can be salvaged. When surgery is delayed, the necrosis may become so extensive that there is no alternative to amputation. Postoperative gas gangrene of the abdominal wall generally requires extensive resection.

The toxemia clears fairly soon after surgery, and most patients who were not comatose, in refractory shock, or in extremis before surgery go on to recover. The surgical wound is left open under sterile dressings for periodic inspection of muscle at the resected margins.

The overall recovery rate in patients who receive competent surgical care is about 75 to 85 per cent (Altemeier and Fullen, 1971; Langley and Winkelstein, 1945). Prognosis is worse in postoperative cases and in patients with advanced age, underlying illness, abdominal wall involvement, and especially, immunocompromised status. Even better recovery rates (85 to 95 per cent) are seen when disease is limited to the extremities.

Surgery must be supplemented with prompt blood, plasma and fluid replacement to correct hypovolemia, which can progress rapidly to refractory hypotension in these critically ill patients. Fluid balance, urine output, central venous pressure, cardiac status, and renal function must be monitored closely.

Aqueous penicillin is recommended in doses of 16 to 24 million units/day. Cephalosporins (cefazolin, 1 gm I.V. every six hours), clindamycin (600 mg I.V. every six hours), or chloramphenicol (1.0 gm I.V. every four to six hours) can be given to patients who are allergic to penicillin. Although antibiotics cannot penetrate the heavily infected necrotic tissues, they help prevent invasion of healthy muscle and can treat bacteremia. An aminoglycoside is needed if gram stains reveal heavy gram-negative rod contamination or if the clinical course raises concern about associated gram-negative bacteremia. Smears of clostridial exudates must be interpreted cautiously, however, because on occasion clostridia do not retain the gram stain and appear as gram-negative rods.

Extensive military experience with polyvalent clostridial antitoxin has shown a high incidence of unpleasant and occasionally dangerous serum sickness reactions without clear-cut therapeutic effect in myonecrosis. Despite intravenous infusion and local infiltration of large amounts of antitoxin, the spread of infection was not prevented and the toxemia was not reversed. Antitoxin is no longer generally recommended for therapy, although some clinicians still favor its use (Altemeier and Fullen, 1971). Antitoxin should be given to the rare patient with associated clostridial septicemia and significant hemolysis.

In some patients the disease is too extensive for resection. This group includes some whose disease has spread extensively despite initial surgery (amputation), some in whom diagnosis or transport was delayed, and a few whose disease progressed very rapidly. In 1961 the use of hyperbaric oxygen (HBO) was reported as a dramatic development for these hopeless cases. The first report in English reviewed two cases with myonecrosis (Brummelkamp et al., 1961). By 1963 a series of 25 cases had been reported, and in 1972 the results of 130 cases treated by HBO therapy in Amsterdam were tabulated (Roding et al., 1972).

The objective of HBO therapy is to raise the Eh of tissues by oxygen saturation to a level at which pathogenic clostridia cannot continue the process of myonecrosis. The inspired partial pressure of oxygen at 3 atmospheres pressure is over 2000 mm Hg; arterial pO_2 reaches 1700 mm Hg, but venous pO_2 values are only about 100 mm Hg. Tissue pO_2 values of 200 to 300 mm Hg have been recorded. Proponents of HBO therapy claim that the hyperoxia reduces toxemia dramatically and terminates the disease process. Experimental studies indicate that *C. perfringens* is inhibited but not killed by oxygen at 3 ATA, and that alpha toxin is not destroyed. One study suggests that the release of alpha toxin is inhibited by HBO (Gottlieb, 1971). Experimental studies in animals have not shown therapeutic effects comparable to the reported clinical experience. There are complications of hyperbaric oxygen therapy related to oxygen toxicity and to hazards of decompression: nausea, vomiting, dizziness, convulsions, tympanic membrane injury, abdominal distention, aeroembolism, and pulmonary complications.

Unfortunately, despite two decades of experience, six international congresses, major expenditures for construction and staffing of hyperbaric facilities, and a reported clinical experience of over 800 cases of "gas gangrene," the exact role of HBO therapy in the management of myonecrosis is still very unclear because it rests on uncontrolled studies and because muscle was not examined in many treated cases. It seems that HBO can arrest disease in some cases, but it is uncertain if it is safe to rely on this therapy instead of surgery in all cases or in any particular case. The documentation of therapeutic effect has been unsatisfactory and does not support the extravagant claims put forth by advocates of this therapy. To resolve this question a large, well-planned and well-monitored collaborative study involving several centers over several years will be required, since myonecrosis is such a rare disease. Since HBO facilities are limited in number and distribution, the questions raised in HBO therapy are academic for much of the world. For the present, prompt surgical excision appears to be the surest therapy for proven myonecrosis.

PROPHYLAXIS. Active immunization is not employed because gas gangrene is so rare (0.5 to 1 case per million per year) and because the incubation period after injury is so short. Toxoids of alpha toxin can be prepared, but the many antigenic subtypes of *C. perfringens*, Type A, limit the development of an effective antibacterial vaccine.

Many cases of gas gangrene have developed despite passive immunization of both military personnel and civilians with polyvalent horse antitoxin shortly after injury. Antitoxin is no longer stocked by the United States military services for prevention (or treatment) of gas gangrene.

Antibiotic prophylaxis is widely practiced for contaminated traumatic injuries. If given early and in large doses, penicillin may offer some degree of protection (Owen-Smith and Matheson, 1968). However, if a wound is not adequately débrided, myonecrosis can develop despite any amount of antibiotic.

Penicillin prophylaxis is strongly recommended to prevent postoperative gas gangrene after mid-thigh amputations for vascular disease and after orthopedic surgery of the hip or femur, both "clean" surgical procedures that carry a special risk (Parker, 1969). The operative site should be prepared with a 30-minute povidone-iodine scrub that can kill the clostridial spores that are so commonly found on the thighs and buttocks. Antimicrobial prophylaxis is also recommended for biliary tract surgery when there is emphysematous cholecystitis, when common duct exploration is planned, or when intraoperative gram stains of bile reveal clostridia. It is less likely that significant anticlostridial protection would be afforded by antibiotics in "contaminated" surgery such as large bowel resection.

Prevention of gas gangrene rests on proper initial surgical care of contaminated traumatic wounds. The wound must be thoroughly cleaned, all foreign material must be removed, dead tissues must be débrided, tissue spaces must be obliterated, compression within fascial compartments must be relieved, arterial injuries should be repaired, primary closure must be avoided, open reduction with prosthetic implantation should be delayed, any casts that are applied should be bivalved, and hypovolemia or shock must be treated promptly. If these principles are followed, over two thirds of cases of clostridial myonecrosis can be prevented.

References

Altemeier, W. A., and Fullen, W. D.: Prevention and treatment of gas gangrene. JAMA 217:806, 1971.

Bornstein, D. L., Weinberg, A. N., Swartz, M. N., and Kunz, L. J.: Anaerobic infections. Review of current experience. Medicine 43:207, 1964.

Brummelkamp, W. H., Hogendijk, J. L., and Boerema, I.: Treatment of anaerobic infections (clostridial myositis) by drenching the tissues with oxygen under high atmospheric pressure. Surgery 49:299, 1961.

Finegold, S. M.: Anaerobic Bacteria in Human Disease. New York, Academic Press, 1977, pp. 386–432.

Gottlieb, S. F.: Effect of hyperbaric oxygen on microorganisms. Ann Rev Microbiol 25:111, 1971.

Langley, F. H., and Winkelstein, L. B.: Gas gangrene. A study of 96 cases treated in an evacuation hospital. JAMA 128:783, 1945.

Ledingham, I. M., and Tehrani, M. A.: Diagnosis, clinical course and treatment of acute dermal gangrene. Br J Surg 62:364, 1975.

MacLennan, J. D.: The histotoxic clostridial infections of man. Bacteriol Rev 26:177, 1962.

Oakley, C. L.: Gas gangrene. Br Med Bull 10:52, 1954.

Owen-Smith, M. S., and Matheson, J. M.: Successful prophylaxis of gas gangrene of the high velocity missile wound in sheep. Br J Surg 55:36, 1968.

Parker, M. T.: Post-operative clostridial infections in Britain. Br Med J 3:671, 1969.

Phillips, J., Heimbach, D. M., and Jones, R. C.: Clostridial myonecrosis of the abdominal wall. Management after extensive resection. Am J Surg 128:436, 1974.

Robb-Smith, A. H. T.: Tissue changes induced by *Clostridium welchii* Type A filtrates. Lancet 2:362, 1945.

Roding, B., Groenveld, P. H. A., and Boerema, I.: Ten years of experience in the treatment of gas gangrene with hyperbaric oxygen. Surg Gynec Obstet 134:579, 1972.

Smith, L. D. S.: Virulence factors of clostridium perfringens. Rev Inf Dis 1:254, 1979.

Strunk, S. W., Smith, C. W., and Blumberg, J. M.: Ultrastructural studies on the lesion produced in skeletal muscle fibers by crude Type A *C. perfringens* toxin and its purified alpha fraction. Am J Pathol 50:89, 1967.

Wilson, T. S.: The significance of *Clostridium welchii* infections and their relationship to gas gangrene. Can J Surg 4:35, 1960.

254 NONCLOSTRIDIAL ANAEROBIC CELLULITIS (SYNERGISTIC NECROTIZING FASCUTIS OR CELLULITES; POLYMICROBIAL GANGRENE)

H. HARLAN STONE, M.D.

Except for clostridial sepsis and rare instances of peptostreptococcal gangrene, anaerobic soft tissue infections are caused by the synergistic action of a mixed bacterial flora, containing several species of aerobic and anaerobic bacteria. Clinical manifestations vary considerably but are primarily determined by the tissue planes involved and the general resistance to infection of the patient. Indeed, specific pathogen combinations appear to be of secondary importance in determining the clinical presentation as well as the final outcome.

As a general rule, the course of the infection is one of progressive tissue destruction, eventually leading to a fatal septicemia caused by the aerobic component, with or without an associated anaerobic bacteremia. Although specific parenteral antibiotic therapy may offer temporary control of the local process as well as the bacteremia, excision of all necrotic tissue and appropriate management of the resultant open contaminated wound are the absolute requisites for survival of the patient.

ETIOLOGY. The usual method for classification of infection on the basis of specific etiologic agent or agents is not practical in the case of nonclostridial anaerobic sepsis because the infectious process is almost always due to a *microbial synergism* between different aerobic and anaerobic bacteria (Giuliano et al., 1977). At times, there may be only one aerobic and one anaerobic species, thereby creating a dual symbiosis, as in Meleney's cellulitis (aerobic *Staphylococcus aureus)* and anaerobic *Peptostreptococcus* (Meleney, 1931). Polymicrobial synergistic infections, however, are far more common and are caused by one or more aerobic gram-negative rods *(Escherichia coli, Klebsiella pneumoniae, Enterobacter aerogenes)* in combination with many different species of anaerobic bacteria, including peptostreptococci, *Bacteroides fragilis, Bacteroides melaninogenicus, Bacteroides corrodens,* and fusobacteria.

PATHOGENESIS. The basic problem is the introduction of a mixture of aerobic and anaerobic bacteria into compromised tissues. The infected tissues often display poor vitality secondary to a generalized illness like diabetes or to local trauma from surgery or accidental causes. The site of infection is often near the rectum, from which the polymicrobial fecal flora can initiate infection.

In a polymicrobial mix, if there are both aerobic and anaerobic bacteria, potentiation of virulence for each component is possible. Aerobic organisms appear to reduce significantly the local redox potential by taking up most if not all of the available tissue oxygen, thereby providing an environment more conducive to anaerobic growth. The greater the quantity of oxygen extracted from tissues infected by aerobic species, the greater the number and the more fastidious the anaerobes that can be supported in a mixed flora. The aerobic gram-negative enteric bacilli are especially well adapted to serve in this capacity because they are facultative organisms that thrive even after tissue oxygen is depleted. In addition, gram-negative bacilli can produce a lethal bacteremia.

Anaerobic organisms bring catabolic enzymes to the bacterial symbiosis. It would seem that gangrene results from the direct action of these exotoxins on host cells or thrombotic occlusion of vessels by these toxins. Since tissue barriers are easily breached and immunoglobulins are probably destroyed by anaerobic proteolysis, it is not surprising that bacteremia is exceedingly common whenever anaerobic organisms participate in an infection.

CLINICAL MANIFESTATIONS

General Features. Anaerobic soft tissue infections characteristically produce a fetid odor. As a general rule, there is spiking fever to 39° or 40° C; leukocytosis exceeds 15,000 mm^3 with a significant shift to immature polymorphonuclear forms; and the patient appears exceedingly toxic and may become irrational as well. The jaundice of a septic hemolytic anemia may likewise be present.

Previously documented or heretofore unsuspected diabetes mellitus often complicates the clinical picture by progressing to overt ketoacidosis. Since renal failure may also pre-exist, development or worsening of antecedent uremia is common. Extremes of nutrition are often noted, with patients being either extremely obese or obviously malnourished. Infants, preschool children, and the elderly are the usual victims of these infections.

Specific Features

Meleney's Cellulitis. The first report of an aerobic-anaerobic symbiosis in clinical infection was made by Meleney in 1924. In this instance, a dual synergism was established between the aerobic *S. aureus* and an anaerobic *Streptococcus,* now classified as *Peptostreptococcus.* The infection is usually a postoperative complication in a compromised patient.

The initial lesion is either an unimpressive cellulitis or a small area of cutaneous gangrene. Over a period of several days, the extent of tissue necrosis enlarges, the more centrally located eschar sloughs, and an ever-expanding ulcer results. Despite relatively healthy appearing granulations in the wound base and at its margin, the lesion steadily progresses.

The infection responds to intravenous oxacillin in a dose of 1.0 g every four hours. Patients allergic to penicillin can be given 600 mg clindamycin every four hours I.V. Wound excision and closure by a delayed split skin graft are usually necessary also.

Polymicrobial Synergistic Gangrene. Most infections caused by a polymicrobial symbiosis of bacteria with strikingly different oxygen requirements harbor one or more facultatively aerobic enteric gram-negative rods, a multitude of various anaerobic species, and often the enterococcus. The enteric bacteria may be *E. coli, K. pneumoniae, E. aerogenes,* and *Proteus mirabilis,* and the anaerobes often consist of *B. fragilis, B. melaninogenicus, Fusobacterium nucleatum, F. necrophorum,* and various peptostreptococci.

The major determinant of which type of septic process

develops is not the inoculum but the resistance of the patient. Diabetes mellitus, renal failure, advanced liver disease, malnutrition, obesity, malignancy, and immunosuppressive therapy are critical factors that promote synergistic gangrene.

The incubation period varies between three and seven days. It is longer than the incubation period for infectious gangrene due to aerobic *Streptococci* or *Clostridia* alone but generally more rapid in onset and progressive than necrosis caused by individual aerobic gram-negative rods, fungi, or the dual symbiosis of Meleney's cellulitis. Only the odor of gas gangrene is more offensive. Often the discharging exudate has the appearance of feces, so much so that a bowel fistula must be ruled out.

Several terms have been used to label these infections. Specific tissue planes along which the process spreads and the region of body involved have been the more popular determinants in classification.

1. Polymicrobial gangrene primarily confined to the skin, subcutaneous fat, and Scarpa's fascia is called *synergistic necrotizing fasciitis* (Defore et al., 1977). Seldom is there deeper penetration unless a surgical or traumatic wound has already bridged the external oblique fascia, as in cases involving the abdominal wall.

2. The same symbiotic infectious gangrene involving those tissues below the deep enveloping fascia is referred to as *synergistic necrotizing cellulitis* (Stone and Martin, 1972). Because there has been no dissection into the superficial subcutaneous fat, the skin overlying the process seldom reflects what is beneath. All soft tissues within the same fascial compartment appear to be equally necrotic, with only vessel and nerve conduits remaining intact. The first observable lesion may be a small skin ulcer that drains a thin brown fluid with a fecal odor and is surrounded by dermal necrosis and sometimes accompanied by crepitation due to gas in the tissues. Fever and toxemia are prominent.

Not only the contained muscle but also all fascial confining walls must be excised. Amputation, even as radical as hip disarticulation and hemipelvectomy, may be required. On occasion, both synergistic necrotizing fasciitis and cellulitis may be present.

3. In *Fornier's cellulitis* there is necrosis of the scrotum, penis, and perineum (Benjamin, 1979; Lee and Oh, 1979). Usually the testicles have been spared.

Most cases of synergistic gangrene are initiated by contamination of adjacent tissues by large bowel contents. A perianal source is common. Trauma or operative perforation of the colon produces synergistic gangrene almost as frequently as does perianal contamination. Similar bacteria may be introduced into a traumatic wound from sources outside the intestinal tract.

DIAGNOSIS. In Meleney's cellulitis the peptostreptococci are best recovered from the advancing edge of the ulcer even though *S. aureus* can be grown from any part of the lesion.

A fetid odor is diagnostic of anaerobic infection in polymicrobial synergistic gangrene. Further insight into the etiology is obtained when bacteria seen in Gram stain of the exudate do not grow in aerobic culture the next day. In fact, peptostreptococci can be identified in smears of fetid drainage if streptococci seen in the Gram stain have not grown aerobically in 48 hours. By then, however, a laboratory with ordinary anaerobic competence can recover peptostreptococci in simple commercial anaerobic jars. *Bacteroides* sp and fusobacteria may be more difficult to isolate and identify.

Clinically, synergistic gangrene must be differentiated from anaerobic streptococcal myonecrosis and clostridial myonecrosis. The last two syndromes, in contrast to synergistic gangrene, are primarily infections of muscles. The purulent drainage from the wound of streptococcal myonecrosis also distinguishes it from synergistic infection, and there is no mixed infection on smear.

TREATMENT. The basic principles of treatment are centered about total excision of all necrotic tissue, maintenance of an open wound with almost daily dressing changes and repeated débridement when necessary, and eventual closure of the surface defect by split-thickness skin graft in cases with a sizable gap, or by delayed primary closure or spontaneous wound contracture if only a small separation persists. Survival can be correlated almost uniformly with the specific anatomic planes involved and thus the potential for all gangrenous tissue to be excised.

Antibiotics are given to control the often attendant bacteremia and to protect fresh tissues exposed to inoculation at the time of surgical débridement. Since exudate smears are not always reliable and since definitive culture data are seldom available for several days, wound appearance is the main determinant by which antibiotics should be selected. In addition, more than one antimicrobial agent may be required, because a polymicrobial flora is often present in the blood as well as within the wound. Systemic antibiotics should be continued until the wound has closed.

The aerobic gram-negative bacilli are treated with tobramycin or gentamicin in a dose of 1.5 mg/kg body weight every eight hours I.V. Penicillin or one of its analogues may be added and should be given intravenously every 4 to 6 hours. For the anaerobic component of the synergism, metronidazole in a dose of 10 mg/kg body weight every 12 hours, intravenously should be selected. At least equally effective, with avoidance of aminoglycoside nephrotoxicity are intravenous moxalactam, 2 g every 6 hours (Winston et al., 1981) or cefotaxime, 2 g every 6 hours (Francke and Neu, 1981).

Topical agents are likewise useful, providing higher concentrations on the wound surface and within the discharging exudate than could be achieved by a parenteral route alone. Local bacterial populations and thus total quantity of necrotizing toxin are thereby reduced.

Antimicrobial agents used for direct application to the wound surface should not freely bind to tissue proteins. Various aminoglycosides, cephaloridine, and mafenide are generally recommended.

PROGNOSIS. Approximately one half of the deaths occur within the first week of therapy from uncontrolled infection. Inability or failure to excise all infected tissue, ineffective antibiotic therapy, and significant impairment in the mechanism of host resistance appear to be the more responsible factors. Although late deaths are sometimes due to recurrent sepsis, the major complications of diabetes mellitus, renal disease, and surgical management of massive tissue defects are the most common reasons for the delayed fatalities.

The overall mortality rate is 40 per cent, being greatest in cases of polymicrobial synergistic gangrene in the elderly compromised patient.

References

Benjamin, B. I.: Fornier's gangrene. Br J Urol 51:312, 1979.

Defore, W. W., Jr., Mattox, K. L., Dang, M. H., Crawford, R., and Jordan, G. L.: Necrotizing fasciitis; a persistent surgical problem. J Am Coll Emerg Phys 6:62, 1977.

Francke, E., and Neu, H.: Use of cefotaxime, a B-lactamase-stable cephalosporin in the therapy of serious infections, including those due to multiresistant organisms. Am J Med 71:435, 1981.

Giuliano, A., Lewis, F., Jr., Hadley, K., and Blaisdell, F. W.: Bacteriology of necrotizing fasciitis. Am J Surg 134:52, 1977.

Lee, C., and Oh, C.: Necrotizing fasciitis of the genitalia. Urology 13:604, 1979.

Meleney, F. L.: Bacterial synergism in disease processes with a confirmation of the synergistic bacterial etiology of a certain type of progressive gangrene of the abdominal wall. Ann Surg 94:961, 1931.

Meleney, F. L.: Hemolytic *Streptococcus* gangrene. Arch Surg 9:317, 1924.

Stone, H. H., and Martin, J. D., Jr.: Synergistic necrotizing cellulitis. Ann Surg 175:702, 1972.

Winston, D., Busuttel, R., Kurtz, T., and Young, L.: Moxalactam therapy for bacterial infections. Arch Int Med 141:1607, 1981.

255

PLEURODYNIA

MELVIN I. MARKS, M.D.

Pleurodynia is an acute viral infection characterized by the sudden onset of pleuritic chest pain, fever, headache, and generalized malaise. Synonyms for this syndrome include Bornholm disease, devil's grip, and epidemic myalgia. Although the infection usually involves the striated intercostal muscles, abdominal pain may be prominent, and other organ systems can be involved.

ETIOLOGY. The most common cause of pleurodynia is an infection due to coxsackievirus B. All six types of the B group viruses have been cultured from patients with this syndrome, and infection with multiple types have been documented as well. Coxsackievirus A, echovirus, and herpes simplex virus infections have also been associated with this syndrome infrequently. Coxsackieviruses A4 and A6 and echovirus Type 8 are recently reported examples.

PATHOGENESIS AND PATHOLOGY. The pathogenesis of this disease is inferred from clinical experience and experimental animal infections. The viruses gain entry via the human gastrointestinal tract. A viremia follows with seeding of virus to the striated intercostal muscles. In some patients the testicles, myocardium, pericardium, and the brain or meninges may also be infected.

IgM is the first class of antibody to increase, and later the IgG level is elevated (Schmidt et al., 1973). These immunoglobulins stop viral replication and terminate the infection. T lymphocytes are stimulated by the viral antigen and appear to contribute to the severity of local inflammation (Woodruff and Woodruff, 1974).

Pathologic studies of human tissues are not available. Coxsackievirus B causes intense myositis in suckling mice and hamsters, and has also been reported in human polymyositis (Schiraldi and Iandolo, 1978). Histopathologic examination of striated muscle lesions reveals necrosis with nuclear pyknosis, loss of cross-striations, fragmentation, and hyaline degeneration.

CLINICAL MANIFESTATIONS. Approximately one-fourth of patients with pleurodynia have prodromal headache, malaise, anorexia, and diffuse myalgia. This prodrome usually lasts two to three days but may be as long as ten days. The incubation period is two to five days. The most common clinical feature is sudden, sharp, paroxysmal pain over the lower ribs or sternum (Sylvest, 1934; Bain et al., 1961). The chest pain is accentuated by deep breathing, coughing, and movement and may radiate to the shoulders, neck, and scapula. A local area of hyperesthesia or tenderness is sometimes present over the painful region. Abdominal pain also occurs frequently and may be the only manifestation, particularly in younger patients. A painful episode may last several seconds to a few minutes, and the patient is remarkably symptom-free between attacks. The pain has been severe enough to simulate coronary occlusion, rib fracture, cholecystitis, or pulmonary embolization.

The fever is occasionally diphasic, as in other enteroviral infections. Nonproductive cough, nausea, vomiting, diarrhea, and shaking chills have also been described.

Despite the severe symptoms in some, most young patients have a mild illness, and coxsackievirus infections may be asymptomatic in one half to two thirds of individuals.

Children and young adults of both sexes seem to be most commonly affected with pleurodynia, although the age range is great (Lau, 1983). Coxsackievirus B infections have been documented in some young infants with only fever, paroxysmal crying, tachycardia, and features suggestive of intussusception in others (Dery et al., 1974).

The physical examination of patients with pleurodynia is often unrewarding. Tachycardia may accompany fever and is occasionally disproportionately severe. A pleural friction rub has been noted in as many as one fourth of patients with pleurodynia; pleural effusion may also be present. Sore throat sometimes occurs and may occasionally be due to exudative pharyngotonsillitis.

The course of pleurodynia is usually benign and lasts three to five days, but symptoms may persist for several months and may cause serious morbidity. Deaths have not been reported.

COMPLICATIONS AND SEQUELAE. Since pleurodynia is one manifestation of systemic coxsackievirus infection, patients may also have meningoencephalitis, myocarditis, pericarditis, pleuritis, hepatitis, or bronchitis. As many as 10 per cent of men may have orchitis, and 30 per cent of these will suffer relapses of testicular pain and swelling one to six months later.

GEOGRAPHIC VARIATIONS IN DISEASE. Pleurodynia is a worldwide disease of the summer and autumn months. The disease is usually sporadic, nevertheless, epidemic outbreaks have been described in several communities in the warmer months. The name Bornholm disease refers to an outbreak of pleurodynia on the Danish island of Bornholm in 1930 (Sylvest, 1934). Person-to-person contact is probably the most critical factor in communicability. Coxsackieviruses have also been isolated from sewage, shellfish, and flies.

DIAGNOSIS. The sudden onset of sharp pain, its intermittent character, location, and the absence of other causes usually make the diagnosis easy. The season and the prevalence of similar illness in family members or in the community are also clues. Preeruptive herpes zoster is differentiated by its more consistent pain, and costochondritis by swelling of the costochondral junction. Although abdominal pain may be severe, physical examination of the abdomen is usually negative. If a pleural effusion is present, pneumonia, malignancy, tuberculosis, pulmonary infarct, and other causes must be excluded.

Laboratory studies are usually normal in pleurodynia. These include chest radiograph, electrocardiogram, and urinalysis. The white blood cell count is usually between 3000 and 8000 cells/mm^3, and polymorphonuclear leukocytes often predominate. Creatine phosphokinase may be elevated as evidence of injury to striated muscle.

Coxsackievirus B and the other viruses causing pleurodynia can be isolated from the throat and/or feces of these patients. Although the recovery rate of viruses is highest in the first week, they may be present in the stools for two to three weeks and sometimes for months. Coxsackie B viruses can be isolated in human diploid fibroblast cell lines as well as in human epithelial and rhesus monkey kidney tissues. Most of the other viruses causing this syndrome can also be cultured in these cell lines; however, certain coxsackieviruses A (Types 9 and 16) require inoculation of suckling mice or other more specialized techniques for cultivation and identification. Coxsackieviruses are serotyped by neutralization, which also serves to characterize the humoral antibody response. Antibody responses to infection are limited to the infecting virus, but occasionally heterotypic booster responses are noted. The virus may be isolated from the cerebrospinal fluid or pericardium in aseptic meningitis or pericarditis.

TREATMENT AND PROPHYLAXIS. Although experimental studies have indicated some activity for thiourea derivatives and other chemical agents against coxsackieviruses, the application of these chemicals to human disease has not yet been reported. Although non-narcotic analgesics may be tried first, codeine and even meperidine may be necessary. Narcotics should be avoided in patients with serious underlying lung disease. Indomethacin may be a useful alternative in these situations.

Prevention of pleurodynia is not possible. However, malnourished individuals, newborns, and immunocompromised hosts should avoid direct contact with patients with pleurodynia or other coxsackievirus infections.

References

Bain, H. W., McLean, D. M., and Walker, S. J.: Epidemic pleurodynia (Bornholm disease) due to coxsackie B-5 virus. Pediatrics 27:889, 1961.

Dery, P., Marks, M. I., and Shapera, R.: Clinical manifestations of coxsackievirus infections in children. Am J Dis Child 128:464, 1974.

Lau, R. C. H.: Coxsackie B virus infection in New Zealand patients with cardiac and noncardiac diseases. J Med Virol 11:131, 1983.

Schiraldi, O., Iandolo, E.: Polymyositis accompanying Coxsackie virus B2 infection. Infection 6.32, 1978.

Schmidt, N., Magoffin, R., and Lennette, E.: Association of group B coxsackieviruses with cases of pericarditis, myocarditis, or pleurodynia by demonstration of immunoglobulin M antibody. Infect Immun 8:341, 1973.

Sylvest, E.: Epidemic myalgia: Bornholm Disease. Copenhagen, Levin and Munksgaard, 1934.

Woodruff, J., and Woodruff, J.: Involvement of T lymphocytes in the pathogenesis of coxsackievirus B, heart disease. J Immunol 113:726, 1974.

J. INFECTIONS ACQUIRED FROM ANIMALS

256

BITES: P. MULTOCIDA, DF-2, S. MONILIFORMIS, AND S. MINOR

J. L. Ryan, Ph.D., M.D.

Animal bites are responsible for approximately 1.2 per cent of the surgical problems handled in hospital emergency rooms in the United States. These bites are due primarily to the more than 100 million canine and feline pets in the United States. Other countries also have significant dog and cat populations, and the problem of domestic animal bites and infections resulting from these bites is therefore international in scope. Studies in the United States and Great Britain indicate that nearly three-fourths of the animal-related injuries are dog bites; cat bites and scratches account for most of the remainder. Most of these bites cause no infections, but many patients have developed cellulitis and lymphangitis. About 5 per cent of dog bites and 29 per cent of cat bites that are severe enough to require medical attention have infectious complications (Kizer, 1979). More invasive infections have also occurred following these bites. The annual incidence of animal bites in the United States has been estimated at 3.5 million; it represents a major medical problem in the United States and very likely in all countries that maintain large pet populations.

P. MULTOCIDA INFECTION. Animal bite wounds are infected by various aerobic and anaerobic bacteria (Goldstein et al., 1978). The pathogen most often isolated has been *Pasteurella multocida* (Arons et al., 1982). This organism was first isolated in 1878 and was recognized for its ability to cause veterinary infections. *P. multocida* is recovered from 50 per cent of infected dog bites and 80 per cent of infected cat bites and scratches (Kizer, 1979; Francis et al., 1975). *P. multocida* is a gram-negative, coccobacillary organism that resides in the oropharynx and gingiva of many animals including dogs, cats, rats, rabbits, opossum, bear, lions, and others (Saphir and Carter, 1977; Owen et al., 1968). Commercial test systems for bacterial speciation frequently fail to identify *P. multocida* (Oberhofer, 1981). At least 50 per cent of dogs and 70 per cent of cats harbor this organism (Saphir and Carter, 1977; Owen et al., 1968; Bailie et al., 1978). In veterinary medicine, *P. multocida* is well known for the infections it causes among birds. Outbreaks of hemorrhagic septicemia due to *P. multocida* have also been reported in horses, cattle, sheep, reindeer, swine, cats, ducks, chickens, rabbits, and mice (Tindall and Harrison, 1972). Similarly, *P. multocida* has been reported to cause a broad spectrum of disease in man (Henderson, 1963). Exposure to animals may result in asymptomatic oropharyngeal carriage of *P. multocida* by man (Jones and Small, 1973).

P. multocida usually has a hyaluronic acid capsule, and at least four antigenic types have been defined. There are also eleven different O antigens. These outer membrane components may increase the pathogenicity of the organism by preventing opsonization and phagocytosis. In animal models of infection, *P. multocida* can multiply rapidly in extracellular spaces and body cavities before phagocytosis begins (Collins, 1977). Defects in humoral (but not cellular) immunity appear to predispose patients to invasive disease. Innate or acquired deficiencies of immunoglobulin or complement may impair opsonization, chemotaxis, and phagocytosis. Chronic liver and pulmonary disease are frequently associated with severe *P. multocida* infection.

P. multocida causes three types of human disease. The first is local soft tissue infection that may become complicated by tenosynovitis or osteomyelitis (Francis et al., 1975; Tindall and Harrison, 1972; Henderson, 1963; Jarvis et al., 1981). This is most frequently a complication of cat bites and scratches or dog bites. Hand infections are particularly common and are often associated with complications (Lucas et al., 1981). Patients with rheumatoid arthritis seem predisposed to joint infections with *P. multocida* following injuries from cats (Spagnuolo, 1978). Soft tissue injuries and septic arthritis have a rapid onset and slow resolution despite specific antimicrobial therapy (Ewing et al., 1980). Abscess formation is frequent in *P. multocida* soft tissue infections.

The second clinical syndrome of *P. multocida* infection is respiratory. It most often occurs with chronic lung disease and may be associated with defects in local humoral immune mechanisms. This syndrome is not directly related to animal bites (Hubbert and Rosen, 1970) and is usually correlated with domestic animal association. Bronchiectasis has been the most common predisposing illness, and the disease occurs after aspiration of secretions. Nosocomial infections have occurred in respiratory care units, suggesting that isolation is indicated for pulmonary infections (Itoh et al., 1980). *P. multocida* may cause pneumonia, pleural effusions, or abscesses (Beyt et al., 1979). Cases of empyema have also been reported (Nelson et al., 1981). These tend to occur in patients with underlying pulmonary disease and are frequently fatal.

The third clinical syndrome is disseminated *P. multocida* infection. It frequently involves the gastrointestinal tract and may spread to many other tissues including the meninges and brain (Whittle et al., 1981). This syndrome has occurred most often in patients with chronic liver disease (Nadler et al., 1979; Stein et al., 1983). In Laennec's cirrhosis and ascites, the syndromes of spontaneous bacterial peritonitis (SBP) and sepsis due to *P. multocida* have been reported following animal bites or scratches (Bearn et al., 1955; Palutke et al., 1973; Normann et al., 1971; Gerding et al., 1976). Since there may be a latent period between the exposure and the clinical presentation, a history of animal bite should always be sought when patients with cirrhosis and ascites present with febrile illness. SBP is felt to be of hematogenous origin, and metastatic infections in multiple other sites including the appendix, joints, and cardiovascular system have occurred (Henderson, 1963; Jones and Small, 1973).

Local infections with *P. multocida* are treated with antimicrobial drugs in addition to débridement and drainage. Penicillin is the drug of choice, given as procaine penicillin 600,000 units intramuscularly twice daily. Ampicillin in an oral dose of 500 mg four times daily or tetracycline in the same oral dosage is also effective. Treatment must be continued for two to four weeks because the organism tends to produce chronic and deep tissue involvement. Relapses may occur when shorter treatment periods are employed (Kam et al., 1980). The median MBC for *P. multocida* is 0.78 μg/ml of penicillin G and 3.12 μg/ml of tetracycline (Stevens et al., 1979). Therapeutic failures have been recorded with both oxacillin and erythromycin. Antimicrobial sensitivity testing is necessary because some strains are resistant to penicillin. Bacteremia is treated with 2,000,000 units of benzylpenicillin intravenously every six hours and meningitis with the same dose every three hours. Patients allergic to penicillin should be given 1.0 g chloramphenicol succinate every four hours intravenously for *P. multocida* meningitis.

Antibiotic prophylaxis for *P. multocida* infection does not appear to be warranted in all dog bite victims. Controlled trials have given conflicting results (Callaham, 1980; Elenbaas et al., 1982). It may be prudent to use prophylactic penicillin or a cephalosporin for high-risk dog bite wounds and for severe cat bites or scratches (Hawkins et al., 1983). Since the rate of infection after cat bites and scratches is much higher than after dog bites prophylactic therapy should be beneficial, but no controlled trials have been reported.

DF-2 INFECTIONS (DOG BITE SEPTICEMIA). Although *P. multocida* is the organism most commonly isolated after dog bites, another gram-negative bacterium, designated dysgonic fermenter type 2, has emerged as a cause of sepsis after contact with dogs. Dysgonic fermenter type 2 (DF-2) has been found in about thirty cases of sepsis, most of which followed dog bites or other exposure to dogs.

The organism is a fastidious gram-negative rod that grows poorly on standard microbiological media, frequently taking seven to ten days to appear in blood cultures. It tends to be of medium length (3 μm) and may be filamentous. The rods appear fusiform when Gram-stained. Growth on solid media may be difficult to obtain. Colonies are small (0.5–1.0 mm) after 72 hours. They are gray, round, convex, translucent, and nonhemolytic (Bobo and Newton, 1976). All isolates are oxidase and catalase positive, but negative for nitrate reduction, motility, urease, and indole. Thus it is relatively easy to differentiate them from other fastidious oxidase-positive gram-negative organisms such as *Brucella* and *Cardiobacterium*. Fermentation cannot usually be determined by standard methods, hence "dysgonic fermenter." In serum-supplemented carbohydrate broth, acid is produced from glucose, maltose, and lactose, but not xylose, mannitol, or sucrose (Smith and Rubin, 1983).

Its distinctive fatty acid composition allows rapid differentiation of DF-2 from other canine flora associated with dog bites. DF-2 contains large amounts of branched chain, 15 carbon fatty acid (i15:0) similar to fatty acids found in *Flavobacterium* (Dees et al., 1981). *Pasteurella multocida* contains 3-OH-myristic acid, which is not in DF-2, and none of the i15:0 acid found in DF-2. Other canine bacteria (EF-4, IIj and M-5) also have distinct fatty acid compositions (Dees et al., 1981).

The estimate that 10 per cent (4/50) of dogs are colonized with DF-2 is probably low because of the difficulties in cultural isolation (Bailie et al., 1978). Growth of DF-2 is optimal in the presence of CO_2 on enriched heart infusion broth. The organism has been detected within 72 hours radiometrically (Smith and Rubin, 1983) and in standard cultures (Schlossberg, 1979), but usually seven to ten days elapse before growth is recognized. Because a gram-stain of cultures will often show the organism before macroscopic growth is evident, it is important that the laboratory staff be alerted to suspicion of infection with this organism.

Infection with DF-2 most often presents as sepsis, but the spectrum may range from a mild febrile illness to fulminant septicemia with disseminated intravascular coagulation. The first comprehensive report of infection with this gram-negative rod described 17 cases referred to the CDC between 1961 and 1975 (Butler et al., 1977). All of the patients had fever, but since that time there have been reports of DF-2 bacteremia and endocarditis occurring without fever. Ten of the original seventeen patients had a recent dog bite and four owned dogs. The association of DF-2 infection with close contact to dogs has continued and recently was strongly supported by the isolation of DF-2 from the gingivae of a dog whose owner became septic secondary to DF-2 infection (Martone et al., 1980).

Underlying diseases predispose to more serious infection with DF-2. Splenectomy appears to offer the greatest risk. Three of the first four cases of DF-2 meningitis occurred in splenectomized patients (Butler et al., 1977). Since then many of the very severe cases of DF-2 septicemia, including a classic case of Waterhouse-Friderichsen syndrome, have been reported in splenectomized patients (Findling et al., 1980; Chaudhuri et al., 1981). In splenectomized patients, the organism has been seen in smears of the buffy coat (Martone et al., 1980). This simple technique should be performed in all splenectomized patients in whom sepsis is suspected. Alcoholism and chronic obstructive pulmonary disease also appear to be significant risk factors for severe DF-2 infection (Butler et al., 1977). Only two of the original seventeen cases reported had no underlying disease. It must be remembered, however, that severe DF-2 infection including meningitis has been reported in previously healthy adults (Orforei-Adjei et al., 1982).

DF-2 infection is probably far more common than is currently appreciated because of the fastidious nature of the organism. Cellulitis is undoubtedly the site of entry in patients who are bitten by dogs. The frequent pulmonary infiltrates associated with DF-2 bacteremia (Butler et al., 1977) may suggest primary pulmonary infection in those not bitten by dogs, but the route is not yet proven by transtracheal aspiration or direct lung aspiration.

DF-2 infection may be self-limited, even in patients with some risk factors. Two patients, one an alcoholic, survived DF-2 bacteremia without antibiotics (Schoen et al., 1980). In contrast, there has been a significant mortality associated with DF-2 infection, particularly in the compromised patient. Three of the original seventeen patients reported in 1977 died and there have been other deaths from overwhelming sepsis since then (Schlossberg, 1979; Butler et al., 1977). IgG, which binds to DF-2, has been noted in the serum of patients with DF-2 sepsis. This antibody does not seem to protect in the splenectomized patients, but may protect most normal people after exposure to DF-2.

Penicillin is the drug of choice for all infections with DF-2. The organism is resistant to aminoglycosides, but all strains tested have been sensitive to penicillin with MIC's in the range of 0.12–0.5 μg/ml (Butler et al., 1977). Up to 24 million units of penicillin G per day (4 million units every four hours) have been given for the most severe cases. Other penicillin derivatives or erythromycin are alternate modes of therapy. Infection with DF-2 should be considered in septic patients who are exposed to dogs, particularly if they lack a spleen or suffer from alcoholism or chronic pulmonary disease.

RAT-BITE FEVER. Infections due to *Streptobacillus moniliformis* and *Spirillum minor* are usually caused by the bite of a rat, and the disease resulting from these infections has been called rat-bite fever. Both organisms are present as normal flora in the oropharynx of many rodents. The clinical syndrome of rat-bite fever caused by each of these organisms overlaps, and it may be difficult to determine the specific etiology of the disease without cultural or serologic information. Rat-bite fever has been known since ancient times in India and has been recognized by the medical community since the early nineteenth century (Roughgarden, 1965).

Streptobacillary Fever. *Streptobacillus moniliformis* is a pleomorphic, gram-negative rod that is a facultative anaerobe and is well known for its ability to convert spontaneously to L-form variants in culture. It grows best in medium supplemented with serum but has frequently been recovered from standard blood culture media. Typical puffball colonies are seen in liquid medium. The organism was studied in some detail after the 1926 outbreak of a febrile disease associated with raw milk consumption in Haverhill, Massachusetts. It was recovered from blood in over half of those in whom blood culture was attempted. It is of interest that cow's milk is a poor medium for growth of *S. moniliformis*, and aside from the epidemiologic association with milk consumption in the affected population, the only direct evidence of milk contamination was the presence of antibody to *S. moniliformis* in one cow from the implicated dairy (Parker and Hudson, 1926). The epidemic was abruptly terminated by pasteurization. It is customary to refer to *S. moniliformis*-caused disease that is not attributable to a rat bite as Haverhill fever (Lambe, 1974). This disease continues to occur in association with the ingestion of raw milk (Shanson, et al., 1983).

The usual incubation time of streptobacillary fever is less than ten and often only two days. Most patients have no evidence of infection at the rat bite when the clinical disease starts. Fever to 40° C (104° F) and a morbilliform or petechial rash are common. The rash is most prominent on the extremities, including the palms and soles, and erupts early in the illness. Polyarthritis occurs in 50 per cent of infected patients and is often the major complaint. Large joints are most frequently affected and are painful and tender. Joint effusions are occasionally present. If untreated, the arthritis may persist for months to years. Mortality is very low in uncomplicated cases, but severe complications including endocarditis, pneumonia, metastatic abscess, and anemia have been reported (Roughgarden, 1965; Taber and Feigen, 1979). Endocarditis of a previously diseased valve has been the most frequent fatal complication of *S. moniliformis* infection, but most reported cases occurred before the modern antibiotic era. The prognosis appears to be much better with antibiotics (McCormack et al., 1967; Hamburger and Knowles, 1953).

In streptobacillary fever there is a mild leukocytosis and a low incidence (15 to 25 per cent) of false-positive serologic tests for syphilis. The therapy of choice is 600,000 units of penicillin per day for at least seven days. Increased doses should be used if a prompt response is not obtained. In complicated cases, such as endocarditis, doses of 10 to 15 million units per day of penicillin have been recommended for four weeks. Streptomycin, tetracycline, and chloramphenicol should be considered when penicillin allergy or a resistant organism is encountered (Stokes et al., 1951).

Streptobacillary fever may occur after a bite from laboratory or pet rats as well as wild rats (Cole et al., 1969). Cases have been reported secondary to bites from other mammals and there are many cases with no history of an animal bite. It may be confused with other diseases, particularly of rickettsial origin, in the absence of cultural or serologic information (Portnoy et al., 1979). Most often, however, it is confused with sodoku.

Sodoku. Sodoku, or spirillary fever, is rat-bite fever secondary to infection with *Spirillum minor*. *S. minor* has not been reproducibly cultured in artificial medium. The organism is a gram-negative spiral rod, relatively short at 2 to 5 μm and containing two to six spirals. It is actively motile. When the diagnosis of spirillary fever is under consideration, the organism should be sought in blood smears and tissue exudates. Animal inoculation is usually necessary to confirm the diagnosis. One ml of blood should be administered intraperitoneally to mice or guinea pigs and the animal blood examined for characteristic organisms one to three weeks later.

Infection with *S. minor* occurs most commonly after rat bites, but as with streptobacillary fever, there are reports of sodoku secondary to the bites of other rodents and animals that eat rodents (Roughgarden, 1965). The incubation period is generally longer than ten days, and inflammation frequently persists at the site of the bite. Regional lymphadenopathy is relatively common but frank arthritis is rare. Criteria in Table 1 may help differentiate spirillary fever from streptobacillary fever. In most patients with sodoku, a macular red-brown rash spreads from the initial lesion. If untreated, the signs and symptoms abate, but relapse occurs with renewed fever, increased local inflammation, and more severe rash. Complications of the disease are rare, but endocarditis has been reported. Uncomplicated disease had a relatively low mortality in the pre-antibiotic era and mortality with penicillin has been negligible. Penicillin is so effective that it is necessary to give procaine penicillin in a dose of 600,000 units intramuscularly twice on only one day. Streptomycin and tetracycline are alternative modes of therapy. Sodoku is rare in the United States; most cases have been reported from Japan.

Table 1. DIFFERENTIAL FEATURES OF STREPTOBACILLARY FEVER AND SODOKU

	Streptobacillary Fever	Sodoku
Isolation of organism	Culture in serum-supplemented medium	Requires animal inoculation
Incubation period	Usually less than ten days	Frequently more than ten days
Local inflammation	Rare	Frequent
Regional lymphadenopathy	Rare	Frequent
Arthritis	Frequent	Rare
Rash	Frequent, morbilliform, petechial	Frequent, macular, red-brown
False-positive serologic test for syphilis	Less than 25 %	At least 50 %
Leukocytosis	Mild	Often absent
Specific serology	Helpful	Unavailable
Complications	Uncommon, severe	Very rare

References

Arons, M. S., Fernando, L., and Polayes, I. M.: *Pasteurella multocida*—the major cause of hand infections following domestic animal bites. J Hand Surg 7:47, 1982.

Bailie, W. E., Stowe, E. C., and Schmitt, A. M.: Aerobic bacterial flora of oral and nasal fluids of canines with special reference to bacteria associated with bites. J Clin Microbiol 7:223, 1978.

Bearn, A. G., Jacobs, K., and McCarty, M.: *Pasteurella multocida* septicemia in man. Am J Med 18:167, 1955.

Beyt, B. E., Sondag, J., Roosevelt, T. S., and Bruce, R.: Human pulmonary pasteurellosis. JAMA 242:1647, 1979.

Bobo, R. A., and Newton, E. J.: A previously undescribed gram-negative bacillus causing septicemia and meningitis. Am J Clin Path 65:564, 1976.

Butler, T., Weaver, R. E., Venkata Ramani, T. K., Uyeda, C. T., Bobo, R. A., Rya, J. S., and Kohler, R. B.: Unidentified gram-negative rod infection. Ann Int Med 86:1, 1977.

Callaham, M.: Prophylactic antibiotics in common dog bite wounds: a controlled study. Ann Emerg Med 9:410, 1980.

Chaudhuri, A. K., Hartley, R. B., and Maddocks, A. C.: Waterhouse-Friderichsen syndrome caused by DF-2 bacterium in a splenectomized patient. J Clin Path 34:172, 1981.

Cole, J. S., Stoll, R. W., and Bulger, R. J.: Rat-bite fever. Am Intern Med 71:979, 1969.

Collins, F. M.: Mechanisms of acquired resistance to *Pasteurella multocida* infection: A review. Cornell Vet 67:103, 1977.

Dees, S. B., Powell, J., Moss, C. W., Hollis, G., and Weaver, R. E.: Cellular fatty acid composition of organisms frequently associated with human infections resulting from dog bites: *Pasteurella multocida* and Groups EF-4, IIj, M-5, and DF-2. J Clin Micro 14:612, 1981.

Elenbaas, R. M., McNabney, W. K. and Robinson, W. A.: Prophylactic oxacillin, in dog bite wounds. Ann Emerg Med 11:248, 1982.

Ewing, R., Fainstein, V., Musher, D. M., Lidsky, M., and Clarridge, J.: Articular and skeletal infections caused by *Pasteurella multocida*. South Med J 73:1349, 1980.

Findling, J. W., Pohlmann, G. P., and Rose, H. D.: Fulminant gram-negative bacillemia (DF-2) following a dog bite in an asplenic woman. Am J Med 68:154, 1980.

Francis, D. P., Holmes, M. A., and Brandon, G.: *Pasteurella multocida:* Infections after domestic animal bites and scratches. JAMA 233:42, 1975.

Gerding, D. N., Khan, M. Y., Ewing, J. E., and Hall, W. H.: *Pasteurella multocida* peritonitis in hepatic cirrhosis with ascites. Gastroenterology 70:413, 1976.

Goldstein, E. J. C., Citron, D. M., Wield, B., Blachman, U., Sutter, V. L., Miller, T. A., and Finegold, S. M.: Bacteriology of human and animal bite wounds. J Clin Microbiol 8:667, 1978.

Hamburger, M., and Knowles, H. C.: *Streptobacillus moniliformis* infection complicated by acute bacterial endocarditis. Arch Intern Med 92:216, 1953.

Hawkins, J., Paris, P. M. and Stewart, R. D.: Mammalian bites: Rational approach to management. Postgrad Med 73:52, 1983.

Henderson, A.: *Pasteurella multocida* infection in man; a review of the literature. Antonie van Leeuwenhoek 29:359, 1963.

Hubbert, W. T., and Rosen, M. A.: *Pasteurella multocida* infection in man unrelated to animal bite. Am J Pub Health 60:1109, 1970.

Itoh, M., Tierno, P. M., Milstoc, M., and Berger, A. R.: A unique outbreak of *Pasteurella multocida* in a chronic disease hospital. Am J Public Health 70:1170, 1980.

Jarvis, W. R., Banko, S., Snyder, E., and Baltimore, R. S.: *Pasteurella multocida* osteomyelitis following dog bites. Am J Dis Child 135:625, 1981.

Jones, F. L., and Small, C. E.: Infections in man due to *Pasteurella multocida*; importance of human carrier. Penn Med 76:41, 1973.

Kam, W. K., Haverkos, H. W., Rodman, H. M., Schmeltz, H. R., and Van Thiel, T. H.: Human pasteurellosis: The first reported case of *Pasteurella multocida* septicemia and peritonitis during pregnancy. Am J Obstet Gynecol 138:351, 1980.

Kizer, K. W.: Epidemiologic and clinical aspects of animal bite injuries. Journal of the American College of Emergency Physicians 8:134, 1979.

Lambe, D. W.: Haverhill fever and rat-bite fever. Am J Clin Pathol 62:444, 1974.

Lucas, G. L., and Bartlett, D. H.: *Pasteurella multocida* infection in the hand. Plast Recons Surg 67:49, 1981.

Martone, W. J., Zuehl, R. W., Minson, G. E., and Scheld, W. M.: Postsplenectomy sepsis with DF-2: Report of a case with isolation of the organism from the patient's dog. Ann Int Med 93:457, 1980.

McCormack, R. C., Kaye, D., and Hooke, E. W.: Endocarditis due to *Streptobacillus moniliformis*. JAMA 200:77, 1967.

Nadler, J. P., Freedman, M. S., and Berger, S. A.: *Pasteurella multocida* septicemia. N Y State J Med 79:1581, 1979.

Nelson, S. C., and Hammer, G. S.: *Pasteurella multocida* empyema: case report and review of the literature. Am J Med Sci 281:43, 1981.

Normann, B., Nilehn, B., Rays, J., and Karlberg, B.: A fatal human case of *Pasteurella multocida* septicemia after cat bite. Scand J Infect Dis 3:251, 1971.

Oberhofer, T. R.: Characteristics and biotypes of *Pasteurella multocida* isolated from humans. J Clin Micro 13:566, 1981.

Oforei-Adjei, D., Blackledge, P., and O'Neill, P.: Meningitis caused by dysgonic fermenter type 2 (DF 2) organism in a previously healthy adult. Brit Med J 285:263, 1982.

Owen, C. R., Buker, E. O., Bell, J. F., and Jellison, W. L.: *Pasteurella multocida* in animal mouths. Rocky Mtn Med J 65:45, 1968.

Palutke, W. A., Boyd, C. B., and Carter, G. R.: *Pasteurella multocida* septicemia in a patient with cirrhosis. Am J Med Sci 266:305, 1973.

Parker, F., and Hudson, N. P.: The etiology of Haverhill fever (erythema arthriticum epidemicum). Am J Pathol 2:357, 1926.

Portnoy, B. L., Satterwhite, T. K., and Dyckman, J. D.: Rat-bite fever misdiagnosed as Rocky Mountain spotted fever. South Med J 72:607, 1979.

Roughgarden, J. W.: Antimicrobial therapy of rat bite fever. Arch Intern Med 116:39, 1965.

Saphir, D. A., and Carter, G. R.: Gingival flora of the dog with special reference to bacteria associated with bites. J Clin Microbiol 3:344, 1977.

Schlossberg, D.: Septicemia caused by DF-2. J Clin Micro 9:297-298, 1979.

Schoen, R. T., Wohlgelernter, D., Barden, G. E., and Swartz, T. J.: Infection with CDC Group DF-2 gram-negative rod. Report of 2 cases. Arch Int Med 140:657, 1980.

Shanson, D. C., Midgley, J., Gazzard, B. G., Dixey, J., Gibson, G. L., Stevenson, J., Finch, R. G., and Cheesbrough, J.: *Streptobacillus moniliformis* isolated from blood in four cases of Haverhill fever. Lancet 2:92, July 9, 1983.

Smith, C., and Rubin, S. J.: DF-2 septicemia. Clin Micro News 15:90, 1983.

Spagnuolo, P. J.: *Pasteurella multocida* infectious arthritis. Am J Med Sci 275:359, 1978.

Stein, A. A., Fialk, M. A., Bievins, A., and Armstrong, D.: *Pasteurella multocida* septicemia. JAMA 249:508, 1983.

Stevens, D. L., Higbee, J. W., Oberhofer, T. R., and Everett, E. D.: Antibiotic susceptibilities of human isolates of *Pasteurella multocida*. Antimicrob Agents Chemother 16:322, 1979.

Stokes, J. F., Gray, I. R., and Stokes, E. J.: *Actinomyces muris* endocarditis treated with chloramphenicol. Br Heart J 13:247, 1951.

Taber, L. H., and Feigen, R. D.: Spirochetal infections. Pediat Clin N Am 26:377, 1979.

Tindall, J. P., and Harrison, C. M.: *Pasteurella multocida* infections following animal injuries, especially cat bites. Arch Dermatol 105:412, 1972.

Whittle, I. R., and Besser, M.: Otogenic *Pasteurella multocida* brain abscess and glomus jugulare tumor. Surg Neurol 17:4, 1982.

257

TULAREMIA

JOSEPH H. BATES, M.D.

Tularemia is an infectious disease caused by endemic *Francisella tularensis*. Although the disease is primarily found in rodents, many cases occur in man and in various kinds of wild life. The first description of a case in man was by Martin, an opthalmic surgeon, in 1907 (Simpson, 1928). The causative organism was reported in 1911 by McCoy and Chapin who described a "plaque-like disease among ground squirrels" in Tulare County, California, and called the organism *Bacterium tularense*. The human disease was called "deer fly fever" in Utah and "rabbit fever" elsewhere. Edward Francis in 1921 recognized the unity of the disease in rodents and man, and gave it the descriptive name tularemia (Francis, 1921). Ohara described an acute febrile disease in Japan transmitted by rabbits in 1925, and working with Francis showed that it was tularemia. In 1928, when Suvorov described tularemia in Astrakhan, the USSR was the scene of several outbreaks.

ETIOLOGY. Although first called *B. tularense*, the organism was soon placed in the genus *Pasteurella* because of similarities with *Pasteurella pestis*. In 1947 a new genus, *Francisella*, was established, since the organism did not belong in any of the genera in which it had been placed previously. (British investigators maintain that the organism belongs to the Brucella group.) *F. tularensis* is a minute, gram-negative, pleomorphic rod that may appear coccoid. It will not grow on ordinary media but will grow on blood-dextrose-cystine agar and other enriched media containing cystine. The disease is endemic on four continents and it appears that variation in the organisms does occur. Tularemia organisms occurring in North America are usually more virulent than the Asian and European varieties, although the less virulent forms are also found in North America. There may be other differences among the varieties, including biochemical reactions, habitat, and mode of transmission.

PATHOGENESIS AND PATHOLOGY. Mechanisms for human infection with *F. tularensis* are highly variable. The earliest descriptions associated the disease with skinning and dressing of wild rabbits and with bites by the deer fly, *Chrysops discalis* commonly found on horses. Careful investigative studies later showed that the common wood tick, *Dermacentor andersoni* harbored tularemia organisms, and presently 11 different species in North America are known to be naturally infected (Hopla, 1974). Transovarial transmission of *F. tularensis* in ticks was long thought to occur and the tick was suspected as being the natural reservoir for the organism, but recent work has shown that this is not true. A more likely natural reservoir is a multiple-host system of disease involving various highly susceptible rabbits, hares, and ticks. The tick is infected after taking a blood meal from an infected animal. The bacteria multiply in the tick, penetrate the gut, and spread to the salivary glands. There they can be injected into the next host along with the saliva or they may persist in the tick gut and be transmitted by tick fecal matter at the time of the blood meal. Naturally infected ticks in the USSR include *Dermacentor sictus* and *Dermacentor marginatus*, in Europe *Ixodes ricinusand*, and in Japan *Haemayshysalis flavis* and *Ixodes japonensia*.

Many vertebrates may become infected and over 100 different species of wild animals, 25 species of birds, and several species of fish and amphibians have been found naturally infected. Cricetine rodents and hares are extremely susceptible; rabbits, squirrels, and beavers are moderately susceptible; and carnivora and domestic animals show low susceptibility. In the USSR the vole, muskrat, mouse, and hamster are the most frequent sources of human infection. In Europe and in Japan it is primarily hares and field mice. In North America, hares, rabbits, voles, muskrats, and sheep are primarily involved in the northern regions, and rabbits and ticks are most important in the south. Minor vectors include fleas, mosquitoes (ten different species), tabanid flies, and mites.

Tularemia may also be acquired by ingestion of infected meat and contaminated water, and by inhalation. The first report of water-borne tularemia and the first major outbreak from water were recognized in the USSR, where infected voles had contaminated the water. The organism has been isolated from thoroughly cooked meat and can penetrate the intact epidermis of humans.

Man-to-man transmission of tularemia has not been proved but the organism can be cultured from the sputum, pharynx, and gastric washings of patients who have tularemic pneumonia. Almost all nonimmune laboratory investigators who study tularemia acquire the disease, most likely by inhalation. Immunized volunteers exposed to aerosol developed chest roentgenographic abnormalities, fever, and malaise after three to five days. An outbreak of an influenza-like illness in northern Sweden turned out to be airborne tularemia from inhalation of dust from dried vole feces in haystacks (Dahlstrand, 1971).

Asymptomatic infection occurs in endemic areas where exposure to ticks and infected animals is common. Sequential serologic surveys among Indians and Eskimos in Alaska and animal trappers in Montana indicate that serologic and skin test conversion occurs without recognized disease. The absence of clinical illness after infection may be explained by decreased strain virulence, a route of infection that discourages asymptomatic infection, and infection in a resistant person.

The most common site for the organism to invade humans is the skin, where an ulcer with surrounding inflammation develops in approximately half of all cases. The ulcer extends deeply and shows coagulation necrosis resembling caseation. About the margins there are polymorphonuclear leukocytes and epithelioid cells. The bacteria in the ulcer and in all other lesions are difficult to demonstrate with routine staining methods. With fluorescent antibody-staining the organisms are readily identified, usually within monocytes, macrophages, and polymorphonuclear leukocytes. Extracellular organisms are uncommon except in necrotic areas, where they are abundant.

Involvement of lymph nodes is characteristically confined to those draining the ulcer, but may become generalized along with hepatic and splenic enlargement. The lesions closely resemble tuberculosis with caseation necrosis, Langhans giant cells, epithelioid cells, and mononuclear cells predominating. At other times acute necrosis and marked suppuration may evolve. Similar lesions may be found in the spleen and liver.

The lung is involved either by inhalation of organisms or by hematogenous dissemination. In experimental animals after inhalation of bacterial aerosol the earliest lesions are collections of polymorphonuclears in the alveolar ducts and alveoli (Baskerville, 1976). This is followed by capillary congestion, bronchial inflammation, and necrosis of bronchial epithelium. Within 72 hours marked arteritis of medium and large vessels occurs. The later changes resemble those in fatal human cases. In experimental respiratory tularemia in the monkey, the primary sites of infection are the respiratory bronchioles and alveolar ducts, where the bacteria are rapidly phagocytized by alveolar macrophages. In man the most frequent pulmonary lesions at autopsy are subpleural foci of necrosis, which may coalesce to produce consolidation of an entire lobe or lung. Abscesses up to 10 centimeters in diameter may occur, and pleural involvement varies from slight thickening to extensive effusion in many nonfatal cases.

The bone marrow, pharynx, esophagus, stomach, ileum, appendix, colon, adrenals, pericardium, kidney, meninges, and brain have been involved with the necrotizing granuloma of tularemia.

CLINICAL MANIFESTATIONS. In North America tularemia shows a remarkable seasonal variation with two peaks during the year. An early spring and summer peak occurs in areas where tularemia is tick-borne, as in the south-central states. Hand contact with blood or tissue of infected animals, especially rabbits, is the most common source of infection in other regions of the United States, and this form peaks between November and February. Most cases can be placed into one of four categories: ulceroglandular, oculoglandular, glandular, and typhoidal (Dienst, 1963). Primary respiratory disease, meningitis, and a gastrointestinal form with severe diarrhea are less common. The incubation period may not be possible to determine, since a specific vector contact cannot be recalled in many cases. In those cases with a reliable vector history the incubation period ranges from a few hours to two weeks, with an average of five days. The clinical type does not alter the incubation period.

The clinical picture is extremely variable owing to the several portals of entry and the great fluctuations in morbidity. Prolonged tularemia with low-grade fever and adenopathy, suggests a lymphoma. The most frequent complaints are chills and fever followed by headache, backache, generalized muscle aches, and weakness. Delirium, stupor, or marked restlessness are frequent in patients with acute toxemia. No central nervous system infection is demonstrated in these patients and the cause for their symptoms is unexplained. Specific treatment clears the central nervous system symptoms rapidly. The liver and spleen enlarge in a few cases. Jaundice is uncommon and seen only in the severely ill patient. Cutaneous manifestations are usually limited to the ulcer and enlarged regional lymph nodes, but in exceptional cases macular, papular, vesicular, and pustular eruptions are prominent. A petechial rash over the trunk and proximal extremities can be seen and typical erythema nodosum is a rare manifestation.

Ulceroglandular Tularemia. This is the most common type and occurs in 50 to 80 per cent of all cases. The primary lesion is a papule at the point of inoculation, usually on the finger or hand if acquired by direct animal contact, but almost anywhere if vector borne. The papule rapidly becomes painful and swollen and suppurates in the center, leaving an ulcer 3 to 5 mm in diameter. Some ulcers may reach 2 cm in diameter. Tenderness and pain in the regional lymph nodes begins about 24 hours later and becomes severe. If untreated or misdiagnosed and improperly treated the overlying skin becomes thin and the nodes drain spontaneously in about one-half of the cases. In a few patients lymphangitic nodules (simulating sporotrichosis) are found along the lymphatics draining the inoculation site. Most ulceroglandular cases do not present the overwhelming toxic infection seen with other forms.

Glandular Tularemia. Glandular tularemia shows no visible primary lesion even upon careful scrutiny. In all other respects, the disease simulates the ulceroglandular type. The glandular form accounts for 10 to 15 per cent of all cases, and most commonly involves axillary nodes. These are the least toxic of all tularemic patients and usually present with fever and localized adenopathy. The involved nodes may be very tender and show marked erythema of the overlying skin.

Oculoglandular Tularemia. This form, which accounts for only 3 to 5 per cent of all cases, enters through the conjunctival sac. Unilateral involvement is usual with associated enlargement of the cervical and preauricular lymph nodes. Photophobia, excessive lacrimation, and decreased visual acuity are common. The conjunctiva is very red and there may be small ulcerations. Membrane formation and corneal ulceration are rare. Late sequelae are seldom seen.

Typhoidal Tularemia. This is the most serious form of tularemia and has the highest mortality. There is no primary lesion and no regional lymphadenopathy. Fever, aching, mental confusion, and extreme toxicity are the primary features. Most cases occurring in laboratory workers are typhoidal. The frequency of this form varies from 10 to 30 per cent. The patients are acutely ill with dehydration, vomiting, and meningismus. Diarrhea is frequent. Pleuropulmonary infection is most frequent in this form and may complicate 40 per cent of cases. In untreated patients, the mortality rate is approximately 30 per cent.

Uncommon Forms. Oropharyngeal tularemia is primarily found in children as exudative pharyngitis (Tyson, 1976). Pustular lesions on the tonsils with membrane formation, cervical lymph node involvement, high fever, and marked difficulty in swallowing is the usual presentation and may progress to tracheal obstruction and death. Infection is probably introduced by ingestion of food or water contaminated with *F. tularensis* or by placing the hand in the mouth after handling an infected animal.

Gastrointestinal tularemia is more common in Europe and the USSR than in North America or Asia. These patients develop acute, watery diarrhea with fever and cramping abdominal pain. Bloody diarrhea or acute hemorrhage with minimal diarrhea secondary to superficial ulcerations in the colon is rare.

COMPLICATIONS AND SEQUELAE. Most observers agree that pleuropulmonary tularemia is usually secondary to hematogenous dissemination of local infection elsewhere in the body (Miller, 1969), but primary respiratory tract infection can also occur. It is a necrotizing process that heals with fibrosis and calcification. Residual pleural thickening is common. The chest roentgenographic features are variable and may be confused with tuberculosis, mycotic infection, acute bacterial pneumonia, lymphoma, and carcinoma of the lung. Almost any roentgenographic pattern may appear and tularemia must be considered in all cases of diagnostically perplexing pneumonia in those regions where tularemia occurs. Lobar consolidation with or without hilar adenopathy, pleural effusion, bronchopleural fistula and empyema, upper lobe interstitial infiltration, and massive mediastinal adenopathy without lung involvement can also occur.

Pneumonia complicates 10 to 30 per cent of cases of tularemia. The most common pulmonary complaints are cough, pleuritic pain, dyspnea, and sputum production. Hemoptysis is rare. A few patients have no respiratory complaints and the pulmonic process is discovered only by roentgenogram.

Pericardial involvement with effusion is usually associated with pneumonia. Cardiac tamponade or constrictive pericarditis may develop, requiring pericardectomy. Rhabdomyolysis may occur in extremely toxic patients.

Tularemic meningitis and encephalitis are rare complications. The symptoms are headache, stiff neck, and delirium. The cerebrospinal fluid usually shows less than 1000 cells per cubic millimeter with lymphocytes predominating. The protein content is elevated above 100 and the sugar is less than 30 mg/ml. Spinal fluid may be bloody. Most reported patients with this complication have succumbed, in part due to a delayed or missed diagnosis.

Acute renal failure secondary to tubular necrosis, exudative glomerulonephritis, or interstitial nephritis is a rare complication.

GEOGRAPHIC VARIATIONS IN DISEASE. The disease in North America is more variable in severity than in Europe or Asia; North American patients may show extreme toxicity or the disease may be mild. Asymptomatic infections occur as evidenced by conversion of serial serologic tests. In Europe and Asia, most illness is mild. In regions where ticks are abundant or where rabbit contact is frequent, ulceroglandular and glandular tularemia are common. In the USSR and eastern European countries water contamination with *F. tularensis* is more common, resulting in water-borne outbreaks in man presenting with gastrointestinal complaints.

DIAGNOSIS. The most important step in making the diagnosis of tularemia is to include it in the differential diagnosis. The initial symptoms simulate those of influenza; after the disease is well advanced with ulceration and adenopathy, streptococcal infection may be considered. When there is nodular lymphangitis, sporotrichosis is mimicked. The uncommon cases that present as generalized lymphadenopathy and fever may suggest lymphoma or infectious mononucleosis. The typhoidal form is similar to typhoid fever, and if pneumonia is present any of a number of acute and chronic bacterial pneumonias must be included as diagnostic possibilities. Sera from patients with tularemia may contain antibodies that cross-agglutinate with *Brucella abortus* and *Brucella melitensis*, but the higher titer is almost always against *F. tularensis*. Upon examination of enlarged lymph nodes the pathologist may suggest a histopathologic diagnosis of tuberculosis or cat-scratch fever.

The clinical diagnosis is relatively easy to confirm or exclude by the serum agglutination test. An agglutination titer of 1:80 or above is highly suspicious. It is always desirable to show a four-fold or greater rise in titer from the acute to the convalescent serum taken ten days to two weeks later. Antibodies first appear about the second week, but in some cases they may not be detectable for up to 30 days or more. The most toxic patients are more likely to show a delayed antibody response. The agglutination titer can reach 1:40,000 and greater but usually peaks near 1:1024. Positive agglutination tests may persist for life, but most patients show a low level of 1:80 or below within three years after recovery.

A tularemia skin test has been primarily an investigative tool. It is read 48 hours after intradermal application and measures delayed hypersensitivity. It is positive in over 90 per cent of cases during the first week of illness even when the agglutination test remains negative.

The organism can be cultured readily from infected tissues such as the skin ulcer, suppurative lymph nodes, and sputum from those with pulmonic involvement; however, it is not routinely isolated in clinical laboratories because laboratory workers who are not specifically immunized are at high risk of acquiring the disease and the special media containing cystine required for the growth of the organism are not utilized. The guinea pig and rabbit can be inoculated with pus, sputum, or infected tissue; the animal will die within one to two weeks and at autopsy focal necrosis of the liver and spleen is evident. Specific staining of infected tissues from inoculated animals or from human tissue by fluorescent antibody techniques will show intracellular organisms within macrophages and polymorphonuclear leukocytes and extracellular organisms in areas where necrosis is marked.

The white blood cell count may range from low normal to marked leukocytosis. The differential count is usually normal and there may be a mild anemia. The sedimentation rate is increased.

TREATMENT. Streptomycin is the drug of choice for treatment of tularemia. The bacteriostatic concentration for most strains of *F. tularensis* is less than 0.4 μg/ml. The dose for adults is generally 1 to 2 g daily with a treatment period of 10 to 14 days. The clinical response is dramatic except in the most advanced cases. If the patient is gravely ill with advanced pneumonia or meningitis at the time chemotherapy is begun, death may not be averted. Frequently streptomycin must be begun on clinical suspicion when serologic proof is lacking. The physician should have no reservation about streptomycin chemotherapy in this situation, since early treatment dramatically reduces the incidence of serious complications and death.

Chloramphenicol and tetracycline are also somewhat effective. Relapses after treatment with these drugs may reach 30 per cent, but retreatment with the same drug is usually effective. Gentamicin is bactericidal for *F. tularensis* and limited clinical experience indicates that this drug may be as effective as streptomycin.

General supportive measures are important in the very ill patient. Most deaths occur from extensive pneumonia producing the "adult respiratory distress syndrome." There are no data to indicate that corticosteroids are effective.

Mortality rates before specific chemotherapy ranged from 7 to 31 per cent; since the advent of streptomycin, the mortality rate has been less than 6 per cent.

PROPHYLAXIS. Strong immunity follows natural infection or immunization with a live attenuated strain of *F. tularensis* (Burke, 1977). The immunity is cell mediated and long lasting. A phenol-killed vaccine has been tried, but the protection that results is very incomplete.

References

Baskerville, A., and Hambleton, P.: Pathogenesis and pathology of respiratory tularemia in the rabbit. Br J Exp Pathol 57:339, 1976.

Burke, S. D.: Immunization against tularemia: Analysis of the effectiveness of liver Francisella tularensis vaccine in prevention of laboratory acquired tularemia. J Infect Dis 135:55, 1977.

Dahlstrand, S., Ringertz, O., and Zetterberg, B.: Airborne tularemia in Sweden. Scand J Infect Dis 3:7, 1971.

Dienst, F. T., Jr., Tularemia: A perusal of three hundred thirty-nine cases. J Louisiana Med Soc 115:114, 1963.

Francis, E. The occurrence of tularemia in nature as a disease of man. Pub Health Dep 36:1731, 1921.

Hopla, C. E.: The ecology of tularemia. Adv Vet Sci Comp Med 18:25, 1974.

Miller, R. P., and Bates, J. H.: Pleuropulmonary tularemia, a review of 29 patients. Am Rev Resp Dis 99:31, 1969.

Simpson, W. M.: Tularemia (Francis' disease). Clinical and pathological study of 48 non-fatal cases and one rapidly fatal case with autopsy occurring in Dayton, Ohio. Ann Int Med 1:1007, 1928.

Tyson, H. K.: Tularemia: An unappreciated cause of exudative pharyngitis. Pediatrics 58:864, 1976.

Wills, P. I., Gedosh, E. A., Nichols, D. R.: Head and Neck Manifestations of Tularemia. Laryngoscope 92:740, 1982.

258

PLAGUE

ALEXANDER L. KISCH, M.D.

Plague is a severe acute or chronic enzootic or epizootic bacterial infection produced by *Yersinia pestis (Y. pseudotuberculosis* subsp. *pestis)* (Williams, J. E., 1983). It is acquired in endemic areas throughout the world (Fig. 1). Over 200 species of wild rodents (e.g., marmots, squirrels, field mice, prairie dogs, and gerbils), commensal rodents (e.g., *Rattus rattus, R. norvegicus, Mus musculus)*, lagomorphs (e.g., rabbits and hares), and certain other mammalian species (e.g., dogs, cats, coyotes, and guinea pigs) are susceptible (Pollitzer, 1954; Rust et al., 1971). Rodents, which are relatively resistant to *Y. pestis*, are the reservoir in which the pathogen is maintained between epidemics of plague. Asymptomatic or, more often, life-threatening infection is sporadically and incidentally transmitted to humans from this natural animal reservoir through the bite of infected fleas (e.g., *Xenopsylla cheopis)* or, rarely, of other ectoparasites (e.g., lice and ticks) when the reservoir host enters the habitat of humans or vice versa. Domestic pet dogs and cats may transmit infection to humans via infected saliva or by transfer of infected fleas. Plague may also be acquired by direct contact with living or dead infected animals or with contaminated rodent burrow soil. Human populations in geographic areas adjoining enzootic regions are at particular risk of epidemic plague during periods when sanitation is disrupted or when rodents are not controlled and there is transmission of *Y. pestis* from

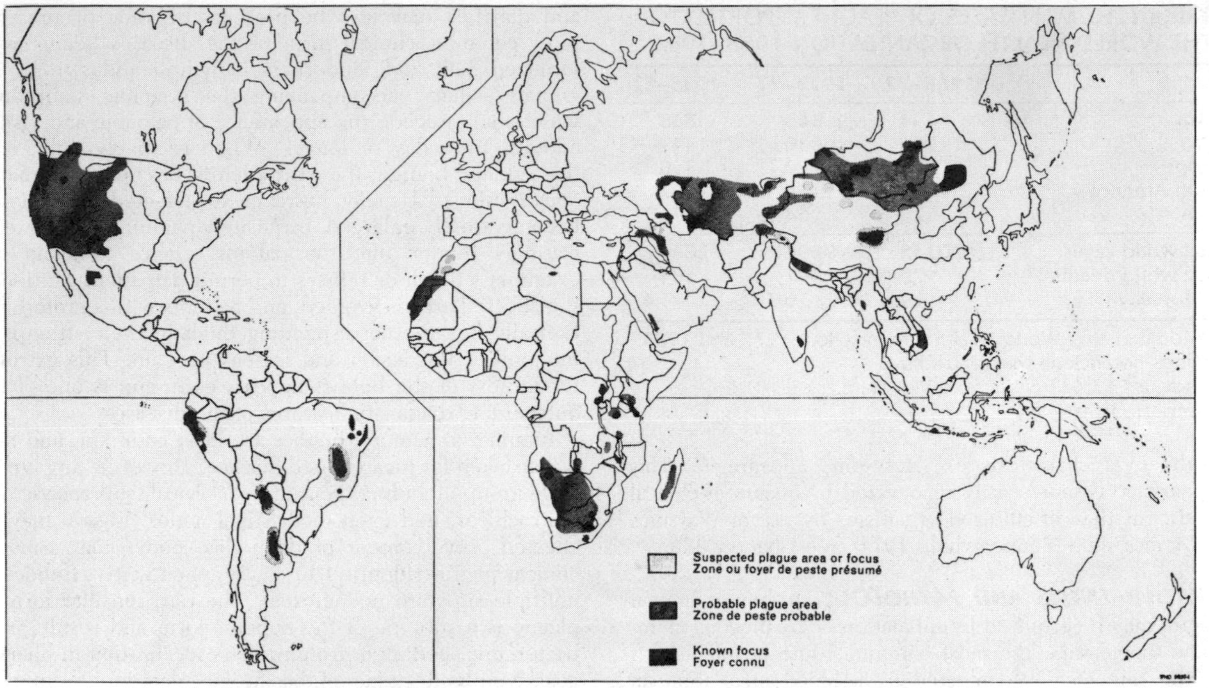

Figure 1. Known and probable foci and areas of plague, 1969. (Reprinted with permission of World Health Organization from WHO Expert Committee on Plague, Fourth Report, WHO Technical Report Series No. 447. Geneva, World Health Organization, 1970.)

sylvatic to urban rat populations. The great historic plague epidemics of mankind have usually occurred when plague-infected rat fleas, deprived of their normal hosts by massive rat epizootics and die-offs, have sought and infected human beings instead. Introduction of unrecognized cases of human or rodent plague into nonendemic areas via air travel and container freighting is an ever-present hazard. Bacteremic pulmonary seeding during the bubonic or septicemic forms of the disease may produce secondary plague pneumonia. Explosive epidemics of highly fatal primary pneumonic plague can then result from human-to-human ("demic") respiratory transmission of *Y. pestis* via droplet aerosols (Fig. 2). There has been an increase in reported cases of plague in the last decade (Table 1).

ETIOLOGY. The causative bacterium of plague, recently reclassified in the genus *Yersinia*, belongs to the family Enterobacteriaceae. Credit for its isolation in Hong Kong during the plague pandemic of 1894 is shared by the French bacteriologist A. E. J. Yersin and the Japanese bacteriologist S. Kitasato (Bibel and Chen, 1976). *Y. pestis* is a gram-negative, nonmotile, aerobic and facultatively anaerobic, nonhemolytic, oxidase-negative, pleomorphic coccobacillus 1 to 2 μm in length whose bipolar staining

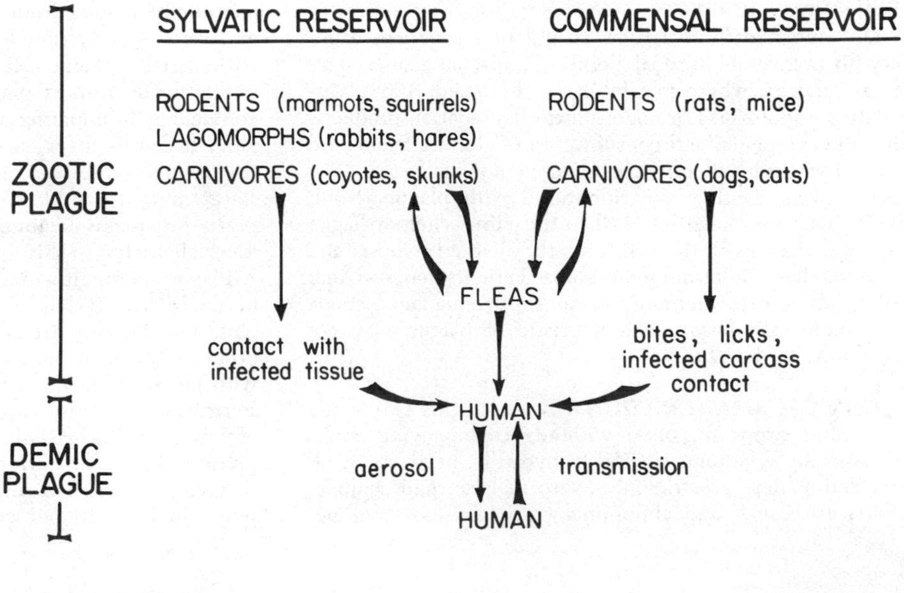

Figure 2. Epidemiologic features of plague.

Table 1. HUMAN CASES OF PLAGUE REPORTED TO THE WORLD HEALTH ORGANIZATION 1968–1982[a]

	1968–72	1973–77	1978–82
Africa	494	645	838
Asia[b]	17986[c]	6030	1449
Europe	1[d]	0	0
South America	1631	1157	507
U.S.A.	24	64	75
Total world cases	20135	7896	2869
Total world deaths	970	497	184
% Mortality	4.8	6.3	6.4

[a]Modified after World Health Organization, 1977 and 1983.
[b]Does not include Mainland China.
[c]Includes 17,437 cases from Viet Nam.
[d]Imported case.

results in a characteristic "safety-pin" appearance. This appearance is more easily recognized in smears of clinical specimens than of cultured organisms by use of Wayson's or Giemsa stain (Sonnenwirth, 1974) (see Chapter 37).

PATHOGENESIS AND PATHOLOGY. Although human plague may be acquired by inhalation or by mucous membrane inoculation, the most common route of infection is by the bite of a flea infected by a blood meal from an infected rodent. *Y. pestis* proliferates in the flea gut, where organisms lacking envelope antigen (Fraction I) replicate and block the proventriculus. Organisms regurgitated by such "blocked fleas" are then inoculated intradermally into human beings when fleas refeed. In some highly immune people, a pustule may develop at the bite but is more often absent. Usually, in less resistant people, the injected organisms spread via lymphatic channels to the regional lymph nodes. These become enlarged due to inflammation, edema, thrombosis, and hemorrhagic necrosis, forming the buboes characteristic of the disease. Bacilli replicating at these sites extracellularly and surviving intracellularly in mononuclear phagocytes (Janssen and Surgalla, 1969) become encapsulated and resistant to phagocytosis. Early bacteremic dissemination establishes suppurative foci throughout the body in the distant lymph nodes, skin, lungs, spleen, liver, and central nervous system. Concentrations of more than 100 *Y. pestis* organisms per ml of blood are common and are associated with a poor prognosis (Butler et al., 1976).

Disseminated intravascular coagulation produces capillary fibrin thrombi in renal glomeruli, adrenal glands, skin, lungs, and elsewhere in fatal cases (Finegold, 1968). Circulating endotoxin, fibrinogen-fibrin degradation products, thrombocytopenia, and consumption of clotting factors are characteristically identifiable even in nonfatal cases. The term "black death," long identified with plague (Nohl, 1961), may well have referred to the diffuse hemorrhagic, necrotic changes in the skin plus the marked hypoxia and cyanosis that result from pneumonia. Patients may succumb so rapidly to overwhelming plague septicemia and toxemia that pathologic lesions characteristic of plague may not have time to develop.

CLINICAL MANIFESTATIONS. Fever begins two to ten days after exposure, often without accompanying chills. Nonspecific symptoms such as tachycardia, headache, generalized aching, prostration, severe malaise, and conjunctivitis are usual, and abdominal pain, nausea, vomiting, and diarrhea may also be present. Bubonic plague, the most common clinical form of the disease, begins with localized pain and tenderness in lymph nodes (e.g., inguinal, axillary) accompanying the systemic symptoms, which may precede the appearance of palpable and visible adenitis by a day or longer. When relatively mild, self-limited, and benign, the early adenitis has been designated "pestis minor." Usually, however, the affected lymph nodes become grossly enlarged, exquisitely painful, and so excruciatingly tender that the patient cringes to avoid the examiner's touch or refuses to permit palpation. Motion of the affected area is avoided, and patients with a groin bubo typically flex the corresponding thigh in their attempt to immobilize the lesion and lessen the pain. This extreme tenderness of the buboes appears early and is one of the outstanding diagnostic features of the disease.

Inguinal or femoral buboes are most common, and may be mistaken for incarcerated herniae. However, any lymph node group including the axillary, cervical, supraclavicular, epitrochlear, and even mediastinal nodes (Fig. 3) may be affected. Involvement of deep iliac nodes may cause a clinical picture identical to acute appendicitis. Buboes at multiple sites are not unusual. The rare tonsillar form of plague is a subtype of the bubonic form and results from bacteremic seeding or from primary localization in pharyngeal lymphoid tissue of bacilli inoculated onto mucous membranes. It has occurred after crushing infected fleas and lice between the teeth.

Fully developed buboes vary in length from 1 to 10 cm, are usually oval or round in shape, and may be formed by the fusion of two or more lymph nodes. With development and progression of periadenitis, the fully developed bubo becomes fixed and doughy or boggy in consistency. The overlying skin may become reddened, edematous, sometimes hemorrhagic, and rarely ulcerated. Bubo suppuration with fluctuance is common, and resolution after institution of specific antibiotic therapy may be slow. Spontaneous drainage is not common in treated cases, and surgical incision and drainage of pus may occasionally become necessary.

In the relatively uncommon primary septicemic form of plague, no obvious focus of lymphadenitis may be evident. The disease may mimic gram-negative rod bacteremia of other etiologies or present as fulminant septic shock, Reyes Syndrome or secondary plague pneumonia. The latter commonly results from bacteremic seeding of the lungs and was recently noted to occur in about 20 per cent of patients with plague (Mann, 1979). Such cases may initiate outbreaks of primary plague pneumonia, a rare but highly contagious fulminating illness, which is virtually always fatal. It causes fever, severe systemic toxicity, and rapidly progressive symptoms and signs of respiratory insufficiency. Large amounts of bloody, frothy sputum teeming with *Y. pestis* organisms beginning 12 to 24 hours after onset of fever characterize this form of the disease.

Plague meningitis may develop from bacteremic seeding of meninges. It has usually occurred in patients, often children, initially treated with penicillin, ampicillin, or other suboptimal antibiotic therapies, and it is observed with increased frequency in patients with axillary buboes. Pericarditis and myocarditis occasionally occur, and signs of congestive heart failure may develop during the acute phase of illness or during convalescence.

Asymptomatic and self-limited pharyngeal carriage of *Y. pestis* in over 10 per cent of healthy contacts of plague

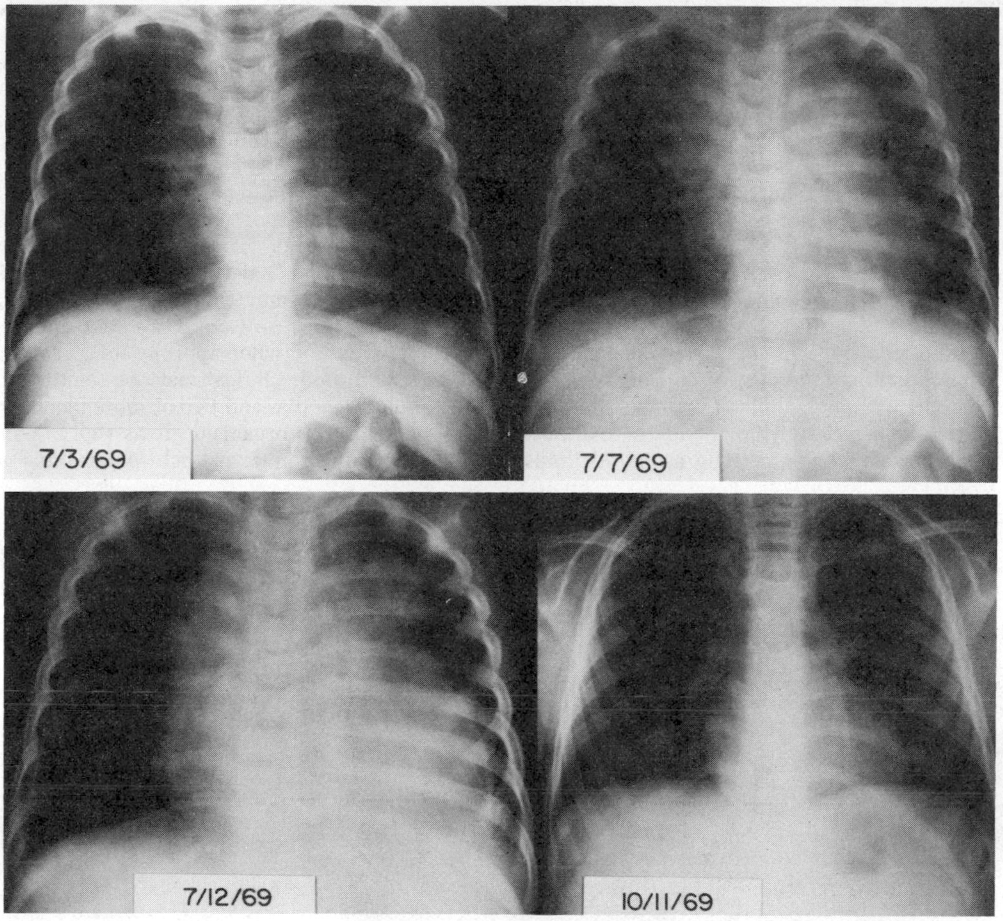

Figure 3. Serial chest roentgenograms taken during the course of bubonic plague in a 3-year-old boy who also exhibited plague meningitis after initial therapy with penicillin. Hilar lymphadenopathy and pulmonary infiltration present on the fourth hospital day (upper left) progressed after four (upper right) and nine (lower left) days, and were associated with clinical evidence of myocarditis. Film three months later (lower right) has reverted to normal appearance. (From Reed, W. P., et al.: Medicine 49:465, 1970. © 1970 The Williams & Wilkins Co., Baltimore.)

cases, as well as in a similar proportion of bubonic plague patients themselves, has been recorded. However, multiple cases of disease within households more likely reflect environmental acquisition than person-to-person respiratory transmission.

COMPLICATIONS AND SEQUELAE. Disseminated intravascular coagulation, bacteremic or endotoxemic shock, and secondary plague pneumonia are the principal early complications of untreated or partially treated plague. The late complications, in some instances attributable to delayed or suboptimal antimicrobial therapy, include *Y. pestis* meningitis, metastatic abscess formation, delayed bubo suppuration, cardiac failure, and, rarely, peripheral symmetrical gangrene.

The case-fatality rate of untreated bubonic plague is between 50 and 80 per cent, while that of the septicemic and meningitic forms of the disease is even higher; untreated plague pneumonia is an almost invariably and rapidly fatal complication.

In recent years overall plague mortality has remained high in various countries of the world, e.g., in excess of 17 per cent in the U.S.A. in the past decade, 22 per cent in the African continent, and up to 42 per cent and even 78 per cent in epidemic outbreaks in Indonesia and Nepal, respectively (Akiev, 1982).

However, with early diagnosis and initiation of antibiotic therapy, survival from bubonic plague approaches 100 per cent (e.g., Brazil) and even in primary pneumonic plague.

GEOGRAPHIC VARIATION IN DISEASE. Differences in the seasonal incidence of bubonic plague outbreaks exist among endemic areas in different parts of the world. The differences appear to be chiefly determined by climatic conditions that may alter the availability and efficiency of insect vectors; plague epidemics are most likely to occur when temperature and humidity are high. Epizootic plague outbreaks in urban rat populations produce die-offs that characteristically result in clustered cases of bubonic plague in the contiguous human settlement. Secondary pneumonic plague cases may then give rise to endemic outbreaks of primary pneumonic plague. In contrast, persistent infection of wild rodents in sylvatic or rural settings results in sporadic cases of human and domestic animal plague. Variations in the clinical features of plague attributable to specific antigenic components of *Y. pestis* or to geography-related strain variation have not been described.

DIAGNOSIS. Bubonic plague must be differentiated from adenitis caused by such other infectious agents as *Staphylococcus aureus, Streptococcus pyogenes, Franciscella tularensis, Pasteurella multocida,* and *Chlamydia trachomatis;* from the etiologic agent of cat-scratch disease; and from a wide variety of other febrile illnesses (Reed et al., 1970). The diagnosis deserves serious consideration in any acutely ill, febrile patient who has tender inguinal or axillary adenopathy and gives a history of possible recent residential, occupational, or recreational exposure to plague-infected rodent fleas or animal carcasses. It should also be considered when cases of pneumonia occur in clusters. Even with a high index of suspicion, the early diagnosis of sporadic cases of septicemic plague, of bubonic plague with occult (e.g., intra-abdominal) adenitis, or of primary pneumonic plague may be extremely difficult or impossible.

Needle aspiration of suspicious lymph nodes (with utmost caution to avoid aerosols when expelling aspirated fluids from syringes) should be performed routinely and usually yields diagnostic material. An 18- or 19-gauge needle on a 10- to 20-ml syringe containing 1 ml of sterile, nonbacteriostatic saline is inserted aseptically into the bubo and aspirated back and forth until a small amount of bloody or purulent fluid is obtained. Smears of lymph fluid, peripheral blood buffy coats, and other body fluids (e.g., sputum, tracheal secretion, and cerebrospinal fluid) should be fixed in absolute methanol to kill the organisms; Giemsa or Wayson's stain then usually reveals the characteristic bipolar staining and "safety-pin" morphology of *Y. pestis* far better than gram stain (Fig. 4). Immunofluorescent staining of methanol-fixed smears is a rapid and highly specific diagnostic method when appropriate reagents are available.

Aspirated body fluids may be cultured on ordinary bacteriologic media, and two or more blood cultures should be obtained. The organism grows well but slowly on solid media, forming convex grayish colonies that are 1 to 3 mm

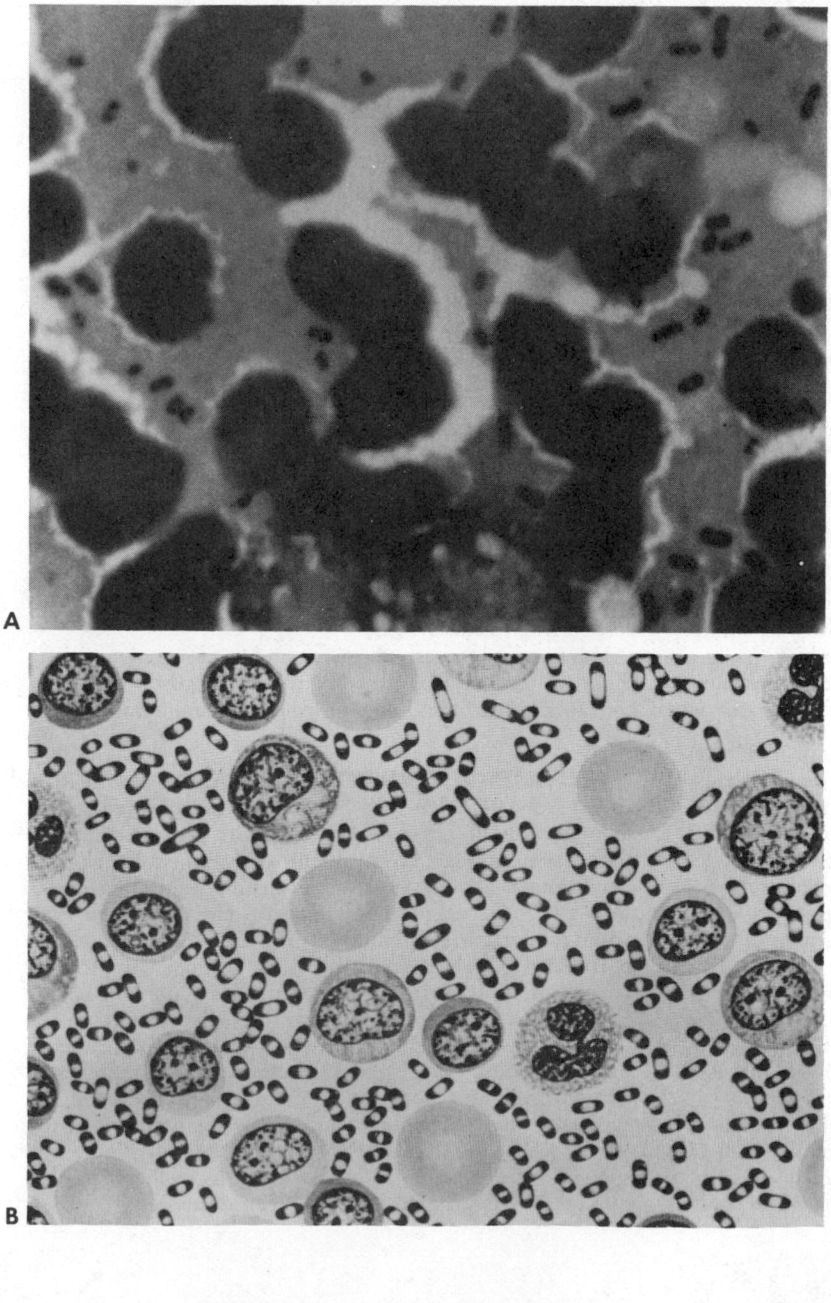

Figure 4. *Yersinia pestis. A,* Gram-stained smear of bubo aspirate reveals many gram-negative bacilli exhibiting characteristic bipolar staining appearance and polymorphonuclear leukocytic exudate. Magnification 960×. (Courtesy of John Ulrich, Ph.D., University of New Mexico, Albuquerque, N.M.) *B,* Drawing of bubo aspirate shows "safety-pin" appearance of *Y. pestis* organisms with Wayson's stain. (From Muir, R.: Bacteriological Atlas. 2nd ed. Edinburgh, E. and S. Livingstone, 1937.)

in diameter after 48 hours. Prior antimicrobial therapy may significantly delay or prevent recovery of *Y. pestis* in cultures. Diagnostic antibody titers in acute and convalescent sera are detectable by the sensitive and specific passive hemagglutination technique of Chen and Meyer (1966) and also by an enzyme linked immunoabsorbent assay (ELISA). The latter is slightly more sensitive and measures specific IgG and IgM immunoglobulin levels (Cavanaugh et al., 1979). Other laboratory methods are of no specific diagnostic value although leukocytosis, disseminated intravascular coagulation, and elevated SGOT levels are common. Roentgenologic evidence of pulmonary infection should be sought (Alsofrom, 1982). *Because of the high mortality and the risk of pneumonic transmission when treatment of plague is delayed, specific presumptive antimicrobial therapy should be urgently instituted on clinical and epidemiologic grounds without awaiting bacteriologic confirmation.*

TREATMENT. Supportive therapy may be needed for hypoxia, hypovolemia, circulatory insufficiency, disseminated intravascular coagulation, and pain. Streptomycin, 30 mg/kg/day should be given intramuscularly in divided doses every 6 to 12 hours for 7 to 10 days, together with tetracycline 0.5 every 6 hours orally, or, if necessary, intravenously. The combination of antibiotics is justified by the intracellular location of *Y. pestis* and by the possibility of rapid development of high level resistance to streptomycin alone. Tetracycline therapy is continued for two weeks. *Y. pestis* may still be cultured from bubo contents after several days of antibiotic administration. Either tetracycline or a sulfonamide has been effective alone in mild to moderately severe cases but is not recommended. Intravenous chloramphenicol (50 to 75 mg/kg/day in six-hourly divided doses) should be substituted for tetracycline in pregnant patients and for treatment of plague meningitis because it readily penetrates the cerebrospinal fluid. Despite the apparent in vitro susceptibility of *Y. pestis* to penicillin and ampicillin, these antibiotics are ineffective in vivo and *have no place in the therapy of plague; Y. pestis* meningitis has frequently been observed as a complication of such treatment. Prolonged fever and an increased incidence of complications have been noted in patients treated with peroral trimethoprim-sulfamethoxazole (Butler et al., 1976). Although gentamicin has cured a few cases of plague septicemia, streptomycin is the antibiotic of choice because the accrued evidence of its efficacy is unequivocal.

Incision and drainage of buboes for diagnostic purposes is not warranted, but may become necessary when fluctuant buboes persist despite adequate antimicrobial therapy.

PROPHYLAXIS. Plague is a quarantinable disease. As soon as the diagnosis is suspected, local and national health agencies must be notified so that epidemiologic investigations may be expedited to define the source of infection and public health measures may be instituted, including rodent and vector control to prevent wider dissemination. Strict hospital isolation of patients suspected of having plague is desirable because cough, sputum production, and auscultatory signs frequently appear late in both primary and secondary plague pneumonia. Strict isolation should be continued until specific antimicrobial treatment has been in effect for 72 hours. The risk of household or nosocomial transmission of *Y. pestis* infection to contacts of patients who have bubonic plague but no pneumonia is minimal, and well-controlled studies of the efficacy of antibiotic prophylaxis of pneumonic spread are not available. Therefore, administration of prophylaxis or "abortive treatment" with oral tetracycline (30 mg/kg) or sulfadiazine (60 mg/kg) daily in six hourly divided doses for ten days should be strictly limited to those believed to have had close and significant exposure to infected respiratory or other secretions. All other case contacts should be placed under surveillance, and their temperatures measured twice daily for ten days. Case contacts who develop fever or other clinical findings compatible with the diagnosis of plague should be hospitalized promptly for confirmation of the diagnosis and for antimicrobial therapy.

All specimens from suspected plague cases should be handled with gloves and transported with extreme caution; attendants as well as laboratory personnel should be alerted to the possible diagnosis. Nosocomially acquired *Y. pestis* infections have occurred only rarely.

In geographic areas in which sylvatic plague is endemic, hunters should avoid direct hand contact with the carcasses of rodents or wild carnivores that are potentially plague-infected or flea-bearing.

Immunization with formalin-killed plague vaccines stimulates production of antibodies. These are detectable by the passive hemagglutination test and afford limited protection against illness and death after *Y. pestis* infection is acquired naturally or in the laboratory. The killed vaccines are preferred to live, attenuated vaccines because they appear to produce greater immunity with fewer and milder local reactions. However, the protection afforded by such vaccines is incomplete and transient, and there is no convincing evidence that vaccination protects against human pneumonic plague. Primary immunization for adults consists of intramuscular injection of 1.0 ml of vaccine followed 4 weeks and 6 months later by additional doses of 0.2 ml. If accelerated immunization is necessary, administration of three intramuscular doses of 0.5 ml each, given at least one week apart, has been recommended. Thereafter, three booster injections of 0.2 ml intramuscularly are required at six-month intervals for maintenance of immunity, followed by additional doses at 1 to 2 year intervals (MMWR, 1982). Vaccination against plague is not required for entry by any country and is not routinely recommended for those living in or traveling to plague-endemic areas unless exposure to plague-infected rodents is specifically anticipated. Laboratory and field personnel engaged in *Y. pestis*-related research should maintain vaccine-induced immunity. A history of plague immunization should under no circumstances eliminate plague from a differential diagnosis when it would otherwise be considered.

References

Akiev, A. K.: Epidemiology and incidence of plague in the world, 1958–1979. Bull WHO 60:165, 1982.

Alsofrom, D. J., Mettler, F. A., Jr., and Mann, J. M.: Radiographic manifestations of plague in New Mexico, 1975–1980. Radiology 139:561, 1981.

Bibel, D. J., and Chen, T. H.: Diagnosis of plague: An analysis of the Yersin–Kitasato controversy. Bacteriol Rev 40:633, 1976.

Butler, T., Levin, J., Linh, N. N., Chan, D. M., Adickman, M., and Arnold, K.: Yersinia pestis infection in Viet Nam. II. Quantitative blood cultures and detection of endotoxin in the cerebrospinal fluid of patients with meningitis. J Infect Dis 133:493, 1976.

Cavanaugh, D. C., Fortier, M. K., Robinson, D. M., Williams, J. E., and Rust, J. H.: Application of the ELISA technique to problems in the serologic diagnosis of plague. Bull Pan Am Health Organ 13:399, 1979.

Chen, T. H., and Meyer, K. F.: An evaluation of Pasteurella pestis Fraction-1-specific antibody for the confirmation of plague infections. Bull WHO 34:911, 1966.
Finegold, M. J.: Pathogenesis of plague. Am J Med 45:549, 1968.
Immunization Practices Advisory Committee (ACIP): Plague vaccine. Morbidity and Mortality Weekly Rep 27:255, 1982.
Janssen, W. A., and Surgalla, M. J.: Plague bacillus: Survival within host phagocytes. Science 163:950, 1969.
Mann, J. M. Plague pneumonia. New Engl J Med 300:1276, 1979.
Nohl, J.: The Black Death. A Chronicle of the Plague. London, Unwin Books, 1961.
Pollitzer, R.: Plague. World Health Organization Monograph No. 22. Geneva, World Health Organization, 1954.
Reed, W. P., Palmer, D. L., Williams, R. C., Jr., and Kisch, A. L.: Bubonic plague in the southwestern United States. Medicine 49:465, 1970.
Rust, J. H., Jr., Cavanaugh, D. C., O'Shita, R., and Marshall, J. D., Jr.: The role of domestic animals in the epidemiology of plague. II. Antibody to *Yersinia pestis* in sera of dogs and cats. J Infect Dis 124:527, 1971.
Sonnenwirth, A. C.: Yersinia. In Lennette, E. H., Spalding, E. H. and Truant, J. P. (eds.): Manual of Clinical Microbiology. Washington, D.C., American Society for Microbiology, 1974, p. 222.
Williams, J. E.: Warning on a new potential for laboratory-acquired infections as a result of the new nomenclature for the plague bacillus. Bull WHO 61:545, 1983.
World Health Organization Expert Committee on Plague: Fourth Report. World Health Organization Technical Report Series No. 447. Geneva, World Health Organization, 1970.
World Health Organization Weekly Epidemiologic Record 52:229, 1977.
World Health Organization Weekly Epidemiologic Record 58:265, 1983.
WHO Informal Consultation. Plague surveillance and control. WHO Chronicle 34:139, 1980.

259
ERYSIPELOID

CHANTAL FRELAND, PH.D.

DEFINITION AND HISTORY. Erysipeloid is a skin infection of man that is acquired by handling infected animal tissues. It is caused by *Erysipelothrix rhusiopathiae,* which also infects many wild and domestic animals. Infections of hogs (swine erysipelas) and poultry cause major economic losses to the agricultural industry. Infection of humans is called erysipeloid because the disease resembles streptococcal erysipelas. Arthritis of the joints underlying erysipeloid lesions is common in humans and is a major manifestation of swine erysipelas. Systemic infection is rare in man, but septicemia and endocarditis have been reported.

In 1873, Fox and Baker described a skin infection of the hands and fingers of butchers and named it erythema serpens. In 1882, Pasteur and Thuillier first isolated *Erysipelothrix* from a diseased pig. Two years later, Rosenbach isolated *E. rhusiopathiae* from erysipeloid lesions of man and proved the existence of a link between the human cutaneous complaint, erythema serpens, and swine erysipelas. Rosenbach named the human disease erysipeloid, but it was often called the "Rouget" of Rosenbach. In 1912, Gunther described the first cases of septicemia with endocarditis caused by *E. rhusiopathiae.*

When the general medical population became aware of the epidemiology of erysipeloid, case reports proliferated (Gilchrist, 1904) until it was realized that erysipeloid was a common occupational disease that was usually self-limited. Since that time, the more unusual manifestations of *Erysipelothrix* infection have been emphasized, and about 60 cases of septicemia or endocarditis have been reported.

ETIOLOGY AND EPIDEMIOLOGY. *E. rhusiopathiae* is a gram-positive bacillus that may be either short and coccobacillary or filamentous. It is nonencapsulated, nonsporulating, and nonmotile regardless of the temperature. Its growth is stimulated by carbon dioxide, reduced oxygen tension, and the addition of blood, serum, or ascitic fluid. Under these conditions, the colonies appear in 24 hours at 37° C as pinpoint, round, regular, smooth colonies that are either transparent or slightly tinged with blue. Rough colonies occasionally occur and are larger and irregular (see Chapter 27).

Erysipelothrix resembles *Listeria,* lactobacilli, and corynebacteria most closely but can be differentiated from these organisms and most other gram-positive bacteria by its production of H_2S. It is also readily differentiated from *Listeria* because it is nonhemolytic and nonmotile. At least 22 serotypes have been reported (Norrung, 1979). Serotypes of *Erysipelothrix* are based on specific polysaccharide antigenic determinants that are associated with the peptidoglycans (Kucsera, 1979). These serotypes, designated by arabic numerals, can be distinguished by bacterial agglutination or by double diffusion gel precipitation. It has been suggested that specific serotypes may differ in the frequency of isolation from different host species, virulence and clinical manifestations of infection. The strongest evidence for this position is that serotypes 1 and 2 are the most common types isolated from swine affected with clinical erysipelas. Other serotypes are relatively uncommon (Wood, 1981).

E. rhusiopathiae is distributed widely in the animal kingdom, where it may behave as either a saprophyte or a pathogen. It has been isolated from the following groups of animals: (1) mammals (swine, sheep, horse, cow, kangaroo, roebuck, mink, wild boar, dolphin, cat, rabbit, rat, and mouse); (2) fish (perch, pike, sardine, and many others); (3) crustaceans (crab, lobster, and shellfish); and (4) domestic and wild birds (turkey, duck, chicken, sparrow, and blackbird).

The susceptibility of animals varies with age, intercurrent disease (enteropathies and parasitic diseases), the season (May to August), and the degree of environmental contamination. *Erysipelothrix* has been isolated from many different tissues of apparently healthy animals, including the tonsils of pigs (Stephenson, 1978) and the slimy surface of fish. These strains are capable of causing disease under appropriate conditions, so these animals and their tissues are reservoirs for *Erysipelothrix.*

The manifestations of *Erysipelothrix* infection vary from animal to animal. Because of its economic importance, swine erysipelas has been described most thoroughly. Four clinical types of disease occur in swine: (1) acute septicemia that is often fatal within three to five days; (2) "diamond-back" or "diamond-skin" disease in which red to purple, rhomboid-shaped skin lesions occur on the back; (3) chronic mitral endocarditis; and (4) arthritis, which may either occur independently or complicate any of the other types of infection (Gledhill, 1948).

The survival of Erysipelothrix in the external environment depends on the temperature and pH. It is sensitive to heat (2 days at 30°C), but resistant to cold (35 days at 3°C). The most favorable pH range is between 5.8 and 8.6. It develops as well in sea water as fresh water.

Erysipelothrix occurs throughout the world but is most prevalent in temperate climates. It is especially common in Germany, France (swine), North America (turkey, fish), South America, and Australia (sheep). Human disease is markedly more common in autumn, just after the peak incidence of animal disease during May to August.

Humans acquire *Erisipelothrix* only from infected animals, their by-products (meat, bones, fish scales, and crustacean shells), and perhaps from plants or soil that have been contaminated by animals. Human-to-human transmission does not occur. Humans are almost always infected through abraded skin, whereas domestic animals are infected by the ingestion of contaminated food; this route of infection remains questionable in man. These observations stress the zoonotic nature of this disease which affects primarily farmers, ranchers butchers, abbatoir workers, veterinarians, fishermen, and housewives. Middle-aged men are most commonly affected (Klauder, 1938).

PATHOGENESIS AND PATHOLOGY. Erysipeloid is characterized by marked inflammation and edema of the skin. The epidermis is edematous, infiltrated with polymorphonuclear leukocytes, and necrotic. The corium is infiltrated with lymphocytes, mast cells, and polymorphonuclears. The bacilli are located throughout the infected skin but are concentrated deep in the corium around the capillaries.

The virulence of *Erysipelothrix* is usually tested in laboratory mice. Most strains kill mice, but there are marked variations in the median lethal dose. The higher neuraminidase activity of virulent strains has led some investigators to conclude that this enzyme is one of the virulence factors (Nikolov, 1978). A glycoprotein extracted from the cell wall of *Erysipelothrix* causes dermal necrosis and high fevers in rabbits (Leimbeck et al., 1975).

Intravenous inoculation of live organisms, dead organisms, and even a cell-free, crude extract of culture filtrates causes polyarthritis in swine, dogs, and rabbits (White et al., 1971). This cell-free extract, which contains murein and many different proteins, binds rapidly to the synovium and persists for many months. It causes cytopathic effects in synovial cell cultures after a single brief exposure (White et al., 1976). Because of clinical and histologic similarities, experimental *Erysipelothrix* arthritis has been used as a model for rheumatoid arthritis.

CLINICAL MANIFESTATIONS, COMPLICATIONS, AND SEQUELAE. **Erysipeloid (Rosenbach's "Rouget").** This common, localized, cutaneous form is by far the most frequent. The lesion follows accidental inoculation along the back of the hand or the thumb, particularly in cases acquired from fish. Clinical manifestations begin within the next 12 to 48 hours around the vestige of the initial injury and consist of a pruritic, purplish-red patch that is slightly indurated and bordered by a clear-cut, slightly raised margin. The lesion gradually spreads over the hand, evolving centrifugally while the center recovers (Erlich, 1946).

Sensations of pressure, itching, and burning are common. Arthralgia of the neighboring small joints occurs occasionally. Lymphangitis and satellite lymphadenopathy occur in about 10 per cent of cases and may be more common in cases of ichthyologic origin. Fever and other signs of systemic involvement are rare. Recovery occurs in two or three weeks, often spontaneously.

In rare cases, localized erysipeloid may spread and cause diffuse generalized skin lesions that are identical to the initial lesion. This rare complication is accompanied by generalized lymphadenopathy and fever.

There is no immunity to erysipeloid; it recurs readily.

Septicemic Form. Only about 60 cases of this serious disease have been reported. Many cases of septicemia (at least ten) have a preceding history of contact and an erysipeloid lesion: there is a latent phase and even apparent recovery before the onset of symptoms. When there is no history of erysipeloid, the earliest symptoms are a low-grade fever, weakness, and malaise. In either case, the fever soon becomes more severe and is accompanied by rigors, generalized myalgia, anorexia, and weight loss. Purpura, splenomegaly, and arthralgia may occur (Coste, 1954).

Endocarditis develops in 75 per cent of septicemic cases. Half of the cases of endocarditis occur on previously normal valves. The aortic valve is commonly affected (Freland, 1977). The symptoms and complications of *Erysipelothrix* endocarditis are not unique. Cerebral (Silberstein, 1965), renal, and pulmonary complications have been described (Proctor, 1965; Russel and Lamb, 1940; and Freland, 1977).

GEOGRAPHIC VARIATIONS IN DISEASE. Most cases of erysipeloid and *Erysipelothrix* endocarditis have been reported from Western Europe, the United States, and other agriculturally developed countries in the temperate zone. The prevalence of infection is directly related to the number of people in close contact with animal reservoirs. There is no apparent geographic variation in the manifestations or severity of infection.

DIAGNOSIS. An individual with a history of contact with an animal reservoir or by-products (meat, bones, crab shells) and an erysipelas-like lesion on the hand is likely to have erysipeloid. Streptococcal erysipelas commonly affects the face and causes bright red lesions that are markedly indurated and spread rapidly. There are usually multiple bullae on the skin. Joints are not affected. Erysipeloid, by contrast, affects the hands, evolves more slowly, causes purplish-red lesions, and frequently causes arthritis of neighboring joints. Bullae are less dramatic and may be absent. Most other causes of dermatitis either differ in appearance or are not localized to the hands.

The definitive diagnosis is made by culture of a skin biopsy. Any coccobacillary, coryneform, or filamentous gram-positive bacillus isolated from such a lesion must be tested for the microbiologic characteristics of *Erysipelothrix*. It can be quickly differentiated from all similar bacteria by the production of H_2S. Its other differential characteristics are given under Etiology and in Chapter 27, Table I.

The diagnosis of septicemia is made by blood culture. It is especially important that *Erysipelothrix* in blood cultures is not misidentified as contaminating coryneform bacteria. The diagnosis of endocarditis in patients with *Erysipelothrix* endocarditis is primarily clinical (see Chapter 213). Immune complex glomerulonephritis, rheumatoid factor, and depression of serum complement levels strongly suggest the diagnosis of endocarditis. The aortic valve is most commonly affected. The vegetations are large and bulky and may be ulcerated.

TREATMENT AND PROPHYLAXIS. Although erysipeloid usually heals spontaneously in a few weeks, recovery is hastened, and complications prevented, by treatment with penicillin. The organism is exquisitely sensitive to penicillin, and infections can usually be cured by injection of 1.2 million units of benzathine penicillin. Oral penicillins (250 mg four times a day for seven days) or daily injections of 600,000 units of procaine penicillin are also effective. One g per day in four divided doses for five to seven days of erythromycin or tetracycline is effective alternate therapy for penicillin-allergic individuals.

Endocarditis has been treated with 10 to 30 million units of penicillin per day for four to five weeks along with streptomycin 1 g per day for ten days. Surgical replacement of the damaged valve is lifesaving in some patients, but the mortality (about 50 per cent) remains high in spite of intensive therapy.

Erysipelothrix infections can be controlled by care in the handling of reservoir animals and their by-products. Gloves and protective aprons are helpful. Control of reservoirs in herds of domestic animals can be achieved by vaccination (see Chapter 27) and by improving techniques of animal husbandry and meat inspection. Except for personal protection, these measures will have little effect on erysipeloid contracted from fish and crustaceans.

References

Coste, F., Domart, A., and Antoine, B.: Manifestations articulaires au cours d'une septicémie à *Erysipelothrix rhusiopathiae*. Rev Rhum 21:47, 1954.

Erlich, J. C.: *Erysipelothrix rhusiopathiae* infection in man. Arch Intern Med 78:565, 1946.

Freland, C.: Les infections à *Erysipelothrix rhusiopathiae*. Revue générale à propos de 31 cas de septicémies avec endocardite relevés dans la littérature. Path Biol 25:345, 1977.

Gilchrist, T. C.: Erysipeloid with a record of 329 cases, of which 323 were caused by crab bites or lesions produced by crabs. J Cutan Dis 22:507, 1904.

Gledhill, A. W.: Swine erysipelas infection *(E. rhusiopathiae)* in man and animals. Proc Roy Soc Med 41:330, 1948.

Klauder, J. V.: Erysipeloid as an occupational disease. JAMA 111:1345, 1938.

Kucsera, G. Y.: Studies on the nature of the type specific antigen of *Erysipelothrix* rhusiopathiae. Acta Vet Acad Sci Hungarica 27:375, 1979.

Leimbeck, R., Bohm, K. H., Ehard, H., and Schulz, L. -C.: Studies of the toxic components of *Erysipelothrix rhusiopathiae:* Detailed characterization of an extracted endotoxin. Zentrabl Bakteriol (Orig A) 232(2–3):266, 1975.

Procter, W. I.: Subacute bacterial endocarditis due to *E. rhusiopathiae*. Report of a case and review of the literature. Am J Med 38:820, 1965.

Nikolov, P., Abrashev, I., Ilieva K., Avramova, T.: Virulence and neuraminidase activity in *Erysipelothrix rhusiopathiae*. Acta Microbiol Bulg 2:62, 1978.

Norrung, V.: Two new serotypes of *Erisipelothrix rhusiopathiae*. Nord Vet Med 31:462, 1979.

Russel, W. O., and Lamb, M. E.: Erysipelothrix endocarditis, a complication of erysipeloid. Report of a case with necropsy. JAMA 114:1045, 1940.

Silberstein, E. B.: Erysipelothrix endocarditis. Report of a case with cerebral manifestations. JAMA 191:862, 1965.

Stephenson, E. H., Berman, D. T.: Isolation of *Erysipelothrix rhusiopathiae* from tonsils of apparently normal swine by two methods. Am J Vet Res 39:187, 1978.

White, T. G., Mirikitani, F. K., and Hargrove, P.: The effects of bacterial extract on synovial cells in tissue culture. In Vitro 12:702, 1976.

White, T. G., Puls, J. L., and Mirikitani, F. K.: Rabbit arthritis induced by cell-free extracts of *Erysipelothrix*. Infect Immun 3:715, 1971.

Wood, R. L., Booth, G. D., Cutlip, R. C.: Susceptibility of vaccinated swine and mice to generalized infection with specific serotypes of *Erysipelothrix rhusiopathiae*. Am J Vet Res 42:608, 1981.

Wood, R. L., Harrington, R., Haubrich, D. R.: Serotypes of previously unclassified isolates of *Erysipelothrix rhusiopathiae* from swine in the United States and Puerto Rico. Am J Vet Res 42:1248, 1981.

260
ANTHRAX

WERNER DUTZ, M.D.

Anthrax (ανθραξ: *charcoal, carbuncle; synonyms: malignant pustule, malignant edema, splenic fever, woolsorters' disease, charbon, Milzbrand)* is caused by *Bacillus anthracis* or its spores, ingested from infected pastures by herbivorous animals or indirectly derived from infected carcasses by carnivorous animals. Man is infected by contaminated products, such as skins, bone, horsehair, bristles, bone meal, or wool. The study of anthrax led to the development of modern bacteriology, serology, and immunology. Microorganisms were first seen in 1863 by Davaine, who proved their infectivity. Robert Koch isolated the bacillus in pure culture in the vitreous of cow's eyes in 1876 and established Koch's postulates. Pasteur performed the first successful vaccination of sheep with attenuated bacilli (Vallery-Radot, 1960).

GEOGRAPHIC VARIATION AND INCIDENCE. The massive plague-like spread of anthrax over the southern part of Europe in the 18th and 19th centuries was stemmed by mandatory vaccination. Anthrax persists in the arid and semi-arid regions of the Middle East, in Africa, Asia, and South America. Wild living animals are often affected. A proper worldwide estimate of disease frequency in animals and man cannot be made. Anthrax is underreported owing to lack of interest, lack of facilities, and sometimes deliberately to prevent economic problems with wool or hide exports (Brachman and Fekety, 1958).

Anthrax epidemics in livestock occur more frequently during draught, when closed-cropped grazing and digging for roots lead to closer contact with spores. Animals feed then on thorny plants that they normally shun. The resulting injuries of the jaws form a portal of entry. Malnutrition reduces resistance. In time of need livestock owners are forced to slaughter animals at the first signs of infection. Farmers, shepherds, butchers, and women spinning wool with hand spindles, carpet weavers, and wool merchants are most frequently infected. Bathhouse epidemics occur in the Middle East, where epilation of the skin is practiced and the body is rubbed down with rough wool that is occasionally contaminated with anthrax spores. Epidemics of inhalation anthrax in woolsorters have been described by Eppinger in Western countries at the turn of the century. Osler noticed that the danger of infection from wool is inversely proportionate to its greasiness. Most infections in the textile industry occur in the carding departments, where the washed and degreased wool is fluffed up. Pulmonary anthrax epidemics occur more frequently in well-ventilated factories, where spores remain longer suspended in the air. Detection of industrial dust contamination is best achieved by the injection of detergent-pretreated, defatted dust material into mice and microscopic examination with fluorescent antianthrax globulin (Brachman and Fekety, 1958). Sporadic infections with infected bristles of shaving brushes, contaminated bone meal fertilizer, or from leather products are continuously reported from all countries of the world (Federation Proceedings, 1967; Dutz and Kohout, 1971).

BACTERIOLOGY AND PATHOPHYSIOLOGY. *B. anthracis* is a large (2.5 × 10 μ) rod-shaped spore-forming gram-positive organism that cannot be differentiated by morphologic criteria or on the usual culture media from the nonpathogenic *B. cereus*. *B. anthracis* lies singly or in pairs in tissue. The characteristic "box car" or "bamboo rod" long chains appear on agar cultures. Stab cultures in gelatin produce the classic inverted fir tree pattern.

Sporulation occurs after the death of the host. The dormant spores are extremely resistant to chemicals, heat, and environmental changes. Pastures once contaminated remain so indefinitely. The transformation of a dormant spore into a vegetative one can be observed under the phase microscope. Dormant spores are refractile, whereas germinated ones are dark and nonrefractile. The growth of the vegetative cell occurs after the germinated spore has been phagocytosed by a macrophage (Federation Proceedings, 1967).

The virulence of *B. anthracis* is proved by animal inoculation. The polysaccharides in the bacillary capsule determine the virulence of the strain. Host phagocytes form a vesicular membrane around avirulent and hypovirulent bacilli, whereas no membrane formation can be detected around virulent ones. The virulence of given strains of *B. anthracis* varies greatly and depends, among other things, on the number of animal passages before sporulation. Growth above or below optimum temperature or on poor nutritional media reduces virulence.

The pathogenicity of a given strain also depends on toxin production (see Chapter 28). The toxins are generated in the bacillary cytoplasm and their release is proportional to the CO_2 tension of the medium. Anthrax toxins cause detachment of cytoplasmic processes of endothelial cells, subsequent increased vascular permeability, platelet thrombi, stasis, and thrombosis. There is extensive edema and hemorrhage owing to capillary wall dissolution and venous obstruction. Injection of pure anthrax toxin into the spinal fluid leads to centrally induced systemic anoxic changes, marked disorganization of the electro-encephalogram pattern, and cerebral death.

The phagocytosis of *B. anthracis* depends on host nutrition. Lysine deficiency leads to phagocytic paralysis (Gray, 1963). Meat-fed rats are resistant to a dosage of bacilli that kills grain-fed littermates (Dutz and Kohout, 1971). Herbivorous animals are therefore more susceptible to infection than carnivores. Most of our own patients with anthrax ate meat very rarely and suffered from relative protein malnutrition. Lysine deficiency after a pure plant-protein diet may explain the particular susceptibility of village populations during times of draught and starvation (Dutz and Kohout, 1971; Gray, 1963).

Experimental infection with a standard toxic strain causes leukocytosis, low plasma pH, hyponatremia, hypocalcemia, and respiratory alkalosis superimposed on metabolic acidosis. Glycogen depletion of the liver, hypoxia, and respiratory failure occur preterminally. Hyperphosphatemia, hyperchloremia, and hyperpotassemia depend on the degree of hemolysis (Federation Proceedings, 1967).

Death in Rhesus monkeys is dosage related. Toxemia and death occur 20 hours after the injection of 10^{10} spores and two hours after 10^{11} spores, if a bacillus of standard virulence and toxicity is used. Lymph nodes may clear up to 10^8 spores from the circulation. Bacillary clearance occurs in some species, predominantly in the spleen. Horses, sheep, and guinea pigs develop splenomegaly and often die after splenic rupture (Federation Proceedings, 1967). Splenomegaly, however, is not a feature of human anthrax (Dutz and Kohout, 1971).

PATHOLOGY. Regardless of portal of entry, virulent strains spread to lymph nodes and produce severe lymphadenitis that is a characteristic feature of all forms of severe anthrax. Septicemia occurs after destruction of the lymph nodes, when bacilli spill into the blood stream. Cutaneous infection is by far the most frequent and occurs in two forms:

1. A *necrotic sore* with little accompanying swelling and tissue reaction. The anthrax bacilli are contained early by macrophages. There is little neutrophilic infiltration. The lesion is characterized by vascular thrombosis, interstitial hemorrhage, and tissue necrosis. (The classic terminology of anthrax pustule or carbuncle is wrong; there is no liquefaction necrosis or pus formation.) The necrotic eschar heals without scarring (Fig. 1).

2. *Malignant edema:* This infection with toxic strains of *B. anthracis* starts with blisters similar to a second degree burn or erysipelas. The blister breaks down rapidly and a necrotic eschar develops surrounded by massive edema, which may distort the face beyond recognition, extend from a primary sore on the eyelid to encompass half the thorax or spread over an entire extremity. The edema in one of our cases with an eschar at the nape of the neck extended to the abdomen and distended the subcutaneous tissue over the sternum to a thickness of 10 cm. The erythrocytes ooze freely out of the vessels and may impart a bluish to black discoloration to the swelling (Fig. 2).

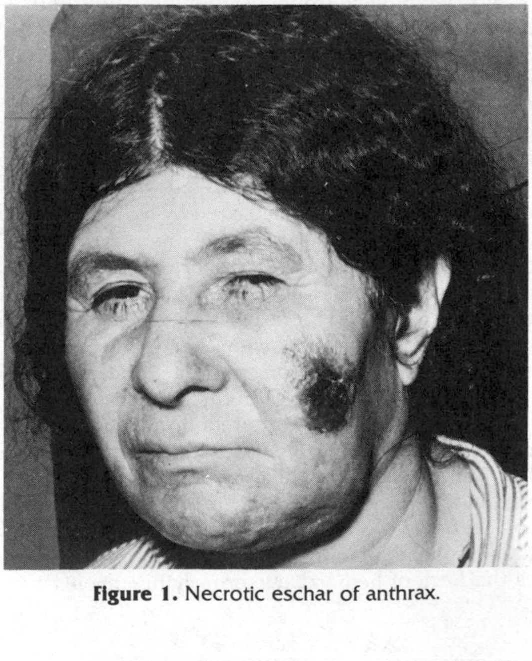

Figure 1. Necrotic eschar of anthrax.

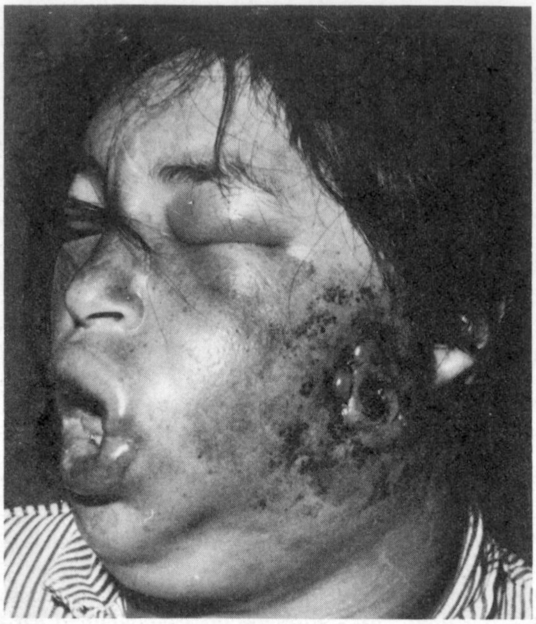

Figure 2. Malignant edema of face. Acute lesion with cutaneous blisters and early eschar formation.

Bacilli spread along the lymphatics and cause lymphadenitis. The phagocytes of the marginal and intermediate sinusoids engulf and kill most of the bacilli. In overwhelming infections, the sinusoids dilate with hemorrhage, the lymph node structure disintegrates and all lymphatics become blocked. Such lymph nodes are swollen, soft, and dark red to blue black. Septicemic dissemination follows the hemorrhagic lymphadenitis (Fig. 3).

Splenic enlargement in man occurs rarely. We found a splenic enlargement to 400 g in only one of 25 deaths from all different forms of anthrax. Bacilli can be found in the Kupffer cells and leukocytosis in the hepatic sinusoids.

Gastrointestinal anthrax develops after ingestion of massively contaminated material deposited in the stomach, or more frequently, the terminal ileum and ileocecal region. There are single or multiple necrotic ulcers up to 5 cm in size, surrounded by massive mucosal edema, which may obstruct the bowel. Fluid may be lost into the abdominal cavity so rapidly and massively that fatal dehydration occurs. The bowel loops may be filled with many liters of fluid. The regional lymph nodes are swollen and hemorrhagic and the entire mesentery may be dark red. Death is usually due to fluid and electrolyte loss.

Inhalation anthrax is characterized by pulmonary edema. Ross showed that the inhaled spores are taken up by the alveolar pneumocytes and transported to the regional lymph nodes (Dutz and Kohout, 1971). Germination occurs during the transport. The result is massive hilar lymphadenopathy with mediastinal edema and hemorrhage, followed by secondary pulmonary edema and hydrothorax. There are no necrotic lesions in the lung or bronchi, since the spores are diffusely scattered throughout the entire lung and are secondarily concentrated in the hilar lymph nodes. Studies in textile factories showed that up to 1300 spores may be inhaled in particles of 5 μ over a five-hour period without infection (Brachman and Fekety, 1958). If anthrax bronchopneumonia follows anthrax septicemia it takes the form of hemorrhagic bronchopneumonia.

Anthrax infections by other routes are rare. Anthrax of the endometrium has followed attempted or completed abortion, and puerperal fever has occurred after delivery in contaminated stables.

One complication of anthrax septicemia is hemorrhagic meningitis. The cerebrospinal fluid is hemorrhagic, and vessels are disrupted and/or thrombosed. The brain substance or the ganglion cells are undisturbed at autopsy because death occurs rapidly after the onset of toxic anthrax meningitis.

CLINICAL PATTERN. Skin lesions occur after abrasions or prolonged contact with infected material. Lesions of the lip are frequent in weavers and spinners who wet the thread with their mouths; infections of the bearded skin occur after shaving. Lesions of the eyelids are frequent in hot arid countries, where the material is rubbed into the skin with the back of the hand (Amidi et al., 1977). Butchers have infections of fingers and forearm; the nape of the neck and back is frequently infected in porters of hides. Lesions of the intertriginous areas between the legs, at the beltline, and in the region of the collar are not infrequent.

The first symptom in cutaneous anthrax is itching at the site of inoculation after two to three hours, followed by a small papule that rapidly becomes vesicular. A dark brown eschar is formed within 36 hours. The necrotic eschar separates within a few days without leaving a scar. This form of the disease has little morbidity, causes no general symptoms, and is rarely seen by physicians. Malignant edema is at the other end of the spectrum of cutaneous

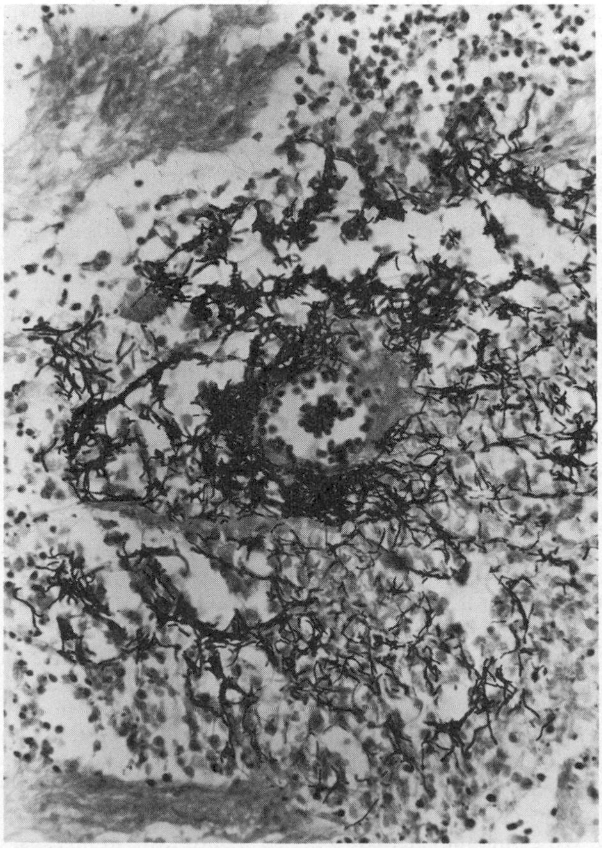

Figure 3. Brown and Bren stain. Magnification 800×. Anthrax bacilli in dilated lymphatics. Note periarteriolar clustering.

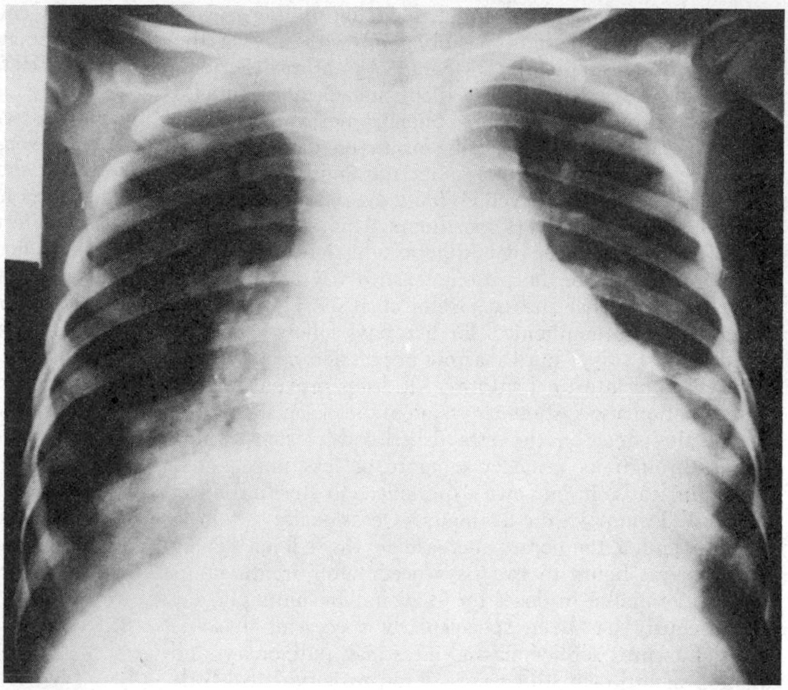

Figure 4. Chest x-ray. Marked mediastinal widening in inhalation anthrax.

anthrax. The lesion starts as one or more small vesicles that may resemble burn blisters. Necrosis follows within one or two days and is surrounded by slightly raised small blisters with a hemorrhagic rim. Subcutaneous edema may distort the features, grotesquely close both eyes, and prevent breathing through the nostrils or eating and drinking with the enlarged lips. All possible transition forms between the two types of cutaneous anthrax may occur.

Leukocytosis with up to 20,000 WBC, 80 per cent neutrophils, and a shift to the left is the earliest systemic manifestation. Moderate fever of 38 to 39° C may accompany severe forms of cutaneous anthrax. Electrolyte disturbances and hemoconcentration are proportionate to the extent of the edema. Renal failure with papillary necrosis and shock precede death by septicemia. The patient is often free of anxiety and his mental state remains clear despite his critical condition.

Gastrointestinal anthrax probably occurs more frequently than stated. Most cases are recognized after death because clinical diagnosis is extremely difficult. We observed one case at laparotomy for bowel obstruction of unknown etiology, who recovered uneventfully after penicillin therapy. Undoubtedly many mild cases escape detection. In gastrointestinal anthrax there are rapidly developing and refilling ascites, cholera-like diarrhea, and moderate to severe fever with chills relatively late in the illness as a sign of septicemia, leukocytosis, and hemoconcentration. Radiographs show signs of intestinal obstruction. Fluid loss from the bowel may reach 12 liters within 24 hours. Hematemesis in gastric anthrax and moderate melena in ileocecal anthrax may occur (Dutz and Kohout, 1971; Nalin et al., 1977).

The initial symptoms of inhalation anthrax are increasing shortness of breath and grippe-like symptoms, with leukocytosis, but fever may be absent. Occasionally there is nonproductive cough. The patient dies after five to seven days in shock with tachypnea, tachycardia, and cyanosis. Fulminating cases present with an onset of chills and high fever, rapidly develop dyspnea, and vascular collapse leading to death within 24 to 48 hours. The massive hilar adenopathy and mediastinal hemorrhage is evident in chest x-rays as a widening of the hilum, followed by massive widening of the mediastinum with clear and sharp borders (Vessal, 1975) (Fig. 4). The absence of pain associated with other forms of rapidly developing mediastinitis, the marked leukocytosis, and the history or possibility of exposure should raise the suspicion of anthrax infection.

Patients with anthrax septicemia should be watched for meningeal irritation, mental changes, delirium, and unconsciousness, which are signs of anthrax meningitis. The spinal fluid is frankly bloody and bacilli may be seen on direct smears or cultured from it.

DIAGNOSIS. The clinical appearance of the eschar and the malignant edema of cutaneous anthrax are characteristic and easy to recognize in endemic areas. It is sometimes difficult to obtain viable bacilli from the eschar or the edematous skin. Perforation of the epidermis with a thin dental root canal needle helps to obtain material from the deeper layers and permits easy inoculation of media as well as the preparation of smears. The finding of single or double gram-positive bacilli in conjunction with the clinical lesion are sufficient evidence for diagnosis. Inhalation anthrax and gastrointestinal anthrax are more difficult to diagnose without invasive methods. Treatment should be started on suspicion alone. Recovery of bacilli from the blood stream in septicemia usually comes too late for clinical purposes. The indirect microhemagglutination test of Buchanan is very specific. A rising titer confirms the identity of the infection after it has run its course.

THERAPY. *B. anthracis* is sensitive to sulfonamides, penicillin, and the broad spectrum antibiotics, but the tetracyclines and erythromycin are the preferred therapy (Gold, 1955). Early diagnosis and treatment before the onset of septicemia are essential. Penicillin is the drug of choice, but good results are obtained with any of the following dosage schedules for cutaneous anthrax (Federation Proceedings, 1967; Gold, 1966): sulfadiazine, initial 3 g, then 1 g every four hours; phenoxymethyl penicillin, 500 mg orally four times daily for seven days; aqueous procaine penicillin, 600,000 units intramuscularly twice daily for five days; tetracycline, 0.5 g every four hours and erythromycin, 0.2 g every four hours. Higher dosages are used if indicated either by antibiotic sensitivity tests or by the clinical status of the patient, particularly in malignant edema and internal anthrax. Nalin et al. (1977) used 6 g per day of chloramphenicol for five days followed by 4 g per day for 18 days until marrow depression occurred, to cure a case of intestinal anthrax. All drugs prevent further dissemination and systemic invasion of the organisms. They have little effect on the established local lesion, which passes through its usual cycle more or less unchanged. Penicillin leads, in our own experience, to sterilization of the local lesion within 24 hours. Occasionally a febrile reaction and a temporary increase in the edema lasting from several hours to two days occur after treatment is started. Penicillin in doses up to 20 million units per day intravenously has been spectacularly successful in some cases of anthrax septicemia and intestinal, pulmonary, and meningeal anthrax with bacteria of low toxicity. It has little effect in well-established toxic septicemic anthrax, where the sudden release of toxins may accelerate death.

Careful monitoring of electrolytes and proper fluid replacement are essential in malignant edema and intestinal and septicemic anthrax. Fluid and electrolyte requirements may approach those in cholera (Dutz and Kohout, 1971; Nalin, 1977). Fluid replacement is particularly important shortly after the start of antibiotic therapy and the subsequent toxin release. Toxemia exhausts the adrenal, and supportive therapy with 100 to 200 mg Solu-Cortef intravenously daily followed by decreasing oral dosage has been recommended (Yeganeh-Doust et al., 1968).

Serum therapy has been superseded by antibiotics and sulfonamides. Topical treatment with antibiotics is useless. Excision and surgical tampering with lesions of the skin should be avoided.

PROPHYLAXIS. Vaccination of occupationally exposed persons is recommended wherever raw materials from countries with endemic anthrax are used. Veterinarians, leather workers, brushmakers, and vendors of bone meal fertilizer should also be protected. The case of a secretary who succumbed to inhalation anthrax although she had never entered the textile factory and worked in a neighboring office building suggests that all employees should be vaccinated. An absorbed anthrax vaccine can be purchased. Three subcutaneous injections of 0.5 cc at two-week intervals followed by boosters after 6, 12, and 18 months, and thereafter once yearly are recommended for complete protection.

The eradication of anthrax depends largely on vaccination of herds of domesticated animals. Burying of the infected carcasses in deep pits and covering them with lime has been recommended, but too many pastures throughout the world are infected for this to be practical. Mass vaccination of humans is cumbersome and therefore only indicated in particularly endangered individuals.

References

Amidi, S., Dutz, W., Kohout, E., and Ronaghy, H. A.: Anthrax in Iran. Z Tropenmed Parasitol 24:250, 1977.
Brachman, P. S., and Fekety, F. R.: Industrial anthrax. Ann NY Acad Sci 70:575, 1958.
Dutz, W., and Kohout, E.: Anthrax. Pathol Annu 6:209, 1971.
Gold, H.: Anthrax: A report of 117 cases. AMA Arch Int Med 96:387, 1955.
Gray, L.: Lysine deficiency and host resistance to anthrax. J Exp Med 117:497, 1963.
Nalin, D. R., et al.: Survival of patient with intestinal anthrax. Am J Med 62:130, 1977.
Proceedings of the conference on progress in the understanding of anthrax. Fed Proc 26:1483, 1967.
Vallery-Radot, R.: The Life of Pasteur. N. Y., Dover Publ., Inc., 1960.
Vessal, K., et al.: Radiological changes in inhalation anthrax. Clin Radiol 26:471, 1975.
Yeganeh-Doust, J., et al.: Corticosteroids in treatment of malignant edema of chest wall and neck (anthrax). Dis Chest 53:773, 1968.

261

GLANDERS (FARCY)

CHARLES E. DAVIS, M. D.

DEFINITION AND HISTORY. Glanders is an infection of horses, mules, and donkeys caused by *Pseudomonas mallei*, the glanders bacillus. Although the natural disease occurs almost exclusively in equines, many other animals and man have occasionally contracted glanders from infected solipeds. Glanders presents in one of three forms: acute fatal septicemia; chronic glanders of the lung and other organs; and farcy, which is the name given to chronic glanders of the skin, subcutaneous tissue, and lymphatics.

Glanders is now primarily of historic interest. It was eliminated from the United States, Canada, and western Europe by 1939. The last known human case in the United States was reported in 1938 (Herold and Erikson, 1938). In fact, *P. mallei* rarely infected man even when it was a common, worldwide disease of horses. In 1906, Robins could find only 156 reported cases in the world literature. The effects of World War I on sanitation and on equine contact in cavalry units temporarily increased the number of cases in the western world, but all industrialized countries had passed effective control acts by 1920 that legislated the destruction of infected equines. This legislation and the replacement of cavalry by motorized vehicles has eliminated glanders from the world except for a few foci in Asia, Africa, and the Middle East.

Despite the fact that it was never common, glanders is one of the oldest diseases known. Hippocrates and Aristotle both described glanders, and Aristotle actually named the disease "malleus," which is derived from the Greek word meaning malignant or epidemic. *P. mallei* was isolated in pure culture and proved to be the etiologic agent of glanders in 1882 by Loeffler and Schutz in Germany and by Bouchard, Charrin, and Capitan in France.

ETIOLOGY. *P. mallei* was originally named *Bacillus mallei* by Zopf in 1885. Since that time, it has been temporarily placed in various ill-defined genera of bacteria including *Pfeifferella, Actinobacillus, Loefferella, Acinetobacter*, and *Malleomyces*. The species name has always been mallei. Because it is a nonfermentative, oxidase-positive, gram-negative bacterium, *P. mallei* seemed most closely related to the pseudomonads but did not fit the definition exactly because of its nonmotility. It was finally placed in the *Pseudomonas* genus in the eighth edition of Bergey's manual because of its many similarities to *P. pseudomallei* (Wetmore and Gochenour, 1956; Redfearn et al., 1966), the cause of meliodosis (a glanders-like disease of man). Among its many similarities to *P. pseudomallei* and the other pseudomonads are its oxidative attack on glucose, reduction of nitrate to nitrite, and its guanine plus cytosine content of 69 $\pm$ 1.0 per cent (Mandel, 1966). An additional significant relationship between *P. mallei* and *P. pseudomallei* is that several temperate phages isolated from *P. pseudomallei* can lyse strains of *P. mallei* but not other pseudomonads (Smith and Cherry, 1957). Finally, it was shown that *P. mallei* and *P. pseudomallei* accumulate poly-B-hydroxybutyrate as a cellular reserve material (Levine and Wolochow, 1960), a common characteristic among the nonfluorescent aerobic pseudomonads.

P. mallei is easily differentiated from *P. pseudomallei* and the other pseudomonads because it is nonmotile, requires 48 hours to form well-developed colonies, and grows best on media supplemented with 4 per cent glycerol.

P. mallei and *P. pseudomallei* also cross-react extensively in serologic reactions. They cross-react almost completely in agglutination (Cravitz and Miller, 1950) and fluorescent antibody (Moody et al., 1956) reactions with serum prepared against whole live or formalin-killed bacteria and also share at least one heat-stable antigen (Fournier, 1967) that is probably located in the lipopolysaccharide. Because the two organisms were so similar but *P. pseudomallei* contained two other heat-stable antigens and was flagellated, Fournier (1967) hypothesized that *P. mallei* evolved from the free-living *P. pseudomallei* when the glanders bacillus adapted to a strict parasitic existence in equines.

PATHOGENESIS AND PATHOLOGY. The virulence of individual strains of *P. mallei* for susceptible laboratory animals varies greatly, but the reasons for this variability are not known. Furthermore, certain animals (cattle and rats) are almost completely resistant to both natural and experimental glanders. Among the equines, horses are the best adapted animal. Chronic infections are common in horses, whereas mules and donkeys usually die of acute disease within 10 to 30 days. Man seems to be fairly resistant to glanders and may develop either acute or chronic disease.

Man acquires glanders by contact with infected nasal secretions of equines. The organism usually enters the body through an abrasion or scratch, but primary nasal infection also occurs. The possibility of aerosol transmission is strongly reinforced by the frequency of laboratory-acquired disease. With the possible exceptions of *Brucella*, the plague bacillus, and *Pasteurella tularensis*, no bacterium is as dangerous to work with in the laboratory as *P. mallei*. Several members of one laboratory became ill a few days after a centrifuge tube was broken (Jennings, 1963). In another laboratory specifically designed to work with *P. mallei*, 50 per cent of the laboratory personnel became ill within one year (Howe and Miller, 1947). Human to human transmission is also well documented.

The classic lesion of glanders is a tuberculoid nodule. In the acute pulmonary form of the disease, diffuse necrotizing pneumonia may accompany multiple abscess-like pulmonary nodules. The acute nodule is 1 to 4 mm in size and dark red because of hemorrhage. As it ages, it becomes gray, firm, and organized. Calcification may occur in old pulmonary nodules (M'Fadyean, 1900).

Nodules occur most commonly in the lungs, mucous membranes of the nose, lymphatics, and skin. The spleen, liver, testes, and bones are less commonly affected. Instead of organizing and healing, nodules may ulcerate and discharge a thick, sticky, purulent, highly infectious exudate into the bronchus or from the skin or the nose (the characteristic nasal discharge of glanders).

The center of acute nodules is thick pus composed of polymorphonuclear leukocytes. In older nodules, the necrotic center is surrounded by epitheliod and giant cells. The entire nodule is surrounded by fibrous tissue.

In farcy, the nodules occur in the skin or subcutaneous tissue and frequently break down and ulcerate. The lymphatics that drain these superficial nodules become firm and stand out as hard cords, the so-called "farcy-pipes." The local lymph nodes, which become firm and enlarge, are referred to as "farcy buds." Farcy can occur in human beings but is much more common in horses.

Very little work has been done on the virulence factors of *P. mallei*. It synthesizes an antigenically complete lipopolysaccharide that presumably contributes to the manifestations of acute, fatal septicemia. Neither capsules nor exotoxins have been described. Mallein, a product obtained by autoclaving, filtering, and concentrating ten-fold a 10- to 14-day culture of *P. mallei*, induces delayed hypersensitivity reactions in the skin of people and animals with glanders. Early investigators were struck with the similarities between glanders and tuberculosis because the growth of *P. mallei* was enhanced by glycerol; mallein induced delayed hypersensitivity reactions in infected animals; and glanders produced pulmonary nodules that were tuberculoid in nature. While the diseases are only slightly similar and the organisms very dissimilar, these characteristics of glanders suggest that some of its pathologic manifestations are characteristic of a facultative intracellular parasite.

CLINICAL MANIFESTATIONS. Untreated glanders in man has been described as an intensely painful, loathsome disease from which few recover (Jennings, 1963). It may be acute or chronic and may be localized primarily either in the respiratory organs or in the skin or subcutaneous tissue. The manifestations are partly determined by the route of infection and, as alluded to in *Pathogenesis and Pathology*, may vary with the virulence of the strain of *P. mallei*. One to five days after accidental inoculation of the skin, the patient develops a nodule with surrounding lymphangitis. As this type of infection progresses, typical "farcy pipes" and "farcy buds" form. If the mucous membranes are involved, mucopurulent drainage from the nose, eye, or lips is soon replaced by extensive, disfiguring granulomatous lesions that may ulcerate and drain tenacious pus.

The septicemic form of the disease may occur either primarily or secondary to localized disease. It is characterized by early onset of anorexia, malaise, fever, nausea, and myalgia. Erysipeloid lesions on the face and limbs develop and are quickly followed by a generalized pustular eruption. Ulcerations of the nasal septum cause a mucopurulent, blood-streaked discharge. Bronchopneumonia or nodular, necrotizing pneumonia occurs very commonly and may cause severe cough and pleuritic pain. Cervical lymphadenopathy, splenomegaly, and jaundice are common. The skin pustules finally become suppurative and metastatic lesions in the muscles, bones, spleen, and liver often precede fatal collapse, which usually occurs within two weeks in untreated patients. A slight leukocytosis and left shift are usual, but leukopenia also occurs.

Chronic disease most commonly involves the skin and musculoskeletal system (83 per cent), the lymphatics (50 per cent), and the nose (50 per cent) (Robins, 1906). Patients who recover from septicemia after developing chronic disease and patients with chronic glanders may develop septicemia at any time during the course of the disease.

COMPLICATIONS AND SEQUELAE. Most patients with untreated, acute septicemia die. The chief complication of chronic glanders is the development of disfiguring lesions of the skin, subcutaneous tissue, and face. The lesions of the nose and lips, which resemble those of cutaneous leishmaniasis and other granulomatous diseases of the mucous membranes, are not only disfiguring but also interfere with breathing, eating, and swallowing. Patients may also live for many years with the nodules of metastatic glanders in the musculoskeletal system or viscera before they finally succumb to a fatal episode of septicemia.

GEOGRAPHIC VARIATIONS IN DISEASE. When glanders was a worldwide disease, there were no known geographic variations in its manifestations or course. Individual variation in the virulence of strains and the variable susceptibility of mammalian species seemed to be independent of geographic location. The only known foci of infection in the 1980s are in remote, underdeveloped areas of Asia, Africa, and the Middle East.

DIAGNOSIS. Microscopic examination of pus from skin or subcutaneous nodules, nasal drainage, or sputum shows polymorphonuclear leukocytes and small gram-negative bacilli that tend to stain irregularly in the Gram and methylene blue stains. The microscopic appearance of *P. mallei* is not distinctive. It cannot be differentiated from *P. pseudomallei* or most other common gram-negative bacilli. The specimen should be inoculated onto nutrient agar, glycerol agar, blood agar, or all three media. If the source of the specimen is likely to be contaminated, it should be inoculated onto agar containing a 1 to 200,000 dilution of crystal violet to suppress gram-positive organisms. Gram-negative colonies that develop after 24 to 48 hours should be worked up as possible *P. mallei*. The fastest way to differentiate *P. mallei* from *P. pseudomallei* is by examination of a hanging-drop preparation of a culture grown at room temperature. *P. mallei* is nonmotile. Either primary material or the isolated, suspected bacterium should also be inoculated intraperitoneally into male guinea pigs. Moderate or large doses produce localized peritonitis that involves the scrotum. The testicles become enlarged and finally form a caseous mass that breaks through the scrotum (Straus' reaction). This reaction is specific for *P. mallei* and *P. pseudomallei*. Organisms can also be identified as either *P. mallei* or *P. pseudomallei* by immunofluorescence with fluoresceinated antiserum against formalinized *P. mallei* or *P. pseudomallei*.

A high percentage of infected people and equines have developed a firm, indurated nodule about 24 to 48 hours after intradermal inoculation of 0.1 ml of commercial mallein at a dilution of 1 to 10,000. False positives are uncommon. Mallein may induce an antibody response and should not be injected until serologic studies are completed.

The complement fixation and bacterial agglutination tests are valuable diagnostic techniques (Cravitz and Miller, 1950). The agglutination test is more sensitive than the complement fixation test (CF), but the CF is more specific. Normal people often have agglutination titers of 1:20 to 1:160, and patients with meliodosis may have high titers. Glanders almost always causes agglutination titers of greater than 1:320. A complement fixation titer of 1:20 or greater is specific for glanders. Patients with meliodosis do not develop CF antibodies to *P. mallei*.

Acute glanders could be confused with any acute bacterial septicemia, especially typhoid, brucellosis, and meliodosis. The blood count may not be high enough to exclude typhoid fever or brucellosis, which usually cause white counts of less than 10,000 per mm^3, and acute meliodosis may closely resemble glanders. Chronic glanders may be confused with sporotrichosis and other mycotic infections of the skin and subcutaneous tissue, with other granulomatous infections of the nose and mouth, and with pulmonary tuberculosis. A history of exposure to equines in an endemic area and proper bacteriologic and serologic techniques should quickly establish the correct diagnosis.

TREATMENT. *P. mallei* is resistant to penicillin but sensitive to sulfonamides, streptomycin, the tetracyclines, and chloramphenicol. The natural disease in man and experimental glanders in laboratory rodents responds to treatment with sulfonamides (Howe and Miller, 1947; Cravitz and Miller, 1950). The optimal dose and duration of therapy is unknown. The results of treatment of experimental glanders with streptomycin and tetracycline are contradictory.

PROPHYLAXIS. Glanders has been virtually eliminated from the developed world by procedures like those laid down in the British Glanders or Farcy Order of 1907 and similar legislation in the United States and Canada at the same time. According to these laws, every animal with clinical evidence of glanders or a positive mallein test was considered a diseased animal and slaughtered. The carcasses were burned, the area disinfected and all equine contacts tested with mallein. Reactors were destroyed. These procedures were effective because of the relatively limited host range of the natural disease.

References

Cravitz, L., and Miller, W. R.: Immunologic studies with *Malleomyces mallei* and *Malleomyces pseudomallei*. J Infect Dis 86:46, 1950.

Fournier, J.: The thermostable antigens of *Pseudomonas pseudomallei* and of *Malleomyces mallei* and their communities. Ann Inst Pasteur 112:93, 1967.

Herold, A. A., and Erikson, C. G.: Human glanders—case report. South Med J 1022, 1938.

Howe, C., and Miller, W. R.: Human glanders: Report of 6 cases. Ann Intern Med 26:93, 1947.

Jennings, W. E.: Glanders. In Hull, T. G. (ed.): Diseases Transmitted from Animals to Man. 5th ed. Springfield, Ill., Charles C Thomas, 1963, p. 264.

Levine, H. B., and Wolochow, H.: Occurrence of poly-B-hydroxybutyrate in *Pseudomonas pseudomallei*. J. Bacteriol 79:805, 1960.

Mandel, M.: Deoxyribonucleic acid base composition in the genus *Pseudomonas.* J Gen Microbiol 43:273, 1966.
M'Fadyean, J.: The curability of glanders. J Comp Pathol Ther 13:55, 1900.
Moody, M. D., Golman, M., and Thomason, B. M.: Staining bacterial smears with fluorescent antibody. J Bacteriol 72:357, 1956.
Redfearn, M. S., Palleroni, N. J., and Stanier, R. Y.: A comparative study of *Pseudomonas pseudomallei* and *Bacillus mallei.* J Gen Microbiol 43:293, 1966.
Robins, G. D.: Chronic glanders in man. Studies from the Royal Victoria Hospital, Montreal 2, No. 1, 1906.
Smith, P. B., and Cherry, W. B.: Identification of malleomyces by specific bacteriophages. J Bacteriol 74:668, 1957.
Wetmore, P. W., and Gochenour, W. S.: Comparative studies of the genus *Malleomyces* and selected *Pseudomonas* species. I. Morphological and cultural characteristics. J Bacteriol 72:79, 1956.

262

TOXOPLASMOSIS

JACK S. REMINGTON, M.D.
RIMA MCLEOD, M.D.

The term toxoplasmosis has been used imprecisely to refer to both infection and disease due to *Toxoplasma gondii.* The distinction between infection and disease caused by this organism is important clinically and epidemiologically. *Toxoplasma* infection refers to the presence of the protozoan in individuals with or without clinical manifestations. Toxoplasmosis refers to the disease caused by the organism. *Toxoplasma* infection is usually asymptomatic in older children and adults; but when signs and symptoms are present, they are usually of short duration (acute) and self-limited. Chronic *Toxoplasma* infection describes persistence of the organism in the cyst form without clinical manifestations. The term chronic toxoplasmosis is best reserved to describe the disease in which active *Toxoplasma* infection is the proven cause of persistent or recrudescent clinical manifestations (e.g., encephalitis in infants; myocarditis, chorioretinitis, or lymphadenopathy). Throughout the world, *Toxoplasma* infection occurs with significantly greater frequency than toxoplasmosis.

ETIOLOGY

Classification of the Organism. *T. gondii* is an obligate intracellular protozoan. It has an enteroepithelial and extraintestinal cycle in members of the cat family and only an extraintestinal cycle in all other mammalian and avian hosts. The organism is classified among the Sporozoa and exists in three forms: trophozoite, cyst, and oocyst (Fig. 1).

Trophozoites (Tachyzoites). The trophozoite (Fig. 1A and B) is crescent or oval, with one end pointed and the other rounded. It measures approximately 3 by 7 μm. It stains well with either Wright's stain or Giemsa stain. The nucleus is centrally located, and there are no flagella, cilia, or pseudopods. Trophozoites are found in tissues during the acute stage of infection and invade all mammalian cells except non-nucleated erythrocytes. Multiplication is by endodyogeny (i.e., two *Toxoplasma* organisms form within each parent cell). Division continues until the host cell ruptures or a tissue cyst forms. Desiccation, freezing and thawing, and gastric secretions kill trophozoites.

Trophozoites can be propagated in the peritoneum of mice, in tissue culture, or in eggs. Antigens of trophozoites are used in complement fixation and hemagglutination tests for diagnosis of *Toxoplasma* infection, and whole trophozoites are used in the Sabin-Feldman dye test, agglutination test, and fluorescent antibody method.

Cysts. The tissue cyst (Fig. 1C) develops within host cells and may contain thousands of organisms. Cysts range in size from 10 to 100 μm and stain well with periodic acid-Schiff (PAS) stain. The cyst wall also stains with silver. Because cysts may be present in tissues ingested by carnivorous animals or humans, they are important in transmission. It seems likely that they are also the likely source of recrudescent disseminated infection in the immunosuppressed individual and in older children and adults who develop chorioretinitis. Cysts are demonstrable as early as the eighth day of infection in animals and may remain viable in multiple tissues throughout the life of the host. Skeletal and heart muscle and brain are the most common sites of chronic (latent) infection in humans, although cysts may exist in virtually every organ. Peptic or tryptic digestive fluids disrupt the cyst wall, thereby liberating viable *T. gondii,* which can survive several hours of exposure to these digestive enzymes. Freezing (−20° C) and thawing, heating to 60° C, or desiccation destroys tissue cysts.

Oocysts. The oocyst (Fig. 1E to H) is oval and measures 10 to 12 μm in diameter. Only members of the cat family have been reported to excrete oocysts (Fig. 2), and cats have systemic infection with *T. gondii* as well. After a cat eats food containing cysts or contaminated with oocysts, *T. gondii* are released into the lumen of the stomach or small intestine. After invasion of the epithelial cells of the small intestine (Fig. 1D) (Dubey et al., 1972), the organism undergoes an asexual cycle (schizogony) and then a sexual cycle (gametogony), resulting in development of the noninfectious, unsporulated oocyst (Fig. 1E and G). A cat begins to excrete oocysts 3 to 24 days after the infection, depending on the form of the infecting organism. This excretion continues for 7 to 20 days, and as many as 10 million oocysts may be shed in the feces in a single day. Renewed oocyst excretion has been reported to occur when a cat becomes reinfected with *Toxoplasma* organisms or is acutely infected with *Isospora.* Maturation (sporulation) (Fig. 1F and H), which is required for the oocyst to become infectious, occurs only after the oocysts have been excreted. Sporulation occurs in 2 to 3 days at 24° C, in 5 to 8 days at 15° C, and in 14 to 21 days at 11° C. Oocysts do not sporulate below 4° C or above 37° C. Under favorable conditions (e.g., warm, moist soil), oocysts remain infectious for several months to over a year. Dry heat (over 66° C) or boiling water renders oocysts noninfectious. Ingestion of oocysts has been shown to cause infection.

Life Cycle and Modes of Transmission of T. gondii. *T. gondii* is ubiquitous and can infect herbivorous, omnivorous, and carnivorous animals, including all orders of mammals, some birds, and some reptiles. Most commonly, *T. gondii* infects man or other animals when organisms are released from ingested cysts or oocysts. The trophozoites invade the intestinal epithelium and spread hematogenously or via lymphatics to tissues, where they form cysts.

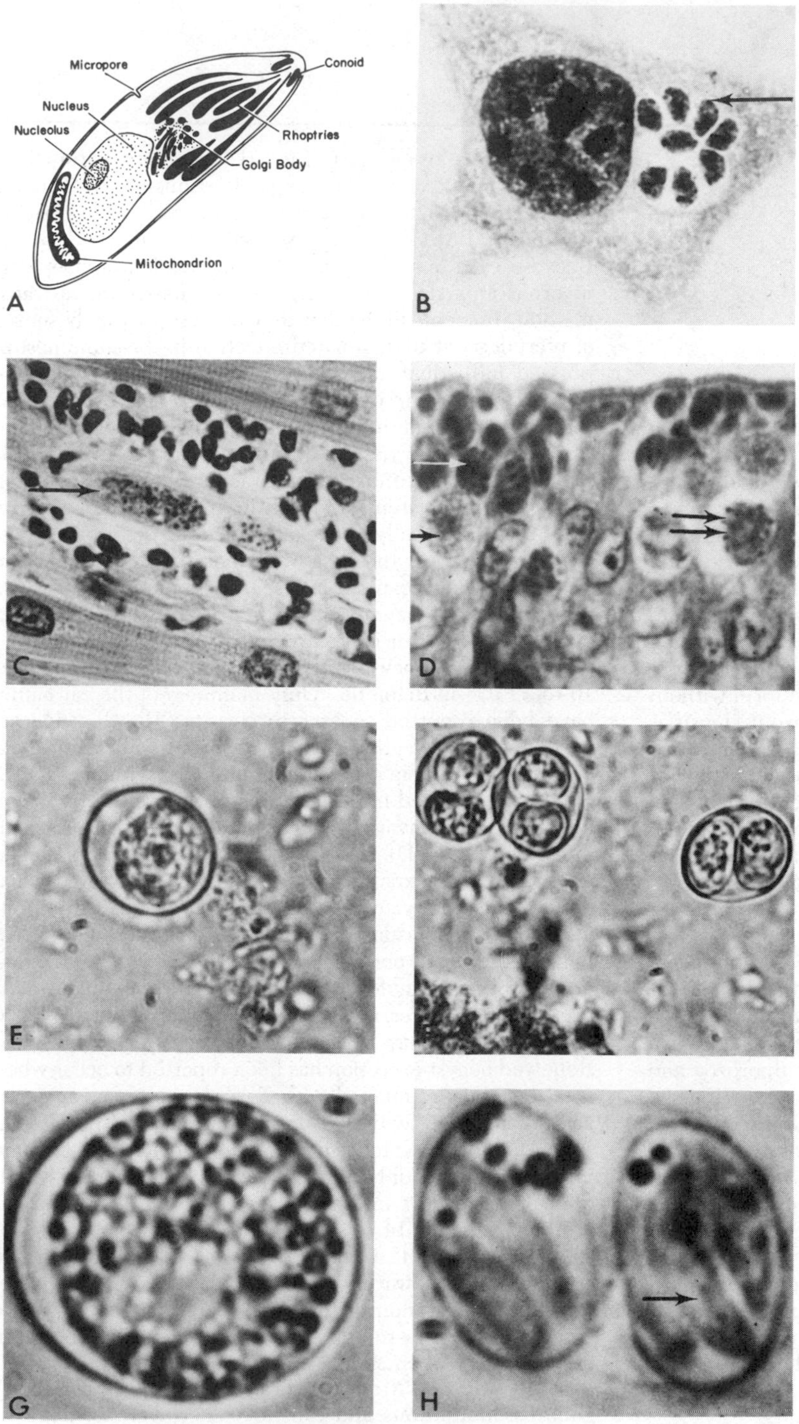

Figure 1. The forms of *Toxoplasma. A,* Trophozoite, schematic representation. (Courtesy of W. M. Hutchinson, Glasgow.) *B,* Trophozoites (arrow) in vacuole in the cytoplasm of cell cultured in vitro. *C,* Tissue cyst (arrow) in human myocardium. Note that cyst conforms to shape of muscle fiber. In brain, cysts are spherical. *D,* Schizonts (white arrow). Male (double arrow) and female (black arrow) gametocytes in the cat ileum. (From Dubey, J., and Frenkel, J. K.: J Protozool 19:155, 1972.) *E,* Unsporulated oocyst. *F,* Sporulated oocyst. *G,* Unsporulated oocyst (higher magnification). *H,* Unsporulated oocyst (higher magnification) in which two sporozoites (arrow) are visible. (From Dubey, J., Miller, N., and Frenkel, J.: J Exp Med 132:636, 1970.)

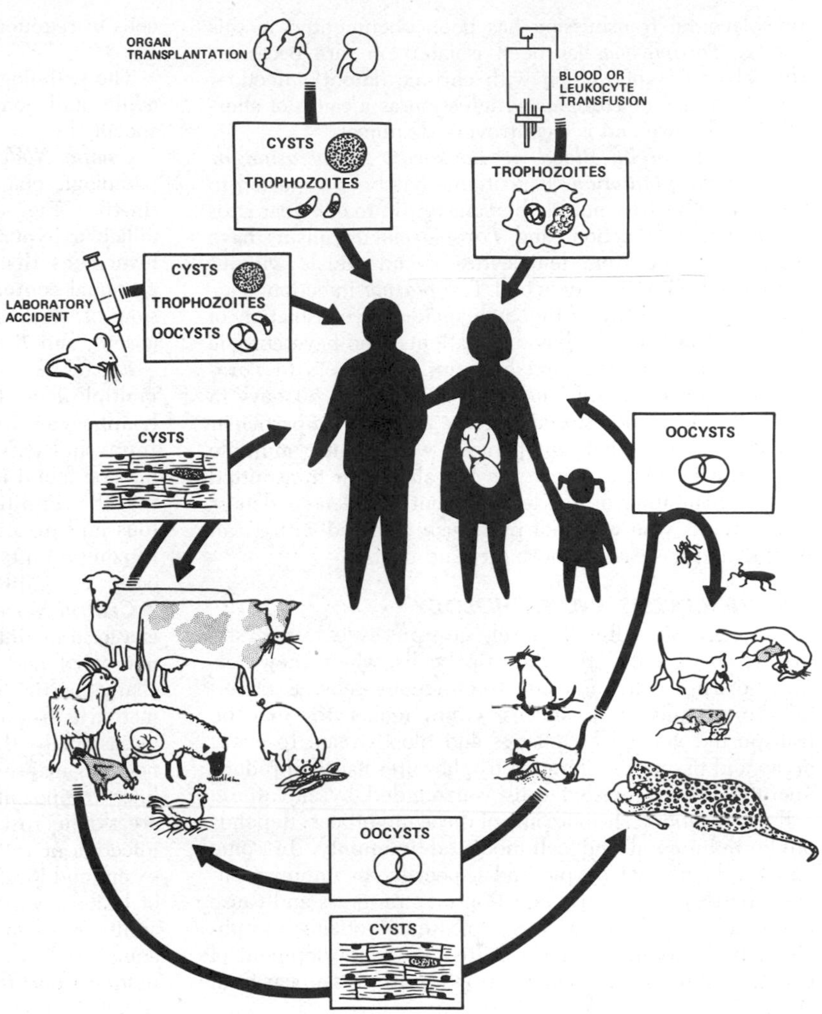

Figure 2. Life cycle and modes of transmission of *Toxoplasma gondii.* Infection in man and other animals occurs primarily after ingestion of either the cyst or the oocyst. Released organisms invade the intestinal epithelium, spread to tissues (either hematogenously or via lymphatics), and form cysts. When man or other animals (including the cat) eat infected tissues (from any animal) or mature oocysts (excreted only by members of the cat family), the life cycle is completed. Laboratory accidents, organ transplantation, and blood and white blood cell transfusion also have beem implicated in transmission of the organism.

When man or other animals (including the cat) eat infected tissues (from any animal) or mature oocysts (excreted only by members of the cat family), the life cycle is completed. Members of the family Felidae, including both domestic and feral cats, appear to be the definitive hosts in this life cycle because they are the only animals that are known to shed oocysts. Oocysts have been found in the feces of approximately 1 per cent of cats in diverse areas of the world (including Costa Rica, Germany, Japan, and the United States).

Toxoplasma organisms are acquired mainly by ingestion and transplacental transmission and less commonly through blood or leukocyte transfusion, organ transplantation, and laboratory accident (Fig. 2). Reinfection from an exogenous source occurs but has not been recognized as a cause of clinical illness.

Ingestion. *T. gondii* is acquired principally by eating food containing cysts or contaminated with oocysts. In most areas of the world, approximately 10 per cent of lamb and 25 per cent of pork contain cysts; the prevalence of cysts in beef is not known. Oocysts are ingested after direct contact with material contaminated by infected cat feces. Flies, cockroaches, and probably other insects can transport oocysts to food. Water, probably contaminated with oocysts, has been implicated as a means of transmission in one outbreak of toxoplasmosis.

Transplacental Transmission. *Toxoplasma* may be transmitted transplacentally to the fetus in utero or at vaginal delivery. This transmission occurs if infection is acquired by the mother during pregnancy. Infection acquired by the mother during the current pregnancy most often results in birth of an uninfected infant but may also result in spontaneous abortion, stillbirth, or birth of a premature or full-term infected infant. Approximately one third of infants born to mothers who acquire infection during pregnancy are infected. In infants born to mothers infected during the first trimester, congenital infection is least common (approximately 17 per cent) but disease is most severe; in infants born to mothers infected during the third trimester, congenital infection is most common (approximately 65 per cent) but is usually asymptomatic. *Toxoplasma* infection that is acquired by the mother during pregnancy is symptomatic in only about 10 to 20 per cent of cases; but whether or not the infection is symptomatic, the fetus is still at risk.

The following are guidelines for ascertaining the risk to the fetus of a woman who has been infected before the pregnancy in question. An immunocompetent woman who acquired *Toxoplasma* infection more than 6 months before gestation will not deliver an infected infant. When conception occurs less than 6 months after acquisition of the infection, the risk to the fetus is exceedingly low, but transplacental transmission has been documented in this setting. *Toxoplasma* has been isolated on rare occasions from abortuses of women with chronic (latent) infection. The frequency of *Toxoplasma* infection as a cause of abortion is unknown and is a controversial subject.

Transmission by Blood or Leukocyte Transfusion or Organ Transplantation. Parasitemia has been reported to persist in otherwise normal persons for up to one year after acquisition of infection, and *Toxoplasma* organisms have been recovered from leukocytes of individuals without recognized clinical evidence of *Toxoplasma* infection. Particularly noteworthy is the high incidence of isolation of the organism from the blood of patients who have chronic myelogenous leukemia and high antibody titers to *Toxoplasma*. The organism can survive for up to 50 days in whole citrated blood stored at 4° C. This poses a particular threat to immunodeficient patients who require multiple blood transfusions. *Toxoplasma* has also been transmitted by transplantation of hearts from acutely infected donors to recipients who were not previously infected with *Toxoplasma* and has caused morbidity and death.

PATHOGENESIS AND PATHOLOGY

Pathogenesis. After their release from cysts or oocysts, the organisms enter gastrointestinal cells, where they multiply, disrupt cells, and infect contiguous cells. Extracellular organisms or organisms within leukocytes may be transported via the lymphatics and bloodstream to every organ and tissue. Proliferating trophozoites usually produce necrotic foci of invaded cells, surrounded by an intense cellular reaction. The outcome of the acute process depends on both humoral and cell-mediated immunity. In some apparently normal people and especially in immunodeficient patients, the acute infection may progress and cause potentially lethal lesions, such as acute necrotizing encephalitis, pneumonitis, or myocarditis. With development of the normal immune response, trophozoites disappear from the tissues.

A unique aspect of the infection is that organisms persist as cysts in multiple organs for the lifespan of the host. The tissue cysts, which are characteristic of chronic infection, provoke little or no inflammatory response. Either rupture of cysts or persistence of viable trophozoites within monocytes and macrophages may be the source of recurrent parasitemias in some asymptomatic individuals with chronic infection. Cysts are the likely source of organisms that cause recrudescent disease in immunocompromised patients or chorioretinitis in older children and adults with congenital toxoplasmosis.

Pathology. The meager information on the pathologic changes of toxoplasmosis in immunologically normal people is derived largely from lymph node biopsy, because most of these infections are asymptomatic and self-limited. There is limited information concerning changes in other organs. Pathology has been defined most clearly in congenitally infected infants and in immunosuppressed patients with disseminated infection.

There are considerable variations in the degree of organ and tissue involvement in infants with congenital infection. In some, autopsy reveals only central nervous system (CNS) and eye involvement, whereas in others there is wide dissemination of lesions and organisms. The central nervous system is never spared. In extraneural organs, whose tissues can regenerate, residual lesions may be so slight that they are easily overlooked. In the central nervous system and eye, on the other hand, the inability of nerve cells to regenerate leads to more severe, permanent damage.

The pathologic changes described below are the same in adults and congenitally infected infants unless otherwise specified.

Lymph Node. In older children and adults, the histopathologic changes in toxoplasmic lymphadenitis are distinctive (Fig. 3). The characteristic lesion is a reactive follicular hyperplasia with irregular clusters of epithelioid histiocytes that encroach upon and blur the margins of germinal centers. There is also an associated focal distension of sinuses with monocytoid cells. Giant cells are absent, and *T. gondii* can be demonstrated only rarely.

Eye. The earliest changes in the eye are single or multiple foci of necrosis. The infiltrate consists largely of lymphocytes, plasma cells, and mononuclear phagocytes. Intra- and extracellular trophozoites and numerous cysts may be found in the retinal lesions. It has been suggested that the retinitis originates from cyst rupture. Granulomatous inflammation of the choroid is secondary to the necrotizing retinitis. Iridocyclitis, glaucoma, and cataracts may occur as complications of the chorioretinitis.

Central Nervous System (CNS). In acute infection, there is a focal or diffuse meningoencephalitis with necrosis and microglial nodules. Multinucleated giant cells are not a characteristic feature. Perivascular mononuclear inflammation is frequent and is contiguous to areas of necrosis. Occasionally there is necrosis of vessel walls. Areas of necrosis may mimic mass lesions, and intra- and extracellular trophozoites are usually found at the periphery of areas of necrosis. Cysts in the brain may occur during acute infection or reflect infection of long duration (Fig. 4). The extent and location of CNS involvement, as well as the size of lesions, vary considerably. The lesions in the CNS in adults and congenitally infected infants are similar. Periaqueductal or periventricular vasculitis with necrosis is a unique aspect of severe congenital infection. Necrotic tissue sloughs into the ventricles, obstructing the aqueduct of Sylvius or the foramen of Monro and causing internal hydrocephalus. Calcification of necrotic areas is especially prominent in congenital infection but may also occur in older children or adults.

Lung. Pulmonary infection may cause clinically significant interstitial pneumonitis in congenitally infected infants and in immunocompromised patients, and uncommonly in individuals without apparent underlying disease. In each of these settings, there are thickened and edematous alveolar septa that, along with peribronchial areas, may be infiltrated with mononuclear cells, occasional plasma cells, and rare eosinophils. The walls of small blood vessels may also be infiltrated with lymphocytes and mononuclear cells, and *Toxoplasma* may be present in endothelial cells. Both trophozoites and cysts have been seen within alveolar lining cells. Necrosis within granulomatous foci is prominent in some patients with disseminated toxoplasmosis and malignancy but is rarely seen in infants or in patients without malignancy. In many cases, there is some bronchopneumonia, often caused by superimposed infection with other organisms.

Heart. Myocarditis is found in congenital infection, in infection of immunocompromised individuals, and rarely in severe acute infection of apparently normal individuals. Cysts and large aggregates of trophozoites occur within muscle fibers (Fig. 1C). Single organisms are found adjacent to and within areas of necrotic tissue. Foci of inflammatory cells (lymphocytes, plasma cells, mononuclear cells, and

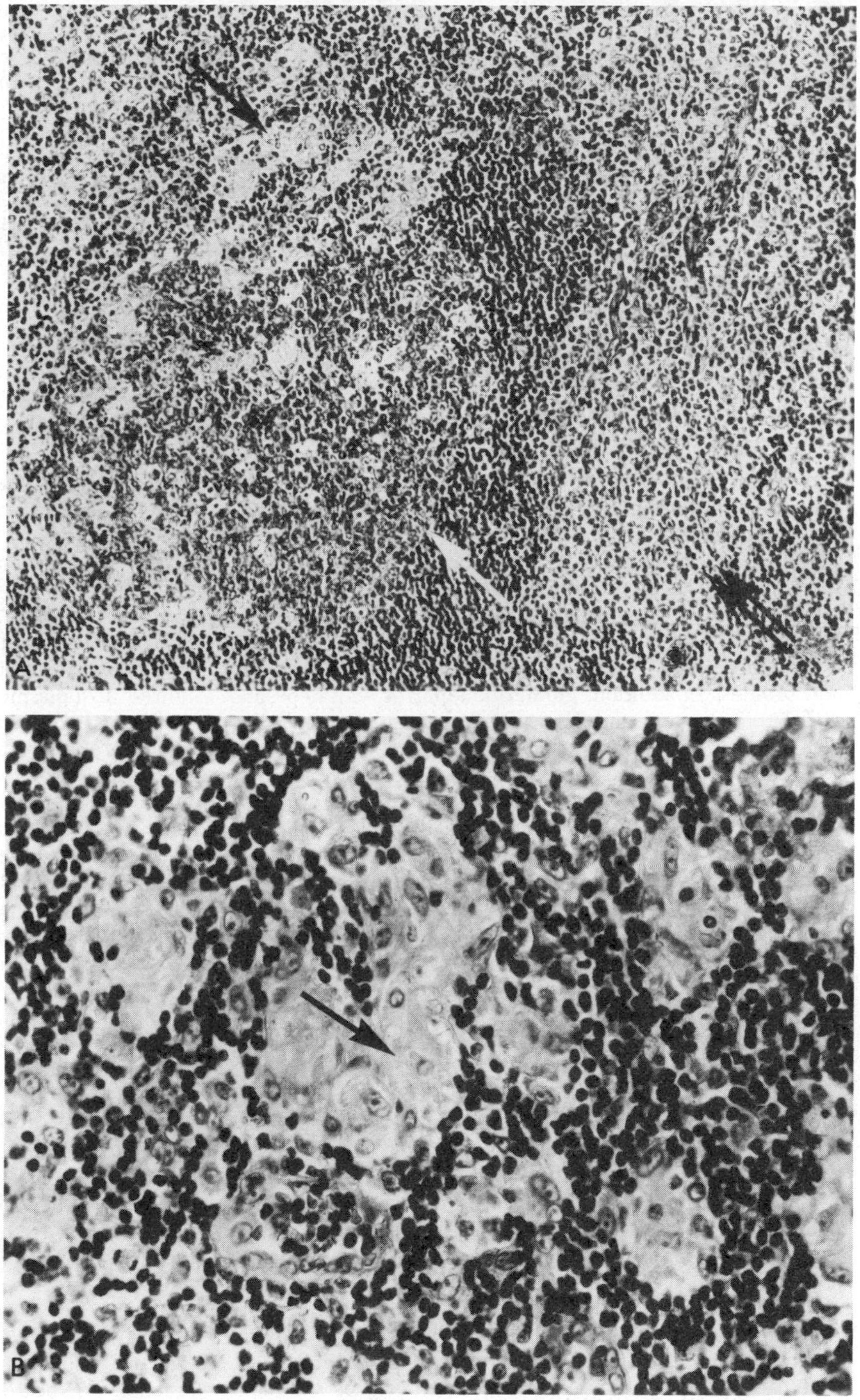

Figure 3. Characteristic lymph node pathology in lymphadenitis due to *Toxoplasma*. *A*, Epithelioid cells (black arrow) encroach upon and blur margins of germinal center (white arrow), and there is focal distension of subcapsular and trabecular sinuses by "monocytoid" cells (double black arrows). *B*, Irregular clusters of epithelioid cells (arrow) scattered throughout paracortical lymphoid stroma. (From Dorfman, R. F., and Remington, J. S.: N Engl J Med 289:878, 1973.)

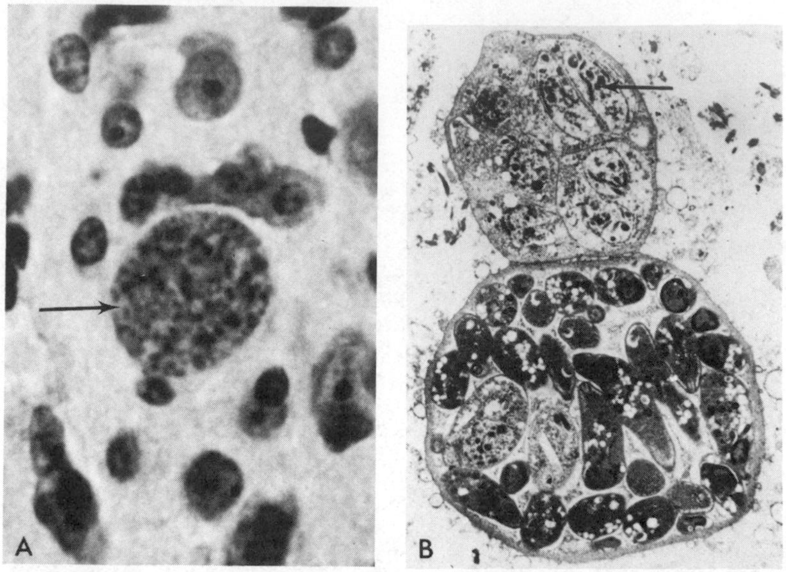

Figure 4. Infection of central nervous system with *Toxoplasma*. *A*, Cyst (arrow) in brain is seen in acute infection as early as eight days, or in chronic (latent) infection. *B*, Electronmicrograph of central nervous system *Toxoplasma* infection. The diagnosis may be established by electronmicroscopic identification of organism (arrow) when light microscopic examination is not definitive. (From Ghatak, N. R., Poon, T. P., and Zimmerman, H. M.: Arch Pathol 89:337, 1970.)

occasional eosinophils) are associated with hyaline necrosis and fragmentation of myocardial cells, usually without organisms. Hemorrhagic pericarditis has also been reported in some patients with toxoplasmosis.

Kidney. In congenital toxoplasmosis and disseminated infection in older children and adults, the pathologic changes in the kidney resemble those in other organs (i.e., necrosis and the presence of cysts, trophozoites, and inflammatory cells). Necrosis may occur in both glomeruli and tubules. In addition, glomerulonephritis with deposits of IgM, fibrinogen, and *Toxoplasma* antigen and antibody has been reported.

Other Sites. The organisms and foci of necrosis have been found in the adrenal cortex, testes, and ovaries of infected infants; and *Toxoplasma*, usually without inflammation, have been found in the pituitary. Cysts or trophozoites with or without inflammation have been reported in multiple organs including liver, spleen, bone marrow, thyroid, pancreas, adipose tissue, and skin in infected infants and adults. Pancreatic involvement has been a prominent finding in infection in immunocompromised patients. Involvement of skeletal muscles varies from parasitized fibers without pathologic changes to focal areas of infiltration or widespread myositis with necrosis.

Immunologic Abnormalities. Monoclonal gammopathy of the IgG class has been described in infants with congenital toxoplasmosis. IgM levels may be elevated in newborns with congenital toxoplasmosis.

Circulating immune complexes have been detected by Clq binding assay in sera from adults with the systemic, febrile, and lymphadenopathic forms of toxoplasmosis and an infant with congenital toxoplasmosis, but not after signs and symptoms resolved.

There are marked and prolonged alterations in T lymphocyte subpopulations associated with *T. gondii* infection that can be correlated with disease syndromes but not necessarily with disease outcome: In some patients with prolonged fever and malaise there is lymphocytosis, increased suppressor T cells and depressed helper-to-suppressor cell ratio. Some of these patients have fewer helper cells even when they are asymptomatic. In some patients with lymphadenopathy helper cells diminish for more than 6 months after onset of infection. Asymptomatic patients have abnormal T cell subpopulations. Some patients with disseminated disease have a marked reduction in the number of T cells and a marked depression in the ratio of helper to suppressor lymphocytes.

CLINICAL MANIFESTATIONS

Lymphadenopathy and Other Manifestations. The most commonly recognized clinical manifestation of acute acquired toxoplasmosis is lymphadenopathy. The cervical nodes (either a single posterior cervical node or multiple nodes) are involved most frequently, and discovery of their involvement is often incidental. Asymptomatic lymphadenopathy may mimic lymphoma. Involvement of a pectoral node may be mistaken for carcinoma of the breast in females. Suboccipital, supraclavicular, axillary, and inguinal nodes are involved frequently. It is important to recognize that the mediastinal, mesenteric, and retroperitoneal nodes may also be involved. With infection of the mesenteric or retroperitoneal nodes, there may be abdominal pain and fever to 40° C. Involved lymph nodes are usually discrete and vary in firmness; they may be tender but do not suppurate. Confusion, malaise, fever, stiff neck, myalgias, arthralgias, headache, sore throat, maculopapular rash (which spares the palms and soles), urticaria, hepatosplenomegaly, hepatitis or reactive lymphocytes may occur. In a recent epidemic, 35 of 37 individuals with serologic evidence of acute acquired *Toxoplasma* infection had signs or symptoms of infection. Although 25 individuals went to physicians, only three were correctly diagnosed as having toxoplasmosis. The lymphadenopathic form of toxoplasmosis is self-limited, but lymphadenopathy and/or malaise may persist or recur for months.

Rarely, someone who seems to be normal immunologically may develop any of the following, alone or in combination: myocarditis, pericarditis, pericardial effusion, polymyositis, hepatitis, pneumonitis, encephalitis, or meningoencephalitis. None of the signs or symptoms from involvement of these organs are specific for infection with *T. gondii*. Some of these patients have died.

Ocular Involvement. *Toxoplasma* has been estimated to cause approximately 35 per cent of cases of chorioretinitis in the United States and Central and Western Europe. In the older child and adult, ocular disease is most frequently a consequence of congenital *Toxoplasma* infection, but chorioretinitis has been estimated to occur in approximately 1 per cent of patients with acute acquired *Toxoplasma* infection.

Active chorioretinitis may produce blurred vision, scotomas, pain, photophobia, or epiphora (O'Connor, 1974). Central vision may be impaired or lost if the macula is involved. Strabismus may be an early sign of chorioretinitis in children. In congenital toxoplasmosis, micropthalmia, small cornea, posterior cortical cataract, anisometropia, strabismus, nystagmus, and leukocoria also occur. Nystagmus may result either from poor fixation due to the chorioretinitis or from involvement of the central nervous system. Convergent or divergent strabismus may be caused by involvement of extraocular muscles or the brain. Associated systemic signs of infection are uncommon. Since ocular involvement may cause the only clinical sign of infection in newborns, newborn infants require ophthalmologic examination to exclude toxoplasmosis. As inflammation subsides, vision improves, but often only incompletely. Episodic flares of chorioretinitis are common and destroy retinal tissue. These multiple recurrences may result in glaucoma.

On ophthalmoscopic examination the acute lesions appear as yellowish white, cotton-like patches that have elevated, indistinct margins surrounded by a zone of hyperemia. The inflammatory exudate in the vitreous may obscure the fundus. Older lesions are atrophic, whitish gray plaques with distinct borders and black spots of choroidal pigment. The lesions may be single or, more commonly, multiple and are usually located near the posterior pole of the retina, although they may be peripheral. Lesions of varying age may be seen simultaneously (Fig. 5). Less commonly, a panuveitis and papillitis with optic atrophy may occur. Isolated anterior uveitis due to toxoplasmosis has never been proved. Bilateral congenital chorioretinitis is the typical ocular lesion of congenital toxoplasmosis. Its distinguishing features in infants are (1) consistent bilateral macular involvement; (2) tendency toward bilateral occurrence of other lesions; (3) tendency toward peripheral involvement in one or more quadrants of the retina and choroid; (4) punched-out lesions in the late phase; (5) massive chorioretinal degeneration; (6) extensive fibrosis and heavy pigmentation, as contrasted with the dissociation of these changes in other chorioretinal lesions; (7) normal retina and vasculature surrounding the lesions throughout the infection; (8) tendency toward associated congenital defects in the eyes; (9) rapid development of sequential optic nerve atrophy; and (10) frequent clarity of the media despite severe chorioretinitis.

Special Considerations

Toxoplasmosis in the Immunocompromised Patient. All forms of toxoplasmosis that occur in normal individuals also occur in immunocompromised individuals (Ruskin and Remington, 1976). Acute toxoplasmosis in the immunocompromised patient may be due to reactivation of latent infection or to acquisition of infection from exogenous sources, including organ transplants and blood or leukocyte transfusions. Immunosuppressed patients with the greatest predilection for life-threatening toxoplasmosis are those receiving immunosuppressive therapy for lymphoproliferative disorders (especially Hodgkin's disease), hematologic malignancy, or prevention of organ graft rejection and individuals with the recently recognized acquired immu-

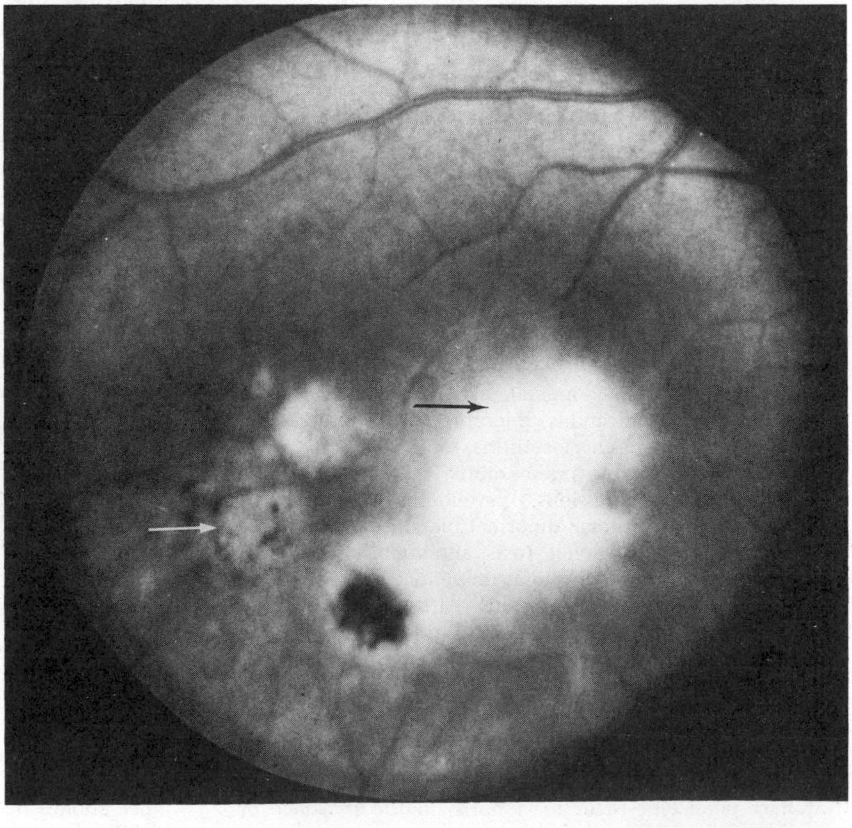

Figure 5. Chorioretinitis due to *Toxoplasma.* The characteristic lesion is a focal necrotizing retinitis with cottonlike patches in the fundus. Note that the acute lesions (black arrow) have indistinct borders and appear soft and white, while older lesions (white arrow) are whitish-gray, sharply outlined, and spotted by accumulations of choroidal pigment. (From O'Connor, G. R.: Ocular toxoplasmosis. In Locatcher-Khorazo, D., and Seegal, B. C. (eds.): Microbiology of the Eye. St. Louis, The C. V. Mosby Company, 1972, p. 199.)

nodeficiency syndrome (AIDS). In immunosuppressed patients the infection is often fulminant and rapidly fatal. Since effective therapy is available, it is incumbent on clinicians to be aware of the clinical presentation in this type of patient.

The most characteristic clinical manifestations of toxoplasmosis in immunocompromised patients result from brain involvement, which is present in over 50 per cent of documented cases. The symptoms and signs are manifestations of diffuse encephalopathy, meningoencephalitis, or cerebral mass lesions and include changes in mental status, headache, seizures, and focal neurologic deficits. In one series of patients with AIDS and toxoplasmic encephalitis, prominent signs and symptoms included fever, chills, headache, seizures, chorioretinitis, depressed mental status and neurologic findings. Computed axial tomography revealed findings of diffuse encephalitis and mass lesions. Brain biopsy revealed organisms in approximately 75 per cent. Individuals who have not been infected previously with Toxoplasma and receive a cardiac transplant from an infected individual often develop signs and symptoms of toxoplasmosis. The diagnosis of brain involvement can be made by finding trophozoites in a biopsy specimen or in material aspirated from mass lesions that resemble a brain abscess on computerized axial tomography scan. The cerebrospinal fluid typically shows a mononuclear pleocytosis, a moderate elevation in protein concentration, and a normal glucose level. In any immunosuppressed patient with symptoms or signs of brain involvement, the diagnosis of toxoplasmosis must be excluded. Other manifestations of the disease in immunocompromised patients may be nonspecific or reflect inflammation and necrosis of the organs involved, particularly the heart and lungs.

Toxoplasmosis and Toxoplasma Infection in the Pregnant Woman. Toxoplasma infection acquired in pregnancy causes symptoms in only about 10 to 20 per cent of mothers; but the fetus is at risk whether symptoms are present or not. Guidelines regarding toxoplasmosis and *Toxoplasma* infection in the pregnant woman have been offered earlier under the heading Transplacental Transmission.

Congenital Toxoplasmosis. Most infected newborns are asymptomatic at birth. Some asymptomatic infants may never suffer untoward sequelae of the infection; others will develop chorioretinitis, strabismus, blindness, epilepsy, or psychomotor or mental retardation at any time (weeks, months, or even years later). Those with clinically apparent infection at birth may have all or any combination of the following: a mild nonspecific illness, fever, hypothermia, vomiting, diarrhea, jaundice, rash (most commonly petechiae due to thrombocytopenia), hydrocephalus, microcephaly, cerebral calcifications, microphthalmia, strabismus, cataracts, glaucoma, chorioretinitis, optic atrophy, deafness, lymphadenopathy, pneumonitis, myocarditis, hepatosplenomegaly, convulsions, psychomotor retardation, other CNS signs, anemia, abnormal bleeding, thrombocytopenia, eosinophilia, monocytosis, and abnormal cerebrospinal fluid with xanthochromia, mononuclear pleocytosis, and high protein (grams per cent). Although not specific for toxoplasmosis in infants, these cerebrospinal fluid changes should make one consider toxoplasmosis even in subclinical cases. *Toxoplasma* does not cause fetal malformations.

COMPLICATIONS AND SEQUELAE. The lymphadenopathic form of acquired toxoplasmosis is usually self-limited but may persist or recur for months in the presence or absence of constitutional symptoms.

Mental retardation, epilepsy, spasticity, palsies, and severe impairment of vision are common when clinical signs of infection are present at birth. Deafness also may occur. Microcephaly has been reported in approximately 13 per cent and hydrocephalus in approximately 28 per cent of infants with signs or symptoms of toxoplasmosis involving the CNS. These serious sequelae are a threat to all congenitally infected infants whether or not they are symptomatic in the newborn period.

Ocular toxoplasmosis is characterized by frequent relapses. It may result in glaucoma or loss of vision and ultimately may necessitate enucleation.

Acute infection is extremely serious in immunodeficient patients. Although mortality is high, the actual death rate is unknown. Relapse is frequent in patients with AIDS.

GEOGRAPHIC VARIATIONS IN DISEASE AND INFECTION. There are considerable geographic variations in prevalence of infection with *Toxoplasma* (Fig. 6). In all areas surveyed, the prevalence of positive serologic reactions increases with age. Generally, there is less human infection in cold regions, in hot and arid areas, and at high elevations. Exceptions do exist: Eskimos, once thought to be free of this infection, have been found to have prevalence rates of 13 to 46 per cent, whereas some isolated tropical communities have little or no *Toxoplasma* infection. It is interesting that these tropical communities do not have known exposure to domestic or feral cats. However, there are also populations who are infected with *T. gondii* and who have no known exposure to cats. Most of the variations in prevalence and incidence of infection from area to area have not been explained. However, personal habits and exposure to cat feces are important in transmission. For example in the United States of America and Europe ingestion of undercooked meat is common and probably important in transmission. In Costa Rica, proximity of the area where cats defecate to human habitation is important in transmission.

The actual incidence of congenital toxoplasmosis is unknown. Approximations per 1000 live births are as follows: Vienna, 6 to 7; Paris, 3; New York City, 1.3; and Mexico City, 2.

No particular genetic susceptibility has been documented for humans. Epidemics of toxoplasmosis have been documented in humans and in domestic animals in several countries including the United States of America, Brazil, and Spain. Simultaneous occurrence of infection in multiple members of the same family living together has been reported.

DIAGNOSIS. The diagnosis of acute infection with *Toxoplasma* is made by isolation of *T. gondii* from blood or body fluids. It is also made by demonstration of trophozoites in sections or preparations of tissues and body fluids; of cysts in the placenta or tissues of a fetus or newborn; and of characteristic lymph node histology. Serologic tests are also useful for diagnosis.

Isolation Procedures. The organism can be isolated by inoculation of body fluids, leukocytes, or tissue specimens into the peritoneal cavity of mice or into tissue cultures. Body fluids should be processed and inoculated immediately; tissues and blood may be stored at 4° C overnight. Freezing or treating specimens with formalin kills the organism.

Mice should be examined for *Toxoplasma* in their peritoneal fluid at six to ten days after inoculation, or earlier if

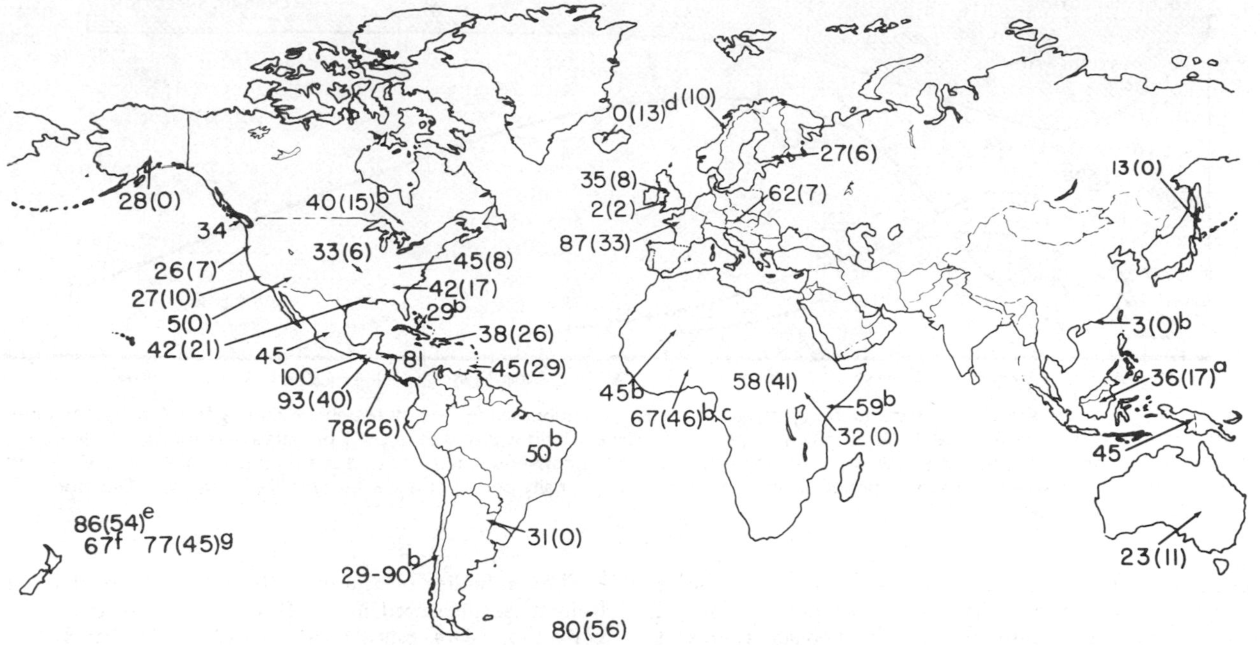

Figure 6. Prevalence of antibodies against *Toxoplasma gondii* in individuals in selected locales. Unless otherwise specified, figures outside parentheses equal per cent of positive adults of approximately 30 to 40 years of age; figures inside parentheses equal per cent of positive children less than 10 years of age. a, IHA antibodies, others were IFA or dye test; b, adults with either age range not clearly specified or wider age range than approximately 30 to 40 years of age; c, "juveniles"; d, although 14 individuals between 30 and 39 years of age had no *Toxoplasma* antibody, 29 per cent of 14 individuals 40 to 49 years of age did have *Toxoplasma* antibody; e, Society Island; f, American Samoa; g, Tahiti.

they die. Mice surviving for six weeks should be tested for *Toxoplasma* antibody in their serum. If antibody is present, definitive diagnosis is made by visualization of *Toxoplasma* cysts in the mouse brain. If no cysts are seen in mice with *Toxoplasma* antibody, portions of brain, liver, and spleen from the mice should be inoculated into other mice.

Isolation of *T. gondii* from body fluids reflects acute infection, as does isolation from the blood in most patients. Persistent parasitemia in asymptomatic people with latent infection appears to be rare, except perhaps in chronic myelogenous leukemia. Isolation from tissues (e.g., skeletal muscle, lung, brain, or eye) obtained by biopsy or at autopsy may reflect the presence of tissue cysts and thus is not proof of acute infection.

Histologic Diagnosis. Demonstration of trophozoites in tissue sections (e.g., endomyocardial biopsy in cardiac transplant recipients) or smears (e.g., brain biopsy, bone marrow aspirate) or in body fluids (e.g., cerebrospinal fluid, amniotic fluid) establishes the diagnosis of acute toxoplasmosis. Although it is difficult to see the trophozoite with ordinary stains, immunofluorescent antibody techniques and a peroxidase-antiperoxidase (PAP) immunohistochemical staining technique have been successful. Demonstration of the tissue cyst is diagnostic of infection with *Toxoplasma* but does not differentiate between acute and chronic infection. Numerous cysts in any organ usually indicate recent acute infection. The presence of cysts in the placenta or tissues of the newborn infant establishes the diagnosis of congenital infection. The characteristic histologic criteria are sufficient to establish the diagnosis of toxoplasmic lymphadenitis (Fig. 3) (Dorfman and Remington, 1973).

Serologic Tests. The Sabin-Feldman dye test, indirect fluorescent antibody (IFA) tests, and the indirect hemagglutination (IHA) test are the methods most widely used for diagnosis of acute toxoplasmosis. Tests for antigenemia are particularly promising (although experimental) for diagnosis in the newborn and in the immunocompromised individual. The immunosorbent assays or radioimmunoassay are potentially valuable because they allow for automation.

The dye test is sensitive and specific and measures primarily IgG antibodies. The World Health Organization (WHO) has recommended that dye test titers be expressed in International Units (IU/ml). An international standard reference serum for this purpose is available on request from WHO.

The IFA test is the most widely available procedure and appears to measure the same antibodies as the dye test. In both tests, the titers tend to be parallel. Dye test and IFA test antibodies usually appear one to two weeks after infection, reach high titers (≥1:1000) in six to eight weeks, and then gradually decline over months to years; low titers (1:4 to 1:64) commonly persist for life (Fig. 7). The antibody titer does not correlate with severity of illness.

The agglutination test is available commercially in Europe (Bio-Merieux, Lyon, France). It employs formalin-preserved whole parasites and detects IgG. "Natural" IgM antibodies frequently cause nonspecific agglutination in serum that is negative by dye and IFA tests, and eliminated with 2-mercaptoethanol. This method should not be used for measurement of IgM antibodies. It is accurate, simple to perform, inexpensive, and excellent for screening pregnant women.

The IgM-fluorescent antibody (IgM-IFA) test is useful for the diagnosis of acute infection with *T. gondii* because IgM antibodies appear faster (as early as five days after infection) and disappear sooner than IgG antibodies. In most cases, IgM-IFA test antibodies rise rapidly (to levels of 1:80 to ≥1:1000) and fall to low titers (1:10 or 1:20) or

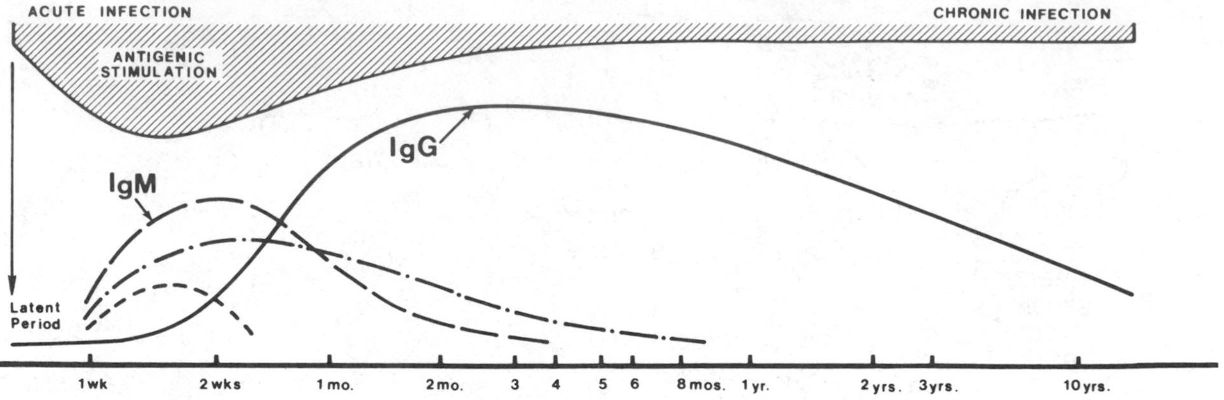

Figure 7. Antibody response of humans to *Toxoplasma* infection. IgM antibodies (— —), detectable by the IgM-IFA test, reach their maximum titer within the first weeks after infection and may decline within a few weeks (- -) or persist for months (—•—). IgG antibodies (—), detectable by either the Sabin-Feldman dye test or the conventional IFA test, reach their maximum titer within two months, maintain a plateau for months or years, and then decline, but usually persist at a low titer for life. (Data from Desmonts, G.: Feuillets de Biologie 16:61, 1975.)

disappear within a few weeks or months (Fig. 7). In some patients, they remain positive at low titers for as long as several years. IgM antibodies in the neonate represent synthesis in utero by the infected fetus because IgM does not normally pass the placental barrier. IgM *Toxoplasma* antibodies may not be demonstrable in some immunodeficient patients with acute toxoplasmosis, most patients with active toxoplasmosis limited to the eye, and approximately 25 per cent of newborns with congenital toxoplasmosis. Antinuclear antibodies may cause false-positive reactions in both the IFA and IgM-IFA tests; rheumatoid factor may cause false-positive reactions in the IgM-IFA test.

Detection of IgM antibodies by the double sandwich enzyme-linked immunosorbent assay (DS-IgM-ELISA) is more sensitive and specific than the IgM-IFA test. Rheumatoid factor and antinuclear antibodies do not cause false positive test results (Naot and Remington, 1980). In the adult, a serum level of IgM antibodies against *Toxoplasma* of 6 to 10 in this test indicates that *Toxoplasma* infection has most likely been acquired within 5 months, levels of 2 or 3 indicates infection acquired within several months or more, 4 or 5 is intermediate, and 0 or 1 is negative. The DS-IgM-ELISA detects approximately 75 per cent of infants with proven congenital infection, whereas the IgM-IFA detects only 25 per cent of such cases. The DS-IgM-ELISA avoids false positives due to rheumatoid factor, which the infant can produce in utero and false negatives due to competition from high levels of maternal IgG antibody, which occur in the IgM-IFA test.

The IgM immunosorbent assay (IgM-ISA), which combines trapping of patient's IgM to a solid surface and formalin-fixed organisms or antigen-coated latex particles to detect the IgM antibodies, is specific and sensitive. The test is read as an agglutination test. It avoids false positive results due to rheumatoid factor or antinuclear antibodies and is more sensitive and specific than the IgM-IFA test. It is used in a major European laboratory for screening pregnant women.

Toxoplasma antigen has been detected in serum of adults with lymphadenopathic form of toxoplasmosis or with other acute *Toxoplasma* infection, but not found in sera of uninfected or chronically infected individuals. It was detected in serum, amniotic fluid, and cerebrospinal fluid from the few congenitally infected infants tested.

The antibodies measured in the IHA test are different from those measured in the IFA and dye tests and may persist for years. Since IHA titers rise later than IFA or dye test titers, the IHA test may be helpful when these titers have stabilized. The IHA test should not be used in infants with suspected congenital infection or in screening for infection acquired during pregnancy, since the test may be negative for too long a period early in the infection. There is a great need for proper standardization of methodology for this and all other serologic tests, and particularly for quality control of commercial kits that are often used by laboratories inexperienced in performing these serologic tests.

Complement fixation (CF) antibodies may appear several weeks later than those measured in the IFA and dye tests and may persist for years. A single positive CF test does not indicate acute infection, nor does a negative CF test exclude toxoplasmosis. A significant rise in CF titer (i.e., two serial dilutions performed in parallel on sera obtained several weeks apart) establishes recent infection.

Guidelines for interpretation of test results are presented in Table 1.

The level of *Toxoplasma* antibody in cerebrospinal fluid or aqueous humor may be used to demonstrate local production of antibody in active ocular or CNS toxoplasmosis. Local antibody production is assessed by application of the following equation:

$$C = \frac{\text{antibody titer in body fluid}}{\text{antibody titer in serum}} \times \frac{\text{concentration of gamma globulin in serum}}{\text{concentration of gamma globulin in body fluid}}$$

A significant correlation coefficient [c] is ≥8 and reflects local antibody production due to active infection of the CNS or eye. If the dye test serum titer is ≥1000, it is usually not possible to demonstrate significant local antibody production by application of this formula. This formula has been applied by using dye test titers and IgM-IFA test titers.

Acute Acquired Toxoplasma Infection in the Immunocompetent Person. In settings in which acute acquired *Toxoplasma* infection is suspected in the immunocompetent person, a negative dye test or IFA test virtually excludes the diagnosis. The diagnosis of recent acute acquired infection is confirmed if there is a seroconversion from a

Table 1. GUIDELINES[a] FOR INTERPRETATION OF COMMONLY EMPLOYED SEROLOGIC TESTS FOR DIAGNOSIS OF TOXOPLASMOSIS

Test (Abbreviation)	Positive Titer	Titer in Acute Infection	Titer in Chronic (Latent) Infection	Duration of Elevation of Titer	Special Considerations
Sabin-Feldman dye test	1:4 undiluted[b]	≥ 1:1000	1:4 to 1:2000	years	(1) There are no known cross-reactions or false-positives in man. (2) The World Health Organization has recommended that titers be expressed in IU/ml.
Indirect fluorescent antibody (IFA) test	1:10[c]	≥ 1:1000	1:8 to 1:2000	years	(1) The same recommendation for expression of test results in IU/ml applies. (2) Antibody measured is the same as that measured in the dye test. (3) Antinuclear antibodies may cause false-positive results.
Indirect fluorescent antibody test for IgM *Toxoplasma* antibodies (IgM-IFA)	1:2 infants[c] 1:10 adults[c]	≥ 1:80	negative to 1:20	weeks to months; occasionally years	(1) Either antinuclear antibodies or rheumatoid factor (IgM) may cause false-positive results. Rheumatoid factor may be absorbed from serum with heat-aggregated IgG.
Indirect hemagglutination (IHA) test	1:16[c]	≥ 1:1000	1:16 to 1:256	years	(1) Not useful for diagnosis of congenital toxoplasmosis. (2) Antibodies by IHA rise later than antibodies measured by dye test and IFA. This test may be especially useful when a rising IHA titer can be demonstrated.
Complement fixation (CF) test	1:4[c]	varies among laboratories	negative to 1:8	years	(1) Antigen preparations used for this test have not been standardized. (2) See (2) under IHA.
Double Sandwich IgM-ELISA (DS-IgM-ELISA)	≥ 2	≥ 6	negative to 1	unknown, often > 1 year	(1) Sensitive and specific
Immunosorbent assay for IgM Toxoplasma antibody (IgM-ISA)	≥ 1	≥ 6	negative to 1	unknown, often > 1 year	
Direct Agglutination test (after treatment of sera with 2-mercaptoethanol)	≥ 1:20	Rising slowly from a negative or low titer (≥ 1:20) to a high titer (≥ 1:512)	Stable (> 1:1000) or slowly decreasing titer	> 1 year	(1) Measures IgG (2) Often less than dye test in early weeks of acute infection. (3) Often slightly more than dye test in older infection and much greater in chronic infection. (4) Striking difference between dye test and agglutination test titers may be observed.

[a]These guidelines are useful in the interpretation of test results, but exceptions to these generalizations may occur.
[b]In some cases of eye disease, the dye test may be positive only in undiluted serum.
[c]These values are representative, but normal values for each laboratory may differ significantly.

negative to a positive titer (in the absence of transfer of antibody by transfusion), or if there is a serial two-tube rise in titer when sera drawn at three-week intervals are run in parallel. Although suggestive of active infection, one high titer in any test is not diagnostic.

The following guidelines are helpful in interpretation of test results, but exceptions may occur. A dye test or IFA test titer of 1:1000 or greater in the presence of a high IgM-IFA test titer (1:80 or greater) or DS-IgM-ELISA or IgM-ISA titer (≥ 6) is probably diagnostic of recent acute infection with or without symptoms. In immunologically normal people with positive titers in the dye test or IFA test, the absence of IgM-IFA test or DS IgM-ELISA or IgM-ISA antibodies almost always excludes the diagnosis of acute infection.

Ocular Toxoplasmosis. The diagnosis of ocular toxoplasmosis in older children and adults is difficult because the titer of antibody in the serum does not necessarily correlate with presence of active lesions in the fundus. Indeed, low serologic test titers (1:4 to 1:64) are usual in patients with active toxoplasmic chorioretinitis. For practical purposes, toxoplasmic chorioretinitis is probably excluded if serologic tests are negative when performed on undiluted serum. If retinal lesions are characteristic and serologic tests are positive, the diagnosis can be made with a high degree of confidence. If the retinal lesion is atypical and the serologic test is positive, the diagnosis of toxoplasmosis is only presumptive; a high prevalence of antibodies in the normal population precludes the assumption of a causal relationship in this situation.

Active Infection in the Immunocompromised Individual. The available diagnostic techniques, including the IgM-IFA test, DS-IgM-ELISA and IgM-ISA are at times insufficient for detection of active infection in immunocompromised patients because antibody responses may be abnormal. For example, in patients with AIDS, dye test antibody titers are low (<1:1000) in approximately half the cases and an IgM response is rarely demonstrable. These patients, however, sometimes make IgG antibody that can be detected by IFA and quite regularly by agglutination tests. Serologic tests in immunocompromised individuals can identify those who are at risk for primary infection or reactivation of latent infection (see also the section Prophylaxis).

Kinetics of serologic responses in cardiac transplant recipients who receive a heart donated by a seropositive individual are variable. In seronegative patients who received hearts donated by seropositive individuals, seroconversion occurred 4 days to 7 weeks and severe illness 1 week to 9 months after transplantation. In approximately 50 per cent of patients who are seropositive before transplantation there is a significant rise in IgG and IgM antibody, although all remain asymptomatic.

Detection of *Toxoplasma* antigen in serum and possibly CSF by ELISA seems promising for identifying disseminated *Toxoplasma* infection in immunocompromised persons.

Toxoplasmosis and Toxoplasma Infection in the Pregnant Woman. Any woman who is considering becoming pregnant should have a *Toxoplasma* serologic test performed to determine whether she has *Toxoplasma* infection before pregnancy. (See Transplacental Transmission for a complete discussion of risks to the fetus in relation to *Toxoplasma* infection acquired by the mother before pregnancy versus during pregnancy.)

In systematic monthly screening of pregnant women serum IgM antibodies usually appeared first, but low titers of IgG antibodies, as measured in the dye test, also appeared early. Sera in which only IgM antibodies were detectable were uncommon. A rise in IgM antibody titer was infrequent, suggesting that its rise was steep and reached its peak in 1 or 2 weeks. In contrast, the rise in IgG antibody was initially very slow. The dye test titer usually remained relatively low (2 to 50 IU/ml or 1:10 to 1:200) for 3 to 6 weeks. Thus acute infection cannot be ruled out when two samples collected 2 or even 3 weeks apart show no significant rise in titer, especially if the dye test is performed with four-fold dilutions of the sera, which would require an eight-fold (two-tube) rise in titer to be considered significant. For this reason, two-fold dilutions are imperative. A four-fold rise is often difficult to detect in the IgG-IFA test. After the initial 3 to 6 weeks, the rise in IgG antibody becomes steeper; and high titers (> 400 IU/ml or ≥ 1:1000) are usually reached within an additional 3 weeks. Thereafter, the rise is slower but still detectable over an additional 3 to 6 weeks by careful methodology avoiding four-fold dilutions of sera. Thus, although the rise in IgG antibody in the dye test differs from case to case, it lasts over 2 months and sometimes 3 months. In the agglutination test with 2-mercaptoethanol, IgG antibody may parallel exactly the dye test response or may rise more slowly, reaching the peak not earlier than 6 months after infection. By 6 months, the IgM-IFA test will be negative in most cases, whereas the DS-IgM-ELISA and the IgM-ISAGA will usually remain positive; in women who become infected during pregnancy, the latter two tests are almost always positive at the time of parturition.

When Toxoplasma infection is treated during the initial antibody response (when the IgG titer is low), the rise in IgG antibody titer slows and the titer (e.g., in the dye test or conventional IFA test) may remain low as long as treatment is continued. A late (delayed) rise often occurs after cessation of treatment.

In the absence of a routine screening program in which *Toxoplasma* serologic tests are performed each month in the pregnant woman, an IgM-IFA or DS-IgM-ELISA or IgM-ISA test should be performed if any other serologic test is positive at any titer. If the IgM-IFA or DS-IgM-ELISA or IgM-ISA test is unavailable, the serologic test should be repeated in three or four weeks with serial two-fold dilutions in order to determine if the titer is stable or rising. If the IgM-IFA test or DS-IgM-ELISA or IgM-ISA is negative and an IFA or dye test titer is stable and less than 1:1000 (300 IU), no further evaluation is necessary. Because titers in the dye test or IFA test usually stabilize at high levels (≥1:1000) six to eight weeks or longer after acquisition of infection, if the dye test or IFA test titer is ≥1:1000 (300 IU) and stable (regardless of titer in the IgM-IFA test or DS-IgM-ELISA or IgM-ISA), the infection was acquired at least four weeks earlier and probably more than eight weeks before the serum was obtained. Thus, for practical purposes, if the dye test or IFA test titer is ≥1:1000 and stable when measured in the first two months of pregnancy, risk to the fetus is very low.

Whereas titers in the dye test or IFA test may have stabilized and peaked by eight weeks after onset of infection, titers in the complement fixation or indirect hemagglutination test may continue to rise for four to six months or longer after acquisition of infection. Therefore, rises in the last two tests may not be helpful in defining when the infection occurred relative to the time of conception.

A common problem is the interpretation of serologic test

results in an asymptomatic woman who is tested for *Toxoplasma* antibody late in the first trimester or in the second trimester of pregnancy. Her IFA or dye test titer is found to be in the range of 1:2000, her IgM-IFA test titer or DS-IgM-ELISA or IgM-ISA is negative, and no significant rise in titer in any test is demonstrable. It is impossible to determine whether her infection occurred before, at, or after conception in this situation. Detection of *Toxoplasma* antigen in amniotic fluid may become useful in determining whether the fetus of a woman who acquired *Toxoplasma* during the current pregnancy is infected, but its use is experimental now.

Congenital Toxoplasmosis. Guidelines for interpreting serologic test results in a mother just delivered of an infant suspected of having congenital toxoplasmosis are given in Table 2. These interpretations are not absolutes but can be used until definitive data become available.

Diagnosis of acute toxoplasmosis in the neonate is based on finding either persistent or rising titers in the dye test or IFA test, or a positive IgM-IFA test (at any titer) in the absence of a placental leak. Since rheumatoid factor may be present in a newborn with congenital infection, it is important to exclude the presence of this antibody in an infant with a positive IgM-IFA test. If a placental leak of maternal blood has occurred, the IgM-IFA test titer in the neonate will fall significantly within a week, since the half-life of IgM is approximately three to five days. Passively transferred maternal antibodies may require six to twelve months or longer, depending on the original titer, to disappear from the infant's serum. Synthesis of *Toxoplasma* antibody by the infected infant is usually demonstrable by the third month of life if the infant is not treated, but it may be delayed until the sixth or ninth month if the infant is treated. Thus, at the time the infant begins to synthesize antibody, infection may be documented serologically even when IgM antibodies are not demonstrable. This may be accomplished by computation of the specific "antibody load," i.e., the ratio of specific serum antibody titer to the level of serum IgG in mother and infant. For example, in an uninfected infant with only maternal antibody, there is no change in antibody load because, as the titer of antibody decreases in the infant's serum, total IgG decreases in a similar manner. During the second and third months, the amount of IgG synthesized by the infant increases. Because this newly synthesized IgG does not contain *Toxoplasma* antibodies, the antibody load decreases and will continue to decrease as IgG synthesis in the child progresses. In congenitally infected infants, the production of antibody may vary considerably from one case to another. Early and delayed antibody production can be demonstrated by increases in antibody load.

Table 2. GUIDELINES FOR INTERPRETATION OF ANTIBODY TEST. RESULTS IN A MOTHER JUST DELIVERED OF A CHILD SUSPECTED OF HAVING CONGENITAL TOXOPLASMOSIS

Congenital Infection in Child	**Serologic Test Results in Mother** *Dye Test*[a]	***IgM Fluorescent Antibody Test***
Most often present	300 to 3000 IU/ml (1:1200 to 1:12,000)	Positive
Often present	1000 to 3000 IU/ml (1:4000 to 1:12,000)[b]	Negative
Seldom present	300 to 1000 IU/ml (1:1200 to 1:4000)[b]	Negative
Possible[c]	< 300 IU/ml	Positive
Excluded	< 300 IU/ml	Negative

[a]Figures in parentheses indicate approximate titers expressed as reciprocal of serum dilution, which correspond to the titers expressed in international units.

[b]There is no information concerning interpretation of high dye test titers in a mother just delivered of a child suspected of having congenital toxoplasmosis in regions in which a significant number of infected mothers have high dye test titers (e.g., Central America).

[c]Usually present if maternal dye test is rising after delivery; usually absent if maternal dye test is not rising.

Adapted from Remington and Desmonts, 1976.

THERAPY

Therapy in Specific Clinical Settings. The need for and duration of therapy are determined by the clinical severity of the illness and by the individual who is infected.

Immunologically normal patients with the lymphadenopathic form of acute toxoplasmosis do not require specific treatment, unless there are severe and persistent symptoms, or evidence of damage to vital organs. Infections acquired in laboratory accidents or via transfusions may be more severe than naturally acquired infections and probably should be treated.

Patients with active chorioretinitis should be treated with specific drug therapy. G. Richard O'Connor (1974) recommends that patients with active ocular toxoplasmosis receive pyrimethamine and sulfadiazine for one month. Within 10 days, the borders of retinal lesions should sharpen and the vitreous haze should disappear. A favorable clinical response is seen in 60 to 70 per cent of cases; if unfavorable, the courses of pyrimethamine and sulfadiazine are repeated. Systemic corticosteroids are administered if vision is endangered by lesions involving the macula, optic nerve head, or papillomacular bundle. Photocoagulation has been used to treat active lesions and to prevent their spread since most new lesions appear contiguous to old ones. Occasionally vitrectomy and removal of the lens may be necessary to restore visual acuity.

Toxoplasmosis should be treated in a patient whose resistance to infection is compromised by an underlying disease or by therapy (e.g., corticosteroids or cytotoxic drugs). Either serologic evidence of acute infection in an immunocompromised patient, whether or not signs and symptoms of infection are present, or the demonstration of trophozoites in tissue, regardless of serologic test titers, is an indication for therapy. In 80 per cent of immunocompromised patients in whom the diagnosis was established antemortem, improvement occurred when specific therapy was administered. The major problem lies in making the diagnosis early enough to institute treatment.

If a pregnant woman who acquires infection at any time during pregnancy is treated, the chance of congenital infection in her infant is decreased but not eliminated. In one series, the incidence of infection was decreased from 17 per cent to 5 per cent, and in another series it was decreased from 60 per cent to 23 per cent. The drugs effective in the only two reported studies were spiramycin in France and pyrimethamine plus sulfonamide in Germany. Because of the potential teratogenicity of pyrimethamine, sulfadiazine (which is highly effective in animal models when used alone) should be used alone if treatment is to be given in the first trimester of pregnancy. Spiramycin (not available in the United States) has also been used safely for treatment during the first trimester of pregnancy.

Because of the high probability of severe damage when infection occurs early in fetal life, therapeutic abortion has been recommended by some authorities. Because the risk of transmission of the infection to the fetus is low (approximately 15 per cent) in the first trimester and because the incidence of congenital toxoplasmosis can be reduced significantly by interpartum therapy, other authorities recommend treatment rather than abortion, reasoning that this would result in saving a significant number of healthy fetuses. The decision about mode of therapy ultimately must be made with the well-informed pregnant patient who is aware of the risks discussed above. There are no carefully controlled studies to support the contention that a pregnant woman who has *Toxoplasma* antibody and a history of habitual abortion will benefit from treatment. We suggest that pregnant women who have depressed cell-mediated immunity (e.g., a pregnant woman with systemic lupus erythematosis who is receiving corticosteroids) and with serologic or other clinical evidence of Toxoplasma infection receive anti-Toxoplasmic therapy in an attempt to prevent transmission to the fetus, whether the infection is acutely acquired or chronic.

Both symptomatic and asymptomatic infants with congenital toxoplasmosis should be treated in an effort to prevent further destruction of vital organs. Guidelines for treatment of congenitally infected infants in whom the diagnosis is strongly suspected are outlined in Table 3. The guidelines are those of Dr. Jacques Couvreur, who has treated over 100 cases of congenital toxoplasmosis using this regimen. Recent data from Europe and the United States suggest that early institution of specific treatment in these infants may prevent some sequelae.

Therapeutic Agents

Pyrimethamine Plus Sulfadiazine or Trisulfapyrimidines. Pyrimethamine and sulfadiazine act synergistically against *Toxoplasma* in vivo with a combined activity that is eight times the amount expected if their effects were merely additive. There are no reports of controlled clinical trials in which adult humans with severe symptomatic toxoplasmosis were treated with this combination; nevertheless, clinical experience confirms their efficacy. There is evidence that treatment of an acutely infected pregnant woman may prevent infection of her fetus (see above under Therapy in Specific Clinical Settings). The simultaneous use of both drugs is indicated except during the first trimester of pregnancy. Comparative tests have shown that sulfapyrazine, sulfamethazine, and sulfamerazine are about as effective as sulfadiazine. All the other sulfonamides tested (sulfathiazole, sulfapyridine, sulfadimetine, and sulfisoxazole) are much less effective.

Pyrimethamine. In adults, a loading dose of 100 to 200 mg pyrimethamine should be given orally in two divided doses on the first day of treatment. In young children, a loading dose of 2 mg/kg body weight should be given for the first two to three days of treatment. Infants are given 1 mg/kg body weight as a loading dose. A maintenance dose for all ages is 1 mg/kg body weight (with a maximum of 25 mg) in one dose. Administration of the maintenance dose at three- to four-day intervals has been suggested in view of the drug's half-life of four to five days. Since there are no data concerning absorption of the drug in the patient who is very ill, daily administration is recommended. Daily therapy is recommended for active ocular infection. Pyrimethamine is available only in tablet form. For infants, this may be crushed and administered with food or fluid.

Table 3. GUIDELINES FOR THERAPY OF CONGENITAL TOXOPLASMOSIS*

Drugs

1. *Pyrimethamine + sulfadiazine or trisulfapyrimidines:* 21-day course.
   a. Pyrimethamine: 1 mg/kg by the oral route every two to three or even four days (since the half-life of pyrimethamine is four to five days).
   b. Sulfadiazine: 50 to 100 mg/kg/day by the oral route in two daily divided doses.
2. *Spiramycin*[a]*:* 30- to 45-day course. 100 mg/kg/day by the oral route in two daily divided doses.
3. *Corticosteroids* (prednisone or methylprednisolone): 1 to 2 mg/kg/day by the oral route in two divided doses. Continued until the inflammatory process (e.g., high cerebrospinal fluid protein, chorioretinitis) has subsided; dosage then to be tapered progressively to nil.
4. *Folinic acid:* 5 mg twice weekly during pyrimethamine treatment.

Indications

1. *Overt congenital toxoplasmosis:* Pyrimethamine + sulfadiazine + folinic acid; 21 days. During the first year of life, the child is given three to four courses of pyrimethamine + sulfadiazine, separated with spiramycin courses of 30 to 45 days.[a] No treatment is usually given after 12 months of age.
2. *Overt congenital toxoplasmosis with evidence of inflammatory process* (chorioretinitis, high cerebrospinal fluid protein content, generalized infection, jaundice): As in (1) above + corticosteroid treatment.
3. *Subclinical congenital toxoplasmosis:* As in (1) above.
4. *Healthy newborn in whom serologic testing has not provided definitive results but maternal infection was acquired during pregnancy:* One course of pyrimethamine + sulfadiazine for 21 days, followed by spiramycin. Then wait for laboratory evidence for diagnosis.

[a]If spiramycin is not available, we recommend continued use of the pyrimethamine-sulfonamide combination for the total period of therapy.

*Courtesy of Dr. Jacques Couvreur, Laboratoire de Sérologie Néonatale et de Recherche sur la Toxoplasmose, Institut de Puériculture, Paris.

Adapted from Remington and Desmonts, 1976.

Pyrimethamine is a folic acid antagonist and therefore produces a dose-related, reversible, and usually gradual depression of the bone marrow. Thrombocytopenia, leukopenia, and anemia may occur. All patients treated with pyrimethamine should have platelet and peripheral blood cell counts twice weekly.

Folinic acid (calcium leucovorin) or Baker's yeast should be administered with pyrimethamine to prevent suppression of the bone marrow. The optimal frequency for administration of folinic acid is unknown. An oral dose of 5 to 10 mg is recommended daily in older children and adults, or 5 mg twice weekly in infants. Bakers' yeast (three to four cakes daily) may be used if folinic acid is not available. Unlike folic acid, neither folinic acid nor Bakers' yeast inhibits the action of pyrimethamine on *T. gondii.*

Sulfadiazine or Trisulfapyrimidines. Sulfadiazine or trisulfapyrimidine is administered to older children and adults, in a loading dose of 50 to 75 mg/kg body weight; thereafter, a daily dose of 75 to 100 mg/kg body weight is administered in four divided doses every six hours. In infants, the loading dose is 50 to 100 mg/kg body weight; thereafter, a total daily dose of 100 to 150 mg/kg is administered in two or four divided doses every six hours.

Tablet and liquid oral forms and intravenous forms are available.

The potential toxic effects of sulfonamides (e.g., crystalluria, hematuria, and rash) must be carefully monitored. Hypersensitivity reactions to sulfonamides may be a particular problem in patients with AIDS.

Other Drugs. Trimethoprim alone or with a sulfonamide has not been proved effective in humans, but the activity of this combination in vitro and in vivo in animal models warrants carefully controlled clinical trials. This combination is significantly less active than is the combination of pyrimethamine with sulfadiazine.

Duration of Therapy. The optimal duration of specific therapy of toxoplasmosis is unknown. Patients who appear to be immunologically normal but have severe and persistent symptoms or damage to vital organs (e.g., chorioretinitis, myocarditis) require specific therapy for at least four to six weeks, or possibly longer.

In the immunocompromised patient, therapy should continue for at least four to six weeks *beyond* complete resolution of all signs and symptoms of active disease. Careful follow-up of these patients is imperative because relapse may occur, requiring prompt reinstitution of therapy. Relapse is frequent in patients with AIDS. There are no data as to whether prolonged prophylaxis should be used. Although therapy may be effective against *T. gondii* trophozoites and may induce a beneficial response clinically, it does not eradicate the cyst form from the CNS and perhaps not from other tissues.

Desmonts and Couvreur treated the acutely infected pregnant woman with 2 to 3 grams spiramycin daily, administered orally in four divided doses, intermittently from the time of diagnosis until term. A three-week course of treatment was alternated with a two-week interval without treatment. Kraubig et al. in Germany gave a course of sulfonamide and pyrimethamine followed by one to two courses of sulfonamide administered alone or in combination with pyrimethamine. Each course was given for approximately two weeks. The courses of treatment were alternated with three- to four-week intervals without treatment. Pyrimethamine was not given in the first trimester of pregnancy.

Infants with congenital toxoplasmosis should be treated as outlined in Table 3.

PROPHYLAXIS. Prophylaxis against *Toxoplasma* involves intervention in the cycle of transmission. Prevention of infection by *T. gondii* is most important in immunodeficient patients and seronegative pregnant women.

Meat should be heated to 60° C to kill cysts. Freezing to −20° C will kill cysts in meat, but commercial freezers in most areas of the world do not reach or maintain this temperature reliably. Hands should be washed after touching uncooked meat. Fruits and vegetables may be contaminated with oocysts and should be washed. Contact with cat feces should be avoided.

Although there are no definitive data on the risks of using seropositive donors, the following are our recommendations: Blood or blood products donated by people with *Toxoplasma* antibody should not be used in immunosuppressed recipients, and organs of those with *Toxoplasma* antibody should not be given to seronegative recipients.

A nontoxic drug that eliminates the organism in the tissue cyst form as well as in the trophozoite form is needed to prevent the devastating complications of recrudescent infection in immunocompromised patients.

For prevention of transmission of *Toxoplasma* to the fetus, see Therapy in Specific Clinical Settings.

There is no effective vaccine to prevent infection with *Toxoplasma*. Because maternal immunity appears to prevent congenital transmission of *T. gondii*, development of a vaccine for use in nonimmune women of childbearing age should be explored. Vaccines that prevent oocyst development in household cats could interrupt the life cycle of *T. gondii*.

References

Araujo, F. G., and Remington, J. S.: Antigenemia in recently acquired acute Toxoplasmosis. J Infect Dis 141:144, 1980.

Conley, F. K., and Remington, J. S.: *Toxoplasma gondii* infection of the central nervous system. Use of the PAP method to demonstrate *Toxoplasma* in formalin-fixed parafin-embedded tissue sections. Hum Pathol 12:690, 1981.

Desmonts, G.: Serodiagnostic de la toxoplasmose. Intérêt et limites des différentes méthodes. Leur application au diagnostic de la toxoplasmose acquise. Feuillets de Biologie 6:61, 1975.

Desmonts, G., and Remington, J. S.: Direct agglutination test for diagnosis of Toxoplasma infection: method for increasing sensitivity and specificity. J Clin Microbiol 11:562, 1980.

Dorfman, R. F., and Remington, J. S.: Value of lymph node biopsy in the diagnosis of acute acquired toxoplasmosis. N Engl J Med 289:878, 1973.

Dubey, J. P., Miller, N. L., and Frenkel, J. K.: Characterization of the new fecal form of *Toxoplasma gondii*. J Parasitol 56:447, 1970.

Dubey, J. P., Swan, G. V., and Frenkel, J, K.: A simplified method for isolation of *Toxoplasma gondii* from the feces of cats. J Parasitol 58:1005, 1972.

Feldman, H. A.: Toxoplasmosis. N Engl J Med 279:1370 and 1431, 1968.

Frenkel, J. K., and Ruiz, A.: Endemicity of Toxoplasmosis in Costa Rica. Amer J Epidemiol 113:254, 1981.

Ghatak, N. R., Poon, T. P., and Zimmerman, H. M.: Toxoplasmosis of the central nervous system in the adult: A light and electron microscopic study of three cases. Arch Pathol 89:337, 1970.

Luft, B. J., Conley, F., and Remington, J. R.: Outbreak of central nervous system Toxoplasmosis in Western Europe and North America. Lancet Apr. 9, 1983.

Luft, B. J., Naot, Y., Araujo, F. G., Stinson, E. B., and Remington, J. S.: Primary and reactivated toxoplasma infection in patients with cardiac transplants. Ann Intern Med 99:27, 1983.

Naot, Y., and Remington, J. S.: An enzyme-linked immunosorbent assay for detection of IgM antibodies to *Toxoplasma gondii*: Use for diagnosis of acute acquired toxoplasmosis. J Infect Dis 142:757, 1980.

O'Connor, G. R.: Ocular toxoplasmosis. In Locatcher-Khorazo, D., and Seegal, B. C. (eds.): Microbiology of the Eye. St. Louis, The C. V. Mosby Company, 1972, p. 199.

O'Connor, G. R.: Manifestations and management of ocular toxoplasmosis. Bull NY Acad Med 50:192, 1974.

Remington, J. S., and Desmonts, G.: Toxoplasmosis. *In* Remington, J. S., and Klein, J. O. (eds.): Infectious Diseases of the Fetus and Newborn Infant. Philadelphia, W. B. Saunders Company, 1983, p. 143.

Ruskin, J., and Remington, J. S.: Toxoplasmosis in the compromised host. Ann Intern Med 84:193, 1976.

Siegel, J. P., and Remington, J. S.: Comparison of methods for quantitating antigen-specific immunoglobulin M antibody with a reverse enzyme-linked immunosorbent assay. J Clin Microbiol 18:63, 1983.

Siim, J. C.: Acquired toxoplasmosis. JAMA 147:1641, 1951.

Townsend, J. J. et al: Acquired toxoplasmosis. Arch Neurol 32:335, 1975.

Wilson, C. B., Remington, J. S., Stagno, S., and Reynolds, D. W.: Development of adverse sequelae in children born with subclinical congenital toxoplasma infection. Pediatrics 66:767, 1980.

263
TRICHINELLOSIS

Z. S. Pawlowski, M.D.

Trichinellosis (trichinosis) is a zoonotic infection caused by *Trichinella spiralis*. Symptomatic infections have an acute allergic phase and a protracted phase with muscle inflammation and degeneration, metabolic disorders, and restoration of damaged muscle tissue. Trichinellosis may be fatal when it is not diagnosed and treated properly (Gould, 1970; Campbell, 1982).

ETIOLOGY. Man may ingest infectious larvae of *T. spiralis* in the incompletely cooked meat of many domestic or wild animals. The most common source of trichinellosis is infected pork; less common sources (Fig. 1) include the meat of wild animals—e.g., polar bear (Alaska, Siberia); wild boar (Europe, Hawaii); brown or black bear (Canada); bush pig or warthog (Africa) and the domesticated dog (Alaska, Indonesia) and horse (Italy) (Pawlowski, 1980).

Within three days, the ingested larvae become adult worms and penetrate into the mucosa of the small intestine. As early as the fifth day after infection, the first newborn *T. spiralis* larvae are produced by fertilized female worms (Fig. 2) (Gould et al., 1963). After migration through lymphatics and blood vessels, the larvae invade the fibers of striated muscles. A few may reach the myocardium or internal organs, but they develop and encyst only in skeletal muscle. Encapsulation of coiled larvae takes a minimum of 17 days after they enter the muscle fibers. One female worm produces about 1500 larvae. In intensive infections more than 1000 larvae may be present per g of human deltoid muscle. Encysted larvae are gradually destroyed by the host and become calcified after six to eight years.

The life cycle is identical in man, hog, rat, and other infected animals. Traditionally, hogs have acquired trichinellosis from uncooked garbage containing infected pork-scraps. Rats can also be infected by uncooked garbage and serve as another source of infection for domestic or wild hogs. With the exceptions of Australasia, the Pacific islands other than Hawaii, China, and Japan, trichinellosis is endemic throughout the temperate regions of the world wherever pork is eaten. Cooking garbage before it is fed to hogs, meat inspection, and public education have greatly reduced the prevalence of trichinellosis in Europe and the United States (Fig. 3) (Zimmerman et al., 1973).

PATHOGENESIS AND PATHOLOGY. Adult worms provoke a mononuclear cellular infiltration of the small intestinal mucosa. Intestinal infection rarely causes abdominal symptoms but plays an important role in stimulating immunologic processes. In an immune host, the life span of adult worms is much shorter, and females produce fewer larvae. When *T. spiralis* larvae invade the muscle, they disturb the ultrastructure and the metabolic process of muscle fiber, resulting in basophilic transformation (Fig. 4). A myositis follows, characterized by muscle fiber damage, cellular infiltration, fibrous tissue production, and finally destruction of muscle fibers and encapsulation of larvae. In the months and years that follow, the encapsulated larvae gradually die, provoking an intense granulomatous reaction or foreign body cellular response that ends in a fibrotic scar or calcification. This process may be responsible for prolonged muscular symptoms.

In early trichinellosis the most severe symptoms are caused by hypersensitivity and inflammatory reactions. Small vessel vasculitis is characterized by hemorrhagic conjunctivitis, splinter hemorrhages under the fingernails

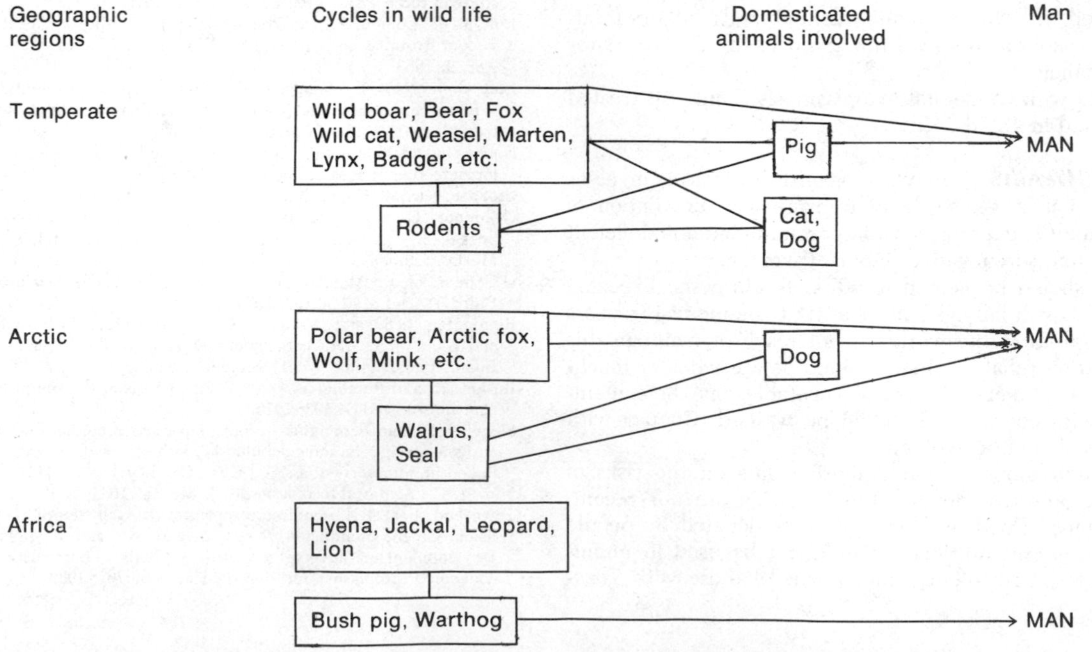

Figure 1. Transmission of trichinellosis to man in different geographic regions.

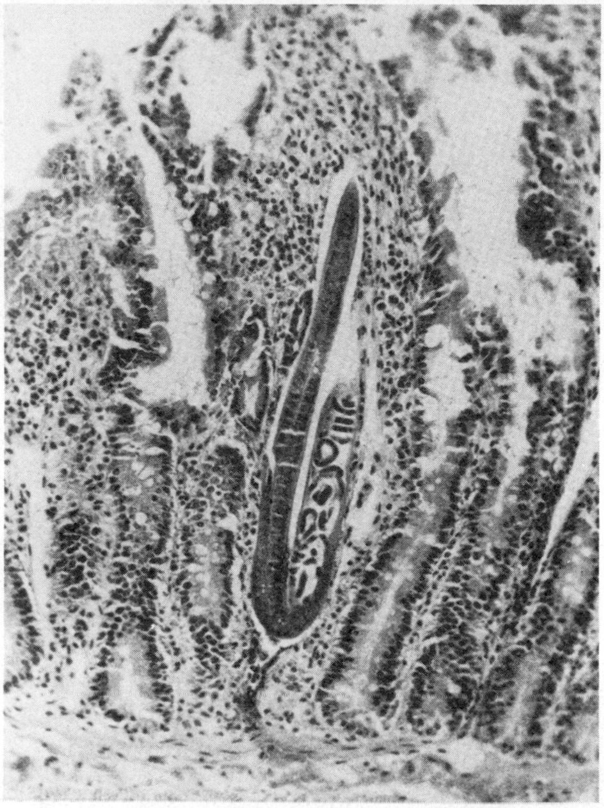

Figure 2. Gravid adult female *Trichina* embedded in a villus of the small intestine. Note second generation filariform larvae within the uterus in the right portion of the segment. × 120 (From Gould, S. E., Hinerman, E. L., Batsakis, J. G., and Beamer, P. R.: Am J Clin Pathol 40:197, 1963.)

and periorbital edema. Fever and malaise are thought to be due to absorption of toxic products of the larvae and to the development of hypersensitivity to these substances. Larvae may induce acute myocarditis, although encystment does not occur in the myocardium.

In the later stages of severe trichinellosis, metabolic disorders characterized by hypoalbuminemia and hypopotassemia secondary to muscle tissue damage may dominate the clinical picture. Muscle contractures and atrophy may follow untreated severe trichinellosis.

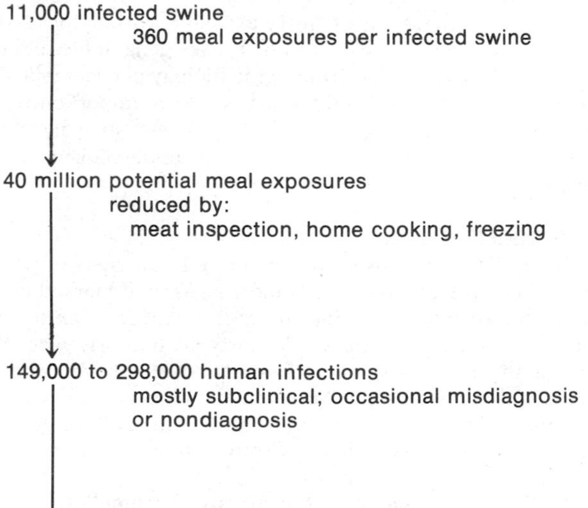

Figure 3. Estimate of transmission rate of trichinellosis in the United States (Zimmerman et al., 1973).

At any stage of trichinellosis, unexpected complications may occur owing to hypersensitivity or migration of *T. spiralis* larvae into tissues other than muscle.

CLINICAL MANIFESTATIONS. Trichinellosis is frequently asymptomatic (Fig. 3) when the intensity of infection is less than 1 larva per g of deltoid muscle tissue. On the other hand, the frequency and severity of allergic reactions may be out of proportion to the size of the inoculum. The incubation period is between 5 and 46 days, but in intensive infections it may be shorter (5 to 10 days). During the incubation period, abdominal pain, diarrhea, and nausea may occur but are uncommon (12 per cent). The disease usually begins with allergic manifestations characterized by fever, malaise, myalgia, periorbital edema, and eosinophilia. Fever is usually over 38° C and may be remittent for one to three weeks. Malaise is often severe and persists longer than fever. Myalgia, which is particularly severe in the ocular, brachial, and crural muscles, may continue for months. Some muscles are painful when examined or used. Periorbital edema is present in 86 per cent of patients and is often complicated by subconjunctival and subungual hemorrhages; all these signs disappear within one to two weeks.

Eosinophilia, which is usually greater than 20 per cent and may be greater than 50 per cent, frequently persists for several months and is often the only sign of trichinellosis. In very serious cases, the number of eosinophils may be low. The blood leukocyte count is usually greater than

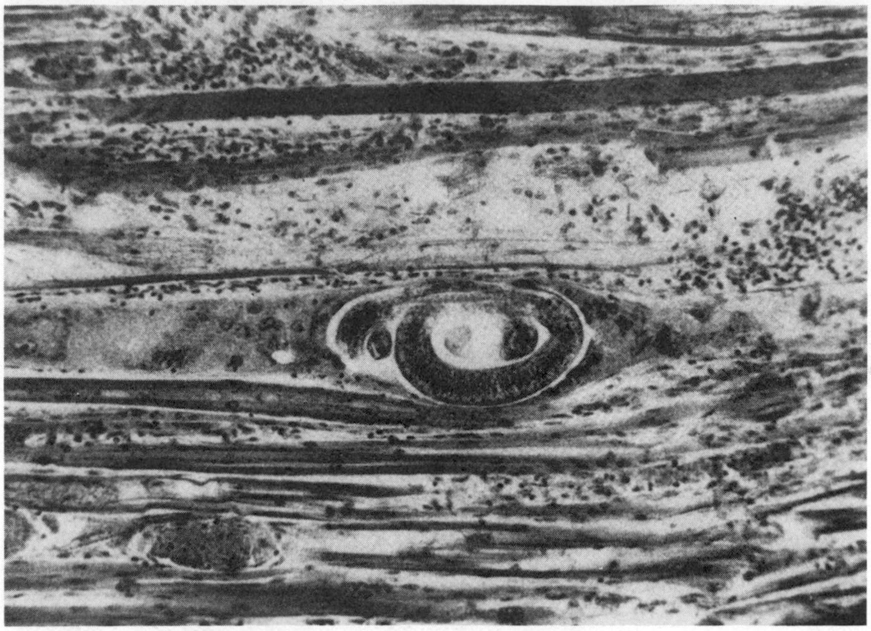

Figure 4. Encysted *Trichina* larva in human skeletal muscle fiber four weeks after infection. The fiber has undergone basophilic transformation, and the muscle nuclei seem to be increased in number. The cyst wall has not yet formed. Note the degeneration of adjacent fibers and infiltration of histiocytes and leukocytes including eosinophils. × 125. (From Gould, S. E., Hinerman, E. L., Batsakis, J. G., and Beamer, P. R.: Am J Clin Pathol 40:197, 1963.)

10,000/mm^3. The first chemical evidence of a muscle disorder is elevation of the serum creatine phosphokinase (CPK) and the serum transaminase levels that may be observed by the second week of the disease. By the third week, hypoalbuminemia may occur with concentrations of as low as 2.5 gm/100 ml. Despite hypergammaglobulinemia, the total serum protein level may be quite low. Severe hypoalbuminemia causes hydrostatic edema, mainly of the back and lower extremities. Hypopotassemia usually accompanies hypoalbuminemia and may cause cardiac disorders in the later stages of trichinellosis. Recovery from these metabolic disorders may take as long as two to four months in patients with untreated severe disease. Muscle atrophy and contractures may also occur.

The course of trichinellosis may be asymptomatic with mild eosinophilia only; abortive with myalgia only; mild with moderate fever and typical symptoms that disappear within three weeks; moderate with high fever and metabolic disorders; or severe with high fever, severe metabolic disorders and cardiac, pulmonary, or cerebral complications.

COMPLICATIONS AND SEQUELAE. Hypersensitivity reactions, intense cardiac involvement, and adrenal cortical insufficiency are responsible for the early deaths in fulminating trichinellosis. Deaths that occur between the third and fifth weeks of disease are usually due to cardiac, pulmonary, or cerebral complications.

In early trichinellosis, myocardial inflammation causes decreased cardiac contractability and conduction disorders. Later in the disease, hypoalbuminemia and hypopotassemia further impair cardiac function. Pneumonitis, bronchitis, and Loeffler's syndrome are unusual complications of early trichinellosis, but secondary bacterial pneumonia is common after the third week of severe disease. Meningitis, encephalopathy, and focal neurologic impairment are rare complications that occur only during the larval migratory phase of severe trichinellosis.

Recovery can be slow. Myalgia, inflammation around encapsulated larvae, and impaired electromyography may last for years after the infection. The symptoms and signs of muscular involvement during severe untreated trichinellosis usually disappear within one to three years. Contractures and atrophy are very rare. Permanent impairment of the eye, central nervous system, heart, or lung can be caused by ectopic localization of larvae but is rare.

GEOGRAPHIC VARIATIONS. In the last two decades, two new strains of *T. spiralis* have been found: *T. spiralis nativa* in the Arctic and *T. spiralis nelsoni* in Africa south of the Sahara. Both strains are less infective for man than classic *T. spiralis*, but the Arctic strain seems to be more immunogenic, more pathogenic, and less sensitive to corticosteroid therapy; the African strain seems to be much less pathogenic. A new species, *T. pseudospiralis*, has been found in wild animals in Asia but not in man. These larvae were less coiled and unencapsulated.

The different range of hosts available within the geographic distribution of *T. spiralis* causes geographic differences in the transmission and epidemiology of trichinellosis (Fig. 1). Infections of wild animals serve an important role as a reservoir and source of infection whenever man joins the natural cycle by eating the raw or undercooked meat of wild animals.

DIAGNOSIS. Fever, malaise, and myalgia are common in many infectious diseases, but the clinical signs of periorbital edema, conjunctival hemorrhages, and marked eosinophilia are more specific for trichinellosis. A group of people, such as a family or a party of hunters, who all ingest the same suspicious food and who present these signs and symptoms can be given the clinical diagnosis of trichinellosis. Food intoxication and acute gastroenteritis must be considered when gastrointestinal symptoms are present.

In the allergic phase of the disease, trichinellosis must be differentiated from typhoid, septicemia, and influenza on the one hand, and serum sickness, drug allergy, and collagen vascular diseases on the other. Trichinellosis is sometimes first diagnosed by an ophthalmologist when eye signs are prominent.

Elevated serum transaminase and creatine phosphoki-

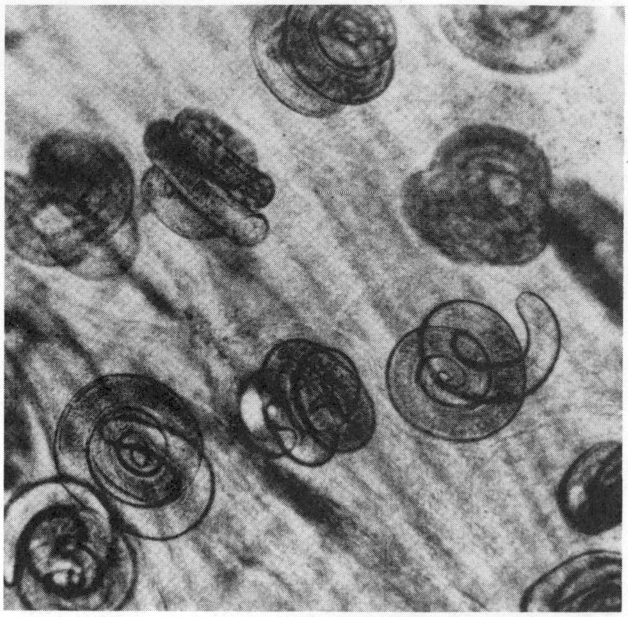

Figure 5. Encysted larvae in compressed, unstained skeletal muscle seen by stereoscopic microscopy (× 75). The cyst walls are transparent. (From Gould, S. E., Hinerman, E. L., Batsakis, J. G., and Beamer, P. R.: Am J Clin Pathol 40:197, 1963.)

nase levels are helpful in establishing the diagnosis. The intradermal skin test, which is read within 15 minutes and reflects immediate hypersensitivity, becomes positive three weeks after infection. If positive, it is helpful, but many false-negative reactions are reported. The most useful

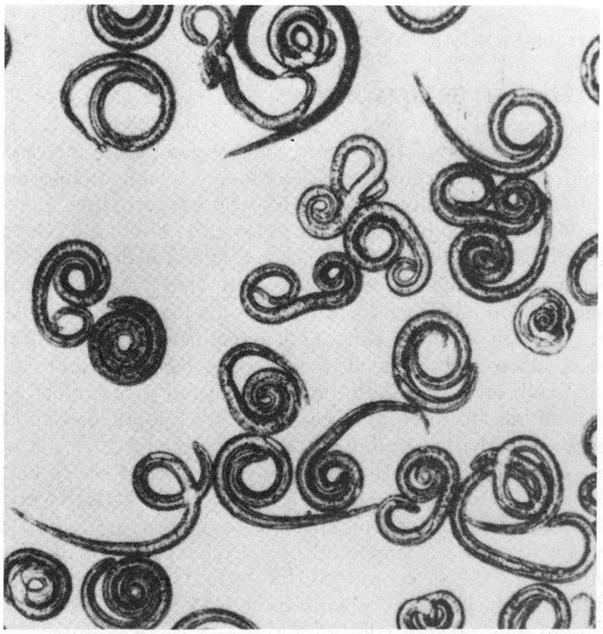

Figure 6. Larvae freed from cysts by digestion of ground muscle at 37° C in 1 per cent HCl and 1 per cent pepsin. The tightly coiled forms are motile. Elongated or partially uncoiled larvae are dead or dying. × 40 (From Gould, S. E., Hinerman, E. L., Batsakis, J. G., and Beamer, P. R.: Am J Clin Pathol 40:197, 1963.)

specific serologic tests for trichinellosis are bentonite flocculation (the bentonite is treated with an extract of muscle larvae) and counterimmunoelectrophoresis of the patient's serum against larval extracts. These tests also become positive three weeks after infection. The indirect fluorescent antibody test becomes positive earlier but is less widely available.

Definitive diagnosis is made by finding *Trichinella* larvae in muscle biopsies or by finding adult worms in the gastrointestinal mucosa at autopsy if early death occurs. The deltoid, biceps, and gastrocnemius muscles yield the highest number of positive biopsies. Part of the biopsy section should be compressed between glass slides for direct microscopic examination (Fig. 5), part should be digested before examination (Fig. 6), and part should be fixed and sectioned for staining (Fig. 4).

TREATMENT. Ethanol may help prevent infection if it is drunk concurrently or a few hours after ingestion of infected meat. Gastric lavage also has some prophylactic value. Saline purgatives and anthelmintics (thiabendazole at daily dose of 25 to 50 mg/kg for 5 days or mebendazole 200 mg per day for 5 days) may prevent the disease if taken a few days after ingestion of infected meat. Later on at any stage of the disease, tetramisole, pyrantel, or mebendazole should be taken to eliminate adult *T. spiralis* (Campbell and Blair, 1974).

In severe allergic trichinellosis, high doses of corticosteroids and circulatory support may save the lives of heavily infected patients. Smaller doses of corticosteroids readily alleviate the symptoms and signs of mild disease. In light or abortive cases, only antipyretics and analgesics are needed. When metabolic disorders dominate, replacement therapy with albumin and potassium may be necessary. Prompt institution of treatment and intensive rehabilitative care accelerate recovery from severe disease.

PROPHYLAXIS. The individual can protect himself from trichinellosis by cooking all meat thoroughly, especially pork, wild boar, or bear meat. Cooking until meat changes from pink to gray (65° C) provides a good margin of safety. Public health control measures include cooking garbage and offal fed to pigs, rodent control, meat inspection, deep-freezing carcasses or canned meat products for at least 36 hours at −30° C, and sanitary education of pigbreeders, hunters, butchers, and consumers.

References

Campbell, W. C. (ed.): Trichinella and Trichinosis. Plenum Press, New York, 1983.

Campbell, W. C., and Blair, L. S.: Chemotherapy of *Trichinella spiralis* infections: A review. Exp Parasitol 35:304, 1974.

Gould, S. E. (ed.): Trichinosis in Man and Animals. Springfield, Ill., Charles C Thomas, 1970.

Gould, S. E., Hinerman, E. L., Batsakis, J. G., and Beamer, P. R.: Diagnostic patterns: *Trichinella spiralis*. Am J Clin Pathol 40:197, 1963.

Kim, C. W. (ed.): Proceedings of the Third International Conference on Trichinellosis. New York, Intext Educational Publishers, 1974.

Kim, C. W. and Pawlowski, Z. (eds.): Proceedings of the Fourth International Conference on Trichinellosis. Warsaw, 1978.

Pawlowski, Z. S.: Control of Trichinellosis. In Proceedings of the Fifth International Conference on Trichinellosis. Noordwijk aan Zee, 1980.

Zimmermann, W. J., Steele, J. H., and Kagan, I. G.: Trichiniasis in the U. S. population, 1966–1970. Prevalence and epidemiologic factors. Health Services Rep 88:606, 1973.

264

VISCERAL LARVA MIGRANS

CAROLYN COKER HUNTLEY, M.D.

Visceral larva migrans (VLM) is a clinical syndrome characterized by eosinophilia and evidence of visceral involvement caused by the larval migratory phase of roundworms indigenous to lower animal species. A similar disease may also occur during the larval migratory phases of *Ascaris lumbricoides*, *Ancylostoma duodenale*, *Necator americanus*, and *Strongyloides stercoralis*, roundworms whose definitive host is man.

ETIOLOGY. *Toxocara canis*, the common roundworm of dogs, has most often been incriminated as the cause of VLM, and the syndrome has become synonymous with *T. canis* infection in the minds of many physicians. Other animal roundworms can, however, cause an illness indistinguishable from *T. canis* infection. These helminths include *Toxocara cati; Ascaris suum*, the pig roundworm; *Capillaria hepatica*, a rat liver parasite requiring another rat or cat as the intermediate host; and *Dirofilaria immitis*, the dog heart worm that is considered to be the most common cause of tropical eosinophilia in the western hemisphere. The role of *T. cati* in VLM is unknown because of the difficulty of distinguishing this parasite from *T. canis* in tissue sections. *Toxascaris leonina* has been suspected as the cause of VLM in northern Canada (Unruh et al., 1973) because of the prevalence of this parasite and the absence of *T. canis* in the dog population of this area.

T. canis is an almost universal infection of puppies owing to transplacental passage of larvae. Ova are found in the stools of the pup by 3 weeks of age. After a period of embryonation in the soil at appropriate conditions of temperature and moisture, ova become infective and may remain viable for years. Dogs are most heavily infected between the ages of 3 weeks and 6 months, after which the worms are often discharged spontaneously. Human beings become infected by ingesting infective ova in soil. The ova are very sticky and cling to the hair of animals and fomites so that transmission can occur without direct contact with contaminated soil.

A. suum, the common roundworm of pigs, may infect farmers who are exposed to infected pigs (Phills et al., 1972). The mode of infection is the same as that for *T. canis*.

C. hepatica, a rat liver parasite, requires a second host (a rat or cat) before becoming infective for man. The intermediate host eats the infected rat and, without acquiring the infection, excretes noninfective ova in the feces. These ova mature in the soil and become infectious for man. The rarity of this infection in man is difficult to understand considering the high prevalence of *C. hepatica* infection in rats.

PATHOGENESIS AND PATHOLOGY. After embryonated ova are ingested, secondstage larvae of *T. canis* are released from the ova in the small bowel. The second stage larvae penetrate the bowel and migrate via the lymphatics and venules to the portal system (Sprent, 1958). *T. canis* larvae do not mature past the second stage in man and therefore remain small. Their average length is 320 μm and their maximum diameter 14 to 20 μm. In primary infections the larvae migrate from the portal system to the lung and from there throughout the body, including the spinal cord and brain. Studies of experimental toxocariasis in mice, which are good models of human disease, show that migration of larvae through the liver of immune mice is slowed and that most larvae remain in the liver. Very large livers are found in children who have been repeatedly infected with *T. canis*.

The microscopic pathology varies with the location of the parasite. Eosinophilic granulomas predominate in the lungs and liver in the early stages of the disease, but intact larvae may be difficult to find in biopsy specimens. Mature granulomas contain a predominance of macrophages, epitheliod cells, and giant cells, rather than eosinophils. The larvae may escape from the granuloma and be found some distance from the site of the original inflammatory reaction. There is little tissue reaction in the central nervous system except for hemorrhagic tracts along the path of larval migration.

The second-stage larvae of *A. suum* also migrate to the liver and lung, where they elicit marked eosinophilic and granulomatous reactions. In the lung they mature to third- and fourth-stage larvae and do not migrate into the systemic circulation, presumably because of their larger size. Although larvae can be found in sputum and are swallowed, they rarely mature to adult worms in the human gastrointestinal tract.

Unlike the other helminths that cause VLM, *C. hepatica* develops into the adult form in the liver (Cochrane et al., 1957). After penetration of the bowel, larvae of *C. hepatica* migrate directly to the liver, where they mature, mate, and produce large numbers of ova. In autopsied cases the liver is massively enlarged with an intense inflammatory reaction consisting of many eosinophils and giant cells surrounding both the adult worms and the ova.

CLINICAL MANIFESTATIONS. The clinical picture of *T. canis* infection depends on the size of the infecting dose. Massive infections that cause the visceral larva migrans syndrome are acquired most commonly by small children between the ages of 1 to 4 years who eat dirt. Boys have VLM more often than girls in a ratio of 2:1. Minor infections are probably much more common than we realize and can occur at any age in individuals who have contact with infected soil and have hand-to-mouth habits such as smoking or nail biting. Minor infections are of no clinical importance unless one of the *T. canis* larvae migrates to the eye (Fig. 1). It is also possible that one or more larvae that migrate to the brain may set up an epileptic focus and lead to idiopathic epilepsy (Glickman et al., 1979). Eye involvement is seen in children older than 4 years and occasionally in adults. There are three basic types of eye lesions: (1) central granulomas, (2) peripheral granulomas, which may be accompanied by elevated retinal folds extending to the disk, and (3) diffuse endophthalmitis with retinal detachment (Wilkinson and Welch, 1971). The patient may present with a blind eye or the lesion may be seen on routine ophthalmoscopic examination. It is not known whether the larva migrates to the eye at the time of initial infection or whether it migrates to the eye from another organ, months or years after the primary infection. It is known that larvae may remain alive in nonhuman

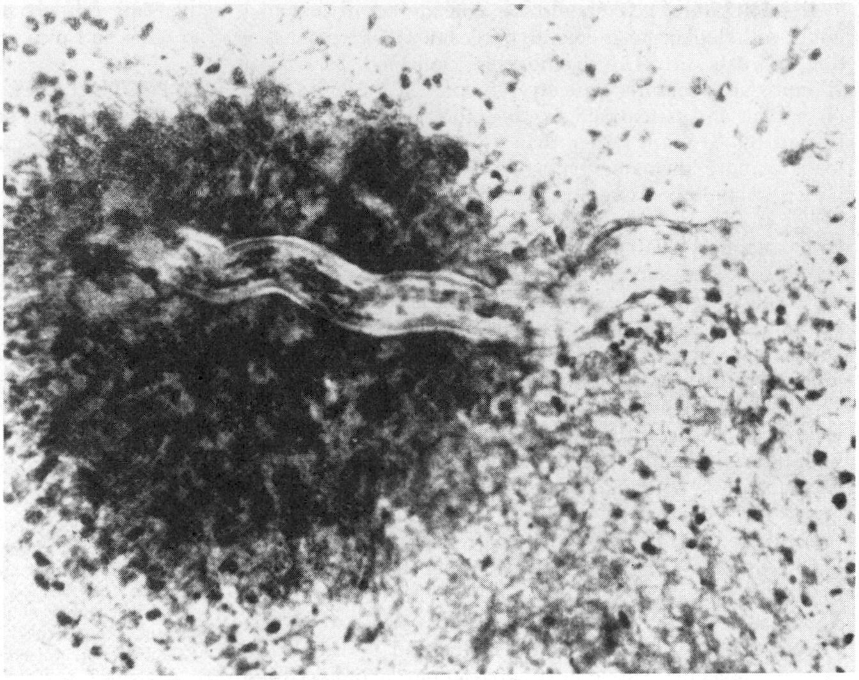

Figure 1. Ocular VLM. Nematode larva in eosinophilic abscess of vitreous membrane × 400. (From Wilder, H. C.: Trans Am Acad Ophthalmol Otolaryngol 55:99, 1950.)

primate hosts for many years following a single infection, but the disease is usually benign and self-limited.

Typical VLM caused by massive infection with *T. canis* is most often characterized by fever, pulmonary symptoms, including cough and/or wheezing, rales, and hepatomegaly (Huntley et al., 1965). A history of pica is usually elicited, and other conditions associated with pica, such as lead poisoning or hydrocarbon ingestion, may coexist. Less common symptoms and signs include abdominal pain, vomiting, papular skin lesions, lymphadenopathy, and muscle pain. Central nervous system symptoms occur in 15 to 20 per cent of the patients and include seizures (Huntley et al., 1965), ataxia, coma, hemiparesis (Anderson et al., 1975), and Guillain-Barré syndrome (Phillips et al., 1969). Fatalities have occurred as a result of myocarditis (Becroft, 1964), a bronchiolitis-like syndrome, and encephalitis (Mikhael et al., 1974).

The marked eosinophilia usually associated with this disease (Beaver et al., 1952) may be discovered accidentally or in association with fever, cough, and wheezing. There is no absolute eosinophil count above which the disease should be considered, since the daily count varies widely in known cases, but spectacularly high counts can be seen with a leukocytosis of above 100,000 and 80 to 90 per cent eosinophils. The eosinophilia of experimental murine toxocariasis is dependent upon intact T lymphocyte function (Kayes and Oaks, 1980). Liver function tests, even in patients with massive hepatomegaly, are only slightly or transiently abnormal. Serum immunoglobulin concentrations are abnormal in most cases. IgE is markedly elevated (Huntley, 1976). IgG and IgM are moderately elevated, but IgA is usually normal. The immunoelectrophoretic pattern is one of a polyclonal hypergammopathy. Antibodies to group A and B human erythrocytes are often of the IgG type, and titers of such antibodies may be extremely high (Huntley et al., 1969). It has been suggested that *T. canis* infection of pregnant women in tropical countries may contribute to the increased incidence of ABO hemolytic disease of newborns in these areas (Huntley et al., 1976). Antibodics to human IgG as determined by the latex agglutination test (rheumatoid factors) are present in half of the cases (Huntley et al., 1966). Antinuclear antibodies are not present, but serum precipitins to proteins of cow's milk are present in 20 per cent of the patients, usually those with iron deficiency anemia. Chest radiographs may be normal, or the lungs may be hyperinflated with or without fluffy infiltrates.

COMPLICATIONS AND SEQUELAE. Ocular *T. canis* infection may be asymptomatic or may lead to a blind eye as the result of retinal detachment. Unnecessary enucleation has been carried out in some cases because of the similarity of this lesion to retinoblastoma. Eye lesions may occur during the acute phase of the disease or as a late complication.

As a generalized *T. canis* infection, VLM is rarely fatal and is usually self-limited. Theoretically, recurrent infections could cause liver failure, but this has not been reported. Persistent myoclonic seizures have killed at least one patient. Serum antibodies to *T. canis* have been reported to be encountered more frequently in children with seizures than in normal children.

Massive *A. suum* infection can lead to respiratory failure, and *C. hepatica* infection to liver failure.

GEOGRAPHIC VARIATIONS IN DISEASE. VLM is a worldwide disease that occurs primarily in tropical and temperate areas. Twenty-four per cent of 800 soil samples from public places in Britain contained viable ova of *T. canis* (Seah et al., 1975). Infections have been reported from all parts of the United States, Canada, Australia, and Great Britain, but the disease is more prevalent in tropical countries where hygienic conditions are poor and dogs are numerous.

DIAGNOSIS. VLM should be considered in a young child with leukocytosis and hypereosinophilia who has a dog and eats dirt. The diagnosis is confirmed if larvae of *T. canis* are identified in a liver biopsy. If the child lives on a farm and is exposed to pigs, the syndrome may be caused by *A. suum* rather than *T. canis*. Since pica may lead to more than one type of parasitic infection, these patients should be examined for other intestinal helminths. *Strongyloides stercoralis* may cause massive eosinophilia and visceral involvement in the elderly and the immunosuppressed and should be considered in these patients, especially if gastrointestinal symptoms are prominent. If routine stool examination is negative for *Strongyloides*, larvae may be seen by direct examination of liquid stools following catharsis. Flotation techniques are ineffective.

Serologic diagnosis has been hampered because of the lack of a specific antigen that does not cross-react either with other helminth antigens, human A and B blood group substances, or Forssman antigen. Larval antigens or whole larvae of *T. canis* have been utilized in immunoprecipitation, tanned cell hemagglutination, enzyme-linked immunosorbent assays (ELISA), and fluorescent antibody techniques (Cypess et al., 1977; Glickman et al., 1978). Secretory-excretory antigens also offer promise for the development of a reliable test (Savigny and Tizard, 1977). A macromolecular antigen extracted in our laboratory from adult *A. suum* worms precipitates the serum from rabbits infected with *T. canis*. It does not precipitate the serum of rabbits infected with *A. suum* nor cross-react with Forssman antigen or A and B blood group substances. The preparation of this antigen, which may be identical to an important *T. canis* larval antigen, does not require working with the infective stage of the worm. Of 50 patients with LVM, 45 had elevated serum titers (>1:160) against this antigen by the ELISA technique. Patients with ocular toxocariasis were identified less frequently (13 of 45), but antibodies were found in the aqueous fluids from 4 of 5 infected eyes and 0 to 11 control fluids obtained at the time of cataract surgery (Huntley, in preparation). In vitro lymphocyte proliferative responses have also been useful in the immunodiagnosis of *T. canis* and other nematode infections (Welch and Dobson, 1981).

TREATMENT. There is no proven effective treatment for *T. canis* infections of humans. Diethylcarbamazine (Hetrazan) decreased the numbers of larvae recovered from whole carcasses of infected mice in several experiments (Dafalla, 1972; Pike 1960; Wiseman et al., 1971) but did not affect the numbers of *T. canis* larvae in the brains of mice in other experiments (Holt et al., 1981). Thiabendazole did not decrease the numbers of larvae in similar experiments Dafalla, 1972; Wiseman et al., 1971). The benzimidazole, fenbendazole, is a potent larvacidal agent for *T. canis* infections of mice. Unfortunately, this drug is impractical in larger animals because it is poorly absorbed (Nicolas and Stewart, 1979). If intestinal infection with *A. lumbricoides* is present in association with *T. canis* in humans, adult *Ascaris* should be eliminated from the gastrointestinal tract before the use of diethylcarbamazine. Diethylcarbamazine causes adult *Ascaris* to migrate, which can cause bowel perforation or obstruction of the intestine or common bile duct. Ocular infections with *T. canis* should be treated with anthelmintic agents cautiously and only in association with steroids. Steroids may be helpful in the treatment of *T. canis* endophthalmitis without other drugs. Severe respiratory symptoms, wheezing, and dyspnea must be treated like any other type of asthma. Iron deficiency should be treated and pica must be strictly prevented.

PROPHYLAXIS. It is not generally appreciated that *T. canis* infection is an increasing problem in the world today because of the burgeoning population of dogs, which are usually infected during the early months of life. The ova are very resistant to destruction, and families sometimes have to move to a new home if dirt-eating by children cannot be prevented. Proper disposal of canine feces combined with frequent worming of dogs during the first 6 months of life would reduce the prevalence of infected soil (Seah et al., 1975). As long as infected animals are allowed to roam free and contaminate the soil in areas frequented by children, the incidence of VLM and serious ocular infections with *T. canis* will continue to increase.

References

Anderson, D. C., Greenwood, R., Fishman, M., and Kagan, I. G.: Acute infantile hemiplegia with cerebrospinal fluid eosinophilic pleocytosis: An unusual case of visceral larva migrans. J Pediatr 86:247, 1975.

Beaver, P. C., Snyder, C. H., Carrera, G. M., Dent, J. H., and Lafferty, J. W.: Chronic eosinophilia due to visceral larva migrans; report of 3 cases. Pediatrics 9:7, 1952.

Becroft, D. M.: Infection by the dog roundworm *Toxocara canis* and fatal myocarditis. N Z Med J 63:729, 1964.

Cochrane, J. C., Sagorin, L., and Wilcocks, M. G.: *Capillaria hepatica* infection in man. S Afr Med J 31:751, 1957.

Cypess, R. H., Karol, M. H., Zidian, J. L., Glickman, L. T., and Gitlin, D.: Larva-specific antibodies in patients with visceral larva migrans. J Infect Dis 135(4):633, 1977.

Dafalla, A. A.: A study of the effect of diethylcarbamazine and thiabendazole on experimental *Toxocara canis* infection in mice. Am J Trop Med Hyg 75:158, 1972.

de Savigny, D. H., and Tizard, I. R.: Toxocaral larva migrans: The use of larval secretory antigens in hemagglutination and soluble antigen fluorescent antibody tests. Trans R Soc Trop Med Hyg 71(6):581, 1977.

Glickman, L., Schantz, P., Domeroske, R., and Cypess, R. H.: Evaluation of serodiagnostic tests for visceral larva migrans. Am J Trop Med Hyg 27(3):492, 1978.

Glickman, L. T., Cypess, R. H., Crumriné, P. K., and Gitlin, D. A.: Toxocara infection and epilepsy in children. J Pediatr 94:75, 1979.

Hogarth-Scott, R. S.: Visceral larva migrans—an immunofluorescent examination of rabbit and human sera for antibodies to the ES antigens of the second stage larvae of *Toxocara canis*, *Toxocara cati* and *Toxascaris leonina* (Nematoda). Immunology 10:217, 1966.

Holt, P. E., Clarkson, M. J., and Kerslake, M.: Anthelmintic tests on *Toxocara canis* infection in mice. Vet Rec 108:308, 1981.

Huntley, C. C.: Of worms and asthma, or Tullis revisited. N Eng J Med 294:1295, 1976.

Huntley, C. C., Costas, M. C., and Lyerly, A.: Visceral larva migrans syndrome: Clinical characteristics and immunologic studies in 51 patients. Pediatrics 36:523, 1965.

Huntley, C. C., Costas, M. C., Williams, R. C., Lyerly, A. D., and Watson, R. G.: Anti-gamma-globulin factors in visceral larva migrans. JAMA 197:552, 1966.

Huntley, C. C., Lyerly, A., and Patterson, M. V.: Isohemagglutinins in parasitic infections. JAMA 208:1145, 1969.

Huntley, C. C., et al.: ABO hemolytic disease in Puerto Rico and North Carolina. Pediatrics 57:875, 1976.

Kayes, S. G., and Oaks, J. A.: *Toxocara canis*: T lymphocyte function in murine visceral larva migrans and eosinophilia onset. Exp Parasitol 49:47, 1980.

Mikhael, N. Z., Montpetit, V. J. A., Orizaga, M., Rowsell, H. C., and Richard, M. T.: *Toxocara canis* infestation with encephalitis. Can J Neurol Sci 1:114, 1974.

Nicolas, W. L., and Stewart, A. C.: The action of benzimidazoles on the larval stage of *Toxocara canis* in the mouse. Ann Trop Med Parasitol 73:57, 1979.

Phillips, J. A., McLean, W. T., and Huntley, C. C.: Letter: Co-existing Guillain-Barré and visceral larva migrans syndromes. Pediatrics 44:142, 1969.

Phills, J. A., Harrold, A. J., Whiteman, G. V., and Perelmutter, L.: Pulmonary infiltrates, asthma and eosinophilia due to *Ascaris suum* infestation in man. N Engl J Med 286:965, 1972.

Pike, E. H.: Effect of diethylcarbamazine, oxophenarsine hydrochloride and

piperazine citrate on *Toxocara canis* larvae in mice. Exp Parasitol 9:223, 1960.
Seah, S. K., Hucal, G., and Law, C.: Dogs and intestinal parasites: A public health problem. Can Med Assoc J 112:1191, 1975.
Sprent, J. F. A.: Observations on the development of *Toxocara canis*. Parasitology 48:184, 1958.
Unruh, D. H. A., King, J. E., Eaton, R. D. P., and Allen, J. R.: Parasites of dogs from Indian settlements in Northwestern Canada: A survey of wide public health implications. Can J Comp Med 27:25, 1973.
Welch, J. S., and Dobson, C.: Immunodiagnosis of parasitic zoonoses: sensitivity and specificity of in vitro lymphocyte proliferative responsiveness using nematode antigens purified by affinity chromatography. Trans R Soc Trop Med Hyg 75:5, 1981.
Wilder, H. C.: Nematode endophthalmitis. Trans Am Acad Ophthalmol Otolaryngol 55:99, 1950.
Wilkinson, C. P., and Welch, R. B.: Intraocular *Toxocara*. Am J Ophthalmol 71:921, 1971.
Wiseman, R. A., Woodruff, A. W., and Pettitt, L. E.: The treatment of toxocaral infection: some experimental and clinical observations. Trans R Soc Trop Med Hyg 65:591, 1971.

265
LEPTOSPIROSIS

GEORGE A. EDWARDS, B.A., M.D.

Leptospirosis is a spirochetal disease of animals and man caused by pathogenic members of the genus *Leptospira*. Several leptospiral serovars have been associated with presumably distinct diseases or syndromes, e.g., *icterohaemorrhagiae* with "Weil's disease," *canicola* with "canicola fever," *pomona* with "swineherd's disease," and *grippotyphosa* with "swamp fever" or "mud fever," but use of such terms as synonyms for leptospiral infections is confusing and inaccurate, as it has become evident that no clinical syndrome is exclusively attributable to a specific serovar and that no serovar invariably causes the same pattern of illness. In the interest of accuracy and clarity, the generic term leptospirosis should be used, regardless of the infecting serovar. The disease is worldwide in distribution and ranks among the most important of the zoonoses.

ETIOLOGY. Landouzy, in 1883, and Weil, in 1886, published clinical accounts of patients with a form of infectious jaundice that appeared to differ from the usual catarrhal jaundice with which they were familiar. The syndrome was later given Weil's name, and cases were reported from various localities in Europe and the Orient. However, the etiologic agent remained unknown until 1915, when Inada and his co-workers isolated a spirochete from the blood of a patient with Weil's syndrome. Noguichi subsequently assigned the organism to a new genus, the *Leptospira*, and named it *Leptospira icterohaemorrhagiae*.

Taxonomy of the leptospires has been troublesome from the beginning and is still evolving. The genus *Leptospira* is now composed of two species: the pathogenic *L. interrogans* and the saprophytic *L. biflexa*. Within the pathogenic species there are some 180 serovars that fall into 20 serogroups on the basis of common antigenic components. The biology of these remarkable pathogens is discussed in Chapter 46.

EPIDEMIOLOGY. All pathogenic leptospires are harbored by animal hosts and are communicated via water and soil (Alston and Broom, 1958). Animals transmit infection primarily by excreting leptospires in urine, although man can acquire the disease through contact with tissues of infected animals as well as urine. Organisms shed in urine can survive in neutral or slightly alkaline water or moist soil for weeks if the temperature exceeds 22° C. In warm seasons, fresh water in ponds, slow-moving streams, drains, canals, and mud may remain infectious for long periods.

The leptospires are essentially parasites of mammals, of which the rodents and a few domestic animals play a dominant role in their transmission to man. Rats and mice are the pre-eminent rodent hosts. Because their close association with man is worldwide, it is not surprising that leptospirosis knows no geographic limits. Dogs, pigs, and cows are the major sources of human infection in the developing countries. Leptospirosis can occur in humans of any age, at any season, and in both sexes, but is primarily a disease of young adults, of warm weather (summer and autumn), and of men (Johnson, 1976). It is a threat to pet owners, certain occupational groups, and those fond of outdoor sports. Hunters, fishermen, and swimmers are at risk because surface waters in rural areas are likely to be contaminated by animal carriers. Among occupational groups most vulnerable to infection are workers in the fish and poultry industries, veterinarians, miners, sewer workers, those engaged in animal husbandry, abattoir workers, and hand laborers in grain, rice, vegetable, and sugar cane fields.

PATHOGENESIS AND PATHOLOGY. The intraperitoneal inoculation of guinea pigs with leptospires is followed by rapid invasion of the bloodstream and, after 24 hours, by the presence of organisms in virtually all organs and tissues (Green and Arean, 1964). As the disease progresses, the organisms spread unchecked through the tissues and can be recovered from the cerebrospinal fluid, brain, and anterior chamber of the eye in the absence of visible irritation or hemorrhage. This observation led Green and Arean (1964) to conclude that leptospires penetrate tissues mechanically and are not necessarily carried into tissues by hemorrhage. Their conclusion is supported by the clinical observation that leptospires regularly invade the subarachnoid space and anterior chamber of the eye without inciting inflammation. The tissue injury caused by virulent leptospires appears to be toxic in nature. Hemorrhage appears to result from damage to endothelial cells by a cytotoxin. Leptospiral virulence appears to depend on toxin production.

Death due to anicteric leptospirosis is exceedingly rare; hence, knowledge of morbid anatomy in leptospirosis has been gained principally from the study of fatal cases of Weil's disease (Arean, 1962). At autopsy, the only gross changes of note are bile staining of tissues and extensive ecchymoses or petechiae in striated muscle, kidneys, adrenals, liver, stomach, spleen, and lungs, with less extensive bleeding elsewhere. The most prominent renal injury is in the tubular epithelium, where damage ranges from cloudy swelling to complete necrosis and desquamation. Tubules may be dilated and the lumina of medullary tubules may contain cellular casts, blood, bile-stained hyaline casts, and other debris. Interstitial edema, scattered hemorrhages, and mononuclear cell infiltration are characteristic. In acute renal failure, there is nonspecific acute tubular necrosis. Liver cords are dissociated with separation of hepatocytes, focal areas of necrosis around central veins, an increase in the number of binucleated liver cells, slight to moderate infiltration by neutrophils and round cells, and inspissation of bile in canaliculi. Overall, the pathologic changes in the liver are nonspecific and unimpressive and show little correlation with the degree of functional impairment. Leptospires are rarely demonstrable in hepatic tissues, and acute yellow atrophy is very uncommon.

In skeletal muscle, there is focal loss of cross-striations, vacuolation, and hyalinization early in the disease, and necrosis in the later stages. Leptospiral antigens can be demonstrated in areas of muscle degeneration. Hemorrhagic pneumonitis in localized or confluent patches is found in patients with pulmonary symptoms. Hemorrhages are the only characteristic lesions in other organs.

CLINICAL CHARACTERISTICS. The manifestations and severity of leptospiral infection can vary greatly. Approximately 10 to 15 per cent of patients present with the distinctive features of Weil's disease—e.g., jaundice, hemorrhage, and renal damage—and virtually all deaths due to leptospirosis occur in this group of patients. Fortunately, the majority of patients experience an acute, benign, anicteric, self-limited illness (Edwards and Domm, 1960).

Incubation Period. The incubation period averages 10 days, with a usual range of 7 to 13 days. However, isolated opportunities for exposure, as in laboratory or water accidents, indicate an extreme range of 2 to 26 days.

Phases of Illness. Leptospirosis is biphasic, a fact that can best be appreciated from observations of anicteric patients (Edwards, 1959). The initial "septicemic" or "leptospiremic" phase is an acute systemic infection with leptospires in the blood and cerebrospinal fluid. Defervescence and symptomatic improvement occur after four to seven days of acute illness, coincident with the disappearance of leptospires from the blood and spinal fluid. Following an asymptomatic interval of 24 to 72 hours, the second, or "immune," phase is ushered in by the reappearance of fever and often by a recurrence or intensification of headache. This phase of illness is characterized by manifestations related to the development of immunity and by the appearance of circulating IgM antibodies. Leptospires usually cannot be recovered from blood or cerebrospinal fluid after the first week but make their appearance in the urine around the middle of the second week. The variable severity, manifestations, and morbidity of the second phase are in sharp contrast to the monotonous clinical picture of the first phase. Many patients experience no symptoms in the second phase; others remain symptomatic for only one to three days; and a few have extended morbidity.

First Phase. Typically, the illness begins with the abrupt onset of headache, chills, fever, severe muscle aching, anorexia, nausea, vomiting, and prostration. Headache is frontal (sometimes bitemporal or occipital) and is intense, unremitting, rarely throbbing, and tends to persist several days. Repeatedly, patients with headache and nuchal rigidity have been found to have normal cerebrospinal fluid when lumbar puncture has been performed in anticipation of finding evidence of meningitis. Muscular discomfort is usually maximal in the calf and lumbar areas; fever is universal and usually spiking, chills may recur over three to five days; anorexia, nausea, and vomiting are common; and constipation is the rule, although a few patients have diarrhea. A significant number of patients complain of abdominal pain, which is probably caused by involvement of muscles of the abdominal wall rather than by inflammation of the gastrointestinal tract. Cough, dyspnea, and chest pain have been prominent symptoms in some reported series but not in others. Nevertheless, involvement of the respiratory system is an important feature of the first phase. Hemoptysis is infrequent.

Patients examined early in the illness are febrile, dehydrated, and lethargic, and may be confused or delirious. Relative bradycardia and normal or low blood pressure are the rule. Muscle tenderness may be marked in the presence of severe myalgia, and nuchal rigidity is often present. The most characteristic and valuable physical sign is suffusion of the conjunctivae, found in 80 to 85 per cent of cases. The eyes have a bright pink appearance similar to that seen after swimming in fresh water. Photophobia and burning are common, but purulent exudate and chemosis are rare. Infrequent findings include splenomegaly, hepatomegaly, lymphadenopathy, rash (macular, maculopapular, blotchy, urticarial, or even hemorrhagic), and rales or signs of pulmonary consolidation. Death is unusual in the first week of illness, even among patients with Weil's disease. The nonspecific manifestations of this phase suggest such diagnoses as bacterial pneumonia, typhus, tularemia, acute bronchitis, and viral infection.

Second Phase—Meningitis. Aseptic meningitis is the principal manifestation of the immune phase of illness. Approximately 50 per cent of all patients exhibit signs and symptoms, but fewer than half of these have the full-blown picture of meningitis, with excruciating headache, stiffness of the neck, and vomiting. Some of these latter patients are prostrated for a week or longer and may require narcotics for relief. Patients with severe headache may experience considerable relief from lumbar puncture. Around 30 to 35 per cent of patients have pleocytosis despite the absence of symptoms and signs of meningitis, while the remaining 15 to 20 per cent have normal spinal fluid throughout the illness.

Neither the development nor the severity of meningitis can be correlated with the severity of other manifestations of leptospirosis. It is not unusual for a patient who has had an insignificant first-phase illness to seek medical attention only following the onset of severe symptoms due to meningitis. Hence, the concept of "pure" leptospiral meningitis has arisen. Fortunately, a careful history usually brings to light an account of the antecedent febrile illness.

In meningitis, the leukocytes in the cerebrospinal fluid range from fewer than 10 to over 1000 per mm^3. Although neutrophils may predominate initially, the percentage of lymphocytes rises thereafter, and lymphocytosis of the spinal fluid may persist six to eight weeks after the patient becomes asymptomatic. Protein values are elevated to the range of 80 to 120 mg per mm^3 early in the course of meningitis but then decline. Glucose values are usually normal but fall occasionally. Xanthochromic spinal fluid may be found in jaundiced patients.

Other Nervous System Lesions. A variety of lesions of the nervous system may develop in the immune phase. Fortunately, these are uncommon, but they may be devastating. They include encephalitis, myelitis, radiculitis, the Guillain-Barré syndrome, and peripheral nerve lesions. The optic, oculomotor, facial, glossopharyngeal, auditory, and spinal nerves may be affected. These lesions resemble those that occur as sequelae of certain infections, vaccinations, and hypersensitivity to antibiotic agents and antisera and are thought to have the same pathogenesis.

Uveitis. Some authors have reported uveal tract involvement in many patients, but others have found it infrequently, apparently because it is easily overlooked. There have been reports of the isolation of viable leptospires from the aqueous humor of patients with lesions of the uveal tract, but it is not certain that uveitis is always due to persistence of organisms in the anterior chamber. It is of interest that no evidence of preceding leptospiral infection was found in many patients with unexplained uveitis. In contrast to other manifestations of leptospirosis, uveitis first becomes evident during convalescence or after a latent period of several weeks or months. The prognosis for cure is excellent, but visual impairment may be permanent.

SPECIAL FEATURES

Weil's Disease. The term Weil's disease is a convenient designation for severe leptospirosis characterized by icterus, azotemia, hemorrhage, anemia, vascular collapse, and disturbances in consciousness. In contrast to benign anicteric leptospirosis, Weil's disease is a dramatic, life-threatening illness. It cannot be equated with illness due to *icterohaemorrhagiae* infection, as every pathogenic serovar can cause such a syndrome. Although fairly insignificant from a numerical standpoint, this variant of leptospirosis far overshadows the anicteric form with respect to morbidity and mortality.

The onset and first phase of Weil's disease, before jaundice appears, are indistinguishable from those of anicteric leptospirosis. The distinctive manifestations of the syndrome (jaundice, hemorrhage and renal damage) first become evident around the third to fifth day of illness and reach their peak in the second week. Nevertheless, a biphasic temperature curve is usually discernible, and leptospires disappear from blood and cerebrospinal fluid around the seventh day. However, fever in the immune phase tends to be more prominent than in anicteric disease and may persist for two to three weeks.

The clinical picture may be dominated by hepatic, renal, or hemorrhagic manifestations, but death usually results from renal failure or hemorrhage rather than from hepatic failure. Fortunately, as methods of management of dehydration, shock, and acute renal failure have improved, the mortality rate of Weil's disease in developed countries has declined in recent years from 25 to 40 per cent to 5 per cent or less.

Hepatic Damage. Hepatic enlargement and tenderness are the rule in the presence of jaundice but are rarely found in its absence. Serum bilirubin levels usually remain below 20 mg per 100 ml, with the conjugated fraction predominating, but extreme hyperbilirubinemia has been recorded in some cases, usually in those with the triad of acute renal failure, hemolytic anemia, and severe liver involvement. There is evidence that bilirubin excretion is blocked at the subcellular level. Prothrombin production is usually normal, but if it is impaired, the deficiency can be corrected with vitamin K or one of its precursors. Complete resolution of hepatic damage is the rule in surviving patients.

Renal Damage. Renal dysfunction is common in leptospirosis. Proteinuria, transient oliguria, microscopic hematuria, and modest elevations of blood urea nitrogen are detected in 70 per cent of patients in the first phase, but with rare exceptions, major renal damage is limited to patients with Weil's disease. Renal injury is aggravated by shock, extreme hyperbilirubinemia, and possibly hemoglobinemia in severely ill patients. Renal failure was once the primary cause of death, but this is no longer necessarily true, as the incidence of acute tubular necrosis can be reduced by vigorous attention to fluid and blood replacement in the first phase of illness, and survival can be enhanced by use of modern methods of managing acute renal failure, including dialysis if necessary. Either peritoneal or extracorporeal dialysis may be utilized, but there are claims that hemodialysis is superior. Plasma exchange has been advocated for treatment of patients with the hepatorenal failure with very high serum bilirubin levels (Landini et al, 1981).

Cardiac Involvement. Electrocardiographic T-wave abnormalities and minor disturbances of conduction are relatively common in leptospirosis, but clinically significant cardiac manifestations are infrequent. Premature ventricular contractions, atrial flutter, ventricular tachycardia, and paroxysmal atrial fibrillation have been described, and patients with evidence of myocardial damage, e.g., dilatation, ventricular gallop rhythm, or frank congestive heart failure, have been reported.

Anemia is common in Weil's disease but rarely occurs without jaundice. It is due to hemolysis, hemorrhage, and azotemia and may be severe.

LABORATORY FEATURES

White blood cell counts vary from low to slightly elevated in anicteric leptospirosis, but jaundiced patients have significant leukocytosis, usually in the range of 15,000 to 30,000 per mm^3, although extreme leukocytosis may occur. Neutrophilia is so characteristic of the first stage that its absence virtually negates the diagnosis of leptospirosis. Anemia is not a feature of anicteric leptospirosis but may be severe in Weil's disease. Thrombocytopenia is rarely clinically significant.

Jaundice occurs in approximately 15 per cent of cases. Bilirubin levels remain below 20 mg per 100 ml in two-thirds of these, but in the remaining cases may reach 40 to 60 mg per 100 ml. Transaminase and alkaline phosphatase levels are usually elevated in jaundiced patients, although rarely more than threefold. In anicteric patients, the values tend to be normal or nearly so. Anicteric patients tend to maintain normal serum urea nitrogen levels, but as many as 25 per cent have elevations in the range of 20 to 60 mg per 100 ml, sometimes in the presence of normal urine. Patients with Weil's disease often have azotemia, and serum urea nitrogen values greater than 100 mg per 100 ml are characteristic in patients with acute tubular necrosis.

Urinalysis often discloses proteinuria, casts, and red and white blood cells early in the disease. However, the urine clears rapidly except in patients who sustain acute tubular necrosis.

PROPHYLAXIS. Leptospiral vaccines for human use were first developed more than 50 years ago, but several important problems remain to be solved. Killed vaccines have received the most attention, but live vaccines composed of virulent strains cultured in special media are being tested. Although the general use of vaccines cannot be justified because of the sporadic nature of leptospirosis, their use for the protection of workers in certain high-risk occupations is probably worthwhile. Unfortunately, the killed vaccines afford minimal protection against heterologous serotypes, and vaccines must be custom manufactured by using the specific serotype to which exposure is anticipated. A recent report (Takafuji et al., 1984) indicated that doxycycline is effective as a prophylactic agent against leptospirosis. Soldiers training in a jungle area who were given 200 mg of the drug by mouth at weekly intervals had an attack rate of 0.2 per cent as compared to 4.2 per cent in placebo-treated troops. Such chemoprophylaxis appears to be feasible in geographic areas where the attack rate is 3 to 5 per cent or higher.

Educational campaigns are needed to alert outdoor recreationalists, pet owners, and certain occupational groups to the hazards of the disease. The danger of swimming or wading in surface waters to which domestic or wild animals have access should be publicized. Pet owners, veterinarians, and livestock workers should be encouraged to protect themselves from contact with the urine or tissues of sick animals by wearing rubber gloves and aprons, and laborers in sugar cane and rice fields, abattoirs, and pig farms should be provided with protective clothing, including shoes. The incidence of infection due to serovar *icterohaemorrhagiae* in urban areas can be reduced by water purification, sewage and waste disposal systems, and vigorous rodent control programs.

COMPLICATIONS AND SEQUELAE. There are few sequelae of leptospiral infections. The liver and kidneys recover full function in patients who survive Weil's disease, except for a few patients left with permanent impairment of renal concentration. Leptospiral uveitis usually resolves completely, although there have been reported instances of blindness and cataract formation. Meningitis clears without residuals, but recovery from the "postinfectious" lesions of the nervous system is prolonged and may be incomplete.

As a statistical possibility, chronic systemic leptospirosis can be ignored. Only one such case has been documented, that of a patient who was probably immunodeficient. Although leptospires may persist in the anterior chamber of the eye and in the renal tubules for many months, little or no damage is caused by their presence in the kidneys, and surprisingly little reaction results from their presence in the eye other than an indolent uveitis.

GEOGRAPHIC VARIATIONS. Published accounts of leptospirosis seem to indicate that the disease is much more severe in some geographic areas than others. Reports from Latin America and the Caribbean islands depict leptospirosis as a serious hepatonephritic syndrome, yet public health authorities believe large numbers of anicteric cases go unrecognized. On the other hand, in developed countries where clinicians are aware of the anicteric form of the disease, patients with Weil's disease constitute a minority of all cases of leptospirosis. Thus, it is probable that the reported geographic variations in severity of leptospirosis are more apparent than real and can be attributed to differences in awareness of the full clinical spectrum of the disease.

It is reasonable to expect the experience of the United States in regard to leptospirosis to be recapitulated in Latin America and other developing countries in the next few decades. Between 1905 and 1974 the percentage of cases of leptospirosis due to serovar *icterohaemorrhagiae* fell from 90 per cent before 1946 to 40 per cent between 1949 and 1961 and to 20 per cent between 1965 and 1974. Before 1948, a total of 299 cases were reported, the vast majority of the patients were jaundiced, and the mortality rate was approximately 25 per cent. In contrast, of the 791 cases reported between 1965 and 1974, less than 15 per cent of the patients were icteric, and of these less than 5 per cent died.

DIAGNOSIS. The laboratory diagnosis of leptospirosis depends on isolation of the organisms by bacteriologic methods or serologic tests. Dark-field microscopy, once widely used for identification of the spirochetes in body fluids, is no longer considered reliable. The blood or cerebrospinal fluid should be cultured in the first week of illness and the urine after the middle of the second week. Leptospiruria is usually limited to two to four weeks but sometimes persists for months. Since only a minority of patients exhibit leptospiruria, failure to recover the organisms from urine does not exclude the diagnosis. A special semisolid medium such as Fletcher's, Korthof's, or Stuart's is required for culture. Inoculation of guinea pigs or hamsters is preferred to culture if specimens are contaminated.

Leptospiral antibodies appear in the blood around the end of the first week and usually reach their peak titer in the third or fourth week. There are a number of satisfactory serologic tests in use, but the microscopic agglutination test is regarded as most specific and is often used in confirming results of other tests. Blood for serologic tests should be collected in both the acute and convalescent phases of illness. A rise in titer of fourfold or greater is considered diagnostic, but if only a single specimen is available, a titer in the range of 1:1600 provides strong presumptive evidence of leptospirosis. Unfortunately, definitive identification of the infecting serotype by serologic test is impossible because of extensive cross-agglutination, nor is there a reliable diagnostic serologic test in the first week of illness.

TREATMENT. Leptospires have in vivo sensitivity to a wide variety of antimicrobial drugs including the penicillins, tetracyclines, and erythromycin. Antibiotic therapy seems to be beneficial if it is initiated within the first four days of illness (Kocen, 1962). Therapy begun after the fifth day cannot be expected to alter the course of illness, and the use of antimicrobials in the treatment of jaundice or meningitis has no rationale. Soluble penicillin in a daily dose of 2.4 million units and tetracycline in a dose of 2 g daily are the most widely used regimens, with penicillin being preferred by most authorities. Headache should be relieved, volume depletion corrected, and blood replaced in Weil's disease.

References

Alston, J. M., and Broom, J. C.: Leptospirosis in Man and Animals. Edinburgh and London, E. & S. Livingstone Ltd., 1958.

Arean, V. M.: The pathologic anatomy and pathogenesis of fatal human leptospirosis (Weil's disease). Am J Pathol 40:393, 1962.

Edwards, G. A.: Clinical characteristics of leptospirosis. Am J Med 27:4, 1959.

Edwards, G. A., and Domm, B. M.: Human leptospirosis. Medicine 39:117, 1960.

VIII Inter-American Meeting on Foot-and-Mouth Disease and Zoonose Control. Pan American Health Organization: Scientific Publication No. 316. Washington, D.C., World Health Organization, 1976.

Green, J. H., and Arean, V. M.: Virulence and distribution of *Leptospira*

icterohaemorrhagiae in experimental guinea pig infections. Am J Vet Res 25:264, 1964.
Johnson, R. C.: The Biology of Parasitic Spirochetes. New York, Academic Press, 1976.
Kocen, R. S.: Leptospirosis: A comparison of symptomatic and penicillin therapy. Br Med J 1:1181, 1962.
Landini, S., Coli, U., Lucatello, S., and Bazzato, G.: Plasma exchange in severe Leptospirosis. Lancet 2:1119, 1981.
Takafuji, E. T., Kirkpatrick, J. W., Miller, R. N., Karwacki, J. J., Kelley, P. W., Gray, M. R., McNeill, K. M., Timboe, H. L., Kane, R. E., and Sanchez, J. L.: An efficacy trial of doxycycline chemoprophylaxis against leptospirosis. New Engl J Med 310:497, 1984.

266

MARBURG VIRUS DISEASE

R. SIEGERT, M.D.

Marburg virus disease is a hemorrhagic fever with a high mortality rate which first appeared in Germany and Yugoslavia in 1967. It is named after the city where most of the cases occurred, and where the etiology of the disease was elucidated. The agent is a coated RNA virus of unusual shape and length. The primary source of infection in 1967 was monkeys imported from Uganda, and at first the disease was also referred to as green or vervet monkey disease. Two minor outbreaks occurred in 1974 in South Africa and in 1980 in Kenya. So far, only 36 cases have been observed.

ETIOLOGY. The clinical symptoms, pathologic and anatomic findings, epidemiology, and fruitless microbiologic and serologic efforts all indicated a hitherto unknown disease. From material obtained from patients, Marburg virus was first grown in guinea pigs and in monkey kidney cell cultures. Cytoplasmic antigen inclusions were demonstrated in organs of guinea pigs and dead patients, and also in infected cell cultures, using immunofluorescence-labeled antisera from guinea pigs and patients. Finally, a virus was revealed by electron microscopy in the sera and tissues of patients and likewise in infected animals, thus meeting the Henle-Koch postulates for an infectious agent (Siegert et al., 1967).

PATHOGENESIS AND PATHOLOGY. Of the 36 known patients 27 were primary cases and nine secondary. Incubation periods for primary infections lasted three to seven days, and five to nine days for secondary infections via human contacts. The most severe symptoms and all fatalities were observed only in primary infections. The main reason for these pathogenic differences is probably that the virus loses its virulence following passage in humans (Siegert, 1978).

All the cases examined revealed viremia, marked by high fever and lasting an average of 14 days. Marburg virus was carried hematogenously to all organs. Virus propagation leads to diffuse necrosis and functional disturbances in various parenchymatous organs. Fatalities occurred only during the acute stage of the disease.

The persistence of the virus in the liver, testes, and eye in the presence of circulating antibodies was of particular pathogenetic interest. It was verified in three patients by isolating the virus in a liver sample, in semen samples, and in ocular fluid two to three months after inception of the disease. Virus persistence was also suggested by the relapsing hepatitis observed in five cases at intervals of four to 73 days after fever had disappeared.

Repeated examinations of all the patients have yielded no signs of late organ damage, so that the prognosis is favorable once the patient has survived the acute stage of the disease. In spite of extensive necrosis, the liver structure can be expected to regenerate.

Frequent testicular and ovarian damage, together with the fact that the disease was transmitted in one case via semen, raised the question whether germinal transmission of Marburg virus to offspring is possible. However, no evidence of this has been found in animal experiments.

The pathologic changes resulting from Marburg virus disease were closely studied in five patients who died between the eighth and sixteenth day after onset of symptoms. Since death occurred at the climax of the disease or at the beginning of the convalescent phase, nothing is known about possible early changes.

Macroscopic findings were noncharacteristic and yielded little information. The important findings in microscopic examination of various tissues were limited to the liver, kidney, and lung. The most striking of these were hemorrhages and parenchymal necroses, which occurred without any appreciable inflammatory reactions (Gedigk et al., 1968).

Liver necrosis was severe. The individual and focal necroses of the liver cells were scattered irregularly over all the zones of the lobes and were characterized by changes in the cytoplasm—partly homogeneous, partly lumpy—and by positive PAS reactions and increased eosin staining. Cytoplasmic degeneration, with nucleolysis and formation of structures resembling Councilman bodies, was noted. Maximal alteration was observed in the second week, after which the cells degenerated rapidly and were resorbed. The defects were replaced by hepatogenic formations, and therefore liver structure can be expected to return to normal. Hepatitis caused by Marburg virus differs in regard to combination, distribution pattern, and development of lesions from classic forms of hepatitis, namely, yellow fever, leptospirosis, and other hemorrhagic fevers.

There were also hemorrhages and necroses in the testes, ovaries, pancreas, and kidneys; in each case, they indicated a severe tubular insufficiency. In addition, follicular necroses and perifollicular hemorrhages were found in the pulp of the spleen and in the medulla of the lymph nodes, which showed a striking paucity of cells and dense deposits of eosinophilic, PAS-positive material. Later, plasma-cellular monocytoid infiltrations were also found. In the lungs, edema was seen, with an accumulation of alveolar macrophages in fluid-filled alveoli.

Most of the fatalities had a glial nodular encephalitis distributed throughout the brain (Jacob, 1971). The process resembled that of other forms of encephalitis, especially louse-borne typhus and infections with arboviruses.

CLINICAL MANIFESTATIONS. All 36 patients were adults aged 18 to 64 years. They were closely observed clinically and showed uniform symptoms (Martini et al.,

1968; Stille and Böhle, 1971; Gear et al., 1975; Smith et al., 1982). Marburg virus disease began suddenly, with brief and noncharacteristic prodromes: marked malaise, torpor, and pain in the head, limbs, and muscles. Within a few hours, body temperature rose to more than 39° C.

The fever, accompanied by relative bradycardia, reached its climax on the third and fourth day, continued between 38° and 40° C up to the second week, and then gradually declined. Some of the patients had a second attack of fever around the twelfth to fourteenth day. Altogether, fever lasted from 12 to 22 days.

Gastrointestinal disturbances were present from the beginning. At first, marked nausea and occasionally uncontrolled vomiting were observed. Later, there was profuse watery diarrhea, which led to extreme dehydration in certain patients.

The most reliable symptom was a maculopapular, nonpruritic rash, which appeared in every patient between the fifth and eighth day, almost always beginning on the face and then spreading to the trunk and extremities. It consisted of livid red pinhead-sized papillae, which then developed into an extensive exanthem. In the more serious cases, the exanthem on the face and trunk merged into a dark red, diffuse erythema. Some of the patients also developed scrotal or labial dermatitis. Petechial skin hemorrhages occurred less frequently. The exanthem disappeared within a few days. After the sixteenth day, all the patients showed a fine exfoliative desquamation, especially on the soles and palms.

Simultaneously, most of the patients developed a dark red enanthem on the hard and soft palates, sometimes with glassy vesicles. In addition, there was noticeable conjunctivitis, with photophobia and increased secretion.

Between the third and sixth day, many of the patients showed a swelling of the lymph nodes in the neck, throat, and axillae. These were pea- to bean-sized, soft, and slightly sensitive to pressure. The spleen was not palpable.

From the fourth day on, half of the patients showed a hemorrhagic diathesis, with spontaneous bleeding from the nose and gums, hematuria, and hemorrhages in the gastrointestinal tract. Younger female patients also had genital hemorrhages. In the severe cases, large hematomas developed at injection sites, and bleeding from the punctures was hard to arrest.

Almost all of the parenchymatous organs were affected. The most obvious alteration was in the liver, which was seriously damaged in all cases. Some showed an extreme increase in the serum transaminase level, although icterus was extremely rare and hepatic coma did not ensue. Electrocardiographic changes indicated myocarditis. When the disease reached its crisis, there were frequent disturbances in heart rhythm and signs of cardiac insufficiency. A drop in blood pressure was observed only in the terminal stage. In severe cases there was considerable kidney damage, with proteinuria, oliguria, and anuria, as well as microhematuria and uremia.

In many of the patients, certain symptoms, including marked restlessness, depressive and sullen behavior, myoclonia, tremor, hyperesthesia, and paresthesia, indicated that the central nervous system was also affected. Some patients became confused, lost consciousness, and died in coma; two of them were convulsive. One woman developed a severe psychosis, and another a postinfectious myelitis with flaccid paralysis of both legs. The cell count and protein content of the cerebrospinal fluid remained within the normal range in the cases examined.

The laboratory findings revealed characteristic changes. A marked increase in serum glutamic oxaloacetic transaminase (SGOT) and serum glutamic pyruvic transaminase (SGPT) was noted in virtually all the patients during the second week. The SGOT values were always higher than the SGPT levels, in extreme cases attaining values of more than 5000 units/ml.

Bilirubin values were slightly increased, if at all, only during the terminal stages of the disease. Creatinine and urea levels increased only in cases of anuria. Hypokalemia appeared in connection with vomiting and diarrhea. The total serum protein concentration occasionally decreased to less than 5 per cent. In a few patients, elevated serum amylase levels were noted.

The hematologic changes consisted of marked leukopenia, with cell counts sometimes as low as 1000/mm^3. Excessive leukocytosis was observed only in patients with pulmonary complications. The blood sedimentation rate was rarely abnormal.

The hemopoietic system in all the patients was affected during the first few days. This was shown mainly by a critical decline in platelets, which sometimes dropped to as low as 10,000/mm^3. Some investigators regard the hematologic picture seen in patients with Marburg disease as characteristic of disseminated intravascular coagulopathy.

COMPLICATIONS AND SEQUELAE. Various complications appeared at the crisis of the disease: bronchopneumonia, edema in the lower leg, unilateral orchitis with painful swelling of the scrotum. There was one case each of pericarditis, psychosis, and postinfectious myelitis and uveitis. Shock and anuria may complicate the terminal picture.

Twenty-five per cent of patients died from cardiac and circulatory failure, renal failure, and cerebral coma.

The prognosis was favorable for all patients who survived the acute phase, even though convalescence was slow. During late convalescence, certain patients suffered a single relapse of hepatitis, with raised transaminase levels and slight fever. Recovery from liver damage, as ascertained by biopsy, was complete in all cases.

Sequelae also appeared: extensive alopecia, sharp pain in the liver region, and inability to tolerate alcohol. These sequelae persisted for some time. Some patients developed unilateral testicular atrophy, with oligospermia, loss of libido, and impotence, although the ketosteroids remained normal. Neurovegetative disturbances such as hyperhidrosis and fatigability lasted for many years.

DIAGNOSIS. All of the recorded outbreaks of Marburg virus disease had a connection with Africa, where the disease probably originated. Therefore, differential diagnostic considerations can be limited mainly to African febrile hemorrhagic diseases.

Protozoal diseases (malaria, trypanosomiasis) can be ruled out by negative blood smears, and bacterial diseases (leptospirosis, shigellosis, typhoid fever, plague) can be eliminated by negative blood or stool cultures as well as by the failure of suspected cases to respond clinically to high doses of broad spectrum antibiotics. Other important possibilities include certain virus diseases (chikungunya and Rift Valley fever, dengue, mononucleosis, hepatitis). The most important differential diagnosis is that between Lassa and yellow fever and Marburg and Ebola virus disease.

The earliest symptom of Lassa fever is a severe sore throat, usually with exudative or ulcerative pharyngitis, which makes it difficult or impossible for the patient to swallow. This severe pharyngitis is generally lacking in Marburg virus disease and yellow fever. Maculopapular rash is a prominent feature of Marburg virus disease but is never seen in yellow fever and only rarely in Lassa fever. Jaundice is common in yellow fever but occurs only rarely in the other diseases. The immediate medical problem in Lassa fever is hypotension and shock, whereas in Marburg virus disease shock appears to be a terminal event resulting from blood loss and/or overwhelming bacterial superinfection.

TREATMENT AND PROPHYLAXIS. Therapy is symptomatic. Antibiotics, singly or combined, had no effect on the viral process. However, their early use is recommended in order to prevent secondary bacterial infections. Convalescent plasma was used in some cases, but its effect is uncertain. The patient must be promptly treated for any complications that may arise; for instance, if the platelet level falls, platelets or fresh blood must be transfused. If disseminated intravascular coagulation sets in, intravenous heparin may be effective. Adequate replacement of fluid and electrolytes was especially important in patients with vomiting and diarrhea. Cardiac and circulatory drugs were necessary in most cases. Hypoproteinemia was treated with up to 30 g of human albumin daily. Corticosteroids had no effect. Therapy with human interferon on a trial basis is advisable.

Prevention and control measures in Marburg and Frankfurt consisted of destroying all monkeys and monkey cell cultures. All animal housing and laboratories were thoroughly disinfected. There were no further primary infections after these steps had been taken (Hennessen et al., 1968).

The patients were kept completely isolated in quarantine wards and were attended by volunteer physicians and nurses. The medical personnel all wore completely protective clothing in order to prevent contact, especially with blood from the patients. The patients were not released until two weeks after complete recovery. The men with orchitis were advised to be sexually continent as a precautionary measure. That this measure was justified is shown by the later seminal infection of a woman by her husband.

All primary and secondary contact persons were kept under observation and were given daily medical examinations. The general public and all medical personnel were kept informed, which proved to be psychologically effective.

The World Health Organization formulated recommendations for the capture, transportation, export and import, buying and selling, quarantine, and veterinary inspection of monkeys. In addition, national regulations were issued for protective measures in monkey and cell experiments.

Preclusion of Marburg virus from all live virus vaccines produced from monkey kidney cells was of particular importance. The 1967 outbreak led to worldwide efforts to find a suitable replacement for monkey kidney cells in vaccine production. As a result, they are no longer used.

Experience so far indicates that Marburg virus disease is very rare. Still, as long as the natural reservoir and means of transmission of the agent are not known, there are no means of primary prevention. No vaccine is available for endangered laboratory personnel.

References

Gear, J. S. S., Cassel, G. A., Gear, A. J., Trappler, B., Clausen, L., Meyers, A. M., Kew, M. C., Bothwell, T. H., Sher, R.; Miller, G. B., Schneider, J., Koornhof, H. J., Gomperts, E. D., Isaäcson, M., and Gear, J. H. S.: Outbreak of Marburg virus disease in Johannesburg. Br Med J 1:489, 1975.

Gedigk, P., Bechtelsheimer, H., and Korb, G.: Die pathologische Anatomie der "Marburg-Virus"-Krankheit (sog. "Marburger Affenkrankheit"). Dtsch Med Wochenschr 93:590, 1968.

Hennessen, W., Bonin, O., and Mauler, R.: Zur Epidemiologie der Erkrankung von Menschen durch Affen. Dtsch Med Wochenschr 93:582, 1968.

Jacob, H.: The neuropathology of the Marburg disease in man. In Martini, G. A., and Siegert, R. (eds.): Marburg Virus Disease. Berlin, Springer-Verlag, 1971, p. 54.

Martini, G. A., Knauff, H. G., Schmidt, H. A., Mayer, G., and Baltzer, G.: Über eine bisher unbekannte, von Affen eingeschleppte Infektionskrankheit: Marburg-Virus-Krankheit. Dtsch Med Wochenschr 93:559, 1968.

Siegert, R.: Marburgvirus-Krankheit. In Röhrer, H. (ed.): Handbuch der Virusinfektionen bei Tieren. Vol. 6. Jena, Gustav Fischer Verlag, 1978, p. 579.

Siegert, R., Shu, H. L., Slenczka, W., Peters, D., and Müller, G.: Zur Ätiologie einer unbekannten, von Affen ausgegangenen menschlichen Infektionskrankheit. Dtsch Med Wochenschr 92:2341, 1967.

Smith, D. H., Isaacson, M., Johnson, K. M., Bagshaire, A., Johnson, B. K., Siranopoel, R., Killey, M., Tarap Siongok, and Koinange Keruga, H.: Marburg-Virus disease in Kenya. Lancet 7:816, 1982.

Stille, W., and Böhle, E.: Clinical course and prognosis of Marburg virus ("green monkey") disease. In Martini, G. A., and Siegert, R. (eds.): Marburg Virus Disease. Berlin, Springer-Verlag, 1971, p. 10.

267
EBOLA VIRUS DISEASE

R. SIEGERT, M.D.

Ebola virus disease is a hemorrhagic fever with a high mortality rate. Clinically, it is extremely similar to Marburg virus disease, and Africa is the natural habitat of both. However, the agent, which is named after a river in Zaire, shares no antigen with Marburg virus, despite their extensive morphologic similarity. Neither the natural hosts of Ebola virus nor its habitat and transmission are known. In 1976 there was an epidemic in southern Sudan and northern Zaire, and approximately 600 cases were identified. Another outbreak occurred in 1979 in the Yambio-Nzara district of southern Sudan, where the first cases were observed in 1976 (World Health Organization, 1979).

ETIOLOGY. The agent was isolated and identified by means of investigations similar to those that clarified the etiology of Marburg virus disease (Bowen et al., 1977; Johnson et al., 1977; Pattyn et al., 1977). Although Ebola virus is an independent agent antigenically of two serotypes (Richman et al., 1983), it is very closely related to Marburg virus in structure and pathogenic properties.

PATHOGENESIS AND PATHOLOGY. Since detailed pathologic and anatomic information is lacking, it has not yet been possible to analyze the pathogenic mechanism. The incubation period is given as 4 to 16 days, with an average of 7 days. Subsequently, viremia always develops, and the virus appears in all organs. Persistence must also be expected, since the virus was isolated in the semen of one patient on the thirty-ninth and the sixty-first day after the onset of the disease. The infection conveys immunity of an undetermined duration.

No representative description of pathologic changes is yet available. So far, histologic examinations have been restricted to liver specimens from three virologically verified patients from Zaire. These specimens showed fatty degeneration and necrosis distributed in a focal pattern. Inflammatory reactions were remarkably slight. Eosinophilic inclusion bodies of varying size were found in the cytoplasm of the hepatocytes. These bodies, together with the presence of structures resembling Councilman bodies, made tentative histologic diagnosis possible.

CLINICAL MANIFESTATIONS. The disease begins suddenly, with fever, gastrointestinal symptoms, and pain in the limbs as prodromes (Brès, 1977; Emond et al., 1977). On the third day, diarrhea, pharyngitis, and a dry cough usually set in, and on the fifth day the characteristic symptoms appear: hepatitis without jaundice, morbilliform exanthems, and, in severe cases, hemorrhagic diathesis with spontaneous bleeding. In pregnant patients there are massive metrorrhagias and miscarriages. Torpor, tremor, and convulsions indicate that the central nervous system is affected. Alopecia and loss of weight are frequent accompanying symptoms. Convalescence is slow. Nothing is known about possible complications or sequelae, nor are any clinicochemical findings available. The mortality resulting from Zaire strains was approximately 90 per cent, from Sudan subtype it was 55 per cent. (One obvious difference from the outbreaks of Marburg fever was the low standard of medical care). When the disease reaches its final stages, death occurs between the fourth and tenth day.

DIAGNOSIS. The principles of differential diagnosis of Marburg virus disease also apply to Ebola virus disease.

TREATMENT AND PROPHYLAXIS. Therapy is symptomatic. A laboratory worker with a relatively light case received more than 80 million units of human interferon and about 800 ml of immune plasma. This serotherapy led to an immediate decrease of the virus titer in the blood, but it is not clear which therapy was responsible for recovery (Emond et al., 1977).

Prevention and control measures were limited mainly to ascertaining and quarantining those with the disease as well as primary contacts (Brès, 1977). In addition, attending physicians and nurses wore protective clothing, and disinfection measures were taken. The above-mentioned laboratory worker was isolated in a low-pressure plastic tent. Vaccines are not yet available.

References

Bowen, E. T. W., Lloyd, G., Harris, W. J., Platt, G. S., Baskerville, A., and Vella, E. E.: Viral haemorrhagic fever in southern Sudan and northern Zaire. Lancet 1:571, 1977.

Brès, P.: WHO report of the informal consultation on the Marburg virus-like disease outbreaks in the Sudan and Zaire in 1976, held at the London School of Hygiene and Tropical Medicine, 4 and 5 January 1977. Geneva, World Health Organization, 1977.

Emond, R. T. D., Evans, B., Bowen, E. T. W., and Lloyd, G.: A case of Ebola virus infection. Br Med J 2:541, 1977.

Johnson, K. M., Lange, J. V., Webb, P. A., and Murphy, F. A.: Isolation and partial characterisation of a new virus causing acute haemorrhagic fever in Zaire. Lancet 1:569, 1977.

Pattyn, S., Groen, G. van der, Jacob, W., Piot, P., and Courteille, G.: Isolation of Marburg-like virus from a case of haemorrhagic fever in Zaire. Lancet 1:573, 1977.

Richman, D., Cleveland, P., McCormick, J., et al.: Antigenic analysis of strains of Ebola virus: identification of two Ebola virus serotypes. J Infect Dis 147:268, 1983.

World Health Organization: Viral haemorrhagic fever surveillance. Weekly Epidem. Rec. 54:319, 1979.

268

CAT SCRATCH DISEASE

WARREN J. WARWICK, M.D.

Cat scratch disease (cat scratch fever, cat scratch syndrome, cat claw fever, benign inoculation lymphoreticulosis, nonbacterial regional lymphadenitis, cat adenitis) is an acute, benign, self-limited disease of the regional lymph nodes. The most specific feature is subacute regional lymphadenitis, almost always preceded by a granulomatous skin reaction at the site of a skin injury, which is usually a scratch by a cat. This skin lesion is important in establishing the diagnosis because no lymphangitis develops between the skin lesion and the enlarged lymph nodes. In one third of cases the enlarged lymph nodes become necrotic and filled with pus. Fever, mild and of short duration, is the only common constitutional symptom.

ETIOLOGY. The causative agent is presumed to be an incompletely identified delicate pleomorphic gram-negative bacillus found by histologic examination in 87 per cent of biopsied lymph nodes from 39 typical cases of cat scratch disease (Wear et al., 1983). While still awaiting confirmation, this apparently will bring to conclusion the search for the agent because reports of isolation of viral or chlamydial agents from cases of cat scratch disease have not been confirmed and tests for antibodies against candidate etiologic agents have been inconclusive (Emmons et al., 1976).

EPIDEMIOLOGY

Subjects. Although cat scratch disease can occur at any age, children and young adults are most often affected. Cat scratch disease affects both sexes equally and all races. Excluding obvious bacterial infections, it is the most common cause of localized lymphadenopathy during the middle years (Carithers et al., 1969).

Seasonal Variation. Cat scratch disease that is severe enough to be diagnosed and reported has a strong seasonal variation. In the temperate zone of Europe and North America three fourths of cases have been observed to occur between September and February (Warwick, 1967). However, factors influencing transmission of cat scratch disease may operate differently in other climates and environments. In the subtropical climate of Florida, three fourths of cases have been seen in the last six months of the year (Carithers et al., 1969), and in temperate-zone Japan most cases have been reported in summer and autumn (Miupa et al., 1975). In tropical areas the seasonal variation may be different or nonexistent.

Cat Scratches and Cat Contact. Cat contact, which was reported early by Daniels and MacMurray (1954) and Debré and Job (1954) to occur in nine tenths of cases, may be of major importance but by itself insufficient, for 90 per cent of children in the United States have similar exposure to cats. Nevertheless, the hallmark of this disease historically (Carithers, 1970) and clinically (Warwick, 1967) has been a preceding cat scratch. Since many of the cases of cat scratch disease that occur without a preceding cat scratch follow a puncture of the skin, the type of injury may be of equal importance. This uncertain significance has been demonstrated by alternative names for the syndrome; i.e., benign inoculation lymphoreticulosis, thereby emphasizing the mode of injury rather than the usual cat contact.

Epidemics. Although familial outbreaks of cat scratch disease occur, infectivity is low, fewer than one fifth of exposed family members acquiring symptomatic disease. Most family outbreaks are associated with a kitten in the household. Epidemics of cat scratch disease occur during the months of greatest likelihood of sporadic occurrence (Warwick, 1967).

CLINICAL MANIFESTATIONS. Cat scratch disease usually begins with an isolated lesion (the primary lesion) at the site of and a week or two after a scratch by a cat. Two or three weeks after the primary lesion the patient notices a slightly painful swollen lymph node and has slight malaise for a few days with a low fever, reduced appetite, and an occasional ache. His white blood count is slightly elevated with slight eosinophilia. The constitutional symptoms and the local discomfort regress rapidly. The lymphadenopathy disappears in another three to four weeks. The patient's symptoms have been so mild that he has not come to his doctor for consultation.

Primary Lesion. Despite early reports that primary lesions were present in only half the cases, with a careful search the primary lesion can be found in 95 per cent of cat scratch disease patients (Carithers et al., 1969). Since the primary lesion usually begins one to two weeks after the inoculating skin injury and lasts a variable period of one to four weeks, it is probably missed when it is looked for late in the course of cat scratch disease. It may begin as early as three days after the cat scratch or as late as a month, and rarely lasts several months. It does not itch. The primary lesion is usually a single papule but may consist of multiple papules along a cat scratch. The early papule is red, 2 to 5 mm in diameter; there is no associated lymphangitis. Later, the papule may be reddish purple, scaly, vesicular, or pustular. All primary lesions are sterile by conventional bacterial and viral cultures. The pathologic sign is granuloma formation that resembles the pathologic process of the lymph nodes. Primary lesions heal without a scar.

Failure to find a primary lesion should alert the clinician to consider another diagnosis.

Regional Lymphadenopathy. Every patient with cat scratch disease has lymphadenopathy. The adenopathy may affect only one node in mild cases but may involve all or most of the lymph nodes in several sequential regional chains in severe cases. Although adenopathy is occasionally painless, a local tenderness usually calls attention to the node enlargement. When the enlargement is rapid, acute tenderness may be present.

The enlargement of the lymph nodes follows the appearance of the primary lesion—in over half of cases it develops between one and two weeks and in two thirds of cases by three weeks after the inoculating cat scratch. Rarely, the lymphadenopathy may not appear for seven to ten weeks. In such cases a primary lesion may be hard to find or even absent.

Once started, the nodal pathology progresses toward suppuration. In mild cases this occurs infrequently, perhaps 10 per cent of the time. In more severe cases with substantial lymph node enlargement, suppuration may occur in half the cases.

Lymph node regression varies directly with severity of illness: in 10 per cent regression occurs by two weeks, in 25 per cent by four weeks, in 50 per cent by six weeks, in 75 per cent by nine weeks, and in 95 per cent by six months after onset of the enlargement.

The site of lymph node involvement parallels the sites of frequency of cat scratches: epitrochlear and axillary nodes in two thirds of cases, cervical and submandibular in one fourth, preauricular (Parinaud's ocular glandular syndrome) in one tenth, and inguinal and femoral nodes in one tenth. Nevertheless, lymph nodes in almost every location in the body, including the mediastinum and the mesentery, may be involved.

Lymphadenopathy in any location, when accompanied by an inoculating skin injury, a primary lesion, and absence of lymphangitis, should alert the physician to a suspicion of cat scratch disease. On the other hand, the diagnosis of cat scratch disease should not be made in the absence of lymphadenopathy.

Parinaud's Oculoglandular Syndrome. Parinaud's syndrome has been found in 2 to 18 per cent of cat scratch disease patients (Carithers, 1978). Cat scratch disease is probably the only cause of this unusual syndrome. Inoculation appears to be in the conjunctiva without the intervention of a cat scratch. Presumably rubbing the eyes after cat contact or rubbing one's face in the cat's fur can inoculate the bacterial agent. This speaks for the agent being in the environment, rather than confined to cat's claws. One or more atypical primary lesions—gray, yellow, or reddish necrotic nodular or granulomatous lesions—develop in the retrotarsal area. When such lesions are associated with preauricular lymph node enlargement, with or without cervical node involvement or constitutional symptoms, a clinical diagnosis of cat scratch disease may be made. The conjunctival lesion heals in one to three weeks without injury to the eye.

Systemic Symptoms. Although over two thirds of diagnosed patients are only mildly ill, constitutional symptoms can be important. In patients with milder lymphadenopathy fever may be associated in one third of cases, whereas in more severe illness fever may be present in three fourths of cases. Fever is usually low, 38° C, but rarely it may exceed 39° C. Generalized or local aching, malaise, anorexia, nausea, and abdominal pain are seen more often in older patients and in patients with extensive lymph node involvement. Although systemic symptoms are most likely due to circulating toxin, observations of fibro-granulomatous lesions with scar formation in a splenectomy specimen eight weeks after cat-scratch disease and occasional splenomegaly in the disease suggest that hematogenous dissemination of the bacterial agent occasionally occurs. (Chelloul et al., 1977).

COMPLICATIONS. Table 1 contains a list of many of the reported atypical manifestations associated with cat scratch disease. These are rare, sometimes only one observation, but they demonstrate the many variations of symptomatology that can make diagnosis difficult. Encephalitis is the most important symptom and has been reported in over 50 patients.

The association of encephalitis (Lyon, 1971; Warwick, 1967) with cat scratch disease is hard to establish in a given case but should be suspected if the neurological signs develop within 6 weeks of unexplained lymphadenopathic or diagnosed cat-scratch disease (Miller and Bell, 1980). The afflicted patients have abrupt onset of convulsions and coma. The clinical impression of encephalitis is supported by findings of mild pleocytosis. The patients regain consciousness within two to ten days and recover completely. About one third have transient neurologic problems lasting a few months to a year. Although not proved beyond a doubt, deaths have been seen in suspected cases of encephalitis attributed to cat scratch disease.

DIAGNOSIS. Since the delicate pleomorphic gram-negative bacillus cannot yet be cultured and no simple serologic test exists, the diagnosis of cat scratch disease requires matching symptoms to a syndrome: (1) There must be regional lymphadenopathy; (2) there must be no other cause for the lymphadenopathy; (3) a primary lesion is present; (4) a cat scratch or other puncture wound precedes the other symptoms; (5) the disease shows a benign course with spontaneous recovery.

When these five criteria are satisfied a presumptive diagnosis of cat scratch disease may be made. When atypical features are present or when the syndrome is incomplete, the diagnosis can usually be confirmed by finding: (6) typical histopathology on biopsy of the primary lesion or the affected lymph node; (7) demonstration of pleomorphic gram-negative bacilli in the walls of the capillaries and macrophages lining the sinuses near or in the lymph node germinal centers with the Warthin-Story silver impregnation stain (Wear et al., 1983); (8) a positive Hanger-Rose skin test.

Biopsy. The pathology of the skin lesion and of the skin test is one of dermal necrosis within a zone of acellular necrobiosis, which is in turn inside a zone of epithelial cells and giant cells surrounded by a thin layer of small lymphocytes (Johnson and Helwig, 1969; Czarnetzki et al., 1975).

The lymph node changes of early lymphoid hyperplasia, later granuloma, and finally microabscess formation are separately characteristic but not diagnostic of cat scratch disease. When all three histologic phases are present in the same lymph node, however, the trio is distinctive (Campbell, 1977). When Campbell's observations of the simultaneous presence of lymphoid hyperplasia, granulomas, and microabscess in the same lymph node are found, the diagnosis of cat scratch disease may be made. The demonstration of intracellular bacilli singly, in chains, or in clusters within the blood vessels of the areas of reaction or within the reactive histocytes is the strongest evidence to date for the diagnosis. (Wear et al., 1983).

Hanger-Rose Skin Test. The development of a skin test antigen by Hanger and Rose (Carithers, 1970) made it possible for clinicians to assign a common cause to many benign lymphadenopathies. The Hanger-Rose antigen is prepared from pus from proven cases of cat scratch disease and varies in sensitivity and specificity from batch to batch.

Not all antigens give positive skin tests in all proven cases of cat scratch disease and a variable proportion of healthy normal subjects have positive skin tests within any batch of Hanger-Rose antigen. The frequency of positive skin tests, a typical delayed-type cutaneous reaction, varies, in healthy normals, from 4 per cent in nonendemic areas to 10 per cent in endemic areas. Almost one fifth of family contacts and one fourth of veterinary workers have positive skin tests.

The relatively high background of positive tests, induration of 5 mm or more or erythema of 10 mm or more after 48 hours, and the substantial number of false-negative tests indicate that the Hanger-Rose skin test is not to be substituted for clinical judgment or pathologic studies and that it cannot be used as the sole arbiter of a diagnosis. The scientific foundation for the Hanger-Rose skin test awaits preparation of antigen from the identified pleomorphic gram-negative bacillus.

Since there is no commercial antigen, persons studying cat scratch disease continue to make their own antigen. In view of the problems of specificity, sensitivity, and safety, new workers in the field of cat scratch disease are advised to collaborate with workers still active in cat scratch disease research in preparation of new Hanger Rose antigens.

Table 1. ATYPICAL SIGNS OF CAT SCRATCH DISEASE

- Parinaud's oculoglandular syndrome
- Lymphadenopathy
  - Bilateral
  - Generalized
  - Mesenteric hilar
- Skin reactions
  - Erythema annulare
  - Erythema multiforme
  - Papular vesicular rash
  - Maculopapular rash
  - Thrombocytopenic purpura
  - Erythema nodosum
  - Nonthrombocytopenic purpura
- Miscellaneous
  - Pneumonia
  - Pharyngitis
  - Osteolytic granuloma
  - Subacute iriditis
  - Nonspecific nongonococcal urethritis
  - Lymphedema
  - Herpes zoster
  - Thyroiditis
  - Anicteric hepatitis
  - Submaxillary and parotid localization
  - Encephalitis
  - Hepatomegaly
  - Splenomegaly
  - Optic neuritis

Despite 35 years of use with no untoward reactions reported, questions of the safety of the Hanger-Rose antigen continue to be raised—especially concerning viral hepatitis, a slow virus, or an incomplete virus. Autoclaving at 4.5 kg, 100° C for 10 minutes (Kalter et al., 1977), heating at 56° C for 12 hours (Carithers, 1977), or sterilizing with gamma radiation (Bradstreet and Gidherd, 1977) has been recommended to make the antigen safe.

Laboratory Studies. Techniques have not yet been developed for culture or serologic recognition of the pleomorphic gram-negative bacillus recently discovered in biopsies. In the meantime laboratory tests are useful only for establishing that a patient with lymphadenopathy does not have another disease. The exclusion of other provable causes of lymphadenopathy is a major step in arriving at a diagnosis.

Cultures for bacteria, fungi, mycobacteria, and viruses are sterile. Agglutination tests for syphilis, *Brucella*, and tularemia are negative, as are the heterophil tests. Skin tests for mycobacteria and fungi are negative. Although low titers against chlamydial antigens develop in many patients who have suppurative lymph nodes, these titers are not helpful in diagnosis. Hematologic studies show no neutropenia, rare leukocytosis, and occasional eosinophilia; the occasionally elevated sedimentation rate is related to fever.

Differential Clinical Diagnosis. The lymphadenopathy of cat scratch disease, especially when suppuration occurs, may be misdiagnosed as a purulent bacterial lymphadenopathy. When cat scratch disease is the cause, antibiotic treatment will not alter the course of the illness, and when the diagnosis is missed, prolonged antibiotic therapy only exposes the patient to the expense and hazards of overtreatment.

On the other hand, when the lymph node enlargement is solid and of long duration, the question of lymphoma may arise. Since the pathology of cat scratch disease may not be specific and since the pleomorphic gram-negative bacilli are not demonstrable in all biopsied nodes, confusion with lymphoma or Hodgkin's disease can lead to serious errors in treatment.

TREATMENT. Supportive symptomatic treatment is indicated. Antibiotics do not change the course of the disease, nor does cortisone. Suppurative nodes should be aspirated. Incision and drainage are contraindicated because draining sinuses frequently result. Excision of the affected nodes may be indicated when a draining sinus is present, when the symptoms are atypical, when constitutional symptoms are severe (i.e., encephalitis), when diagnosis is urgent, or when malignancy is suspected. As excision of affected nodes promptly halts systemic symptoms, these are presumably usually due to locally produced toxins.

References

Bradstreet, C. M., and Digherd, N. W.: Cat-scratch fever skin-test antigen (letter). Lancet 1:913, 1977.

Campbell, J. A.: Cat-scratch disease. Pathol Annu 12:277, 1977.

Carithers, H. A.: Cat-scratch disease; notes on its history. Am J Dis Child 119:200, 1970.

Carithers, H. A.: Cat-scratch skin test antigen; purification by heating. Pediatrics 60:928, 1977.

Carithers, H. A.: Oculoglandular disease of Parinaud. A manifestation of cat-scratch disease. Am J Dis Child 132:1195, 1978.

Carithers, H. A., Carithers, C. M., and Edwards, R. O., Jr.: Cat-scratch disease: Its natural history. JAMA 207:312, 1969.

Chelloul, N., Briere, J., Schaison, G. and Vorhauer, W.: (Splenic lesions during benign inoculation lymphoreticulosis), Sem Hop Paris 53:2182, 1977.

Daniels, W. B., and MacMurray, F. G.: Cat-scratch disease; report of 160 cases. JAMA 154:1247, 1954.

Debré, R., and Job, J. C.: La maladie des griffes de chat. Acta Paediat Suppl Upps 43:1, 1954.

Emmons, R. W., Riggs, J. L. and Schachter, J.: Continuing search for the etiology of cat scratch disease. J Clin Microbiol 4:112, 1976.

Johnson, W. T., and Helwig, E. B.: Cat-scratch disease. Histopathologic changes in the skin. Arch Dermatol 100:148, 1969.

Kalter, S. S., Rodriguez, A. P., and Heberling, R. L.: Cat-scratch disease skin-test antigen preparation (letter). Lancet 2:606, 1977.

Lyon, L. W.: Neurologic manifestations of cat-scratch disease. Report of a case and review of the literature. Arch Neurol 25:23, 1971.

Margileth, A. M.: Cat-scratch disease: Nonbacterial regional lymphadenitis. The story of 145 patients and a review of the literature. Pediatrics 42:803, 1968.

Miller, P. and Bell, W. C.: Cat-scratch disease with encephalopathy. Clin Pediatr 106:306, 1980.

Miupa, T., Topinuki, T. W., and Tanahashi, Y.: Cat-scratch disease. J Exp Med 117:373, 1975.

Warwick, W. J.: The cat-scratch syndrome, many diseases or one disease. Prog Med Virol 9:256, 1967.

Wear, D. J., Margileth, A. M., Hadfield, T. L., Fischer, G. W., Schlogel, C. J., and King, F. M.: Cat Scratch Disease: A bacterial infection. Science 221:1403, 1983.

269

COLORADO TICK FEVER

ALAN G. BARBOUR, M. D.

SPOTSWOOD L. SPRUANCE, M. D.

Colorado tick fever is a viral disease characterized by a biphasic course and leukopenia. It is transmitted by ticks in the Rocky Mountain area and the Pacific slope of the United States and Canada.

ETIOLOGY AND EPIDEMIOLOGY. At the end of the 19th century, physicians in the newly settled Rocky Mountain region of the United States recognized a mild, tick-borne disease that was distinct from Rocky Mountain spotted fever. In 1944, Florio reported the successful transmission of Colorado tick fever to human volunteers and to hamsters by the injection of serum from patients with the disease. Florio later noted that the agent would pass through bacterial filters and the causative organism was subsequently shown to be a double-stranded RNA virus with 12 discrete RNA segments. Colorado tick fever virus is classified in the genus *Orbivirus* of the family Reoviridae. Human virus isolates have been of one major serotype. An unclassified tick-borne virus, the Eyach virus, isolated in the Federal Republic of Germany, has partial antigenic cross-reactivity with the Colorado tick fever virus.

Colorado tick fever is acquired from the bite of infected ticks. The disease occurs almost exclusively in the area of distribution of the wood tick, *Dermacentor andersoni* (Fig. 1). Infection of travelers and vacationers may lead to the appearance of the disease outside of western North America. The virus has been recovered from other ticks in the

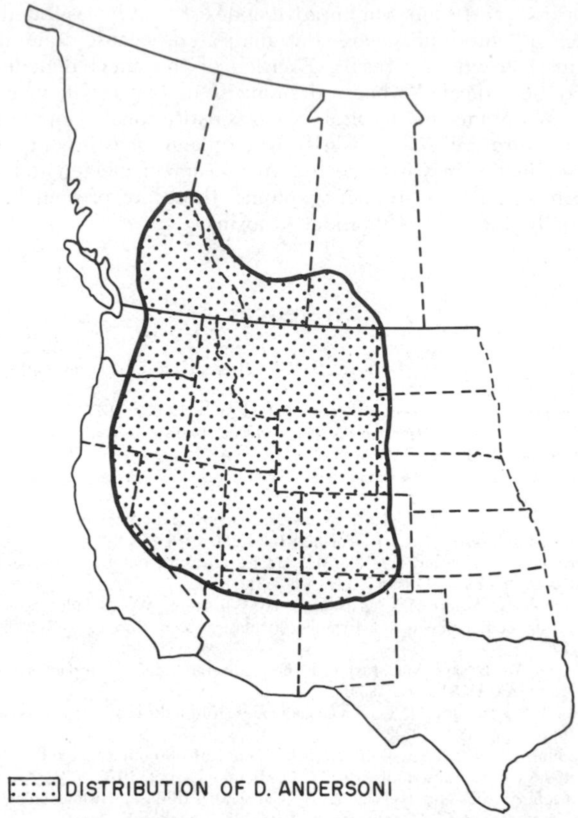

Figure 1. Distribution of *Dermacentor andersoni* in the western United States and Canada. (Adapted from Eklund, C. M., Kohls, G. M., and Brennan, J. M.: JAMA 157:335, 1955.)

endemic area, but *D. andersoni* is the only tick known to transmit the disease to man (Eklund et al., 1955).

D. andersoni, a hard-body tick, resides at 1200 to 3300 meters altitude in regions of brushy and evergreen vegetation, such as sagebrush and juniper. It is scarce in heavy timber or open grassland. Female ticks lay their eggs under dead vegetation. The six-legged larvae that emerge find a small mammal such as a ground squirrel, feed for a few days, and drop off to molt into nymphs. The eight-legged nymphs hibernate unfed and seek another small mammal in the spring. After feeding for four to nine days, the nymphs fall off and molt into adults. The adults seek larger mammal hosts, including deer and man. Female ticks attach and feed for 6 to 13 days, drop off to lay eggs, and die. The male may feed only briefly before seeking an attached female to mate. A cycle of inapparent infections between the immature stages of the tick and small mammals maintains the virus in the endemic area. The virus overwinters in nymphal ticks and may also persist in hibernating animals. Transovarial passage of the virus by the tick has not been demonstrated.

Man acquires infected adult ticks by contact with grass stalks and low shrubs while hiking, camping, or engaging in other outdoor activities. Although most patients with Colorado tick fever report possible exposure to ticks, only one half have been aware of a tick bite or attachment. Prolonged feeding by the tick is not necessary for transmission. The high proportion of Colorado tick fever patients who are men reflects their more frequent exposure to the vector. As many as 15 per cent of individuals in high-risk occupations, such as forest rangers, may possess neutralizing antibody against the virus.

Colorado tick fever occurs in the late spring and summer (Fig. 2), the seasons when adult *D. andersoni* ticks are most active. The peak incidence of human cases occurs during April and May at lower altitudes and during June and July at higher elevations. Rarely, cases may occur at atypical times of the year in recipients of infected blood, in laboratory workers who are accidentally inoculated, or in individuals to whom the virus has been mechanically transmitted from a viremic mammal by a mosquito or biting fly.

PATHOGENESIS AND PATHOLOGY. Viremia is a regular occurrence in Colorado tick fever. The virus can be recovered from the plasma for approximately one week and from the erythrocyte fraction of blood for up to 120 days after onset of the disease. The duration of viremia corresponds with the lifespan of red cells. Its intra-erythrocytic location protects the virus from neutralizing antibody. Because the mature erythrocyte lacks functional ribosomes that are essential to viral replication, it is likely that infection of red cells begins in hematopoietic cells. Virions and evidence of viral replication have been seen by electronmicroscopy within erythrocyte precursors in the bone marrow of infected patients.

Leukopenia with the nadir at the beginning of the second febrile episode is characteristic of Colorado tick fever. Neutrophils and lymphocytes both decrease. Because lymphocytes appear to recover more quickly, neutropenia is observed more commonly. There is an increase in the proportion of immature neutrophils in the peripheral blood and a maturation arrest in the neutrophil series in the marrow. The white cell count may remain depressed for up to seven days after clinical recovery. The pathogenesis of the leukopenia is unknown, but it may be caused by infection of stem cells in the bone marrow. Alternatively, because Colorado tick fever virus is an interferon inducer, high systemic or local hematopoietic tissue levels of interferon may depress the white cell count.

Thrombocytopenia, disseminated intravascular coagula-

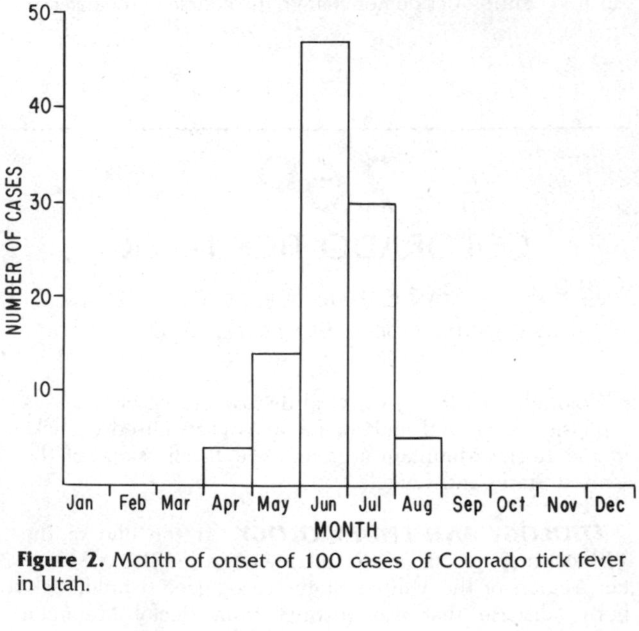

Figure 2. Month of onset of 100 cases of Colorado tick fever in Utah.

tion, and hemorrhage occur rarely. Focal necrosis and swelling of the capillary epithelium were seen on postmortem examination of one patient. Meningitis and encephalitis occur rarely and are probably the result of infection rather than immunologic injury. The virus has been recovered from the cerebrospinal fluid of one patient with encephalitis and from the CSF of experimentally infected volunteers without neurologic symptoms. There were intracytoplasmic inclusion bodies in the Purkinje cells and neurons of the midbrain in one fatal case. In mice, there is an apparent predilection of the virus for brain as well as for heart muscle, spleen, lymphoid tissue, and bone marrow.

CLINICAL MANIFESTATIONS. The incubation period is usually three to five days, but it may be as long as ten days. There are no prodromal manifestations. The onset is sudden, and symptoms are commonly maximal within hours. Patients often report chilliness without true rigors. The triad of fever, headache, and myalgia, notably of the back and legs, is usual. Retro-orbital pain and pain elicited by ocular movements are other common complaints. Respiratory symptoms are very rare. Abdominal pain and vomiting occur occasionally.

The course of Colorado tick fever is distinctive (Fig. 3). Most patients experience a biphasic fever in which a two- to three-day febrile period is followed by a remission of one or two days before the onset of another two- to three-day febrile period ("saddle-back" fever). The remaining patients have a single febrile episode or, more rarely, three bouts of fever.

Physical findings are meager. A mild, transient rash occurs in approximately 5 to 10 per cent of patients; it may be macular, maculopapular, or petechial. Tachycardia, a flushed face, injection of the conjunctiva and pharynx, and a palpable spleen are other findings that may be observed. There is usually no unusual local reaction at the site of the tick bite.

COMPLICATIONS AND SEQUELAE. Complications of Colorado tick fever are rare and usually occur only in children. Encephalitis, meningitis, meningoencephalitis, and a hemorrhagic state resembling the hemorrhagic syndrome of dengue have occurred. Adults have developed pericarditis and myocarditis.

Many patients, especially those over 30 years of age, experience a prolonged convalescence with complaints of malaise and weakness. There is no apparent association between the length of convalescence and the duration of viremia. Immunity is usually life-long, but there is one documented case of reinfection (Goodpasture et al., 1978).

In laboratory animals, Colorado tick fever virus crosses the placenta and is teratogenic. Of the six known cases of Colorado tick fever in pregnant women, one woman aborted, four delivered normal infants, and one delivered an infant with multiple congenital abnormalities.

DIAGNOSIS. Usually the biphasic course and the leukopenia should suggest Colorado tick fever, particularly if there is a history of tick exposure. Dengue is the closest clinical analog of Colorado tick fever but can be distinguished by the mutually exclusive epidemiologic features of the two diseases. Dengue is transmitted by *Aedes* mosquitoes in tropic and subtropic regions. Influenza may have a similar abrupt onset and may also be accompanied by leukopenia but usually causes prominent respiratory complaints such as sore throat, cough, and chest pain. In areas that are endemic for Colorado tick fever, the disease is commonly confused with Rocky Mountain spotted fever

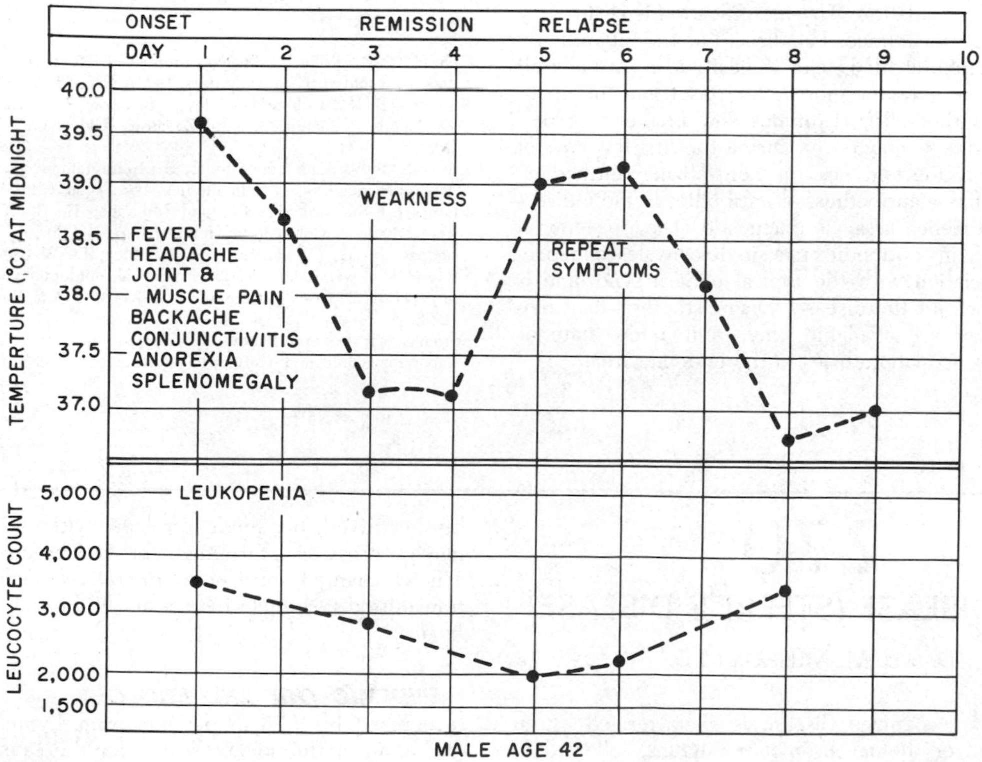

Figure 3. Temperature curve, clinical findings, and leukocyte count during the course of Colorado tick fever. (Adapted from Johnson, E. S., Napoli, V. M., and White, W. C.: Am J Clin Pathol 34:118, 1960.)

(Spruance and Bailey, 1973). Although this rickettsial disease is not as frequently diagnosed now in the Rocky Mountain area as in decades past, the agent is still recoverable from *D. andersoni* ticks. Rocky Mountain spotted fever can often be distinguished by the progressive rash that appears two to four days after onset, a tendency to cause leukocytosis, and a more severe, unremitting course. Tick-borne relapsing fever, caused by *Borrelia* species and transmitted by soft-body ticks of the genus *Ornithodoros*, can closely mimic Colorado tick fever. In relapsing fever, the leukocyte count is usually within normal limits, and the spirochete can be seen in blood smears obtained from the patient during a febrile episode or from weanling mice inoculated with the patient's blood. Specific serologic tests are available for Rocky Mountain spotted fever. Tularemia may be tick-borne but is usually accompanied by an ulcer at the tick bite and by lymphadenopathy. The agglutination test for tularemia is positive after 10 to 14 days.

Leukopenia, as noted above, is very common during Colorado tick fever. Leukocyte counts of between 2000 and 3000 per mm^3 are common. The lowest values occur during the beginning of the second febrile period. The white cell count may be normal during the initial stages of the illness. On blood smear, "toxic" neutrophils and atypical lymphocytes may be seen.

The diagnosis is confirmed by isolating the virus from blood, by identifying the agent in red cells by fluorescent antibody staining, or by serology. Because the viremia is cell-associated and because neutralizing antibody may be present in the plasma, a blood clot or erythrocytes washed free of plasma is the appropriate specimen for virus isolation and fluorescent antibody studies (Emmons, 1979). Red cells are homogenized and injected intraperitoneally or intracerebrally into suckling mice for virus isolation. The injection is usually lethal for mice, but serial passage may be necessary for isolation. The identification is verified by neutralization tests in mice. The direct fluorescent antibody stain of a peripheral blood clot is positive in virtually all human cases six days or more after onset and for up to several weeks thereafter (Emmons and Lennette, 1966). False-negative tests may occur during the first few days of the disease. A fourfold rise in neutralizing antibodies, complement-fixing antibodies, or antibodies in the indirect immunofluorescence assay is diagnostic. The presence of complement-fixing antibodies in a single convalescent specimen in association with the typical clinical syndrome is strong evidence for the disease. Diagnostic tests for Colorado tick fever are available only from a few state or regional reference laboratories in the endemic area.

TREATMENT. Treatment is symptomatic. Analgesics and antipyretics such as salicylates are usually adequate for control of headache and myalgia. When a patient with tick exposure is seriously ill, one should consider other tick-borne diseases such as Rocky Mountain spotted fever, relapsing fever, and tularemia.

PREVENTION. The cornerstone of prevention is avoidance of tick bites. Individuals who are outdoors in the endemic area during spring and summer should inspect their clothing, hair, and skin periodically with special attention to the hairline and axillae. If an attached tick is discovered, it can be removed by gentle backward traction. Trying to "unscrew" the tick will often only break off the body and leave the mouth parts embedded. A physician removing a tick from a patient should insert the tip of a needle under the head of the tick before applying traction with forceps. Application of an organic solvent such as alcohol or nail polish remover to the tick may aid detachment. A lighted match or other flame should not be used.

An experimental vaccine has been prepared from inactivated virus. Immunized volunteers developed high titers of neutralizing antibody. Vaccination would appear to be justifiable only for laboratory personnel and outdoor workers at high risk of exposure in the restricted ecologic niche of *D. andersoni*.

The Colorado tick fever patient is not contagious and need not be isolated at home or in the hospital. However, the patient's blood products should be considered potentially hazardous and should not be used for transfusion for at least six months after recovery.

References

Eklund, C. M., Kohls, G. M., and Brennan, J. M.: Distribution of Colorado tick fever and virus-carrying ticks. JAMA 157:335, 1955.

Emmons, R. W.: Colorado tick fever. In Beran, G. (ed.): CRC Handbook of Zoonoses. Section B: Viral Zoonoses. Cleveland, CRC Press, Inc., 1981.

Emmons, R. W., and Lennette, E. H.: Immunofluorescent staining in the laboratory diagnosis of Colorado tick fever. J Lab Clin Med 68:923, 1966.

Florio, L., Steward, M. O., and Mugrage, E. R.: The experimental transmission of Colorado tick fever. J Exp Med 80:165, 1944.

Goodpasture, H. C., Poland, J. D., Francy, D. B., Bowen, G. S., and Horn, K. A.: Colorado tick fever: Clinical, epidemiologic, and laboratory aspects of 228 cases in Colorado in 1973–1974. Ann Intern Med 88:303, 1978.

Spruance, S. L., and Bailey, A.: Colorado tick fever: A review of 115 laboratory confirmed cases. Arch Intern Med 131:288, 1973.

270

LYME DISEASE (STEERE'S DISEASE)

DANIEL M. MUSHER, M.D.

This newly recognized disease is characterized by an initial bout of erythema chronicum migrans, followed in some cases by neurologic or cardiac manifestations and frequently culminating in frank arthritis. The disease may be short lived, but tends to relapse without treatment and may progress to deforming arthritis. The etiologic agent is a newly named spirochete, *Borrelia burgdorferi*, that is transmitted to human beings by the bite of a tick, species *Ixodes*.

EPIDEMIOLOGY AND ETIOLOGY. Lyme disease was recognized in 1975 in patients from Lyme, Connecticut during an epidemiologic search for the cause of a cluster of cases of arthritis, often preceded by distinctive expanding annular skin lesions called erythema chronicum migrans.

This infection was later found to occur along the northeastern seaboard of the United States and isolated cases have been identified in north, central, and western states, as well as in France, Germany, Switzerland, and Australia. The etiology was discovered by Steere and his coworkers through application of classical epidemiologic techniques. Cases appeared between May 1 and November 30, with 80 per cent having their onset in June or July. The rural setting of case clusters and the identification of erythema chronicum migrans as a feature of the disease raised the possibility of an insect vector. The location of the skin lesions on the thigh, groin, and axilla suggested an arthropod vector, and one-fifth to one-third of patients gave the history of a tick bite. Examination of *Ixodes* ticks from endemic areas revealed that 20 to 80 per cent harbored a spirochete. A morphologically identical organism has been grown from mice and deer that are preferred hosts for the ticks and from skin lesions, blood, and/or cerebrospinal fluid of a few patients with the disease. This spirochete has recently been named *Borrelia burgdorferi*.

PATHOGENESIS AND PATHOLOGY. Three to 32 days after a tick bite (median, 7 days) a papule appears at the site, promptly followed by an expanding ringlike lesion called erythema chronicum migrans. In the center of the lesion there is acanthosis, spongiosis, parakeratosis, and/or keratinocyte necrosis of the epidermis with an intact basal layer. In the dermis, perivascular infiltrates are seen with lymphocytes and histiocytes predominating; edema is characteristic and nuclear fragments are also present. At the periphery of the lesions only the dermis is involved. Additional lesions that resemble the primary ones but are smaller and less aggressive, appear in about one-half of patients. Without treatment the median duration of the skin lesions is 28 days, but they may persist for one year; after resolution a recurrence is seen in one-fourth of patients.

About 3 to 4 weeks after the onset of erythema chronicum migrans, neurologic and cardiologic manifestations develop. Because of their resemblance to serum sickness and rheumatic fever, respectively, a pathogenetic role has been proposed for circulating immune complexes which are often present in these patients. Arthritis develops weeks to months after the onset of the skin lesions; its pathogenesis is obscure, but immune complexes are present in the joint fluid of such patients. Patients with severe and prolonged arthritis have a greatly increased likelihood of possessing the DR2 alloantigen, giving further support for an immunologic basis for the clinical manifestations. Histologic examination of affected joints reveals pannus formation with synovial proliferation. There is hypertrophy of synovial cells, vascular proliferation, and infiltration by lymphocytes and plasma cells.

CLINICAL ILLNESS

Early Infection. Lyme disease begins with erythema chronicum migrans, accompanied (and in one-third of cases, actually preceded) by generalized, systemic symptoms suggesting an acute infection. The skin lesions are distinctive and suggest the diagnosis. A flat, red, ringlike lesion begins around the papule caused by the tick bite and expands (Fig. 1). The central area may clear, remain red, or become more red with induration. Almost one-half of patients develop other lesions elsewhere on the body but not the palms and soles; there may be a few or up to 100 of these so-called secondary lesions, which resemble the initial one

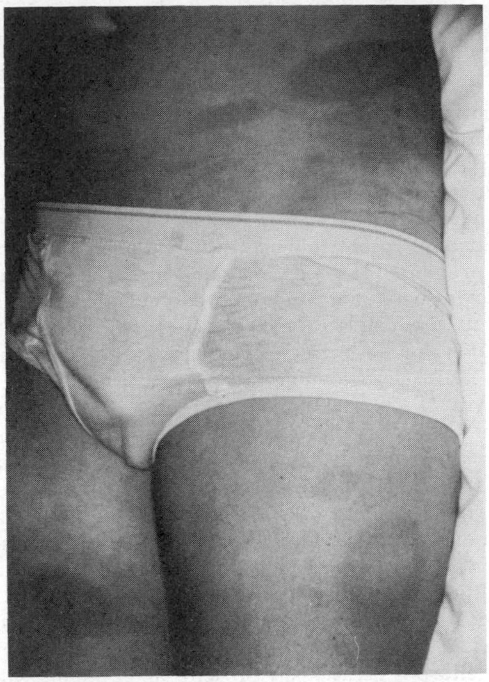

Figure 1. Flat red ring-like skin lesions of early Lyme disease. (Kindly provided by Dr. A. C. Steere, New Haven, Connecticut.)

except they lack a central papule or central induration. Systemic symptoms include malaise, fatigue, lethargy (in 80 per cent of cases), headache and/or stiff neck, (70 per cent) and fever (60 per cent); migratory arthralgias, myalgias, backache, anorexia, and sore throat are also present in decreasing frequency. The fever is usually low-grade in adults but may be high in children. The headache, somnolence and/or mental changes may suggest aseptic meningitis or even meningoencephalitis. About 10 per cent of patients have a hepatitis-like syndrome with nausea, vomiting and/or abdominal pain. An interesting feature of the early phase of Lyme disease is that different organ systems may be involved sequentially, giving a pleomorphic appearance to the clinical picture. In an undetermined number of patients, systemic symptoms and the later features may appear without the characteristic skin lesions. Although erythema chronicum migrans persists for up to 1 year without treatment, its mean duration is 28 days. After the lesions seem to have disappeared spontaneously, relapses develop in one-quarter of patients, sometimes triggered by exposure to sun or cold.

Physical findings in early infection, aside from the skin eruption, are unremarkable. Lymph nodes enlarge only in erythematous areas in 40 per cent of cases. In 20 per cent the node enlargement is generalized and suggests infectious mononucleosis. A malar rash, red throat, conjunctivitis, or enlarged liver and/or spleen are seen in less than 10 per cent of cases.

Except for a mild anemia, leukocytosis and/or hematuria in a few cases, blood counts and urinalyses are normal. The erythrocyte sedimentation rate is elevated in one-half of cases, and liver enzymes in one-fifth. Cerebrospinal fluid (CSF) has been normal in a few subjects who have undergone lumbar puncture in the early stage of infection.

Later Infection. About 3 to 4 weeks after the onset of erythema chronicum migrans, neurologic or cardiac manifestations may develop in 15 or 8 per cent of patients, respectively. Given the highly variable course of the erythema chronicum migrans, it is not surprising that the skin lesions may still be present, may have vanished, or may have disappeared and recurred. Most patients with neurologic involvement have symptoms of aseptic meningitis or meningoencephalitis. About one-half have mononeuritis multiplex, characterized by weakness or sensory changes in one or more cranial or peripheral nerves. Chorea or cerebellar ataxia is seen in some cases. Papilledema is occasionally present, and may occur even without increased CSF pressure. The CSF contains up to a few hundred leukocytes with mononuclears predominant, a slightly lowered glucose and a protein elevated to 2 to 5 times the normal value. Electroencephalograms are abnormal in some cases. Cryoglobulins are present in the serum in 80 per cent of cases and total IgM may also be elevated. Serum C3 and C4 levels are normal. The sedimentation rate is again elevated in one-half of cases. Most patients with neurologic manifestations of Lyme disease recover fully within 6 to 8 months, but weakness, sensory changes, and mental or behavioral abnormalities may persist in a few.

The heart rate shows either brady- or tachycardia. Fluctuating atrioventricular conduction block is the commonest finding in patients with cardiac involvement. Congestive heart failure is occasionally present, and patients who lack signs of failure may still have a decreased left ventricular ejection fraction. Nonspecific electrocardiographic findings suggesting diffuse myocardial involvement are found in one-half of patients with cardiologic involvement. Unlike neurologic findings, cardiac signs tend to resolve within 3 to 4 weeks and do not recur.

In contrast to the neurologic and cardiologic manifestations of Lyme diseases, which always appear within a few weeks of the onset of infection, arthritis may develop weeks to months or even years later. If not treated, about 60 per cent of those with Lyme disease develop arthritis. Within the first few months after infection the clinical picture is that of migratory polyarthritis or brief attacks of oligoarthritis in any joint. After 4 to 24 months of this intermittent arthritis, chronic arthritis develops, in a few patients most frequently in, but not restricted to, one or both knees. There is a thickened synovium with pannus and popliteal cysts may form and rupture. The disease resembles rheumatoid or juvenile rheumatoid arthritis but the laboratory and clinical signs of rheumatoid arthritis (symmetrical polyarthritis with morning stiffness or nodules) or other rheumatologic syndromes such as Reiter's disease or psoriasis are absent. This arthritis persists, and in affected joints, may cause all the disabilities that characterize rheumatoid disease.

DIAGNOSIS. Lyme disease is recognized by the presence of erythema chronicum migrans, which is not thought to occur in any other condition, especially in an area where this infection is present. Cardiologic or neurologic complaints following closely upon such a characteristic skin lesion should reinforce the diagnosis. Lyme disease must also be considered in patients from endemic areas who suddenly develop arthritic complaints and a history of the characteristic antecedent skin rash should be sought. Since Lyme arthritis may meet criteria for rheumatoid arthritis, differentiation must be made on epidemiologic considerations and the relation of its onset to erythema chronicum migrans. The test for rheumatoid factor is usually negative. The joint fluid usually has 10,000 to 25,000 cells (range 500 to 100,000) and most are polymorphonuclear leukocytes. Complement levels in the joint are not as low as in rheumatoid arthritis. Antibody determinations for the causative spirochete are the most helpful tests for differentiating Lyme arthritis from rheumatoid arthritis.

TREATMENT. Treatment of early Lyme disease with penicillin V or tetracycline, 500 mg orally four times daily for 10 days shortens the illness to a mean of about 5.5 days compared to 9.2 days for erythromycin and 2 to 3 weeks for untreated subjects. A few (5 to 10 per cent) require a second course of therapy for failure to respond or for relapse. In one study (Steere et al., 1983) of relatively few patients, treatment with penicillin reduced, but tetracycline eliminated cardiologic, neurologic, or arthritic sequelae, although some systemic symptoms of infection, such as lethargy and arthralgias recurred transiently in 50 per cent of subjects treated with either regimen. Thus, tetracycline is considered the preferred drug for treating Lyme disease in its early stages. A reaction resembling the Jarisch-Herxheimer reaction occurs in 15 per cent of treated patients.

In late disease, glucocorticosteroids appear to suppress neurologic and, to a lesser extent, cardiologic manifestations. Meningitis appears to respond well to penicillin, and 12,000,000 units intravenously daily is recommended. The mononeuritis multiplex is unaffected by antibiotic therapy but may respond at least partially to glucocorticosteroids. Antibiotics and aspirin are generally recommended for cardiac involvement although steroids are given for congestive heart failure or atrioventricular block in order to reduce myocardial inflammation.

Intraarticular injection of corticosteroids is recommended as needed. In some patients with progressive joint disease synovectomy has produced seemingly good results. The problem with interpreting the results of treatment is that, over a period of several years, the arthritis remits spontaneously in most cases.

References

Reik, L., Steere, A. C., Bartenhagen, N. H., Shope, R. E., and Malawista, S. E.: Neurologic abnormalities of Lyme disease. Medicine 58:281, 1979.

Steere, A. C., Gibofsky, A., Patarroyo, M. E., Winchester, R. J., Hardin, J. A., and Malawista, S. E.: Chronic Lyme arthritis: clinical and immunogenetic differentiation from rheumatoid arthritis. Ann Intern Med 90:896, 1979.

Steere, A. C., Batsford, W. P., Weinberg, M., Alexander, J., Berger, H. J., Wolfson, S., and Malawista, S. E.: Lyme carditis: cardiac abnormalities of Lyme disease. Ann Intern Med 93:8-16, 1980.

Steere, A. C., Bartenhagen, N. H., Craft, J. E., Hutchinson, G. J., Newman, J. H., Rahn, D. W., Sigal, L. H., Spieler, P. N., Stenn, K. S., and Malawista, S. E.: The early clinical manifestations of Lyme disease. Ann Intern Med 99:76, 1983.

Steere, A. C., Hutchinson, G. J., Rahn, D. W., Sigal, L. H., Craft, J. E., DeSanna, E. T., and Malawista, S. E.: Treatment of the early manifestations of Lyme disease. Ann Intern Med 99:22, 1983.

Steere, A. C., Grodzicki, R. L., Kornblatt, A. N., Craft, J. E., Barbour, A. G., Burgdorfer, W., Schmid, G. P., Johnson, E., and Malawista, S. E.: The spirochetal etiology of Lyme disease. N Engl J Med 308:733, 1983.

271
RELAPSING FEVER

Philip Higginbottom, M.D.

Relapsing fever is an acute febrile systemic disease caused by spirochetes of the genus *Borrelia,* which are transmitted to man by lice or soft back ticks. After a sudden attack of fever lasting 3 to 5 days, a series of fevers recur but are usually less intense and shorter.

The first well-documented epidemic of louse-borne relapsing fever occurred in 1739 in Ireland. It was first found in America in 1844 (Felsenfeld, 1971). During World War I, the incidence of louse-borne relapsing fever rose to unprecendented levels due to human crowding in military trenches and prison camps. Tick-borne relapsing fever was first recognized in 1857 and occurs endemically where man encounters infected *Ornithodoros* ticks.

ETIOLOGY AND TRANSMISSION. *Borrelia* are unicellular spiral organisms which stain easily with aniline dyes such as Wright and Giemsa stains (Fig. 1). They are usually 10 to 20μ long with 4 to 30 uneven coils. They multiply by transverse fission. Although lipopolysaccharide has not been demonstrated in borreliae, they do possess endotoxin-like activity (Butler, 1979). *Borreliae* are very difficult to cultivate on artificial media. As a consequence, the biochemistry, the immune response, and the genetics of the organisms are obscure. Current classification acknowledges multiple species of borreliae, but evidence that these species are antigenically and genetically distinct is lacking. Thus, they may eventually all be called *Borrelia recurrentis* when appropriate studies can be done. *Borrelia* are differentiated from the other two pathogenic spirochetes (*Treponema* and *Leptospira*) by the loose, irregularly spaced coils on borreliae. The number of axial fibrils is the other characteristic that separates the three genera of spirochetes. *Treponema pallidum* contains 6 to 10 axial fibrils, *Borrelia* species 30 to 40, and leptospirae only 2 (Felsenfeld, 1971). It is customary to accept *B. recurrentis* as the only species that causes louse-borne (epidemic) relapsing fever, but many species of borreliae cause tick-borne (endemic) relapsing fever. The species names of these borreliae are usually derived from the 15 species of soft back ticks which transmit them to man (Table 1).

Two different vectors transmit borreliae to man. *Pediculis humanis* spreads *B. recurrentis*. The crab louse, *Phthirus pubis*, cannot transmit this organism. *B. recurrentis* has no natural animal reservoir and cannot be passed transovarially to louse progeny. Thus, human crowding and weather cool enough to require clothing are important features of epidemics. Lice are host-specific; after they feed on infected human blood, 12 to 50 per cent become infected (Felsenfeld, 1971). Borreliae find their way from the gut of the louse to the coelomic cavity (hemolymph) where they multiply throughout the several week life span of the louse. The louse must die in order to transmit *Borrelia* to man because the coelomic fluid does not flow out unless the louse is crushed, usually when the victim scratches his bite. Within five to eight days, clinical illness begins.

Tick-borne relapsing fever is transmitted by a number of *Ornithodoros* species that feed exclusively on blood. In addition to man, chipmunks and other rodents act as reservoirs. The ticks are also often found in caves or on walls of primitive wooden cabins. The painless bite of ticks is critical for transmission of tick-borne relapsing fever. Bites usually occur at night. All species of ticks transmit borreliae to their ova but the penetration of larvae by borreliae varies markedly from 2 to 100 per cent of eggs, depending on the species of tick. Thus, although the average lifespan of ticks is only 2 years, there is always a new population of infected ticks that transmit the organism among natural animal reservoirs, making tick-borne borreliosis an endemic zoonotic disease. Domestic animals in the U. S. are not hosts for these specific tick vectors. Consequently, most infections are acquired in rural settings where man enters the natural habitat of the rodent reservoirs. Because ticks, unlike lice, do not have to be damaged, crushed, or killed to infect man, a single tick can infect multiple animals or people. Adult ticks usually transfer borreliae through their coxal fluid, which is excreted during or after a 30-minute feeding.

Borreliae also can be transmitted by blood transfusion (Wang, 1936) and by transplacental transmission (Fuchs, 1969). These routes are rare because of the care taken to

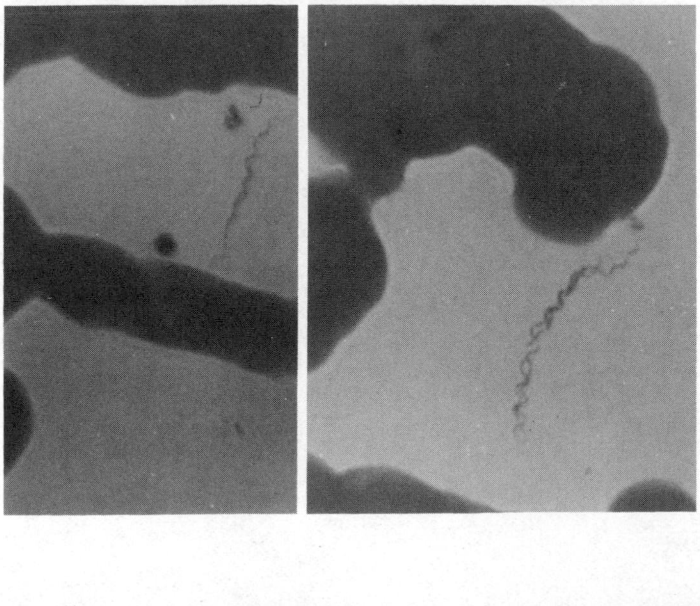

Figure 1. *Borrelia recurrentis* in smear of peripheral blood of patient with relapsing fever in San Diego. The spirochetes have loose coils (Wright stain × 1800).

Table 1. GEOGRAPHIC DISTRIBUTION OF BORRELIAE CAUSING RELAPSING FEVER

Major Geographic Locations	*Vector*	*Borrelia*
Western North and South America, and Central America	O. turicata	B. turicatae
	O. talaje	B. mazzottii
	O. talaje	B. dugesii
Western North America	O. parkeri	B. parkerii
	O. hermsi	B. hermsii
South America	O. rudis	B. venezolensis
Asia, Africa, and the Mediterranean	O. moubata	B. duttonii
	O. tholozani	B. persica
	O. tartakovskyi	B. latyschewii
	O. erraticus sonrai	B. crocidurae
		B. microti
		B. merionesi
		B. dipodilli
	O. erraticus erraticus	B. hispanica
World Wide	Pediculus humanus	B. recurrentis

exclude febrile blood donors and because pregnant women who develop relapsing fever usually abort.

PATHOGENESIS AND PATHOLOGY. Borreliae, like trypanosomes, can change their antigenic structure so that they escape the immune response and cause a relapse of fever every 7 to 9 days. The exact mechanism of this antigenic variation is not known. Early investigators (Cunningham, 1925) found that peak antibody titers to relapse spirochetes appeared in the order in which the spirochete populations were isolated from blood. It was felt that growth of a new population of organisms accounted for each relapse. The demonstration of elevated antibody titers just before the termination of the first attack added support to this hypothesis (Calabi, 1959). Recently, Barbour (1982) used serotype-specific antisera and monoclonal antibodies to demonstrate a variable protein in the cell lysates of *B. hermsii.* This protein appears to be the surface antigen that changes in each relapse population of organisms originally derived from a single *Borrelia.*

The bulk of borreliae remain inside the vasculature with particular predilection for terminal arterioles, capillaries, small veins, and the sinusoids of the liver, spleen, and bone marrow. The central nervous system is also penetrated and may be the reservoir for relapse in some cases. Bleeding and thrombocytopenia are common in relapsing fever. These manifestations and fever may be caused by a pyrogenic portion of the spirochete that is not a true endotoxic lipopolysaccharide (Butler, 1979).

Pathologic differences between tick-borne and louse-borne disease are minimal. Nervous system involvement seems to be more prominent in tick-borne disease. Extensive hepatitis and hepatocellular damage are reflected in rises in the transaminase levels to three times normal. Total bilirubin usually rises to about 5 to 7 mg % but can go higher. Renal function may be mildly compromised. A mild myocarditis may occur and focal areas of myocardial necrosis appear in fatal cases. Primary involvement of the lungs is rare. When the central nervous system is involved, the spinal fluid may contain 3 to 1400 white cells with equal numbers of polymorphonuclear leukocytes and lymphocytes (Hawking, 1941). The spinal fluid glucose and protein are usually normal.

The events that terminate the fever and clear the bloodstream of spirochetes are not clear. Most early authors felt that immobilizing or lytic antibody was responsible. Recently, in vitro studies have demonstrated that both phagocytes and antibody attack *B. recurrentis* (Spagnuolo, 1982). The organism probably induces the production of both IgM and IgG antibody. IgM may act as a lytic antibody in the presence of complement. IgM antibody and the third component of complement may act as opsonins that enable polymorphonuclear leukocytes and macrophages to engulf borreliae via the C3b receptor. IgG may also be opsonic via the Fc receptor of phagocytes. When a relapse occurs, the new wave of organisms usually has a different serotype-specific protein (Barbour, 1982) and phagocytosis and lysis may become ineffective until new specific antibody directed against that protein is generated.

CLINICAL MANIFESTATIONS. Louse-borne and tick-borne disease cannot be differentiated clinically. Although tick-borne relapsing fever is more severe, the epidemiologic setting of the disease is the most helpful clue in separating the two. The clinical syndrome of relapsing fever is separable into three phases: the incubation phase, the acute attack, and the relapse. Five to ten days after a tick or louse bite, symptoms start abruptly with frank, violent chills and severe headache (Southern, 1969 and Bryceson, 1970). Photophobia, joint pains, cough, and muscle tenderness are present in more than half of the patients. Fever persists for 3 to 5 days. Bleeding, usually epistaxis or purpura, occurs in a quarter of patients. None of these symptoms are specific for borreliosis and the diagnosis rests on examination of the blood for *Borreliae.*

During the acute attack, the patient is toxic with dry skin and fever to 39.4 to 40°C. Blood pressure is normal, but the sensorium is dull. The insect bite is almost never apparent, but if present, a small hemorrhage surrounds it. Meningismus is common. Tender splenomegaly, found in 40 to 70 per cent of cases, is the hallmark of the disease and parallels the necrotic miliary splenic foci (Russell, 1932). The liver is large and tender in half the patients and there is biochemical evidence of hepatocellular necrosis.

The crisis starts abruptly about 5 days after the initial rigor. It may be heralded by a maculopapular rash most prominent over the shoulders. Profuse diaphoresis and extreme weakness develop suddenly and severe fatigue persists for several days. In most patients, no fever is reported once this phase begins but low-grade pyrexia may persist in rare patients. The first relapse of tick-borne disease begins suddenly and occurs six days after the crisis.

In louse-borne disease, relapse is slightly later. Three to five relapses ensue in untreated, tick-borne relapsing fever. Louse borne disease usually only relapses once or twice. In both the symptoms become progressively less intense with each relapse and the duration of fever is shortened to two days or less. Eventually, even untreated patients usually recover.

COMPLICATIONS AND SEQUELAE. Death is uncommon in sporadic relapsing fever but mortality rates can reach 30 per cent during epidemics. The variation in mortality rates probably reflects not only differences in the parasites, but also differences in host nutrition and general health. Non-fatal sequelae lasting more than 6 weeks are unusual. Rupture of the spleen is the most catastrophic, but is extremely rare. Iritis and iridocyclitis are not uncommon; 61 carefully documented cases have been reported (Gaud, 1947/48). Scarring, synechiae, and decreased visual acuity are the major sequelae.

Hemorrhage, secondary to thrombocytopenia, is usually manifested by epistaxis, but gastrointestinal blood loss can occur. Abortion is the rule in infected pregnant women and is thought to be due to retroplacental hemorrhage. Endocardial involvement and heart murmurs were described frequently in one outbreak but have been uncommon in others. Neurologic sequelae such as paralysis, cranial nerve palsies, and psychoses are infrequent, and other causes should be sought before they are attributed to borreliosis.

GEOGRAPHIC VARIATIONS IN DISEASE. Epidemics of louse-borne relapsing fever can occur anywhere since there are no countries without lice. Ethiopia harbors the only endemic focus of *B. recurrentis* (Bryceson, 1970). Migratory labor continuously provides a new nonimmune population in Ethiopia and the shortage of water for laundering and bathing during several months of the year promotes the spread of lice. Small outbreaks of louse-borne relapsing fever can occur whenever the spirochete is introduced into a lice-infested population.

Tick-borne borreliosis is a much more restricted disease in man. Its geographic location coincides with the habitat of *Ornithodoros* ticks. In the United States, this tick is most common at altitudes of at least 5,000 feet, but it is occasionally found as low as 3,000 feet above sea level. In Africa, the extent of *B. duttoni*, transmitted by *Ornithodoros moubata*, is incompletely defined. Eastern Africa reported large epidemics during World War II. Subsequently, the use of pesticides has significantly decreased the incidence of tick-borne disease, but it is still present in Kenya, Tanzania, and Southwest Africa (Walton, 1964). Tick-borne disease is still endemic in Asia where the species is *B. persica* transmitted by *Ornithodoros tholozani*. Because the walls of crude buildings are the sites where most ticks are found, the use of insecticides around the base of the walls has reduced human disease. Panama and much of the West Coast of South America are also endemic areas. Australia may be the only part of the world free of human borreliosis.

DIAGNOSIS. Relapsing fever is easily diagnosed in the midst of an epidemic. The sporadic case of tick-borne disease in a camper, a hunter, or a traveler is more difficult. The differential diagnosis of borreliosis is very narrow when the appropriate history is taken; malaria and typhus are the major considerations.

The peripheral bloodsmear stained by the Wright or Giemsa method will often establish the diagnosis. Loosely coiled spirochetes in the stained smear are diagnostic (Fig. 1). Thick smears are made with three to four times as much blood and thus increase the likelihood of a positive smear. Dark field examination is preferred by some because borreliae are easily spotted in their live, motile state. To examine dark field slides, a drop of blood on a glass slide is covered with a glass cover slip and sealed with mounting media or paraffin. Borreliae remain viable and motile for several hours. If tissue is obtained, silver stains such as the Dieterle or Warthin-Starry are excellent for demonstrating spirochetes. This silver method worked well on splenic tissue, reviewed 11 years after an autopsy when an astute pathologist reconsidered the diagnosis (Cleland, 1938).

Intraperitoneal inoculation of 1 to 2 ml of blood or spinal fluid into 6-to-8-week-old mice increases the chances of establishing the diagnosis in difficult cases with negative blood smears. After 48 to 72 hours spirochetes can usually be demonstrated in smears of blood obtained from the heart or tail vein of infected mice. This method may demonstrate spirochetemia during apyrexic periods of the disease.

Xenodiagnosis has been used widely but the problems of maintaining a tick colony make it impractical. Serologic studies are not helpful.

TREATMENT. Untreated borreliosis resolves by crisis 5 to 10 days after the onset of spirochetemia. Convalescent immune human serum in a dose of 20 ml intravenously was effective treatment in a North African outbreak where 32 treated patients exhibited a prompt crisis within 5 hours (Gaud, 1947/48).

Crises brought on by antibiotics or immune serum are initiated by the Jarisch-Herxheimer reaction, i.e., paradoxical exacerbation of clinical signs. Careful study of these reactions (Bryceson, 1970, Warrell, 1983) has not revealed circulating endotoxin despite the fact that their hallmarks are hypotension, transient leukopenia, and fever, which are classic manifestations of endotoxemia. The Herxheimer reaction is treated with at least 2000 ml of 0.9 per cent saline intravenously before antibiotic therapy. Neither acetaminophen nor hydrocortisone have aborted the reaction, but the opioid antagonist Meptazinol reduced its clinical severity (Teklu, 1983).

Tetracycline is the drug of choice for the treatment of both tick and louse-borne relapsing fever. A seven-day oral course of 500 mg four times a day is effective. Single dose oral therapy has been used in louse-borne disease, in the form of either doxycycline 100 mg, tetracycline 500 mg, or erythromycin 500 mg. For patients with vomiting, Bryceson (1970) preferred an initial intravenous dose of 250 mg of tetracycline followed by oral therapy (Bryceson, 1970).

Many authors suggest longer treatment of tick-borne disease, usually 10 days. The drug of choice remains tetracycline, which clears the nervous system and the reticulo-endothelial infection. Oral chloramphenicol at 500 mg four times daily for 10 days is effective but marrow toxicity is a risk. Pregnant women and children should be given erythromycin 500 mg orally 4 times a day for 10 days to avoid permanent dental staining.

PROPHYLAXIS. Immunization is not practical because so little is known of the biology of the parasite. In endemic regions of Africa, some natives are said to carry with them a tick that they allow to feed on them sporadically. It is unclear whether this aids in the development of natural immunity. Prophylaxis with doxycycline or similar drugs has not been studied. It is likely that prophylaxis would be effective in travelers planning short trips to known endemic areas.

The most useful preventive measure has been the application of insecticides around the inner walls of the crude buildings that often harbor ticks. Insecticides and the avoidance of human crowding brought about by war and other disasters will limit this disease more than antibiotics in the next decade.

REFERENCES

Barbour, A. G., Tessier, S. L., and Stoenner, H. G.: Variable major proteins of Borrelia hermsii. J. Exp. Med. 156:1312, 1982.

Bryceson, A. D. M., Parry, E. H. O., Perine, P. L., Warrell, D. A., Vukovich, D., and Leithead, C. S.: Louse-borne relapsing fever: a clinical and laboratory study of 62 cases in Ethiopia and a reconsideration of the literature. QJM 39:129, 1970.

Butler, T., Hazen, P., Wallace, C. K., Awoke, S., and Habte-Michael, A.: Infection with Borrelia recurrentis: pathogenesis of fever and petechiae. J. Inf. Dis. 140:665, 1979.

Calabi, Ornella: The presence of plasma inhibitors during the crisis phenomenon in experimental relapsing fever (Borrelia novyi). J. Exp. Med. 110:811, 1959.

Cleland, J. B.: A death from relapsing fever in Australia. Med. J. Australia 1:820–21, 1938.

Cunningham, J.: Serologic observations on relapsing fever in Madras. Royal Soc. Trop. Med. and Hyg. 19:11, 1925.

Felsenfeld, O.: Borrelia: strains, vectors, human and animal borrelosis. St. Louis, Warren H. Green, 1971.

Fuchs, P. C., Oyama, A. A.: Neonatal relapsing fever due to transplacental transmission of Borrelia. JAMA 208:690, 1969.

Gaud, M., and Morgan, M. T.: Epidemiological study of relapsing fever in North Africa (1943–1945). Bull. World Health Org. 1:69, 1947/48.

Hawking, Frank: Relapsing fever: cerebrospinal fluid and therapy. J. Trop. Med. and Hyg. 44:104–5, 1941.

Russell, H.: The pathology of the spleen in relapsing fever. Trans. Roy. Soc. Trop. Med. and Hyg. 26:259, 1932.

Southern, P. M., Jr., and Sanford, J. P.: Relapsing fever: a clinical and microbiologic review. Medicine 48:129, 1969.

Spagnuolo, P. J., Butler, T., Bloch, E. H., Santoro, C. Tracy, J. W., and Johnson, R. C.: Opsonic requirements for phagocytosis of Borrelia hermsii by human polymorphonuclear leukocytes. J. Inf. Dis. 145:358, 1982.

Teklu, B., Habte-Michael, A., Warrell, D. A., White, N. J., and Wright, D. J. M.: Meptazinol diminishes the Jarisch-Herxheimer reaction of relapsing fever. Lancet 1:835, 1983.

Walton, G. A.: The *Ornithodoros* "Moubata" group of ticks in Africa: Control problems and implications. J. Med. Ent. 1:53–64, 1964.

Wang, C. W., and Lee, C. U.: Malaria and relapsing fever following blood transfusion. Chinese Med. J., 50:241, 1936.

Warrell, D. A., Perine, P. L., Krause, D. W., Bing, D. H., and MacDougal, S. J.: Pathophysiology and immunology of the Jarisch-Herxheimer-like reaction in louse-borne relapsing fever: comparison of tetracycline and slow-release penicillin. J. Inf. Dis. 147:898, 1983.

K. ILLNESSES SIMULATING INFECTIONS

272

FACTITIOUS AND DELUSIONAL ILLNESSES SIMULATING INFECTIONS

J. ALLEN MCCUTCHAN, M.D.

Certain illnesses simulate infections but are self-inflicted or delusional. In order to deceive their physicians, psychologically disturbed patients may injure themselves by causing factitious infections. These patients sometimes present additional signs or symptoms of other hereditary, metabolic, immunologic, or traumatic conditions (Aduan et al., 1979; Petersdorf and Bennett, 1957; Rumans and Vosti, 1978; Reich and Gottfried, 1983). Because of the multiple and sometimes exotic agents and syndromes of infection, the possibility of deception is often overlooked until extensive diagnostic evaluations have been repeated several times.

Factitious illnesses seen at three major medical centers in the United States have been recently reviewed (Aduan et al., 1979; Rumans and Vosti, 1978; Reich and Gottfried, 1983). The cases collected in these series suggest that these diseases are uncommon but not rare. For example, factitious fever accounted for 32 of 342 (9 per cent) cases referred to the National Institutes of Health for evaluation of prolonged, unexplained fever. The first part of this chapter describes the clinical syndromes, psychopathology, diagnosis, and management of these difficult and confounding patients. The second part deals with delusional illnesses that simulate infection.

DEFINITIONS. *Factitious illness* is the simulation or production of illnesses with the intent of deception. In *simulated disease*, data or symptoms are falsified to mimic illness when none exists (for example, heating a thermometer to simulate fever). *Self-inflicted disease* is unacknowledged self-injury that produces real illness. Although illnesses (for example, lung cancer) may result from chronic self-injury (smoking), the intent is not to injure or defraud, and activity is not concealed. In contrast to those who intentionally deceive their physicians, patients with delusional illnesses believe they have a disease when none exists. Thus, *delusional disease* is obsessive belief in a nonexistent illness (for example, delusions of parasitosis) after reassurance by a physician. Rarely, parents cause simulated disease in their children, medical personnel falsify clinical data about patients, and groups of patients may share delusions (epidemic hysteria).

Several conditions related to factitious illness require definition and differentiation. *Malingering* refers to fraudulent illness practiced for some clear gain (Asher, 1959). Because the gain may be socially acceptable (for example, escape from prison camps in wartime), malingerers are not necessarily psychologically disturbed or sociopathic. Physicians can usually recognize malingering easily because the motive (for example, transfer from jail to the hospital) is obvious. *Munchausen's syndrome* refers to a distinct subgroup of chronic fraudulent illnesses in which wandering, homeless men repeatedly simulate dramatic acute illnesses (Cramer et al., 1971).

PATHOGENESIS. Factitious illnesses occur in patients who have both the motivation and skills to simulate or produce illness. The motivation is not well understood, and the degree of psychological disturbance varies widely. Psychiatric diagnoses in these patients range from malingering to schizophrenia, but many patients lack easily recognizable psychological disturbances. Malingerers achieve secondary gains from their illness, which most physicians recognize in obviously sociopathic persons. When apparently well-adjusted people use self-inflicted illness to avoid responsibility, gain attention, or manipulate others, malingering is not so obvious. Patients with chronic factitious illness include several groups with moderately severe psychological disturbances often described as "borderline personalities" (Asher, 1959). Munchausen's syndrome describes a group of male wanderers who present in dramatic fashion to hospital emergency rooms with elaborate false medical histories and assumed identities. They often submit to extensive, invasive, and potentially dangerous diagnostic and therapeutic procedures and then abruptly leave against medical advice. Their motivation and psychopathology are not understood. More common, but less easily recognized, are young, usually female, medical and paramedical personnel. For example, Reich and Gottfried found that 28 of 41 patients diagnosed in a Boston teaching hospital with factitious illnesses were in medically related occupations; 39 were female and they ranged in age from 16 to 51 (mean 33). Twenty five of the 41 had illnesses suggesting infection such as sepsis (12), non-healing wounds (8), fever (4), or urinary tract infection (1). These patients have a variety of psychiatric syndromes ranging from neuroses, conversion reactions, borderline personalities, and transient psychoses. Many of them appear to have an underlying personality disorder characterized by hostility, dependency, hysteria, and self-destruction. On the other hand, many are conscientious workers without obvious psychological problems. Because psychopathology in these patients is usually not obvious, their physicians often fail to consider the possibility of fraudulent illness and to deny it when consultants suggest it. Further self-destructive behavior in the form of suicide is unusual but must be borne in mind.

Medical and paramedical workers are heavily represented among patients with factitious illnesses for several reasons. They have the necessary skills, knowledge, and access to equipment. They may have selected a medical career because of the need to form dependent relationships with physicians. Moreover, their hostility and dependency toward physicians may have developed because of their relative occupational status or individual relationships with physicians. Other persons with the equipment and skills necessary for self-infection are intravenous drug users and insulin-dependent diabetics.

CLINICAL SYNDROMES. Factitious illnesses can be classified by the methods of deception, the diseases they mimic, or the psychopathology of the patients. The following classification divides these illnesses by clinical syndrome.

Factitious Fever

Simulated Fever. Falsification of temperatures to mimic prolonged unexplained fever is the most widely recognized factitious infectious disease. By definition, real fever and its symptoms are absent, but some of these patients deliberately prolong a real febrile illness. Objective evidence of a real disease early in its course often dissuades the physician from considering the diagnosis of factitious prolongation of the fever.

The two major techniques for falsifying fever are warming the thermometer or substituting thermometers with preset recordings. Various sources of heat (water, light bulbs, cigarette lighters, and hair dryers) have been used. Patients may also submit fraudulent temperature records taken at home or in other hospitals. The major clues to the diagnosis are lack of objective signs of disease, bizarre temperature patterns, other factitious symptoms, and manipulative behavior during temperature recording. When these patients are examined immediately after a high temperature is recorded, they have neither the tachycardia, skin warmth, and flushing of high fever, nor the cool, wet skin found after recent defervescence. Temperature readings more than 41.1° C and rapid, nonphysiologic changes in fever should arouse suspicion. Carefully monitored temperature recordings show no fever. This syndrome occurs most commonly in paramedical personnel whose knowledge of hospital routine makes it easy for them to deceive the nursing staff. Other factitious diseases may coexist with fever but usually do not.

The first two illustrative cases outlined below were reported by Rumans and Vosti (1978). The first patient's age, sex, occupation, history of emotional problems, and methods of deception are typical of factitious fever in paramedical personnel. The second case illustrates the problem of factitious prolongation of fever after a real febrile illness in a school-age adolescent. The third case (communicated from Lausanne, Switzerland, by M. Potin, M. P. Glauser, and C. L. Regamey) illustrates the difficulty in diagnosis when serious diseases that cause fever coexist with factitious fever.

Case 1. **A 28-year-old registered nurse was admitted after a 10-day course of pain in the right lower abdominal quadrant. Her intrauterine contraceptive (Dalkon shield) was removed without improvement. Admission temperature was 37.0° C with a pulse of 70. Pelvic exam revealed only minimal tenderness; complete blood count was normal; cultures of blood, urine, and cervix were negative; and radiologic examination of colon and intravenous pyelogram were normal. Laparoscopy and cystoscopy discovered no disease. On oral cephalosporin therapy, she had repeatedly elevated temperatures as high as 40° C without accompanying tachycardia. The nursing staff was instructed to measure the temperature very carefully with a nurse in attendance at the bedside. Despite these instructions, the patient was able repeatedly to manipulate those responsible for obtaining an accurate record of her temperature; that is, she would leave the bed to go to the bathroom with the thermometer in place or she would wear electric hair curlers while her temperature was taken. Frequent measurements gave the following pattern of temperature: 10:15 A.M., 38.6° C; 10:45 A.M., 36.6° C; 11:15 A.M., 37.2° C; 12 Noon, 39.5° C; 12:30 P.M., 37.3° C. Corresponding pulse rates were 80 to 94/minute. No antipyretics were given.**

The patient was confronted with these findings by her private gynecologist. She denied any attempted manipulation of the thermometer. A significant past history for emotional problems was obtained, including a history of child abuse. In addition, she had recently experienced a stormy breakup with a boyfriend of long standing and described marked distress with her job. She was discharged with no antibiotics and subsequently returned to work. There has been no recurrence of fever or abdominal pain.

Case 2. **A 16-year-old woman student had persistent fever for 6 months following acute right otitis media with drainage. Ampicillin for 2 months failed to affect the fevers (38.5 to 39.0° C), and the patient stayed home from school. After stopping ampicillin, her fevers increased to between 39 and 40° C, but diaphoresis, chills, weight loss, and drainage were absent. The patient attended school but went to bed promptly on arriving home. Admission temperature was 39.0° C with pulse of 70/minute. The right ear canal was red, but the tympanic membrane was normal. CBC was normal, sedimentation rate was 27 mm/minute. Radiographic exam of mastoids and chest, blood cultures, and bone marrow exam were normal. When rectal temperature measurements were carefully monitored because of the lack of tachycardia with fever, she remained afebrile.**

Case 3 (Fig. 1). **A 45-year-old healthy white man was admitted to the Central Hospital of the University of Vaud, Lausanne, Switzerland, after three weeks of exertional dyspnea, cough, alternating sweats and chills, loss of about 5 kg body weight, and pulsatile headaches. Admission fever was 39.7° C, and pulse was 135/min. He also had meningismus but the rest of the examination was unremarkable. The sedimentation rate was 68 mm, and leukocyte count 19.900/mm^3 with a left shift (30% bands). There were 52 leukocytes in his cerebrospinal fluid of which 47 per cent were polymorphonuclear leukocytes. Cerebral CT showed pansinusitis without cerebral abscess. Group C streptococcus was recovered from the blood and maxillary sinus pus. The maxillary sinuses were surgically drained and the patient was given ampicillin (12 g per day) and chloramphenicol (4 g per day) with resolution of fevers.**

Two months after the admission, a lymph node biopsy revealed Hodgkin's disease (nodular sclerosing stage Ib), following which the patient became increasingly febrile to 38 to 38.5°C. Radiotherapy of 4,500 rads over a period of five weeks was delivered to all nodal regions above the diaphragm. Because fever continued, an exploratory laparotomy and splenectomy was performed, but no sub-diaphragmatic spread of the tumor was found. Fever did not abate one month after his laparotomy and he was given a trial of chemotherapy for occult tumor. After two weeks of treatment, the patient remained febrile.

While frontal osteitis was being considered, the patient was found manipulating his thermometer. Temperatures taken under strict supervision always remained less than 37.0°C (Fig. 1). Retrospectively, it was discovered that the patient was observed manipulating his thermometer early in his hospitalization, but the physicians were not informed. On several occasions physicians had asked his nurses to remain next to the patient while taking his temperature and they claimed to have done so. It was only when the physician himself took the temperature that the fraud was discovered. The nurses had such confidence in the patient's veracity after his several months in the hospital that they considered it unnecessary to supervise him.

Self-Inflicted Fever. Fever, without local signs of infection, may result from skillful intravenous injection of sterile pyrogens, cultures of bacteria, other contaminated material (such as sputum, urine, or feces), or allergens such as foreign proteins. Blood cultures may document the presence of bacteremia. Repeated isolation of the same organism may simulate endocarditis. Polymicrobial bacteremia might suggest an occult biliary tract, gastrointestinal, or genitourinary infection. Ingestion or intravenous injection of allergens is a less common method of producing fever and may simulate febrile rheumatologic, metabolic, or infectious diseases. Since the fever is real, these patients have the usual signs and symptoms of fever and defervescence.

The cases below were reported by Aduan and his colleagues at the National Institutes of Health in Bethesda (Aduan et al., 1979). The patient described in Case 4 produced polymicrobial bacteremia probably by intravenous injection of feces. In Case 5, a patient with access to pure cultures of bacteria injected herself subcutaneously many times. In the hospital, she produced *Staphylococcus aureus* and *Pseudomonas* bacteremia with hypotension probably by deep subcutaneous or intravenous self-injection.

Case 4. **A 25-year-old, white licensed practical nurse was admitted with fever and abdominal pain for 10 months. Nine years before admission, the patient had suffered right lower quadrant pain and had undergone an exploratory laparotomy with removal of a right ovarian cyst and a normal appendix. One year before admission, because of recurrent abdominal pain, she underwent a second exploratory laparotomy with**

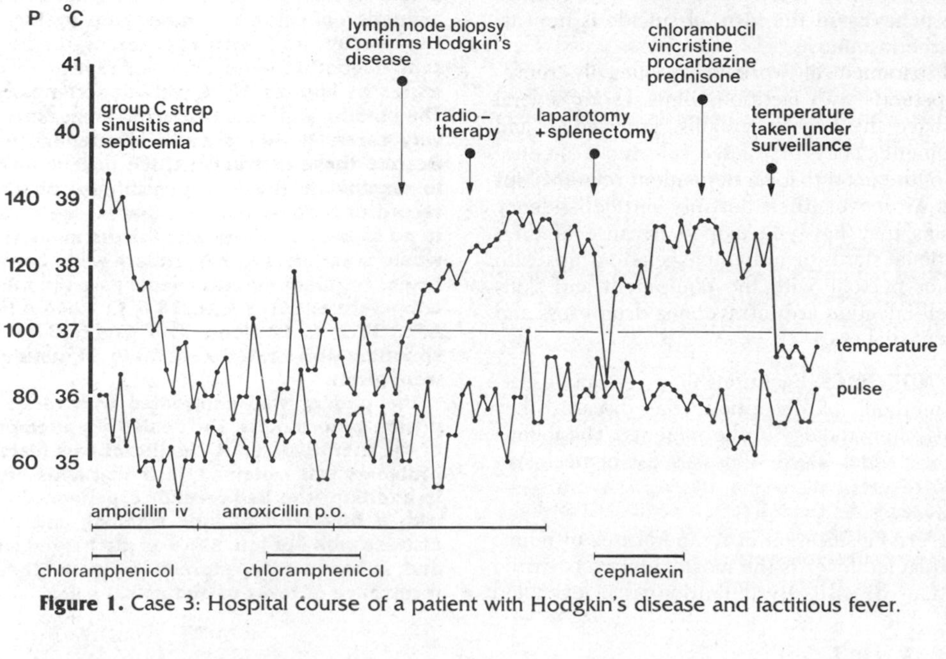

Figure 1. Case 3: Hospital course of a patient with Hodgkin's disease and factitious fever.

a right oophorectomy and removal of a left ovarian cyst. Ten months before admission, she developed fever and abdominal pain. Initial urine and blood cultures grew *Klebsiella* species. Subsequent blood cultures grew *Clostridia* species, *E. coli,* anaerobic diphtheroids, and another species of *Klebsiella.* Because a pelvic abscess was suspected, the patient underwent her third exploratory laparotomy, which revealed only splenomegaly. Seven months before admission, she was evaluated at a major hospital center. Blood cultures were again positive for multiple different organisms including *E. coli,* two *Bacillus* species, *Pseudomonas maltophilia,* and *Klebsiella* sp. Celiac angiography suggested a splenic abscess, and the patient underwent her fourth exploratory laparotomy. Again, only splenomegaly was found. Four months before admission, she again developed abdominal pain, fever, and shock. Repeat celiac angiography was negative, but subsequent abdominal radiographic contrast studies suggested a pancreatic cyst. Because of continued episodes of pain, she required three additional hospitalizations and large doses of narcotic analgesics. Factitious fever had been considered by this patient's referring physician but was not proved.

At admission, her temperature was 37.2° C rectally. Physical examination revealed numerous areas of induration on her buttocks and anterior thighs bilaterally from intramuscular injections of analgesics. A grade 2/6 systolic murmur was heard. Multiple well-healed surgical scars were noted on the abdomen. Leukocyte count was 4000/mm with a normal differential count; erythrocyte sedimentation rate was 70 mm/hour. Other laboratory serologic tests were negative. The patient complained of severe abdominal pain and had multiple temperature spikes up to 40° C rectally. Two days after admission, she had an episode of polymicrobial bacteremia with blood cultures growing *Klebsiella, E. coli, Proteus morgani,* and Group D streptococcus. Subsequent blood cultures were negative. Extensive diagnostic evaluation failed to reveal a septic focus. Because of the high index of suspicion of factitious fever or self-induced bacteremia, the patient's room was searched. Several syringes, needles, and an open bottle of local anesthetic (lidocaine) were found.

A psychiatric consultant made a diagnosis of borderline personality disorder. The patient denied self-injection or possession of needles and syringes and never admitted to inducing either her fevers or infections. She was referred for inpatient psychiatric care at another institution.

During the next 3 months, she had an unsuccessful trial of psychotherapy. Hypnosis, with posthypnotic suggestion, was used unsuccessfully to treat her persistent abdominal pain (conversion reaction). She made four suicide attempts during this period and underwent 14 electroconvulsive treatments. Some progress was made by using behavior modification. The final psychiatric diagnosis was (1) hysterical personality, severe, with depressive neurosis, or (2) borderline state with hysterical features.

Case 5. A 28-year-old, white laboratory technologist had a 5-year history of fever and recurrent skin lesions. She claimed to have a lifelong history of skin lesions attributed to "staphylococcal infections." At age 15, she had an apparent episode of acute rheumatic fever manifested by arthritis and a heart murmur. Over the next 6 years, she received penicillin prophylaxis. Her heart murmur was subsequently not heard. Five years before admission, she developed the first of many episodes of fever, chills, and erythematous skin lesions on the extremities. Blood cultures were negative, a heart murmur was again heard, however, and a presumptive diagnosis of subacute bacterial endocarditis was made. The patient was treated for 4 weeks with antibiotics. Her fever and skin lesions recurred when the antibiotics were withdrawn, and the patient was treated for an additional 6 weeks with antibiotics for a presumed relapse of endocarditis.

Intermittent fever and erythematous skin lesions continued, and the patient was referred to a major hospital center for evaluation of a possible immune deficiency. No clear-cut abnormalities were found. During that hospitalization, the patient had two subcutaneous abscesses that required incision and drainage.

At admission, she was afebrile (37° C rectally). Physical examination revealed well-healed sites of prior incision and drainage procedures on the left lower extremity and upper extremities. She had no acute or chronic skin lesions. A grade 1/6 systolic murmur was heard. Routine evaluations were unrevealing, with the exception of an elevated antistreptolysin-O titer of 500 Todd units.

The patient had no fever or skin lesions during a 10-day hospitalization and was discharged, only to return 6 days later with a 2-day history of fever to 38.3° C. At readmission, the patient noted the spontaneous development of a tender posterior calf lesion associated with fever of 38.9° C to 39.4° C. She had a temperature of 38.2° C rectally. A 1-cm, raised, erythematous lesion with 8 cm of surrounding induration was present on the left posterior calf. There appeared to be a pinpoint-sized break in the skin at the center of the lesion. Leukocyte count was 16,000/mm^3 with a left shift; erythrocyte sedimentation rate was 102 mm/hour. Blood cultures obtained at admission were negative. The patient was treated with heat and elevation of the extremity and intravenous antibiotics.

Because the skin lesion appeared to have been self-induced, psychiatric consultation was obtained. A diagnosis was made of borderline personality disorder with self-destructive behavior. The patient was confronted with the suspicion that her fever and skin lesions were self-induced, and she vehemently denied these charges. The next day she developed fever and hypotension. Physical examination was unrevealing. Leukocyte count was 27,000/mm with a left shift. Blood cultures subsequently grew *S. aureus* and *Pseudomonas diminuta.* She was treated with intravenous fluids and antibiotics and made an uneventful recovery.

A second psychiatric consultation was obtained. The patient eventually admitted that she had been inducing the recurrent episodes of fever and skin lesions over the past 2 years. In fact, she further admitted to having falsified or induced episodes of "fever" since age 12. She stated that she had obtained pure cultures of streptococcus from the hospital laboratory in which she worked. Upon returning home, she would inject the culture material into the deep subcutaneous tissues with a needle and syringe. She did not, however, admit any responsibility for the episode of sepsis noted above. The patient was referred for outpatient psychotherapy.

Self-Inflicted Local Infections

Skin and Subcutaneous Tissues. Infections of the skin or subcutaneous tissues are simulated or actually produced by injections, excoriation, or repeated wounding with heat, chemicals, or instruments. *Dermatitis artefacta* was recognized and described early in this century (Sneddon and Sneddon, 1975). Either infectious or noninfectious skin diseases are simulated, and inadvertent superinfections are not unusual. *Subcutaneous abscesses* may be mistaken for erythema nodosum, Weber-Christian's disease, immune deficiency, recurrent furunculosis, or thrombophlebitis. Cellulitis combined with subcutaneous injection of air may simulate gas gangrene.

Case 6. A right-handed, 20-year-old man was transferred from jail to University Hospital in San Diego for left knee arthritis and fever. He reported progressive pain in the knee since "bumping" it on a bed in jail. On examination, he had needle tracks consistent with a history of heroin addiction and numerous, amateur tatoos in the form of swasticas. Temperature was 102° F, WBC was 10,400, and sedimentation rate was 8. There was minimal swelling of the medial left knee centered on three small puncture wounds. Aspira-

tion of the joint was unsuccessful and 5 cc of sterile fluid was washed into the joint and cultured. This fluid grew scant amounts of nonpathogenic *Neisseria, Gaffkya,* diphtheroids, *Streptococcus viridans,* and *Hemophilus parahemolyticus.* On high-dose intravenous penicillin for possible gonococcal arthritis, swelling and erythema progressed and an x-ray showed gas under the patella. On the third hospital day, frank pus was aspirated during arthrocentesis and the knee was surgically explored. A necrotizing fasciitis of the capsular fascia was drained of foul-smelling pus containing gram-negative rods, gram-positive cocci, and polymorphonuclear leukocytes. Cultures of necrotic tissue grew heavy, β-hemolytic streptococci (not Groups A, B, D, E, or F), moderate *Streptococcus viridans,* and scant penicillin-sensitive *Bacteroides.* Exploration revealed no necrosis or obvious infection of the knee joint, and sterile effusion was aspirated from the joint. The patient was treated with high-dose penicillin, chloramphenicol, and multiple drainage procedures. He was discharged on the twenty-fourth day with a healing wound. Mild joint dysfunction remained 3 years later. The patient was questioned several times by his physicians but denied injecting anything into his leg.

This patient's infection with mixed anaerobic and aerobic mouth flora was almost certainly the result of injecting his saliva into the periarticular and subcutaneous tissues of his knee. When this flora is inoculated into tissues (for example, with human bites), it typically produces the necrotizing, gas-producing, subcutaneous, and fascial infection seen in this patient. The diagnosis of self-injection is supported by his sociopathic personality, the secondary gain afforded by hospitalization, his familiarity with needles, and his history of self-injection as evidenced by tatooing.

Septic Arthritis. The following patient illustrates that septic arthritis may be produced by injection of body fluids into the joint space rather than near the joint as in the previous example.

***Case 7.* A 32-year-old, insulin-dependent, diabetic woman with multiple complications was admitted to University Hospital in San Diego for 3 days of fever to 103° F, chills, and left leg swelling. Four months before admission, an "insect bite" had resulted in a large abscess over the lateral left leg that grew only *S. aureus* and responded to surgical drainage and cephalosporins. The wound healed well, leaving only a small, shallow ulcer in the wound scar over the knee laterally. On admission, she appeared chronically ill with fever of 100.5° F and multiple signs of her diabetic complications, including retinopathy, cataracts, peripheral neuropathy, and generalized weakness. Her skin had multiple 1 to 3 cm ulcers on arms, legs, face, and chest. The back was spared. The lesions were excoriated but not infected, and they resembled lesions seen during an earlier admission. There was brawny pitting edema of both legs, which was greater on the left. The left leg was slightly warm and tender, and Homans' sign was present. Laboratory studies revealed leukocytosis of 12,700, mild azotemia (creatinine = 1.9), and hyperglycemia (glucose = 437). Culture of urine grew 20,000 *Candida parapsilosis,* and the left leg ulcer was sterile. On the second hospital day, a left-knee effusion developed and was aspirated of grossly purulent fluid containing 198,000 leukocytes that were 98 per cent neutrophils. Gram stain revealed budding yeast and large gram-positive rods. *Candida parapsilosis* and *Lactobacillus* were grown in moderate amounts from repeated aspirates. Her arthritis ultimately required surgical drainage of the knee joint and subcutaneous tissues. The patient responded slowly to cefazolin, gentamicin, 5-fluorocytosine, and local instillation of amphotericin B. Cultures at 17 days were sterile.**

Because the excoriated skin lesions and the unusual microbiology of the arthritis suggested self-injection, she was asked if she had injected the knee. She admitted to exploring the overlying wound on multiple occasions with her insulin needle "to help it drain," but not to injecting anything.

Psychiatric evaluation revealed a history of attempted suicide, depression over recent death of a diabetic roommate, and the long-held expectation that she would "die in my twenties" from diabetes. In addition, she related "riding with Hell's Angels" and working as a prostitute in the past, but said she was no longer sexually active because of fecal incontinence.

This young woman with a history of self-destructive behavior and advanced diabetes had two organisms *(Candida* and *Lactobacillus)* only rarely found in infected joints. Because the overlying ulcer was sterile and did not communicate with the joint, she appears to have injected urine or vaginal flora into the joint. Simultaneous hematogenous seeding of the joint with these organisms is unlikely. Her familiarity, as a diabetic, with needles and urine collections probably provided her the means for further self-destructive behavior.

DIAGNOSIS. Factitious diseases are often difficult to recognize because the patient may not appear overtly disturbed, and the illness may seem plausible. Physicians justifiably fear overlooking rare or unfamiliar diseases when an illness is atypical. Recurrent bacterial infections may suggest one of the rare genetic defects of cellular or humoral immunity. Abnormal numbers or functions of leukocytes, antibody production, or complement components do predispose to recurrent bacterial infections. Before undertaking an exhaustive search for such defects, however, consideration should be given to fraudulent disease. In addition to fear of missing a diagnosis, many physicians have difficulty believing that a patient is intentionally deceiving them. Recognition of fraudulent diseases requires both a knowledge of fraudulent syndromes and a willingness to entertain the diagnosis. Systematic attempts to find objective evidence of fraud can confirm the diagnosis and save the patient from unnecessary and dangerous diagnostic tests and therapy.

Atypical clinical or microbiologic features are the most important clue to fraudulent infectious diseases. Knowledge of the pathogenesis of most infections is enough to alert well-informed physicians that many fraudulent diseases "don't make sense." For instance, polymicrobial bacteremia in patients without compromised immunity or an identifiable site of infection suggests intravenous injection of bacteria. This suspicion is strengthened by the isolation of organisms that make up the flora found in feces, saliva, vaginal secretions, or on the skin. Fever without changes in other vital signs, rapid defervescence without diaphoresis, temperature of 41.1° C or higher, or prolonged fevers without objective signs of inflammation should suggest simulated fever.

Age, sex, occupation, and psychiatric history are helpful in diagnosis. Young, female medical and paramedical workers (for example, nurses and laboratory technicians) or students are the most frequently represented groups. Self-injection requires experience with and access to needles and syringes. Medical and paramedical personnel, laboratory workers, diabetics, and intravenous drug abusers are the groups with such experience. Atypical illness in these groups should arouse suspicion of self-inoculation. In persons with a knowledge of microbiology and access to pure cultures, self-injection may lead to repeated isolation of the same organism from blood or from recurrent subcutaneous abscesses.

Motivation in the form of secondary gain is an important clue. Adolescent students who have been legitimately ill may prolong convalescence to avoid returning to school or home. Prisoners may use factitious or self-inflicted illness to escape the dangers or tedium of jail, or addicts may seek opiates. In many patients, however, the motivation is not so clear.

A number of techniques are useful to detect simulated fevers. The most effective is immediate measurement of fever at several sites with a responsible observer continuously present. Assessment of other vital signs, skin warmth and moisture, and measurement of the temperature of freshly voided urine can also help. Checking the serial number of glass thermometers makes substitution of preheated ones more difficult.

Major corroborative evidence of self-injection can be found by searching the patient's room for the apparatus used (syringe and needle, bacterial cultures). Additional clues are needle marks over veins or sites of infection and the resolution of chronic infections when they are rendered inaccessible by casting the affected limb.

The diagnosis of fraudulent disease is made by careful exclusion of other explanations for the patient's illness and enough positive evidence that the means is clear. It is often hard to understand the patient's motivation, and most patients are unwilling to admit to fraud even if confronted with the evidence.

When the diagnosis cannot be made with certainty, physicians may wish to explore the patient's social and psychiatric history for psychopathology. The value of this approach to diagnosis and therapy has not been determined. Techniques such as Amytal interviews, projective psychometric testing, hypnosis, or analytic psychotherapy have not been systematically applied to these patients, and aggressive attempts to explore the patient's psychopathology may be contraindicated.

MANAGEMENT. Most physicians experienced with this problem agree on the basic principles of management when the diagnosis of fraudulent illness is made. The first step is to ask for psychiatric help to evaluate the patient's psychopathology with emphasis on their potential for self-destruction. Next, the physicians, nurses, and others involved in the patient's care should be told the diagnosis and plan of management. Since these patients may arouse strong emotional reactions in those caring for them, an opportunity to deal with these feelings away from the patient is thereby provided. The need to maintain a nonjudgmental, supportive attitude should be emphasized to the staff. Next, the patient is confronted with the evidence for fraudulent illness in a sympathetic, but realistic, manner. Those involved must be prepared for anger and hostility as a result of confrontation and not attack the patient's defenses in reaction. The possibility of flight (almost invariable in Munchausen's syndrome) or even suicide should be recognized, but should not deter the physician from this approach. Confrontation frequently ends the deceptive practices despite denial by the patients that they are involved in deception. By expressing concern for the patient's medical and emotional problems, the physician may be able to redefine the illness and direct therapy at the underlying psychopathology. Practical and emotional support, limitation of self-destructive behavior, and exploration of the social pressures on the patient are the immediate goals. Strengthening and preserving the patient's fragile defenses is the ultimate goal.

Self-inflicted illness requiring further medical therapy can be treated on a medical ward. When outpatient therapy is arranged and the immediate consequences of confrontation have passed, patients may be discharged. The medical consequences of self-inflicted disease can be serious and even life-threatening. Careful medical management of infections and, when possible, measures to prevent further manipulation are mandatory. In doing so, the physician communicates his continuing support for the patient and emphasizes the importance of stopping the injurious behavior.

After the diagnosis of factitious infection is made, it is important to entertain alternative diagnoses. Obviously a correct diagnosis of factitious disease does not protect the patient from developing "real" complications or unreleated naturally occurring illnesses. The consequences of incorrect diagnosis or inadequate treatment of self-inflicted diseases are potentially severe. Jokes about the high mortality of malingering and hysteria abound.

Delusional Illnesses

DELUSIONAL INFESTATIONS (DELUSIONS OF PARASITOSIS)

Delirious or psychotic patients may suffer hallucinations or delusions of infestation that are dramatic and easily recognized. In contrast, other patients with delusions of infestation by worms or insects ("parasitosis") are otherwise not obviously psychotic. They cling tenaciously to their delusion despite reassurance and can sometimes involve others in their delusion. They present their physicians with evidence of the infestations in the form of household or bodily detritus (vegetable material from their stools, bits of skin, nasal mucus, thread, and so on). When the nonparasitic nature of this material is demonstrated, they often collect more and may refer themselves to specialists in parasitology or infectious diseases or to entomologists. Most patients localize the infestation to the skin or hair, but the mouth, nose, subcutaneous tissues, bowel, or internal organs may be involved. In some cases, insects are described as biting, rather than infesting the patient. Another variation is that parasites are feared obsessively, but delusions are absent. Excoriation and artifactual dermatitis may result from scratching or attempts to remove the "parasites" with instruments, heat, or caustics. Real arthropod infestations may precede and trigger the delusional one. Real cutaneous or systemic diseases (especially if pruritic) may be misinterpreted by the patient as caused by parasites. Medications (for example, monoamine oxidase inhibitors) or psychostimulants (for example, amphetamines, cocaine, or methylphenidate) may cause delusions of parasitosis. In addition, a variety of social or psychological stresses may be linked to the delusion. An illustrative example of social stress leading to similar delusions in three housewives was observed by Wilson (1952) in Los Angeles during the Second World War. Each had unwillingly yielded to social pressure by allowing soldiers or defense workers to share their homes during the wartime housing shortage. They became convinced that the unwanted houseguests had brought insects into their homes and that these insects were attacking them.

The psychiatric diagnosis underlying delusions of parasitosis and the degree of psychopathology are controversial. "Monosymptomatic hypochondriacal psychosis" describes the major elements of the syndrome. These anxious patients suffer a persistent, unshakable delusion, but reject psychiatric diagnoses or therapy, retain their underlying personality, continue to function socially, and rarely become severely depressed or overtly schizophrenic. Diagnosis of delusory infestation is made when the patient repeatedly rejects alternative explanations for the "parasites" or for his symptoms. Obviously, examination of the patient for real infestations or other diseases must precede attempts at reassurance. Scabies is notoriously deceptive and should be excluded if itching and unusual skin lesions are present, regardless of how bizarre the patient's explanations for these findings may seem.

Treatment for delusions of infestation has been frustrating to both physicians and psychiatrists. The recognition that these patients refuse referral and do not benefit from psychotherapy has led some physicians to attempt supportive, informal psychotherapy bolstered by antipsychotic agents (Gould and Gragg, 1976). Pimoxide, a diphenyl butylpiperidine antipsychotic agent, may have specific value for them (Munro, 1978).

DELUSIONAL EPIDEMICS (EPIDEMIC HYSTERIA)

Rapidly developing epidemics usually result from exposures of groups to toxins or microorganisms. Contagious spread of delusional or hysterical symptoms within groups can simulate infections or intoxications. A number of such outbreaks of subjective symptoms within closed groups are best explained as mass hysteria (Sirois, 1974). Typically, young women in institutions (for example, schools or hospitals) rapidly develop similar, dramatic, subjective symptoms (for example, fainting, hyperventilation, or weakness). In one case, fainting, headache, nausea, and weakness spread rapidly within an American high school marching band after a moderate heat stress (Levine, 1977).

These epidemics may have several patterns. Sudden, explosive outbreaks spread within minutes and may be preceded by a few cases during slower, prodromal stages. A small outbreak may be followed in hours or days by a second, more prominent wave. Cumulative epidemics may build over several weeks, usually within closed institutional settings. The inciting event may be a real or hysterical illness within a group predisposed to hysteria by anxiety. The role of anxiety is illustrated by outbreaks of symptoms simulating poliomyelitis (benign myalgic encephalomyelitis or Icelandic disease) in nurses during epidemics of poliomyelitis (McEvedy and Beard, 1970).

The diagnosis should be considered when dramatic, subjective symptoms spread within a group under stress. Various combinations of weakness, headache, hyperventilation, myalgias, fainting, abnormal movements, tremor, globus, pain, nausea, and vomiting have been reported. Objective signs of disease such as fever or diarrhea are absent. Careful clinical and epidemiologic investigations eliminate the possibility of infection or intoxication.

Management of epidemic hysteria is dispersion of the group, isolation of affected individuals, and careful search for objective signs of illness. Confrontation or exhortation has not been effective and may aggravate the outbreak.

References

Aduan, R. P., Fauci, A. S., Dale, D. C., Herzberg, J. H., and Wolff, S. M.: Factitious fever and self-induced infection. Ann Intern Med 90:230, 1979.

Asher, R.: Malingering. Trans Med Soc Lond 75:145, 1959.

Cramer, B., Gershberg, M. R., and Stern, M.: Munchausen Syndrome. Arch Gen Psychiatry 24:573, 1971.

Gould, W. M., and Gragg, T. M.: Delusions of parasitosis. Arch Dermatol 112:1745, 1976.

Levine, R. J.: Epidemic faintness and syncope in a school marching band. JAMA 238:2373, 1977.

McEvedy, C. P., and Beard, A. W.: Concept of benign myalgic encephalomyelitis. Br Med J 1:11, 1970.

Munro, A.: Two cases of delusions of worm infestation. Am J Psychiatry 135:2, 1978.

Petersdorf, R. G., and Bennett, I. L.: Factitious fever. Ann Intern Med 46:1039, 1957.

Reich, P., and Gottfried, L. A.: Factitious disorders in a teaching hospital. Ann Intern Med 99:240, 1983.

Rumans, L. W., and Vosti, K. L.: Factitious and fraudulent fever. Am J Med 65:745, 1978.

Sirois, F.: Epidemic hysteria. Acta Psychiatrica Scandinavia Supplementum 252, 1974.

Sneddon, I., and Sneddon, J.: Self-inflicted injury: a follow-up study of 43 patients. Br Med J 3:527, 1975.

Wilson, J. W.: Delusions of parasitosis (Acarophobia). Arch Dermatol Syphilis 66:577, 1952.

273
ACQUIRED IMMUNODEFICIENCY SYNDROME

J. ALLEN McCUTCHAN, M.D., M.Sc. (EPID.)
W. CHRISTOPHER MATHEWS, M.D.

DEFINITION. *Acquired immunodeficiency syndrome (AIDS)* is an epidemic, transmissible retroviral disease, manifested in severe cases as a profound depression of cell-mediated immunity. The clinical consequences of this defect in immune function are a variety of unusual opportunistic infections (most commonly *Pneumocystis carinii* pneumonia) and neoplasia (especially Kaposi's sarcoma). For purposes of epidemiological surveillance the Centers for Disease Control (CDC, Atlanta, Georgia, USA) has formulated a definition ("CDC/AIDS"), which seeks to detect the majority of severe cases:

> A person (adult or child) who has had a reliably diagnosed disease that is at least moderately indicative of an underlying cellular immune deficiency, but who, at the same time, has had no known underlying cause of cellular immune deficiency nor any other cause of reduced resistance reported to be associated with that disease.

Those diseases that indicate depressed cell-mediated immunity are listed below with the required method of diagnosis in parentheses.

A. Protozoal and Helminthic Infections:

1. *Cryptosporidiosis*, intestinal, causing diarrhea for over one month (on histology or stool microscopy);

2. *Pneumocystis carinii pneumonia*, (on histology, or microscopy of a "touch" preparation or bronchial washings);

3. *Strongyloidiasis*, causing pneumonia, central nervous system infection, or disseminated infection, (on histology);

4. *Toxoplasmosis*, causing pneumonia or central nervous system infection (on histology or microscopy of a "touch" preparation).

B. Fungal Infections:

1. *Aspergillosis*, causing central nervous system or disseminated infection (on culture or histology);

2. *Candidiasis*, causing esophagitis (on histology, or microscopy of a "wet" preparation from the esophagus, or endoscopic findings of white plaques on an erythematous mucosal base);

3. *Cryptococcosis*, causing pulmonary, central nervous system or disseminated infection (on culture, antigen detection, histology, or India ink preparation of CSF).

C. Bacterial Infections:

1. *Atypical mycobacteriosis* (species other than tuberculosis or lepra), causing disseminated infection (on culture).

D. Viral Infections:

1. *Cytomegalovirus*, causing pulmonary, gastrointestinal tract, or central nervous system infection (on histology);

2. *Herpes simplex virus*, causing chronic mucocutaneous infection with ulcers persisting more than 2 months, or pulmonary, gastrointestinal tract, or disseminated infection (on culture, histology, or cytology);

3. *Progressive multifocal leukoencephalopathy* (presumed to be caused by a papovavirus) (on histology).

E. Neoplasia:

1. *Kaposi's sarcoma* (on histology);

2. *Lymphoma limited to the brain* (on histology).

This list of infectious diseases and neoplasia should not be viewed as the only complications of AIDS. Instead, they are diseases that usually occur in patients with recognized forms of immunosuppression and thus are good indicators of severe immune disturbances. The CDC definition is apparently fairly specific because 94 per cent of the cases it has detected have occurred in persons in a few high-risk groups and many of the remainder are connected epidemiologically to persons in these high risk groups. It is probably not very sensitive for detecting persons infected with the microbial agent of AIDS, however, because an epidemic of less severe illness resembling CDC/AIDS, but not meeting these diagnostic criteria, has appeared simultaneously in persons in the high-risk groups. In recognition of this less severe form of AIDS, the CDC and the National Institutes of Health, Bethesda, Maryland have defined *AIDS-related complex* for epidemiological purposes as:

An illness characterized by 1) at least two clinical signs or symptoms listed below persisting for more than 3 months, and 2) at least two or more of the listed laboratory abnormalities occurring in patients without other known infections who are at increased risk of AIDS.

SIGNS AND SYMPTOMS OF AIDS-RELATED COMPLEX

1) Fever >100°; 2) Weight loss of >10 per cent of body weight or of more than 15 lbs; 3) Adenopathy in 2 lymph node chains excluding femoral or inguinal chains; 4) Diarrhea; 5) Fatigue interfering with normal functioning; 6) Night sweats.

LABORATORY ABNORMALITIES IN AIDS-RELATED COMPLEX

1) Cytopenias (low numbers of circulating erythrocytes, total leukocytes, or platelets); 2) Depressed T_H/T_S (ratio of helper to suppressor T lymphoctyes >2 S.D. below mean of normal controls); 3) Depressed T_H (helper T lymphocyte numbers >2 S.D. below mean of normal control); 4) Depressed lymphocyte blastogenesis in response to mitogens; 5) Elevated immunoglobulins; 6) Cutaneous anergy to multiple skin tests.

Healthy persons in several groups at increased risk of AIDS, such as male homosexuals and men receiving replacement therapy for hemophilia, have abnormalities of lymphocytes similar to patients with AIDS and AIDS-related complex (Stahl et al., 1982). Whether these abnormalities are a direct result of preclinical or subclinical infection by the agent of AIDS or are unrelated to AIDS in these patients is unclear. Since most infectious agents provoke a broad spectrum of clinical illnesses, the AIDS agent probably produces disturbances ranging from asymptomatic to fatal.

EPIDEMIOLOGY. AIDS was first recognized as a new disease by American physicians who noted clusters of Pneumocystis pneumonia and Kaposi's sarcoma in urban male homosexuals and documented an underlying defect in immunity (Gottlieb et al., 1981; Masur et al., 1981; Siegal et al., 1981). The possibly infectious nature of this condition led the CDC to establish a working epidemiological definition and search both retrospectively and prospectively for other cases (Centers for Disease Control, 1982). Figure 1 shows the early history of the epidemic in the United States as reconstructed by the CDC. In the United States it is clear that AIDS, at least in epidemic form, is a new disease. Retrospective analysis of Kaposi's sarcoma in tumor registries in epidemic areas and of requests to the CDC for pentamidine to treat pneumocystis pneumonia show that these manifestations of AIDS first began to appear in 1978–1979. Figure 2 shows that the incidence of AIDS rose exponentially in the United States from 1981 to mid-1983 with a doubling of the number of newly reported cases about every six months. Should the incidence of AIDS continue in this pattern, the total number of cases in 1985 is projected at 10,000.

The distinctive geographical distribution and groups at risk of AIDS offer clues to its etiology and transmission. In the United States, AIDS first appeared in homosexual men in New York City, and slightly later in San Francisco and Los Angeles, and then slowly spread to other urban areas where homosexual men, intravenous drug users, or Haitians are concentrated. Figure 2 shows that areas like Europe (represented by the Federal Republic of Germany) have similar epidemic curves to New York and San Francisco, but that the onset is delayed by about 1 to 2 years. Spread among intravenous drug users has been limited geographically to the East Coast of the United States despite the large population of intravenous drug users on the West Coast. Beginning in 1981 cases were recognized in Europe and Haiti, and more recently in both Europeans and Africans who have lived in Central Africa. By October 1983, over 250 cases had been recognized in 10 European countries (Figure 3), 110 cases had been diagnosed in Haiti, and a quarter of European cases (>60) were Central

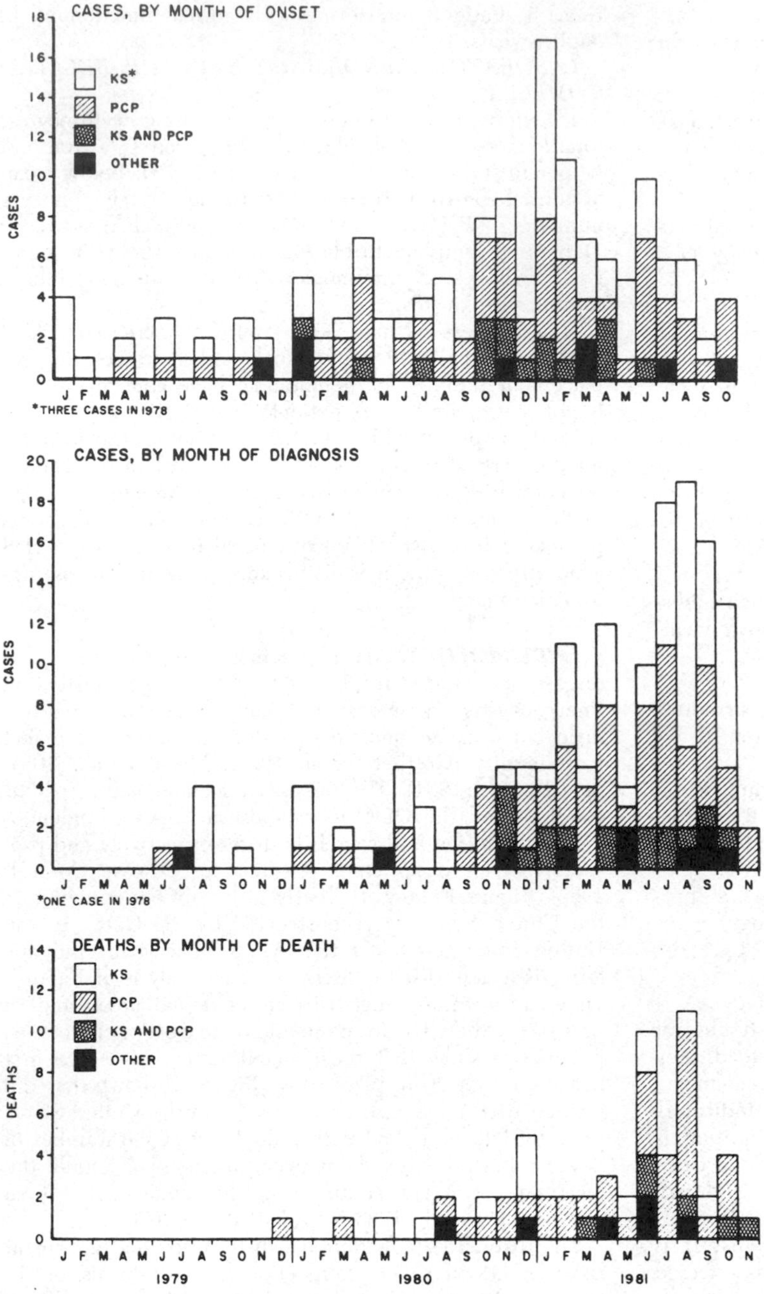

Figure 1. Reconstruction of the early history of the AIDS epidemic in the United States. Using the CDC definition of AIDS, medical records in epidemic cities indicate that the symptoms in the earliest cases appeared in 1979, patients were diagnosed soon thereafter, and significant mortality caused by AIDS appeared in 1980. (Reproduced from a review of AIDS epidemiology by CDC in N Engl J Med 306:248, 1982.)

Africans who had reached Europe for medical care. Because the difficulty and expense of coming to Europe probably selected only a minority of African cases, the total number of cases in Central Africans is almost certainly many-fold greater. Figure 4 shows the distribution of 2,259 cases in the United States as of September 1983. Note that nearly half the cases had been seen in New York. California with large populations of homosexual men, New Jersey with a large population of intravenous drug abusers, and Florida where a majority of recent Haitian immigrants reside accounted together for another one-third of the total cases.

The major groups affected (Table 1) have been American and European male homosexuals, American intravenous drug-users, hemophiliacs (Centers for Disease Control, 1983) and Haitians living in both the United States and Haiti (Moskowitz et al., 1983; Pape et al., 1983), and persons recently residing in Central Africa (especially Zairians). Additionally, smaller numbers of cases are reported in female sexual contacts of men in high risk groups (Harris et al., 1983), children born to mothers at high risk (Olleske et al., 1983; Rubinstein et al., 1983; Scott et al., 1984), and transfusion recipients (Curran et al., 1984). Equally important for understanding the mode of transmission are groups that do not appear to be at increased risk. Early in the epidemic, many medical and laboratory workers helped to care for patients without taking special precautions, but have not been affected. Co-workers and family members of persons at high risk do not appear to be at risk. Thus, the most likely routes of spread appear to be sexual (homosexual more efficiently than heterosexual) and

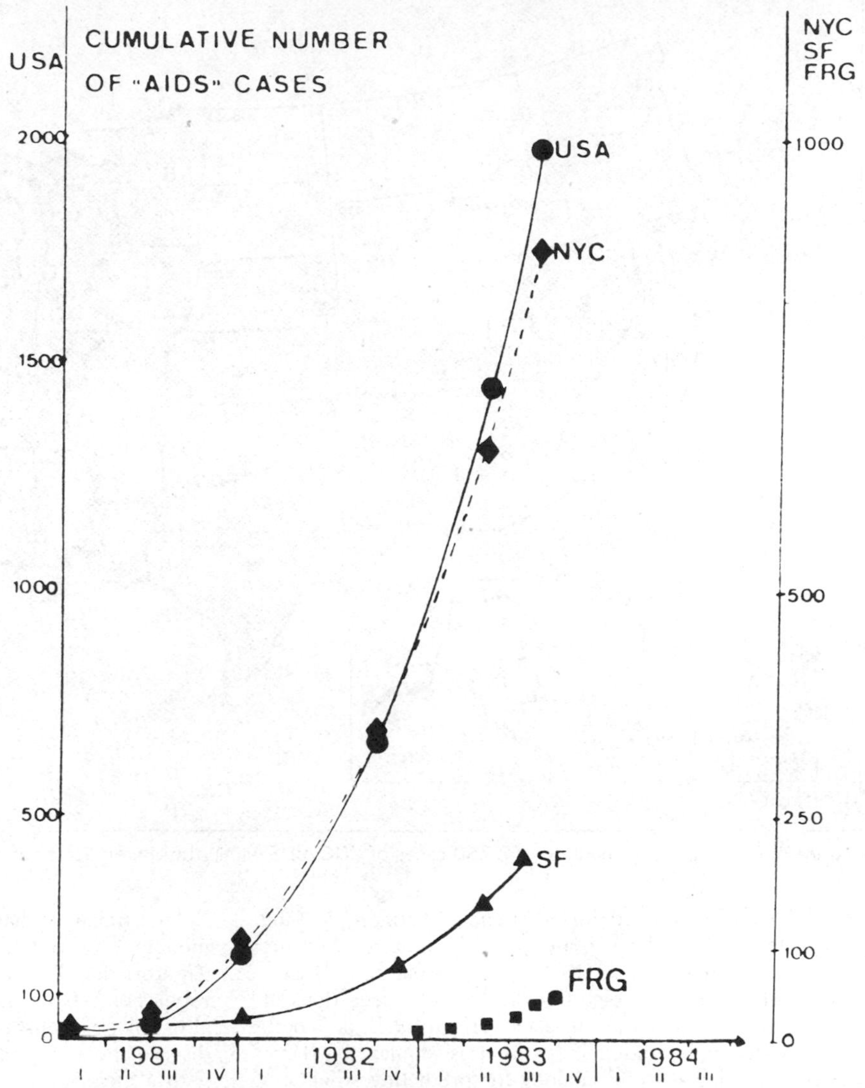

Figure 2. Epidemic curves for CDC/AIDS in the United States, two U.S. cities, and the Federal Republic of Germany. Total U.S. cases (circles and solid line referred to ordinate at the left) have followed an exponentially increasing curve dominated by cases seen in New York City (diamond and broken line referred to right ordinate). The epidemic reached San Francisco later, but has pursued a similar curve. Experience in other American cities (e.g., San Diego) is similar to that shown for Germany. (Reproduced from Lancet ii:1370, 1983.)

Reported AIDS Cases in Europe

Source: The World Health Organization

	Before 1979	'79	'80	'81	'82	'83	Total by country
Austria						7	7
Belgium			2	4	8	24	38
Britain				2	5	17	24
Czechoslovakia					1	1	2
France	6	1	5	5	30	47	94
Ireland						2	2
Italy					2		2
The Netherlands					3	9	12
Scandinavia			1	2	5	13	21
Spain				1	1	4	6
Switzerland			2	3	5	7	17
West Germany	1	1			7	33	42
European total	**7**	**2**	**10**	**17**	**67**	**164**	**267**

Figure 3. Cases of AIDS reported from Europe to the World Health Organization. Cases fall into five broad risk groups: homosexual men, persons who have lived in Central Africa, Haitians, hemophiliacs, and intravenous drug abusers. The large number of Zairian cases seen in Francophone countries in Europe suggest that a major epidemic of AIDS is occurring in Central Africa.

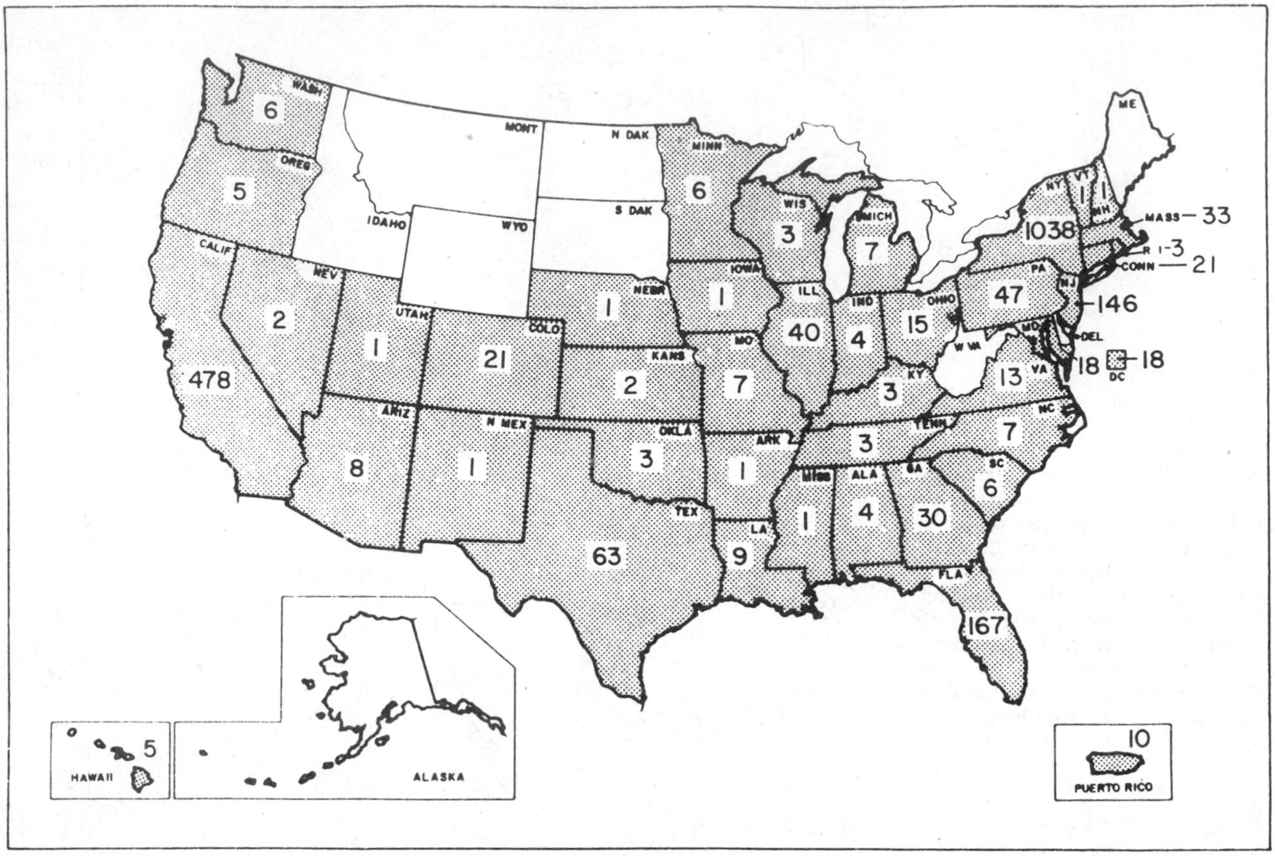

Figure 4. Geographic distribution of 2,250 cases of CDC/AIDS within the United States as of September 1983 by state of residence.

through transfer of blood during medical treatment, sharing of needles by drug abusers, and possibly in utero or during parturition. Spread of AIDS through sexual contact may also involve serum or blood cells in genital secretions or on traumatized mucosal surfaces. Hepatitis B, a blood-borne virus with epidemiology that is similar to AIDS, appears to offer a useful analogy for predicting what precautions are necessary to prevent further spread of AIDS and what future patterns of transmission are likely (Conte et al., 1983).

An extensive chain of transmission among homosexual men in Los Angeles was mapped early in the epidemic (Centers for Disease Control, 1982). From that study, reports of AIDS in infants, and reports of AIDS developing after blood transfusions, the incubation period of this disease appears to range from six months to over four years with a mean of about two years. This unusually long and variable incubation period renders contact tracing of sexual partners or of blood donors very difficult. It also provides a prolonged period of potential infectivity during which the

Table 1. HIGH RISK GROUPS IN CDC/AIDS AS OF 1 OCTOBER 1984

	Total		Males		Females	
Patient Groups	***Number***	***%***	***Cases***	***% of Total***	***Cases***	***% of Total***
Adult-Adolescent						
Homosexual or bisexual men	4503	73	4503	78	—	—
IV drug user	1061	17	835	14	226	57
Haitian	230	4	195	3	35	9
Hemophiliac	42	1	42	1	0	0
Heterosexual contact	46	1	2	0	44	11
Transfusions with blood products	72	1	42	1	30	8
None of the above	228	4	164	3	64	16
Total	6182	100	5783	100	399	100
Pediatric						
Parent with AIDS or at increased risk of AIDS	44	64	21	53	23	79
Hemophiliac	4	6	4	10	0	0
Transfusion with blood products	12	17	10	25	2	7
None of the above	9	13	5	13	4	14
Total	69	100	40	100	29	100

carrier may spread the disease through sexual encounters or repeated blood or plasma donations. For example, none of seven donors who were implicated as the source of transfusion-acquired AIDS had CDC/AIDS, but all had abnormal Th/Ts ratios and four had lymphadenopathy (Curran et al., 1984).

A case-control study by the CDC identified a number of risk factors in homosexual men, which occurred more frequently in patients with AIDS than in controls matched for age, sexual orientation, and place of residence (Jaffe et al., 1983a). While factors associated with sexual exposures (especially number of sexual partners) were the most powerful risk factors, use of nitrite inhalants was also implicated. This association of AIDS with drug use and the large number of known sexually transmitted agents infecting some homosexual men has suggested to some observers alternative explanations for the AIDS epidemic aside from an infectious agent. They have proposed that exposures to drugs, sperm, and a variety of venereal diseases might alone or in combination produce the immunosuppression that is the central feature of AIDS. Because no sudden change in promiscuity or drug use among homosexual men was apparent in the late 1970's and other risk groups don't share these practices, "toxic" or "immune overload" hypotheses are regarded by most epidemiologists as unlikely explanations for a rapidly increasing epidemic. The available evidence implicates a new, transmissible (infectious) agent that spreads during intimate (possibly necessarily sexual) contact and circulates in the blood.

The epidemiology of Kaposi's sarcoma suggests that it is an "opportunistic" tumor in AIDS patients that arises most frequently in immunosuppressed persons with a genetic predisposition. Kaposi's sarcoma is the most common neoplasm arising in AIDS patients and is several times more common in homosexual men with AIDS than in other high risk groups. Before AIDS, Kaposi's sarcoma was known to occur in three groups: elderly men often of Mediterranean ancestry who were not immunosuppressed; young, mostly male, Black Central Africans; and renal homograft recipients on immunosuppressive drugs. The relationship of the endemic form of Kaposi's sarcoma that has been documented for many decades in Central Africa (Hutt, 1981) and the current epidemic of both Kaposi's sarcoma and opportunistic infections (AIDS) in Zairians is unclear. Immunity in those with the endemic form of African Kaposi's has not been well investigated. Physicians in Europe (especially in Belgium) are certain that the large number of Zairians presenting to their hospitals with AIDS is unprecedented. This new development suggests that the older, endemic form of Kaposi's sarcoma in Africa is epidemiologically distinct from AIDS.

A genetic predisposition to Kaposi's sarcoma is suggested by the known ethnic predisposition in elderly men of Italian and Jewish descent, by increased risk of Kaposi's sarcoma in American homosexuals of Italian descent (Jaffe et al., 1983), and by the greater than expected frequency of HLA DR5 in American Kaposi's sarcoma patients with AIDS (Stahl et al., 1982). The higher frequency of HLA-DR5 in healthy Mediterranean Europeans and Blacks compared to other ethnic groups could account for increased susceptibility to Kaposi's sarcoma in those ethnic groups. An increased frequency of HLA-DR5 is also seen in homosexual men with chronic lymphadenopathy (AIDS-related complex) (Metroka, 1983). A relationship of HLA-DR5 to susceptibility to the AIDS agent or to the clinical expression of infection is suggested by these associations.

Most of the opportunistic infections in CDC/AIDS are common, latent infections that reactivate when immunity declines. Table 2 shows the relative incidence of agents in AIDS patients reported to the CDC. These reports are subject to considerable error, because 1) diagnosis of many of these infections requires sophisticated methods, 2) serodiagnosis of infections in AIDS is unreliable, 3) patients are often infected with multiple pathogens, and 4) reporting of opportunistic infections is incomplete. Clinical reports to the CDC and series from large teaching hospitals in the United States indicate that *Pneumocystis carinii* pneumonia is by far the most common serious opportunistic infection. Conversely, AIDS is also the most common underlying immunosuppressive disease found in patients with Pneumocystis pneumonia in areas where AIDS is epidemic. All of the human herpesviruses appear to reactivate frequently in AIDS patients. Cytomegalovirus and Epstein-Barr virus can be grown from the blood of about half of AIDS patients and may be implicated in both the etiology and pathogenesis of AIDS (see below). Although it is difficult to document, reactivation of *Herpes zoster* infections seems more frequent than expected in homosexual men in areas where AIDS is occurring and may precede development of AIDS. *Herpes simplex* of both types I and II frequently reactivate in severely ill AIDS patients to produce relapsing or chronic invasive ulcers. Mycobacteria, especially the *M. avium-intracellulare* group of atypical mycobacteria, commonly disseminate in the blood and reach high numbers in multiple tissues. The predominance of *M. avium-intracellulare* in AIDS, in contrast to its lower frequency in other severely immunosuppressed patients, suggests a specific failure of immunity to this widely distributed bacterium. *M. tuberculosis* has been most common in Haitians with AIDS (infecting 36/117 = 31 per cent). After pneumocystis, the protozoan parasite causing problems most often in AIDS is *Toxoplasma gondii*, another widespread, common, latent infection that occasionally reactivates in other immunosuppressed patients. The two fungi strongly associated with AIDS are *Candida albicans* and *Cryptococcus neoformans*. Mucocutaneous candidiasis is very common in AIDS and is frequently the first opportunistic infection to appear in AIDS patients, but is seldom life-threatening. *Cryptococcus neoformans*, a soil fungus acquired primarily through inhalation, may appear first in the lung or may disseminate to the meninges, skin, or other organs in a

Table 2. SEVERE OPPORTUNISTIC INFECTIONS IN CDC/AIDS AS OF 12 DEC 1983

Opportunistic Infections		**Number**	**% of Pts**
Pneumocystis pneumonia		1783	58.2
Esophageal candidiasis		226	9.0
Cryptococcus of CNS		136	5.4
Cytomegalovirus infections		106	4.2
Cerebral toxoplasmosis		103	4.1
Mycobacterium tuberculosis		68	2.7
Atypical mycobacteria		65	2.6
avium-intracellulare	- 60		
other	- 5		
Chronic herpes simplex		63	2.5
Cryptosporidium		60	2.4
Progressive multifocal leukoencephalopathy (J.C. virus)		15	.05

(Data courtesy of Ken Castro, M.D., CDC, Atlanta, Georgia)

variety of immunosuppressive conditions including AIDS. *Cryptosporidium enteriditis*, a rare cause of self-limited diarrhea in healthy persons, produces severe, intractable diarrhea in at least 2 per cent of AIDS patients. The epidemiology of infection with this sporozoan parasite of mammals is not well understood, but limited serological surveys suggest that a large proportion of Western European adults have been infected.

The feature of CDC/AIDS that distinguishes it from most other epidemic or sexually transmitted diseases is the high case fatality rate. Because the epidemic has not yet provided long periods of observation, only preliminary estimates of mortality are available over unspecified periods of time; thus, the overall cross-sectional mortality of 20 per cent for Kaposi's sarcoma and 50 per cent for opportunistic infections in AIDS patients reported to the CDC seriously underestimates ultimate mortality. Review of cases diagnosed early in the epidemic suggests that the ultimate mortality in CDC/AIDS approaches 100 per cent. Confirmed cases of AIDS who have regained normal immunological function have not been published. This extremely poor prognosis has been documented only in those with CDC/AIDS and should not be assumed to apply to AIDS-related complex.

Summary of the Epidemiology of AIDS in Early 1985. The sudden emergence of both an unusual tumor, Kaposi's sarcoma, and unusual opportunistic infections in previously healthy, American homosexuals has alerted physicians to a new, transmissible, and frequently fatal form of immunosuppression. Less severe illness probably caused by the same agent has been defined and the likely modes of transmission in developed countries have been identified. The incubation period has been estimated and evidence for transmission by asymptomatic carriers has accumulated. Longitudinal studies of the natural history of AIDS and AIDS-related complex and investigation of the epidemiology of this disease in Haiti and Zaire are underway. The similarity of AIDS to hepatitis B, a viral infection of high prevalence in many tropical areas, and the appearance of epidemic AIDS in two tropical populations in Central Africa and Haiti raises the possibility of widespread dissemination of AIDS throughout the tropical world. The study of the epidemiology of AIDS through surveillance, description of its natural history, and analytical investigations of its cause and transmission have permitted the identification of an etiological agent.

ETIOLOGY. The human T cell leukemia viruses (HTLV), a recently discovered family of retroviruses, have been linked to a minority of unusual and epidemiologically distinct T cell leukemias and lymphomas and more recently to AIDS. Similar viruses of this family have been isolated from homosexual men with lymphadenopathy (LAV) (Barre-Sinoussi et al., 1983) and from patients with AIDS (HTLV-3) (Papovic et al., 1984). HTLV-3 has been detected in 23 of 64 (36 per cent) adults with AIDS, 18 of 21 (86 per cent) patients with "pre-AIDS", but in only 1 of 22 (5 per cent) of homosexual controls (Gallo et al., 1984). Seroepidemiological studies support this strong association of both HTLV-3 and LAV with AIDS. Antibody to HTLV-3 was detected by ELISA in 43 of 49 (88 per cent) of AIDS patients and 11 of 14 (79 per cent) with pre-AIDS compared to 6 of 17 (25 per cent) homosexual controls and 1 of 164 (0.6 per cent) healthy heterosexual controls. Antibody to LAV was found less frequently (38 per cent) in AIDS patients, but as frequently (75 per cent) in pre-AIDS patients (Brun-Vezinet et al., 1984). LAV selectively infects helper cells, resulting in impaired proliferation and cytopathic effects in vitro (Klatzmann et al., 1984). This in vitro behavior of LAV may indicate the mechanism by which it produces profound immunosuppression, that is, destruction of the helper subset of T lymphocytes.

Additional support for the retroviral etiology of human AIDS is the proven retroviral etiology of Simian AIDS (SAIDS). Epidemics of opportunistic infections, Kaposi's-like sarcomas, and lymphomas have been documented since 1969 in various species of macaques held in several primate centers in the United States (Hendrickson et al., 1983, Letvin et al., 1983). Healthy macaques inoculated with tissue extracts and serum from primates with SAIDS have become infected and developed both neoplasia and immunosuppression (Letvin et al., 1983, London et al., 1983). A type D retrovirus related to the Mason Pfizer virus of monkeys has been isolated from two *Macaca cyclopis* monkeys with the syndrome (Daniel et al., 1984). Reports of transmission of SAIDS by purified preparations of this virus (Marx et al., 1984) and the identification of LAV as a type D retrovirus (Cherman et al., 1984) lends credibility to the central role of a retrovirus in human AIDS.

This concept is strengthened by findings of integrated HTLV-1 sequences in splenocytes of an AIDS patient who lacked antibody to HTLV proteins and from whom the virus could not be grown (Erhlich et al., 1984). Expansion of these observations to other AIDS patients (7/8) by using a subgenomic DNA probe suggests that proviral DNA sharing nucleic acid sequences with HTLV-1 can be found in lymphocytes of most AIDS patients regardless of serological status. Because this portion of the HTLV-1 genome may be highly conserved among human retroviruses, this finding implicates the family of HTLV, but not necessarily HTLV-1, as the cause of AIDS.

Given the strong evidence for a human retrovirus as the primary cause of AIDS, the possible role of drugs and coinfections as additional risk factors should not be ignored. Thus, it is necessary to view several known viruses as potential secondary infections contributing to immunosuppression, oncogenesis, or clinical manifestations. Sufficient evidence has accumulated to implicate two herpesviruses, cytomegalovirus (CMV) and Epstein-Barr virus (EBV).

CMV commonly infects homosexual men (Mintz et al., 1983; Drew et al., 1981), causes immunosuppression (Rinaldo et al., 1983), reactivates during drug-induced immunosuppression (Schooley et al., 1983), contributes to morbidity and mortality in AIDS (Mildvan et al., 1982), and is associated with Kaposi's sarcoma. EBV causes heterophile-positive mononucleosis, which resembles features of AIDS-related complex and is associated with reversed helper/suppressor T lymphocyte ratios (DeWaele et al., 1981). EBV is the possible cause of two neoplasms (Burkitt's lymphoma and nasopharyngeal carcinoma), has been isolated from Burkitt-like tumors in AIDS patients (Magrath et al., 1983), and is a risk factor (history of infectious mononucleosis) for AIDS (Jaffe et al., 1983). Gay men with AIDS and with asymptomatic immune disturbances have high titers of antibody to EBV viral capsid antigen (Rogers et al., 1983). Nearly all CDC/AIDS patients reactivate both CMV and EBV (Fauci et al., 1984). CMV was found in the blood of 5 of 10 patients and in blood or secretions of 9 of 10. EBV was grown from throat washings of 17 of 18 patients. Because these two herpesviruses have frequently infected homosexual men and the general population for many years it seems unlikely that they could account for the outbreak of a new disease. Their reactivation could account for many of the symptoms of AIDS-related complex that resemble symptoms of CMV or EBV mononucleosis. Furthermore, the oncogenic potential of these agents, suggested by their association with Kaposi's sarcoma (CMV) and Burkitt's lymphoma (EBV), makes them good candidates for a role in causing tumors associated with AIDS.

Several electron microscopic studies have described structures that could be related to the AIDS agents. Both "tubuloreticular structures" of the type seen in systemic lupus erythematosis and "test tube and ring forms" have been described in multiple tissues from a majority of 64 AIDS patients (Sidhu et al., 1983). The latter structure had previously been seen in a single Japanese patient with HTLV-associated T lymphoma and in chimpanzees infected with non-A, non-B hepatitis. "Vesicular rosettes" have been reported in the cytoplasm of lymphocytes from 17 of 18 homosexual men with unexplained lymphadenopathy (Ewing et al., 1983). The nature of these structures and their relationship to AIDS remains to be determined.

PATHOGENESIS. The infectious complications of AIDS point to a severe disorder of cell-mediated immunity. The infections that reactivate in AIDS patients are often caused by latent agents that require intact T lymphocyte function for their containment. Virtually all the infectious complications of AIDS also occur in patients with other diseases of abnormal T lymphocyte function (e.g., lymphomas, Hodgkin's disease, congenital T cell defects). Adults with AIDS do not seem especially susceptible to infections with the encapsulated pyogenic bacteria, which afflict patients with diseases of the B lymphocytes (e.g., multiple myeloma or the congenital and acquired immunoglobulin deficiencies). Nor do they have frequent problems with gram-negative bacteremia or with invasive infections by environmental molds both of which occur frequently in agranulocytic patients. In contrast to adults with AIDS, fatal gram-negative bacteremias do occur frequently in infants with AIDS and are a major cause of death. Thus, most adult AIDS patients have dysfunction of T lymphocytes with clinically adequate antibody and phagocyte function.

The immunological correlates of these clinical observations are marked depression of both the number and function of "helper" and an increased number of "suppressor" T lymphocytes. A variety of lymphocyte membrane antigens can be demonstrated by staining with commercially-available, monoclonal antibodies and then by counting under microscopy or on fluorescence-activated cell sorters. These antigens can be used to quantify the number of B and T lymphocytes as well as functional subsets of "helper" and "suppressor" T lymphocytes. Broadly, the helper subset (T_H, OKT4, or Leu3) is thought to enhance the function of both B cells and other T cells and the suppressor cells (T_S, OKT8, or Leu 2) to inhibit their function. Both subsets act as regulatory as well as effector cells in assays of cytotoxicity that measure the destruction of cells displaying foreign antigens. The normal percentages of T_H and T_S cells as determined by monoclonal antibodies are shown in Figure 5. The numbers of T_H are markedly reduced and of T_S are increased in AIDS patients. Patients with AIDS-related complex have less severe abnormalities. Healthy homosexual or hemophiliac men have similar changes, but these are less marked than in patients. As a group, patients with opportunistic infections are more abnormal than those with Kaposi's sarcoma. Similar, but transient, changes also occur during primary infections (mononucleosis) caused by EBV and CMV (Dewaele et al., 1981; Rinaldo et al., 1983). Thus, while not specific for AIDS, these changes in lymphocyte subsets, often expressed as the ratio T_H/T_S, appear to correlate with the severity of clinical illness and to reflect progressive destruction of a functionally important subset of T lymphocytes during evolution of the disease. In vitro functional assays are also abnormal. Proliferative responses to both specific and nonspecific mitogens by B cells and T cells from AIDS patients are markedly depressed (Stahl et al., 1982; Lane et al., 1983).

Both the opportunistic infections and changes in the

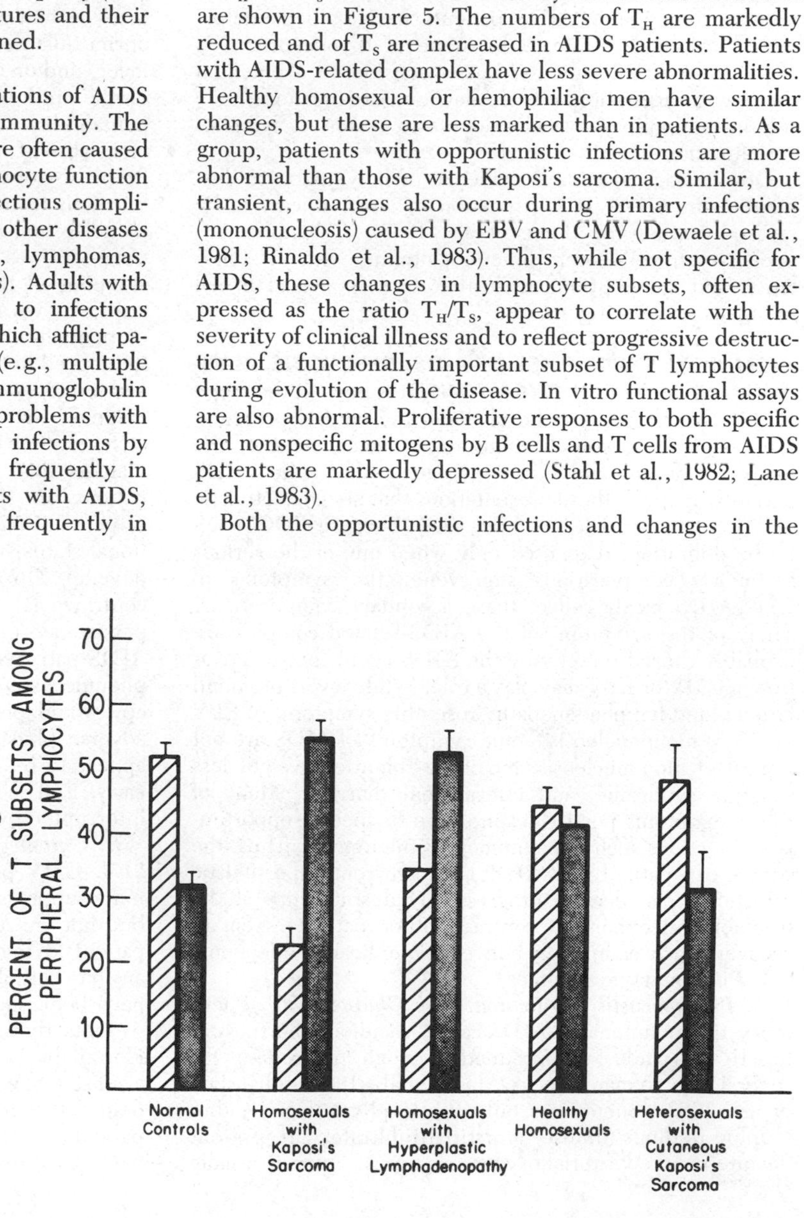

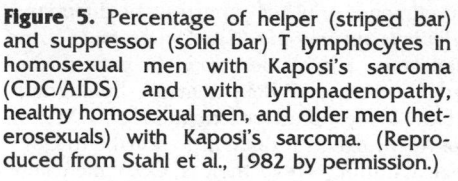

Figure 5. Percentage of helper (striped bar) and suppressor (solid bar) T lymphocytes in homosexual men with Kaposi's sarcoma (CDC/AIDS) and with lymphadenopathy, healthy homosexual men, and older men (heterosexuals) with Kaposi's sarcoma. (Reproduced from Stahl et al., 1982 by permission.)

distribution of T lymphocyte subsets suggest that depletion of helper T lymphocytes is central to the pathogenesis of AIDS, but a variety of other immune disturbances have been described. In the absence of longitudinal studies of these abnormalities it is difficult to fit them into a comprehensive model of pathogenesis. A practical approach to these questions has been therapeutic trials of available immune mediators such as interferon, interleukin II, and alpha-thymosin given to AIDS patients to correct postulated deficiencies. Interferons, a complex family of immunoregulatory peptides, are abnormal in several respects. For example, an abnormal, acid-labile form of alpha interferon is elevated in AIDS (Destefano et al., 1982; Eyster et al., 1983). While interferons have produced remissions in a minority of patients with Kaposi's sarcoma, the underlying immune deficiency has not been improved in patients with AIDS or AIDS-related complex (Krown et al., 1983; Metroka et al., 1983). Interleukin II, also called T cell growth factor, has been shown to restore the function of lymphocytes from AIDS patients in vitro (Rook et al., 1983), but the therapeutic effect of interleukin II on immune function in AIDS patients has not been determined. Alpha-thymosin, a hormone of thymic origin, is elevated in AIDS patients, but is considered a potential therapeutic agent on the basis that "end organ failure" may require supraphysiological amounts to restore T lymphocyte function (Hersh et al., 1983).

Despite lack of clinical evidence of B lymphocyte dysfunction in AIDS, B cell function in vitro appears to be markedly abnormal (Lane et al., 1983). B lymphocytes appear to hyper-secrete immunoglobulins without stimulation and fail to stimulate further in response to B cell mitogens or neoantigens.

CLINICAL SYNDROMES OF AIDS—DIAGNOSIS, MANAGEMENT, AND COMPLICATIONS. It is beyond the scope of this chapter to describe in detail the clinical presentations, diagnosis, complications, and management of the many neoplasms and infectious agents that afflict AIDS patients. Instead, those presentations that are characteristic of AIDS patients will be emphasized. Because CDC/AIDS is, by definition, diagnosed only when one of the serious secondary complications supervene, the symptoms of CDC/AIDS partly reflect these secondary complications. Many of the symptoms of the AIDS-related complex are probably caused directly by the AIDS agent, but reactivation of CMV or EBV may play a role. While fever, profound fatigue, and lymphadenopathy resemble symptoms of EBV or CMV mononucleosis, some symptoms of AIDS are not typical of mononucleosis, including relentless weight loss (wasting syndrome) and intermittent diarrhea. Many of these symptoms persist despite cure of specific opportunistic infections such as pneumocystis pneumonia. Thus, the course of a patient with AIDS and recurrent opportunistic infections may decline progressively despite cure of the treatable infections. In contrast, other patients seem to recover nearly completely between complicating infections.

I. Pulmonary Syndromes

A. Pneumocystis Pneumonia. (See Chapter 130). Pneumocystis pneumonia in AIDS causes insidious shortness of breath and mild, non-productive cough progressing for several days to many weeks (Masur et al., 1981; Follansbee et al., 1982). Sometimes only subtle physical and radiographic findings (diffuse interstitial infiltrates) are present despite lowered arterial oxygen pressures. Fever is usually present and may be the most dramatic symptom. Chest pain, pleural effusions, and productive cough, are distinctly unusual. Asymmetrical or localized changes on x-ray of the chest occur, but are not the rule and suggest other diagnoses. Although organisms can sometimes be seen in respiratory secretions, either endoscopic transbronchial biopsy, brushings, or washings or surgical lung biopsy are necessary to make the specific diagnosis in most patients. Consensus favors a three step procedure in diagnosis of patients with AIDS suspected of having opportunistic pulmonary infections. First, examine sputum, if available, to rule out easily diagnosed bacterial pneumonias. Second, perform endoscopy with transbronchial biopsy, brushing, and high volume (>100 ml) saline lavage. Impression smears of material obtained should be stained and examined. Finally, perform open surgical biopsy when the former procedures are unrevealing. Therapy for pneumocystis can be started before diagnostic procedures because treatment doesn't eliminate cysts immediately.

Most patients respond clinically within a week of beginning either high doses of cotrimoxazole or pentamidine. As many as half of those treated with cotrimoxazole (trimethoprim/sulfamethoxazole) develop a diffuse macular rash, fever, and/or depression of granulocyte or platelet counts on the ninth or tenth day of treatment and are switched to pentamidine for the remainder of their 10 to 21 day course of treatment (Jaffe et al., 1983). In contrast to the high frequency of reactions to cotrimoxazole in AIDS, adverse reactions to pentamidine are not increased in AIDS compared to non-AIDS patients. The consequences of continuing cotrimoxazole in the face of leukopenia or rash or of stopping all therapy after only 7 or 10 days of treatment are unknown. The decision whether to use cotrimoxazole or pentamidine to treat pneumocystis in AIDS has been influenced in the United States by the investigational status and limited availability of pentamidine. There is developing evidence that cotrimoxazole may produce faster resolution of fever, impaired gas diffusion, and radiographic abnormalities than pentamidine. In many American hospitals, patients are treated first with cotrimoxazole and switched to pentamidine, which has been removed from investigational status, when the reversible side effects listed above develop. Duration of therapy (conventionally 14 days) is controversial because repeated lung biopsy has shown persistence of cysts after two weeks of therapy in many AIDS patients and some patients have second episodes of pneumocystis pneumonia. Whether more prolonged therapy would prevent these problems is not yet clear. The adverse physiological effects of pneumocystis pneumonia appear to be reversible in most patients who are treated early. Full recovery may require 2 to 6 weeks and may be interrupted by recurrence or other opportunistic infections.

B. Cytomegalovirus pneumonia (See Chapters 117 and 217). CMV pneumonia is well described in patients immunosuppressed for renal and bone marrow homografts, but not in AIDS. Widespread reactivation of CMV in patients dying of AIDS makes it difficult to ascribe to CMV any one pathological finding. Nevertheless, CMV inclusions have been seen and the virus grown from lungs of AIDS patients dying of progressive pneumonias without other identifiable pathogens. Antiviral drugs with specific activity against CMV are under development. They may help to define the role of CMV in fatal pneumonias in AIDS patients.

C. Cryptococcal pneumonia (See Chapter 122). The

environmental fungus, *Cryptococcus neoformans*, produces primary focal pneumonia in healthy persons. In immunosuppressed patients, it may disseminate to the meninges, skin, or other sites. Too few cases of cryptococcal disease have been described in AIDS patients to allow a description of the full clinical spectrum. The high incidence of positive blood cultures for cryptococci is a striking feature of the disease in AIDS. Patients with disseminated disease have been cured by the combination of amphotericin B and 5-fluorocytosine for 6 weeks, the recommended regimen for cryptococcal meningitis, but relapses are common.

D. Mycobacterial disease (See Chapters 120 and 121). Both *Mycobacterium tuberculosis* and *M. avium-intracellulare* (MAI) occur at increased frequency in AIDS patients and are usually disseminated (Greene et al., 1982, Zakowski et al., 1982). Widely disseminated infections with the environmental, slow growing, mycobacteria of the avium-intracellulare group have been commonly found at autopsy. Enormous numbers of these acid-fast bacilli may pack the macrophages in lung, spleen, liver, lymph nodes, kidney, the gastrointestinal tract and bone marrow simulating lepromatous leprosy histologically. The organisms can be grown from the blood if proper techniques and long incubation are employed (Pierce et al., 1983). Lesions in the GI tract may resemble Whipple's disease both morphologically and clinically, but can be differentiated because the bacilli filling mucosal histocytes in classical Whipple's disease are not acid-fast (Strom et al., 1983, Roth et al., 1983). Parenchymal disease of the lung is uncommon, but enlarging hilar adenopathy may signify reactivation of latent MAI followed by dissemination. Treatment of MAI is unsatisfactory in AIDS as in other conditions. New drugs with greater potency against MAI such as ansamycin and clofazamine may soon become available through the CDC.

II. Gastrointestinal Syndromes. Diarrheal illnesses are common in those homosexual men whose sexual practices involve fecal-oral exposures to multiple partners and have been associated with a variety of bacterial *(Shigella, Campylobacter, Salmonella)* and protozoal (*Giardia, amoeba*) pathogens (Quinn et al., 1983). In addition to these recognized causes of sexually-transmitted diarrheas, five other gastrointestinal syndromes are recognized in AIDS patients.

A. Kaposi's Sarcoma. At least half of AIDS patients with Kaposi's sarcoma have gastrointestinal lesions if carefully examined with panendoscopy and radiographic contrast studies and most of these lesions are asymptomatic (Stahl et al., 1982; Rose et al., 1982). They range from nodular tumors to flat, red to purple, submucosal patches. The flat lesions are not visible on routine contrast studies of the bowel. Lesions occur throughout the GI tract from the mouth to the rectum and may initially present only in a GI site.

B. Cryptosporidiosis and Isosporiosis (See Chapter 140 and 141). The zoonotic sporozoan parasites *Cryptosporidium enteriditis* and, less commonly, *Isospora belli* cause diarrhea and malabsorption in AIDS patients. Cryptosporidiosis in healthy persons is a self-limited infection of lesser severity than, but similar symptoms to, giardiasis (Jokipii et al., 1983). At least 60 cases of cryptosporidiosis, (Table 2) many with severe, intractable, high volume diarrhea, have been reported to the CDC (Center for Disease Control, 1982). Symptoms may include nausea, vomiting, anorexia, low grade fever, abdominal cramps and pain, and multiple (5 to 25) watery, frothy bowel movements daily. Because malabsorption and fluid loss may be profound (mean 3 to 5 liters daily), patients may require total parenteral nutrition. Diagnosis can be made easily by observing the small cysts in stools by modified acid-fast or auramine staining (Ma et al., 1983; Payne et al., 1983). The most striking feature of this parasite is its resistance to many agents that have failed to cure AIDS patients and animals with the disease.

Isospora belli, another coccidial parasite of animals, has produced chronic, severe, but treatable, diarrheas in a small number of AIDS patients and apparently normal patients. This organism has responded to combinations of anti-folate drugs such as pyrimethamine and sulfadiazine or cotrimoxazole.

C. Ulcerative esophagitis (See Chapters 104 and 105). *Candida albicans, Herpes simplex*, and cytomegalovirus alone or in combination have been associated with ulcerative lesions of the esophagus in AIDS patients. Substernal pain or dysphagia from candida esophagitis, usually in association with oral thrush may be the first manifestation of AIDS. Both herpes simplex and cytomegalovirus have been seen in and grown from biopsies or at autopsy in patients with extensive ulcers of the esophagus. Diagnosis of esophagitis can be made radiographically or specifically by endoscopic appearance, cultures, and biopsy. Candida esophagitis responds to systemic antifungals (amphotericin ± 5 fluorocytosine or oral ketoconazole alone) and *Herpes simplex* may be treated with acyclovir.

D. Ulcerative enteritis and colitis. In patients with AIDS as well as other immunosuppressed persons ulcers of the bowel have been described in which cytomegalovirus may play a role (Guttmann et al., 1983). These multiple discreet ulcers of the large or small bowel (especially caecum) have typical cytomegalovirus cells in perivascular distribution suggesting a vasculitis, but the role of CMV in this syndrome is not clear because of widespread dissemination of CMV in uninflamed tissues of the same patients.

E. Proctitis. Various infectious agents cause proctitis in homosexual men, but AIDS patients are subject to chronic, progressive, destructive *Herpes simplex* infections of the perianal skin and rectum (Siegal, et al., 1981). These lesions, like other herpetic infections in AIDS have responded to intravenous acyclovir.

III. Neurological Syndromes. Many different opportunistic infections produce focal and diffuse encephalitis and meningitis in AIDS patients, but tumors (especially primary lymphomas), vascular complications, and peripheral neuropathies also occur. In a review of the experience at Memorial Hospital in New York (Snider et al., 1983), the wide variety of neurological complications shown in Table 3 were documented in 50 of 160 patients with AIDS.

A. Opportunistic Infections. The most common syndrome was progressive subacute encephalitis of unknown cause, insidious onset, and relentless progression. Patients developed initial subtle cognitive changes and psychomotor retardation suggesting depression, but progressed to dementia, focal neurological defect, or seizures. Mild cerebrospinal pleocytosis, elevated protein, and/or lowered glucose occurred in 12 of 16 patients. Computerized tomography (CT) scans often showed diffuse cerebral atrophy. Postmortem examination of the brain showed microglial nodules without inflammation in gray matter and poorly defined foci of demyelination in white matter. No infectious cause was found for these changes.

Toxoplasma gondii caused intracerebral abscesses in 5

Table 3. NEUROLOGICAL COMPLICATIONS OF ACQUIRED IMMUNE DEFICIENCY SYNDROME IN 50 PATIENTS (FROM SNIDER ET AL., 1983)

Central nervous system infections	
Subacute encephalitis	18
Toxoplasma gondii	5
Progressive multifocal leukoencephalopathy	2
Cryptococcal meningitis	2
? *M. avium intracellulare*	3
Candida albicans	1
Total	31
Neoplasms	
Primary lymphoma of brain	3
Meningeal lymphoma	4
Epidural (thoracic) lymphoma	1
Epidural (thoracic) plasmacytoma	1
Total	9
Vascular complications	
Nonbacterial thrombotic endocarditis	2
Cerebral hemorrhage	3
? Parainfectious cerebral arteritis	1
Total	6
Peripheral neuropathy	8
Other conditions	
Focal mass lesions of unknown cause	3
Aseptic meningitis	4
Polymyositis	1
Retinopathy	10

patients, usually with focal neurological signs (See also Wong et al., 1984). CT scans showed contrast-enhancing lesions that were often multiple and located in basal ganglia. Serological diagnosis was not possible because patients failed to show rises in or high levels of IgG antibody or to develop IgM antibody during infection (Luft et al., 1983). Biopsy of the brain can provide definitive diagnosis and treatment with pyrimethamine and sulfadiazine has improved some patients.

Progressive multifocal leukoencephalopathy (PML), an opportunistic, reactivated infection in immunosuppressed patients caused by the papovavirus, J.C., produced focal lesions and dementia in two patients (also Miller et al., 1982). Cryptococcal meningitis, a frequent opportunist in other diseases of depressed cellular immunity, was seen in two patients who responded to therapy.

B. Neoplastic, vascular, and peripheral lesions. Primary CNS lymphomas (7) and a variety of lymphatic neoplasms that invaded the CNS (6) constituted the neoplastic complications of AIDS in the nervous system. Two patients developed nonbacterial thrombotic endocarditis with embolic lesions to the CNS. Two thrombocytopenic men had cerebral hemorrhage, one each related to brain biopsy and subarachnoid hemorrhage. Progressive peripheral polyneuropathy characterized in most by painful dysthesias, distal sensory loss and weakness, and slowing of nerve conduction velocity consistent with demyelination were seen in 8 patients. Transient aseptic meningitis of unknown cause was found in four patients. Chorioretinitis was attributed to CMV and toxoplasma in one patient each, but a variety of retinal findings have been described (Newman et al., 1983).

IV. Hematological Syndromes and Lymphomas. Unexplained thrombocytopenia, neutropenia, and anemia are frequent complications of AIDS. An epidemic, immunologically-distinct form of idiopathic thrombocytopenia purpura (ITP) has been reported in male homosexuals and hemophiliacs (Morris et al., 1982, Ratnoff et al., 1983). While clinically similar to classic autoimmune thrombocytopenia purpura, ITP in patients with AIDS and in homosexual men without CDC/AIDS is mediated by circulating immune complexes rather than by antiplatelet antibodies (Walsh and Karpatkin, 1983). The relationship of ITP to AIDS has been strengthened by the observation that homosexual men with ITP have developed CDC/AIDS and that most have lymphocyte abnormalities and impaired cellular immunity similar to patients with CDC/AIDS (Walsh and Karpatkin, 1983). Many of these patients have responded to steroids, but some have required splenectomy.

Granulocytopenia in the range of 1.5 to 4.0×10^9 neutrophils/liter is very common in AIDS patients. More profound neutropenia has been described (Zauber et al., 1983) in association with Coomb's positive hemolytic anemia. In two patients with AIDS and severe granulocytopenia, granulocyte production appeared to be suppressed by inhibitory T lymphocytes (Bagby et al., 1983).

The frequent development of cytopenias (especially granulocytopenia) during high dose cotrimoxazole therapy for pneumocystis pneumonia appears to be immunologically mediated because it often occurs in combination with fever or skin rashes on the ninth day of therapy and does not usually respond to folinic acid.

In twenty-three homosexual men living in the AIDS epidemic areas, B cell lymphomas appeared mainly in extranodal sites (Levine et al., 1984; Ziegler et al., 1983; Snider et al., 1983). These tumors have been called immunoblastic sarcomas, Burkitt-like lymphomas, and plasmacytoid lymphocytic leukemias. Most have had markedly abnormal ratios of helper to suppressor T lymphocytes and generalized lymphadenopathy. Many, but not all, have also had opportunistic infections suggestive of AIDS.

V. Mucocutaneous Syndromes

A. Kaposi's Sarcoma. The mucocutaneous lesions of Kaposi's sarcoma are very common in AIDS patients, may be the only manifestation of AIDS for prolonged periods, and are only occasionally symptomatic, usually because of mechanical effects. The problems caused for the patient are psychological, social, and medical. Because they often appear on the face, they raise questions that may make it difficult for the patient to continue working or socializing. The lesions may be superficial macules, papules, or deep subcutaneous nodules. Color ranges from colorless in deep, nodular, subcutaneous lesions to red or purple in more superficial ones. Lesions are usually oblong, oriented with their long axis along skin cleavage lines, and multiple with approximately symmetrical distribution over the body. They frequently involve the mouth and especially the hard palate. Definitive diagnosis requires biopsy, but their appearance, distribution, and development in the setting of established AIDS is often sufficiently characteristic for tentative clinical diagnosis by experienced physicians.

Therapy of Kaposi's sarcoma in AIDS is controversial given the minority of responsive patients, short duration of remission, and concerns about the immunosuppressive effects of chemotherapy (Volberding et al., 1983; Fauci et al., 1984). Treatment of Kaposi's limited to the skin or gastrointestinal tract may not be indicated.

B. Mucocutaneous Candidiasis. Oropharyngeal or intertriginous thrush is a very common manifestation of AIDS and is, with candida esophagitis, often the first opportunistic infection in AIDS patients. Patients with other syndromes of generalized or candida-specific loss of T lymphocyte-mediated immunity share this susceptibility. AIDS patients are not as susceptible to disseminated candidiasis as patients with neutropenia or intravenous catheters. Both topical and systemic therapy may provide relief and some patients require chronic topical or systemic prophylaxis.

C. Chronic Herpes Simplex. Herpetic lesions of unusual chronicity, destructiveness, and extent are common and may be difficult to recognize if not found in their usual facial, genital, or perirectal sites (Siegal et al., 1981). These lesions may deeply erode normal tissues, simulate pyogenic infections by forming pus and becoming superinfected (especially with *Staphylococcus aureus*), and persist for months if untreated. They respond poorly to topical antivirals, but most respond to intravenous acyclovir.

D. Herpes zoster. As expected, reactivation of dermatomal zoster is common in AIDS, but fortunately dissemination or poor resolution is not. The need for routine treatment of zoster in AIDS with antivirals has not yet been demonstrated. The value of routine adenine arabinoside or acyclovir treatment of zoster in other immunosuppressive diseases has been established in controlled studies (Whitley et al., 1982; Balfour et al., 1983). Dissemination or poor resolution would appear to be a clear indication for antiviral therapy.

E. Disseminated Fungal Infections. Cryptococcosis and coccidioidomycosis may involve the skin when pulmonary infections disseminate and require systemic therapy.

VI. AIDS-Related Complex. An epidemic syndrome of less severe, but related abnormalities has been recognized simultaneously with CDC/AIDS. The features of this syndrome, recently designated AIDS-related complex, are chronic generalized lymphadenopathy; fatigue, weight loss and fevers; prolonged diarrhea; and minor opportunistic infections (e.g., thrush or herpetic dermatitis). Laboratory findings are cytopenias and the T lymphocyte abnormalities associated with CDC/AIDS. AIDS-related complex is a less severe form of HTLVIII LAV infection and progresses to CDC/AIDS in a minority of patients. CDC/AIDS patients who have been successfully treated for opportunistic infections frequently continue to suffer from symptoms of AIDS-related complex suggesting that these symptoms are caused directly by the AIDS agent. On the other hand, many persons with AIDS-related complex have been followed for several years without developing CDC/AIDS.

The CDC first called attention to chronic generalized lymphadenopathy (CGL) in homosexual males, a subgroup of patients with AIDS-related complex, in May, 1982 (Centers for Disease Control, 1982). Enlarged lymph nodes involving two or more groups of nodes (excluding femoral or inguinal regions), persisting for 3 or 6 months without evidence of CDC/AIDS, and unexplained by any known illness or drug have qualified patients for inclusion in a number of prospective, ongoing studies. Two of these have been reported (Metroka et al., 1983; Abrams et al., 1984). These studies and others have demonstrated that chronic generalized lymphadenopathy (CGL) is common in AIDS, but is not necessary for development of CDC/AIDS. A minority (~10 to 20 per cent) of CGL patients have developed CDC/AIDS in the first years of follow-up. Hepatosplenomegaly, hematological abnormalities, dermatological problems, mild hepatitis, and elevated viral (CMV and EBV) antibody titers are common, and so are less severe opportunistic infections (thrush, herpes zoster, recurrent or chronic herpes simplex infections).

Abnormalities of immune function similar to those in CDC/AIDS (abnormal lymphocyte subsets, anergy to skin tests, depressed lymphocyte proliferation in vitro) occur in most patients with CGL. A "wasting syndrome" consisting of relentless weight loss with variable degrees of anorexia, diarrhea, fever, or CGL identifies a subset of patients at high risk of CDC/AIDS. Lymph nodes from the vast majority of CGL patients exhibit florid follicular hyperplasia, but a few have involution or depletion of follicles which is associated with a high risk (~60 per cent) of subsequent development of CDC/AIDS (Fernandez et al., 1983).

Management of AIDS-related complex is difficult because the diagnosis, natural history, and prognostic indicators are not well defined. The following practical approach to management of these patients stratifies them into groups requiring various degrees of laboratory evaluation, surveillance, and counselling regarding potential infectivity. Stratification is based on the following evaluation:

1) *History* focuses on a) non-AIDS-related causes of lymphadenopathy such as heroin use, phenytoin and other drugs, secondary syphilis, etc. b) risk factors for AIDS such as homosexual exposures, intravenous drug use, transfusion therapy, or exposures to others in high risk groups, and c) infections suggestive of decreased cell-mediated immunity such as zoster or thrush.

2) *Physical Examination* emphasizes inspection of skin and mucous membranes (including proctoscopy), funduscopic examination, and careful search for enlarged lymph nodes and hepatosplenomegaly.

3) *Laboratory Examination* at minimum includes complete blood count with differential, cultures and ova and parasite examinations of stool if diarrhea is present, and a serological test for syphilis. Patients with objective constitutional symptoms, history of opportunistic infections, cytopenias, or prolonged adenopathy (>3 months) have skin tests placed [PPD-S, coccidiodin, candida extract, tetanus toxoid (diluted 1/5), mumps and trichophyton]. Patients with persistent cytopenias or prolonged fevers have their bone marrow examined and cultured if blood cultures are unrevealing. Lymph nodes are biopsied if history, physical exam, or constitutional symptoms suggest possible lymphoma, but criteria for increased risk of lymphoma in AIDS have not been established. Lymphocyte subsets are enumerated when there is strong suspicion (medium or high risk) of CDC/AIDS, but their value in diagnosis or prognosis is not established. Nevertheless, persistently reduced T_H (helper cell) percentages (<10 per cent) are associated with a bad prognosis.

Based on this evaluation patients can be designated as *low risk* if they have no or only "soft" constitutional symptoms (fatigue, malaise, undocumented sensation of fevers, or mild diarrhea), *medium risk* if they have "hard" constitutional symptoms (fevers, mild weight loss, or persistent diarrhea), or *high risk* if they have severe weight loss, opportunistic infections not meeting CDC/AIDS definitions, or profound cytopenias. This stratification of risk of CDC/AIDS is used to determine the extent of initial immunological evaluation, the frequency of follow-up visits, the threshold for investigation of subsequent complaints, and the extent of counseling about measures to reduce transmission.

PREVENTION. Because the AIDS agent appears to be transmitted only by sexual intimacy and transfer of blood or blood products, measures to prevent its spread focus on reducing dangerous sexual or drug habits and eliminating blood donation by persons in high risk groups. An effect of the widespread publicity about AIDS on behavior of homosexual men who have been highly promiscuous can be inferred from declining rates of gonorrhea. Blood banks in most epidemic areas have asked that persons in high risk groups refrain from donating blood or identify themselves if they do.

Available evidence indicates that the risk of contracting AIDS through even close, nonsexual contacts with AIDS patients or persons in high risk groups is minimal. Specifically, roommates, family members, and providers of medical care are at extremely low (undemonstrated) risk from AIDS patients and need not take precautions beyond avoiding exposure to blood or body fluids containing blood (Conte et al., 1983). Certain opportunistic infectious agents such as *Herpes zoster* and *H. simplex, Cytomegalovirus, M. tuberculosis,* and *Cryptosporidium* are potentially transmissible and require precautions.

Specific advice to persons in high risk groups must be based on the incomplete knowledge about transmission, incubation period of AIDS, and period of infectivity before symptoms develop. All persons at *high risk* of AIDS should be considered potentially infectious and measures designed to reduce risk of transmission by sexual routes or blood products should be based broadly on high risk groups rather than patients with CDC/AIDS. For homosexual men, this means reducing the number of sexual partners and avoiding traumatic sexual practices. For intravenous drug users, it means not sharing needles or eliminating intravenous injections. For recipients of blood transfusions or blood products (e.g., hemophiliacs) it means using products derived from a minimum number of donors who are, if possible, unpaid volunteers. The risk for female sexual partners of men in high risk groups appears to be increased, but the exact mode of spread is unknown. A prudent precaution, short of terminating sexual intimacy, would be use of condoms to eliminate exposure to semen.

Appropriate precautions for medical and clinical laboratory personnel, as well as researchers, have been published by the Centers for Disease Control (1982). In general, these recommendations are those appropriate to handling material from patients with any blood-borne infectious agent such as hepatitis B. Although medical personnel have been diagnosed with AIDS, most have been in high risk groups and probably did not acquire the disease occupationally. The few medical personnel who may have contracted AIDS at work had not had direct contact with AIDS patients (Centers for Disease Control, 1983).

References

Abrams, D. I., Lewis, B. J., Beckstead, J. H., Casavant, C. A., and Drew, W. L.: Persistent diffuse lymphadenopathy in homosexual men: endpoint or prodrome. Ann Intern Med (In Press, 1984).

Bagby, G. C., Lawrence, H. J., and Neerhout, R. C.: T-lymphocyte-mediated granulopoietic failure. N Engl J Med 309:1073, 1983.

Balfour, H. H. Jr., Bean, B., Laskin, O. L. et al.: Acyclovir halts progression of herpes zoster in immunocompromised patients. N Engl J Med 308:1448, 1983.

Barre-Sinoussi, F., et al.: Isolation of a T-lymphotropic retrovirus from a patient at risk for acquired immunodeficiency syndrome (AIDS). Science 220:868, 1983.

Blun-Vezinet, F., Barre-Sinoussi, F., Rouzioux, C., et al.: Detection of IgG antibodies to lymphadenopathy-associated virus in patients with AIDS or lymphadenopathy syndrome. Lancet 1: 1253, 1984.

Centers for Disease Control: A cluster of Kaposi's sarcoma and *Pneumocystis carinii* pneumonia among homosexual male residents of Los Angeles and Orange Counties, California. Morbid Mortal Weekly Rep 3:305, 1982.

Centers for Disease Control: Acquired immunodeficiency syndrome (AIDS): Precautions for clinical and laboratory staffs. Morbid Mortal Weekly Rep 31:557, 1982.

Centers for Disease Control: An evaluation of acquired immunodeficiency syndrome (AIDS) reported in health care personnel—United States. Morbid. Mortal. Weekly Rep. 32:358, 1983.

Centers for Disease Control: Cryptosporidiosis: assessment of chemotherapy of males with acquired immunodeficiency syndrome (AIDS). Morbid Mortal Weekly Rep 31:589, 1982.

Centers for Disease Control: Persistent, generalized lymphadenopathy among homosexual males. Morb Mortal Weekly Rep 31:249, 1982.

Centers for Disease Control: Epidemiological aspects of the current outbreak of Kaposi's sarcoma and opportunistic infections. N Engl J Med 306:248, 1982.

Centers for Disease Control: Acquired immunodeficiency syndrome among patients with hemophilia—United States. Morbid Mortal Weekly Rep 32:615, 1983.

Cherman, J. C., Barre-Sinoussi, F., Dauguet, C., et al.: Characterization of a new type of retrovirus isolated from patients with AIDS and from patients at risk of AIDS. J Cell Biochem Abstract 0008, Supplement 8A, 1984.

Conte, J. E., Hadley, W. K., Sande, M. et al.: Infection control guidelines for patients with the acquired immunodeficiency syndrome (AIDS). N Engl J Med 309:740, 1983.

Curran, J. W., Lawrence, D. N., Jaffe, H., et al.: Acquired immunodeficiency syndrome (AIDS) associated with transfusions. N Engl J Med 310:69, 1984.

Daniel, M. D., King, N. W., Letvin, N. L., et al. A new type D retrovirus isolated from macaques with an immunodeficiency syndrome. Science 223:602, 1984.

Destefano, E., Friedman, R. M., Friedman-Kien, A. E., et al.: Acid-labile leukocyte interferon in homosexual men with Kaposi's sarcoma and lymphadenopathy. J Infect Dis 146:451, 1982.

DeWaele, M., Thielemans, C., and VanCamp, B. K. G.: Characterization of immunoregulatory T cells in EBV-induced infectious mononucleosis by monoclonal antibodies. N Eng J Med 304:640, 1981.

Drew, W. L., Mintz, L., Miner, R. C., et al.: Prevalence of cytomegalovirus infection in homosexual men. J Infect Dis 143:188, 1981.

Ehrlich, G., Moore, J., Tomas, R., et al.: Integrated HTLV proviral DNA in splenocytes of a patient with AIDS. J Cell Biochem. Abstract 0039 Supplement 8A 1984.

Essex, M., et al.: Antibodies to cell membrane antigens associated with human T-cell leukemia virus in patients with AIDS. Science 220:859, 1983.

Ewing, E. P., Spira, T. J., Chandler, F. W., et al.: Unusual cytoplasmic body in lymphoid cells of homosexual men with unexplained lymphadenopathy. N Engl J Med 308:819, 1983.

Eyster, E. M., Goedert, J. J., Poon, M. C., and Prebel, O. T.: Acid-labile alpha interferon. N Engl J Med 309:584, 1983.

Fauci, A. S., Macher, A. M., Longo, D. L., et al.: Acquired immunodeficiency syndrome: epidemiologic, clinical, immunologic, and therapeutic considerations. Ann Intern Med 100:92, 1984.

Fernandez, R., Mouradian, J., Metroka, C., and Davis, J.: The prognostic value of histopathology in persistent generalized lymphadenopathy in homosexual men. N Engl J Med 309:185, 1983.

Follansbee, S. E., Busch, D. F., Wofsy, C. B., et al.: An outbreak of *Pneumocystis carinii* pneumonia in homosexual men. Ann Intern Med 96:705, 1982.

Gallo, R. C., Sarahudpin, S. Z., Papovic, M., et al.: Frequent detection and isolation of cytopathic retroviruses (HTLV-III) from patients with AIDS and at risk of AIDS. Science 224:500, 1984.

Gelmann, E. P., et al.: Proviral DNA of a retrovirus, human T-cell leukemia virus, in two patients with AIDS. Science 220:862, 1983.

Giraldo, G., Beth, E., and Kyalwazi, S. K.: Etiological implications on Kaposi's sarcoma. In *Antibiotics Chemotherapy* (Karger, Basel, 1981) vol. 29, pp 12-29.

Gottlieb, M. S., Schroff, R., Schanker, H. M., et al.: *Pneumocystis carinii* pneumonia and mucosal candidiasis in previously healthy homosexual men: evidence of a new acquired cellular immunodeficiency. N Engl J Med 305:1425, 1981.

Greene, J. B., Sidhu, G. S., Lewin, S., et al.: *Mycobacterium avium-intracellulare:* a cause of disseminated life-threatening infection in homosexuals and drug abusers. Ann Intern Med 97:539, 1982.

Guttmann, D., Raymond, A., Gelb, A., et al.: Virus-associated colitis in homosexual men: two case reports. Am J Gastroenterol 78:167, 1983.

Harris, C., Small, C. B., Klein, R. S. et al. Immunodeficiency in female sexual partners of men with the acquired immunodeficiency syndrome. N Engl J Med 308:1181, 1983.

Hendrickson, R. V., Maul, D. H., Osborn, K. G.: Epidemic of acquired immunodeficiency in *Rheusus*. Lancet i:388, 1983.

Hersh, E. M., Reuben, J. M., Rios, A., et al.: Elevated serum thymosin −1 levels associated with evidence of immune dysregulation in male homosexuals with a history of infectious or Kaposi's sarcoma (Letter) N Engl J Med 308:45, 1983.

Hutt, M. S. R.: The epidemiology of Kaposi's sarcoma. In *Antibiotics Chemotherapy* (Karger, Basel) 29:3, 1981.

Jaffe, H. S., Abrams, D. I., Amman, A. J., Lewis, B. J., and Golden, J. A.: Complications of co-trimoxazole in treatment of AIDS-associated Pneumocystis pneumonia in homosexual men. Lancet ii:1109, 1983.

Jaffe, H. W., Choi, K., Thomas, P. A., et al.: National case-control study of Kaposi's sarcoma and *Pneumocystic carinii* pneumonia in homosexual men: Part I, Epidemiologic results. Ann Intern Med 99:145, 1983.

Jokipii, L., Pohjola, S., and Jokipii, A. M. M.: Cryptosporidium: a frequent finding in patients with gastrointestinal symptoms. Lancet ii:358, 1983.

Klatzman, D., Barre-Sinoussi, F., Nugeyre, M. T., et al.: Selective tropism of lymphadenopathy associated virus (LAV) for helper-inducer T lymphocytes. Science 125:59, 1984.

Krown, S. E., Real, F. X., Cunningham-Rundles, S., et al.: Preliminary observations on the effect of recombinant leukocyte A interferon in homosexual men with Kaposi's sarcoma. N Engl J Med 308:1071, 1983.

Lane, H. C., Masyr, H., Edgar, L. C., et al.: Abnormalities of B cell activation and immunoregulation in patients with acquired immunodeficiency syndrome. N Engl J Med 308:453, 1983.

Letvin, N. L., Aldrich, W. R., King, N. W., et al.: Experimental transmission of macaque AIDS by means of inoculation of macaque lymphoma tissue. Lancet ii:599, 1983.

Letvin, N. L., Eaton, K. A., Aldrich, W. R.: Acquired immunodeficiency syndrome in a colony of macaque monkeys. Proc Nat Acad Sci 80:2718, 1983.

Levine, A. M., Meyer, P. R., Begandy, M. K., et al.: Development of B-cell lymphoma in homosexual men clinical and immunological findings. Ann Intern Med 100:7, 1984.

London, W. T., Sever, J. L., Madden, D. L., et al.: Experimental transmission of simian acquired immunodeficiency syndrome (SAIDS) and kaposi-like skin lesions. Lancet ii:869, 1983.

Luft, B. J., Conley, F., Remington, J. S. et al.: Outbreak of central nervous system toxoplasmosis in Western Europe and North America. Lancet i:781, 1983.

Magrath, I., Erickson, J., Whang-Peng, J., et al.: Synthesis of kappa light chains by cell lines containing an 8:22 chromosomal translocation derived from a male homosexual with Burkitt's lymphoma. Science 222:1094, 1983.

Marx, P. A., Maul, D. H., Osborn, K. G., et al.: Simian AIDS: isolation of a type D retrovirus and transmission of the disease. Science 223:1083, 1984.

Masur, H., Michelis, M. A., Greene, J. B., et al.: An outbreak of community-acquired *Pneumocystis carinii* pneumonia: initial manifestation of cellular immune dysfunction. N Engl J Med 305:1431, 1981.

Metroka, C. E., Cunningham-Rundles, S., Pollack, M. S. et al.: Generalized lymphadenopathy in homosexual men. Ann Intern Med 99:585, 1983.

Mildvan, D., Mathur, U., Enlow, R. W., et al.: Opportunistic infections and immune deficiency in homosexual males. Ann Intern Med 96:700, 1982.

Miller, J. R., Barrett, R. E., Britton, C. B., et al.: Progressive multifocal leukoencephalopathy in a male homosexual with T-cell immune deficiency. N Engl J Med 307:1436, 1982.

Mintz, L., Drew, W. L., Miner, R. C., and Braff, E. H.: Cytomegalovirus infections in homosexual men. Ann Intern Med 99:326, 1983.

Morris, L., Distenfeld, A., Amorisi, E., and Karpatkin, S.: Autoimmune thrombocytopenia purpura in homosexual men. Ann Intern Med 96:714, 1982.

Ma, P., Soave, R.: Three-step stool examination for cryptosporidiosis in ten homosexual men with protracted watery diarrhea. J Infect Dis 147:824, 1983.

Moskowitz, L. B., Kory, P., Chan, J. C., et al.: Unusual causes of death in Haitians residing in Miami. JAMA 250:1187, 1983.

Newman, N., Mandel, M. R., Gullett, J., and Fujikawa, L.: Clinical and histological findings in opportunistic ocular infections. Arch Ophthalmol 101:396, 1983.

Olleske, J., Minnefor, A., Cooper, R., et al.: Immune deficiency syndrome in children. JAMA 249:2345, 1983.

Pape, J. W., Liautaud, B., Thomas, F.: Characteristics of the acquired immunodeficiency syndrome (AIDS) in Haiti. N Engl J Med 309:945, 1983.

Papovic, M., Sarngadharan, M. G., Read, E., and Gallo, R. C.: Frequent detection and isolation of cytopathic retroviruses (HTLV-III) from patients with AIDS and at risk for AIDS. Science 224:497, 1984.

Payne, P., Lancaster, L. A., Heinzman, M., and McCutchan, J. A.: Identification of Cryptosporidium in patients with the acquired immunodeficiency syndrome. N Engl J Med 309:613, 1983.

Pierce, P. F., Deyoung, D. R., Roberts, G. D.: Mycobacteremia and the new blood culture systems. Ann Intern Med 99:786, 1983.

Quinn, T. C., Stamm, W. E., Goodell, S. E., et al.: The polymicrobial origin of intestinal infections in homosexual men. N Engl J Med 309:576, 1983.

Ratnoff, O. D., Menitove, J. E., Aster, R. H., Lederman, M. M.: Coincident classic hemophilia and "idiopathic" thrombocytopenic purpura in patients under treatment with concentrates of antihemophilic factor (factor VIII). N Engl J Med 308:439, 1983.

Rinaldo, C. R., Ho, M., Hamoudi, W. H., Gui, X., Debiasio, L.: Lymphocyte subsets and natural killer cell responses during cytomegalovirus mononucleosis. Infect and Immun 40:472, 1983.

Rogers, M. F., Morens, D. M., Steward, J. A., et al.: National case-control study of Kaposi's sarcoma and *Pneumocystis carinii* pneumonia in homosexual men: Part 2, Laboratory results. Ann Intern Med 99:151, 1983.

Rook, A. H., Masur, H., Lane, C. H., et al.: Interleukin-2 enhances the depressed natural killer and cytomegalovirus-specific cytotoxic activities of lymphocytes from patients with the acquired immune deficiency syndrome. J Clin Invest 72:398, 1983.

Rose, H. S., Balthazar, E. J., Megibow, A. J., Horowitz, L., and Laubenstein, L. J.: Alimentary tract involvement in Kaposi's sarcoma. Amer J Roent 139:661, 1982.

Roth, R. I., Owen, R. L., and Keren, D. F.: AIDS with *Mycobacterium avium* intracellulare lesions resembling those of Whipple's disease. N Engl J Med 309:1324, 1983.

Rubinstein, A., Sicklick, M., Gupta, A., et al.: Acquired immunodeficiency with reversed T4/T8 ratios in infants born to promiscuous and drug-addicted mothers. JAMA 249:2350, 1983.

Sarngadharan, M. G., Papovic, M., Bruch, L., et al.: Antibodies reactive with human T lymphotropic retroviruses (HTLV III) in the serum of patients with AIDS. Science 24:506, 1984.

Schooley, R. T., Hirsch, M. S., Colvin, R. B. et al.: Association of herpesvirus infections with T-lymphocyte-subset alterations, glomerulopathy, and opportunistic infections after renal transplantation. N Engl J Med 308:307, 1983.

Scott, G. B., Buck, B. E., Leterman, J. G., et al.: Acquired immunodeficiency syndrome in infants. N Engl J Med 310:76, 1984.

Sidhu, G. P., Stahl, R. E., Sadr, W. E., and Zolla Pazner, S.: Ultrastructural markers of AIDS. Lancet i:990, 1983.

Siegal, F. P., Lopez, C., Hammer, G. S. et al.: Severe acquired immunodeficiency in male homosexuals manifested by chronic perianal ulcerative herpes simplex lesions. N Engl J Med 305:1439, 1981.

Snider, W. D., Simpsom, D. M., Aronyk, K. E., Nielsen, S. L.: Primary lymphoma of the nervous system associated with acquired immune deficiency syndrome [letter]. N Engl J Med 308:45, 1983.

Snider, W. D., Simpsom, D. M., Nielsen, S. et al.: Neurological complications of acquired immune deficiency syndrome: analysis of 50 cases. Ann Neurol 14:403, 1983.

Stahl, R. E., Friedman-Kien, A., Durbin, R., Marmor, M., Zolla-Pazner, S.: Immunologic abnormalities in homosexual men: Relationship to Kaposi's sarcoma. Am J Med 73:171, 1982.

Strom, R. L. and Gruninger, R. P.: AIDS with *Mycobacterium avium intracellulare* lesions resembling those of Whipple's disease. N Engl J Med 309:1323, 1983.

Volberding, P., Conant, M. A., Stricker, R. B., and Lewis, B. J.: Chemotherapy in advanced Kaposi's sarcoma. Am J Med 74:652, 1983.

Walsh, C. and Karpatkin, S.: On the mechanism of thrombocytopenia purpura in sexually active homosexuals. Clin Res 31:325A, 1983.

Whitley, R. J., Soong, S. J., Dolin, R., et al.: Early vidarabine therapy to control the complications of herpes zoster in immunocompromised patients. N Engl J Med 307:971, 1982.

Wong, B., Gold, J. W. M., Brown, A., et al.: Central nervous system toxoplasmosis in homosexual men and parenteral drug abusers. Ann Intern Med 100:36, 1984.

Zakowski, P., Fligiel, S., Berlin, G. W., Johnson, B. L. Jr.: Disseminated *Mycobacterium avium intracellulare* intracellulare infection in homosexual men dying of acquired immunodeficiency. JAMA 248:2980, 1982.

Zauber, P. and Park, Y. K.: Neutropenia and hemolytic anemia in a homosexual man. N Engl J Med 309:1029, 1983.

Ziegler, J. L., Drew, W. L., Miner, R. C., et al.: Outbreak of Burkitt-like lymphoma in homosexual men. Lancet ii:631, 1982.

M. TOXIC SHOCK

274

STAPHYLOCOCCAL TOXIC SHOCK SYNDROME

MARIAN E. MELISH, M. D.

Toxic Shock Syndrome (TSS) is an acute febrile exanthematous illness involving multiple systems with the potential for developing hypotension, shock, and profound cardiovascular collapse. The illness was first recognized as a distinct entity and described as TSS in 1977 (Todd, 1978) but suddenly became more prevalent in 1980 in certain areas of the United States and Europe. It is characteristically associated with focal staphylococcal infection without positive blood cultures. Because the impressive multisystem manifestations and shock occur in the absence of septicemia, these severe physiologic changes are thought to be mediated by a hematogenously disseminated staphylococcal toxin or toxins produced at the site of infection.

ETIOLOGY. Coagulase-positive staphylococci (*Staphylococcus aureus*) were implicated as the possible etiologic agent in the first report by Todd and associates. Further strong support for a staphylococcal etiology was provided by cases occurring in men and children who had focal staphylococcal infections including cutaneous infections, subcutaneous abscesses, surgical wound infections, adenitis, pneumonia, empyema, and septic arthritis. Blood cultures are generally negative but a few patients have had either bacteremia associated with a severe focal infection or nonfocal bacteremia. To date TSS has been most common among menstruating women who are using vaginal tampons. *S. aureus* is found in the vagina of nearly all these patients, while bacteremia is almost never encountered.

Staphylococci recovered from TSS patients are uniformly coagulase positive and resistant to penicillin. They belong to multiple phage types, although strains lysed by the group I phages especially 29/52, are dominant. TSS-associated staphylococci are less likely to produce alpha toxin than other clinical isolates. Nearly all TSS strains produce the Toxic Shock Syndrome Toxin 1 (TSST-1), which is now used to identify TSS strains.

The acute onset, rapid progression, multisystem involvement, and the occurrence of shock in the absence of bacteremia have suggested that many of the manifestations of TSS may be caused by a hematogenously disseminated staphylococcal toxin or toxins. To date, none has been proven to be the mediator of shock and multisystem disease. Kapral first reported that TSS strains elaborate a factor that causes cellular disruption deep in the epidermis of neonatal mice (Todd, 1978, Kapral, 1982). It is chemically different from the epidermolytic toxins and affects a different site. This material has not been isolated nor chemically identified and is not produced by all TSS strains so that its relationship to TSS is doubtful. The extracellular protein with the strongest claim to be the etiologic agent is TSST-1. This exoprotein was identified independently by different means by Bergdoll (1981) and Schlievert (1981). First called staphylococcal Enterotoxin F and Pyrogenic Exotoxin C, respectively, the proteins identified by these two researchers have been found to be the same material by independent laboratories. TSST-1, a 24 kilodalton protein, is a reliable marker identifying well over 90 per cent of TSS-associated staphylococci in blinded testing. Depending on the source, from 3 to 20 per cent of other clinical or epidemiologic collections of staphylococci produce this protein. Properties of TSST-1 confirmed to date include abilities to produce fever on intravenous infusion in rabbits and to enhance the effects of sublethal doses of endotoxin in rabbits. Preliminary reports also indicate that intravenous infusion in rabbits and primates causes hypotension, azotemia, lymphopenia, and liver damage similar to that seen in human TSS. Although a convincing animal model that reproduces all of the clinical features of TSS has not yet been presented, work from several laboratories indicates that TSST-1 is likely to be the major mediator of the shock, renal, hepatic and muscle damage characteristic of TSS.

EPIDEMIOLOGY. Although TSS was first recognized among children with focal staphylococcal infection, it has subsequently become clear that the group at highest risk are young women using tampons during their menstrual periods. More than 80 per cent of recorded cases of TSS have occurred in young women during the menstrual period or the post-partum period. The remainder (nonmenstrual TSS) occur in adults or children with focal infections at sites other than the vagina. For both sexes the mean age is in the third decade with a range from the newborn to advanced age. The age-specific attack rate in menstrual TSS is highest in the youngest women with one-third of cases in women less than 19. The overwhelming majority of patients with TSS in the United States have been Caucasian, but it is unknown whether Caucasians are at greatest risk or whether this is an artifact of reporting. To date, TSS has been reported primarily from North America and Europe. In the United States the highest incidence has occurred in 3 states with active surveillance programs, Wisconsin, Minnesota, and Utah. It is not yet clear whether there are true geographic differences in incidence. Such differences could be due to regional variation in the prevalence of staphylococci with TSS marker protein or in the availability and use patterns of menstrual hygiene products.

TSS was only sporadically diagnosed in the United States from the time of its first description in 1978 until 1980. From January to May, 1980, 55 cases were reported to the Centers for Disease Control and the epidemiologic case definition was formulated. Widespread publicity about this disease during 1980 undoubtedly spurred reporting of further cases. Cases reported to the Centers for Disease Control of the United States peaked in August and September 1980 and have declined since that time (Reingold, 1982). TSS has been reported from other countries of North America, Europe, and Australia. In the State of Minnesota, U.S.A., where active surveillance has continued, there has not been an appreciable decline in incidence rates or total numbers of cases but the severity of illness has decreased with earlier diagnosis and treatment. The annual incidence rate of TSS among menstruating women is 8.9/100,000 (Osterholm, 1982).

By mid-1980, it became apparent that the overwhelming majority of cases of TSS were menstrually associated and that nearly all victims were using tampons at the onset of symptoms. Two rapidly performed telephone survey case control studies performed by the U.S. Centers for Disease Control established that tampon users were at higher risk and implicated a single tampon brand, a newly introduced highly absorbent tampon that was subsequently removed from the market in October 1980 (Reingold, 1982). A more thorough case control study conducted in Wisconsin, Minnesota, and Iowa demonstrated that the odds ratio for developing TSS with any use of tampons was 18 compared with no use, that odds ratios for individual brands ranged from 5.8 to 27.5 compared with no use of tampons, and that the risk of developing TSS was directly associated with the absorbancy of tampons (Osterholm, 1982).

Recently, interest in nonmenstrual TSS has increased. The proportion of nonmenstrual cases reported to the U.S. Centers for Disease Control has risen from 7 per cent in 1980 to 22 per cent in 1983. Nonmenstrual TSS is generally a sporadic event of low frequency, but apparent nosocomial transmission of TSS associated with surgical wound infections on a post-operative hospital ward, TSS in a mother-infant pair, and apparent vertical transmission of TSS-positive staphylococci have been documented.

PATHOGENESIS AND PATHOLOGY. The acute onset and widespread multisystem involvement in TSS is presumed to be the effect of hematogenous dissemination of one or more toxins produced at and liberated from a site of focal staphylococcal infection or colonization. Although the target tissue of this toxin(s) has not been defined, it is likely to affect the autonomic nervous system causing vomiting and diarrhea, the muscles causing myolysis with liberation of muscle enzymes and myoglobin, hepatic cells, and the vascular system causing changes in permeability and vascular tone that result in hypotension. Changes in renal function may be primary or secondary to alterations in the circulation. Complete elucidation of the pathogenesis of TSS awaits analysis of convincing animal models of the disease and complete study of the biologic effects of the putative toxins.

Pathologic changes in fatal TSS are largely nonspecific and appear to be secondary to changes caused by prolonged or profound hypotension. The most specific changes among 21 fatal cases of menstrual associated TSS in two series were fatty metamorphosis, of the liver with periportal inflammation, pronounced hemophagocytosis and ulcerative desquamation of cervical and vaginal mucosa. All had changes presumed to be secondary to hypoperfusion including pulmonary damage consisting of capillary congestion, intraalveolar hemorrhage and edema and hyaline membrane formation, and renal damage compatible with acute tubular necrosis (Paris, 1982, Larkin, 1982).

CLINICAL FINDINGS. TSS is an acute rapidly progressive disease characterized by precipitous onset of fever, chills, myalgia, nausea and vomiting. It may progress to oliguria and hypotension within 48 hours. Most patients develop a diffuse, but faint, blanching erythroderma rash but it is frequently inapparent in poor light or in the dark-skinned. Mucous membrane involvement consisting of conjunctival and oropharyngeal hyperemia with or without a "strawberry" appearance of the tongue is extremely common. The *epidemiologic* case definition used by the Centers for Disease Control is given in Table 1. It is an accurate description of the major abnormalities of TSS and will identify definite cases. The clinical course of severely ill patients is presented in Figure 1.

Constitutional Symptoms. Fever is characteristically of sudden onset, remarkably elevated, and associated with chills. Most patients experience some degree of headache, confusion, disorientation, or hallucinations. "Light headedness", orthostatic dizziness, and fainting are frequent signs of impending or actual hypotension. Most patients note decreased frequency of urination after the onset of fever. Edema of hands, feet, face, and eyelids is common but may not be noted until fluid replacement is begun.

Skin Manifestations. The initial rash, which occurs within 3 days of onset and may be very faint, consists of nonpainful, nonpruritic flushing of the skin either in a diffuse pattern or localized to the lower abdomen, thighs, and peripheral extremities. A positive Nicolsky sign has been reported in a few patients. Petechiae may accompany thrombocytopenia during the first 4 days of illness. Approximately one-third of patients develop a more distinctive and discrete generalized erythematous maculopapular rash from 5 to 10 days after onset of fever. Full thickness desquamation beginning at finger and toe tips and pro-

Table 1. EPIDEMIOLOGIC CASE DEFINITION OF TOXIC SHOCK SYNDROME[1]

Fever: temperature ≥ 38.9° C (102° F)

Rash: Diffuse macular erythroderma

Desquamation 1 to 2 weeks after onset of illness, particularly of palms and soles

Hypotension: systolic blood pressure ≤ 90 mm Hg for adults or below fifth percentile by age for children below 16 years of age, orthostatic drop in diastolic blood pressure ≥15 mm Hg from lying to sitting, orthostatic syncope, or orthostatic dizziness

Multisystem involvement—three or more of the following:
- Gastrointestinal: vomiting or diarrhea at onset of illness
- Muscular: severe myalgia or creatine phosphokinase level at least twice the upper limit of normal for laboratory
- Mucous membrane: vagina, oropharyngeal, or conjunctival hyperemia
- Renal: blood urea nitrogen or creatinine at least twice the upper limit of normal for laboratory or urinary sediment with pyuria (≥ 5 leukocytes per high-power field) in the absence of urinary tract infection.
- Hepatic: total bilirubin, SGOT[2], SGPT[3] at least twice the upper limit of normal for laboratory
- Hematologic: platelets ≥ 100,000/mm^3
- Central nervous system: disorientation or alterations in consciousness without focal neurologic signs when fever and hypotension are absent.

Negative results on the following tests, if obtained:
- Blood, throat, or cerebrospinal fluid cultures (blood culture may be positive for *Staphylococcal aureus*)
- Rise in titer to Rocky Mountain spotted fever, leptospirosis, or rubeola

[1]Centers for Disease Control (Reingold, et al., 1981)
[2]SGOT denotes serum aspartate transaminase.
[3]SGPT denotes serum alanine transaminase.

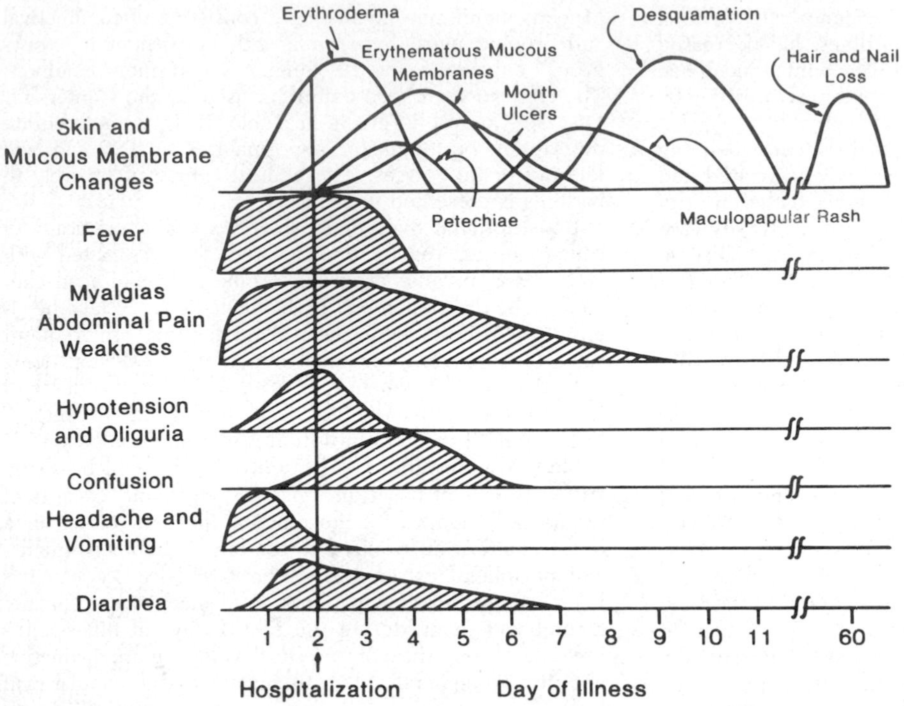

Figure 1. The clinical course of patients with severe toxic shock syndrome. Reproduced with permission from Chesney (1981).

gressing to involve both palms and soles is an uniform finding from 7 to 14 days after onset. Loss of hair and nails (telogen effluvium) occurs from 30 to 60 days after onset.

Gastrointestinal Involvement. Vomiting is a consistent early symptom that appears within 1 day of fever. It persists for 1 to 2 days and consists of less than 3 to over 25 discrete episodes. It is frequently accompanied by moderate abdominal pain and followed by a period of watery diarrhea, of variable severity and frequency and associated with occult but not gross blood in stools. Moderate hepatic tenderness to palpation may be noted. Liver function tests are frequently abnormal; serum bilirubin and transaminase levels are elevated in more than half of patients.

Renal Involvement. Oliguria is extremely common by the time patients seek medical attention and decreased urine volume is routinely documented during the first 8 hours of hospital admission. Most patients have evidence of prerenal azotemia and some develop renal failure with markedly reduced creatinine clearance. The urine sediment is abnormal in most patients. Pyuria (usually with sterile urine) is very common during the first 3 days. Microscopic hemoglobinuria and mild proteinuria are also common; occasional patients have myoglobinuria. Blood urea nitrogen and creatinine values are elevated in the majority of patients. Renal failure, both oliguric and nonoliguric, is directly correlated with the presence of shock. Most patients make a full recovery with supportive care but chronic renal failure has occurred.

Cardiopulmonary Involvement. Cardiopulmonary involvement forms a spectrum from mild orthostatic hypotension, orthostatic dizziness or syncope to profound and irreversible shock complicated by secondary adult respiratory distress syndrome. Hypotension is positively correlated with evidence of oliguric renal failure and decreased peripheral circulation. Nearly all recorded deaths have been associated with profound hypotension and pulmonary failure persisting despite intravenous fluid therapy and vasopressors. Severely hypotensive patients have been demonstrated to have high cardiac output, low peripheral resistance, and normal pulmonary artery wedge pressure and pulmonary resistance. Profound abnormalities of peripheral circulation and gangrene have been observed.

Hematologic Manifestations. TSS causes important and dynamic changes in the hematologic system. Platelet counts are decreased to 150,000 or less in more than 70 per cent of patients at the time of presentation. Thrombocytopenia and prolonged prothrombin and partial thromboplastin times are common and occasionally accompanied by hemorrhagic manifestations. Profound lymphocytopenia in nearly all patients at the time of presentation resolves by the fourth day of treatment.

Musculoskeletal Involvement. Two-thirds of patients have evidence of myositis with diffuse muscle pain, tenderness to palpation and elevated creatine phosphokinase. Myoglobinemia and myoglobinuria may occur and lead to further renal damage. Moderate to severe muscle weakness in the early recovery period may persist for several weeks.

Arthralgias of multiple joints are common; approximately one-quarter of patients develop objective signs of arthritis including warmth, erythema or swelling of joints. Arthritis usually resolves in one to several weeks.

DIAGNOSIS. The diagnosis of TSS requires that the diagnostic criteria (Table 1) be fulfilled and that coagulase-positive staphylococci be isolated. It is also necessary to exclude other diagnoses. In order to treat early or mild cases, one must be prepared to make the diagnosis and start therapy in the absence of some of the typical diagnostic features. It should be noted that not all patients have a discernible rash and that measured hypotension may not have developed at the time the patient is first seen. Bacteremia occurs in some cases so that its presence does not exclude the diagnosis. Scarlet fever, bacterial sepsis, and shock and rickettsial infections such as Rocky Mountain spotted fever must be excluded. Although Kawasaki syndrome is another multisystem disease with compatible clinical features, the clinical course and epidemiology are markedly different. Kawasaki syndrome usually causes a more impressive exanthem and a much less acute and rapidly progressive clinical course. Unlike TSS, Kawasaki syndrome is virtually restricted to children under 8 years.

TREATMENT. Prompt institution of intensive supportive measures and antistaphylococcal antibiotics is essential. Nearly all patients will require fluid replacement to restore central venous pressure and arterial pressure to normal. Vasopressors will be needed by all patients with hypotension refractory to simple volume expansion. Patients may require ventilator support for respiratory failure secondary to shock and the adult respiratory distress syndrome. Supportive care will also be necessary to correct hypocalcemia, myocardial irritability, acute renal failure, and thrombocytopenia with bleeding diatheses.

Specific therapy at the present involves vigorous treatment of the focus of staphylococcal infection with systemic administration of antibiotics and drainage of purulent abscesses. Because nearly all TSS-associated staphylococci are resistant to penicillin, semisynthetic beta-lactamase-resistant penicillins such as methicillin, oxacillin, and cloxacillin or cephalosporins are required.

At present, methods for the removal of the responsible toxin or toxins are limited to drainage of focal infections or tampon removal followed by vaginal lavage in menstrual TSS. In the future, toxin inactivation by specific antitoxin and methods to enhance toxin elimination may become available.

Corticosteroids have been administered in massive doses to some extremely ill patients. The benefit, if any, of high dose glucocorticoid therapy cannot be assessed at this time.

COMPLICATIONS AND SEQUELAE. With early recognition, prompt therapy, and provision of intensive supportive care, the case fatality rate has declined from 15 per cent to less than 3 per cent from 1979 to 1984. Death is usually caused by irreversible hypotension, renal failure, or adult respiratory distress syndrome. Earlier recognition of disease by both patient and primary physician has also resulted in a change in the clinical spectrum of disease toward milder cases with fewer serious sequelae.

TSS is primarily an acute episodic illness. The vast majority of patients make a full recovery. The early convalescent period, however, is complicated by arthritis, which may last for several weeks, diffuse or localized myopathy, which persists for weeks to months, and loss of hair and nails beginning 3 to 4 weeks after onset and persisting for several weeks.

Long-term or permanent sequelae have been most common in patients with severe shock during the acute illness. These serious consequences include chronic or permanently decreased renal function, cyanotic extremities or peripheral gangrene with loss of digits, amenorrhea or menstrual abnormalities and neuromuscular and neuropsychiatric disease. There is at present no reliable information from controlled systematic follow-up studies of adequate numbers of patients about the incidence of these sequelae.

Recurrent menstrual associated TSS is not uncommon. Among patients in the Tri-State epidemiologic studies who did not receive antistaphylococcal antibiotics and who continued to use tampons, the recurrence rate of TSS in subsequent menstrual periods was 60 per cent. The risk was reduced to 35 to 50 per cent in patients who had either received a course of anti-staphylococcal antibiotics during or after their episode of TSS but continued to use tampons *or* had discontinued the use of tampons but had not received anti-staphylococcal antibiotics. For patients who had *both* received anti-staphylococcal antibiotics and discontinued the use of tampons, recurrences were reduced to 17 per cent. Recurrences tend to occur with the succeeding menstrual period and to become milder with the passage of time. Five or more recurrences in succeeding menstrual periods have been documented in some patients (Osterholm, 1982). There is preliminary evidence that patients with a history of TSS do not develop antibody to the Toxic Shock Antigen even though this antibody is extremely common among normal individuals. Failure to develop protective anti-toxic immunity is the most likely explanation for recurrent disease. Recurrent disease has not yet been documented in non-menstrual TSS.

PREVENTION. The prevelance of TSS in a community will be dependent upon the prevalence of staphylococci possessing TSS antigen in that community. Some geographic areas that have yet to record their first cases may experience sporadic cases or outbreaks of disease. While anti-toxic immunization for high risk groups or populations may be available and effective in the future, only limited strategies for prevention are currently available. Women are at greatest risk and young women are the most susceptible. All women who develop the symptom complex of early TSS during menses: fever, myalgia, and gastroenteritis should discontinue using tampons and seek immediate medical attention. Any woman with a history of TSS should avoid the use of intravaginal devices and undergo a course of therapy with anti-staphylococcal antibiotics.

References

Bergdoll, M. S., Crass, B. A., Reiser, R. F., Robbins, R. N., Davis, J. P.: A new staphylococcal enterotoxin, enterotoxin F, associated with Toxic Shock Syndrome *Staphylococcal aureus* isolates. Lancet 1:1017–21, 1981.

Chesney, P. J., Davis, J. P., Purdy, W. K., Wand, P. J., Chesney, R. W.: Clinical manifestations of the Toxic Shock Syndrome. JAMA 246:741–8, 1981.

Kapral, F. A.: Epidermal toxin production by *Staphylococcus aureus* strains from patients with Toxic Shock Syndrome. Ann Intern Med 96:972–974, 1982.

Larkin, S. M., Williams, D. N., Osterholm, M. T., Tofte, R. W., Posalaky, Z.: Toxic Shock Syndrome: Clinical, Laboratory and Pathologic Findings in nine fatal cases. Ann Intern Med 96:858–864, 1982.

Osterholm, M. T., Davis, J. P., Gibson, R. W., Mandel, J. S., Wistermeyer, L. A., Helms, C. M., Forfang, J. C., Rondeau, J., Vergeront, J. M., and the Investigation Team, Tri-State Toxic Shock Syndrome Study I. Epidemiologic Findings. J Infect Dis 145:431–440, 1982.

Osterholm, M. T., forfang, J. C.: Toxic Shock Syndrome in Minnesota: Results of an active-passive surveillance system. J Infect Dis 145:458–464, 1982.

Paris, A. L., Herwaldt, L. A., Blum, D., Schmid, G. P., Shands, K. N., Broome, C. V.: Pathologic findings in twelve fatal cases of Toxic Shock Syndrome. Ann Intern Med 96:852–857, 1982.

Reingold, A. L., Hargrett, N. T., Shands, K. N., Dan, B. B., Schmid, G. P., Struckland, B. Y., Broome, C. V.: Toxic Shock Syndrome surveillance in the United States, 1980 to 1981. Ann Intern Med 96:875–880, 1982.

Schlievert, P. M., Shands, K. N., Dan, B. B., Schmid, G. P., Nishimura, R. D.: Identification and characterization of an exotoxin from *Staphylococcus aureus* associated with Toxic Shock Syndrome. J Infect Dis 143:509–16, 1981.

Todd, J., Fishaut, M., Kapral, F., Welch, T.: Toxic Shock Syndrome associated with phage group II staphylococci. Lancet 2:1116–8, 1978.

Index

Note: Page numbers in *italic* refer to illustrations; page numbers followed by t indicate tables.